VOLUME I

FIELDS
VIROLOGY

SIXTH EDITION

VOLUME I

FIELDS VIROLOGY

SIXTH EDITION

EDITORS-IN-CHIEF

David M. Knipe, PhD
Higgins Professor of Microbiology and Molecular Genetics
Department of Microbiology and Immunobiology
Chair, Harvard Program in Virology
Harvard Medical School
Boston, Massachusetts

Peter M. Howley, MD
Shattuck Professor of Pathological Anatomy
Department of Microbiology and Immunobiology
Harvard Medical School
Boston, Massachusetts

ASSOCIATE EDITORS

Jeffrey I. Cohen, MD
Chief
Laboratory of Infectious Diseases
National Institute of Allergy and Infectious Diseases
National Institutes of Health
Bethesda, Maryland

Diane E. Griffin, MD, PhD
Professor and Chair
W. Harry Feinstone Department of Molecular Microbiology and Immunology
Johns Hopkins Bloomberg School of Public Health
Baltimore, Maryland

Robert A. Lamb, PhD, ScD
John Evans Professor of Molecular and Cellular Biology
Investigator, Howard Hughes Medical Institute
Department of Molecular Biosciences
Northwestern University
Evanston, Illinois

Malcolm A. Martin, MD
Chief
Laboratory of Molecular Microbiology
Division of Intramural Research
National Institute of Allergy and Infectious Diseases
National Institutes of Health
Bethesda, Maryland

Vincent R. Racaniello, PhD
Higgins Professor
Department of Microbiology and Immunology
Columbia University
College of Physicians and Surgeons
New York, New York

Bernard Roizman, ScD
Joseph Regenstein Distinguished Service Professor
Departments of Microbiology and Molecular Genetics and Cell Biology
University of Chicago
Chicago, Illinois

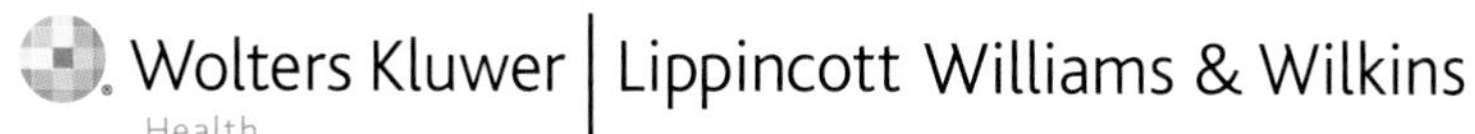

Philadelphia • Baltimore • New York • London
Buenos Aires • Hong Kong • Sydney • Tokyo

Acquisitions Editor: Julie Goolsby
Product Manager: Tom Gibbons
Project Manager: David Saltzberg
Manufacturing Manager: Beth Welsh
Marketing Manager: Kimberly Schonberger
Design Coordinator: Steve Druding
Production Service: Aptara, Inc.

Two Commerce Square
2001 Market Street
Philadelphia, PA 19103 USA
LWW.com

Printed in China

Library of Congress Cataloging-in-Publication Data

Fields virology/editors-in-chief, David M. Knipe, Peter M. Howley. – 6th ed.
p. ; cm.
Includes bibliographical references and index.
ISBN-13: 978-1-4511-0563-6 (alk. paper)
ISBN-10: 1-4511-0563-0
I. Fields, Bernard N. II. Knipe, David M. (David Mahan), 1950- III. Howley, Peter M.
[DNLM: 1. Viruses. 2. Virus Diseases. QW 160]
QR360
616.9′101–dc23

2013003842

Care has been taken to confirm the accuracy of the information presented and to describe generally accepted practices. However, the authors, editors, and publisher are not responsible for errors or omissions or for any consequences from application of the information in this book and make no warranty, expressed or implied, with respect to the currency, completeness, or accuracy of the contents of the publication. Application of the information in a particular situation remains the professional responsibility of the practitioner.

The authors, editors, and publisher have exerted every effort to ensure that drug selection and dosage set forth in this text are in accordance with current recommendations and practice at the time of publication. However, in view of ongoing research, changes in government regulations, and the constant flow of information relating to drug therapy and drug reactions, the reader is urged to check the package insert for each drug for any change in indications and dosage and for added warnings and precautions. This is particularly important when the recommended agent is a new or infrequently employed drug.

Some drugs and medical devices presented in the publication have Food and Drug Administration (FDA) clearance for limited use in restricted research settings. It is the responsibility of the health care provider to ascertain the FDA status of each drug or device planned for use in their clinical practice.

To purchase additional copies of this book, call our customer service department at (800) 638-3030 or fax orders to (301) 223-2320. International customers should call (301) 223-2300.

Visit Lippincott Williams & Wilkins on the Internet: at LWW.com. Lippincott Williams & Wilkins customer service representatives are available from 8:30 am to 6 pm, EST.

10 9 8 7 6 5 4 3 2 1

CCS0413

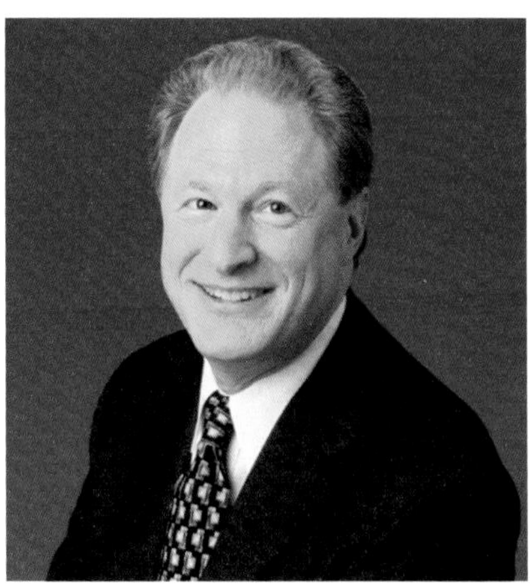

Stephen E. Straus, 1946–2007

Steve Straus was the consummate physician–scientist with broad interests in the basic science and clinical aspects of viral and immunological diseases and therefore was an ideal person to serve as clinical virology editor for *Fields Virology*. We were fortunate to work with him in his role as associate editor for the third through fifth editions of *Fields Virology*. However, unfortunately, with Steve's premature death in 2007, we lost our friend, colleague, and fellow editor. Steve's medical training and accomplishments are detailed elsewhere (*J Infect Dis* 2007;196:963–964). His research interests were broad and included the molecular biology and pathogenesis of varicella-zoster and herpes simplex viruses, acyclovir suppression of oral and genital herpes simples viruses, antiviral drug resistance, clinical testing of herpes simplex virus and varicella zoster virus vaccines, chronic active Epstein–Barr virus, chronic fatigue syndrome, and autoimmune lymphoproliferative syndrome. Steve was one of the leading scientists in the National Institutes of Health intramural program, serving as chief of the Laboratory of Clinical Investigation at the National Institute of Allergy and Infectious Diseases and the founding director of the National Center for Complementary and Alternative Medicine.

Steve cowrote the chapter on varicella zoster virus, and additionally worked effectively as an associate editor, for the third to fifth editions of *Fields Virology*. He seemed to read and edit the chapters immediately upon their submission, amazing us with his ability to do all of this on top of his other responsibilities. Steve was diagnosed with brain cancer in 2004 but insisted on editing chapters for the fifth edition right through the compiling of the chapters. The book was published in early 2007, not long before his death in May 2007.

On behalf of everyone who contributed to the sixth edition of *Fields Virology*, we dedicate this book to the memory of Stephen E. Straus, MD.

CONTRIBUTORS

Carlos F. Arias, MD
Professor
Department of Developmental Genetics and Molecular Physiology
Instituto de Biotecnologia
Universidad Nacional Autonoma de Mexico
Cuernavaca, Morelos, Mexico

Ann M. Arvin, MD, PhD
Lucile Salter Packard Professor
Departments of Pediatrics and Microbiology and Immunology
Stanford University School of Medicine
Stanford, California

Justin R. Bailey, MD, PhD
Assistant Professor
Department of Medicine
Johns Hopkins University School of Medicine
Baltimore, Maryland

Arnold J. Berk, MD
Professor and UCLA Presidential Chair in Molecular Cell Biology
Molecular Biology Institute
Department of Microbiology, Immunology, and Molecular Genetics
University of California, Los Angeles
Los Angeles, California

Kenneth I. Berns, MD, PhD
Distinguished Professor Emeritus
Department of Molecular Genetics and Microbiology
University of Florida College of Medicine
Gainesville, Florida

Thomas J. Braciale, MD, PhD
Beirne B. Carter Professor in Immunology
Director, Carter Immunology Center
Professor of Pathology and Molecular Medicine
Professor of Microbiology, Immunology, and Cancer Biology
University of Virginia School of Medicine
Charlottesville, Virginia

Thomas Briese, PhD
Associate Professor
Department of Epidemiology
Associate Director
Center for Infection and Immunity
Mailman School of Public Health
Columbia University
New York, New York

Christopher C. Broder, PhD
Professor and Emerging Infectious Diseases
Graduate Program Director
Department of Microbiology and Immunology
Uniformed Services University
Bethesda, Maryland

Michael J. Buchmeier, PhD
Deputy Director
Pacific Southwest Center for Biodefense and Emerging Infectious Diseases
Professor
Division of Infectious Disease
Professor
Department of Molecular Biology and Biochemistry
University of California, Irvine
Irvine, California

Dennis R. Burton, PhD
Professor
Department of Immunology and Microbial Science
Center for HIV/AIDS Vaccine Immunology and Immunogen Disccovery and IAVI Neutralizing Consortium
Scripps Research Institute
La Jolla, California

Kathryn M. Carbone, MD
Deputy Scientific Director
Division of Intramural Research
National Institute of Dental and Craniofacial Research
National Institutes of Health
Bethesda, Maryland

Ethel Cesarman, MD, PhD
Professor
Department of Pathology and Laboratory Medicine
Weill Cornell Medical College
New York, New York

Donald M. Coen, PhD
Professor
Department of Biological Chemistry and Molecular Pharmacology
Harvard Medical School
Boston, Massachusetts

Jeffrey I. Cohen, MD
Chief
Laboratory of Infectious Diseases
National Institute of Allergy and Infectious Diseases
National Institutes of Health
Bethesda, Maryland

Peter L. Collins, PhD
Chief
RNA Viruses Section
Laboratory of Infectious Diseases
National Institute of Allergy and Infectious Diseases
National Institutes of Health
Bethesda, Maryland

Philippe Colson, PharmD, PhD
Associate Professor
URMITE UM 63 CNRS 7278 IRD 198 INSERM U1095
Aix-Marseille Université
Facultés de Médecine et de Pharmacie
Pôle des Maladies Infectieuses et Tropicales Clinique et Biologique
Fédération de Bactériologie-Hygiène-Virologie
IHU Méditerranée Infection
Centre Hospitalo-Universitaire Timone, Assistance Publique-Hôpitaux de Marseille
Marseille, France

Richard C. Condit, PhD
Professor
Department of Molecular Genetics and Microbiology
University of Florida
Gainesville, Florida

James E. Crowe Jr., MD
Ingram Professor of Research
Departments of Pediatrics and Pathology, Microbiology, and Immunology
Director, Vanderbilt Vaccine Center
Vanderbilt University
Nashville, Tennessee

Blossom A. Damania, PhD
Professor
Department of Microbiology and Immunology
Lineberger Comprehensive Cancer Center
University of North Carolina at Chapel Hill
Chapel Hill, North Carolina

Inger K. Damon, MD, PhD
Chief
Poxvirus and Rabies Branch
Division of High-Consequence Pathogens and Pathology
Centers for Disease Control and Prevention
Atlanta, Georgia

Juan-Carlos de la Torre, PhD
Professor
Department of Immunology and Microbial Science
The Scripps Research Institute
La Jolla, California

James A. DeCaprio, MD
Associate Professor of Medicine
Department of Medicine
Harvard Medical School
Associate Professor of Medicine
Dana-Farber Cancer Institute
Boston, Massachusetts

Terence S. Dermody, MD
Dorothy Overall Wells Professor of Pediatrics and Pathology, Microbiology, and Immunology
Director, Division of Pediatric Infectious Diseases
Director, Medical Scientist Training Program
Lamb Center for Pediatric Research
Vanderbilt University School of Medicine
Nashville, Tennessee

Ronald C. Desrosiers, PhD
Professor
New England Primate Research Center
Harvard Medical School
Southborough, Massachusetts

Michael S. Diamond, MD, PhD
Professor
Departments of Medicine, Molecular Microbiology, and Pathology and Immunology
Washington University School of Medicine
St. Louis, Missouri

Daniel DiMaio, MD
Waldemar Von Zedtwitz Professor
Department of Genetics
Yale School of Medicine
Scientific Director
Yale Cancer Center
Yale University
New Haven, Connecticut

John H. Elder, PhD
Professor
Department of Immunology and Microbial Science
The Scripps Research Institute
La Jolla, California

Richard M. Elliott, DPhil
Chair of Infectious Diseases
Centre for Virus Research
University of Glasgow
Glasgow, Scotland, United Kingdom

Suzanne U. Emerson, PhD
Chief
Molecular Hepatitis Laboratory
Laboratory of Infectious Diseases
National Institutes of Health
Bethesda, Maryland

Lynn W. Enquist, PhD
Professor
Department of Molecular Biology
Princeton University
Princeton, New Jersey

Mary K. Estes, PhD
Professor
Department of Molecular Virology and Microbiology
Baylor College of Medicine
Houston, Texas

David T. Evans, PhD
Associate Professor
Department of Microbiology and Immunobiology
Harvard Medical School
Southborough, Massachusetts

Hung Fan, MD
Professor and Director
Cancer Research Institute
Department of Molecular Biology and Biochemistry
University of California, Irvine
Irvine, California

Patrizia Farci, MD
Senior Investigator and Chief
Hepatic Pathogenesis Section, Laboratory of Infectious Diseases
National Institute of Allergy and Infectious Diseases
National Institutes of Health
Bethesda, Maryland

Heinz Feldmann, MD
Chief
Laboratory of Virology
Division of Intramural Research
National Institute of Allergy and Infectious Diseases
National Institutes of Health
Hamilton, Montana

Eric O. Freed, PhD
Head, Virus-Cell Interaction Section
HIV Drug Resistance Program
Frederick National Laboratory for Cancer Research
National Cancer Institute
National Institutes of Health
Frederick, Maryland

Paul D. Friesen, PhD
Professor
Institute for Molecular Virology
University of Wisconsin, Madison
Madison, Wisconsin

Masahiro Fujii, MD, PhD
Professor
Division of Virology
Niigata University Graduate School of Medical and Dental Sciences
Niigata, Japan

Thomas W. Geisbert, PhD
Professor
Departments of Microbiology and Immunology
University of Texas Medical Branch at Galveston
Galveston, Texas

James E. Gern, MD
Professor of Pediatrics and Medicine
Department of Pediatrics
University of Wisconsin School of Medicine and Public Health
Medical Staff, Department of Pediatrics
University of Wisconsin Hospital and Clinics
American Family Children's Hospital
Madison, Wisconsin

Don Gilden, MD
Louise Baum Endowed Chair and Professor
Department of Neurology
University of Colorado School of Medicine
Neurologist
University of Colorado Denver
Aurora, Colorado

Stephen P. Goff, PhD
Higgins Professor of Biochemistry
Department of Biochemistry and Molecular Biophysics
Columbia University and Howard Hughes Medical Institute
New York, New York

Barney S. Graham, MD, PhD
Senior Investigator
Chief, Viral Pathogenesis Laboratory
Chief, Clinical Trials Core
Vaccine Research Center
National Institute of Allergy and Infectious Diseases
National Institutes of Health
Bethesda, Maryland

Kim Y. Green, PhD
Senior Investigator
Caliciviruses Section, Laboratory of Infectious Diseases
National Institute of Allergy and Infectious Diseases
National Institutes of Health
Bethesda, Maryland

Harry B. Greenberg, MD
Joseph D. Grant Professor
Departments of Medicine and Microbiology and Immunology
Stanford University School of Medicine
Stanford, California

Diane E. Griffin, MD, PhD
Professor and Chair
W. Harry Feinstone Department of Molecular Microbiology and Immunology
Johns Hopkins Bloomberg School of Public Health
Baltimore, Maryland

Paul D. Griffiths, MD, DSc
Professor of Virology
Centre for Virology
University College London
Professor of Virology
Royal Free London NHS Foundation Trust
London, United Kingdom

Young S. Hahn, PhD
Professor
Department of Microbiology, Immunology, and Cancer Biology
University of Virginia School of Medicine
Charlottesville, Virginia

Stephen C. Harrison, PhD
Giovanni Armenise–Harvard Professor of Basic Biomedical Sciences
Department of Biological Chemistry and Molecular Pharmacology
Harvard Medical School and Howard Hughes Medical Institute
Boston, Massachusetts

Mark T. Heise, PhD
Associate Professor
Department of Genetics, Microbiology, and Immunology
University of North Carolina
Chapel Hill, North Carolina

Ari Helenius, PhD
Professor
Institute of Biochemistry
ETH Zurich
Zurich, Switzerland

Roger W. Hendrix, PhD
Distinguished Professor
Department of Biological Science
University of Pittsburgh
Pittsburgh, Pennsylvania

Christiane Herden, Prof Dr habil
Full Professor
Institute of Veterinary Pathology
Justus-Liebig-University Giessen
Giessen, Germany

Tom C. Hobman, PhD
Professor
Department of Cell Biology
University of Alberta
Edmonton, Alberta, Canada

F. Blaine Hollinger, MD
Professor of Medicine, Molecular Virology, and Epidemiology
Director, Eugene B. Casey Hepatitis Research Center
Departments of Molecular Virology and Microbiology and Medicine
Baylor College of Medicine
Houston, Texas

Edward C. Holmes, MD
NHMRC Australia Fellow
School of Biological Sciences and Sydney Medical School
The University of Sydney
Sydney, New South Wales, Australia

Peter M. Howley, MD
Shattuck Professor of Pathological Anatomy
Department of Microbiology and Immunobiology
Harvard Medical School
Boston, Massachusetts

Eric Hunter, PhD
Professor
Department of Pathology and Laboratory Medicine
Emory University
Atlanta, Georgia

Michael J. Imperiale, PhD
Arthur F. Thurnau Professor
Department of Microbiology and Immunology
University of Michigan
Ann Arbor, Michigan

Michael G. Ison, MD, MS, FIDSA
Associate Professor
Divisions of Infectious Diseases and Organ Transplantation
Northwestern University Feinberg School of Medicine
Director
Northwestern University Comprehensive Transplant Center
Northwestern Memorial Hospital
Chicago, Illinois

Akiko Iwasaki, PhD
Professor
Departments of Immunobiology and Molecular, Cellular, and Developmental Biology
Yale University School of Medicine
New Haven, Connecticut

Ruth A. Karron, MD
Professor
Department of International Health
Director, Center for Immunization Research
Johns Hopkins Bloomberg School of Public Health
Baltimore, Maryland

Yoshihiro Kawaoka, DVM, PhD
Professor
Influenza Research Institute
Department of Pathobiological Sciences
School of Veterinary Medicine
University of Wisconsin, Madison
Madison, Wisconsin
Director and Professor
International Research Center for Infectious Diseases
Division of Virology, Department of Microbiology and Immunology
Institute of Medical Sciences
University of Tokyo
Tokyo, Japan

Elliott Kieff, MD, PhD
Albee Professor of Microbiology and Immunobiology
Harvard Medical School
Channing Laboratory
Albee Professor of Infectious Diseases
Department of Medicine
Brigham and Women's Hospital
Boston, Massachusetts

Marjolein Kikkert, PhD
Associate Professor
Department of Medical Microbiology
Leiden University Medical Center
Leiden, The Netherlands

David M. Knipe, PhD
Higgins Professor of Microbiology and Molecular Genetics
Department of Microbiology and Immunobiology
Chair, Harvard Program in Virology
Harvard Medical School
Boston, Massachusetts

Richard A. Koup, MD
Chief
Immunology Laboratory
Vaccine Research Center
National Institute of Allergy and Infectious Diseases
National Institutes of Health
Bethesda, Maryland

Richard J. Kuhn, PhD
Professor and Head
Department of Biological Sciences
Purdue University
West Lafayette, Indiana

Daniel R. Kuritzkes, MD
Professor of Medicine
Harvard Medical School
Chief, Division of Infectious Diseases
Brigham and Women's Hospital
Boston, Massachusetts

Ivan V. Kuzmin, PhD
Director
Aravan, LLC (Biomedical Consulting)
Lilburn, Georgia

Robert A. Lamb, PhD, ScD
John Evans Professor of Molecular and Cellular Biology
Investigator, Howard Hughes Medical Institute
Department of Molecular Biosciences
Northwestern University
Evanston, Illinois

Julie E. Ledgerwood, DO
Senior Clinician
Deputy Chief, Clinical Trials Core
Vaccine Research Center
National Institute of Allergy and Infectious Diseases
National Institutes of Health
Bethesda, Maryland

Dirk Lindemann, PhD
Professor
Institute of Virology
Technische Universität Dresden
Dresden, Germany

Brett D. Lindenbach, PhD
Associate Professor
Department of Microbial Pathogenesis
Yale University School of Medicine
New Haven, Connecticut

W. Ian Lipkin, MD
John Snow Professor of Epidemiology and Director
Center for Infection and Immunity
Mailman School of Public Health
Professor of Pathology and Neurology
College of Physicians and Surgeons
Columbia University
New York, New York

Richard M. Longnecker, PhD
Dan and Bertha Spear Research Professor
Department of Microbiology and Immunology
Northwestern University Medical School
Chicago, Illinois

Douglas R. Lowy, MD
Chief
Laboratory of Cellular Oncology
Center for Cancer Research
Deputy Director, National Cancer Institute
Bethesda, Maryland

Douglas S. Lyles, PhD
Professor and Chair
Department of Biochemistry
Wake Forest School of Medicine
Winston-Salem, North Carolina

John S. Mackenzie, PhD
Professor of Tropical Infectious Diseases
Faculty of Health Sciences
Curtin University
Perth, Western Australia
Honorary Senior Principal Fellow
Burnet Institute
Melbourne, Australia

Eugene O. Major, PhD
Senior Investigator
Laboratory of Molecular Medicine and Neuroscience
National Institute of Neurological Disorders and Stroke
National Institutes of Health
Bethesda, Maryland

Annette Martin, PhD
Senior Scientist and Principal Investigator
Department of Virology
Institut Pasteur
Paris, France

Malcolm A. Martin, MD
Chief
Laboratory of Molecular Microbiology
Division of Intramural Research
National Institute of Allergy and Infectious Diseases
National Institutes of Health
Bethesda, Maryland

William S. Mason, PhD
Professor
Department of Virology
Fox Chase Cancer Center
Philadelphia, Pennsylvania

Paul S. Masters, PhD
Chief
Laboratory of Viral Replication and Vector Biology
Division of Infectious Diseases
Wadsworth Center
New York State Department of Health
Associate Professor
Department of Biomedical Sciences
School of Public Health
University at Albany
State University of New York
Albany, New York

Masao Matsuoka, MD, PhD
Professor and Director
Institute for Virus Research
Kyoto University
Kyoto, Japan

Ruslan Medzhitov, PhD
David W. Wallace Professor of Immunobiology
Investigator, Howard Hughes Medical Institute
Chevy Chase, MD

Ernesto Méndez, PhD (deceased)
Associate Professor
Department of Developmental Genetics and Molecular Physiology
Instituto de Biotecnologia
Universidad Nacional Autonoma de Mexico
Cuernavaca, Morelos, Mexico

Xiang-Jin Meng, MD, PhD
Professor of Molecular Virology
Department of Biomedical Sciences and Pathobiology
Virginia Polytechnic Institute and State University
Blacksburg, Virginia

W. Allen Miller, PhD
Professor
Department of Plant Pathology and Microbiology
Iowa State University
Ames, Iowa

Edward S. Mocarski Jr., PhD
Robert W. Woodruff Professor
Department of Microbiology and Immunology
Emory University School of Medicine
Atlanta, Georgia

Yasuko Mori, MD, PhD
Professor
Department of Microbiology and Infectious Diseases
Division of Clinical Virology
Kobe University Graduate School of Medicine
Kobe, Japan

Bernard Moss, MD, PhD
Chief
Laboratory of Viral Diseases
National Institute of Allergy and Infectious Diseases
National Institutes of Health
Bethesda, Maryland

William J. Moss, MD, MPH
Professor
Departments of Epidemiology, International Health, and Molecular Microbiology and Immunology
Johns Hopkins Bloomberg School of Public Health
Baltimore, Maryland

Catherine L. Murray, PhD
Novartis Institutes for BioMedical Research
Infectious Disease Area
Emeryville, California

Neal Nathanson, MD
Associate Dean, Global Health Programs
University of Pennsylvania School of Medicine
Philadelphia, Pennsylvania

Gabriele Neumann, PhD
Research Professor
Influenza Research Institute
Department of Pathobiological Sciences
School of Veterinary Medicine
University of Wisconsin, Madison
Madison, Wisconsin

M. Steven Oberste, PhD
Chief
Polio and Picornavirus Laboratory Branch
Centers for Disease Control and Prevention
Atlanta, Georgia

Peter Palese, PhD
Professor and Chair
Department of Microbiology
Mount Sinai School of Medicine
New York, New York

Mark A. Pallansch, PhD
Director
Division of Viral Diseases
Centers for Disease Control and Prevention
Atlanta, Georgia

Ann C. Palmenberg, PhD
Professor
Institute for Molecular Virology
University of Wisconsin, Madison
Madison, Wisconsin

John S. L. Parker, BVMS, PhD
Associate Professor
Baker Institute for Animal Health
Cornell University
Ithaca, New York

Griffith D. Parks, PhD
Professor and Chair
Department of Microbiology and Immunology
Wake Forest School of Medicine
Winston-Salem, North Carolina

Colin R. Parrish, PhD
Professor of Virology
Baker Institute for Animal Health
College of Veterinary Medicine
Cornell University
Ithaca, New York

Robert F. Pass, MD
Professor
Departments of Pediatrics and Microbiology
University of Alabama at Birmingham
Director, Hospital Medicine
Department of Pediatrics
Children's of Alabama
Birmingham, Alabama

Philip E. Pellett, PhD
Professor
Department of Immunology and Microbiology
Wayne State University
Detroit, Michigan

Stanley Perlman, MD, PhD
Professor
Departments of Microbiology and Pediatrics
University of Iowa
Iowa City, Iowa

Clarence J. Peters, MD
Professor
Department of Microbiology and Immunology
University of Texas Medical Branch
Galveston, Texas

Theodore C. Pierson, PhD
Senior Investigator
Laboratory of Viral Diseases
National Institute of Allergy and Infectious Diseases
National Institutes of Health
Bethesda, Maryland

Stanley B. Prusiner, MD
Director
Institute for Neurodegenerative Diseases
Professor
Department of Neurology
University of California, San Francisco
San Francisco, California

Robert H. Purcell, MD (Retired)
Distinguished Investigator
Laboratory of Infectious Diseases
National Institute of Allergy and Infectious Diseases
National Institutes of Health
Bethesda, Maryland

Vincent R. Racaniello, PhD
Higgins Professor
Department of Microbiology and Immunology
Columbia University
College of Physicians and Surgeons
New York, New York

Didier Raoult, Professor, MD, PhD
Professor
URMITE, Inserm 1095
Aix Marselle Université
Professor
Pôle Infectieux
CHU de la Timone
Marseille, France

Stuart C. Ray, MD
Professor
Fellowship Program Director
Department of Medicine, Infectious Diseases
Johns Hopkins Medical Institutions
Baltimore, Maryland

Axel Rethwilm, MD
Head of Institute
Institute for Virology
University of Wuerzburg
Wuerzburg, Germany

Charles M. Rice, PhD
Professor and Head
Laboratory of Virology and Infectious Disease
Rockefeller University
New York, New York

Douglas D. Richman, MD
Florence Seeley Riford Distinguished Professor
Director, Center for AIDS Research
Departments of Pathology and Medicine
University of California, San Diego
La Jolla, California

Jürgen A. Richt, DVM, PhD
Regents Distinguished Professor
Department of Diagnostic Medicine/Pathobiology
College of Veterinary Medicine
Kansas State University
Manhattan, Kansas

Bernard Roizman, ScD
Joseph Regenstein Distinguished Service Professor
Departments of Microbiology and Molecular Genetics and Cell Biology
University of Chicago
Chicago, Illinois

Polly Roy, MSc, PhD, FMed Sci
Professor
Department of Infectious and Tropical Diseases
London School of Hygiene and Tropical Medicine
London, United Kingdom

Steven A. Rubin, PhD
Senior Investigator
Center for Biologics Evaluation and Research
U.S. Food and Drug Administration
Bethesda, Maryland

Charles E. Rupprecht, VMD, MS, PhD
Director of Research
The Global Alliance for Rabies Control
Manhattan, Kansas

Anthony Sanchez, PhD
Associate Director for Laboratory Science
Division of High-Consequence Pathogens and Pathology
Centers for Disease Control and Prevention
Atlanta, Georgia

Christian J. Sauder, PhD
Staff Scientist
Center for Biologics Evaluation and Research
U.S. Food and Drug Administration
Bethesda, Maryland

John T. Schiller, PhD
Senior Investigator
Laboratory of Cellular Oncology
National Cancer Institute
National Institutes of Health
Bethesda, Maryland

Connie S. Schmaljohn, PhD
Senior Scientist, Infectious Diseases
U.S. Army Medical Research Institute of Infectious Diseases
Ft. Detrick, Frederick, Maryland

Christoph Seeger, PhD
Professor
Department of Virology
Fox Chase Cancer Center
Philadelphia, Pennsylvania

Megan L. Shaw, PhD
Associate Professor
Department of Microbiology
Mount Sinai School of Medicine
New York, New York

Thomas Shenk, PhD
Professor
Department of Molecular Biology
Princeton University
Princeton, New Jersey

Barbara Sherry, PhD
Professor
Department of Molecular Biomedical Sciences
North Carolina State University
Raleigh, North Carolina

Eric J. Snijder, PhD
Professor of Molecular Virology
Department of Medical Microbiology
Leiden University Medical Center
Leiden, The Netherlands

Gregory A. Storch, MD
Ruth L. Siteman Professor of Pediatrics
Professor of Medicine and of Molecular Microbiology
Department of Pediatrics
Washington University in St. Louis School of Medicine
Medical Director, Clinical Laboratories
St. Louis Children's Hospital
St. Louis, Missouri

John M. Taylor, PhD
Professor Emeritus
Fox Chase Cancer Center
Philadelphia, Pennsylvania

Prof. Dr. Heinz-Jürgen Thiel
Professor
Institute of Virology
Justus-Liebig University
Head of Institute
Veterinary Medicine
Giessen, Germany

David L. Thomas, MD, MPH
Chief
Division of Infectious Diseases
Stanhope Baine Jones Professor of Medicine
Johns Hopkins School of Medicine
Baltimore, Maryland

Herbert W. Virgin IV, MD, PhD
Edward Mallinckrodt Professor and Head
Department of Pathology and Immunology
Washington University School of Medicine
St. Louis, Missouri

David Wang, PhD
Associate Professor
Departments of Molecular Microbiology and Pathology and Immunology
Washington University in St. Louis
St. Louis, Missouri

Lin-Fa Wang, PhD
Science Leader
CSIRO Australian Animal Health Laboratory
Geelong, Australia
Director and Professor
Program in Emerging Infectious Diseases
Duke–NUS Graduate Medical School
Singapore

Sean Whelan, PhD
Professor
Department of Microbiology and Immunobiology
Harvard Medical School
Boston, Massachusetts

Steven A. Whitham, PhD
Professor
Department of Plant Pathology and Microbiology
Iowa State University
Ames, Iowa

Richard J. Whitley, MD
Distinguished Professor
Department of Pediatrics
Division Director
Department of Pediatric Infectious Diseases
Vice Chair
Department of Pediatrics
University of Alabama at Birmingham
Birmingham, Alabama

J. Lindsay Whitton, MD, PhD
Professor
Department of Immunology and Microbial Science
Scripps Research Institute
La Jolla, California

Reed B. Wickner, MD
Chief
Laboratory of Biochemistry and Genetics
National Institute of Diabetes and Digestive and Kidney Diseases
National Institutes of Health
Bethesda, Maryland

William S.M. Wold, PhD
Professor and Chairman
Department of Molecular Microbiology and Immunology
Saint Louis University
St. Louis, Missouri

Peter F. Wright, MD
Professor
Department of Pediatrics
Geisel School of Medicine at Dartmouth University
Lebanon, New Hampshire

Koichi Yamanishi, MD, PhD
Director General
National Institute of Biomedical Innovation
Osaka, Japan

Fabien Zoulim, MD
Professor and Head of Laboratory
Viral Hepatitis Laboratory
INSERM Unit 1052
Professor and Head of Department
Department of Hepatology
Hospices Civils de Lyon
Lyon, France

PREFACE

In the early 1980s, Bernie Fields originated the idea of a virology reference textbook that combined the molecular aspects of viral replication with the medical features of viral infections. This broad view of virology reflected Bernie's own research, which applied molecular and genetic analyses to the study of viral pathogenesis, providing an important part of the foundation for the field of molecular pathogenesis. Bernie led the publication of the first three editions of *Virology* but unfortunately died soon after the third edition went into production. The third edition became *Fields Virology* in his memory, and it is fitting that the book continues to carry his name.

We are pleased that the printed book of the sixth edition of *Fields Virology* contains four-color art throughout and that an e-book version accompanies the printed book as well. We have increased the numbers of figures in each chapter, and with the color and availability of the figures from the e-book for use as slides, most chapters should have sufficient figures for slides for one lecture. There have been continued significant advances in virology since the previous edition 6 years ago, and all of the chapters have been updated to reflect these advances. Our increased knowledge of virology has caused us to use shortened lists of key references (up to 200 in most cases) in the printed book to save space, whereas complete reference lists appear as part of the e-book. We have retained the general organization of the earlier editions for the sixth edition of *Fields Virology*. Section I contains chapters on general aspects of virology, and Section II contains chapters on replication and medical aspects of specific virus families and specific viruses of medical importance. In Section I, we have added a new emphasis on virus discovery in the Diagnostic Virology chapter and emerging viruses in the Epidemiology chapter to address the interest in discovery of new viruses and emerging viruses. In Section II, we have added new chapters on circoviruses and mimiviruses and have added a new section on Chikungunya virus to the alphavirus chapter.

Numerous chapters have been updated to include the latest information on outbreaks during the past 5 years, including pandemic H1N1 influenza, new adenovirus serotypes, noroviruses, human polyomaviruses, the re-emergence of West Nile virus in North America, novel coronaviruses, novel Coxsackie and rhino viruses, and other emerging and re-emerging viruses. Important advances in antivirals, including new hepatitis C virus protease inhibitors and HIV integrase inhibitors, have been described. As with the previous edition, we have continued to combine the medical and replication chapters into a single chapter to eliminate duplication and to present a more coherent presentation of that specific virus or virus family. The main emphasis continues to be on viruses of medical importance and interest; however, other viruses are described in specific cases where more is known about their mechanisms of replication or pathogenesis. Although not formally viruses, prions are still included in this edition for historical reasons and because of the intense interest in the infectious spongiform encephalopathies.

We wish to thank Lisa Holik of Harvard Medical School, Richard Lampert of Lampert Consultancy, Grace Caputo of Dovetail Content Solutions, Chris Miller of Aptara, and Leanne Vandetty and Tom Gibbons and all of the editorial staff members of Lippincott Williams & Wilkins for all their important contributions to the preparation of this book.

David M. Knipe, PhD
Peter M. Howley, MD
Jeffrey I. Cohen, MD
Diane E. Griffin, MD, PhD
Robert A. Lamb, PhD, ScD
Malcolm A. Martin, MD
Vincent R. Racaniello, PhD
Bernard Roizman, ScD

CONTENTS

General Virology

SECTION I

CHAPTER 1

Lynn W. Enquist • Vincent R. Racaniello

Virology: From Contagium Fluidum to Virome

Virology has had a remarkable history. Even though humans did not realize viruses existed until the late 1880s, viral diseases have shaped the history and evolution of life on the planet. As far as we know, all living organisms, when studied carefully, are infected by viruses. These smallest microbes exert significant forces on every living thing, including themselves. The consequences of viral infections have not only altered human history, they have powerful effects on the entire ecosystem. As a result, virologists have gone to extraordinary lengths to study, understand, and eradicate these agents. It is noteworthy that just as the initial discovery of viruses required new technology (porcelain filters), uncovering the amazing biology underlying viral infections has gone hand in hand with new technology developments. Indeed, virologists have elucidated new principles of life processes and have been leaders in promoting new directions in science. For example, many of the concepts and tools of molecular biology and cell biology have been derived from the study of viruses and their host cells. This chapter is an attempt to review selected portions of this history as it relates to the development of new concepts in virology.

THE CONCEPT OF VIRUSES AS INFECTIOUS AGENTS

A diverse microbial world of bacteria, fungi, and protozoa had been widely accepted by the last half of the 19th century. An early proponent of the germ theory of disease was the noted German anatomist Jacob Henle of Gottingen (the discoverer of Henle's loop and the grandfather of 20th-century virologist Werner Henle). He hypothesized in 1840 that specific diseases were caused by infectious agents that were too small to be observed with the light microscope. However, he had no evidence for such entities, and consequently his ideas were not generally accepted. It would take the work of Louis Pasteur and Henle's student, Robert Koch, before it became evident that microbes could cause diseases.

Three major advances in microbiology came together to set the stage for the development of the concept of a submicroscopic agent that would come to be called a virus (e-Table 1.1). The first advance concerned spontaneous generation of organisms, which for years had been both supported and refuted by a variety of experiments. Louis Pasteur (1822–1895) used his swan-neck flasks to strike a mortal blow to the concept of spontaneous generation. Afterward Pasteur went on to study fermentation by different microbial agents. From his work he concluded that "different kinds of microbes are associated with different kinds of fermentations," and he soon extended this concept to diseases. Pasteur's reasoning strongly influenced Robert Koch (1843–1910), a student of Jacob Henle and a country doctor in a small German village. Koch developed solid media to isolate colonies of bacteria to produce pure cultures, and stains to visualize the microorganisms. With these tools in hand, Koch identified the bacterium that causes anthrax (*Bacillus anthracis,* 1876) and tuberculosis (*Mycobacterium tuberculosis,* 1882). Joseph Lister (1827–1912), a professor of surgery in Glasgow, had heard about Pasteur's work, and he surmised that a sterile field should be maintained during surgery. Although many other scientists of that day contributed tools and concepts, it was principally Pasteur, Lister, and Koch who put together a new experimental approach for medical science.

These observations led Robert Koch to formalize some of Jacob Henle's original ideas for defining whether a microorganism is the causative agent of a disease. Koch's postulates state that (a) the organism must be regularly found in the lesions of the disease, (b) the organism must be isolated in pure culture, (c) inoculation of such a pure culture of organisms into a host should initiate the disease, and (d) the organism must be recovered once again from the lesions of the host. By the end of the 19th century, these concepts outlined an experimental method that became the dominant paradigm of medical microbiology. It was only when these rules broke down and failed to yield a causative agent that the concept of a virus was born.

THE BIRTH OF VIROLOGY

Pathogen Discovery, 1886–1903 (e-Table 1.1)

Adolf Mayer (1843–1942) was a German agricultural chemist and director of the Agricultural Experiment Station at Wageningen in The Netherlands when he was asked to investigate a disease of tobacco. He named the affliction tobacco mosaic disease after the dark and light spots that appeared on infected leaves (e-Fig. 1.1). To investigate the nature of the disease, Mayer inoculated healthy plants with the juice extracted from diseased plants by grinding up the infected leaves in water. Mayer reported that, "in nine cases out of ten (of inoculated plants), one will be successful in making the healthy plant...heavily diseased".[131] Although these studies established the infectious nature of the tobacco mosaic disease, neither a bacterial agent nor a fungal agent could be consistently cultured or detected in these extracts, so Koch's postulates could not be satisfied. In a preliminary communication in 1882,[130] Mayer speculated that the cause could be a "soluble, possibly enzyme-like contagium, although almost any analogy for such a supposition is failing in science." Later Mayer concluded that the mosaic disease "is bacterial, but that the infectious forms have not yet been isolated, nor are their forms and mode of life known".[131]

A few years later, Dimitri Ivanofsky (1864–1920), a Russian scientist working in St. Petersburg, was commissioned by the Russian Department of Agriculture to investigate the cause of a tobacco disease on plantations in Bessarabia, Ukraine, and the Crimea. Ivanofsky repeated Mayer's observations by showing that the sap of infected plants contained an agent that could transmit the disease to healthy plants. But he added an important step—before the inoculation step, he passed the infected sap through a Chamberland filter (e-Fig. 1.2). This device, made of unglazed porcelain and perfected by Charles Chamberland, one of Pasteur's collaborators, contained pores small enough to retard most bacteria. Ivanofsky reported to the Academy of Sciences of St. Petersburg on February 12, 1892, that "the sap of leaves infected with tobacco mosaic disease retains its infectious properties even after filtration through Chamberland filter candles".[94]

Ivanofsky, like Mayer before him, failed to culture an organism from the filtered sap and could not satisfy Koch's postulates. Consequently he suggested that a toxin (not a living, reproducing substance) might pass through the filter and cause the disease. As late as 1903, when Ivanofsky published his thesis,[95] he still believed that he had been unable to culture the bacteria that caused this disease. Bound by the dogma of Koch's postulates, Ivanofsky could not make a conceptual leap. It is therefore not surprising that Pasteur, who worked on the rabies vaccine[145] at the same time (1885), never investigated the unique nature of the infectious agent.

The conceptual leap was provided by Martinus Beijerinck (1851–1931), a Dutch soil microbiologist who collaborated with Adolf Mayer at Wageningen. Unaware of Ivanofsky's work, in 1898 Beijerinck independently found that the sap of infected tobacco plants could retain its infectivity after passage through a Chamberland filter. But he also showed that the filtered sap could be diluted and regain its "strength" after replication in living, growing tissue of the plant. This observation showed that the agent could reproduce (therefore, it was not a toxin) but only in living tissue, not in the cell-free sap of the plant. Suddenly it became clear why others could not culture the pathogen outside its host. Beijerinck called this agent a *contagium vivum fluidum,*[10] or a contagious living liquid. He sparked a 25-year debate about whether these novel agents were liquids or particles. This conflict was resolved when d'Herelle developed the plaque assay in 1917[36] and when the first electron micrographs were taken of tobacco mosaic virus (TMV) in 1939.[104]

Mayer, Ivanofsky, and Beijerinck each contributed to the development of a new concept: a novel organism smaller than bacteria—an agent defined by the pore size of the Chamberland filter—that could not be seen in the light microscope, and could multiply only in living cells or tissue. The term *virus,* from the Latin for slimy liquid or poison,[89] was at that time used interchangeably for any infectious agent, and so the agent of tobacco mosaic disease was called tobacco mosaic virus, or TMV. The literature of the first decades of the 20th century often referred to these infectious entities as filterable agents, and this was indeed the operational definition of viruses. Sometime later, the term *virus* became restricted in use to those agents that fulfilled the criteria developed by Mayer, Ivanofsky, and Beijerinck, and that were the first agents to cause a disease that could not be proven by using Koch's postulates.

Shortly after this pioneering work on TMV, the first filterable agent from animals was identified by Loeffler and Frosch—foot-and-mouth disease virus.[122] The first human virus discovered was yellow fever virus (1901), by Walter Reed and his team in Cuba.[154]

The years from 1930 to 1956 were replete with the discovery of a plethora of new viruses (e-Table 1.2). In fact, in this short time, virologists found most of the viruses we now know about. More fascinating perhaps is that these studies laid the groundwork for the birth of molecular virology.

Plant Viruses and the Chemical Period: 1929–1956

For the next 50 years, TMV played a central role in research that explored the nature and properties of viruses. With the development of techniques to purify proteins in the first decades of the 20th century came the appreciation that viruses were proteins and so could be purified in the same way. Working at the Boyce Thompson Institute in Philadelphia, Vinson and Petre (1927–1931) precipitated infectious TMV—using an infectivity assay developed by Holmes[88]—from the crude sap of infected plants using selected salts, acetone, or ethyl alcohol.[193] They showed that the infectious virus could move in an electric field, just as proteins did. At the same time, H. A. Purdy-Beale, also at the Boyce Thompson Institute, produced antibodies in rabbits that were directed against TMV and could neutralize the infectivity of this agent.[151] This observation was taken as further proof of the protein nature of viruses, although it was later realized that antibodies recognize chemicals other than proteins. With the advent of purification procedures for viruses, both physical and chemical measurements of the virus became possible. The strong flow birefringence of purified preparations of TMV was interpreted (correctly) to show an asymmetric particle or rod-shaped particle.[180] Max Schlesinger,[167] working on purified preparations of bacteriophages in Frankfurt, Germany, showed that the virions were composed of proteins and contained phosphorus and ribonucleic acid. This observation led to the first suggestion that viruses were composed of nucleoproteins. The crystallization of TMV in 1935 by Wendell Stanley,[173] working at the Rockefeller Institute branch in Princeton, New Jersey, brought this infectious agent into the world of the chemists. Within a year, Bawden and Pirie[8,9] had demonstrated that crystals of TMV contained 0.5% phosphorus and 5% RNA. The first "view" of a virus came from x-ray crystallography using these crystals to show rods of a constant diameter aligned in hexagonal arrays containing RNA and protein.[16] The first electron micrographs of any virus were of TMV, and they confirmed that the virus particle is shaped like a rod[105] (e-Fig. 1.3).

The x-ray diffraction patterns[16] suggested that TMV was built from repeating subunits. These data and other considerations led Crick and Watson[33] to realize that most simple viruses had to consist of one or a few species of identical protein subunits. By 1954–1955, techniques had been developed to dissociate TMV protein subunits, allowing reconstitution of infectious TMV from its RNA and protein subunits[64] and leading to an understanding of the principles of virus self-assembly.[25]

The concept that viruses contained genetic information emerged as early as 1926, when H. H. McKinney reported the isolation of "variants" of TMV with a different plaque morphology that bred true and could be isolated from several geographic locations.[132,133] Seven years later, Jensen confirmed McKinney's observations[101] and showed that the plaque morphology phenotype could revert. Avery's DNA transformation experiments with pneumococcus[5] and the Hershey-Chase experiment with bacteriophages,[83] both demonstrated that DNA was genetic material. TMV had been shown to contain RNA, not DNA, and this nucleic acid was shown to be infectious, and therefore comprise the genetic material of the virus, in 1956[64,72]—the first demonstration that RNA could be a genetic material. Studies on the nucleotide sequence of TMV RNA confirmed codon assignments for the genetic code, added clear evidence for the universality of the genetic code, and helped to elucidate the mechanisms of mutation by diverse agents.[63] Research on TMV and related plant viruses has contributed significantly to both the origins of virology and its development as a science.

BACTERIOPHAGES

Early Years: 1915–1940

Frederick W. Twort was superintendent of the Brown Institution in London when he discovered viruses of bacteria in 1915. In his research, Twort was searching for variants of vaccinia virus (the smallpox vaccine virus), which would replicate in simple defined media outside living cells. In one of his experiments, he inoculated nutrient agar with an aliquot of the smallpox vaccine. The virus failed to replicate, but bacterial contaminants flourished on the agar medium. Twort noticed that some of these bacterial colonies changed visibly with time and became "watery looking" (i.e., more transparent). The bacteria within these colonies were apparently dead, as they could no longer form new colonies on fresh agar plates. He called this phenomenon glassy transformation. Simply adding the glassy transforming principle could rapidly kill a colony of bacteria. It readily passed through a porcelain filter, could be diluted a million-fold, and when placed upon fresh bacteria would regain its strength, or titer.[188–190]

Twort published these observations in a short note[190] in which he suggested that a virus of bacteria could explain glassy transformation. He then went off to serve in World War I, and when he returned to London, he did not continue this research.

While Twort was puzzled by glassy transformation, Felix d'Herelle, a Canadian medical bacteriologist, was working at the Pasteur Institute in Paris. When a *Shigella* dysentery infection devastated a cavalry squadron of French soldiers just outside of Paris in August 1915, d'Herelle readily isolated and cultured the dysentery bacillus from filtered fecal emulsions. The bacteria multiplied and covered the surface of his agar plates, but occasionally d'Herelle observed clear circular spots devoid of growth. He called these areas *taches vierges*, or plaques. He followed the course of an infection in a single patient, noting when the bacteria were most plentiful and when the plaques appeared.[35,36] Plaques appeared on the fourth day after infection and killed the bacteria in the culture dish, after which the patient's condition began to improve.

d'Herelle found that a filterable agent, which he called a bacteriophage, was killing the *Shigella* bacillus. In the ensuing years he developed fundamental techniques in virology that are utilized to this day, such as the use of limiting dilutions to determine the virus titer by plaque assay. He reasoned that the appearance of plaques showed that the virus was particulate, or "corpuscular," and not a liquid as Beijerinck had insisted. d'Herelle also found that if virus was mixed with a host cell and then subjected to centrifugation, the virus was no longer present in the supernatant fluid. He interpreted this to mean that the first step of a virus infection is attachment, or adsorption, of virus to the host cell. Furthermore, viral attachment occurred only when bacteria sensitive to the virus were used, demonstrating that host specificity can be conferred at a very early step in infection. Lysis of cells and the release of infectious virus were also described in startlingly modern terms. d'Herelle clearly established many of the principles of modern virology.[34,35]

Although d'Herelle's bacteriophages lysed their host cells, by 1921 it had become apparent that under certain situations the virus and cell existed peacefully—a condition called lysogeny. In some experiments it became impossible to separate the virus from its host. This conundrum led Jules Bordet of the Pasteur Institute in Brussels to suggest that the transmissible agent described by d'Herelle was nothing more than a bacterial enzyme that stimulates its own production.[22] Although incorrect, the hypothesis has remarkable similarities to modern ideas about prion structure and replication (see Chapter 77).

During the 1920s and 1930s, d'Herelle sought ways to use bacteriophages for medical applications, but he never succeeded. Furthermore, the basic research of the era was frequently dominated by the interpretations of scientists with the strongest personalities. Although it was clear that there were many diverse bacteriophages, and that some were lytic while some were lysogenic, their interrelationships remained ill defined. The highlight of this period was the demonstration by Max Schlesinger that purified phages had a maximum linear dimension of 0.1 micron and a mass of about 4×10^{-16} grams, and that they were composed of protein and DNA in roughly equal proportions.[166,167] In 1936, no one quite knew what to make of that observation, but over the next 20 years it would begin to make a great deal of sense.

Phages and the Birth of Molecular Biology: 1938–1970 (e-Table 1.3)

Max Delbrück was trained as a physicist at the University of Göttingen, and his first position was at the Kaiser Wilhelm Institute for Chemistry in Berlin. There he joined a diverse group of individuals who were actively discussing how quantum physics related to an understanding of heredity. Delbrück's interest in this area led him to develop a quantum mechanical model of the gene, and in 1937 he moved to the biology division at the California Institute of Technology to study genetics of *Drosophila*. Once there, he became interested in bacteria and their viruses, and teamed up with another research fellow, Emory Ellis,[51] who was working with the T-even group of bacteriophages, T2, T4, and T6. Delbrück soon appreciated that these viruses were ideal for the study of virus replication, because they allowed analysis of how genetic information could determine the structure and function of an organism. Bacteriophages were also viewed as model systems for understanding cancer viruses or even for understanding how a sperm fertilizes an egg and a new organism develops. Together with Ellis, Delbrück showed that viruses reproduced in one step, in contrast to the multiplication of other organisms by binary fission.[52] This conclusion was drawn from the elegant one-step growth curve experiment, in which an infected bacterium liberates hundreds of phages synchronously after a half-hour period during which viral infectivity was lost (e-Fig. 1.4). The one-step growth curve became the experimental paradigm of the phage group.

When World War II erupted, Delbrück remained in the United States (at Vanderbilt University) and met an Italian refugee, Salvador E. Luria, who had fled to America and was working at Columbia University in New York (on bacteriophages T1 and T2). After their encounter at a meeting in Philadelphia on December 28, 1940, they went to Luria's laboratory at Columbia where they spent 48 hours doing experiments with bacteriophages. These two scientists eventually established the "phage group," a community of researchers focused on using bacterial viruses as a model for understanding life processes. Luria and Delbrück were invited to spend the summer of 1941 at Cold Spring Harbor Laboratory, where they pursued research on phages. The result was that a German physicist and an Italian geneticist joined forces during the war years to travel throughout the United States and recruit a new generation of biologists (e-Fig. 1.5).

When Tom Anderson, an electron microscopist at the RCA Laboratories in Princeton, New Jersey, met Delbrück, the result was the first clear pictures of bacteriophages.[126] At the same time, the first phage mutants were isolated and characterized.[125] By 1946, the first phage course was being taught at Cold Spring Harbor, and in March 1947, the first phage meeting attracted eight people. From these humble beginnings grew the field of molecular biology, which focused on the bacterial host and its viruses.

Developing the Modern Concept of Virology (see e-Tables 1.3 to 1.5)

The next 25 years (1950–1975) was an intensely productive period of bacteriophage research. Hundreds of virologists produced thousands of publications that covered three major areas: (a) lytic infection of *Escherichia coli* with the T-even phages; (b) the nature of lysogeny, using lambda phage; and (c) the replication and properties of several unique phages such as ϕX174 (single-stranded circular DNA), the RNA phages, and T7. This work set the foundations for modern molecular virology and biology.

The idea of examining, at the biochemical level, the events occurring in phage-infected cells during the latent period had come into its own by 1947–1948. Impetus for this work came from Seymour Cohen, who had trained first with Erwin Chargaff at Columbia University, studying lipids and nucleic acids, and then with Wendell Stanley working on TMV RNA. His research direction was established when after taking Delbrück's 1946 phage course at Cold Spring Harbor, Cohen examined the effects of phage infection on DNA and RNA levels in infected cells using a colorimetric analysis. The results showed a dramatic alteration of macromolecular synthesis in infected cells. This included cessation of RNA accumulation, which later formed the basis for detecting a rapidly turning-over species of RNA and the first demonstration of messenger RNA (mRNA).[4] DNA synthesis also halted, but for 7 minutes, followed by resumption at a 5- to 10-fold increased rate. At the same time, Monod and Wollman showed that the synthesis of a cellular enzyme, the inducible β-galactosidase, was inhibited after phage infection.[134] Based on these observations, the viral eclipse period was divided into an early phase, prior to DNA synthesis, and a late phase. More importantly, these results demonstrated that a virus could redirect cellular macromolecular synthetic processes in infected cells.[32]

By the end of 1952, two experiments had a critical effect on virology. First, Hershey and Chase asked whether viral genetic information is DNA or protein. They differentially labeled viral proteins ($^{35}SO_4$) and nucleic acids ($^{32}PO_4$), and allowed the "tagged" particles to attach to bacteria. When they sheared the viral protein coats from the bacteria using a Waring blender, only DNA was associated with the infected cells.[83] This result proved that DNA had all the information needed to reproduce new virus particles. A year later, the structure of DNA was elucidated by Watson and Crick, a discovery that permitted full appreciation of the Hershey-Chase experiment.[195] The results of these two experiments formed a cornerstone of the molecular biology revolution.[26]

While these blockbuster experiments were being carried out, G. R. Wyatt and S. S. Cohen were quietly making another seminal finding.[207] They identified a new base, hydroxymethylcytosine, in the DNA of T-even phages, which replaced cytosine. This began a 10-year study of how deoxyribonucleotides were synthesized in bacteria and phage-infected cells, and it led to the critical observation that the virus introduces genetic information for a new enzyme into the infected cell.[60] By 1964, Mathews and colleagues had proved that hydroxymethylase does not exist in uninfected cells and must be encoded by the virus.[32] These experiments introduced the concept of early enzymes, utilized in deoxypyrimidine biosynthesis and DNA replication,[109] and provided biochemical proof that viruses encode new information that is expressed as proteins in an infected cell. At the same time, phage genetics became extremely sophisticated, allowing mapping of the genes encoding these viral proteins. Perhaps the best example of genetic fine structure was done by Seymour Benzer, who carried out a genetic analysis of the rII A and B cistrons of T-even phages with a resolution of a single nucleotide (without doing any DNA sequencing!).[13] Studies on viral DNA synthesis, using phage mutants and cell extracts to complement and purify enzyme activities *in vitro,* contributed a great deal to our understanding of DNA replication.[1] A detailed genetic analysis of phage assembly, utilizing the complementation of phage assembly mutants *in vitro,* revealed how complex structures are built by living organisms using the principles of self-assembly.[47] The genetic and biochemical analysis of phage lysozyme helped to elucidate the molecular nature of mutations,[176] and the isolation of phage amber mutations (nonsense mutations) provided a clear way to study second-site suppressor mutations at the molecular level.[14] The circular genetic map of the T-even phages[176] was explained by the circularly permuted, terminally redundant (giving rise to phage heterozygotes) conformation of these DNAs.[186]

The remarkable reprogramming of viral and cellular protein synthesis in phage-infected cells was dramatically revealed by an early use of sodium dodecyl sulfate (SDS)–polyacrylamide gels,[112] showing that viral proteins are made in a specific sequence of events. The underlying mechanism of this temporal regulation led to the discovery of sigma factors modifying RNA polymerase and conferring gene specificity.[75] The study of gene regulation at almost every level (transcription, RNA stability, protein synthesis, protein processing) was revealed from a set of original contributions derived from an analysis of phage infections.

Although this remarkable progress had begun with the lytic phages, no one knew quite what to make of the lysogenic phages. This situation changed in 1949 when André Lwoff began his studies with *Bacillus megaterium* and its lysogenic phages at the Pasteur Institute. By using a micromanipulator, Lwoff could show that single lysogenic bacteria divided up to 19 times without liberating a virus particle. No virions were detected when lysogenic bacteria were broken open by the investigator. But from time to time a lysogenic bacterium spontaneously lysed and produced many viruses.[128] Ultraviolet light was found to induce the release of these viruses, a key observation that began to outline this curious relationship between a virus and its host.[129] By 1954, Jacob and Wollman[97,98] at the Pasteur Institute had made the important observation that a genetic cross between a lysogenic bacterial strain and a nonlysogenic recipient resulted in the induction of the virus after conjugation, a process they called zygotic induction. In fact, the position of the lysogenic phage or prophage in the chromosome of its host *E. coli* could be mapped by interrupting mating between two strains.[98] This experiment was crucial for our understanding of lysogenic viruses, because it showed that a virus behaved like a bacterial gene on a chromosome in a bacterium. It was also one of the first experimental results to suggest that the viral genetic material was kept quiescent in bacteria by negative regulation, which was lost as the chromosome passed from the lysogenic donor bacteria to the nonlysogenic recipient host. This conclusion helped Jacob and Monod to realize as early as 1954 that the "induction of enzyme synthesis and of phage development are the expression of one and the same phenomenon".[128] These experiments laid the foundation for the operon model and the nature of coordinate gene regulation.

Although the structure of DNA was elucidated in 1953[195] and zygotic induction was described in 1954, the relationship between the bacterial chromosome and the viral chromosome in lysogeny was still referred to as the attachment site and literally thought of in those terms. The close relationship between a virus and its host was appreciated only when Campbell proposed the model for lambda integration of DNA into the bacterial chromosome,[27] based on the fact that the sequence of phage markers was different in the integrated state than in the replicative or vegetative state. This model led to the isolation of the negative regulator or repressor of lambda, a clear understanding of immunity in lysogens, and one of the early examples of how genes are regulated coordinately.[150] The genetic analysis of the lambda bacteriophage life cycle is one of the great intellectual adventures in microbial genetics.[82] It deserves to be reviewed in detail by all students of molecular virology and biology.

The lysogenic phages such as P22 of *Salmonella typhimurium* provided the first example of generalized transduction,[210] whereas lambda provided the first example of specialized transduction.[137] The finding that viruses could not only carry within them cellular genes, but transfer those genes from one cell to another, provided not only a method for fine genetic mapping but also a new concept in virology. As the genetic elements of bacteria were studied in more detail, it became clear that there was a remarkable continuum from lysogenic phages to episomes, transposons and retrotransposons, insertion elements, retroviruses, hepadnaviruses, viroids, and prions. Genetic information moves between viruses and their hosts to the point where definitions and classifications begin to blur. The genetic and biochemical concepts that emerged from the study of bacteriophages made the next phase of virology possible. The lessons of the lytic and lysogenic phages were often relearned and modified as the animal viruses were studied.

ANIMAL VIRUSES

Cell Culture Technology and Discovery: 1898–1965 (see e-Tables 1.1 to 1.3)

Once the concept of viruses as filterable agents took hold, many diseased animal tissues were subjected to filtration to determine if a virus were involved. Filterable agents were found that were invisible in a light microscope, and replicated only in living animal tissue. There were some surprises, such as the transmission of yellow fever virus by a mosquito vector,[154] specific visible pathologic inclusion bodies (virions and subviral particles) in infected tissue,[95,142] and even viral agents that can "cause cancer".[50,159]

Throughout this early time period (1900–1930), a wide variety of viruses were found (see e-Tables 1.1 and 1.2) and characterized with regard to their size (using the different pore sizes of filters), resistance to chemical or physical agents (e.g., alcohol, ether), and pathogenic effects. Based on these properties alone, it became clear that viruses were a very diverse group of agents. Some were even observable in the light microscope (vaccinia in dark-field optics). Some were inactivated by ether, whereas others were not. Viruses were identified that affected every tissue type. They could cause chronic or acute disease; they were persistent agents or recurred in a periodic fashion. Some viruses caused cellular destruction or induced cellular proliferation. For the early virologists, unable to see their agents in a light microscope and often confused by this great diversity, their studies certainly required an element of faith. In 1912, S. B. Wolbach, an American pathologist, remarked, "It is quite possible that when our knowledge of filterable viruses is more complete, our conception of living matter will change considerably, and that we shall cease to attempt to classify the filterable viruses as animal or plant".[204]

The way out of this early confusion was led by the plant virologists and the development of techniques to purify viruses and characterize both the chemical and physical properties of these agents (see previous section, The Plant Viruses and the Chemical Period: 1929–1956). The second path out of this problem came from the studies with bacteriophages, where single cells infected with viruses in culture were much more amenable to experimental manipulation than were virus infections of whole animals. Whereas the plant virologists of that day were tethered to their greenhouses, and the animal virologists were bound to their animal facilities, the viruses of bacteria were studied in Petri dishes and test tubes. Nevertheless, progress was made in the study of animal viruses one step at a time: from studying animals in the wild, to laboratory animals, such as the mouse[66] or the embryonated chicken eggs,[205] to the culture of tissue, and then to single cells in culture. Between 1948 and 1955, a critical transition converting animal virology into a laboratory science came in four important steps: Sanford and colleagues at the National Institutes of Health (NIH) overcame the difficulty of culturing single cells[163]; George Gey at Johns Hopkins Medical School cultured and passaged human cells for the first time and developed a line of immortal cells (HeLa) from a cervical carcinoma[71]; and Harry Eagle at the NIH developed an optimal medium for the culture of single cells.[46] In a demonstration of the utility of all these advanced, Enders and his colleagues showed that poliovirus could replicate in a nonneuronal human explant of embryonic tissues.[54]

These ideas, technical achievements, and experimental advances had two immediate effects on the field virology. They led to the development of the polio vaccine, the first ever produced in cell culture. From 1798 to 1949, all the vaccines in use (smallpox, rabies, yellow fever, influenza) had been grown in animals or embryonated chicken eggs. Poliovirus was grown in monkey kidney cells that were propagated in flasks.[84,117] The exploitation of cell culture for the study of viruses began the modern era of molecular virology. The first plaque assay for an animal virus in culture was done with poliovirus,[43] and it led to an analysis of poliovirus every bit as detailed and important as the contemporary work with bacteriophages. The simplest way to document this statement is for the reader to compare the first edition of *General Virology* by S. E. Luria in 1953[124] to the second edition by Luria and J. E. Darnell in 1967,[127] and to examine the experimental descriptions of poliovirus infection of cells. The modern era of virology had arrived, and it would continue to be full of surprises.

The Molecular and Cell Biology Era of Virology (see e-Tables 1.4 to 1.6)

The history of virology has so far been presented chronologically or according to separate virus groups (plant viruses, bacteriophages, animal viruses), which reflects the historical separation of these fields. In this section, the format changes as the motivation for studying viruses began to change. Virologists began to use viruses to probe questions central to understanding all life processes. Because viruses replicate in and are dependent on their host cells, they must use the rules, signals, and regulatory pathways of the host. By using viruses to probe cells, virologists began to make contributions to all facets of biology. This approach began with the phage group and was continued by the animal virologists. The recombinant DNA revolution also took place during this period (1970 to the present), and both bacteriophages and animal viruses played a critical and central role in this revolution. For these reasons, the organization of this section focuses on the advances in cellular and molecular biology made possible by experiments with viruses. Some of the landmarks in virology since 1970 are listed in e-Tables 1.4 to 1.6.

The Role of Animal Viruses in Understanding Eukaryotic Gene Regulation

The closed circular and superhelical nature of polyomavirus DNA was first elucidated by Dulbecco and Vogt[42] and Weil and Vinograd.[197] This unusual DNA structure was intimately related to the structure of the genome packaged in virions of simian vacuolating virus 40 (SV40). The viral DNA is wound around nucleosomes[70]; when the histones are removed, a superhelix is produced. The structure of polyoma viral DNA served as an excellent model for the *E. coli* genome[206] and the mammalian chromosome.[113] Viral genomes have unique configurations not found in other organisms, such as single-stranded DNA (ssDNA),[171] plus or minus strand RNA, or double-stranded RNA (dsRNA) as modes of information storage.

Many elements of the eukaryotic transcription machinery have been elucidated with viruses. The first transcriptional enhancer element (acts in an orientation- and distance-independent fashion) was described in the SV40 genome,[76] as was a distance- and orientation-dependent promoter element observed with the same virus. The transcription factors that bind to the promoter, SP-1,[44] or to the enhancer element, such as AP-1 and AP-2,[116] and which are essential to promote transcription along with the basal factors, were first described with SV40. AP-1 is composed of fos and jun family member proteins, demonstrating the role of transcription factors as oncogenes.[21] Indeed, the great majority of experimental data obtained for basal and accessory transcription factors come from *in vitro* transcription systems using the adenovirus major late promoter or the SV40 early enhancer–promoter.[196] Our present-day understanding of RNA polymerase III promoter recognition comes, in part, from an analysis of the adenovirus *VA* gene transcribed by this polymerase.[62]

Almost everything we know about the steps of messenger RNA (mRNA) processing began with observations made with viruses. RNA splicing of new transcripts was first described in adenovirus-infected cells.[15,31] Polyadenylation of mRNA was first observed with poxviruses,[102] the first viruses shown to have a DNA-dependent RNA polymerase in the virion.[103] The signal for polyadenylation in the mRNA was identified using SV40.[59] The methylated cap structure found at the 5′ end of most mRNAs was first discovered on reovirus mRNAs.[67] What little is known about the process of RNA transport out of the nucleus has shown a remarkable discrimination of viral and cellular mRNAs by the adenovirus E1B-55 Kd protein.[147]

Most of our understanding of translational regulation has come from studies of virus infected cells. Recruitment of ribosomes to mRNAs was shown to be directed by the 5′ cap structure first discovered on reovirus mRNAs. The nature of the protein complex that allows ribosomes to bind the 5′ cap was elucidated in poliovirus-infected cells, because viral infection leads to cleavage of one of the components, eIF4G. Internal initiation of translation was discovered in cells infected with picornaviruses (poliovirus and encephalomyocarditis virus).[99,146] Interferon, discovered as a set of proteins that inhibits viral replication, was subsequently found to induce the synthesis of many antiviral gene products that act on translational regulatory events.[92,93] Similarly, the viral defenses against interferon by the adenovirus VA RNA has provided unique insight into the role of eIF-2 phosphorylation events.[108] Mechanisms for producing more than one protein from a eukaryotic mRNA (there is no "one mRNA one protein" rule in bacteria) were discovered in virus-infected cells, including polyprotein synthesis, ribosomal frameshifting, and leaky scanning. Posttranslational processing of proteins by proteases, carbohydrate addition to proteins in the Golgi apparatus, phosphorylation by a wide variety of important cellular protein kinases, or the addition of fatty acids to membrane-associated proteins have all been profitably studied using viruses. Indeed, a good deal of our present-day knowledge of how protein trafficking occurs and is regulated in cells comes from the use of virus-infected cell systems. The field of gene regulation has derived many of its central tenets from the study of viruses.

Animal Viruses and the Recombinant DNA Revolution

The discovery of the enzyme reverse transcriptase,[6,185] not only elucidated the replication cycle of retroviruses, but also provided an essential tool to convert RNA molecules to DNA, which could then be cloned and manipulated. The first restriction enzyme map of a chromosome was done with SV40 DNA, using the restriction enzymes HindII plus HindIII DNA,[37,38] and the first demonstration of restriction enzyme specificity was carried out with the same viral DNA cleaved with EcoRI.[136,138] Some of the earliest DNA cloning experiments involved insertion of SV40 DNA into lambda DNA, or human β-hemoglobin genes into SV40 DNA, yielding the first mammalian expression vectors.[96] A debate about whether these very experiments were potentially dangerous led to a temporary moratorium on all such recombinant experiments following the scientist-organized Asilomar Conference. From the earliest experiments in the field of recombinant DNA, several animal viruses had been developed into expression vectors to carry foreign genes, including SV40,[74] the retroviruses,[198] the adenoviruses,[69,78] and adeno-associated virus.[162] which has the remarkable property of preferential integration into a specific genomic site.[110] Modern-day strategies of gene therapy rely on some of these recombinant viruses. Hemoglobin mRNA was first cloned using lambda vectors, and the elusive hepatitis virus C (non-A, non-B) viral genome was cloned from serum using recombinant DNA techniques, reverse transcriptase, and lambda phage vectors.[30]

Animal Viruses and Oncology

Much of our present understanding of the origins of human cancers is a consequence of work on two major groups of animal viruses: retroviruses and DNA tumor viruses. Oncogenes were first discovered in the genome of Rous sarcoma virus, and subsequently shown to exist in the host cell genome.[174] Since those seminal studies, virologists have identified a wide variety of oncogenes that have been captured by retroviruses (see Chapter 8). Additional oncogenes were identified when they were activated by insertion of the proviral DNA of retroviruses into the genomes of cells.[77] The second group of genes that contribute to the origins of human cancers, the tumor suppressor genes,[118] has been shown to be intimately associated with the DNA tumor viruses. Genetic alterations at the p53 locus are the single most common mutations known to occur in human cancers—they are found in 50% to 80% of all cancers.[119] The p53 protein was first discovered in association with the SV40 large T-antigen.[115,120] SV40, the human adenoviruses, and the human papillomaviruses all encode oncoproteins that interact with and inactivate the functions of two tumor suppressor gene products, the retinoblastoma susceptibility gene product (Rb) and p53.[40,44,115,120,164,200,201] Our understanding of the roles of cellular oncogenes and the tumor suppressor genes in human cancers would be far less significant without the insight provided by studies with these viruses. Curiously, none of the four human polyoma viruses central to these studies was associated with human cancers. However, in 2008, a new polyomavirus associated with Merkel cell carcinoma was discovered.[57]

Viruses that cause cancers have provided some of the most extraordinary episodes in modern animal virology.[135] The recognition of a new disease and the unique geographic distribution of Burkitt's lymphoma in Africa[20] set off a search for viral agents that cause cancers in humans. From D. Burkitt[24] to Epstein, Achong, and Barr[56] to W. Henle and G. Henle,[81] the story of the Epstein-Barr virus and its role in several cancers, as well as in infectious mononucleosis, is a science detective story without rival. Similarly, the identification of a new pathologic disease, adult T-cell leukemia, in Japan by K. Takatsuki[181,191] led to the isolation of a virus that causes the disease by I. Miyoshi and Y. Hinuma[208] and the realization that this virus (human T-cell leukemia virus type 1 [HTLV-1]) had been identified previously by Gallo and his colleagues.[149] Even with the virus in hand, there is still no satisfactory explanation of how this virus contributes to adult T-cell leukemia.

An equally interesting detective story concerns hepatitis B virus and hepatocellular carcinoma. By 1967, S. Krugman and his colleagues[111] had strong evidence indicating the existence of distinct hepatitis A and B viruses, and in the same year B. Blumberg[20] had identified the Australia antigen. Through a tortuous path, it eventually became clear that the Australia antigen was a diagnostic marker—the coat protein—for hepatitis B virus. Although this discovery freed the blood supply of this dangerous virus, Hilleman at Merck Sharp & Dohme and the Chiron Corporation (which later isolated the hepatitis C virus) went on to produce the first human vaccine that prevents hepatitis B infections and very likely hepatocellular carcinomas associated with chronic virus infections (see Chapter 69). The idea of a vaccine that can prevent cancer—first proven with the Marek's disease virus and T-cell lymphomas in chickens,[18,49]—comes some 82 to 85 years after the first discoveries of tumor viruses by Ellerman, Bang, and Rous. An experiment is under way in Taiwan, where 63,500 newborn infants have been inoculated to prevent hepatitis B infections. Based on the epidemiologic predictions, this vaccination program should result in 8,300 fewer cases of liver cancer in that population in 35 to 45 years.

Vaccines and Antivirals

Among the most remarkable achievements of our century is the complete eradication of smallpox, a disease with a greater than 2,000-year-old history.[79] In 1966, the World Health Organization began a program to immunize all individuals who had come into contact with an infected person. This strategy was adopted because it simply was not possible to immunize entire populations. In October 1977, Ali Maolin of Somalia was the last person in the world to have a naturally occurring case of smallpox (barring laboratory accidents). Because smallpox has no animal reservoir and requires person-to-person contact for its spread, most scientists agree that we are free of this disease, at least as a natural infection.[79] As a consequence, most populations have not maintained immunity to the virus and the world's populations are becoming susceptible to infection. Many governments now fear the use of smallpox virus as a weapon of bioterrorism, and the debate continues over whether to destroy the two known stocks of smallpox virus in the United States and Russia.[80] As a consequence, the development of new, more effective vaccines and safe anti-smallpox virus drugs has risen high on the list of priorities for some countries, and such vaccines have already been stockpiled in the United States. It is paradoxical that humankind's most triumphant medical accomplishment is now tarnished by the spectre of biowarfare.

The Salk and Sabin poliovirus vaccines were the first products to benefit from the cell culture revolution. In the early 1950s in the United States, just before the introduction of the Salk vaccine, about 21,000 cases of poliomyelitis were reported annually. Today, thanks to aggressive immunization programs, polio has been eradicated from the United States (see Chapters 18 and 19).[141] As of this writing, only three countries have seen interruption of wild-type poliovirus circulation: Nigeria, Afghanistan, and Pakistan. With the substantial financial support of the Gates Foundation, there is hope that global immunization campaigns can lead to eradication of poliomyelitis from the planet.

The first viral vaccines deployed included infectious vaccines, attenuated vaccines, inactivated virus vaccines, and subunit vaccines. Both the Salk inactivated virus vaccine and the recombinant hepatitis B virus subunit vaccine were products of the modern era of virology. Today many new vaccine technologies are either in use or are being tested for future deployment.[3,23,168] These include recombinant subunit vaccines, virus-like particle vaccines, viral antigens delivered in viral vectors comprising vaccinia virus or adenovirus, and DNA plasmids that express viral proteins from strong promoters. Therapeutic vaccines boost the immune system using specific cytokines or hormones in combination with new adjuvants to stimulate immunity at specific locations in the host or to tailor the production of immune effector cells and antibodies. Considering that the first vaccines for smallpox were reported in the Chinese literature of the 10th century,[58] vaccinology has clearly been practiced well before the beginning of the field of virology.

Although vaccines have been extraordinarily successful in preventing specific diseases, up until the 1960s, few natural products or chemotherapeutic agents that cured or reduced viral infections were known. That situation changed dramatically with the development of Symmetrel (amantadine) by Dupont in the 1960s as a specific influenza A virus drug. Soon after, acyclovir, an inhibitor of herpesviruses, was developed by Burroughs-Wellcome. Acyclovir achieves its remarkable specificity because to be active, it must be phosphorylated by the viral enzyme thymidine kinase before it can be incorporated into viral DNA by the viral DNA polymerase. This drug blocks herpes simplex virus type 2 (HSV-2) replication after reactivation from latency and stopped a growing epidemic in the 1970s and 1980s (Chapter 14). The development of other nucleoside analogs has led to many compounds effective against DNA viruses. Until the human immunodeficiency virus (HIV) epidemic, few drugs effective against RNA viruses other than the influenza A virus were known. As natural products, the interferons (Chapter 9) are used successfully in the clinic for hepatitis B and C infections, cancer therapy, and multiple sclerosis. The interferons, novel cytokines found in the course of studying virus interference,[23,92,93] modulate the immune response and continue to play an increasing role in the treatment of many clinical syndromes.

Virology and the Birth of Immunology

Edward Jenner was a British surgeon who is credited with making the first smallpox vaccine in 1796, and has also been called the "father of immunology." Jenner began a long tradition of virology providing seminal discoveries about the immune response. Two examples will serve to illustrate this pattern.

Alick Issacs and Jean Lindenmann, while working at the National Institute for Medical Research in London, found that addition of heat-inactivated influenza virus to the chorioallantoic membrane of chicken eggs interfered with the replication of influenza virus. When they published this observation in 1957, they coined the term *interferon* (IFN).[92] In the 1970s the protein was purified from cells by Sidney Pestka and Alan Waldman,[161] and subsequently the genes encoding the proteins were cloned.[73] This allowed formal proof that IFN—by that time known to comprise a variety of different proteins—could interfere with viral replication. Extensive work with viruses showed that IFNs bind to cell-surface receptors, and through the JAK-STAT signal transduction pathway, induce the synthesis of more than 1,000 mRNAs that establish an antiviral state.[39] IFNs protect against both viral and bacterial infections, and also play a role in tumor clearance.

While working at the John Curtin School of Medical Research in Australia, Rolf Zinkernagel and Peter Doherty provided seminal insight into how cytotoxic T cells (CTLs) recognize virus-infected cells. They were studying infection of mice with lymphocytic choriomeningitis virus (LCMV). Because this virus is noncytopathic, they hypothesized that brain damage in infected mice was a consequence of CTLs attacking virus-infected cells. They made the observation that CTLs isolated from LCMV-infected mice lysed virus-infected target cells *in vitro* only if both cell types had the same major histocompatibility complex (MHC) haplotype. This requirement was termed MHC restriction.[211] In other words, a CTL must recognize two components on a virus-infected cell: one virus specific and one from the host. Subsequent research revealed that CTLs recognize a short viral peptide bound to MHC class I (MHC-I) proteins on the surface of target cells. These observations revolutionized our understanding of T-cell–mediated killing, thereby establishing a foundation for understanding the general mechanisms used by the immune system to recognize both foreign microorganisms and self-molecules. The results have had wide implications for clinical medicine, not only in infection but also in areas such as cancer and autoimmune reactions in inflammatory diseases.

Emerging Viruses

In general, emerging viruses cause human infections that have not been seen or reported before. They usually attract the public's attention, often by media sound bites like "killer viruses emerge from the jungle." The fact is that spread of infections through different hosts is well known in virology. Most so-called emerging infections represent zoonotic infections: infection of humans by a virus that normally exists in an animal population in nature.[187]

Perhaps the most infamous emerging virus infection of the 20th century is the human immunodeficiency virus type 1, HIV-1, a retrovirus.[85] Progenitor HIV viruses exist in primates, and we now believe they infected humans as a result of hunting and slaughter for food.[170] HIV was first recognized as a new disease entity by clinicians and epidemiologists in the early 1980s, and they rapidly tracked down the venereal mode of virus transmission. The virus was detected in blood products and transplant tissue. The immune system of HIV-infected individuals is severely compromised, which results in a variety of infections by usually benign microbes. The first published report of acquired immunodeficiency syndrome (AIDS) was in June 1981. Possible causative agents were first suggested in 1983.[7] and then 1984.[68] Had this pandemic occurred in 1961 instead of 1981, neither the nature of retroviruses nor the existence of its host cell (CD4 helper T cell) would have been understood. HIV is a lentivirus (*lenti* is Latin for slow) and despite its recent appearance in humans, lentiviruses have been around for a long time. In fact, one of the first animal viruses to be identified in 1904 was the lentivirus that causes infectious equine anemia.

Many other examples of emerging viruses have attracted global concern and an exceptional rapid response of scientists and health officials.[187] The severe acute respiratory syndrome (SARS) and West Nile virus epidemics revealed the presence of a new human coronavirus (SARS), identified with unprecedented speed, and the invasion of an Old World virus into the Western hemisphere (West Nile virus).[90,140] In 2006, chikungunya virus (an endemic virus infection in Africa) spread explosively to several countries where it was hitherto unknown.[169] On La Reunion Island, more than 40% of the population of 800,000 people was infected. The first appearance of avian influenza A (H5N1) virus in humans in 1997 produced fears of a pandemic of serious proportions because humans had no immunological history of infection by this avian strain.[182] Soon thereafter, the emergence of the pandemic H1N1 influenza virus in 2009 produced similar worries because of the relationship of the virus to the deadly 1918 influenza epidemic.[184] The mobilization of world health networks, public health officials, vaccine producers, veterinarians, clinicians, and molecular virologists marked a new chapter in dealing with emerging diseases.

Epidemiology of Viral Infections

The study of the incidence, distribution, and control of disease in a population is an integral part of virology. The technology advancements of the last 50 years have provided epidemiology with a terrific boost. The discovery of specific molecular reagents (e.g., recombinant DNA technology, antibodies, polymerase chain reaction [PCR], rapid diagnostic tests, high volume DNA and RNA sequencing) now enables detection of virions, proteins, and nucleic acids in body fluids, tissue samples, or in the environment. Moreover, we now can compare and classify viral isolates rapidly, determine the relationships between virus strains, and track the spread of infections around the world. The marriage of behavioral, geographic, and molecular epidemiology made this a most powerful science.[87]

The understanding of epidemics and pandemics of our most common viral infections such as influenza requires the perspectives of ecology, population biology, and molecular biology.[106,182] G. Hirst and his colleagues (1941–1950) developed the diagnostic tools that permitted both the typing of the hemagglutinin (HA protein) of influenza A strains and the monitoring of the antibody response to this antigen in patients (see Chapters 42 and 43). These observations have been expanded, with more and more sophisticated molecular approaches, to prove the existence of animal reservoirs for influenza viruses, the reassortment of viral genome segments between human and animal virus strains (antigenic shift), and a high rate of mutation (antigenic drift) caused by RNA-dependent RNA synthesis with no known RNA editing or corrective mechanisms.[153,184] These molecular events that lead to episodic local epidemics and worldwide pandemics are understood in broad outline. Many viruses are now known to evolve at high rates following basic Darwinian principles in a time frame shorter than that of any other organism. Indeed, we now understand that RNA virus populations exist as a quasispecies or a swarm of individual viral genomes where every member is unique. Influenza viruses are successful because they have evolved to carry the very engines of evolution: mechanisms of mutation and recombination (reassortment), Influenza A virus has not been eliminated even with effective vaccines and antiviral drugs. Variants always arise that escape effective immune responses thorough high mutation (drift), and when co-infection occurs with viruses spreading from nonhuman hosts, new reassortants regularly arise. Expression of these new combinations of viral genes can change the pattern of infection from local to pandemic via an antigenic shift of its HA and NA subunit proteins. These studies (Chapters 42 and 43) have revealed an extraordinary lifestyle that reverberates around the planet in birds, farm animals, and humans. The study of the mechanisms of viral pathogenesis and modulation of the immune system have led to new insights in the virus–host relationship.

New technology discovered and developed over the last 35 years is changing the way viral infections are studied in the laboratory and in the field, and is changing our appreciation of epidemiology and virus ecology.[183] Amplification technologies such as PCR permit rapid sampling of viral nucleic acids without growth in culture or plaque purification. Microarray technology where discriminatory DNA sequences from all sequenced viral genomes are put on a single array enables rapid classification of PCR-amplified nucleic acids.[194] Rapid genome sequencing has revealed hitherto described viral genomes, relationships among viruses, and sequence heterogeneity within a virus population.[123] Mutations can be detected rapidly, documented, and localized in the viral genome. Importantly, the biological consequences can be monitored quickly. For example, in the late 1970s, viral epidemiologists were confronted with a highly transmissible, lethal infection of puppies.[144] In record time, scientists found that just two mutations in the capsid gene of feline parvovirus altered the host range such that the mutant could infect dogs. In less than a year, a completely new, highly pathogenic virus called canine parvovirus spread all around the world. Its evolution has continued to be monitored, and a highly effective vaccine was developed. A similar type of molecular archeology enabled scientists to analyze serum samples collected from patients in the 1950s in efforts to understand the origins of HIV.[85] Sequence analysis of the HIV genome from one sample (ZR 1959) suggested that the virus may have emerged in the 1940s to 1950s. Field studies in Africa of viruses present in primate feces indicated that HIV most likely derived from a chimpanzee lentivirus in Africa.[170] After the initial human infection, rapid mutation and selection established the first human variants of this lentivirus that replicated and continued to evolve as they spread through their new human hosts.

The advances in our understanding of the viral etiology of tumors pay tribute to the modern epidemiology strategy by D. Burkitt and K. Takatsuki, leading to the identification of Epstein-Barr virus (EBV) and HTLV-1. Similarly, the recombinant DNA revolution overcame the problems of propagating human papillomaviruses. The human papillomaviruses (see Chapter 56) differ in transmission, location on the body, their nature of pathogenesis, and persistence. New technology permitted the identification of new virus serotypes, triggering epidemiologic correlations for high- or low-risk cancer viruses.[212] The same technology enabled the development and use of an effective vaccine against cervical cancer. We cannot forget the considerable impact of veterinary virus epidemiology on our understanding of complicated human diseases. For example, careful epidemiologic work by Sigurdsson and colleagues on unusual diseases of sheep[175] provided the first understanding of slow infections in sheep (Visna-Maedi virus; a lentivirus) and infectious proteins (prions), which cause spongiform encephalopathies (Chapter 78).

As we describe in the next section, molecular epidemiology is reaching new levels of sophistication, not only in detecting new viruses, but also taking inventory of the viral ecosystem. Whether the next human epidemic will result from a novel variant of Ebola virus, coronavirus, or Norwalk virus, or the more likely possibility of a new pandemic variant of influenza virus, remains to be seen. The new technologies also enable analysis of virus populations in natural communities of nonhuman animals. For example, we can now monitor pandemic spread of avian influenza virus in wild birds and other nonhuman hosts.[153] These alternative hosts have never been sampled for virus populations in such molecular detail. New insights into the selection pressures and bottlenecks are emerging almost faster than the viruses. What is abundantly clear, however, is that the demographics of the human population on earth are changing at unprecedented rates (Table 1.1). Even as birth rates slow, our planet will house 8 to 10 billion people by 2050 to 2100. For the first time, there will be three to four times more people older than the age of 60 than younger than 3 to 4 years of age. Not only are we an aging population, we are moving to urban environments, with more than 20 to 30 cities containing more than 10 million people. Clearly, patterns of human behavior (increased population density, increased travel, increased ages of the population) will provide the environment for the selection of emerging viruses and the challenges to the new field of molecular epidemiology.

HOST–VIRUS INTERACTIONS AND VIRAL PATHOGENESIS

The technologies that contributed most to the modern era of virology (1960 to present), were advances in cell culture and molecular biology.[55] Virologists were able to describe the replicative cycles of viruses in great detail under well-defined conditions, and they demonstrated the elaborate interactions between viral genomes, viral proteins, and the cellular machinery of the host. As indicated previously, these advances resulted in an extraordinary inquiry into the functions of infected or uninfected host cells using the tools of both molecular biology and cell biology. As this approach matured, it became more reductionist in nature, and the questions became more detailed. However, some virologists used the new knowledge to move back to more complicated *in vivo* systems to study previously difficult problems in host–virus

TABLE 1.1 Advances and Challenges

Vaccines	Yellow fever virus vaccine, live attenuated Salk and Sabin vaccines for poliovirus, killed and live attenuated Recombinant hepatitis B vaccine, subunit Vaccinia virus vaccine to eradicate natural smallpox virus from the planet Influenza virus vaccines, inactivated and live attenuated Varicella-zoster virus vaccines, live attenuated Rotavirus vaccines, live attenuated Measles vaccines, live attenuated Recombinant human papillomavirus vaccine, subunit; prevents cancers and virus infections
Antiviral drugs	Acyclovir against herpes simplex type 1 and type 2 Combination therapy: Protease, reverse transcriptase, and integrase inhibitors against HIV Interferon therapy for hepatitis B and C Amantadine against influenza A virus Neuraminidase inhibitors against influenza virus
Epidemiologic advances	Understanding the molecular basis of antigenic shift and drift in influenza viruses Identification of the causes of AIDS and SARS Prion diseases recognized and mechanisms elucidated Deep sequencing, genome analysis; pathogen discovery, uncovering the molecular nature of epidemic and pandemic infections Recognition of the role of zoonotic infections in the emergence of new viral diseases Recognition of specific viruses as causative agents in human cancers Elucidation of the concept of viral quasispecies and the molecular biology of viral populations
Viral pathogenesis	Identification of viral virulence genes Identification of host genes affecting virus replication and spread Identification of the molecular bases for antiviral immune defenses (adaptive immunity) Identification of the molecular basis of front-line cellular defenses (intrinsic and innate immunity) including apoptosis and induction of defensive cytokines Understanding of the molecular basis for viral tropism Elucidation of the mechanisms involved in viral quiescence and persistence
The challenges (societal)	Population explosion: more people now live on the planet than at any time in our existence (predicted to be 8 to 10 billion in the next few decades) Population concentration: world populations are concentrating in large urban centers of 10 to 20 million people or more
The challenges (scientific)	Population demographics: for the first time there are more people older than the age of 60 than younger than the age of 4 Population interactions: world populations interact physically at rates and extents never before possible Pandemic viral diseases and bioterrorism provide continuing challenges for human survival Research costs money: how do we alleviate the pressures on funding and support of fundamental research Discoveries cannot be predicted: how to balance true discovery research with applied (translational) research Public support: how do we develop support and advocacy for virology research Policy makers need to understand virology: more engagement of scientists with lawmakers and the general public Public education about vaccination and other public health issues Discovering an effective vaccine against HIV Developing vaccines against persistent viruses Discovering and developing new antiviral drugs Development of rapid viral diagnostic and identification strategies Coupling new technology with established procedures Balancing risks and benefits of dangerous pathogen research Developing surrogates for Koch's postulates in modern pathogen discovery programs Defining and understanding the composition and interplay of microbial communities inside and outside hosts (natural versus unnatural flora)

AIDS, acquired immunodeficiency syndrome; HIV, human immunodeficiency virus; SARS, severe acute respiratory syndrome.

interactions involving the natural host or animal models of infection. Chief among these new questions was, how does a virus cause disease processes in the animal? How do we quantitate viral virulence and what is the genetic basis of an attenuated virus? These studies have identified, in selected viruses, a set of genes and functions that broadly influence our understanding of pathogenesis.

Despite an abundance of data, we have distilled six general categories relating to viral pathogenesis. Four of these involve viral gene products and two involve the hosts.

1. Mutations in genes that impair virus replication in the host, lower the threshold of pathogenesis by reducing the number of progeny produced. These mutations are found in essential genes (essential for life) *in vivo.*
2. A second class of mutations impairs virulence (reduces the degree of pathogenicity), but does not alter normal virus replication (at least in some cell or tissue types). Here, host- or tissue-range mutations are most common. Mutations can change the pattern of virion adsorption to a particular cell type and so prevent viral entry into a cell. Mutations in viral enhancer elements can alter viral transcription in selected cell types. In some viral genomes, mutations affect rates of translation such that virulence is reduced. A classic example comes from analysis of the attenuated strains of poliovirus in the Sabin vaccine. All three strains of the Sabin poliovirus vaccine contain mutations in the 5′ untranslated region of the viral RNA genome, which impair translation of these RNAs, and as a consequence virus yields are reduced. As a result, after infection, viral replication occurs, the host is immunized, but disease does not occur.
3. A third class of genes affecting virulence is involved in producing products that modify the host defenses. Intrinsic host defenses depend on receptors inside and on the surface of cells that detect viral gene products. When these receptors are activated, cytokines can be produced to alert more global innate immune defenses, the cell may die by apoptosis, or autophagy may be induced to engulf virus particles. It is likely that every successful virus can bypass or modulate these most fundamental cell-autonomous defenses. Mutations in these primary defense systems or viral proteins that block them affect virulence and spread. Some viruses encode genes that produce viral homologs of host cytokines (virokines). These proteins are secreted from infected cells and modify the immune response to infection. Other viruses encode decoy receptors that bind host-produced cytokines and reroute the immune response as a result. Many viral genomes encode genes whose products block infected cells from undergoing apoptosis in response to a virus infection. Some viruses, such as African swine fever virus, secrete a pro-apoptotic factor that kills lymphocytes and enhances its virulence. Many viruses produce proteins that alter the MHC proteins (MHC-I and MHC-II; also known as human leukocyte antigens or HLA proteins). These complex proteins display on the cell surface, short peptides derived from newly made or newly ingested proteins inside the cell. T cells detect these complexes and respond if non–self-peptides are detected. Many viral infections alter the expression or function of these MHC proteins. Other viruses encode superantigens that stimulate or eliminate lymphoid cells of a selected specificity or with a class of receptors. HIV infection kills CD4 T cells and disrupts the immune response.
4. A fourth class of viral virulence genes enhances the spread of a virus in the host. Some viruses are released from infected cells at the apical or basolateral surface, permitting selected spread *in vivo.* Some RNA viruses acquire infectivity (maturation) only after specific proteolytic cleavage of their structural proteins. In some cases, maturation is accomplished by a viral protease and in others by a cellular protease, each with a specific amino acid sequence required for proper cleavage and resulting spread of the virus. Altering this sequence will affect virulence and overall transmissibility of the infection in a host population.
5. A fifth class involves host gene products. A wide variety of polymorphisms or mutations in the host result in modulated resistance or virulence of a virus. These host mutations can even be selected during viral epidemics, changing the gene pool of the surviving host population. In humans, polymorphisms in a chemokine receptor gene (a co-receptor) impart resistance to HIV infection at the level of viral absorption. New antiviral drugs have been designed to target this viral–cytokine interaction. Variations in the immune responses of diverse hosts in a population will result in large variations in viral virulence. The host mechanisms that minimize viral diseases after infection are certainly major topics in viral pathogenesis.
6. The final class involves the society and interaction of hosts. Changes in population density, lifestyles, cultural traditions, and economic factors all play a major role in viral virulence. Poliovirus was a minor endemic virus infection for 3,000 years before the introduction of improved sanitation in the last century. As a result, human populations were infected for the first time at a later age and large poliovirus epidemics resulted. It may not have been a coincidence that the worst influenza epidemic in the century, killing 20 to 40 million people, started in about 1918 toward the end of World War I, with so many people dislocated and moving about the world in very crowded and poor conditions. If there is a general lesson from history it is that cultural and environmental changes will surely play a role in the virulence of viruses in the future.

THE FUTURE OF VIROLOGY? (E-TABLE 1.7 AND TABLE 1.1)

The future of virology is unpredictable, but it is guaranteed to be exciting. Who knows what discoveries remain? Certainly, the number of astounding and groundbreaking discoveries in biology over the last 50 years is remarkable.[55] Most could not have been predicted or even imagined, prior to their discovery. That virologists participated in making many of these discoveries is no accident: Viral gene products have evolved to engage all the key nodes of biology ranging from the atomic to the organismal. We only have to be smart enough to figure out how to identify these nodes. The forces that will drive our field are technology development, public health, information processing, and, of course, personal curiosity. Indeed new life science technologies invariably will give rise to new, unexpected insights in virology to meet our current challenges. That has been, and continues to be, the future of virology (see Table 1.1).

Despite a cloudy crystal ball, three general trends are likely to rise to the forefront of virology research over the next 10 years.

1. **The detailed understanding of the systems biology inherent in virus–host interactions.** Although virus particles are inanimate, it is the living, infected cell that delivers the phenotype promoted by the viral genome. The change of state of a cell or tissue from uninfected to infected is fertile ground for modern systems biology. The constellation of new gene products (viral and host) and altered host pathways produced in an infected cell give rise to biological outputs that go far beyond the single cell in the laboratory. Viruses offer useful modalities for the systems biologist. One can synchronize an infection and go from the uninfected to infected state within minutes, or use the same virus to produce an acute or a quiescent infection. Regulatory circuits, modulation of host defenses, emergence of pathogenesis, and modes of efficient transmission in a hostile environment, are all inherent in the nanobiology of viruses. How can a viral genome with so few genes relative to the host, dominate a cell and the host so quickly and dynamically? How does it all work? How has evolution produced such diversity of infected cell phenotypes? Microarrays, PCR, mass spectroscopy, microfluidics, large-scale nucleic-acid sequencing, massive database assembly, and computer modeling are what toothpicks and Petri dishes were to the students of the Delbrück phage school 60 years ago.
2. **The understanding of viruses as integral participants in the ecosystem.** Such knowledge means uncovering the multiple interrelationships and interactions of all viruses and their hosts. This is ecology, but on a scale that has hitherto been unimaginable for virologists. Viruses exist wherever life is found, and they are the most abundant entities on the planet. Indeed their biomass rivals that of the prokaryotes. Estimates are that we know less than 1% of the viral genomes on the planet, but first principles inform us that there can be only a limited number of genome strategies for replication and expression of information. Therefore, despite what appears to be incredible diversity, we will be able to identify new viruses by the unique signatures of a viral genome. The viral ecology problem, therefore, is one of knowing what is out there and why. The powerful techniques of interrogating virus populations in the wild for their RNA, DNA, proteins, and unique small molecules have changed the worldview of ecologists and molecular biologists alike. The new biology will require the intellectual firepower of computer scientists, engineers, chemists, and physicists, as well as biologists. As part of this growing knowledge of the viral ecosystem, virologists will come to be more ecumenical in their studies and not balkanize the field into animal and plant virology or viruses of single cell hosts.
3. **Health of humans and the world.** The fundamental need for public health measures is unprecedented, as the human population is now greater than ever before. However, despite all attempts to prove otherwise, humans are not the top of the food chain. Every living thing ultimately engages every other entity directly or indirectly—and, as far as we know, every living thing is infected with viruses. These infections shape human existence on the planet. A human centric view of public health is short-sighted. First principles tell us that all successful viruses today carry a collection of genes that have survived the best defenses that hosts can muster. Our knowledge of the microbial world must be used to inform our national and international health policies. The bedrock of old-fashioned public health policies cannot be ignored: clean water, sewage treatment, proper nutrition, and management of epidemic childhood disease by vaccines. However, the continuing divide between rich and poor nations, the conflicts among ethnic and religious groups, the changing climate, and resulting calamities of drought and other natural disasters stress even these most basic attempts at maintaining public health. Certainly the high-tech approach to public health of developed counties will find no purchase in those countries where the basics of survival are lacking.

Intrinsic and Extrinsic Defenses Against Viral Infections

It is likely that considerable work in the future will be directed to the host defenses that meet viral infections in the first minutes to hours. All viral infections begin as individual, single-cell events that either are resolved or expand to produce the characteristic phenotypes of the persistent or acute infection. Ancient single-cell pathways of response to external stimuli have been honed over millions of years to provide cells and communities of cells, a repertoire of defensive actions that are now being revealed. Every cell is capable of responding to infection immediately (so-called intrinsic resistance) by processes whose nature and actions will fuel discovery research in the near future.[17,61] These processes act immediately upon infection, before the so-called innate and adaptive immune responses are called into action. We understand some of these processes, such as apoptosis in some detail, but others, including RNA interference (RNAi), autophagy, DNA repression, and the restriction factors first defined by retrovirologists, remain fertile ground for discovery.[28,29,41] The interaction between signals of early warning from single cells with the local multicellular innate immune response and the global adaptive immune response are likely to be key to recognizing and responding to the various patterns of viral infections that arise in nature. Primary questions concerning the molecular biology and cellular biology of persistent and latent infection cannot be answered without knowledge of early defense responses of single cells and local tissues.

DNA microarray technology has enabled the measurement of the whole genome responses of single cells exposed to a wide variety of viral infections.[100] The systematic profiling of gene-expression changes has provided an exceptionally rich database from which we now are learning of cell-common and cell-specific responses to infection. The differences and similarities are proving to be the proverbial gold mine of information on the definition of evolutionarily conserved host-defense components and viral gene products that counter them. Understanding the relationship of common cell-stress responses and pathogen-specific responses and counter-responses will certainly provide insights into potential diagnostic and therapeutic targets for viral infections.[100]

Viruses and Cancer

Since the 1960s, seven different human viruses have been isolated, identified, and shown to be associated with the etiology of human cancer.[135] Surprisingly, even after 50 years, we have only a rudimentary understanding of the oncogenic pathogenesis of these infectious agents.[135] The first cancer-associated virus was discovered in 1964 when Epstein, Achong, and Barr[56] detected herpesvirus particles in cells obtained from a Burkitt's lymphoma.[24] The DNA episomes of the Epstein-Barr virus (or EBV) have been consistently found to be associated with some types of B-cell lymphomas. Despite this 40-year period, it remains unclear how or even if this virus actually causes this lymphoma. Although it is certain that the EBV genome contains one or more oncogenes (latent membrane protein 1, LMP-1), they are not expressed in the lymphoma cells. The only viral gene product expressed in these lymphoma cells is Epstein-Barr nuclear antigen 1 (EBNA-1), and its possible role of contributing to lymphomas is still controversial. Similarly the HTLV-1 viral genome does not contain a cellular oncogene, and it does not integrate into the host-cell DNA near a cellular proto-oncogene in a consistent fashion. Therefore, HTLV-1 does not employ the two most common mechanisms for tumor formation observed with the retroviruses. There is no clear association of any hepatitis B or C gene products in the causation of liver cancers. Rather it appears that immune destruction of liver cells followed by the regeneration of this tissue activates several growth factors made by the surrounding tissue resulting in fibrosis. The local milieu of inflammation and the positive feedback loop for growth drives the division of liver cells and hepatocellular carcinoma. This complex mix of infection, immune-mediated cell death, and chronic inflammation in a tissue with regenerative capacity is challenging to analyze. Although Kaposi's sarcoma herpesvirus also encodes potential oncogenes, no clear mechanism of how it initiates or propagates cancer is available. On the other hand, studies of the human papillomaviruses[45] have provided a mechanistic understanding of how these viruses transform cells. The viral E7 protein binds to the cellular retinoblastoma protein and inactivates its function, thereby initiating entry of the cell into the cell cycle and division. The viral E6 protein binds the cellular p53 protein and promotes its ubiquitylation and proteolytic degradation, thereby preventing cellular apoptosis.[165] More research is needed to fully understand the mechanisms that lead to cancers after infection by these viruses.[199]

A Role for Systems Biology in Virology

Not too long ago, molecular virology was limited to studies of one virus and one gene or gene product at a time. More complex studies often were seen as "descriptive." Times have changed! New technology enables virologists to interrogate simultaneously many viruses and large groups of genes or gene products in ever-expanding environments and biological networks. In this context, a network is defined as the interconnected intracellular processes that control everything within a cell, for example, DNA replication, processes of gene expression, organelle biogenesis, and metabolism to name a few.[139] The definition also encompasses networks of intercellular communication at the tissue, organ, and whole-organism level. Virologists are beginning to embrace a tenet of systems biology where information flows through these networks and disease arises when these networks are perturbed. Viral gene products cause changes in network architecture and thereby alter the dynamics of information flow. Future studies of viral pathogenesis are likely to involve identification and understanding of specific viral signatures of network imbalance that do not affect just one pathway but alter the fundamental homeostatic balance.[19,55,152,179]

Genomics and the Predictive Power of Sequence Analysis

The development of technologic advances in biology often drives new approaches and permits one to ask novel questions that could not even be framed in the past. In the last decade of the 20th century, rapid and inexpensive DNA-sequencing methods paved the way to sequence the genomes of many viruses and their hosts. This created large databases containing information about the variation of DNA or RNA sequences within a single virus (e.g., HIV, influenza) and permitted predictions about the nature of the mutations that were driving selective changes, mutation frequencies of different viruses, and evolutionary changes from isolates around the world. The correlations of these sequence variations with drug resistance, changes in the genetic background of the host, and virulence have been informative. By combining this information with the three-dimensional structure of the influenza A hemagglutinin (HA) protein, J. Plotkin and colleagues have examined codon use in this gene and suggested that the degeneracy of codon use was being optimized to permit changes in amino acids at critical positions in this protein, so as to reduce the impact of the immune response to this virus.[148] Although this concept has been controversial, it has permitted a set of predictions of the direction of future changes in these codons as the host develops its immune response and immunity of the population. Predicting the future changes in influenza strains provides a testable hypothesis and might then impact how we prepare for genetic drift in virus populations by designing vaccines.[184]

The degeneracy of the genetic code means that there are different codons that encode the same amino acid. As a result, many sequences can encode the same protein. This choice of sequences is constricted by several selective forces such as restrictions on transfer RNA (tRNA) availability in a host, giving rise to preferential codon use, the overall G-C content of a genome, the frequency in which two or three amino acids appear next to each other in proteins encoded by the virus, or the avoidance of some sequence contexts due to a high mutational load.[158] The low level of CpG dinucleotides in some genomes may result because a C-residue can be methylated. This change is mutagenic because methyl-C will pair with a T residue, causing a C to T transition in the genome. Once these restrictions on the frequency of certain dinucleotide to septanucleotide sequences are appreciated, they can be factored into a calculation of whether certain nucleotide sequences are over-represented or under-represented in a genome despite these selected pressures observed in a particular genome.

Algorithms have been designed to accomplish this, and it is clear from an analysis of 209 prokaryotic genomes and 90 bacteriophages that replicate in these hosts, that selected sequences of di-septanucleotides are over-represented and others are under-represented in these viral and bacterial genomes.[157] Having factored out the genetic codon preferences in this algorithm, these preferences represent a second code of under- or over-represented frequencies of nucleotide sequences, and the available data indicate that these sequences are functional and are selected for over evolutionary time scales. First, coding regions of a genome have been shown to have different over- or under-represented sequences in a genome. Second, if these coding regions sequences are employed to assemble a phylogenetic tree, these sequences do an excellent job in reconstructing the known evolutionary relationships of these 209 prokaryotic genome sequences (done originally by aligning the ribosomal gene sequences). Third, about 80% of the viruses in these databases can be correctly assigned to their hosts by matching the over- and under-represented sequences in their viral and host genomes. The same selection pressure acting upon this second code in a host genome also acts upon the genomes of their parasites. We now await the application of this algorithm to the more complex genomes and viruses of eukaryotes. Host genomes contain an amazing number of viral or viral-related sequences. More than 50% of the DNA sequences found in the human genome were derived from retroviruses, retrotransposons, DNA transposons and randomly amplified sequences of genes (short interspersed nuclear element [SINES] and the 7S RNA gene), pseudogenes, and repetitive DNA sequences.[114,192] Viruses certainly have left a major mark upon the evolution of their host's genomes in addition to the selective pressures they exert via virus infections and deaths. During the evolution of humans from their ancestral line, retroviruses and retro-transposons (the long interspersed nuclear element [LINE-1]) have entered the germ line, amplified their copy numbers, and integrated at various sites in the genome. This process introduces mutations, alters patterns of gene expression, and creates new interactions of viruses with their hosts. This is clearly one of the drivers of host evolution. Over time these retroviruses (human endogenous retroviruses, or HERVs) accumulate mutations in their genes, and some recombine out of the genome leaving only the long terminal repeats (LTRs) as a remnant marking their past insertion. Although humans no longer contain viable HERVs, the multiple copies of HERV–H or HERV-K viruses when transcribed in cells, produce functional viral proteins from different copies of these viruses, and the viral particles that are produced are defective and very poorly transmitted. Cellular transcription factors regulate the expression of the HERVs, and the p53 transcription factor (activated by stress and DNA damage) transcribes the HERV-H genome and produces particles in response to such stress.[209] Similarly the LINE-1 retrotransposons, which have about 300 viable and movable elements in the human genome today, are responsible for about 1% of the mutations found in each generation. LINE-1 transposons also contain p53 DNA response elements[86] and thus are also regulated by stress responses recorded by the host. Although it is clear that retroviruses and transposons can shape the host genome, it is equally clear that the host genome is a place for new viral genomes to evolve, recombine with exogenous viral genomes, and possibly produce a new agent optimized for replication in its host. Understanding of the dynamics of these vestiges of viruses that reside in our genome is a challenge for the future.

With many host-genome sequences representing all kingdoms of life in the databases, it has been possible to do some rather eye-opening analyses. For example, the resurrection of endogenous retroviruses from inactive sequences in host DNA has allowed the investigation of interactions between extinct pathogens called paleoviruses and their hosts that occurred millions of years ago.[53] By cloning these sequences, it has been possible to identify the cellular receptor of these extinct retroviruses.[172] Perhaps more amazing is that similar "viral genome fossils" representing DNA copies of filoviruses and bornaviruses as well as parvoviruses and circoviruses have been found in a variety of host genomes.[11,12] When the evolutionary history of various host genomes harboring these viral sequences were compared, it was possible to deduce that ancestors of modern viruses were in existence millions of years ago. What is even more curious is that these genome-insertion events seemed to happen around the same time in a wide variety of mammals. What global event could have stimulated such activities?

The Virome: How Many Viruses Are There? Where Are They? Why Are They There?

Virus ecology, as a result of modern virus discovery technology, is posing many questions (see 106,183). In 1977, when Fred Sanger sequenced the DNA genome of coliphage phiX174, many virologists were impressed with the wealth of information contained in a "simple" DNA sequence and the congruence of genetic and biochemical data with the genome structure. In fewer than 25 years, sampling, sequencing, and computer technology now provide the wherewithal to identify and sequence entire viral communities from their natural environment without the intervention of time-held techniques of isolation and characterization of individual viruses.[48,178,194] In early 2003, a novel viral DNA microarray was used to reveal and partially sequence a previously uncharacterized coronavirus in a viral isolate cultured from a patient with SARS. This chip technology has advanced to the point that essentially all the known viral genomes can be represented on a single microarray. New techniques for discovery and analysis of viral populations are certain to be found. As can be expected in this "omics" era, the identification and study of an entire community of viruses in their natural habitat has been called metagenomics.[2,156,202] The diversity of viruses in the environment is essentially unknown, as we have been limited to studying only those viruses that are easy to work with in the laboratory or those that have major impact on human health. The first metagenomic studies on viruses have revealed stunning diversity of genes and gene products that remain to be understood even in principle.[178,203] The combination of host and bacteriophage genome sequencing in the bacteria has proved to be an exceptional window on genome evolution and gene transfer. The practical value of identifying new gene products with novel functions cannot be overestimated. The repertoire of tactics for gene control and regulation is far more extensive than any of us imagined before the era of metagenomics. We can only expect that as the metagenomics of animal and plant viruses advances, the effect of knowing everything that is out there and the resulting knowledge of the dynamics of host–parasite interactions will be mind-boggling.[177]

Pathogen Discovery

Historically, discovery of new viral pathogens followed identification of diseases of consequence to humans, animals, and plants. Field biologists, clinicians, veterinarians, and the lay public noted syndromes, unusual behaviors, or drastic changes of animal and plant populations, which motivated scientists to discover the cause. The early days of virology were all "translational research." Koch's postulates were developed to identify the causative agent for a given disease. Advances in virus identification were driven in large part by technology developments such as porcelain filters, animal models, tissue and cell culture, microscopic visualization of cytopathic effect, serology, immunoassays, hybridization, western blotting, PCR, sequencing, microarrays, and imaging technology. These advances paved the way to our current understanding of viral pathogens and provided the data to advance our current understanding of mechanisms of pathogenesis. Modern pathogen discovery has entered a new phase where via sequencing technology, virologists can detect and identify viral nucleic acids with unprecedented sensitivity in essentially any sample.[123] We no longer need to be able to grow a virus stock to be able to identify it and develop diagnostic reagents, vaccines, or antiviral drugs.

The discovery of new viral genomes is proceeding at an amazing pace.[143] Although the discovery process is straightforward, understanding what these viruses are doing is a serious challenge.[91,155] If one finds novel viral genomes in samples from patients with disease, are these viruses the cause of the disease? Is it possible that they may be part of the normal flora of an individual (the microbiome;[107])? There are many populations of microbes in and on various parts of the body. Just identifying the microbiome differences in body sites of a single individual is challenging enough; cataloging the microbiome variation from individual to individual is even more difficult.[156] What functions does the microbiome have? There is evidence that our normal microbial flora stimulates local and systemic immune responses that protect against or suppress responses that contribute to pathogenesis by more-virulent microbes. Future virologists will have to unravel these heretofore unknown microbial relationships, and to do so we will need new technology. Whatever we find will undoubtedly reveal unanticipated insights about viruses and their hosts. Modern pathogen discovery will require the interaction of infectious disease specialists, epidemiologists, and bioinformatics specialists; virologists will have to be professionally "multilingual".[121]

Perhaps of fundamental importance is that proof of causation can no longer rely on the time-honored Koch's postulates.[91] This assertion is made not only because it may be difficult to propagate new viruses and find models to test their pathogenicity, it also is likely that many diseases will involve the interaction of multiple microbial communities (viruses, bacteria, fungi) that will be difficult to reproduce in the laboratory. Pathogen discovery will require new biomarkers of health and disease, methods to improve sampling and stability of samples, technology to record relevant data, and capacity to associate all this data with the sample. In the past, pathogen identification methods were slow and tedious, and working with multiple samples was difficult if not impossible. It is now possible to collect and analyze serial samples over time as patients move from health to disease. Assembling data, maintaining databases, and providing access for analysis will also involve advances in software and bioinformatics. In the end, the fundamental challenge will be how one moves from correlation of the presence of an agent or agents in disease to proof of causation.

REFERENCES

1. Alberts BM, Bedinger BP, Formosa T. Studies on DNA replication in the bacteriophage T4 in vitro systems. *Cold Spring Harbor Symp Quant Biol* 1982;47:655–668.
2. Angly F, Felts B, Breitbart M, et al. The marine viromes of four oceanic regions. *PLoS Biol* 2006;4:e368.
3. Arvin A, Greenberg HB. New viral vaccines. *Virology* 2006;344:240–249.
4. Astrachan L, Volkin E. Properties of ribonucleic acid turnover in T2-infected Escherichia coli. *Biochim Biophys Acta* 1958;29:536–544.
5. Avery OT, Macleod CM, McCarty M. Studies on the Chemical nature of the substance inducing transformation of pneumococcal types: induction of transformation by a desoxyribonucleic acid fraction isolated from pneumococcus type III. *J Exp Med* 1044;79:137–158.
6. Baltimore D. RNA-dependent DNA polymerase in virions of RNA tumour viruses. *Nature* 1970;226:1209–1211.
7. Barre-Sinoussi F, Chermann JC, Rey F, et al. Isolation of a T-lymphotropic retrovirus from a patient at risk for acquired immune deficiency syndrome (AIDS). *Science* 1983;220:868–871.
8. Bawden FC, Pirie NW. The isolation and some properties of liquid crystalline substances from solanaceous plants infected with three strains of tobacco mosaic virus. *Proc R Soc Med* 1937;123:274–320.
9. Bawden FC, Pirie NW, Bernal JD, et al. Liquid crystalline substances from virus infected plants. *Nature* 1939;138:1051–1052.
10. Beijerinck M. Concerning a contagium vivum fluidum as a cause of the spot-disease of tobacco leaves. *Verh Akad Wetensch, Amsterdam, II* 1898; 6:3–21.
11. Bely V, Levine A, Skalka A. Sequences from ancestral single-stranded DNA viruses in vertebrate genomes: the parvoviridae and Circoviridae are more than 40-50 million years old. *J Virol* 2010;84:12458–12464.
12. Bely V, Levine A, Skalka A. Unexpected inheritance: multiple integrations of ancient bornavirus and ebola/marburgvirus sequences in vertebrate genomes. *PLoS Pathogens* 2010;6:e1001030.
13. Benzer S. Fine Structure of a Genetic Region in Bacteriophage. *Proc Natl Acad Sci U S A* 1955;41:344–354.
14. Benzer S, Champe SP. Ambivalent rII Mutants of Phage T4. *Proc Natl Acad Sci U S A* 1961;47:1025–1038.
15. Berget SM, Moore C, Sharp PA. Spliced segments at the 5′ terminus of adenovirus 2 late mRNA. *Proc Natl Acad Sci U S A* 1977;74:3171–3175.
16. Bernal JD, Fankuchen I. X-ray and crystallographic studies of plant virus preparations. *J Gen Physiol* 1941;25:147–165.
17. Bieniasz PD. Intrinsic immunity: a front-line defense against viral attack. *Nat Immunol* 2004;5:1109–1115.
18. Biggs PM, Payne LN, Milne BS, et al. Field trials with an attenuated cell associated vaccine for Marek's disease. *Vet Rec* 1970;87:704–709.
19. Biurungi G, Chen S, Loy B, et al. Metabolomics approach for investigation of effects of dengue fever infection using the EA.hy926 cell line. *J Proteome Res* 2010;9:6523–6534.
20. Blumberg BS, Gerstley BJ, Hungerford DA, et al. A serum antigen (Australia antigen) in Down's syndrome, leukemia, and hepatitis. *Ann Intern Med* 1967;66:924–931.
21. Bohmann D, Bos TJ, Admon A, et al. Human proto-oncogene c-jun encodes a DNA binding protein with structural and functional properties of transcription factor AP-1. *Science* 1987;238:1386–1392.
22. Bordet J. Concerning the theories of the so-called "bacteriophage". *Br Med J* 1922;2:296.

23. Buonaguro L, Pulendran B. Immunogenomics and systems biology of vaccines. *Immunol Rev* 2011;1:197–208.
24. Burkitt D. A children's cancer dependent on climatic factors. *Nature* 1962; 194:232–234.
25. Butler PJ, Klug A. Assembly of the particle of tobacco mosaic virus from RNA and disks of protein. *Nat New Biol* 1971;229:47–50.
26. Cairns J, ed. *The Autoradiography.* Cold Spring Harbor, NY: Cold Spring Harbor Laboratory Press; 1966.
27. Campbell AM. Episomes. *Adv Genet* 1962;11:101–145.
28. Chakrabarti A, Jha B, Silverman R. New insights into the role of Rnase L in innate immunity. *J Interferon Cytokine Res* 2011;31:49–57.
29. Chiu Y-L, Greene W. APOBEC3G: an intracellular centurion. *Philos Trans R Soc Lond B Biol Sci* 2009;364:689–703.
30. Choo QL, Kuo G, Weiner AJ, et al. Isolation of a cDNA clone derived from a blood-borne non-A, non-B viral hepatitis genome. *Science* 1989; 244:359–362.
31. Chow LT, Gelinas RE, Broker TR, et al. An amazing sequence arrangement at the 5′ ends of adenovirus 2 messenger RNA. *Cell* 1977; 12:1–8.
32. Cohen SS. *Virus-induced Enzymes.* New York: Columbia University Press; 1968.
33. Crick FH, Watson JD. Structure of small viruses. *Nature* 1956;177: 473–475.
34. d'Herelle F. *The Bacteriophage and Its Behavior.* Baltimore: Williams & Wilkins; 1926.
35. d'Herelle F. Le microbe bactériophage, agent d'immunité dans la peste et le barbone. *C R Hebd Seances Acad Sci Paris* 1921;72:99.
36. d'Herelle F. Sur un microbe invisible antagoniste des bacilles dysentériques. *C R Hebd Seances Acad Sci Paris* 1917;1:72–99.
37. Danna K, Nathans D. Specific cleavage of simian virus 40 DNA by restriction endonuclease of Hemophilus influenzae. *Proc Natl Acad Sci U S A* 1971;68:2913–2917.
38. Danna KJ, Sack GH Jr, Nathans D. Studies of simian virus 40 DNA. VII. A cleavage map of the SV40 genome. *J Mol Biol* 1973;78: 363–376.
39. Darnell JE Jr, Kerr IM, Stark GR. Jak-STAT pathways and transcriptional activation in response to IFNs and other extracellular signaling proteins. *Science* 1994;264:1415–1421.
40. DeCaprio JA, Ludlow JW, Figge J, et al. SV40 large tumor antigen forms a specific complex with the product of the retinoblastoma susceptibility gene. *Cell* 1988;54:275–283.
41. Ding S-W, Voinet O. Antiviral immunity directed by small RNAs. *Cell* 2007;130:413–426.
42. Dulbecco R, Vogt M. Evidence for a Ring Structure of Polyoma Virus DNA. *Proc Natl Acad Sci U S A* 1963;50:236–243.
43. Dulbecco R, Vogt M. Some problems of animal virology as studied by the plaque technique. *Cold Spring Harb Symp Quant Biol* 1953;18: 273–279.
44. Dynan WS, Tjian R. The promoter-specific transcription factor Sp1 binds to upstream sequences in the SV40 early promoter. *Cell* 1983;35: 79–87.
45. Dyson N, Howley PM, Munger K, et al. The human papilloma virus-16 E7 oncoprotein is able to bind to the retinoblastoma gene product. *Science* 1989;243:934–937.
46. Eagle H. The specific amino acid requirements of a human carcinoma cell (Stain HeLa) in tissue culture. *J Exp Med* 1955;102:37–48.
47. Edgar RS, Wood WB. Morphogenesis of bacteriophage T4 in extracts of mutant-infected cells. *Proc Natl Acad Sci U S A* 1966;55: 498–505.
48. Edwards RA, Rohwer F. Viral metagenomics. Nature reviews. *Microbiology* 2005;3:504–510.
49. Eidson CS, Kleven SH, Anderson DP. *Vaccination Against Marek's Disease.* Lyon: Oncogenesis and Herpesvirus; 1972.
50. Ellermann V, Bang O. Experimentelle Leukamie bei Huhnern. *Zentralbl Bakteriol Alet I* 1908;46:595–597.
51. Ellis EL, ed. *Bacteriophage: One-step Growth.* Cold Spring Harbor, NY: Cold Spring Harbor Laboratory Press; 1966.
52. Ellis EL, Delbruck M. The Growth of Bacteriophage. *J Gen Physiol* 1939; 22:365–384.
53. Emerman M, Malik H. Paleovirology- modern consequences of ancient viruses. *PLoS Biology* 2010;8:e1000301.
54. Enders JF, Weller TH, Robbins FC. Cultivation of the Lansing strain of poliomyelitis virus in cultures of various human embryonic tissues. *Science* 1949;109:85–87.
55. Enquist L. Virology in the 21st Century. *J Virol* 2009;83:5296–5308.
56. Epstein MA, Achong BG, Barr YM. Virus Particles in Cultured Lymphoblasts from Burkitt's Lymphoma. *Lancet* 1964;1:702–703.
57. Feng H, Shuda M, Chang Y, et al. Clonal integration of a polyomavirus in human Merkel cell carcinoma. *Science* 2008;319:1096–1100.
58. Fenner F, Nakano JJ. Poxviridae: The poxviruses. In: Lennette EH, Halonen P, Murphy FA, ed. *The Laboratory Diagnosis of Infectious Diseases: Principles and Practice, Viral, Rickettsial, and Chlamydial Diseases,* vol. 2. New York: Springer-Verlag; 1988.
59. Fitzgerald M, Shenk T. The sequence 5′-AAUAAA-3′forms parts of the recognition site for polyadenylation of late SV40 mRNAs. *Cell* 1981; 24:251–260.
60. Flaks JG, Cohen SS. Virus-induced acquisition of metabolic function. I. Enzymatic formation of 5-hydroxymethyldeoxycytidylate. *J Biol Chem* 1959;234:1501–1506.
61. Flint SJ, Enquist LW, Racaniello VR, et al. *Principles of Virology.* Washington, DC: ASM Press; 2009.
62. Fowlkes DM, Shenk T. Transcriptional control regions of the adenovirus VAI RNA gene. *Cell* 1980;22:405–413.
63. Fraenkel-Conrat H, Singer B. The chemical basis for the mutagenicity of hydroxylamine and methoxyamine. *Biochim Biophys Acta* 1972;262: 264–268.
64. Fraenkel-Conrat H, Singer B, Williams RC. Infectivity of viral nucleic acid. *Biochim Biophys Acta* 1957;25:87–96.
65. Freeman VJ. Studies on the virulence of bacteriophage-infected strains of Corynebacterium diphtheriae. *J Bacteriol* 1951;61:675–688.
66. Furth J, Strumia M. Studies on Transmissible Lymphoid Leucemia of Mice. *J Exp Med* 1931;53:715–731.
67. Furuichi Y, Morgan M, Muthukrishnan S. Reovirus messenger RNA contains a methylated, blocked 5′-terminal structure: m-7G(5′)ppp(5′) G-MpCp. *Proc Natl Acad Sci U S A* 1975;72:362–366.
68. Gallo RC, Salahuddin SZ, Popovic M, et al. Frequent detection and isolation of cytopathic retroviruses (HTLV-III) from patients with AIDS and at risk for AIDS. *Science* 1984;224:500–503.
69. Gaynor RB, Hillman D, Berk AJ. Adenovirus early region 1A protein activates transcription of a nonviral gene introduced into mammalian cells by infection or transfection. *Proc Natl Acad Sci U S A* 1984;81: 1193–1197.
70. Germond JE, Hirt B, Oudet P, et al. Folding of the DNA double helix in chromatin-like structures from simian virus 40. *Proc Natl Acad Sci U S A* 1975;72:1843–1847.
71. Gey GO, Coffman WD, Kubicek MT. Tissue culture studies of the proliferative capacity of cervical carcinoma and normal epithelium. *Cancer Res* 1952;12:264–265.
72. Gierer A, Schramm G. Infectivity of ribonucleic acid from tobacco mosaic virus. *Nature* 1956;177:702–703.
73. Goeddel DV, Shepard HM, Yelverton E, et al. Synthesis of human fibroblast interferon by E. coli. *Nucleic Acids Res* 1980;8:4057–4074.
74. Goff SP, Berg P. Construction of hybrid viruses containing SV40 and lambda phage DNA segments and their propagation in cultured monkey cells. *Cell* 1976;9:695–705.
75. Gribskov M, Burgess RR. Sigma factors from E. coli, B. subtilis, phage SP01, and phage T4 are homologous proteins. *Nucleic Acids Res* 1986;14: 6745–6763.
76. Gruss P, Dhar R, Khoury G. Simian virus 40 tandem repeated sequences as an element of the early promoter. *Proc Natl Acad Sci U S A* 1981;78: 943–947.
77. Hayward WS, Neel BG, Astrin SM. Activation of a cellular onc gene by promoter insertion in ALV-induced lymphoid leukosis. *Nature* 1981; 290:475–480.
78. Hearing P, Shenk T. Sequence-independent autoregulation of the adenovirus type 5 E1A transcription unit. *Mol Cell Biol* 1985;5:3214–3221.
79. Henderson DA. Principles and lessons from the smallpox eradication programme. *Bull World Health Organ* 1987;65:535–546.

80. Henderson DA. Smallpox Virus Destruction and the Implications of a New Vaccine. *Biosecur Bioterror* 2011;9(2)163–168.
81. Henle G, Henle W, Diehl V. Relation of Burkitt's tumor-associated herpes-ytpe virus to infectious mononucleosis. *Proc Natl Acad Sci U S A* 1968;59:94–101.
82. Hershey AD. *The Bacteriophage Lambda.* Cold Spring Harbor, NY: Cold Spring Harbor Laboratory Press; 1971.
83. Hershey AD, Chase M. Independent functions of viral protein and nucleic acid in growth of bacteriophage. *J Gen Physiol* 1952;36:39–56.
84. Hilleman MR. Historical and contemporary perspectives in vaccine developments: from the vantage of cancer. *Prog Med Virol* 1992;39: 1–18.
85. Ho D, Bieniasz P. HIV at 25. *Cell* 2008;454:236–240.
86. Hoh J, Jin S, Parrado T, et al. The p53MH algorithm and its application in detecting p53-responsive genes. *Proc Natl Acad Sci U S A* 2002;99: 8467–8472.
87. Holmes E. The evolutionary genetics of emerging viruses. *Ann Rev Ecol Evol Syst* 2009;40:353–372.
88. Holmes FA. Local lesions in tobacco mosaic. *Bot Gaz* 1929;87:39–55.
89. Hughes SS. *The Virus: A History of the Concept.* London: Heinemann Education Books; 1977.
90. Hui D, Chan P. Severe acute respiratory syndrome and coronavirus. *Infect Dis Clin North Am* 2010;24:619–638.
91. Inglis T. Principia aetiologica: taking causality beyond Koch's postulates. *J Med Micro* 2007;56:1419–1422.
92. Isaacs A, Lindenmann J. Virus interference. I. The interferon. *Proc R Soc Lond B Biol Sci* 1957;147:258–267.
93. Isaacs A, Lindenmann J, Valentine RC. Virus interference. II. Some properties of interferon. *Proc R Soc Lond B Biol Sci* 1957;147:268–273.
94. Ivanofsky D. Concerning the mosaic disease of the tobacco plant. *St. Petersburg Acad Imp Sci Bull* 1892;35:67–70.
95. Ivanofsky D. On the mosaic disease of tobacco. *Zeitschrift fur Pfanzenkrankheit* 1903;13:1–41.
96. Jackson DA, Symons RH, Berg P. Biochemical method for inserting new genetic information into DNA of Simian Virus 40: circular SV40 DNA molecules containing lambda phage genes and the galactose operon of Escherichia coli. *Proc Natl Acad Sci U S A* 1972;69:2904–2909.
97. Jacob F, Wollman E. Etude génétique d'un bactériophage tempéré d'Escherichia coli. I. Le système génétique du bactériophage l. *Ann Inst Pasteur* 1954;87:653–673.
98. Jacob F, Wollman E. *Sexuality and the Genetics of Bacteria.* New York: Academic Press; 1961.
99. Jang SK, Davies MV, Kaufman RJ, et al. Initiation of protein synthesis by internal entry of ribosomes into the 5' nontranslated region of encephalomyocarditis virus RNA in vivo. *J Virol* 1989;63:1651–1660.
100. Jenner RG, Young RA. Insights into host responses against pathogens from transcriptional profiling. Nature reviews. *Microbiology* 2005;3: 281–294.
101. Jensen JH. Isolation of yellow-mosaic virus from plants infected with tobacco mosaic. *Phytopathology* 1933;23:964–974.
102. Kates J, Beeson J. Ribonucleic acid synthesis in vaccinia virus. II. Synthesis of polyriboadenylic acid. *J Mol Biol* 1970;50:19–33.
103. Kates JR, McAuslan BR. Poxvirus DNA-dependent RNA polymerase. *Proc Natl Acad Sci U S A* 1967;58:134–141.
104. Kausche G. Die Sichtbarmachung von PF lanzlichem Virus in Ubermikroskop. *Naturwissenschaften* 1939;27:292–299.
105. Kausche G, Ankuch PF, Ruska H. Die Sichtbarmachung von PF lanzlichem Virus in Ubermikroskop. *Naturwissenschaften* 1939;27:292–299.
106. Keesing F, Belden L, Daszak P, et al. Impacts of biodiversity on the emergence and transmission of infectious diseases. *Nature* 2010;468: 647–652.
107. Kinross J, Darzi A, Nicholson J. Gut microbiome-host interactions in health and disease. *Genome Med* 2011;3:14.
108. Kitajewski J, Schneider RJ, Safer B, et al. An adenovirus mutant unable to express VAI RNA displays different growth responses and sensitivity to interferon in various host cell lines. *Mol Cell Biol* 1986;6:4493–4498.
109. Kornberg A. Biologic synthesis of deoxyribonucleic acid. *Science* 1960; 131:1503–1508.
110. Kotin RM, Siniscalco M, Samulski RJ, et al. Site-specific integration by adeno-associated virus. *Proc Natl Acad Sci U S A* 1990;87:2211–2215.
111. Krugman S, Giles JP, Hammond J. Infectious hepatitis. Evidence for two distinctive clinical, epidemiological, and immunological types of infection. *JAMA* 1967;200:365–373.
112. Laemmli UK. Cleavage of structural proteins during the assembly of the head of bacteriophage T4. *Nature* 1970;227:680–685.
113. Laemmli UK, Cheng SM, Adolph KW, et al. Metaphase chromosome structure: the role of nonhistone proteins. *Cold Spring Harb Symp Quant Biol* 1978;42(Pt 1):351–360.
114. Lander ES, Linton LM, Birren B, et al. Initial sequencing and analysis of the human genome. *Nature* 2001;409:860–921.
115. Lane DP, Crawford LV. T antigen is bound to a host protein in SV40-transformed cells. *Nature* 1979;278:261–263.
116. Lee W, Haslinger A, Karin M, et al. Activation of transcription by two factors that bind promoter and enhancer sequences of the human metallothionein gene and SV40. *Nature* 1987;325:368–372.
117. Levine AJ. The origins of the small DNA tumor viruses. *Adv Cancer Res* 1994;65:141–168.
118. Levine AJ. The tumor suppressor genes. *Annu Rev Biochem* 1993;62: 623–651.
119. Levine AJ, Momand J, Finlay CA. The p53 tumour suppressor gene. *Nature* 1991;351:453–456.
120. Linzer DI, Levine AJ. Characterization of a 54K dalton cellular SV40 tumor antigen present in SV40-transformed cells and uninfected embryonal carcinoma cells. *Cell* 1979;17:43–52.
121. Lipkin I. Pathogen discovery. *PLoS Pathogens* 2008;4:31000002.
122. Loeffler F, Frosch P. Zentralbl Bakteriol 1. *Orig* 1898;28:371.
123. Long C, Turner-Shelef K, Relman D. Building a better virus trap. *Trends Biotechnol* 2007;12:535–538.
124. Luria SE. *General Virology.* New York: Wiley; 1953.
125. Luria SE. Mutations of Bacterial Viruses Affecting Their Host Range. *Genetics* 1945;30:84–99.
126. Luria SE, Anderson TF. The Identification and Characterization of Bacteriophages with the Electron Microscope. *Proc Natl Acad Sci U S A* 1942;28:127–130 1.
127. Luria SE, Darnell JE. *General Virology.* New York: J. Wiley and Sons; 1967.
128. Lwoff A, ed. *The Prophage and I.* Cold Spring Harbor, NY: Cold Spring Harbor Laboratory Press; 1961.
129. Lwoff A, Siminovitch L, Kjeldgaard N. Induction de la lyse bactériophagique de la totalité d'une population microbienne lysogène. *C R Hebd Seances Acad Sci Paris* 1950;231:190–191.
130. Mayer A. On the mosaic disease of tobacco: prelminary communication. *Tijdschr Landbouwk* 1882;2:359–364.
131. Mayer A. On the mosaic disease of tobacco. *Landwn VerSStnen* 1886;32: 451–467.
132. McKinney HH. Factors affecting the properties of a virus. *Phytopathology* 1926;16:753–758.
133. McKinney HH. Mosaic diseases in the Canary Islands. *J Agric Res* 1929; 39:557–578.
134. Monod J, Wollman E. L'inhibition de la croissance et de l'adaption enzymatique chez les bactéries infectées par le bactériophage. *Ann Inst Pasteur* 1947;73:937–957.
135. Moore P, Chang Y. Why do viruses cause cancer? Highlights of the first century of human tumor virology. *Nat Rev Cancer* 2010;12:878–889.
136. Morrow JF, Berg P. Cleavage of Simian virus 40 DNA at a unique site by a bacterial restriction enzyme. *Proc Natl Acad Sci U S A* 1972;69:3365–3369.
137. Morse ML, Lederberg EM, Lederberg J. Transduction in Escherichia Coli K-12. *Genetics* 1956;41:142–156.
138. Mulder C, Delius H. Specificity of the break produced by restricting endonuclease R1 in Simian virus 40 DNA, as revealed by partial denaturation mapping. *Proc Natl Acad Sci U S A* 1972;69:3215–3219.
139. Munger J, Bennett B, Parkikh A, et al. Systems-level metabolic flux profiling identifies fatty acid synthesis as a target for antiviral therapy. *Nat Biotechnol* 2008;10:1179–1186.
140. Murray K, Mertens E, Despres P. West Nile virus and its emergence in the United States of America. *Vet Res* 2010;41:67.
141. Nathanson N, Kew OM. From emergence to eradication: the epidemiology of poliomyelitis deconstructed. *Am J Epidemiol* 2010;172: 1213–1229.
142. Negri A. Beitrag zum Stadium der Aetiologie der Tollwuth. *Z Hyg Infektkrankh* 1903;43:507–528.

143. Palacio G, Briese T, Lipkin I. Microbe hunting in laboratory animal research. *ILAR J* 2010;51:245–254.
144. Parrish C, Kawaoka Y. The origins of new pandemic viruses: the acquisition of new host ranges by canine parvovirus and influenza A viruses. *Annu Rev Microbiol* 2005;59:553–586.
145. Pasteur L. Méthode pour prévenir la rage apres morsure. *CR Acad Sci* 1885; 101:765–772.
146. Pelletier J, Sonenberg N. Internal binding of eucaryotic ribosomes on poliovirus RNA: translation in HeLa cell extracts. *J Virol* 1989;63: 441–444.
147. Pilder S, Moore M, Logan J, et al. The adenovirus E1B-55K transforming polypeptide modulates transport or cytoplasmic stabilization of viral and host cell mRNAs. *Mol Cell Biol* 1986;6:470–476.
148. Plotkin JB, Dushoff J. Codon bias and frequency-dependent selection on the hemagglutinin epitopes of influenza A virus. *Proc Natl Acad Sci U S A* 2003;100:7152–7157.
149. Poiesz BJ, Ruscetti FW, Gazdar AF, et al. Detection and isolation of type C retrovirus particles from fresh and cultured lymphocytes of a patient with cutaneous T-cell lymphoma. *Proc Natl Acad Sci U S A* 1980; 77:7415–7419.
150. Ptashne M. *A Genetic Switch, Gene Control and Phage Lambda*. Palo Alto, CA: Blackwell Science; 1987.
151. Purdy-Beale HA. Immunologic reactions with tobacco mosaic virus. *J Exp Med* 1929;49:919–935.
152. Qian X, Yoon B. Comparative analysis of protein interaction networks reveals that conserved pathways are susceptible to HIV-1 interception. *BMC Bioinformatics* 2011;12(Suppl 1):S19.
153. Rambaut A, Pybus O, Nelson M, et al. The genomic and epidemiological dynamics of human influenza A virus. *Nature* 2008;453:615–619.
154. Reed W, Carroll J, Agramonte A, et al. Senate Documents 1901;66:156.
155. Relman D. 'Til death do us part': coming to terms with symbiotic relationships. *Nat Rev Microbio* 2008;10:721–724.
156. Reyes A, Haynes M, Hanson N, et al. Metagenomic analysis of viruses in the fecal microbiota of monozygotic twins and their mothers. *Nature* 2010;466:334–340.
157. Robins H, Krasnitz M, Barak H, et al. A Relative Entropy Algorithm for Genomic Fingerprinting Captures Host-Phage Similarities. *J Bacteriol* 2005;187:8370–8374.
158. Robins H, Krasnitz M, Levine A. The Computational Detection of Functional Nucleotide Sequence Motifs in the Coding Regions of Organisms. *Exp Biol Med* 2008;233:665–673.
159. Rous P. A Sarcoma of the Fowl Transmissible by an Agent Separable from the Tumor Cells. *J Exp Med* 1911;13:397–411.
160. Roux E. Sur les microbes dits invisible. *Bull Inst Pasteur Paris* 1903;1:49–56.
161. Rubinstein M, Rubinstein S, Familletti PC, et al. Human leukocyte interferon purified to homogeneity. *Science* 1978;202:1289–1290.
162. Samulski RJ, Chang LS, Shenk T. Helper-free stocks of recombinant adeno-associated viruses: normal integration does not require viral gene expression. *J Virol* 1989;63:3822–3828.
163. Sanford KK, Earle WR, Likely GD. The growth in vitro of single isolated tissue cells. *J Natl Cancer Inst* 1948;9:229–246.
164. Sarnow P, Ho YS, Williams J, et al. Adenovirus E1b-58kd tumor antigen and SV40 large tumor antigen are physically associated with the same 54kd cellular protein in transformed cells. *Cell* 1982;28:387–394.
165. Scheffner M, Werness BA, Huibregtse JM, et al. The E6 oncoprotein encoded by human papillomavirus 16 and 18 promotes the degradation of p53. *Cell* 1990;63:1129–1136.
166. Schlesinger M. Die Bestimmung von Teilchengrïsse und Spezifischem gewicht des Bakteriophagen durch Zentrifugierversuche. *Z Hyg Infektionskrankh* 1932;114:161.
167. Schlesinger M. Zur Frage der chemischen Zusammensetzung des Bakteriophagen. *Biochem Z* 1934;273:306–311.
168. Schultz-Cherry S, Jones J. Influenza vaccines: the good, the bad, and the eggs. *Adv Virus Res* 2010;77:63–84.
169. Schwartz O, Albert M. Biology and pathogenesis of chikungunya virus. *Nat Rev Microbio* 2010;8:491–500.
170. Sharp P, Hahn B. The evolution of HIV-1 and the origin of AIDS. *Philos Trans R Soc Lond B Biol Sci* 2010;365:2487–2494.
171. Sinsheimer RL. A single-stranded DNA from bacteriophage phi X174. *Brookhaven Symp Biol* 1959;12:27–34.
172. Soll S, Stuart J, Neil D, et al. Identification of a receptor for an extinct virus. *Proc Natl Acad Sci U S A* 2010;107:19496–19501.
173. Stanley W. Isolation of a crystaline protein possessing the properties of tobacco-mosaic virus. *Science* 1935;81:644–645.
174. Stehelin D, Varmus HE, Bishop JM, et al. DNA related to the transforming gene(s) of avian sarcoma viruses is present in normal avian DNA. *Nature* 1976;260:170–173.
175. Straub O. Maedi-visna virus infection in sheep. History and present knowledge. *Comp Immunol Microbiol Infect Dis* 2004;27:1–5.
176. Streisinger G, Edgar RS, Denhardt GH. Chromosome Structure in Phage T4. I. Circularity of the Linkage Map. *Proc Natl Acad Sci U S A* 1964; 51:775–779.
177. Suttle C. Marine viruses-major players in the global ecosystem. *Nat Rev Microbiol* 2007;5:801–812.
178. Suttle CA. Viruses in the sea. *Nature* 2005;437:356–361.
179. Szpara M, Kobiler O, Enquist L. A Common Neuronal Response to Alphaherpesvirus Infection. *J Neuroimmune Pharmacol* 2010;5:418–427.
180. Takahashi WN, Rawlins RE. Method for determining shape fo colloidal particles: Applications in study of tobacco mosaic virus. *Proc Natl Acad Sci U S A* 1932;30:155–157.
181. Takatsuki K, Uchuyama T, Ueshima Y. Adult T-cell leukemia: Proposal as a new disease and cytogenetic, phenotypic and function studies of leukemic cells.*Gann Monogr Cancer Res* 1982;28:13–22.
182. Tang J, Shetty N, Lam T, et al. Emerging, novel, and known influenza virus infections in humans. *Infect Dis Clin North Am* 2010;24:603–617.
183. Tang P, Chiu C. Metagenomics for the discovery of novel human viruses. *Future Microbiol* 2010;5:177–189.
184. Taubenberger J, Kash J. Influenza virus evolution, host adaptation, and pandemic formation. *Cell Host Microbe* 2010;7:440–451.
185. Temin HM, Mizutani S. RNA-dependent DNA polymerase in virions of Rous sarcoma virus. *Nature* 1970;226:1211–1213.
186. Thomas CA Jr. The arrangement of information in DNA molecules. *J Gen Physiol* 1966;49:143–169.
187. Tulsiani S, Graham G, Moore P, et al. Emerging tropical diseases in Australia. Part 5, Hendra virus. *Ann Trop Med Parasitol* 2011;105:1–11.
188. Twort FW. The bacteriophage: The breaking down of bacteria by associated filter-passing lysins. *Br Med J* 1922;2:293.
189. Twort FW. The discovery of the bacteriophage. *Sci News* 1949;14:33.
190. Twort FW. An investigation on the nature of the ultramicroscopic viruses. *Lancet* 1915;189:1241–1243.
191. Uchiyama T, Yodoi J, Sagawa K, et al. Adult T-cell leukemia: clinical and hematologic features of 16 cases. *Blood* 1977;50:481–492.
192. Venter JC, Adams MD, Myers EW, et al. The sequence of the human genome. *Science* 2001;291:1304–1351.
193. Vinson CG, Petre AW. Mosaic disease of tobacco. *Botan Gaz* 1929;87: 14–38.
194. Wang D, Urisman A, Liu YT, et al. Viral discovery and sequence recovery using DNA microarrays. *PLoS Biol* 2003;1:E2.
195. Watson JD, Crick FH. Molecular structure of nucleic acids; a structure for deoxyribose nucleic acid. *Nature* 1953;171:737–738.
196. Weil PA, Luse DS, Segall J, et al. Selective and accurate initiation of transcription at the Ad2 major late promotor in a soluble system dependent on purified RNA polymerase II and DNA. *Cell* 1979;18:469–484.
197. Weil R, Vinograd J. The Cyclic Helix and Cyclic Coil Forms of Polyoma Viral DNA. *Proc Natl Acad Sci U S A* 1963;50:730–738.
198. Weiss R, Teich N, Varmus H, et al. *RNA Tumor Viruses.* Cold Spring Harbor, NY: Cold Spring Harbor Laboratory Press; 1982.
199. Weitzman M, Lilley C, Chaurushiya M. Genomes in conflict: maintaining genome integrity during virus infection. *Annu Rev Microbiol* 2010;13: 61–81.
200. Werness BA, Levine AJ, Howley PM. Association of human papillomavirus types 16 and 18 E6 proteins with p53. *Science* 1990;248:76–79.
201. Whyte P, Buchkovich KJ, Horowitz JM, et al. Association between an oncogene and an anti-oncogene: the adenovirus E1A proteins bind to the retinoblastoma gene product. *Nature* 1988;334:124–129.
202. Willner D, Furlan M, Haynes M, et al. Metagenomic analysis of respiratory tract DNA viral communities in Cystic Fibrosis and Non-Cystic Fibrosis individuals. *PLoS One* 2009;4:1–12.

203. Willner D, Thurber R, Rohwer F. Metagenomic signatures of 86 microbial and viral metagenomes. *Env Micro* 2009;16:75–84.
204. Wolbach SB. The Filterable Viruses, a Summary. *J Med Res* 1912;27:1–25.
205. Woodruff AM, Goodpasture EW. The susceptibility of the chorio-allantoic membrane of chick embryos to infection with the fowl-pox virus. *Am J Pathol* 1931;7:209–222.5.
206. Worcel A, Burgi E. On the structure of the folded chromosome of Escherichia coli. *J Mol Biol* 1972;71:127–147.
207. Wyatt GR, Cohen SS. The bases of the nucleic acids of some bacterial and animal viruses: the occurrence of 5-hydroxymethylcytosine. *Biochem J* 1953;55:774–782.
208. Yoshida M, Miyoshi I, Hinuma Y. Isolation and characterization of retrovirus from cell lines of human adult T-cell leukemia and its implication in the disease. *Proc Natl Acad Sci U S A* 1982;79:2031–2035.
209. Zhao R, Gish K, Murphy M, et al. Analysis of p53-regulated gene expression patterns using oligonucleotide arrays. *Genes Dev* 2000;14:981–993.
210. Zinder ND, Lederberg J. Genetic exchange in Salmonella. *J Bacteriol* 1952;64:679–699.
211. Zinkernagel RM, Doherty PC. Restriction of in vitro T cell-mediated cytotoxicity in lymphocytic choriomeningitis within a syngeneic or semiallogeneic system. *Nature* 1974;248:701–702.
212. zur Hausen H. Viruses in human cancers. *Science* 1991;254:1167–1173.

CHAPTER 2

Richard C. Condit

Principles of Virology

Viruses are unique in nature. They are the smallest of all self-replicating organisms, historically characterized by their ability to pass through filters that retain even the smallest bacteria. In their most basic form, viruses consist solely of a small segment of nucleic acid encased in a simple protein shell. Viruses have no metabolism of their own but rather are obliged to invade cells and parasitize subcellular machinery, subverting it to their own purposes. Many have argued that viruses are not even living,[128] although to a seasoned virologist, they exhibit a life as robust as any other creature.

The apparent simplicity of viruses is deceptive. The truth is that as a group, viruses infect virtually every organism in nature, they display a dizzying diversity of structures and lifestyles, and they embody a profound complexity of function.

The study of viruses—virology—must accommodate both the uniqueness and the complexity of these organisms. The singular nature of viruses has spawned novel methods of classification and experimentation entirely peculiar to the discipline of virology. The complexity of viruses is constantly challenging scientists to adjust their thinking and their research to describe and understand some new twist in the central dogma revealed in a *simple* virus infection.

This chapter explores several concepts fundamental to virology as a whole, including virus taxonomy, virus cultivation and assay, and virus genetics. The chapter is not intended as a comprehensive or encyclopedic treatment of these topics, but rather as a relatively concise overview with sufficient documentation for more in-depth study. In addition to primary resources and practical experience, the presentation draws heavily on previous editions of *Fields Virology*[35–37] for the taxonomy and genetics material, plus several excellent texts for material on virus cultivation and assay.[20,34,41,59,70,76,81] It is hoped that this chapter will be of value to anyone learning virology at any stage: a novice trying to understand basic principles for the first time, an intermediate student of virology trying to understand the technical subtleties of virological protocols in the literature, or a bewildered scientist in the laboratory wondering why the host-range virus mutant received from a colleague does not seem to manifest the described host range.

VIRUS TAXONOMY

A coherent and workable system of classification—a taxonomy—is a critical component of the discipline of virology. However, the unique nature of viruses has defied the strict application of many of the traditional tools of taxonomy used in other disciplines of biology. Thus, scientists who concern themselves with global taxonomy of organisms have traditionally either ignored viruses completely as nonliving entities or left them scattered throughout the major kingdoms, reasoning that viruses have more in common with their individual hosts than they do with each other.[82,90] By contrast, for practical reasons at least, virologists agree that viruses should be considered together as a separate group of organisms regardless of host, be it plant, animal, fungus, protist, or bacterium, a philosophy borne out by the observation that in several cases viruses now classified in the same family—for example, family *Reoviridae*—infect hosts from different kingdoms. Interestingly, the discipline of virus taxonomy brings out the most erudite and thought-provoking, virtually philosophical discussions about the nature of viruses, probably because the decisions that must be made to distinguish one virus from another require the deepest thought about the nature of viruses and virus evolution. In the end, all of nature is a continuum, and the business of taxonomy has the unfortunate obligation of drawing boundaries within this continuum, an artificial and illogical task but necessary nevertheless. The execution of this obligation results today in a free-standing virus taxonomy, overseen by the International Committee on Taxonomy of Viruses (ICTV), with rules and tools unique to the discipline of virology. The process of virus taxonomy that has evolved uses some of the hierarchical nomenclature of traditional taxonomy, identifying virus species and grouping these into genera, genera into families, and families into orders, but at the same time, to cope with both the uniqueness and diversity of viruses as a group, the classification process has been deliberately nonsystematic and thus is "based upon the opinionated usage of data".[92]

Most importantly, the virus taxonomy that has been developed works well. For the trained virologist, the mention of a virus family or genus name, such as "family *Herpesviridae*" or "genus *Rotavirus*" immediately conjures forth a set of characteristics that form the basis for further discussion or description. Virus taxonomy serves an important practical purpose as well, in that the identification of a limited number of biological characteristics, such as virion morphology, genome structure, or antigenic properties, quickly provides a focus for identification of an unknown agent for the clinician or epidemiologist and can significantly impact further investigation into treatment or prevention of a virus disease. Virus taxonomy is an evolving field, and what follows is a summary of the state of the art, including important historical landmarks that influenced the present system of virus taxonomy, a description of the system used for virus taxonomy and the means for implementation of that system, and a very brief overview of the taxonomy of viruses that infect humans and animals.

History and Rationale

Virology as a discipline is scarcely 100 years old, and thus the discipline of virus taxonomy is relatively young. In the early 1900s, viruses were initially classified as distinct from other organisms simply by virtue of their ability to pass through unglazed porcelain filters known to retain the smallest of bacteria. As increasing numbers of filterable agents became recognized, they were distinguished from each other by the only measurable properties available, namely the disease or symptoms caused in an infected organism. Therefore, animal viruses that caused liver pathology were grouped together as hepatitis viruses, and viruses that caused mottling in plants were grouped together as mosaic viruses. In the 1930s, an explosion of technology spawned a description of the physical properties of many viruses, providing numerous new characteristics for distinguishing viruses one from another. The technologies included procedures for purification of viruses, biochemical characterization of purified virions, serology, and perhaps most importantly, electron microscopy, in particular negative staining, which permitted detailed descriptions of virion morphology, even in relatively crude preparations of infected tissue. In the 1950s, these characterizations led to the distinction of three major animal virus groups, the myxoviruses, the herpesviruses, and the poxviruses. By the 1960s, because of the profusion of data describing numerous different viruses, it became clear that an organized effort was required to classify and name viruses, and thus the ICTV (originally the International Committee on Nomenclature of Viruses [ICNV]) was established in 1966. The ICTV functions today as a large, international group of virologists organized into appropriate study groups, whose charge it is to develop rules for the classification and naming of viruses and to coordinate the activities of study groups in the implementation of these rules.

Early in its history, the ICTV wrestled with the fundamental problem of developing a taxonomic system for classification and naming of viruses that would accommodate the unique properties of viruses as a group and that could anticipate advancements in the identification and characterization of viruses. Perhaps the most critical issue was whether the classification of viruses should consider virus properties in a monothetical, hierarchical fashion or a polythetical, hierarchical fashion. A *monothetic* system of classification is defined as a system based on a single characteristic or a series of single characteristics. *Polythetic* is defined as sharing several common characteristics without any one of these characteristics being essential for membership in the group or class in question. Thus, a monothetical, hierarchical classification, modeled after the Linnaean system used for classification of plants and animals, would effectively rank individual virus properties, such as genome structure or virion symmetry, as being more or less important relative to each other and use these individual characteristics to sort viruses into subphyla, classes, orders, suborders, and families.[79] Although the hierarchical ordering of viruses into groups and subgroups is desirable, a strictly monothetical approach to using virus properties in making assignments to groups was problematic because both the identification of individual properties to be used in the hierarchy and the assignment of a hierarchy to individual properties seemed too arbitrary. A polythetic approach to classification would group viruses by comparing simultaneously numerous properties of individual viruses without assigning a universal priority to any one property. Thus, using the polythetic approach, a given virus grouping is defined by a collection of properties rather than a single property, and virus groups in different branches of the taxonomy may be characterized by different collections of properties. One argument against the polythetic approach is that a truly systematic and comprehensive comparison of dozens of individual properties would be at least forbidding if not impossible. However, this problem could be avoided by the adoption of a nonsystematic approach, namely, using study groups of virologists within the ICTV to consider together numerous characteristics of a virus and make as rational an assignment to a group as possible. Therefore, the system that is currently being used is a nonsystematic, polythetical, hierarchical system. This system differs from any other taxonomic system in use for bacteria or other organisms; however, it is effective, useful, and has withstood the test of time.[91] As our understanding of viruses increases, and as new techniques for characterization are developed, notably comparison of gene and genome sequences, the methods used for taxonomy will undoubtedly continue to evolve.

As a consequence of the polythetic approach to classification, the virus taxonomy that exists today has been filled initially from the middle of the hierarchy by assigning viruses to genera, and then elaborating the taxonomy upward by grouping genera into families and, to a limited extent, families into orders. By 1970, the ICTV had established two virus families each containing 2 genera, 24 floating genera, and 16 plant *groups*.[133] A rigorous species definition,[126] discussed later, was not approved by the ICTV until 1991 but has now been applied to the entire taxonomy and has become the primary level of classification for viruses. As of this writing, the currently accepted taxonomy recognizes 6 orders, 87 families, 19 subfamilies, 348 genera,

TABLE 2.1 Summary Characteristics of Vertebrate Virus Families

Family	Nucleocapsid morphology	Envelope	Virion morphology	Genome[a]	Host[b]
dsDNA viruses					
Adenoviridae	Icosahedral	No	Icosahedral	1 ds linear, 26–48 kb	V
Alloherpesviridae	Icosahedral	Yes	Spherical, tegument	2 ds linear, 135–294 kb	V
Asfaviridae	Icosahedral	Yes[c]	Icosahedral	1 ds linear, 165–190 kb	V, I
Herpesviridae	Icosahedral	Yes	Spherical, tegument	1 ds linear, 125–240 kb	V
Iridoviridae	Icosahedral	No[d]	Icosahedral	1 ds linear, 140–303	V, I
Papillomaviridae	Icosahedral	No	Icosahedral	1 ds circular, 7–8 kb	V
Polyomaviridae	Icosahedral	No	Icosahedral	1 ds circular, 5 kb	V
Poxviridae	Ovoid	Yes	Ovoid	1 ds linear, 130–375 kb	V, I
ssDNA viruses					
Anellovirus	Icosahedral	No	Icosahedral	1 – circular, 2–4 kb	V
Circoviridae	Icosahedral	No	Icosahedral	1 – or ± circular, 2 kb	V
Parvoviridae	Icosahedral	No	Icosahedral	1 +, – or ± linear, 4–6 kb	V, I
dsDNA reverse transcribing viruses					
Hepadnaviridae	Icosahedral	Yes	Spherical	1 ds circular, 3–4 kb	V
ssRNA reverse transcribing viruses					
Metaviridae	Spherical	Yes	Spherical	1 + linear, 4–10 kb	F, I, P, V
Retroviridae	Spherical, rod or cone shaped	Yes	Spherical	1 + linear dimer, 7–13 kb	V
dsRNA viruses					
Birnaviridae	Icosahedral	No	Icosahedral	2 ds linear, 5–6 kb	V, I
Picobirnaviridae	Icosahedral	No	Icosahedral	3 ds linear, 4 kb	V
Reoviridae	Icosahedral	No	Icosahedral, layered	10–12 ds linear, 19–32 kb	V, I, P, F
Negative sense ssRNA viruses					
Bornaviridae	ND[e]	Yes	Spherical	1 – linear, 9 kb	V
Deltavirus[f]	Isometric	Yes	Spherical	1 – circular, 2 kb	V
Filoviridae	Helical filaments	Yes	Bacilliform, filamentous	1 – linear, 19 kb	V
Orthomyxoviridae	Helical filaments	Yes	Pleomorphic, spherical	6–8 – linear, 10–15 kb	V
Paramyxoviridae	Helical filaments	Yes	Pleomorphic, spherical, filamentous	1 – linear, 13–18 kb	V
Rhabdoviridae	Coiled helical filaments	Yes	Bullet shaped	1 – linear, 11–15 kb	V, I, P
Positive sense ssRNA viruses					
Arteriviridae	Linear, asymmetric	Yes	Spherical	1 + linear, 13–16 kb	V
Astroviridae	Icosahedral	No	Icosahedral	1 + linear, 6–8 kb	V
Caliciviridae	Icosahedral	No	Icosahedral	1 + linear, 7–8 kb	V
Coronaviridae	Helical	Yes	Spherical	1 + linear, 26–32 kb	V
Flaviviridae	Spherical	Yes	Spherical	1 + linear, 9–13 kb	V, I
Hepevirus[e]	Icosahedral	No	Icosahedral	1 + linear, 7 kb	V
Nodaviridae	Icosahedral	No	Icosahedral	2 + linear, 4–5 kb	V, I
Picornaviridae	Icosahedral	No	Icosahedral	1 + linear, 7–9 kb	V
Togaviridae	Icosahedral	Yes	Spherical	1 + linear, 10–12 kb	V, I
Ambisense ssRNA viruses					
Arenaviridae	Filamentous	Yes	Spherical	2 ± linear, 11 kb	V
Bunyaviridae	Filamentous	Yes	Spherical	3 – or ± linear, 11–19 kb	V, I, P
Subviral agents: prions					
Prions	—	—	—	—	V, F

[a]Number of segments, polarity (ds, double stranded; +, mRNA like; –, cRNA like; ±, ambisense), conformation, size.
[b]V, vertebrate; P, plant; I, insect; F, fungus.
[c]Contains both an outer envelope plus a lipid membrane internal to the capsid.
[d]Contains a membrane internal to the capsid.
[e]ND, not determined.
[f]*Deltavirus* represents an unassigned genus.

and 2,290 species. The complete virus taxonomy is far too extensive to relate here; however, examples of the results of the taxonomy are offered in Tables 2.1 and 2.2. Table 2.1 lists the distinguishing characteristics of the vertebrate animal virus families, whereas Table 2.2 provides an example of the entire taxonomic classification of one virus order, namely order *Mononegavirales*.

The International Committee on Taxonomy of Viruses Universal System of Virus Taxonomy

Structure and Function

The ICTV is a committee of the Virology Division of the International Union of Microbiological Societies. The objectives of the ICTV are to develop an internationally agreed taxonomy

TABLE 2.2 Taxonomy of the Order *Mononegavirales*

Order	Family	Subfamily	Genus	Type species	Host
Mononegavirales	*Bornaviridae*		*Bornavirus*	*Borna disease virus*	V
	Rhabdoviridae		*Vesiculovirus*	*Vesicular stomatitis Indiana virus*	V, I
			Lyssavirus	*Rabies virus*	V
			Ephemerovirus	*Bovine ephemeral fever virus*	V, I
			Novirhabdovirus	*Infectious hematopoietic necrosis virus*	V
			Cytorhabdovirus	*Lettuce necrotic yellows virus*	P, I
			Nucleorhabdovirus	*Potato yellow dwarf virus*	P, I
	Filoviridae		*Marburgvirus*	*Lake Victoria marburgvirus*	V
			Ebolavirus	*Zaire ebolavirus*	V
	Paramyxoviridae	*Paramyxovirinae*	*Rubulavirus*	*Mumps virus*	V
			Avulavirus	*Newcastle disease virus*	V
			Respirovirus	*Sendai virus*	V
			Henipavirus	*Hendra virus*	V
			Morbillivirus	*Measles virus*	V
		Pneumovirinae	*Pneumovirus*	*Human respiratory syncytial virus*	V
			Metapneumovirus	*Avian metapneumovirus*	V

V, vertebrate; I, insect; P, plant.

and nomenclature for viruses, to maintain an index of virus names, and to communicate the proceedings of the committee to the international community of virologists. The ICTV publishes an update of the taxonomy at approximately 3-year intervals.[32,33,39,85,86,92,133] At the time of this writing, the ninth report is being completed. The official taxonomy is also available on line at the ICTV website: http://www.ictvonline.org.

Virus Properties and Their Use in Taxonomy

As introduced previously, the taxonomic method adopted for use in virology is polythetic, meaning that any given virus group is described using a collection of individual properties. The description of a virus group is nonsystematic in that there exists no fixed list of properties that must be considered for all viruses and no strict formula for the ordered consideration of properties. Instead, a set of properties describing a given virus is simply compared with other viruses described in a similar fashion to formulate rational groupings. Characters such as virion morphology, genome organization, method of replication, and the number and size of structural and nonstructural viral proteins are used for distinguishing different virus families and genera. Characters such as genome sequence relatedness, natural host range, cell and tissue tropism, pathogenicity and cytopathology, mode of transmission, physicochemical properties of virions, and antigenic properties of viral proteins are used for distinguishing virus species within the same genus.[127]

The Hierarchy

The ICTV has adopted a universal classification scheme that employs the hierarchical taxonomic levels of order, family, subfamily, genus, and species. Because the polythetic approach to classification introduces viruses into the middle of the hierarchy, and because the ICTV has taken a relatively conservative approach to grouping taxa, levels higher than order are not currently used. Interestingly, groupings above the level of order may prove to be inappropriate: Higher taxons imply a common ancestry for viruses, whereas multiple independent lineages for viruses now seems the more likely evolutionary scenario.[32] Taxonomic levels lower than species, such as clades, strains, and variants, are not officially considered by the ICTV but are left to specialty groups.

A virus species is defined as "a polythetic class of viruses that constitutes a replicating lineage and occupies a particular ecological niche".[126] The formal definition of a polythetic class is "a class whose members always have several properties in common although no single common attribute is present in all of its members".[127] Thus, no single property can be used to define a given species, and application of this formal definition of a polythetic class to species accounts nicely for the inherent variability found among members of a species. The qualification of a replicating lineage implies that members of a species experience evolution over time with consequent variation, but that members share a common ancestor. The qualification of occupation of an ecological niche acknowledges that the biology of a virus, including such properties as host range, pathogenesis, transmission, and habitat, are fundamental components of the characterization of a virus. A *type species* has been identified for each genus. The type species is not necessarily the best characterized or most representative species in a genus; rather, it is usually the virus that initially necessitated the creation of the genus and therefore best defines or identifies the genus.

Taxonomic levels higher than species are formally defined by the ICTV only in a relative sense, namely a genus is a group of species sharing certain common characters, a subfamily is a group of genera sharing certain common characters, a family is a group of genera or subfamilies sharing certain common characters, and an order is a group of families sharing certain common characters. As the virus taxonomy has evolved, these higher taxa have acquired some monothetic character. They remain polythetic in that they may be characterized by more than one virus property; however, they violate the formal definition of a polythetic class in that one or more defining properties may be required of all candidate viruses for membership in the taxon. Not all taxonomic levels need be used for a given grouping of viruses, thus whereas most species are grouped into genera and genera into families, not all families contain subfamilies, and only a few families have been grouped into orders. Consequently, the family is the highest consistently used taxonomic grouping, it therefore carries the most generalized description of a given virus group, and as a result has become the benchmark of the taxonomic system. Most families have distinct virion morphology, genome structure, and/or replication strategy (see Table 2.1).

Nomenclature

The ICTV has adopted a formal nomenclature for viruses, specifying suffixes for the various taxa, and rules for written descriptions of viruses. Names for genera, subfamilies, families, and orders must all be single words, ending with the suffixes -virus, -virinae, -viridae, and -virales, respectively. Species names may contain more than one word and have no specific ending. In written usage, the formal virus taxonomic names are capitalized and written in italics, and preceded by the name of the taxon, which is neither capitalized nor italicized. For species names that contain more than one word, the first word plus any proper nouns are capitalized. As an example, the full formal written description of human respiratory syncytial virus is as follows: order *Mononegavirales,* family *Paramyxoviridae,* subfamily *Pneumovirinae,* genus *Pneumovirus,* species *Human respiratory syncytial virus.* The ICTV acknowledges that vernacular (informal) taxonomic names are widely used; however, they should not be italicized or capitalized. For example, the vernacular name "herpesvirus" refers to a member of the family *Herpesviridae.*

Informal Groupings and Alternate Classification Schemes

For convenience in presenting or tabulating the virus taxonomy, informal categorical groupings of taxa are often used. The criteria applied for such groupings typically include nature of the viral genome (DNA or RNA), strandedness of the viral genome (single stranded or double stranded), polarity of the genome (positive sense, negative sense, or ambisense), and reverse transcription. Separate categories accommodate subviral agents (including viroids, satellites, and prions) and unassigned viruses. The Baltimore classification system, named after its creator David Baltimore, is a widely used scheme based on the nature of the genome packaged in virions and the pathway of nucleic acid synthesis that each group takes to accomplish messenger RNA (mRNA) synthesis.[1] This classification divides viruses into seven categories as depicted in Figure 2.1. Most usages of this system group ambisense virus families (family *Arenaviridae*

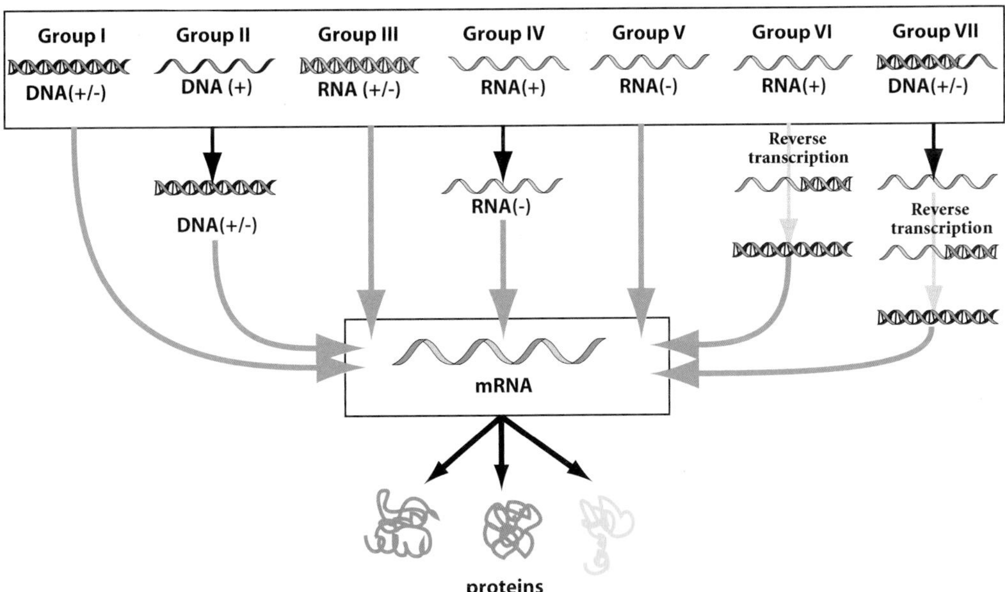

FIGURE 2.1. The Baltimore classification, a virus classification scheme based on the form of nucleic acid present in virion particles and the pathway for expression of the genetic material as messenger RNA.[1] The original scheme contained groups I through VI and has been expanded to accommodate DNA-containing, reverse transcribing viruses. Viruses containing ambisense single-stranded RNA genomes are grouped under negative sense single-stranded RNA viruses. (Reprinted from Hulo C, de Castro E, Masson P, et al. ViralZone: a knowledge resource to understand virus diversity. *Nucleic Acids Res* 2011;39 (Database issue):D576–D582; ViralZone, Swiss Institute of Bioinformatics, http://www.expasy.ch/viralzone/, with permission.)

and family *Bunyaviridae*) along with negative sense, single-stranded RNA (ssRNA) viruses. The families of vertebrate viruses listed in Table 2.1 have been grouped according to the Baltimore classification, with ambisense viruses split into an eighth genome category.

Universal Virus Database

To facilitate the management and distribution of virological data, the ICTV has established the universal virus database of the ICTV (ICTVdB). The ICTVdB is accessible on the Internet at http://www.ictvdb.org. Constructed from virus descriptions in the published reports of the ICTV, the database comprises searchable descriptions of all virus families, genera, and type species, including microscopic images of many viruses. The ICTVdB is a powerful resource for management of and access to virological data, and promises to considerably extend the reach and capability of the ICTV.

VIRUS CULTIVATION AND ASSAY

Different branches of science are defined in large part by their techniques, and virology is no exception. Whereas the study of viruses uses some general methods that are common to other disciplines, the unique nature of viruses and virus infections requires a unique set of technical tools designed specifically for their investigation. Conversely, what we know and *can* know about viruses is delimited by the techniques used; therefore, a genuine understanding of virology requires a clear understanding of virological methods. What follows is a summary of the major techniques essential and unique to all of virology, presented as fundamental background for understanding the discipline.

Initial Detection and Isolation

The presence of a virus is evidenced initially by effects on a host organism or, in the case of a few animal viruses, by effects on cultured cells. Effects on animal hosts obviously include a broad spectrum of symptoms, including skin and mucous membrane lesions; digestive, respiratory, or neurological disorders; immune dysfunction; specific organ failure such as hepatitis or myocarditis; and death. Effects on cultured cells include a variety of morphological changes in infected cells, termed *cytopathic effects* and described in detail later in this chapter and in Chapter 15. Both adenovirus[108] and the polyomavirus SV40[121] were discovered as cell culture contaminants before they were detected in their natural hosts.

Viruses can be isolated from an infected host by harvesting excreted or secreted material, blood, or tissue and testing for induction of the original symptoms in the identical host, or induction of some abnormal pathology in a substitute host or in cell culture. Historically, dogs, cats, rabbits, rats, guinea pigs, hamsters, mice, and chickens have all been found to be useful in laboratory investigations,[70] although most animal methods have now been replaced by cell culture methods.[81] Once the presence of a virus has been established, it is often desirable to prepare a genetically pure clone, either by limiting serial dilution or by plaque purification.

Viruses that are cultivated in anything other than the natural host may adapt to the novel situation through acquisition of genetic alterations that provide a replication advantage in the new host. Such adaptive changes may be accompanied by a loss of fitness in the original host, most notably by a loss of virulence or pathogenicity. Whereas this adaptation and attenuation may present problems to the basic scientist interested in understanding the replication of the virus in its natural state, it also forms the basis of construction of attenuated viral vaccines.

Hosts for Virus Cultivation

Laboratory Animals and Embryonated Chicken Eggs

Prior to the advent of cell culture, animal viruses could be propagated only on whole animals or embryonated chicken eggs. Whole animals could include the natural host or laboratory animals such as rabbits, mice, rats, and hamsters. In the case of laboratory animals, newborn or suckling rodents often provide the best hosts. Today, laboratory animals are seldom used for routine cultivation of virus; however, they still play an essential role in studies of viral pathogenesis.

The use of embryonated chicken eggs was introduced to virology by Goodpasture et al[44] in 1932 and developed subsequently by Beveridge and Burnet.[4] The developing chick embryo, 10 to 14 days after fertilization, provides a variety of differentiated tissues, including the amnion, allantois, chorion, and yolk sac, which serve as substrates for growth of a wide variety of viruses, including orthomyxoviruses, paramyxoviruses, rhabdoviruses, togaviruses, herpesviruses, and poxviruses.[70] Members of each of these virus families may replicate in several tissues of the developing egg, or replication may be confined to a single tissue. Several viruses from each of the previously mentioned groups cause discrete and characteristic foci when introduced onto the chorioallantoic membrane of embryonated eggs, thus providing a method for identification of virus types, or for quantifying virus stocks or assessing virus pathogenicity (Fig. 2.2). Although embryonated eggs have been almost wholly replaced by cell culture techniques, they are still the most convenient method for growing high titer stocks of some viruses and thus continue to be used both in research laboratories and for vaccine production.

Cell Culture

The growth and maintenance of animal cells *in vitro,* described generally (albeit incorrectly) as tissue culture, can be formally divided into three different techniques: organ culture, primary explant culture, and cell culture. In *organ culture,* the original three-dimensional architecture of a tissue is preserved under culture conditions that provide a gas–liquid interface. In *primary explant culture,* minced pieces of tissue placed in liquid medium in a culture vessel provide a source for outgrowth of individual cells. In *cell culture,* tissue is disaggregated into individual cells prior to culturing. Only cell culture will be discussed in detail here, because it is the most commonly used tissue culture technique in virology.

Cultured cells currently provide the most widely used and most powerful hosts for cultivation and assay of viruses. Cell cultures are of three basic types—primary cell cultures, cell strains, and cell lines—that may be derived from many animal species and that differ substantially in their characteristics. Viruses often behave differently on different types of cultured cells; in addition, each of the culture types possess technical

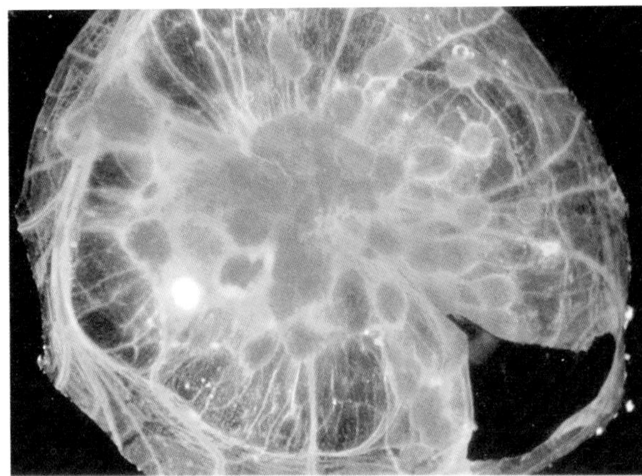

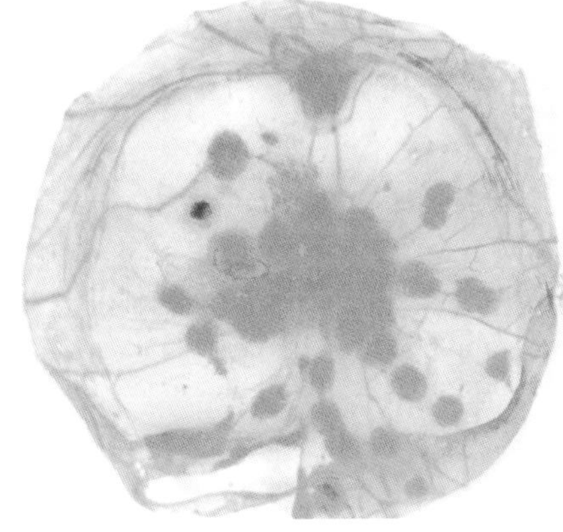

FIGURE 2.2. Cowpox-induced pock formation on the chorioallantoic membrane of chick embryos. The chorioallantoic membrane of intact chicken embryos, 11 days old, were inoculated with cowpox, and the eggs were incubated for an additional 3 days at 37.5°C. Chorioallantoic membranes were then dissected from the eggs and photographed. The membrane shown in **A** was untreated, whereas the membrane in **B** was stained with NBT, an indicator of activated heterophils.[40] Wild-type cowpox forms red hemorrhagic pocks on the membrane (**A** and **B**). Spontaneous deletion mutants of cowpox virulence genes occur at a high frequency, resulting in infiltration of inflammatory cells into the pock. The infiltration of inflammatory cells causes the pocks to appear white in unstained membrane preparations or dark blue on NBT-stained membranes. The unstained membrane preparation **(A)** contains a single white pock, whereas the NBT-stained preparation **(B)** contains a single blue pock. NBT, nitroblue tetrazolium. (Courtesy of Dr. R. Moyer.)

advantages and disadvantages. For these reasons, an appreciation of the use of cultured cells in animal virology requires an understanding of several fundamentals of cell culture itself. A detailed description of the theory and practice of cell and tissue culture is provided by Freshney,[41] and several additional texts provide excellent summaries of cell culture as it specifically applies to virology.[20,34,59]

Primary Cell Culture

A primary cell culture is defined as a culture of cells obtained from the original tissue that have been cultivated *in vitro* for the first time and that have not been subcultured. Primary cell cultures can be established from whole animal embryos or from selected tissues from embryos, newborn animals, or adult animals of almost any species. The most commonly used cell cultures in virology derive from primates, including humans and monkeys; rodents, including hamsters, rats, and mice; and birds, most notably chickens. Cells to be cultured are obtained by mincing tissue and dispersing individual cells by treatment with proteases and/or collagenase to disrupt cell–cell interactions and interactions of cells with the extracellular matrix. With the exception of cells from the hemopoietic system, normal vertebrate cells will grow and divide only when attached to a solid surface. Dispersed cells are therefore placed in a plastic flask or dish, the surface of which has been treated to promote cell attachment. The cells are incubated in a buffered nutrient medium in the presence of blood serum, which contains a complex mixture of hormones and factors required for the growth of normal cells. The blood serum may come from a variety of sources, although bovine serum is most commonly used. Under these conditions, cells will attach to the surface of the dish, and they will divide and migrate until the surface of the dish is covered with a single layer of cells, a monolayer, whereupon they will remain viable but cease to divide. If the cell monolayer is "wounded" by scraping cells from an isolated area, cells on the border of the wound will resume division and migration until the monolayer is reformed, whereupon cell division again ceases. These and other observations lead to the conclusion that the arrest of division observed when cells reach confluency results from cell–cell contact and therefore is called *contact inhibition.* Primary cultures may contain a mixture of cell types and retain the closest resemblance to the tissue of origin.

Subcultivation

Cells from a primary culture may be subcultured to obtain larger numbers of cells. Cells are removed from the culture dish and disaggregated by treating the primary cell monolayer with a chelating agent, usually EDTA, or a protease, usually trypsin, or both, giving rise to a single cell suspension. This suspension is then diluted to a fraction of the original monolayer cell density and placed in a culture dish with fresh growth medium, whereupon the cells attach to the surface of the dish and resume cell division until once again a monolayer is formed and cell division ceases. Cultures established in this fashion from primary cell cultures may be called *secondary cultures.* Subsequently, cells may be repeatedly subcultured in the same fashion. Each subculturing event is called a *passage,* and each passage may comprise several cell generations, depending on the dilution used during the passage. Most vertebrate cells divide at the rate of approximately one doubling every 24 hours at 37°C. Thus, a passage performed with an eightfold dilution will require three cell doublings over 3 days before the cells regain confluency.

Cell Strains

Normal vertebrate cells cannot be passaged indefinitely in culture. Instead, after a limited number of cell generations, usually 20 to 100 depending on the age and species of the original animal, cultured normal cells cease to divide, then degenerate and die, a phenomenon called *crisis* or *senescence*[51] (Fig. 2.3). Starting with the establishment of a secondary culture and until cells either senesce or become transformed as described later, the culture is termed a *cell strain* to distinguish it from a primary culture

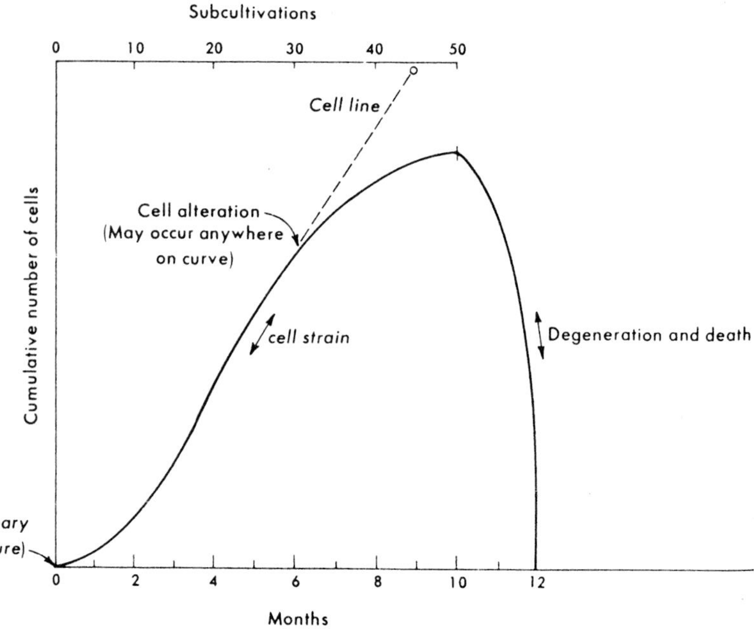

FIGURE 2.3. Growth of cells in culture. A primary culture is defined as the original plating of cells from a tissue, grown to a confluent monolayer, without subculturing. A cell strain (*solid line*) is defined as a euploid population of cells subcultivated once or more *in vitro,* lacking the property of indefinite serial passage. Cell strains ultimately undergo degeneration and death, also called *crisis* or *senescence.* A cell line (*dashed line*) is an aneuploid population of cells that can be grown in culture indefinitely. Spontaneous transformation or alteration of a cell strain to an immortal cell line can occur at any time during cultivation of the cell strain. The time in culture and corresponding number of subcultivations or passages are shown on the abscissas. The ordinate shows the total number of cells that would accumulate if all were retained in culture. (Reprinted from Animal cells: cultivation, growth regulation, transformation. In: Davis BD, Dulbecco R, Eisen HN, et al, eds. *Microbiology.* 4th ed. Philadelphia: J. B. Lippincott Company.)

on the one hand, or a transformed, immortal cell line on the other hand. During culture, cells in a strain retain their original karyotype and are thus called *euploid;* however, culturing induces profound changes in the composition and characteristics of the cell strain, which are manifested early during the passage history and may continue during passage. Whereas primary cell cultures may contain a mixture of cell types that survive the original plating of cells, only a few cell types survive subculturing; thus, by the second or third passage, typically only one cell type remains in the cell strain. Cell strains are usually composed of one of two basic cell types—fibroblast-like or epithelial-like—characterized based on their morphology and growth characteristics (Fig. 2.4). Fibroblasts have an elongated, spindle shape, whereas epithelial cells have a polygonal shape. Although after only a few passages only one cell type may remain in a cell strain, continued passage may select for faster-growing variants, such that the

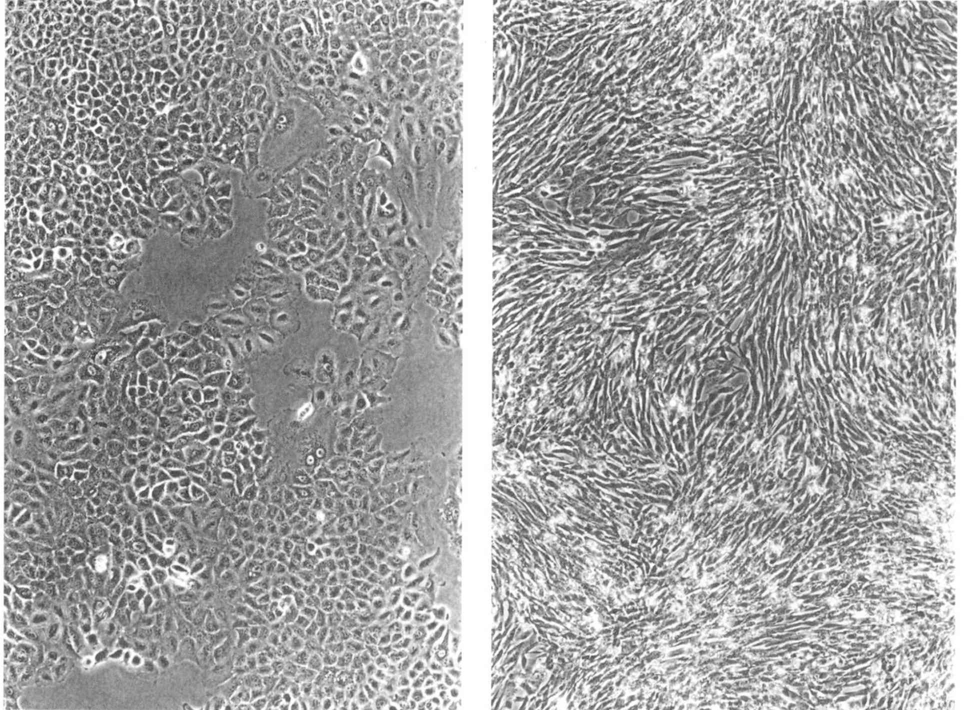

FIGURE 2.4. Cultured cell types. Phase contrast photomicrographs are shown. **A:** Epithelial-like cells, A549, a human lung carcinoma cell line, a slightly subconfluent monolayer. **B:** Fibroblast-like cells, BHK, a baby hamster kidney cell line. (A549 cell culture courtesy of J. I. Lewis. BHK cell culture courtesy of D. Holmes and Dr. S. Moyer.)

characteristics of a cell strain may change with increasing passage number. Despite the fact that normal cell strains experience senescence in culture, they may be maintained for many years by expanding the culture to a large number of cells early during the passage history and storing numerous small samples of low passage cells by freezing. Therefore, as a given strain approaches high passage number and senescence, low passage cells of the same strain may be thawed and cultured.

Cell Lines

At any time during the culture of a cell strain, cells in the culture may become *transformed* such that they are no longer subject to crisis and senescence but can be passaged indefinitely. Transformation is a complex phenomenon, discussed in more detail later and in Chapter 7; however, in the context of cell culture, the most important characteristic of transformation is that the transformed cells become immortalized. Immortal cell cultures are called *cell lines,* or sometimes *continuous cell lines,* to distinguish them from primary cultures and cell strains. Immortalization can occur spontaneously during passage of a cell strain, or it can be induced by treatment with chemical mutagens, infection with tumorigenic viruses, or transfection with oncogenes. In addition, cells cultured from tumor tissue frequently readily establish immortal cell lines in culture. Spontaneous immortalization does not occur in cultured cells from all animal species. Thus, immortalization occurs frequently during culture of rodent cells (e.g., in mouse and hamster cell strains), and it has been observed in monkey kidney cells, although it occurs rarely, if at all, during the culture of chicken or human cells. Immortalization is typically accompanied by genetic changes such that cells become aneuploid, containing abnormalities in the number and structure of chromosomes relative to the parent species, and not all cells in a culture of a continuous cell line necessarily display the same karyotype. Like cell strains, cell lines are usually composed of cells that are either fibroblast-like or epithelial-like in morphology.

As with the propagation of cell strains, continued culture of a cell line may result in selection of specific variants that outgrow other cells in the culture over time, and thus with passage the character of a cell line may change substantially, and cell lines of the same origin cultured in different laboratories over a period of years may have significantly different characteristics. It is prudent, therefore, to freeze stocks of cell lines having specific desirable properties so that these cells can be recovered if the properties disappear during culture. Likewise, it makes sense to obtain a cell line showing certain desired characteristics directly from the laboratory that described those characteristics, because cells from alternate sources may differ in character.

Transformation

Transformed cells are distinguished from normal cells by myriad properties that can be grouped into three fundamental types of changes: immortalization, aberrant growth control, and malignancy. *Immortalization* refers simply to the ability to be cultured indefinitely, as described previously. *Aberrant growth control* comprises a number of properties, several of which have relevance to experimental virology, including loss of contact inhibition, anchorage independence, and tumorigenicity. Loss of contact inhibition means that cells no longer cease to grow as soon as a monolayer is formed, and cells will now grow on top of one another. Anchorage independence means that the cells no longer need to attach to a solid surface to grow. Anchorage independence is often assayed as the ability to form colonies suspended in a semisolid medium such as agar, and a practical consequence of anchorage independence is the ability to grow in liquid suspension. Tumorigenicity refers to the ability of cells to form a tumor in an experimental animal, and *malignancy* refers to the ability to form an invasive tumor *in vivo.* While malignancy is obviously of vital importance as a phenomenon in its own right, it has limited application in virology except within the specific discipline of tumor virology (Chapter 7). Importantly, the many properties of transformed cells are not necessarily interdependent, and no one property is an absolute prerequisite for another. Thus, transformation is thought to be a multistep genetic phenomenon, and varying degrees of transformation are measurable. Tumorigenicity is often regarded as the most stringent assay for a fully transformed cell and is most closely correlated with anchorage independence.

The fact that the various characteristics of transformed cells are not interdependent has important consequences for experimental virology, especially in the assay of tumor viruses. Specifically, a transformed cell line that is immortalized but still contact inhibited may be used in a viral transformation assay that measures the further transformation to loss of contact inhibition. When cells in a monolayer are transformed by a tumor virus and lose contact inhibition, they grow on top of a confluent monolayer, forming a *focus,* literally a pile of cells, which is readily distinguishable from the rest of the monolayer. This property forms the basis for quantitative biological assay of tumor viruses,[129] described in more detail later.

Advantages and Disadvantages of Different Cultured Cell Types

The various types of cultured cells described previously have specific application to different problems encountered in experimental virology. For most applications, an adherent cell line provides the most useful host cell. Cell lines are relatively easy to maintain because they can be passaged indefinitely, and adherence is a prerequisite for a plaque assay, described later. A distinct technical advantage of adherent cells is that the culture medium can easily be changed for the purposes of infection or metabolic labeling by simply aspirating and replacing fluid from a monolayer, a process that requires repeated centrifugations with suspension cells. By contrast, relative to adherent cell lines, suspension cell lines are easier to sample than adherent cells, and they produce large numbers of cells from a relatively small volume of medium in a single culture vessel, which has significant advantages for some high-volume applications in virology. Unfortunately, not all viruses will grow on a cell line, and often under these circumstances, a primary cell culture will suffice. This may reflect a requirement for a particular cell type found only under conditions of primary cell culture, or it may reflect a requirement for a state of metabolism or differentiation closely resembling the *in vivo* situation, which is more likely to exist in a primary culture than it is in a cell line.

Lastly, some viruses do not grow in cell culture at all. In such cases, investigators are reliant either on the old expedients of natural hosts, laboratory animals, or embryonated eggs, or on some more modern advances in tissue culture and recombinant DNA technology. The papillomaviruses, which cause warts, provide an enlightening example of this situation (Chapter 54). Although the viral nature of papillomatosis was demonstrated more than 90 years ago, progress on the study of papillomaviruses was seriously hampered in the virology heyday of the mid 20th century because the viruses grow well only on the natural host; they do not grow in culture. The inability to grow in culture is now reasonably well understood, and results from a tight coupling of the regulation of viral gene expression with the differentiation state of the target epithelial cell, which in turn is tightly coupled to the three-dimensional architecture of the epidermis, which is lost in culture. Specialized tissue culture techniques have now been developed that result in the faithful reconstruction of an epidermis by seeding primary keratinocytes on a "feeder" layer composed of an appropriate cell line and incubating these cells on a "raft" or grid at a liquid–air interface. On these raft cultures, the entire replication cycle of a papillomavirus can be reproduced *in vitro,* albeit with difficulty.[7] In the meantime, it is significant that a large fraction of the genetics and biology of papillomaviruses was determined primarily through the use of recombinant DNA technology, without ever growing virus in culture. Thus, the genetic structure of both the model bovine papillomavirus and many human papillomaviruses has been determined by cloning genomic DNA from natural infections, and regulation and function of many genes can be gleaned from sequence alone, from *in vitro* assays on individual gene products expressed *in vitro,* and from cell transformation assays that use all or parts of a papillomavirus genome. In summary, the inability to grow a virus in culture, although it increases the challenge, no longer presents an insurmountable impediment to understanding a virus.

Recognition of Viral Growth in Culture

Two principal methods exist for the recognition of a virus infection in culture: cytopathic effect and hemadsorption. *Cytopathic effect* comprises two different phenomena: (a) morphological changes induced in individual cells or groups of cells by virus infection that are easily recognizable under a light microscope, and (b) inclusion bodies, which are more subtle alterations to the intracellular architecture of individual cells. *Hemadsorption* refers to indirect measurement of viral protein synthesis in infected cells, detected by adsorption of erythrocytes to the surface of infected cells. Cytopathic effect is the simplest and most widely used criterion for infection; however, not all viruses cause a cytopathic effect, and in these cases, other methods must suffice.

Morphological changes induced by virus infection comprise a number of cell phenomena, including rounding, shrinkage, increased refractility, fusion, aggregation, loss of adherence or lysis. Morphological changes caused by a given virus may include several of these phenomena in various combinations, and the character of the cytopathic effect may change reproducibly during the course of infection. Morphological changes caused by a given virus are very reproducible and can be so precisely characteristic of the virus type that significant clues to the identity of a virus can be gleaned from the cytopathic effect alone (Chapter 15). Figure 2.5 depicts different cytopathic effects caused by two viruses—measles and vaccinia. Most important to the trained virologist, a simple microscopic examination of a cell culture can reveal whether an infection is present, what fraction of cells are infected, and how advanced the infection is. In addition, because cytopathology results directly from the action of virus gene products, virus mutants can be obtained that are altered in cytopathology, yielding either a conveniently marked virus or a tool to study cytopathology *per se.*

The term *inclusion bodies* refers generally to the observation of intracellular structures specific to an infected cell and discernible by light microscopy. The effects are highly specific for a particular virus type so that, as with morphological alterations, the presence of a specific type of inclusion body can be diagnostic of a specific virus infection. Electron microscopy, combined with a more detailed understanding of the biology of many viruses, reveals that inclusion bodies usually represent focal points of virus replication and assembly, which differ in appearance depending on the virus. For example, Negri bodies formed during a rabies virus infection represent collections of virus nucleocapsids[84] (Chapter 31).

Hemadsorption refers to the ability of red blood cells to attach specifically to virus-infected cells.[111] Many viruses synthesize cell attachment proteins, which carry out their function wholly or in part by binding substituents such as sialic acid that are abundant on a wide variety of cell types, including erythrocytes. Often, these viral proteins are expressed on the surface of the infected cell—for example, in preparation for maturation of an enveloped virus through a budding process. Thus, a cluster of infected cells may be easily detectable to the naked eye as areas that stain red after exposure to an appropriate preparation of red blood cells. Hemadsorption can be a particularly useful assay for detecting infections by viruses that cause little or no cytopathic effect.

Virus Cultivation

From the discussion presented previously, it may be obvious that ultimately the exact method chosen for growing virus on any particular occasion will depend on a variety of factors, including (a) the goals of the experiment, namely whether large amounts of one virus variant or small amounts of several variants are to be grown; (b) limitations in the *in vitro* host range of the virus, namely whether it will grow on embryonated eggs, primary cell cultures, continuous adherent cell lines, or suspension cell lines; and (c) the relative technical ease of alternative possible procedures. Furthermore, the precise method for harvesting a virus culture will depend on the biology of the virus—for example, whether it buds from the infected cell, lyses the infected cell, or leaves the cell intact and stays tightly cell associated. As a simple example, consider cultivation of a budding, cytopathic virus on an adherent cell line. Confluent monolayers of an appropriate cell line are exposed to virus diluted to infect a fraction of the cells, and progress of the infection is monitored by observing the development of the cytopathic effect until the infection is judged complete based on experience with the relationship between cytopathic effect and maximum virus yield. A crude preparation of virus can be harvested simply by collecting the culture fluid; it may not even be necessary to remove cells or cell debris. Most viruses can be stored frozen indefinitely either as crude or purified, concentrated preparations.

Quantitative Assay of Viruses

Two major types of quantitative assays for viruses exist: physical and biological. *Physical* assays, such as hemagglutination, electron microscopic particle counts, optical density measurements, or immunological methods, quantify only the presence of virus particles whether or not the particles are infectious. *Biological* assays, such as the plaque assay or various endpoint

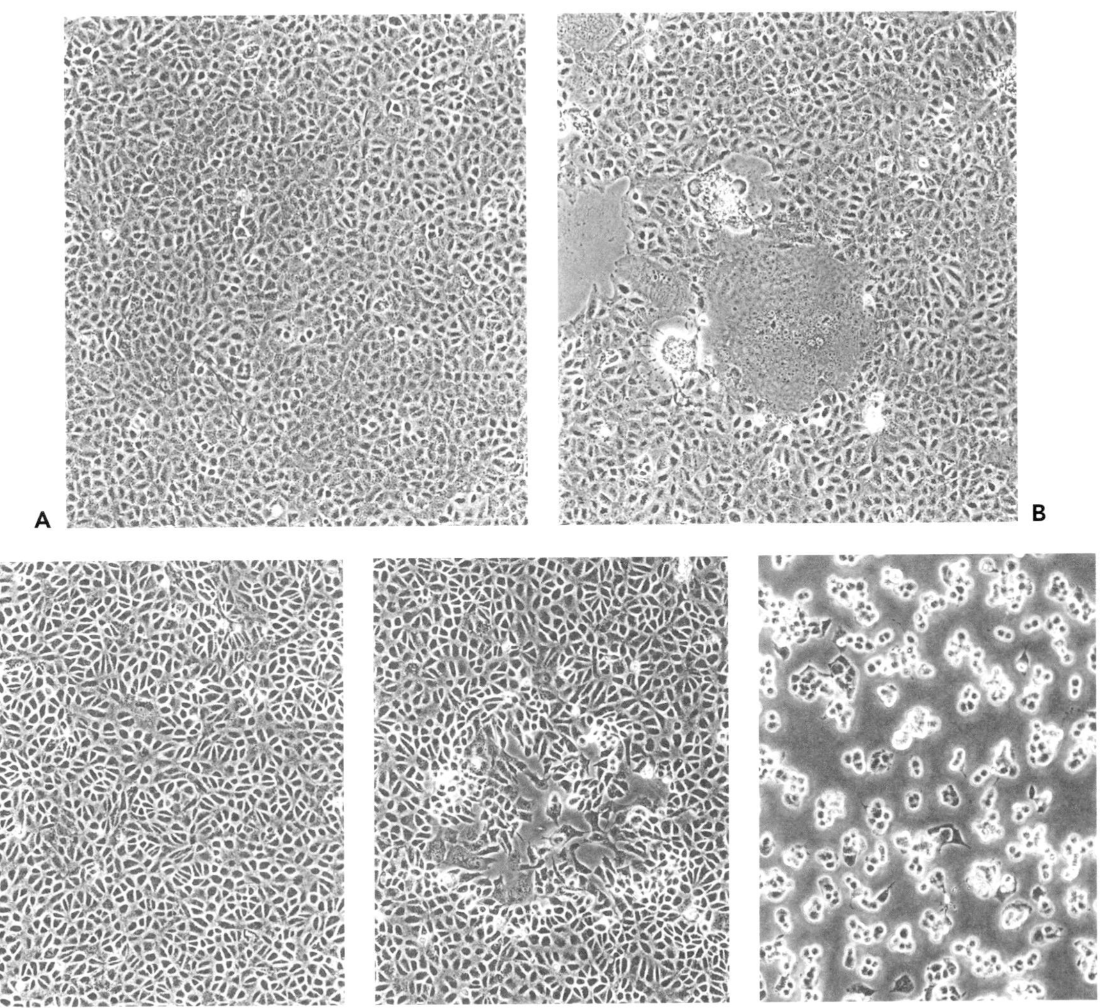

FIGURE 2.5. Virus-induced cytopathic effects. Phase contrast photomicrographs are shown. **A:** Uninfected A549 cells, a human lung carcinoma cell line. **B:** A549 cells infected with measles virus at a moi of less than 0.01 pfu/cell. Individual plaques can be discerned. Measles fuses cells, causing formation of syncytia. In mid field is a large syncytium containing multiple nuclei. Surrounding this area are additional syncytia, including two that have rounded and are separating from the dish. **C:** Uninfected BSC40 cells, an African green monkey cell line. **D:** BSC40 cells infected with vaccinia virus at a moi of less than 0.01 pfu/cell. A single plaque is shown in the middle of the field. **E:** BSC40 cells infected with vaccinia virus at a moi of 10 pfu/cell, 48 hours after infection. All cells are infected and display complete cytopathic effect. (Cultures of vaccinia infections courtesy of J. I. Lewis. Cultures of measles infections courtesy of S. Smallwood and Dr. S. Moyer.)

methods that have in common the assay of infectivity in cultured cells or *in vivo,* measure only the presence of infectivity and may not count all particles present in a preparation, even many that are in fact infectious. Thus, a clear understanding of the nature and efficiency of both physical and biological quantitative virus assays is required to make effective use of the data obtained from any assay.

Biological Assays

The Plaque Assay

The plaque assay is the most elegant, the most quantitative, and the most useful biological assay for viruses. Developed originally for the study of bacteriophage by d'Herelle[18] in the early 1900s, the plaque assay was adapted to animal viruses by Dulbecco and Vogt[28] in 1953, an advance that revolutionized animal virology by introducing a methodology that was relatively simple and precisely quantitative, which enabled the cloning of individual genetic variants of a virus, and which permitted a qualitative assay for individual virus variants that differ in growth properties or cytopathology.

The plaque assay is based simply on the ability of a single infectious virus particle to give rise to a macroscopic area of cytopathology on an otherwise normal monolayer of cultured cells. Specifically, if a single cell in a monolayer is infected with a single virus particle, new virus resulting from the initial infection can infect surrounding cells, which in turn produce virus that infects additional surrounding cells. Over a period of days (the exact length of time depending on the particular virus), the initial infection thus gives rise through multiple rounds of infection to an area of infection, called a *plaque.* Photomicrographs of plaques are shown in Figure 2.5, and stained monolayers containing plaques are shown in Figure 2.6.

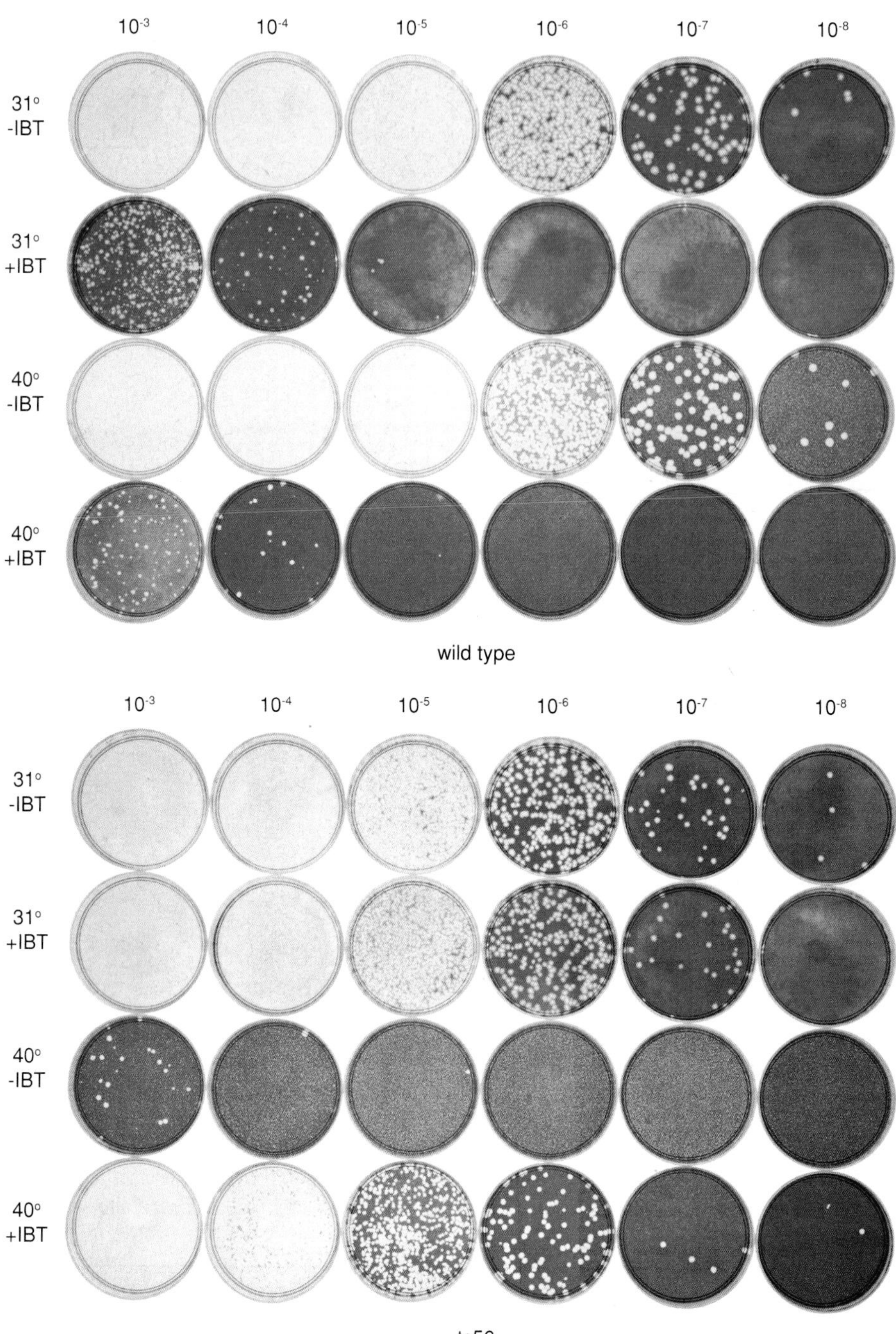

FIGURE 2.6. Plaque assay. Monolayers of the African green monkey kidney cell line BSC40 were infected with 0.5-mL portions of 10-fold serial dilutions of wild-type vaccinia virus or the temperature-sensitive vaccinia mutant, ts56, as indicated. Infected monolayers were overlayed with semisolid medium and incubated at 31°C or 40°C, the permissive and nonpermissive temperatures for *ts*56, in the presence of 45 μM isatin-β-thiosemicarbazone (IBT) or in the absence of drug as indicated, for 1 week. Overlays were removed, and monolayers were stained with crystal violet. Wild-type vaccinia virus forms plaques at both 31°C and 40°C; however, plaque formation is inhibited by IBT. Spontaneous IBT-resistant mutants in the wild-type virus stock are revealed as plaques forming at 10^{-3}, 10^{-4}, and 10^{-5} dilutions in the presence of IBT. *ts*56 carries a single-base missense mutation in the vaccinia gene *G2R*.[87] *G2R* is an essential gene that when completely inactivated renders virus dependent on IBT; hence, *ts*56 is not only temperature sensitive, forming plaques at 31°C but not at 40°C in the absence of IBT, but it is also IBT dependent at 40°C, forming plaques in the presence but not the absence of IBT. *ts*56 is slightly defective at 31°C; it forms smaller than wild-type plaques and is IBT resistant, forming plaques both in the presence and absence of drug, a phenotype intermediate between the wild-type IBT-sensitive phenotype and the null *G2R* mutant IBT-dependent phenotype. Wild-type, temperature-insensitive revertants present in the *ts*56 stock are revealed as plaques growing on the 10^{-3} plate at 40°C. Based on this assay, the titer of the wild-type stock is 2.0×10^9 pfu/mL, and the titer of the *ts*56 stock is 6.0×10^8 pfu/mL. IBT, isatin-β-thiosemicarbazone.

The plaque assay can be used to quantify virus in the following manner (see Fig. 2.6). A sample of virus of unknown concentration is serially diluted in an appropriate medium, and measured aliquots of each dilution are seeded onto confluent monolayers of cultured cells. Infected cells are overlayed with a semisolid nutrient medium usually consisting of growth medium and agar. The semisolid medium prevents formation of secondary plaques through diffusion of virus from the original site of infection to new sites, ensuring that each plaque that develops in the assay originated from a single infectious particle in the starting inoculum. After an appropriate period of incubation to allow development of plaques, the monolayer is stained so that the plaques can be visualized. The precise staining technique depends on the cytopathology; however, vital dyes such as neutral red are common. Neutral red is taken up by living cells but not by dead cells; thus, plaques become visible as clear areas on a red monolayer of cells. In cases where the virus cytopathology results in cell lysis or detachment of cells from the dish, plaques exist literally as holes in the monolayer, and a permanent record of the assay can be made by staining the monolayer with a general stain such as crystal violet, prepared in a fixative such as formalin. The goal of the assay is to identify a dilution of virus that yields 20 to 100 plaques on a single dish—that is, a number large enough to be statistically significant yet small enough such that individual plaques can be readily discerned and counted. Usually, a series of four to six 10-fold dilutions is tested, which are estimated to bracket the target dilution. Dishes inoculated with low dilutions of virus will contain only dead cells or too many plaques to count, whereas dishes inoculated with high dilutions of virus will contain very few, if any, plaques (see Fig. 2.6). Dishes containing an appropriate number of plaques are counted, and the concentration of infectious virus in the original sample can then be calculated taking into account the serial dilution. The resulting value is called a *titer* and is expressed in plaque-forming units per milliliter (pfu/mL) to emphasize specifically that only viruses capable of forming plaques have been quantified. Titers derived by serial dilution are unavoidably error prone, owing simply to the additive error inherent in multiple serial pipetting steps. Errors of up to 100% are normal; however, titers that approximate the real titer to within a factor of two are satisfactory for most purposes.

A critical benefit of the plaque assay is that it measures infectivity, although it is important to understand that infectivity does not necessarily correspond exactly to the number of virus particles in a preparation. In fact, for most animal viruses, only a fraction of the particles—as few as 1 in 10 to 1 in 10,000—may be infections as judged by comparison of a direct particle count, described later, with a plaque assay. This low *efficiency of plating,* or high particle to infectivity ratio, may have several causes. First, to determine a particle to infectivity ratio, virus must be purified to determine the concentration of physical particles and then subjected to plaque assay. If the purification itself damages particles, the particle to infectivity ratio will be increased. Second, some viruses produce empty particles, or particles that are for other reasons defective during infection, resulting in a high particle to infectivity ratio. Lastly, it is possible that not all infectious particles will form plaques in a given plaque assay. For example, infectious virus may require that cells exist in a specific metabolic state or in a specific stage of the cell cycle; thus, if not all cells in a culture are identical in this regard, only a fraction of the potentially infectious virions may be able to successfully launch an infection and form a plaque.

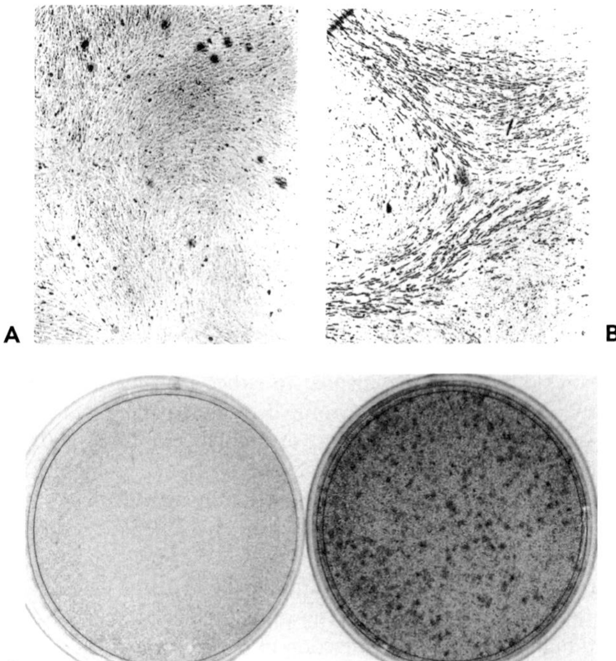

FIGURE 2.7. Focus assay. Monolayers of the NIH3T3 mouse fibroblast cell line were infected with Maloney murine sarcoma virus. **A, B:** Photomicrographs of uninfected cells **(A)** and a single virus-induced focus **(B). C:** Stained dishes of uninfected **(left)** and infected **(right)** cells. Foci are clearly visible as darker areas on the infected dish. (Courtesy of Dr. D. Blair.)

In addition to its utility as a quantitative assay, the plaque assay also provides a way to detect genetic variants of a virus that possess altered growth properties, and it provides a very convenient method to clone genetically unique variants of a virus (see Fig. 2.6). Genetic variants are considered in detail in the Virus Genetics section; in brief, they may comprise viruses that plaque only under certain conditions of temperature or drug treatment, or form plaques of altered size or shape. Because each plaque results from infection with a single infectious virus particle, unique genetic variants of a virus can be cloned simply by picking plaques—that is, literally excising a small plug of semisolid medium and infected cells from a plaque using a Pasteur pipette.

The Focus Assay

Some tumor viruses, most notably retroviruses, normally transform cells rather than killing them but can nevertheless be quantified by taking advantage of the transformation cytopathology.[116,129] For example, retrovirus transformed cells may lose contact inhibition and therefore grow as foci, literally piles of transformed cells, on top of a contact-inhibited cell monolayer. Dense foci of transformed cells stain more darkly than cells in a monolayer and thus can be quantified on treatment of an infected monolayer with an appropriate stain. Otherwise, the focus assay is similar to the plaque assay in both technique and function. Photomicrographs of foci and stained monolayers containing foci are shown in Figure 2.7.

Pock Formation

As mentioned previously in the discussion of embryonated eggs, many viruses will cause focal lesions on the chorioallantoic membrane of eggs. While cumbersome, this assay can be used to quantify virus in a fashion similar to a plaque assay. The pock assay found utility before the adaptation of the plaque assay to animal virology, although now it has largely been replaced with other assays utilizing cultured cells and is used only for specialized purposes as noted in Figure 2.2.

The Endpoint Method

Viruses that cannot be adapted to either a plaque or a focus assay but nevertheless cause some detectable pathology in cultured cells, embryonated eggs, or animals can be quantified using an endpoint method. Briefly, virus is serially diluted, and multiple replicate samples of each dilution are inoculated into an appropriate assay system. After a suitable incubation period, an absolute judgment is made as to whether or not an infection has taken place. The dilution series is constructed such that low dilutions show infection in all replicate inoculations, and high dilutions show infection in none of the inoculations, although some dilutions result in infection in some but not all inoculations. Statistical methods, described in more detail later, have been devised to calculate the dilution of virus that results in infection in 50% of replicate inoculations, and titers are expressed as the infectious dose 50 (ID_{50}). Assay systems are various and include, for example, observation of cytopathic effect in cultured cells, yielding tissue culture infective dose 50 ($TCID_{50}$); cytopathology or embryonic death in inoculated embryonated chicken eggs, yielding egg infective dose 50 (EID_{50}); or death of an experimental laboratory animal, yielding lethal dose 50 (LD_{50}). As with the plaque assay, the focus assay, and the pock assay, the endpoint method has the advantage of measuring infectivity; however, importantly, the unit of infectivity measured by the endpoint method may require more than one infectious particle. A sample determination of a $TCID_{50}$ is provided in the eBook.

Physical Assays

Direct Particle Count

The concentration of virus particles in a sample of purified virus can be counted directly using an electron microscope.[78,131] Briefly, a purified preparation of virus is mixed with a known concentration of microscopic marker particles such as latex beads, which can be easily distinguished from virus particles in the electron microscope. Samples of the solution containing virus and beads are then applied to an electron microscope grid and visualized following shadowing or staining. The volume of liquid applied to a given area of the grid can be determined by counting the beads. The virus particles in the same area can then be counted, resulting in an accurate determination of the concentration of virus particles in the original solution. An example of an electron microscopic count of vaccinia virus is shown in Figure 2.8. Given a solution of virus with a known concentration determined by microscopic particle count, the same solution can be subjected to any number of chemical or spectrophotometric analyses to yield a conversion from protein, nucleic acid, or simply absorbance at a fixed wavelength to a concentration of virus in particles per unit volume.

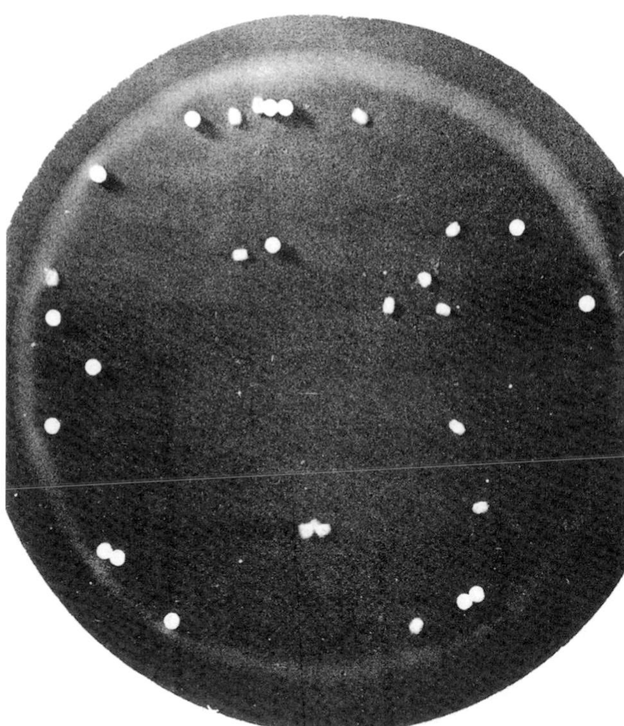

FIGURE 2.8. Direct electron microscopic particle count. An electron micrograph of a spray droplet containing 15 latex beads (spheres) and 14 vaccinia virus particles (slightly smaller brick-shaped particles). (Reprinted from Dumbell KR, Downie AW, Valentine RC. The ratio of the number of virus particles to infective titer of cowpox and vaccinia virus suspensions. Virology 4(3):467–482, © 1957 with permission from Elsevier.)

Thus, once a microscopic particle count has been performed, future quantitative assays of purified virus are greatly simplified. Importantly, the direct particle count does not distinguish infectious from noninfectious particles.

Hemagglutination

As noted previously in the discussion of hemadsorption, many viruses express cell attachment proteins, which carry out their function wholly or in part by binding substituents such as sialic acid that are abundant on a wide variety of cell types, including erythrocytes. Because these cell attachment proteins decorate the surface of the virion, virions may bind directly to erythrocytes. Because both the virions and the erythrocytes contain multiple binding sites for each other, erythrocytes will agglutinate, or form a network of cells and virus, when mixed with virus particles in sufficiently high concentration. Agglutinated erythrocytes can be easily distinguished from cells that are not agglutinated, and thus hemagglutination can be used as a simple quantitative assay for the presence of a hemagglutinating virus.

In practice, a hemagglutination assay is carried out as follows (Fig. 2.9). Virus is serially diluted, mixed with a fixed concentration of erythrocytes, and the mixture is allowed to settle in a specially designed hemagglutination tray, containing wells

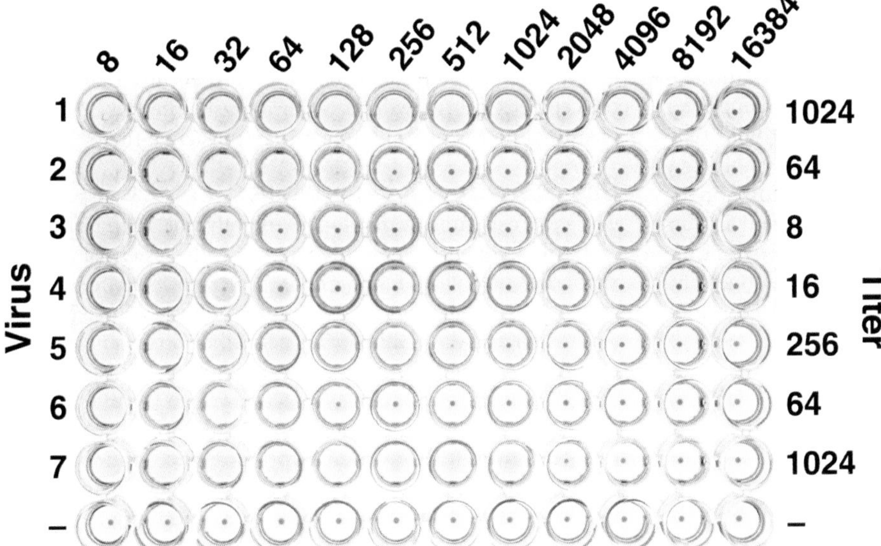

FIGURE 2.9. Hemagglutination assay. Seven different samples of influenza virus, numbered 1 through 7 at the **left**, were serially diluted as indicated at the **top**, mixed with chicken RBCs, and incubated on ice for 1 to 2 hours. Wells in the **bottom row** contain no virus. Agglutinated RBCs coat wells evenly, in contrast to nonagglutinated cells, which form a distinct button at the bottom of the well. The hemagglutination titer, shown at the **right** is the last dilution that shows complete hemagglutination activity. RBCs, red blood cells. (Courtesy of Drs. J. Talon and P. Palese.)

with rounded bottoms. Erythrocytes that are not agglutinated are free to roll to the bottom of the well, forming a dense, easily recognizable button, or cluster of cells. Erythrocytes that are agglutinated are not free to roll to the bottom of the well but instead evenly coat the bottom surface of the well to form what is called a *shield*. One hemagglutination unit is defined as the minimum amount of virus required to cause agglutination, and the titer of the virus solution, expressed as hemagglutination units per milliliter (HA units/mL), can be calculated taking into account the serial dilution. It is noteworthy that, such as with the direct particle count assay, the hemagglutination assay does not distinguish infectious from noninfectious particles. In addition, because it may require many particles to cause a detectable hemagglutination, one HA unit may represent many physical particles.

Quantitative Considerations in Virus Assay, Cultivation, and Experimentation

Dose Response in Plaque and Focus Assays

With few exceptions, the number of infectious units observed on a given plate in a plaque assay is a linear function of the dilution of the virus; thus, the development of plaques follows single-hit kinetics, proving that each plaque results from infection with a single virus particle. Exceptions include the murine sarcoma viruses, assayed in a focus assay, which require co-infection with both a defective transforming virus and a nondefective helper virus, in which case the number of foci observed relative to the dilution used follows two-hit kinetics.[46]

Comparison of Quantitative Assays

As noted in the previous individual descriptions, the various quantitative assays of viruses measure different physical and biological properties, and a one-to-one correlation between assays cannot be assumed. Table 2.3 summarizes the titers of an influenza virus preparation as measured by several different assays and thus provides an example the magnitude of differences that might be expected in the various assays. Hence, relative to a direct particle count, the efficiency of virus detection in the influenza sample shown in Table 2.3 is 10^{-1} as assayed in eggs, 10^{-2} as assayed in a plaque assay, and 10^{-7} as assayed in a hemagglutination assay. As indicated in the foregoing discussion, some differences result from different properties being measured (e.g., physical particles versus infectivity), and some differences result from differences in the sensitivity of the assay (e.g., direct particle count versus assay of particles by hemagglutination).

Multiplicity of Infection

Multiplicity of infection, often abbreviated "moi," measures the average amount of virus added per cell in an infection. Multiplicity of infection can be expressed using any quantitative measure of virus titer—for example, particles/cell, HA units/cell, $TCID_{50}$/cell, or pfu/cell. Because the efficiency of plating varies depending on the method of quantitation used, some knowledge of the infectivity of the sample or the efficiency

TABLE 2.3 Comparison of Quantitative Assay Efficiency

Method	Amount (per mL)
Direct electron microscope count	10^{10} EM particles
Quantal infectivity assay in eggs	10^{9} egg ID_{50}
Quantal infectivity assay by plaque formation	10^{8} pfu
Hemagglutination assay	10^{3} HA units

EM, electron microscopy; ID_{50}, infective dose 50; pfu, plaque-forming unit; HA, hemagglutination assay.

Reprinted from Fenner F, McAuslan BR, Mims CA, et al. *The Biology of Animal Viruses*. New York: Academic Press, © 1974, with permission from Elsevier.

of plating is required to correctly anticipate the consequences of the use of a particular moi. The multiplicity of infection used in different protocols can have a profound outcome on the procedure. For example, some viruses, if serially passaged at a moi of greater than 1 infectious unit/cell, will accumulate spontaneously deleted defective particles that are maintained during passage by the presence of complementing wild-type helper virus.[130] Passage of the same virus at very low moi (e.g., 0.01 infectious units/cell) discourages the accumulation of defective particles because few cells will be co-infected with an infectious and a defective particle, and defective particles cannot replicate in the absence of a wild-type helper. Conversely, most metabolic labeling experiments are done at a high moi (e.g., 10 infectious units/cell) to ensure that all cells in the culture are infected and that the infection is as synchronous as possible. For such experiments, use of too low a moi may result in an apparently asynchronous infection and a high background owing to the presence of uninfected cells in the culture.

The Poisson distribution can be used to predict the fraction of cells in a population infected with a given number of particles at different multiplicities of infection. As applied to virus infections, the Poisson distribution can be written as:

$$P(k) = e^{-m}\, m^k / k!,$$

where P(k) equals the probability that any cell is infected with k particles, m equals moi, and k equals the number of particles in a given cell.

To determine the fraction of uninfected cells in any experiment—that is, when k = 0—the equation simplifies to:

$$P(0) = e^{-m}$$

For practical purposes, solution of this equation for given values of m and k (other than 0) is most easily accomplished using published tables.[142] Sample solutions are shown in Table 2.4 for commonly used multiplicities of infection. Inspection of this table and consideration of the error inherent in any virus titration involving a serial dilution leads to some significant practical guides in experimental design. Note first that in a culture infected at a moi of 1 pfu/cell, 37% of cells remain uninfected—an unacceptably high number for an experiment designed to measure a single round of synchronous infection. A moi of at least 3 is required to infect 95% of the cells in culture. Given that titers can easily be inaccurate by a factor of two, the use of a calculated moi of 10 ensures that 99% of the cells in a culture will be synchronously infected even if the measured titer is twofold higher than the actual titer.

TABLE 2.4 The Poisson Distribution: Values of P(k) for Various Values of m and k

	moi (m)			
#/cell (k)	1	3	5	10
0	0.37	0.05	0.01	0.00
1	0.37	0.15	0.03	0.00
2	0.18	0.22	0.08	0.00
3	0.06	0.22	0.14	0.01
4	0.02	0.17	0.18	0.02
5	0.00	0.10	0.18	0.04
6	0.00	0.05	0.15	0.06
7	0.00	0.02	0.10	0.09
8	0.00	0.00	0.07	0.11
9	0.00	0.00	0.04	0.13
10	0.00	0.00	0.02	0.13

moi, multiplicity of infection.

One-Step Growth Experiment

A classic experiment developed initially for bacteriophage[29] and still frequently used to determine the essential growth properties of a virus is the one-step growth experiment. The goal of this experiment is to measure the time course of virus replication and the yield of virus per cell during a single round of infection. The experiment is carried out as follows. Several dishes containing confluent monolayers of an appropriate cultured cell are infected simultaneously with virus at a high moi (e.g., 10 pfu/cell). After an adsorption period, monolayers are washed to remove unabsorbed virus and then incubated in culture medium. At various times after infection, virus from individual dishes is harvested, and at the completion of the experiment, the virus titer in samples representing each time point is determined. The virus yield at each point can be converted to pfu/cell (also called *burst size*) by dividing the total amount of virus present in the sample by the number of cells originally infected in the sample.

The results from one example of a one-step growth experiment, in this case comparing growth of wild-type vaccinia virus and a temperature-sensitive mutant at permissive and nonpermissive temperatures, are shown in e-Figure 2.1. Several features of the growth curve are noteworthy. First, during the first several hours of the wild-type infection or the *ts*56 infection at the permissive temperature, the titer in the cultures decreases and then increases. This dip in the growth curve is called *eclipse* and results from the fact that early during the experiment, virus attached to the cell surface but not uncoated remains infectious; however, infectivity is lost following uncoating during the first few hours of infection, and infectivity is recovered only after new virus is produced. The infection then enters a rapid growth phase, followed by a plateau. The plateau results from the fact that all infected cells have reached the maximum yield of virus, or have died or lysed, depending on the type of virus infection. The time interval from infection to plateau represents the time required for a single cycle of growth, and the yield of virus at plateau shows the amount of virus produced per cell. The experiment in e-Figure 2.1 demonstrates the utility of the one-step growth experiment. As judged by this experiment, wild-type virus grows with identical kinetics and to the identical yields at both 31°C and 40°C, which are permissive and nonpermissive temperatures for the temperature-sensitive mutant, respectively. The temperature-sensitive mutant, *ts*56,[87] grows more slowly than wild-type virus at 31°C, indicating some defective character even at the permissive temperature, although at plateau the yields of mutant virus at 31°C are equivalent to wild-type virus. The experiment demonstrates conclusively that the mutant does not grow at all at the nonpermissive temperature of 40°C.

Multiplicity of infection is a critical factor in the design of a virus growth experiment. A true one-step growth experiment can only be done at high moi. If the moi is too low and a large fraction of cells are left uninfected, then virus produced during the first round of infection will replicate on previously uninfected cells, and thus multiple rounds of infection rather than one round will be measured. A growth experiment done at low moi has utility in that it measures both growth and spread of a virus in culture; however, the time from infection to plateau does not accurately reflect the time required for a single cycle of infection. It is also noteworthy that some mutant phenotypes are multiplicity dependent.[6]

VIRUS GENETICS

Viruses are subject to the same genetic principles at work in other living systems, namely mutation, selection, complementation, and recombination. Genetics impacts all aspects of virology, including the natural evolution of viruses, clinical management of virus infections, and experimental virology. For example, antigenic variation, which is a direct result of mutation and selection, plays a prominent role in the epidemiology of influenza virus and human immunodeficiency virus (HIV) in the human population, and mutation to drug resistance offers a significant challenge to the clinical management of virus infections with antiviral drugs. This section deals primarily with the application of experimental genetic techniques to basic virology.

The ultimate goal of experimental virology is to understand completely the functional organization of a virus genome. In a modern context, this means determination of the structure of a virus genome at the nucleotide sequence level, coupled with isolation of mutational variants of the virus altered in each gene or control sequence, followed by analysis of the effects of each mutation on the replication and/or pathogenesis of the virus. Thus, genetic analysis of viruses is of fundamental importance to experimental virology.

Before the advent of modern nucleic acid technology—that is, during a *classical* period of *forward* genetics—genetic analysis of viruses consisted of the random, brute force isolation of large numbers of individual virus mutants, followed first by complementation analysis to determine groupings of individual mutants into genes, then recombination analysis to determine the physical order of genes on the virus genome, and finally the phenotypic analysis of mutants to determine gene function. This approach, pioneered in the 1940s through the 1960s in elegant studies of several bacteriophage, notably lambda, T4, and T7 (Chapter 75), was the primary method for identifying, mapping, and characterizing virus genes. The application of cell culture techniques to animal virology opened the door to classical genetic analysis of animal viruses, resulting in a flurry of activity in the 1950s through the 1970s, during which time hundreds of mutants were isolated and analyzed in prototypical members of most of the major animal virus families.[38] Modern nucleic acid technology introduced in the 1970s brought with it a variety of techniques for physical mapping of genomes and mutants, including restriction enzyme mapping, marker rescue, and DNA sequence analysis, which together replaced recombination analysis as an analytic tool. Mutants and techniques from the classical period continue to be of enormous utility today; however, recombinant DNA technology has brought with it *reverse* genetics, in which the structure of the genome is determined first using entirely physical methods, then the function of individual genetic elements is determined by analyzing mutants constructed in a highly targeted fashion.

The genetic approach to experimental virology, or any field of biology for that matter, has the profound advantage of asking of the organism under study only the most basic question—What genes do you need to survive, and why do you need them?—without imposing any further bias or assumptions on the system. Happily, organisms often respond with surprises that the most ingenious biochemist or molecular biologist would never have imagined. What follows is a summary of the critical elements of both the classical and modern approaches to virus genetics as applied to experimental virology.

Mutants

Wild-type Virus

It is important to understand that in the context of experimental virus genetics, a virus designated as *wild-type* can differ significantly from the virus that actually occurs in nature. For example, virus genetics often relies heavily on growth and assay of viruses in cell culture, and as noted previously, natural isolates of viruses may undergo significant genetic change during adaptation to cell culture. In addition, viruses to be designated as wild-type should be plaque purified before initiating a genetic study to ensure a unique genetic background for mutational analysis. Lastly, viruses may be specifically adapted for use in genetic analysis—for example, by passage under conditions that are to be restrictive for conditionally lethal mutants so that the analysis can be initiated with a preparation free from spontaneous mutants.

Fundamental Genetic Concepts

Concepts fundamental to genetic analysis of other organisms apply to genetic analysis of viruses, and a clear understanding of these concepts is essential to understanding virus genetics. The most important of these concepts, including distinctions between genotype and phenotype, a selection and a screen, and essential versus nonessential genes, are briefly summarized next.

Genotype and Phenotype

Genotype refers to the actual genetic change from wild-type in a particular virus mutant, whereas *phenotype* refers to the measurable manifestation of that change in a given assay system. This distinction is emphasized by the fact that a single genotype may express different phenotypes depending on the assay applied. Thus, for example, the same missense mutation in a virus gene may cause temperature sensitivity in one cell line but not another, or a deletion in another virus gene may have no effect on the replication of virus in culture but may alter virulence in an animal model.

Selection and Screen

Selection and screen refer to two fundamentally different methods of identifying individual virus variants contained in a mixed population of viruses. *Selection* implies that a condition exists where only the desired virus will grow, and growth of unwanted viruses is suppressed. Thus, a drug-resistant virus can be identified by plating a mixture of wild-type, drug-sensitive, and mutant, drug-resistant viruses together on the same cell monolayer in the presence of the inhibitory drug, thereby selecting for drug-resistant viruses that grow, and selecting against wild-type viruses that do not grow (see Fig. 2.6). A *screen* implies that both the desired virus variant and one or several other unwanted virus types grow under a given condition, such that many viruses must be analyzed individually to identify the desired variant. For example, in searching for a temperature-sensitive mutant (i.e., a virus whose growth is inhibited relative to wild-type virus at an elevated temperature), no condition exists under which the mutant alone will grow. Therefore, virus must be plated at a low temperature where both wild-type and mutant virus will grow, and plaques tested individually for temperature sensitivity. Sometimes a screen can be streamlined by introducing a phenotypic marker into the variant of choice. For example, a knockout virus might be constructed by inserting the β-galactosidase gene into the virus gene to be inactivated. In the presence of an appropriate chromophoric substrate, viruses containing the insertional knockout produce blue-colored plaques and can therefore be distinguished from unmodified viruses, which form clear plaques, growing on the same plate.[139] This latter example is still a screen, because both wild-type and mutant viruses grow under the conditions used; however, the screen is simplified because mutant viruses can be readily identified by their color, obviating the need to pick and test individual plaques. Selections have considerable advantages over screens but are not always possible.

Essential and Nonessential

The terms *essential* and *nonessential* describe phenotypes, specifically whether a given gene is required for growth under a specific condition. Most viruses are finely tuned through selection to fit a specific niche. Not all viral genes are absolutely required for virus replication in that niche; some may simply confer a subtle selective advantage. Furthermore, if the niche is changed—such as from a natural animal host to a cell line in a laboratory—some genes that may have been essential for productive infection in the animal may not be required for replication in cell culture. Genes that are required for growth under a specific condition are termed *essential,* and those that are not required are termed *nonessential.* Because as a phenotype essentiality may be a function of the specific test conditions, the test conditions need to be specified in describing the mutation. As an example, the herpesvirus thymidine kinase gene is nonessential for virus replication in cell culture. Genes that are either essential or nonessential under a given condition present unique characteristics for analysis. Thus, mutants in nonessential genes may be easy to isolate because the gene can be deleted, although the function of the gene may be difficult to determine because, by definition, nonessential genes have no phenotype. Conversely, genes that are essential can be used to study gene function by characterizing the precise replication defect caused by a mutation in the gene; however, acquiring the appropriate mutant is confounded by the necessity for identifying a condition that will permit growth of the virus for study.

Mutation

Spontaneous Mutation

Spontaneous mutation rates in viruses are measured by fluctuation analysis,[60] a technique pioneered by Luria and Delbruck[77] for analysis of mutation in bacteria, and later adapted to viruses by Luria.[75] Fluctuation analysis consists of measuring the proportion of spontaneous mutants with a particular phenotype in many replicate cultures of virus and applying the Poisson distribution to these data to calculate a mutation rate. Importantly, because spontaneous mutations occur at random and may occur only rarely, the raw data in a fluctuation analysis displays enormous scatter, with some cultures containing a high proportion of mutants and some containing no mutants. Thus, from a practical perspective, although the proportion of mutants in a single culture of virus may reflect the mutation rate, it does not necessarily provide an accurate measure of mutation rate.

Both DNA and RNA viruses undergo spontaneous mutation; however, the spontaneous mutation rate in RNA viruses is usually much higher than in DNA viruses. In general, the mutation rate at a specific site in different DNA viruses ranges from 10^{-8} to 10^{-11} per replication, whereas in RNA viruses it is at least hundred-fold higher, between 10^{-3} and 10^{-6} per replication. The difference in mutation rate observed between RNA and DNA viruses is thought to result primarily from differences in the replication enzymes. Specifically, the DNA-dependent DNA polymerases used by DNA viruses contain a proofreading function, whereas the reverse transcriptases used by retroviruses and RNA-dependent RNA polymerases used by RNA viruses lack a proofreading function. The difference in spontaneous mutation rate has profound consequences for both the biology of the viruses and for laboratory genetic analysis of viruses. Specifically, RNA viruses exist in nature as *quasispecies*[25]—that is, populations of virus variants in relative equilibrium with the environment but capable of swift adaptation owing to a high spontaneous mutation rate (Chapter 11). Conversely, DNA viruses are genetically more stable but less adaptable. In the laboratory, the high mutation rate in RNA viruses presents difficulties in routine genetic analysis because mutants easily revert to wild-type virus that can outgrow the mutant virus.

It is noteworthy that whereas the actual mutation rate at a single locus is probably relatively constant for a given virus, the apparent mutation rate to a given phenotype depends on the nature of the mutation(s), which can give rise to that phenotype. For example, spontaneous mutation to bromodeoxyuridine (BrdU) resistance in vaccinia virus may occur at least 10 to 100 times more frequently than spontaneous reversions of temperature-sensitive mutations to a wild-type, temperature-insensitive phenotype. In the case of BrdU resistance, any mutation that inactivates the thymidine kinase causes resistance to BrdU, and thus there are literally hundreds of different ways in which spontaneous mutation can give rise to BrdU resistance. By contrast, a temperature-sensitive mutation is usually a single-base missense mutation, in which may exist only one possible mutational event that could cause reversion to the wild-type phenotype; thus, the apparent spontaneous mutation rate for the revertant phenotype is lower than the apparent spontaneous mutation rate to the BrdU-resistant phenotype. From a practical perspective, the apparent spontaneous mutation rate for specific selectable phenotypes may be sufficiently high such that induction of mutants is unnecessary for their isolation. Note, for example, that the wild-type vaccinia virus culture titered in Figure 2.6 contains numerous spontaneous isatin-β-thiosemicarbazone (IBT)-resistant viruses that could easily be plaque purified from assays done in the presence of IBT. However, for most mutants (e.g., temperature-sensitive mutants), where the desired mutational events are rare and a screen must be used rather than a selection, induced mutation is required for efficient isolation of mutants.

Induced Mutation

Under most circumstances, the incidence of spontaneous mutations is low enough so that induction of mutation is a practical prerequisite for isolation of virus mutants. It is usually desirable to induce limited, normally single-base changes, and for this purpose, chemical mutagens are most appropriate. Commonly used chemical mutagens are of two types: *in vitro* mutagens and *in vivo* mutagens.[26] *In vitro mutagens* work by chemically altering nucleic acid and can be applied by treating virions in the absence of replication. Examples of *in vitro* mutagens include hydroxylamine, nitrous acid, and alkylating agents, which through chemical modification of specific bases cause mispairing leading to missense mutations. *In vivo* chemical mutagens comprise compounds such as nucleoside analogs that must be incorporated during viral replication and thus must be applied to an infected cell. One of the most effective mutagens is the alkylating agent nitrosoguanidine, which although is capable of alkylating nucleic acid *in vitro* is most effective when used *in vivo,* where it works by alkylating guanine residues at the replication fork, ultimately causing mispairing.

The effectiveness of a mutagenesis is often assayed by observing the killing effect of the mutagen on the virus, the assumption being that many mutational events will be lethal and thus an effective mutagenesis will decrease a virus titer relative to an untreated control. However, killing does not always correlate precisely with mutagenesis, especially with an *in vitro* mutagen that can damage virion structure without necessarily causing mutation. An alternative method for assessing mutagenesis is to monitor an increase in the mutation frequency to a selectable phenotype where possible. For example, in vaccinia virus, mutagenesis causes a dose-dependent increase in resistance to phosphonoacetic acid, a drug that prevents poxvirus replication by inhibiting the viral DNA polymerase.[12] In summary, the use of mutagens can increase the mutation frequency several hundred–fold, such that desired mutants may comprise as much as 0.5% of the total virus population.

Double Mutants and Siblings

The existence of *double mutants* and *siblings* can theoretically complicate genetic analysis of a virus. A double (or multiple) mutant is defined as a virus that contains more than one mutation contributing to a phenotype. Theoretically, because the probability that a double mutant will be created increases as the dose of a mutagen is increased, there is a practical limit to the amount of induced mutation that is desirable. Double mutants are usually revealed as mutants that are noncomplementing with more than one mutant or are impossible to map by recombination or physical methods. Siblings result from replication of mutant virus either through amplification of a mutagenized stock or during an *in vivo* mutagenesis. The only completely reliable method to avoid isolation of sibling mutants is to isolate each mutant from an independently plaque-purified stock of wild-type virus.

Mutant Genotypes

There exist two basic categories of mutation: base substitution and deletion/insertion mutations. Both mutation types can occur with consequence in either a protein coding sequence or in a control sequence, such as a transcriptional promoter, a replication origin, or a packaging sequence. *Base substitution* mutations consist of the precise replacement of one nucleotide with a different nucleotide in a nucleic acid sequence. In coding sequences, base substitution mutations can be silent, causing no change in amino acid sequence of a protein; they can be missense, causing replacement of the wild-type amino acid with a different residue; or they can be nonsense, causing premature translation termination during protein synthesis. *Deletion and insertion* mutations comprise deletion or insertion of one or more nucleotides in a nucleic acid sequence. In a coding sequence, deletion or insertion of multiples of three nucleotides can result in precise deletion or insertion of one or more amino acids in a protein sequence. In a coding sequence, deletions or insertions that do not involve multiples of three nucleotides result in a shift in the translational reading frame, which almost invariably results in premature termination at some distance downstream of the mutation. In general, nonsense mutations, frameshift mutations, or large in-frame insertions or deletions are expected to inactivate a gene, whereas missense mutations may cause inactivation or much more subtle phenotypes such as drug resistance or temperature sensitivity.

Mutant Phenotypes

In the context of experimental virology where the goal is to understand the function of individual virus genes, the most useful mutants are those that inhibit virus replication by inactivating a virus gene. The nonproductive infections with these lethal mutants can be studied in detail to determine the precise aspect of virus replication that has been affected, thus providing information about the normal function of the affected gene. However, one must be able to grow the mutant to conduct experiments. Thus, a condition must be found where the mutation in question is not lethal—hence, the general class of mutant phenotypes, *conditional lethal.* Conditional lethal mutants comprise by far the largest and most useful class of mutant phenotypes, consisting of host-range, nonsense, temperature-sensitive, and drug-dependent phenotypes, described individually in the next section. Two additional classes of mutant phenotypes—resistance and plaque morphology—have very specific application to genetic analysis of viruses and are also described.

Host Range

A host-range virus mutant is broadly defined as a mutant that grows on one cell type and not on another, in contrast to wild-type virus, which grows on both cell types. Two general subcategories of host-range mutants exist: natural and engineered. *Natural* host-range virus mutants are relatively rare, primarily because they must be identified by brute force screen or serendipity, in many cases in the absence of a viable rationale for the targeted host range. The existence of a host-range phenotype implies that a specific virus–host interaction is compromised, which also implies that for any specific host-range phenotype, only one or a limited number of virus genes will be targeted. A classic example of a natural host-range mutant would be the host range-transformation (hr-t) mutants of mouse polyoma virus, which affect both small and middle T antigens and grow on primary mouse cells but not continuous mouse 3T3 cell lines.[3] *Engineered* host-range mutants are constructed by deleting an essential gene of interest in the virus while at the same time creating a cell line that expresses the gene. The engineered cell line provides a permissive host for growth of the mutant virus because it complements the missing virus function, whereas the normal host lacking the gene of interest provides a nonpermissive host for study of the phenotype of the virus. This technology has been useful for study of a variety of viruses, notably adenovirus and herpes simplex virus, where it has facilitated study of several essential virus genes.[21,61]

Nonsense Mutants

Nonsense mutants contain a premature translation termination mutation in the coding region of the mutant gene. They are formally a specific class of conditionally lethal, host-range mutants. Specifically, the permissive host is one that expresses a transfer RNA (tRNA) containing an anticodon mutation that results in insertion of an amino acid in response to a nonsense codon, thus restoring synthesis of a full-length polypeptide and suppressing the effects of the virus nonsense mutation. The nonpermissive host is a normal cell in which a truncated, nonfunctional polypeptide is made. In practice, most nonsense mutants in existence have been isolated by random mutagenesis followed by a brute force screen for host range. Nonsense mutants have three distinct advantages for the conduct of virus genetics: (a) mutants can be isolated in virtually any essential virus gene using one set of permissive and nonpermissive hosts and one set of techniques; (b) the mutations result in synthesis of a truncated polypeptide, thereby facilitating identification of the affected gene; and (c) virus mutants can be engineered relatively easily because the exact sequence of the desired mutation is predictable. Nonsense mutants have provided the single most powerful genetic tool in the study of bacteriophage, where efficient, viable nonsense suppressing bacteria are readily available. Unfortunately, attempts to isolate nonsense-suppressing mammalian cells have met with only limited success, probably because the nonsense-suppressing tRNAs are lethal in the eukaryotic host.[110]

Temperature Sensitivity

Temperature sensitivity is a type of conditional lethality in which mutants can grow at a low temperature but not a high temperature, in contrast to wild-type virus, which grows at both temperatures (see Fig. 2.6). Genotypically, temperature-sensitive mutations result usually from relatively subtle single amino acid substitutions that render the target protein unstable and hence nonfunctional at an elevated or nonpermissive temperature while leaving the protein stable and functional at a low, permissive temperature. In practice, temperature-sensitive mutants are usually isolated by random mutagenesis followed by brute force screening for growth at two temperatures. Screening can be streamlined by a plaque enlargement technique in which mutagenized virus is first plated at a permissive temperature, then stained and shifted to a nonpermissive temperature after marking the size of plaques, to screen for plaques that do not increase in size at the nonpermissive temperature.[112] Replica plating techniques that permit relatively straightforward screening of thousands of mutant candidates in yeast and bacteria have not been successfully adapted to virology; thus, a screen for temperature sensitivity, even when streamlined with plaque enlargement, ultimately depends on the laborious but reliable process of picking and testing individual plaques. Temperature-sensitive mutants have the profound advantage of theoretically accessing any essential virus gene using a single set of protocols. Temperature-sensitive mutants have proved enormously useful in all branches of virology but have been particularly useful for the study of animal viruses, where nonsense suppression has not been a viable option. Cold-sensitive mutants (i.e., mutants that grow at a high but not a low temperature) comprise a relatively rare but nevertheless useful alternate type of temperature-sensitive mutants.

Temperature-sensitive mutants can actually be divided into two subclasses: thermolabile and temperature sensitive for synthesis (tss) mutants.[140] *Thermolabile mutants* are those in which the gene product can be inactivated following synthesis by a shift from the permissive to the nonpermissive temperature. *Tss* mutants display gene dysfunction only if the infection is held at the nonpermissive temperature during synthesis of the mutant gene product; if the gene product is made at the permissive temperature, it cannot be inactivated by raising the temperature. Clearly, the two mutant types can be distinguished by performing appropriate temperature shift experiments. Thermolability obviously implies that a protein preformed at the permissive temperature is directly destabilized by raising the temperature. Tss mutations commonly involve multisubunit structures or complex organelles, where theoretically the quaternary structure of a complex formed correctly at the permissive temperature stabilizes the mutant protein, making the mutation resistant to temperature shift. If a tss mutant protein is synthesized at the nonpermissive temperature, it may be degraded before assembly or may not assemble properly because of misfolding. For most purposes, the thermolabile and tss mutant types are equally useful.

Drug Resistance and Dependence

Several antiviral compounds have now been identified, and virus mutants that are resistant to or depend on these compounds have found utility in genetic analysis of viruses. A few compounds have been identified that target similar enzymes in different viruses, including phosphonoacetic acid, which inhibits DNA polymerases[50,114] and BrdU, which targets thymidine kinases.[27,119] More often, however, antiviral drugs are highly specific for a gene product of one particular virus—for example, guanidine, which targets the polio 2C NTPase[98,99]; acyclovir, which targets the herpes simplex virus thymidine kinase and DNA polymerase[9,109]; amantadine, which targets the influenza virus M2 virion integral membrane ion channel protein[49]; or isatin-β-thiosemicarbazone, which is highly specific for poxviruses and targets at least two genes involved in viral transcription.[11,17,87] The most useful drugs are those that inhibit wild-type virus growth in a plaque assay without killing cells in a monolayer, such that resistant or dependent viruses can be selected by virtue of their ability to form plaques on a drug-treated monolayer. Examples of both drug resistance and drug dependence are shown in Figure 2.6.

Drug-resistant or drug-dependent virus mutants have two general uses in virus genetics. First, they can be useful in identifying the target or mechanism of action of an antiviral drug. For example, studies of influenza virus mutants resistant to amantadine were of importance in characterizing both the *M2* gene and the mechanism of action of amantadine.[100] Second, resistant or dependent mutants provide selectable markers for use in recombination mapping, for the assessment of specific genetic protocols, or for selection of recombinant viruses in reverse genetic protocols. For example, guanidine resistance has been used as a marker for use in three-factor crosses in recombination mapping of poliovirus temperature-sensitive mutants[16]; phosphonoacetic acid resistance and isatin-β-thiosemicarbazone dependence has been used in vaccinia virus to assess the efficiency of marker rescue protocols[31,47]; and acyclovir resistance and BrdU resistance, resulting from mutation of the herpesvirus or poxvirus thymidine kinase genes, has been used in both herpesviruses and in poxviruses to select for insertion of engineered genes into the viral genome.[10,80,94]

Plaque Morphology

Plaque morphology mutants are those in which the appearance of mutant plaques is readily distinguishable from wild-type plaques. Most commonly, the morphological distinction is plaque size (i.e., mutant plaques may be larger or smaller than wild-type plaques); however, other morphological distinctions are possible, such as formation of clear versus turbid bacteriophage plaques. Most plaque morphology mutants affect very specific virus functions, which in turn affect the virus–host relationship in a fashion that impacts on the appearance of a plaque. Notable examples from bacteriophage research include clear plaque mutants of bacteriophage lambda and rapid lysis mutants of the T-even bacteriophage. Wild-type lambda forms turbid plaques because some percentage of cells are lysogenized and thus survive the infection, leaving intact bacteria within a plaque. Clear mutants of lambda typically affect the lambda repressor such that lysogeny is prevented and all infected bacteria lyse, resulting in a clear plaque.[63] Wild-type T-even phages produce small plaques with a turbid halo because only a fraction of infected bacteria lyse during a normal infection, a phenomenon called *lysis inhibition.* Rapid lysis mutants, which affect a phage membrane protein, do not display lysis inhibition and as a result form large, clear plaques.[53] Examples from animal virus research include large plaque mutants of adenovirus and syncytial mutants of herpes simplex virus. The large plaque phenotype in adenovirus results from faster than normal release of virus from infected cells.[68] Syncytial mutants of herpesvirus express altered virus surface glycoproteins and result in fusion of infected cells, whereas wild-type virus causes cells to round and clump without significant fusion. Thus, syncytial mutants form large plaques readily distinguishable from the smaller dense foci caused by wild-type virus.[107] All of these specific plaque morphology mutants have value either in the study of the actual functions affected or as specific phenotypic markers for use in recombination studies, where they can be used in the same fashion as drug resistance markers, described previously.

In addition to the existence of specific plaque morphology loci in several viruses, it is noteworthy that any mutation that affects virus yield or growth rate may result in production of a smaller than wild-type plaque, which can be useful in genetic experiments. Thus, many temperature-sensitive mutants form smaller than wild-type plaques even at the permissive temperature because the mutant gene may not be fully functional even under permissive conditions, and this property is often useful in mutant isolation or for distinguishing wild-type from mutant virus in plaque assays involving several virus variants. Note, for example, in Figure 2.6 that the vaccinia virus temperature-sensitive mutant *ts*56 forms smaller than wild-type plaques at the permissive temperature of 31°C. Lastly, intragenic or extragenic suppressors of conditional lethal virus mutants may grow poorly relative to wild-type virus and form small plaques as a result, facilitating their isolation from a mixture containing true wild-type revertant viruses.[14]

Neutralization Escape

Neutralization escape mutants are a specific class of mutants selected as variant viruses that form plaques in the presence of neutralizing antibodies. Such mutants affect the structure or modification of viral surface proteins and have been of value in studies of virus structure, antigenic variation, and virus–cell interactions.[43,55]

Reversion

Reversion may be defined as mutation that results in a change from a mutant genotype to the original wild-type genotype. Accordingly, revertants in a stock of mutant virus are revealed as viruses that have acquired a wild-type phenotype. For example, Figure 2.6 shows that when the vaccinia virus temperature-sensitive mutant *ts*56 is plated at the nonpermissive temperature, plaques with wild-type morphology, probably revertants, are detectable at low dilutions of virus. Spontaneous reversion of missense mutations probably results from misincorporation during replication, because the reversion frequency of different viruses often reflects the error rate of the replication enzyme. Spontaneous reversion of significant deletion mutations occurs rarely, if at all, because reversion would require replacement of missing nucleotides with the correct sequence. Reversion impacts on viral genetics in two ways. First, in any genetic experiment involving mixed infections with two genetically different viruses, wild-type viruses can arise either through reversion or recombination; in most cases, it is important to be able to distinguish between these two processes. This is discussed in more detail in the later sections describing complementation and recombination. Second, as described earlier in the description of spontaneous mutation, if the spontaneous reversion rate is extremely high, revertants can easily come to dominate a mutant virus stock, thus obscuring the mutant phenotype and causing serious difficulties in both genetic and biochemical analysis of mutants.

Leakiness

Not all conditionally lethal mutants are completely defective in replication under nonpermissive conditions, and leakiness is a quantitative measure of the ability of a mutant virus to grow under nonpermissive conditions. Leakiness can be quantified with a one-step growth experiment. To quantify leakiness of a temperature-sensitive mutant, for example, cells are infected at a high moi with wild-type or mutant virus, infected cells are incubated at either permissive or nonpermissive temperatures, and maximum virus yields are then determined by plaque titration under permissive conditions so that the growth of mutant and wild-type virus can be quantitatively compared. Ideally, for wild-type virus, the ratio of the yield for infections done at the nonpermissive temperature relative to the permissive temperature should be one—that is, the virus should grow equally well at both temperatures. For mutant viruses, the ratio of the yield for infections done at the nonpermissive temperature relative to the permissive temperature may range from less than 10% to as much as 100%, even for mutants that are clearly defective in plaque formation under nonpermissive conditions. Mutants that are *tight*—or grow poorly under nonpermissive conditions—are desirable for phenotypic characterization relative to leaky mutants, because leaky mutants will logically display considerable wild-type phenotypic behavior. Special cases exist where extreme leakiness is an expected and desirable trait. Specifically, virus mutants that are wild-type for replication and production of infectious virions but defective in cell-to-cell spread have a phenotype characterized by defective plaque formation, which requires spread, but 100% leakiness, which does not require spread if assayed in a high moi one-step growth protocol.[5]

Genetic Analysis of Mutants

Complementation

Complementation analysis provides a general method for determining whether two different virus mutants affect the same or different genes. The quantitative test to determine complementation is a two-step procedure in which co-infections are first done to induce an interaction between two mutants, and the results of those infections are quantitatively assessed by plaque titration. The test compares the ability of two mutants to grow in mixed relative to single infections done under nonpermissive conditions. Specifically, cells are first infected with two different virus mutants at high moi so that all cells are co-infected with both mutants, and infected cells are incubated under nonpermissive conditions where neither mutant alone can replicate, for an interval sufficient to achieve maximum virus yield. Single high moi infections under nonpermissive conditions are performed as controls. Virus is then harvested, yields are quantified by plaque titration under both permissive and nonpermissive conditions, and a complementation index (CI) is calculated according to the following formula:

$$\frac{\text{yield}(A+B)_p - \text{yield}(A+B)_{np}}{\text{yield}(A)_p + \text{yield}(B)_p} = \text{CI},$$

where A and B represent individual virus mutants, and the subscripts p and np represent the conditions, either permissive or nonpermissive, under which the virus yields were plaque titrated. Because both mutant and wild-type viruses will be counted in plaque titrations done at the permissive temperature, the first term in the numerator, $\text{yield}(A + B)_p$, measures the yield of all viruses, both mutant and wild-type, from the initial high moi mixed infections done under nonpermissive conditions. The second term in the numerator, $\text{yield}(A + B)_{np}$, measures the yield of wild-type viruses, mostly recombinants, from the high moi mixed infections done under nonpermissive conditions, because only wild-type viruses will be counted in plaque titrations done at the nonpermissive temperature. Subtraction of the wild-type viruses from the total viruses leaves a count of only the mutant viruses in the numerator. The denominator measures the ability of each of the mutants to grow in single high moi infections done initially under nonpermissive conditions. If the two mutants, A and B, are in different virus genes, then in the mixed infection done under nonpermissive conditions, mutant A can contribute wild-type B gene product and mutant B can contribute wild-type A gene product. Thus, the mutants can help or complement each other, resulting in a high yield of mutant virus in the mixed infection compared to the single infections, and a CI significantly greater than one. If the two mutants, A and B, affect the same gene, then the wild-type gene product will be lacking in the mixed infection. In this case, the yield from the mixed infection will be equivalent to the yield from the single infections, and the CI should not exceed one. In practice, owing to error in plaque assays and from other sources, mixed infections with mutants in the same viral gene will often yield CIs of slightly greater than one, and the practical cutoff must be determined empirically for a given viral system. An example of complementation analysis is provided in the eBook.

Qualitative complementation tests have also been devised for use with both bacterial and mammalian viruses.[8,12,71,118] These qualitative tests are much easier to perform than quantitative tests and in practice are just as reliable. In general, the tests are designed such that bacterial lawns or eukaryotic cell monolayers are infected either singly or with two viruses under nonpermissive conditions and at relatively low moi. The moi must be high enough so that numerous cells are doubly infected in the mixed infection, although low enough so that most cells are uninfected and a lawn or monolayer is maintained. Complementing mutant pairs produce plaques or cleared areas under nonpermissive conditions, whereas noncomplementing mutant pairs do not. An example of a qualitative complementation test is shown in Figure 2.10. A theoretical disadvantage of the qualitative test is that it does not discriminate between complementation and recombination. In some cases, recombination between mutants in the same complementation group under nonpermissive conditions is sufficiently rare, thus the qualitative test is reliable.[13] If recombination does occur under nonpermissive conditions, false positives occur in the qualitative test and the number of complementation groups is overestimated.[65] Nevertheless, negative tests are still a reliable measure of noncomplementation.

Complementation analysis has been of tremendous benefit in sorting mutants in most, but not all, viral systems. A notable exception is poliovirus, where complementation between temperature-sensitive mutants *in vivo* is not observed. The lack of complementation in picorna viruses may be related to the unique mechanism of viral gene expression, in which all protein products are produced from a polyprotein precursor by proteolytic cleavage. If individual temperature-sensitive mutants affect structure, synthesis, or cleavage of the polyprotein precursor, they may behave as if they all belong to a single complementation group, even though they may map to different protein end products.

As a concept, complementation impacts broadly on virology and is not limited simply to the grouping of conditionally lethal mutants into genes. For example, the growth of engineered host-range deletion mutants in essential virus genes, discussed previously, relies on complementation of the missing viral function by an engineered cell line that expresses the wild-type viral gene product. In addition, the accumulation of defective virus genomes at high multiplicity passage, also discussed earlier, results from a complementing helper function provided by wild-type virus.

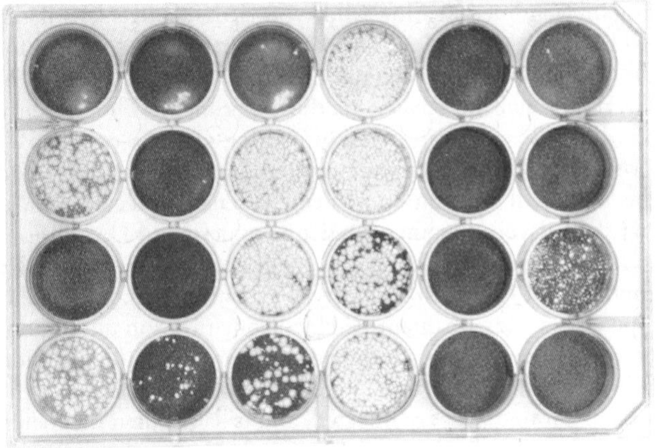

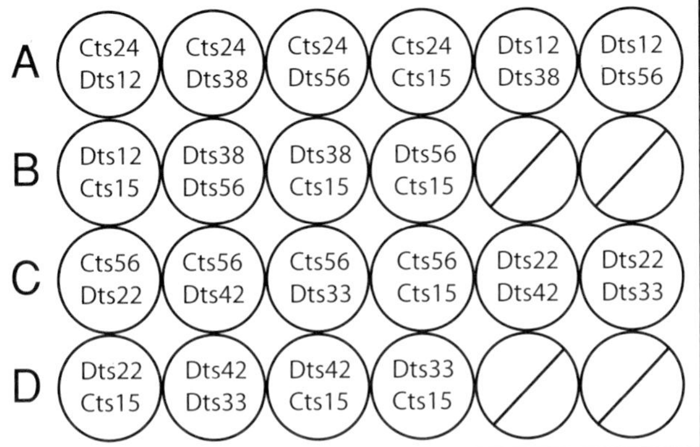

FIGURE 2.10. Qualitative complementation test. This test was done to confirm the composition of two different complementation groups in vaccinia virus, one in gene *D5* (*rows A* and *B*) and one in gene *G2* (*rows C* and *D*). Candidate mutants in gene *D5* are C*ts*24, D*ts*12, D*ts*38, and D*ts*56. Candidates in gene *G2* are C*ts*56, D*ts*22, and D*ts*42. C*ts*15 and D*ts*33 were known to map to different genes and were used as positive controls for complementation. Monolayers of the African green monkey kidney cell line BSC40 grown in a 24-well dish were infected at very low moi (~0.03 pfu/cell) with individual mutants or mutant pairs. The dish was incubated at a nonpermissive temperature (40°C) for 3 days and stained with crystal violet. The stained dish is shown at the **top**, and a key to the infections is shown at the **bottom**. Mixed infections in *rows A* and *B* represent all possible pairwise combinations of gene *D5* temperature-sensitive mutants along with the C*ts*15 positive control, and mixed infections in *rows C* and *D* represent all possible pairwise combinations of gene *G2* temperature-sensitive mutants along with C*ts*15 and D*ts*33 positive controls. The absence of plaques confirms that mutants reside in the same complementation group. Control single infections produced no plaques (not shown). (Reprinted from Lackner CA, D'Costa SM, Buck C, et al. Complementation analysis of the dales collection of vaccinia virus temperature-sensitive mutants. *Virology* 2003;305:240–259, © 2003, with permission from Elsevier.)

Recombination and Reassortment

Recombination describes a process by which nucleic acid sequences from two genotypically different parental viruses are exchanged so that the progeny contain sequences derived from both parents. In viral systems, there exist three distinct mechanisms of recombination, dictated by the structures of the viral genomes. For DNA viruses, recombination occurs by the physical breakage and rejoining of parental DNA molecules through regions of sequence homology, in a fashion similar or identical to the same process in bacteria or higher organisms. For RNA viruses containing segmented genomes, gene exchange occurs primarily through reassortment of individual parental genome segments into progeny viruses, although intragenic recombination has been reported for orthomyxoviruses, reoviruses, and bunyaviruses.[97,101,103,115,120] For most nonsegmented RNA viruses, recombination appears to be a much less frequent event compared with DNA viruses. Recombination has been observed in several ssRNA virus families representing both positive and negative sense genomes; picornaviruses, coronaviruses, togaviruses, and retroviruses display relatively efficient recombination.[2,45,56,66,67,73,74,136] Recombination in RNA viruses is thought to occur during replication via *copy choice,* namely switching templates during replication such that the newly synthesized genome contains sequence from two different parental molecules.[16] Historically, recombination has been used to construct genetic maps of virus mutants and to construct novel virus genotypes. Although recombination mapping has been largely replaced by physical mapping techniques such as marker rescue, a technical knowledge of recombination mapping can contribute to an appreciation of the complexity of genetic interactions between viruses.

The methods used to determine recombination frequencies are the same regardless of genome structure or mechanism of recombination. As with complementation, the quantitative test to determine recombination frequency between two mutants, called a *two-factor cross,* is a two-step procedure, but in this case co-infections are first done under conditions permissive for replication, then the fraction of recombinants relative to the total virus yield is quantitatively assessed by plaque titration. Specifically, cells are first infected with two different virus mutants at high moi so that all cells are co-infected with both mutants, and infected cells are incubated under permissive conditions so that both mutants have maximum opportunity for interaction, for an interval sufficient to achieve maximum virus yield. Single high moi infections under permissive conditions are performed as controls. Virus is then harvested, yields are quantified by plaque titration under both permissive and nonpermissive conditions, and a recombination frequency (RF) is calculated according to the following formula:

$$\frac{\text{yield}(A+B)_{np} - \text{yield}(A)_{np} - \text{yield}(B)_{np}}{\text{yield}(A+B)_{p}} \times 2 \times 100\% = \text{RF},$$

where A and B represent individual virus mutants, and the subscripts p and np represent the conditions, permissive or nonpermissive, under which the virus yields were plaque titrated. The first term in the numerator, $\text{yield}(A + B)_{np}$, quantifies wild-type virus emerging from the mixed infection, including both recombinants and revertants, because only wild-type virus will grow in the plaque assay done under nonpermissive conditions. The second and third terms in the numerator, $\text{yield}(A)_{np}$ and $\text{yield}(B)_{np}$, quantify wild-type virus emerging from the control single infections, providing a measure of reversion in each of the two mutants. Subtraction of the revertants from the total yield of wild-type virus leaves a measure of recombinants only in the numerator. The denominator, yield$(A + B)_p$, quantifies the total virus yield from the mixed infection including both wild-type and mutant virus, because all input virus types will grow in the plaque assay done under permissive conditions. The quotient is multiplied by a factor of two to account for unscored progeny representing the reciprocal of the wild-type recombinants, namely double mutants, and converted to a percent.

Recombination mapping in DNA viruses relies on the assumption that the frequency of recombination between two genetic markers is proportional to the distance between the two markers. For several DNA viruses, observed recombination frequencies comprise a continuous range from less than 1% up to a theoretical maximum of 50%, allowing for construction of linear genetic maps.[38]

In viruses with segmented genomes, recombination between markers on the same segment is rare but reassortment of segments is extremely efficient; thus, recombination is effectively an all or none phenomenon, with markers on the same segment displaying no recombination, and markers on different segments displaying very high levels of recombination.[102] For these reasons, genetic exchange in segmented RNA viruses is commonly referred to as reassortment rather than recombination. Reassortment analysis for segmented viruses is useful for determining whether or not two mutants map to the same genome segment but cannot be used to determine the order of markers on a given segment. Mutants can be mapped to individual RNA segments by performing *intertypic* crosses between virus types that differ in the electrophoretic mobility of each RNA segment. Specifically, if crosses are performed between a wild-type virus of one type and a mutant virus of another type and numerous wild-type progeny analyzed, one segment bearing the wild-type allele will be conserved among all the progeny, whereas all other segments will display reassortment.[102]

Marker Rescue

Marker rescue is a physical mapping technique that measures directly whether a given virus mutation maps within a specific subfragment of a virus genome. The use of marker rescue is confined to DNA viruses where homologous recombination takes place and has been of enormous value in these systems. The application of the technique varies somewhat depending on the virus system under study; however, the general principles are the same. Specifically, full-length mutant viral genomic DNA plus a wild-type DNA genomic subfragment, either a cloned DNA molecule or a PCR product, are introduced into cells under conditions permissive for recombination and for wild-type virus replication. For viruses that contain infectious DNA, such as herpesviruses,[117] adenoviruses,[42] and polyomaviruses,[72,89] the mutant genomic DNA and the wild-type genomic subfragment may be co-transfected into cells. For viruses containing noninfectious genomic DNA, such as poxviruses,[122] the mutant DNA must be introduced into cells by infection with the mutant virus, which is then followed by transfection with the wild-type DNA subfragment. In either case, the protocol allows for homologous recombination between the mutant genome and the wild-type DNA subfragment. If the wild-type DNA subfragment contains the wild-type allele for the mutation, the recombination can exchange the wild-type for the mutant sequence in the mutant genome, creating wild-type virus. Conversely, if the wild-type fragment does not contain the wild-type allele for the mutation, no wild-type virus, above a background of revertants, will be created in the experiment. The presence of wild-type virus can be assayed using either a two-step or a one-step protocol. In the two-step protocol, depending on the nature of the mutation being rescued, infected and/or transfected cells are incubated under permissive conditions to facilitate recombination and replication, or nonpermissive conditions to select for wild-type recombinants, then wild-type virus yields are quantified by plaque titration under nonpermissive conditions. In the one-step protocol, the infection and/or transfection is done so that only a small fraction of the cells in a monolayer are infected, and cells are then incubated under nonpermissive conditions such that wild-type virus formed during a successful rescue will form plaques on the monolayer.[122] In short, regardless of the precise method used, conversion or *rescue* of mutant virus to wild-type with a given wild-type DNA fragment means that the mutation maps within that fragment. Initial marker rescue mapping experiments may be facilitated by the use of a few large but overlapping wild-type DNA fragments, and fine mapping may be accomplished with fragments as small as a few hundred nucleotides. Marker rescue mapping has completely replaced recombination mapping as a method for mapping mutations in DNA viruses, and precise genetic maps of several DNA viruses have now been constructed.

Reverse Genetics

Prior to the advent of recombinant DNA and DNA sequencing technologies, classical genetic analysis, namely random isolation and characterization of virus mutants, was one of the few effective methods for identifying, mapping, and characterizing virus genes, and the only method for obtaining virus mutants. With the current ready availability of genomic sequences for virtually all prototypical members of each virus family and a versatile package of genetic engineering tools, the experimental landscape has changed completely. One can now conduct a genetic analysis with a reasonably complete foreknowledge of the genetic structure of the virus, focus attention on individual genes of interest, and deliberately engineer mutations in genes to study their function. Termed *reverse genetics,* this process has come to dominate the genetic analysis of viruses. Reverse genetics covers a broad range of activities ranging from engineering a single nucleotide substitution in a target gene to engineering chimeric viruses to be used as gene therapy vectors, oncolytic vectors, or vaccines. Currently, virtually every significant human viral pathogen can be engineered using reverse genetic approaches. Perhaps one of the most impressive feats in reverse genetics is the resurrection of the deadly 1918 pandemic strain of influenza using genome sequences derived from archived formalin-fixed lung autopsy materials and from frozen, unfixed lung tissues from an Alaskan influenza victim who was buried in permafrost.[125]

Reverse genetic analysis involves two distinct considerations: strategies for design of a given mutation and strategies for incorporation of mutations into virus. The principles governing these strategies highly depend on the structure of a given viral genome and the strategy of virus replication, and thus vary in the extreme. However, some general principles can be identified, which are discussed next, accompanied by a few specific examples to illustrate the general principles.

Incorporation of Mutations into Virus

The methods used for incorporation of mutations into a virus depend on several features of the individual virus under consideration, including genome size, whether or not the nucleic acid is infectious, whether the genome is composed of DNA or RNA or replicated via reverse transcription, and whether replication is nuclear or cytoplasmic.

DNA Viruses and Reverse Transcribing Viruses

With the exception of poxviruses, which because of their cytoplasmic site of replication must carry virion-encapsidated transcription enzymes into cells during infection, virtually all DNA virus genomes (see Table 2.1) are infectious. Likewise, double-stranded DNA (dsDNA) comprising the genomic sequences of reverse transcribing viruses that package RNA (retroviruses) or DNA (hepadnaviruses) genomes are also infectious. Thus, in these cases, the incorporation of a mutation into the virus genome is essentially an exercise in molecular cloning, and pure mutant virus is produced by transfection of the cloned mutant genome into cultured cells. In practice, the herpesvirus genome is sufficiently large such that manipulation as a full-length genomic clone presents some difficulties, and therefore incorporation of mutations into the viral genome is often done by co-transfecting cells with full-length genomic viral DNA along with a DNA fragment containing the desired mutant allele flanked by wild-type DNA sequences. Replication is launched from the transfected infectious wild-type genomic DNA, and homologous recombination between the co-transfected mutant DNA fragment and the wild-type genome incorporates the mutant allele into a fraction of the replicating wild-type genomes[139] (Fig. 2.11). A similar protocol is applied to engineering poxviruses; however, because poxvirus DNA is noninfectious, virus replication must be initiated by infection with intact virus. In its simplest form, this protocol entails infection with virus bearing the wild-type target genome followed by transfection with a DNA fragment containing the desired mutation flanked by wild-type DNA sequences[95] (Fig. 2.12; identical to the protocol for marker rescue described earlier). Similar to the herpesvirus co-transfection protocol just described, homologous recombination catalyzed by viral enzymes results in incorporation of the mutant allele into a fraction of the wild-type infecting genomes. An alternate protocol for constructing poxvirus recombinants involves first infecting cells with a replication defective, nonhomologous helper poxvirus, followed by transfection with either a cloned full-length mutant genome or a mixture of fragments comprising the desired engineered genome.[23,105,137] The helper virus provides

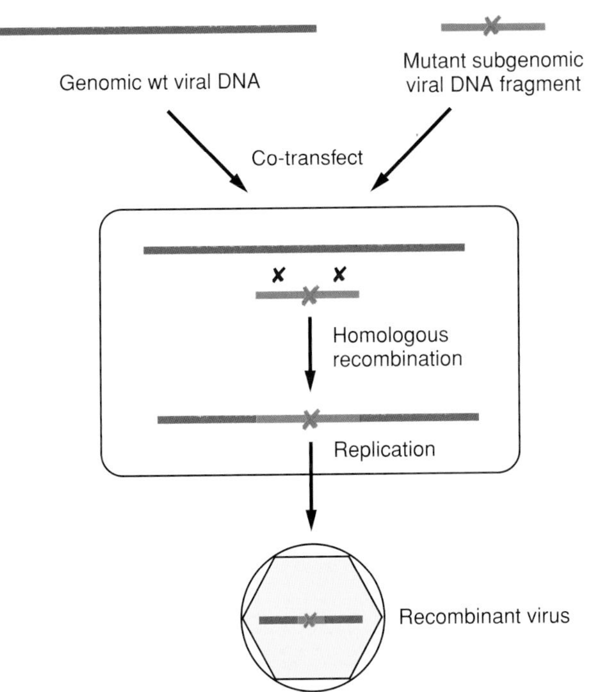

FIGURE 2.11. Reverse genetics with large double-stranded DNA viruses containing infectious genomes. Wild-type full-length infectious genomic viral DNA (*blue line*) is co-transfected into cells along with a subgenomic viral DNA fragment (*green line*) containing the desired mutation (*red X*). Homologous recombination between the co-transfected viral DNAs takes place within the cell catalyzed by viral and/or cellular enzymes. The recombinant genome is replicated and packaged to yield recombinant virus (mixed with wild-type virus replicated from unrecombined genomes).

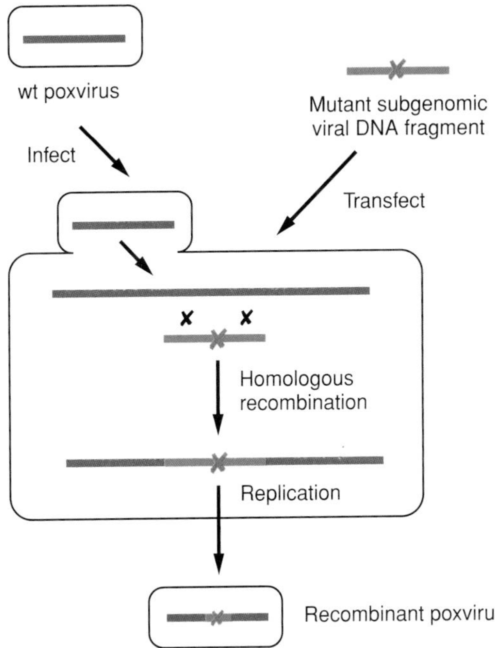

FIGURE 2.12. Reverse genetics with large double-stranded DNA viruses containing noninfectious genomes (poxviruses). Cells are infected with virus containing a wild-type DNA genome (*blue line*) and transfected with a subgenomic viral DNA fragment (*green line*) containing the desired mutation (*red X*). Homologous recombination between the infecting viral DNA and co-transfected fragment takes place within the cell catalyzed by viral enzymes. The recombinant genome is replicated and packaged to yield recombinant virus (mixed with wild-type virus replicated from unrecombined genomes).

enzymes critical for launching replication of the transfected full-length mutant viral DNA genome, or for homologous recombination among transfected subgenomic fragments to assemble and launch replication of the desired virus.

When mutants are engineered in cloned, infectious genomes, only the mutant allele of the target gene is present in the construction, all virus recovered from the transfection will be mutant, and no selection or screen for mutants is required. However, in situations where *in vivo* homologous recombination has been used to incorporate the cloned mutation into a wild-type genome, such as in poxviruses or herpesviruses, both mutant and wild-type viruses emerge from the mutant construction protocol, and thus a screen or selection is required to identify the mutant of interest. For mutations in nonessential genes, this may be a relatively straightforward matter of inserting into the target gene a color marker such as β-galactosidase[139] or green fluorescent protein[19] to facilitate a screen, or inserting a dominant selectable marker such as *Escherichia coli* guanine phosphoribosyltransferase,[30] to facilitate a selection. For conditionally lethal phenotypes such as temperature sensitivity, although techniques exist that enrich for recombinant viruses, mutant isolation ultimately relies on a screen of individual mutants for differential growth under permissive and nonpermissive conditions .[47] The use of full-length clones of herpesvirus and vaccinia virus obviates the need for *in vivo* recombination, and thus only mutant virus will be recovered after transfection or reactivation of an engineered, mutant genome, and no mutant screen or selection is necessary.[24,88]

RNA Viruses

The genomes of positive sense, ssRNA viruses (see Table 2.1) are infectious; therefore, as with most DNA viruses, the engineering of mutant viruses is largely an exercise in molecular cloning, yet formidable for large RNA viruses such as coronaviruses.[138] To recover infectious virus, complementary DNA (cDNA) clones of mutant genomes may be transfected directly into cultured cells or transcribed *in vitro* into positive sense RNA that is then transfected into cells. Virus replication is launched by translation of the transfected RNA *in vivo,* resulting in recovery of only mutant virus. A good example of the application of this technology is the directed construction of temperature-sensitive mutants in poliovirus.[22]

Negative sense ssRNA viruses must package in the virion a virus-coded RNA-dependent RNA polymerase so that the genome, in the form of a nucleocapsid, can be transcribed into mRNA immediately following infection. Thus, negative sense ssRNA virus genomes are not infectious, and engineering these viruses becomes more of a challenge. Generally, the strategy consists of transfection of cells with multiple plasmids, some of which are transcribed into genome-length RNAs (encoding the desired genotype) and some of which direct expression of proteins required for genome replication, specifically a nucleocapsid protein and proteins comprising the viral RNA-dependent RNA polymerase. The expressed nucleocapsid protein encapsidates the transcribed genomic RNA, and this nucleocapsid can then be transcribed into mRNA by the expressed viral RNA polymerase, thus launching the infection and ultimately yielding pure virus of the desired genotype. Historically, the requirements for "rescue" of virus from cloned fragments are different for the segmented negative sense ssRNA orthomyxoviruses compared to most nonsegmented negative sense ssRNA viruses, namely rhabdoviruses, paramyxoviruses, and filoviruses, comprising most of the order *Mononegavirales.* The differences are attributable, at least in part, to the fact that the orthomyxoviruses replicate in the nucleus, whereas most of the viruses in the order *Mononegavirales* replicate in the cytoplasm. Specifically, for the orthomyxoviruses,[93] genome segments are cloned so that they are transcribed from a polymerase I promoter to yield the negative sense genomic RNA, and the replication proteins are cloned so that they are transcribed from a polymerase II promoter to yield mRNA. Both polymerases are expressed in the cell nucleus so that after transfection of the plasmids, the viral RNAs are synthesized in the appropriate cellular compartment. The number of plasmids required for rescue can be minimized by flanking each genome segment with a polymerase I promoter at the 3′end and a polymerase II promoter at the 5′end so that each plasmid yields both a negative sense genomic RNA and a positive sense mRNA (Fig. 2.13). For most *Mononegavirales* viruses,[15] rescue is best achieved if synthesis of both the genomic RNA and the replication proteins are driven by the bacteriophage T7 RNA polymerase, which localizes efficiently to the cell cytoplasm. The T7 RNA polymerase can be supplied either by infection with a poxvirus expressing T7 RNA polymerase, by using a cell line containing a stably integrated copy of the T7 RNA polymerase gene, or by transfection of an additional plasmid designed to express the enzyme. An additional (counterintuitive) requirement for rescue of *Mononegavirales* viruses is that the plasmid encoding the genomic RNA is configured so that it is initially transcribed to yield positive sense, antigenomic RNA, which is then encapsidated with expressed nucleocapsid protein, and replicated into encapsidated negative sense genomic RNA, which is in turn transcribed into mRNAs to launch the infection (Fig. 2.14). The use of a plasmid that expresses the negative sense genomic RNA compromises the rescue, presumably because the negative sense genomic RNA will hybridize in the cytoplasm with the positive sense mRNAs for replication proteins, thus repressing their expression. Despite these generalities, examples exist of rescue of cytoplasmic *Mononegavirales* viruses using polymerase I or polymerase II promoters.[83]

The segmented, double-stranded (dsRNA)-containing, cytoplasmic reoviruses can be rescued using a protocol similar to that used for *Mononegavirales.*[69] Specifically, cDNAs of individual segments are cloned downstream from a bacteriophage T7 promoter, each yielding an RNA product that doubles as mRNA and the positive strand template for genomic dsDNA. Transfection of these plasmids into cells expressing T7 RNA polymerase results in synthesis of genomic segments and replication proteins, ultimately yielding pure virus of the desired genotype. T7 RNA polymerase can be supplied by any of the previously mentioned methods: co-transfection of an expression plasmid, expression from a stably integrated chromosomal gene, or infection with a poxvirus expressing the enzyme. Interestingly, this protocol does not work for all reoviruses, most notably the important human pathogen rotavirus, which must still be engineered using more complex helper-mediated protocols.[124]

Mutation Design

Design of mutations for use in virology is problematic only if the gene in question is essential, necessitating isolation of

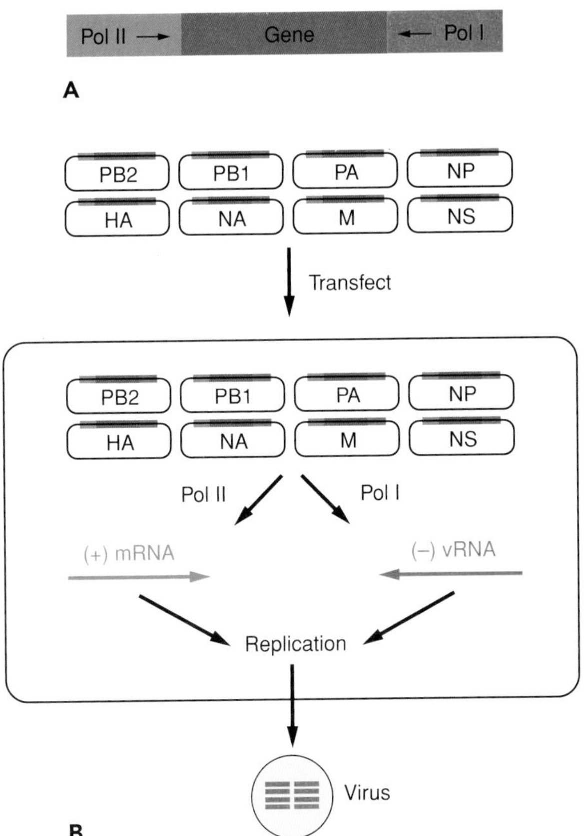

FIGURE 2.13. Reverse genetics with orthomyxoviruses (influenza). **A:** Detailed structure of cloned viral genes. Coding sequences for each viral gene (*blue*) are cloned flanked by an RNA polymerase II transcriptional promoter (*green*) at the upstream (5′) end and an RNA polymerase I transcriptional promoter (*red*) at the downstream (3″) end. **B:** Reverse genetic protocol. Cells are transfected with eight plasmids together representing the entire complement of virus genes. Transcription in the nucleus with polymerase II produces positive sense messenger RNAs (*green*) that are translated into viral proteins including the polymerase (PB1, PB2, PA) and nucleocapsid protein (NP). Transcription from the polymerase I promoter produces negative sense genomic viral RNAs (*red*), which are then replicated by the viral replication proteins. Further transcription, replication, and encapsidation produces virus.

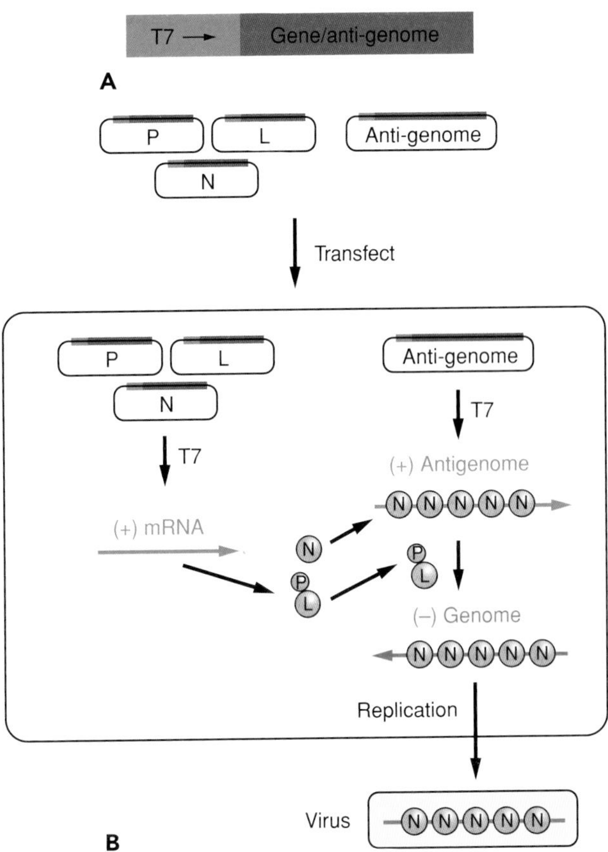

FIGURE 2.14. Reverse genetics with viruses in the order *Mononegavirales*. **A:** Detailed structure of cloned genes. Coding sequences for replication proteins or the full-length viral genome (*blue*) are cloned downstream from a bacteriophage T7 transcriptional promoter (*green*). **B:** Reverse genetic protocol. Cells are transfected with four plasmids, three of which encode replication proteins (P, L, and N) and one of which contains the full-length viral genome oriented such that transcription yields a positive sense antigenomic RNA. Transcription by T7 RNA polymerase (usually encoded by an engineered stably integrated copy in the cell nucleus) yields messenger RNA for the replication proteins (*green*) plus positive sense antigenomic viral RNA (*green*). Translation of the messenger RNAs provides nucleocapsid protein (N), which encapsidates the antigenomic RNA. Antigenomic nucleocapsid is replicated by the viral polymerase (L and P) to yield negative sense genomic viral nucleocapsid (red viral RNA encapsidated with brown N protein), which can be further transcribed and replicated to yield recombinant virus.

a conditionally lethal mutation. For genes that are nonessential, mutation design is a simple matter of engineering a null mutation (e.g., a deletion, insertion, or nonsense mutation) into the cloned gene sequence. Three basic types of engineered conditionally lethal mutations are currently in use: host-range deletion mutants, which rely on the availability of a complementing host cell; temperature-sensitive mutants constructed by clustered charge to alanine scanning; and artificially induced gene regulation. For host-range deletion mutants, the primary problem is construction of a host cell that expresses the target gene in a fashion appropriate for complementation of a null mutant in the virus. Once a cell line has been isolated, construction of the cloned mutation in the virus gene follows the same principles governing construction of a null mutation in a nonessential gene. The fundamental problem in creating temperature-sensitive mutations is that it is currently impossible to predict from primary amino acid sequence or even from three-dimensional protein structure what type of mutation will render a protein temperature sensitive. This difficulty has been partially overcome with the use of clustered charge to alanine scanning mutagenesis, in which clusters of three or more charged residues in the primary amino acid sequence of a protein are all changed to alanine.[132] In theory, charge clusters are likely to reside on the surface of the protein where they may facilitate protein–protein interactions, and neutralization of the charge by replacement with alanine may weaken such interactions without seriously disrupting the three-dimensional conformation of the protein. In practice, as much as 30% of clustered charge to alanine scanning mutants prove to be temperature sensitive *in vivo*, and this mutagenesis technique has been successfully used to construct temperature-sensitive mutants of both picornaviruses and poxviruses.[22,48] Lastly, conditionally lethal mutants have been constructed in poxviruses by placing essential genes under bacterial operator-repressor control in the viral genome.[52,106,123]

Defective Interfering Particles

Interference refers generally to a phenomenon whereby infection by one virus results in inhibition of replication of another virus.[34] Defective interfering (DI) particle-mediated interference was first described by von Magnus,[130] who noted that serial undiluted passage of influenza virus resulted in a dramatic decrease in infectious titer while the number of particles remained constant. Essentially the same phenomenon was subsequently observed in a wide variety of RNA and DNA animal viruses, as well as in plant and bacterial viruses.[57] The mechanism of interference in each case is similar, namely virus stocks accumulate *DI particles.* DI particles are virus particles that contain genomes that are grossly altered genetically, usually by significant deletion of essential functions, but nevertheless retain critical replication origins and packaging signals, allowing for amplification and packaging in co-infections with complementing wild-type *helper* virus. DI particles usually display a replication advantage relative to wild-type virus, resulting from increases in the copy number or efficiency of replication origins. DI particles actively inhibit replication of wild-type virus, presumably by competing for limiting essential replication factors. Study of DI particles has provided significant insight into the viral replication, particularly structure and function of replication origins.

Phenotypic Mixing and Pseudotypes

If two heterologous viruses infect the same cell, then depending on the relatedness of the two viruses, the opportunity exists for packaging of either virus genome into a nucleocapsid or envelope comprised wholly or in part of structural proteins encoded by the heterologous virus. This phenomenon, termed *phenotypic mixing,* has been observed in mixed infections in a laboratory setting using both nonenveloped and enveloped viruses. Phenotypic mixing is a transient phenomenon, because infection of a cell with a single phenotypically mixed particle will result in replication and assembly only of viruses that reflect the infecting genome. In mixed infections with nonenveloped viruses, phenotypic mixing has been observed between closely related adenoviruses, reoviruses, and picornaviruses.[54,103,135] Phenotypic mixing has been observed between picornaviruses as distantly related as echovirus 7 and coxsackievirus A9.[58] In the case of enveloped viruses, phenotypic mixing consists of packing the nucleocapsid of one virus within an envelope of a heterologous virus, and the resulting viruses are called *pseudotypes.* Pseudotype formation among enveloped viruses is relatively promiscuous, especially among retroviruses and rhabdoviruses.[141] For example, pseudotypes have been formed that contain retrovirus envelope antigens combined with genomes from rhabdoviruses, paramyxoviruses, orthomyxoviruses, or herpesviruses. Conversely, pseudotypes have been formed that contain a rhabdovirus genome combined with envelope antigens from togaviruses, retroviruses, bunyaviruses, arenaviruses, paramyxoviruses, orthomyxoviruses, herpesviruses, or poxviruses. Historically, phenotypic mixing experiments have contributed to understanding virus structure and assembly. Currently, the concept of phenotypic mixing and pseudotype formation is of critical utility in packaging and delivery of virus vectors, particularly because phenotypic mixing permits the tropism of a virus particle to be manipulated.[62] Lastly, there has been some speculation that phenotypic mixing may actually play a role in a natural setting, serving to maintain otherwise unfit genomes within a quasispecies over time.[134]

REFERENCES

1. Baltimore D. Expression of animal virus genomes. *Bacteriol Rev* 1971; 35:235–241.
2. Barr JN, Fearns R. How RNA viruses maintain their genome integrity. *J Gen Virol* 2010;91:1373–1387.
3. Benjamin TL. Host-range mutants of polyoma virus. *Proc Natl Acad Sci U S A* 1970;67:394–401.
4. Beveridge WIB, Burnet FM. *The Cultivation of Viruses and Rickettsiae in Chick Embryo.* Special Report Series, Medical Research Council (Great Britain). London: HM Stationery Office; 1946:256.
5. Blasco R, Moss B. Extracellular vaccinia virus formation and cell-to-cell virus transmission are prevented by deletion of the gene encoding the 37,000-Dalton outer envelope protein. *J Virol* 1991;65:5910–5920.
6. Cai W, Schaffer PA. Herpes simplex virus type 1 ICP0 regulates expression of immediate- early, early, and late genes in productively infected cells. *J Virol* 1992;66:2904–2915.
7. Chow LT, Broker TR. In vitro experimental systems for HPV: epithelial raft cultures for investigations of viral reproduction and pathogenesis and for genetic analyses of viral proteins and regulatory sequences. *Clin Dermatol* 1997;15:217–227.
8. Chu CT, Schaffer PA. Qualitative complementation test for temperature-sensitive mutants of herpes simplex virus. *J Virol* 1975;16:1131–1136.
9. Coen DM, Schaffer PA. Two distinct loci confer resistance to acycloguanosine in herpes simplex virus type 1. *Proc Natl Acad Sci U S A* 1980;77: 2265–2269.
10. Coen DM, Weinheimer SP, McKnight SL. A genetic approach to promoter recognition during trans induction of viral gene expression. *Science* 1986;234:53–59.
11. Condit RC, Easterly R, Pacha RF, et al. A vaccinia virus isatin-beta-thiosemicarbazone resistance mutation maps in the viral gene encoding the 132-kDa subunit of RNA polymerase. *Virology* 1991;185:857–861.
12. Condit RC, Motyczka A. Isolation and preliminary characterization of temperature-sensitive mutants of vaccinia virus. *Virology* 1981;113:224–241.
13. Condit RC, Motyczka A, Spizz G. Isolation, characterization, and physical mapping of temperature-sensitive mutants of vaccinia virus. *Virology* 1983;128:429–443.
14. Condit RC, Xiang Y, Lewis JI. Mutation of vaccinia virus gene G2R causes suppression of gene A18R ts mutants: implications for control of transcription. *Virology* 1996;220:10–19.
15. Conzelmann KK. Reverse genetics of mononegavirales. *Curr Top Microbiol Immunol* 2004;283:1–41.
16. Cooper PD. Genetics of picornaviruses. In: Fraenkel-Conrat H, Wagner RR, eds. *Comprehensive Virology.* New York: Plenum Press; 1977: 133–207.
17. Cresawn SG, Prins C, Latner DR, et al. Mapping and phenotypic analysis of spontaneous isatin-beta-thiosemicarbazone resistant mutants of vaccinia virus. *Virology* 2007;363:319–332.
18. d'Herelle F. *The Bacteriophage and Its Behavior.* Baltimore: Williams & Wilkins; 1926.
19. Da FF, Moss B. Poxvirus DNA topoisomerase knockout mutant exhibits decreased infectivity associated with reduced early transcription. *Proc Natl Acad Sci U S A* 2003;100:11291–11296.

20. Davis BD, Dulbecco R, Eisen HN, Ginsberg HS. *Microbiology.* 4th ed. Philadelphia: J. B. Lippincott; 1990.
21. DeLuca NA, McCarthy AM, Schaffer PA. Isolation and characterization of deletion mutants of herpes simplex virus type 1 in the gene encoding immediate-early regulatory protein ICP4. *J Virol* 1985;56:558–570.
22. Diamond SE, Kirkegaard K. Clustered charged-to-alanine mutagenesis of poliovirus RNA-dependent RNA polymerase yields multiple temperature-sensitive mutants defective in RNA synthesis. *J Virol* 1994;68: 863–876.
23. Domi A, Moss B. Cloning the vaccinia virus genome as a bacterial artificial chromosome in *Escherichia coli* and recovery of infectious virus in mammalian cells. *Proc Natl Acad Sci U S A* 2002;99:12415–12420.
24. Domi A, Moss B. Engineering of a vaccinia virus bacterial artificial chromosome in *Escherichia coli* by bacteriophage lambda-based recombination. *Nat Methods* 2005;2:95–97.
25. Domingo E, Holland JJ, Biebricher C, et al. Quasi-species: the concept and the word. In: Gibbs A, Calisher CH, Garcia-Arenal F, eds. *Molecular Basis of Virus Evolution.* Cambridge: Cambridge University Press; 1995: 181–191.
26. Drake JW, Baltz RH. The biochemistry of mutagenesis. *Annu Rev Biochem* 1976;45:11–37.
27. Dubbs DR, Kit S. Isolation and properties of vaccinia mutants deficient in thymidine kinase inducing activity. *Virology* 1964;22:214–225.
28. Dulbecco R, Vogt M. Some problems of animal virology as studied by the plaque technique. *Cold Spring Harb Symp Quant Biol* 1953;18:273–279.
29. Ellis EL, Delbruck M. The growth of bacteriophage. *J Gen Physiol* 1939;22:365–384.
30. Falkner FG, Moss B. *Escherichia coli* gpt gene provides dominant selection for vaccinia virus open reading frame expression vectors. *J Virol* 1988;62:1849–1854.
31. Fathi Z, Sridhar P, Pacha RF, et al. Efficient targeted insertion of an unselected marker into the vaccinia virus genome. *Virology* 1986;155:97–105.
32. Fauquet CM, Mayo MA, Maniloff J, et al. *Virus Taxonomy: Eighth Report of the International Committee on Taxonomy of Viruses.* London: Elsevier; 2005.
33. Fenner F. The classification and nomenclature of viruses: second report of the International Committee on Taxonomy of Viruses. *Intervirology* 1976;7:1–115.
34. Fenner F, McAuslan BR, Mims CA, et al. *The Biology of Animal Viruses.* New York: Academic Press; 1974.
35. Fields BN, Knipe DM, Chanock RM, et al. *Fields Virology.* New York: Raven Press; 1985.
36. Fields BN, Knipe DM, Chanock RM, et al. *Fields Virology.* 2nd ed. New York: Raven Press; 1990.
37. Fields BN, Knipe DM, Howley PM, et al. *Fields Virology.* 3rd ed. Philadelphia: Lippencott-Raven; 1996.
38. Fraenkel-Conrat H, Wagner RR. *Comprehensive Virology.* New York: Plenum Press; 1977.
39. Francki RIB, Fauquet CM, Knudson DL, et al. *The Classification and Nomenclature of Viruses: Fifth Report of the International Committee on Taxonomy of Viruses.* Vienna: Springer-Verlag; 1991.
40. Fredrickson TN, Sechler JM, Palumbo GJ, et al. Acute inflammatory response to cowpox virus infection of the chorioallantoic membrane of the chick embryo. *Virology* 1992;187:693–704.
41. Freshney RI. *Culture of Animal Cells: A Manual of Basic Technique.* 4th ed. New York: Wiley-Liss; 2000.
42. Frost E, Williams J. Mapping temperature-sensitive and host-range mutations of adenovirus type 5 by marker rescue. *Virology* 1978;91:39–50.
43. Gerhard W, Webster RG. Antigenic drift in influenza A viruses. I. Selection and characterization of antigenic variants of A/PR/8/34 (HON1) influenza virus with monoclonal antibodies. *J Exp Med* 1978;148: 383–392.
44. Goodpasture EW, Woodruff AM, Buddingh GJ. Vaccinal infection of the chorio-allantoic membrane of the chick embryo. *Am J Pathol* 1932; 8:271–281.
45. Hahn CS, Lustig S, Strauss EG, et al. Western equine encephalitis virus is a recombinant virus. *Proc Natl Acad Sci U S A* 1988;85:5997–6001.
46. Hartley JW, Rowe WP. Production of altered cell foci in tissue culture by defective Maloney sarcoma virus particles. *Proc Natl Acad Sci U S A* 1966;55:780–786.
47. Hassett DE, Condit RC. Targeted construction of temperature-sensitive mutations in vaccinia virus by replacing clustered charged residues with alanine. *Proc Natl Acad Sci U S A* 1994;91:4554–4558.
48. Hassett DE, Lewis JI, Xing X, et al. Analysis of a temperature-sensitive vaccinia virus mutant in the viral mRNA capping enzyme isolated by clustered charge-to-alanine mutagenesis and transient dominant selection. *Virology* 1997;238:391–409.
49. Hay AJ, Wolstenholme AJ, Skehel JJ, et al. The molecular basis of the specific anti-influenza action of amantadine. *EMBO J* 1985;4:3021–3024.
50. Hay J, Subak-Sharpe JH. Mutants of herpes simplex virus types 1 and 2 that are resistant to phosphonoacetic acid induce altered DNA polymerase activities in infected cells. *J Gen Virol* 1976;31:145–148.
51. Hayflick L, Moorhead PS. The serial cultivation of human diploid cell strains. *Exp Cell Res* 1961;25:585–621.
52. Hedengren-Olcott M, Hruby DE. Conditional expression of vaccinia virus genes in mammalian cell lines expressing the tetracycline repressor. *J Virol Methods* 2004;120:9–12.
53. Hershey AD. Spontaneous mutations in bacterial viruses. *Cold Spring Harb Symp Quant Biol* 1946;11:67.
54. Holland JJ, Cords CE. Maturation of poliovirus RNA with capsid protein coded by heterologous enteroviruses. *Proc Natl Acad Sci U S A* 1964; 51:1082–1085.
55. Holland TC, Sandri-Goldin RM, Holland LE, et al. Physical mapping of the mutation in an antigenic variant of herpes simplex virus type 1 by use of an immunoreactive plaque assay. *J Virol* 1983;46:649–652.
56. Hu WS, Temin HM. Effect of gamma radiation on retroviral recombination. *J Virol* 1992;66:4457–4463.
57. Huang AS, Baltimore D. Defective interfering animal viruses. In: Fraenkel-Conrat H, Wagner RR, eds. *Comprehensive Virology.* New York: Plenum Press; 1977:73–116.
58. Itoh H, Melnick JL. Double infections of single cells with ECHO 7 and Coxsackie A9 viruses. *J Exp Med* 1959;109:393–406.
59. Joklik WK, Willett HP, Amos DB, et al. *Zinsser Microbiology.* 20th ed. Norwalk, CT: Appleton & Lange; 1992.
60. Jones ME, Thomas SM, Rogers A. Luria-Delbruck fluctuation experiments: design and analysis. *Genetics* 1994;136:1209–1216.
61. Jones N, Shenk T. An adenovirus type 5 early gene function regulates expression of other early viral genes. *Proc Natl Acad Sci U S A* 1979; 76:3665–3669.
62. Kafri T. Gene delivery by lentivirus vectors an overview. *Methods Mol Biol* 2004;246:367–390.
63. Kaiser AD. Mutations in a temperate bacteriophage affecting its ability to lysogenize *E. coli. Virology* 1957;3:42.
64. Karber G. Beitrag zur kollektiven Behandlung pharmakologischer Reihenversuche. *Arch Exp Path Pharmakol* 1931;162:480–483.
65. Kato SE, Moussatche N, D'Costa SM, et al. Marker rescue mapping of the combined Condit/Dales collection of temperature-sensitive vaccinia virus mutants. *Virology* 2008;375:213–222.
66. Keck JG, Stohlman SA, Soe LH, et al. Multiple recombination sites at the 5'-end of murine coronavirus RNA. *Virology* 1987;156:331–341.
67. Kirkegaard K, Baltimore D. The mechanism of RNA recombination in poliovirus. *Cell* 1986;47:433–443.
68. Kjellen LE. A variant of adenovirus type 5. *Arch Ges Virusforsch* 1963; 13:482–488.
69. Kobayashi T, Antar AA, Boehme KW, et al. A plasmid-based reverse genetics system for animal double-stranded RNA viruses. *Cell Host Microbe* 2007;1:147–157.
70. Kuchler RJ. *Biochemical Methods in Cell Culture and Virology.* Stroudsburg, PA: Dowden, Hutchingon & Ross; 1977.
71. Lackner CA, D'Costa SM, Buck C, et al. Complementation analysis of the dales collection of vaccinia virus temperature-sensitive mutants. *Virology* 2003;305:240–259.
72. Lai CJ, Nathans D. Mapping temperature-sensitive mutants of simian virus 40: rescue of mutants by fragments of viral DNA. *Virology* 1974; 60:466–475.
73. Lai MM. Genetic recombination in RNA viruses. *Curr Top Microbiol Immunol* 1992;176:21–32.
74. Lai MM. RNA recombination in animal and plant viruses. *Microbiol Rev* 1992;56:61–79.

75. Luria SE. The frequency distribution of spontaneous bacteripohage mutants as evidence for the exponential rate of phage reproduction. *Cold Spring Harb Symp Quant Biol* 1951;16:463–470.
76. Luria SE, Darnell JE, Baltimore D, et al. *General Virology.* 3rd ed. New York: John Wiley & Sons; 1978.
77. Luria SE, Delbruck M. Mutations of bacteria from virus sensitivity to virus resistance. *Genetics* 1943;28:491–511.
78. Luria SE, Williams RC, Backus RC. Electron micrographic counts of bacteriophage particles. *J Bacteriol* 1951;61:179–188.
79. Lwoff A, Horne R, Tournier P. A system of viruses. *Cold Spring Harb Symp Quant Biol* 1962;27:51–55.
80. Mackett M, Smith GL, Moss B. Vaccinia virus: a selectable eukaryotic cloning and expression vector. *Proc Natl Acad Sci U S A* 1982;79:7415–7419.
81. Mahy BWJ, Kangro HO. *Virology Methods Manual.* San Diego: Academic Press; 1996.
82. Margulis L. *Five Kingdoms: An Illustrated Guide to the Phyla of Life on Earth.* 3rd ed. New York: W. H. Freeman; 1998.
83. Martin A, Staeheli P, Schneider U. RNA polymerase II-controlled expression of antigenomic RNA enhances the rescue efficacies of two different members of the Mononegavirales independently of the site of viral genome replication. *J Virol* 2006;80:5708–5715.
84. Matsumoto S. Rabies virus. *Adv Virus Research* 1970;16:257–302.
85. Matthews REF. Classification and nomenclature of viruses: third report of the International Committee on Taxonomy of Viruses. *Intervirology* 1979;12:132–296.
86. Matthews REF. Classification and nomenclature of viruses: fourth report of the International Committee on Taxonomy of Viruses. *Intervirology* 1982;17:1–199.
87. Meis RJ, Condit RC. Genetic and molecular biological characterization of a vaccinia virus gene which renders the virus dependent on isatin-beta-thiosemicarbazone (IBT). *Virology* 1991;182:442–454.
88. Messerle M, Crnkovic I, Hammerschmidt W, et al. Cloning and mutagenesis of a herpesvirus genome as an infectious bacterial artificial chromosome. *Proc Natl Acad Sci U S A* 1997;94:14759–14763.
89. Miller LK, Fried M. Construction of the genetic map of the polyoma genome. *J Virol* 1976;18:824–832.
90. Mindell DP, Villarreal LP. Don't forget about viruses. *Science* 2003; 302:1677.
91. Murphy FA. Virus taxonomy. In: Fields BN, Knipe DM, Howley PM, et al, eds. *Fields Virology.* 3rd ed. Philadelphia: Lippincott-Raven; 1996:15–57.
92. Murphy FA, Fauquet CM, Bishop DHL, et al. *Virus Taxonomy: The Classification and Nomenclature of Viruses. The Sixth Report of the International Committee on Taxonomy of Viruses.* Vienna: Springer-Verlag; 1995.
93. Neumann G, Kawaoka Y. Reverse genetics systems for the generation of segmented negative-sense RNA viruses entirely from cloned cDNA. *Curr Top Microbiol Immunol* 2004;283:43–60.
94. Panicali D, Paoletti E. Construction of poxviruses as cloning vectors: insertion of the thymidine kinase gene from herpes simplex virus into the DNA of infectious vaccinia virus. *Proc Natl Acad Sci U S A* 1982;79:4927–4931.
95. Perkus ME, Goebel SJ, Davis SW, et al. Deletion of 55 open reading frames from the termini of vaccinia virus. *Virology* 1991;180:406–410.
96. Pfefferkorn ER. Genetics of togaviruses. In: Fraenkel-Conrat H, Wagner RR, eds. *Comprehensive Virology.* New York: Plenum Press; 1977:209–238.
97. Phan TG, Okitsu S, Maneekarn N, et al. Evidence of intragenic recombination in G1 rotavirus VP7 genes. *J Virol* 2007;81:10188–10194.
98. Pincus SE, Diamond DC, Emini EA, et al. Guanidine-selected mutants of poliovirus: mapping of point mutations to polypeptide 2C. *J Virol* 1986;57:638–646.
99. Pincus SE, Rohl H, Wimmer E. Guanidine-dependent mutants of poliovirus: identification of three classes with different growth requirements. *Virology* 1987;157:83–88.
100. Pinto LH, Holsinger LJ, Lamb RA. Influenza virus M2 protein has ion channel activity. *Cell* 1992;69:517–528.
101. Plyusnin A, Kukkonen SK, Plyusnina A, et al. Transfection-mediated generation of functionally competent Tula hantavirus with recombinant S RNA segment. *EMBO J* 2002;21:1497–1503.
102. Ramig RF, Fields BN. Genetics of reoviruses. In: Joklik WK, ed. *The Reoviridae.* New York: Plenum Press; 1983:197–228.
103. Ramig RF, Ward RL. Genomic segment reassortment in rotaviruses and other reoviridae. *Adv Virus Res* 1991;39:163–207.
104. Reed LJ, Muench H. A simple method for estimating 50% endpoints. *Amer J Hyg* 1932;27:493–497.
105. Rice AD, Gray SA, Li Y, et al. An efficient method for generating poxvirus recombinants in the absence of selection. *Viruses* 2011;3:217–232.
106. Rodriguez JF, Smith GL. Inducible gene expression from vaccinia virus vectors. *Virology* 1990;177:239–250.
107. Roizman B. Polykaryosis: results from fusion of nononucleated cells. *Cold Spring Harb Symp Quant Biol* 1962;27:327–342.
108. Rowe WP, Huebner RJ, Gilmore LK, et al. Isolation of a cytopathogenic agent from human adenoids undergoing spontaneous degeneration in tissue culture. *Proc Soc Exp Biol Med* 1953;84:570–573.
109. Schnipper LE, Crumpacker CS. Resistance of herpes simplex virus to acycloguanosine: role of viral thymidine kinase and DNA polymerase loci. *Proc Natl Acad Sci U S A* 1980;77:2270–2273.
110. Sedivy JM, Capone JP, RajBhandary UL, et al. An inducible mammalian amber suppressor: propagation of a poliovirus mutant. *Cell* 1987; 50:379–389.
111. Shelokov A, Vogel JE, Chi L. Hemadsorption (adsorption-hemagglutination) test for viral agents in tissue culture with special reference to influenza. *Proc Soc Exp Biol Med* 1958;97:802–809.
112. Simpson RW, Hirst GK. Temperature-sensitive mutants of influenza A virus: isolation of mutants and preliminary observations on genetic recombination and complementation. *Virology* 1968;35:41–49.
113. Spearman C. The method of right and wrong cases (constant stimuli) without Gauss's formulae. *Br J Psychol* 1908;2:227–242.
114. Sridhar P, Condit RC. Selection for temperature-sensitive mutations in specific vaccinia virus genes: isolation and characterization of a virus mutant which encodes a phosphonoacetic acid-resistant, temperature-sensitive DNA polymerase. *Virology* 1983;128:444–457.
115. Steinhauer DA, Skehel JJ. Genetics of influenza viruses. *Annu Rev Genet* 2002;36:305–332.
116. Stoker MGP, Macpherson I. Transformation assays. In: Maramorosch K, Koprowski H, eds. *Methods in Virology.* New York: Academic Press; 1967:313–336.
117. Stow ND, Subak-Sharpe JH, Wilkie NM. Physical mapping of herpes simplex virus type 1 mutations by marker rescue. *J Virol* 1978;28: 182–192.
118. Studier FW. The genetics and physiology of bacteriophage T7. *Virology* 1969;39:562–574.
119. Summers WP, Wagner M, Summers WC. Possible peptide chain termination mutants in thymide kinase gene of a mammalian virus, herpes simplex virus. *Proc Natl Acad Sci U S A* 1975;72:4081–4084.
120. Suzuki Y, Gojobori T, Nakagomi O. Intragenic recombinations in rotaviruses. *FEBS Lett* 1998;427:183–187.
121. Sweet BH, Hilleman MR. The vacuolating virus SV40. *Proc Soc Exp Biol Med* 1960;105:420–427.
122. Thompson CL, Condit RC. Marker rescue mapping of vaccinia virus temperature-sensitive mutants using overlapping cosmid clones representing the entire virus genome. *Virology* 1986;150:10–20.
123. Traktman P, Liu K, DeMasi J, et al. Elucidating the essential role of the A14 phosphoprotein in vaccinia virus morphogenesis: construction and characterization of a tetracycline-inducible recombinant. *J Virol* 2000;74:3682–3695.
124. Trask SD, Taraporewala ZF, Boehme KW, et al. Dual selection mechanisms drive efficient single-gene reverse genetics for rotavirus. *Proc Natl Acad Sci U S A* 2010;107:18652–18657.
125. Tumpey TM, Basler CF, Aguilar PV, et al. Characterization of the reconstructed 1918 Spanish influenza pandemic virus. *Science* 2005;310: 77–80.
126. Van-Regenmortel MH. Virus species, a much overlooked but essential concept in virus classification. *Intervirology* 1990;31:241–254.
127. Van-Regenmortel MH, Fauquet CM, Bishop CM, et al. *Virus Taxonomy: The Seventh Report of the International Committee on Taxonomy of Viruses.* San Diego: Academic Press; 2000.
128. Villarreal LP. Are viruses alive? *Sci Am* 2004;291:100–105.

129. Vogt PK. Focus assay of Rous sarcoma virus. In: Habel K, Salzman NP, eds. *Fundamental Techniques in Virology.* New York: Academic Press; 1969: 198–211.
130. Von Magnus P. Incomplete forms of influenza virus. *Adv Virus Research* 1954;2:59–78.
131. Watson DH, Russell WC, Wildy P. Electron microscopic particle counts on herpes virus using phosphotungstate staining technique. *Virology* 1963; 19:250–260.
132. Wertman KF, Drubin DG, Botstein D. Systematic mutational analysis of the yeast ACT1 gene. *Genetics* 1992;132:337–350.
133. Wildy P. Classification and nomenclature of viruses: first report of the International Committee on Taxonomy of Viruses. *Monogr Virol* 1971; 5:1–181.
134. Wilke CO, Novella IS. Phenotypic mixing and hiding may contribute to memory in viral quasispecies. *BMC Microbiol* 2003;3:11.
135. Williams J, Young H, Austin P. Complementation of human adenovirus type 5 ts mutants by human adenovirus type 12. *J Virol* 1975;15:675–678.
136. Worobey M, Holmes EC. Evolutionary aspects of recombination in RNA viruses. *J Gen Virol* 1999;80 (Pt 10):2535–2543.
137. Yao XD, Evans DH. High-frequency genetic recombination and reactivation of orthopoxviruses from DNA fragments transfected into leporipoxvirus-infected cells. *J Virol* 2003;77:7281–7290.
138. Yount B, Denison MR, Weiss SR, et al. Systematic assembly of a full-length infectious cDNA of mouse hepatitis virus strain A59. *J Virol* 2002;76:11065–11078.
139. Yu D, Sheaffer AK, Tenney DJ, et al. Characterization of ICP6::lacZ insertion mutants of the UL15 gene of herpes simplex virus type 1 reveals the translation of two proteins. *J Virol* 1997;71:2656–2665.
140. Yu MH, King J. Surface amino acids as sites of temperature-sensitive folding mutations in the P22 tailspike protein. *J Biol Chem* 1988;263:1424–1431.
141. Zavada J. The pseudotypic paradox. *J Gen Virol* 1982;63(Pt 1):15–24.
142. Zwillinger D. *CRC Standard Mathematical Tables and Formulae.* 30th ed. Boca Raton, FL: CRC Press; 1996.

CHAPTER 3

Stephen C. Harrison

Principles of Virus Structure

Virus particles are carriers of genetic material from one cell to another. They are, in effect, extracellular organelles. They contain most or all of the molecular machinery necessary for efficient and specific packaging of viral genomes, escape from an infected cell, survival of transfer to a new host cell, attachment, penetration, and initiation of a new replication cycle. In many cases, the molecular machinery works in part by subverting more elaborate elements of a host cell's apparatus for carrying out related processes.

A number of organizational modes have evolved to perform the functions just outlined. The most critical distinction, from a structural perspective, is between *enveloped* viruses—those with lipid-bilayer membranes—and *nonenveloped* viruses—those without such membranes. Both categories include well-known human pathogens. Examples of the former are human immunodeficiency virus (HIV) and influenza virus; examples of the latter, poliovirus and papillomavirus. Enveloped viruses have, in their lipid bilayer, an impermeable barrier between their genomes and the outside environment, reducing the need for continuity of any protein layer. Nonenveloped viruses require a tightly packed shell to exclude nucleases or other sources of genomic damage.

For the structure of any virus particle, a central constraint is that the information needed to specify its macromolecular components must not exhaust the genetic capacity of the packaged genome. This requirement for genetic economy is in practice quite stringent. For example, consider a very simple genome of 5 kb, enough to encode about 1,600 amino acid residues, if reading frames do not overlap. A tightly condensed single-stranded RNA or DNA of this size will occupy a spherical volume about 90 Å in radius. To protect it with a gap-free protein shell, 30 Å thick, would require roughly 25,000 amino acid residues—far more than the viral nucleic acid can encode. The shell of a nonenveloped virus with even a very small genome must therefore contain a large number of identical protein subunits—at least 60, if the coat-protein gene is to use up less than 25% of the coding capacity in the enclosed nucleic acid. As explained later, an important consequence of this observation (first made by Crick and Watson[56] even before a triplet code had been established) is that virus particles, or their substructures, are usually highly symmetric.

HOW VIRUS STRUCTURES ARE STUDIED

Electron microscopy is the most direct way to determine the general morphology of a virus particle. Traditional thin-sectioning methods are useful for examining infected cells and larger, isolated particles. The thickness of a section and the coarseness of staining methods limit resolution to about 50 to 75 Å, even in the best cases. (*Resolution* means the approximate minimum size of a substructure that can be separated in an image from its neighbor. Recall that one atomic diameter is 2.3 Å; an α-helix, 10 Å; and a DNA double helix, 20 Å.) Negative staining, with uranyl acetate, potassium phosphotungstate, or related electron-dense compounds, gives somewhat more detailed images of isolated and purified virus particles. Viruses embedded in negative stain are often relatively well preserved. The electron beam destroys the particle itself very rapidly, but it leaves the dense "cast" of stain undamaged for much longer. If the particle is fully covered by the negative stain, the image contains contrast from both the upper and the lower surface of the particle, and visual interpretation of finer aspects of the image can be difficult.[57]

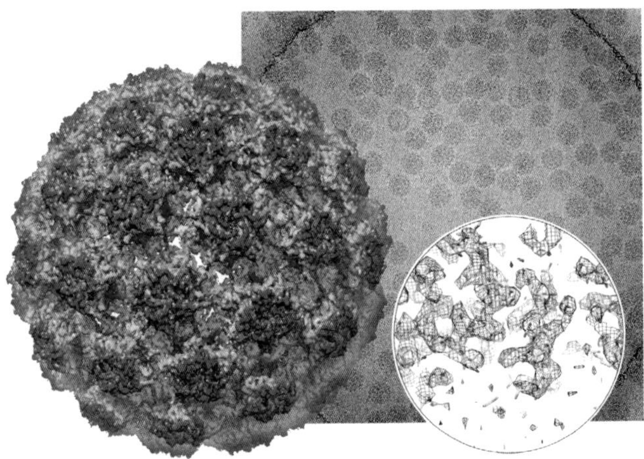

FIGURE 3.1. Bovine papillomavirus (BPV), as seen by electron cryomicroscopy (cryoEM). In the foreground is a color rendering of the three-dimensional image reconstruction, based on the kinds of micrographs shown in the background picture. The circular inset at **lower right** illustrates that this reconstruction provides information that extends to a nearly atomic level of detail (*resolution*); it shows a small part of the density map that resulted from the image analysis and the fit to that map of parts of the L1 polypeptide chain. (See Grigorieff and Harrison[94] and Wolf et al.[246])

Methods for preserving viruses and other macromolecular assemblies by rapid freezing to liquid nitrogen or liquid helium temperatures have permitted visualization of electron-scattering contrast from the structures in the particle itself and not just from the cast created by a surrounding layer of negative stain.[10] Moreover, quantitative methods for image analysis, originally developed for studying negatively stained particles, have been applied effectively to such images. An advantage of such electron cryomicroscopy (cryoEM) is that regular images can be selected from a heterogeneous field, allowing study of unstable or relatively impure preparations. Advances during the decade preceding the current revision of this chapter have enabled cryoEM three-dimensional density maps at resolutions that reveal molecular details—the tracing of a polypeptide chain and the orientations of large amino acid side chains.[94] One example is illustrated in Figure 3.1.[246] Such *image reconstructions* are obtained by combining information from hundreds or thousands of different images of individual particles. The combination is possible because the particles of these viruses are all the same. When such uniformity is not present, for example, as in the case of a complete herpesvirus particle rather than an isolated nucleocapsid, then information from different particles cannot be combined. A *tomographic* tilt series of images from a single particle can be obtained (analogous to a computed tomography [CT] scan in medical radiography), but the resulting three-dimensional image is of much lower resolution, as electron damage limits its quality, even when the data are taken at liquid nitrogen or liquid helium temperatures (electron cryotomography, or cryoET). Tomographic reconstructions can nonetheless be very useful, as illustrated in Figure 3.2. In some cases, averaging the images of defined substructures within a tomogram or among many tomograms (e.g., the "spikes" on the surface of certain enveloped viruses) can yield a more detailed representation.

The information obtained from even the most elegant of electron microscopy methods still falls short of the atomic detail that often can be obtained by x-ray diffraction methods, if single crystals of the relevant structure can be prepared. It has been known since the 1930s that simple plant viruses, such as tomato bushy stunt virus (TBSV), can be crystallized,[13] and the first x-ray diffraction patterns of such crystals were recorded as early as 1938.[17] Crystallization of poliovirus and other important animal viruses showed that the approach could be extended to human pathogens.[213] The first complete high-resolution structure of a crystalline virus was obtained from TBSV in 1978,[107] and since then the structures of a number of animal, plant, and insect pathogens have been determined (for a compilation, see the VIPER website: http://viperdb.scripps.edu). Only very regular structures can form single crystals, and in order to study the molecular details of larger and more complex virus particles, it is necessary to "dissect" them into well-defined subunits or substructures. This dissection was originally done with proteases, by disassembly, or by isolation of substructures from infected cells. For example, the structure of the influenza virus hemagglutinin[244]—the first viral glycoprotein for which atomic details were visualized—was obtained from crystals of protein cleaved from the surface of purified virions[243]; the structure of the adenovirus hexon was obtained from excess unassembled protein derived from adenovirus-infected cells.[189] In the past two decades, this dissection has more commonly been carried out using recombinant expression (e.g., of a fragment of gp120 from HIV-1[131]). Most of the high-resolution structures of enveloped virus components described in this chapter—both surface glycoproteins and internal proteins—come from x-ray crystallographic analysis of recombinant gene products, often suitably truncated or otherwise modified to enable crystallization. A handful of atomic-level structures of virus components have come from nuclear magnetic resonance (NMR) spectroscopy,[178,200] but application of that technique is limited to relatively small proteins or protein complexes.

SYMMETRY OF VIRUSES

Virus particles must assemble specifically and rapidly in an infected cell, as directed by the mutual interactions among their component protein subunits. Specificity requires a defined stereochemical relationship between contacting proteins. Because there are many copies of the same subunit, there must also be many repeating instances of the same kind of contact. This repetition—a consequence of the requirement for genetic economy described in the introductory section of this chapter—implies symmetry.

A rigorous definition of symmetry involves an operation, such as a rotation, that brings an object into self-coincidence. For example, if the ring of three commas in Figure 3.3A is rotated by 120 or 240 degrees, it will not be possible to recognize that a rotation has occurred (assuming that the commas are truly indistinguishable). The full symmetry of an object is defined by the collection of such operations that apply to it. In the case of protein assemblies, these operations can be rotations, translations, or combinations of the two. A symmetry axis that includes rotation by 180 degrees is called a *twofold axis* or a *dyad;* one with a 120-degree rotation (and, of course,

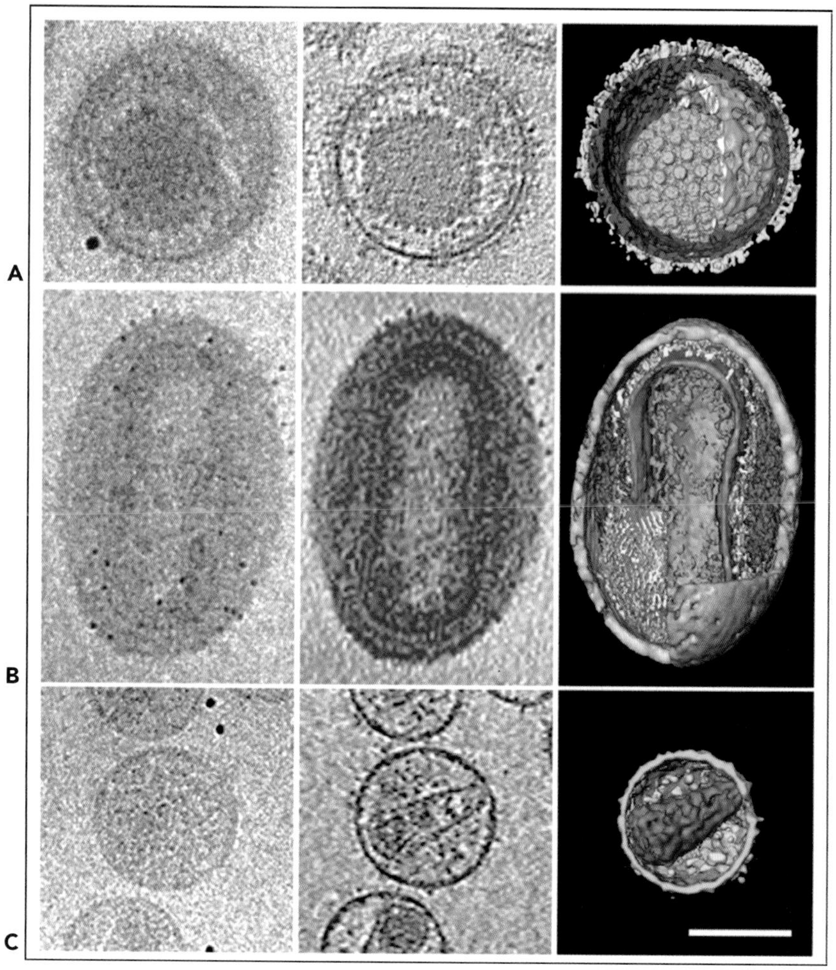

FIGURE 3.2. **Electron cryotomography (cryoET) of herpes simplex virus type 1 (A),[98] vaccinia intracellular mature virion (B),[58] and HIV-1 (C).[23]** Images in the **left-hand column** are single, projected images; those in the **middle column**, slices through the reconstructed tomogram; those on the **right**, cut-away surface renderings of the three-dimensional tomographic reconstructions. (Adapted from Cyrklaff M, Risco C, Fernandez JJ, et al. Cryo-electron tomography of vaccinia virus. *Proc Natl Acad Sci U S A* 2005;102:2772–2777.)

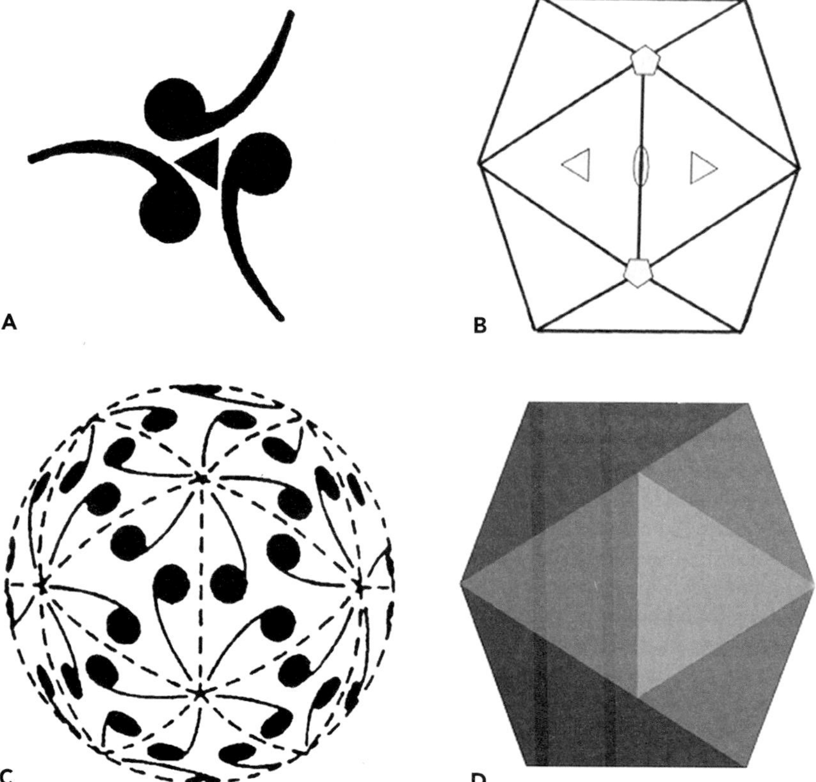

FIGURE 3.3. **Icosahedral symmetry. A:** Threefold symmetry: the three commas are related to each other by 120-degree rotations about the central axis, marked by a small triangle. **B:** Outline of an icosahedron, showing positions of some of the symmetry axes (imagined to extend from the center of the icosahedral to the point on the surface marked by the symbol): fivefold, threefold, and twofold axes are marked by pentagons, triangles, and an oval, respectively. **C:** An icosahedrally symmetric arrangement of commas on the surface of a sphere. For locations of symmetry axes, compare with panel **B. D:** Shaded surface view of an icosahedron.

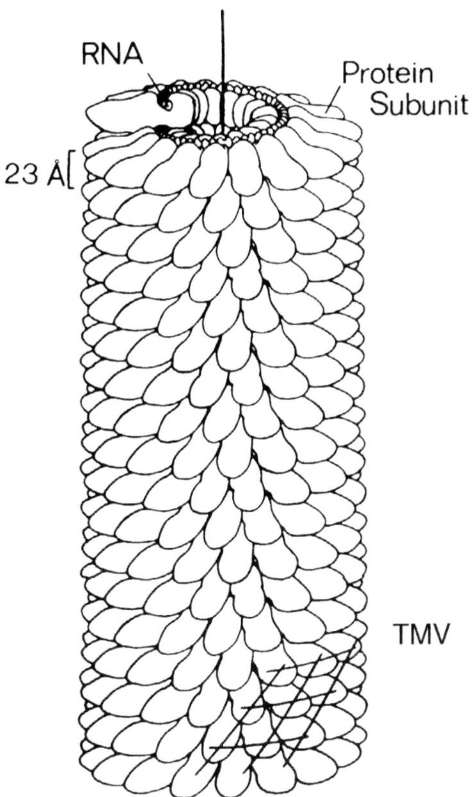

FIGURE 3.4. Diagram of the tobacco mosaic virus (TMV) particle. The elongated "loaves," with a groove for the RNA, represent the protein subunits. Three RNA nucleotides fit into the groove on each subunit. There are 16 ⅓ subunits per turn of the right-handed helix (i.e., 49 subunits in three turns), with a rise of 23 Å as indicated. At the **lower right**, the *surface lattice* is drawn onto the outer particle. (Adapted from Caspar DL. Assembly and stability of the tobacco mosaic virus particle. *Adv Protein Chem* 1963;18:37–121.)

a 240-degree rotation as well) is called a *threefold axis*; and so forth. Note the distinction between shape and symmetry: the *shape* of an object refers to the geometry of its outline, whereas its *symmetry* refers to the operations that describe it. The set of commas in Figure 3.3A has threefold symmetry; so does an equilateral triangle, the beer-company symbol with three interlocked rings, and countless other objects with unrelated shapes.

As a first example, consider the rod-like coat of tobacco mosaic virus (TMV)[125] (Fig. 3.4). The helical arrangement of its protein subunits illustrates that symmetry is an important consequence of its assembly from many identical building blocks. If we look at the model of TMV, we find that a rotation of 22 degrees and a translation of 1.4 Å along the particle axis will superpose subunit 1 on subunit 2. But if the surfaces of subunit 2 are the same as those of subunit 1, the same rotation and translation must superpose subunit 2 on subunit 3, and so forth. The combination of rotation and translation that effects this superposition is a *screw axis.* Strictly speaking, the screw axis of TMV would only be an ideal symmetry operation if the helix were infinite. In practice, it is so long that we can neglect end effects.

In TMV, and probably in the nucleocapsids of negative-strand RNA viruses such as influenza and vesicular stomatitis virus (VSV), the RNA winds in a helical path that follows the protein.[125] That is, the tubular package does not simply contain the RNA; it co-incorporates it. There are exactly three nucleotides per subunit in TMV, and they fit into a defined groove between the helically arrayed proteins. By contrast, the protein coat of a filamentous, single-stranded DNA (ssDNA) phage, such as M13, forms a sleeve that surrounds and constrains the closed, circular genome, without there being a specific way in which each subunit contacts one or more nucleotides.[87] Thus, there can be a nonintegral ratio of nucleotides to protein monomers.

The length of the packaged nucleic acid determines the length of virus particles such as TMV or M13. Structures such as the tail of bacteriophage lambda or T4 have a protein component that extends from the initiating structure at the base of the tail to the end connected to the head.[3] The number of such polypeptide chains corresponds to the rotational symmetry of the tail.

Rod-like structures are not very efficient ways to package long genomes. At least one dimension of a helical assembly such as TMV grows linearly with the length of the packaged viral DNA or RNA, leading to awkwardly elongated particles. The number of subunits is likewise proportional to length. *Isometric* (i.e., essentially spherical) particles are more compact and more economical: if the nucleic acid condenses into the interior of the particle, then the diameter increases as the cube root of the genome length, and the number of required subunits as the genome length to the two-thirds power. Most animal viruses are roughly isometric.

Closed, isometric shells composed of identical subunits that interact through conserved, specific interfaces can have one of only three symmetries: the symmetry of the regular tetrahedron, the cube, or the regular icosahedron. These shells will accommodate 12, 24, or 60 subunits, respectively. The icosahedral shells are obviously the most efficient of the three designs: they use the largest number of subunits to make a container of a given size, and hence they use subunits of the smallest size and the smallest coding requirement. Tetrahedral and cubic symmetries have not appeared in any naturally occurring virus assemblies. Note the distinction between icosahedral symmetry and icosahedral shape. Not all objects with icosahedral symmetry have even the vague outline of an icosahedron; conversely, painting a single asymmetric object, such as a comma, on each face of an icosahedron, rather than three such objects related by the threefold axis through the middle of the face, would destroy the symmetry of the decorated object but would not affect its shape.

The diagram in Figure 3.3B shows the operations that belong to an icosahedrally symmetric object. They are a collection of twofold, threefold, and fivefold rotation axes. Placement of a single, asymmetric object on a surface governed by this symmetry leads to the generation of 59 others, when the various rotations are applied (Fig. 3.3C). One such object, one-sixtieth of the total shell, can therefore be designated as an *icosahedral asymmetric unit,* the fundamental piece of structure from which all the rest can be produced by the operations of icosahedral symmetry.

STRUCTURES OF CLOSED SHELLS

With a typical, compact protein domain of 250 to 300 amino acid residues, close to the upper limit for most single-protein

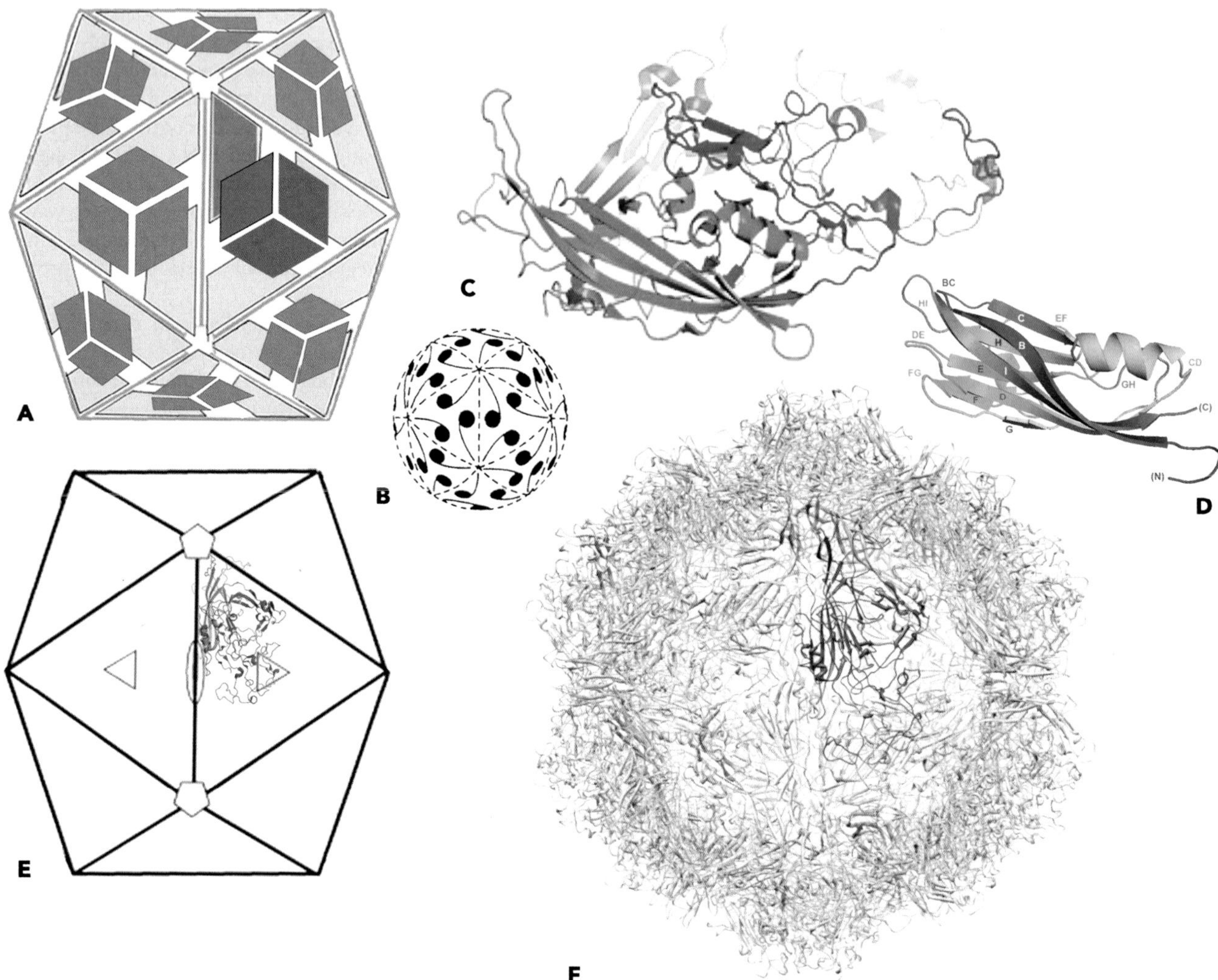

FIGURE 3.5. Canine parvovirus (CPV): a simple, icosahedrally symmetric virion. A: Icosahedron, viewed along a twofold axis, with diagrammatic representations of a protein subunit with a core domain (colored red on one of the subunits) and a projecting region (blue). Compare the subunits with the representation of commas in **B**, repeated from Figure 3.3 C. **C:** Ribbon diagram of the CPV protein subunit; the core domain (red) is a β-jelly-roll, from which emanate several loops that cluster to form a complex projecting region (blue). The simplified representation of the β-jelly-roll in **D** is in rainbow coloring, from blue at its N-terminus to red at its C-terminus. The eight strands are lettered B–I; the loops have the letters of the strands they connect. The projecting region of the CPV subunit comprises loops BC, EF, and GH. **E:** Icosahedron, as in **A**, but with a ribbon representation of one subunit; symbols for symmetry axes as in Figure 3.3B. **F:** Ribbon representation of all 60 subunits, with the subunit from E in blue and all others in gray.

domains, what sort of icosahedrally symmetric container can we construct? Suppose that the protein is so shaped that 60 copies fit together into a 30-Å thick shell with no significant gaps. Then the cavity within that shell will have a radius of about 80 Å, which can contain a 3- to 4-kb piece of single-stranded DNA or RNA, tightly condensed. A few, very simple virus particles indeed conform to this description. The parvoviruses (see Chapter 57) contain a 5.3-kb ssDNA genome, and their shells have 60 copies of a protein of approximately 520 residues (Fig. 3.5). The capsid protein therefore uses up about one-third of the genome. ("Capsid," from the Latin *capsa,* "box," designates the protein shell that directly packages DNA or RNA; "nucleocapsid" refers to the shell plus its nucleic acid contents.) Likewise, the satellite of tobacco necrosis virus (STNV) contains 60 copies of a 195-residue subunit and a 1,120-bp single-stranded RNA (ssRNA) genome, of which over half is used for the coat protein.[141] As the name implies, however, STNV is actually a defective virus, and it requires tobacco necrosis virus co-infection to propagate.

More complex viruses have evolved ways to make larger, icosahedrally symmetric shells without expending unnecessary genetic resources. The simplest, but least economical, is just to use several different subunits, each of "garden variety" size, to make up one icosahedral asymmetric unit. The picornaviruses (polioviruses, rhinoviruses, etc.) have 60 copies of three distinct proteins, VP1, VP2, and VP3, each between 230 and 300 amino acid residues, as well as 60 copies of a small internal peptide, VP4 (see Fig. 3.6). The shell has a cavity about 95 Å

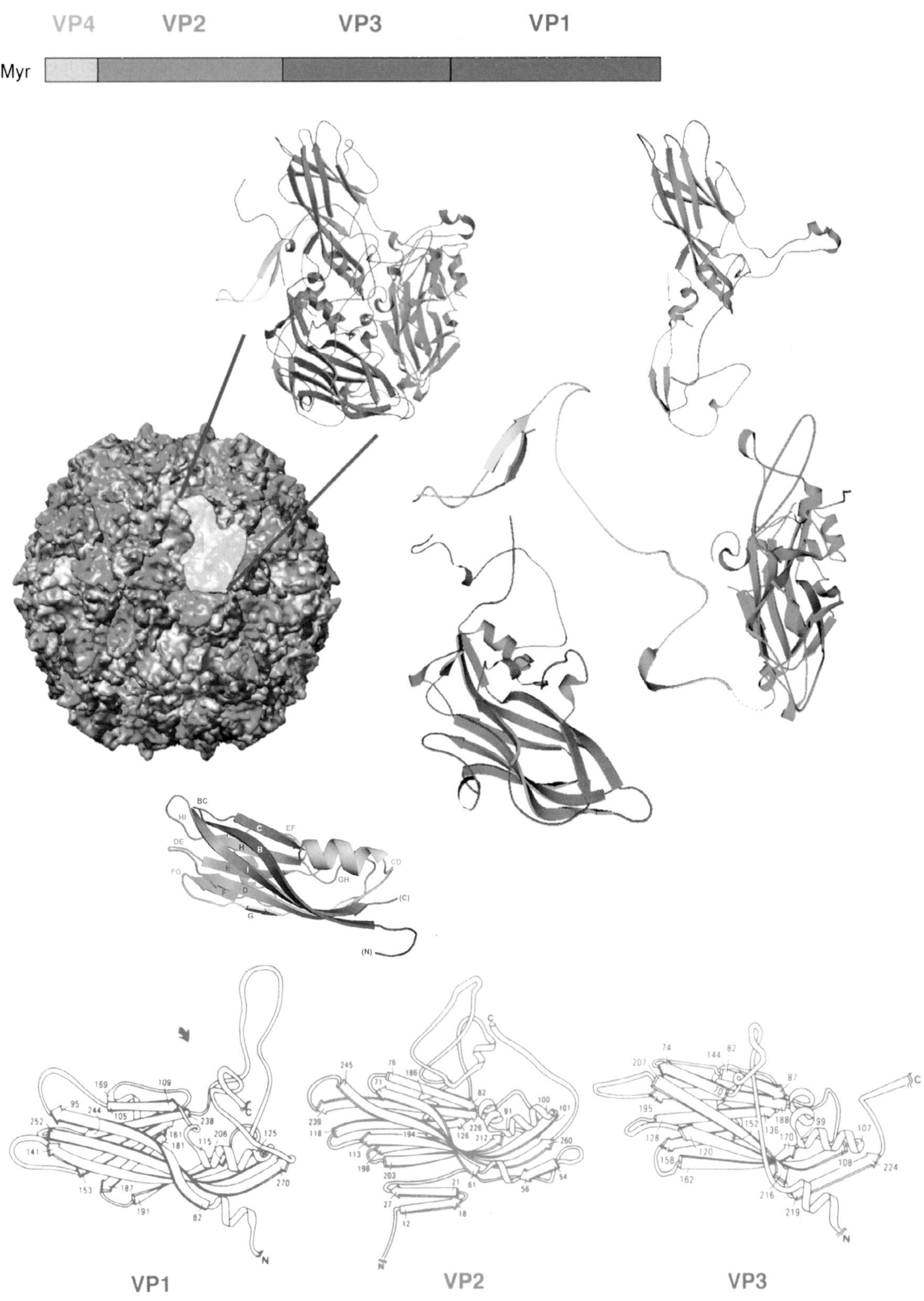

FIGURE 3.6. Poliovirus. Top: The order of structural proteins in the polyprotein encoded by the viral RNA. These domains are at the N-terminal end of the polyprotein, which is modified by myristoylation (Myr). The viral protease that cleaves between VP0 (= VP4 + VP2) and VP3 and between VP3 and VP1 is encoded by a region 3′ to the region that encodes the structural proteins; the VP4-VP2 cleavage is autolytic and occurs only after assembly of the virion precursor. **Middle:** Surface representation of the virus particle, with colors as in the diagram at the top. Two successively "exploded" views of an icosahedral asymmetric unit (*protomer*) are shown next to the surface rendering. VP1, VP2, and VP3 each have a central β-jelly-roll, with variable interstrand loops and variable N- and C-terminal extensions. The rainbow-colored β-jelly-roll below the surface view is repeated from Figure 3.5D. **Bottom:** Side-by-side views of the β-jelly-roll domains of VP1, VP2, and VP3 to illustrate their congruence.

in radius, which holds an RNA genome of 7.5 to 8 kb. The picornaviruses thus expend about one-third of their genome to encode the structural proteins of the virion. (The term *virion* means *virus particle*, generally implying the mature, infectious structure.) We note here two other important features of picornavirus molecular architecture. First, the folded structures of VP1, VP2, and VP3 all have the same kernel—a domain known as a *jelly-roll β-barrel* (Figs. 3.5 and 3.6). The single subunits of the parvoviruses and of STNV have the same basic fold. It is a module particularly well suited to the formation of closed, spherical shells because of its block-like, trapezoidal outline, but its prevalence among viral subunits may be evidence of a deeper evolutionary relationship. A second noteworthy feature of picornavirus design is that arm-like extensions of the subunits tie together the assembled particle (Fig. 3.6). The importance of scaffold-like intertwining of subunit arms was first discovered in the simple plant viruses.[107] In effect, folding of part of the subunit and assembly of the shell are concerted processes.

Quasiequivalent Icosahedral Arrangements

A more economical way to build shells from more than 60 average-sized, identical subunits was described by Caspar and Klug[35] in 1961. It is illustrated by the diagram of 180 commas in Figure 3.7. The commas have similar interactions (head-to-head in pairs; neck-to-neck in rings of three; tail-to-tail in rings of five or six), but they fall into three sets, designated A, B, and C. If the commas are taken to represent proteins, then the conformational differences between A and B positions, for example, involve the differences between rings of five and rings of six, for contacts involving the parts of the proteins symbolized by the tails. Caspar and Klug[35] suggested that protein subunits might have the sort of flexibility or capacity for conformational switching needed to accommodate somewhat different packing environments without sacrificing specificity. They postulated that viruses with more than 60 chemically and genetically identical subunits might exhibit the sort of near equivalence seen in the A, B, and C conformers in the comma illustration. They called this sort of local distortability, which might conserve much of the specificity and character of the protein contacts, *quasi-equivalence.*

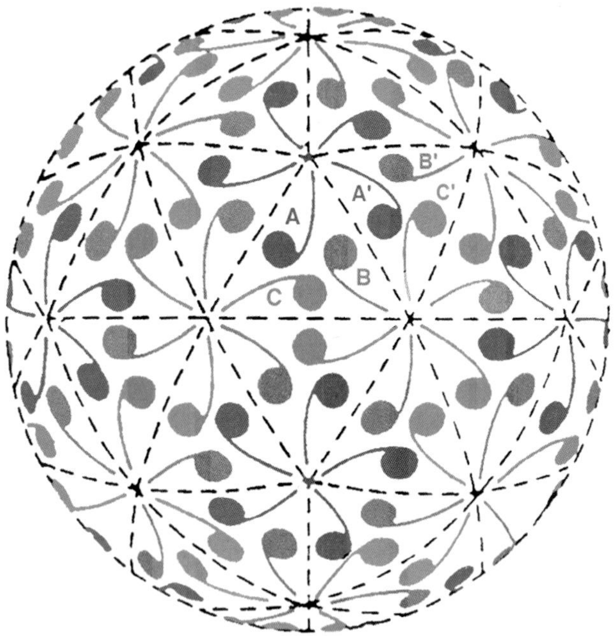

FIGURE 3.7. Quasiequivalent arrangement of 180 commas, in a T = 3 icosahedral surface lattice on a sphere. Compare Figure 3.3C, a T = 1 arrangement of 60 commas with icosahedral axes oriented similarly. The three quasiequivalent positions within a single icosahedral asymmetric unit are shown in blue, red, and green and labeled A, B, and C, respectively, in two of the asymmetric units.

A number of plant and animal viruses, such as TBSV[107] and Norwalk virus,[182] conform to this description of quasiequivalent arrangements (Fig. 3.8). In TBSV and Norwalk virus, there are 180 genetically and chemically identical subunits in the capsid. The subunits are actually larger than those of the picornaviruses, but most of the extra size comes from a second, projecting domain that serves functions other than the construction of a closed shell. The size of the *shell domain* (S domain) in both cases is just about 200 residues, and the folded structure of the domain is again a jelly-roll β-barrel. The important feature of the packing of these 180 S domains is illustrated by the TBSV diagram in Figure 3.8. The contents of an icosahedral asymmetric unit can be described as three chemically identical subunits, with somewhat different conformations. These conformers are denoted A, B, and C, echoing the designation of commas in Figure 3.7. The differences among the conformers reside principally in an ordered or disordered conformation for part of the N-terminal arm and in the angle of the hinge between the S domain and the projecting, *P domain.* The A and B conformations are nearly identical, with disordered arms and similar hinge angles. The C conformation has an ordered arm and a different hinge angle from A and B. The ordered arms extend along the base of the S domain and intertwine with two others around the icosahedral threefold axis. Thus, the whole collection of 60 C-subunit arms forms a coherent inner scaffold.

How equivalent or nonequivalent are the actual intersubunit contacts in TBSV and related structures? Most of the interfaces are well conserved, with very modest local distortions that do not significantly change the way individual amino acid side chains contact each other. The interfaces between conformers that do exhibit noteworthy differences are those that include the ordered arms in one of the quasiequivalent locations (the C-conformer). At these interfaces, there is a discrete switch between two states, with ordering and disordering of the arm as the toggle. Nonetheless, many side chain contacts are conserved around the fulcrum that relates an A/B dimer to a C/C dimer (Fig. 3.8).

Only certain multiples of 60 subunits can pack with quasiequivalent contacts; they are given by the formula $T = h^2 + hk + k^2$, where h and k are any integer or zero.[125] The multiple T is known as the *triangulation number,* because, as illustrated by comparison of the 60- and 180-comma structures in Figures 3.3 and 3.7, they correspond to subtriangulations of an icosahedral net on the surface of a sphere. Such nets are known as *surface lattices.* If we think of an icosahedrally symmetric structure as a folded-up hexagonal net (Fig. 3.9), then 12 uniformly spaced sixfold vertices are transformed into fivefold vertices.

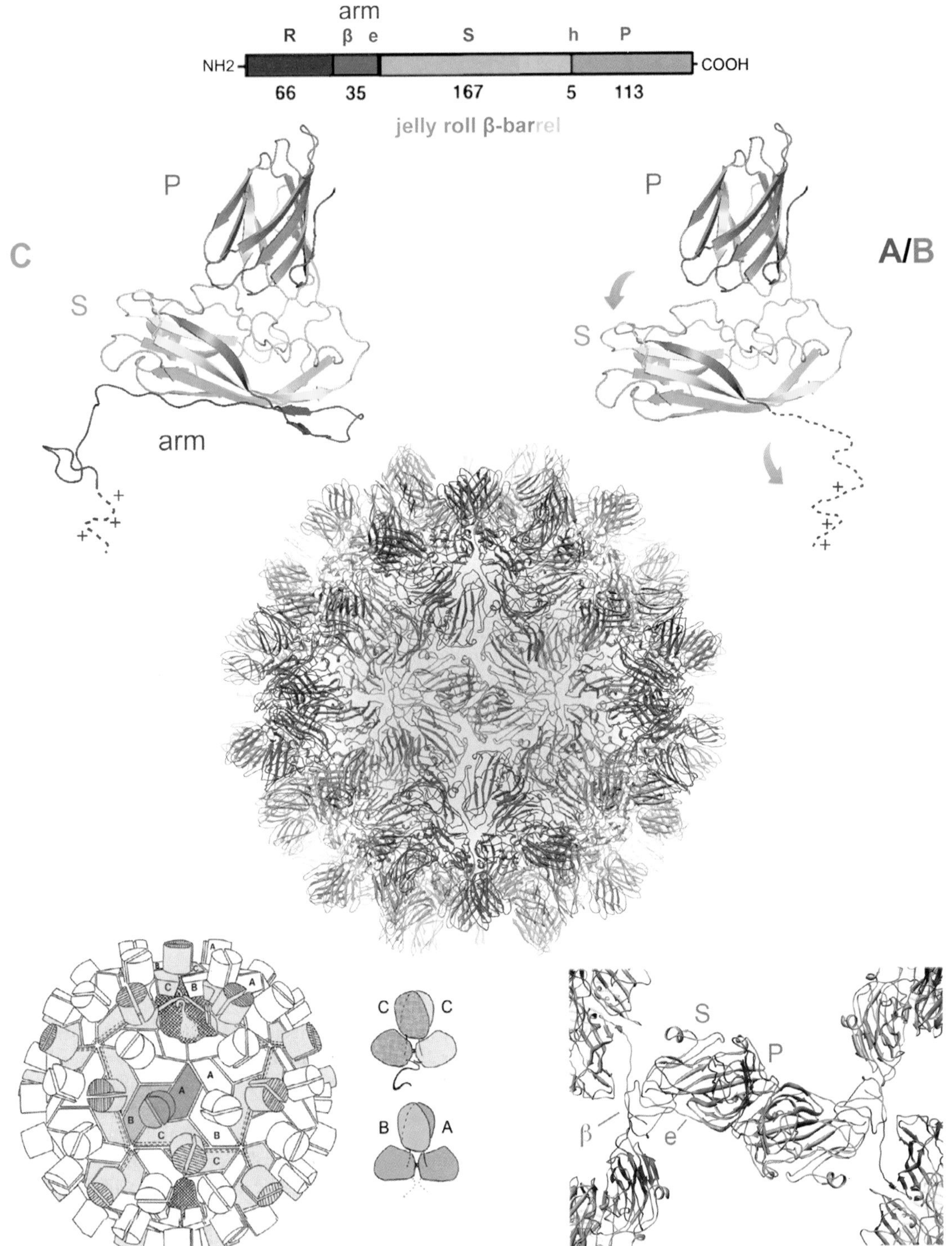

FIGURE 3.8. Tomato bushy stunt virus (TBSV), a T = 3 icosahedral structure. Top: Modular organization of the TBSV coat-protein polypeptide chain. R: unstructured, positively charged N-terminal region. β, e: segments of the "arm," ordered on the C-conformation subunits and unstructured on the A- and B-conformation subunits; when ordered, the β segment forms an interdigitated β-*annulus* with corresponding segments from two other chains, and the e segment extends along the base of the subunit (see panel at **bottom, left**). S: shell domain, a β-jelly-roll. P: projecting domain, a β-sandwich of somewhat different fold from the jelly-roll S domain. h: hinge between the S and P domains. The color coding in the bar representation of the chain is repeated in the ribbon diagrams of the C (**left**) and A/B (**right**) conformations. Note that the two conformations differ in two respects: the ordering of the arm and the hinge angle between S and P domains (curved arrows on the **right-hand ribbon diagram**). **Center:** Ribbon representation of the entire protein coat of the virus; the colors of the A-, B-, and C-conformation subunits are as in Figure 3.7. **Bottom left:** Schematic figure, showing that the arms of the C-subunits (green) interdigitate around threefold axes of the icosahedral symmetry, forming a coherent inner framework. **Bottom right:** Magnified view of some of the C-subunits from the coat seen in the central part of the figure, illustrating the β-annulus (β) and the extended part of the arm (e). In the **bottom center** are schematic views of the C-C and A-B dimers, showing how the hinge between S and P domains correlates with the ordering of the arms (inserted into the slot between S domains, which have rotated away from the contact that they have when the arms are unfolded into the particle interior).

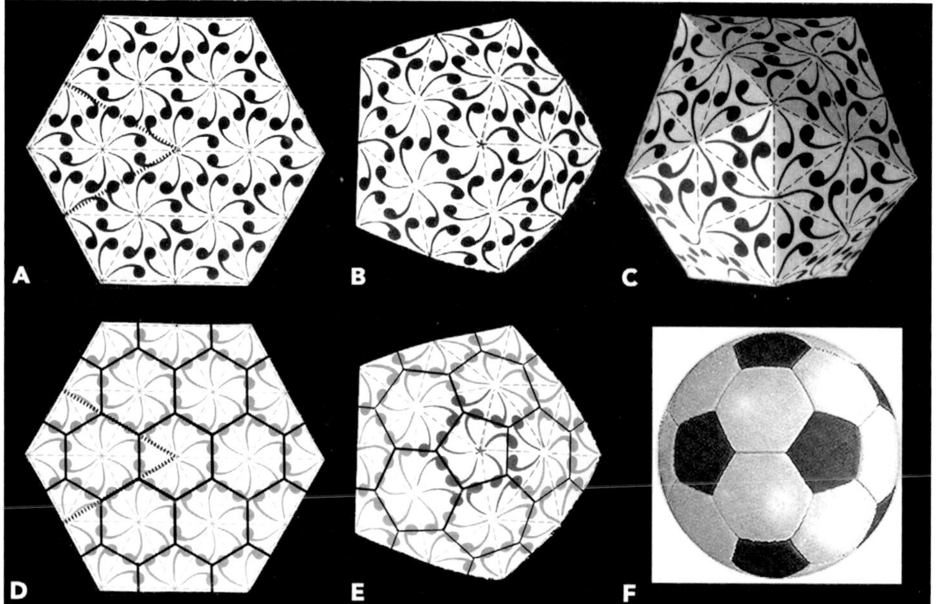

FIGURE 3.9. Generation of curved structures from planar lattices. A: Portion of a hexagonal lattice. Six triangular cells of the lattice meet at each lattice point, and each triangular cell contains three "subunits" (commas). Thus, there is a sixfold symmetry axis at each lattice point, a threefold symmetry axis at the center of each triangle, and a twofold axis at the midpoint of each edge. Imagine that the lattice extends indefinitely in all directions. **B:** Curvature can be introduced by transforming one of the sixfold positions into a fivefold **(center)**. A 60-degree "pie slice" has been removed from the object in **A** by cutting along the heavy dotted lines, and the cut edges have been joined to generate the curved lattice shown here. **C:** If further cuts are made at regular intervals in an extended lattice, such as the one in **A**, and the edges joined as in **B**, a closed solid can be produced. In the case of the icosahedral solid shown here, vertices of the lattice separated by two cell edges have been transformed into fivefolds, while the intervening lattice points have been left as local sixfolds, producing a T = 4 (h = 2, k = 0) structure. Notice that the local sixfolds are actually only approximately sixfold in character; they correspond strictly to the twofold axes of the icosahedral object. **D:** Lines joining the centers of the triangular cells in **A** create a pattern of hexagons. **E:** When a sixfold is transformed into a fivefold, a hexagon becomes a pentagon. **F:** If second nearest-neighbor lattice points are all transformed into pentagons, a soccer-ball figure results. This is a T = 3 structure. A description of the lattice as a network of hexagons and pentagons is complementary to its description as a network of triangles. The representations in Figures 3.3, 3.5, 3.13, and 3.16 **(left)** use triangles. The representation in Figure 3.16 **(right)** uses hexagons and pentagons. One representation for a given lattice can easily be derived from the other.

Nonequivalent Icosahedral Surface Packings

Hexagonal packing is an efficient way to tile a surface (think of hexagonal floor tiles), even if the building blocks themselves do not have sixfold symmetry and hence do not interact identically with their neighbors. In many larger, icosahedrally symmetric virus particles, the outer-shell building blocks are centered at the vertices of an icosahedral surface lattice, subtriangulated as anticipated by Caspar and Klug, but the oligomeric building blocks themselves are not hexamers. In some cases, for example, adenoviruses (Fig. 3.10), they are trimers, with a chemically distinct, pentameric building block on the fivefold vertices; in other cases, for example, the polyoma- and papillomaviruses, the building blocks are all identical pentamers (Fig. 3.1). Viewed at low resolution (e.g., by negative-stain electron microscopy), all of these viruses have globular "lumps" at the vertices of a lattice with one of the allowed triangulation numbers (T = 25 for the adenoviruses: Fig. 3.10; T = 7 for the polyoma- and papillomaviruses: Fig. 3.1), but when seen at higher resolution, the six-coordinated lumps are actually trimers or pentamers, and in the former case, the five-coordinated lumps are pentamers of a related but distinct polypeptide chain. Special mechanisms (either involving other structural proteins or flexible intersubunit connections) are needed to hold the particle together because a single set of repeating, quasiequivalent intersubunit contacts is not possible. Before the molecular principles of virus structure were fully understood, the globular lumps seen by low-resolution electron microscopy were called *capsomeres,* meaning the *structural units* of the *capsid.* This word is still used when referring to apparent morphologic units on the surface of a virus shell, but it is best reserved for cases where all capsomeres are the same and hence represent a defined oligomer, as in the pentameric units of papovaviruses (see later).

The flaviviruses and picobirnaviruses illustrate yet another adaptation to icosahedral packing. As illustrated in Figure 3.7, the asymmetric unit of an icosahedral surface lattice can be represented by a (spherical) triangle with a fivefold axis and two adjacent threefold axes as its vertices. The flavivirus envelope protein (E) is a flat, elongated dimer; three such dimers neatly fill a twofold-related pair of asymmetric-unit triangles, with the dyad of the central dimer coincident with the icosahedral twofold (Fig. 3.11).[128] The shell contains 180 subunits, but not in a T = 3 arrangement. The picobirnavirus coat protein

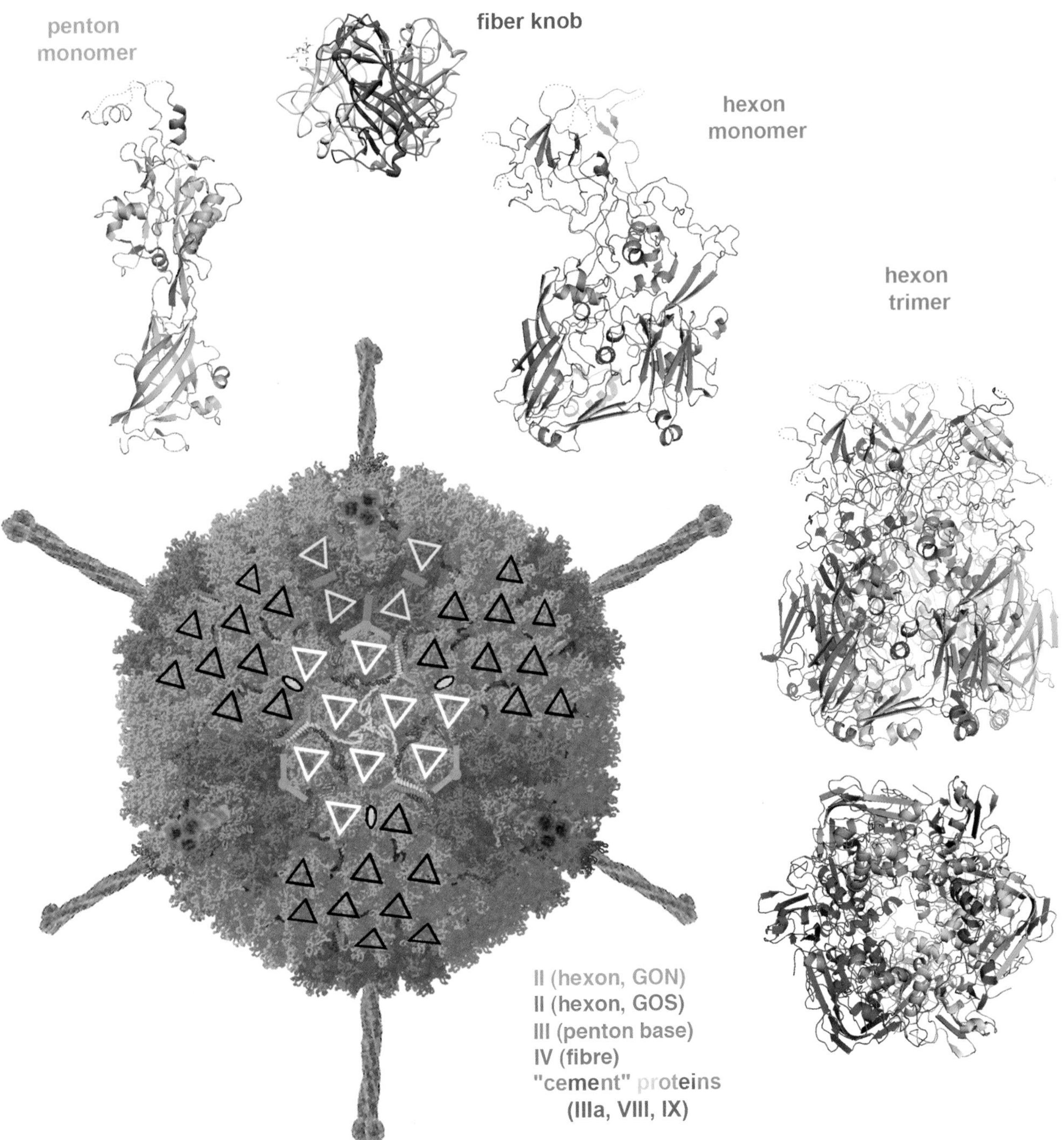

FIGURE 3.10. Adenovirus structure. A representation of the complete particle, based on a high-resolution electron cryomicroscopy (cryoEM) image reconstruction,[142] is at the **lower left**, surrounded by ribbon representations of a number of the component proteins. The view of the particle is along a threefold symmetry axis. The hexons (light and medium blue) and the pentons (brown) lie on vertices of a T = 25 icosahedral lattice, but the hexons are actually trimers with a pseudohexameric character, as illustrated by the "bottom view" (as if from the particle interior) at the **lower right**. Three species of so-called cement proteins (IIIa, VIII, and IX) retain the hexons and pentons in the shell and determine its fixed geometry. One of them (various chains in red, dark blue, yellow, and light green) fits into the crevices between the hexons and organizes them into *groups of nine* (GON)—as shown by the sets of white and black triangles on the hexon surfaces. The other two are on the inner surface of the hexon–penton shell and cement five "peripentonal" hexons and the penton base into a *group of six* (GOS); locations of some of them are shown here simply as magenta and orange lines, because they are not visible from the outside of the particle. The trimeric fibers project from each penton base, with a receptor-binding knob **(top of figure)** at their tip. Each hexon monomer (see red ribbon diagram, **upper right**) has two jelly-roll β-barrels, in parallel orientation, imparting a pseudohexagonal character to the trimer. The penton base **(upper left)** has a single β-jelly roll. (Image reconstruction courtesy Z. H. Zhou; see also Harrison[103]).

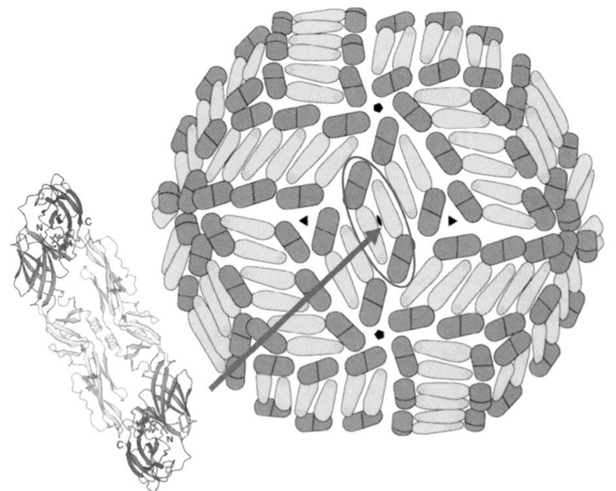

FIGURE 3.11. Organization of a flavivirus particle. Ninety dimers of the E protein tile the surface as shown. E is an elongated, three-domain protein **(lower left)**, oriented with its long axis parallel to the surface of the virion. At the tip of domain II (yellow) is a hydrophobic *fusion loop* (orange, shown also as an asterisk on the larger schematic).

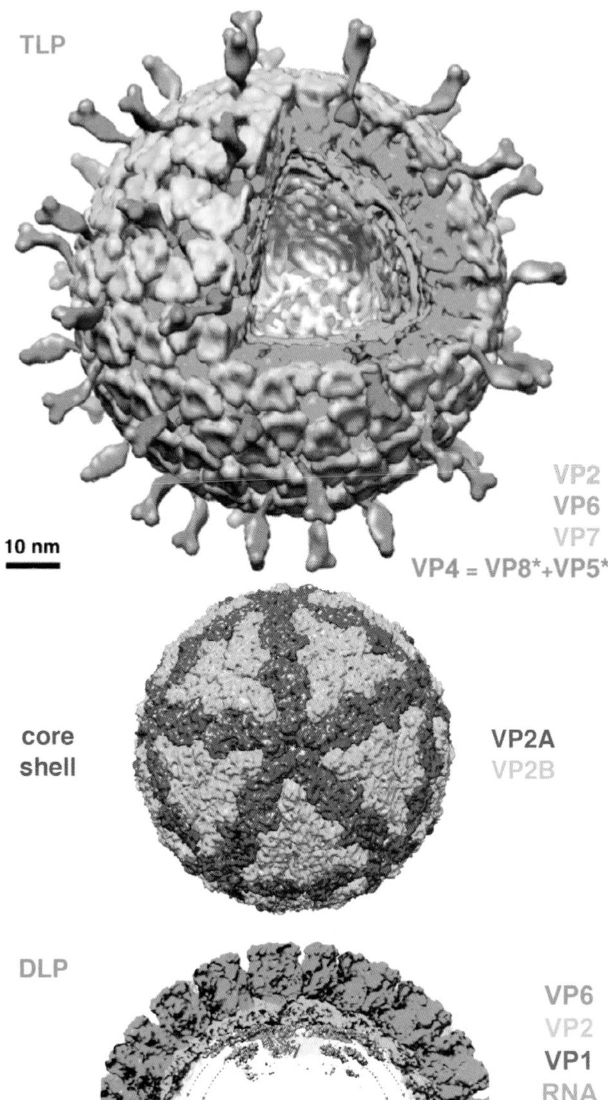

FIGURE 3.12. Molecular organization of a rotavirus particle, illustrating the multiple concentric protein shells.[42,202,259] The complete virion **(top)** or *triple-layered particle* (TLP) has an outer layer composed of VP7 (yellow) and VP4 (red: cleaved during maturation into two parts, VP8* and VP5*, which remain associated). The *double-layered particle* or DLP **(bottom)** has a core shell **(center)** with 120 VP2 subunits (blue) surrounded by a layer of 290 VP6 trimers (green) in a T = 13 icosahedral lattice. The VP6 layer in turn dictates the organization of the VP7 layer, which clamps into place 60 VP4 trimers projecting from a particular set of six-coordinated positions. The locations of the VP1 polymerase (purple, ribbon representation)[72] and of tightly wound, double-stranded RNA (dsRNA) (magenta)[151] are also shown in the bottom cutaway. The icosahedrally symmetric core shell has 120 VP2 subunits in two sets (designated A and B, dark blue and light blue, respectively), with completely nonequivalent contacts and only slightly different conformations. This type of shell is characteristic of many groups of dsRNA viruses.

is so shaped that two dimers can fill a similar (smaller) rhombic unit; the icosahedral twofold lies between the two dimers, and the complete coat contains 120 subunits.[66] Recombinant brome mosaic virus coat-protein dimer, expressed in yeast cells, packs in a closely related way when it assembles into 120-subunit virus-like particles.[126]

The arrangement of 120 copies of the inner- (core-) shell protein in double-stranded RNA (dsRNA) viruses is a particularly striking example of nonequivalent packing (Fig. 3.12). There are two completely distinct environments for this protein (designated A and B in Fig. 3.12, center): two is not a permitted triangulation number, and quasiequivalent packing of 120 proteins in an icosahedral array is not possible. The amino acid side chains on the lateral surface of the core-shell protein have different partners, depending on the interface in which they lie. The distortion of the subunit itself, when the two environments are compared, is quite small.

Frameworks and Scaffolds

The protein subunits of TBSV or picornaviruses have extended N- or C-terminal arms augmenting a central jelly-roll β-barrel. These arms are essential for building a stable coat. They form an internal framework, such as the one illustrated for TBSV in Figure 3.9. In TBSV, the *assembly unit*—the oligomer of the coat subunit that forms spontaneously in solution (and by inference, in the cell following its synthesis)—is a dimer, which can have two conformations: an "A/B" dimer, with disordered N-terminal arms, and a "C/C" dimer, with folded arms.[105] The local curvature of those two conformations is different, and the framework of C/C arms fixes the overall diameter of the particle. Removal of the N-terminal arms of TBSV-like subunits leads to self-assembly of a small, 60-subunit icosahedrally symmetric particle that cannot package RNA.[88] That is, without the arms, there is no mechanism for a conformational switch.

In the papilloma- and polyomaviruses, N- and C-terminal extensions (principally the latter) of the subunit globular domains tie together the pentameric building blocks, which have almost no contacts except through these extensions (Fig. 3.13).[139,246] Flexibility of the arms allows formation of the different kinds of contacts required to surround a pentamer with six other pentamers (i.e., to position a pentamer at the

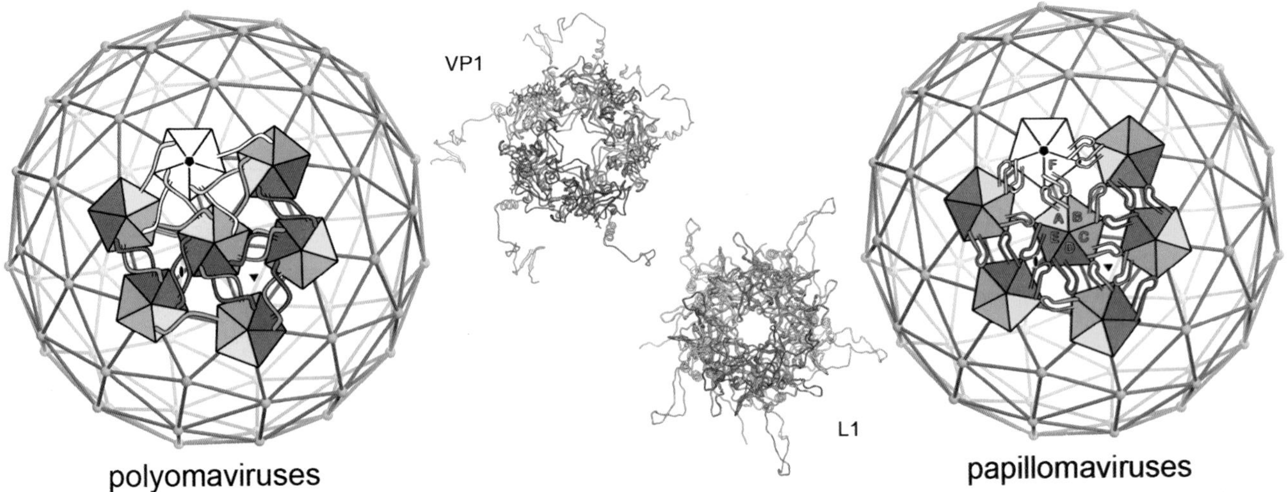

FIGURE 3.13. Packing of pentamers in the capsids of polyoma- and papillomaviruses. The ribbon diagrams in the center show pentamers of VP1 (polyomaviruses) and L1 (papillomaviruses), viewed from their outward-facing surfaces. Note the C-terminal arms of the subunits, which extend away from the pentamers in VP1 but loop back to it in L1. The schematic diagrams to the left and right illustrate the packing of these pentamers in the virion shell. The framework shows a T = 7 icosahedral lattice; VP1 or L1 pentamers are centered on both six- and five-coordinated positions.

six- as well as at the five-coordinated vertices of a T = 7 subtriangulated icosahedral lattice). The C-terminal arms emanate from one pentamer and dock into another. The way they dock is the same for all 360 arms, with identical interactions locking them in place; their configurations differ, however, between the point at which they emerge from the globular domain of their subunit of origin and the point at which they dock into their target subunit.

Larger and more complex structures, such as adenoviruses, have separate framework proteins. The principal outer-shell components of adenoviruses are *hexons* (trimers of a subunit with two similar jelly-roll β-barrel domains) and *pentons* (pentamers of a subunit with a single jelly-roll β-barrel domain); a set of additional proteins cement the structure together and determine its size (Fig. 3.10).[80,214,215] The elaborate interaction patterns of these *cement* proteins stabilize a *group of nine* hexons, centered on the icosahedral threefold axis, and a *group of six* (five hexons and a penton), centered on the icosahedral fivefold axis.[134,142] The structure of an adenovirus-like bacteriophage, PRD1,[16] shows a somewhat simpler size-determining and stabilizing framework: a *tape-measure protein* extends from the penton toward the icosahedral twofold axis, where it interacts with an identical protein running toward it from the twofold-related penton (Fig. 3.14).[2] Unlike adenoviruses, PRD1 has a lipid-bilayer membrane between the P3 layer and the internally coiled DNA.[11,49]

During assembly of the heads of most double-stranded DNA (dsDNA) bacteriophages, an internal scaffold protein directs formation of a *prohead*.[33] Signals related to initiation of DNA packaging trigger release and recycling (P22) or degradation (T4) of the scaffold, accompanied by a reorganization and expansion of the head (Fig. 3.15A,B).[68,119] DNA is pumped into the empty head until it reaches a tightly coiled state, as illustrated in Figure 3.15C.[69,70,211] In these examples, *scaffold* is a good description of the internal protein, because it is removed once the structure is complete.

The fundamental principle embodied in all the various structures just described is one of mass production. One or more standard building blocks assemble into the larger structure. In simple (T = 1) cases, such as the parvoviruses and picornaviruses, a repeating set of identical interactions determines the final structure. Even in many of these cases, however, extended arms form an interconnecting framework. In more elaborate cases, framework elements, either permanent or transient, ensure a unique outcome.

Elongated Shells

The examples in Figure 3.16 illustrate elongated particles with caps at either end. In many of the dsDNA bacteriophages, the shell looks like a familiar icosahedral design at the poles. As the lattice approaches the equator, however, the regular interspersion of fivefolds and local sixfolds gives way to local sixfolds only, so that there is a tubular region around the middle of the particle (Fig. 3.16A–C).[224] The tubular region can be of varying extent; in extreme cases, it can be much longer than the caps themselves. A further variation on this theme is found in the shells formed by the CA fragment of the lentivirus Gag protein. Conical structures seen within HIV-1 particles have been shown to be based on the sort of arrangement shown in Figure 3.16D, where one cap has more than six fivefolds and the other has less, so that the diameters of the two caps are different.[83] (Note that if there are only sixfold and fivefold vertices in a closed surface lattice, there will always be exactly 12 of the latter.)

Multishelled Particles

Most dsRNA viruses have a genuinely multishelled icosahedral organization, with some common features and some variation from group to group (see Chapters 44–46). In virions of the mammalian dsRNA virus groups (reoviruses, rotaviruses, and orbiviruses), the innermost protein shell contains 120 copies of

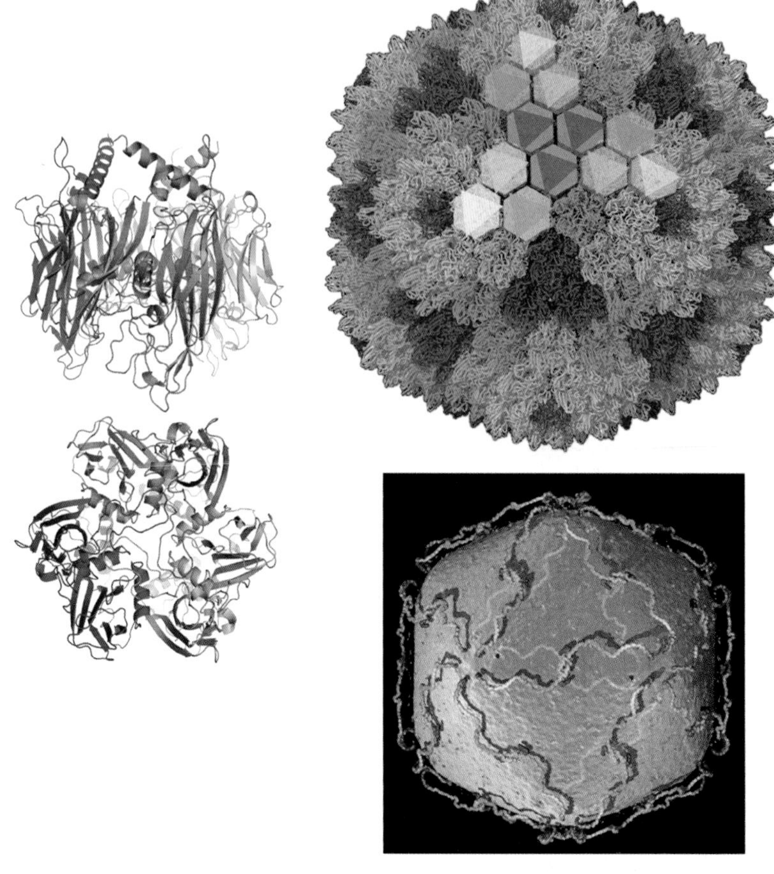

FIGURE 3.14. Bacteriophage PRD1. Left: Side and bottom views of the *hexon* protein, P3. The colors correspond to those in the ribbon diagrams of the adenovirus hexon trimer in Figure 3.10. Like the adenovirus hexon, P3 has two jelly-roll β-barrels, but the loops that project outward are much less elaborate.[16] (The variable adenovirus hexon loops probably evolved as a means of immune evasion, not relevant for a bacteriophage.) The image on the **upper right**, based on a crystal structure of the intact phage particle,[2] is a view along a twofold axis. One threefold set of P3 trimers is highlighted by triangles. The pentons (P31) are in red. At the **lower right** is a view with the outer layer stripped away, to show the extended *tape-measure* protein, P30, which helps determine the size of the shell, and the lipid bilayer just beneath it. There are 60 copies of P30; each chain extends from a twofold axis (N-terminal end, blue) to the inner surface of a penton (C-terminal end, red). At the twofold axis, one P30 associates with a second, twofold-related P30, which projects toward the opposite icosahedral vertex. (Courtesy D. Stuart, Oxford University.)

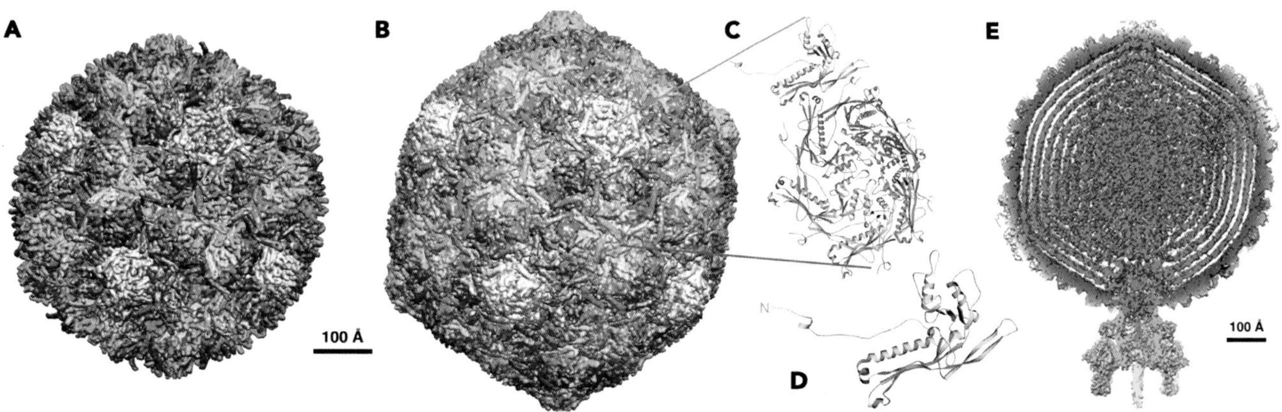

FIGURE 3.15. Capsid reorganization and DNA packaging in tailed bacteriophages.[119] **A:** Surface of the HK97 procapsid. The surface organization is a locally distorted T = 7 arrangement, with fivefold symmetric association of the subunit at the fivefold positions (beige) but a skewed arrangement in the rings of six subunits that surround a local six-coordinated position (colored in magenta, blue, red, green, yellow, and cyan, in clockwise order).[53] An N-terminal extension of the head subunit is the scaffold for prohead assembly; its cleavage by a co-assembled protease triggers rearrangement of the subunits into the expanded, thinner, more angular shell illustrated in **B**.[65] **B:** Capsid (head) of the mature HK97 particle; molecular surface, based on crystallographic model, colored as in **A**.[242] This view is oriented so that a fivefold axis is vertical. The image is derived from the structure of an empty capsid with 420 subunits in a T = 7 icosahedral lattice. In a wild-type bacteriophage particle, one of the rings of five subunits is replaced with a portal protein connected to a tail (see E). **C:** Expanded view in ribbon representation of one icosahedral asymmetric unit (i.e., one of the five subunits in the pentameric ring and one each of the quasiequivalent subunits in the hexameric ring). All subunits are chemically identical. In HK97, but not in many related bacteriophages, an intersubunit isopeptide bond, which forms during maturation, crosslinks the entire coat.[65] **D:** A further enlarged view of a single, 31-kD subunit. The 105-residue N-terminal extension that functions as an assembly scaffold is indicated schematically by a dotted line. **E:** Cutaway representation of a three-dimensional electron cryomicroscopy (cryoEM) image reconstruction of bacteriophage P22. Its assembly is formally similar to that of HK97, but there is a distinct, recycled scaffold protein[33] and no covalent crosslinking of the head.[173] The packaged DNA (green) winds tightly around an internal extension of the portal protein (red).[169,222] The axis of DNA winding is vertical in this view; averaging of many particles in the reconstruction produces concentric shells of density, because the exact register of the DNA coils varies from particle to particle. (Images in **A–D** from VIrus Particle ExploreR [VIPERdb] Web Site, http://viperdb.scripps.edu/.)

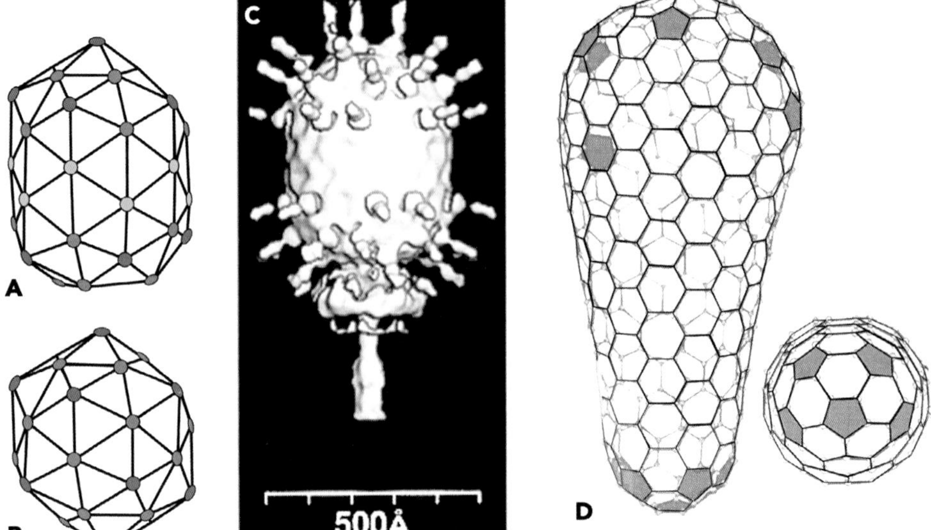

FIGURE 3.16. Elongated shells. A–C: Bacteriophage ϕ29.[224] The surface lattice of the φ 29 capsid **(A)** has the equivalent of a T = 3 icosahedral cap **(B)** at either pole with an equatorial insertion of two rows of six-coordinated positions (i.e., six, locally sixfold-related, coat-protein subunits). The blue dots are at five-coordinated positions (five, locally fivefold-related, coat-protein subunits); the red dots are at the six-coordinated positions of a T = 3 lattice in the cap; the orange dots are at the inserted six-coordinated positions. The cap at the "south pole" is further modified by replacement of the axial pentameric cluster of coat subunits with the collar and tail structure, as shown in the surface view in **C. D:** The conical structure of the mature capsid of HIV-1.[83] The capsid subunit, CA, cleaved from the Gag precursor, forms a structure with two unequal caps, one with seven five-coordinated positions and one with five. In the former, the five-coordinated positions have more intervening six-coordinated lattice points than in the latter, so that the radius of the one is larger than the radius of the other. The shaft of six-coordinated positions is wrapped in such a way that a circumference includes increasing numbers of subunits as one traces from the "bottom" to the "top" of the conical capsid, as illustrated here. The two caps have a five-coordinated lattice point at the apex, but immediately deviate from an icosahedral arrangement, as shown in the end-on view of the lower cap **(bottom left)**.

a large, rather plate-like protein[96,151,186] (Fig. 3.12). Surrounding the inner shell is a second characteristic layer. In most cases, it contains 780 copies of a trimeric protein with a radially directed jelly-roll β-barrel and inwardly directed N- and C-termini, which together form an extensive and largely α-helical "base" domain.[95,140,149] This second layer corresponds closely to a "classical," quasiequivalently packed, T = 13 icosahedral shell—all the interactions between adjacent trimers are variations on the same set of contacts.

Various elaborations and simplifications of the two-layer design just described differentiate the families of dsRNA viruses. For example, in the reoviruses, the T = 13 layer has gaps, through which pentameric "turrets" of yet another protein, anchored on the inner shell, project; only 600 of the potential 780 subunits are actually present.[27,64,186] The birnaviruses lack the 120-subunit layer altogether and have instead 780 copies of a single major capsid protein, with a shell domain that resembles those of plant and insect viruses and a trimer-clustered projecting domain that resembles the jelly-roll β-barrel in the T = 13 shell of rotaviruses and orbiviruses.[54] The T = 13 packing of the shell domain so closely recalls that of its counterparts in T = 3 and T = 4 positive-strand RNA virus structures that a bridge between the two families seems plausible. Similarities in the RNA-dependent RNA polymerases of these viruses also suggest some common ancestry. The dsRNA bacteriophages such as φ6 contain the 120-subunit, inner-shell layer and a fenestrated, T = 13 layer (rather like reoviruses), contained within a lipid-bilayer membrane.[27,112,114,236]

Rearrangements in Surface Lattices

Icosahedral surface lattices can undergo rearrangements, which preserve the overall symmetry of the structure but change the pattern of specific intersubunit contacts. There can be an accompanying change in the diameter of the shell. These rearrangements are cooperative—that is, they occur more or less simultaneously across the whole structure. As illustrated in Figure 3.14, when dsDNA bacteriophages such as P22 insert their genomic DNA into a preformed prohead, the outer shell of the prohead expands as its subunits shift around to form the mature structure.[33,53,117,133] Another well-characterized example is expansion of the T = 3 plant viruses, which occurs when the calcium ions that stabilize a particular set of subunit interfaces are removed[190] (Fig. 3.17). This swelling is believed to be the first step in disassembly; plant viruses are injected by their vectors directly into the cytoplasm of the recipient cell, where they are exposed to a low Ca^{2+} environment. A similar, but transient, expansion occurs when poliovirus binds its receptor.[15] In both the T = 3 plant viruses and the picornaviruses, internally directed "arms" of the protein subunits move outward from the interior as expansion creates gaps in the shell. Exposure of the arms may be part of the uncoating process in the case of the plant viruses or of the penetration

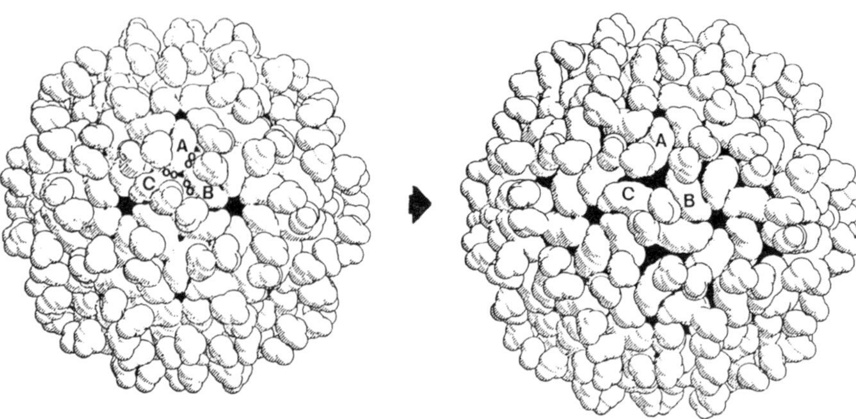

FIGURE 3.17. Expansion of tomato bushy stunt virus (TBSV).[190] The mature, compact particle **(upper left)** expands when Ca^{2+} ions (small circles) are removed. The expanded form **(upper right)** is reached by a smooth transition, in which many of the intersubunit contacts are conserved. The contacts that included the ions in the compact state have separated substantially, creating a fenestrated shell.

process in the case of the picornaviruses. Cooperativity of these rearrangements implies that a few points of inhibition can prevent the change. For example, only a few intersubunit crosslinks from bound neutralizing antibodies are sufficient to block infection by a picornavirus particle.[71] The same may be true of small molecules that inhibit the subunit conformational changes needed for the receptor-triggered expansion of picornaviruses.[8,177,212]

Helical surface lattices can also rearrange without dissociating. Contraction of bacteriophage tail sheaths is a good example.

Two Recurring Globular Domains in Icosahedral Capsid Proteins

The icosahedrally symmetric shells of nearly all well-characterized, nonenveloped viruses contain one of two types of globular domain. (The known exceptions at the time of writing this chapter are the RNA bacteriophages—R17, Qβ, and their relatives[229]—and the dsRNA picobirnaviruses.[66]) One is the jelly-roll β-barrel in viruses of animals and plants, which we have described in various examples of viruses of animals and plants; it is also the principal component of icosahedral ssDNA bacteriophage capsids (e.g., ϕX174).[152] The various ways this module can form a coat are quite different, of course, and we have emphasized earlier the importance of framework components (either as extensions of the polypeptide chain of the β-barrel or as separate protein species) in directing or regulating coat assembly. What sort of evolutionary parsimony resulted in such widespread appearance of a single kind of protein module is not evident. Viruses can jump from plants to insects and from insects to vertebrates, so the recurrence of the jelly-roll β-barrel is unlikely to reflect a common origin for all these viruses that antedates host divergence, but rather the result of more recent selection and genetic exchange. Cellular fusion proteins acquired from viral fusion proteins through retrotransposons illustrate one way in which such exchange can occur.

Figure 3.14 shows the second basic building block, discovered initially in the coat of dsDNA bacteriophages such as HK97 and subsequently found in most other dsDNA bacteriophages (T4, lambda, P22, etc.). This *HK97 fold* is also the core of the herpesvirus capsid subunit.[9] Like their bacteriophage cousins, herpesviruses pump their genome DNA into a preformed shell through a specialized icosahedral vertex and a dodecameric *portal protein*.[39,163,164] Adenoviruses, and probably their bacteriophage cousins like PRD1, with hexon-like capsid subunits, are also thought to insert DNA into a preassembled empty capsid, but the motors that effect the insertion seem to be different from those in the herpesviruses.[113,170,256,257] Thus, the structures of the coat proteins of two major classes of dsDNA viruses appear to correlate with the machinery by which members of each of these classes package DNA.

SELF-ASSEMBLY AND CLEAVAGE STEPS

Some of the simplest virus particles can assemble spontaneously from their dissociated or recombinant components, in the absence of any further modifications or scaffolds. These particles are said to *self-assemble,* because they do not require additional activities (encoded either by the virus or by the host cell) to form. In an infected cell, however, host chaperones, such as Hsc70 and its paralogs, may enhance efficiency of subunit folding or subunit assembly, even when they are not absolutely essential.

Most viruses, and nearly all viruses that infect animal cells, cannot reassemble from dissociated particles, because one or more irreversible steps intervene in forming the mature, infections virion. The picornaviruses, already described, illustrate one kind of irreversible step. In an infected cell, the principal structural proteins are cleaved from a polyprotein precursor (by a viral protease) before particle assembly, but one final, autocatalytic cleavage step occurs after assembly—the scission of a peptide bond between VP4 and VP2 (see Chapter 16 and caption to Fig. 3.7). The cleavage depends on the three-dimensional arrangement of the scissile bond, as found in a newly assembled precursor particle. Rearrangements of parts of the subunits following the cleavage stabilize the now mature, infectious virion. Proteolytic cleavages by cellular or extracellular host proteases are critical steps in the maturation of many types of virus particles, even when processing of a precursor polyprotein is not involved. For example, many of the surface glycoproteins that facilitate membrane fusion during entry of enveloped viruses require activation by a furin-like protease late in the secretory pathway.

Specific, postassembly proteolytic cleavage usually has two consequences. First, as in poliovirus or many viral fusion proteins (see later), it leads to a local rearrangement of polypeptide chains that stabilizes the structure. Second, it allows the structure to undergo a much larger reorganization when "triggered" by binding of a specific ligand. Thus, when a mature poliovirus particle binds its receptor, an expansion occurs that allows VP4 to escape and to interact with adjacent membrane—a critical first step for translocating the particle (or its genome) from an endocytic compartment into the cytosol.[21,100,157] Likewise, many fusion proteins of enveloped viruses undergo large-scale, fusion-promoting conformational changes when they bind protons in acidic endosomes—but again, only if the critical cleavage has occurred.[209] In physicochemical terms, the cleaved structure is *metastable:* a large kinetic barrier separates it from its true energy minimum. The barrier can be so large that the virus remains infectious for many weeks or months. Ligand binding (receptors, protons, etc.) lowers the kinetic barrier, leading to a rapid conformational rearrangement, coupled in most cases to an important step in viral entry.

GENOME PACKAGING

Incorporation of viral nucleic acid must be specific, but it must also be independent of most of the base sequence of the genome. Therefore, viral genomes generally have a *packaging signal*—a short sequence or set of sequences that directs encapsidation. Recognition of the packaging signal depends on the nature of the genome and on the complexity of the assembly mechanism. In many cases, there is a direct interaction between the packaging signal and the capsid protein. Some complex viruses insert genomic nucleic acid into a preformed shell, and genome recognition is a property of the packaging system. If replication and packaging are closely coupled, as they are in picornaviruses,[168] flaviviruses,[121] and at least some RNA plant viruses,[5] a specific packaging signal may be less essential.

Positive-Strand RNA Genomes

Viruses with ssRNA genomes (e.g., most icosahedral plant viruses; picornaviruses; alphaviruses; flaviviruses) require no definite overall secondary or tertiary fold for the genomic RNA, aside from the restriction that it fit within the shell. This restriction is actually quite severe, and the RNA is packed very tightly, approximating the density of RNA in crystals.[160] Even random-sequence RNA contains about 60% to 70% of its nucleotides in base-paired stems,[91] and to fit efficiently within the interior of a capsid, these RNA stems must pack tangentially, not radially, with many of the stems in contact with the inward-facing surface of the shell. Such packing can be achieved by assembly around the RNA, without definite capsid–RNA interactions, other than those of a few subunits with a packaging signal (if present). In some viruses, segments of partially ordered RNA can be detected, tucked into shallow grooves on the inner capsid surface.[44,74] The ordered positions of these segments probably result just from the shapes of the grooves and the possible structures that a tightly packed polynucleotide chain can adopt; there do not appear to be any base-specific contacts.

In a few cases, we know the molecular details of RNA packaging-signal recognition. A translational regulatory sequence that is probably also the packaging signal of RNA bacteriophages such as MS2 and R17 folds into a stem-loop structure (Fig. 3.18A), recognized by a dimer of the coat protein (the assembly unit for this $T = 3$ particle).[30,230,231] Bases in the loop and a looped-out base in the stem fit into a groove on the inward-facing surface of the subunit dimer; conserved bases make defined protein contacts.

Many nonenveloped, positive-stranded RNA viruses of eukaryotes recognize their genomic RNA, not through a groove-like site on the protein, but rather through a flexibly extended, positively charged protein arm, often at the N-terminus of the coat protein. There is an interaction of this kind between the coat protein of alfalfa mosaic virus and a 3′-terminal segment of RNA.[99] A bound coat-protein dimer is essential for replication—probably to recruit the RNA-dependent RNA polymerase. The same interaction is also likely to initiate packaging. The dimer contacts a pair of tandem RNA hairpins through a 26-residue, N-terminal arm. The two arms and the two RNA stem loops fold together into a well-defined structure, cross-strutted by base pairing between conserved AUCG sequences that follow each stem (Fig. 3.18B). There are six such stem loops in the 3′ segment of the viral genome; it is possible that binding of three coat-protein dimers initiates shell assembly.

The enveloped alphaviruses also have a multi-stem-loop packaging signal, recognized (with structural details not yet determined) by an extended N-terminal arm of the nucleocapsid subunit.[122] There appears to be some redundancy in the stem loops, all of which contain a GGG trinucleotide in the loop, as deletion of several of the eight stem loops does not compromise the efficiency of RNA packaging and virion assembly.

Retroviral packaging signals, known as *psi* sequences, are recognized by the nucleocapsid (NC) domain of the Gag protein. The HIV-1 psi element has a stem-loop structure that associates with two *zinc-knuckle* modules in HIV-1 NC[60] (Fig. 3.18C). The two zinc modules are flexibly linked in unbound NC, but they adopt a defined, three-dimensional organization in complex with the RNA. Thus, the structure of the RNA imparts additional order to the protein element with which it binds (just as in alfalfa mosaic virus).

Assembly of helical structures requires unwinding of any base-paired stems in the RNA genome being packaged. TMV has evolved an assembly-driven helix-breaking feature into its packaging pathway. Viral assembly begins at an internal origin sequence, about 1 kb from the 3′ end of the genome.[227,261] A 75-base sequence containing a presumptive stem-loop structure is sufficient to initiate specific encapsidation (Fig. 3.18D), which proceeds by a mechanism that requires the 5′ end of the RNA to be drawn through a channel along the axis of the assembling particle.[28]

The mechanism of overall condensation of a viral genome is in general distinct from the specific recognition just discussed, unless, as in TMV, there is a regular, repeated interaction between coat protein and genomic RNA. There are various strategies for neutralizing the net negative charge on the nucleic acid. Those icosahedral viruses with inwardly projecting, positively charged arms use most of their arms for nonspecific interactions with RNA and only a few for specific recognition. In the picornaviruses, polyamines are incorporated to achieve charge neutralization.

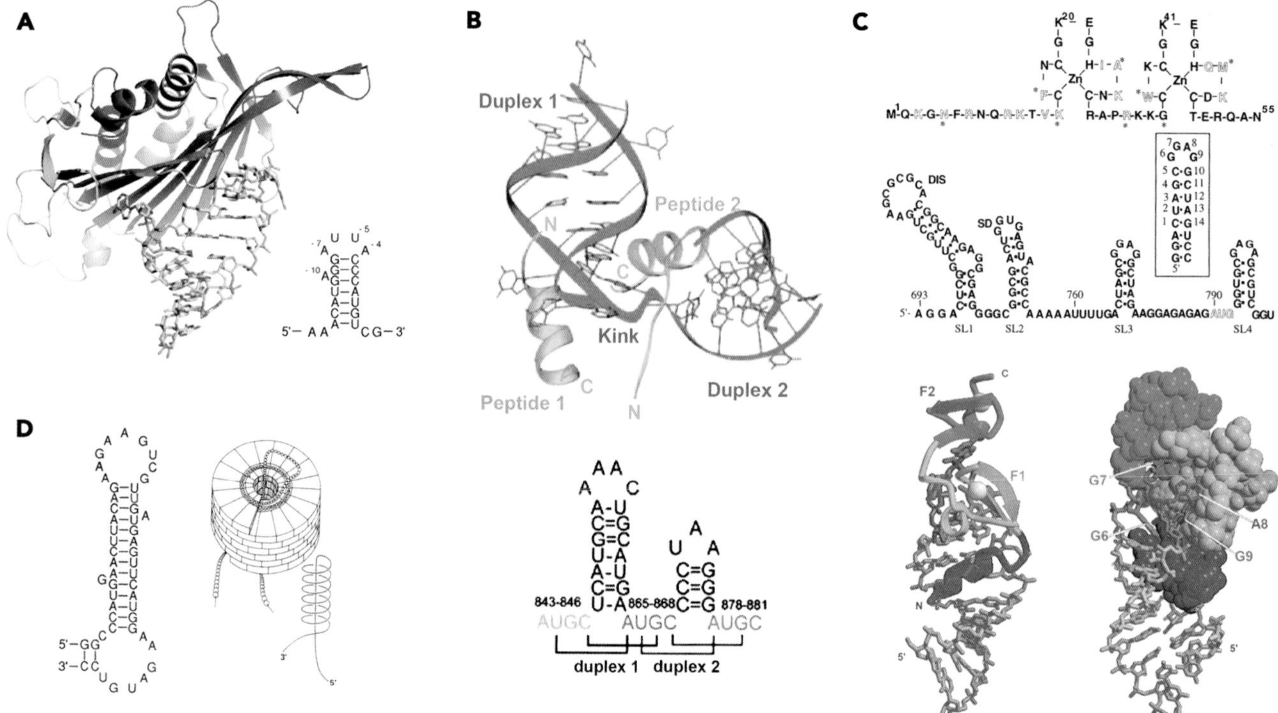

FIGURE 3.18. Various modes of single-stranded RNA (ssRNA) recognition and packaging. A: RNA bacteriophage. A stem-loop (sequence shown as inset) packs against the inward-facing surface of a protein-subunit dimer; there are specific contacts between residues in the protein and four unpaired bases (-4, -5, -7, -10). **B:** Alfalfa mosaic virus. A folded, stem-loop, RNA structure (green) is a docking site for two N-terminal subunit arms (gold). The arms are unstructured until they associate with the RNA. **C:** HIV-1. Two *zinc-knuckle* domains (labeled F1 and F2 in the ribbon representation at the **lower left**), near the C-terminal end of the Gag polyprotein (sequences shown at the **top**), bind a stem-loop structure in the packaging signal of the genomic RNA **(center and bottom)**. Purine bases that have conserved stacking interactions are labeled in the surface representation at the **lower right. D:** Tobacco mosaic virus.[28,227,261] The sequence at which RNA packaging initiates, shown on the **left**, is roughly 500 nucleotides from the 3′ end of the genome, and assembly of the helical particle proceeds by addition of subunits at one end of the growing helix, drawing the 5′ end up through the center of the particle, as shown on the **right**. Coating of the 3′ overhang proceeds more slowly at the other end of the particle. (**A** adapted from Valegard K, Murray JB, Stonehouse NJ, et al. The three-dimensional structures of two complexes between recombinant MS2 capsids and RNA operator fragments reveal sequence-specific protein-RNA interactions. *J Mol Biol* 1997;270:724–738. **B** modified from Guogas LM, Filman DJ, Hogle JM, et al. Cofolding organizes alfalfa mosaic virus RNA and coat protein for replication. *Science* 2004;306:2108–2111.) **C** adapted from De Guzman RN, Wu ZR, Stalling CC, et al. Structure of the HIV-1 nucleocapsid protein bound to the SL3 psi-RNA recognition element. *Science* 1998;279:384–388.

dsDNA Genomes

The best-understood dsDNA packaging mechanisms are those of the tailed bacteriophages.[97] DNA inserts into a preformed prohead, from which the scaffold has been lost by triggered release or by proteolysis.[14,33] Removal of the scaffold leads in most cases to a substantial expansion of the head, accomplished through conformational rearrangements in the major capsid protein.[68,119] The head itself is either an isometric icosahedral shell (e.g., lambda, P22, or HK97; Fig. 3.15) or a prolate one (e.g., T4 or ϕ29; Fig. 3.16). In the latter cases, the scaffold protein directs the elongation. DNA packaging depends on adenosine triphosphatase (ATP) hydrolysis by a multicomponent motor. The *connector* or *portal protein,* which connects head to tail in the completed particle, is part of the motor complex, but the ATPase itself is shed from the prohead after DNA packaging is complete.[97] The ϕ29 connector is a dodecameric ring attached at a fivefold symmetric vertex.[207] The substantial internal pressure of the packaged DNA[211] may help drive injection into a target bacterium.

Various models have been proposed for the coupling of ATP hydrolysis by the five ATPase subunits that surround the connector with the concomitant transport of DNA into the head.[1,156,207,217–219] To avoid entanglement, it is possible that the leading end of the DNA attaches to the head interior.[104] In P22, a tube-like, inward-projecting extension of the portal may also help direct coiling and prevent tangles[222]; closely related viruses lack the prominent tube, however. DNA insertion leads to formation of a tight, uniform coil (Fig. 3.15C). Because the DNA is tightly wound, the side-to-side spacing of adjacent segments is very regular; the value of this spacing is determined by the precise volume of the head and by the length of the inserted genome.[69] Viruses such as bacteriophage lambda that replicate their DNA in a rolling-circle mode couple DNA packaging with cleavage of the replicated concatemer. Others, such as

ϕ29, have a virally encoded protein that primes synthesis of both DNA strands and that remains attached to the ends of the encapsidated genome.

DNA packaging into herpesvirus capsids resembles the process just described for the tailed bacteriophages (see Chapter 75). Not only does the shell-forming domain of the major capsid protein appear to have the HK97 fold,[9] as described earlier, but also the portal protein, attached to a unique vertex, likewise resembles its tailed-phage counterpart.[113,164] Rolling-circle DNA replication late in infection yields a concatemer, and cleavage of the DNA into a single "head-full" accompanies encapsidation.

Adenoviruses have, near the left-hand end of their linear genome, a set of AT-rich repeats that determines DNA incorporation into virions (see Chapter 55). Virions contain about 1,000 copies of a protein (VII) with strong positive charge, and it is believed that this protein condenses the viral DNA within the virion core and that it may remain associated with the DNA after uncoating. In the adenovirus-like bacteriophage PRD1, there is a unique vertex defined by the presence of proteins required for DNA packaging and injection.[90] One of these, the ATPase, is distantly related to protein IVa2 of adenoviruses and more closely related to candidate packaging ATPases for other dsDNA viruses with internal membranes.[113]

Papovaviruses incorporate cellular histones, so that the closed, circular DNA comprises about 20 to 25 nucleosomes (see Chapters 53 and 54). This minichromosome is further condensed as the capsid assembles around it. Packaging appears to be directed by sequences in a histone-free region.

dsRNA Genomes

RNA packaging by dsRNA viruses presents several puzzles, the most important of which is selection of RNA segments (see Chapters 44–46). Reoviruses have 10 RNA segments, and rotaviruses, 11. Random incorporation would lead to a vanishingly small proportion of fully infectious particles. Moreover, the range of segment sizes is substantial, and a capsid-full of RNA accommodates just one of each size. The RNA must wind tightly into nonentangled spools to enable the many rounds of transcription of each gene segment that occur when the inner capsid particle is released into the cytoplasm of an infected cell.[223]

Some molecular details of assembly have been worked out for the dsRNA bacteriophage, φ6, and its relatives.[153,180] A procapsid assembles, into which each of the three positive-stranded RNA segments inserts sequentially, in a specific order. Minus-strand synthesis occurs inside the shell. The procapsid includes the major shell protein (similar to that of reovirus or rotavirus, Fig. 3.12), the polymerase, an ATPase, and a protein thought to serve as an assembly "clamp." One copy of the hexameric ATPase, which may be a packaging helicase analogous in function to the packaging proteins of dsDNA bacteriophages, lies at each fivefold vertex[61]; RNA insertion appears to occur at only 1 of these 12 positions, even though all are occupied by an ATPase.

Assembly of other dsRNA viruses probably exhibits some similar features, but it seems likely that the inner shell co-assembles with the polymerase and the various plus-strand RNA segments.[175] The rotavirus polymerase, VP1, recognizes a conserved sequence at the 3′ end of the plus strand (the template for dsRNA synthesis); this interaction may direct specific packaging of viral RNA.[146] VP1 requires association with the shell protein, VP2, for activity, and it is plausible to infer that one copy of VP1 and 10 copies of VP2 (together with one copy of the capping enzyme, VP3) make up the inner-core assembly unit. The ssRNA template could extend away from the incomplete particle, with dsRNA synthesis as the driving force to reel it into the shell,[82,151,174] or it could condense into the interior of the assembling shell, as in the ssRNA viruses. Packaging of the genome as ssRNA, rather than as completed dsRNA segments, has an attractive feature: the tightly wound dsRNA spools required to fit the full genome into the shell could be generated readily during synthesis[223] (Fig. 3.12). The presence of an RNA cap-binding site on the surface of the polymerase provides a mechanism for associating a particular polymerase molecule with a particular gene segment during subsequent rounds of transcription, which occurs without disassembly.[223]

Reoviruses and rotaviruses have a nonstructural protein, designated σNS and NSP2, respectively, that appears to have a role in RNA packaging. NSP2 is an octamer with a central channel that could accommodate ssRNA.[116,118,129,225] A second nonstructural protein, NSP5, appears to compete with RNA for binding to NSP2, suggesting it may have some sort of co-chaperone–like activity.[118]

The central question remains: how does packaging of the *n*th RNA segment lead to selection of segment n + 1? The most likely mechanism involves RNA–RNA recognition: for example, when the *n*th RNA has been partially packaged, a single-strand region near its trailing edge will be exposed and perhaps unwound from internal secondary structural interactions with regions already packaged. This trailing segment could then recognize some feature—base sequence or three-dimensional structure—of segment n + 1. An allosteric mechanism involving protein conformational changes has been proposed for packaging the three segments of φ6,[153] but extending such a picture to 10 or 11 distinct states seems unlikely.

Negative-Strand RNA Genomes

The nucleocapsid proteins (N) of three negative-strand RNA viruses with single-segment genomes (VSV and rabies virus, both rhabdoviruses, and borna disease virus) all have closely related structures.[4,93,197] Recombinant N proteins from VSV and rabies viruses bind nonspecific RNA from the expression host and form rings of 10 to 14 subunits, with an N-terminal arm that embraces one neighbor in the ring and a loop near the C-terminus that extends into the other neighbor. The subunits have two lobes with a groove between them that faces the center of the ring and binds the RNA—nine bases per subunit. The VSV-N ring is evidently a more tightly wound and circularized version of the helical ramp that the nucleocapsid forms in the bullet-shaped rhabdoviruses (see Fig. 3.19). Sequences at the 5′ end of the negative-strand RNA, not present in the crystal structures, participate in specific packaging, but the structures do not indicate any preferential base recognition in the RNA grooves. One possibility is that there are distinct recognition events at the 5′ end, which can contact the lateral surface of the initial N-protein subunit in the ribonucleoprotein complex (RNP), and at the 3′ end, for polymerase entry.[4] The polymerase must withdraw the RNA from the groove in the RNP.[4,93]

Influenza, like other orthomyxoviruses, has an eight-segment genome. The eight RNPs resemble rods folded back on themselves and coiled.[51] The rod lengths, from 300 to 1,200 Å,

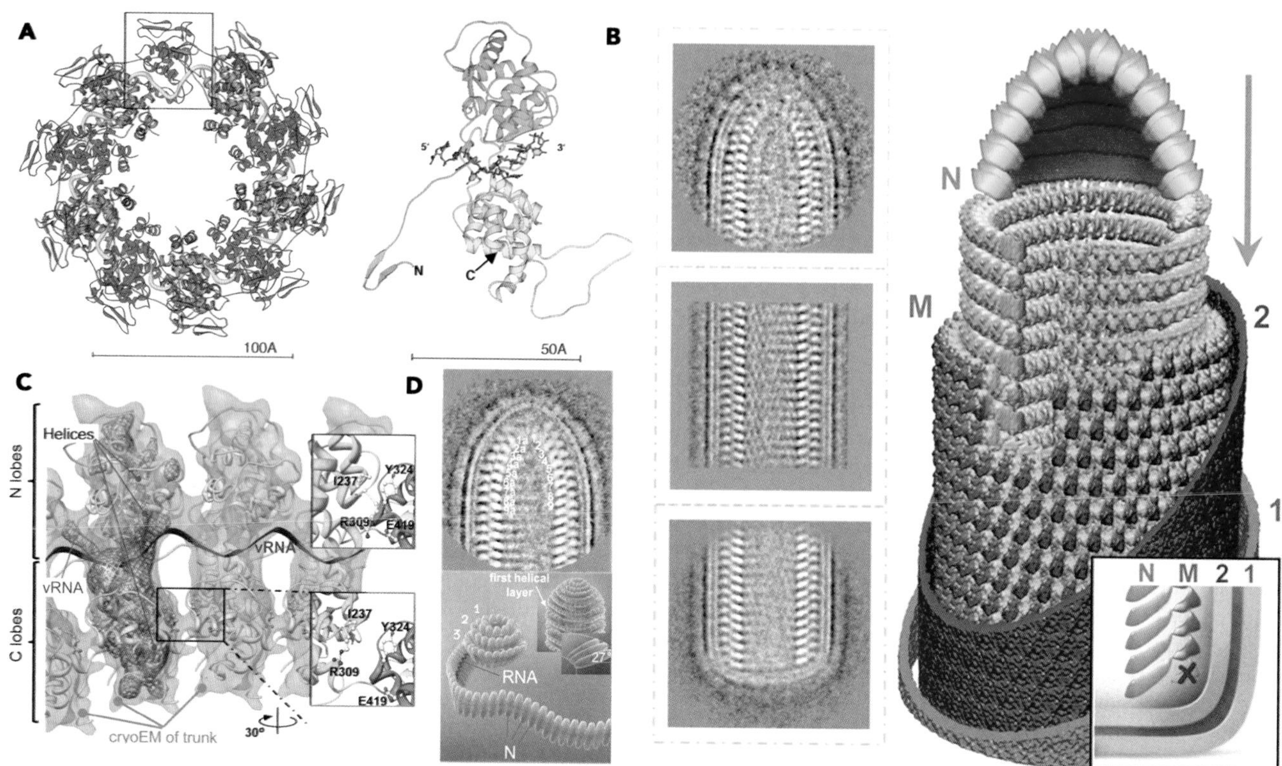

FIGURE 3.19. RNA binding and organization of the ribonucleoprotein complex (RNP) in vesicular stomatitis virus. A: Binding of RNA by N. **Left:** A ring of 10 recombinant nucleocapsid (N) protein subunits (alternating red and blue) binds a 90-nucelotide RNA segment (yellow). Recombinant N forms rings of various sizes, which take up random fragments of cellular RNA tightly enough to withstand purification. The view of the ring is from the "bottom" (C-terminal lobe) of the subunit; this lobe has been removed from one of the subunits (boxed), to show the (yellow) RNA more clearly. **Right:** One subunit from the ring, with a nine-nucleotide RNA segment in the groove between the two lobes of the protein. N- and C-terminal extensions project laterally and interact with neighboring subunits: the radius of the ring can vary, because these links are flexible. **B:** Image reconstruction, from electron cryomicroscopy (cryoEM) images (averaged projections of which are shown on the **left**), of the bullet-shaped vesicular stomatitis virus (VSV) particle. The outer glycoprotein (G) layer is not well-enough ordered to appear as discrete density in the map, but a fuzzy "halo" on the surface of the particle is evident in the projections. The nucleocapsid (green) winds into a shallow helix, guided by association with the matrix protein (M, blue), which in turn contacts the membrane (purple and magenta for the inner and outer headgroup layers, respectively). **C:** View from the inside of the RNP helix. The two insets illustrate the relationship between the subunits seen from the inside of the 10-subunit ring **(upper box)** and as they "unwrap" to form the larger-diameter helix in the virion **(lower box)**. **D:** Color-coded interpretation of the upper projection in **B**, with colors as in the surface representation in **B**, and diagram showing wrapping of the RNP into the particle. The inner diameter of the helical coil formed by the RNP is about 450 Å and the rise per turn, about 50 Å. (**A** adapted from Green TJ, Zhang X, Wertz GW, et al. Structure of the vesicular stomatitis virus nucleoprotein-RNA complex. *Science* 2006;313:357–360. **B–D** adapted from Ge P, Tsao J, Schein S, et al. Cryo-EM model of the bullet-shaped vesicular stomatitis virus. *Science* 2010;327:689–693.)

correspond to the various genome segment lengths, when coiled as described; their diameter is about 120 Å.[167] A superhelical organization of the RNP probably determines the dimensions. Partially complementary sequences in the 5′ and 3′ noncoding regions probably dictate the folded-back arrangement; sequences at either end of the coding region also contribute to specific packaging.[161] Serial transverse sections through elongated buds of the WSN strain of influenza A show eight rods, seven around one, about 120 Å in diameter, extending for variable distances from the tip of the bud toward its proximal end; the distances correspond to the lengths of the various genome segments.[167] Tomographic reconstructions of purified filamentous influenza virus particles show that this internal organization is retained in the budded particle.[29] Interfering with packaging of one segment reduces packaging of others.[161] Thus, there appears to be a sequential recognition mechanism to ensure a proper complement of genome segments, perhaps formally (although not structurally) analogous to the selection mechanism in dsRNA viruses. The RNA that forms the central element in the seven-around-one arrangement may have a particularly critical role; some evidence suggests that this segment is the one that encodes polymerase subunit PB2.[161]

The influenza N-protein, like those of the single-segment negative-strand RNA viruses, has two lobes with an RNA-binding groove between them, but the folded structures are not identical.[248] The recombinant N forms trimers in a tight association determined by a loop, toward the C-terminus of the polypeptide chain, that inserts into a neighboring subunit as two antiparallel strands. The groove likely to accept RNA faces away from the threefold axis of the trimer. The relationship

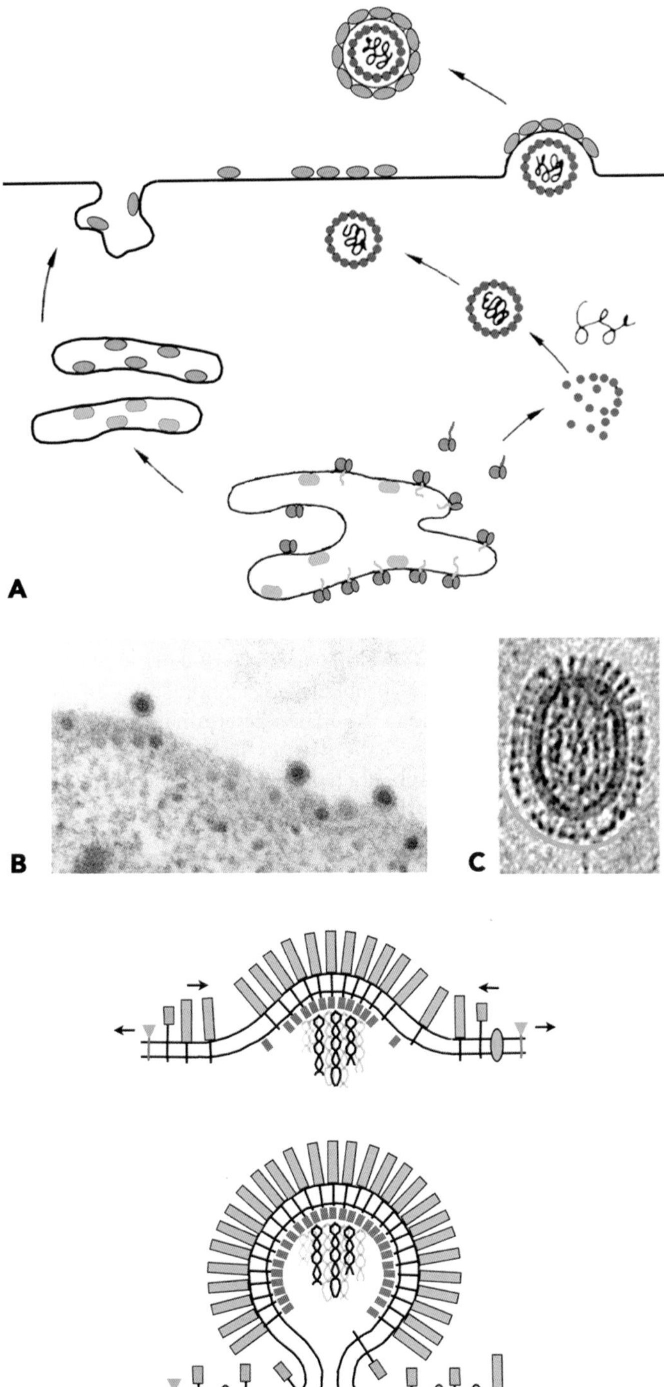

FIGURE 3.20. **Budding of enveloped viruses. A:** Schematic of alphavirus maturation and budding. The core protein, C (blue), synthesized on cytosolic ribosomes, assembles with viral RNA into T = 4 nucleocapsids. The envelope proteins, E1 and pE2 (red), synthesized on endoplasmic reticulum (ER)-bound ribosomes, mature as they pass through the ER and Golgi, and pE2 is cleaved as it passes the trans-Golgi network to the cell surface. The nucleocapsid organizes the E1-E2 heterodimers into a T = 4 lattice as the particle buds. **B:** Electron micrograph of budding Semliki Forest virus. Arrow: complete virus particle just released. Arrowhead: nucleocapsid in the cytosol. Bar = 1,000 Å. **C:** Section through a tomogram of an isolated influenza virus particle. The hemagglutinin (HA) and neuraminidase (NA) spikes, which project from the membrane bilayer, have distinct outlines, and the blue curve at the bottom of the figure illustrates that the NA concentrates at one end of the particle. The M1-protein lines the inner membrane surface; the ribonucleoprotein complexes (RNPs) pack in longitudinal orientation inside the particle. Bar = 1,000 Å. **D:** Diagram of influenza virus budding. The HA (red), NA (blue), M2 proton channel (yellow), M1 protein (purple), and eight RNPs (gray and black) co-assemble at the site of budding. Host cell proteins (green) are excluded. NA and M2 enter the particle late in the process and cluster toward one end. (**B** adapted from Sjoberg M, Garoff H. Interactions between the transmembrane segments of the alphavirus E1 and E2 proteins play a role in virus budding and fusion. *J Virol* 2003;77:3441–3450. **C** adapted from Calder LJ, Wasilewski S, Berriman JA, et al. Structural organization of a filamentous influenza A virus. *Proc Natl Acad Sci U S A* 2010;107:10685–10690.)

of the trimer configuration to N-protein interactions in the double-helical nucleocapsid has not yet been determined.

VIRAL MEMBRANES

Budding

Most enveloped viruses (except for the large and very complex poxviruses and probably some of the membrane-containing bacteriophages) acquire their membrane, a lipid bilayer with associated proteins, by budding through some cellular membrane—the plasma membrane in many cases, the endoplasmic reticulum (ER), Golgi, or nuclear membrane in others (Fig. 3.20). These viruses direct insertion of their surface glycoproteins into the relevant membrane of the cell, through the usual cellular compartmentalization pathways. The driving force for budding then comes either from interactions between cytoplasmic tails of the glycoproteins and assembling or preassembled internal structures, from lateral interactions between glycoprotein subunits, or from a combination of both. Retroviruses can bud without any glycoprotein at all: interactions between the myristoylated Gag protein and the lipid bilayer are sufficient to induce formation of a bud. Pinching off from the cell surface, or into the lumen of the ER or Golgi, appears in some cases (alphaviruses and flaviviruses) not to require a cellular pinching activity; assembly of viral components provides the force needed to distort the membrane bilayer. In many other cases, however, completion of budding requires that the virus recruit components of a cellular budding machinery.[181] In the examples that have been studied in some detail (retroviruses, especially HIV), the virus redirects to the cell surface a set of protein complexes (the ESCRT machinery) that normally function at late endosomes, where they generate pinched-off invaginations into the endosomal lumen to create *multivesicular bodies*.[85,216] The topology of viral budding from the cell surface is the same as the topology of luminal vesicle formation (away from the cytosol).

The lipids in the viral membrane derive from the cell, whereas the viral genome encodes the proteins. To a first approximation, the incorporated lipids represent a sample of those in the membrane through which the virus budded.[124] Viruses that emerge through the plasma membrane contain phospholipid and cholesterol in characteristic proportions, whereas those that emerge into the lumen of the ER contain almost no cholesterol. Cholesterol tends to increase the thickness of a bilayer by restricting free rotation about single bonds in the fatty acid chains of adjacent phospholipids.[183] The lengths of α-helical transmembrane segments in viral glycoproteins vary accordingly: from about 26 residues in flu (which buds at the cell surface) to 18 to 20 in yellow fever (which buds into the ER). Viral envelope proteins can also specify detailed specificities in lipid incorporation. For example, when present on a cell surface, the influenza virus envelope proteins (hemagglutinin [HA] and neuraminidase [NA]) associate with lipids characteristic of cholesterol-rich microdomains, and the lipid composition of the virus reflects this bias.[199,221,254] The differential lipid composition of the viral membrane may contribute to membrane scission, which is ESCRT independent.[40] The viral M2 protein, a small, tetrameric ion channel that does not partition into microdomain lipids, incorporates at the base of the bud; an amphipathic helix in M2 appears to participate in pinching off the nascent virion.[194] The N protein also incorporates selectively at the base.[29]

The two examples in Figure 3.20 illustrate features of the budding process. The structure of the nucleocapsid varies with virus type. It is a compact, spherical particle in the alphaviruses; a filamentous, helical nucleocapsid in paramyxoviruses and rhabdoviruses; and a multisegmented helical nucleocapsid in the orthomyxoviruses. The viral glycoproteins are anchored in the cellular membrane by a transmembrane hydrophobic segment (in some cases, a hydrophobic hairpin), and there is a small cytoplasmic domain. In alphaviruses (Fig. 3.20A), a core particle (nucleocapsid) assembles independently in the cytoplasm. Interactions between the core and the cytoplasmic tail of the glycoproteins then determine the location of budding. Lateral interactions of the glycoproteins probably assist the budding process. In orthomyxoviruses such as influenza (Fig. 3.20C), the M (*matrix*) protein associates with the nucleocapsid segments and with the inner face of the membrane, presumably by interaction with the cytoplasmic domains of the glycoproteins. M organizes both the glycoproteins and the nucleocapsids. Budding then proceeds by co-assembly of structures on both surfaces of the membrane. The two patterns of budding shown in Figure 3.20 are not fundamentally different; rather, they depend on the relative strength of core–core, envelope–envelope, and core–envelope contacts. In at least one case, a mutation has been shown to convert budding from one mode to the other.[188] Absolute specificity is sometimes violated in viral budding, leading to cases of phenotypic mixing, in which, for example, simian virus type 5 (SV5) glycoproteins can be found in the membrane of VSV. HIV buds with only a few copies of its glycoprotein on the virion surface, and some host–cell membrane proteins tend to incorporate nonspecifically into the particle.

The simplest enveloped virus particles—those of the alphaviruses and the flaviviruses—are icosahedrally symmetric.[45,128,179,232,233] In these positive-strand RNA viruses, one-to-one interactions between the envelope glycoprotein and the nucleocapsid subunit appear to ensure coherence between external and internal structures (Figs. 3.20A and 3.21). The larger, negative-strand RNA bunyaviruses also have an icosahedrally symmetric envelope (a T = 12 lattice), but their internal structures are probably not icosahedrally organized, and the outer lattice is the major determinant of symmetry and stability.[234] The rhabdoviruses have a helically organized shaft with a (probably hemi-icosahedral) cap at one end (Fig. 3.19). The orthomyxoviruses, like influenza A, bud out as variable, round or elongated structures with no overall symmetry, although there is probably considerable local order.[167] Retrovirus particles also appear to have no global symmetry.[79] The fluid character of a lipid bilayer means that the virus can form a closed structure without a perfect surface lattice. Defects in a protein layer that would produce unacceptable holes in a nonenveloped virus are tolerable if the barrier protecting the genome is a lipid membrane rather than a protein shell.

Internal Structures

The proteins on the internal side of viral envelopes are significantly more varied in design than those in the shells of nonenveloped viruses. The alphaviruses have subverted a serine protease to serve as the principal domain of the capsid subunit (C)[46] (Fig. 3.21). The protease is functional in the single step required to cleave C from the nascent polyprotein of these positive-strand RNA viruses. The core, sealed within the bilayer, can afford to be fenestrated. The hexamer and pentamer clusters of the protease domains do not contact each other, and interacting N-terminal arms maintain coherence of the T = 4 icosahedral lattice.[258] These positively charged arms, like those of TBSV (Fig. 3.7), appear to knit the core together as well as to recognize and neutralize RNA. The hepatitis B capsid is also an open, almost lattice-like, structure, formed by a largely α-helical subunit that can assemble into either T = 3 or T = 4 shells.[20] The retroviral Gag precursor is usually anchored by an N-terminal myristoyl group to the membrane bilayer, and successive domains are separated by cleavage into radially organized layers[84,247] (see Chapter 47). The structures of the various domains from HIV-1 Gag are known,[77] as are those of certain domains from a few other retroviruses.

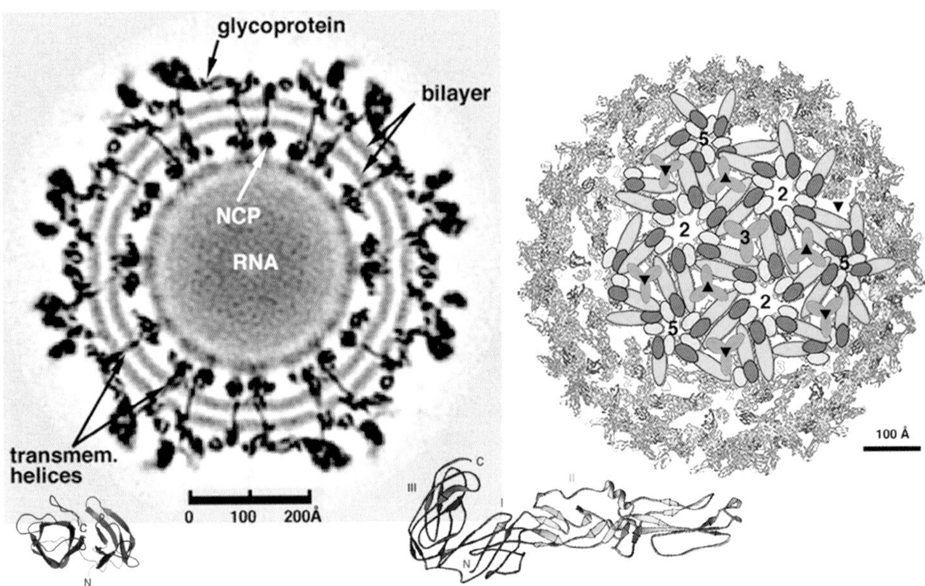

FIGURE 3.21. Molecular organization of alphavirus particles. Left: Cross-section through an electron cryomicroscopy (cryoEM) three-dimensional image reconstruction of Sindbis virus.[258] The labels point out the glycoprotein layer (E1 and E2) on the outside, anchored into the lipid bilayer through C-terminal transmembrane helices, with a short segment at the C-terminus of E2 in contact with the nucleocapsid protein (NCP). **Right:** The T = 4 glycoprotein surface lattice of the closely related Semliki Forest virus.[136] Superposed on a ribbon representation of the lattice of 240 E1 subunits is a more schematic diagram of the packing of E1 and E2. The E1 subunits are in red, yellow, and blue, representing respectively the three subdomains of the E1 ectodomain (see ribbon representation at **bottom, center**, in the same colors; the three subdomains are labeled I, II, and III). The approximate location of the E2 ectodomain is in green. The numerals 5, 3, and 2 designate positions of fivefold, threefold, and twofold icosahedral symmetry axes; black triangles designate local threefold positions in the T = 4 surface lattice. The E2 subunits clamp the E1 subunits in place; exposure to low pH releases the clamp. At the bottom left is a ribbon representation (blue) of the nucleocapsid protein (an autoprotease with a trypsin-chymotrypsin–like fold; the cleavage generates its C-terminus, which remains bound in the catalytic cleft as an inhibitor); N and C designate its termini.[46]

Surface Envelope Proteins

Most viral envelope proteins are so-called type I membrane proteins, with a single transmembrane α-helix linking an N-terminal ectodomain and a C-terminal tail inside the membrane. Some (e.g., the influenza virus neuraminidase) have the opposite polarity (type II). In flavivirus structural proteins, which derive from a polyprotein precursor (as in most positive-strand RNA viruses), the anchor is an α-helical hairpin that traverses the membrane twice.[36] The transmembrane helices have been resolved in cryoEM studies of alphaviruses and flaviviruses[159,255,258] (Fig. 3.21). Contacts between the cytoplasmic tails of viral envelope glycoproteins and target sites on the underlying core of matrix subunits generally determine specificity of envelope protein incorporation (Figs. 3.20D and 3.21). These interactions often involve a short segment of envelope polypeptide, fitting against a site on the internal protein.[19,135,171] Individual interactions are weak, and bilayer disruption by nonionic detergents readily dissociates them.

The proteins on the outer surface of an enveloped virus must carry out at least two functions: receptor binding and fusion. In addition, there may be a receptor-destroying enzyme (e.g., the influenza virus neuraminidase or the coronavirus esterase) to promote viral release. The membrane of influenza A contains a fourth activity: a proton channel that assists uncoating and transcriptase activation (M2). In certain cases (e.g., rhabdoviruses and retroviruses), the receptor-binding and fusion activities are combined in a single protein; in others (e.g., paramyxoviruses), there are two distinct proteins to carry out these functions. Structures of viral fusion proteins are described later in the subsection on membrane fusion.

STRUCTURAL BIOLOGY OF VIRUS ENTRY

Receptor Binding

There are no simple generalizations about virus receptors and how they bind with viral surfaces (Fig. 3.22). We note two points here. The first is that most viruses have evolved a mechanism to avoid "getting stuck" at the cell surface when emerging from an infected cell. Many viruses simply bind weakly to their receptors, and thus can dissociate in a reasonable time. The virulence of polyomavirus in mice is inversely related to viral affinity for its sialoglycoconjugate receptor (Fig. 3.22A), demonstrating that spread in the animal host, rather than entry into cells, is the principal correlate of pathogenesis.[12] Like polyoma, influenza virus recognizes a sialic acid–containing carbohydrate for cell attachment[176] (Fig. 3.22B). A receptor-destroying enzyme (neuraminidase) is present on the surface of the virion; its activity allows release of newly assembled virions from the cell surface through which they have budded.[172] The neuraminidase is thus required for effective spread of the virus, and the enzyme is the target of anti-influenza drugs, developed

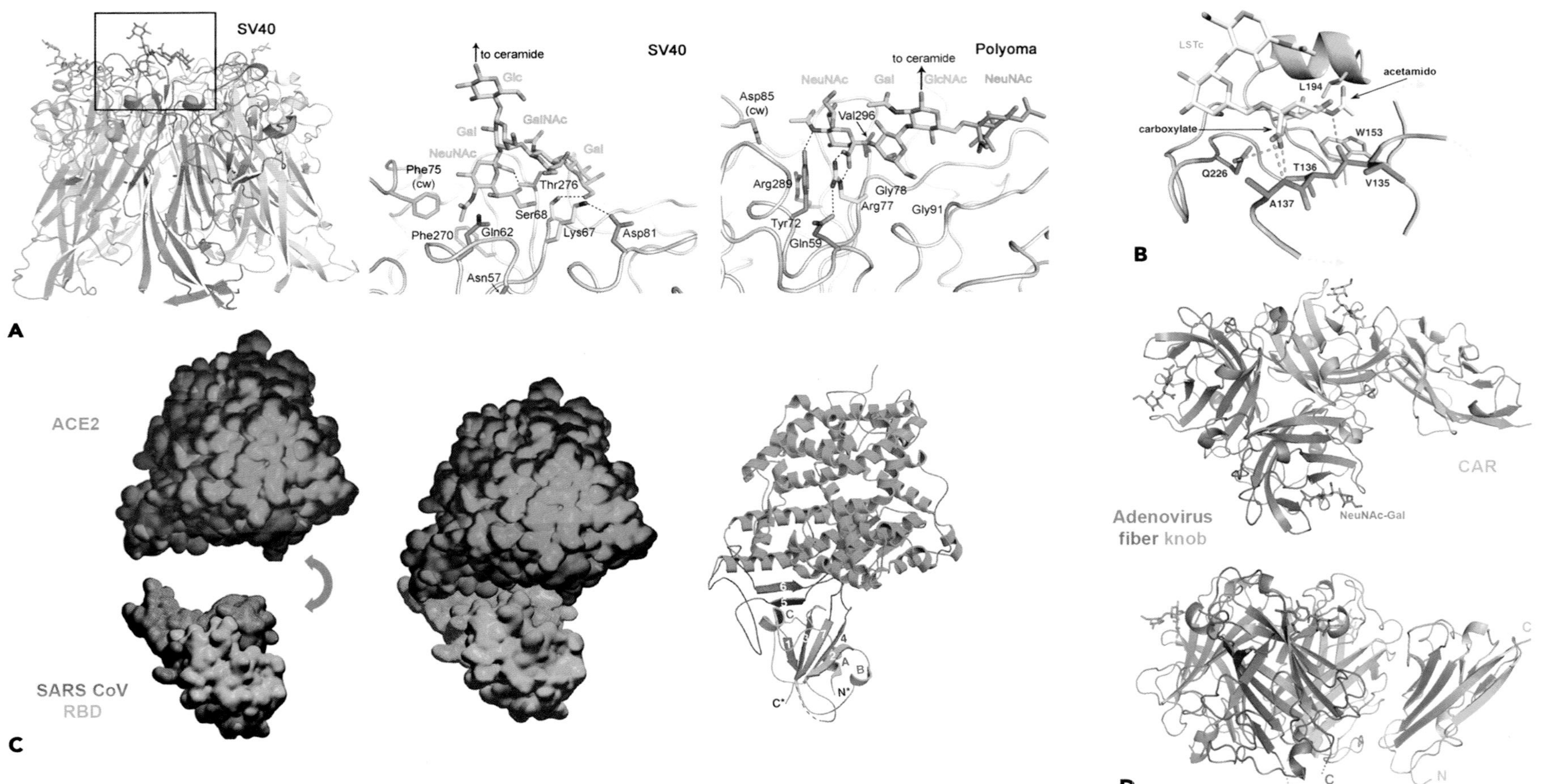

FIGURE 3.22. Examples of virus–receptor interactions. A: Simian virus type 40 (SV40) and polyomavirus. **Left:** Pentamer of SV40 VP1, showing location of the interaction on the outward-facing surface of the subunit. **Right:** Detailed views of the receptor-binding sites for the two viruses (boxed region in the **left-hand panel**), showing interactions of distinct glycan structures (from glycolipid headgroups) with homologous sites on the VP1 subunits. **B:** Influenza virus: sialic acid–binding site on the HA1 "head." **C:** Severe acute respiratory syndrome (SARS) coronavirus: docking of the ACE2 receptor with the receptor-binding domain (RBD) of the viral glycoprotein spike.[137] **D:** Adenovirus penton-fiber knob **(top view)**, bound with domain 1 of the multi-Ig domain receptor, CAR (coxsackievirus-adenovirus receptor), and with sialic acid **(side view)**, which helps recruit type 2 adenovirus to cell surfaces.[201] (**A** adapted from Neu U, Woellner K, Gauglitz G, et al. Structural basis of GM1 ganglioside recognition by simian virus 40. *Proc Natl Acad Sci U S A* 2008;105:5219–5224. **B** adapted from Whittle JR, Zhang R, Khurana S, et al. Broadly neutralizing human antibody that recognizes the receptor-binding pocket of influenza virus hemagglutinin. *Proc Natl Acad Sci U S A* 2011;108:14216–14221.)

in part by exploiting knowledge of the NA structure.[235] HIV-1 has several mechanisms for down-regulating its receptor (CD4) after infection, both to avoid envelope–receptor interactions within the secretory pathway and to facilitate viral release after budding (see Chapter 49).

The second general point is that some viruses require a cascade of at least two distinct receptors—one for initial cell attachment and a second for triggering fusion or penetration. The receptor used for initial attachment may be a widely distributed molecule, such as sialic acid or other glycans (heparan sulfate for herpes simplex virus-1), or it may be a quite specific protein, such as the adenovirus receptor, CAR, or the HIV-1 receptor, CD4 (Fig. 3.22C). The molecule that triggers fusion or penetration is sometimes called a *co-receptor*—for example, the chemokine receptors for HIV-1. In the case of HIV-1, CD4 primes the envelope glycoprotein to bind the co-receptor, which in turn induces fusion activation. An obligate order of this sort may turn out to be relatively common.

Viruses that mutate to avoid recognition by the immune system (e.g., influenza, HIV) have sometimes evolved structural features to sequester their conserved, receptor-binding surface from interaction with antibodies. The footprint of an antibody-combining site is substantial, and thus even if a receptor site is exposed, it rarely matches the full extent of the surface within which amino acid residue changes will lower antibody affinity and hence escape neutralization.[50] While some viral receptor sites (e.g., those on certain picornaviruses: Fig. 3.4) lie within a groove or pocket too narrow to admit the antigen-combining end of an antibody (sometimes called a "canyon"[195,196]), others are fully exposed or even protruding (Fig. 3.22D).[137] Moreover, antibodies with unusually long or prominent heavy-chain CDR3 loops can penetrate relatively tight cavities.

An Irreversible Step Between Assembly and Entry

Assembly of TMV protein and RNA into infectious particles was among the key observations that triggered thinking about viral symmetry.[56] *In vitro* self-assembly of components from the mature virion into complete infectious particles is, however, an exceptional characteristic of the simplest plant and bacterial RNA viruses. A far more general property of virus assembly pathways is a modification, often a simple proteolytic cleavage, that "primes" the particle for large-scale, irreversible events accompanying entry. Loss of a scaffolding protein is a particularly extreme example of such a modification. Poliovirus and other picornaviruses assemble from VP0, VP1, and VP3, but autolytic cleavage of VP0 into VP4 (an internal peptide) and VP2 accompanies assembly (see Chapter 16). When receptor binding triggers expansion of the viral shell, exit of VP4 renders the rearrangement irreversible.[15,100] The receptor is a catalyst that lowers the energy barrier to an irreversible reorganization.[226] The function of this reorganization is viral entry, and the triggering mechanism has evolved to occur only in an appropriate location. Reoviruses have an outer protein, $\sigma3$, that caps the penetration protein, $\mu1$.[64,140] Proteolytic removal of $\sigma3$ is required to render the particle competent to attach and penetrate (see Chapter 44). There is, in addition, an essential autolytic cleavage of $\mu1$.[165] The HA of influenza virus folds in the ER into a stable, trimeric structure. Cleavage of one peptide bond in HA by the protease furin in a compartment late in the secretory pathway primes the

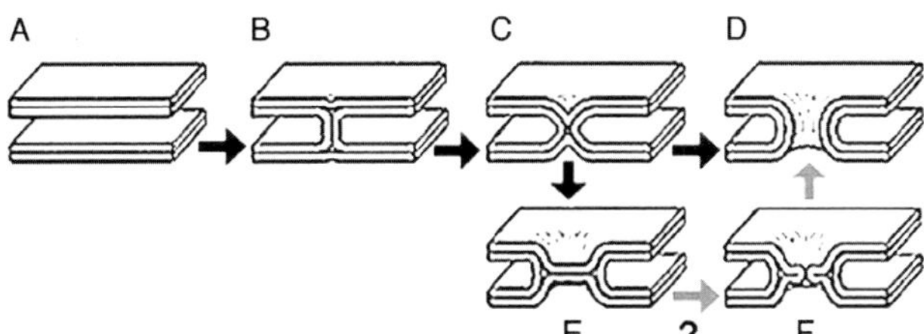

FIGURE 3.23. Fusion of two lipid bilayers. A: Two parallel bilayer membranes. There is a substantial barrier to close approach. **B:** Hemifusion stalk. **C:** Proposed transition structure. **D:** Fusion pore (before lateral expansion). **E:** Hemifusion diaphragm. **F:** Some models include perforation of the hemifusion diaphragm as a productive step toward fusion-pore formation, but diaphragm formation is more often considered a dead end. (Adapted from Jahn R, Lang T, Sudhof TC. Membrane fusion. *Cell* 2003; 112:519–533.)

protein to undergo a dramatic, low-pH-triggered rearrangement, which mediates fusion of viral and target cell membranes. In effect, cleavage renders the virion form of HA metastable, but the barrier to rearrangement is so great at neutral pH that no conformational change occurs. Proton binding in the low pH environment of the endosome removes this barrier and triggers a refolding of the HA protein. Protons have the role taken in other cases by a co-receptor (e.g., the chemokine receptors for HIV-1). The expression "spring loaded" has been used to describe the state of HA at neutral pH after cleavage to HA_1 and HA_2.[32] *Jack-in-the-box* might be a comparable image for poliovirus after cleavage of VP0.

Membrane Fusion

Bilayer Fusion

The bilayer fusion reaction common to all the enveloped viral entry pathways is shown schematically in Figure 3.23. It is believed to pass through an intermediate known as a *hemifusion stalk* (Fig. 3.23, top center), in which the two apposed leaflets have fused, but not the distal ones.[130,147,184,205] Hemifused bilayers can then form either a *fusion pore* (Fig. 3.24, right) or a structure in which the two distal leaflets create a single bilayer. This state, which can spread laterally, is called a *hemifusion diaphragm* (Fig. 3.23, bottom center). Bilayers do not fuse spontaneously (e.g., concentrated liposomes are quite stable), because the reaction in Figure 3.23 has a high activation barrier, both at the step between the precursor bilayers and the hemifusion stalk and at the step between the hemifusion stalk and the fusion pore. A newly opened pore may revert to a hemifusion structure (*flickering*), and the largest kinetic barrier may be for the step in which the pore dilates rather than reverts.[148,184]

Conformational Rearrangements in Viral Fusion Proteins

Viral fusion proteins must lower the kinetic barriers to fusion of viral and cellular membranes. They do so by undergoing dramatic conformational rearrangements that lead to tight apposition of the two membranes.[106] We can thus distinguish *prefusion* and *postfusion* conformations, as well as potential intermediates. The viral fusion proteins analyzed in detail at the time this

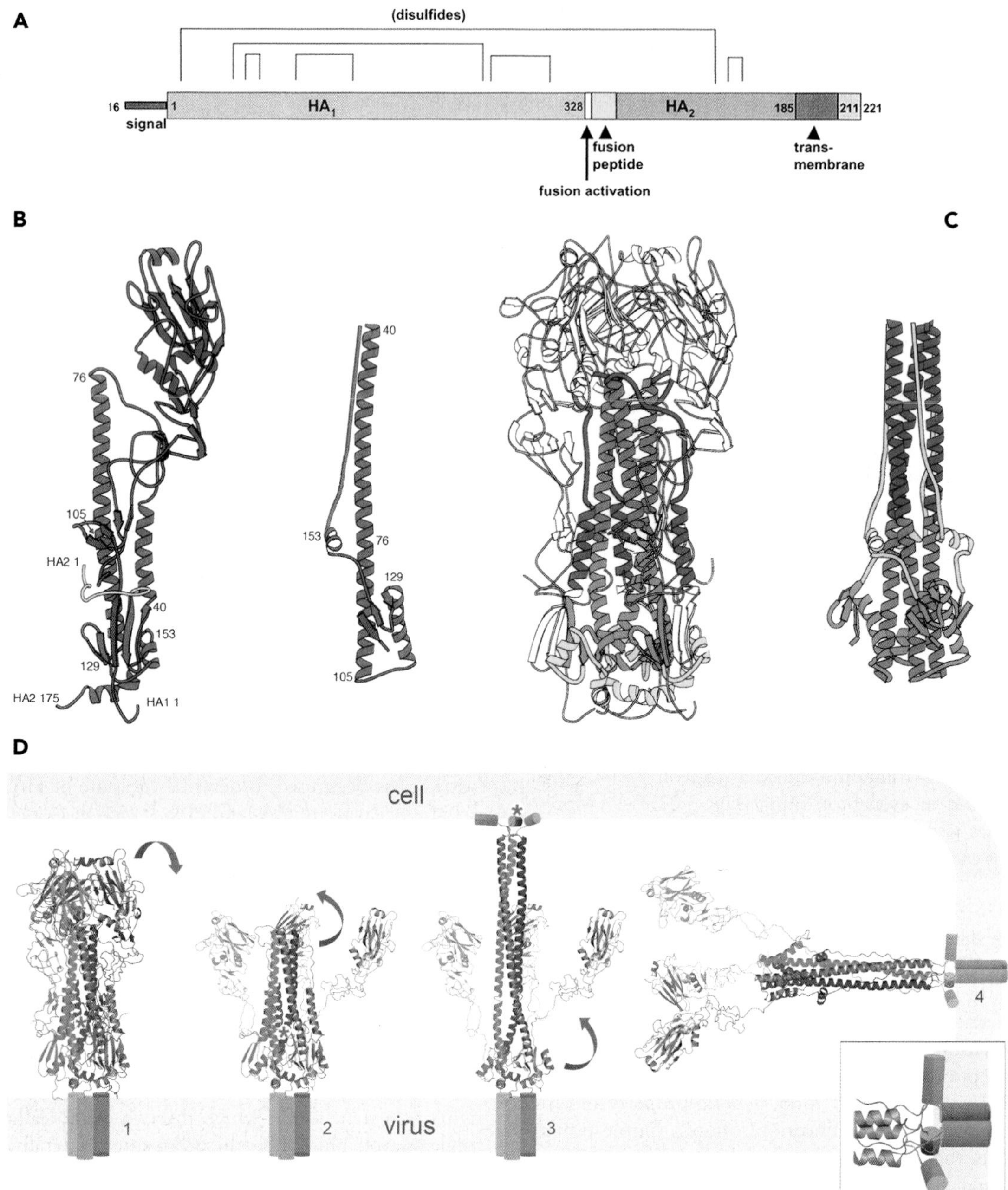

FIGURE 3.24. Influenza virus hemagglutinin (HA): structure and fusion-promoting conformational change. A: The HA polypeptide chain. HA_1 in blue; HA_2 in yellow (fusion peptide), red (remainder of ectodomain), and gray (transmembrane and internal segments). The position of the fusion activation cleavage between HA_1 and HA_2 is a narrow white stripe, indicating excision of a single residue in many cases. The location of disulfide bonds is shown schematically above the bar. Residue numbers correspond to positions in the HA of strain X-31. **B:** The HA ectodomain monomer, in prefusion and postfusion (the latter, HA_2 only) conformations to the left and right, respectively. HA_1 in blue; HA_2 in red. The postfusion HA_2 structure illustrated here lacks the fusion peptide as well as additional residues at both ends of the chain. **C:** The HA ectodomain trimer, in prefusion and postfusion (the latter, HA_2 only) conformations, to the left and right, respectively. HA_1 in black and white; HA_2 in colors showing various segments of the ectodomain, so that their reconfiguration during the transition from the pre- to the postfusion structure is evident. Note the loop-to-helix transition in the C-terminal portion of the red segment. **D:** Model for the coupling of the fusion-promoting conformational change in HA to the fusing membranes. **Stage 1:** Prefusion conformation. Red asterisk shows position of fusion peptide at N-terminus of HA_2. Engagement with a sialic acid receptor in the target membrane is not shown. **Stages 2 and 3:** Transition to an extended intermediate, in which the three fusion peptides of the trimer associate tightly with the target cell membrane. The fusion peptide is shown schematically as an amphipathic helix in the membrane surface—the actual structure is probably an amphipathic helical hairpin.[143,144] Proton binding at low pH dissociates HA_1 from HA_2, although the two fragments remain tethered by a disulfide bond. **Stage 4:** During the transition of HA_2 from intermediate to postfusion conformation, the fusion peptide and transmembrane segment come together, thereby bringing the two membranes close enough to fuse. The final, postfusion conformation of HA_2 is locked in place by the "cap," shown in the **inset**, in which residues near the C-terminus of the HA_2 ectodomain interact with residues between the fusion peptide and the long, central α-helix.[41]

chapter went to press fall into three structural classes, generally designated I, II, and III. Common characteristics of fusion by all three classes are insertion of a segment of the fusion protein into the target membrane and refolding of the protein so that this inserted segment and the transmembrane anchor are adjacent, thereby bringing together cell and viral membranes. The three structural classes probably represent meaningful evolutionary categories, as a cellular representative of at least one of the classes very closely resembles its viral orthologs.

Influenza Virus Hemagglutinin, a Class I Viral Fusion Protein

The defining characteristics of class I fusion proteins are synthesis as a precursor that requires a proteolytic cleavage for activation (often, but not always, by a furin-like enzyme in the trans-Golgi network); trimeric oligomerization in both pre- and postfusion conformations, based on a central, three-chain α-helical coiled-coil in the postfusion conformation; and presence of a hydrophobic *fusion peptide* near the N-terminus created by the activating cleavage. The fragment C-terminal to the cleavage, with the viral transmembrane segment, is the fusogen; the fragment N-terminal to the cleavage, in many but not all cases, is a receptor-binding structure, which generally dissociates when suitably triggered, releasing its grip on the fusogenic fragment. The final, postfusion structure is a *trimer of hairpins,* as described later.

Influenza virus HA is the best-studied class I fusion protein.[244] HA_0, the uncleaved precursor, and HA_1/HA_2, the cleavage product, are almost identical in structure, except for a local shift that tucks the fusion peptide (the N-terminus of HA_2) between the splayed helices of the central coiled-coil (Fig. 3.24B). Unless induced to refold by lowered pH or by heat, HA_1/HA_2 is very stable. HA_1 forms a globular domain at the "top" of the molecule, with a binding pocket (Fig. 3.24B,C) for the receptor, sialic acid.[237] Proton-induced rearrangement of HA (Fig. 3.24B–D) has two essential features. The first is ejection of the protected hydrophobic fusion peptide (Fig. 3.24D, transition from stage 2 to stage 3). The second is folding back of the fusion protein (HA_2) so that the N-terminus (the fusion peptide) and the C-terminus (the viral membrane anchor) come together (Fig. 3.24D, transition from stage 3 to stage 4).[26,41,210] A likely intermediate state, for which there is experimental evidence in the case of HIV-1 gp41,[62,81,108] is an extended structure with the fusion peptide buried in one membrane and the anchor in the other (Fig. 3.24D, stage 3). Zipping up of the C-terminal part of the HA_2 ectodomain along the core of this *prefusion intermediate* will cause the transmembrane anchor and the fusion peptide to approach each other. Formation of an intricate "cap" on the three-helix core snaps the refolded structure in place (Fig. 3.24D, inset).[41] Note that the zipping-up process cannot be symmetrical, because the trimer would otherwise encase itself in lipid. The C-terminal outer-layer segments are long enough, in their unfolded state, to reach around the core of the refolding trimer. Contacts between the three outer-layer chains in the refolded structure are minimal, so that the three can zip up independently and at different rates. Several rearranged fusion proteins might be required to surround and induce a hemifusion stalk. Estimates from measurements of fusion by HA expressed on a cell surface and of fusion of virions with a supported bilayer *in vitro* indicate that on average, three HA trimers participate in fusion pore formation.[59,76]

Other Class I Fusion Proteins

The postfusion conformation of HA is a trimer of hairpins. The N- and C-termini of each subunit lie at the same end of the elongated protein, and the polypeptide chain traverses the length of the molecule just twice—once from the N-terminus to the distal end, and once back to the C-terminus—with some modest complexity in the distal loop. The *inner core* is a trimeric coiled-coil; the *outer layer* of each subunit is largely extended chain, with a short helical segment. Other class I fusion proteins have the same postfusion characteristics (Fig. 3.25), the structure in the case of HIV-1 being particularly simple, as both inner core and outer layer are helical.[18,37,145,239] The two helices are sometimes designated HR1 or HRA and HR2 or HRB (*helical region 1* or *A* and *helical region 2* or *B,* respectively), but the postfusion HA structure illustrates that identification of two helical regions may not always be informative. Moreover, a major part of the central coiled-coil in postfusion HA_2 is not even helical in the prefusion trimer—another reason why "HR1" and "HR2" are partly misleading designations. Note further that in influenza HA, the N-terminal parts of HA_2 are on the outside of the spike in the prefusion conformation and on the inside in the postfusion conformation (Fig. 3.24). The protein turns itself inside out during the refolding.

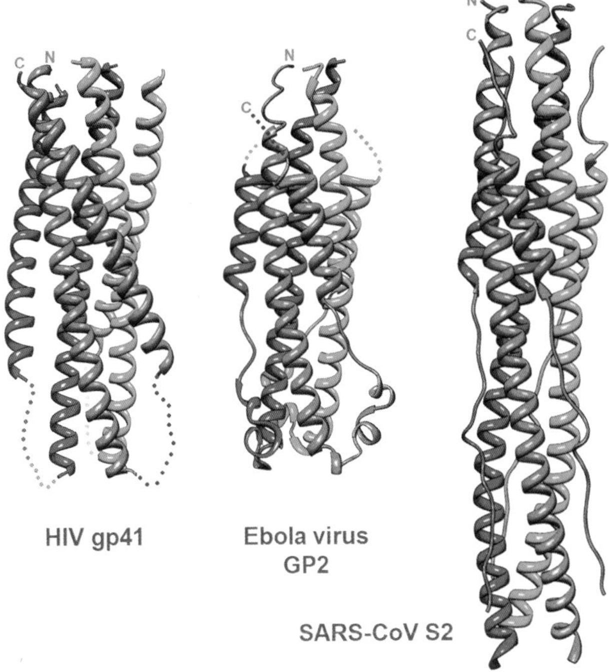

FIGURE 3.25. Postfusion conformations of three class I fusion-protein ectodomains.[37,220,238,239,260] Only the folded-back cores of the proteins are shown. The fusion peptide extends from the N-terminus of the trimeric bundle; the transmembrane segment is at its C-terminus. Compare with the postfusion conformations of influenza virus HA_2 in Figure 3.24C and of the paramyxovirus human parainfluenzavirus 3 (hPIV3) F2 protein in Figure 3.26B. The HIV gp41 structure is particularly simple: a six-helix bundle with a relatively short loop (dotted lines) between the inner (N-terminal) and outer (C-terminal) helices (HR1 or HRA and HR2 or HRB, respectively). A 200-residue domain intervenes between the postfusion inner and outer layers of severe acute respiratory syndrome virus-coronavirus (SARS-CoV) S2.

The postfusion conformation of a class I fusion protein is the most stable one it can adopt when constraints such as the covalent linkage between the two fragments have been removed, and proteins in this conformation have therefore been easier to prepare and study than have prefusion conformers or protein models for intermediate structures. It is important to emphasize, however, that no inferences can be drawn about the prefusion structures of these proteins from their trimer-of-hairpins postfusion conformers.

One other class I fusion protein for which both pre- and postfusion structures have been determined is paramyxovirus F[43,52,132,249,250] (Fig. 3.26). It has a cleavage site just N-terminal to a fusion peptide, which resembles (in being hydrophobic and relatively glycine-rich) the fusion peptides in gp160 and HA_0. Cleavage is essential for fusion activity, but not for the fusion-promoting conformational change. In the mushroom-like, prefusion conformation, a three-strand α-helical coiled-coil, the stem of the mushroom, is the C-terminal part of the ectodomain. It connects directly (in the intact protein) to the transmembrane segment. The strap between the coiled-coil stem and the head of the mushroom is an ordered, but very extended, stretch of polypeptide chain, which wraps around the outside of the globular cap. The cap also presents a groove to accommodate the fusion peptide. A separate protein (designated HN, H, or G in various paramyxoviruses) binds receptor and triggers the conformational rearrangement of F (see Chapter 33). In the refolded state, no parts of the protein dissociate (as they do from HA and gp120/gp41), but a long, three-strand coiled-coil forms from segments (all C-terminal to the cleavage site) that are part of the globular "cap" in the prefusion structure.[249] The C-terminal coiled-coil comes apart so that the C-terminal helices can fold back up along the outside of the newly formed coiled-coil. The length of the strap between the globular domains and these helices, which probably dissociate, unfold, translocate, and refold as they zip along the coiled-coil core, allows sufficient flexibility for this transition. None of the trimer contacts in the prefusion state are fully conserved in the postfusion structure, raising the possibility of a monomeric intermediate, but the overall geometry does permit the assembly to refold as a trimer without such dissociation.

The Flavivirus Envelope Subunit (E), a Class II Fusion Protein

Class II fusion proteins have been found only on alphaviruses, flaviviruses, and bunyaviruses, all of which have compact, icosahedrally symmetric virions. The defining characteristics of fusion

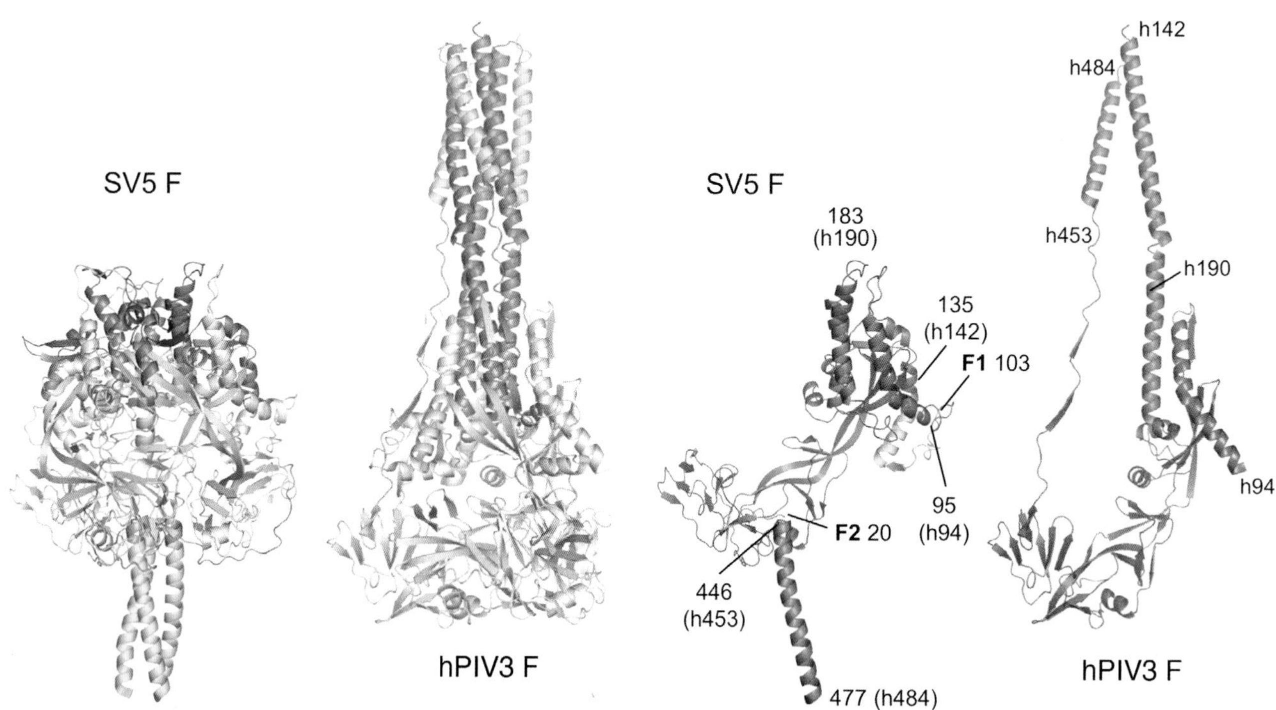

FIGURE 3.26. The paramyxovirus fusion protein (F). A: The ectodomain trimer of simian virus type 5 (SV5) F in its prefusion conformation. F1 is in black and white; F2, in color. The order of colors corresponds to the order of colors in influenza HA_2 in Figure 3.24C. The viral membrane would be at the bottom of the figure: the polypeptide chain of F2 enters the membrane immediately following the yellow segment, which forms a three-chain coiled-coil in the prefusion conformation. **B:** The postfusion conformation of F from another paramyxovirus, human parainfluenzavirus 3 (hPIV3). Color scheme as in **A.** Note that the red and blue segments toward the N-terminus of F2 have refolded into a three-chain coiled-coil, projecting the fusion peptide (not shown) toward the "top" of the trimer. Compare these segments with those of corresponding color in Figure 3.24 C. Also note that the yellow segments at the C-terminus of the F2 ectodomain no longer form a coiled-coil, but rather align along the outside of the coiled-coil generated by the (red and blue) N-terminal region. **C, D:** Pre- and postfusion conformations of monomers, with F1 in blue, F2 in red, and fusion peptide (N-terminus of F2) in yellow. Numbers in **C** correspond to SV5 F; numbers with "h" in C and D, to hPIV3 F. (Courtesy of Ted Jardetzky, Stanford University.)

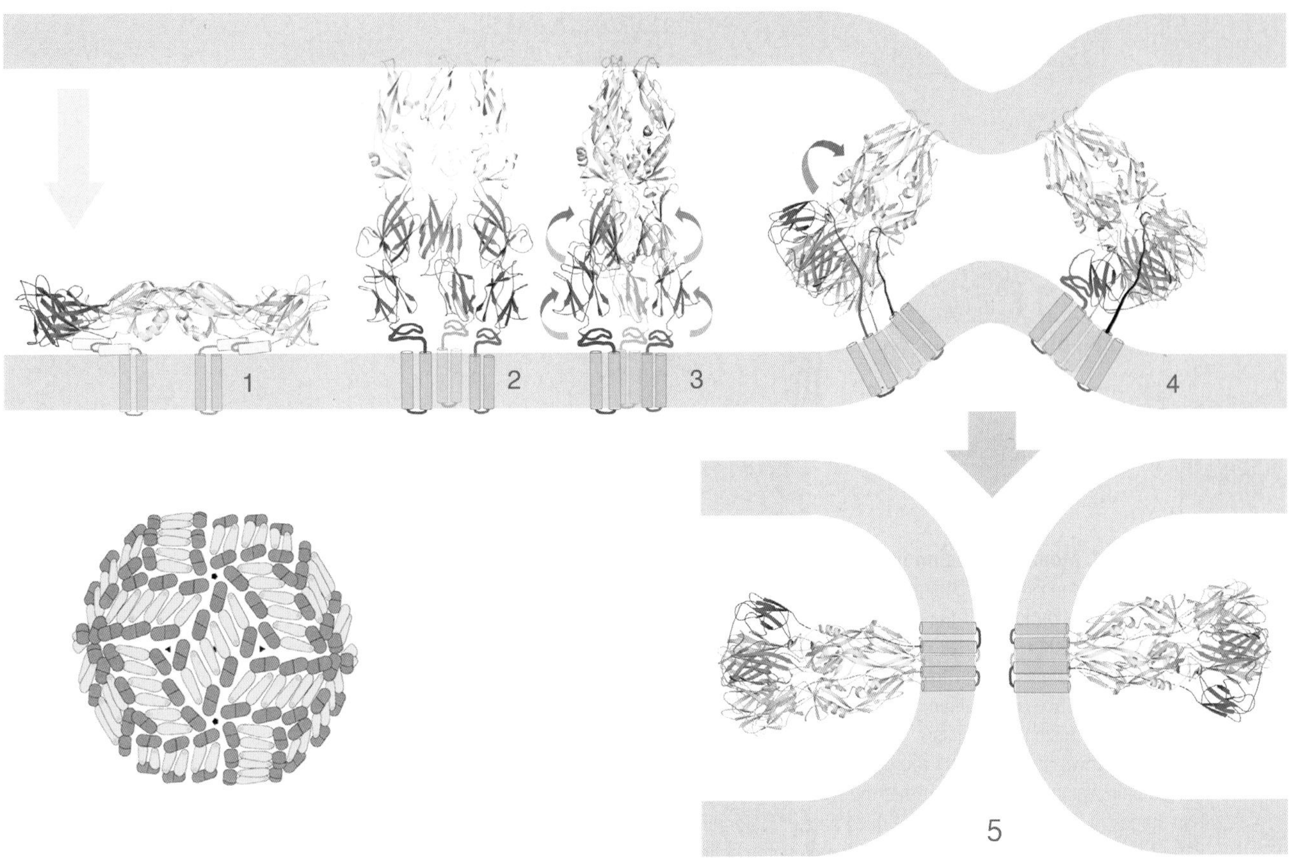

FIGURE 3.27. Membrane fusion induced by the flavivirus envelope protein, E. Diagram lower left: Dimer-clustered packing of E on the virion surface. The three domains of each protein ectodomain are in red, yellow, and blue. **Numbered sequence:** likely series of conformational states of E and their links to viral and cellular membranes. Structures for states 1 and 5 are known; those for states 2 to 4 are inferred from indirect data. One subunit in each dimer or trimer is colored as in the schematic; its partner(s) are in gray. **1:** E dimer on the virion surface. The ectodomain terminates in a helical hairpin called the *stem* (light blue) on the surface of the viral membrane (lower gray bar) and connects with a transmembrane helical hairpin. Blue arrow from above symbolizes a receptor interaction with domain III (blue). **2:** Exposure to low pH (in endosomes) dissociates the E dimer, allowing the subunits to project outward, so that the fusion loops (tip of the yellow domain II) encounter the endosomal membrane (upper gray bar). **3:** Initial trimer association, requiring some rearrangement across the surface of the virion. Arrows show presumed pattern of folding back; upper arrows: domain III (blue) flips over against domain I (red); lower arrows: the stem refolds to "zip up" alongside the trimer clustered domain II (yellow). **4:** Stem continues to reorganize (asymmetrically), pulling the two membranes together. The fusion loops must be firmly anchored in the target membrane. **5:** Formation of a fusion pore allows the refolding to finish, so that all three stems and all three fusion loops cluster together, restoring full threefold symmetry.

proteins in this class are a three-domain subunit, with an internal, hydrophobic *fusion loop* at the tip of the elongated second domain; association with a viral "chaperone" protein, which must be cleaved to prime the fusion process; and formation of a stable trimer in the postfusion state, with the three fusion loops and the three C-terminal, transmembrane anchors clustered at one end (Fig. 3.27). The fusion proteins are known, respectively, as E1 and E in alphaviruses and flaviviruses; the chaperones, as pE2 and prM. Cleavage of the latter proteins generates E2 and M, with release (at some point in the fusion process) of a "pre" fragment, which covers the fusion loop of E1 or E in the unprimed state.

The flavivirus E protein tiles the surface of the virion as a tightly associated dimer[128] (Fig. 3.11). There are 90 such dimers; their packing is not a quasiequivalent, T = 3 arrangement, but a herringbone-like pattern. On an immature particle, before cleavage of prM (the chaperone), E forms heterodimers with prM rather than homodimers with itself.[128] Substantial structural rearrangements accompany maturation and dissociation of the "pre" fragment.[138,252,253] Likely steps in the fusion process, deduced from comparison of the pre- and postfusion conformations,[22,154,155,187] are illustrated in Figure 3.27. The underlying similarity of class I– and class II–mediated fusion should be evident. The fusion loops insert only partway into the outer leaflet of the target membrane.

VSV-G, a Class III Fusion Protein

Class III fusion proteins mediate penetration of particles as distinct as the rhabdoviruses[191,193] and herpesviruses,[7,109] as well as the insect baculoviruses.[6,120] There appears to be no proteolytic cleavage, either of the fusion protein itself or of a chaperone, required for priming, and the fusion-inducing conformational

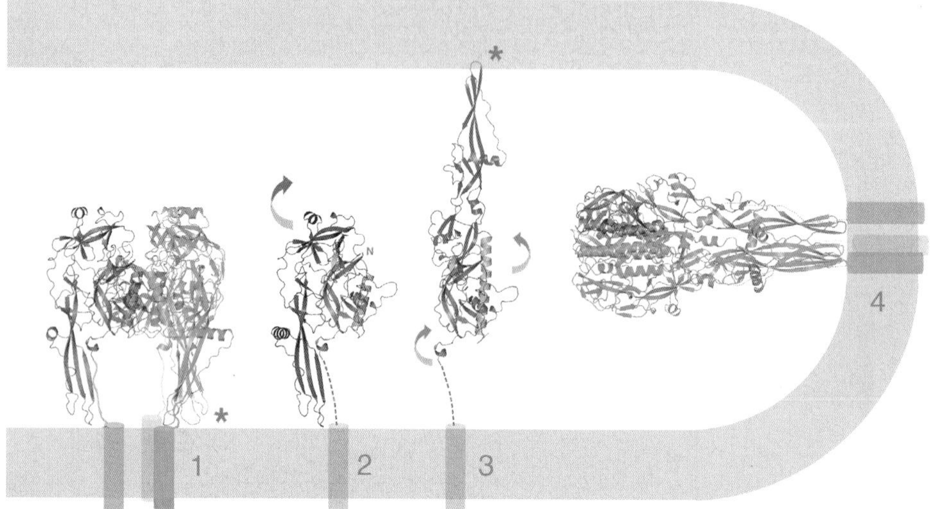

FIGURE 3.28. Membrane fusion induced by the vesicular stomatitis virus (VSV) glycoprotein (G). Sequence of conformational events as in Figures 3.24 and 3.27. **1:** Prefusion trimer of VSV G on the virion surface. Subunits colored in red, blue, and green. Red asterisk: fusion loops of the green and blue subunits. **2:** Conformation of one subunit of the trimer in **1**, now colored to show a central, red domain and a set of peripheral, blue domains. An axial helix (lighter blue) joins part of the central domain to the set of peripheral domains. In the low-pH-triggered rearrangement, the blue regions reorient with respect to the red domain (arrow). **3:** Presumed initial rearrangement, in which the domain bearing the fusion loops projects toward the cellular (endosomal) membrane, into which the fusion loops insert. The axial helix remains, augmented by a segment derived from its connection to the peripheral domains. Arrows indicate likely reorganization that follows: the central domain flips over and the *stem* at the C-terminus of the ectodomain zips up, bringing together the two membranes. **4:** Formation of a fusion pore (not shown explicitly—compare the last two stages in Figure 3.27) allows the three sets of fusion loops and the membrane-proximal segments of the ectodomain to cluster. Part of the stem rearrangement includes formation of a helical segment, which forms a six-helix bundle with the central-region helix. The conformational details thus have features of both class I fusion proteins (formation of a six-helix bundle) and of class II fusion proteins (preconfigured, internal fusion loops that insert into the target membrane).

change is in at least some cases reversible.[192] That is, virions inactivated by prolonged incubation at pH less than 6 can be reactivated by raising the pH to neutral or above, and both conformations of the multidomain, trimeric protein can be obtained from the same protein preparation.

VSV-G, the only protein on the surface of the virion, has two hydrophobic loops that can interact with membrane lipids[67] (Fig. 3.28). The connectivity of the strands joined by these fusion loops is different from the connectivity in domain II of the class II proteins (i.e., the domains themselves have different folds), but the general picture is quite similar: hydrophobic residues (including at least one tryptophan) are displayed on tightly structured loops at the tip of an elongated domain. In the prefusion conformation of VSV-G, these domains face the viral membrane around the periphery of the trimer.[193] In the postfusion conformation, they cluster around the threefold axis[191] (Fig. 3.28; compare the "inside-out" transition in influenza HA, Fig. 3.25).

In the rhabdovirus G protein, a core domain contains residues from the N-terminal segment of the polypeptide chain and residues from near the C-terminal part of the chain: it is a framework around which the rest of the molecule reorients. Two other domains form a jointed, two-part fusion machinery. The result of their rotations relative to the core domain (and to each other) is to move the fusion loops away from the viral membrane and toward the target membrane. In a likely extended intermediate conformation (shown in Fig. 3.29, but for which there are no direct structural data), the C-terminal segment still connects toward the viral membrane in one direction, while the fusion loops interact with the target membrane in the opposite direction. In the fully rearranged, low-pH conformation, the C-terminal segment has zipped up along the fusion domains, much like in the flavivirus fusion transition.

The herpesvirus fusion protein, gB, looks like an elongated version of VSV-G.[109] This unexpected similarity between fusion proteins of a DNA virus and a negative-strand RNA virus has allowed information about one protein (e.g., the identification of the rhabdovirus fusion loops) to be carried over to the other.[102] Only the postfusion structure of gB has been determined so far. The gB conformational transition is triggered not by changes in pH, but rather by receptor binding to another surface protein, gD.[31,127] A binding-induced conformational change in gD leads to the reorganization of gB, with participation of yet another protein, the gH/gL heterodimer.[48,150]

Penetration by Nonenveloped Viruses

Nonenveloped viruses must breach a membrane to access the cytoplasm or nucleus of a cell, but unlike their enveloped cousins, they cannot do so by membrane fusion. One can imagine two classes of models by which a nonenveloped particle, bound at the surface of a cell or taken up into an endosome or other internal compartment, translocates itself (or its genome) across the intervening lipid bilayer (i.e., *penetrates*). Models of one class (*pore formation*) invoke creation of a pore, through which the viral genome is drawn into the cell. Those of the other class (*membrane perforation*) postulate a more extensive, transient disruption of a cellular membrane (e.g., the membrane of an endosome), in order to admit the virion (in altered form) into the cytosol. Either of these models is consistent with a variety of distinct molecular mechanisms. In all well-studied cases, binding of a receptor, co-receptor, or some other ligand induces a conformational change in the virus particle, with consequent exposure of previously buried, hydrophobic structures. Examples of the exposed components are a pore-forming peptide or protein, frequently N-terminally myristolated; a protein with membrane-interacting, hydrophobic loops; and a lipase. Certain bacterial viruses, such as the T-even bacteriophages, have much more elaborate injection structures that couple the induced conformational change to mechanical force generation.

Released or exposed virion components that bear an N-terminal myristoyl group include VP4 of picornaviruses,[47] VP2 of polyomaviruses,[198] and μ1N of reoviruses.[166] Myristoyl groups target proteins to membranes, and it is logical to suppose that exposure of the myristolated peptide protein leads it to associate with membranes and ultimately to contribute to penetration. In at least one case (reovirus μ1N), pore-forming activity has been shown directly.

Receptor binding by picornaviruses triggers a rearrangement or destabilization of the virion, exposing the myristoylated VP4 as well as a hydrophobic N-terminal segment of VP1.[24,78,89,100,101] Evidence from electron microscopy suggests that a poliovirus particle, bound to membrane-anchored receptors and therefore altered in this way, interacts closely with the receptor-bearing membrane.[25,228] In one proposed model, the exposed hydrophobic segments form a pore in the endosomal membrane, through which the genomic RNA passes.[24,110] This model requires a mechanism for destabilizing secondary-structural elements in the RNA in order to make translocation possible. One candidate helicase would be a ribosome or ribosome-associated factor, by analogy with an uncoating mechanism established (*in vitro*) for certain positive-strand RNA plant viruses. With those viruses, exposure of the 5′ end of the RNA (e.g., through expansion of the virion induced by intracellular ionic conditions) leads to association of ribosomes with the still largely packaged RNA genome, and progress of the ribosome along the message-sense genome appears to uncoat the particle.[203,204,245] A similar mechanism could, in principle, draw RNA through a membrane pore as well as through an opening in the viral shell. An alternative model for picornavirus penetration would involve membrane disruption (a "large" pore). If receptor binding and subsequent endocytosis caused the shell to dissociate, rather than just to expand or reorganize, components of the dissociated shell could be the agents of membrane disruption, and concomitant RNA unwinding would not be required.

For adenoviruses, the entry route is endosomal uptake; penetration proceeds by disruption of the endosome containing the virion.[75,92] The subviral particle admitted to the cytoplasm lacks pentons as a result of events triggered by receptor and co-receptor binding. Exposure of an internal viral protein, pVI, which depends on the activity of a packaged viral protease, leads to perforation of the endosomal membrane.[206,241] The membrane-disrupting properties of pVI may come from an N-terminal amphipathic α-helix.[158] Following penetration, the partially stripped virion migrates to a nuclear pore, where it disassembles and liberates its DNA for nuclear import.

Like adenoviruses, the dsRNA viruses release into the cytoplasm an intact, roughly 700-Å-diameter subviral particle (called the *core* in the case of reoviruses and the *double-layered particle* in the case of rotaviruses). This inner capsid particle never uncoats, however, as it contains all the enzymes necessary for messenger RNA (mRNA) synthesis and modification (see Chapters 44–46). The penetration protein of reoviruses is the outer-shell trimer, μ1.[38,111,165] On the virion, this protein is associated with a "chaperone" subunit, σ3; degradation of σ3 (by proteases in the gut or by cathepsins in endosomes) and autocleavage of μ1 allows μ1 to release a myristoylated, N-terminal peptide (μ1N). The released peptide, up to 600 copies of which could emerge from a single virion, forms membrane pores. The penetration protein of rotaviruses is VP4, which must also be cleaved (by intestinal trypsin) to activate entry. VP4 is not a homolog of μ1, although rotaviruses do have such a homolog, VP6, which appears to have a purely structural role.[149] The conformation of VP4 changes quite dramatically when cleaved to VP8* and VP5* by trypsin: the initially disordered "spikes" of this protein become rigid projections,[55,202] which rearrange further in subsequent, penetration-inducing steps.[63,251] VP5* presents a set of hydrophobic loops, noticeably similar to the fusion loops of class II and class III fusion proteins, that direct membrane association.[123] The observed conformational transitions of VP5* resemble the folding back of fusion proteins, but there is yet no evidence for a direct coupling of these rearrangements to membrane breakage.

Parvoviruses have a single kind of coat subunit (see Fig. 3.5), but a few of the 60 copies of this protein have an extra, N-terminal domain, which is sequestered within the virion. This domain is a phospholipase A_2. During entry, it moves to the outside of the particle, to which it nonetheless remains tethered. Its lipase activity is essential for entry.[73]

Disruption of the membrane of an endosome or other intracellular compartment is a relatively nonspecific process, in the sense that other particles within the same compartment can accompany the active particle into the cytosol, once the membrane is breached. Thus, several of the viruses described earlier mediate penetration of bacterial toxins that lack their own cell-entry mechanism, and other viruses (e.g., adenoviruses or nondefective parvoviruses) can complement a phospholipase-deficient parvovirus.

REFERENCES

1. Aathavan K, Politzer AT, Kaplan A, et al. Substrate interactions and promiscuity in a viral DNA packaging motor. *Nature* 2009;461:669–673.
2. Abrescia NG, Cockburn JJ, Grimes JM, et al. Insights into assembly from structural analysis of bacteriophage PRD1. *Nature* 2004;432: 68–74.
3. Abuladze NK, Gingery M, Tsai J, et al. Tail length determination in bacteriophage T4. *Virology* 1994;199:301–310.
4. Albertini AA, Wernimont AK, Muziol T, et al. Crystal structure of the rabies virus nucleoprotein-RNA complex. *Science* 2006;313:360–363.
5. Annamalai P, Rao AL. Packaging of brome mosaic virus subgenomic RNA is functionally coupled to replication-dependent transcription and translation of coat protein. *J Virol* 2006;80:10096–10108.

6. Backovic M, Jardetzky TS. Class III viral membrane fusion proteins. *Curr Opin Struct Biol* 2009;19:189–196.
7. Backovic M, Longnecker R, Jardetzky TS. Structure of a trimeric variant of the Epstein-Barr virus glycoprotein B. *Proc Natl Acad Sci U S A* 2009; 106:2880–2885.
8. Badger J, Minor I, Kremer MJ, et al. Structural analysis of a series of antiviral agents complexed with human rhinovirus 14. *Proc Natl Acad Sci U S A* 1988;85:3304–3308.
9. Baker ML, Jiang W, Rixon FJ, et al. Common ancestry of herpesviruses and tailed DNA bacteriophages. *J Virol* 2005;79:14967–14970.
10. Baker TS, Olson NH, Fuller SD. Adding the third dimension to virus life cycles: three-dimensional reconstruction of icosahedral viruses. *Microbiol Mol Biol Rev* 1999;63:862–922.
11. Bamford DH, Caldentey J, Bamford JK. Bacteriophage PRD1: a broad host range DSDNA tectivirus with an internal membrane. *Adv Virus Res* 1995;45:281–319.
12. Bauer PH, Cui C, Stehle T, et al. Discrimination between sialic acid-containing receptors and pseudoreceptors regulates polyomavirus spread in the mouse. *J Virol* 1999;73:5826–5832.
13. Bawden FC, Pirie NW. Crystalline preparations of tomato bushy stunt virus. *Br J Exp Pathol* 1938;29:251–263.
14. Bazinet C, King J. The DNA translocating vertex of dsDNA bacteriophage. *Annu Rev Microbiol* 1985;39:109–129.
15. Belnap DM, Filman DJ, Trus BL, et al. Molecular tectonic model of virus structural transitions: the putative cell entry states of poliovirus. *J Virol* 2000;74:1342–1354.
16. Benson SD, Bamford JK, Bamford DH, et al. Viral evolution revealed by bacteriophages PRD1 and human adenovirus coat protein structures. *Cell* 1999;98:825–833.
17. Bernal JD, Fankuchen I. Structure types of protein "crystals" from virus-infected plants. *Nature (London)* 1939;139:923–924.
18. Blacklow SC, Lu M, Kim PS. A trimeric subdomain of the simian immunodeficiency virus envelope glycoprotein. *Biochemistry* 1995;34:14955–14962.
19. Bottcher B, Tsuji N, Takahashi H, et al. Peptides that block hepatitis B virus assembly; analysis by cryomicroscopy, mutagenesis and transfection. *EMBO J* 1998:23.
20. Bottcher B, Wynne SA, Crowther RA. Determination of the fold of the core protein of hepatitis B virus by electron cryomicroscopy. *Nature* 1997; 386:88–91.
21. Brandenburg B, Lee LY, Lakadamyali M, et al. Imaging poliovirus entry in live cells. *PLoS Biol* 2007;5:e183.
22. Bressanelli S, Stiasny K, Allison S.L, et al. Structure of a flavivirus envelope glycoprotein in its low-pH-induced membrane fusion conformation. *EMBO J* 2004;23:728–738.
23. Briggs JA, Grunewald K, Glass B, et al. The mechanism of HIV-1 core assembly: insights from three-dimensional reconstructions of authentic virions. *Structure* 2006;14:15–20.
24. Bubeck D, Filman DJ, Cheng N, et al. The structure of the poliovirus 135 S cell entry intermediate at 10-angstrom resolution reveals the location of an externalized polypeptide that binds to membranes. *J Virol* 2005; 79:7745–7755.
25. Bubeck D, Filman DJ, Hogle JM. Cryo-electron microscopy reconstruction of a poliovirus-receptor-membrane complex. *Nat Struct Mol Biol* 2005;12:615–618.
26. Bullough PA, Hughson FM, Skehel JJ, et al. The structure of influenza haemagglutinin at the pH of membrane fusion. *Nature* 1994;371:37–43.
27. Butcher SJ, Dokland T, Ojala PM, et al. Intermediates in the assembly pathway of the double-stranded RNA virus phi6. *EMBO J* 1997;16: 4477–4487.
28. Butler PJ, Finch JT, Zimmern D. Configuration of tobacco mosaic virus, RNA during virus assembly. *Nature* 1977;265:217–219.
29. Calder LJ, Wasilewski S, Berriman JA, et al. Structural organization of a filamentous influenza A virus. *Proc Natl Acad Sci U S A* 2010;107:10685–10690.
30. Carey J, Cameron V, de Haseth PL, et al. Sequence-specific interaction of R17 coat protein with its ribonucleic acid binding site. *Biochemistry* 1983;22:2601–2610.
31. Carfi A, Willis SH, Whitbeck JC, et al. Herpes simplex virus glycoprotein D bound to the human receptor HveA. *Mol Cell* 2001;8:169–179.
32. Carr CM, Kim PS. A spring-loaded mechanism for the conformational change of influenza hemagglutinin. *Cell* 1993;73:823–832.
33. Casjens S, King J. Virus assembly. *Ann Rev Biochem* 1975;44:555–611.
34. Caspar DL. Assembly and stability of the tobacco mosaic virus particle. *Adv Protein Chem* 1963;18:37–121.
35. Caspar DLD, Klug A. Physical principles in the construction of regular viruses. *Cold Spr Harb Symp Quant Biol* 1962;27:1–24.
36. Chambers TJ, Hanh CS, Galler R, et al. Flavivirus genome organization, expression, and replication. *Ann Rev Microbiol* 1990;44:649–688.
37. Chan DC, Fass D, Berger JM, et al. Core structure of gp41 from the HIV envelope glycoprotein. *Cell* 1997;89:263–273.
38. Chandran K, Walker SB, Chen Y, et al. In vitro recoating of reovirus cores with baculovirus-expressed outer-capsid proteins mu1 and sigma3. *J Virol* 1999;73:3941–3950.
39. Chang JT, Schmid MF, Rixon FJ, et al. Electron cryotomography reveals the portal in the herpesvirus capsid. *J Virol* 2007;81:2065–2068.
40. Chen BJ, Lamb RA. Mechanisms for enveloped virus budding: can some viruses do without an ESCRT? *Virology* 2008;372:221–232.
41. Chen J, Skehel JJ, Wiley DC. N- and C-terminal residues combine in the fusion-pH influenza hemagglutinin HA(2) subunit to form an N cap that terminates the triple-stranded coiled coil. *Proc Natl Acad Sci U S A* 1999;96:8967-8972.
42. Chen JZ, Settembre EC, Aoki ST, et al. Molecular interactions in rotavirus assembly and uncoating seen by high-resolution cryo-EM. *Proc Natl Acad Sci U S A* 2009;106:10644–10648.
43. Chen L, Gorman JJ, McKimm-Breschkin J, et al. The structure of the fusion glycoprotein of Newcastle disease virus suggests a novel paradigm for the molecular mechanism of membrane fusion. *Structure* 2001;9:255–266.
44. Chen ZG, Stauffacher C, Li T, et al. Protein-RNA interactions in an icosahedral virus at 3.0 A resolution. *Science* 1989;245:154–159.
45. Cheng RH, Kuhn RJ, Olson NH, et al. Nucleocapsid and glycoprotein organization in an enveloped virus. *Cell* 1995;80:621–630.
46. Choi H-K, Tong L, Minor W, et al. Structure of sindbis virus core protein reveals a chymotrypsin-like serine proteinase and the organization of the virion. *Nature* 1991;354:37–43.
47. Chow M, Newman JF, Filman D, et al. Myristylation of picornavirus capsid protien VP4 and its structural significance. *Nature* 1987;327:482–486.
48. Chowdary TK, Cairns TM, Atanasiu D, et al. Crystal structure of the conserved herpesvirus fusion regulator complex gH-gL. *Nat Struct Mol Biol* 2010;17:882–888.
49. Cockburn JJ, Abrescia NG, Grimes JM, et al. Membrane structure and interactions with protein and DNA in bacteriophage PRD1. *Nature* 2004;432:122–125.
50. Colman PM. Virus versus antibody. *Structure* 1997;5:591–593.
51. Compans RW, Content J, Duesberg PH. Structure of the ribonucleoprotein of influenza virus. *J Virol* 1972;10:795–800.
52. Connolly SA, Leser GP, Yin HS, et al. Refolding of a paramyxovirus F protein from prefusion to postfusion conformations observed by liposome binding and electron microscopy. *Proc Natl Acad Sci U S A* 2006; 103:17903–17908.
53. Conway JF, Wikoff WR, Cheng N, et al. Virus maturation involving large subunit rotations and local refolding. *Science* 2001;292:744–748.
54. Coulibaly F, Chevalier C, Gutsche I, et al. The birnavirus crystal structure reveals structural relationships among icosahedral viruses. *Cell* 2005; 120:761–772.
55. Crawford SE, Mukherjee SK, Estes MK, et al. Trypsin cleavage stabilizes the rotavirus VP4 spike. *J Virol* 2001;75:6052–6061.
56. Crick FHC, Watson JD. Structure of small viruses. *Nature (London)* 1956; 177:473–375.
57. Crowther RA, Klug A. Structural analysis of macromolecular assemblies by image reconstruction from electron micrographs. *Annu Rev Biochem* 1975;44:161–182.
58. Cyrklaff M, Risco C, Fernandez JJ, et al. Cryo-electron tomography of vaccinia virus. *Proc Natl Acad Sci U S A* 2005;102:2772–2777.
59. Danieli T, Pelletier SL, Henis YI, et al. Membrane fusion mediated by the influenza virus hemagglutinin requires the concerted action of at least three hemagglutinin trimers. *J Cell Biol* 1996;133:559–569.
60. De Guzman RN, Wu ZR, Stalling CC, et al. Structure of the HIV-1 nucleocapsid protein bound to the SL3 psi-RNA recognition element. *Science* 1998;279:384–388.

61. de Haas F, Paatero AO, Mindich L, et al. A symmetry mismatch at the site of RNA packaging in the polymerase complex of dsRNA bacteriophage phi6. *J Mol Biol* 1999;294:357–372.
62. de Rosny E, Vassell R, Jiang S, et al. Binding of the 2F5 monoclonal antibody to native and fusion-intermediate forms of human immunodeficiency virus type 1 gp41: implications for fusion-inducing conformational changes. *J Virol* 2004;78:2627–2631.
63. Dormitzer PR, Nason EB, Prasad BV, et al. Structural rearrangements in the membrane penetration protein of a non-enveloped virus. *Nature* 2004;430:1053–1058.
64. Dryden KA, Wang G, Yeager M, et al. Early steps in reovirus infection are associated with dramatic changes in supramolecular structure and protein conformation: analysis of virions and subviral particles by cryoelectron microscopy and image reconstruction. *J Cell Biol* 1993;122:1023–1041.
65. Duda RL, Hempel J, Michel H, et al. Structural transitions during bacteriophage HK97 head assembly. *J Mol Biol* 1995;247:618–635.
66. Duquerroy S, Da Costa B, Henry C, et al. The picobirnavirus crystal structure provides functional insights into virion assembly and cell entry. *EMBO J* 2009;28:1655–1665.
67. Durrer P, Gaudin Y, Ruigrok RW, et al. Photolabeling identifies a putative fusion domain in the envelope glycoprotein of rabies and vesicular stomatitis viruses. *J Biol Chem* 1995;270:17575–17581.
68. Earnshaw W, Casjens S, Harrison SC. Assembly of the head of bacteriophage P22: x-ray diffraction from heads, proheads and related structures. *J Mol Biol* 1976;104:387–410.
69. Earnshaw WC, Harrison SC. DNA arrangement in isometric phage heads. *Nature* 1977;268:598–602.
70. Earnshaw WC, King J, Harrison SC, et al. The structural organization of DNA packaged within the heads of T4 wild-type, isometric and giant bacteriophages. *Cell* 1978;14:559–568.
71. Emini EA, Ostapchuk P, Wimmer E. Bivalent attachment of antibody onto poliovirus leads to conformational alteration and neutralization. *J Virol* 1983;48:547–550.
72. Estrozi LF, Navaza J. Ab initio high-resolution single-particle 3D reconstructions: the symmetry adapted functions way. *J Struct Biol* 2010;172:253–260.
73. Farr GA, Zhang LG, Tattersall P. Parvoviral virions deploy a capsid-tethered lipolytic enzyme to breach the endosomal membrane during cell entry. *Proc Natl Acad Sci U S A* 2005;102:17148–17153.
74. Fisher AJ, Johnson JE. Ordered duplex RNA controls capsid architecture in an icosahedral animal virus. *Nature* 1993;361:176–179.
75. FitzGerald DJ, Padmanabhan R, Pastan I, et al. Adenovirus-induced release of epidermal growth factor and pseudomonas toxin into the cytosol of KB cells during receptor-mediated endocytosis. *Cell* 1983;32:607–617.
76. Floyd DL, Ragains JR, Skehel JJ, et al. Single-particle kinetics of influenza virus membrane fusion. *Proc Natl Acad Sci U S A* 2008;105:15382–15387.
77. Frankel AD, Young JA. HIV-1: fifteen proteins and an RNA. *Ann Rev Biochem* 1998;67:1–25.
78. Fricks CE, Hogle JM. Cell-Induced conformational change in poliovirus: externalization of the amino terminus of VP1 is responsible for liposome binding. *J Virol* 1990;64:1934–1945.
79. Fuller SD, Wilk T, Gowen BE, et al. Cryo-electron microscopy reveals ordered domains in the immature HIV-1 particle. *Curr Biol* 1997;7:729–738.
80. Furciniti PS, Van Oostrum J, Burnett RM. Adenovirus polypeptide IX revealed as capsid cement by difference images from electron microscopy and crystallography. *EMBO J* 1989;8:3563–3570.
81. Furuta RA, Wild CT, Weng Y, et al. Capture of an early fusion-active conformation of HIV-1 gp41. *Nat Struct Biol* 1998;5:276–279.
82. Gallegos CO, Patton JT. Characterization of rotavirus replication intermediates: a model for the assembly of single-shelled particles. *Virology* 1989;172:616–627.
83. Ganser BK, Li S, Klishko VY, et al. Assembly and analysis of conical models for the HIV-1 core. *Science* 1999;283:80–83.
84. Ganser-Pornillos BK, Yeager M, Sundquist WI. The structural biology of HIV assembly. *Curr Opin Struct Biol* 2008;18:203–217.
85. Garrus JE, von Schwedler UK, Pornillos OW, et al. Tsg101 and the vacuolar protein sorting pathway are essential for HIV-1 budding. *Cell* 2001;107:55–65.
86. Ge P, Tsao J, Schein S, et al. Cryo-EM model of the bullet-shaped vesicular stomatitis virus. *Science* 2010;327:689–693.
87. Glucksman MJ, Bhattacharjee S, Makowski L. Three-dimensional structure of a cloning vector. X-ray diffraction studies of filamentous bacteriophage M13 at 7 A resolution. *J Mol Biol* 1992;226:455–470.
88. Golden JS, Harrison SC. Proteolytic dissection of turnip crinkle virus subunit in solution. *Biochemistry* 1982;21:3862–3866.
89. Gomez Yafal A, Kaplan G, Racaniello VR, et al. Characterization of poliovirus conformational alteration mediated by soluble cell receptors. *Virology* 1993;197:501–505.
90. Gowen B, Bamford JK, Bamford DH, et al. The tailless icosahedral membrane virus PRD1 localizes the proteins involved in genome packaging and injection at a unique vertex. *J Virol* 2003;77:7863–7871.
91. Gralla J, DeLisi C. mRNA is expected to form stable secondary structures. *Nature* 1974;248:330–332.
92. Greber UF, Willetts M, Webster P, et al. Stepwise dismantling of adenovirus 2 during entry into cells. *Cell* 1993;75:477–486.
93. Green TJ, Zhang X, Wertz GW, et al. Structure of the vesicular stomatitis virus nucleoprotein-RNA complex. *Science* 2006;313:357–360.
94. Grigorieff N, Harrison SC. Near-atomic resolution reconstructions of icosahedral viruses from electron cryo-microscopy. *Curr Opin Struct Biol* 2011;21:265–273.
95. Grimes J, Basak AK, Roy P, et al. The crystal structure of bluetongue virus VP7. *Nature* 1995;373:167–170.
96. Grimes JM, Burroughs JM, Gouet P, et al. The atomic structure of the bluetongue virus core. *Nature* 1998;395:470–478.
97. Grimes S, Jardine PJ, Anderson D. Bacteriophage phi 29 DNA packaging. *Adv Virus Res* 2002;58:255–294.
98. Grunewald K, Desai P, Winkler DC, et al. Three-dimensional structure of herpes simplex virus from cryo-electron tomography. *Science* 2003;302:1396–1398.
99. Guogas LM, Filman DJ, Hogle JM, et al. Cofolding organizes alfalfa mosaic virus RNA and coat protein for replication. *Science* 2004;306:2108–2111.
100. Guttman N, Baltimore D. A plasma membrane component able to bind and alter virions of poliovirus type 1: studies on cell-free alteration using a simplified assay. *Virology* 1977;82:25–36.
101. Hall L, Rueckert RR. Infection of mouse fibroblasts by cardioviruses: premature uncoating and its prevention by elevated pH and magnesium chloride. *Virology* 1971;43:152–165.
102. Hannah BP, Heldwein EE, Bender FC, et al. Mutational evidence of internal fusion loops in herpes simplex virus glycoprotein B. *J Virol* 2007;81:4858–4865.
103. Harrison SC. Looking inside adenovirus. *Science* 2010;329:1026–1027.
104. Harrison SC. Packaging of DNA into bacteriophage heads: a model. *J Mol Biol* 1983;171:577–580.
105. Harrison SC. Protein interfaces and intersubunit bonding. The case of tomato bushy stunt virus. *Biophys J* 1980;32:139–153.
106. Harrison SC. Viral membrane fusion. *Nat Struct Mol Biol* 2008;15:690–698.
107. Harrison SC, Olson A, Schutt CE, et al. Tomato bushy stunt virus at 2.9 Å resolution. *Nature (London)* 1978;276:368–373.
108. He Y, Vassell R, Zaitseva M, et al. Peptides trap the human immunodeficiency virus type 1 envelope glycoprotein fusion intermediate at two sites. *J Virol* 2003;77:1666–1671.
109. Heldwein EE, Lou H, Bender FC, et al. Crystal structure of glycoprotein B from herpes simplex virus 1. *Science* 2006;313:217–220.
110. Hogle JM. Poliovirus cell entry: common structural themes in viral cell entry pathways. *Annu Rev Microbiol* 2002;56:677–702.
111. Hooper JW, Fields BN. Role of the mu 1 protein in reovirus stability and capacity to cause chromium release from host cells. *J Virol* 1996;70:459–467.
112. Huiskonen JT, de Haas F, Bubeck D, et al. Structure of the bacteriophage phi6 nucleocapsid suggests a mechanism for sequential RNA packaging. *Structure* 2006;14:1039–1048.
113. Iyer LM, Makarova KS, Koonin EV, et al. Comparative genomics of the FtsK-HerA superfamily of pumping ATPases: implications for the origins of chromosome segregation, cell division and viral capsid packaging. *Nucleic Acids Res* 2004;32:5260–5279.

114. Jaalinoja HT, Huiskonen JT, Butcher SJ. Electron cryomicroscopy comparison of the architectures of the enveloped bacteriophages phi6 and phi8. *Structure* 2007;15:157–167.
115. Jahn R, Lang T, Sudhof TC. Membrane fusion. *Cell* 2003;112:519–533.
116. Jayaram H, Taraporewala Z, Patton JT, et al. Rotavirus protein involved in genome replication and packaging exhibits a HIT-like fold. *Nature* 2002;417:311–315.
117. Jiang W, Li Z, Zhang Z, et al. Coat protein fold and maturation transition of bacteriophage P22 seen at subnanometer resolutions. *Nat Struct Biol* 2003;10:131–135.
118. Jiang X, Jayaram H, Kumar M, et al. Cryoelectron microscopy structures of rotavirus NSP2-NSP5 and NSP2-RNA complexes: implications for genome replication. *J Virol* 2006;80:10829–10835.
119. Johnson JE. Virus particle maturation: insights into elegantly programmed nanomachines. *Curr Opin Struct Biol* 2010;20:210–216.
120. Kadlec J, Loureiro S, Abrescia NG, et al. The postfusion structure of baculovirus gp64 supports a unified view of viral fusion machines. *Nat Struct Mol Biol* 2008;15:1024–1030.
121. Khromykh AA, Varnavski AN, Sedlak PL, et al. Coupling between replication and packaging of flavivirus RNA: evidence derived from the use of DNA-based full-length cDNA clones of Kunjin virus. *J Virol* 2001;75:4633–4640.
122. Kim DY, Firth AE, Atasheva S, et al. Conservation of a packaging signal and the viral genome RNA packaging mechanism in alphavirus evolution. *J Virol* 2011;85:8022–8036.
123. Kim IS, Trask SD, Babyonyshev M, et al. Effect of mutations in VP5 hydrophobic loops on rotavirus cell entry. *J Virol* 2010;84:6200–6207.
124. Klenk HD, Choppin PW. Lipids of plasma membranes of monkey and hamster kidney cells and of parainfluenza virions grown in these cells. *Virology* 1969;38:255–268.
125. Klug A, Caspar DL. The structure of small viruses. *Adv Virus Res* 1960;7:225–325.
126. Krol MA, Olson NH, Tate J, et al. RNA-controlled polymorphism in the in vivo assembly of 180-subunit and 120-subunit virions from a single capsid protein. *Proc Natl Acad Sci U S A* 1999;96:13650–13655.
127. Krummenacher C, Supekar VM, Whitbeck JC, et al. Structure of unliganded HSV gD reveals a mechanism for receptor-mediated activation of virus entry. *EMBO J* 2005;24:4144–4153.
128. Kuhn RJ, Zhang W, Rossmann MG, et al. Structure of dengue virus: implications for flavivirus organization, maturation, and fusion. *Cell* 2002;108:717–725.
129. Kumar M, Jayaram H, Vasquez-Del Carpio R, et al. Crystallographic and biochemical analysis of rotavirus NSP2 with nucleotides reveals a nucleoside diphosphate kinase-like activity. *J Virol* 2007;81:12272–12284.
130. Kuzmin PI, Zimmerberg J, Chizmadzhev YA, et al. A quantitative model for membrane fusion based on low-energy intermediates. *Proc Natl Acad Sci U S A* 2001;98:7235–7240.
131. Kwong PD, Wyatt R, Robinson J, et al. Structure of an HIV gp120 envelope glycoprotein in complex with the CD4 receptor and a neutralizing human antibody. *Nature* 1998;393:648–659.
132. Lamb RA, Jardetzky TS. Structural basis of viral invasion: lessons from paramyxovirus F. *Curr Opin Struct Biol* 2007;17:427–436.
133. Lata R, Conway JF, Cheng N, et al. Maturation dynamics of a viral capsid: visualization of transitional intermediate states. *Cell* 2000;100:253–263.
134. Laver WG, Wrigley NG, Pereira HG. Removal of pentons from particles of adenovirus type 2. *Virology* 1969;39:599–604.
135. Lee S, Owen KE, Choi HK, et al. Identification of a protein binding site on the surface of the alphavirus nucleocapsid and its implication in virus assembly. *Structure* 1996;4:531–541.
136. Lescar J, Roussel A, Wien MW, et al. The fusion glycoprotein shell of Semliki Forest virus: an icosahedral assembly primed for fusogenic activation at endosomal pH. *Cell* 2001;105:137–148.
137. Li F, Li W, Farzan M, et al. Structure of SARS coronavirus spike receptor-binding domain complexed with receptor. *Science* 2005;309:1864–1868.
138. Li L, Lok SM, Yu IM, et al. The flavivirus precursor membrane-envelope protein complex: structure and maturation. *Science* 2008;319:1830–1834.
139. Liddington RC, Yan Y, Zhao HC, et al. Structure of simian virus 40 at 3.8 Å resolution. *Nature* 1991;354:278–284.
140. Liemann S, Chandran K, Baker TS, et al. Structure of the reovirus membrane-penetration protein, Mu1, in a complex with is protector protein, Sigma3. *Cell* 2002;108:283–295.
141. Liljas L, Unge T, Jones TA, et al. Structure of satellite tobacco necrosis virus at 3.0 A resolution. *J Mol Biol* 1982;159:93–108.
142. Liu H, Jin L, Koh SB, et al. Atomic structure of human adenovirus by cryo-EM reveals interactions among protein networks. *Science* 2010;329:1038–1043.
143. Lorieau JL, Louis JM, Bax A. Helical hairpin structure of influenza hemagglutinin fusion peptide stabilized by charge-dipole interactions between the N-terminal amino group and the second helix. *J Am Chem Soc* 2011;133:2824–2827.
144. Lorieau JL, Louis JM, Bax A. The complete influenza hemagglutinin fusion domain adopts a tight helical hairpin arrangement at the lipid:water interface. *Proc Natl Acad Sci U S A* 2010;107:11341–11346.
145. Lu M, Blacklow SC, Kim PS. A trimeric structural domain of the HIV-1 transmembrane glycoprotein. *Nat Struct Biol* 1995;2:1075–1082.
146. Lu X, McDonald SM, Tortorici MA, et al. Mechanism for coordinated RNA packaging and genome replication by rotavirus polymerase VP1. *Structure* 2008;16:1678–1688.
147. Markin VS, Kozlov MM, Borovjagin VL. On the theory of membrane fusion. The stalk mechanism. *Gen Physiol Biophys* 1984;3:361–377.
148. Markosyan RM, Cohen FS, Melikyan GB. HIV-1 envelope proteins complete their folding into six-helix bundles immediately after fusion pore formation. *Mol Biol Cell* 2003;14:926–938.
149. Mathieu M, Petitpas I, Navaza J, et al. Atomic structure of the major capsid protein of rotavirus: implications for the architecture of the virion. *EMBO J* 2001;20:1485–1497.
150. Matsuura H, Kirschner AN, Longnecker R, et al. Crystal structure of the Epstein-Barr virus (EBV) glycoprotein H/glycoprotein L (gH/gL) complex. *Proc Natl Acad Sci U S A* 2010;107:22641–22646.
151. McClain B, Settembre E, Temple BR, et al. X-ray crystal structure of the rotavirus inner capsid particle at 3.8 A resolution. *J Mol Biol* 2010;397:587–599.
152. McKenna R, Xia D, Willingman P, et al. Atomic structure of single-stranded DNA bacteriophage ϕX174 and its functional implications. *Nature* 1992;355:137–143.
153. Mindich L. Packaging, replication and recombination of the segmented genome of bacteriophage Phi6 and its relatives. *Virus Res* 2004;101:83–92.
154. Modis Y, Ogata S, Clements D, et al. A ligand-binding pocket in the dengue virus envelope glycoprotein. *Proc Natl Acad Sci U S A* 2003;100:6986–6991.
155. Modis Y, Ogata S, Clements D, et al. Structure of the dengue virus envelope protein after membrane fusion. *Nature* 2004;427:313–319.
156. Moffitt JR, Chemla YR, Aathavan K, et al. Intersubunit coordination in a homomeric ring ATPase. *Nature* 2009;457:446–450.
157. Moscufo N, Yafal AG, Rogove A, et al. A mutation in VP4 defines a new step in the late stages of cell entry by poliovirus. *J Virol* 1993;67:5075–5078.
158. Moyer CL, Wiethoff CM, Maier O, et al. Functional genetic and biophysical analyses of membrane disruption by human adenovirus. *J Virol* 2011;85:2631–2641.
159. Mukhopadhyay S, Zhang W, Gabler S, et al. Mapping the structure and function of the E1 and E2 glycoproteins in alphaviruses. *Structure* 2006;14:63–73.
160. Munowitz MG, Dobson CM, Griffin RG, et al. On the rigidity of RNA in tomato bushy stunt virus. *J Mol Biol* 1980;141:327–333.
161. Muramoto Y, Takada A, Fujii K, et al. Hierarchy among viral RNA (vRNA) segments in their role in vRNA incorporation into influenza A virions. *J Virol* 2006;80:2318–2325.
162. Neu U, Woellner K, Gauglitz G, et al. Structural basis of GM1 ganglioside recognition by simian virus 40. *Proc Natl Acad Sci U S A* 2008;105:5219–5224.
163. Newcomb WW, Homa FL, Thomsen DR, et al. Assembly of the herpes simplex virus capsid: characterization of intermediates observed during cell-free capsid formation. *J Mol Biol* 1996;263:432–446.

164. Newcomb WW, Juhas RM, Thomsen DR, et al. The UL6 gene product forms the portal for entry of DNA into the herpes simplex virus capsid. *J Virol* 2001;75:10923–10932.
165. Nibert ML, Fields BN. A carboxy-terminal fragment of protein ml/m1 C is present in infectious subvirion particles of mammalian reoviruses and is proposed to have a role in penetration. *J Virol* 1992;66:6408–6418.
166. Nibert ML, Schiff LA, Fields BN. Mammalian reoviruses contain a myristoylated structural protein. *J Virol* 1991;65:1960–1967.
167. Noda T, Sagara H, Yen A, et al. Architecture of ribonucleoprotein complexes in influenza A virus particles. *Nature* 2006;439:490–492.
168. Nugent CI, Johnson KL, Sarnow P, et al. Functional coupling between replication and packaging of poliovirus replicon RNA. *J Virol* 1999; 73:427–435.
169. Olia AS, Prevelige PE Jr, Johnson JE, et al. Three-dimensional structure of a viral genome-delivery portal vertex. *Nat Struct Mol Biol* 2011; 18:597–603.
170. Ostapchuk P, Almond M, Hearing P. Characterization of empty adenovirus particles assembled in the absence of a functional adenovirus IVa2 protein. *J Virol* 2011;85:5524–5531.
171. Owen KE, Kuhn RJ. Alphavirus budding is dependent on the interaction between the nucleocapsid and hydrophobic amino acids on the cytoplasmic domain of the E2 envelope glycoprotein. *Virology* 1997;230: 187–196.
172. Palese P, Tobita K, Ueda M, et al. Characterization of temperature sensitive influenza virus mutants defective in neuraminidase. *Virology* 1974;61: 397–410.
173. Parent KN, Khayat R, Tu LH, et al. P22 coat protein structures reveal a novel mechanism for capsid maturation: stability without auxiliary proteins or chemical crosslinks. *Structure* 2010;18:390–401.
174. Patton JT, Gallegos CO. Rotavirus RNA replication: single-stranded RNA extends from the replicase particle. *J Gen Virol* 1990;71(Pt 5):1087–1094.
175. Patton JT, Vasquez-Del Carpio R, Tortorici MA, et al. Coupling of rotavirus genome replication and capsid assembly. *Adv Virus Res* 2007; 69:167–201.
176. Paulson JC, Sadler JE, Hill RL. Restoration of specific myxovirus receptors to asialoerythrocytes by incorporation of sialic acid with pure sialyltransferases. *J Biol Chem* 1979;254:2120–2124.
177. Pevear DC, Fancher MJ, Felock PJ, et al. Conformational change in the floor of the human rhinovirus canyon blocks adsorption to HeLa cell receptors. *J Virol* 1989;63:2002–2007.
178. Pielak RM, Oxenoid K, Chou JJ. Structural investigation of rimantadine inhibition of the AM2-BM2 chimera channel of influenza viruses. *Structure* 2011;19:1655–1663.
179. Pletnev SV, Zhang W, Mukhopadhyay S, et al. Locations of carbohydrate sites on alphavirus glycoproteins show that E1 forms an icosahedral scaffold. *Cell* 2001;105:127–136.
180. Poranen MM, Tuma R, Bamford DH. Assembly of double-strand RNA viruses. In: Roy P, ed. *Virus Structure and Assembly.* Vol. 64. San Diego: Elsevier Academic Press; 2005:15–43.
181. Pornillos O, Garrus JE, Sundquist WI. Mechanisms of enveloped RNA virus budding. *Trends Cell Biol* 2002;12:569–579.
182. Prasad BV, Hardy ME, Dokland T, et al. X-ray crystallographic structure of the Norwalk virus capsid. *Science* 1999;286:287–290.
183. Rand RP, Luzzati V. X-ray diffraction study in water of lipids extracted from human erythrocytes: the position of cholesterol in the lipid lamellae. *Biophys J* 1968;8:125–137.
184. Razinkov VI, Melikyan GB, Cohen FS. Hemifusion between cells expressing hemagglutinin of influenza virus and planar membranes can precede the formation of fusion pores that subsequently fully enlarge. *Biophys J* 1999;77:3144–3151.
185. Reddy VS, Natarajan P, Okerberg B, et al. Virus Particle Explorer (VIPER), a website for virus capsid structures and their computational analyses. *J Virol* 2001;75:11943–11947.
186. Reinisch K, Nibert M, Harrison SC. The reovirus core: structure of a complex molecular machine. *Nature* 2000;404:960–967.
187. Rey FA, Heinz FX, Mandl C, et al. The envelope glycoprotein from tick-borne encephalitis virus at 2 Å resolution. *Nature* 1995;375:291–298.
188. Rhee SS, Hunter E. A single amino-acid substitution within the matrix protein of a type D retrovirus converts its morphogenen's to that of a type C retrovirus. *Cell* 1990;63:77–86.
189. Roberts MM, White JL, Grütter MG, et al. Three-dimensional structure of the adenovirus major coat protein hexon. *Science* 1986;232:1148–1151.
190. Robinson IK, Harrison SC. Structure of the expanded state of tomato bushy stunt virus. *Nature (London)* 1982;297:563–568.
191. Roche S, Bressanelli S, Rey FA, et al. Crystal structure of the low-pH form of the vesicular stomatitis virus glycoprotein G. *Science* 2006;313: 187–191.
192. Roche S, Gaudin Y. Characterization of the equilibrium between the native and fusion-inactive conformation of rabies virus glycoprotein indicates that the fusion complex is made of several trimers. *Virology* 2002; 297:128–135.
193. Roche S, Rey FA, Gaudin Y, et al. Structure of the prefusion form of the vesicular stomatitis virus glycoprotein G. *Science* 2007;315:843–848.
194. Rossman JS, Jing X, Leser GP, et al. Influenza virus M2 protein mediates ESCRT-independent membrane scission. *Cell* 2010;142:902–913.
195. Rossmann MG. The canyon hypothesis. Hiding the host cell receptor attachment site on a viral surface from immune surveillance. *J Biol Chem* 1989;264:14587–14590.
196. Rossmann MG, He Y, Kuhn RJ. Picornavirus-receptor interactions. *Trends Microbiol* 2002;10:324–331.
197. Rudolph MG, Kraus I, Dickmanns A, et al. Crystal structure of the borna disease virus nucleoprotein. *Structure* 2003;11:1219–1226.
198. Sahli R, Freund R, Dubensky T, et al. Defect in entry and altered pathogenicity of a polyoma virus mutant blocked in VP2 myristylation. *Virology* 1993;192:142–153.
199. Scheiffele P, Rietveld A, Wilk T, et al. Influenza viruses select ordered lipid domains during budding from the plasma membrane. *J Biol Chem* 1999;274:2038–2044.
200. Schnell JR, Chou JJ. Structure and mechanism of the M2 proton channel of influenza A virus. *Nature* 2008;451:591–595.
201. Seiradake E, Henaff D, Wodrich H, et al. The cell adhesion molecule "CAR" and sialic acid on human erythrocytes influence adenovirus in vivo biodistribution. *PLoS Pathog* 2009;5:e1000277.
202. Settembre EC, Chen JZ, Dormitzer PR, et al. Atomic model of an infectious rotavirus particle. *EMBO J* 2010;30:408–416.
203. Shaw JG, Plaskitt KA, Wilson TMA. Evidence that tobacco mosaic virus particles disassemble cotranslationally in vivo. *Virology* 1986;148:326–336.
204. Shields SA, Brisco MJ, Wilson TM, et al. Southern bean mosaic virus RNA remains associated with swollen virions during translation in wheat germ cell-free extracts. *Virology* 1989;171:602–606.
205. Siegel DP. Energetics of intermediates in membrane fusion: comparison of stalk and inverted micellar intermediate mechanisms. *Biophys J* 1993;65:2124–2140.
206. Silvestry M, Lindert S, Smith JG, et al. Cryo-electron microscopy structure of adenovirus type 2 temperature-sensitive mutant 1 reveals insight into the cell entry defect. *J Virol* 2009;83:7375–7383.
207. Simpson AA, Tao Y, Leiman PG, et al. Structure of the bacteriophage phi29 DNA packaging motor. *Nature* 2000;408:745–750.
208. Sjoberg M, Garoff H. Interactions between the transmembrane segments of the alphavirus E1 and E2 proteins play a role in virus budding and fusion. *J Virol* 2003;77:3441–3450.
209. Skehel JJ, Bayley PM, Brown EB, et al. Changes in the conformation of influenza virus haemagglutinin at the pH optimum of virus-mediated membrane fusion. *Proc Natl Acad Sci U S A* 1982;79:968–972.
210. Skehel JJ, Wiley DC. Receptor binding and membrane fusion in virus entry: the influenza hemagglutinin. *Annu Rev Biochem* 2000;69: 531–569.
211. Smith DE, Tans SJ, Smith SB, et al. The bacteriophage straight phi29 portal motor can package DNA against a large internal force. *Nature* 2001;413: 748–752.
212. Smith TJ, Kremer MJ, Luo M, et al. The site of attachment in human rhinovirus 14 for antiviral agents that inhibit uncoating. *Science* 1986;233: 1286–1293.
213. Steere RL, Schaffer FL. The structure of crystals of purified mahoney poliovirus. *Acta Biochem Biophys* 1958;28:241.
214. Stewart PL, Burnett RM, Cyrklaff M, et al. Image reconstruction reveals the complex molecular organization of adenovirus. *Cell* 1991;67:145–154.
215. Stewart PL, Fuller SD, Burnett RM. Difference imaging of adenovirus: bridging the resolution gap between X-ray crystallography and electron microscopy. *EMBO J* 1993;12:2589–2599.

216. Strack B, Calistri A, Accola MA, et al. A role for ubiquitin ligase recruitment in retrovirus release. *Proc Natl Acad Sci U S A* 2000;97:13063–13068.
217. Sun S, Kondabagil K, Draper B, et al. The structure of the phage T4 DNA packaging motor suggests a mechanism dependent on electrostatic forces. *Cell* 2008;135:1251–1262.
218. Sun S, Kondabagil K, Gentz PM, et al. The structure of the ATPase that powers DNA packaging into bacteriophage T4 procapsids. *Mol Cell* 2007;25:943–949.
219. Sun S, Rao VB, Rossmann MG. Genome packaging in viruses. *Curr Opin Struct Biol* 2010;20:114–120.
220. Supekar VM, Bruckmann C, Ingallinella P, et al. Structure of a proteolytically resistant core from the severe acute respiratory syndrome coronavirus S2 fusion protein. *Proc Natl Acad Sci U S A* 2004;101:17958–17963.
221. Takeda M, Leser GP, Russell CJ, et al. Influenza virus hemagglutinin concentrates in lipid raft microdomains for efficient viral fusion. *Proc Natl Acad Sci U S A* 2003;100:14610–14617.
222. Tang J, Lander GC, Olia AS, et al. Peering down the barrel of a bacteriophage portal: the genome packaging and release valve in p22. *Structure* 2011;19:496–502.
223. Tao Y, Farsetta DL, Nibert ML, et al. RNA synthesis in a cage–structural studies of reovirus polymerase lambda3. *Cell* 2002;111:733–745.
224. Tao Y, Olson NH, Xu W, et al. Assembly of a tailed bacterial virus and its genome release studied in three dimensions. *Cell* 1998;95:431–437.
225. Taraporewala ZF, Jiang X, Vasquez-Del Carpio R, et al. Structure-function analysis of rotavirus NSP2 octamer by using a novel complementation system. *J Virol* 2006;80:7984–7994.
226. Tsang SK, McDermott BM, Racaniello VR, et al. Kinetic analysis of the effect of poliovirus receptor on viral uncoating: the receptor as a catalyst. *J Virol* 2001;75:4984–4989.
227. Turner DR, Joyce LE, Butler PJG. The tobacco mosaic virus assembly origin RNA. *J Mol Biol* 1988;203:531–547.
228. Tuthill TJ, Bubeck D, Rowlands DJ, et al. Characterization of early steps in the poliovirus infection process: receptor-decorated liposomes induce conversion of the virus to membrane-anchored entry-intermediate particles. *J Virol* 2006;80:172–180.
229. Valegard K, Liljas L, Fridborg K, et al. The three-dimensional structure of the bacterial virus MS2. *Nature* 1990;345:36–41.
230. Valegard K, Murray JB, Stockley PG, et al. Crystal structure of an RNA bacteriophage coat protein-operator complex. *Nature* 1994;371:623–626.
231. Valegard K, Murray JB, Stonehouse NJ, et al. The three-dimensional structures of two complexes between recombinant MS2 capsids and RNA operator fragments reveal sequence-specific protein-RNA interactions. *J Mol Biol* 1997;270:724–738.
232. Vogel RH, Provencher SW, von Bonsdorff CH, et al. Envelope structure of Semliki Forest virus reconstructed from cryo-electron micrographs. *Nature* 1986;320:533–535.
233. Von Bonsdorff CH, Harrison SC. Sindbis virus glycoproteins form a regular icosahedral surface lattice. *J Virol* 1975;16:141–145.
234. Von Bonsdorff CH, Pettersson RF. Surface structure of Uukuniemi virus. *J Virol* 1975;16:1296–1307.
235. von Itzstein M, Wu W-Y, Kok GB, et al. Rational design of potent sialidase-based inhibitors of influenza virus replication. *Nature* 1993;363:418–423.
236. Wei H, Cheng RH, Berriman J, et al. Three-dimensional structure of the enveloped bacteriophage phi12: an incomplete T = 13 lattice is superposed on an enclosed T = 1 shell. *PLoS One* 2009;4:e6850.
237. Weis W, Brown J, Cusack S, et al. The structure of the influenza virus haemagglutinin complexed with its receptor, sialic acid. *Nature (London)* 1988;333:426–431.
238. Weissenhorn W, Carfi A, Lee KH, et al. Crystal structure of the Ebola virus membrane fusion subunit, GP2, from the envelope glycoprotein ectodomain. *Mol Cell* 1998;2:605–616.
239. Weissenhorn W, Dessen A, Harrison SC, et al. Atomic structure of the ectodomain from HIV-1 gp41. *Nature* 1997;387:426–430.
240. Whittle JR, Zhang R, Khurana S, et al. Broadly neutralizing human antibody that recognizes the receptor-binding pocket of influenza virus hemagglutinin. *Proc Natl Acad Sci U S A* 2011;108:14216–14221.
241. Wiethoff CM, Wodrich H, Gerace L, et al. Adenovirus protein VI mediates membrane disruption following capsid disassembly. *J Virol* 2005;79:1992–2000.
242. Wikoff WR, Liljas L, Duda RL, et al. Topologically linked protein rings in the bacteriophage HK97 capsid. *Science* 2000;289:2129–2133.
243. Wiley DC, Skehel JJ. Crystallization and x-ray diffraction studies on the haemagglutinin glycoprotein from the membrane of influenza virus. *J Mol Biol* 1977;112:343–347.
244. Wilson IA, Skehel JJ, Wiley DC. Structure of the haemagglutinin membrane glycoprotein of influenza virus at 3 Å resolution. *Nature (London)* 1981;289:366–373.
245. Wilson TMA. Cotranslational disassembly of tobacco mosaic virus in vitro. *Virology* 1984;137:255–265.
246. Wolf M, Garcea RL, Grigorieff N, et al. Subunit interactions in bovine papillomavirus. *Proc Natl Acad Sci U S A* 2010;107:6298–6303.
247. Wright ER, Schooler JB, Ding HJ, et al. Electron cryotomography of immature HIV-1 virions reveals the structure of the CA and SP1 Gag shells. *EMBO J* 2007;26:2218–2226.
248. Ye Q, Krug RM, Tao YJ. The mechanism by which influenza A virus nucleoprotein forms oligomers and binds RNA. *Nature* 2006;444:1078–1082.
249. Yin HS, Paterson RG, Wen X, et al. Structure of the uncleaved ectodomain of the paramyxovirus (hPIV3) fusion protein. *Proc Natl Acad Sci U S A* 2005;102:9288–9293.
250. Yin HS, Wen X, Paterson RG, et al. Structure of the parainfluenza virus 5 F protein in its metastable, prefusion conformation. *Nature* 2006;439:38–44.
251. Yoder JD, Dormitzer PR. Alternative intermolecular contacts underlie the rotavirus VP5(*) two- to three-fold rearrangement. *EMBO J* 2006;25:1559–1568.
252. Yu IM, Holdaway HA, Chipman PR, et al. Association of the pr peptides with dengue virus at acidic pH blocks membrane fusion. *J Virol* 2009;83:12101–12107.
253. Yu IM, Zhang W, Holdaway HA, et al. Structure of the immature dengue virus at low pH primes proteolytic maturation. *Science* 2008;319:1834–1837.
254. Zhang J, Pekosz A, Lamb RA. Influenza virus assembly and lipid raft microdomains: a role for the cytoplasmic tails of the spike glycoproteins. *J Virol* 2000;74:4634–4644.
255. Zhang W, Chipman PR, Corver J, et al. Visualization of membrane protein domains by cryo-electron microscopy of dengue virus. *Nat Struct Biol* 2003;10:907–912.
256. Zhang W, Imperiale MJ. Requirement of the adenovirus IVa2 protein for virus assembly. *J Virol* 2003;77:3586–3594.
257. Zhang W, Low JA, Christensen JB, et al. Role for the adenovirus IVa2 protein in packaging of viral DNA. *J Virol* 2001;75:10446–10454.
258. Zhang W, Mukhopadhyay S, Pletnev SV, et al. Placement of the structural proteins in Sindbis virus. *J Virol* 2002;76:11645–11658.
259. Zhang X, Settembre E, Xu C, et al. Near-atomic resolution using electron cryomicroscopy and single-particle reconstruction. *Proc Natl Acad Sci U S A* 2008;105:1867–1872.
260. Zheng Q, Deng Y, Liu J, et al. Core structure of S2 from the human coronavirus NL63 spike glycoprotein. *Biochemistry* 2006;45:15205–15215.
261. Zimmern D, Wilson TMA. Location of the origin for viral reassembly on tobacco mosaic virus RNA and its relation to stable fragment. *FEBS Lett* 1976;71:294–298.

CHAPTER 4

Ari Helenius

Virus Entry and Uncoating

Viral particles have a single mission: to transport the viral genome from an infected host cell to a noninfected host cell and to deliver it into the cytoplasm or the nucleus in a replication-competent form. The target can be a neighboring cell, a cell elsewhere in the host organism, or a cell in another organism. The process starts in an infected cell with the packaging of the viral genome and accessory proteins into a new virus particle, which is released into the extracellular space. When the virus contacts the surface of a new host cell, a complex series of events ensues tightly coordinated in time and space. These events include binding to receptors and signaling, often followed by endocytic internalization, vesicular trafficking, membrane penetration, cytosolic transport, and nuclear import (Fig. 4.1). Uncoating is an integral part of the process; the virus particle is modified, destabilized, disassembled, and eventually the genome, present in a protected and condensed form in the virion, is decondensed and exposed in a replication- or transcription-competent form. The progression of a virus particle through its entry program depends critically on cellular functions. The *Trojan horse strategy* that is used is necessary because the particles are simple and capable of limited independent functions.

This chapter describes some of the general concepts that govern cellular entry of animal viruses. For information about the entry of specific viruses and virus families, the reader is referred to the virus chapters. Information relevant to the topics covered here also can be found in numerous reviews that cover early virus cell interactions.[43,81,100,109,110,124,150,167,212]

THE BARRIERS

The first barrier that incoming viruses must overcome is the glycocalyx, a layer of glycoconjugates that covers the external surface of cells. It is composed of glycoproteins, glycolipids, and proteoglycans. The composition and thickness of this layer is variable. By binding to oligosaccharides, many viruses make use of the glycocalyx for initial attachment.

The next barrier is the plasma membrane. Responsible for the cell's exchanges with the environment, it is the most complex and most dynamic of all cell membranes. The composition and properties are regulated by the endocytic and secretory pathways and by a continuous association and disassociation of proteins that interact with the cytosolic leaflet. The plasma membrane is a highly sensitive organ for recognizing and responding to external stimuli. Viruses take advantage of this during entry.

After clearing the plasma membrane by direct penetration or by exploiting endocytic pathways, viruses and viral capsids have to reach sites deeper in the cytoplasm. The cortical actin network underneath the plasma membrane and extreme crowding constitute major barriers to movement within the cytoplasm.[184] Finally, because many viruses replicate in the nucleus, the genome and accessory proteins must travel to the nucleus and cross the nuclear envelope. This requires cooperation between the incoming virus and the nuclear import machinery.[211]

VIRUS BINDING TO THE CELL SURFACE

Viruses can only infect cells to which they can bind. Binding occurs to *attachment factors* and *virus receptors* on the surface of the cell. To a large extent, the identity, distribution, and behavior of these cellular components determine which cell types, tissues, and organisms a virus can infect. The receptors also define, in part, the pathogenic potential of a virus as well the nature of the disease that it causes.

Virus *receptors* can be defined as cell surface molecules that bind the incoming viruses to the cell, and, in addition, promote entry by (a) inducing conformational changes in the virus that lead to priming, association with other receptors, membrane fusion, and penetration; (b) transmitting signals through the plasma membrane that lead to virus uptake or penetration and prepare the cell for the invasion; or (c) guiding bound virus particles into a variety of endocytic pathways.[124] *Attachment factors* help to concentrate the particles on the cell's

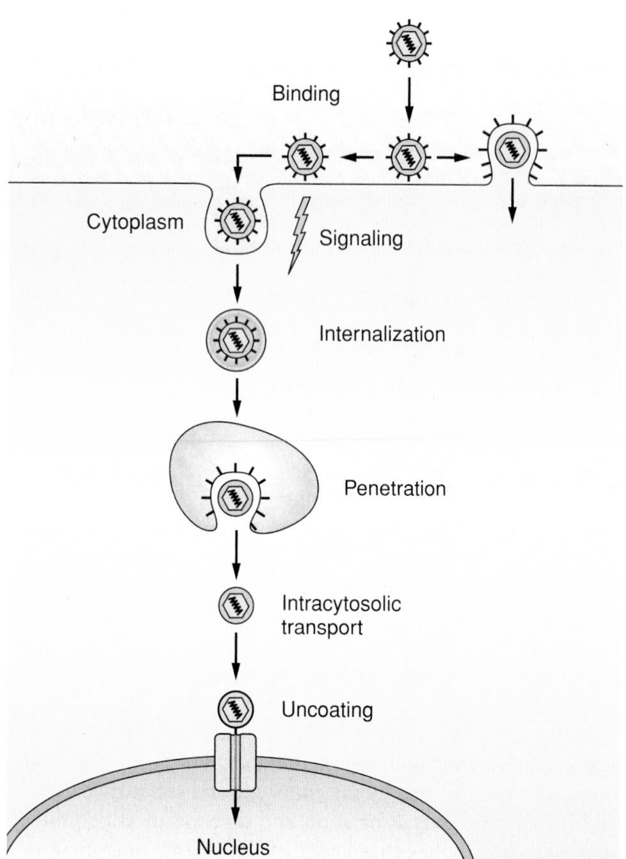

FIGURE 4.1. Stepwise entry of animal viruses. The entry of animal viruses involves a series of steps that start with virus binding to the cell surface. Binding is multivalent and involves cell surface molecules serving as passive attachment factors or receptors that are more active in that they activate signaling pathways, induce conformational changes in the virus, or mediate endocytic internalization. Although some enveloped viruses are able to fuse with the plasma membrane, the majority of viruses rely on internalization by different endocytic mechanisms. Internalization is followed by transport to secondary organelles (usually endosomes), where the virus receives cues to trigger the penetration process. After reaching the cytosol, the viruses or viral capsids are transported to the site of genome uncoating and replication. For most DNA viruses and a few RNA viruses, this site is the nucleus. Many viruses have evolved mechanisms that allow them to deliver their genome and accessory proteins through the nuclear pore complexes.

surface, thus enhancing entry and infection. Unlike receptors, however, they do not actively promote entry and mediate signals. Often, the interactions with attachment factors are not highly specific. In practice, the distinction between a receptor and an attachment factor is not always straightforward because the consequences of virus binding to a given surface component are difficult to assess experimentally and can vary depending on cell type and conditions.

Receptors and attachment factors constitute a diverse collection of proteins, carbohydrates, and lipids with physiologic functions unrelated to pathogen interaction. Ranging from abundant and ubiquitous to rare and species specific, they differ from one virus to the next. In the past few decades, an impressive number have been identified in different virus and host cell systems. As shown in Table 4.1, which gives a partial list, receptors include ligand-binding receptors, glycoproteins, ion channels, gangliosides, carbohydrates, proteoglycans, and so on. Some families of surface molecules seem to be favored; the immunoglobulin-G superfamily of transmembrane proteins, proteoglycans, and glycoconjugates with terminal sialic acid residues, belong to these. In addition, a large group of viruses use integrins as their receptors.[190]

Many viruses use multiple attachment factors and receptors. They interact with them in parallel or in series, or they use different receptors for entry into different cell types. When multiple receptors are required for productive entry, it is the convention to call the one contacted first a *receptor* and the subsequent ones *coreceptors.* A good example is human immunodeficiency virus type 1 (HIV-1), which makes use of heparan sulfate proteoglycans as attachment factors, CD4 as a receptor,[25] and CXCR4 and CCR5 (or a related chemokine receptor) as coreceptors.[13,127] In this case, the two receptors are used to induce stepwise conformational changes in the spike glycoprotein. In other cases (e.g., adenovirus 2 and coxsackie B virus), two receptors seem to be needed to overcome anatomic and topological barriers.[39,131] Herpes viruses are able to infect a variety of cell types, probably in part because they possess proteins that can bind to several different receptors.[185] Cases are also seen where unrelated viruses make use of the same receptors. One well-studied example is coxsackie and adenovirus receptor (CAR) (Table 4.1), which is used as a receptor both by adenovirus 2 and 5 and coxsackie B viruses.[219]

The interaction between a viral surface protein and a receptor can be highly specific, but the affinity is often low. However, the presence of multiple, closely spaced binding sites on the surface of the virus particle allows multivalent binding, and the avidity is therefore frequently high. The affinity of influenza hemagglutinin for sialic acid containing glycoconjugates is, for example, in the millimolar range, but virus binding to cells is virtually irreversible.[180] That most receptor molecules are laterally mobile in the plasma membrane allows, moreover, the formation of a local *microdomain* rich in receptors under the bound virus with a composition and properties different from that in the surrounding membrane.[52] The consequences can be the inclusion of the virus in lipid rafts, or entrapment in caveolae, coated pits, and other membrane specializations. Receptor clustering can also lead to transmembrane signaling, changes in the actin cytoskeleton, and recruitment of cytosolic factors such as a clathrin coat to the plasma membrane.

Although the interaction between a virus and its receptors is generally direct, there are cases where adaptor proteins are involved. For example, binding of antibodies to dengue virus allows infection of macrophages via Fc receptors on the surface of these cells.[143] In this case, the virus particle is internalized as an immune complex. Instead of neutralizing the virus, the antibodies mediate expansion of the host cell repertoire.

In enveloped viruses, the spike glycoproteins are responsible for receptor binding. Typically, these are oligomeric type 1 integral membrane proteins that have the bulk of their mass outside the membrane with the receptor-binding domain exposed. Other external domains in the same protein may be responsible for membrane fusion and receptor destruction. In some spike proteins (e.g., the HIV-1 glycoprotein), the receptor-binding moiety is not covalently connected to the rest, which allows its dissociation

TABLE 4.1 Receptor Proteins for Some Viruses

Virus	Family	Receptor	Function	References
G-protein-coupled receptors				
HIV	*Retroviridae*	CXCR4,CCR3,CCR2b,CCR8 CCR5	Chemokine receptors	2,32,47,163
HIV/SIV	*Retroviridae*	CCR5, Bonzo/STRL-33/ TYMSTR, BOB/GPR15, GPR1	Chemokine receptors	3,56,99
Proteins with multiple membrane-spanning domains				
GALV/FeLV-B/SSAV	*Retroviridae*	PiT-1	Phosphate transport	137,196
MLV-E	*Retroviridae*	MCAT-1	Cationic amino acid transport	1
MLV-A	*Retroviridae*	PiT-2	Phosphate transport	125,205
MLV-X/MLV-P	*Retroviridae*	XPR1/Rmc1/SYG1	Transporter	8,195
HCV	*Flaviviridae*	CD81	Tetraspanin membrane protein	147
Immunoglobulin-related proteins				
Poliovirus	*Picornaviridae*	PVR (CD155)	Adhesion receptor	121
PRV/BHV-1	*Herpesviridae*	PVR (CD155)	Adhesion receptor	67
HSV-1/HSV-2/PRV	*Herpesviridae*	Prr2/HveB/nectin-2	Adhesion	55
HSV-/HSV-2/	*Herpesviridae*	Prr1/HveC/nectin-1	Adhesion	67
Coxsackie B	*Picornaviridae*	CAR	Homotypic cell interaction	9,198
Ad-2/Ad-5	*Adenoviridae*	CAR	Homotypic cell interaction	10,198
MHV-A59	*Coronaviridae*	MHVR/Bgp1 (a)	Biliary glycoprotein	49
Human rhinoviruses (type B, and A major group)	*Picornaviridae*	ICAM-1	Cell adhesion/signaling	71,188
HIV/SIV	*Retroviridae*	CD4	T-cell signaling	106
HHV-7	*Herpesviridae*	CD4	T-cell signaling	104
Low-density lipoprotein receptor–related proteins				
Rous Sarcoma virus (type A)	*Retroviridae*	LDLR	Lipoprotein receptor	7
Human rhinoviruses (type A, minor group)	*Picornaviridae*	LDLR/α 2MR/LRP	Lipoprotein receptors	80
Integrins				
Adenovirus	*Adenoviridae*	$\alpha v\beta 3$	Vitronectin binding	213
Coxsackie A9	*Picornaviridae*	$\alpha v\beta 3$	Vitronectin binding	159
Adenovirus	*Adenoviridae*	$\alpha v\beta 5$	Vitronectin binding	214
Echoviruses-1/-8	*Picornaviridae*	$\alpha 2\beta 1$	Collagen/laminin binding	12
Foot-and-mouth-disease virus	*Picornaviridae*	$\alpha 2\beta 1$, $\alpha v\beta 3$, $\alpha v\beta 6$	Vitronectin binding	14,84
Hantaan virus	*Bunyaviridae*	$\alpha 3$ integrins		65
Rotavirus	*Reoviridae*	$\alpha 4\beta 1$, $\alpha v\beta 3$, $\alpha 2\beta 1$		78
Cytomegalovirus	*Herpesviridae*	$\alpha v\beta 3$, $\alpha 2\beta 1$, $\alpha 6\beta 1$		58
Tumor necrosis factor receptor–related proteins				
ALV-B/D/E	*Retroviridae*	TVB	Apoptosis-inducing receptor	17
Herpes simplex virus 1	*Herpesviridae*	HveA	LIGHT receptor	26,115
Small consensus repeat–containing proteins				
Epstein-Barr virus	*Herpesviridae*	CR2	C3d/C3dg/iC3b binding	59,60
Measles	*Paramyxoviridae*	CD46	Complement inhibition	48
Echoviruses	*Picornaviridae*	CD55	Complement inhibition	9
Coxsackie B-1/-3/-5	*Picornaviridae*	CD55	Complement inhibition	11,173
Miscellaneous				
Coronavirus-229E/TGEV	*Coronaviridae*	Aminopeptidase-*N*	Metalloproteinase	11,217
LCMV/Lassa fever virus	*Arenaviridae*	α-Dystroglycan	Laminin/agrin binding	24

TABLE 4.2 pH-Dependence of Virus Families

Low pH-dependent	pH-independent
Adeno	Corona (majority)
Alpha	Retroviruses (majority)
Borna	Herpes (majority)
Bunya	Paramyxo
Corona (some)	Hepadna
Filo	Pox (some)
Flavi	Rota
Orthomyxo	Picorna (most)
Parvo	Noro
Papilloma	
Picorna (some)	
Pesti	
Pox (some)	
Rhabdo	
Arena	
Arteri	
Hepaci	

once receptor interaction has occurred. X-ray crystal structures of spike glycoprotein–receptor complexes exist for several enveloped viruses (see Chapter 3).

In nonenveloped viruses, the structures that bind receptors are projections or indentations in the capsid surface. Adenoviruses have trimeric fiber proteins with globular knobs that project from the vertices.[15] The penton base protein of many adenovirus subfamilies contains in addition an exposed Arg-Gly-Asp (RGD) sequence that associates with integrins.[189] Many enterovirus receptors bind in a cleft in the capsid surface called the *canyon,* the molecular features of which have been analyzed in great detail.[161]

ROLE OF CARBOHYDRATES

Glycoconjugates on the cell surface have an important role during entry of many viruses as receptors and attachment factors. Glycoproteins and glycolipids, with terminal sialic-acid residues, serve as specific receptors for a variety of viruses, including orthomyxo-, paramyxo-, and polyoma viruses. The HA1 subunits of influenza A virus hemaglutinin (HA) bind terminal sialic acid residues associated with galactose through either a Neu5Ac α(2,3)-Gal or Neu5Ac α(2,6)-Gal bond.[180] Human influenza recognizes the α(2,6) linkage; avian and equine viruses, the α(2,3) linkages, whereas porcine viruses appear to recognize both. These specificities reflect the structure of the glycans expressed in the different species and play a central role in limiting cross-species transmission. The tetrameric hemagglutinin-neuraminidase (HN) proteins of parainfluenza virus 5, has specificity for α(2,3)-sialyllactose,[218] and polyomaviruses bind to specific saccharide residues in the glycan moieties of various gangliosides.[201] A difference limited to a single atom in sialic acids plays a major role in species specificity of simian virus 40 (SV40), because it binds better to the simian GM1 ganglioside, which has a *N*-glycolylneuraminic acid, than to the human, which has a *N*-acetylneuraminic acid.[23]

The list of viruses recognized as binding to glycosaminoglycan (GAG) chains (e.g., heparan sulfate) is steadily growing.[6] It now includes several herpes-, alpha-, flavi-, retro-, parvo-, picorna-, and papillomaviruses. Binding often involves positively charged patches in viral surface proteins. In some cases, viruses adopt GAGs as receptors when grown in tissue culture; their surface proteins mutate and express more basic residues.[22,181] In contrast to tissue culture-adapted strains, natural isolates do not necessarily bind to heparan sulfate. Indeed, adaptation of different glycan receptors is likely part of the age-old war against pathogens, including viruses and their hosts, a war in which the diversity of surface carbohydrates plays an important role.

In most cases, it is the viruses that recognize host cell glycans. However, the reverse is true when cell surface lectins bind to glycans present in the envelope proteins of incoming viruses. One such lectin is DC-SIGN, a tetrameric, C-type lectin present on the surface of immature dendritic cells. It binds *N*-linked glycans of the high-mannose type,[57] such as in glycans that have failed to undergo terminal glycosylation in the Golgi complex of the infected cells. Because glycoproteins synthesized in insect cells have exclusively high-mannose glycans, viruses introduced into the skin via insect bites are often recognized by DC-SIGN, resulting in the infection of dendritic cells. Viruses that bind to these lectins include HIV-1, Sindbis, human cytomegalovirus, dengue, and severe acute respiratory syndrome (SARS) viruses.[66,91,103,149,178,197] Thus cells that our body uses in the front-line defense against pathogens end up serving the interests of viruses instead by spreading the infection.

MOBILITY OF CELL-ASSOCIATED VIRUSES

The encounter between individual viruses and the cell can be visualized live by light microscopy using fluorescent viruses. What happens depends on the virus, the receptor, and the host cell. Parvovirus particles undergo rapid binding and release events that eventually result in permanent attachment and endocytic internalization.[171] Polyomavirus particles bind firmly and diffuse laterally in the membrane for 5 to 10 seconds, after which they are arrested in confinement zones defined by the cortical actin network and eventually internalized.[54] Reoviruses do not show lateral motion after binding.[50] In the case of a bunyavirus, Uukuniemi virus, the rapid clustering of receptor molecules (GFP-tagged DC-SIGN) can be seen to occur at the site of virus binding.[102]

Filopodia have been shown to play an active role by providing directed transport of surface-associated virus particles toward the cell body.[96] They are thin, mobile extensions of the plasma membrane stabilized by an actin filament bundle. Such "virus surfing" occurs at a rate of 1 to 2 μm/min, mirroring the rate of retrograde actin flow from the tip of the filopodia inward.[168] It is actin dependent and inhibited by inhibitors of myosin II. Although such motility of viruses is not essential for infection in tissue culture cells, it may play a role in tissues.

After endocytosis, the actin- and microtubule-dependent movement of intracellular vacuoles, viruses, and naked capsids inside the cell can also be visualized.[50,77,95,164,207] This is illustrated by fluorescent influenza A viruses, which after a slow period of actin-restricted motion in the cell periphery, undergo rapid microtubule-mediated transport toward the perinuclear space where penetration by membrane fusion occurs.[95,164] In the case of adenovirus 2, the transport of capsids along microtubules is both plus- and minus-end directed, but net transport in the minus-end direction allows the virus to reach the nucleus.[193] The entry of parvovirus adeno-associated virus 2 has been traced all the way to the nucleus, inside of which it moves unidirectionally along well-defined pathways.[171]

VIRUS-INDUCED SIGNALS

Many viruses use the host cell's signaling systems to promote entry and optimize infection.[68,124,131] Viruses take advantage of the fact that cells are exquisitely sensitive to ligands that bind to the plasma membrane, particularly if they induce clustering of surface components. More specifically, signaling is used to trigger access to coreceptors, to induce endocytic responses, to reprogram endocytic pathways, and to induce favorable intracellular conditions for infection.

Signaling starts at the plasma membrane after binding of the virus to receptors and formation of receptor clusters. Depending on the virus, receptors, and host cells, initial binding can lead to activation of tyrosine or other kinases, which, in turn, trigger cascades of downstream responses at the plasma membrane, in the cytoplasm, and, in some cases, in the nucleus. Virus-induced signaling depends on the usual panel of second messengers (phosphatidylinositides, diacylglycerides, and calcium), and on numerous regulators of membrane trafficking and actin dynamics.

One well-studied case that demonstrates the complexity of virus-induced signaling is provided by adenoviruses 2 and 5, which use CAR and integrin $\alpha v\beta 3$ as receptors.[68,131] Endocytic internalization occurs via clathrin-coated vesicles, and penetration takes place in endosomes. The interaction with the integrin triggers activation of p85/p110, a PI(3) kinase. The synthesis of PI(3,4)P_2 and PI(3,4,5)P_3 activates protein kinase C. Small GTPases (e.g., Rab and Rho family members) are also activated. One of the downstream responses is the transient activation of macropinocytosis, an actin-dependent process that results in a rapid increase in internalization of fluid.[118] This response seems to promote subsequent penetration of adenovirus from endocytic vacuoles by virus-induced rupture.

Another example is SV40, which is entirely dependent on signaling for entry. After binding to GM1 gangliosides, the virus induces local activation of tyrosine kinases, which results in actin filament reorganization, activation of caveolar dynamics, internalization of the virus in caveolar or lipid raft vesicles, and induction of long-distance transport of the virus-containing vesicles.[44,135,145,187] More than 50 different kinases were shown to regulate the entry and early steps in the infection of HeLa cells by this virus.[144]

A final example involves Kaposi's sarcoma–associated herpesvirus (human herpesvirus 8).[28] The glycoprotein gB of this virus possesses an RGD sequence in the ectodomain that allows it to bind to the integrin $\alpha 3\beta 1$. Binding activates focal adhesion kinase (FAK) and Src kinases, which, in turn, activate PI(3) kinases and Rho GTPases. Furthermore, via the PI(3) K-PKCzeta-mitogen activated or extracellular regulated kinase (MEK) pathway, the virus induces the extracellular signal-regulated kinase 1 and 2 (ERK1/2). Activation of these pathways leads to major alterations in the actin cytoskeleton, and the virus is internalized by macropinocytosis in human fibroblasts.

ENDOCYTIC PATHWAYS OF INFECTION

Whether viruses penetrate into the cytosol directly through the plasma membrane or after endocytosis has been a hotly debated issue from the beginning of animal virology. It is now recognized that a majority of animal viruses—whether enveloped or nonenveloped—make use of endocytosis for productive infection. They exploit one or more of several endocytic mechanisms offered by cells (Fig. 4.2), and most of them enter endocytic vacuoles where penetration into the cytosol occurs often triggered by low pH. Enveloped virus families (e.g., paramyxo-, herpes-, and retroviruses) that can penetrate directly through the plasma membrane because they do not require endocytosis for fusion may still depend on endocytosis for productive infection at least in some cell types.[92,133] Here, the reason may be that fusion at the plasma membrane remains nonproductive because it does not ensure passage of the capsids through further barriers such as the actomyosin cortex.[108]

The main reason why endocytosis is a preferred mode of entry is most likely that endocytic vesicles offer viruses a free ride through the cortical cytoskeleton and other barriers that encumber movement of virus-sized particles in the cytoplasm. By delaying their penetration, viruses can in this way get a ride to the perinuclear region of the cell. In endocytic vacuoles, viruses can, moreover, count on receiving specific cues such as a drop in pH and exposure to proteases to trigger penetration

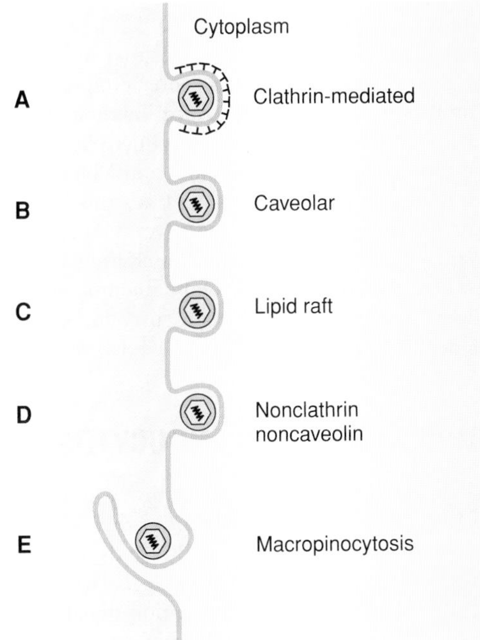

FIGURE 4.2. Mechanisms of endocytosis used for virus entry. Viruses can use different mechanisms of endocytosis. The majority of animal viruses enter cells by endocytosis. The mechanisms include **(A)** clathrin-mediated endocytosis, the most commonly used mechanism for virus entry; **(B)** caveolar endocytosis, a caveolin and lipid raft-dependent mechanism mainly used by polyomaviruses; **(C)** a caveolin-independent, lipid raft-mediated mechanisms with many similarities to the caveolar mechanism; **(D)** various caveolin- and clathrin-independent mechanisms often with similarities to macropinocytosis; and **(E)** macropinocytosis, a transient, ligand-induced, actin-dependent mechanism.

and uncoating. Because no trace of the virus is left exposed on the plasma membrane, immunorecognition of infected cell is delayed. Moreover, for nonenveloped viruses that use membrane lysis or pore formation for penetration, it may be essential to cross membranes of intracellular organelles to minimize damage to the cell.

In recent years, the landscape of endocytosis research has expanded dramatically beyond phagocytosis and the classic clathrin-mediated endocytosis pathway. New mechanisms include caveolar or lipid raft-mediated endocytosis, macropinocytosis, and several other clathrin- and caveolae-independent pathways (Fig. 4.2).[46,116,123,141,203] The situation is often confusing because the mode of uptake of a virus can vary between cell types and strains, and many viruses can make use of multiple receptors and parallel routes of endocytosis in the same cell. In addition to caveolae, SV40 can, for example, utilize a related, noncaveolar pathway.[44] Influenza A uses both clathrin-mediated and clathrin-independent pathways,[112,164,175] and HIV-1, which can fuse with the plasma membrane, can in some cell lines also make efficient use of an endocytic pathway for entry.[42] The use of multiple receptors and redundant endocytic pathways provides viruses with a degree of flexibility and adaptability that make entry a difficult step for host organisms to protect themselves against.

The cell biology of endocytosis and its regulation is complex.[35,98] Not surprisingly, the analysis of virus entry by high throughput siRNA silencing screens have led to the identification of hundreds of genes involved as critical factors in early infection of tissue culture cells.[31,79,144] Entry studies are often further complicated by the fact that only a small fraction of the cell-associated viruses enter productively. Because most morphological and biochemical methods fail to distinguish between particles that enter productively and those that do not, studies using these methods must be complemented with readouts based on infection (i.e., the biological outcome of successful entry). This involves the use of inhibitors, dominant negative mutants, small interfering RNAs, mutant viruses, and mutant cell lines. Only a combination of methods allows pathways of productive entry to be charted with confidence.

CLATHRIN-MEDIATED ENDOCYTOSIS

The clathrin-mediated endocytic pathway is used by many viruses (Figs. 4.2 and 4.3). It is a process that cells use to internalize a spectrum of receptor-bound ligands, fluid, membrane proteins, and lipids for recycling or degradation. By binding to receptors that have the internalization signals necessary for inclusion in clathrin-coated pits, viruses make use of this pathway as opportunistic ligands. Uptake is characterized by rapid kinetics (viruses are generally internalized within a few minutes after binding) and by high capacity (3,000 virus particles or more per minute).[109] With a diameter up to 120 nm, coated vesicles are large enough for the endocytosis of most animal viruses. Sometimes larger particles (e.g., vesicular stomatitis virus [VSV]) can be accommodated.[113]

Although clathrin-mediated endocytosis is a continuously ongoing process, it is under stringent control. Interestingly, when the uptake of VSV, influenza, and reovirus particles has been followed in live cells, it has been observed that most are internalized by clathrin-coated pits that form *de novo* under the virus particles.[41,85,164] Only a few enter via pre-existing clathrin-coated pits. Exactly how the virus induces a transbilayer signal to direct the assembly of the clathrin coat remains to be defined.

A role for clathrin-coated pits in internalization and infection can be demonstrated by inhibiting clathrin function using dominant negative mutants or depletion of adaptors such as epsin, eps15, AP2, or the clathrin chains themselves.[37,175] Inhibition of dynamin 2, a scission factor in clathrin vesicle formation, is not a sufficient indicator for clathrin involvement because dynamin 2 is also involved in other forms of endocytosis.

MACROPINOCYTOSIS

Among the clathrin-independent mechanisms, macropinocytosis and related processes are commonly used by larger viruses such as vaccinia, herpes, adeno 3, and Ebola virus, but evidently also in some cases by smaller viruses such as HIV-1 and influenza A.[4,87,107,122,165] Macropinocytosis is ligand triggered, transient, actin dependent, and regulated by a complex signaling pathway.[123,194] The physiological cargo is mainly composed of extracellular fluid that is trapped in large vacuoles, the formation of which depends on plasma membrane ruffling. The process differs from phagocytosis in the signaling pathways used and in that it can be activated in most cell types, not only in specialized cells.[194] In addition, by serving as a major mechanism in the elimination of apoptotic debris in tissues, macropinocytosis differs from phagocytosis by failing to activate innate immune responses and inflammation.

In macropinocytosis, the interaction of viruses with the plasma membrane induces a rapid activation of receptor tyrosine kinases or integrins. This leads to a signaling cascade that usually involves the activation of GTPases Rac1 or cdc42, the p21-activated kinase (PAK1), myosin II, and numerous other kinases and signaling factors.[123] A change in the dynamics of cortical actin leads to ruffling of the plasma membrane, where the ruffles can take the form of lamellipodia, filopodia, and blebs. In the case of vaccinia virus and Kaposi's sarcoma virus, internalization by macropinocytosis occurs during bleb retraction, and the viruses enter macropinosomes from which they escape by membrane fusion.[122,202] As more is learned about the mechanisms underlying macropinocytosis, it is becoming increasingly clear that there are variations of the general themes. Differences between cell lines and signaling pathways lead to a complex spectrum of related activities.

CAVEOLAR AND LIPID RAFT-MEDIATED ENDOCYTOSIS

The caveolar and lipid raft-mediated pathways of endocytosis were first observed for SV40 and mouse polyomavirus[5,44,158,187] (Figs. 4.2 and 4.3). They are cholesterol dependent, tyrosine kinase activated, cargo induced, and involve small endocytic vesicles. The cholesterol dependence reflects a central role of lipid rafts. Three variants of caveolar or lipid raft endocytosis are currently recognized[94]: (a) endocytosis via classical caveolae, dynamin 2 dependent; (b) noncaveolar, lipid raft-mediated

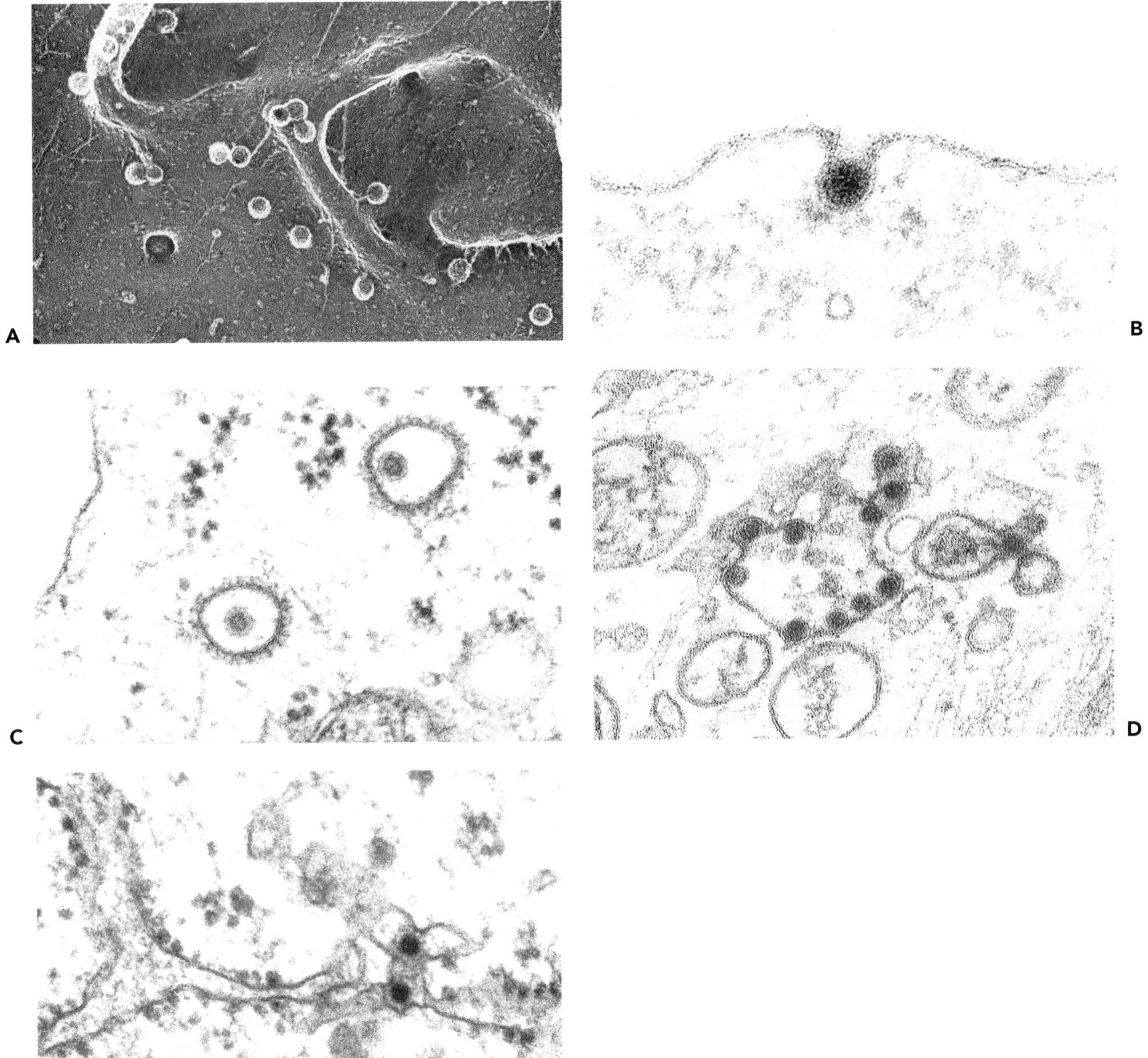

FIGURE 4.3. Electron microscopy of virus endocytosis. A: A surface replica of a BHK21-cell with Semliki Forest virus (SFV) particles attached. Some particles are bound to microvilli, and one is about to be endocytosed inside a coated vesicle (Courtesy of J. Heuser and A. Helenius). **B:** Internalization of a SV40 particle by caveolar- or raft-mediated endocytosis. The tight fitting vesicle in which the virus is internalized has a diameter of about 60 to 70 nm, and it has no visible coat (Courtesy of J. Kartenbeck and A. Helenius). **C:** SFV particles in clathrin-coated vesicles (Courtesy of *J Cell Biol*). **D:** SV40 particles in an early endosome. **E:** Incoming SV40 particles in a smooth membrane section of the endoplasmic reticulum, which they reach via the endocytic pathway. (From Kartenbeck J, Stukenbrok H, Helenius A. Endocytosis of simian virus 40 into the endoplasmic reticulum. *J Cell Biol* 1989;109(6 PE1): 2721–2729, with permission.)

endocytosis, dynamin 2 dependent; and (c) noncaveolar, lipid raft-mediated endocytosis, dynamin independent.

Caveolae constitute 70-nm flask-shaped indentations that contain caveolins and cavins as major protein components and a membrane enriched in cholesterol and sphingolipids.[141,156] Most cell surface caveolae are stationary, with a minority population undergoing a local cycle of fission and fusion with the plasma membrane.[146,204] When local tyrosine phosphorylation is activated by a virus such as SV40, caveolae become more dynamic.[94,141] With a virus particle trapped inside, the caveolae pinch off and move into the cytoplasm where they fuse with endosomes.

SV40 and other polyomaviruses also enter in vesicles devoid of caveolar proteins.[44] After association with lipid rafts in the plasma membrane or artificial liposomes, the binding of SV40 to multiple receptor gangliosides, GM1, leads to the induction membrane curvature following the shape of the virus and the formation of tight-fitting indentations of variable depth.[53] For detachment of a vesicle, these inward-oriented,

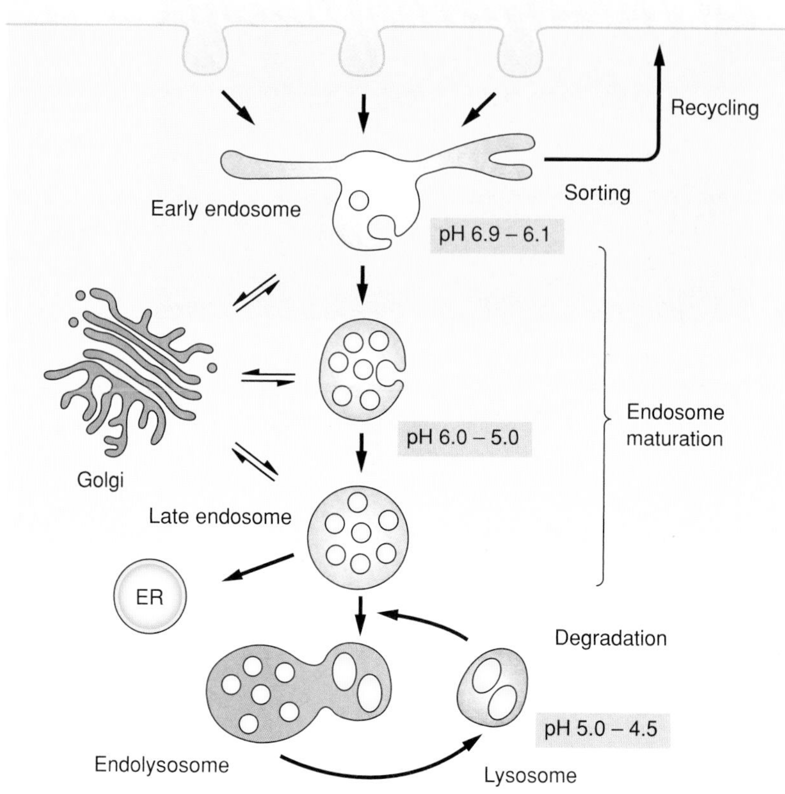

FIGURE 4.4. The endosomal pathway. The pathway functions as two interconnected cycles of membrane trafficking. One involves the plasma membrane, early endosomes, and a variety of carrier vesicles. Its major role is the sorting and recycling of incoming membrane components, ligands, and fluid via the endosome back to the cell surface. In this pathway, the pH does not drop below about 6.0, and the cargo is not exposed to a spectrum of lysosomal enzymes. The main function of the second cycle, the lysosome cycle, is degradative (i.e., the down-regulation of receptor-ligand complexes, degradation, and processing of incoming nutrients and their carriers, digestion of autophagic substrates, elimination of incoming pathogens, etc.). The endocytic cargo to be degraded, including viruses, is sorted from early endosomes into late endosomes, and these deliver the cargo to lysosomes 10 to 40 minutes after formation by fusing with them to form endolysosomes. The late endosomes undergo a complex maturation process, acquire intraluminal vesicles, and move along microtubules to the perinuclear region of the cells. Degradation occurs in the endolysosomes through the action of soluble hydrolases. Endolysosomes and lysosomes keep fusing with new late endosomes in a continuous cycle. Early and late endosomes communicate via vesicle trafficking with the Golgi complex, and late endosomes and endolysosomes have a poorly understood connection to the endoplasmic reticulum.

virus-containing "buds" require the activation of kinases and other cellular factors. The process shares many features with the endocytic mechanism triggered by certain bacterial toxins, such as shiga and cholera.[160]

THE ENDOCYTIC PATHWAY

The early endosomes in the periphery of the cytoplasm receive incoming viruses a few minutes after internalization (Figs. 4.4 and 4.5). Early endosomes constitute complex, heterogeneous organelles with tubular and vacuolar elements. They are mildly acidic (pH 6.6 to 6.0), which is enough to activate viruses with a high pH threshold for penetration, and these viruses are thought to penetrate from early endosomes.[110] Most viruses are not activated in this pH range and continue deeper into the degradative arm of the endocytic pathway in order to penetrate from late endosomes or endolysosomes. In exceptional cases, such as some of the polyomaviruses, viruses continue even farther, using a poorly characterized transport system that brings them to the endoplasmic reticulum (ER).[51,152] Their penetration occurs through the ER membrane. In the case of macropinocytosis, the penetration is likely to occur in macropinosomes, but there is not much information available about macropinosome maturation and fate.

To understand virus entry, it is important to understand the cell biology of endosomes. There are numerous reviews that provide insights into this important topic.[63,73,120,166,170] One of the central topics is the maturation of late endosomes, a program of changes that prepares them for fusion with lysosomes.[82] The changes include a further drop in pH, a switch of predominant Rabs from Rab5 to Rab7, a switch from phosphatidylinosides (PI(3)P to PI(3,5)P_2, exchange of tethering factors for fusion, exchange of microtubule-dependent motors, formation of intralumenal vesicles, and accumulation of lysosomal membrane proteins and hydrolases. It is a complex process where the various alterations are coordinated and interdependent. The key factors include small GTPases of the Rab, Arf, and Rho families and their effectors, phosphatidylinositides and their kinases and phosphatases, protein ubiquitination and the endosomal sorting complex required for transport machinery responsible for the formation of intralumenal vesicles in endosomes, the vacuolar ATPase responsible for acidification, and various soluble *N*-ethylmaleimide-sensitive factor attachment protein receptors and tethering factors required for selective fusion events.

Late penetrating viruses such as influenza virus, minor group rhinoviruses, polyomaviruses, and bunyaviruses depend on a smoothly functioning maturation program. They require the formation of late endosomes, the reduction in pH, and transport of the endosome to the perinuclear region.[63,72,101,174] Infection can be blocked by interfering with the maturation program using inhibitors, dominant negative mutants, and siRNA depletion of endocytosis factors.

The significance of low pH in endosomes as a cue for the activation of virus penetration was discovered a long time ago.[76] It is now clear that for the majority of animal viruses, low pH is needed to trigger conformational changes in metastable viral particles and fusion proteins, thus activating membrane

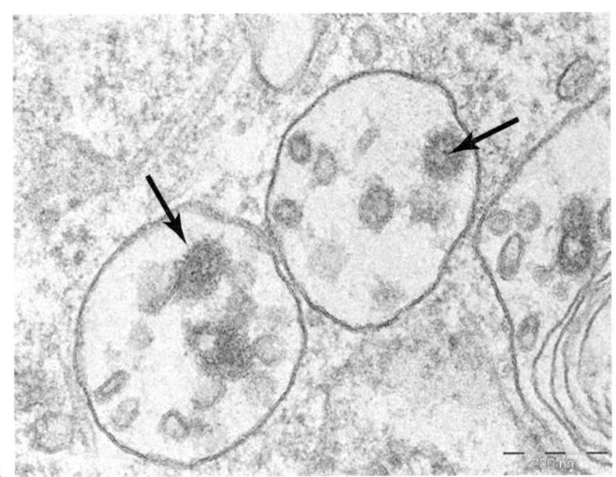

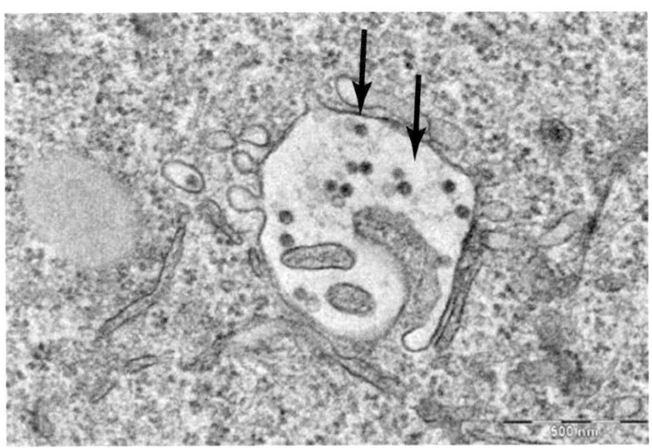

FIGURE 4.5. Viruses enter endosomes. Endosomes are cytoplasmic vacuoles with complex and quite heterogeneous morphology. Thin section electron microscopy reveals that many of them are filled with intracellular vesicles and membrane lamellae. **A:** Influenza A viruses (*arrow heads*) are here seen in multivesicular endosomes closely connected to microtubules. **B:** Human papilloma-16 pseudovirus particles are here seen in an endosome with tubular extensions. (Courtesy of Roberta Mancini.)

penetration mechanisms (see Chapter 3). Viruses with a relatively high pH threshold (pH 6.5 to 6.0) such as VSV are activated 3 to 10 minutes after internalization in early endosomes.[109] Viruses with a lower pH threshold are sorted from early endosomes into the degradative branch and penetrate later (10 to 50 minutes or even longer after infection) and less synchronously in late endosomes or endolysosomes that have a pH of 6.0 to 4.9. For example, influenza A virus, with a pH threshold of 5.6 to 4.9, passes via early endosomes to perinuclear late endosomes before membrane fusion and penetration occurs.[176]

PENETRATION BY MEMBRANE FUSION

The membrane of an enveloped virus is a *de facto* transport vesicle designed for intercellular membrane traffic (Fig. 4.6). Like intracellular transport vesicles, the transport process relies on budding, fission, and fusion. The cargo is the viral capsid, which does not have to cross the hydrophobic barrier of a membrane. The fusion reaction during entry can occur with the plasma membrane or with the limiting membrane of an endosome. On the basis of studies with VSV, it has been proposed that a virus can also fuse with lumenal membrane vesicles inside multivesicular endosomes followed by a delayed second fusion event between the vesicle and the limiting membrane of late endosomes.[72,162] The second fusion would have to depend on a cellular rather than viral fusion machinery.

As described in Chapter 3, viral fusion proteins are integral membrane proteins, with the bulk of their mass external to the viral envelope. They are usually glycoproteins and occur as homo- or hetero-oligomers. Many of them combine fusion and receptor-binding activities in the same molecule. To become

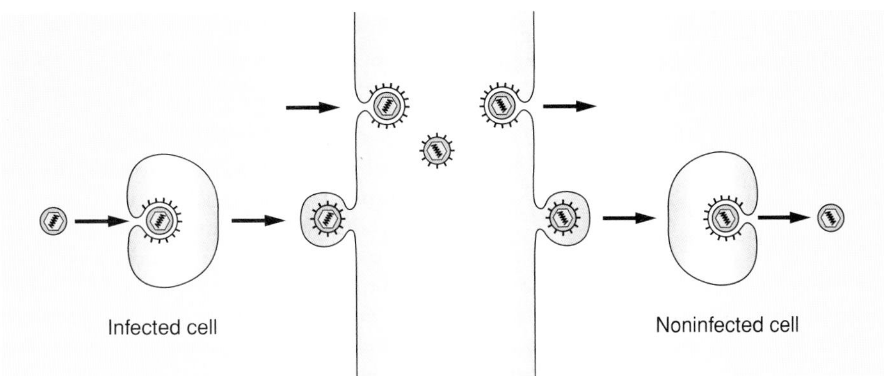

FIGURE 4.6. Enveloped viruses use a vesicle shuttle mechanism. They transport the capsids and the viral genome from cell to cell using a vesicle transport strategy based on membrane fission and fusion. The viral envelope constitutes the transport vesicle, and the capsid is the cargo. The vesicle is formed after capsid loading and glycoprotein sorting in the infected cell by budding and membrane fission at the plasma membrane or internal membranes. The viral envelope membrane protects the capsid during the voyage through the extra cellular space. After associating with a new host cell, the virus delivers the capsid into the cytosol by membrane fusion, either at the plasma membrane or after endocytosis, at the limiting membranes of intracellular organelles. The advantage of this strategy is the viral genome, and accessory proteins can be transferred from cytosol to cytosol without the need of translocation directly across the hydrophobic barrier of any membrane.

fusion competent after folding and assembly in the ER, they are often primed by proteolytic cleavage during transit through the trans-Golgi network (TGN). Typically, the proteases responsible for priming are furin family convertases that cleave either the chains involved in fusion directly (i.e., in myxo-, retro-, and paramyxoviruses) or the companion proteins in the spike protein complex (i.e., alpha- and flaviviruses).[90,186,208] If virus assembly and budding occurs intracellularly, as for flaviviruses, the activating cleavages take place as the assembled viral particles pass through the TGN.[75] In some cases, such as Ebola virus, proteolytic activation can occur as part of the entry program by proteases present in endocytic vacuoles.[30]

Proteolytic priming renders fusion proteins metastable and, thus, competent to undergo large, irreversible conformational changes without added energy.[27] This is important because, to elicit fusion, they must undergo changes that dramatically alter their quaternary or tertiary structure. As a result, they expose previously hidden hydrophobic peptide segments (fusion peptides) that interact with the target membrane, and in doing so allow the proteins to be hydrophobically anchored in both membranes.[210] The conformational change is thought to provide the energy required to overcome the so-called *hydration force* that prevents biological membranes from fusing spontaneously.[155]

The changes in conformation are triggered either by low pH in endosomes or by interaction between viral proteins and receptors in the plasma membrane. Sometimes receptor binding followed by low pH is needed. This type of receptor-mediated priming, observed for some retroviruses,[128] may allow the virus particle to limit conversion of spike glycoproteins to the site most intimately in contact with the target membrane. The priming and activation of viral membrane fusion proteins as well as the mechanisms of fusion are discussed in greater detail in Chapter 3.

PENETRATION BY NONENVELOPED VIRUSES

Nonenveloped viruses penetrate into the cytosol through the limiting membranes of internal organelles (e.g., endosomes, lysosomes, the ER). The cues that trigger penetration are similar to those used by enveloped viruses (e.g., receptor-binding, low pH, redox environment). These viruses must, however, transfer their capsids, genomes, and associated proteins through a cellular membrane without the convenience of the membrane-fusion mechanism.

The mechanisms involved have proved challenging and remain incompletely understood. It seems, however, that nonenveloped viruses can use three general strategies:

(a) *Membrane puncture.* The virus particle generates a pore in the membrane through which the genome is selectively released into the cytosol. The viral capsid does not enter the cytosol, and release of fluid phase markers from the lumen of the organelle is either undetectable or limited to small molecular weight compounds.
(b) *Perforation.* The entire capsid is transferred through the membrane without major lysis of the membrane and little loss of lumenal fluid markers.
(c) *Lysis.* The virus particles induce breakage of the membrane of cytoplasmic organelles, allowing the virus and other lumenal contents to be released into the cytosol.

The puncture or pore mechanism is favored for picornaviruses.[64,81] Some rhinoviruses and foot-and-mouth disease virus are acid-activated and penetrate from endosomes, whereas others (e.g., polio, coxsackie B, and echovirus 1) are pH independent but penetrate from endosomes or other intracellular organelles. In the case of poliovirus, which is one of the best characterized, penetration is induced by binding of a cluster of poliovirus receptor (PVR) molecules to "canyons" in the capsid surface. This triggers a large, concerted, irreversible change in the particle, the so-called *eclipse,* which leads to the formation of a penetration competent conformation. An internal protein, VP4, is released, and the myristylated *N*-terminus of VP1 inserts into the endosomal membrane.[16,61] The RNA is most likely released to the cytosolic side of the membrane through a narrow pore.[199] According to this view, penetration and uncoating occur simultaneously, and the capsid does not enter the cytosol. Recently, cryo-electron microscopy (cryoEM) studies have shown that one of the icosahedral vertices interacts with five receptors that connect the modified particle intimately with the membrane.[19]

Adenoviruses make use of a lytic mechanism.[172] The best studied are adenoviruses 2 and 5, which penetrate by acid-activated rupture of the endosomal membrane.[117,119] The lytic effect is thought to involve a change in the penton base and exposure of an amphipathic helix in protein VI, but the mechanism is unclear.[130] Altogether, the process is complex; it depends on low pH, the integrin receptors, cleavages in structural proteins induced by the L3/p23 viral protease, the release of fiber proteins, activation of macropinocytosis, and signaling through protein kinase C.[117,119,131]

For parvoviruses, evidence is accumulating that the *N*-terminal domain of VP1 possesses a phospholipase 2 domain activated by low pH.[38,74] It is likely that this promotes membrane penetration of the intact virus by modifying the permeability of endosomal and lysosomal membranes. Lysis of the membrane is not detected.

INTRACELLULAR TRAFFICKING

Before they can replicate, viruses and capsids delivered into the cytosol must be transported to the correct location before uncoating and replication can take place. Within the nucleus, replication usually occurs in defined foci. In the cytosol, it is often associated with specific membrane organelles (e.g., the ER or the ER-Golgi intermediate compartment) or with virus factories in the perinuclear space.[136,215]

Given the extreme crowding in the cytoplasm that prevents diffusion of virus- and capsid-sized particles as well as uncondensed forms of DNA or RNA, it is not surprising that viruses rely on cytoplasmic transport systems offered by the cell.[45,70,105,182] For long-distance transport, viruses mainly exploit microtubule-mediated mechanisms. When actin filaments play a role, it is usually in short-distance movement close to the plasma membrane. Although viruses can undergo partial disassembly *in transit* through the cytosol, they postpone final uncoating of the condensed genome until they have reached their final destination. Viruses travel variable distances. To reach the cell body, neurotropic viruses that enter via axons may have to move in a retrograde direction over the full length of axons, which can be more than 1 m in length.

To move through the cytoplasm, incoming viruses have two options. They can postpone penetration into the cytosol and move as cargo in endocytic vesicles and thus benefit from the motor-driven transport of vesicles and organelles through the cytoplasm. Alternatively, they can penetrate early into the cytosol, in which case the viruses or their capsids are themselves responsible for associating with molecular motors and adaptors (e.g., dynein and kinesins). The former strategy is used by viruses that enter by endocytosis, the latter by viruses that prefer to penetrate through the plasma membrane. Many viruses make use of both; part of the journey is mediated by vesicular traffic, the rest by cytosolic transport. Thus, viruses (e.g., adeno- and parvoviruses) that enter by endocytosis have been shown to use microtubule-mediated transport after penetration into the cytosol.[171,192,193] Although transport of capsids along microtubules is often bidirectional and characterized by stops, restarts, and changes in direction, net transport generally occurs in the minus-end direction toward the microtubule organizing center, where viruses and capsids are often found to accumulate before transport to the nucleus.[154] Whether they switch to plus-end directed motors for the final leg of transport is not known.

UNCOATING

The entry of viruses includes partial or full disassembly as an essential, integrated part of the program. For enveloped viruses, uncoating involves loss of the envelope during membrane fusion. Often, the capsid thus released undergoes further stepwise uncoating steps. Once the capsids have reached the correct location within the cell, then, and only then, they release the replication competent form of the genome. In some cases (e.g., retro-, reo-, and poxviruses), the cytosolic capsids serve as a protected site for reverse transcription of the genome or transcription of messengers following entry into the cytosol.[88,134]

In the case of nonenveloped viruses, the uncoating process involves conformational changes, progressive loss of structural proteins, proteolytic cleavages, isomerization of intermolecular disulfide bonds, and weakening of intermolecular interactions.[69,81,117,132,169] For adenovirus 2, disassembly starts already at the cell surface with loss of some of the fibers followed by activation of a viral protease (the L3/p23 protease, located within the virion), proteolytic cleavage of capsid proteins, and loss of stabilizing capsid components. Final disassembly of the particle and DNA release occurs at the nuclear pore complex (NPC).

The conformational changes that accompany penetration and uncoating of polio and other picronaviruses have been extensively analyzed.[64,81,100] Depending on the virus, the initial uncoating event is triggered by receptor association, low pH, or both. Conversion from a 150S to 160S particle to a slower sedimenting 135S particle occurs with elimination of the internal VP4 protein and externalization of the myristylated *N*-terminus of VP1. This leads to membrane association, followed by the release of the RNA, resulting in the RNA-free 80S particle. The single-stranded viral RNA is likely to escape through one of the 12 vertices, possibly aided by the VPg protein covalently linked to the 5′ end of the viral RNA.[18,89]

The capsids of viruses with a double-stranded RNA genome (e.g., reoviruses) undergo many alterations in transit into the cell, but instead of releasing their genomic RNA in free form into the cytosol, they retain it in a modified capsid, which serves as an RNA-replication and transcription factory.[29,177]

TRIGGERING THE UNCOATING PROGRAM

Penetration brings many viruses and viral capsids for the second time into a cytosolic environment. The first time is when they assemble in the cytosol of an infected cell or when they pass through the cytosol on their way from the nucleus to the extracellular space. During entry into a new host cell, the agenda involves disassembly and uncoating instead of assembly. This means that, in the entry phase, something must be profoundly different either about the virus itself or the cell.

Usually, the difference is in the virus or the capsid because it has undergone structural alterations *in transit*. After release from the infected cell or during earlier stages of entry, the viruses are structurally *reset* so they can respond to cellular cues according to requirements of the uncoating program. The best illustration of this is provided by retroviruses, in which the viral protease induces a series of cleavages in Gag and Gag-Pol proteins during and after virus budding. The capsid is reorganized and ready for reverse transcription and for the formation of functional preintegration complexes (PICs) in the cytosol of a new target cell.[134]

Another example is influenza A, in which the switch involves a change in the properties of the matrix protein (M1). M1 serves as an adaptor between the virus ribonucleoproteins (vRNPs) and the viral membrane as well as between the vRNPs, and it plays a crucial role during assembly of these components during virus assembly and budding.[157,220] During entry, dissociation of these interactions is induced by an irreversible conformational change in M1 triggered by acid exposure in endosomes.[20] To acidify the internal space of the virus, where the M1 and the vRNPs are located, the viral membrane possesses acid-activated proton channels in the form of M2 protein complexes.[148,191] If the M2 proton channel is blocked using amantadine, a specific M2 channel blocker used as an anti-influenza drug; HA-mediated fusion occurs normally in endosomes, but the vRNP and M1 fail to dissociate from each other, and transport of vRNP to the nucleus is inhibited.[21,111]

Alphaviruses seem to use an altogether different strategy. Here the *switch* seems to involve a change in the cell rather than in the viral capsid. A cellular factor required for uncoating of incoming capsids is inactivated during the course of infection, thus allowing assembly of progeny capsids. The factor in question is the 60S ribosomal subunit, which has high affinity binding sites for the viral capsid protein.[179,209] Incoming capsids rapidly lose capsid proteins to ribosomal subunits, and the viral RNA is thus liberated. When synthesis of structural protein starts later in an infection, newly synthesized capsid proteins bind to the ribosomal subunits and the ribosomal subunits can no longer interfere with assembly of progeny capsids.

NUCLEAR IMPORT

Most DNA viruses and a few negative-stranded RNA viruses replicate in the nucleus. To enter the nucleus, they can make use of the NPC for transport of the genome and accessory proteins into the nucleoplasm[34,40,69,211,212] (Fig. 4.7). Alternatively, the viruses may enter by rupturing the nuclear envelope, a process for which there is some evidence in the parvovirus field. These

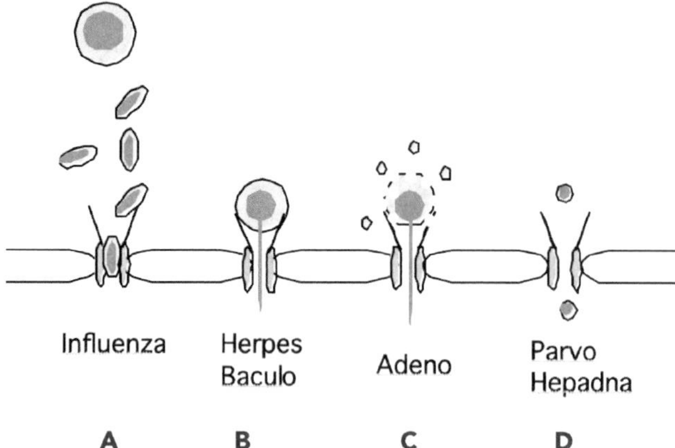

FIGURE 4.7. Import of viruses and subviral particles through the nuclear pore complex. To circumvent the size limitation (diameter 35 to 40 nm) of particle transport through the nuclear pore complex (NPC), viruses have evolved different strategies. **A:** The genome of a virus can be divided in multiple subgenomic particles with an elongated shape thin enough for individual entry (e.g., influenza virus). **B:** Limited uncoating takes place in the cytosol with the generation of an opening in the capsid wall that allows the DNA to escape, leaving an empty capsid at the NPC (e.g., herpes simplex virus 1). **C:** The virus dissembles after association with the NPC, allowing the genome and accessory proteins to pass through the NPC (e.g., adenoviruses). **D:** The virus particles or capsids are small enough to enter as spherical particles without uncoating or major deformation with uncoating occurring in the nucleoplasm.

two entry routes allow infection of nondividing, terminally differentiated, interphase cells in which the nuclear envelope represents a permanent barrier. Finally, viruses and viral capsids may wait in the cytosol for the dissolution of the nuclear envelope during cell division. This mechanism is used by most retroviruses with the exception of lentiviruses (and possibly papilloma viruses)[151] and restricts infection to cell populations that undergo division. In principle, a fourth possibility would be penetration directly from the lumen of the ER through the inner nuclear membrane because the lumen of the ER is continuous with the space between the membranes in the nuclear envelope. Although some incoming viruses do pass through the ER and incoming viral particles have been occasionally seen between the two membranes of the nuclear envelope,[114] no evidence currently indicates that any viruses use this pathway.

Nuclear import via the NPC involves several steps: binding of import receptors, transport through the cytosol, association with the NPC, and transfer of the intact virus, a subviral complex, or a nucleic acid through the pore. To be recognized by the cellular import machinery, viruses and viral capsids make use of nuclear localization signals (NLSs) similar to those present on cellular proteins and ribonucleoprotein complexes. These signals in viral proteins are recognized by soluble receptor proteins (importins or karyopherins) that mediate recognition, transport, and docking of the viral capsids to the NPC. In some cases, the NLS and the importins involved have been identified. Exposure of the NLS is sometimes modulated by phosphorylation-induced conformational modifications to avoid premature capsid import in the infected cell,[86] and some viruses are thought to be processed by proteasomes.[206] It is also possible that viruses bind directly to the NPC without interaction with importins. This seems to be the case for adenovirus 2, which binds directly to the CAN/Nup214 nucleoporin.[200]

The size limitation for transport through the NPC is an obvious problem. Although estimates of the functional pore diameter have been adjusted upward to 39 nm,[140] only the smallest viruses and capsids are likely to enter intact without modifications. These include parvoviruses and the capsids of hepatitis B virus (HBV).[153,206] When nuclear import of injected HBV capsids through the NPC are imaged by electron microscopy, the capsids can be seen to line up on the cytosolic fibers of the NPC and inside the central channel (Fig. 4.8). Uncoating of these capsids occurs in the basket, a structure located on the nucleoplasmic side of the NPC.[153]

Being too large, most viruses and capsids must undergo shape changes or disassembly before passage of the genome through the NPC. Partially uncoated and modified adenovirus 2 particles bind to the CAN/Nup214 nucleoporins on the outer surface of the NPC, where they break apart, releasing the linear, double-stranded viral DNA for transport through the NPC.[200] A histone protein, H1, has been implicated as a disassembly factor and a trans-NPC *guide* for the released DNA.

Binding of herpes simplex virus capsids to the NPC is mediated by capsid and tegument proteins.[139,142] After association with CAN/Nup214 and another NPC protein, hCG1, through the minor capsid protein pUL25, and after opening of the portal structure at one of the vertexes of the capsid, the viral DNA escapes into the nucleus, leaving an empty capsid behind at the mouth of the NPC (Fig. 4.9). Influenza A viruses deal with the problem of size limits by having a segmented

FIGURE 4.8. Herpes simplex virus 1 (HSV-1) entry at the plasma membrane level and the nuclear envelope. A: In HSV-1, virus can fuse with the plasma membrane and release the capsid and the tegument into the cytosol. A large part of the tegument can be seen separating from the capsid. **B:** After binding to the cytosolic fibers attached to the nuclear pore complex (NPC), the viral capsid releases its DNA genome through one of the pentameric facets, and an intact-looking empty capsid shell remains bound to the NPC for some time. PM, plasma membrane; NE, nuclear envelope. Space bar, 100 nm. (Courtesy of B. Sodeik and A. Helenius.)

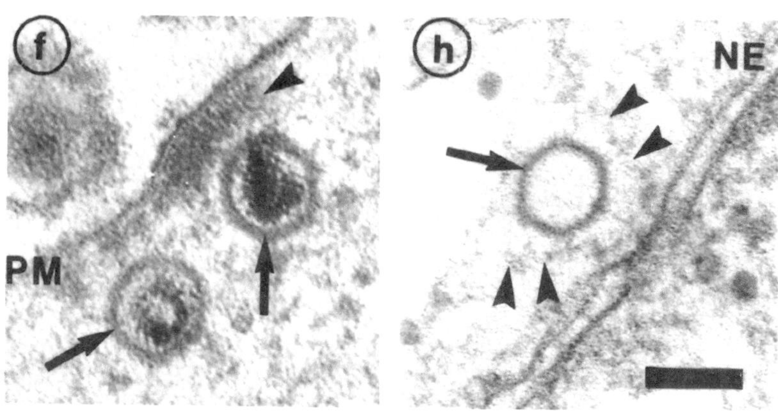

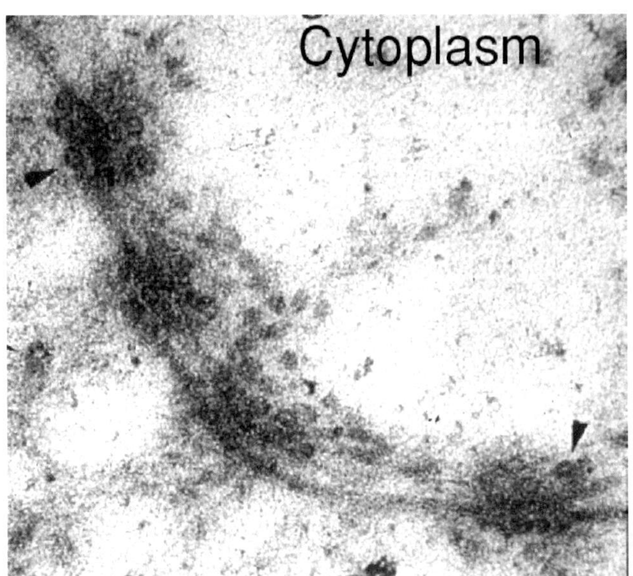

FIGURE 4.9. Import of hepatitis B virus (HBV) capsids through the nuclear pore complex (NPC). After injection into *Xenopus oocytes,* isolated HBV cores can be seen binding to fibers at the mouth of the NPC, and to line up in a row inside the channel of the pore. Uncoating of this capsid occurs in the basket on the nucleoplasmic side of the NPC. (Courtesy of N. Pante and M. Kann.)

genome. The eight subgenomic RNA are individually packaged into viral vRNP complexes. When interactions with the M1 protein are dissociated after exposure of the virus to low pH in endosomes, the vRNP can interact with importins, travel to the nucleus, and enter individually through the NPC (Fig. 4.7).[20,111,138] The vRNPs are rod shaped and, although variable in length, have a thickness of only 10 to 20 nm.[36]

The PIC of retroviruses has been reported to be about 50 to 60 nm in diameter.[126] Too big to enter the nuclei without conformational adjustments, they remain in the cytosol until the breakdown of the nuclear envelope occurs during cell division.[97] Being capable of entering interface nuclei, the PIC of HIV-1 and other lentiviruses are exceptions. The details of how and in which form lentivirus PICs are imported into the nucleus remain controversial.

TRANSMISSION DIRECTLY FROM CELL TO CELL

Discussion so far has focused on the mechanisms of entry by free viral particles attaching to the surface of cells. It is increasingly clear that there are situations in which infection occurs from cell to cell without participation of free virus particles[129,167] (Fig. 4.10). One mechanism involves fusion of an infected cell's plasma membrane with the membrane of a neighboring cell. In infected tissues and cultures, the result is the formation of multinucleated cells (i.e., syncytia). Fusion in this case is mediated by viral fusion proteins expressed on the surface of the infected cell with receptors present on the noninfected cell. Commonly observed with paramyxovirus, herpesvirus, and other viruses with pH-independent fusion proteins, cell

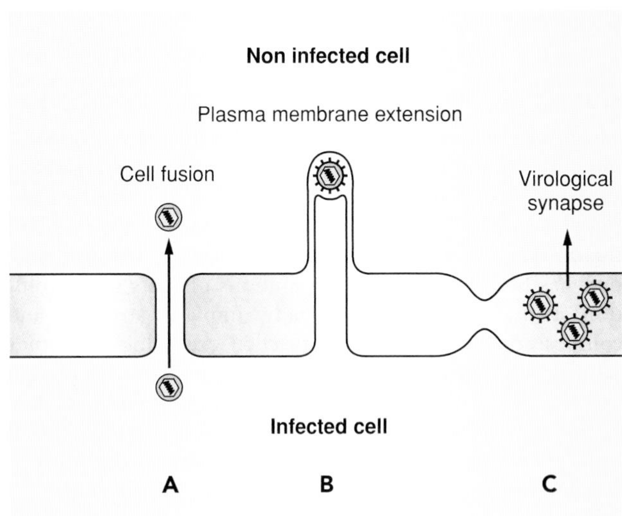

FIGURE 4.10. Direct cell-to-cell transmission. Several mechanisms allow infection to be transmitted via cell contacts without the release of free virus particles into the extracellular space. **A:** Due to the presence of viral fusion proteins on the surface of the infected cells and virus receptors on the noninfected cells, fusion of two cells can occur without producing virus particles. This results in the formation of syncytia. This mechanism is often seen with enveloped viruses and with fusion proteins that do not require low pH for fusion. **B:** In the case of poxviruses, extracellular viruses belonging to the so-called extracellular class of virions remain attached to the surface of the infected cell, where they trigger the formation of a motile, actin-containing, extension of the plasma membrane. This extension is thought to promote contact of the virus with the surface of a neighboring cells. **C:** The infected cells can undergo polarization so that progeny viruses are selectively released into a region of the cell periphery intimately in contact with another cell. Such specialized regions are called virological synapses.

fusion provides a mechanism for transmitting infection independently of virus particle assembly.[33]

Other mechanisms of cell-to-cell transmission require the formation of virus particles, but these are not released freely into the extracellular space. Poxviruses such as vaccinia virus generate infectious particles called external enveloped viruses, most of which not only remain attached to the cell surface after formation, but also induce the formation of a motile surface extensions through the polymerization of actin inside the cytoplasm.[62,70,183,216] The actin polymerization reaction helps to form membrane extensions that push the virus into contact with the neighboring cell, thus generating an efficient mechanism for local dissemination in infected tissues.

Structures termed infectious or virological synapses were first described for the transmission of the human T-cell leukemia virus type 1 (HTLV-1).[83] These are areas of intimate contact between infected and uninfected cells reminiscent of immunological synapses. They provide a domain where virus assembly and release are focused with efficient targeting of the virus particles to the next host cell without access of antibodies from the outside.[129] Similar means of transfer have been described for herpesviruses and for the T-cell to T-cell transfer of HIV. Dendritic cells that bind HIV-1 via DC-SIGN help to transport the virus to lymph nodes where they present the virus to T cells, providing an efficient system for targeted infection of host cells through virological synapses.[66,93]

PERSPECTIVES

The entry and uncoating mechanisms and strategies are highly variable depending on the virus and the target cell. They have in common that the viruses depend critically on the host cell and its activities. To extract the necessary assistance from the cell, viruses make use of the detailed *insider information* they have about the host organisms, their tissues, the cells, and a variety of molecular processes. This information has been acquired during millions of years of coevolution. Thus, although exceptionally simple in structure and composition, viruses are able to elicit exceedingly complex cellular responses. The induction of signals, the activation of endocytic pathways, the exploitation of intracellular targeting systems and molecular motors, and the cell-assisted mechanisms of uncoating provide examples of the ways in which viruses make use of cellular machinery during entry. As details unfold, interesting and important insights about the viruses and their hosts continue to emerge.

The entry program involves the transport of the incoming viruses and capsids through the membranes and the compartments of the cell, the stepwise dismantling of the virus particle, and the release of the genome. Entry and uncoating involve *switches* in particle structure and properties that have to occur in the right place at the right time. It is remarkable how little seems to be left to chance. In the future, these switches need more attention because they provide powerful targets for therapeutic and prophylactic intervention. Also, the cellular defenses against virus entry, ranging from degradation of incoming viruses to interferon-induced expression of interception proteins in the cytosol, deserve thorough study. After all, it is clear that, of the incoming cell-associated viruses, only a small fraction generally reach the intended goal.

It will be important to focus on the cellular factors involved in infection (i.e., on the Trojans and not only on the Trojan horses). They represent new targets for antiviral strategies. How viruses enter tissues and cells in intact organisms remains for the most part territory uncharted. New technologies and model systems are emerging that allow work at the whole animal level. A multidisciplinary approach that combines cell and molecular biology, structural biology, biochemistry, physiology, systems biology, and medicine as central disciplines is required. As important as knowing the pathogens, it will also be important in the spirit of an ancient greek aphorism to know ourselves (i.e., to understand the cell and molecular biology of the host cells).

REFERENCES

1. Albritton LM, Tseng L, Scadden D, et al. A putative murine ecotropic retrovirus receptor gene codes a multiple membrane spanning protein and confers susceptibility to virus infection. *Cell* 1989;57:659–666.
2. Alkhatib G, Combadiere C, Broder CC, et al. CC CKR5: a RANTES, MIP-1alpha, MIP-1beta receptor as a fusion cofactor for macrophage-tropic HIV-1. *Science* 1996;272:1955–1958.
3. Alkhatib G, Liao F, Berger EA, et al. A new SIV co-receptor, STRL33. *Nature* 1997;388:238.
4. Amstutz B, Gastaldelli M, Kalin S, et al. Subversion of CtBP1-controlled macropinocytosis by human adenovirus serotype 3. *EMBO J* 2008;27: 956–969.
5. Anderson HA, Chen Y, Norkin LC. Bound simian virus 40 translocates to caveolin-enriched membrane domains, and its entry is inhibited by drugs that selectively disrupt caveolae. *Mol Biol Cell* 1996;7:1825–1834.
6. Bartlett AH, Park PW. Proteoglycans in host-pathogen interactions: molecular mechanisms and therapeutic implications. *Expert Rev Mol Med* 2010;12:e5.
7. Bates P, Young JA, Varmus HE. A receptor for subgroup A Rous sarcoma virus is related to the low density lipoprotein receptor. *Cell* 1993;74: 1043–1051.
8. Battini JL, Rasko JE, Miller AD. A human cell-surface receptor for xenotropic and polytropic murine leukemia viruses: possible role in G protein-coupled signal transduction. *Proc Natl Acad Sci U S A* 1999;96: 1385–1390.
9. Bergelson JM. Virus interactions with mucosal surfaces: alternative receptors, alternative pathways. *Curr Opin Microbiol* 2003;6:386–391.
10. Bergelson JM, Cunningham JA, Droguett G, et al. Isolation of a common receptor for coxsackie B viruses and adenoviruses 2 and 5. *Science* 1997; 275:1320–1323.
11. Bergelson JM, Mohanty JG, Crowell RL, et al. Coxsackievirus B3 adapted to growth in RD cells binds to decay-accelerating factor (CD55). *J Virol* 1995;69:1903–1906.
12. Bergelson JM, Shepley MP, Chan BM, et al. Identification of the integrin VLA-2 as a receptor for echovirus 1. *Science* 1992;255:1718–1720.
13. Berger EA, Murphy PM, Farber JM. Chemokine receptors as HIV-1 coreceptors: roles in viral entry, tropism, and disease. *Annu Rev Immunol* 1999;17:657–700.
14. Berinstein A, Roivainen M, Hovi T, et al. Antibodies to the vitronectin receptor (integrin alpha V beta 3) inhibit binding and infection of foot-and-mouth disease virus to cultured cells. *J Virol* 1995;69:2664–2666.
15. Bewley MC, Springer K, Zhang YB, et al. Structural analysis of the mechanism of adenovirus binding to its human cellular receptor, CAR. *Science* 1999;286:1579–1583.
16. Brandenburg B, Lee LY, Lakadamyali M, et al. Imaging poliovirus entry in live cells. *PLoS Biol* 2007;5:e183.
17. Brojatsch J, Naughton J, Rolls MM, et al. CAR1, a TNFR-related protein, is a cellular receptor for cytopathic avian leukosis-sarcoma viruses and mediates apoptosis. *Cell* 1996;87:845–855.
18. Bubeck D, Filman DJ, Cheng N, et al. The structure of the poliovirus 135S cell entry intermediate at 10-angstrom resolution reveals the location of an externalized polypeptide that binds to membranes. *J Virol* 2005;79:7745–7755.
19. Bubeck D, Filman DJ, Hogle JM. Cryo-electron microscopy reconstruction of a poliovirus-receptor-membrane complex. *Nat Struct Mol Biol* 2005;12:615–618.
20. Bui M, Whittaker G, Helenius A. The effect of M1 protein and low pH on nuclear import of influenza virus vRNPs. *J Virol* 1996;70:8391–8401.
21. Bukrinskaya AG, Vorkunova NK, Kornilayeva GV, et al. Influenza virus uncoating in infected cells and effect of rimatidine. *J Gen Virol* 1982; 60:49–59.
22. Byrnes AP, Griffin DE. Large-plaque mutants of Sindbis virus show reduced binding to heparan sulfate, heightened viremia, and slower clearance from the circulation. *J Virol* 2000;74:644–651.
23. Campanero-Rhodes MA, Smith A, Chai W, et al. N-glycolyl GM1 ganglioside as a receptor for simian virus 40. *J Virol* 2007;81:12846–12858.
24. Cao W, Henry MD, Borrow P, et al. Identification of alpha-dystroglycan as a receptor for lymphocytic choriomeningitis virus and Lassa fever virus [see comments]. *Science* 1998;282:2079–2081.
25. Capon DJ, Ward RH. The CD4-gp120 interaction and AIDS pathogenesis. *Annu Rev Immunol* 1991;9:649–678.
26. Carfi A, Willis SH, Whitbeck JC, et al. Herpes simplex virus glycoprotein D bound to the human receptor HveA. *Mol Cell* 2001;8:169–179.
27. Carr CM, Kim PS. A spring-loaded mechanism for the conformational change of influenza hemagglutinin. *Cell* 1993;73:823–832.
28. Chandran B. Early events in Kaposi's sarcoma-associated herpesvirus infection of target cells. *J Virol* 2010;84:2188–2199.
29. Chandran K, Farsetta DL, Nibert ML. Strategy for nonenveloped virus entry: a hydrophobic conformer of the reovirus membrane penetration protein micro 1 mediates membrane disruption. *J Virol* 2002;76:9920–9933.
30. Chandran K, Sullivan NJ, Felbor U, et al. Endosomal proteolysis of the Ebola virus glycoprotein is necessary for infection. *Science* 2005;308: 1643–1645.
31. Cherry S. Genomic RNAi screening in Drosophila S2 cells: what have we learned about host-pathogen interactions? *Curr Opin Microbiol* 2008;11: 262–270.

32. Choe H, Farzan M, Sun Y, et al. The beta-chemokine receptors CCR3 and CCR5 facilitate infection by primary HIV-1 isolates. *Cell* 1996;85: 1135–1148.
33. Choppin PW, Compans RW. Replication of paramyxoviruses. In: Fraenkel-Conrat H, Wagner RR, eds. *Comprehensive Virology*, Vol. 4. New York: Plenum; 1975:94–178.
34. Cohen S, Au S, Pante N. How viruses access the nucleus. *Biochim Biophys Acta* 2010;1813:1634–1645.
35. Collinet C, Stoter M, Bradshaw CR, et al. Systems survey of endocytosis by multiparametric image analysis. *Nature* 2010;464:243–249.
36. Compans RW, Content J, Duesberg PH. Structure of the ribonucleoprotein of influenza virus. *J Virol* 1972;10:795–800.
37. Conner SD, Schmid SL. Regulated portals of entry into the cell. *Nature* 2003;422:37–44.
38. Cotmore SF, Tattersall P. Parvoviral host range and cell entry mechanisms. *Adv Virus Res* 2007;70:183–232.
39. Coyne CB, Bergelson JM. Virus-induced Abl and Fyn kinase signals permit coxsackievirus entry through epithelial tight junctions. *Cell* 2006;124: 119–131.
40. Cullen B. Journey to the center of the cell. *Cell* 2001;105:697–700.
41. Cureton DK, Massol RH, Saffarian S, et al. Vesicular stomatitis virus enters cells through vesicles incompletely coated with clathrin that depend upon actin for internalization. *PLoS Pathog* 2009;5:e1000394.
42. Daecke J, Fackler OT, Dittmar MT, et al. Involvement of clathrin-mediated endocytosis in human immunodeficiency virus type 1 entry. *J Virol* 2005;79:1581–1594.
43. Dales S. Early events in cell-animal virus interactions. *Bacteriol Rev* 1973; 37:103–135.
44. Damm EM, Pelkmans L, Kartenbeck J, et al. Clathrin- and caveolin-1-independent endocytosis: entry of simian virus 40 into cells devoid of caveolae. *J Cell Biol* 2005;168:477–488.
45. Dohner K, Nagel CH, Sodeik B. Viral stop-and-go along microtubules: taking a ride with dynein and kinesins. *Trends Microbiol* 2005;13: 320–327.
46. Donaldson JG, Porat-Shliom N, Cohen LA. Clathrin-independent endocytosis: a unique platform for cell signaling and PM remodeling. *Cell Signal* 2009;21:1–6.
47. Doranz BJ, Rucker J, Yi Y, et al. A dual-tropic primary HIV-1 isolate that uses fusin and the beta-chemokine receptors CKR-5, CKR-3, and CKR-2b as fusion cofactors. *Cell* 1996;85:1149–1158.
48. Dorig RE, Marcil A, Chopra A, et al. The human CD46 molecule is a receptor for measles virus (Edmonston strain). *Cell* 1993;75:295–305.
49. Dveksler GS, Pensiero MN, Cardellichio CB, et al. Cloning of the mouse hepatitis virus (MHV) receptor: expression in human and hamster cell lines confers susceptibility to MHV. *J Virol* 1991;65:6881–6891.
50. Ehrlich M, Boll W, Van Oijen A, et al. Endocytosis by random initiation and stabilization of clathrin-coated pits. *Cell* 2004;118:591–605.
51. Engel S, Heger T, Mancini R, et al. The role of endosomes in SV40 entry and infection. *J Virol* 2011;85:4198–4211.
52. English TJ, Hammer DA. The effect of cellular receptor diffusion on receptor-mediated viral binding using Brownian adhesive dynamics (BRAD) simulations. *Biophys J* 2005;88:1666–1675.
53. Ewers H, Römer W, Smith AE, et al. GM1 structure determines SV40-induced membrane invagination and infection. *Nat Cell Biol* 2010;12: 11–18.
54. Ewers H, Smith AE, Sbalzarini IF, et al. Single-particle tracking of murine polyoma virus-like particles on live cells and artificial membranes. *Proc Natl Acad Sci U S A* 2005;102:15110–15115.
55. Fadok VA, Bratton DL, Frasch SC, et al. The role of phosphatidylserine in recognition of apoptotic cells by phagocytes. *Cell Death Differ* 1998; 5:551–562.
56. Farzan M, Choe H, Martin K, et al. Two orphan seven-transmembrane segment receptors which are expressed in CD4-positive cells support simian immunodeficiency virus infection. *J Exp Med* 1997;186: 405–411.
57. Feinberg H, Mitchell DA, Drickamer K, et al. Structural basis for selective recognition of oligosaccharides by DC-SIGN and DC-SIGNR. *Science* 2001;294:2163–2166.
58. Feire AL, Koss H, Compton T. Cellular integrins function as entry receptors for human cytomegalovirus via a highly conserved disintegrin-like domain. *Proc Natl Acad Sci U S A* 2004;101:15470–15475.
59. Fingeroth JD, Weis JJ, Tedder TF, et al. Epstein-Barr virus receptor of human B lymphocytes is the C3d receptor CR2. *Proc Natl Acad Sci U S A* 1984;81:4510–4514.
60. Frade R, Barel M, Ehlin-Henriksson B, et al. gp140, the C3d receptor of human B lymphocytes, is also the Epstein-Barr virus receptor. *Proc Natl Acad Sci U S A* 1985;82:1490–1493.
61. Fricks CE, Hogle JM. Cell-induced conformational change in poliovirus: externalization of the amino terminus of VP1 is responsible for liposome binding. *J Virol* 1990;64:1934–1945.
62. Frischknecht F, Way M. Surfing pathogens and the lessons learned for actin polymerization. *Trends Cell Biol* 2001;11:30–38.
63. Brabec-Zaruba M, Pfanzagl B, et al. Site of human rhinovirus RNA uncoating revealed by fluorescent in situ hybridization. *J Virol.* 2009:83: 3770–3777.
64. Fuchs R, Blaas D. Uncoating of human rhinoviruses. *Rev Med Virol* 2010; 20:281–297.
65. Gavrilovskaya IN, Shepley M, Shaw R, et al. beta3 Integrins mediate the cellular entry of hantaviruses that cause respiratory failure. *Proc Natl Acad Sci U S A* 1998;95:7074–7079.
66. Geijtenbeek TB, Kwon DS, Torensma R, et al. DC-SIGN, a dendritic cell-specific HIV-1-binding protein that enhances trans-infection of T cells. *Cell* 2000;100:587–597.
67. Geraghty RJ, Krummenacher C, Cohen GH, et al. Entry of alphaherpesviruses mediated by poliovirus receptor-related protein 1 and poliovirus receptor. *Science* 1998;280:1618–1620.
68. Greber U. Signalling in viral entry. *Cell Mol Life Sci* 2002;59:608–626.
69. Greber UF, Fassati A. Nuclear import of viral DNA genomes. *Traffic* 2003; 4:136–143.
70. Greber UF, Way M. A superhighway to virus infection. *Cell* 2006;124: 741–754.
71. Greve JM, Davis G, Meyer AM, et al. The major human rhinovirus receptor is ICAM-1. *Cell* 1989;56:839–847.
72. Gruenberg J. Viruses and endosome membrane dynamics. *Curr Opin Cell Biol* 2009;21:582–588.
73. Gruenberg J, Stenmark H. The biogenesis of multivesicular endosomes. *Nat Rev Mol Cell Biol* 2004;5:317–323.
74. Harbison CE, Chiorini JA, Parrish CR. The parvovirus capsid odyssey: from the cell surface to the nucleus. *Trends Microbiol* 2008;16:208–214.
75. Heinz FX, Allison SL. The machinery for flavivirus fusion with host cell membranes. *Curr Opin Microbiol* 2001;4:450–455.
76. Helenius A, Kartenbeck J, Simons K, et al. On the entry of Semliki forest virus into BHK-21 cells. *J Cell Biol* 1980;84:404–420.
77. Helmuth JA, Burckhardt CJ, Greber UF, et al. Shape reconstruction of subcellular structures from live cell fluorescence microscopy images. *J Struct Biol* 2009;167:1–10.
78. Hewish MJ, Takada Y, Coulson BS. Integrins alpha2beta1 and alpha4beta1 can mediate SA11 rotavirus attachment and entry into cells. *J Virol* 2000;74:228–236.
79. Hirsch AJ. The use of RNAi-based screens to identify host proteins involved in viral replication. *Future Microbiol* 2010;5:303–311.
80. Hofer F, Gruenberger M, Kowalski H, et al. Members of the low density lipoprotein receptor family mediate cell entry of a minor-group common cold virus. *Proc Natl Acad Sci U S A* 1994;91:1839–1842.
81. Hogle JM. Poliovirus cell entry: common structural themes in viral cell entry pathways. *Annu Rev Microbiol* 2002;56:677–702.
82. Huotari J, Helenius A. Endosome maturation. *EMBO J* 2011;30:3481–3500.
83. Igakura T, Stinchcombe JC, Goon PK, et al. Spread of HTLV-I between lymphocytes by virus-induced polarization of the cytoskeleton. *Science* 2003;299:1713–1716.
84. Jackson T, Blakemore W, Newman JW, et al. Foot-and-mouth disease virus is a ligand for the high-affinity binding conformation of integrin alpha5beta1: influence of the leucine residue within the RGDL motif on selectivity of integrin binding. *J Gen Virol* 2000;81:1383–1391.
85. Johannsdottir HK, Mancini R, Kartenbeck J, et al. Host cell factors and functions involved in vesicular stomatitis virus entry. *J Virol* 2009; 83:440–453.
86. Kann M, Sodeik B, Vlachou A, et al. Phosphorylation-dependent binding of Hepatitis B virus core particles to the nuclear pore complex. *J Cell Biol* 1999;145:45–55.

87. Karjalainen M, Kakkonen E, Upla P, et al. A Raft-derived, Pak1-regulated entry participates in alpha2beta1 integrin-dependent sorting to caveosomes. *Mol Biol Cell* 2008;19:2857–2869.
88. Kates J, Beeson J. Ribonucleic acid synthesis in vaccnina virus. I. The mechanism of synthesis and release of RNA in vaccinia cores. *J Mol Biol* 1970;50:1–18.
89. Kienberger F, Zhu R, Moser R, et al. Monitoring RNA release from human rhinovirus by dynamic force microscopy. *J Virol* 2004;78:3203–3209.
90. Klenk HD, Rott R, Orlich M, et al. Activation of influenza A viruses by trypsin treatment. *Virology* 1975;68:426–439.
91. Klimstra WB, Nangle EM, Smith MS, et al. DC-SIGN and L-SIGN can act as attachment receptors for alphaviruses and distinguish between mosquito cell- and mammalian cell-derived viruses. *J Virol* 2003;77:12022–12032.
92. Kolokoltsov AA, Deniger D, Fleming EH, et al. Small interfering RNA profiling reveals key role of clathrin-mediated endocytosis and early endosome formation for infection by respiratory syncytial virus. *J Virol* 2007;81:7786–7800.
93. Kwon DS, Gregorio G, Bitton N, et al. DC-SIGN-mediated internalization of HIV is required for trans-enhancement of T cell infection. *Immunity* 2002;16:135–144.
94. Lajoie P, Nabi IR. Regulation of raft-dependent endocytosis. *J Cell Mol Med* 2007;11:644–653.
95. Lakadamyali M, Rust MJ, Babcock HP, et al. Visualizing infection of individual influenza viruses. *Proc Natl Acad Sci U S A* 2003;100:9280–9285.
96. Lehmann MJ, Sherer NM, Marks CB, et al. Actin- and myosin-driven movement of viruses along filopodia precedes their entry into cells. *J Cell Biol* 2005;170:317–325.
97. Lewis PF, Emerman M. Passage through mitosis is required for oncoretroviruses but not for the human immunodeficiency virus. *J Virol* 1994; 68:510–516.
98. Liberali P, Ramo P, Pelkmans L. Protein kinases: starting a molecular systems view of endocytosis. *Annu Rev Cell Dev Biol* 2008;24:501–523.
99. Loetscher M, Amara A, Oberlin E, et al. TYMSTR, a putative chemokine receptor selectively expressed in activated T cells, exhibits HIV-1 coreceptor function. *Curr Biol* 1997;7:652–660.
100. Lonberg-Holm K, Philipson L. Early interaction between animal viruses and cells. *Monogr Virol* 1974;9:1–149.
101. Lozach PY, Huotari J, Helenius A. Late-penetrating viruses. *Curr Opin Virol* 2011;1:35–43.
102. Lozach PY, Kuhbacher A, Meier R, et al. DC-SIGN as a receptor for phleboviruses. *Cell Host Microbe* 2011;10:75–88.
103. Lozach PY, Lortat-Jacob H, de Lacroix de Lavalette A, et al. DC-SIGN and L-SIGN are high affinity binding receptors for hepatitis C virus glycoprotein E2. *J Biol Chem* 2003;278:20358–20366.
104. Lusso P, Secchiero P, Crowley RW, et al. CD4 is a critical component of the receptor for human herpesvirus 7: interference with human immunodeficiency virus. *Proc Natl Acad Sci U S A* 1994;91:3872–3876.
105. Lyman MG, Enquist LW. Herpesvirus interactions with the host cytoskeleton. *J Virol* 2009;83:2058–2066.
106. Maddon P, Dalgleish A, McDougal J, et al. The T4 gene encodes the AIDS virus receptor and is expressed in the immune system and the brain. *Cell* 1986;47:333–348.
107. Marechal V, Prevost MC, Petit C, et al. Human immunodeficiency virus type 1 entry into macrophages mediated by macropinocytosis. *J Virol* 2001;75:11166–11177.
108. Marsh M, Bron R. SFV infection in CHO cells: cell-type specific restrictions to productive virus entry at the cell surface. *J Cell Sci* 1997;110(Pt 1): 95–103.
109. Marsh M, Helenius A. Virus entry into animal cells. *Adv Virus Res* 1989; 36:107–151.
110. Marsh M, Helenius A. Virus entry: open sesame. *Cell* 2006;124:729–740.
111. Martin K, Helenius A. Nuclear transport of influenza virus ribonucleoproteins: the viral matrix protein (M1) promotes export and inhibits import. *Cell* 1991;67:117–130.
112. Matlin KS, Reggio H, Helenius A, et al. Infectious entry pathway of influenza virus in a canine kidney cell line. *J Cell Biol* 1982;91:601–613.
113. Matlin KS, Reggio H, Helenius A, et al. The pathway of vesicular stomatitis virus entry leading to infection. *J Mol Biol* 1982;156:609–631.
114. Maul GG, Rovera G, Vorbrodt A, et al. Membrane fusion as a mechanism of Simian Virus 40 entry into different cellular compartments. *J Virol* 1978;28:936–944.
115. Mauri DN, Ebner R, Montgomery RI, et al. LIGHT, a new member of the TNF superfamily, and lymphotoxin alpha are ligands for herpesvirus entry mediator. *Immunity* 1998;8:21–30.
116. Mayor S, Pagano RE. Pathways of clathrin-independent endocytosis. *Nat Rev Mol Cell Biol* 2007;8:603–612.
117. Medina-Kauwe LK. Endocytosis of adenovirus and adenovirus capsid proteins. *Adv Drug Deliv Rev* 2003;55:1485–1496.
118. Meier O, Boucke K, Hammer SV, et al. Adenovirus triggers macropinocytosis and endosomal leakage together with its clathrin-mediated uptake. *J Cell Biol* 2002;158:1119–1131.
119. Meier O, Greber UF. Adenovirus endocytosis. *J Gene Med* 2003;5:451–462.
120. Mellman I. Endocytosis and molecular sorting. *Annu Rev Cell Dev Biol* 1996;12:575–625.
121. Mendelsohn CL, Wimmer E, Racaniello VR. Cellular receptor for poliovirus: molecular cloning, nucleotide sequence, and expression of a new member of the immunoglobulin superfamily. *Cell* 1989;56:855–865.
122. Mercer J, Helenius A. Vaccinia virus uses macropinocytosis and apoptotic mimicry to enter host cells. *Science* 2008;320:531–535.
123. Mercer J, Helenius A. Virus entry by macropinocytosis. *Nat Cell Biol* 2009;11:510–520.
124. Mercer J, Schelhaas M, Helenius A. Virus entry by endocytosis. *Annu Rev Biochem* 2010;79:803–833.
125. Miller D, Miller A. A family of retroviruses that utilize related phosphate transporters for cell entry. *J Virol* 1994;68:8270–8276.
126. Miller M, Farnet C, Bushman F. Human immunodeficiency virus type 1 preintegration complexes: studies of organization and composition. *J Virol* 1997;71:5382–5390.
127. Mondor I, Ugolini S, Sattentau QJ. Human immunodeficiency virus type 1 attachment to HeLa CD4 cells is CD4 independent and gp120 dependent and requires cell surface heparans. *J Virol* 1998;72:3623–3634.
128. Mothes W, Boerger AL, Narayan S, et al. Retroviral entry mediated by receptor priming and low pH triggering of an envelope glycoprotein. *Cell* 2000;103:679–689.
129. Mothes W, Sherer NM, Jin J, et al. Virus cell-to-cell transmission. *J Virol* 2010;84:8360–8368.
130. Moyer CL, Wiethoff CM, Maier O, et al. Functional genetic and biophysical analyses of membrane disruption by human adenovirus. *J Virol* 2011;85:2631–2641.
131. Nemerow GR. Cell receptors involved in adenovirus entry. *Virology* 2000;274:1–4.
132. Neu U, Stehle T, Atwood WJ. The Polyomaviridae: contributions of virus structure to our understanding of virus receptors and infectious entry. *Virology* 2009;384:389–399.
133. Nicola AV, Hou J, Major EO, et al. Herpes simplex virus type 1 enters human epidermal keratinocytes, but not neurons, via a pH-dependent endocytic pathway. *J Virol* 2005;79:7609–7616.
134. Nisole S, Saib A. Early steps of retrovirus replicative cycle. *Retrovirology* 2004;1:9.
135. Norkin LC. Caveolae in the uptake and targeting of infectious agents and secreted toxins. *Adv Drug Deliv Rev* 2001;49:301–315.
136. Novoa RR, Calderita G, Arranz R, et al. Virus factories: associations of cell organelles for viral replication and morphogenesis. *Biol Cell* 2005; 97:147–172.
137. O'Hara B, Johann S, Klinger H, et al. Characterization of a human gene conferring sensitivity to infection by gibbon ape leukemia virus. *Cell Growth Differ* 1990;1:119–127.
138. O'Neill RE, Jaskunas R, Blobel G, et al. Nuclear import of influenza virus RNA can be mediated by viral nucleoprotein and transport factors required for protein import. *J Biol Chem* 1995;270:22701–22704.
139. Ojala PM, Sodeik B, Ebersold MW, et al. Herpes simplex virus type 1 entry into host cells: reconstitution of capsid binding and uncoating at the nuclear pore complex in vitro. *Mol Cell Biol* 2000;20:4922–4931.
140. Pante N, Kann M. Nuclear pore complex is able to transport macromolecules with diameters of about 39 nm. *Mol Biol Cell* 2002;13:425–434.
141. Parton RG, Simons K. The multiple faces of caveolae. *Nat Rev Mol Cell Biol* 2007;8:185–194.
142. Pasdeloup D, Blondel D, Isidro AL, et al. Herpesvirus capsid association with the nuclear pore complex and viral DNA release involve the nucleoporin CAN/Nup214 and the capsid protein pUL25. *J Virol* 2009;83:6610–6623.
143. Peiris JSM, Porterfileld JS. Antibody mediated enhancement of flavivirus replication in macrophage-like cell lines. *Nature* 1979;282:509–511.

144. Pelkmans L, Fava E, Grabner H, et al. Genome-wide analysis of human kinases in clathrin- and caveolae/raft-mediated endocytosis. *Nature* 2005; 436:78–86.
145. Pelkmans L, Puntener D, Helenius A. Local actin polymerization and dynamin recruitment in SV40-induced internalization of caveolae. *Science* 2002;296:535–539.
146. Pelkmans L, Zerial M. Kinase-regulated quantal assemblies and kiss-and-run recycling of caveolae. *Nature* 2005;436:128–133.
147. Pileri P, Uematsu Y, Campagnoli S, et al. Binding of hepatitis C virus to CD81. *Science* 1998;282:938–941.
148. Pinto LH, Holsinger LJ, Lamb RA. Influenza virus M2 protein has ion channel activity. *Cell* 1992;69:1–20.
149. Pohlmann S, Baribaud F, Doms RW. DC-SIGN and DC-SIGNR: helping hands for HIV. *Trends Immunol* 2001;22:643–646.
150. Poranen MM, Daugelavicius R, Bamford DH. Common principles in viral entry. *Annu Rev Microbiol* 2002;56:521–538.
151. Pyeon D, Pearce SM, Lank SM, et al. Establishment of human papillomavirus infection requires cell cycle progression. *PLoS Pathog* 2009;5: e1000318.
152. Qian M, Cai D, Verhey KJ, et al. A lipid receptor sorts polyomavirus from the endolysosome to the endoplasmic reticulum to cause infection. *PLoS Pathog* 2009;5:e1000465.
153. Rabe B, Vlachou A, Pante N, et al. Nuclear import of hepatitis B virus capsids and release of the viral genome. *Proc Natl Acad Sci U S A* 2003; 100:9849–9854.
154. Radtke K, Kieneke D, Wolfstein A, et al. Plus- and minus-end directed microtubule motors bind simultaneously to herpes simplex virus capsids using different inner tegument structures. *PLoS Pathog* 2010;6:e1000991.
155. Rand RP. Interacting phospholipid bilayers: measured forces and induced structural changes. *Annu Rev Biophys Bioeng* 1981;10:277–314.
156. Razani B, Woodman SE, Lisanti MP. Caveolae: from cell biology to animal physiology. *Pharmacol Rev* 2002;54:431–467.
157. Rees PJ, Dimmock NJ. Electrophoretic separation of influenza virus ribonucleoproteins. *J Gen Virol* 1981;53:125–132.
158. Richterova Z, Liebl D, Horak M, et al. Caveolae are involved in the trafficking of mouse polyomavirus virions and artificial VP1 pseudocapsids toward cell nuclei. *J Virol* 2001;75:10880–10891.
159. Roivainen M, Piirainen L, Hovi T, et al. Entry of coxsackievirus A9 into host cells: specific interactions with alpha v beta 3 integrin, the vitronectin receptor. *Virology* 1994;203:357–365.
160. Römer W, Berland L, Chambon V, et al. Shiga toxin induces tubular membrane invaginations for its uptake into cells. *Nature* 2007;450:670–675.
161. Rossmann MG, He Y, Kuhn RJ. Picornavirus-receptor interactions. *Trends Microbiol* 2002;10:324–331.
162. Roth SL, Whittaker GR. Promotion of vesicular stomatitis virus fusion by the endosome-specific phospholipid bis(monoacylglycero)phosphate (BMP). *FEBS Lett* 2011;585:865–869.
163. Rucker J, Edinger AL, Sharron M, et al. Utilization of chemokine receptors, orphan receptors, and herpesvirus-encoded receptors by diverse human and simian immunodeficiency viruses. *J Virol* 1997;71:8999–9007.
164. Rust MJ, Lakadamyali M, Zhang F, et al. Assembly of endocytic machinery around individual influenza viruses during viral entry. *Nat Struct Mol Biol* 2004;11:567–573.
165. Saeed MF, Kolokoltsov AA, Albrecht T, et al. Cellular entry of Ebola virus involves uptake by a macropinocytosis-like mechanism and subsequent trafficking through early and late endosomes. *PLoS Pathog* 2010;6: e1001110.
166. Saftig P, Klumperman J. Lysosome biogenesis and lysosomal membrane proteins: trafficking meets function. *Nat Rev Mol Cell Biol* 2009;10:623–635.
167. Sattentau Q. Avoiding the void: cell-to-cell spread of human viruses. *Nat Rev Microbiol* 2008;6:815–826.
168. Schelhaas M, Ewers H, Rajamaki ML, et al. Human papillomavirus type 16 entry: retrograde cell surface transport along actin-rich protrusions. *PLoS Pathog* 2008;4:e1000148.
169. Schelhaas M, Malmstrom J, Pelkmans L, et al. Simian virus 40 depends on ER protein folding and quality control factors for entry into host cells. *Cell* 2007;131:516–529.
170. Scott CC, Gruenberg J. Ion flux and the function of endosomes and lysosomes: pH is just the start: the flux of ions across endosomal membranes influences endosome function not only through regulation of the luminal pH. *Bioessays* 2011;33:103–110.
171. Seisenberger G, Ried MU, Endress T, et al. Real-time single-molecule imaging of the infection pathway of an adeno-associated virus. *Science* 2001;294:1929–1932.
172. Seth P, FitzGerald DJP, Willigham MC, et al. Role of a low-pH environment in adenovirus enhancement of the toxicity of a *Pseudomonas* exotoxin-epidermal growth factor conjugate. *J Virol* 1984;51:650–655.
173. Shafren DR, Bates RC, Agrez MV, et al. Coxsackieviruses B1, B3, and B5 use decay accelerating factor as a receptor for cell attachment. *J Virol* 1995;69:3873–3877.
174. Sieczkarski SB, Brown HA, Whittaker GR. Role of protein kinase C beta II in influenza virus entry via late endosomes. *J Virol* 2003;77:460–469.
175. Sieczkarski SB, Whittaker GR. Influenza virus can enter and infect cells in the absence of clathrin-mediated endocytosis. *J Virol* 2002;76:10455–10464.
176. Sieczkarski SB, Whittaker GR. Differential requirements of Rab5 and Rab7 for endocytosis of influenza and other enveloped viruses. *Traffic* 2003;4:333–343.
177. Silverstein SC, Astell C, Levin DH, et al. The mechanisms of reovirus uncoating and gene activation in vivo. *Virology* 1972;47:797–806.
178. Simmons G, Reeves JD, Grogan CC, et al. DC-SIGN and DC-SIGNR bind ebola glycoproteins and enhance infection of macrophages and endothelial cells. *Virology* 2003;305:115–123.
179. Singh I, Helenius A. Role of ribosomes in Semliki Forest virus nucleocapsid uncoating. *J Virol* 1992;66:7049–7058.
180. Skehel JJ, Wiley DC. Receptor binding and membrane fusion in virus entry: the influenza hemagglutinin. *Annu Rev Biochem* 2000;69:531–569.
181. Smit JM, Waarts BL, Kimata K, et al. Adaptation of alphaviruses to heparan sulfate: interaction of Sindbis and Semliki Forest viruses with liposomes containing lipid-conjugated heparin. *J Virol* 2002;76:10128–10137.
182. Smith GA, Enquist LW. Break ins and break outs: viral interactions with the cytoskeleton of mammalian cells. *Annu Rev Cell Dev Biol* 2002; 18:135–161.
183. Smith GL, Murphy BJ, Law M. Vaccinia virus motility. *Annu Rev Microbiol* 2003;57:323–342.
184. Sodeik B. Mechanisms of viral transport in the cytoplasm. *Trends Microbiol* 2000;8:465–472.
185. Spear PG, Eisenberg RJ, Cohen GH. Three classes of cell surface receptors for alphaherpesvirus entry. *Virology* 2000;275:1–8.
186. Stadler K, Allison SL, Schalich J, et al. Proteolytic activation of tick-borne encephalitis virus by furin. *J Virol* 1997;71:8475–8481.
187. Stang E, Kartenbeck J, Parton RG. Major histocompatibility complex class I molecules mediate association of SV40 with caveolae. *Mol Biol Cell* 1997;8:47–57.
188. Staunton DE, Merluzzi VJ, Rothlein R, et al. A cell adhesion molecule, ICAM-1, is the major surface receptor for rhinoviruses. *Cell* 1989; 56:849–853.
189. Stewart PL, Dermody TS, Nemerow GR. Structural basis of nonenveloped virus cell entry. *Adv Protein Chem* 2003;64:455–491.
190. Stewart PL, Nemerow GR. Cell integrins: commonly used receptors for diverse viral pathogens. *Trends Microbiol* 2007;15:500–507.
191. Sugrue RJ, Hay AJ. Structural characteristics of the M2 protein of influenza A viruses: evidence that it forms a tetrameric channel. *Virology* 1991; 180:617–624.
192. Suikkanen S, Saajarvi K, Hirsimaki J, et al. Role of recycling endosomes and lysosomes in dynein-dependent entry of canine parvovirus. *J Virol* 2002;76:4401–4411.
193. Suomalainen M, Nakano MY, Keller S, et al. Microtubule-dependent plus- and minus end-directed motilities are competing processes for nuclear targeting of adenovirus. *J Cell Biol* 1999;144:657–672.
194. Swanson JA, Watts C. Macropinocytosis. *Trends Cell Biol* 1995;5: 424–428.
195. Tailor CS, Nouri A, Lee CG, et al. Cloning and characterization of a cell surface receptor for xenotropic and polytropic murine leukemia viruses. *Proc Natl Acad Sci U S A* 1999;96:927–932.
196. Takeuchi Y, Vile RG, Simpson G, et al. Feline leukemia virus subgroup B uses the same cell surface receptor as gibbon ape leukemia virus. *J Virol* 1992;66:1219–1222.
197. Tassaneetrithep B, Burgess TH, Granelli-Piperno A, et al. DC-SIGN (CD209) mediates dengue virus infection of human dendritic cells. *J Exp Med* 2003;197:823–829.

198. Tomko RP, Xu R, Philipson L. HCAR and MCAR: the human and mouse cellular receptors for subgroup C adenoviruses and group B coxsackieviruses. *Proc Natl Acad Sci U S A* 1997;94:3352–3356.
199. Tosteson MT, Chow M. Characterization of the ion channels formed by poliovirus in planar lipid membranes. *J Virol* 1997;71:507–511.
200. Trotman L, Mosberger N, Fornerod M, et al. Import of adenovirus DNA involves the nuclear pore complex receptor CAN/Nup214 and histone H1. *Nat Cell Biol* 2001;3:1092–1100.
201. Tsai B, Inoue T. A virus takes an "L" turn to find its receptor. *Cell Host Microbe* 2010;8:301–302.
202. Valiya Veettil M, Sadagopan S, Kerur N, et al. Interaction of c-Cbl with myosin IIA regulates bleb associated macropinocytosis of Kaposi's sarcoma-associated herpesvirus. *PLoS Pathog* 2010;6:e1001238.
203. van Deurs B, Petersen OW, Olsnes S, et al. The ways of endocytosis. *Int Rev Cytol* 1989;117:131–177.
204. van Deurs B, Roepstorff K, Hommelgaard AM, et al. Caveolae: anchored, multifunctional platforms in the lipid ocean. *Trends Cell Biol* 2003;13: 92–100.
205. van Zeijl M, Johann S, Closs E, et al. A human amphotropic retrovirus receptor is a second member of the gibbon ape leukemia virus receptor family. *Proc Natl Acad Sci U S A* 1994;91:1168–1172.
206. Vihinen-Ranta M, Suikkanen S, Parrish CR. Pathways of cell infection by parvoviruses and adeno-associated viruses. *J Virol* 2004;78:6709–6714.
207. Vonderheit A, Helenius A. Rab7 associates with early endosomes to mediate sorting and transport of Semliki Forest virus to late endosomes. *PLoS Biol* 2005;3:e233.
208. Wengler G. Cell-associated West Nile flavivirus is covered with E+pre-M protein heterodimers which are destroyed and reorganized by proteolytic cleavage during virus release. *J Virol* 1989;63:2521–2526.
209. Wengler G. The regulation of disassembly of alphavirus cores. *Arch Virol* 2009;154:381–390.
210. White J, Kielian M, Helenius A. Membrane fusion proteins of enveloped animal viruses. *Q Rev Biophys* 1983;16:151–195.
211. Whittaker GR. Virus nuclear import. *Adv Drug Deliv Rev* 2003;55: 733–747.
212. Whittaker GR, Kann M, Helenius A. Viral entry into the nucleus. *Annu Rev Cell Dev Biol* 2000;16:627–651.
213. Wickham TJ, Filardo EJ, Cheresh DA, et al. Integrin alpha v beta 5 selectively promotes adenovirus mediated cell membrane permeabilization. *J Cell Biol* 1994;127:257–264.
214. Wickham TJ, Mathias P, Cheresh DA, et al. Integrins alpha v beta 3 and alpha v beta 5 promote adenovirus internalization but not virus attachment. *Cell* 1993;73:309–319.
215. Wileman T. Aggresomes and pericentriolar sites of virus assembly: cellular defense or viral design? *Annu Rev Microbiol* 2007;61:149–167.
216. Wolffe EJ, Weisberg AS, Moss B. Role for the vaccinia virus A36R outer envelope protein in the formation of virus-tipped actin-containing microvilli and cell-to-cell virus spread. *Virology* 1998;244:20–26.
217. Yeager CL, Ashmun RA, Williams RK, et al. Human aminopeptidase N is a receptor for human coronavirus 229E. *Nature* 1992;357:420–422.
218. Yuan P, Thompson TB, Wurzburg BA, et al. Structural studies of the parainfluenza virus 5 hemagglutinin-neuraminidase tetramer in complex with its receptor, sialyllactose. *Structure (Camb)* 2005;13:803–815.
219. Zhang Y, Bergelson JM. Adenovirus receptors. *J Virol* 2005;79:12125–12131.
220. Zvonarjev AY, Ghendon YZ. Influence of membrane (M) protein on influenza A virus virion transcriptase activity in vitro and its susceptibility to rimantadine. *J Virol* 1980;33:583–586.

CHAPTER 5

Sean Whelan

Viral Replication Strategies

INTRODUCTION

Replication of genetic information is the single most distinctive characteristic of living organisms, and nowhere in the biosphere is replication accomplished with greater economy and apparent simplicity than among viruses. To achieve the expression, replication, and spread of their genes, different virus families have evolved diverse genetic strategies and replicative cycles to exploit the biology of their hosts. Despite their comparatively limited genetic repertoire, viruses encode the information necessary to rewire their hosts to become viral factories. The intimacy of this relationship and the co-evolution of virus and host continue to provide unique mechanistic insights into host biology at the molecular, cellular, organismal, and population levels. Understanding this interplay enriches our understanding of the biosphere in general and virus–host relationships in particular, but also creates opportunities for the rational development of antiviral drugs, and for domesticating viruses as expression vectors, live-attenuated vaccines, and pesticides. This chapter provides an overview of the replication strategies of the major virus families that infect vertebrates, attempting where possible to emphasize the general principles that guide and constrain virus replication and evolution.

Viral Genome Diversity and Replication Strategies

Perhaps the most striking aspect of viruses at the molecular level is the diversity of their genome structures and replication strategies. Unlike cellular genomes, which consist uniformly of double-stranded DNA (dsDNA), viral genomes provide examples of almost every structural variation imaginable. As shown in Table 5.1, different families of viruses have genomes made of either double-stranded (ds) or single-stranded (ss) DNA or RNA; of either positive, negative, or ambisense polarity; of either linear or circular topology; and comprising either single or multiple segments. Each variation has consequences for the pathways of genome replication, viral gene expression, and virion assembly. This diversity argues strongly that viruses had several different evolutionary origins and can be thought of in D. J. McGeoch's evocative phrase as "mistletoe on the tree of life." Accordingly, viral taxonomy above the family level is patchy, with only 22 of 87 families assigned to the six orders that are currently recognized.[57] However, it is likely that more distant phylogenetic relationships will emerge as the number of genome sequences and protein structures increase, and as more powerful comparison algorithms become available.

Unique Biology of Virus Replication

As obligate intracellular parasites, all viruses depend heavily on functions provided by their host cells. This dependence, as well as the extensive metabolic overlap between host and parasite, limits the number of possible targets for antiviral therapy. Nevertheless, almost all viruses encode and express unique proteins, including enzymes, and many viruses exploit pathways of information transfer that are unknown elsewhere in the biosphere. This is particularly evident among the RNA

Updated from the previous text by L. Andrew Ball.

TABLE 5.1 Families and Genera of Viruses that Infect Vertebrates

Virus family or genera	Genome				Genome replication	
	Type	Polarity[a]	Topology[b]	Segments	Enzyme	Intracellular site
Adenoviridae	dsDNA	Both	Linear	1	Viral DdDp	Nucleus
Anelloviridae	ssDNA	Negative	Circular	1	Cellular DdDp	Nucleus
Asfarviridae	dsDNA	Both	Linear	1	Viral DdDp	Cytoplasm
Circoviridae	ssDNA	Negative or ambisense	Circular	1	Cellular DdDp	Nucleus
Hepadnaviridae	dsDNA	Both	Linear	1	Virion RdDp	Nucleus/cytoplasm
Herpesviridae	dsDNA	Both	Linear	1	Viral DdDp	Nucleus
Iridoviridae	dsDNA	Both	Linear	1	Viral DdDp	Nucleus/cytoplasm
Papillomaviridae	dsDNA	Both	Circular	1	Cellular DdDp	Nucleus
Parvoviridae	ssDNA	Either	Linear	1	Cellular DdDp	Nucleus
Polyomaviridae	dsDNA	Both	Circular	1	Cellular DdDp	Nucleus
Poxviridae	dsDNA	Both	Linear	1	Viral DdDp	Cytoplasm
Arenaviridae	ssRNA	Ambisense	Linear	2	Virion RdRp	Cytoplasm
Arteriviridae	ssRNA	Positive	Linear	1	Viral RdRp	Cytoplasm
Astroviridae	ssRNA	Positive	Linear	1	Viral RdRp	Cytoplasm
Birnaviridae	dsRNA	Both	Linear	2	Virion RdRp	Cytoplasm
Bornaviridae	ssRNA	Negative	Linear	1	Virion RdRp	Nucleus
Bunyaviridae	ssRNA	Negative or ambisense	Linear	3	Virion RdRp	Cytoplasm
Caliciviridae	ssRNA	Positive	Linear	1	Viral RdRp	Cytoplasm
Coronaviridae	ssRNA	Positive	Linear	1	Viral RdRp	Cytoplasm
Deltavirus genus	ssRNA	Negative	Circular	1	RNA pol II	Nucleus
Filoviridae	ssRNA	Negative	Linear	1	Virion RdRp	Cytoplasm
Flaviviridae	ssRNA	Positive	Linear	1	Viral RdRp	Cytoplasm
Hepeviridae	ssRNA	Positive	Linear	1	Viral RdRp	Cytoplasm
Nodaviridae	ssRNA	Positive	Linear	2	Viral RdRp	Cytoplasm
Orthomyxoviridae	ssRNA	Negative	Linear	6–8	Virion RdRp	Nucleus
Paramyxoviridae	ssRNA	Negative	Linear	1	Virion RdRp	Cytoplasm
Picornaviridae	ssRNA	Positive	Linear	1	Viral RdRp	Cytoplasm
Reoviridae	dsRNA	Both	Linear	10–12	Virion RdRp	Cytoplasm
Retroviridae	ssRNA	Positive	Linear	2 identical	Virion RdDp	Nucleus/cytoplasm
Rhabdoviridae	ssRNA	Negative	Linear	1	Virion RdRp	Cytoplasm
Togaviridae	ssRNA	Positive	Linear	1	Viral RdRp	Cytoplasm

DdDp, DNA-dependent DNA polymerase; ds, double-stranded; RdDp, RNA-dependent RNA polymerase; ss, single-stranded.

[a]Polarity of the encapsidated genome.

[b]Topology of the encapsidated genome—note that some circularize during replication.

viruses, which are the only organisms that are known to store their genetic information in the form of RNA. They accomplish this by replicating their genomes via one of two unique biochemical pathways—either by RNA-dependent RNA synthesis (RNA replication), or, among the retroviruses, by RNA-dependent DNA synthesis (reverse transcription) followed by DNA replication and transcription. Both pathways require enzymatic activities that are not usually found in uninfected host cells and must therefore be encoded by the viral genome and expressed during infection. Furthermore, in some families of RNA-containing viruses those unique synthetic processes are required right at the start of the infectious cycle. This necessitates co-packaging of the corresponding polymerase and other associated enzymes with the viral genome during the assembly of viral particles in preparation for the next round of infection.

Whatever the structure and replication strategy of their genomes, all viruses must express their genes as functional messenger RNAs (mRNAs) early in infection in order to direct the cellular translational machinery to make viral proteins. The various genomic strategies employed by viruses can therefore be organized around a simple conceptual framework centered on viral mRNA (Figs. 5.1 and 5.2). By convention, mRNA is defined as positive-sense and its complement as negative-sense. The pathways leading from genome to message vary widely among the different virus families and form the basis of viral taxonomy. Although it is generally believed that viruses originated from cellular organisms, perhaps fairly recently in evolutionary times, it remains possible that some RNA viruses are descended directly from a primordial "RNA world" or "ribonucleoprotein world," which may have predated the emergence of DNA and cells.

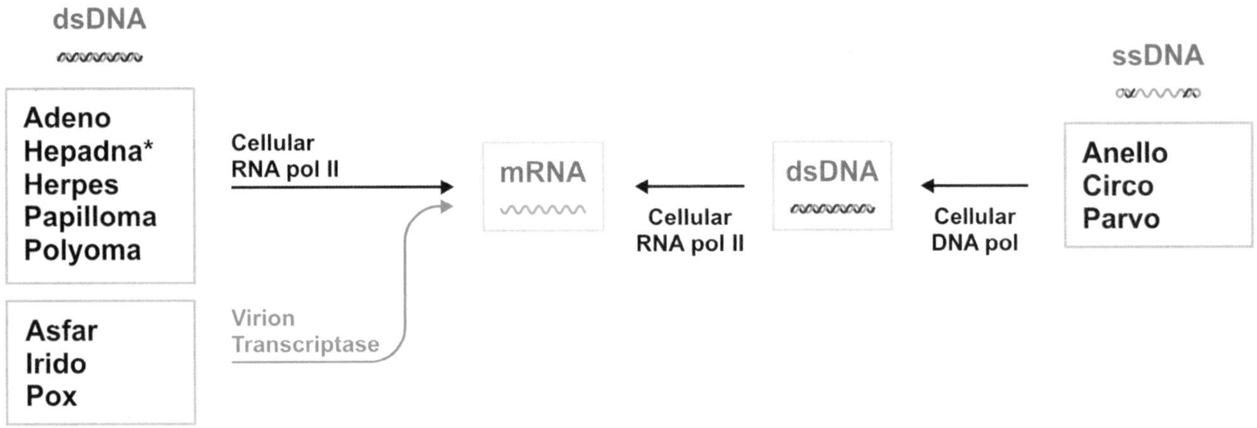

FIGURE 5.1. Pathways of primary mRNA synthesis by DNA viruses of animals. Hepadnaviruses replicate via reverse transcription of an ssRNA intermediate.

Subcellular Sites of Viral Replication

Most DNA viruses of eukaryotes transcribe and replicate their genomes and assemble progeny in the nucleus, the site of cellular DNA transcription and replication. The exceptions are the poxviruses, iridoviruses, and African swine fever virus, which replicate their DNA genomes partly or completely in the cytoplasm. In contrast, most RNA viruses replicate their genomes in the cytoplasm. However, in addition to the retroviruses that integrate DNA copies of their genomes into the host chromosomes, other notable exceptions to this generalization are the orthomyxoviruses, bornaviruses, and many plant-infecting rhabdoviruses, whose linear negative-sense RNA genomes replicate in the nucleus. The circular RNA genome of hepatitis delta virus (HDV), also replicates in the nucleus (Table 5.1). Each site of replication presents distinct opportunities and challenges in terms of which cellular components and pathways are available to be co-opted, and how the synthesis and trafficking of viral proteins, genome replication, virion assembly, and the release of progeny can be coordinated. For example, RNA splicing occurs only in the nucleus, so among the RNA viruses,

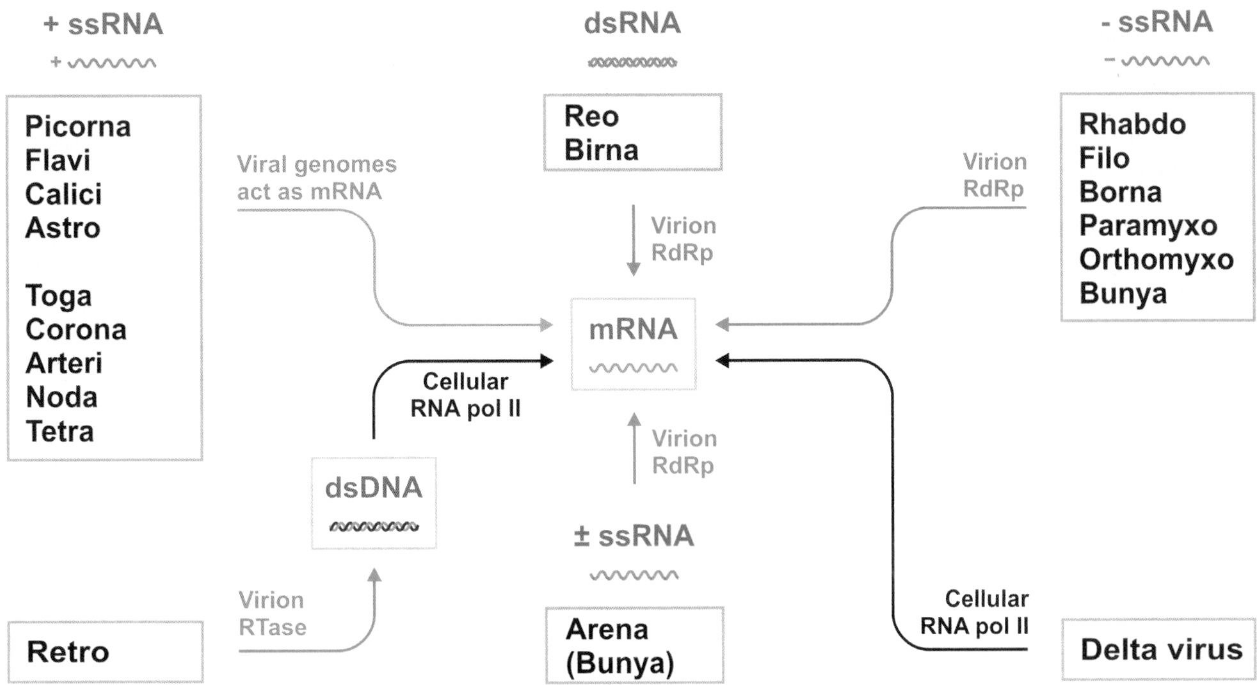

FIGURE 5.2. Pathways of primary mRNA synthesis by RNA viruses of animals. How RNA viruses produce mRNA at the start of infection depends upon the nature of the viral genome.

this mechanism of accessing more than one open-reading frame in a single transcript can be employed by only the retro-, orthomyxo-, and bornaviruses that transcribe there. It is remarkable that the paramyxoviruses that replicate in the cytoplasm have evolved a transcriptional editing mechanism that achieves a similar result.[99] Irrespective of the site of replication (nuclear or cytoplasmic) the viral replication machinery itself is frequently compartmentalized within specific structures or viral-induced organelles. For example, herpesviruses form replication compartments within the nucleus at nuclear speckles,[16,88] and many RNA viruses that replicate in the cytoplasm do so in association with membranes or an inclusion-like structure that contains the viral replication machinery.[25]

Evasion of Host Response to Infection

To ensure their survival, host organisms have evolved a variety of responses to combat viral infection. In turn, many viruses express specific gene products that act to circumvent one or more of those antiviral defense mechanisms. Examination of these measures and countermeasures provides a revealing glimpse into the heart of the host–parasite relationship as it plays out in nature. Host-defense mechanisms can be categorized as innate or adaptive. Among the former, which operate at the cellular level, are apoptosis (programmed cell suicide that limits the spread of infection, see Chapter 8), the induction and action of interferons in vertebrates (inducible cytokines that render cells resistant to infection by inducing a multifaceted antiviral state, see Chapter 8), and RNA interference in plants and invertebrates (a sequence-specific mechanism of RNA degradation, see Chapter 8). Adaptive immune mechanisms operate at the organismal level, and include the cell- and antibody-mediated immune response (see Chapter 9). Increasingly, specific restriction factors have been identified that limit the replication of subsets of viruses. Such factors include tripartite motif containing protein 5 (TRIM5), which appears to trigger the premature disassembly of the incoming human immunodeficiency virus type 1 (HIV-1) capsid to limit the establishment of infection; the apolipoprotein B mRNA editing, enzyme catalytic (APOBEC) family, which induces a biased hypermutation in RNA through its cytidine deaminase activity that converts C to U; and bone marrow stromal antigen 2 (Bst2)/Tetherin, which is incorporated into the membranes of some enveloped viruses resulting in a linking together of budding viral particles. Although a number of other cellular proteins have been termed "restriction factors," they are distinguished by their dependence on induction by interferon and are therefore not considered here. In different viruses, mechanisms and gene products have been identified that inhibit apoptosis, intercept interferons or suppress their activities, obstruct RNA interference, either evade or suppress different arms of the adaptive immune response, or block intrinsic restriction factors.[4,36,46,47,63,70,90,92,93,100]

Viruses are sensed by the host in ways that appear to involve recognition of unique signatures present in viral genomes or gene products. Such signatures are termed pathogen-associated molecular patterns (or PAMPS), and are recognized by an array of host pathogen-recognition receptors (or PRRs). Those PRRs include the toll-like receptors (TLRs), which are membrane-associated molecules that sense invading pathogens directly at the plasma membrane or during endosomal transit. The retinoic acid inducible gene (RIG)-like receptors (RLRs), which are cytoplasmic RNA helicases that recognize the products of RNA viral nucleic-acid replication, and the absent in melanoma 2-like receptors that recognize cytoplasmic DNA. Although viral ligands have not been defined, the NOD-like receptors (NLRs), which sense bacterial peptidoglycan, appear to also detect some viruses. A striking example of such PRR function is the detection of off-pathway products of replication such as abortive initiation products, dsRNA, and defective viral genomes, which can serve as ligands for the cytoplasmic sensors RIG-I and melanoma differentiation association protein 5 (MDA-5) to engage in a signaling cascade that leads to the activation of interferon.[40] The net result of interferon activation is both the blocking of infection within the cell, and the preactivation of defense mechanisms in neighboring cells to render them less susceptible to infection. The latter is accomplished by the transcription of interferon (IFN)–stimulated genes (ISG), which themselves act to block various steps in the replication cycle of DNA and RNA viruses[93] (see Chapter 8). In turn, viruses themselves have evolved countermeasures to such host-defense mechanisms that act to block the induction of IFN itself, or to interfere with specific ISG function.[22,43] The elaborate arms race between viruses and their hosts is described in more detail in Chapter 8 and Chapter 9, as well as within the specific chapters dealing with individual virus families. Molecular signatures of this arms race throughout evolution are also visible in the sequences of virus and host genes. Retroviruses provide a unique insight into this, since they integrate into the host genome. Evidence for integration of portions of other viral genomes into the host chromosome including RNA viruses such as bornavirus, and lymphocytic choriomeningitis virus, has also emerged.[33,80]

Error Prone Nature of RNA Replication

The polymerases that catalyze RNA replication and reverse transcription have minimal proofreading activities. The polymerase error rate of such RNA-dependent RNA polymerases (RdRp's) and reverse transcriptases is approximately three orders of magnitude higher than that of DNA-dependent DNA polymerases, and approaches the reciprocal of their genome length.[28,52,74] The net result is that the genomes of RNA viruses evolve at a much faster rate than those of their hosts. Biologically, RNA viruses therefore represent a swarm of sequences around a consensus sequence or master sequence.[31,62] This molecular swarm provides a fertile source of phenotypic variants that can respond rapidly to changing selection pressures by shifting its composition. As a consequence, RNA viruses can evolve up to 1 million times faster than DNA-based organisms. The error prone nature of RNA virus replication is also critical for pathogenesis in infected hosts. The diversity of viral sequences regenerated following bottleneck transmission of HIV in humans,[89] and experimental poliovirus infection of mice,[84,101] provide striking examples of this *in vivo*. In the case of HIV, the resulting sequence variation achieved following transmission of a limited number of genomes is enormous and accounts for—among other phenotypes—the rapid escape of the virus from neutralizing antibody, and the escape from antiviral monotherapy.

Such rapid rates of evolution are not without cost for the RNA viruses, however, because higher polymerase error rates impose upper limits on genome size. The combination of replicative error rate and genome size defines an "error threshold" above which a virus cannot maintain even the sequence integrity of its quasispecies.[31] As a result, few RNA virus genomes contain more than 30 kilobases (kb) and most have between 5 and 15 kb. RNA genomes of this size are poised just below their error thresholds, and although their genetic diversity inevitably wastes individual progeny that carry deleterious mutations, the cost is offset by the potential for rapid evolutionary response to changing selective pressures. This positioning of RNA viruses—just below their error threshold—may also present an opportunity for antiviral development. Specifically, therapeutics that lead to an increase in error rate can shift the balance beyond the error threshold toward "error catastrophe." Indeed evidence has accumulated that this is one such mechanism by which ribavirin, an adenosine analog, may inhibit the replication of some RNA viruses.[21] The largest RNA virus genomes currently recognized are those of the coronaviruses, which approach a size of 30 kb. Strikingly, it appears that for coronaviruses the nonstructural protein nsp14 functions as an RNA exonuclease that may function as a proofreading mechanism that could help maintain genome integrity.[27]

Levels of Segmentation

Another distinctive feature of eukaryotic cells—besides their partitioning into nuclear and cytoplasmic compartments—has a profound influence on the biology of their viruses. On most mRNAs, eukaryotic ribosomes require a methylated mRNA cap structure at the 5′ end that plays a critical role in signaling the initiation of protein synthesis. As a result, eukaryotes typically conform to the "one mRNA one polypeptide chain" rule; with very few exceptions, each message operates as a single translational unit. Similarly, viral RdRp's generally appear somewhat restricted in their ability to access internal promoter elements on RNA templates, and this creates a problem of how an RNA virus can derive several separate protein products from a single genome.

Through evolution, different RNA virus families have found three different solutions: fragmentation at the level of proteins, mRNAs, or genes, with some viruses using more than one of those solutions. For example, RNA viruses in the picorna- toga-, flavi-, and retrovirus families rely on extensive proteolytic processing of polyprotein precursors to derive their final protein products.[29] Others (in the orders *Mononegavirales* and *Nidovirales*) depend on complex transcriptional mechanisms to produce several monocistronic mRNAs from a single RNA template.[1,91] Still others (in the reo-, orthomyxo-, bunya-, and arenavirus families, among others) have solved the problem by fragmenting their genomes and assembling virions that contain multiple genome segments, each often representing a single gene.[34,69,76] Among plant viruses, such RNA genome segments are often packaged into separate virions, necessitating co-infection by several virus particles to transmit infectivity,[107] but the genome segments of animal viruses are typically co-packaged into single virions. In contrast, DNA viruses seldom use either genome segmentation or polyprotein processing. This is likely due to the relative ease with which monocistronic mRNAs can be transcribed from internal promoter elements of dsDNA, and the extensive use of differential splicing of nuclear transcripts to express promoter-distal open-reading frames.

Host Cell Components for Replication

Viruses depend on their host cells to support their replication, and this degree of dependency—to some extent—reflects their genome size. Although all viruses depend on the host translational machinery, large DNA viruses, such as mimivirus, may encode specific initiation factors that may provide a translational advantage for viral genes.[18] Entry of viruses into cells usually requires specific host-cell factors, and can require co-opting of cellular endocytic pathways.[71] The end point of entry is the release of the minimal viral replication machinery into the host-cell cytoplasm to initiate infection. How viruses establish infection in the hostile environment of the host cell remains one of the least understood steps of the viral replication cycle. The input genomes must either associate directly with ribosomes in the case of positive-strand RNA viruses, or be copied into mRNA, in the case of the negative-strand RNA viruses, dsRNA viruses, and DNA viruses. Because the particle-to-infectivity ratio of some viruses approaches 1:1, this process must be highly efficient despite its inherent challenges. Our knowledge of the subsequent viral rewiring of host-cell structures to establish replication compartments, traffic viral proteins and nucleic acids, and assemble viral particles is also far from complete, but has yielded a wealth of information into host biology as well as that of the viruses themselves. Indeed, study of viruses has contributed enormously to our understanding of promoters, transcriptional enhancers, the mRNA cap structure, RNA splicing, and mechanism of translation. Similarly, critical discoveries in host-cell transport and trafficking pathways including endocytosis, exocytosis, and secretory transport were achieved because of the ability to synchronize infections with viruses. Although systematic approaches including RNA interference (RNAi), proteomics, gene-knockout studies, and microarrays are helping to further transform our understanding of the virus–host interaction at the molecular level, we have yet to understand fully the complexities of the interactions of any virus with its host. Zoonotic viruses must strike a balance for optimal replication in often quite disparate hosts, likely adding further complexity to this intimate relationship. Striking examples of this are provided by members of the *Flaviviridae,* such as Dengue virus (which replicates in both its mosquito host and animals), and experimentally with many viruses including vesicular stomatitis virus (which replicates in virtually all eukaryotic cells in culture).

STRUCTURES AND ORGANIZATION OF VIRAL GENOMES

DNA versus RNA Genomes

Among families of viruses that infect vertebrates, those with RNA genomes outnumber those with DNA genomes by about 2 to 1 (Table 5.1); among viruses infecting plants the disparity is even greater. Indeed, no dsDNA viruses of plants are known except for those that like the hepadnaviruses of vertebrates, replicate via reverse transcription (see Chapter 68). This remarkable observation remains to be explained, but it may suggest that non–RT dsDNA viruses arose only after animals and plants diverged. Be that as it may, the prevalence of RNA viruses attests to the evolutionary success and versatility of RNA as genetic material for smaller genomes. As discussed previously, the high error rates of RNA replication restrict RNA genome sizes to 30 kb or less, whereas proofreading and error repair ensure sufficiently accurate replication of DNA virus genomes as large as that of the 1200-kb megaviruses.[3] In addition, the fact that DNA is more chemically stable than RNA likely explains why all known viruses of thermophilic hosts have dsDNA genomes.[57]

Single- and Double-Stranded Genomes

Although all viral genomes replicate via conventional Watson-Crick base pairing between complementary template and daughter strands, viruses that belong to different families encapsidate and transmit different molecular stages of the genome replication cycle. Families of ssRNA viruses outnumber families of dsRNA viruses by almost 10 to 1, roughly the inverse of the ratio between ssDNA and dsDNA viruses. In view of the greater chemical stability of double-stranded nucleic acids of both types, this difference calls for an explanation. Two possibilities seem plausible: First, dsRNA viruses must somehow circumvent the translational suppression that can result from the coexistence of equimolar amounts of the sense and antisense RNAs. How the dsRNA reoviruses solve this problem is addressed in Chapter 44. Second, dsRNA is widely recognized by the cells of higher eukaryotes as a signal for the induction of defense mechanisms that act to suppress viral replication, such as the IFN system in vertebrates (see also Chapter 8), gene silencing in plants, and RNAi in a variety of organisms.[15,40,93,106] These effects probably suffice to explain the relative scarcity of dsRNA virus families.

For these same reasons, it is important even for ssRNA viruses to limit the accumulation of replicative intermediates that contain regions of dsRNA, and the strategies to ensure this differs between the positive- and negative-sense RNA viruses. All known positive-strand RNA viruses synthesize disproportionately low amounts of the negative-strand RNA—typically 1% to 5% of the levels of the positive-strand—and thereby minimize the potential for dsRNA accumulation. Moreover, because the replication of these viruses appears to universally occur in sequestered membranous compartments, there appears to be a physical separation of the replicative intermediates from the host-cell cytoplasm, likely reducing the chances of detection.[25] In contrast, negative-strand RNA viruses, which need substantial amounts of both positive- and negative-sense RNAs to use as messages and progeny genomes, respectively, prevent the complementary RNAs from annealing to one another by encasing the genomic and antigenomic RNAs with a viral nucleocapsid protein.[2,44] Here, RNA synthesis also appears confined at some stages of infection to specific subcellular compartments that may help serve to limit detection of viral products of RNA synthesis by the innate immune system.

Positive, Negative, and Ambisense Genomes

The differences between positive- and negative-strand RNA viruses extend beyond the polarity of the RNA assembled into virions. Positive-sense RNA genomes exchange their virion proteins for ribosomes and cellular RNA binding proteins at the onset of infection. Once synthesized and assembled the virus-specified RdRp and other nonstructural proteins replace the ribosomes to accomplish RNA replication. Virion structural proteins are reacquired during the assembly of progeny virions. In contrast, negative-strand RNA genomes and their antigenomic complements remain associated with their nucleocapsid proteins, both within the viral particles and throughout the viral replication cycle, even during RNA replication. These fundamentally different adaptations can be attributed to the fact that whereas positive-sense RNA genomes must satisfy criteria for translation that are dictated by the host cell, negative-sense RNA genomes must only satisfy the template requirements for the virus-specified RdRp because they are replicated but never translated. Although the precise mechanism by which the protein-coated templates of negative-strand RNA genomes are copied by their cognate polymerases is not fully understood, short naked RNAs that correspond to the terminal promoters can be copied by their viral polymerases.[26,59,73] Such experimental evidence is consistent with a model for RNA synthesis in which the nucleocapsid protein is transiently displaced from the template RNA during copying of the genome.

The dsRNA virus genomes are intermediates between the two. The parental genome remains sequestered within a subviral particle during the synthesis of the unencapsidated positive-sense mRNA transcripts, which are replicated to produce progeny dsRNAs only after being assembled into subviral core particles.[81] Although the core RdRp's of each of these viruses are structurally as well as functionally analogous, the distinctions in the genomic structure likely place additional structural constraints on the viral polymerase complexes.

Linear and Circular Genomes

Genome replication not only requires an acceptable error rate as described previously, but must also avoid the systematic deletion or addition of nucleotides. Genome termini are particularly troublesome in this respect, a fact that has been dubbed "the end problem." For DNA replication, the end problem is exacerbated by the fact that DNA polymerases cannot initiate the synthesis of daughter strands and must therefore use primers, thus creating additional complications of replicating the primer-binding site(s). Among several known solutions, the most economical and widespread in nature is to eliminate the ends altogether by covalently circularizing the genomic DNA, as occurs in the genomes of prokaryotes. Polyoma-, papilloma-, circo-, and anellovirus genomes follow this model, and the dsDNA genomes of herpes and hepadnaviruses, although linear, in virions are covalently circularized before replication. Poxviruses and asfiviruses also have linear dsDNA genomes, but in these cases the individual complementary strands are covalently continuous at the termini of the duplex, which provides another solution to the end problem. A similar close-ended duplex DNA is generated during the replication of the ssDNA genomes of parvoviruses (Chapter 57). Terminal redundancy (iridoviruses), inverted terminal repeats (adenoviruses), and the use of protein primers that do not occlude the binding site (adenoviruses and hepadnaviruses) represent the other ways that DNA viruses have evolved to ensure accurate and complete replication of their genome termini.

Unlike DNA polymerases, most RNA polymerases do not require primers, so RNA genomes are less susceptible to the end problem. Accordingly, most RNA genomes are linear molecules. Covalently closed circular RNAs are found only in HDV in animals (Table 5.1) as well as among the viroids and other subviral RNA pathogens that infect plants. Nevertheless the termini of linear RNA genomes are vulnerable to degradation, and their replication is likely to be particularly error prone. Consequently, every family of RNA viruses has features designed to preserve the termini of the genome.[6] For example, many positive-strand RNA viruses have a 5′ cap structure and 3′ polyadenylate tail that serve to protect eukaryotic RNAs against degradation, and a similar role is likely played by the VPg that is covalently linked to the 5′ end of the picornavirus genomes,[64] and by the stable RNA secondary structures present at the 3′ end of the flaviviral RNA and other genomes. The 3′ ends of many plant virus RNAs form clover leaf structures that resemble transfer RNAs (tRNAs) so closely that they are recognized by the cellular tRNA charging and modifying enzymes.[30] In addition to playing protective roles, terminal modifications of positive-sense RNAs may also serve to bring their ends together by binding to interacting cellular proteins such as the poly(A) binding protein and cap-binding complex, thereby forming noncovalent functionally circular complexes that may promote repetitive translation by ribosomes and repetitive replication by RdRp's.[49,102]

Unlike the genomes of positive-sense RNA viruses, negative-sense and ambisense RNA virus genomes rarely carry covalent terminal modifications. Those RNA genomes show some degree of terminal sequence complementarity that is thought to lead to the formation of a panhandle type of structure that, in the case of the segmented viruses, favors RNA replication. Because the templates are encapsidated by the viral nucleocapsid protein, it is not clear how the RNA bases can engage in base-pairing interactions between the termini. However, complementarity between the genomic termini favors replication and likely promotes polymerase transfer during RNA synthesis to ensure efficient reinitiation of replication. In other solutions to the end problem among the RNA viruses, retroviral genomes are terminally redundant and have direct repeats of 12 to 235 nucleotides at each end that maintain and restore the integrity of the termini during reverse transcription and virus replication (see Chapter 47).

Segmented and Nonsegmented Genomes

As discussed previously, segmentation of RNA genomes is one way to facilitate the production of multiple gene products in eukaryotic cells, but it also means that the various segments must each contain appropriate *cis*-acting signals to mediate their expression, replication, and assembly into virions. In some virus families whose members have segmented genomes (e.g., the orthomyxoviruses and some reoviruses), these signals comprise conserved sequences at the RNA termini, but in others (e.g., the bipartite nodaviruses and tetraviruses) sequence conservation between the segments is minimal. In these latter cases, the specificity of RNA replication and assembly is presumably dictated by conserved RNA secondary or tertiary structures. Moreover, segmentation of the viral genome requires a level of coordination to ensure that the correct amounts of viral gene products are expressed and to ensure the packaging of multiple genome segments to form infectious virus particles. How such coordination is achieved is not understood. Furthermore, in the case of the negative-sense, ambisense, and dsRNA viruses that have segmented genomes, a mechanism is required to ensure that the polymerase is packaged into the virus particle so that the incoming segments can be transcribed into mRNA. For the dsRNA viruses the polymerase is an integral structural component of the core transcribing particle ensuring that the polymerase and capping machinery are present within the incoming particle. In the case of the arenavirus, Machupo, this is a function of a small viral protein Z, which locks the polymerase on the promoter in an inactive form.[60]

Evidently, the evolutionary barrier between viruses with segmented and nonsegmented RNA genomes is readily transversed because both genome types occur in members of the alphaviruslike supergroup, a taxonomic cluster based on phylogenetic comparisons of nonstructural protein sequences. Indeed, among the tetraviruses, segmented and nonsegmented genomes can even be found in the same family. Furthermore, the genomes of some togaviruses, rhabdoviruses, and paramyxoviruses, which are naturally nonsegmented, have been experimentally divided into segmented genomes without destroying viral infectivity,[38,96] thus confirming the flexibility of RNA genomes in this regard. Nevertheless, genome segmentation has major effects on the biology of a virus because individual segments can reassort between dissimilar strains in co-infected cells, which enables segmented genome viruses to make substantial evolutionary leaps by horizontal gene transfer. This mechanism underlies the antigenic shifts that produce new pandemic strains of the orthomyxovirus influenza virus (see Chapter 40 and Chapter 41).

As discussed previously, genome segmentation is almost unknown among DNA viruses, most likely because internal initiation of transcription and alternative splicing provide more facile ways to access multiple open-reading frames. Only the polydnaviruses, a family of dsDNA viruses that infect parasitic wasps and participate in a complex and unusual host–parasite relationship, show extensive DNA segmentation.[7]

Cis-Acting RNA Signals and Specificity

Replication and packaging of viral RNAs display striking specificity; both processes unerringly pick the correct viral molecules from among thousands of cellular RNAs that may be much more abundant. This is generally attributed to the presence of *cis*-acting signals that selectively channel the viral RNAs into replication and assembly complexes, but in most RNA virus genomes these signals remain to be clearly identified. Those that have been characterized most, comprise not linear nucleotide stretches, but RNA secondary structures such as bulged stem-loops, tRNA-like cloverleaves, and pseudoknots, which are believed to create distinctive three-dimensional molecular shapes that interact specifically with the viral enzymes and structural proteins. Although high-resolution structures have been determined for some RdRp's, reverse transcriptases, and several viral capsids, our understanding of the molecular basis of specificity in RNA replication and virus assembly is limited by the scant knowledge of the three-dimensional structures of viral RNA and its *cis*-acting signals. However, the structural basis of RNA specificity during replication and assembly has often proved elusive, perhaps because the specificity determinants can be redundant, dispersed, or global properties of the viral genome. Furthermore, in both RNA replication and assembly, specific interaction is followed by less-specific RNA–protein interactions that propagate the reactions. The transitions between these different stages are largely unexplored, and much remains to be learned concerning the recognition of *cis*-acting RNA signals and how they promulgate RNA replication and assembly. In the case of some viruses, the products of replication are selectively channeled into the assembly pathway, thereby diminishing the need for separate assembly signals.

Promising advances in our understanding of *cis*-acting regions of RNA viral genomes have recently come from the application of a chemical probing methodology termed selective 2′ hydroxyl acetylation analyzed by primer extension (SHAPE), first applied to provide an overview of the complete genome of HIV-1.[103] In addition to correctly identifying known structures within the HIV-1 genome, several structures were identified within the coding regions at regions close to the positions of polyprotein processing. Such structured elements are thought to lead to a slowing of ribosomes to facilitate the correct folding of the preceding region of the polypeptide chain, although data proving this are lacking. Whatever the function of such structured elements, application of this methodology promises to improve our definition of the *cis*-acting elements within RNA virus genomes as well as the overall structure of viral genomes.

Satellite, Dependent, and Defective Genomes

Occasionally, subviral genomes arise that are neither independently infectious nor essential for infectivity, but nevertheless contain *cis*-acting signals that promote their own replication and/or packaging by the proteins encoded by another virus. Such satellite nucleic acids are parasitic on the parental virus and can modulate its replication and virulence.[94] Most commonly, they are ssRNAs, but dsRNA and ssDNA satellites are also known. Among the RNA viruses of animals, a prime example is hepatitis delta virus (or HDV), which packages its ssRNA genome in virion proteins encoded by the hepadnavirus hepatitis B virus and can severely exacerbate its pathogenicity.[97] Dependence of an RNA satellite on a DNA virus parent is unusual; more commonly satellite, RNAs are replicated and encapsidated by the proteins of an RNA virus parent with which they share at least some sequence homology. In some instances, satellite RNAs encode their own distinct capsid proteins, or proteins required for RNA replication (as in the case of HDV), but in others they are translationally silent. Satellite RNAs are much more common among the viruses of plants than those of animals (see Chapter 72), perhaps because the transmission of animal viruses between hosts generally involves narrower bottlenecks that select against the spread of satellites. Dependence of one virus on another is also found occasionally among viruses with DNA genomes. For example, adeno-associated virus (family *Parvoviridae,* genus *Dependovirus*) requires coinfection of host cells by adenoviruses or herpesvirus to provide helper functions necessary for its replication.

In contrast to the transmission of viral infection between hosts, the spread of infection within a single animal usually involves successive episodes of localized viral replication that resemble the conditions of plaque formation and serial high multiplicity passage in cell culture. These conditions favor the generation and amplification of defective viral genomes, which can arise from a simple internal deletion of genes as well as more complex genome rearrangements that occur during RNA replication. Like satellite RNAs, defective RNAs parasitize the parent virus and usually interfere with its replication, but because they also depend upon it for their own survival, they typically establish a fluctuating coexistence. Most families of animal RNA viruses readily generate defective interfering (DI) RNAs in cell culture, but their influence on viral disease and evolution is less well understood.

EXPRESSION AND REPLICATION OF DNA VIRUS GENOMES

DNA Virus Genome Strategies

Viral DNA genomes range in size from the 1.8-kb circoviruses to the 1,200-kb genomes of the *Megaviridae.*[3] This difference in the coding capacity means that viruses from different families vary widely in how many of the functions necessary for viral replication they can encode themselves. For example, DNA viruses with small genomes such as the polyoma-, papilloma-, and parvoviruses use host-cell enzymes for transcription and replication (Figs. 5.3 and 5.4). Those with intermediate-size genomes (up to 35 kb) such as adenoviruses, encode much of their DNA replication machinery including a DNA polymerase, terminal protein and ssDNA binding protein, but they employ cellular RNA polymerase II and III for transcription (Fig. 5.5). Those with larger genomes (150 to 350 kb), such as the herpesviruses and poxviruses, encode DNA polymerases and binding proteins. In the case of herpesviruses, multiple specific transcription factors serially modify the promoter specificity of RNA polymerase II (Fig. 5.6), or in the case of the poxviruses multi-subunit transcriptase complexes perform all the functions of capping and polyadenylation as well as RNA transcription (Fig. 5.7). Hepadnaviruses buck this general trend in that they are small genomes (3 kb) but encode the DNA polymerase/reverse transcriptase that executes their unique mechanism of DNA replication via an ssRNA intermediate (Fig. 5.8).

Because cellular DNA synthesis occurs during the S phase of the cell cycle and not at all in terminally differentiated G0 cells, viruses that depend on the host DNA polymerase must either wait for the infected cell to enter S phase spontaneously, as in the case of parvoviruses, or early in infection, they must express one or more viral oncogenes to override the regulation of the cell-cycle control proteins p53 or pRb and thereby stimulate infected cells to enter S phase, as in polyomaviruses and papillomaviruses. Inactivation of pRb releases cellular transcription factor E2F, which induces expression of the cellular DNA polymerase α primase, DNA polymerase δ, ssDNA binding protein, and several critical cellular enzymes that are involved in both the *de novo* and the salvage pathways of deoxynucleotide triphosphate (dNTP) biosynthesis, including ribonucleotide reductase, thymidylate synthetase, dihydrofolate reductase, deoxyuridine triphosphate nucleotidohydrolase (dUTPase), and thymidine and thymidylate kinases. Viruses with large DNA genomes (e.g., herpesviruses and poxviruses) encode some of those enzymes themselves and can thus replicate in nondividing cells and other environments that would not normally support DNA replication, such as terminally differentiated cells of the nervous system (some herpesviruses) or even the cytoplasm (poxviruses). Although these viral genes are often dispensable for virus replication in actively dividing cells in culture, they can exert a profound influence on viral virulence in infected organisms and thus provide targets for chemotherapeutic intervention. For example, the thymidine kinase gene of some herpesviruses (but not the host enzyme) phosphorylates the prodrug acyclovir to generate a dNTP analog that terminates nascent strands during DNA synthesis.[32]

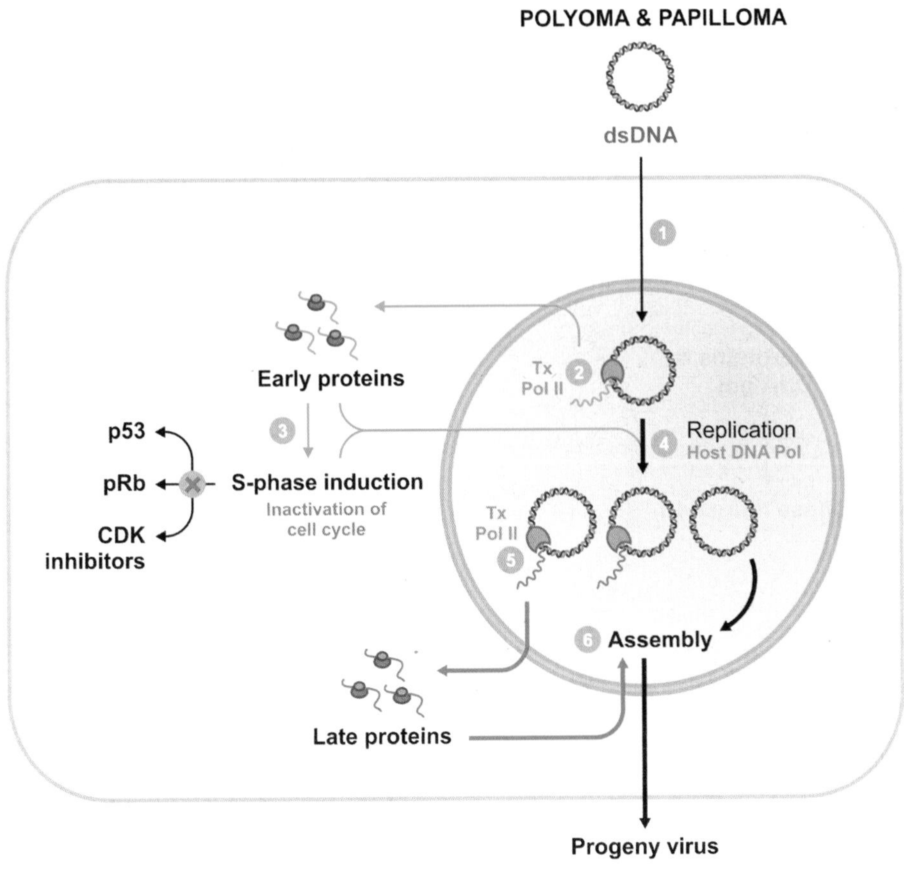

FIGURE 5.3. Simplified view of the replication scheme of *Polyomaviridae* and *Papillomaviridae*. The circular dsDNA genome is transported to the nucleus (step 1) where cellular RNA polymerase II transcribes the early genes (step 2) that encode the viral oncoproteins or transforming (T) antigens. The products of step 2 interfere with the host-cell cycle control proteins p53 and pRb or interact with inhibitors of cyclin-dependent kinases (CDKs) to stimulate cellular DNA replication (step 3). In nonpermissive cells that cannot support the vegetative replication cycles and therefore survive the infection, these early events can lead to neoplastic transformation. In permissive cells, the viral DNA is replicated by the host-cell DNA polymerase (step 4), following which cellular RNA pol II can transcribe the late genes that encode viral structural proteins (step 5). The assembly of viral particles occurs in the nucleus (step 6). The thickness and color intensity of the arrows signifies the predominant events.

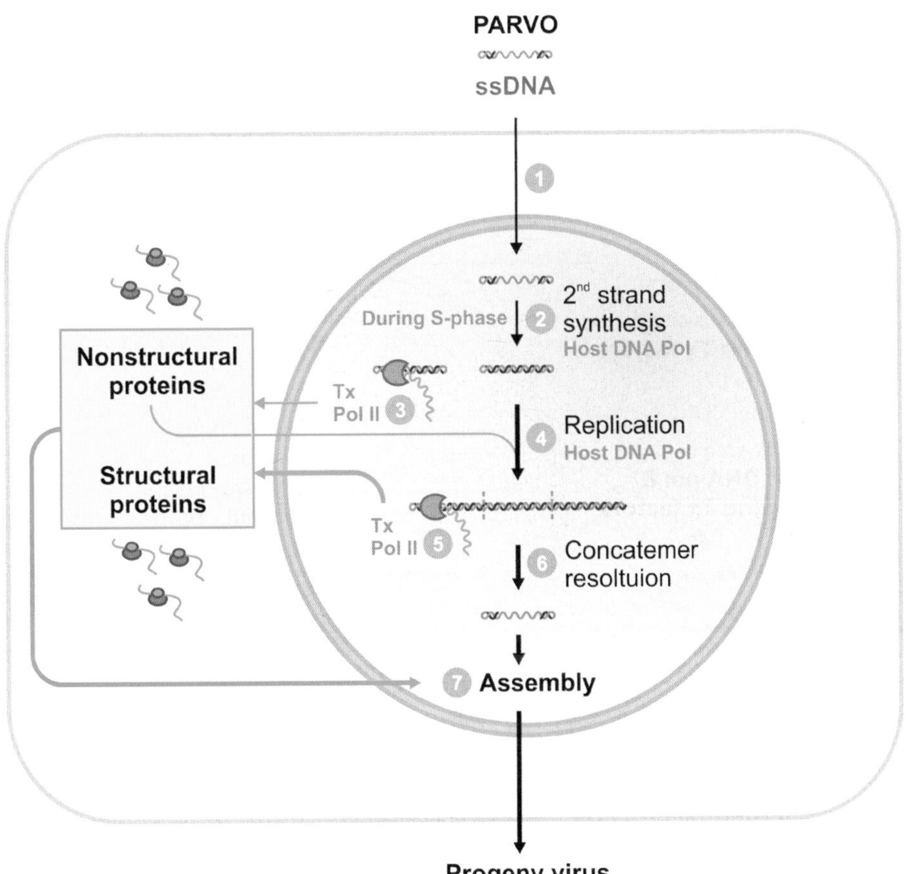

FIGURE 5.4. Simplified view of the replication scheme of *Parvoviridae*. Following entry, the linear ssDNA genome is delivered to the nucleus (step 1) where self-primed second strand synthesis is mediated by the host DNA polymerase during the S phase of the cell cycle (step 2). The resulting dsDNA hairpin is transcribed by the cellular RNA polymerase II (step 3) to produce mRNAs that encode viral nonstructural and structural proteins, and is ligated to form a covalently continuous duplex. The nonstructural proteins promote further DNA replication by the host DNA polymerase, which occurs via a rolling hairpin mechanism to produce double-stranded concatamers of the viral genome (step 4). The concatamers are templates for transcription by host RNA polymerase II to produce further viral proteins (step 5), and they are resolved (step 6) prior to assembly (step 7) into viral particles.

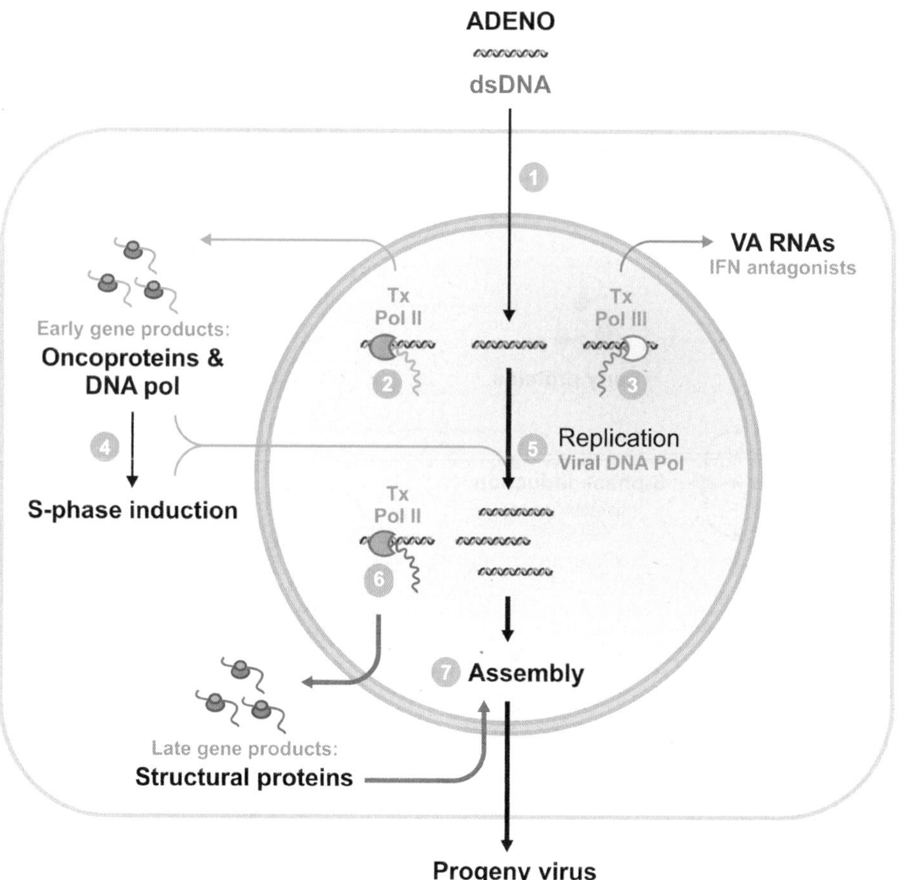

FIGURE 5.5. Simplified overview of the replication scheme of *Adenoviridae*. The linear dsDNA genome is delivered into the nucleus (step 1), where it is transcribed by the host cell RNA polymerase II (step 2) to produce the early gene products including oncoproteins and the viral DNA polymerase. In adenoviruses of primates, the host RNA polymerase III also transcribes the genome to produce VA RNAs that act as interferon antagonists (step 3). The early gene products override cell cycle controls and inhibit apoptosis (step 4) as well as provide the essential viral polymerase components for genome replication (step 5). Following DNA replication, the late genes are transcribed by the host RNA polymerase II from a single major late promoter, and following extensive differential splicing provide the viral structural proteins (step 6). Virus assembly (step 7) occurs in the nucleus.

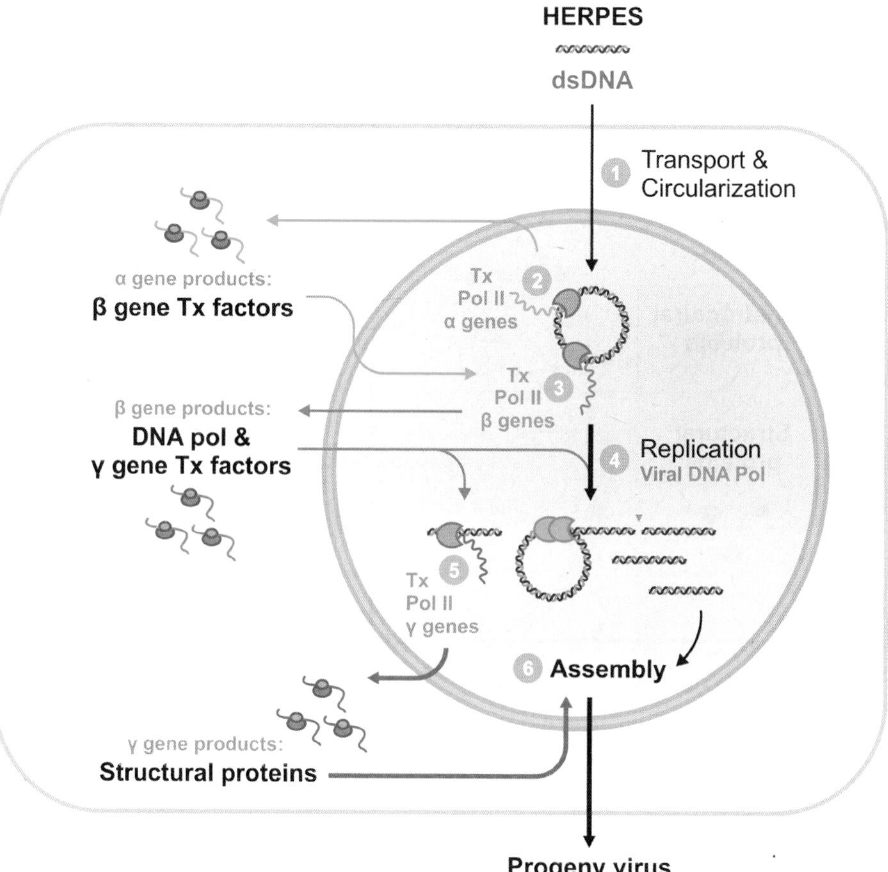

FIGURE 5.6. Simplified overview of the replication scheme of *Herpesviridae*. The linear genomic dsDNA genome is delivered to the nucleus, where it undergoes covalent circularization (step 1). Cellular RNA polymerase II transcribes the immediate-early α genes (step 2) that encode transcription factors that mediate the host RNA polymerase II recognition of the promoters for the delayed-early β genes (step 3). Those genes encode the viral DNA polymerase and other proteins required for genome replication (step 4) as well as transcription factors required for the pol II–mediated expression of the late γ genes that encode most of the structural proteins (step 5). Virions assemble in the nucleus (step 6) and exit through the nuclear pore. The assembled virion contains the necessary transcription factors for expression of the immediate-early α genes on infection of the next cell. Note that this scheme represents only the vegetative cycle of *Herpesviridae* replication. Readers are referred to the individual *Herpesviridae* chapters regarding the establishment, maintenance of, and reactivation from latency.

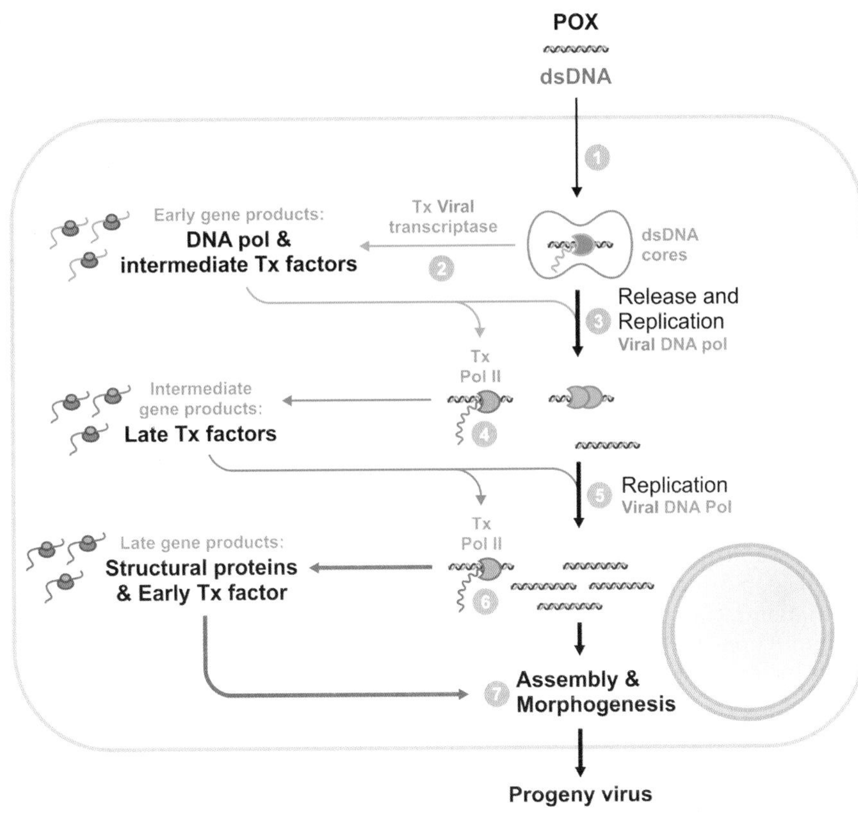

FIGURE 5.7. Simplified scheme of the replication of *Poxviridae*. Entry delivers the viral core containing the dsDNA genome into the cytoplasm—the site of viral RNA synthesis (step 1). In the cytoplasm the multisubunit virion DNA-dependent RNA polymerase transcribes the early viral genes (step 2), which comprise approximately 50% of the genome. The early gene products include factors that mediate the release of the dsDNA into the cytoplasm (second stage uncoating), the viral DNA polymerase and associated enzymes required for replication (step 3), and transcription factors that direct the viral RNA polymerase to transcribe a limited number of intermediate genes (step 4). DNA replication proceeds via a rolling hairpin mechanism (step 3 and 5) similar to that for parvoviruses, and is concurrent with the expression of the intermediate gene products (step 4). The intermediate gene products include transcription factors required for late gene expression (step 6). The products of late gene expression encode most of the structural proteins as well as the viral transcriptase and associated factors that will be required at the start of a new infection. Progeny genomes, viral structural proteins, and membranes of the host cell participate in the assembly of viral particles that undergo extensive morphogenesis and maturation (step 7) prior to release.

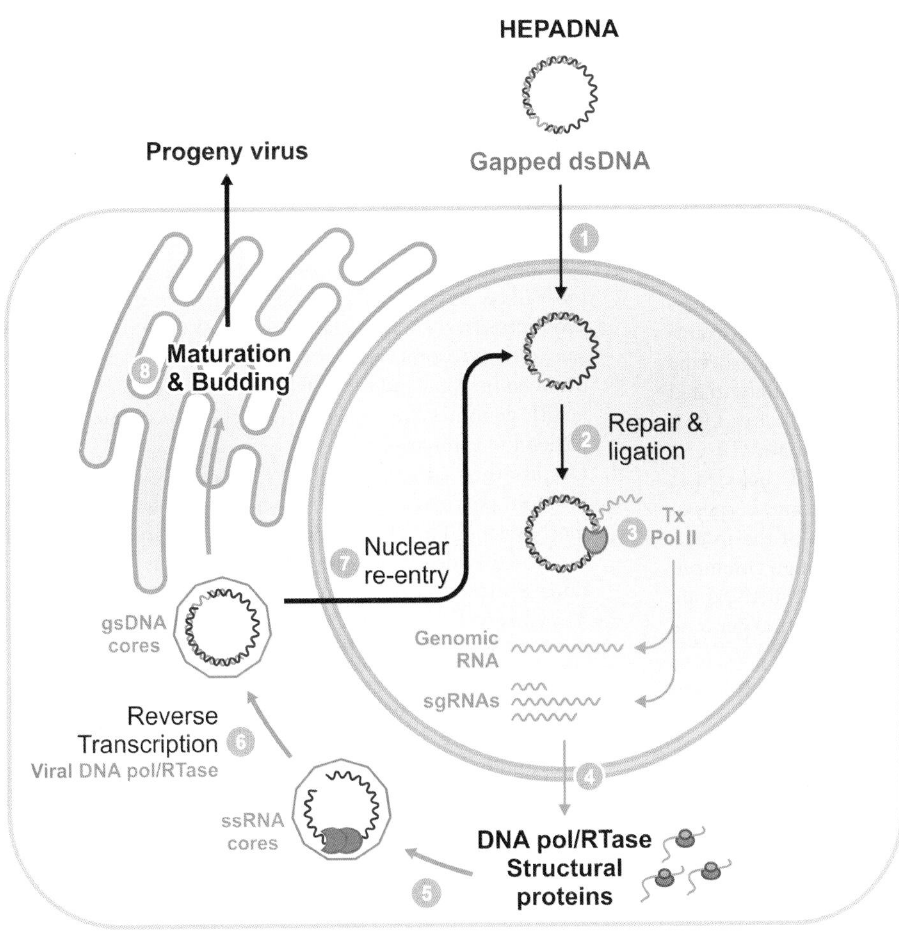

FIGURE 5.8. Simplified replication scheme for hepadnaviruses. Following entry and partial uncoating (step 1), viral cores containing the gapped dsDNA genome migrate to the nucleus where the dsDNA genome is repaired and ligated into a covalently closed circle (steps 1 and 2). This repaired genome is transcribed by the host-cell RNA polymerase II (step 3) to yield terminally redundant pregenomic RNA and subgenomic RNAs for the viral structural and nonstructural proteins (step 4). In the cytoplasm, the viral DNA polymerase, reverse transcriptase (RTase), and core proteins associate with the pregenomic RNA to form immature cores (step 5) that mediate polymerase-primed reverse transcription of the pregenomic RNA to yield gapped dsDNA genomes (step 6). The progeny cores either then enter the nucleus (step 7) to repeat the cycle or can bud through the endoplasmic reticulum to yield viral particles (step 8).

Regulation of Viral Gene Expression

During the early, prereplicative phase of the infectious cycle of a typical DNA virus, a subset of so-called immediate early viral genes is expressed to produce mostly catalytic quantities of nonstructural proteins required for DNA replication and host-cell manipulation. After DNA replication, a different set of genes is expressed (late genes) that direct the synthesis of stoichiometric amounts of the structural proteins required for viral assembly. Expression of the early genes is often concomitantly repressed. This early/late switch, which is a common feature of many DNA virus families, can be understood as an evolutionary adaptation that gives viruses an advantage in competing with the host cell for gene expression: Early gene expression is modest, whereas later during the postreplicative stage of the infectious cycle, increased gene copy numbers enable the virus to dominate the protein synthesis capacity of the cell. In addition to the early and late genes, sets of intermediate genes have been identified in the poxviruses and herpesviruses, with each temporal class encoding factors that switch on the next in a transcriptional cascade (Figs. 5.6 and 5.7). For the viruses in these families, transcription factors for immediate early genes are expressed late in infection and assembled into progeny virions in preparation for the next infectious cycle.

At the start of infection, immediate early viral promoters face stiff competition from overwhelming numbers of cellular promoters. To successfully recruit RNA pol II and other components of the transcriptional machinery, many DNA viral genomes contain enhancers: *cis*-acting regulatory elements that facilitate the assembly of transcription complexes by binding multiple cellular transcription factors and other accessory proteins. A defining feature of enhancers, which were first identified in the genome of the polyomavirus simian vacuolating virus 40 (SV40), is that they exert their effects from either upstream or downstream of promoters and can act over distances of several kilobases.

Efficient transcription from late promoters usually requires one or more early gene products, as well as cellular transcription factors that may differ from those used by the early promoters. Dependence on specific cellular transcription factors can limit the expression of late genes to particular cells or tissues where the necessary factors are naturally expressed. For example, transcription of late papillomavirus genes requires a specific transcription factor that is expressed only in fully differentiated skin cells. As a result the replication cycle is stalled after DNA replication (Fig. 5.3, step 4) until the cell differentiates.

Infection of cells with herpesviruses and poxviruses increases the rate of mRNA degradation.[19] In some herpesviruses, that is mediated by a protein component of the infecting virions called vhs (virion host shutoff). Although enhanced turnover is not specific for cellular mRNAs, viral mRNAs are readily replenished by robust transcription of the viral genome so that the net result is the selective suppression of host protein synthesis. In addition, the rapid turnover of viral mRNAs accelerates the transitions in the transcriptional cascade.

Mechanisms of DNA Replication and Transcription

Most DNA viruses produce functional viral mRNAs by usurping the transcriptional machinery of the cell (Fig. 5.1). This machinery includes RNA pol II, multiple transcription factors, poly(A) polymerase, guanylyltransferase, methyltransferases, and the pathway of mRNA export from the nucleus. Even viruses with unusual genome structures such as parvoviruses and hepadnaviruses use these cellular components because their genomes are rendered into dsDNA before transcription (Figs. 5.4 and 5.8). Only DNA viruses that replicate in the cytoplasm (pox-, irido-, and asfiviruses) use virus-specific enzymes for transcription and posttranscriptional modification of their mRNAs (Fig. 5.7). Because these enzymes are virion structural components, they can often be purified more readily than their cellular counterparts, and in the case of the vaccinia poxvirus and Chlorella virus, their reactions and structural properties have been well studied.[45,51,53] The majority of RNA viruses also replicate in the cytoplasm and employ virus-specific enzymes to synthesize and modify their mRNA.[24]

Viral DNA genomes replicate by at least five different mechanisms, which are summarized as follows (for more details readers are referred to the chapters that describe each viral family).

1. The circular dsDNA genomes of polyomaviruses and papillomaviruses (Fig. 5.3) replicate bidirectionally from a single AT-rich origin via the RNA-primed synthesis of continuous leading strands and discontinuous lagging strands at both replication forks. Circularity of the genome aside, the reactions at the replication forks closely resemble how the host chromosome is replicated.[35,68]
2. In stark contrast, the linear dsDNA genome of adenoviruses (Fig. 5.5) is replicated by a protein-primed synthesis of only the leading strand, resulting in displacement of ssDNA from each end of the parental duplex. The termini of the displaced strands anneal via inverted terminal repeats, creating duplex panhandle structures that serve as secondary origins of replication. The primer (preterminal protein) is the product of an early gene, and a copy of this protein is covalently bound to the 5′ end of each of the daughter strands.[23,67]
3. The linear dsDNA of herpesvirus genomes is first circularized and then replicated from one or more internal origins, most likely by an RNA-primed mechanism that eventually produces dsDNA concatamers (Fig. 5.6). Progeny DNA can undergo isomerization by homologous recombination between internal and terminal repeated sequences, and unit length genomes are resolved from the concatamers during packaging into virions.[75]
4. Despite their different structures and sizes, poxvirus (Fig. 5.7) and parvovirus (Fig. 5.4) genomes replicate by similar mechanisms. The close-ended duplex poxvirus genome (or the closed-ended duplex intermediate in parvovirus replication) is nicked near its terminus, and the newly generated 3′ end serves to prime DNA synthesis using the complementary strand of the duplex as template. This initial self-priming event is reproduced by partially base-paired hairpin structures located at each end of the duplex genome, resulting in so called "rolling hairpin" replication. For both poxviruses and parvoviruses, the product is a dsDNA concatamer from which unit length genomes are excised by resolution of concatamer junctions.[9,20,104]
5. Finally, in the most tortuous mechanism of all, hepadnaviruses (Fig. 5.8) replicate their dsDNA genome by a

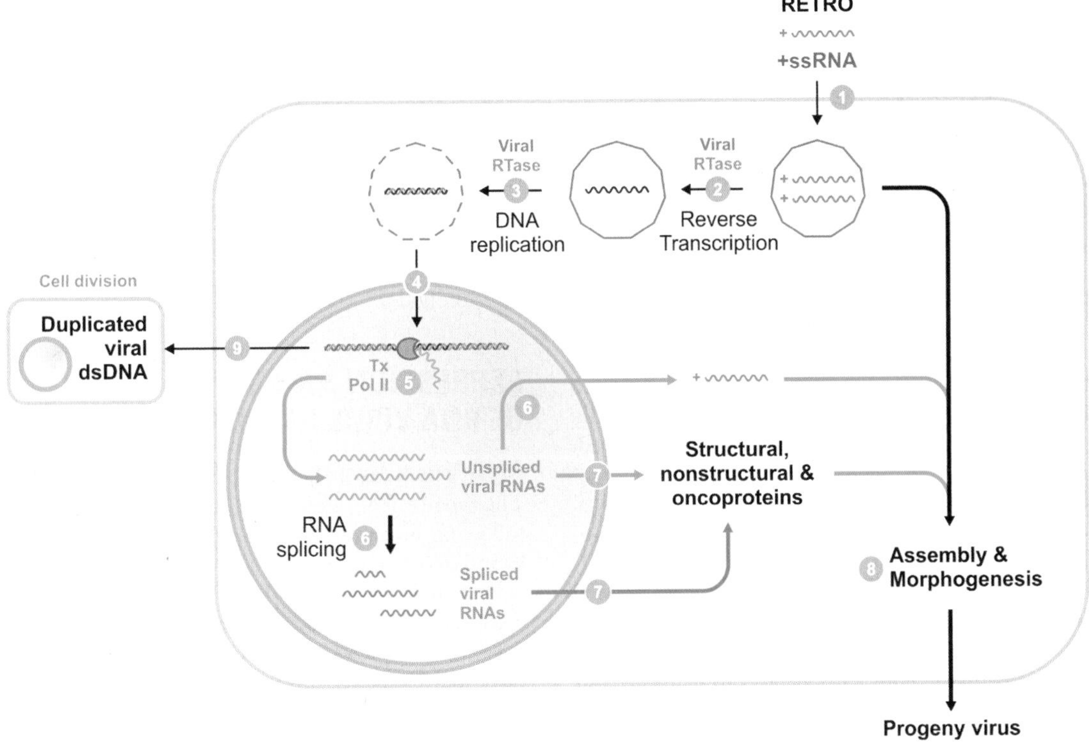

FIGURE 5.9. Simplified replication scheme of *Retroviridae*. Following entry and partial uncoating (step 1), the viral genome is copied into dsDNA by the reverse transcriptase (step 2 and 3) and integrated into the host chromosome by the virion DNA integrase (step 4). The integrated viral genome (provirus) is transcribed by the host-cell RNA polymerase II (step 5) to produce viral transcripts that function as precursors to the mRNA for the viral proteins (steps 6 and 7) as well as progeny genomes for assembly into infectious particles (step 8).

full-length pregenomic ssRNA transcript made by RNA polymerase II. Pregenomic RNA is then reverse transcribed by the viral encoded DNA polymerase/reverse transcriptase to produce dsDNA progeny. In contrast to retroviruses (Fig. 5.9), DNA integration is not required for hepadnavirus replication, the genome being maintained as a circular episome in the nucleus of infected cells. Caulimoviruses—the only dsDNA viruses that infect plants—use a similar reverse transcriptase (RT)-mediated replication strategy. To prime first strand DNA synthesis, hepadnavirus RTase uses a domain of the polymerase itself. This differs from the tRNA-primed strategy employed by retroviruses and caulimoviruses.

The polymerases employed for these strategies of replication are structurally and functionally homologous—yet they accomplish replication via very distinct mechanisms. Thus the evolutionary origin of such disparate mechanisms of replication remains uncertain.

Remarkably protein-primed replication is discontinuous. In the three known examples—adenovirus, poliovirus, and hepadnaviruses—the first few nucleotides of the genome are templated from an internal motif rather than at the very 3′ end of the parental genome. This necessitates a jump or realignment of the protein-primer product together with the polymerase to the 3′ end of the parental genome to complete synthesis of the daughter strand. In the case of adenovirus, the first templated nucleotides added to the primer are positions 4–6 of the genome, which then realigns with the 3′ end of the genome to complete daughter-strand synthesis following annealing of the nascent strand to the first three nucleotides of the parental genome.[23] For hepadnaviruses, the first four nucleotides are added to the RTase from a stem loop positioned at the 5′ end of the pregenomic RNA. The RTase nascent strand RNA product leaps almost 3 kb and then continues processively to complete synthesis of the daughter strand. Among the RNA viruses, the picornaviruses employ an internal stem loop termed the *cis*-acting replication element (cre) within the parental strand to template the uridylylation of a protein primer, VPg.[82] This primer is then repositioned together with polymerase at the 3′ end of the genome to prime synthesis of the new strand. Such protein-primed mechanisms likely aid in maintaining the integrity of the genome ends, which contain vital signals for replication.

Latent and Persistent Infections

In addition to the typical vegetative replication cycles illustrated in Figures 5.3 through 5.8, many DNA viruses establish latent or persistent infections of their hosts. Several distinct mechanisms of persistence have been identified with different viruses, but they all involve suppression of viral cytopathic effects, long-term maintenance of the viral genome, and evasion of the cellular and organismal defences. For example, herpesviruses typically establish latent infections in which the viral genome is maintained as a circular episome in the nucleus, expressing at most only a few viral genes and yielding no infectious virus. Such latent herpesvirus infections persist throughout the life of the host, successfully evading host immune surveillance, yet able to reemerge at intervals as productive lytic infections. Because of its importance for human health, understanding the establishment and maintenance of herpesvirus latency and the mechanisms that regulate the reemergence of infectious virus are the subject of intense study (see Chapters 59 to 65). In the case of human herpesvirus 4 (Epstein-Barr virus), which infects B lymphocytes and causes mononucleosis, latent infections can be established and maintained in cell culture; this has greatly facilitated experimental study of the mechanisms involved. For other herpesviruses, the establishment and maintenance of latency occur in less-accessible cell types and are much less well understood.

Viral Oncogenes and Neoplastic Transformation

In cells that somehow survive DNA virus infection, such as nonpermissive cells that express early genes but cannot replicate viral DNA or produce infectious progeny, the expression of viral oncogenes and the consequent loss of cell cycle control can lead to neoplastic transformation and the formation of tumors in infected animals (see Chapter 7). Unlike typical retrovirus-induced tumors, where the entire viral genome is integrated into the host chromosome as an essential step of the viral replication cycle, tumors induced by DNA viruses rarely contain a complete viral genome or produce infectious virus. Instead, they typically express only the viral oncogenes from integrated copies, disrupting cell cycle control by inactivating p53/pRb or by activating cyclin-dependent kinases, for example. Alone among the DNA viruses that replicate in the nucleus, parvoviruses do not induce tumors because they are unable to override cell cycle controls. Some poxviruses induce the formation of self-limiting benign tumors when they secrete a virus-encoded growth factor that induces surrounding cells to divide.

EXPRESSION AND REPLICATION OF RNA VIRUS GENOMES

RNA Virus Genome Strategies

The type of RNA genome dictates the first biosynthetic steps following infection. For example, the message sense positive-strand RNA viruses, excluding the retroviruses, all initially deliver their genomes to ribosomes to ensure the synthesis of essential proteins to establish viral replication (Figs. 5.10 and 5.11). Consequently the viral genomic RNA alone is infectious once delivered into a host cell—a fact that greatly facilitated the genetic manipulation of such viruses. That the RNA alone was infectious was first shown for tobacco mosaic virus, in experiments that helped establish that genes were comprised of nucleic acids.[41] By contrast to the genomes of positive-sense RNA viruses, those of the negative-strand RNA viruses, retroviruses, and double-stranded RNA viruses all must deliver into

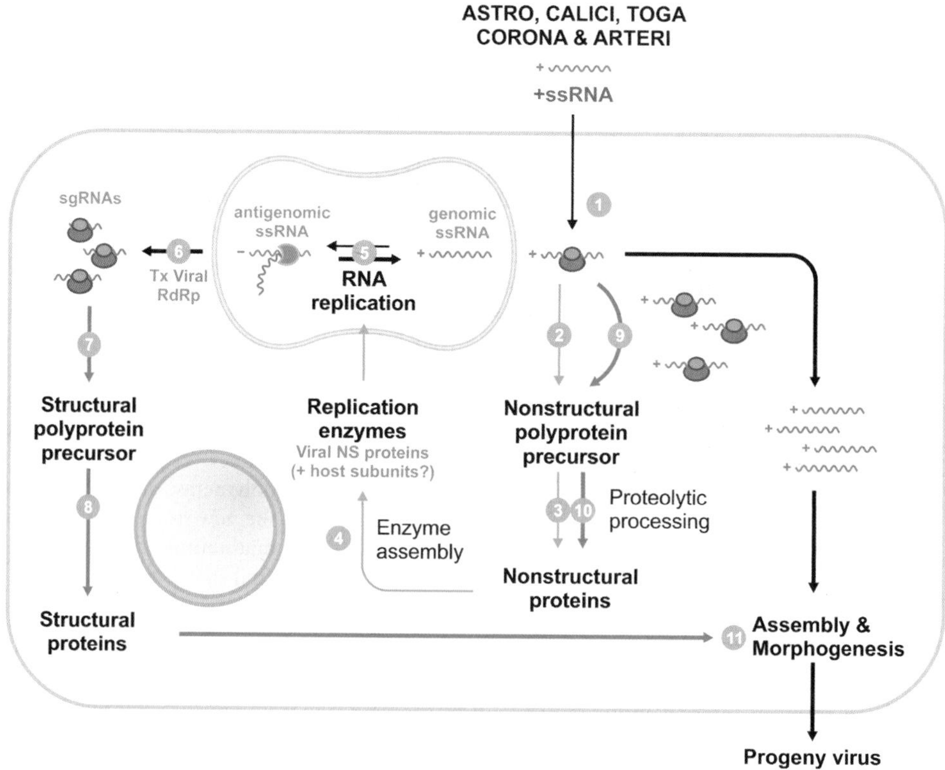

FIGURE 5.10. Simplified replication scheme of positive-strand RNA viruses that produce subgenomic RNA. Following entry and uncoating (step 1), the genomic RNA is engaged by the host-cell ribosome to produce the nonstructural proteins including the RdRp (steps 2 and 3). The viral replication enzymes together with host components form replication compartment in which the genomic RNA is replicated into an antigenome and progeny genomes (steps 4 and 5). The viral RdRp also transcribes one or more subgenomic RNAs (step 6) that encode viral structural proteins (steps 7 and 8). Replicated genomes are translated to amplify the production of viral proteins (steps 9 and 10) and may be used as templates for further replication. The genomes are assembled with viral structural proteins (step 11) to yield progeny virions. The scheme by which the *Coronaviridae* and *Arteriviridae* synthesize their subgenomic RNA is different from that employed by the *Toga-*, *Astra-*, and *Caliciviridae*.

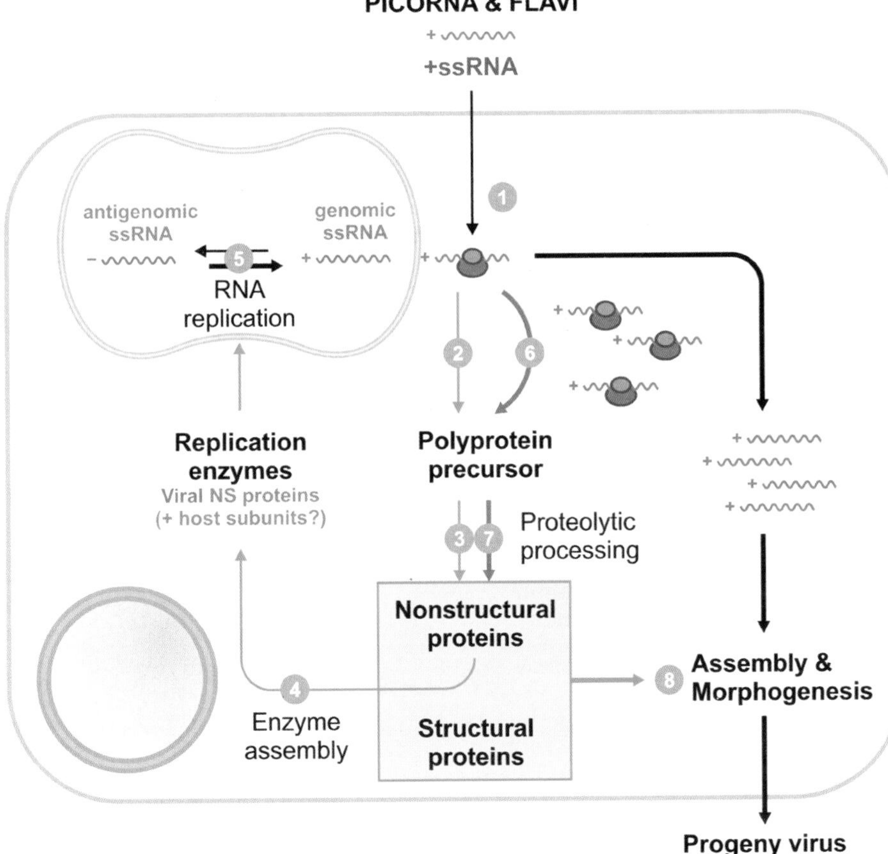

FIGURE 5.11. Schematic of the replication cycle of positive-strand RNA viruses that do not make subgenomic RNA. Following entry and uncoating (step 1), the genomic RNA is used directly as an mRNA to synthesize both structural and nonstructural proteins (steps 2 and 3). The nonstructural proteins, including the RdRp and host components, establish a membrane-associated replication compartment in which the genomic RNA is copied into antigenomic RNA and progeny genomes (steps 4 and 5). Replication produces additional genomic RNA that can be used for further translation and genomic amplification (steps 6, 7, and 5) as well as assembly with the viral structural proteins (step 8) to yield progeny virions.

the cell a protein RNA complex that contains within it the viral polymerase.

The positive-sense RNA viruses fall into two general groups, those that transcribe subgenomic RNAs (Fig. 5.10) and those that do not (Fig. 5.11). Viruses that do not transcribe subgenomic RNA are translated by the host ribosomes to produce one or more polyprotein precursors that undergo a set of in *cis* and in *trans* cleavage reactions by viral encoded proteases.[29] Those cleavage reactions result in the production of the individual non-structural proteins essential for the replication of the viral genome, including the establishment of the site of viral replication. For viruses that produce a single polyprotein the precursors of the catalytic components are generated in equimolar amounts to the structural proteins. In some cases, control over the abundance of the catalytic components is provided by the accumulation of intermediates in the processing cascade in which one or more of the catalytic activities are absent.[95] Such components can play crucial structural or regulatory roles in the establishment of replication compartments. Viruses that produce two polyprotein precursors always employ an internal ribosome entry site (IRES) to drive the expression of the second polyprotein. Because the translation of the second polyprotein is independent of the first, the proteins are not produced in equimolar amounts, allowing for some regulation of the abundance of the different proteins.[50] For viruses that produce subgenomic RNAs, the input genome is first translated into a precursor of the nonstructural proteins that includes the RdRp. The genome is then subsequently copied into one or more subgenomic mRNAs that encode the structural proteins. The production of subgenomic mRNAs facilitates the synthesis of distinct amounts of the structural and nonstructural proteins—such that the structural proteins are often produced in vast molar excess of the catalytically essential nonstructural proteins.

In contrast to the naked RNA of the positive-sense RNA viruses, that of the negative-sense, ambisense, and dsRNA viruses is noninfectious (Figs. 5.12–5.14). This is because the infectious unit is a ribonucleoprotein complex comprising the genomic RNA associated with the necessary viral polymerase components for synthesis of mRNA.[76,105] In the case of the negative-sense and ambisense RNA viruses, the input genomic RNA is copied by the viral polymerase complex into mRNA (Figs. 5.12 and 5.13). The input genomes are then replicated to yield antigenomes, a process that requires newly synthesized viral nucleocapsid protein to coat the nascent RNA strand.[76,105] For the negative-sense RNA viruses (Fig. 5.12), the antigenomes are positive sense, but they do not serve as templates for translation, rather they function exclusively as templates for genomic replication.[76,105] The negative-sense orthomyxoviruses and bornaviruses replicate within the host-cell nucleus, whereas the mammalian infecting rhabdoviruses as well as the paramyxoviruses and filoviruses replicate in the cytoplasm. A further important distinction is that the rhabdo-, filo-, paramyxo-, and bornaviruses sequentially transcribe a series of 5 to 10 monocistronic mRNAs from a single genomic template, whereas the orthomyxoviruses synthesize only a single mRNA from each segment. In the case of the ambisense RNA viruses, the genomic and antigenomic RNAs have both message and

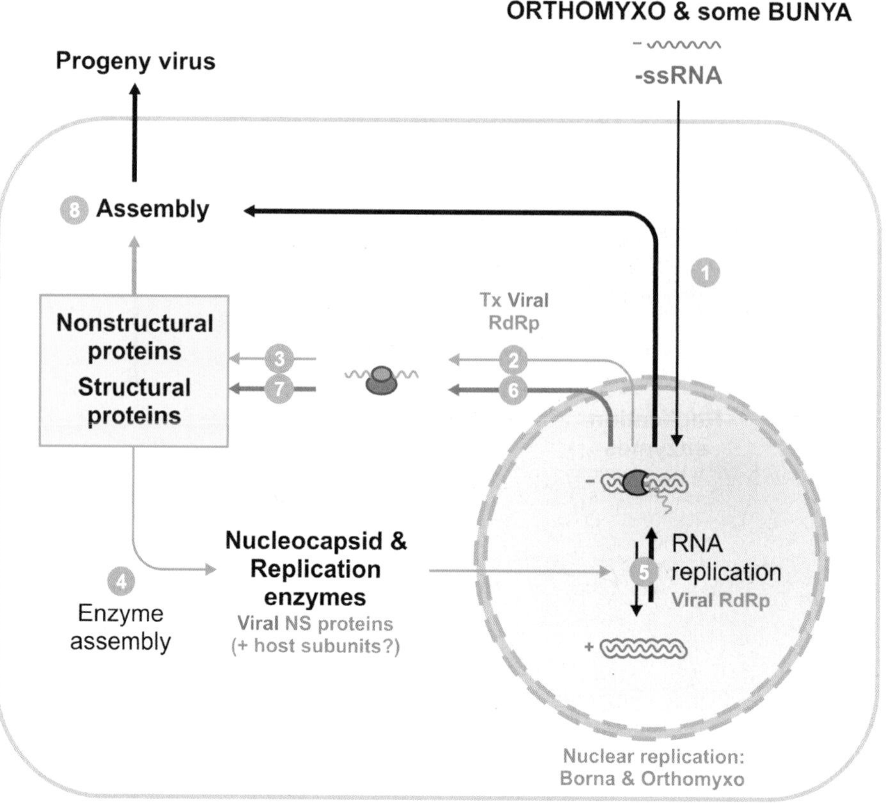

FIGURE 5.12. Simplified replication scheme for negative-sense RNA viruses. Following entry and partial uncoating (step 1), the encapsidated viral genomic RNAs are transcribed by the virion RdRp into mRNAs (step 2) that encode the viral structural and nonstructural proteins (step 3). For the *Orthomyxoviridae* and *Bornaviridae*, transcription occurs in the nucleus (reflecting their need for splicing), whereas for the *Rhabdo, Filo, Paramyxo,* and *Bunyaviridae* this occurs in the cytoplasm. Replication is concomitant with encapsidation of the genomic and antigenomic RNAs (steps 4 and 5), and the newly produced genomic RNAs serve as templates for further mRNA production (step 6) as source of further viral proteins (step 7) as well as for assembly of progeny virions (step 8). The segmented negative-sense RNA viruses transcribe each genomic segment into a single transcript (which can be alternately spliced in the case of the orthomyxoviruses). The nonsegmented negative-sense RNA viruses sequentially transcribe a series of 5 to 10 monocistronic mRNAs from the genomic template.

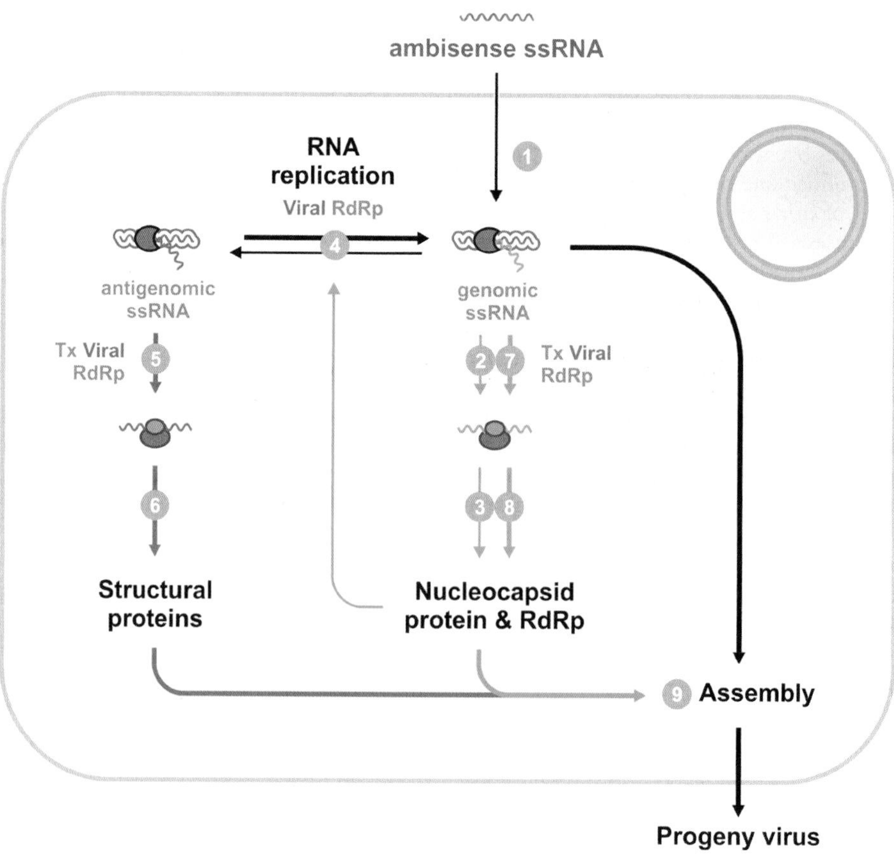

FIGURE 5.13. Replication scheme for the ambisense RNA viruses. Following entry and partial uncoating (step 1), the encapsidated genomic RNAs are transcribed by the virion RdRp to yield mRNAs (step 2) that encode the viral nucleocapsid protein and RdRp (step 3). These proteins catalyze the synthesis of antigenomic RNA (step 4), which serves both as templates for transcription of additional mRNAs (step 5) that encode the remaining viral proteins (step 6), as well as templates for production of more genomic RNA (step 4). The replication products (both genomic and antigenomic) can serve as further templates for transcription of mRNA that encode both viral structural and nonstructural proteins (steps 5 through 8). The genomic RNAs are also assembled together with the structural proteins into infectious viral particles (step 9). Note some bunyaviruses are also simply negative-sense.

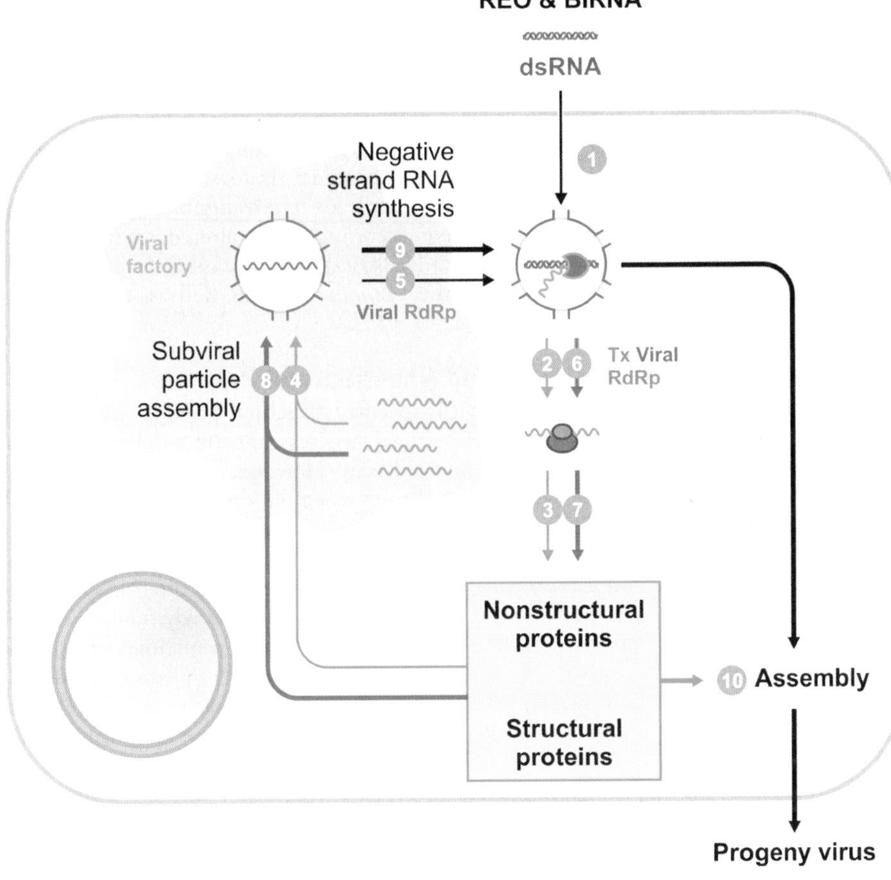

FIGURE 5.14. Simplified replication scheme for dsRNA viruses. Following entry and partial uncoating (step 1), the dsRNA segments within viral cores are transcribed by the core associated RdRp to produce mRNA (step 2) for the viral proteins (step 3). These form subviral particles around the mRNA (step 4), which are then copied to produce genomic dsRNAs (step 5). RNA synthesis and replication likely occur within a specific cytoplasmic factory established by the viral proteins. Progeny subviral particles contribute to viral gene expression (steps 6 and 7) and replication (steps 8 and 9) and assemble with outer shell proteins to form progeny virus particles (step 10).

anti-message polarity. However, those RNAs serve exclusively as templates for both mRNA transcription and replication (Fig. 5.13) rather than translation.[34] In contrast to all other negative-strand RNA viruses, the circular ssRNA genome of HDV does not require a specialized viral polymerase for copying. Rather, the HDV genome is transcribed and replicated by the host DNA-dependent RNA polymerase II in a unique RNA-templated reaction.[97]

For the dsRNA viruses, the segmented genomes are delivered into the cell as a subviral particle that remains intact for transcription of the mRNA (Fig. 5.14). The polymerase and RNA-modifying enzymes form a structural element through which the nascent mRNA strand passes and is cotranscriptionally modified. The ssRNA and their encoded proteins reassemble into new subviral particles that can direct the synthesis of antigenome RNA and form a dsRNA genome. Those progeny subviral particles can serve as templates for the production of further mRNA, and the viral protein or can be packaged into new virions.[69]

The positive-sense RNA genomes of retroviruses (Fig. 5.9) use a distinct mechanism for replication. Here, the incoming ssRNA is copied into a dsDNA provirus using the virally encoded reverse transcriptase—an essential component of the incoming virion.[5,98] This dsDNA is integrated into the host genome, where it is copied into differentially spliced transcripts that either serve as template for production of viral proteins or for production of viral progeny.

Regulation of Gene Expression

In contrast to DNA viruses, which exhibit clearly demarked early/late-phase gene expression, most RNA viruses show little differentiation between the pre- and postreplicative phases of the infectious cycle, and express their genes at roughly the same relative levels throughout infection. In cases such as the togaviruses and orthomyxoviruses (e.g., the influenza viruses) where some temporal regulation of gene expression occurs, the differences are subtle and mostly accompanied at the transcriptional level by modulation of mRNA levels.

Although DNA viruses utilize alternate translational control mechanisms as well as RNA viruses, translational control is especially prevalent among RNA viruses. The rate-limiting step for translation of cellular mRNA by the ribosome is at the process of initiation, and more specifically recognition of the mRNA cap structure by the cap-recognition protein eIF-4E, part of a multi-subunit complex. The cap-recognition complex then facilitates the recruitment of the small subunit of the ribosome in complex with other initiation factors. This complex then scans to the first AUG on the template RNA, typically localized within 100 or so nucleotides of the mRNA cap structure. Following this scanning to the AUG, the small subunit is joined by the large ribosomal subunit, and polypeptide chain synthesis is initiated. The poly(A) tail present at most cellular mRNA structures stimulates translation, as it is bound by the poly(A)-binding protein that bridges interactions with the eIF-4G component of the cap-recognition complex. This may serve to functionally circularize the mRNA to facilitate ongoing translation. There are many notable exceptions to this general mechanism that have been exploited by RNA viruses. This reflects the fact that although superficially many RNA virus positive-sense transcripts resemble cellular mRNAs, there are distinctions at both the 5′ and 3′ ends of the RNA that are accompanied frequently by an altered mechanism of translational initiation.

One of the best known examples of an altered mechanism of translational initiation was provided by studies of how the genomes of picornaviruses—which lack a 5′ mRNA cap structure and instead contain a genome-linked protein VPg—are expressed. The 5′ untranslated regions of picornavirus genomes are unusually long (several 100s of nucleotides, including several AUG-specifying triplet) and are highly structured. Those structured elements termed internal ribosome entry sites (or IRES) serve to recruit the ribosome directly to the viral RNA,[83] without the need for a full complement of initiation factors for translation. Indeed in some viruses, such as cricket paralysis virus, the ribosome is recruited to the IRES without the need for any of the initiation factors that are essential for conventional translation. Such altered mechanisms are exploited by viruses to facilitate the efficient translation of the viral mRNA, thereby outcompeting cellular transcripts for translation ensuring the robust synthesis of viral proteins.

There are also many RNA viruses that produce mRNAs that lack a polyadenylate tail, the dsRNA reoviruses and rotaviruses, many of the ambisense arenaviruses and bunyaviruses, as well as numerous positive-strand RNA viruses. On most cellular mRNAs, the polyadenylate tail is generally thought to function as an element that stabilizes the mRNA and additionally favors translation by facilitating recycling of ribosomes through a protein-mediated bridging mechanism that brings the 5′ and 3′ ends of the mRNA together. Such circularization is likely achieved by direct RNA–RNA interactions in the case of some positive-strand RNA plant viruses—such as the luteovirus, barley yellow dwarf virus.[58] A similar mechanism has been postulated to function for the flavivirus, Dengue virus, although direct evidence for this is lacking.

A further mechanism of regulation of translation initiation exploited by RNA viruses is a translation termination–reinitiation strategy. This strategy involves the termination of translation of an upstream open-reading frame followed by the reinitiation at a proximal (<40 nt away) downstream open-reading frame. The stop and start codons are frequently found in an overlapping arrangement, but in distinct reading frames to one another, and termination is essential for the subsequent reinitiation. This strategy is exploited by the positive-strand RNA calciviruses, such as feline calicivirus and murine norovirus; as well as the negative-strand RNA viruses influenza B virus and respiratory syncytial virus.[86] Although the mechanism is not well understood, evidence from studies of calicivirus translation implicates the presence of a secondary structure in the mRNA that may function to "tether" the small ribosomal subunit to the transcript before reengagement of the large subunit.

Suppression of termination is also exploited during the translation of many viral mRNAs, notably those of the alphavirus and retrovirus families, as a mechanism of producing a protein with an extended C-terminus. In the case of some retroviruses, a *cis*-acting regulatory element at the Gag-Pol junction functions to suppress termination of translation by leading to the misreading of the UAG termination codon to form the Gag-Pol polyprotein. Processing of this polyprotein then provides the viral reverse transcriptase and integrase. A second strategy is used by Rous sarcoma virus as well as other retroviruses, termed ribosomal frameshifting. A slippery sequence in the template leads to a realignment of the tRNA and the subsequent accessing of an altered reading frame. Such a mechanism is also exploited by other positive-strand viruses (notably the *Coronaviridae*) as well as several DNA viruses.

Structural and Nonstructural Proteins

By definition, virus-specified structural proteins are incorporated into virus particles, whereas nonstructural proteins are found only in infected cells. However, negative-sense, ambisense, and dsRNA viruses assemble their RdRp's and associated enzymes into progeny virions and therefore encode predominantly or exclusively structural proteins. In addition to the polymerase, virus-encoded enzymes often include one or more proteases, an RNA helicase, guanylyltransferase and methyltransferases, poly(A) polymerase, sometimes a nuclease, and in the case of retroviruses, a DNA integrase. However, for several RNA viruses, the evidence that these enzymes are virally encoded is only circumstantial or based on inconclusive sequence homologies.

The proteases process the primary translation products of which they are a part by cleaving them at highly specific target sequences, and in some picornavirus-infected cells they also selectively inhibit host-cell protein synthesis by cleavage of the eIF-4G component of the cap-recognition complex. Particularly among the larger RNA viruses, RNA helicases may be required to disrupt intermolecular or intramolecular base pairing during RNA synthesis, although some RdRp's are capable of melting RNA duplexes without help. Guanylyl and methyltransferases construct the 5′ caps found on the mRNAs of most eukaryotic RNA viruses,[24,37] except for the picornaviruses, which are uncapped, and the orthomyxoviruses, arenaviruses and bunyaviruses, which acquire their caps by stealing them from the host using a virus-encoded cap-dependent endonuclease.[72,85] The cap structures of the *Mononegavirales* are formed by an altered mechanism involving a guanosine diphosphate (GDP)—polyribonucleotidyltransferase that is found within the same polypeptide chain that contains the polymerase and mRNA cap methylase activities.[65,66,77,78] At their 3′ ends, most animal virus mRNAs carry untemplated poly(A) tails, although 3′ tRNA-like structures are common among plant RNA viruses (see Chapter 72). Polyadenylation is usually ascribed to a stuttering side reaction of the viral RdRp rather than to a separate poly(A) polymerase, as found in poxviruses, although the enzymology of the reaction remains to be clearly defined.[76,105]

Comparisons among the amino acid sequences of viral RdRp's establish clear phylogenetic relationships that also reflect other differences in viral genome structures and strategies. Moreover, the x-ray crystal structures of the polio-, hepatitis C, reo-, rota-, phi6- and other RdRp's show clear resemblance to one another as well as to reverse transcriptases and DNA-dependent RNA and DNA polymerases. Although the overall levels of amino acid sequence homology among these diverse polymerases are statistically insignificant, RdRp's share many of the characteristic polymerase motifs that occupy critical positions in the three-dimensional architecture of the polymerase active site. Taken together the structural similarities of their RdRp's firmly anchor the RNA viruses to the rest of the biosphere, and suggest that despite their diversity these viruses probably escaped from cellular origins to establish a horizontally transmissible parasitic existence using polymerases that radiated from a common ancestor.

Host Cell Factors

Proteins provided by the host undoubtedly play essential roles in RNA virus replication, although different cellular proteins have been implicated in different virus systems. The clearest example comes from the RNA replicase enzymes of the RNA bacteriophages Qβ and MS2, which, in addition to the single phage-specified polypeptide that provides the polymerase active site, contain four cell-specified subunits: the *Escherichia coli* ribosomal protein S1, two translation elongation factors (EF-Tu and EF-Ts), and a strand-specific RNA-binding protein, host factor 1.[8] In view of the similarity of their host components, the distinct specificities of the Qβ and MS2 replicases for their cognate RNA templates must be determined by their unique viral subunits. The unexpected recruitment of translation factors to assist RNA replication—despite the evident differences between these two processes—may reflect underlying biochemical similarities in the RNA–protein interactions involved.

Translation factors have also been implicated in the replication of RNA viruses of eukaryotes. For example, a subunit of the initiation factor eIF-3 binds to the brome mosaic virus RdRp and increases its activity,[87] and several other host proteins have been found to associate with viral RNAs in infected cells. One of the difficulties in definitively assigning whether such proteins are just passengers, or active players in the replication of the viral genome, is often the lack of *in vitro* replication assays and/or genetically tractable host systems. Substantial progress has been made in this regard with the use of genetic, chemical, RNAi, as well as proteomic screens to hunt for host factors that are required for viral replication. Reconstructing the replication cycle of viruses in yeast,[54,79] has permitted screens in collections of gene knockouts in *Saccharomyces cerevisiae,* and the application of RNAi has extended such screens to invertebrate and vertebrate cells.[17] More recently the use of haploid human cells and gene-trap retroviruses has allowed the discovery of host-cell factors that are essential for the entry into cells of a number of viral pathogens.[13,14] Although in some cases the overlap of "hits" between seemingly similar screens is low—likely reflecting technical difficulties of such large scale screens—the convergence on specific pathways exploited by viruses for their replication is generally high.[42] Such systematic analyses provide a potentially fertile source for understanding the virus–host relationship; however, the detailed mechanistic understanding of how specific host proteins mediate viral replication lags behind.

In addition to host proteins, host nucleic acids also appear to participate directly in the replication of some RNA viruses. One such example is provided by host micro RNA's that function to titrate cellular gene expression by promoting transcript turnover or by sequestration. Work with hepatitis C virus (HCV) identified a liver specific microRNA-122—which regulates cholesterol biosynthesis—that binds to two sites at the 5′ end of the viral genome and enhances HCV replication.[55] Such control of viral replication only further serves to underscore the intimate relationship between viruses and their host cells.

Compartmentalization of Replication Sites

Unlike the phage replicases, the RdRp's of eukaryotic viruses are invariably found associated with some type of supramolecular assembly: host-cell membranes for positive-sense RNA viruses, nucleocapsids frequently found as inclusion-like structures for the negative-sense RNA viruses, and subviral particles arranged as factories for the dsRNA viruses. The positive-strand RNA viruses (Figs. 5.10 and 5.11) represent the best-characterized examples of membrane-associated replication complexes, with most information being available for the picornavirus and nodavirus families.[25] In most cases, the membranes are extensively rearranged, often—although not exclusively—derived from the endoplasmic reticulum, and invariable topologically arranged as an invagination of the membrane of the endoplasmic reticulum (ER) to form an open-necked crucible. Within each vesicle are a relatively small number of genomic templates—possibly as few as one, along with the viral replication machinery and cellular proteins that appear to play a role in the formation of the vesicular structure. The prevailing model is that such vesicular structures represent the sites of viral RNA replication, and that the nascent RNA chains are rapidly exported to the cytoplasm. In many cases, virion assembly sites are juxtaposed to such compartmentalized replication sites, which likely facilitates the coordination of the replication and assembly of viral particles. In the case of some positive-strand RNA viruses, notably the coronaviruses, the vesicles that are formed by the replication machinery appear to be closed from the cytoplasm. Whether specific viral protein(s), or a complex of viral and cellular proteins, are required to exchange nucleoside triphosphates and progeny genomes is not yet certain.

In the case of the negative-sense RNA viruses that replicate in the cytoplasm (Fig. 5.12), the viral replication machinery is typically found in inclusion-like structures that are often rich in cellular chaperones such as heat shock protein (hsp)70.[61] Although such inclusion-like structures are not essential for RNA synthesis—as they are absent at the onset of infection and at a time at which the intracellular environment is likely most hostile for viral replication—such structures have been shown to be active sites of RNA transcription and seem to be sites of genome replication.[48,61] Likewise, dsRNA viruses establish factories or viroplasms (Fig. 5.13) in the infected cell that are sites of RNA synthesis and assembly.[10] Such compartmentalization of the replication machinery is therefore a conserved theme across a spectrum of viruses. Although it is clear that replication can occur in such sites, and this sequestration may both facilitate catalysis and sequester the viral replication machinery from surveillance by host defense machinery, it is largely uncertain what events lead to the establishment of such sites. Although there is a strong correlation between compartment formation and viral replication, examination of the very initial replication events including establishment of such sites remains challenging.

Mechanisms of RNA Replication and Transcription

The simplest mechanism of RNA replication is that used by HDV in which rolling circle synthesis by RNA polymerase II makes multimeric RNAs of both positive and negative polarity. *cis*-Acting ribozymes then cleave linear RNA monomers from these concatamers and covalently circularize them to produce mature antigenomes and genomes, respectively[97] (see Chapter 69). Although this simple mechanism is shared by several viroids and other subviral RNA pathogens of plants, HDV is the only RNA pathogen of vertebrates known to replicate by a rolling circle mechanism. Far more commonly, ssRNA genomes are replicated via the synthesis of complementary RNA monomers produced by successive rounds of strand displacement during end-to-end copying of linear templates.[11] However, both ends of the RNA are generally required for template activity, suggesting that even linear RNAs may be functionally circularized, perhaps to facilitate reiterative replication and hinder erosion of the termini.

The relative abundance of the genomic and antigenomic RNAs is regulated in different ways in different virus families. In the case of Qβ, negative-strand RNA synthesis is limited by the requirement for an additional host subunit that is not required for positive-strand RNA synthesis.[8] In other virus systems, distinct *cis*-acting RNA signals are largely responsible for determining the relative template activities of the complementary strands, although it is possible that different host factors are involved here as well. For the togavirus Sindbis, negative-sense RNA is synthesized only by a short-lived version of the RdRp, which is an intermediate in the proteolytic processing pathway of the viral nonstructural proteins.[56] As infection proceeds, increased viral protease activity cleaves this transient intermediate and thereby switches the template specificity of the RdRp to the synthesis of positive-strand RNA (see Chapter 22).

There are two general mechanisms of initiation by RdRp's: primer dependent and primer independent mechanisms. The majority of RNA viruses appear to employ a primer independent mechanism. Some of the best studied examples of this are provided by the bacteriophages Qβ, MS2, and φ6, as well as by eukaryotic viruses HCV, and reo-, rota-, and vesicular stomatitis virus. The general mechanism by which *de novo* initiation occurs is that the RdRp initiates synthesis by forming a phosphodiester bond between the initiation nucleoside triphosphate (iNTP) and a second NTP.[12] Atomic structures of polymerases engaged in the steps of initiation have provided remarkable insights into this process. The second general mechanism is a primer-dependent mechanism of initiation. The primers themselves can come in different flavors, for example, the picornavirus RdRp's use a small viral-encoded protein, VPg, that is covalently uridylylated by the polymerase on an internal RNA structure at a single A residue.[82] This primer, polymerase complex then relocalizes to the terminus to prime the initiation reaction. Nucleic acids can also serve as primers for RNA synthesis, and here there are two currently known variations of this mechanism of primed initiation. The first of these is exploited by the RdRp's of the segmented negative-strand RNA viruses: *Orthomyxo-*, *Bunya-*, and *Arenaviridae* to prime messenger RNA synthesis. Here a virally encoded endonuclease cleaves a short capped primer from either host-cell pre-mRNA in the case of the *Orthomyxoviridae,* or mature cytoplasmic mRNA in the case of the *Arena-* and *Bunyaviridae.*[85] Such primers then base pair with the ends of the template to prime synthesis of the viral mRNA. Remarkably the polymerases of those viruses also initiate "*de novo*". However, the available evidence supports that this reaction occurs not by initiation of synthesis opposite the terminal nucleotide, but by initiation at the penultimate nucleotide followed by a subsequent realignment of the nascent strand to "prime" the process of replication.[39] This strategy, termed "prime and realign" may help ensure the integrity of the termini are maintained during copying.

SUMMARY AND PERSPECTIVES

Mechanistic studies of viral replication have led us to some of the most fundamental discoveries in biology as well as provided critical knowledge to facilitate the development of vaccines and antiviral therapeutics to combat disease. The global burden of infectious disease caused by existing viruses and the ongoing threat of emerging viral infections further emphasizes the need to fully understand the mechanisms by which viruses replicate. Such studies promise to continue to uncover strategies to combat disease, and to harness viral replication for beneficial purposes both in the laboratory as expression vectors, gene knockout tools, neural circuit tracers, and probes of cellular, organismal, and population biology, but also in the clinic as potential vaccines, delivery vehicles, and imaging tools. The industrial applications of viruses are equally profound—as polymers, as well as tools to make microcircuits and even as potential fuel cells. All these applications of viruses have depended on our current understanding of the replication machinery and the strategies of viral replication. With the ability to simply manipulate viral genomes combined with the new burst in discovery of viruses from large scale sequencing projects, the future of fundamental studies of viral replication promises to be even more informative than the exciting past.

ACKNOWLEDGMENT

The author gratefully acknowledges the expert help of Silvia Piccinotti with the diagrams.

REFERENCES

1. Albertini AA, Ruigrok RW, Blondel D. Rabies virus transcription and replication. *Adv Virus Res* 2011;79:1–22.
2. Albertini AA, Wernimont AK, Muziol T, et al. Crystal structure of the rabies virus nucleoprotein-RNA complex. *Science* 2006;313:360–363.
3. Arslan D, Legendre M, Seltzer V, et al. Distant Mimivirus relative with a larger genome highlights the fundamental features of Megaviridae. *Proc Natl Acad Sci U S A* 2011;108:17486–17491.
4. Bahar MW, Graham SC, Chen RA, et al. How vaccinia virus has evolved to subvert the host immune response. *J Struct Biol* 2011;175:127–134.
5. Baltimore D. RNA-dependent DNA polymerase in virions of RNA tumour viruses. *Nature* 1970;226:1209–1211.
6. Barr JN, Fearns R. How RNA viruses maintain their genome integrity. *J Gen Virol* 2010;91:1373–1387.
7. Bezier A, Herbiniere J, Lanzrein B, et al.. Polydnavirus hidden face: the genes producing virus particles of parasitic wasps. *J Invertebr Pathol* 2009;101:194–203.
8. Blumenthal T, Carmichael GG. RNA replication: function and structure of Qbeta-replicase. *Annu Rev Biochem* 1979;48:525–548.

9. Boyle KA, Stanitsa ES, Greseth MD, et al. Evaluation of the role of the vaccinia virus uracil DNA glycosylase and A20 proteins as intrinsic components of the DNA polymerase holoenzyme. *J Biol Chem* 2011;286:24702–24713.
10. Broering TJ, Kim J, Miller CL, et al. Reovirus nonstructural protein mu NS recruits viral core surface proteins and entering core particles to factory-like inclusions. *J Virol* 2004;78:1882–1892.
11. Buck KW. Comparison of the replication of positive-stranded RNA viruses of plants and animals. *Adv Virus Res* 1996;47:159–251.
12. Butcher SJ, Grimes JM, Makeyev EV, et al. A mechanism for initiating RNA-dependent RNA polymerization. *Nature* 2001;410:235–240.
13. Carette JE, Guimaraes CP, Varadarajan M, et al. Haploid genetic screens in human cells identify host factors used by pathogens. *Science* 2009;326:1231–1235.
14. Carette JE, Raaben M, Wong AC, et al. Ebola virus entry requires the cholesterol transporter Niemann-Pick C1. *Nature* 2011;477:340–343.
15. Chakrabarti A, Jha BK, Silverman RH. New insights into the role of RNase L in innate immunity. *J Interferon Cytokine Res* 2011;31:49–57.
16. Chang L, Godinez WJ, Kim IH, et al. Herpesviral replication compartments move and coalesce at nuclear speckles to enhance export of viral late mRNA. *Proc Natl Acad Sci U S A* 2011;108:E136–144.
17. Cherry S, Doukas T, Armknecht S, et al. Genome-wide RNAi screen reveals a specific sensitivity of IRES-containing RNA viruses to host translation inhibition. *Genes Dev* 2005;19:445–452.
18. Claverie JM, Abergel C, Ogata H. Mimivirus. *Curr Top Microbiol Immunol* 2009;328:89–121.
19. Clyde K, Glaunsinger BA. Getting the message direct manipulation of host mRNA accumulation during gammaherpesvirus lytic infection. *Adv Virus Res* 2010;78:1–42.
20. Cotmore SF, Tattersall P. High-mobility group 1/2 proteins are essential for initiating rolling-circle-type DNA replication at a parvovirus hairpin origin. *J Virol* 1998;72:8477–8484.
21. Crotty S, Cameron CE, Andino R. RNA virus error catastrophe: direct molecular test by using ribavirin. *Proc Natl Acad Sci U S A* 2001;98:6895–6900.
22. Daffis S, Szretter KH, Schriewer J, et al. 2′-O methylation of the viral mRNA cap evades host restriction by IFIT family members. *Nature* 2010;468:452–456.
23. de Jong RN, van der Vliet PC, Brenkman AB. Adenovirus DNA replication: protein priming, jumping back and the role of the DNA binding protein DBP. *Curr Top Microbiol Immunol* 2003;272:187–211.
24. Decroly E, Ferron F, Lescar J, et al. Conventional and unconventional mechanisms for capping viral mRNA. *Nat Rev Microbiol* 2011;10:51–65.
25. den Boon JA, Ahlquist P. Organelle-like membrane compartmentalization of positive-strand RNA virus replication factories. *Annu Rev Microbiol* 2010;64:241–256.
26. Deng T, Vreede FT, Brownlee GG. Different de novo initiation strategies are used by influenza virus RNA polymerase on its cRNA and viral RNA promoters during viral RNA replication. *J Virol* 2006;80:2337–2348.
27. Denison MR, Graham RL, Donaldson EF, et al. Coronaviruses: an RNA proofreading machine regulates replication fidelity and diversity. *RNA Biol* 2011;8:270–279.
28. Domingo E, Holland JJ. RNA virus mutations and fitness for survival. *Annu Rev Microbiol* 1997;51:151–178.
29. Dougherty WG, Semler BL. Expression of virus-encoded proteinases: functional and structural similarities with cellular enzymes. *Microbiol Rev* 1993;57:781–822.
30. Dreher TW. Role of tRNA-like structures in controlling plant virus replication. *Virus Res* 2009;139:217–229.
31. Eigen M. Viral quasispecies. *Sci Am* 1993;269:42–49.
32. Elion GB, Furman PA, Fyfe JA, et al. Selectivity of action of an antiherpetic agent, 9-(2-hydroxyethoxymethyl) guanine. *Proc Natl Acad Sci U S A* 1977;74:5716–5720.
33. Emerman M, Malik HS. Paleovirology—modern consequences of ancient viruses. *PLoS Biol* 2010;8:e1000301.
34. Emonet SE, Urata S, de la Torre JC. Arenavirus reverse genetics: new approaches for the investigation of arenavirus biology and development of antiviral strategies. *Virology* 2011;411:416–425.
35. Fanning E, Zhao K. SV40 DNA replication: from the A gene to a nanomachine. *Virology* 2009;384:352–359.
36. Favoreel HW, Van de Walle GR, Nauwynck HJ, et al. Virus complement evasion strategies. *J Gen Virol* 2003;84:1–15.
37. Furuichi Y, Shatkin AJ. Viral and cellular mRNA capping: past and prospects. *Adv Virus Res* 2000;55:135–184.
38. Gao Q, Park MS, Palese P. Expression of transgenes from newcastle disease virus with a segmented genome. *J Virol* 2008;82:2692–2698.
39. Garcin D, Kolakofsky D. Tacaribe arenavirus RNA synthesis in vitro is primer dependent and suggests an unusual model for the initiation of genome replication. *J Virol* 1992;66:1370–1376.
40. Gerlier D, Lyles DS. Interplay between innate immunity and negative-strand RNA viruses: towards a rational model. *Microbiol Mol Biol Rev* 2011;75:468–490, second page of table of contents.
41. Gierer A, Schramm G. Infectivity of ribonucleic acid from tobacco mosaic virus. *Nature* 1956;177:702–703.
42. Goff SP. Knockdown screens to knockout HIV-1. *Cell* 2008;135:417–420.
43. Goodbourn S, Randall RE. The regulation of type I interferon production by paramyxoviruses. *J Interferon Cytokine Res* 2009;29:539–547.
44. Green TJ, Zhang X, Wertz GW, et al. Structure of the vesicular stomatitis virus nucleoprotein-RNA complex. *Science* 2006;313:357–360.
45. Hakansson K, Doherty AJ, Shuman S, et al. X-ray crystallography reveals a large conformational change during guanyl transfer by mRNA capping enzymes. *Cell* 1997;89:545–553.
46. Haller O, Weber F. Pathogenic viruses: smart manipulators of the interferon system. *Curr Top Microbiol Immunol* 2007;316:315–334.
47. Hay S, Kannourakis G. A time to kill: viral manipulation of the cell death program. *J Gen Virol* 2002;83:1547–1564.
48. Heinrich BS, Cureton DK, Rahmeh AA, et al. Protein expression redirects vesicular stomatitis virus RNA synthesis to cytoplasmic inclusions. *PLoS Pathog* 2010;6:e1000958.
49. Herold J, Andino R. Poliovirus RNA replication requires genome circularization through a protein-protein bridge. *Mol Cell* 2001;7:581–591.
50. Hertz MI, Thompson SR. Mechanism of translation initiation by Dicistroviridae IGR IRESs. *Virology* 2011;411:355–361.
51. Hodel AE, Gershon PD, Quiocho FA. Structural basis for sequence-nonspecific recognition of 5′-capped mRNA by a cap-modifying enzyme. *Mol Cell* 1998;1:443–447.
52. Holland JJ, De La Torre JC, Steinhauer DA. RNA virus populations as quasispecies. *Curr Top Microbiol Immunol* 1992;176:1–20.
53. Hu G, Gershon PD, Hodel AE, et al. mRNA cap recognition: dominant role of enhanced stacking interactions between methylated bases and protein aromatic side chains. *Proc Natl Acad Sci U S A* 1999;96:7149–7154.
54. Janda M, Ahlquist P. RNA-dependent replication, transcription, and persistence of brome mosaic virus RNA replicons in S. cerevisiae. *Cell* 1993;72:961–970.
55. Jopling CL, Yi M, Lancaster AM, et al. Modulation of hepatitis C virus RNA abundance by a liver-specific MicroRNA. *Science* 2005;309:1577–1581.
56. Kim KH, Rumenapf T, Strauss EG, et al. Regulation of Semliki Forest virus RNA replication: a model for the control of alphavirus pathogenesis in invertebrate hosts. *Virology* 2004;323:153–163.
57. King AMQ, Adams MJ, Carstens EB, et al. (eds.). *Virus Taxonomy: Classification and Nomenclature of Viruses: Ninth Report of the International Committee on Taxonomy of Viruses.* San Diego: Elsevier Academic Press, 2011.
58. Kneller EL, Rakotondrafara AM, Miller WA. Cap-independent translation of plant viral RNAs. *Virus Res* 2006;119:63–75.
59. Kranzusch PJ, Schenk AD, Rahmeh AA, et al. Assembly of a functional Machupo virus polymerase complex. *Proc Natl Acad Sci U S A* 2010;107:20069–20074.
60. Kranzusch PJ, Whelan SP. Arenavirus Z protein controls viral RNA synthesis by locking a polymerase-promoter complex. *Proc Natl Acad Sci U S A* 2011;108:19743–19748.
61. Lahaye X, Vidy A, Pomier C, et al. Functional characterization of Negri bodies (NBs) in rabies virus-infected cells: Evidence that NBs are sites of viral transcription and replication. *J Virol* 2009;83:7948–7958.
62. Lauring AS, Andino R. Quasispecies theory and the behavior of RNA viruses. *PLoS Pathog* 2010;6:e1001005.
63. Lee HR, Kim MH, Lee JS, et al. Viral interferon regulatory factors. *J Interferon Cytokine Res* 2009;29:621–627.
64. Lee YF, Nomoto A, Detjen BM, et al. A protein covalently linked to poliovirus genome RNA. *Proc Natl Acad Sci U S A* 1997;74:59–63.

65. Li J, Fontaine-Rodriguez EC, Whelan SP. Amino acid residues within conserved domain VI of the vesicular stomatitis virus large polymerase protein essential for mRNA cap methyltransferase activity. *J Virol* 2005;79:13373–13384.
66. Li J, Rahmeh A, Morelli M, et al. A conserved motif in region v of the large polymerase proteins of nonsegmented negative-sense RNA viruses that is essential for mRNA capping. *J Virol* 2008;82:775–784.
67. Liu H, Naismith JH, Hay RT. Adenovirus DNA replication. *Curr Top Microbiol Immunol* 2003;272:131–164.
68. McBride AA. Replication and partitioning of papillomavirus genomes. *Adv Virus Res* 2008;72:155–205.
69. McDonald SM, Patton JT. Assortment and packaging of the segmented rotavirus genome. *Trends Microbiol* 2011;19:136–144.
70. McFadden G, Mohamed MR, Rahman MM, et al. Cytokine determinants of viral tropism. *Nat Rev Immunol* 2009;9:645–655.
71. Mercer J, Schelhaas M, Helenius A. Virus entry by endocytosis. *Annu Rev Biochem* 2010;79:803–833.
72. Morin B, Coutard B, Lelke M, et al. The N-terminal domain of the arenavirus L protein is an RNA endonuclease essential in mRNA transcription. *PLoS Pathog* 2010;6:e1001038.
73. Morin B, Rahmeh AA, Whelan SP. Mechanism of initiation of RNA synthesis by the RNA dependent RNA polymerase of vesicular stomatitis virus. *EMBO J* 2012;31:1320–1329.
74. Moya A, Elena SF, Bracho A, et al. The evolution of RNA viruses: A population genetics view. *Proc Natl Acad Sci U S A* 2000;97:6967–6973.
75. Muylaert I, Tang KW, Elias P. Replication and recombination of herpes simplex virus DNA. *J Biol Chem* 2011;286:15619–15624.
76. Neumann G, Brownlee GG, Fodor E, et al. Orthomyxovirus replication, transcription, and polyadenylation. *Curr Top Microbiol Immunol* 2004;283:121–143.
77. Ogino T, Banerjee AK. Unconventional mechanism of mRNA capping by the RNA-dependent RNA polymerase of vesicular stomatitis virus. *Mol Cell* 2007;25:85–97.
78. Ogino T, Kobayashi M, Iwama M, et al. Sendai virus RNA-dependent RNA polymerase L protein catalyzes cap methylation of virus-specific mRNA. *J Biol Chem* 2005;280:4429–4435.
79. Panavas T, Serviene E, Brasher J, et al. Yeast genome-wide screen reveals dissimilar sets of host genes affecting replication of RNA viruses. *Proc Natl Acad Sci U S A* 2005;102:7326–7331.
80. Patel MR, Emerman M, Malik HS. Paleovirology—Ghosts and gifts of viruses past. *Curr Opin Virol* 2011;1:304–309.
81. Patton JT, Vasquez-Del Carpio R, Tortorici MA, et al. Coupling of rotavirus genome replication and capsid assembly. *Adv Virus Res* 2007;69:167–201.
82. Paul AV, Rieder E, Kim DW, et al. Identification of an RNA hairpin in poliovirus RNA that serves as the primary template in the in vitro uridylylation of VPg. *J Virol* 2000;74:10359–10370.
83. Pelletier J, Sonenberg N. Internal initiation of translation of eukaryotic mRNA directed by a sequence derived from poliovirus RNA. *Nature* 1988;334:320–325.
84. Pfeiffer JK, Kirkegaard K. Bottleneck-mediated quasispecies restriction during spread of an RNA virus from inoculation site to brain. *Proc Natl Acad Sci U S A* 2006;103:5520–5525.
85. Plotch SJ, Bouloy M, Ulmanen I, et al. A unique cap(m7GpppXm)-dependent influenza virion endonuclease cleaves capped RNAs to generate the primers that initiate viral RNA transcription. *Cell* 1981;23:847–858.
86. Powell ML. Translational termination-reinitiation in RNA viruses. *Biochem Soc Trans* 2010;38:1558–1564.
87. Quadt R, Kao CC, Browning KS, et al. Characterization of a host protein associated with brome mosaic virus RNA-dependent RNA polymerase. *Proc Natl Acad Sci U S A* 1993;90:1498–1502.
88. Quinlan MP, Chen LB, Knipe DM. The intranuclear location of a herpes simplex virus DNA-binding protein is determined by the status of viral DNA replication. *Cell* 1984;36:857–868.
89. Quinones-Mateu ME, Arts EJ. Virus fitness: concept, quantification, and application to HIV population dynamics. *Curr Top Microbiol Immunol* 2006;299:83–140.
90. Randow F, Lehner PJ. Viral avoidance and exploitation of the ubiquitin system. *Nat Cell Biol* 2009;11:527–534.
91. Sawicki SG, Sawicki DL, Siddell SG. A contemporary view of coronavirus transcription. *J Virol* 2007;81:20–29.
92. Schutz S, Sarnow P. Interaction of viruses with the mammalian RNA interference pathway. *Virology* 2006;344:151–157.
93. Sen GC, Sarkar SN. The interferon-stimulated genes: targets of direct signaling by interferons, double-stranded RNA, and viruses. *Curr Top Microbiol Immunol* 2007;316:233–250.
94. Simon AE, Roossinck MJ, Havelda Z. Plant virus satellite and defective interfering RNAs: new paradigms for a new century. *Annu Rev Phytopathol* 2004;42:415–437.
95. Strauss JH, Strauss EG. The alphaviruses: gene expression, replication, and evolution. *Microbiol Rev* 1994;58:491–562.
96. Takeda M, Nakatsu Y, Ohno S, et al. Generation of measles virus with a segmented RNA genome. *J Virol* 2006;80:4242–4248.
97. Taylor JM. Chapter 3. Replication of the hepatitis delta virus RNA genome. *Adv Virus Res* 2009;74:103–121.
98. Temin HM, Mizutani S. RNA-dependent DNA polymerase in virions of Rous sarcoma virus. *Nature* 1970;226:1211–1213.
99. Thomas SM, Lamb RA, Paterson RG. Two mRNAs that differ by two nontemplated nucleotides encode the amino coterminal proteins P and V of the paramyxovirus SV5. *Cell* 1988;54:891–902.
100. Versteeg GA, Garcia-Sastre A. Viral tricks to grid-lock the type I interferon system. *Curr Opin Microbiol* 2010;13:508–516.
101. Vignuzzi M, Stone JK, Arnold JJ, et al. Quasispecies diversity determines pathogenesis through cooperative interactions in a viral population. *Nature* 2006;439:344–348.
102. Villordo SM, Gamarnik AV. Genome cyclization as strategy for flavivirus RNA replication. *Virus Res* 2009;139:230–239.
103. Watts JM, Dang KK, Gorelick RJ, et al. Architecture and secondary structure of an entire HIV-1 RNA genome. *Nature* 2009;460:711–716.
104. Weitzman MD, Lilley CE, Chaurushiya MS. Genomes in conflict: maintaining genome integrity during virus infection. *Annu Rev Microbiol* 2010;64:61–81.
105. Whelan SP, Barr JN, Wertz GW. Transcription and replication of nonsegmented negative-strand RNA viruses. *Curr Top Microbiol Immunol* 2004;283:61–119.
106. Wu Q, Wang X, Ding SW. Viral suppressors of RNA-based viral immunity: host targets. *Cell Host Microbe* 2010;8:12–15.
107. Zaccomer B, Haenni AL, Macaya G. The remarkable variety of plant RNA virus genomes. *J Gen Virol* 2005;76(Pt 2):231–247.

CHAPTER 6

Eric Hunter

Virus Assembly

Virus assembly, a key step in the replication cycle of any virus, involves a process in which chemically distinct macromolecules are transported, often through different pathways, to a point within the cell where they are assembled into a nascent viral particle. A diversity of strategies and intracellular assembly sites are employed by members of the various virus families to ensure the efficient production of fully infectious virions. Nevertheless, a virus, irrespective of its molecular structure (membrane enveloped or nonenveloped) or the symmetry with which it assembles (icosahedral, spherical, or helical), must be able to take advantage of the intracellular transport pathways that exist within the cell if it is to achieve this goal. The end product of this selection process is assembly of each virus at a defined point within the cell. This chapter will focus on the cell biology of these intracellular targeting events, the intermolecular interactions that mediate targeting, and the assembly steps themselves.

Most viruses encode a very limited number of gene products. They therefore depend on the cell not only for biosynthesis of the macromolecules that constitute the virus particle but also for the pre-existing intracellular sorting mechanisms that the virus utilizes to achieve delivery of those macromolecules to the sites of virion assembly. Because these are the same sorting mechanisms that the cell uses to delineate its subcellular organelles, the viral macromolecules must possess targeting signals similar to those of the components of those organelles. For a virus such as adenovirus, which assembles its nonenveloped capsids in the nucleus, this means that, following translation in the cytoplasm, each of the structural proteins of the mature virus must have the necessary protein-targeting information to be efficiently routed through the nuclear membrane to the assembly site. The situation is more complicated for a membrane-enveloped virus, such as influenza virus. For this virus, which assembles and releases virions from the apical surface of the epithelial cells that it infects, there is a necessity to ensure that the surface glycoproteins of the virus are correctly sorted by the secretory pathway of the cell to apical membranes. In addition, nucleocapsids, assembled in the nucleus, must be transported into and through the cytoplasm to the same location. As will be discussed later, the intracellular site at which the final phase of assembly and budding of an enveloped virus takes place is most often defined by the accumulation of the viral glycoproteins at a specific point in the secretory pathway of the cell. This also implies that there is specific molecular recognition of the virally encoded, membrane-spanning envelope components by the cytoplasmic nucleocapsids for a productive budding process to occur. Thus, interactions between proteins of viral and cellular origin, between viral proteins and nucleic acids and lipids, and between the viral proteins themselves are at the heart of the assembly process.

PARTITIONING OF PROTEINS WITHIN THE CELL

For an actively growing eukaryotic cell, there is a constant need to transport proteins and nucleic acids from their site of synthesis to the specific intracellular domains where they must function (Fig. 6.1). Proteins synthesized on cytosolic ribosomes, for example, must be transported to specific regions of the cytoplasm, to mitochondria and into the nucleus, whereas those synthesized on membrane-bound ribosomes will enter the secretory pathway and be targeted to specific organelles along the way. At the same time, messenger RNAs (mRNAs) and integral RNA components of the ribosome, or ribosomal RNAs (rRNAs), must be transported out of the nucleus. Proteins that participate in these intracellular trafficking processes have evolved to contain specific motifs that ensure the correct localization of the protein within the cell. Viruses have similarly evolved to take advantage of these pre-existing

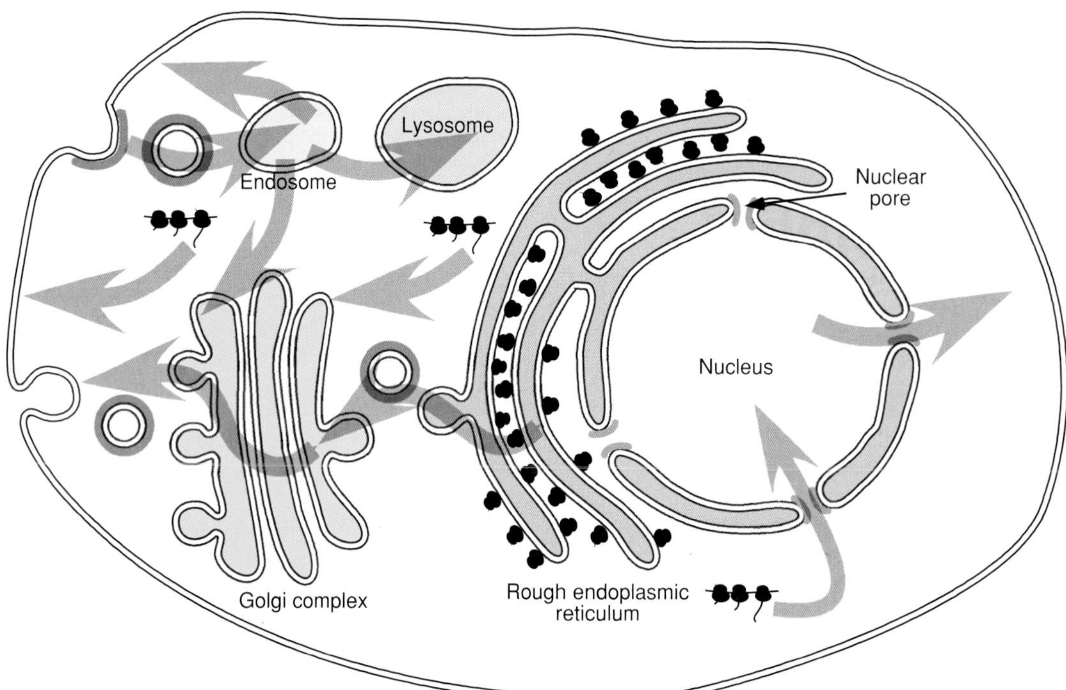

FIGURE 6.1. Protein localization in a mammalian cell. Proteins destined for the plasma membrane traverse the secretory pathway of the cell. They associate with the endoplasmic reticulum co-translationally and are translocated across the ER membrane via a proteinaceous pore—the translocon. Proteins are transported from the ER to the Golgi complex and on to the plasma membrane unless they contain specific amino acid motifs that localize or retain them at an intermediate location. Transport from one compartment to the next is via coated vesicles. Some membrane-spanning (integral membrane) proteins contain endocytosis motifs in their cytoplasmic domain that facilitate incorporation into clathrin-coated endocytic vesicles. Such proteins can be sorted back to the plasma membrane, to the trans-Golgi compartment of the secretory pathway, or to a lysosome for degradation. Proteins destined for the nucleus contain nuclear localization signals. These are short amino acid sequences that allow interaction with the nuclear pore machinery for transport across the nuclear membrane. Some proteins shuttle between the nucleus and cytoplasm and contain in addition a nuclear export signal. ER, endoplasmic reticulum.

pathways to accumulate, in specific locations, the necessary components for assembly of a nascent virus.

Nuclear Import and Export of Proteins and Nucleic Acids

The Nuclear Pore Complex

The nucleus is segregated from the cytoplasm by an inner and outer membrane; thus, access to and egress from this subcellular domain is mediated by specialized structures termed *nuclear pore complexes* (NPCs).[202] There are approximately 3,000 NPCs on the nuclear envelope of an animal cell, and each provides a proteinaceous channel between the nucleus and cytosol. The NPC itself is a very large structure, with a molecular mass exceeding 50 mDa that exhibits eightfold symmetry and is constructed of multiple copies of approximately 30 different proteins called *nucleoporins* (Nups). Negative stain and cryoelectron microscope reconstructions of these complexes reveal a 125-nm diameter core structure in which eight spokes in a radially symmetrical arrangement join to form three main rings surrounding a central channel of approximately 35 nm.[3] Attached to both faces of the central framework are peripheral structures, cytoplasmic filaments, and a nuclear basket assembly, which interact with molecules that transit the NPC.[58] The channel is filled with flexible, filamentous FG-Nups, which are characterized by regions of multiple Phe-Gly repeats and form a *virtual gate* restricting transport into and out of the nucleus.[181] Small molecules and proteins may be able to passively diffuse through the NPC; however, it acts as a molecular sieve for macromolecules. Larger proteins and macromolecular assemblages must be actively moved through what is clearly a dynamic, malleable transporter structure that has the capacity to accommodate macromolecular complexes with diameters of up to nearly 35 nm.[154]

Nuclear Localization Signals

Proteins that are actively transported into or out of the nucleus are characterized by the presence of amino acid motifs that allow them to interact with the nuclear transport machinery. For import into the nucleus, these motifs are termed *nuclear localization signals* (NLS) and for export, *nuclear export signals* (NES). NLS motifs, such as that first identified in the SV40 T antigen,[95] are not only necessary for nuclear localization of the proteins in which they are present but are also sufficient to actively direct large foreign proteins, such as β-galactosidase, into the nucleus. Although there is no conservation of sequence in different NLS motifs, they are generally short (<20 amino acids), rich in basic amino acids, and

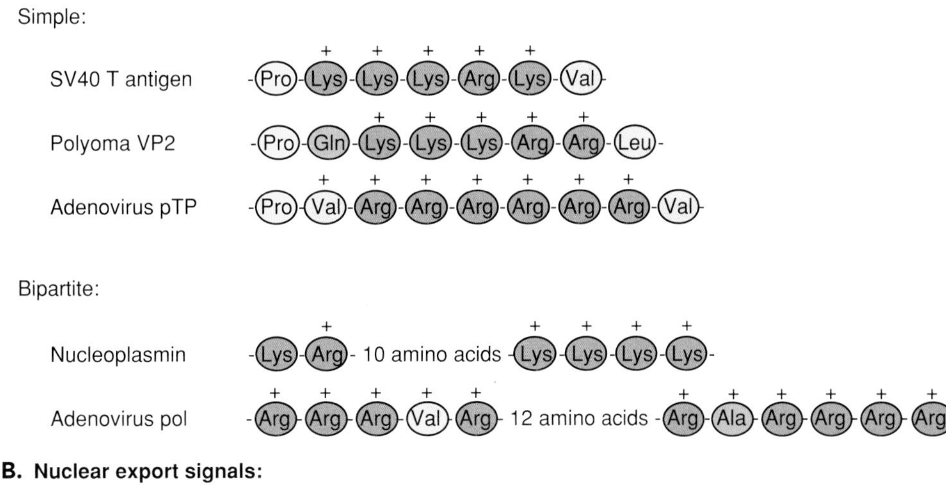

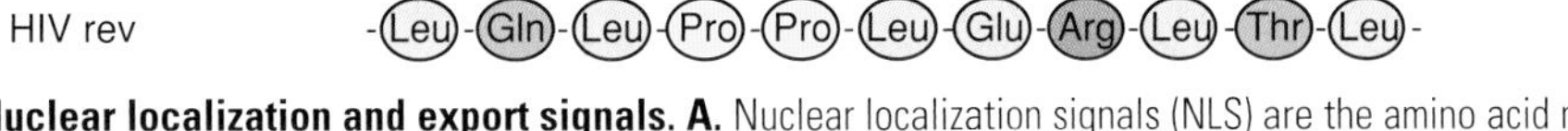
HIV rev
-Leu-Gln-Leu-Pro-Pro-Leu-Glu-Arg-Leu-Thr-Leu-

FIGURE 6.2. Nuclear localization and export signals. A. Nuclear localization signals (NLS) are the amino acid motifs that direct proteins into the nucleus. Simple NLS sequences, such as those present in the SV40 virus T antigen or polyoma virus VP2, often contain a proline residue followed by a stretch of basic residues. This short sequence can relocate large proteins such as β-galactosidase into the nucleus. Bipartite NLS sequences, such as those present in nucleoplasmin or the adenovirus polymerase, are characterized by two stretches of basic amino acids separated by a variable spacer sequence. These NLS sequences are recognized by import receptor molecules such as importin-α. **B.** Proteins that shuttle into and out of the nucleus, such as Rev, possess a second motif, the nuclear export signal. These motifs are characterized by a pattern of conserved leucine residues.

frequently preceded by proline residues (Fig. 6.2A). Some NLS, such as that in the adenovirus DNA-binding protein, are bipartite and require two separate short clusters of basic residues to be functional.[238]

To be exported from the nucleus, proteins contain an NES. This nuclear transport signal is also short (~10 amino acids) and contains a pattern of conserved leucines[134] (Fig. 6.2B). Some proteins, such as Rev of human immunodeficiency virus type 1 (HIV-1), possess both an NLS and an NES and appear to shuttle back and forth between the cytoplasm and the nucleus.[124]

Nuclear Transport Pathways: In and Out

Nuclear import is a two-stage process. In the first stage, the newly synthesized NLS-containing protein interacts with cytosolic receptor proteins that then bind to phenylalanine-glycine (FG) repeat containing Nups (FG-Nups) that make up the filaments on the cytoplasmic side of the NPC - a process referred to as docking. This complex is then translocated, in an energy-independent process, through the nuclear pore into the nucleus, where the complex is disassembled, allowing the transported protein to become functional.

The best-characterized protein import receptor is importin-α (also named karyopherin-α). After binding its NLS-containing cargo, importin-α interacts with importin-β, which then mediates docking with the NPC.[98] Most nuclear transport receptors belong to one large family of proteins (karyopherins), all of which share homology with importin-β (also named karyopherin-β). Members of this family have been classified as importins or exportins on the basis of the direction that they carry their cargo. Importins and exportins are regulated by the small guanosine triphosphatease (GTPase), Ran, which is highly enriched in the nucleus in its GTP-bound form. Importins recognize their substrates in the cytoplasm and transport them through nuclear pores into the nucleus. In the nucleoplasm, RanGTP binds to importins, inducing the release of their cargoes. In contrast, exportins interact with their substrates only in the nucleus in the presence of RanGTP and release them after GTP hydrolysis in the cytoplasm, causing disassembly of the export complex (Fig. 6.3).[204] Thus, the directionality of transport is regulated by whether Ran is complexed with guanosine diphosphate (GDP) or GTP.

Active transport of large molecules in either direction across the nuclear pore involves interaction with the FG-Nups. The FG repeats in these filamentous proteins provide binding sites for the nuclear transport receptors as well as other molecules, such as nuclear transport factor 2 (NTF2), involved in this process. The exact mechanism by which the importin-cargo complex is carried through the nuclear pore is not known. It is likely, however, that the process involves a series of docking and release cycles with the FG-Nup proteins that make up the transporter machinery within the nuclear pore channel.[199,202]

The Secretory Pathway of the Cell

Proteins of both viral and cellular origin that are destined for the outer membrane of the cell travel along a highly conserved route known as the secretory pathway. This complex series of membrane-bound subcellular compartments, through which proteins pass sequentially, includes the endoplasmic reticulum (ER), an intermediate membrane compartment, and the cis-, medial-, and trans-compartments of the Golgi apparatus

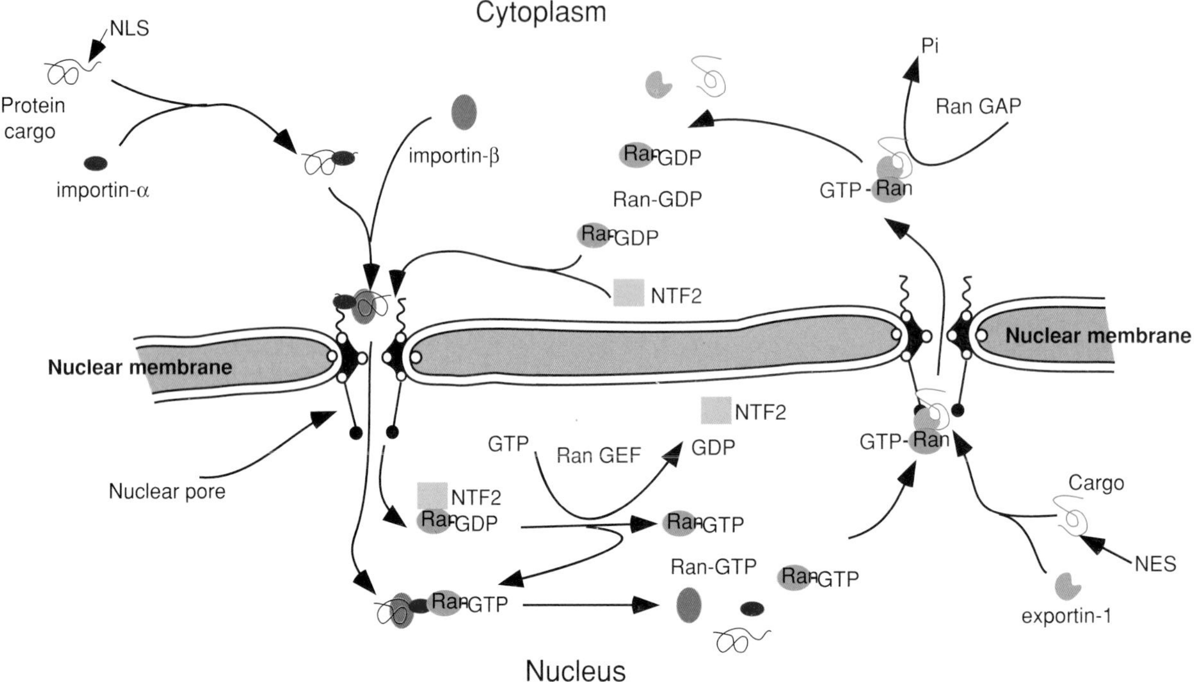

FIGURE 6.3. Nuclear import and export pathways. A protein bearing a nuclear localization signal is recognized and bound by importin-α. Importin-β binds to this complex and carries it to the cytoplasmic filaments of the nuclear pore, where together they mediate translocation of the protein complex into the nucleus in an energy-independent process. In the nucleus, Ran-GTP binds to the importin complex, and it dissociates delivering the protein cargo into the nucleus. Proteins destined for export out of the nucleus bind to exportin-1 via their nuclear export signal. This complex, together with Ran-GTP, binds to nucleoporins localized to the nuclear basket of the pore complex and initiates translocation into the cytoplasm. Once there, Ran-GTP is converted to Ran-GDP by a Ran-GTPase-activating protein (RanGAP-1), causing the cargo-exportin-1-Ran complex to dissociate, thereby delivering the cargo to the cytoplasm. GTP, guanosine triphosphate; GDP, guanosine diphosphate.

(see Fig. 6.1). Proteins that traverse this pathway, such as the envelope glycoproteins of viruses, enter via the ER. Insertion of proteins into the ER occurs during translation through a process termed *translocation.* The ER network of tubules and sacs defines a unique environment in which protein modification and folding can occur isolated from the cytoplasm. Because polyribosomes, in the process of translating proteins that are translocating into the secretory pathway, are bound tightly to the ER membrane, regions containing them are known as the rough ER.

Translocation

Translating ribosomes are directed to the ER membrane by a short sequence in the nascent polypeptide known as the signal sequence. In most proteins, this 15 to 30 amino acid sequence, which contains a core of hydrophobic amino acids, is located at the N-terminus of the protein. Shortly after the signal peptide emerges from the ribosome, it is bound by a ribonucleoprotein (RNP) complex known as the signal recognition particle (SRP). Binding of SRP transiently arrests any further translation and directs the ribosome to an SRP-receptor on the ER (Fig. 6.4). Both SRP and its receptor have GTP-binding components, and the presence of this nucleotide is essential for efficient targeting.[187]

Following the initial docking of the translationally arrested complex, the ribosome becomes tightly associated with the ER membrane via the translocon—a gated, aqueous, protein channel that spans the ER membrane. Concomitant with this process, the SRP and its receptor are released, the signal peptide is introduced into the channel, and translation resumes. The components of the translocon have been identified through biochemical approaches in mammalian cells and genetic approaches in yeast and are comprised of a heterotrimeric complex known as the Sec61p (composed of Sec61 alpha, beta, and gamma chains). Based on the crystal structure of the archaebacterial Sec61 homolog, SecY$\beta\gamma$, this complex forms a 40 Å × 40 Å structure with a pore-like central cavity and a single potential lateral opening to allow transition of membrane-spanning domains into the lipid bilayer.[195,239] Additional proteins (e.g., the translocating chain-association membrane or TRAM protein) are necessary for optimal translocation. It is unlikely that the central pore of the translocon ever allows free diffusion between the cytosol and the lumen of the ER, because these compartments are chemically distinct. A constriction in the channel appears to be plugged by a short helix, and widening of the constriction as well as displacement of the plug have been linked to conformational changes induced by SRP binding to the complex.[219] GRP78 (BiP), a member of the Hsp70 family of chaperone proteins located in the lumen of the ER, plays multiple roles in gating the channel and facilitating translocation. The chaperone is then poised to facilitate the folding of the nascent polypeptide chain as it emerges from the pore, although

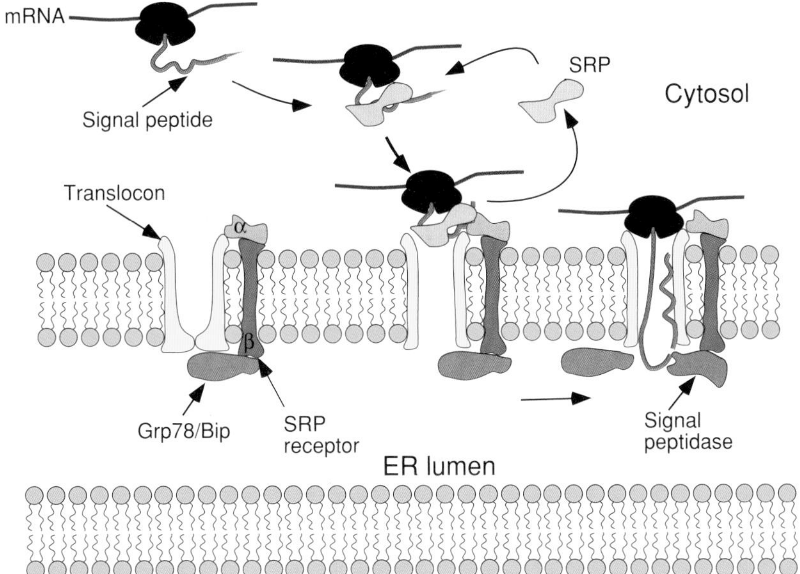

FIGURE 6.4. Protein translocation into the secretory pathway. Translation of a protein destined for the secretory pathway proceeds until the signal peptide exits the ribosome. The SRP binds to the signal peptide and the ribosome and arrests translation. The ribosome-SRP complex moves to the ER membrane, where SRP binds to its receptor (SRP receptor). This interaction, with concomitant hydrolysis of bound GTP, releases SRP and mediates a tight interaction between the ribosome and a proteinaceous channel—the translocon. The release of SRP and binding of the signal peptide to components of the translocon induces a conformational change that widens a constriction in the channel and allows resumption of translation to occur. The chaperone protein, Grp78 (BiP), present in the lumen, is poised to facilitate the folding of the nascent polypeptide chain as it emerges from the pore. The signal peptidase complex removes the signal peptide co-translationally from those proteins that have a cleavable signal peptide. Secreted proteins will continue to traverse the translocon until they are completely located in the lumen of the ER. In contrast, for integral membrane proteins, translocation will stop following introduction of the hydrophobic anchor domain into the translocon, and transition into the lipid bilayer occurs through a single lateral opening in the pore. SRP, signal recognition particle; ER, endoplasmic reticulum; GTP, guanosine triphosphate.

this binding is not essential for translocation to proceed. The signal peptide, in those proteins with a transient N-terminal sequence, is cleaved from the rest of the polypeptide by a complex of five proteins called the *signal peptidase* shortly after it enters the lumen of the ER (see Fig. 6.4).

For secreted proteins, translocation of the polypeptide through the translocon continues until the entire protein is present in the lumen of the ER. In contrast, integral membrane proteins, such as the envelope glycoproteins of viruses, contain a stop-transfer, membrane-anchor sequence that is generally located toward the C-terminus of the protein. Following the translation of this short (~25 amino acids) and mostly hydrophobic sequence, the translocon undergoes a conformational change that allows the membrane-spanning domain to be associated directly with the lipid bilayer. The product of this process is a type I integral membrane protein (Fig. 6.5), such as the influenza virus hemagglutinin (HA), in which the N-terminal ectodomain is in the lumen of the ER and the C-terminus is in the cytoplasm. In some proteins, such as the influenza virus neuraminidase (NA), a longer N-terminal signal peptide also functions as the membrane anchor. In this case, the signal peptide is not cleaved from the polypeptide chain and the sequences C-terminal to it are translocated into the ER lumen, resulting in a type II orientation. Multiple membrane-spanning proteins, such as the M protein of the coronaviruses, appear to possess hydrophobic sequences that are alternatively recognized as signal and stop-transfer sequences, and translocation of such proteins may involve multiple Sec61 heterotrimers.[195]

Posttranslational Modifications

Protein Folding and Quality Control. Proteins enter the lumen of the ER in an unfolded state and the process of folding into a transport-competent conformation is facilitated by interactions with molecular chaperones and folding enzymes located there. This collection of proteins includes BiP, calnexin (Cnx), calreticulin (Crt), GRP94, and protein disulfide isomerase (PDI). In addition to assisting in folding the nascent molecules, these proteins retain incompletely folded molecules in the lumen and act as a quality control system for the secretory pathway.[20] Oligomeric proteins, such as the receptor/fusion proteins of enveloped viruses, also assemble into their quaternary conformation in this compartment. For many of these molecules, oligomerization appears to be a prerequisite for transport out of the ER.

Glycosylation. Most proteins that traverse the secretory pathway are modified by the addition of oligosaccharide side chains either to the amino group of asparagines (N-linked glycosylation) or through the hydroxyl group of serines or threonines (O-linked glycosylation). N-linked moieties are added co-translationally in the lumen of the ER, where mannose-rich

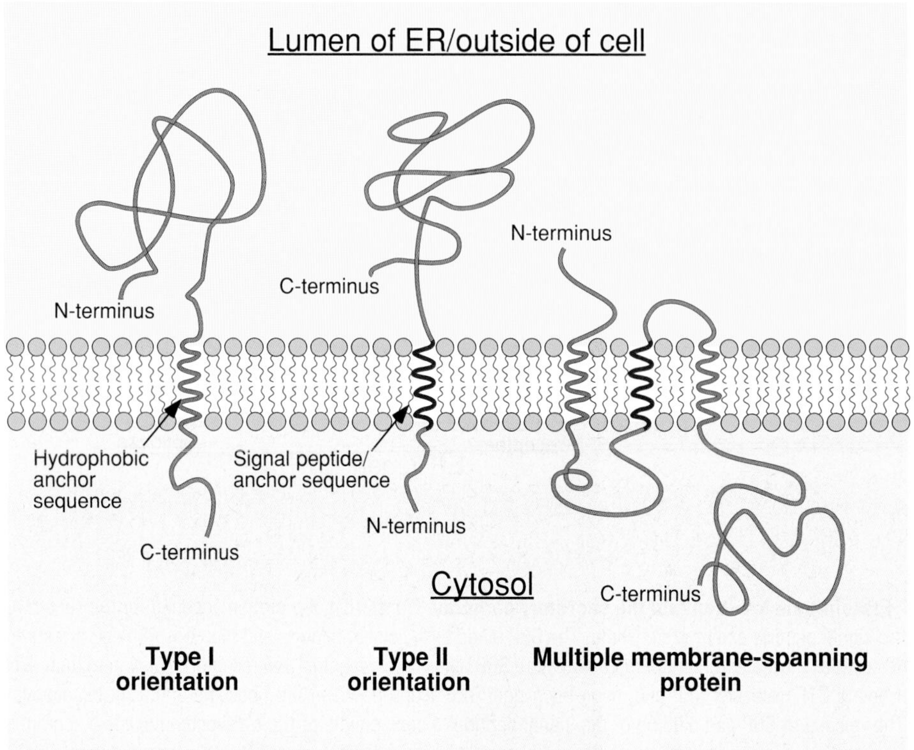

FIGURE 6.5. Protein topology. Proteins with type I orientation generally have a cleavable N-terminal signal peptide that is removed co-translationally from the nascent protein. The protein continues to be transferred into the lumen of the ER until a hydrophobic anchor sequence is translated and enters the translocon. Translocation then stops, and the protein transitions from the protein pore into the lipid bilayer. Thus, type I integral membrane proteins, such as the hemagglutinin of influenza virus, have their C-terminus in the cytoplasm and their N-terminus in the lumen of the ER (topologically equivalent to outside the cell). In type II proteins, such as the influenza virus neuraminidase, the signal peptide forms the membrane anchor domain; thus, at the end of translation, the C-terminal sequences are translocated into the lumen of the ER, leaving the N-terminus in the cytoplasm. For multiple membrane-spanning proteins, such as the M protein of the coronaviruses, translocation is initiated at the first signal peptide sequence and continues until the first anchor domain. It is reinitiated following translation of a subsequent signal sequence and stopped again following translation of a second anchor. The exact mechanism by which this is accomplished without dismantling the translocon at intermediate steps in the process is not understood. ER, endoplasmic reticulum.

oligosaccharides are transferred by oligosaccharyltransferase from a lipid (dolichol) carrier to asparagine residues present in NXS/T motifs (where X is any amino acid but proline) within the protein. Trimming of terminal glucose and mannose residues from the branched oligosaccharide occurs in the ER and is closely linked with the Cnx- and Crt-mediated quality control process.[20] Further trimming of mannose residues followed by addition of other sugars (N-acetylglucosamine, galactose, fucose, and sialic acid), to yield complex oligosaccharide structures, occurs in the Golgi complex. O-linked oligosaccharides are also added in this organelle.

Transport Through the Secretory Pathway

Transport of soluble and membrane-spanning proteins from one compartment of the secretory pathway to the next is mediated by the formation of coated membrane vesicles that travel to and fuse with the target organelle. Thus, once the process of protein folding and quality control has been completed in the ER, proteins are sequestered into these transport vesicles prior to transit to the Golgi complex. The processes of cargo protein selection, budding, targeting, and fusion are probably all mediated by specific protein constituents that define the different transport vesicles involved in shuttling proteins between components of the secretory pathway.[86,210] In the case of ER-to Golgi-transport, the vesicles have coat protein complex II (COPII),[43] whereas retrograde transport of vesicles from the Golgi to the ER, as well as anterograde transport through the Golgi, is mediated by COPI coats.[149] Budding is initiated at specialized regions of the ER (transitional ER) when a small myristoylated protein (SAR1) is converted to the GTP-bound form, allowing it to bind to the membrane and recruit coat proteins (Sec23, Sec24, Sec13, and Sec31) in a stoichiometric manner.[43] Formation of the coat itself induces membrane curvature and vesicle budding. Sorting signals displayed on the cytosolic surfaces of transmembrane protein cargo direct it into COPII vesicles, in some instances through physical association of the Sec23/Sec24 components in a sorting signal-dependent manner.[100] Soluble proteins and transmembrane proteins lacking COPII sorting signals depend on a diversity of transmembrane adaptor proteins that can link them to the budding machinery. These include the endoplasmic reticulum–Golgi intermediate compartment-53 (ERGIC-53) and p24 family of receptor proteins, as well as a set of multiple membrane-spanning ER vesicle (Erv14p, 26p, and 29p) proteins that can facilitate concentration of soluble proteins in COPII vesicles.[43]

Membrane receptors that mediate docking of the transport vesicle with the target organelle are also incorporated into the coat and appear to define the specificity with which the cargo protein is delivered. Rab-GTPases and tethering proteins appear to play an important role in defining the initial vesicle-target interactions,[79,210] whereas soluble N-ethylmaleimide-sensitive factor (Nsf) attachment protein receptors (SNAREs) are generally accepted to mediate the final stage of vesicle docking and the subsequent membrane fusion events that are critical to transport.[16,79] A vesicle-specific SNARE (v-SNARE) interacts with a target-membrane–specific SNARE (t-SNARE) complex (generally comprised of three peptides) during this process. Two additional proteins, the Nsf and soluble Nsf attachment proteins (SNAPs), act to disassemble the complex following fusion, allowing the SNARE components to be recycled.[79,86]

Protein Localization

Subcellular localization of proteins within the secretory pathway appears to be determined by a combination of sorting/targeting signals that mediate interactions with the coat complex for inclusion in a transport vesicle and retention signals that localize the protein to a specific compartment within the secretory pathway. Localization is enhanced by the interplay of anterograde and retrograde transport that allows retrieval of proteins inadvertently transported beyond their target location. The classical example of this is the KDEL peptide sequence found on soluble proteins that are localized to the lumen of the ER.[131] Proteins containing this sequence are efficiently retrieved from the cis-Golgi by the KDEL receptor, which is incorporated into COPI vesicles for trafficking back to the ER. Similarly, membrane-spanning proteins localized to the ER have, at the C-terminus of the cytoplasmic domain, a dilysine (KKXX) COPI-binding motif, which ensures their efficient retrieval from the Golgi complex.[84] This type of motif is utilized by the primate foamy viruses to concentrate the envelope glycoprotein complex (gp80/gp48) in the ER/intermediate compartment (IC), where virus budding occurs.[66] For integral membrane proteins, retention signals often appear to be associated with the membrane-spanning domain(s) of the protein, as is the case for the coronavirus M protein, and may reflect preferred association with specific lipid compositions of the membrane within a particular component of the secretory pathway.

The Golgi Complex

The Golgi complex represents a unique organelle within the secretory pathway in that it is comprised of a series of membrane-bound compartments that are the sites for specific biochemical modifications to proteins and oligosaccharides, as well as locations where specific protein-sorting decisions are made. Proteins transported from the ER enter the Golgi complex via the cis-Golgi network and, after traversing the cis-, medial-, and trans-cisternae, exit via the trans-Golgi network.[179] Each of the compartments provides a spatially distinct site for maintaining an ordered set of enzymes involved in the process of oligosaccharide maturation. They are also the sites at which proteins undergo O-linked glycosylation, through the addition, at certain serines and threonines, of monomeric sugar residues. It is in the trans-Golgi cisternae and trans-Golgi network where viral glycoprotein precursors, such as the Env polyprotein of the retroviruses, are cleaved to their mature forms through the action of members of the furin family of proteinases—enzymes that normally function to process cellular substrates such as polypeptide hormone precursors. This cleavage event is critical for the generation of a biologically functional glycoprotein and thus for virus infectivity.

INTRACELLULAR TARGETING AND ASSEMBLY OF VIRION COMPONENTS

Viruses can be nominally divided into two groups based on the presence or absence of a lipid bilayer envelope. The nonenveloped viruses can assemble in the cytoplasm or nucleus and generally, for those that propagate in animal cells, exhibit icosahedral symmetry (Chapter 3). For these viruses, the viral structural proteins and genomic nucleic acid must be targeted to or retained at the subcellular domain at which assembly occurs. Enveloped viruses, by their very nature, must acquire a lipid bilayer from one of the cell's membranes during the process of assembly. In some viruses, such as the herpesviruses and some retroviruses, this envelopment step takes place after the assembly of an intact capsid shell, whereas for others the processes of envelopment and capsid assembly occur concomitantly. Some viruses undergo transient envelopment and in some cases re-envelopment during the process of assembly.

For nonenveloped viruses, the tightly assembled structure of the icosahedral shell forms a protective coat that prevents degradation of the genome by environmental factors. For enveloped viruses, the integrity of the nucleocapsid structure is less critical because the membrane provides a barrier to external degradative enzymes.

Assembly of Nonenveloped Viruses in the Nucleus

Adenoviruses are nonenveloped icosahedral viruses, 70 to 100 nm in diameter, that have a protein shell surrounding a DNA core. The protein shell (capsid) is composed of 252 capsomeres, of which 240 are hexons and 12 are pentons. Each penton consists of a five-subunit base (polypeptide III) and a trimeric fiber (polypeptide IV) that extends out and away from the shell. The hexon capsomeres are comprised of trimers of three tightly associated molecules of polypeptide II (Fig. 6.6).

For a nonenveloped virus such as adenovirus, which replicates exclusively in the nucleus, there is a strong dependence on nuclear targeting/transport pathways to export newly synthesized mRNAs out of the nucleus and to import structural proteins back into the nucleus. Nuclear import of the major capsid protein—hexon or polypeptide II—depends on the involvement of a second adenovirus protein, the pVI (precursor) polypeptide, which acts as a nucleocytoplasmic shuttling adapter and provides the necessary NLS for transporting the hexon into the nucleus.[229] Trimer formation, in turn, depends on yet another virus-encoded, chaperone-like protein—L4 100K—which transiently binds to the newly synthesized hexon monomer and mediates its association with two additional monomers.[24] Thus, the most abundant structural protein of the adenovirus capsid needs to interact with two additional virus-encoded factors to attain the correct tertiary structure and subcellular location for assembly.

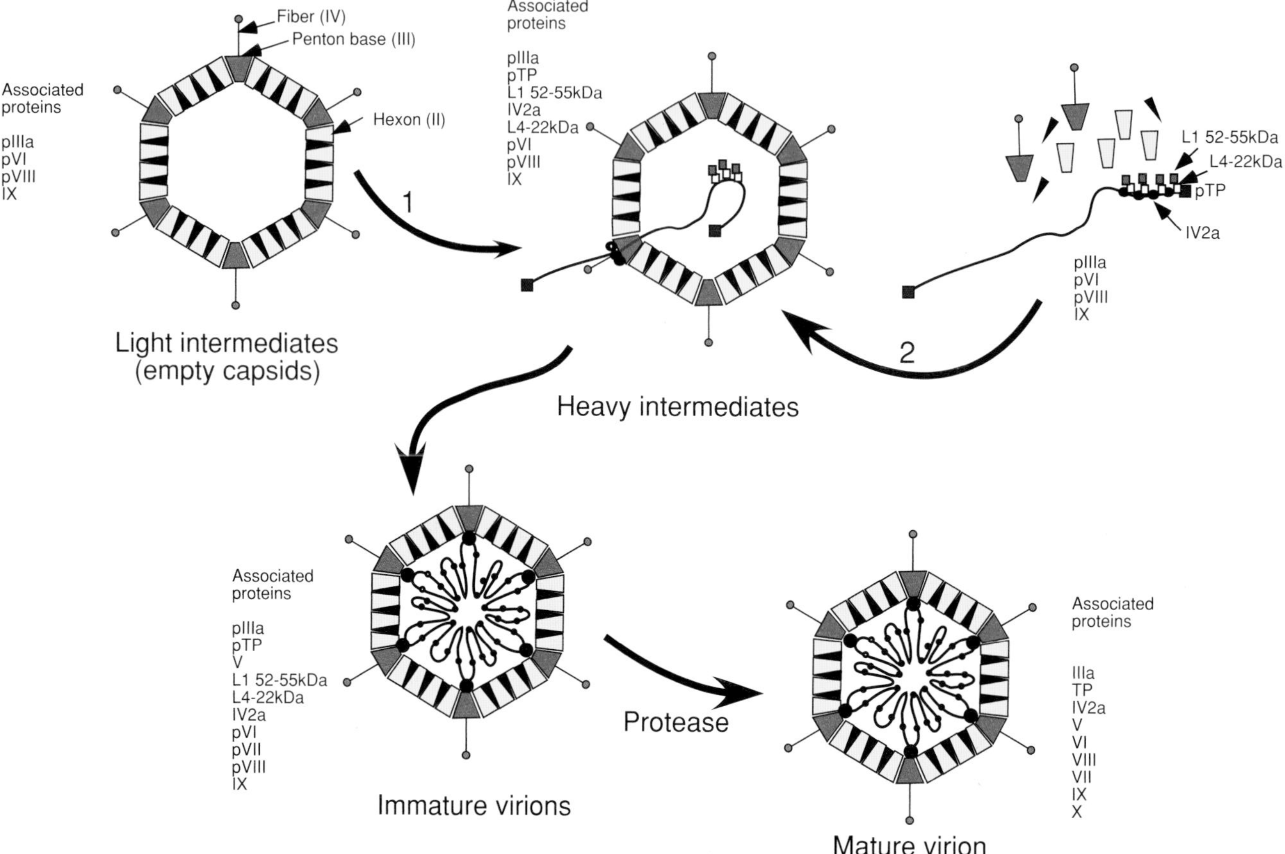

FIGURE 6.6. Assembly pathway for adenoviruses. Following transport into the nucleus, the hexons and pentons are proposed to assemble into empty capsids (previously known as light intermediates of assembly) around scaffolding proteins. These nonstructural scaffolding proteins are lost on packaging of viral DNA, which is inserted into this structure via a packaging sequence at the left end of the genome. The mechanism of insertion appears to be similar to DNA phages and involves a portal complex. The pIV2a protein may represent the ATP-hydrolyzing component required to drive DNA through the portal structure in the procapsid. Heavy intermediate forms of the capsid probably represent those in which DNA packaging is incomplete and the DNA is fragmented. Precursor core proteins would be packaged into the empty capsid along with the genome to form immature virions. Proteolytic cleavage of the precursor proteins by the viral proteinase yields the mature virion. ATP, adenosine 5′-triphosphate.

The two other proteins that form the 12 vertices of the capsid—penton and fiber—appear to assemble independently in the cytoplasm. Mutations in the C-terminus of the penton that block assembly into pentamers do not prevent transport into the nucleus,[96] indicating that each monomer has an active NLS. In contrast, the fiber must form trimers to be efficiently transported to the nucleus,[146] even though this protein has an active NLS located at its N-terminus. It seems likely that the penton base and fibers are transported independently into the nucleus and assemble into the intact penton at the site of assembly.

Although two distinct pathways for adenovirus capsid assembly have been postulated from a large body of work in this area, it now appears that an empty procapsid is first formed around scaffolding proteins, in a manner similar to that observed with DNA phages. Results from experiments that combined kinetic labeling with temperature-sensitive replication mutants and additional site-directed mutants have yielded the assembly scheme shown in Figure 6.6. Several viral products appear to act as scaffolding proteins, around which shells are assembled and that facilitate the encapsidation process. These proteins are present in the intermediate capsid-like particles but are absent once DNA has been encapsidated.[39] Disruption of adenovirus capsids with denaturants results in the release of groups of nine hexons that are associated with the faces of the icosahedron and lack the peripentonal hexons. Under acidic conditions, these nanomers can reassemble to form icosahedral shells that lack the 12 vertices, which would normally be composed of the penton and the five peripentonal hexons, raising the possibility that hexon nanomers are intermediates of adenovirus capsid assembly. Following procapsid assembly, DNA and associated core proteins are then subsequently packaged into these empty shells to yield immature virions that then undergo proteolytic maturation. Recent studies have demonstrated that the approximately six to eight copies of the pIV2a protein, which binds to the packaging sequence, are present at a single apex of the mature virion.[29] This, and the fact that the pIV2a protein contains motifs (the Walker A and B boxes) associated with the binding and hydrolysis of adenosine 5′triphosphate (ATP), suggests that it may represent the ATP-hydrolyzing component required to drive DNA through a portal structure in the procapsid. Consistent with this, mutations that either prevent synthesis of pIV2a or prevent binding of ATP to the protein block genomic packaging and result in the assembly of empty procapsids.[150]

Assembly of Enveloped Viruses in the Nucleus

Two enveloped animal virus families—the herpesviruses and the orthomyxoviruses—utilize cell components that are located within the nucleus in their replication and initiate their assembly within that compartment. In addition to importing into the nucleus the necessary components for assembly, these viruses must also export large nucleoprotein complexes back out into the cytoplasm.

In some respects, the herpesviruses represent a hybrid between a nonenveloped virus, such as adenovirus, and a more conventional enveloped virus, such as a retrovirus, in that they utilize the compartments of the secretory pathway to transport large capsid structures from the nucleus to the outside of the cell. Members of this group of large viruses assemble, within the nucleus, an icosahedral capsid shell that is 160 Å thick and 1,250 Å in diameter. The major component of this protein shell is pUL19, which forms both the pentameric and hexameric capsomeres necessary to assemble the icosahedral structure. Associated with the outer surface of the hexamers is the abundant small protein pUL35. Two additional proteins—pUL38 and pUL18—in a 1:2 ratio, form heterotrimeric triplexes that fit between and link together adjacent capsomeres.[140] Scaffolding proteins are essential for herpes simplex virus type 1 (HSV-1) capsid assembly/maturation; in their absence, incomplete and aberrantly shaped capsids are assembled. As with adenovirus, the major capsid protein lacks a nuclear targeting signal, and its transport into the nucleus requires an interaction with either the scaffolding protein (pUL26.5) or the triplex protein pUL38, which presumably provide the necessary NLS. pUL18 similarly requires pUL38 for nuclear localization, whereas pUL35 appears to be directed there via its interaction with pUL19.[170]

Studies of virus-infected cells together with *in vitro* assembly studies have provided valuable insights into the assembly process.[123,142] These studies point to a pathway in which pUL19, pUL38, and pUL18 assemble around a scaffold to form an icosahedral but predominantly spherical procapsid—the *B-capsids* identified by electron microscopy. Although not required for capsid formation, in its presence the portal complex apparently initiates capsid formation leading to its incorporation into the nascent capsid.[141] Cleavage of the scaffolding protein at a site near its C-terminus by the viral protease removes a 25 amino acid sequence that is necessary for binding to pUL19. The resulting disassociation and release of scaffold allows for packaging of the viral DNA genome and induction of maturation of the capsid into a more angular icosahedral structure, the previously identified *C-capsids*. DNA enters the procapsid through a unique vertex composed of the portal protein pUL6, which is assembled into rings composed of 12 subunits to form the portal complex.[143] The pUL6 portal resembles the connector or portal complexes employed for DNA encapsidation by double-stranded DNA bacteriophages such as φ29, T4, and P22. In the absence of an active proteinase, the scaffolding proteins remain associated with the protein shell, preventing packaging of the viral DNA, and the procapsid is unable to mature.[144]

Unlike adenoviruses, which accumulate in the nucleus and are released on lysis of the cell, herpesviruses exit the nucleus by budding into the lumen of the nuclear membrane. This process depends on the products of two highly conserved genes—UL31 and UL34—that encode a phosphoprotein and a type II membrane protein, respectively. Nuclear localization of pUL31 depends on its interaction with pUL34.[97] Although both proteins are present in the primary enveloped virions present in the lumen of the nuclear membrane, they are absent from mature virions, consistent with a model in which herpesvirus virions are first enveloped at the inner nuclear membrane, de-envelop by budding through the outer nuclear membrane and are re-enveloped by Golgi membranes in the cytoplasm. The complexities of this interaction and subsequent steps in assembly will be discussed later in this chapter.

For influenza virus to take advantage of its unusual capacity to "steal" the capped 5′ ends of host cell mRNAs to initiate its own mRNA synthesis, transcription and viral RNA replication must occur in the nucleus (Chapters 5, 40 and 41). Genomic (minus sense) RNAs are replicated by a different mechanism to yield templates for mRNA synthesis as well as progeny viral genomes. The eight viral RNA segments of this virus are packaged into individual RNPs containing the four proteins of the transcriptase complex (PB1, PB2, PA, and NP, each containing a functional NLS sequence) and the nuclear export protein (NEP, previously NS2), but are not exported into the cytosol until late in infection when the viral matrix protein begins to be synthesized.[113] Under conditions where matrix synthesis is inhibited, the viral ribonucleoproteins (vRNPs) accumulate in the nucleus, tightly associated with the nuclear matrix. The block to export can be relieved by expression of matrix from an independent vector.[22] It has also been shown that the vRNPs remain in the nucleus of cells if NEP is not encoded by the virus. NEP does not interact directly with vRNPs; rather, it mediates (RanGTP-dependent) formation of a bridge between the cellular export receptor Crm1 and the N-terminal domain of M1, which in turn binds to the vRNP via its C-terminal domain. This *daisy-chain* complex of (Crm1–RanGTP)–NEP–M1–vRNP is likely what mediates the export of vRNP across the nuclear envelope.[2,137] Matrix association with the vRNPs also appears to be important for preventing their re-entry into the nucleus, because conditions such as acidification or mutations that promote dissociation of M1 allow the RNPs to be reimported.[228] Thus, the matrix protein of influenza virus is a key modulator of vRNP transport into and out of the nucleus.

Assembly of Viruses in the Cytoplasm

Targeting and import of proteins into the nucleus or secretory pathway involves well-characterized motifs on the proteins involved; therefore, the processes by which proteins are targeted to destinations within the cytoplasm remains for the most part obscure. Nevertheless, most viruses, even those that are nonenveloped, initiate or complete their assembly in association with membranes of the secretory or endocytic pathways, although the intracellular pathways that function to transport their capsid components and genomes to these sites have not been defined. Reoviruses are the only animal viruses that appear to complete their assembly entirely in the cytoplasm without the involvement of membranes. Genome replication and virus assembly both occur in specialized areas of the cytoplasm known as virus factories or viroplasms. The virus nonstructural proteins NSP2 and NSP5 appear to play a critical role in establishing these sites of virus replication and can form morphologically similar structures when expressed in the absence of other viral proteins.[158] It is likely that they are responsible for recruitment of the other viral proteins and viral nucleic acid to these sites, thereby avoiding the complexities of transporting virion components to multiple separate cytoplasmic assembly sites following translation.

Intracytoplasmic Transport and Assembly of Retroviral Capsids

Retroviruses are enveloped viruses that, for the most part, complete their assembly by budding through the plasma membrane of the infected cell. For these viruses, the immature capsid of the virus is assembled from polyprotein precursors that must be transported through the cytoplasm to the inner leaflet of the membrane. The viral glycoproteins, on the other hand, must be transported through the secretory pathway of the cell to the cell surface, where they co-localize with the nascent, membrane-extruding capsid (Fig. 6.7). All replication competent retroviruses contain four genes that encode the structural and enzymatic components of the virion. These are *gag* (capsid protein), *pro* (aspartyl proteinase), *pol* (reverse transcriptase and integrase enzymes) and *env* (envelope glycoprotein) (Chapter 47). However, the product of the *gag* gene has been shown to possess the necessary structural information to mediate intracellular transport, to direct self-assembly into the capsid shell, and to catalyze the process of membrane extrusion known as budding.[183] For most retroviruses, the nascent Gag polyproteins are transported to the plasma membrane, where assembly of the capsid shell and envelopment occur simultaneously (see Fig. 6.7, Pathway 1). Viruses that undergo this *type C* form of morphogenesis include members of the alpha- and

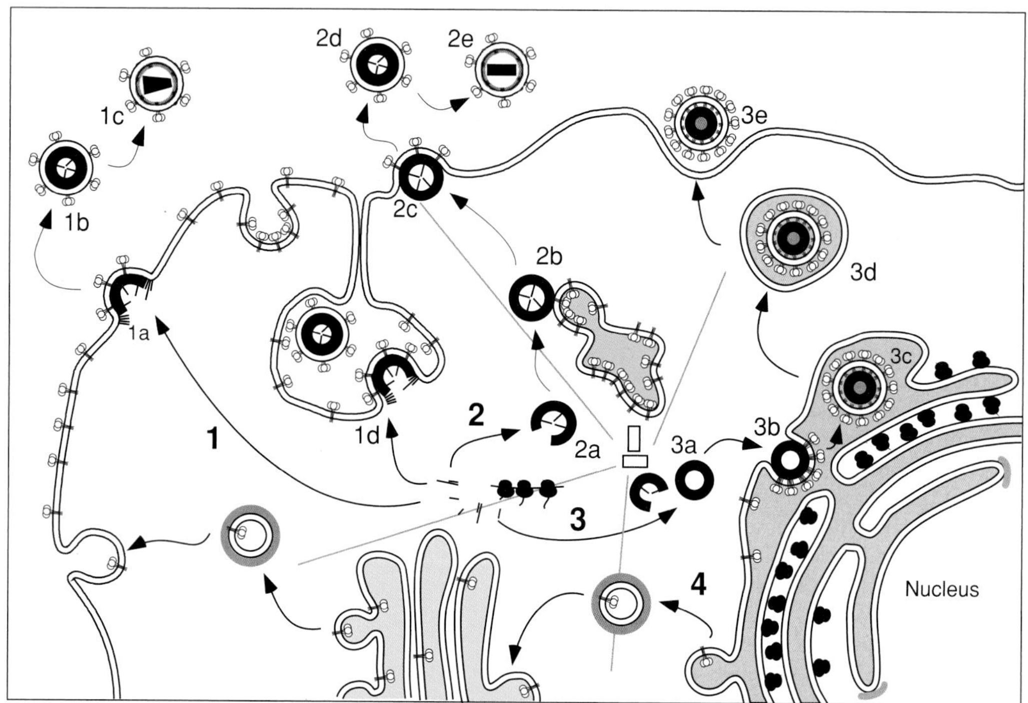

FIGURE 6.7. Assembly of retroviruses. The assembly pathways of retroviruses that exhibit C type morphogenesis (*Pathway 1*), B-/D-type morphogenesis (*Pathway 2*), and that of the foamy viruses (*Pathway 3*) are shown. The envelope glycoproteins are translated on membrane-bound polysomes and, for most retroviruses, are transported to the cell surface through the cell's secretory pathway (*Pathway 4*). For all morphogenic classes, the Gag proteins are synthesized on free polysomes. In the case of the C-type morphogenic viruses (i.e., RSV and HIV), the Gag and Gag-Pol proteins migrate either individually or in small multimers to the plasma membrane, where immature capsid assembly and envelopment occurs concurrently (1a). At some point in this pathway, the viral genomic RNAs associate with the Gag and Gag-Pol precursors and are incorporated into the developing capsid. For HIV in macrophages, assembly can occur on deep invaginations of the plasma membrane to which Env has been targeted (1d). In the case of the B-/D-type viruses, polysomes translating Gag and Gag-Pol precursors are first transported via microtubules to an intracytoplasmic, pericentriolar assembly site (2a), where they assemble into immature capsids. The immature structures are then transported, most likely in association with endosomal vesicles (2b), to the plasma membrane (2c), where they associate with the envelope glycoproteins and induce viral budding. For both classes of retroviruses, the capsids of the nascent immature particles appear as doughnut-shaped structures and contain unprocessed Gag and Gag-Pol precursors (1b and 2d). The mature virus particles contain electron-dense cores with morphologies characteristic of the virus (1c and 2e). The maturation step is required for infectivity and is the result of the activation of the viral protease, which cleaves the Gag and Gag-Pol precursors into the internal structural and enzymatic proteins of the virus. For the foamy viruses, Gag and Pro-Pol precursors also assemble into immature capsids in a pericentriolar site (3a); however, budding primarily occurs at the ERGIC compartment, where the viral glycoproteins are retained (3b). The enveloped virion is presumably transported to the plasma membrane by transport vesicles (3d). Maturational cleavage of the immature core is limited to removal of 4kd from the C-terminus of the precursor; the mature infectious virion maintains an immature morphology (3e). RSV, Rous sarcoma virus; HIV, human immunodeficiency virus; ERGIC, endoplasmic reticulum–Golgi intermediate compartment.

gammaretroviruses. Lentiviruses and deltaretroviruses assemble their capsids in a similar fashion in most cell types. In the second morphogenic class of retroviruses, the *type B/D* class, the Gag precursors are targeted first to an intracytoplasmic site, where capsid assembly occurs. These assembled immature capsids are then transported to the plasma membrane, where they undergo budding and envelopment (see Fig. 6.7, Pathway 2). Viruses that undergo this process of assembly and release include members of the betaretroviruses. Members of the spumavirus family also assemble immature capsids in the cytoplasm but are targeted to the ER or ERGIC for envelopment (see Fig. 6.7, Pathway 3).

Whereas the size and protein content of the precursor varies between different retroviral families, at least three *gag*-encoded proteins are found in all retroviruses: the matrix protein (MA), the capsid protein (CA), and the nucleocapsid protein (NC). In addition to these functionally conserved domains, the Gag precursor can, depending on the virus encoding it, contain additional peptide sequences (Fig. 6.8) whose functions in virus assembly and future cycles of infection are only now being resolved.

The detailed mechanisms by which the capsid precursor proteins are directed to the site of assembly are only now starting to be elucidated in molecular detail; however, the process is mediated primarily by the MA domain of the Gag precursor. In most retroviruses, the matrix protein contains two elements involved in plasma membrane targeting. The first of these is

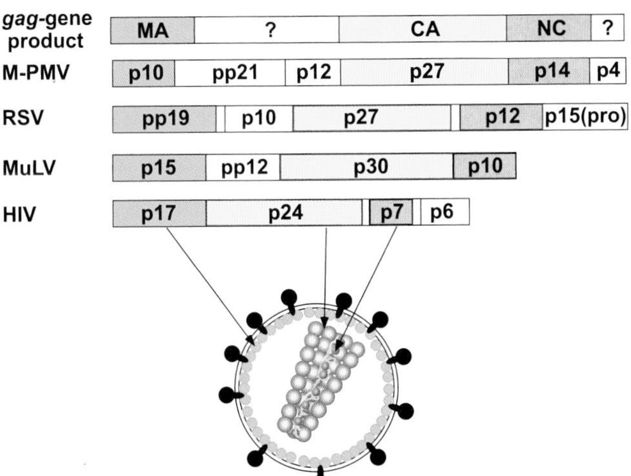

FIGURE 6.8. Organization of the retroviral Gag precursor. The Gag precursor polyproteins of all retroviruses contain, beginning at the N-terminus, matrix (*MA*), capsid (*CA*), and nucleocapsid (*NC*) domains linked in this order. The *gag* gene products of the betaretrovirus Mason-Pfizer monkey virus (*M-PMV*), the alpharetrovirus Rous sarcoma virus (*RSV*), the gammaretrovirus murine leukemia virus (*MuLV*), and the lentivirus human immunodeficiency virus (*HIV*) are shown. The unshaded boxes represent regions of the Gag precursor for which no common functions or locations in the mature virion have been established. However, for the three representatives of the alpha-, beta-, and gammaretroviruses, a *late domain* function required for pinching off of the virus particle from the cell is located between the MA and CA domains. The specific name associated with the Gag cleavage products is derived from their respective apparent molecular weights ($\times 10^{-3}$).

an N-terminal myristic acid, which is thought to insert into the hydrophobic lipid bilayer. The second is a surface patch of basic amino acids that are hypothesized to mediate the initial interaction of Gag with the negatively charged, phospholipid head groups of the membrane. Mutations that interfere with either myristoylation or the charged residues can abrogate plasma membrane targeting, and in some instances, the mutated Gag precursors are targeted to internal membranes.[57]

In the betaretroviruses, where capsid assembly and virus budding are discrete events, a genetic dissection of this process has shown that Gag-containing precursors express a dominant sorting signal (the cytoplasmic targeting/retention signal [CTRS]) that targets the proteins to the initial assembly site.[28] Recent studies suggest that the CTRS interacts with Tctex-1, a light chain of the microtubule-associated dynein motor, and directs nascent Gag proteins and translating polysomes to the centriolar region of the cell, where capsid assembly occurs.[194,222] A point mutation within the Mason-Pfizer monkey virus (M-PMV) CTRS domain can abrogate intracytoplasmic targeting and results in the type C–like transport of precursors to the plasma membrane, where efficient capsid assembly occurs.[81] Efficient transport of wild-type capsids out of the assembly site depends on both the presence of the M-PMV Env protein and endosomal trafficking, and appears to reflect a requirement for Gag-Env interactions at the pericentriolar recycling endosome.[193] Interestingly, studies in murine leukemia virus (MuLV), in which the viral RNA was tagged for visualization by fluorescence microscopy, have suggested that prebudding complexes of Env, Gag, and RNA associate with late endosomes and are routed in this way to the plasma membrane.[8] It is likely that similar preassembly complexes also participate in the intracellular transport of HIV-1 Gag proteins, because their transport is modulated by the cellular adaptins AP-1, AP-2, and AP-3, and intracellular interactions with Env direct Gag assembly to specific plasma membrane regions of the cell.[5,49] Although in macrophages HIV-1 Gag was initially thought to be targeted to a late endosomal compartment for intracellular assembly and budding, more recent studies suggest that these compartments are derived from deep invaginations of the plasma membrane[5,11] (see Fig. 6.7, Pathway 1d). Targeting of the plasma membrane by HIV-1 Gag for assembly in part reflects specific MA domain recognition of phosphatidylinositol 4,5-bisphosphate [PI(4,5)P_2], which is enriched there. Depletion of this lipid component by overexpression of the cognate phosphatase (5-phosphatase IV) redirects HIV-1 assembly away from the plasma membrane to internal membranes.[5]

Irrespective of the assembly site, Gag precursor proteins must associate in a reproducible fashion to assemble into the nascent capsid. Mutational analyses of *gag* genes, as well as *in vitro* assembly studies, have shown that the CA and NC domains of Gag play a critical role in assembly; MA is dispensable for this process.[36,57] NC binding to RNA may act to nucleate the capsid assembly process, whereas CA forms a symmetrical hexameric network of proteins. *In vitro,* the CA protein alone can assemble into tubes that exhibit local sixfold symmetry (hexamers), and cryo-electron tomography studies of immature HIV-1 capsids have revealed a similar but distinct arrangement of the CA domain of Gag. A striking observation in the context of HIV-1 is that released immature virus particles have an incomplete protein shell, with the ordered

Gag lattice covering, on average, only two-thirds of the membrane surface.[19,231]

For most retroviruses, capsid assembly drives the process of membrane extrusion known as budding. As we will discuss later, for an infectious virus to be formed, the Gag precursors (or for other viruses, NPs) and surface glycoproteins of the virus must be targeted to the same region of the same membrane. In this way, during virus budding, a proper complement of glycoproteins can be incorporated into the nascent virion.

Assembly of Enveloped Viruses at Cellular Membranes

For most enveloped viruses, the location within the cell at which envelopment takes place is determined by the targeting to or retention of the viral glycoproteins at that site. Indeed, with the exception of the retroviruses, the efficiency of virus budding and particle release highly depends on the presence of the envelope glycoprotein(s), and in its absence, few particles are produced. Because the glycoproteins define the site of virus budding, specific interactions between the viral NP and the glycoproteins, sometimes mediated by a matrix protein, must take place to ensure that the genome of the virus is incorporated. For each of the viruses that assemble at intermediate points within the secretory pathway, fully assembled viruses must traverse the remainder of the pathway to be released from the cell (Fig. 6.9). Glycoproteins on these released viruses have complex oligosaccharides and are most likely modified by the Golgi-localized enzymes on the way to the cell surface.

Assembly at the Endoplasmic Reticulum–Golgi Intermediate Compartment

The coronaviruses are positive-stranded RNA viruses with large (30-kb) genomes packaged in a helical nucleocapsid. The nucleocapsid acquires its envelope by budding into the lumen of the ERGIC, a pre-Golgi compartment of the secretory pathway. Coronaviruses invariably encode three envelope proteins. The spike protein (S), which determines the host range of the virus, is a type I glycoprotein that forms the distinct bulbous peplomers of the virus. Expressed independently of the other glycoproteins, infectious bronchitis virus (IBV) S is transported to the plasma membrane, although it does contain both ER retention and endocytosis signals that can redirect it to the ERGIC.[106] The most abundant virion protein is the membrane (M) glycoprotein. M spans the lipid bilayer three times, exposing a short N-terminal domain outside the virus and a long C-terminus inside the virion. Because of its abundance and because M is transported to the Golgi complex but not to the surface, it was initially thought to define the site at which this family of viruses was enveloped. Studies, however, have shown that the small envelope protein (E), which is only

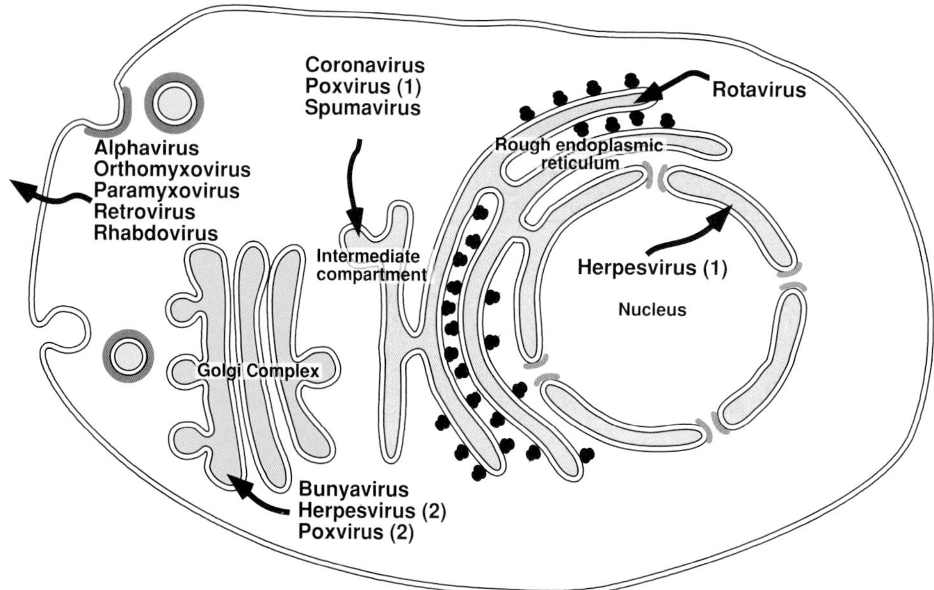

FIGURE 6.9. Viral assembly at cellular membranes. Schematic representation shows the intracellular locations at which enveloped virus assembly takes place. For each virus that is enveloped at organelles within the secretory pathway, the virions must traverse the remainder of the pathway to be released from the cell. Rotaviruses appear to utilize the ER membrane as a scaffold for assembly of virion proteins—the capsids that form during the assembly process are only transiently enveloped, and nonenveloped particles accumulate in the lumen of the ER. Coronaviruses localize the three membrane proteins (E, M, and S) in the ER–Golgi intermediate compartment, and virus budding occurs into the lumen of this compartment of the secretory pathway. In contrast, the vaccinia virus nucleocapsid appears to be wrapped by a double membrane derived from this compartment [Poxvirus (1)] but remains free in the cytoplasm so that it can then be further enveloped by Golgi-derived membranes [Poxvirus (2)]. Similarly, herpesviruses initially bud into the lumen of the nuclear membrane [Herpesvirus (1)]; however, after fusion and release of the capsid into the cytoplasm, it is re-enveloped by Golgi membranes [Herpesvirus (2)]. The G1 and G2 glycoproteins of bunyaviruses co-localize in the trans-Golgi compartment to direct budding of nucleocapsids at this location. For the retroviruses, which can assemble and release virus particles in the absence of envelope glycoproteins, the envelope glycoproteins appear to direct virus budding to the basolateral plasma membrane of polarized epithelial cells. ER, endoplasmic reticulum.

a minor component of virions, is the key to defining the site and nature of coronavirus envelopment.[77] E is a hydrophobic type I membrane protein that localizes to the ERGIC and induces the formation of tubular, convoluted membrane structures characteristic of virus infection.[34,166] The E protein of IBV appears to be retained in the ERGIC by a novel ER retrieval signal (RDKLYS-COOH) and localizes M to this site through intermolecular interactions.[102] Co-expression of E, M, and S results in the assembly and release from cells of virus-like particles (VLPs) containing these three viral membrane proteins. The enveloped particles produced by this system form a homogeneous population of spherical particles indistinguishable from authentic virions in size and shape.[221] Only M and E are required for efficient particle formation, and expression of E alone can mediate particle release.[110] The S glycoprotein is thus dispensable for virus particle assembly but is retained in the Golgi by the M protein, which appears to direct its assembly into virions. M protein also directs the incorporation of nucleocapsids containing the genome-length RNA into virions, and nucleocapsids associated with newly synthesized M protein have been localized to the budding site in the ERGIC.[135]

Although most retroviruses are enveloped at the plasma membrane of the cell, for most members of the spumavirus genus, this occurs on internal membranes. In human fibrosarcoma cells, primate foamy virus (FV) Gag and Env appear to co-localize predominantly in the trans-Golgi region of the cell;[235] however, in other cells, immature capsids appear to bud into the ERGIC region of the secretory pathway. This is consistent with the observation that expression of the primate FV Env complex, gp80/gp48, in the absence of other structural proteins, results in its localization to the ER. A di-lysine ER retrieval motif at the C-terminus of gp48 is responsible for this localization, and mutation of either lysine results in efficient transport of the protein to the plasma membrane. Although a greater fraction of capsids bud from the plasma membrane in mutant virus–infected cells, envelopment of capsids at the ER is still observed.[66] A second distinguishing feature of foamy viruses is the dependence of capsid envelopment on Env expression.[6] As with the betaretroviruses, assembly of immature FV capsids is targeted to the pericentriolar region of the cell by a CTRS located around an arginine residue at position 50 in Gag.[235] They are then transported to the ER (or plasma membrane) for envelopment. In the absence of FV Env, these preassembled capsids do not associate with membranes or initiate budding. Recent experiments have shown that it is the posttranslationally cleaved (148 amino acids long), membrane-spanning, signal peptide domain of the FV Env that mediates capsid membrane association/envelopment; they have also shown that this protein is incorporated into the virus in the process.[103]

Assembly in the Golgi Complex

Bunyaviruses are negative-stranded, enveloped viruses with a segmented genome that assembles in tube-like virus factories that are built around the Golgi complex and are connected to mitochondria and rough ER[226] (see Fig. 6.9). By physically juxtaposing viral RNA replication and assembly, these factories appear to allow accumulation of RNPs that can associate with viral glycoproteins and bud into the lumen of swollen Golgi stacks. The glycoprotein spikes of the best-characterized member of this family, Uukuniemi virus, are comprised of two type I glycoproteins—Gn (previously G1) and Gc (G2)—that determine the site of virus budding. Gn and Gc are cotranslationally cleaved from a single precursor protein by signal peptidase, which cleaves after the internal signal sequence that mediates translocation of Gc. The two proteins have been shown to fold with distinctly different kinetics, but once properly folded, they form a Gn-Gc heterodimer that is transported to the Golgi complex. Gc expressed in the absence of Gn is retained in the ER, whereas Gn expressed alone is targeted to the Golgi.[71] The Uukuniemi virus Golgi localization signal of Gn has been mapped, through analysis of mutations and glycoprotein chimeras, to the membrane proximal half of the 98 amino acid long cytoplasmic tail of the protein. Glycoprotein retention in this case appears, therefore, to depend on interactions between the cytoplasmic tail of Gn in the Gn-Gc heterodimer with components residing on the cytoplasmic side of the Golgi membrane. However, although all bunyavirus Gn-Gc complexes accumulate in the Golgi, the exact location and nature of the signal(s) that ensure this do appear to differ among the genera.[226]

During assembly of bunyaviruses, the helical nucleoproteins, consisting of the three single-stranded genomic RNA segments and the associated nucleocapsid (N) protein, accumulate in the Golgi component of the virus factories and through interactions with the Gn and Gc cytoplasmic domains initiate the budding of virus particles into the Golgi lumen. The region of the secretory pathway at which Gn-Gc heterodimers accumulate clearly defines the budding site, because in the presence of brefeldin, a drug that redistributes Golgi components to the ER, virus budding occurs into the ER.[71]

Assembly at the Plasma Membrane

Members of several virus families undergo their envelopment at the plasma membrane. These families include the togaviruses, the rhabdoviruses, the para- and orthomyxoviruses, and the retroviruses. In each of these cases, the viral glycoproteins, either as hetero-oligomeric complexes or homo-oligomers, have traversed the entire secretory pathway to be delivered to the plasma membrane of the cell. Assembly at the plasma membrane obviates the need for the assembled virus to navigate additional compartments of the secretory pathway, because virions are released directly into the external milieu of the cell. Alphaviruses are among the best characterized of these different viral systems, because a combination of biochemical, genetic, and structural information has been amassed to shed light on the complexity of this assembly process. The major glycoproteins E1 and E2 of the alphaviruses are translated from a subgenomic 26S RNA as a pE2, 6K, E1 precursor complex. The 6K and E1 proteins are released from the precursor by signal peptidase but remain in a complex with pE2. Following transport to the Golgi, pE2 is processed to E2 and E3. Stable trimers of E1-E2 heterodimers are then transported to the plasma membrane, where they associate with nucleocapsids formed from the capsid (C) protein and genome-length RNA. The 6K protein travels to the plasma membrane with the E1-E2 complex but is inefficiently incorporated into virions.[62,89] Cryo-electron microscopy analyses of mature alphavirus particles have revealed a detailed structure of this enveloped virion (Chapters 3 and 23). These studies have shown that both the envelope and the core display icosahedral symmetry. Surprisingly, however, the trimers of E1 and E2 are located at the threefold and quasi-threefold symmetry axes of the pentameric and hexameric order of the nucleocapsid. Moreover, the heterodimers of each spike splay out above the membrane in a skirt-like fashion, traverse the lipid bilayer individually, and interact with three underlying capsid (C) proteins that belong to three separate capsomeres. This creates a complex network of molecular interactions where the glycoprotein–capsid protein interactions mediate not only the binding of the nucleocapsid to the spikes but also stabilize the connections between the capsomeres.[89] Above the membrane, the skirts formed by the E1-E2 heterodimers form lateral connections that mimic the pentameric and hexameric arrangement of the capsid. These interactions may facilitate the process of budding by providing a multivalent binding site for the capsid, as well as by providing a force for membrane bending. Budding, however, requires a cooperative interaction between the glycoproteins and the capsid protein, because in the absence of either, budding does not occur. Moreover, mutations in the cytoplasmic tail of the E2 protein alone can abrogate budding. Two models have been proposed for assembly.[62] In the first, glycoprotein trimers assemble around a preformed nucleocapsid that is associated with the inner leaflet of the plasma membrane. The second hypothesizes that it is through interactions between E1-E2 heterotrimers that the icosahedral structure of the virus is established and that interactions between the E1-E2 heterodimers and C proteins organize the nucleocapsid similarly. Evidence for the latter model came from deletion mutants in C that are defective in the formation of intracellular capsids but that nevertheless can associate with E1-E2 to facilitate the release of $T = 4$ icosahedral capsids.[56]

For the negative-strand RNA viruses, orthomyxoviruses, paramyxoviruses, and rhabdoviruses, an additional protein, the matrix protein, mediates the interactions between the viral glycoproteins and the RNP and appears to play a key role in envelopment. These proteins are able to bind to membranes through hydrophobic domains or, as with the retroviruses, through a cluster of positively charged residues that initiate electrostatic interactions with the plasma membrane. Cross-linking studies have demonstrated that these M proteins form homo-oligomers in the virus and can self-associate *in vitro* or when expressed at high levels in cells. As discussed earlier, the M1 protein of influenza virus acts to mediate the transport of RNPs from the nucleus to the site of virus assembly on the plasma membrane, and it seems likely that the intracytoplasmic transport pathway for this M1-vRNP complex involves interactions with cytoskeletal components of the cell.[4] The importance of the M protein in the paramyxovirus budding process was inferred from the defective measles viruses found in subacute sclerosing pan-encephalitis that are unable to assemble virus particles and that have mutations in the M protein coding region.[13] However, the development of reverse genetics systems for the negative-stranded viruses, in which mutations can be reintroduced into the viral genome, has allowed a more rational approach to examining these questions. Construction of rhabdovirus genomes that lack the M coding region resulted in a dramatic (more than 10^5-fold) decrease in the release of virus particles, and those that were released lacked the characteristic bullet-shape morphology. The defect could be complemented by expression of M in trans.[120] Thus, in the rhabdoviruses, the M protein condenses the helical RNP into its characteristic shape and mediates the envelopment process. Similarly, for the orthomyxoviruses, M1 can define whether spherical or filamentous forms of the virus particle are produced[17]; although in the absence of M1 particles can be released, this is a much less efficient process.[178]

Reverse genetics approaches have also shed light on the role of the G glycoprotein in rhabdovirus assembly and of the HA and NA in orthomyxovirus assembly. Rhabdoviruses that lack the G-protein coding domain do assemble and release bullet-shaped particles but at only 3% to 10% the efficiency of wild-type.[119,173] Initial studies with G proteins lacking a cytoplasmic tail have suggested that this domain might be important in the budding process; however, more recent studies have shown that although there is a general requirement for a short cytoplasmic tail, it is amino acid sequence independent, and that G proteins with large C-terminal extensions can be efficiently incorporated into virions, thereby leaving the basis for M protein interactions with G unresolved.[88] Although foreign glycoproteins can be efficiently incorporated into rhabdovirus particles (creating pseudotype particles), they do not stimulate budding.[171] This is consistent with experiments that have identified a domain within the extracellular membrane-proximal stem (GS) of vesicular stomatitis virus (VSV) G that is required for efficient VSV budding. Recombinant viruses encoding glycoprotein chimeras with 12 or more membrane-proximal residues of the GS, as well as the G protein transmembrane and cytoplasmic tail domains, produced near-wild-type levels of particles. In contrast, those with shorter regions produced 10- to 20-fold fewer particles. It is possible, therefore, that this region of the G protein membrane-proximal domain modifies the membrane to facilitate the budding process.[173] Recent cryo-electron microscopy studies of VSV suggest that assembly begins with the formation of an RNA-N protein nucleocapsid ribbon, which, after forming a tight ring that represents the tip of the bullet-shaped particle, is forced to curl into larger rings that eventually tile the helical trunk. The assembling structure would be stabilized by the binding of M protein to the outside of the nucleocapsid, which in turn forms a triangular platform for binding G-trimers and the lipid membrane.[64]

In influenza virus, the fact that the cytoplasmic domains of all three membrane proteins (HA, NA, and M2) are highly conserved in all isolates of the virus pointed to a role for these domains in assembly of enveloped virus. Early studies indicated that HA proteins with foreign cytoplasmic tails are not incorporated into virions, although HAs lacking this domain can be incorporated at levels 50% that of wild-type.[133] Studies using reverse genetics have confirmed these findings and have shown that the short (six amino acid) cytoplasmic domain of NA also plays an important role in morphogenesis. Viruses encoding the truncated NA protein were released less efficiently and were larger and more filamentous. However, in viruses encoding tailless versions of both HA and NA, a 10-fold reduction in virus release was observed and morphogenesis was drastically altered. Virus particles released from these cells were greatly elongated with an extended irregular shape and a reduced level of viral RNA. Similarly, truncation of the cytoplasmic tail of M2, which binds to M1, results in much reduced virus infectivity, coupled with reduction in the amount of packaged RNA and budding efficiency.[118] Thus, it appears that for influenza virus, the interactions between M1 and the viral membrane-spanning proteins are so important for envelopment and morphogenesis that the virus has developed redundant interaction domains in these proteins.[136,178]

With the exception of the spumaviruses, glycoprotein–capsid interactions are not absolutely required for the assembly and release of enveloped retrovirus particles; the Gag precursor alone contains the information necessary to be specifically targeted to the plasma membrane and to drive budding. Nevertheless, for members of the lentivirus family, such as HIV and simian immunodeficiency virus (SIV), that encode envelope glycoproteins with a long (150+ amino acid) cytoplasmic domain, a specific interaction between this region of the transmembrane component of Env and the MA domain of the Gag precursor appears to be necessary for Env incorporation. For these viruses, mutations in MA or in the cytoplasmic tail can abrogate Env incorporation.[26] Whereas viral glycoproteins are not required for assembly and budding of most retroviruses, in the case of M-PMV, Env appears to facilitate the intracellular transport of Gag molecules to the plasma membrane.[193] An understanding of the process by which Gag is transported to the plasma membrane remains incomplete; however, there is a growing body of evidence that Gag and Env may interact at intracellular sites and utilize components of the endocytic pathway to target these structural gene products, as well as genomic RNA, to an assembly site on the plasma membrane. Further evidence for an Env–Gag interaction is derived from polarized epithelial cells, where retroviral glycoproteins define the plasma membrane domain at which virus budding and release occur (see later discussion).

Several viruses appear to make use of cholesterol- and sphingolipid-rich domains on the plasma membrane known as lipid rafts to assist in the concentration and organization of viral components for assembly.[25] These rafts are characterized by their insolubility in detergent at low temperatures (4°C), and proteins associated with them remain in the insoluble fraction following extraction from cells. Both HA and NA of influenza virus cluster in lipid rafts via targeting signals that have been mapped to both their transmembrane and cytoplasmic domains, and it is hypothesized that through interactions with the clustered glycoproteins, M1 and the vRNPs are organized for budding.[137] Consistent with these observations, the lipid bilayer of influenza virions is enriched in cholesterol and sphingolipids and appears also to be in ordered domains.[189] Similarly, the glycoproteins and capsid precursors of HIV-1 have been shown to associate with lipid rafts, and depletion of cholesterol from the plasma membrane impairs HIV-1 particle production.[225] Gag-Env interactions appear to be required for Env association with lipid rafts, as mutations in either MA or the cytoplasmic domain of the gp41transmembrane protein that interfere with Gag-gp41 interactions prevent Env association with rafts.[10] Although it was initially assumed that VSV assembled independently of rafts, it has been shown that G clusters in microdomains and can co-localize on the plasma membrane with proteins known to be located in rafts.[163] Thus, it is possible that VSV also utilizes rafts to organize its components for assembly.

Targeting of Viral Glycoproteins in Polarized Epithelial Cells Defines the Site of Budding

Many viruses initiate their infection of a host by interacting with cells at an epithelial surface. Individual cells within an epithelial layer are tightly connected by junction complexes that form a barrier to diffusion of molecules throughout the cell membrane and divide the cell surface into two distinct plasma membrane domains: the apical domain, which faces the exterior, and the basolateral domain, which faces the interior. As a result of differential targeting of lipids and protein components to apical and basolateral membranes, epithelial cells in tight monolayers are highly polarized with each plasma membrane domain having a distinct lipid and protein composition.[175] The assembly and release of many viruses from epithelial cells is also highly polarized, occurring selectively at either the apical or basolateral surface. Influenza virus releases newly assembled virions from the apical surface of polarized epithelial cells, whereas VSV and many retroviruses are released from the basolateral membrane. In the absence of other viral proteins, VSV G protein and several retroviral Env proteins are transported to the basolateral surface, whereas HA, NA, and M2 are targeted to the apical membrane.[32,136] Sorting of proteins to one or the other domain occurs in the trans-Golgi network, and recent evidence suggests that proteins destined for the basolateral surface contain within their cytoplasmic domain motifs that direct the protein to that membrane. In the VSV G protein, a tyrosine-based motif within the cytoplasmic tail appears to be critical for basolateral targeting.[214] Similarly, tyrosine-based endocytosis motifs in the cytoplasmic domain of both the MuLV and HIV Env proteins are important for their polarized expression and for basolateral budding of their cognate viruses.

Apical transmembrane proteins appear to contain two signals that probably act cooperatively in targeting to the apical surface. Glycosylation in the ectodomain and a signal in the membrane-spanning domain function together to ensure association with sphingolipid-cholesterol–enriched membrane domains or rafts, which have been proposed to mediate apical transport in polarized epithelial cells.

In the absence of a basolateral targeting signal, retroviral Env proteins are delivered to and virus buds from both membranes with equal efficiency, arguing that interactions with Env guide Gag to the basolateral surface.[105] The rhabdoviruses differ in this regard, in that even when the basolateral targeting signal for G has been mutated such that G is transported to the apical surface, virus assembly still occurs predominantly at the basolateral surface. Similarly, under conditions where the influenza virus HA is directed to the basolateral surface, virus budding remains predominantly apical. In these viruses, therefore, it appears that the internal components of the virion possess independent targeting signals that direct them to their respective membranes.[136] Polarized virus assembly and release may be important in determining the pathogenesis of viral infections, as it can influence, in a major fashion, the pattern of virus spread in the infected host.[32]

Complex Interactions with the Secretory Pathway

Whereas most enveloped viruses undergo assembly and envelopment at a single site within the secretory pathway, some viruses have a more complex interaction that can involve de-envelopment or re-envelopment as part of their assembly pathway.

Rotavirus Assembly Within the Endoplasmic Reticulum

Rotaviruses are nonenveloped viruses that undergo transient envelopment at the ER as an essential step in the formation of the mature double-shelled (triple-layered) virus that is retained within the lumen of the ER until cell lysis. As with the reoviruses, the nucleocapsid, in this case containing

11 double-stranded RNA segments, is assembled in electron-dense areas of the cytoplasm, located close to the ER membrane, known as viroplasm. This assembly domain depends on expression of two nonstructural proteins—NS2 and NS5—and mutations or silencing of either gene product results in its abrogation.[55,107,159] The nucleocapsids that assemble have an outer icosahedral shell assembled from VP6, the most abundant protein of the virus, surrounding an inner core (Chapters 44 and 45). They appear to bud directly into regions of the ER that contain the two outer shell proteins VP7 and VP4. A nonstructural protein, NSP4, which forms hetero-oligomers with the two outer shell proteins, mediates the interaction of the immature particle with the ER membrane.[125,147,212]

The exact topology of VP7 in the ER is not known. The mature protein has a cleaved signal peptide but is retained in the ER as if it were an integral membrane protein.[94,200] VP4 is thought to associate with VP7 and NSP4 just prior to budding of the nucleocapsid into the ER. Enveloped particles can be observed in the lumen of the ER, which then undergo a process of calcium-dependent de-envelopment, forming in the process an outer icosahedral shell of VP7 and VP4.[165] This process seems to be directed by VP7 because the silencing of this protein has not blocked the budding of double-layered particles into the ER but instead has arrested maturation at the membrane-enveloped particle stage in this compartment.[182] The rapid association of VP4 with lipid rafts and the nonlytic release of rotaviruses from the apical plasma membrane of gut epithelial cells has led to the suggestion that the site of budding might be the ERGIC and that rafts may play a role in transport of virus directly from this region to the plasma membrane.[37,47] Thus, this nonenveloped icosahedral virus appears to transiently utilize membranes of the secretory pathway as a scaffold on which to assemble an icosahedral shell and a nontraditional vesicle-mediated route to the plasma membrane.

Herpesvirus Transport from the Nucleus

As we described previously, the end product of herpesvirus capsid assembly is a large icosahedral structure that is too large to transit the nuclear pore. Members of this family have therefore evolved to utilize a complex envelopment/de-envelopment/re-envelopment strategy that allows the final acquisition of a lipid envelope to occur at a late compartment of the secretory pathway[121] (Fig. 6.10). The first evidence for this initially controversial pathway came from electron microscopic observations of infected cells.[71,169] Capsids that have assembled in the nucleus acquire an envelope derived from the inner leaflet of the nuclear membrane as they bud into the lumenal space (termed *primary envelopment*). Products of the UL31 and UL34 genes are involved in this process—the former encoding a nuclear phosphoprotein and the latter encoding a type II membrane protein. Both proteins are located on the nuclear membrane; however, the UL31 protein requires UL34 for nuclear targeting. Absence of either protein abrogates primary envelopment and results in capsid accumulation in the nucleus.[167] Although these proteins are components of the primary enveloped virions, they are absent from mature virions. Primary envelopment does not occur in the absence of the pUL25 capsid-associated protein and thus appears to be required for the budding process.[97] The initially enveloped virions lack proteins that are abundant in mature virus particles (e.g., pUL47 or pUL49), indicating that the most prominent components of the viral tegument have to be added during later steps of virion morphogenesis.[123]

In the de-envelopment step, the newly enveloped virus fuses with the outer nuclear membrane to release the capsid into the cytoplasm. It is here that tegument proteins of the mature virus, a collection of proteins including transcription factors located between the viral capsid and its lipid bilayer in the mature particle, are proposed to associate with the capsid prior to its re-envelopment by Golgi-derived membrane vesicles.[123] For herpes simplex virus and pseudorabies virus, glycoproteins of the gE/I complex together with gM appear to be essential for the re-envelopment step, and in their absence, intracytoplasmic aggregates of tegument-associated capsids are formed.[18]

Some of the clearest evidence for this complex assembly pathway comes from studies of human cytomegalovirus (HCMV) and human herpesvirus 6 (HHV-6). In these viruses, the tegument is a dense structure that can be observed in electron micrographs. Enveloped virions in the lumen of the nuclear membrane display no evidence of tegument but acquire this layer following loss of the nuclear-derived envelope and subsequent release into the cytoplasm.[176,216] Studies of the glycoproteins of the gamma herpesvirus, Epstein-Barr virus, also support this model. Distribution of the viral glycoproteins gp110 and gp350/220 is consistent with the former being incorporated in virions at the nuclear membrane and then lost on budding into the cytoplasm, whereas the latter is acquired only during re-envelopment in the Golgi.[67] Similarly, studies of the lipid composition of extracellular HSV-1 virions indicate that it is similar to that of the Golgi complex and distinct from that of the nucleus.[220] Why would viruses evolve to utilize such

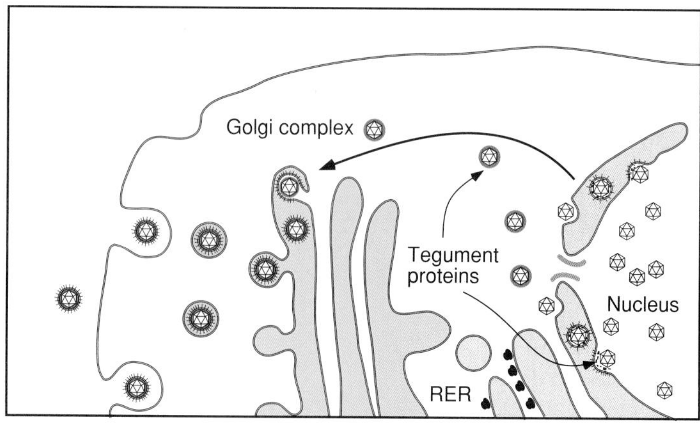

FIGURE 6.10. Herpesvirus assembly. In the re-envelopment pathway, nascent assembled capsids bud into the lumen of the nuclear membrane utilizing a subset of virally encoded glycoproteins. These enveloped particles then fuse with and are released from the outer nuclear membrane into the cytoplasm. There they associate with the tegument proteins and are transported through the cytoplasm to be enveloped by Golgi-derived membranes that contain the full complement of virion glycoproteins.

a complex assembly strategy? Perhaps the most persuasive argument comes from the perspective of the neurotropic alphaherpesviruses. These viruses infect nerve endings in the periphery; however, DNA replication and capsid assembly must occur in the cell body. To initiate a second round of infection at the nerve synapse, viral components must be transported down the axon. Thus, by separately transporting the viral capsids on microtubules and viral glycoproteins by the vesicular pathway, the site at which infectious virus is assembled can be much more accurately controlled.[120,215]

Poxvirus Acquisition of Multiple Membranes

Poxviruses, exemplified by vaccinia virus, exhibit an equally complex interaction with the secretory pathway. These large DNA viruses, which encode all of the machinery necessary for genomic replication and transcription, propagate entirely in the cytoplasm in specialized areas designated as virus factories (Chapters 66 and 67). The assembly and envelopment of these viruses is particularly complex because they apparently can be enclosed by multiple lipid bilayers.[33,172] The first recognizable structure is a crescent-shaped membrane that appears to be comprised of a single lipid bilayer with an external protein lattice constituted of trimers of the D13 protein.[76,209] Initial electron microscopy studies suggested that the crescent membranes that wrap the immature virions (IV) are formed *de novo* within the virus factories,[42] and additional high-resolution electron microscopy experiments have been interpreted as support for the conclusion that the crescents are formed from a single membrane.[78] Nevertheless, the origin, mode of formation, and composition of these crescent membranes remains controversial. Several investigators have provided evidence that these envelopes are composed of two closely apposed membranes, which are derived from the IC of the secretory pathway.[168,198] Co-localization of IC resident cellular proteins with several vaccinia virus membrane proteins (A17L, A14L, and A13L) known to be critical for the formation of IV membranes have supported this model.[99,185] However, subsequent studies have shown that transport of proteins from the ER to the IC and Golgi is not necessary for IV formation and that there is a transport pathway from the ER to the assembling IV.[82] Moreover, epitope tagging of the L2 protein, an early poxvirus protein essential for crescent formation, showed that it was associated with the ER tubules throughout the cytoplasm and in some instances appeared to be continuous with the membrane crescents.[116] The D13 protein, which forms a honeycomb lattice on the outer surface of the IVs, is critical for crescent formation and appears to act as a scaffold for their formation through its interaction with the N-terminus of the membrane-spanning A17 protein.[14] Interestingly, Rouiller et al[180] have reported that the virus core of the related African swine fever virus core is also wrapped by specialized regions of the ER.

The process by which the nucleoprotein/transcription machinery is targeted into the immature envelopes is unclear; however, a multiprotein complex of seven viral proteins—A15, A30, D2, D3, F10, G7, and J1—appears to be critical. Repression of several of these viral products yields the same phenotype-the failure of viral membranes and viroplasm to associate with each other.[208] Maturation of the IV to the infectious intracellular mature virus (IMV) involves a series of proteolytic cleavages of vaccinia structural proteins.[33] The mature virus particles are transported out of the assembly areas toward the periphery of the cell, where additional membranes that are derived from the trans-Golgi or early endosomal compartments wrap them to form the intracellular enveloped virus (IEV).[196,197] The membranes of these compartments contain vaccinia proteins that will be present in the external enveloped virus (EEV). Wrapping requires the participation of at least one protein present on the IMV and two EEV membrane proteins. It thus appears to be driven by interactions between vaccinia-encoded membrane proteins.[15,174] It is likely then that the IEV contains at least three concentric membranes, one derived from the ER and two from the Golgi/endosome. These particles are then transported via a reorganized actin cytoskeleton (so-called actin-tails) to the plasma membrane,[38] where membrane fusion releases the infectious EEV form of the virus.

Modification of the Secretory Pathway

Transcription and Assembly of Poliovirus on a Disassembled Secretory Pathway

Poliovirus is a nonenveloped positive sense RNA virus that modifies the host cell extensively during its replication. Once introduced into a target cell, the genomic RNA is translated into a long polyprotein precursor that contains both structural and replicative proteins of the virus (Fig. 6.11). Early in the replication of the virus, there is a massive rearrangement of the intracellular membranes into clusters of vesicles that are 200 to 400 nm in diameter.[186] The altered membranes appear to have characteristics of autophagosomal vesicles; they have two membranes and contain, in addition to the viral RNA replication machinery, several autophagosomal proteins, including LAMP1 and LC3. Moreover, stimulation of autophagy has been shown to increase poliovirus yield, and inhibition of the autophagosomal pathway decreased virus yield, suggesting subversion of this pathway by poliovirus.[85,213] Electron microscopy and inhibitor studies have suggested that the induced vesicles are derived from the host cell secretory pathway, as they appear to be connected to ER membranes and both their formation and poliovirus replication are blocked by Brefeldin A.[83] Viral RNA transcription occurs in close association with these vesicles, and both viral RNA and viral proteins known to be required for RNA replication have been shown by electron microscopy to be associated with their cytoplasmic surface.[12,217] Similarly, priming of RNA synthesis by the protein primer VPg appears to require membranes.[211] For poliovirus, the viral precursor protein 2BC, when expressed alone, was shown to cause both membrane vesiculation and the formation of multilamellar structures[27]; however, it is in combination with poliovirus protein 3A, which causes the inhibition of ER-to-Golgi protein traffic,[50] that membrane alterations most consistent with the pattern in poliovirus-infected cells are observed.[206]

The formation of vesicular platforms for transcription may also be necessary for efficient capsid assembly. The poliovirus capsid appears to be assembled in a sequential process in which the 5S protomers containing VP1, VP3, and VP0 assemble to form 14S pentamers, which in turn are assembled into virus capsids (see Fig. 6.11). Pentamers may associate with newly synthesized genomic RNA on intracytoplasmic vesicles and then assemble to form RNA-containing capsids on completion of the RNA. This assembly pathway is supported by immunoelectron microscopy studies showing that pentamers associated with the replication complex can, if released by detergent, rapidly assemble into empty capsids—arguing that the vesicle

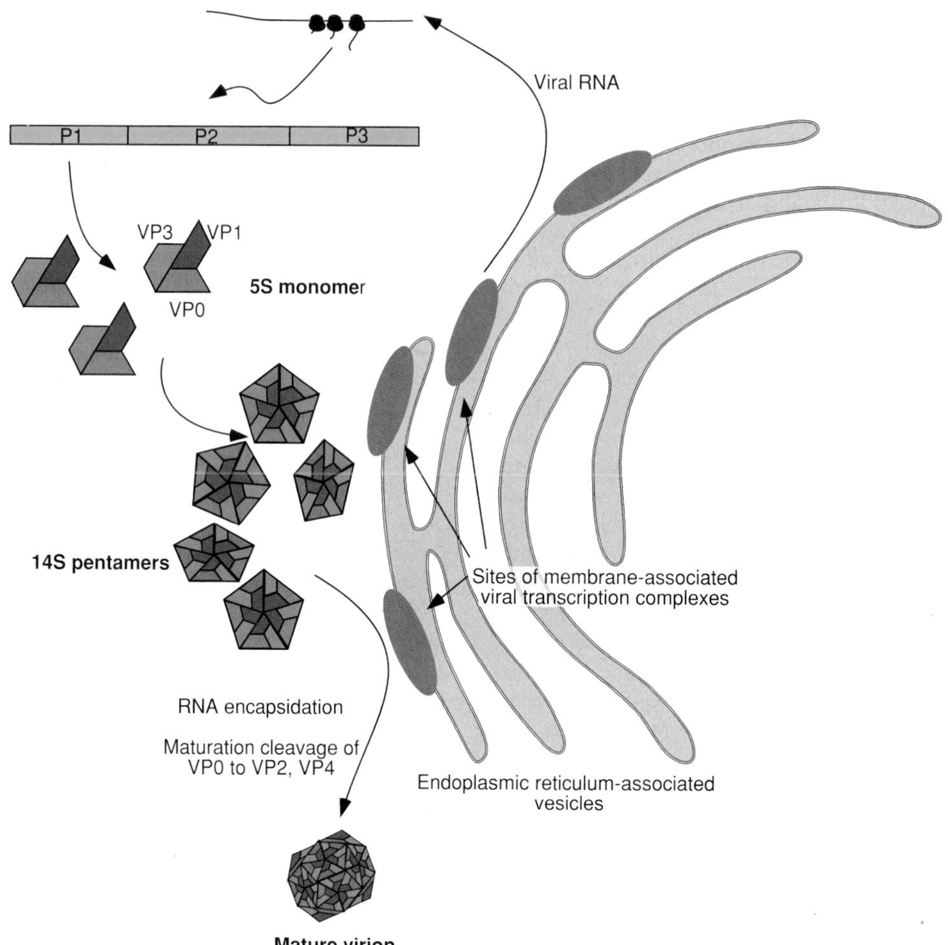

FIGURE 6.11. Poliovirus assembly. The P1 precursor protein is cleaved via an autocatalytic event from the nascent polyprotein and is then cleaved twice by the 3CD-protease to yield VP1, VP2, and VP0. This cleavage is essential for assembly of the 5S monomers into 14S pentamers. It is likely that 12 of these pentamers associate directly with nascent genomic RNA that is being transcribed from membrane-bound transcriptional complexes to assemble an immature 150S provirion. Maturation cleavage of VP0 to yield VP2 and VP4 results in conversion of these immature provirions into the 160S mature virion.

prevents assembly of the capsid and keeps the pentamer in an appropriate configuration for association with the RNA.[162] In this instance, poliovirus appears to have circumvented the problems of intracytoplasmic localization of replicative and structural components by utilizing a membranous organizing center.

Modification of Post-Golgi Vesicle pH by the Influenza Virus M2 Protein

The influenza HA is synthesized as a precursor protein (HA0) that in the case of the avian influenza viruses is cleaved in the trans-Golgi by furin-like proteinases to the biologically functional HA1-HA2 heterodimer, three of which in turn form the trimeric HA complex (Chapters 3, 40 and 41). The influenza virus HA present on an infecting virion is activated to its fusogenic state by the low pH of the endosome. Thus, the similarly low pH of the trans-Golgi network and post-Golgi vesicles poses a problem for the virus during the assembly phase of its life cycle, if it is to maintain HA in a functional prefusogenic form. This is apparently solved by the action of the M2 protein, a small tetrameric protein that forms cation-selective ion channels that can reduce the pH of the trans-Golgi network by pumping out hydrogen ions.[164,205]

INCORPORATION OF THE NUCLEIC ACID GENOME DURING THE ASSEMBLY PROCESS

The processes involved in the assembly of structural components of a virus are complex and interplay intimately with those of the host cell; thus, they merely provide a mechanism by which the genomic information of the virus can be packaged into a protective environment for transfer to additional host cells. As such, the assembling virus must have evolved to efficiently select its genomic nucleic acid out of the pools of RNA and/or DNA that are present at the assembly site. Packaging of viral genomes generally involves a cis-acting sequence in the nucleic acid—the so-called packaging sequence—and a structural component(s) of the virus that can recognize and bind this element.

DNA Viruses

As described previously, for adenovirus, an empty procapsid is first formed around scaffolding proteins in a manner similar to that observed with DNA phages. Following procapsid assembly, DNA and associated core proteins are then subsequently packaged into these empty shells to yield "immature virions" that then undergo proteolytic maturation.

Early studies indicated that *light* virus particles contain subgenomic-length viral DNA with an overrepresentation of left-end sequences. Subsequent studies showed that a cis-acting packaging sequence that is absolutely required for encapsidation of viral DNA is located within the left 390 bp of the genome. This region is highly conserved between different adenovirus subtypes and, in Ad 5, overlaps with two distinct enhancer elements for E1A transcription. Deletion of the packaging domain abrogates viability; however, infectivity can be restored by substitution of the left-end sequences at the right end of the genome.[73,74] The packaging sequence only functions if it is within 600 bp of the inverted terminal repeat (ITS) but does not depend on the ITS itself.[152] Mutational analyses showed that this packaging region contains at least seven functional AT-rich units called *A-repeats.* These repeats are functionally redundant but not functionally equivalent. Moreover, a sequence homology shared by the most important A-repeats, 5′-TTTG-N_8-CG-3′, is essential for packaging domain function. Overexpression of an A-repeat multimer competes in *trans* resulting in a dramatic decrease in viral yield without affecting DNA replication or late transcription, suggesting the involvement of limiting viral protein components in packaging.[69,191] It seems likely from a variety of genetic analyses, *in vitro* DNA-binding studies, and chromatin immunoprecipitation approaches that the viral IVa2 protein together with the L4-22K protein bind directly to the A-repeat sequences to initiate packaging.[54,151,153] The L1 52/55K protein, which is also critical for DNA packaging, is a part of this complex perhaps through interactions with IVa2 or L4-22K.[153,161]

Packaging of the herpesvirus genome is equally complex. As with the large DNA phages, herpesvirus DNA replicates to yield concatemers of genomes in a head-to-tail arrangement, thus packaging must be linked to the generation of genomic-length units of DNA. In this virus, two packaging sequences—*pac1* and *pac2*—located within the terminally repeated *a* sequences appear to be important for both recognition and cleavage of the DNA (Chapters 59 and 60). As with the DNA phages, a combination of cleavage recognition sequences and *head-full* packaging appears to ensure the incorporation of unit-length genomes into the procapsid. Studies utilizing a temperature-sensitive protease mutant of HSV-1, which accumulates procapsids (containing an uncleaved scaffolding protein) at the nonpermissive temperature, although can remove the scaffold and package DNA on temperature shift to the permissive temperature, have shown that ATP is necessary for DNA packaging to occur but DNA synthesis is not.[30,44] At least seven viral proteins—products of the genes UL6, UL15, UL17, UL25, UL28, UL32, and UL33—are required for cleavage and packaging of HSV-1 DNA. When cells are infected with HSV-1, mutants lacking the function of any of the seven genes, capsid formation, and DNA replication occur normally; however, no packaging takes place. By analogy with the DNA bacteriophages such as P22, the portal vertex, which is assembled from 12 copies of the *UL6* gene product, likely forms the docking site for these packaging proteins. Sequence analysis reveals that another critical component, encoded by the *UL15* gene, shares homology with gp17, the large catalytic subunit of the bacteriophage T4 terminase. Thus, the product of this gene, together with that of UL28, which can specifically recognize the *pac* site, may play a direct role in the cleavage of viral DNA replication intermediates into monomers.[1,234]

RNA Viruses

For retroviruses, genomic packaging represents a particularly difficult problem because the assembling capsid must select genomic RNAs from a large pool of viral and cellular mRNAs that are also present in the cytoplasm. Viral RNAs to be specifically packaged are identified by the presence of an RNA sequence named the packaging signal or psi (ψ) and are selected from the cytoplasmic pool by a specific interaction with the zinc knuckle motif(s) of the NC domain of the Gag precursor.[41,108] The cis-acting RNA element is located at the 5′ end of the viral genome, has the capacity to mediate the packaging of heterologous RNAs, and appears to be comprised of a series of stem-loop structures that each contribute to the strength and specificity of the signal. One of the best characterized, although perhaps most complex, ψ-sequence is that of HIV-1, which is now known to span the 5′ untranslated region of the genome, as well as downstream nucleotides in the Gag region for optimal packaging efficiency. This 5′ untranslated region, which can confer packaging specificity on foreign RNAs, includes the TAR sequence that is important in Tat-mediated transcriptional control, the adjacent poly-A loop, and four stem loops that incorporate the primer binding site (PBS), the dimerization sequence (DIS), the 5′-splice donor (SD) and the packaging signal (ψ), respectively. Gag has been shown to bind specifically to this region, with PBS, DIS, and ψ stem loops each providing independent high-affinity binding sites. Disruptive and compensatory mutations within the TAR, Poly(A), PBS, DIS, and ψ elements indicate that the structure of the stem loops is important for packaging.[31,117] NMR analyses of SL3 in the presence and absence of the NC protein have shown that tight binding is mediated by specific interactions between the amino- and carboxyl-terminal CCHC-type zinc knuckles of the NC protein and nucleotide bases of the RNA loop.[45,108,237]

Regions of retroviral genomes that promote genome packaging often overlap with segments that promote the RNA dimerization, which is necessary for packaging of the diploid genome. Moreover, there is mounting evidence that dimerization and packaging events are intimately coupled. An elegant structural analysis by D'Souza and Summers[40] showed that dimerization of the MuLV genome results in an altered secondary structure in the psi region of the RNA, which exposes conserved UCUG elements that bind NC with high affinity. These elements are base paired and do not bind NC in the monomeric structure. Thus, for MuLV, the problem of ensuring the encapsidation of two genomic RNAs has been solved by linking exposure of the packaging recognition sequence to dimer formation itself. It seems likely that HIV and other retroviruses will utilize similar switches for this purpose.[148]

Given its role in specifying genomic RNA packaging, one might expect the ψ-sequence to be located downstream of the SD site for subgenomic mRNAs. This is the case for the MuLV and reticuloendotheliosis virus ψ-sequences but not the case for HIV-1, as described earlier, or for Rous sarcoma virus (RSV). The major RNA packaging signal for HIV-2 is present on all RNA species, although this virus appears to overcome the lack of packaging signal location specificity by two novel mechanisms—co-translational packaging and competition for limiting Gag polyprotein.[70]

The cellular location in which Gag:RNA recognition occurs remains an unanswered question. Parent et al[156] have provided strong evidence that for RSV, genome packaging depends on Gag trafficking through the nucleus, a process that is mediated by NLS and NES signals in the MA domain of Gag.[60,72] However, the role of nuclear trafficking of HIV-1 Gag in RNA packaging remains unresolved and controversial.[108,156] Recent experiments by Moore et al suggest that HIV-1 RNAs form dimers preferentially in the cytoplasm and that dimerization, mediated by the DIS sequence in the genome, is critical to efficient packaging into virions.[126,127] The incorporation of genomic RNA into assembling virions was recently imaged in live cells and showed that in the absence of Gag, genomic RNA molecules were highly dynamic and did not localize at specific sites at or near the plasma membrane. In contrast, in the presence of Gag, genomes were targeted to specific sites on the plasma membrane, where after initially exhibiting slow lateral movement they became fixed and were the site for accumulation of additional Gag molecules.[90,92]

Genomic RNA packaging signals in other RNA viruses are less well defined. In the alphaviruses, this appears to involve direct binding of genomic RNA by the capsid protein. A short (132-nt) segment of RNA in the region of the genome encoding the nonstructural protein NS1 is critical for this interaction and for packaging of genomic RNA. As with the retroviral psi-sequence, it has also been predicted to form a series of stem-loop structures. The N-terminal third of the capsid protein is basic and unstructured in the current crystal structure. Nevertheless, a 32 amino acid region (residues 76 to 107) has been shown to be essential for RNA binding in a gel shift assay.[190]

For segmented viruses, such as the orthomyxoviruses or the reoviruses, genomic packaging requires that a complete set of segments be packaged together in a single virus particle. For influenza virus, reverse genetic approaches have shown that the signals for transcription and replication of an RNA segment are located in the 22 5′ terminal and the 26 3′ terminal nucleotides of the RNA.[109] These studies do not, however, address how a full complement of RNAs is selected during assembly. Two models have been proposed to accomplish this. The random incorporation model assumes a common structural feature in all vRNPs, which enables them to be incorporated randomly into virions. Support for this model comes from the observation that an influenza A virion can possess more than eight vRNPs.[7,52] The selective-incorporation model predicts the presence of specific structures in each vRNA segment, leading to their individual incorporation into virions. Two lines of evidence support this hypothesis: the first was data showing that defective RNA segments could inhibit the packaging of the parental segment into virions,[51] and the second was the finding that viruses grown in the presence of bacterial NA and antibody to NA retained an extensively deleted NA vRNA, suggesting that the altered NA segment participates in viral replication and carries structural features required for its incorporation into virions.[80,232] Experiments utilizing reverse genetics approaches have further supported the selective-incorporation model by demonstrating that all eight vRNA segments must be present for efficient virion formation and that sequences within the coding region of the NA vRNA encode a signal that drives incorporation of this segment into virions.[59,101,132] Electron microscopic studies of serially sectioned influenza virus A particles, which showed the RNPs organized in a distinct pattern (seven segments of different lengths surrounding a central segment), also support a model where the eight segments are specifically packaged.[145]

POSTASSEMBLY MODIFICATIONS AND VIRUS RELEASE

Proteolytic Cleavage and Virus Maturation

Virus-encoded proteolytic enzymes play important roles in the process of assembly for many viruses and in a postassembly maturation step that is required for the development of an infectious particle for others. These cleavage events can act as molecular switches that introduce flexibility, as well as irreversibility, into the assembly process.

Proteolytic cleavage in the case of the alphaviruses, for example, is used to allow protein domains, translated from a single mRNA, to enter different transport pathways in the cell. The C protein, which is encoded at the 5′ end of the subgenomic 26S mRNA, folds co-translationally into an active serine proteinase that cleaves itself from the growing polypeptide chain. This releases the C protein into the cytoplasm for capsid assembly while freeing up the N-terminus of the signal peptide for the p62 glycoprotein precursor, which can then bind SRP and direct the ribosome to the ER.[62]

In the herpesviruses, proteolytic cleavage of the scaffolding protein occurs after assembly of the procapsid is complete and is a prerequisite for DNA packaging. The scaffolding proteins of HSV-1 are encoded by a pair of overlapping genes—UL26 and UL26.5—in which the open reading frame of UL26 is an in-frame N-terminal extension of that of UL26.5. The product of the smaller gene is the abundant scaffolding protein pre-VP22a, whereas the larger gene encodes a protease precursor, which cleaves itself internally to give the proteins VP24 (protease) and VP21. Temperature-sensitive mutants in UL26 that have an inactive proteinase at the nonpermissive temperature are blocked at the procapsid stage of assembly.[169]

A somewhat more complex proteolytic pathway is utilized by the picornaviruses to regulate the release of both structural and replicative protein components from the single polyprotein precursor that is translated from its positive-stranded RNA genome (see Fig. 6.11). The initial event in this proteolytic cascade is the primary cleavage in which the P1 structural protein precursor is separated from the P2-P3 precursor. This reaction is catalyzed by the 2A proteinase, which hydrolyzes a Tyr-Gly bond at its own amino-terminus. Whereas cleavage of the P2-P3 region is carried out by the 3C proteinase at Gln-Gly bonds, the efficient cleavage of the structural protein precursor at the VP0-VP3 and VP3-VP1 boundaries is catalyzed specifically by the 3CD precursor that includes the viral polymerase. Cleavage of the P1 precursor appears to be a prerequisite for entry of the capsid proteins into the assembly pathway. The final processing step is cleavage of VP0 to VP4 and VP2. This autocatalytic, maturational cleavage occurs late in the assembly pathway and appears to be linked to encapsidation of the viral RNA genome. It is likely that the structural alterations that accompany the cleavage event both stabilize the capsid and irreversibly commit the virus to the conformational changes induced on receptor binding that are necessary for productive infection of cells.[75]

A similar maturational cleavage is required following assembly and envelopment of retroviral capsids. As we described earlier, the retroviral capsid is assembled from polyprotein precursors that are encoded by the *gag* gene. The viral aspartyl proteinase is encoded by the *pro* region of the genome and is translated from unspliced, genome-length RNA by a ribosomal frameshift mechanism as a Gag-Pro or Gag-Pro-Pol precursor protein (Chapters 47 and 49). The presence of the Gag sequences ensures that this key enzyme is targeted to and incorporated into the assembling capsid. The mechanism by which the protease is activated late in the assembly process (most probably after envelopment is complete) is not known. Because the active enzyme is a homodimer of two protease subunits, it has been postulated that dimerization of proteinase precursors in the nascent capsid might allow a functional enzyme to form. However, in the betaretroviruses, the immature capsid contains a full complement of proteinase precursors, which are not activated until late in envelopment at the plasma membrane. Immature capsids of the betaretrovirus M-PMV are stable when isolated from infected cells; however, the protease can be activated to cleave the assembled precursors to their mature products by treatment with the reducing agent dithiothreitol, suggesting that modification of cysteine residues might act to regulate the initiation of proteolysis.[157]

Cleavage of the Gag precursors in the immature capsid is accompanied by a major morphological rearrangement in which the mature NC protein condenses the genomic RNA inside a CA shell (see Fig. 6.7)—the electron dense core structure of the virus seen in electron micrographs.[65] Cleavage at the N-terminus of CA induces a conformational change in the protein that allows the newly freed N-terminal proline to form a charge pair with a nearby aspartic acid, redirecting assembly from a *spherical* immature capsid to assembly of the cylindrical or cone-like core shell structure.[139,223] Maturational cleavage, as in the case of poliovirus, results in an irreversible commitment to the entry pathway. It prevents a simple reversal of the assembly process and presumably, through the formation of the core, allows the rearrangement of RNA and the reverse transcriptase into a conformation that is optimal for reverse transcription of the genome. In the absence of cleavage, reverse transcription cannot occur and the virions are noninfectious.[207]

Adenoviruses, like retroviruses, undergo a maturational cleavage after assembly that is essential for infectivity. The immature virions formed after DNA packaging contain five precursor proteins that must be processed before the mature infectious virion is produced. These include components of the core and the preterminal protein (pTP) used to initiate DNA synthesis. The 23kD adenovirus proteinase, which is encoded by the L3 region of the genome, is inactive in its purified form. It requires an 11 amino acid peptide present at the carboxy-terminus of pVI and viral DNA as co-factors for its activity. This unique use of DNA as a co-factor ensures that proteolytic maturation of the virus cannot take place until packaging of DNA is complete.[39,112]

Budding: Role of Viral and Cellular Proteins in Membrane Extrusion

It is clear from the discussions in previous sections that various strategies are utilized by different enveloped viruses to mediate the process of membrane extrusion that we have termed *budding*. Envelopment by a lipid bilayer fulfills two functions for a virus: it provides a protective outer layer into which can be embedded the necessary machinery for target cell attachment and entry, and, in most cases, it releases the virus into an environment that is topologically equivalent to the exterior of the cell. The strategies used to drive the budding process can be classified into three general mechanisms.[61] In the first, membrane extrusion is driven by envelope glycoproteins alone. This is exemplified by the E protein of the coronaviruses that is capable of inducing the release of VLPs in the absence of an RNP. The second strategy is that used by the retroviruses where the capsid precursors, in the absence of the viral glycoproteins, are able to efficiently induce membrane extrusion and particle release. In this instance, it is hypothesized that the tight interaction between the MA domain of Gag and the lipid bilayer, coupled with the force of Gag-Gag interactions in assembly, drives the budding process. The third mechanism is that of the alphaviruses, which involves interactions between the viral glycoprotein spikes and the assembled capsid. In this case, neither the glycoproteins nor the capsid alone can mediate budding. It appears that lateral interactions between the glycoproteins, coupled with cytoplasmic domain-capsid connections, progressively bend the membrane to form the spherical particle.[62]

For all of these mechanisms, the final step of budding—the process of pinching off—requires a membrane fusion event. For several viruses, it is now clear that this is a separable event that requires the involvement of both viral and host components. Experiments in HIV have shown that deletion of the p6 domain at the C-terminus of Gag results in a block to virus release at the pinching off stage,[68] and it is now understood that diverse retroviruses encode functionally equivalent Gag *late function* or L domains that are required for efficient release of virions.[48,130] Viral L domains fall into three classes based on their characteristic tetrapeptide sequence motifs—Pro-Thr/Ser-Ala-Pro (PTAP or PSAP), Pro-Pro-X-Tyr (PPXY), and Tyr-Pro-$(X)_n$-Leu [$YP(X)_nL$]. In many instances, these viral L domains are functionally interchangeable and can mediate pinching off of the virion even when positioned at different locations in Gag.[155,236] Evidence has accumulated over the past several years that these motifs interact with components of a complex cellular machinery that is used in the biogenesis of an endosomal compartment known as the multivesicular body (MVB). Unlike other mechanisms used by the cell to form and pinch off vesicles into the cytoplasm, this machinery facilitates the pinching off into the MVB of exosomes that have the same topology as virus. This process is mediated by a complex and highly conserved protein network—the endosomal sorting complex required for transport (ESCRT) machinery—which exists in all eukaryotes and consists of five hetero-oligomeric complexes (ESCRT-0, ESCRT-1, ESCRT-II, ESCRT-III, and VPS-4).[11,114,227] Components of this complex also appear to be involved in the last stage of cytokinesis, termed *abscission,* where, as with virus release, a membranous stalk must undergo membrane fission to release the two daughter cells.[23,128] Recent studies have shown that the ESCRT-0 complex functions to concentrate ubiquitinated cargo on endosomal membranes; the ESCRT-I and -II complexes together induce bud formation while remaining outside the vesicle; and the ESCRT-III complex mediates membrane scission from the cytosolic side of the bud.[230] Mammalian ESCRT-III is formed by charged multivesicular body proteins (CHMPs), a family of structurally related but highly divergent α-helical proteins that has 12 known members in humans.[114,227]

The initial indication that retroviral budding and this machinery were linked came from the observation that the ESCRT-I component Tsg101 interacted with p6 and that this interaction depended on the PTAP motif.[63] A Tsg101 interacting protein, AIP1, which can also interact directly with ESCRT-III, has been shown to interact with the $YP(X)_nL$ motif in both equine infectious anemia virus and HIV.[115,201] It is less clear how Gag proteins, which contain the PPXY motif, enter the pathway. These proteins interact with Nedd4 family members that are ubiquitin E3 ligases involved in the covalent attachment of ubiquitin to membrane-associated proteins.[184,233] Monoubiquitination has been shown to direct the modified protein to the MVB and likely functions to link PPXY L-domain proteins to the ESCRT machinery.[130]

In addition to those L-domains that play a major role in virus release, it is becoming clear that in several viruses, multiple auxiliary L-domains are present that can augment the process. In HIV-1, for example, there is evidence that the PTAP motif acts synergistically with ALIX-binding sequences at the C-terminus of p6 to optimize release.[114] Through these disparate and still incompletely understood mechanisms[114,227] viruses recruit components of ESCRT-III to the site of budding to mediate the process of membrane scission. Only a subset of the 12 proteins known to make up the ESCRT-III complex may be involved, as a recent study demonstrated that the co-depletion of CHMP2 or CHMP4 family members profoundly impairs HIV-1 release, whereas other CHMPs are not required.[129]

The ATPase vacuolar protein sorting 4 (VPS4) acts at a late stage of ESCRT function, providing energy for ESCRT dissociation. Recent live cell imaging studies reveal that ESCRT-III and VPS4 are rapidly and transiently recruited before HIV-1 particle release, supporting the notion that VPS4 has a direct role in HIV-1 budding.[9,93] Overexpression of a dominant negative mutant of this protein inhibits the budding of several retroviruses that encode each of the tetrapeptide motifs, arguing that divergent retroviruses all depend on the ESCRT sorting complex.[115,224]

What is now clear is that retroviruses are not the only virus family that interact with this cellular pathway. Late domain motifs that facilitate release of virions have been identified in the structural proteins of the filoviruses,[87] rhabdoviruses,[35] arenaviruses,[160,203] and paramyxoviruses,[192] suggesting that divergent virus families have adopted a common mechanism for this late stage in enveloped virus budding.

Influenza virus is an exception to this widespread dependence on the ESCRT machinery.[21] Rossman et al[177] showed that for this virus, it is the viral M2 protein, rather than a host component, that mediates virus membrane scission. During morphogenesis, the M2 protein localizes to the neck of budding virions, and a highly conserved amphipathic helix in the cytoplasmic tail appears to mediate a cholesterol-dependent alteration in membrane curvature. Mutation of the amphipathic helix results in failure of the virus to undergo membrane scission and virion release.[177,178] Thus, it is possible that viral proteins such as M2 are able to mimic the functions of the ESCRT III machinery by constricting the viral membrane and inducing the scission events required for virus release.

Mechanisms to Facilitate the Release of Nascent Particles

If viruses are to efficiently travel to an uninfected target cell, they face one last hurdle following envelopment and release. This is the need to avoid rebinding to receptors on the producing cell. For viruses such as the ortho- and paramyxoviruses, which utilize sialic acid as a receptor on the cell surface, this problem is circumvented by the incorporation of a receptor-destroying enzyme, a sialidase, which can remove these residues during transit through the secretory pathway. For influenza virus, the NA is critical for virus release because, in its absence, nascent virus binds to both the cell surface and other virions in large aggregates.[104]

Retroviruses have similarly evolved mechanisms to facilitate release and thereby reduce superinfection of a cell. Cells infected with one retrovirus are generally resistant to subsequent infection by a second virus of the same receptor class. The presumed mechanism for this viral interference is the synthesis of viral glycoproteins in large excess over the levels that are incorporated into virions with the effect that cellular receptors that are transported to the cell surface are already occupied by their ligand. This results in removal or down-regulation of the receptor from the cell surface. For HIV-1, down-regulation of the primary receptor CD4 seems to be crucial, because the virus has evolved two additional mechanisms to ensure this. Two of the accessory proteins encoded by HIV—Vpu and Nef—act by binding CD4 in the ER and at the cell surface, respectively, and targeting the receptor for degradation (Chapter 49).

Independent of this need to down-regulate viral receptors, recent work has demonstrated that virus escape from the cell surface, the last step of the replication cycle, is effectively targeted by a host cell restriction factor, tetherin (also known as BST2 or CD317). This protein was initially identified as the factor responsible for the block to virion release from certain cell types infected by HIV-1 mutants lacking the accessory gene *vpu*.[11,114,138,218] Tetherin can be induced by type I interferon and other proinflammatory stimuli and has an unusual topology in which the extracellular domain forms an extended parallel coiled-coil that is anchored at the N-terminus by a protein transmembrane domain and at the C-terminus by a glycosyl phosphatidylinositol GPI anchor. Biochemical and structural data favor a model where parallel tetherin dimers crosslink virions to the plasma membrane or the membrane of other virions.[11,114] Tetherin can restrict the release of all retroviral particles tested to date, including those of the spumavirus and betaretrovirus families, which preassemble capsids in the cytoplasm. In addition, mammalian tetherins block release of a variety of membrane viruses, including filoviruses, arenaviruses, rhabdoviruses, and at least one herpesvirus.[53,91] In turn, viruses have evolved countermeasures that have allowed them to overcome this inhibition of release. The Vpu protein of HIV-1 is the prototypical antagonist to tetherin and interacts through the transmembrane region to mediate down-regulation and lysosomal degradation of the host restriction factor. In the case of SIVs, this function is primarily carried out by the Nef protein, although in some instances, as in HIV-2 or Ebola virus, it can be mediated by the viral glycoprotein.[53] Given the diversity of mechanisms utilized to counteract tetherin, it is clear that this last step of the life cycle is critical to the virus. Indeed, the evolution of primate lentiviruses, particularly pandemic HIV-1, has been shaped by species-specific differences in this host cell restriction factor.[188]

REFERENCES

All cited references are available in the e-book.

1. Adelman K, Salmon B, Baines JD. Herpes simplex virus DNA packaging sequences adopt novel structures that are specifically recognized by a component of the cleavage and packaging machinery. *Proc Natl Acad Sci U S A* 2001;98:3086–3091.
2. Akarsu H, Burmeister WP, Petosa C, et al. Crystal structure of the M1 protein-binding domain of the influenza A virus nuclear export protein (NEP/NS2). *EMBO J* 2003;22:4646–4655.
3. Alber F, Dokudovskaya S, Veenhoff LM, et al. The molecular architecture of the nuclear pore complex. *Nature* 2007;450:695–701.
5. Balasubramaniam M, Freed EO. New insights into HIV assembly and trafficking. *Physiology (Bethesda)* 2011;26:236–251.
6. Baldwin DN, Linial ML. The roles of Pol and Env in the assembly pathway of human foamy virus. *J Virol* 1998;72:3658–3665.
7. Bancroft CT, Parslow TG. Evidence for segment-nonspecific packaging of the influenza a virus genome. *J Virol* 2002;76:7133–7139.
8. Basyuk E, Galli T, Mougel M, et al. Retroviral genomic RNAs are transported to the plasma membrane by endosomal vesicles. *Dev Cell* 2003; 5:161–174.
9. Baumgartel V, Ivanchenko S, Dupont A, et al. Live-cell visualization of dynamics of HIV budding site interactions with an ESCRT component. *Nat Cell Biol* 2011;13:469–474.
10. Bhattacharya J, Repik A, Clapham PR. Gag regulates association of human immunodeficiency virus type 1 envelope with detergent-resistant membranes. *J Virol* 2006;80:5292–5300.
11. Bieniasz PD. The cell biology of HIV-1 virion genesis. *Cell Host Microbe* 2009;5:550–558.
14. Bisht H, Weisberg AS, Szajner P, et al. Assembly and disassembly of the capsid-like external scaffold of immature virions during vaccinia virus morphogenesis. *J Virol* 2009;83:9140–9150.
15. Blasco R, Moss B. Extracellular vaccinia virus formation and cell-to-cell virus transmission are prevented by deletion of the gene encoding the 37,000-Dalton outer envelope protein. *J Virol* 1991;65:5910–5920.
16. Bonifacino JS, Glick BS. The mechanisms of vesicle budding and fusion. *Cell* 2004;116:153–166.
17. Bourmakina SV, Garcia-Sastre A. Reverse genetics studies on the filamentous morphology of influenza A virus. *J Gen Virol* 2003;84:517–527.
18. Brack AR, Dijkstra JM, Granzow H, et al. Inhibition of virion maturation by simultaneous deletion of glycoproteins E, I, and M of pseudorabies virus. *J Virol* 1999;73:5364–5372.
19. Briggs JA, Krausslich HG. The molecular architecture of HIV. *J Mol Biol* 2011;410:491–500.
20. Brodsky JL, Skach WR. Protein folding and quality control in the endoplasmic reticulum: recent lessons from yeast and mammalian cell systems. *Curr Opin Cell Biol* 2011;23:464–475.
21. Bruce EA, Medcalf L, Crump CM, et al. Budding of filamentous and non-filamentous influenza A virus occurs via a VPS4 and VPS28-independent pathway. *Virology* 2009;390:268–278.
22. Bui M, Wills EG, Helenius A, et al. Role of the influenza virus M1 protein in nuclear export of viral ribonucleoproteins. *J Virol* 2000;74:1781–1786.
23. Carlton JG, Martin-Serrano J. Parallels between cytokinesis and retroviral budding: a role for the ESCRT machinery. *Science* 2007;316:1908–1912.
24. Cepko CL, Sharp PA. Assembly of adenovirus major capsid protein is mediated by a nonvirion protein. *Cell* 1982;31:407–415.
26. Checkley MA, Luttge BG, Freed EO. HIV-1 envelope glycoprotein biosynthesis, trafficking, and incorporation. *J Mol Biol* 2011;410:582–608.
27. Cho MW, Teterina N, Egger D, et al. Membrane rearrangement and vesicle induction by recombinant poliovirus 2C and 2BC in human cells. *Virology* 1994;202:129–145.
28. Choi G, Park S, Choi B, et al. Identification of a cytoplasmic targeting/retention signal in a retroviral Gag polyprotein. *J Virol* 1999;73:5431–5437.
29. Christensen JB, Byrd SA, Walker AK, et al. Presence of the adenovirus IVa2 protein at a single vertex of the mature virion. *J Virol* 2008;82: 9086–9093.
30. Church GA, Dasgupta A, Wilson DW. Herpes simplex virus DNA packaging without measurable DNA synthesis. *J Virol* 1998;72:2745–2751.
31. Clever JL, Eckstein DA, Parslow TG. Genetic dissociation of the encapsidation and reverse transcription functions in the 5′ R region of human immunodeficiency virus type 1. *J Virol* 1999;73:101–109.
32. Compans RW. Virus entry and release in polarized epithelial cells. *Curr Top Microbiol Immunol* 1995;202:209–219.
33. Condit RC, Moussatche N, Traktman P. In a nutshell: structure and assembly of the vaccinia virion. *Adv Virus Res* 2006;66:31–124.
34. Corse E, Machamer CE. Infectious bronchitis virus E protein is targeted to the Golgi complex and directs release of virus-like particles. *J Virol* 2000;74:4319–4326.
36. Craven RC, Parent LJ. Dynamic interactions of the Gag polyprotein. *Curr Top Microbiol Immunol* 1996;214:65–94.
37. Cuadras MA, Greenberg HB. Rotavirus infectious particles use lipid rafts during replication for transport to the cell surface in vitro and in vivo. *Virology* 2003;313:308–321.
38. Cudmore S, Reckmann I, Griffiths G, et al. Vaccinia virus: a model system for actin-membrane interactions. *J Cell Sci* 1996;109:1739–1747.
40. D'Souza V, Summers MF. Structural basis for packaging the dimeric genome of Moloney murine leukaemia virus. *Nature* 2004;431:586–590.
41. D'Souza V, Summers MF. How retroviruses select their genomes. *Nat Rev Microbiol* 2005;3:643–655.
42. Dales S, Mosbach EH. Vaccinia as a model for membrane biogenesis. *Virology* 1968;35:564–583.
43. Dancourt J, Barlowe C. Protein sorting receptors in the early secretory pathway. *Ann Rev Biochem* 2010;79:777–802.
44. Dasgupta A, Wilson DW. ATP depletion blocks herpes simplex virus DNA packaging and capsid maturation. *J Virol* 1999;73:2006–2015.
45. De Guzman RN, Wu ZR, Stalling CC, et al. Structure of the HIV-1 nucleocapsid protein bound to the SL3 psi-RNA recognition element. *Science* 1998;279:384–388.
46. Deiss LP, Chou J, Frenkel N. Functional domains within the a sequence involved in the cleavage-packaging of herpes simplex virus DNA. *J Virol* 1986;59:605–618.
48. Demirov DG, Freed EO. Retrovirus budding. *Virus Res* 2004;106:87–102.
49. Deschambeault J, Lalonde JP, Cervantes-Acosta G, et al. Polarized human immunodeficiency virus budding in lymphocytes involves a tyrosine-based signal and favors cell-to-cell viral transmission. *J Virol* 1999;73:5010–5017.
50. Doedens JR, Giddings TH Jr, Kirkegaard K. Inhibition of endoplasmic reticulum-to-Golgi traffic by poliovirus protein 3A: genetic and ultrastructural analysis. *J Virol* 1997;71:9054–9064.
52. Enami M, Sharma G, Benham C, et al. An influenza virus containing nine different RNA segments. *Virology* 1991;185:291–298.
53. Evans DT, Serra-Moreno R, Singh RK, et al. BST-2/tetherin: a new component of the innate immune response to enveloped viruses. *Trends Microbiol* 2010;18:388–396.
54. Ewing SG, Byrd SA, Christensen JB, et al. Ternary complex formation on the adenovirus packaging sequence by the IVa2 and L4 22-kilodalton proteins. *J Virol* 2007;81:12450–12457.
55. Fabbretti E, Afrikanova I, Vascotto F, et al. Two non-structural rotavirus proteins, NSP2 and NSP5, form viroplasm-like structures in vivo. *J Gen Virol* 1999;80:333–339.
56. Forsell K, Xing L, Kozlovska T, et al. Membrane proteins organize a symmetrical virus. *EMBO J* 2000;19:5081–5091.
57. Freed EO. HIV-1 gag proteins: diverse functions in the virus life cycle. *Virology* 1998;251:1–15.
59. Fujii K, Fujii Y, Noda T, et al. Importance of both the coding and the segment-specific noncoding regions of the influenza A virus NS segment for its efficient incorporation into virions. *J Virol* 2005;79:3766–3774.
60. Garbitt-Hirst R, Kenney SP, Parent LJ. Genetic evidence for a connection between Rous sarcoma virus gag nuclear trafficking and genomic RNA packaging. *J Virol* 2009;83:6790–6797.

61. Garoff H, Hewson R, Opstelten DJE. Virus maturation by budding. *Microbiol Mol Biol Rev* 1998;62:1171–1190.
62. Garoff H, Sjoberg M, Cheng RH. Budding of alphaviruses. *Virus Res* 2004;106:103–116.
63. Garrus JE, von Schwedler UK, Pornillos OW, et al. Tsg101 and the vacuolar protein sorting pathway are essential for HIV-1 budding. *Cell* 2001;107:55–65.
64. Ge P, Tsao J, Schein S, et al. Cryo-EM model of the bullet-shaped vesicular stomatitis virus. *Science* 2010;327:689–693.
66. Goepfert PA, Shaw K, Wang G, et al. An endoplasmic reticulum retrieval signal partitions human foamy virus maturation to intracytoplasmic membranes. *J Virol* 1999;73:7210–7217.
67. Gong M, Kieff E. Intracellular trafficking of two major Epstein-Barr virus glycoproteins, gp350/220 and gp110. *J Virol* 1990;64:1507–1516.
70. Griffin SD, Allen JF, Lever AM. The major human immunodeficiency virus type 2 (HIV-2) packaging signal is present on all HIV-2 RNA species: cotranslational RNA encapsidation and limitation of Gag protein confer specificity. *J Virol* 2001;75:12058–12069.
71. Griffiths G, Rottier P. Cell biology of viruses that assemble along the biosynthetic pathway. *Semin Cell Biol* 1992;3:367–381.
72. Gudleski N, Flanagan JM, Ryan EP, et al. Directionality of nucleocytoplasmic transport of the retroviral gag protein depends on sequential binding of karyopherins and viral RNA. *Proc Natl Acad Sci U S A* 2010; 107:9358–9363.
73. Hammarskjold ML, Winberg G. Encapsidation of adenovirus 16 DNA is directed by a small DNA sequence at the left end of the genome. *Cell* 1980;20:787–795.
74. Hearing P, Samulski RJ, Wishart WL, et al. Identification of a repeated sequence element required for efficient encapsidation of the adenovirus type 5 chromosome. *J Virol* 1987;61:2555–2558.
75. Hellen CUT, Wimmer E. Enterovirus structure and assembly. In: Robart HA, ed. *Human Enterovirus Infections.* Washington, DC: American Society for Microbiology; 1995:155–174.
76. Heuser J. Deep-etch EM reveals that the early poxvirus envelope is a single membrane bilayer stabilized by a geodetic "honeycomb" surface coat. *J Cell Biol* 2005;169:269–283.
77. Hogue BG, Machamer CE. Coronavirus structural proteins and virus assembly. In: Perlman S, Gallaher T, Snijder EJ, eds. *Nidoviruses.* Washington, DC: American Society for Microbiology; 2007:179–200.
78. Hollinshead M, Vanderplasschen A, Smith GL, et al. Vaccinia virus intracellular mature virions contain only one lipid membrane. *J Virol* 1999; 73:1503–1517.
81. Hunter E. Macromolecular interactions in the assembly of HIV and other retroviruses. *Semin Virol* 1994;5:71–83.
82. Husain M, Weisberg AS, Moss B. Existence of an operative pathway from the endoplasmic reticulum to the immature poxvirus membrane. *Proc Natl Acad Sci U S A* 2006;103:19506–19511.
84. Jackson MR, Nilsson T, Peterson PA. Identification of a consensus motif for retention of transmembrane proteins in the endoplasmic reticulum. *EMBO J* 1990;9:3153–3162.
85. Jackson WT, Giddings TH Jr., Taylor MP, et al. Subversion of cellular autophagosomal machinery by RNA viruses. *PLoS Biol* 2005;3:e156.
88. Jayakar HR, Jeetendra E, Whitt MA. Rhabdovirus assembly and budding. *Virus Res* 2004;106:117–132.
89. Jose J, Snyder JE, Kuhn RJ. A structural and functional perspective of alphavirus replication and assembly. *Future Microbiol* 2009;4:837–856.
90. Jouvenet N, Bieniasz PD, Simon SM. Imaging the biogenesis of individual HIV-1 virions in live cells. *Nature* 2008;454:236–240.
91. Jouvenet N, Neil SJ, Zhadina M, et al. Broad-spectrum inhibition of retroviral and filoviral particle release by tetherin. *J Virol* 2009;83: 1837–1844.
92. Jouvenet N, Simon SM, Bieniasz PD. Imaging the interaction of HIV-1 genomes and Gag during assembly of individual viral particles. *Proc Natl Acad Sci U S A* 2009;106:19114–19119.
93. Jouvenet N, Zhadina M, Bieniasz PD, et al. Dynamics of ESCRT protein recruitment during retroviral assembly. *Nat Cell Biol* 2011;13: 394–401.
94. Kabcenell AK, Poruchynsky MS, Bellamy AR, et al. Two forms of VP7 are involved in assembly of SA11 rotavirus in endoplasmic reticulum. *J Virol* 1988;62:2929–2941.
95. Kalderon D, Roberts BL, Richardson WD, et al. A short amino acid sequence able to specify nuclear location. *Cell* 1984;39:499–509.
96. Karayan L, Gay B, Gerfaux J, et al. Oligomerization of recombinant penton base of adenovirus type 2 and its assembly with fiber in baculovirus-infected cells. *Virology* 1994;202:782–795.
97. Klupp BG, Granzow H, Keil GM, et al. The capsid-associated UL25 protein of the alphaherpesvirus pseudorabies virus is nonessential for cleavage and encapsidation of genomic DNA but is required for nuclear egress of capsids. *J Virol* 2006;80:6235–6246.
98. Kohler A, Hurt E. Exporting RNA from the nucleus to the cytoplasm. *Nat Rev Mol Cell Biol* 2007;8:761–773.
99. Krijnse-Locker J, Schleich S, Rodriguez D, et al. The role of a 21-kDa viral membrane protein in the assembly of vaccinia virus from the intermediate compartment. *J Biol Chem* 1996;271:14950–14958.
100. Kuehn MJ, Herrmann JM, Schekman R. COPII-cargo interactions direct protein sorting into ER-derived transport vesicles. *Nature* 1998;391: 187–190.
101. Liang Y, Hong Y, Parslow TG. cis-Acting packaging signals in the influenza virus PB1, PB2, and PA genomic RNA segments. *J Virol* 2005;79: 10348–10355.
102. Lim KP, Liu DX. The missing link in coronavirus assembly. Retention of the avian coronavirus infectious bronchitis virus envelope protein in the pre-Golgi compartments and physical interaction between the envelope and membrane proteins. *J Biol Chem* 2001;276:17515–17523.
103. Lindemann D, Goepfert PA. The foamy virus envelope glycoproteins. *Curr Top Microbiol Immunol* 2003;277:111–129.
105. Lodge R, Delamarre L, Lalonde JP, et al. Two distinct oncornaviruses harbor an intracytoplasmic tyrosine-based basolateral targeting signal in their viral envelope glycoprotein. *J Virol* 1997;71:5696–5702.
106. Lontok E, Corse E, Machamer CE. Intracellular targeting signals contribute to localization of coronavirus spike proteins near the virus assembly site. *J Virol* 2004;78:5913–5922.
107. Lopez T, Camacho M, Zayas M, et al. Silencing the morphogenesis of rotavirus. *J Virol* 2005;79:184–192.
108. Lu K, Heng X, Summers MF. Structural determinants and mechanism of HIV-1 genome packaging. *J Mol Biol* 2011;410:609–633.
109. Luytjes W, Krystal M, Enami M, et al. Amplification, expression, and packaging of foreign gene by influenza virus. *Cell* 1989;59:1107–1113.
110. Maeda J, Maeda A, Makino S. Release of coronavirus E protein in membrane vesicles from virus-infected cells and E protein-expressing cells. *Virology* 1999;263:265–272.
111. Mancini EJ, Clarke M, Gowen BE, et al. Cryo-electron microscopy reveals the functional organization of an enveloped virus, Semliki Forest virus. *Mol Cell* 2000;5:255–266.
112. Mangel WF, Baniecki ML, McGrath WJ. Specific interactions of the adenovirus proteinase with the viral DNA, an 11-amino-acid viral peptide, and the cellular protein actin. *Cell Mol Life Sci* 2003;60:2347–2355.
113. Martin K, Helenius A. Nuclear transport of influenza virus ribonucleoproteins: the viral matrix protein (M1) promotes export and inhibits import. *Cell* 1991;67:117–130.
114. Martin-Serrano J, Neil SJ. Host factors involved in retroviral budding and release. *Nat Rev Microbiol* 2011;9:519–531.
115. Martin-Serrano J, Zang T, Bieniasz PD. Role of ESCRT-I in retroviral budding. *J Virol* 2003;77:4794–4804.
116. Maruri-Avidal L, Domi A, Weisberg AS, et al. Participation of vaccinia virus l2 protein in the formation of crescent membranes and immature virions. *J Virol* 2011;85:2504–2511.
118. McCown MF, Pekosz A. Distinct domains of the influenza a virus M2 protein cytoplasmic tail mediate binding to the M1 protein and facilitate infectious virus production. *J Virol* 2006;80:8178–8189.
120. Mebatsion T, Weiland F, Conzelmann KK. Matrix protein of rabies virus is responsible for the assembly and budding of bullet-shaped particles and interacts with the transmembrane spike glycoprotein G. *J Virol* 1999; 73:242–250.
121. Mettenleiter TC. Budding events in herpesvirus morphogenesis. *Virus Res* 2004;106:167–180.
122. Mettenleiter TC. Herpesvirus assembly and egress. *J Virol* 2002;76: 1537–1547.
123. Mettenleiter TC, Klupp BG, Granzow H. Herpesvirus assembly: an update. *Virus Res* 2009;143:222–234.

124. Meyer BE, Malim MH. The HIV-1 Rev trans-activator shuttles between the nucleus and the cytoplasm. *Genes Dev* 1994;8:1538–1547.
125. Meyer JC, Bergmann CC, Bellamy AR. Interaction of rotavirus cores with the nonstructural glycoprotein NS28. *Virology* 1989;171:98–107.
127. Moore MD, Nikolaitchik OA, Chen J, et al. Probing the HIV-1 genomic RNA trafficking pathway and dimerization by genetic recombination and single virion analyses. *PLoS Pathog* 2009;5:e1000627.
129. Morita E, Sandrin V, McCullough J, et al. ESCRT-III protein requirements for HIV-1 budding. *Cell Host Microbe* 2011;9:235–242.
130. Morita E, Sundquist WI. Retrovirus budding. *Annu Rev Cell Dev Biol* 2004;20:395–425.
131. Munro S, Pelham HR. A C-terminal signal prevents secretion of luminal ER proteins. *Cell* 1987;48:899–907.
132. Muramoto Y, Takada A, Fujii K, et al. Hierarchy among viral RNA (vRNA) segments in their role in vRNA incorporation into influenza A virions. *J Virol* 2006;80:2318–2325.
134. Nakielny S, Dreyfuss G. Nuclear export of proteins and RNAs. *Curr Opin Cell Biol* 1997;9:420–429.
135. Narayanan K, Maeda A, Maeda J, et al. Characterization of the coronavirus M protein and nucleocapsid interaction in infected cells. *J Virol* 2000; 74:8127–8134.
136. Nayak DP, Balogun RA, Yamada H, et al. Influenza virus morphogenesis and budding. *Virus Res* 2009;143:147–161.
137. Nayak DP, Hui EK, Barman S. Assembly and budding of influenza virus. *Virus Res* 2004;106:147–165.
138. Neil SJ, Zang T, Bieniasz PD. Tetherin inhibits retrovirus release and is antagonized by HIV-1 Vpu. *Nature* 2008;451:425–430.
139. Nermut MV, Bron P, Thomas D, et al. Molecular organization of Mason-Pfizer monkey virus capsids assembled from Gag polyprotein in Escherichia coli. *J Virol* 2002;76:4321–4330.
141. Newcomb WW, Homa FL, Brown JC. Involvement of the portal at an early step in herpes simplex virus capsid assembly. *J Virol* 2005;79: 10540–10546.
142. Newcomb WW, Homa FL, Thomsen DR, et al. Assembly of the herpes simplex virus capsid: characterization of intermediates observed during cell-free capsid formation. *J Mol Biol* 1996;263:432–446.
143. Newcomb WW, Juhas RM, Thomsen DR, et al. The UL6 gene product forms the portal for entry of DNA into the herpes simplex virus capsid. *J Virol* 2001;75:10923–10932.
144. Newcomb WW, Trus BL, Cheng N, et al. Isolation of herpes simplex virus procapsids from cells infected with a protease-deficient mutant virus. *J Virol* 2000;74:1663–1673.
145. Noda T, Sagara H, Yen A, et al. Architecture of ribonucleoprotein complexes in influenza A virus particles. *Nature* 2006;439:490–492.
147. O'Brien JA, Taylor JA, Bellamy AR. Probing the structure of rotavirus NSP4: a short sequence at the extreme C terminus mediates binding to the inner capsid particle. *J Virol* 2000;74:5388–5394.
148. Ooms M, Huthoff H, Russell R, et al. A riboswitch regulates RNA dimerization and packaging in human immunodeficiency virus type 1 virions. *J Virol* 2004;78:10814–10819.
149. Orci L, Glick BS, Rothman JE. A new type of coated vesicular carrier that appears not to contain clathrin: its possible role in protein transport within the Golgi stack. *Cell* 1986;46:171–184.
150. Ostapchuk P, Almond M, Hearing P. Characterization of empty adenovirus particles assembled in the absence of a functional adenovirus IVa2 protein. *J Virol* 2011;85:5524–5531.
151. Ostapchuk P, Anderson ME, Chandrasekhar S, et al. The L4 22-kilodalton protein plays a role in packaging of the adenovirus genome. *J Virol* 2006;80:6973–6981.
152. Ostapchuk P, Hearing P. Control of adenovirus packaging. *J Cell Biochem* 2005;96:25–35.
153. Ostapchuk P, Yang J, Auffarth E, et al. Functional interaction of the adenovirus IVa2 protein with adenovirus type 5 packaging sequences. *J Virol* 2005;79:2831–2838.
155. Parent LJ, Bennett RP, Craven RC, et al. Positionally independent and exchangeable late budding functions of the Rous sarcoma virus and human immunodeficiency virus Gag proteins. *J Virol* 1995;69:5455–5460.
156. Parent LJ, Gudleski N. Beyond plasma membrane targeting: role of the MA domain of Gag in retroviral genome encapsidation. *J Mol Biol* 2011;410:553–564.
157. Parker SD, Hunter E. Activation of the Mason-Pfizer monkey virus protease within immature capsids in vitro. *Proc Natl Acad Sci U S A* 2001; 98:14631–14636.
158. Patton JT, Silvestri LS, Tortorici MA, et al. Rotavirus genome replication and morphogenesis: role of the viroplasm. *Curr Top Microbiol Immunol* 2006;309:169–187.
159. Patton JT, Vasquez-Del Carpio R, Tortorici MA, et al. Coupling of rotavirus genome replication and capsid assembly. *Adv Virus Res* 2007; 69:167–201.
162. Pfister T, Pasamontes L, Troxler M, et al. Immunocytochemical localization of capsid-related particles in subcellular fractions of poliovirus-infected cells. *Virology* 1992;188:676–684.
163. Pickl WF, Pimentel-Muinos FX, Seed B. Lipid rafts and pseudotyping. *J Virol* 2001;75:7175–7183.
164. Pinto LH, Holsinger LJ, Lamb RA. Influenza virus M2 protein has ion channel activity. *Cell* 1992;69:517–528.
165. Poruchynsky MS, Maass DR, Atkinson PH. Calcium depletion blocks the maturation of rotavirus by altering the oligomerization of virus-encoded proteins in the ER. *J Cell Biol* 1991;114:651–656.
166. Raamsman MJ, Locker JK, de Hooge A, et al. Characterization of the coronavirus mouse hepatitis virus strain A59 small membrane protein E. *J Virol* 2000;74:2333–2342.
167. Reynolds AE, Ryckman BJ, Baines JD, et al. U(L)31 and U(L)34 proteins of herpes simplex virus type 1 form a complex that accumulates at the nuclear rim and is required for envelopment of nucleocapsids. *J Virol* 2001;75:8803–8817.
168. Risco C, Rodriguez JR, Lopez-Iglesias C, et al. Endoplasmic reticulum-Golgi intermediate compartment membranes and vimentin filaments participate in vaccinia virus assembly. *J Virol* 2002;76:1839–1855.
169. Rixon FJ. Structure and assembly of herpesviruses. *Semin Virol* 1993; 4:135–144.
170. Rixon FJ, Addison C, McGregor A, et al. Multiple interactions control the intracellular localization of the herpes simplex virus type 1 capsid proteins. *J Gen Virol* 1996;77:2251–2260.
172. Roberts KL, Smith GL. Vaccinia virus morphogenesis and dissemination. *Trends Microbiol* 2008;16:472–479.
173. Robison CS, Whitt MA. The membrane-proximal stem region of vesicular stomatitis virus G protein confers efficient virus assembly. *J Virol* 2000;74:2239–2246.
174. Rodriguez JF, Smith GL. IPTG-dependent vaccinia virus: identification of a virus protein enabling virion envelopment by Golgi membrane and egress. *Nucleic Acids Res* 1990;18:5347–5351.
177. Rossman JS, Jing X, Leser GP, et al. Influenza virus M2 protein mediates ESCRT-independent membrane scission. *Cell* 2010;142:902–913.
178. Rossman JS, Lamb RA. Influenza virus assembly and budding. *Virology* 2011;411:229–236.
179. Rothman JE, Wieland FT. Protein sorting by transport vesicles. *Science* 1996;272:227–234.
180. Rouiller I, Brookes SM, Hyatt AD, et al. African swine fever virus is wrapped by the endoplasmic reticulum. *J Virol* 1998;72:2373–2387.
182. Ruiz MC, Leon T, Diaz Y, et al. Molecular biology of rotavirus entry and replication. *ScientificWorldJournal* 2009;9:1476–1497.
183. Sakalian M, Hunter E. Molecular events in the assembly of retrovirus particles. *Adv Exp Med Biol* 1998;440:329–339.
185. Salmons T, Kuhn A, Wylie F, et al. Vaccinia virus membrane proteins p8 and p16 are cotranslationally inserted into the rough endoplasmic reticulum and retained in the intermediate compartment. *J Virol* 1997; 71:7404–7420.
186. Salonen A, Ahola T, Kaariainen L. Viral RNA replication in association with cellular membranes. *Curr Top Microbiol Immunol* 2005;285:139–173.
187. Saraogi I, Shan SO. Molecular mechanism of co-translational protein targeting by the signal recognition particle. *Traffic* 2011;12:535–542.
188. Sauter D, Schindler M, Specht A, et al. Tetherin-driven adaptation of Vpu and Nef function and the evolution of pandemic and nonpandemic HIV-1 strains. *Cell Host Microbe* 2009;6:409–421.
189. Scheiffele P, Rietveld A, Wilk T, et al. Influenza viruses select ordered lipid domains during budding from the plasma membrane. *J Biol Chem* 1999;274:2038–2044.
191. Schmid SI, Hearing P. Bipartite structure and functional independence of adenovirus type 5 packaging elements. *J Virol* 1997;71:3375–3384.

193. Sfakianos JN, Hunter E. M-PMV capsid transport is mediated by Env/Gag interactions at the pericentriolar recycling endosome. *Traffic* 2003; 4:671–680.
194. Sfakianos JN, LaCasse RA, Hunter E. The M-PMV cytoplasmic targeting-retention signal directs nascent Gag polypeptides to a pericentriolar region of the cell. *Traffic* 2003;4:660–670.
195. Skach WR. The expanding role of the ER translocon in membrane protein folding. *J Cell Biol* 2007;179:1333–1335.
196. Smith GL, Law M. The exit of vaccinia virus from infected cells. *Virus Res* 2004;106:189–197.
198. Sodeik B, Krijnse-Locker J. Assembly of vaccinia virus revisited: de novo membrane synthesis or acquisition from the host? *Trends Microbiol* 2002;10:15–24.
199. Stewart M. Molecular mechanism of the nuclear protein import cycle. *Nat Rev Mol Cell Biol* 2007;8:195–208.
200. Stirzaker SC, Whitfeld PL, Christie DL, et al. Processing of rotavirus glycoprotein VP7: implications for the retention of the protein in the endoplasmic reticulum. *J Cell Biol* 1987;105:2897–2903.
201. Strack B, Calistri A, Craig S, et al. AIP1/ALIX is a binding partner for HIV-1 p6 and EIAV p9 functioning in virus budding. *Cell* 2003;114: 689–699.
202. Strambio-De-Castillia C, Niepel M, Rout MP. The nuclear pore complex: bridging nuclear transport and gene regulation. *Nat Rev Mol Cell Biol* 2010;11:490–501.
204. Strom AC, Weis K. Importin-beta-like nuclear transport receptors. *Genome Biol* 2001;2:reviews3008.1–reviews3008.9.
205. Sugrue RJ, Bahadur G, Zambon MC, et al. Specific structural alteration of the influenza haemagglutinin by amantadine. *EMBO J* 1990;9:3469–3476.
206. Suhy DA, Giddings TH Jr, Kirkegaard K. Remodeling the endoplasmic reticulum by poliovirus infection and by individual viral proteins: an autophagy-like origin for virus-induced vesicles. *J Virol* 2000;74:8953–8965.
207. Swanstrom R, Wills JW. Synthesis, assembly and processing of viral proteins. In: Coffin JM, Hughes SH, Varmus HE, eds. *Retroviruses.* New York: Cold Spring Harbor Laboratory Press; 1997:263–334.
208. Szajner P, Jaffe H, Weisberg AS, et al. A complex of seven vaccinia virus proteins conserved in all chordopoxviruses is required for the association of membranes and viroplasm to form immature virions. *Virology* 2004; 330:447–459.
209. Szajner P, Weisberg AS, Lebowitz J, et al. External scaffold of spherical immature poxvirus particles is made of protein trimers, forming a honeycomb lattice. *J Cell Biol* 2005;170:971–981.
210. Sztul E, Lupashin V. Role of tethering factors in secretory membrane traffic. *Am J Physiol Cell Physiol* 2006;290:C11–C26.
212. Taylor JA, O'Brien JA, Yeager M. The cytoplasmic tail of NSP4, the endoplasmic reticulum-localized non-structural glycoprotein of rotavirus, contains distinct virus binding and coiled coil domains. *EMBO J* 1996;15:4469–4476.
213. Taylor MP, Kirkegaard K. Potential subversion of autophagosomal pathway by picornaviruses. *Autophagy* 2008;4:286–289.
214. Thomas DC, Roth MG. The basolateral targeting signal in the cytoplasmic domain of glycoprotein G from vesicular stomatitis virus resembles a variety of intracellular targeting motifs related by primary sequence but having diverse targeting activities. *J Biol Chem* 1994;269:15732–15739.
215. Tomishima MJ, Smith GA, Enquist LW. Sorting and transport of alpha herpesviruses in axons. *Traffic* 2001;2:429–436.
216. Torrisi MR, Gentile M, Cardinali G, et al. Intracellular transport and maturation pathway of human herpesvirus 6. *Virology* 1999;257: 460–471.
217. Troxler M, Egger D, Pfister T, et al. Intracellular localization of poliovirus RNA by in situ hybridization at the ultrastructural level using single-stranded riboprobes. *Virology* 1992;191:687–697.
218. Van Damme N, Goff D, Katsura C, et al. The interferon-induced protein BST-2 restricts HIV-1 release and is downregulated from the cell surface by the viral Vpu protein. *Cell Host Microbe* 2008;3:245–252.
219. Van den Berg B, Clemons WM Jr, Collinson I, et al. X-ray structure of a protein-conducting channel. *Nature* 2004;427:36–44.
220. Van Genderen IL, Brandimarti R, Torrisi MR, et al. The phospholipid composition of extracellular herpes simplex virions differs from that of host cell nuclei. *Virology* 1994;200:831–836.
221. Vennema H, Godeke GJ, Rossen JW, et al. Nucleocapsid-independent assembly of coronavirus-like particles by co-expression of viral envelope protein genes. *EMBO J* 1996;15:2020–2028.
222. Vlach J, Lipov J, Rumlova M, et al. D-retrovirus morphogenetic switch driven by the targeting signal accessibility to Tctex-1 of dynein. *Proc Nat Acad Sci U S A* 2008;105:10565–10570.
223. Von Schwedler UK, Stemmler TL, Klishko VY, et al. Proteolytic refolding of the HIV-1 capsid protein amino-terminus facilitates viral core assembly [published erratum appears in *EMBO J* 2000;19(10):2391]. *EMBO J* 1998;17:1555–1568.
224. Von Schwedler UK, Stuchell M, Muller B, et al. The protein network of HIV budding. *Cell* 2003;114:701–713.
225. Waheed AA, Freed EO. The role of lipids in retrovirus replication. *Viruses* 2010;2:1146–1180.
226. Walter CT, Barr JN. Recent advances in the molecular and cellular biology of bunyaviruses. *J Gen Virol* 2011;92:2467–2484.
227. Weiss ER, Gottlinger H. The role of cellular factors in promoting HIV budding. *J Mol Biol* 2011;410:525–533.
228. Whittaker GR, Helenius A. Nuclear import and export of viruses and virus genomes. *Virology* 1998;246:1–23.
229. Wodrich H, Guan T, Cingolani G, et al. Switch from capsid protein import to adenovirus assembly by cleavage of nuclear transport signals. *EMBO J* 2003;22:6245–6255.
230. Wollert T, Hurley JH. Molecular mechanism of multivesicular body biogenesis by ESCRT complexes. *Nature* 2010;464:864–869.
231. Wright ER, Schooler JB, Ding HJ, et al. Electron cryotomography of immature HIV-1 virions reveals the structure of the CA and SP1 Gag shells. *EMBO J* 2007;26:2218–2226.
232. Yang P, Bansal A, Liu C, et al. Hemagglutinin specificity and neuraminidase coding capacity of neuraminidase-deficient influenza viruses. *Virology* 1997;229:155–165.
233. Yasuda J, Hunter E, Nakao M, et al. Functional involvement of a novel Nedd4-like ubiquitin ligase on retrovirus budding. *EMBO Rep* 2002;3: 636–640.
234. Yu D, Weller SK. Herpes simplex virus type 1 cleavage and packaging proteins UL15 and UL28 are associated with B but not C capsids during packaging. *J Virol* 1998;72:7428–7439.
235. Yu SF, Eastman SW, Linial ML. Foamy virus capsid assembly occurs at a pericentriolar region through a cytoplasmic targeting/retention signal in Gag. *Traffic* 2006;7:966–977.
237. Zeffman A, Hassard S, Varani G, et al. The major HIV-1 packaging signal is an extended bulged stem loop whose structure is altered on interaction with the gag polyprotein. *J Mol Biol* 2000;297:877–893.
238. Zhao LJ, Padmanabhan R. Three basic regions in adenovirus DNA polymerase interact differentially depending on the protein context to function as bipartite nuclear localization signals. *New Biol* 1991;3: 1074–1088.
239. Zimmermann R, Eyrisch S, Ahmad M, et al. Protein translocation across the ER membrane. *Biochim Biophys Acta* 2011;1808:912–924.

CHAPTER 7

Daniel DiMaio • Hung Fan

Viruses, Cell Transformation, and Cancer

GENERAL PRINCIPLES OF VIRAL TRANSFORMATION

In 1908, Ellerman and Bang[143] reported that cell-free filtrates from chickens with leukemia could transmit the disease to healthy birds. The ability of the causative agent to pass through a fine filter identified it as a virus, providing the first evidence that viruses could cause cancer as well as acute contagious diseases. Three years later, Peyton Rous[382] showed that a solid tumor in chickens, sarcoma, could also be transmitted by cell-free filtrates. In the 100 years since these discoveries, tumor viruses have been studied intensely in the belief that thorough understanding of these relatively simple agents would provide mechanistic insight into carcinogenesis, identify the causes of some human malignancies, and suggest novel strategies to prevent and treat cancer. All of these expectations have been met. Tumor viruses dysregulate or exploit crucial regulatory nodes in cells in order to replicate and persist in their host. Because these nodes regulate cell proliferation and survival, these viruses can cause cancer. Furthermore, because of their intimate association with this central cellular machinery, tumor viruses have proven to be prime tools for unraveling the complexities of all human cancers, not just those induced by viruses themselves. For example, studies of tumor viruses led to the discovery of cellular oncogenes and tumor suppressor proteins and to the elucidation of many important aspects of signal transduction, cell cycle control, cellular biochemistry, and carcinogenesis. Indeed, the concept that cancer is a genetic disease emerged largely from studies of tumor viruses. We have also learned that tumor viruses are associated with specific types of human cancer and that tumor virus infection is responsible for approximately 15% of human cancer deaths.[310] Vaccines have been developed and deployed that prevent infection by certain tumor viruses and inhibit the formation of precancerous lesions or cancers.[403] The remarkable success of these endeavors is due to the efforts of generations of virologists, biochemists, molecular biologists, epidemiologists, and clinicians, and to the favorable properties of the viruses themselves.

Cell Transformation

Early studies of tumor viruses focused on isolation of viruses from naturally occurring tumors in animals and description of the effects of these viruses in experimental animals. These studies revealed that a wide variety of viruses can induce tumors (Table 7.1). Diverse taxonomic groups of viruses with DNA genomes can cause tumors: polyomaviruses, papillomaviruses, adenoviruses, herpesviruses, hepadnaviruses, and poxviruses. Among the RNA viruses, a subset of retroviruses cause tumors in animals, and Hepatitis C virus has been implicated in human cancer. Thus, the ability to induce tumor formation is not associated with a particular class of virus or mode of virus replication. The types of tumors induced by viruses are also diverse and include sarcomas (tumors of mesenchymal cells), leukemias and lymphomas (tumors of hematopoietic cells), and carcinomas (tumors of epithelial cells).

Although such experimental pathogenesis studies revealed many fascinating and complex features of viral tumorigenesis, experiments in animals are cumbersome, slow, expensive, and often poorly suited for biochemical and mechanistic analysis. Therefore, cultured cell models of tumorigenesis are widely used. Cells explanted from tumors display many properties that

TABLE 7.1 Oncogenic Viruses

Taxonomic grouping	Examples	Primary tumor types
RNA viruses		
Flaviviridae	Hepatitis C virus (HCV)	Hepatocellular carcinoma
Retroviridae		
Alpharetroviruses	Avian leukosis and sarcoma viruses	
	Rous sarcoma virus (RSV)	Sarcoma
	Rous-associated viruses (RAV)	B-cell lymphoma, erythroleukemia
	Avian acute leukemia viruses	
	Avian myeloblastosis virus (AMV)	Myeloid and/or erythroid leukemia
	Avian erythroblastosis virus (AEV)	Erythroid leukemia
	Myelocytoma virus MC29	Myeloid leukemia
Betaretroviruses	Mouse mammary tumor virus (MMTV)	Mammary carcinoma
	Jaagsiekte sheep retrovirus	Lung carcinoma
Gammaretroviruses	Murine leukemia viruses (MuLVs)	Leukemias and lymphomas
	Moloney MuLV	T lymphoma, also B-lymphoma and myeloid leukemia
	Murine sarcoma viruses (MuSVs)	Sarcoma
	Harvey MuSV	
	Feline leukemia viruses	Leukemias and lymphosarcomas
	Feline sarcoma viruses	Sarcomas
	Simian sarcoma virus	Sarcomas
	Gibbon ape leukemia virus	Leukemia
	Koala retrovirus	T-cell leukemia
Deltaretroviruses	Human T-lymphotropic virus (HTLV)	Adult T-cell leukemia
	Bovine leukemia virus	B-cell leukemia
Epsilonretroviruses	Walleye dermal sarcoma virus	Sarcoma
DNA viruses		
Adenoviridae	All types	Various solid tumors
Hepadnaviridae	Hepatitis B virus (HBV)	Hepatocellular carcinoma
Herpesviridae	Epstein-Barr virus (EBV)	Burkitt lymphoma (African)
		Nasopharyngeal carcinoma
	Kaposi sarcoma herpesvirus (KSHV)	Kaposi sarcoma
Polyomaviridae	SV40, polyomavirus	Various solid tumors (parotid gland tumors, mammary carcinoma)
Papillomaviridae	Human papillomavirus (HPV), bovine papillomavirus	Papillomas, carcinomas
Poxviridae	Shope fibromavirus	Myxomas, fibromas

distinguish them from normal cells. Collectively, these properties are referred to as the transformed phenotype (Table 7.2), and cells displaying these properties are called transformed cells. Infection of normal cells in culture with many (but not all) tumor viruses can cause the rapid acquisition of the transformed phenotype, a process called transformation. The most commonly used cell types for transformation studies are rodent fibroblasts, which in general are easier to transform *in vitro* than human cells.

The most striking property of transformed cells is their ability to form tumors when inoculated into animals. Experiments in animals have classically been used to determine whether a virus can cause a tumor in a living organism and to identify the viral gene(s) responsible for this activity. Although mice are used for the vast majority of such experiments, other commonly used hosts are rats, hamsters, rabbits, and monkeys. Immunodeficient animals (e.g., athymic nude mice) are frequently used in order to avoid immune rejection of the inoculated cells.

In addition to tumorigenicity, transformed cells display a variety of features in culture that distinguish them from normal cells. These include changes in growth, morphology, metabolism, and intracellular and cell surface biochemistry. Normal cells have very stringent requirements for growth. To proliferate in culture, normal cells require peptide growth factors, commonly supplied as fetal bovine serum. When plated on plastic, normal adherent cells typically divide to fill the available space on the surface of the culture vessel until they become a confluent monolayer of cells and then cease proliferation, even if supplied with adequate amounts of nutrients and growth factors. The cessation of growth at confluence is known as density-dependent growth inhibition or contact inhibition. Most normal cells also require attachment to a solid substrate and are unable to grow when suspended in semisolid medium such as agarose or methylcellulose, a property known as anchorage dependence. Finally, normal cells usually display a limited life span in culture after isolation from an animal and can be serially passaged for no more than a few months before they

TABLE 7.2 Properties of Transformed Cells

	Normal cells	Transformed cells	Behavior of transformed cells in the laboratory
Growth	Nontumorigenic	Tumorigenic	Form tumors upon inoculation into susceptible animal hosts
	Finite life span	Immortal	Indefinite life span in culture
	Contact inhibition	Loss of contact inhibition	Increased saturation density Focus formation
	Anchorage dependent	Anchorage independent	Colony formation in semisolid medium
	Growth factor dependent	Growth factor independent	Growth in reduced concentration of growth factors or serum DNA synthesis despite nutrient deprivation
Biochemical	Normal nutrient transport	Increased nutrient transport	
	Oxidative respiration	Aerobic glycolysis (Warburg effect)	Acidification of culture medium

Other changes in transformed cells include:

- Decreased levels of fibronectins, decreased adhesion to solid substrates, and loss of stress fibers
- Increased agglutination by lectins and synthesis of cell surface proteases
- Redistribution of microfilaments and altered morphology

cease proliferation and adopt a permanently growth-arrested state called senescence.

Transformed cells display strikingly different growth properties than normal cells (Table 7.2). Transformed cells have minimal requirements for growth factors and can proliferate in low concentrations of serum (or even in its absence). Transformed cells continue to proliferate after reaching confluence and display a multilayered, piled-up appearance and higher saturation densities than normal cells (Fig. 7.1). If a transformed cell is present in an excess of normal cells in a culture, it will override contact inhibition at confluence and continue to proliferate locally, forming a discrete, clonal group of transformed cells known as a focus (Fig. 7.1).[198] Because each focus originates from a single transformed cell, the number of foci formed provides a convenient measure of the number of transforming viruses in an inoculum. In addition, because foci are readily apparent on a background monolayer of cells, focus formation provides a simple means of identifying and isolating transformants. Transformed cells also display anchorage independence and can form colonies in semisolid medium without adhering to a solid surface.[294] Anchorage independence is the property of transformed cells that is most closely associated with the ability to form tumors in animals. Finally, in contrast to normal cultured cells, transformed cells that divide indefinitely in culture are said to be immortal.

Transformed cells can also display striking morphologic differences from normal cells due to changes in the cellular cytoskeleton, extracellular matrix, and cell surface.[226,371] Transformed cells also switch from oxidative respiration to aerobic glycolysis, a phenomenon known as the Warburg effect. The resulting lactic acid production and acidification of the culture medium (and the tell-tale yellow of medium containing phenol red, a pH indicator) allows the rapid identification of transformed cultures.

It should be noted that transformation is not an all-or-nothing phenomenon. Some transformed cells display only a subset of these properties. For example, in some cases cells can form foci but fail to display anchorage independence or tumorigenicity, or they can display reduced serum requirements but not form foci. It is therefore important to specify the assay used to assess transformation. "Normal" established cell lines, such as murine NIH3T3 cells, are immortal but do not display other features of transformed cells and thus can be regarded as being minimally transformed.

Identification of Viral Oncogenes

To determine whether a virus has tumorigenic or transforming activity, host animals or cells are infected and the appearance of tumors or the acquisition of a transformed phenotype in culture is measured. Acute transforming retroviruses cause the rapid formation of tumors in animals and rapidly transform cells in culture because they carry genetic information known as oncogenes. In contrast, retroviruses that lack oncogenes cause tumors in animals many months after infection and do not transform cells in culture. Most DNA tumor viruses contain oncogenes and can transform cells in culture and induce tumors in animals.

For viruses that contain oncogenes, cell transformation typically occurs within a few days or weeks of infection, although some measures of transformation, such as cell immortalization, take months to assess. When infected at high multiplicity of infection (moi), the entire culture of cells may undergo transformation, which can allow biochemical characterization of cell transformation. Infections at low moi require the use of quantal measures of transformation, such as focus formation or colony formation in agarose, to score transformation because most cells in the culture remain normal.

Although acute properties of transformation are fairly easy to elicit, for some viruses stable transformation that persists in culture is a very rare event. In addition, for lytic DNA viruses, where replication is cytocidal, transformation can only occur when the virus life cycle cannot go to completion. Transformation by these viruses is commonly studied following infection of nonpermissive cells that cannot support a full virus life cycle. In these cells, the initial steps (the early phase) of virus infection take place—virus attachment to cells, penetration into the cells, virion uncoating, and expression of the early proteins—but then

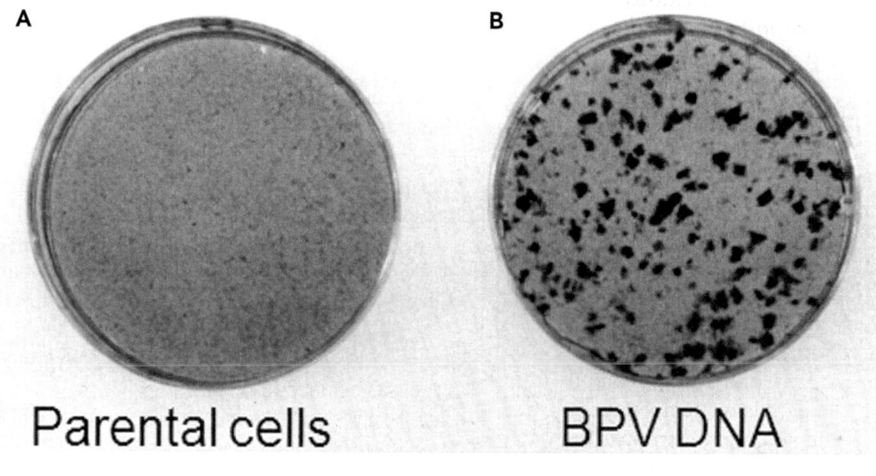

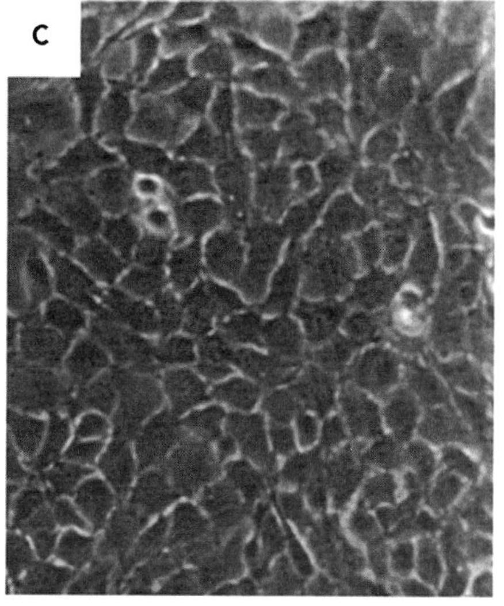

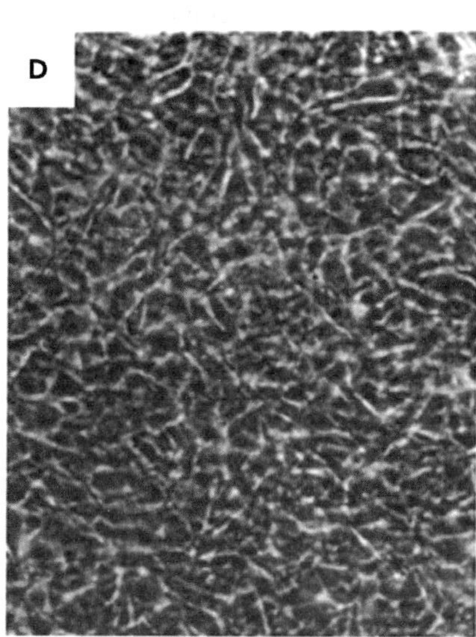

FIGURE 7.1. Appearance of transformed cells. A: Plate showing a monolayer of normal murine C127 fibroblasts. **B:** Plate of fibroblasts showing transformed foci induced by transfection with bovine papillomavirus DNA. **A** and **B** were stained 12 days after transfection. **C:** Micrograph of a monolayer of normal murine fibroblasts, showing flat, spread-out morphology. **D:** Culture of murine fibroblasts transformed by the bovine papillomavirus E5 protein. Note the piled-up, refractile appearance of small, transformed cells.

productive infection is aborted before the onset of vegetative viral DNA replication. For example, rat and mouse cells are nonpermissive for replication by simian virus 40 (SV40), a monkey virus, so many transformation assays are conducted in these cells. Alternatively, permissive cells, in which the wild-type virus can complete its life cycle, can be transformed if viral replication is blocked. Infection with replication-defective viral mutants or transfection with nonreplicating, subgenomic viral DNA fragments that contain viral oncogenes can transform permissive cells.[299] In addition, some tumor viruses (such as herpesviruses) can establish latency in permissive cells, and in some cases expression of a subset of viral genes in the latently infected cells can lead to transformation. Infection by acute transforming retroviruses usually does not result in cell death, and stable transformation is very efficient, with virtually every infected cell becoming transformed.

An oncogene can display potent activity in one transformation assay but be totally devoid of activity in another assay, even in the same host cell, because it may modulate multiple independent cellular signaling pathways. Host-specific differences can also greatly influence transforming activity, so a variety of host animals or cells are commonly tested to assess transforming activity. Some oncogenes have potent transforming activity in numerous assays but are unable to cause cell immortalization. Therefore, transformation is often studied in established cell lines that are already immortal.

Viral mutants can be used to identify specific viral genes with transforming activity. In early experiments, mutagenized viral stocks were tested for loss of transforming activity or for the acquisition of temperature-sensitive transforming activity. The generation and analysis of conditional mutants were particularly useful for identifying and studying transforming genes, especially those that are essential for virus replication.[380,467] In these situations, the virus is first propagated under permissive conditions, and then the virus is used to infect cells under nonpermissive conditions and transformation is assessed. Genetic mapping approaches can then be used to identify the mutant viral gene responsible for the transformation defect. More recently, specific mutations were constructed in individual viral open reading frames, and the resulting virus mutants were assayed for transforming activity. Alternatively, individual viral genes or subgenomic segments can be introduced into cells or transgenic animals and assessed for transforming activity or tumorigenicity.[192,420] This approach is complicated when more than one viral oncogene is required for transformation, because no single gene displays activity. In these situations, combinations of viral genes can be transferred into cells, or the ability of viral genes to cooperate with cellular oncogenes can be tested.

The analysis of murine polyomavirus transforming functions illustrates some of the power and pitfalls of these approaches. Murine polyomavirus (hereafter called polyomavirus) is related to SV40. SV40 and polyomavirus express the early protein, large T antigen (LT), which is required for viral DNA replication. Certain mutations in the SV40 *LT* gene caused temperature-sensitive defects in cell transformation as well as viral DNA replication, identifying the *LT* gene as the major oncogene of SV40.[2] However, the equivalent polyomavirus LT mutants were temperature sensitive for virus replication but, at least under some conditions, able to transform cells at the nonpermissive temperature. In addition, the polyomavirus *LT* gene was often disrupted in transformed cells. These findings suggested that, in contrast to SV40, LT was not the major transforming protein of polyomavirus. Indeed, Benjamin[26] isolated transformation-defective polyomavirus mutants that could replicate in mouse cells that had been transformed by wild-type polyomavirus, but not in normal mouse cells, so-called *h*ost-*r*ange–restricted and *t*ransformation-defective (hr-T) mutants. Genetic mapping revealed that the hr-T mutant phenotype resulted not from mutations in the *LT* gene but rather from mutations in an alternative open reading frame in the early region of polyomavirus, which encoded a distinct protein, middle T antigen (mT) (e-Fig. 7.1). SV40 does not encode mT. These findings indicated that SV40 and polyomavirus, though genetically similar, used different mechanisms to transform cells.

To determine the activities of the individual early proteins of polyomavirus, a panel of complementary DNA (cDNA) clones that each expressed a single viral protein was assayed in rat1 cells, an established cell line. The clone expressing polyomavirus mT antigen alone was the only one that displayed transforming activity: cells expressing mT antigen formed foci, appeared morphologically transformed, and formed tumors in animals.[468] These results implied that mT is the major transforming protein of polyomavirus. However, cells transformed by mT antigen were unable to grow in low serum and were thus only partially transformed. On the other hand, cells expressing polyomavirus LT alone were able to grow in low serum, even though they did not display other properties of transformed cells.[373] By using a different assay to study polyomavirus transformation, namely, the ability of the viral genes to convert primary rat embryo fibroblasts into immortalized cells, Rassoulzadegan et al[374] found that LT was active while mT was not. Furthermore, sequential transfer of the *LT* and *mT* genes could convert primary cells into immortal, fully transformed cells. Thus, the individual oncogenes of polyomavirus displayed different transforming activities. Together, these important experiments identified the polyomavirus oncogenes, revealed that they had different effects on cell growth, demonstrated that oncogenes can cooperate to generate fully transformed cells, and highlighted the critical importance of the particular assays used to assess transformation.

Another approach to identify viral oncogenes rests on the finding that genes responsible for transformation are frequently retained in transformed cells, whereas the other viral genes can be lost. Thus, DNA virus genes that are uniformly expressed in transformed cells are likely to be viral oncogenes. Experiments searching for viral DNA and RNA in transformed cells led to the presumptive identification of E1A and E1B as the primary adenovirus oncogenes.[123,167] As the roster of viral and cellular oncogenes has expanded, it is now often possible to identify viral oncogenes by comparing the sequences of viral genes to sequence databases, because novel viral oncogenes are often homologous to validated oncogenes.

The mapping experiments outlined previously demonstrated that DNA tumor viruses typically contain multiple oncogenes. In contrast, acute transforming retroviruses usually contain one oncogene, although there are examples of retroviruses with two (e.g., avian erythroblastosis virus [AEV] ES4 contains both ErbA and ErbB oncogenes). Nonacute retroviruses lack oncogenes.

Maintenance of Transformation

Is continuous expression of viral oncogenes required to maintain the transformed phenotype, or do tumor virus oncogenes only initiate cell transformation, after which they are not required (a hit-and-run–type mechanism)? If viral genes are required to maintain transformation, then they will be expressed in stably transformed cells. Biochemical and immune-based analysis can detect the presence of viral genes and proteins in cells transformed by many viruses, but often only a subset of viral genes is expressed in these cells. The production of infectious virus by transformed cells would provide definitive evidence for the presence of an intact, functional viral genome in the cells, but one of the striking properties of virally transformed cells is that they often do not produce infectious virus. This is not surprising for viruses, including many of the DNA tumor viruses, whose transforming activity is typically studied in nonpermissive cells unable to support virus replication. In contrast, cells transformed by Rous sarcoma virus or some other retroviruses produce infectious virus.

The presence of wild-type virus genomes in transformed cells was demonstrated by virus rescue experiments. In a typical experiment, SV40-transformed mouse cells (which are nonpermissive for replication of SV40) were fused to nontransformed, permissive monkey cells (e-Fig. 7.2). The fused cells produced infectious wild-type SV40, which could be detected by plaque formation assays in permissive cells.[266] This demonstrated that transformed cells could contain full-length, infectious virus genomes in a latent state, which could be activated by replication factors present in permissive cells. We now know that the inability of mouse cells to support SV40 replication is due to the inability of murine DNA polymerase-α/primase to interact with SV40 LT.[408]

The study of conditional viral mutants and expression constructs proved that viral genes expressed in transformed cells are required to maintain the transformed state. In these experiments, cells transformed under the permissive condition when the viral oncoprotein was active often reverted to normal under nonpermissive conditions that inactivated the oncoprotein. This was initially shown with temperature-sensitive mutants of viral oncogenes, where transformation was extinguished at the higher, nonpermissive temperature.[27,302,416] More recently, individual oncogenes driven by inducible/repressible promoters or maneuvers such as RNA interference were used to show that viral oncogene expression was required to maintain the transformed phenotype. Ongoing oncogene expression is not required in cells transformed by all viruses, but it is commonly observed for cells transformed by a variety of DNA viruses and acute transforming retroviruses.

Continuous oncogene expression is also required for cells derived from some virally induced human tumors. For example, repression of human papillomavirus (HPV) oncogene expression in cervical cancer cells causes the rapid cessation of proliferation or the induction of apoptosis (e.g., reference [225]). Thus, even though mutations presumably accumulated in these cells during the extended period of human carcinogenesis, these mutations are not sufficient to maintain the transformed phenotype in the absence of viral oncogene expression. This finding raises the hope that it will be possible to treat virally induced cancers by interfering with the expression or action of viral oncogenes.

To continuously provide viral oncogene products in stably transformed cells, the viral genome must persist. Most commonly, the viral DNA is covalently integrated into the cellular DNA and replicates passively with the host genome. For retroviruses, integration of an essentially intact viral genome is an integral step in the viral life cycle, but for most DNA viruses, integration is incidental (and indeed inimical) to normal viral DNA replication. For these viruses, integration does not occur at specific sites in the cellular genome, and often only portions of the viral genome containing the viral oncogenes are present in the cell. Integration of DNA virus genomes is a rare event, which may explain at least in part why stable transformation by these viruses is so inefficient. Papillomavirus and herpesvirus genomes stably replicate as plasmids in transformed cells, but the DNA of these viruses can be integrated in cancer cells.

Origin of Viral Oncogenes

Where do viral oncogenes come from? Initial studies with retroviruses were conducted with Rous sarcoma virus (RSV). Cells transformed by infection with a mutant RSV carrying a temperature-sensitive *src* gene rapidly reverted to a nontransformed phenotype when shifted to the nonpermissive temperature, but the mutant was replication competent at both high and low temperatures.[74,302] Similarly, transformation-defective RSV deletion mutants were isolated that retained the ability to replicate.[27] These important results indicated that a specific gene (*src*) was responsible for RSV transformation but not for virus replication. Stehelin, Varmus, and Bishop[441] later used molecular hybridization to show that *src* sequences were actually derived from chicken cell DNA. We now know that acute transforming retroviruses such as RSV incorporate altered versions of cellular genes into the viral genomes, a process known as transduction. These transduced genes typically encode constitutively active versions of cellular signal transduction components, such as growth factor receptors and other signaling proteins (see next section). The cellular versions of these genes (designated by the prefix *c*, e.g., c-*src*) are known as the proto-oncogenes, whereas the active viral versions (e.g., v-*src*) are called oncogenes.[86] In contrast, the nonacute retroviruses induce tumors by integrating near-cellular proto-oncogenes and activating their expression.

The discovery that cellular proto-oncogenes can be activated by viruses to generate cancer suggested that nonviral cancers might also arise by activation of proto-oncogenes. Indeed, spontaneously arising human tumors frequently contain altered or overexpressed versions of the proto-oncogenes targeted by oncogenic retroviruses. In several cases, drugs have been developed that specifically inhibit activated proto-oncogene products and provide substantial clinical benefit to cancer patients (e.g., in chronic myelogenous leukemia and lung cancer). Thus, the practical legacy of tumor virology extends far beyond virally induced tumors.

In contrast to most retroviral oncogenes, the oncogenes of the small DNA tumor viruses are intrinsic viral genes required for virus replication, and mutations that interfere with transforming activity usually also inhibit viral replication. In some cases, phylogenetic analysis shows that these genes have been essential for virus replication for millions of years. DNA virus oncogenes usually encode proteins that bind and modulate cellular proteins that regulate cell growth. Most commonly, nuclear oncoproteins of a number of DNA tumor viruses bind to the p53 and retinoblastoma (Rb) tumor suppressor proteins and neutralize their growth inhibitory activity, but the oncoproteins of DNA tumor viruses can modulate other cellular targets as well. Some DNA virus oncoproteins mimic constitutively active forms of a cellular regulatory protein.

p53 and Rb are not only targets of viral tumorigenesis. Most sporadic human cancers, as well as some inherited cancers, contain inactivating mutations in the *p53* and *Rb* genes and in genes in the pathways they control.[284] As was the case with the discovery of cellular proto-oncogenes, studies of DNA tumor viruses identified cellular proteins and pathways crucial for understanding the genetic basis of naturally occurring, nonviral tumors.

Although retroviral oncogenes usually have cellular origins and DNA tumor virus oncogenes typically have viral origins, these distinctions are not absolute. The Jaagsiekte sheep retrovirus envelope protein is required for both virus replication and cell transformation, and the gp55P oncoprotein of the Friend erythroleukemia retrovirus is a mutant retroviral envelope protein that contributes to erythroleukemia in mice.[285,296] On the other hand, the genome of Kaposi sarcoma herpesvirus (KSHV), a large DNA-containing virus, contains a number of genes essential for viral replication and cell transformation that appear to have been acquired from the cellular genome in relatively recent evolutionary times.[328,389]

Cellular Targets of Viral Oncogenes

The great majority of viral oncogenes stimulate cell proliferation (most of the others inhibit cell death). In untransformed cells, the cell division cycle is regulated by intrinsic oscillators, which ensure the orderly progression of the cell cycle, and by external growth factors, which indirectly affect the activity of the cell cycle machinery. Like serum growth factors, many viral oncogenes can stimulate DNA synthesis in normal cells made quiescent by serum starvation. Thus, the signal transduction pathways activated by growth factors provide a useful framework to understand the function of viral oncogenes (Fig. 7.2).

Serum contains polypeptide growth factors such as platelet-derived growth factor (PDGF) and epidermal growth factor (EGF), which bind to specific cell surface receptors to initiate mitogenic signaling. These growth factor receptors are often transmembrane proteins with an extracellular ligand binding domain, a membrane-spanning domain, and an intracellular signaling domain. Ligand binding induces dimerization and/or reorientation of the receptors, initiating intracellular signaling cascades.[407] Many of these receptors are tyrosine kinases or associate with tyrosine kinases. The molecular events induced by ligand binding result in activation of the intrinsic tyrosine kinase activity of the receptors (or of the associated kinases) and in tyrosine phosphorylation of the receptor itself. Phosphorylation on

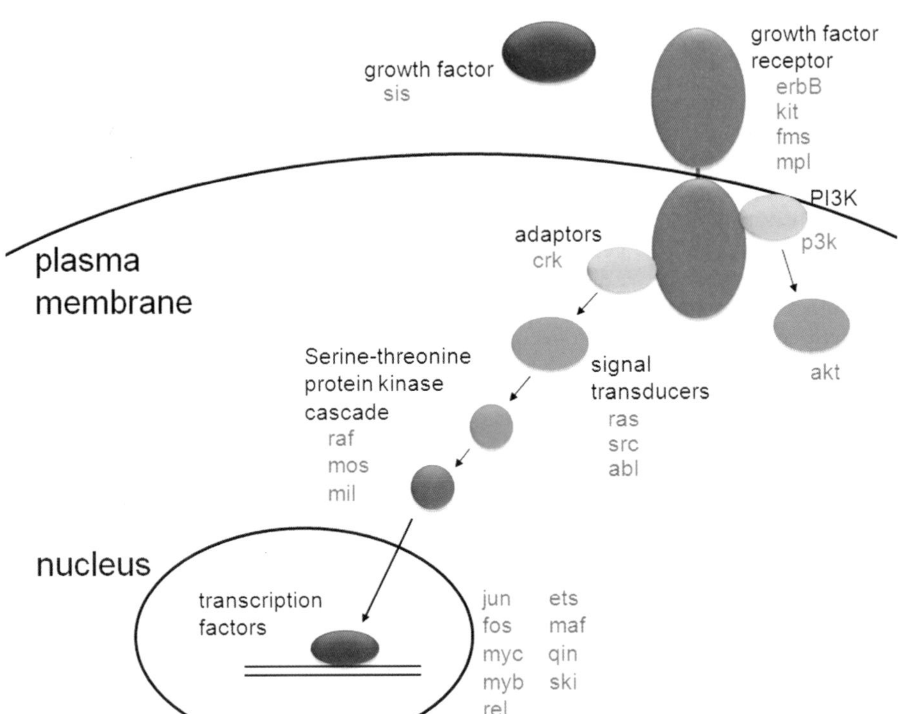

FIGURE 7.2. Mitogenic signal transduction pathways and retroviral oncogenes. This figure shows a schematic representation of mitogenic signal transduction. Binding of a growth factor to a growth factor receptor initiates signal transduction pathways involving adaptor proteins, signal transducing proteins, and serine/threonine kinases. This results in the phosphorylation of transcription factors to alter gene expression and execute pro-proliferative or antiapoptotic signals. Components of this pathway that were transduced by acute transforming retroviruses are listed in red.

tyrosine in turn generates specific binding sites for a variety of signaling proteins that contain SH2 (*src* homology region 2) or other protein–protein interaction domains, which themselves may be tyrosine phosphorylated after binding the activated receptor.[386] Among the targets of these signaling proteins are intracellular guanine nucleotide exchange factors (GEFs) that activate signal transducing molecules such as p21^{ras}.[39] This then initiates a cytoplasmic signaling cascade involving a series of serine/threonine kinases (the mitogen-activated protein [MAP] kinase cascade) that ultimately results in the phosphorylation and activation of nuclear transcription factors, such as AP1 (composed of jun and fos subunits) and c-myc, allowing them to stimulate the expression of various cellular genes.[34,36,80] Growth factor treatment also activates phosphotidylinositol 3-kinase (PI3K) signaling, which generates antiapoptotic and pro-growth signals mediated by the downstream kinase, akt.

A major target of transcriptional activation following growth factor treatment is the cyclin D gene.[306] Cyclins, including cyclin D, are regulatory subunits of the cyclin-dependent kinases (cdks), which directly regulate the cell cycle by allowing cells to move past specific cell cycle checkpoints (e.g., the G1/S boundary) (Fig. 7.3). Cyclin concentrations vary periodically throughout the cell cycle, and association of cyclins with cdks stimulates the activity of the cdk complexes, which catalyze the phosphorylation of nuclear substrates. For example, association of cyclin D with cdk4 results in phosphorylation of members of the Rb family (Fig. 7.3). Phosphorylation of Rb proteins causes their release from E2F proteins, a family of transcription factors that was first identified because E2F is required for activation of the adenovirus E2 promoter.[268] Rb release increases transcription of a set of E2F-dependent cellular genes that encode proteins required for cellular DNA synthesis, including DNA polymerases, topoisomerases, and enzymes involved in nucleotide synthesis.[114] Thus, growth factor treatment triggers a signal transduction cascade that results in the inactivation of the Rb family and stimulation of the G1 to S phase transition and cellular DNA synthesis.

Cdks are also regulated by the p53 pathway.[284] The p53 protein is a transcription factor that can stimulate or repress the expression of various genes. Typically present at low levels

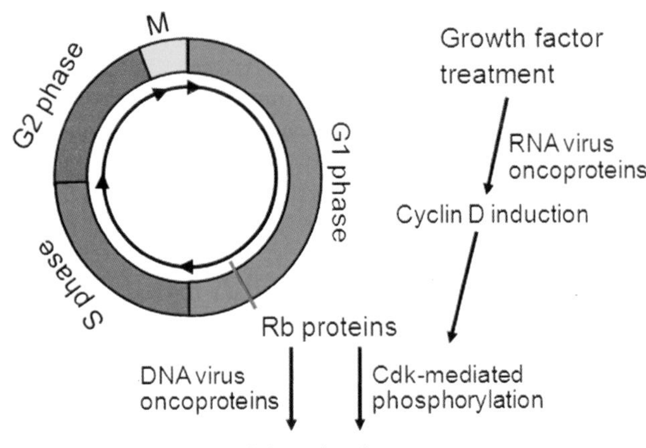

FIGURE 7.3. The cell cycle. The figure shows a simplified version of the cell cycle. The active form of the retinoblastoma family members prevents progression through the G1 phase. Rb-mediated inhibition is abrogated by growth factor treatment, which results in accumulation of cyclin D, stimulation of cyclin-dependent kinases (cdks), and Rb phosphorylation. Rb can also be inhibited by the expression of several DNA virus oncoproteins, such as adenovirus E1A, human papillomavirus (HPV) E7, or simian virus 40 (SV40) large T antigen (see Fig. 7.12).

and inactive, the expression and activity of p53 is induced by a variety of stresses, including DNA damage. An important target of p53-mediated transcriptional activation is $p21^{WAF1/CIP1}$, an inhibitor of cdk activity and cell cycle progression.[139] Therefore, a direct consequence of p53 activation is $p21^{WAF1/CIP1}$ induction and the inhibition of cdk activity. This causes the retention of the Rb family in the underphosphorylated form, which inhibits cell cycle progression by preventing E2F-mediated gene activation. Conversely, inhibition of p53 reduces the levels of $p21^{WAF1/CIP1}$, and the resulting increase in cdk activity and Rb phosphorylation dissociates E2F and Rb, allowing DNA synthesis to occur.

According to this simplified view of cell cycle control, proliferation can be stimulated by activation of mitogenic signaling or by inhibition of tumor suppressor proteins. Not surprisingly, most viral oncogenes function in just this way, either by activating signal transduction cascades or by inhibiting tumor suppressor pathways.[31,47] Indeed, much of our molecular understanding of mitogenic signal transduction and the role of tumor suppressor proteins in cell proliferation and cancer is derived from genetic and biochemical analysis of viral oncoproteins.

Cells not only respond to mitogenic signals but also possess intrinsic pathways that limit cell proliferation in response to a variety of stresses. DNA damage elicits cell cycle arrest (via p53 activation) to allow cells time to repair the damage. If the damage is extensive, apoptosis will result. Virus infection or oncogene action can also activate checkpoints that block cell proliferation. For example, replicating viral DNA itself can be recognized as foreign and trigger a DNA damage response.[488] In addition, the aberrant activation of mitogenic signaling pathways by viral oncoproteins can cause unscheduled DNA synthesis, which in turn induces apoptosis or senescence.[137] Because such premature cell death or inhibition of proliferation will reduce virus yield, these cellular responses can be viewed as antiviral defense mechanisms. In many cases, the p53 and the Rb pathways are required for the execution of these antiviral processes. Neutralization of these tumor suppressor pathways by viral oncoproteins will not only directly stimulate cell proliferation but also interfere with these checkpoints and remove these barriers to transformation and tumorigenesis. Furthermore, when the checkpoint fails, the resulting inaccurate DNA repair or unscheduled DNA synthesis allows the accumulation of mutations in cellular regulatory genes or global genomic instability, which further contribute to the erosion of cell growth control.

TRANSFORMATION BY RETROVIRUSES

Retroviruses were discovered because they caused cancers in animals. The first transmissible tumors associated with retroviruses were avian myeloblastosis in 1908[143] and avian sarcomas in 1911,[382] caused by avian myeloblastosis virus (AMV) and RSV, respectively. Other early retroviruses associated with cancers include murine mammary tumor virus (MMTV, mammary carcinomas)[60] and murine leukemia viruses (MuLVs, lymphomas and leukemias).[195] Of the seven retrovirus genera, viruses from five (alpha, beta, gamma, delta and epsilon) are associated with cancers. Only lentiviruses and foamy viruses have not been found to directly induce cancer—and for human immunodeficiency virus type 1 (HIV-1), a lentivirus, a major clinical manifestation of acquired immunodeficiency syndrome (AIDS) is development of cancer.

Most oncogenic retroviruses can be divided into two categories, based on the rapidity with which they induce tumors. *Acute transforming* retroviruses induce tumors rapidly (often within weeks in experimental animals) and can often transform cells in culture. As mentioned earlier, acute transforming retroviruses carry additional genetic information beyond the standard genes for retroviral replication (*gag, pol,* and *env;* see Chapter 47). These additional sequences, the viral oncogenes, are responsible for rapid and efficient tumorigenesis and cell transformation. *Nonacute* retroviruses induce tumors in animals more slowly, do not carry oncogenes, and usually do not transform cells in culture. Nevertheless, these viruses often induce tumors with high efficiency, typically by causing transcriptional activation of cellular proto-oncogenes.

Acute Transforming Retroviruses and Viral Oncogenes

Acute transforming retroviruses belong to the alpha- and gammaretrovirus genera (Table 7.1). The first acute transforming retroviruses to be studied were avian alpharetroviruses, beginning with RSV and avian acute leukemia viruses such as AMV. Acute transforming gammaretroviruses include murine and rat sarcoma viruses, murine acute leukemia viruses, and feline and simian sarcoma viruses. Study of acute transforming retroviruses and their cognate proto-oncogenes has provided numerous important insights into pathways of growth regulation. Indeed, some of the most important proteins in signal transduction and cancer were first identified through study of retroviral oncogenes, including *Ras, Src, Abl, Myc, Fos,* and *Jun.*

RSV and src. Infection of chick embryo fibroblasts with RSV results in cell transformation; a focus-formation assay can be used to quantify the amount of transforming virus present.[463] After the original isolation of RSV, several different strains of related transforming viruses were developed. Some of these strains (e.g., Schmidt-Ruppin [SR-RSV] and Prague [Pr-RSV]) are replication competent. Others, such as the Bryan high-titer strain, consist of a replication-defective RSV genome, which carries the viral oncogene, as well as a related replication-competent "helper" virus genome (e.g., Rous-associated virus [RAV]). In a mixed infection, this helper virus encodes viral replication proteins *in trans* to allow the production of infectious virus.[204]

Passage of replication-competent RSV occasionally results in loss of transforming capacity without affecting viral replication—such variants are termed *t*ransformation-*d*efective RSV (tdRSV).[130] Thus, oncogenesis and transformation are not required for RSV replication. The size of the tdRSV genome was smaller than wild-type RSV, suggesting that viral genomic sequences responsible for transforming activity were missing from tdRSV. These deleted sequences were mapped to the 3′ end of the RSV genome,[484] and they were eventually termed *src*,[86] providing the first example of a retroviral oncogene (Fig. 7.4). *Src* is expressed via a spliced messenger RNA (mRNA) from the splice donor site at the 5′ end of the genome and an acceptor site at the 5′ end of the *src* gene.[202]

Antisera from RSV-infected rabbits were used to identify the protein product of the *src* oncogene as a 60-kD phosphoprotein designated $pp60^{v\text{-}src}$.[50] When an anti-*src* antibody was incubated with a cell lysate from RSV-transformed cells and

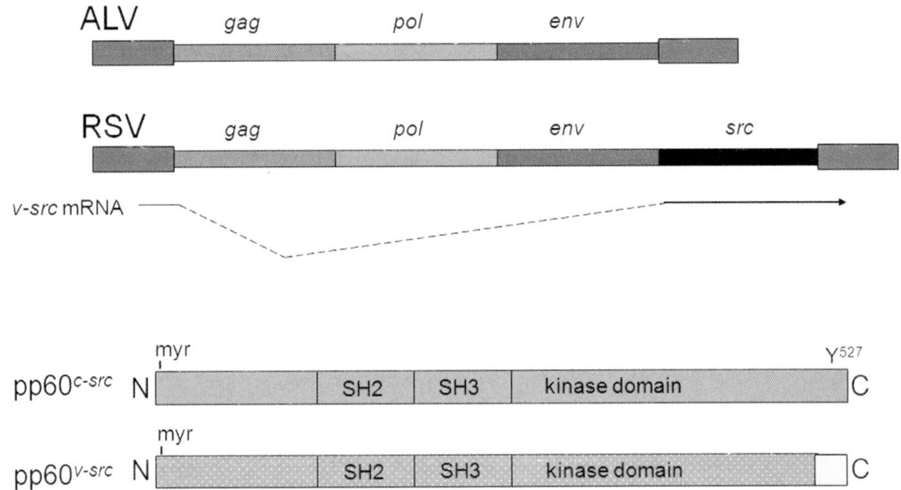

FIGURE 7.4. Structure of Rous sarcoma virus (RSV) and pp60^{src}. The **top part** of the figure shows the proviral structure of avian leukosis virus containing the three retroviral genes required for virus replication, *gag, pol,* and *env.* The long terminal repeats (LTRs) are shown in red. The second provirus shows RSV with the *src* gene located at the 3′ end of the viral genome. A schematic picture of spliced *v-src* messenger RNA (mRNA) is shown below the RSV provirus, with spliced-out introns depicted as dashed lines. The **bottom part** of the figure shows schematic diagrams of pp60$^{v\text{-}src}$ and pp60$^{c\text{-}src}$. Both proteins contain conserved SH2 and SH3 protein–protein interaction domains, tyrosine kinase domains, and an amino-terminal myristal (myr) group. A regulatory tyrosine at position 527 in pp60$^{c\text{-}src}$ (Y^{527}) is also shown. pp60$^{v\text{-}src}$ contains several amino acid substitutions compared to pp60$^{c\text{-}src}$, represented by the stippling, as well as a frameshift mutation that replaces the 19 carboxyl-residues of pp60$^{c\text{-}src}$, including the Y527, with 12 unrelated amino acids.

γ–^{32}P-adenosine triphosphate (ATP) as a phosphate donor, ^{32}P was transferred to the antibody heavy chain, thus identifying pp60$^{v\text{-}src}$ as a protein kinase.[88] Subsequently it was shown that pp60$^{v\text{-}src}$ is a tyrosine-specific protein kinase; that is, it phosphorylates tyrosine residues in its substrate proteins.[89,223] Phosphorylation of proteins on tyrosines is a relatively rare modification (compared to phosphorylation on serine and threonine), and *pp60$^{v\text{-}src}$* was the first tyrosine kinase discovered. Tyrosine phosphorylation is now known to be a major mechanism to regulate protein activity.

Another key discovery was the determination of the origins of the RSV *src* gene. Hybridization experiments with radioactive *src*-specific DNA probes revealed the presence of homologous sequences in DNA from uninfected chickens.[441] The *src*-specific DNA also hybridized with DNA of other species, and the extent of hybridization correlated with the evolutionary distance from chickens. Thus, the *src* gene of RSV, *v-src,* was derived by capture of a normal cell gene, *c-src,* referred to as a proto-oncogene.

The domains of pp60$^{v\text{-}src}$ are shown in Figure 7.4. The protein is modified by myristoylation at the N-terminus, which anchors it to the inner surface of the plasma membrane.[52] Membrane attachment is necessary for transformation, although not for kinase activity.[243] The kinase domain is located in the internal region of pp60$^{v\text{-}src}$. Two adjacent domains are "*src homology*" domains—SH2 and SH3. These domains were originally identified as regions of homology between *v-src* and *src*-related oncogenes of other avian acute transforming retroviruses.[393] The SH2 and SH3 domains mediate the specific interaction of pp60$^{v\text{-}src}$ (and other proteins) with cellular proteins, including regulatory proteins and substrates for phosphorylation.[261,319] SH2 and SH3 domains are present in many cellular proteins, and they are important protein–protein interaction motifs. SH2 domains bind phosphotyrosine residues in specific sequence contexts in their target proteins, while SH3 domains bind proline-rich regions.[261]

The *c-src* proto-oncogene encodes a similar protein, pp60$^{c\text{-}src}$, which differs from pp60$^{v\text{-}src}$ by several amino acid substitutions throughout the protein and by a different C-terminal sequence due to a frameshift mutation in *v-src* (Fig. 7.4).[454,460] The C-terminus of pp60$^{c\text{-}src}$ is a regulatory domain that contains a crucial tyrosine residue at position 527 (Y^{527}). When Y^{527} is phosphorylated, it binds the SH2 domain on the same molecule of pp60$^{c\text{-}src}$, resulting in a closed conformation in which the kinase is inactive.[503] Dephosphorylation of Y^{527} displaces the SH2 domain, resulting in activation of *src* kinase.[94] Of note, the viral protein pp60$^{v\text{-}src}$ lacks the regulatory Y^{527} and is thus constitutively in the open, kinase-active form where it signals for cell transformation by catalyzing high-level phosphorylation of substrates.

Substrates phosphorylated by pp60$^{v\text{-}src}$ provide the key to understanding transformation and oncogenesis by RSV. Various substrates have been identified by searching for proteins that show enhanced levels of tyrosine phosphorylation in RSV-transformed cells compared to normal cells.[91,97,367,381,398,415] pp60$^{v\text{-}src}$ substrates whose phosphorylation is important for RSV transformation include the mitogen-activated protein kinase (MAPK) Erk-1/2,[381] focal adhesion kinase (FAK),[398] and Connexin43, a tight junction protein.[98]

Overview of Other Retroviral Oncogenes. The basic principles elucidated by analysis of RSV also apply to the other acute transforming retroviruses and are summarized here. With a few exceptions described below, acute transforming retroviruses contain viral oncogenes resulting from capture of cellular proto-oncogenes (Table 7.3), although the location

TABLE 7.3 Oncogenes Transduced by Acute Transforming Retroviruses

Oncogene	Retrovirus	Oncoprotein[a]	Identity
Growth factor			
sis	Simian sarcoma virus	$p28^{env\text{-}sis}$	Platelet-derived growth factor-B
Receptor tyrosine kinases			
*erb*B	AEV-ES4, AEV-R, AEV-H	$gp65^{erbB}$	Epidermal growth factor receptor
fms	McDonough FeSV	$gp180^{gag\text{-}fms}$	Colony stimulating factor-1 receptor
sea	S13 AEV	$gp160^{env\text{-}sea}$	Macrophage-stimulating protein receptor
kit	Hardy-Zuckerman-4 FeSV	$gp80^{gag\text{-}kit}$	Stem cell factor receptor
ros	UR2 ASV	$p68^{gag\text{-}ros}$	Ligand unknown
eyk	Avian retrovirus RPL30	$gp37^{eyk}$	Gas6 receptor
Cytokine receptor			
mpl	Mouse myeloproliferative leukemia virus	$p31^{env\text{-}mpl}$	Thrombopoietin receptor
Hormone receptor			
*erb*A	AEV-ES4, AEV-R	$p75^{gag\text{-}erbA}$	Thyroid hormone receptor
Lipid kinase			
p3k	ASV16	$p150^{gag\text{-}p3k}$	Catalytic subunit of PI3K
Ubiquitin ligase			
cbl	Cas NS-1 MuLV	$p100^{gag\text{-}cbl}$	
G proteins			
H-*ras*	Harvey MSV	$p21^{H\text{-}ras}$	
K-*ras*	Kirsten MSV	$p21^{K\text{-}ras}$	
Adaptor protein			
crk	CT10, ASV-1	$p47^{gag\text{-}crk}$	
Nonreceptor tyrosine kinases			
src	Rous sarcoma virus	$pp60^{src}$	
abl	Abelson MuLV	$p160^{gag\text{-}abl}$	
fps[b]	Fujinami ASV	$p130^{gag\text{-}fps}$	
	PRC 11 ASV	$p105^{gag\text{-}fps}$	
fes[b]	Snyder-Theilen FeSV	$p85^{gag\text{-}fes}$	
	Gardner-Arnstein FeSV	$p110^{gag\text{-}fes}$	
fgr	Gardner-Rasheed FeSV	$p70^{gag\text{-}actin\text{-}fgr}$	
yes	Y73 ASV	$p90^{gag\text{-}yes}$	
	Esh ASV	$p80^{gag\text{-}yes}$	
Serine-threonine kinases			
akt	AKT8 MuLV	$p105^{gag\text{-}akt}$	
mos	Moloney MSV	$p37^{env\text{-}mos}$	Cytostatic factor component
raf[c]	3611-MSV	$p75^{gag\text{-}raf}$	
mil[c]	MH2 avian myelocytoma virus	$p100^{gag\text{-}mil}$	
Transcription factors			
jun	ASV17	$p65^{gag\text{-}jun}$	AP1 component
fos	Finkel-Biskis-Jenkins MSV	$p55^{fos}$	AP1 component
myc	MC29 avian myelocytoma virus	$p100^{gag\text{-}myc}$	
	CMII avian myelocytoma virus	$p90^{gag\text{-}myc}$	
	OK10 avian leukemia virus	$p200^{gag\text{-}pol\text{-}myc}$	
	MH2 avian myelocytoma virus	$p59^{gag\text{-}myc}$	
myb	AMV BAI A	$p45^{myb}$	
	AMV-E26	$p135^{gag\text{-}myb\text{-}ets}$	
ets	AMV-E26	$p135^{gag\text{-}myb\text{-}ets}$	
rel	Avian reticuloendotheliosis virus T	$p64^{rel}$	NF-κB component
maf	Avian retrovirus AS42	$p100^{gag\text{-}maf}$	
ski	SKV ASV	$p110^{gag\text{-}ski\text{-}pol}$	
qin	ASV31	$p90^{gag\text{-}qin}$	

AEV, avian erythroblastoma virus; AMV, avian myeloblastoma virus; ASV, avian sarcoma virus; FeSV, feline sarcoma virus; MSV, murine sarcoma virus; MuLV, murine leukemia virus; NF-κB, nuclear factor-κB; PI3K, phosphotidylinositol 3-kinase.

[a]The nomenclature of viral oncoproteins refer to basic structural data: p, protein; gp, glycoprotein; pp, phosphoprotein; the numbers designate the molecular weight in kilodaltons; the superscript indicates the genes from which the coding information is derived in a 5′ to 3′ direction.

[b]*fps* and *fes* are the same oncogene derived from the avian and feline genomes, respectively.

[c]*raf* and *mil* are the same oncogene derived from the murine and avian genomes, respectively.

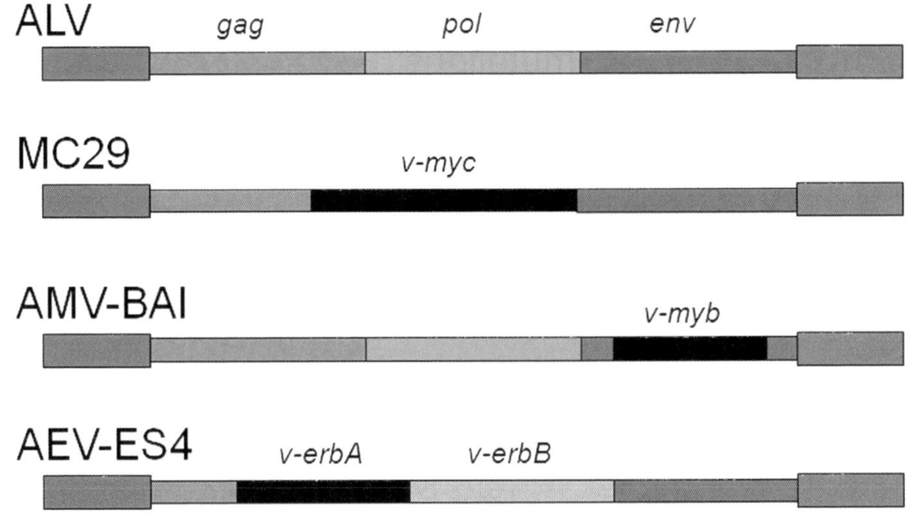

FIGURE 7.5. Genome maps of avian acute transforming retroviruses. The genome structures of the following avian acute transforming viruses are shown: ALV, avian leukosis virus; MC29, avian myelocytoma virus MC29; AMV-BAI, avian myeloblastosis virus BAI; AEV-ES4, avian erythroblastosis virus ES4. The proviral long terminal repeats (LTRs) are shown in red, and the retroviral structural genes *gag, pol,* and *env* are shown in blue, green, and lavender, respectively. Transduced oncogenes are shown in black or gray.

of the oncogene in the viral genome can vary (Fig. 7.5). In some cases the same proto-oncogene has been captured independently by several different viruses. For example, the avian retroviruses Fujinami sarcoma virus and PRC-II both captured the *c-fps* proto-oncogene from the chicken genome, and the Snyder-Theilen strain of feline sarcoma virus captured the homologous gene (*c-fes*) from the cat genome.[194] Proto-oncogene proteins, which generally play positive roles in stimulation of cell growth or division, are typically tightly regulated. The viral oncogene proteins often differ from their parent proteins by amino acid substitutions, deletions, and/or fusion to an intrinsic viral replication protein, most commonly gag. These differences lead to activation of the viral oncogene proteins compared to the proto-oncogene proteins by allowing the viral proteins to escape from the tight regulatory control imposed on the normal cellular homologs. For example, deletions may lead to loss of regulatory regions present in the normal proto-oncogene protein (e.g., $pp60^{v\text{-}src}$ vs. $pp60^{c\text{-}src}$ as described earlier). Amino acid substitutions can also result in loss of regulatory mechanisms (e.g., the *v-ras* proteins), and fusion of viral sequences to the oncogene protein can enhance activity (e.g., the *v-abl* protein). In other cases, the viral oncogene product may be identical to the proto-oncogene product but delivers a sustained or enhanced signal because it is overexpressed. In either case, the viral oncogene proteins signal for cell proliferation by the same molecular mechanisms as the proto-oncogene proteins, but in a constitutive or uncontrolled manner (see Fig. 7.2).

Most acute transforming retroviral genomes are replication defective, because capture of the proto-oncogene sequences generally results in loss of part of the viral genome (Fig. 7.5). Therefore, in order to produce infectious virus, these viruses require co-infection with a helper virus that supplies replication functions. Infection of cells with low concentrations of an acute transforming virus stock can generate foci of transformed cells harboring only the acute transforming viral genome (and not the helper virus genome). Cells from these foci express the viral oncogene, but they do not produce infectious virus—they are called nonproducer cells. Infectious transforming virus can be recovered from these nonproducer cells by infecting them with a replication-competent helper virus to provide replication functions.

Retroviral oncogenes also differ from their corresponding proto-oncogenes because they lack introns. This likely reflects the mechanism of oncogene capture, which is thought to be initiated by integration of a retroviral provirus upstream from a cellular proto-oncogene.[454] Read-through transcription from the retrovirus into the proto-oncogene causes the production of a fusion transcript containing 5′ retroviral sequences and 3′ proto-oncogene sequences. The fusion transcript is then processed by mRNA splicing to remove the proto-oncogene introns, followed by packaging into virions. In a subsequent infection, recombination during reverse transcription presumably results in recovery of the 3′ end of the viral genome and the generation of an acute transforming retroviral genome containing a captured oncogene lacking introns.

Mechanism of Action of Retroviral Cytoplasmic and Membrane-Associated Oncogene Products (see Fig. 7.2). Many oncogenes encode membrane-associated proteins that are derived from RTKs and other growth factor receptors. For example, the *v-erbB* oncogene of AEV ES4 is a transduced version of the EGF receptor.[125] In comparison to the wild-type EGF receptor, the *v-erbB* protein of AEV lacks the extracellular growth factor binding domain, as well as a tyrosine-containing inhibitory autoregulatory domain at the C-terminus (analogous to Y^{527} of $pp60^{c\text{-}src}$).[210] As a result, the truncated *v-erbB* protein delivers downstream signals in an EGF-independent manner. Other RTKs captured and constitutively activated by acute transforming retroviruses include the stem cell factor receptor (*v-kit*) and the colony-stimulating factor 1 receptor (*v-fms*).[219,425,517] The *v-mpl* oncogene encodes a constitutively active version of the thrombopoietin receptor, which lacks intrinsic kinase activity but associates with intracellular tyrosine kinases.[109,249,291] The *v-cbl* oncogene encodes a ubiquitin ligase that can regulate receptor abundance and activity.[239] On the other hand, the *v-sis* oncogene of simian sarcoma virus is a transduced version of a growth factor itself, the platelet-derived growth factor B chain (PDGF-B) gene.[79,338] Thus, *v-sis* can transform only cells that express the PDGF receptor.

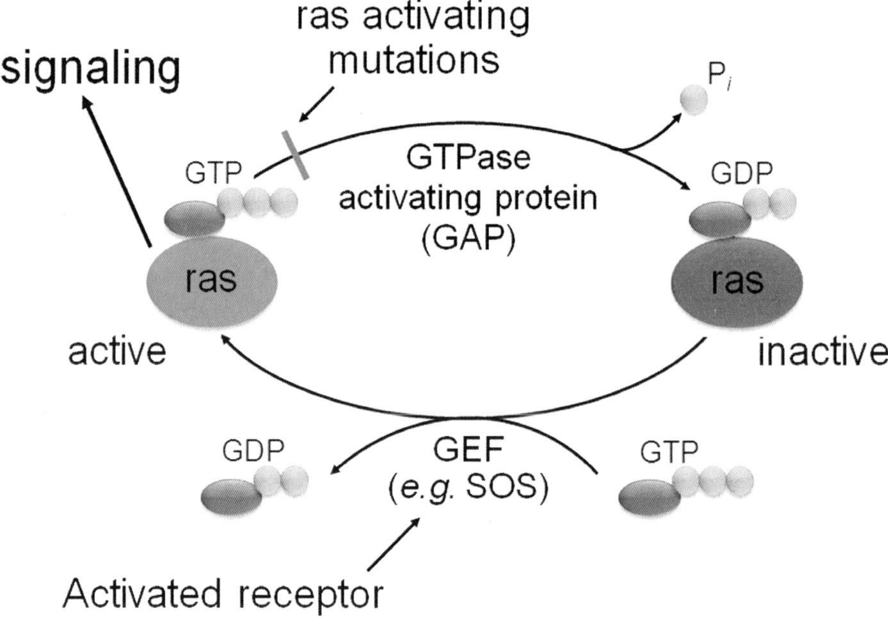

FIGURE 7.6. The ras cycle. Cellular ras proteins exist in two different forms, active guanosine triphosphate (GTP)-bound ras (green) and inactive GDP-bound ras (red). Inactive ras is activated by guanine nucleotide exchange factors (GEFs, such as SOS) that load GTP onto ras; GEFs are activated by growth factor receptor signaling. Active ras is inactivated by its intrinsic GTPase activity, which hydrolyzes bound GTP to guanosine diphosphate (GDP). GTPase activity is stimulated by GTPase activating proteins (GAPs). Activating point mutations at particular positions in v-ras cause the accumulation of ras in the active form, usually by preventing GAP action. Active ras induces signaling by binding and activating effector proteins such as raf.

The *src* family constitutes a class of membrane-associated tyrosine kinases that function in the cytoplasm and lack a ligand binding domain. Thus, *src* family members are not RTKs. In addition to *v-src* itself, other avian acute transforming retroviruses contain the *v-fps*/*v-fes* oncogene and the *v-yes* oncogene.[194] These oncogene proteins share substantial homology with pp60$^{v\text{-}src}$ in the kinase domain as well as in other domains.[261,393] There are other cellular tyrosine protein kinases in the *src* family that function in different signal transduction pathways (e.g., *lck,* whose protein is important for signaling in B lymphocytes[478]), but they have not been captured by acute transforming retroviruses. The genes encoding other cytoplasmic tyrosine kinases unrelated to *src* have been transduced and activated by other acute transforming retroviruses, such as the *v-abl* oncogene of Abelson murine leukemia virus.[496,497]

The cytoplasmic products of other retroviral oncogenes are kinases that phosphorylate protein substrates on serines or threonines, rather than tyrosines. Three oncogenes in this class are *v-raf* (of murine sarcoma virus 3611 [and the homologous *v-mil* from an avian virus]),[234,372] *v-mos* (of Moloney murine sarcoma virus),[413] and *v-akt* (of Akt murine leukemia virus).[24] The corresponding cellular proto-oncogene proteins function in different signaling pathways. Cellular Raf protein is a mediator in signal transduction from RTKs and Ras (see later), initiating a cascade of protein phosphorylations that ultimately leads to phosphorylation and nuclear translocation of MAPKs of the extracellular signal-regulated kinase (ERK) family.[262,514] Cellular Mos protein is required for meiosis and is a component of cytostatic factor (CSF).[508] *v-mos* is activated primarily by overexpression from the viral long terminal repeat (LTR).[33] Cellular Akt protein is a key intermediate in downstream signaling from PI3 kinase, which is also coupled to RTK signaling (see Fig. 7.2). Akt activation delivers survival and proliferative signals to cells. In addition, PI3 kinase itself has been captured by an avian acute transforming retrovirus (AS-16) as the *v-p3 k* oncogene.[64] For the viral oncogenes that encode protein kinases, constitutive, unregulated enzyme activity causes overactive signaling through the corresponding signal transduction pathways, leading to transformation and tumorigenesis.

Other important cytoplasmic oncogenes are the *ras* oncogenes, *v-Hras* and *v-Kras,* identified in Harvey and Kirsten murine sarcoma viruses, respectively.[86,145] These viruses were generated by the capture of two closely related cellular proto-oncogenes, *c-Hras* and *c-Kras,* when MuLVs were passaged through rats. The cellular Hras and Kras proteins, which play critical roles in signal transduction, are guanosine triphosphatases (GTPases) (known as G proteins) that bind guanine nucleotides (guanosine diphosphate [GDP] or guanosine triphosphate [GTP]). In the GTP-bound form, Ras proteins induce signals that result in cell proliferation (e.g., by binding and activating Raf kinase), but they are inactive when bound to GDP (Fig. 7.6).[39,44] Guanine nucleotide exchange factors (GEFs), which stimulate replacement of GDP with GTP, cause inactive Ras to cycle to GTP-bound, active Ras. GEFs include adaptor proteins such as Grb-2 or Sos, which are mobilized by RTK activation.[136,292] The active GTP-bound Ras cycles back to the inactive form by hydrolysis of the bound GTP to GDP by the intrinsic GTPase activity of the Ras protein, which is stimulated by GTPase activating proteins (GAPs).[35] The v-Hras and v-Kras proteins contain missense mutations at key residues (e.g., amino acids 12 and 59 for v-Hras)[459] that reduce the ability of GAP to stimulate GTP hydrolysis.[1] Therefore, the v-Ras proteins accumulate in the active, GTP-bound form because they are unable to cycle to the inactive form, and they signal constitutively for cell growth.

The avian sarcoma virus CT10 and its transduced oncogene, *v-crk,*[307] have provided insight into a family of cellular proteins known as adaptor proteins. The proto-oncogene protein c-crk (*crkI*), along with proteins from related proto-oncogenes *crkII* and *crkL,* contain SH2 and SH3 domains, but they do not have enzymatic activity. Rather, they function as adaptor proteins that assemble proteins into signal transduction complexes by way of interactions via the SH2 and SH3 domains. Cellular signaling proteins that interact with Crk family proteins include Abl, Sos, and FAK.[304]

Mechanism of Action of Retroviral Nuclear Oncogene Products (see Fig. 7.2). The nuclear oncogenes of retroviruses are largely derived from proto-oncogenes that encode DNA binding proteins, many of which act as transcription factors. The *v-myc* oncogene, originally identified in the avian acute leukemia virus MC29 (but also captured by other avian acute transforming viruses), was one of the first studied.[421,476] The c-myc protein (Myc) is involved in early responses to mitogenic stimuli and binds E-box motifs in promoters/enhancers of target genes.[138] Myc exists as a homodimer or as a heterodimer with a related protein, Max. The Myc-Myc homodimers bind E-boxes with low affinity, while Myc-Max heterodimers bind with high affinity.[32] Early after a mitogenic stimulus, levels of Myc transiently rise, leading to activation of E-box–containing genes such as those encoding E2F and cyclin D and repression of genes including those encoding cdk inhibitors.[138] *v-myc* appears to transform cells because of its constitutive overexpression of the retroviral LTR.

The *v-myb* oncogene was also discovered in two different avian acute leukemia viruses (AMV BAI A and AMV E26).[258] It is derived from *c-myb,* which encodes a cellular DNA binding protein that acts as a transcription factor important in hematopoietic cell development.[28] Structural alterations in v-myb appear to be responsible for activation.[28,193]

The oncogene of acute transforming viruses of the Finkel-Biskis-Jinkins (FBJ) murine osteosarcoma virus complex is *v-fos,*[472] and *v-jun* is the oncogene of avian sarcoma virus S17 ("jun" is 17 in Japanese).[297] The *c-fos* and *c-jun* proto-oncogenes encode nuclear DNA binding proteins that are subunits of the transcription factor, activator protein-1 (AP1).[375] Jun can homodimerize, or it can heterodimerize with Fos. Jun-Jun homodimers bind AP1 sites in DNA with low affinity, while Fos-Jun heterodimers bind these sites with high affinity. Activation of Fos transcription from undetectable levels is one the earliest events after mitogenic stimulation—levels of Fos protein rise within 15 minutes of bombesin stimulation in fibroblasts.[324] In contrast, Jun protein is present in the absence of mitogenic stimulation, and Jun levels do not change substantially in response to growth factor treatment. As a result, early after mitogenic stimulation, there is a shift from Jun-Jun homodimers to Fos-Jun heterodimers, resulting in activation of promoters/enhancers containing AP1 sites.[329] Expression of these target genes (e.g., *c-myc*)[227] is important for cell division and growth. Both the v-jun and the v-fos proteins contain structural alterations responsible for oncogenic activation. For example, v-jun contains missense mutations and a deletion that removes an auto-inhibitory segment, resulting in constitutive activation.[41]

Another nuclear oncogene is *v-erbA* of AEV. The *c-erbA* proto-oncogene encodes the thyroid hormone receptor-α (THR-α), a sequence-specific DNA binding protein.[395,487] In contrast to wild-type THR-α, which binds DNA and activates transcription of target genes, the *v-erbA* protein consists largely of the DNA binding domain.[105,395] As a result, it binds to DNA nonproductively and acts as a dominant negative form by inhibiting transcription of THR-α–responsive genes. This leads to a block in erythroid cell differentiation, which in turn results in enhanced proliferation of undifferentiated erythroid progenitors.

The *v-rel* oncogene was initially identified in avian reticuloendotheliosis virus.[73,443] The *c-rel* proto-oncogene encodes a member of the nuclear factor-κB (NFκB) transcription factor family and is important for B-cell development.[180] C-Rel can homodimerize or heterodimerize with the p50 NFκB protein and bind NFκB sites in target genes. Point mutations and amino acids derived from env are required for v-rel activation.[172,457]

Tumorigenesis by Nonacute Retroviruses

Oncogenic nonacute retroviruses belong to the alpha-, beta-, and gammaretrovirus genera. Prototypic nonacute retroviruses include avian leukosis virus (ALV), MMTV, and various MuLVs. These viruses are replication competent, lack viral oncogenes, and do not transform cultured cells. In contrast to tumors induced by acute transforming retroviruses, which are often polyclonal, tumors induced by nonacute retroviruses are monoclonal or oligoclonal (i.e., derived from one or a few transformed cells). Another feature of these viruses is that high-level infection in animals typically occurs many months before development of tumors. Thus, infection is not synonymous with oncogenic transformation for nonacute viruses. The common mechanism by which most nonacute retroviruses induce tumors is insertional activation of cellular proto-oncogenes by the integrated retroviral genome.

B Lymphomas Induced by ALV and Activation of c-myc. Pioneering experiments investigating tumorigenesis by nonacute retroviruses were conducted on chicken B-cell lymphomas induced by ALV. Neel et al[331] analyzed DNA from these tumors and found that many of them did not contain intact integrated ALV proviruses, although each tumor contained at least some segment of viral DNA. They studied tumor RNA by northern blot analysis by using two different radioactive viral cDNA hybridization probes, one representing the entire viral coding region and another representing only the ends of the viral RNA including portions of the viral LTR. The full-length probe did not detect viral RNAs in all tumors; however, the LTR probe invariably detected transcripts in tumors, and different tumors gave transcripts of similar sizes. This led Neel et al[331] to propose the *promoter insertion* model of ALV tumorigenesis, in which transcription from the downstream ALV LTR continues into adjacent cellular sequences (Fig. 7.7). Furthermore, the similar sizes of the transcripts suggested that the ALV proviruses were inserted into the same chromosomal locus in different tumors. Further experiments showed that the ALV LTR was indeed inserted into the same chromosomal region in independent tumors, adjacent to the *c-myc* proto-oncogene.[211] This placed *c-myc* under control of the strong ALV promoter/enhancer, resulting in read-through transcription into the proto-oncogene. Thus, *c-myc* can be activated either by transduction by the acute transforming retroviruses or by proviral insertion by the nonacute retroviruses. Many ALV-induced tumors contain a deletion of a portion of integrated proviral ALV DNA, resulting in loss of the upstream LTR, so that most of the viral DNA is not transcribed. Deletion of the upstream LTR likely stimulates the activity of the downstream LTR, which drives enhanced transcription of *c-myc.*

In some ALV-induced B lymphomas overexpressing *c-myc,* the relative transcriptional orientations of ALV DNA and *c-myc* were not consistent with the promoter insertion model.[352] For example, some tumors contained proviral DNA

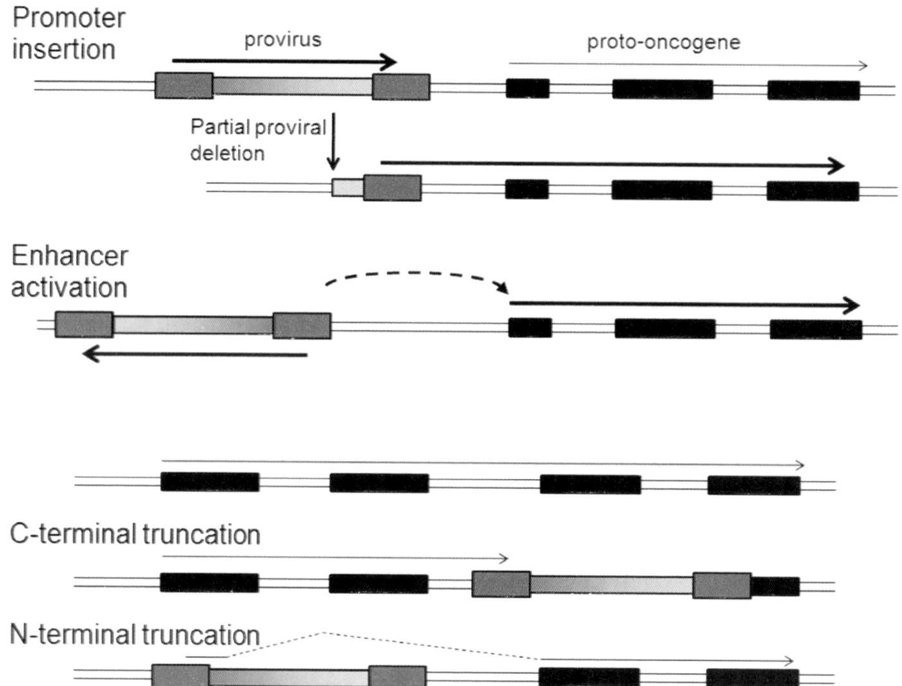

FIGURE 7.7. Insertional activation of cellular proto-oncogenes by retroviruses. The **top two diagrams** show proto-oncogene activation by promoter insertion. The **top diagram** shows a provirus integrated upstream of a proto-oncogene in the same transcriptional orientation. The thickness of the horizontal arrows indicates the relative level of expression. Partial deletion of the provirus activates the downstream long terminal repeat (LTR), which results in read-through transcription into the proto-oncogene. The **third diagram** shows proto-oncogene activation by enhancer activation. In the example shown, the provirus integrates farther upstream from the proto-oncogene in the opposite transcriptional orientation, and the enhancer in the viral LTR activates expression from the proto-oncogene promoter (dashed arrow). Proviruses inserted downstream of a proto-oncogene can also enhance expression. The **bottom three diagrams** show a proto-oncogene with four exons. Proviral insertion in the same transcriptional orientation in the 3′ portion of the proto-oncogene could result in synthesis of a C-terminally truncated protein product due to cleavage/polyadenylation sequences in the LTR. A provirus inserted in the 5′ portion of the proto-oncogene could be transcribed into downstream proto-oncogene exons followed by splicing from a viral splice donor site to a proto-oncogene splice acceptor site. This could result in the deletion or splicing out of proto-oncogene exons and expression of an N-terminally truncated protein product. If the deleted portions regulate the activity of the wild-type protein, these deletions might result in proto-oncogene activation.

inserted upstream of *c-myc* but in the opposite orientation, whereas in other cases the provirus was inserted downstream of *c-myc* (Fig. 7.7). Activation of c-myc expression in these cases can be explained by activation of the endogenous *c-myc* promoter by the enhancer sequences in the ALV LTR, which can activate adjacent promoters in an orientation- and position-independent manner. Thus, activation of proto-oncogenes by nonacute retroviruses can be considered as LTR activation, either by promoter insertion or by enhancer activation. Insertional activation of proto-oncogenes has proven to be a common mechanism of tumorigenesis by nonacute retroviruses. Other variations of these mechanisms are described in the next sections.

MMTV Tumorigenesis. MMTV (a betaretrovirus) also employs insertional activation. Common proviral insertion sites (CISs) were identified[340] in independently arising MMTV-induced mammary tumors. For MMTV, the first CIS did not correspond to any proto-oncogene known at the time, but by analogy to ALV-induced B lymphomas, it was hypothesized that the CIS marked a cellular gene that was activated by the MMTV provirus. This gene was named *int-1* (integration site-1), and *int-1* RNA was overexpressed in tumors. Subsequently *int-1* was renamed *wnt-1* because the *Drosophila* homolog had been identified by the developmental mutation *wingless.*[378] *Wnt-1* is an important molecule in the *Wnt-β-catenin* signal transduction pathway, which is mutated in a wide variety of human cancers, most notably colorectal cancer.[254] Thus, CISs initially identified in nonacute retroviral tumors led to discovery of new proto-oncogenes (Table 7.4). In contrast to ALV-induced B lymphomas where the provirus was integrated quite near *c-myc,* the MMTV provirus in most cases was inserted farther from *Wnt-1.*[340] Activation of *Wnt-1* likely occurs by enhancer activation, because transcriptional enhancers can work over relatively long distances (kilobases). Other CISs in MMTV-induced tumors include *int-2* (FGF-3),[120] *int-3,* and *int-4.*[247]

MuLV Leukemogenesis. MuLVs are gammaretroviruses and include Moloney MuLV (M-MuLV), SL3-3 MuLV, and radiation leukemia virus (RadLV), which induce T lymphoma, and Friend MuLV (F-MuLV), which induces erythroid or myeloid leukemia. Activation of *c-myc* commonly occurs in leukemias induced by M-MuLV.[417,440] Other M-MuLV

TABLE 7.4 Proto-Oncogenes Identified As Common Insertion Sites

Virus	Disease	Common insertion site or activated proto-oncogene
Moloney MuLV	T lymphoma	
	In mice	*c-myc, pim-1, pvt-1/mis-1/mlvi-1, lck, pim-2,*[a] *n-myc,*[a] *bmi-1,*[a] *frat-1,*[a] *pal-1/gfi-1*[a]
	In rats	*c-myc, pvt-1/mis-1/mlvi-1, mlvi-2, mlvi-3, mlvi-4, dsi-1, lck, tpl-1/ets-1,*[a] *tpl-2,*[a] *gfi-1/pal-1,*[a] *gfi-2/IL-9R*
	Myeloid leukemia	*c-myb, mml-1*
AKR MuLV/Gross Virus; SL3-3 MuLV	T lymphoma	*c-myc, gin-1, n-ras*
RadLV	T lymphoma	*c-myc, pim-1, vin-1/cyclinD2, notch1, kis-1, kis-2*
Friend MuLV	Erythroleukemia	*fli-1, fre-2*
	Myeloid leukemia	fis-1, fim-1, evi-1/fim-3, c-fms/fim-2
Endogenous MuLV	Myeloid leukemia	evi-1/fim-3, evi-2, meis-1, and others
(AKXD, BXH-2 recombinant inbred mice)	B lymphoma	*evi-3* and others
Abelson MuLV[b]	B-lymphoma	*ahi-1, ahi-2*[c]
Friend SSFV[d]	Erythroleukemia	*Spi-1, p53*[e]

MuLV, murine leukemia virus; RadLV, radiation leukemia virus.

Data from retroviral tagging of mice genetically predisposed to cancer (e.g., *myc* transgenic mice) are not included here. They can be found in the Mouse Retrovirus Tagged Cancer Gene (RTCG) database at http://RTCGD.ncifcrf.gov.

[a]Insertions associated with tumor progression or that collaborate with other proto-oncogene activations.

[b]Also contains v-abl oncogene.

[c]Common proviral insertion site of helper virus.

[d]Also contains gp55 oncogene.

[e]Insertion at *p53* inactivates its function.

tumors contained novel CISs that led to the discovery of new proto-oncogenes such as the cytoplasmic serine/threonine protein kinases, *pim-1* and *pim-2*[48,99] (Table 7.4). A number of other CISs have been identified in T lymphomas induced by M-MuLV or RadLV, some of which correspond to known cellular genes such as cyclin D2.[205] F-MuLV–induced tumors show activation of a different set of proto-oncogenes than those activated by M-MuLV. Proto-oncogenes commonly activated by F-MuLV include *fli-1* (a nuclear DNA binding protein of the *ets* family), *fim-1*,[435] and *fim-2* (M-CSF).[182] In rapidly arising erythroid leukemias induced by the Friend virus complex, a provirus activates the *spi-1* proto-oncogene, which encodes another *ets* family transcription factor.[320,350] In addition, an acute transforming retrovirus has also been identified in the Friend virus complex: spleen focus-forming virus (SFFV), which contains an oncogene encoding gp55. Gp55 is unusual in that it is not derived from a cellular proto-oncogene, but rather is a deleted form of an endogenous (genetically transmitted) MuLV *env* gene that recombined into the F-MuLV genome.[498]

The different activated proto-oncogenes in leukemias induced by M-MuLV and F-MuLV likely reflect the fact that different signaling pathways are important for transformation of lymphoid versus erythroid/myeloid cells. Studies of MuLV leukemogenesis revealed that the viral LTRs played critical roles in leukemogenicity. First, exchange of the U3 regions of the LTRs between an oncogenic MuLV (e.g., M-MuLV or SL3-3) and a nononcogenic virus (e.g., an endogenous MuLV) demonstrated that leukemogenicity was lost when the U3 region of the LTR was derived from the nononcogenic MuLV.[118,281] Furthermore, substitution of the enhancer region of the F-MuLV LTR into M-MuLV shifted the disease spectrum from T-lymphoid to erythroid/myeloid tumors.[68] This finding reflects the fact that enhancers are often tissue specific; that is, they specifically bind transcription factors present in a subset of differentiated cells. Indeed, in reporter assays, the M-MuLV LTR is most active in T-lymphoid cell lines and less so in erythroid/myeloid cells, while F-MuLV LTR is most active in erythroid/myeloid cells.[428] Taken together, these results indicate that in order for an MuLV to induce tumors, it must have LTRs that efficiently activate cellular proto-oncogenes in the target cells.

Recombinant inbred strains of mice have also been used to study MuLV leukemogenesis. Certain strains of mice genetically transmit replication-competent endogenous MuLVs to their offspring. Crossing such strains with other mouse strains, followed by in-crossing, yields recombinant inbred lines. Some of these lines have high rates of leukemia development due to activation of the endogenous virus, which in turn infects cells and activates cellular proto-oncogenes. Leukemias in such lines have been used to identify new proto-oncogenes that are activated in the tumors, such as *evi-1* (endogenous virus insertion site-1) and *evi-2*, associated with myeloid leukemias.[92]

Another feature of leukemogenesis by MuLVs is the formation of recombinants between these viruses and endogenous MuLV proviruses present in the mouse germline. The genomes of most higher eukaryotes carry retroviral DNA that was introduced by germline infection by retroviruses sometime during evolution. This endogenous retroviral DNA is transmitted vertically from parents to offspring, and multiple endogenous proviruses have accumulated over time. Indeed, approximately 8%

of the human genome is derived from endogenous retroviruses. Many endogenous retroviruses are replication defective, perhaps reflecting evolutionary selection against genetically transmitted, replication-competent viruses, but some can still be expressed. When mice are infected with MuLVs, recombination between the incoming MuLV and endogenous MuLVs can occur to generate mink cell focus-inducing (MCF) recombinant viruses.[207] MCFs express an endogenous MuLV-derived envelope protein that allows them to infect cells by using a different cellular receptor than the original MuLV. Most MuLVs that infect mice or mouse cells are ecotropic and bind to the ecotropic receptor murine cationic amino acid transporter 1 (MCAT-1) on mouse cells; in contrast, MCFs infect via the xenotropic and polytropic retrovirus receptor (XPR-1) receptor. MCFs have been suggested to be the *proximal leukemogens* for some MuLVs (e.g., in AKR mice that develop spontaneous leukemia by activation of a ecotropic endogenous MuLV [Akv-MuLV]),[207] although for other MuLVs MCF recombinants may play early roles in disease.[148] For MuLVs with weak LTR enhancer activity (e.g., Akv-MuLV), MCF recombinants also acquire a stronger LTR by recombination with a second endogenous provirus.[448]

Other Mechanisms of Insertional Oncogenesis. While the predominant mechanisms of oncogenesis by nonacute retroviruses are LTR-mediated activation of proto-oncogenes by promoter insertion or enhancer activation, several related mechanisms have also been identified, all of which involve integration of proviral DNA into the genome at specific places, leading to changes in cellular gene expression and development of tumors.

In one such mechanism, a provirus is inserted upstream of a proto-oncogene or within a proto-oncogene in the same transcriptional orientation as the cellular gene. The viral genome is transcribed beginning in the upstream LTR, but transcription continues past the poly(A) signal in the downstream LTR into the proto-oncogene (Fig. 7.7). Splicing of the fusion transcript from the viral splice donor into downstream proto-oncogene splice acceptor sites can generate mRNAs that encode truncated proto-oncogene proteins. This has been observed in erythroid leukemias induced by ALV in line 15_1 chickens, where a truncated c-ErbB (EGF receptor) protein is produced,[164] and in myeloid leukemias induced by M-MuLV in pristane-primed Balb/c mice, where a truncated c-Myb protein is generated.[330] Similarly, transcription of a proto-oncogene could terminate at the LTR of a provirus inserted into a downstream portion of the proto-oncogene, resulting in a C-terminal truncation (Fig. 7.7). In these cases, the truncations remove regulatory domains from the proto-oncogene proteins, leading to the synthesis of unregulated, growth stimulatory proteins.

As mentioned earlier, inoculation of chicken embryos with ALV leads to rapid development of B lymphomas harboring proviral activation of *c-myc*. In addition, some ALV-induced lymphomas contain proviruses at both *c-myc* and a novel CIS, *bic-1*.[84] Although *bic-1* RNA was overexpressed in these tumors, presumably due to provirus insertion, *bic-1* does not contain protein-coding sequences. Rather, *bic-1* encodes the precursor for microRNA (miRNA) miR155—a so-called onco-miR that is overexpressed in a variety of human cancers.[149] miR155 causes the down-regulation of growth inhibitory genes, which presumably accounts for its oncogenic potential.[38] Insertional activation of other miRNAs has also been observed in retrovirally induced tumors. The miR-103-363 cluster is activated in RadLV-induced T lymphomas,[275] and miR-106 a is activated in SL3-3 MuLV-induced T lymphomas.[293]

Another mechanism of insertional oncogenesis involving miRNAs has been described for T lymphomas induced by SL3-3 MuLV. In these tumors, the provirus is inserted into downstream noncoding sequences of the *gfi-1* proto-oncogene.[100] These sequences contain binding sites for several miRNAs, including miRNA-155. This results in overexpression of a truncated *gfi-1* mRNA, presumably because the inserted provirus eliminates binding sites for inhibitory miRNAs.

Finally, insertions of the SFFV provirus into the p53 tumor suppressor gene occur in erythroleukemia cell lines established from tumors induced by the acute transforming Friend SFFV/F-MuLV complex.[25,323] The insertions inactivate p53, and in these tumors the normal *p53* gene is generally lost. Similarly, in BXH2 recombinant inbred mice, proviral insertion occurs in *evi-2*, which encodes the NF-1 tumor suppressor.[277] In these cases, then, rather than activating proto-oncogenes, proviral insertion inactivates tumor suppressor genes.

Multiple Changes in Nonacute Retrovirus-Induced Tumors. Multiple genetic changes may be involved in some tumors induced by nonacute retroviruses. Proviral insertions next to more than one proto-oncogene have been observed in some MMTV-induced mammary tumors and M-MuLV–induced T lymphomas (e.g., *wnt-1* and *int-2* for MMTV and *c-myc* and *pim-1* for M-MuLV).[311,417] Although in some cases this reflects two independent tumors, each containing an insertion event near a different proto-oncogene, in other cases the same tumor cell harbors both of the activated proto-oncogenes, suggesting that the proto-oncogenes cooperate in tumorigenesis. This notion has been further developed by studying leukemogenesis in transgenic mice. For example, mice with a *pim-1* transgene under expression of a T-cell–specific promoter develop lymphomas very inefficiently. However, if these mice are infected with M-MuLV, tumors develop extremely rapidly, and analysis of the tumors revealed proviral activations of both *c-myc* and *n-myc*.[473] This result provided direct evidence that overexpressed *pim* family members and *myc* family members can cooperate in T lymphomagenesis. In later experiments, several additional pairs of cooperating proto-oncogenes have been identified.[474]

Secondary events may also be important in tumors induced by acute transforming retroviruses. Abelson MuLV (carrying the *v-abl* gene) induces B-cell lymphomas when it is co-infected with an M-MuLV helper virus but not with other helper MuLVs, suggesting that M-MuLV also contributes to tumor development. The critical region for this activity was localized to the M-MuLV LTR, and a CIS for the M-MuLV helper in Abelson MuLV tumors was identified adjacent to the *ahi-1* gene.[361] Thus, expression of the *v-abl* oncogene along with *ahi-1* protein[238] is required for efficient lymphomagenesis.

Another approach to identify activated proto-oncogenes that contribute to later steps in tumorigenesis involves *in vitro* or *in vivo* passage of tumors. For example, *in vitro* passage of rat T lymphomas induced by M-MuLV results in acquisition of additional proviral CISs, which have been termed tumor progression loci (e.g., *tpl-1* and *tpl-2*).[20,349] Likewise, *in vitro* infection of growth factor–dependent M-MuLV–induced

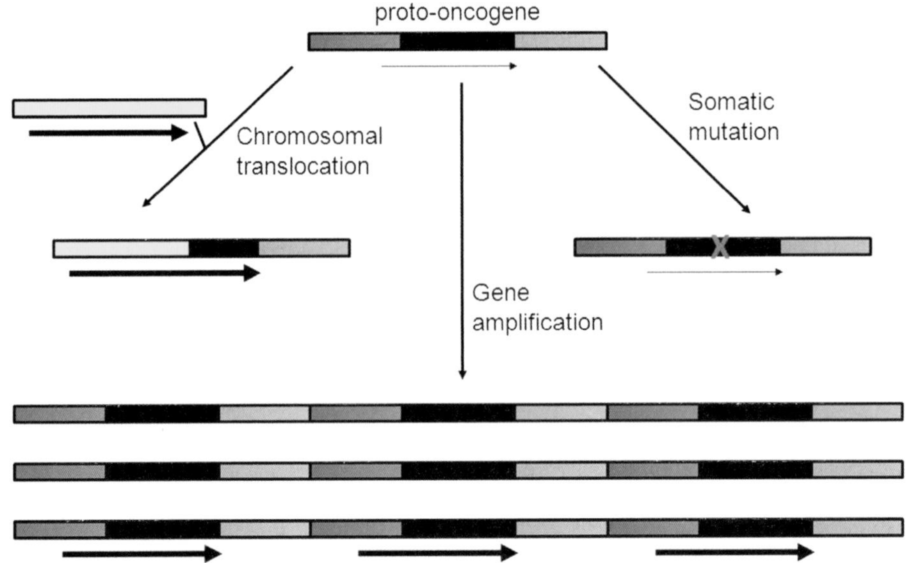

FIGURE 7.8. Proto-oncogene activation in nonviral tumors. The figure shows three mechanisms of proto-oncogene activation in tumors of nonviral origin: tandem amplification of the oncogene and flanking cellular DNA, resulting in overexpression of the oncogene; chromosomal translocation resulting in overexpression and/or structural alteration of the oncogene, leading to its constitutive activation; and point mutations in the coding region of an oncogene, resulting in constitutive activation. The thickness of the horizontal arrows indicates the relative level of expression. Black, proto-oncogene; blue, flanking normal cell DNA; yellow, translocated chromosome. Red X indicates mutation.

lymphomas with a second MuLV (MCF-MuLV) resulted in the generation of factor-independent cells, which contained proviral activation of new proto-oncogenes (e.g., *gfi-1*).[159,179] Finally, as described earlier, insertional inactivation of p53 occurs during *in vitro* passage of erythroleukemia cell lines from Friend virus complex–infected mice, so it is a late step in the development of these lines.[25]

Proto-Oncogene Discovery in the Age of Genomics. The initial discovery of CISs and activated proto-oncogenes was very labor intensive and typically required identifying virus-induced tumors harboring a small number of proviruses, followed by generating a lambda phage library of tumor DNA and cloning all of the proviruses. Adjacent cell sequences from each provirus were then used as hybridization probes on Southern blots of DNA from other virus-induced tumors to identify additional tumors that harbored proviral insertions in the same cellular site.[211,352] The availability of whole genome sequences substantially increased the pace of CIS discovery, particularly in mice.[422] New cloning techniques such as inverse polymerase chain reaction (PCR) facilitated the cloning of proviral DNA and viral–host junctions.[422] Sequencing of the adjacent cellular DNA in these clones, followed by alignment of the cellular DNA sequence with the host genome, allowed rapid localization of each proviral insertion site within host cell DNA. Common insertion sites could be readily identified by insertions into similar chromosomal locations in different tumors.

The advent of high-throughput DNA sequencing has further enhanced the efficiency of CIS discovery. In a recent approach, linker-ligated PCR techniques are used to amplify viral–cellular junctions from tumor samples, and then the entire reactions are analyzed by deep sequencing.[265] This provides high-resolution analysis of all of the proviral insertions in a tumor, and then comparison with other tumors induced by the same virus is used to identify CISs. In a recently published study, over 9,000 insertion sites were analyzed in a collection of 476 murine tumors, and multiple new CISs were identified.[265]

Activation of Proto-Oncogenes in Nonviral Tumors

Studies of retroviral oncogenes and their corresponding proto-oncogenes led to the first discoveries of molecular genetic alterations in human cancers, namely, activation of proto-oncogenes. Genetic alterations in cancer are now major subjects of study in cancer research. The basic mechanisms of proto-oncogene activation in tumor cells—gene amplification, chromosomal translocation, and missense mutations—mirror the consequences of retroviral activation of oncogenes (Fig. 7.8).

Gene amplification in tumor cells is manifested by tandem head-to-tail duplication of chromosomal regions (up to several hundred kilobases in length), resulting in as many as ~10 additional copies of the amplified region of the chromosome. Amplified regions typically contain a proto-oncogene (as well as flanking genes) and were originally detected on Southern blots by cross-hybridization with viral oncogene probes. For example, *c-myc* is amplified in several kinds of tumors such as lung cancer and neuroblastoma.[410,411] Amplification leads to overexpression of the protein product of the proto-oncogene and excessive stimulation of growth. Early studies on *c-myc* amplification led to the discovery of *c-myc*–related genes that were also amplified in tumors (e.g., *n-myc* in neuroblastomas and *l-myc* in lung cancers). These findings expanded the concept of proto-oncogenes beyond those that had been captured by acute transforming viruses: proto-oncogenes are cellular genes that are activated in tumors and stimulate growth or division.

Chromosomal translocations have also been observed in tumors; for example, the 9:22 translocation (the Philadelphia chromosome) is pathognomonic for chronic myelogenous leukemia (CML).[385] The first molecular description of such translocations was in Burkitt lymphoma (of B-cell origin), where *c-myc* is characteristically present at an 8:14 translocation breakpoint,[103] which moves *c-myc* on chromosome 8 next to the immunoglobulin heavy chain gene. In other cases, Burkitt lymphoma cells harbor a translocation of the *c-myc* gene into the immunoglobulin light chain locus on chromosome 22. In B lymphocytes, whose function is to produce antibodies, the immunoglobulin genes are highly expressed. Therefore, translocation of *c-myc* into these regions leads to *c-myc* overexpression and growth stimulation. Similarly, the 9:22 translocation in CML juxtaposed *c-abl* from chromosome 9 next to the Bcr (breakpoint cluster region) on chromosome 22.[108] This translocation results in a novel Bcr-abl fusion protein, which exhibits elevated tyrosine kinase activity compared to the normal Abl protein.[264] Thus, chromosomal translocations can have the same consequences as proviral insertion and proto-oncogene transduction. Characteristic translocations have been detected in various additional tumors (particularly of hematopoietic lineage, but also in prostate and lung carcinoma), and genes at the translocation junctions either are overexpressed or have altered signaling properties.[257] These genes are now considered proto-oncogenes as well.

Missense mutations in proto-oncogenes in tumors were first detected by DNA transfection experiments. When naked DNA from certain tumor cell lines or primary tumors was introduced into mouse NIH-3T3 fibroblasts, foci of transformed cells appeared, whereas DNA from normal cells was, in general, devoid of transforming activity.[426] Thus, these tumor cells contained a genetic change that could be transferred to other cells to cause transformation. Molecular cloning from the EJ bladder carcinoma cell line identified the transforming gene as cellular *H-ras.*[346] The *H-ras* gene in the EJ cells had a missense mutation at residue 12 (G12V) of the protein,[458] resulting in inhibition of GTPase activity and constitutive signaling, similar to changes in the *v-ras* proteins described earlier. Other tumors had missense mutations in the *K-ras* gene[117] or in a third homolog, *N-ras.*[168] *Ras* mutations are some of the most frequent genetic alterations in human tumors (e.g., they are present in greater than 90% of pancreatic cancers), but this assay has identified other transforming genes in human tumor DNA as well. Activating mutations have also been found by direct sequencing of cellular proto-oncogenes (e.g., EGF receptor mutations in lung cancer, c-kit mutations in gastrointestinal stromal tumors, and B-raf mutations in melanoma).

Other Mechanisms of Retroviral Oncogenesis

While transduction of oncogenes by acute transforming retroviruses and insertional activation of proto-oncogenes by nonacute retroviruses are the most common mechanisms of retroviral oncogenesis, a few retroviruses induce tumors by other mechanisms. These mechanisms involve replication-competent retroviruses, which carry genes that function as oncogenes, although they are not derived from cellular genes.

HTLV-I and BLV. Human T-cell leukemia virus type I (HTLV-I) and bovine leukemia virus (BLV) induce adult T-cell leukemia (ATL) in humans and bovine B-cell leukemia, respectively. These deltaretroviruses are covered in Chapter 48 in detail. *In vitro* infection of T lymphocytes with HTLV-I leads to immortalization, suggesting that the virus carries an oncogene.[245] Deltaretroviruses contain additional genes not found in other retroviruses, which encode regulatory proteins such as Tax, encoded by alternatively spliced mRNA within the *X* region of the virus, downstream of *env.* The Tax protein is a transcriptional transactivator of the HTLV-I LTR.[57,153] It can also transactivate or inhibit cellular promoters by affecting the activity of the NFκB pathway, various transcriptional co-activators, and interleukin-2 (IL-2) signaling,[72,283,333,430] and it induces defects in DNA replication and repair by nontranscriptional mechanisms.[288,300] *Tax* has many properties of an oncogene; for instance, it can transform rodent fibroblasts in culture, and mice harboring a *tax* transgene develop tumors of mesenchymal origin.[333] Tax can also up-regulate telomerase expression, inactivate p53, and immortalize human T cells in the presence of IL-2.

WDSV and Dermal Sarcomas. Walleye dermal sarcomavirus (WDSV) is an epsilonretrovirus that induces dermal sarcomas in walleye pike.[383] Related viruses (WEHV-1 and -2) induce epidermal hyperplasia in these fish, and similar viruses induce tumors in other fish. Tumors arise only during the winter; during spring spawning the tumors are shed, where the released virus presumably infects new hatchlings. WDSV and other epsilonretroviruses carry three additional reading frames besides the standard retroviral genes—*orf A,* *orf B,* and *orf C.* During the winter, the tumors do not express infectious virus, and the only transcripts present are for *orf A* and *orf B,* so the proteins encoded by these genes are likely involved in tumorigenesis.[383] *Orf A* encodes a viral cyclin, rvCyclin, which binds cellular cdk8 and cdk3 and affects viral transcription and transformation. rvCyclin in complex with cdk8 negatively regulates transcription from the WDSV LTR and may be involved in inhibiting viral expression in the winter. rvCyclin can also affect expression of cellular genes, and it may positively affect cell transformation and tumorigenesis. Mice transgenic for rvCyclin develop squamous epithelial hyperplasia and dysplasia,[274] but tumors do not form in transgenic rvCyclin fish.[351] *Orf B* may also contribute to tumorigenesis. This gene appears to have an antiapoptotic function, and *orf B* can transform cells in culture.[383]

JSRV and Env as an Oncogene. Jaagsiekte sheep retrovirus (JSRV) and the related enzootic nasal tumor virus (ENTV-1 and -2) are betaretroviruses. JSRV causes a transmissible lung cancer (ovine pulmonary adenocarcinoma) in sheep, and ENTV-1 and -2 cause adenocarcinoma of nasal epithelial cells in goats.[216] Interestingly, the native envelope protein of these viruses not only mediates viral entry but also functions as an oncogene. Expression of Env protein can transform various fibroblast and epithelial cells *in vitro*[296] and induce tumors in mice or sheep.[59,78,102,500]

As is the case for all retroviruses, there are two Env proteins, which are derived by cleavage from a polyprotein precursor—the SU (surface) protein on the exterior of virions and the TM (transmembrane) protein that spans the lipid bilayer of the viral envelope. In JSRV-transformed cells, the SU protein is presumably extracellular and the TM spans the plasma membrane. The intracellular cytoplasmic tail (CT) of TM is necessary for transformation, and a specific required tyrosine residue in CT might serve as a docking site for PI3K.[343] Signal transduction pathways important for JSRV transformation include PI3K/Akt/mammalian target of rapamycin (mTOR) and Ras/Raf-MEK/MAPK.[295] In addition to TM, the SU region of JSRV Env is also important for transformation.

Studies in a human lung epithelial line (BEAS-2B) suggested another mechanism for JSRV transformation. In these cells, JSRV Env binds hyaluronidase 2 (Hyal2), which itself binds and inactivates the Ron RTK (also known as STK).[106] Expression of JSRV Env leads to binding and degradation of Hyal-2, releasing Ron from inhibition. Signaling downstream from Ron involves the PI3K/Akt/mTOR and Ras/Raf-

MEK/MAPK pathways. However, JSRV Env is able to transform cells such as mouse fibroblasts, whose Hyal-2 does not bind Env and where Ron is not expressed.[289] Thus, while binding and inactivation of Hyal-2 may participate in transformation of lung epithelial cells, this interaction is not required for transformation of other cell types.

As described earlier, MMTV induces mammary tumors by insertional activation of proto-oncogenes. However, MMTV envelope may also have oncogenic properties. MMTV-infected cell lines are not transformed when grown in monolayer culture. However, MMTV-infected MCF10 mammary epithelial cells show enhanced and disorganized growth when cultured in three dimensions, whereas normal MCF10 cells form well-organized spheres consisting of a single layer of polarized epithelial cells.[248] This transforming activity requires an immunoreceptor tyrosine-based activation motif (ITAM) in the MMTV Env TM protein, which leads to signaling through pathways used for ITAM signaling in lymphocytes.[248]

Finally, as mentioned earlier, the oncogene of the acute transforming Friend SFFV virus encodes an internally deleted form of an endogenous MuLV Env protein recombined into F-MuLV, designated gp55.[85] Gp55 protein binds two growth factor receptors on the surface of erythroid cells: the erythropoietin receptor (EpoR)[285] and the short form of STK (sfSTK)/Ron.[339] Binding leads to constitutive downstream signaling from these receptors through signaling molecules such as Stat 3, Ras/Raf-MEK/MAPK, and PI3K/Akt.[85] Signaling through sfSTK appears to be more important for oncogenic transformation in some cell types, although in others EpoR signaling is sufficient.

MECHANISMS OF DNA VIRUS ONCOGENE ACTION

Overview

As shown in Table 7.1, several families of DNA-containing viruses induce transformation in cell culture or tumors in animals or humans. The DNA tumor viruses with the smallest genomes and clearly defined oncogenes are the polyomaviruses, including murine polyomavirus and SV40 (a polyomavirus of African green monkeys). Polyomaviruses have circular double-stranded DNA genomes of ca. 5,200 base pairs (bp) that encode two or three oncoproteins—the tumor (T) antigens (large T [LT], small T [sT], and in the case of murine polyomavirus, middle T [mT]). Papillomaviruses have slightly larger circular double-stranded genomes (ca. 8,000 kb) and cause warts in various species. Major oncogenic papillomaviruses include bovine papillomavirus (BPV) and oncogenic strains of HPV. Papillomaviruses encode three oncoproteins: E6, E7, and E5. Adenoviruses are common respiratory viruses with intermediate-sized, linear double-stranded DNA genomes (ca. 30 kb). Certain strains of human adenoviruses can induce tumors in rodents and transform rodent cells in culture. The major oncoproteins of adenovirus are encoded by the E1 region. In addition, adenoviruses express some less well-studied oncogenes, including adenovirus type 9 E4-orf1, which is a major determinant of estrogen-dependent mammary tumor formation in female rats.[235] Herpesviruses are enveloped viruses with large double-stranded DNA genomes (100–150 kb). Several viruses of the gammaherpesvirus genus induce tumors in their host species including humans. Oncogenic human herpesviruses include Epstein-Barr virus (EBV—primarily lymphomas and nasopharyngeal carcinomas) and KSHV (primarily Kaposi's sarcoma). Herpesviruses encode multiple oncoproteins. Another virus with a small DNA genome, hepatitis B virus, can cause tumors, but its mode of action remains poorly defined.

The mechanisms of action of many DNA tumor virus oncogene products are known in considerable detail, and several common features of DNA virus transformation have emerged. DNA virus oncoproteins are required for normal virus replication, typically acting during the early phase of infection prior to the onset of viral DNA replication or active in replication itself. Most DNA viruses encode more than one oncoprotein, which often cooperate to transform cells, in some cases because one protein negates the deleterious effects of the other one. Most commonly, these oncoproteins function by binding to cellular proteins and modulating their activities (Table 7.5). Often, a single viral oncoprotein can bind to numerous cellular targets. As is the case for transduced retroviral oncogenes, some DNA tumor virus oncoproteins stimulate cellular mitogenic

TABLE 7.5 DNA Virus Oncoproteins and Their Major Targets

Adenovirus E1A	Rb family members, p300/CBP, CtBP
Adenovirus E1B 19K	Bak, Bax
Adenovirus E1B 55K	p53
Adenovirus E4orf6	p53
Bovine papillomavirus E5	PDGF-β receptor
Epstein-Barr virus EBNA2	RBP-Jκ/CBF1, glycogen synthetase kinase
Epstein-Barr virus LMP1	Tumor necrosis factor signaling components, PI3K
Epstein-Barr virus LMP2	*Src* family members
Hepatitis B virus X protein	p53
Herpesvirus saimiri STP	Tumor necrosis factor signaling components *Src* family members
Herpesvirus saimiri Tip	*Src* family members
Human papillomavirus E5	EGF receptor
Human papillomavirus E6	p53, PDZ proteins, E6-AP, DNA repair and apoptosis machinery
Human papillomavirus E7	Rb family members, p21, p27, p600
KSHV K-bZIP	p53
KSHV ORF 50	p53
KSHV vCyclin	Cyclin-dependent kinase 6
Polyomavirus large T antigen	p53 (not murine polyomavirus), Rb family members
Polyomavirus middle T antigen	*Src* family members, PI3K, PP2A, shc
Polyomavirus small T antigen	PP2A

EBNA, Epstein-Barr virus nuclear antigen; EGF, epidermal growth factor; KSHV, Kaposi sarcoma herpesvirus; LMP, latent membrane protein; PDGF, platelet-derived growth factor; PI3K, phosphotidylinositol 3-kinase; PP2A, protein phosphatase 2A.

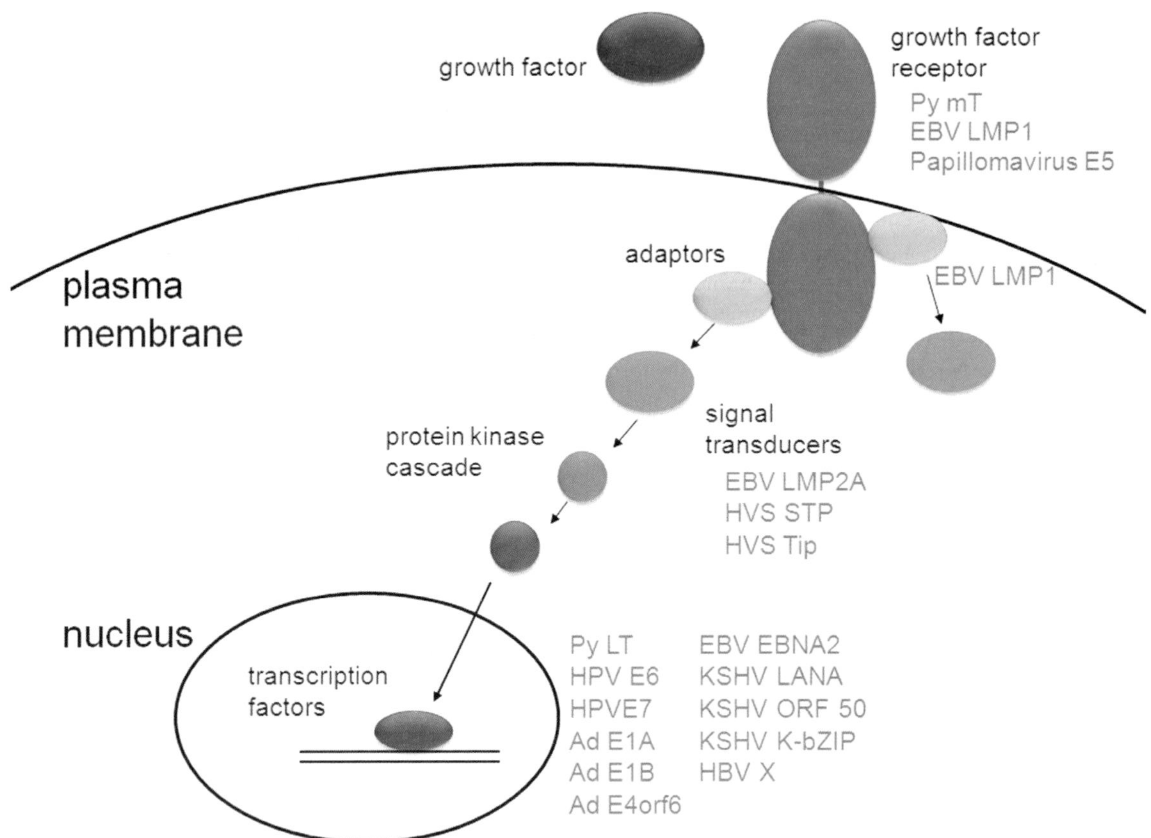

FIGURE 7.9. Mitogenic signal transduction pathways and DNA virus oncogenes. In this diagram of mitogenic signal transduction, DNA tumor virus oncoproteins that mimic or modulate cellular signaling components are listed in red.

signal transduction pathways (Fig. 7.9), and these examples are described first. In a mechanism of action that is shared among several DNA viruses, other oncoproteins inactivate the Rb and p53 cellular tumor suppressor pathways (Fig. 7.9). It is striking that diverse DNA tumor viruses modulate a limited number of common cellular targets, implying that there are relatively few crucial nodes that regulate cell proliferation (Table 7.6).

DNA Virus Oncoproteins That Stimulate Mitogenic Signaling Pathways

Polyomavirus Middle T Antigen. mT is responsible for the major transforming activity of murine polyomavirus in established lines of rodent cells and can induce a variety of cancers in animals.[468] mT is also important for productive polyomavirus infection by regulating viral DNA replication, transcription, and virion assembly.[160]

mT is a 55-kD, largely cytoplasmic protein that is anchored in the plasma membrane by a C-terminal transmembrane segment (Fig. 7.10). Membrane association is required for mT activity, but the native mT transmembrane domain can be replaced by certain other membrane-targeting sequences.[144] The first clue to the mechanism of mT function came from biochemical studies showing that mT associates with protein kinase activity.[134] Further analysis revealed that mT is not an enzyme, but rather associates with a cellular nonreceptor tyrosine kinase. This cellular enzyme turned out to be none

TABLE 7.6 Common Targets of DNA Virus Oncogenes

p53	SV40 large T antigen High-risk HPV E6 Adenovirus E1B 55K and E4orf6 KSHV K-bZIP, LANA, and ORF 50 Hepatitis B virus X protein
Rb family members	Polyomavirus large T antigens (e.g., murine polyomavirus, SV40, Merkel cell polyomavirus) High-risk HPV E7 Adenovirus E1A KSHV LANA
Src family members	Middle T antigen EBV LMP2A HVS STP and Tip
PI3K	Polyomavirus middle T antigen, EBV LMP1
PP2A	Polyomavirus small T antigen and middle T antigen

EBV, Ebstein-Barr virus; HPV, human papillomavirus; HVS, *Herpesvirus saimiri;* KSHV, Kaposi sarcoma herpesvirus; LANA, latency-associated nuclear antigen; LMP1, latent membrane protein 1; PI3K, phosphotidylinositol 3-kinase; PP2A, protein phosphatase 2A; SV40, simian virus 40.

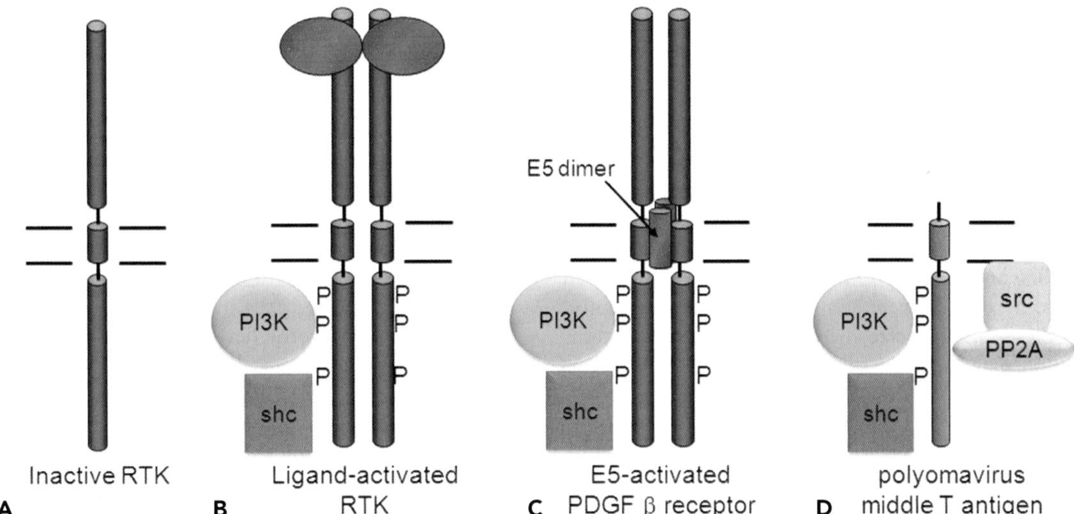

FIGURE 7.10. DNA virus oncoproteins and receptor tyrosine kinases. A: An unstimulated receptor tyrosine kinase (RTK) exists as unphosphorylated monomer with an extracellular ligand binding domain, a membrane-spanning segment, and an intracellular catalytic domain. Horizontal lines represent the plasma membrane. **B:** Treatment with ligand induces receptor dimerization and tyrosine phosphorylation, which recruits various signaling proteins to the receptor. To simplify the drawing, only a single molecule of two substrates is shown. **C:** A dimer of the bovine papillomavirus E5 oncoprotein interacts the transmembrane domain of two molecules of the platelet-derived growth factor-*β* (PDGF-*β*) receptor, resulting in receptor dimerization, autophosphorylation, and recruitment of signaling proteins. **D:** Murine polyomavirus middle T antigen (mT) is anchored into the plasma membrane by a carboxyl-terminal transmembrane domain. Protein phosphatase 2A (PP2A) binds to the cytoplasmic domain of mT and recruits $pp60^{c\text{-}src}$ (src), which catalyzes mT tyrosine phosphorylation and generates binding sites for signaling proteins.

other than $pp60^{c\text{-}src}$, the product of the *c-src* proto-oncogene![96] mT also associates with some other members of the *src* kinase family.[160] Biochemical studies showed that mT activated the tyrosine kinase activity of $pp60^{c\text{-}src}$ by preventing an inhibitory phosphorylation event at Y^{527}.[37,94] These experiments drew the first connection between RNA and DNA tumor viruses and suggested that DNA viruses transformed cells, at least in this case, by causing biochemical activation of a cellular proto-oncogene product. This, of course, is what happens during oncogene transduction by the acute transforming retroviruses, but in the case of mT, activation was induced by binding to a viral protein and not by structural alterations in the proto-oncogene product itself. Nevertheless, these results provided a satisfyingly unified view of tumor virus action.

The importance of c-*src* for mT transformation was illustrated by experiments showing that down-regulation of c-*src* expression by RNA interference attenuated mT-mediated transformation.[3] Similarly, knockout of *src* family members can inhibit tumor formation in mice expressing mT, but the interpretation of these experiments is complicated by redundancy between different members of the *src* family.[160,464]

mT also binds to protein phosphatase 2A (PP2A), an important regulatory serine/threonine kinase.[342,480] The major role of PP2A in mT function appears to be as a scaffolding factor that recruits *src* family members to the mT/PP2A complex. Consequently, mT mutants unable to bind PP2A are defective for $pp60^{c\text{-}src}$ binding and transformation. Once bound to wild-type mT, activated $pp60^{c\text{-}src}$ phosphorylates mT on several cytoplasmic tyrosine residues, thereby generating specific binding sites for cellular signaling proteins including PI3K, phospholipase C*γ*, and shc, many of which are then tyrosine phosphorylated and activated by the *src* family kinase.[95,462] Although the results are complex and influenced by the cell type studied, mutating these phosphorylation sites on mT often caused transformation and tumor-forming defects, suggesting that these binding partners are important for transformation.[160] For example, mutation of an asparagine-proline-threonine-tyrosine (NPTY) sequence in mT prevented transformation, but insertion of an ectopic NPTY motif elsewhere in mT restored the activity to the original transformation-defective mutant, suggesting that this motif functions as a modular protein–protein interaction motif.[126] Biochemical studies demonstrated that phosphorylation of the tyrosine in the NPTY motif generates a binding site for the adaptor protein shc.[56,121] Once bound to mT, shc is tyrosine phosphorylated by $pp60^{c\text{-}src}$, allowing it to bind the SH2 domain of Grb2. Grb2 then recruits Sos to the mT signaling complex, and ras-MAPK signaling is activated.

Another major phosphorylation-dependent binding partner of mT is the p85 regulatory subunit of PI3K.[246,493] Indeed, it was through studies of mT that PI3K was identified as a lipid kinase that phosphorylated phosphotidylinositol bisphosphate (PIP2) to generate the second messenger, PIP3. In mouse models of mT-mediated tumorigenesis, genetic knockout of the p110*α* catalytic subunit of PI3K prevented tumor formation, highlighting the importance of PI3K signaling in mT transformation.[471] The main role of PIP3 is to activate proteins that contain pleckstrin homology (PH) domains by recruiting them to the plasma membrane. Targets of this mechanism include the kinases PDK1 and Akt, which in turn phosphorylate their own substrates and regulate numerous important cellular processes, including apoptosis and cell growth.[101]

On the basis of these experiments, the following view of mT action has emerged. Membrane-anchored mT binds to PP2A, which allows it to bind and activate pp60$^{c\text{-}src}$, which in turn catalyzes tyrosine phosphorylation of the cytoplasmic domain of mT. This results in the recruitment and activation of a constellation of signaling molecules, which activate ras-MAPK signaling and block apoptosis. mT, then, can be viewed as a mimic of a constitutively active growth factor receptor, which assembles a phosphotyrosine-dependent signaling complex containing many of the same proteins at the cell membrane (Fig. 7.10).

Papillomavirus E5 Proteins. The BPV *E5* gene can cause morphologic and tumorigenic transformation of cultured fibroblasts, reflecting the ability of BPV to cause fibroblastic tumors in animals. Only 44 amino acids long, E5 is the smallest autonomous oncoprotein. Even more strange is its extremely hydrophobic amino acid composition, resembling a membrane-anchoring domain of a transmembrane protein. Indeed, the E5 protein is essentially an isolated transmembrane domain that exists in the intracellular membranes of transformed cells as a disulfide-linked dimer.[51,406,461] The role of E5 in the BPV life cycle is not known.

Analysis of transformed cells revealed that the E5 dimer simultaneously binds to the transmembrane domains of two molecules of the PDGF-β receptor, causing ligand-independent receptor dimerization and activation[185,273,356,357] (Fig. 7.10). This results in tyrosine phosphorylation of the cytoplasmic domain of the receptor, recruitment and activation of cellular signaling proteins, and mitogenic signaling.[127] Thus, like *v-sis,* the oncogene of the simian sarcoma retrovirus, the E5 protein causes constitutive activation of the PDGF receptor. However, E5 does not resemble the natural ligand and uses entirely different biochemical interactions to drive receptor activation.

Numerous genetic, biochemical, and pharmacologic studies demonstrated the importance of PDGF-β receptor activation for transformation by the E5 protein.[461] Most notably, cells lacking PDGF-β receptor expression are not susceptible to E5-mediated transformation unless the receptor gene is introduced into the cells.[127,187,337,461] Interestingly, the E5 protein activates an immature, intracellular form of the PDGF-β receptor, suggesting that signaling occurs from an intracellular location.[51,357]

The ability of the BPV E5 protein to activate the PDGF-β receptor by transmembrane interactions suggested that it might be possible to reprogram the E5 protein to bind to other transmembrane protein targets by changing the sequence of its transmembrane domain.[161] Indeed, by screening a library expressing several hundred thousand E5-like proteins with randomized transmembrane domains, Cammett et al[55] isolated an artificial 44-amino acid transmembrane protein that caused ligand-independent activation of the human erythropoietin receptor, a cytokine receptor unrelated to the PDGF-β receptor. Even though this small transmembrane activator bears no biochemical resemblance to erythropoietin, it is able to stimulate erythroid differentiation of primary human hematopoietic cells *in vitro.* It may be possible to extend this approach to isolate artificial small transmembrane proteins that interact with many other transmembrane targets, providing a new approach to modulate cell activity.

The BPV E5 protein also associates with a 16-kD transmembrane subunit of the vacuolar H^+-ATPase and appears to inhibit its ability to acidify intracellular organelles.[186,399] It has not been firmly established if this E5 activity, which is shared with HPV E5 proteins,[90] is required for E5-mediated cell transformation.

The high-risk HPV E5 proteins display weak transforming activity in cultured cells and can induce epithelial hyperplasia and contribute to the development of cancer in transgenic mice. These proteins are also hydrophobic and short (about twice the size of their BPV counterpart). The HPV E5 proteins appear to increase the sensitivity of the EGF receptor to EGF, but the biochemical mechanism for this activity remains obscure.[449] A functional interaction of the HPV16 E5 protein and the EGF receptor is responsible for the growth-promoting effects of the HPV16 E5 protein in transgenic mice.[175] The B-cell–associated protein, Bap31, has also been implicated in the proliferative effects of the HPV16 E5 protein.[377] Although the role of E5 in HPV replication is poorly defined, it appears to be required for efficient, differentiation-dependent viral DNA replication and expression of the late viral genes.[150,174]

Epstein-Barr Virus and *Herpesvirus Saimiri*. Although herpesviruses normally grow lytically, they can also establish a state of viral latency in which a limited subset of genes (the latency genes) are expressed. Latently infected cells do not produce progeny virus, but the viral genome is maintained in the cells as an extrachromosomal plasmid. In some circumstances, latently infected cells can reactivate lytic viral gene expression and produce infectious virus. The cells in which lytic infection takes place can be different from those where latency is established. For example, EBV replicates lytically in epithelial cells of the oropharynx, whereas latency is established in infected lymphocytes. Tumors induced by the gammaherpesvirus, such as EBV and KSHV, often express the latency genes.

EBV can convert primary B lymphocytes into long-term lymphoblastoid cell lines.[213,362,451] It can also transform rodent fibroblasts growing in culture. Like the small DNA tumor viruses, EBV contains multiple oncogenes. The first EBV oncogene identified was latent membrane protein 1 (LMP1), which can transform established lines of rodent fibroblasts.[481] LMP1 is also essential for EBV-mediated transformation of human B lymphocytes.[250,354] In transgenic mice, LMP1 can induce epithelial and B-lymphocytic hyperplasia, which can progress to lymphoma.[271]

LMP1 is a dimeric, integral membrane protein with six membrane-spanning domains and a 200-amino acid cytoplasmic, carboxyl-terminal tail (Fig. 7.11). Sequences in the carboxyl-terminal tail of LMP1 that are required for lymphocyte transformation bind to several proteins that mediate signaling by the tumor necrosis factor-α (TNF-α) receptor.[230,231,322] These proteins include several TNF receptor–associated factors (TRAFs), receptor interacting protein (RIP), and a TNF receptor–associated death domain (TRADD) protein.[229,230,231,322] Constitutive association of these proteins with LMP1 activates a number of cellular transcription factors, including NFκB, c-Jun N-terminal kinase (JNK), and p38, resulting in up-regulation of several antiapoptotic proteins

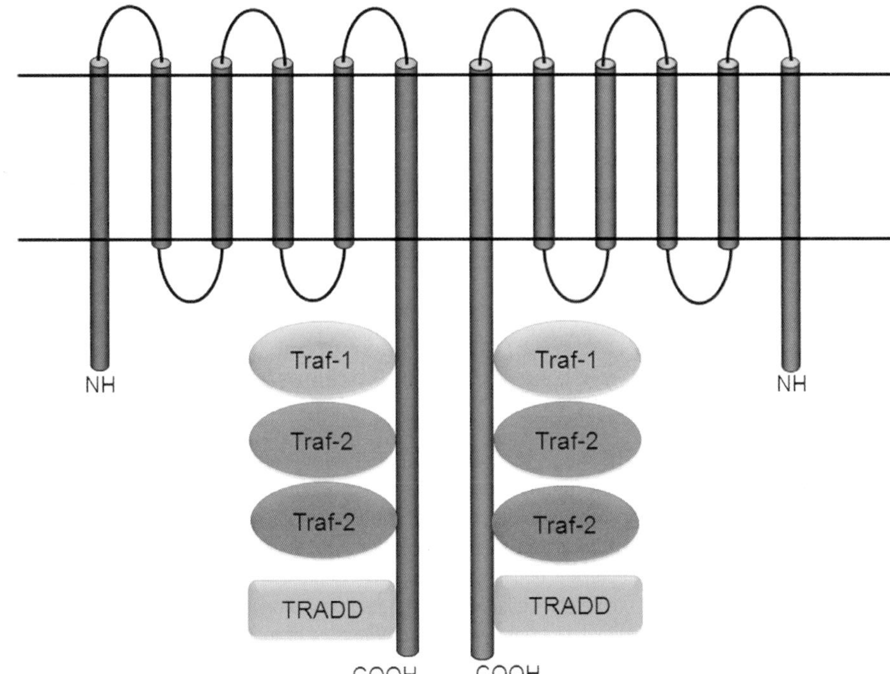

FIGURE 7.11. Structure of latent membrane protein 1 (LMP1). The figure shows a schematic diagram of a dimer of Epstein-Barr virus LMP1 protein, a multipass, transmembrane protein (blue). The carboxyl-terminal segment of LMP1 binds to a number of cellular signal transduction proteins in the tumor necrosis factor-α pathway. Horizontal lines represent the plasma membrane.

including Bcl-2 and survivin.[140,141,384] The LMP1 sequences bound by the TNF signaling proteins are homologous to binding sites in the pro-survival CD40 form of the TNF receptor active in B lymphocytes. Thus, LMP1 mimics a constitutively active CD40 TNF receptor to deliver a pro-survival signal.[469] The cytoplasmic tail of LMP1 also binds the p85 subunit of PI3K, which may contribute to its pro-survival effects by activating akt.[107]

EBV also expresses a structurally related protein, LMP2A, which contains 12 transmembrane segments. In epithelial cells, LMP2A can induce features of transformation, but most studies of LMP2A have been carried out in lymphocytes. LMP2A binds to the *lyn* tyrosine kinase, a member of the *src* family, resulting in inhibition of B-cell antigen receptor signaling.[54,313,314] Because B-cell receptor signaling induces EBV to enter the lytic replication cycle, LMP2A can inhibit viral reactivation and allow the persistence of latently infected cells. LMP2A also mediates B-lymphocyte survival by activating akt signaling.[363,456]

Studies of replication-competent EBV strains unable to transform lymphocytes revealed that the Epstein-Barr virus nuclear antigen 2 (*EBNA2*) gene is required for lymphocyte transformation.[87,190,203] The EBNA2 protein is a nuclear phosphoprotein that transactivates the expression of several EBV genes, including LMP1, as well as numerous cellular genes involved in cell proliferation, including *c-Myc* and *CD23*.[482] EBNA2 acts by forming a complex with the cellular site-specific DNA binding protein, RBP-Jκ/CBF1.[197,286] Once bound to DNA, EBNA2 recruits additional transcription factors to promoters to mediate gene induction.[240] The activated cellular receptor for Notch also stimulates transcription through RBP-Jκ, so EBNA2 can be regarded as a mimic of a constitutively active Notch receptor. Consistent with this view, activated Notch can partially restore B-cell–transforming activity to EBV lacking EBNA2.[189]

EBV expresses additional antiapoptotic proteins that can contribute to tumorigenesis. For example, the *BHRF1* gene product is homologous to the cellular antiapoptotic protein, Bcl-2, and binds and inhibits the pro-apoptotic activities of a number of cellular pro-apoptotic proteins including Bim, Bak, and Puma.[214]

Herpesvirus saimiri (HVS) infects nonhuman primates and causes T-cell lymphomas in new world monkeys. The STP oncogene of HVS, like EBV LMP1, transforms lymphocytes by activating NFκB via TNF receptor signaling molecules.[104] The STP protein of subgroup A HVS also associates with pp60$^{c\text{-}src}$. The HVS Tip oncoprotein interacts with *lck*, another *src* family kinase, and inhibits T-cell receptor signaling.[29]

DNA Virus Oncoproteins That Inactivate Rb or p53

As described in this section, several DNA tumor viruses inactivate the Rb pathway. This induces a p53-dependent stress response that can result in growth arrest or apoptosis, either of which would limit virus production.[137,445] There are multiple pathways that lead to p53 activation. In one such pathway, E2F1 released by Rb neutralization increases expression of p19^{ARF}.[515] p19 in turn stabilizes p53 by interfering with mdm2, a ubiquitin ligase that would otherwise destabilize p53.[447] To inhibit the antiviral response elicited by Rb inactivation, viruses engage mechanisms to block p53 function. Thus, many DNA tumor viruses inactivate p53 as well as Rb to neutralize the pro-apoptotic signals initiated by Rb inactivation. The one known apparent exception to this shared strategy among the small DNA tumor viruses is murine polyomavirus. Polyomavirus LT binds Rb but does not bind p53. mT also lacks p53 binding. Therefore, this virus evidently has developed a strategy to overcome the deleterious effects of Rb neutralization without expressing a protein that directly inactivates p53. Viral oncogenes that target Rb and p53 are described in the following sections.

Adenovirus Oncogenes. Early studies revealed that adenovirus-transformed cells invariably retained only the *E1A* and *E1B* genes at the left end of the viral genome, suggesting that these were the major viral oncogenes.[123,167] Indeed, transfection studies demonstrated that these genes had transforming activity and that full transformation required both E1A and E1B.[242] The 12S E1A gene product can stimulate cellular DNA synthesis and immortalize cells on its own, but it requires a cooperating oncogene such as E1B or activated *ras* to cause full transformation of primary rat embryo fibroblasts.[388] As is the case for most DNA tumor virus oncogenes, E1A and E1B are required for normal productive infection.

Adenovirus E1A. Comparison of the amino acid sequences of E1A proteins from various strains of adenoviruses revealed that they shared a number of conserved motifs including conserved region 2 (CR2), which contains the sequence leucine-X-cysteine-X-glutamic acid, where X can be any amino acid (the LXCXE motif) (e-Fig. 7.3). Mutational analysis demonstrated that CR2 was required for transformation. Strikingly, SV40 LT and HPV E7 proteins also contain required LXCXE motifs,[242,495] even though they are otherwise unrelated to E1A or each other (e-Fig. 7.3). Substitution of the LT CR2 region into a transformation-defective E1A mutant lacking its own CR2 restored transforming activity, suggesting that CR2 might constitute a discrete binding site for a cellular protein required for transformation.[318] Based on the precedent of the association of mT and *src,* it seemed plausible that the CR2 motif of E1A bound to the product of a cellular oncogene and activated it, resulting in transformation.

To identify cellular proteins that bind to E1A and possibly mediate transformation, E1A antibodies were used to immunoprecipitate E1A and associated cellular proteins from infected cell extracts.[206,507] A 105-kD E1A-associated protein was soon identified as the product of the *RB1* gene.[494] *RB1* encodes the retinoblastoma tumor suppressor protein, $p105^{Rb}$, and had been previously implicated in retinoblastoma, a hereditary cancer of the eye. Notably, in retinoblastoma, *RB1* acts not as an oncogene, but rather as a tumor suppressor gene, whose loss predisposes individuals to tumor development. Mutations in E1A CR2 that blocked $p105^{Rb}$ binding also inhibited transformation.[376] Biochemical and gene transfer experiments showed that the association of E1A and $p105^{Rb}$ freed E2F from repressive Rb/E2F complexes, resulting in increased transcription of E2F-regulated genes[16,71,376] (Fig. 7.12). These seminal and at the time surprising findings showed that viral oncogenes can transform cells not only by activating the products of cellular proto-oncogenes but also by inactivating cellular proteins that inhibit cell proliferation. The ability of E1A to inactivate $p105^{Rb}$ was foreshadowed by the observation that injection of adenovirus type 12 into the eyes of newborn rats caused retinoblastoma.[260]

Two additional members of the retinoblastoma tumor suppressor family, p107 and p130, also bind E1A. Because all three Rb family members evidently share a structural pocket that binds to the LXCXE motif on various viral oncoproteins, these Rb family members are sometimes referred to as the pocket proteins.

In addition to CR2, conserved sequences in the amino-terminus of E1A (CR1) are also required for induction of DNA synthesis and transformation (but not for Rb binding),

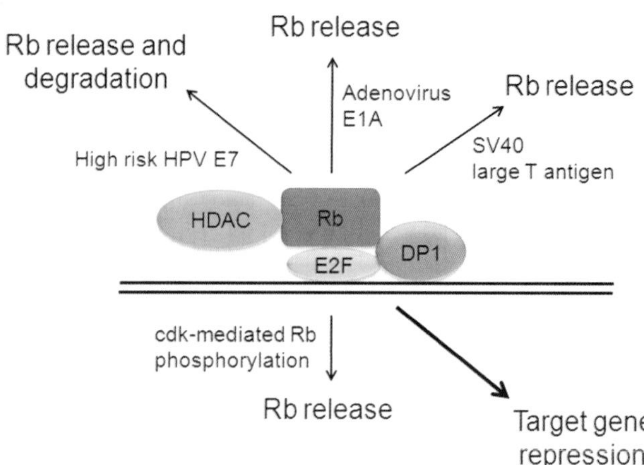

FIGURE 7.12. Interaction between retinoblastoma proteins and DNA tumor virus oncoproteins. Retinoblastoma (Rb) family members in complex with an E2F/DP1 heterodimer recruit histone deacetylases (HDACs) to promoters, resulting in their repression. Horizontal lines represent double-stranded DNA. Repressive complexes are disrupted in uninfected cells by cdk-mediated phosphorylation of Rb, allowing E2F to stimulate transcription. The effects of oncoproteins from three unrelated DNA tumor viruses are shown above the DNA.

implying that there are additional cellular targets of E1A involved in transformation.[495] These sequences bind to p300 and CBP, closely related histone acetyl transferases that are co-activators for the CREB transcription factor.[6] These proteins presumably contribute to transformation by directly regulating the activity of cellular genes. SV40 LT and high-risk HPV E7 also bind p300/CBP, as well as Rb. The extreme C-terminus of E1A binds a cellular protein, CtBP, a transcriptional co-repressor.[397] Deletion of this binding site affects the ability of E1A to cooperate with other oncogenes.[77]

Adenovirus E1B. Co-expression of adenovirus *E1A* and *E1B* genes can cause cell transformation.[242] However, in the absence of E1B, acute expression of E1A causes a burst of cellular DNA synthesis followed by a dramatic cellular phenotype involving degradation of viral and cellular DNA and cell death.[8,359,370,491] This phenotype is now recognized as apoptosis and is a response in large part to the unscheduled DNA synthesis elicited by the inactivation of Rb by E1A. Thus, a major function of E1B is to counter E1A-induced apoptosis.[110,370] How does E1B accomplish this? There are two unrelated E1B protein products encoded by alternatively spliced mRNAs, each of which can independently cooperate with E1A. The 55-kD E1B product of adenovirus binds to p53, which is required for E1A-induced apoptosis, and neutralizes its activity.[110,390,391,396] The importance of p53 inactivation for transformation was shown by the ability of dominant-negative p53 (see next section) to cooperate with E1A in inducing transformation of primary cells.[388] The adenovirus E4orf6 protein can also cooperate with E1A to transform cells by inhibiting p53 function, and in cooperation with E1B-55K causes the degradation of p53.[438] The complete absence of amino acid sequence homology between E1B-55K, E4orf6, SV40 LT, and HPV E6, proteins that all inactivate p53, is a striking example of convergent evolution and highlights the need of diverse DNA tumor viruses to interfere with p53 activity.

The smaller E1B gene product, E1B-19K, also inhibits E1A-mediated apoptosis.[370,492] E1B-19K is homologous to the cellular *Bcl-2* gene family that regulates apoptosis.[423] E1B-19K inhibits apoptosis by sequestering the pro-apoptotic family members Bak and Bax and preventing the formation of pores in the mitochondrial outer membrane and the release of pro-apoptotic proteins such as cytochrome c.[492]

SV40 Large T Antigen. LT is a multifunctional protein required for SV40 DNA replication, late gene expression, and other aspects of the viral lytic life cycle.[2] It is also the major oncoprotein of SV40, and expression of LT in transgenic mice can give rise to a number of tumors including choroid plexus tumors, retinoblastoma, pancreatic carcinoma, and intestinal hyperplasia. At least three segments of LT are required for transforming activity: a J domain and a conserved LXCXE motif in the amino-terminal half of the protein, and a distinct segment in the carboxyl-terminal half.[2] The relative importance of these segments depends on the transformation assay employed, but in some assays the amino-terminal half of LT was sufficient for transformation. In addition, a second early protein of SV40, small t antigen, which shares amino acid sequences with the amino-terminus of LT, can contribute to transformation under some conditions, apparently by inhibiting PP2A.[30,392,505,510]

Soon after it was discovered that adenovirus E1A bound p105[Rb], LT was also found to bind the Rb family.[112] Furthermore, assay of a series of point mutations in the LT LXCXE motif demonstrated that Rb binding was required for transformation. The molecular chaperone function of the J domain of LT is also required for Rb inactivation by recruiting an Hsp70 activity to remodel the Rb/E2F complexes and release free E2F to activate cellular genes required for cell proliferation.[111,424,450] Thus, two otherwise unrelated transforming proteins, adenovirus E1A and SV40 LT, shared a common property, namely, the ability to bind to and neutralize Rb proteins (Fig. 7.12).

Rb family members are not the only cellular proteins bound by LT. In fact, the well-known tumor suppressor protein, p53, was first discovered as an LT binding protein. The analysis of p53 was initially confusing and is a tale worth telling. Antibodies that recognized LT also co-immunoprecipitated a cellular protein called p53.[276,287] In general, p53 levels were high in LT-transformed cells. p53 binding mapped to the C-terminal segment of LT required for transformation, and LT mutants unable to bind p53 were transformation defective.[2,516] In addition, molecular clones of the *p53* gene from immortalized mouse cell lines displayed transforming activity in cooperation with validated oncogenes such as v-*ras,* and the *p53* gene was amplified in human sarcomas.[142,236,341,345] These results strongly suggested that p53 was an oncogene product. This led to the conclusion that LT bound and activated the product of a cellular oncogene (namely, p53), resulting in transformation.

Results soon accumulated that challenged this apparently straightforward interpretation. First, some proviral integration sites in retrovirus-induced leukemias actually disrupted the *p53* gene, rather than activated it.[241] Second, inactivating p53 mutations were frequently found in naturally arising sporadic human tumors, as well as in some familial cancers, where mutant p53 displayed a pattern of inheritance consistent with tumor suppressor function.[284,298] Mice engineered to lack p53 displayed a higher incidence of spontaneous tumor formation.[124] In addition, the interaction with LT did not stimulate the transcriptional activity of p53 but rather blocked it.[312] Finally, independent molecular clones of the *p53* gene from primary, nonimmortalized cells did not display transforming activity, but inhibited cell growth.[11,156] The role of p53 was finally resolved with the discovery that the original cloned *p53* genes that displayed transforming activity were actually mutants. The wild-type *p53* gene acts not as an oncogene but as a tumor suppressor gene.[284] Thus, as was the case with E1A or LT with Rb, LT transforms cells in part by inactivating the tumor suppressor activity of p53 (Fig. 7.13).

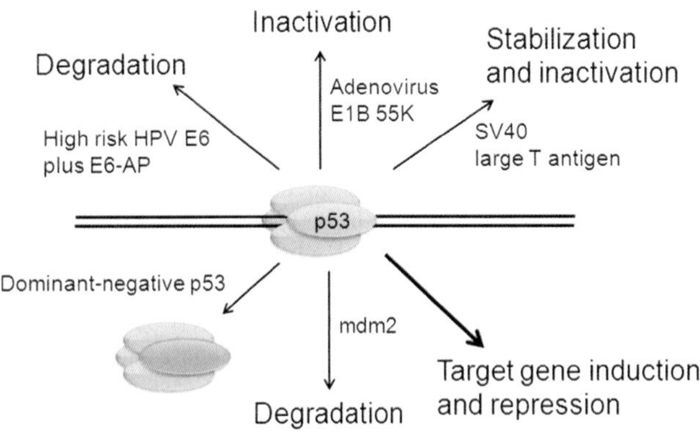

FIGURE 7.13. Interaction between p53 and DNA tumor virus oncoproteins. A tetramer of p53 bound to double-stranded DNA is shown in blue at the middle. The ability of p53 to regulate gene expression can be inactivated in uninfected cells by mdm2-mediated p53 degradation or by expression of a dominant negative mutant of p53, which forms an inactive tetramer. The effects of three oncoproteins from unrelated DNA tumor viruses are shown above the DNA.

Certain p53 mutants with transforming activity are said to be dominant negative, because they hetero-oligomerize with the wild-type version of p53 and neutralize its activity.[284] Expression of such a mutant effectively titrates active p53 from the cell and is functionally equivalent to the loss of both p53 alleles, as is the case for a classic inherited tumor suppressor gene. Such p53 mutations are some of the most common genetic alterations in human cancer.

Human Papillomavirus Nuclear Oncogenes. E6 and E7 encode short nuclear proteins (~100 amino acids), which are required for productive infection.[158] The high-risk HPV *E6* and *E7* genes cooperate to immortalize primary human keratinocytes, the progenitor cells of cervical and other squamous cell cancers; block the terminal differentiation of these cells; and disrupt genomic integrity.[22,209,325,405,490] The ability of HPV to immortalize cultured cells correlates with their oncogenic potential in patients—proteins from the high-risk HPV types have increased activity in comparison to the low-risk proteins.[17,353,446,499] The *E6*/*E7* genes from high-risk HPV can also induce a variety of tumors in transgenic mice, including cervical cancer in mice chronically treated with estrogen.[7] In addition, the high-risk but not low-risk E7 protein can stimulate DNA synthesis in resting cells and transform rodent cells either on its own or in cooperation with the v-*ras* oncogene.[244,479] As is the case for LT and E1A/E1B, a major activity of E6 and E7 is to neutralize p53 and Rb.

Human Papillomavirus E7. The E7 protein is not an enzyme, but rather modulates the activity of regulatory proteins encoded by the host cell. Like LT and E1A, the HPV E7 protein contains an LXCXE motif that binds to the Rb family pocket proteins.[133,326] This results in the displacement of Rb proteins from E2F family members and in degradation of Rb[45,71] (Fig. 7.12). Although the LXCXE motif is sufficient for Rb binding, sequences outside of this motif are required for degradation and complete inactivation of Rb. The mechanism of Rb degradation is not understood completely but appears to involve the assembly of a cullin 2 ubiquitin ligase complex with Rb, followed by proteosomal degradation.[220]

Repression of E7 expression in cervical cancer cells results in the loss of hyperphosphorylated Rb and the induction of the hypophosphorylated, growth inhibitory form of Rb that binds E2F.[188] This in turn results in repression of E2F-responsive genes and growth arrest, demonstrating that continuous association with E7 is required for sustained Rb inhibition.

Several lines of evidence suggest that the transforming activities of E7 depend on its ability to neutralize the Rb family. Both high-risk and low-risk E7 proteins contain the LXCXE motif, but the affinity of HPV E7 proteins for $p105^{Rb}$ correlates with the oncogenic potential of the virus: high-risk E7 binds $p105^{Rb}$ tightly; low-risk E7 binds it poorly.[166,326] These differences map to a single amino acid immediately adjacent to the LXCXE motif, which determines the ability of E7 to transform rat kidney cells in cooperation with the *ras* oncogene.[212] In addition, E7 can be replaced in an E6-dependent keratinocyte immortalization assay by down-regulation of the cdk inhibitor $p16^{INK4a}$, a manipulation that also inactivates $p105^{Rb}$ by allowing its phosphorylation and release from E2F.[255] These results suggest that inactivation of the Rb family by E7 is important for cell transformation, keratinocyte immortalization, and cervical carcinogenesis. On the other hand, transformation assays carried out with E7 mutants defective for various activities have not yielded consistent results, although some experiments suggest that Rb binding is essential for transformation.[237,309] In transgenic mice, the ability of E7 to neutralize Rb function is tightly linked to its ability to support DNA synthesis in differentiating epithelial cells, but not for cervical carcinogenesis.[13,14]

The E7 proteins can also affect cellular checkpoint control. High-risk E7 interacts with two cdk inhibitors, $p21^{CIP1}$ and $p27^{KIP1}$, and abrogates their growth inhibitory effects.[116,165,432,513] These E7 activities may also contribute to the ability of E7 to induce resistance to growth inhibitory cytokines such as transforming growth factor-β, tumor necrosis factor, and interferon.[18,19,348,358] The signals mobilized by the E7 protein maintain the proliferative status of suprabasal keratinocytes, which otherwise undergo terminal differentiation and become unable to support DNA synthesis. These signals thereby allow viral DNA replication and the production of progeny virus in the stratified epithelium.[14,76]

The E7 proteins bind to a large number of additional cell proteins.[309] Some of these binding partners, such as various cyclins and E2F family members, are likely to reinforce the activities mentioned previously. p600, an Rb-associated protein, associates with both high-risk and low-risk E7 and appears to allow the survival of cells in the absence of anchorage and may thus contribute to malignancy.[115,221] Other E7 binding partners include histone-modifying enzymes and members of the polycomb group transcriptional repressor complexes, suggesting that E7 may affect epigenetic status.[309] However, the biological relevance of most of the interactions of the E7 protein with cellular proteins is not known.

Cervical cancer cells are often aneuploid and contain other chromosomal abnormalities, which presumably play a role in malignant progression. The high-risk E7 protein induces genomic instability in part by interfering with the synthesis or function of centrosomes, the subcellular structures that form the poles of the mitotic spindle to ensure proper chromosome segregation during mitosis.[128] Primary human epithelial cells expressing E7 often contain abnormal or supernumerary centrosomes due to the uncoupling of centriole synthesis from cell cycle progression. The molecular mechanism by which E7 interferes with centrosome synthesis is not known in detail, but it is at least in part independent of Rb targeting and may involve interactions with cellular proteins involved in centrosome activity or mitosis.[129,334]

Human Papillomavirus E6. Like the E7 protein, the HPV E6 protein lacks enzymatic activity and functions by modulating the activity of cellular proteins.[218] The high-risk E6 protein is able to immortalize human mammary epithelial cells on its own,[15] but most analyses of E6 have been conducted in keratinocytes and focus on its ability to cooperate with E7. A number of the signaling pathways stimulated by the E7 protein, including unscheduled DNA synthesis due to Rb inactivation, tend to drive cells into apoptosis.[137,445] A major role of E6 is to limit this deleterious cellular response to E7 expression.

The E6 protein from the high-risk HPV types binds to a number of cellular proteins and induces their ubiquitin-mediated degradation.[218] The proximal target of the E6 protein is the E3 ubiquitin ligase, E6-associated protein (E6-AP).[222,402] The direct binding of E6 to a leucine-X-X-leucine-leucine motif on E6-AP reprograms it to ubiquitylate a number of cell proteins, which leads to their proteosome-mediated degradation.[400,402] The most prominent target of E6/E6-AP is p53, which is normally a substrate of a different ubiquitin ligase, mdm2, not E6-AP[74,208,489,502] (Fig. 7.13). Although p53 is wild type in most cervical carcinoma cell lines, it has a short half-life and its levels are low in these cells because of E6-mediated degradation.[312,401] As a consequence, p53-dependent checkpoint controls, for example, in response to Rb inactivation or DNA damage, are blunted although not necessarily eliminated in cells expressing high-risk E6 proteins.[53,490] The low-risk E6 proteins do not induce p53 degradation. Mutant p53 can replace HPV16 E6 in inducing keratinocyte immortalization, implying that E6-mediated p53 inactivation is important for this activity.[414] In addition to E6-AP–mediated degradation, there appear to be several other mechanisms utilized by E6 to attenuate p53 activity.[218] Repression of E6 expression in cervical cancer cells results in the elevation of p53 levels and restoration of p53 signaling, indicating that continuous association with E6 is required for sustained p53 inhibition.[113]

The E6 proteins also exert p53-independent antiapoptotic effects.[272] High-risk E6 blocks several steps in the extrinsic apoptosis signaling cascade by interacting with a death receptor (tumor necrosis factor receptor-1), the FAS-associated via death domain (FADD) adaptor protein, and caspase-8.[155] E6 also inhibits the intrinsic apoptotic pathway by binding to the pro-apoptotic molecule Bak and inducing its proteosome-dependent degradation, thereby blocking release of apoptotic mediators from mitochondria.[465] In addition, HPV16 E6 and E7 can up-regulate two cellular inhibitors of apoptosis, c-IAP2 and survivin, which act farther downstream in the apoptosis signaling cascade.[40,233,512] In concert, this barrage of antiapoptotic action prevents cell death and sets the stage for ongoing proliferation in response to E7 signals. Indeed, the ability of E6 from some HPVs to inhibit ultraviolet light–induced apoptosis has been proposed to be a prime contributor in HPV-associated skin cancer.[232]

In E6-expressing cells, E6-AP (and possibly other ubiquitin ligases) also ubiquitylates and causes the degradation of a series of PDZ domain–containing proteins[171,303] (Fig. 7.13). These proteins are recruited to the E6/E6-AP ubiquitylation complex by binding to a serine/threonine-X-valine consensus PDZ domain binding motif at the extreme C-terminus of high-risk E6 proteins.[256,280] These PDZ proteins include a number of proteins with presumed tumor suppressor activity, including Scribble, hDlg, and MAGI-1, which regulate signal transduction, cell–cell contact, and cell polarity. Loss of these proteins disrupts the formation of epithelial tight junctions and may contribute to the invasiveness of cervical cancer cells.[269,486] E6 also promotes the degradation of several PDZ domain–containing protein tyrosine phosphatases, which regulate growth factor signaling pathways.[436] The biological importance of PDZ binding was demonstrated by the finding that deletion of the PDZ binding motif from E6 affected viral genome replication and abrogated its ability to transform keratinocytes and stimulate epithelial hyperplasia in transgenic mice.[278,335,486] Other viral oncoproteins, such as rhesus papillomavirus E7 (but not E6) and adenovirus E4-orf1, also bind PDZ proteins.[466]

Another consequence of E6 expression is transcriptional induction of the gene encoding hTERT, the catalytic subunit of telomerase, the ribonucleoprotein that maintains the ends of chromosomes.[259,475] Introduction of hTERT can replace E6 in a keratinocyte immortalization assay,[255] suggesting that hTERT induction is a crucial activity of E6. It has been proposed that E6-AP–mediated degradation of NFX1-91, a transcriptional repressor of the *hTERT* gene, is involved in hTERT induction by E6, although E6 probably exerts additional layers of control on telomerase.[177] Indeed, E6 also interacts with the telomerase complex and activates it posttranscriptionally.[290] Other targets of E6-AP–mediated degradation include several GAPs, which regulate the activity of ras-like proteins, and proteins involved in DNA replication and repair.[218] E6 also inhibits O(6)-methylguanine-DNA methyltransferase, a crucial DNA repair enzyme,[437] and the DNA repair scaffolding protein, XRCC1.[228]

In summary, it appears that the main biochemical activity of E6 is to redirect the E6-AP ubiquitin ligase to a number of cellular proteins with tumor suppressor or related activity, inducing their degradation. Knockout of the *E6-AP* gene in transgenic mice prevents the development of E6-mediated cervical cancer, demonstrating that E6-AP is required for this biological activity of HPV E6.[419]

KSHV Oncogenes. Cells latently infected with KSHV express latency-associated nuclear antigen (LANA), a large, multifunctional nuclear protein required for the establishment and maintenance of the extrachromosomal viral genome.[12,93] LANA can transform cultured fibroblasts in cooperation with activated *ras* and extend the life span of human endothelial cells. In transgenic mice, LANA causes lymphocyte hyperplasia and, rarely, the development of lymphomas.[147,368,485] Like the oncoproteins of many other DNA tumor viruses, LANA binds and neutralizes p53 and Rb.[162,368,379] In addition, by binding to glycogen synthetase kinase 3β, LANA modulates β-catenin and up-regulates expression of genes involved in cell proliferation such as cyclin D and c-myc.[163] The KSHV ORF50 and K-bZIP proteins also interfere with p53 activity.[200,347]

The KSHV K1 protein contains two ITAM motifs and mimics signaling by the B-cell antigen receptor by activating the src family kinase *lyn*.[365] The signals constitutively emanating from K1 inhibit apoptosis and can transform cells in a variety of settings.[279,366] Another KSHV gene with transforming activity is *K12*, which encodes a series of active gene products.[327] These include kaposin B, a mixture of short polypeptides that appear to function by activating the p38-MK2 pathway and stabilizing cellular mRNAs encoding pro-proliferative cytokines.[308]

In addition to the genes mentioned above, the KSHV genome also contains numerous genes that are clear homologs of cellular genes that stimulate proliferation or block apoptosis.[328] These encode proteins that function as cytokines, a cyclin (v-Cyc), a constitutively active G-protein–coupled receptor (vGPCR), and a variety of other regulatory proteins. v-Cyc activates cdks that allow cell cycle progression.[67,184] v-Cyc appears to be resistant to cdk inhibitors, and a v-Cyc/cdk6 complex can phosphorylate and inactivate $p27^{KIP1}$, itself a cdk inhibitor, thus reinforcing the pro-proliferative response caused by cdk-mediated phosphorylation of Rb.[455] vIRF and vIL-6, homologous to interferon regulatory factors and interleukin-6, respectively, can also promote cell growth.[69,169] vGPCR displays transforming activity in cultured fibroblasts and primary endothelial cells, and it can induce tumors that resemble KS in mice.[9] Biochemical studies showed that vGPCR activates various mitogenic and pro-survival signaling pathways.[58,316] KSHV also expresses at least three additional gene products that inhibit apoptosis: v-Bcl, which is homologous to Bcl-2 and acts by maintaining mitochondrial integrity; vIAP (viral inhibitor-of-apoptosis protein), which is homologous to a different cellular antiapoptotic protein, survivin; and vFLIP, which is thought to block apoptosis by inhibiting the Fas death receptor pathway or up-regulating NKκB.[23,70,75,122,183,199,453,483] These activities contribute to lymphomagenesis in transgenic mice.[83] Several KSHV gene products also stimulate angiogenesis[43] in this highly vascularized tumor. For example, vGPCR signaling induces the expression of the angiogenic factor vascular endothelial growth factor (VEGF),[506] and the KSHV chemokine viral macrophage inflammatory protein-I (v-MIP-I) promotes angiogenesis by inducing VEGF expression and stimulating the chemotaxis of endothelial cells.[444] Finally, it should be noted that herpesviruses express many gene products that down-regulate the innate and adaptive immune response. These activities are presumably of critical importance for tumor formation in otherwise immunocompetent animals.

Noncoding RNAs and Transformation. Many DNA tumor viruses express microRNAs and other noncoding RNAs (ncRNAs). EBER1 and EBER2, ncRNAs expressed by Epstein-Barr virus, can induce several features of transformation in cultured lymphocytes, including tumorigenicity in immunodeficient mice.[263,387,504] The biochemical activities of the EBERs responsible for transformation are not known. KSHV encodes miR-K12-11 microRNA, which shows many similarities to the growth-promoting cellular microRNA, miR-155.[191] HVS encodes five small ncRNAs that form ribonucleoprotein complexes and induce the expression of numerous T-cell activation genes, at least in part by causing the degradation of specific cellular microRNAs.[63]

VIRUSES AND HUMAN CANCER

Because viruses cause cancer in animals, it was natural to ask if they cause cancer in humans. The search for human tumor viruses began in earnest with the discovery of murine leukemia virus in the early 1950s[196] and took on special urgency in the 1960s with the startling discovery that some early stocks of the poliovirus vaccine were contaminated with live SV40, which has potent tumor-inducing activity in newborn hamsters.[135,176,181] The SV40 contamination resulted from growing poliovirus in primary African green monkey kidney cells, some of which harbored SV40. Despite the suspected association between viruses and cancer, it took many years to assemble convincing evidence that viruses play an etiologic role in human cancer. Epidemiologic and laboratory studies designed to implicate viruses in human cancer were difficult because human tumor viruses do not act rapidly or efficiently. Rather, cancer arises only years or even decades after the initial infection, and most infected people do not get cancer, suggesting that virus infection represents only one step in carcinogenic progression and that additional cellular alterations must occur for cancer formation. In addition, many tumor virus infections (e.g., EBV, HPV, and HBV) are quite common, complicating attempts to forge epidemiologic links to specific cancers. Finally, virally induced tumors usually do not produce virus particles, obscuring the viral cause of some cancers.

Despite these challenges, six viruses are now generally recognized as playing causal roles in cancers that account for approximately 15% of all human cancer deaths worldwide[310,317] (Table 7.7). These virus-induced cancers tend to be much more common in the developing world, where they can be the most common cause of cancer death. Virus-induced cancers also occur relatively frequently in immunosuppressed individuals. Because viruses provide well-defined targets for prevention and therapy, virally associated cancers appear to represent a class of tumors that are particularly susceptible to rational prevention and treatment approaches.

TABLE 7.7 Human Tumor Viruses

Epstein-Barr virus	Burkitt lymphoma Nasopharyngeal carcinoma Hodgkin disease Gastric carcinoma
Hepatitis B virus	Hepatocellular carcinoma
Hepatitis C virus	Hepatocellular carcinoma Non-Hodgkin lymphoma
Human papillomaviruses	Cervical carcinoma Other anogenital carcinomas Oropharyngeal carcinoma Nonmelanoma skin cancer
Human T-lymphotropic retrovirus	Adult T-cell leukemia/lymphoma
Kaposi sarcoma-associated herpesvirus	Kaposi sarcoma Multicentric Castleman disease Primary effusion lymphoma

Human Papillomaviruses

The HPVs cause papillomas or warts, benign tumors of epithelial cells in the skin and mucous membranes. Although warts are usually self-limited, genital warts (condyloma acuminata) and laryngeal papillomas can be serious medical conditions. The main medical importance of the HPVs derives from their association with human cancer.[518] High-risk strains of HPV such as HPV16 and HPV18, which were first discovered in cervical cancer samples,[42,132] are responsible for virtually all cancers of the uterine cervix and a substantial fraction of other anogenital and oropharyngeal cancers in both men and women. Additional HPV types are associated with severe warts and skin cancer in immunosuppressed individuals.

As described earlier, the major oncogenes of the high-risk genital HPV are the *E6* and *E7* genes, which are continuously expressed in cancer cells.[10,412] However, keratinocytes transformed *in vitro* by E6/E7 are not initially tumorigenic in experimental animals, implying that HPV-infected cells must accumulate additional mutations or other events to form cancers.[131,224] This requirement for additional, presumably rare events may account for the observation that most people infected with high-risk HPV do not develop cancer. It is also likely to account for the long period of time that usually passes between infection and development of cancer. In most cervical cancers, the gene encoding the HPV E2 transcription factor is disrupted or its action is inhibited by mutation or epigenetic modification.[81] This prevents E2-mediated repression of the promoter driving E6 and E7 transcription, and the resulting increased expression of the oncogenes presumably plays a role in carcinogenesis.

The finding that the E6 and E7 proteins from the high-risk HPV types are more effective at inhibiting the p53 and Rb tumor suppressor pathways than are the low-risk types, such as HPV6 and HPV11, implies that these interactions are important in human carcinogenesis.[166,326] Similarly, the presence of wild-type *p53* and *Rb* genes in most cervical cancers implies that these pathways are neutralized by a nonmutational mechanism in these cells (i.e., by the expression of the viral oncoproteins).[401,501] Continuous expression of the HPV *E6* and *E7* genes is required to maintain the Rb and p53 pathways in an inactive state in cervical carcinoma cells, and repression of E6/E7 rapidly activates these pathways and inhibits cell survival and proliferation.[188,225,439,477] The third viral oncogene, the *E5* gene, is expressed in some but not all cervical cancers, and its role in human carcinogenesis is unclear.

Prophylactic vaccines formulated from virus-like particles (VLPs) composed of L1, the major HPV capsid protein, are very effective at raising neutralizing antibodies to the HPV types in the vaccine and preventing infection with these HPV types.[267,403] These vaccines are likely to prevent many cases of HPV-associated cancers, but because of the long lag between the time of initial infection and cancer development, it will take many years to document this effect. In addition, a therapeutic vaccine composed of HPV16 E7 peptides has shown promise in treating women suffering from HPV16-associated vulvar neoplasia.[253]

HPV-associated squamous cell carcinoma of the head and neck primarily occurs in the oropharynx and tonsils, and its incidence is rising rapidly. HPV-associated cancer appears to be less aggressive than classic head and neck cancer, which is associated with tobacco and alcohol use, p53 mutations, and low levels of the cdk inhibitor p16.[4] HPV16 DNA is the predominant HPV type found in these cancers, and repression of HPV16 E6/E7 in head and neck cancer cell lines can inhibit their proliferation.[369] Prophylactic VLP vaccines developed to prevent cervical cancer are likely to be effective in preventing head and neck cancer as well.

Epstein-Barr Virus

EBV virus is a ubiquitous human gammaherpesvirus that causes infectious mononucleosis and a variety of cancers including Burkitt lymphoma in Africa and nasopharyngeal cancer (NPC) in certain areas in Southeast Asia.[418] EBV also causes lymphoproliferative disease in individuals with congenital or acquired immunodeficiency, including central nervous system lymphomas in patients with acquired immunodeficiency syndrome (AIDS) and posttransplant lymphoproliferative disease in patients undergoing bone marrow or stem cell transplantation. EBV also appears to play a role in additional cancers including a substantial fraction of Hodgkin disease and some gastric cancers. EBV was the first human virus shown to cause tumors in nonhuman primates.[427]

A number of viral genes have been implicated in transformation by EBV including LMP1, which mimics an activated TNF receptor, and EBNA2, a transcription factor involved in lymphocyte immortalization. The LMP1 oncoprotein is often expressed in NPC specimens.[49] Because the EBV genome replicates as a plasmid in latently infected cells and tumors, the viral DNA replication factor EBNA1 is required for persistence of the viral genome. Studies in Burkitt lymphoma cell lines indicate that ongoing expression of EBV genes is required for the survival of these cells.[252] Further interesting features of Burkitt lymphoma include its association with malaria and with the consistent presence of chromosomal translocations in the tumor cells, which result in increased expression of the *c-Myc* proto-oncogene by fusing it to regulatory elements of immunoglobulin genes.

Kaposi Sarcoma Herpesvirus

KSHV, also known as human herpesvirus type 8 (HHV-8), is associated with Kaposi Sarcoma (KS), a systemic disease affecting multiple cell types and organs including the skin, with a prominent vascular endothelial component.[5] In fact, the KSHV genome was first identified by molecular cloning from KS.[66] Unlike many other tumors, KS lesions are not monoclonal and display features consistent with paracrine signaling, and cells derived from them often lack properties of transformed cells.

KS, previously a very rare disease, is associated with immunosuppression and appeared in an aggressive form in a relatively high proportion of AIDS patients.[146] In fact, KS was the most common cause of cancer death in this population, but its incidence dropped dramatically with the use of highly active antiretroviral therapy (HAART) for HIV infection. However, because HIV-infected individuals on HAART are now surviving longer, the number of patients with KS and other HIV-associated cancers may increase in the future. KSHV is also associated with primary effusion lymphoma and some cases of multicentric Castleman disease, a polyclonal lymphoid malignancy. The KSHV genome contains numerous homologs of cellular genes implicated in growth control and evasion of the host cell innate and adaptive immune response, but the pathogenesis of KS and other KSHV-associated cancer is undoubtedly complex and poorly understood.[328]

A number of drugs in clinical use inhibit herpesvirus DNA replication. The appearance of new KS lesions in AIDS patients was significantly suppressed by treatment with ganciclovir, a modified nucleoside that is phosphorylated by KSHV thymidine kinase and inhibits the viral DNA polymerase.[61,301] This finding generates optimism that antiviral drugs have a role in the prevention and treatment of virally induced cancer.

Human T-Cell Leukemia Virus

HTLV-I was the first retrovirus implicated in human disease. Approximately 20 million people are infected with HTLV-I worldwide, with high endemic areas in Latin America, the Caribbean, Africa, and Japan. Infection is associated with adult T-cell leukemia/lymphoma (ATL), a relatively rare tumor, as well as some neurologic diseases.[178,360,509] ATL typically arises decades after infection and occurs in only a small fraction of infected individuals. As described earlier, Tax protein appears to play a role in latently transforming T lymphocytes. It has multiple effects on transcription of cellular genes, and it affects a variety of other cellular processes as well.[364,434] Despite the presence of *Tax,* ATL takes many years to develop. An explanation for the long latency of ATL could be that HTLV-I establishes a pool of T lymphocytes with enhanced proliferative potential, but that additional events (likely nonviral), such as accumulation of cellular mutations, are required for development of leukemia. The Tax protein is often not expressed in end-stage ATLs.[245] This may reflect immunological selection against continued expression of this viral protein as the tumors progress. ATLs do express another viral protein, HBZ, encoded by an mRNA from the opposite strand of viral DNA.[173,305] HBZ may contribute to the late stage of tumorigenesis (including downregulation of Tax expression), while Tax may be involved in early preleukemic steps.[245]

Hepatitis B Virus

HBV infects more than 1 billion people worldwide and is associated with acute and chronic hepatitis, as well as with the majority of hepatocellular carcinoma (HCC).[21] Although HBV contains a DNA genome, it undergoes an unusual replication cycle that involves RNA replicative intermediates.[452] Unlike the other DNA tumor viruses, HBV does not contain well-defined oncogenes, although the *X* gene has been implicated in cell transformation and tumorigenesis in transgenic mice.[119,431] *X* affects cellular gene expression and may interfere with p53 function.[152]

In some HBV-infected individuals (particularly those infected as infants), infection becomes persistent. Over time, persistent infection can lead to chronic liver damage (chronic active hepatitis [CAH]), which has a significant likelihood of progressing to HCC. In individuals with CAH, the liver injury caused by HBV replication and the resulting inflammation and rounds of hepatocyte proliferation and mutagenesis during liver regeneration are thought to cause the accumulation of cellular mutations that lead to cancer formation. Reactive oxygen species produced by inflammatory cells recruited to sites of liver injury are also likely to cause DNA damage and mutagenesis. Moreover, segments of the HBV genome can show monoclonal integration patterns in HCC, raising the possibility that the viral genome also plays a *cis*-acting role in hepatic carcinogenesis.[151] A recombinant HBV subunit vaccine has been deployed for decades and is reducing the incidence of HBV-mediated HCC.[65]

Hepatitis C Virus

HCV is an RNA-containing virus of the *Flavivirus* family. HCV causes viral hepatitis and HCC and is also associated with non-Hodgkin B-cell lymphoma.[82,332,355,394] HCV lacks a clearly defined viral oncogene, but HCV structural genes have transforming activity in various assays.[282,321,433] Like HBV, HCV can establish persistent infections and CAH, leading to HCC. The carcinogenic potential of HCV is thought to derive primarily from its cytolytic activity in hepatocytes and the resulting inflammation and regeneration. However, unlike HBV, whose genome is relatively stable, even in a single infected individual the HCV genome is highly variable and constitutes a swarm of closely related viral variants, complicating attempts to develop an effective HCV vaccine. There are reports that successful antiviral treatment of HCV infection can also provide benefit for HCV-associated lymphomas.[215]

Retroviral Oncogenesis in Human Gene Therapy Trials

Because retroviruses can stably deliver genes into host cell DNA, they have been used as gene transfer vectors in clinical trials to correct inherited genetic defects, most notably of the hematopoietic system.[336] In one trial, an MuLV-based vector expressing the cytokine receptor common γ-chain was used to treat patients with X-linked severe combined immunodeficiency (X-SCID).[201] In this trial, hematopoietic progenitor cells from X-SCID patients were transduced with the vector *ex vivo* and then infused back into the same individuals. This approach corrected the SCID defect, but several of the treated individuals subsequently developed T-cell lymphoma.[201] Molecular analysis of the lymphomas revealed that the retroviral gene transfer vector caused insertional activation of the LMO2 proto-oncogene, as well as of other proto-oncogenes. Vector-induced malignancies or premalignant conditions have also arisen in similar trials for correction of chronic granulomatous disease and Wiskott-Aldrich syndrome.[46,270,442] These findings raise cautions about the use of retroviral vectors for gene correction in humans.

In response to these findings, second- and third-generation retroviral vectors have been developed for human gene transfer. The enhancer sequences have been removed from the upstream LTR of the vector to generate a vector that has inactive LTRs after reverse transcription (a self-inactivating or SIN vector).[511] The absence of functional viral enhancers in the transduced cells is designed to reduce the likelihood of insertional activation of cellular proto-oncogenes. A second approach has been to use retroviral vectors based on lentiviruses such as HIV-1, because lentiviruses have not been shown to induce cancer. Moreover, while MuLV has a preference for integration near the transcription start sites of genes (and thus may more efficiently activate adjacent genes), HIV-1 tends to integrate within the bodies of genes.[315,409] A recent human clinical trial to correct β-thalassemia employed an HIV-1–based SIN vector expressing human β-globin.[62] In the first treated patient, the clinical symptoms of thalassemia were relieved, but there was an expansion of a clone of cells where the vector was inserted into the gene for HMG2A, which is overexpressed in certain malignancies. Molecular analysis of the integration site in these cells demonstrated that insertion of the provirus truncated the 3′ noncoding region of HMG2A mRNA, resulting in removal of binding sequences for a regulatory miRNA and upregulation of HMG2A mRNA. This is reminiscent of tumors in SL3-3 MuLV-induced T-lymphomas, where *gfi-1* was activated by removal of miRNA binding sequences from the mRNA.[100]

Additional Viruses Implicated in Human Cancer

In addition to the six viruses firmly implicated in naturally occurring cancer, it is likely that additional viruses will be shown to be involved in cancer causation in humans, particularly for cancers associated with immunosuppression. Rapid improvements in DNA sequencing technology suggest that sequencing-based efforts are likely to be the prime method of detecting new candidate tumor viruses, as they were in the identification of KSHV and MCV (see next paragraph). Rigorous genetic, cell biological, and epidemiologic studies must be performed to confirm the role of any new candidates in human carcinogenesis.

The next virus likely to be recognized as a human tumor virus is Merkel cell polyomavirus (MCV). Merkel cell carcinoma is a rare but aggressive tumor of neuroendocrine cells in the skin, and it is often associated with sunlight exposure and immunosuppression. Through extensive sequencing of Merkel cell carcinoma RNA, in 2008 Feng et al[154] identified sequences that were homologous to known polyomaviruses. Further analysis showed that up to 80% of Merkel cell carcinomas worldwide contain an intact, integrated polyomavirus genome, designated MCV. Like all known polyomaviruses, the MCV genome encodes LT that binds Rb family members and sT that binds PP2A. Tumors contain monoclonal integrations of MCV DNA in the cellular genome that disrupt the DNA replication activity of LT but leave the Rb binding activity intact,[429] providing a plausible mechanism of tumor suppressor inactivation and cell transformation. Recent experiments indicate that Merkel cell carcinoma cell lines require MCV early region expression for continued proliferation[217] and that sT can transform rodent cells in culture. Taken together, these results provide strong evidence that MCV is the seventh human tumor virus. Similar to other oncogenic human DNA viruses, MCV infection appears to be fairly common,[251] even though Merkel cell cancers are rare.

SV40 itself has been implicated in a number of human cancers, including non-Hodgkin lymphoma, mesothelioma, and childhood brain tumors.[170] However, the evidence in support of these claims, and even of the conclusion that SV40 infection can occur in humans, remains controversial. Two pathogenic human polyomaviruses closely related to SV40, JC virus and BK virus, have also been implicated in human cancer, but the evidence for oncogenic activity in humans is inconclusive.

A retroviral genome closely related to MuLV genomes has been detected in human prostate carcinoma DNA and named xenotropic murine leukemia virus–related virus (XMRV). XMRV DNA was originally found in patients with hereditary prostate cancer, and the viral genome was detected in stromal cells, not epithelial tumor cells.[470] Some subsequent reports have detected XMRV DNA and proteins in prostate cancer specimens, but the association of the virus with the hereditary form of prostate cancer and its restriction to stromal cells has not been confirmed.[157,404] Other groups have failed to detect any association of XMRV with prostate cancer. Recent molecular studies suggest that XMRV was generated by recombination between two endogenous MuLV-related retroviruses during passage of a human prostate cancer in nude mice.[344] As a consequence, the prostate cancer cell 22Rv.1 produces high amounts of XMRV, which replicates efficiently in certain human prostate cancer cell lines and appears to have been detected as a contaminant during surveys of prostate cancer tissues by highly sensitive PCR amplification techniques. Viruses related to MMTV have been suggested to play a role in the etiology of human breast cancer, but convincing candidate viruses have not yet emerged.

The foregoing discussion assumes that tumor virus gene products persist in tumor cells. If a virus can cause cancer through a true "hit-and-run" mechanism, there may be many more human tumor viruses than are currently recognized.

Finally, although HIV is not regarded as a tumor virus, the immunosuppression caused by HIV plays an important role in the genesis of many virally induced tumors. AIDS is associated with increased frequencies of many of the virus-associated human cancers (e.g., HPV-associated cancer of the cervix and anus, EBV-associated lymphomas, and Kaposi sarcoma). This suggests that the increased cancer incidence in AIDS patients results from reduced immunological control of the oncogenic virus. However, the incidence of some nonviral cancers is also elevated in individuals with AIDS. Improved prevention and control of HIV infection will reduce worldwide cancer prevalence.

WHY DO VIRUSES TRANSFORM CELLS?

The preceding sections describe how viruses transform cells. But why do so many diverse viruses transform cells and cause tumors? Evolution selects for the ability of viruses to replicate, avoid host cell defenses, and spread to new hosts. Many viruses accomplish these tasks without displaying transforming or tumor-forming activity, so transforming activity *per se* is not essential for virus replication.

Retrovirus transformation is incidental to virus replication. The absence of oncogenes in the replication-competent nonacute retroviruses demonstrates that these genes are not required for virus replication. Rather, the appearance of monoclonal tumors in animals many months after infection indicates that tumorigenic transformation by these viruses is an exceedingly rare event at the cellular level. This conclusion is supported by the inability of these viruses to transform cultured cells. It is only because of the huge number of infected cells in animals and the dramatic consequences of *in vivo* transformation, namely, tumor formation, that these events are even observed by scientists and studied. Presumably, proviruses integrate near many cellular genes, but the vast majority of these integration events do not provide a growth advantage to the cells, and therefore they are not detected. For the acutely transforming retroviruses, oncogenes are acquired from the host cell genome extremely infrequently during virus propagation. But once incorporated in an active form into the viral genome, the transduced gene is introduced into every newly infected cell and is a potent and rapidly acting carcinogen, allowing scientists to capture these viruses. Tumor-forming activity confers no replication advantage to these viruses, and in fact the acquisition of an oncogene is in almost all cases associated with virus replication defects.

The peculiar lifestyle of retroviruses, involving integrated proviruses that stably persist in infected cells, explains why these viruses are unique among RNA viruses in having transforming potential in cultured cells, because the provirus allows the sustained expression of the viral oncogene or acts *in cis* to regulate the expression of cellular proto-oncogenes or tumor suppressor genes.

DNA tumor virus oncogenes typically are essential, intrinsic viral genes. The biochemical activities of the proteins encoded by these genes were selected during virus evolution for their roles in virus replication and persistence, not for their ability to transform cells. In order for viruses to synthesize the large amounts of viral DNA needed to sustain a productive infection, up to 100,000 or more progeny genomes per infected cell, the cell must be reprogrammed into a DNA replication factory to provide an abundant supply of DNA polymerases and other replication factors. Most cells are resting and not able to support high-level DNA replication when initially exposed to a virus. Therefore, the virus must stimulate the cell to enter S phase to generate a cellular environment conducive to viral DNA replication. What better way to generate this state than to exploit the intrinsic cellular machinery that controls cell cycle progression? Thus, it is no accident that DNA virus oncoproteins stimulate cell proliferation. And when virus replication is aborted, in nonpermissive cells for example, and the viral genome undergoes rare recombination events to integrate into cellular DNA, the ongoing proliferative stimulus may result in cell transformation or tumor formation. According to this view, transformation by DNA viruses is an accidental byproduct of their need to drive the cell into S phase for viral DNA replication. Consistent with this hypothesis is the observation that parvoviruses, which do not stimulate S phase and can only replicate in cells induced by other means to enter the cell cycle, are one of the few DNA virus groups devoid of transforming activity.

This aspect of viral oncogene action can be seen clearly with the E7 protein of HPV, because the cells undergoing various responses in stratified squamous epithelia are physically separated. HPV initially infects basal epithelial cells. Normally, when basal cells divide and migrate away from the basement membrane, they undergo a process of terminal differentiation and growth arrest, which is incompatible with vegetative viral DNA replication. However, high-level viral DNA replication must be able to take place in the suprabasal cells because keratinocyte differentiation is required for the virus life cycle to proceed. Therefore, the viral E7 protein inactivates the Rb pathway in suprabasal cells to maintain the DNA replication machinery in an active state without preventing keratinocyte differentiation.[76] The ability of the E7 protein to inhibit the activity of $p21^{WAF1}$, which is implicated in keratinocyte differentiation, may assist in this process.[165,242]

Another aspect of viral tumorigenesis is suggested by the presence of immune evasion genes in the larger DNA viruses such as the herpesviruses. This model posits that transforming activity and tumorigenesis are indirect consequences of viral countermeasures to defense mechanisms erected by the host cell.[317] Upon initial confrontation with a virus, and even in response to latent infection, cells mobilize innate immune signaling pathways to block virus replication. In some cases, these pathways activate tumor suppressor pathways or interferon signaling, resulting in growth arrest or apoptosis, which restricts virus replication or spread. The transforming proteins of some viruses may have evolved to neutralize tumor suppressor pathways and thereby circumvent these cell defenses and other innate immune pathways. By removing these blocks to virus propagation, the blocks to cell proliferation are removed as well. Virus genes that inhibit these host defenses thus exert a proliferative and eventually a transforming effect on the cells.

Neither transforming activity nor tumorigenicity is required for replication of RNA and DNA tumor viruses, and these activities have not been directly selected for during evolution. Rather, transforming activity is an accident or at most an unintended consequence of the complex biochemistry of viral genome integration, replication, and persistence. From the scientific and medical point of view, we are the beneficiary of these accidents, because they have generated a set of biological reagents, the viruses themselves, which have provided unprecedented insights into such fundamental cellular and pathologic processes as signal transduction, cell cycle control, and above all carcinogenesis. The dependence of nonviral tumorigenesis on the same pathways mobilized by tumor viruses emphasizes the central role of the regulatory pathways targeted by these viruses and highlights the value of tumor viruses as uniquely powerful probes of cell function.

REFERENCES

All cited references are available in the e-book.

2. Ahuja D, Saenz-Robles MT, Pipas JM. SV40 large T antigen targets multiple cellular pathways to elicit cellular transformation. *Oncogene* 2005;24:7729–7745.
4. Ang KK, Harris J, Wheeler R, et al. Human papillomavirus and survival of patients with oropharyngeal cancer. *N Engl J Med* 2010;363:24–35.
5. Antman K, Chang Y. Kaposi's sarcoma. *N Engl J Med* 2000;342:1027–1038.
7. Arbeit JM, Howley PM, Hanahan D. Chronic estrogen-induced cervical and vaginal squamous carcinogenesis in human papillomavirus type 16 transgenic mice. *Proc Natl Acad Sci U S A* 1996;93:2930–2935.
9. Bais C, Santomasso B, Coso O, et al. G-protein-coupled receptor of Kaposi's sarcoma-associated herpesvirus is a viral oncogene and angiogenesis activator. *Nature* 1998;391:86–89.
16. Bandara LR, La Thangue NB. Adenovirus E1A prevents the retinoblastoma gene product from complexing with a cellular transcription factor. *Nature* 1991;351:494–497.
20. Bear SE, Bellacosa A, Lazo PA, et al. Provirus insertion in Tpl-1, an Ets-1-related oncogene, is associated with tumor progression in Moloney murine leukemia virus-induced rat thymic lymphomas. *Proc Natl Acad Sci U S A* 1989;86:7495–7499.
21. Beasley RP, Hwang LY, Lin CC, et al. Hepatocellular carcinoma and hepatitis B virus. A prospective study of 22 707 men in Taiwan. *Lancet* 1981;2:1129–1133.
22. Bedell MA, Jones KH, Grossman SR, et al. Identification of human papillomavirus type 18 transforming genes in immortalized and primary cells. *J Virol* 1989;63:1247–1255.
25. Ben-David Y, Lavigueur A, Cheong GY, et al. Insertional inactivation of the p53 gene during friend leukemia: a new strategy for identifying tumor suppressor genes. *New Biologist* 1990;2:1015–1023.
31. Bishop JM. Viral oncogenes. *Cell* 1985;42:23–38.
34. Blenis J. Signal transduction via the MAP kinases: proceed at your own RSK. *Proc Natl Acad Sci U S A* 1993;90:5889–5892.
36. Bohmann D, Bos TJ, Admon A, et al. Human proto-oncogene c-jun encodes a DNA binding protein with structural and functional properties of transcription factor AP-1. *Science* 1987;238:1386–1392.
37. Bolen JB, Thiele CJ, Israel MA, et al. Enhancement of cellular src gene product associated tyrosyl kinase activity following polyoma virus infection and transformation. *Cell* 1984;38:767–777.
39. Bollag G, McCormick F. Regulators and effectors of ras proteins. *Annu Rev Cell Biol* 1991;7:601–632.
43. Boshoff C, Endo Y, Collins PD, et al. Angiogenic and HIV-inhibitory functions of KSHV-encoded chemokines. *Science* 1997;278:290–294.
44. Bourne HR, Sanders DA, McCormick F. The GTPase superfamily: conserved structure and molecular mechanism. *Nature* 1991;349:117–127.
45. Boyer SN, Wazer DE, Band V. E7 protein of human papilloma virus-16 induces degradation of retinoblastoma protein through the ubiquitin-proteasome pathway. *Cancer Res* 1996;56:4620–4624.
46. Boztug K, Schmidt M, Schwarzer A, et al. Stem-cell gene therapy for the Wiskott-Aldrich syndrome. *N Engl J Med* 2010;363:1918–1927.
48. Breuer ML, Cuypers HT, Berns A. Evidence for the involvement of pim-2, a new common proviral insertion site, in progression of lymphomas. *Embo J* 1989;8:743–748.
50. Brugge JS, Erikson RL. Identification of a transformation-specific antigen induced by an avian sarcoma virus. *Nature* 1977;269:346–348.
56. Campbell KS, Ogris E, Burke B, et al. Polyoma middle tumor antigen interacts with SHC protein via the NPTY (Asn-Pro-Thr-Tyr) motif in middle tumor antigen. *Proc Natl Acad Sci U S A* 1994;91:6344–6348.
59. Caporale M, Cousens C, Centorame P, et al. Expression of the jaagsiekte sheep retrovirus envelope glycoprotein is sufficient to induce lung tumors in sheep. *J Virol* 2006;80:8030–8037.
62. Cavazzana-Calvo M, Payen E, Negre O, et al. Transfusion independence and HMGA2 activation after gene therapy of human beta-thalassaemia. *Nature* 2010;467:318–322.
65. Chang MH, Chen CJ, Lai MS, et al. Universal hepatitis B vaccination in Taiwan and the incidence of hepatocellular carcinoma in children. Taiwan Childhood Hepatoma Study Group. *N Engl J Med* 1997;336:1855–1859.
66. Chang Y, Cesarman E, Pessin MS, et al. Identification of herpesvirus-like DNA sequences in AIDS-associated Kaposi's sarcoma. *Science* 1994;266:1865–1869.
67. Chang Y, Moore PS, Talbot SJ, et al. Cyclin encoded by KS herpesvirus. *Nature* 1996;382:410.
68. Chatis PA, Holland CA, Silver JE, et al. A 3′ end fragment encompassing the transcriptional enhancers of nondefective Friend virus confers erythroleukemogenicity on Moloney leukemia virus. *J Virol* 1984;52:248–254.
71. Chellappan S, Kraus VB, Kroger B, et al. Adenovirus E1A, simian virus 40 tumor antigen, and human papillomavirus E7 protein share the capacity to disrupt the interaction between transcription factor E2F and the retinoblastoma gene product. *Proc Natl Acad Sci U S A* 1992;89:4549–4553.
72. Chen IS, Wachsman W, Rosenblatt JD, et al. The role of the x gene in HTLV associated malignancy. *Cancer Surv* 1986;5:329–342.
76. Cheng S, Schmidt-Grimminger DC, Murant T, et al. Differentiation-dependent up-regulation of the human papillomavirus E7 gene reactivates cellular DNA replication in suprabasal differentiated keratinocytes. *Genes Dev* 1995;9:2335–2349.
79. Chiu IM, Reddy EP, Givol D, et al. Nucleotide sequence analysis identifies the human c-sis proto-oncogene as a structural gene for platelet-derived growth factor. *Cell* 1984;37:123–129.
80. Chiu R, Boyle WJ, Meek J, et al. The c-Fos protein interacts with c-Jun/AP-1 to stimulate transcription of AP-1 responsive genes. *Cell* 1988;54:541–552.
84. Clurman BE, Hayward WS. Multiple proto-oncogene activations in avian leukosis virus-induced lymphomas: evidence for stage-specific events. *Mol Cell Biol* 1989;9:2657–2664.
86. Coffin JM, Varmus HE, Bishop JM, et al. Proposal for naming host cell-derived inserts in retrovirus genomes. *J Virol* 1981;40:953–957.
87. Cohen JI, Wang F, Mannick J, et al. Epstein-Barr virus nuclear protein 2 is a key determinant of lymphocyte transformation. *Proc Natl Acad Sci U S A* 1989;86:9558–9562.
88. Collett MS, Erikson RL. Protein kinase activity associated with the avian sarcoma virus src gene product. *Proc Natl Acad Sci U S A* 1978;75:2021–2024.
89. Collett MS, Purchio AF, Erikson RL. Avian sarcoma virus-transforming protein, pp60src shows protein kinase activity specific for tyrosine. *Nature* 1980;285:167–169.

92. Copeland NG, Jenkins NA. Myeloid leukemia: disease genes and mouse models. *Prog Exp Tumor Res* 1999;35:53–63.
94. Courtneidge SA. Activation of the pp60 c-src kinase by middle T antigen binding or by dephosphorylation. *EMBO J* 1985;4:1471–1477.
96. Courtneidge SA, Smith AE. Polyoma virus transforming protein associates with the product of the c-src cellular gene. *Nature* 1983;303:435–439.
98. Crow DS, Kurata WE, Lau AF. Phosphorylation of connexin43 in cells containing mutant src oncogenes. *Oncogene* 1992;7:999–1003.
99. Cuypers HT, Selten G, Quint W, et al. Murine leukemia virus-induced T-cell lymphomagenesis: integration of proviruses in a distinct chromosomal region. *Cell* 1984;37:141–150.
100. Dabrowska MJ, Dybkaer K, Johnsen HE, et al. Loss of MicroRNA targets in the 3′ untranslated region as a mechanism of retroviral insertional activation of growth factor independence 1. *J Virol* 2009;83:8051–8061.
103. Dalla-Favera R, Bregni M, Erikson J, et al. Human c-myc onc gene is located on the region of chromosome 8 that is translocated in Burkitt lymphoma cells. *Proc Natl Acad Sci U S A* 1982;79:7824–7827.
104. Damania B, Lee H, Jung JU. Primate herpesviral oncogenes. *Mol Cells* 1999;9:345–349.
106. Danilkovitch-Miagkova A, Duh FM, Kuzmin I, et al. Hyaluronidase 2 negatively regulates RON receptor tyrosine kinase and mediates transformation of epithelial cells by jaagsiekte sheep retrovirus. *Proc Natl Acad Sci U S A* 2003;100:4580–4585.
108. de Klein A, van Kessel AG, Grosveld G, et al. A cellular oncogene is translocated to the Philadelphia chromosome in chronic myelocytic leukaemia. *Nature* 1982;300:765–767.
109. de Sauvage FJ, Hass PE, Spencer SD, et al. Stimulation of megakaryocytopoiesis and thrombopoiesis by the c-Mpl ligand. *Nature* 1994; 369:533–538.
110. Debbas M, White E. Wild-type p53 mediates apoptosis by E1A, which is inhibited by E1B. *Genes Dev* 1993;7:546–554.
112. DeCaprio JA, Ludlow JW, Figge J, et al. SV40 large tumor antigen forms a specific complex with the product of the retinoblastoma susceptibility gene. *Cell* 1988;54:275–283.
113. DeFilippis RA, Goodwin EC, Wu L, et al. Endogenous human papillomavirus E6 and E7 proteins differentially regulate proliferation, senescence, and apoptosis in HeLa cervical carcinoma cells. *J Virol* 2003; 77:1551–1563.
117. Der CJ, Krontiris TG, Cooper GM. Transforming genes of human bladder and lung carcinoma cell lines are homologous to the ras genes of Harvey and Kirsten sarcoma viruses. *Proc Natl Acad Sci U S A* 1982; 79:3637–3640.
118. DesGroseillers L, Jolicoeur P. Mapping the viral sequences conferring leukemogenicity and disease specificity in Moloney and amphotropic murine leukemia viruses. *J Virol* 1984;52:448–456.
128. Duensing S, Lee LY, Duensing A, et al. The human papillomavirus type 16 E6 and E7 oncoproteins cooperate to induce mitotic defects and genomic instability by uncoupling centrosome duplication from the cell division cycle. *Proc Natl Acad Sci U S A* 2000;97:10002–10007.
130. Duesberg PH, Kawai S, Wang LH, et al. RNA of replication-defective strains of Rous sarcoma virus. *Proc Natl Acad Sci U S A* 1975;72:1569–1573.
133. Dyson N, Howley PM, Munger K, et al. The human papilloma virus-16 E7 oncoprotein is able to bind to the retinoblastoma gene product. *Science* 1989;243:934–937.
134. Eckhart W, Hutchinson MA, Hunter T. An activity phosphorylating tyrosine in polyoma T antigen immunoprecipitates. *Cell* 1979;18:925–933.
138. Eilers M, Eisenman RN. Myc's broad reach. *Genes Dev* 2008;22:2755–2766.
143. Ellermann V, Bang O. Experimentelle Leukamie bei Huhnern. *Zentralb Bakteriol* 1908;46:595–609.
145. Ellis RW, Defeo D, Shih TY, et al. The p21 src genes of Harvey and Kirsten sarcoma viruses originate from divergent members of a family of normal vertebrate genes. *Nature* 1981;292:506–511.
154. Feng H, Shuda M, Chang Y, et al. Clonal integration of a polyomavirus in human Merkel cell carcinoma. *Science* 2008;319:1096–1100.
156. Finlay CA, Hinds PW, Levine AJ. The p53 proto-oncogene can act as a suppressor of transformation. *Cell* 1989;57:1083–1093.
160. Fluck MM, Schaffhausen BS. Lessons in signaling and tumorigenesis from polyomavirus middle T antigen. *Micro Molec Biol Rev* 2009;73: 542–563.
164. Fung YK, Lewis WG, Crittenden LB, et al. Activation of the cellular oncogene c-erbB by LTR insertion: molecular basis for induction of erythroblastosis by avian leukosis virus. *Cell* 1983;33:357–368.
165. Funk JO, Waga S, Harry JB, et al. Inhibition of CDK activity and PCNA-dependent DNA replication by p21 is blocked by interaction with the HPV-16 E7 oncoprotein. *Genes Dev* 1997;11:2090–2100.
171. Gardiol D, Kuhne C, Glaunsinger B, et al. Oncogenic human papillomavirus E6 proteins target the discs large tumour suppressor for proteasome-mediated degradation. *Oncogene* 1999;18:5487–5496.
173. Gaudray G, Gachon F, Basbous J, et al. The complementary strand of the human T-cell leukemia virus type 1 RNA genome encodes a bZIP transcription factor that down-regulates viral transcription. *J Virol* 2002; 76:12813–12822.
175. Genther Williams SM, Disbrow GL, Schlegel R, et al. Requirement of epidermal growth factor receptor for hyperplasia induced by E5, a high-risk human papillomavirus oncogene. *Cancer Res* 2005;65: 6534–6542.
178. Giam CZ, Jeang KT. HTLV-1 Tax and adult T-cell leukemia. *Front Biosci* 2007;12:1496–1507.
185. Goldstein DJ, Andresson T, Sparkowski JJ, et al. The BPV-1 E5 protein, the 16 kDa membrane pore-forming protein and the PDGF receptor exist in a complex that is dependent on hydrophobic transmembrane interactions. *EMBO J* 1992;11:4851–4859.
186. Goldstein DJ, Finbow ME, Andresson T, et al. Bovine papillomavirus E5 oncoprotein binds to the 16 K component of vacuolar H(+)-ATPases. *Nature* 1991;352:347–349.
188. Goodwin EC, DiMaio D. Repression of human papillomavirus oncogenes in HeLa cervical carcinoma cells causes the orderly reactivation of dormant tumor suppressor pathways. *Proc Natl Acad Sci U S A* 2000; 97:12513–12518.
191. Gottwein E, Mukherjee N, Sachse C, et al. A viral microRNA functions as an orthologue of cellular miR-155. *Nature* 2007;450:1096–1099.
195. Gross L. Development and serial cellfree passage of a highly potent strain of mouse leukemia virus. *Proc Soc Exp Biol Med* 1957;94:767–771.
201. Hacein-Bey-Abina S, von Kalle C, Schmidt M, et al. A serious adverse event after successful gene therapy for X-linked severe combined immunodeficiency. *N Engl J Med* 2003;348:255–256.
203. Hammerschmidt W, Sugden B. Genetic analysis of immortalizing functions of Epstein-Barr virus in human B lymphocytes. *Nature* 1989; 340:393–397.
207. Hartley JW, Wolford NK, Old LJ, et al. A new class of murine leukemia virus associated with development of spontaneous lymphomas. *Proc Natl Acad Sci U S A* 1977;74:789–792.
209. Hawley-Nelson P, Vousden KH, Hubbert NL, et al. HPV16 E6 and E7 proteins cooperate to immortalize human foreskin keratinocytes. *EMBO J* 1989;8:3905–3910.
210. Hayman MJ, Enrietto PJ. Cell transformation by the epidermal growth factor receptor and v-erbB. *Cancer Cells* 1991;3:302–307.
211. Hayward WS, Neel BG, Astrin SM. Activation of a cellular onc gene by promoter insertion in ALV-induced lymphoid leukosis. *Nature* 1981; 290:475–480.
216. Hofacre A, Fan H. Jaagsiekte sheep retrovirus molecular biology and oncogenesis. *Viruses* 2010;2:2618–2648.
218. Howie HL, Katzenellenbogen RA, Galloway DA. Papillomavirus E6 proteins. *Virology* 2009;384:324–334.
219. Huang E, Nocka K, Beier DR, et al. The hematopoietic growth factor KL is encoded by the Sl locus and is the ligand of the c-kit receptor, the gene product of the W locus. *Cell* 1990;63:225–233.
222. Huibregtse JM, Scheffner M, Howley PM. A cellular protein mediates association of p53 with the E6 oncoprotein of human papillomavirus types 16 or 18. *EMBO J* 1991;10:4129–4135.
223. Hunter T, Sefton BM. Transforming gene product of Rous sarcoma virus phosphorylates tyrosine. *Proc Natl Acad Sci U S A* 1980;77:1311–1315.
242. Jones NC. Transformation by the human adenoviruses. *Semin Cancer Biol* 1990;1:425–435.
245. Kannian P, Green PL. Human T lymphotropic virus type 1 (HTLV-1): molecular biology and oncogenesis. *Viruses* 2010;2:2037–2077.
248. Katz E, Lareef MH, Rassa JC, et al. MMTV Env encodes an ITAM responsible for transformation of mammary epithelial cells in three-dimensional culture. *J Exp Med* 2005;201:431–439.

249. Kaushansky K, Lok S, Holly RD, et al. Promotion of megakaryocyte progenitor expansion and differentiation by the c-Mpl ligand thrombopoietin. *Nature* 1994;369:568–571.
250. Kaye KM, Izumi KM, Kieff E. Epstein-Barr virus latent membrane protein 1 is essential for B-lymphocyte growth transformation. *Proc Natl Acad Sci U S A* 1993;90:9150–9154.
255. Kiyono T, Foster SA, Koop JI, et al. Both Rb/p16INK4 a inactivation and telomerase activity are required to immortalize human epithelial cells. *Nature* 1998;396:84–88.
256. Kiyono T, Hiraiwa A, Fujita M, et al. Binding of high-risk human papillomavirus E6 oncoproteins to the human homologue of the Drosophila discs large tumor suppressor protein. *Proc Natl Acad Sci U S A* 1997;94:11612–11616.
258. Klempnauer KH, Gonda TJ, Bishop JM. Nucleotide sequence of the retroviral leukemia gene v-myb and its cellular progenitor c-myb: the architecture of a transduced oncogene. *Cell* 1982;31:453–463.
259. Klingelhutz AJ, Foster SA, McDougall JK. Telomerase activation by the E6 gene product of human papillomavirus type 16. *Nature* 1996;380: 79–82.
261. Koch CA, Anderson D, Moran MF, et al. SH2 and SH3 domains: elements that control interactions of cytoplasmic signaling proteins. *Science* 1991;252:668–674.
262. Kolch W, Heidecker G, Lloyd P, et al. Raf-1 protein kinase is required for growth of induced NIH/3T3 cells. *Nature* 1991;349:426–428.
264. Konopka JB, Watanabe SM, Witte ON. An alteration of the human c-abl protein in K562 leukemia cells unmasks associated tyrosine kinase activity. *Cell* 1984;37:1035–1042.
265. Kool J, Uren AG, Martins CP, et al. Insertional mutagenesis in mice deficient for p15Ink4b, p16Ink4a, p21Cip1, and p27Kip1 reveals cancer gene interactions and correlations with tumor phenotypes. *Cancer Res* 2010;70:520–531.
271. Kulwichit W, Edwards RH, Davenport EM, et al. Expression of the Epstein-Barr virus latent membrane protein 1 induces B cell lymphoma in transgenic mice. *Proc Natl Acad Sci U S A* 1998;95:11963–11968.
280. Lee SS, Weiss RS, Javier RT. Binding of human virus oncoproteins to hDlg/SAP97, a mammalian homolog of the Drosophila discs large tumor suppressor protein. *Proc Natl Acad Sci U S A* 1997;94:6670–6675.
281. Lenz J, Celander D, Crowther RL, et al. Determination of the leukaemogenicity of a murine retrovirus by sequences within the long terminal repeat. *Nature* 1984;308:467–470.
283. Leung K, Nabel GJ. HTLV-1 transactivator induces interleukin-2 receptor expression through an NF-kappa B-like factor. *Nature* 1988;333: 776–778.
284. Levine AJ. p53, the cellular gatekeeper for growth and division. *Cell* 1997;88:323–331.
285. Li JP, D'Andrea AD, Lodish HF, et al. Activation of cell growth by binding of Friend spleen focus-forming virus gp55 glycoprotein to the erythropoietin receptor. *Nature* 1990;343:762–764.
296. Maeda N, Palmarini M, Murgia C, et al. Direct transformation of rodent fibroblasts by jaagsiekte sheep retrovirus DNA. *Proc Natl Acad Sci U S A* 2001;98:4449–4454.
297. Maki Y, Bos TJ, Davis C, et al. Avian sarcoma virus 17 carries the jun oncogene. *Proc Natl Acad Sci U S A* 1987;84:2848–2852.
301. Martin DF, Kuppermann BD, Wolitz RA, et al. Oral ganciclovir for patients with cytomegalovirus retinitis treated with a ganciclovir implant. Roche Ganciclovir Study Group. *N Engl J Med* 1999;340:1063–1070.
302. Martin GS. Rous sarcoma virus: a function required for the maintenance of the transformed state. *Nature* 1970;227:1021–1023.
305. Matsuoka M, Green PL. The HBZ gene, a key player in HTLV-1 pathogenesis. *Retrovirology* 2009;6:71.
307. Mayer BJ, Hanafusa H. Association of the v-crk oncogene product with phosphotyrosine-containing proteins and protein kinase activity. *Proc Natl Acad Sci U S A* 1990;87:2638–2642.
309. McLaughlin-Drubin ME, Munger K. The human papillomavirus E7 oncoprotein. *Virology* 2009;384:335–344.
310. McLaughlin-Drubin ME, Munger K. Viruses associated with human cancer. *Biochim Biophys Acta* 2008;1782:127–150.
317. Moore PS, Chang Y. Why do viruses cause cancer? Highlights of the first century of human tumour virology. *Nat Rev Cancer* 2010;10: 878–889.
321. Moriya K, Fujie H, Shintani Y, et al. The core protein of hepatitis C virus induces hepatocellular carcinoma in transgenic mice. *Nat Med* 1998;4:1065–1067.
322. Mosialos G, Birkenbach M, Yalamanchili R, et al. The Epstein-Barr virus transforming protein LMP1 engages signaling proteins for the tumor necrosis factor receptor family. *Cell* 1995;80:389–399.
323. Mowat M, Cheng A, Kimura N, et al. Rearrangements of the cellular p53 gene in erythroleukaemic cells transformed by Friend virus. *Nature* 1985;314:633–636.
325. Munger K, Phelps WC, Bubb V, et al. The E6 and E7 genes of the human papillomavirus type 16 together are necessary and sufficient for transformation of primary human keratinocytes. *J Virol* 1989;63: 4417–4421.
326. Munger K, Werness BA, Dyson N, et al. Complex formation of human papillomavirus E7 proteins with the retinoblastoma tumor suppressor gene product. *EMBO J* 1989;8:4099–4105.
328. Murphy PM. Pirated genes in Kaposi's sarcoma. *Nature* 1997;385:296–297, 299.
330. Nason-Burchenal K, Wolff L. Activation of c-myb is an early bone-marrow event in a murine model for acute promonocytic leukemia. *Proc Natl Acad Sci U S A* 1993;90:1619–1623.
331. Neel BG, Hayward WS, Robinson HL, et al. Avian leukosis virus-induced tumors have common proviral integration sites and synthesize discrete new RNAs: oncogenesis by promoter insertion. *Cell* 1981;23:323–334.
333. Nerenberg M, Hinrichs SH, Reynolds RK, et al. The tat gene of human T-lymphotropic virus type 1 induces mesenchymal tumors in transgenic mice. *Science* 1987;237:1324–1329.
335. Nguyen ML, Nguyen MM, Lee D, et al. The PDZ ligand domain of the human papillomavirus type 16 E6 protein is required for E6's induction of epithelial hyperplasia in vivo. *J Virol* 2003;77:6957–6964.
338. Niman HL. Antisera to a synthetic peptide of the sis viral oncogene product recognize human platelet-derived growth factor. *Nature* 1984; 307:180–183.
339. Nishigaki K, Thompson D, Hanson C, et al. The envelope glycoprotein of friend spleen focus-forming virus covalently interacts with and constitutively activates a truncated form of the receptor tyrosine kinase Stk. *J Virol* 2001;75:7893–7903.
340. Nusse R, Varmus HE. Many tumors induced by the mouse mammary tumor virus contain a provirus integrated in the same region of the host genome. *Cell* 1982;31:99–109.
342. Pallas DC, Shahrik LK, Martin BL, et al. Polyoma small and middle T antigens and SV40 small t antigen form stable complexes with protein phosphatase 2A. *Cell* 1990;60:167–176.
344. Paprotka T, Delviks-Frankenberry KA, Cingoz O, et al. Recombinant origin of the retrovirus XMRV. *Science* 2011;333:97–101.
346. Parada LF, Tabin CJ, Shih C, et al. Human EJ bladder carcinoma oncogene is homologue of Harvey sarcoma virus ras gene. *Nature* 1982; 297:474–478.
352. Payne GS, Bishop JM, Varmus HE. Multiple arrangements of viral DNA and an activated host oncogene in bursal lymphomas. *Nature* 1982; 295:209–214.
355. Perz JF, Armstrong GL, Farrington LA, et al. The contributions of hepatitis B virus and hepatitis C virus infections to cirrhosis and primary liver cancer worldwide. *J Hepatol* 2006;45:529–538.
356. Petti L, DiMaio D. Stable association between the bovine papillomavirus E5 transforming protein and activated platelet-derived growth factor receptor in transformed mouse cells. *Proc Natl Acad Sci U S A* 1992; 89:6736–6740.
357. Petti L, Nilson LA, DiMaio D. Activation of the platelet-derived growth factor receptor by the bovine papillomavirus E5 transforming protein. *EMBO J* 1991;10:845–855.
361. Poirier Y, Kozak C, Jolicoeur P. Identification of a common helper provirus integration site in Abelson murine leukemia virus-induced lymphoma DNA. *J Virol* 1988;62:3985–3992.
364. Pozzatti R, Vogel J, Jay G. The human T-lymphotropic virus type I tax gene can cooperate with the ras oncogene to induce neoplastic transformation of cells. *Mol Cell Biol* 1990;10:413–417.
367. Radke K, Gilmore T, Martin GS. Transformation by Rous sarcoma virus: a cellular substrate for transformation-specific protein phosphorylation contains phosphotyrosine. *Cell* 1980;21:821–828.

368. Radkov SA, Kellam P, Boshoff C. The latent nuclear antigen of Kaposi sarcoma-associated herpesvirus targets the retinoblastoma-E2F pathway and with the oncogene Hras transforms primary rat cells. *Nat Med* 2000;6:1121–1127.
370. Rao L, Debbas M, Sabbatini P, et al. The adenovirus E1A proteins induce apoptosis, which is inhibited by the E1B 19-kDa and Bcl-2 proteins. *Proc Natl Acad Sci U S A* 1992;89:7742–7746.
372. Rapp UR, Goldsborough MD, Mark GE, et al. Structure and biological activity of v-raf, a unique oncogene transduced by a retrovirus. *Proc Natl Acad Sci U S A* 1983;80:4218–4222.
373. Rassoulzadegan M, Cowie A, Carr A, et al. The roles of individual polyoma virus early proteins in oncogenic transformation. *Nature* 1982; 300:713–718.
374. Rassoulzadegan M, Naghashfar Z, Cowie A, et al. Expression of the large T protein of polyoma virus promotes the establishment in culture of "normal" rodent fibroblast cell lines. *Proc Natl Acad Sci U S A* 1983;80:4354–4358.
375. Rauscher FJ 3rd, Cohen DR, Curran T, et al. Fos-associated protein p39 is the product of the jun proto-oncogene. *Science* 1988;240:1010–1016.
381. Rossomando AJ, Payne DM, Weber MJ, et al. Evidence that pp42, a major tyrosine kinase target protein, is a mitogen-activated serine/threonine protein kinase. *Proc Natl Acad Sci U S A* 1989;86:6940–6943.
382. Rous P. A sarcoma of the fowl transmissible by an agent separable from the tumor cells. *J Exp Med* 1911;13:397–411.
383. Rovnak J, Quackenbush SL. Walleye dermal sarcoma virus: molecular biology and oncogenesis. *Viruses* 2010;2:1984–1999.
387. Ruf IK, Rhyne PW, Yang C, et al. Epstein-Barr virus small RNAs potentiate tumorigenicity of Burkitt lymphoma cells independently of an effect on apoptosis. *J Virol* 2000;74:10223–10228.
388. Ruley HE. Adenovirus early region 1A enables viral and cellular transforming genes to transform primary cells in culture. *Nature* 1983; 304:602–606.
389. Russo JJ, Bohenzky RA, Chien MC, et al. Nucleotide sequence of the Kaposi sarcoma-associated herpesvirus (HHV8). *Proc Natl Acad Sci U S A* 1996;93:14862–14867.
390. Sabbatini P, Chiou SK, Rao L, et al. Modulation of p53-mediated transcriptional repression and apoptosis by the adenovirus E1B 19K protein. *Mol Cell Biol* 1995;15:1060–1070.
393. Sadowski I, Stone JC, Pawson T. A noncatalytic domain conserved among cytoplasmic protein-tyrosine kinases modifies the kinase function and transforming activity of Fujinami sarcoma virus P130gag-fps. *Mol Cell Biol* 1986;6:4396–4408.
395. Sap J, Munoz A, Damm K, et al. The c-erb-A protein is a high-affinity receptor for thyroid hormone. *Nature* 1986;324:635–640.
398. Schaller MD, Borgman CA, Cobb BS, et al. pp125FAK a structurally distinctive protein-tyrosine kinase associated with focal adhesions. *Proc Natl Acad Sci U S A* 1992;89:5192–5196.
400. Scheffner M, Huibregtse JM, Vierstra RD, et al. The HPV-16 E6 and E6-AP complex functions as a ubiquitin-protein ligase in the ubiquitination of p53. *Cell* 1993;75:495–505.
402. Scheffner M, Werness BA, Huibregtse JM, et al. The E6 oncoprotein encoded by human papillomavirus types 16 and 18 promotes the degradation of p53. *Cell* 1990;63:1129–1136.
403. Schiller JT, Lowy DR. Vaccines to prevent infections by oncoviruses. *Annu Rev Microbiol* 2010;64:23–41.
405. Schlegel R, Phelps WC, Zhang YL, et al. Quantitative keratinocyte assay detects two biological activities of human papillomavirus DNA and identifies viral types associated with cervical carcinoma. *EMBO J* 1988;7: 3181–3187.
407. Schlessinger J. How receptor tyrosine kinases activate Ras. *Trends Biochem Sci* 1993;18:273–275.
410. Schwab M, Alitalo K, Klempnauer KH, et al. Amplified DNA with limited homology to myc cellular oncogene is shared by human neuroblastoma cell lines and a neuroblastoma tumour. *Nature* 1983;305:245–248.
419. Shai A, Pitot HC, Lambert PF. E6-associated protein is required for human papillomavirus type 16 E6 to cause cervical cancer in mice. *Cancer Res* 2010;70:5064–5073.
421. Sheiness D, Fanshier L, Bishop JM. Identification of nucleotide sequences which may encode the oncogenic capacity of avian retrovirus MC29. *J Virol* 1978;28:600–610.
422. Shen H, Suzuki T, Munroe DJ, et al. Common sites of retroviral integration in mouse hematopoietic tumors identified by high-throughput, single nucleotide polymorphism-based mapping and bacterial artificial chromosome hybridization. *J Virol* 2003;77:1584–1588.
424. Sheng Q, Denis D, Ratnofsky M, et al. The DnaJ domain of polyomavirus large T antigen is required to regulate Rb family tumor suppressor function. *J Virol* 1997;71:9410–9416.
425. Sherr CJ, Rettenmier CW, Sacca R, et al. The c-fms proto-oncogene product is related to the receptor for the mononuclear phagocyte growth factor, CSF-1. *Cell* 1985;41:665–676.
426. Shih C, Shilo BZ, Goldfarb MP, et al. Passage of phenotypes of chemically transformed cells via transfection of DNA and chromatin. *Proc Natl Acad Sci U S A* 1979;76:5714–5718.
428. Short MK, Okenquist SA, Lenz J. Correlation of leukemogenic potential of murine retroviruses with transcriptional tissue preference of the viral long terminal repeats. *J Virol* 1987;61:1067–1072.
430. Siekevitz M, Feinberg MB, Holbrook N, et al. Activation of interleukin 2 and interleukin 2 receptor (Tac) promoter expression by the trans-activator (tat) gene product of human T-cell leukemia virus, type I. *Proc Natl Acad Sci U S A* 1987;84:5389–5393.
431. Singh M, Kumar V. Transgenic mouse models of hepatitis B virus-associated hepatocellular carcinoma. *Rev Med Virol* 2003;13:243–253.
441. Stehelin D, Varmus HE, Bishop JM, et al. DNA related to the transforming gene(s) of avian sarcoma viruses is present in normal avian DNA. *Nature* 1976;260:170–173.
443. Stephens RM, Rice NR, Hiebsch RR, et al. Nucleotide sequence of v-rel: the oncogene of reticuloendotheliosis virus. *Proc Natl Acad Sci U S A* 1983; 80:6229–6233.
448. Stoye JP, Moroni C, Coffin JM. Virological events leading to spontaneous AKR thymomas. *J Virol* 1991;65:1273–1285.
454. Swanstrom R, Parker RC, Varmus HE, et al. Transduction of a cellular oncogene: the genesis of Rous sarcoma virus. *Proc Natl Acad Sci U S A* 1983;80:2519–2523.
458. Tabin CJ, Bradley SM, Bargmann CI, et al. Mechanism of activation of a human oncogene. *Nature* 1982;300:143–149.
459. Tabin CJ, Weinberg RA. Analysis of viral and somatic activations of the cHa-ras gene. *J Virol* 1985;53:260–265.
460. Takeya T, Hanafusa H. Structure and sequence of the cellular gene homologous to the RSV src gene and the mechanism for generating the transforming virus. *Cell* 1983;32:881–890.
462. Talmage DA, Freund R, Young AT, et al. Phosphorylation of middle T by pp60 c-src: a switch for binding of phosphatidylinositol 3-kinase and optimal tumorigenesis. *Cell* 1989;59:55–65.
467. Toyoshima K, Vogt PK. Temperature sensitive mutants of an avian sarcoma virus. *Virology* 1969;39:930–931.
469. Uchida J, Yasui T, Takaoka-Shichijo Y, et al. Mimicry of CD40 signals by Epstein-Barr virus LMP1 in B lymphocyte responses. *Science* 1999;286:300–303.
470. Urisman A, Molinaro RJ, Fischer N, et al. Identification of a novel Gammaretrovirus in prostate tumors of patients homozygous for R462Q RNASEL variant. *PLoS Pathog* 2006;2:e25.
472. Van Beveren C, van Straaten F, Curran T, et al. Analysis of FBJ-MuSV provirus and c-fos (mouse) gene reveals that viral and cellular fos gene products have different carboxy termini. *Cell* 1983;32:1241–1255.
473. van Lohuizen M, Verbeek S, Krimpenfort P, et al. Predisposition to lymphomagenesis in pim-1 transgenic mice: cooperation with c-myc and N-myc in murine leukemia virus-induced tumors. *Cell* 1989;56:673–682.
476. Vennstrom B, Sheiness D, Zabielski J, et al. Isolation and characterization of c-myc, a cellular homolog of the oncogene (v-myc) of avian myelocytomatosis virus strain 29. *J Virol* 1982;42:773–779.
477. von Knebel Doeberitz M, Oltersdorf T, Schwarz E, et al. Correlation of modified human papilloma virus early gene expression with altered growth properties in C4-1 cervical carcinoma cells. *Cancer Res* 1988;48: 3780–3786.
481. Wang D, Liebowitz D, Kieff E. An EBV membrane protein expressed in immortalized lymphocytes transforms established rodent cells. *Cell* 1985;43:831–840.
484. Wang LH, Duesberg P, Beemon K, et al. Mapping RNase T1-resistant oligonucleotides of avian tumor virus RNAs: sarcoma-specific oligonucleotides are near the poly(A) end and oligonucleotides common to

sarcoma and transformation-defective viruses are at the poly(A) end. *J Virol* 1975;16:1051–1070.

485. Watanabe T, Sugaya M, Atkins AM, et al. Kaposi's sarcoma-associated herpesvirus latency-associated nuclear antigen prolongs the life span of primary human umbilical vein endothelial cells. *J Virol* 2003;77:6188–6196.
488. Weitzman MD, Carson CT, Schwartz RA, et al. Interactions of viruses with the cellular DNA repair machinery. *DNA Repair (Amst)* 2004; 3:1165–1173.
489. Werness BA, Levine AJ, Howley PM. Association of human papillomavirus types 16 and 18 E6 proteins with p53. *Science* 1990;248:76–79.
493. Whitman M, Kaplan DR, Schaffhausen B, et al. Association of phosphatidylinositol kinase activity with polyoma middle-T competent for transformation. *Nature* 1985;315:239–242.
494. Whyte P, Buchkovich KJ, Horowitz JM, et al. Association between an oncogene and an anti-oncogene: the adenovirus E1A proteins bind to the retinoblastoma gene product. *Nature* 1988;334:124–129.
496. Witte ON, Dasgupta A, Baltimore D. Abelson murine leukaemia virus protein is phosphorylated in vitro to form phosphotyrosine. *Nature* 1980; 283:826–831.
497. Witte ON, Goff S, Rosenberg N, et al. A transformation-defective mutant of Abelson murine leukemia virus lacks protein kinase activity. *Proc Natl Acad Sci U S A* 1980;77:4993–4997.
498. Wolff L, Scolnick E, Ruscetti S. Envelope gene of the Friend spleen focus-forming virus: deletion and insertions in 3′ gp70/p15E-encoding region have resulted in unique features in the primary structure of its protein product. *Proc Natl Acad Sci U S A* 1983;80:4718–4722.
500. Wootton SK, Halbert CL, Miller AD. Sheep retrovirus structural protein induces lung tumours. *Nature* 2005;434:904–907.
503. Xu W, Harrison SC, Eck MJ. Three-dimensional structure of the tyrosine kinase c-Src. *Nature* 1997;385:595–602.
504. Yajima M, Kanda T, Takada K. Critical role of Epstein-Barr Virus (EBV)-encoded RNA in efficient EBV-induced B-lymphocyte growth transformation. *J Virol* 2005;79:4298–4307.
508. Yew N, Strobel M, Vande Woude GF. Mos and the cell cycle: the molecular basis of the transformed phenotype. *Curr Opin Genet Dev* 1993; 3:19–25.
513. Zerfass-Thome K, Zwerschke W, Mannhardt B, et al. Inactivation of the cdk inhibitor p27KIP1 by the human papillomavirus type 16 E7 oncoprotein. *Oncogene* 1996;13:2323–2330.
514. Zhang XF, Settleman J, Kyriakis JM, et al. Normal and oncogenic p21ras proteins bind to the amino-terminal regulatory domain of c-Raf-1. *Nature* 1993;364:308–313.
517. Zsebo KM, Williams DA, Geissler EN, et al. Stem cell factor is encoded at the Sl locus of the mouse and is the ligand for the c-kit tyrosine kinase receptor. *Cell* 1990;63:213–224.

CHAPTER 8

Akiko Iwasaki • Ruslan Medzhitov

Innate Responses to Viral Infections

The innate immune system provides a universal form of host protection from infectious diseases. It detects the presence of pathogens using several recognition strategies. The best-characterized innate microbial sensing mechanism is based on pattern recognition receptors (PRRs). These receptors detect conserved microbial structures shared by entire classes of microorganisms. The targets of PRRs are commonly products of metabolic pathways unique to a particular class of microbes, such as lipopolysaccharide in the case of Gram-negative bacteria. In the case of viral pathogens, however, all viral molecular constituents are produced in the host cell. Consequently, the major targets of innate immune recognition are viral nucleic acids. Whenever possible, the innate immune system detects structural features of viral RNA and DNA that are distinct from the host nucleic acid. These include long double-stranded RNA, RNAs containing 5′-triphosphate, and unmethylated CpG motifs in viral DNA genomes. Detection of these structural features, however, is insufficient to reliably distinguish the host and viral nucleic acids. Therefore, additional factors help to determine their origin. For example, viral but not host nucleic acids are normally found in the endolysosomes and viral but not host DNA is present in the cytosol. Innate immune sensors of viral RNA and DNA are present in these locations, where they can be triggered to activate the antiviral responses. In addition to pattern recognition, viral pathogens might be detected indirectly, through alteration in normal cellular processes, such as acute decline in host protein synthesis, altered activity of ion channels, or ER stress. These forms of recognition are still incompletely understood and remain to be fully characterized in future studies.

Detection of viral pathogens by the innate immune system has two major consequences: first, it leads to the induction of the innate antiviral mechanisms, most of which are mediated primarily by type-I interferons (IFNs). Second, it leads to the activation of the adaptive immune response that can provide a more directed, antigen-specific, and long-lasting antiviral immunity. The main host defense strategy against viral pathogens is the elimination of the infected cells. This can be achieved by cell-intrinsic mechanisms that are induced by type-I IFNs and operate in the infected cells, or with the help of cytotoxic lymphocytes: natural killer (NK) cells and CD8 T cells. Another important host defense mechanism is the blockade of viral entry into the host cells. This is primarily a function of neutralizing antibodies. Many additional mechanisms exist that interfere with viral replication, gene expression, virion assembly, and exit from the infected cells. The relative contribution of these defense mechanisms varies depending on the virus and host. Detailed knowledge of the specific antiviral defense mechanisms is difficult to establish due in large part to a high degree of redundancy between different mechanisms.

In this chapter, we will focus on the better-characterized viral sensing mechanisms of the innate immune system and discuss the major defense mechanisms utilized in mammalian hosts.

SENSING VIRAL INFECTIONS

Viral Sensing Through Pattern Recognition Receptors

The mammalian immune system detects the presence of viruses through multiple mechanisms. The best understood mechanisms involve various PRRs. Most common molecular patterns associated with virus infection are the features associated with viral nucleic acids. Innate immune recognition can be cell intrinsic or cell extrinsic, depending on whether it is mediated by infected or non-infected cells. Cell-intrinsic innate immune recognition is mediated by cytosolic sensors, including the NOD-like receptors (NLRs) and RIG-I-like receptors (RLRs). Activation of these receptors generally occurs in infected cells. Accordingly, PRRs involved in cell-intrinsic recognition are broadly expressed because viral pathogens target a variety of cell types for replication. In contrast, cell-extrinsic innate immune recognition is mediated by transmembrane receptors (including Toll-like receptors (TLRs) and C-type lectins [CLRs]); their activation does not require the cells expressing these receptors to be infected. Cell-extrinsic recognition is mainly mediated by specialized cells of the immune system, such as the plasmacytoid dendritic cell (pDC), macrophage, and dendritic cell (DC).

PRRs involved in microbial recognition have modular structures and share several structurally related domains for innate recognition, multimerization, interaction with adaptor molecules, and signaling (Fig. 8.1).

CELL-AUTONOMOUS VIRUS RECOGNITION

RIG-I-Like Receptors (RLRs)

RNA viruses are recognized by the cytoplasmic RNA helicases, retinoic acid–inducible gene-I (RIG-I), and melanoma differentiation–associated gene 5 (MDA5).[198] The RIG-I-like receptors (RLRs) are expressed by most cell types, and both RIG-I and MDA5 recognize viral RNA through their helicase domains. RIG-I also contains the repressor domain (RD) at its C-terminus, which inhibits the activation of RIG-I at steady state. Binding to viral RNA catalyzes a conformational rearrangement, which exposes a caspase activation and recruitment domain (CARD) to initiate antiviral signaling[152,199] (Fig. 8.1). Both RIG-I and MDA5 utilize a common adaptor molecule called mitochondria antiviral signaling protein (MAVS)[162]—also known as IPS-1,[93] Cardif,[127] or VISA[194]—that localizes to the mitochondrial membrane[162] and to the peroxisomes.[47] MAVS activates two protein kinase complexes, one consisting of FADD and caspases 8/10[175] and the other containing TANK and NAP1[155] (Fig. 8.2). The former activates the IKKα/IKKβ/IKKγ complex while the latter activates the TBK1-IKKi complex, leading to the activation and nuclear translocation of transcription factors NF-κB and IRF3, respectively. In addition, the TRAF6-dependent pathway involving MEKK1 is essential to activate the MAP kinase and NF-κB pathways.[201] Despite similarity in overall structure and signaling mechanisms, RIG-I and MDA-5 have important differences in their mechanisms of activation. For example, RIG-I but not MDA5 requires ubiquitination by E3 ligase TRIM25 for its activity.[58] Additional differences in the function of RIG-I and MDA-5 likely exist and may reflect distinct features of viral pathogens that they recognize.

Analysis of animals deficient in the RLRs revealed important and distinct roles for these sensors in innate immunity. These molecules cumulatively provide the host with the ability to recognize a large group of viral pathogens in infected cells and mediate a critical aspect of innate antiviral defense.

RIG-I

RIG-I consists of two N-terminal CARDs, a central DExH box RNA helicase/adenosine triphosphatase (ATPase) domain, and a C-terminal regulatory domain (RD) (Fig. 8.1). RIG-I functions as a critical PRR for a number of viruses including Sendai virus (SeV), vesicular stomatitis virus (VSV), influenza, hepatitis C virus, Japanese encephalitis virus, as well as small RNA encoded by the DNA virus, Epstein-Barr virus.[92] RIG-I

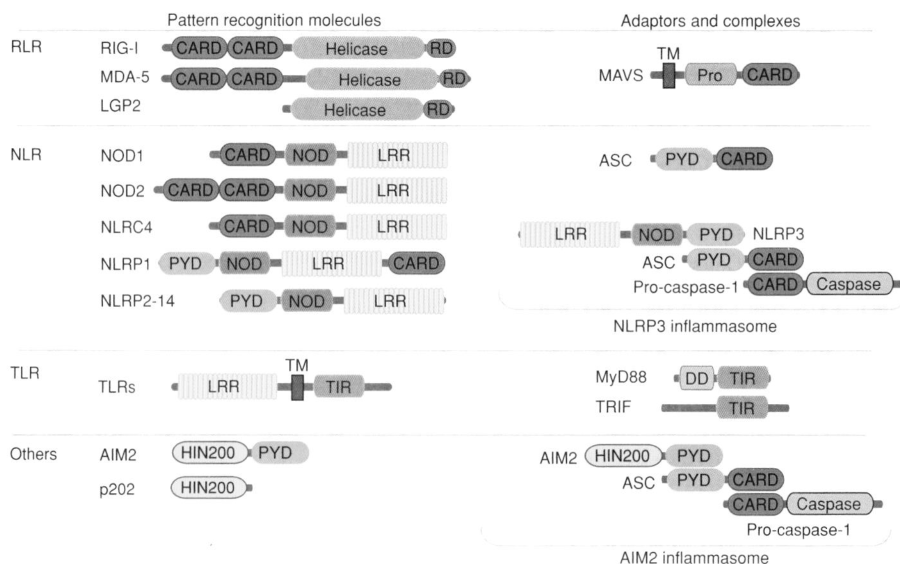

FIGURE 8.1. Domain structure of viral sensors and adaptor molecules. Pattern recognition molecules involved in viral sensing contain distinct domains, some of which are shared by different classes of receptors. These domains include: CARD, caspase activation and recruitment domain; DD, death domain; HIN200, hemopoietic IFN-inducible nuclear proteins is a 200-amino acid motif; LRR, leucine-rich repeat; NOD, nucleotide-binding oligomerization domain; Pro, proline-rich region; PYD, pyrin domain; caspase domain; TIR, toll/interleukin-1 receptor; TM, transmembrane region. Many of these domains can be used for homotypic oligomerization. Examples of molecular complexes are depicted for NLRP3 and AIM2 inflammasomes.

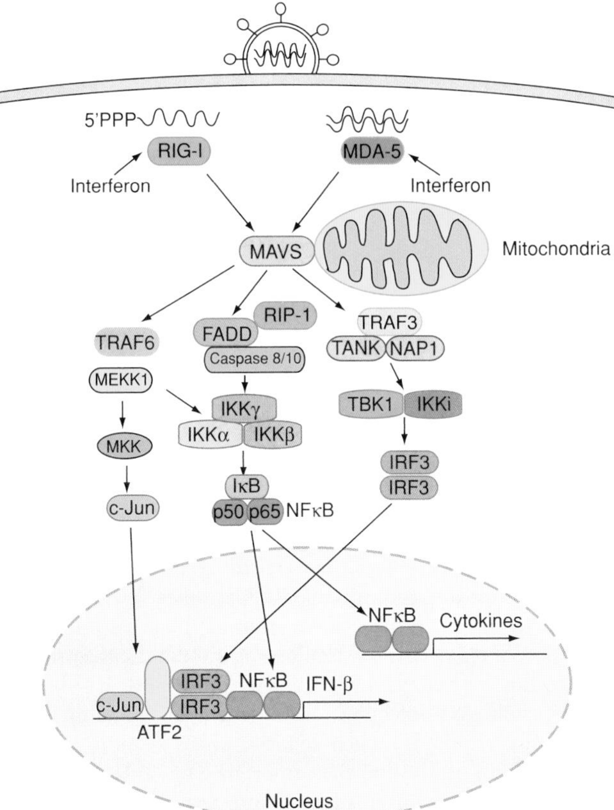

FIGURE 8.2. RIG-I and MDA-5 virus recognition pathways. In a virally infected cell, RNA structures that are unique to viruses are recognized by RIG-I and MDA-5. RIG-I detects ssRNA containing 5′ triphosphate, while MDA-5 recognizes a long stretch of dsRNA. RNA binding to RLRs induces conformational changes, enabling their binding to MAVS adaptor protein expressed on the surface of mitochondria and peroxisomes. MAVS activates signaling to activate NF-κB, MAP kinases, and IRF3, leading to target gene expression including IFN-β and cytokines. Type I IFNs increase the levels of RLRs in bystander cells, enabling robust antiviral signaling upon infection.

recognizes single-stranded (ssRNA) that contains 5′ triphosphate end, but not 5′ OH or a 5′-methylguanosine cap[73,144] that is longer than 23 nucleotides[123] and contains a uridine- or adenosine-rich ribonucleotide sequence[153] (Fig. 8.2). RIG-I can also recognize double-stranded (dsRNA) in the absence of 5′ triphosphate in some cases with a preference for shorter-length dsRNA compared to those recognized by MDA-5.[91] Analysis of the central DExH box RNA helicase/ATPase domain of RIG-I revealed an ATP-powered dsRNA translocation activity. The CARD domains suppress translocation in the absence of 5′-triphosphate, and the activation by 5′-triphosphate triggers RIG-I to translocate preferentially on dsRNA in *cis*.[130] This ATPase activity is required for RIG-I signaling, indicating that RIG-I recognizes two distinct features of viral RNA simultaneously: triphosphate at the 5′ end and dsRNA. RIG-I indeed selectively detects blunt, short, double-stranded 5′-triphosphate RNA, which is common in the panhandle region of ssRNA viral genomes.[157]

MDA5

MDA5 serves as a sensor of picornaviruses and can be activated by cytosolic synthetic dsRNA, such as polyinosinic-polycytidylic acid (poly I:C).[60,92] There appears to be some level of redundancy in RIG-I and MDA5 in recognition of certain viruses. Dengue virus and West Nile virus are recognized by both MDA5 and RIG-I; either of these sensors is sufficient to induce type I IFN production.[115] Comparison of synthetic and viral dsRNA revealed that MDA-5 preferentially recognizes longer dsRNA that is at least 2 k bp in length, while RIG-I is activated by a wider range of dsRNA sizes (400 bp–4 kbp).[91] Many viruses that replicate in the cytoplasm express their own 2′-*O*-methyltransferases to autonomously modify their messenger RNA (mRNA). Interestingly, infection with viruses deficient in 2′-*O*-methyltransferase leads to robust activation of MDA5, indicating that lack of ribose 2′-*O*-methylation is used as a signature of viral RNA for recognition by MDA5.[205] Therefore, MDA5 likely recognizes large dsRNA structures lacking 2′-*O*-methylation generated in the cytosol during virus infection. Of note, 2′-*O*-methylation is also used by viruses to evade restriction by IFN-induced proteins with tetratricopeptide repeats (IFIT) proteins.[36,205]

LGP2

The third member of the RLR family, laboratory of genetics and physiology 2 (LGP2), displays sequence homology to the helicase domains of RIG-I and MDA5. It lacks a CARD domain, however, and therefore has been proposed to serve as a negative regulator of both sensors. Overexpression studies indicated that LGP2 does not activate the production of type I IFNs on its own, but inhibits RIG-I- and MDA5-mediated signaling in a dose-dependent manner.[98,149,200] Interestingly, studies of *lgp2* knockout mice indicated that LGP2 may play both positive and negative regulatory roles in MDA5- and RIG-I-mediated innate immunity.[189] This study found that the loss of lgp2 augments type I IFN production in response to transfected poly I:C (MDA-5 agonist) or VSV infection (RIG-I agonist). In contrast, LGP2 is required for efficient antiviral responses following EMCV infection (MDA5 agonist). Therefore, LPG2 can serve as a positive or negative regulator of RLR signaling depending on the type of viral infection. The precise mechanism underlying the opposing functions of LPG2 is still unclear.

NOD-Like Receptors (NLRs)

NLRs comprise a large family of intracellular PRRs that regulates innate immunity in response to recognition of various PAMPs and stress signals.[125] The NLR family consists of multidomain proteins that contain a C-terminal LRR domain, a central NOD domain and an N-terminal effector domain. NLR proteins can be subdivided into three subfamilies depending on the structure of N-terminal domains: CARD-containing subfamily (NOD1, NOD2, NLRCs, CIITA), pyrin domain (PYD)–containing subfamily (NLRPs) (Fig. 8.1), and BIR domain–containing subgroup (NAIPs) (not shown). Both NOD and NLRP members contribute to antiviral defense. The PYD subfamily of NLRPs consists of 14 members. Although the functions of many of the NLRPs are largely unknown, several NLRPs play a key role in the activation of caspase-1 by forming a multiprotein complex known as the

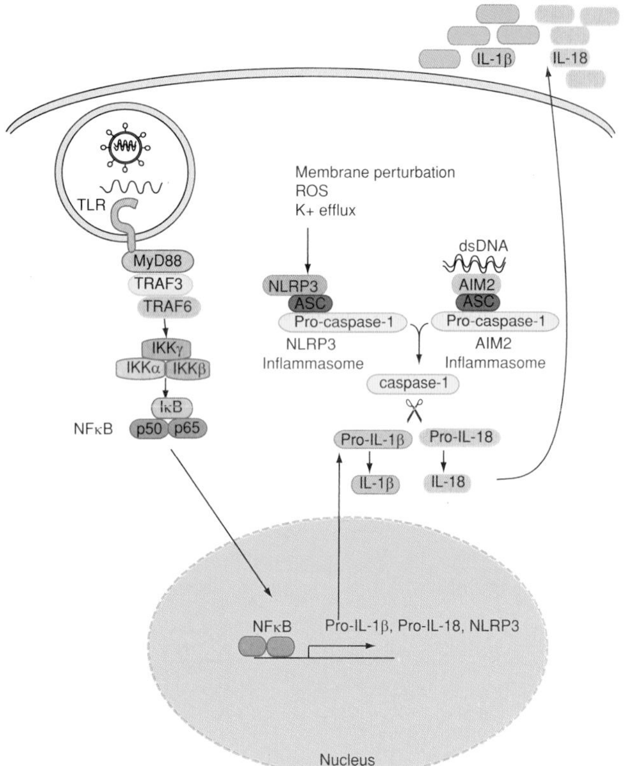

FIGURE 8.3. Inflammasome activation by virus infection. Virus infection can lead to inflammasome activation through two separate pathways. NLRP3 inflammasome is activated upon infection by adenovirus or influenza virus. This pathway is initiated by membrane perturbation, K^+ efflux, and reactive oxygen species (ROS). The second pathway involves AIM2, which is activated by dsDNA in the cytosol. Both NLRP3 and AIM2 form a complex with ASC and pro-caspase-1 (inflammasome), leading to the self-cleavage and activation of caspase-1. Pro-forms of IL-1*β* and IL-18 induced by TLR signals are cleaved by activated caspase-1. Mature forms of these cytokines are then released to the extracellular space.

"inflammasome"[124] (Fig. 8.3). Caspase-1 is an essential mediator of inflammatory response through its capacity to cleave and generate active forms of IL-1*β* and IL-18. IL-1*β* and IL-18 are potent proinflammatory cytokines, as described below. Formation and secretion of mature IL-1*β* and IL-18 require a two-step activation mechanism: first, transcriptional and translational upregulation of the pro-forms of these cytokines are induced by TLR signaling, and a second signal that leads to the proteolytic activation of caspase-1. The latter process is mediated by the inflammasome. Inflammasome complexes that are important in antiviral defense are described below.

NLRP3-ASC Inflammasome

NLRP3, also known as NALP3/Cryopyrin/CIAS1/PYPAF1,[181] forms an ASC-dependent inflammasome (Fig. 8.3). The NLRP3 inflammasome can be activated by a variety of stimuli including endogenous signals from dying cells (uric acid), crystals (asbestos, silica, alum), as well as microbial signals such as whole bacteria, bacterial RNA, extracellular ATP, pore-forming toxins, or viral infections.[125] It is unclear whether microbial ligands can directly activate the NLRP3 inflammasome. Instead, the NLRP3 inflammasomes likely sense cellular stress such as disruption in membrane integrity and extracellular ATP released from stressed or damaged cells. Virus infection also results in the activation of inflammasomes. Both SeV and influenza virus activated the NLRP3 inflammasome in macrophages pulsed transiently with ATP (signal 2) *in vitro*.[90] DNA viruses such as adenovirus stimulate the NLRP3-ASC-caspase-1 inflammasomes *in vivo*.[129] However, inflammasomes are not activated by transfection of RNA, poly I:C, or infection with reovirus (dsRNA virus) or VSV (ssRNA virus),[129] indicating that viral RNAs are insufficient to trigger inflammasome activation. Influenza virus activates the inflammasome through the activity of the M2 ion channel.[79] The M2 channel of influenza A virus is a homotetrameric integral membrane protein that associates to form a highly specific proton channel,[145] and is essential for influenza A virus infection and replication.[179] Among other things, the M2 channel exports protons in the acidic trans-Golgi network (TGN) to neutralize the pH of the lumen of the TGN in order to prevent the premature maturation of hemagglutinin to its low-pH fusogenic form.[32] Within influenza virus–infected cells, NLRP3 complex detects changes in ionic imbalance in the TGN to activate the inflammasomes. *In vivo, NLRP3* deficiency resulted in increased susceptibility to high-dose flu challenge.[4,180] In addition, after a sublethal dose of influenza infection, ASC-dependent inflammasome activation is required to elicit adaptive protective immunity to influenza virus, indicating the importance of NLRs in linking innate viral recognition to adaptive immunity.[78]

AIM2-ASC Inflammasome

Not all inflammasomes are activated by NLRPs. Recent studies showed that AIM2 couples cytosolic dsDNA recognition to ASC-caspase-1 inflammasome.[25,53,72,148] AIM2 is an HIN200 family of protein that contains a dsDNA binding domain (HIN domain) and the PYD domain, which promotes interaction with the PYD domain of ASC (Fig. 8.1). AIM2 recognizes dsDNA in the cytosol and induces oligomerization of ASC and caspase-1, leading to activation of caspase-1 and cleavage of pro-forms of cytokines including IL-1*β*, IL-18, and IL-33 (Fig. 8.3). Vaccinia virus, which contains a dsDNA genome, was shown to require AIM2 for recognition and activation of caspase1 inflammasomes.[72] It is interesting to note that different classes of dsDNA viruses are recognized by NLRP3 (adenovirus) or AIM2 (vaccinia virus) for inflammasome activation. This likely depends on both the accessibility of the dsDNA genome to intracellular sensors and the viral-induced cellular stress responses. While cytosolic dsDNA can bind to AIM2 directly and activate inflammasomes, how and where exactly NLRP3 becomes activated by dsDNA viruses is yet to be determined.

p202

Mouse HIN200 protein, p202, is a negative regulator of the AIM2 inflammasome.[148] No orthologs of p202 have been found in humans. p202 contains two HIN domains but no PYD domain, and binds specifically to dsDNA. Unlike AIM2, p202 cannot bind ASC and therefore appears to function as an inhibitor of AIM2, presumably by limiting its access to DNA.

Cytosolic DNA Sensors

The existence of a cytoplasmic DNA sensing molecule leading to type I IFN production was suggested from studies of infection by DNA viruses and bacteria.[82,170] It is now clear that there are likely multiple sensors that recognize distinct types of DNA. These DNAs include DNA from viruses, bacteria, apoptotic host cells, and synthetic B-form DNAs—particularly poly(dA:dT) and interferon stimulatory DNA (ISD). ISDs are dsDNA containing >25 base-pair oligonucleotides, which in sequence-independent manner, trigger stimulation of type I IFNs through a pathway involving TBK1 and IRF3, but not MAVS.[170] Interestingly, ISD does not engage NK-κB or MAPK pathways, thus activating only IRF3-induced pathways. ISD recognition pathway exists only in primary cells but is lost from transformed cells.[170] However, the sensor for ISD still remains to be identified. TREX1, an exonuclease, was identified to be a negative regulator of ISD pathway by inhibiting excess accumulation of DNA products from endogenous retroelements.[169] TREX1-deficient humans and mice suffer from autoimmune disease due to hyperstimulation of ISD pathway. TREX1 is also involved in degrading nonproductive RT products generated during HIV-1 infection, enabling HIV-1 to remain undetected by the ISD sensor.[195]

In contrast, B-form DNA—or poly(dA-dT)·poly(dT-dA) dsDNA—triggers type I IFNs via IRF3 and NK-κB, suggesting that this form of DNA triggers a separate sensor from ISD.[81] The sensor(s) for cytosolic DNA remained elusive until recently. First, a molecule called DAI (also known as DLM-1/ZBP1) was identified as a candidate intracellular DNA sensing molecule.[176] IFN induction following poly(dA-dT)·poly(dT-dA) DNA treatment was abrogated by a small interfering RNA (siRNA) directed against DAI, suggesting that DAI is a critical cytoplasmic DNA sensor.[176] However, DAI is not the sole sensor of DNA in the cytosol, as DAI-knockout mice still responded to B-DNA or plasmid DNA.[83] More recent studies showed that poly(dA-dT)·poly(dT-dA) DNA is recognized by RIG-I upon transcription by RNA polymerase III (Pol III).[1,30] Pol III synthesizes 5′-triphosphate RNA using AT-rich dsDNA as a template, generating an RIG-I agonist in the cytosol. Therefore, RIG-I is the sensor for cytosolic poly(dA-dT)·poly(dT-dA) dsDNA upon transcription by Pol III. In addition to the indirect sensing of poly(dA-dT)·poly(dT-dA) by RIG-I, IFI16, a PYHIN protein, can bind to poly(dA-dT)·poly(dT-dA), and knockdown of IFI16 expression led to reduction in IFN-β production.[186]

Cyclophilin A

While most pattern recognition of virus infection involves detection of nucleic acids, there are few exceptions in which viral protein serves as a signature for viral infection. Cyclophilin A is a peptidylprolyl isomerase that can catalyze *cis/trans* isomerization of X-Proline epitopes on target proteins. Innate response to HIV-1 in DCs depends on interaction between the newly synthesized HIV-1 capsid and cellular cyclophilin A, leading to activation of type I IFNs through IRF-3-dependent mechanisms.[122] Human DCs, but not CD4 T cells, have intrinsic machinery for responding to HIV-1 infection through cyclophilin A. However, infected humans are unable to utilize the cyclophilin A–dependent pathway of IFN induction against HIV-1 infection because DCs are resistant to HIV-1 infection. In addition, cyclophilin A is also known to be incorporated into the HIV-1 virions by binding to capsid protein. Virions lacking cyclophilin A possess normal morphology and can penetrate host cells, but are defective in the reverse transcription of viral RNA.[22] Therefore, HIV-1 utilizes cyclophilin A for its infectivity, and renders cyclophilin A useless in antiviral defense by avoiding infection in the relevant cell type.

CELL-EXTRINSIC VIRUS RECOGNITION

Toll-Like Receptors (TLRs)

TLRs are the best characterized members of the PRR family, which recognize evolutionarily conserved molecular patterns associated with a large variety of microorganisms.[87] There are 11 functional TLRs in mice (TLR1–7, 9, 11–13) and 10 functional TLRs in humans (TLR1–10). All TLRs are type I transmembrane proteins with ectodomains containing leucine rich repeat (LRR) that mediate the recognition of PAMPs. Some TLRs recognize bacterial, fungal, and protozoan pathogens, while others are dedicated for viral recognition.[177] This chapter will focus on the TLRs that recognize viral pathogens.

The transmembrane domains of TLRs dictate the localization of the receptor, and the cytosolic domain contains the toll/interleukin-1 receptor (TIR) domain, which binds to adaptor proteins and ultimately leads to expression of a variety of genes.[2] TLR activation, following virus detection, catalyzes a complex signaling cascade that bifurcates into two main pathways, culminating in the synthesis of proinflammatory cytokines (NF-κB-dependent) and antiviral cytokines, type I interferons (IFNs) (IRF-dependent). In addition, TLR signaling results in the activation of the mitogen-activated protein kinases (MAPKs) (see Fig. 8.5). Type I IFNs in turn induce a battery of genes that directly suppress viral replication. Other cytokines and chemokines efficiently recruit immune cells to sites of virus infection. In particular, TLR recognition by DCs, the most potent antigen-presenting cells, enables their activation and antigen-presenting function, effectively linking innate recognition to the induction of adaptive immunity.[86]

TLRs are distributed on specific subcellular locations and are specifically expressed by different cell types. TLRs can be categorized into two major types: those that are expressed on the cell surface (TLR1, 2, 4, 5, 6, 11, and 12) and those that are expressed in the endolysosomes (TLR3, 7, 8, and 9). Although virus–TLR interaction can occur with both types of TLRs, many of the virus interactions with surface TLRs represent viral invasion mechanism (beneficial to the virus) rather than PAMP recognition by TLRs (beneficial to the host) (see discussion under Virus Manipulation of Innate Immunity). In this section, we will discuss the latter type of TLR-virus PAMP recognition leading to antiviral defense.

Viruses are recognized by a group of TLRs that reside in the endosomal membrane—namely, TLR3, 7, 8, and 9—where they can gain access to viral nucleic acids upon endocytosis of virions. A major advantage of this strategy of viral recognition is that the viral sensing and subsequent induction of type I IFN genes are not subjected to viral evasion mechanisms. In addition, since all viruses contain genomes consisting of RNA or DNA, such molecular patterns can be surveyed by a very limited number of receptors. These endosomal TLRs require trafficking by the endoplasmic reticulum (ER) membrane protein, UNC-93B.[24,174] UNC-93B physically interacts with TLR3, 7, and 9 via the transmembrane domain,[24] and transports these TLRs from the ER to the endosome (Fig. 8.4). Mutations in the *Unc93b1* gene were found in two patients with severe HSV encephalitis,[26] indicating the importance of transport of endosomal TLRs via

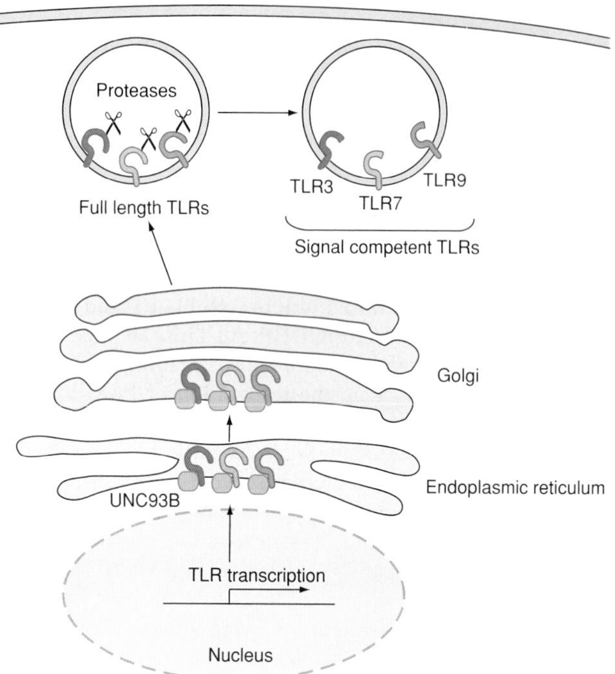

FIGURE 8.4. Endosomal TLR trafficking and processing. Endosomal TLRs, TLR3, TLR7, and TLR9, are synthesized in the ER, transported through Golgi, and are sorted into endosomes. UNC93B is an ER-resident protein, which facilitates TLR transport to the endolysosomes. Once in the endosomes, TLR3, 7, and 9 undergo proteolytic cleavage by proteases, which makes these receptors competent for signaling.

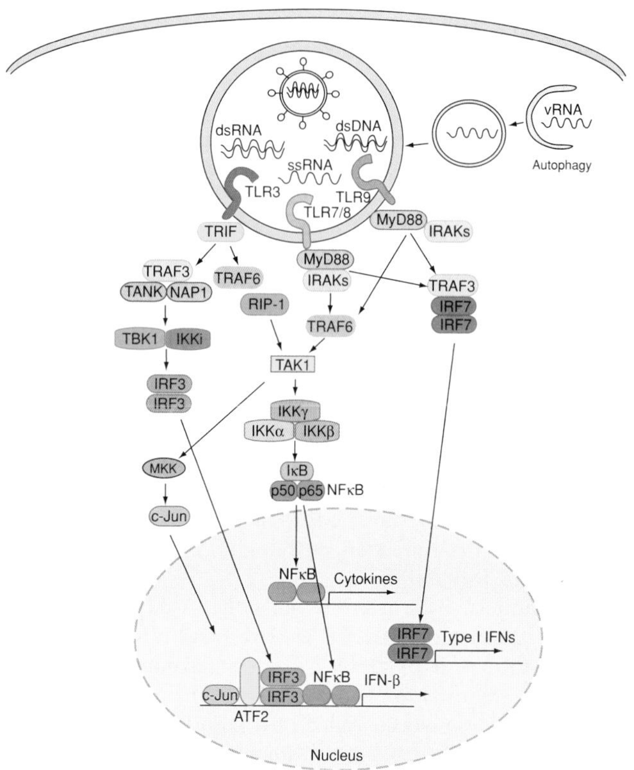

FIGURE 8.5. Endosomal TLR virus recognition and signaling. Viruses or virus-infected cells are endocytosed, and signatures of virus infection become accessible to TLRs upon digestion of membranes and nucleocapsid. TLR3 recognizes dsRNA, TLR7 and TLR8 recognize ssRNA, and TLR9 recognizes DNA. In addition, autophagy delivers TLR7 ligand (cytosolic viral replication intermediate) by fusion with the endosomes containing TLR7. Proteolytically activated TLRs in the endosomes recruit adaptor proteins and induce downstream signaling to activate a variety of transcription factors. IRF3 in combination with NF-κB, c-Jun, and ATF bind to the promoter and induce IFN-β expression. IRF7 homodimer binds to promoter regions of *IFN-a* genes and induces IFN-a expression. In addition, NF-κB activates transcription of a large number of genes, including cytokines.

UNC93B in antiviral defense. Upon arrival in the endosomal compartment, these TLRs undergo processing by endosomal proteases. While full-length and cleaved forms of TLR9 are capable of binding ligands, only the processed form recruits MyD88 upon activation.[52,140] The ectodomain of TLR9, and likely TLR3 and TLR7,[52] must first be cleaved in the endolysosomes by cathepsins in order to become competent for signaling (Fig. 8.4). Dependence of TLR9 activation on proteolytic processing in the endolysosomes ensures that aberrant activation of TLR9 from cell surface (for example, upon recognition of self DNA) is avoided.

TLR3

TLR3 is expressed by a variety of cells in human and mice, including conventional DCs, B cells, fibroblasts, and epithelial cells but not in plasmacytoid DCs (pDCs). Upon PAMP recognition, TLR3 recruits TRIF via its TIR domain (Fig. 8.5). TRIF is responsible for activation of both NF-κB and IRF3, leading to proinflammatory cytokines and type I IFN gene expression, respectively. TRIF binds to TRAF6, which is a RING-domain E3 ubiquitin ligase capable of polyubiquitinylating TRAF6 and IKKγ. Ubiquitinylated TRAF6 and IKKγ recruit TAK1 complex (consisting of TAK1 and TAB proteins), leading to the activation of MAPK. TRIF also binds to receptor-interacting protein (RIP)1 to initiate NF-κB activation. To activate the type I IFN genes, TRIF also recruits TRAF3, which engages TBK1 and subsequent activation of IRF3. IRF-3 translocates to the nucleus and binds to promoters of type I IFN genes.

dsRNA intermediates are produced during the replication cycle of most RNA viruses (except for retroviruses). DNA viruses also produce dsRNA by convergent transcription of their genomes.[193] It has long been known that dsRNA triggers IFN production. The first TLR implicated in viral nucleic acid recognition was TLR3.[3] TLR3 responds to the artificial dsRNA mimic, poly I:C, when it is provided extracellularly.[60,92] However, evidence supporting TLR3-mediated recognition of authentic viral replication intermediates remains elusive, possibly due to overlapping recognition pathways that can compensate for the loss of TLR3. TLR3 may be involved in recognizing virus-produced dsRNA in the context of phagocytized apoptotic cells.[159] Humans with dominant negative mutations in the *tlr3* gene suffer from neonatal herpes infection,[202] indicating the importance of this receptor in protection against HSV-1 in the CNS.

TLR7/8

In humans, TLR7 is expressed in plasmacytoid DCs and B cells, while TLR8 is expressed by myeloid DCs and monocytes. In mice, TLR7 is expressed by pDCs, conventional DCs (except for CD8α^+ DCs), and B cells. The function of the mouse TLR8 is still poorly understood. However TLR8-deficient mice develop autoimmunity due to hyperstimulation of TLR7.[39] TLR7, 8, and 9 are all expressed in the endosomes and share similar signaling pathways. Upon engagement, these receptors recruit MyD88 via the TIR domain. MyD88 subsequently interacts with the death domain of several IRAK proteins to induce both NF-κB and IRF7 activation. IRAK4 is required for activation of NF-κB pathway by interacting with TRAF6, which in turn activates the TAK1 complex, leading to activation of NF-κB and MAPK pathways (Fig. 8.5). NF-κB activation follows the recruitment of IRF5 to the MyD88 complex. On the other hand, MyD88 also recruits IRF7, which forms a signaling complex with IRAK4 and TRAF6. TRAF3 also binds MyD88 and IRAK1 to induce IRF7 activation. Unlike TLR3, TLR7 and 9 utilize IRF7 and not IRF3 for activation of type I IFN genes in pDCs. Interestingly, in conventional DCs, TLR7 and 9 utilize MyD88 and IRF1 to induce IFN-β but not IFN-α genes.[143]

TLR7 and 8 recognize ssRNA and induce innate immune responses to ssRNA viruses. TLR7 is required for type I IFN and cytokine responses to influenza, SeV, and VSV.[44,117] Uridine and ribose, the defining signatures of RNA, are both necessary and sufficient for TLR7 stimulation.[45] Furthermore, viral fusion and/or uncoating and endosomal acidification are required for TLR7-dependent recognition.[117] Viral RNA, synthetic poly U RNA, and even nonviral, cellular RNA in the endosome is sufficient to stimulate TLR7-dependent cytokine production,[44,68] indicating that any RNA localized to the endosome is able to trigger TLR7 activation. While influenza virus is recognized upon endocytosis by TLR7, other viruses such as VSV and SeV require replication in the cytosol prior to recondition by TLR7. The latter type of viruses are recognized by TLR7 in the endosome upon delivery of cytosolic viral replication intermediates through the process of autophagy[106] (see below).

TLR9

TLR9 is expressed in pDCs and B cells in humans. Mice express TLR9 in pDCs, B cells, macrophages, and conventional DCs. TLR9 is located in the endosome and mediates recognition of viral DNA. Originally, bacterial DNA sequences containing hypomethylated CpG motifs were shown to activate TLR9.[69] More recent studies showed that TLR9 might recognize the sugar-base-backbone, 2-deoxyribose, of phosphodiester DNA irrespective of the CpG content.[61] TLR9 is the principal means by which HSV-1 and HSV-2 stimulate type I IFNs in pDCs *in vivo.*[100,116] Interestingly, a TLR9 molecule "retargeted" to the plasma membrane, unable to respond to viral nucleic acids, however now responded to self DNA that did not stimulate wild-type TLR9.[15] These results suggest that not only is endosomal localization important to trigger TLR-viral nucleic acid interactions, but that endosomal TLRs may limit access to nonviral nucleic acids via an active sequestering mechanism in the endosome.

C-Type Lectins

In addition to TLRs, C-type lectin receptors (CLRs) expressed on the plasma membrane can bind to certain viruses. Classical CLRs contain carbohydrate recognition domain responsible for the Ca2$^+$-dependent binding to their ligands. However, carbohydrate-recognition domains of many CLRs do not bind to Ca2$^+$.[8] CLRs can be classified into those that are used solely for endocytosis of pathogens and those that are used for inducing signaling. The endocytic CLRs include mannose receptor DEC205 and Langerin, which are expressed on CD8α^+ DCs and Langerhans cells, respectively. Langerin on Langerhans cells are capable of clearing HIV by receptor-mediated endocytosis and degradation in Birbeck granules.[37]

The signaling CLRs include Dectin-1 and DC-SIGN.[40] Dectin-1, which is a receptor for fungal β-glucans, contains an ITAM motif in the cytosolic domain, and engages Syk tyrosine kinase and CARD9, leading to NF-kB activation.[95] Dectin-1 plays an important role in antifungal defense, but it is not known to have antiviral functions. DC-SIGN binds to HIV-1 and Ebola virus. Signaling through DC-SIGN alone does not lead to the activation of NF-κB or expression of cytokines, but can modulate signaling through other PRRs. DC-SIGN engagement by viruses leads to serine/threonine kinase Raf-1 activation. After translocation of NF-κB by TLR-stimulation, DC-SIGN-activated Raf-1 mediates the phosphorylation of NF-κB subunit p65, which in turn leads to p65-acetylation. Acetylation of p65 both prolongs and increases IL-10 transcription, resulting in increased IL-10 production. However, the majority of C-type lectin–virus interactions reflect a viral invasion mechanism. A clear example of this is DC-SIGN signaling by HIV-1. This interaction results in impaired DC maturation, enhanced T-cell proliferation and transmission of HIV-1 to T cells, thereby promoting systemic infection of the host. DC-SIGN and a related C-type lectin, DC-SIGNR, also enhance infection by Ebola virus.[13] Another example is Dengue virus, which binds to CLEC5A and induces signaling through DAP12 to induce proinflammatory cytokines. This leads to lethality, not protection, in mice.[29]

Other Strategies of Viral Recognition

In addition to PRR-based viral recognition, non-PRR-based, cell-autonomous virus sensing mechanisms exist in mammalian hosts. While molecular mechanisms for such pathways are not yet understood, these pathways likely involve sensing various forms of cellular stresses inflicted by virus infection. One of the hallmarks of virus infection is the production of large amounts of viral proteins. This often leads to ER overload, leading to ER stress and unfolded protein response (UPR) induction. Virus infection also often leads to the generation of reactive oxygen species (ROS) by interfering with proper mitochondrial function. In addition, as discussed below, most viruses express molecules that inhibit vital cellular functions such as transcription, translation and secretion. These types of stress that accompany virus infections might be seen by the mammalian host as a signature of virus infection. In conjunction with pattern recognition, such stress sensing pathways can engage signals leading to type I IFNs synthesis, cell-cycle arrest or cell death to avoid further viral replication and spread.

INNATE ANTIVIRAL CYTOKINES

Type I Interferons

Antiviral mechanisms in vertebrates are highly dependent on the action of type I IFNs. Type I IFNs are a family of cytokines that act early in the innate immune response and are key cytokines capable of inducing an antiviral state in infected and uninfected neighboring cells.[80] In addition to this antiviral activity, the interferon cytokines have a role in regulating the ensuing adaptive immune response.[171] While type II and type III IFNs also have antiviral activities, in this chapter we will focus on the role of type I IFNs in innate antiviral defense. In humans, the type I IFNs consist of 13 α-genes coding for 12 IFN-α subtypes, one β-gene encoding a single IFN-β subtype and a single gene encoding IFN-ω. Type I IFNs bind to IFN-$\alpha\beta$R, which is a heterodimer of IFN-αR1 and IFN-αR2 chains. High levels of IFN-α subtypes are rapidly secreted from pDCs upon viral recognition, whereas IFN-β can be induced from most virus-infected cell types.

Type I IFN Induction

As described in detail above, stimulation of various PRRs including TLRs (TLR3, 4, 7, 8, and 9), RLRs (RIG-I, MDA-5), and cytosolic DNA sensor(s) leads to the production of type I IFNs. Most virally infected cells trigger the cell intrinsic pathway of type I IFN production through activation of RLRs or DNA sensors. In contrast, pDCs recognize viral genomes within the endosome via TLR7 or TLR9 and induce robust secretion of IFN-α and IFN-β. pDCs are thought to express high constitutive levels of IRF7 and are the only cells capable of coupling TLRs to IRF7 directly, thereby leading to rapid and robust transcription of type I IFN genes.

Amplification of IFN Production by IRF7

In the cytosol of most cells, IRF3 is constitutively expressed while very low levels of IRF7 are found.[71] While *IFN-α* genes contain ISREs, the *IFN-β* gene also contains binding sites for NF-κB and activator protein 1 (AP1). IRF3 is a potent activator of the *IFN-β* and *IFN-α4* gene but not the *IFN-α* genes, whereas IRF7 efficiently activates both *IFN-α* and *IFN-β* genes. Thus, upon activation of RLRs or TLR3, IFN-β and IFN-α4 production is immediately triggered by the IRF3 homodimer binding to the promoter regions of these genes, while the production of other members of IFN-α occurs at a later time point upon IFN-$\alpha\beta$R-induced production of IRF7. In addition, IFN-$\alpha\beta$R signaling increases PRR expression (TLRs and RLRs), leading to further amplification of antiviral signaling pathways.

IFN-$\alpha\beta$R Signaling

The IFN-$\alpha\beta$R utilizes the so-called JAK-STAT signaling pathway, which is used by many other cytokine receptors. This pathway consists of a receptor, JAK family tyrosine kinases (JAK1, JAK2, JAK3, and Tyk2), and transcription factors (STAT1–6). The receptor complex typically consists of two or three distinct polypeptides that contain in their cytoplasmic domain binding sites for different combinations of JAK and STAT proteins. Upon receptor engagement by its ligand, the receptor complex is assembled, resulting in activation of JAK kinases with subsequent tyrosine phosphorylation of STAT proteins, leading to their dimerization, nuclear translocation, and activation of target genes (Fig. 8.6).

Thus, upon engagement of Type I IFN receptor complex IFN-αR1 and IFN-αR2 by IFN-α, IFN-β or IFN-ω, these receptor subunits dimerize, resulting in phosphorylation of Tyk2, which is associated with the IFN-αR1, by Janus kinase (JAK) 2. Activated Tyk2 subsequently phosphorylates JAK1, which is coupled to the IFN-αR2 chain. Signal transducer and activator of transcription (STAT) 1 and 2 are prebound to the IFN-αR2 chain. Activated JAK1 binds to STAT2 and phosphorylates it, creating a binding site for STAT1, causing their dimerization and transport to the nucleus. The STAT1–2 heterodimer forms a transcription complex, ISGF3, with IRF9 to facilitate transcription of ISGs by binding to the sequence motif called interferon simulated response element (ISRE). In addition, STAT1 homodimers bind to the IFN-γ-activated site (GAS) sequence motif and induce a different set of ISGs (Fig. 8.6).

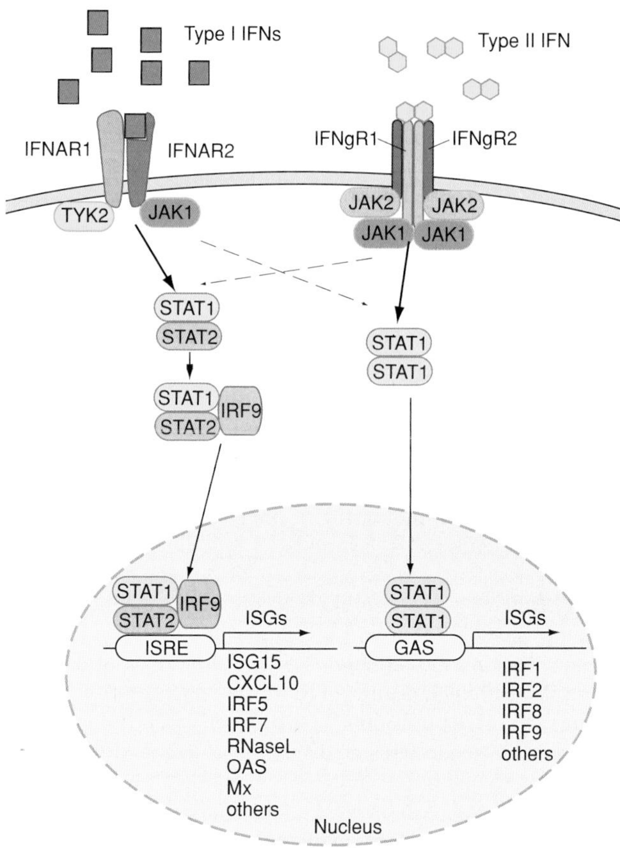

FIGURE 8.6. Type I and type II IFN receptor signaling. Type I and type II IFN receptors consist of IFNAR1 + IFNAR2, and IFNgR1 + IFNgR2, respectively. Engagement of the receptors by cognate cytokines induces activation of prebound kinases (Tyk2 and JAK), leading to phosphorylation of STAT proteins. Phosphorylated STAT molecules form dimers, which translocate into the nucleus to initiate transcription of genes. STAT1/STAT2 dimers recruit IRF9, forming ISGF3, which binds to ISRE sequence found in the promoter of many ISGs. STAT1 homodimer binds to the GAS sequence on different sets of ISGs and induces their transcription.

Inflammatory Cytokines

In addition to type I IFNs, many inflammatory cytokines play an important role in antiviral defense, by directly inducing antiviral effector molecules or indirectly by stimulating cellular recruitment, phagocytosis of infected cells, and activating adaptive immune responses such as cytotoxic T lymphocytes and neutralizing antibodies. Cytokines can act locally through autocrine and paracrine mechanisms or, if produced at high enough levels, they can gain access to the circulation and induce systemic effects, such as acute-phase response or fever. The major inflammatory cytokines IL-6, IL-1β, and TNF are produced by virally infected DCs and macrophages, and act systemically with a wide spectrum of biological activities that help to coordinate the body's response to infections. These cytokines are responsible for causing fever by inducing prostaglandin E2, which acts on the hypothalamus, causing increased heat production from brown fat and by inducing vasoconstriction to prevent heat loss through the skin. Fever is thought to be generally beneficial to host defense, because some pathogens may replicate less efficiently at high temperatures. However, the role of fever in host defense is still incompletely understood. IL-6, IL-1β, and TNF also stimulate the acute-phase response in the liver. Acute-phase proteins secreted by hepatocytes can have direct antiviral effects, for example, by promoting their killing by complement or phagocytes. Finally, IL-6, IL-1β, and TNF induce leukocytosis, leading to an increase in circulating neutrophils, which are phagocytes that help to clear virally infected cells.

Interleukin 6

IL-6R belongs to the hemopoietin family of receptors, which are tyrosine kinase–associated receptors that form dimers upon binding their cytokine ligand. IL-6R consists of IL-6Rα and gp130 chains. IL-6 bound to the IL-6Rα chain causes the association of the complex with gp130, resulting in the activation of Jak1, Jak2 and Tyk2, followed by the phosphorylation of Stat3. Phospho-Stat3 dimerizes and translocates into the nucleus, where it activates transcription of target genes. IL-6 is a pleiotropic cytokine with a wide range of biological activities in immune regulation, hematopoiesis, inflammation, and oncogenesis.[96] IL-6 is induced by a variety of signals including TLR, NLR, and RLR signaling, and is a key cytokine that triggers the acute-phase response, as well as activation of T cells and antibody-producing plasma cells.

Interleukin 1-β and Interleukin-18

As described above, secretion of IL-1β and IL-18 requires the activation of inflammasomes. Both IL-1R and IL-18R are heterodimers of a ligand-binding α chain and a coreceptor accessory protein (AcP). Both chains contain a TIR domain in the cytoplasmic tail. As such, these receptors recruit MyD88 and induce NF-κB signaling (Fig. 8.7). IL-1β through binding to IL-1R induces the expression of hundreds of genes, including cytokines (IL-6 and TNF-α), chemokines (e.g., IL-8), and adhesion molecules that are important for leukocyte trafficking.[46] In adaptive antiviral immunity, IL-1β plays an important role in the antigen-driven expansion and differentiation of CD4 T cells.[16] While IL-1R is widely expressed by many cell types, IL-1β is mainly produced by the sentinel cells of the innate immune system, including macrophages and DCs, although fibroblasts and keratinocytes can also synthesize this cytokine in response to tissue injury or stress signals.[46,168] On the other hand, IL-18, which is expressed mainly by macrophages and DCs, work alone or in combination with IL-15 prime NK cells for the production of IFN-γ and enhance their cytolytic activity.[55,76,178] IL-18 in combination with IL-12 or IL-2 alone can also induce differentiation of either Th1 or Th2 cell types depending on the cytokine milieu.[75,136] IL-18 is also required for optimal cytokine production by CTLs, including IFN-γ, TNF-α, and IL-2.[41]

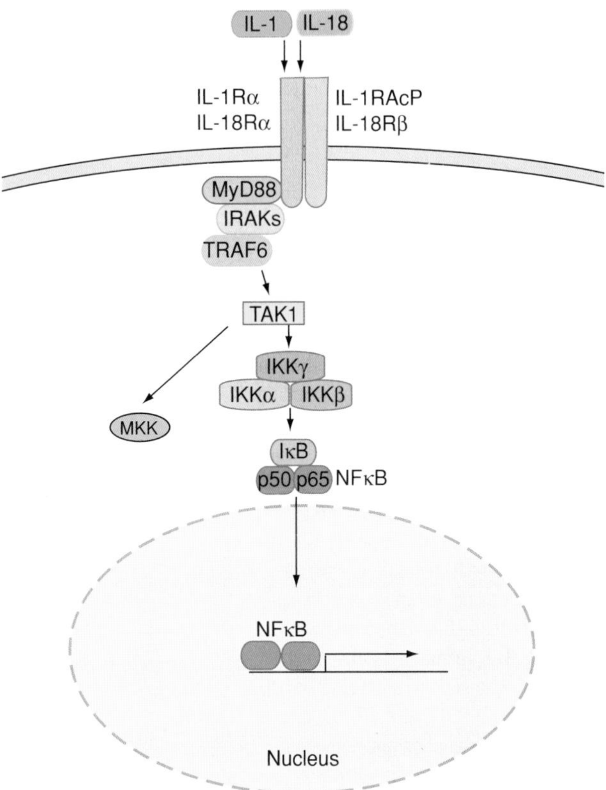

FIGURE 8.7. IL-1R and IL-18R signaling. IL-1R consists of the IL-1Rα and IL-1RAcP chains, while IL-18R consists of the IL-18Rα and IL-18Rβ chains. Each chain contains a TIR domain in the cytoplasmic region and, upon receptor engagement by IL-1 or IL-18, recruits MyD88 and induces signaling, resulting in NF-κB and MAPK activation.

IL-1β plays an integral role in antiviral immunity against influenza A virus infection. IL-1R$^{-/-}$ mice infected with influenza virus have impaired leukocyte recruitment to the lung, diminished CD4 and CD8 T cell responses, impaired immunoglobulin responses, and succumb to virus-induced fatality.[78,158] On the other hand, mice deficient in IL-18 were found to have a transient increase in viral titer due to defective NK cytotoxicity after influenza A virus infection but otherwise had normal adaptive immunity to influenza infection.[110]

Tumor Necrosis Factor (TNF)

TNFR belongs to a group of receptors known as TNFR family, characterized by a cysteine-rich common extracellular binding domain. Upon engagement of the ligand TNF, TNFR forms a trimer (Fig. 8.8). TNFRI contains a cytoplasmic death domain, which recruits the adaptor TRADD through its death domain. TRADD can assemble two different signaling complexes, involving FADD pro-caspase 8 or RIP1 and TRAF2. RIP1 activates IKK, resulting in the activation of NF-κB, while TRAF2 stimulates the JNK signaling pathway. Similar to IL-1 and IL-6, TNF is involved in induction of a stereotypic inflammatory response that promotes host defense from a broad range of pathogens, including viruses. Recent studies revealed an additional pathway activated by TNFR—the induction of cell necrosis via the protein kinase RIP3. This TNF-induced necrosis was shown to be important for immune defense against vaccinia virus and CMV.[31,187]

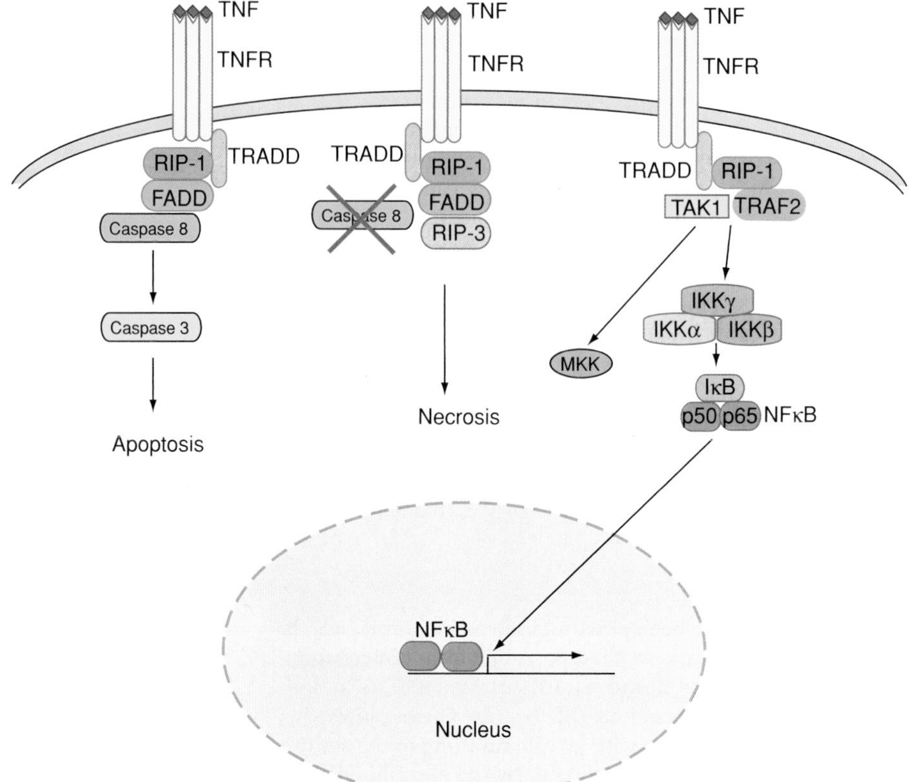

FIGURE 8.8. TNFR signaling leads to three distinct cell fates. TNF binding trimerizes the TNFR. Through the cytoplasmic death domain, TNFR recruits TRADD, which also contains a DD. TRADD can assemble different signaling complexes. TRADD can recruit FADD through DD–DD interaction, which results in caspase-8 activation, leading to apoptosis. In cells in which caspase-8 is rendered nonfunctional, RIP-3 is recruited to the complex to induce necrosis. In addition, TRADD can also recruit RIP-1 and TRAF2, resulting in signal transduction and activation of NF-κB and MAP kinase pathways.

Interleukin 15

IL-15 is produced by DCs and macrophages upon viral infection. IL-15R is a trimer of the IL-15Rα chain, which is specific to IL-15, and β, and the common γ chains that are shared with IL-2 and other cytokines. An unusual feature of IL-15R complex is that the IL-15Rα chain is expressed on the cells that produce IL-15, rather than on the target cell that responds to IL-15. IL-15 forms a complex with the IL-15Rα chain in the ER and the two proteins are transported to the cell surface, where they remain associated and function as a ligand for the IL-15Rβ and the common γ chains expressed on target cells. IL-15R induces activation of STAT5, resulting in expression of anti-apoptotic and growth-promoting genes in target cells.[120] The main target-cell types of IL-15 are cytotoxic lymphocytes: IL-15 is an important growth and survival factor for CD8 T cells, NK cells, and a subset of NKT cells. Importantly, IL-15 can function downstream of type I IFNs in antiviral immune responses.[133]

Interferon γ

IFN-γ is secreted mainly by three lymphocyte types, NK cells (during early phase of viral infection), CD8 T cells, and Th1 cells (after induction of adaptive immunity). IFN-γR, like IFN-$\alpha\beta$R, belongs to the type II cytokine receptor family (Fig. 8.6). IFN-γR is expressed by most cells, and consists of two subunits: IFN-γR1, the ligand-binding chain, and IFN-γR2, the signal-transducing chain. As the ligand-binding IFN-γR1 chains interact with IFN-γ, they dimerize and become associated with two signal-transducing IFN-γR2 chains. Receptor assembly leads to activation of the JAK1 and JAK2 and phosphorylation of a tyrosine residue on the intracellular domain of IFN-γR1. This leads to the recruitment and phosphorylation of STAT1, which forms homodimers and translocates to the nucleus to bind to GAS elements, activating a wide range of IFN-γ–responsive genes. IFN-γ has a potent antiviral function, by inducing transcription of genes encoding antiviral effectors such as PKR and viperin. Note that some antiviral effectors are induced only by type I IFNs and not by IFN-γ, including 2′5′OAS, Mx1, Mx2, and RNaseL.[42] Instead, IFN-γR signaling induces activation of genes involved in antigen processing and presentation, facilitating the activation of virus-specific T cells.

CELL-AUTONOMOUS ANTIVIRAL DEFENSE MECHANISMS

Type I IFN-Dependent Antiviral Defense

IFN-$\alpha\beta$R signaling leads to the expression of over 300 ISGs. Although the functions of majority of these genes are currently unknown, they are all thought to participate in antiviral defense. The effect of IFN-$\alpha\beta$R signaling is different in infected and noninfected cells. In infected cells IFN-$\alpha\beta$ signals in an autocrine fashion to induce ISGs involved in cell autonomous antiviral defenses. These ISG encode proteins that interfere with multiple steps of viral infection cycles. In specialized noninfected cells, such as APCs and cytotoxic lymphocytes, IFN-$\alpha\beta$ promotes antigen processing and presentation, along with cytotoxic activity of NK cells and CD8 T cells. In addition, IFN-$\alpha\beta$ signals in a paracrine fashion to induce an antiviral state in neighboring cells, thereby minimizing the spread of viral infection. Only a handful of ISGs that have direct antiviral effects have been characterized in detail. Their functions are described below.

2′-5′ Oligoadenylate Synthetase (OAS) and Ribonuclease L (RNase L)

OAS and RNase L act in concert to degrade viral RNA in the cytosol. While basal levels of OAS and RNase L are found constitutively, stimulation through IFN-$\alpha\beta$R dramatically increases their expression levels. Activated by dsRNA, (2′-5′) OAS converts ATP into 2′-5′ oligoadenylate, which functions as a second messenger to activate latent ribonuclease RNase L. Activated RNase L degrades viral and cellular ssRNAs, inhibiting protein synthesis and viral growth (Fig. 8.9). Mice deficient in RNase L suffer from increased susceptibility to RNA viruses including Picornaviridae, Reoviridae, Togaviridae, Paramyxoviridae, Orthomyxoviridae, Flaviviridae, and Retroviridae families.[167] However, the roles of OAS and RNase L pathway in defense against DNA viruses remain less clear. Interestingly, the cleavage products of RNase L can serve as ligands for RIG-I and MDA5, leading to amplification of the RLR pathway.[121]

Protein Kinase R (PKR)

PKR is a serine/threonine kinase that phosphorylates the α-subunit of eukaryotic translation initiation factor 2 α (eIF2α). PKR becomes activated through homodimerization upon binding to viral dsRNA structures via its dsRNA binding domains. This results in inhibition of translation and a decrease in total cellular and viral protein synthesis, effectively reducing viral production. In addition to its translational regulatory function, PKR has a role in signal transduction and transcriptional control through the IκB/NF-κB pathway.[102] PKR can also mediate apoptosis, cell-growth arrest, and autophagy, all of which curb viral replication and spread in the host.[151] In addition to the virus-restricting function of PKR, recent studies indicate that PKR functions to stabilize IFN-α and IFN-β mRNA, thereby ensuring robust IFN protein production.[160] Mice genetically deficient in PKR are susceptible to infection with viruses including rhabdovirus, orthomyxovirus, and orthobunyavirus.

Orthomyxovirus Resistance Gene (Mx) Proteins

Mx proteins belong to a family of GTPases consisting of MxA and MxB in humans and Mx1 and Mx2 in mice.[63] The Mx

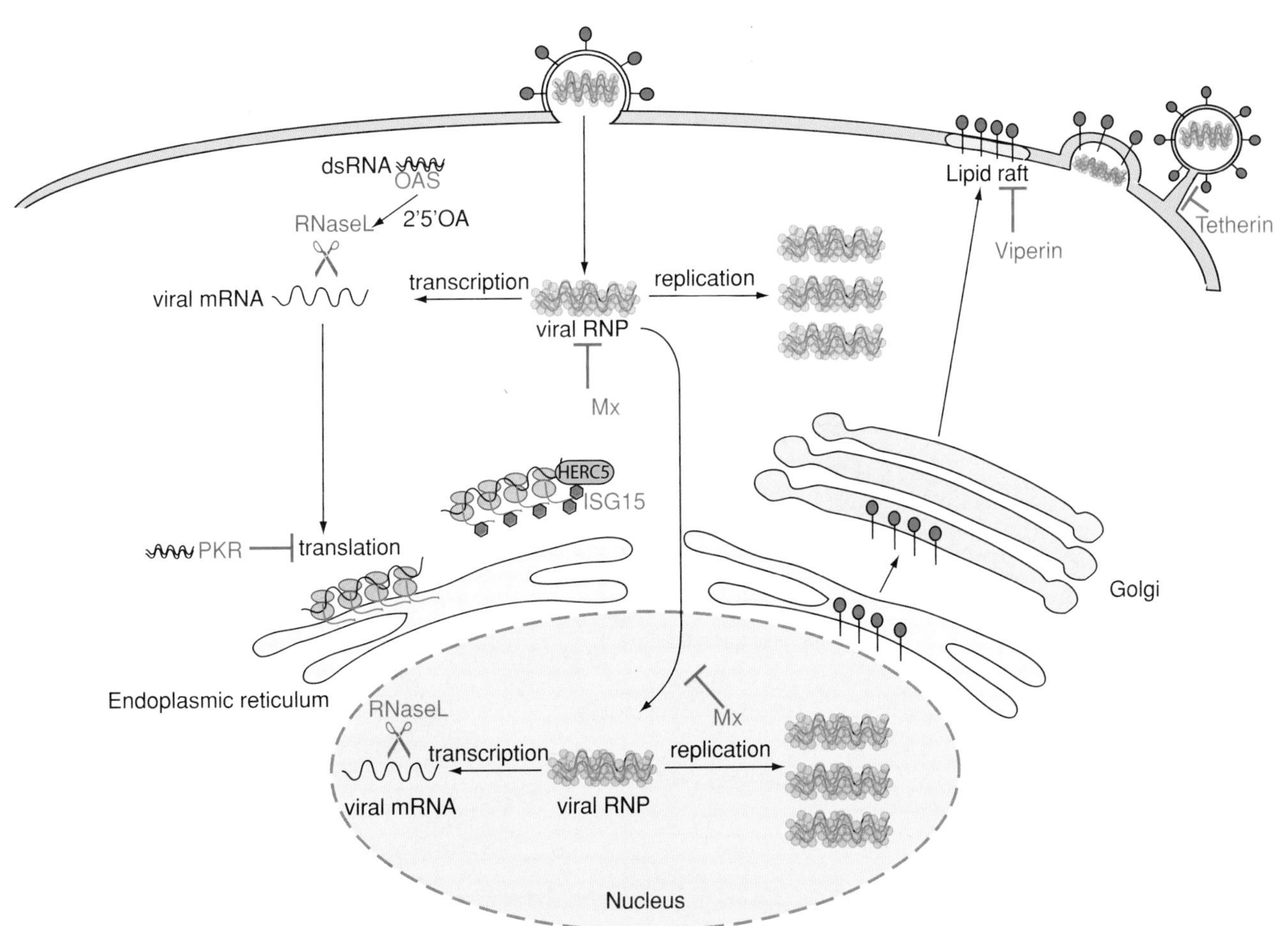

FIGURE 8.9. Type I IFN–induced antiviral mechanisms. Type I IFNs induce over 300 genes, many of which are antiviral effectors. When an IFN-stimulated cell encounters a virus, viral dsRNA activates OAS and PKR. OAS produces 2′5′ oligoadenylate from ATP, which activates a latent ribonuclease RNaseL. RNaseL can cleave viral mRNA (as well as host mRNA). PKR activated by dsRNA inhibits translation, thereby impairing viral protein synthesis. Mx gene products trap viral RNP in the cytosol and prevent its nuclear import. ISG15 modifies newly synthesized proteins (most of these are viral proteins) by forming a complex with HERC5. Viperin impairs viral budding by disrupting lipid rafts. Tetherin inhibits viral particle release.

proteins have a large N-terminal GTPase domain, a central interacting domain (CID) and a C-terminal leucine zipper (LZ) domain. Both the CID and LZ domains are required to recognize target viral structures. Viruses targeted by Mx proteins include orthomyxomaviruses, paramyxomaviruses, rhabdoviruses, togaviruses, and bunyaviruses. Remarkably, transgenic expression of human MxA in IFN-$\alpha\beta$R–deficient mice confers full resistance to otherwise fatal infection with Thogoto virus, influenza virus, VSV, LaCrosse virus or, Semliki Forest virus,[67,142] indicating that this effector molecule is sufficient for protective innate defense against these viruses. The main viral targets seems to be the viral nucleocapsid-like structures.[97] Mx proteins are thought to survey exocytic events and mediate vesicle trafficking to trap essential viral components. It is interesting to note that most inbred strains of mice harbor defective Mx1 gene.[63] Therefore, studies using inbred mice must be interpreted with the caveat that they are Mx-1 deficient.

ISG15

ISG15 is an ubiquitin-like molecule that can be covalently attached to target proteins using E1-, E2-, and E3-like enzymes. UBE1L (E1-like ubiquitin-activating enzyme) was shown to be the specific ISG15-activating enzyme.[147] Two E2 ubiquitin-conjugating enzymes, UBCH6 and UBCH8, serve as ISG15 carriers. Subsequently, two E3 ubiquitin ligases—HERC5 (homologous to the E6-associated protein C terminus (HECT) domain and RCC1-like domain containing protein 5) and TRIM25—conjugate ISG15 to protein substrates. All enzymes identified in the ISGylation pathway are coordinately induced by type I IFNs. There are over 150 targets of ISGylation: RIG-I and STAT1, as well as several IFN-induced antiviral effector proteins. Interestingly, by physically associating with polyribosomes, HERC5 ensures that ISG15 conjugation is restricted to the newly synthesized pool of proteins, which in infected cells will consist primarily of newly translated viral proteins.[49] Further, ISGylation of a small percentage of human papillomavirus (HPV) L1 capsid protein has a dominant inhibitory effect on the infectivity of HPV16 pseudoviruses. Given that acute viral replication in general requires a vast amount of *de novo* protein synthesis, ISG15 modification of newly synthesized viral protein might be a powerful virus restriction mechanism that can be broadly applicable to many viruses.

Tetherin and Viperin

Tetherin (also known as BST-2, PDCA-1, and CD317) is a GPI-anchored protein that is highly expressed upon type I IFN stimulation. Tetherin associates with lipid rafts and inhibits retrovirus particle release in the absence of Vpu.[132] Vpu utilizes the beta-TrCP E3 ubiquitin ligase complex to induce endosomal trafficking events that remove tetherin from the cell surface, rendering it incapable of restricting the release of enveloped viruses.[128] Thus far, tetherin has been implicated in restricting the release of members of the retrovirus, filovirus, and arenavirus families. Viperin (*v*irus *i*nhibitory *p*rotein, *e*ndoplasmic *r*eticulum-associated, *in*terferon inducible) is another IFN-inducible protein that is known to prevent replication of a variety of viruses including HCMV, influenza virus, hepatitis C virus (HCV), dengue virus, alphaviruses, and HIV-1.[54] Viperin impairs the release of influenza virus by disrupting lipid rafts via suppression of the activity of farnesyl diphosphate synthase,

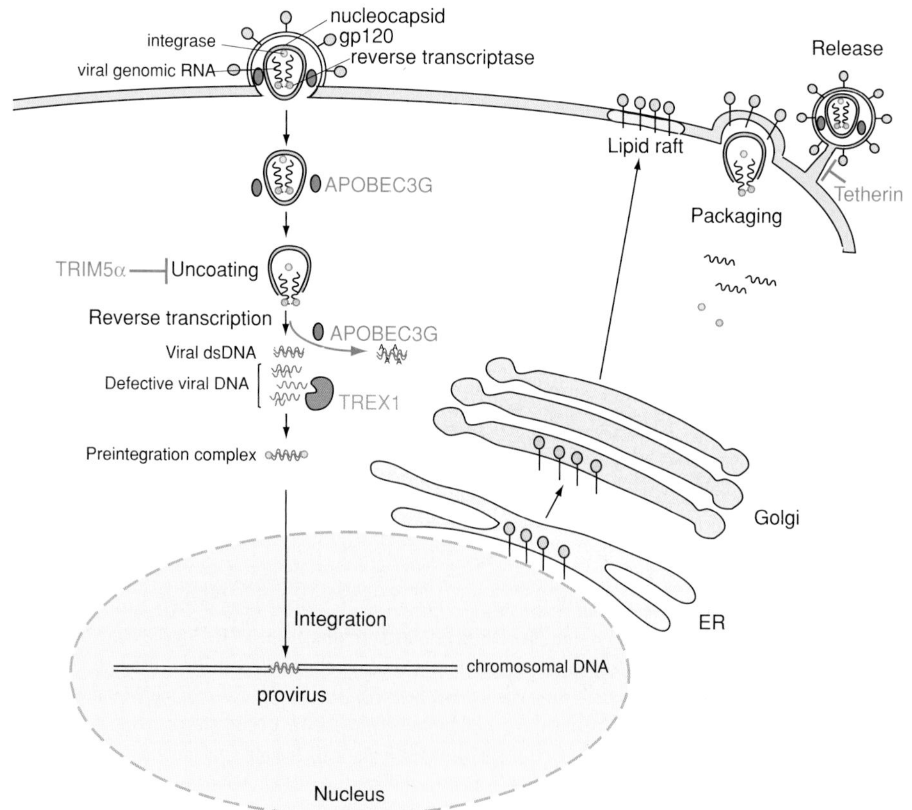

FIGURE 8.10. Innate restriction of retroviruses. TRIM5α perturbs the controlled uncoating of the subviral particle prior to reverse transcription. APOBEC3G deaminates cytosine residues in nascent retroviral cDNA, causing C/G to T/A hypermutation and degradation of viral cDNA. Tetherin inhibits retroviral particle release. In contrast, TREX1, an exonuclease, inhibits innate immune detection of HIV DNA by degrading nonproductive RT products.

a key enzyme in isoprenoid biosynthesis[191] (Fig. 8.9). In addition, viperin localizes to the lipid droplets[54] and through a yet undefined pathway interferes with replication of other viruses that do not require lipid rafts for synthesis.

Retroviral Restriction Factors

In addition to the IFN-inducible antiviral molecules described above, cells are equipped with "host restriction" factors that are constitutively expressed in some cell types and are induced by IFNs in others.[18] The host restriction factors that specifically counter retrovirus infections are described below.

TRIM5α

Members of the tripartite motif (TRIM) protein family are involved in various cellular processes, including cell proliferation, differentiation, development, oncogenesis, and apoptosis.[134] There are 66 known members of TRIM proteins in humans, characterized by the presence of RING, B-box, and coiled-coil domains. Many of the TRIM proteins display antiviral properties, particularly against retrovirus entry and release.[184] TRIM5α has been extensively studied as a key factor responsible for antiretroviral activities. TRIM5α is thought to perturb the controlled uncoating of the subviral particle prior to reverse transcription by recognizing and degrading the capsid protein of retroviruses, resulting in a block of viral replication (Fig. 8.10). Interestingly, TRIM5α from Old World monkeys confers potent resistance to HIV-1, but not SIV, while the human ortholog of TRIM5a is unable to specifically target HIV. Strikingly, the differential ability of human and monkey TRIM5α to restrict HIV hinges on a single amino acid, R332 (human) vs. P332 (monkey).[109] It is likely that HIV and SIV have evolved in their natural hosts to evade interaction with TRIM5α.

APOBEC Family

APOBEC (apolipoprotein BmRNA-editing catalytic polypeptide) proteins are a group of cytidine deaminases. Members of the APOBEC family contain either one or two catalytic deaminase domains. APOBEC is constitutively expressed in various cell types but its expression can be enhanced by type I and type II IFNs. APOBEC3G becomes encapsidated into retroviral virions in infected cells. Upon viral fusion and entry into the new host cell, APOBEC3G deaminates cytosine residues in nascent retroviral cDNA[65] (Fig. 8.10). The resulting uracil residues function as a template for the incorporation of adenine, which, in turn, can result in strand-specific C/G to T/A transition mutations that affect virus viability. The antiviral activity of APOBEC3G is strongly inhibited by HIV-1 Vif protein, allowing the virus to replicate virtually unimpaired in APOBEC3G-expressing host cells. Vif induces the ubiquitin-dependent degradation of some of the APOBEC proteins. However, Vif is also able to prevent encapsidation of APOBEC3G and APOBEC3F through degradation-independent mechanisms.

Type I IFN-Independent Antiviral Defense

Type I IFN-dependent antiviral mechanisms are only known to exist in vertebrates. Other animals rely on more ancient forms of antiviral defenses, including RNA interference and autophagy.

RNA Interference

RNAi was first identified as a potent antiviral defense mechanism in plants, then subsequently in fungi, nematodes, and insects.[108] The mechanism of RNAi involves two steps (Fig. 8.11). First, viral dsRNA is recognized by members of the Dicer endonuclease family, which processes it into siRNA. Second, these siRNA are incorporated into RNA-induced silencing complex (RISC), which guides the RNase enzyme AGO to complementary sequences in viral RNA for cleavage and degradation. In plants and nematodes, but not in insects, this antiviral response is further amplified through a secondary wave of siRNAs generated by RNA-dependent RNA polymerases (RdRPs), which greatly increases the pool of siRNAs available to RISC. To combat antiviral RNAi responses, many plant and invertebrate viruses have evolved to encode proteins that act as suppressors of RNA silencing. Interestingly, in addition to generating RNAi, Dicer-2 was shown to trigger a signaling pathway, resulting in the expression of antiviral genes in *Drosophila*. The latter function requires the helicase domain of Dicer-2, and given its phylogenic relation to RIG-I, suggests a parallel role of Dicer-2 to mammalian RIG-I in the induction of antiviral genes.[38] In mammalian cells, RNAi has not been found in virally infected cells. Further, mammalian cells lack the RdRPs to amplify the siRNA and fail to mount a systemic antiviral RNAi response. Therefore, with the evolution of the potent type I IFN system, the RNAi mechanism may have become obsolete for antiviral defense in mammals.

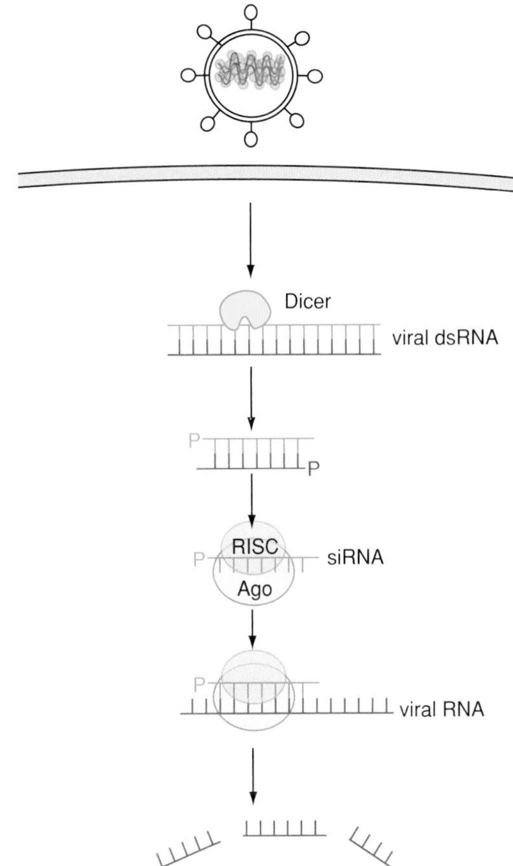

FIGURE 8.11. RNA interference is an ancient antiviral defense mechanism. In plants and invertebrates, the RNAi pathway plays a major role in the recognition and destruction of viral RNA. Viral dsRNA is recognized by Dicer, which processes such RNA into short RNAi (~20 bp). The processed RNAi is incorporated into the RISC complex, which serves as the guide strand. The guide strand base pairs with a complementary sequence of a viral RNA molecule and induces its cleavage by AGO, the catalytic component of the RISC complex.

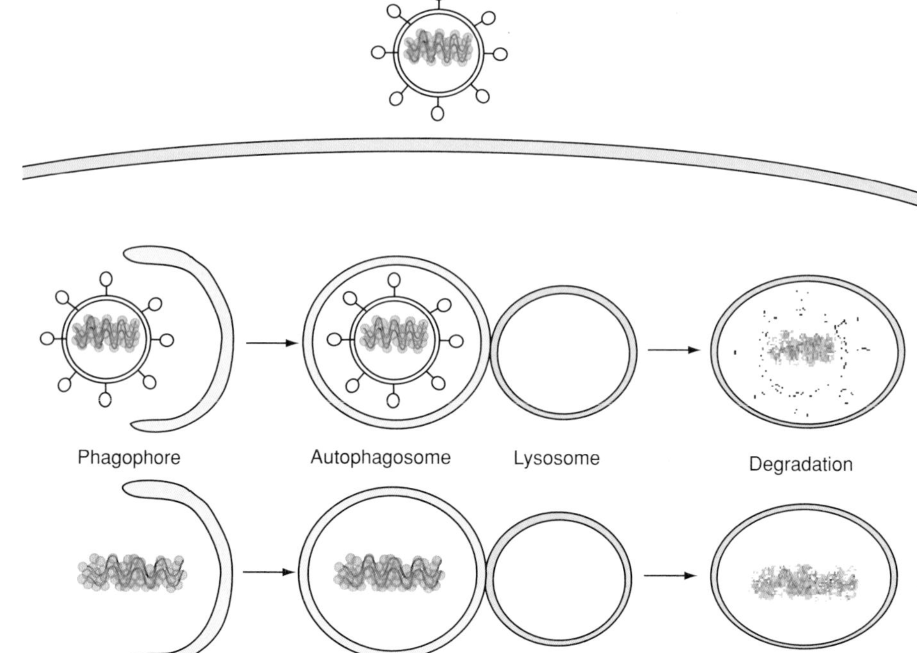

FIGURE 8.12. Autophagy as innate antiviral defense mechanism. From insects to humans, xenophagy is used to limit viral replication in the cytosol. A double membrane structure called a phagophore forms around the invading or replicating virus, engulfing either the virion or replication intermediate into autophagosomes. Contents are degraded when autophagosomes fuse with lysosomes.

Xenophagy

Autophagy is an ancient, highly conserved pathway responsible for the lysosomal degradation of cytosolic constituents and organelles that is critical in maintaining cellular homeostasis. Recent studies have illustrated an important interplay between autophagy and the innate immune system. Signaling through PRRs can lead to the induction of autophagy. Clearance of intracellular pathogens via autophagy followed by degradation in the lysosome is referred to as "xenophagy" and presents an important mechanism of antiviral defense.[107] Upon xenophagocytosis, virions or viral replication products in the cytosol are engulfed into autophagosomes and degraded in the lysosome for clearance (Fig. 8.12). This pathway of viral clearance was shown to be important in protection of *Drosophila* from VSV infection.[163] Intracranial HSV-1 infection of mice defective in autophagy results in uncontrolled virus replication and neuropathogenesis.[137] In addition to xenophagic removal of virions within the cytosol, autophagic clearance of viral proteins or other viral products plays a key role in protection of infected cells, particularly terminally differentiated cell types such as neurons.[138] Given that multiple human viruses—including HSV-1, HCMV, HIV-1, and gamma herpesviruses—have evolved evasion mechanisms to escape destruction by xenophagy,[43] this pathway likely plays an important role in viral sequestration and clearance of viruses in humans.

CELL TYPES INVOLVED IN INNATE ANTIVIRAL RESPONSES

NK Cells

NK cells are cytotoxic lymphocytes that play an important role in antiviral immunity. NK cells detect and eliminate virally infected cells and produce IFN-γ to induce other antiviral mechanisms. The importance of NK cells and antiviral immunity, particularly against Herpesviridae, is highlighted by the fact that an individual identified to have isolated NK deficiency with no other identifiable deficiency suffered from disseminated, life-threatening varicella infection, followed by cytomegalovirus (CMV) pneumonitis and cutaneous HSV infection.[19] A similar observation was reported for a 2 year old who died of recurrent severe varicella infections.[50]

NK cells express two classes of receptors, known as activating and inhibitory receptors. These receptors induce or inhibit the target cell lysis and IFN-γ production upon recognition of their cognate ligands on target cells (Fig. 8.13). The ligands for activating NK receptors are induced in virally infected cells. The ligands for NK inhibitory receptors are MHC class I molecules and other molecules constitutively expressed on most cells and downregulated upon viral infection. The ligands for inhibitory receptors can be downregulated either as a result of sensing the viral infection in the cell or, in the case of MHC-I, as a result of viral downregulation of MHC-I. Many DNA viruses encode molecules dedicated for evasion of MHC I processing and presentation of viral antigens in order to avoid recognition by CD8 T cells.[64] Through their ability to detect missing self (reduction in MHC class I molecules on the cell surface), NK cells fulfill the gap in immunosurveillance by CD8 T cells. Thus NK cell recognition of infected cells relies on both the sensing of "induced self" (by activating receptors) and the "missing self" (by inhibitory receptors)[146] (Fig. 8.13). The net effect of these changes is detected by NK cells. Only when positive signals dominate, NK cells induce apoptotic death of target cells by unleashing their cytotoxic granules.

NK receptors fall into two structurally distinct families. One group belongs to the killer inhibitory receptor (KIR) family of proteins, which contains immunoglobulin-like domains. Another group of receptors is known as killer lectin-like receptors (KLRs), and contains C-type lectin domains.[197] Both groups of receptors contain activating and inhibitory receptors. The signaling property is defined by the sequence motifs found in cytoplasmic tails of the receptors or their signaling adaptors. Activating receptors typically contain a short (few

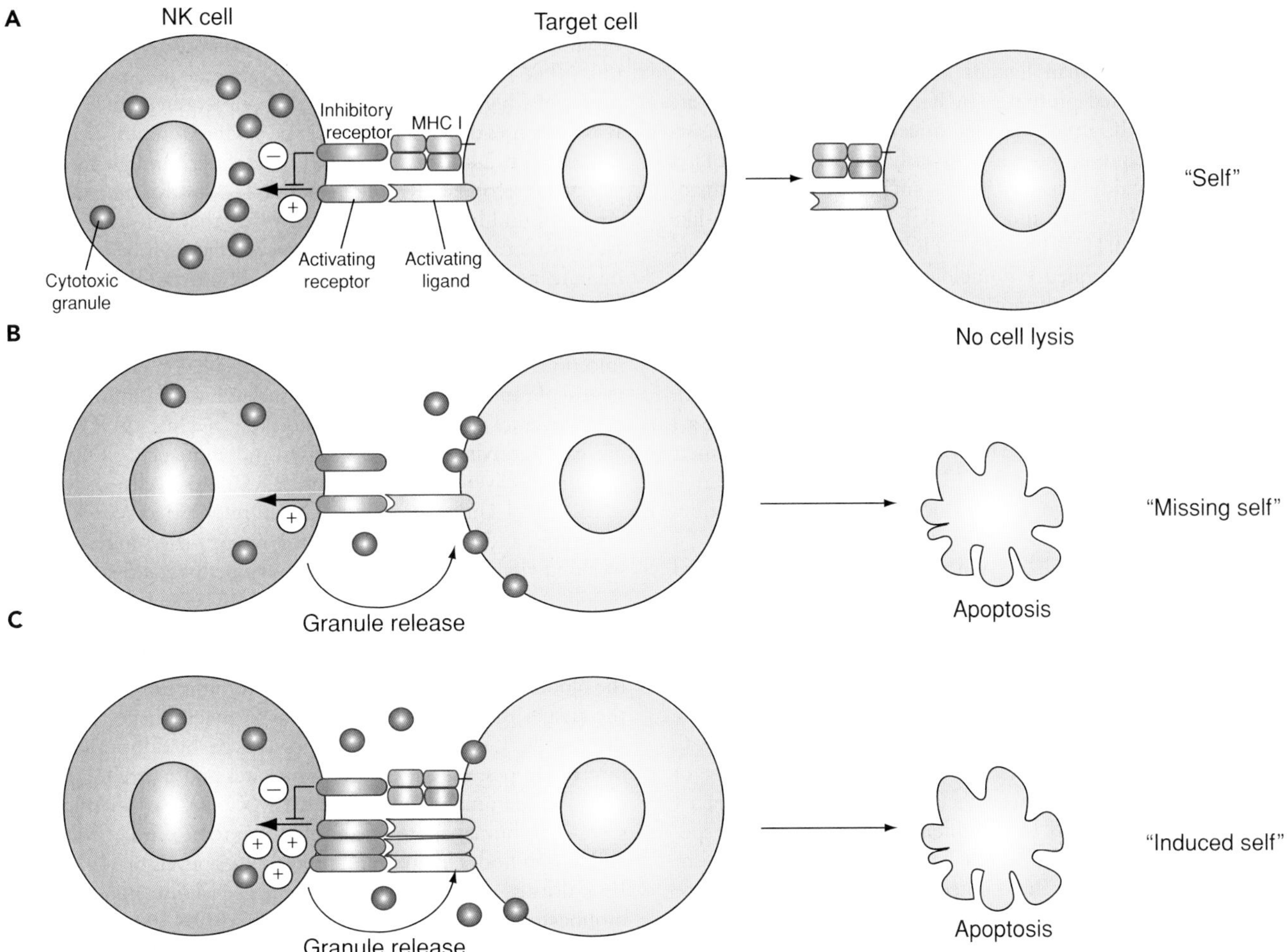

FIGURE 8.13. Natural killer cell activation and inhibition. NK cell recognition of infected cells relies on both the sensing of "induced self" (by activating receptors) and the "missing self" (by inhibitory receptors). NK cells contain cytosolic lytic granules that mediate apoptosis in target cells. **(A)** When an NK cell recognizes a healthy cell, NK cell lysis of the target cell is prevented by engagement of the inhibitory receptor by anormal level of MHC class I on the target cell. **(B)** When an NK cell interacts with virally infected cells that have reduced MHC class I on the cell surface ("missing self"), NK cells induce apoptosis in the target cell. **(C)** When an NK cell recognizes stressed virally infected cell expressing high levels of stimulating ligands ("induced self"), negative signals from inhibitory receptor is overridden by the activating signal, leading to lysis of target cells.

amino acids) cytoplasmic tail and are associated with signaling adaptors via ionic interactions of charged residues within their transmembrane regions. Several adaptor proteins are known to associate with activating receptors: DAP12 (DNAX-activating protein of 12 kDa), which contains the so-called immunoreceptor tyrosine-based activation motif (ITAM), which is a phosphotyrosine signaling module that recruits and activates Syk-72 tyrosine kinase upon recognition of the ligand by the ectodomain of the receptor complex. Another adaptor protein, called DAP10, has a distinct sequence motif that engages the PI3K signaling pathway. This adaptor is used exclusively by the NKG2D receptor, which is discussed in more detail below. In contrast to activating receptors, the inhibitory receptors contain the ITIM motif in their cytoplasmic regions.[114] ITIM motifs recruit either tyrosine phosphatase SH2-domain-containing protein tyrosine phosphatase 1 (SHP1) or lipid phosphatase SH2-domain-containing inositol polyphosphate 5′ phosphatase (SHIP1), which counter the effects of activating receptors. The opposing effects of ITAM and ITIM motifs explain how the balance of activating and inhibitory receptor ligands determines the outcome of NK cell recognition.

Both humans and mice express the NKG2 family of KLRs, which heterodimerizes with CD94 and interact with nonpolymorphic MHC molecules such as HLA-E (human) and Qa-1 (mouse). In humans, the NKG2 family consists of NKG2A, B, C, D, E, and F, of which NKG2A and B are inhibitory and C is D are activating. In mice, the Ly49 family of KLR proteins is inhibitory except for Ly49H.

NK-activating receptors include the immunoglobulin domain containing proteins NKp30, NKp44, and NKp46, along with the KLR, NKG2D. The NKp proteins associate with CD3ζ homodimers or the Fc receptor γ chain to induce activating signals. NKG2D is unique among the NKG2 family members in that it recognizes non-MHC ligands and associates with DAP10 and DAP12 signaling molecules, and provides activating signals to NK cells.

The ligands for activating receptors are generally absent or expressed at a low level on normal uninfected cells. Their expression is upregulated in response to viral infection and cellular stress. The best characterized activating ligands are recognized by NKG2D.[104] Human ligands for NKG2D include MHC class-I-chain–related protein A (MICA) and MICB, which are nonclassical MHC I molecules. In mice, NKG2D binds to several ligands including retinoic acid early transcript 1 (Rae1), a glycosylphosphatidylinositol (GPI) anchored protein, histocompatibility 60 (H60), and mouse UL16-binding protein-like transcript 1 (Mult1). While Rae1, H60, and Mult1 only share 20% amino acid sequence homology, they share a structurally related domain that is distantly related to the MHC I $\alpha 1$ and $\alpha 2$ domains. Inducible expression of these ligands can overcome inhibitory signals provided by recognition of normally expressed MHC class I molecules, resulting in target cell lysis (Fig. 8.13C).

NK inhibitory receptors sense the level of MHC class I molecules on target cells. The CD94:NKG2A heterodimers recognize nonpolymorphic MHC class I molecules HLA-E in humans and Qa-1 in mice, which present leader peptides from classical MHC class-I proteins. Thus, when the MHC-I level decreases as a result of viral manipulation, it is reflected in the decreased level of HLA-E/Qa-1 expression, resulting in disengagement of the CD94:NKG2A inhibitory receptor. Not surprisingly, several viruses mimic the activity of HLA-E. UL40 of HCMV confers protection in infected cells by encoding the same leader sequence that can be presented on HLA-E,[182] while HIV-1 selectively avoids downregulation of HLA-E and HLA-C to prevent NK-mediated lysis.[33] The mouse Ly49 family of inhibitory receptors recognizes the polymorphic MHC class I molecules. There are 18 Ly49 proteins in mice that have specificity to different MHC class I haplotypes. This mechanism of NK inhibition has been co-opted by MCMV, which encode m157, which stimulates Ly49I to inhibit NK activation.[7]

Plasmacytoid DCs

Among the leukocytes, pDCs are considered professional viral sensors for several reasons.[111] First, pDCs are equipped with special cellular machinery to endocytose many types of viruses and transport them to the endolysosomal compartment, whereupon uncoating of viral envelope and capsid, viral genomic DNA or RNA can be detected through TLR9 or TLR7, respectively. Second, pDCs constitutively express molecules involved in signaling to induce type I IFN genes. For instance, these cells express constitutively high levels of IRF7[94] and utilize IRAK1,[185] TRAF3,[62,135] IKKα,[74] osteopontin,[164] and PDC TREM[192] to induce IRF7-dependent IFN transcription. Third, pDCs form specialized lysosome-related organelles from which TLR9 and TLR7 can engage IRF7 activation to trigger transcription of type I IFN genes. The formation of IFN-inducing organelles depends on the presence of adaptor protein 3 (AP-3).[154]

Consequently, pDCs were originally known as IFN-producing cells (IPC), characterized by its potent ability to secrete type I IFNs in response to viruses.[9,23,59,85] The phenotype of these type I IFN–producing pDCs has been found to differ by species, as they are $CD4^{+}CD11c^{-}BDCA\text{-}2^{+}$ $CD123^{+}$ in humans[166] and $CD11c^{int}CD11b^{-}Gr\text{-}1^{+}B220^{+}SiglecH^{+}$ in mice.[9,131] Whereas DCs as a class are thought to be the professional antigen presenting cells specializing in antigen uptake, processing, and presentation to T cells, the predominant role of the pDCs appears to be the secretion of type I IFNs. In particular, pDCs can be induced to secrete large amounts of IFNα when stimulated with viruses including SeV,[85] influenza,[9] and HSV-1.[23,59] However, this situation may not be universal, as inflammatory monocytes after vaccinia virus infection,[12] and alveolar macrophages after respiratory NDV infection,[101] but not pDCs, are the predominant IFN producers, highlighting a differential cell requirement for type I IFN responses dependent on the type of viral stimulus. The pDCs express both L-selectin and CCR7 and enter through the blood vessel into secondary lymphoid tissues.[27] At steady state, these cells are not found in peripheral tissues, where they can come in contact with local viral infections. However, they can be induced to migrate into peripheral tissues and secrete antiviral IFNs *in situ*.[118] In mice that are depleted of pDCs, reduced early IFN-I production and augmented viral burden was observed after MCMV infection. During VSV infection, pDC depletion enhanced early viral replication and impaired the survival and accumulation of virus-specific cytotoxic T lymphocytes.[172] Thus, pDCs mediate early antiviral IFN-I responses and influence CD8 T cell responses. Given the location of pDCs, these cells likely serve as the initial source for type I IFNs in response to systemic viral infections, and as a secondary source of type I IFNs in response to localized viral infections restricted to the peripheral tissues.

Monocytes

Monocytes are a population of circulating leukocytes that patrol the blood stream and peripheral tissue for infection. Once inside the tissue, monocytes can give rise to macrophages and dendritic cells. Circulating monocytes can be broadly categorized into two types: inflammatory monocytes and patrolling monocytes.[10] Inflammatory monocytes ($Ly6C^{+}$ $CCR2^{+}$ in mice and $CD14^{+}$ in humans) are selectively recruited to inflamed tissues and lymph nodes in vivo, and produce high levels of TNF-α and IL-1 during infection or tissue damage. Mouse inflammatory monocytes express TLR2 and recognize dsDNA viruses such as vaccinia virus and MCMV, and secrete large amounts of type I IFNs.[12] Interestingly, monocyte recognition of viruses by TLR2 requires endocytosis while recognition of bacterial TLR2 ligands does not. While the exact viral ligands for TLR2-dependent detection by monocytes is unclear, TLR2 is known to be triggered by a variety of viruses including human cytomegalovirus,[34] mouse cytomegalovirus (MCMV),[173] herpes simplex virus types 1 and 2,[103,156] hepatitis C virus,[28] lymphocytic choriomeningitis virus,[203] measles virus,[17] and vaccinia virus.[204]

The other subset of monocytes ($Ly6C^{-}$ in mice and $CD14^{dim}$ in humans) patrols the blood vasculature, can differentiate into macrophages after extravasation into tissues, and has been suggested to be associated with tissue repair.[10] The human $CD14^{dim}$ monocytes do not express cell surface TLRs but express endosomal TLR7 and TLR8, and after recognition of viral nucleic acids, produce TNF, IL-1β, and chemokine (C-C motif) ligand 3 (CCL3), but not type I IFNs.[35]

Macrophages

Macrophages are versatile cells that play central roles in inflammation, wound healing, tissue homeostasis, and tissue remodeling. Macrophages are professional phagocytes, clearing dying cells and pathogens. Macrophage can be found in most organs as specialized cell types, such as Kupffer cells (liver), microglia (neuronal tissue), and osteoclasts (bone). Macrophages are well known in their defense against bacterial and protozoan pathogens, as they are the chief phagocytes that engulf and degrade these types of pathogens upon activation with IFN-γ. Recent studies highlight the importance of macrophages in antiviral defense. Macrophages are situated at the forefront of mucosal barriers. In the lung, alveolar macrophages sample and degrade incoming pathogens. In addition, alveolar macrophages become highly infected with respiratory viruses such as Newcastle disease virus (NDV), and produce the highest levels of type I IFNs locally that prevent other cells from becoming infected.[101] Not only do macrophages provide the initial type I IFNs in infected tissue, they also serve as "viral sink" to prevent more vulnerable cell types from becoming infected. Subcutaneous injection of VSV results in selective and productive infection of subcapsular sinus macrophages in the draining lymph nodes. These macrophages secrete high levels of type I IFNs that prevent infection of neurons. In mice depleted of such macrophages, local injection of VSV results in infection of innervating neurons in the lymph node and neuropathogenesis and death of mice.[77] It is interesting to speculate how virus replication niche is supported by the subcapsular macrophages in the face of large amounts of type I IFNs secreted by these cells. Perhaps these subcapsular macrophages have a unique mechanism of resisting viral and IFN-induced cell death.

Dendritic Cells

Dendritic cells are professional antigen-presenting cells capable of stimulating naïve antigen-specific lymphocytes in secondary lymphoid organs. Dendritic cells play an important role in immune responses at multiple levels. First, they are situated at various sites of pathogen entry, and are among the first cells to recognize the incoming pathogens through a set of PRRs. Engagement of PRRs upon viral recognition induces the expression of genes required to both eliminate the pathogens (innate effectors) and to initiate adaptive immune responses.[126] Second, DCs are the only cell type capable of initiating adaptive immune responses by activating naïve T lymphocytes. Pathogen recognition through PRRs activates DCs to increase their expression of the chemokine receptor, CCR7, which enables them to migrate from the site of infection to the secondary lymphoid tissues, where naïve lymphocytes recirculate (Fig. 8.14). On transit, DCs undergo a maturation program that results in the upregulation of costimulatory molecules and translocation of their MHC class II to the cell surface.[183] Once in the lymph node, DCs can present antigens derived from the pathogens to naïve T cells and induce their activation (through costimulation) and differentiation (through secretion of appropriate cytokines)[11] (Fig. 8.15). A naïve T cell requires three kinds of signals for activation and differentiation. First, a T cell must recognize viral peptides presented by the MHC molecules (signal 1). CD4 T cells bind to peptides presented by MHC class II, while CD8 T cells bind to peptides presented by MHC class I. Second, T cells must receive signals from costimulatory molecules on APCs. PRR stimulation of APCs results in the expression of costimulatory molecules including CD80 and CD86, which bind to CD28 on naïve T cells and provide this second signal that allows optimal clonal expansion. The third signal dictates the differentiation of a naïve T cell into different effector types. CD4 T cells can differentiate into Th1, Th2, and Th17 cells depending on the cytokines provided by the APCs or other accessory cell types. Antiviral responses are mediated by Th1 cells, as they are uniquely capable of secreting IFN-γ.

DCs can be broadly divided into two types, those that reside in the peripheral tissues (mucosa, skin, internal organs; tissue DCs) and those that reside in the blood and lymphoid

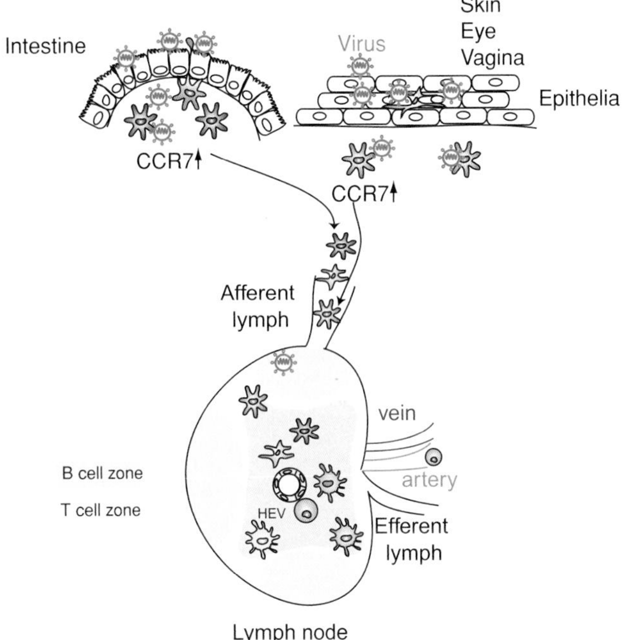

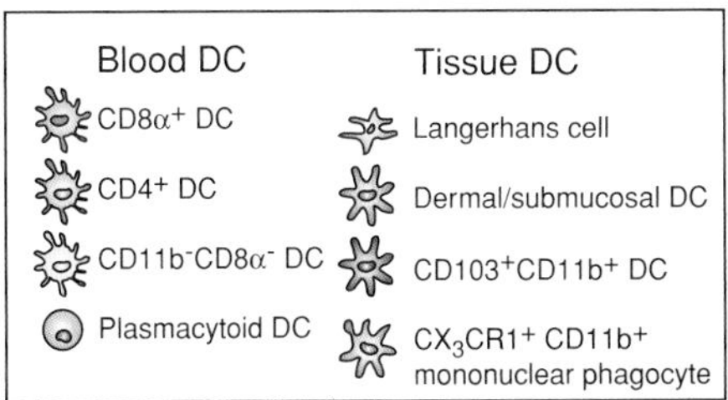

FIGURE 8.14. Dendritic cell populations in the peripheral tissues and in the secondary lymphoid organs. At the mucosal surfaces and in skin, distinct DC populations are found. In intestinal mucosa, CX3CR1$^+$ mononuclear phagocytes extend their dendrites and survey the environment just beneath the epithelial layer, while CD103$^+$ CD11b$^+$ DCs in the lamina propria can take up antigens and migrate to the mediastinal lymph node to prime T cells. In the epithelial layer of the mucosa of the vagina and eye or in the skin, Langerhans cells are the only DCs present in this layer. In the submucosal or dermis, submucosal/dermal DCs survey the environment for pathogen invasion. Both Langerhans cells and submucosal/dermal DCs are able to migrate to the draining lymph node. In most cases, the latter DC populations are required for T-cell priming. Within the lymph nodes, four different DC subsets appear to perform distinct functions. CD8α^+ DCs are specialized in cross presentation of viral antigens to CD8 T cells, while CD11b$^+$ and DN cells are capable of priming CD4 T cells. Plasmacytoid DCs do not participate in induction of effector T cell responses but serve as a key producer of type I IFNs.

tissues (blood DCs).[84] The blood DCs differentiate from precursors that enter these tissues from peripheral blood. In the mouse lymph nodes and spleen, the blood DCs can be divided into CD8α^+ DC (CD8α^+ CD11b$^-$), CD4$^+$ DC (CD4$^+$ CD11b$^+$), DN DC (CD4$^-$ CD8$^-$), and plasmacytoid DCs (pDCs).[66,165] In cutaneous lymph nodes or lymph nodes draining vaginal or eye mucosae, two extra DC subsets exist that are derived from the tissue, the Langerhans cells (LCs) and dermal or submucosal DCs[6,70,150] (Fig. 8.13). In the intestinal lamina propria, a distinct set of tissue DCs surveys the environment.[188] Just beneath

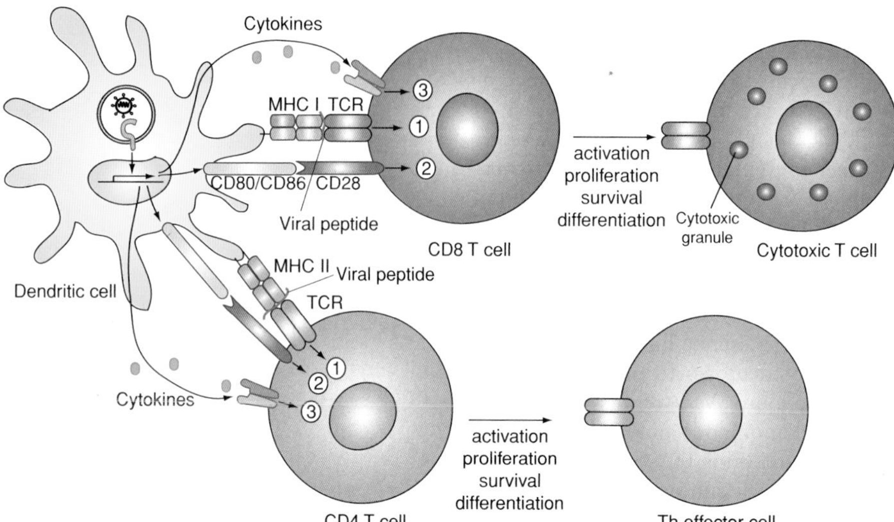

FIGURE 8.15. Innate instruction of adaptive immunity. Within the lymph node, DCs presenting viral antigenic peptides on MHC class I and MHC class II are able to interact with naïve CD8 T and CD4 T cells whose T cell receptors (TCR) are specific to the peptide presented by MHC molecules. PRR engagement (shown here for an endosomal TLR) by viral PAMPs induce expression of costimulatory molecules CD80 and CD86, as well as cytokines that stimulate naïve T cells, providing second and third signals needed for robust T-cell activation and differentiation. T cells receiving all three signals can proliferate and differentiate to become effector T cells. Depending on the cytokines secreted by DCs, CD4 T cells can become various effector Th types including Th1, Th2, or Th17.

the villous epithelial layer, CX_3CR1^+ mononuclear phagocytes extend their dendrites into the lumen. These cells do not migrate to the lymph node, but play an important role in intestinal homeostasis. In the lamina propria, $CD103^+$ $CD11b^+$ DCs pick up ingested antigens, and migrate to the mesenteric lymph node to prime immune responses. DC subsets are equipped with specialized cellular machinery to perform distinct functions. For instance, among the blood DC groups, $CD8^+$ DCs are equipped with machinery to carry out cross-priming to activate naïve CD8 T cells, while $CD8^-$ DCs express proteins involved in the MHC class II presentation pathway leading to the activation of naïve CD4 T cells.[48] However, migratory DCs from the infected tissues are required to elicit immune responses to localized infections, indicating that both tissue-resident and lymphoid-resident DCs cooperate to prime a robust immune response to pathogens.[105] In contrast, pDCs are specialized in recognizing viruses and secreting high levels of type I IFNs, but are not involved in activation of naïve T cells. Different DC subsets orchestrate innate and adaptive immune responses to viruses, depending on the type of PRR engaged by a given virus infection.

VIRUS MANIPULATION OF INNATE IMMUNITY

Virus–TLR Interaction as Viral Pathogenesis Mechanism

A virus–host PRR interaction reflects either host recognition of viruses to elicit appropriate antiviral defense, or viral strategy to infect the host. As discussed in the previous section, an example of the former is TLR9 recognition of viral DNA within the endosomes. This interaction leads to the activation of type I IFNs and prevention of viral replication in neighboring cells. However, most TLR-virus interactions that occur at the cell surface belong to the latter category, with the exception of TLR2-mediated recognition of viruses by monocytes (see Cell Types Involved in Innate Antiviral Responses). In fact, certain viruses rely on TLR signaling as a survival mechanism.[17,89] MMTV persists indefinitely in WT mice, but is rapidly cleared in mice deficient in TLR4 by cytotoxic T-cell response.[89] MMTV stimulates IL-10 production by B cells through dendritic cell and macrophage activation mediated by TLR4 signaling. IL-10, which is an immune suppressive cytokine, protects the MMTV-infected B cells from removal by cytotoxic T cells. It has been suggested that IL-10 may serve as a master regulator of chronic vs. acute viral infections,[20] thus it warrants analyzing whether TLR-dependent IL-10 production plays an important role in the pathogenesis of other chronic viral systems, such as HIV and HCV. Another example in which TLR-virus interaction benefits the virus is the measles virus. The HA protein of measles virus induces cytokine secretion in a TLR2-dependent manner. Interestingly, this interaction also results in upregulated expression of the MV receptor, CD150, suggesting that HA-TLR2 interactions in fact benefit the virus at the expense of the host.[17]

Viral Evasion of the Innate Immune System

Virtually all viruses encode factors to counteract the induction, signaling, or antiviral effector functions induced by the type I IFNs.[190] While viruses employ distinct molecules to achieve blockade of the antiviral effects of type I IFNs, these can be categorized into four major strategies: (1) global inhibition of cellular gene expression, (2) evasion from innate recognition, (3) inhibition of molecules involved in the IFN induction and signaling (Fig. 8.16), and (4) inactivation of the IFN-induced effector molecules (Fig. 8.17). A common strategy

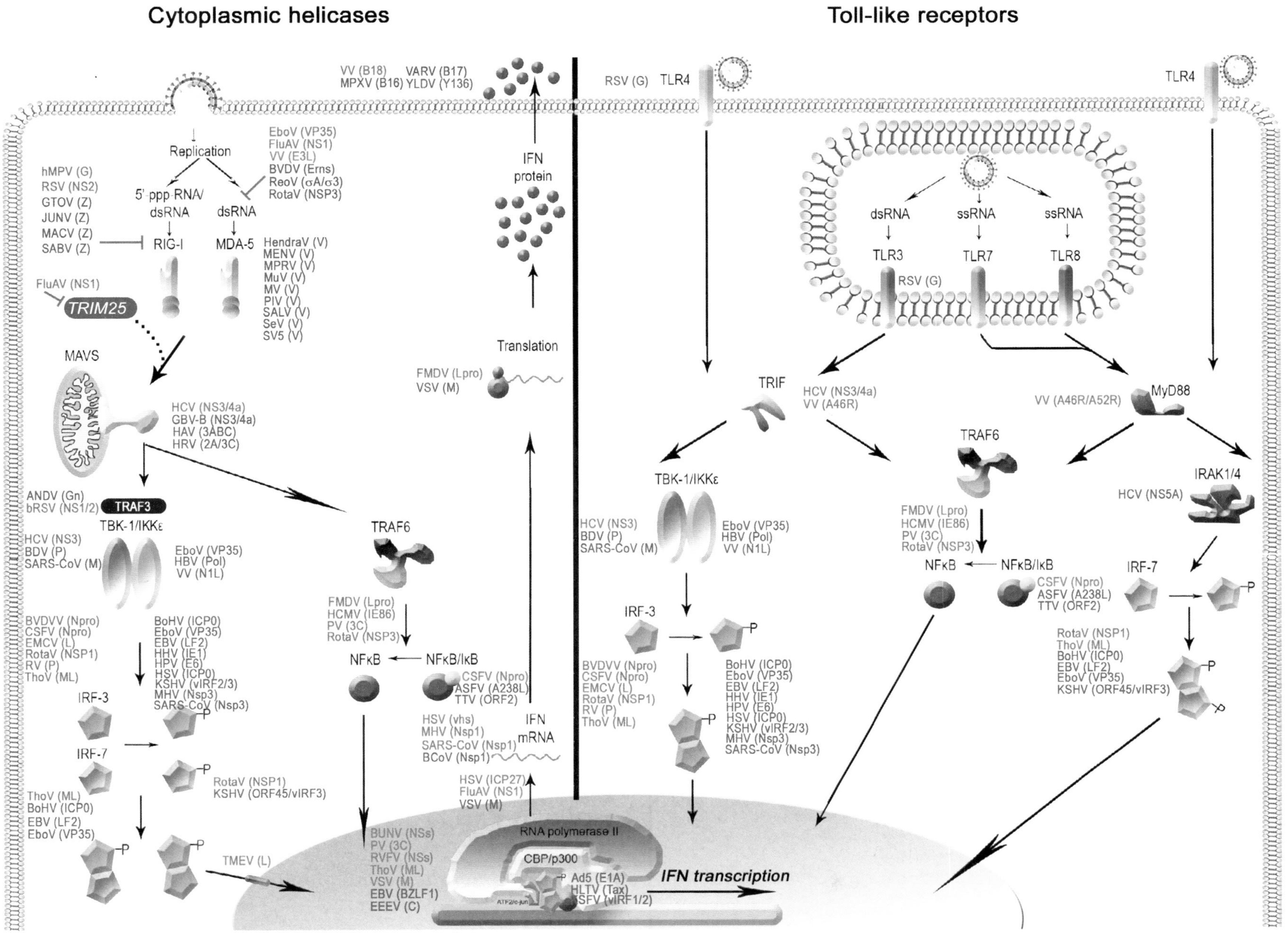

FIGURE 8.16. Viral evasion strategies that interfere with RLR and TLR pathways. Viruses and their proteins are indicated at the steps at which they interfere with innate receptor signaling. *Red letters* indicate proof for antagonism by recombinant viruses lacking the specific molecule, and *blue letters* indicate proof by overexpression and/or wild-type virus infection. (From Versteeg, GA, Garcia-Sastre A. Viral tricks to grid-lock the type I interferon system. *Curr Opin Microbiol* 2010;13:508–516, © 2010 with permission.)

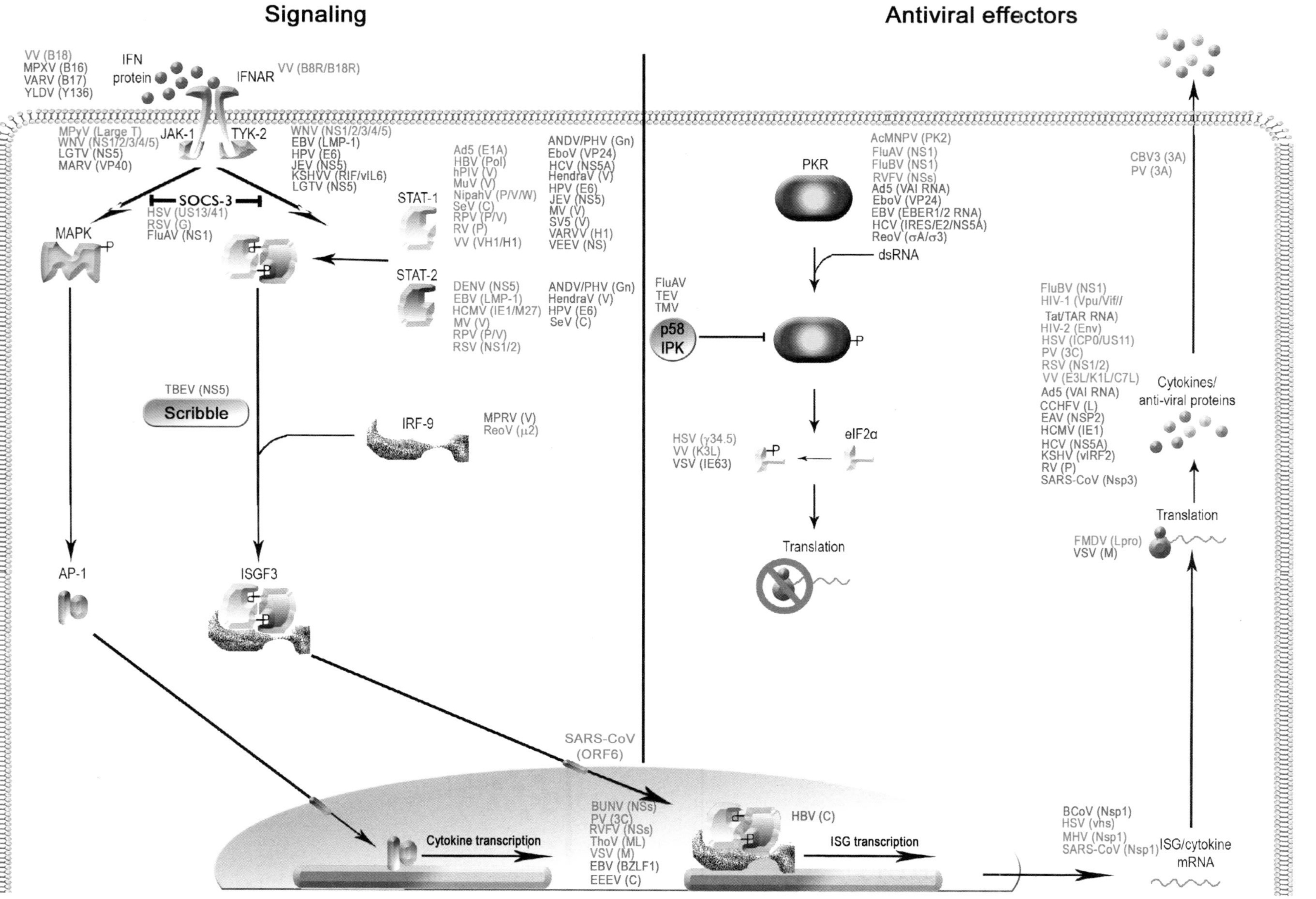

FIGURE 8.17. Viral evasion strategies that interfere with IFN signaling and antiviral effectors. Viruses and their antagonistic proteins are indicated at the steps of the IFN pathway. *Red letters* indicate proof for IFN antagonism by recombinant viruses lacking the specific molecule, and *blue letters* indicate proof by overexpression and/or wild-type virus infection. (From Versteeg, GA, Garcia-Sastre A. Viral tricks to grid-lock the type I interferon system. *Curr Opin Microbiol* 2010;13:508–516, © 2010 with permission.)

employed by many viruses is to inhibit cellular gene expression by interfering with host transcription and/or translation. Viruses that replicate in the cytosol that do not require host transcription for replication often employ strategies to block host transcription altogether. Poliovirus 3C protease and the VSV matrix (M) protein inhibit host gene expression by inactivating transcription initiation factor, TFIID.[119] The cleavage of translation initiation factor eIF4G in picornavirus-infected cells is a classic example of virus-induced inhibition of host translation. For this group of viruses, the inhibition of cap-dependent translation has no effect on translation of viral mRNAs because they depend on an internal ribosome entry site (IRES) for translation. Other viruses block the earliest steps in innate recognition by interfering with the function of innate sensors such as MDA-5 and RIG-I. Paramyxovirus V protein prevents MDA-5 dimerization,[5] and influenza A and B viruses express an NS1 protein preventing the activation of RIG-I by binding and inhibiting the actions of the E3 ligase TRIM25.[57] A common viral strategy to interfere with IFN gene induction is represented by viral inhibitors of IRF3 and IRF7, master transcription factors of type I IFN genes. Examples include KSHV vIRF3, that block host IRF7 activity,[88] and rotavirus NSP1, that block IRF3 and IRF7.[14,161]

Finally, even if the infected cells are able to produce type I IFNs, many viruses encode factors that inhibit signaling through the IFN-$\alpha\beta$R. SARS-CoV ORF6 protein is involved in preventing nuclear translocation of STAT1 by sequestering nuclear import factors on the ER/Golgi membrane.[56] Even if the infected cells manage to induce and respond to type I IFNs, influenza virus,[141] RSV,[139] HCV,[21] and HSV[196] induce SOCS-1 and SOCS-3 expression, which negatively regulates the JAK–STAT pathway.

Differences between Evasion Strategy Mechanisms of DNA vs. RNA Viruses

Even though all viruses encode factors that interfere with host antiviral defense mechanisms, different classes of viruses appear to target different stages in antiviral defense. Nearly all viruses with (–)ssRNA genomes interfere with the innate sensors themselves. By contrast, (+)ssRNA and dsDNA viruses target the downstream IRFs as the means to interfere with IFN induction.[190] Another intriguing feature shared among the dsDNA viruses, particularly poxviruses, is that they encode soluble decoy receptors that bind to secreted type I IFNs and prevent IFN-$\alpha\beta$R signaling. A key advantage of this strategy, compared to the others, is to be able to prevent neighboring cells from becoming resistant to viral infection.

Another striking difference between the host evasion mechanisms employed by different virus groups is that RNA viruses encode often only one or two molecules dedicated to inhibiting host response, usually through interception at the initiation of innate immune responses. Such a viral factor is usually a nonstructural protein that is expressed in infected cells, and has multiple functions in inhibiting the antiviral mechanisms of the host cells. A good example of this is influenza virus NS1. Despite being only 230aa long, NS1 inhibits almost all stages of antiviral pathways: through sequestration of viral RNA from innate recognition, blocking RIG-I function, inhibition of host mRNA processing and export, inhibition of innate effectors PKR and OAS, and IFN-$\alpha\beta$R signaling.[190]

In contrast, many dsDNA viruses, because of their large genome size, can accommodate multiple genes to specifically inhibit pathways that are useful for their own replicative niche. By expressing soluble IFN-binding proteins that compete with the cellular IFN receptor for its ligand, dsDNA viruses allow for infection and spread to cells that would otherwise be prevented from infection. Another feature associated with dsDNA viruses is their ability to establish latency. To this end, almost all herpesviruses encode molecules that specifically block PKR and its downstream target to block cell-mediated arrest of translation. This strategy is particularly important to ensure survival of the latently infected cells. Other dsDNA viruses have as narrow a target as to inhibit one specific NK receptor ligand. MCMV encodes three proteins—m152, m145, and m155—that reduce surface expression of NKG2D ligands, RAE-1,[112] MULT-1,[99] and H60,[113] respectively, in infected cells. Chronicity of virus infection may result from the ability of dsDNA viruses to manipulate the host immune response by interfering with specific effector mechanisms of various host cell types.

CONCLUSION

In the past 10 years, there has been a tremendous progress in characterization of the innate immune recognition of viral pathogens. The role of type-I IFNs, NK cells, TLRs, and RLRs in antiviral defense is now well appreciated and understood in considerable detail. There are some obvious gaps remaining, such as better characterization of intracellular DNA recognition pathways and their role in immunity to DNA viruses. Most IFN-induced antiviral gene products still have to be functionally characterized. These proteins likely interfere with multiple steps in viral infection cycles. This functional redundancy makes the analysis of their contribution to antiviral defense particularly challenging. Other outstanding questions include the elucidation of the mechanisms that control the expression of ligands for activating and inhibitory NK receptors. These ligands may be regulated by cellular stresses associated with viral infection or by signals from cell-intrinsic pattern recognition receptors. Finally, in the next few years we will likely witness continuous progress in understanding the role of noncoding RNAs, such as micro RNAs and piwi-interacting RNAs in antiviral immunity. Ultimately, the greatest challenge lies with the application of the accumulating knowledge to the management, and potentially even eradication, of major viral infections that continue to threaten our well being.

REFERENCES

1. Ablasser A, Bauernfeind F, Hartmann G, et al. RIG-I-dependent sensing of poly(dA:dT) through the induction of an RNA polymerase III-transcribed RNA intermediate. *Nat Immunol* 2009.
2. Akira S, Takeda K. Toll-like receptor signalling. *Nat Rev Immunol* 2004; 4:499–511.
3. Alexopoulou L, Holt AC, Medzhitov R, et al. Recognition of double-stranded RNA and activation of NF-kappaB by Toll-like receptor 3. *Nature* 2001;413:732–738.
4. Allen IC, Scull MA, Moore CB, et al. The NLRP3 inflammasome mediates in vivo innate immunity to influenza A virus through recognition of viral RNA. *Immunity* 2009;30:556–565.

5. Andrejeva J, Childs KS, Young DF, et al. The V proteins of paramyxoviruses bind the IFN-inducible RNA helicase, mda-5, and inhibit its activation of the IFN-beta promoter. *Proc Natl Acad Sci U S A* 2004; 101:17264–17269.
6. Anjuere F, Martin P, Ferrero I, et al. Definition of dendritic cell subpopulations present in the spleen, Peyer's patches, lymph nodes, and skin of the mouse. *Blood* 1999;93:590–598.
7. Arase H, Mocarski ES, Campbell AE, et al. Direct recognition of cytomegalovirus by activating and inhibitory NK cell receptors. *Science* 2002;296:1323–1326.
8. Areschoug T, Gordon S. Pattern recognition receptors and their role in innate immunity: focus on microbial protein ligands. *Contrib Microbiol* 2008;15:45–60.
9. Asselin-Paturel C, Boonstra A, Dalod M, et al. Mouse type I IFN-producing cells are immature APCs with plasmacytoid morphology. *Nat Immunol* 2001;2:1144–1150.
10. Auffray C, Sieweke MH, Geissmann F. Blood monocytes: development, heterogeneity, and relationship with dendritic cells. *Annu Rev Immunol* 2009;27:669–692.
11. Banchereau J, Steinman RM. Dendritic cells and the control of immunity. *Nature* 1998;392:245–252.
12. Barbalat R, Lau L, Locksley RM, et al. Toll-like receptor 2 on inflammatory monocytes induces type I interferon in response to viral but not bacterial ligands. *Nat Immunol* 2009;10:1200–1207.
13. Baribaud F, Doms RW, Pohlmann S. The role of DC-SIGN and DC-SIGNR in HIV and Ebola virus infection: can potential therapeutics block virus transmission and dissemination? *Expert Opin Ther Targets* 2002; 6:423–431.
14. Barro M, Patton JT. Rotavirus NSP1 inhibits expression of type I interferon by antagonizing the function of interferon regulatory factors IRF3, IRF5, and IRF7. *J Virol* 2007;81:4473–4481.
15. Barton GM, Kagan JC, Medzhitov R. Intracellular localization of Toll-like receptor 9 prevents recognition of self DNA but facilitates access to viral DNA. *Nat Immunol* 2006;7:49–56.
16. Ben-Sasson SZ, Hu-Li J, Quiel J, et al. IL-1 acts directly on CD4 T cells to enhance their antigen-driven expansion and differentiation. *Proc Natl Acad Sci U S A* 2009;106:7119–7124.
17. Bieback K, Lien E, Klagge IM, et al. Hemagglutinin Protein of Wild-Type Measles Virus Activates Toll-Like Receptor 2 Signaling. *J Virol* 2002; 76:8729–8736.
18. Bieniasz PD. Intrinsic immunity: a front-line defense against viral attack. *Nat Immunol* 2004;5:1109–1115.
19. Biron CA, Byron KS, Sullivan JL. Severe herpesvirus infections in an adolescent without natural killer cells. *N Engl J Med* 1989;320: 1731–1735.
20. Blackburn SD, Wherry EJ. IL-10, T cell exhaustion and viral persistence. *Trends Microbiol* 2007;15:143–146.
21. Bode JG, Ludwig S, Ehrhardt C, et al. IFN-alpha antagonistic activity of HCV core protein involves induction of suppressor of cytokine signaling-3. *FASEB J* 2003;17:488–490.
22. Braaten D, Franke EK, Luban J. Cyclophilin A is required for an early step in the life cycle of human immunodeficiency virus type 1 before the initiation of reverse transcription. *J Virol* 1996;70:3551–3560.
23. Brawand P, Fitzpatrick DR, Greenfield BW, et al. Murine plasmacytoid pre-dendritic cells generated from flt3 ligand-supplemented bone marrow cultures are immature APCs. *J Immunol* 2002;169:6711–6719.
24. Brinkmann MM, Spooner E, Hoebe K, et al. The interaction between the ER membrane protein UNC93B and TLR3, 7, and 9 is crucial for TLR signaling. *J Cell Biol* 2007;177:265–275.
25. Burckstummer T, Baumann C, Bluml S, et al. An orthogonal proteomic-genomic screen identifies AIM2 as a cytoplasmic DNA sensor for the inflammasome. *Nat Immunol* 2009;10(3)266–272.
26. Casrouge A, Zhang SY, Eidenschenk C, et al. Herpes simplex virus encephalitis in human UNC-93B deficiency. *Science* 2006;314:308–312.
27. Cella M, Jarrossay D, Facchetti F, et al. Plasmacytoid monocytes migrate to inflamed lymph nodes and produce large amounts of type I interferon. *Nat Med* 1999;5:919–923.
28. Chang S, Dolganiuc A, Szabo G. Toll-like receptors 1 and 6 are involved in TLR2-mediated macrophage activation by hepatitis C virus core and NS3 proteins. *J Leukoc Biol* 2007;82:479–487.
29. Chen ST, Lin YL, Huang MT, et al. CLEC5A is critical for dengue-virus-induced lethal disease. *Nature* 2008;453:672–676.
30. Chiu YH, Macmillan JB, Chen ZJ. RNA polymerase III detects cytosolic DNA and induces type I interferons through the RIG-I pathway. *Cell* 2009;138(3):576–591.
31. Cho YS, Challa S, Moquin D, et al. Phosphorylation-driven assembly of the RIP1-RIP3 complex regulates programmed necrosis and virus-induced inflammation. *Cell* 2009;137:1112–1123.
32. Ciampor F, Bayley PM, Nermut MV, et al. Evidence that the amantadine-induced, M2-mediated conversion of influenza A virus hemagglutinin to the low pH conformation occurs in an acidic trans Golgi compartment. *Virology* 1992;188:14–24.
33. Cohen GB, Gandhi RT, Davis DM, et al. The selective downregulation of class I major histocompatibility complex proteins by HIV-1 protects HIV-infected cells from NK cells. *Immunity* 1999;10:661–671.
34. Compton T, Kurt-Jones EA, Boehme KW, et al. Human Cytomegalovirus Activates Inflammatory Cytokine Responses via CD14 and Toll-Like Receptor 2. *J Virol* 2003;77:4588–4596.
35. Cros J, Cagnard N, Woollard K, et al. Human CD14dim monocytes patrol and sense nucleic acids and viruses via TLR7 and TLR8 receptors. *Immunity* 2010;33:375–386.
36. Daffis S, Szretter KJ, Schriewer J, et al. 2′-O methylation of the viral mRNA cap evades host restriction by IFIT family members. *Nature* 2010; 468:452–456.
37. de Witte L, Nabatov A, Pion M, et al. Langerin is a natural barrier to HIV-1 transmission by Langerhans cells. *Nat Med* 2007;13:367–371.
38. Deddouche S, Matt N, Budd A, et al. The DExD/H-box helicase Dicer-2 mediates the induction of antiviral activity in drosophila. *Nat Immunol* 2008;9:1425–1432.
39. Demaria O, Pagni PP, Traub S, et al. TLR8 deficiency leads to autoimmunity in mice. *J Clin Invest* 2010;120:3651–3662.
40. den Dunnen J, Gringhuis SI, Geijtenbeek TB. Innate signaling by the C-type lectin DC-SIGN dictates immune responses. *Cancer Immunol Immunother* 2009;58:1149–1157.
41. Denton A, Doherty P, Turner S, et al. IL-18, but not IL-12, is required for optimal cytokine production by influenza virus-specific CD8+ T cells. *Eur J Immunol* 2007;37:368–375.
42. Der SD, Zhou A, Williams BR, et al. Identification of genes differentially regulated by interferon alpha, beta, or gamma using oligonucleotide arrays. *Proc Natl Acad Sci U S A* 1998;95:15623–15628.
43. Deretic V, Levine B. Autophagy, immunity, and microbial adaptations. *Cell Host Microbe* 2009;5:527–549.
44. Diebold SS, Kaisho T, Hemmi H, et al. Innate antiviral responses by means of TLR7-mediated recognition of single-stranded RNA. *Science* 2004;303:1529–1531.
45. Diebold SS, Massacrier C, Akira S, et al. Nucleic acid agonists for Toll-like receptor 7 are defined by the presence of uridine ribonucleotides. *Eur J Immunol* 2006;36:3256–3267.
46. Dinarello CA. Biologic basis for interleukin-1 in disease. *Blood* 1996; 87:2095–2147.
47. Dixit E, Boulant S, Zhang Y, et al. Peroxisomes are signaling platforms for antiviral innate immunity. *Cell* 2010;141:668–681.
48. Dudziak D, Kamphorst AO, Heidkamp GF, et al. Differential antigen processing by dendritic cell subsets in vivo. *Science* 2007;315: 107–111.
49. Durfee LA, Lyon N, Seo K, et al. The ISG15 conjugation system broadly targets newly synthesized proteins: implications for the antiviral function of ISG15. *Mol Cell* 2010;38:722–732.
50. Etzioni A, Eidenschenk C, Katz R, et al. Fatal varicella associated with selective natural killer cell deficiency. *J Pediatr* 2005;146:423–425.
51. Ewald SE, Engel A, Lee J, et al. Nucleic acid recognition by Toll-like receptors is coupled to stepwise processing by cathepsins and asparagine endopeptidase. *J Exp Med* 2011;208:643–651.
52. Ewald SE, Lee BL, Lau L, et al. The ectodomain of Toll-like receptor 9 is cleaved to generate a functional receptor. *Nature* 2008;456:658–662.
53. Fernandes-Alnemri T, Yu JW, Datta P, et al. AIM2 activates the inflammasome and cell death in response to cytoplasmic DNA. *Nature* 2009; 458(7237):509–513.
54. Fitzgerald KA. The interferon inducible gene: Viperin. *J Interferon Cytokine Res* 2011;31:131–135.

55. French AR, Holroyd EB, Yang L, et al. IL-18 acts synergistically with IL-15 in stimulating natural killer cell proliferation. *Cytokine* 2006; 35:229–234.
56. Frieman M, Yount B, Heise M, et al. Severe acute respiratory syndrome coronavirus ORF6 antagonizes STAT1 function by sequestering nuclear import factors on the rough endoplasmic reticulum/Golgi membrane. *J Virol* 2007;81:9812–9824.
57. Gack MU, Albrecht RA, Urano T, et al. Influenza A virus NS1 targets the ubiquitin ligase TRIM25 to evade recognition by the host viral RNA sensor RIG-I. *Cell Host Microbe* 2009;5:439–449.
58. Gack MU, Shin YC, Joo CH, et al. TRIM25 RING-finger E3 ubiquitin ligase is essential for RIG-I-mediated antiviral activity. *Nature* 2007;446:916–920.
59. Gilliet M, Boonstra A, Paturel C, et al. The development of murine plasmacytoid dendritic cell precursors is differentially regulated by FLT3-ligand and granulocyte/macrophage colony-stimulating factor. *J Exp Med* 2002;195:953–958.
60. Gitlin L. Essential role of mda-5 in type I IFN responses to polyriboinosinic: polyribocytidylic acid and encephalomyocarditis picornavirus. *Proc Natl Acad Sci U S A* 2006;103:8459.
61. Haas T, Metzger J, Schmitz F, et al. The DNA sugar backbone 2′ deoxyribose determines toll-like receptor 9 activation. *Immunity* 2008;28:315–323.
62. Hacker H, Redecke V, Blagoev B, et al. Specificity in Toll-like receptor signalling through distinct effector functions of TRAF3 and TRAF6. *Nature* 2006;439:204–207.
63. Haller O, Staeheli P, Kochs G. Interferon-induced Mx proteins in antiviral host defense. *Biochimie* 2007;89:812–818.
64. Hansen TH, Bouvier M. MHC class I antigen presentation: learning from viral evasion strategies. *Nat Rev Immunol* 2009;9:503–513.
65. Harris RS, Liddament MT. Retroviral restriction by APOBEC proteins. *Nat Rev Immunol* 2004;4:868–877.
66. Heath WR, Carbone FR. Dendritic cell subsets in primary and secondary T cell responses at body surfaces. *Nat Immunol* 2009;10:1237–1244.
67. Hefti HP, Frese M, Landis H, et al. Human MxA protein protects mice lacking a functional alpha/beta interferon system against La crosse virus and other lethal viral infections. *J Virol* 1999;73:6984–6991.
68. Heil F, Hemmi H, Hochrein H, et al. Species-specific recognition of single-stranded RNA via toll-like receptor 7 and 8. *Science* 2004;303: 1526–1529.
69. Hemmi H, Takeuchi O, Kawai T, et al. A Toll-like receptor recognizes bacterial DNA. *Nature* 2000;408:740–745.
70. Henri S, Vremec D, Kamath A, et al. The dendritic cell populations of mouse lymph nodes. *J Immunol* 2001;167:741–748.
71. Honda K, Taniguchi T. IRFs: master regulators of signalling by Toll-like receptors and cytosolic pattern-recognition receptors. *Nat Rev Immunol* 2006;6:644–658.
72. Hornung V, Ablasser A, Charrel-Dennis M, et al. AIM2 recognizes cytosolic dsDNA and forms a caspase-1-activating inflammasome with ASC. *Nature* 2009;458(7237):514–518.
73. Hornung V, Ellegast J, Kim S, et al. 5′-Triphosphate RNA is the ligand for RIG-I. *Science* 2006;314:994–997.
74. Hoshino K, Sugiyama T, Matsumoto M, et al. IkappaB kinase-alpha is critical for interferon-alpha production induced by Toll-like receptors 7 and 9. *Nature* 2006;440:949–953.
75. Hoshino T, Kawase Y, Okamoto M, et al. Cutting edge: IL-18-transgenic mice: in vivo evidence of a broad role for IL-18 in modulating immune function. *J Immunol* 2001;166:7014–7018.
76. Hyodo Y, Matsui K, Hayashi N, et al. IL-18 up-regulates perforin-mediated NK activity without increasing perforin messenger RNA expression by binding to constitutively expressed IL-18 receptor. *J Immunol* 1999;162: 1662–1668.
77. Iannacone M, Moseman EA, Tonti E, et al. Subcapsular sinus macrophages prevent CNS invasion on peripheral infection with a neurotropic virus. *Nature* 2010;465:1079.
78. Ichinohe T, Lee HK, Ogura Y, et al. Inflammasome recognition of influenza virus is essential for adaptive immune responses. *J Exp Med* 2009; 206(1):79–87.
79. Ichinohe T, Pang IK, Iwasaki A. Influenza virus activates inflammasomes via its intracellular M2 ion channel. *Nat Immunol* 2010;11:404–410.
80. Isaacs A, Lindenmann J. Virus interference. I. The interferon. *Proc R Soc Lond B Biol Sci* 1957;147:258–267.
81. Ishii KJ, Akira S. Innate immune recognition of, and regulation by, DNA. *Trends Immunol* 2006;27:525.
82. Ishii KJ, Coban C, Kato H, et al. A Toll-like receptor-independent antiviral response induced by double-stranded B-form DNA. *Nat Immunol* 2006;7:40–48.
83. Ishii KJ, Kawagoe T, Koyama S, et al. TANK-binding kinase-1 delineates innate and adaptive immune responses to DNA vaccines. *Nature* 2008; 451:725–729.
84. Itano AA, Jenkins MK. Antigen presentation to naive CD4 T cells in the lymph node. *Nat Immunol* 2003;4:733–739.
85. Ito T, Amakawa R, Kaisho T, et al. Interferon-alpha and interleukin-12 are induced differentially by Toll-like receptor 7 ligands in human blood dendritic cell subsets. *J Exp Med* 2002;195:1507–1512.
86. Iwasaki A, Medzhitov R. Toll-like receptor control of the adaptive immune responses. *Nat Immunol* 2004;5:987–995.
87. Janeway CA Jr. Approaching the asymptote? Evolution and revolution in immunology. *Cold Spring Harb Symp Quant Biol* 1989;54 Pt 1:1–13.
88. Joo CH, Shin YC, Gack M, et al. Inhibition of interferon regulatory factor 7 (IRF7)-mediated interferon signal transduction by the Kaposi's sarcoma-associated herpesvirus viral IRF homolog vIRF3. *J Virol* 2007; 81:8282–8292.
89. Jude BA, Pobezinskaya Y, Bishop J, et al. Subversion of the innate immune system by a retrovirus. *Nat Immunol* 2003;4:573–578.
90. Kanneganti TD, Body-Malapel M, Amer A, et al. Critical role for Cryopyrin/Nalp3 in activation of caspase-1 in response to viral infection and double-stranded RNA. *J Biol Chem* 2006;281:36560–36568.
91. Kato H, Takeuchi O, Mikamo-Satoh E, et al. Length-dependent recognition of double-stranded ribonucleic acids by retinoic acid-inducible gene-I and melanoma differentiation-associated gene 5. *J Exp Med* 2008;205:1601–1610.
92. Kato H, Takeuchi O, Sato S, et al. Differential roles of MDA5 and RIG-I helicases in the recognition of RNA viruses. *Nature* 2006;441:101.
93. Kawai T, Takahashi K, Sato S, et al. IPS-1, an adaptor triggering RIG-I- and Mda5-mediated type I interferon induction. *Nat Immunol* 2005; 6:981–988.
94. Kerkmann M, Rothenfusser S, Hornung V, et al. Activation with CpG-A and CpG-B oligonucleotides reveals two distinct regulatory pathways of type I IFN synthesis in human plasmacytoid dendritic cells. *J Immunol* 2003;170:4465–4474.
95. Kerrigan AM, Brown GD. Syk-coupled C-type lectin receptors that mediate cellular activation via single tyrosine based activation motifs. *Immunol Rev* 2010;234:335–352.
96. Kishimoto T. Interleukin-6: from basic science to medicine–40 years in immunology. *Annu Rev Immunol* 2005;23:1–21.
97. Kochs G, Haller O. Interferon-induced human MxA GTPase blocks nuclear import of Thogoto virus nucleocapsids. *Proc Natl Acad Sci U S A* 1999;96:2082–2086.
98. Komuro A, Horvath CM. RNA- and virus-independent inhibition of antiviral signaling by RNA helicase LGP2. *J Virol* 2006;80:12332–12342.
99. Krmpotic A, Hasan M, Loewendorf A, et al. NK cell activation through the NKG2D ligand MULT-1 is selectively prevented by the glycoprotein encoded by mouse cytomegalovirus gene m145. *J Exp Med* 2005; 201:211–220.
100. Krug A, Luker GD, Barchet W, et al. Herpes simplex virus type 1 activates murine natural interferon-producing cells through toll-like receptor 9. *Blood* 2004;103:1433–1437.
101. Kumagai Y, Takeuchi O, Kato H, et al. Alveolar macrophages are the primary interferon-alpha producer in pulmonary infection with RNA viruses. *Immunity* 2007;27:240–252.
102. Kumar A, Haque J, Lacoste J, et al. Double-stranded RNA-dependent protein kinase activates transcription factor NF-kappa B by phosphorylating I kappa B. *Proc Natl Acad Sci U S A* 1994;91:6288–6292.
103. Kurt-Jones EA, Chan M, Zhou S, et al. Herpes simplex virus 1 interaction with Toll-like receptor 2 contributes to lethal encephalitis. *Proc Natl Acad Sci U S A* 2004;101:1315–1320.
104. Lanier LL. NK cell recognition. *Annu Rev Immunol* 2005;23:225.
105. Lee HK, Iwasaki A. Innate control of adaptive immunity: dendritic cells and beyond. *Semin Immunol* 2007;19:48–55.

106. Lee HK, Lund JM, Ramanathan B, et al. Autophagy-dependent viral recognition by plasmacytoid dendritic cells. *Science* 2007;315:1398–1401.
107. Levine B, Deretic V. Unveiling the roles of autophagy in innate and adaptive immunity. *Nat Rev Immunol* 2007;7:767–777.
108. Li F, Ding SW. Virus counterdefense: diverse strategies for evading the RNA-silencing immunity. *Annu Rev Microbiol* 2006;60:503–531.
109. Li Y, Li X, Stremlau M, et al. Removal of arginine 332 allows human TRIM5alpha to bind human immunodeficiency virus capsids and to restrict infection. *J Virol* 2006;80:6738–6744.
110. Liu B, Mori I, Hossain MJ, et al. Interleukin-18 improves the early defence system against influenza virus infection by augmenting natural killer cell-mediated cytotoxicity. *J Gen Virol* 2004;85:423–428.
111. Liu YJ. IPC: professional type 1 interferon-producing cells and plasmacytoid dendritic cell precursors. *Annu Rev Immunol* 2005;23:275–306.
112. Lodoen M, Ogasawara K, Hamerman JA, et al. NKG2D-mediated natural killer cell protection against cytomegalovirus is impaired by viral gp40 modulation of retinoic acid early inducible 1 gene molecules. *J Exp Med* 2003;197:1245–1253.
113. Lodoen MB, Abenes G, Umamoto S, et al. The cytomegalovirus m155 gene product subverts natural killer cell antiviral protection by disruption of H60-NKG2D interactions. *J Exp Med* 2004;200:1075–1081.
114. Long EO. Negative signaling by inhibitory receptors: the NK cell paradigm. *Immunol Rev* 2008;224:70–84.
115. Loo YM, Fornek J, Crochet N, et al. Distinct RIG-I and MDA5 signaling by RNA viruses in innate immunity. *J Virol* 2008;82:335–345.
116. Lund J, Sato A, Akira S, et al. Toll-like receptor 9-mediated recognition of Herpes simplex virus-2 by plasmacytoid dendritic cells. *J Exp Med* 2003;198:513–520.
117. Lund JM, Alexopoulou L, Sato A, et al. Recognition of single-stranded RNA viruses by Toll-like receptor 7. *Proc Natl Acad Sci U S A* 2004;101:5598–5603.
118. Lund JM, Linehan MM, Iijima N, et al. Cutting Edge: Plasmacytoid dendritic cells provide innate immune protection against mucosal viral infection in situ. *J Immunol* 2006;177:7510–7514.
119. Lyles DS. Cytopathogenesis and inhibition of host gene expression by RNA viruses. *Microbiol Mol Biol Rev* 2000;64:709–724.
120. Malamut G, El Machhour R, Montcuquet N, et al. IL-15 triggers an antiapoptotic pathway in human intraepithelial lymphocytes that is a potential new target in celiac disease-associated inflammation and lymphomagenesis. *J Clin Invest* 2010;120:2131–2143.
121. Malathi K, Dong B, Gale M Jr, et al. Small self-RNA generated by RNase L amplifies antiviral innate immunity. *Nature* 2007;448:816.
122. Manel N, Hogstad B, Wang Y, et al. A cryptic sensor for HIV-1 activates antiviral innate immunity in dendritic cells. *Nature* 2010;467:214–217.
123. Marques JT, Devosse T, Wang D, et al. A structural basis for discriminating between self and nonself double-stranded RNAs in mammalian cells. *Nat Biotechnol* 2006;24:559–565.
124. Martinon F, Burns K, Tschopp J. The inflammasome: a molecular platform triggering activation of inflammatory caspases and processing of proIL-beta. *Mol Cell* 2002;10:417–426.
125. Martinon F, Mayor A, Tschopp J. The inflammasomes: guardians of the body. *Annu Rev Immunol* 2009;27:229–265.
126. Medzhitov R, Janeway CA Jr. Innate immune induction of the adaptive immune response. *Cold Spring Harb Symp Quant Biol* 1999;64:429–435.
127. Meylan E, Curran J, Hofmann K, et al. Cardif is an adaptor protein in the RIG-I antiviral pathway and is targeted by hepatitis C virus. *Nature* 2005;437:1167–1172.
128. Mitchell RS, Katsura C, Skasko MA, et al. Vpu antagonizes BST-2-mediated restriction of HIV-1 release via beta-TrCP and endo-lysosomal trafficking. *PLoS Pathog* 2009;5:e1000450.
129. Muruve DA, Petrilli V, Zaiss AK, et al. The inflammasome recognizes cytosolic microbial and host DNA and triggers an innate immune response. *Nature* 2008;452:103–107.
130. Myong S, Cui S, Cornish PV, et al. Cytosolic viral sensor RIG-I is a 5′-triphosphate-dependent translocase on double-stranded RNA. *Science* 2009;323:1070–1074.
131. Nakano H, Yanagita M, Gunn MD. CD11c(+)B220(+)Gr-1(+) cells in mouse lymph nodes and spleen display characteristics of plasmacytoid dendritic cells. *J Exp Med* 2001;194:1171–1178.
132. Neil SJ, Zang T, Bieniasz PD. Tetherin inhibits retrovirus release and is antagonized by HIV-1 Vpu. *Nature* 2008;451:425–430.
133. Nguyen KB, Salazar-Mather TP, Dalod MY, et al. Coordinated and distinct roles for IFN-alpha beta, IL-12, and IL-15 regulation of NK cell responses to viral infection. *J Immunol* 2002;169:4279–4287.
134. Nisole S, Stoye JP, Saib A. TRIM family proteins: retroviral restriction and antiviral defence. *Nat Rev Microbiol* 2005;3:799–808.
135. Oganesyan G, Saha SK, Guo B, et al. Critical role of TRAF3 in the Toll-like receptor-dependent and -independent antiviral response. *Nature* 2006;439:208–211.
136. Okamura H, Tsutsi H, Komatsu T, et al. Cloning of a new cytokine that induces IFN-gamma production by T cells. *Nature* 1995;378:88–91.
137. Orvedahl A, Alexander D, Talloczy Z, et al. HSV-1 ICP34.5 Confers Neurovirulence by Targeting the Beclin 1 Autophagy Protein. *Cell Host Microbe* 2007;1:23.
138. Orvedahl A, MacPherson S, Sumpter R Jr, et al. Autophagy protects against Sindbis virus infection of the central nervous system. *Cell Host Microbe* 2010;7:115–127.
139. Oshansky CM, Krunkosky TM, Barber J, et al. Respiratory syncytial virus proteins modulate suppressors of cytokine signaling 1 and 3 and the type I interferon response to infection by a toll-like receptor pathway. *Viral Immunol* 2009;22:147–161.
140. Park B, Brinkmann MM, Spooner E, et al. Proteolytic cleavage in an endolysosomal compartment is required for activation of Toll-like receptor 9. *Nat Immunol* 2008;9:1407–1414.
141. Pauli EK, Schmolke M, Wolff T, et al. Influenza A virus inhibits type I IFN signaling via NF-kappaB-dependent induction of SOCS-3 expression. *PLoS Pathog* 2008;4:e1000196.
142. Pavlovic J, Arzet HA, Hefti HP, et al. Enhanced virus resistance of transgenic mice expressing the human MxA protein. *J Virol* 1995;69:4506–4510.
143. Pichlmair A, Reis e Sousa C. Innate Recognition of Viruses. *Immunity* 2007;27:370–383.
144. Pichlmair A, Schulz O, Tan CP, et al. RIG-I-mediated antiviral responses to single-stranded RNA bearing 5′-phosphates. *Science* 2006;314:997–1001.
145. Pinto LH, Lamb RA. The M2 Proton Channels of Influenza A and B Viruses. *J Biol Chem* 2006;281:8997–9000.
146. Raulet DH. Missing self recognition and self tolerance of natural killer (NK) cells. *Semin Immunol* 2006;18:145–150.
147. Ritchie KJ, Zhang DE. ISG15: the immunological kin of ubiquitin. *Semin Cell Dev Biol* 2004;15:237–246.
148. Roberts TL, Idris A, Dunn JA, et al. HIN-200 proteins regulate caspase activation in response to foreign cytoplasmic DNA. *Science* 2009:323(5917):1057–1060.
149. Rothenfusser S, Goutagny N, DiPerna G, et al. The RNA helicase Lgp2 inhibits TLR-independent sensing of viral replication by retinoic acid-inducible gene-I. *J Immunol* 2005;175:5260.
150. Ruedl C, Koebel P, Bachmann M, et al. Anatomical origin of dendritic cells determines their life span in peripheral lymph nodes. *J Immunol* 2000;165:4910–4916.
151. Sadler AJ, Williams BR. Structure and function of the protein kinase R. *Curr Top Microbiol Immunol* 2007;316:253–292.
152. Saito T, Hirai R, Loo YM, et al. Regulation of innate antiviral defenses through a shared repressor domain in RIG-1 and LGP2. *Proc Natl Acad Sci U S A* 2007;104:582.
153. Saito T, Owen DM, Jiang F, et al. Innate immunity induced by composition-dependent RIG-I recognition of hepatitis C virus RNA. *Nature* 2008;454:523–527.
154. Sasai M, Linehan MM, Iwasaki A. Bifurcation of Toll-like receptor 9 signaling by adaptor protein 3. *Science* 2010;329:1530–1534.
155. Sasai M, Shingai M, Funami K, et al. NAK-associated protein 1 participates in both the TLR3 and the cytoplasmic pathways in type I IFN induction. *J Immunol* 2006;177:8676–8683.
156. Sato A, Linehan MM, Iwasaki A. Dual recognition of herpes simplex viruses by TLR2 and TLR9 in dendritic cells. *Proc Natl Acad Sci U S A* 2006;103:17343–17348.
157. Schlee M, Roth A, Hornung V, et al. Recognition of 5′ triphosphate by RIG-I helicase requires short blunt double-stranded RNA as contained in panhandle of negative-strand virus. *Immunity* 2009;31:25–34.

158. Schmitz N, Kurrer M, Bachmann MF, et al. Interleukin-1 is responsible for acute lung immunopathology but increases survival of respiratory influenza virus infection. *J Virol* 2005;79:6441–6448.
159. Schulz O, Diebold SS, Chen M, et al. Toll-like receptor 3 promotes cross-priming to virus-infected cells. *Nature* 2005;433:887.
160. Schulz O, Pichlmair A, Rehwinkel J, et al. Protein kinase R contributes to immunity against specific viruses by regulating interferon mRNA integrity. *Cell Host Microbe* 2010;7:354–361.
161. Sen A, Feng N, Ettayebi K, et al. IRF3 inhibition by rotavirus NSP1 is host cell and virus strain dependent but independent of NSP1 proteasomal degradation. *J Virol* 2009;83:10322–10335.
162. Seth RB, Sun L, Ea CK, et al. Identification and characterization of MAVS, a mitochondrial antiviral signaling protein that activates NF-kappaB and IRF 3. *Cell* 2005;122:669–682.
163. Shelly S, Lukinova N, Bambina S, et al. Autophagy is an essential component of Drosophila immunity against vesicular stomatitis virus. *Immunity* 2009;30:588–598.
164. Shinohara ML, Lu L, Bu J, et al. Osteopontin expression is essential for interferon-alpha production by plasmacytoid dendritic cells. *Nat Immunol* 2006;7:498–506.
165. Shortman K, Liu Y-J. Mouse and human dendritic cell subtypes. *Nature Rev Immunol* 2002;2:153–163.
166. Siegal FP, Kadowaki N, Shodell M, et al. The nature of the principal type 1 interferon-producing cells in human blood. *Science* 1999;284:1835–1837.
167. Silverman RH. Viral encounters with 2′,5′-oligoadenylate synthetase and RNase L during the interferon antiviral response. *J Virol* 2007;81:12720–12729.
168. Sims JE, Smith DE. The IL-1 family: regulators of immunity. *Nat Rev Immunol* 2010;10:89–102.
169. Stetson DB, Ko JS, Heidmann T, et al. Trex1 prevents cell-intrinsic initiation of autoimmunity. *Cell* 2008;134:587–598.
170. Stetson DB, Medzhitov R. Recognition of cytosolic DNA activates an IRF3-dependent innate immune response. *Immunity* 2006;24:93–103.
171. Stetson DB, Medzhitov R. Type I Interferons in Host Defense. *Immunity* 2006;25:373.
172. Swiecki M, Gilfillan S, Vermi W, et al. Plasmacytoid dendritic cell ablation impacts early interferon responses and antiviral NK and CD8(+) T cell accrual. *Immunity* 2010;33:955–966.
173. Szomolanyi-Tsuda E, Liang X, Welsh RM, et al. Role for TLR2 in NK cell-mediated control of murine cytomegalovirus in vivo. *J Virol* 2006; 80:4286–4291.
174. Tabeta K, Hoebe K, Janssen EM, et al. The Unc93b1 mutation 3d disrupts exogenous antigen presentation and signaling via Toll-like receptors 3, 7 and 9. *Nat Immunol* 2006;7:156–164.
175. Takahashi K, Kawai T, Kumar H, et al. Roles of caspase-8 and caspase-10 in innate immune responses to double-stranded RNA. *J Immunol* 2006;176:4520–4524.
176. Takaoka A. DAI (DLM-1/ZBP1) is a cytosolic DNA sensor and an activator of innate immune response. *Nature* 2007;448:501.
177. Takeda K, Kaisho T, Akira S. Toll-like receptors. *Annu Rev Immunol* 2003;21:335–376.
178. Takeda K, Tsutsui H, Yoshimoto T, et al. Defective NK cell activity and Th1 response in IL-18-deficient mice. *Immunity* 1998;8:383–390.
179. Takeda M, Pekosz A, Shuck K, et al. Influenza a virus M2 ion channel activity is essential for efficient replication in tissue culture. *J Virol* 2002;76:1391–1399.
180. Thomas PG, Dash P, Aldridge JR Jr, et al. The intracellular sensor NLRP3 mediates key innate and healing responses to influenza A virus via the regulation of caspase-1. *Immunity* 2009;30:566–575.
181. Ting JP, Lovering RC, Alnemri ES, et al. The NLR gene family: a standard nomenclature. *Immunity* 2008;28:285–287.
182. Tomasec P, Braud VM, Rickards C, et al. Surface expression of HLA-E, an inhibitor of natural killer cells, enhanced by human cytomegalovirus gpUL40. *Science* 2000;287:1031.
183. Trombetta ES, Mellman I. Cell biology of antigen processing in vitro and in vivo. *Annu Rev Immunol* 2005;23:975–1028.
184. Uchil PD, Quinlan BD, Chan W-T, et al. TRIM E3 Ligases Interfere with Early and Late Stages of the Retroviral Life Cycle. *PLoS Pathog* 2008;4:e16.
185. Uematsu S, Sato S, Yamamoto M, et al. Interleukin-1 receptor-associated kinase-1 plays an essential role for Toll-like receptor (TLR)7- and TLR9-mediated interferon-{alpha} induction. *J Exp Med* 2005;201: 915–923.
186. Unterholzner L, Keating SE, Baran M, et al. IFI16 is an innate immune sensor for intracellular DNA. *Nat Immunol* 2010;11:997–1004.
187. Upton JW, Kaiser WJ, Mocarski ES. Virus inhibition of RIP3-dependent necrosis. *Cell Host Microbe* 2010;7:302–313.
188. Varol C, Zigmond E, Jung S. Securing the immune tightrope: mononuclear phagocytes in the intestinal lamina propria. *Nat Rev Immunol* 2010;10:415–426.
189. Venkataraman T, Valdes M, Elsby R, et al. Loss of DExD/H box RNA helicase LGP2 manifests disparate antiviral responses. *J Immunol* 2007; 178:6444.
190. Versteeg GA, Garcia-Sastre A. Viral tricks to grid-lock the type I interferon system. *Curr Opin Microbiol* 2010;13:508–516.
191. Wang X, Hinson ER, Cresswell P. The interferon-inducible protein viperin inhibits influenza virus release by perturbing lipid rafts. *Cell Host Microbe* 2007;2:96–105.
192. Watarai H, Sekine E, Inoue S, et al. PDC-TREM, a plasmacytoid dendritic cell-specific receptor, is responsible for augmented production of type I interferon. *Proc Natl Acad Sci U S A* 2008;105:2993–2998.
193. Weber F, Wagner V, Rasmussen SB, et al. Double-stranded RNA is produced by positive-strand RNA viruses and DNA viruses but not in detectable amounts by negative-strand RNA viruses. *J Virol* 2006;80: 5059–5064.
194. Xu LG, Wang YY, Han KJ, et al. VISA is an adapter protein required for virus-triggered IFN-beta signaling. *Mol Cell* 2005;19:727–740.
195. Yan N, Regalado-Magdos AD, Stiggelbout B, et al. The cytosolic exonuclease TREX1 inhibits the innate immune response to human immunodeficiency virus type 1. *Nat Immunol* 2010;11:1005–1013.
196. Yokota S, Yokosawa N, Okabayashi T, et al. Induction of suppressor of cytokine signaling-3 by herpes simplex virus type 1 contributes to inhibition of the interferon signaling pathway. *J Virol* 2004;78:6282–6286.
197. Yokoyama WM, Plougastel BF. Immune functions encoded by the natural killer gene complex. *Nat Rev Immunol* 2003;3:304–316.
198. Yoneyama M. The RNA helicase RIG-I has an essential function in double-stranded RNA-induced innate antiviral responses. *Nature Immunol* 2004;5:737.
199. Yoneyama M, Fujita T. Structural Mechanism of RNA Recognition by the RIG-I-like Receptors. *Immunity* 2008;29:178.
200. Yoneyama M, Kikuchi M, Matsumoto K, et al. Shared and unique functions of the DExD/H-box helicases RIG-I, MDA5, and LGP2 in antiviral innate immunity. *J Immunol* 2005;175:2851.
201. Yoshida R, Takaesu G, Yoshida H, et al. TRAF6 and MEKK1 play a pivotal role in the RIG-I-like helicase antiviral pathway. *J Biol Chem* 2008; 283:36211–36220.
202. Zhang SY, Jouanguy E, Ugolini S, et al. TLR3 deficiency in patients with herpes simplex encephalitis. *Science* 2007;317:1522–1527.
203. Zhou S, Kurt-Jones EA, Mandell L, et al. MyD88 is critical for the development of innate and adaptive immunity during acute lymphocytic choriomeningitis virus infection. *Eur J Immunol* 2005;35:822–830.
204. Zhu J, Martinez J, Huang X, et al. Innate immunity against vaccinia virus is mediated by TLR2 and requires TLR-independent production of IFN-beta. *Blood* 2007;109:619–625.
205. Zust R, Cervantes-Barragan L, Habjan M, et al. Ribose 2′-O-methylation provides a molecular signature for the distinction of self and non-self mRNA dependent on the RNA sensor Mda5. *Nat Immunol* 2011;12: 137–143.

CHAPTER 9

Thomas J. Braciale • Young S. Hahn • Dennis R. Burton

Adaptive Immune Response to Viral Infections

INTRODUCTION

Viruses have been part of human ecology since the human species first evolved on the plains of East Africa. As humans moved out of Africa to populate the continental landmasses, viruses—already adapted to the human species—were carried along with other microorganisms as part of the human ecological baggage. With the migration of humans around the world, we were exposed to new viruses present in the animal species that humans encountered. Some viruses, such as the herpesviridae family members, Epstein-Barr virus (EBV), and herpes simplex virus (HSV), have co-evolved with humans and have developed complex mechanisms (e.g., latency) to subvert the host defense mechanisms and sustain themselves in the human population. These viruses generally produce mild disease, except where host defenses are absent or weakened (e.g., in immune-deficient or immune-suppressed individuals). Other human viruses (e.g., measles virus) appear to have evolved mechanisms to persist at low levels in some infected individuals and sustain themselves by infecting previously unexposed individuals (typically children) who then go on to develop mild to severe illness and, in turn, serve as reservoirs for further virus propagation. Animal viruses can also *jump* from their host reservoir to infect humans and produce devastating diseases of potentially pandemic proportions. Notable examples of zoonotic viral diseases are the following: (a) the acquired immunodeficiency syndrome (AIDS) pandemic produced by the human immunodeficiency virus (HIV); (b) the outbreak of severe acute respiratory syndrome (SARS) in 2002 produced by the SARS coronavirus; (c) the 2009 H1N1 swine origin influenza A virus pandemic arising from the genetic reassortment in pigs of viruses with donated genes of human, swine, and avian flu origin; and (d) the periodic outbreaks of highly pathogenic avian influenza infection in poultry since 1997 in Asia and most recently in Africa and Europe, which have resulted in sporadic direct infections of humans with mortality rates approaching 50%. Indeed, the recent reconstruction and analysis of the genome of the influenza virus that caused the 1918 *Spanish flu* pandemic suggest that this virus may have been an avian influenza virus that spread directly to humans (without modification of virus in an intermediate host or the acquisition of genetic information from then-circulating human influenza strains).[288]

Virus infection can result in acute or chronic disease in virtually any organ and tissue of the body. Furthermore, infection with human papillomavirus (HPV), human herpesvirus 8 (HHV-8), and hepatitis B virus (HBV) and hepatitis C virus (HCV) have been directly linked to the development of cervical cancer, Kaposi's sarcoma, and hepatocellular carcinoma, respectively. Given the pandemic outbreak of the swine origin A/California/2009 (H1N1) virus infection, the possibility of another human influenza pandemic from an avian influenza source, as well as the devastating effects of HIV infection all suggest, virus infection represents a continuing threat to human health. We can point to some notable successes in the struggle against viruses (e.g., the eradication of smallpox in the 1970s, and the effectiveness of the live attenuated oral polio vaccine in eliminating paralytic polio in the developing world, raising the prospect of eradicating polio worldwide). Both of these vaccination successes rely on the mobilization of the body's major defense against virus infection—the adaptive immune system. Our enthusiasm about these *successes* must be tempered, however. Because of the success of smallpox eradication, mandatory smallpox vaccination was discontinued in the United States in the early 1970s, making a large fraction of the population (i.e., those younger than age 40) now susceptible to smallpox. This fact, along with the advances in poxvirus genetics and genetic engineering, now makes smallpox a major bioterrorism threat. Similarly, administration of live oral polio vaccine to children in underdeveloped countries whose immune function is compromised by malnutrition or HIV infection can result in outbreaks of paralytic polio caused by infection with virulent mutants (revertants) of the live attenuated vaccine strain. This realization has prompted a modification of the guidelines for oral polio vaccine administration in the United States and a reevaluation of the prospect of global polio eradication using current vaccination strategies. To counter the continuing threat posed by viruses, it is essential to understand the body's primary defense against virus infection in the immune system.

OVERVIEW OF THE ADAPTIVE IMMUNE RESPONSE TO VIRUS INFECTION

Viruses are obligatory intracellular parasites; that is, they replicate within cells of the infected host and use the cell's biosynthetic machinery for replication and production of progeny virions. Furthermore, most viruses replicate rapidly in infected cells (i.e., within hours) producing progeny virions capable of infecting additional cells, thereby propagating and sustaining infection in the host. These properties of infection by viruses dictate how the immune system must respond to counterinfection. In acute virus infection, the race between the replication of the virus and the host response will result either in the death of the host or in virus clearance and the termination of infection. The tissue injury produced by viruses at the site(s) of infection results both from the cytopathic effects of virus replication and, equally importantly, from the host immune response to infection. In general, therefore, the greater the extent of virus replication in the infected host, the greater the tissue injury and illness severity.

In chronic infection, the time scale of virus replication in the host is not measured in days (as in acute infection) but in weeks, months, or even years, with the host immune response likewise continuing over the same prolonged time scale. Viruses that produce chronic, persistent infection have evolved mechanisms to suppress or alter the immune response (allowing these viruses to persist in the infected host). The tissue injury produced by the immune response to virus infection (termed, *immunopathology*) occurs with both acute and chronic virus infection. In many chronic virus infections (e.g., HCV infection); however, immune-mediated tissue injury predominates (rather than direct virus-mediated injury).[38] Furthermore, the clinical manifestations of virus infection (e.g., fever, headache, myalgia, anorexia) are caused primarily by inflammatory mediators (e.g., cytokines) released by cells of the immune system in response to infection. Undoubtedly, chronic (persistent) virus infection also alters or modifies the immune system and its capacity to respond to microbes and environmental antigens.[297] Finally, the triggering of the immune system by virus infection can result in the induction of aberrant immune responses directed both to the virus, and to self-cellular constituents, resulting in autoimmune disease.[143]

The primary host defenses against virus infection are physical/chemical barriers to infection and the immune system. The immune system can be divided into two components: the innate immune system (see Chapter 8) and the adaptive immune system. This division is based on the properties of

TABLE 9.1 Cells of the Immune System

Type	Subtype	Onset of effect
Innate immune Cell		
Granulocytic	Neutrophil, basophil, eosinophil	Immediate/inducible (hr)
Monocytic	Macrophage, DCs	Immediate/inducible (hr)
Lymphocytic[a]	NK cell, NK T cell	Immediate/inducible (hr)
Somatic cell (nonhematopoietic)	Epithelial, endothelial cell, etc.	Immediate/inducible (hr)
Adaptive immune Cell		
B Lymphocyte	—	Inducible (d)
T Lymphocyte	$CD4^+$, $CD8^+$, T_{reg}	Inducible (d)

DC, dendritic cell; NK, natural killer; TCR, T-cell antigen receptor; T_{reg}, regulatory T-cells; hr, hour; d, day.

[a]Specific subtypes of T lymphocytes [e.g., $\gamma\delta$ T cells and intraepithelial (IEL) $CD8^+\alpha\alpha$ T lymphocytes] are considered to be part of the innate immune system. These cell types with lymphocytic morphology employ a TCR-type antigen recognition system, but differ in their function and strategy of antigen recognition from conventional T cells.

the immune cell types and molecules involved in the response to infection and the tempo of the response (Table 9.1). The response of the innate immune system to virus infection is either immediate (i.e., constitutively active) or rapidly induced (i.e., typically within hours of infection). The innate immune response is triggered in two ways: first, through recognition of viral constituents (e.g., viral nucleic acids) by a limited set of cellular pattern recognition receptors for foreign molecules displayed on innate immune cells; and, second, through the activation of intracellular signaling mechanisms following virus entry into cells and the initiation of virus replication. Importantly, a defining feature of the innate immune response is that repeat exposure to a particular virus generally evokes an identical response from the innate immune system (although a form of that enhanced efficiency of pathogen recognition has recently been reported for natural killer (NK) cells.[298] The genes encoding these receptors and associated signaling mechanisms within innate immune cells are encoded within the germline (i.e., fixed in the genome).

By contrast, the response of the adaptive immune system to a first encounter with a virus takes days to evolve. The response of the cells of the adaptive immune system (i.e., B lymphocytes and T lymphocytes) is triggered by viral constituents, primarily through the engagement of highly specific cell-surface recognition receptors generated by somatic gene rearrangement and displayed by a minuscule fraction of the total repertoire of adaptive immune cells for any given virus. These receptors only recognize the constituents (antigens) of that particular virus. Importantly, this arm of the immune system *adapts* to repeat exposure to a particular virus or viral protein; this results in a more rapid response of higher magnitude by the specific adaptive immune cells on repeat exposure/infection—a phenomenon called *immunological memory*, the basis for vaccination.

The constituents of the innate immune response include proteins of the complement system, and so called *acute phase proteins* (e.g., members of the collectin protein family).[251] These molecules are present *constitutively* in the blood and tissue fluids or are induced rapidly in the liver following infection and can bind directly to certain viruses, thereby inhibiting virus infection. Leukocytes, in particular, neutrophils, blood monocytes, tissue macrophages, dendritic cells, NK cells and NK T cells are the dominant, innate immune cell types responding to virus infection. They are triggered/activated through the engagement of pattern recognition receptors (e.g., Toll-like receptors [TLRs], C-type lectins) expressed on their cell surface, which recognize viral constituents (e.g., viral nucleic acids), and in the case of NK and NK T cells, alterations of the cell surface of infected cells. These cells reside in the tissues, and they respond there or are recruited to sites of infection from the bloodstream through the action of cytokines/chemokines released during infection.

Nonhematopoietic body cells (e.g., epithelial cells, endothelial cells, fibroblasts) that are targets of virus infection, must also be considered part of the innate immune response because, on infection, they are triggered to secrete antiviral proinflammatory mediators such as type 1 interferons and certain cytokines/chemokines (the production of which can initiate and amplify the innate immune response to infection). The induction of the innate immune response and the role of innate immune cells and molecules in controlling virus infection are discussed in detail elsewhere (Chapter 8). One of these innate immune cell types, the dendritic cell (DC), however, bridges the innate and adaptive immune response, and its role in the initiation of the adaptive immune response is discussed in a later section of this chapter.

A hallmark of the adaptive immune response is the exquisite specificity of adaptive immune cells for a particular foreign viral antigen, and the capacity of this system to recognize and respond to a myriad of viruses (or other antigens). This remarkable property of the adaptive immune cells is achieved by the generation of a correspondingly diverse array of cell surface recognition receptors, which are randomly generated within the lymphocytes of every individual and clonally distributed among the adaptive immune cells. As a consequence, in a nonimmune individual, only an extremely small fraction of the adaptive immune cell repertoire (e.g., one cell in a million or less) will have an antigen receptor capable of recognizing a specific virus (viral antigen). Understanding how this diverse array of clonally distributed antigen receptors is generated during lymphocyte development and how that rare adaptive immune cell directed to particular virus finds virus or infected cells in a peripheral site of infection (e.g., the skin or lungs) is critical to the understanding of the adaptive immune response to virus infection.

Viruses, because they exist as extracellular virion particles and replicate/assemble within infected cells, pose a unique recognition problem for the adaptive immune system (i.e., how

TABLE 9.2 Properties of T and B Lymphocytes

General properties	B lymphocytes	T lymphocytes
Origin	Bone marrow	Bone marrow
Self/non–self-discrimination	Bone marrow	Thymus
Activation	BCR and other ligand receptors	TCR and other ligand receptors
Antigen recognition	Native (3D) conformation	Nonnative fragments
Antigen receptor	**B lymphocytes**	**T lymphocytes**
Somatically generated	+	+
High specificity	+	+
Clonally represented	+	+
Localization	Cell surface/secreted (Ab)	Cell surface only

BCR, B-cell antigen receptor; TCR, T-cell antigen receptor; 3D, three-dimensional; Ab, antibody.

to recognize the virus [viral proteins or genome] both outside of the cell and within the infected cell). The elegant solution to this problem employed by the adaptive immune system is the partitioning of the adaptive immune system into two distinct cell types: B and T lymphocytes (Table 9.2). B lymphocytes displaying a receptor specific for a particular virus will, on encounter with the virus and activation, release their antigen receptor in a soluble form (i.e., as antibody molecules) capable of binding free (extracellular) virions in a highly specific matter. This interaction typically results in virus neutralization and/or elimination. Antiviral B-lymphocyte responses are exquisitely sensitive to the three-dimensional confirmation of the virus (and its constituents), and they play a dominant role in clearing virus during infection, in preventing or limiting reinfection (after previous virus infection), and in vaccination against a specific virus.

Activated antiviral T lymphocytes retain their antigen-specific receptors on the cell surface and are responsible for recognizing and eliminating virus-infected cells. T lymphocytes, however, do not recognize viral proteins in their native conformation. Rather, the antigen receptors on the T lymphocytes recognize *processed* peptide fragments of viral proteins displayed on the infected cell surface bound to cell-surface molecular recognition platforms (i.e., the major histocompatibility complex [MHC] locus gene products). Activated virus-specific T lymphocytes halt the spread of infection by killing virus-infected cells through direct cell-to-cell contact and by the release of soluble mediators (e.g., cytokines, such as IFN-γ and tumor necrosis factor α [TNF-α]). By releasing these and other soluble mediators, the activated T lymphocytes recruit and orchestrate the response of the innate immune cells which, in turn, act to clear infection. Understanding how and where B and T lymphocytes activate, the mechanism of antigen presentation to the cells, and the range of effector activities that these cells use to control and eliminate virus is essential for understanding the adaptive immune response to virus infection. These important topics are reviewed in this chapter.

Finally, the importance of the immune system in general and the adaptive immune response in particular in controlling virus clearance and promoting recovery from infection is exemplified by the fact that viruses have evolved a variety of mechanisms to inhibit or alter the host immune response. Whereas the virus immune evasion strategies are best considered in the context of viral pathogenesis (Chapter 10) and are addressed in chapters dealing with individual viruses, this chapter highlights some of the viral evasion strategies directed to the adaptive immune response.

ARCHITECTURE OF THE ADAPTIVE IMMUNE SYSTEM

Generation of T and B Lymphocytes: Primary Lymphoid Organ

Unlike the cells of the innate immune system, T and B lymphocytes possess one unique and profoundly important property. On their surfaces, these cells also display a receptor complex capable of recognizing foreign (nonself) structures—with exquisite specificity. This receptor complex is both randomly generated (by somatic recombination of genetic elements ultimately encoding the mature receptors) and clonally distributed among progeny lymphocytes during their differentiation from progenitor cells. Therefore, of the approximate 10^9 naive T and B lymphocytes in the human adaptive immune system, each cell may, in principle, display a unique receptor directed to a specific foreign antigenic structure. This common property of the antigen receptor on T and B lymphocytes (i.e., random generation by somatic DNA recombination and clonal receptor display) immediately raises two important questions. First, if these antigen receptors are stochastically generated, how is the generation of lymphocytes with receptors to self-structures (e.g., tissue proteins) avoided/prevented? Second, if the frequency of lymphocytes with a receptor directed to a specific foreign antigen (e.g., the coat proteins of an invading virus) is extremely low (1 in 10^7 lymphocytes), how can those rare lymphocytes locate the antigen quickly enough to respond before the infection is beyond control? As is discussed below, it is the unique structure of the primary (central) lymphoid organs where lymphocyte progenitors develop into mature T and B lymphocytes, and of the secondary (peripheral) lymphoid organs where mature T and B lymphocytes respond to invading microorganisms that provides the answers to these questions.

Mature T and B lymphocytes are derived from lymphoid progenitors present in the bone marrow, as well as in sites of hematopoiesis in developing fetus (e.g., the liver) through a process of differentiation and selection linked to, and driven by, the antigen receptors displayed by these cells.[221,233] As described in Table 9.2, B-lymphocyte lineage development occurs in the bone marrow and follows a well-defined, step-wise program of gene activation (e.g., expression of the recombination activating gene 1 and 2 [*RAG1* and *2*], lymphoid DNA-specific recombinases), and sequential rearrangement of immunoglobulin (Ig) V_H, D_H, J_H, and C_H heavy (H) chain genetic elements (by random somatic recombination), followed by rearrangement of the Ig K/λ V_L-J_L-$C_{LK/\lambda}$ light (L) chain locus elements. Then B-lymphocyte progenitors transit from the pro-B, through the pre-B, and to the surface immunoglobulin-positive immature B-lymphocyte stage. It is during this development/differentiation program that the B-lymphocyte receptor (B-cell receptor [BCR]) diversification occurs through random association of one of the 40 V_H gene segments with one of the 25 D_H and 6 J_H and 70 V_L with 9 J_L to yield (after nucleotide addition and/or excision at the site of gene segment recombination) 10^7 or more different potential BCR H and L chain combinations. During this development process in the bone marrow, T-Lymphocytes expressing a BCR with reactivity to self-molecules (i.e., proteins, lipids, carbohydrates, nucleic acids) will, as a result of BCR engagement, undergo a process of negative selection. These *self-reactive* B cells are largely eliminated/deleted through interaction of the BCR on the developing cells, with self-constituents resulting in apoptosis or in activation ("anergy") of self-reactive B lymphocytes. The immature B lymphocytes that escape negative selection undergo final maturation, migrate from the bone marrow to join the pool of mature B lymphocytes that circulate through the blood, and populate the secondary lymphoid organs. B lymphocytes ultimately express their effector activity by releasing the BCR of the mature B lymphocyte in a secreted form as immunoglobulin (antibody) molecules. This fact has the following two important implications for the recognition of viruses by B lymphocytes: (a) the B-lymphocyte response to viruses will be particularly effective when interacting with free/extracellular virus constituents (e.g., virions); and (b) the BCR and its antibody product will be sensitive to the conformation of viral constituent recognized.

T-Lymphocyte lineage development follows a program similar to that of B lymphocytes. The T-cell antigen receptor (TCR) is also a heterodimer consisting of two polypeptide chains, each of which is formed by somatic recombination of variable (V), diversity (D), and joining (J) segments encoding the variable portion of one chain (or V and J joining for the other chain) to a constant (C) gene segment. As in B lymphocytes, the randomly recombined gene segments encoding the V region gene segment joined to the respective C region gene segment for the two TCR chains encodes the TCR on the developing T lymphocyte. Unlike the BCR, however, the TCR always remains cell associated. Therefore, the TCR is normally directed to foreign antigens (or self-structures) that are cell associated. Consequently, T lymphocytes are uniquely suited to recognize cells that have been invaded by microorganisms (e.g., viruses and intracellular bacteria). Unlike the BCR, the TCR does not recognize intact microbial products, but rather recognizes small fragments of molecules—typically, short peptide fragments of microbial or self-proteins bound to protein products of the mammalian MHC genetic locus (e.g., the classically defined major human transplantation antigens). These MHC gene products expressed on cell surfaces serve as molecular platforms, both selecting and displaying the self-peptides involved in TCR selection during T-lymphocyte precursor development, and presenting microbial peptides to mature T lymphocytes responding to uptake/infection of cells by the microbes. The steps in the processing (fragmenting) and presentation of both self and microbial gene products by the MHC locus protein, and the structure of the major classes of MHC locus proteins (i.e., MHC class I and II proteins) are discussed below.

The generation of mature T lymphocyte from committed lymphocyte progenitors (arising in the bone marrow) occurs primarily in the thymus (Fig. 9.1). Here, immature thymocytes undergo the developmental program resulting in the formation of mature T lymphocytes, which then leave the thymus, enter the circulation, and ultimately populate secondary lymphoid organs. Two classes of mature T lymphocytes are produced in the thymus. The major population (~80% of the peripheral T lymphocyte pool) are the $\alpha^+\beta^+$ T cells (because their heterodimeric TCR express two chains encoded by TCR α and β loci). The second minor population of mature T cells are the $\gamma^+\delta^+$ T cells (because they express a related two-chain TCR derived from the TCR γ and δ loci). Much of our current information on T-lymphocyte development comes from analysis of $\alpha^+\beta^+$ T-cell development. These T lymphocytes represent the T-cell subset that responds primarily to viral infection, and the selection process of these T cells in the thymus will be emphasized here. The $\gamma^+\delta^+$ T-cell subset likely plays a secondary role in the adaptive response to most virus infections, and the properties/function of this T-cell subset is summarized below.

T-Lymphocyte development in the thymus proceeds in a stepwise fashion with the sequential generation and expression of one (i.e., TCR-β or TCR-δ), and then the other (i.e., TCR-α or TCR-γ) TCR chain by random somatic recombination as thymocytes mature. A complex of four cell-surface molecules called CD3 (CD3 γ, δ, ε, and ξ), which are noncovalently associated with the TCR and are critical for signaling through the TCR, are also expressed during T-lymphocyte development. Specific antigen recognition by the TCR-α:β (or γ:δ) heterodimer is transduced into the cells by the CD3 complex. Concomitant with the expression of the rearranged TCR chains and the signal transducting CD3 complex, the developing thymocytes simultaneously express two co-receptor molecules, CD4 and CD8. Early in the developmental program, thymocytes do not express CD4 or CD8, and they are classified as immature, *double-negative* thymocytes. As thymic development/differentiation proceeds, immature thymocytes that express both CD4 and CD8 co-receptors (as well as CD3 complex and the TCR-α and β chains) and, at this point, are classified as are $CD4^+/CD8^+$ *double-positive* thymocytes. CD4 and CD8 molecules recognize structurally conserved domains on the MHC class II and I molecules, respectively. As a result of binding to MHC molecules displaying self-peptides on the surface of thymic stromal cells, CD4 or CD8 also delivers signals to the developing immature thymocytes. The combined signaling by TCR/CD3 complex and the CD4 or CD8 co-receptor directs the development of the immature thymocytes into *single-positive* $CD4^+$ or $CD8^+$ mature thymocytes (expressing TCR, CD3, and either CD4 or CD8).

Because the TCR does not recognize foreign molecules directly (but rather small fragments of molecules bound to MHC molecules), the TCR generated and expressed on developing thymocytes must recognize both MHC molecules and the peptide fragments bound to these molecules. The source of these peptides bound by MHC class I and class II molecules are self-proteins expressed by several different cell types in the thymus. The selection of the thymocytes that ultimately become mature co-receptor *single-positive* T lymphocytes ($CD4^+$ or $CD8^+$) and populate the secondary lymphoid organs is a process in the thymus of positive and negative selection.

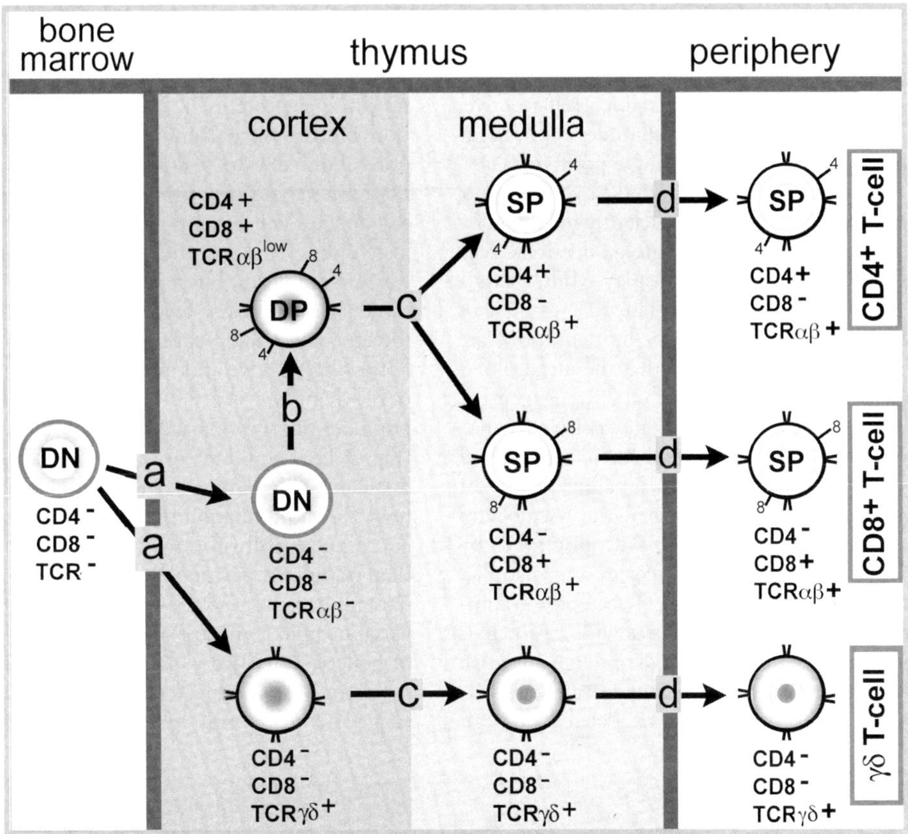

FIGURE 9.1. T-Lymphocyte development and selection in the thymus. The progenitors of mature peripheral T lymphocytes arise in the bone marrow as mononuclear stem cell progenitors committed to T-cell lineage development, but lacking cell surface receptors characteristic of T-lymphocyte lineage (e.g., T-cell receptors [TCRs] or the co-receptors CD4 and CD8). These TCR- and co-receptor–deficient "double negative" (DN) cells enter the thymic cortex **(a)** from the bloodstream as CD4/CD8-deficient DN lymphocytes. In the case of conventional TCR$\alpha\beta$ T cells, the DN cells also lack antigen receptor. The cells then undergo a multistep differentiation process **(b)**, which results in cells simultaneously expressing both CD4 and CD8 as well as a low level expression of the TCR$\alpha\beta$ receptor complex—so-called double-positive (DP) thymocytes. Within the thymic cortex and medulla **(c)**, the DP cells first undergo "positive selection"—that is, selection for those cells with TCR$\alpha\beta$ and CD4 or CD8 co-receptor complexes capable of interaction with self-peptide/major histocompatibility complex (MHC) ligands. DP thymocytes that interact with self-peptide/MHC ligand with insufficient avidity die (undergo apoptosis). The surviving DP thymocytes then transition into either CD4$^+$ or CD8$^+$ single-positive (SP) thymocytes, which then undergo a process of "negative selection." In this case, only those SP thymocytes with an appropriate immediate affinity for self-peptide/MHC complexes survive and go on to traffic through the thymus into the bloodstream to ultimately proceed to the secondary lymphoid organs **(d)** as mature peripheral CD4$^+$ or CD8$^+$ T cells. The TCR$\gamma\delta$ T cells likewise arrive in the thymus **(a)** as DN progenitors, which eventually upregulate the $\gamma\delta$ TCR **(b)** and undergo a form of positive and negative selection **(c)** without upregulation of the canonical co-receptors through a selection process that is not well understood. The TCR$\gamma\delta$ T cells will exit the thymus **(d)** and populate peripheral sites including mucosal surfaces and secondary lymphoid organs. Natural regulatory T-cells (T_{reg}) cells (not shown) undergo selection for recognition of self-peptide/MHC class II ligands late in thymocyte differentiation by a selection process poorly understood that this time.

At a specific development stage, immature double-positive thymocytes (expressing the randomly generated $\alpha{:}\beta$ TCR, CD3, and both CD4/CD8) encounter, within the thymic cortex, thymic cortical epithelial cells displaying MHC class I and II molecules complexed with self-peptides. Most of these thymocytes (~80%) have randomly generated TCR that are unable to bind to the self-peptide/MHC molecular complexes. In the absence of a signal delivered through the TCR, these thymocytes will die by apoptosis. Those double-positive thymocytes whose TCR can bind the self-peptide/MHC complexes above a threshold avidity augmented by either a CD4 or a CD8 co-receptor binding to the MHC molecule will undergo positive selection and survive. If the thymocyte TCR can bind peptides bound to MHC class II molecules in association with the CD4 co-receptor, this interaction will result in the silencing of the CD8 co-receptor gene. This signaling event results in the development of a CD4$^+$ single-positive thymocyte whose TCR recognizes (is restricted to) peptides bound to MHC class II molecules. Similarly, the double-positive thymocytes whose TCR and associated CD8 molecule can recognize MHC class I/self-peptide complexes with sufficient avidity to survive (i.e., those that are positively-selected) will give rise to MHC class I–restricted CD8$^+$ single-positive thymocytes by a similar silencing mechanism of the *CD4* gene.

After undergoing positive selection, the surviving single-positive thymocytes are all auto-reactive (i.e., directed to self-peptide/MHC complexes). Therefore, a process of negative selection must then ensue to eliminate/reduce self-reactive, mature peripheral T cells. Although less well understood, negative selection of the $\alpha:\beta$ TCR-expressing single-positive ($CD4^+$ or $CD8^+$) thymocytes probably occurs in both the thymus cortex and medulla. Negative selection is most efficiently mediated by mononuclear cells of hematopoietic origin (e.g., dendritic cells and macrophages) that simultaneously display MHC class I and II molecules expressing self-peptides. The 10% to 20% of thymocytes that survive positive selection, by definition, are auto-reactive. It is likely (but not certain) that the intracellular signal transduction cascade associated with TCR engagement is altered in the cortical and medullary single-positive thymocytes following positive selection. As a result these cortical and medullary thymocytes acquire the TCR-signaling profile of mature T lymphocytes. Consequently, when the thymocytes encounter the self-peptide/MHC complexes displayed by hematopoietic origin cells like DC in the cortex and medulla, those thymocytes whose TCR/CD4 or CD8 co-receptor complex recognizes self-peptide/MHC complexes with a sufficient avidity to activate will be eliminated (i.e., undergo negative selection—death by apoptosis). Thymocytes directed to self-"tissue specific" molecules (e.g., insulin) are deleted through the action of the autoimmune regulator (*AIRE*) gene. This gene is expressed in thymic medullary stromal cells and triggers the transient low level expression of many extrathymic tissue-specific self-proteins in these cells resulting in negative selection of tissue-reactive single-positive thymocytes. Therefore, only about 2% to 5% of immature thymocytes will survive the positive and negative selection processes. These remaining thymocytes will have the properties of mature $CD4^+$ or $CD8^+$ T lymphocytes (i.e., they have TCR that recognize peptide/MHC complexes, but will only interact with the MHC molecules with sufficient avidity to activate when the appropriate foreign [microbial] peptides are bound to the MHC molecule). Following positive and negative selection, these single-positive $\alpha:\beta$ T lymphocytes ($CD4^+$ or $CD8^+$) will leave the thymus to populate the secondary lymphoid organs as peripheral T cells (Fig. 9.1). The $CD4^+$ or $CD8^+$ $\alpha:\beta$ T cells represent 70% to 80% of the circulating extrathymic T-cell population—the primary T-cell population that responds to virus infection.

The second (minor) population of thymus-derived cells that populates peripheral sites is that of the $\gamma:\delta$ T cells, so named because they employ a heterodimeric TCR whose variable (and constant) region is encoded by a distinct set of genetic loci (the γ locus and the δ locus) homologous to the α and β TCR loci[103] (Table 9.3). These *TCR* genes rearrange in the thymus in a manner analogous to that of the

TABLE 9.3 T Lymphocyte Subsets

TCR $\alpha:\beta$	Dominant T-cell Type Responding to Virus Infection		
	$CD8^+$	Recognize major histocompatibility complex (MHC) class I viral peptide complexes, and are important adaptive immune antiviral effector cells	
	$CD4^+$	Recognize MHC class II viral peptide complexes, and regulate B-cell differentiation and host inflammatory responses to infection	
		T_H1	Effector $CD4^+$ T cells that produce proinflammatory antiviral cytokines (e.g., IFN-γ) characterized by mononuclear cell inflammatory infiltrates
		T_H2	Effector $CD4^+$ T cells that produce cytokines linked to allergic responses (e.g., IL-4, IL-5)
		T_H17	Effector $CD4^+$ T cells that produce pro-inflammatory cytokines (e.g., IL-17A/F, IL-6) associated with antibacterial responses and characterized by neutrophil-rich inflammatory infiltrates
		T_{FH}	Activated $CD4^+$ T cells that produce cytokines /chemokines (e.g., IL-21), which facilitate B-cell differentiation in SLO and which are retained in the SLO
TCR $\gamma:\delta$	Play a prominent role as "innate-like" effector cells –Express the CD3 complex, but usually not CD4 or CD8 –The generation process of $\gamma:\delta$ TCR chains in the thymus is similar to that of the dominant TCR $\alpha:\beta$ T-cell TCR –Present in the circulation and lymphoid organs and prominently expressed at body surfaces (e.g., gut, skin) –Recognize products of stressed cells—no restriction in recognition by MHC class I/II molecules, but can recognize lipid complexed to MHC class Ib molecules		
NKT	Act as "innate-like" immune effectors early in immune responses –Express conventional TCR $\alpha:\beta$ chains, and can use a restricted number of possible TCR genes (i.e., invariant NK T-cells [iNK T cells]) –Express CD4 molecules (most NK T cells) and NK cell markers, but not CD8 molecules –Recognize products of stressed cells and can recognize lipid moieties displayed by MHC class Ib–related molecules on cell surfaces –Activation of TCR triggers release of regulatory cytokines (e.g., IL-4)		
T_{reg}	Conventional TCR $\alpha:\beta$ T cells that control the response of T and B lymphocytes to foreign (e.g., viral) antigens and self-proteins –Dominant population expresses CD4 and CD25 –May occur spontaneously during T-cell differentiation (natural Treg cells) or after exposure to foreign (e.g., viral) antigen (inducible Treg cells) –Regulates (usually suppresses) the response of $CD4^+$ T cells and $CD8^+$ T cells to infectious agents and self-constituents		

IFN, interferon; TCR, T-cell receptor; IL, interleukin; NKT, natural killer T cells.

dominant $\alpha:\beta$ TCR T-cell homolog. The generation of $\gamma:\delta$ T cells in the thymus precedes $\alpha:\beta$ T-cell development. The $\gamma:\delta$ T cells are generated in two waves during T-cell development in the fetus. The first wave of maturing thymocytes consists of cells with limited TCR V gene diversity (i.e., utilize one or few $V\gamma$ and $V\delta$ rearrangement in their TCR). After selection, these $\gamma:\delta$ T cells leave the thymus, traffick through the circulation, and preferentially localize to epithelial surfaces, particularly the skin, gut, and urogenital tract. The second wave of $\gamma:\delta$ T cells, as with $\alpha:\beta$ T cells, displays a highly diverse TCR array, and these cells localize to the secondary lymphoid tissues. Unlike the $\alpha:\beta$ TCR, however, the $\gamma:\delta$ TCR does not recognize peptides bound to the MHC class I or II locus products. Rather, $\gamma:\delta$ T cells either directly recognize structures such as heat shock proteins displayed on the surface of the infected cells, or recognize lipid or glyco/phospholipids moieties bound to MHC-like molecules (e.g., nonpolymorphic MHC Ib molecules) on the surface of stressed (infected) cells. The subset of intraepithelial $\gamma:\delta$ T cells, in particular, differs from the $\alpha:\beta$ T cells, and appears to function like cells of the innate immune system, recognizing not a specific pathogen, but alterations in epithelial cells induced by infection with microbes such as bacteria. At present, no direct role for $\gamma:\delta$ T cells in the control of virus infection has been firmly established although this T-cell subset has been implicated in the control of HIV and herpesvirus infection in humans.[5]

Among the other T-lymphocyte subsets (Table 9.3) generated during development are NK T cells, so-called because these $\alpha:\beta$ TCR-expressing T cells display cell-surface markers shared with NK cells, most notably the C-type lectin NK 1.1. NK T cells are divided into two subsets $CD4^+$ $CD8^-$ or $CD4^-CD8^-$ based on co-receptor expression. One subset of NK T cells employs a range of $\alpha:\beta$ V gene combinations in their expressed TCR. The other NK T-cell subset is similar to $CD4^-$ and $CD8^-$ $\gamma:\delta$ T cells, in that the cells utilize a limited number of TCR $\alpha:\beta$ V genes in receptor generation and are classified as invariant NK T cells (iNK T cells). The iNK T cells recognize foreign and self-lipid/glycolipid bound to MHC-like cell-surface CD1 molecules. The NK T cells with diverse TCR usage by contrast, directly recognize self- or microbial gene products rather than peptide/MHC complexes. Although not as yet certain, the CD1/lipid complexes and the self-moieties (e.g., heat shock proteins) recognized by NK T cells are likely produced or upregulated by cells in response to virus infection.

One T-lymphocyte subset has recently been recognized as a critical regulator of the adaptive immune responses to both infectious agents and self-molecules: the regulator T lymphocyte (T_{reg}) subset. The TCR on T_{reg} cells utilize rearranged $\alpha:\beta$ TCR gene products, and appear (at least in experimental animals) to arise late in thymic development (i.e., after the major wave of both $\gamma:\delta$ $\alpha v \delta \alpha:\beta$ T-cell generation). As mature thymocytes, T_{reg} cells appear able to recognize self-peptides bound to MHC molecules and directly activate without undergoing negative selection. Therefore, T_{reg} cells that display primarily the CD4 co-receptor exist both in the thymus (as mature thymocytes) and in the periphery (i.e., in secondary lymphoid organs) as *activated* $CD4^+$ T cells. The encounter with self and the resulting activation of T_{reg} cells, however, does not result in autoimmunity. Rather, recent evidence suggests that these T cells suppress/downregulate the activity of conventional $CD4^+$ and $CD8^+$ T cells responding to viral infection. Although both the role of T_{reg} cells in adaptive immune responses and their mechanism of action are not yet fully understood, these cells may prevent the development of excessive injury during T-cell responses to infection, and suppress the development of autoimmune responses during viral infection. Recent emerging information on the role of T_{reg} cells in virus infection is discussed in a separate section below.

Secondary Lymphoid Organs: Structure and Function

The mature naïve (resting) B and T lymphocytes that egress from their development site (bone marrow and thymus, respectively) enter the blood, and then migrate to secondary (peripheral) lymphoid organs (SLOs). The SLOs play a critical role in the initiation of the adaptive (T- and B-cell) immune response to viruses and other microbes. The major SLOs are the lymph nodes (LNs), the spleen, and the so-called mucosal-associated lymphoid tissue (MALT). LNs are highly organized structures located at vessel convergence points in the lymphatic system, a system that collects fluids and cells from the tissues of most internal organs (e.g., liver, stomach) and body surfaces (e.g., skin, mucosa of the gastrointestinal [GI], genitourinary [GU], and respiratory tracts). The capacity of lymphatic vessels to collect antigen (e.g., virus, viral constituents) from the body surfaces/tissues, and deliver them to the LNs (where antigen concentrates) is essential for the efficient triggering of the adaptive immune response to microbes. The spleen plays a role similar to that of the LN network; however, the spleen is uniquely suited to collect antigen (virus) directly from the bloodstream, because of its unique architecture and extensive blood circulation. The third class of SLOs, the MALT, is composed of specialized lymphoid aggregates associated with major mucosal surfaces and sites of microbial invasions (e.g., the GI, GU, and respiratory tracts). The gut-associated MALT (also called GALT) includes tonsils, adenoids, appendix, and Peyer's patches in the small intestine. In the respiratory tract are similar, but more diffuse, aggregates of lymphoid tissues associated with the epithelium of small/medium airways (i.e., bronchial-associated lymphoid tissue [BALT]). As with the other SLOs, the MALTs are sites of antigen localization where the initiation/induction of the adaptive immune response can occur.

The common feature of SLOs is the localization of adaptive immune cells (i.e., T and B cells) to distinct regions of the SLOs. For example, most B cells are localized in distinct follicles within the LN cortex. Activation of B cells specific for a pathogen/antigen leads to their proliferation and formation of a germinal center within the LN cortex. T cells within the LN localize to, and are diffusely distributed within, the LN paracortical areas. Other cell types are also distributed within the outer cortex and central medulla of the normal LN. These include stromal cells and cells of macrophage and DC lineage. These cells (particularly DC) play a crucial role in the induction of the adaptive immune response, and serve to direct T-cell/B-cell localization to distinct LN regions through the constitutive release of small (low molecular weight) chemotactic proteins—chemokines. A similar segregation of B cells/T cells to distinct regions occurs within the white pulp of the spleen and the MALT (likewise, under control of chemokines elaborated by SLO-resident cells).

Induction of Adaptive Immune Responses in the Secondary Lymphoid Organs

The body's complement of B and T cells consists of more than 10^9 cells, each of which may display a unique antigen receptor directed to a specific epitope. Therefore, the frequency of B or T cells directed to a specific pathogen is extremely low (e.g., a frequency of 1 of 10^4 to 10^6 naïve B or T cells). The problem faced by the adaptive immune systems is that these rare, antigen-specific cells are distributed randomly throughout the body, and must be rapidly mobilized to respond to invading organism. These rare antigen-specific cells must first contact antigen, then activate and generate effector cells capable of eliminating the pathogen. The solution to this problem is achieved through the process of lymphocyte recirculation through the SLO.[57,273]

Naïve (primary) T cells and most naïve B cells do not permanently reside in the SLOs. Rather, the T and B cells are constantly migrating from the blood through the SLOs and back to the bloodstream. Lymphocyte recirculation is controlled by the expression of distinct homing receptors (adhesion molecules) whose ligands are expressed on cells within the SLO. Naïve $CD4^+$ and $CD8^+$ T cells within the bloodstream express on their surface the adhesion/homing receptor, CD62L (L-selectin). T cells entering the blood vessels encounter the CD62L ligands—the mucin-like moieties CD34 and GlyCam-1 that are constitutively displayed in the endothelium of specialized high endothelial venules (HEVs) within the LN cortex. The interaction of CD62L (on the T cell) with its endothelial cell ligands arrests the T cell's migration through the blood vessel, which results in its binding to the HEV endothelial cell. Other adhesion receptors displayed on endothelial cells that recognize carbohydrate ligands displayed on the surface of lymphocytes (as well as the $\alpha_L\beta_2$ integrin, lymphocyte function-associated antigen 1 [LFA-1] displayed on lymphocytes) also contribute to the arrest of T-cell migration. The naïve circulating T cells also constitutively express a chemokine receptor (CCR7) that recognizes specific chemokines (CCL19, CCL21) displayed on the surface of the HEV endothelial cells. These chemokines are produced by the HEV cells and by cell types within the LN (e.g., DC and stromal cells). The chemokines produced by the latter cell types diffuse into the HEV and are bound to/displayed on, the surface of the HEV endothelial cell. The interaction between the CCR7 receptor on the arrested T cells and its chemokine ligand triggers the migration of the naïve T cells through the HEV and into the LN cortex (parafollicular T-cell region). If the T cells do not encounter antigen, they traffic through the LN cortex to the LN medulla, and then exit the LN though the efferent lymphatic vessels, and ultimately return to the bloodstream where the process of recirculation though the SLO begins again. The egress of naïve T cells from the LN is as noted above, controlled by a chemotactic receptor S1P1R for the lipid sphingosine-1-P (S1P). S1P is present at higher concentrations in lymph and blood than in the LN. S1P1R engagement attracts naïve T cells away from the LN and back into the circulation. Antigen recognition by T cells transiently downregulates S1P1R retaining the antigen detecting T cells in the LN.

Naïve B cells traffic through the LN by similar mechanisms and transiently localize to the lymphoid follicles along a chemokine gradient mediated by a specific chemokine receptor, CXCR5, displayed on the surface of circulating naïve B cells. Lymphocyte trafficking through the spleen and MALT are likewise regulated by the interplay of adhesion receptor/ligand interactions and chemokines constitutively expressed in these SLOs. In the case of MALT, a set of unique receptor/ligand interactions (restricted to these sites) guides the trafficking of adaptive immune cells to these specialized mucosal sites.

Afferent lymphatic vessels are localized in all body surfaces/tissues, and they drain into the LN. Virus infection of a body surface/tissue triggers the innate immune system—the initial defense against infection. Innate immune cells located at the body surfaces/tissues (specifically, DC and monocyte/macrophages) encounter pathogen, take up virus/viral antigen, and then activate/migrate through the afferent lymphatics to the draining LN. In the draining LN, these migrating cells (along with DC and, to a lesser extent, monocyte/macrophages present in the LN cortex) serve as antigen-bearing presenting cells (APCs) to the naïve B and T lymphocytes trafficking through the LN. As a result of encounter with antigen displayed on the APCs, the lymphocytes with antigen receptors specific for the antigen or pathogen will no longer traffic through the LN, but rather will be retained in the LN (due to S1P1R downregulation) and initiate the process of activation and differentiation, leading to the generation of specific effector B and T cells directed to the pathogen. Therefore, the SLO concentrate antigen in a specific site where the rare antigen-specific, naïve B and T cells circulating through the body can encounter and respond to the pathogen. Afferent lymphatics can also carry large particulates (e.g., viruses as well as "soluble" viral proteins) directly to the LN where the particulates can be captured by macrophages lining subcapsular lymph node sinuses and subsequently delivered to DC or presented to naïve T cells, as well as directed along with soluble antigens through fibroreticular conduits to B cells and a lymphoid follicles.[95,125]

If infection by a virus is localized to the body surface (e.g., papillomavirus infection of the skin or influenza virus infection of the respiratory tract), then the adaptive immune response to that pathogen will be induced primarily in the LN draining these sites. Virus infections that result in systemic spread (i.e., viremia) will also induce adaptive immune responses in the spleen. Viruses that infect sites where MALT is prominent (e.g., rotavirus infection in the Peyer's patches of the small intestine) will trigger the local induction of the adaptive immune responses at the site of MALT localization.[196]

ANTIGEN PRESENTING CELLS AND THE INDUCTION OF ADAPTIVE IMMUNE RESPONSES

As with most microorganisms, viruses enter the body surfaces where the initial encounter with the immune system occurs. These body surfaces (e.g., skin and mucosa of the GI, GU, and respiratory tracts) contain epithelial lining cells, which can serve as the initial cells supporting virus replication. The epithelial surfaces also contain DC, specialized cells of bone marrow origin, which serve as both infection sentinels and APCs, which migrate to the SLOs and deliver antigen to the adaptive immune cells that are trafficking from the blood to the SLOs. A large body of evidence now suggests that DCs are critical APCs for the induction of the primary adaptive immune (T cell) response.[184]

For our purposes, two classes or types of DCs, conventional DCs (cDCs) and plasmacytoid DCs (pDCs) can be distinguished. cDCs are localized to the body surfaces and SLOs where they exist as immature (inactive) DCs prior to infection and carry out the aforementioned sentinel and APC function. As discussed below, a subset of cDCs identified by expression of CD8α in the SLO and αE integrin CD103 in mucosal tissue has the capacity to efficiently take up and present cellular material—for example, apoptotic-infected cells, particulates like viruses, and soluble proteins—to naïve CD8$^+$ T cells without direct infection of the DC. pDCs, so-called because of their plasma cell–like morphology are derived from blood monocyte precursors and recruited to sites of inflammation/infection where, following activation, they are major producers of type 1α-interferons.[80] In most circumstances these important innate immune effectors cells have limited capacity to act as APC for naïve T cells.

cDCs localize to the epithelium within the epithelial cell layer (e.g., Langerhans' cells in the skin) at the junction of the epithelial basement membrane in GI and respiratory tracts, as well as in the mucosa and submucosa underlying the epithelial surface. The cDCs at body surfaces are derived from circulating monocytic progenitors originating in the bone marrow, which are present in the blood and migrate to the body surfaces and differentiate into peripheral (tissue) DCs. These tissue DCs exist as immature (inactive) DCs at these sites, turn over at a low variable rate, and are replenished by the circulating blood monocyte progenitors that enter the tissues.

Immature DCs are sessile cells that have a particular set of phenotypic markers or characteristics. They express low to intermediate levels of cell-surface MHC class I and class II molecules; the latter (class II) molecules are found predominately not on the DC surface, but within specialized endocytic vesicles. Immature DCs also express low levels of cell-surface molecules, which serve as co-stimulatory ligands for naïve lymphocytes (e.g., CD80, CD86, CD40, CD83).[272] These molecules play a critical accessory role in the triggering of naïve antigen-specific (e.g., virus-specific) T cells, ultimately leading to the generation of effector (i.e., antiviral) T and B cells, and the formation of memory T and B cells directed to the pathogen. In addition, immature DCs have the ability to take up particulate and fluid-phase antigen into pinocytic/phagocytic vesicles with high efficiency. The enhanced capacity of these DCs to take up material (including the remains of infected apoptotic cells) likely accounts for their unique capacity to serve as APCs.[185]

The initiation of an inflammatory response at the body surface (as produced by virus infection) triggers the DC activation (maturation) process. Activation of the tissue-resident DC results in the *de novo* expression/upregulation of chemokine receptors (notably, CCR7), which renders the activated DCs capable of migrating from the peripheral tissue, primarily through lymphatic vessels along a gradient of constitutively expressed CCR7 ligands, the CCL19/CCL21 chemokines produced by lymphatic endothelial cells. Activation of the tissue DCs is also accompanied by upregulated expression of MHC class I/II molecules, and co-stimulatory ligands resulting in the maturation of the DCs, which, on activation/maturation, characteristically express high cell-surface levels of MHC class I/II molecules and the co-stimulatory ligands, CD80/86, CD40, and CD83. Mature DCs migrate to the SLOs where they act as the principal APCs for the induction of the adaptive immune response. Therefore, DCs (and to a lesser extent macrophages) serve the dual role of delivery (concentration) of antigen to the SLOs and acting as APCs to retain/activate the rare antigen-specific adaptive immune cell entering the SLOs from the circulation.

Immature DCs can be triggered to activate by virus infection through at least three mechanisms:

1. *Direct infection* of immature DCs. The stimulus for DC activation/maturation is provided primarily by the interaction of viral nucleic acids with (and signaling through) microbial pattern-recognizing Toll-like receptors (TLRs) displayed by DC,[129] and/or activation of intracellular antiviral signaling mechanisms mediated by the RNA-activated protein kinase (PKR kinase),[240] the retinoic-acid–inducible protein I (RIG-I) helicase systems,[130] and for some viruses the caspase/IL-1β–associated inflammasome.[289]
2. *Uptake of virus* and soluble antigen (or more likely the remnant of infected epithelial cells that have undergone apoptosis in response to infection) with activation of immature DC through binding to one or more scavenger or C-type lectin receptor(s), for example, dendritic and epithelial cells, 205 kDa (DEC-205); dendritic cell-specific intercellular adhesion molecule-3 grabbing non-integrin (DC-SIGN) displayed on DC with specificity for carbohydrates on viral glycoproteins/glycolipids[274] or through the process of phagocytic uptake.
3. Dendritic cell activation/maturation induced by *inflammatory mediators* (i.e., cytokines, such as TNF-α) released by infected epithelial cells and tissue macrophages in response to TLR and/or intracellular antiviral signaling.

The first two types of virus encounters with immature DC will result in the initiation of the adaptive immune response by delivery of virus/viral antigen to the SLO presented by the activated/mature DC. The significance of inflammatory mediator–induced DC maturation in the induction of the antiviral immune response is still not clear, because the activated, mature DC would not directly deliver viral antigen and would not serve as an APC.

Direct infection of immature DCs and the subsequent migration of the activated/mature DCs to the SLOs would appear to be the most likely mechanism to ensure the induction of an effective antiviral adaptive immune response. Whereas this mechanism of viral antigen delivery to T and B lymphocytes in the SLO occurs,[36] it raises the important question: *How do viruses with a very narrow cell tropism, which are unable to either infect or express viral genes in hematopoietic cells like DC (e.g., papillomaviruses) initiate an immune response?*

The capacity of certain immature cDCs to take up and internalize cellular debris such as apoptotic remnants of infected epithelial cells provides the most likely mechanism for triggering adaptive immune T-cell responses. This process of the uptake of infected cell material with presentation to T cells by cDCs is called cross-presentation[259] and is carried out by CD8α^+ cDCs in SLO and by CD103$^+$ cDCs at mucosal surfaces. Indeed, the speculation based on evidence from experimental viral infection is that endocytic uptake of virions or material from virus-infected cells may be the primary/sole mechanism of viral antigen presentation—at least to virus-specific naïve CD8$^+$ T cells.[230] The relative contribution of direct presentation (virus infection of DC), and *cross-presentation* of viral antigen remains controversial[296] and will differ for different viruses.

Naïve (primary) T lymphocytes have stringent requirements for activation that include both TCR antigen receptor engagement by the appropriate processed antigenic peptide/MHC complexes and engagement of co-stimulatory receptors (e.g., CD28) displayed on naïve T cells by their corresponding ligands (e.g., CD80/86) along with peptide/MHC complexes by APC. Mature, antigen-bearing DCs are uniquely suited to carry out this process. The inflammatory response triggered by virus infection triggers DC maturation/migration. Virus infection also results in the infection of and/or antigen uptake by tissue macrophages. However, the migration of infected DC and macrophages along with infectious virions (either cell-associated or free) from the body surface to the SLO, not only initiates an immune response in the SLO, but also can in many instances spread infection to other sites in the body. One classic example of this is the dissemination of poxvirus from a peripheral infection site (body surface) to the SLOs, where free (infectious) virions and infected cells carried from the inoculation site to the SLOs can result in additional virus replication there, followed by virus entry into the bloodstream.[78] Migrant macrophages are probably not as efficient as mature DCs in triggering primary immune response, but they may also serve as a potential APC in the induction of recall memory (secondary) immune responses where the requirements for memory T- and B-lymphocyte activation are less stringent.[71] In this regard, it should also be noted that the mature migrant DCs that have entered the SLOs in response to virus infection may not be the primary APCs for T-cell activation. Several lines of evidence suggest the LN-resident DCs (particularly, CD8α expressing cDCs) can capture viral antigen delivered by migrant DCs (or macrophages), and present that antigen to naïve (primary) T lymphocytes in the SLOs—not by direct infection, but by the transfer of viral antigen from migrant antigen-bearing DCs to SLO-resident DCs through cross-presentation.[296] Intact virions and/or soluble (free, intact) viral antigen, however, undoubtedly contribute to the induction of effective antiviral antibody response by B lymphocytes (as discussed in a later section of this chapter).

Studies examining the induction of adaptive immune responses using confocal and intravital multiphoton microscopy in intact viable LN have provided new insight into the early interaction events between DC-APCs and antigen-specific B and T lymphocytes.[27,255] Some studies indicate that, on entering the draining LN, activated (mature) DCs migrate under a chemokine gradient stimulus to the paracortical T-cell regions in the vicinity of the HEV.[35] Therefore, antigen-bearing DCs would be in the precise location to interact with naïve virus-specific B and T lymphocytes that have entered the draining LN from the circulation and, thereby, initiate the adaptive immune response. However, soluble antigens (viral proteins) and particulates such as virions that entered the LN via lymphatics may be presented to T cells, and particularly B cells, by mechanisms not involving DC migration from the site of infection.[94]

Activation of T and B Lymphocytes in the Secondary Lymphoid Organs

The precise localization of T cells, B cells, DCs, and macrophages within the SLOs is controlled by chemokines, which are largely produced by stromal cells of the SLOs, and by bone marrow–derived cells (e.g., SLO-resident DCs). In draining LN, naïve (primary) T cells that are present in the circulation will enter the LN through the specialized HEV, where they encounter mature DCs (and macrophages) displaying processed antigen bound to MHC molecules, which are localized to sites in the parafollicular cortex of the LN facilitate interaction with T cells. Most naïve CD8$^+$ T cell and CD4$^+$ T cells entering the LN will not recognize the antigen (i.e., they have TCRs that fail to recognize the processed antigen with sufficient avidity to activate the cells). These T cells will ignore the DCs and migrate from the LN cortex to the medulla, then enter the efferent lymphatics, and ultimately return to the bloodstream to continue their perpetual search for relevant antigen.[273] A similar process of lymphocyte egress through the HEV occurs in the MALT; for example, Peyer's patches of the small intestine where antigen uptake by mucosal DCs and direct viral antigen transfer to the gut MALT through specialized intestinal epithelial cells, called M cells, result in antigen delivery to these mucosal lymphoid aggregates.[150] Viruses that enter the bloodstream (i.e., produce viremia) as well as any antigen-bearing tissue DCs that, on maturation, bypass the LN and gain access to the circulation will localize to the splenic white pulp. Here, circulating T and B lymphocytes enter the splenic white pulp by transiting through splenic arterioles where viral antigen-bearing DCs can encounter lymphocytes. The lymphocytes that do not recognize antigen will exit the splenic white pulp by entering trabecular veins, and re-enter the circulation.

The rare naïve CD8$^+$ T cells and CD4$^+$ T cells that recognize processed antigenic peptides displayed on the APC surface in the SLO do so through TCR engagement. The activation of naïve T cells leading to the induction of the adaptive immune response is a multistep process (at both the molecular and cellular level).[112] For induction of antigen-specific (virus-specific) CD8$^+$ T-cell responses, the activation process requires both interaction of the antigen-specific TCR $\alpha{:}\beta$ chain complex with *processed* antigen fragments bound to MHC class I molecules on the APC surface, with sufficient avidity and interaction of the CD8 molecule on the T cell with a region of the MHC class I molecule distant from the site of peptide binding. To fully activate the naïve CD8$^+$ (or CD4$^+$) T cells, additional signaling events must occur, including binding of the co-stimulatory receptor, the CD28 molecule, displayed on naïve T lymphocytes with its ligands, CD80/86, which are displayed at high levels on mature (activated), antigen-bearing DCs. The sequence of events resulting in the activation of antigen-specific naïve CD4$^+$ T cells parallels the steps in CD8$^+$ T-cell activation, except that the antigen-recognizing TCR $\alpha{:}\beta$ chain complex must bind (with sufficient avidity) the antigenic peptides bound to MHC class II molecules displayed by APC; and the CD4 co-receptor on CD4$^+$ T cells, in turn, must interact with a distinct site (outside of the region of peptide binding) on the MHC class II molecule. One important early consequence of CD4$^+$ T-cell activation by antigen is the upregulation of the expression of the CD154 molecule on activated CD4$^+$ T cells. CD154 (also called CD40 ligand or CD40L) is a member of the *TNF* gene family, and, as its name implies, is a ligand for CD40 (a TNF receptor gene family member). CD40 is expressed on both activated/mature DCs and antigen-activated B cells. Engagement of CD40 on DCs and B cells by CD154 (CD40L) on activated CD4$^+$ T cells has important consequences for the function of these cells. Engagement of CD40 on DCs results in increased synthesis of certain cytokines (notably IL-12) by the antigen-bearing DCs in the SLO, which promotes CD4$^+$ and CD8$^+$

T-cell differentiation into effectors.[142] For B cells, the interaction between CD40-activated B cells and CD40L expressed on activated CD4+ T cells is critical for B-cell differentiation into antibody-secreting effector B cells (plasma cells).[182] Strategies to modulate the CD40/CD40L interaction *in vivo* may have important consequences in vaccine development.

The engagement of the TCR/co-receptor complex, and the CD28 co-stimulatory receptor on T cells in the SLO are the first two critical steps in the induction of a T-cell response to a foreign antigen. This initial antigen encounter by the TCR on specific T cells is called *signal 1* in the lexicon of lymphocyte activation/differentiation. The engagement of the CD28 co-stimulatory receptor is designated as *signal 2*. As a consequence of their interaction with antigen and co-stimulatory ligand displaying DC APC, the naïve T cells halt their transit through the SLO (i.e., downregulation of S1P1R, and are retained there). The APC/T cell encounter leading to signal 1 and 2 transmission in the T cells appears to be of short duration (from 6 to 24 hours), after which the initial programming for T-cell activation/differentiation is independent of additional interaction with antigen.[174,293] Delivery of signals 1 and 2, although necessary, is not sufficient in itself, however, to ensure full T-cell activation/differentiation and the generation of effector and memory T cells to the antigen. A third signal, signal 3, is required to complete the T-cell activation/differentiation program in the SLO. Signal 3 is delivered by soluble mediators (i.e., cytokines and chemokines) produced primarily by cells of the innate immune system (e.g., pDCs mature/activated in cDCs, NK cells, NK T cells), which enter the SLO in response to infection/antigen deposition in the SLO. IL-12 produced by mature (activated) DC in the SLO is a particularly critical type of signal 2 in T-cell responses to virus, because engagement of the IL-12 receptor on activated CD8+ T cell and CD4+ T cells promotes their differentiation into effector T cells with potent antiviral activity (e.g., the generation of cytolytic T cells).[199]

Other cytokines produced during T-cell activation (e.g., type 1 and type II/III IFNs [IFN-α, β, IFN-γ, IFN-*l*, respectively], IL-1, IL-4, IL-6, IL-10 and so on) by innate immune cells responding in the SLOs to virus infection will dramatically modulate the magnitude and type of both the effector and memory T-cell responses. These and other soluble mediators modify the course of T-cell activation/differentiation during the T cell's residence in the SLO.[142]

Similarly, in addition to CD28, other co-stimulatory receptors belonging (like CD28) to the Ig receptor gene family (e.g., Cytolytic T-Lymphocyte antigen-4 [CTL A-4]; inducible T-cell co-stimulator [ICOS]; programmed death-1 [PD-1]) and the TNF receptor gene family (e.g., CD27, OX40, 4-1BB, CD40L) whose expression on activated T cells is temporarily regulated following T-cell activation in the SLO, can either positively (ICOS, CD27) or negatively (PD-1, CTLA-4) regulate the tempo and magnitude of T-cell activation and differentiation into effector cells in the SLO or in peripheral sites of virus infection following interaction with their perspective ligands on APC.[248,252]

The temporal sequence of signal 1, 2, and 3 delivery to T lymphocytes in the SLO is reflected in the morphologic change of the naïve (primary) T cells from small, resting cells to activated lymphoblasts. This is followed by proliferative expansion of the antigen-specific T-cell *clones* in the SLO, and their differentiation into both effector T cells and an expanded population of memory CD8+ T cell and CD4+ T cells. T-cell proliferation is extremely rapid (cell cycle time of ≤6 hours and in one report ≤2 hours,[317] with estimates of individual naïve T-cell precursors undergoing 8 to 20 divisions during this programmed proliferation.[137] During their proliferative expansion and differentiation in the SLO, the responding T cells lose cell-surface adhesion molecules (e.g., CD62L) and receptors (e.g., CCR7) necessary for naïve T-cell circulation, and they upregulate the expression or express *de novo* adhesion molecules (e.g., the β2 integrin, LFA-1, and β1 integrin, very late antigen 4 [VLA-4], respectively), and chemokine receptors (e.g., CCR5, CXCR3) essential for effector T cells to localize to sites of inflammation.[165] At the end of the proliferation/differentiation sequence, most activated antigen-specific effector T cells will upregulate S1P1R and exit the SLO (through the efferent lymphatics in the case of T cells responding in the draining LN), enter the circulation, and traffic to the site of infection/inflammation. The homing of activated T cells is controlled by chemokines released by innate immune cells (as well as by epithelial and endothelial cells and fibroblasts) at the site of inflammation/infection (e.g., CXCL9 [Mig/CXCL9 (Monocline Induced by Gamma interferon)], CXCL10 [IP-10 (Interferon gamma induced Protein-10)], and CXCL11 [I-TAC (Interferon-inducible T cell Alpha Chemoattractant)] for CXCR3; and CCL3 [macrophage inflammatory protein-1α; MIP-1α] and CCL4 [MIP-1β] for CCR5). This homing is also controlled by the inflammation-induced upregulation of integrin ligands (e.g., intercellular adhesion molecule-1 [ICAM-1] for LFA-1, and vascular adhesion molecule [VCAM] for VLA-4) and adhesion receptors (P-selectin, E-selectin) on endothelial/epithelial cells at these sites.

The generation of effector T cells in the SLOs responding to infection can occur in as few as 5 to 7 days in both experimental models and human viral infection.[68] Given the rapid replication of most viruses, it is obviously essential to get specific T cells activated and mobilized as soon as possible through the concentration of antigen and the accumulation of the rare antigen-specific T cells in the SLO, followed by rapid proliferative expansion/differentiation of these cells into effectors in the SLO. The rapid induction of an adaptive immune response to virus infection is not a foregone conclusion, however. The process of T- and B-cell activation can be delayed for weeks to months in the case of infection with viruses such as HIV and HCV, which induce chronic infection.[111,187] In these instances, the virus has the capacity to suppress/delay the induction of the adaptive immune response.

The process of naïve B-cell activation in the SLOs is similar to that of naïve T-cell activation. In the case of B-cell responses to viruses and other T cell–dependent antigens, however, antigen-specific CD4+ T cells play a critical role in driving B-cell activation/differentiation. As with naïve T cells, naïve B cells enter the LN though the HEV; unlike T cells, however, the B cells migrate from the paracortical (T-cell rich) area of the LN and into the B cell–enriched LN cortical follicle. This migration is controlled by the chemokine CXCL13, produced by a stromal cell type resident in the follicle (called a *follicular DC* because of its dendritic morphology, but not of hematopoietic origin). CXCL13 is the ligand for CXCR5 chemokine receptor that is constitutively expressed by naïve B cells. If the B cell does not encounter antigen in the follicle, it will ultimately migrate out of the cortical follicle to the medulla, then enter the efferent lymphatics, and rejoin the circulating pool of B cells in the bloodstream.

The B cells that display a BCR antigen receptor (i.e., the cell-surface membrane-bound form of the immunoglobulin molecule that recognizes antigen) for an antigen present in the LN would encounter this antigen immediately after migrating out of the HEV in the parafollicular (T-cell rich area) of the LN. In the case of viral antigen, the relative contribution of free virus, soluble viral proteins, and viral proteins transported by migrant DC/macrophages from the infection site to the reservoir of antigen present in the SLO and available to specific B cells is not certain. However, it has been recently appreciated that structures (i.e., conduits) within the SLO (in the case of LN) direct particulates like viruses and soluble proteins directly to regions of naïve B-cell accumulation in the SLOs.[125] Binding of antigen to the BCR (i.e., cross-linking cell surface immunoglobulin) provides the initial stimulus (signal 1) for specific B-cell activation. Signal 1 delivery halts the constitutive migration of the B cell from the paracortical T-cell zone to the LN follicle, and activates the chemokine-dependent migration of the B cells to the junction between the T-cell zone and the follicle. The strength of signal 1 can be greatly enhanced if the BCR co-receptor complex[201] is ligated simultaneously with the BCR by interaction with complement components bound to antigen or antigen–antibody complexes. In addition, cross-linking of the immunoglobulin receptor induces internalization of the antigen–immunoglobulin complex into an endosomal compartment where the antigen is fragmented and associates with MHC class II molecules that are constitutively expressed by B cells. The antigen/MHC class II complexes are then cycled to the B-cell surface, where they are available for recognition by antigen-specific $CD4^+$ T cells. Another consequence of signal 1 delivery (by antigen to B cells) is CD40 upregulation. The $CD4^+$ T cells, which interact with antigen-stimulated B cells, are themselves activated by prior encounter with antigen/MHC class II complexes on APC (i.e., mature, antigen-bearing DC), and have upregulated CD154 (CD40L) expression. The activated antigen-specific $CD4^+$ T cells recognize the antigen/MHC complexes on the antigen-stimulated B cells, and deliver signal 2 to the B cells in two forms: interaction of CD40L (on T cells) with CD40 (on B cells), and the release of T-cell–derived cytokines (notably, IL-4, IL-21, and/or IFN-γ) whose synthesis is triggered in the $CD4^+$ T-cell TCR recognition of antigenic peptides displayed by the B cells. Antigen-activated $CD4^+$ T cells in LN may support B cell responses by differentiating into so-called T follicular helper (T_{FH}) cells. These activated $CD4^+$ T cells appear to represent a distinct CXCR 5^+/PD-1^+ $CD4^+$ T-cell subset, the generation of which is in part regulated by IL-6 produced within the responding LN. The cells secrete IL-21 in response to TCR engagement and also express CD154 (CD40L). The interaction of the T_{FH} with the naïve parafollicular B cells through CD40 engagement (on B cells) by CD40L on the T cells, and IL-21 signaling through its receptor on naïve T cells helps support the formation of B-cell germinal centers.

The fully activated (signals 1^+2^+) B-cell lymphoblasts undergo programmed proliferation after migration to the follicles to produce germinal center, which are follicular structures consisting primarily of responding/proliferating B-cell lymphoblasts. The proliferation/differentiation of the germinal center B-cell lymphoblasts results in the formation of antibody-secreting plasma cells, which migrate from the LN to the sites of infection/inflammation, and more importantly to the bone marrow where the plasma cells serve as a depot of long-lived antibody-secreting cells.[167] B cells that encounter antigen without $CD4^+$ T-cell *help* (i.e., receive signal 1, but not signal 2) are capable of producing specific secreted antibodies; however, these antibodies will be of the immunoglobulin M (IgM) isotype and of low affinity. The isotype switch of antibody production from IgM to the IgG, IgA, and so on isotypes, as well as, the process of antibody affinity maturation requires T-cell help (signal 2).[167]

VIRAL ANTIGEN RECOGNITION BY B CELLS

Viral antigens are found on virions, on virus-infected cells, as soluble molecules produced by virally infected cells, and as breakdown products from virions and infected cells. These antigens can be recognized by antibodies in soluble form in plasma or tissues and by antibodies on the surface of B cells (i.e., BCR). If the individual has had previous exposure to viral antigen(s) through infection or vaccination, then specific soluble high-affinity antibodies will likely be present in the plasma. A minority of these antibodies will be reactive with viral antigens presented on virions and virally infected cells and able to function antivirally. Many will be directed to a range of nonsurface viral antigens; that is, they will be functionally inert, but may be useful in the diagnosis of viral infection. In the case of prior infection or vaccination, memory B cells that express specific antibody will be activated on contact with viral antigen, leading to the production of soluble, specific high-affinity antibody and the increase of specific serum antibody levels. In the absence of a previous encounter with viral antigen, antibodies on the surface of naïve B cells will bind antigen with relatively low affinity, setting in motion antibody affinity maturation and class-switching processes, which are discussed below.

NATURE OF B-CELL EPITOPES

Most of what is known about how antibodies recognize antigens has been determined from studies on the interaction of soluble antibodies or antibody fragments with antigen.[61,208,308] Given that B-cell surface antibody is essentially identical to soluble monomeric antibody, with an extra segment ensuring membrane localization, the conclusions should apply broadly to cell surface antibody. Antibodies recognize molecular shapes, termed epitopes, on the surface of antigens. The antibody-combining site makes multiple contacts with the surface of the antigen to form complementary surfaces. The more complementary these surfaces are to one another—in terms of geometry and chemical character—the more favorable interactions will be formed between the antibody and antigen and the higher will be the affinity of the antibody for antigen. The affinity of the antibody for the antigen is one of the most important factors in determining the efficacy of the antibody *in vivo.*

The antibody-combining site is made up of residues contributed primarily from six highly variable segments or loops referred to as hypervariable loops or complementary determining regions (CDRs). The site can vary greatly in shape and character depending on the length and characteristics of the CDRs. Generally, most or all of the CDRs contribute to antigen binding, but their relative contributions vary. The heavy chain CDRs (particularly the third heavy chain CDR [CDR H3]) tend to contribute disproportionately to antigen binding. The CDR H3 in human antibodies can be very long, with distinctive shapes such as fingers and hammerheads that contact viral epitopes. The combining site of antibodies against smaller molecules such as carbohydrates and organic groups (haptens) are often more obviously grooves or pockets, rather than the extended surfaces typically found in antiprotein antibodies.

On the antigen, epitopes come in as many different shapes and sizes as do antibody-combining sites. The area of antigen that contacts antibody, referred to as a footprint, is typically between about 400 and 1,000 Å^2. All antibodies recognize a topographic surface of a protein antigen. Most usually, key residues in the epitope will arise from widely different positions in the linear amino acid sequence of the protein because of the manner in which proteins are folded. The linear sequence typically traverses from one side of the protein to the other a number of times. Such epitopes are described as discontinuous. Occasionally, key residues arise from a linear amino acid sequence. In such cases, the antibody may bind with relatively high affinity to a peptide incorporating the appropriate linear sequence from the antigen. Furthermore, the peptide may inhibit the antigen binding to the antibody. The epitope in such cases is described as continuous. An example of a continuous epitope would be a loop on the surface of the protein for which an antibody recognized successive residues in the loop. It should be noted, however, that an antibody that recognizes a continuous epitope does not bind a random or disordered structure. Rather, it recognizes a defined structure that is found in the complete protein but can be readily adopted by the shorter peptide.

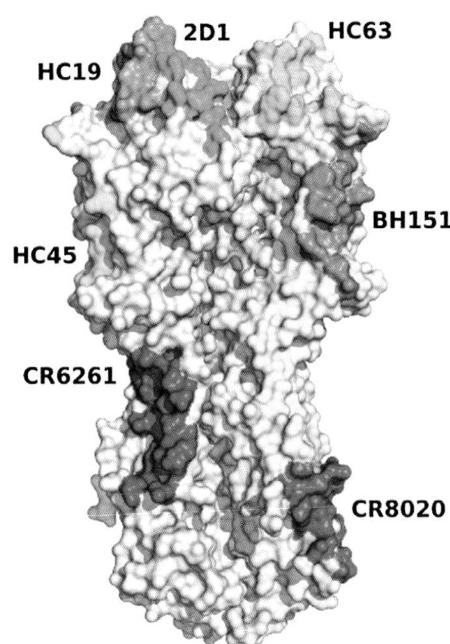

FIGURE 9.2. Neutralizing epitopes on influenza hemagglutinin (HA). The epitopes were determined from crystal structures of neutralizing Fab fragments in complex with HA. The viral membrane is at the **bottom** of the figure. Most of the epitopes toward the top of the HA molecule are relatively variable in different influenza strains. The epitopes defined by the antibodies CR6261 and CR8020 in the stem of the HA molecule are conserved and might be targeted by a universal influenza vaccine. (Courtesy of Damian Ekiert and Ian Wilson.)

ANTIGENICITY AND IMMUNOGENICITY

A clear distinction is seen between the ability of an epitope to be recognized by antibody (antigenicity) and its ability to stimulate an antibody response when presented to a host antibody system (immunogenicity). A number of factors appear to be involved in how well a given epitope elicits an antibody response. Perhaps one of the most important factors is the accessibility of the epitope on the protein surface. Loops that protrude from the surface of the folded protein tend to elicit particularly good antibody responses. Figure 9.2 shows epitopes on the hemagglutinin (HA) protein from the surface of the influenza virus, with those at the "top" of the molecule distant from the viral membrane and most accessible to antibody. Natural infection and classical vaccination strategies typically induce antibodies to the top of the HA and mostly to variable regions that are therefore strain specific. Changes within these immunodominant variable regions allow neutralization escape and dictate repeated annual influenza vaccinations to provide robust protection to large populations. More conserved regions in the stem region of the HA appear to induce weaker antibody responses, but if these could be presented in a more immunodominant format they might induce broadly neutralizing antibodies and thereby provide a universal influenza vaccine that would replace the current annual vaccines. HIV is another virus in which highly exposed variable regions on the viral surface glycoprotein are immunogenic.[313] Following primary infection, it takes some time (weeks) for neutralizing antibodies to reach a level where they interfere with virus replication.[229,303] These antibodies are typically elicited to exposed variable loops on the virus. While these antibodies are being elicited, the virus has diversified (i.e., it has become a swarm of related viruses through the errors associated with reverse transcription of this RNA retrovirus). Among this swarm is a virus that has sequence changes in the epitopes targeted by the neutralizing antibody response that allows it to escape from the response. This new virus becomes predominant. Eventually, a response is mounted to this virus and a second new virus emerges and so on. The antibody response chases the virus over many years but never appears to gain control.

An important consideration in relation to viral surface antigens and immunogenicity is the spacing of the antigens on the virion surface.[12] It is well established that haptenated polymers, in which the haptens are spaced at 5 to 10 nm, can induce antibody responses in the absence of T-cell help. For vesicular stomatitis virus (VSV), in which the G protein is found in a highly organized quasicrystalline state on the virion surface, a strong immunodominant T-cell–independent neutralizing antibody response is induced by infection. A poorly organized recombinant form of VSV-G expressed in micelles induces a weaker B-cell response that is partially T-cell dependent. Soluble VSV-G alone, in the absence of adjuvant, fails to induce a B-cell response.

GENERATION OF THE PRIMARY B-CELL REPERTOIRE

The humoral immune system first senses the presence of novel viral antigens through the interaction of B-cell surface antibody (monomeric IgM and/or IgD) with antigen. Individual B cells possess multiple BCRs of identical specificity, which when occupied by antigen, are activated to divide and differentiate. The final results include the production of large amounts of specific, soluble high-affinity antibody and the generation of memory B cells that can be readily triggered to produce high-affinity antibody on repeated encounter with viral antigen.[226] The first encounter of viral antigen is with the primary B-cell repertoire of the individual. This repertoire is large, allowing recognition with low affinity of essentially any molecular shape and, therefore, any viral variant. It is produced in B cells by recombination of a limited set of germline segments.[121,134,169,175] Hence, an individual's primary repertoire is unique to that individual and is in a constant state of flux. Briefly, the variable regions of antibody heavy and light chains are produced by V(D)J recombination in which numerous unique immunoglobulin genes can be made by joining different combinations of the V, D, and J segments at the heavy, and V and J segments at the light, chain loci. In humans, the potential heavy chain repertoire is approximately 50 VH × 27 DH × 6 JH = 8 × 103 different combinations. Similarly, approximately 165 (33 Vλ × 5 Jλ) and 200 (40 Vκ × 5 Jκ) different combinations exist, for a total of 365 light chain (λ and κ) combinations. If we consider that each heavy chain could potentially pair with each light chain, then the diversity of the immunoglobulin repertoire is of the order of 10^6 possible combinations. Further diversity (junctional diversity) is generated because the joining of the V, D, and J gene segments is imprecise.

Although mice and humans use combinatorial and junctional diversity as a mechanism to generate a diverse repertoire, in many species, including birds, cattle, swine, sheep, horses, and rabbits, V(D)J recombination results in assembly and expression of a single functional gene.[169,179] Repertoire diversification is then achieved by gene conversion, a process in which pseudo-V genes are used as templates to be copied into the assembled variable region exon. For example in the chicken, during B-cell development in the bursa of Fabricius, rapidly proliferating B cells undergo gene conversion to diversify the antibody repertoire. Stretches of sequences from germline variable region pseudogenes, located upstream of the functional V genes, are introduced into the VL and VH regions. This process takes place in the ileal Peyer's patches of cattle, swine, and horses, and in the appendix of rabbits.

B-CELL ACTIVATION BY VIRAL ANTIGENS

B cells can recognize and respond to both soluble and membrane-bound viral antigens, although it is likely that, in vivo, the most relevant interaction is with antigen on the surface of APCs.[14,15] The encounter of viral antigens with BCR has two consequences. First, a signal is transmitted into the B cell that is amplified via intracellular pathways and results in the activation of transcription factors such as nuclear factor-kappaB (NF-κB) and AP-1. These factors act to induce specific gene transcription promoting B-cell proliferation and differentiation. Second, the BCR delivers viral antigens to intracellular sites where they are proteolytically cleaved and some viral peptides are bound to MHC class II molecules. The peptide/MHC II complexes are returned to the B-cell surface where they can be recognized by viral-specific TCR on specialized $CD4^+$ T cells (T helper cells), known as TFH or T follicular helper cells.[52,200] These TFH cells are then stimulated to produce cytokines and provide surface costimulatory molecules that promote B-cell proliferation and act on later generations of these B cells to promote differentiation to antibody-producing and memory B cells. Some viral antigens, as described above, can activate B cells directly in the absence of T-cell help (so-called T-independent antigens).

Cell signaling from the BCR occurs when multiple antigen contacts lead to clustering of cell surface IgM molecules.[219] In the BCRs, IgM monomer is associated with a heterodimer of membrane-bound Igα and Igβ molecules, which bear immunoreceptor tyrosine activation motifs (ITAM) on their cytoplasmic domains. Following BCR clustering, tyrosines in the ITAM become phosphorylated to trigger a series of events that eventually lead to activation of transcription factors. Signaling by the BCR is modulated by co-receptors, most notably Fc receptor IIB for IgG (FcRγIIB) and CD19. FcRγIIB is a potent inhibitor of B-cell signaling[197] by reversing protein kinase activities and by inhibiting the formation of BCR microclusters. CD19 is an activating coreceptor[64] that functions to recruit activating molecules to the BCR. In addition, CD19 occurs on the surface of B cells alone and is linked to CD21, a receptor for the complement fragment C3d. If, following complement activation, C3d has been linked to viral antigen or to antibody–virus complex, the co-receptor complex can be linked to the BCR and BCR activation enhanced. The involvement of complement can be crucial in the development of normal B-cell memory responses (see below). Mice with deficiency in C3, C4, or CD21/CD35 and infected with HSV show a reduction in specific IgG and germinal centers compared to normal mice.[59]

The interaction of B cells with viral-specific TFH cells in lymphoid tissue leads to B-cell activation and proliferation and differentiation. It is important to note that the B-cell surface antibody and the TCR must recognize epitopes from the same molecular complex for the help signal to be delivered and B-cell activation to occur. Therefore, a B cell that is expressing surface antibody to the surface protein of a virus could be activated by a T helper cell expressing a TCR to an internal viral protein if antigen challenge involved whole virions.[241] A subunit vaccine consisting only of the envelope protein could not obtain help from such a T helper cell. The process is as follows. The B cell binds a virion through antibody recognizing surface protein. The whole virion is internalized and degraded, and peptides displayed on MHC class II molecules are carried to the B cell surface. Specific TFH cells that have previously been primed by DCs recognize the peptide-MHC class II complex on B cells through specific TCRs.[44] Antigen recognition results in T-cell adhesion to the B cell and the provision of "help" to the B cell via a range of transmembrane costimulatory receptors and cytokines. TFHs are highly enriched for selective expression of an array of cell surface molecules, reflecting their specialized role for cell–cell interaction with B cells.[52] The most critical cell–cell interaction is CD40–CD40L. CD40 on B cells engages CD40 ligand (denoted CD40L and also known as CD154) on TFH cells, driving B-cell proliferation. The combination of B- and T-cell interactions and locally released cytokines can further enhance B-cell proliferation or direct differentiation, depending on the signals provided by the TFH cell and the cell surface molecules expressed by the B cell. Of interest, the process of shared CD4 T-cell help to B cells specific for a different viral protein may occur only for small viruses, as the B cell and antibody responses to infection with vaccinia virus (a large poxvirus used as the smallpox vaccine) are strictly dependent on matched CD4 T-cell help.[254] This likely reflects a limit on the pathogen or particle size that a B cell can endocytose whole.

There are two pathways for B cells that have contacted specific T cells. In the first, after several rounds of proliferation, B cells differentiate into plasma cells in extrafollicular foci[168] and secrete relatively large amounts of soluble antibody to the virion surface protein of our example. This antibody is encoded by the unmutated germline repertoire and of the IgM isotype or class-switched to IgG or IgA. The plasma cells are short-lived with a lifespan of a few days. This early antibody is believed to be important as a first-line humoral response against viral infection.

In the second pathway involving germinal centers (GCs) in lymphoid tissues (see Section 2), the quality and versatility of the antibody to the virion surface protein can be improved by affinity maturation and isotype switching.[40,73,154,166,172,182,188,195] In GCs, B cells divide very rapidly, every 6 to 8 hours. CD4 T cells are required for the formation and maintenance of GCs. GC TFH cells provide signals that regulate maintenance of GC B cells and GC B-cell differentiation into plasma cells and memory B cells.[52] GC TFH cells critically stimulate somatic hypermutation and selection of high affinity clones. Somatic hypermutation[177] involves the introduction of nontemplated point mutations into V regions of the rapidly proliferating B cells at a rate on the order of 1×10^{-3} mutations per base pair per generation, which is approximately 10^6 times higher than the mutation rate of cellular housekeeping genes. The enzyme activation–induced cytidine deaminase (AID) has been demonstrated to be essential for somatic hypermutation. AID is a cytidine deaminase capable of carrying out targeted deamination of C to U, and shows strong homology with the RNA-editing enzyme APOBEC-1. It seems that AID directly deaminates DNA to produce U:G mismatches that ultimately can result in sequence changes in the V regions. Selection from the array of B cells expressing slightly different mutated forms of cell surface antibody was thought to occur based directly on the ability of higher affinity clones to compete for antigen and receive stronger BCR signals and survive. More recently however,[56,294] a somewhat different view has emerged in which B cells gather antigen as they move over the network of follicular DCs in GCs. Cells with the highest affinity for antigen acquire the most antigen, thereby leading to greater presentation of peptide/MHC II complexes to T cells, which in turn provide the requisite cytokine signals for B-cell survival and selection.

Isotype switching, in which the constant region of IgM is replaced by that of another isotype, also occurs in germinal centers. This might lead for example to a switch from IgM to IgG or IgA antibodies against a virion surface protein. Switching occurs through deletional DNA recombination events and involves repetitive DNA sequences or switch regions. The enzyme AID, described above, appears to be critically involved in the process. Cytokines such as IFN-γ and IL-17, which are expressed by germinal center TFH cells in a context-dependent manner, control appropriate isotype switching to different pathogens.

The B cells surviving the germinal center differentiate into plasma cells or memory B cells.[97,171,182,304] Plasma cells accumulate in the spleen or draining lymph nodes during the early stages of acute infection, but as the immune responses subside, the majority of plasma cells are found in the bone marrow.[11,124,267,318] These cells no longer express surface antibody but are committed to the secretion of soluble antibody—up to 10,000 antibody molecules per second.[113,118] Because the half-life of IgG is on the order of 1 to 3 weeks, but specific antibody can be present for many years after antigen exposure, it appears that plasma cells maintain serum antibody levels. A favored hypothesis is that plasma cells are very long-lived and continue secreting antibody long after antigen has disappeared (see below). The half-lives of antibody responses in humans to measles and mumps viruses for example are estimated at more than 200 years.[6] Memory B cells can also last for many decades.[54,319] Memory B cells maintain surface antibody but secrete little if any antibody, unless activated. They divide slowly if at all. B-cell memory is considered in greater detail below.

VIRAL ANTIGEN RECOGNITION BY T CELLS

The T-cell response to viruses is largely mediated by T cells that utilize the TCR $\alpha{:}\beta$ chain heterodimer to recognize a foreign antigen. T cells, which employ the $\gamma{:}\delta$ chain complex (the gamma/delta cells), as well as certain rare TCR $\alpha{:}\beta$ expressing T cells with restricted variable α (or β) gene segment usage in TCR generation (e.g., NK T cells) have a less clearly defined role in the adaptive immune response to viruses (and will be briefly discussed below). The conventional TCR $\alpha{:}\beta$ T cells, which have left the thymus and populated the SLOs and bloodstream, express, along with their TCRs, either the CD4 or the CD8 co-receptor molecules. One defining feature of the response of these cells is that $\alpha{:}\beta$ antigen receptors recognize nonnative peptide fragments of foreign antigen (including viral polypeptides). Therefore, in contrast to the immunoglobulin receptor (BCR), which is sensitive to antigen conformation, T-cell recognition of antigen is insensitive to three-dimensional antigen structure. Furthermore, T-cell recognition of antigens (e.g., viruses) is limited primarily to the polypeptide constituents of the virus or, more precisely, to viral gene products expressed in infected cells (although some rare exceptions exist to this general rule, which are noted later in this chapter).

A second defining feature of the $\alpha{:}\beta$ TCR is that the antigen receptor recognizes these antigenic peptides bound to MHC molecules displayed on the surface of the antigen-containing (e.g., virus-infected) cells. Therefore, $CD4^+$ and $CD8^+$ T cells are restricted in their recognition of foreign antigen to cells displaying the foreign peptide complexed to the MHC molecule to which that T cell was selected during development in the thymus. This is the phenomenon of MHC restriction[324] that defines antigen recognition by T cells. $CD8^+$ T cells will recognize cells displaying the foreign antigen peptide bound to one of several distinct MHC class I molecules expressed on the cell surface. $CD4^+$ T cells, likewise, are restricted in foreign peptide recognition by the cell surface MHC class II molecule to which the peptide fragment is bound.

The implications of MHC-restricted recognition of processed peptide fragments by T cells for virus recognition are immediate and profound. Conventional TCR $\alpha{:}\beta$ T cells responding to virus infection will recognize infected cells and not free virions or soluble viral proteins. Therefore, the activation of naïve T cells and the expression of the effector activity of activated T cells responding to virus infection will be primarily mediated through cell-to-cell contact (i.e., contact between naïve T cells and APCs or the infected cell targets of effector T cells, such as epithelial cells). In addition, T cells have the potential to recognize any viral gene product (structural or nonstructural) that can be fragmented into peptides, and bound to/displayed by MHC molecules on the surface of infected cells. Consequently, $CD8^+$ T cells will only recognize virus-infected cells that display peptide fragments of viral protein bound to cell surface MHC class I molecules, whereas $CD4^+$ T cells will recognize only those cells in which display viral peptide/MHC class II complexes. The differences in the cell types that display MHC class I and II molecules, and the distinct mechanisms by which foreign polypeptides are processed (fragmented) and bound to/presented by MHC class I and II molecules determine how $CD8^+$ and $CD4^+$ T cells respond to virus infection.

The function of the MHC molecules is to bind peptide fragments from pathogens, and to display them on the cells harboring the pathogen for recognition by T cells expressing the appropriate (i.e., specific) TCR. The consequences of this MHC-TCR–dependent cell–cell interaction are almost always deleterious to the pathogen: virus-infected cells are killed; macrophages are activated to destroy intracellular bacteria living within their intracellular vesicles; and B cells are activated to produce antibodies that eliminate or neutralize extracellular forms of pathogens. The MHC locus is located on chromosome 17 in the human (chromosome 4 in the mouse), and extends over approximately 4 centimorgans of DNA ($\sim 4 \times 10^6$ base pairs). Two properties of the MHC locus product make it difficult for pathogens to evade the adaptive immune response. First, the MHC locus is polygenic.[258] It encodes several different MHC class I and II gene products, and these differences in nucleotide/amino acid sequence control the range of peptide fragments that an individual MHC molecule can bind, so that every individual possesses a set of MHC molecules with a different range of peptide-binding specificity. Second, the MHC locus is highly polymorphic. Multiple versions (alleles) exist of each MHC gene product expressed in the population as a whole. In fact, the MHC genes are the most polymorphic genes in the human genome.[258]

The MHC locus contains three major classes of genes: class I, II, and III. The MHC class I and II genes (and their products) were first identified because of their critical role as targets in graft rejection. Hence, the name for the human MHC locus, HLA, (for human leukocyte antigen locus), and H-2 (histocompatability-2 locus) for the corresponding genes in the mouse. The MHC class I genes (or more precisely MHC class Ia genes) consist of eight exons and encode a 45-kD protein containing three external domains (α_1, α_2, α_3), along with a membrane-spanning segment and a short cytoplasmic tail. The α_1 and α_2 domains fold to form a molecular platform on the upper, outer surface of the molecule, with a *groove* or cleft to accommodate peptide fragments from pathogens.[83] Amino acid differences in the α_1 and α_2 domains among several class I molecules encoded within the MHC locus genes of an individual and between the numerous alleles of the gene encoding a given MHC class I gene product among humans dictate the types of peptides that can be accommodated in the peptide-binding groove. The α_3 domain contains the site for the binding CD8 molecules to the MHC class I. The MHC class I molecule is a heterodimer consisting of the MHC encoded 45-kD heavy (H) chain complexed noncovalently with a non-MHC locus-encoded small molecule, β-2 microglobulin (β-2M), which interacts with the H chain α_3 domain. Stable cell surface expression of the MHC class I molecule usually requires β-2M association. Importantly, MHC class I molecules are expressed at varying levels on most cells of the body, with neurons being a notable exception.[218] The expression levels of class I molecules on the cell surfaces can be upregulated by exposure of the cell to inflammatory mediators (e.g., type I and II IFN, TLR agonist, and so on).[85,141] Therefore, the T cells that recognize peptide/MHC class I complexes (i.e., the $CD8^+$ T cells) have the capacity to survey most body cells and interact with/destroy cells displaying the appropriate peptide/MHC class I complex. Three class I genes (more precisely, three class Ia genes) exist in the human: HLA-A, HLA-B, and HLA-C (H-2K, H-2D, and H-2L in the mouse), and each gene is polymorphic (i.e., displays multiple different alleles) within the human population.

The MHC class II molecules are also heterodimers, consisting of two chains (α and β), each encoded by a separate gene. These genes have a similar exon–intron structure, with the class II α chain genes encoding two extracellular domains (α_1 and α_2), and the class II β chain gene likewise encoding two extracellular domains (β_1 and β_2). The α_1 and β_1 domains of the class II molecules interact to form a molecular platform with a groove to accommodate the foreign peptide, which is like the α_1 and α_2 domain of the class I molecule on the upper outer surface of the molecule and, therefore, available for recognition by the TCR on $CD4^+$ T cells. The CD4 molecule on the T cell interacts with the surface of the β_2 domain, distal to (away from) the TCR binding site. The class II heterodimer is anchored to the cell membrane by transmembrane segments of both chains, and each chain contains a short cytoplasmic tail. In contrast to class I molecules, the expression of class II molecules is largely restricted to immune system cells: B cells, macrophages, DCs, and activated T cells in the human (and to a lesser extent, for activated at T cells in the mouse), as well as specialized epithelial cells in the thymus and type II alveolar epithelial cells in the lungs. The expression of MHC class II molecules on these cells can be upregulated by cytokines (in particular, IFN-γ)[64]; evidence indicates that certain somatic (nonimmune) cells can be induced to express MHC class II molecules in response to inflammation.[85] Three pairs of MHC class II α and β chain genes exist, which are called HLA-DR, HLA-DP, and HLA-DQ (two pairs in the mouse: $H\text{-}2^{I\text{-}A}$ and $H\text{-}2^{I\text{-}E}$). In some instances, the DR cluster contains the genes for two β chains (DRβ_1, DRβ_2), each of which can pair with the DRα chain. Again, multiple alleles exist for each gene pair. The amino acid differences among the alleles are localized primarily to the α_1 and β_1 domains, where these residue differences control the range of foreign peptide bound by the various MHC class II allelic gene products.[66]

Although both MHC class I and II molecules are similar in structure and function (i.e., presenting foreign peptides), the difference in the cellular distribution of these molecules points to the role of the T-cell subsets ($CD8^+$ and $CD4^+$ T cells) that recognize these molecules in the function of the adaptive immune system. For example, viruses have the potential to infect most nucleated body cells. Because these cells also express (to a varying degree) MHC class I molecules, they would be susceptible to recognition and destruction by activated effector T cells that are restricted by class I molecules in antigen recognition (i.e., $CD8^+$ T cells). This simple association suggests an important role of $CD8^+$ T cells in eliminating virus-infected cells and recovery from infection.[70] By contrast, MHC class II molecules are displayed primarily on cells of the immune system. Therefore, the main role of $CD4^+$ T cells, which recognize these molecules and the bound foreign peptides, is to activate and regulate the effector response of the other immune cells (e.g., the recognition by activated $CD4^+$ T cells of peptide/MHC class II complexes on B cells to stimulate antibody production, the recognition of peptide/MHC class II complexes on macrophages harboring pathogens within intracellular vesicles to stimulate macrophage activation and pathogen destruction, and the recognition of peptide/MHC class II complexes on DCs to stimulate cytokine production during the induction of adaptive immune responses).

Of course, the ability of $CD8^+$ and $CD4^+$ T cells to interact with cells displaying foreign peptide/MHC complexes also depends on the ability of these foreign antigens to provide peptides to complex with the MHC class I and II molecules. As will be discussed, the pathways by which foreign antigens gain access to and charge MHC class I and II molecules is distinctly different, and dictates the contribution of $CD8^+$ T cell and $CD4^+$ T cells in the adaptive immune response to invading microorganisms.

ANTIGEN PROCESSING AND PRESENTATION TO T CELLS

The pathways of antigen processing and peptide presentation by MHC class I and II molecules to $CD8^+$ and $CD4^+$ T cells are historically called the *endogenous* and *exogenous* presentation pathways. In the most basic terms, protein antigens, such as viral polypeptides, which gain access to the cell cytoplasm, have the potential to efficiently enter the MHC class I processing/presentation pathway—that is, produce peptides that can charge MHC class I molecules in the cells for subsequent recognition by antigen-specific $CD8^+$ T cells. During viral infection, access to the cell cytoplasm is perhaps most effectively achieved by infection of the cell that is by *de novo* synthesis of viral gene products.[92] This endogenous presentation pathway (i.e., infection of the cells) is the typical way that most virus-infected body cells are sensitized for recognition by activated $CD8^+$ T cells. Certain bacteria (e.g., *Listeria monocytogenes, Salmonella*) and parasites (e.g., malaria) that can gain access to the infected cell cytoplasm can provide protein antigens, which enter the class I presentation pathway, as can strategies that introduce proteins directly into the cytosol of cells (e.g., liposome-cell fusion).[99,306] Certain cell types that act as professional APCs (most notably, DCs) have the capacity to take up soluble or aggregated antigenic material (i.e., apoptotic, infected cell debris), and process/present antigenic peptide by MHC class I molecules to $CD8^+$ T cells by one of several different cross-presentation mechanisms that have been elucidated.[259]

Protein antigens, both soluble and particulate (e.g., bacteria, virions), which are internalized into the endocytic compartment of cells expressing MHC class II molecules, have the potential to enter the class II processing/presentation pathway and charge MHC class II molecules for recognition by $CD4^+$ T cells. This exogenous presentation pathway (i.e., uptake from without) characterizes the handling of soluble antigen (e.g., intact, inactivated virons and subunit vaccines and extracellular bacteria) by the adaptive immune system, leading to the production of activated $CD4^+$ T cells and antibodies. Any foreign protein (including a viral membrane glycoprotein) expressed on an infected MHC class II–expressing cell can enter the class II pathway, however, if it can gain access to the endocytic compartment where processing/presentation occurs (Table 9.4).

This somewhat simplified distinction between endogenous (class I) and exogenous (class II) processing/presentation pathways highlights the importance of antigen presentation in dictating the action or effector activity of the T-cell arm of the adaptive immune system. Generally, pathogens that gain access the cell cytoplasm will generate peptide/MHC class I complexes and trigger a $CD8^+$ T-cell response, whereas pathogens/pathogen

TABLE 9.4 Features of Viral Antigen Processing by the Major Histocompatibility Complex Class I and Class II Presentation Pathways

	Location	Proteolysis	MHC loading peptides
MHC Class I Pathway	Cytoplasm[a]	Proteosome[b] neutral pH	Endoplasmic reticulum
MHC Class II Pathway	Endosome[c]	Acid proteases low pH	Endosome[d]

[a]Viral proteins gain access to the cytoplasm by (a) de novo expression of viral proteins in infected cells; (b) direct virus-cell fusion at plasma membrane or in endosomes; (c) in specialized antigen-bearing presenting cells (APCs) (i.e., dendritic cells) by phagocytic uptake of virus or virus-infected cellular material into endosomes followed by endosome–endoplasmic reticulum (ER) fusion with or without retrograde transport of viral proteins into the cytoplasm.

[b]Other proteases in the cytoplasm and ER can modify the length of the viral peptide fragment produced by the proteosome before or after transport of the peptide into the ER by the transporter associated with antigen processing (TAP) transporter complex.

[c]Viral proteins in the form of virions and soluble and membrane-associated viral proteins must gain access to the endosome for fragmentation and binding to major histocompatibility complex (MHC) class II molecules.

[d]Newly synthesized MHC class II molecules are blocked from loading peptides in the ER by the class II-associated invariant (Ii) complex which is dissociated from class II molecules in the endosome by step-wise proteolytic cleavage of the Ii chain.

products that remain exclusively in the specialized endocytic compartment of MHC class II–expressing cells will typically trigger a $CD4^+$ T-cell response. The steps in the processing (fragmentation) of polypeptides into peptides, as well as the transport and interaction of peptides with MHC molecules, not surprisingly, are different in the class I and class II presentation pathways. Examination of these steps merits review because viruses have developed strategies to suppress the T-cell response by subverting the steps along these pathways.

ANTIGEN PRESENTATION BY THE MAJOR HISTOCOMPATIBILITY COMPLEX CLASS I PATHWAY

Antigenic peptides usually bind newly synthesized MHC class I molecules in the endoplasmic reticulum (ER) of the antigen-bearing/infected cells. Therefore, in most cell types, the foreign polypeptide must be fragmented in the cytoplasm, transported from the ER, and associate with a newly synthesized class I 45-kD heavy chain/β_2M chain complex before transport of the MHC/peptide complex from the ER through the secretory pathway to the cell surface (Fig. 9.3). Antigenic peptide production through fragmentation of cytosolic proteins is primarily carried out by the multisubunit, multicatalytic 20S/26S proteosome complex present in the cell cytoplasm.[231] This enzyme complex accounts for most of the cytosolic protein degradation in all cells, and the proteasome is probably responsible for the generation of most self-peptides involved in T-cell selection in the thymus through the turnover (degradation) of cellular proteins in the thymic cortical epithelial cells and medullary DCs. Two important sources of proteasome substrates are newly synthesized self- or foreign (e.g., *de novo*) expressed gene products, such as viral proteins in an infected cell and preformed foreign microbes/microbial proteins that have gained access to the cell cytoplasm. The proteasome recognizes and degrades polyubiquinated proteins. This protein tagging involves the sequential action of the ubiquitin-activating enzyme (E3), several ubiquitin-conjugating enzymes (E2), and substrate-specific ubiquitin ligases (E3)[231] to form the polyubiquinated substrate of the proteasome. Some evidence suggests that enhancing ubiquination of a protein may increase the amount of antigenic peptides generated for loading into MHC class I molecules. Furthermore, a significant fraction of newly synthesized proteins are ubiquinated during the normal turnover of cellular protein, and evidence suggests that defective ribosomal translation products (i.e., products of premature ribosome termination and/or misfolded translation products) are a major source of the protein substrates for MHC class I peptide epitopes.[316] Therefore, the rate of protein synthesis rather than turnover or expression level would be critical for the loading of MHC I molecules with appropriate antigenic peptides. Such a strategy favors the generation and recognition of newly synthesized viral proteins in infected cells.

The core proteasome cleaves polypeptide substrates after hydrophobic and basic residues.[256] Exposure of cells to certain cytokines (particularly, IFN-γ) induces the expression of three new proteasome subunits: b1i, b5i, and b2i (formally called LMP-2, LMP-7, and MECL-7, respectively). These subunits replace existing subunits in the core proteasome, producing a second proteasome form, the immunoproteasome present in IFN-treated cells.[314] This replacement of the constitutive proteasome subunits with these inducible subunits changes the proteasome cleavage specificity, thereby increasing the cleavage of polypeptides after hydrophobic and basic residues and decreasing the cleavage after acidic residues (i.e., peptides with acidic C-termini). This is noteworthy because MHC class I molecules preferentially bind peptides (in an MHC class I allele-dependent manner) with hydrophobic or basic *anchor* residues at their C-termini.[29]

Two of the IFN-γ–inducible proteasome subunits, b1i and b5i, are encoded by genes within the MHC locus,[258] suggesting a strong evolutionary selective pressure for the immunoproteasome in MHC function. IFN-γ also increases the production of antigenic peptides by inducing the expression of a multisubunit proteasome adaptor complex PA28 which, on binding to the ends of the core proteasomes/immunoproteasome cylinder, increases the peptide efflux rate from the proteasome. Therefore, a cytokine product, IFN-γ, produced by an innate immune cell type (NK cells) or adaptive immune effector cells (antigen-specific $CD4^+$ effector T cells) can enhance the display of antigen peptide fragments recognized by effector $CD8^+$ T cells. Proteasomes generate peptides 3 to 20 amino acids (a.a.) in length.[93] Studies in which peptide fragments bound to MHC class I molecules isolated from cell surfaces were extracted and analyzed, however, revealed that these class I–bound peptides, in general, are 8 to 10 a.a. in length. Therefore, the proteasome peptide products that have the appropriate C-termini for MHC class I binding must also undergo cleavage at their N-termini. Several cytosolic (and one ER resident) aminopeptidases have been implicated in carrying out this process.[93,126,159] N-Terminal trimming in the ER of transported peptides having an extended (greater than 8–10 a.a.) length is carried out in this compartment by the ER-associated amino peptidase (ERAAP). One cytosolic peptidase, tripeptidyl peptidase II (TPPII), may be capable of generating a limited range of peptides in the absence of proteasome function.[147] Overall, several studies have suggested that modifications of the proteasome core by inflammatory cytokines, combined with the action of cytosolic proteases, can affect antigenic peptide generation, including the production of antigenic peptides (in cells infected with several different viruses), the recognition of which by $CD8^+$ T cells is dependent on these proteasome modifications and/or action of other cytosolic and ER proteases.[261,290]

Peptides generated in the cytosol are transported to the ER by the heterodimeric transporters associated with antigen presentation (TAP)-1/TAP-2 protein complex. This transporter complex is located within the ER membrane, forming a pore/channel there.[96] Both proteins are members of the ABC family of ATP-dependent small molecule transporters, and are also encoded by genes mapping to the MHC locus. This transporter complex preferentially translocates peptide of 8 to 16 a.a. in length with hydrophobic or basic C-termini, and the TAP complex exhibits some restriction in transport efficiency of peptides with certain residues at the N-termini. Peptides gaining ER access through the TAP pore encounter the MHC class I peptide loading complex.[291]

Newly synthesized MHC class I molecules must bind to β-2M and have a stably bound peptide (of self or foreign origin) in their peptide binding groove to retain the stable

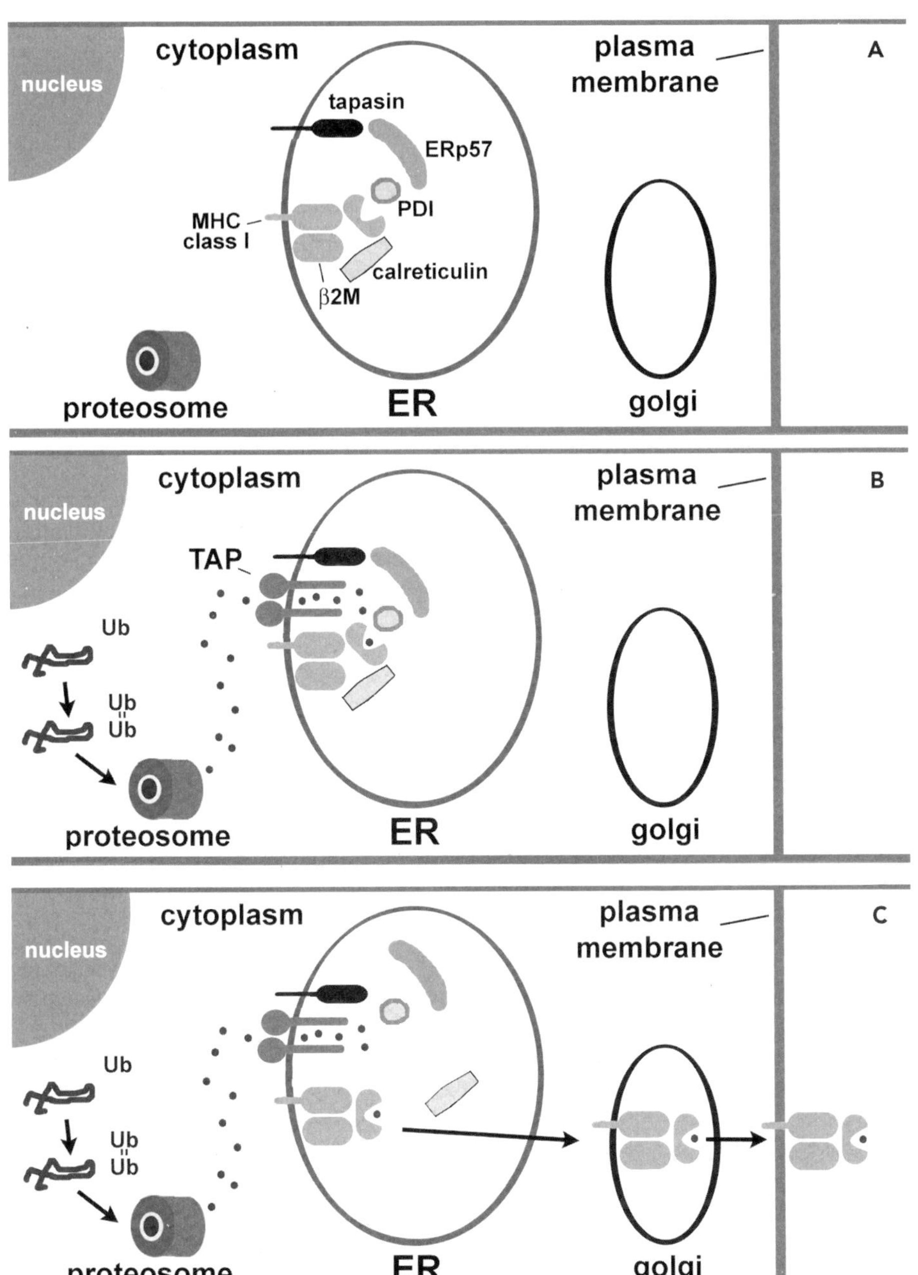

FIGURE 9.3. **Major histocompatibility (MHC) class I presentation pathway. A:** Following their co-translational translocation into the endoplasmic reticulum (ER), newly synthesized MHC class I forms a complex consisting of the ER scaffolding protein calreticulin (and calnexin—not shown), peptide and protein modifying enzymes (ERp57, protein disulfide isomerase [PDI]), the antigen presentation transporter associated with antigen presentation (TAP) transporter targeting molecule tapasin and a weak interaction with beta 2 microglobulin (β2M). **B:** Processing/presentation through the classical MHC class I pathway requires that a target protein (e.g. viral polypeptide) gain access to the cell cytoplasm where it is ubiquinated before fragmentation by the cytosolic protein complex, the proteosome. Peptide fragments are then transferred from the cytoplasm to the ER through the TAP transporter complex. The MHC class I complex is targeted to the TAP through the action of tapasin, and here the MHC class I and associated molecules come in contact with transported peptides. Peptides with the appropriate amino acid sequence (binding motif) and length/conformation (following modification by enzymes within the ER) will associate with the nascent MHC lass I molecules/β2M to form a stable complexes. **C:** The new stable MHC class I/peptide/β2M complexes dissociate from scaffolding proteins and are transported via the secretory pathway to the cell surface where interaction with the CD8+ T-lymphocyte antigen receptor occurs.

conformation necessary for it to exit the ER.[291] Within the ER, nascent class I α chain molecules are bound to the ER chaperone, calnexin, until the 12-kD β-2M molecule binds, and calnexin is then replaced by the calreticulin scaffolding protein and the tapasin molecule (an MHC locus–encoded protein that forms a bridge between the class I α chain/β-2M complex and the TAP transporter). The binding of calreticulin and tapasin to the nascent MHC class I molecule stabilizes the complex, allowing the partially folded class I/β-2M complex to maintain a conformation (while it awaits a soluble peptide from the cytosol). The partially folded MHC class I molecule will selectively bind (select) only those peptides containing certain motifs; that is, common or conserved amino acid sequences distributed along the length of the peptide fragment. Each allelic form of the class I molecule has specificity for (binds to) a peptide containing an MHC class I allele, a specific peptide binding motif. The ability of a specific MHC class I allelic variant to capture peptides displaying this conserved amino acid motif is dictated by the presence of polymorphic amino acid residues in the binding cleft formed by the α_1 and α_2 domains. A third component of the peptide loading complex is the ERp57 thioreductase and protein disulfide isomerase (PDI, which presumably catalyzes disulfide interchange in the class I α chain during peptide loading). In certain cells (e.g., macrophages, DCs), the aforementioned ER amino-peptidase, ERAAP,[246] is associated with the loading complex, and acts to trim the N-termini of long peptide (i.e., $\geq$10 a.a.) down to size before final folding of the complex. After proper peptide loading and folding, the stable class I/β-2M/peptide complex is freed from the chaperones, and migrates from the ER to the cell surface. Note that in the uninfected cells, class I molecules still require a stably bound peptide to exit the ER and traffic to the cell surface. The source of these *antigenic* peptides is degraded cellular (self) proteins.[28]

The classic MHC class I presentation pathway would appear to be a restricted to proteins synthesized/retained in the cytosol. However, this is not the case. Numerous examples are found of secreted and membrane proteins/glycoproteins that contain peptides that are recognized by $CD8^+$ T cells and, therefore, bound to MHC class I molecules. The most likely way that these proteins may be degraded is if the polypeptide chains are generated in the cytosol as defective or mistranslated ribosomal products, DRiPs).[315] Another way is retrograde transport of defective (misfolded) translation products that have been co-translationally translocated into the ER by the Sec61-dependent transport mechanism.[1] Sec61 normally acts in the translocation of the translation products of membrane-bound ribosomes into the ER, but can also shuttle intact (presumably defective) proteins in a retrograde fashion into the cytosol from the ER for degradation by the proteasome.[1] The unique ability of professional APCs (particularly $CD8\alpha^+$ and $CD103^+$ cDCs) to "cross-present" cellular constituents/fragments of virus-infected cells may reflect the use of such a mechanism (i.e., uptake of virions, infected cellular material, and so on into endosomes followed by retrograde transport of this cargo into the ER) preferentially. Protein processing and peptide presentation to MHC class I molecules may also occur by direct loading peptides into the MHC molecules within endosomes, but the mechanistic basis for this processing pathway is poorly understood, and its *in vivo* significance for virus infection is uncertain.[259]

ANTIGEN PRESENTATION BY THE MAJOR HISTOCOMPATIBILITY COMPLEX CLASS II PATHWAY

Antigen processing and presentation along the MHC class II pathway differs from class I presentation in several ways (Table 9.4). First, the class II pathway focuses primarily on antigens (both soluble and particulate) that enter cells by endocytosis/phagocytosis, and are retained in endocytic compartments for subsequent processing (fragmentation) and loading of the peptide fragments into class II molecules. These endocytic compartments include early and late endosomes and, in certain instances, lysosomes.[301] Second, antigen fragmentation occurs in the low pH environment of the endosome (rather than in the neutral pH of the cytosol where proteasome-dependent MHC class I binding peptides are generated). Third, both newly synthesized and recycled (from the cell surface) MHC class II molecules can capture and present peptide fragments to $CD4^+$ T cells. Fourth, unlike the strict length constraints (i.e., 8 to 10 a.a.) for peptides bound to MHC class I molecules, peptides bound to class II molecules are at least 13 amino acids long, and can be longer (i.e., up to 20 a.a.). As with the class I molecules, however, specific class II molecules (alleles) will selectively bind (select) peptides containing particular a.a. motifs (i.e., peptides containing common/conserved a.a. distributed along the length of the peptide). As for class I molecules, these peptide-binding motifs are dictated by the presence of polymorphic a.a. residues in the class II binding cleft (which differ for each class II locus gene product allele). In summary, class II molecules bind peptides produced from soluble or particulate antigen taken up by endocytosis in the same low pH compartment where protein fragmentation occurs. How then is class II processing achieved?

The MHC class II α and β chains, as with other membrane glycoproteins, are synthesized in the ER. After synthesis, the $\alpha{:}\beta$ chain heterodimer engages a type II membrane protein, the MHC class II–associated invariant (Ii) chain—invariant because the Ii gene is nonpolymorphic. The invariant chain forms a trimer complex consisting of three class $\alpha{:}\beta$ heterodimers and three Ii subunits, with each Ii subunit binding noncovalently to a class $\alpha{:}\beta$ heterodimer. This interaction of the class II $\alpha{:}\beta$ heterodimer with Ii serves two important functions. First, a region of Ii binds (with low affinity) to the peptide binding groove/cleft of the nascent class II molecule in the ER, and prevents the loading of peptides transported into the ER from binding to class II in this compartment. Therefore, class II molecules do not bind the same spectrum of peptides as class I molecules, because they do not bind peptides in the ER. Second, Ii targets the class II molecules to the cell's low pH endosomal compartment (rather than the cell surface via the secretory pathway) where protein antigen fragmentation and peptide loading into the class II peptide biding groove occurs.[106]

Processing (fragmentation) of protein antigens in the MHC class II pathway is carried out by a variety of acid proteases, and at least one IFN-γ–induced lysosomal thiol reductase (GILT) located in the low pH endosomal compartment. Several related cathepsin cysteine proteases (e.g., cathepsins S, L, B, F), and the unrelated cysteine protease, asparagineendopeptidase (AEP), have been implicated in antigen processing (fragmentation) in endosomes as inhibition of, or deficiency in, one or more of these proteases that can affect the generation of certain antigenic epitopes recognized by $CD4^+$ T cells.[295]

To bind peptides in the endosome, class II molecules must be liberated from Ii. This is achieved by the sequential cleavage of Ii by endosomal proteases (including, AEP, cathepsin S, and cathepsin L), freeing the class II $\alpha{:}\beta$ heterodimer from the membrane portion of the Ii, and leaving a short fragment of Ii (called *CLIP* for class II-associated invariant chain peptide), which remains bound to the peptide-binding groove of the class II molecule. CLIP must be removed from the class II molecule to make the class II binding groove accessible to peptide fragmentation in the endosome, which is achieved through the action of a MHC-like molecule, DM (HLA-DM for human, H-2M for mouse) and which is encoded in the MHC locus and resides in the endosome. DM catalyzes the dissociation of CLIP from the class II $\alpha{:}\beta$ heterodimer. As with Tapasin for class I molecules, DM stabilizes the class II molecule as the class II molecule interacts with and sorts through the myriad of antigenic peptides in the endosome, selecting those peptides displaying the correct motif to allow these peptides to stably bind to the class II molecule. This peptide selection process by class II molecules typically occurs in 2 to 4 hours (during the time that the class II molecules reside in the endosome). Once a stable peptide/class II complex forms, DM dissociates; and the complex transits to the cell surface of MHC class II–expressing cells. *Empty* class II molecules (i.e., lacking a peptide in the binding groove) are unstable. Consequently, in the absence of infection or specific exposure to foreign antigen (e.g., vaccination), it is self-peptides derived from the endosomal proteolysis of cellular proteins (e.g., soluble proteins taken up from the extracellular space by pinocytosis or the residues of phagocytosed apoptotic cell) that are bound to the MHC class II molecules on the surface of uninfected, class II-expressing cells.

Although *de novo* synthesized MHC class II molecules likely play a major role in capturing/presenting processed antigen to CD4$^+$ T cells, class II molecules can cycle back into the endosomes from the cell surface, and these *recycled* class II molecules may also capture/present antigenic peptide. Class II molecules containing self-peptides (or less frequently, class II molecules that escape the endosome and exit to the cell surface with CLIP peptide in their groove) appear able to re-enter the endocyte compartment, exchange the bound peptide for a new peptide, and cycle back to the cell surface. By employing this recycling mechanism, MHC class II–expressing cells (in particular, professional APC, as with DC) would increase their chances of capturing and displaying foreign antigenic peptides to CD4$^+$ T cells. In immature DCs, endosomal/lysosomal proteolytic activity is weak and newly synthesized MHC class II/Ii complexes are shunted to and retained in the endosome where they will be eventually degraded unless the DC are activated.

ANTIGEN PRESENTATION AND PROFESSIONAL ANTIGEN-PRESENTING CELLS

The hallmark of the adaptive immune system is specificity of foreign antigen recognition. For T cells, this means recognition of antigenic peptides bound to MHC class I or II molecules displayed on the cell surface. The T-cell response proceeds, as we have seen, in two phases. First is the inductive phase: the activation of quiescent primary (or memory) T cells in response to recognition of specialized APC displaying the peptide/MHC complex, resulting in the generation of armed effector T cells. Second is the effector phase, where cells displaying the appropriate peptide/MHC complexes are recognized by the activated T cells. The *classic* class I presentation pathway (which utilizes peptides derived from proteins synthesized *de novo* in the cell) is ideally suited to generate the antigenic peptide/MHC class I complexes recognized by CD8$^+$ effectors in response to viral infection of any body cell type. Virus infection of a cell leads to the generation of an ample supply of viral protein substrates for processing by the proteasome. The expression of MHC class I molecules, and the molecular machinery of processing (i.e., the TAP transporter complexes and immunoproteasome subunits) are upregulated by type I and, in particular, type II IFN induced during virus infection by infected cells and by responding NK and effector CD4$^+$ T cells (increasing the efficiency of infected cell recognition by CD8$^+$ T cells). Furthermore, because antigenic peptide/MHC class I complexes are extremely stable,[250] viral peptides bound to MHC class I molecules displayed on the surface infected cells are not transferred to surrounding uninfected cells. Consequently, the resulting destruction of bystander cells by CD8$^+$ T cells is negligible. Evidence accumulated over several decades suggests that this classic pathway of cytoplasmic generation of viral peptides and loading of viral peptides into class I molecules in the ER is employed in the recognition of virus-infected cells by CD8$^+$ T cells. As discussed below, many viruses have evolved strategies to disrupt the class I presentation pathway to prevent effector CD8$^+$ T-cell recognition of infected cells and sustain virus infection.

Due to the more stringent requirements for the activation of resting naïve T cells, there has been considerable attention given over the last decade to the process of antigen processing and/or presentation by professional APCs (in particular DCs) in the generation of peptide/MHC complexes during the inductive phase of the T-cell response. Although a number of DC subsets had been identified and categorized, as noted above, DC can be conveniently divided into two main subsets: cDC (conventional/myeloid DC) and plasmacytoid (lymphoid) DC (based on the bone marrow progenitor cell types that give rise to these two DC subsets and on the expression of certain DC lineage-specific cell surface molecules.[260] The cDCs are the primary APCs, which stimulate antiviral T-cell responses.[17] The DC subset derived from lymphoid progenitors, the plasmacytoid DCs (pDCs), has received considerable scrutiny. pDCs, so called because of their plasma cell–like morphology and surface expression of a CD45 isoform (i.e., the B220 molecule, which, characteristically, is found only in B cells) have weak APC activity but have been demonstrated to be the major source of IFN-α produced early (24 to 48 hours) after inflammatory stimuli, including virus infection.[49] Therefore, in addition to serving as a potential, albeit weak APC for T cells, the pDCs may serve as a major early innate immune defense against virus infection.[80]

In support of their essential role in immune response induction, DCs (when activated/mature) are 10 to 100 times more potent on a per cell basis as activators of naïve T cells when compared with other immune cell APCs (e.g., macrophages, B cells).[2] Immature DCs can take up virus by the following several mechanisms:

1. Binding of viruses to their cognate receptors displayed on the DC surface with direct fusion or uptake of bound virus into endosomes, and subsequent release of the viral genome to initiate infection.
2. Phagocytosis of virions using a range of lectin-like, innate immune pathogen pattern recognition receptors displayed by DCs (e.g., DEC 205, DC-SIGN). Although triggering of phagocytosis and the likely engagement of TLR capable of recognizing viral nucleic acids/proteins (i.e., TLR-3, 7, 9) should result in DC activation/maturation, engagement of certain lectin receptors by particular viruses (e.g., HIV interaction with DC SIGN) may induce an inhibitory signal suppressing DC activation.[79]
3. DC uptake of virus nonspecifically by fluid phase macropinocytosis. This bulk uptake of fluid phase soluble and particulate material is a characteristic property of immature DCs.
4. For viruses capable of directly activating the complement cascade (i.e., without prior antibody binding) (e.g., HIV), DCs expressing the complement receptor CR3 (i.e., the integrin complex, CD11b/CD18) can take up (by receptor-mediated endocytosis) virions displaying the activated complement C3 product, iC3b.

Any or all of these uptake mechanisms can directly or indirectly deliver viral polypeptides to the MHC class II and classic class I presentation pathways in DC.

Given the critical role of cDCs in the induction of the T-cell response (in particular, the antiviral $CD8^+$ T-cell response,[144] viruses might be expected to have evolved strategies to inhibit the induction of $CD8^+$ T-cell responses in virus-infected DCs. As discussed elsewhere in this text, for individual virus genera, evidence indicates that infection of DCs by certain viruses may inhibit the APC capacity of DCs.[242,253] Furthermore, productive virus infection of tissue DCs at body surfaces could also result in virus dissemination when the DCs traffic to the SLOs. These considerations, as well as the fact that certain viruses with narrow cellular tropism (e.g., papillomavirus), therefore, are not capable of infecting DCs and providing polypeptides for processing via the classic class I pathway, led to the concept of cross-presentation of antigen (including, viral polypeptides) by DCs to $CD8^+$ T cells. As discussed above, the likely mechanism(s) of antigen cross-presentation by DCs involves phagocytic uptake by DCs of virus or, more likely, of fragments of productively infected apoptotic cells. Recent evidence points to several potential mechanisms of cross-presentation by DCs, including a mechanism where the DC phagosomes containing viral antigen (taken into the DCs by phagocytosis of virus/virus-infected cellular material) fuses with the ER; therefore, viral polypeptides in this ER/phagosome complex would be available for transport through the Sec61 retrograde transport mechanism into the cytosol for proteasome-dependent proteolysis and subsequent transport of viral peptide into the ER for loading onto nascent MHC class I molecules.[180] Cross-presentation of antigens to naïve T cells is believed to be limited to professional APCs, that is, cDCs and possibly certain macrophage subsets that function at the inductive phase of T-cell responses. The concept of cross-presentation as the mechanism of viral antigen presentation to naïve $CD8^+$ T cells, is gaining general acceptance, particularly because it solves several of the nagging issues concerning the induction of $CD8^+$ T-cell response to viruses such as papilloma and polio viruses, which presumably do not infect DCs (and to tumor cells that cannot serve as professional APCs). It remains uncertain, however, why most pathogens (e.g., extracellular bacteria, fungi) only trigger $CD4^+$ T-cell responses (i.e., do not activate the MHC class I presentation pathway) despite the potential for these antigens to enter the phagocytic compartment of DC.

CYTOKINES AND CHEMOKINES

Many cytokines and chemokines act to orchestrate the innate and adaptive immune responses. The cellular and molecular biology of these molecules have been extensively reviewed.[175,184] Several of the cytokines also play an important role in T-cell activation and are worth consideration. Interleukin-12 (IL-12) is primarily a product of activated DCs and macrophages, and exists in two forms: IL-12p70 (a heterodimer consisting of the p40 and p35 subunits), and a homodimer of IL-12p40. (The p40 subunit is also part of the heterodimer making up the cytokine IL-23-an important regulator of CD4 Th-17 effector T-cell responses as discussed below.) IL12p70 interacts with its receptor on naïve and activated T cells, providing *signal 3* in the naïve T-cell activation sequence through recruitment and activation of signal transducers and activators of transcription 4 (STAT-4). The outcome of this signaling process is to promote the differentiation of $CD8^+$ T cells into activated cytolytic effector cells, and to help drive the differentiation of $CD4^+$ T cells along a pathway leading to effector $CD4^+$ T cells capable of secreting IFN-γ on TCR engagement (i.e., the generation of T_H1, T *helper* 1 effector T cells). The effect of IL-12p70 on T cells is to generate activated effector T cells that are efficient at viral clearance.

IL-2 is a cytokine produced by both $CD4^+$ T cells and, to a lesser extent, $CD8^+$ T cells, during the initial phase of T-cell activation and differentiation.[132] Engagement of the high affinity IL-2 receptor (expressed only after T-cell activation) by IL-2 drives T-cell proliferative expansion. Although IL-2 was initially believed to be the primary T-cell growth factor (acting in an autocrine fashion to stimulate T-cell proliferation), T-cell activation and proliferative expansion occur normally in the absence of IL-2 (e.g., in IL-2–deficient patients or experimental animals with a targeted disruption of the IL-2 gene). Therefore, it appears that, in the absence of IL-2, other cytokines (e.g., IL-15) can support the normal T-cell expansion in response to antigenic stimulation. As with many cytokines, IL-15 can be produced by a variety of cell types, both constitutively and in response to inflammation. A genetic deficiency in IL-2 results not in a defective T-cell response to antigen, but rather paradoxically, in exaggerated T-cell proliferation (lymphoproliferative disease) and the development of autoimmune responses caused by the defective generation of regulatory T cells.[237] Recently, IL-2 produced by effector $CD4^+$ T cells has been shown to regulate the production by $CD8^+$ T effector cells of the regulatory cytokine IL-10 during respiratory virus infection.[123]

Other cytokines, for example, IFN-γ, IL-4, IL-6, and transforming growth factor β (TGF-β) are, like IL-12, sources of *signal 3* and therefore are important regulators of the adaptive immune system and immune cell function during the adaptive immune response to virus infection. IFN-γ is the product of a single gene with minimal allelic variation in the coding sequence of the gene. It is produced during virus infection primarily by activated $CD4^+$ T cell and $CD8^+$ T cells (and some NK T cells) in response to TCR engagement and by NK cells after engagement of stimulatory NK cell receptors. The role of IFN-γ in augmenting antigen presentation (i.e., upregulation of MHC class I and II expression, immunoproteasome subunit induction) has been discussed earlier. IFN-γ also plays a critical role in activating mononuclear phagocytes (macrophages) to destroy infected intracellular bacteria, and it presumably plays a similar role in the destruction of virus and, possibly, virus-infected cells when armed effector T cells respond to viral antigen at peripheral sites of virus infection. The early production of IFN-γ (likely produced by NK cells entering the SLO in response to infection) during the initiation of T-cell responses to antigen can drive T-cell differentiation to a type 1 (T_H1) pathway (characteristic of antiviral T-cell responses). The IFN-γ gene is rendered transcriptionally active by exposure of responding primary T cells to IL-12p70, resulting in IFN-γ production by activated effector T cells on subsequent TCR engagement by antigen.[193] IFN-γ signaling through its receptor is mediated primarily by STAT-1.

Interleukin-4 is produced at high levels by activated $CD4^+$ T cells that have differentiated along the type 2 (T_H2) pathway.[193]

IL-4 may also be produced at low levels in primary T cells early in the response to antigen and by NKT cells and NK cells. Exposure of responding CD4+ T cells to IL-4 early in the activation/differentiation sequence is essential for the generation of T_H2 effector T cells in the SLO. The early low-level production of IL-4 by activated T cells (or by NKT cells and NK cells recruited to the SLO) before their commitment to T_H1 or T_H2 differentiation may be sufficient to render the IL-4 gene locus capable of high-level IL-4 production by CD4+ T_H2 effectors on TCR engagement.[283] The NKT-cell subset, which rapidly produces high levels of IL-4 early in the response to pathogens, has been suggested to be a potential source of IL-4, which can regulate conventional α:β:TCR T-cell differentiation in the SLO in response to antigen. IL-4 produced by activated T cells serves both as a B-cell growth-promoting factor and also triggers immunoglobulin type switching during B-cell activation/differentiation. Engagement of the IL-4 receptor activates STAT-6 to mediate the effect of IL-4 on responding B and T cells. As will be discussed, IL-4 and IFN-γ act antagonistically to regulate T-cell differentiation and T-cell effector generation into T_H1 or T_H2 effectors.

The cytokines IL-6 and TGF-β play a critical role in driving naïve CD4 T-cell differentiation into IL-17–producing effector T cells, and in the case of TGF-β, an essential role in the development of T regulatory cells. IL-6 is a proinflammatory cytokine, the expression of which is upregulated following an inflammatory stimulus such as virus infection, and signaling through the IL-6 receptor is mediated by STAT-3. TGF-β exists on cell surfaces in an inactive form and its expression is regulated at the level of transcription, translation, and posttranslation modifications.[245] Signaling through of the TGF-β receptor is signal transducing mothers against decapentapeligic protein (SMAD) dependent. Both cytokines can be produced by hematopoietic and nonhematopoietic origin cells. Production of IL-6 and TGF-β in the SLO at the time of infection will trigger naïve CD4+ T-cells to differentiate into T_H17 T_E as discussed below (see text under heading "CD4+ Te Effector Mechanisms").

EFFECTOR ACTIVITIES OF B CELLS

The antiviral activities of B cells are largely mediated by antibodies,[32,72,91,139,305,325] although B cells may also have modulating effects on innate immunity. Antibodies are distinguished from T-cell effectors in that they have activity against free virus particles as well as against virally infected cells. They are the first line of defense against viral infection. In a very real sense, the adaptive antiviral activities of antibodies and T cells are complementary and should be considered together in attempting to understand immune responses to viruses.[8] Nevertheless, it is revealing to consider the antiviral activities of antibodies at different layers of complexity[32]: *in vitro, in vivo* in the absence of other adaptive immune effectors as revealed by passive antibody transfer studies; and *in vivo* in the presence of T-cell responses as in natural infection or following some vaccination strategies.

ANTIVIRAL ACTIVITIES OF ANTIBODY *IN VITRO*

As stated earlier, antibody can act against both free virus and infected cells. This is presented schematically in Figure 9.4 for an enveloped virus. Probably the most studied antiviral activity of antibody in vitro and the one most important for antibody protection in vivo is neutralization of free virus particles. Neutralization has been defined as the loss of infectivity that ensues when antibody molecule(s) bind to a virus particle, and usually occurs without the involvement of any other agency. As such, this is an unusual activity of antibody paralleled only by the inhibition of toxins and enzymes.[67] The mechanism(s) of neutralization have been much debated over the years. The simplest models are based on steric obstruction of virus attachment or virus entry by the antibody molecule.[116,145,215,269] The relatively large bulk of the antibody molecule, very roughly similar to that of a typical viral spike for an enveloped virus, is suggested to be critical. Such models predict that the neutralizing efficacy of an antibody should be related primarily to its affinity for antigen on the virion surface, and the precise epitope recognized should be of lesser, but potentially significant, importance. Indeed, clear evidence exists that antibodies can neutralize viruses without binding directly to functional sites on the virion surface.[22,228] The models described can be very loosely termed occupancy or coating models, where the degree of coating of the virus surface by antibody to achieve neutralization differs between models. One model noted a striking linear relationship between the surface area of a set of viruses and the number of antibody molecules bound to virus at neutralization.[212] This implied that, for these viruses at least, a coating density corresponding to about half the available antibody sites occupied on the virus produced neutralization. This model is likely to be less applicable to complex viruses expressing multiple surface proteins (e.g., the herpes or pox viruses). A related model of neutralization of flaviviruses proposes that highly accessible epitopes may require lower occupancy than poorly accessible epitopes to reach a threshold for neutralization.[220] Further models taking into account kinetic factors in virus neutralization are being developed.

Alternative neutralization models suggest that (a) viruses are neutralized by the binding of one or only a few antibody molecules to critical sites on the virion surface; (b) conformational changes in envelope or capsid molecules are crucial to neutralization; and (c) viral inactivation by antibody can occur following entry to infected cells, for example, by blocking virus uncoating[67] or by interaction of the Fc of IgG with TRIM21.[169a] Considerable debate remains in the area of antibody neutralization mechanism and, furthermore, it may be that different mechanisms are operative for different viruses under differing conditions.

Antibody activity against free virus particles can be augmented by Fc-mediated effector systems in several ways. First, complement activation[271] by virion-bound antibody and deposition of complement components on the virion surface can enhance neutralization.[183] Occupancy/coating models argue that this reflects an increased coating of molecules on the virion that hinders productive interaction of virion and target cell. Second, complement activation can lead directly to virolysis by deposition of the terminal components of complement in the viral membrane. Third, Fc and complement receptors can bind antibody or complement-coated virions, leading to phagocytosis followed by inactivation in an intracellular compartment within the phagocyte. This process has been described in vitro for the picornavirus foot-and-mouth disease virus (FMDV) and is believed to be important in vivo in protection against FMDV.[181] It is likely that neutralizing antibodies, which tend

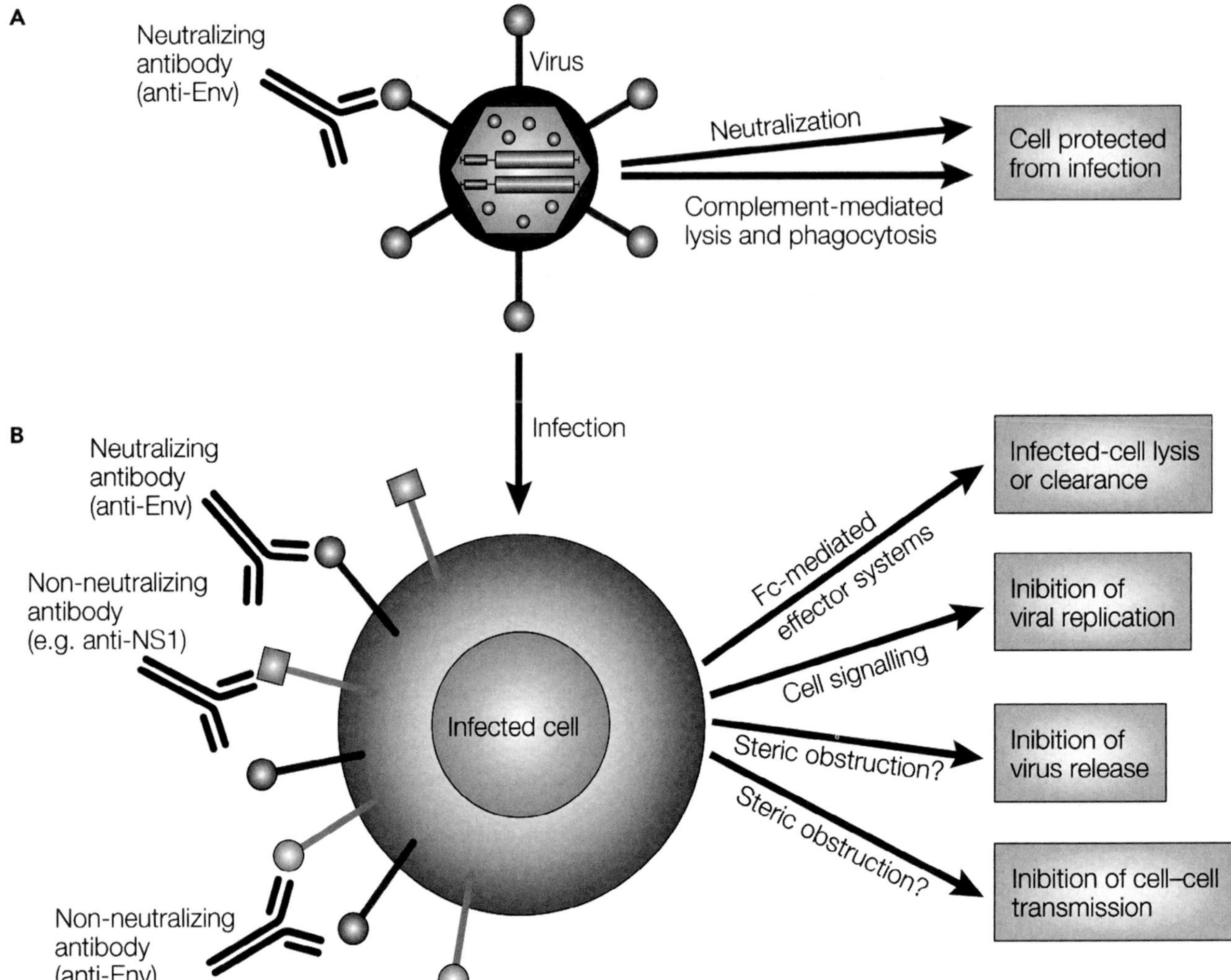

FIGURE 9.4. Antibody activities against free virus particles and virally infected cells. A: Activities against free virus particles. The primary activity is probably neutralization, whereby antibody molecules bind to virion surface proteins and block infection. Virion-bound antibody molecules may also trigger lysis of virions via complement or phagocytosis of virions. An enveloped virus expressing only one surface protein is shown. A virus expressing multiple surface proteins (e.g., a herpes or poxvirus) may not be neutralized by antibody saturation of a single surface protein. Non-functional surface molecules may also be present on infectious virions for some viruses such as HIV.[224] Nonneutralizing antibodies may bind to such molecules and trigger the elimination of infectious virions by effector systems or perhaps trap virus in vivo and prevent contact with target cells. **B:** Activities against virally infected cells. Neutralizing antibodies will bind to the proteins that are also expressed on virions (typically Env proteins). Nonneutralizing antibodies will bind to proteins that are expressed on infected cells but not virions (e.g., NS1 protein of dengue virus) or that are also expressed on virions but whose blockade does not lead to neutralization (e.g., neuraminidase on influenza virions). (Reproduced from Burton DR. Antibodies, viruses and vaccines. *Nat Rev Immunol* 2002;2:706–713, with permission.)

to coat the viral surface, will be most effective in triggering virolysis or phagocytosis. An antigen present at relatively low density on the surface of a virion could, however in principle, bind antibody without mediating neutralization. Such nonneutralizing antibody could nevertheless trigger virolysis or phagocytosis.

Antibodies can act, not only against free virions, but also against infected cells by binding to viral proteins expressed on the surface of virally infected cells (Fig. 9.4). Fc-mediated effector systems can lead to cell lysis or clearance via complement-dependent cytotoxicity (CDC) or antibody-dependent cellular cytotoxicity (ADCC). In the case of CDC, activation of the classic pathway by antibody that complexes arrayed viral proteins on the infected cell surface can lead to C3b deposition and uptake by effector cells or the deposition of the terminal complement components in the infected cell membrane resulting in lysis.[18] For ADCC, the antibody array on the infected cell surface is recognized by Fc receptors on effector cells, triggering killing of the infected cells. Antibody can also inhibit (a) virus release from infected cells[91] by simply binding to viral proteins at the infected cell surface and (b) cell-to-cell transmission of virus[30,211] by mechanisms that are thought to be very similar to those that lead to virus neutralization. Binding of antibody to the infected cell surface, particularly of neurons, has also been suggested to inhibit viral replication inside cells, presumably via signaling mechanisms.[87,160]

Generally, it appears that antibody is less effective against infected cells than against free virions. For instance, higher concentrations of neutralizing antibody are required to inhibit cell-to-cell transmission than are required to inhibit infection by free virions.[119,211] Similarly, a higher concentration of antibody has been associated with effective CDC and ADCC than has neutralization.[117] It is expected that neutralizing antibodies will be effective against infected cells if they bind to envelope molecule presentations on free infected cells that are also expressed on virions. Antibodies that bind to molecules expressed on infected cells but not virions, for example, the NS1 protein of dengue virus,[114] can be effective against infected cells, although they are nonneutralizing.

Polymeric IgA and IgM have been shown to be capable of intracellular neutralization of virus. These antibodies are actively transported over the mucosal epithelium after binding to the polymeric immunoglobulin receptor and may, during transport, contact and neutralize transcytosing viruses.[25,88,139,178]

Finally, antibody can enhance viral infection *in vitro* under certain circumstances, generally in the presence of subneutralizing concentrations of neutralizing antibodies. Enhancement is mediated by Fc receptors in some cases (e.g., dengue virus),[16,104,109,191] but not in other cases where enhancement is observed with antibody Fab fragments.[277] The occupancy model of neutralization described above explains enhancement of infection as an effect that occurs at low occupancy of virion sites in the presence of permissive cells (e.g., those bearing Fc receptors). As antibody concentrations increase, coating of the virus increases, eventually resulting in neutralization.

ANTIVIRAL ACTIVITIES OF ANTIBODY *IN VIVO*

The classic approach to determine the protective activities of antibody *in vivo* is to passively transfer immune sera or monoclonal antibodies to a naïve animal, challenge with virus, and observe the outcome. This approach has consistently shown—for many different viruses, animal models, and challenge routes—a good correlation between the protection achieved and antibody serum neutralizing activity measured in vitro.[212] It should be noted that this does not necessarily mean that neutralization is the mechanism of protective activity. Neutralizing antibodies are probably those that bind most effectively to free virions and to virus-infected cells (at least for many enveloped viruses) so that, in principle at least, any of the mechanisms of antiviral activity presented in Figure 9.4 could be operative in protection.

Generally speaking, protection in animal models is achieved when neutralizing titers in the serum of the animal at the time of virus challenge are relatively high, often of the order of 1:100 or higher. In other words, the serum of the animal can be diluted 100-fold and 50% to 90% (depending on the study and assay) neutralization achieved *in vitro.* In some instances, protection can be described as sterilizing in that no evidence is seen of viral replication following challenge. Serum neutralizing titers (80%) of 1:380 or greater provide sterilizing immunity in the lungs of cotton rats challenged with respiratory syncytial virus (RSV),[225] and titers as high as 1:400 (90%) and 1:38 (~100%) or as low as 1:1 (90%) provide sterilizing immunity against challenge of macaques with chimeric simian-human immunodeficiency virus (SHIV)[115,198,214] In other instances, such as challenge with lymphocytic choriomeningitis virus (LCMV) in a mouse model[312] and with Ebola virus in a guinea pig model,[213] high titers of neutralizing antibody do not provide sterilizing immunity but do prevent disease. In the latter case, similar titers prevent disease due to Ebola virus in guinea pigs but have no effect on disease course in macaques.[205] However, more recently, a cocktail of neutralizing antibodies has been shown to protect macaques against disease due to Ebola virus infection.[225a] In most instances, however, it has not been established whether sterilizing immunity has been achieved.

A number of possible explanations exist for the neutralizing titers required for protection in many animal studies. If the assumption is that neutralization is the dominant protective mechanism, then for some viruses/animal models/challenge routes it may be necessary for protection for antibody to mop up essentially every last virus particle requiring an excess of antibody. With the same assumption, the protective activity may be achieved at a tissue site with a lower antibody concentration than that of serum, again leading to an apparent overcapacity. Alternatively, protection may require an additional activity of neutralizing antibody distinct from neutralization. For instance, it may be that activity against infected cells, as well as (or in some cases even instead of) activity against free virions, is needed to provide protection. This would be consistent with observations that antibody concentrations required for activities against infected cells (e.g., blocking cell-to-cell transmission) are typically higher than required for neutralization of free virus particles. A further alternative explanation is that the neutralization *in vitro* is not reflective of the process *in vivo,* for example the target cell type used *in vitro* may have important differences from the target cell *in vivo.*

Animal model studies do provide evidence that mechanisms other than neutralization can be important in protection by neutralizing antibodies. In some cases, protection is found to be as effective with F(ab′)2 fragments, which lack the Fc domain and, therefore, are unable to trigger effector functions, as the corresponding whole IgG molecule. In other cases, however, F(ab′)2 fragments that are equally active as whole IgG molecules at neutralization *in vitro* are ineffective at protection. For yellow fever virus,[243] it has been shown that neutralizing mouse IgG1 antibodies (poor activators of effector functions) are ineffective at protection, whereas IgG2a molecules (good activators) of the same specificity are effective. Similarly for vaccinia virus,[18] it has been shown that human IgG1 but not IgG4 isotypes of human mAbs are effective. In many of the examples in mouse models in which the Fc part of IgG is important, protection is independent of complement.[212] This implies that protection by neutralizing antibodies in these cases may require activity against infected cells and involves ADCC or phagocytosis. Many examples of protective activity due to passively transferred nonneutralizing antibodies have been described. The activity appears to be directed at infected cells (Fig. 9.4) and generally appears to be somewhat less potent than that due to neutralizing antibodies. For instance, a number of cases have been reported where neutralizing antibodies are protective against higher challenge doses or more pathogenic viruses than nonneutralizing antibodies. In many cases, protection by nonneutralizing antibodies is shown to depend critically on the Fc part of the antibody molecule and to occur in complement-deficient mice, suggesting that ADCC (or phagocytosis) may be crucial in clearing antibody-complexed infected cells. Protection with nonneutralizing antibodies is mostly restricted to those antibodies directed against enveloped viruses.

Passive transfer of antibodies to humans has been shown to provide protection against disease caused by a number of viruses, including hepatitis B, hepatitis A, measles, polio, and RSV.[39] Indeed, a humanized, neutralizing anti-RSV monoclonal antibody is in clinical use to protect at-risk infants.[101] In some or many of these cases, it is unlikely that the titers of passively transferred neutralizing antibody achieve the levels necessary to offer sterilizing immunity, although this has not been widely studied. Rather, it would seem that neutralizing antibody sufficiently blunts the infection to allow the development of other protective mechanisms, presumably a $CD8^+$ T-cell response, active antibody responses, and innate immunity (see below). The protection of young infants by maternal neutralizing antibodies likely falls into this category. Maternal antibodies may "attenuate infection during the initial months of life, thereby creating optimal conditions for the natural immunization of the child as a result of infection".[323] In some instances (e.g., rabies virus infection), passive antibody has been shown to protect against disease after exposure, when some measure of infection is clearly established. Once infection is clearly established, however, reports of beneficial effects of passive antibody are limited.

Many important human viral pathogens gain entry to the host via mucosal surfaces. Passive transfer studies show that antibodies present in the mucosal compartments at the time of exposure can protect against viral challenge.[139,202] Both mucosal secretory IgA (sIgA) and systemic IgG have been shown to be effective. Dramatically, classically nonneutralizing IgA can protect against rotavirus challenge in mice by an intracellular "neutralization" mechanism.[31] A recent study elegantly shows how different antibody specificities can interfere with HPV infection *in vivo* in a cervicovaginal mouse model at two stages: first to prevent virion binding to the basement membrane and second to prevent virion association with the epithelial cell surface.[62]

Evidence for the importance of antibody enhancement of viral infection *in vivo* is limited.[277] Early observations on dengue virus infection in humans[146] are the most convincing, and the case for antibody enhancement leading to dengue-associated disease has been strengthened by recent observations in animal models.[13,321]

In terms of human vaccination, it is often stated that neutralizing antibodies are the best correlate of protection.[7,222] This is not to argue that neutralizing antibodies are the sole or even necessarily the most important mechanism of protection, although the circumstantial evidence in many cases is quite strong. For smallpox, neutralizing titers of 1:20 to 1:32 indicate protective immunity.[105] For measles, low titers of neutralizing antibody (<120 mIU/ml) are strongly associated with clinical disease, intermediate titers (~200 to 900) are associated with a substantial proportion of subclinical infections reflected in boosting of antibody titers following exposure and high titers (>~1,000) with no indication of subclinical infection and possible sterilizing immunity.

EFFECTOR ACTIVITIES OF T CELLS

The categorization of $\alpha{:}\beta$ TCR T cells into $CD8^+$ and $CD4^+$ subsets not only demarcates the MHC molecules that restrict recognition (i.e., class I or class II), but also has functional significance at the effector level (Table 9.5). $CD8^+$ T-cell effector cells ($CD8^+$ T_E) are capable of destroying antigen-displaying cells (e.g., virus-infected cells expressing the appropriate peptide/MHC class I complex) by direct cell-to-cell contact. $CD8^+$ T_E also produce/secrete several cytokines with antiviral activity (e.g., IFN-γ, TNF-α) on TCR engagement. $CD4^+$ T-cell effectors ($CD4^+$ T_E) primarily function by release of cytokines (notably, IFN-γ, and/or IL-4, IL-5) in response to antigenic stimulation. $CD4^+$ T_E, however, in rare instances, can also acquire killing capacity by direct contact with cells displaying the appropriate peptide/MHC class II ligand recognized by the TCR/CD4 complex. The differentiation of the naïve T cells into T_E, in particular naïve $CD4^+$ T-cell differentiation into T_H1, T_H2, or T_H17 effector cells, is regulated by a variety of factors (as discussed below).

TABLE 9.5 Effector Activation of Activated $CD8^+$ and $CD4^+$ T Cells

Effector type	Target cell	Effector mechanism
$CD8^+$ T cell	MHC class I^+	–Direct cytolysis (cell–cell contact) –Granule exocytosis (perforin/granzyme) –FasL (T cell) – Fas (infected target cell) interaction Cytokine synthesis –IFN-γ, TNF-α, chemokines
$CD4^+$ T-cell – T_H1	MHC class II^+	Cytokine synthesis –IFN-γ, TNF-α, chemokines
$CD4^+$ T-cell – T_H2	MHC class II^+	Cytokine synthesis –IL-4, IL-5, IL-13
$CD4^+$ T-cell – T_H17	MHC class II^+	Cytokine synthesis –IL-17A/F, IL-6, +/-IL-21

MHC, major histocompatibility complex; IFN, interferon; TNF, tumor necrosis factor.

CD8$^+$ T$_E$ EFFECTOR MECHANISMS

The CD8$^+$ T$_E$ destroy *target* cells (e.g., virus-infected cells) following direct cell-to-cell contact, by two distinct mechanisms. One mechanism is by granule exocytosis.[161] Mature (fully differentiated) CD8$^+$ T$_E$ contain lytic granules within their cytoplasm, and TCR engagement on the T$_E$ by peptide/MHC class I complexes on the target cell results in the formation of intermolecular signaling clusters (consisting of TCRα:β, CD3, and integrins, e.g., LFA-1). In response to TCR engagement, and signal transduction, the cytoplasmic granules are directed by the cellular microtubule-organizing center along actin filaments to the site of TCR aggregation where the granules are then released onto the surface of the target cell. The adhesive interaction between the T$_E$ and the target cell is stabilized/strengthened through the interaction of LFA-1 (on T$_E$) with its ligand, ICAM-1 (on the target cell). The lytic granules contain a protein, perforin, which has a sequence homology to the complement component C9. The granules also contain a set of serine proteases, known as *granzymes* (for granule enzymes), which are present in a proenzyme form within the T$_E$ granule as part of a multimeric complex with perforin imbedded within a scaffold consisting of proteoglycan, serglycin, which are activated (by granule-associated cathepsin C) on granule exocytosis. Because of its homology to C9, the perforin monomer released onto the target cell was believed to intercalate and polymerize (in the presence of extracellular Ca^{2+}), forming a pore within the target cell plasma membrane that allows the granzymes access to the target cell cytoplasm. More recent evidence suggests that released granzymes bind directly to target cells, possibly through cell surface receptors, and either gain direct access to the cell cytoplasm or are first internalized into endosomes.[28] Perforin may act by facilitating the transfer of granzymes from the cell surface or endosome into the cytoplasm. The granzyme family of serine proteases consists of at least five members in the human (granzyme A, B, C).[235] They are believed to function by activating cell death pathways in the target cells, including both direct activation of the caspase-dependent cell death mechanism, and the caspase-independent mitochondrial death pathway associated with granzyme-dependent activation of proapoptotic Bcl-2 family members (e.g., BID, BAX).[10] Although the mechanism of action and function of each granzyme is not completely understood at present, at least one granzyme, granzyme B, is present in both CD8$^+$ T$_E$ and NK cell lytic granules, and acts by proteolytic cleavage and activation of procaspases (procaspase 3 caspase 3) and proapoptotic Bcl2 family members (e.g., BID $\rightarrow$ BID*) resulting in the indicative DNA fragmentation and mitochondrial damage characteristic of apoptosis. An additional granule-associated lytic molecule, granulysin (present in human T$_E$), can form pores in membranes and may play a role in the destruction of certain bacteria by direct lysis.[151]

The CD8$^+$ T$_E$ can also destroy target cells by the upregulation (in response to TCR engagement) of the TNF family protein, CD154 (FasL, CD95L) on the T$_E$, and engagement of its receptor, the TNF receptor family member, CD95 (Fas), on the infected target cell.[65] CD95 engagement results in the recruitment/activation of caspases and apoptotic death of target cells. Studies in experimental models of virus infection suggest that both the Fas/FasL and the granule exocytosis mechanisms can contribute to the elimination of virus-infected cells, and virus clearance by CD8$^+$ T$_E$.[28,286] The relative contribution of each lytic mechanism to virus clearance differs for different viruses.

The CD8$^+$ T$_E$ also produce a number of cytokines in response to TCR engagement by antigen, most notably IFN-γ and TNF-α. The production/secretion of these effector cytokines appears to be tightly regulated and typically requires TCR-dependent signaling in the CD8$^+$ T$_E$.[268] IFN-γ exhibits its antiviral effects through upregulation of MHC molecule expression and stimulation of the MHC class I processing/presentation pathway in infected cells. Because IFN-γ is a potent activator of tissue macrophages, activated macrophages would also have the capacity to take up and destroy virus/virus-infected cells. TNF-α, as can the other member of the TNF ligand family, CD154 (FasL), induces apoptosis of infected cells expressing the receptor for TFNα, and in addition can signal the production of proinflammatory/anti-viral cytokines through receptor-dependent NF-κB activation. In addition, recent evidence has emerged from the analysis of experimental models of acute virus infection that CD8$^+$ T$_E$ responding to infection can serve as a major source of the regulatory cytokine IL-10.[278] This T-cell derived IL-10 may act to attenuate excess inflammation associated with T cell–dependent virus clearance mechanisms.[278]

CD4$^+$ T$_E$ EFFECTOR MECHANISMS

An essential role of activated CD4$^+$ T cells in antiviral immunity is to provide *help* for responding B cells in the SLOs in the production of anti-viral antibody. Emerging evidence suggests that CD4$^+$ T cells (presumable CD4$^+$ T$_E$ effectors) also play a role, not yet completely defined, in the development and maintenance of the memory CD8$^+$ T-cell response during virus infection.[264,304] CD4$^+$ T$_E$ express effector activity through the release of cytokines on TCR engagement (i.e., recognition of specific peptide/MHC class II complexes on target cells). CD4$^+$ T$_E$ had originally been categorized as T$_H$1 (type 1 or T helper 1) or T$_H$2 (type 2 or T helper 2) T$_E$, based on the constellation of cytokines produced. More recently a third major CD4$^+$ effector T-cell subset or lineage has been identified, the T$_H$17 CD4$^+$ TE. Among these CD4$^+$ T-cell subsets, the T$_H$1 CD4$^+$ T$_E$, which produce IFN-γ and to a lesser extent TNF, serve the most prominent role as the critical CD4$^+$ T$_E$ in virus infection. The hallmark of T$_H$1–induced inflammation is accumulation of mononuclear cells (inflammatory macrophages, monocytes, DCs, lymphocytes, etc.) at sites of infection. The IL-4, IL-5, IL-13 producing T$_H$2 CD4$^+$ T cells are recognized as a major T$_E$ responding to helminth (worm) and certain parasitic infections, and they play a pivotal role in orchestrating the allergic responses to nonpathogenic environmental antigens. The response of T$_H$2 T$_E$ is characterized by the development of IgE antibody to antigens and an inflammatory response rich in eosinophils.[307]

As their name implies, the T$_H$17 T$_E$ produce IL-17A/F (as well as IL-6 and in some instances IL-21). T$_H$17 T$_E$ release these cytokines at sites of infection following TCR engagement by antigen. Because of the ability of these cytokines, in particular IL-17, to activate epithelial cells to produce chemokines that are chemotactic for neutrophils, T$_H$17 T$_E$ are potent inducers of neutrophil recruitment to sites of infection. In keeping with the neutrophil-rich inflammatory response induced by these

T_E, they have been implicated as important adaptive immune effectors in the host response to extracellular bacteria and fungi, as well as in the pathogenesis of certain autoimmune diseases previously believed to be orchestrated by T_H1 T_E. The contribution of T_H17 T_E to the adaptive immune response to the virus infection has yet to be firmly established—although, not surprisingly, T_H17 responses have been reported to be dysregulated in HIV-infected patients,[192] and in one model of experimental virus infection in the CNS, the development of a T_H17 T_E response has been reported to suppress the expression of $CD8^+$ T-cell effector activity.[98]

The strict classification of $CD4^+$ T_E responses into T_H1, T_H2, or T_H17 categories is somewhat artificial and based largely on *in vitro* studies where differentiation of naïve $CD4^+$ T cells into one of these $CD4^+$ effector cell subsets can be skewed to produce a single T_E subset exclusively. During the course of antigen exposure/infection *in vivo,* $CD4^+$ T_E capable of producing both the T_H1 and T_H2 cytokines (or T_H1 and T_H17 cytokines) are generated; and it is the relative proportion of the T_H1 (IFN-γ, TNF-α) or T_H2 (IL-4, IL-5) or T_H17 (IL-17, IL-6) T_E subsets in the T cells responding to infection that dictates the overall balance of the $CD4^+$ T_E response. As noted, it is the milieu in which $CD4^+$ T cells activate or differentiate in response to antigen in the SLOs that dictates the balance between T_H1, T_H2, or T_H17 $CD4^+$ T_E generation.[50] Numerous factors control the $CD4^+$ T-cell differentiation program, and the relative proportion of T_H1 or T_H2 T_E generated. Among these factors are (a) the form and dose of antigen/pathogen; (b) the APC response (in particular, DC) that express cell surface molecules after antigen encounter that can influence $CD4^+$ T-cell differentiation; and (c) cytokine production by APCs (e.g., IL-12p70) and by innate immune cells present in the SLO (e.g., IFN-γ from NK cells, IL-4 from NK T cells, and IL-6 and TGF-β from mononuclear phagocytes and stromal cells). Detailed discussion of the contribution of these T_H1/T_H2/ T_H17 differentiation influences is beyond the scope of this chapter but has been reviewed by others.[50,270] Whereas virus infection, in general, drives $CD4^+$ T-cell differentiation toward the development of T_H1 $CD4^+$ T_E responses, evidence indicates that, in certain chronic human infections, T_H2 $CD4^+$ T_E responses may predominate.[34,270] Because the induction of the T_H2 $CD4^+$ T_E response with IL-4 (and IL-10) production can suppress the development of a T_H1 $CD4^+$ T_E response characteristic of the adaptive immune response to virus infection, this form of virus-induced immune deviation could potentially result in the inhibition of virus clearance, leading to the development of persistent infection. Although virus infection typically results in the development of $CD8^+$ T_E, which are *T_H1-like* (i.e., producing IFN-γ, TNF-α), differentiating $CD8^+$ T cells may also be deviated toward the T_H2 effector response (i.e., weakly cytolytic T_E producing IL-4, IL-5), potentially resulting in decreased virus clearance efficiency by these antiviral T_E.[310]

Whether two other recognized subsets of $CD4^+$ T lymphocytes, the recently appreciated T follicular helper (T_{FH}) T cells and T_{reg} cells can be classified as T_E is up for debate and may simply be a matter of semantics, that is, how one defines an "effector" cell. The factors controlling the differentiation of naïve $CD4^+$ T cells into these various activated T-cell subsets as well as their cytokine profile and role in adaptive immune responses are summarized in Table 9.5. The properties of T_{reg} cells and their role in virus infection are discussed in the next section.

REGULATORY T-CELL FUNCTION IN ANTIVIRAL ADAPTIVE IMMUNE RESPONSES

T_{reg} cells are a subset of $CD4^+$ T cells that express the FoxP3 lineage commitment transcription factor and are crucial for maintaining self-tolerance in the periphery.[81,236] Despite the fact that CD25 and FoxP3 expression are reliable markers for T_{reg} cells in mice, both FoxP3 and CD25 are also expressed by activated T cells in humans. Therefore, FoxP3 expression alone does not serve a reliable T_{reg} marker. Recently additional markers, such as CTLA-4 and lymphocyte activation gene-3 associated protein (LAP), have been identified as human T_{reg} markers: CTLA-4 is known to be functionally active for T_{reg} cells[84] and LAP (a TGF-β binding protein) surface expression is enhanced on functional human T_{reg}.[287] In addition, although lower expression of CD127 has been correlated with FoxP3 expression and suppression in humans,[164] activation of T_{reg} is recently shown to result in an increase in CD127 expression.[262] Nevertheless, a combination of these markers can allow for improved identification of T_{reg} in humans.

The various regulatory T cells are categorized as (a) naturally occurring, thymus-derived $CD4^+CD25^+$ T cells (named as $CD4^+CD25^+$ T_{reg})[122,207]; or (b) induced, peripheral T cells, which include $CD4^+CD25^-$ T cells, T_H3 cells, and $CD8^+$ T cells.[55] T_{reg} subsets are defined by differences in their cell surface marker expression, their cytokine secretion patterns, and their mode of suppression. There is evidence of the generation of $FoxP3^+$ suppressive cells from $FoxP3^-$ nonsuppressive cells both *in vivo* and *in vitro.* These cells are referred to as inducible T_{reg}, adaptive T_{reg}, or iT_{reg}. The factors involved in *in vivo* conversion are not precisely defined. However, TCR activation in the presence of TGF-β has successfully induced T_{reg} development *in vitro.* Two other types of peripherally induced regulatory cells are named Tr1 and Th3. Tr1 causes immunosuppression by secretion of large amounts of IL-10; whereas Tr1 cells develop in the presence of IL-10, IL-15 promotes the survival of these cells. Tr1 cells have regulatory function, but do not express FoxP3. Th3 cells are developed in the presence of TGF-β and also produce a large quantity of this cytokine. Importantly, T_{reg} activity can be modulated by exposure to costimulatory molecules. For instance, activation of OX40 and 4-1BB on $CD4^+CD25^+$ T_{reg} results in increased proliferation; and stimulation of 4-1BB has also been implicated in the maintenance of suppressive function.

T_{reg} cells play a critical role in the regulation of immune responses to viral infection as well as the prevention of tissue damage caused by viral infection. Particularly, T_{reg} cells are involved in suppressing effector T cells in chronic viral infections such as HSV, Epstein-Barr virus (EBV), and HCV, having the appearance of $CD4^+$ regulatory T cells in chronic viral infection. In case of HCV infection, the frequency of $CD4^+CD25^+$ regulatory T cells in chronic patients is greater than those in recovered or healthy patients,[24,33,276] suggesting that natural T_{regs} are associated with the establishment of HCV persistent infection. Apparently, the suppressor function of $CD4^+CD25^+$ T cells derived from chronic HCV patients does not rely on soluble mediator(s) (i.e., cytokines) because neutralizing antibodies to either IL-10 or TGF-β do not reverse suppression.[24] In addition, the frequency of $CD4^+CD25^{hi}$ T cells in patients with hepatocellular carcinoma is greater than in individuals who are chronically infected with HCV.[204]

Besides the role of regulatory T cells in suppression of host immune responses to viral infection, T_{reg} cells are paradoxically essential to control tissue damage caused by host immune responses to viral infection. Direct evidence of a role for regulatory T cells in preventing immunopathology has come from studies using murine models of viral infection. Theiler's murine encephalomyelitis virus (TMEV) infection induces $CD4^+$ T cell–mediated demyelinating disease[110] such that TMEV-specific $CD4^+$ T cells transferred into susceptible, irradiated C/cByJ mice accelerate clinical disease and enhance TMEV-specific delayed-type hypersensitivity (DTH). Importantly, $CD8^+$ T cells from infected C/cByJ mice suppress the *in vivo* disease progression as well as virus-specific T-cell responsiveness in recipients of TMEV-specific $CD4^+$ T-cell blasts. So, the transfer of virus-specific $CD8^+$ regulatory T cells at the time of Theiler's virus infection reduced tissue damage by preventing the pathogenic role of $CD4^+$ T cells. In case of HSV infection, depletion of $CD4^+CD25^+$ T cells before viral infection increases the generation of virus-specific $CD8^+$ T-cell responses and viral clearance.[280,281] In contrast, the severity of T cell–mediated lesions in the cornea of HSV-infected mice was increased upon removal of $CD4^+CD25^+$ T cells. Therefore, $CD4^+CD25^+$ T_{reg} cells are likely involved in reducing the severity of immune-mediated inflammatory lesions by preventing the pathogenic effects of $CD4^+$ T_H1 cells as well as limiting the migration of these cells to inflammatory sites. During chronic viral infections, T_{reg} cells might be beneficial to the host by maintaining a balance between efficient effectors and memory responses, but with a low level of inflammation to limit host tissue damage.

Numerous mechanisms are utilized by eliciting suppressive function of T_{reg} cells. One way is through the production of the suppressive cytokines such as TGF-β and IL-10. Although most studies indicate that the suppressive effect of T_{reg} cells is not mediated by soluble factors,[257] that does not exclude the possibility of contribution of cytokines acting in proximity or cell-bound cytokines. In fact, TGF-β blockade appears to reduce the suppressive function of T_{reg} cells following the administration of high amounts of TGF-β antibodies,[194] and T_{reg} production of IL-10 is also necessary for protection in a murine colitis model.[279] Another way for suppressive function of T_{reg} is mediated by cell surface molecule such as CTLA-4 to negatively regulate T-cell activity and proliferation. The importance of CTLA-4 to T_{reg} suppressive function is evidenced by the development of fatal autoimmune disease as a result of reduced suppressor function in CTLA-4–deficient mice[309] as well as treatment of CTLA-4 blocking antibodies for the action of human T_{reg}.[322] Finally, the induction of effector cell apoptosis as a result of IL-2 consumption is proposed for suppressive function of T_{reg}. T_{reg} cells such as effector T cells require IL-2 to survive and highly express the high-affinity IL-2 receptor containing CD25. However, T_{reg} cells produce no IL-2 and therefore are reliant on other sources of IL-2 for survival. In one study, IL-2 consumption by T_{reg} cells resulted in increased Bim-dependent T-cell apoptosis,[209] whereas other modes of T_{reg}-mediated apoptosis include perforin production by natural T_{reg} cells[100] and FasL expression by inducible T_{reg} cells.[302]

Furthermore, recent studies indicate that T_{reg} cells exert a suppressive effect through modulation of APCs rather than directly modulating effector T cells; a CTLA-4–dependent reduction in CD80/CD86 expression on DCs by T_{reg} cells,[309,189] but other studies show that T_{reg} cells exert no change in the expression of costimulatory molecules on APCs and addition of functional APCs did not overcome T_{reg} suppression.[285] Direct T-cell to T-cell suppression was demonstrated using peptide-MHC tetramer stimulation in the absence of APCs.[217] Further research may clarify possible contributions of APCs to act as target for T_{reg} suppression; however, it is evident that T_{reg} cells can suppress T cells directly.

ADAPTIVE IMMUNE MEMORY

Two features that define the adaptive immune system and distinguish it from the innate immune system are (a) the exquisite specificity for antigen and (b) the establishment of immunologic memory. Immunologic memory is perhaps the most important consequence of the induction of an adaptive immune response. As a result of clonal expansion of antigen-specific B or T lymphocytes, and a lower activation threshold for memory cells, the immune system can respond more rapidly and efficiently to previously encountered pathogens. This capacity of B and T cells to adapt to a previously encountered antigen is the basis for vaccination. Memory B and T cells generated after infection or vaccination are generally long-lived. In humans, memory T-cell responses (or circulating antibody titer) can be detected decades after pathogen exposure, under conditions where subsequent reexposure to (subclinical infection with) the organism or persistent infection is unlikely. Memory B and T cells directed to an antigen are usually present at a frequency 100 to 1,000 times higher than the corresponding naïve immune cell precursors of memory T and B cells. The factors controlling the formation/duration of the memory immune responses are not yet well understood, but several cytokines may play an important role in maintaining the viability and basal (homeostatic) proliferation of memory cells.

B-CELL MEMORY

The phrase "B cell memory" is often used as shorthand for the mechanisms that lead to long-term humoral immunity. The following two principal mechanisms exist: (a) specific memory B cells expressing BCR to viral antigens, so that viral infection leads to activation of specific B cells and ultimately the production of high-affinity, class-switched antibody to virus; and (b) preexisting serum and tissue high-affinity, class-switched antibody to virus, probably from long-lived plasma cells in the bone marrow. We consider each in turn.

MEMORY B CELLS

Memory B cells express class-switched, somatically mutated surface antibody and can be detected as antigen-specific cells using labeled antigen and a technique such as flow cytometry.[182] They are in a resting state and do not secrete antibodies unless stimulated by antigen. When this stimulation is carried out *in vitro,* memory B cells can be readily detected by enzyme-linked immunospot (ELISPOT) assays. In mice, multiple subtypes of memory B cells have been defined by a number of cell surface markers and gene activation markers.[182] After clearance of virus on first exposure, memory B cells accumulate in the spleen and other lymphoid tissues. Reexposure to virus leads to rapid secondary antibody responses to viral antigens. This response arises because of rapid proliferation and differentiation of memory B cells in a CD4+ T-cell–dependent manner. The specific B-cell population of spleen and lymph nodes expands massively, and differentiation to plasma cells generates a burst in specific antibody production and in antibody levels. Therefore, repeated exposure to antigen is one way in which memory B cell levels can be maintained.

Although controversies have existed over the years, it appears that memory B cells can be long-lived, even in the absence of antigen. An elegant experiment by Maruyama et al.[173] is persuasive. Mice were engineered so the memory B cells expressing a BCR against antigen 1 could be switched *in vivo* to express a BCR specific for antigen 2. B cells expressing BCR to antigen 2 were identified as persisting in the mice as well as B cells expressing BCR to antigen 1, although the mice had never encountered antigen 2. It should also be noted that BCR expression is required for B-cell survival,[153] so the possibility exists that nonspecific BCR stimulation, perhaps via a low affinity antigen interaction, is needed for persistence of B-cell memory. Alternatively, the BCR may receive a signal from another molecule such as a cytokine or a molecule such as a B-cell activating factor (BAFF).

One interesting phenomenon related to memory B cells is that of original antigenic sin, (OAS), which was first proposed to describe a phenomenon whereby an individual, originally infected with a virus and then later with variant of this virus, makes an antibody response during the second viral infection that reacts more strongly to the original virus than the newer variant.[60] It is suggested that boosting of memory B cells against the first virus may interfere with the activation of naïve B cells to the second virus by an undefined mechanism, resulting in a condition that specific antibody responses against the second virus will not be as great compared with a naïve host that has never encountered the first virus. OAS has been reported in both humans[76,102] and animals,[77] although a recent study found no evidence of OAS in healthy adults receiving influenza vaccination.[311]

LONG-LIVED PLASMA CELLS

Plasma cells are terminally differentiated, nondividing cells able to secrete relatively large amounts of antibody. Two populations of plasma cells exist. Short-lived plasma cells survive for only a few days, produce antibody in extrafollicular foci, and are probably crucial in the very early response to pathogen.[168] In mice, a second population of plasma cells, secreting high-affinity antibody, is long-lived. Irradiation experiments show that the half-life of plasma cells secreting antibody to LCMV was 94 days in the bone marrow and 172 days in the spleen.[266] Pulse chase experiments show that plasma cells secreting specific antibody to ovalbumin survived without cell division for a minimum of 3 months.[171] These half-lives constitute a sizable proportion of the total lifespan of the mouse. It may be that plasma cells live for many years in humans and contribute to the maintenance of antibody levels over decades.[97] The bone marrow niche appears to provide survival signals to plasma cells, because *in vitro* such cells survive for only a few days. Another hypothesis is that the pool of plasma cells is being continually replenished from specific memory B cells that are undergoing antigen-independent or bystander activation.[19] These two hypotheses are not mutually exclusive, and it is possible that multiple mechanisms are involved in maintaining serum antibody levels.

LONG-TERM HUMORAL IMMUNITY

Humoral responses can be measured in the sera of humans many years after the last known contact with the pathogen (Table 9.6). Similarly, many vaccines induce serum antibody responses that are present decades later.[223] A key question has been: Are these responses maintained by intrinsic mechanisms or is there a periodic boosting of immunity through contact with antigen? This question can be difficult to answer given the

TABLE 9.6 Humoral Response to Acute Viral Infection in Humans

Example	Virus family	Persistence of antibody
Systemic infections		
Chikungunya	*Alphaviridae*	30 yr
Rift Valley fever	*Bunyaviridae*	12 yr
Dengue	*Flaviviridae*	32 yr
Yellow fever	*Flaviviridae*	75 yr
Measles	*Paramyxoviridae*	65 yr
Mumps	*Paramyxoviridae*	12 yr
Polio	*Picornaviridae*	40 yr
Hepatitis A	*Picornaviridae*	25 yr
Smallpox	*Poxviridae*	40 yr
Vaccinia	*Poxviridae*	75 yr
Rubella	*Togaviridae*	14 yr
Mucosal infections		
Coronavirus	*Coronaviridae*	12 mo
Influenza	*Orthomyxoviridae*	30 mo
RSV	*Paramyxoviridae*	3 mo
Rotavirus	*Reoviridae*	12 mo

RSV, respiratory syncytial virus; yr, year; mo, month.

Modified from Slifka MK, Ahmed R. Long-term humoral immunity against viruses: revisiting the issue of plasma cell longevity. Trends Microbiol 1996;4:394–400.

unknowns associated with typical human contacts with pathogens. For at least two vaccines, serum antibody levels appear to be maintained in the absence of antigen boosting.[53]

A large cross-sectional study of poliovirus immunity in Sweden, a country from which the virus has been eradicated, and which used inactivated poliovirus only as a vaccine, showed substantial anti-poliovirus antibody titers in all age groups.[26] Virtually no differences in titers were found in the different age groups, indicating the maintenance of antibody titers over decades in the absence of further vaccination or exposure to live virus. Notably, in the same study, declining antibody titers against tetanus and diphtheria were observed.

Two studies have looked at smallpox vaccination using vaccinia virus.[54,105] Vaccinia is an excellent model for investigating immune memory, because the virus is typically cleared from the site of infection within a month, does not persist, and does not spread systemically in healthy individuals. Immunization with vaccinia ceased in 1972 and smallpox has been eradicated. Specific memory B cells could be detected more than 60 years after vaccination.[53,54] Furthermore, memory B cells seemed to show a bimodal kinetics. A drop from peak responses occurred at vaccination to an approximately 10-year time point, but stable levels were seen between 10 and 60 years. Serum antibody responses could be identified at 60 to 75 years after vaccination.[54,75,105] Because overall antivaccinia antibody levels correlated well with neutralizing antivaccinia antibody levels, it was postulated that different specificities may be equally well preserved. Furthermore, the results suggest, as originally posited by Jenner more than 200 years ago, that protective immunity against lethal smallpox infection may be lifelong.

Finally, it is apparent from Table 9.6, that mucosal antibody responses are much shorter-lived than are serum responses. This may indicate that plasma cells initially produced at mucosal sites migrate to the bone marrow and contribute less to mucosal antibody production.

T-CELL MEMORY

Unlike the immunoglobulin receptors on B cells, the genes encoding the TCR on $CD4^+$ T cell and $CD8^+$ T cells do not undergo any additional somatic mutations, and memory T cells do not, therefore, exhibit affinity maturation after antigen encounter. Memory T cells distinguished functionally from their naïve precursors by being present at increased frequency (a result of clonal expansion of naïve antigen-specific T cells), and by their lower activation threshold (i.e., decreased requirement for CD28 co-stimulation) to trigger cell proliferation and differentiation.[247] Certain memory T cells can also rapidly express effector activity (e.g., proinflammatory/antiviral cytokines, such as IFN-γ and TNF-α) within hours after TCR engagement on these T cells, and without DNA synthesis (additional cell proliferation). Naïve T-cell activation and proliferation and memory T-cell population formation and maintenance are controlled by three cytokines: IL-2, IL-7, and IL-15.[244] The receptors on T cells for these three cytokines have a common feature—these heterodimeric and trimeric receptors have a common signaling subunit, the so-called *γ chain* (γ_c), which participates in both ligand (cytokine) binding and Janus Kinase (JAK)/STAT–dependent signal transduction.[149] IL-2/IL-15 can drive proliferation of activated naïve T cells after TCR engagement (IL-4, which engages another member of the γ_c family of cytokine receptors, will also support proliferation of differentiating T_H2 $CD4^+$ T cells). Current evidence suggests that once memory T cells are formed, they can undergo basal/homeostatic low-level proliferation, which is IL-15-dependent, and long-term memory T-cell viability (i.e., suppression of apoptosis) is supported by IL-7, which upregulates/sustains the expression of anti-apoptotic Bcl-2 gene family members in the developing memory T cells.

Although activated naïve T cells give rise to both effector (T_E) and memory (T_M) T cells, the relationship of the two naïve T-cell products is unclear (i.e., we do not know if T_E give rise to T_M in a linear progression, or if T_E and T_M are separate cellular subsets).[247] T_M can be distinguished from naïve T cells and, to a lesser extent, from T_E by the expression of certain cell surface molecules (e.g., isoforms of CD45) differentially expressed on T_M and naïve T cells. Several lines of recent evidence indicate that a further subdivision may exist of $CD4^+$ T cell and $CD8^+$ T cell T_M into central memory (T_{CM}) and peripheral effector memory (T_{EM}) populations.[155] T_{CM} express cell surface molecules such as CD62L and the chemokine receptor CCR7, which would facilitate the circulation of T_{CM} from the blood into the SLOs (particularly the lymph nodes). So, T_{CM} would mimic the circulation pattern of naïve T cells (from the blood into secondary lymphoid organs (SLO) and then back into the bloodstream), and would respond to antigen delivered to the SLO; and, as with naïve T cells, T_{CM} may require both activation and cell division to express effector activity. By contrast, T_{EM} do not display the homing receptors for the SLOs, and have been suggested to reside primarily in the blood and peripheral tissues, where they can rapidly respond to a pathogen at the initial site of pathogen entry in the periphery. Unlike T_{CM}, the T_{EM} appear to undergo limited proliferation in response to antigen, but rapidly express antimicrobial effector activity in response to infection. Although this classification of memory T cells (T_{CM}/T_{EM}) based on cell surface markers is useful as an experimental framework, evidence from the analysis of the immune response to virus infection in humans suggests that considerable heterogeneity exists in cell surface marker expression on circulating T cells in the peripheral blood.[292] Therefore, under conditions of natural infection (and possible vaccination) the memory T-cell response may consist of a continuum of activation and differentiation states—at least, based on activation/differentiation marker expression.

MEMORY $CD8^+$ T CELL DIFFERENTIATION

Memory $CD8^+$ T cells are characterized by distinct features in terms of quantity and quality of responses from their naïve precursors.[3,21,136] Substantial progress has been made in defining the phenotypic and functional changes involved in the course of memory $CD8^+$ T-cell differentiation. During the acute phase of viral infection, antigen recognition and inflammatory signals such as type I IFN and IL-12 induce a rapid and substantial clonal expansion of naïve antigen-specific T cells, which develop into effector T cells at 1 to 2 weeks after infection.[133,148] In this expansion phase, there are several changes in phenotype and function of antigen-specific T cells to acquire memory T cells. At the peak of $CD8^+$ T cell responses, naïve T-cell expansion leads to two distinct subsets (short-liver effector cells and memory precursor effector cells). These cells can be defined by expression of the cell surface markers CD127 and KLRG1.[135,239] CD127 is highly expressed on naïve T cells but appears to be downregulated on all antigen-specific $CD8^+$ T cells after activation. These $CD127^{lo}$ T cells consist of $KLRG1^{hi}$ and $KLRG1^{lo/int}$. Memory $CD8^+$ T cells arise from $KLRG1^{lo/int}$ populations by subsequent reexpression of CD127. However, these memory precursor effector cells ($CD127^{hi}KLRG1^{lo/int}$) efficiently survive the contraction phase, memory T-cell properties, and constitute the majority of the memory T-cell pool. These memory $CD8^+$ T cells further differentiate into self-renewing memory T cells, and the extended lifespan depends partly on IL-7/IL-15–dependent homeostatic proliferation having slow cell division and minimal cell number changes.

Recently, factors involved in controlling the differentiation of effector and memory $CD8^+$ T cells have been demonstrated. First, T box expressed in T-cells (T bet) has been identified as a transcription factor regulating the differentiation of effector and memory $CD8^+$ T-cell responses[133]: the high levels of inflammation and T-bet promoted effector cell differentiation, whereas mild inflammation and low T-bet generated memory cells. Another T-box transcription factor, Eomesodermin (Eomes), is expressed in a reciprocal manner to T-bet such that it is repressed by inflammatory cytokine, IL-12[284] and may play a role in promoting memory responses.[127] In addition, genetic studies reveal that their function is redundant by promoting both killer T-cell fate and $CD8^+$ memory homeostasis.[126] Lastly, Blimp-1, a regulator of plasma cell differentiation, is required for $CD8^+$ T cell differentiation into functional killer cells and is crucial for recall response to reinfection. However, Blimp-1 is not essential for the generation of memory T cells.[138]

VIRAL STRATEGIES TO EVADE THE ADAPTIVE IMMUNE RESPONSE

The immune responses to virus involve complex molecular and cellular interaction between the virus and its host. Therefore, any stage in this interaction could be targeted by a pathogen and used for its own benefit. The systematic study of viral genomes reveals that most viruses have evolved means of escaping or subverting immune defenses, and that some of them have many genes devoted to this purpose. Although the large, more complex DNA viruses encode viral proteins to avoid immune recognition, RNA viruses usually generate small numbers of proteins as compared to DNA virus with large genomic materials. Regardless of whether they are DNA and RNA viruses, it seems that many, and possibly all, pathogens that cause chronic infections have evolved strategies to subvert the immune responses of the host as listed in Table 9.7. These strategies include evasion of humoral and cellular immunity by antigen variation, interference with antigen processing and presentation, and modulating the production of cytokines. Viral proteins that interfere with class I MHC antigen presentation and modulate inflammatory cytokines are listed in Tables 9.8 and 9.9. Understanding of the complex interactions between the immune system of the host and the invading viral pathogen will eventually enable researchers to devise better strategies for preventing viral diseases.

As described above, effector function of $CD8^+$ T cells and $CD4^+$ T_H1 cells plays a pivotal role in controlling viral infection. One critical way to induce virus-specific T-cell responses deals with the generation of antigenic peptides derived from viral products to $CD8^+$ T cells and $CD4^+$ T_H1 cells. The generation of antigenic peptides also involves the

TABLE 9.7 Viral Strategies to Avoid Host Adaptive Immunity

- Escape by mutations
- Escape by latency
- Escape by destruction of immune cells
- Escape by subverting antigen processing and presentation
- Inhibition of T cell–mediated target cell lysis
- Inhibition of inflammatory responses via modulation of cytokine action
- Inhibition of humoral immunity by virally encoded Fc receptor, complement receptor/control protein

TABLE 9.8 Inhibition of Antigen Presentation Via the Major Histocompatibility Complex Class I Pathway

Steps to Interfere with MHC class I pathway	Virus-encoded proteins
Inhibit MHC class I synthesis	Lentivirus (Vpu)
Inhibit transporter associated with antigen processing (TAP)	
–Expression	EBV (vIL-10), HCMV (UL111A)
–Function	HCMV (US6), HSV (ICP47)
Inhibit MHC class I transport	
–Retain MHC class I in the ER	HCMV (US3), adenovirus (E3-19K)
–Retain MHC class I in the pre-Golgi compartment	MCMV (m152)
–Dislocate MHC class I to the cytoplasm	HCMV (US11, US2)
–Dislocate MHC class I to lysosomes	MCMV (m6/gp48)
–Bind to cell surface MHC class I molecules	MCMV (gp34)
–Increase endocytosis of MHC class I molecules	HIV (nef), HHV-8 (K3, K4)

EBV, Epstein-Barr virus; ER, endoplasmic reticulum; MHC, major histocompatibility complex; HCMV, human cytomegalovirus; HSV, herpes simplex virus; MCMV, murine cytomegalovirus; HIV, human immunodeficiency virus; HHV, human herpesvirus.

TABLE 9.9 Viral Modulation of the Cytokine System

Ways to interfere with cytokine function
Interrupt cytokine production
–Interfere with cytokine and chemokine synthesis
–Inhibit the generation of functional cytokines
Interfere with cytokine action
–Encode homologs of cytokines and cytokine receptors
–Type I interferon (IFN) homolog: VV (B18R)
–IFN-γ homolog: VV (B8R)
–Interleukin (IL)-6: KSHV (K2)
–IL–8 homolog: HCMV (UL146, 147)
–IL–10 homolog: EBV (BCRF1), HCMV (UL111A)
–Generate soluble cytokine receptors to neutralize cytokines
–IFN-γ receptor: myxoma virus (MT–7)
–IL-1βR: VV WR (B15R)
–TNFR homolog: orthopoxvirus (CrmB, CrmD)
Interfere with cytokine effector function
–Alter cytokine signaling pathway

HCMV, human cytomegalovirus; EBV, Epstein-Barr virus; IFN, interferon; IL, interleukin; TNFR, tumor necrosis factor receptor; Crm, cytokine response modifier.

class I II MHC-dependent presentation of antigenic peptides to $CD8^+$ and $CD4^+$ T cells. The details for virus-mediated class I MHC and class II MHC antigen presentation is well described in.[131,162] A second critical way for successful induction of antiviral T-cell responses involves the production of cytokines such as IFN-γ, which is pivotal for protective $CD8^+$ T cells and $CD4^+$ T_H1 cells. It has been well established that IFN-γ production is positively influenced by IL-12, but is negatively regulated by IL-10. It is conceivable that viruses exploit strategies to mimic the immunomodulatory cytokines, IL-12 and IL-10, to modulate virus-specific T-cell responses.[4] Among the multiple ways to subvert adaptive T-cell responses, we will describe viral immune evasion strategies to evade innate immunity by interfering with the recognition of viral constituents by pattern-recognition receptor (PPR) and the initiation of inflammatory responses.

Innate immunity consists of multiple cellular sensors and signaling pathways, which lead to activation of early host defense mechanisms in response to viral invasion. These early antiviral responses result in the production of type I IFN that activates numerous transcription factors to induce the inflammatory gene expression.[23,128,140] Thereby the early detection of viruses is the main role of innate immune cells by sensing virus-derived molecules and triggering host defense mechanisms. These sensors include the RIG-I–like helicase family for recognition of viral RNA as well as TLR and NOD-like receptor pathways for sensing various virus-derived molecules.

Activation of the interferon response is triggered by the detection of viral pathogen-associated patterns. All of the PRRs initiate signaling pathways that converge at the activation of transcription factors, IRF-3, IRF-7, and NF-κB. The activation of these transcription factors leads to the expression of IFN-β. IFN-β initiates an anti-viral effector program in the infected cells and neighboring cells by the expression of numerous IFN-stimulated genes (ISGs). Because the host has evolved strategies for detecting and responding to viral infection, viruses constantly evade TLR signaling to inhibit antiviral IFN action. One best example is the cleavage of IPS1 by HCV NS3/4a protease to block RIG-I signaling.[82,90] The influenza A virus NS1 protein inhibits RIG-I–mediated PRR signaling by direct interaction,[89,206] whereas paramyxovirus V protein binds and inhibits MDA-5 to abrogate PPR signaling.[42,43]

VIRAL EVASION OF HUMORAL (B CELL) IMMUNITY

Viruses use a number of mechanisms to evade humoral immune responses, and viral neutralizing antibodies in particular (reviewed in[156]). Viral strategies to evade neutralizing antibody responses to the viral surface proteins include (a) mutation of surface proteins by antigenic drift and shift, and recombination, most notably for highly variable viruses such as influenza virus, HIV and HCV; (b) masking of conserved epitopes; (c) glycan shielding as seen for HIV and Ebola viruses for example; (d) surface protein decoys that may "mop up" neutralizing antibodies under certain conditions, for example as with HBV; (e) original antigenic sin; (f) irregular surface protein spacing that tends to reduce immunogenicity; and (g) multiple surface proteins and virus forms, for example poxviruses encode multiple proteins for entry. Viruses can also evade humoral responses by spreading directly between cells, upregulating and hijacking host complement regulatory proteins, encoding antagonistic Fc and complement receptors and inducing immunosuppression.

VIRAL EVASION OF CELLULAR (T CELL) IMMUNITY

Escape by Subverting Antigen Processing and Presentation

A number of viruses have devised strategies to impair presentation of their antigens by the MHC class I pathway, thereby reducing activation of antigen-specific $CD8^+$ T cells as well as recognition of virus-infected cells by $CD8^+$ T cells. This stresses the importance of this cell subset for antiviral defense. Nearly every step of the MHC class I presentation pathway can be interfered with, and some viruses encode multiple proteins that act at different levels of the MHC class I processing pathway (Table 9.8): (a) inhibition of MHC class I synthesis, (b) antigenic peptide generation, (c) transporter associated with antigen processing, and (d) the cell surface expression of MHC class I molecule expression. Although interference of the MHC class II antigen processing pathway by virus is less common, some evidence indicates that viruses are able to inhibit this pathway.

Inhibition of Class I or II Major Histocompatibility Complex Synthesis

Viral proteins, including HIV Tat protein, have been reported to suppress or inhibit MHC gene promoter activity.[120] It has been shown for HIV Tat protein that the activity of the MHC class I gene promoter was decreased up to 12 times. With respect to the inhibition of MHC class II expression, human cytomegalovirus (HCMV) can impair MHC class II expression through two distinct pathways. MHC class II molecules are expressed only on a subset of cells, and this expression is regulated at the transcriptional level through control elements that include those that allow both constitutive and cytokine-induced transcription of the MHC class II genes. The MHC class II transactivator (CIITA) is essential for constitutive and induced transcription, and is the rate-limiting factor of MHC class II production. One of the four promoters controlling CIITA production is activated by IFN-γ, which, on binding to its receptors, triggers a signaling cascade through Janus kinases, leading to transcription of IFN-inducible genes. The inhibition of IFN-γ–stimulated MHC class II expression occurs by two different mechanisms: (a) decreased Janus kinases[186] and (b) interference with the CIITA promoter.[158]

INHIBITION OF ANTIGENIC PEPTIDE GENERATION

The metalloproteases, CD10 (endopeptidase) and CD13 (aminopeptidase N), are downregulated during HCMV infection.[216] CD10 expression is apparently blocked at the transcriptional or translational level, whereas CD13 seems to be retained within the ER compartment. These endopeptidases play a role in peptide processing in both MHC class I and II antigen presentation pathways. Both CD10 and CD13 peptidases are expressed on the cell surface and trim antigenic peptides to a size that allows their binding to the groove of class I or II molecules.

Inhibition of Transporter Associated with Antigen Processing

The peptide transporter TAP is needed to shuttle peptides from the cytoplasm to the ER, in which they associate with MHC class I determinants. TAP peptide transport is inhibited by a protein of HCMV, US6, which acts from the luminal site of the ER. HCMV US6 protein specifically binds at the ER-luminal loops of TAP signals across the membrane to the nucleotide-binding domains. This binding prevents ATP hydrolysis of TAP, which is necessary for peptide transport.

The ICP47 polypeptide from HSV inhibits TAP by binding to TAP's peptide binding site, thus preventing its association with other peptides. This results in an insufficient number of peptides in the ER for binding to MHC class I molecules. In contrast, TAP-independent peptide loading of MHC class I molecules is not affected by US6 or ICP47. As described below, EBV encodes a protein that weakly binds the IL-10 receptor. As with cellular IL-10, the EBV protein reduces expression of TAP and of MHC class II.

INHIBITION OF MAJOR HISTOCOMPATIBILITY COMPLEX CLASS I CELL SURFACE EXPRESSION

Modulation of MHC class I expression has been reported in at least three viral systems: adenoviruses, HCMV, and HSV. HCMV US3 protein, a type I membrane protein, prevents maturation of MHC class I molecules by retaining them in the ER compartment. US3 protein binds to MHC class I molecules in a transient fashion, but retains them efficiently in the ER. The US3 luminal domain is responsible for ER retention of US3 itself, whereas both the US3 luminal and transmembrane domains are necessary for retaining MHC class I in the ER. In contrast to HCMV US3 protein, HCMV US2 and US11 catalyze the dislocation of MHC class I products, resulting in their rapid degradation. US11 protein uses its transmembrane domain to recruit MHC class I products to human homologue of yeast Der1p, a protein essential for the degradation of MHC class I molecules catalyzed by US11, but not by US2. HCMV US2 has been shown to differentially affect surface expression of MHC class I but only targets membrane-bound (not soluble) HLA-G1 antigen for degradation.

Adenovirus expresses a protein E3/19K, which is an ER-retained protein; it has a cytosolic ER-retention signal in the C-terminus of its cytoplasmic tail (-DEKKMP). The 19K binds certain murine MHC class I molecules (e.g., A2, K^d, L^d, but not K^k, or D^d) and holds them in the ER. This results in decreased MHC class I expression and decreased CTL recognition. An immediate early gene product of HSV, the ICP47 gene product, interferes with transport of peptides from the cytoplasm to the ER, thereby depriving MHC class I molecules in the ER of peptides. This results in both the ER peptides and destabilization and retention of MHC class I molecules in the ER.

VIRAL EVASION OF IMMUNE EFFECTOR MECHANISMS

Interference with Cytokine Functions

Cytokines (e.g., IFN and TNF) induce intracellular pathways that activate an antiviral stage or apoptosis, and thereby limit viral replication. A large number of cytokines induce mechanisms that enhance immune recognition and/or immune responses that protect against viral infection. In addition, antiviral cytokines play a pivotal role in removal of infected cells by NK cells or CTL. Therefore, it is not surprising that viruses use immune evasion strategies to control the function of cytokines.

Recently, viral modulation of cytokines by several viruses has been reported. Three different mechanisms have been shown to affect the activity of cytokines (Table 9.9). Viruses produce cytokine homologs, which bind to the same cytokine receptors. Alternatively, viruses generate antigens that mimic cytokine receptors and, thus, neutralize the corresponding factors. Finally, they can directly interfere with the action of cytokines by generating soluble cytokine-binding proteins. The functions of viral homologues of cytokine and their receptors are diverse. The virus-encoded cytokine homologs might be involved in inactivating inflammatory cytokines or redirecting the immune responses.

Inhibition of cytokine production has been shown by poxvirus; cowpox virus (CPV) cytokine response modifier A (CrmA) protein inhibits the production of caspase-1, which prevents the proteolytic cleavage of prointerleukin-1β (pro–IL-1β) to mature IL-1β. In addition, the attachment of measles virus to its cellular receptor, CD46, a complement regulatory protein, inhibits the production of IL-12. Many virus-encoded mechanisms are involved in blocking the effector functions of cytokines, such as the antiviral state induced by IFN or apoptosis triggered by TNF, and intracellular antagonists of TNF or IL-1/Toll-like receptor (TLR) signaling. Interestingly, LMP-1 of EBV recruits components of tumor necrosis factor receptor (TNFR) and CD40 signal-transduction machinery, which induces biological responses to help viral replication.

RECEPTOR BINDING AND MODULATION OF IMMUNE CELL FUNCTION

Measles virus binds to, and enters, monocyte/macrophages using the CD46 molecule (a C3b receptor) as its receptor for entering cells; cross-linking CD46 inhibits the production of IL-12 by macrophages. Therefore, measles-induced immune suppression may be related to the failure of infected APCs to make the proinflammatory cytokine IL-12. Another IL-12 homolog, UL111A, is encoded by HCMV.

CYTOKINE AND CYTOKINE RECEPTOR HOMOLOGS

Alterations in cytokine function represent a newly appreciated mechanism of evasion. One of the most striking examples of this mechanism has been reported for EBV, has apparently cannibalized the gene for the human IL-10 cytokine. The viral genome, gene BCRF1, encodes a protein with 70% amino acid homology to human IL-10, which inhibits cytokine production by T_H1 type T cells and monocytes (macrophages) through its action on macrophage function. IL-10 also activates B lymphocytes and upregulates BCL-2. The viral IL-10 has all of the same activities as human IL-10.

Our understanding of the role of viral immunomodulatory proteins in the context of infection is limited, mainly because of the lack of appropriate experimental models of infection. In many cases, we can only predict the *in vivo* function of a viral protein in view of a known function of cytokines. As expected, inactivation of poxvirus-soluble cytokine receptors (e.g., the myxoma virus vTNFR and vIFN-γR, or the vaccinia virus vIFN-α/βBP) leads to virus attenuation. The attenuated phenotype of the myxoma virus vIFN-γR (M-T7) mutant might also be attributed to the ability of M-T7 virus to bind chemokines, which is consistent with increased leukocyte recruitment to sites of infection. The consequences of the inactivation of a viral immunomodulatory protein on the outcome of infection, however, might be unpredictable. Deletion of vaccinia vIL-1βR exacerbates vaccinia virus infection in a mouse intranasal model because of enhanced systemic activity of the proinflammatory cytokine IL-1β, which might cause increased fever and weight loss, leading to enhanced mortality of the infected host. This indicates that some viral immunomodulatory proteins might downregulate immune-mediated pathology to favor equilibrium with the host, rather than to increase viral replication.

VIRUS-INDUCED IMMUNE DYSREGULATION AND AUTOIMMUNE DISEASE

Chronic diseases can result when the immune system is overly active, often causing the affected tissues to be inflamed and abnormally infiltrated by lymphocytes and other leukocytes. However, no active infection is associated with such diseases. Therefore, these diseases are caused by the immune system itself, which attacks cells and tissues of the body. Chronic diseases of this kind are known as autoimmune diseases, as they are caused by immune responses directed toward self-components of the body. Several genetic risk factors and protective elements have shown to influence the susceptibility of autoimmune disease.[74] However, a considerable discordance in incidence of autoimmune disease comparing identical twins indicates that, in many cases, additional factors such as environment modulators could influence the incidence of autoimmune diseases.[47]

Indeed, viral infections, particularly chronic viruses, are shown to enhance autoimmune disease in susceptible individuals, as infections frequently induce strong inflammatory responses in various organs.[203,210] There are several major pathways through which viruses can initiate or more likely modulate autoimmunity: (a) direct infection of target cells/organs can cause the release of sequestered autoantigens and enhance antigen presentation; (b) local inflammation might alter the repertoire of self-epitopes presented by APCs by altering Ag degradation properties of the proteasome; (c) Presentation of pathogen epitopes with structural or sequential similarity to self-epitopes might specifically activate autoreactive lymphocytes. However, some viral infections can also act to ameliorate autoimmunity. There are several reports supporting the association of autoimmune diseases with viral infection. Indeed, associations with infectious agents have been suggested for a multitude of autoimmune diseases, including type 1 diabetes (TID), multiple sclerosis (MS), and ankylosing spondylitis. However, attempts to establish a direct epidemiological, statistically relevant association between microbial infections and various autoimmune disorders have been unsuccessful thus far.

Recently, several animal models for human autoimmune diseases have been established to elucidate the role of molecular mimicry in initiating autoimmune diseases. In transgenic animals that express specific target antigens, challenge with pathogens containing identical or similar antigens act as a triggering factor for the autoimmune disease process.[46] The induction of autoimmune disease in these models requires sufficient numbers of autoaggressive lymphocytes. Thereby, it is likely that infection with a pathogen having molecular identity to a target self antigen can result in the generation of more lymphocytes with high avidity to the identical transgenic target antigen. In the rat insulin promotor (RIP)-LCMV model for type 1 diabetes, the avidity of self-reactive lymphocytes has been demonstrated to determine the course of disease. RIP-LCMV mice express the glycoprotein or nucleoprotein of LCMV under the control of the RIP, specifically in the β cell of the pancreatic islets of Langerhans.[299] However, even in the absence of possible thymic expression of target antigen, mechanism of peripheral tolerance can result in a certain degree of unresponsiveness to the identical antigen present on the triggering virus that might prevent aggressive immune responses. In addition, infection with pathogens with similar but not identical structures might overcome tolerance induced by the host. This has been demonstrated in the development of autoimmune hepatitis in the CYP2D6 mouse model, which is associated with the molecular mimicry. In the model of CYP2D6, adenovirus (Ad-2D6) expressing human cytochrome P450 (CYP) 2D6 (CYP2D6) was used to trigger autoimmune liver damage, and CYP2D6 is a major natural autoantigen in autoimmune hepatitis type 2.[170,320] As targets, wild-type FVH mice, which express mouse CYP isoenzymes with a structural and sequential similarity to human CYP2D6 (molecular mimicry), or transgenic CYP2D6 mice, which express additional human CYP2D6 (molecular identity). However, it is yet to be known whether autoimmunity initiated by the molecular mimicry generates enough autoaggressive lymphocytes with sufficient avidity to cross the threshold for clinical autoimmune disease.

REFERENCES

All cited references are available in the e-book.

1. Ackerman AL, Cresswell P. Cellular mechanisms governing cross-presentation of exogenous antigens. *Nat Immunol* 2004;5:678–684.
3. Ahmed R, Gray D. Immunological memory and protective immunity: understanding their relation. *Science* 1996;272:54–60.
4. Alcami A. Viral mimicry of cytokines, chemokines and their receptors. *Nat Rev Immunol* 2003;3:36–50.
6. Amanna IJ, Carlson NE, Slifka MK. Duration of humoral immunity to common viral and vaccine antigens. *N Engl J Med* 2007;357:1903–1915.
8. Amanna IJ, Slifka MK. Contributions of humoral and cellular immunity to vaccine-induced protection in humans. *Virology* 2011;411: 206–215.
10. Ashton-Rickardt PG. The granule pathway of programmed cell death. *Crit Rev Immunol* 2005;25:161–182.
11. Bachmann MF, Kundig TM, Odermatt B, et al. Free recirculation of memory B cells versus antigen-dependent differentiation to antibody-forming cells. *J Immunol* 1994;153:3386–3397.
13. Balsitis SJ, Williams KL, Lachica R, et al. Lethal antibody enhancement of dengue disease in mice is prevented by Fc modification. *PLoS Pathog* 2010;6:e1000790.
14. Batista FD, Harwood NE. The who, how and where of antigen presentation to B cells. *Nat Rev Immunol* 2009;9:15–27.
16. Beltramello M, Williams KL, Simmons CP, et al. The human immune response to Dengue virus is dominated by highly cross-reactive antibodies endowed with neutralizing and enhancing activity. *Cell Host Microbe* 2010;8:271–283.
17. Belz GT, Smith CM, Kleinert L, et al. Distinct migrating and nonmigrating dendritic cell populations are involved in MHC class I-restricted antigen presentation after lung infection with virus. *Proc Natl Acad Sci U S A* 2004;101:8670–8675.
18. Benhnia MR, McCausland MM, Moyron J, et al. Vaccinia virus extracellular enveloped virion neutralization in vitro and protection in vivo depend on complement. *J Virol* 2009;83:1201–1215.
19. Bernasconi NL, Traggiai LE, Lanzavecchia A. Maintenance of serological memory by polyclonal activation of human memory B cells. *Science* 2002;298:2199–2202.
21. Bevan MJ. Helping the CD8(+) T-cell response. *Nat Rev Immunol* 2004; 4:595–602.
23. Blasius AL, Beutler B. Intracellular toll-like receptors. *Immunity* 2010; 32:305–315.
24. Boettler T, Spangenberg HC, Neumann-Haefelin C, et al. T cells with a CD4+CD25 +regulatory phenotype suppress in vitro proliferation of virus-specific CD8+ T cells during chronic hepatitis C virus infection. *J Virol* 2005;79:7860–7867.
26. Bottiger M, Gustavsson O, Svensson A. Immunity to tetanus, diphtheria and poliomyelitis in the adult population of Sweden in 1991. *Int J Epidemiol* 1998;27:916–925.
28. Bouvier M. Accessory proteins and the assembly of human class I MHC molecules: a molecular and structural perspective. *Mol Immunol* 2003;39:697–706.
31. Burns JW, Siadat-Pajouh M, Krishnaney AA, et al. Protective effect of rotavirus VP6-specific IgA monoclonal antibodies that lack neutralizing activity. *Science* 1996;272:104–107.
32. Burton DR. Antibodies, viruses and vaccines. *Nat Rev Immunol* 2020; 2:706–713.
33. Cabrera R, Tu Z, Xu Y, et al. An immunomodulatory role for CD4(+) CD25(+) regulatory T lymphocytes in hepatitis C virus infection. *Hepatology* 2004;40:1062–1071.
34. Cacciarelli TV, Martinez OM, Gish RG, et al. Immunoregulatory cytokines in chronic hepatitis C virus infection: pre- and posttreatment with interferon alfa. *Hepatology* 1996;24:6–9.
35. Cahalan MD, Parker I. Close encounters of the first and second kind: T-DC and T-B interactions in the lymph node. *Semin Immunol* 2005; 17:442–451.
38. Chang KM. Immunopathogenesis of hepatitis C virus infection. *Clin Liver Dis* 2003;7:89–105.
39. Chanock RM, Crowe JE Jr, Murphy BR, et al. Human monoclonal antibody Fab fragments cloned from combinatorial libraries: potential usefulness in prevention and/or treatment of major human viral diseases. *Infect Agents Dis* 1993;2:118–131.
42. Childs K, Stock N, Ross C, et al. mda-5, but not RIG-I, is a common target for paramyxovirus V proteins. *Virology* 2007;359:190–200.
43. Childs KS, Andrejeva J, Randall RE, et al. Mechanism of mda-5 Inhibition by paramyxovirus V proteins. *J Virol* 2009;83:1465–1473.
44. Choi YS, Kageyama R, Eto D, et al. ICOS receptor instructs T follicular helper cell versus effector cell differentiation via induction of the transcriptional repressor Bcl6. *Immunity* 2011;34:932–946.
45. Choudhuri K, Dustin ML. Signaling microdomains in T cells. *FEBS Lett* 2010;584:4823–4831.
46. Christen U, Hintermann E, Holdener M, et al. Viral triggers for autoimmunity: is the 'glass of molecular mimicry' half full or half empty? *J Autoimmun* 2010;34:38–44.
47. Christen U, von Herrath MG. Initiation of autoimmunity. *Curr Opin Immunol* 2004;16:759–767.
49. Colonna M, Trinchieri G, Liu YJ. Plasmacytoid dendritic cells in immunity. *Nat Immunol* 2004;5:1219–1226.
50. Constant SL, Bottomly K. Induction of Th1 and Th2 CD4+ T cell responses: the alternative approaches. *Annu Rev Immunol* 1997;15:297–322.
52. Crotty S. Follicular helper CD4 T cells (TFH). *Annu Rev Immunol* 2011; 29:621–663.
53. Crotty S, Ahmed R. Immunological memory in humans. *Semin Immunol* 2004;16:197–203.
54. Crotty S, Felgner P, Davies H, et al. Cutting edge: long-term B cell memory in humans after smallpox vaccination. *J Immunol* 2003;171: 4969–4973.
55. Curotto de Lafaille MA, Lafaille JJ. Natural and adaptive foxp3+ regulatory T cells: more of the same or a division of labor? *Immunity* 2009; 30:626–635.
56. Cyster JG. B cell follicles and antigen encounters of the third kind. *Nat Immunol* 2010;11:989–996.
57. Cyster JG. Chemokines, sphingosine-1-phosphate, and cell migration in secondary lymphoid organs. *Annu Rev Immunol* 2005;23:127–159.
59. Da Costa XJ, Brockman MA, Alicot E, et al. Humoral response to herpes simplex virus is complement-dependent. *Proc Natl Acad Sci U S A* 1999; 96:12708–12712.
62. Day PM, Kines RC, Thompson CD, et al. In vivo mechanisms of vaccine-induced protection against HPV infection. *Cell Host Microbe* 2010;8:260–270.
64. Depoil D, Fleire S, Treanor BL, et al. CD19 is essential for B cell activation by promoting B cell receptor-antigen microcluster formation in response to membrane-bound ligand. *Nat Immunol* 2008;9:63–72.
65. Depraetere V, Golstein P. Fas and other cell death signaling pathways. *Semin Immunol* 1997;9:93–107.
66. Dessen A, Lawrence CM, Cupo S, et al. X-ray crystal structure of HLA-DR4 (DRA*0101, DRB1*0401) complexed with a peptide from human collagen II. *Immunity* 1997;7:473–481.
68. Doherty PC, Christensen JP. Accessing complexity: the dynamics of virus-specific T cell responses. *Annu Rev Immunol* 2000;18:561–592.
73. Dudley DD, Chaudhuri J, Bassing CH, et al. Mechanism and control of V(D)J recombination versus class switch recombination: similarities and differences. *Adv Immunol* 2005;86:43–112.
74. Ebers GC, Bulman DE, Sadovnick AD, et al. A population-based study of multiple sclerosis in twins. *N Engl J Med* 1996;315:1638–1642.
75. el-Ad B, Roth Y, Winder A, et al. The persistence of neutralizing antibodies after revaccination against smallpox. *J Infect Dis* 1990;161:446–448.

78. Fenner F. Adventures with poxviruses of vertebrates. *FEMS Microbiol Rev* 2000;24:123–133.
81. Fontenot JD, Rasmussen JP, Williams LM, et al. Regulatory T cell lineage specification by the forkhead transcription factor foxp3. *Immunity* 2005;22:329–341.
82. Foy E, Li K, Sumpter R Jr, et al.. Control of antiviral defenses through hepatitis C virus disruption of retinoic acid-inducible gene-I signaling. *Proc Natl Acad Sci U S A* 2005;102:2986–2991.
84. Friedline RH, Brown DS, Nguyen H, et al. CD4+ regulatory T cells require CTLA-4 for the maintenance of systemic tolerance. *J Exp Med* 2009;206:421–434.
85. Fruh K, Yang Y. Antigen presentation by MHC class I and its regulation by interferon gamma. *Curr Opin Immunol* 1999;11:76–81.
87. Fujinami RS, Oldstone MB. Antiviral antibody reacting on the plasma membrane alters measles virus expression inside the cell. *Nature* 1979; 279:529–530.
89. Gack MU, Albrecht RA, Urano T, et al. Influenza A virus NS1 targets the ubiquitin ligase TRIM25 to evade recognition by the host viral RNA sensor RIG-I. *Cell Host Microbe* 2009;5:439–449.
90. Gale M Jr, Foy EM. Evasion of intracellular host defence by hepatitis C virus. *Nature* 2005;436:939–945.
92. Germain RN. MHC-dependent antigen processing and peptide presentation: providing ligands for T lymphocyte activation. *Cell* 1994;76: 287–299.
94. Gonzalez SF, Degn SE, Pitcher LA, et al. Trafficking of B cell antigen in lymph nodes. *Annu Rev Immunol* 2011;29:215–233.
95. Gonzalez SF, Pitcher LA, Mempel T, et al. B cell acquisition of antigen in vivo. *Curr Opin Immunol* 2009;21:251–257.
98. Gris D, Ye Z, Iocca HA, et al. NLRP3 plays a critical role in the development of experimental autoimmune encephalomyelitis by mediating Th1 and Th17 responses. *J Immunol* 2010;185:974–981.
99. Gromme M, Neefjes J. Antigen degradation or presentation by MHC class I molecules via classical and non-classical pathways. *Mol Immunol* 2002;39:181–202.
100. Grossman WJ, Verbsky JW, Barchet W, et al. Human T regulatory cells can use the perforin pathway to cause autologous target cell death. *Immunity* 2004;21:589–601.
104. Halstead SB. Immune enhancement of viral infection. *Prog Allergy* 1982; 31:301–364.
105. Hammarlund E, Lewis MW, Hansen SG, et al.. Duration of antiviral immunity after smallpox vaccination. *Nat Med* 2003;9:1131–1137.
110. Haynes LM, Vanderlugt CL, Dal Canto MC, et al. CD8(+) T cells from Theiler's virus-resistant BALB/cByJ mice downregulate pathogenic virus-specific CD4(+) T cells. *J Neuroimmunol* 2000;106:43–52.
112. Healy JI, Goodnow CC. Positive versus negative signaling by lymphocyte antigen receptors. *Annu Rev Immunol* 1998;16:645–670.
113. Helmreich E, Kern M, Eisen HN. The secretion of antibody by isolated lymph node cells. *J Biol Chem* 1961;236:464–473.
115. Hessell AJ, Rakasz EG, Poignard P, et al. Broadly neutralizing human anti-HIV antibody 2G12 is effective in protection against mucosal SHIV challenge even at low serum neutralizing titers. *PLoS Pathog* 2009; 5:e1000433.
117. Hezareh M, Hessell AJ, Jensen RC, et al. Effector function activities of a panel of mutants of a broadly neutralizing antibody against human immunodeficiency virus type 1. *J Virol* 2001;75:12161–12168.
120. Howcroft TK, Strebel K, Martin MA, et al. Repression of MHC class I gene promoter activity by two-exon Tat of HIV. *Science* 1993;260:1320–1322.
122. Hsieh CS, Zheng Y, Liang Y, et al.. An intersection between the self-reactive regulatory and nonregulatory T cell receptor repertoires. *Nat Immunol* 2006;7:401–410.
127. Intlekofer AM, Takemoto N, Wherry EJ, et al. Effector and memory CD8+ T cell fate coupled by T-bet and eomesodermin. *Nat Immunol* 2005; 6:1236–1244.
128. Iwasaki A, Medzhitov R. Regulation of adaptive immunity by the innate immune system. *Science* 2010;327:291–295.
129. Iwasaki A, Medzhitov R. Toll-like receptor control of the adaptive immune responses. *Nat Immunol* 2004;5:987–995.
130. Johnson CL, Gale M Jr. CARD games between virus and host get a new player. *Trends Immunol* 2006;27:1–4.
131. Johnson DC, Hegde NR. Inhibition of the MHC class II antigen presentation pathway by human cytomegalovirus. *Curr Top Microbiol Immunol* 2002;269:101–115.
133. Joshi NS, Cui W, Chandele A, et al. Inflammation directs memory precursor and short-lived effector CD8(+) T cell fates via the graded expression of T-bet transcription factor. *Immunity* 2007;27:281–295.
134. Jung D, Alt FW. Unraveling V(D)J recombination; insights into gene regulation. *Cell* 2004;116:299–311.
135. Kaech SM, Tan JT, Wherry EJ, et al. Selective expression of the interleukin 7 receptor identifies effector CD8 T cells that give rise to long-lived memory cells. *Nat Immunol* 2003;4:1191–1198.
136. Kaech SM, Wherry EJ. Heterogeneity and cell-fate decisions in effector and memory CD8+ T cell differentiation during viral infection. *Immunity* 2007;27:393–405.
138. Kallies A, Xin A, Belz GT, et al. Blimp-1 transcription factor is required for the differentiation of effector CD8(+) T cells and memory responses. *Immunity* 2009;31:283–295.
139. Kato H, Kato R, Fujihashi K, et al. Role of mucosal antibodies in viral infections. *Curr Top Microbiol Immunol* 2001;260:201–228.
140. Kawai T, Akira S. The roles of TLRs, RLRs and NLRs in pathogen recognition. *Int Immunol* 2009;21:317–337.
143. Kim B, Kaistha SD, Rouse BT. Viruses and autoimmunity. *Autoimmunity* 2006;39:71–77.
144. Kim TS, Braciale TJ. Respiratory dendritic cell subsets differ in their capacity to support the induction of virus-specific cytotoxic CD8+ T cell responses. *PLoS One* 2009;4:e4204.
145. Klasse PJ, Sattentau QJ. Occupancy and mechanism in antibody-mediated neutralization of animal viruses. *J Gen Virol* 2002;83:2091–2108.
146. Kliks SC, Nimmanitya S, Nisalak A, et al. Evidence that maternal dengue antibodies are important in the development of dengue hemorrhagic fever in infants. *Am J Trop Med Hyg* 1998;38:411–419.
147. Kloetzel PM. Generation of major histocompatibility complex class I antigens: functional interplay between proteasomes and TPPII. *Nat Immunol* 2004;5:661–669.
148. Kolumam GA, Thomas S, Thompson LJ, et al. Type I interferons act directly on CD8 T cells to allow clonal expansion and memory formation in response to viral infection. *J Exp Med* 2005;202:637–650.
149. Kovanen PE, Leonard WJ. Cytokines and immunodeficiency diseases: critical roles of the gamma(c)-dependent cytokines interleukins 2, 4, 7, 9, 15, and 21, and their signaling pathways. *Immunol Rev* 2004;202:67–83.
150. Kraehenbuhl JP, Neutra MR. Epithelial M cells: differentiation and function. *Annu Rev Cell Dev Biol* 2000;16:301–332.
151. Krensky AM, Clayberger C. Granulysin: a novel host defense molecule. *Am J Transplant* 2005;5:1789–1792.
153. Lam KP, Kuhn R, Rajewsky K. In vivo ablation of surface immunoglobulin on mature B cells by inducible gene targeting results in rapid cell death. *Cell* 1997;90:1073–1083.
154. Lanzavecchia A, Sallusto F. Progressive differentiation and selection of the fittest in the immune response. *Nat Rev Immunol* 2002;2:982–987.
155. Lanzavecchia A, Sallusto F. Understanding the generation and function of memory T cell subsets. *Curr Opin Immunol* 2005;17:326–332.
156. Law M, Sanna PP, Burton DR. Viral subversion of humoral immune responses. In: Lachmann PJ, ed. *Microbial Subversion of Immunity: Current Topics.* Norwich, UK: Caister Academic Press, 2006;177–210.
158. Le Roy E, Muhlethaler-Mottet A, Davrinche C, et al. Escape of human cytomegalovirus from HLA-DR-restricted CD4(+) T-cell response is mediated by repression of gamma interferon-induced class II transactivator expression. *J Virol* 1999;73:6582–6589.
159. Lehner PJ, Cresswell P. Recent developments in MHC-class-I-mediated antigen presentation. *Curr Opin Immunol* 2004;16:82–89.
160. Levine B, Hardwick JM, Trapp BD, et al. Antibody-mediated clearance of alphavirus infection from neurons. *Science* 1991;254:856–860.
161. Lieberman J. The ABCs of granule-mediated cytotoxicity: new weapons in the arsenal. *Nat Rev Immunol* 2003;3:361–370.
162. Lilley BN, Ploegh HL. Viral modulation of antigen presentation: manipulation of cellular targets in the ER and beyond. *Immunol Rev* 2005;207:126–144.
164. Liu W, Putnam AL, Xu-Yu Z, et al. CD127 expression inversely correlates with FoxP3 and suppressive function of human CD4+ T reg cells. *J Exp Med* 2006;203:1701–1711.

167. MacLennan IC, Gulbranson-Judge A, Toellner KM, et al. The changing preference of T and B cells for partners as T-dependent antibody responses develop. *Immunol Rev* 1997;156:53–66.
168. MacLennan IC, Toellner KM, Cunningham AF, et al. Extrafollicular antibody responses. *Immunol Rev* 2003;194:8–18.
170. Manns MP, Johnson EF, Griffin KJ, et al. Major antigen of liver kidney microsomal autoantibodies in idiopathic autoimmune hepatitis is cytochrome P450db1. *J Clin Invest* 1989;83:1066–1072.
172. Martin A, Scharff MD. AID and mismatch repair in antibody diversification. *Nat Rev Immunol* 2002;2:605–614.
173. Maruyama M, Lam KP, Rajewsky K. Memory B-cell persistence is independent of persisting immunizing antigen. *Nature* 2000;407:636–642.
177. Maul RW, Gearhart PJ. AID and somatic hypermutation. *AdvImmunol* 2010;105:159–191.
179. McCormack WT, Tjoelker LW, Thompson CB. Avian B-cell development: generation of an immunoglobulin repertoire by gene conversion. *Annu Rev Immunol* 1991;9:219–241.
180. McCracken AA, Brodsky JL. Evolving questions and paradigm shifts in endoplasmic-reticulum-associated degradation (ERAD). *Bioessays* 2003; 25:868–877.
181. McCullough KC, Parkinson D, Crowther JR. Opsonization-enhanced phagocytosis of foot-and-mouth disease virus. *Immunology* 1998;65: 187–191.
183. Mehlhop E, Nelson S, Jost CA, et al. Complement protein C1q reduces the stoichiometric threshold for antibody-mediated neutralization of West Nile virus. *Cell Host Microbe* 2009;6:381–391.
185. Mellman I, Turley SJ, Steinman RM. Antigen processing for amateurs and professionals. *Trends Cell Biol* 1998;8:231–237.
186. Miller DM, Rahill BM, Boss JM, et al. Human cytomegalovirus inhibits major histocompatibility complex class II expression by disruption of the Jak/Stat pathway. *J Exp Med* 1998;187:675–683.
189. Misra N, Bayry J, Lacroix-Desmazes S, et al. Cutting edge: human CD4+CD25+ T cells restrain the maturation and antigen-presenting function of dendritic cells. *J Immunol* 2004;172:4676–4680.
192. Munz C, Lunemann JD, Getts MT, et al. Antiviral immune responses: triggers of or triggered by autoimmunity? *Nature Rev Immunol* 2009; 9:246–258.
193. Murphy KM, Reiner SL. The lineage decisions of helper T cells. *Nat Rev Immunol* 2002;2:933–944.
194. Nakamura K, Kitani A, Strober W. Cell contact-dependent immunosuppression by CD4(+)CD25(+) regulatory T cells is mediated by cell surface-bound transforming growth factor beta. *J Exp Med* 2001;194: 629–644.
195. Neuberger MS, Harris RS, Di Noia J, et al. Immunity through DNA deamination. *Trends Biochem Sci* 2003;28:305–312.
196. Neutra MR, Mantis NJ, Kraehenbuhl JP. Collaboration of epithelial cells with organized mucosal lymphoid tissues. *Nat Immunol* 2001;2:1004–1009.
197. Nimmerjahn F, Ravetch JV. Fcgamma receptors as regulators of immune responses. *Nature Rev Immunol* 2008;8:34–47.
198. Nishimura Y, Igarashi T, Haigwood N, et al. Determination of a statistically valid neutralization titer in plasma that confers protection against simian-human immunodeficiency virus challenge following passive transfer of high-titered neutralizing antibodies. *J Virol* 2002;76:2123–2130.
203. Oldstone MB. Molecular mimicry and autoimmune disease. *Cell* 1997;50:819–820.
204. Ormandy LA, Hillemann T, Wedemeyer H, et al. Increased populations of regulatory T cells in peripheral blood of patients with hepatocellular carcinoma. *Cancer Res* 2005;65:2457–2464.
205. Oswald WB, Geisbert TW, Davis KJ, et al. Neutralizing antibody fails to impact the course of Ebola virus infection in monkeys. *PLoS Pathog* 2007;3:e9.
206. Pachler K, Vlasak R. Influenza C virus NS1 protein counteracts RIGI-mediated IFN signalling. *Virology J* 2011;8:48.
207. Pacholczyk R, Kern J, Singh N, et al. Nonself-antigens are the cognate specificities of Foxp3+ regulatory T cells. *Immunity* 2007;27:493–504.
209. Pandiyan P, Zheng L, Ishihara S, et al. CD4+CD25+Foxp3+ regulatory T cells induce cytokine deprivation-mediated apoptosis of effector CD4+ T cells. *Nat Immunol* 2007;8:1353–1362.
210. Panoutsakopoulou V, Sanchirico ME, Huster KM, et al. Analysis of the relationship between viral infection and autoimmune disease. *Immunity* 2001;15:137–147.
211. Pantaleo G, Demarest JF, Vaccarezza M, et al. Effect of anti-V3 antibodies on cell-free and cell-to-cell human immunodeficiency virus transmission. *Eur J Immunol* 1995;25:226–231.
212. Parren PW, Burton DR. The antiviral activity of antibodies in vitro and in vivo. *Adv Immunol* 2001;77:195–262.
213. Parren PW, Geisbert TW, Maruyama T, et al. Pre- and postexposure prophylaxis of Ebola virus infection in an animal model by passive transfer of a neutralizing human antibody. *J Virol* 2002;76:6408–6412.
214. Parren PW, Marx PA, Hessell AJ, et al. Antibody protects macaques against vaginal challenge with a pathogenic R5 simian/human immunodeficiency virus at serum levels giving complete neutralization in vitro. *J Virol* 2001;75:8340–8347.
215. Pestka S, Krause CD, Walter MR. Interferons, interferon-like cytokines, and their receptors. *Immunol Rev* 2004;202:8–32.
216. Phillips AJ, Tomasec T, Wang EC, et al. Human cytomegalovirus infection downregulates expression of the cellular aminopeptidases CD10 and CD13. *Virology* 1998;250:350–358.
219. Pierce SK, Liu W. The tipping points in the initiation of B cell signalling: how small changes make big differences. *Nat Rev Immunology* 2010;10:767–777.
220. Pierson TC, Fremont DH, Kuhn RJ, et al. Structural insights into the mechanisms of antibody-mediated neutralization of flavivirus infection: implications for vaccine development. *Cell Host Microbe* 2008;4:229–238.
222. Plotkin SA. Correlates of protection induced by vaccination. *Clin Vaccine Immunol* 2010;17:1055–1065.
225. Prince GA, Horswood RL, Chanock RM. Quantitative aspects of passive immunity to respiratory syncytial virus infection in infant cotton rats. *J Virol* 1985;55:517–520.
228. Ren X, Sodroski J, Yang X. An unrelated monoclonal antibody neutralizes human immunodeficiency virus type 1 by binding to an artificial epitope engineered in a functionally neutral region of the viral envelope glycoproteins. *J Virol* 2005;79:5616–5624.
235. Russell JH, Ley TJ. Lymphocyte-mediated cytotoxicity. *Annu Rev Immunol* 2002;20:323–370.
236. Sakaguchi S. Naturally arising CD4+ regulatory t cells for immunologic self-tolerance and negative control of immune responses. *Annu Rev Immunol* 2004;22:531–562.
237. Sakaguchi S. Naturally arising Foxp3-expressing CD25+CD4+ regulatory T cells in immunological tolerance to self and non-self. *Nat Immunol* 2005;6:345–352.
239. Sarkar S, Kalia V, Haining WN, et al. Functional and genomic profiling of effector CD8 T cell subsets with distinct memory fates. *J Exp Med* 2008;205:625–640.
240. Saunders LR, Barber GN. The dsRNA binding protein family: critical roles, diverse cellular functions. *FASEB J* 2003;17:961–983.
241. Scherle PA, Gerhard W. Functional analysis of influenza-specific helper T cell clones in vivo. T cells specific for internal viral proteins provide cognate help for B cell responses to hemagglutinin. *J Exp Med* 1986; 164:1114–1128.
242. Schlender J, Hornung V, Finke S, et al. Inhibition of toll-like receptor 7- and 9-mediated alpha/beta interferon production in human plasmacytoid dendritic cells by respiratory syncytial virus and measles virus. *J Virol* 2005;79:5507–5515.
243. Schlesinger JJ, Chapman S. Neutralizing F(ab')2 fragments of protective monoclonal antibodies to yellow fever virus (YF) envelope protein fail to protect mice against lethal YF encephalitis. *J Gen Virol* 1995;76(Pt 1): 217–220.
244. Schluns KS, Lefrancois L. Cytokine control of memory T-cell development and survival. *Nat Rev Immunol* 2003;3:269–279.
245. Schmierer B, Hill CS. TGFbeta-SMAD signal transduction: molecular specificity and functional flexibility. *Nat Rev Mol Cell Biol* 2007;8:970–982.
247. Seder RA, Ahmed R. Similarities and differences in CD4+ and CD8+ effector and memory T cell generation. *Nat Immunol* 2003;4:835–842.
250. Sercarz EE, Maverakis E. Mhc-guided processing: binding of large antigen fragments. *Nat Rev Immunol* 2003;3:621–629.
251. Sereti I, Rodger AJ, French MA. Biomarkers in immune reconstitution inflammatory syndrome: signals from pathogenesis. *Curr Opin HIV AIDS* 2010;5:504–510.

252. Serghides L, Vidric M, Watts TH. Approaches to studying costimulation of human antiviral T cell responses: prospects for immunotherapeutic vaccines. *Immunol Res* 2006;35:137–150.
254. Sette A, Moutaftsi M, Moyron-Quiroz J, et al. et al. Selective CD4+ T cell help for antibody responses to a large viral pathogen: deterministic linkage of specificities. *Immunity* 2008;28:847–858.
255. Shakhar G, Lindquist RL, Skokos D, et al.Stable T cell-dendritic cell interactions precede the development of both tolerance and immunity in vivo. *Nat Immuno*l 2005;6:707–714.
256. Shastri N, Schwab S, Serwold T. Producing nature's gene-chips: the generation of peptides for display by MHC class I molecules. *Annu Rev Immunol* 2002;20:463–493.
257. Shevach EM. CD4+ CD25+ suppressor T cells: more questions than answers. *Nat Rev Immunol* 2002;2:389–400.
259. Shortman K, Heath WR. The CD8+ dendritic cell subset. *Immunol Rev* 2010;234:18–31.
262. Simonetta F, Chiali A, Cordier C, et al. Increased CD127 expression on activated FOXP3+CD4+ regulatory T cells. *Eur J Immunol* 2010;40: 2528–2538.
264. Slifka MK. Immunological memory to viral infection. *Curr Opin Immunol* 2004;16:443–450.
265. Slifka MK, Ahmed R. Long-term humoral immunity against viruses: revisiting the issue of plasma cell longevity. *Trends Microbiol* 1996;4:394–400.
266. Slifka MK, Antia R, Whitmire JK, et al. Humoral immunity due to long-lived plasma cells. *Immunity* 1998;8:363–372.
267. Slifka MK, Matloubian M, Ahmed R. Bone marrow is a major site of long-term antibody production after acute viral infection. *J Virol* 1995; 69:1895–1902.
268. Slifka MK, Rodriguez F, Whitton JL. Rapid on/off cycling of cytokine production by virus-specific CD8+ T cells. *Nature* 1999;401:76–79.
270. Sobue S, Nomura T, Ishikawa T, et al. Th1/Th2 cytokine profiles and their relationship to clinical features in patients with chronic hepatitis C virus infection. *J Gastroenterol* 2001;36:544–551.
271. Spear GT, Hart M, Olinger GG, et al. The role of the complement system in virus infections. *Curr Top Microbiol Immunol* 2001;260: 229–245.
272. Sperling AI, Bluestone JA. The complexities of T-cell co-stimulation: CD28 and beyond. *Immunol Rev* 1996;153:155–182.
276. Sugimoto K, Ikeda F, Stadanlick J, et al. Suppression of HCV-specific T cells without differential hierarchy demonstrated ex vivo in persistent HCV infection. *Hepatology* 2003;38:1437–1448.
277. Sullivan NJ. Antibody-mediated enhancement of viral disease. *Curr Top Microbiol Immunol* 2001;260:145–169.
278. Sun J, Madan R, Karp CL, et al. Effector T cells control lung inflammation during acute influenza virus infection by producing IL-10. *Nat Med* 2009;15:277–284.
279. Suri-Payer E, Cantor H. Differential cytokine requirements for regulation of autoimmune gastritis and colitis by CD4(+)CD25(+) T cells. *J Autoimmun* 2001;16:115–123.
280. Suvas S, Azkur AK, Kim BS, et al. CD4+CD25+ regulatory T cells control the severity of viral immunoinflammatory lesions. *J Immunol* 2004; 172:4123–4132.
281. Suvas S, Kumaraguru U, Pack CD, et al. CD4+CD25+ T cells regulate virus-specific primary and memory CD8+ T cell responses. *J Exp Med* 2003;198:889–901.
283. Szabo SJ, Sullivan BM, Peng SL, et al. Molecular mechanisms regulating Th1 immune responses. *Annu Rev Immunol* 2003;21:713–758.
284. Takemoto N, Intlekofer AM, Northrup JT, et al. Cutting Edge: IL-12 inversely regulates T-bet and eomesodermin expression during pathogen-induced CD8+ T cell differentiation. *J Immunol* 2006;177:7515–7519.
285. Thornton AM, Shevach EM. Suppressor effector function of CD4+CD25 +immunoregulatory T cells is antigen nonspecific. *J Immunol* 2000; 164:183–190.
286. Topham DJ, Tripp RA, Doherty PC. CD8+ T cells clear influenza virus by perforin or Fas-dependent processes. *J Immunol* 1997;159:5197–5200.
287. Tran DQ, Andersson J, Hardwick D, et al. Selective expression of latency-associated peptide (LAP) and IL-1 receptor type I/II (CD121a/ CD121b) on activated human FOXP3+ regulatory T cells allows for their purification from expansion cultures. *Blood* 2009;113:5125–5133.
288. Tumpey TM, Basler CF, Aguilar PV, et al. Characterization of the reconstructed 1918 Spanish influenza pandemic virus. *Science* 2005;310:77–80.
289. van de Veerdonk FL, Netea MG, Dinarello CA, et al. Inflammasome activation and IL-1beta and IL-18 processing during infection. *Trends Immunol* 2011;32:110–116.
290. van Hall T, Sijts A, Camps M, et al. Differential influence on cytotoxic T lymphocyte epitope presentation by controlled expression of either proteasome immunosubunits or PA28. *J Exp Med* 2000;192:483–494.
292. van Lier RA, ten Berge IJ, Gamadia LE. Human CD8(+) T-cell differentiation in response to viruses. *Nat Rev Immunol* 2003;3:931–939.
294. Victora GD, Schwickert TA, Fooksman DR, et al. Germinal center dynamics revealed by multiphoton microscopy with a photoactivatable fluorescent reporter. *Cell* 2010;143:592–605.
297. Virgin HW, Wherry EJ, Ahmed R. Redefining chronic viral infection. *Cell* 2009;138:30–50.
298. Vivier E, Raulet DH, Moretta A, et al. Innate or adaptive immunity? The example of natural killer cells. *Science* 2011;331:44–49.
299. von Herrath MG, Dockter J, Oldstone MB. How virus induces a rapid or slow onset insulin-dependent diabetes mellitus in a transgenic model. *Immunity* 1994;1:231–242.
301. Watts C. The exogenous pathway for antigen presentation on major histocompatibility complex class II and CD1 molecules. *Nat Immunol* 2004;5:685–692.
302. Weber SE, Harbertson J, Godebu E, et al. Adaptive islet-specific regulatory CD4 T cells control autoimmune diabetes and mediate the disappearance of pathogenic Th1 cells in vivo. *J Immunol* 2006;176:4730–4739.
306. Williams A, Peh CA, Elliott T. The cell biology of MHC class I antigen presentation. *Tissue Antigens* 2002;59:3–17.
309. Wing K, Onishi Y, Prieto-Martin P, et al. CTLA-4 control over Foxp3+ regulatory T cell function. *Science* 2008;322:271–275.
310. Woodland DL, Dutton RW. Heterogeneity of CD4(+) and CD8(+) T cells. *Curr Opin Immunol* 2003;15:336–342.
311. Wrammert J, Smith K, Miller J, et al. Rapid cloning of high-affinity human monoclonal antibodies against influenza virus. *Nature* 2008; 453:667–671.
312. Wright KE, Buchmeier MJ. Antiviral antibodies attenuate T-cell-mediated immunopathology following acute lymphocytic choriomeningitis virus infection. *J Virol* 1991;65:3001–3006.
313. Wyatt R, Sodroski J. The HIV-1 envelope glycoproteins: fusogens, antigens, and immunogens. *Science* 1998;280:1884–1888.
314. Yewdell JW. Immunoproteasomes: regulating the regulator. *Proc Natl Acad Sci U S A* 2005;102:9089–9090.
315. Yewdell JW, Reits E, Neefjes J. Making sense of mass destruction: quantitating MHC class I antigen presentation. *Nat Rev Immunol* 2003;3: 952–961.
316. Yewdell JW, Schubert U, Bennink JR. At the crossroads of cell biology and immunology: DRiPs and other sources of peptide ligands for MHC class I molecules. *J Cell Sci* 2001;114:845–851.
317. Yoon H, Kim TS, Braciale TJ. The cell cycle time of CD8+ T cells responding in vivo is controlled by the type of antigenic stimulus. *PLoS One* 2010;5:e15423.
318. Youngman KR, Franco MA, Kuklin NA, et al. Correlation of tissue distribution, developmental phenotype, and intestinal homing receptor expression of antigen-specific B cells during the murine anti-rotavirus immune response. *J Immunol* 2002;168:2173–2181.
319. Yu X, Tsibane T, McGraw PA, et al. Neutralizing antibodies derived from the B cells of 1918 influenza pandemic survivors. *Nature* 2008;455: 532–536.
320. Zanger UM, Hauri HP, Loeper J, et al. Antibodies against human cytochrome P-450db1 in autoimmune hepatitis type II. *Proc Natl Acad Sci U S A* 1998;85:8256–8260.
321. Zellweger RM, Prestwood TR, Shresta S. Enhanced infection of liver sinusoidal endothelial cells in a mouse model of antibody-induced severe dengue disease. *Cell Host Microbe* 2010;7:128–139.
323. Zinkernagel RM. Maternal antibodies, childhood infections, and autoimmune diseases. *N Engl J Med* 2001;345:1331–1335.
324. Zinkernagel RM, Doherty PC. MHC-restricted cytotoxic T cells: studies on the biological role of polymorphic major transplantation antigens determining T-cell restriction-specificity, function, and responsiveness. *Adv Immunol* 1979;27:51–177.

CHAPTER 10

Mark T. Heise • Herbert W. Virgin

Pathogenesis of Viral Infection

INTRODUCTION TO VIRAL PATHOGENESIS

Viral pathogenesis is the series of steps that occurs when a virus infects the host. Viruses are obligate parasites of living cells that cannot live independent of an intricate relationship with an infected cell. The cells targeted by viruses during infection survive, differentiate, and function in a tissue that has an intimate relationship with other tissues and physiologic processes in the body. Thus, in the same sense that viruses are obligate parasites of living cells, they are obligate parasites of tissues in living organisms. Living in tissues and spreading from host to host represent processes only approximated in cell culture or biochemical experimentation. The study of viral pathogenesis elucidates this special relationship between the virus and the intact host.

The term *pathogenesis* refers to the processes related to disease induction; therefore, *viral pathogenesis* often refers to disease induction by a virus rather than the process of infection *per se*. However, viral infection does not always result in apparent or immediate disease, and the border between infection and disease becomes less clear as we learn more. It is most useful to consider the pathogenesis of infection independently of whether or not severe or immediate disease is induced. As the pathogenesis of infection is analyzed, the pathogenesis of disease can be considered as a subset of events that occur *in vivo* during infection. Fundamentally important mechanisms are revealed when one considers how the pathogenesis of infection differs between the host with asymptomatic infection or minimal disease and the host doomed to suffer severe consequences of viral infection.

Viral pathogenesis is the integrated result of many complex factors unique to a particular virus, a particular species, and an individual host. The interplay of these factors determines the nature of infection, whether disease occurs, and the severity of disease. In many cases, individual factors involved in pathogenesis can be studied in detail. For example, the crystal structure of a viral immune evasion protein allows predictions as to protein function during infection *in vivo*. However, definitive pathogenesis experiments often falsify such predictions. Thus, all conclusions derived from reductionist experiments utilizing molecular and biochemical approaches need to be validated in living organisms to understand viral pathogenesis.

The complexity of directly testing molecular mechanisms *in vivo* has been a significant stumbling block for pathogenesis research. The difficulty of doing definitive pathogenesis experiments that prove a molecular mechanism *in vivo* has resulted in pathogenesis research being relegated at times to a lesser status as a phenomenological science when compared to studies of molecular and biochemical mechanisms. However, in the end, infection occurs in the intact host; thus, events *in vivo* are highly relevant. With the development of new tools, in particular those that allow genetic analysis of pathogenesis from both the viral and host standpoint, pathogenesis research has rapidly evolved into a mechanistic science. Moreover, classical studies of pathogenesis have often stood the test of time and are useful at a minimum for defining the fundamental questions to be addressed using molecular pathogenesis approaches.

Goals of This Chapter

This chapter will focus on integrating classical concepts of pathogenesis with more current molecular understanding of viruses. Viral pathogenesis is the subject of many authoritative texts, and the reader is referred to one such text for detailed treatment of many of the important concepts developed here in necessarily shorter form.[195,196] There is a rich history of how the initial observations that form the basis for our current understanding of viral pathogenesis were made.[196] These founding studies are important to our understanding of the pathogenesis of infection as well as to major advances in human health such as the elimination of smallpox and the development of vaccines against diseases such as polio, measles, mumps, rubella, hepatitis B virus (HBV), and human papillomavirus. Exposure to the historical roots of pathogenesis research is strongly recommended for those who wish to delve into viral pathogenesis as a career or avocation.

Because it is impossible to provide a detailed description of the pathogenesis of all viral infections in a single chapter, the goal of this chapter is to provide a conceptual framework for understanding viral pathogenesis. Principles will be defined and then examples provided from a broad range of infections. For details of specific viral infections, refer to chapters on individual viruses. This chapter will specifically focus on the pathogenesis of infection with nucleic acid–containing viruses in mammals. There is a rich body of knowledge on plant viral diseases and prion diseases that will not be addressed in this chapter.

DEFINITIONS AND CONCEPTS IN VIRAL PATHOGENESIS

The literature on pathogenesis is extensive and more than 100 years old. A search of the recent literature accessed by Entrez using the term *viral pathogenesis* pulls up more than 426,000 references, whereas a search of *viral disease* pulls up more than 695,000 references. Within this complex and voluminous literature, terms are used in multiple ways. Often the utilization of terms is predicated on historical factors rather than more up-to-date considerations. We will therefore begin by defining terms as they will be used in this chapter.

Productive, Abortive, and Latent Infection

Infection is the process by which a virus introduces its genome into a cell. Infection is *productive* if new infectious virus is made and *abortive* if no new infectious virus is produced. Infection is *latent* if the production of infectious virus does not occur immediately but the virus retains the potential to initiate productive infection at a later time. The process of reinitiating a productive infection cycle from the latent state is termed *reactivation*. Latency is not merely a slow productive replication cycle; latency represents a unique transcriptional and translational state where infectious virus is not present, but where a productive replication cycle can be reinitiated when the need arises. A cell is permissive if it can support productive infection and nonpermissive if infection cannot occur at all or is abortive.

Acute Versus Chronic or Persistent Infection

Acute infection occurs when a virus first infects a susceptible host (Fig. 10.1). *Chronic* or *persistent infection* is the continuation of infection beyond the time when the immune system might reasonably be expected to clear acute infection. The

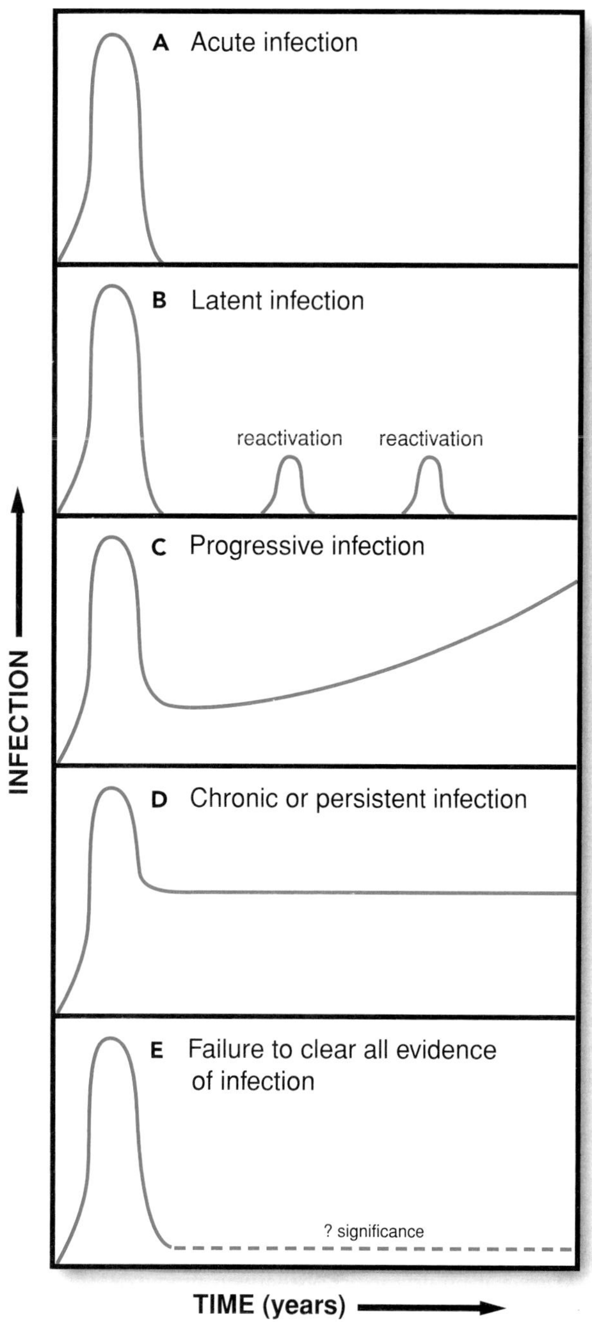

FIGURE 10.1. Schematic of different patterns of viral infection.

terms *chronic* and *persistent* have been used interchangeably for many years; we will continue this convention. It is important to note that these terms denote the presence of viral infection in the host for long periods but do not provide insight as to the mechanism(s) responsible for prolonged survival of the virus in the host. Mechanisms responsible for chronic infection include persistence of nucleic acid, continuous replication, latency, and reactivation. More than one of these processes may occur at the same time. In some cases, viral nucleic acid can be detected in the host for prolonged periods, although the nature of the infectious process has not been defined (see Fig. 10.1). In such cases, chronic infection may represent continuous replication, latent infection, abortive infection without clearance of residual nucleic acid, or perhaps some as-yet-unidentified form of viral infection.

In some cases, as for HBV or hepatitis C virus (HCV), a proportion of persons become chronically infected while others are cured. In these cases, the transition from acute to chronic is arbitrarily defined as the time when most patients have cleared acute infection. In other cases, essentially all hosts become chronically infected, as is seen with herpesviruses or lentiviruses such as human immunodeficiency virus (HIV). In this case, the transition between acute and chronic infection is defined as the time required for clearance of the initial burst of viral replication and establishment of equilibrium between the host and the virus.

There are two primary mechanisms for establishment of chronic infection: *continuous replication* and *establishment of latency.* During latent viral infection, the virus has a genomic and transcriptional strategy, often involving restricted viral gene expression, which allows the genome to survive even when lytic replication is not occurring. Examples include the proviral form of retroviruses or the circular episomal form with selective expression of viral genes observed for herpesviruses such as Epstein-Barr virus (EBV) and herpes simplex virus (HSV). Often, latently infected cells express no viral proteins, making latency immunologically silent. This is the ultimate form of immune evasion, as the host has no known mechanisms for sensing the presence of the virus. To survive and spread from the latently infected cell, the virus must be able reactivate and reinitiate the lytic cycle of gene expression, potentially generating antigens that the immune system can respond to.

To succeed via continuous replication, a virus must generate new infectious virions despite ongoing innate and adaptive immune responses. Even for viruses that utilize the establishment of latency as a primary strategy, intermittent reactivation and replication may be required to maintain latency and to spread from host to host. Some viruses, such as HIV, persist via both continuous replication and establishment of latency, presenting a particularly difficult challenge for the host immune system.[107,301]

Quasispecies

The mixture of viruses present in the host at a given time is a *quasispecies.* Although it is convenient to think of a virus as a single homogeneous agent, this is not true because both viral RNA and DNA polymerases make errors that generate mutant viruses during infection. The polymerases of RNA viruses are generally less accurate in copying template molecules than those of DNA viruses; mutation may therefore play a greater role in RNA than DNA virus pathogenesis. However, mutation may play a role in the pathogenesis of any virus. The quasispecies generated by mutation is acted on by complex and powerful selective pressures in the host, with some viruses having a survival or fitness advantage over others. The nature of these selective pressures and the pathogenic potential of the selected viruses are important determinants of viral pathogenesis.

Control of Acute Versus Chronic Infection

The distinctions between acute and chronic or persistent infection are very important. The viral genes and host immune factors that foster or control acute versus chronic infection are distinct. For example, the cytokine interferon-γ (IFNγ) regulates latency and continuous replication of the murine γHV68 (also referred to as MHV-68) but has at most a minimal effect during acute infection.[16] This indicates that certain host responses are more relevant to chronic than acute infection. Control of either acute or chronic infection may involve responding to viral quasispecies. This is the case for both HIV and HCV infection, presenting the infected host with the overwhelming problem of dealing with many antigenically distinct viruses with different pathogenic strategies. Many viruses, including herpesviruses, papillomaviruses, and retroviruses, use different gene or gene expression patterns to succeed during acute versus chronic infection. For these reasons, it is fundamentally important not to consider chronic infection as a mere continuation of acute infection.

Equilibrium and Nonequilibrium States in Pathogenesis

A fundamental concept in pathogenesis is that acute infection is a nonequilibrium state, whereas chronic infection is a metastable equilibrium between virus and host. During acute infection, both the host response and virus infection change continuously until infection is resolved or progresses to death of the host or establishment of chronic infection. In contrast, chronic infection, once established, is an equilibrium process with viral and host processes balancing each other. In particular, the immune system of the host brings the acute infection under control and delays or prevents a chronic infection from killing the host. Progression of chronic infection to disease often reflects a change in this equilibrium (see Fig. 10.1). Even when the host and virus are in a stable equilibrium, the infectious process is dynamic with host and viral processes balanced on a knife-edge such that small changes in either virus or host can disrupt the equilibrium with devastating consequences.

An example of nonequilibrium and equilibrium states during acute and chronic infection is provided by EBV, a γ-herpesvirus that causes acute mononucleosis in humans. During the acute stage of infection, EBV causes rapid B-cell expansion (a nonequilibrium process) that is then brought under control by the expansion of virus-specific T cells, which act to maintain the virus in a latent state (an equilibrium process). When levels of latently infected B cells are assessed, significant individual-to-individual variation is observed but levels are remarkably constant within a given individual over time. However, when patients are immune suppressed, the level of latently infected B cells increases,[12] suggesting that interactions between the virus-specific T cells and the virus maintain equilibrium during the chronic stage of infection. This balance between immune and viral processes during chronic infection is incompletely understood in most cases and yet is fundamentally important for understanding many human diseases.

Disease

Disease is a harmful pathologic consequence of infection. In many cases, infection is apparently harmless to the host and does not result in disease. One of the most important goals of pathogenesis research is to define in molecular terms what determines the difference between infection and disease. Even highly virulent viruses often establish infection in a greater number of hosts than they cause disease. Viruses such as rabies, Ebola, or HIV, which cause significant disease in nearly all infected persons, are the exception.

Disease may be associated with cell and tissue destruction (as in rabies virus killing neurons), induction or secretion of inflammatory cytokines (as in the induction of fever by many viruses), cellular dysfunction induced by viral infection (as in the case with lymphocytic choriomeningitis virus [LCMV] infection of the pituitary), paracrine effects of viral gene products (as in induction of angiogenesis by Kaposi's sarcoma herpesvirus [KSHV]), and the induction of malignant tumors to the effects of the immune system as it responds to infection (as in immunopathology seen with many viruses) or to the presence of a specific virus interacting with allelic polymorphisms in the host to trigger disease.[40,300]

In many cases, virus-associated disease is defined as a series of nonspecific symptoms or signs such as fever, malaise, or anorexia. The presence of these symptoms and signs is common to infection with many different pathogens and therefore provides little insight into the mechanisms of viral pathogenesis. Recent work with microarray technology suggests that even the nonspecific syndromes associated with acute virus infection with different viruses may be distinguished by the pattern of host gene expression. It is likely that pathogenesis researchers will use such molecular signatures to distinguish between infections with different viruses and to define host genes involved in viral pathogenesis.

In contrast to the nonspecific syndromes commonly associated with virus infection, the presence of specific symptoms or signs of disease such as hepatitis, immunodeficiency, pocks on the skin, or paralysis provides important clues as to the nature of the pathogenic process. It is this relationship between the signs and symptoms of disease and the presence of infection with specific viruses that has led to the close link between clinical observations of the natural history of disease and the science of viral pathogenesis.

Virulence

Virulence—the relative capacity of a virus to cause disease—determines the relationship between infection and disease. Virulent viruses cause disease in a greater proportion of infected hosts, and cause more severe disease, than viruses of lower virulence. Virulence comes in many forms, from the induction of rapid death as for variola major (the causative agent in smallpox) to the induction of tumors over prolonged periods, as is the case with certain papillomaviruses or herpesviruses, to the induction of organ failure over many years, as is the case with chronic HBV or HCV infection. Thus, the manifestations of virulence highly depend on the strategies that a given virus uses during infection.

The determination of whether one virus (e.g., Ebola virus) is more virulent than another virus (e.g., papillomavirus) represents a qualitative judgment, because it involves determining whether virus-induced hemorrhagic fever (as is seen with Ebola virus) is worse than metastatic cancer (as is seen with papillomaviruses). To avoid biases inherent in comparing different types of disease, virulence is properly used to compare the disease-inducing capacity of related viruses, such as different strains of the same virus. For example, Ebola Reston, which is not associated with human disease, is less virulent in humans than Ebola Zaire.

It is commonly assumed that viruses that replicate efficiently in the host are more virulent than viruses that replicate less efficiently, and indeed replication is an important determinant of the severity of disease in many cases. However, virulence is much more complex than simply the efficacy of replication. Other aspects of pathogenesis, including tropism, the host response to infection, and interactions between the virus and host tissues, play key roles in viral virulence. Therefore, virulence reflects host resistance to infection functioning in counterpoint to viral virulence genes and determinants with the outcome for the host hanging in the balance.

Invasiveness

Invasiveness is the capacity of a virus to enter into and damage a tissue, a property that distinguishes viruses with high potential virulence but differ in the efficiency with which they enter target tissues. For example, a virus may be highly virulent if directly inoculated into the central nervous system (CNS) but unable to cause disease if inoculated into the periphery, whereas a related virus with a mutation allowing it to cross the blood–brain barrier into the CNS can cause lethal disease following either peripheral or intracranial inoculation. This concept is nicely exemplified by the identification of neuroinvasiveness determinants in Sindbis virus that confer the capacity to cause lethal encephalitis.[66]

Cell-Intrinsic Versus Cell-Extrinsic Mechanisms

Because infected cells live in a tissue in the host, they are affected both by events that occur inside the cell and by events that influence the cell from the outside. Events that occur in a cell independent of events outside of the infected cell are termed *cell intrinsic*. Some cell-intrinsic determinants of infection are owing to intrinsic cellular resistance to infection conferred by the presence of molecules that block viral infection. Events that are dictated by processes that occur outside of the cell are termed *cell extrinsic*. Many cell-extrinsic events are owing to innate and adaptive immunity. It is often the case that processes occurring in infected cells or tissues are affected by both cell-intrinsic and cell-extrinsic mechanisms. An example is the induction of death of infected cells that may be owing to cell-intrinsic induction of programmed cell death or cell-extrinsic immune factors such as cytokines or perforin and granzymes.

Evasion of Host Molecules and Mechanisms

Most viruses have evolved mechanisms to counter host innate and adaptive immunity or to bypass intrinsic cellular resistance molecules so that the virus can complete the infectious process and spread to a new host. These mechanisms constitute viral *evasion* of host responses. Often, evasion strategies involve viral genes with close homology to host genes, as when a virus encodes a host cytokine or cytokine receptor mimic. Other evasion strategies utilize molecules with novel structures to avoid host responses. Because the mechanisms responsible for acute and chronic infection differ, both with regard to viral and host factors, it follows that immune evasion mechanisms are different for acute versus chronic infection. During acute infection, viral immune evasion strategies commonly focus on the host innate immune response, whereas evasion of adaptive immunity is more important for maintaining chronic infection. When analyzing immune evasion mechanisms, it is therefore important to identify the aspects of the infectious process for which a given molecule is important.

Subversion of Host Molecules and Mechanisms

Viruses must be able to utilize host metabolic and regulatory systems to optimize their growth, survival, and spread. In some cases, the normal functions of the host cell may be sufficient for the virus to replicate. In other cases, host cellular processes may be insufficient or have deleterious effects on the virus. *Subversion* refers to the ability of a virus to redirect or alter normal host processes to the advantage of the virus. For example, some viruses subvert the function of chemokine receptors or other immune-signaling proteins to supply intracellular signals that regulate viral gene expression or encode molecules that subvert the cyclin-dependent progression of cell cycle. There are many different signaling pathways and cellular processes that are subverted by viruses; in fact, it is reasonable to presume that essentially every pathway and process within the cell is subverted by one virus or another. This is the inevitable consequence of the obligate intracellular lifestyle of viruses and their capacity to evolve more rapidly than the mammalian host.

Tropism

Tropism is the capacity of a virus to infect or damage specific cells, tissues, or species. It is a fundamentally important contributor to viral pathogenesis and virulence, as the capacity to induce disease depends on the cell and tissue infected. For example, a neurotropic virus such as West Nile Virus can cause encephalitis or paralysis, whereas a virus with tropism for CD4 T cells such as HIV causes immunodeficiency.

One key determinant of viral tropism is the cognate interaction between the viral cell attachment protein(s) and receptor(s) present on host cells. However, there are many additional factors that determine cell, tissue, and species tropism. The concept of tropism is rapidly evolving with the recognition that essentially every aspect of the viral infectious process within a cell or tissue can be a determinant of tropism. Both cell-intrinsic and cell-extrinsic factors may alter viral tropism.

Essential Genes, Virulence Genes, and Virulence Determinants

Virulence is determined by the capacity of a virus to grow, be invasive, infect vulnerable cells, evade the immune system, subvert cellular processes, and cause tissue damage. These capacities are encoded in the viral genome, by alleles of individual *virulence genes*. That viral genotype confers pathogenic capacity was proven by studies using reassortant viruses, mutant viruses, or molecularly cloned viruses to show that alterations in genotype confer virulence phenotype (e.g., 10,55,56,66,69,121, 168,229,265,287,291,308). Subsequent studies have shown that different viral genes can confer capacities for infection in different tissues, indicating that viral virulence genes are tissue specific.[109,175] Consistent with this, viral variants that arise during chronic infection are often cell and tissue specific.[2,3,108,143,189]

Any gene essential for replication contributes to virulence, because viruses must replicate to complete their life cycle. In this sense, all viral genes involved in replication are virulence genes. As this is not a very useful concept, viral genes essential for replication in permissive cells are termed *essential genes* rather than virulence genes. Virulence genes are not required for replication *per se* but are important for virulence in the host. Although the distinction between an essential gene and a virulence gene is useful, it is important to recognize that allelic variations in the function of essential genes can be important determinants of viral virulence. In this case, the specific property associated with virulence is termed a *virulence determinant*. Thus, virulence determinants can be allelic variants of essential genes that confer significant differences in pathogenesis.

The size of the viral genome puts boundaries on the number of genes that a virus can use for pathogenesis and replication. For example, smaller RNA viruses often have genomes of less than 10,000 nucleotides, whereas poxviruses or herpesviruses may have genomes greater than 200,000 nucleotides in length. However, viral proteins often have multiple independent functions—a property particularly well documented for RNA viruses. Thus, the pathogenic capacity of a virus with a small genome should not be underestimated.

Virus particles can contain virulence determinants that are not encoded in their genomes. For example, vaccinia virus incorporates host complement regulatory proteins into its envelope, thereby becoming resistant to inactivation by host complement proteins.[294] Another type of epigenetic mechanism is exemplified by herpesviruses such as human cytomegalovirus (HCMV) and HSV that can package host and viral messenger RNAs (mRNAs) into the virion.[36,93,251,282] Although their role in pathogenesis is not yet clearly defined, carryover of these mRNAs can result in synthesis of viral proteins before the traditional transcription program of the virus is initiated.[251,282]

It is not necessarily true that viral virulence determinants exert their effects in host cells actually infected by the virus. One example of this is paracrine regulation of tissue pathology by virus-encoded cytokines. Another example is the movement of viral proteins from an infected to an uninfected cell. For example, the HSV protein VP22 can efficiently move from an infected cell to the nucleus of uninfected cells,[68] can carry other proteins between cells,[224] and can transport mRNAs from one cell to the next.[251] This is a fascinating example of how a viral virulence determinant can act on uninfected cells to contribute to viral pathogenesis.

Virulence Genes and Determinants May Not Encode Proteins

Virulence can be conferred by viral promoters or other cis elements in the viral genome or noncoding RNAs. For example, EBV infection is associated with the development of B-cell lymphomas. The EBV EBNA1 protein plays an important role in the maintenance of latent EBV infection in B lymphocytes. EBNA1 can be expressed from any of four promoters—Cp, Wp, Fp, and Qp—each of which is regulated in distinct ways by viral and host proteins,[264] ensuring that EBNA1 is expressed at the appropriate place and time in B cells. These finely tuned promoters are therefore properly considered virulence determinants for EBV-associated malignancies. Another example of non–protein-coding virulence determinants are virally encoded microRNAs, which are expressed by a number of mammalian viruses, including herpesviruses, adenoviruses, and polyomaviruses.[228,257] These noncoding RNAs target multiple cellular processes, including cell cycle regulators, apoptotic machinery, or virus-encoded transcript, and play a role in promoting viral persistence. Noncoding elements also play important roles in the pathogenesis of several RNA viruses. For example, attenuating mutations within the internal ribosomal entry site (IRES) of the Sabin vaccine strain of poliovirus are important for replication in neurons and neurovirulence in mice and primates.[97,99,141,149] It is becoming increasingly clear that the transcriptional complexity of a broad range of organisms is considerably higher than previously believed,[23,117] and it is now recognized that this is also the case for viruses such as herpesviruses.[46,47,133] It is likely that virulence genes that do not encode proteins will increasingly be recognized in many viruses.

CONCEPTUALIZING VIRAL PATHOGENESIS

Every fact or principle presented in this textbook relates in some way to the pathogenesis of infection or disease. Thus, it may seem that pathogenesis is too complex to be studied in any mechanistic detail, or that viruses differ so significantly that common principles do not exist. This problem is further compounded because many events and processes are going on at the same time *in vivo*. Furthermore, processes that occur *in vivo* are nonlinear (e.g., unrestricted viral replication may be exponential) or even stochastic (e.g., whether a mutation occurs when a genome is replicated), or otherwise are the results of as-yet-unidentified allelic variations in host genes that influence pathogenesis.[1,300]

Given this complexity, it is worth considering how the questions of pathogenesis are formulated and placed in context for interpretation. There are many ways to look at infection—three of which are presented here as a basis for understanding viral pathogenesis. Pathogenesis may be conceptualized as an organized process consisting of sequential stages, as the result of stochastic events under selection by bottlenecks in infection, or as the integration of host allelic variations in genes that determine resistance to infection. Each view of pathogenesis has its limitations and benefits as a basis for understanding the nature and mechanisms of viral infection.

Clinical Observations Define Fundamental Pathogenesis Questions

Viral pathogenesis has been studied for longer than any other aspect of virology; however, in many ways, we know less about pathogenesis than we do about other aspects of virology. The pathogenesis of viral disease was studied before viruses were even identified. Smallpox was known before variola virus was identified, and rabies virus was propagated in animals and an effective vaccine was developed by Pasteur before the virus was characterized.[131] It was known that chickenpox infection conferred lifelong resistance to disease before varicella-zoster virus (VZV) was identified. A study of measles in 1886 in the Faroe Islands identified the incubation period between exposure and disease, resistance of previously exposed individuals to reinfection, and the susceptibility of the very young to disease.[95,96] These clinical observations often identify the questions that must be answered in pathogenesis studies. For example, mosquito-borne alphaviruses such as chikungunya virus cause severe acute and persistent arthralgia in infected humans, raising the question of how these viruses cause joint pain and whether chronic disease is associated with viral persistence. Through the careful analysis of human clinical samples and the use of appropriate animal models, the viral pathogenesis researcher can begin to define the molecular mechanisms underlying a disease process.

Conceptualizing Viral Pathogenesis as a Series of Sequential Stages in Infection

A very useful way to conceptualize viral pathogenesis is as a series of sequential stages resulting in survival and spread of a virus through the infected host and on to a new host (Figs. 10.2 and 10.3). Different viruses may utilize distinct molecular mechanisms to accomplish each of these stages. For example, all viruses must infect cells on entry into the host and must spread to new hosts. As the host has mechanisms to inhibit each of these stages of infection, the stages of infection may be considered as hurdles over which the virus must jump to survive.

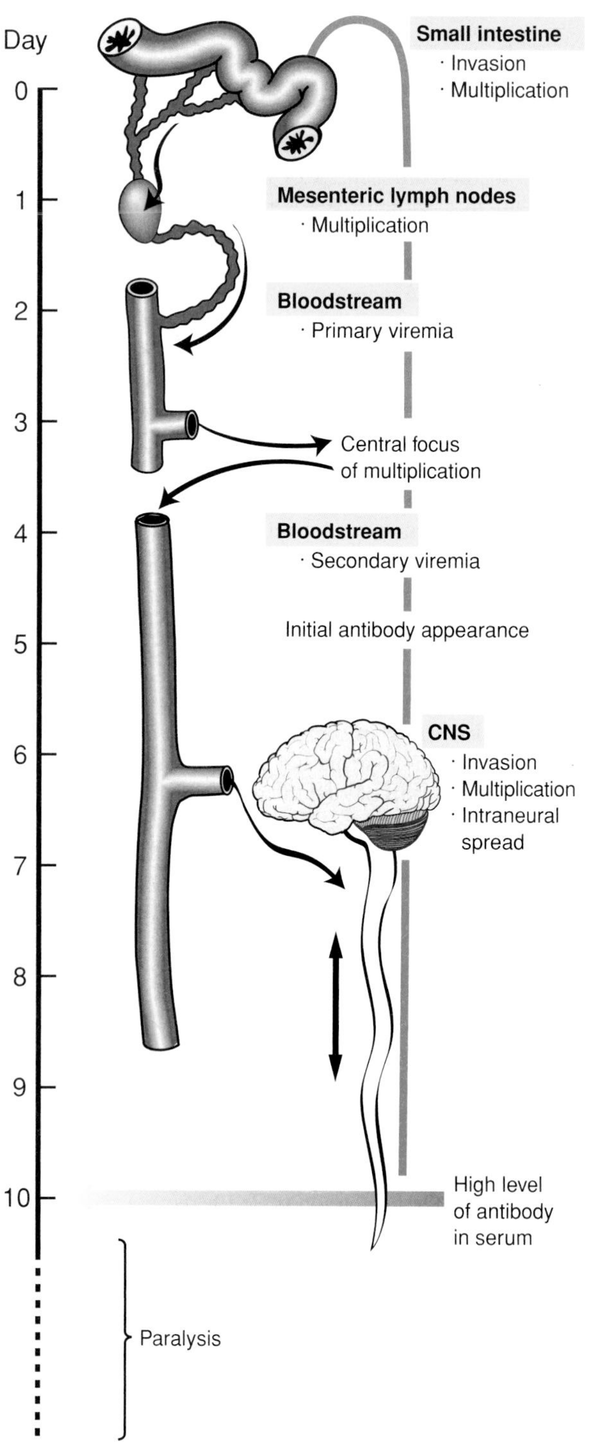

FIGURE 10.2. Model of poliovirus pathogenesis as a series of sequential stages. The steps in poliovirus infection of a human are schematized.

There may be more than one way for a virus to overcome such a hurdle; however, different viruses may utilize the same strategy to overcome a given hurdle. An example of a common strategy is the relative resistance of some viruses to inactivation in water or sewage, allowing them to spread between hosts by fecal–oral transmission. Another example is infection of the thymus resulting in deletion of virus-specific T cells as *self*-antigens. Yet another common strategy is evading immunity via the establishment of latent infection. Thus, there are many common strategies for infection shared by different viruses.

Dividing viral pathogenesis into stages is a very useful way to conceptualize the infectious process but has significant limitations. First, dividing pathogenesis into stages creates the impression that events are both sequential and depend on each other. This is not always the case; many independent events may be going on at the same time in the host. Second, this conceptual framework suggests that completion of a stage is associated with initiation of the next stage; a significant oversimplification. For example, viremia may continue after a virus has entered the CNS to cause encephalitis. The utility of considering viral pathogenesis as a series of sequential events must be balanced against how well this conceptual framework fits actual events during infection.

Poliovirus pathogenesis provides an excellent example of how pathogenesis can be broken down into a series of steps that culminate in either virus-induced disease or viral control. Clinical questions that drove poliovirus pathogenesis research through the first half of the past century included why poliomyelitis emerged in the 20th century, what mechanisms were responsible for paralysis, and how did protective immunity work.[183,234,235,274] Solving these questions was central to combating a very important and pressing public health problem. Infection with poliovirus in humans has a wide range of possible outcomes from asymptomatic infection to meningoencephalitis with or without paralysis.[183,234,235,274]

Studies over many years identified and analyzed a series of stages of poliovirus infection, leading to a relatively simple model for the pathogenesis of disease that elegantly explains paralysis, the low proportion of infected hosts paralyzed, and the lifelong immunity conferred by prior infection. This model, one of the most useful ever constructed, provided a basis for developing the poliovirus vaccines that have largely, although not completely, eliminated paralytic poliomyelitis as a scourge of humanity.

The stages in poliovirus pathogenesis according to this model are outlined in Figure 10.2.[24,183,234,235] The virus enters the intestine via the fecal–oral route, binds to M cells overlying the Peyer's patch, is transported into the intestinal wall, and then replicates in lymphoid cells, leading to a primary viremia and infection of secondary sites. Replication in secondary sites gives rise to a secondary viremia that reaches a level capable of initiating CNS infection.[234,235] CNS infection involves passage of the virus across the blood–brain barrier to infect neurons within the CNS. The blood–brain barrier is viewed as an

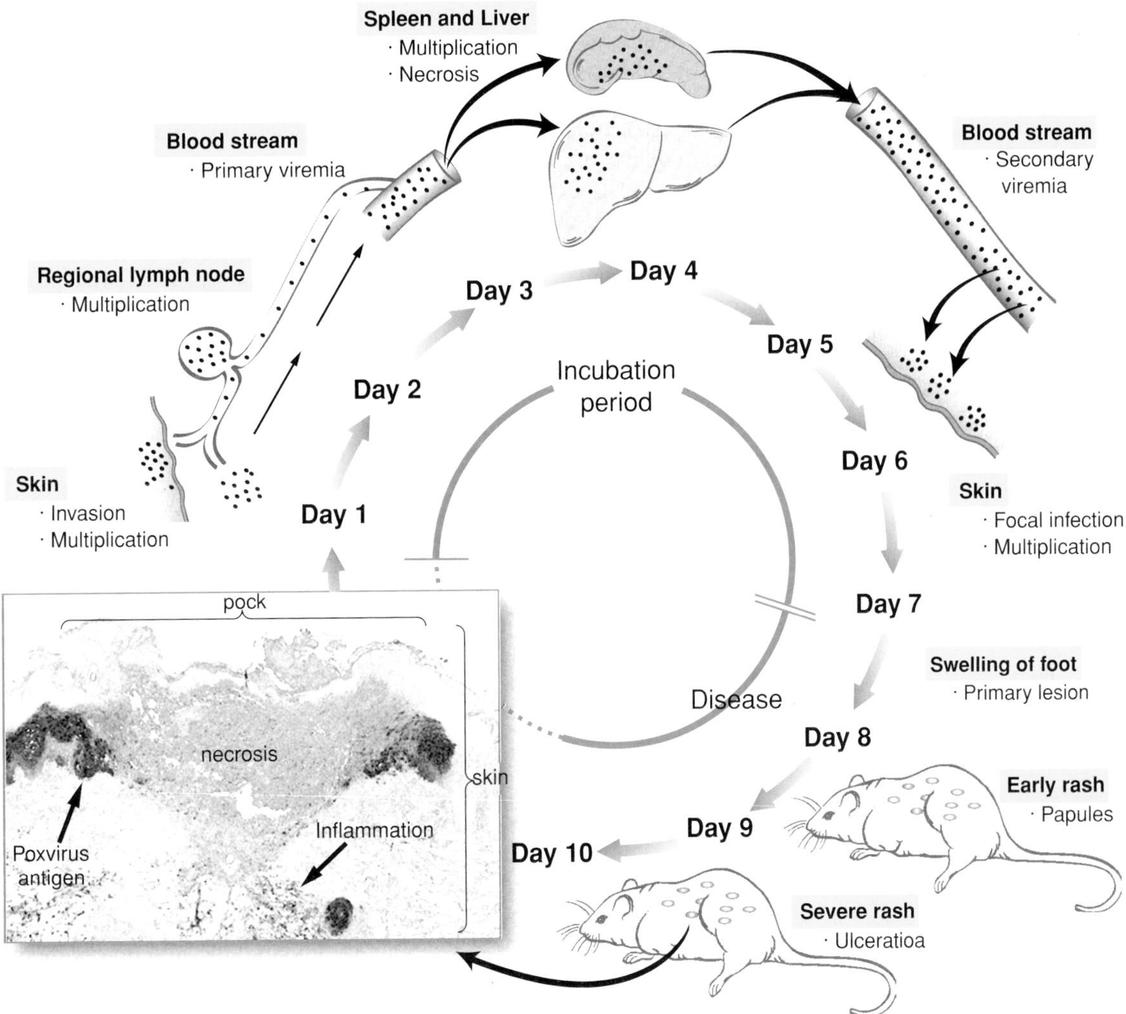

FIGURE 10.3. Model of poxvirus pathogenesis as a series of sequential stages. The steps in ectromelia virus pathogenesis are schematized. The outcome of ectromelia infection varies with mouse and viral strain.[39,75] The viremia is thought to be cell associated. The histopathologic image of a pock was provided by Drs. Mark Martinez and Peter Jahrling and is skin from a variola-infected monkey stained with specific antisera to identify the infected cells shown as *poxvirus antigen* in the inset image. (Adapted from Fenner F, Buller RM. Mousepox. In: Nathanson N, Ahmed R, Gonzalez-Scarano F, et al, eds. *Viral Pathogenesis*. Philadelphia: Lippincott-Raven, 1997:535–553.)

important anatomic barrier to infection of the CNS, and passage across this barrier is poorly understood. Alternatively, the virus may spread via the blood to peripheral nerves and then spread up the nerves to enter the CNS.[98,185,205,235,241] Within the CNS, the virus infects motor neurons; destruction of these cells leads to paralysis. Certain motor neurons are hypothesized to more susceptible to poliovirus infection than others, and some poliovirus strains are either more invasive or more likely to kill neurons than others; these variables contribute to variation in disease penetrance and severity.

Concurrent with entry into the lymphatic system, an immune response is generated (see Fig. 10.2). It is hypothesized in this model that immune antibody limits access to the CNS and prevents paralytic disease.[183,235] Antibody might act by preventing virus in the circulation from crossing the blood–brain barrier and entering the CNS. However, antibody is capable of inhibiting neural spread of viruses and can inhibit viral infection by acting directly on or within neurons.[160,183,290,292,299] Regardless of the mechanisms by which antibody protects, the outcome of infection is a race between the virus and the immune system, presenting another explanation for variations in clinical outcome. The immune system wins if antibody is made early enough to prevent spread to the CNS and neuronal destruction. The virus wins if infection of motor neurons occurs prior to development of protective antibody responses.

This model provides a basis for understanding many aspects of poliovirus infection, disease, immunity, and vaccination; however, many questions are left open. Questions that remain unanswered at the molecular level include how the virus enters the body, the molecular basis of cell and tissue tropism, the mechanism by which antibody acts to prevent CNS disease, the mechanisms of induction of immunity, and the route(s) by which the virus spreads.

Importantly, although the mechanistic details underpinning the pathogenesis of different viruses will differ significantly, the broad stages of the systemic infection process outlined for poliovirus pathogenesis are also relevant for a wide array of other viral pathogens. For example, although poxviruses are very different from small RNA viruses, such as poliovirus, there are remarkable parallels between the models of poliovirus infection (see Fig. 10.2) and those for poxviruses (Fig. 10.3). This includes the concept that both viruses must reach a threshold of viremia to facilitate viral invasion into target organs and that the disease process represents a race between the virus and the host immune response, where the outcome of that race plays a major role in determining whether the virus is controlled or if disease results. Refer to the eBook for a more complete description of poxvirus pathogenesis as a stepwise process. These general principles extend to a wide array of viral pathogens, including arboviruses, herpesviruses, and lentiviruses.

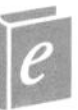

Conceptualizing Viral Pathogenesis as the Interaction Between Stochastic Events and Bottlenecks in Infection

It is important to recognize that the process of infection has, in addition to a series of predictable events that occur in sequence, an element of stochastic variation that contributes to real variability to the outcome of infection. Thus, viral pathogenesis can be conceptualized as a series of stochastic events with the process of infection determined by strong selective pressures in the host referred to as bottlenecks in infection (Fig. 10.4). These bottlenecks can be thought of as analogous to the rate-limiting step in a chemical reaction. Stochastic events such as mutations or the random success of a given virus at a stage in infection provide variation in the substrates for these rate-limiting steps.

The concept that random events contribute to pathogenesis is not a comfortable one for investigators. However, even using clonal virus stocks for inoculation of genetically identical mice of the same sex and age results in viral titers in tissues that vary considerably (even by orders of magnitude) from one mouse to the next. This variation is not experimental error or noise but is rather a real phenomenon relevant to understanding infection. During natural infection of genetically variable hosts with viral quasispecies, the variation is likely to be much larger.[297]

The reasons for the occurrence of significant variations even when conditions of infection are apparently homogeneous are not clear but likely involve several different factors, including epigenetic changes within the host, specific interactions between viruses and certain host genes that confer disease,[44,300] environmental variables, and viral factors such as viral mutation rates that drive the generation of mutants with selective advantages in the host. This latter process, which involves the random generation of mutant viruses—a subset of which may provide a selective advantage that allow the virus to overcome bottlenecks and efficiently spread throughout the host—represents an important component of viral pathogenesis. For example, polioviruses that have high-fidelity polymerases, and therefore are less able to generate mutant viruses, are less efficient in infecting target tissues and causing disease, suggesting that the generation of viral quasispecies allows the virus to overcome bottlenecks and is essential for disease pathogenesis.[296]

Selective pressures at bottlenecks in infection can select mutants from within the viral quasispecies that have a fitness advantage (see Fig. 10.4). This is illustrated experimentally by studies with Venezuelan equine encephalitis virus (VEE), an equine pathogen that infects both humans and mice. Following subcutaneous inoculation, VEE initially replicates in the draining lymph node before seeding a serum viremia that leads to viral dissemination and ultimately viral entry into the CNS. Studies that compared molecularly clones of wild-type VEE to a mutant virus with a defined mutation at position 76 in the E2 envelope protein demonstrated that the mutant virus replicated within the draining lymph node but failed to spread systemically. Importantly, infection with the mutant virus led to the rapid generation of viruses that were able to efficiently spread within the host, and characterization of these viruses found that some contained a reversion of the original E2 mutation to wild-type. However, other viruses maintained the original E2 mutation but developed second site mutations that conferred the ability to disseminate systemically.[10,94] These results demonstrate that there may be many ways to overcome

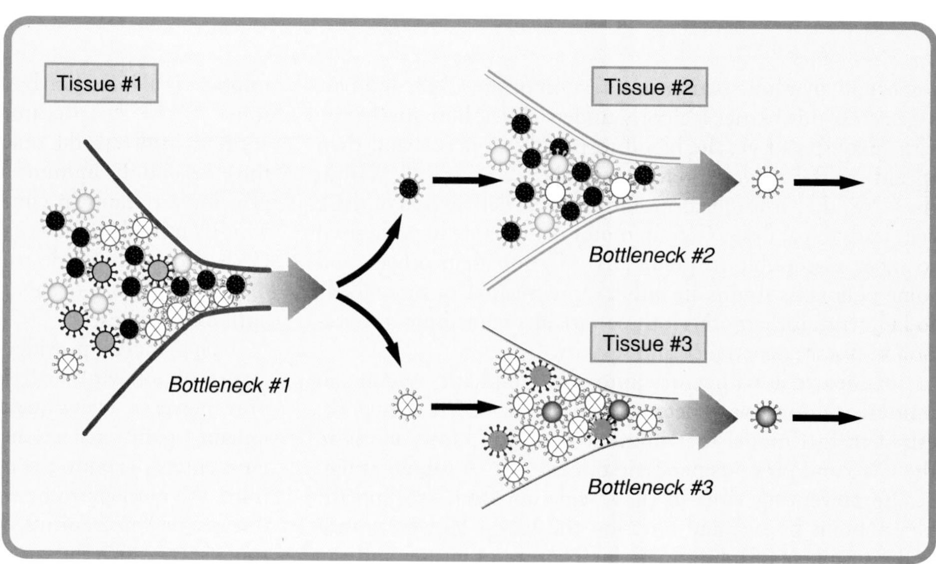

FIGURE 10.4. Viral pathogenenesis as stochastic events followed by selection by bottlenecks in infection. Shown is a representation of a viral quasispecies, only two of which are fit to pass through an initial bottleneck in infection. Subsequent replication of these viruses in different tissues generates further quasispecies that are again acted in by selective forces at further bottlenecks in infection.

a specific bottleneck. Bottlenecks may also be responsible for significant variations in the kinetics of infection between hosts. For example, a variant capable of bypassing a given bottleneck may arise sooner in one host than in another. Refer to the eBook for an expanded discussion of how VEE rapidly mutates to overcome bottlenecks in infection.

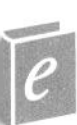

An example of a bottleneck in infection exerting a selective pressure comes from HIV infection. When an infected person exposes an uninfected person to the diverse HIV quasispecies that develops during chronic infection, the viruses that emerge in the new host represents only a subset of the viruses in the inoculum.[106,301] This suggests the existence of a bottleneck early in infection through which some viruses selectively pass. Detailed study shows that HIV viruses that utilize the CCR5 co-receptor are more efficient at spread and initial replication in both men and women than viruses that utilize CXCR4 as a co-receptor.[167,214,231] This suggests that co-receptor utilization is a critical event for passing through a bottleneck during the initial stages of infection. After passage through this bottleneck, HIV isolates that utilize CCR5 are less fit for later events in infection leading to selection of viruses utilizing CXCR4 as a co-receptor. Thus, a virus that is more effective at passing one bottleneck in infection can be replaced, via mutation and selection, by viruses more fit for bypassing subsequent bottlenecks in infection. For these reasons, one must not assume that the virus initially entering the host is the virus responsible for viral disease but must consider stochastic events and selective pressures in models of pathogenesis.

An important consequence of passage through a bottleneck is contraction of quasispecies heterogeneity. When a mutant virus is selected, allelic variations in regions of the genome that are not under selective pressure are carried along through the bottleneck. Thus, random mutation followed by selection can generate novel viruses with properties that are not selected for at all and may therefore have unique pathogenic properties. For example, a virus may mutate sequences encoding a T-cell epitope to escape control by T lymphocytes, and this new sequence may confer previously unexpected properties to the virus. Therefore, selective pressure may result in the emergence of different viruses in different hosts, providing a mechanism for the emergence of viruses with new properties in a population of susceptible individuals.

Conceptualizing Viral Pathogenesis as the Integrated Effects of Host Genetic Variation

The previously discussed ways to conceptualize viral pathogenesis are highly focused on the virus, but it has been clear since the earliest studies of viral pathogenesis that hosts differ significantly in genetic susceptibility to infection.[44,301] The major host determinant of viral virulence and pathogenesis is innate and adaptive immunity, but host genes not involved immunity also play a role. Allelic variations in these host genes can alter viral pathogenesis (Fig. 10.5).

The extent to which allelic variations in host genes control viral pathogenesis is only now being appreciated. Some examples are well established, whereas others come from single studies and await confirmation. Mutations in CCR5 confer resistance to HIV infection.[57,164,248] Human noroviruses (type virus Norwalk) are responsible for more than 90% of the epidemic nonbacterial gastroenteritis in the world.[61,90] Norwalk virus susceptibility is determined by blood group secretor status conferred by the presence of the FUT2 fucosyltransferase.[127,163] Among human norovirus strains, there are multiple patterns of virus-like particle (VLP) binding to blood group carbohydrates, suggesting that allelic variation in human blood groups contribute to susceptibility to a variety of norovirus strains. Patients with mutations in the IFNγ receptor have been reported to have unusual viral syndromes.[226] Autosomal dominant mutations in the chemokine receptor CXCR4 have been associated with severe warts,[154] and mutations in *EVER1* and *EVER2* have been associated with an unusual clinical presentation of papillomavirus infection called *epidermodysplasia verruciformis*.[237] Allelic variations in mannose-binding lectin and FcγRIIA have been linked to the severity of severe acute respiratory syndrome (SARS).[130,320] A relationship between expression of certain KIR genes, encoding NK cell receptors, and severity and chronicity of infection with HIV, HCV, and EBV have been reported.[43] Responsiveness to hepatitis B vaccine may be linked to allelic variations in complement genes.[25,119] Thus, a significant number of allelic variations in

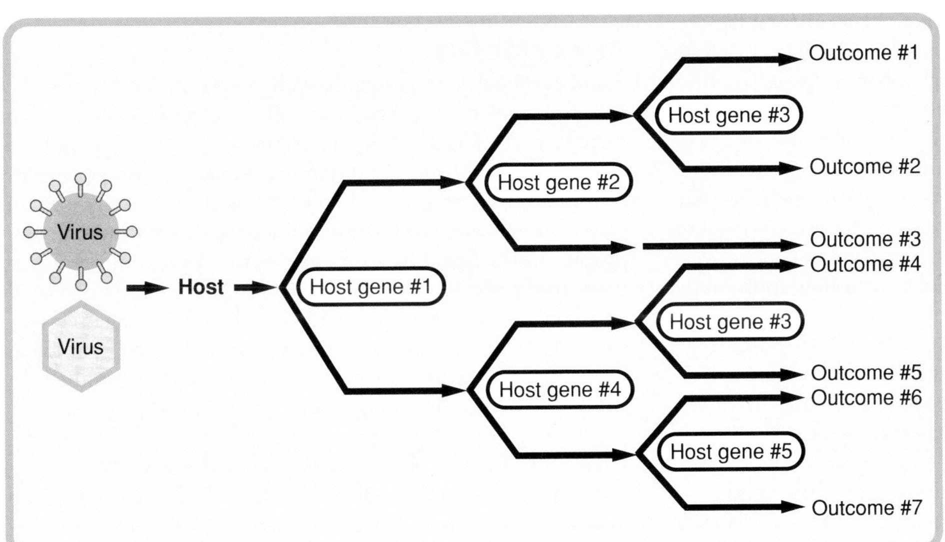

FIGURE 10.5. Viral pathogenesis as the result of the action of a series of host genes. Shown is a representation of infection with different viruses progressing through the host as acted on by host genes that confer either resistance or susceptibility to infection. Depending on the effects of host gene 1, one of two different patterns of infection emerges. In turn, additional host genes interact with the virus, resulting in different outcomes for the host. Note that the more host genes play a determining role, the greater the number of possible outcomes.

humans are important determinants of viral pathogenesis, and additional candidates for such variation are being found at a high rate. Refer to the eBook for further discussion of how variation in blood group secretor status affects susceptibility to human norovirus infection.

Although many studies have focused on the impact of variation in a single gene on viral susceptibility, it is clear that susceptibility or resistance to viral infections is a complex phenotype regulated by multiple interacting genes and gene networks. For example, studies designed to identify genes that regulate resistance to influenza infection between two mouse strains have identified multiple quantitative trait loci (QTL) that contribute to disease susceptibility.[28] Although the full number of host genes that vary between susceptible and resistant hosts for a single virus is only beginning to be understood, it is likely that variation in hundreds of different genes may contribute to disease resistance or susceptibility.[44,302] Recent advances in the area of host genetics, including the application of genome-wide association studies (GWAS), which scan the genome for allelic variants, such as single nucleotide polymorphisms (SNPs), associated with specific phenotypes, as well as whole exome and whole genome sequencing, promise to further enhance our understanding of how different polymorphic genes contribute to disease susceptibility. For example, recent application of GWAS approaches to identify genes that associate with HIV control identified a major association between polymorphisms in the human leukocyte antigen (HLA) locus that affect class I peptide presentation to CD8 T cells and an individual's ability to control HIV.[221] These approaches have also been extended to HCV and recently identified a polymorphism within the *IL28B* gene (interferon λ3) that associates with viral clearance following therapy with interferon.[84] These types of findings have direct implications for predicting treatment outcomes for infection in patient populations, as has been suggested for inflammatory diseases.[300]

The examples outlined previously illustrate that allelic variants in host genes can have a significant impact on the pathogenesis of infection (see Fig. 10.5). As multiple independently segregating genes contribute to the susceptibility or resistance to a viral pathogen, many human genotypes exist that may vary significantly in their resistance to even a single viral infection. Therefore, even without considering the impact of viral virulence determinants or other environmental factors, much of the variation in viral pathogenesis within a diverse population could be explained by polymorphisms in host genes. This has implications not only for viral pathogenesis in human populations but also for studying viral pathogenesis in animal models. Although GWAS and candidate gene studies in humans can establish an association between a polymorphic gene and susceptibility to a viral infection, the investigation of the mechanisms by which a polymorphic gene or genes affects pathogenesis requires additional tools, including appropriate animal models. However, pathogenesis studies are often performed in genetically homogeneous experimental hosts (e.g., inbred mouse strains), which results in the loss of any significant effect of host genetic variation on viral pathogenesis and limits investigation of how allelic variants affect pathogenesis outcomes. New model systems that more accurately model the genetic diversity that is present in human populations, such as the Collaborative Cross mouse RI panel,[11] as well as classical mouse genetics systems, including BXD recombinant inbred lines,[28] should enhance studies of the role of host variation and gene:gene interactions in viral pathogenesis.

THE STUDY OF VIRAL PATHOGENESIS

Many different tools must be used to understand the complex process of viral pathogenesis. Some of these tools have played essential roles in understanding pathogenesis and will continue to be useful. Examples include assays for infectious virus and histopathologic evaluation of infected tissues. Others are more recently developed and have only been applied in limited circumstances. Understanding the tools of experimental pathogenesis research is essential to understanding the interpretation of experiments that have contributed to our current understanding of virus infection.

Epidemiology

Epidemiology is an essential tool for pathogenesis research for defining patterns of disease and infection and the mode of transmission between hosts. Together with assays for prior infection such as serology or molecular detection of chronic virus infection, epidemiology can define the relationship between infection, immunity, and disease. Epidemiologic studies link a virus to a specific disease and allow formulation of the fundamental questions that must be answered to understand viral pathogenesis. This is nicely illustrated by the identification of Kaposi's sarcoma (KS) herpesvirus, where epidemiology studies suggested that HIV status alone was not an accurate predictor of KS risk, indicating that an additional co-factor was responsible for KS.[48,250] Following the discovery of KSHV,[48] additional epidemiologic investigations convincingly linked KSHV infection with KS via demonstration that KSHV sequences were present almost universally in KS lesions and that seroconversion to KSHV preceded the development of KS.[174]

In some cases, epidemiologic investigation finds that known viruses explain but a part of the disease burden, leaving open the question of whether unknown agents contribute to disease. The process of associating new viruses with both viral and nonviral diseases continues to this day, with new viruses constantly emerging or being identified as responsible for already described diseases.

Animal Models

Animal models are fundamentally important tools for the study of viral pathogenesis. The need to understand human infection, combined with the complexities of doing human studies, has led to the use of animal models to ask pathogenesis questions that cannot be effectively answered via human studies. There are two types of animal models for human viral disease. In the first, one studies a human virus in infected animals. In the second, one studies an animal virus that is related to a human virus in its animal host. There is an essential tension between these two approaches; in one the "real" pathogen is studied, and in the other a "natural" infection is studied. In truth, each has its advantages and each its limitations.

Study of Human Viruses in Animal Models

Human viruses can be studied in animals that are susceptible to infection either because the virus does not exhibit species tropism or because tropism restrictions are overcome via genetic manipulation of the host or virus. An important caveat of such studies is that human viruses seldom or never behave in an experimental animal exactly as they do in humans. Nevertheless, this is a very valuable approach. Examples include the use of mice to study HSV, Sindbis virus, yellow fever virus, VEE, LCMV, or chikungunya viruses; the use of humanized mouse models to study HCV and HIV; and the use of primates to study poliovirus, variola, HIV, and Ebola virus.

Excellent examples of this approach are the analysis of infection with filoviruses such as Ebola or Marburg that are very difficult to study in infected patients. However, these viruses cause disease in macaques with significant similarities to human disease, including a striking hemorrhagic diathesis including disseminated intravascular coagulation.[85–87] These animal models have been used to demonstrate that it is possible to vaccinate against filovirus infection[136,270,319] and that passive transfer of antibody can be partially protective.[105,216]

Not all human viruses can replicate in animals. Five approaches have been taken to overcome this hurdle. These approaches are, first, passage-based adaptation of the human virus to growth in an experimental animal; second, engineering of the host to accommodate all or part of the pathogenesis of the human infection; third, expressing the virus as a transgene in an experimental animal; fourth, the creation of humanized mice where immunodeficient mice are reconstituted with aspects of the human immune system and components of the human target organ (e.g., the liver for HCV); and fifth, targeted modification of viruses to allow replication in a model host. Increasing knowledge of the mechanisms of viral pathogenesis and immunity holds out great hope for generations of better animal models.

1. In the first approach, a human virus is adapted to growth in an animal model. Ebola has adapted to infect guinea pigs and mice.[35,52,89] Ebola infection of small animals is similar to primate and human Ebola infections in some ways. For example, dendritic cells (DCs) and monocytes are early targets of infection in all of the different models. However, mice and guinea pigs do not show the hemorrhagic diathesis seen in humans and macaques, which is a significant limitation for pathogenesis studies.[35,52,85,89]
2. In the second approach, the host is genetically engineered to allow analysis of a human virus. For example, transgenic expression of the poliovirus or measles virus receptors in mice confers susceptibility to intracerebral infection with poliovirus or measles virus.
3. In the third approach, the virus is expressed as a transgene in a live animal, allowing the replication cycle of the virus to proceed in certain cells even though the host is nonpermissive for infection. This has been accomplished for HBV with mice engineered to generate infectious virus from a transgenic viral genome.[103,104]
4. In the fourth approach, mice are used as hosts for human tissue allografts that can then be infected with human viruses. This approach is particularly useful for viruses that fail to replicate in nonhuman systems and has been applied to viruses such as HIV[155] and VZV.[14,249,321]
5. In the fifth approach, the virus is manipulated in a specific way to allow infection of the animal to be used as a model. For example, based on an intimate knowledge of the mechanisms of lentivirus species tropism, it has been possible via manipulation of the HIV *vif* gene to create an HIV isolate that can replicate in macaques.[113]

Study of Animal Virus Infections That Resemble Human Infection

It is often impossible to approximate all aspects of the pathogenesis of a human virus in an animal model. An important alternative approach is to study the pathogenesis of an animal virus that is related to a human virus in an animal host. Examples include the study of murine cytomegalovirus (MCMV) as a model for HCMV, simian immunodeficiency virus (SIV) as a model for HIV, murine γHV68 as a model for human γ-herpesvirus infection, myxoma virus and ectromelia virus as models for smallpox, and murine norovirus infection as a model for human noroviruses. These models provide, especially in the murine system, tools for doing pathogenesis and host genetics that are unavailable in any other model.

An important caveat of this approach is that animal viruses seldom faithfully reproduce in every detail of a human disease. This is not surprising; after all, animals are not humans and animal viruses are not identical to human viruses. These dissimilarities are often used to argue against the utility of such animal models. However, many principles and mechanisms of viral pathogenesis have first been described in animal models and later proven relevant in humans.

Viral Genetics as a Tool for Analysis of Pathogenesis

Studies taking advantage of genetic differences between viral strains are as old as the study of pathogenesis itself. Comparisons between viral strains can identify correlates of virulence or attenuation but do not necessarily shed light on the mechanisms responsible for the phenomena observed. Reliance on naturally occurring strains of virus has strict limitations for defining pathogenesis mechanisms, because it is only by luck that genetic variation occurs between strains in a manner that allows a specific hypothesis to be tested. Thus, advent of sequencing, structural biology, and directed mutagenesis of viral genomes as tools for pathogenesis research has been a turning point for pathogenesis as an experimental science. Infectious clone technology now exists for most virus families, and by applying directed mutagenesis strategies to these molecularly cloned viruses, mechanistic hypotheses can be tested directly. Often, this is done using a loss-of-function genetic approach in which an entire viral gene is deleted or in which a mutation is used to ablate a specific biochemical function of a viral protein. By evaluating such viruses, one can link structural and biochemical properties of a protein to specific aspects of pathogenesis, thus making loss-of-function genetic approaches a fundamental part of current pathogenesis research.

It is important to understand the limitations of viral mutagenesis as an approach. First, loss-of-function genetic analysis depends on whether a viral property can truly be attributed to a specific mutation. Further, it is necessary to prove that a phenotype is not an artifact of changes that occur during manipulation of the viral genome. This is often accomplished by *marker-rescue,* in which the mutant virus is repaired to wild-type status and the resulting virus characterized. If this marker-rescued virus is different from the wild-type virus, it indicates that other mutations have occurred during the process of mutant generation, thereby invalidating conclusions drawn using the mutant. This can be particularly problematic for rapidly evolving RNA viruses that may select compensatory mutations during generation of viral stocks. An alternative is to fully sequence the viral mutant—an approach that is now increasingly practical for even the largest viruses.

It is also necessary to prove that a phenotype is owing to a change in a viral protein and not to alterations in cis-elements in the viral genome or in adjacent genes that may confer phenotypes. For example, mutating a residue in a protein might alter a promoter for another viral gene or change the processing of a viral polyprotein. These problems are addressed by studying multiple distinct mutations in a protein, analysis of the expression of other viral proteins, or, when possible, complementing the mutation by expressing the protein in trans from another location in the virus.

A second limitation of loss-of-function genetics is that linking a mutation in a virus to a specific alteration in pathogenesis shows that the gene in question is necessary but does not indicate that the gene is sufficient for the virus to perform a specific task. For example, several genes might be important for an aspect of pathogenesis such that mutation of any one of them would give a phenotype; however, no single gene is independently sufficient for the virus to perform a certain task *in vivo*.

A third limitation of loss-of-function genetics is that the identification of an important role for a gene at a given step in pathogenesis does not provide information on the mechanisms responsible for the phenotype observed. In the absence of additional studies, one can only make correlative statements about the relationship between the behavior of a mutant virus and the biochemical properties of the protein encoded by the altered gene. For example, if a certain amino acid is important for binding of a host protein by a viral protein, and that same mutation causes the virus to be defective in pathogenesis, it is plausible that the phenotype observed *in vivo* relates to the binding between the host and viral protein. Proof of mechanism *in vivo* requires additional studies.

Interactions Between Host and Viral Genes in the Study of Pathogenesis

Defining the mechanism of action of a viral protein or gene *in vivo* is much more complex than showing that the gene is important, requiring that one determine experimentally why pathogenesis is altered by a specific mutation. It is this latter level of analysis that provides the greatest challenges. The attribution of changes in pathogenesis to a specific biochemical property of either the host or the virus is a complex task. The most important question is whether a change in the behavior of a virus *in vivo* is attributable to direct effects of a given mutation or is owing to indirect effects of the mutation. To exemplify this problem, consider the case of a mutant virus that both grows more poorly and induces a lesser inflammatory response than the wild-type virus. One interpretation of such data might be that the mutation influences the function of a gene that evades or subverts the host inflammatory response. A more trivial interpretation is that the host responds to a virus that grows poorly with a lesser inflammatory response. In this situation, one cannot cleanly attribute an immune evasion property to the viral protein in the absence of additional data.

This problem is conceptually similar to the Heisenberg uncertainty principle in physics in which detecting an electron requires the use of a particle that in turn changes the location of the electron. Analogously, one determines the function of the viral gene by mutating the gene; however, mutating the gene can change the process of infection sufficiently to complicate interpretation of any differences observed in pathogenesis.[297] A major challenge in defining mechanisms of viral pathogenesis is then to identify genetic, structural, and pathogenesis approaches that allow attribution of events *in vivo* to specific biochemical mechanisms.

One method for doing this involves using a combination of host and viral genetics in a process termed *host complementation*. For example, the *ICP34.5* gene of HSV is essential for viral virulence.[27,50] One activity of ICP34.5 is to bind protein phosphatase 1A (PP1A) and to redirect PP1A phosphatase activity to dephosphorylation of eIF2α, thereby reversing the eIF2α-dependent antiviral effects of PKR.[51,115,116,245,277] If ICP34.5 is acting to promote virulence through interactions with PKR, the ICP34.5 mutant should exhibit restored virulence specifically in mice lacking PKR, but not mice lacking other antiviral effector molecules. In fact, deletion of PKR, but not RNAse L, from mice fully restores the virulence of an ICP34.5 mutant virus,[156] thereby establishing that ICP34.5 interacts with PKR *in vivo*. Other examples of this approach include the role of the influenza virus *NS1* gene in countering STAT-1 dependent innate immunity,[83] the role of the murine γHV68 complement regulatory protein v-RCA in evasion of complement responses,[138] and the role of the *m157* gene of MCMV as natural killer (NK) cell–activating receptor ligand.[9,78,260] In all of these studies, deletion of a host gene or cell type has been used to define the mechanisms of action of a viral gene during infection.

It is important to note that this approach is limited to analysis of host genes that do not play an essential role in development or the ontogeny of the animal or the immune system. Moreover, it is essential to use controls including a viral mutant that is unaffected by mutation of a host pathway and a host mutant in which the viral mutant maintains its attenuated phenotype. Simply showing that a mutant virus regains growth or virulence in an immunocompromised host does not constitute genetic proof that a viral gene is countering a specific host pathway.

An important correlate of these experiments is that one must interpret studies of wild-type viruses in animals lacking specific genes with caution. For example, if a mouse lacking a certain gene is capable of resisting infection normally, it is often concluded that the host gene is unimportant. An alternative interpretation is that the virus encodes a molecule that effectively inhibits the host pathway in question, making even a wild-type host effectively deficient in the pathway. The erroneous conclusion that a host pathway cannot play a role in infection has important consequences. For example, inhibiting the viral protein responsible for evading a protective host response might allow the host to effectively control infection. Thus, potential therapeutic approaches for viral infection may be missed by ignoring the possible presence of effective viral strategies for evading host responses.

Cell Culture

Cell culture is an essential tool for the study of viral replication and tropism. However, conditions in cell culture are not representative of conditions *in vivo,* and thus hypotheses from cell culture experiments must be validated *in vivo.* One obvious limitation to cell culture studies is the absence of a cellular immune response. There are additional important limitations to cell culture studies. Often, a small proportion of cells in a tissue are actually infected at a given time, whereas cell culture is often optimized for synchronized infection of all cells. This obviates effects of infected cells on as-yet-uninfected cells—a fundamentally important part of what happens in tissues. For example, interferon released from one infected cell can protect uninfected cells from viral infection. As interferon effects generally require induction of gene expression, pretreatment of cells in culture is usually required to see full effects of interferon on viral infection, effects that are lost if all cells are simultaneously infected. Furthermore, cultured cells are often transformed or continuous lines whose behavior is at most distantly related to the behavior of primary cells. Even when primary cells are used in tissue culture, it is unlikely that the biology of these cells is the same as the biology of cells residing in a tissue in contact with physiologic extracellular matrix, the circulatory system, the endocrine system, and other primary cells.

DETERMINANTS OF CELL, ORGAN, AND TISSUE TROPISM

One of the most important concepts for understanding pathogenesis is the concept of cell, organ, and species tropism. Tropism is determined by many factors in both the virus and the host, including how the virus enters the host, how the virus spreads within the host (lymphatic, neural, or hematogenous spread), the permissiveness of specific cell types for the virus (as defined by receptors, cellular differentiation, and intrinsic cellular resistance to infection), the nature of innate and adaptive immune responses, and specific properties of tissues such as accessibility and effectiveness of the immune system (immunoprivilege). Each of these factors can play a determining role during viral infection and must be considered when defining mechanisms of viral pathogenesis.

Entry into the Host

A virus must access permissive cells to establish infection and therefore must overcome a series of anatomic and innate immune barriers to enter the host. The route of entry and the mechanisms of spread are therefore important determinants of viral tropism. The route and tissue through which a virus infects the host may be clear from epidemiologic studies. For example, both measles virus and VZV spread by the respiratory route, and polioviruses and noroviruses spread fecal–orally. However, even when the route of infection is known, the precise events involved in entry into the host are mostly unknown. Addressing this apparently simple question is a major challenge for pathogenesis research. The lack of knowledge of this critical step in pathogenesis is owing to the difficulties in studying viral spread under natural infection conditions when only a few infectious virus particles are sufficient to establish infection.

The critical determinants of viral spread include the form of the virus that spreads, the capacity of the virus to survive in the environment, the route of natural exposure to the virus, the mechanisms by which the virus gains entry, and the nature of host barriers to infection. Host barriers may include nonspecific barriers, barriers based on pattern recognition by the immune system, and barriers based on pre-existing adaptive immune responses.

Viruses may enter the body in different forms and via different vehicles.[198] The viral strategy for overcoming host barriers to entry is tightly linked to the form of the virus that spreads and how the virus is shed from the previously infected host. For example, viruses may enter carried in infected cells, may be injected via the mouth parts of arthropods,[307] may be contained in droplets or fomites shed from an infected host, or may be ingested as free virus. To spread in a population, viruses may benefit from survival in the environment. For example, HIV is relatively unstable in the environment and does not effectively spread via environmental surfaces. This contrasts dramatically with noroviruses such as Norwalk virus that can spread via contact with contaminated environmental surfaces.[126]

There are six primary portals of entry for viruses, each used by a variety of viruses. Five of these are epithelial surfaces: skin, conjunctiva, respiratory tract, gastrointestinal tract, and genitourinary tract. The sixth is the unique interface between the mother and the germ cell or the developing fetus.

Penetration Through Epithelial Barriers

The body is covered by epithelia, presenting a large surface for viruses to access. However, epithelia share several properties that inhibit viral entry. For example, epithelial cells are constantly turning over and being replenished; thus, cells that are contacted by a virus are shed continuously. The skin has an added protective mechanism, being many cells deep with the surface comprised of metabolically inactive cells that cannot support viral replication. In addition, barriers may be protected by low pH or secretions, including mucus.

Epithelial tissues are highly active immune organs. In all epithelia, DCs (e.g., Langerhans cells in the skin) serve as sentinels for invasion, having the capacity to, when activated, move to lymph nodes to induce immune responses. These sentinel cells play a dual role in infection, both as critical for induction of immunity and as cells targeted by viruses as an initial site of infection. For example, when VEE is inoculated into mice, the first cells infected are DCs; these cells rapidly move to draining lymph nodes, providing the virus access to the lymphatic system but potentially at the cost of the induction of immunity[171] (Fig. 10.6). DCs lie beneath the intestinal columnar epithelium, and thus the intestine, as with skin, has a resident DC population plausibly involved in sentinel functions.[146,202]

Intraepithelial lymphocytes are present in subepithelial and epithelial tissues, providing cells capable of protective immune responses in the most superficial layers of the body. In addition, epithelial cells themselves may be activated to express interferons or other antiviral molecules. In many sites, an invading virus is subject to inactivation by antibodies and complement. Even when a virus passes superficial epithelial barriers, the virus must confront the innate and adaptive immune response as well as an increasingly well understood set of intracellular barriers to infection collectively referred to as intrinsic cellular resistance to infection.

Viruses cross epithelial barriers through mechanical breaches (e.g., vectorborne delivery of arboviruses or bite wound delivery of rabies) or by accessing specialized cells

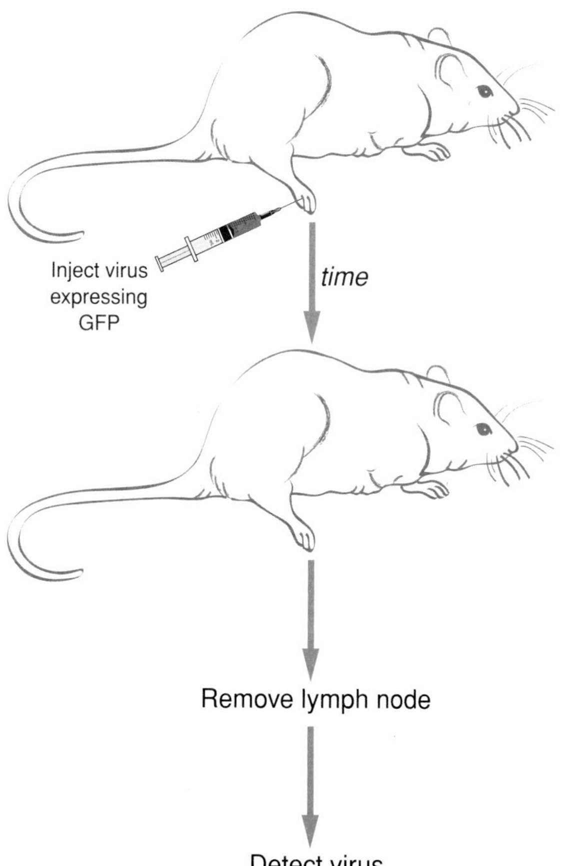

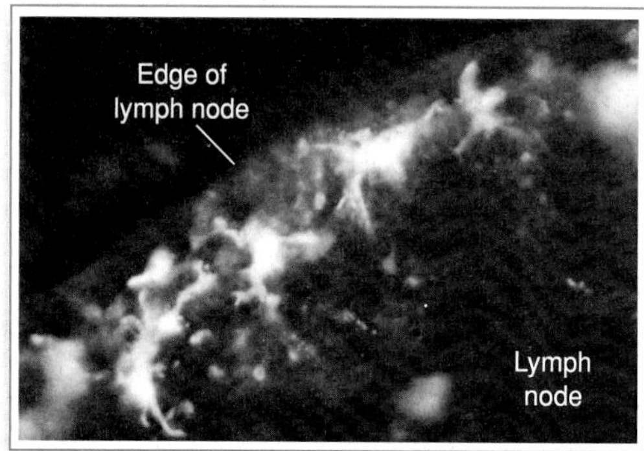

Viral GFP expression

FIGURE 10.6. Infection of dendritic cells early after virus infection. To determine which cells are initially infected with VEE, a mutant virus expressing GFP was constructed and inoculated into the hindlimb (as described in reference 171). This mutant is capable of only a single round of infection; thus, GFP expression is restricted to cells infected by virus in the inoculum. Twelve hours later, the draining lymph node was resected and imaged for GFP expression. In the bottom image, dendritic cells within the lymph node express GFP, demonstrating that dendritic cells are initial targets of VEE infection. VEE, Venezuelan equine encephalitis virus; GFP, green fluorescent protein. (GFP image courtesy of Dr. Robert Johnston.)

within the epithelium. An excellent example of this latter situation is provided by reovirus, which accesses the Peyer's patch through specialized epithelial cells called M cells.[54,147,200] Upon entry into the intestine, the reovirus virion is proteolyzed, triggering a remarkable structural transition with cleavage and loss of $\sigma 3$, cleavage of $\mu 1$, and conformational changes in both $\sigma 1$ and $\lambda 2$ that generate the infectious subviral particle (ISVP) (Fig. 10.7). The ISVP binds to M cells, which then transport the virus into the Peyer's patch where productive infection occurs.

Vertical Spread of Viruses

Many viruses infect either the immature fetus or the newborn during the birth—a process referred to as vertical transmission. There are two mechanisms for entry into the developing fetus. The first is via placental penetration, as when a virus enters the fetus after invasion of the fetal circulation or amniotic fluid. Viruses such as HCMV and rubella can spread transplacentally,[22,201] with devastating consequences for the developing fetus. Viruses such as human endogenous retroviruses (HERVs) can also be vertically transmitted via the germ line and constitute a significant fraction of the human genome.[132,140] HERVs continue to proliferate within the genome and are likely to exert both beneficial and detrimental effects on their hosts. Refer to the eBook for more discussion of the vertical spread of viral elements encoded in the host genome.

Systemic Spread of Virus Infection

Once a virus has passed through epithelia or penetrated the placenta, the virus may still be far from its target cells and tissue(s). Viruses spread via three host systems that can provide access to a large number of tissues and cells: blood, lymphatics, and nerves. Although the blood is a major highway for spread of viruses through the host, many viruses use nerves or a combination of hematogenous and neural spread to access host tissues.

The level of viremia has been correlated with the severity of acute viral disease, the prognosis of chronic viral disease (as in HIV), the extent of viral dissemination, and the efficiency of viral spread between hosts.[198,307] The level of viremia is a function of viral access to the blood, viral clearance from the blood, and the vehicle (plasma vs. cell associated) that the virus uses to travel through the blood. Viruses can access the blood either directly via introduction into the circulation, as by a needle or an insect bite, or indirectly after entering into and replicating in tissues. A very common finding is the rapid appearance of a virus in draining lymph nodes or in lymphoid structures such as Peyer's patches or tonsils. The connection between viral spread to lymphoid structures and subsequent spread to the rest of the host was recognized early on.[73,182]

Entry into lymphoid tissue is a two-edged sword for the virus, as a facile route to access the viscera of the host but one that passes through the very tissues that generate adaptive antiviral immune responses. For viruses that primarily infect mucosal surfaces such as influenza virus, rotavirus, papillomaviruses, rhinoviruses, and noroviruses, it is likely that the primary effect of entry into the lymphoid system is the induction of antiviral immune responses. However, there are clear advantages for lymphoid invasion if the virus has tropism for cells of the immune system that are capable of circulating and entering tissues. For example, HIV and EBV each have tropism for lymphocytes for latent and/or productive infection, and both MCMV and HCMV can spread through the body in infected cells of the monocyte-macrophage lineage.

In many cases, viruses can access the nervous system by infecting neurons in the periphery and then spreading along

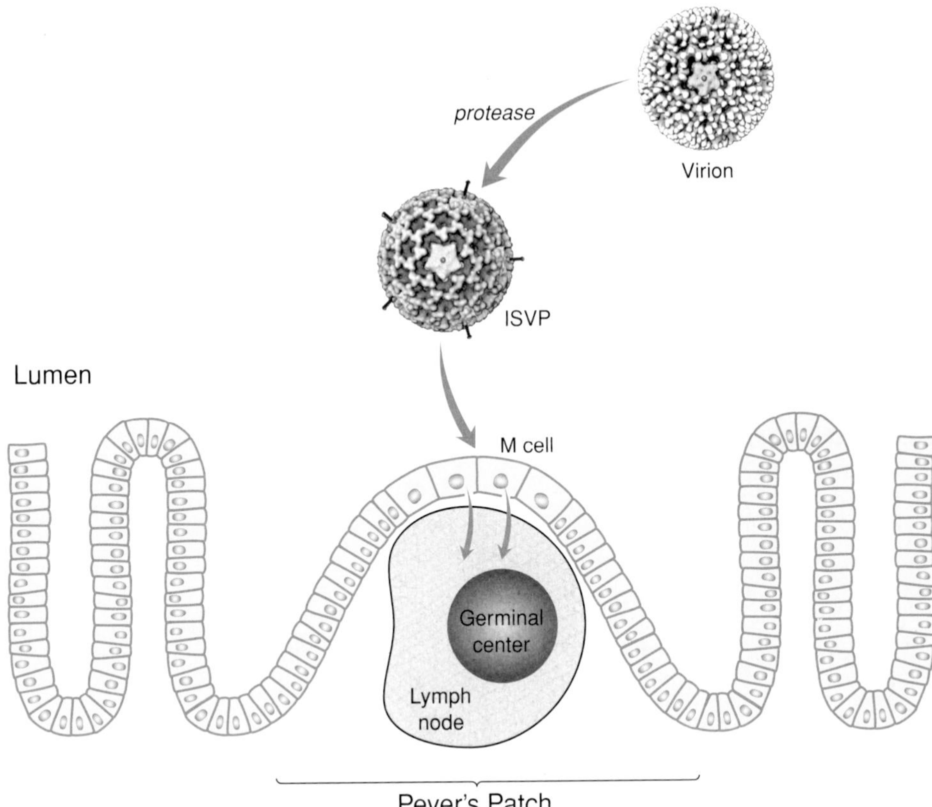

FIGURE 10.7. Reovirus entry into Peyer's patches in the intestine. Reovirus enters the body as an intact virion. The action of proteases in the intestinal lumen cleaves proteins on the surface of the virion, generating a highly infectious form of the virus—the intermediate subviral particle—which interacts with the microfold or M cell overlying the Peyer's patch and is transported into the Peyer's patch where infection is established. From this point, the virus may enter the bloodstream or enter nerves for spread to organs such as the brain and spinal cord. (Reovirus images courtesy of Dr. Terrence Dermody.)

axons toward the CNS.[198] The classical example of this strategy is rabies virus, which spreads along nerves from the area of inoculation to the CNS.[131] The time between inoculation and development of signs and symptoms of rabies encephalitis depends on the length of the nerves between the site of inoculation and the CNS. The virus travels up nerves toward the CNS at a rate of 50 to 100 mm/day, and the disease can be cured by surgical removal of the infected limb as long as the virus has not entered the CNS.[13,131] For example, if the initial bite is on a lower extremity, there is a longer time within which vaccination and passive transfer of rabies-immune antibody can be effective than if the bite is on the face.[131] Studies with several viruses, including HSV, pseudorabies virus, and reoviruses, have been used to elucidate the viral and cellular determinants that regulate viral spread through neural tissues, including sophisticated genetic and molecular mechanisms that regulate viral anterograde and retrograde axonal transport. Importantly, the immune system can also modulate neural spread. For example, antibodies can interrupt many of the steps in neural spread of reoviruses to and within the CNS

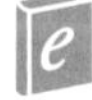

(Fig. 10.8). Refer to the eBook for an expanded discussion of the mechanisms of neural spread of viruses.

Determinants of Cell, Tissue, and Species Tropism

Once a virus has spread via lymphatic, hematogenous, or neural routes, a fundamental determinant of viral pathogenesis becomes the distribution of the virus between and within tissues of the host. Distribution of virus in tissues is a dynamic process determined by competing processes, including the speed of viral replication, the presence of specific viral receptors or other pro-viral factors the permit viral entry or replication, viral mutation rate, viral virulence genes, host susceptibility and resistance genes, and innate and adaptive immunity. It is useful to think of tissue distribution of a virus as an ongoing battle between the virus and the host being played out in different tissues. This battle has very local aspects, such as the contact between a virus and a specific cell or the contact between an NK cell or cytolytic T cell and a virus-infected cell. However, the outcome of this battle is also determined by effects over short distances in tissues, as, for example, the effects of host cytokines or virus-encoded soluble proteins that evade or subvert host responses. Lastly, there are long-range effects of host responses on infection, including production of antibody, synthesis of stress steroids, activation of the bone marrow to produce inflammatory cells, stimulation of the liver to synthesize and release acute-phase reactants such as complement proteins, and stimulation of autonomic centers in the brain to produce fever.

The Role of Viral Receptors in Cell, Tissue, and Species Tropism

An important step in viral infection, and a primary determinant of the distribution of virus between and within tissues, is the interaction of a virus with specific receptors on permissive cells. Receptor expression plays a major role in determining the tropism of several viruses, including poliovirus and measles virus, and the use of molecular tools, including transgenic mice, expressing the virus-specific receptors provides key insights into the role of receptors in regulating viral tissue tropism and pathogenesis. The importance of viral–receptor interactions is further illustrated by the fact that zoonotic viruses must often

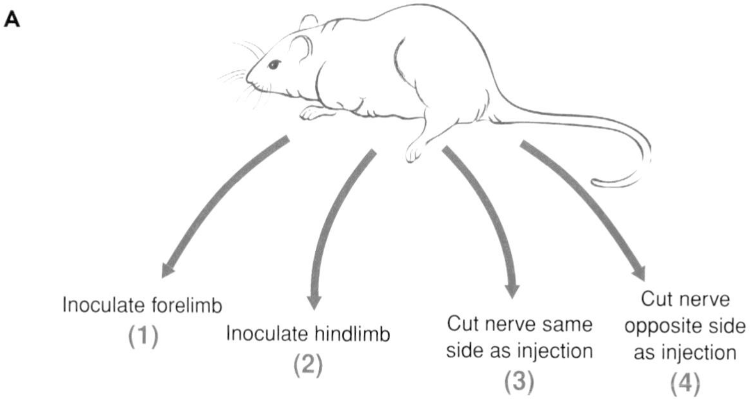

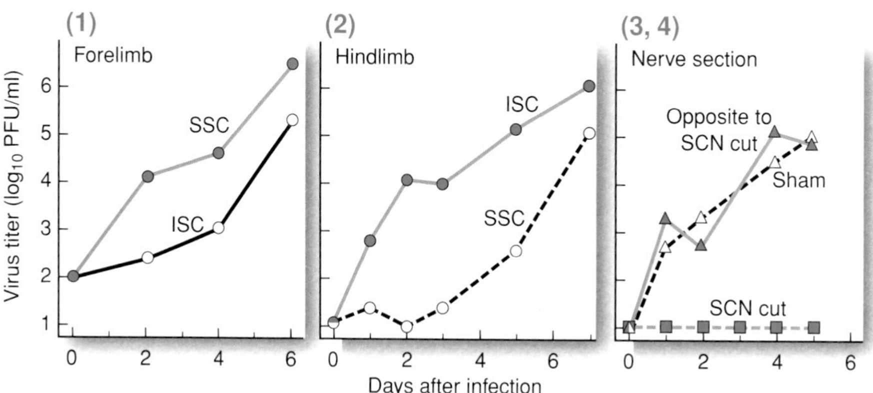

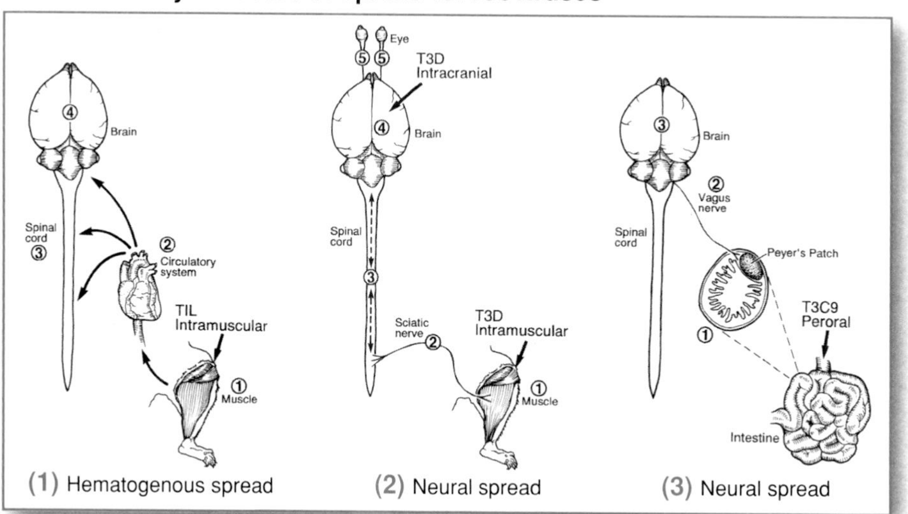

FIGURE 10.8. Neural versus hematogenous spread of reoviruses. A: Experimental design. **B:** Viral titrations after various experimental manipulations. **C:** Summary of the routes of spread of reovirus serotype 1 strain Lang (T1L), serotype T3 strain Dearing (T3D), and serotype 3 clone 9 (T3C9). (Adapted from Tyler KL, McPhee DA, Fields BN. Distinct pathways of viral spread in the host determined by reovirus S1 gene segment. *Science* 1986;233: 770–774, and from Nathanson N, Murphy FA. Evolution of viral disease. In: Nathanson N, Ahmed R, Gonzalez-Scarano F, et al, eds. *Viral Pathogenesis.* Philadelphia: Lippincott-Raven; 1997:353–369.)

adapt to receptors in their new host species to effectively cause disease and disseminate, as was the case with SARS.[161] These binding interactions are necessary for infection but are often not sufficient to explain all aspects of cell, species, and tissue tropism. For example, CD4 and chemokine receptors such as CCR5 or CXCR4 confer susceptibility to HIV infection; however, permissiveness is also controlled by cytoplasmic proteins that restrict HIV infection.

Often, viruses use a binding receptor to increase the concentration of virus at the cell surface and one or more entry receptors. An example of this latter strategy is HSV, which interacts with specific sulfated sugars on heparan sulfate[255] in a process that enhances infection but is not required if a cell expresses an entry receptor such as the appropriate nectin.[88,263,269] Another example of this strategy is utilized by serotype 3 reoviruses, which interact with sialic acid via one portion of their cell attachment protein $\sigma1$ and the protein JAM1 via another portion of the $\sigma1$ protein.[54] Importantly, the interaction with the broadly expressed carbohydrate sialic acid has been shown to be important in the tropism of the reovirus *in vivo,* indicating that even interactions with ubiquitously expressed molecules can play a role in cell and tissue tropism.[54] Tropism can also be conferred by interactions between viral cell attachment proteins and proteases, as is seen with Newcastle disease and influenza viruses.[41,191]  Refer to the eBook for a more extensive discussion of how receptor tropism affects viral pathogenesis using poliovirus infection as an example.

Innate Immunity and Intrinsic Cellular Resistance to Infection Determine Tropism

Factors in addition to specific receptors play a major role in determining viral tropism. Tropism can be determined by proteins responsible for cell-intrinsic defense against viral infection, transcription factors, cell cycle regulators, and microRNAs. For example, the liver-specific host microRNA miR-122 is essential for robust HCV replication,[137] and inhibition of miR-122 in nonhuman primates limits HCV replication.[151]

Once a virus has bound to a cell and delivered its genome or capsid to the cytoplasm, a series of events occur that can have a profound effect on the viral cell tropism. These events likely explain why receptor expression does not always explain the cell and tissue tropism of a virus. The host cell expresses on its cell surface and in its cytoplasm molecules that can either directly inhibit viral replication (intrinsic cellular resistance to infection) or can induce a signaling cascade that in turn generates antiviral molecules (innate immune responses). Together, these molecules and pathways are determinants of both the permissiveness of cells for viral replication and species tropism. It is likely that mechanistic relationships will be discovered between molecules involved in innate immunity and intrinsic cellular resistance to infection as more is learned about each of these two important processes.

Molecules involved in innate immunity can be important components of tissue and species tropism. This is illustrated by myxoma virus, which does not normally infect mice but readily infects murine cell lacking type I interferon responses and causes lethal disease in STAT-1 deficient mice.[305] Intrinsic cellular resistance to infection is also conferred by molecules such as the TRIM or APOBEC proteins that restrict retrovirus infection. Importantly, allelic variations in the genes involved in these processes may contribute to regulation of viral pathogenesis.

Immunoprivilege

One important determinant of viral tropism is the fact that the innate and adaptive immune systems are not equally efficacious at clearing virus infection from all tissues. The concept that the immune system is selectively ineffective at clearing virus infection from specific tissues is referred to as immunoprivilege. Immunoprivilege plays a significant part in the pathogenesis of many viruses but has been best studied in experimental murine pathogenesis models. For example, in studies of LCMV infection of mice,[32,38] many organs including liver, spleen, lung, and pancreas are cleared relatively efficiently within 30 days of transfer of immune cells. However, virus persists in the CNS for up to 90 days and in the kidney and genitourinary system for more than 200 days, indicating that both the CNS and the genitourinary tract are immunoprivileged. These data also show that immunoprivilege is a relative term, with the efficacy of the immune system varying depending on when infection is analyzed. Analysis of the mice at a time point more than 90 days after transfer of immune cells identifies only the genitourinary tract as immunoprivileged (Fig. 10.9).

It is likely that the selective inability of the immune system to clear virus infection from certain tissues is owing to a combination of two interrelated factors. The first is intrinsic limitations of immune system function in certain tissues or to limited capacity to address infection of certain cell types. For example, CD8 T cells may be more effective at eliminating infection from major histocompatibility complex (MHC) class I–expressing hepatocytes than from neurons that do not express MHC class I molecules. The second factor is viral evasion of immunity. An example of this is the capacity of HSV to evade clearance by the host immune system via establishment of latency in neurons. It is plausible that in most cases immunoprivilege is owing to a combination of both viral strategies and cell- or tissue-specific limitations in the efficacy of the immune response. The mechanisms responsible for immunoprivilege are poorly defined at the cellular and molecular level.

Cellular Differentiation as a Determinant of Viral Tropism and Pathogenesis

Another important determinant of viral tissue distribution is cellular differentiation. Thus, cells at different stages of differentiation may have specific properties that favor or disfavor viral infection or replication. This is especially true in a tissue responding to virus-induced damage. For example, when hepatocytes are damaged during chronic HBV or HCV infection, the liver regenerates, providing viruses with access to cells in different differentiation states.

Many viruses take advantage of differentiated functions of the cells that they target. For example, HSV establishes latency in fully differentiated neurons, and EBV latently infects memory B cells; in each case, the reservoir for chronic infection is a particularly long-lived cell type. The lytic cycle of gene expression for both HIV and EBV is triggered by induction of lymphocyte activation and differentiation. In each case, a specific relationship between a virus and a certain differentiation state of an infected cell contributes to viral pathogenesis.

Papillomavirus infection of the skin provides an outstanding example of the impact of cellular differentiation on pathogenesis[26,190] (Fig. 10.10). In normal skin, basal stem cells give rise to ever more differentiated cells that move toward the skin surface, lose their nucleus, become cornified, and are finally

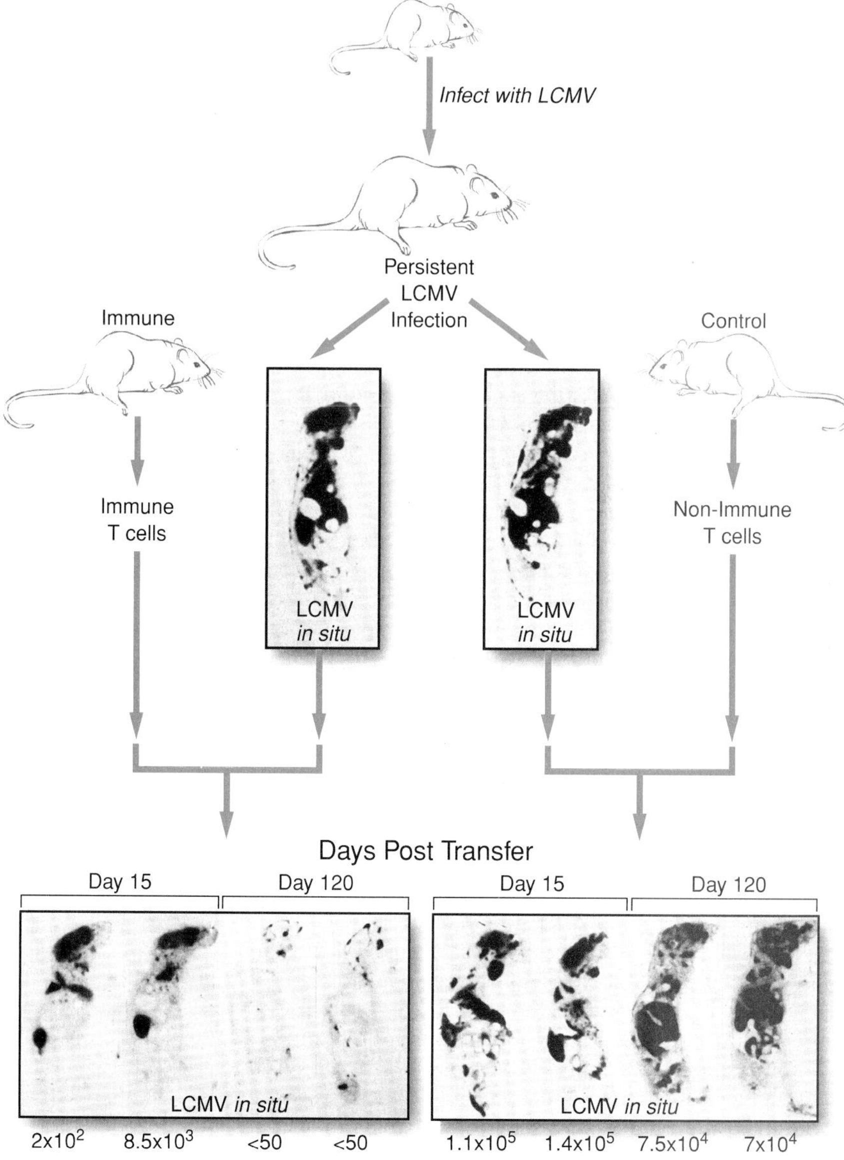

FIGURE 10.9. LCMV clearance by immune T cells reveals immunoprivileged tissues. Shown is the pattern of clearance of LCMV after transfer of either immune or control T cells into mice with persistent LCMV infection as described in reference 208. The clearance of virus is indicated both by the viral titers shown and by the *in situ* hybridization signal from cross sections of the whole mouse. LCMV, lymphocytic choriomeningitis virus. (Adapted from Oldstone MB, et al. Cytoimmunotherapy for persistent virus infection reveals a unique clearance pattern from the central nervous system. *Nature* 1986;321:239–243; courtesy of Dr. Michael Oldstone.)

shed. Papillomaviruses infect basal stem cells of the skin, where they can persist in a latent state for prolonged periods. Activation of a program of gene expression initially involving the expression of E6 and E7 proteins results in cell cycle progression, inhibition of apoptosis, and viral replication. As infected cells differentiate and move toward the skin surface, they become permissive for expression of genes involved in viral replication and assembly (see Fig. 10.10). The normal differentiation process is subverted by the virus, resulting in retention of the nucleus and synthesis of proteins required for viral DNA and protein synthesis. The virus assembles and is released from the skin in shed cells.

The principle that cellular differentiation is a determinant of viral pathogenesis is very important and general. When tissues are damaged, stem cells are activated to generate new cells with consequent proliferation of somatic cells and differentiation into cells such as hepatocytes, endothelial cells, or epithelial cells. These processes are plausibly subverted by several viruses, many of which grow optimally in replicating cells. One consequence of this principle is that the full potential of a virus's genetic program may not be revealed in a cell line that is transformed or represents a single differentiation state within a particular cell lineage. It is plausible that, as with papillomaviruses, many viruses have genes that play specific roles in the cell at certain stages of differentiation and thereby contribute to pathogenesis.

FATE OF THE INFECTED CELL, TISSUE, AND HOST

The presence of a virus in a tissue may or may not result in damage. The variables that determine the fate of the infected tissue

Virus Infection Changes with Differentiation of a Cell

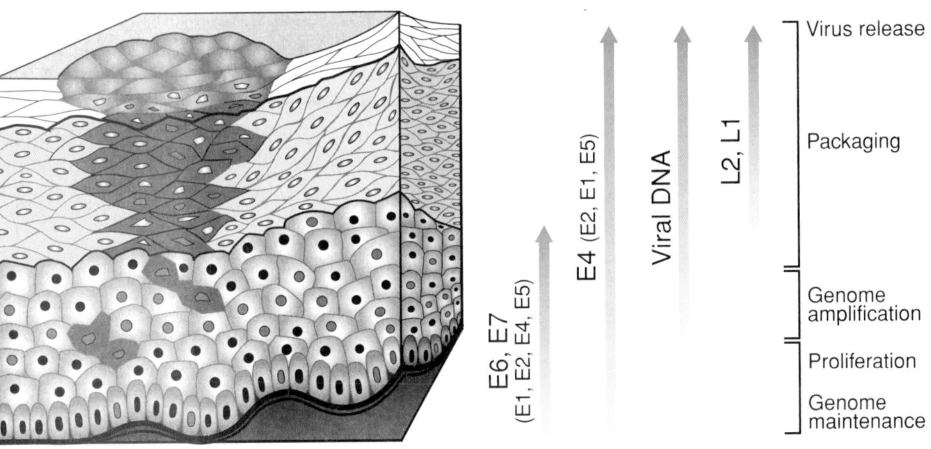

FIGURE 10.10. Critical role of differentiation in papillomavirus pathogenesis. Shown are the relationships between stages in the replication of a papillomavirus on the **far right,** the nature of the progressions of infection through the layers of the skin on the **left,** and the patterns of papillomavirus gene expression as shown by the labeled *blue arrows* in the **center**. Within the skin, virus-infected cells are designated in *dark grey.* (Adapted from Doorbar J. The papillomavirus life cycle. *J Clin Virol* 2005;32:S7–S15.)

and host are complex and involve the interplay between the virus and its cytopathic potential; the age, sex, and nutritional status of the host; the regenerative capacities of different primary cell types; whether the immune system damages the tissue as part of the protective response; whether the virus induces autoimmune responses; and perhaps most importantly, whether the virus is ever cleared from the tissue and, if not, the nature of residual virus infection. Determinants of tissue damage may be local in nature, such as the death of infected cells owing to viral cytopathicity or killing by immune cells, or operative over longer distances, as in the case of vascular damage leading to ischemia, systemic hormonal and cytokine responses, induction of fever or cachexia, cytokine induction of the death of uninfected cells, metastatic tumors, or virus-induced autoimmunity.

Although viruses can directly kill infected cells as they replicate, one is always confronted with the question of whether tissue damage is directly caused by the virus or is indirectly caused by the immune system; what is the balance between the protective and destructive capacities of the immune system? Additionally, viruses can damage the host indirectly by making the host susceptible to secondary infections or by altering fluid and electrolyte balance, as in the case of dehydration induced by gastroenteritis. It has recently been found that virus infection can trigger, in a host with a specific genetic makeup, novel disease phenotypes in uninfected cells,[40] and therefore that a virus can have a substantial effect on diseases that are highly specific to a given constellation of genes in the host. Thus, in many situations, the pathogenesis of disease may be independent of whether virus replication *per se* induces the death of infected cells.

Age as a Determinant of Susceptibility to Viral Infection

Many viral infections are far more severe in young than older hosts[159,256]—an increase in severity that often correlates with increased replication and dissemination of virus. For example, suckling mice have long been used to isolate new viruses because they have greater susceptibility to virus infection than mature mice. The susceptibility of young mice to Sindbis virus infection is a striking example.[150] Intracerebral inoculation of 1-day-old mice with most strains of Sindbis virus results in rapid death, extensive neuronal apoptosis, and high levels of viral replication. In contrast, the same viral inoculum in 4-week-old mice results in a nearly 10-fold lower viral replication, no death, and no neuronal apoptosis. This observation extends to many other viruses, including poliovirus, where 2-week-old poliovirus receptor transgenic mice are 10,000-fold more susceptible to paralytic disease than adult mice.[53] All measles virus receptor transgenic mice inoculated at 1 to 6 days of age succumb to lethal infection, whereas mice aged 30 to 60 days at inoculation survive.[153,236]

The practical importance of this principle is reflected in studies in primates with potential live attenuated SIV vaccines and in the epidemiology of human HBV infection. Vaccination of an adult monkey with live attenuated SIV viruses lacking nef or combinations of nef and other genes significantly protects against SIV challenge.[311] However, inoculation of neonatal animals with the same live attenuated vaccine virus results in progressive immunodeficiency. Similarly, whereas adults infected with HBV often clear the infection, exposure of human neonates to HBV results in a very high level of chronic infection.[315] Age dependence of virus resistance does not always favor older hosts. For example, West Nile virus encephalitis is more common and more severe in older hosts,[114] and lethality after SARS infection is significantly higher in people older than 60 years of age than in younger people.[62,219] This is also the case in mouse models of SARS infection.[244,246]

Together, these data indicate that age plays a critical role in determining viral virulence. The mechanism(s) responsible for this are incompletely understood. It is commonly considered that maturation of the immune system explains increased resistance to infections seen in older hosts. However, this has not been rigorously demonstrated as the reason for age-dependent susceptibility to viral infection. Other age-dependent processes, such as cellular differentiation and proliferation, may play a role as large as that of the immune system in age-related susceptibility. For example, the genes expressed in the nervous system during infection of younger versus older hosts differ,[150,213] indicating that there are fundamental differences in how older and younger tissues respond to viral infection.

Fate of Infected and Uninfected Cells in Tissues

A primary determinant of the tissue damage and pathology observed after viral infection is the fate of the infected cell. It is often unclear why cells in tissues die when infected by viruses, and the extent to which cell death is destructive or protective in tissues is often uncertain. On the one hand, death of infected cells is harmful if those cells are essential to the host; on the other hand, death of an infected cell may inhibit viral replication with the sacrifice of one cell contributing to the protection of other cells. The immune system has many mechanisms for killing infected cells, arguing that the death of infected cells can benefit the host (Chapters 8 and 9). The death of cells in an infected tissue may be indirect, with uninfected cells dying owing to cytokines, bystander killing by leukocytes, or ischemia. The consequences of viral infection range from rapid destruction of tissue cells, as seen with variola or Ebola viruses, to continuous replication in the absence of severe cytopathology, as seen with LCMV, to the establishment of latency, as seen with herpesviruses.

Direct Killing of Cells by Viruses

Cytopathic effect is defined as the destructive consequences of virus infection on cells. Direct killing of cells by viruses may be attributable to viral subversion of cell metabolism for replication or to cell-intrinsic programmed cell death pathways such as necrosis, apoptosis, or nonnecrotic and nonapoptotic cell death. Despite the great importance of understanding the specific mechanisms responsible for virus-induced tissue damage, the balance between virus-induced cell death and cell death owing to host programs induced by the presence of the virus is very poorly understood in most cases.

The term *cytopathic effect* is most commonly used to describe the consequences of infection in cultured cells. Cell death that occurs in a cultured cell may or may not reflect the process of cell death that occurs *in vivo*. An advantage of studying cell death and cytopathicity in cultured cells is that the interaction between the virus and the cell occurs without cell-extrinsic factors, with exception of those owing to autocrine stimulation (e.g., the expression of interferons by infected cells). A disadvantage of this approach to studying cell death is that events in cultured cells may have little relationship to what happens in primary cells in an infected tissue.

It is easiest to ascribe cell killing to direct viral effects, rather than immunopathology or ischemia, when death of virus-infected cells occurs in the absence of inflammation or extensive tissue damage. For example, in both Sindbis and rabies, virus kill neurons in the absence of extensive inflammation. Further proof that viruses can directly damage tissue without invoking indirect effects of immunopathology comes from the susceptibility of SCID mice and *RAG* gene–deficient mice, which cannot mount adaptive T- or B-cell responses, to several different viruses. In these cases, death of host cells cannot be attributed to the immunopathologic consequences of adaptive immunity, although contributions from innate immunity cannot be ruled out. It is important to remember that the presence of inflammation does not necessarily indicate the participation of inflammatory cells in the killing of infected cells. Inflammatory cells may be beneficial or present as a host response to killed cells and tissue damage rather than being participants in the death of infected cells.

Killing of Cells by Cell-Extrinsic Effects of the Immune System

Not all cell death in an infected tissue is a result of direct viral effects or cell-intrinsic mechanisms of programmed cell death triggered by the presence of the virus. The host has many cell-extrinsic mechanisms for initiating apoptosis or lysis of infected cells via cytokines, serum proteins such as complement, and proteins such as the granzymes that are injected via perforin into infected cells by leukocytes (Chapters 8 and 9).

The role of cell killing by the lytic activity of granzymes is important because perforin- and/or granzyme-deficient mice are susceptible to coronaviruses, West Nile virus, LCMV, ectromelia virus, HSV, Theiler's virus, MCMV, and murine γHV68,[165,166,188,220,254] and a human with a mutation in perforin has been described with chronic active EBV infection.[139] As detailed later, these cell killing pathways can contribute to virus-induced immune pathology, as studies in HBV transgenic mice in which cytolytic antiviral CD8 T cells mediate liver disease show that both perforin- and FAS-dependent pathways contribute to liver destruction.[193]

The complement cascade is a two-edged sword important for antiviral immunity but can also contribute to virus-induced tissue damage.[25,268] Complement proteins are involved in induction of antibody and T-cell responses, trapping of viral antigen on antigen-presenting cells, induction of chemotactic and vascular permeability changes in infected tissues, and activation of leukocytes. In addition to being immunoregulatory, complement can lyse both virus-infected cells and lyse or neutralize virions.[25,79,178,294]

Clearance of Virus Infection and Chronic Viral Infection

A fundamentally important variable in viral pathogenesis is whether the immune system can clear a virus from the body. Some viruses are readily cleared but can do significant damage to the host during their brief time of residence in the body. An example is variola virus, which causes smallpox. This pattern of acute infection (see Figs. 10.1 and 10.3) is associated with development of sterilizing immunity and effective resistance to reinfection. Many viruses for which effective vaccines are available fall into this category. Other viruses are less amenable to elimination by the immune system, resulting in latent, chronic, or progressive infection (see Fig. 10.1). Examples of chronic viral infections of great medical significance are those caused by HIV, HCV, and HBV. Other chronic infections are less consistently harmful to their hosts but do cause significant disease. Examples include herpesviruses such as EBV, VZV, HCMV, and HSV, each of which permanently infects most human beings. It is possible that such chronic infection can, in addition to causing disease in rare cases, provide a symbiotic benefit to the host via chronic stimulation of the innate immune system, including macrophages and NK cells.[17,302,310,326,327]

Between the extremes of complete clearance and establishment of chronic infection, there are viruses that persist in a small proportion of hosts. For example, measles virus persists in the CNS of a small proportion of infected persons, causing subacute sclerosing panencephalitis (SSPE). In SSPE, a chronic CNS infection with measles leads to a progressive destruction of neurons and often to death. Importantly, SSPE is associated with an unusual pattern of mutations in defective measles viruses that persists in the CNS, with mutations in several proteins and a bias toward U to C mutations in the matrix protein.[45,209,243] In the murine measles virus receptor transgenic system, transient infection with LCMV predisposes to development of an SSPE-like disease.[209] This is a paradigmatic example of how a common infection (measles) may cause pathology triggered by a second infection.

Whereas persistence of certain viruses is related to disease in a proportion of infected hosts, the role of persistent infection is more controversial for many other viruses (see Fig. 10.1). For example, coxsackievirus RNA persists in the hearts of some persons with chronic myocarditis, and poliovirus RNA may persist in the CNS of a proportion of persons who develop "postpolio" syndrome.[142,312] These situations are not as well understood as SSPE or chronic infections with herpesviruses, retroviruses, HCV, or HBV. However, the data suggests the hypothesis that persistence of either virus or viral genomes may contribute to disease in some cases, and it seems highly likely that additional examples of similar phenomena will be detected as unbiased and highly sensitive next-generation sequencing technologies are applied in clinical settings to detect viral genomes.

Tissue Damage During Beneficial Immune Responses Is a Necessary Evil

Certain viruses, such as HCV, HBV, HIV, SIV, and LCMV, can persistently replicate in tissues despite an active adaptive immune response. Although the immune response is ineffective at clearing the virus, activated immune cells and cytokines are still capable of killing host cells. Even when the immune system can clear a virus, these adaptive immune mechanisms may cause significant damage to host tissues. Importantly, the innate immune system can also contribute to host disease in the setting of acute infection, as has been shown, for example, for influenza.[281]

Although there are clear examples in which the immune system is primarily responsible for virus-induced tissue pathology, and thus disease is immunopathologic, the situation is seldom that simple. The antiviral immune response has two faces: a beneficial face as the host system responsible for curing infection and a harmful face via induction of tissue pathology and systemic toxicity. This sets the stage for consideration of one of the most complex topics in viral pathogenesis: the relationship between immune-mediated damage and clearance of infection.

It is not always true that the function of the immune system causes pathology. For example, protective effects of antibody that do not damage tissues are seen in most if not all viral infections. Sindbis virus is cleared from neurons by antibody to the E2 envelope glycoprotein in the absence of neuronal loss,[160] and antibody to measles virus can alter expression of measles proteins in infected cells.[80,82] Antibody can inhibit the neural spread of viruses, such as reovirus, and can act inside cells to inhibit reovirus and West Nile virus replication.[283,298,299] Whereas immunity can be beneficial without harming host cells, in other cases, the more harmful face of the immune system is prominent and tissue injury is associated with immune-mediated clearance of infection.

A clear example of the two-faced nature of immunity comes from studies of HBV. HBV DNA replication occurs for weeks before induction of a significant immune and inflammatory response or significant release of serum alanine aminotransferase (sALT), a marker of hepatocyte lysis, into the circulation[314,315] (Fig. 10.11). Damage to the liver does occur during the latter stages of clearance of HBV DNA from the liver, as evidenced by increases in both sALT and the number of apoptotic hepatocytes, and the induction of this damage correlates with the appearance of CD8 T cells and IFNγ mRNA in the liver[314,316] (see Fig. 10.11). Thus, active immune responses and clearance of the last vestiges of infection are associated with significant tissue injury.

The mechanisms underlying these processes have been further elucidated using transgenic mice that express viral antigen and nucleic acids in all hepatocytes and produce infectious HBV in serum. Using these mice, it has been shown that virus replication can be limited and viral protein and nucleic acid can be cleared from hepatocytes without killing the hepatocytes[100–103,286] via a mechanism that depends on interferons and tumor necrosis factor (TNF). However, these same studies also demonstrated that virus-specific T cells can contribute to the induction of liver injury. These results were further validated by studies in chimpanzees, where depletion of CD8 T cells resulted in delayed viral clearance, and the kinetics of viral clearance and alanine aminotransferase (ALT) induction suggested that virus was cleared in large part by noncytolytic mechanisms but that the CD8 T cells also drove final resolution of infection and subsequent liver damage through cytolytic mechanisms. These studies illustrate the potential dual nature of the immune response in mediating viral clearance while also causing tissue pathology during the clearance process.

Immunopathology Occurs When the Immune System Goes Too Far

In some cases, the balance between the protective effects of immunity and the harmful effects of immunity clearly shifts to immunity being the primary cause of tissue pathology and even death of the host.[32,323] These processes can be driven by overactive innate immune responses, which result in inflammatory responses that drive virus-induced tissue pathology and disease,[328] nonspecific cell killing, or even induction of autoimmunity by the host adaptive immune response. The balance between acceptable tissue damage associated with viral clearance and immunopathology is determined by the effectiveness of the immune system in clearing the infection. For example, even severe hepatitis would be an acceptable outcome of HCV infection if the virus could be cleared; however, the immune response to HCV infection is often ineffective. Immunopathology can be attributable to either T- or B-cell responses or to innate immunity and may be the consequence of virus-induced immune responses to either viral antigens or, in the case of induced autoimmunity, host antigens.

An excellent example of immunopathology owing to B-cell responses is the kidney damage done by immune complexes generated during the continuous replication of viruses such as LCMV, lactic dehydrogenase virus, Aleutian disease of mink, HBV, HCV, or murine retroviruses.[110,118,210,211,232,295] In these cases, circulating immune complexes containing viral antigen are deposited in the kidney with consequent activation of complement and cellular inflammation that results in damage to the renal filtration apparatus of the glomerulus.

The existence of T-cell–mediated immune pathology was first demonstrated using the LCMV system.[32,38] Infection of adult mice by the intracerebral route with LCMV

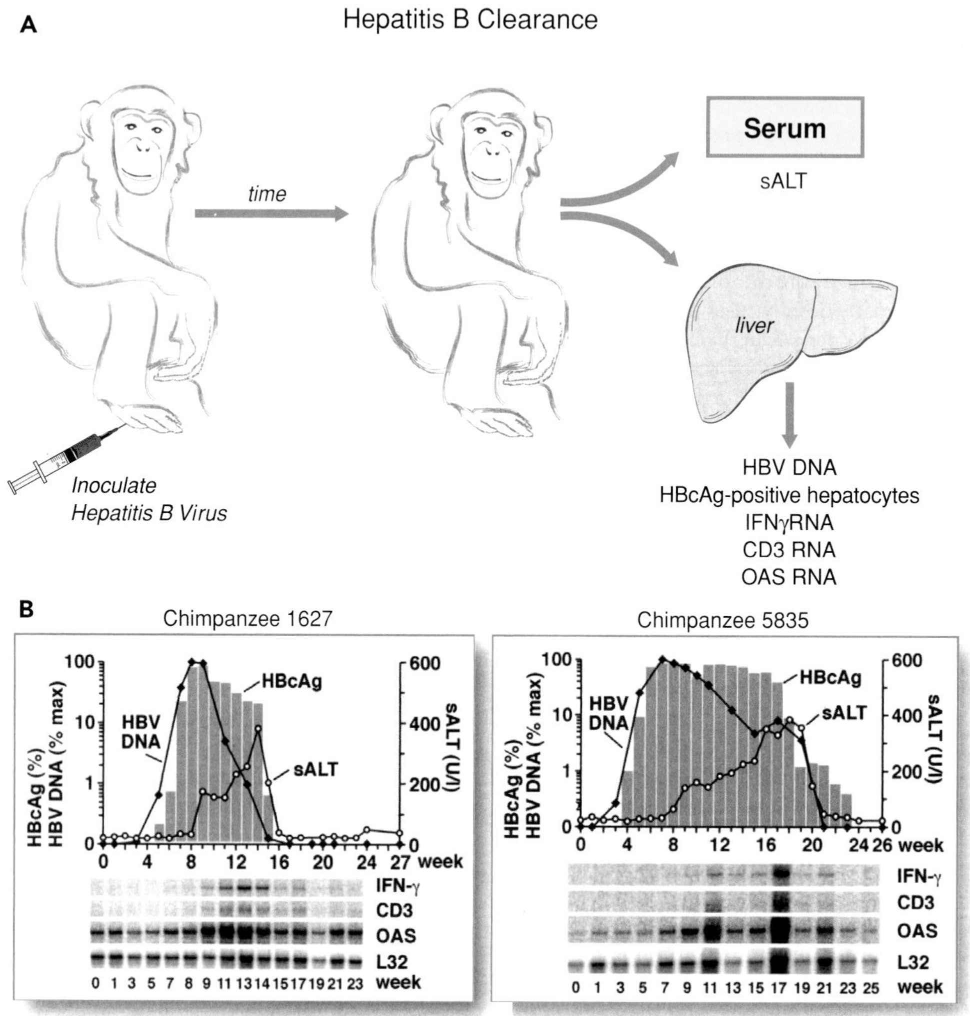

FIGURE 10.11. Clearance of HBV is associated with liver damage. Chimpanzees were infected as shown in **panel A** as described in detail in reference 314; at various times after infection, serum samples or liver biopsies were taken and analyzed for sALT and various parameters of HBV infection. Intrahepatic HBV DNA (*black squares*) is expressed as a percentage (% max) of the peak HBV DNA levels in the liver of each animal. Hepatitis B core antigen–positive hepatocytes (*gray bars*) are expressed as percentage of the total number of hepatocytes. sALT (*open circles*) is expressed in units per liter. Intrahepatic expression profiles for IFNγ, CD3, and 2′5′OAS were determined by RNase protection assay. HBV, hepatitis B virus; sALT, serum alanine aminotransferase; IFNγ, interferon-γ. (Adapted from Wieland S, Thimme R, Purcell RH, et al. Genomic analysis of the host response to hepatitis B virus infection. *Proc Natl Acad Sci U S A* 2004;101:6669–6674.)

results in death attributable to inflammation of the meninges and choroid plexus termed *choriomeningitis*.[32,38,177] The importance of this model is that, as opposed to most viral infections in which depletion of T cells worsens infection, for LCMV depletion of T cells protects against disease.[32,38,157,186] Further studies have demonstrated that LCMV-specific CD8 T cells were responsible for virus-induced immune pathology.[325]

These experiments in the LCMV system show that CD8 T cells, in addition to their protective capacities, can be responsible for destruction of many different types of virus-infected cells. Why is the balance of protection versus immunopathology tipped toward immunopathology for LCMV? The most obvious reason is that the virus is largely noncytopathic, thus the presence of the virus in the host even over long periods does limited direct cellular damage. In this view, CD8 T cells kill virus-infected cells that would not otherwise die, resulting in immunopathology. This makes a plausible case for a key role for immunopathology in chronic diseases attributed to largely noncytopathic viruses such as HBV and HCV.

Virus-Induced Autoimmunity

A variant mechanism of immunopathology is the induction of autoimmunity by virus infection.[21,181,207,304] The contributions of autoimmunity to tissue pathology associated with viral infection, or putatively associated with viral vaccination, remain quite controversial. The role of autoimmunity in virus infection and postinfection syndromes has been studied in several systems, and viruses have at one time or another been candidate etiologic agents for many autoimmune or inflammatory diseases in humans, including rheumatoid arthritis, multiple sclerosis, Crohn's disease, myocarditis, uveitis, hepatitis, Sjögren's syndrome, and type 1 diabetes.

To date, unequivocal proof of the role of a specific virus in a human autoimmune disease has been lacking, although this is an important area of interest. The presence of immune responses to self-antigens after virus infection is common; however, these responses should not be confused with a pathological role for self-responses in virus-induced pathology. Moreover, when studies in some viral models that have been touted to represent autoimmunity are examined very carefully, the persistence of viral genome, and perhaps protein, provides a plausible alternative to autoimmunity as a mechanism. This is true for coxsackievirus-induced myocarditis,[313] underlining the importance of careful virologic assessment of potentially autoimmune phenomena.

A proposed mechanism for the induction of autoimmunity is molecular mimicry between virus and host antigens leading to a breakdown of self-tolerance.[207] This might plausibly occur in the setting of virus-induced tissue damage and inflammation. Since the first proof that this can happen, numerous experiments supporting the concept that molecular mimicry can trigger autoimmunity have been published. The opportunity for molecular mimicry for T cells is provided by the degenerate recognition of peptides by even clonally expanded antigen-specific T cells, making it more likely that antiviral T cells could recognize peptides derived from the host proteome.

The potential for molecular mimicry to cause virus-associated pathology has been proven using transgenic mice engineered to express the LCMV nucleoprotein or glycoprotein under the control of the insulin promoter in the insulin-producing islet cells of the pancreas.[81,204,206,212,303,304] Infection of these mice with LCMV can trigger diabetes. In this case, LCMV infection triggers a T-cell response to the viral protein expressed in the pancreas as a pseudo–self-antigen. Autoimmune T-cell responses can also develop during persistent virus infection when viral and self-proteins do not demonstrably cross-react—a process termed *epitope spreading.*[181,222] In this process, it may be that the inflammatory response to chronic infection results in the induction of T-cell responses to self-proteins via breakdown in self-tolerance and expansion of rare clones of autoreactive T cells that escape negative selection in the thymus. Although these studies demonstrate that a virus can induce disease by inducing responses to proteins expressed in a host tissue, studies proving that this mechanism is responsible for a specific human disease have not been published.

VIRAL DETERMINANTS OF VIRULENCE

Niche-Specific Virulence Genes

Viral genes and virulence determinants are important indicators of viral pathogenesis and viral virulence. Examples of specific properties of viruses that contribute to virulence abound in the literature, and many—including tropism, the capacity to persist, and the capacity to kill cells—have already been discussed. *Virulence* is a general term representing the severity of viral infection for the host. However, specific viral genes and properties most often play a role in a very specific tissue, at a certain time, at a very specific bottleneck in infection, or to counter a very specific host response to infection. A useful concept is that such genes are niche specific, having functions in a single aspect of infection defined by time, tissue, and stage of infection or host response. Thus, virulence is the sum of the actions of multiple niche-specific viral genes and virulence determinants that play their specific roles in limited settings *in vivo.*

The concept that viral virulence genes and virulence determinants have niche-specific roles *in vivo* during infection is important for understanding experimental pathogenesis research. *In vivo* readouts of infection often depend on a single route and dose of infection, are often measured in a genetically homogeneous host, and commonly rely on a limited set of assays for viral infection such as death of the infected host, growth of virus in a certain tissue at a certain time, or severity of tissue pathology. The experimentalist is rarely able to mimic the entire process of pathogenesis under physiologic conditions, and so the virus is not asked to perform all of the tasks for which it has evolved in nature. Experiments performed under such conditions may reveal a minor, or even no, contribution of a niche-specific viral virulence gene or allele to infection as measured by a limited set of assays in a given experiment. This type of negative data is fundamentally unrevealing. The gene or allele under study may have a significant role that would be revealed by further experimentation that quantitatively evaluated the niche within which the gene functions. It is plausible that every viral gene has been under considerable evolutionary pressure and that the mere presence of the gene indicates that the gene has an important function for the virus. Exceptions may be found when a virus has recently jumped from one species to another; however, even in that setting, the pressure to utilize the limited viral genome parsimoniously likely results in rapid selection against useless genes.

It is therefore true that niche-specific functions of viral genes may only be identified in specific experimental conditions. Examples of this phenomenon abound and include the role of the *M3* gene of murine γHV68 that encodes a chemokine scavenger. M3 mutant viruses are completely normal in a broad range of properties *in vivo* in mice, including replication in many tissues and the establishment of viral latency. However, the gene contributes significantly to virulence after intracranial inoculation.[293] Similarly, a comparison of vaccinia virus mutants inoculated either intranasally or in the pinna of the ear revealed that fully half of a panel of 16 different mutants had a phenotype in only one of the two inoculation models.[285] Other examples of niche-specific virulence genes include herpesvirus genes associated with chronic infection or latency. These genes may be dispensable for the lytic phase of the life cycle but then play an essential role in promoting or maintaining the chronic stage of the viral infection. For example, γHV68 viruses lacking either the *v-cyclin* or *v-Bcl-2* genes have limited or no phenotype during acute infection or in the establishment of latency.[16] However, these genes play an important role in reactivation from latency and in the capacity to continuously replicate in immunocompromised mice. Therefore, when considering the function of a gene or virulence determinant *in vivo,* it is necessary to consider the limitations of the experimental system for revealing the role of a niche-specific viral gene.

Mutation and Selection of Viral Variants

Although viruses have niche-specific genes specialized for specific tasks *in vivo,* it is also possible for mutation and selection to meet specific needs during infection. For this reason, the error-prone RNA polymerases of viruses such as HCV and HIV play a role in viral pathogenesis. Viral RNA polymerases can make a mistake every 10^3 to 10^5 nucleotides while copying an RNA.[59,60,65,223] In addition, point mutations, duplications, deletions, recombination events, and even acquisition of host mRNAs into RNA and DNA viral genomes have occurred in different viruses. Thus, the total mutational capacity of viruses is very high. It is plausible that a virus with a nearly 9,700-bp genome, such as HCV, will have a large number of mutations generated during replication even in a single cell. However, the variation actually observed *in vivo* or in serial passage in cultured cells is much lower than predicted from this argument. For example, comparison of the sequences of HCV over 13 years of infection of a single host revealed a mutation rate of 1.92×10^{-3} base substitution per genome site per year.[203] Because the observed variation is low compared to the potential variation, it is plausible that the strength of the selective pressure applied to a viral population determines the nature of viruses present in the host at a given time. The capacity of mutation to provide the substrate on which selective pressure operates to generate new viral strains with altered pathogenic capacity has significant implications for understanding and controlling viral infections.

An excellent example of a mutation contributing to the pathogenesis of viral infection is the emergence of immune escape mutants. The principle that viral escape mutants can evade CD8 responses was first identified by study of murine LCMV infection.[227] In this study, investigators created T-cell receptor transgenic (LCMV TCRtg) mice containing a large number of T cells specific for the epitope containing amino acids 32-42 of the LCMV glycoprotein. Within 8 days of infection, many LCMV isolates were no longer recognized by TCRtg T cells and contained mutations in the 32-42 epitope.[227] Importantly, mutations in other T-cell epitopes that were not recognized by TCRtg T cells were not selected, indicating specificity of the selective pressure.

The relevance of this initial observation to events during infection in normal hosts is now well established.[34,72,225] Both HIV and SIV accumulate mutations in CD8 T-cell epitopes over time, which is associated with progression of disease, escape from vaccine-mediated control of SIV infection, and escape from control of infection by adoptively transferred HIV-specific T cells.[7,15,31,72,92,144,225] Similar observations have been made during chronic HCV infection, viruses such as MCMV develop mutations that enable escape from NK cell–mediated control, and genetic drift in seasonal influenza virus strains is in large part driven by selective pressure from antiviral antibodies.

Virus-Induced Immunosuppression

Virus infection is often associated with the induction of an immunosuppressed state. Immunosuppression is defined as a virus infection-associated decrease in the capacity of the immune system to respond to antigen. The phenomenon of immunosuppression was first noted as inhibition of tuberculin skin test reactivity during measles virus infection.[95,96,187,218] That initial observation has been followed by a deluge of reports of altered immune reactivity in virus-infected hosts.

An immunosuppressed state may benefit a virus by inhibiting antiviral responses; however, it is important to distinguish between immunosuppression and viral immune evasion that occurs without inducing a general deficiency in immune function. It is also important not to confuse immunosuppression with the normal down-regulation of virus-specific responses that occurs as viral infection is cleared. There are three categories of immunosuppressive mechanisms.[194] In the first, virus kills significant numbers of critical immune system cells; an example of this is HIV-associated depletion of CD4 T cells. Likewise, LCMV clone 13 causes immunodeficiency owing to destruction of DCs that are critical antigen-presenting cells. In this case, activated CD8 T cells that recognize viral antigens expressed by infected DCs damage the immune system.[8,30,158,324] A second potential mechanism involves alterations in cytokine secretion by infected cells or the induction of secreted molecules that inhibit immune responses. This mechanism, however, does not provide a clear explanation for a case in which immunosuppression persists long after infection is thought to be cleared. A third but largely speculative potential mechanism only now being explored is viral induction of regulatory T cells that may inhibit the immune response.

Viral Evasion and Subversion of Host Cytokine Responses

Host molecules present in the extracellular fluid including cytokines, prostaglandins, steroid hormones, peptide hormones, growth factors, and serum components such as complement provide important targets for viral evasion and subversion strategies. Viruses encode molecules that evade or subvert host hormonal and cytokine responses that regulate both innate and adaptive immunity, such as interferons, TNF, IL18, IL6, IL10, complement, and chemokines. These viral evasion and subversion molecules have been studied in detail for herpesviruses and poxviruses, including via the use of viral mutants lacking these proteins to determine their specific role *in vivo.*

The remarkable sophistication of viral cytokine evasion proteins is exemplified by the structure of the γHV68 chemokine-binding protein M3, which alters the inflammatory response to viral infection[6,293] (Fig. 10.12). Chemokines are a large group of polypeptides that regulate immune cell trafficking, cell differentiation, and tissue development. The M3 protein has evolved to mimic both the chemokine receptor of the host and the dimer interface between chemokines as a way to bind a broad array of chemokines with a very high affinity. It is likely that similar molecules and mechanisms will be discovered in other viruses and that additional host cytokine systems will be discovered that are targeted by viral immune evasion and/or subversion molecules. In addition, viruses can increase inflammation to foster infection and can induce tissue damage via paracrine effects of virus-infected cells.

Virus–Host Co-Evolution Drives the Host–Pathogen Interaction

The interactions between viral immune evasion proteins in host cytokine networks are highly sophisticated. Given this capacity to manipulate the host, one may question why viruses are not more virulent. A common belief is that the most dangerous and virulent viruses are those that have recently jumped from one species to another—the idea being that virulence *per se* can be the result of incomplete adaptation of the virus to the host. Implicit in this view of viral pathogenesis and evolution is the

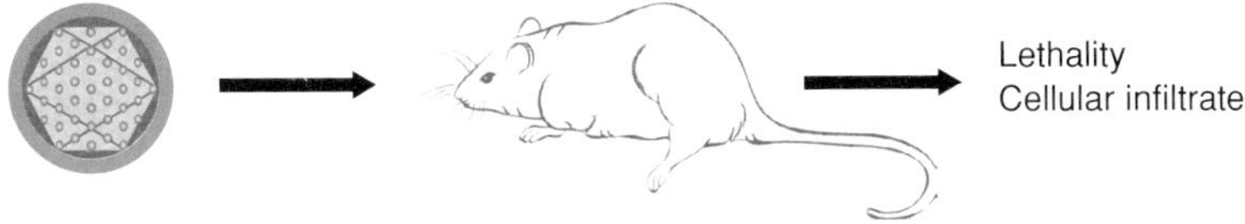

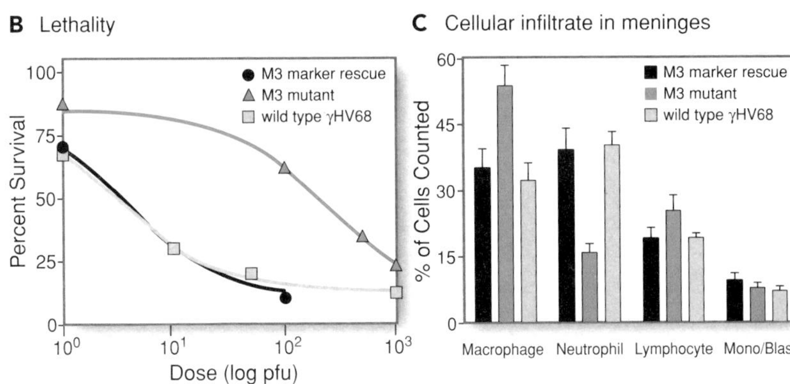

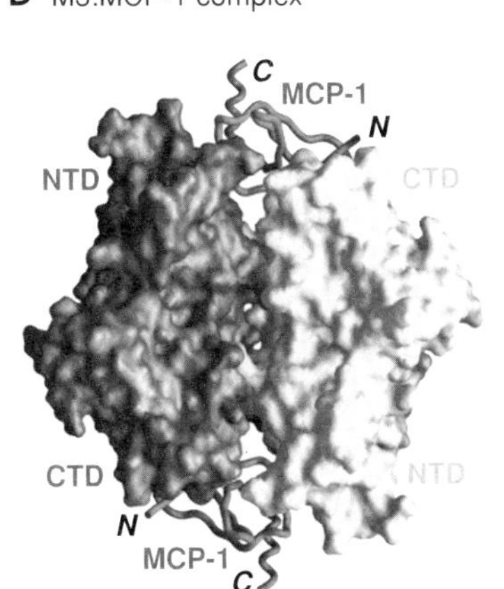

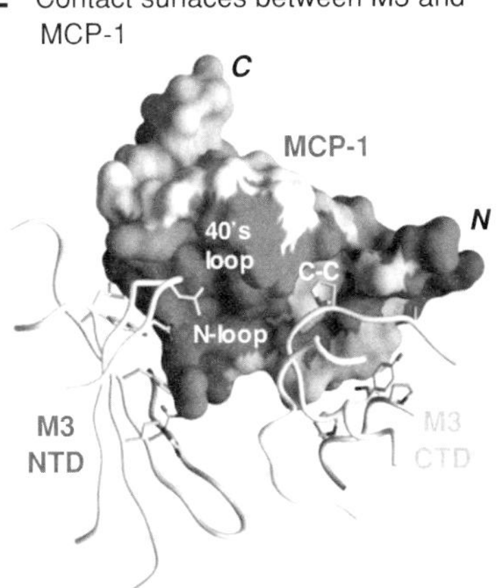

FIGURE 10.12. Role of a viral chemokine-binding protein in herpesvirus pathogenesis. **A:** Experimental protocol for analysis of the pathogenesis of an M3 mutant in murine γHV68 derived from reference 293. **B:** Lethality observed at different doses of virus administered intracranially. *Marker rescue* refers to a control virus generated by restoring wild-type γHV68 sequences to the M3 mutant virus. **C:** The nature of the meningeal cellular infiltrate of mice infected with the indicated viruses. Note that inflammation induced by the M3 mutant virus shows increased macrophages and decreased neutrophils compared to wild-type and control viruses. **D:** Three-dimensional structure of M3 homodimer (*solid*) in complex with the chemokine MCP-1 (*tubes*) bound at either end of the M3 homodimer in a 2:2 stoichiometry. Note that the M3 dimer is arranged in an antiparallel fashion with the M3 N- and C-terminal domain packed together to form the chemokine-binding niche. **E:** The interfaces between M3 and MCP-1 are shown in more detail than in **D.** M3 chemokine-binding regions are shown as tubes, whereas the sequestered MCP-1 is depicted with its solvent accessible surface. M3 acts as a competitive inhibitor of chemokine function, shown here engaging the same interface of MCP-1 employed to bind the host chemokine receptor CCR2. (**D** and **E** adapted from Alexander JM, Nelson CA, van Berkel V, et al. Structural basis of chemokine sequestration by a herpesvirus decoy receptor. *Cell* 2002;111:343–356; courtesy of Drs. Jennifer Alexander-Brett and Daved Fremont.)

concept that viruses benefit from adapting to lesser virulence. Examples of the virulence of viruses that have recently entered a new host population abound, with the influenza pandemic of 1918, Ebola virus, and HIV being outstanding examples. Each of these virulent viruses has entered humans from another species and is more virulent in the newly invaded species than in the original host species.

What really happens to the virus and the host species as an emergent virus spreads? In a classic series of experiments analyzing the epidemiology, pathogenesis, and virology of myxomatosis in rabbits, Fenner et al. demonstrated virus–host co-evolution. The natural history and evolution of both a virus and its host were followed in real time after the introduction of a virulent virus into a highly susceptible population. Importantly, although both the host and virus evolved in this enormous experiment of nature, this work does not support the concept that viruses necessarily evolve to become completely avirulent in a new species.

The introduction of European rabbits into Australia by European settlers provided the substrate for both an ecological disaster and a series of fundamentally important experiments in viral pathogenesis. Absent natural predators, European rabbits expanded rapidly in Australia with severe ecological consequences, creating a need for a pest control strategy. Myxomatosis is a relatively benign disease in *Sylvilagus* rabbits from South America but is almost uniformly lethal in the European rabbit *Oryctolagus*.[74,76] Recognizing that an infection that spread quickly and killed rabbits might be an effective biological weapon, investigators released myxoma virus into the Australian rabbit population in 1950. Initially, the kill rate was calculated as 99.4% to 99.8%, with most surviving rabbits being uninfected.

Over the next several years, a remarkable process of evolution of both the virus and the rabbit host occurred and was experimentally documented.[76,77] Similar evolution of the rabbit host was observed in laboratory experiments.[262] Over the course of a single year, the virus became less virulent, killing only 90% of laboratory European rabbits[74] (Table 10.1). It is hypothesized that this initial decrease in virulence allowed enough rabbits to survive and breed to allow selection of rabbits capable of resisting virulent myxoma. The virulence of isolates was categorized into five classes, with grade 1 killing more than 99% of rabbits and grade 5 killing less than 50% of rabbits[74,77] (see Table 10.1). By 1975, less than 2% of isolates were highly virulent class I viruses, whereas more than 60% of isolates were class III viruses. Notably, the distribution of isolates with

TABLE 10.1 Virulence of Field Isolates of Myxoma Virus, 1951–1981

	Virulence grade					
	I	II	III	IV	V	
Fatality rate (%)	>99	95–99	70–95	50–70	<50	
Mean survival time (d)	<13	14–16	17–28	29–70	NA	
Years	% of isolates					**Number of samples**
1950–1951	100	0.0	0.0	0.0	0.0	1
1952–1955	13	20	53	13	0.0	60
1955–1958	0.7	5	55	24	15	432
1959–1963	1.7	11	61	22	5	449
1964–1966	0.7	0.3	64	34	1.3	306
1967–1969	0.0	0.0	62	36	1.7	229
1970–1974	0.6	5	74	21	0.0	174
1975–1981	1.9	3	67	28	0.0	212

NA, not applicable.

Adapted from Nathanson N, Ahmed R, Gonzalez-Scarano F, et al, eds. *Viral Pathogenesis*. Philadelphia: Lippincott-Raven, 1997, and based on data from Fenner F. Biological control, as exemplified by smallpox eradication and myxomatosis. *Proc R Soc Lond B* 1983;218:259–285.

differing virulence was relatively stable from about 1955 onward, indicating that equilibrium between rabbit and virus was established. The rabbit population similarly evolved. Whereas wild rabbits initially exhibited more than 90% lethality when challenged with a virulent isolate of myxoma virus, after multiple epidemics only 30% of challenged rabbits died and 46% suffered mild to moderate disease (Table 10.2).

Given this evidence for evolution toward resistance in the rabbit population and toward lower virulence in the virus, why didn't myxomatosis become a benign disease in European rabbits? Evolution of the virus to lower virulence, but not avirulence, occurred (see Table 10.1). There were other selective pressures at work in this evolutionary experiment. Field experiments showed that virulent viruses were at a disadvantage compared to less virulent naturally occurring isolates.[74] Even when virulent isolates were introduced into areas in which attenuated viruses were endemic, the attenuated viruses were dominant. Very virulent viruses plausibly were at a disadvantage as they killed their hosts rapidly, allowing less time for natural transmission by mosquitoes. Thus, the capacity to persistently infect some hosts or to slow the infectious process might have fostered the capacity to infect new hosts over longer periods, thereby providing a selective advantage. However, the virus had to spread efficiently to survive, and experiments showed that viruses with midrange virulence were present in skin at sufficient levels to spread via mosquitoes. It is believed that selective pressure retained a level of virulence associated with replication to high enough levels to spread,[74] explaining why the outcome was not evolution to avirulence.

Virus Genes That Inhibit Pathogenesis of Disease

It is a common misconception that viruses primarily encode molecules to cause disease. Although retention of some level

TABLE 10.2 The Susceptibility of Nonimmune Wild Rabbits After Successive Epidemics of Myxomatosis

	Severity of disease (%)[a]			
Number of epidemics	**Fatality rate**	**Severe disease including fatalities**	**Moderate disease**	**Mild disease**
0	90	93	5	2
2	88	95	5	0
3	80	93	5	2
4	50	61	26	12
5	53	75	14	11
7	30	54	16	30

[a]Rabbits were challenged with a virus of grade III (intermediate) virulence. (See Table 10.1.)

Adapted from Nathanson N, Ahmed R, Gonzalez-Scarano F, et al, eds. *Viral Pathogenesis*. Philadelphia: Lippincott-Raven, 1997, and based on data from Fenner F. Biological control, as exemplified by smallpox eradication and myxomatosis. *Proc R Soc Lond B* 1983;218:259–285.

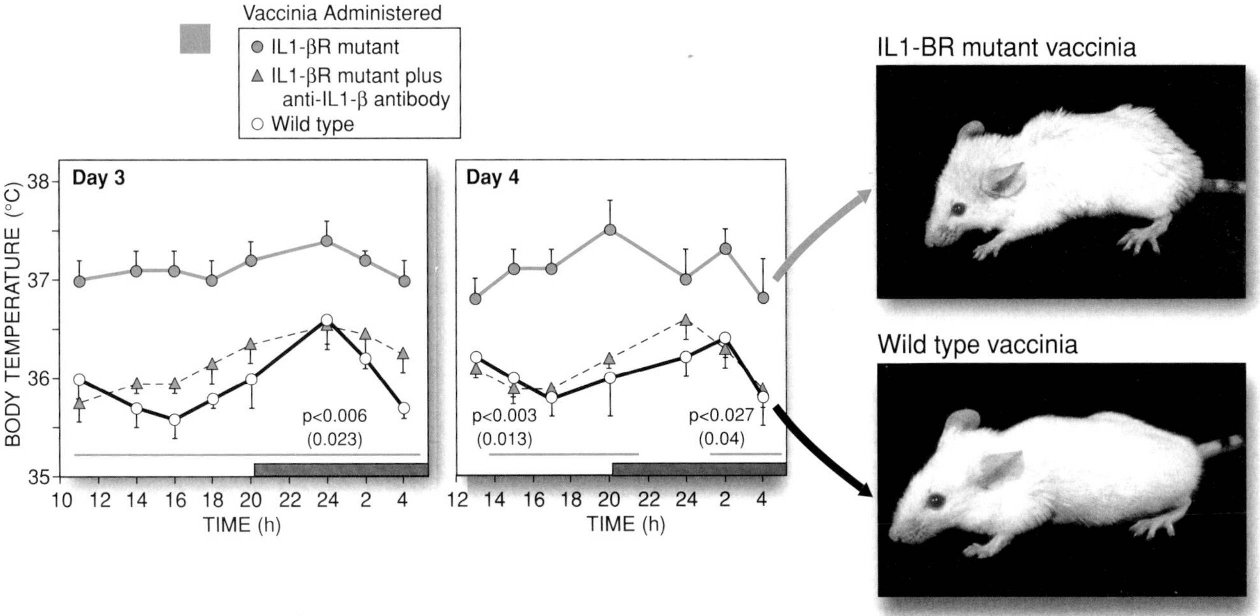

FIGURE 10.13. Protection of the host by the vaccinia virus IL-1β receptor gene. Shown are body temperatures and clinical appearance of mice infected with the indicated viruses and either left untreated or treated with antibody specific for IL-1β. IL, interleukin. (Adapted from Alcami A, Smith GL. A mechanism for the inhibition of fever by a virus. *Proc Natl Acad Sci U S A* 1996;93: 11029–11034; images of mice courtesy of Dr. Antonio Alcami.)

of virulence during adaptation within a host species can be an advantage, evolution to lower virulence did occur in the example presented earlier.[74,197] One way to lose virulence would be to sequentially lose or inactivate virulence genes or determinants. A second nonexclusive mechanism would be to select for genes that actually protect the host from lethal infection—a prediction borne out by studies of vaccinia virus showing that some viral genes protect their hosts from virus-induced disease.[4,5] Vaccinia virus expresses a secreted IL-1β receptor homolog that neutralizes the effects of IL-1β. Although this gene might plausibly contribute to virulence, instead a mutant virus induced fever and the wild-type virus did not despite similar levels of replication (Fig. 10.13).[5] The fever induced by the mutant virus was attributed to IL-1 secretion by the host because anti-IL-1 antibody blocked fever induced by the mutant virus (see Fig. 10.13). Expression of the soluble IL-1β receptor also decreased clinical signs of illness and decreased weight loss. Repair of a nonsense mutation in the soluble IL-1β receptor in a vaccine strain of vaccinia resulted in a virus that did not induce fever. These data demonstrate that protection of the host can be an active result of viral gene expression rather than a passive process of loss of virulence factors, suggesting that viruses have the capacity to precisely balance virulence and avirulence strategies to foster their survival.

FUTURE OF VIRAL PATHOGENESIS RESEARCH

The study of viral pathogenesis promises to be as important in the future as it has been in the past for understanding fundamental biological and biochemical mechanisms of disease. Understanding the process of infection is increasingly recognized as the best, and perhaps the only, approach to understanding how to vaccinate against and treat severe unconquered infections such as HIV and HCV and emerging viruses such as Ebola and H5N1 bird influenza. New developments in human genomics combined with ever-improving methods for manipulation of both viral and host genomes will continue to accelerate progress in this critical field of biology. The progress made in other fields as unbiased genetic screens are applied to cell biological problems is breathtaking. In recent years, we have seen the application of these approaches to virology, where whole genome RNA interference (RNAi) screens provide new insights into which host genes are essential for viral replication. Similar approaches are now being applied to identify antiviral and viral restriction factors that regulate the control, tissue tropism, and host range of a wide range of viruses. To date, many of these approaches have been restricted to cell culture–based studies; however, the broadening availability of large panels of genetically modified mice, including knockout and transgenic animals, should continue to facilitate major advances in viral pathogenesis from the standpoint of virus–host interactions.

We have also seen unprecedented progress in our ability to perform studies in genetically complex populations, including the use of GWAS and whole exome and whole genome sequencing to identify polymorphic host genes that are associated with specific phenotypes, including susceptibility to viral infection. The application of these approaches in humans, as well as newly developed mouse models designed to model genetically diverse populations, to the study of viral pathogenesis is likely to revolutionize our understanding of how viral interactions with genetically diverse populations result in different pathogenic outcomes.

Related to these latter approaches, the power of mathematical methods for modeling complex phenomena is improving rapidly and will ultimately be applied to viral pathogenesis. It will be important to apply these tools with a rigorous understanding of the clinical context of disease and an awareness of both the benefits and limitations of studying viral infection in the live host. *In vivo veritas.*

REFERENCES

All cited references are available in the e-book.

1. Abel L, Casanova JL. Human genetics of infectious diseases: fundamental insights from clinical studies. *Semin Immunol* 2006;18:327–329.
3. Ahmed R, Oldstone MB. Organ-specific selection of viral variants during chronic infection. *J Exp Med* 1988;167:1719–1724.
4. Alcami A, Smith GL. A mechanism for the inhibition of fever by a virus. *Proc Natl Acad Sci U S A* 1996;93:11029–11034.
5. Alcami A, Smith GL. A soluble receptor for interleukin-1 beta encoded by vaccinia virus: a novel mechanism of virus modulation of the host response to infection. *Cell* 1992;71:153–167.
6. Alexander JM, Nelson CA, van Berkel V, et al. Structural basis of chemokine sequestration by a herpesvirus decoy receptor. *Cell* 202;111:343–356.
7. Allen TM, O'Connor DH, Jing P, et al. Tat-specific cytotoxic T lymphocytes select for SIV escape variants during resolution of primary viraemia. *Nature* 2000;407:386–390.
9. Arase H, Mocarski ES, Campbell AE, et al. Direct recognition of cytomegalovirus by activating and inhibitory NK cell receptors. *Science* 2002;296:1323–1326.
10. Aronson JF, Grieder FB, Davis NL, et al. A single-site mutant and revertants arising in vivo define early steps in the pathogenesis of Venezuelan equine encephalitis virus. *Virology* 2000;270:111–123.
11. Aylor DL, Valdar W, Foulds-Mathes W, et al. Genetic analysis of complex traits in the emerging Collaborative Cross. *Genome Res* 2011;21:1213–1222.
14. Baiker A, Fabel K, Cozzio A, et al. Varicella-zoster virus infection of human neural cells in vivo. *Proc Natl Acad Sci U S A* 2004;101:10792–10797.
15. Barouch DH, Kunstman J, Kuroda MJ, et al. Eventual AIDS vaccine failure in a rhesus monkey by viral escape from cytotoxic T lymphocytes. *Nature* 2002;415:335–339.
16. Barton E, Mandal P, Speck SH. Pathogenesis and host control of gammaherpesviruses: lessons from the mouse. *Annu Rev Immunol* 2011;29:351–397.
17. Barton ES, White DW, Cathelyn JS, et al. Herpesvirus latency confers symbiotic protection from bacterial infection. *Nature* 2007;447:326–329.
21. Benoist C, Mathis D. Autoimmunity provoked by infection: how good is the case for T cell epitope mimicry? *Nat Immunol* 2001;2:797–801.
23. Birney E, Stamatoyannopoulos JA, Dutta A, et al. Identification and analysis of functional elements in 1% of the human genome by the ENCODE pilot project. *Nature* 2007;447:799–816.
25. Blue CE, Spiller OB, Blackbourn DJ. The relevance of complement to virus biology. *Virology* 2004;319:176–184.
26. Bodily J, Laimins LA. Persistence of human papillomavirus infection: keys to malignant progression. *Trends Microbiol* 2011;19:33–39.
28. Boon AC, deBeauchamp J, Hollmann A, et al. Host genetic variation affects resistance to infection with a highly pathogenic H5N1 influenza A virus in mice. *J Virol* 2009;83:10417–10426.
30. Borrow P, Evans CF, Oldstone MB. Virus-induced immunosuppression: immune system–mediated destruction of virus-infected dendritic cells results in generalized immune suppression. *J Virol* 1995;69:1059–1070.
32. Borrow P, Oldstone MBA. Lymphocytic choriomeningitis virus. In: Nathanson N, Ahmed R, Gonzalez-Scarano F, et al, eds. *Viral Pathogenesis.* Philadelphia: Lippincott-Raven; 1997:593–627.
36. Bresnahan WA, Shenk T. A subset of viral transcripts packaged within human cytomegalovirus particles. *Science* 2000;288:2373–2376.
38. Buchmeier MJ, Welsh RM, Dutko FJ, et al. The virology and immunobiology of lymphocytic choriomeningitis virus infection. *Adv Immunol* 1980;30:275–331.
39. Buller RM, Palumbo GJ. Poxvirus pathogenesis. *Microbiol Rev* 1991;55:80–122.
40. Cadwell K, Patel KK, Maloney NS, et al. Virus-plus-susceptibility gene interaction determines Crohn's disease gene Atg16L1 phenotypes in intestine. *Cell* 2010;141:1135–1145.
43. Carrington M, Martin MP. The impact of variation at the KIR gene cluster on human disease. *Curr Top Microbiol Immunol* 2006;298:225–257.
44. Casanova JL, Abel L. Human genetics of infectious diseases: a unified theory. *EMBO J* 2007;26:915–922.
50. Chou J, Kern ER, Whitley RJ, et al. Mapping of herpes-simplex virus-1 neurovirulence to gamma-134.5, a gene nonessential for growth in culture. *Science* 1990;250:1262–1266.
52. Connolly BM, Steele KE, Davis KJ, et al. Pathogenesis of experimental Ebola virus infection in guinea pigs. *J Infect Dis* 1999;179(Suppl 1):S203–S217.
53. Crotty S, Hix L, Sigal LJ, et al. Poliovirus pathogenesis in a new poliovirus receptor transgenic mouse model: age-dependent paralysis and a mucosal route of infection. *J Gen Virol* 2002;83:1707–1720.
54. Danthi P, Guglielmi KM, Kirchner E, et al. From touchdown to transcription: the reovirus cell entry pathway. *Curr Top Microbiol Immunol* 2010;343:91–119.
62. Donnelly CA, Ghani AC, Leung GM. Epidemiological determinants of spread of causal agent of severe acute respiratory syndrome in Hong Kong. *Lancet* 2003;361:1761–1766.
63. Doorbar J. The papillomavirus life cycle. *J Clin Virol* 2005;32:S7–S15.
66. Dubuisson J, Lustig S, Ruggli N, et al. Genetic determinants of Sindbis virus neuroinvasiveness. *J Virol* 1997;71:2636–2646.
69. Endres MJ, Griot C, Gonzalez-Scarano F, et al. Neuroattenuation of an avirulent bunyavirus variant maps to the L RNA segment. *J Virol* 1991;65:5465–5470.
73. Fenner F. Mouse-pox; infectious ectromelia of mice; a review. *J Immunol* 1949;63:341–373.
74. Fenner F. The Florey lecture, 1983: biological control, as exemplified by smallpox eradication and myxomatosis. *Proc R Soc Lond B Biol Sci* 1983;218:259–285.
75. Fenner F, Buller RM. Mousepox. In: Nathanson N, Ahmed R, Gonzalez-Scarano F, et al, eds. *Viral Pathogenesis.* Philadelphia: Lippincott-Raven; 1997:535–553.
76. Fenner F, Poole WE, Marshall ID, et al. Studies in the epidemiology of infectious myxomatosis of rabbits. VI. The experimental introduction of the European strain of myxoma virus into Australian wild rabbit populations. *J Hyg (Lond)* 1957;55:192–206.
77. Fenner F, Woodroofe GM. Changes in virulence and antigenic structure of strains of myoma virus recovered from Australian wild rabbits between 1950 and 1964. *Aust J Exp Biol Med Sci*1965;43:359–370.
79. Friedman HM, Wang L, Fishman NO, et al. Immune evasion properties of herpes simplex virus type 1 glycoprotein gC. *J Virol* 1996;70:4253–4260.
80. Fujinami RS, Oldstone MB. Alterations in expression of measles virus polypeptides by antibody: molecular events in antibody-induced antigenic modulation. *J Immunol* 1980;125:78–85.
82. Fujinami RS, Oldstone MB. Antiviral antibody reacting on the plasma membrane alters measles virus expression inside the cell. *Nature* 1979;279:529–530.
83. Garcia-Sastre A, Egorov A, Matassov D, et al. Influenza A virus lacking the NS1 gene replicates in interferon-deficient systems. *Virology* 1998;252:324–330.
84. Ge D, Fellay J, Thompson AJ, et al. Genetic variation in IL28B predicts hepatitis C treatment-induced viral clearance. *Nature* 2009;461:399–401.
85. Geisbert TW, Hensley LE, Larsen T, et al. Pathogenesis of Ebola hemorrhagic fever in cynomolgus macaques: evidence that dendritic cells are early and sustained targets of infection. *Am J Pathol* 2003;163:2347–2370.
86. Geisbert TW, Young HA, Jahrling PB, et al. Mechanisms underlying coagulation abnormalities in ebola hemorrhagic fever: overexpression of tissue factor in primate monocytes/macrophages is a key event. *J Infect Dis* 2003;188:1618–1629.
87. Geisbert TW, Young HA, Jahrling PB, et al. Pathogenesis of Ebola hemorrhagic fever in primate models: evidence that hemorrhage is not a direct effect of virus-induced cytolysis of endothelial cells. *Am J Pathol* 2003;163:2371–2382.

89. Gibb TR, Bray M, Geisbert TW, et al. Pathogenesis of experimental Ebola Zaire virus infection in BALB/c mice. *J Comp Pathol* 2001;125: 233–242.
90. Glass RI, Parashar UD, Estes MK. Norovirus gastroenteritis. *N Engl J Med* 2009;361:1776–1785.
95. Griffin DE. Immune responses during measles virus infection. *Curr Top Microbiol Immunol* 1995;191:117–134.
96. Griffin DE. Virus-induced immune suppression. In Nathansen N, Ahmed R, Gonzalez-Scarano F, et al, eds. *Viral Pathogenesis.* Philadelphia: Lippincott-Raven; 1997:207–233.
98. Gromeier M, Wimmer E. Mechanism of injury-provoked poliomyelitis. *J Virol* 1998;72:5056–5060.
100. Guidotti LG, Ando K, Hobbs MV, et al. Cytotoxic T lymphocytes inhibit hepatitis B virus gene expression by a non-cytolytic mechanism in transgenic mice. *Proc Natl Acad Sci U S A* 1994;91:3764–3768.
101. Guidotti LG, Borrow P, Brown A, et al. Noncytopathic clearance of lymphocytic choriomeningitis virus from the hepatocyte. *J Exp Med* 1999; 189:1555–1564.
102. Guidotti LG, Guilhot S, Chisari FV. Interleukin-2 and alpha/beta interferon down-regulate hepatitis B virus gene expression in vivo by tumor necrosis factor-dependent and -independent pathways. *J Virol* 1994;68:1265–1270.
103. Guidotti LG, Ishikawa T, Hobbs MV, et al. Intracellular inactivation of the hepatitis B virus by cytotoxic T lymphocytes. *Immunity* 1996;4:25–36.
104. Guidotti LG, Rochford R, Chung J, et al. Viral clearance without destruction of infected cells during acute HBV infection. *Science* 1999; 284:825–829.
105. Gupta M, Mahanty S, Bray M, et al. Passive transfer of antibodies protects immunocompetent and immunodeficient mice against lethal Ebola virus infection without complete inhibition of viral replication. *J Virol* 2001;75:4649–4654.
106. Haase AT. Perils at mucosal front lines for HIV and SIV and their hosts. *Nat Rev Immunol* 2005;5:783–792.
107. Haase AT. Targeting early infection to prevent HIV-1 mucosal transmission. *Nature* 2010;464:217–223.
108. Haller BL, Barkon ML, Li X-Y, et al. Brain and intestine-specific variants of reovirus serotype 3 strain Dearing are selected during chronic infection of severe combined immunodeficient mice. *J Virol* 1995;69:3933–3937.
109. Haller BL, Barkon ML, Vogler G, et al. Genetic mapping of reovirus virulence and organ tropism in severe combined immunodeficient mice: organ specific virulence genes. *J Virol* 1995;69:357–364.
110. Han SH. Extrahepatic manifestations of chronic hepatitis B. *Clin Liver Dis* 2004;8:403–418.
113. Hatziioannou T, Ambrose Z, Chung HP, et al. A macaque model of HIV-1 infection. *Proc Natl Acad Sci U S A* 2009;106:4425–4429.
114. Hayes EB, Komar N, Nasci RS, et al. Epidemiology and transmission dynamics of West Nile Virus disease. *Emerg Infect Dis* 2005;11:1167–1173.
118. Hirsch MS, Allison AC, Harvey JJ. Immune complexes in mice infected neonatally with Moloney leukaemogenic and murine sarcoma viruses. *Nature* 1969;223:739–740.
119. Hohler T, Stradmann-Bellinghausen B, Starke R, et al. C4A deficiency and nonresponse to hepatitis B vaccination. *J Hepatol* 2002;37:387–392.
126. Hutson AM, Atmar RL, Estes MK. Norovirus disease: changing epidemiology and host susceptibility factors. *Trends Microbiol* 2004;12: 279–287.
127. Hutson AM, Atmar RL, Graham DY, et al. Norwalk virus infection and disease is associated with ABO histo-blood group type. *J Infect Dis* 2002;185:1335–1337.
130. Ip WK, Chan KH, Law HK, et al. Mannose-binding lectin in severe acute respiratory syndrome coronavirus infection. *J Infect Dis* 2005;191: 1697–1704.
131. Jackson AC. Rabies. In: Nathanson N, Ahmed R, Gonzalez-Scarano F, et al, eds. *Viral Pathogenesis.* Philadelphia: Lippincott-Raven; 1997: 575–591.
132. Jern P, Coffin JM. Effects of retroviruses on host genome function. *Annu Rev Genet* 2008;42:709–732.
133. Johnson LS, Willert EK, Virgin HW. Redefining the genetics of murine gammaherpesvirus 68 via transcriptome-based annotation. *Cell Host Microbe* 2010;7:516–526.
137. Jopling CL, Yi M, Lancaster AM, et al. Modulation of hepatitis C virus RNA abundance by a liver-specific MicroRNA. *Science* 2005;309: 1577–1581.
138. Kapadia SB, Levine B, Speck SH, et al. Critical role of complement and viral evasion of complement in acute, persistent, and latent gamma-herpesvirus infection. *Immunity* 2002;17:143–155.
139. Katano H, Ali MA, Patera AC, et al. Chronic active Epstein-Barr virus infection associated with mutations in perforin that impair its maturation. *Blood* 2004;103:1244–1252.
146. Kraehenbuhl JP, Corbett M. Immunology. Keeping the gut microflora at bay. *Science* 2004;303:1624–1625.
149. La Monica N, Almond JW, Racaniello VR. A mouse model for poliovirus neurovirulence identifies mutations that attenuate the virus for humans. *J Virol* 1987;61:2917–2920.
150. Labrada L, Liang XH, Zheng W, et al. Age-dependent resistance to lethal alphavirus encephalitis in mice: analysis of gene expression in the central nervous system and identification of a novel interferon-inducible protective gene, mouse ISG12. *J Virol* 2002;76:11688–11703.
151. Lanford RE, Hildebrandt-Eriksen ES, Petri A, et al. Therapeutic silencing of microRNA-122 in primates with chronic hepatitis C virus infection. *Science* 2010;327:198–201.
153. Lawrence DMP, Vaughn MM, Belman AR, et al. Immune response-mediated protection of adult but not neonatal mice from neuron-restricted measles virus infection and central nervous system disease. *J Virol* 1999;73:1795–1801.
154. Lawrence T, Puel A, Reichenbach J, et al. Autosomal-dominant primary immunodeficiencies. *Curr Opin Hematol* 2005;12:22–30.
155. Legrand N, Ploss A, Balling R, et al. Humanized mice for modeling human infectious disease: challenges, progress, and outlook. *Cell Host Microbe* 2009;6:5–9.
156. Leib DA, Machalek MA, Williams BR, et al. Specific phenotypic restoration of an attenuated virus by knockout of a host resistance gene. *Proc Natl Acad Sci U S A* 2000;97:6097–6101.
159. Lennette EH, Koprowski H. Influence of age on the susceptibility of mice to infection with certain neurotropic viruses. *J Immunol* 1944;49: 175–191.
160. Levine B, Hardwick JM, Trapp BD, et al. Antibody-mediated clearance of alphavirus infection from neurons. *Science* 1991;254:856–860.
161. Li W, Zhang C, Sui J, et al. Receptor and viral determinants of SARS-coronavirus adaptation to human ACE2. *EMBO J* 2005;24:1634–1643.
163. Lindesmith L, Moe C, Marionneau S, et al. Human susceptibility and resistance to Norwalk virus infection. *Nat Med* 2003;9:548–553.
165. Loh J, Chu DT, O'Guin AK, et al. Natural killer cells utilize both perforin and gamma interferon to regulate murine cytomegalovirus infection in the spleen and liver. *J Virol* 2005;79:661–667.
166. Loh J, Thomas DA, Revell PA, et al. Granzymes and caspase 3 play important roles in control of gammaherpesvirus latency. *J Virol* 2004;78: 12519–12528.
171. MacDonald GH, Johnston RE. Role of dendritic cell targeting in Venezuelan equine encephalitis virus pathogenesis. *J Virol* 2000;74:914–922.
175. Matloubian M, Kolhekar SR, Somasundaram T, et al. Molecular determinants of macrophage tropism and viral persistence: importance of single amino acid changes in the polymerase and glycoprotein of lymphocytic choriomeningitis virus. *J Virol* 1993;67:7340–7349.
181. Miller SD, Vanderlugt CL, Begolka WS, et al. Persistent infection with Theiler's virus leads to CNS autoimmunity via epitope spreading. *Nat Med* 1997;3:1133–1136.
182. Mims CA, Dimmock N, Nash A, et al, eds. The spread of microbes through the body. In: *Mims' Pathogenesis of Infectious Disease.* San Diego: Academic Press; 1995:106–135.
183. Minor PD. Poliovirus. In: Nathanson N, Ahmed A, Gonzalez-Scarano F, et al, eds. *Viral Pathogenesis.* Philadelphia: Lippincott-Raven; 1997:555–574.
190. Munger K, Howley PM. Human papillomavirus immortalization and transformation functions. *Virus Res* 2002;89:213–228.
191. Nagai Y. Protease-dependent virus tropism and pathogenicity. *Trends Microbiol* 1993;1:81–87.
193. Nakamoto Y, Guidotti LG, Pasquetto V, et al. Differential target cell sensitivity to CTL-activated death pathways in hepatitis B virus transgenic mice. *J Immunol* 1997;158:5692–5697.
194. Naniche D, Oldstone MB. Generalized immunosuppression: how viruses undermine the immune response. *Cell Mol Life Sci* 2000;57:1399–1407.

195. Nathanson N. Introduction and history. In: Nathanson N, Ahmed R, Gonzalez-Scarano F, et al, eds. *Viral Pathogenesis.* Philadelphia: Lippincott-Raven; 1997:3–11.
196. Nathanson N, Ahmed R, Gonzalez-Scarano F, et al, eds. *Viral Pathogenesis.* Philadelphia: Lippincott-Raven; 1997.
197. Nathanson N, Murphy FA. Evolution of viral disease. In: Nathanson N, Ahmed R, Gonzalez-Scarano F, et al, eds. *Viral Pathogenesis.* Philadelphia: Lippincott-Raven; 1997:353–369.
198. Nathanson N, Tyler KL. Entry, dissemination, shedding, and transmission of viruses. In: Nathanson N, Ahmed R, Gonzalez-Scarano F, et al, eds. *Viral Pathogenesis.* Philadelphia: Lippincott-Raven; 1997:13–33.
201. Newell ML, McIntyre J. *Congenital and Perinatal Infections.* Cambridge: Cambridge University Press; 2000.
202. Niess JH, Brand S, Gu X, et al. CX3CR1-mediated dendritic cell access to the intestinal lumen and bacterial clearance. *Science* 2005;307:254–258.
203. Ogata N, Alter HJ, Miller RH, et al. Nucleotide sequence and mutation rate of the H strain of hepatitis C virus. *Proc Natl Acad Sci U S A* 1991;88:3392–3396.
208. Oldstone MB, Blount P, Southern PJ, et al. Cytoimmunotherapy for persistent virus infection reveals a unique clearance pattern from the central nervous system. *Nature* 1986;321:239–243.
210. Oldstone MB, Dixon FJ. Lactic dehydrogenase virus-induced immune complex type of glomerulonephritis. *J Immunol* 1971;106:1260–1263.
211. Oldstone MB, Dixon FJ. Pathogenesis of chronic disease associated with persistent lymphocytic choriomeningitis viral infection. I. Relationship of antibody production to disease in neonatally infected mice. *J Exp Med* 1969;129:483–505.
213. Oliver KR, Scallan MF, Dyson H, et al. Susceptibility to a neurotropic virus and its changing distribution in the developing brain is a function of CNS maturity. *J Neurovirol* 1997;3:38–48.
214. Overbaugh J, Bangham CR. Selection forces and constraints on retroviral sequence variation. *Science* 2001;292:1106–1109.
216. Parren PW, Geisbert TW, Maruyama T, et al. Pre- and postexposure prophylaxis of Ebola virus infection in an animal model by passive transfer of a neutralizing human antibody. *J Virol* 2002;76:6408–6412.
219. Peiris JSM, Yuen KY, Osterhaus ADME, et al. Current concepts: the severe acute respiratory syndrome. *N Engl J Med* 2003;349:2431–2441.
220. Pereira RA, Simon MM, Simmons A. Granzyme A, a noncytolytic component of CD8(+) cell granules, restricts the spread of herpes simplex virus in the peripheral nervous systems of experimentally infected mice. *J Virol* 2000;74:1029–1032.
221. Pereyra F, Jia X, McLaren PJ, et al. The major genetic determinants of HIV-1 control affect HLA class I peptide presentation. *Science* 2010;330:1551–1557.
223. Pfeiffer JK, Kirkegaard K. Increased fidelity reduces poliovirus fitness and virulence under selective pressure in mice. *PLoS Pathog* 2005;1:e11.
225. Phillips RE, Rowland-Jones S, Nixon DF, et al. Human immunodeficiency virus genetic variation that can escape cytotoxic T cell recognition. *Nature* 1991;354:453–459.
226. Picard C, Casanova JL. Novel primary immunodeficiencies. *Adv Exp Med Biol* 2005;568:89–99.
227. Pircher H, Moskophidis D, Rohrer U, et al. Viral escape by selection of cytotoxic T cell-resistant virus variants in vivo. *Nature* 1990;346:629–633.
228. Plaisance-Bonstaff K, Renne R. Viral miRNAs. Methods. *Mol Biol* 2011;721:43–66.
232. Porter DD, Larsen AE, Porter HG. The pathogenesis of Aleutian disease of mink. I. In vivo viral replication and the host antibody response to viral antigen. *J Exp Med* 1969;130:575–593.
234. Racaniello VR. One hundred years of poliovirus pathogenesis. *Virology* 2006;344:9–16.
235. Racaniello VR, Ren R. Poliovirus biology and pathogenesis. *Curr Top Microbiol Immunol* 1996;206:305–325.
236. Rall GF, Manchester M, Daniels LR, et al. A transgenic mouse model for measles virus infection of the brain. *Proc Natl Acad Sci U S A* 1997;94:4659–4663.
237. Ramoz N, Rueda LA, Bouadjar B, et al. Mutations in two adjacent novel genes are associated with epidermodysplasia verruciformis. *Nat Genet* 2002;32:579–581.
241. Ren R, Racaniello VR. Poliovirus spreads from muscle to the central nervous system by neural pathways. *J Infect Dis* 1992;166:747–752.
243. Rima BK, Duprex WP. Molecular mechanisms of measles virus persistence. *Virus Res* 2005;111:132–147.
244. Roberts A, Paddock C, Vogel L, et al. Aged BALB/c mice as a model for increased severity of severe acute respiratory syndrome in elderly humans. *J Virol* 2005;79:5833–5838.
246. Rockx B, Sheahan T, Donaldson E, et al. Synthetic reconstruction of zoonotic and early human severe acute respiratory syndrome coronavirus isolates that produce fatal disease in aged mice. *J Virol* 2007;81:7410–7423.
248. Samson M, Libert F, Doranz BJ, et al. Resistance to HIV-1 infection in caucasian individuals bearing mutant alleles of the CCR-5 chemokine receptor gene. *Nature* 1996;382:722–725.
251. Sciortino MT, Taddeo B, Poon AP, et al. Of the three tegument proteins that package mRNA in herpes simplex virions, one (VP22) transports the mRNA to uninfected cells for expression prior to viral infection. *Proc Natl Acad Sci U S A* 2002;99:8318–8323.
254. Shrestha B, Samuel MA, Diamond MS. CD8+ T cells require perforin to clear West Nile virus from infected neurons. *J Virol* 2006;80:119–129.
255. Shukla D, Spear PG. Herpesviruses and heparan sulfate: an intimate relationship in aid of viral entry. *J Clin Invest* 2001;108:503–510.
256. Sigel MM. Influence of age on suceptibility to virus infection with particular reference to laboratory animals. *Annu Rev Microbiol* 1952;6:247–280.
257. Skalsky RL, Cullen BR. Viruses, microRNAs, and host interactions. *Annu Rev Microbiol* 2010;64:123–141.
262. Sobey WR. Selection for resistance to myxomatosis in domestic rabbits (Oryctolagus cuniculus). *J Hyg (Lond)* 1969;67:743–754.
263. Spear PG. Herpes simplex virus: receptors and ligands for cell entry. *Cell Microbiol* 2004;6:401–410.
264. Speck SH. Regulation of EBV latency-associated gene expression. In: Robertson ES, ed. *Epstein-Barr Virus.* Norfolk, England: Caister Academic Press; 2005:403–427.
268. Stoermer KA, Morrison TE. Complement and viral pathogenesis. *Virology* 2011;411:362–373.
270. Sullivan NJ, Sanchez A, Rollin PE, et al. Development of a preventive vaccine for Ebola virus infection in primates. *Nature* 2000;408:605–609.
281. Teijaro JR, Walsh KB, Cahalan S, et al. Endothelial cells are central orchestrators of cytokine amplification during influenza virus infection. *Cell* 2011;146:980–991.
285. Tscharke DC, Reading PC, Smith GL. Dermal infection with vaccinia virus reveals roles for virus proteins not seen using other inoculation routes. *J Gen Virol* 2002;83:1977–1986.
290. Tyler KL, Mann MA, Fields BN, et al. Protective anti-reovirus monoclonal antibodies and their effects on viral pathogenesis. *J Virol* 1993;67:3446–3453.
292. Tyler KL, Virgin HW, Bassel Duby R, et al. Antibody inhibits defined stages in the pathogenesis of reovirus serotype 3 infection of the central nervous system. *J Exp Med* 1989;170:887–900.
293. Van Berkel V, Levine B, Kapadia SB, et al. Critical role for a high affinity chemokine binding protein in lethal meningitis caused by a g-herpesvirus. *J Clin Invest* 2002;109:905–914.
294. Vanderplasschen A, Mathew E, Hollinshead M, et al. Extracellular enveloped vaccinia virus is resistant to complement because of incorporation of host complement control proteins into its envelope. *Proc Natl Acad Sci U S A* 1998;95:7544–7549.
296. Vignuzzi M, Stone JK, Arnold JJ, et al. Quasispecies diversity determines pathogenesis through cooperative interactions in a viral population. *Nature* 2006;439:344–348.
297. Virgin HW. In vivo veritas: pathogenesis of infection as it actually happens. *Nat Immunol* 2007;8:1143–1147.
298. Virgin HW, Bassel Duby R, Fields BN, et al. Antibody protects against lethal infection with the neurally spreading reovirus type 3 (Dearing). *J Virol* 1988;62:4594–4604.
299. Virgin HW, Mann MA, Tyler KL. Protective antibodies inhibit reovirus internalization and uncoating by intracellular proteases. *J Virol* 1994;68:6719–6729.
300. Virgin HW, Todd J. Metagenomics and personalized medicine. *Cell* 2011;147:44–56.
301. Virgin HW, Walker BD. Immunology and the elusive AIDS vaccine. *Nature* 2010;464:224–231.

302. Virgin HW, Wherry EJ, Ahmed R. Redefining chronic viral infection. *Cell* 2009;138:30–50.
304. Von Herrath MG, Fujinami RS, Whitton JL. Microorganisms and autoimmunity: making the barren field fertile? *Nat Rev Microbiol* 2003;1: 151–157.
306. Wang G, Barrett JW, Nazarian SH, et al. Myxoma virus M11L prevents apoptosis through constitutive interaction with Bak. *J Virol* 2004;78: 7097–7111.
307. Weaver SC, Barrett AD. Transmission cycles, host range, evolution and emergence of arboviral disease. *Nat Rev Microbiol* 2004;2:789–801.
310. White DW, Keppel CR, Schneider SE, et al. Latent herpesvirus infection arms NK cells. *Blood* 2010;115:4377–4383.
311. Whitney JB, Ruprecht RM. Live attenuated HIV vaccines: pitfalls and prospects. *Curr Opin Infect Dis* 2004;17:17–26.
312. Whitton JL, Cornell CT, Feuer R. Host and virus determinants of picornavirus pathogenesis and tropism. *Nat Rev Microbiol* 2005;3: 765–776.
313. Whitton JL, Feuer R. Myocarditis, microbes and autoimmunity. *Autoimmunity* 2004;37:375–386.
314. Wieland S, Thimme R, Purcell RH, et al. Genomic analysis of the host response to hepatitis B virus infection. *Proc Natl Acad Sci U S A* 2004; 101:6669–6674.
315. Wieland SF, Chisari FV. Stealth and cunning: hepatitis B and hepatitis C viruses. *J Virol* 2005;79:9369–9380.
316. Wieland SF, Spangenberg HC, Thimme R, et al. Expansion and contraction of the hepatitis B virus transcriptional template in infected chimpanzees. *Proc Natl Acad Sci U S A* 2004;101:2129–2134.
319. Xu L, Sanchez A, Yang Z, et al. Immunization for Ebola virus infection. *Nat Med* 1998;4:37–42.
320. Yuan FF, Tanner J, Chan PKS, et al. Influence of Fc gamma RIIA and MBL polymorphisms on severe acute respiratory syndrome. *Tissue Antigens* 2005;66:291–296.
323. Zinkernagel RM. Virus-induced immunopathology. In: Nathanson N, Ahmed R, Gonzalez-Scarano F, et al, eds. *Viral Pathogenesis.* Philadelphia: Lippincott-Raven; 1997:163–181.
324. Zinkernagel RM, Hengartner H. Virally induced immunosuppression. *Curr Opin Immunol* 1992;4:408–412.
325. Zinkernagel RM, Pfau CJ, Hengartner H, et al. Susceptibility to murine lymphocytic choriomeningitis maps to class I MHC genes—a model for MHC/disease associations. *Nature* 1985;316:814–817.
326. Nguyen L, Knipe DM, Finberg RW. Mechanism of virus-induced Ig subclass shifts. *J Immunol* 1994;152(2):478–484
327. Ahmed R, Morrison LA, Knipe DM. Persistence of viruses. In: Fields BN, Knipe DM, Howley PM, eds. *Virology.* 3rd ed. Philadelphia: Lippincott-Raven; 1996:219–249.
328. Kurt-Jones EA, Chan M, Zhou S, et al. Herpes simplex virus 1 interaction with toll-like receptor 2 contributes to lethal encephalitis. *Proc Natl Acad Sci U S A* 2004;101(5):1315–1320.

CHAPTER 11

Edward C. Holmes

Virus Evolution

Although Charles Darwin preempted many of the great questions in evolutionary biology, he wrote little about viral infections. Of course, viruses were not formally identified until a full decade after Darwin's death, and, aside from some brief discussion of the origins of yellow fever, his writings make scant reference to what we now know are diseases caused by viruses. This is a great historical shame because it seems certain that Darwin would have held viruses up as some of the best exemplars of evolution by natural selection, and in the case of RNA viruses the evolutionary process is so rapid that it can be effectively followed in "real time".[123,204]

Although evolutionary analysis arrived relatively late in the science of virology, the study of virus evolution has become one of the most rapidly growing and successful aspects of modern microbiology. The blossoming of evolutionary virology is largely due to two developments. First, viruses, and especially those that possess RNA genomes, have become remarkably powerful research tools for the study of evolutionary processes. The utility of RNA viruses in this respect is a function of the fact that they evolve extremely rapidly, are easy to manipulate *in vitro* and sometimes *in vivo,* often have large and measurable effects on phenotype, and possess such small genomes that the mutations associated with any phenotype change can be determined relatively easily.[60] It is therefore no surprise that a growing number of evolutionary researchers are turning to viruses as model systems. For example, studies of viruses represent one of the few cases in which biologists have been able to achieve two of the great aims of modern evolutionary genetics: to measure the fitness effects of individual mutations[195] and to determine the nature of the epistatic interactions between these mutations.[197] Second, the rapidity of RNA virus evolution has acted as a direct stimulus for the development of phylogenetic and coalescent methods that are able to incorporate information on the exact time of sampling of the sequences in question, in turn revolutionizing molecular epidemiology.[49,132] Indeed, many of the computer programs designed for the evolutionary analysis of gene sequence data were first applied to viruses, such that determining the origin and pathways of spread of specific viruses over epidemiologic time has become a relatively exact science with a myriad of potential applications. The advent of next-generation sequencing promises even more rapid advances in this area, potentially enabling the analysis of many thousands of sequences with detailed associated metadata.[95] An important spinoff from these studies has been new insights into the patterns and processes of virus evolution.[79,92] In sum, although their focus is very different, the combination of experimental analyses of model viruses as a means to understand the intricacies of the evolutionary process and studies of molecular epidemiology based on the comparative analysis of virus gene sequence data to document patterns of virus spread has told us a great deal about the nature of virus evolution. Evolutionary virology has blossomed into a well-developed science.

Despite advances on multiple fronts, some fundamental aspects of viral evolution remain unknown, contentious, or both, which will be highlighted in this chapter. For example, there are still major debates over some of the key mechanisms of evolutionary change in RNA viruses, particularly whether their populations routinely form quasispecies, which reflects a wider uncertainty on the roles of mutation, natural selection, and genetic drift as forces of evolutionary change.[92] For example, it is striking that precise estimates of mutation rates are absent from some important groups of viruses even though they represent a sort of "ground zero" in studies of evolutionary change. Similarly, although we know a great deal more about the origin of viruses than we did 10 years ago, particularly since the discovery and analysis of highly conserved protein structures, exactly when and how viruses first evolved, whether this occurred before or after the appearance of the first cellular organisms, what a precellular world might have looked like, and even if viruses should be classified as living are sources of major debate.[71,121,138,159] In part, this debate highlights our profound ignorance of the virosphere. For example, does the apparent absence of RNA viruses in *Archaea* mean that they never existed in these species, that they have been selectively removed, or that we have simply not looked hard enough? Another important issue is that in some respects our knowledge of DNA virus evolution lags behind what we know of the evolution of RNA viruses. We remain ignorant of a number of key aspects of the patterns and processes of DNA virus evolution, particularly whether common principles can be applied to DNA viruses that differ so greatly in size and genome structure. It is hoped that the rise of metagenomics, such that we will sample far more of the virosphere, likely leading to the discovery of a multitude of diverse viruses, will stimulate many advances in this area. Finally, the time scale of evolutionary history in many viruses is unclear, with very different inferences drawn from either the study of endogenous viruses, which are usually indicative of ancient origins, or the molecular clock analysis of recently sampled and often rapidly evolving viral genomes, which usually paints a picture of very recent origins.[80,94] Advances in this area may require the development of a new class of analytical methods.

Aside from their ability to inform on evolutionary processes, there are a number of practical reasons that the study of virus evolution deserves attention. It is likely that a better understanding of the exact processes of evolutionary change in viruses will assist in the development of improved strategies for their treatment and control and for predicting the spread of newly emerged pathogens. For example, knowing whether natural selection or genetic drift largely controls how mutations spread through a population is essential to understanding the likelihood and rate that a specific drug resistance mutation will become established,[131] while a knowledge of the factors that control how viruses diffuse at the epidemiologic scale represents useful information for any emergent virus.[95] Similarly, it is likely that a better understanding of the origin of viruses will be essential to obtaining a more precise picture of the earliest events in the early history of life on earth, including the genesis of both RNA and DNA, as it seems reasonable to suppose that some of the earliest replicators resemble what we now know as viruses.

The future of evolutionary virology appears strong. The development and continued refinement of next-generation sequencing methods will doubtless provide unprecedented amounts of data for evolutionary study and stimulate the development of new analytical methods for use in all genetic systems. Innovations in experimental studies of virus evolution will continue, addressing ever more intricate questions, increasingly considering *in vivo* systems, and providing broad-scale evolutionary insights. Metagenomic studies of the virosphere will provide a powerful new perspective on virus biodiversity, in turn bringing important new information on virus ecology, origins, and cross-species transmission and emergence. It therefore seems easy to predict that our understanding of viral evolution 10 years from now will be very different, and more complete, than it is today.

THE ORIGIN AND TIME SCALE OF VIRUS EVOLUTION

The Origins of Viruses

Of all topics in the study of virus evolution, determining exactly how and when viruses first evolved is perhaps the most difficult. The main hindrance to progress in this area is that viruses likely originated so long ago, and perhaps even before the first cellular species, that the signal of ancient evolutionary history that can be recovered through phylogenetic analysis has largely been eroded. This is particularly true for RNA viruses where rapid rates of evolutionary change ensure that the phylogenetic signal is quickly lost. Accordingly, each individual amino acid and nucleotide site in a viral genome has accumulated so many substitutions since its origin that accurate phylogenetic inference becomes an impossible task. For this reason sequence-based phylogenies have proven to be blunt tools for the study of viral origins, although signs of common ancestry may still reside in aspects of protein structure.

Despite the inherent limitations to understanding viral origins, a number of important theories have been proposed for the genesis of both RNA and DNA viruses, which continue to be debated to this day. Currently two such theories dominate discussions in this area; first, that viruses have a precellular origin, such that they are billions of years old, and may have even contributed to some of the fundamental architecture of the first cells; second, that viruses evolved after the first cellular organisms as "escaped genes" that acquired capsid proteins and the ability to replicate autonomously (Fig. 11.1). Although a third hypothesis—that viruses are regressed copies of cellular species that have shed those genes whose functions are provided by the host—has also been proposed, most notably in the case of the giant mimivirus and megavirus of amoeba,[9,128] it does appear to be of general applicability. For example, the gene contents of RNA viruses and cellular species have almost no overlap, whereas under the regressive theory virus genes should have their ancestries in cellular genomes. In addition, although often discussed as such, these theories of viral origins are not mutually exclusive, and it is plausible that while some viruses predate the appearance of the first cells, others appeared more recently.

For many years the escaped gene theory dominated discussions on virus origins.[160] Support for this theory was often based on the idea that as viruses are obligate parasites of host cells now, they must have always been so in the past, such that cells must have evolved before viruses. However, this idea is easy to refute. Because it is commonly thought that the first replicating molecules resided in an "RNA world" that existed before the evolution of DNA, it is easy to believe that modern RNA viruses originated from such ancient self-replicating RNA molecules and parasitized cells at a later date. Important recent evidence for the existence of an RNA world was the demonstration that ribonucleotides could be synthesized *de novo* under conditions that might replicate those of early earth.[179] In most cases the escaped gene theory was also taken to mean that viruses could have escaped from host cells on multiple occasions. This is an attractive idea given the huge phenotypic diversity seen in viruses and that there is no one gene that characterizes all viruses. For example, an early idea was that eukaryotic viruses had escaped from eukaryotic cells, while bacteriophages had escaped from bacterial cells.[180] Similarly, it is possible that RNA, DNA, and perhaps retroviruses represent independent episodes of host gene escape, as could the single- (ss) and double-stranded (ds) versions of RNA and DNA viruses, particularly as small ssDNA and large dsDNA viruses clearly have little in common.

However many different origins are postulated, the same general mechanisms are thought to have occurred: that a host

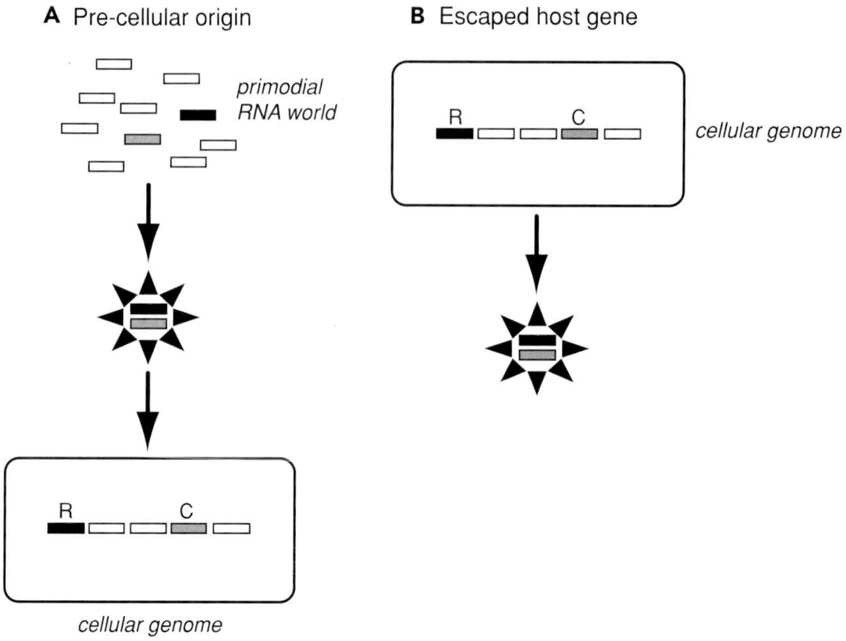

FIGURE 11.1. Schematic representation of two competing models for the origin of viruses. A: The precellular origin theory (in this case depicting the origin of RNA viruses). **B:** The escaped gene theory. Cellular genomes are represented by rounded rectangles, and the simplest model virus is shown here to comprise replicase (R) and capsid (C) genes only. (From Holmes EC. *The Evolution and Emergence of RNA Viruses.* Oxford: Oxford University Press, 2009, by permission of Oxford University Press.)

gene that possessed or acquired the ability to self-replicate escaped from the cell, acquiring a protein coat on the way, eventually evolving into an autonomously replicating entity. For example, single-strand positive-sense RNA (ssRNA+) viruses might be descended from escaped cellular messenger RNA (mRNA) molecules that either possessed or evolved RNA polymerase activity, while DNA viruses could be descended from DNA transposable elements or bacterial plasmids. It is also the case that all forms of the escaped gene theory make two important predictions: first, that most virus genes, including the capsid and replicase proteins, ultimately have their ancestries in cellular genomes, and second, because escape events could have occurred multiple times, viruses do not have a single (i.e., monophyletic) origin. In other words, there is no single phylogeny linking all types of virus, as is easily argued from the huge diversity of viruses described today. In theory, both of these predictions are testable, although in practice this is greatly inhibited by the enormous sequence divergence among viruses.

A number of pieces of data have been used to support the idea that viruses had multiple origins after the appearance of cells. At the level of primary amino acid sequence, there is no robust sequence-based phylogeny for either RNA or DNA viruses, nor any gene that contains statistically significant sequence similarity at such vast evolutionary distances. Although there have been attempts to infer the evolutionary history of RNA viruses based on phylogenetic analyses of the RNA-dependent RNA polymerase (RdRp), the phylogenies in question are highly uncertain at the interfamily level where there is often no more sequence similarity than expected by chance alone.[92,236] However, lack of phylogenetic resolution is not the same thing as an absence of common ancestry, and it is more likely that the inability to accurately infer the evolutionary history of all RNA viruses simply reflects extreme levels of sequence divergence. Indeed, it is striking that the RdRp sequences assigned to different RNA virus families still share a number of short, signature, amino acid motifs (such as a highly conserved GDD motif), some of which are also found in the reverse transcriptase (RT) protein used by retroviruses.[81,120] Such conservation, albeit fragmentary, suggests that these replicatory proteins are distantly related. Unfortunately, these motifs are too short to allow the inference of reliable phylogenetic trees. Even more notable is that recent analyses of protein structure have revealed strong similarities between viruses that exhibit no primary sequence similarity, including between RNA and DNA viruses (see later).

In the case of RNA viruses, early phylogenetic analyses of RdRp sequences combined with information on gene order and content were used to construct *supergroup* classification schemes encompassing multiple viral families. For example, one such study suggested that RNA viruses be classified into the alpha-like, carmo-like, corona-like, flavi-like, picorna-like, and sobemo-like supergroups, each of which is characterized by a conserved gene order, distinctive 5′ and 3′ genome structures, as well as a putative clustering in RdRp phylogenies.[81] However, as noted earlier, extreme sequence divergence means that these RdRp phylogenies are of debatable validity,[236] and it is difficult to construct trees on gene order and content when these differ so dramatically among viral families and in genomes as small as those of RNA viruses. As a consequence, these deep interfamily phylogenies have in reality told us little about virus origins. However, a number of higher-order viral groupings, usually referred to as *orders,* do receive strong phylogenetic support, such that some aspects of the early evolutionary history of RNA viruses can be resolved. These groupings are (a) the *Mononegavirales,* which comprises four families of unsegmented ssRNA− viruses—the *Bornaviridae, Filoviridae, Paramyxoviridae,* and *Rhabdoviridae* (and the *Mononegavirales* clearly cluster together in RdRp trees); (b) the *Nidovirales,* comprising the *Arteriviridae, Coronaviridae,* and *Roniviridae* families of ssRNA+ viruses; and (c) the *Picornavirales,* comprising the *Picornaviridae, Comoviridae, Dicistroviridae, Marnaviridae,* and *Sequiviridae* families of ssRNA+ viruses.

Interfamily phylogenetic analyses of DNA viruses have generally proven more successful, in large part because the reliance on high-fidelity DNA polymerases for replication means that dsDNA viruses exhibit lower rates of nucleotide substitution and hence preserve the phylogenetic signal for longer time periods. For example, a number of families of large dsDNA viruses (i.e., those with genomes greater than 100 kb) clearly possess common ancestry such that they can be classified as nucleocytoplasmic large DNA viruses (NCLDVs), comprising ascoviruses, asfarviruses, iridoviruses, phycodnaviruses, and poxviruses.[104] More recent analyses extended the NCLDV group to include the giant amoebal mimivirus, which is most closely related to the phycodnaviruses,[105] as well as the recently described Marseillevirus, which was isolated from the same amoebal host as mimivirus.[235] In other DNA viruses elements of capsid protein structure have been used to link herpesviruses with tailed bacteriophages,[149] while there are clear evolutionary links between the *Papillomaviridae* and *Polyomaviridae* families of small dsDNA viruses.[232] However, there is no phylogeny that encompasses both single- and double-stranded DNA viruses, which again reflects the great divergence between these very different types of virus (which differ massively in genome size) that share no genes in common. More starkly, it is even difficult to infer phylogenetic trees that link all the large dsDNA viruses that infect eukaryotes.[105]

The second prediction of the escaped gene theory—that most virus proteins ultimately have a host origin—is equally difficult to resolve. The two most important proteins in this respect, as they essentially define viruses, are the polymerase (a defining feature of all RNA viruses that carry an RdRp or RT) and those that make up the capsid (a defining feature of viruses). The case of the DNA polymerases used by DNA viruses is the easiest to discuss in this context as these enzymes are of the same form, and hence ancestry, as those used by cellular species (i.e., they are classified within the same polymerase families), and small DNA viruses utilize the host DNA polymerases for replication. However, while it is clear that these host and virus DNA polymerases are related,[65,103] the position of the root, and therefore the direction of evolutionary change, in phylogenetic trees of DNA polymerases is uncertain. Hence, it is difficult to determine whether DNA polymerases are ultimately of host or viral origin,[200] particularly as DNA polymerases may also have been involved in ancient lateral gene transfer events.[65]

A similar discussion can be mounted in the case of reverse transcriptase. Proteins that function as reverse transcriptase are a common component of cellular genomes in the form of telomerase, the group II (self-replicating) introns observed in a variety of bacterial species, not to mention the abundant retroelements found in many cellular species, as well as a variety of other genetic elements. Importantly, there are recognizable sequence similarities between the RTs of viruses and those that reside in host genomes such that it is possible to infer phylogenetic trees containing both.[32,54] These trees have revealed a number of interesting features, including a major division between the long terminal repeat (LTR) and non-LTR retrotransposons, with retroviruses most closely related to the LTR retrotransposons, and that hepadnaviruses and caulimoviruses (small dsDNA viruses that utilize RT) have independent origins and are probably from LTR retrotransposons. However, as with the case of the DNA polymerases, the lack of an outgroup makes the rooting of these phylogenies uncertain, so whether viral RT genes preceded those present in cells or vice versa is difficult to determine.[55]

The situation is far more complex when it comes to the origin of the RdRp used by RNA viruses. Although the cells of some eukaryotic species contain proteins that function as RdRps, particularly those involved in the production of microRNAs, these exhibit little similarity with the RdRps encoded by viruses, even at the structural level.[106] Similarly, cellular DNA polymerase (Pol) II, which catalyzes the synthesis of RNA from DNA, possesses RdRp activity[130] yet shares little similarity with the RdRp utilized by RNA viruses, such that their evolutionary origins are currently impossible to resolve. Clearly, determining the evolutionary relationships among these highly diverse polymerase proteins represents a major technical challenge.

While the evidence from phylogenetic trees is ambiguous at best, other pieces of data do provide some support for the escaped gene theory. The most compelling of these is that there is at least one example of a virus whose origins likely lie with a host cellular protein, demonstrating that this mode of viral genesis is possible. The case in point involves hepatitis delta virus (HDV) agent, the ribozyme of which is related to the CPEB3 ribozyme found in a human intron sequence.[192] That HDV is only found in humans and requires hepatitis B virus (HBV) for replication strongly suggests that its origins lie with the human genome.[192]

There has also been considerable debate over the significance of the giant amoebal mimivirus for theories of viral origins and evolution. Although phylogenetic analysis has shown that a small proportion (less than 1%) of mimivirus genes are of host origin, which has been used as support for the idea that viruses are "gene pickpockets" that originated after cellular species,[158,159] at least 25% of the approximately 1,000 genes in mimivirus clearly link it to the NCLDV group of large DNA viruses,[105] while an even larger set of genes (~70% at the time of writing) have no known homologs, in either viral or cellular genomes, such that they can be regarded as orphans.[64]

Finally, it is striking that, at the time of writing, no RNA viruses have been discovered in *Archaea*. This could mean that either RNA viruses arose as escaped genes after the divergence of *Archaea* from other cellular species or that temperature constraints have led to a major reduction in the frequency of RNA viruses in hyperthermophilic *Archaea*,[237] although this does not explain their absence in nonthermophiles. An alternative, and perhaps more likely, explanation is that RNA viruses do exist in *Archaea* but have simply not been detected as yet.

The competing theory for the origin of viruses, and one that is growing in popularity, is that they originated before the last universal cellular ancestor (LUCA) and represent the modern descendants of the earliest time in earth's history. Hence, modern RNA viruses would be descendants of replicating elements from the RNA world, while DNA viruses would be remnants of the first DNA replicators, and retroviruses perhaps descendants of the first molecules that made the transition from RNA to DNA. For example, because they lack protein-coding regions, possess ribozyme activity, exhibit complex secondary structures, and mutate very rapidly, viroids are potential candidates for extant descendants of the RNA world.[59] However, although the earliest RNA replicators may share some features with contemporary viroids, because viroids are only seen in plants and likely replicate with the assistance of host cellular

DNA Pol II makes it more likely that they represent escaped host genes or introns that never acquired protein coats.

There are a number of theories for what the pre-LUCA world may have looked like, although all reasonably assume that this precellular stage of evolutionary history contained genetic elements less complex than the viruses we see today. One theory is that there was an *ancient virus world* of primordial replicators that existed before any cellular organisms and that both RNA (first) and DNA (later) viruses originated at this time.[121] A version of this view of virus origins is shown in Figure 11.2. These ancient "viruses" may even have provided some of the features that characterized the first cellular organisms. For example, it has been proposed that the eukaryotic cell nucleus is derived from a virus envelope (the so-called viral eukaryogenesis hypothesis).[13] An alternative theory for the pre-LUCA world is that RNA cells existed before the LUCA, that RNA viruses parasitized these hypothetical RNA cells, and that DNA evolved later as a way of escaping host cell responses.[70] Although fascinating, such theories are unfortunately extremely difficult to test.

As sequence-based phylogenetic trees cannot provide insights into the pre-LUCA world, the main evidence for the precellular theory of virus origins is the presence of conserved genes, and more notably protein structures, among divergent viruses. In fact, arguably one of the most important advances in viral evolution in recent years has been the discovery of protein structures that are conserved among diverse viruses that possess little, if any, primary sequence similarity.[11] For example, a conserved palm subdomain protein structure, consisting of a four-stranded antiparallel β-sheet and two α-helices, is found in both RNA-dependent and DNA-dependent polymerases.[84] A more important case in point concerns the jelly-roll capsid, a tightly structured protein barrel that forms the major capsid subunit of virions with an icosahedral structure. Remarkably, the jelly-roll capsid is found in the virions of both RNA and DNA viruses, including such diverse groups as herpesviruses (dsDNA), picornaviruses (ssRNA+), and birnaviruses (dsRNA).[11,41] Such conservation is strongly suggestive of an ancient common ancestry. Other highly conserved capsid architectures that strongly argue for ancient origins include the PRD1-adenovirus lineage, which is characterized by a double β-barrel fold and found in dsDNA viruses as diverse as bacteriophage PRD1, human adenovirus, and a variety of archaean viruses; the BTV-like lineage, which is found in some dsRNA viruses including members of the *Reoviridae* and *Totiviridae;* and the HK97-like lineage, which encompasses tailed dsDNA viruses that infect archaea, bacteria, and eukaryotes.[16,17,124] Finally, a common virion architecture has been proposed for some viruses that do not possess an icosahedral capsid, including the archaean virus *Halorubrum* pleomorphic virus type 1 (HRPV-1).[176]

Although such structural conservation seems to provide a compelling argument for the antiquity of viruses, it has been proposed that any similarities in protein structure could have arisen more recently due to either strong convergent evolution or lateral gene transfer.[159] While it is theoretically possible that convergent evolution may occur relatively frequently in viral capsid proteins that may be subject to strong selection to be small and perhaps of a specific shape, such large-scale convergence seems highly unlikely given that the similarity in capsid structure covers a huge range of viral taxa. As a consequence, multiple convergent events need to be invoked from very different starting points, and the more convergent evolution that is required, the less likely it becomes. Frequent lateral gene transfer also seems unlikely. As noted later, current data suggest that lateral gene transfer is relatively rare in RNA viruses (although commonplace in large DNA viruses), in large part because of major selective pressures against the expansion of genome sizes.[92] As the earliest replicating RNAs likely possessed higher error rates than those of contemporary RNA viruses, the first genomes would have been even more restricted in size, such that lateral gene transfer without exact gene replacement must also have been uncommon at this time. Hence, although DNA viruses may be habitual gene pickpockets, RNA viruses do not seem to be. In conclusion, while not conclusive, the presence of structural similarities among highly divergent viruses currently constitutes the strongest evidence that viruses have a precellular origin.

The Time Scale of Virus Evolution

As our understanding of viral origins is vague, so is our knowledge of the antiquity of those families of viruses that circulate today, in part because viruses lack any sort of fossil record. In general, there are three ways in which the evolutionary history of viruses can be placed on a chronological scale. First, if there is a strong match between the phylogenetic tree of viruses and that of their hosts, such that they have *co-diverged,* then it is possible to use the divergence times of hosts to calibrate the time scale of virus evolution. Second, for viruses that evolve rapidly such that there is *measurable evolution* (i.e., mutations are fixed in viral populations during the time frame of human observation), which has been clearly demonstrated in both RNA viruses and ssDNA viruses, it is possible to determine the number of substitutions that have occurred between viruses sampled at known times (heterochronous samples) and use this information to calibrate the time scale of virus evolution under the assumption of a molecular clock (i.e., that there is an approximately constant rate of nucleotide or amino acid fixation). Third, for viruses where endogenous genome copies are present in the host, it is possible to use the substitution rate of the host to determine when these genome integration events occurred, especially if the endogenous sequences also co-diverge with their host species. All three approaches have limitations and can lead to wildly different interpretations of evolutionary time scales, the resolution of which has yet to be achieved.

Dating the time scale of virus evolution through the use of host divergence times (i.e., co-divergence) is perhaps the simplest and most robust approach to this form of molecular archaeology. This approach has been particularly successful in the study of DNA virus evolution. Good examples of its utility are the dating of herpesvirus evolution through an examination of the phylogenetic relationships of their vertebrate hosts, in which virus–host co-divergence may extend to some 400 million years[148,149]; of the animal iridoviruses[107]; of the baculoviruses of insects[90]; and of the papillomaviruses sampled from a number of vertebrates including humans.[19] Clearly, although each of these virus families can be considered as "ancient," they are in no way of sufficient age to inform on the question of virus origins. In addition, in some other large DNA viruses, with the poxviruses a good example, frequent host-jumping means that patterns of host–virus co-divergence can be difficult to infer,

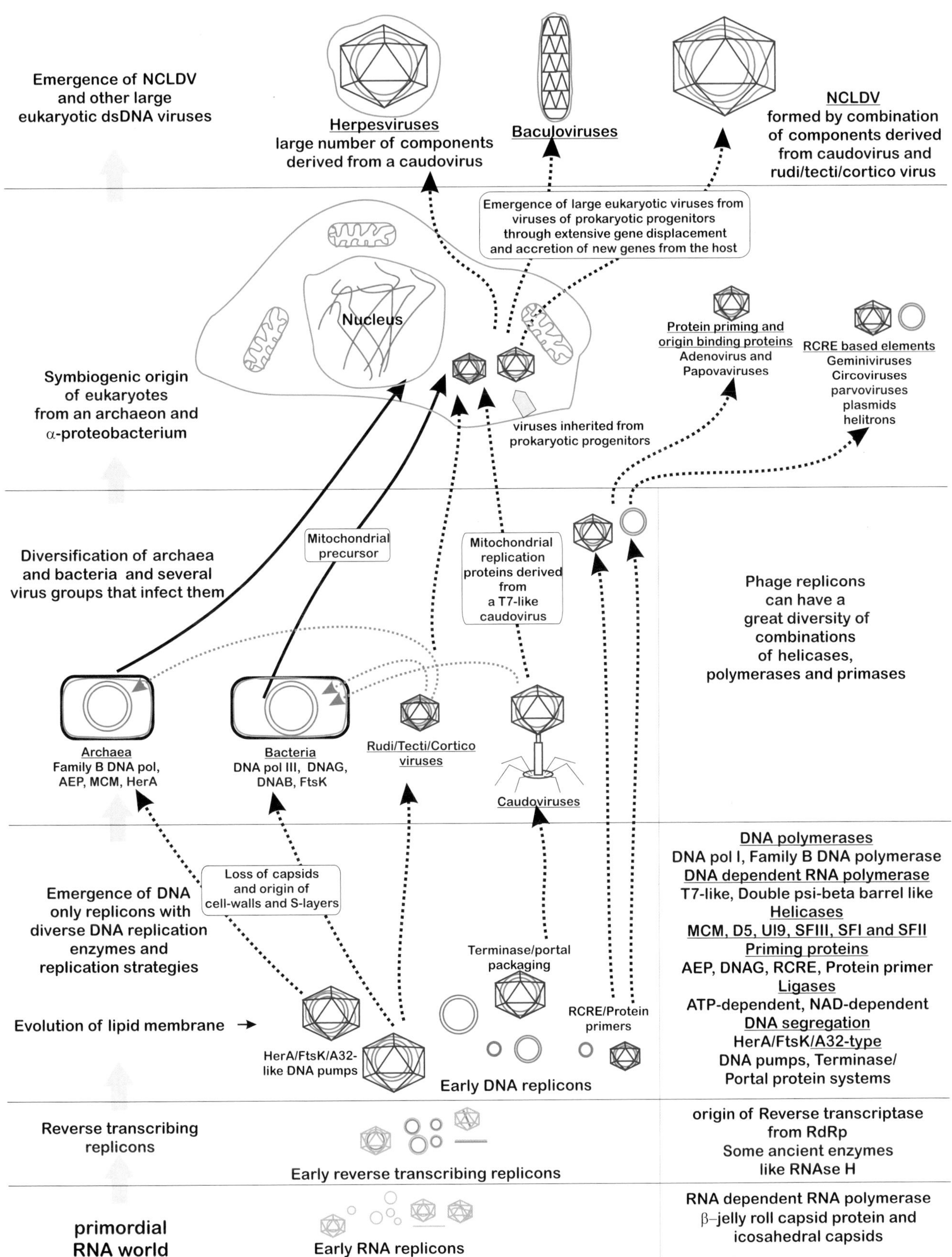

FIGURE 11.2. A plausible scenario for the origin of viruses. Major evolutionary transitions are shown on the **left** of the figure, while the innovations that occurred at each of these transitions are listed on the **right.** Colors are as follows: blue, RNA genomes; red, DNA genomes; green, lipid membranes. (Reprinted from Iyer LM, Balaji S, Koonin EV, et al. Evolutionary genomics of nucleo-cytoplasmic large DNA viruses. *Virus Res* 2006;117:156–184, with permission from Elsevier. Figure kindly provided by Eugene Koonin.)

so that the times of origin of key human pathogens like variola virus (VARV; the agent of smallpox) are still the source of considerable debate.[102,135,206]

Virus–host co-divergence has also been used to date the origin of a number of RNA viruses and retroviruses, although these estimates have sometimes proven controversial. Perhaps the most compelling case to date concerns the retrovirus simian foamy virus (SFV), where a statistically significant match between the phylogenetic trees of host and virus may extend to at least 30 million years[137,217] (Fig. 11.3), and where the analysis of endogenous foamy viruses places their evolutionary history in mammals to over 100 million years.[114]

While *bona fide* examples of virus–host co-divergence constitute a powerful way to date the age of specific viruses, it is also the case that co-divergence is sometimes claimed without any associated statistical test, especially when a small number of taxa are involved such that any resemblance between host and virus phylogeny could occur by chance alone. Given that

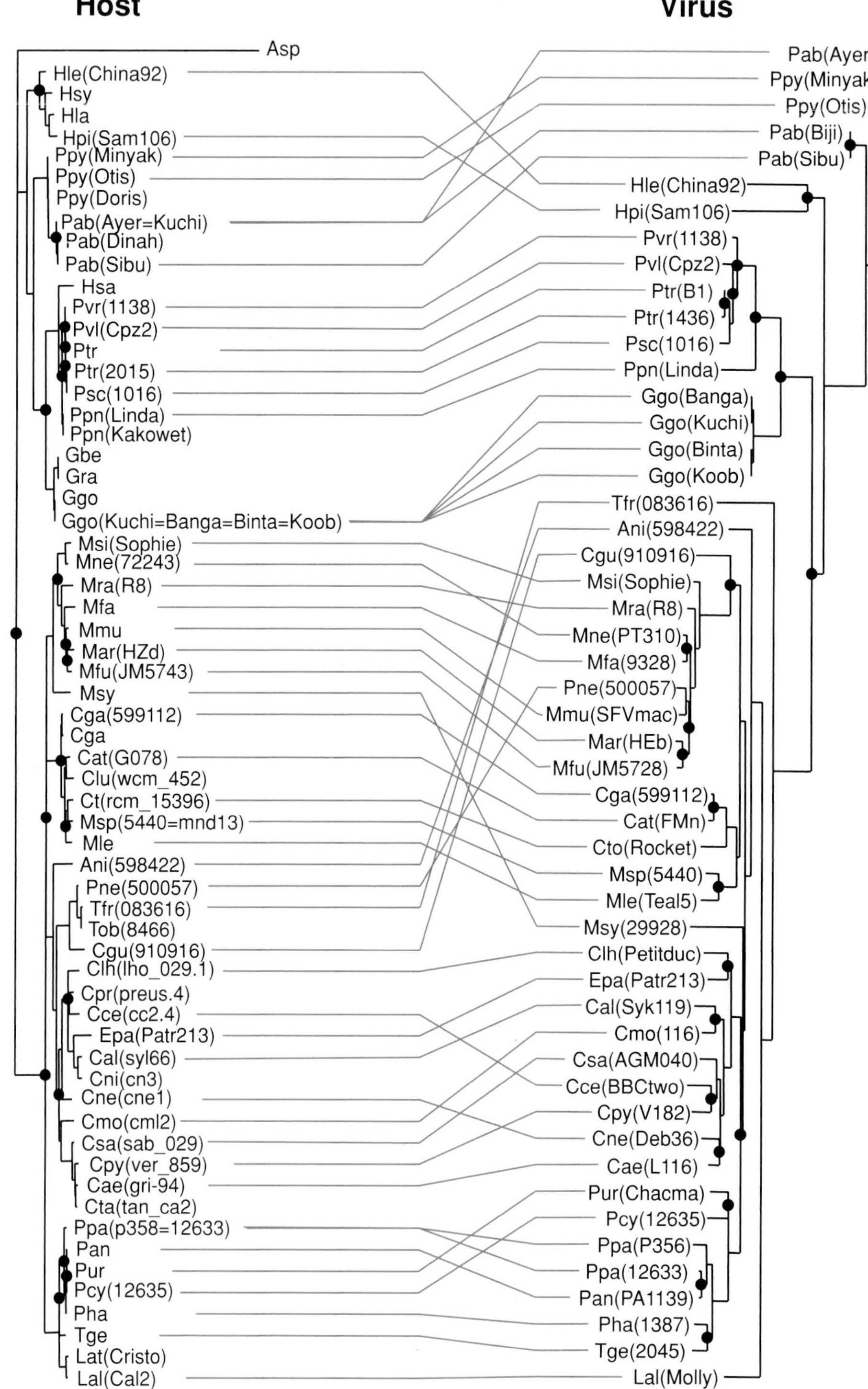

FIGURE 11.3. Long-term co-divergence between simian foamy virus (SFV) and its primate hosts. The tree on the **left** comprises 55 primate species and was inferred using mitochondrial COII sequences. The tree on the **right** contains 44 SFV sequences and was inferred using the viral *pol* gene. Strong host–virus associations are shown as horizontal lines, while incongruent relationships (i.e., host jumps) are shown as crossed lines (note that some hosts have no SFV associated with them). Host–virus co-divergence events are depicted by solid circles at the nodes. The match between the host and virus trees is far stronger than expected by chance ($p = 0.007$). Branch lengths are drawn to scale of nucleotide substitutions per site. (From Switzer WM, Salemi M, Shanmugam V, et al. Ancient co-speciation of simian foamy viruses and primates. *Nature* 2005;434:376–380; reprinted by permission from Macmillan Publishers Ltd.)

cross-species transmission is a very common mode of virus macroevolution, it can be dangerous to construct a time scale of virus evolution without statistically significant co-divergence. In addition, there are a number of other evolutionary processes that can lead to a match between host and virus phylogenies that do not entail co-divergence. For example, it could be that cross-species transmission occurs more often among closely related host species.[215] This *preferential host switching*[36] may produce phylogenetic patterns that are difficult to distinguish from those of co-divergence. A good example is provided by the primate lentiviruses that infect humans (human immunodeficiency virus [HIV]), chimpanzees (simian immunodeficiency virus [SIV] cpz), and gorillas (SIVgor). That these three viruses are very closely related and infect related hosts might at face value be taken to mean that host and virus have co-diverged for several million years. However, closer inspection of the relevant virus phylogenies revealed that the genetic diversity in each case was in fact due to more recent cross-species transmission. Indeed, cross-species transmission involving very closely related host species appears to be common in viruses.[119]

Using heterochronous samples to calibrate the virus molecular clock is an extremely powerful and increasingly popular way to study the time scale of virus evolution in the recent past and is the most common method used with RNA viruses where measurable sequence evolution is a routine observation. However, it is also an approach where erroneous conclusions can be drawn if not performed with care. Because large numbers of gene sequences where the precise date of sampling is known are now available, and because virus evolution is often relatively clock-like, it is a straightforward exercise to date the age of samples of genetic diversity.[49] In some cases divergence times estimated in this manner can be very accurate. For example, an analysis of heterochronous samples of human influenza A virus was able to accurately reconstruct the seasonal peaks and troughs in the population size of this virus.[184] However, while these molecular clock approaches can work well for recent virus evolution—that is, for time scales covering that last few hundred years—they are prone to error at far deeper divergence times, providing a picture of virus evolution that is far too recent. An illustrative example of this effect is provided by the case of the SIVs. While molecular clock studies of SIV evolution using heterochronous samples place this on a time scale of hundreds of years, a calibration based on the biogeographic separation of Bioko Island from the coast of West Africa gave dates of at least 32,000, and perhaps over 100,000 years.[233] More generally, there are cases in the literature where sensible preconception says that a specific virus should be a certain age, usually because it is thought to have diverged with a particular host species or is associated with a particular event in human history, yet molecular clock studies present a far more recent depiction of its origin.[91]

More difficult to explain is precisely why recently calibrated molecular clocks fail so badly in the estimation of ancient divergent times. The most likely explanation is that the statistical models used to estimate the number of nucleotide substitutions separating any two sequences fail to adequately account for all the details of virus evolution, thereby greatly underestimating the true numbers of mutations that have accumulated.[91,94] In short, there has been excessive site saturation that leads to erroneous estimates of divergence times. At present there is no clear way to resolve this problem, although a likely path for the future is the development of more sophisticated models of nucleotide and amino acid substitution.

The final, and most recently developed, way to infer the time scale of virus evolution involves the use of endogenous viral sequences that are a common component of eukaryotic genomes. Endogenous genomic copies of exogenous viruses that have entered the germline are particularly commonplace in retroviruses, and it is estimated that approximately 5% to 8% of the human genome is composed of endogenous retrovirus, comprising at least 31 distinct families.[115] In addition, there is a growing list of endogenous RNA and small DNA viruses, also referred to as endogenous viral elements (EVEs), usually composed of partial virus genome sequences.[94,113]

The importance of endogenous viruses is that they represent a sort of "fossil record" of past viral infections; once integrated into host genomes they cease to evolve like viruses and instead assume the low rates of nucleotide substitution that characterize their hosts, replicating using high-fidelity host DNA polymerases and likely experiencing fewer replications per unit time (Fig. 11.4). Consequently, if the mutational differences between endogenous viruses are known to occur postintegration, such as those observed between the LTRs of a single endogenous retrovirus, between duplicated EVEs, or when there is clear evidence for co-divergence, then divergence times can be estimated in a relatively straightforward manner using host substitution rates.

Molecular clock dating in this manner suggests that the exogenous ancestors of some human retroviruses may have diversified relatively early on in mammalian evolution.[115] Most dramatic are cases of when both exogenous and endogenous copies of the same virus exist, which have generally resulted in a radically different picture of the time scale of viral evolution than using clock estimates based on heterochronous samples. For example, estimates of the age of primate lentiviruses based on the use of heterochronous sequences generally results in time scales of thousands of years at most,[205] while the presence of endogenous lentiviruses in lemurs suggests that these viruses have circulated in primates for at least several million years.[116] The same is true of endogenous viruses that are not retroviruses. Perhaps the most compelling of these are the avian hepadnaviruses, in which the observation of EVEs integrated at the same genomic positions in bird species that diverged at least 19 million years ago strongly suggests that hepadnaviruses are at least of the same age.[80] This antiquity sits in stark contrast to studies of hepadnavirus evolution based on the use of heterochronous sequences, in which divergence times are measured on scales of a few thousand years.[240] The same phenomenon has been proposed for a variety of other RNA viruses, including bornaviruses and filoviruses,[14,97,113,218] as well as ssDNA viruses of the families *Circoviridae* and *Parvoviridae*.[15,111,113,136] In each case, integrated copies of these viruses are observed in diverse host species, for example, comprising both placental and marsupial mammals in the case of the filoviruses, and sometimes showing virus–host co-divergence such that they are clearly millions of years old.[113] However, there are also many cases where the phylogenies of the endogenous viruses and their hosts do not match, which complicates estimates of virus divergence times. As more host genomes are sequenced, it is certain that more endogenous viral elements will be discovered, which will undoubtedly shed new light on the true time scale of virus evolution.

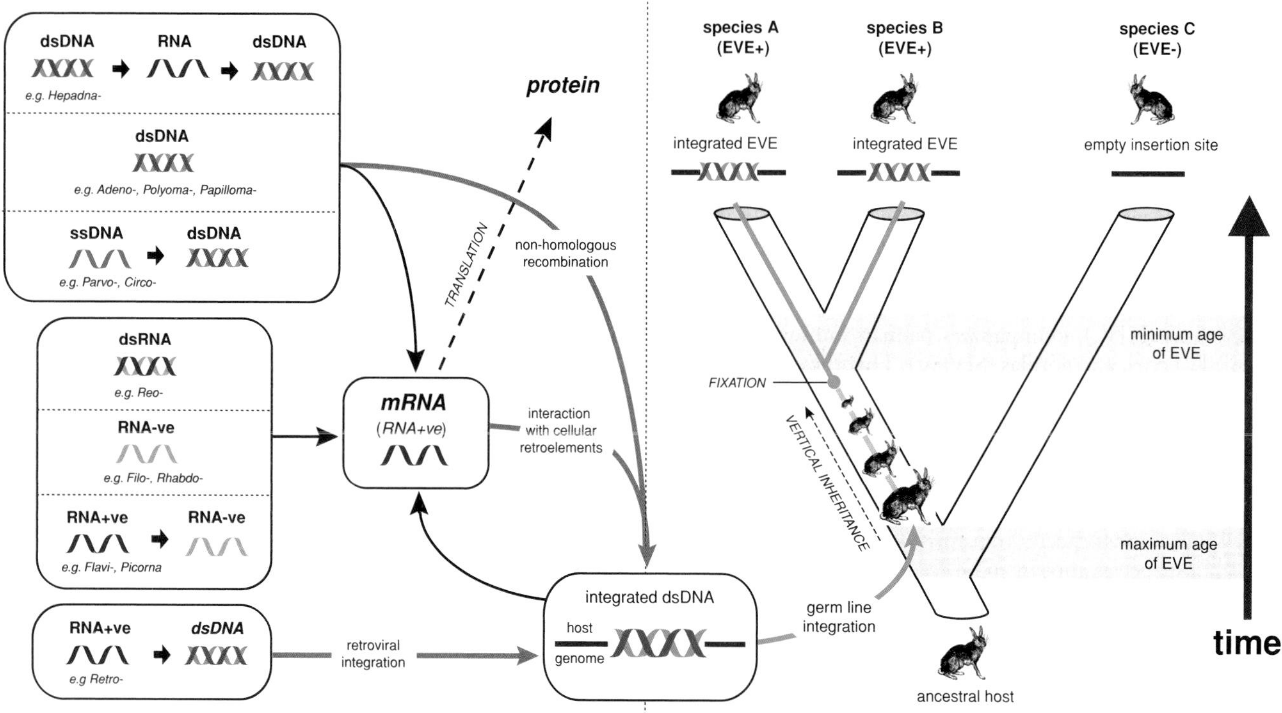

FIGURE 11.4. How endogenous virus elements (EVEs) are generated and can be used to estimate the age of viral families. Examples of different types of mammalian RNA and DNA viruses are shown. Critically, the presence of EVEs in related host species A and B and integrated into the same genomic position indicates that this integration event occurred prior to the divergence of these two species, such that its minimum age can be estimated if it is known when the host species diverged. (From Katzourakis A, Gifford RJ. Endogenous viral elements in animal genomes. *PLoS Genet* 2010;6:e1001191. Original figure kindly provided by Rob Gifford.)

Virus Classification

Finally, and as a brief digression, it is useful to discuss the schemes used for virus classification, ranging from orders to species and genotypes, and what they mean in an evolutionary context, particularly as they indirectly relate to the issue of virus origins. The main points to make here are that although a useful and important aspect of comparative biology, all such classification schemes have a large arbitrary component to them, are not based on a specific evolutionary pattern or process, and do not necessarily mean that the viruses in question exhibit a specific set of biological differences. Indeed, these limitations are likely to apply to most microorganisms. To some extent, this arbitrariness sits in contrast to what is seen in sexually reproducing eukaryotes, where *species* represents a distinct and clearly definable evolutionary group—a population of interbreeding individuals. Hence, although what are termed virus *species* may possess phenotypic characteristics that can be defined for each group and form well-supported clusters on phylogenetic trees, this should not be taken as evidence that they have been formed by a distinct evolutionary process that is analogous to reproductive isolation in eukaryotes. The same is also true of the higher-order classifications proposed for viruses (e.g., supergroups, orders, genera) and for those below the level of species (e.g., genotypes or subtypes). All these groupings can be thought of as points in phylogenetic space rather than describing taxonomic groups that have attained a specific level of phenotypic divergence. In other cases viruses are classified simply through estimates of pairwise genetic diversity, with different levels of diversity signifying the division into species, genotypes, and so forth. Although simple, classification schemes constructed in this manner similarly have no basis in evolutionary theory and may be biased if different lineages evolve at different rates. In sum, it is overly simplistic to think that nature will generate clear-cut divisions in phenotypic and genotypic space that can be used to construct meaningful classification schemes, and hence that systematics tells us anything about virus origins and evolution.

PROCESSES OF VIRUS EVOLUTION

Irrespective of debates over whether viruses are alive, it is clear that they are subject to the same forces that shape the evolution of cellular species, that is, mutation, natural selection, genetic drift, recombination (and reassortment), and migration. I will discuss the first four of these processes in this chapter. Migration, in the guise of viral epidemiology, is discussed elsewhere in this volume.

Mutation and Nucleotide Substitution in Viruses

The simplest way to examine the role of mutation in virus evolution is to measure the rate of its occurrence. Indeed, understanding the factors that shape the speed at which genetic variation is generated in viruses is central to understanding many aspects of their evolution. For RNA viruses mutation can in some ways be thought of as their defining evolutionary feature, as it occurs at a pace that greatly exceeds that observed in other organisms.

Although mutation is the ultimate source of genetic variation, the pace of evolutionary change can in fact be measured in two rather different ways. One method is to estimate, experimentally, the rate at which mutations are generated *de novo*. Such rates have usually been presented as the number of mutations per nucleotide, per replication or the number of mutations per genome, per replication. However, because of the inherent complexities and biases in making these estimates, it has been suggested that estimates of mutation rate per nucleotide, per cell infection may be more informative.[196] For example, one important complicating factor is that some viruses employ so-called stamping machine replication, in which a single virus acts as the template for all progeny genomes, so that mutations accumulate linearly, while others utilize "geometric" replication, in which some of the early progeny genomes are used as templates to produce further progeny, in turn increasing the rate of mutation accumulation.[52]

The power of mutation rate estimates is that they reveal the intrinsic error dynamics of the RNA or DNA polymerases used in viral replication and in theory allow a count of each type of mutation—advantageous, neutral, or deleterious—before they have been shaped by natural selection, although it is always difficult to accurately count the number of lethal mutations that are rapidly removed by purifying selection. A detailed compilation of mutation rate estimates for 23 viruses, and accounting for many of the complexities inherent in analyses of this kind, revealed that these rates varied from 10^{-6} to 10^{-4} mutations/nucleotide/cell infection for RNA viruses to 10^{-8} to 10^{-6} mutations/nucleotide/cell infection for DNA viruses[196] (Fig. 11.5). For RNA viruses that replicate with RdRp, an enzyme that lacks a proofreading or repair function, this equates to mutation rates that are usually a little below approximately one per genome, per replication.[47,48,52] Similarly, the lower mutation rates observed in large DNA viruses clearly reflect the higher fidelity of the DNA polymerases employed in their replication cycle. Of particular note is that mutation rate estimates in ssDNA viruses (a maximum of 1.1×10^{-6}, although only two estimates are available) are higher than those of large dsDNA viruses (which range from 5.9×10^{-8} to 5.4×10^{-7}), even though ssDNA viruses have such small genomes that they use host DNA polymerases for replication. It is therefore possible that the relatively high mutation rates in ssDNA viruses reflect less efficient proofreading and excision repair on ssDNA and/or frequent deamination.[51] The study of Sanjuán et al.[196] was also of note in that it revealed that retroviruses such as HIV have error rates that overlapped with those of RdRp-utilizing viruses, even though earlier studies suggested that RT exhibits higher fidelity than RdRp.[47,48,143]

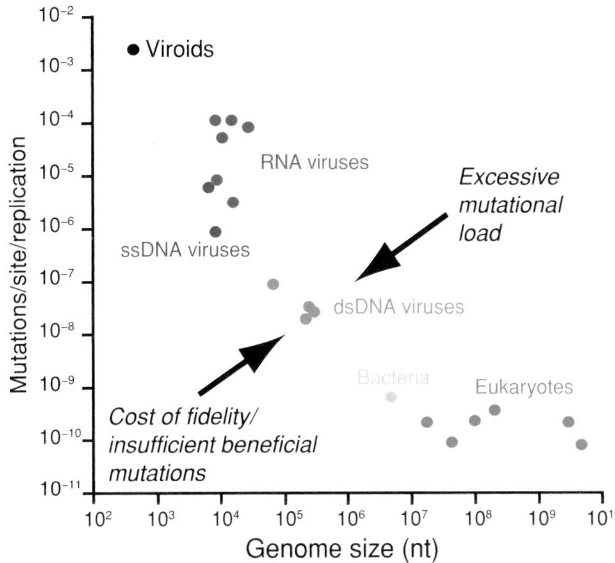

FIGURE 11.6. Relationship between mutation rate and genome size in diverse organisms including RNA and DNA viruses and viroids. The competing evolutionary forces that might be responsible for the limited range of observed error rates and genome sizes are shown. For details see reference 93. Data from reference 75. (From Holmes EC. What does virus evolution tell us about virus origins? *J Virol* 2011;85:5247–5251.)

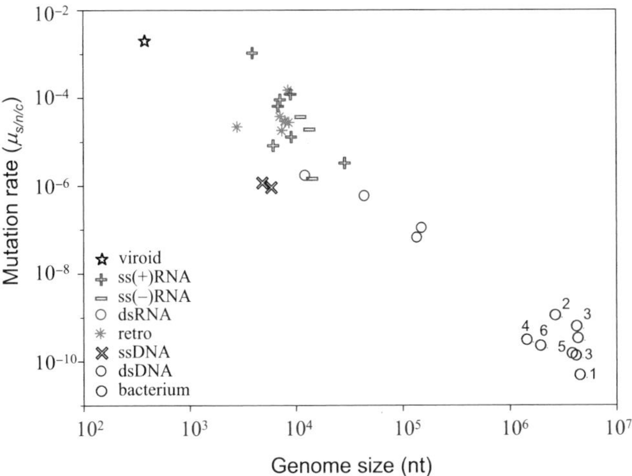

FIGURE 11.5. Comparative rates of mutation in different types of virus and their relationship to genome size. Comparable values from bacteria are also shown. Mutation rates (y-axis) are given per nucleotide per cell infection (s/n/c). See reference 196 for more details including the taxa analyzed. (From Sanjuán R, Nebot MR, Chirico N, et al. Viral mutation rates. *J Virol* 2010;84:9733–9748. Figure kindly provided by Rafa Sanjuán.)

From a broader perspective these estimates of mutation rate are compatible with the idea that for all living systems there is a strongly inverse relationship between mutation rate and genome size (Fig. 11.6).[75,93] It also seems likely that the systematic difference in mutation rate and genome size between RNA and DNA viruses is associated with many of the main evolutionary distinctions between these two types of infectious agents that are discussed throughout this chapter, such that they can be thought of as occupying very different regions of evolutionary parameter space (Table 11.1).

Although they utilize related DNA polymerases, mutation rates in large DNA viruses are higher than those of bacteria and eukaryotes, which may reflect an absence of the full set of repair enzymes and pathways in the former. However, there are two possible exceptions to this rule. First, there is currently no estimate of mutation rates in mimivirus or megavirus, although these are expected to fall within the bacterial range (as the genome sizes of these viruses overlap with those of bacteria), and hence are lower than that observed in any virus to date.

TABLE 11.1 The Differing Evolutionary Parameter Spaces Occupied by RNA and DNA Viruses[a]

Characteristic	RNA (and ssDNA) viruses	dsDNA viruses
Mutation rate (per nt)	High	Low
Genome size	Small (<32,000 nt)	Can be large (>100,000 nt)
Population sizes	Usually large	Can be small
Recombination	Often low rates	Often high rates
Epistasis	Antagonistic	Synergistic[b]
Gene duplication	Apparently rare	Common
Lateral gene transfer	Apparently rare	Common
Overlapping reading frames	Common	Relatively rare

dsDNA, double-stranded DNA; ssDNA, single-stranded DNA.

[a]Note that the properties shown are "average" ones, and cannot be applied to every taxon in each category (particularly for DNA-based organisms).

[b]By inference only: the extent and sign of epistasis has not been measured in dsDNA viruses.

Second, we similarly lack an estimate of mutation rate in the small dsDNA viruses, such as the papillomaviruses. Although the relationship depicted in Figures 11.5 and 11.6 implies that these viruses will mutate rapidly, most estimates of substitution rate in papillomaviruses are in a similar range to those of large DNA viruses.[68,187] This implies that papillomaviruses similarly mutate relatively slowly, which would break the simple relationship between mutation rate and genome size.

The relationship between mutation rate and genome size is of twofold importance. First, because it incorporates genetic systems ranging from viroids to eukaryotes, it covers at least eight orders of magnitude of both genome size and mutation rate, and few things in biology encompass such diversity. Second, it implies that mutation rates that are either too high or too low are selected against.[93] With respect to the latter, a popular idea is that viral mutation rates (and particularly the high mutation rates of RNA viruses) are the result of an evolutionary trade-off, either between replication rate and replication fidelity[74] or between the rates of deleterious and advantageous mutation.[52,213] Data can be cited in support of both relationships.[92,144,224] The possible trade-off between the rates of deleterious and advantageous mutation seems particularly compelling. On the one hand, as viruses will be commonly exposed to changing environments (i.e., different hosts, a variety of cell types, frequent immune pressure), the generation of some genetic variation via mutation is likely to be selectively advantageous. This idea also has experimental support; RNA polymerases with lower fidelity are sometimes selectively favored over those with higher fidelity.[92,144,224] On the other hand, there must be an upper limit on the mutation rates experienced by viruses (and all living systems), as excessive error will result in major fitness losses. Powerful evidence for this ceiling on mutation rates is provided by experiments invoking *lethal mutagenesis* (see later), in which artificially increasing error rates with mutagens such as 5-fluorouracil and ribavirin result in an excessive mutational load.[26,171] It is therefore likely that RNA viruses exist close to their maximum tolerable mutation rates, which in turn imposes an upper limit on genome size. However, it is also likely that RNA viruses are mechanistically unable to reduce their error rates to the levels associated with DNA polymerases. A higher-fidelity RNA polymerase would need to be more complex, and hence longer, than those that currently exist, yet this cannot evolve because, by increasing genome length, it will result in too many deleterious mutations. This evolutionary conundrum is commonly referred to as *Eigen's paradox* and is a key element in theories for the early evolution of genomic complexity.

The second measure of the pace of virus evolution is the rate of nucleotide substitution per nucleotide site, per year (subs/site/year). As this measure reflects the population success of any mutation, it by necessity incorporates the action of natural selection. Accordingly, deleterious mutations that have been removed by purifying selection will not be counted, while advantageous mutations will be fixed more rapidly than neutral ones. Nucleotide substitution rates are usually far easier to estimate than mutation rates and as such provide a simple and powerful means to compare patterns of virus evolution.

As with rates of mutation, rates of nucleotide substitution vary markedly among viruses. Across RNA and DNA viruses as a whole, nucleotide substitution rates vary by over five orders of magnitude, in large part reflecting the differences in background mutation rate described earlier. Hence, most substitution rates in RNA viruses fall within an order of magnitude of a value of 1×10^{-3} subs/site/year,[87,110] while the rates in many dsDNA viruses are closer to 1×10^{-8} subs/site/year.[89,145,148,187] Undoubtedly, our understanding of viral substitution rates would be improved by measures of evolutionary dynamics in the smallest (i.e., viroids) and largest (i.e., mimivirus) viral systems.

Most of the variance in the substitution rates in both RNA and DNA viruses likely reflects virus-specific differences in either mutation rate, replication rate, or both. Mutation rates have been discussed earlier, and some studies have revealed that substitution rates in RNA viruses are negatively associated with genome size as expected if background mutation is the main determinant of substitution rate.[110] Although few direct estimates of replication rate are available, they likewise clearly play a major role in shaping substitution rates. For example, although the retrovirus SFV likely has an RT-associated error rate that is similar to those of other retroviruses, its co-divergence with primates for over 30 million years (Fig. 11.3) leads to estimates of the substitution rate of only 1.7×10^{-8} subs/site/year.[217] This most likely reflects a low rate of replication, although this merits further investigation. Similarly, replication rates appear to be low in papillomaviruses, in which virus replication occurs simultaneously with the division of host epithelial cells, at approximately 10 to 100 generations per year,[19] which likely contributes to the low substitution rates estimated in this virus. In contrast, that DNA viruses often replicate more rapidly than their hosts may in part explain why virus substitution rates are higher than host substitution rates even though they utilize similar polymerases. For example, the Bo17 protein of bovine herpesvirus 4 represents a viral capture of the mammalian 2β-1,6-N-acetylglucosaminyltransferase-mucin protein.[145] As a phylogenetic analysis revealed that this gene was captured from the host after the split between cattle and African buffalo approximately 1.5 million years ago, it was possible to estimate that the viral gene had evolved 20 to 30 times faster than its cellular homolog.[145] Finally, for persistently infecting viruses, substitution rates may also differ between periods of intra- and interhost evolution. For example, HIV-1 substitution rates are higher within than among hosts.[142] This may be because intrahost HIV evolution is dominated by the positive selection of immune escape mutations or because some of the mutations that occur within hosts are purged at interhost transmission, thereby reducing the substitution rate.

Although most estimates of substitution rate suggest a fundamental division in virus evolution in which RNA viruses evolve rapidly and DNA viruses evolve slowly, there are a number of important exceptions. First, a number of RNA viruses are reported to evolve anomalously slowly.[99,216] A much debated example is the rodent hantaviruses (*Bunyaviridae*), which are often claimed to have co-diverged with their murid hosts over many millions of years, which would lead to rates of nucleotide substitution in the range of 10^{-7} subs/site/year.[178] Clearly, these substitution rates are far closer to those of dsDNA viruses than to other RNA viruses. However, there are also important mismatches between the virus and host phylogenies, most notably that hantavirus sequences from various insectivores are mixed with those sampled from rodents,[6] and hantavirus substitution rates estimated over the short term fall within the usual RNA virus range.[185] As a consequence, the true rate of nucleotide substitution in the rodent hantaviruses is uncertain. Second, ssDNA viruses exhibit substitution rates—often in the realm of 10^{-4} subs/site/year—that are closer to those of RNA viruses than to large DNA viruses. Such high rates have now been described in both carnivore[203] and human[167,201] parvoviruses, in porcine circovirus,[67] and in plant geminiviruses.[51,222] Although the mutation rates of ssDNA viruses are higher than those of large DNA viruses, they do not fully explain the elevated substitution rates.[196] It is therefore possible that rapid nucleotide substitution in ssDNA viruses reflects short generation times and/or strong positive selection, the latter of which is well documented in the carnivore parvoviruses following cross-species transmission.[172,203] An important caveat is that both endogenous circoviruses and parvoviruses have now been documented, which suggests that these viruses are ancient.[111,113] Unfortunately, however, the sequences of these endogenous viruses are often so divergent as to challenge any attempt to reliably estimate rates of evolutionary change.

Finally, there are also cases in which large DNA viruses evolve more rapidly than might be expected. A case in point is VARV, in which estimates of the substitution rate fall between 10^{-6} and 10^{-5} subs/site/year, and hence are far higher than those observed in other large DNA viruses where evolutionary rates have been inferred, particularly the herpesviruses.[68,102,206] In addition, VARV exhibits a strongly linear relationship between genetic distance and time of sampling (i.e., measurable evolution) that is also indicative of a high substitution rate.[68] It is therefore possible that VARV has been subject to strong positive selection (at least in the recent past) and that this has elevated the substitution rate to above that expected by neutral mutation pressure alone. Such strong positive selection may be a characteristic common to the orthropoxviruses.[151]

Natural Selection and Genetic Drift in Virus Evolution

Despite long-standing debates over whether natural selection or genetic drift is the more important process of evolutionary change at the molecular level, there is little doubt that viruses provide some of the very best examples of natural selection in action. The literature contains numerous examples of natural selection for such properties as immune evasion (of antibody, T-cell, or innate responses), antiviral resistance, and the adaptation to new cell types and host species. The strength of these selection pressures is readily apparent in the fact that the genomes of large DNA viruses such as poxviruses and herpesviruses contain many genes dedicated to immune evasion. As there are numerous examples of each of these types of positive (i.e., Darwinian) selection for both RNA and DNA viruses, and they are generally not contentious, I will not discuss them here. A more pressing question is, what proportion of all the mutations that arise and are fixed in viral genomes are entirely free of natural selection and hence evolve in a strictly neutral manner, compared to the proportion that are fixed because they are selectively advantageous? Simple population genetic theory predicts that natural selection should be a potent force in viral evolution. Natural selection dominates molecular evolution when the product $N_e s >> 1$, where N_e is the effective population size, and s the selection coefficient (i.e., the fitness of the mutation in question). Although easy to state, estimating these parameters is usually thwarted with difficulties, such that the measures obtained are often only approximate. As a consequence, conclusively determining the role of natural selection versus genetic drift in viral evolution is inherently difficult, although a number of important generalities can be made.

In the case of RNA viruses, it is likely that few amino acid mutations are strictly neutral (i.e., $s = 0$), with most clearly deleterious. In particular, their small genomes ensure there is extensive pleiotropy, epistasis, and multifunctionality such that there is little evolutionary elbow room. Indeed, mutagenesis studies of vesicular stomatitis virus (VSV) revealed that nearly 40% of random mutations are lethal, another 29% deleterious, a further 27% neutral, and only 4% beneficial,[195] although these estimates only relate to fitness effects in a single cell and a far larger proportion of mutations are expected to be deleterious (or lethal) when considering the entirety of the virus life cycle. In addition, as recombination is infrequent in many RNA viruses (see later), there will be strong linkage between neutral mutations and those that are either fixed or purged by natural selection, such that their evolutionary fates will be linked. The same is also likely to be true of ssDNA viruses, which are also characterized by very small genome sizes. Accordingly, most estimates of the ratio of nonsynonymous (d_N) to synonymous (d_S) nucleotide substitutions per site (ratio

d_N/d_S, a common measure of selection pressures, with $d_N/d_S = 1$ indicative of selective neutrality) in RNA and ssDNA viruses suggest that purifying selection is the most common evolutionary force (i.e., $d_N/d_S < 1$).[92,101] However, the case of large DNA viruses is far less clear, in large part because relatively few studies of their molecular evolution have been undertaken. One comparative study of d_N/d_S revealed weaker purifying selection in DNA than RNA viruses,[101] suggesting that the former may possess a class of neutrally evolving amino acid sites. Although the explanation for this effect is unclear, it may be a function of the large genome sizes in large dsDNA viruses, which allow more genetic redundancy through the presence of duplicated genes (see later). Alternatively, it may be indicative of greater levels of positive selection in DNA viruses, as also suggested by the high rates of nucleotide substitution documented in some.[68] Determining the exact nature of the selection pressures acting on large DNA viruses, including the fitness of individual mutations, is clearly an area where a combination of experimental study and evolutionary analysis will be of fundamental importance.

Obviously, the most likely class of neutral sites in viral genomes is those that do not code for protein. For RNA viruses it is debatable how many nucleotide sites fall into this category, particularly as these viruses contain very few, if any, clear-cut examples of "functionless" noncoding RNA, such as pseudogenes and introns. A similar story can be told for small DNA viruses, either single or double stranded, which can be considered as exemplars of genomic efficiency. Indeed, many small DNA viruses, such as circoviruses, parvoviruses, and hepadnaviruses, contain extensive overlapping reading frames, suggesting that they are under strong selective pressure to maximize the phenotypic diversity they can produce from a restricted genomic space. Importantly, the existence of overlapping reading frames changes the selective regime acting on many nucleotide sites. In particular, synonymous sites in one reading frame are likely to be nonsynonymous in another, such that they must be subject to some sort of purifying selection. Similarly, although some pseudogenes are present in the genomes of large DNA viruses,[76] there are relatively few gene overlaps, and it is unclear whether they contain stretches of purely nonfunctional DNA. For example, although the genomes of herpesviruses and poxviruses contain many regions that do not code for protein (~5% to 15% of the genome in the case of poxviruses), these may still encode promoters, transcription termination signals, functional RNA molecules, or other functional elements. One candidate for truly nonfunctional sequences is the imperfect tandem repeat seen in the intergenic regions of some poxviruses and that exhibit various deletions and duplications. Understanding the potential functions, if any, of these noncoding regions is an important goal for the future.

Evolution of Synonymous Sites

Perhaps the most intense debates on the nature of selection pressures acting on viral genomes concern synonymous (silent) nucleotide sites. In eukaryotes, and particularly mammals, there is good evidence that many synonymous nucleotides are subject to only weak (if any) selection pressures and therefore evolve in an effectively neutral manner, although selection on silent sites is being increasingly documented[31] and can take a variety of forms (Fig. 11.7). Under neutral evolution the nucleotide composition of synonymous sites tends to match that of the genome region in which they are located, reflecting the action of background mutation pressure. That in all viruses genome-scale levels of synonymous variation are far higher than those observed at nonsynonymous sites indicates that the fitness effects of synonymous mutations are usually less than those of nonsynonymous mutations (as is true of all living systems). However, this does not necessarily mean that

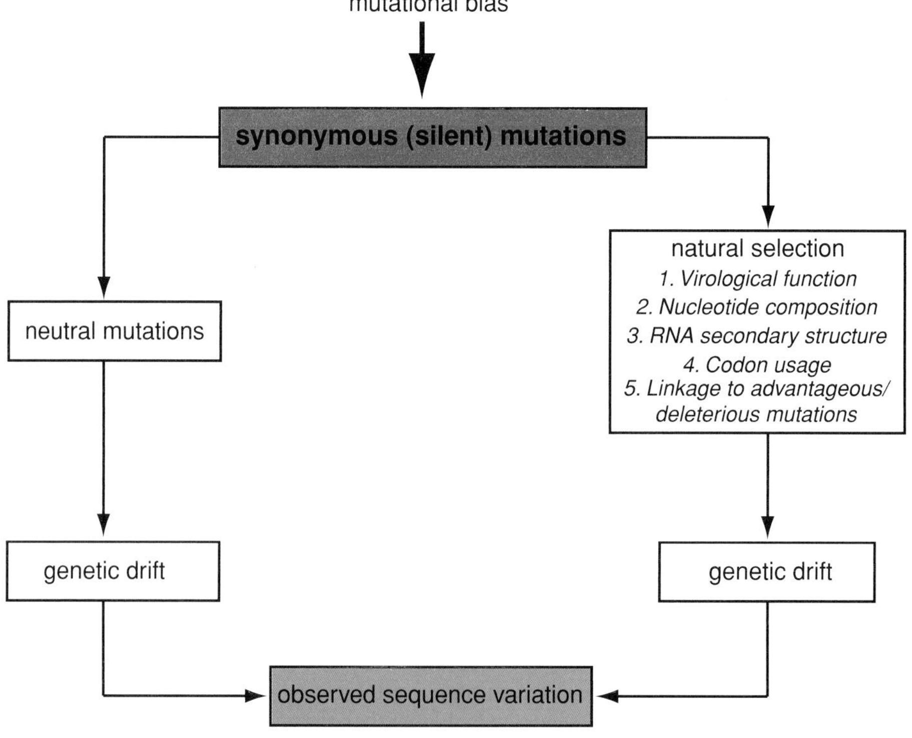

FIGURE 11.7. Evolutionary processes acting on synonymous (silent) nucleotide sites in viruses. The first bias is generated by the basic process of mutation, which may make some types of mutation (e.g., specific nucleotide transitions) more frequent than others. Those synonymous mutations that do arise may either be neutral, so that they are not subject to natural selection, or exhibit fitness differences (listed), in which case they are put through the sieve of natural selection. Both neutral and advantageous mutations are also subject to random genetic drift.

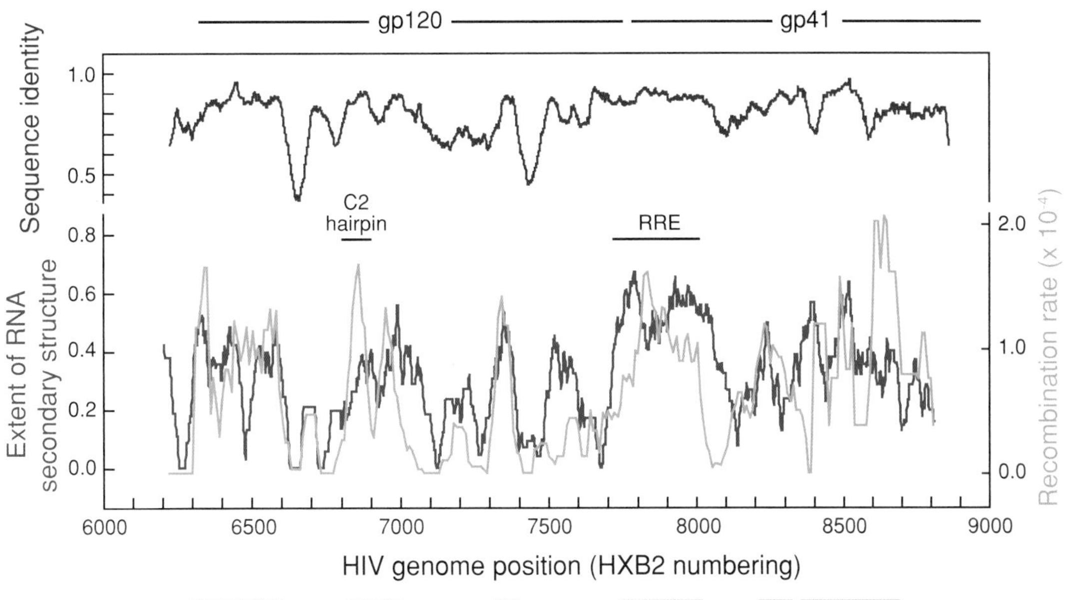

FIGURE 11.8. The relationship between recombination rate, sequence similarity, and RNA secondary structure in the *env* (envelope) gene of human immunodeficiency virus type 1 (HIV-1). Recombination rates are shown in light blue, conserved RNA structures in dark blue, and sequence similarity (identity) in brown. The location of recombination hotspots are marked by light blue bars at the bottom of the figure. (Adapted from Simon-Loriere E, Martin DP, Weeks KM, et al. RNA structures facilitate recombination-mediated gene swapping in HIV-1. *J Virol* 2010;84:12675–12682, which should be consulted for more details. Figure kindly provided by Etienne Simon-Loriere.)

synonymous mutations are strictly neutral, particularly at large effective population sizes where natural selection is especially potent. In fact, there is mounting experimental evidence that synonymous mutations can sometimes have a major effect on viral fitness, as they contain the signals for such processes as promotion, transcription, and encapsidation,[147,168] which means that all studies of d_N/d_S should be interpreted with care.

The most discussed ways in which natural selection might act on synonymous sites are through RNA secondary structures and codon usage. RNA secondary structures are a common feature of many RNA viruses, can occur in both untranslated regions and coding regions, and can comprise genome-scale interactions.[210,226] It is well established that these RNA secondary structures can have a major impact on key elements of virus function, such as containing important signals for such processes as replication and translation. RNA secondary structures may impact on other aspects of virus evolution including shaping, to some extent, genome-wide recombination frequencies[212] (Fig. 11.8). Similarly, functional RNA structures have been noted in a number of DNA viruses.[156] Evidently, the presence of RNA secondary structures strongly argues against the selective neutrality of many synonymous sites,[209] although their precise effects on fitness have rarely been documented.

The second form of natural selection that may act on synonymous sites is codon usage. As with RNA secondary structure, changing codon usage may have a profound effect on fitness. As a dramatic case in point, experimental alteration of synonymous codon usage resulted in the attenuation of poliovirus.[39] When genetic drift dominates molecular evolution, synonymous codon usage is set by the background (i.e., neutral) mutational bias in the organism in question. In contrast, natural selection could shape codon choice by optimizing the match between codon and anticodon so as to increase the accuracy and/or efficiency of protein translation (although a variety of other selective explanations exist[177]). While viruses often exhibit strong biases in codon usage, the explanations for these biases have usually not been resolved. Many RNA viruses utilize synonymous codons that tend to match the nucleotide composition of the viral genome as a whole, suggesting that selection on codon choice is likely to be relatively weak and mainly set by background mutational pressure[108] or that selection is acting on the overall nucleotide composition (see later). However, direct selection for a specific pattern of codon usage seems to characterize other viruses. For example, codon usage bias in Epstein-Barr virus is associated with levels of viral gene expression, varying between the latent and productive phases,[112] while there is a strong match between codon usage and host transfer RNA (tRNA) availability in papillomavirus, which determines the levels of capsid protein expression.[239] Similarly, a study of honeybee viruses revealed the same pattern of codon usage in unrelated RNA viruses, indicative of a bee-specific selection pressure.[33] More interesting is the case of hepatitis A virus in which codon usage seems to be set by the kinetics (rather than the accuracy) of protein translation such that rare codons that utilize nonabundant tRNAs are used, which slows down the translation process to ensure proper protein folding.[5]

As noted earlier, it is also possible that overall nucleotide composition is the selectively determined trait, which has a secondary effect on codon usage bias. Evidence for such a process is the major host-specific differences in nucleotide composition observed in some viruses.[10,109] For example, nucleotide composition noticeably changes in influenza A virus following host jumps from birds to mammals, although precisely why is unclear.[85] Systematic differences in nucleotide composition also characterize DNA viruses, and nucleotide compositions can vary enormously even at the intrafamily level.[149] For example, CpG nucleotide frequency was observed to be the major correlate of codon usage bias in vertebrate DNA viruses, again pointing to the importance of genome-wide mutation pressure.[202] However, small DNA viruses were observed to have CpG contents far below that expected given their overall nucleotide composition, in contrast to the situation in large DNA viruses, although the explanations for this difference are unclear.[202]

Effective Population Size and Population Bottlenecks

After the selective coefficient of mutations, the second factor that determines the respective roles of natural selection and genetic drift in virus evolution is the effective population size (N_e), which is usually far lower than the census population size, N. Available data indicate that N_e fluctuates dramatically during the life cycle of most viruses. For all exogenous viruses, large values of N_e are most likely observed within an individual host following multiple rounds of replication and at the epidemiologic scale. Natural selection is expected to be an efficient force in these cases. For example, perhaps 10^{10} virions are produced by HIV-1 replication per day in every infected individual,[175] with some 10^7 human hosts HIV-infected on a global scale. In addition, the burst sizes of many acute viruses will be large, such that within-host values of N_e are expected to be high for at least some parts of the virus life cycle. The exception to this rule may be latent viruses, in which effective population sizes are often likely to be relatively small, reflecting a lack of active replication.

Conversely, low values of N_e, reflecting the time when genetic drift is strongest and perhaps overriding the action of natural selection, will generally occur at interhost transmission. At this point in the virus life cycle a major population bottleneck may be a common occurrence, although this is also likely to be at least in part determined by the mode of transmission and hence the infecting dose; for example, vertical transmission (wide bottleneck) might be expected to be associated with the transfer of more viruses between hosts than sexual transmission (narrow bottleneck).[134] In some cases, including HIV-1, it is possible that the transmission bottleneck is so extensive that new infections are initiated by a single virus particle,[69] which would obviously result in a major stochastic effect on virus genetic diversity. Similarly, experimental studies of plant viruses have commonly revealed the existence of extensive population bottlenecks, both at interhost transmission and as the virus moves through an individual plant[3,191] and which may also be true of vector-borne viruses of animals.[214] In these cases the stochastic effects of genetic drift are expected to be strong, even to the extent of allowing many slightly deleterious mutations to rise to appreciable frequencies, although to date there have been few *in vivo* experiments to address this issue. Interestingly, some comparative sequencing studies have suggested that interhost transmission might be associated with relatively wide population bottlenecks. For example, multiple viral lineages passed among horses during experimental transmissions with equine influenza virus,[162] while the occurrence of mixed infections in viruses such as influenza[78,162] and dengue[1] also suggests that transmission bottlenecks might be relatively broad. Overall, it is evident that a great deal more work is needed to fully understand the nature and scale of population bottlenecks in viruses and what this means for the relative frequencies of natural selection versus genetic drift, particularly in natural as opposed to experimental infections.

Evolutionary Interactions: Epistasis, Defecting Interfering Particles, and Complementation

A common assumption in many evolutionary studies is that nucleotide sites evolve independently. However, this assumption is often highly simplistic as epistatic interactions among mutations are a regular occurrence in viral genomes. Not only might such epistasis be of great functional importance, such as that resulting from RNA or protein secondary structure, but it may also tell us a great deal about the basic mechanics of virus evolution.

Epistatic effects can be antagonistic (positive), in which case they reduce the effect of combined mutations on fitness, or synergistic (negative), in which case they increase this effect. Although determining the nature of epistasis represents a major technical challenge because it entails a precise measurement of the combined fitness effects of multiple mutations, there is growing evidence for epistasis in viruses, and particularly in RNA viruses where experimental studies are rather easier to perform. Importantly, most of the epistatic interactions determined to date in RNA viruses are antagonistic rather than synergistic,[20,125,197] which has major implications for understanding why recombination evolved in viruses (see later). Similar epistatic effects have been observed in small ssDNA viruses.[174]

It is useful to discuss the extent of epistasis in the context of mutational robustness, which is a way in which phenotypes can be "protected" against the adverse effects of deleterious mutation pressure. Robustness can be generated in a number of ways, including through genetic redundancies such as duplicated genes, through the creation of neutral spaces as might be contained in RNA or protein secondary structure, or by complementation.[45,157] There is a strong relationship between the level of genetic redundancy and epistasis, such that antagonistic epistasis is most common in genomes that are characterized by little redundancy and weak robustness, as is the case for RNA and ssDNA viruses (Fig. 11.9).[58,194] Hence, when mutations occur in viruses with small genomes, which contain many overlapping reading frames and functions, they will tend to repeatedly damage the same functions, leading to antagonistic epistasis.[229] Conversely, synergistic epistasis is more commonplace in larger DNA-based organisms that exhibit a greater level of genetic redundancy and robustness, of which duplicated genes are a good example, which allows them to tolerate a certain number of deleterious mutations (Fig. 11.9). Where large DNA viruses fall on this spectrum is uncertain, as there have been no experimental measures of the rate and sign of epistasis in these organisms to date. However, that multigene families are a common occurrence in large DNA viruses, resulting in a level of genetic redundancy, suggests that most of the epistatic interactions that occur in these viruses will be synergistic.

While individual mutations in viruses can interact through epistasis, whole virus genomes can interact through the presence of defective interfering (DI) particles and complementation.

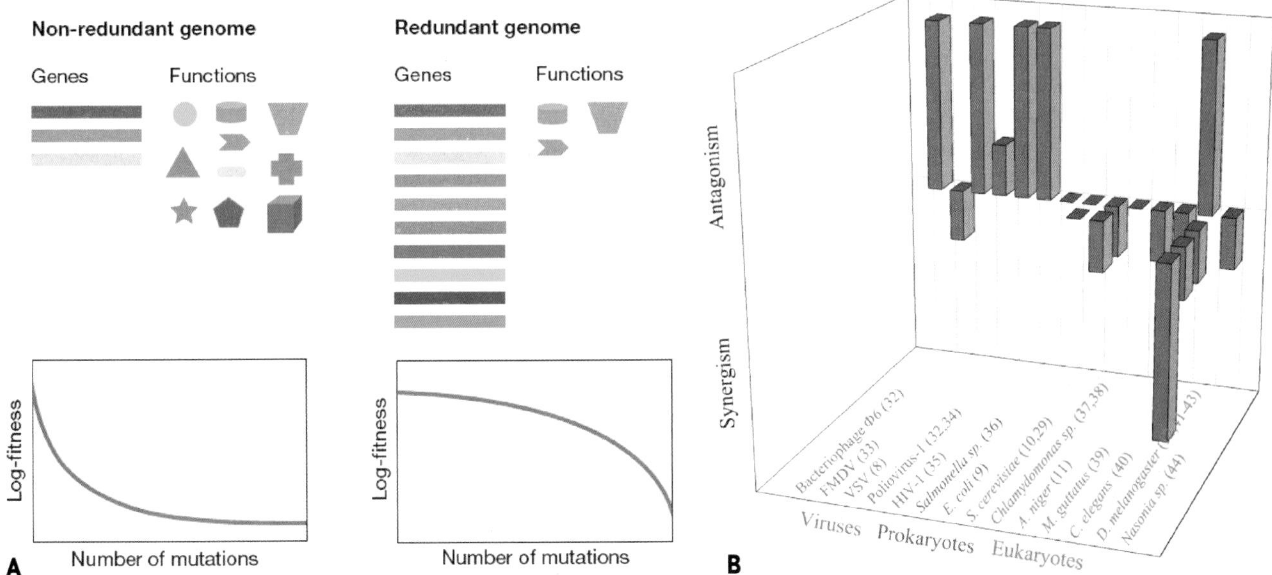

FIGURE 11.9. Redundancy and epistasis in viruses. A: Differing properties of robust (redundant) and nonrobust (nonredundant) genetic systems. In robust genetic systems that contain many genes, which may include large DNA viruses, the presence of genetic redundancy means that individual mutations have weak fitness effects and interact through synergistic epistasis. In contrast, in nonrobust systems such as RNA viruses and single-stranded DNA (ssDNA) viruses, there are few genes, and hence little genetic redundancy, so that single genes have multiple functions and single mutations have strong fitness effects. This results in antagonistic epistasis. (From Elena SF, Carrasco P, Daròs JA, et al. Mechanisms of genetic robustness in RNA viruses. *EMBO Rep* 2006;7:168–173.) **B:** The type of epistasis seen in a variety of organisms: long bars, significant epistasis; short bars, nonsignificant epistasis; flat bars, no evidence for epistasis. For details see reference 92. (From Sanjuán R, Elena SF. Epistasis correlates to genomic complexity. *Proc Natl Acad Sci U S A* 2006;103:14402–14405; copyright 2006 National Academy of Sciences, U.S.A.)

DI particles are a common observation in many virus families[98] and have been implicated in a number of virological traits, including persistence.[190] DI particles often harbor large genomic deletions and compete with fully functional viruses during replication because they are able to replicate faster. DI particles have a number of interesting evolutionary consequences, although these will usually be short term. First, the high frequency of DI particles further illustrates the high rate at which deleterious mutations are produced in virus populations, including large-scale deletions. Second, as noted later, the polymerase error process that generates DI particles also has important implications for the evolution of recombination in viruses. Third, because they are able to replicate more rapidly than full-length viral genomes, DI particles may theoretically inhibit the spread of the advantageous mutations that are present on full-length viral genomes, if only transiently.

DI particles are likely to be maintained in virus populations through complementation, which is predicted to be a common occurrence at high multiplicity of infection, and which has been relatively frequently documented in both RNA (e.g., references 77, 221) and DNA viruses (e.g., references 37, 150). Perhaps the most interesting evolutionary consequence of complementation is that it allows deleterious mutations to persist for extended periods.[73] Until relatively recently, complementation was a process that had only been observed *in vitro,* such that DI particles were thought to survive just a few generations and therefore had little long-term evolutionary consequence. However, more recent analyses reveal that complementation may be frequent in nature[72] and may extend over very long time periods.[1] As a consequence, complementation may play more of a role in virus evolution than is usually envisioned, particularly in the context of how deleterious and advantageous mutations interact with each other, although this will evidently require further study.

The Evolution of Viral Recombination

A combination of comparative genomics and experimental study has provided growing evidence for the action of recombination, and its sister process reassortment, in viral genomes, although rates of virus recombination are often far lower than those documented in many cellular species. At the sequence level recombination is commonly apparent as incongruent phylogenetic trees, in which phylogenies inferred on either side of a recombination breakpoint differ significantly in topology, reflecting the contrasting evolutionary histories of these gene regions. Although such phylogenetic approaches can be biased in two ways—false positives caused by mixed infection or experimental error[21] and that tree-based methods only detect recombination when there is measurable sequence diversity—they represent a simple means to detect recombination in a wide range of viruses and in doing so allow a direct comparison of recombination frequency.

Mechanisms of recombination differ markedly between viruses, reflecting the very different types of replication strategy employed, although all require co-infection of a single cell by two or more viruses. In the case of dsDNA viruses, recombination likely occurs in a manner analogous to that observed in other DNA-based organisms, although the precise mechanisms of recombination are not known in all cases. Hence, recombination will involve the occurrence and repair of double-stranded breaks and, in the case of large dsDNA viruses, the presence of multiple recombination enzymes.[105] Recombination appears to be particularly commonplace in poxviruses, an apparent outcome of the form of DNA strain invasion used in replication,[63,64] as well as in herpesviruses.[23] Recombination in large DNA viruses can be both homologous, in that it occurs at regions exhibiting strong sequence identity, and nonhomologous, involving divergent gene sequences (usually occurring as lateral gene transfer) and can occur at the intra- and interspecific levels.[219] It therefore plays a major role in shaping genomic architecture.[151] For example, in poxviruses recombination may be more commonplace at the extremities of the genome, as these contain most of the species-specific genes, than in the central genomic regions that are conserved among viruses.[62,151] Rather less is known about the mechanics of recombination in ssDNA viruses, although it is likely to occur as a consequence of the rolling circle replication employed by these viruses,[199] which may both determine the distribution of recombination breakpoints[223] and result in frequent genome rearrangements, as in the case of Torque teno (TT) virus.[133]

Evolutionary aspects of recombination are better studied in RNA viruses. Recombination in this case occurs by two rather different mechanisms. The first, sometimes called RNA recombination, occurs when two viruses co-infect a single host cell and a hybrid molecule is produced, most likely through a process of *copy-choice replication*,[127] although other mechanisms have been proposed. Under the copy-choice model the viral polymerase is thought to jump templates during negative strand synthesis, generating a chimeric RNA molecule.[127] Although this process is usually homologous, template switching can also occur among genomic regions that do not share sequence similarity. In theory, RNA recombination can occur in any type of RNA virus, irrespective of their genome structure or orientation, although rates vary hugely among viruses (see later). The second process of recombination in RNA viruses is reassortment, which only occurs in RNA viruses that possess segmented genomes, such that a progeny virus packages segments with different ancestries. Rates of reassortment also vary markedly among RNA viruses, from very frequent in the case of influenza A virus[182] to far less so in the case of hantaviruses.[165]

Clearly, recombination can be of great evolutionary importance for viruses[211] and has been associated with such features as the evasion of host immunity,[141] the development of antiviral resistance,[166] the ability to infect new hosts,[96] increases in virulence,[118] and even the creation of new viruses.[227] As a consequence, it is important to document cases of viral recombination and reveal the determinants of this process. However, the occasional occurrence of beneficial traits arising from recombination does not necessarily mean that recombination evolved for this purpose, as recombination is as likely to break up beneficial genotypic configurations as create them. Indeed, explaining why recombination has evolved is one of the outstanding questions in evolutionary biology.

For viruses, clues for the reasons underlying the evolution of recombination are provided by the huge variation in recombination rates, from effectively clonal (i.e., asexual) to cases in which the recombination rate per nucleotide exceeds that of mutation. This extensive rate variation is particularly true of RNA viruses. The most common theory for the evolution of recombination is that it functions as a form of sexual reproduction in viruses and as such has been selectively optimized to either create advantageous genetic configurations or remove deleterious mutations (Fig. 11.10). However, this seems unlikely on first principles as high rates of recombination are only seen in a relatively small fraction of virus taxa, such that high recombination rates cannot be universally advantageous.[211] This patchy distribution sits in marked contrast to theories for the evolution of sex in eukaryotes, the aim of which is to explain common recombination and sporadic asexuality.[189] Similarly, the patchy distribution of recombination

Evolutionary Benefit of Recombination

(1) Creation of beneficial genotypes:
Recombination increases the rate of adaptive evolution compared to clonal evolution. It also disassociates advantageous from deleterious mutations, allowing the former to spread.

(2) Purging of deleterious mutations:
Recombination enables deleterious mutations to be placed into a single genome which can be removed by purifying selection. This can be selectively favored if deleterious mutations occur at a high rate (i.e. $U > 1$) and interact through synergistic epistasis.

Schematic Representation

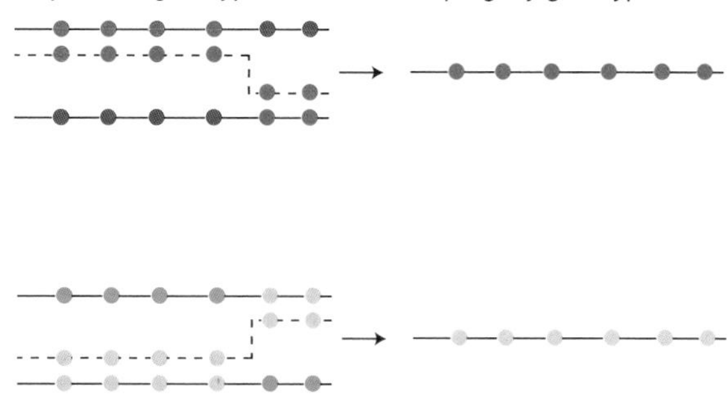

FIGURE 11.10. Potential evolutionary benefits of viral recombination (and reassortment) that might be favored by natural selection and that are commonly invoked in discussions of the evolution of sex. Accordingly, recombination can either (1) create advantageous genetic configurations (red circles), and also disassociate advantageous from deleterious mutations, or (2) purge deleterious mutations (green circles) by placing them in a single individual, which can be removed by purifying selection. In both cases the hatched line denotes the recombination event. (Adapted from Simon-Loriere E, Holmes EC. Why do RNA viruses recombine? *Nat Rev Microbiol* 2011;9:617–626, which should be consulted for more details.)

means that it is unlikely to universally have evolved as a form of repair.[153]

It is obvious that recombination allows viruses to create potentially beneficial genetic configurations more rapidly than asexual populations, and there are many documented cases in viruses in which recombination has been associated with the generation of advantageous characteristics, such as drug-resistant genotypes. However, there are a number of viruses where rates of recombination are very low but where adaptive evolution is extremely common, with hepatitis C virus (HCV) a good case in point.[188] Hence, it may be that RNA viruses create a sufficient number of beneficial genotypes through mutation alone to offset the need for recombination. Recombination has two other important consequences for adaptive evolution. First, it disassociates advantageous from linked deleterious mutations,[189] and second, it prevents *clonal interference.* The latter describes a competition between beneficial mutations as they go to fixation in asexual populations, such that their rate of adaptation is retarded compared to that of sexual populations. Although both these processes are likely to occur in virus populations,[155] their overall importance is unclear.

The second advantage of recombination over purely clonal evolution is that it facilitates the efficient removal of deleterious mutations. This is often called the *mutational deterministic hypothesis* and is a hotly debated theory for the evolution of sex in a wide range of species.[117,122] The central idea is that rather than many individuals (or genomes) carrying deleterious mutations, which would have a major negative impact on fitness, recombination allows these injurious mutations to be placed in a single individual whose selective removal greatly reduces fitness costs. A related theory is that of Muller's ratchet, which describes a progressive decrease in fitness due to the gradual accumulation of deleterious mutations in asexual populations of finite size and where genetic drift accelerates the loss of mutation-free individuals. Muller's ratchet has been observed in laboratory populations of RNA viruses[34,35,50] and may therefore play some role when clonal viruses experience small population sizes, such as during transmission bottlenecks, although its effects are likely to be negated when viruses reach large population sizes.

For the mutational deterministic hypothesis to explain the origin of recombination, it is essential that the deleterious mutation per genome replication (U) is greater than 1, and hence very high, and that these deleterious mutations interact through synergistic epistasis.[122] For RNA viruses $U > 1$ may be attained relatively regularly.[52,61] This may also be true of ssDNA viruses, which similarly possess small genomes and genes that encode multiple overlapping reading frames and functions. Unfortunately, there are currently no estimates of U in large DNA viruses. However, there is little good evidence for synergistic epistasis in RNA viruses, with most studies undertaken to date suggesting that epistatic interactions are antagonistic rather than synergistic.[20,28,197] In contrast, the greater genetic redundancy in large DNA viruses makes antagonistic epistasis a more likely occurrence in this instance. In addition, sequence comparisons suggest that the burden of deleterious mutation is high for all RNA viruses studied, irrespective of background recombination rate.[181] Hence, it is not recombination that saves RNA viruses from an excessive mutational load, but rather their large population sizes that provide a form of *population robustness* that offsets the effects of deleterious mutation.[58]

An opposing theory for the evolution of viral recombination is that rather than being optimized by natural selection as a form of sexual reproduction, it is simply a mechanistic by-product of differing types of genome architecture, replication strategy, and polymerase processivity.[211] The principal evidence for this theory is that there is an apparent association between recombination frequency and virus genome structure. Hence, recombination is relatively frequent in some retroviruses, and as is reassortment in viruses with segmented genomes. Far more variable recombination rates are observed in ssRNA+ viruses, for example, frequently in coronaviruses and enteroviruses, sporadically in flaviviruses, and currently absent in *Leviviridae* and *Narnaviridae* (although this may be a function of sample size). Finally, recombination is far less common in ssRNA– viruses. A simple example of the disparity of recombination rates is provided by a comparison of HIV-1 and HCV. In the former, recombination rates have been estimated at between 1.38×10^{-4} and 1.4×10^{-5} recombination events per site, per generation,[164,207] while the equivalent estimates for HCV are only 4×10^{-8}.[188] The low rate in HCV means that recombination is unlikely to be of great evolutionary significance for this virus. Most DNA viruses studied to date seem to experience relatively high levels of recombination (including through lateral gene transfer in the case of large DNA viruses), although there have been few attempts to estimate rates of recombination relative to those of mutation.[23] One DNA virus in which recombination has been particularly well studied is HBV, along with related hepadnaviruses. In this case recombination is commonly depicted using phylogenetic methods and likely represents one of the main reasons that the evolutionary history of this virus has been so hard to determine.[208]

In each case mentioned previously the frequency of recombination seems to reflect the genome structure of the virus in question.[211] Hence, the high recombination rates of retroviruses are likely a function of the fact that their virions carry two RNA molecules, such that *heterozygous* progeny will be produced when viruses with different ancestries are packaged together. Copy-choice recombination, which is common in this virus, may then produce genetically distinct progeny during reverse transcription. However, not all retroviruses recombine at the same rate as HIV. For example, recombination rates in murine leukemia virus (MLV) are up to 100 times lower than those observed in HIV, despite very similar rates of template switching. The difference between these two viruses is that while HIV genome dimerization occurs randomly in the cytoplasm, genome dimerization in MLV takes place in the nucleus and generally leads to self-associations, rather than to those involving genetically different parental molecules.[170]

That heterozygous viral progeny cannot be produced when the genomic material is present as a single molecule obviously acts to reduce recombination rates in most RNA viruses. However, in some cases specific genome organizations can facilitate frequent recombination. Case in point are the coronaviruses, such as murine hepatitis virus (MHV), where up to 25% of the progeny of co-infected cells may be recombinant. Such a high recombination rate reflects the mechanisms controlling gene expression in coronaviruses, in which discontinuous transcription leads to the production of subgenomic RNAs through a copy-choice mechanism.[198] An even more dramatic example of how replication strategy and genome organization may shape recombination rate occurs in the ssRNA– viruses, in which recombination is relatively infrequent. In these viruses the genomic and antigenomic RNA molecules are quickly bound to multiple nucleoprotein subunits, as well as to other proteins, to form ribonucleoprotein (RNP) complexes from which viral replication and transcription can proceed. However, this tight complex of RNA and protein necessarily limits the probability of hybridization of complementary sequences between the nascent and acceptor nucleic acid molecules, and hence the probability of template switching, and also reduces the potential number of substrates for this process.[211] Accordingly, those phylogenetic studies undertaken to date have revealed relatively few cases of recombination in ssRNA– viruses.[7,231]

The RNA Virus Quasispecies

One of the most contentious issues in the study of virus evolution is whether RNA viruses evolve according to a particular population genetic model known as the *quasispecies*.[92] In some aspects, this debate merely reflects a semantic point about how best to describe the intrahost genetic variation commonly seen in RNA viruses. However, a far more important issue, and the true essence of the quasispecies debate, is how natural selection acts on virus genomes.

Quasispecies theory was originally developed by Manfred Eigen and colleagues as a model of the evolution of self-replicating RNA molecules that likely represent the first replicators.[56,57] The theory was first applied to RNA viruses after genetic variation was observed in a number of experimental systems, beginning with the bacteriophage Qβ.[46] Since this time the quasispecies has become a popular descriptor of intrahost RNA virus evolution, particularly because widespread gene sequencing has uncovered abundant genetic diversity. However, because the theory is based on high mutation rates (see later), it should not be applied to large DNA viruses where error frequencies are lower.

Although commonly used simply as a synonym for genetic variation, quasispecies in fact describes a specific type of mutation-selection balance. Mutation-selection balances are commonly invoked in population genetics and describe an evolutionary equilibrium between the generation of new mutations and their removal by purifying selection. The form of mutation-selection balance invoked in quasispecies theory is based on the occurrence of an extremely high mutation rate, which ensures that the frequency of any variant in the population is a function of both its individual fitness *plus* the frequency at which it is produced by the erroneous replication of other variants in the population that are linked to it in mutational space. This *mutational coupling* means that viral genomes are not independent entities, such that natural selection favors the entire population as opposed to individual variants. In this manner the group, rather than the individual, becomes the unit of selection.[57]

The central tenet of quasispecies theory is thus that natural selection acts on the viral population as a whole, rather than on individual variants. As a consequence, the entire quasispecies evolves to maximize its average fitness, rather than that of individual variants as is the case in other population genetic models. The most interesting outcome of this particular evolutionary process is that low fitness variants can sometimes outcompete those of higher individual fitness if the former are surrounded by beneficial mutational neighbors. This is sometimes referred to as the *quasispecies effect* or the *survival of the flattest*[230] and describes a situation in which a population whose component mutants have a similar mean fitness can outcompete a population that has a lower average fitness even though it contains variants of higher individual fitness. Under classic *survival of the fittest* population genetic models, these individual high-fitness variants are selectively favored, whereas under *survival of the flattest* (i.e., quasispecies) models, the flatter population is selectively superior as it possesses a higher mean fitness (Fig. 11.11). This can also be thought of as a form of mutational robustness.

A key component of quasispecies theory is that intrahost populations of RNA viruses harbor abundant genetic diversity. There is no doubt that this specific aspect of quasispecies theory is correct, and even so for acute infections, as intrahost genetic variation is commonly observed in RNA viruses.[44,92] In particular, studies using next-generation sequencing, in which the sequencing coverage of individual nucleotides is very high, have revealed extensive genetic diversity, with HIV-1[69] and foot-and-mouth disease virus (FMDV)[234] serving as good examples.

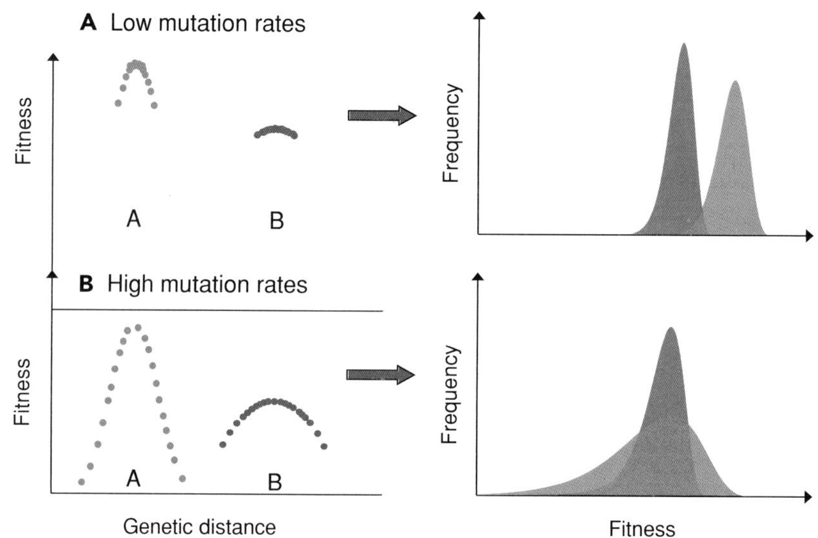

FIGURE 11.11. The quasispecies effect (*survival of the flattest*) in experimental populations of RNA viruses. The red population **(A)** has a high replication rate (i.e., fitness) but low mutational robustness, while the blue population **(B)** has a lower replication rate but greater mutational robustness. Dots depict mutational variants located on each peak at low and high mutation rates, and the expected distribution of individual fitness values for the two populations is shown on the **right** of the figure. At low mutation rates, population **A** will always outcompete the flatter population **B** as it contains the variant of highest individual fitness. However, at very high mutation rates natural selection favors the flatter population **(B)** as predicted under quasispecies theory. (From Sanjuán R, Cuevas JM, Furió V, et al. Selection for robustness in mutagenized RNA viruses. *PLoS Genet* 2007;3:e93.)

However, a very important caveat is that many estimates of intrahost genetic diversity are likely to have been inflated by erroneous polymerase chain reaction (PCR) and sequencing.[140] Indeed, RT-PCR is a notoriously error-prone process, with artificially induced mutations an inevitable consequence, and different sequencing systems are also characterized by specific error rates. In addition, intrahost genetic diversity in nature is not simply the product of *de novo* mutation because the mixed infection of individual hosts may also play an important role in shaping levels of intrahost genetic variation (see later). More importantly, although the observation of intrahost genetic variation is a necessary criterion for an RNA virus population to be thought of as a quasispecies, it is not sufficient in itself as intrahost genetic diversity is expected under any evolutionary model if the mutation rate is high enough. The quasispecies is therefore not simply another word for intrahost genetic variation.

Both *in silico* and *in vitro* studies have provided some evidence for the existence of quasispecies dynamics defined correctly. As an example of the former, computational studies using *digital organisms* revealed that the survival of the flattest could be induced at very high mutation rates.[40,230] However, as the mutation rates involved were always higher than one mutation per genome replication, it is uncertain whether such mutation rates could ever be attained for sustained periods in RNA viruses in nature. Similar results have been obtained from some experimental analyses of RNA virus evolution. Studies using both viroids of plants and VSV showed that viral populations with lower replication rates were able to outcompete those with higher replication rates, as expected under the quasispecies model, although this again requires the elevation of mutation rate (by either chemical mutagens or ultraviolet C light) to levels that may not commonly occur in RNA viruses in nature.[38,193] Additional experimental evidence for the existence of RNA virus quasispecies was the observation that high-fitness clones of bacteriophage $\phi6$ evolved to a lower mean fitness because their mutational neighbors were of low fitness,[27] and that strains of poliovirus that possessed higher fidelity than the wild type, such that the virus population carried less genetic diversity, were unable to infect the full range of tissues that are associated with severe disease.[224] This in turn suggested that quasispecies dynamics might be a central determinant of viral pathogenesis.[224]

Another class of experimental studies that have been cited in support of the quasispecies model involves lethal mutagenesis. This entails treating virus populations with mutagens, such as 5-fluorouracil and ribavirin, that increase the error rate to the extent that so many deleterious mutations are produced that fit genotypes are never able to regenerate themselves. Although lethal mutagenesis can clearly result in virus extinction, especially if mutagens are used in combination with more standard antiviral inhibitors,[4,171] the basis of this effect is more complex. Quasispecies theory predicts that virus extinction in this instance occurs because of an *error catastrophe,* which is the point at which the fittest genotype suffers so many deleterious mutations that it cannot sustain itself in the population (i.e., it has breached an *error threshold*). However, another interpretation is that the virus has instead crossed an *extinction threshold,* the point at which deleterious mutations accumulate faster than they can be eliminated by natural selection, which will also lead to population extinction.[26] Importantly, error catastrophe requires a fundamental shift in viral genotype that is independent of population size, whereas extinction threshold entails a major decline in viral population size.

Studies of RNA virus evolution based on the comparative analysis of gene sequence data have provided less support for the existence of quasispecies. Indeed, there is currently no clear evidence that selection acts on groups rather than individual variants in natural populations of RNA viruses, although this may reflect the fact that even with the most sophisticated tools of gene sequence analysis it is difficult to discern the effects of all but the most strongly favored and disfavored variants. For example, although natural selection is very commonly documented in HIV, the adaptive process always seems to involve the fitness advantage of individual mutants over others in the population, rather than group selection. Similar points can be made for other RNA viruses.[92] Again, though, it is arguable that natural selection is so strong in these cases as to obscure any quasispecies effect, and that the latter model is a far better description of mutations subject to weaker positive selection, as most natural selection will be in nature. This is clearly a major area for further study.

To conclude, given a sufficiently high mutation rate, quasispecies is a viable and extremely interesting evolutionary model. However, it is less clear whether the quasispecies concept can be successfully applied to RNA viruses in nature, where to date there has been no convincing evidence for its occurrence. This does not necessarily mean that the quasispecies model is wrong, but rather that too few RNA viruses have been studied in sufficient detail through deep amplicon sequencing and precise fitness assays to determine whether they form quasispecies, exemplified by a process of natural selection acting on the virus population as a whole.

PATTERNS AND PROCESSES OF VIRAL GENOME EVOLUTION

The Evolution of Virus Genome Size

Viruses possess a remarkable range of genome sizes (Fig. 11.12). This is especially so for DNA viruses in which genome sizes range from only 1,758 nt in *Porcine circovirus* (ssDNA) to a remarkable 1,259,197 nt in the case of the megavirus *Megavirus chilensis* (dsDNA),[9] hence covering approximately three orders of magnitude, although all ssDNA viruses have genomes less than 11,000 nt in length. A far narrower range of genome sizes is observed in RNA viruses. The smallest RNA virus currently known is *Ophiostoma novo-ulmi mitovirus* 6-Ld, at only 2,343 nt, while the largest RNA viruses are the coronaviruses and roniviruses (order *Nidovirales*), which have genome sizes of approximately 30,000 nt. Mean genome sizes in RNA viruses are around 10,000 nt. Interestingly, there does not appear to be a major difference in genome size between segmented and unsegmented RNA viruses,[92] with, for example, the unsegmented *Coronaviridae* and *Roniviridae* possessing larger genomes than all segmented RNA viruses. This strongly suggests that genome segmentation has not evolved as a way to increase virus genome sizes.

A variety of theories have been proposed to explain the evolution of genome sizes in viruses. One theory is that virus genome sizes are constrained by the maximum size of the

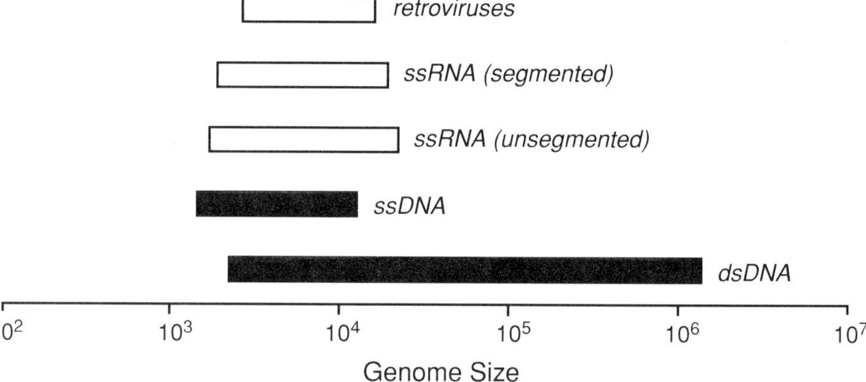

FIGURE 11.12. Distribution of genome sizes in RNA and DNA viruses. Note the similarity in (small) genome sizes between RNA viruses, retroviruses, and single-stranded DNA (ssDNA) viruses.

genetic material that can be contained within a single capsid protein.[238] However, the huge range of genome sizes, especially in DNA viruses, argues against this. The genome content of large DNA viruses in part reflects often frequent lateral gene transfer and gene duplication (see later). In particular, the central part of the genome of many large DNA viruses is composed of a set of core genes that control basic biochemical functions, including replication, while the outer, flanking genes distinguish individual viruses and are often responsible for modulating immunity, host range, and virulence, and it is these that have often been captured from host genomes. This process of gene birth and depth has resulted in a great variation in genome sizes, with, for example, a massive increase in genome size from the ancestral NCLDV to those circulating today.[105] This evolutionary process, combined with the discovery of the giant viruses of algae and amoeba, suggests that there are unlikely to be strict constraints against genome sizes in large DNA viruses. Similarly, that bacteriophages are able to transiently carry large parts of bacterial genomes, which evidently plays a key role in lateral gene transfer among bacterial species,[169] also argues against strict constraints on genome size.

However, it is also the case that certain structural features must constrain genome sizes to some extent. First, longer viral genomes are expected to cause an increase in replication times, which may be disadvantageous. Second, in the case of RNA viruses, it is possible that the difficulty in unwinding potentially long regions of dsRNA during replication inhibits the maximum genome size attainable.[186] For example, it has been argued that the unwinding of dsRNA in RNA viruses with genomes greater than 6,000 nt is controlled by the presence of a helicase (HEL) domain,[83] the evolution of which allowed RNA viruses to greatly increase their genome size.[82]

A more plausible explanation for the range of viral genome sizes is that they reflect background mutation rates. As noted previously, there is a fundamental relationship between mutation rate and genome size that seemingly applies to all living systems (Fig. 11.6). Accordingly, dsDNA viruses with relatively low mutation rates will be able to attain relatively large genome sizes, while the small genomes observed in RNA and ssDNA viruses reflect the higher error rates seen in these systems. Perhaps paradoxically, the idea that mutation rates set genome size can be extended to explain the very large (by RNA virus standards) genomes seen in the coronaviruses and roniviruses. The major part of the genomes of these families is composed of a large (greater than 20,000 nt) replicase gene that contains an ExoN domain encoding a 3′ to 5′ exoribonuclease. As this ExoN domain is homologous to cellular proteins of the DEDD superfamily of exonucleases that are involved in proofreading and repair,[154] it is possible that coronaviruses and roniviruses reduce their error rate through some sort of proofreading activity of the 3′ to 5′ exoribonuclease.[53] This, in turn, will reduce mutational load and allow larger genome sizes.

A final important difference between RNA and dsDNA viruses with respect to genome size is that the former (as well as ssDNA viruses) frequently utilize overlapping open reading frames, whereas these are less common in the latter (although, for example, the M065R and M066R genes of the poxvirus myxoma virus overlap by ~100 bp). Belshaw et al.[12] noted 819 cases of gene overlap among 701 RNA virus genomes; 56% of the viruses examined possessed some degree of overlap, which nearly always involved a +1 or −1 frame shift. In addition, RNA viruses with longer genomes tend to show less gene overlap than those with shorter genomes.[12] Although the exact evolutionary processes responsible for the evolution of overlapping reading frames are uncertain, they clearly allow an increase in the amount of protein diversity encoded by a single nucleotide sequence.

The Evolution of Genome Organization

It is arguable that viruses contain a greater diversity of genome structures and organizations than any other group of organisms. As well as the obvious division into RNA viruses, DNA viruses, and retroviruses, distinct genome structures include viruses in positive and negative sense orientations, those with single or double strands of the nucleic acid, those with single or multiple segments (which are usually multicomponent in the case of ssRNA+ viruses from plants), those that utilize subgenomic RNAs, and those like the coronaviruses that utilize ribosomal frame shifting. A key challenge for evolutionary virologists is therefore to explain why such a diverse array of structures exists.

One of the most debated issues with respect to the evolution of genome structures in RNA viruses is why some are segmented and others not. As noted previously, one theory for the evolution of segmentation is that it evolved as a way of facilitating reassortment, although this seems unlikely.[211] Similarly, there is no good evidence that segmentation allows the evolution of longer genomes. Another possibility is that genome segmentation, particularly in multicomponent viruses, resulted from the intracellular selection for smaller RNAs that, because they are shorter, would have had a replication advantage over their full-length counterparts.[163] However, this theory cannot easily explain why multicomponent viruses are nearly all restricted to plants.

A competing theory for the evolution of genome segmentation is that it allows greater control over gene expression. Clearly, all RNA viruses need to control the levels of each protein they produce. For many ssRNA+ viruses such control occurs at the level of translation as this is necessarily the first step in the virus life cycle. Additional constraints faced by viruses of this type are that eukaryotic ribosomes only recognize the 5′ regions of mRNA molecules, so that internal start codons are not utilized, and mRNAs are usually monocistronic.[92] Many ssRNA+ viruses therefore simply translate a single polyprotein that is proteolytically cleaved into individual protein products, which may represent the ancestral type of genome organization in ssRNA viruses. Although this genomic structure allows efficient replication, similar amounts of each protein product are produced, so that there is relatively little control over gene expression. As a consequence, other ssRNA+ viruses have evolved a variety of more complex ways to control gene expression, all of which can be envisioned as ways of dividing the viral genome into individual *transcriptional units,* within which transcription (and translation) can occur at different rates. Such a division can involve the creation of multiple genome segments, the utilization of subgenomic RNAs, and the use of a −1 ribosomal frameshift to produce multiple open reading frames as in the case of the coronaviruses and roniviruses[92] (Fig. 11.13).

The situation is rather different in the case of ssRNA− viruses. Because ssRNA− viruses by necessity transcribe their genomes before translating them, some control over gene expression can occur at the level of transcription; multiple mRNAs can be produced and there will be a transcriptional gradient from the first (i.e., 3′) mRNA, of which most is produced, to the last (5′) mRNA, of which least is produced. It is therefore possible that the ability to better control gene expression, itself through the control of transcription, represents the reason that negative-sense genomes evolved in the first instance. In this respect it is significant that the genomes of unsegmented ssRNA− viruses possess a highly conserved gene order, cluster together on polymerase phylogenies, and can easily be classified within the *Mononegavirales.* Moreover, this genome order seems to be a function of the amount of each

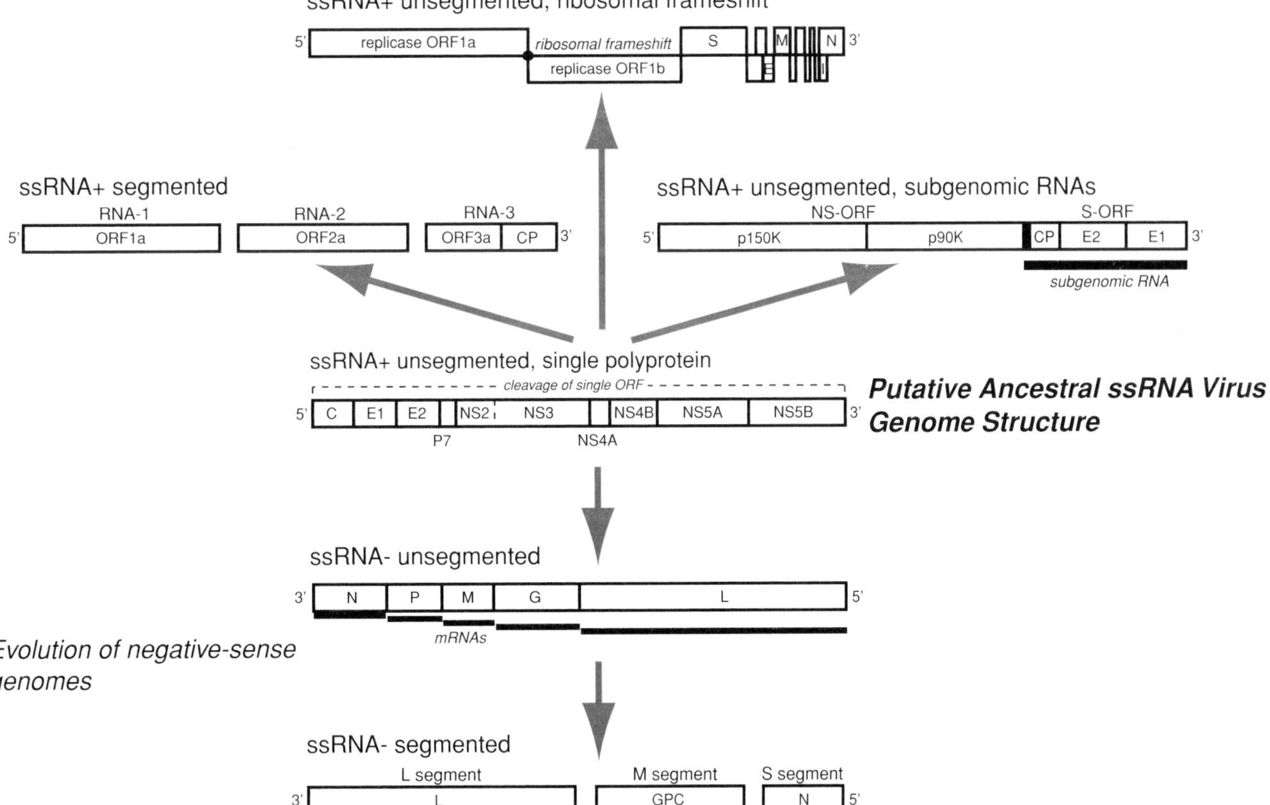

FIGURE 11.13. Schematic representation of the major types of genome organization and replication strategy in RNA viruses and a scenario for their evolutionary origin. Each of these organizations results in a different way to control gene expression, although they should not be considered as mutually exclusive. Unsegmented single-stranded RNA-positive (ssRNA+) viruses that produce a single polyprotein are considered here to be the ancestral type, although this is debatable. Gene and segment sizes are drawn approximately to scale within each of the six organizations, but not among them, and the 5′ and 3′ terminal sequences have been excluded. (From Holmes EC. *The Evolution and Emergence of RNA Viruses.* Oxford: Oxford University Press, 2009, by permission of Oxford University Press.)

protein product required, such that the 3′ gene encodes the nucleocapsid while the 5′ gene encodes the RNA polymerase, again suggesting that it is an adaptation to facilitate the control of gene expression.

Gene Duplication in Virus Evolution

One of the most important processes of genome evolution in eukaryotes is gene duplication. This represents an important way in which these organisms create evolutionary novelty; gene duplication is a simple way to create new genes that, following subsequent mutation and adaptation, can exhibit different but related functions, which often appear as multigene families. Because of the evolutionary importance of gene duplication in molecular evolution, it is important to determine its frequency in viruses. Such an analysis again reveals a major division between RNA and ssDNA viruses on the one hand and large dsDNA viruses on the other.

While gene duplication must be responsible for at least some of the genome size variation observed in RNA viruses, particularly during their early evolution, it is striking how rarely this process has been observed in RNA viruses.[92] An important caveat to make here is that because RNA virus evolution is so rapid and phylogenetic signals lost so quickly, it is possible that gene duplication has occurred more frequently in the past but that the footprints of this process are hidden by frequent multiple substitution. Those gene duplication events documented thus far in RNA viruses tend to occur as short duplications in untranslated or intragenic regions and often result in defective viruses.[29] Only occasionally have gene duplication events been described that produce two complete (and sometimes tandemly repeated) genes,[24,225] although improvements in computational analysis are likely to reveal more. The difficulties in analyzing divergent sequences notwithstanding, there are good reasons for the relative rareness of gene duplication in RNA (and ssDNA) viruses. In particular, given the size limit on virus genome discussed throughout this chapter, increasing genome size through gene duplication is likely to result in major fitness losses through an increase in the load of deleterious mutations.

The situation is very different in large dsDNA viruses, where cases of gene duplication, as well as gene loss, are a common observation and are evidently responsible for some of the size variation among viruses[100,200] (Fig. 11.14). Gene duplication can occur in both the core and species-specific genes of large DNA viruses as signified by the presence of related gene pairs and multigene families.[149] For example, gene duplication has been commonplace in the E4 region of some adenoviruses[43] and in the terminal inverted repeats of the poxvirus myxoma virus,[126] although many other examples exist. The process of gene duplication may also be related to that of recombination. For example, in some poxviruses recombination seems to have resulted in the duplication, inversion, and transposition of genes to opposite ends of the genome.[161] Finally, the analysis of protein structure suggests that some of these gene duplication events may have occurred in the distant past and assisted in the production of very distinct proteins, such as the head–tail connector protein and tail tube protein of bacteriophage lambda.[30]

Lateral Gene Transfer and Modular Evolution

A major way for bacteria to create evolutionary novelty is through lateral (or horizontal) gene transfer (LGT), which can sometimes result in genes being transferred for large phylogenetic distances.[169] As LGT will also result in an increase in virus genome size, unless the original gene is directly replaced by the invading gene (which is unlikely unless an exact excision is made, as faulty excision will result in deleterious mutants), it is not surprising that this process has to date only been rarely described in RNA viruses and ssDNA viruses, although it is again important to recall that inferences are compromised by extreme phylogenetic distance. One well-documented case of LGT in an RNA virus involves the acquisition by influenza C virus of the hemagglutinin-esterase (*HE*) gene of coronaviruses.[139]

Lateral gene transfer can occur among viruses and between viruses and hosts. In the case of RNA viruses there are sporadic reports of these infectious agents transiently incorporating host genome sequences. A famous example is provided by the integration of ubiquitin into the genomes of bovine viral diarrhea virus.[152] Similarly, the sequence similarity between the 65-kD protein of closteroviruses (ssRNA+) and the cellular heat shock protein hsp70[2] may indicate an early LGT event, while the capture of the ExoN domain by coronaviruses has been discussed in more detail earlier. In reality, however, there are few reports of the stable integration of cellular sequences into the genomes of RNA viruses, although more are likely to be documented with the acquisition of increasing numbers of host genome sequences.

In contrast, the capture of host genes is very well documented in the case of large DNA viruses, including those from

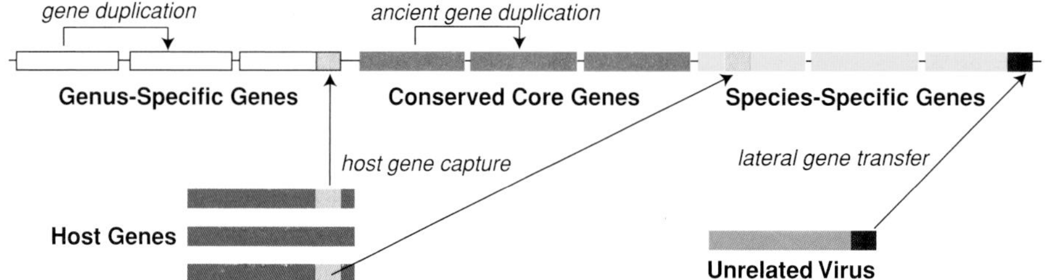

FIGURE 11.14. Processes of lateral gene transfer, from both hosts and other viruses, and gene duplication in large double-stranded DNA (dsDNA) viruses. Core viral genes, which are conserved across divergent taxa, are shown in red and often located in the central part of the genome. Genus and species-specific genes are shown as white and yellow, respectively, and more often located at the terminal regions of the genome. Refer to Figure 11.15 for a real data example. (Adapted from Shackelton LA, Holmes EC. The evolution of large DNA viruses: combining genomic information of viruses and their hosts. *Trends Microbiol* 2004;12:458–465.)

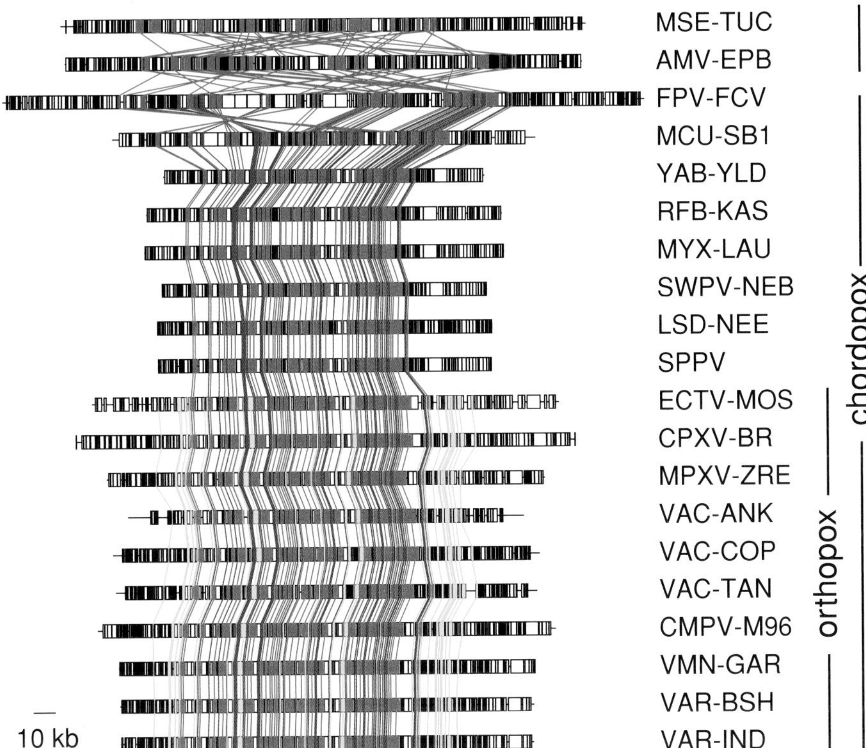

FIGURE 11.15. Comparative genomics of poxviruses. The figure shows a comparison of 92 gene families from 20 different poxviruses. Genes present in all the poxviruses analyzed are shown in red and are located in the central genomic regions. Those genes present in chordopox viruses only are shown in blue, while those present in orthopoxviruses only are shown in yellow. Vertical lines link orthologous genes. Horizontal differences are drawn proportional to genetic distances. (From McLysaght A, Baldi PF, Gaut BS. Extensive gene gain associated with adaptive evolution of poxviruses. *Proc Natl Acad Sci U S A* 2003;100:14960–14965. Figure kindly provided by Aoife McLysaght.)

both bacteria[173] and eukaryotes,[105] although the complex phylogenetic shadows cast by gene birth and gene loss means that it is sometimes difficult to determine from which host species and when these gene transfer events occurred. The poxviruses have been very well studied in this respect, with the interleukin-10 (*IL-10*) gene family and the vertebrate vascular endothelial growth factor (*VEGFA*) genes, which are distributed among both poxviruses and a range of vertebrates, as well as the DNA ligases, acting as good examples (and the IL-10 family is also observed in herpesviruses).[25,102,151] In fact, LGT is a common occurrence in all NCLDVs and covers an enormous taxonomic range of hosts.[66,105] For example, mimivirus may have acquired perhaps 10% of its total gene content from bacterial species, including a number of mobile genetic elements.[64] In poxviruses gene content seems to change more rapidly than gene order, reflecting the fact that species-specific genes tend to get added to the extremities of genomes (Figs. 11.14 and 11.15). That the flanking genes of large DNA viruses are often the ones captured by the host in turn suggests that internal gene orders are optimized to the extent that disrupting them may result in major fitness losses. Similarly, human herpesviruses contain homologs to such important immune genes as those that encode cytokines, chemokines, and complement system proteins, as well as those of the immunoglobulin superfamily.[145,183] These genes may modulate the immune response of the host, often by interfering or mimicking their cellular homologs. However, it is not only host immune genes that are acquired by dsDNA viruses. As a case in point, iridoviruses encode a number of cellular proteins that seem essential for virus replication.[220]

It is also the case that LGT has occurred among large DNA viruses and is particularly well documented in bacteriophage, where it appears to be a common mode of molecular evolution[86] (and phage-mediated LGT is of course a key process of bacteria evolution[169]), as well as in a number of eukaryotic viruses.[43] As another example, the entomopoxvirus *Amsacta moorei* virus (AMV) contains a number of genes that have been acquired from baculoviruses.[105] However, as with the case of LGT among viruses and hosts, it is often hard to pinpoint the exact origin and direction of any gene transfer event.

Less clear is exactly how viruses capture host genes. Although such an event could obviously occur through direct recombination, this would require entry into the nucleus and would result in virus genes containing introns. An alternative possibility is that complementary DNA (cDNA) copies of spliced cellular mRNAs, which do not contain introns, have been inserted into virus genomes, perhaps utilizing the RTs present in cellular retroelements.[200] On the other hand, LGT that occurs among viruses, or between viruses and bacteria, most likely occurs during host co-infections.

One of the most interesting developments in studies of virus evolution in recent years is the observation of segments of RNA virus genomes incorporated into host cellular genomes. For retroviruses that make dsDNA and enter the cell nucleus, as well as small ssDNA viruses that are so restricted in size that they do not carry their own polymerase genes and similarly must enter the cell nucleus, the presence of these integrated virus genes is perhaps not a surprise. Indeed, it has been known for many years that much of the eukaryotic genome was composed of endogenous retroviruses.[18,228] More surprising was the discovery that RNA viruses, which do not make a DNA genomic copy and often replicate in the cytoplasm, could also become integrated into host genomes (in the form of EVEs; see earlier). The first clear-cut case of virus-to-host

LGT to be documented involved sequences closely related to those of insect flaviviruses and found to be integrated into the genomes of *Aedes* mosquitoes.[42] Since this time a number of other examples have been discovered, including bornavirus,[97] filoviruses,[218] and rhabdoviruses,[113] often comprising a very wide range of hosts.[94] Similarly, EVEs have also been documented in a number of small DNA viruses, including circoviruses, parvoviruses,[15,111,136] and hepadnaviruses.[80]

As noted at the start of this chapter, the presence of these endogenous virus elements has changed our perspective of the time scale of virus evolution, indicating that some virus families may be far older than previously anticipated. However, these sequences raise other interesting questions, most notably by what mechanisms single-stranded RNA is converted into double-stranded DNA. The most plausible answer involves interaction with the cellular retroelements that are an abundant component of eukaryotic genomes, with the L1 long interspersed nucleotide elements a notable example[97] (Fig. 11.4). In addition, some EVEs appear to be more conserved than expected if they were evolving in a strictly neutral manner, free of all selective constraints.[113] As such, some of these endogenous virus copies may be of functional importance, perhaps because they confer resistance against related exogenous viruses.[8]

Finally, one process of genome evolution that is mechanistically similar to that of lateral gene transfer, and that has been of great historical importance in studies of virus evolution, is that of *modular evolution*.[22] This theory posits that viral genomes can be thought of as comprising a series of functional modules, such as those containing the capsid and the polymerase, that can be exchanged through recombination, and in doing so sometimes create entirely new viruses. For example, it has been suggested that some RNA viruses were created through a process of modular evolution.[88] In addition, there is evidence that recombination may occasionally reflect aspects of genome modularity in some small DNA viruses,[129,146] as well as some RNA viruses, which is compatible with a form of modular evolution. However, this pattern more likely reflects essentially random LGT across the viral genome with natural selection then filtering out those transfers that reduce fitness, which tend to occur at intragenic locations, rather than LGT occurring at specific genomic sites as specified in the original modular evolution model.[173] Similarly, although LGT is a common occurrence in dsDNA viruses, it is another thing to say that these transfer events involve distinct functional *modules*, rather than occasional genes, and there is as yet no good evidence that new DNA viruses have been created by LGT. In sum, the role of modular evolution in the generation of virus diversity remains uncertain.

REFERENCES

All cited references are available in the e-book.

1. Aaskov J, Buzacott K, Thu HM, et al. Long-term transmission of defective RNA viruses in humans and *Aedes* mosquitoes. *Science* 2006;311:236–238.
3. Ali A, Li H, Schneider WL, et al. Analysis of genetic bottlenecks during horizontal transmission of *Cucumber mosaic virus*. *J Virol* 2006;80:8345–8350.
4. Anderson JP, Daifuku R, Loeb LA. Viral error catastrophe by mutagenic nucleosides. *Annu Rev Microbiol* 2004;58:183–205.
5. Aragonès L, Guix S, Ribes E, et al. Fine-tuning translation kinetics selection as the driving force of codon usage bias in the hepatitis A virus capsid. *PLoS Pathog* 2010;6:e1000797.
7. Archer AM, Rico-Hesse R. High genetic divergence and recombination in arenaviruses from the Americas. *Virology* 2002;304:274–281.
8. Arnaud F, Caporale M, Varela M, et al. A paradigm for virus-host coevolution: sequential counter-adaptations between endogenous and exogenous retroviruses. *PLoS Pathog* 2007;3:e170.
9. Arslan D, Legendre M, Seltzer V, et al. Distant mimivirus relative with a larger genome highlights the fundamental features of Megaviridae. *Proc Natl Acad Sci U S A* 2011;108:17486–17491.
11. Bamford DH, Grimes JM, Stuart DI. What does structure tell us about viral evolution? *Curr Op Struct Biol* 2005;15:1–9.
12. Belshaw R, Pybus OG, Rambaut A. The evolution of genome compression in RNA viruses. *Genome Res* 2007;17:1496–1504.
13. Bell PJ. The viral eukaryogenesis hypothesis: a key role for viruses in the emergence of eukaryotes from a prokaryotic world environment. *Ann N Y Acad Sci* 2009;1178:91–105.
14. Belyi VA, Levine AJ, Skalka AM. Unexpected inheritance: multiple integrations of ancient bornavirus and ebolavirus/marburgvirus sequences in vertebrate genomes. *PLoS Pathog* 2010;6:e1001030.
15. Belyi VA, Levine AJ, Skalka AM. Sequences from ancestral single-stranded DNA viruses in vertebrate genomes: the *Parvoviridae* and *Circoviridae* are more than 40 to 50 million years old. *J Virol* 2010;84:12458–12462.
16. Benson SD, Bamford JKH, Bamford DH, et al. Viral evolution revealed by bacteriophage PRD1 and human adenovirus coat protein structures. *Cell* 1999;98:825–833.
17. Benson SD, Bamford JKH, Bamford DH, et al. Does common architecture reveal a viral lineage spanning all three domains of life. *Mol Cell* 2004;16:673–685.
18. Benveniste RE, Todaro GJ. Evolution of C-type viral genes: inheritance of exogenously acquired viral genes. *Nature* 1974;252:456–459.
19. Bernard H-U, Calleja-Macias IE, Dunn ST. Genome variation of human papillomavirus types: phylogenetic and medical implications. *Int J Cancer* 2006;118:1071–1076.
20. Bonhoeffer S, Chappey C, Parkin NT, et al. Evidence for positive epistasis in HIV-1. *Science* 2004;306:1547–1550.
22. Botstein D. A theory of modular evolution for bacteriophages. *Ann N Y Acad Sci* 1980;354:484–490.
23. Bowden R, Sakaoka H, Donnelly P, et al. High recombination rate in herpes simplex virus type 1 natural populations suggests significant co-infection. *Infect Genet Evol* 2004;4:115–123.
24. Boyko VP, Karasev AV, Agranovsky AA, et al. Coat protein gene duplication in a filamentous RNA virus of plants. *Proc Natl Acad Sci U S A* 1992;89:9156–9160.
25. Bratke KA, McLysaght A. Identification of multiple independent horizontal gene transfer events into poxviruses using a comparative genomics approach. *BMC Evol Biol* 2008;8:67.
26. Bull JJ, Sanjuan R, Wilke CO. Theory of lethal mutagenesis for viruses. *J Virol* 2007;81:2930–2939.
27. Burch CL, Chao L. Evolvability of an RNA virus is determined by its mutational neighbourhood. *Nature* 2000;406:625–628.
28. Burch CL, Turner PE, Hanley KA. Patterns of epistasis in RNA viruses: a review of the evidence from vaccine design. *J Evol Biol* 2003;16:1223–1235.
30. Cardarelli L, Pell LG, Neudecker P, et al. Phages have adapted the same protein fold to fulfill multiple functions in virion assembly. *Proc Natl Acad Sci U S A* 2010;107:14384–14389.
31. Chamary JV, Parmley JL, Hurst LD. Hearing silence: non-neutral evolution at synonymous sites in mammals. *Nat Rev Genet* 2006;7:98–108.
32. Chang GS, Hoon Y, Ko KD, et al. Phylogenetic profiles reveal evolutionary relationships within the 'twilight zone' of sequence similarity. *Proc Natl Acad Sci U S A* 2008;105:13474–13479.
34. Chao L. Fitness of RNA virus decreased by Muller's ratchet. *Nature* 1990;348:454–455.
35. Chao L, Tran TT, Tran TT. The advantage of sex in the RNA virus phi6. *Genetics* 1997;147:953–959.
36. Charleston MA, Robertson DL. Preferential host switching by primate lentiviruses can account for phylogenetic similarity with the primate phylogeny. *Syst Biol* 2002;51:528–535.

37. Cicin-Sain L, Podlech J, Messerle M, et al. Frequent coinfection of cells explains functional in vivo complementation between cytomegalovirus variants in the multiply infected host. *J Virol* 2005;79:9492–9502.
38. Codoñer FM, Daros JA, Sole RV, et al. The fittest versus the flattest: experimental confirmation of the quasispecies effect with subviral pathogens. *PLoS Pathog* 2006;2:e136.
39. Coleman JR, Papamichail D, Skiena S, et al. Virus attenuation by genome-scale changes in codon pair bias. *Science* 2008;320:1784–1787.
40. Comas I, Moya A, Gonzalez-Candelas F. Validating viral quasispecies with digital organisms: a re-examination of the critical mutation rate. *BMC Evol Biol* 2005;5:5.
41. Coulibaly F, Chevalier C, Gutsche I, et al. The birnavirus crystal structure reveals structural relationships among icosahedral viruses. *Cell* 2005; 120:761–772.
42. Crochu S, Cook S, Attoui H, et al. Sequences of flavivirus-related RNA viruses persist in DNA form integrated in the genome of *Aedes* spp. mosquitoes. *J Gen Virol* 2004;85:1971–1980.
43. Davison AJ, Telford EA, Watson MS, et al. The DNA sequence of adenovirus type 40. *J Mol Biol* 1993;234:1308–1316.
45. de Visser JA, Hermisson J, Wagner GP, et al. Evolution and detection of genetic robustness. *Evolution* 2003;57:1959–1972.
46. Domingo E, Sabo D, Taniguchi T, et al. Nucleotide sequence heterogeneity of an RNA phage population. *Cell* 1978;13:735–744.
47. Drake JW. Rates of spontaneous mutation among RNA viruses. *Proc Natl Acad Sci U S A* 1993;90:4171–4175.
48. Drake JW, Charlesworth B, Charlesworth D, et al. Rates of spontaneous mutation. *Genetics* 1998;148:1667–1686.
49. Drummond AJ, Pybus OG, Rambaut A, et al. Measurably evolving populations. *Trends Ecol Evol* 2003;18:481–488.
50. Duarte E, Clarke D, Moya A, et al. Rapid fitness losses in mammalian RNA virus clones due to Muller's ratchet. *Proc Natl Acad Sci U S A* 1992; 89:6015–6019.
52. Duffy S, Shackelton LA, Holmes EC. Rates of evolutionary change in viruses: patterns and determinants. *Nat Rev Genet* 2008;9:267–276.
54. Eickbush TH. Origin and evolutionary relationships of retroelements. In: Morse SS, ed. *The Evolutionary Biology of Viruses.* New York: Raven Press, 1994:121–157.
55. Eickbush TH. Telomerase and retrotransposons: which came first? *Science* 1997;277:911–912.
56. Eigen M. Self-organization of matter and the evolution of biological macromolecules. *Naturwissenschaften* 1971;58:465–523.
57. Eigen M. *Steps Towards Life.* New York: Oxford University Press, 1996.
58. Elena SF, Carrasco P, Daròs JA, et al. Mechanisms of genetic robustness in RNA viruses. *EMBO Rep* 2006;7:168–173.
59. Elena SF, Dopazo J, Flores R, et al. Phylogeny of viroids, viroidlike satellite RNAs, and the viroidlike domain of hepatitis δ virus RNA. *Proc Natl Acad Sci U S A* 1991;88:5631–5634.
60. Elena SF, Lenski RE. Evolution experiments with microorganisms: the dynamics and genetic bases of adaptation. *Nat Rev Genet* 2003;4: 457–470.
61. Elena SF, Moya A. Rate of deleterious mutation and the distribution of its effects on fitness in vesicular stomatitis virus. *J Evol Biol* 1999;12: 1078–1088.
62. Esposito JJ, Sammons SA, Frace AM, et al. Genome sequence diversity and clues to the evolution of variola (smallpox) virus. *Science* 2006; 313:807–812.
63. Evans DH, Stuart D, McFadden G. High levels of genetic recombination among cotransfected plasmid DNAs in poxvirus-infected mammalian cells. *J Virol* 1988;62:367–375.
64. Filée J, Chandler M. Gene exchange and the origin of giant viruses. *Intervirology* 2010;53:354–361.
65. Filée J, Forterre P, Sen-Lin T, et al. Evolution of DNA polymerase families: evidences for multiple gene exchange between cellular and viral proteins. *J Mol Evol* 2002;54:763–773.
66. Filée J, Pouget N, Chandler M. Phylogenetic evidence for extensive lateral acquisition of cellular genes by nucleocytoplasmic large DNA viruses. *BMC Evol Biol* 2008;8:320.
68. Firth C, Kitchen A, Shapiro B, et al. Using time-structured data to estimate evolutionary rates of double-stranded DNA viruses. *Mol Biol Evol* 2010;27:2038–2051.
69. Fischer W, Ganusov VV, Giorgi EE, et al. Transmission of single HIV-1 genomes and dynamics of early immune escape revealed by ultra-deep sequencing. *PLoS One* 2010;5:e12303.
70. Forterre P. The two ages of the RNA world, and the transition to the DNA world: a story of viruses and cells. *Biochimie* 2005;87:793–803.
71. Forterre P, Prangishvili D. The origin of viruses. *Res Microbiol* 2009;160: 466–472.
72. Froissart R, Michalakis Y, Blanc S. Helper component-transcomplementation in the vector transmission of plant viruses. *Phytopathology* 2002; 92:576–579.
73. Froissart R, Wilke CO, Montville R, et al. Co-infection weakens selection again epistatic mutations in RNA viruses. *Genetics* 2004;168:9–19.
74. Furió V, Moya A, Sanjaun R. The cost of replication fidelity in an RNA virus. *Proc Natl Acad Sci U S A* 2005;102:10233–10237.
75. Gago S, Elena SF, Flores R, et al. Extremely high mutation rate of a hammerhead viroid. *Science* 2009;323:1308.
77. García-Arriaza J, Manrubia SC, Toja M, et al. Evolutionary transition toward defective RNAs that are infectious by complementation. *J Virol* 2004;78:11678–11685.
78. Ghedin E, Fitch A, Boyne A, et al Mixed infection and the genesis of influenza diversity. *J Virol* 2009;83:8832–8841.
79. Gibbs AJ, Ohshima K, Phillips MJ, et al. The prehistory of potyviruses: their initial radiation was during the dawn of agriculture. *PLoS One* 2008; 3:e2523.
80. Gilbert C, Feschotte C. Genomic fossils calibrate the long-term evolution of hepadnaviruses. *PLoS Biol* 2010;8:e1000495.
81. Goldbach R, de Haan P. RNA viral supergroups and evolution of RNA viruses. In: Morse SS, ed. *The Evolutionary Biology of Viruses.* New York: Raven Press, 1994:105–119.
82. Gorbalenya AE, Enjuanes L, Ziebuhr J, et al. *Nidovirales:* evolving the largest RNA virus genome. *Virus Res* 2006;117:17–37.
83. Gorbalenya AE, Koonin EV. Viral proteins containing the purine NTP-binding sequence pattern. *Nuc Acids Res* 1989;17:8413–8440.
84. Gorbalenya AE, Pringle FM, Zeddam JL, et al. The palm subdomain-based active site is internally permuted in viral RNA-dependent RNA polymerases of an ancient lineage. *J Mol Biol* 2002;324:47–62.
85. Greenbaum BD, Levine AJ, Bhanot G, et al. Patterns of evolution and host gene mimicry in influenza and other RNA viruses. *PLoS Pathog* 2008; 4:e1000079.
86. Hambly E, Suttle CA. The viriosphere, diversity, and genetic exchange within phage communities. *Curr Opin Microbiol* 2005;8:444–450.
88. Haseloff J, Goelet P, Zimmern D, et al. Striking similarities in amino acid sequence among nonstructural proteins encoded by RNA viruses that have dissimilar genomic organization. *Proc Natl Acad Sci U S A* 1984; 81:4358–4362.
89. Hatwell JN, Sharp PM. Evolution of human polyomavirus JC. *J Gen Virol* 2000;81:1191–1200.
90. Herniou EA, Olszewski JA, O'Reilly DR, et al. Ancient coevolution of baculoviruses and their insect hosts. *J Virol* 2004;78:3244–3251.
91. Holmes EC. Molecular clocks and the puzzle of RNA virus origins. *J Virol* 2003;77:3893–3897.
92. Holmes EC. *The Evolution and Emergence of RNA Viruses.* Oxford: Oxford University Press, 2009.
93. Holmes EC. What does virus evolution tell us about virus origins? *J Virol* 2011;85:5247–5251.
94. Holmes EC. The evolution of endogenous viral elements. *Cell Host Microbe* 2011;10:368–377.
95. Holmes EC, Grenfell BT. Discovering the phylodynamics of RNA viruses. *PLoS Comput Biol* 2009;5:e1000505.
96. Hon CC, Lam TY, Shi ZL, et al. Evidence of the recombinant origin of a bat severe acute respiratory syndrome (SARS)-like coronavirus and its implications on the direct ancestor of SARS coronavirus. *J Virol* 2008; 82:1819–1826.
97. Horie M, Honda T, Suzuki Y, et al. Endogenous non-retroviral RNA virus elements in mammalian genomes. *Nature* 2010;463:84–87.
98. Huang AS, Baltimore D. Defective viral particles and viral disease processes. *Nature* 1970;226:325–327.
100. Hughes AL, Friedman R. Poxvirus genome evolution by gene gain and loss. *Mol Phylogenet Evol* 2005;35:186–195.
101. Hughes AL, Hughes MA. More effective purifying selection on RNA viruses than in DNA viruses. *Gene* 2007:404:117–125.

102. Hughes AL, Irausquin S, Friedman R. The evolutionary biology of poxviruses. *Infect Genet Evol* 2010;10:50–59.
104. Iyer LM, Aravind L, Koonin EV. Common origin of four diverse families of large eukaryotic viruses. *J Virol* 2001;75:11720–11734.
105. Iyer LM, Balaji S, Koonin EV, et al. Evolutionary genomics of nucleo-cytoplasmic large DNA viruses. *Virus Res* 2006;117:156–184.
106. Iyer LM, Koonin EV, Aravind L. Evolutionary connection between the catalytic subunits of DNA-dependent RNA polymerases and eukaryotic RNA-dependent RNA polymerases and the origin of RNA polymerases. *BMC Struct Biol* 2003;3:1.
107. Jancovich JK, Bremont M, Touchman JW, et al. Evidence for multiple recent host species shifts among the Ranaviruses (family *Iridoviridae*). *J Virol* 2010;84:2636–2647.
108. Jenkins GM, Holmes EC. The extent of codon usage bias in human RNA viruses and its evolutionary origin. *Virus Res* 2003;92:1–7.
109. Jenkins GM, Pagel M, Gould EA, et al. Evolution of base composition and codon usage bias in the genus *Flavivirus*. *J Mol Evol* 2001;52: 383–390.
110. Jenkins GM, Rambaut A, Pybus OG, et al. Rates of molecular evolution in RNA viruses: a quantitative phylogenetic analysis. *J Mol Evol* 2002; 54:152–161.
111. Kapoor A, Simmonds P, Lipkin WI. Discovery and characterization of mammalian endogenous parvoviruses. *J Virol* 2010;84:12628–12635.
112. Karlin S, Blaisdell BE, Schachtel GA. Contrasts in codon usage of latent versus productive genes of Epstein-Barr virus: data and hypotheses. *J Virol* 1990;64:4264–4273.
113. Katzourakis A, Gifford RJ. Endogenous viral elements in animal genomes. *PLoS Genet* 2010;6:e1001191.
114. Katzourakis A, Gifford RJ, Tristem M, et al. Macroevolution of complex retroviruses. *Science* 2009;325:1512.
116. Katzourakis A, Tristem M, Pybus OG, et al. Discovery and analysis of the first endogenous lentivirus. *Proc Natl Acad Sci U S A* 2007;104: 6261–6265.
118. Khatchikian D, Orlich M, Rott R. Increased viral pathogenicity after insertion of a 28S ribosomal RNA sequence into the haemagglutinin gene of an influenza virus. *Nature* 1989;340:156–157.
119. Kitchen A, Shackelton L, Holmes EC. Family level phylogenies reveal modes of macroevolution in RNA viruses. *Proc Natl Acad Sci U S A* 2011; 108:238–243.
120. Koonin EV. The phylogeny of RNA-dependent RNA polymerases of positive-strand RNA viruses. *J Gen Virol* 1991;72:2197–2206.
121. Koonin EV, Senkevich TG, Dolja VV. The ancient virus world and evolution of cells. *Biol Direct* 2006;1:29.
123. Korber B, Muldoon M, Theiler J, et al. Timing the ancestor of the HIV-1 pandemic strains. *Science* 2000;288:1789–1796.
124. Krupovic M, Bamford DH. Virus evolution: how far does the double beta-barrel viral lineage extend? *Nat Rev Microbiol* 2008;6:941–948.
125. Kryazhimskiy S, Dushoff J, Bazykin GA, et al. Prevalence of epistasis in the evolution of influenza A surface proteins. *PLoS Genet* 2011;7: e1001301.
127. Lai MMC. RNA recombination in animal and plant viruses. *Microbiol Rev* 1992;56:61–79.
128. La Scola B, Audic S, Robert C, et al. A giant virus in amoebae. *Science* 2003;299:2033.
129. Lefeuvre P, Lett JM, Reynaud B, et al. Avoidance of protein fold disruption in natural virus recombinants. *PLoS Pathog* 2007;3:e181.
130. Lehmann E, Brueckner F, Cramer P. Molecular basis of RNA-dependent RNA polymerase II activity. *Nature* 2007;450:445–459.
131. Leigh Brown AJ, Richman DD. HIV-1: Gambling on the evolution of drug resistance? *Nat Med* 1997;3:268–271.
132. Lemey P, Rambaut A, Drummond AJ, et al. Bayesian phylogeography finds its roots. *PLoS Comput Biol* 2009;9:e1000520.
133. Leppik L, Gunst K, Lehtinen M, et al. In vivo and in vitro intragenomic rearrangement of TT viruses. *J Virol* 2007;81:9346–9356.
134. Li H, Bar KJ, Wang S, et al. High multiplicity infection by HIV-1 in men who have sex with men. *PLoS Pathog* 2010;6:e1000890.
135. Li Y, Carroll DS, Gardner SN, et al. On the origin of smallpox: correlating variola phylogenics with historical smallpox records. *Proc Natl Acad Sci U S A* 2007;104:15787–15792.
136. Liu H, Fu Y, Xie J, et al. Widespread endogenization of densoviruses and parvoviruses in animal and human genomes. *J Virol* 2011;85:9863–9876.
137. Liu W, Worobey M, Li Y, et al. Molecular ecology and natural history of simian foamy virus infection in wild-living chimpanzees. *PLoS Pathog* 2008;4:e1000097.
138. Ludmir EB, Enquist LW. Viral genomes are part of the phylogenetic tree of life. *Nat Rev Microbiol* 2009;7:615.
140. Malet I, Belnard M, Agut H, et al. From RNA to quasispecies: a DNA polymerase with proofreading activity is highly recommended for accurate assessment of viral diversity. *J Virol Methods* 2003;109:161–170.
141. Malim MH, Emerman M. HIV-1 sequence variation: drift, shift, and attenuation. *Cell* 2001;104:469–472.
142. Maljkovic Berry I, Ribeiro R, Kothari M, et al. Unequal evolutionary rates in the human immunodeficiency virus type 1 (HIV-1) pandemic: the evolutionary rate of HIV-1 slows down when the epidemic rate increases. *J Virol* 2007;81:10625–10635.
143. Mansky LM. Retrovirus mutation rates and their role in genetic variation. *J Gen Virol* 1998;79:1337–1345.
144. Mansky LM, Cunningham KS. Virus mutators and antimutators: roles in evolution, pathogenesis and emergence. *Trends Genet* 2000;16:512–517.
145. Markine-Goriaynoff N, Georgin JP, Goltz M, et al. The core 2 β-1,6-N-acetylglucosaminyltransferase-mucin encoded by bovine herpesvirus 4 was acquired from an ancestor of the African buffalo. *J Virol* 2003; 77:1784–1992.
146. Martin DP, van der Walt E, Posada D, et al. The evolutionary value of recombination is constrained by genome modularity. *PLoS Genet* 2005; 51:475–479.
147. Marsh GA, Rabadán R, Levine AJ, et al. Highly conserved regions of influenza a virus polymerase gene segments are critical for efficient viral RNA packaging. *J Virol* 2008;82:2295–2304.
148. McGeoch DJ, Gatherer D. Integrating reptilian herpesviruses into the family Herpesviridae. *J Virol* 2005;79:725–731.
149. McGeoch DJ, Rixon FJ, Davison AJ. Topics in herpesvirus genomics and evolution. *Virus Res* 2006;117:90–104.
151. McLysaght A, Baldi PF, Gaut BS. Extensive gene gain associated with adaptive evolution of poxviruses. *Proc Natl Acad Sci U S A* 2003;100: 14960–14965.
152. Meyers G, Rumenapf T, Thiel HJ. Ubiquitin in a togavirus. *Nature* 1989;341:491.
154. Minskaia E, Hertzig T, Gorbalenya AE, et al. Discovery of an RNA virus 3′->5′ exoribonuclease that is critically involved in coronavirus RNA synthesis. *Proc Natl Acad Sci U S A* 2006;103:5108–5113.
155. Miralles R, Gerrish PJ, Moya A, et al. Clonal interference and the evolution of RNA viruses. *Science* 1999;285:1745–1747.
156. Mitton-Fry RM, DeGregorio SJ, Wang J, et al. Poly(A) tail recognition by a viral RNA element through assembly of a triple helix. *Science* 2010;330:1244–1247.
157. Montville R, Froissart R, Remold SK, et al. Evolution of mutational robustness in an RNA virus. *PLoS Biol* 2005;3:e381.
158. Moreira D, López-Garcia P. Comment on 'The 1.2-megabase genome sequence of mimivirus'. *Science* 2005;308:1114a.
159. Moreira D, López-Garcia P. Ten reasons to exclude viruses from the tree of life. *Nat Rev Micro* 2009;7:306–311.
160. Morse SS. Toward an evolutionary biology of viruses. In: Morse SS, ed. *The Evolutionary Biology of Viruses*. New York: Raven Press, 1994:1–28.
161. Moyer RW, Graves RL, Rothe CT. The white pock (mu) mutants of rabbit poxvirus. III. Terminal DNA sequence duplication and transposition in rabbit poxvirus. *Cell* 1980;22:545–553.
162. Murcia PR, Baillie GJ, Daley J, et al. The intra- and inter-host evolutionary dynamics of equine influenza virus. *J Virol* 2010;84:6943–6954.
163. Nee S. The evolution of multicompartmental genomes in viruses. *J Mol Evol* 1987;25:277–281.
164. Neher RA, Leitner T. Recombination rate and selection strength in HIV intra-patient evolution. *PLoS Comput Biol* 2010;6:e1000660.
166. Nora T, Charpentier C, Tenaillon O, et al. Contribution of recombination to the evolution of human immunodeficiency viruses expressing resistance to antiretroviral treatment. *J Virol* 2007;81:7620–7628.
167. Norja P, Eis-Hübinger AM, Söderlund-Venermo M, et al. Rapid sequence change and geographical spread of human parvovirus B19: comparison of B19 virus evolution in acute and persistent infections. *J Virol* 2008;82:6427–6433.
168. Novella IS. Contributions of vesicular stomatitis virus to the understanding of RNA virus evolution. *Curr Opin Microbiol* 2003;6:399–405.

170. Onafuwa-Nuga A, Telesnitsky A. The remarkable frequency of human immunodeficiency virus type 1 genetic recombination. *Microbiol Mol Biol Rev* 2009;73:451–480.
171. Pariente N, Sierra S, Lowenstein PR, et al. Efficient virus extinction by combinations of a mutagen and antiviral inhibitors. *J Virol* 2001; 75:9723–9730.
172. Parrish CR. Emergence, natural history, and variation of canine, mink, and feline parvoviruses. *Adv Virus Res* 1990;38:403–450.
173. Pedulla ML, Ford ME, Houtz JM, et al. Origins of highly mosaic mycobacteriophage genomes. *Cell* 2003;113:171–182.
174. Pepin KM, Wichman HA. Variable epistatic effects between mutations at host recognition sites in phiX174 bacteriophage. *Evolution* 2007;61: 1710–1724.
175. Perelson AS, Neumann AU, Markowitz M, et al. HIV-1 dynamics in vivo: virion clearance rate, infected cell life-span, and viral generation time. *Science* 1996;271:1582–1586.
176. Pietilä MK, Roine E, Paulin L, et al. An ssDNA virus infecting archaea: a new lineage of viruses with a membrane envelope. *Mol Microbiol* 2009; 72:307–319.
177. Plotkin JB, Kudla G. Synonymous but not the same: the causes and consequences of codon bias. *Nat Rev Genet* 2011;12:32–42.
178. Plyusnin A, Morzunov SP. Virus evolution and genetic diversity of hantaviruses and their rodent hosts. *Curr Top Microbiol Immunol* 2001; 256:47–75.
179. Powner MW, Gerland B, Sutherland JD. Synthesis of activated pyrimidine ribonucleotides in prebiotally plausible conditions. *Nature* 2009; 459:239–242.
180. Prangishvili D, Forterre P, Garrett RA. Viruses of the Archaea: a unifying view. *Nat Rev Microbiol* 2006;4:837–848.
181. Pybus OG, Rambaut A, Freckleton RP, et al. Phylogenetic evidence for deleterious mutation load in RNA viruses and its contribution to viral evolution. *Mol Biol Evol* 2007;24:845–852.
184. Rambaut A, Pybus OG, Nelson MI, et al. The genomic and epidemiological dynamics of human influenza A virus. *Nature* 2008;453:615–619.
186. Reanney DC. The evolution of RNA viruses. *Annu Rev Microbiol* 1982; 36:47–73.
187. Rector A, Lemey P, Tachezy R, et al. Ancient papillomavirus-host cospeciation in *Felidae*. *Genome Biol* 2007;8:R57.
188. Reiter J, Pérez-Vilaró G, Scheller N, et al. Hepatitis C virus RNA recombination in cell culture. *J Hepatol* 2011;55:777–783.
191. Sacristán S, Malpica JM, Fraile A, et al. Estimation of population bottlenecks during systemic movement of Tobacco mosaic virus in tobacco plants. *J Virol* 2004;77:9906–9911.
192. Salehi-Ashtiani K, Lupták A, Litovchick A, et al. A genomewide search for ribozymes reveals an HDV-like sequence in the human CPEB3 gene. *Science* 2006;313:1788–1792.
193. Sanjuán R, Cuevas JM, Furió V, et al. Selection for robustness in mutagenesized RNA viruses. *PLoS Genet* 2007;3:e93.
194. Sanjuán R, Elena SF. Epistasis correlates to genomic complexity. *Proc Natl Acad Sci U S A* 2006;103:14402–14405.
195. Sanjuán R, Moya A, Elena SF. The distribution of fitness effects caused by single-nucleotide substitutions in an RNA virus. *Proc Natl Acad Sci U S A* 2004;101:8396–8401.
196. Sanjuán R, Nebot MR, Chirico N, et al. Viral mutation rates. *J Virol* 2010; 84:9733–9748.
197. Sanjuán R, Moya A, Elena SF. The contribution of epistasis to the architecture of fitness in an RNA virus. *Proc Natl Acad Sci U S A* 2004; 101:15376–15379.
198. Sawicki SG, Sawicki DL, Siddell SG. A contemporary view of coronavirus transcription. *J Virol* 2007;81:20–29.
200. Shackelton LA, Holmes EC. The evolution of large DNA viruses: combining genomic information of viruses and their hosts. *Trends Microbiol* 2004;12:458–465.
202. Shackelton LA, Parrish CR, Holmes EC. Striking differences in codon usage bias and nucleotide composition among small and large DNA viruses. *J Mol Evol* 2006;62:551–563.
203. Shackelton LA, Parrish CR, Truyen U, et al. High rate of viral evolution associated with the emergence of canine parvoviruses. *Proc Natl Acad Sci U S A* 2005;102:379–384.
204. Sharp PM. Origins of human virus diversity. *Cell* 2002;108:305–312.
205. Sharp PM, Bailes E, Chaudhuri RR, et al. The origins of acquired immune deficiency syndrome viruses: where and when? *Phil Trans Roy Lond B* 2001;356:867–876.
207. Shriner D, Rodrigo AG, Nickle DC, et al. Pervasive genomic recombination of HIV-1 in vivo. *Genetics* 2004;167:1573–1583.
208. Simmonds P, Midgley S. Recombination in the genesis and evolution of hepatitis B virus genotypes. *J Virol* 2005;79:15467–15476.
209. Simmonds P, Smith DB. Structural constraints on RNA virus evolution. *J Virol* 1999;73:5787–5794.
210. Simmonds P, Tuplin A, Evans DJ. Detection of genome-scale ordered RNA structure (GORS) in genomes of positive-stranded RNA viruses: implications for virus evolution and host persistence. *RNA* 2004;10: 1337–1351.
211. Simon-Loriere E, Holmes EC. Why do RNA viruses recombine? *Nat Rev Microbiol* 2011;9:617–626.
212. Simon-Loriere E, Martin DP, Weeks KM, et al. RNA structures facilitate recombination-mediated gene swapping in HIV-1. *J Virol* 2010;84: 12675–12682.
213. Sniegowski PD, Gerrish PJ, Johnson T, et al. The evolution of mutation rates: separating causes from consequences. *BioEssays* 2000;22:1057–1066.
214. Smith DR, Adams AP, Kenney JL, et al. Venezuelan equine encephalitis virus in the mosquito vector *Aedes taeniorhynchus:* infection initiated by a small number of susceptible epithelial cells and a population bottleneck. *Virology* 2008;372:176–186.
215. Streicker DG, Turmelle AS, Vonhof MJ, et al. Host phylogeny constrains cross-species emergence and establishment of rabies virus in bats. *Science* 2010;329:676–679.
217. Switzer WM, Salemi M, Shanmugam V, et al. Ancient co-speciation of simian foamy viruses and primates. *Nature* 2005;434:376–380.
218. Taylor DJ, Leach RW, Bruenn J. Filoviruses are ancient and integrated into mammalian genomes. *BMC Evol Biol* 2010;10:193.
220. Tidona CA, Darai G. Iridovirus homologues of cellular genes - implications for the molecular evolution of large DNA viruses. *Virus Genes* 2000; 21:77–81.
223. van der Walt E, Rybicki EP, Varsani A, et al. Rapid host adaptation by extensive recombination. *J Gen Virol* 2009;90:734–746.
224. Vignuzzi M, Stone JK, Arnold JJ, et al. Quasispecies diversity determines pathogenesis through cooperative interactions in a viral population. *Nature* 2005;439:344–348.
226. Watts JM, Dang KK, Gorelick RJ, et al. Architecture and secondary structure of an entire HIV-1 RNA genome. *Nature* 2009;460:711–716.
227. Weaver SC. Evolutionary influences in arboviral disease. *Curr Top Microbiol Immunol* 2006;299:285–314.
228. Weiss RA, Mason WS, Vogt PK. Genetic recombinants and heterozygotes derived from endogenous and exogenous avian RNA tumor viruses. *Virology* 1973;52:535–552.
229. Wilke CO, Lenski RE, Adami C. Compensatory mutations cause excess of antagonistic epistasis in RNA secondary structure folding. *BMC Evol Biol* 2003;3:3.
230. Wilke CO, Wang JL, Ofria C, et al. Evolution of digital organisms at high mutation rates leads to survival of the flattest. *Nature* 2001;412:331–333.
231. Wittmann TJ, Biek R, Hassanin A, et al. Isolates of Zaire ebolavirus from wild apes reveal genetic lineage and recombinants. *Proc Natl Acad Sci U S A* 2007;104:17123–17127.
233. Worobey M, Telfer P, Souquière S, et al. Island biogeography reveals the deep history of SIV. *Science* 2010;329:1487.
234. Wright CF, Morelli MJ, Thébaud G, et al. Beyond the consensus: dissecting within-host viral population diversity of foot-and-mouth disease virus by using next-generation genome sequencing. *J Virol* 2011;85:2266–2275.
236. Zanotto PM de A, Gibbs MJ, Gould EA, et al. A reevaluation of the higher taxonomy of viruses based on RNA polymerases. *J Virol* 1996; 70:6083–6096.
238. Zhang Z, Kottadiel VI, Vafabakhsh R, et al. A promiscuous DNA packaging machine from bacteriophage T4. *PLoS Biol* 2011;9:e1000592.
239. Zhou J, Liu WJ, Peng SW, et al. Papillomavius capsid protein expression level depends on the match between codon usage and tRNA availability. *J Virol* 1999;73:4972–4982.

CHAPTER 12

Neal Nathanson • William J. Moss

Epidemiology

BASIC DEFINITIONS AND METHODS

Epidemiology deals with the occurrence of diseases in populations. Historically, epidemics of viral disease were recognized long before their causal agents were discovered, and viral epidemiology was one of the first aspects of the science of virology to be developed. Evolving insights into the pathogenesis and molecular aspects of virology have provided an increasingly rational basis for understanding the epidemiology of viruses. In this chapter, the biology of viral infections is used to explain the essentials of viral epidemiology.

Incidence and Prevalence

The quantification of disease occurrence is the cardinal feature of epidemiology. To accomplish this, the concept of rates was introduced, and rates have become the basic coinage of epidemiology (Fig. 12.1). Rates are fractions in which the numerator is the number of cases of disease and the denominator is a measure of the population. The *incidence rate* (also called the *attack rate* for acute infectious diseases) is used to quantify the number of new infections. A population and a time frame are defined, and the number of new cases in that population during that interval of time is counted. Note that the denominator includes both the size of population and time frame, and is often expressed as person-years (or any other standard interval of time; e.g., "thousand person-years" or "hundred person-weeks"). The incidence rate is then expressed as "cases per thousand person-years" or a similar term. Also note that the time element may be omitted in expressing incidence; the reader must then determine by context the time frame used.

Prevalence, technically not a rate but a ratio, refers to the total number of cases present within a specified time interval. Thus, the numerator in prevalence includes not just new cases but cases carried forward from the period prior to the specified time interval. When point prevalence is computed, a particular narrow time frame is selected, and the population recorded for that time frame constitutes the denominator. All cases "prevalent" on that date constitute the numerator. Prevalence is expressed as a ratio such as "cases per million"; note that there is no time parameter in this ratio.

Changes in incidence and prevalence may be divergent. A control program for human immunodeficiency virus (HIV) infection, for example, could decrease HIV incidence within a population through effective preventative measures but increase the prevalence of HIV infection through access to antiretroviral therapy and improved survival.

In epidemiology, consistency is a virtue. When cases and populations are counted prior to computing rates, care must be

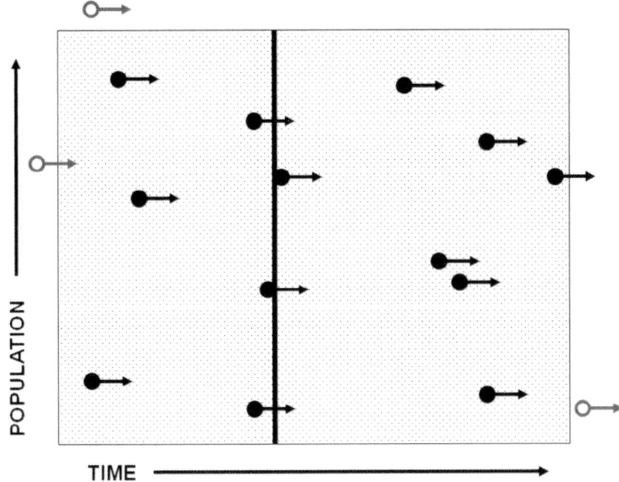

FIGURE 12.1. Computation of incidence rate and prevalence ratio. The *shaded area* defines a population and a time frame that can be expressed as person-time units. Cases of disease are indicated by *circles* (placed according to the date of their onset) and *arrows* for duration of illness. *Solid circles* would be counted for computation of incidence, whereas *open circles* would be excluded because they had onset outside the designated time frame or were resident outside the population boundaries. Incidence equals the number of cases divided by population-time units. Prevalence would be determined by a *single vertical line* across the hatched area: Cases active at that time point would be divided by the size of the population to compute the prevalence.

taken to use the same definition for numerator and denominator. Persons counted in the denominator should be at risk to be a case in the numerator if infected. For instance, if incidence is computed for the population of Philadelphia for 2011, a case hospitalized in the city but resident outside the city would not be counted. A case with onset in December 2010 but still ill in 2011 would not be counted as an incident case but would be a prevalent case.

What distinguishes infectious disease epidemiology from chronic disease epidemiology is that the former accounts for *dependent happenings,* a term introduced by Ronald Ross,[102] in which the incidence of a disease depends on its prevalence within a population.[45] Traditional epidemiologic and statistical methods that infer relationships between exposure and disease outcome assume that the outcome in one individual is independent of the outcome in other individuals, an assumption that is invalid for communicable viral infections.[54,82]

Sources of Data

In practice, the accurate collection of data for the computation of rates is often a major undertaking, whereas the computations are relatively simple. Furthermore, the practicing epidemiologist must frequently work with incomplete and inaccurate information. In most developed countries, denominator (population) information is usually good, and numerator (case) information is the major problem. In resource-limited settings, accurate population data may be unavailable.

For infectious (viral) diseases, there are several sources of case data. Passive surveillance denotes the continuous reporting of disease by healthcare workers. By law, many viral diseases are designated as "reportable," and in theory, the reporting of all cases is required. Cases are reported by practicing physicians, hospitals, or laboratories to local health jurisdictions, which in turn relay reports to a central state office whence they are transmitted to a national center (e.g., the U.S. Centers for Disease Control and Prevention). The weakest link is the initial report; in practice, only a small fraction of cases of many common viral diseases (such as 10%–15% of measles or hepatitis B cases) are reported to the national center (called the *reporting efficiency*). However, if the proportion of cases reported is consistent between geographic locales and between years, these reports may be used to monitor trends. Consistency is an important caveat, because the proportion of cases reported may increase if the absolute number of cases decreases. Changes in the case definition also may result in spurious changes in surveillance data. Reporting of certain rare or serious diseases, such as poliomyelitis or acquired immunodeficiency syndrome (AIDS), is often close to 100%; in such instances, reported cases can be used with much greater confidence for calculation of rates. Within increasing interest in the pandemic spread of respiratory viruses and the emergence of new zoonotic viral pathogens, global disease surveillance networks have been established to provide data on disease incidence and transmission in real time,[14] including the Program for Monitoring Emerging Diseases (ProMED) and the World Health Organization's Global Outbreak Alert and Response Network (GOARN).

Active case detection through epidemic investigation is the traditional approach to collecting information on outbreaks of disease. Such investigations are usually initiated by public health authorities but may be instigated by healthcare workers or patient families. The investigation is tailored to the situation and to the resources at hand, although experience has set certain guidelines, particularly for recurring outbreaks such as food-borne diseases. The purpose of such studies is several: (a) to classify the illness and determine the causative organism, (b) to assess the extent of the outbreak and its economic and health impact, (c) to abort the outbreak or prevent recurrent episodes, and (d) to inform or reassure the public. The first recognition of a new disease or isolation of a previously unknown virus has been accomplished as a result of an epidemic investigation. Examples are the identification of Lassa virus; Marburg virus; Sin Nombre virus (SNV), a hantavirus that is the cause of acute pulmonary syndrome; severe acute respiratory syndrome (SARS)-coronavirus; and the 2009 H1N1 influenza virus.

Serological surveys may be used to detect the footprints that a virus leaves in a population. Serosurveys are particularly useful for viruses because most viral infections leave an imprint on all infected individuals—that is, the presence of immunoglobulin G (IgG) antibody, which often is life long. Because many viruses cause asymptomatic infections or nondescript illnesses in addition to diagnosable diseases, serological surveys identify inapparent as well as apparent infections. Incident viral infection can be identified using assays for immunoglobulin M (IgM) antibody or antibody avidity, whereas IgG antibodies indicate prior infection or vaccination.

Cohort and Case-Control Study Designs

Modern epidemiology has made one outstanding contribution to the discipline—namely, the extension of hypothesis testing from the laboratory to populations. In general, the epidemiologist

TABLE 12.1 Hypothetical Data to Illustrate Computations for a Cohort and a Case-Control Study of Vaccine Efficacy

Group	2012 Cases	Population	Rate per 100,000 person-years	Relative risk
Cohort study[a]				
Vaccinated	100	1,000,000	10	0.33
Unvaccinated	900	3,000,000	30	
Group	**Cases**	**Controls**	**Odds**	**Odds ratio**
Case-control study[b]				
Vaccinated	10	25	10/90	0.33
Unvaccinated	90	75	25/75	

Vaccine efficacy = 1 − Relative risk = 0.67.

[a]Cohort study: Two populations, vaccinated and not vaccinated, are followed for 1 year, and cases occurring in each group are recorded. Rates are calculated, and the ratio of rates gives the relative risk for those who were vaccinated. In this instance, relative risk is lower for those with than without the attribute (immunization). The validity of this design depends on the assumption that vaccinated and not vaccinated groups would be at equal risk except for the attribute under study.

[b]Case-control study: A group of 100 cases and 100 controls are randomly picked to be representative of the groups from which they are drawn. Subjects in each group are classified as vaccinated or not vaccinated, and two ratios are computed: vaccinated cases/vaccinated controls and unvaccinated cases/unvaccinated controls. The odds of a case being exposed (vaccinated) and the odds of the control being exposed are used to compute the odds ratio, which provides an estimate of the relative risk. The validity of the case-control design depends on two assumptions: (a) the case and control groups are representative of the larger groups from which they are drawn, and (b) the number of cases is very small (<1/10) relative to the total population.

attempts to test the hypothesis that one or more population variables influence the occurrence of a specified disease and, if so, to quantify this effect and estimate confidence limits. There are two general designs used for such studies: *cohort* and *case-control* studies. The essence of these designs is summarized next, and the reader is referred to appropriate texts for methodological exposition.[35]

Cohort Studies

In a cohort study, which may be conducted prospectively or retrospectively, the population is divided into two groups, one with and one without a specified exposure or attribute. Both groups are followed prospectively for the *incidence* of the disease under study, and incidence rates for both groups are then computed. A hypothetical example is shown in Table 12.1. In this example, the population attribute is immunization against a specified viral disease, and the attack rate in the immunized population is one-third the rate in the unimmunized control group. The *relative risk* (RR) associated with immunization is 0.33, and vaccine efficacy is 67% [(1 − RR) × 100]. There is one important assumption underlying the validity of such a study: The immunized and unimmunized groups are at equal risk of disease. For various reasons, this assumption may not be correct. Differences in the risk of disease between two study groups may be minimized by random allocation of the exposure (in this case, the vaccine) when that is deemed ethical. However, random allocation of exposure is not possible unless the study is of an intervention. Stratifying each study arm according to parameters such as age, race, and socioeconomic status and then comparing rates for each subgroup can be used to identify inequalities between the two groups. Table 12.2 summarizes one such study of polio vaccine and documents the problems of comparing groups (in this instance, vaccinated and unvaccinated) that are not at equivalent risk of disease (in this instance, poliomyelitis).

More complex study designs are used to measure indirect effects of vaccines or other interventions that affect the transmission of viral pathogens. Such indirect effects include protection of non-vaccinated individuals through decreased transmission from vaccinated individuals, referred to as herd immunity.[27] Cluster randomized trials—for example, cohort studies in which communities rather than individuals are randomized to receive the intervention—allow direct measurement of the indirect effects of vaccines by comparing the risk of disease outcomes in nonvaccinated individuals residing in intervention and control communities.[44,46]

Case-Control Studies

Cohort studies usually require extensive resources and time because they necessitate the enrollment of large numbers of subjects who must be followed for a period of months or years; the less frequent the expectation of disease, the larger the population or longer the follow-up needed. Needless to say, the costs of prospective cohort studies can be great, limiting them to situations such as the introduction of a new drug or vaccine, as illustrated in Table 12.2. Case-control studies can be more cost-effective because they involve smaller numbers of subjects and do not require longitudinal follow-up, particularly if the disease outcome is rare. Table 12.1 shows a simplified version of such a study. In this instance, 100 cases of the study disease and 100 unaffected control subjects are identified and classified according to the exposure or attribute (vaccination) under study. For both vaccinated and unvaccinated individuals, an odds ratio is computed. Because, under certain assumptions, the odds ratios have the same relationship as the rates computed in the prospective study shown in the upper half of Table 12.1,

TABLE 12.2 The 1954 Field Trial of Poliomyelitis Vaccine: Comparison of Attack Rates for Vaccinated and Unvaccinated Children[a]

Study area	Vaccination group	Population	Paralytic cases	Rate per 100,000	Estimated efficacy
Placebo areas	Vaccinated	201,000	33	16	72%
	Placebo	201,000	115	57	
	Not inoculated	339,000	121	36	
Observed areas	Vaccinated	222,000	38	17	63%
	Controls	725,000	330	46	
	2nd grade, not inoculated	124,000	43	35	

[a]Vaccine was administered in the spring of 1954, and children were followed prospectively through the summer poliomyelitis season. Placebo areas were divided into volunteers who were vaccinated, volunteers who received placebo inoculations, and nonvolunteers (not inoculated). Observed areas were divided into second-grade volunteers (vaccinated), second-grade nonvolunteers (not inoculated), and first and third graders (controls).

From Francis T, Jr., Napier JA, Voight RB, et al. *Evaluation of the 1954 Field Trial of Poliomyelitis Vaccine. Final Report.* Ann Arbor: University of Michigan; 1957.

the relative risk can be estimated as the ratio of the two odds (0.4/1.2 = 0.33). Two assumptions underlie the validity of the case-control design and analysis, specifically the use of the odds ratio as an estimate of relative risk: The two samples (cases and controls) must be representative of the population from which they are drawn, and the incidence of disease must be low so that cases comprise less than 10% of the total population. Because case-control studies are particularly useful to study risk factors for rare diseases, the second assumption is usually correct. The main challenge in designing case-control studies is the choice of a valid and representative control group, a subject considered in depth in epidemiologic texts.[35]

BASIC BIOLOGICAL CONCEPTS

Susceptibility and Immunity

Many acute viral infections confer lifelong immunity. Upon re-exposure after initial infection, there is often reinfection but with minimal virus replication and an anamnestic immune response. Such reinfections are usually covert and almost never severe, resulting in minimal or no shedding of infectious virus. For certain viruses, such as poliovirus or rhinovirus, immunity is type specific and confers little protection against exposure to a different serotype. These simple facts have profound implications for viral epidemiology. For epidemiologic purposes, a population may be divided into three groups: susceptible, infected (and infectious), and immune. Persons infected at any time in the past may be considered immune (recovered) and are exempt from disease and unable to act as links in a transmission chain, whereas susceptible individuals can be infected, become infectious, and experience disease. This compartmentalization of the population is the basis for simple SIR (susceptible, infectious, recovered) models of virus transmission[4] that can explain the periodicity in incidence as the outcome of the buildup and decline of susceptible individuals.

Susceptibility may not be present immediately after birth. IgG antibodies are actively transported across the placenta, conferring protective immunity to neonates and young infants. For such viral infections, individuals move from a protected state to a susceptible one in the first year of life. Immunity can then be conferred by vaccination or infection.

Persistent viral infections differ from acute infections because the infected individual may be capable of transmitting infection over many years and may develop disease at any time during virus persistence. In the instance of persistent viruses, the population may be divided into uninfected susceptibles and immune-but-infectious persons who carry serological markers of prior infection but who are still capable of acting as links in the chain of infection. Important examples are hepatitis B virus, HIV, and several herpesviruses (herpes simplex virus, varicella-zoster virus, and cytomegalovirus) that establish latent infection capable of reactivation.

Parameters That Determine Incidence

For acute viral infections, the following three parameters determine incidence: the proportion of the population susceptible, the proportion of the population that is infectious, and the rate of contact between susceptible and infectious individuals, with *contact* defined as an encounter sufficient for transmission. The proportion of infected persons who become ill—the case infection ratio—determines the proportion of infected persons detected through case surveillance.

Proportion Susceptible

When a population is exposed to an infectious individual with a specific virus, the susceptible part of the population will determine the spread of the agent and account for all new cases. The proportion susceptible will reflect the past history of infection with the specific virus in the population and the past history of immunization for vaccine-preventable viral infections.

Proportion Infectious

The proportion of susceptibles who become infected, and subsequently infectious, during a fixed period of time (e.g., year or season) can vary widely, depending on the dynamics of transmission, which is influenced by the density of susceptibles and contact patterns between susceptible and infectious individuals.

TABLE 12.3 Estimated Case Infection and Case Fatality Ratios for Selected Viral Infections

Virus	Cases per 100 infections	Fatalities per 100 cases	Comment
Smallpox	>95	<1	Variola minor
	>95	25	Variola major
Measles	>95	0.1	United States, 1970
	>95	2	Africa, 1988
Poliomyelitis	<1	5	United States, 1955
Hepatitis B	50	3	United States, adults
	<1	<0.1	Taiwan, infants

Rate of Contact Between Susceptible and Infectious Individuals

The rate of contact between susceptible and infectious individuals determines the dynamics of viral spread within a population. This rate depends on the mode of transmission (e.g., respiratory, oral–fecal, sexual, or vector-borne), age-specific contact patterns or networks between individuals, and the distribution of susceptible and infectious individuals within a population. Spatial clustering of susceptible individuals can result in outbreaks despite a high proportion of immune individuals within the population.

Case Infection and Fatality Ratios

The proportion of infections resulting in overt disease—the pathogenicity of the organism—is characteristic for each virus and is strikingly different for different agents. One of the most important contributions of modern laboratory methods to viral epidemiology was the identification of inapparent or subclinical infections and the insight that most infections caused by some viruses were asymptomatic. The relative frequency of subclinical infections is expressed as the *case infection ratio*—that is, the number of clinical cases per 100 infections. The lethality of disease is a different parameter that represents the virulence of the organism and is designated as the *case fatality ratio.* The case fatality ratio is the number of deaths attributable to an infection per 100 cases. Table 12.3 lists selected common viral infections and shows estimated case infection ratios and case fatality ratios for each. It is noteworthy that there is no regular relationship between the case infection ratio and severity of illness (i.e., between pathogenicity and virulence). For instance, measles has a very high case infection ratio (>95:100) but a low case fatality ratio in developed countries (<1:1000 in the United States). Conversely, poliomyelitis has a low case infection ratio (<1:100) but a higher case fatality ratio (~5:100). Determining the case infection ratio is an important objective of outbreak investigations of novel pathogens, such as severe acute respiratory syndrome (SARS)-coronavirus and the 2009 pandemic H1N1 influenza virus. Typically, early in an outbreak, only cases that come to clinical attention are counted as incident cases, resulting in an underestimate of the true incidence. Accurate measurement of subclinical infection requires population-based surveys with laboratory confirmation (e.g., serological surveys).

Incubation, Latent, and Infectious Periods

The course of infection in a single individual can be conveniently divided into several periods.[29] The interval from acquisition of infection to onset of illness is the *incubation period.* Note that "onset of illness" must be explicitly defined for each disease and is often measured by the first day on which pathognomonic signs or symptoms are reported. The interval from acquisition of infection to onset of infectiousness is the *latent period.* For most viral diseases, the latent period is shorter than the incubation period. Consequently, the infected individual begins to shed virus prior to the onset of illness (smallpox is a notable exception) and continues to shed during and sometimes after recovery from the acute illness. The effectiveness of quarantine measures is reduced when the latent period is significantly shorter than the incubation period as the infectious individual goes unrecognized. The period during which the infected person is potentially infectious for others is the *infectious period.*

Incubation periods for any viral disease vary around the mean, as illustrated in Figure 12.2. When a frequency distribution of individual incubation periods is plotted, it usually has a longer tail at the high end of the distribution (right skewed). If the frequency is plotted against the logarithm of time, the data often approximate a normal distribution.[104] This log-normal distribution is characteristic of the incubation periods of many viral infections.[60]

Generation Time and Serial Interval

The average period between infection of an individual and transmission to others is the *generation time* or transmission interval. From studies of selected outbreaks, the average interval between onsets of successive waves of cases (called the *serial interval*) has been determined, and the generation time is often assumed to be equal to this interval as the best approximation available. This is because it is often impossible to know the exact time of infection. These relationships are shown in Figure 12.3 for a typical acute viral infection.

TRANSMISSION OF VIRUSES

There are two major patterns of transmission into which viruses may be classified: viruses maintained in a single species and viruses that alternately infect different host species. There

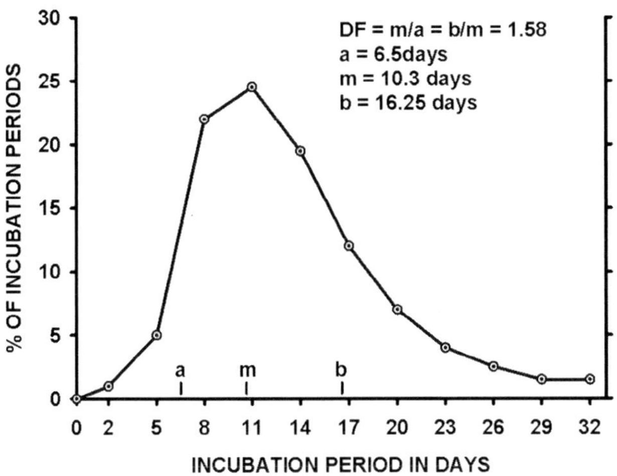

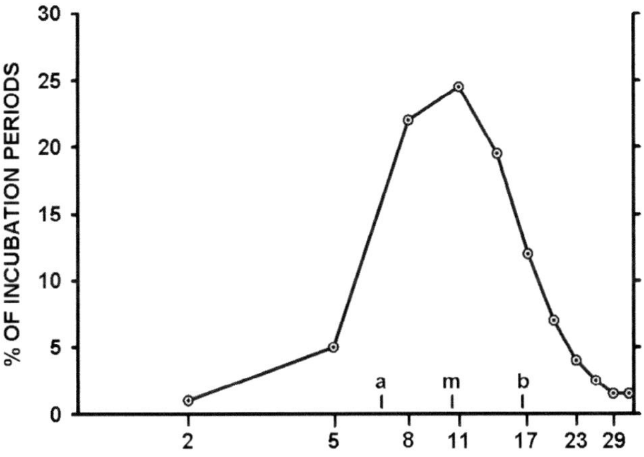

FIGURE 12.2. Log-normal distribution of incubation periods. Upper panel: Incubation period distribution is shown for poliomyelitis; there is a right-hand tail. **Lower panel:** The same incubation periods when plotted on a logarithmic scale. Logarithmic incubation period approximates a normal distribution, and the standard deviation may be computed (on the logarithmic scale). The dispersion factor (*DF*), a measure of the variation of incubation periods, is the antilogarithm of the standard deviation. The mean (*m*) is shown, together with the standard deviation (points *a* and *b* on the graph). The log DF equals the interval (log *m* to log *a*) or the interval (log *b* to log *m*). In this instance, *m* is about 10.3 days, *a* is 6.5 days, *b* is 16.25 days, and DF is 1.58—that is, about two-thirds of the incubation periods fall into the range (1.58 × mean) to (mean/1.58). (Data from Aycock WL, Luther EH. The incubation period of poliomyelitis. *J Prev Med* 1929;3:103–120; Casey AE. The incubation period in epidemic poliomyelitis. *JAMA* 1942;120:805–807; Horstmann DM, Paul JR. The incubation period in human poliomyelitis and its implications. *JAMA* 1947;135:11–14; Nathanson N, Langmuir AD. The Cutter incident. *Am J Hyg* 1963;78:16–28; and Sartwell PE. The incubation period of poliomyelitis. *Am J Public Health Nations Health* 1952;42:1403–1408, with permission.)

are a few apparent exceptions, such as rabies and influenza viruses, which spread across species boundaries; however, even in these instances, cycles of transmission between different species may be self-contained. For agents that infect humans, a second distinction may be made between those viruses that rely on human transmission for their perpetuation (the majority)

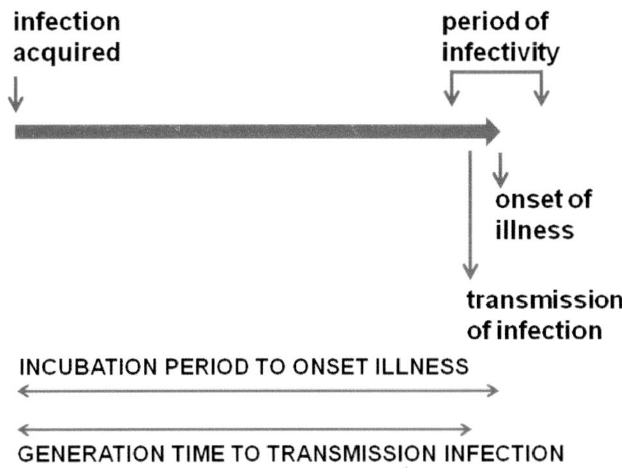

FIGURE 12.3. Incubation period and generation time. Incubation period is the interval between acquisition of infection and onset of illness, whereas generation time is the interval between acquisition of infection and transmission to another person. This diagram shows the mean for each parameter; in practice, there is a spread around this mean.

and those viruses maintained in an extrahuman cycle for which humans are a dead-end host. Examples of these patterns are set forth in Table 12.4.

Viruses Maintained Within a Single Host Population

Each virus has characteristic modes of host-to-host transmission: (a) direct person-to-person transmission through respiratory, fecal–oral, sexual, blood, or from mother to child, or (b) indirect transmission through fomites or vectors. Viruses that cause acute short-term infections require efficient transmission to subsequent hosts. Such infections are characterized by a relatively short infectious period and the excretion of high titers of infectious agent over a limited period of time, as in the instance of influenza, measles, and smallpox viruses. Viruses that cause persistent infections do not require such highly efficient modes of transmission, because they are excreted continuously or intermittently for many years and thus have a long infectious period to maintain virus

TABLE 12.4 Major Transmission Patterns of Viral Infections of Humans

Transmission pattern	Maintenance cycle	Example
Human to human	Human to human	Measles virus Hepatitis A virus Human immunodeficiency virus
Animal to human	Animal to animal	Rabies virus Hantavirus
Vector to human	Vector to human	Dengue virus Urban yellow fever virus
Vector to human	Vector to vertebrate	St. Louis encephalitis virus Western encephalitis virus

TABLE 12.5 Transmission Mechanisms of Human Viruses Maintained by the Person-to-Person Route

General category	Transmission mechanism	Example
Horizontal	Respiratory	Influenza virus
	Fecal–oral	Rotavirus
Vertical	Placental–fetal	Rubella virus
	Maternal parturition	Herpes simplex virus
		Human immunodeficiency virus
	Maternal breast milk	Human immunodeficiency virus
	Germ line	Unknown

transmission. Horizontal transmission is often used to designate these modes of transmission from person to person.

Vertical transmission is used to denote transmission between parent and offspring. Such transmission may occur during gestation, by passage of virus across the placenta (e.g., rubella virus and HIV); perinatally during birth (e.g., herpes simplex or hepatitis B viruses); or from the mother via colostrum or milk (e.g., HIV). Germline transmission, another mode of vertical spread, is seen with certain animal retroviruses such as murine leukemia virus, which are transmitted as an integrated provirus that may be transcribed into infectious virus. Although retroviral sequences are carried in the human genome, there are presently no proven instances where these have been shown to function as infectious virions. Selected examples of horizontal and vertical transmission are listed in Table 12.5.

Viruses That Alternately Infect Different Host Species

Arthropod-borne viruses (arboviruses) are usually maintained by continuously cycling between an insect host and a vertebrate host. In most instances, the virus replicates optimally in a single species or in a few closely related species of insects, which constitute the major, if not exclusive, vectors. Because most blood-feeding insects have a clear feeding preference for a few vertebrate species, this determines and limits the vertebrate species involved in the maintenance cycle. For some arboviruses, alternate maintenance cycles are limited to the insect host, with transovarial or sexual transmission from generation to generation of insects. These insect cycles may be critical to perpetuation of the virus during adverse conditions, such as overwintering, but otherwise play a minor role in viral dissemination.

There are only two arboviruses—dengue and urban yellow fever—of which humans are the major vertebrate host. In other instances, such as St. Louis encephalitis and La Crosse encephalitis, humans are accidentally infected when the vector mosquito happens to feed on humans as an alternate to the preferred vertebrate blood source, such as birds or woodland rodents.

Terminal Hosts

A *dead end* or *terminal host* is one not involved in maintaining viral transmission. Humans are occasional terminal hosts for several viruses maintained in extrahuman cycles. These include arbovirus infections, with the exceptions of dengue and yellow fever viruses noted earlier. In addition, there are several zoonotic infections, most notably rabies, in which humans are terminal hosts. Transmission of rabies is often by bite, although for most other terminal infections in this group (such as Korean and Bolivian hemorrhagic fever viruses), environmental exposure to fomites is responsible. Table 12.4 lists examples of viral infections in which humans are terminal hosts.

Transmission of Persistent Viral Infections

The transmission of persistent viral infections differs from that of classic acute infections. Those persistent infections that can become latent, such as the herpesviruses, are transmissible intermittently during periods of activation. Thus, one individual may be infected in childhood and transmit infection 50 years later during a recrudescence. The ability for a single link in the infection chain to extend over such an interval has important implications for perpetuation and eradication of infection. Infections such as those caused by hepatitis B virus and HIV, which are transmissible over many years, are often transmitted very inefficiently. Thus, hepatitis B is transmitted to susceptible household contacts at a frequency of less than 1 per 100 person-years exposure, and HIV is transmitted to sexual contacts at a rate of approximately 1 transmission per 100 to 1,000 contact episodes, with the risk of transmission directly correlated with HIV viral load.[36] For such infections, transmission requires passage of body fluids or of viable infected cells. Despite inefficient transmission, the number of new infections initiated by each persistent infection may be high because of the long infectious period. An epidemic curve caused by such a virus may stretch over years rather than weeks, and the mathematical modeling of such persistent viral infections is profoundly different from acute infections because infectious individuals are not rapidly converted to noninfectious immunes but continue to accumulate.[8]

Quantitation of Transmission and the Basic Reproductive Rate

The transmissibility of viral infections may be quantified by the basic reproductive rate (R_0), defined as the average number of new infections initiated by a single infectious individual in a completely susceptible population over the course of that individual's infectious period.[48] The reproductive rate of a pathogen is a function of pathogen characteristics as well as contact patterns within the community. Examples of R_o are 12 to 18 for measles virus, 5 to 7 for poliovirus and smallpox virus, and 1.5 to 2.0 for influenza viruses.[4]

R_o is determined by (a) the number of contacts between an infected individual and others, (b) the proportion of these contacts that are susceptible (assumed 100%), and (c) the probability of transmission per susceptible contact. The effective or net reproductive number (R) is the actual average number of secondary cases that occur and equals the product of R_o and the proportion of susceptible individuals in the population. R is smaller than R_o because not all individuals in real populations are susceptible, because of either prior infection or immunization. When R is greater than 1, the incidence of infection increases; when R is less than 1, the incidence wanes. When R equals 1, the number of infections is constant. Control programs aim to reduce R to below 1 to achieve disease elimination.

A simple mathematical expression that captures the three parameters for a directly transmitted pathogen is R = βXD, where β represents the transmission coefficient (a measure of the rate of contact between individuals and the likelihood of transmission during that contact per unit time), X is the proportion of susceptible individuals, and D is the duration of infectiousness. As can be seen from this simple formulation, elimination of a viral infection could be achieved by reducing effective contacts (e.g., quarantine), reducing the proportion of susceptible individuals (e.g., through vaccination), or reducing the infectious period (e.g., treatment to reduce viral load).

Modeling Viral Dynamics

Mathematical models of viral dynamics with varying degrees of sophistication are widely used by infectious disease epidemiologists to understand temporal and spatial patterns of virus transmission within populations and to evaluate the potential impact of control strategies. Mathematical models help to quantify our understanding of infectious disease dynamics and can be used to assess interventions for which epidemiologic studies are not feasible or ethical (e.g., strategies to contain a smallpox outbreak as a result of bioterrorism).[54] The use of mathematical models in infectious disease epidemiology has a long history, with one of the earliest successful approaches being the model of malaria transmission dynamics developed by Sir Ronald Ross in the early 20th century.[103] Subsequent models of infectious disease dynamics were developed by Wade Hampton Frost and Lowell Reed (the Reed-Frost model), in which the incidence of newly infected persons was based on the probability of contact between susceptible and infectious hosts.[2] The models developed by W. O. Kermack and A. G. McKendrick were the first to divide the population into the three classes of individuals discussed earlier (susceptibles, infectious, and recovered; hence, SIR models) and estimated the number of new infections as a function of the number of susceptible and infectious individuals.[52] These deterministic, compartmental models (based on difference or differential equations depending on whether time is treated as a discrete or continuous variable) were expanded and popularized by Roy Anderson and Robert May[4] and became the basis for much infectious disease modeling. Variations on the basic SIR model include the addition of other compartments or classes of individuals (e.g., infected but not infectious or a period of maternally acquired protection), age-specific contact patterns, and stochastic processes. Useful models balance the goals of realism and simplicity, as more complex models require a greater number of underlying assumptions and parameter estimates. Useful models clarify our conceptual framework of viral transmission dynamics, suggest which variables are most important for transmission and require careful measurement, and generate new hypotheses. In addition, models can be used to estimate the likely size of an epidemic, its time course and periodicity, the reproductive number R, and the expected impact of various interventions. Finally, model validation against epidemiologic data is a critical component of model building and use.

Measles has long been a favored disease by infectious disease modelers because of the simple transmission dynamics and the long time series available as a result of the readily distinguishable clinical characteristics. Mathematical models of measles virus transmission allow for exploration of the impact of various vaccination strategies, including the optimum age at measles vaccination and the use of mass vaccination campaigns,[59,74] that would otherwise be difficult to evaluate in epidemiologic studies. Model results suggest that the best age at which to vaccinate against measles depends critically on the age distribution of cases of infection prior to the introduction of control measures,[74] the introduction of mass vaccination will induce a temporary phase of low incidence of infection before the system settles to a new pattern of recurrent epidemics,[74] and that frequent, relatively low coverage mass vaccination campaigns are effective in reducing measles virus transmission.[59]

DESCRIPTIVE EPIDEMIOLOGY

A hallowed maxim in epidemiology is that a complete description of epidemic or endemic disease must include the parameters person, place, and time. The collection and display of this descriptive information is a necessary first step in understanding the epidemiologic mechanisms leading to occurrence, distribution, and course of an epidemic. This simple, systematic approach is a surprisingly powerful tool in analysis. A few selected examples are presented in this section to demonstrate the application of descriptive epidemiology to the understanding of virus transmission.

Person

In tabulating cases of viral infection, the epidemiologist looks for features that distinguish affected persons from the general population to identify risk factors for infection and disease. Clues may exist in demographic features and behavioral characteristics, such as age, sex, race, occupation, residence, or any aspect of personal conduct. Such variables are frequently the most important initial step in understanding an outbreak.

The first recognized outbreak of St. Louis encephalitis in 1933 involved a classical exercise in "shoe leather" epidemiology,[69] the finding of which led to the proposal that the disease was transmitted by an arthropod vector rather than by person-to-person contact. When this outbreak occurred, neither the disease nor the causal agent was known. Because it was an acute neurological disease, occurring in the summer, it was first thought to be a form of poliomyelitis or to be transmitted in the same manner through the fecal–oral route. The characteristic encephalitic manifestations made it relatively easy to identify many of the cases clinically. When these cases were assembled, and rates estimated, it became apparent that the incidence was greater in the suburbs of St. Louis than in the city proper. Furthermore, there was a striking concentration of cases among the inhabitants of one institution located in the suburbs; however, a comparison of several adjacent institutions revealed even more dramatic discrepancies, illustrated in Table 12.6. First, there were no cases in the personnel in an infectious disease hospital caring for many acute encephalitis cases—strong evidence against person-to-person transmission. Second, there were high rates in an almshouse but very low rates in two insane asylums. Investigation revealed that the almshouse lacked screens, whereas the other three institutions were screened. These observations were strongly reminiscent of the classic findings of the Reed commission investigating yellow fever in Havana[98] and suggested mosquito transmission. Finally, it was observed that the suburbs of St. Louis, although home to many affluent residents, lacked the system of storm

TABLE 12.6 Attack Rates for St. Louis Encephalitis in Four Institutions in the Suburbs of St. Louis During the Epidemic of 1933[a]

Institution	Population	Cases	Rate per 100,000
Mental hospital	400	0	—
Hospital for the insane	4,000	0	—
Isolation hospital	500	0	—
Almshouse (infirmary)	1,200	13	10,800

[a]Of these four institutions, three had adequate screening, whereas one (infirmary) did not. The isolation hospital cared for 300 patients with St. Louis encephalitis, but no cases occurred among the staff, estimated at 500.

From Lumsden LL. St. Louis encephalitis in 1933: observations on epidemiological features. *Public Health Rep* 1958;73:340–353.

sewers present in the city. More sites with standing groundwater existed in the suburbs, and in the hot, dry summer of 1933, these sites were prime mosquito breeding sites. These observations suggested the mechanisms of transmission to the investigating epidemiologists.

The "Cutter incident" offers another example where descriptive epidemiology defined an unusual distribution of disease in a population, leading directly to the cause.[86] In mid-April 1955, newly approved inactivated poliomyelitis vaccine was distributed throughout the United States for immunization of children 5 to 9 years of age—the age group considered the highest risk and therefore given preference in the utilization of limited vaccine supplies. About 2 weeks later, at the end of April, reports were received of cases of acute paralytic poliomyelitis occurring in a small number of recently immunized children. Because this was close to the seasonal trough in poliomyelitis incidence, relatively few cases of poliomyelitis were occurring in the general population, thus a small number of vaccine-associated cases were particularly striking. Furthermore, vaccine-associated cases were confined to a few of the western states. It quickly became apparent that this geographic distribution was related to the manufacturer of vaccine. Vaccine had been produced by five manufacturers, and most cases were associated with vaccine produced by Cutter Laboratories, which produced the vaccine mainly used in western states. When rates were tabulated for different production pools of Cutter vaccine, the association focused on two high rate pools, as indicated in Table 12.7. Subsequent investigations showed that there were inadequacies in the inactivation and safety testing protocols recommended by the government, permitting the release of vaccine lots containing residual infectious virulent virus.

Age Distribution

The age distribution of viral infection reflects differences in risk. For many endemic human viruses, the cumulative incidence of infection reaches 100% of the population. In such instances, disease is confined to children or to children and young adults, because older individuals are immune as a result of prior subclinical or apparent infection. Poliomyelitis prior to the introduction of vaccine is such an example, and differences in age distribution of disease in different regions or in the same population in different eras reflect differing transmission rates.[87] Where this enterovirus is transmitted readily, cases are confined to young children; contrariwise, in countries with more rigorous personal hygiene, infection may be delayed so that poliomyelitis occurs up to age 30 or older.[84] Figure 12.4 compares these age distributions and shows the parallelism with the acquisition of immunity.

For viruses that never infect more than a small proportion of a population, the age distribution of cases reflects differences in exposure or case infection ratio rather than immunity. An example is St. Louis encephalitis, which produces unpredictable outbreaks in different areas of the central United States and is infrequent enough so that most of all age groups are susceptible. Attack rates are typically lower in children and higher in the elderly (10-fold differences). A classic investigation of an epidemic in Houston, Texas, showed that, surprisingly, the frequency of infection was very similar for all ages, indicating that age-specific differences in the case infection ratio accounted for age-specific clinical attack rates.[95]

Age-specific differences in case infection ratios can be a key determinant of epidemiologic patterns of disease. In some instances, infants experience much more severe disease than do adults. A classical example is the outbreak of measles that

TABLE 12.7 The Cutter Incident: Attack Rates Among Children Receiving Cutter Vaccine According to Production Pool, United States, Spring 1955[a]

Production pool	Number of inoculations	Paralytic poliomyelitis cases	Rates per 100,000
468	73,700	34	46.1
746	48,000	17	35.4
460	34,100	0	—
463	63,400	1	1.5
467	56,700	1	1.8
762	54,400	1	1.8
766	57,200	0	—
767	3,100	0	—

[a]Cutter vaccine was administered April 18 through 27, and this table is limited to cases with onset between April 18 and May 14, 1955.

From Nathanson N, Langmuir AD. The Cutter incident. *Am J Hyg* 1963;78:16–28.

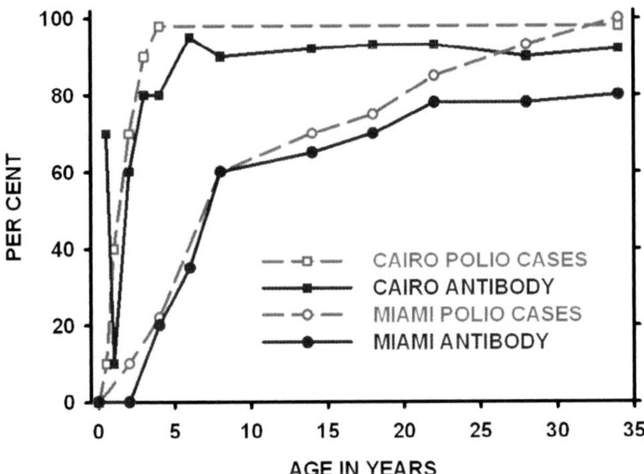

FIGURE 12.4. Age distribution of poliomyelitis cases and immunity. A comparison of cumulative distribution of cases of poliomyelitis and prevalence of antibodies to type 2 poliovirus in two populations, Cairo and Miami, to show that the age distribution of cases reflects the ages at which infection is acquired. There are few cases above age 3 years in Cairo and above age 30 years in Miami—the ages at which cumulative infection prevalence reaches 100%. (Data from Paul JR. Epidemiology of poliomyelitis. In: *Poliomyelitis*. Geneva: World Health Organization; 1955:9.)

occurred in the Faroe Islands in 1846.[93] Because measles had not occurred in this isolated site for more than 50 years, women of childbearing age were seronegative, and their infants lacked maternal antibody. During the epidemic, the case fatality ratio was about 20% in infants and below 1% in children and young adults (Table 12.8). This episode illustrates the biological role of passively acquired maternal antibody. On the other hand, hepatitis B virus causes inapparent but persistent infection in infants but acute liver disease followed by immunity in adults. In developing countries, infections are frequently transmitted from persistently infected mothers to their newborns, whereas infection in developed countries is mainly transmitted to older children and adults. These differences account for the paradox that the attack rates for hepatitis B are higher in developed countries, whereas cumulative infection rates are much higher and the virus carrier state is more frequent in developing countries, as illustrated in Table 12.9.

Networks

In addition to identifying individual characteristics associated with viral infection or disease, epidemiologists increasingly are interested in transmission networks critical to the dynamics of viral infections within populations.[68] Network theory and analysis is a complex subject with a long history in mathematics and sociology but has recently been developed by infectious disease epidemiologists, in part because of the ability to characterize complex social networks, such as large-scale social and sexual networks.[62] The epidemiologic study of social networks is facilitated by unique sampling strategies, including snowball sampling or respondent-driven sampling in which study participants are asked to recruit additional participants among their social contacts. For example, concurrent partnerships (as opposed to serial monogamy) can amplify the spread of HIV and other sexually transmitted infections.[78] Social networks were shown to affect transmission of 2009 H1N1 influenza virus and were responsible for cyclical patterns of transmission between the school, community, and household.[15]

Place

Historically, mapping the distribution of disease preceded the development of epidemiology and became more significant with the introduction of place-specific rates. A famous example is John Snow's mapping of cholera cases during the Broad Street outbreak in London. Mapping spatial patterns of disease distribution remains one of the most powerful and intriguing aspects of descriptive epidemiology and has been enhanced by remote sensing technologies[101] and sophisticated spatial analysis tools, including patch and network models.[100]

TABLE 12.8 Age-Specific Mortality Rates on the Faroe Islands During the Measles Epidemic of 1846 Compared to Years 1835–1845[a]

	Annual mortality per 100		
Age group (Years)	**1835–1845**	**1846**	**Excess in 1846**
<1	10.8	30.0	19.2
1–9	0.5	0.5	—
10–19	0.5	0.4	—
20–29	0.5	0.7	0.2
30–39	0.8	2.1	1.3
40–49	1.1	2.7	1.6
50–59	0.9	4.4	3.5
60–69	2.0	7.7	5.7
70–79	6.5	13.1	6.6
80–100	16.8	26.0	9.2

[a]The mortality for 1846 is for January through August, the period of the epidemic. The excess mortality provides a crude estimate of measles-specific mortality during the epidemic. At least 80% of the population had measles during the epidemic, which was the first to occur since 1781.

From Panum PL. *Observations Made During the Epidemic of Measles on the Faroe Islands in the Year 1846*. New York: Delta Omega Society; 1940.

TABLE 12.9 Prevalence of Hepatitis B in the United States and in Taiwan, Measured by Anti-HBs and HBs Antigenemia[a]

Population	Age group (Years)	Anti-HBs (%)	HBs (%)
New York City blood donors (white)	<25	2	<0.1
	25–34	4	0.2
	35–44	3	0.2
	>44	8	<0.1
Taiwan (Chinese)	<10	28	23.0
	10–19	50	20.0
	20–29	48	18.0
	30–39	52	16.0
	40–49	48	15.0
	50–59	48	15.0
	60–69	48	10.0
	>69	48	7.0

Anti-HBs, hepatitis B antibodies; HBs, hepatitis B surface antigen.

[a]The prevalence of antibody and antigen expressed as a percentage of those tested.

From Szmuness W, Harley EJ, Ikram H, et al. Sociodemographic aspects of the epidemiology of hepatitis. In: Vyas GN, ed. *Viral Hepatitis*. Philadelphia: Franklin Institute Press; 1978:297–320.

Two outbreaks of St. Louis encephalitis in two cities of Texas illustrate the complexities of geographic epidemiology. A large outbreak in Houston in 1964 was concentrated in the center of the city with decreasing rates toward the outskirts (Table 12.10). Subsequent serological surveys showed that infection rates paralleled cases and also showed that high rates were associated with the lowest economic strata, open foundations, unscreened windows, and lack of air-conditioning, as well as with areas of standing water close to the banks of the river that flowed through center city. Conversely, in Corpus Christi, attack rates were highest in the suburbs, as shown in Table 12.11. In Corpus Christi, the determining factor was mosquito breeding in pools of standing water associated with lack of a storm sewer system rather than with reduced protection from mosquito attack.

Spatial Patterns and Traveling Waves

Spatial patterns of viral infections are not static but display complex dynamics,[100] one of which is traveling waves of transmission. Measles virus transmission was shown to exhibit spatiotemporal traveling wave patterns in England and Wales, with regional movement from large cities to small towns.[39] The incidence of dengue hemorrhagic fever, a mosquito-borne disease caused by dengue virus, in Thailand was characterized by a spatiotemporal traveling wave emanating from the capital Bangkok.[18] The spatiotemporal dynamics of rotavirus infection in the United States prior to the introduction of rotavirus vaccine, which typically started in the Southwest in late fall and ended in the Northeast 3 months later, was explained by spatiotemporal variation in birth rates and thus the introduction of susceptible hosts.[96]

Time

Seasonality

Many acute viral infections exhibit striking seasonal patterns in incidence.[30] In temperate climates, some viral infections peak in the winter, whereas others peak in the summer. In general, respiratory infections spread more readily in the winter, although they may peak at different times. Conversely, the incidence of enteroviral infections peak in the summer, although rotaviruses are a striking exception, as noted earlier. Arbovirus infections are confined to the summer months, when their vectors are active.

TABLE 12.10 Regional and Socioeconomic Differences in Attack Rates (per 100,000) for St. Louis Encephalitis, Houston, Texas, 1964[a]

Circle	White upper class	White middle class	White lower class	Nonwhite	Totals
1 (innermost)	—	70	102	77	77
2	34	73	51	50	50
3	14	20	30	20	20
4	2	10	6	7	7
5 (outermost)	3	8	—	6	6

[a]The city was divided into concentric circles and into socioeconomically and racially stratified census tracts within each circle prior to computation of rates.

From Luby JP. St. Louis encephalitis. *Epidemiol Rev* 1979;1:55–73.

TABLE 12.11 Regional and Socioeconomic Differences in Attack Rates for St. Louis Encephalitis, Corpus Christi, Texas, 1966[a]

Circle	Socioeconomic stratum	Population	Cases	Rates per 100,000
4 (innermost)	Lower	46,000	5	11
3	Lower middle	49,000	19	39
2	Upper middle	45,000	20	63
1 (outermost)	Upper	46,000	24	52

[a]The city was divided into four zones; zones 4 and 3 were concentric circles, whereas zones 2 and 1 were extensions to the South. Each zone contained a single socioeconomic stratum.

From Williams KH, Hollinger FB, Metzger WR, et al. The epidemiology of St. Louis encephalitis in Corpus Christi, Texas, 1966. *Am J Epidemiol* 1975;102:16–24.

In the tropics, seasonal patterns of viral infections differ from patterns in temperate climates. Influenza virus transmission in the tropics can be either seasonal or relatively constant throughout the year.[118] Strong seasonal transmission of measles virus in sub-Saharan Africa generates large, irregular measles outbreaks and is an example of nonlinear, chaotic viral dynamics.[26]

The underlying explanations for seasonal differences remain elusive. In general, three types of mechanisms have been hypothesized to explain the seasonality of viral infections.[64] First are seasonal cycles in host resistance to infection, including seasonal differences in vitamin D levels.[22] The second involves changes in host behavior and contact patterns, particularly the role of schools as shown for measles virus.[28] Third is the role of climatic factors, particularly temperature and humidity. An example is the seasonality of poliomyelitis in the northeastern United States, which contrasts with the relative absence of seasonality for poliomyelitis in islands of Hawaii, where humidity remains relatively constant throughout the year (Fig. 12.5). This observation led to the hypothesis that viruses differ in their sensitivity to humidity,[120] with, for example, poliovirus rapidly inactivated during winter months of low humidity,[87] whereas influenza virus remains viable under similar conditions.[132] More recently, influenza virus transmission was shown to decrease as vapor pressure (a measure of absolute moisture in air) increases, likely mediated by increased virus survival at low levels of vapor pressure.[110,111]

The Impact of Viral Pandemics on Secular Trends in Life Expectancy

On rare occasions, the emergence of a new virus may initiate a pandemic so severe that it reduces the life expectancy of the human population. Although exceptional, such events deserve

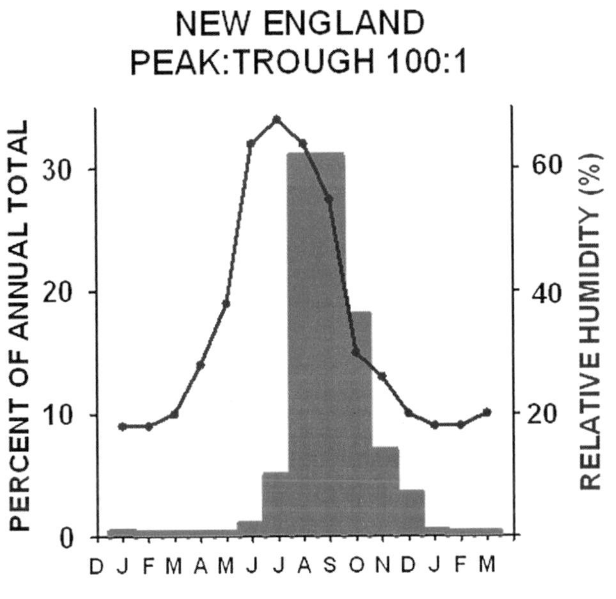

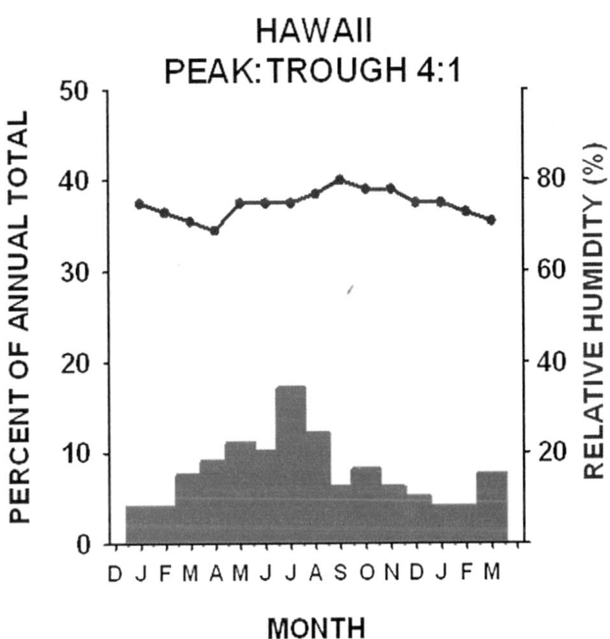

FIGURE 12.5. Seasonal distribution of poliomyelitis in New England and Hawaii, and the seasonal variation in relative humidity. Upper panel: Cases for 1942–1951 for New England. **Lower panel:** Cases for 1938–1952 for Hawaii. (Data from Enright JR. Epidemiology of poliomyelitis. *Hawaii Med J* 1954;13:350–354; Nathanson N, Martin JR. The epidemiology of poliomyelitis: enigmas surrounding its appearance, epidemicity, and disappearance. *Am J Epidemiol* 1979;110:672–692; and Serfling RE, Sherman IL. Poliomyelitis distribution in the United States. *Public Health Rep* 1953;68:453–466.)

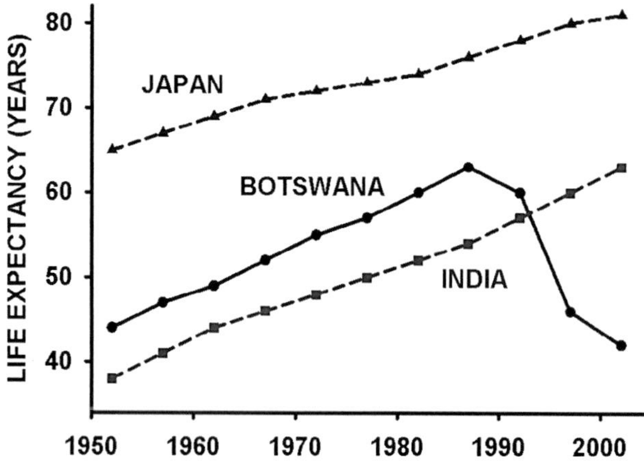

FIGURE 12.6. The drastic effect of the acquired immunodeficiency syndrome pandemic on life expectancy in Botswana, compared with Japan and India. Life expectancy is computed from the age-specific mortality rates for each calendar year, which are averaged to obtain the expectancy for that calendar year. (Data from McMichael AJ, McKee M, Shkolnikov V, et al. Mortality trends and setbacks: global convergence or divergence? *Lancet* 2004;63:1155–1159.)

mention because of their enormous impact. The global influenza pandemic of 1918 was such an event.[92] A type A influenza virus with an H1N1 genotype emerged, likely a recombinant between an avian and a human influenza virus. Because the human population under age 25 years was negative for H1 antibodies, this virus spread rapidly around the world and is estimated to have caused an excess mortality of about 40 million deaths in less than 1 year, sufficient to cause a transient reduction in life expectancy of about 15 years. Viral archaeology led to reconstruction of the genetic sequence of this virus and the generation of infectious virus through reverse genetics[125]; however, its apparent high virulence has yet to be fully explained in molecular terms.[121] A second striking instance is the impact of HIV/AIDS on life expectancy in some countries of sub-Saharan Africa (Fig. 12.6). In Botswana, for instance, AIDS reduced life expectancy by about 20 years, from age 63 to age 42—an effect whose magnitude has not been seen in recorded medical history.[75]

VIRAL EMERGENCE

One of the most dramatic aspects of historical epidemiology is the appearance of a new viral disease. This may reflect (a) the true appearance of a new virus in the population, a rare but real possibility; (b) an increase in the case infection ratio so that an endemic infection is associated with a marked increase in disease incidence; or lastly, (c) the recognition of an existing but previously unidentified disease that can now be clearly diagnosed owing to new laboratory tests accompanied by heightened practitioner awareness.

Emergence of Novel Viruses

AIDS and other diseases associated with HIV are an only too familiar example of the emergence of a virus new to the population. AIDS first appeared in the United States and Europe around 1979, and serological studies demonstrated that infection first occurred in the gay population of San Francisco 1 to 2 years prior to the recognition of the disease. The emergence of AIDS was re-enacted in India and Southeast Asia in the mid-1980s, when newly developed serologic and virologic methods permitted the infection to be followed from its earliest entry into the population. Evidence suggests that HIV-2 was derived from viruses indigenous to sooty mangabeys[112] and that HIV-1 originated in simian immunodeficiency virus (SIV) strains circulating in chimpanzees.[113]

Bovine spongiform encephalopathy (BSE) was first detected in the United Kingdom in the mid-1980s and was quickly identified as a spongiform encephalopathy similar to scrapie, an endemic disease of sheep. Detailed epidemiologic investigation strongly suggested that BSE represented a common source epidemic owing to the contamination of meat and bone meal nutritional supplements routinely fed to dairy cattle.[99] Scrapie-infected sheep tissues were included in the raw material used to produce the feed supplement, and a change (introduced in the late 1970s) in the production methods permitted scrapie infectivity to survive the production process at a residual level. The rapidly evolving epidemic (Fig. 12.7) led to the exclusion of ruminant tissues from feed supplements, a step that was predicted to terminate the epidemic. However, the long incubation period (averaging about 5 years with a range of 3–9 years) of BSE indicated that the epidemic would continue to evolve. The relatively long tail to the declining epidemic reflected a delay in implementation of the feed ban and a low level of direct cow-to-cow transmission, similar to that observed in scrapie of sheep.

In April 2009, a novel influenza A virus was identified from two children with respiratory symptoms in southern California as a consequence of field epidemiologic investigations.[116] Within the first few weeks of identification, field and epidemiologic studies lead to the initial genetic characterization of the virus,[34] a description of the clinical and epidemiologic features of infected persons,[20] characterization of viral transmission (including the serial interval) within different populations, and assessments of population susceptibility through serological surveys.[47]

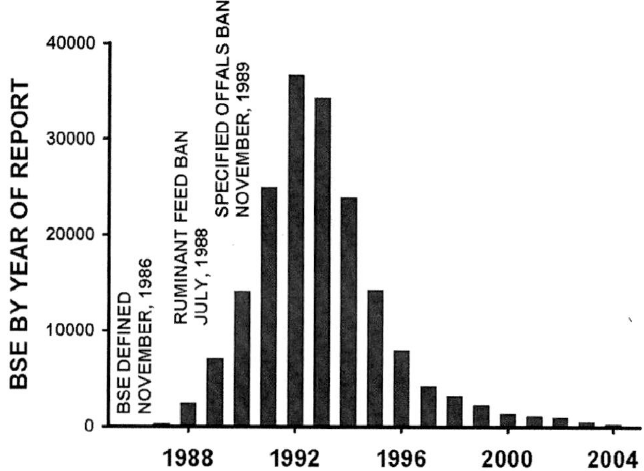

FIGURE 12.7. The course of the epidemic of bovine spongiform encephalopathy (BSE) in Great Britain, with confirmed cases by year of report. (Data from Department of Environment, Food and Rural Affairs. *BSE: Statistics*. 2011, available at http://archive.defra.gov.uk/foodfarm/farmanimal/diseases/atoz/bse/)

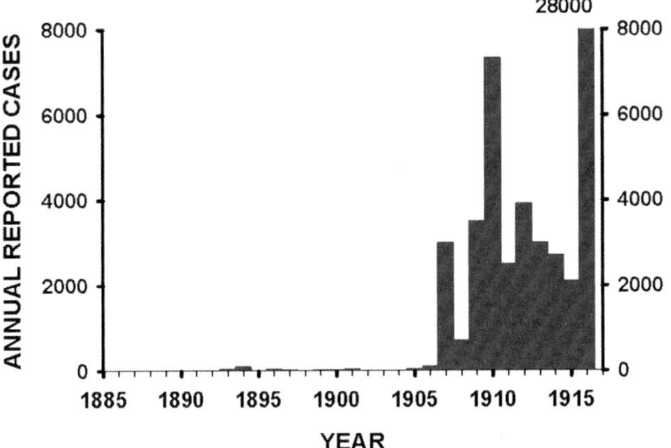

FIGURE 12.8. The appearance of epidemic poliomyelitis in the United States from 1885 to 1916. The graph is based on reported cases (mainly paralytic) during an era when reporting was estimated at about 50%. (Data from Lavinder CH, Freeman SW, Frost WH. Epidemiologic studies of poliomyelitis in New York City and the northeastern United States during the year 1916. *USPHS Hyg Lab Bull* 1918;91:1–150; and Nathanson N, Martin JR. The epidemiology of poliomyelitis: enigmas surrounding its appearance, epidemicity, and disappearance. *Am J Epidemiol* 1979;110:672–692.)

Increase in the Case Infection Ratio

The dramatic appearance of epidemic poliomyelitis (then known as *infantile paralysis*) in Europe and the United States in the 19th century is illustrated in Figure 12.8.[87] In retrospect, it is clear that polioviruses had been endemic for millennia but that cases of paralysis were few and sporadic. The likely explanation is that an improvement in standards of personal hygiene reduced the transmission of this enterovirus, delaying infection of young children beyond the age during which they were protected by maternal antibody (see Fig. 12.4), and resulting in the first epidemics of infantile paralysis.[90] Support for this view was the re-enactment of the appearance of poliomyelitis in other countries (in the Middle East and Africa) during the 20th century. In such instances, it was possible to conduct serological studies that demonstrated the high prevalence of antibodies prior to the appearance of clinical epidemics. Furthermore, the secular trend continued in the United States, with a gradual stepwise increase in the age distribution of paralytic poliomyelitis (Table 12.12) so that by the time of vaccine introduction in 1955, the term *infantile paralysis* had become outmoded.

New Recognition of an Existing Virus

La Crosse virus is a mosquito-transmitted bunyavirus that causes La Crosse encephalitis. The causal agent was first isolated from a fatal case in 1964[123] and led to the ability to distinguish this disease from the rubric of "arbovirus encephalitis, etiology unknown." Beginning in 1964, about 100 cases have been reported annually, mainly from the midwestern United States. It is likely that the "emergence" of this disease reflected the ability to make the specific diagnosis, because the incidence did not change and serological studies indicate that infections were occurring at a similar frequency long before isolation of the virus was reported in 1965.[41]

A striking acute pulmonary syndrome with high mortality was first reported in the southwestern United States in 1993, and combined epidemiologic and laboratory investigation indicated that the agent, SNV, was a previously unknown bunyavirus belonging to the *Hantavirus* genus.[88] SNV is an indigenous virus of deer mice (*Peromyscus maniculatus*), in which it causes a persistent infection accompanied by virus excretion leading to production of virus-infected aerosols and exposure of humans. The emergence of SNV was the result of the recognition of a long-existing agent and disease that was brought to attention because of an unusual cluster of cases associated with a transient increase in the deer mouse population.

Possible Increased Frequency of Viral Disease Emergence

New viral diseases may be emerging as zoonoses at an increasing frequency.[129] Several secular trends have enhanced the probability of emergence of new viral diseases[127] (Fig. 12.9). First, the population of the world has inexorably continued to increase, and urbanization has concentrated a higher proportion of people in densely populated areas, facilitating the transmission of any new infection. Second, modern transportation permits the carriage of infections around the globe within a single incubation period. Third, man-made perturbations of the environment are occurring at an increasing pace, thus increasing the likelihood of transmission of zoonotic and arboviral infections

TABLE 12.12 Age Distribution of Poliomyelitis in Massachusetts, 1912–1952[a]

Years	Age 0–4 years (%)	Age 5–9 years (%)	Age ≥10 years (%)
1912–1916	70	18	12
1920–1924	48	24	28
1925–1929	40	30	30
1930–1934	28	38	34
1935–1939	28	28	44
1940–1944	22	28	50
1948–1952	18	27	55

[a]Includes paralytic and nonparalytic cases.

From Dauer CC. The changing age distribution of paralytic poliomyelitis. *Ann N Y Acad Sci* 1955;61:943–955; and Nathanson N, Martin JR. The epidemiology of poliomyelitis: enigmas surrounding its appearance, epidemicity, and disappearance. *Am J Epidemiol* 1979;110:672–692.

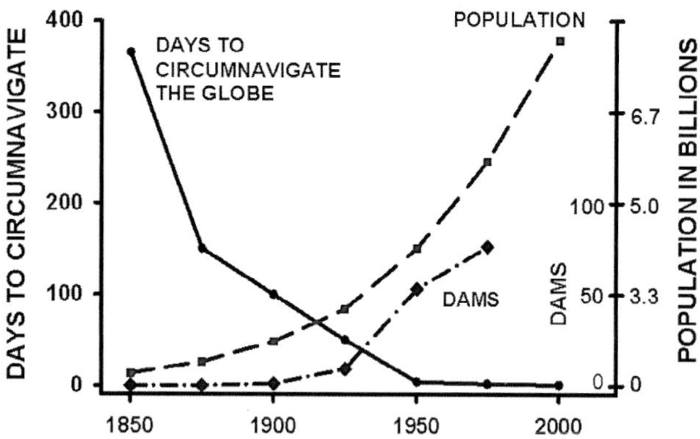

FIGURE 12.9. Since the middle of the 19th century, many global changes have enhanced the probability of the emergence of new viral diseases of humans and animals. This chart depicts three examples of such trends. The rise in the human population has been accompanied by a massive increase in large urban populations, markedly increasing the risk of epidemic spread of infection. Dramatic reductions in the time to travel over long distances have increased the possibility of global transport of infectious agents over short periods of time. The number of large dams (dams >75 meters high built in the United States from 1890 to 1975) exemplifies increases in man-made manipulation of the environment. (Data from Anonymous. *Atlas of World Population History*. New York: Penguin Books and Allen Lane; 1978; Anonymous. *Statistical Yearbook, 38th Issue, 1990/1991*. New York: United Nations Publications; 1993; and Mandzhavidze NF, Mamradze GP. *The High Dams of the World*. Springfield, VA: Academy of the Sciences of the Georgian SSR and Clearinghouse for Federal Scientific and Technical Information; 1994.)

to humans. Finally, advances in fundamental virology have made available a new armamentarium of methods for the detection of previously unknown pathogenic viruses, although numerous challenges are raised by these methods in establishing causal relationships between pathogens and disease.[63] The current controversy over the potential association between xenotropic murine leukemia virus-related virus (XMRV) and chronic fatigue syndrome represents an example where the initial report of a causal association between a pathogen and disease based on molecular methods was not confirmed in subsequent studies.[3,65]

An example that illustrates these forces is the emergence of West Nile virus (WNV) in the United States.[55] WNV, a mosquito-transmitted flavivirus, was endemic in northern and eastern Africa, the Middle East, and eastern Europe. However, WNV had been limited to these contiguous geographic areas, which is characteristic of the regional distribution of most arboviruses, in contrast to the global distribution of viruses endemic to humans. In 1999, an outbreak of arboviral encephalitis occurred in and around New York City, which was first thought to be caused by St. Louis virus, a flavivirus endemic to the United States. Further study showed that the outbreak was caused by WNV, which had never been found in North America. Although speculative, it appears that WNV was imported from the Middle East, likely by infected mosquitoes that were unpaid passengers on an incoming airliner. Because of the presence of vector mosquitoes permissive for WNV and susceptible avian hosts, WNV spread rapidly and is now endemic across the United States.[81]

EPIDEMICS

No medical phenomenon is more dramatic than the occurrence of an epidemic. The immediate cause of any viral epidemic is heightened transmission of the causal agent. Epidemics can be classified according to their principal mode of transmission as either common source or propagated.

Common Source Epidemics

Common source outbreaks are, as the term implies, owing to exposure to the virus from a common source, usually either in food, water, aerosol, or injected product. Common source outbreaks have the potential to be explosive because of the simultaneous exposure of many individuals; however, because the exposure is frequently limited in time, such outbreaks may be of relatively short duration. Finally, common source outbreaks challenge the epidemiologist, because unraveling the source may lead to termination of an ongoing outbreak or prevention of recurrences.

Two examples illustrate common source epidemics. At the beginning of World War II, the military decided to immunize a large number of troops against yellow fever because it was clear that there would be action in several tropical theaters where jungle yellow fever might be encountered. The attenuated 17D strain of yellow fever virus was a newly developed vaccine considered to be a safe and effective immunogen. Because vaccine efficacy depended on the infectivity of 17D virus, its stability was enhanced by including serum in the final formulation. Human serum was used (to avoid serum sickness), and almost 1,000 donors were recruited, most of whom were medical students at Johns Hopkins University. Unfortunately, at least one individual was a carrier of hepatitis B virus. As a result, over 400,000 troops received contaminated vaccine, causing a massive epidemic of hepatitis B infection (about 20,000 cases) in the spring of 1942.[106] Although disease onset was spread over time, when the common source was recognized and cases were plotted from the time of initial immunization with 17D vaccine, they formed a classical log-normal distribution (Fig. 12.10) that provided a definitive estimate of the distribution of incubation period for hepatitis B. Although this epidemic was originally considered to be one of hepatitis A, the great length of the incubation period (mean of 14 weeks) and the absence of secondary spread to contacts provided strong epidemiologic evidence that this disease was a distinct entity.

An outbreak of hepatitis A occurred in 1961 in Pascagoula, Mississippi.[73] In some cases, detailed food histories were taken that showed, by comparison with controls, that there was an association with raw oysters. Subsequent investigation disclosed that certain oyster beds in Pascagoula Bay were located near the discharge point for inadequately treated sewage from the city, and cases were associated with oysters supplied from these beds. This was one of the first instances of shellfish-associated hepatitis A, and it was later demonstrated that oysters, through their siphoning system, are capable of concentrating virus up to 1,000-fold. One of the largest outbreaks of hepatitis A virus infection associated with shellfish in the United States within the past two decades occurred in 2005 and involved 39 people.[10] This was the first such outbreak in which identical viral genetic sequences were demonstrated in both cases and food products.

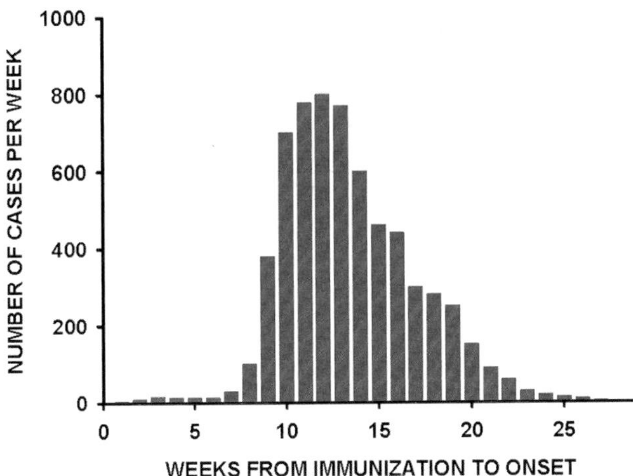

FIGURE 12.10. Distribution of incubation periods for a common source epidemic of vaccine-associated hepatitis B. The graph shows cases of jaundice tabulated by weeks from immunization with 17D yellow fever vaccine to onset for military units in California. (Data from Sawyer WA, Meyer KF, Eaton MD, et al. Jaundice in army personnel in the western region of the United States and its relation to vaccination against yellow fever. *Am J Hyg* 1944;39:337–387.)

Propagated Epidemics

Propagated epidemics, as the term implies, involve host-to-host spread of virus. The occurrence of an epidemic is therefore owing to the action of three parameters that determine clinical disease incidence—namely, the proportion of the population susceptible, the proportion of infected (and infectious) individuals, and the case infection ratio. To produce the unusually high incidence that defines an epidemic, at least one of these parameters must be operating above its usual level. In some but not all outbreaks, it is possible to implicate a specific parameter.

Measles incidence in Iceland over a 50-year period is shown in Figure 12.11, during which epidemics alternated with periods of complete absence of measles. In this extreme situation, the virus invades the population, spreads widely and quickly, and fades out when the concentration of susceptibles drops below the level needed to perpetuate the virus. The virus disappears entirely, allowing susceptibles to accumulate as new cohorts of infants are born. Once enough susceptibles have accumulated, a single importation of measles can initiate a new epidemic. In this situation, the parameter critical for epidemic initiation is the proportion of susceptible individuals in the population.

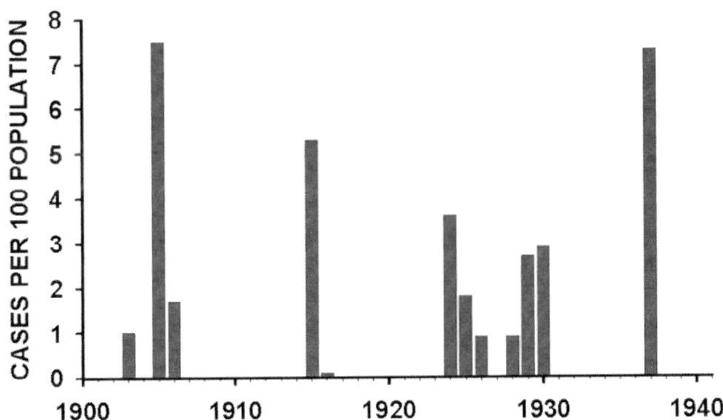

FIGURE 12.11. Measles incidence in Iceland from 1900 to 1940. (Data from Tauxe R. Measles incidence in Iceland, 1900–1940. Unpublished report. 1979.)

By contrast, outbreaks of arbovirus disease are unrelated to the proportion of susceptibles, because infection is infrequent and a high proportion of the population is always susceptible (areas with hyperendemic yellow fever or dengue may represent exceptions). Epidemics are a reflection of the proportion of susceptibles who become infected. Because humans are terminal hosts who do not act as links in the infection chain, the key determinants are ecological factors that result in a high concentration of vectors and a high infection rate in the vector population. Epidemics are most commonly preceded by those climatic conditions (rainfall, temperature, and the like) that maximize the vector population.

In some instances, an outbreak is clearly associated with an increase in the ratio of cases to infections, often associated with a virus strain of high pathogenicity. Such occurrences are probably quite frequent but are rarely well documented. One well-studied example is the pandemic of avian influenza that overwhelmed the poultry industry of Pennsylvania in 1983. In this instance, there was a sudden increase in the virulence of an influenza virus, already enzootic in the poultry population, resulting in a pandemic that led to major commercial losses and was only controlled by a widespread slaughter program. Unusually, isolates of the virus from before and after the epidemic were available for analysis, and a classical series of studies showed that a point mutation in the viral hemagglutinin enhanced the replication ability and virulence of the virus.[126]

Epidemics, Viral Pathogenesis, and Molecular Epidemiology

Expanding knowledge of basic virology provides molecular insights into the determinants of viral epidemics. In certain instances, it is possible to identify some of the molecular determinants of each of three parameters (proportion immune, proportion infected, and case infection ratio) that are responsible for propagated epidemics.

The proportion of the population immune is a relatively inflexible parameter for most viruses, with the exception of those against which vaccine exist. Influenza virus is a special instance. This virus is transmitted so effectively that it nearly exhausts the supply of susceptible hosts. The major antigenic protein of influenza virus is the viral hemagglutinin, which serves as the viral attachment protein and the target for neutralizing antibodies. Influenza virus has a genome composed of eight segments, and these segments may reassort when two type A influenza viruses co-infect the same cells, with the creation of viruses containing a mixture of segments from the two parents. On rare occasions, a human strain of virus reassorts with an animal strain and acquires the hemagglutinin of the animal virus. This leads to major shifts in the antigenicity of the virus, such as occurred in 1957, with the appearance of the Asian strain, which had an H2 hemagglutinin whereas previous influenza viruses had an H1 hemagglutinin, and in 2009, resulting in a complex, triple-reassortment H1N1 influenza virus.[20] Such a radical shift in antigenicity provides the newly created virus with a global population that is relatively susceptible; as a result, a worldwide influenza pandemic may occur.

TABLE 12.13 Comparison of Case Fatality Rates for Severe (Variola Major) and Mild (Variola Minor) Forms of Smallpox

Disease	Place and years	Cases	Deaths	Case fatality ratio per 100 (%)
Variola major	Minneapolis, 1924–1925	1,430	365	25.5
Variola minor	London, 1928–1934	13,686	34	0.2

From Marsden JP. A critical review of the clinical features of 13,686 cases of smallpox (variola minor). *Bull Hyg* 1948;23:735–746; and Sweitzer SE, Ikeda K. Variola, a clinical study of the Minneapolis epidemic of 1924–1925. *Arch Derm Syph* 1927;15:19–29.

The proportion of susceptibles infected will be determined by two characteristics of a given virus—namely, the generation time and the transmissibility. A virus with a relatively short generation time, such as influenza virus, can spread more rapidly than a virus such as poliovirus despite its lower transmissibility (R_0 for influenza virus is approximately 2 compared to 5–7 for polioviruses). Generation time and transmissibility determine the kinetics of the infection and are related to the titers of virus excreted; these parameters may be influenced by specific viral genes. Analysis of the genetic determinants of reovirus transmission demonstrated that the λ2 spike protein encoded by the L2 gene segment is a major determinant of transmissibility.[53] Likewise, the transmission of California serogroup bunyaviruses, by their mosquito vector, *Aedes triseriatus*, is determined by the middle RNA segment, which encodes the viral glycoproteins.[42]

A major determinant of the case infection ratio is viral pathogenicity. Most viruses exhibit great natural variation in pathogenicity. One classical example is variola virus, which caused virulent forms of smallpox (variola major) in India and Africa and much milder disease (alastrim or variola minor) in South America (Table 12.13). It was known for many years that natural isolates of poliovirus varied greatly in their neurovirulence, and attenuated isolates were the starting point for the development of avirulent vaccine strains. Molecular analysis identified the genomic determinants of virulence, which are located both in the structural genes and in the noncoding 5′ region of the genome.[83] This natural variation might have been a factor in the severity of poliomyelitis epidemics of the past. Another example is the 1983 pandemic of avian influenza cited previously, which was traced to a point mutation that increased the cleavability of the hemagglutinin molecule, thereby enhancing viral maturation and infectiousness with dramatic epidemiologic consequences.[126]

Molecular epidemiology has permitted the unraveling of otherwise enigmatic epidemiologic events. Poliomyelitis was eradicated from many countries, and outbreaks were relatively unusual. However, numerous outbreaks have been traced to revertant strains of oral poliovirus vaccine (OPV), resulting in vaccine-associated poliomyelitis. The genealogy of these revertant viruses was determined by their genomic sequences to be closely aligned with OPV strains but were distinctly different from circulating strains of wild-type poliovirus.[76]

Phylodynamics

Infectious disease epidemiologists are increasingly interested in linking evolutionary and epidemiologic processes, a field referred to as phylodynamics.[40] Because of the high mutation rates of viral pathogens, evolutionary and epidemiologic processes take place on a similar time scale.[97] According to this framework, phylodynamic processes that determine the degree of viral diversity are a function of host immune selective pressures and epidemiologic patterns of transmission.

PERPETUATION AND ERADICATION OF VIRUSES

All viruses, whether they cause acute or chronic infections, are capable of persisting in populations because perpetuation is a requirement for survival. Eradication is the converse of perpetuation and represents the ultimate method for control of an infectious disease. To determine the potential for eradication, it is necessary first to understand the requirements for perpetuation.

The principal ecological patterns of viruses in host populations have been discussed previously, with emphasis on human viruses. In most instances, a virus is perpetuated in a single species, and discussion will be limited to this dominant ecological pattern. Parameters that determine perpetuation include population variables and viral variables.[4] Population determinants include (a) the size of the population, (b) the turnover rate (rate at which susceptibles are introduced), (c) the density of the population, and (d) the proportion of the population susceptible. Viral determinants include (a) transmissibility, (b) generation time, and (c) duration of infectiousness (acute or persistent). These three viral variables determine the rate of spread of a virus through a population (for a given set of population parameters). Paradoxically, an agent that spreads rapidly may exhaust susceptibles and disappear more quickly from a small population than a virus that moves indolently through the same population. Perpetuation will be discussed separately for large and small populations, because population size is such an important determinant.

Small Populations

For small populations, a crude prediction of perpetuation may be made by determining the number of susceptibles entering the population per generation period. If this number is less than one, persistence will almost certainly not occur.[132]

Isolated Human Populations

Small primitive human populations that have minimal contact with the outside world are occasionally available for serological

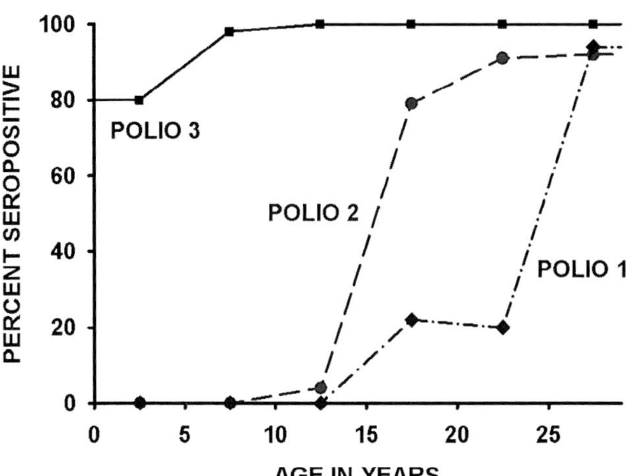

FIGURE 12.12. Age-specific prevalence of antibodies to poliovirus types 1, 2, and 3 in an isolated Eskimo village in Greenland. (Data from Paffenbarger RS, Jr., Bodian D. Poliomyelitis immune status in ecologically diverse populations, in relation to virus spread, clinical incidence, and virus disappearance. *Am J Hyg* 1961;74:311–325.)

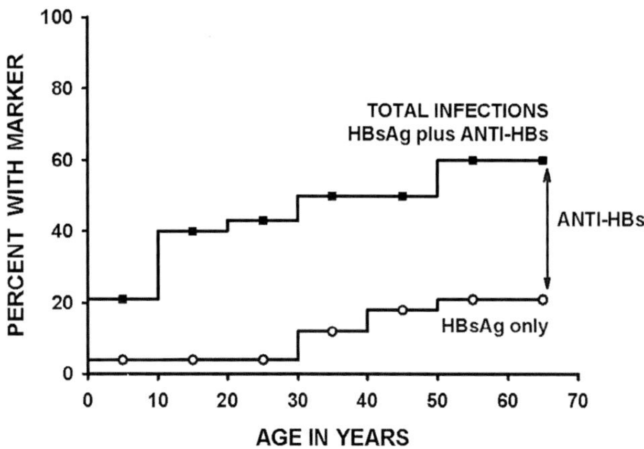

FIGURE 12.13. Age-specific prevalence of hepatitis B antibodies (*anti-HBs*) and hepatitis B surface antigen (*HBsAg*) in Eskimos in southwest Greenland. (Data from Skinhoj P. Hepatitis and hepatitis B-antigen in Greenland. II: Occurrence and interrelation of hepatitis B associated surface, core, and "e" antigen-antibody systems in a highly endemic area. *Am J Epidemiol* 1977;105:99–106.)

study. These populations provide a unique opportunity to determine the ability of viruses to perpetuate in their natural hosts. There are two principal patterns.[11] Viruses that cause acute short-term infections produce abrupt outbreaks after introduction into human populations and then die out until reintroduced. Viruses that are capable of persisting in individual hosts are able to perpetuate in small isolated groups.

Figure 12.12 presents the age distribution of antibodies to poliovirus types 1, 2, and 3 in an isolated Eskimo village. The profiles show that type 1 virus had infected essentially the entire population 25 years before the study, type 2 virus had caused a similar wave of infections 15 years before the study, and type 3 virus had been present shortly before the collection of sera. In addition, it is clear that following its intrusion, each virus disappeared from the population, because there were few people younger than 25 years of age with type 1 antibody (the few seropositive individuals probably represent cross-reacting antibody following type 2 infection) and few younger than 15 years of age with type 2 antibody.

In contrast, hepatitis B virus produces a considerable proportion of persistent infections, particularly in primitive populations, where infection occurs early in life. Figure 12.13, from another study of Eskimos, shows that infections occurred at all ages, with a gradual rise in cumulative incidence to 60% by 60 years of age, with no evidence of disappearance of virus from the population or of exhaustion of susceptibles. The curve for hepatitis B surface antigen indicates that there were many persistently infected carriers in the population accounting for perpetuation in this small community.

Small Animal Populations

Animal populations differ radically from human populations in their relatively rapid rate of turnover—a critical variable in virus perpetuation. Mean life expectancy in many animal populations ranges from 6 to 12 months, in contrast to a range of 30 to 70 years for humans. However, the kinetics of infection are similar in an individual human or animal host. For instance, the median incubation period (to rash) is about 14 days in smallpox and 10 days in mousepox. The consequence is that perpetuation may occur in animal populations (with rapid turnover) that are much smaller than the minimum human population required to sustain a similar virus.

Laboratory animal colonies have provided an opportunity to document the quantitative impact of population turnover. Perpetuation in such colonies is of more than academic interest, because enzootic infections present an important practical problem that frequently confounds biomedical research. One documented example is ectromelia (mousepox) that closely resembles variola in humans.[24] Infection is initiated either by entry through the skin or by inhalation and results in a generalized pox-like rash of the skin from which aerosolized virus is transmitted. As in smallpox, infections can be fatal, although recovered mice are solidly immune. Ectromelia is a relatively infectious agent and a notorious cause of acute and devastating epizootics. When a few infected mice are placed in a larger group of susceptible animals, the virus spreads rapidly, all mice are infected within two incubation periods, and many mice die.

In these circumstances, ectromelia would not be expected to perpetuate in a small mouse population. However, a series of classical studies demonstrated that this virus was readily perpetuated in a population of 100 to 200 animals.[37] In one representative experiment, a mouse colony was established with 25 normal and 20 infected mice, and 3 uninfected mice were added daily; animals were removed only if dead. During a 30-month observation period, the total colony size gradually rose to a constant level of about 230 animals. The infection was maintained throughout the observation period; at equilibrium, about one-fifth of the mice were uninfected, one-fifth were actively infected (mortality rate, 50% to 60%), and three-fifths were recovered immune animals. It was possible to maintain this acute highly lethal virus over long periods of time in mouse populations with as few as 70 animals, demonstrating that high turnover markedly reduces the population size required for perpetuation.

TABLE 12.14 Fadeouts of Measles in North American Cities, 1921–1940[a]

Size of city (millions)	Number of cities	Average annual measles reports (thousands)	Years of study	Years with fadeout
1.0–7.5	6	3.5–21	120	0
0.5–0.9	9	2.8–4.0	180	1
0.2–0.3	5	0.9–2.1	100	56

[a]Estimate of reporting ranged from 14% to 55% of measles incidence. *Large cities:* New York, Chicago, Philadelphia, Detroit, Los Angeles, Montreal; *medium cities:* Cleveland, Baltimore, Boston, Toronto, Washington, Pittsburgh, Milwaukee, Buffalo, Minneapolis; *small cities:* Vancouver, Rochester, Dallas, Akron, Winnipeg.

From Bartlett MS. The critical community size for measles in the United States. *J R Stat Soc A* 1960;123:37–44; and Yorke JA, London WP. Recurrent outbreaks of measles, chickenpox and mumps. II. Systematic differences in contact rates and stochastic effects. *Am J Epidemiol* 1973;98:469–482.

Large Populations

To follow the pattern of viral infection in large populations, it is generally necessary to rely on reportable diseases that can be identified from clinical observations and that exhibit relatively high case infection ratios. Measles is one of the few viral diseases that meets these criteria; however, even measles surveillance has its limitations, considering only a fraction (usually 10%–50%) of cases are reported. Table 12.14 shows that in cities of 200,000 to 300,000, measles faded out for at least 1 month in 56 of the 100 years recorded. Because a population of 300,000 might be expected to experience about 5,000 cases of measles in an average year, it is initially surprising that this would be insufficient to maintain measles virus transmission. The explanation becomes more apparent when the seasonal cycle of measles is examined.[66,131,132] Data for the city of Baltimore (population 900,000) for 32 years of observation showed that annual reports averaged about 5,000 cases, representing about 35% of cases; incidence rates ranged more than 100-fold from the peak in March to the seasonal low in August, when about 10 cases were reported. Because there were about three generation periods per month, this represents no more than 3 cases per generation period, which is barely sufficient to perpetuate the virus. A similar city of 300,000 would experience only 1 case per generation period at the seasonal trough; in such an instance, it is quite plausible that periodic fadeouts would occur.

This analysis suggests that persistence of a short-cycle infection in a large population depends on the relationship between incidence during the seasonal trough and the generation time. Influenza virus, with a generation time of 1 to 3 days, has difficulty persisting in human populations through the seasonal trough but circumvents the problem by shuttling between Northern and Southern hemispheres each year.

Requirements for Eradication

The history of smallpox, and more recently rinderpest virus, demonstrates that eradication is an attainable objective for selected human and animal viral infections. The salient epidemiologic features that made smallpox eradication possible were its relatively long incubation period (about 14 days) and low infectiousness, the near equivalent durations of the latent and incubation periods, its marked seasonality, a case to infection ratio approaching 1, and the lack of an extrahuman reservoir.[49] These features made it possible to abandon mass vaccination in favor of a search-and-containment strategy in which local outbreaks were identified and aborted by intensive immunization around each focus.[31] The few local outbreaks during the seasonal trough were essential to the success of this strategy.

Eradication of Polioviruses

Two poliovirus vaccines (inactivated poliovirus vaccine [IPV] and OPV) were introduced in the period from 1955 to 1963 in the United States, and their application led to the elimination of circulating wild polioviruses around 1970.[84,85] Wild polioviruses were eliminated from the Western Hemisphere by 1990 as a result of immunization programs in Latin America, and the World Health Organization set a goal of global eradication in 1988. Worldwide efforts reduced polio cases from an estimated 350,000 in 1988 to fewer than 1,000 in 2000. However, since then, elimination efforts have stalled at a level of 1,000 to 2,000 cases annually, owing to the persistence of wild polioviruses in a few countries: Nigeria and a belt extending from Afghanistan east across Pakistan to northern India. There have been two major impediments in these countries, first the failure to immunize a sufficiently high proportion of infants and young children in settings where transmission of enteric infections is very intense and, second, a low "take" rate of OPV, owing in part to competition between the three serotypes in the vaccine. The latter problem was solved in part by the introduction of monovalent (type 1) and bivalent (types 1 and 3) OPV, whereas concentrated efforts to increase immunization rates have reduced circulating polioviruses in Nigeria and India.[16] At this writing (2011), it is unclear whether these efforts will eliminate residual circulation wild polioviruses, particularly in areas of Pakistan and Afghanistan where there is a breakdown of civil society.

OPV presents another complicating issue, namely the tendency to revert to a more virulent phenotype on human enteric passage. Vaccine-derived polioviruses have caused about 15 documented outbreaks of poliomyelitis in settings where weak immunization programs have left many children susceptible and capable of spreading OPV shed by those who were immunized. Most of these outbreaks have been quite small; however, an outbreak in Nigeria attributable to revertant type 2 vaccine-derived poliovirus has caused nearly 300 paralytic cases over a period of 5 years.[124] The potential dangers of OPV have led many industrialized countries to shift from OPV to IPV, and some experts believe that the world will not be freed from paralytic poliomyelitis until immunization with OPV is ended.[85]

Eradication of Measles Virus

Remarkable progress has been made in reducing global measles incidence and mortality as a consequence of measles vaccination. In the Americas, intensive vaccination and surveillance efforts interrupted endemic transmission of measles virus, in part based on the successful Pan American Health Organization strategy of periodic nationwide measles vaccination campaigns and high routine measles vaccine coverage. In the United States, high coverage with two doses of measles vaccine eliminated endemic measles virus transmission in 2000. More recently, progress in reducing measles incidence and mortality has been made in sub-Saharan Africa and Asia as a consequence of increasing routine measles vaccine coverage and provision of a second opportunity for measles vaccination through mass measles vaccination campaigns. The feasibility of measles eradication has been discussed for more than 30 years, beginning in the late 1960s when the long-term protective immunity induced by measles vaccines was becoming evident.[108] Three biological criteria are deemed important for disease eradication, including measles virus: (a) humans are the sole pathogen reservoir; (b) accurate diagnostic tests exist; and (c) an effective, practical intervention is available at reasonable cost.[1] Interruption of transmission in large geographical areas for prolonged periods further supports the feasibility of eradication. Measles is thought by many experts to meet these criteria.[89]

Several potential biological obstacles to measles eradication should be considered.[79] Persistent infection with transmissible measles virus would pose a biological barrier to eradication. Measles virus is known to establish persistent infection in persons with subacute sclerosing panencephalitis (SSPE); however, virion assembly and budding is defective and multiple mutations occur throughout the measles virus genome.[33] As a consequence, infectious measles virus is not present. Theoretically, selective pressure on measles viruses to mutate neutralizing epitopes and escape protective immune responses induced by vaccines could be a biological obstacle to measles eradication. However, despite the high degree of genetic variation expected of an RNA virus, mutations in the measles virus genome have not reduced the protective immunity induced by measles vaccines.[119] Subclinical infection resulting in sustained measles virus transmission also could pose a barrier to eradication,[80] as it has for polioviruses. However, sustained measles virus transmission among partially immune individuals without clinical disease would be highly unlikely.[61]

Eradication of Rinderpest Virus

Rinderpest virus, a pathogen of cattle and many other domestic and wild artiodactyl species, was declared eradicated on May 25, 2011, following widespread vaccination and control efforts coordinated by the Global Rinderpest Eradication Programme.[77] Rinderpest virus is a *Morbillivirus* closely related to measles virus, transmitted by close contact with an infected animal via inhalation of virus-containing nasal, oral, or fecal secretions. Infection resulted in severe diarrhea leading to dehydration and death. Rinderpest impacted on human health in Europe and Africa by decimating cattle populations, leading to famine, disease, and death.

What is remarkable about rinderpest eradication is that the virus has many potential reservoirs, both domestic and wild, and yet the goal of eradication was achieved through widespread vaccination of cattle and buffalo, establishment of effective surveillance programs, and regional coordination of control efforts.

APPLICATIONS OF EPIDEMIOLOGY

Identification of Etiological Agents

Viruses that cause acute infections, are readily transmitted, and cause intense outbreaks, are often first identified as distinct clinical entities during epidemiologic studies. Examples include HIV (AIDS), hantavirus (pulmonary syndrome), WNV (encephalitis), SARS-coronavirus, and the 2009 H1N1 influenza virus. Epidemiologically, it may be difficult to infer whether the cause is a virus or other infectious agent. Epidemiologic observations, however, may suggest the portal of virus shedding and the period of infectiousness, which is important for the collection of specimens for isolation.

Epidemiologic observations may also contribute insights into more obscure persistent infections associated with atypical chronic diseases. The spongiform encephalopathies or prion diseases are an example. This group of agents includes scrapie of sheep, kuru and Creutzfeldt-Jakob disease of humans, and BSE.[17] The initial definitive evidence that scrapie, a chronic degenerative neurological disease, could be transmitted by an infectious agent and occurred as an unwanted complication of the use of louping ill vaccine in Scotland in 1935.[38] Table 12.15 shows that three lots of vaccine against louping ill, a flavivirus, were injected into sheep in Scotland. Unexpectedly, there was a very high incidence of scrapie in recipients of one of the three lots. Subsequent epidemiologic investigation showed that louping ill vaccine was prepared by formalin treatment of virus grown in sheep brain and that several of the sheep used were probably incubating scrapie because their parents subsequently came down with the disease. Prions are extremely resistant to inactivation by formalin; thus, contamination of the vaccine was readily explained. Prior to this episode, it was not generally accepted that scrapie was attributable to a transmissible agent with an incubation period of several years.

TABLE 12.15 Occurrence of Scrapie in Sheep Immunized with Louping Ill Vaccine, Scotland, 1935[a]

Vaccine batch	Number of sheep vaccinated	Percentage with scrapie
1	>22,000	<0.1%
2	18,000	5%
3	>4,000	<0.1%

[a]Batch 2 was prepared from 122 sheep infected with louping ill; of these, 8 were offspring of scrapie-affected ewes. Interval between subcutaneous injection of vaccine and onset was 20 months or longer.

From Greig JR. Scrapie in sheep. *J Comp Pathol* 1950;60:263–266.

Evaluation of Vaccine Efficacy and Safety

The ultimate test of viral vaccines is their efficacy and safety in humans. Epidemiology provides well-established methods for the design and analysis of prospective studies of vaccine efficacy.[44] These are illustrated by the 1954 field trial of poliomyelitis vaccine.[71] In this trial, a large number of children in the first three grades of elementary school were enrolled. As shown in Table 12.2, the trial comprised two different study designs—namely, placebo and observed. In the placebo design, children fell into three categories: vaccinated, placebo inoculated, and nonvolunteers (uninoculated). In the observational study, the three groups were vaccinated second graders, nonvolunteer second graders (unvaccinated), and controls (all children in the first and third grades). The most valid comparison was between vaccinated and placebo-inoculated children in the placebo areas: This group yielded an estimated efficacy of 72% for paralytic poliomyelitis, whereas the observed control area yielded an efficacy of 63%. The discrepancy was explained by the fact that the nonvolunteer children in both areas experienced an attack rate that was considerably lower than that of the placebo controls or the observed controls. Apparently, volunteer children were at higher risk (presumably because they included a higher percentage of susceptibles) than were nonvolunteer children. Thus, the strict placebo control was the best comparison group. When the placebo study was further refined by limiting the analysis to laboratory-confirmed cases, the estimated efficacy was even higher (85%), underlining the importance of etiology-proven cases in vaccine evaluation.

Epidemiologic studies can also play a vital role in documenting vaccine complications. The occurrence of Guillain-Barré syndrome associated with the use of swine influenza virus vaccine in the fall of 1976 provides a good illustration.[107] About 40 million people received influenza vaccine in a mass campaign. Cases of a relatively rare neurological disease, Guillain-Barré syndrome, were reported in vaccinees at a frequency considered excessive, and the vaccine was withdrawn. When vaccine-associated cases were compiled by interval after immunization (Fig. 12.14), they exhibited a log-normal distribution typical of many incubation periods. This pathognomonic epidemiologic feature, along with the excessive rates seen during the early weeks after immunization, provided strong evidence of an association and justified termination of the vaccine program. Epidemiologic evidence was the key in this episode because the association (<1 case per 100,000 vaccinees) was only detectable in a massive field study. Because Guillain-Barré syndrome occurs at a baseline rate in the population and those cases associated with the vaccine were not clinically distinguishable from the baseline cases, this episode presented a special epidemiologic challenge. The occurrence of Guillain-Barré syndrome was not predictable by any small-scale human trial or laboratory test, and the biological explanation is still unclear. In fact, epidemiologic studies conducted with influenza vaccines used after 1976 have demonstrated that these vaccines (produced from nonswine strains of virus) apparently carry no risk of Guillain-Barré syndrome.[58] Nevertheless, the importance of epidemiologic studies to determine background rates of disease remains critical to assessing the risk of adverse events associated with vaccines. In considering mass vaccination against the 2009 H1N1 influenza virus, it was estimated that if a cohort of 10 million individuals were

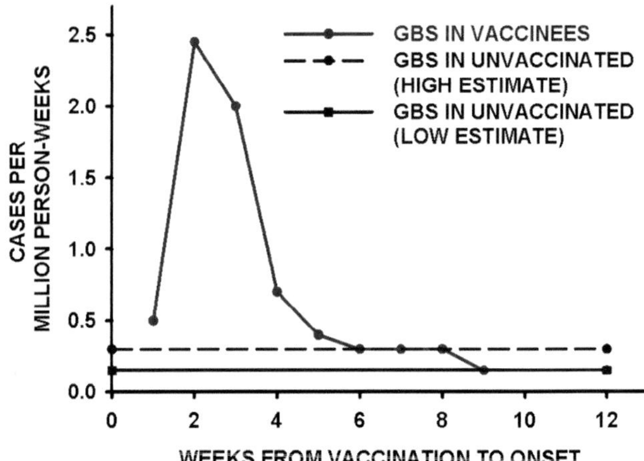

FIGURE 12.14. Guillain-Barré syndrome (limited to cases with extensive involvement) associated with swine influenza vaccine, according to the interval between immunization and onset in the United States in 1976. Two baseline rates are shown to define the expected rate of spontaneous Guillain-Barré syndrome. The period of the epidemic is readily defined (1–6 weeks after immunization) and the intervals during this period of excess incidence form a classical log-normal curve. (Data from Langmuir AD, Bregman DJ, Kurland LT, et al. An epidemiologic and clinical evaluation of Guillain-Barre syndrome reported in association with the administration of swine influenza vaccines. *Am J Epidemiol* 1984;119:841–879.)

vaccinated in the United Kingdom, 21.5 cases of Guillain-Barré syndrome and 5.75 cases of sudden death would be expected to occur within 6 weeks of vaccination as coincident background cases.[12]

Development and Assessment of Control Measures

In addition to vaccines, other control measures are sometimes useful against viral infections. Such approaches seek to reduce the risk of exposure and are usually suggested by epidemiologic studies of transmission mechanisms. Examples include reduction of risk associated with blood or blood products for viruses such as hepatitis B and hepatitis C, HIV, and human T-cell leukemia viruses I and II. Another classical example is the reduction of urban yellow fever and dengue through control of *Aedes aegypti* mosquito populations. The use of epidemiologic management of viral infection is illustrated by a study of Bolivian hemorrhagic fever—an arenavirus that was endemic in certain rural villages.[51] Ecological studies suggested that this virus was enzootic in one species of peridomestic house-dwelling mouse—*Calomys callosus*—and was transmitted by aerosolized fomites. Table 12.16 shows a study in which rodent control was initiated in one-half of a village and then extended to the other half. The dramatic effect of rodenticides confirmed the hypothesis of the virus reservoir and its transmission mechanism and provided a practical approach to control of a serious viral infection. More recently, sophisticated mathematical models have been used to evaluate control measures that cannot be tested in epidemiologic studies, including containment of a potential bioterrorist use of smallpox virus[43] and containment of pandemic influenza virus through vaccination[130] and the use of prophylactic antivirals.[25]

TABLE 12.16 Control of Bolivian Hemorrhagic Fever by Reduction of the Rodent Reservoir, San Joaquin, Bolivia, 1964[a]

Ten-day period beginning	New cases, east sector	New cases, west sector
April 1	12	9
11	8	17
21	12	8
May 1	7	18
11	4	14
21	2	9
31	3	12
June 10	0	10
20	5	7
30	0	0
July 10	0	0

[a]Rodents were controlled by trapping and poisoning, beginning in the East sector on May 1 and in the West sector on June 15.

From Johnson KM, Halstead SB, Cohen SN. Hemorrhagic fevers of Southeast Asia and South America: a comparative appraisal. *Prog Med Virol* 1967;9:105–158.

ACKNOWLEDGMENTS

We wish to acknowledge our mentors in epidemiology, Alexander Langmuir and Philip Sartwell for N.N. and Leon Gordis for W.J.M., on whose teachings much of this chapter is based.

REFERENCES

1. *The Eradication of Infectious Diseases: Report of the Dahlem Workshop on the Eradication of Infectious Diseases, Berlin, March* 16-22, 1997. In: Dowdle WR, Hopkins DR, eds. New York: John Wiley & Sons; 1998.
2. Abbey H. An examination of the Reed-Frost theory of epidemics. *Hum Biol* 1952;24:201–233.
3. Alberts B. Editorial expression of concern. *Science* 2011;333:35.
4. Anderson RM, May RM. *Infectious Diseases of Humans. Dynamics and Control.* Oxford: Oxford University Press; 1992.
5. Anonymous. *Atlas of World Population History.* New York: Penguin Books and Allen Lane; 1978.
6. Anonymous. *Statistical Yearbook, 38th Issue, 1990/1991.* New York: United Nations Publications; 1993.
7. Aycock WL, Luther EH. The incubation period of poliomyelitis. *J Prev Med* 1929;3:103–120.
8. Baggaley RF, Fraser C. Modelling sexual transmission of HIV: testing the assumptions, validating the predictions. *Curr Opin HIV AIDS* 2010;5:269–276.
9. Bartlett MS. The critical community size for measles in the United States. *J R Stat Soc A* 1960;123:37–44.
10. Bialek SR, George PA, Xia GL, et al. Use of molecular epidemiology to confirm a multistate outbreak of hepatitis A caused by consumption of oysters. *Clin Infect Dis* 2007;44:838–840.
11. Black FL. Infectious diseases in primitive societies. *Science* 1975;187:515–518.
12. Black S, Eskola J, Siegrist CA, et al. Importance of background rates of disease in assessment of vaccine safety during mass immunisation with pandemic H1N1 influenza vaccines. *Lancet* 2009;374:2115–2122.
13. Casey AE. The incubation period in epidemic poliomyelitis. *JAMA* 1942;120:805–807.
14. Castillo-Salgado C. Trends and directions of global public health surveillance. *Epidemiol Rev* 2010;32:93–109.
15. Cauchemez S, Bhattarai A, Marchbanks TL, et al. Role of social networks in shaping disease transmission during a community outbreak of 2009 H1N1 pandemic influenza. *Proc Natl Acad Sci U S A* 2011;108:2825–2830.
16. Centers for Disease Control and Prevention. Tracking progress toward global polio eradication—worldwide, 2009-2010. *MMWR Morb Mortal Wkly Rep* 2011;60:441–445.
17. Collins SJ, Lawson VA, Masters CL. Transmissible spongiform encephalopathies. *Lancet* 2004;363:51–61.
18. Cummings DA, Irizarry RA, Huang NE, et al. Travelling waves in the occurrence of dengue haemorrhagic fever in Thailand. *Nature* 2004;427:344–347.
19. Dauer CC. The changing age distribution of paralytic poliomyelitis. *Ann N Y Acad Sci* 1955;61:943–955.
20. Dawood FS, Jain S, Finelli L, et al. Emergence of a novel swine-origin influenza A (H1N1) virus in humans. *N Engl J Med* 2009;360:2605–2615.
21. Department of Environment, Food and Rural Affairs. *BSE: Statistics.* 2011, available at http://archive.defra.gov.uk/foodfarm/farmanimal/diseases/atoz/bse/.
22. Dowell SF. Seasonal variation in host susceptibility and cycles of certain infectious diseases. *Emerg Infect Dis* 2001;7:369–374.
23. Enright JR. Epidemiology of poliomyelitis. *Hawaii Med J* 1954;13:350–354.
24. Fenner F. Mouse-pox; infectious ectromelia of mice: a review. *J Immunol* 1949;63:341–373.
25. Ferguson NM, Cummings DA, Cauchemez S, et al. Strategies for containing an emerging influenza pandemic in Southeast Asia. *Nature* 2005;437:209–214.
26. Ferrari MJ, Grais RF, Bharti N, et al. The dynamics of measles in sub-Saharan Africa. *Nature* 2008;451:679–684.
27. Fine P, Eames K, Heymann DL. "Herd immunity": a rough guide. *Clin Infect Dis* 2011;52:911–916.
28. Fine PE, Clarkson JA. Measles in England and Wales—I: An analysis of factors underlying seasonal patterns. *Int J Epidemiol* 1982;11:5–14.
29. Fine PEM. The interval between successive cases of an infectious disease. *Am J Epidemiol* 2003;158:1039–1047.
30. Fisman DN. Seasonality of infectious diseases. *Annu Rev Public Health* 2007;28:127–143.
31. Foege WH. *House on Fire. The Fight to Eradicate Smallpox.* Berkeley: University of California Press; 2011.
32. Francis T, Jr., Napier JA, Voight RB, et al. *Evaluation of the 1954 Field Trial of Poliomyelitis Vaccine. Final Report.* Ann Arbor: University of Michigan; 1957.
33. Garg RK. Subacute sclerosing panencephalitis. *J Neurol* 2008;255:1861–1871.
34. Garten RJ, Davis CT, Russell CA, et al. Antigenic and genetic characteristics of swine-origin 2009 A(H1N1) influenza viruses circulating in humans. *Science* 2009;325:197–201.
35. Gordis L. *Epidemiology.* Philadelphia: Saunders Elsevier; 2009.
36. Gray RH, Wawer MJ, Brookmeyer R, et al. Probability of HIV-1 transmission per coital act in monogamous, heterosexual, HIV-1-discordant couples in Rakai, Uganda. *Lancet* 2001;357:1149–1153.
37. Greenwood M, Bradford Hill A, Topley WWC. *Experimental Epidemiology.* Special Report Series No. 209. Medical Research Council. London: His Majesty's Stationery Office; 1936.
38. Greig JR. Scrapie in sheep. *J Comp Pathol* 1950;60:263–266.
39. Grenfell BT, Bjornstad ON, Kappey J. Travelling waves and spatial hierarchies in measles epidemics. *Nature* 2001;414:716–723.
40. Grenfell BT, Pybus OG, Gog JR, et al. Unifying the epidemiological and evolutionary dynamics of pathogens. *Science* 2004;303:327–332.
41. Grimstad PR, Barrett CL, Humphrey RL, et al. Serologic evidence for widespread infection with La Crosse and St. Louis encephalitis viruses in the Indiana human population. *Am J Epidemiol* 1984;119:913–930.
42. Griot C, Gonzalez-Scarano F, Nathanson N. Molecular determinants of the virulence and infectivity of California serogroup bunyaviruses. *Annu Rev Microbiol* 1993;47:117–138.
43. Halloran ME, Longini IM, Jr., Nizam A, et al. Containing bioterrorist smallpox. *Science* 2002;298:1428–1432.
44. Halloran ME, Longini IM, Jr., Struchiner CJ. *Design and Analysis of Vaccine Studies.* New York: Springer; 2010.
45. Halloran ME, Struchiner CJ. Study designs for dependent happenings. *Epidemiology* 1991;2:331–338.

46. Halloran ME, Struchiner CJ, Longini IM, Jr. Study designs for evaluating different efficacy and effectiveness aspects of vaccines. *Am J Epidemiol* 1997;146:789–803.
47. Hancock K, Veguilla V, Lu X, et al. Cross-reactive antibody responses to the 2009 pandemic H1N1 influenza virus. *N Engl J Med* 2009;361:1945–1952.
48. Heesterbeek JA. A brief history of R_0 and a recipe for its calculation. *Acta Biotheor* 2002;50:189–204.
49. Henderson DA. *Smallpox— The Death of a Disease: The Inside Story of Eradicating a Worldwide Killer.* Amherst, NY: Promethius Books; 2009.
50. Horstmann DM, Paul JR. The incubation period in human poliomyelitis and its implications. *JAMA* 1947;135:11–14.
51. Johnson KM, Halstead SB, Cohen SN. Hemorrhagic fevers of Southeast Asia and South America: a comparative appraisal. *Prog Med Virol* 1967;9:105–158.
52. Kermack WO, McKendrick AG. Contributions to the mathematical theory of epidemics—I. 1927. *Bull Math Biol* 1991;53:33–55.
53. Keroack M, Fields BN. Viral shedding and transmission between hosts determined by reovirus L2 gene. *Science* 1986;232:1635–1638.
54. Koopman J. Modeling infection transmission. *Annu Rev Public Health* 2004;25:303–326.
55. Lanciotti RS, Roehrig JT, Deubel V, et al. Origin of the West Nile virus responsible for an outbreak of encephalitis in the northeastern United States. *Science* 1999;286:2333–2337.
56. Langmuir AD, Bregman DJ, Kurland LT, et al. An epidemiologic and clinical evaluation of Guillain-Barre syndrome reported in association with the administration of swine influenza vaccines. *Am J Epidemiol* 1984;119:841–879.
57. Lavinder CH, Freeman SW, Frost WH. Epidemiologic studies of poliomyelitis in New York City and the northeastern United States during the year 1916. *USPHS Hyg Lab Bull* 1918;91:1–150.
58. Lehmann HC, Hartung HP, Kieseier BC, et al. Guillain-Barre syndrome after exposure to influenza virus. *Lancet Infect Dis* 2010;10:643–651.
59. Lessler J, Moss WJ, Lowther SA, et al. Maintaining high rates of measles immunization in Africa. *Epidemiol Infect* 2011:1–11.
60. Lessler J, Reich NG, Brookmeyer R, et al. Incubation periods of acute respiratory viral infections: a systematic review. *Lancet Infect Dis* 2009;9:291–300.
61. Lievano FA, Papania MJ, Helfand RF, et al. Lack of evidence of measles virus shedding in people with inapparent measles virus infections. *J Infect Dis* 2004;189(Suppl 1):S165–S170.
62. Liljeros F, Edling CR, Amaral LA, et al. The web of human sexual contacts. *Nature* 2001;411:907–908.
63. Lipkin WI. Microbe hunting. *Microbiol Mol Biol Rev* 2010;74:363–377.
64. Lipsitch M, Viboud C. Influenza seasonality: lifting the fog. *Proc Natl Acad Sci U S A* 2009;106:3645–3646.
65. Lombardi VC, Ruscetti FW, Das Gupta J, et al. Detection of an infectious retrovirus, XMRV, in blood cells of patients with chronic fatigue syndrome. *Science* 2009;326:585–589.
66. London WP, Yorke JA. Recurrent outbreaks of measles, chickenpox and mumps. I. Seasonal variation in contact rates. *Am J Epidemiol* 1973;98:453–468.
67. Luby JP. St. Louis encephalitis. *Epidemiol Rev* 1979;1:55–73.
68. Luke DA, Harris JK. Network analysis in public health: history, methods, and applications. *Annu Rev Public Health* 2007;28:69–93.
69. Lumsden LL. St. Louis encephalitis in 1933: observations on epidemiological features. *Public Health Rep* 1958;73:340–353.
70. Mandzhavidze NF, Mamradze GP. *The High Dams of the World.* Springfield, VA: Academy of the Sciences of the Georgian SSR and Clearinghouse for Federal Scientific and Technical Information; 1994.
71. Marks HM. The 1954 Salk poliomyelitis vaccine field trial. *Clin Trials* 2011;8:224–234.
72. Marsden JP. A critical review of the clinical features of 13,686 cases of smallpox (variola minor). *Bull Hyg* 1948;23:735–746.
73. Mason JO, McLean WR. Infectious hepatitis traced to the consumption of raw oysters. An epidemiologic study. *Am J Hyg* 1962;75:90–111.
74. McLean AR, Anderson RM. Measles in developing countries. Part II. The predicted impact of mass vaccination. *Epidemiol Infect* 1988;100:419–442.
75. McMichael AJ, McKee M, Shkolnikov V, et al. Mortality trends and setbacks: global convergence or divergence? *Lancet* 2004;63:1155–1159.
76. Minor P. Vaccine-derived poliovirus (VDPV): impact on poliomyelitis eradication. *Vaccine* 2009;27:2649–2652.
77. Morens DM, Holmes EC, Davis AS, et al. Global rinderpest eradication: lessons learned and why humans should celebrate too. *J Infect Dis* 2011;204:502–505.
78. Morris M, Kretzschmar M. Concurrent partnerships and the spread of HIV. *AIDS* 1997;11:641–648.
79. Moss WJ, Strebel P. Biological feasibility of measles eradication. *J Infect Dis* 2011;204(Suppl 1):S47–S53.
80. Mossong J, Nokes DJ, Edmunds WJ, et al. Modeling the impact of subclinical measles transmission in vaccinated populations with waning immunity. *Am J Epidemiol* 1999;150:1238–1249.
81. Murray KO, Mertens E, Despres P. West Nile virus and its emergence in the United States of America. *Vet Res* 2010;41:67.
82. Mutapi F, Roddam A. p values for pathogens: statistical inference from infectious-disease data. *Lancet Infect Dis* 2002;2:219–230.
83. Nathanson N. The pathogenesis of poliomyelitis: what we don't know. *Adv Virus Res* 2008;71:1–50.
84. Nathanson N, Kew OM. From emergence to eradication: the epidemiology of poliomyelitis deconstructed. *Am J Epidemiol* 2010;172:1213–1229.
85. Nathanson N, Kew OM. Poliovirus vaccines: past, present, and future. *Arch Pediatr Adolesc Med* 2011;165:489–490.
86. Nathanson N, Langmuir AD. The Cutter incident. *Am J Hyg* 1963;78:16–28.
87. Nathanson N, Martin JR. The epidemiology of poliomyelitis: enigmas surrounding its appearance, epidemicity, and disappearance. *Am J Epidemiol* 1979;110:672–692.
88. Nichol ST, Spiropoulou CF, Morzunov S, et al. Genetic identification of a hantavirus associated with an outbreak of acute respiratory illness. *Science* 1993;262:914–917.
89. Orenstein WA, Strebel PM, Papania M, et al. Measles eradication: is it in our future? *Am J Public Health* 2000;90:1521–1525.
90. Oshinsky DM. *Polio. An American Story.* New York: Oxford University Press; 2005.
91. Paffenbarger RS, Jr., Bodian D. Poliomyelitis immune status in ecologically diverse populations, in relation to virus spread, clinical incidence, and virus disappearance. *Am J Hyg* 1961;74:311–325.
92. Palese P. Influenza: old and new threats. *Nat Med* 2004;10:S82–S87.
93. Panum PL. *Observations Made During the Epidemic of Measles on the Faroe Islands in the Year 1846.* New York: Delta Omega Society; 1940.
94. Paul JR. Epidemiology of poliomyelitis. In: *Poliomyelitis.* Geneva: World Health Organization; 1955:9.
95. Phillips CA, Melnick JL. Community infection with St. Louis encephalitis virus. Serologic study of the 1964 epidemic in Houston. *JAMA* 1965;193:207–211.
96. Pitzer VE, Viboud C, Simonsen L, et al. Demographic variability, vaccination, and the spatiotemporal dynamics of rotavirus epidemics. *Science* 2009;325:290–294.
97. Pybus OG, Rambaut A. Evolutionary analysis of the dynamics of viral infectious disease. *Nat Rev Genet* 2009;10:540–550.
98. Reed W. Recent researches concerning the etiology, propagation, and prevention of yellow fever, by the United States Army Commission. *J Hyg (Lond)* 1902;2:101–119.
99. Ricketts MN. Public health and the BSE epidemic. *Curr Top Microbiol Immunol* 2004;284:99–119.
100. Riley S. Large-scale spatial-transmission models of infectious disease. *Science* 2007;316:1298–1301.
101. Rogers DJ, Randolph SE. Studying the global distribution of infectious diseases using GIS and RS. *Nat Rev Microbiol* 2003;1:231–237.
102. Ross R. An application of the theory of probabilities to the study of *a priori* pathometry, Part I. *Proc R Soc Series A* 1916;92:204–230.
103. Ross R. *Report on the Prevention of Malaria in Mauritius.* London: Waterlow & Sons Ltd.; 1908.
104. Sartwell PE. The incubation period and the dynamics of infectious disease. *Am J Epidemiol* 1966;83:204–206.
105. Sartwell PE. The incubation period of poliomyelitis. *Am J Public Health Nations Health* 1952;42:1403–1408.
106. Sawyer WA, Meyer KF, Eaton MD, et al. Jaundice in army personnel in the western region of the United States and its relation to vaccination against yellow fever. *Am J Hyg* 1944;39:337–387.

107. Schonberger LB, Bregman DJ, Sullivan-Bolyai JZ, et al. Guillain-Barre syndrome following vaccination in the National Influenza Immunization Program, United States, 1976–1977. *Am J Epidemiol* 1979;110: 105–123.
108. Sencer DJ, Dull HB, Langmuir AD. Epidemiologic basis for eradication of measles in 1967. *Public Health Rep* 1967;82:253–256.
109. Serfling RE, Sherman IL. Poliomyelitis distribution in the United States. *Public Health Rep* 1953;68:453–466.
110. Shaman J, Goldstein E, Lipsitch M. Absolute humidity and pandemic versus epidemic influenza. *Am J Epidemiol* 2011;173:127–135.
111. Shaman J, Kohn M. Absolute humidity modulates influenza survival, transmission, and seasonality. *Proc Natl Acad Sci U S A* 2009;106: 3243–3248.
112. Sharp PM, Bailes E, Chaudhuri RR, et al. The origins of acquired immune deficiency syndrome viruses: where and when? *Philos Trans R Soc Lond B Biol Sci* 2001;356:867–876.
113. Sharp PM, Hahn BH. The evolution of HIV-1 and the origin of AIDS. *Philos Trans R Soc Lond B Biol Sci* 2010;365:2487–2494.
114. Skinhoj P. Hepatitis and hepatitis B-antigen in Greenland. II: Occurrence and interrelation of hepatitis B associated surface, core, and "e" antigen-antibody systems in a highly endemic area. *Am J Epidemiol* 1977; 105:99–106.
115. Sweitzer SE, Ikeda K. Variola, a clinical study of the Minneapolis epidemic of 1924–1925. *Arch Derm Syph* 1927;15:19–29.
116. Swerdlow DL, Finelli L, Bridges CB. 2009 H1N1 influenza pandemic: field and epidemiologic investigations in the United States at the start of the first pandemic of the 21st century. *Clin Infect Dis* 2011;52(Suppl 1): S1–S3.
117. Szmuness W, Harley EJ, Ikram H, et al. Sociodemographic aspects of the epidemiology of hepatitis. In: Vyas GN, ed. *Viral Hepatitis.* Philadelphia: Franklin Institute Press; 1978:297–320.
118. Tamerius J, Nelson MI, Zhou SZ, et al. Global influenza seasonality: reconciling patterns across temperate and tropical regions. *Environ Health Perspect* 2011;119:439–445.
119. Tamin A, Rota PA, Wang ZD, et al. Antigenic analysis of current wild type and vaccine strains of measles virus. *J Infect Dis* 1994;170:795–801.
120. Tang JW. The effect of environmental parameters on the survival of airborne infectious agents. *J R Soc Interface* 2009;6(Suppl 6):S737–S746.
121. Taubenberger JK. The origin and virulence of the 1918 "Spanish" influenza virus. *Proc Am Philos Soc* 2006;150:86–112.
122. Tauxe R. Measles incidence in Iceland, 1900-1940. Unpublished report. 1979.
123. Thompson WH, Kalfayan B, Anslow RO. Isolation of California encephalitis group virus from a fatal human illness. *Am J Epidemiol* 1965; 81:245–253.
124. Wassilak S, Pate MA, Wannemuehler K, et al. Outbreak of type 2 vaccine-derived poliovirus in Nigeria: emergence and widespread circulation in an underimmunized population. *J Infect Dis* 2011;203:898–909.
125. Watanabe T, Kawaoka Y. Pathogenesis of the 1918 pandemic influenza virus. *PLoS Pathog* 2011;7:e1001218.
126. Webster RG, Kawaoka Y, Bean WJ, Jr. Molecular changes in A/Chicken/ Pennsylvania/83 (H5N2) influenza virus associated with acquisition of virulence. *Virology* 1986;149:165–173.
127. Weiss RA, McMichael AJ. Social and environmental risk factors in the emergence of infectious diseases. *Nat Med* 2004;10:S70–S76.
128. Williams KH, Hollinger FB, Metzger WR, et al. The epidemiology of St. Louis encephalitis in Corpus Christi, Texas, 1966. *Am J Epidemiol* 1975;102:16–24.
129. Wolfe ND, Dunavan CP, Diamond J. Origins of major human infectious diseases. *Nature* 2007;447:279–283.
130. Yang Y, Sugimoto JD, Halloran ME, et al. The transmissibility and control of pandemic influenza A (H1N1) virus. *Science* 2009;326:729–733.
131. Yorke JA, London WP. Recurrent outbreaks of measles, chickenpox and mumps. II. Systematic differences in contact rates and stochastic effects. *Am J Epidemiol* 1973;98:469–482.
132. Yorke JA, Nathanson N, Pianigiani G, et al. Seasonality and the requirements for perpetuation and eradication of viruses in populations. *Am J Epidemiol* 1979;109:103–123.

CHAPTER 13

Donald M. Coen • Douglas D. Richman

Antiviral Agents

OVERVIEW

Medical Importance of Antiviral Drugs and Barriers to Their Development

Viruses are a leading cause of disease and death worldwide. Although public health measures and vaccines are the most effective ways to control many viral infections, preventive measures have not succeeded for numerous viral diseases. For some of these diseases, antiviral drugs have been developed. A number of these drugs have been highly successful, saving lives and relieving suffering. This has been most dramatic with drugs that are active against human immunodeficiency virus (HIV). In the developed world, these drugs have transformed a progressive fatal disease into a manageable condition, in which virus replication can be suppressed presumably for a lifetime as long as antiretroviral therapy is maintained. These dramatic benefits had been extended to more than 7 million people globally by 2011.[182]

Despite these successes, there are still relatively few diseases for which highly effective antiviral drugs have been developed. There are several factors that contribute to this. With very few exceptions, such as the polymerases of related viruses, drug targets are virus specific, and therefore only a few antiviral drugs developed against one virus have been active against other viruses. Some viruses (e.g., herpesviruses, HIV) establish latent infections, so treating active infections does not cure the patient. Different viruses, especially respiratory viruses, can cause similar symptoms, making diagnosis difficult. Often, treatment must begin early to be beneficial, sometimes because the viral diseases are quickly controlled by immune responses.

On top of these factors are economic issues that have often discouraged pharmaceutical companies from developing antiviral drugs. For example, any individual virus disease may represent a relatively small potential market. It is not surprising then that companies have focused mainly on easily diagnosed and chronic viral diseases that require prolonged drug administration and that are relatively widespread in developed countries, because these are diseases for which treatment would earn substantial profits. Perhaps ironically, these diseases are often caused by viruses that establish latent infections and are not curable.

The first highly successful antiviral drug was acyclovir (ACV), initially developed in the late 1970s against herpes simplex virus (HSV) 1 and 2 and varicella zoster virus (VZV).[91] Antiviral drug discovery expanded markedly with the acquired immunodeficiency syndrome (AIDS) epidemic, which led to a variety of drugs against HIV and opportunistic pathogens such as human cytomegalovirus (HCMV). This coincided with expanding knowledge about virus genetics, molecular biology, enzymology, and protein structure, which permitted modern, more rational approaches, to drug discovery. Indeed, antiviral drugs have been a proving ground for these approaches.

The Process of Antiviral Drug Development

Older antiviral drugs such as amantadine and ACV were discovered by the testing of chemicals for their ability to inhibit virus replication in labor- and time-intensive assays of viral replication, such as assays of cytopathic effect or plaque assays.[75,327] These chemicals had typically been synthesized for some other purpose, and discovery of their antiviral activities was often serendipitous. When particular chemicals were known to have antiviral activity, a variety of other chemicals with similar structures were tested for activity. Several examples of this somewhat more rational procedure can be found in the sections on specific drugs.

The more modern and rational approach of high-throughput screening of large libraries of chemicals has been used to discover some newer drugs. High throughput screens can be "target-based" or "cell-based." Target-based screens start with the identification of a viral gene product that would make a good drug target (see below for discussion). It is important that the target protein can be expressed at high levels and purified, and that it can be assayed rapidly with high-throughput robotic technology. Such target-based screens can examine more than one million chemical compounds in no more than a few weeks. Most nonnucleoside reverse transcriptase inhibitors (NNRTIs), which are active against HIV-1, were discovered using this approach (e.g., nevirapine[246]). Cell-based high-throughput screens are slower, more cumbersome, and more expensive. However, such assays permit interrogation of multiple and unappreciated mechanisms of action, and can be performed relatively rapidly using robots (i.e., within one to a few days per assay). In addition, they automatically identify compounds that can enter cells and block a step of virus replication. Highly potent compounds that target a poorly understood function of hepatitis C virus (HCV) and block HCV replication in vivo have been discovered using a cell-based screen.[110]

A still more rational approach is to exploit detailed knowledge about a viral protein to design drugs that will inhibit its activity. In particular, knowledge of the three-dimensional structure of the protein can enable visualization of its active site and understanding of its mechanism of action, and can also be used to design or refine small molecules that can block the active site and the protein's action. An example of a drug discovered using this approach is the neuraminidase inhibitor, zanamivir, which is active against influenza A and B viruses.[370]

The approaches outlined in the preceding text result in what is called a "hit"; however, a hit is only an inhibitor of the function of a viral protein or of viral replication in cell culture. The next steps involve using medicinal chemistry to convert the hit into a compound with high potency and desirable pharmacological properties (e.g., bioavailability, long elimination half-life, low toxicity), not to mention patentability. If the structure of the hit compound bound to its target is available, this information can be used to help generate additional compounds to be tested. This process will be illustrated below with the example of the anti-HIV protease inhibitor, ritonavir. Simultaneously, studies to demonstrate the mechanism(s) of action of the compounds are undertaken (see section on antiviral drug mechanisms and drug resistance below). A key, but often overlooked aspect of drug development is developing optimal methods for synthesis of pure compound on a large scale and formulation of the compound for administration to humans.

When a candidate compound with desirable properties has been developed, clinical trials begin. There is no rigid formula by which an antiviral candidate is assessed after it enters the clinic. Typically, the process of clinical development starts with the administration of drug in escalating doses to small cohorts of volunteers to assess pharmacokinetics and tolerability (phase I trials). With some virus infections, these studies may be performed in patients in whom drug activity can also be assessed, for example by quantifying reductions of chronic HCMV shedding in the genitourinary tract or of HCV in the plasma (proof-of-concept studies). Substantial reductions in viral load encourage progression to more advanced clinical trials. However, with an infection such as HIV, the risk of selecting for drug resistance that might compromise future treatment options often restricts phase I trials to studies of HIV-seronegative subjects. This issue may become important for other viruses (e.g., HCV).

A major advantage of antiviral drug development, compared to drug development for many other diseases, is that quantitative reductions in virus shedding are a precise measure of activity and in general correlate with clinical end points. These quantitative reductions can be measured quickly (days) and permit determination of whether drugs work and of appropriate doses and dosing intervals. Phase II clinical trials assess this antiviral activity along with additional pharmacological and safety information in dozens to several hundred subjects. The data from phase II trials permit the design of larger phase III registrational studies, which provide statistically robust results that fulfill regulatory requirements for drug approval. Trials for drugs for influenza and herpesviruses infections require clinical end points (i.e., amelioration of disease), with virological data supporting those. For HIV, and increasingly for hepatitis B virus (HBV) and HCV, the correlations between levels of viremia and disease, and the correlations between drug-induced reductions in viremia and improvement of disease have resulted in virological end points (quantitative reduction and proportion of patients below the limit of detection) as criteria for drug approval.

Phase III studies of a new antiretroviral drug can pursue two general indications. For patients who failed prior regimens because of drug-resistant virus and who have limited treatment options, an accelerated approval process is available with shorter trials to document efficacy. Historically, patients were randomized to an optimized regimen based on the results of a drug resistance test with or without the addition of the test drug that presumably has activity against drug-resistant virus. Demonstration of superior virological end points after 24 weeks with continued follow-up for at least a year was considered supportive of an unmet medical need to fulfill criteria for registrational approval. Repeated demonstrations that this approach worked have led to the sense that placebo arms were no longer ethically defensible. The proper design of future trials for these patients remains unclear.[206]

Development of a drug for first-line (initial) therapy faces higher hurdles. Patients starting antiretroviral therapy are now usually asymptomatic and must plan for decades of successful suppression of virus replication. Therefore, a new drug must offer superiority to the current standard of care, and a combination including a new drug "X" (for example, tenofovir and emtricitabine [FTC] plus drug X) might be compared to tenofovir and FTC plus efavirenz. Hundreds of subjects in each arm must be followed for at least 2 years for efficacy and safety to fulfill regulatory criteria for approval of a drug for use in initial treatment. A predefined statistical definition of "noninferiority" is the criterion for approval of candidate drugs for which there is an approved drug in the same class,

Should the clinical trials yield the desired results, the "hit" will have turned into an approved drug. Even then, its efficacy and safety will be put to the test in much larger populations, and new indications for its use may emerge.

Importance of Antiviral Drugs for Basic Science

Aside from their importance in treating viral diseases, antiviral drugs make excellent laboratory tools. As is illustrated in detail later in this chapter, drugs can block the functions of specific viral proteins and thus specific stages in viral replication. This is crucial for understanding the timing of particular events in the virus replication cycle and which proteins are needed for each step. Studies using selective antiviral drugs, coupled with viral mutations that confer drug resistance, can help to identify the roles of viral proteins and dissect the details of how these proteins function. Drug-resistance mutations can provide selectable markers for engineering interesting mutant viruses and performing viral genetics.

Examples of how studies of antiviral drugs and drug resistance can illuminate virus biology and biochemistry include the role of amantadine in the discovery of an influenza A ion channel and its function in virus uncoating,[142,289] and the role of ganciclovir in the discovery of an unusual HCMV protein kinase that can phosphorylate nucleoside analogs.[350] Crystal structures of drug targets with bound inhibitors have yielded important insights into structure and function of these targets. For example, the first structure of a retroviral (HIV) reverse transcriptase was obtained in complex with nevirapine.[193] Similarly, clinical investigation has been greatly abetted by antiviral drugs. Intensive monitoring of the dynamics of HIV replication following the administration of drug has permitted important insights about rates of virus production, virus clearance, and cellular sources of virus replication.[129,282] Studies of patients receiving HIV therapy have elucidated much of our understanding of HIV latency, evolution, and fitness.[50,98,390] Finally, the remarkable restoration of CD4 cell numbers and function with HIV therapy provides insights regarding both lymphocyte dynamics and immune function.[7,129]

General Aspects of Antiviral Drug Mechanisms and Drug Resistance

Drug Selectivity, Resistance, and Drug Targets

The value of antiviral drugs to basic science depends on how selective they are and on how well their mechanisms are understood. Selectivity and mechanism are also crucial for the clinical use of antiviral drugs. Biologically, selectivity is the difference between the dose of the drug that exerts its antiviral effect (usually quantified as the dose that reduces viral activity by 50%) and the dose that exerts its cytotoxic effect (or more subtle impairments of the host). Examples of how selectivity is achieved biochemically can be found among the descriptions of the mechanisms of specific antiviral drugs.

It is generally agreed that the best way to understand antiviral selectivity and mechanism is through the study of drug resistance. Because viruses are obligate intracellular parasites, the detection of resistance to an antiviral drug implies that the drug is selective. That is, the drug acts at least in part by interfering directly with a virus-specific process, rather than by incapacitating the host cell.[157] In much the same way, a mutation in a viral gene that confers resistance to an antiviral drug implies that the gene or its product is necessary for at least part of the selective action of the drug. It is not enough to identify a mutation in a drug-resistant mutant to show that the mutation confers resistance. It is crucial to perform a genetic experiment (e.g., reconstruct a virus with the mutation [and no other] and show that the reconstructed virus is drug-resistant).

In most cases, drug-resistant mutations identify targets of antiviral drugs. However, not all drug-resistant mutations identify drug targets. For example, inhibitors of influenza virus neuraminidase (e.g., zanamivir) can select for mutations in the gene encoding hemagglutinin.[125,241,341] These mutations would be expected to result in a hemagglutinin that binds less avidly to cell surface glycoproteins. This in turn could result in a reduced requirement for neuraminidase to release the virion from the cell, and thus resistance to the neuraminidase inhibitor. Accordingly, genetics alone is not sufficient to identify a drug target. Ideally, one should also show that the drug interacts with the target, and that the resistance mutation results in a target with an altered interaction with the drug that explains the resistance phenotype. This usually requires biochemical studies, and the analyses are not always straightforward.

Genetics alone is also not sufficient to reveal the detailed mechanism of action of an inhibitor. Mapping a resistance mutation that results in a single amino acid change in the target protein identifies that residue as being necessary for sensitivity to the drug. Other genetic approaches, such as the generation of chimeric genes from closely related viruses that are susceptible or resistant to a drug (e.g., HIV-1 and HIV-2, and NNRTIs[67]), can identify residues that are sufficient to confer susceptibility to the drug to an otherwise resistant protein. However, these results do not identify residues that interact with the drug. Identification of a drug-binding site requires methods such as photoaffinity cross-linking and x-ray crystallography. These two methods have identified the binding site for the NNRTI, nevirapine, on HIV-1 reverse transcriptase (RT).[62,193,392] Mapping a drug binding site is valuable, but does not tell us how drug binding exerts its physiologic action. In the case of NNRTIs, pre–steady-state kinetic analyses of HIV-1 RT were used to show that the drug slows the enzyme's incorporation of deoxynucleoside triphosphates (dNTPs) into DNA,[313,338] presumably by altering the orientation of catalytic residues, as suggested by the location of the drug binding site.[193] Therefore, solving the mechanism of action of an antiviral drug requires multidisciplinary approaches.

For a number of antiviral drugs, we still lack a complete understanding of their mechanisms of action and resistance, and, in some cases, there is considerable controversy regarding these mechanisms. This can even be true for drugs that are designed against a specific target. For example, fomivirsen is an oligonucleotide drug that is designed to inhibit HCMV replication by its complementarity to messenger RNA (mRNA) for an important regulatory protein.[3,8] However, studies of a drug-resistant mutant did not confirm this mechanism of action.[262] Therefore, the mechanism of fomivirsen remains unknown. We will not discuss this and certain other drugs such as the anti-HSV topical treatment, docosanol, whose mechanisms are unknown.

General Aspects of Antiviral Drug Targets

There are two major kinds of virus proteins that serve as antiviral drug targets. In general, it is easier to inhibit a protein's function (with an antagonist) than to promote its function (with an agonist). Therefore, the most common antiviral drug target is a virus-encoded protein that can be inhibited by a drug. Ideally, this kind of target should be essential for viral replication. Less ideally, it should at least be very important for replication and pathogenesis in the human host. The target should also be sufficiently different from any important host proteins to permit selectivity. It should be *druggable*; that is, a small molecule should be able to inhibit it. Enzymes make especially good targets for inhibition because they are usually at low concentrations inside cells, they are relatively well-understood mechanistically, they often interact with small-molecule substrates, and, as catalysts, their inhibition interrupts multiple reactions. Furthermore, pharmaceutical companies have a great deal of experience in developing enzyme inhibitors as drugs. It is therefore not surprising that most antiviral drug targets are virus-encoded enzymes. A second kind of target is a virus-encoded protein that can activate the drug to make it inhibitory to the virus (*lethal synthesis*), and that is sufficiently different from host counterparts to permit selectivity. An example is HSV thymidine kinase (TK), which activates ACV and its congeners.[108]

Host proteins may also serve as antiviral drug targets, if they have an activity that is more important for viral replication than for host functions. A successful example of this approach is targeting the cell surface molecule, C-C chemokine receptor type 5 (CCR5), which led to the development of the anti-HIV drug maraviroc.[207,297] Targeting of host functions is inherently more likely to result in toxicity than is targeting of viral functions. Conversely, it has been argued that viruses should be less likely to develop resistance against drugs that target host functions. Regardless, such mutants certainly can develop (e.g.,[328,366]).

Factors Affecting the Development of Drug Resistance

If a drug acts selectively against a virus, the virus will generally be able to develop resistance to it. However, the frequency of drug-resistant mutants in a population, and how rapidly they arise depend on several factors: The first is the mutation rate of the virus. The higher the mutation rate, the more rapidly resistance can develop. Viral mutation rates are largely controlled by the fidelity of the polymerases that replicate the viral genomes. RNA viruses, which replicate using low-fidelity RNA polymerases, usually have the highest mutation rates, averaging one mutation per genome per replication cycle,[87,232] whereas DNA viruses, whose DNA polymerases include proofreading 3′ to 5′ exonucleases that contribute to fidelity,[172] have lower mutation rates. However, other factors, including nucleotide pools, which can be modulated by both viral and cellular factors, also contribute to mutation rate.

The second factor is the target size for mutation. The more sites where mutations can confer drug resistance, the more rapidly resistance can arise. For some drugs, such as ACV, many mutations can confer resistance, as any mutation that substantially reduces viral TK activity results in resistance. In addition, some sites within a gene are more or less likely to mutate than others. Homopolymeric runs in the HSV *tk* gene (e.g., a run of seven G's) are hot spots for frameshift mutations that confer ACV resistance.[170]

The third factor is magnitude of replication of the virus. The more copies of viral genomes produced, the more opportunities for resistance to arise. The fourth factor is the preexisting size of the virus population. The more virus present, even in the absence of drug selection, the more likely that drug-resistant mutants will be present among the array of genetic variants. Examples of these two factors that have an impact on HIV drug resistance are provided below in the section on drug resistance in antiviral therapy.

The fifth factor involves fitness (i.e., how well a genetic variant reproduces relative to other genetic variants, which can include "wild-type"). The more fit, the more likely resistance will occur. This is especially important for clinically significant drug resistance. For a virus to cause disease that is resistant to an antiviral drug, it must mutate not only to evade drug action, but also to retain pathogenicity. In vivo fitness and pathogenicity can be inferred from clinical studies, but can be assessed more directly in animal models. Although there is always the question of whether animal models are predictive of human disease, in most cases, there has been an excellent correlation between how drug-resistant mutants behave in clinical and animal studies. Some drug-resistant mutants, such as influenza viruses that are resistant to adamantanes, can be highly fit, both in cell culture and in animal models.[15,355] Moreover, such mutants appear to be highly fit in human infections as well (reviewed in 144). Most ACV-resistant HSV mutants are highly fit in cell culture, but are much less so in animal models, which correlates with the low frequency that these mutants are recovered in immunocompetent humans (reviewed in 58 and 199). Still other drug-resistant mutants, such as certain HCMV mutants that are resistant to the drug foscarnet, can be less fit in cell culture, but not so impaired that they do not cause disease in patients.[12] Relative fitness is important both in the absence and in the presence of drug. If wild-type virus can replicate relatively well in the presence of drug (e.g., at subtherapeutic concentrations), then resistant mutants will be less likely to predominate. These various factors—mutation rate, target size, replication rate, pre-existing population, and fitness—can be taken into account in mathematical formulas and used to model the emergence of drug resistance (e.g.[61]).

In addition, these factors influence how different viral infections are treated. For example, HIV infections are now treated with combinations of antiviral drugs, whereas HSV infections are treated with single agents. This is discussed later in the sections on antiviral therapy.

MECHANISMS OF SPECIFIC ANTIVIRAL DRUGS

This section mainly considers agents that are currently approved for clinical use. No endorsement of the therapeutic value of these drugs is intended. For certain viruses that can be studied usefully in animal models, we discuss the effects of drug-resistant mutations on replication and pathogenesis in vivo.

Targeting Drugs to Specific Stages of Virus Infection

As detailed throughout this book, the infection of cells by viruses can be broken down into a common set of steps or stages, and most of these stages have been targeted by approved antiviral drugs (Fig. 13.1). The order of stages can differ for different viruses, and some viruses have stages that are not

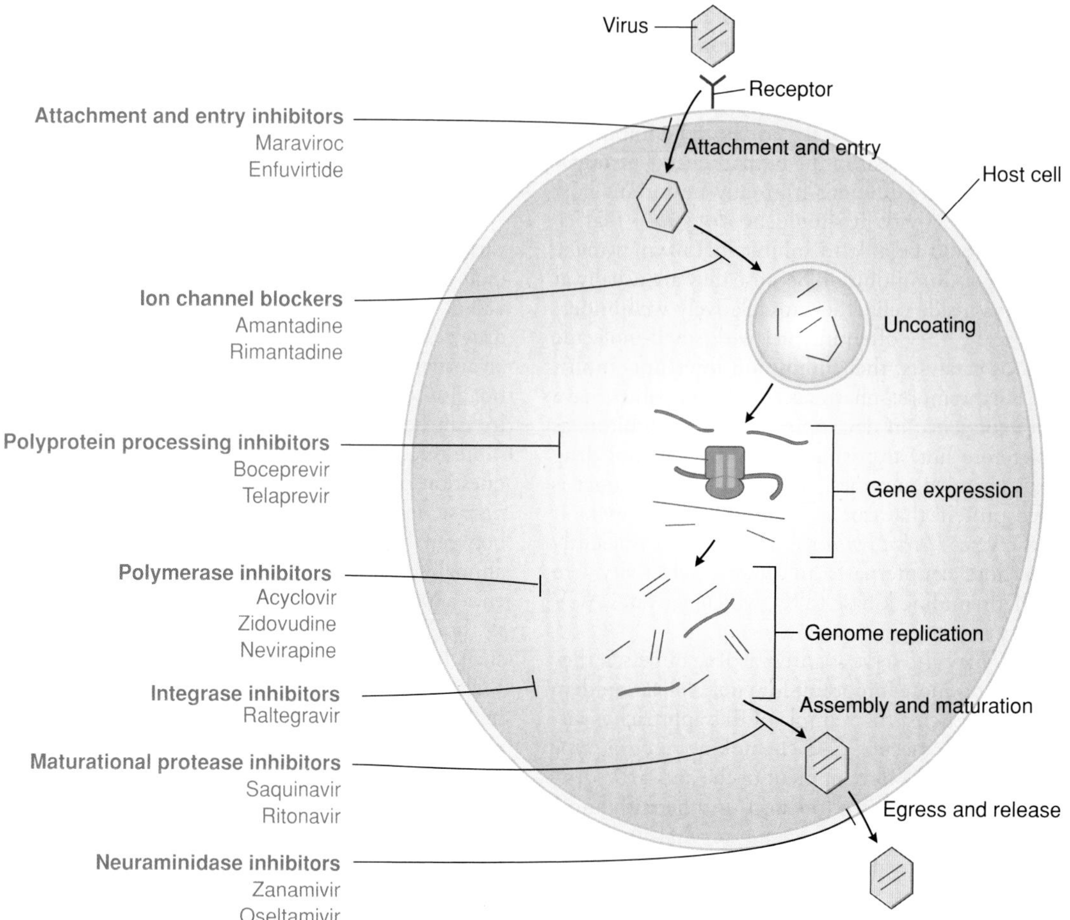

FIGURE 13.1. Antiviral drugs block various stages of viral replication. A generic replication cycle of viruses in cells is cartooned, showing the stages of infection, which different drug classes block. These include attachment and entry, uncoating, gene expression, genome replication, assembly and maturation, and egress and release. Examples of specific drug classes are provided. For some viruses (e.g., human immunodeficiency virus [HIV]), the order of the stages differs from that in this cartoon (see Fig. 13.2). Some viruses lack stages shown here (e.g., release), whereas other viruses have additional stages. (Modified from Yeh RW, Coen DM. Pharmacology of viral infections. In: Golan DE, Tashjian AH, Jr., Armstrong EJ, et al., eds. *Principles of Pharmacology: The Pathophysiologic Basis of Drug Therapy.* Third edition. Philadelphia: Lippincott Williams & Wilkins, 2012:649–673.)

shared with other viruses. For example, the replication of HIV and the stages that have been targeted by approved antiviral drugs are illustrated in Figure 13.2. In principle, any stage can be targeted for inhibition. There are potential advantages to targeting very early or late stages such as attachment, entry, and release, because inhibitors of these stages do not have to enter cells to exert activity. Stages such as genome replication, assembly, and maturation often require specific viral enzymes, which, as described earlier, are attractive drug targets. Indeed, most antiviral drugs currently available inhibit genome replication. Nevertheless, there are antiviral drugs that act at nearly every stage of viral infection.

Inhibition of Viral Attachment and Entry

Inhibition of attachment and entry prevents all subsequent steps in virus infection and permits the virion to be cleared by immune and other mechanisms. There have been two general approaches for drugs that inhibit attachment and entry, which thus far have resulted in two approved anti-HIV drugs: maraviroc and enfuvirtide. Both of these drugs have unusual properties; maraviroc targets a host protein, whereas enfuvirtide is a peptide.

CCR5 Blockers

Maraviroc (Fig. 13.3) is a CCR5 blocker; it inhibits binding of HIV to the CCR5 co-receptor. CCR5 is the co-receptor used by the most commonly transmitted HIV-1 strains (R5 tropic), which predominate during the early stages of HIV-1 infection.[26] There are several attractive features to CCR5 as a target for anti-HIV drugs: Knockout mice lacking CCR5, and humans with homozygous deletions in the gene encoding CCR5 (CCR5Δ32) lack detectable abnormalities, suggesting that blocking this host function might not have adverse consequences.[38] Certain of these CCR5Δ32 homozygotes who have been highly exposed to HIV have remained uninfected, and their cells are resistant to R5-tropic strains of HIV *in vitro.*[221] Blockade of CCR5 with a natural ligand (e.g., RANTES) or antibody inhibits R5-tropic HIV replication (e.g.,[56]). These observations suggested that

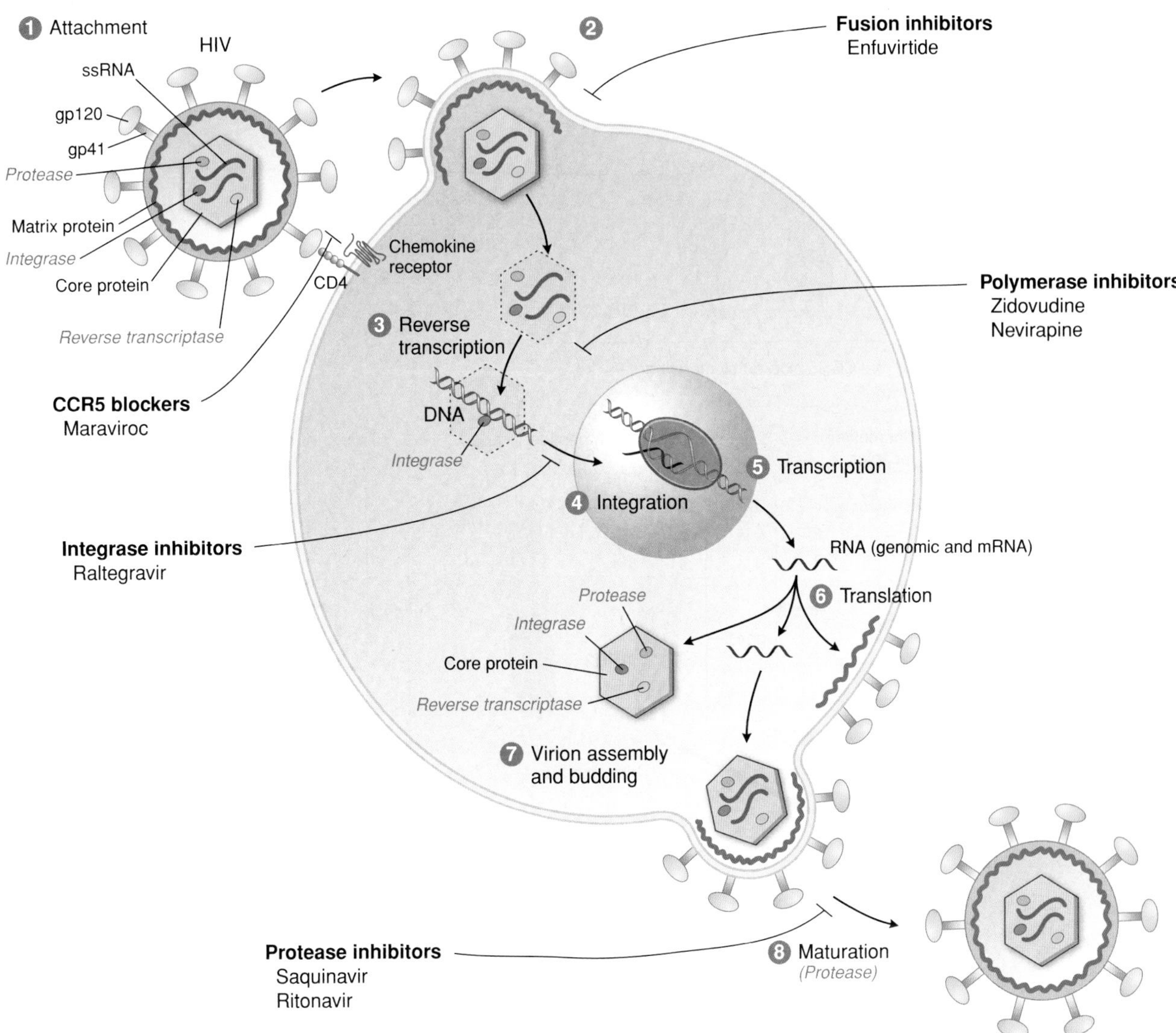

FIGURE 13.2. Stages of HIV infection blocked by different classes of antiviral drugs. The lifecycle of HIV is cartooned, showing the following. **1:** Virus attachment is dependent on binding interactions between viral gp160 (composed of gp41 and gp120 proteins) and host cell CD4 and certain chemokine receptors. **2:** Fusion of the viral membrane (envelope) with the host cell plasma membrane allows the human immunodeficiency (HIV) genome complexed with certain virion proteins to enter the host cell. **3:** Uncoating permits the single-stranded RNA (ssRNA) HIV genome to be copied by reverse transcriptase into double-stranded DNA. **4:** The HIV DNA is integrated into the host cell genome, in a reaction that depends on HIV-encoded integrase. **5:** Gene transcription and posttranscriptional processing by host cell enzymes produce genomic HIV RNA and viral messenger RNA (mRNA). **6:** The viral mRNA is translated into proteins on host cell ribosomes. **7:** The proteins and genomic RNA assemble into immature virions that bud from the host cell membrane. **8:** The virions undergo proteolytic cleavage, maturing into fully infective virions. The steps at which classes of anti-HIV drugs act (attachment, fusion, reverse transcription, integration, and maturation) are indicated, with examples from specific drug classes provided. (Modified from Yeh RW, Coen DM. Pharmacology of viral infections. In: Golan DE, Tashjian AH, Jr., Armstrong EJ, et al., eds. *Principles of Pharmacology: The Pathophysiologic Basis of Drug Therapy.* Third edition. Philadelphia: Lippincott Williams & Wilkins, 2012:649–673.)

blocking CCR5 could be efficacious against R5-tropic HIV without causing much toxicity.

Maraviroc was discovered using high-throughput screening for small molecules that block binding of CCR5 to a natural ligand, followed by medicinal chemistry efforts to improve upon a hit from the screen.[83] Modeling and mutational studies suggest that maraviroc and several other CCR5 blockers bind to a pocket on CCR5 formed by transmembrane domains,[195] and allosterically inhibit binding to HIV gp120, thereby blocking HIV entry (Fig. 13.3).[9,83,112,374] R5 tropic HIV mutants resistant to CCR5 blockers including maraviroc contain altered gp120 molecules that are able to bind to the drug-bound form of CCR5.[366,374] Maraviroc was approved in 2007 for use in combination with other anti-HIV drugs in patients with R5-tropic

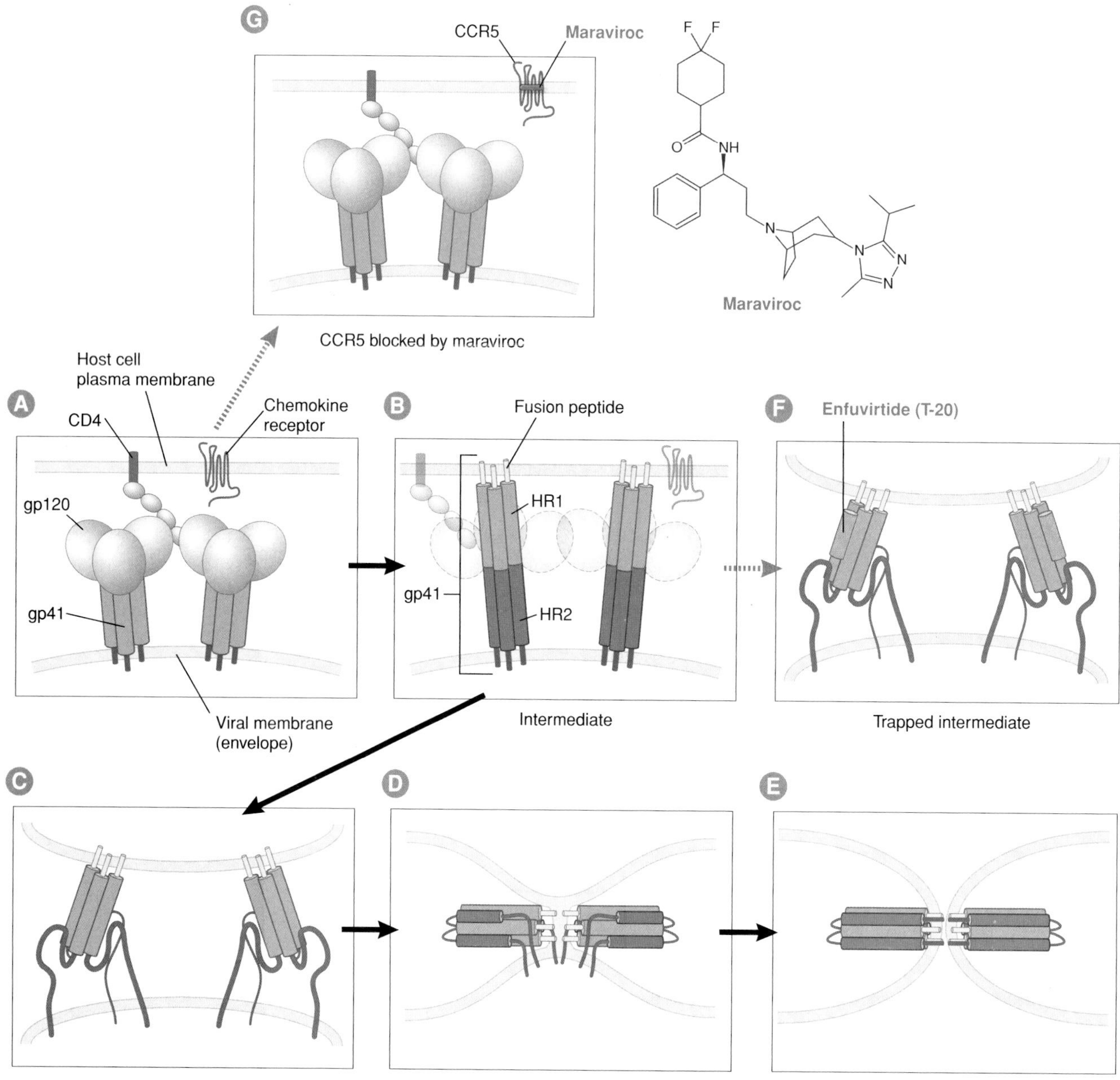

FIGURE 13.3. Model for HIV gp41-mediated fusion and maraviroc and enfuvirtide (T-20) action. A: Human immunodeficiency virus (HIV) glycoproteins exist in trimeric form in the viral envelope. Each gp120 molecule is depicted as a ball attached noncovalently to gp41. The CD4 receptor and a chemokine receptor that serves as a co-receptor in the host cell plasma membrane are shown. **B:** The binding of gp120 to CD4 and the co-receptor causes a conformational change in gp41 that exposes the fusion peptide, heptad-repeat region 1 (HR1) and heptad-repeat region 2 (HR2). The fusion peptide inserts into the host cell plasma membrane. **C:** gp41 undergoes further conformational changes, characterized by unfolding and refolding of the HR2 segments. **D:** Completed refolding of the HR regions creates a hemifusion stalk in which the outer leaflets of the viral and host cell membranes are fused. **E:** Formation of a complete fusion pore allows viral entry into the host cell. **F:** Enfuvirtide (T-20) is a synthetic peptide that mimics HR2 and binds to HR1. It prevents the HR1–HR2 interaction (dashed arrow). The drug, therefore, traps the virus–host cell interaction at the attachment stage, preventing membrane fusion and viral entry. **G:** Maraviroc is a small molecule antagonist of the CCR5 chemokine receptor; the drug blocks cellular infection of HIV strains that use CCR5 for attachment and entry (dashed arrow from **A** to **G.** The structure of maraviroc is shown). (From Yeh RW, Coen DM. Pharmacology of viral infections. In: Golan DE, Tashjian AH, Jr., Armstrong EJ, et al., eds. *Principles of Pharmacology: The Pathophysiologic Basis of Drug Therapy.* Third edition. Philadelphia: Lippincott Williams & Wilkins, 2012:649–673.)

strains. Therefore, patients must be tested to determine if they harbor virus that utilizes a different co-receptor (i.e., CXCR4). Maraviroc treatment failures are more frequently attributable to preexisting minority populations of CXCR4-tropic virus than to selection of R5-tropic virus that is resistant to maraviroc.[259] Resistance to CCR5 blockers has not resulted thus far from R5-tropic virus evolving to use a different co-receptor. Nevertheless, this possibility and the effects of antagonizing a host function remain potential issues for the long-term clinical use of maraviroc and other CCR5 blockers, which are in development (e-Table 13.1).

Fusion Inhibitors: Enfuvirtide

Although compounds that bind to virus particles and block attachment and entry have been investigated in the laboratory and clinic for decades (e.g., the anti-picornavirus drug, pleconaril), enfuvirtide was the first drug approved for clinical use that acts this way. This agent was discovered by a rational, directed approach that examined the ability of peptides to inhibit HIV infection in cell culture.[385,386] The peptide that was most potent (T-20) is similar to a segment of gp41, the HIV protein that mediates membrane fusion. The proposed mechanism for gp41-mediated membrane fusion and T-20 action is illustrated in Figure 13.3: The gp41 protein in the virion is ordinarily trapped in a metastable conformation so that it cannot fuse membranes or bind T-20. Binding of HIV to its cellular receptors triggers a conformational change that exposes the segment of gp41 that is thought to insert into host cell membranes (fusion peptide), a heptad repeat region (HR-1), and the segment that T-20 resembles, which is a second heptad repeat (HR-2). The gp41 then rearranges so that HR-1 and HR-2 bind to each other. If the fusion peptide has inserted into the host cell membrane, this refolding brings the virion envelope and the cell membrane in proximity, thereby allowing membrane fusion to occur (by mechanisms that remain incompletely understood). When T-20 is present, however, it binds to HR-1 and prevents the refolding process, thereby preventing fusion of the HIV envelope with the host cell membrane.

Although this model requires an exogenous peptide to compete with an intramolecular interaction to bind to a target that is available only transiently, it is supported by a number of observations. These include the crystal structure of the rearranged form of gp41, which shows the HR-1–HR-2 interaction[41,357,373] and evidence that T-20 interacts with HR-1 containing peptides.[42,205,384] Genetic studies show that HR-1 and HR-2 are crucial for fusion.[88,383] Perhaps the strongest evidence that T-20 inhibits HIV replication by binding to HR-1 is that HIV mutations that confer resistance to T-20 alter HR-1 residues, and that these alterations weaken binding of T-20 to HR-1.[312]

Not only is the mechanism of T-20 remarkable, but so is its development into a drug. Because it is a peptide, there were major obstacles to its large-scale synthesis and manufacture, and outpatients must mix the drug and inject it themselves. Regardless, it proved that inhibitors of attachment and entry can be effective antiviral agents.

Inhibition of Viral Uncoating: Adamantane Derivatives

The adamantanes, amantadine and rimantadine (Fig. 13.4), are active exclusively against influenza A virus (and not influenza B or C viruses). In most influenza A virus strains, these drugs inhibit virus uncoating. It took decades to identify the target of these drugs. A key finding[142,143] was that amantadine has an unusual dose–response curve, at least for some strains of influenza A virus. It inhibits viral replication at concentrations of approximately 1 μM, which are those attained in patients treated with the drugs; however, at somewhat higher concentrations, it loses antiviral activity. It then regains antiviral activity at concentrations greater than 100 μM. Hay and colleagues[142] then showed that mutants that could replicate in 5 μM amantadine were resistant due to point mutations within the M segment of influenza RNA gene, in an open reading frame that had only recently been recognized. This open reading frame encodes a small membrane protein known as M_2 (the M segment also encodes the long-recognized matrix [M_1] protein.) Subsequent biochemical and electrophysiologic experiments showed that the M^2 protein forms a tetrameric, pH-gated channel for H^+ ions and that amantadine and rimantadine block this channel.[17,89,163,289,349]

The manner in which amantadine and rimantadine block the M_2 ion channel has been investigated intensively. Viral mutations conferring resistance to these drugs alter any of five residues in the transmembrane segment of the protein that are predicted to be within the pore of the channel, suggesting that the drugs bind to these residues and "plug" the channel.[141] Structural studies of drug-bound versions of M_2 followed by electrophysiologic assays using Xenopus oocytes and assays of engineered viral mutants support this suggestion.[36,180,270,343] However, evidence from nuclear magnetic resonance (NMR) studies and liposomal proton flux assays supported the suggestion that these drugs do not act as "plugs," but instead bind to the outside of the channel and stabilize its closed conformation.[287,330] This controversy appears to have been resolved in favor of the pore-binding site being the one that mediates drug action, with the NMR structure of rimantadine bound within the pore of a drug-sensitive chimeric M_2 derived from influenza A and B viruses.[286]

How would blocking an ion channel lead to inhibition of uncoating? A reasonable but not completely verified model is diagrammed in Figure 13.4. Influenza A virus attaches to sialic acid moieties on cell surface glycoproteins, and then, bound to its receptor, is internalized, surrounded by a cell membrane–bounded compartment, the endosome, which normally participates in membrane protein recycling. As part of its normal function, the endosome becomes acidified. During influenza virus entry, this reduction in pH causes a conformational change in the virion hemagglutinin protein, and fusion of the virion envelope and the endosomal membrane via a mechanism similar to that of HIV gp41 (Fig. 13.3). By itself, this action would release viral ribonucleoprotein into the cytoplasm. However, in the presence of amantadine or rimantadine, the matrix protein, M_1, does not dissociate from the ribonucleoprotein, which remains in the cytoplasm instead of entering the nucleus.[34,236] Low pH can promote the dissociation of M_1, and allow nuclear entry of the ribonucleoprotein.[33] Therefore, M2 in the virion envelope functions to let H^+ ions from the acidified endosome enter the virion, and dissociate M_1 from the ribonucleoprotein. Amantadine and rimantadine would block the entry of H^+ ions, thereby preventing this uncoating event.

With certain influenza A virus strains, amantadine and rimantadine also block late events in virus replication, in particular,

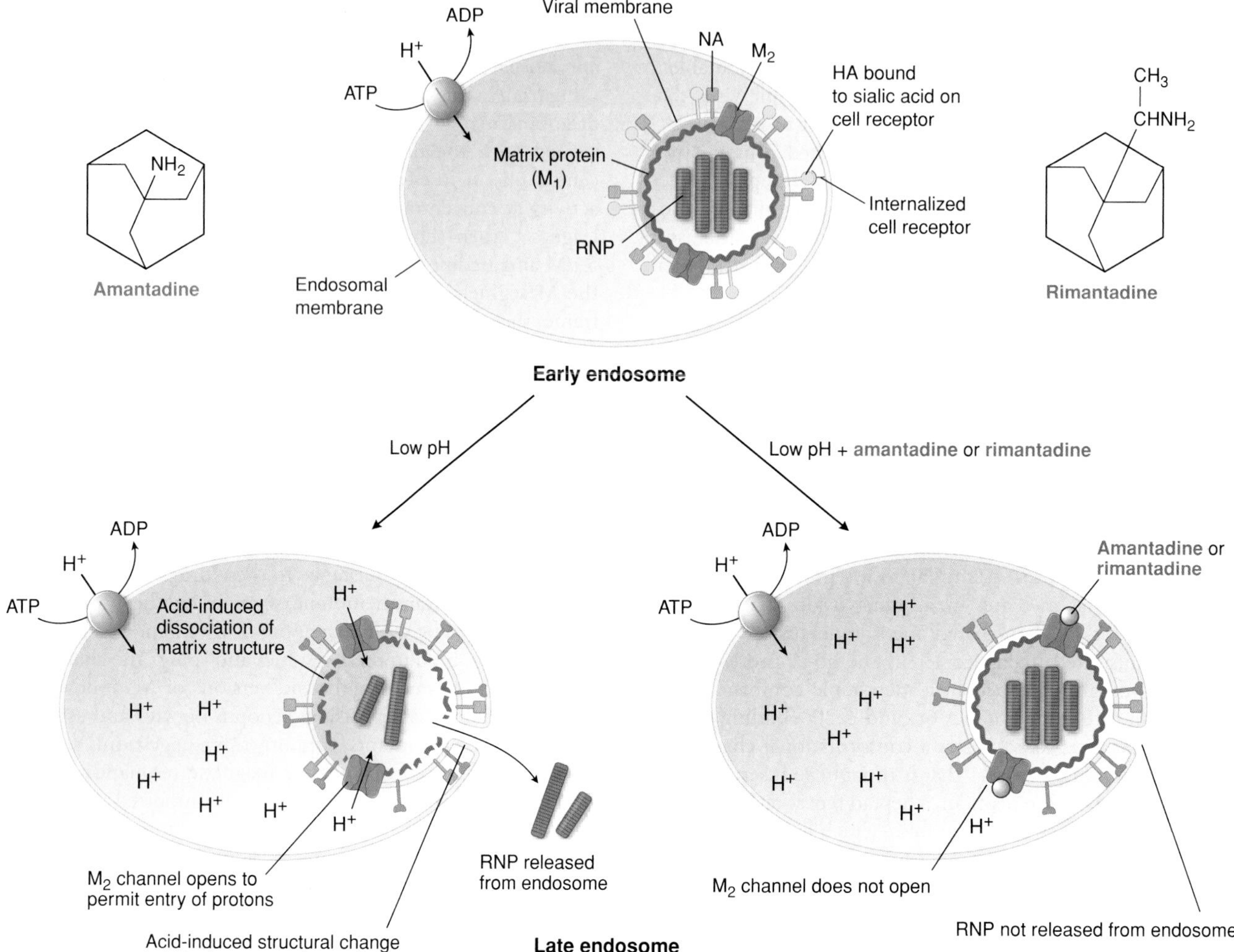

FIGURE 13.4. Model for uncoating of influenza A virus and effect of amantadine or rimantadine. The structures of amantadine and rimantadine are shown. The process of influenza A virus uncoating and drug action is depicted. The virus enters host cells by receptor-mediated endocytosis (not shown) and is contained within an early endosome. The early endosome contains a H^+-ATPase that acidifies the endosome by pumping protons from the cytosol into the endosome. A low pH-dependent conformational change in the envelope protein, hemagglutinin (HA), triggers fusion of the viral membrane with the endosomal membrane. This fusion event, however, is not sufficient to cause viral uncoating. In addition, protons from the late endosome must enter the virion through the M_2 proton channel, which is a virion envelope protein that opens in response to acidification (pH-gated ion channel). The entry of protons into the virion causes dissociation of the M_1 matrix protein from the influenza A ribonucleoprotein (RNP), releasing it into the cytoplasm. The dissociation of matrix is required for RNP to be transported to the nucleus, where it is transcribed and replicated. Amantadine and rimantadine block M_2 ion channel function and thereby inhibit acidification of the interior of the virion, matrix dissociation, and uncoating. NA, neuraminidase. (Modified from Yeh RW, Coen DM. Pharmacology of viral infections. In: Golan DE, Tashjian AH, Jr., Armstrong EJ, et al., eds. *Principles of Pharmacology: The Pathophysiologic Basis of Drug Therapy.* Third edition. Philadelphia: Lippincott Williams & Wilkins, 2012:649–673.)

maintenance of hemagglutinin in a proper conformation for infectivity.[141]

Influenza virus mutants that are resistant to amantadine and rimantadine due to altered M_2 have been assayed in animal models including mice and ferrets, and show little or no diminution in their replication or pathogenesis.[15,273,355] This correlates well with their behavior in human infections.[144] Since the discoveries of the mechanism of adamantanes and the function of M_2, a number of other viruses have been found to encode proteins that can form ion channels. These also might serve as good drug targets.

Inhibition of Viral Gene Expression: NS3/4A Protease Inhibitors

Viral gene expression entails not only the transcription of the viral genome into mRNA, the translation of mRNA into protein, and the stabilities of RNA and protein gene products, but can also include a variety of processing events including capping, splicing, and polyadenylation of viral mRNAs, and proteolytic cleavage of viral polyproteins into their individual protein units. Many viruses encode functions that execute or abet one or more of these steps in gene expression, and much

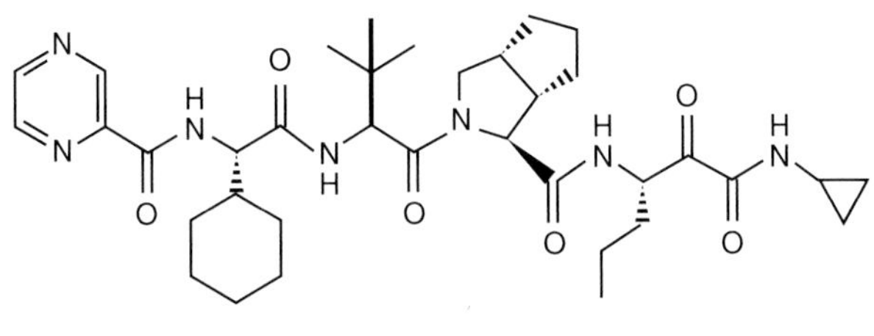

Telaprevir

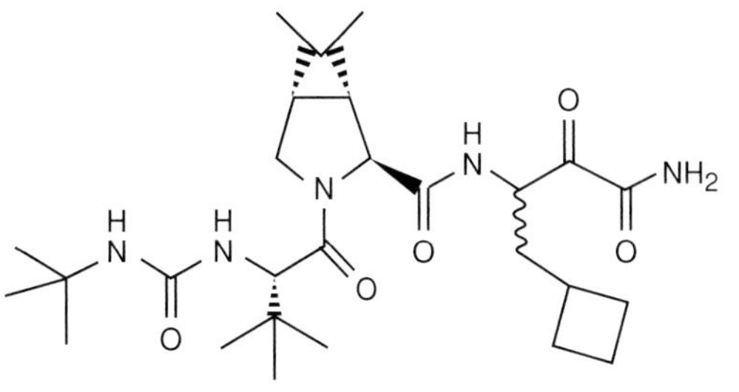

Boceprevir

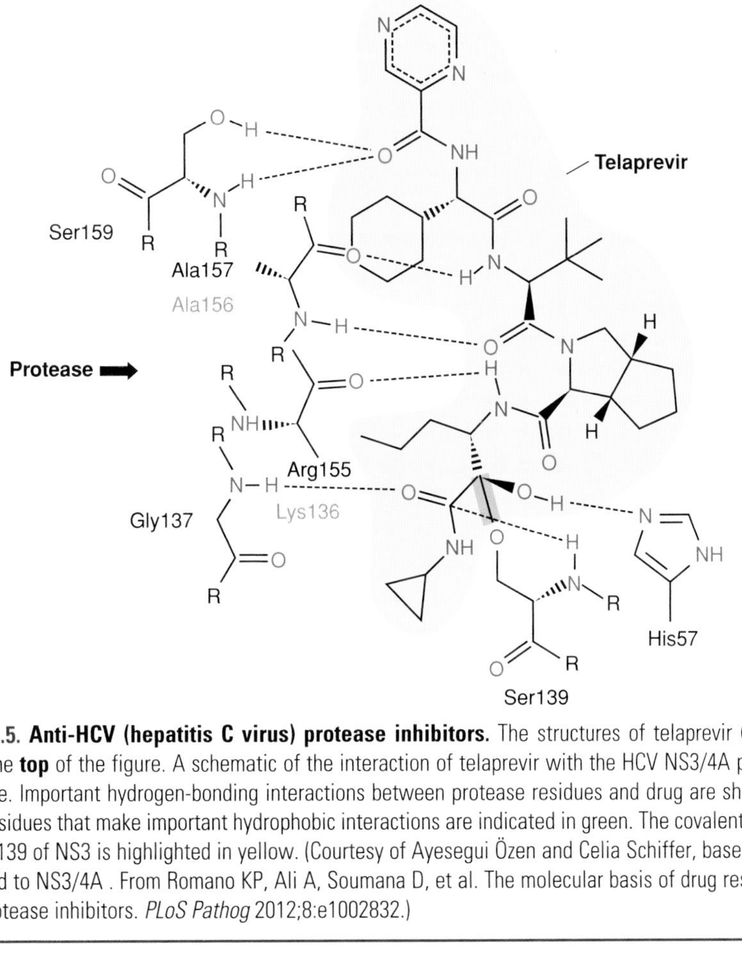

FIGURE 13.5. Anti-HCV (hepatitis C virus) protease inhibitors. The structures of telaprevir **(left)** and boceprevir **(right)** are shown at the **top** of the figure. A schematic of the interaction of telaprevir with the HCV NS3/4A protease is shown at the **bottom** of the figure. Important hydrogen-bonding interactions between protease residues and drug are shown with dashed lines, whereas protease residues that make important hydrophobic interactions are indicated in green. The covalent bond formed between telaprevir and serine 139 of NS3 is highlighted in yellow. (Courtesy of Ayesegui Özen and Celia Schiffer, based on the crystal structure of telaprevir bound to NS3/4A . From Romano KP, Ali A, Soumana D, et al. The molecular basis of drug resistance against hepatitis C virus NS3/4A protease inhibitors. *PLoS Pathog* 2012;8:e1002832.)

effort has gone into targeting these functions for development of antiviral drugs. In particular, viral proteases that generate individual viral proteins have been targeted. The activity of one of these, the HIV protease, is not required until the viral particle is fully assembled, and thus will be discussed under the heading Inhibition of Viral Assembly and Maturation below. The activity of the HCV NS3/4A protease, however, is required for proper expression of viral gene products for essentially all subsequent steps in viral infection. In 2011, the first drugs that target this stage of viral replication were approved by the U.S. Food and Drug Administration (FDA). These two drugs—telaprevir and boceprevir (Fig. 13.5)—are peptidomimetics that inhibit the NS3/4A protease.

Following entry and uncoating of HCV, its genome serves as an mRNA that is translated into a very large (~3,000 residue) polyprotein. This polyprotein is processed into 10 individual proteins by cellular and viral proteases. One viral protease, which is especially important for generating nonstructural (NS) proteins, is NS3. NS3 contains an N-terminal protease domain and a C-terminal helicase domain. A second protein, NS4A, forms a complex with NS3 (NS3/NS4A), and enhances its protease activity. During polyprotein processing, NS3 autoproteolytically cleaves between NS3 and NS4A, and then cleaves to generate NS4A (its co-factor), NS4B, NS5A, and NS5B. The NS proteins are essential for HCV genome replication and production of infectious virus. These proteins, especially NS3, are also thought to counteract the innate immune response.[109]

Given the success of drugs that inhibit the HIV protease (see below), investigators launched efforts to develop drugs that inhibit the NS3 protease. As described below in more detail for the HIV protease inhibitors, the development process was iterative involving the synthesis of candidate inhibitors, solving the structures of these inhibitors bound to the protease, and then designing new compounds with higher potency and better pharmacological properties based on those structures.[213,266] Several features of the HCV NS3/4A protease and its inhibitors differ from those of their HIV counterparts, however. The HIV protease is an aspartyl protease, whereas the NS3/4A protease is a serine protease. The HIV protease's substrate binding pocket is deep, so that there are multiple opportunities for interactions with a small molecule inhibitor, whereas the NS3/4A binding pocket is shallow, with relatively few obvious sites for binding a small molecule. Despite this obstacle, structure-based medicinal chemistry efforts identified sites on NS3 that could mediate tight and selective binding of inhibitors (Fig. 13.5).[213,266] The anti-HIV protease inhibitors are largely symmetrical, mimicking the protein substrate on both sides of the protease cleavage site, whereas the anti-NS3/4A inhibitors are relatively asymmetric, mainly mimicking the N-terminal product of protease cleavage. The anti-HIV protease inhibitors contain CHOH moieties that mimic the transition state of protease catalysis to achieve tight, but noncovalent binding to the enzyme (transition state analogs). In contrast, the anti-NS3/4A inhibitors contain ketoamide groups that react with the catalytic serine of the enzyme to form a covalent bond with the enzyme (Fig. 13.5), which only very slowly reverses, resulting in time-dependent inhibition of the enzyme (mechanism-based inhibitors) and inhibition constants of ~10 nM.[213,266]

Both boceprevir and telaprevir exhibit submicromolar potencies (concentrations that inhibit replication by 50%) for inhibition of replication of HCV genomes in a cell-based replicon system.[214,229] Interestingly, telaprevir was considerably less potent in these assays than a macrocyclic NS3/4A inhibitor, BILN 2061, which binds tightly but noncovalently; yet both drugs eliminated HCV replicons (10^4-fold reductions) from cells at similar concentrations, which may relate to the very slow reversibility of telaprevir.[214] This observation helps to illustrate the concept that efficacy (how much viral replication is reduced) is likely to be more important than potency in antiviral development. Both boceprevir and telaprevir inhibit HCV genome replication, at least additively in combination with interferon α (IFN-α).[214,229] These findings are important due to the use of boceprevir and telaprevir in combination with IFN-α for HCV therapy, and they may relate to a role for NS3 in counteracting IFN action.[109] Once a suitable cell culture system that supports complete replication of HCV was devised, it was shown that NS3/4A inhibitors block production of infectious virus.[215] Finally, as was first strikingly demonstrated with BILN 2061, NS3/4A inhibitors can drastically reduce levels of HCV in the plasma of patients.[197]

HCV replication is rapid and error-prone; therefore, it is not surprising that resistance to NS3/4A protease inhibitors arises rapidly both in cell culture systems and in patients.[82] Indeed, resistant variants preexist in untreated patients.[14] The different subtypes of HCV complicate HCV drug resistance, with protease inhibitors having different potencies against different subtypes, and with different subtypes requiring different numbers of mutations to achieve resistance.[132]

Several mutations confer resistance to boceprevir and telaprevir, with some altering NS3 residues that make direct contacts with drug and others altering more distant residues that contact amino acids close to the drug, such as the catalytic serine.[132] Certain mutations confer differing degrees of resistance to the two drugs. Notably, some mutations that confer resistance to boceprevir and telaprevir do not confer resistance to newer macrocyclic NS3/4A inhibitors that are in development (e-Table 13.1), and certain mutations that are resistant to the macrocyclic inhibitors do not confer resistance to boceprevir and telaprevir. However, other mutations confer resistance to both classes of NS3/4A drugs.[132] The effects of the different mutations on fitness vary as measured in cell culture systems for genome replication and production of infectious virus or in human hepatocyte chimeric mice, with some mutations being clearly impaired and others having very little impact.[158,334,363] Mathematical modeling of HCV infections in humans suggests that at least some protease inhibitor–resistant mutations retain substantial fitness.[316] These features of resistance to boceprevir and telaprevir are an impetus for continued development of anti-HCV drugs that can be used in combination (e-Table 13.1).

Inhibition of Viral Genome Replication

Most antiviral drugs inhibit viral genome replication, and nearly all of these inhibit a viral polymerase. Those viruses whose genome replication has been successfully targeted to yield FDA-approved drugs include certain human herpesviruses, the retrovirus HIV, and the hepadnavirus HBV. Several inhibitors of the polymerase of the flavivirus HCV are in clinical development. Most of the approved drugs are nucleoside analogs (Figure 13.6). Some of these nucleoside analogs actually mimic nucleoside monophosphates, so they are actually nucleotide analogs. A few approved drugs are nonnucleoside inhibitors of DNA polymerase or reverse transcriptase that act by binding at a site other than the dNTP-binding site, and one approved drug inhibits HIV integrase.

Nucleoside Analogs

Nucleoside analogs that clearly act by inhibiting viral polymerases are approved for treatment of herpesviruses, HBV, and HIV, and several are in development for treatment of HCV. Another nucleoside analog, ribavirin, is used clinically against HCV and respiratory syncytial virus, but its mechanism of action against those viruses is not well understood (see below). All nucleoside and nucleotide analogs must be activated by phosphorylation, usually to the triphosphate form, to exert their effect. Phosphorylated nucleoside analogs inhibit polymerases by competing with the natural substrate (dNTP for DNA polymerase) and are usually also incorporated into the growing nucleic acid chain, where they often terminate elongation. Either or both of these features—inhibition and incorporation—can be important for antiviral activity.

The more efficiently cellular enzymes phosphorylate the nucleoside analog and the more potently the phosphorylated forms act against cellular enzymes, the more toxic the nucleoside analog will be. Selectivity, therefore, is dependent upon how much more potently and effectively viral genome replication is inhibited than are cellular functions, and for the herpesviruses, how much more efficiently viral enzymes phosphorylate the drug than do cellular enzymes.

Anti-Herpesvirus DNA Polymerase Inhibitors

The various human herpesviruses encode both kinases and DNA polymerases. The kinases are usually not essential for viral

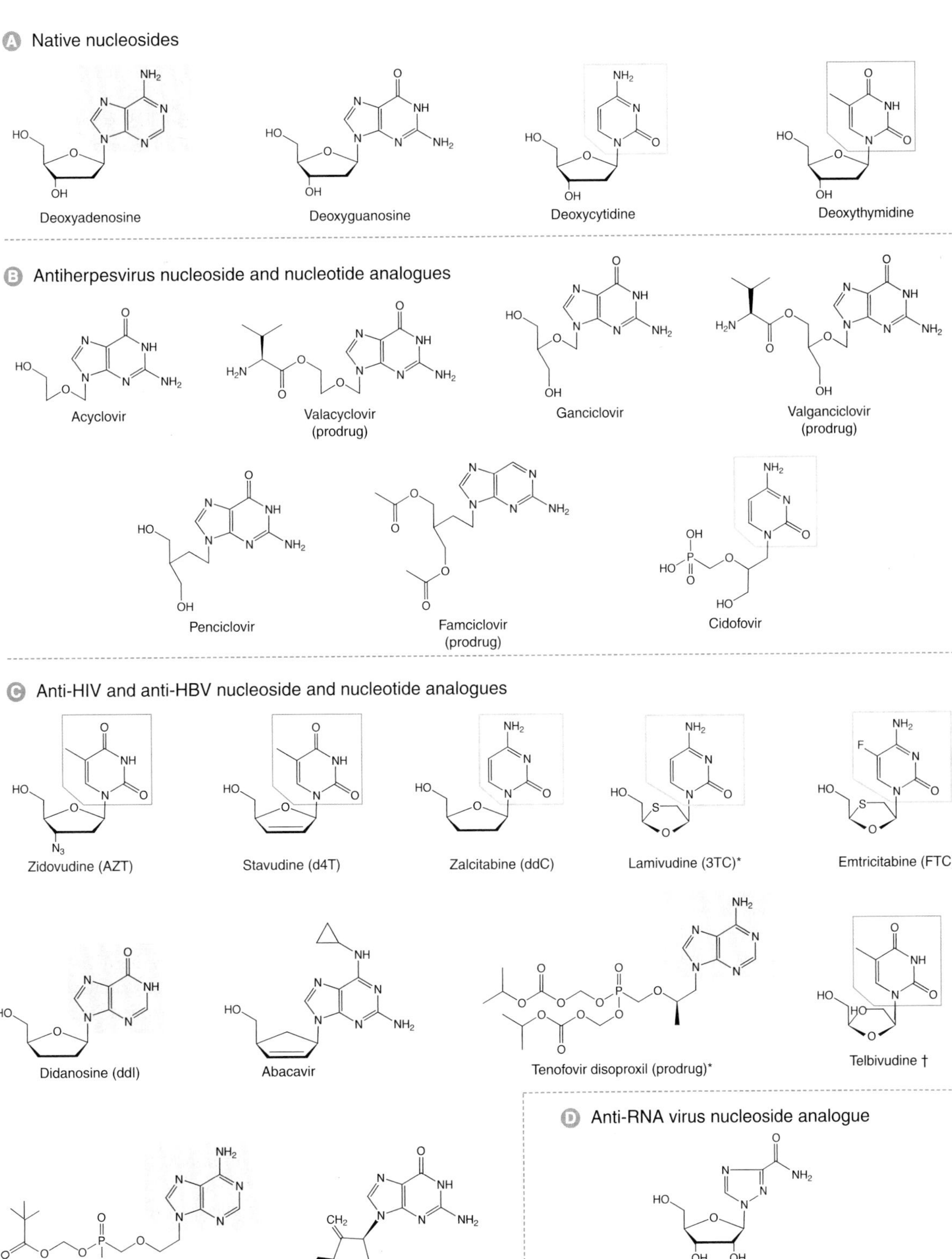

FIGURE 13.6. Structures of antiviral nucleoside analogues. A: The deoxynucleosides used as precursors for DNA synthesis are depicted in their *anti* configurations. The base moieties are shaded. **B:** Anti-herpesvirus nucleoside analogs mimic the deoxynucleoside, deoxyguanosine, except for cidofovir, which mimics the deoxynucleotide dCMP. The compounds shown here all contain acyclic moieties that mimic deoxyribose. Valacyclovir and famciclovir are prodrugs of acyclovir (ACV) and penciclovir, respectively. **C:** Anti-HIV (human immunodeficiency virus) and anti-HBV (hepatitis B virus) nucleoside analogs mimic dT, dC, dA, and dG except for tenofovir, and adefovir, which mimic dAMP. All of the analogs contain a base found in **A,** except for didanosine, which mimics deoxyinosine and is converted to dideoxyadenosine, and abacavir, which contains a cyclopropyl-modified guanine. Tenofovir and adefovir are shown as their disoproxil and dipivoxil prodrugs, respectively. Lamivudine, emtricitabine, and telbivudine are L-stereoisomers, whereas the other nucleoside analogs and dT, dC, dA, and dG are D-stereoisomers. All of the compounds shown except entecavir contain deoxyribose mimics that lack the equivalent of a 3′-hydroxyl, and thus are obligate chain terminators. The anti-HIV nucleoside analogs, lamivudine and tenofovir(*), and telbivudine, adefovir, and entecavir (†) are approved for use against HBV. **D:** Ribavirin, which contains a purine mimic attached to ribose, is approved for use against the RNA viruses hepatitis C virus and respiratory syncytial virus. (Modified from Yeh RW, Coen DM. Pharmacology of viral infections. In: Golan DE, Tashjian AH, Jr., Armstrong EJ, et al., eds. *Principles of Pharmacology: The Pathophysiologic Basis of Drug Therapy.* Third edition. Philadelphia: Lippincott Williams & Wilkins, 2012:649–673.)

replication, but the catalytic subunits of the polymerases (Pols) are. These enzymes differ enough from their cellular counterparts to permit development of selective antiviral nucleoside analog.

A number of antiviral nucleoside analogs including vidarabine, idoxuridine, and trifluridine, were developed and used against HSV infections. However, these drugs have been superseded by more selective compounds, and their mechanisms will not be discussed further.

Acyclovir and Related Drugs

ACV is the paradigmatic antiviral nucleoside analog that illustrates many of the principles of nucleoside analogs. It consists of a guanine base attached to an acyclic sugar-like molecule (Fig. 13.6). ACV and its more orally available valine ester, valacyclovir, and the related drugs, penciclovir and its orally available derivative, famciclovir (structures in Fig. 13.6) have similar mechanisms of action against HSV and VZV. ACV was originally synthesized at Burroughs Wellcome as part of a program to discover adenosine deaminase inhibitors, and only later was it tested for antiviral activity. The mechanism of ACV action[91] is presented in Figure 13.7. The TK encoded by HSV and VZV phosphorylates ACV, despite its differences from the natural substrate of this enzyme, thymidine (also known as deoxythymidine; see Fig. 13.6). Crystal structures of HSV TK in complex with thymidine or ACV[29,40,387] show that the guanine moiety of ACV interacts with the same residues as does the thymine moiety of thymidine, albeit with differences in water-mediated binding and bond angles. Despite this, ACV is not a particularly good substrate for HSV or VZV TK. Nevertheless, no mammalian enzyme phosphorylates ACV nearly as efficiently as the HSV and VZV TKs. Accordingly, HSV- and VZV-infected cells contain 30- to 100-fold more phosphorylated ACV than do uninfected cells, which accounts for much of ACV's antiviral selectivity.

Phosphorylation of ACV by the viral TK produces the compound ACV-monophosphate, which is converted sequentially to ACV-diphosphate and ACV-triphosphate (ACV-TP) by cellular enzymes.[252,253] ACV-TP then inhibits HSV and VZV DNA polymerases. Inhibition of HSV DNA polymerase *in vitro* is a three-step process (Fig. 13.7).[300] In the first step, ACV-TP competitively inhibits deoxyguanosine triphosphate (dGTP) incorporation (high concentrations of dGTP can reverse inhibition at this early step). Next, ACV-TP acts as a substrate and is incorporated into the growing DNA chain opposite a C residue. Finally, the polymerase translocates to the next position on the template, but cannot add a new deoxynucleoside triphosphate because ACV contains no 3′-hydroxyl; hence ACV-TP is an obligate chain terminator. Provided that the next dNTP is present, the viral polymerase freezes at this final step in a "dead-end complex," leading to apparent inactivation of the enzyme. There is biochemical evidence for selectivity at each of these steps, especially the third.[174,235,299] The results of enzymological studies of viral polymerases from ACV-resistant mutants[167] argue that in infected cells, as *in vitro,* ACV-TP is not simply a competitive inhibitor of viral DNA polymerase, but rather that its incorporation is crucial, consistent with the three step model (Fig. 13.7).

Stocks of most HSV-1 strains contain ACV-resistant mutants at a level of about 0.01% to 0.1% (reviewed in 57). For at least certain HSV-2 strains, mutation frequencies are an order of magnitude higher.[323] Compared with the drugs discussed so far, there is considerable variety in ACV-resistant mutants. ACV selects mainly for *tk* mutants[60,324,354] that ablate (TK-negative) or reduce (TK-partial) TK activity or alter TK so that it fails to phosphorylate ACV, but continues to phosphorylate dT (TK-altered). ACV-resistance mutations can also alter the viral polymerase to be less inhibited by the drug (reviewed in **199**). Crystallographic studies have provided details on how *tk* and *pol* mutations affect binding and catalysis.[29,40,102,167,222,387]

Nearly all ACV-resistant HSV mutants exhibit some degree of attenuation in assays of pathogenesis in animal models (reviewed in **58 and 199**). TK-negative mutants are generally the most attenuated, especially for replication in sensory ganglia and reactivation from latency in those ganglia. However, certain clinical isolates are able to reactivate despite being TK negative.[123,164] TK-partial mutants are less attenuated. As little as 5% to 10% of wild-type levels of TK activity permit normal ganglionic replication and reactivation from latency,[44,59] and very low levels of TK produced via these translational mechanisms can suffice to permit some reactivation from latency.[19,123] Interestingly, certain nonsense and frameshift mutations that might be expected to inactivate TK do not do so. This "leakiness" can result from translational mechanisms, including reinitiation and ribosomal frameshifting, that permit low levels of TK despite these mutations.[124,165,171,176] Therefore, several mutants that would be expected to be TK negative are actually TK partial. TK-altered and *pol* mutants include the most pathogenic drug-resistant mutants, but some *pol* mutants are highly attenuated.

This picture becomes even more complicated when mixtures of drug-resistant mutants with each other or with drug-sensitive virus are considered, as these can complement each other for both drug resistance and pathogenicity.[58,199] In addition, *tk* frameshift mutations in homopolymeric sequences, which are the most common drug-resistance mutations, tend to revert, sometimes at remarkably high rates, resulting in mixed populations that reactivate from latency.[122,124,326] Therefore, it is important to consider heterogeneity as a factor influencing drug resistance and pathogenicity.

Ganciclovir and Valganciclovir

Although ACV has been highly successful in treating HSV and VZV disease, it is much less potent against HCMV,[74] which causes serious diseases in immunocompromised persons. This is primarily because much less phosphorylated ACV accumulates in HCMV-infected cells than in HSV- or VZV-infected cells.[106] This helped spur the development of ganciclovir. Ganciclovir is much more potent against HCMV than is ACV[47,336] and was the first drug approved for use against HCMV. Ganciclovir is now also produced as the more orally available agent valganciclovir (see Fig. 13.6).

Ganciclovir, unlike ACV, but like penciclovir, has the equivalent of a 3′-OH moiety (see Fig. 13.6). Much as phosphorylated ACV accumulates in HSV-infected cells, phosphorylated ganciclovir accumulates in HCMV-infected cells.[21,104] However, as HCMV does not encode a TK, this phosphorylation was initially thought to be due to induction of a host cell kinase. However, studies of a ganciclovir-resistant mutant led to the discovery that an unusual HCMV protein kinase (UL97) phosphorylates ganciclovir in infected cells.[152,219,248,350,356] Cellular kinases can convert ganciclovir monophosphate to ganciclovir triphosphate. Like ACV triphosphate, ganciclovir

A

Acyclovir

HSV or VZV thymidine kinase

Acyclovir monophosphate

Cellular kinase

Acyclovir diphosphate

Cellular kinase

Acyclovir triphosphate (pppACV)

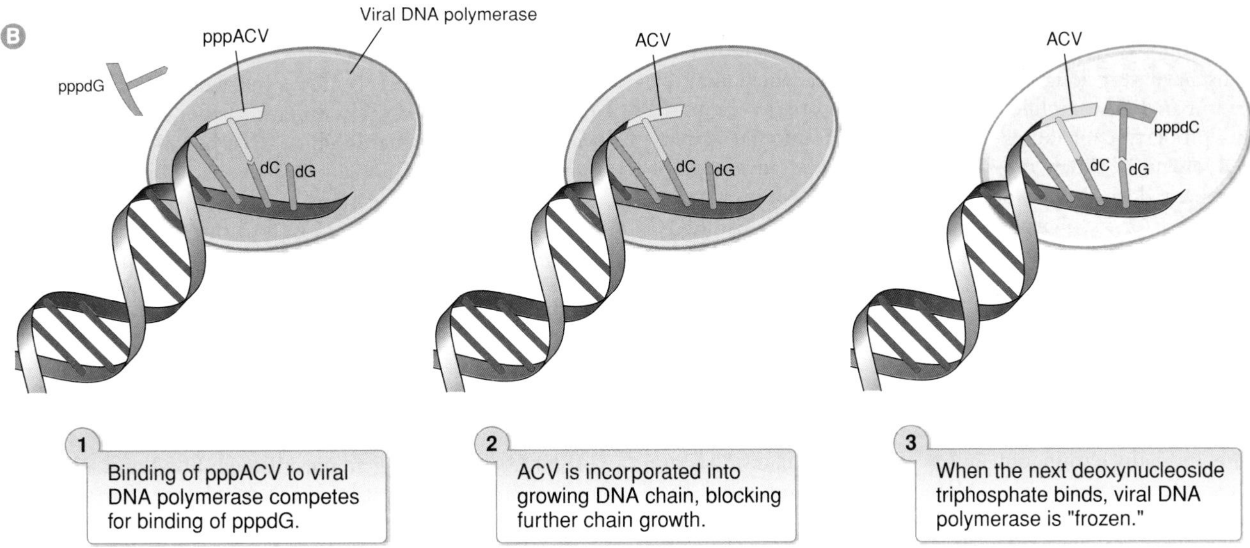

FIGURE 13.7. Mechanism of action of acyclovir (ACV). A: ACV is selectively phosphorylated by herpes simplex virus (HSV) or varicella zoster virus (VZV) thymidine kinase to generate ACV monophosphate. Host cellular enzymes then sequentially phosphorylate the drug monophosphate to the diphosphate and triphosphate (pppACV) forms. **B:** ACV triphosphate has a three-step mechanism of inhibition of herpesvirus DNA polymerase *in vitro:* (1) The drug triphosphate acts as a competitive inhibitor of deoxyguanosine triphosphate (dGTP) (pppdG) binding; (2) the drug triphosphate acts as a substrate and is incorporated into the growing DNA chain across from dC in the template, terminating elongation; and (3) the polymerase becomes trapped on the ACV-terminated DNA chain when the deoxynucleotide triphosphate (dNTP) binds (here shown as pppdC, dCTP, which would be templated by dG). (From Yeh RW, Coen DM. Pharmacology of viral infections. In: Golan DE, Tashjian AH, Jr., Armstrong EJ, et al., eds. *Principles of Pharmacology: The Pathophysiologic Basis of Drug Therapy.* Third edition. Philadelphia: Lippincott Williams & Wilkins, 2012:649–673.)

triphosphate is both a selective competitive inhibitor and substrate for viral DNA polymerase.[21,115,233,235,303,339] Unlike ACV triphosphate, ganciclovir triphosphate is not an obligate chain terminator. Nevertheless, after incorporating ganciclovir monophosphate, HCMV DNA polymerase can stall after incorporating one additional nucleotide.[303] However, biochemical and genetic studies indicate that selectivity at the phosphorylation step and the DNA polymerase inhibition step for HCMV are not as great as the selectivity of ACV against HSV. Accordingly, the drug is more toxic than ACV. Toxicity is most commonly manifested in patients as bone marrow suppression, especially neutropenia.[267]

Most ganciclovir-resistant mutants contain *UL97* mutations, but these have a limited distribution in the gene.[11,118]

Unlike HSV TK, HCMV UL97 protein kinase is very important for viral replication (i.e., null mutants are much less fit[296]). It seems likely that clinical *UL97* drug-resistance mutations would affect recognition of ganciclovir without gravely compromising activity on the physiologic protein substrates of UL97 such as retinoblastoma protein and lamin A.[135,169,185] However, this has not yet been demonstrated. Numerous different *pol* mutations have been shown to confer ganciclovir resistance (reviewed in 11 and 118). Interestingly, some lie in or near regions not altered in ACV-resistant HSV mutants, but in regions that are thought to be important for 3′ to 5′ exonuclease activity. How these mutations confer ganciclovir resistance is not yet known.

Cidofovir and Other Nucleotide Analogs

Cidofovir, a phosphonate-containing acyclic cytosine analog, is approved for use against HCMV, and represents a variation on the mechanism of action of nucleoside analogs. Cidofovir, with its phosphonate group, is a nucleotide analog that mimics deoxycytidine monophosphate (dCMP) (see Fig. 13.6). This charged moiety likely accounts for the relatively poor uptake of cidofovir into cells,[161] and poor oral bioavailability. Once inside the cell, cidofovir is metabolized via cellular enzymes to its monophosphate (akin to a diphosphate) and diphosphate (akin to a triphosphate), and to a third phosphorylated form that contains a choline adduct.[52,161] These phosphorylated forms have very long intracellular half-lives, which may be due in part to the choline metabolite serving as a reservoir.[1,161] This property contributes to the prolonged antiviral activity of cidofovir,[260] which provides the therapeutic advantage of infrequent dosing. In addition, because cidofovir uses cellular kinases for its phosphorylation, it is active against *UL97* mutants that are resistant to ganciclovir,[225] although this also removes the selectivity gained by requiring a viral kinase for efficient phosphorylation.

The diphosphorylated form of cidofovir is an analog of dCTP that inhibits HCMV DNA polymerase more potently than it does various cellular DNA polymerases.[48,161,394] It is also incorporated into DNA, which slows elongation, but does not result in chain termination unless two cidofovir residues are incorporated in a row.[393,394] Many of the *pol* mutations that confer resistance to ganciclovir confer resistance to cidofovir.

Two related phosphonate-containing drugs are the acyclic deoxyadenosine monophosphate analogues, tenofovir, which is used against HIV and HBV, and adefovir, which has been used against HBV (see Fig. 13.6). The mechanisms of action of these drugs against their respective viruses are similar to those of cidofovir against HCMV, except that these drugs are chain-terminators of DNA synthesis. (See below for discussions of nucleoside analogs active against HIV and HBV.) These two drugs are administered as orally available prodrugs (Fig. 13.6). In contrast, there is currently no such approved prodrug for cidofovir, which must be administered intravenously. Orally available prodrugs of cidovir are being developed with the added potential benefit of activity against poxviruses, adenoviruses, polyomaviruses, and papillomaviruses[166] (e-Table 13.1).

Nonnucleoside Inhibitors of Herpesvirus DNA Polymerase: Foscarnet

As described above, nucleoside analogs can inhibit cellular as well as viral enzymes, and viruses can mutate to resist these drugs. As a result, efforts have been made to discover compounds that might inhibit viral polymerases by other mechanisms. The first of these to be approved for clinical use was foscarnet (phosphonoformic acid, PFA; structure in Fig. 13.8). Although it is not orally available so that intravenous administration is required, and it is nephrotoxic, it is approved for treatment of severe HSV, VZV, and HCMV infections that are resistant to front-line drugs.

Foscarnet is an analog of pyrophosphate, which is a product of polymerization of nucleic acids. Unlike the nucleoside analogs described above, it does not require activation by either cell or viral enzymes but rather inhibits HCMV DNA polymerase directly and selectively. Inhibition is not competitive with deoxynucleoside triphosphates. Rather, it appears that foscarnet acts as a product analog, preventing normal pyrophosphate release so the polymerase cannot complete the catalytic cycle.[93,271] The structure of foscarnet bound to a DNA polymerase that is a chimera of a bacteriophage DNA polymerase and segments of HCMV polymerase that are important for foscarnet sensitivity has been solved.[398] In the structure, the drug binds to highly conserved basic residues in a closed form of the enzyme that has not translocated to the next base on the template. The drug occupies the position of the beta and gamma phosphates of an incoming dNTP. The structure suggests that foscarnet stabilizes this untranslocated state, thus stalling the polymerase.

Because foscarnet is not a nucleoside analog, HSV *tk* mutants and HCMV *UL97* mutants are not resistant to it. However, although foscarnet inhibits DNA polymerase by a mechanism that differs substantially from the nucleoside analogs, many *pol* mutants that are resistant to nucleoside analogs are resistant to foscarnet. Moreover, most foscarnet-resistant mutants are resistant to one or more nucleoside analogs (reviewed in 118). Therefore, there are patients with serious herpesvirus infections for whom there are no viable treatment options. This should be an impetus to further drug development.

Anti-HIV and HBV Polymerase Inhibitors

The retrovirus HIV and the hepadnavirus hepatitis B virus (HBV) replicate their genomes through DNA and RNA intermediates, respectively, using a DNA polymerase that can copy RNA. The HIV RT and the HBV DNA polymerase are thus essential for viral replication, and differ substantially from cellular polymerases, making them excellent targets for antivirals. The success of anti-herpesvirus nucleoside analogs provided a rationale for the development of nucleoside analogs active against HIV. Within 2 years of the identification of HIV as the etiologic agent of AIDS, a nucleoside analog, zidovudine (AZT), was shown to have antiviral activity in patients.[395] Shortly thereafter AZT therapy was shown to have an impact on mortality in the short term.[100] The success of AZT, but also its limitations, led to the development of other anti-HIV nucleoside analogs. These, in turn, provided an impetus for the development of nucleoside analogs against HBV, and, with the RT validated as a target, the nonnucleoside reverse transcriptase inhibitors (NNRTIs) against HIV.

Numerous nucleoside analogs have been approved to treat HIV (see Fig. 13.6). Many of the principles that govern their mechanisms of action and resistance are similar to those of the anti-herpesvirus nucleoside analogs. For the sake of brevity, this chapter focuses on only two anti-HIV nucleoside analogs,

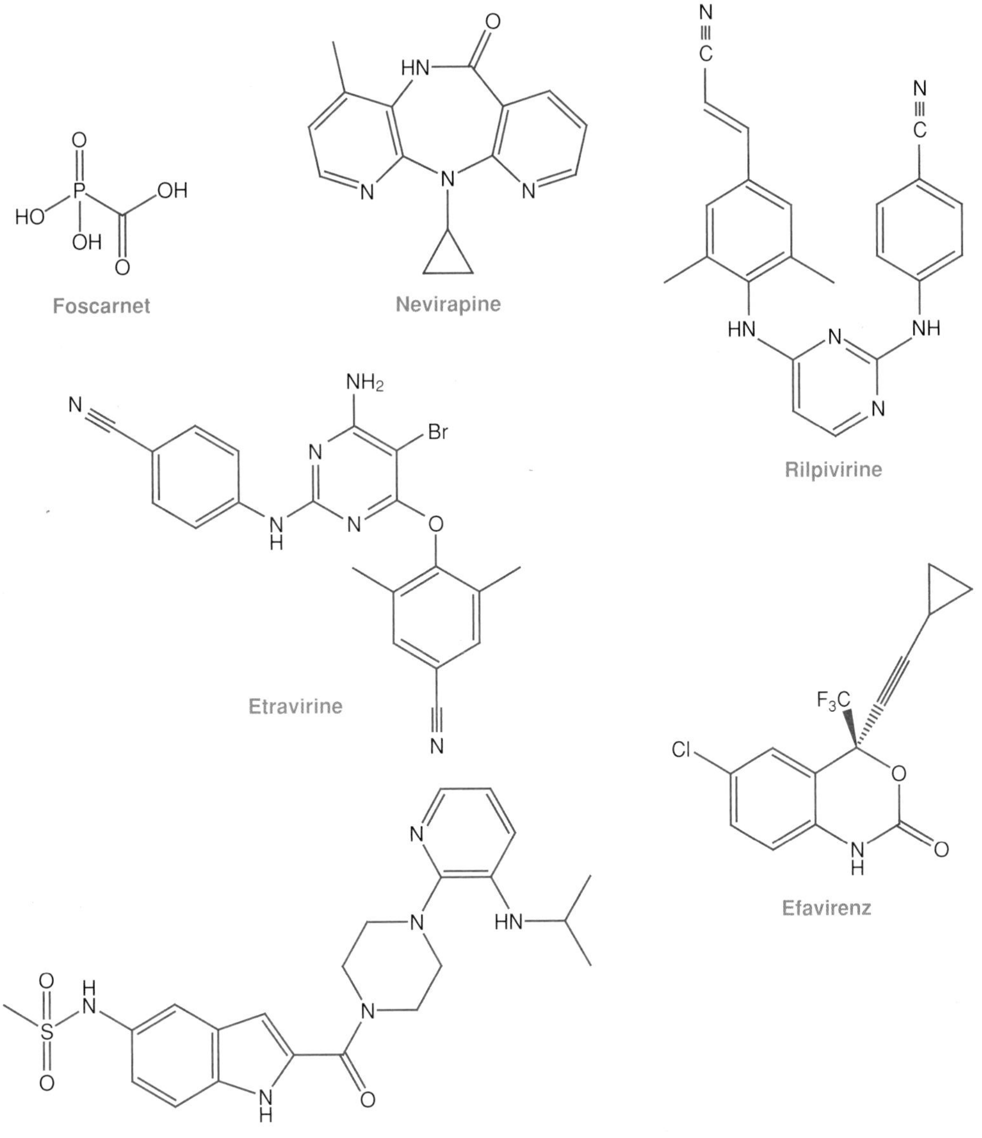

Foscarnet

Nevirapine

Rilpivirine

Etravirine

Efavirenz

Delavirdine

FIGURE 13.8. Nonnucleoside DNA polymerase inhibitors (foscarnet and nonnucleoside reverse transcriptase inhibitors [NNRTIs]). Foscarnet is a pyrophosphate analog that inhibits viral polymerases. It is approved for treatment of herpes simplex virus (HSV) and human cytomegalovirus (HCMV) infections that are resistant to other drugs. Nevirapine, delavirdine, efavirenz, etravirine, and rilpivirine, which do not mimic any known ligands of DNA polymerases, inhibit HIV-1 reverse transcriptase and are approved for treatment of HIV-1 in combination with other drugs. (Modified from Yeh RW, Coen DM. Pharmacology of viral infections. In: Golan DE, Tashjian AH, Jr., Armstrong EJ, et al., eds. *Principles of Pharmacology: The Pathophysiologic Basis of Drug Therapy*. Third edition. Philadelphia: Lippincott Williams & Wilkins, 2012:649–673.)

zidovudine and lamivudine (which also is an anti-HBV drug), and compares and contrasts their mechanisms with each other and with the anti-herpesvirus drugs.

Zidovudine (AZT)

Zidovudine (azidothymidine, AZT) was synthesized years before the AIDS epidemic as a potential anticancer drug. It was first reported to have anti-HIV activity in 1985.[255] Like the anti-herpesvirus drugs described earlier, AZT is a nucleoside analog with an altered sugar moiety. In this case, it is a thymine base attached to a sugar in which the normal 3′ hydroxyl has been replaced by an azido group (see Fig. 13.6). Indeed, all of the currently approved anti-HIV nucleoside analogs lack a 3′-hydroxyl or its equivalent. (This contrasts with penciclovir and ganciclovir.)

Unlike herpesviruses, HIV does not encode kinases that can phosphorylate nucleoside analogs. AZT is an excellent substrate for cellular thymidine kinase, which phosphorylates AZT to AZT-monophosphate.[107] AZT-monophosphate is then converted to the diphosphate form by cellular thymidylate kinase and to the triphosphate form by cellular nucleoside diphosphate kinase.[107] Therefore, unlike ACV and ganciclovir, there is no selectivity at the activation step, and phosphorylated AZT accumulates in almost all dividing cells in the body, not just infected cells. Moreover, the activity of AZT and other anti-HIV nucleoside analogs can vary depending on the activity of cellular kinases in the infected cell. For example activated lymphocytes upregulate thymidine kinase, which is needed for DNA replication and cellular proliferation; thymidine analogs are thus more potent in activated than in quiescent CD4 lymphocytes.[335]

AZT-triphosphate (AZT-TP) is a substantially more potent inhibitor and better substrate of HIV RT than of the human DNA polymerases that have been tested.[46,107,340] This biochemical selectivity is reflected in the degree of resistance of AZT-resistant mutants, which can be greater than 100-fold in some cell types.[200] Like ACV triphosphate, AZT-TP lacks a 3′-hydroxyl, and is an obligatory chain terminator (see Fig. 13.6). The details of the inhibition of RT by AZT-TP are not entirely resolved, but given that AZT resistance acts on incorporated drug (see below), it is clear that the efficient incorporation of AZT-TP is crucial for its selectivity. Therefore, the potency of AZT and other nucleoside analogs depends on the levels of dNTPs that compete with the drug triphosphates for the RT.

Especially given that phosphorylated AZT accumulates in almost all dividing cells in the body, its toxicity is a serious clinical issue. In particular, AZT causes bone marrow suppression that manifests most commonly as neutropenia and anemia.[308] AZT toxicity appears to be due not only to the effects of AZT-TP on cellular polymerases, but also to the effects of AZT-monophosphate, which is both a substrate for cellular thymidylate kinase, and an inhibitor of this essential enzyme.[107] For a number of other anti-HIV nucleoside analogs, a key determinant of toxicity appears to be the mitochondrial DNA polymerase (DNA polymerase γ).[43,209,235]

The first AZT-resistant mutants of HIV were obtained from patients who had been treated with the drug for months.[200] AZT-resistance mutations accumulate in the HIV *pol* gene that encodes RT[24,53,187,203] (Fig. 13.9). Interestingly, four or more mutations are required to confer high-level resistance, but some of the mutations confer little or no resistance on their own.[187,202,203] These latter mutations appear to be selected because they boost resistance by the other mutations or compensate for fitness costs of certain mutations. The requirement for multiple mutations for high-level resistance likely explains the relatively slow emergence of AZT resistance in patients and during selection in cell culture.[111,201] Based on sequencing of virus isolated from patients following cessation of AZT therapy or in individuals newly infected with resistant virus, and of virus from replication competition experiments *in vitro,*

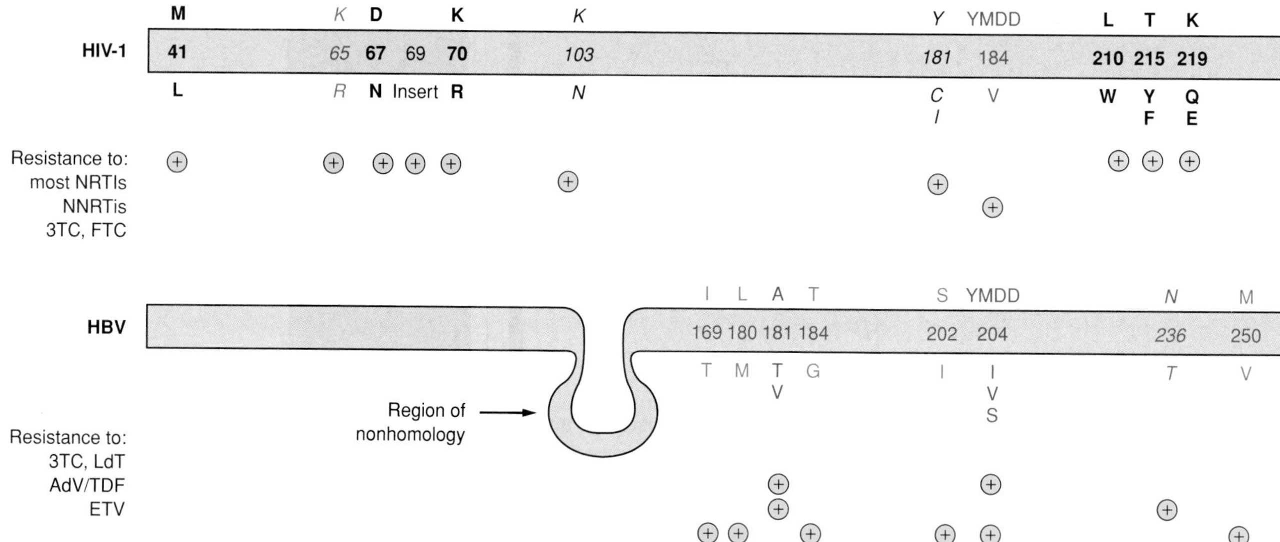

FIGURE 13.9. Locations of drug-resistance alterations in the human immunodeficiency virus type 1 (HIV-1) and hepatitis B virus (HBV) polymerases. The HIV-1 reverse transcriptase (RT) **(top)** and the HBV DNA polymerase **(bottom)** are related enzymes with sequence and predicted structural homology, and are cartooned as bars. The HBV enzyme has a segment that is unrelated to the HIV enzyme, which is depicted here as looping out. The positions of selected substitutions and insertions that confer drug resistance are indicated in single letter code with the wild-type residue above the bar, the residue number within the bar, and mutant residues or inserts below the bar. Methionine 184 in HIV RT and methionine 204 in HBV polymerase are embedded within a YMDD motif (green) that is important for polymerase catalysis. Alterations in this methionine confer resistance to 3TC and related L-stereoisomer drugs, as does alteration of alanine 181 in HBV polymerase (also green). Boldfaced residues in HIV RT indicate the positions of thymidine analog-associated mutations that affect susceptibility to all anti-HIV nucleoside analogues. An insertion at residue 69 in HIV RT (blue) together with other alterations including M41L, K70R, L210W, T215Y, and K219Q also affect susceptibility to these drugs. Substitution of arginine for lysine 65 (purple) in HIV RT confers resistance to all nucleoside analogs except zidovudine (AZT). Substitutions of lysine 103 and tyrosine 181 (italics) confer resistance to nonnucleoside reverse transcriptase inhibitors (NNRTIs). Alterations of isoleucine 169, threonine 184, serine 202, or methionine 250 (red), together with a leucine-to-methionine substitution at residue 180 (orange) plus a methionine 204 substitution in HBV polymerase can result in entecavir resistance. A threonine for asparagine 236 substitution in HBV polymerase (blue) can result in resistance to adefovir (high-level) and tenofovir (intermediate).

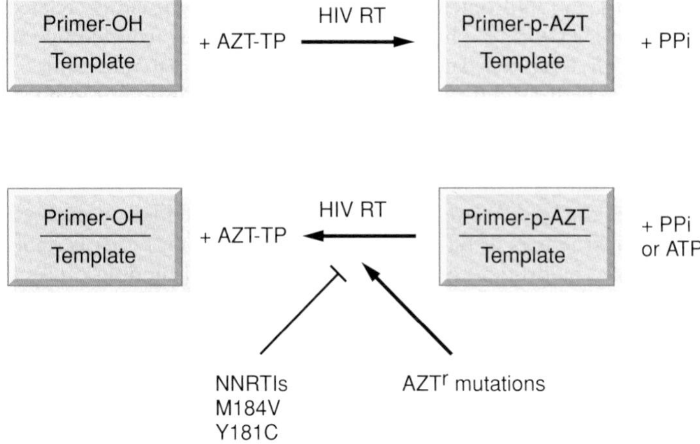

FIGURE 13.10. Biochemical mechanism of resistance to zidovudine (AZT). During synthesis of human immunodeficiency virus (HIV) DNA by HIV reverse transcriptase (RT), AZT-TP (triphosphate) is incorporated into the growing primer strand (Primer-p-AZT), generating pyrophosphate (PPi). This reaction is reversible, so that RT can excise AZT-MP (monophosphate) from the primer terminus and combine it with PPi, regenerating AZT-TP and primer/template. ATP can substitute for PPi in this excision reaction by donating two phosphates to AZT-MP. The excision reaction is enhanced by AZT-resistance mutations, but impaired by NNRTIs and certain HIV RT substitutions that confer resistance to 3TC (e.g., M184V) and NNRTIs (e.g., Y181C).

AZT-resistant mutants appear to be modestly less fit than wild-type virus.[77,120,121,138,217]

The mechanism of AZT resistance remained elusive for over a decade. In 1998, two sets of investigators explained the mystery.[5,249] Chain elongation by 3′-5′ phosphodiester bond formation with an incoming dNTP is a reversible process. In the presence of pyrophosphate or ATP, RT can catalytically excise the terminal nucleotide by a process termed pyrophosphorolysis (Fig. 13.10). Given the K_m's of pyrophosphate and ATP for this reaction, and the concentrations of these species in cells, ATP is the likely substrate *in vivo.* The viral DNA chain is now free to resume elongation with the removal of the chain terminating nucleoside analog. AZT-resistance mutations facilitate this reverse reaction of excision repair.[210,250] Modeling of HIV RT (based on crystal structure) with an AZT-terminated primer/template suggests that the incorporated AZT residue would occupy the site normally used by the next incoming dNTP, and that AZT-resistance mutations, particularly those affecting codon 215, enhance binding of ATP.[25]

AZT-resistance mutations are also selected by another thymidine analog, stavudine (d4T) (see Fig. 13.6), which has led them to be called *thymidine-associated mutations* (TAMS) (see Fig. 13.9). However, the resistance mechanism of excision repair actually applies to most, if not all, anti-HIV nucleoside analogs, with AZT-terminated primer being the most readily excised by this mechanism.[376] Therefore, these mutations have also been termed *nucleoside-associated mutations* (NAMS). The excision repair mechanism accounts for many examples of cross-resistance of HIV toward various nucleoside analogs. Regardless of mechanism, various combinations of mutations affecting HIV RT can confer resistance to every approved nucleoside analog (see Fig. 13.9).[181]

The limited clinical effectiveness of AZT and problems with toxicity and resistance led to the development of other anti-HIV drugs and the use of combination chemotherapy.

Lamivudine (3TC)

Lamivudine (3TC) was reported to exhibit anti-HIV activity in 1992.[54,55,329] Lamivudine and its close relative emtricitabine (FTC) appear to exhibit the least toxicity of the anti-HIV nucleoside analogs. This seems to be related to their highly unusual structures: They have an unusual sugar moiety that contains a sulfur atom and is an L-stereoisomer, not the standard D-stereoisomer of normal nucleosides (see Fig. 13.6). Lamivudine is sequentially phosphorylated by cellular enzymes to its triphosphate.[37] Like AZT-triphosphate, 3TC-triphosphate is both a competitive inhibitor and a substrate for RT, and once incorporated, is an obligate chain-terminator of DNA synthesis. It is a more potent inhibitor of HIV RT than cellular polymerases.[139] The lack of toxicity of 3TC may be due to the negligible inhibition of host polymerases including mitochondrial DNA polymerase by 3TC-triphosphate.[139]

High-level resistance to 3TC develops rapidly both in cell culture and in patients treated with this drug alone (reviewed in **79**). A single mutation at codon 184 from Met to Val (M184V) or to Ile (M184I) confers a high degree of resistance to 3TC. M184 is within the conserved YMDD motif, in which the two Asp (D) residues are involved in catalysis of polymerization (see Fig. 13.9). M184I is less fit than M184V, which likely explains the dominance of the M184V mutant in 3TC-treated patients. Nevertheless, the M184V mutant is also less fit than wild-type virus, which may be due to decreased processivity, primer use, or initiation by the mutant enzyme or some combination of these (reviewed in **79**). The crystal structure of a 3TC-resistant RT was used to develop a molecular model that posits that codon 184 mutations result in steric hindrance that obstruct incorporation of 3TC-triphosphate, but not normal nucleotides.[320]

The M184V mutation also has a number of other interesting effects, including conferring low level resistance to some (e.g. abacavir; see Fig. 13.6) or hypersensitivity to other nucleoside analogs (e.g. AZT and tenofovir; reviewed in **79**). This hypersensitivity to AZT and other drugs in the absence of other mutations is also observed in the presence of known drug resistance mutations such that levels of resistance are reduced with the addition of M184V. This phenotypic suppression is best explained by the M184V mutation reducing the excision repair of AZT-terminated primers (Fig. 13.10).[79] Nevertheless, an accumulation of multiple mutations can result in high level resistance to both AZT and 3TC, and other single mutations such as K65R can confer resistance to 3TC (and most other nucleoside analogs) (see Fig. 13.9).[251]

The mechanisms of action and resistance of FTC are very similar to those of 3TC; however, it may be slightly more potent and have a longer intracellular half-life.[307] Its co-formulation with tenofovir has made this combination the nucleoside analog backbone of combination antiretroviral therapy.

Anti-HBV Drugs

Five nucleoside analogs—lamivudine (3TC) and tenofovir (both also approved for use against HIV), adefovir, telbivudine, and entecavir (see Fig. 13.6)—have been approved for the treatment of HBV. The structures of lamivudine, tenofovir, and adefovir were described above. Telbivudine is simply L-thymidine (see Fig. 13.6), thus sharing this isomeric configuration with 3TC and FTC. Entecavir is an unusual deoxyguanosine nucleoside analog in which the ether oxygen of the sugar is replaced with an exo carbon-carbon double bond (see Fig. 13.6). The mechanisms of action of anti-HBV nucleoside analogs are very similar to those of anti-HIV nucleoside analogs: They are converted to triphosphates by cellular enzymes, and the triphosphates inhibit HBV DNA polymerase (which is also a reverse transcriptase). All are incorporated into the growing DNA chain and cause chain termination, even those that are not obligate chain-terminators. Of note, entecavir-triphosphate has a higher affinity for HBV polymerase than does dGTP.[331]

The similarities in mechanisms of action of these drugs against the two viruses extend to some similarities in mechanisms of resistance, but there are also important differences.[223] For example, a mutation in the methionine codon in the HBV *pol* gene that corresponds to codon M184 in the HIV *pol* gene can confer high-level resistance to 3TC and telbivudine (see Fig. 13.9); however, in this case, the methionine to isoleucine mutant retains fitness, whereas methionine to valine or serine substitutions are usually only found in the presence of additional mutations. There is little if any evidence for HBV drug-resistance mutations resulting in increased excision of incorporated drug as do AZT-resistance mutations of HIV; rather the mutations appear to affect incorporation of drug-triphosphate by various mechanisms. Interestingly, drug resistance that requires only a single mutation develops relatively quickly, but still more slowly *in vivo* with HBV than with HIV. In at least some cases, this may be because sites of mutation also encode residues in an overlapping reading frame that affect HBV surface antigen.

As is the case with AZT resistance, multiple mutations are required to confer high level resistance to entecavir, and some of these mutations confer little resistance on their own.[223] This correlates with slow development of resistance *in vivo*. The greater potency and slower rates of resistance to entecavir and tenofovir has led to these drugs becoming preferred for treatment of HBV.[223] FTC and tenofovir are often used in patients who are infected with both HIV and HBV, because they are active against both viruses (even though FTC is not currently FDA approved for treating HBV infections).

Anti-HIV Nonnucleoside Reverse Transcriptase Inhibitors (NNRTIs)

Five NNRTIs—efavirenz, nevirapine, delavirdine, etravirine and, in 2011, rilpivirine (see Fig. 13.8)—have been approved by the FDA for treatment of HIV infections. The first NNRTIs were discovered using high-throughput screening for inhibition of HIV-1 RT (e.g. nevirapine[246]). Candidate compounds were tested for specificity in a counterscreen by checking their ability to inhibit an unrelated polymerase. The compounds that emerged were then chemically modified to improve their antiviral activities, stabilities, and pharmacokinetics, and to reduce their toxicities. The NNRTIs are highly specific, inhibiting HIV-1 RT at low concentrations while not inhibiting human DNA polymerases or even the RT of the closely related virus HIV-2.[246] This biochemical selectivity is reflected by the high level resistance conferred by HIV-1 *pol* mutations.[305] These drugs directly inhibit RT. The NNRTIs do not mimic a natural ligand of a polymerase. Each NNRTI appears to share a polycyclic structure that tends to form a "butterfly wings" conformation upon binding to RT. NNRTIs bind to a pocket near the catalytic Asp residues of RT.[193] This pocket is not observed in structures of RT in the absence of drug, but rather is stabilized by drug binding.[314] Therefore, NNRTI binding causes a substantial conformational change in RT, including distortion of the catalytic Asp residues, and slows the enzyme's incorporation of dNTPs into DNA.[313,338] NNRTIs inhibit pyrophosphorolysis and the excision of AZT from primer termini by RT (see Fig. 13.10; [269]), which likely accounts for synergy of these drugs against HIV.[304]

As with 3TC, resistance to NNRTIs develops quickly both *in vitro* and in patients, with single amino acid substitutions conferring high-level resistance.[243,305,310] Common resistance mutations arise in codon 181 (see Fig. 13.9), changing Tyr to Cys (Y181C) or to Ile (Y181I), and cause high-level resistance.[243,305] This change alters a residue known to interact with NNRTIs,[62,193,392] and thus reduces drug binding. The Y181C mutant is relatively fit in infected cells,[63,173] and in patients. Some but not all other NNRTI-resistant mutants exhibit reduced fitness in cells and in patients.[217] The Y181C mutation, like the M184V mutation, sensitizes otherwise AZT-resistant mutants to AZT due to suppression of excision repair (see Fig. 13.10; [332]).

The different mechanisms of action and resistance of the anti-HIV nucleoside analogs and NNRTIs help provide the rationales for various combinations of these drugs in treating HIV (see section on HIV therapies).

Ribavirin, a Nucleoside Analog Active Against RNA Viruses

Ribavirin (see Fig. 13.6) is a nucleoside analog that has been touted as a "broad spectrum antiviral".[348] Indeed it exhibits its activity against many viruses *in vitro* and efficacy against certain RNA viruses *in vivo*. In patients, however, it has been approved only as monotherapy for severe respiratory syncytial virus (RSV) infections, and in combination with IFNs for chronic HCV infections (see below for discussion of IFNs). Ribavirin monotherapy results in little reduction in HCV levels in plasma,[78] but when added to IFNs, substantially increases the success rate of therapy.[293]

Structurally, ribavirin differs from the other nucleoside analogs discussed thus far, in that it has a normal sugar moiety (ribose) attached to a base-like moiety, which most resembles a purine (see Fig. 13.6). Its mechanism of action is still not well understood, especially for HCV. Ribavirin is converted to a monophosphate by cellular adenosine kinase and is known to inhibit cellular inosine monophosphate dehydrogenase (IMPDH), thereby lowering GTP pools.[348] This could, in principle, confer selective antiviral activity if certain viral functions have higher K_m values for GTP than do most cellular enzymes. Inhibitor and RNA interference experiments suggest that IMPDH inhibition could be important for the anti-HCV activity of ribavirin.[261,405] A second possible selective mechanism for ribavirin action could be inhibition of viral RNA polymerase. A related possible mechanism, called "error catastrophe," is that ribavirin incorporation by viral RNA polymerase increases the already high mutation rate of the virus[87] "over the edge" of an "error threshold" so that few or no functional viral genomes are produced. This has been investigated most thoroughly with poliovirus,[72,73,284] but similar studies have been performed with HCV.[68,198,226,405] This is an appealing concept, but remains unproven, particularly for RSV and HCV. In HCV replicons, ribavirin resistance was found to be due to mutations affecting the NS5A protein rather than polymerase,[285] and studies of viral mutagenesis in patients treated with ribavirin have not provided definitive answers.[227,281] A fourth possible mechanism is that ribavirin induces IFN-stimulated genes, which may be particularly relevant to the use of ribavirin in combination with IFNs.[96,361] A fifth possible mechanism involves stimulatory effects on T helper cell 1 responses involved in clearing virus from the liver.[162] If anything, there is even less known about the mechanism of ribavirin action against RSV. Further investigations of the mechanisms of ribavirin action and resistance may yield interesting new insights into virus biology and biochemistry.

New nucleoside analog and nonnucleoside inhibitors of viral polymerases are being developed. For example, as of late 2012, several such inhibitors of HCV RNA polymerase were in phase II clinical trials (e-Table 13.1). Therefore, this area of antiviral agents remains highly active.

Anti-Human Immunodeficiency Virus Integrase Inhibitors

A crucial stage in the replication of HIV and other retroviruses is integration of the linear, dsDNA product of reverse transcription into the host genome. The protein that carries out this step, integrase, is an essential enzyme. Integrase assembles onto sequences from the ends of HIV DNA, cleaves dinucleotides from each 3′ strand, and transfers these strands to covalently link them with target DNA (Fig. 13.11). The catalytic core of integrase includes three conserved acidic residues called the DDE motif (Fig. 13.11), which binds Mg^{2+} that is essential for integrase activity. Efforts to identify specific inhibitors of HIV integrase that could serve as effective antiviral drugs commenced in the early 1990s. A breakthrough came when Daria Hazuda and her colleagues at Merck developed an assay selective for DNA strand transfer.[151] Using this assay, they identified integrase inhibitors that act much more potently at this step than at prior steps (Fig. 13.11). These inhibitors contained a diketoacid moiety, which binds to the metal coordinated by the DDE motif, and additional moieties that bind to the enzyme. Medicinal chemistry studies of various classes of diketoacid scaffolds led to the development of raltegravir (Fig. 13.11).[351] Raltegravir was tested against a variety of enzymes that are Mg^{2+}-dependent (e.g., HIV RT), and was highly selective for integrase. Its selectivity for the strand-transfer step seems to depend on binding to a conformation of integrase that is stable only after processing of 3′ ends. Indeed, viral DNA may form part of the binding site for the drug.[2,45,238]

Raltegravir inhibits HIV replication at low nanomolar concentrations. As expected, HIV mutants resistant to raltegravir contain mutations in sequences encoding the integrase, with most mutations that confer resistance altering residues close to the inhibitor binding site.[238] Of mechanistic interest, one mutation alters a residue that, in the crystal structure, makes contact with a nucleotide corresponding to the 5′ terminus of viral DNA. There are also mutations that do not themselves confer resistance, but increase the effects of other mutations. Similar mutations are selected by raltegravir in cell culture and in patients. Single mutations seem to be sufficient to confer clinically significant resistance, but most of these mutations decrease HIV fitness at least modestly.[238]

In 2012 elvitegravir, another integrase inhibitor, was approved, and dolutegravir, which is active against many raltegravir-resistant mutants, was in late-stage clinical trials. It seems likely that this class of drugs will become increasingly important for HIV therapy.

Inhibition of Viral Assembly and Maturation

Protease Inhibitors

Virus assembly and subsequent events to form an infectious virion are attractive targets for drug discovery because they are unique to virus biology. For many viruses, including HIV, mere assembly of proteins and nucleic acid into particles is not sufficient to produce an infectious virion. For such viruses, an additional step—maturation—is required. In most cases, these viruses encode proteases that are essential for maturation. The approved antiviral drugs that target HIV protease are saquinavir, ritonavir (which is now used mainly at low dose to boost plasma drug levels of other protease inhibitors), lopinavir, amprenavir and its prodrug fosamprenavir, indinavir, nelfinavir, atazanavir, darunavir, and tipranavir (Fig. 13.12).

Several features gleaned from a variety of studies established HIV protease as an attractive target for drug discovery and design. Molecular genetic studies showed that the protease is essential for HIV replication, and that a point mutation is sufficient to inactivate the enzyme and viral infectivity, suggesting that a small molecule could be effective.[192] The cleavage sites in the viral polypeptide substrates of HIV protease are conserved and somewhat unusual, suggesting both specificity and a starting point for drug design.[283,292] Unlike the human proteases most closely related to it, HIV protease is a symmetric homodimer, and each subunit contributes to the active site, again suggesting both specificity and a starting point for drug design.[263] The enzyme can be easily overexpressed and assayed, and its crystal structure has been solved,[263,389] all aiding drug discovery.

The HIV protease inhibitors are paradigms of rational drug design. For simplicity, only the development of ritonavir will be detailed. Ritonavir and the other protease inhibitors are peptidomimetics. Indeed, all but tipranavir retain peptide bonds. Ritonavir's design began with the recognition that a natural substrate of the protease contains a phenylalanine-proline (Phe-Pro) bond; mammalian enzymes rarely if ever cleave at such a site. The transition state of this substrate during cleavage was then modeled (Fig. 13.13, top). Knowing that HIV protease is a symmetric dimer, an analog of the transition state was modeled, using the same residue, phenylalanine, on both sides, and with a CHOH group that mimics the transition state as the center of symmetry. This molecule, A-74702, was a very weak inhibitor of HIV protease, but adding groups symmetrically to both ends to form A-74704, resulted in a greater than 40,000-fold increase in potency ($Ki \sim 5$ nM).[92]

Attempts to modify A-74074 to improve solubility reduced potency, so a related potent inhibitor, A-75925, in which the center of symmetry was a C-C bond between two CHOH groups, became the scaffold for further additions to both ends.[190] This resulted in a soluble, highly potent inhibitor,

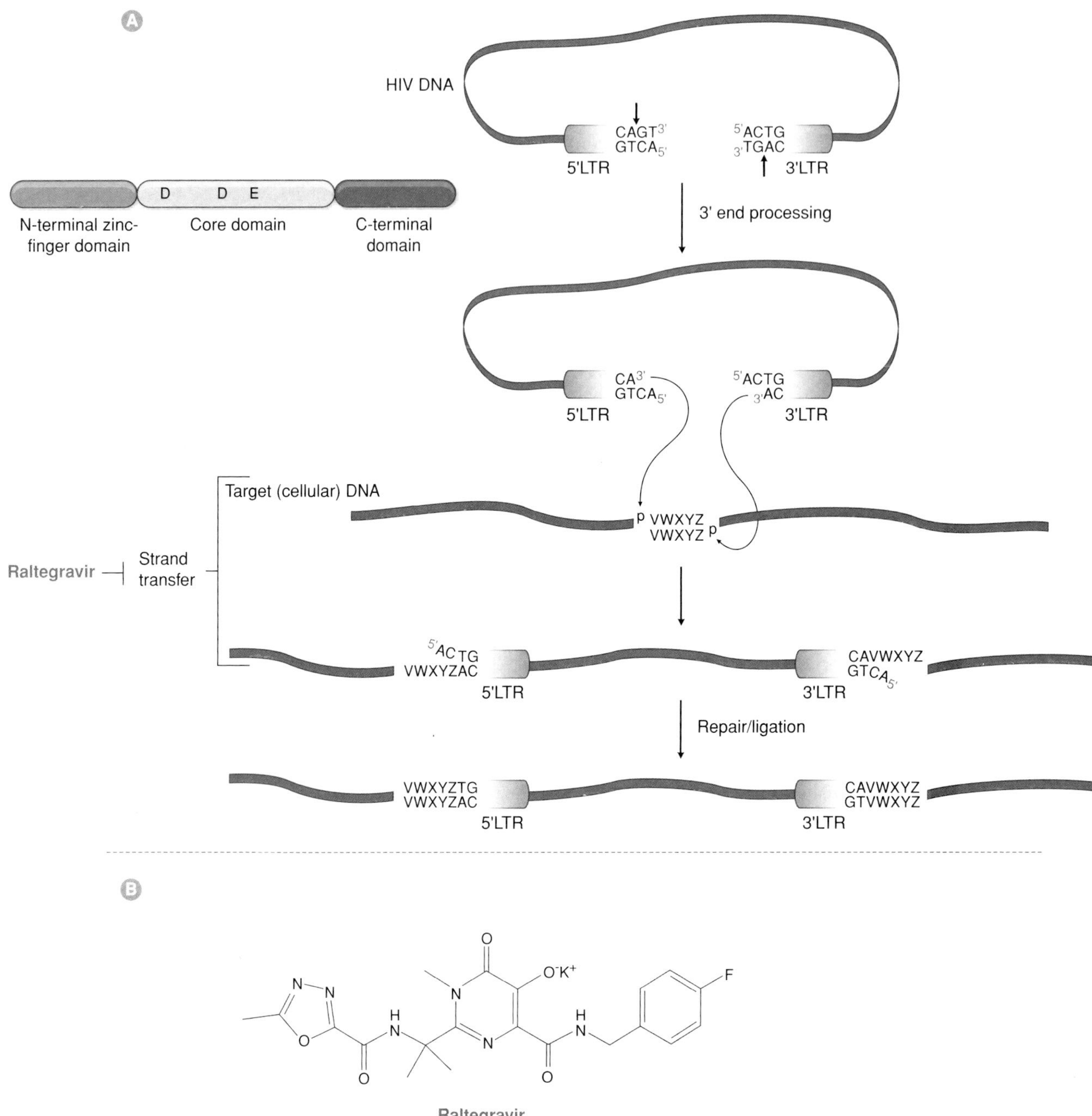

FIGURE 13.11. Human immunodeficiency virus (HIV) integrase and raltegravir action. A: Linear, double-stranded HIV DNA, generated by reverse transcription, contains a four-base sequence at each of its ends, as part of its long terminal repeat (LTR). Integrase (IN), which contains an N-terminal zinc-finger domain important for DNA binding, a C-terminal domain, and an internal core domain containing three acidic residues (DDE) that coordinate magnesium ions important for catalysis, binds to HIV DNA (as part of a larger complex) and cleaves a dinucleotide from the 3' strand at each end of viral DNA (3' end processing). The integrase-viral DNA complex then catalyzes the attack of the recessed 3' ends of viral DNA on phosphodiester bonds of target (cellular DNA) (strand transfer). The product results in 5' flaps of viral DNA and gaps in cellular DNA. Integrase releases, and host enzymes remove the flaps and repair the gaps, resulting in integrated viral DNA flanked by duplicated host sequences. Raltegravir inhibits the strand transfer step of this process. (Modified from Yeh RW, Coen DM. Pharmacology of viral infections. In: Golan DE, Tashjian AH, Jr., Armstrong EJ, et al., eds. *Principles of Pharmacology: The Pathophysiologic Basis of Drug Therapy*. Third edition. Philadelphia: Lippincott Williams & Wilkins, 2012:649–673 and Freed EO, Martin MA. HIVs and their replication. In: Knipe DM, Howley PM, Griffin DE, et al., eds. *Fields Virology*. Fifth edition. Philadelphia: Lippincott Williams & Wilkins, 2007.) **B:** Structure of raltegravir.

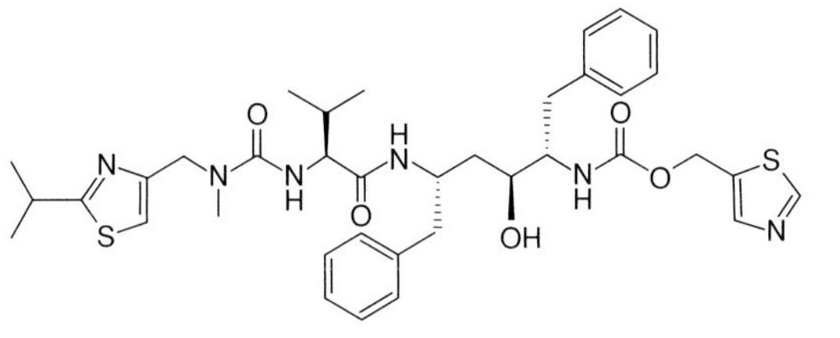

Ritonavir

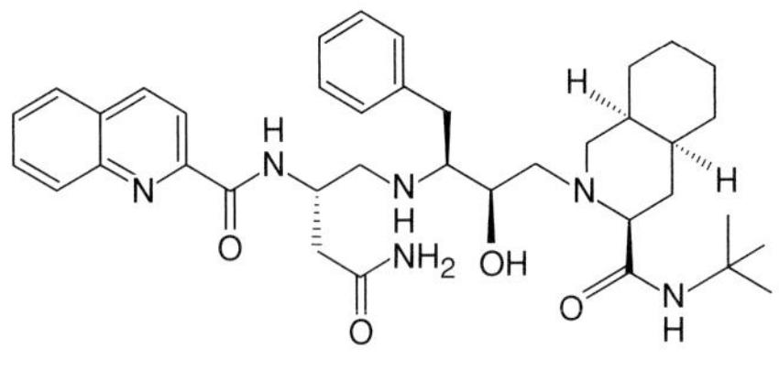

Saquinavir

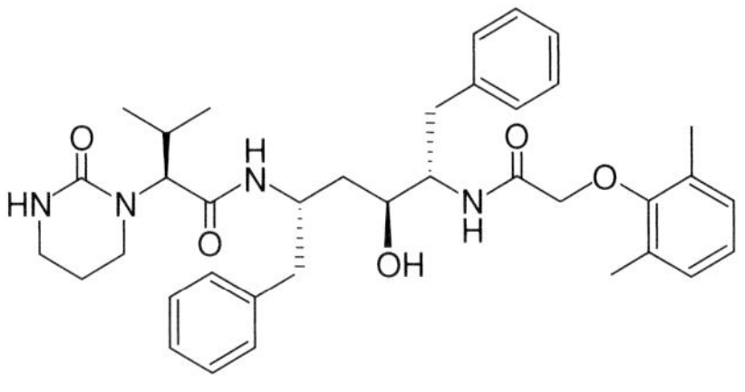

Lopinavir

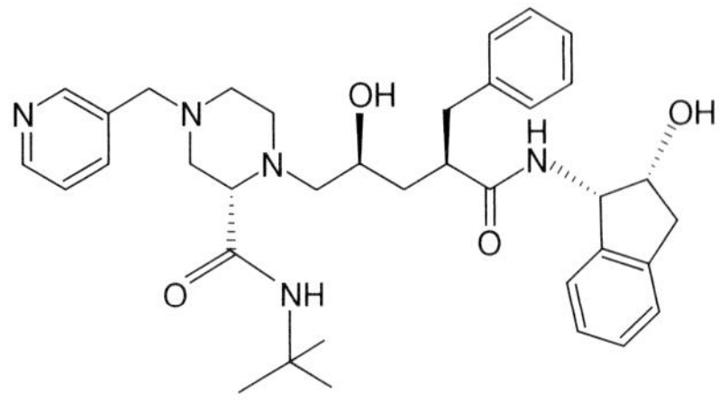

Indinavir

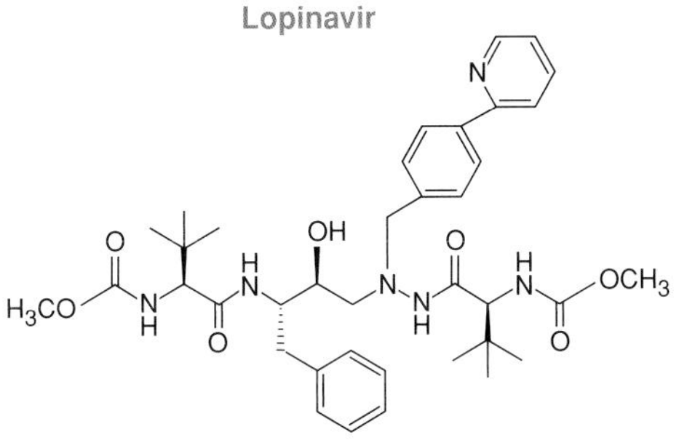

Atazanavir

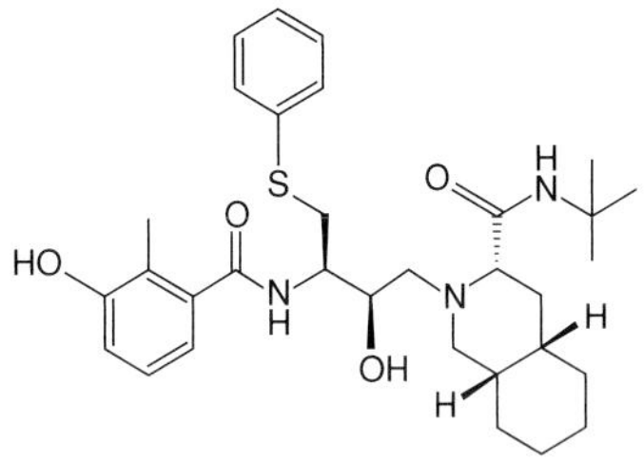

Nelfinavir

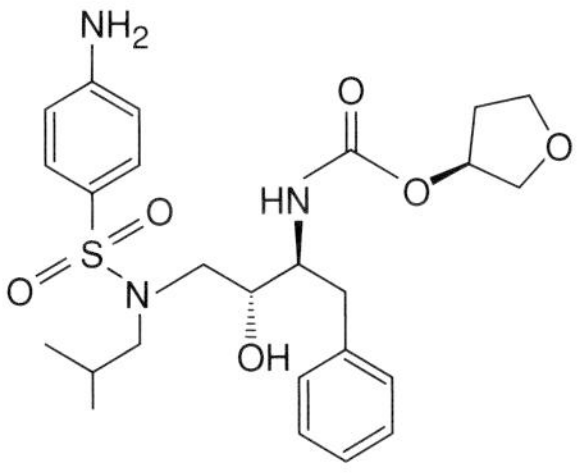

Amprenavir

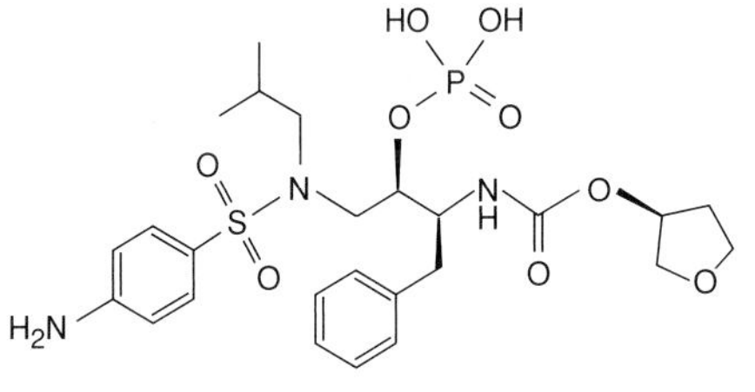

Fosamprenavir

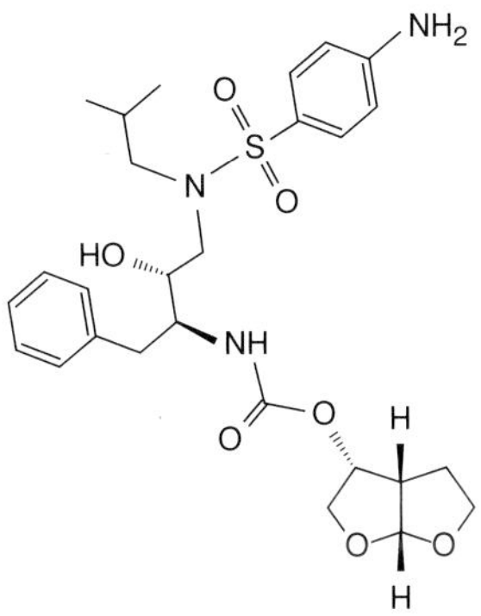

Darunavir

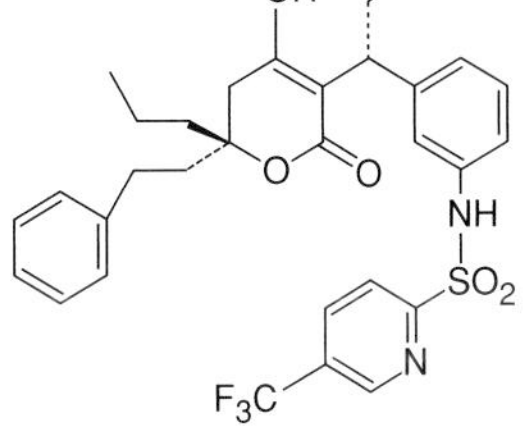

Tipranavir

FIGURE 13.12. Anti-HIV (human immunodeficiency virus) protease inhibitors. The structures of approved anti-HIV protease inhibitors ritonavir, saquinavir, lopinavir, indinavir, atazanavir, nelfinavir, amprenavir, its prodrug, fosamprenavir, darunavir, and tipranavir are shown.

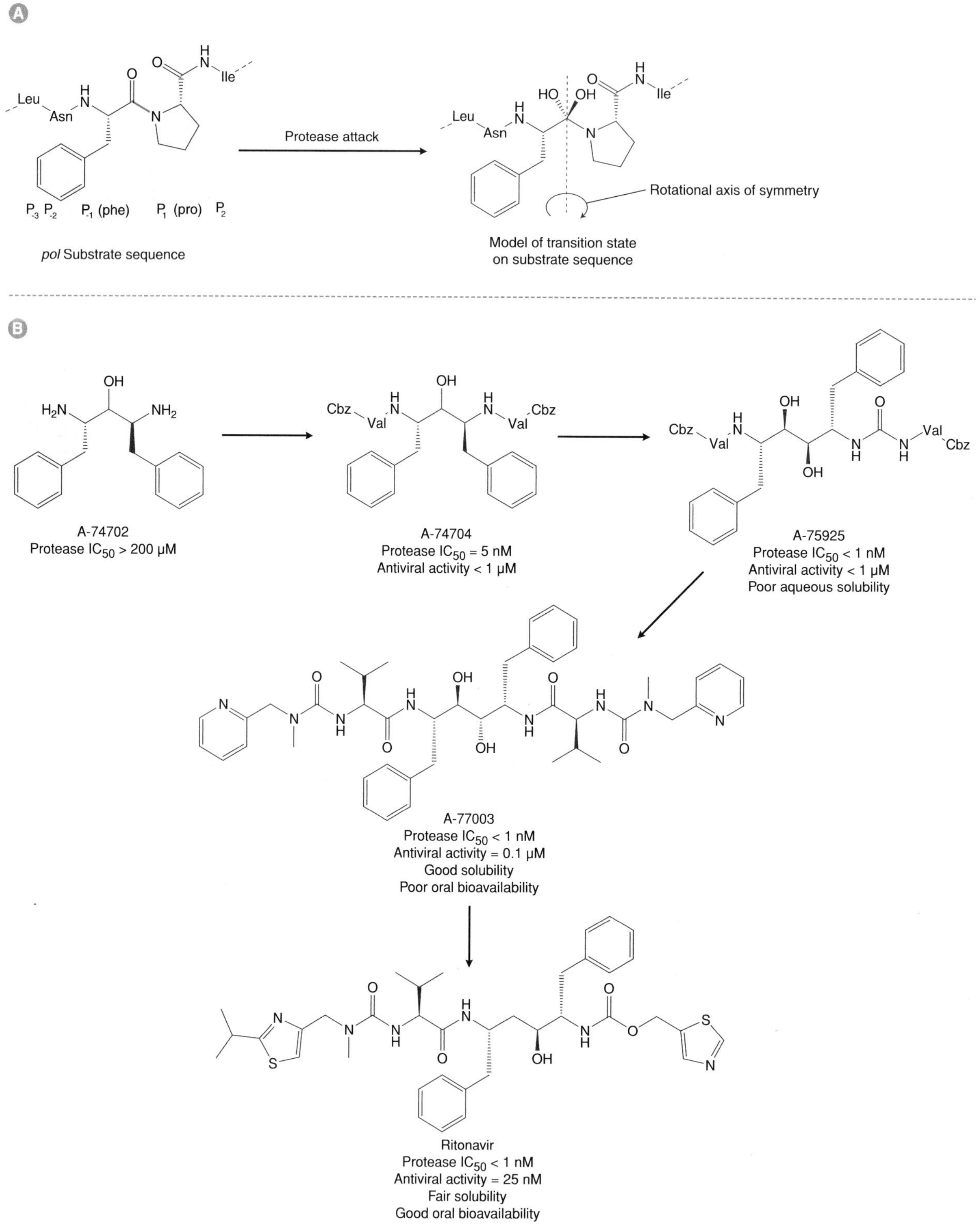

FIGURE 13.13. Steps in the development of ritonavir. A: On the left is shown a substrate sequence that is cleaved by human immunodeficiency virus (HIV) protease between a phenylalanine (phe) on the N-terminal side of the cleavage (P_{-1}) and a proline (pro) on the C-terminal side (P_1). On the right, the transition state of this sequence during protease cleavage is modeled. The transition state contains a rotational axis of symmetry **B:** Structure-based development of ritonavir began with A-74072 **(top left)** that mimics the transition state with a single CHOH moiety between two phenylalanines (to maximize symmetry). This compound, which had weak inhibitory activity, was modified by symmetric addition of other groups to yield A-74074, which was more potent (CBZ, carboxybenzyl), but was insufficiently soluble. This was modified to mimic the transition state with CHOH groups on each side of the axis of symmetry (A-75925, **top right**). This was also poorly soluble, but could be improved by adding more groups (A-77003, **middle**). That compound was not very orally available, so additional modifications, including the removal of a central OH group, were made, resulting in ritonavir **(bottom)**. The choices of modifications were aided by crystal structures of intermediate compounds bound to HIV-1 protease. For each compound, the inhibitory potencies against HIV-1 protease *in vitro* (IC_{50}) and against HIV in infected cells (antiviral activity) are provided.

A-77003 (Fig. 13.13, bottom). However, this compound was not absorbed orally.[189] It was modified by removing a central OH group and altering other moieties at each end (Fig. 13.13, bottom). This resulted in less solubility, but improved antiviral activity and good oral bioavailability.[188] These improvements took advantage of the x-ray structure of HIV protease complexed with each version of the inhibitors (reviewed in **4 and 388**). By examining these structures, chemists were able to make informed guesses about what groups to add or subtract. The result was ritonavir.

Crystallographic studies reveal that upon binding of protease inhibitors, the enzyme assumes a conformation with closed "flaps" that are unable to undergo conformational changes that help form the active site (reviewed in **4 and 388**). The drugs work in cell culture as expected: HIV-infected cells exposed to protease inhibitors continue to make viral proteins, but these proteins are not processed efficiently.[70] Viral particles bud from the infected cells, but they are immature and noninfectious.[114] Mutations conferring drug-resistance map to HIV sequences encoding the protease, confirming that protease is the target.[272]

Resistance to protease inhibitors has taught us a great deal about both the drugs and the virus.[23,66,181] Mutations in more than 30 of the 99 amino acid residues of protease have been selected with the different protease inhibitors, with as many as 24 conferring resistance to any one drug. Some of the mutations affect the active site or sites known to interact with the inhibitors, and thus the mechanism of resistance can be readily understood. However, other mutations affect more distal sites, and it is not clear how they confer resistance. Resistance is often cumulative. In some patients, after failing multiple regimens containing protease inhibitors, more than 20 of these mutations have accumulated in their virus, demonstrating the remarkable plasticity of this enzyme.[159,181] There is even an example of a virus whose replication is enhanced by subinhibitory concentrations of a protease inhibitor.[237]

Different protease inhibitors tend to select different mutations, at least initially. Therefore, although the drugs all work by similar mechanisms, the first mutation selected for resistance to one protease inhibitor often does not confer resistance to another. This can be understood by considering that although the different drugs tend to share similar functionalities that interact with the protease active site, each drug has a different functionality that confers high affinity binding via interactions with a particular site specific to the drug. Therefore, a single mutation that interferes with binding of one drug will not necessarily affect binding of the other. As mutations accumulate, however, cross-resistance develops among the protease inhibitors. Mutations affecting protease cleavage sites can also confer resistance.[86] These result in more easily cleaved precursor substrates for the protease. Different protease mutations also have differing effects on viral fitness. Certain mutations can be readily found in untreated patients, suggesting high fitness, whereas others are not detected except following drug treatment, and often decrease fitness. Cleavage site mutations can improve the fitness of protease mutants.[86,230,399] These different features of resistance to protease inhibitors have important clinical implications (see section on anti-HIV therapy).

Inhibition of Viral Release: Influenza Virus Neuraminidase Inhibitors

Inhibitors of influenza virus neuraminidases block viral release of influenza A and B viruses. The rationale for their action follows from the mechanism of viral attachment. Influenza attaches to cells via interactions between the virion hemagglutinin and sialic acid, which is present on many cellular membrane glycoproteins. However, upon egress of influenza virus from cells at the end of a round of replication, hemagglutinin on nascent virions again binds to sialic acid and tethers virions, preventing release and initiation of new rounds of infection. To overcome this problem, influenza virus encodes a virion neuraminidase, which cleaves sialic acid from the membrane glycoproteins. Studies using influenza virus mutants or an early neuraminidase inhibitor showed that without neuraminidase, the virus remains tethered and cannot spread to other cells.[220,275,276] In 1992, structures of the neuraminidase-sialic acid cleavage product were solved.[35,369] The structure showed that sialic acid occupied two of three well-formed pockets on the enzyme. Based largely on this structure, a new sialic acid transition state analog was designed to make energetically favorable interactions in all three of the pockets, principally by adding a guanidino group[370] (Fig. 13.14). This compound, zanamivir, inhibits neuraminidase with a Ki of about 0.1 nM. Zanamivir is active against both influenza A and influenza B viruses with potencies of about 30 nM. However, it is not orally bioavailable, and must be administered as an aerosol.

Efforts to obtain a neuraminidase inhibitor with better pharmacokinetic properties than zanamivir resulted in oseltamivir (Fig. 13.14).[191,211] Oseltamivir makes use of a carbocyclic ring based on a transition state analog of sialic acid. Rather than use a guanidino group to occupy a third pocket, it makes stronger contacts with one of the two pockets bound by sialic acid by adding a hydrophobic group (Fig. 13.13). Oseltamivir's high oral bioavailability depends in part on its being an ester prodrug, which when cleaved gives rise to the active carboxylate (Fig. 13.14).

Most neuraminidase resistance mutations result in an enzyme that is less inhibited by the drug.[245] As would be expected by the differences in drug binding to the enzyme (Fig. 13.14), mutants resistant to one drug are not necessarily resistant to the other. This phenomenon gained worldwide notice when a human who became ill with virulent, avian H5N1 influenza A virus despite prophylaxis with oseltamivir was found to harbor oseltamivir-resistant, but zanamivir-sensitive virus.[228] Still, compared with amantadine, for many years it was relatively difficult to generate mutants resistant to zanamivir or oseltamivir in the laboratory, and they appeared less frequently in the clinic. This was due in part to most such mutants, such as those containing the H275Y substitution that confers oseltamivir-resistance, being less fit than wild-type virus.[177] Indeed, the oseltamivir-resistant H5N1 just mentioned replicated less well in ferrets than did a drug sensitive virus from the same patient.[228]

However, during the 2007–2008 influenza season, virulent, readily transmitted H275Y viruses began to appear among seasonal H1N1 isolates, even in the absence of oseltamivir therapy.[146] These viruses containing Y275 appear just as fit *in vitro* as controls containing H275.[22,298] The fitness of these H1N1 mutants can be attributed to permissive secondary mutations that allow increased expression of the H275Y mutants on the surface of the infected cell.[22] As described in the Overview section of this chapter, another class of mutants resistant to the neuraminidase inhibitors contains altered hemagglutinins.

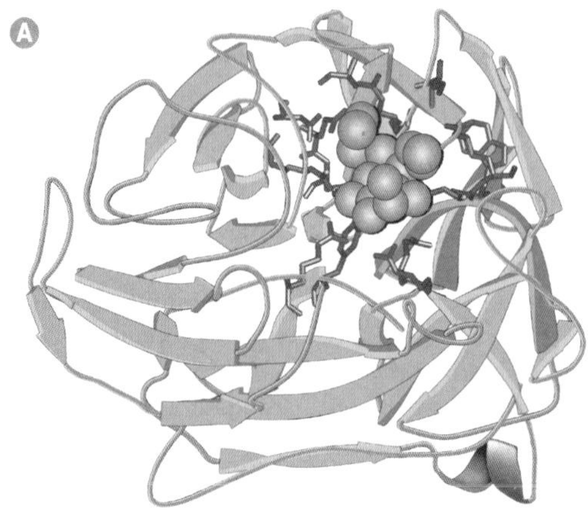

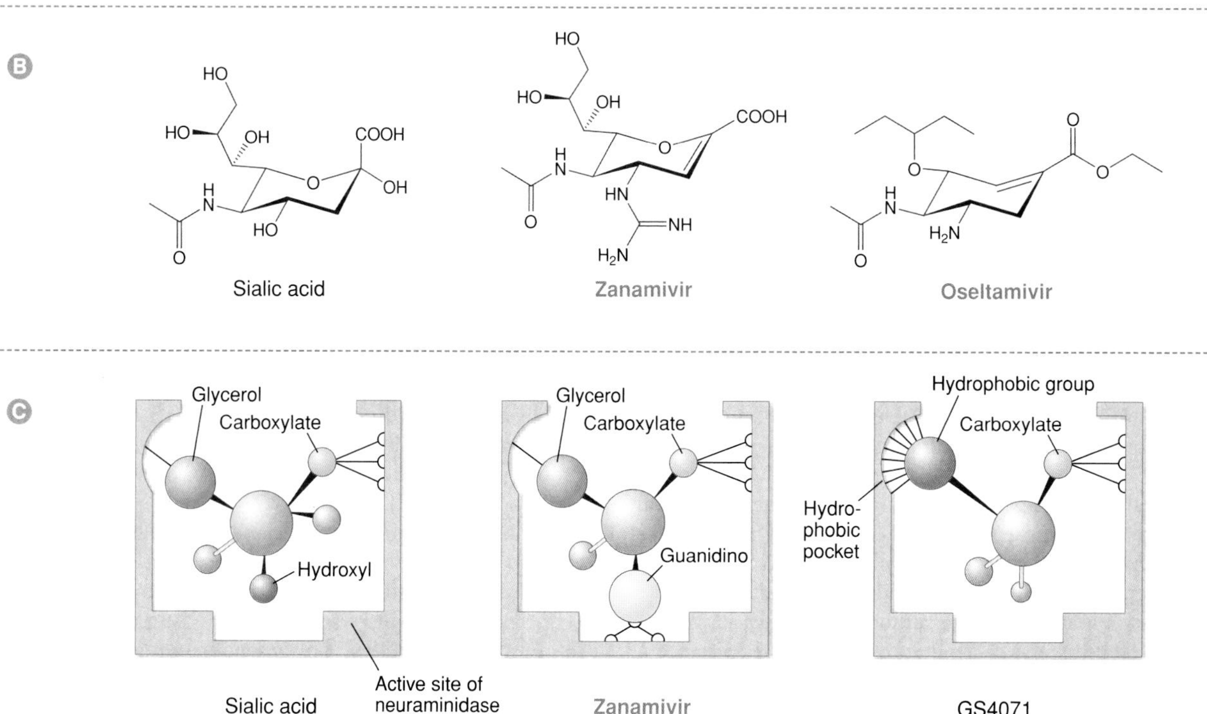

FIGURE 13.14. Structure-based design of inhibitors of influenza A and B virus neuraminidase. A: Shown is a model of sialic acid (space-filling structure in dark purple) bound to the influenza neuraminidase (green and light purple), with the amino acids that bind sialic acid shown in stick form. This structure was used to design transition state inhibitors that bind with higher affinity than sialic acid. **B:** Structures of sialic acid and the neuraminidase inhibitors oseltamivir and zanamivir. **C:** Diagram of the active site of influenza virus neuraminidase, showing the binding of sialic acid, zanamivir, and GS 4071 (oseltamivir is the ethyl ester of this compound), showing how the different ligands interact with pockets in the active site. Note that the compounds in **C** are flipped 180 degrees relative to how they are shown in **A** and **B**. (A and B, from Yeh RW, Coen DM. Pharmacology of viral infections. In: Golan DE, Tashjian AH, Jr., Armstrong EJ, et al., eds. *Principles of Pharmacology: The Pathophysiologic Basis of Drug Therapy.* Third edition. Philadelphia: Lippincott Williams & Wilkins; 2012:649–673. **C,** modified from Laver WG, Bischofberger N, Webster RG. Disarming flu viruses. *Sci Am* 1999;280:78–87.)

Other neuraminidase inhibitors are in clinical development. One of these, peramivir, is approved in Japan and Korea, but not yet in the United States (e-Table 13.1). Nevertheless, in 2009, it was authorized for emergency use in severe cases of pandemic H1N1 influenza in hospitalized patients, because it can be administered intravenously. The H275Y mutation confers resistance to peramivir, limiting its use against oseltamivir-resistant virus.

With increasing concerns regarding influenza pandemics, the mechanisms of action and resistance of neuraminidase inhibitors have become very important, as has the development of new anti-influenza drugs that are active against mutants resistant to neuraminidase inhibitors.

Antiviral Therapies That Target Immune Processes

Two types of drugs approved for treatment of viral infections—imiquimod and IFNs—do not inhibit virus replication directly. Rather, they enhance innate host immune responses to viral infection. Imiquimod (e-Fig. 13.1), which is approved for treating certain diseases caused by human papillomaviruses, interacts with Toll-like receptors TLR7 and TLR8 to boost innate immunity, including secretion of IFNs.[117,155,183] Interferon alpha is approved for treating HCV; HBV; condyloma acuminata, which is caused by certain human papillomaviruses; and Kaposi's sarcoma, which is caused by Kaposi's sarcoma–associated herpesvirus (human herpesvirus 8). The actions of IFNs are reviewed in Chapter 8. However, which of the many activities induced by IFNs contribute to their therapeutic effects (e.g., against HCV; reviewed in 95) remain poorly understood. Interestingly, genetic polymorphisms in a region encoding certain type III IFNs, which are induced by IFN-α, are associated with response of HCV infections to IFN-α and ribavirin, with lower expression of these interferons associated with lower responses to therapy.[113,352,358] Follow-up studies of this observation and greater understanding of mechanisms by which viruses inhibit interferon action (e.g., HCV; reviewed in 95) may facilitate the development of more targeted therapies.

PRINCIPLES OF ANTIVIRAL THERAPY

General Concepts

Viral Dynamics and the Role of the Immune System in Antiviral Therapy

Different viruses can have very different dynamics of infection, and these differences have major impacts on the goals and effects of antiviral therapy. Many of these differences relate to the interplay between antiviral therapy and in the immune system. Acute viral infections of immunocompetent patients are usually cleared by the immune system in a matter of days. It is not surprising then that treatment of most acute influenza virus infections in immunocompetent patients with drugs such as oseltamivir reduces the duration of fever and other symptoms by only a day or so. A corollary is that treatment must be started as soon as possible to obtain clinical benefits. Indeed, prophylaxis can be the most effective approach. Many of the same considerations apply to recurrent disease caused by reactivation of latent viral infections in immunocompetent patients. In the case of frequently recurring herpes genitalis, suppressive therapy is much more effective than treating each episode. Another issue in acute infections can be the extent to which symptoms are due to viral replication rather than the immune response to the virus. For example, most of the symptoms of mononucleosis caused by Epstein-Barr virus (EBV) infections occur when viral replication has subsided. As a result, even though several antiviral drugs that are clinically useful against other herpesviruses are potent inhibitors of EBV replication, they are ineffective at treating mononucleosis.

Many of the viruses for which antiviral drugs have been developed cause persistent infections. The primary goal in the management of persistent viral infections with antiviral therapy is sustained suppression of viral replication. In contrast with acute infections, antiviral therapy can be effective when initiated well after symptoms have appeared. In some cases, such as HCV infections, persistent viral replication occurs in the face of an immune response that usually is incapable of clearing the virus by itself. However, HCV does not form latent infections, and thus can be cured by inhibiting viral replication. In other cases, such as reactivating HCMV in transplant patients, the immune system cannot control virus replication. Antiviral drugs cannot cure HCMV infections, but they can stave off viral disease until an effective immune response is restored. Prophylactic approaches against HCMV are used very selectively in immunosuppressed patients because of the toxicities of anti-HCMV drugs. Physicians often opt for preemptive therapy when a certain level of replicating virus is detected, but before disease symptoms are manifest.

The interplay between antiviral therapy, viral dynamics, and the immune response, and the roles of tissue compartments and cellular reservoirs has been investigated in the most detail with HIV, and is discussed below.

Interplay between Anti-HIV Therapy, Viral Dynamics, and the Immune System

The generation of virions in chronic HIV infection is enormous, and the goal of antiviral therapy is to suppress this. With the initiation of effective treatment, the clearance of virions from the plasma is rapid (minutes to hours). The clearance rate constant varies little among individuals and different stages of disease.[282] The steady state levels of viral nucleic acid in the blood are thus determined by the rates of virus production. For HIV these rates of production are a function of the number of infected lymphocytes in the lymphoid tissue.[129,130] The rate of decline of CD4 lymphocytes is thus directly related to the steady state level of plasma HIV RNA. The higher the RNA levels, the faster the loss of CD4 cells, and the shorter the duration of HIV infection before death.[244] Because the CD4 count determines the risk of disease and death, and the level of HIV RNA determines the rate of CD4 cell decline, these values have been routinely used clinically to assess clinical status and urgency to initiate therapy.[362]

When potent combination antiretroviral therapy is effectively administered, levels of HIV RNA in both plasma and infected cells in lymphoid tissue rapidly decrease. The rapid, first phase clearance is attributable to the death of infected, activated CD4 lymphocytes and the prevention of infection of new cells.[282] The second phase clearance rate is lower and more variable in slope among individuals. It has been attributed to clearance of infected macrophages or to chronically infected CD4 lymphocytes with lower rates of cell death, but may also result from the clearance of the large burden of virions bound to dendritic cells in the germinal centers of lymph nodes.[39,280,403] Failure to reduce plasma HIV RNA levels to below the limit of detection (20–75 copies/ml with the currently available assays) indicates inadequate suppression and a risk for the outgrowth of resistant virus.[362] Even in patients sustaining suppression below this level for 10 years or more, very low levels of viral RNA can often be detected in tissues and blood. This low level viremia is sustained at steady state levels of less than 50 copies of HIV RNA/ml plasma as measured following ultracentrifugation and using very sensitive assays. Although ongoing replication may be occurring in some patients, several lines of evidence would argue that activation of latently infected CD4+ lymphocytes or long-lived persistently infected cells like macrophages or pluripotent multiprogenitor cells are the source of this viremia. Notably, no new drug-resistance mutations emerge, no nucleotide sequence evolution can be discerned, and treatment intensification with additional potent antiretroviral drugs fails to perturb the viremia.[242,277]

The immunologic consequences of suppressing HIV replication are dramatic. The increase in CD4 lymphocyte numbers has two phases. In the first month or two the increase is often large (20–100 cells per μl blood).[7,18,128] The magnitude is proportional to the steady state HIV RNA levels before treatment, which drives the level of generalized activation of the immune system. The normal distribution of lymphocytes is 2% in the circulation and 98% in the lymphoid tissues. With the immune activation of HIV infection, the distribution shifts to 1% and 99%.[129,404] Therapy largely corrects this shift, and results in redistribution of mostly $CD45RO^+$ memory T cells from the lymphoid tissue back to the circulation.[31,274,404] Production of new cells, mostly of the CD45RA-naïve phenotype, is generated both by restored thymic mass and function, which is age related, and by peripheral proliferation.[84,239]

The generation of cell numbers is not sufficient to account for the success of antiretroviral therapy. It is the restoration of immune function that has transformed the natural history of AIDS. Both CD4 and CD8 T-cell responses to recall antigens are regenerated.[7,140,194] Persistent opportunistic infections are often resolved. Occasionally, subclinical chronic infections with *Mycobacterium avium complex* (MAC) or HCMV, for example, are manifested when a restored immune response produces a local inflammatory reaction. Patient care has been transformed with the ability to withdraw prophylactic or suppressive therapy for various opportunistic infections, which had previously been lifelong commitments.

The probability of success of suppressing HIV replication and of preventing the emergence of resistance (see below) is significantly impacted by the level of CD4 cells and of HIV RNA in the blood. This relationship is a practical argument to avoid treating before it is too late, but it also points out that the imperfect efficacy of drug treatments is complemented by having more immunity and less virus. It is noteworthy that the success of treatment of opportunistic infections in AIDS patients, including antiviral therapy for HSV, VZV, and HCMV infections, also is similarly affected by CD4 cell count.

Compartments and Reservoirs

Treatment of HIV is complicated by the existence of tissue compartments and cellular reservoirs. Although there is trafficking between the blood and central nervous system (CNS), much virus in the CNS evolves independently.[346] Similar observations have been made with virus in semen.[288] Drug penetration into these compartments differs from the circulation and lymphoid tissue, and varies with each drug. Latently infected CD4 lymphocytes represent a small fraction of infected cells during active infection, but they have long half-lives,[97,311,345] and may be sustained for life by homeostatic proliferation of latently infected memory CD4+ lymphocytes.[49] Consequently, virus archived at any time during infection can reemerge and propagate after the withdrawal of therapy.

Drug Resistance in Antiviral Therapy

The speed, magnitude, and clinical impact of the emergence of resistance differ among antivirals and viruses. As summarized earlier in the chapter, the rate at which mutants that are resistant to a given drug will emerge is a function of mutation rate, target size for mutation, replication rate, preexisting size of the population, and fitness. All of these factors can have clinical impact. For example, at presentation, an HIV-infected individual contains 10^{11} virions,[130] more than 10 billion (10^{10}) HIV-1 virions are generated daily,[282] and on average one mutation is generated for each newly generated genome.[232] Therefore, genomes with each possible mutation, as well as many with double mutations, are likely generated daily. Moreover, during HIV infection, drug-resistant virus is readily archived in latently infected cells to confound treatment modifications for the remainder of the patient's life.[98,390,311] Therefore, an HIV-infected individual is highly likely to develop an infection that is resistant to any given antiviral drug. In contrast, ACV resistance almost never develops during treatment of HSV or VZV in immunocompetent patients. These patients contain much less virus, and the virus replicates and mutates at a much lower rate than HIV. Nevertheless, ACV resistance does occur more often in immunocompromised patients in whom virus replicates to higher levels and more persistently.

Of particular clinical relevance to antiviral resistance are drug concentrations attained in patients that achieve therapeutic effects. In this regard, fitness is highly important. With increasing drug exposure in a patient, the selective pressure on the replicating virus population increases to promote the more rapid emergence of drug resistant mutants; that is, as drug-sensitive viruses become less fit. For example, higher doses of AZT or ritonavir monotherapy tend to select for drug-resistant HIV more readily than do lower doses.[256,309] As drug concentrations of monotherapy increase, the likelihood that resistant mutants will arise increases, as long as significant levels of virus replication persist. This can occur through improper dosing, suboptimal adherence, pharmacologic hurdles, and ineffectively treated compartments. Incompletely suppressed viral replication with drug regimens sufficient to exert selective pressure drive the evolution and fixation of drug-resistant virus at a rate Darwin himself never imagined. This scenario may explain the emergence of an oseltamivir-resistant H5N1 influenza virus in a patient who had been given relatively low doses of drug as prophylaxis.[228] With further increases in concentration of antiviral drugs, especially in combination, the amount of virus replication diminishes to the point where the likelihood of emergence of resistance begins to diminish, and becomes nil when virus replication is completely inhibited.[306] The ultimate goal of antiviral therapy, especially for viruses like HIV, HBV, and HCV, which have high mutation rates, high replication rates, and high preexisting populations, is to apply drug regimens that completely inhibit virus replication.

Clinical Impact of Drug Resistance

It may seem obvious that drug resistance is important clinically. However, many treatment failures are not due to drug resistance, and many drug-resistant viruses do not cause treatment failures. To demonstrate thoroughly that drug resistance is clinically important, it is necessary to have evidence of treatment failure, to isolate drug-resistant virus, and to successfully treat the disease with a second drug to which the virus is susceptible.

For acute infections like influenza, which are largely controlled by the immune system, antiviral drug resistance is generally not a major problem in the patient in whom it arises. Therefore, during monotherapy with adamantanes or neuraminidase inhibitors, variants probably emerge in all patients within a week, but in immunocompetent patients, that is when the infection has largely resolved. Transmission of resistant virus to others can occur, however, and the antiviral efficacy will be impaired in these secondary cases. In persistent infections, antiviral drug resistance can be a matter of life and death. As resistance mutations accumulate, drug susceptibility diminishes, progressively reducing the efficacy of antiviral regimens. Continued replication in the presence of drug selects for even greater levels of resistance to each administered drug and progressive cross-resistance to drugs of the same class. This drives a vicious cycle of treatment failure and yet more difficult treatment challenges. Regimens for patients who are failing treatment, while constrained to more limited options by resistance, must still contend with the same obstacles of adherence, pharmacology, and tolerability that challenged the first regimen.

Drug-resistant herpesviruses and HIV can establish latent infections. Drug-resistant HIV, HBV, and influenza A viruses have been transmitted to other individuals. In the case of HIV, resistant virus in blood or genital secretions can be transmitted during sex, needle sharing, or childbirth.[216] Rates of transmission of drug-resistant HIV appear to have increased, with 5% to 20% of primary infections caused by drug-resistant virus in developed countries.[216,218] Such patients are more likely to fail their first treatment regimen. Resistance in developing countries has become increasingly appreciated with the rollout of treatment access.[295]

Strategies to Combat Drug Resistance

The increasing prevalence of antiviral drug resistance raises challenges to the effective treatment of individuals and to the public health similar to those that have resulted from widespread antibiotic resistance. One strategy to combat this problem is to test viruses for drug resistance before choosing antiviral regimens. Resistance testing can help determine which drugs will not work (thereby diminishing cost, toxicity, and inconvenience) and which drugs are most likely to be effective. Such testing is rapidly being incorporated into standard HIV care,[160] and is certain to become part of the management of HBV and HCV. These tests can be performed most rapidly if they are genotypic (i.e., detecting mutations at the level of DNA or RNA) rather than phenotypic (i.e., measuring changes in drug susceptibility). Genotypic assays are much easier to develop if only a few mutations confer clinically relevant resistance. As reviewed in the sections on mechanisms of specific antiviral drugs, this is more likely to be true for some drugs (e.g., lamivudine) than others (e.g. ACV). As numerous mutations in various combinations accumulate, as occurs during treatment of HIV with RT and protease inhibitors, the interpretation of genotypic assays can become very difficult, and phenotypic assays may be required.

A second key strategy is combination chemotherapy. This strategy combats resistance on several levels. First, the probability of a virus being resistant to multiple different drugs (with different mutations conferring resistance) is the product of the probabilities of resistance to each drug. This makes it much less likely that a preexisting virus in the patient will be resistant to all of the drugs. Second, the combination is likely to suppress replication more completely than would any of the drugs alone. This would provide less chance for resistance to develop. Third, members of the combination might synergize, thereby providing even greater efficacy. It is crucial that drugs in the combination not antagonize each other's activities by mechanism of action or pharmacologic interaction. Fourth, a mutation conferring resistance to one drug in a combination might yield clinical advantages, for example, by making the virus less fit or by sensitizing otherwise resistant viruses to a second drug. Such advantages have been invoked for the M184V mutation in HIV and the M204V/I mutation in HBV that confer resistance to 3TC and FTC (reviewed in **79**).

Why not always use combination chemotherapy? Additional drugs add costs, toxicities, and pharmacological interactions, which sometimes exacerbate those of the first drug. Combination regimens can be difficult for the patient, reducing adherence with the regimen. Sometimes too few drugs are available to combine, or if there are multiple drugs, they entail similar mechanisms of action and resistance. Drug resistance is relatively uncommon with certain virus infections, such as herpesvirus infections in the immunocompetent. These points help explain why combination chemotherapy is rarely used for treating herpesvirus or influenza virus infections.

The history and clinical practices as of 2012, and issues particular to therapies of different viruses will now be reviewed.

HIV Therapy

In the 27 years since AZT was first clinically evaluated, 25 drugs have been approved for treating HIV (Fig. 13.15). This remarkable drug development experience helped elucidate many of the principles of antiviral therapy described earlier. A review of the clinical evaluation of each of the anti-HIV drugs and each of the combinations of these drugs for patients in various stages of disease is beyond the scope of this chapter. Guidelines summarizing the practical use of currently available antiretrovirals are frequently updated.[359,362] With the availability of these treatment alternatives and with an appreciation of the principles of antiviral therapy, HIV has been transformed into a manageable condition for most patients in the developed world and encouraging inroads have been made for millions in resource-limited settings. AIDS mortality and morbidity from opportunistic conditions have been dramatically diminished for those with access to care.

The initial use of AZT monotherapy in patients with late-stage HIV disease had a dramatic effect on mortality over the first several months of follow-up.[100] The benefits dissipated with the emergence of drug-resistant virus.[99,134,200] The availability of additional nucleoside analog RT inhibitors, as replacement therapy on those failing AZT monotherapy and in combination with AZT in previously untreated patients, provided incremental efficacy.[64,65,136,184] The use of nucleoside analogs in various combinations and regimens reduced morbidity and prolonged life. However, for most patients, drug resistance and loss of control ultimately ensued.

The approval of the first drugs in additional classes (NNRTIs and protease inhibitors) permitted the trials of two nucleosides and initially either indinavir or nevirapine, which changed the treatment paradigm.[128,137,257,342] When patients

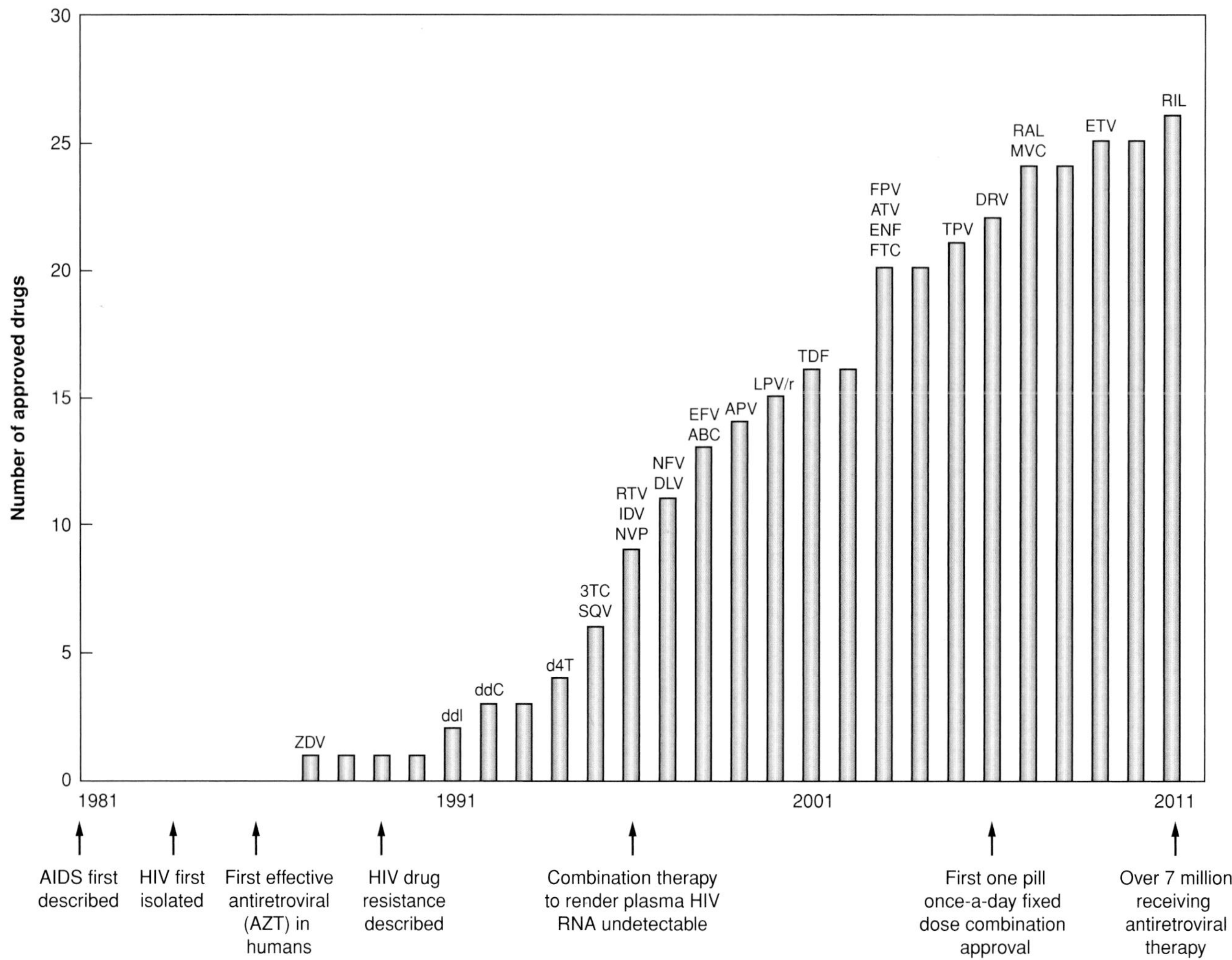

FIGURE 13.15. Time-line of acquired immunodeficiency syndrome (AIDS) therapies. The dates of important events in the understanding and therapy of AIDS are provided together with the dates of U.S. Food and Drug Administration (FDA) approval of antiretroviral drugs. The bars represent the progressive accrual of approved drugs. Abbreviations: ZDV, zidovudine (AZT); ddI, didanosine; ddC, zalcitabine; d4T, stavudine; 3TC, lamivudine; SQV, saquinavir; RTV, ritonavir; IDV, indinavir; NVP, nevirapine; NFV, nelfinavir; DLV, delavirdine; EFV, efavirenz; ABC, abacavir; APV, amprenavir; LPV/r; lopinavir/ritonavir; TDF, tenofovir; FPV, fosamprenavir; ATV, atazanavir; ENF, enfuvirtide; FTC, emtricitabine; TPV, tipranavir; DRV, darunavir; RAL, raltegravir; MVC, maraviroc; ETV, etravirine; RIL, rilpivirine. Elvitegravir was approved in 2012.

who had not yet acquired too many compromising drug-resistance mutations received these triple combinations, they experienced suppression below assay detection for plasma HIV RNA. Many patients are now well into their second decade of HIV RNA suppression and immune restoration. AIDS-related morbidity and mortality are seen primarily in those without access to care. In those who are receiving effective antiretrovirals, the primary complications are related to chronic hepatitis, malignancies, or the accidents and illnesses facing the general population.

The chronic use of antiretrovirals revealed toxicities often not appreciated in the initial preclinical toxicologic assessment of the drugs or clinical trials. Side effects due to nucleoside analogs include bone marrow toxicity (AZT), pancreatitis (ddI), myopathy (AZT), fat wasting in face and limbs (d4T, AZT), lactic acidosis (AZT, d4T, ddI, zalcitabine [ddC]) and peripheral neuropathy (ddC, ddI, d4T, ddC[28,69]). Most protease inhibitors were observed to induce hyperlipidemia and insulin resistance.[268] The availability of more drug alternatives has led to the gradual selection of regimens that minimize toxicity, maximize potency, and improve convenience in terms of pill burden and dosing frequency to facilitate adherence.[359,362] As the regimens become more convenient, more efficacious, and less toxic, the proportions of patients whose circulating HIV becomes fully suppressed is approaching 90% and the mortality curves continue to improve each year.[119,224]

These increasing rates of successful initial treatment diminish the proportion of patients who newly acquire drug resistance. Moreover, the proportion of patients with long-standing resistance to nucleoside analogs acquired before the availability of effective combination therapy is diminishing. The numbers of patients with transmitted drug resistance, after initially rising, now appears to be stable or even diminishing, with improved suppression of ongoing replication in increasing proportions of the population.[119] The availability of multiple alternative drugs is important to address the needs of patients requiring treatment of drug-resistant virus. The phenomenon of cross-resistance within drug classes still leaves many patients with few or no options; however, with newer drugs this number is diminished in developed countries. Therapy for HIV thus requires continuing efforts in drug resistance testing and drug development to contend with a virus so proficient at latency, evolution, and escape.

With the appreciation that treatment is more likely to be effective and less toxic when initiated early, and there is risk with delaying therapy at almost any stage of HIV infection, treatment guidelines have shifted to recommending almost universal treatment if feasible.[362] It has been proposed that this practice can also reduce HIV transmission.[119]

Herpesviruses Therapy

HSV and VZV Therapies

The first effective application of antiviral therapy for a herpesvirus infection was the local application of the nucleoside analog, 5′-iodo-2′-deoxyuridine, for the topical treatment of HSV keratitis.[186] This application has the advantage of permitting high local concentrations of antiviral at the site of infection without the risk of systemic toxicity. Other anti-HSV drugs are now used for this application. The first effective antiviral for systemic use against HSV was vidarabine, a nucleoside analog converted by cellular enzymes to an inhibitor of HSV DNA polymerase. This intravenously administered drug improved biopsy-proven HSV encephalitis in a double-blind, placebo-controlled trial in 1977[382] and subsequently was shown to be effective against neonatal herpes and VZV infection in immunocompromised patients.[379,381]

ACV, the mechanism of which is detailed in this chapter, heralded the second generation of antivirals for herpesviruses and set the standard for the development of antiviral drugs. It became the standard care after randomized, controlled trials of intravenous drug for serious systemic infections such as herpes encephalitis, neonatal herpes, and varicella zoster in immunocompromised hosts.[13,377,378–379] In addition, it was shown to be effective for the prophylaxis of HSV and VZV in transplant patients.[321,322] As an orally available agent with negligible toxicity, it has become widely used for the treatment of primary and recurrent HSV-1 and HSV-2, the prophylaxis of recurrent HSV, and the treatment of uncomplicated VZV.[85,90,168,247,254,265,302,347,371] The earlier in the presentation of symptoms, the more effective the treatment, and prophylaxis is more dependable than treatment. The appearance of resistant isolates has been remarkably rare in immunocompetent patients and occurs in a minority of immunocompromised patients. ACV-resistant HSV and VZV did become a significant challenge in patients with AIDS preceding the availability of combination antiretroviral therapy.[317] The expanded number of resistant infections reflected the number of patients with AIDS, the prevalence of recurrent HSV and VZV infection in these patients, and the duration and magnitude of these opportunistic infections, because of the severely reduced antiviral immunity in these hosts. In many, but not all of these patients, cidofovir or foscarnet showed activity against resistant infections,[318] but resistance to these DNA polymerase inhibitors has developed as well.[118,319]

Two limitations of oral ACV have been its limited oral bioavailability (~15%) and short half-life. These limitations require administration of large pills as often as every 4 hours. As described earlier in this chapter, valacyclovir and famciclovir overcome these limitations, and would have completely displaced the use of ACV except for the expiration of the ACV patent resulting in the availability of low-cost generic drug. Both valacyclovir and famciclovir can be used for applications of oral ACV. In addition, because of the more prolonged maintenance of higher levels of antiviral activity, they are also used for the treatment of serious but not immediately life-threatening infections previously treated with intravenous ACV, for example, herpes zoster in the immunocompromised host.[20,367]

HCMV Therapies

As reviewed earlier in the chapter, the lack of potency of ACV against HCMV led to the development of ganciclovir. Ganciclovir is more toxic than ACV. However, it is the first-line therapy for HCMV disease in the immunocompromised host.

The most common opportunistic complication of HCMV in AIDS is retinitis.[178] Ganciclovir clears viremia and arrests the progression of destructive retinitis.[32,178,360] HCMV disease develops in patients with AIDS who have fewer than 100 CD4 cells per ml; however, before reconstitution of the immune system with combination antiretroviral therapy, these patients uniformly reactivated disease with withdrawal of treatment, thus requiring chronic suppressive maintenance treatment with the consequences of drug toxicity and emergence of resistant virus.[380] Ganciclovir is similarly effective for the treatment of colitis, esophagitis, polyradiculitis, and ventriculitis in patients with AIDS,[80] and HCMV pneumonia in renal transplant patients.[154]

With the difficulties of daily intravenous ganciclovir for maintenance therapy, oral ganciclovir was studied despite its low bioavailability, which resulted in limited efficacy and selection for drug resistance. Some significant benefit for the management of retinitis was the local administration in the eye of ganciclovir (and some other anti-HCMV drugs) by injection or implant.[234] This approach protects the eye with high local concentrations, but fails to address HCMV disease in the rest of the body.[380] The eventual development of valganciclovir has now provided an orally bioavailable drug for HCMV that can achieve levels approaching those of intravenous ganciclovir without the cost, inconvenience, and complications. Although a significant advance, the introduction of effective combination antiretroviral therapy was more crucial, as it dramatically diminished the prevalence of HCMV disease and essentially eliminated the need of maintenance therapy for retinitis.

Foscarnet, cidofovir, and fomivirsen are also approved for the treatment of HCMV. Although equally effective for the treatment of HCMV retinitis, foscarnet is used only for ganciclovir-resistant HCMV infections because of inconvenience and toxicity.[360] Cidofovir is also used for the treatment of ganciclovir-resistant HCMV, with the advantage of requiring administration only every 1 or 2 weeks due to its very prolonged intracellular half-life, but the disadvantage of renal toxicity.

Antiviral therapy has not yet been shown to significantly impact disease attributable to the other human herpesviruses, EBV, and HHV6, HHV7, and HHV8. Various explanations include the limited activity against these viruses of available drugs, the undesirability of testing a difficult drug like foscarnet that might nevertheless have activity, the difficulty of conducting clinical trials for some of these infections, and the relatively small size of the perceived market. Aside from therapies against these other herpesviruses, there remains considerable need for new anti-herpesvirus drugs to combat infections resistant to the current drugs, and to overcome the pharmacological and toxicity limitations of the current anti-HCMV drugs. No available anti-herpesvirus drug effectively addresses the problem of viral latency.

Therapy of Viral Hepatitis

HBV Therapy

The complex natural history of HBV infection is described elsewhere in this text. Criteria based on disease stage and level of HBV viremia, and the availability of more effective drugs, have increased the treatment indications and the long-term success of therapy.[94,391] An important complication is that chronic HBV infection implies that immune responses toward the virus are impaired. In addition, chronic HBV entails the existence of large numbers of cells containing covalently closed circular HBV DNA, a situation akin to herpesvirus latency. For all practical purposes, this may preclude eradication of HBV infection. Therefore, for therapy to be successful, the immune response must be restored, chronic antiviral suppression must be maintained, or both.

A significant proportion, but not all, carriers of HBV progress to cirrhosis, hepatic failure, or hepatocellular carcinoma. Antiviral therapy has been shown to prevent the development of these complications and, in fact, to reverse cirrhotic histopathology.[353] Whom, when, and how to treat are decisions based on risk of progression and therapeutic index of the various treatments.[94,391] Treatment efficacy is impacted by the regimen used as well as viral genotype, host genetics including ethnic background, disease and virologic status, age, and comorbidities such as HIV co-infection.

The therapy for HBV infections has evolved.[94,391] The first effective antiviral therapy for HBV infection was recombinant IFN-α, initially injected three times weekly. Daily injections proved more effective. Pegylation of IFN-α to permit effective levels when injected once weekly improved both acceptance and efficacy. Interferon therapy does not suppress plasma HBV DNA in as high a proportion of patients as does therapy with nucleoside analogs when administered for 12 to 24 weeks. Following the cessation of treatment, however, patients receiving nucleoside analogue therapy only rarely sustain responses, whereas a small subset of patients treated with interferon maintain durable responses. Interferon therapy, in contrast to nucleoside analogs, has not been shown to select for resistant mutants. The use of interferon therapy is limited, however, by its cost, inconvenience, and substantial side-effect profile (fatigue, depression, leukopenia).

Five nucleoside analogs have been approved for the treatment of hepatitis B. The experiences with these drugs recapitulate many of the experiences of HIV therapy. 3TC, telbivudine, and adefovir reduce plasma HBV DNA levels an average of 4 logs over a period of 12 weeks, associated with improvements of liver inflammation and progression of disease. Unfortunately, continuing use was associated with increasing proportions of patients with resistant mutants who experience treatment failure.[223] Entecavir and tenofovir have displaced other drugs for HBV infection because of their high rates of virus suppression with monotherapy and the low rates of emergence of drug-resistant virus during treatment.[94,337,391] The combination of tenofovir and emtricitabine, which is active against HBV, has been approved for the treatment of HIV and is used routinely in patients who are co-infected with HIV and HBV.

HCV Therapy

The same issues regarding who and when to treat that apply to HBV apply to HCV. Factors include impact on response of viral genotype, age, sex, disease stage, host genotype, and co-factors like concurrent HIV infection, renal disease, or alcohol use.[116] One critical difference is that HCV has no DNA intermediate that precludes eradication. HCV is thus curable.

IFN-α administered three times weekly was the first treatment shown to be effective against HCV; however, only 15% to 20% of patients achieved a sustained response with 48 weeks of therapy.[293,401] An analysis of viral dynamics concluded that the three-times weekly regimen of IFN-α provided waning activity between doses and that progressively increasing doses provided progressively increasing efficacy,[264] leading to incrementally better rates of sustained virological response with daily dosing.[153,401]

The introduction of pegylated IFN-α, permitting weekly dosing, and provided yet another increment in these rates. The addition of ribavirin added yet another increment to the rates of sustained virology responses.[105,196,231,240,301] Approximately one-half of patients achieved sustained virological responses with this latter regimen; however, genotypes 2 and 3 respond appreciably better, whereas genotype 1 and patients with HIV co-infection respond less well.[51,131,364] Other factors including disease stage, viral load, race, age, sex, and weight impact this regimen, as they do all preceding regimens.[344] The remarkable impact of the IL-28b genotype on host responsiveness to IFN efficacy provides a substantial explanation for much of the individual variation in treatment responses.[116] It is noteworthy that the treatment of HCV, as with HBV, can reverse liver fibrosis and reduce rates of hepatocellular carcinoma.[175,294]

The resources and commitment to discovery and development of small molecules targeting HCV, called direct acting antivirals (DAAs), has surpassed that directed against HIV. Potent inhibitors of protease, RNA polymerase (both nucleoside analogs and nonnucleosides), NS5A, and other targets have been identified, and entered clinical trials.[279,290,325] The dynamics of response to treatment are faster with HCV than HIV with as much as 3 to 5 $\log_{10}$ reductions with many drugs in a matter of days. Similarly, with the high levels of HCV replication, drug-resistant mutants emerge with monotherapy in a matter of days. The initial clinical studies thus required examination of the incremental benefit of adding a candidate drug to the standard regimen of pegylated IFN plus ribavirin. The first HCV DAAs to be approved in 2011 were the NS3 protease inhibitors, telaprevir and boceprevir.[10,179,291,333,400] These drugs have similar efficacies, and increase the sustained virological response (basically a cure) by approximately 25% to 30% over the proportion with such a response with IFN and ribavirin alone. These improved responses are encouraging; however, a substantial proportion of treated subjects fail (and often with protease-resistant virus). Moreover, the regimen still requires the relatively toxic combination of IFN and ribavirin.

The development of drugs with activities against a broad range of genotypes and targeting multiple targets, which include nucleoside NS3 polymerase inhibitors, nonnucleoside NS3 polymerase inhibitors of targeting multiple different sites,

NS5A inhibitors and nonimmunosuppressive cyclophilin-binding compounds among others provide promise for potent combination regimens that could cure HCV infection in 8 to 24 weeks without the need for IFN or ribavirin. The field of HCV antivirals has accelerated remarkably and developments were occurring at an encouraging pace by 2012, such that the state of the field will certainly be transformed. Should this promise be achieved, earlier and more comprehensive treatment would be indicated. One could even imagine efforts to systematically find asymptomatic carriers of HCV and treat them. This might dramatically reduce transmission, chronic hepatic disease, and liver transplantation, approximately one-half of which is attributable to HCV.[30]

Influenza Therapy

Both the adamantane derivatives and the neuraminidase inhibitors have utility for both prophylaxis and treatment of influenza. The adamantanes, amantadine and rimantadine, reduce rates of illness by 70% to 90% when used prophylactically for influenza A.[6,71,81,212] They have some quantitative activity in reducing viral shedding and diminishing the duration and severity of symptoms when used early after the onset of illness.[133,368,397] These treatment effects are limited. Moreover no data have been generated on the treatment of severe disease requiring hospitalization.

Rimantadine has fewer CNS side effects than amantadine, especially in the elderly. In addition, rimantadine is not renally excreted, and thus requires no dosing adjustments in renal impairment. Neither drug is active against influenza B. Moreover, resistance has developed into a major problem. Resistant virus is often shed after several days of treatment and when illness is resolving.[149] This virus can be transmitted, thus eliminating prospects for prophylaxis of contacts of the treated patient. Because of the limited therapeutic efficacy of the adamantanes and their ready selection for resistance, recommendations for the use of the adamantanes have been primarily as prophylaxis for influenza A. Several subtypes of influenza A have become predominantly amantadine resistant, having first been seen in China where amantadine is included in over-the-counter cold remedies,[27] and allegations of its use on chicken farms have been made.[278] Recent isolates of avian influenza (H5N1) have also been amantadine resistant.[16]

The neuraminidase inhibitors, zanamivir and oseltamivir, are effective for prophylaxis[147,150,258] and treatment[145,148,365] of both influenza A and B. Zanamivir requires inhalational administration, risks of uneven distribution in the respiratory tract, and occasionally bronchospasm. Moreover, should systemic activity be needed, especially with H5N1 disease,[76] oseltamivir is the only option, although parenteral preparations of zanamivir and newer neuraminidase inhibitors are in development.[16] Although the efficacy of neuraminidase inhibitors has not been documented for the treatment of complicated influenza requiring hospitalization, it is recommended as the agent for treatment and prophylaxis of influenza A and B, especially with the expanding prevalence of adamantane resistance. It was stockpiled for a possible epidemic of H5N1 infection for which oseltamivir has been shown to be effective in animal models,[16] and for the pandemic H1N1 epidemic of 2009.

High-level resistance due to His to Tyr mutation in codon 275 of the N1 neuraminidase can emerge during treatment of H1N1 in children and in several patients treated for H5N1 infection.[372] This mutation does not confer cross-resistance to zanamivir.[127,375] By itself, the H275Y (H274Y in N2) mutation reduces fitness *in vitro* and *in vivo,*[177] although it is transmissible to ferrets.[156] However, as reviewed earlier in the section on neuraminidase inhibitor mechanisms, oseltamivir-resistant H1N1 viruses containing H275Y and secondary mutations that increase fitness have emerged, increasing the need for new therapeutic options and engendering intense interest in the epidemiology of resistance to anti-influenza drugs.[146]

Conclusion and Future Directions

Antiviral drugs ameliorate viral disease and save lives. Understanding viral replication and virus–host interactions is crucial for understanding the mechanisms of antiviral agents and for the discovery of new ones. Likewise, antiviral agents provide the virologist with excellent tools with which to investigate viral biology and biochemistry, and the biology and biochemistry of virus hosts. Of the antivirals available today, most inhibit viruses at the genome replication stage. This stage will doubtless continue to be the target for new drugs that become approved for use in patients. However, more and more drugs that target other stages are entering clinical use (e-Table 13.1). There is still a great deal of unmet medical need that can be served by antiviral drugs, and we are still learning how to use them.

REFERENCES

All cited references are available in the e-book.

2. Alian A, Griner SL, Chiang V, et al. Catalytically-active complex of HIV-1 integrase with a viral DNA substrate binds anti-integrase drugs. *Proc Natl Acad Sci U S A* 2009;106:8192–8197.
4. Appelt K. Crystal structures of HIV-1 protease-inhibitor complexes. *Perspect Drug Disc Design* 1993;1:23–48.
5. Arion D, Kaushik N, McCormick S, et al. Phenotypic mechanism of HIV-1 resistance to 3′-azido-3′-deoxythymidine (AZT): increased polymerization processivity and enhanced sensitivity to pyrophosphate of the mutant viral reverse transcriptase. *Biochemistry* 1998;37:15908–15917.
7. Autran B, Carcelain G, Li TS, et al. Positive effects of combined antiretroviral therapy on CD4+ T cell homeostasis and function in advanced HIV disease. *Science* 1997;277:112–116.
9. Baba M, Nishimura O, Kanzaki N, et al. A small-molecule, nonpeptide CCR5 antagonist with highly potent and selective anti-HIV-1 activity. *Proc Natl Acad Sci U S A* 1999;96:5698–5703.
10. Bacon BR, Gordon SC, Lawitz E, et al. Boceprevir for previously treated chronic HCV genotype 1 infection. *N Engl J Med* 2011;364:1207–1217.
13. Balfour HH Jr, Bean B, Laskin OL, et al. Acyclovir halts progression of herpes zoster in immunocompromised patients. *N Engl J Med* 1983;308:1448–1453.
22. Bloom JD, Gong LI, Baltimore D. Permissive secondary mutations enable the evolution of influenza oseltamivir resistance. *Science* 2010;328:1272–1275.
25. Boyer P, Sarafianos S, Arnold E, et al. Selective excision of AZTMP by drug-resistant human immunodeficiency virus reverse transcriptase. *J Virol* 2001;75:4832–4842.
28. Brinkman K, ter Hofstede HJ, Burger DM, et al. Adverse effects of reverse transcriptase inhibitors: mitochondrial toxicity as common pathway. *AIDS* 1998;12:1735–1744.
29. Brown DG, Visse R, Sandhu G, et al. Crystal structures of the thymidine kinase from herpes simplex virus type-1 in complex with deoxythymidine and ganciclovir. *Nat Struct Biol* 1995;2:876–880.
36. Cady SD, Schmidt-Rohr K, Wang J, et al. Structure of the amantadine binding site of influenza M2 proton channels in lipid bilayers. *Nature* 2010;463:689–692.
39. Cavert W, Notermans DW, Staskus K, et al. Kinetics of response in lymphoid tissues to antiretroviral therapy of HIV-1 infection. *Science* 1997;276:960–964.

40. Champness JN, Bennett MS, Wien F, et al. Exploring the active site of herpes simplex virus type-1 thymidine kinase by X-ray crystallography of complexes with aciclovir and other ligands. *Proteins* 1998;32:350–361.
41. Chan DC, Fass D, Berger JM, et al. Core structure of gp41 from the HIV envelope protein. *Cell* 1997;89:263–273.
47. Cheng Y-C, Huang E-S, Lin J-C, et al. Unique spectrum of activity of 9-(1,3-dihydroxy-2-propoxymethyl)guanine against herpesviruses *in vitro* and its mode of action against herpes simplex virus type 1. *Proc Natl Acad Sci U S A* 1983;80:2767–2770.
49. Chomont N, El-Far M, Ancuta P, et al. HIV reservoir size and persistence are driven by T cell survival and homeostatic proliferation. *Nat Med* 2009;15:893–900.
50. Chun T-W, Stuyver L, Mizel lSB, et al. Presence of an inducible HIV-1 latent reservoir during highly active antiretroviral therapy. *Proc Natl Acad Sci U S A* 1997;94:13193–13197.
51. Chung RT, Andersen J, Volberding P, et al. Peginterferon alfa-2a plus ribavirin versus interferon alfa-2a plus ribavirin for chronic hepatitis C in HIV-coinfected persons. *N Engl J Med* 2004;351:451–459.
56. Cocchi F, DeVico AL, Garzino-Demo A, et al. Identification of RANTES, MIP-1α, and MIP-1β as the major HIV-suppressive factors produced by CD8$^+$ T cells. *Science* 1995;270:1811–1815.
58. Coen DM. Acyclovir-resistant, pathogenic herpesviruses. *Trends Microbiol* 1994;2:481–485.
61. Coffin JM. Population dynamics of HIV drug resistance. In: Richman DD, ed. *Antiviral Drug Resistance.* Chichester: John Wiley & Sons; 1996: 279–303.
62. Cohen KA, Hopkins J, Ingraham RH, et al. Characterization of the binding site for nevirapine (BI-RG-587), a nonnucleoside inhibitor of human immunodeficiency virus type-1 reverse transcriptase. *J Biol Chem* 1991;266:14670–14674.
64. Committee CC. Randomised trial of addition of lamivudine or lamivudine plus loviride to zidovudine-containing regimens for patients with HIV-1 infection: the CAESAR trial. *Lancet* 1997;349:1413–1421.
65. Committee DC. Delta: a randomized double-blind controlled trial comparing combinations of zidovudine plus didanozine or zalcitabine with zidovudine alone in HIV-infected individuals. *Lancet* 1996;348:283–291.
67. Condra JH, Emini EA, Gotlib L, et al. Identification of the human immunodeficiency virus reverse transcriptase residues that contribute to the activity of diverse non-nucleoside inhibitors. *Antimicrob Agents Chemother* 1992;36:1441–1446.
72. Crotty S, Cameron CE, Andino R. RNA virus error catastrophe: direct molecular test by using ribavirin. *Proc Natl Acad Sci U S A* 2001;98: 6895–6900.
75. Davies WL, Grunert RR, Haff RF, et al. Antiviral activity of 1-adamantanamine (amantadine). *Science* 1964;144:862–863.
79. Diallo K, Götte M, Wainberg MA. Molecular impact of the M184V mutation in human immunodeficiency virus type 1 reverse transcriptase. *Antimicrob Agents Chemother* 2003;47:337–3383.
81. Dolin R, Reichman RC, Madore HP, et al. A controlled trial of amantadine and rimantadine in the prophylaxis of influenza A infection. *N Engl J Med* 1982;307:580–584.
83. Dorr P, Westby M, Dobbs S, et al. Maraviroc (UK-427,857), a potent, orally bioavailable, and selective small-molecule inhibitor of chemokine receptor CCR5 with broad-spectrum anti-human immunodeficiency virus type 1 activity. *Antimicrob Agents Chemother* 2005;49:4721–4732.
84. Douek DC, McFarland RD, Keiser PH, et al. Changes in thymic function with age and during the treatment of HIV infection. *Nature* 1999;396:690–695.
85. Douglas JM, Critchlow C, Benedetti J, et al. A double-blind study of oral acyclovir for suppression of recurrences of genital herpes simplex virus infection. *N Engl J Med* 1984;310:1551–1556.
86. Doyon L, Croteau G, Thibeault D, et al. Second locus involved in human immunodeficiency virus type 1 resistance to protease inhibitors. *J Virol* 1996;70:3763–3769.
87. Drake JW, Holland JJ. Mutation rates among RNA viruses. *Proc Natl Acad Sci U S A* 1999;96:13910–13913.
90. Dunkle LM, Arvin AM, Whitley RJ, et al. A controlled trial of acyclovir for chickenpox in normal children. *N Engl J Med* 1991;325:1539–1544.
91. Elion GB, Furman PA, Fyfe JA, et al. Selectivity of action of an antiherpetic agent, 9-(2-hydroxyethoxymethyl)guanine. *Proc Natl Acad Sci U S A* 1977;74:5716–5720.
93. Eriksson B, Öberg B, Wahren B. Pyrophosphate analogs as inhibitors of DNA polymerases of cytomegalovirus, herpes simplex virus and cellular origin. *Biochim Biophys Acta* 1982;696:115–123.
94. European Association for the Study of the Liver. EASL clinical practice guidelines: management of chronic hepatitis B. *J Hepatol* 2009;50: 227–242.
95. Feld JJ, Hoofnagle JH. Mechanism of action of inteferon and ribavirin in treatment of hepatitis C. *Nature* 2005;436:967–972.
97. Finzi D, Blankson J, Siliciano JD, et al. Latent infection of CD4+ T cells provides a mechanism for lifelong persistence of HIV-1, even in patients on effective combination therapy. *Nat Med* 1999;5:512–517.
98. Finzi D, Hermankova M, Pierson T, et al. Identification of a reservoir for HIV-1 in patients on highly active antiretroviral therapy. *Science* 1997; 278:1295–1300.
100. Fischl MA, Richman DD, Grieco MH, et al. The efficacy of azidothymidine (AZT) in the treatment of patients with AIDS and AIDS-related complex. A double-blind, placebo-controlled trial. *N Engl J Med* 1987;317:185–191.
103. Freed EO, Martin MA. HIVs and their replication. In: Knipe DM, Howley PM, Griffin DE, et al., eds. *Fields Virology.* 5th ed. Philadelphia: Wolters Kluwer/Lippincott Williams & Wilkins; 2007.
105. Fried MW, Shiffman ML, Reddy RK, et al. Peginterferon alfa-2a plus ribavirin for chronic hepatitis C virus infection. *N Engl J Med* 2002;347: 975–982.
107. Furman PA, Fyfe JA, St. Clair MH, et al. Phosphorylation of 3′-azido-3′-deoxythymidine and selective interaction of the 5′-triphosphate with human immunodeficiency virus reverse transcriptase. *Proc Natl Acad Sci U S A* 1986;83:8333–8337.
108. Fyfe JA, Keller PM, Furman PA, et al. Thymidine kinase from herpes simplex virus phosphorylates the new antiviral compound 9-(2-hydroxyethoxymethyl)guanine. *J Biol Chem* 1978;253:8721–9727.
110. Gao M, Nettles RE, Belema M, et al. Chemical genetics strategy identifies an HCV NS5A inhibitor with a potent clinical effect. *Nature* 2010; 465:96–100.
113. Ge D, Fellay J, Thompson AJ, et al. Genetic variation in IL28B predicts hepatitis C treatment-induced viral clearance. *Nature* 2009;461:399–401.
116. Ghany M, Nelson DR, Strader DB, et al. An update on treatment of genotype 1 chronic hepatitis C virus infection: 2011 practice guidelines by the American Association for the Study of Liver Diseases. *Hepatology* 2011;54(4):1433–1444.
119. Gill VS, Lima VD, Zhang W, et al. Improved virological outcomes in British Columbia concomitant with decreasing incidence of HIV type 1 drug resistance detection. *Clin Infect Dis* 2010;50:98–105.
123. Griffiths A, Chen S-H, Horsburgh BC, et al. Translational compensation of a frameshift mutation affecting herpes simplex virus thymidine kinase is sufficient to permit reactivation from latency. *J Virol* 2003;77: 4703–4709.
128. Gulick RM, Mellors JW, Havlir D, et al. Treatment with indinavir, zidovudine, and lamivudine in adults with human immunodeficiency virus infection and prior antiretroviral therapy. *N Engl J Med* 1997;337: 734–739.
129. Haase AT. Population biology of HIV-1 infection: viral and CD4+ T cell demographics and dynamics in lymphatic tissues. *Annu Rev Immunol* 1999;17:625–626.
130. Haase AT, Henry K, Zupancic M, et al. Quantitative image analysis of HIV-1 infection in lymphoid tissue. *Science* 1996;274:985–989.
131. Hadziyannis SJ, Sette H Jr, Morgan TR, et al. Peginterferon-alpha2a and ribavirin combination therapy in chronic hepatitis C: a randomized study of treatment duration and ribavirin dose. *Ann Intern Med* 2004;140: 346–355.
132. Halfon P, Locarnini S. Hepatitis C virus resistance to protease inhibitors. *J Hepatol* 2011;55:192–206.
136. Hammer SM, Katzenstein DA, Hughes MD, et al. A trial comparing nucleoside monotherapy with combination therapy in HIV-infected adults with CD4 cell counts from 200 to 500 per cubic millimeter. *N Engl J Med* 1996;335:1081–1090.
137. Hammer SM, Squires KE, Hughes MD, et al. A controlled trial of two nucleoside analogues plus indinavir in persons with human immunodeficiency virus infection and CD4 cell counts of 200/μL or less. *N Engl J Med* 1997;337:725–733.
139. Hart GJ, Orr DC, Penn CR, et al. Effects of (-)-2′-deoxy-3′-thiacytidine (3TC) 5′ triphosphate on human immunodeficiency virus reverse

transcriptase and mammalian DNA polymerases alpha, beta, and gamma. *Antimicrob Agents Chemother* 1992;36:1688–1694.
141. Hay AJ. Amantadine and rimantadine - mechanisms. In: Richman DD, ed. *Antiviral Drug Resistance.* Chichester: John Wiley & Sons; 1996: 43–58.
142. Hay AJ, Wolstenholme AJ, Skehel JJ, et al. The molecular basis of the specific anti-influenza action of amantadine. *EMBO J* 1985;4:3021–3024.
144. Hayden FG. Amantadine and rimantadine resistance in influenza A viruses. *Curr Opinion Infect Dis* 1994;7:674–677.
145. Hayden FG, Atmar RL, Schilling M, et al. Use of the selective oral neuraminidase inhibitor oseltamivir to prevent influenza. *N Engl J Med* 1999; 341:1336–1343.
147. Hayden FG, Gubareva LV, Monto AS, et al. Inhaled zanamivir for the prevention of influenza in families. Zanamivir Family Study Group. *N Engl J Med* 2000;343:1282–1289.
148. Hayden FG, Osterhaus AD, Treanor JJ, et al. Efficacy and safety of the neuraminidase inhibitor zanamivir in the treatment of influenzavirus infections. GG167 Influenza Study Group. *N Engl J Med* 1997;337: 874–880.
149. Hayden FG, Sperber SJ, Belshe RB, et al. Recovery of drug-resistant influenza A virus during therapeutic use of rimantadine. *Antimicrob Agents Chemother* 1991;35:1741–1747.
151. Hazuda DJ, Felock P, Witmer M, et al. Inhibitors of strand tranfer that prevent integration and inhibit HIV-1 replication in cells. *Science* 2000;287:646–650.
153. Heathcote EJ, Shiffman ML, Cooksley WG, et al. Peginterferon alfa-2a in patients with chronic hepatitis C and cirrhosis. *N Engl J Med* 2000; 343:1673–1680.
155. Hemmi H, Kaisho T, Takeuchi O, et al. Small anti-viral compounds activate immune cells *via* the TLR7 MyD88-dependent signaling pathway. *Nat Immunol* 2002;3:196–200.
157. Herrmann EC Jr, Herrmann JA. A working hypothesis - virus resistance development as an indicator of specific antiviral activity. *Ann N Y Acad Sci* 1977;284:632–637.
160. Hirsch MS, Gunthard HF, Schapiro JM, et al. Antiretroviral drug resistance testing in adult HIV-1 infection: 2008 recommendations of an International AIDS Society-USA panel. *Clin Infect Dis* 2008;47: 266–285.
161. Ho H-T, Woods KL, Bronson JJ, et al. Intracellular metabolism of the antiherpes agent (*S*)-1-[3-hydroxy-2-(phosphonylmethoxy)propyl]cytosine. *Mol Pharmacol* 1992;41:197–202.
162. Hofmann WP, Herrmann E, Sarrazin C, et al. Ribavirin mode of action in chronic hepatitis C: from clinical use back to molecular mechanisms. *Liver Int* 2008;28:1332–1343.
165. Horsburgh BC, Kollmus H, Hauser H, et al. Translational recoding induced by G-rich mRNA sequences that form unusual structures. *Cell* 1996;86:949–959.
166. Hostetler KY. Synthesis and antiviral evaluation of broad spectrum orally active analogs of cidofovir and other acyclic nucleoside phosphonates. In: DeClercq E, ed. *Advances in Antiviral Drug Design.* Vol 5. Oxford: Elsevier; 2007:167–184.
167. Huang L, Ishii KK, Zuccola H, et al. The enzymological basis for resistance of herpesvirus DNA polymerase mutants to acyclovir: relationship to the structure of α-like DNA polymerases. *Proc Natl Acad Sci U S A* 1999;96:447–452.
171. Hwang CBC, Horsburgh B, Pelosi E, et al. A net +1 frameshift permits synthesis of thymidine kinase from a drug-resistant herpes simplex virus mutant. *Proc Natl Acad Sci U S A* 1994;91:5461–5465.
172. Hwang YT, Liu B-Y, Coen DM, et al. Effects of mutations in the Exo III motif of the herpes simplex virus DNA polymerase gene on enzyme activities, viral replication, and replication fidelity. *J Virol* 1997;71:7791–7798.
175. Imai Y, Kawata S, Tamura S, et al. Relation of interferon therapy and hepatocellular carcinoma in patients with chronic hepatitis C. Osaka Hepatocellular Carcinoma Prevention Study Group. *Ann Intern Med* 1998; 129:94–99.
179. Jacobson IM, McHutchison JG, Dusheiko G, et al. Telaprevir for previously untreated chronic hepatitis C virus infection. *N Engl J Med* 2011; 364:2405–2416.
180. Jing X, Ma C, Ohigashi Y, et al. Functional studies indicate amantadine binds to the pore of the influenza A virus M2 proton-selective ion channel. *Proc Natl Acad Sci U S A* 2008;105:10967–10972.
182. Joint United Nations Programme on HIV/AIDS. UNAIDS Report on the global AIDS epidemic. Available at: http://www.unaids.org/globalreport/Global_report.htm.
183. Jurk M, Heil F, Vollmer J, et al. Human TLR7 or TLR8 independently confer responsiveness to the antiviral compound R-848. *Nat Immunol* 2002;3:499.
184. Kahn JO, Lagakos SW, Richman DD, et al. A controlled trial comparing continued zidovudine with didanosine in human immunodeficiency virus infection. *N Engl J Med* 1992;327:581–587.
186. Kaufman H, Martola EL, Dohlman C. Use of 5-iodo-2′-deoxyuridine (IDU) in treatment of herpes simplex keratitis. *Arch Ophthalmol* 1962; 68:235–239.
188. Kempf DJ, Marsh KC, Denissen JF, et al. ABT-538 is a potent inhibitor of human immunodeficiency virus protease and has high oral bioavailability in humans. *Proc Natl Acad Sci U S A* 1995;92:2484–2488.
192. Kohl NE, Emini EA, Schleif WA, et al. Active human immunodeficiency virus protease is required for viral infectivity. *Proc Natl Acad Sci U S A* 1988;85:4686–4690.
193. Kohlstaedt LA, Wang J, Friedman JM, et al. Crystal structure at 3.5 Å resolution of HIV-1 reverse transcriptase complexed with an inhibitor. *Science* 1992;256:1783–1790.
194. Komanduri KV, Viswanathan MN, Wieder ED, et al. Restoration of cytomegalovirus-specific CD4+ T-lymphocyte responses after ganciclovir and highly active antiretroviral therapy in individuals infected with HIV-1. *Nat Med* 1998;4:953–956.
196. Lai MY, Kao JH, Yang PM, et al. Long-term efficacy of ribavirin plus interferon alfa in the treatment of chronic hepatitis C. *Gastroenterology* 1996;111:1307–1312.
197. Lamarre D, Anderson PC, Bailey M, et al. An NS3 protease inhibitor with antiviral effects in humans infected with hepatitis C virus. *Nature* 2003; 426:186–189.
199. Larder BA, Darby G. Virus drug-resistance: mechanisms and consequences. *Antiviral Res* 1984;4:1–42.
200. Larder BA, Darby G, Richman DD. HIV with reduced sensitivity to zidovudine (AZT) isolated during prolonged therapy. *Science* 1989; 243:1731–1734.
203. Larder BA, Kemp SD. Multiple mutations in HIV-1 reverse transcriptase confer high-level resistance to zidovudine (AZT). *Science* 1989; 246:1155–1158.
204. Laver WG, Bischofberger N, Webster RG. Disarming flu viruses. *Sci Am* 1999;280:78–87.
211. Li W-X, Escarpe PA, Eisenberg EJ, et al. Identification of GS4104 as an orally bioavailable prodrug of the influenza neuraminidase inhibitor GS4701. *Antimicrob Agents Chemother* 1998;42:647–653.
213. Lin C, Kwong AD, Perni RB. Discovery and development of VX-950, a novel, covalent, and reversible inhibitor of hepatitis NS3-4A serine protease. *Infect Disord Drug Targets* 2006;6:3–16.
214. Lin K, Perni RB, Kwong AD, et al. VX-950, a novel hepatitis C virus (HCV) NS3-4A protease inhibitor, exhibits potent antiviral activities in HCV replicon cells. *Antimicrob Agents Chemother* 2006;50:1813–1822.
218. Little SJ, Holte S, Routy JP, et al. Antiretroviral-drug resistance among patients recently infected with HIV. *N Engl J Med* 2002;347:385–394.
219. Littler E, Stuart AD, Chee MS. Human cytomegalovirus UL97 open reading frame encodes a protein that phosphorylates the antiviral nucleoside analogue ganciclovir. *Nature* 1992;358:160–162.
221. Liu R, Paxton WA, Choe S, et al. Homozygous defect in HIV-1 coreceptor accounts for resistance of some multiply-exposed individuals to HIV-1 infection. *Cell* 1996;86:367–378.
222. Liu S, Knafels JD, Chang JS, et al. Crystal structure of the herpes simplex virus 1 DNA polymerase. *J Biol Chem* 2006;281:18193–18200.
223. Locarnini S, Bowden S. Drug resistance in antiviral therapy. *Clin Liver Dis* 2010;14:439–459.
224. Lohse N, Hansen AB, Pedersen G, et al. Survival of persons with and without HIV infection in Denmark, 1995-2005. *Ann Intern Med* 2007; 146:87–95.
228. Mai Le Q, Kiso M, Someya K, et al. Isolation of drug-resistant H5N1 virus. *Nature* 2005;437:1108.
229. Malcolm BA, Liu R, Lahser F, et al. SCH 503034, a mechanism-based inhibitor of hepatitis C virus NS3 protease, suppresses polyprotein maturation and enhances the antiviral activity of alpha interferon in replicon cells. *Antimicrob Agents Chemother* 2006;50:1013–1020.

231. Manns MP, McHutchison JG, Gordon SC, et al. Peginterferon alfa-2b plus ribavirin compared with interferon alfa-2b plus ribavirin for initial treatment of chronic hepatitis C: a randomized trial. *Lancet* 2001; 358:958–965.
232. Mansky LM, Temin HM. Lower in vivo mutation rate of human immunodeficiency virus type 1 than that predicted from the fidelity of purified reverse transcriptase. *J Virol* 1995;69:5087–5094.
237. Matsuoka-Aizawa S, Sato H, Hachiya A, et al. Isolation and molecular characterization of a nelfinavir (NFV)-resistant human immunodeficiency virus type 1 that exhibits NFV-dependent enhancement of replication. *J Virol* 2003;77:318–327.
238. McColl DJ, Chen X. Strand transfer inhibitors of HIV-1 integrase: bringing IN a new era of antiretroviral therapy. *Antiviral Res* 2010;85: 101–118.
239. McCune JM, Loftus R, Schmidt DK, et al. High prevalence of thymic tissue in adults with human immunodeficiency virus-1 infection. *J Clin Invest* 1998;101:2301–2308.
240. McHutchison JG, Gordon SC, Schiff ER, et al. Interferon alfa-2b alone or in combination with ribavirin as initial treatment for chronic hepatitis C. Hepatitis Interventional Therapy Group. *N Engl J Med* 1998; 339:1485–1492.
242. McMahon D, Jones J, Wiegand A, et al. Short-course raltegravir intensification does not reduce persistent low-level viremia in patients with HIV-1 suppression during receipt of combination antiretroviral therapy. *Clin Infect Dis* 2010;50:912–919.
246. Merluzzi VJ, Hargrave KD, Labadia M, et al. Inhibition of HIV-1 replication by a nonnucleoside reverse transcriptase inhibitor. *Science* 1990;250:1411–1413.
249. Meyer PR, Matsuura SE, So AG, et al. Unblocking of chain-terminated primer by HIV-1 reverse transcriptase through a nucleotide-dependent mechanism. *Proc Natl Acad Sci U S A* 1998;95:13471–13476.
255. Mitsuya H, Weinhold KJ, Furman PA, et al. 3′-azido-3′-deoxythymidine (BW A509U): an antiviral agent that inhibts the infectivity and cytopathic effect of human T-lymphotropic virus type III/lymphadenopathy-associated virus *in vitro*. *Proc Natl Acad Sci U S A* 1985;82:7096–7100.
256. Molla A, Korneyeva M, Gao Q, et al. Ordered accumulation of mutations in HIV protease confers resistance to ritonavir. *Nat Med* 1996; 2:760–766.
259. Moore JP, Kuritzkes DR. A pièce de resistance: how HIV-1 escapes small molecule CCR5 inhibitors. *Curr Opin HIV AIDS* 2009;4:118–124.
263. Navia MA, Fitzgerald PM, McKeever BM, et al. Three-dimensional structure of aspartyl protease from human immunodeficiency virus HIV-1. *Nature* 1989;337:615–620.
264. Neumann AU, Lam PYS, Dahlberg JE, et al. Hepatitis C viral dynamics *in vivo* and the antiviral efficacy of interferon-α therapy. *Science* 1998; 282:103–107.
265. Nilsen AE, Aasen T, Halsos AM, et al. Efficacy of oral acyclovir in the treatment of initial and recurrent genital herpes. *Lancet* 1982;2:571–573.
266. Njoroge FG, Chen KX, Shih N-Y, et al. Challenges in modern drug discovery: a case study of boceprevir, an HCV protease inhibitor for the treatment of hepatitis C virus infection. *Acc Chem Res* 2008;41:50–59.
268. Nolan D, Reiss P, Mallal S. Adverse effects of antiretroviral therapy for HIV infection: a review of selected topics. *Expert Opin Drug Saf* 2005; 4:201–218.
269. Odriozola L, Cruchaga C, Andréola M, et al. Non-nucleoside inhibitors of HIV-1 reverse transcriptase inhibit phosphorolysis and resensitize the 3′-azido-3′-deoxythymidine (AZT)-resistant polymerase to AZT-5′-triphosphate. *J Biol Chem* 2003;278:42710–42716.
272. Otto MJ, Garber S, Winslow DL, et al. *In vitro* isolation and identification of HIV-1 variants with reduced sensitivity to C_2 symmetrical inhibitors of HIV type 1 protease. *Proc Natl Acad Sci U S A* 1993;90:7543–7547.
273. Oxford JS, Potter CW. Aminoadamantane-resistant strains of influenza A2 virus. *J Hyg Camb* 1973;71:227–236.
274. Pakker NG, Notermans DW, de Boer RJ, et al. Biphasic kinetics of peripheral blood T cells after triple combination therapy in HIV-1 infection: a composite of redistribution and proliferation. *Nat Med* 1998; 4:208–214.
277. Palmer S, Maldarelli F, Wiegand A, et al. Low-level viremia persists for at least 7 years in patients on suppressive antiretroviral therapy. *Proc Natl Acad Sci U S A* 2008;105:3879–3884.
279. Pawlotsky J-M. Treatment failure and resistance with direct-acting antiviral drugs against hepatitis C virus. *Hepatology* 2011;53:1742–1751.
280. Perelson AS, Essunger P, Cao Y, et al. Decay characteristics of HIV-1-infected compartments during combination therapy. *Nature* 1997; 387:188–191.
282. Perelson AS, Neumann AU, Markowit M, et al. HIV-1 dynamics in vivo: virion clearance rate, infected cell lifetime, and viral generation time. *Science* 1996;271:1582–1586.
285. Pfeiffer JK, Kirkegaard K. Ribavirin resistance in hepatitis C virus replicon-containing cell lines conferred by changes in the cell line or mutations in the replicon RNA. *J Virol* 2005;79:2346–2355.
286. Pielak RM, Oxenoid K, Chou JJ. Structural investigation of rimantadine inhibition of the AM2-BM2 chimera channel of influenza viruses. *Structure* 2011;19:1655–1663.
287. Pielak RM, Schnell JR, Chou JJ. Mechanism of drug inhibition and drug resistance of influenza A M2 channel. *Proc Natl Acad Sci U S A* 2009; 106:7379–7384.
288. Pillai SK, Good B, Pond SK, et al. Semen-specific genetic characteristics of human immunodeficiency virus type 1 *env*. *J Virol* 2005;79:1734–1742.
289. Pinto LH, Holsinger LJ, Lamb RA. Influenza virus M_2 protein has ion channel activity. *Cell* 1992;69:517–528.
290. Pockros PJ. New direct-acting antivirals in the development for hepatitis C virus infection. *Therap Adv Gastroenterol* 2010;3:191–202.
291. Poordad F, McCone J Jr, Bacon BR, et al. Boceprevir for untreated chronic HCV genotype 1 infection. *N Engl J Med* 2011;364:1195–1206.
294. Poynard T, McHutchison J, Manns M, et al. Impact of pegylated interferon alfa-2b and ribavirin on liver fibrosis in patients with chronic hepatitis C. *Gastroenterology* 2002;122:1303–1313.
295. Price MA, Wallis CL, Lakhi S, et al. Transmitted HIV type 1 drug resistance among individuals with recent HIV infection in East and Southern Africa. *AIDS Res Hum Retroviruses* 2011;27:5–12.
300. Reardon JE, Spector T. Herpes simplex virus type 1 DNA polymerase. Mechanism of inhibition by acyclovir triphosphate. *J Biol Chem* 1989; 264:7405–7411.
301. Reichard O, Norkans G, Fryden A, et al. Randomized double-blind, placebo-cotrolled trial of interferon alpha-2b with and without ribavirin for chronic hepatitis C. The Swedish Study Group. *Lancet* 1998;351:83–87.
303. Reid R, Mar EC, Huang ES, et al. Insertion and extension of acyclic, dideoxy, and ara nucleotides by herpesviridae, human alpha and human beta polymerases. A unique inhibition mechanism for 9-(1,3-dihydroxy-2-propoxymethyl)guanine triphosphate. *J Biol Chem*1988;263: 3898–3904.
306. Richman DD. The implications of drug resistance for strategies of combination antiviral chemotherapy. *Antiviral Res* 1996;29:31–33.
308. Richman DD, Fischl MA, Grieco MH, et al. The toxicity of 3′-azido-3′deoxythymidine (azidothymidine) in the treatment of patients with AIDS and AIDS-related complex. *N Engl J Med* 1987;317:192–197.
309. Richman DD, Grimes JM, Lagakos SW. Effect of stage of disease and drug dose on zidovudine susceptibilities of isolates of human immunodeficiency virus. *J Acquir Immune Defic Syndr* 1990;3:743–746.
311. Richman DD, Margolis DM, Delaney M, et al. The challenge of finding a cure for HIV infection. *Science* 2009;323:1304–1307.
312. Rimsky LT, Shugars DC, Matthews TJ. Determinants of human immunodeficiency virus type 1 resistance to gp41-derived peptides. *J Virol* 1998; 72:986–993.
313. Rittinger K, Divita G, Goody RS. Human immunodeficiency virus reverse transcriptase substrate-induced conformational changes and the mechanism of inhibition by nonnucleoside inhibitors. *Proc Natl Acad Sci U S A* 1995;92:8046–8049.
314. Rogers DW, Gamblin SJ, Harris BA, et al. The structure of unliganded reverse transcriptase from human immunodeficiency virus type 1. *Proc Natl Acad Sci U S A* 1995;92:1222–1226.
315. Romano KP, Ali A, Soumana D, et al. The molecular basis of drug resistance against hepatitis C virus NS3/4A protease inhibitors. *PLos Pathog* 2012;8:e1002832.
318. Safrin S, Crumpacker C, Chatis P, et al. A controlled trial comparing foscarnet with vidarabine for acyclovir-resistant mucocutaneous herpes simplex in the acquired immunodeficiency syndrome. The AIDS Clinical Trials Group. *N Eng J Med* 1991;325:551–555.
321. Saral R, Ambinder RF, Burns WH, et al. Acyclovir prophylaxis against herpes simplex virus infection in patients with leukemia. A randomized,

double-blind, placebo-controlled study. *Ann Intern Med* 1983;99:773–776.

322. Saral R, Burns WH, Laskin OL, et al. Acyclovir prophylaxis of herpes-simplex-virus infections. *N Engl J Med* 1981;305:63–67.
325. Sarrazin C, Zeuzem S. Resistance to direct antiviral agents in patients with hepatitis C virus infection. *Gastroenterology* 2010;138:447–462.
327. Schaeffer HJ, Beauchamp L, de Miranda P, et al. 9-(2-hydroxyethoxymethyl)guanine activity against viruses of the herpes group. *Nature* 1978; 272:583–585.
328. Scheidel LM, Durbin RK, Stollar V. Sindbis virus mutants resistant to mycophenolic acid and ribavirin. *Virology* 1987;158:1–7.
330. Schnell JR, Chou JJ. Structure and mechanism of the M2 proton channel of influenza A virus. *Nature* 2008;451(7178):591–595.
331. Seifer M, Hamatake RK, Colonno RJ, et al. In vitro inhibition of hepadnavirus polymerases by the triphosphates of BMS-200475 and lobucavir. *Antimicrob Agents Chemother* 1998;42:3200–3208.
332. Selmi B, Deval J, Alvarez K, et al. The Y181C substitution in 3′-azido-3′-deoxythymidine-resistant human immunodeficiency virus, type 1, reverse transcriptase suppresses the ATP-mediated repair of the 3′-azido-3′-deoxythymidine 5′-monophosphate-terminated primer. *J Biol Chem* 2003;278:40464–40472.
333. Sherman KE, Flamm SL, Afdhal NH, et al. Response-guided telaprevir combination treatment for hepatitis C virus infection. *N Engl J Med* 2011; 365:1014–1024.
336. Smee DF, Martin JC, Verheyden JPH, et al. Anti-herpesvirus activity of the acyclic nucleoside 9-(1,3-dihydroxy-2propoxymethyl)guanine. *Antimicrob Agents Chemother* 1983;23:676–682.
337. Snow-Lampart A, Chappell B, Curtis M, et al. No resistance to tenofovir disoproxil fumarate detected after up to 144 weeks of therapy in patients monoinfected with chronic hepatitis B virus. *Hepatology* 2011;53:763–773.
338. Spence RA, Kati WM, Anderson KS, et al. Mechanism of inhibition of HIV-1 reverse transcriptase. *Science* 1995;267:988–993.
341. Staschke KA, Colacino JM, Baxter AJ, et al. Molecular basis for the resistance of influenza viruses to 4-guanidino-Neu5Ac2en. *Virology* 1995; 214:642–646.
343. Stouffer AL, Acharya R, Salom D, et al. Structural basis for the function and inhibition of an influenza virus proton channel. *Nature* 2008; 451:596–599.
345. Strain MC, Günthard HF, Havlir DV, et al. Heterogeneous clearance rates of long-lived lymphocytes infected with HIV: intrinsic stability predicts lifelong persistence. *Proc Natl Acad Sci U S A* 2003;100:4819–4824.
346. Strain MC, Letendre S, Pillai S, et al. Genetic composition of human immunodeficiency virus type 1 in cerebrospinal fluid and blood without treatment and during failing antiretroviral therapy. *J Virol* 2005; 79:1772–1788.
348. Streeter DG, Witkowski JT, Khare GP, et al. Mechanism of action of 1-β-ribofuranosyl-1,2,4-triazole-3-carboxamide, a new broad spectrum antiviral agent. *Proc Natl Acad Sci U S A* 1973;70:1174–1178.
349. Sugrue RJ, Hay AJ. Structural characteristics of the M_2 protein of influenza A viruses: evidence that it forms a tetrameric channel. *Virology* 1991; 180:617–624.
350. Sullivan V, Talarico CL, Stanat SC, et al. A protein kinase homologue controls phosphorylation of ganciclovir in human cytomegalovirus-infected cells. *Nature* 1992;358:162–164.
351. Summa V, Petrocchi A, Bonelli F, et al. Discovery of raltegravir, a potent, selective orally bioavailable HIV-integrase inhibitor for the treatment of HIV-AIDS infection. *J Med Chem* 2008;51:5843–5855.
352. Suppiah V, Moldovan M, Ahlenstiel G, et al. IL28B is associated with response to chronic hepatitis C interferon-alpha and ribavirin therapy. *Nat Genet* 2009;41:1100–1104.
353. Suzuki Y, Kumada H, Ikeda K, et al. Histological changes in liver biopsies after one year of lamivudine treatment in patients with chronic hepatitis B infection. *J Hepatol* 1999;30:743–758.
357. Tan K, Liu JH, Want JH, et al. Atomic structure of a thermostable subdomain of HIV-1 gp41. *Proc Natl Acad Sci U S A* 1997;94:12303–12308.
358. Tanaka Y, Nishida N, Sugiyama M, et al. Genome-wide association of IL28B with response to pegylated interferon-alpha and ribavirin therapy for chronic hepatitis C. *Nat Genet* 2009;41:1105–1109.
359. The panel on antiretroviral guidelines for adults and adolescents. Guidelines for the use of antiretroviral agents in HIV-1 infected adults and adolescents. Available at: http://www.aidsinfo.nih.gov/guidelines/
362. Thompson M, Aberg J, Hoy J, et al. Antiretroviral Treatment of Adult HIV Infection: 2012 Recommendations of the International Antiviral Society—USA Panel. *JAMA* 2012;308:387–402.
364. Torriani FJ, Rodriguez-Torres M, Rockstroh JK, et al. Peginterferon alfa-2a plus ribavirin for chronic hepatitis C virus infection in HIV-infected patients. *N Engl J Med* 2004;351:438–450.
366. Trkola A, Kuhmann SE, Strizki JM, et al. HIV-1 escape from a small molecule, CCR5-specific entry inhibitor does not involve CXCR4 use. *Proc Natl Acad Sci U S A* 2002;99:395–400.
370. von Itzstein M, Wu WY, Kok GB, et al. Rational design of potent sialidase-based inhibitors of influenza virus replication. *Nature* 1993; 363:418–423.
373. Weissenhorn W, Dessen A, Harrison SC, et al. Atomic structure of the ectodomain from HIV-1 gp41. *Nature* 1997;387:426–430.
374. Westby M, Smith-Burchnell C, Mori J, et al. Reduced maximal inhibition in phenotypic susceptibility assays indicates that viral strains resistant to the CCR5 antagonist maraviroc utilize inhibitor-bound receptor for entry. *J Virol* 2007;81:2359–2371.
377. Whitley RJ, Alford CA, Hirsch MS, et al. Vidarabine versus acyclovir therapy in herpes simplex encephalitis. *N Engl J Med* 1986;314: 144–149.
380. Whitley RJ, Jacobson MA, Friedberg DN, et al. Guidelines for the treatment of cytomegalovirus diseases in patients with AIDS in the era of potent antiretroviral therapy: recommendations of an international panel. *Arch Intern Med* 1998;158:957–969.
382. Whitley RJ, Soong SJ, Dolin R, et al. Adenine arabinoside therapy of biopsy-proven herpes simplex encephalitis. National Institute of Allergy and Infectious Disease collaborative antiviral study. *N Engl J Med* 1977; 297:289–294.
385. Wild C, Oas T, McDanal C, et al. A synthetic peptide inhibitor of HIV replication: correlation between solution structure and viral inhibition. *Proc Natl Acad Sci U S A* 1992;89:10537–10541.
386. Wild C, Shugars DC, Greenwell TK, et al. Peptides corresponding to a predictive alpha-helical domain of HIV-1 gp41 are potent inhibitors of virus infection. *Proc Natl Acad Sci U S A* 1994;91:9770–9774.
388. Wlodawer A, Erickson JW. Structure based inhibitors of HIV-1 protease. *Annu Rev Biochem* 1993;62:543–580.
389. Wlodawer A, Miller M, Jaskólski M, et al. Conserved folding in retroviral proteases: crystal structure of a synthetic HIV-1 protease. *Science* 1989;245:616–621.
390. Wong JK, Hezareh M, Günthard HF, et al. Recovery of replication-competent HIV despite prolonged suppression of plasma viremia. *Science* 1997;278:1291–1294.
391. Woo G, Tomlinson G, Nishikawa Y, et al. Tenofovir and entecavir are the most effective antiviral agents for chronic hepatitis B: a systematic review and Bayesian meta-analyses. *Gastroenterology* 2010;139: 1218–1229.
392. Wu JC, Warren TC, Adams J, et al. A novel dipyridodiazepinone inhibitor of HIV-1 reverse transcriptase acts through a nonsubstrate binding site. *Biochemistry* 1991;30:2022–2026.
394. Xiong X, Smith JL, Kim CU, et al. Kinetic analysis of the interaction of cidofovir diphosphate with human cytomegalovirus DNA polymerase. *Biochem Pharmacol* 1996;51:1563–1567.
396. Yeh RW, Coen DM. Pharmacology of viral infections. In: Golan DE, Tashjian AH Jr, Armstrong EJ, et al, eds. *Principles of Pharmacology: The Pathophysiologic Basis of Drug Therapy.* 3rd ed. Philadelphia: Wolters Kluwer/Lippincott Williams & Wilkins; 2012:649–673.
398. Zahn KE, Tchesnokov EP, Gotte M, et al. Phosphonoformic acid inhibits viral replication by trapping the closed form of the DNA polymerase. *J Biol Chem* 2011;286:25246–25255.
400. Zeuzem S, Andreone P, Pol S, et al. Telaprevir for retreatment of HCV infection. *N Engl J Med* 2011;364:2417–2428.
401. Zeuzem S, Feinman SV, Rasenack J, et al. Peginterferon alfa-2a in patients with chronic hepatitis C. *N Engl J Med* 2000;343: 1666–1672.
403. Zhang Z, Schuler T, Zupancic M, et al. Sexual transmission and propagation of SIV and HIV in resting and activated CD4+ T cells. *Science* 1999;286:1353–1357.
404. Zhang Z-Q, Notermans DW, Sedgewick G, et al. Kinetics of CD4+ T cell repopulation of lymphoid tissues after treatment of HIV-1 infection. *Proc Natl Acad Sci U S A* 1998;95:1154–1159.

CHAPTER 14

Barney S. Graham • James E. Crowe, Jr. • Julie E. Ledgerwood

Immunization Against Viral Diseases

Both innate and adaptive immune responses mediate host resistance to virus infection. Elements of the innate immune system, especially type I interferons (IFNs), strongly influence the clinical outcome of a virus infection. Many viruses have evolved mechanisms to inhibit or evade innate immune responses, indicating the importance of those defenses in limiting virus infection. Innate immune responses also mediate important effects during the induction phase of an immune response and may influence the magnitude and composition of adaptive immune responses. Although memory or "training" of natural killer (NK) cells may occur in response to some antigens (Ags), NK cells do not have mechanisms for somatic diversification of their recognition receptors and are limited to germline sequence.[315,343] The capacity for somatic diversification of B-cell receptors (BCRs) and T-cell receptors (TCRs), selection, and long-term memory are central properties of adaptive immunity. Therefore, vaccine-induced immunity that is established in advance of virus infection relies primarily on adaptive immune responses for protective efficacy. Vaccination depends critically on the properties of Ag recognition, activation, expansion, memory, trafficking, and effector functions inherent to lymphocytes. Subtle influences of vaccination on the timing, magnitude, specificity, quality, and location of responding lymphocytes and their effector molecules determine whether exposure to a viral pathogen results in infection, protection, subclinical infection, mild disease, or exaggerated disease expression. The extent to which vaccine-induced immunity is successful in an individual can determine the spread of virus within a population (e-Fig. 14.1). Thus, vaccines have a profound effect on public health through the control of epidemics (e-Fig. 14.2). An antigenic stimulus that elicits a virus-specific adaptive immune response that can be recalled during subsequent virus infection defines it as an immunization. A vaccination is an antigenic stimulus delivered by intention.

VIRAL ANTIGENS RECOGNIZED BY THE IMMUNE SYSTEM

Development of an immune response to Ags present on the surface of virions or virus-infected cells is often critical for immunity against virus infection. Antibody (Ab) responses to surface viral protein or glycoprotein Ags often effectively limit infection of new cells and thus spread of the virus. Internal viral Ags can be important targets for T-lymphocyte responses that clear virus-infected cells; however, these responses alone cannot prevent subsequent infections (e-Fig. 14.3). The relative importance of Abs to surface proteins and of T-cell responses to internal proteins in influenza virus was illustrated by studies of the 1957 Asian influenza pandemic and the 1977 "Russian" influenza epidemic. The 1957 Asian influenza A (H2N2) virus contained surface glycoproteins (the hemagglutinin [HA] and the neuraminidase [NA]) that were novel, such that the human population had not been exposed to strains containing these or related surface Ags. In contrast, the major internal proteins of the new H2N2 virus, the nucleoprotein and the matrix protein, were closely related to corresponding Ags of previous strains of subtype H1N1 to which most individuals had been exposed. Although recent infection with heterotypic viruses may have diminished the level of illness severity in adults,[126] the population's prior immunological experience with related internal Ags did not prevent the 1957 Asian H2N2 influenza A virus from causing a major pandemic.[303] In contrast to this experience, observations following the re-emergence of the H1N1 virus in 1977 indicated that homotypic humoral immunity provided a high level of resistance that lasted for decades. Similarly, humans exposed to the 1918 influenza H1N1 virus as infants sustained circulating memory B cells encoding neutralizing Abs to the HA into the 10th decade of life,[467] and these Abs cross-reacted with the 2009 H1N1 pandemic strain and provided protection.[233,462] Induction of cross-reactive Abs to influenza may sometimes be harmful. For example, immune complexes with complement deposition have been demonstrated in lung tissues of victims of pandemic influenza.[287] Additional evidence for the importance of responses to influenza A surface glycoproteins was provided by passive and active immunization studies in mice. Monoclonal antibodies (mAbs) directed against the HA or NA proteins protected mice against challenge with virulent wild-type virus, whereas mAbs specific for the internal nucleoprotein or matrix protein did not alter the course of disease.[303] Immunization with recombinant vaccinia viruses expressing each of the 10 known influenza A gene products showed that only recombinants expressing the HA or the NA glycoprotein induced resistance to virus challenge.[124] Whereas the vaccinia vector-induced CD8 T-cell–mediated immunity specific for internal viral proteins provided some measure of heterosubtypic cross-reactivity against influenza challenge,[125] the aggregate data suggest that a successful strategy of immunoprophylaxis against most virus infections requires the generation of an immune response to the surface Ags displayed on virions and on virus-infected cells. Other viruses (such as poxviruses, herpesviruses, filoviruses, some respiratory viruses, and lentiviruses) that have a more complex pathogenesis may require vaccines that induce more complex immune responses for protection from infection or control of disease. Many of these viruses possess the capacity for persistence, infect immunoprivileged sites, use sophisticated immune evasion strategies, directly infect their target organ without a requirement for viremia, or cause disease by eliciting an aberrant host response. Vaccine development for these viruses probably will require the induction of neutralizing Abs against surface proteins to protect against infection in addition to T-cell responses against structural and regulatory proteins to control virus spread and to modulate the composition of the immune response.[167]

The surface glycoproteins of enveloped viruses and the capsid proteins of nonenveloped viruses are the primary target Ags for Ab-mediated protection. The following generalizations can be made about the nature of Abs and their interaction with virus surface proteins. First, antiviral Abs against the extracellular domain of surface proteins predominantly recognize conformational epitopes. Such conformational epitopes are difficult to mimic with peptides or proteins that have had the structure of antigenic sites modified by vaccine preparation and formulation. Presentation of the native Ag structure in its authentic conformation is critical for induction of neutralizing Abs. Even when the structure is mimicked with atomic-level precision and elicits Abs that bind the epitope, the property of viral neutralization may not be achieved.[274,326] Most viral surface proteins assemble into oligomeric states on virions, typically dimers, trimers, or tetramers; however, the monomeric form of the protein is also present in cell debris or shed proteins. The principal neutralizing determinant may be present only in quaternary structures; thus, Abs binding to monomeric protein do not recognize or neutralize virions. In addition, many surface proteins that are targets of neutralizing Abs are fusion proteins present in a metastable state on virions. During the attachment and fusion process, the fusion proteins transition from prefusion to postfusion forms, in some cases drastically altering the structure of neutralizing epitopes. Second, Abs recognize many major antigenic sites on each viral protein, and within each of these antigenic sites, there may be multiple epitopes. For example, the parainfluenza virus attachment glycoprotein (HN) has at least six antigenic sites, three of which are recognized by neutralizing Abs.[85] After infection, individuals often develop Abs only to a subset of the antigenic sites of the infecting virus.[86] After one or more reinfections, the Ab response broadens to recognize more antigenic sites. These findings provide a partial explanation for the failure of immunization to induce complete immunity in certain circumstances and also provide a rationale for recommending multiple immunizations to achieve optimal protection. Third, the large size of immunoglobulin (Ig) molecules often precludes direct access to functional sites on viral surface proteins, such as the receptor binding site, sites with enzymatic activity, or fusion peptides. Such domains can be buried within the protein structure of the surface protein or masked by carbohydrate molecules, variable loops, or conformational flexibility.[236] As a consequence, the critical sites vulnerable to Ab-mediated neutralization can remain relatively inaccessible. Therefore, Abs usually exert their antiviral activities by mechanisms other than direct inactivation of functional sites on the surface proteins. Instead, Abs most often act directly or indirectly to impede attachment of virus to the cell or to prevent uncoating of virus that has attached to or entered the cell. Unfortunately, effective Ab-mediated protection against virus infection is not always achievable. For example, the Ab response to the envelope glycoprotein of human immunodeficiency virus (HIV) evolves over time similar to the response elicited by repeated infections with parainfluenza virus; however, the elaboration of the envelope-specific Ab repertoire is not able to keep pace with the rapid genetic evolution of the virus. The Abs present at a given point in time may neutralize virus isolated from the subject 6 months earlier, although they have very low neutralization activity against current strains that have mutated extensively.[368] Sufficiently high levels of passively administered broadly neutralizing mAbs can prevent simian-human immunodeficiency virus (SHIV) infection of macaques in some settings.[265] SHIV is a chimeric lentivirus with the internal and regulatory proteins of simian immunodeficiency virus (SIV) and the surface glycoprotein (gp160) of HIV-1. However, immunization with currently available HIV-1 envelope Ags does not elicit Abs with these neutralizing properties. There are also examples from Ebola virus,[445] vaccinia virus,[31,271] and lentivirus[393] models that demonstrate settings in which both Ab and T-cell responses contribute to vaccine-induced protection. Ags for eliciting T-cell responses can be surface proteins, internal structural proteins, or regulatory proteins. For example, the major CD8 T-cell responses to HIV-1 are directed toward Gag, Pol, and Nef proteins.[36] Often, the nucleocapsid and matrix proteins of viruses are found to encode important cytotoxic T lymphocyte (CTL) epitopes,[428] perhaps because they are typically more abundant, more conserved, and produced earlier in the virus life cycle than surface proteins.

VACCINE-INDUCED IMMUNITY

Immune mechanisms have evolved to protect the host against a diverse assortment of viral pathogens. Viruses and their hosts co-evolve; viruses find ways to evade host defenses, and hosts adapt mechanisms to control virus replication. The host is equipped with mechanical barriers and innate immune mechanisms that can limit the initial encounter with a virus and adaptive immune mechanisms that provide immunity against repeated exposures to the same viral pathogen. Although innate responses are important during the induction phase of vaccine-induced immunity, humoral and cellular adaptive responses are the primary effector mechanisms of protection from future infection (e-Fig. 14.4). Humoral and cellular responses are complementary in that Ab is able to prevent infection by free virus; however, when infection occurs despite innate defenses and the presence of neutralizing Abs, T-cell responses are designed to eliminate virus-infected cells and diminish the subsequent release of infectious virus. The repertoires of BCRs and TCRs have also evolved complementary strategies to deal with genetic variation in viruses. For a given antigenic site on a viral protein, most hosts can expand a B-cell population that can recognize the structure. This leads to population-wide protection against reinfection with a particular virus. In turn, this forces antigenic change in the virus, often resulting in a new serotype, which is not recognized by the original Ab. Therefore, the host has to start over in the generation of Ab-mediated type-specific protection. In contrast, T-cell epitopes are not shared between hosts unless they happen to share the same major histocompatibility complex (MHC)-restricting allele. Consequently, each infected host generates T-cell responses against a limited number of viral epitopes that are largely determined by human leukocyte antigen (HLA) haplotype. Unlike Ab epitopes, T-cell epitopes are often cross-reactive between viral serotypes and thereby provide the Ag-experienced host with partial protection against new virus strains until the Ab responses can adapt (e-Fig. 14.5).

When virus breaches the physical and innate barriers and infects a target cell, several rounds of replication may occur in a primary infection before the adaptive immune responses are established (e-Fig. 14.6A). Depending on the virus, this may result in spread to the target organ of disease and/or establishment of a persistent infection. The timing, magnitude, location, and qualitative features of the host response will determine the clinical outcome of infection. In persistent virus infections (e.g., HIV, hepatitis C virus [HCV], or herpes simplex virus [HSV]), the disease manifestations are often congruent with virus replication. In self-limited infections (e.g., influenza, respiratory syncytial virus [RSV], or dengue), the bulk of disease is often after the peak of viral replication, although in some cases disease can also be temporally associated with viral load (e-Fig. 14.6B). In cases of persistent or latent virus infection, the immune response attempts to limit virus replication or spread. Control of the magnitude and composition of complex immune responses is critical to avoid immunopathology. Fortunately, there is considerable redundancy inherent in immunity to viruses. For example, while CD8 T cells are the primary mediator of cytolytic activity, this function also can be accomplished by complement or by NK cells targeting the Fc portion of Ab labeling virus-infected cells. Another well-studied example of this redundancy involves CD4 and CD8 T cells, either of which are sufficient to achieve clearance of virus, as shown in studies of influenza A virus or poxviruses in mice. Animals lacking CD8 T cells readily clear influenza virus or vaccinia virus from the lungs, indicating that CD4 T cells and Ab are sometimes sufficient for viral clearance.[271,390] The therapeutic efficacy of Abs acting in the absence of other immune functions has also been demonstrated in experimental influenza A virus infection of mice. Abs to the influenza A virus surface HA have cleared virus from the lungs of persistently infected severe combined immunodeficiency (SCID) mice.[390] Whereas CD8 T cells are specialized in recognition and clearance of virus-infected cells, CD4 T cells (plus the Abs secreted by B cells for which they provide help) and CD8 T cells can mediate viral clearance independently. The relative importance of these two arms of the immune response varies in the resolution of particular virus infection. Even in the case of lymphocytic choriomeningitis virus (LCMV), the prototypic arenavirus, which in the murine model is a paradigm for CD8 T-cell–mediated immunity, Abs and CD4 T cells each make a significant contribution to the resolution of primary virus infection.[21] In general, Abs are the major mediator of resistance to reinfection with virus, and CD8 T cells are the major mediator of clearing virus-infected cells. CD4 T cells are critical for the induction of robust Ab responses and important for "helping" CD8 T-cell responses; they also have potential for direct antiviral effector functions. Abs work best when the target organ for disease pathogenesis is distinct from the initial site of infection, particularly in cases where the virus has to travel through the bloodstream to reach its target organ. For example, in diseases such as measles, polio, hepatitis, or the viral encephalitides, where viremia must be established to cause disease, it often takes very small concentrations of preexisting Abs to achieve clinical protection. Because it is rarely possible to elicit sufficient Ab through vaccination to prevent virus infection completely, other immune mechanisms must contribute to vaccine-induced immunity.

One reason why live virus vaccines are so effective is that many components of both innate and adaptive immunity are engaged. The protein, nucleic acid, carbohydrate, and lipid components of viruses induce innate responses through a variety of toll-like receptor (TLR) and other pathogen-associated molecular pattern (PAMP) receptor interactions. Virus infection induces all components of the adaptive immune response—Ab responses are induced against viral surface proteins in their native conformation, CD4 T cells are stimulated, and importantly, viral proteins are produced in the cytoplasm, processed, and presented in MHC class I molecules for induction of CD8 CTL responses. All of these responses are needed to achieve the optimal clinical outcome from a virus infection. Abs and innate defenses provide the initial barrier to infection by neutralizing incoming virus. After the virus has infected a cell, however, it is then incumbent on the innate defenses to control the virus until the adaptive cellular immune response can be activated, expand, and traffic to the affected tissues. In the immune host, the pre-existing Ab will prevent or limit the number of infected cells, and rapid mobilization of memory T-cell responses will rapidly clear virus-infected cells (e-Fig. 14.7A). Although cytolytic T cells are potent in their ability to clear virus-infected cells and reduce the spread of virus, it comes at a cost. The T-cell response can injure the host as it clears the virus and is thus tightly regulated. Turning the immune response off is just as important as turning it on for the well-being of the host. The system is biased toward controlling inflammation, and that may be a reason why the T-cell response is regulated to require several days to activate and expand. Influencing the events in this period between virus exposure and the fully activated primary T-cell response is one of the key factors in determining the efficacy of vaccine-induced immunity, for which the goal is to prevent, abort, or control virus infection to avoid clinical disease (e-Fig. 14.7B).

Vaccine-Induced Cellular Immunity

MHC class I–restricted CD8 cytotoxic CTLs and MHC class II–restricted CD4 helper T cells (Th cells) each function independently as Ag-specific antiviral effector cells (Chapter 9). Intact cellular immunity is critical for protection against some types of viruses. For example, most herpesvirus infections become more severe and destructive when cellular immunity is compromised. Vaccinia can cause progressive tissue invasion in persons with cell-mediated immune deficiencies. RSV and parainfluenza type 3 often become lethal infections in the setting of SCID or in patients who have undergone bone marrow transplantation. In contrast, patients with Ab deficiencies experience more severe disease only from selected viruses, particularly picornaviruses.

CD8 T Lymphocytes

CD8 T cells are the major T-cell effectors of antiviral activity. They are often referred to as CTLs, although they can clear virus-infected cells by both lytic and noncytolytic mechanisms. The CD8 TCR recognizes a short peptide derived from an endogenously produced viral protein in the context of the MHC class I β2-microglobulin heterodimer expressed on the surface of an infected cell. Ag presentation by the MHC class I β2-microglobulin heterodimer is restricted to viral peptides that are produced and processed during infection. Therefore, the major CTL functions are to eliminate infected cells[134] or to inhibit virus replication by the elaboration of soluble mediators such as cytokines[138,299,425] or chemokines.[77,464] The net effect of CTL activity is to prevent further spread of virus and to terminate infection in cells that are already infected. The importance of CTLs in recovery from virus infection is indicated not only by the association of cellular immune deficiencies with severe virus infection but also by the diverse strategies that viruses use to escape from CTL immunity.[408] Viruses such as herpesviruses, poxviruses, and lentiviruses in particular have evolved strategies for interfering with Ag presentation pathways or CD8 T-cell effector molecules that compromise CTL activity. Lentiviruses are prototypes for escaping CTL killing by genetic variation and selecting mutations of key epitopes. CD8 T-cell activity is critical for controlling SIV replication.[393] When that control is mediated by a dominant CTL response to a single epitope, immune control of viremia is lost when that epitope is altered by mutation.[24]

Although CTL antiviral activity generally is associated with the clearance of virus and the reduction of virus-associated pathology, disease enhancement can be observed under experimental conditions in which CTLs have been transferred passively to virus-infected recipients.[58,121,293] Therefore, one can view the immunopathology caused by the T-cell response to virus infection as the cost for virus clearance. A major goal of vaccination is to induce CD8 T cells with properties to clear virus-infected cells efficiently and rapidly to minimize the immunopathology associated with virus infections.

The time course of CTL activation during virus infection in the lungs is consistent with its important role in clearance of primary virus infection. Primary CD8 CTL activity in lung peaks at about day 7 during acute virus infection, such as that produced by influenza A virus, LCMV, or RSV.[14,134,209] The naive CD8 T cell in the LCMV model undergoes a process of activation and expansion during that time of 10,000- to 50,000-fold.[40] After about 40 days, the level of detectable virus-specific memory CD8 CTL is about 10% of that during acute infection and is then maintained at constant levels for years even in the absence of Ag.[209] Each successive virus infection adds an expanded set of specificities to the pool of memory CD8 T cells over time and shapes the capacity of the host to respond to selected viruses.[398,399] The memory CD8 T-cell pool not only has an increased precursor frequency against virus-specific epitopes; those cells also have a faster response time. The influence of CD8 CTL memory on the outcome of a subsequent virus exposure can be subtle and may depend on the absence or presence of other components of the immune response. For viruses in which a significant component of the clinical syndrome is related to the immune response clearing the virus, having memory CD8 T-cell responses will result in reduced virus replication a day or two earlier than in primary infection, an earlier peak illness time point, and a lower peak magnitude of illness.[138,168] In a setting where there is a large viral load (e.g., high inoculum challenge) and an absence of pre-existing neutralizing Abs to diminish the number of virus-infected cells, a large CTL response or infusion of excessive CD8 T cells can result in more severe disease.[59]

To date, T-cell response has not been used successfully as a correlate of immunity that is the basis for licensure of a vaccine. However, the incorporation of CTL epitopes into viral vaccines has been considered valuable because of the important role that CTLs play in clearance of established virus infections. The following characteristics of the CTL response *in vivo* should be kept in mind when designing a vaccine for viruses that may require a CTL component of immunity. First, the ability of a CTL epitope to induce an immune response is MHC dependent. Therefore, the incorporation of large antigenic content is important so that multiple CD8 T-cell specificities can be elicited by the vaccine to allow selection of epitopes by the diverse repertoire of human MHC class I alleles and to reduce the possibility of immune escape through genetic mutation. Second, when considering vaccine-induced immune protection, CTLs represent a second line of defense against virus infection because they cannot prevent infection and are only effective against infected cells. The localization and phenotype of CD8 T cells can influence the timing and efficiency of viral clearance. For example, immunization of macaques with a recombinant CMV vector that induces a sufficiently high frequency of intraepithelial effector memory CD8 T cells can rapidly clear virus-infected cells following SIV challenge, leading to abortive infection.[185] Technologies such as polychromatic flow cytometry,[348] MHC class I tetramer reagents that provide the means to sort epitope-specific T cells,[108] the ability to define functional subsets of T cells with more precision,[105] sequencing technology that allows single-cell clonotyping of epitope-specific cells, and correlation of the TCR-peptide-MHC biophysical interaction and structure with T-cell functions[37] may provide the necessary information to harness CD8 T cells more effectively in the future.

CD4 T Cells

CD4 T cells provide a variety of functions, including help to B cells and CD8 T cells, thereby augmenting the two major effector mechanisms of the adaptive immune response. CD4 T cells can also mediate direct antiviral activity *in vivo*[188,262,296,426]; however, this is not their major function as it is for CD8 T cells. The MHC class II, $\alpha\beta$ heterodimer—the restricting element for CD4 T cells—is present predominantly on antigen-presenting cells (APCs) such as dendritic cells, macrophages, monocytes, and B cells. However, during inflammation, even epithelial cells can express MHC class II molecules, and CD4 T cells have been shown to have compensatory viral clearance capacity in the absence of CD8 T cells. In addition to having antiviral and helper activity, CD4 T cells can mediate immunopathology[12,279,422] and have been shown to have regulatory and other specialized functions[476] (e-Fig. 14.8).

The CD4 T-cell response to certain internal viral proteins may play a cooperative role in the development of effective resistance by augmenting the Ab response to a major surface protein.[380] For example, immunization with the membrane (M) protein of influenza A virus can prime for a subsequent augmented Ab response to the HA glycoprotein on virus particles.[380] In this manner, the entire CD4 T-cell repertoire developed against the viral surface and internal proteins can be called into play to amplify a B-cell response to a surface protein. Because MHC class II–restricted T-cell epitopes tend to be more numerous on viral proteins than MHC class I–restricted epitopes,[234] the repertoire of CD4 T cells capable of augmenting the Ab response is large. Although CD4 T cells are typically thought to provide indirect helper functions to improve CD8 T-cell and Ab responses, there is evidence that they may also contribute direct effector functions to virus clearance. CD4 T cells have been shown to have cytolytic function against HIV.[329] Viral Ags can induce a protective immune response mediated by CD4 T cells in the absence of B cells or CTLs,[262] indicating that this arm of the immune response can make an independent contribution to resistance against both acute and chronic virus infections.[188] CD4 T cells also secrete IFN-γ, tumor necrosis factor (TNF)-α, and other soluble factors that may directly inhibit virus replication.[322,323] For these reasons, it is advisable to include virus Ags capable of inducing CD4 T-cell responses in viral vaccines to achieve maximal immunogenicity. The processes involved in CD4 T-cell memory induction are distinct from the processes involved in establishing CD8 T-cell memory responses[397] and more complex in some ways. Ag processing and presentation in MHC class II molecules can occur through the endocytic pathway; therefore, unlike CD8 T cells, CD4 T cells can be induced by killed virus vaccines or even purified proteins and do not require live virus or gene delivery approaches to allow Ag to reach the cytoplasm. CD4 T cells do not proliferate to the same extent as CD8 T cells during primary infection, and those producing IFN-γ do not survive as long-lived memory cells.[472]

CD4 T cells have traditionally been considered "helper" T cells (Th), and indeed their activities can improve the potency of B-cell and CD8 T-cell responses. In addition to the original subsets Th1 and Th2, there are now many subpopulations of T cells defined with distinct functions, some of which can alter or diminish effector function. For example, CD4+FoxP3+ T cells have been found to have inhibitory effects on other immune effector functions, hence the name T-regulatory cells, or Tregs.[30] The extent to which vaccines induce CD4+FoxP3+ T cells with T-regulatory activity is not well defined. In addition, there are other subsets of CD4 T cells that produce interleukin (IL)-17 and other proinflammatory cytokines that have been associated with immune-mediated pathology but are also important for immunity against some pathogens. More recently, a CD4+CXCR5+ subset of CD4 T cells designated T-follicular helper (Tfh) cells has been identified that resides primarily in lymph node germinal centers and promotes B-cell memory and plasma cell differentiation.[95] The role of each CD4 T-cell subset in vaccine-induced protection and optimal balance is an area that needs more investigation.

Vaccine-Induced Humoral Immunity

The correlates of immunity that have been established to date for licensed viral vaccines have been associated with Ab responses. In fact, the rationale for development of many of the vaccines in use today was the evidence derived from clinical trials of Ab treatments showing that Abs could mediate protection against disease. Passive transfer studies established the efficacy of Abs in preventing or treating virus infections and disease caused by a wide variety of viruses belonging to diverse RNA or DNA virus families that include the orthomyxoviruses, paramyxoviruses, alphaviruses, flaviviruses, arenaviruses, lentiviruses, picornaviruses, hepadnaviruses, and herpesviruses. Examples of the licensed clinical use of Abs include preparations for hepatitis A and B viruses, measles virus, poliovirus, VZV, rabies virus, RSV, and cytomegalovirus (CMV). A large number of new human mAbs have been discovered in the past decade, and some are under development as prophylactic agents.

A long history of Ab treatments laid the groundwork for current vaccine strategies. Commercial human gamma globulin, which usually contains 16% to 18% immunoglobulin G (IgG) is highly effective in preventing hepatitis A disease and was used widely for that purpose during the past 50 years, even though only a small proportion of the Abs in the preparations are specific for that virus.[89] Currently, inactivated or recombinant protein vaccines for hepatitis A are licensed and thought to work by inducing serum Abs to the virus. A historic double-blind, prospective clinical trial performed in 1951–1952 showed that human IgG also was effective in preventing

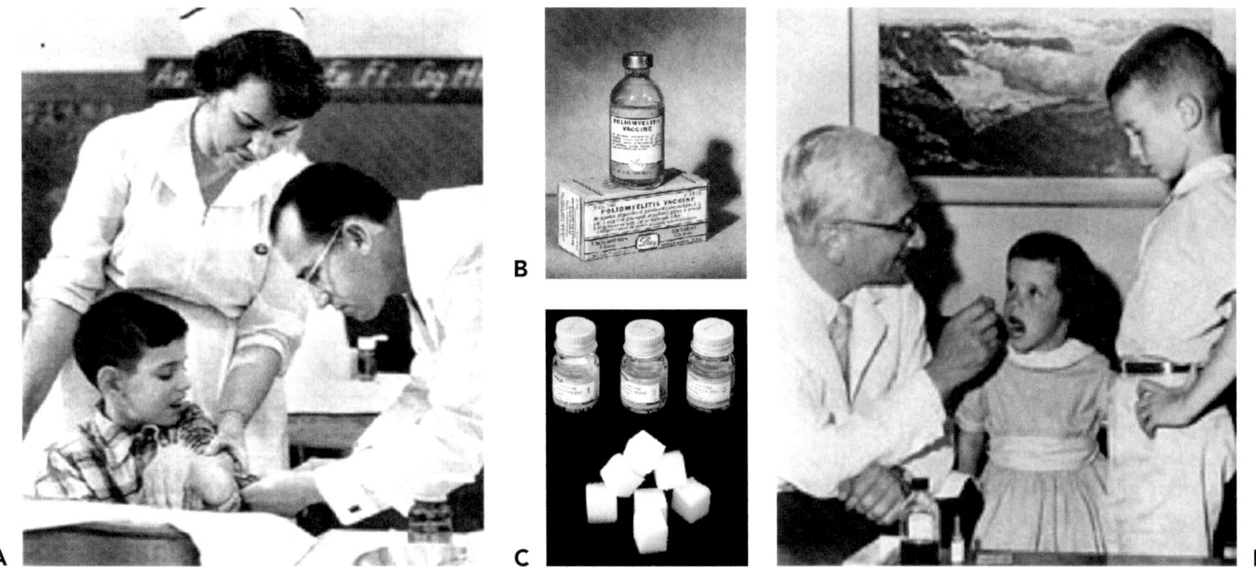

FIGURE 14.1. Polio vaccine development. The development of vaccines for polio brought the process of vaccine development into the public eye and was the first licensed vaccine that relied on mammalian cell culture. Jonas Salk **(A)** spearheaded the development of the inactivated polio vaccine **(B)**. The development of the oral polio vaccine **(C)** was headed by Albert Sabin **(D)**. These two vaccines are still in use today and over the past 50 years have nearly eliminated poliovirus, making the goal of global eradication feasible. (**A,** © AP Wide World Photos; **C** and **D** courtesy Hauck Center for the Albert B. Sabin Archives, Henry R. Winkler Center for the History of the Health Professions, University of Cincinnati.)

paralytic disease caused by poliovirus.[181] Intramuscular inoculation of 0.3 mL of IgG/kg conferred significant resistance that lasted for at least 5 weeks. This seminal observation showed that Abs alone can confer resistance to poliomyelitis and suggested that vaccines inducing such Abs might protect against the disease. Subsequent field trials of inactivated vaccines by Salk and live attenuated vaccines by Sabin validated this view, leading to implementation of universal immunization against poliovirus and ultimately the current worldwide campaign for elimination of polio disease (Fig. 14.1). Before the live measles virus vaccine was licensed for routine use in immunization of young children, human IgG was used for passive prophylaxis and was the mainstay for prevention of disease. IgG given at a dose of 0.5 mL/kg prevented measles, even when administered to exposed individuals as late as 3 days after inoculation with virus.[202] Human IgG prepared from pooled plasma selected for a high titer of varicella-zoster virus (VZV) Abs (varicella-zoster immune globulin [VZIG]) is licensed in the United States for use in prevention of severe varicella in immunosuppressed children.[471] Most of the exposed immunosuppressed children receiving treatment still become infected; however, most exhibit attenuated disease or subclinical infection. Live attenuated varicella virus vaccine was licensed and recommended for universal immunization in 1995. Human IgG was effective in preventing chronic hepatitis B virus (HBV) infection in high-risk infants following maternal exposure.[28] Hepatitis B immune globulin and subunit vaccine are now used in concert to protect infants in this setting.

Preclinical studies in animals suggested that serum RSV-neutralizing Abs above a threshold titer were protective against lower respiratory tract infection, and this observation was validated during a clinical trial of human IgG containing a high titer of RSV-neutralizing Abs that led to licensure in 1995.[1,359] Of interest, the level of serum RSV-neutralizing Abs required for reduction of hospitalization was similar to that needed to prevent infection in cotton rats. A second-generation approach—the use of a humanized murine-neutralizing mAb to RSV—was licensed in 1998.[2] To date, this is the only mAb licensed for prevention of an infectious disease. These clinical applications strongly suggest that neutralizing Abs are an important correlate of protection for RSV vaccines, which are under development. Immunosuppressed patients who have not been infected previously with CMV, a herpesvirus, are at high risk of developing severe life-threatening disease following exposure to the virus, especially when they receive an organ transplant from a CMV-infected donor. Administration of CMV IgG, prepared from pooled units of plasma selected for a high Ab titer, prevents approximately half of the serious illnesses attributable to CMV but does not prevent infection.[405] This finding is interesting because the mode of action suggests that Abs suppress disease by their action on CMV-infected cells and that Abs with these properties should be a target for CMV vaccines under development.

Mechanisms of Virus Neutralization

Abs may render free virus noninfectious, principally through neutralization of infectivity. Virus-neutralizing activity typically is measured by *in vitro* assays in which Ab and infectious virus are incubated and then inoculated onto cell culture. Residual infectivity is quantified by plaque count, infectious foci, signal from recombinant reporter virus, percent of infected cells detected by flow cytometry or other methods and compared to untreated suspensions. Viruses are neutralized *in vitro* by Abs by a wide variety of mechanisms. Important Ab characteristics include affinity/avidity, isotype, concentration, Ab-to-virus ratio, valency, state of polymerization, ability to bind the polyimmunoglobulin receptor (pIgR), ability to fix complement, and specificity for the virus protein and epitope of interest. Virus-related factors important to neutralization include general aspects of the replication cycle of the virus under consideration (receptor use, mode of entry into the cell, pH dependence of fusion, site of replication) and individual characteristics of the specific virus strain (antigenic subgroup and amino acid sequence of viral surface proteins). Host factors influencing the mechanism of neutralization include the type and origin of cells and the level of expression of membrane receptors. The most potent mechanisms of neutralization act prior to infection of cells. First, free infectious virions in solution can be aggregated by multivalent Abs directed against surface glycoproteins.[17,331] The consolidation of multiple infectious virions into an aggregate reduces the number of available infectious units. Second, Abs can inhibit virus attachment to cells, usually by binding directly to virus attachment proteins. Abs to attachment proteins often are poorly neutralizing *in vitro,* effecting only partial neutralization even at high concentration.[211] This effect may be caused by virus heterogeneity owing to a variable extent of glycosylation that occurs during posttranslational processing at the numerous glycosylation sites on these proteins, or because of multiple routes of entry or mechanisms of attachment. Third, viruses can be neutralized following attachment, at the cell surface prior to cell entry, suggesting that immune serum contains Abs capable of inhibiting entry into the cell. For example, Abs to human papillomavirus (HPV) can interrupt infection at two stages of attachment and entry: the first an initial association with the acellular basement membrane that induces conformational changes in the virion and second the association of virus with the keratinocyte cell surface.[104] Some neutralizing Abs decrease infectivity by inhibition of virus–cell fusion at the plasma membrane. Fusion inhibition (FI) activity for some Abs has been inferred from *in vitro* assays in which Ab is incorporated into overlay medium after virus absorption and penetration, and activity measured by inhibition of postinfection cell-to-cell fusion. Additionally, Abs can inhibit the release of progeny viruses from infected cells. There is even evidence that some influenza virus–specific Abs inhibit virus replication by preventing the primary uncoating of virus that is associated with low-pH membrane fusion in the endosome or at the step of the secondary uncoating of the virion core structure—a step required for primary transcription of the virus genome.[330,332] Our current understanding of the induction of such Ab functions is not sufficient to allow us to design specific vaccine strategies to induce them.

Structural and Biochemical Features of Antibodies Important to Affinity

Abs induced by primary infection or immunization are generally of low affinity for the target Ag. Affinity maturation of Abs is mediated by somatic mutation of the genes encoding B-cell receptors, which occurs in germinal centers, most prominently following second infections or booster doses of vaccine. Somatic hypermutation (SHM) coupled with B-cell selection results in the promulgation of high-affinity Abs in the antiviral repertoire. Increases in affinity likely increase neutralizing potency for most antiviral Abs directed to surface proteins. Although the molecular basis for affinity maturation during secondary responses was not understood during the development of early vaccines, the enhanced efficacy of multiple-dose vaccine regimens in clinical trials pointed the way to a practical use of this principle. Most licensed viral vaccines are administered using multiple-dose regimens to enhance the quality, magnitude, and durability of the immune response.

Increased affinity is widely believed to confer enhanced functional competence on Abs. Work using HIV-1–specific Abs derived from combinatorial phage display Ab libraries demonstrated improvements in neutralization associated with affinity maturation caused by SHM.[427] The fusion (F) protein—the major protective Ag of RSV—has at least four antigenic sites, each with a differing capacity as a target for virus neutralization.[29] Recombinant derivatives of a humanized RSV mAb containing random mutations in the combining site have shown that mutations enhancing the association rate improved neutralization and efficacy, whereas mutations improving the dissociation rate did not, despite their contribution to improved steady-state affinity.[458] Somatic mutations in human rotavirus Abs have been shown to enhance affinity and inhibitory function, with individual mutations in Ab combining sites conferring several hundred-fold increases in affinity and function.[211] The broadest and most potent human Abs to HIV and influenza virus isolated to date are distinguished by exceptional numbers of somatic mutations in the Ab sequences (on the order of about one-third of nucleotides altered).[467,474] Hypermutation introduces not only point mutations that enhance function, but in some cases nontemplated insertions of sequences encoding new amino acids that mediate neutralization.[233] In the vesicular stomatitis virus (VSV) mouse model, investigators have shown only modest increases in the affinities of hypermutated Abs compared with those in germline configuration over the course of infection and after repeated booster injections.[210] The VSV G glycoprotein is unusual in that it contains only a single immunodominant antigenic site that reliably induces neutralizing Abs. Neutralization activity also is determined by the number of times the neutralizing determinant is displayed on the surface of the virion, and some studies suggest that virion particles may be dynamic in their display of epitopes.[112] Understanding the relationship of affinity and neutralization is needed so that we can better appreciate the B-cell response to exposure with foreign Ags in a physiologic context. Furthermore, elucidation of the role of affinity in antiviral Ab function is critical for designing new active and passive immunization strategies against pathogenic human viruses. The absence of somatic mutations in the virus-specific Ab sequences of infants probably accounts for the difficulty in inducing high-affinity, high-potency Abs in this population after a single vaccination.[448]

CDR3 Loops of the Antibody Variable Region in Antigen Binding

A combining site formed by the variable heavy (V_H) and variable light (V_L) domains of the Ab fragment (Fab) mediates Ag recognition. Both the V_H and the V_L chains have three noncontiguous linear sequences of greatest variability—CDRs—that result in flexible loops in the Ig protein and form the classical Ag binding site. HCDR3 shows the greatest variability in terms of length and sequence, particularly in human Abs. Several crystal structures of Abs have demonstrated that human CDRs tend to adopt a limited number of canonical conformations, with the exception of HCDR3.[75] In each of the crystal structures of human Abs complexed with Ags, HCDR3 has been shown to make important contacts in every case.[23,401] Diverse CDR length and gene family usage have been shown to be essential features of immunological health and functional antiviral immune responses.[153,228,389] Vaccinations that induce a broad Ab repertoire that is rich in CDR diversity are more likely to succeed than highly focused vaccinations inducing limited Ab repertoires. Although not universal, long HCDR3 regions are common in highly active Abs to HIV, and they may facilitate high-affinity binding to complex viral antigenic sites. For example, the crystal structure of the 17b mAb complexed with CD4-triggered HIV gp120 reveals a complex interaction that is accomplished only by the unique long HCDR3 region of this Ab.[235] High-throughput screening for broadly reactive high-potency HIV-neutralizing Abs has isolated two unusual Abs with the longest CDRs ever identified,[440] and the HCDR3s of these Abs possess fascinating secondary structural elements.[346] In contrast, identification of another broadly neutralizing mAb specific for the CD4 binding site has a CDR3 loop of only 13 amino acids, although the variable region of the heavy chains is more than 30% somatically mutated from germ line.[459]

The Role of Isotype in Additional Mechanisms of Antibody-Mediated Virus Neutralization

The complement system is activated by the classical (Ab-dependent), alternative (Ab-independent), and lectin-binding pathways. Viral neutralization by specific Abs is concentration dependent and is often enhanced by complement activation. It has been reported that even apparently "nonneutralizing" Abs can acquire neutralizing activity with the addition of complement—for example, a nonneutralizing RSV murine mAb was shown to exhibit complement-enhanced neutralization *in vivo* in the presence of complement.[92] Complement fixation is mediated by the C_H2 region of the Ab Fc domain of immunoglobulin M (IgM), IgG1, and IgG3 subclasses in humans and the IgM, IgG2a, and IgG2b subclasses in mice.[328] Understanding the role of complement in enhancing the functional capacity of Abs to neutralize viruses has broad implications for vaccine design, because the cytokine milieu induced by infection or immunization affects the isotype and subclass of the Ab response to the viral Ags by activating selective promoters in the appropriate Ig heavy chain locus. B cells triggered in an environment with high IFN-γ concentrations tend to produce IgG1 and IgG3 Abs. In contrast, in the presence of a dominant IL4 response, B cells produce immunoglobulin E (IgE) and IgG4 Abs. IgE participates in allergic diseases, and it is generally considered desirable to avoid strong IgE responses following vaccination. The Fc region of Abs also mediates some cellular activities, termed *Ab-dependent cell-mediated cytotoxicity* (ADCC), which are discussed below.

Structural Features of Antigens Critical for Inducing Efficient Antibody Interactions

The conformation of epitopes on viral surface proteins often is critical to the ability of vaccine Ags to induce or bind neutralizing Abs. Most neutralizing Abs bind to conformationally dependent epitopes on surface proteins. Linear peptide vaccine candidates derived from the sequence of the natural Ag rarely recapitulate the conformation of the protective Ag, which is why most peptide-based vaccines are poor immunogens for humoral immunity. Many subunit Ags comprising purified or recombinant viral proteins that have been developed as vaccine candidates contain the full polypeptide sequence of the Ag; however, the protein emerges from the purification process in a conformationally relaxed state that resembles the natural Ag only in part. Such Ags may induce high levels of Abs that bind the vaccine Ag but low levels of Abs that bind or neutralize virus.[385] Some viruses appear to present highly antigenic surface loops to the immune system that are structurally nonessential, causing immune focusing on hypervariable domains of viral proteins, such as the influenza HA variable loops surrounding the sialic acid receptor–binding domain or the third variable (V3) region of HIV gp120. Recent studies, however, reveal that some subjects make broadly neutralizing Abs that recognize these hypervariable domains.[156] Many structurally critical domains of viral surface proteins are hidden from B cells because they are buried in the interior of viral molecules or oligomers of molecules, or they are exposed only briefly during rapid conformational changes required for virus attachment or virus–cell membrane fusion. For example, viral hydrophobic fusion peptides, receptor-binding domains, heptad repeats, and other critical regions of fusion proteins usually are not accessible to Abs. Most fusion proteins require cleavage by proteases before they are competent to fuse, and Abs to the precursor protein may not bind the cleaved protein in the mature virus particle.[336] Posttranslational modifications of surface proteins, especially glycosylation, can present a challenge for Ab recognition of protein because of the highly varied nature of the glycoprotein population. Deglycosylated protein Ags may enhance induction of protein-specific Ags; however, these Abs may not efficiently recognize glycosylated proteins *in vivo*. Some virus-neutralizing Abs are directed specifically to carbohydrates on virus glycoproteins.[56] Some broadly neutralizing Abs to HIV, such as PG9 and PG16, recognize a conformational epitope that depends on glycosylation at specific variable loop N-linked sites.[111] Posttranslational modification of Abs also can affect the interaction of Ab and virus. For instance, several human Abs to HIV gp120 are sulfated in the combining site, which allows the Ag-combining sites to mimic the structure of the virus coreceptor CCR5, which is sulfated.[74] These Abs inhibit infectivity by binding to the co-receptor-binding domain on HIV gp120.

Antibody Escape Mechanisms

Viruses, especially RNA viruses with error-prone RNA-dependent RNA polymerases, exhibit facility in generating genetic diversity during multiple replicative cycles. During chronic infections, such as those with HBV, HCV, or retroviruses such as HIV, viruses that accumulate amino acid changes in epitopes that are targets of Abs owing to point missense mutations in the corresponding genes can escape neutralization by reduction or loss of binding. Some viruses easily shed surface glycoproteins (e.g., HIV gp120 or Ebola GP)[187] or encode soluble forms of surface glycoproteins using alternative start codons (e.g., RSV G protein),[369] in part as a decoy mechanism, targeting Abs away from infectious virions. The immunity induced by experimental vaccine candidates that are narrowly targeted to single epitopes or single proteins are susceptible to rapid viral escape. To avoid such Ab-resistant mutants, optimal vaccines should induce broad humoral responses to a diversity of antigenic sites.

Antibodies Active Against Virus-Infected Cells

Viruses that mature at the cell surface by budding or that insert viral glycoprotein(s) into the cell surface membrane render the infected cell susceptible to lysis by Ab-dependent complement-mediated lysis or ADCC mechanisms. This lysis is mediated by cytolytic cells, including NK cells, neutrophils, and eosinophils, in an Fc region–dependent manner. Ab-dependent cell-mediated virus inhibition (ADCVI) activity is similar but is typically measured with a readout of reduction of virus replication instead of lysis of target cells. Cytophilic Abs can arm leukocytes in the ADCC reaction, which has been shown to be important in the resistance of infant mice to herpes infection and for clearance of a retrovirus.[87,226] Fc receptor–mediated mechanisms appear important to neutralization of HIV.[191] Some herpesviruses encode an IgG Fc receptor homolog, which enables the virus to evade ADCC by binding Abs, especially virus-specific Abs if they bind virus proteins on infected cells, suggesting the importance of the ADCC effector or other Fc-mediated mechanisms *in vivo.*[115] RSV ADCC activity mediated by NK cells has been detected in monkey or human peripheral blood using Abs in serum.[216,277,395] Because infection of cells must occur for these immune mechanisms to act, these mechanisms represent a second line of defense against infection or disease.

Inadvertent Induction of Antibodies to Host Antigens

Immunization of monkeys with formalin-inactivated SIV produced in human cells induced Abs directed at Ags originating from the cells used to produce the virus.[407] These anticellular Abs can neutralize the infectivity of SIV produced in human cells, although not virus produced in monkey cells, by interacting with human Ags incorporated into the virion outer membrane. This form of neutralization, which is mediated by complement-mediated virolysis, can yield an overestimate of vaccine immunogenicity. Hence, an effort should be made to avoid immunization with virions into which foreign host cell Ags have become incorporated.[407] In some cases, even the native virion proteins may mimic structures associated with host cell proteins. For example, many of the original broadly neutralizing mAbs specific for the HIV-1 gp160 envelope glycoprotein have been shown to cross-react with host cell proteins.[190]

Inhibitory Antibodies That Lack Classical *In Vitro* Neutralizing Activity

Some Abs that do not exhibit neutralizing activity *in vitro* can mediate resistance to virus infections, although typically they are less effective than neutralizing Abs.[297] Such Abs can be directed against Ags on the surface of virus particles or against virion or nonstructural proteins displayed on the surface of infected cells. *In vivo,* these Abs mediate antiviral activities by several different mechanisms. First, virus particles coated with nonneutralizing Abs can undergo accelerated clearance from the bloodstream. Second, Abs directed at surface glycoproteins such as the NA of influenza A virus or the HA-esterase protein of coronavirus (CoV) can decrease the level of virus replication in the target organ, presumably by inhibiting the release of virus from infected cells.[46,466] Third, Abs can lyse virus-infected cells via IgG Fc-dependent mechanisms.[92,391]

Antiviral Activity of Antibodies *In Vivo*

Resolution of infection generally depends on CTLs, which reduce infection by lysing virus-infected cells. However, virus-specific Abs also can exert a therapeutic effect. Dramatic clinical therapeutic effect of viral Abs has been observed in patients with Argentine hemorrhagic fever, which is caused by Junin virus (an arenavirus). This disease has a high mortality; however, death can be prevented with a preparation of pooled human serum with a high titer of Junin virus–neutralizing Abs administered within 8 days of onset of symptoms.[123,261] Mucosal virus infections that are limited to the cells that line the lumen of the respiratory tract also can be cleared by specific Abs that are delivered by parenteral inoculation or by direct instillation into the lungs. RSV immune globulin or RSV-neutralizing Abs protect against severe lower respiratory tract disease.[1,2] These Abs also reduce established infection in animal models; however, therapeutic trials in humans have not revealed a clinical benefit of treatment of active infection. Influenza A virus HA-specific IgG Abs cleared the lungs of influenza-infected SCID mice in the absence of other recognized immune functions.[334] Abs can exert a therapeutic effect in privileged sites where CD8 CTLs are not active. Central nervous system (CNS) neurons are not good targets for CD8 CTLs, because they have highly regulated expression of class I MHC glycoproteins. Nevertheless, in SCID mice, persistent infection of brain neurons by the alphavirus Sindbis virus can be cleared rapidly by parenteral inoculation of envelope-glycoprotein–specific Abs without causing obvious cell damage.[248] Some patients with underlying X-linked agammaglobulinemia complicated by chronic enteroviral meningoencephalitis have been treated successfully with human IgG that contains Abs specific for the infecting virus. A therapeutic effect was achieved with IgG administered by the intravenous or intraventricular routes.[118,275] Failure of human IgG to alter chronic enteroviral meningoencephalitis in some patients suggests that the concentration of enterovirus-specific Abs in human IgG is often inadequate.

Mucosal Antibodies

Abs have been shown to function within mucosal epithelium.[268,269] Dimeric immunoglobulin A (IgA) secreted at the basolateral surface of cells or from plasma is transcytosed to the apical surface in association with polymeric Ig receptor to which dimeric IgA with J chain binds. During transcytosis through cells infected with the Sendai virus, virus-specific IgA can reduce intracellular virus and infectivity. The mechanism responsible for this effect is not clear, although it is possible that the endocytic pathway used for IgA transport and the exocytic pathways used for transport of viral glycoproteins intersect at some location within the cell, possibly the apical recycling endosome.[142] Similar studies with IgA Abs to rotavirus and measles virus suggest that IgA molecules may inhibit viruses inside epithelial cells or after transcytosis.[50,463] Induced IgA molecules to HIV gp41 appear to block transcytosis across genital epithelial surfaces.[42] The FcRn receptor for IgG also is present in some epithelial cells and could participate in transport or retention of IgG at mucosal surfaces.

Abs present in the systemic circulation efficiently protect internal organs against viruses that are introduced directly into the bloodstream (e.g., HBV and HIV) or that spread via the bloodstream from primary sites of replication such as the respiratory or gastrointestinal mucosa. As mentioned previously, diseases produced by viruses that fall into the latter category (i.e., measles, polio, hepatitis A, rubella, smallpox, and varicella) can be prevented or modified by Ig prophylaxis, often with small amounts of Ab that are difficult to detect in the blood of recipients. Such Abs are relatively easy to induce by parenteral immunization with live or inactivated virus vaccines. In contrast, Abs present in the systemic circulation do not provide efficient protection against viral diseases that are limited to mucosal surfaces unless these Abs are present in high titer. This is because only a small proportion of such Ig molecules traffic from the plasma to the lumenal surface of the mucosal epithelium by transudation. Therefore, to prevent viral diseases that are limited to mucosal tissue, two different strategies can be employed. The first is to induce Abs such as secretory IgA at the mucosal site by virus replication or immunization at that site. The second, and less efficient, strategy is to stimulate a high titer of serum IgG Abs that can protect mucosal surfaces following transudation.

When IgG Abs present in the blood are passively transferred to mucosal surfaces by transudation where they can exert antiviral activity, there is a gradient regarding the ability of serum IgG-derived Abs to restrict virus replication on mucosal surfaces. This gradient is less in lung than it is in the nasopharynx. IgG Abs, if present in the serum in high enough titer, can provide almost complete resistance to pulmonary replication of RSV; however, resistance in the upper respiratory tract is more difficult to achieve. Transudation of IgG also probably occurs in the intestine, especially in inflammatory states, although IgG is more easily subjected to proteolytic degradation in the intestinal lumen than in the respiratory tract. Immunization of the female genital tract with a live virus vaccine can induce the local synthesis of IgG antiviral Abs such that the specific activity of mucosal IgG Abs significantly exceeds that of serum, indicating that IgG Abs present on a mucosal surface can come either from serum via transudation or from IgG Ab-secreting cells present in the submucosal tissues.[340] Although passively transferred IgG Abs can provide mucosal immunity in the lower respiratory tract, the major mediators of resistance to virus infection of the upper respiratory tract, the larger airways of the lungs, and the gastrointestinal tract are mucosal Abs, many of which are IgAs selectively transported across mucosal surfaces to exert antiviral effects on the lumenal surface. Both nonneutralizing[50] and neutralizing[379] IgA Abs have antiviral effects on mucosal surfaces, with the former active intracellularly during transcytosis and the latter active both intracellularly and on the lumenal side of the epithelium. Antiviral IgA Abs function to clear virus infections, to modify the severity of disease on reinfection, and to prevent infection on re-exposure to virus. The level of antiviral IgA Abs, as well as the number of virus-specific IgA-secreting cells, often correlates with resistance to virus infection.[83,469] The advantages of IgAs in the mucosal fluids are that they are transported more efficiently, they resist proteolytic degradation better than IgG, and the dimeric nature of secretory IgA enhances avidity.

The primary mucosal IgA response peaks within the first 6 weeks after infection and usually decreases to a low, often barely detectable, level by 3 months. The transient nature of the primary mucosal Ab response is a factor in the ability of many viruses to reinfect mucosal surfaces and underlies the need for two or more doses of vaccine to efficiently immunize mucosal surfaces. The virus-specific IgA Ab response is greater at the site of virus replication or of Ag administration than at distal sites, suggesting that mucosal immunity is best induced by antigenic stimulation of sites directly involved in replication of the wild-type virus.

Adverse Effects of Antibodies

Abs can contribute to the potentiation of disease. For example, heterotypic Abs to the envelope glycoprotein of dengue virus appear to play a role in the severe clinical entity known as dengue hemorrhagic fever/shock syndrome.[231] Dengue viruses replicate primarily in cells of the mononuclear phagocyte lineage, and subneutralizing amounts of dengue virus Abs enhance dengue virus infection of these cells *in vitro* by increasing uptake of virus via IgG Fc receptors present on these cells.[180] However, the mechanism by which augmented disease results from enhanced access of dengue virus into mononuclear cells remains unclear.[377] Immune complexes were detected in the lung tissues of fatal cases of influenza during the 1957 and 2009 pandemics, suggesting a potential role for enhancing Abs in severe influenza disease.[287]

OBSTACLES TO IMMUNIZATION IN EARLY LIFE AND IN THE ELDERLY

Immunization of Infants

The developmental immaturity of the immune response to viruses in the very young is seen clearly in the difficulty to immunize neonates and infants.[402] Young infants are a preferred target population for immunization, because most children present to health systems with the highest frequency at birth or shortly after. A high level of access to infants allows universal immunization, and many viral diseases are most severe early in life. Many obstacles arise, however, in attempts to immunize infants in the first several weeks or months of life against disease caused by viruses.

First, most infants possess maternal Abs that can interfere with response to infection or the infectivity or immunogenicity of primary immunization. Live attenuated measles virus cannot be given effectively prior to 1 year of age, because many infants possess maternal Abs until that time that reduce or eliminate immunogenicity of the vaccine.[10] Ab-mediated suppression can be overcome in some instances by increasing the dose of the vaccine—for example, the inactivated hepatitis A vaccine or a replicating influenza vaccine.[84,101] The immune suppression by maternal Abs is more potent against B-cell responses than against induction of virus-specific T cells, possibly because the Ab response generally depends more on Ag dose than T-cell responses.[97]

Second, the ability to respond to viral surface proteins with a protective Ab response is acquired gradually over the first year of life, reflecting developmental maturation of the neonatal immune system. Responses of seronegative infants to live measles vaccine remain relatively poor during the second 6 months of life.[144] Responses to live VZV vaccine also are reduced in the first year of life.[436] The youngest infants mount Ab responses to experimental mucosal immunization with live influenza, RSV, or parainfluenza virus vaccines that are low in magnitude, quality, and durability.[84,213,214] The molecular and cellular basis for immunological immaturity is not fully defined. Infant virus-specific Ab sequences are characterized by marked lack of somatic mutations, resulting in low-affinity Abs of low function.[448] Infant B cells exhibit limited capability to switch isotype from IgM to IgG2 Abs, and the isotype profile of circulating Abs differs from adults until age 5 to 6 years. Infants possess reduced levels of some components of the complement cascade, especially C8 and C9 that participate in membrane attack complexes, leading to impaired complement-mediated reactions. Infants exhibit a high proportion of transitional immature B cells and poor organization of the splenic marginal zone.

The Ab responses that young infants make to respiratory virus surface glycoproteins are significantly lower in quality than those of adults. Studies have described a dissociation of the level of neutralizing and binding Abs in the very young infant.[457] This dissociation may be of functional significance, because neutralizing Ab titers correlate well with protective efficacy in studies of protection for viruses. Dissociation between neutralizing and binding Abs also characterized the serum Abs induced by the ill-fated formalin-inactivated RSV experimental vaccine of the 1960s and probably accounts for the lack of protective efficacy of Abs induced by that vaccine candidate.[301] Ab responses induced by infections of infants are less durable than those of older subjects. Postinfection serum Ab levels to respiratory viruses often wane significantly several months after primary infection, especially if infection occurs at a very young age. Animal models suggest that B-cell priming occurs effectively early in life or in the presence of suppressive Abs[96,97]; however, the deficient maintenance of long-lived plasma cells in the bone marrow may lead to rapid waning of humoral immunity.[349] Reduced humoral immunity to vaccines early in life also may reflect reduced T-helper cell function and altered dendritic cell function. Neonatal CD4 T cells exhibit reduced ability to secrete IFN-γ, reflecting limited secretion of IFN-α and IL-12 by dendritic cells.[106,155]

Immunization of the Elderly

Obstacles to effective immunization also arise late in life owing to immune senescence. Immune senescence in the elderly is marked by a decrease in the magnitude, quality, and duration of Ab responses and a reduction in functional T cells, especially CD8 T cells. Elderly T cells are distinguished by alterations in cytokine production, co-stimulatory molecule expression, susceptibility to apoptosis, and changes in the level of DNA damage and repair and telomerase length.[145] Chronic virus infection may contribute to immune senescence. For example, CMV-specific T cells progress to a differentiated state in the elderly owing to chronic antigenic stimulation.[344] This syndrome has been described as an immune risk phenotype in the elderly, reflecting the accumulation of a high percentage of circulating CMV-specific CD8 T cells at a terminal stage of differentiation that may detract from the flexibility of the T-cell repertoire to respond to other Ags. The CD4 T-cell responses of healthy elderly individuals appear to sustain a good level of function until late in life. Waning immunity to latent viruses may be boosted in the elderly in some cases. Immunization of the elderly with live attenuated varicella virus vaccine reduces the incidence of shingles in that population.[333]

Aging has varying effects on the response to different Ags. For example, the immunogenicity of recombinant hepatitis B vaccine is reduced starting in the fifth decade and is poor in the elderly.[455] Ab responses to influenza virus vaccine also are reduced in the elderly. Practically speaking, however, although vaccination in the elderly may be reduced in efficacy and may require frequent boosters or other alterations in strategy, the effectiveness of many vaccines such as influenza virus vaccine are reasonable enough to support vaccination of this group. It also may be possible to improve the immune responses in the elderly by utilizing adjuvants or alternative vaccination strategies. Investigational gene-based vaccines have been shown to be highly immunogenic in older adults compared to the typical age-related decrease in responses seen with many traditional vaccines.[243]

GOALS OF IMMUNIZATION AGAINST VIRAL DISEASES

Prevention

The major goals of immunization against viruses are the prevention or modification of disease in an individual and the control of epidemic infection within populations. Most viral vaccines prevent or modify disease without necessarily preventing infection. The ways in which this objective is achieved are diverse. Whereas most viral vaccines are administered before infection occurs, prevention of CNS disease in individuals inoculated with rabies virus by an animal bite can be achieved by administration of a vaccine regimen initiated shortly after infection has occurred. This postexposure prophylaxis is possible because the long incubation period of the infection permits the development of an effective immune response in time to modify infection and prevent disease. Interestingly, even for viruses with a more rapid course, such as variola, individuals can be protected against a fatal outcome if vaccinia virus vaccine is administered up to 4 days after the initial exposure to the virus. This effect may be attributable to augmented innate immune responses or more rapid induction of adaptive immune responses.

The major goal of immunization against rubella virus is the prevention of fetal abnormalities caused by intrauterine infection. To achieve this goal, both males and females are immunized in the United States. Immunization of males has little direct benefit to the vaccinee other than prevention of the relatively mild illness caused by the rubella virus, and males are not targeted in all national vaccine programs. The fetus of a vaccinated female is protected by immunization of the mother before pregnancy. Herd immunity resulting from extensive immunization of males and females provides some protection to the fetus of an unvaccinated female by decreasing the circulation of virus in the community. An example of herd immunity was seen early after introducing the mumps vaccine. The incidence of mumps declined precipitously before vaccine coverage was significantly expanded. A modest reduction in the number of susceptible persons and transmitters had a significant impact on the epidemic (Fig. 14.2) and e-Fig. 14.2.

In addition to reducing the frequency of susceptible persons and transmitters, some live viral vaccines can improve herd immunity by the spread of vaccine from recipients to contacts. This phenomenon has been observed with oral live poliovirus vaccine[383] resulting in the indirect immunization of a significant proportion of the population and a marked reduction in the incidence of poliomyelitis in both vaccinated and "unvaccinated"

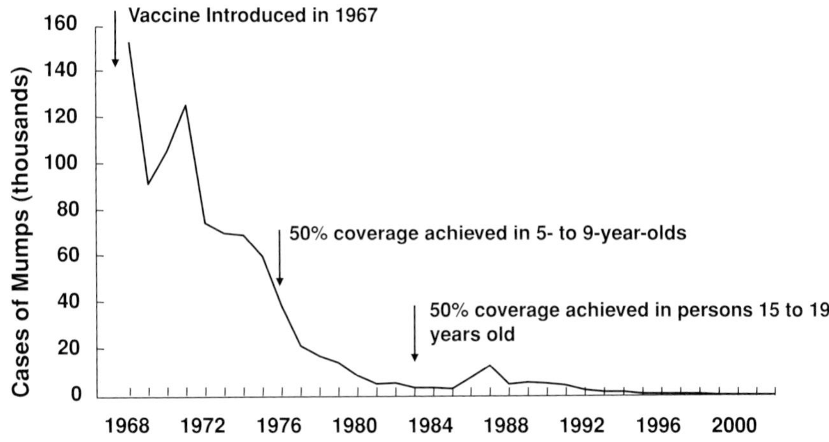

FIGURE 14.2. Incidence of mumps in the United States after introduction of vaccine. The number of mumps cases in the United States began diminishing shortly after the introduction of the vaccine. This effect is considered to be an example of herd immunity, because vaccine distribution and coverage was less than 50% for about 10 years and was not a formal recommendation in the United States until 1976. (Adapted from Cochi SL, Preblud SR, Orenstein WA. Perspectives on the relative resurgence of mumps in the United States. *Am J Dis Child* 1988;142(5):499–507.) Also see e-Fig. 14.2.

individuals. Spread of vaccine virus has been viewed by many as a desirable property because this transmission confers the benefits of immunization on many individuals who were not vaccinated. However, spread of vaccine in the population also raises concern because of the rare occurrence of vaccine-associated paralytic disease among contacts of vaccinees, and immunization of persons without their prior consent presents ethical issues.

Although most vaccines in use today are effective in preventing disease, they usually are inefficient at completely preventing infection. Prevention of infection is a desirable property for specific vaccines such as HBV and HIV. Infection with HBV during the neonatal period is associated with an increased risk of progression to the chronic carrier state and associated with the development of chronic liver disease and hepatocellular carcinoma later in life. Therefore, a major goal of HBV vaccination is to prevent transmission of infection from persistently infected mothers to their infants during the neonatal period. Considerable success in this effort has been achieved through the use of hepatitis B surface antigen (HBsAg) vaccine or hyperimmune HBV antiserum plus vaccine immediately after delivery.[195] HIV is a lentivirus, and the possibility of progression to AIDS can occur many years after initial infection. Therefore, it is desirable to develop a vaccine that induces immunity to prevent infection or result in an abortive or transient HIV infection.

The vaccine for HPV was licensed based on its ability to prevent cervical neoplasia.[4] In addition to preventing the acute effects of virus infection, the HBV vaccine is also given with the goal of preventing hepatomas.[195]

Immunotherapy

Herpes simplex virus type 1 (HSV-1) or type 2 (HSV-2) and VZV produce latent infections in sensory ganglia that periodically reactivate, resulting in development of new lesions and increased opportunity for transmission of virus. Therefore, a goal of immunization of persons previously infected with these viruses is to prevent or ameliorate recurrent disease caused by reactivation of their latent infection.[35] This form of immunization is referred to as immunotherapy. Other illnesses that are candidates for immunotherapeutic vaccines include warts and cancer caused by HPV and chronic hepatitis caused by HBV or HCV. HIV-1 has also been considered as a target for immunotherapy to prevent the long-term consequences of chronic infection or to reduce the requirements for ongoing antiretroviral drug therapy. Because of the extent of repeated Ag exposure and damage to many elements of the adaptive immune system, it may be difficult to elicit new immune responses to effectively control virus.[62] Effective immunotherapeutic vaccines for recurrent HSV face a similar challenge because the vaccinees previously infected by wild-type virus are repeatedly reimmunized during each recurrence. However, for a related herpesvirus, VZV, where recurrence is relatively uncommon, immunization with live attenuated vaccine reduces the incidence of herpes zoster and postherpetic neuralgia.[333]

Eradication or Elimination

Appropriate use of a highly effective vaccine can help to eradicate a major disease when humans are the only natural host for the virus and there is no natural reservoir or intermediate host. During the 1970s, this goal of eradication was achieved for smallpox largely through the use of live vaccinia virus vaccine. This campaign ranks as one of the major public health achievements in all history. Two other human viruses have been targeted similarly for eradication, namely poliovirus and measles virus, and significant progress toward these goals has been made for both viral pathogens. The United Nations officially declared eradication of the morbillivirus animal pathogen rinderpest in 2011, after a concerted worldwide eradication program. Unfortunately, eradication of viral pathogens usually is an elusive goal because of setbacks from social instability, anti-vaccine sentiments, the threat of bioterrorism, and the potential for intentional reintroduction or resurrection of previously eradicated viral pathogens. Therefore, it will be prudent to find ways of maintaining immunity to serious virus pathogens even after eradication of virus in the natural reservoir has been achieved. The new technologies that have improved our ability to identify emerging pathogens and to develop biologics for vaccines and therapeutics have also created an intellectual reservoir that is a formidable barrier to true eradication efforts. Elimination of a virus pathogen suggests that epidemic and endemic disease is controlled and no active cases are present. However, setting the goal of elimination acknowledges the possibility of re-emergence and would include maintenance of active vaccine-induced immunity.

HISTORY OF VIRAL VACCINE DEVELOPMENT AND FUTURE PROSPECTS

The history of discovery and development for each viral vaccine is unique and instructional. Although space limitations prevent the full description of each vaccine, some of the major events are outlined. Although each vaccine development story is different, there are common events and themes that have been catalogued in a supplementary table (e-Table 14.1) that includes (a) disease description and virus discovery, (b) vaccine discovery and/or proof of concept, (c) vaccine licensure or first human use, and (d) unique or unanticipated events.

Origins of Vaccinology

Origin of Live Virus Vaccination

Most viral vaccines were developed as a result of both fortuitous events and empirical findings. The origin of modern vaccinology, and particularly live virus vaccination, is based on the practice of variolization (mechanical attenuation and

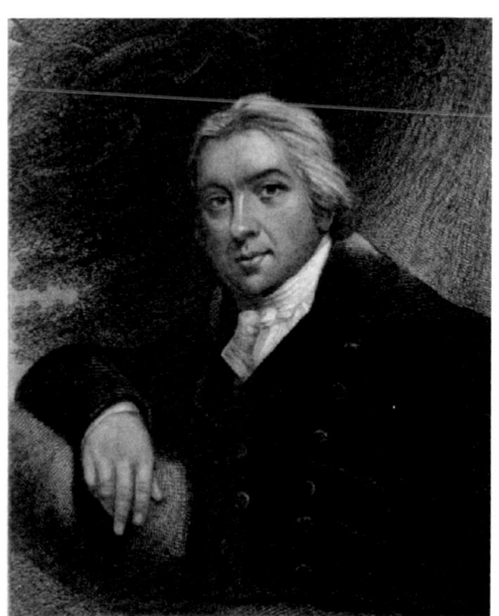

A

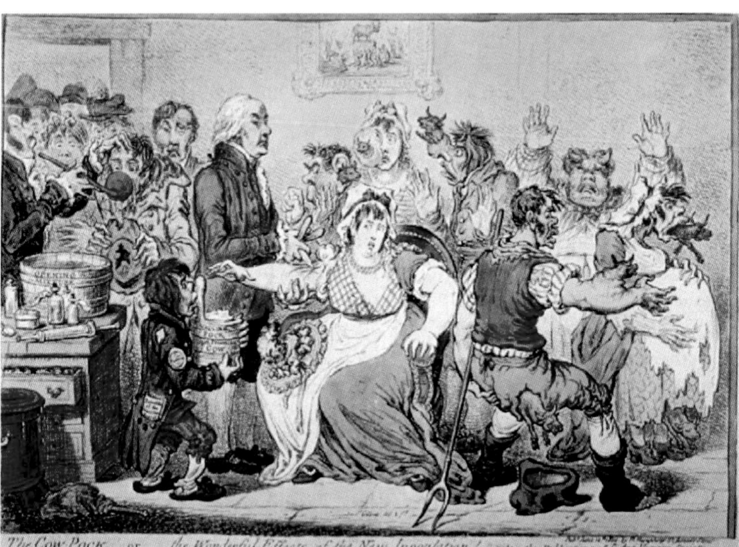
The Cow-Pock—or—the Wonderful Effects of the New Inoculation!

B

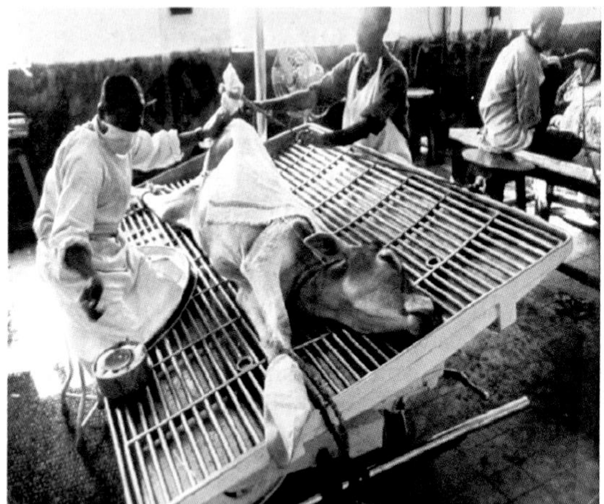

C

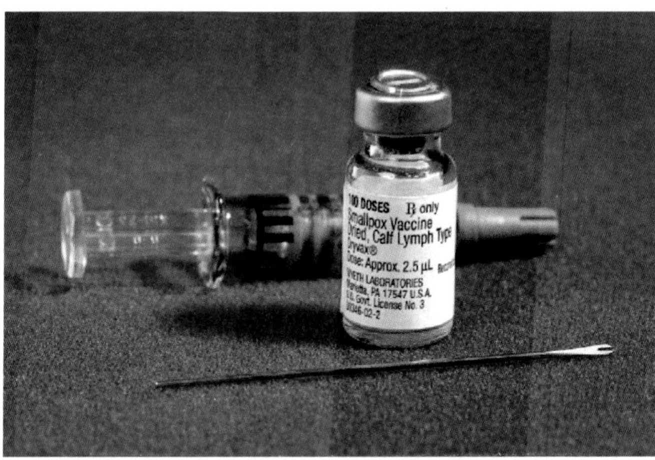

D

FIGURE 14.3. Origins of live attenuated viral vaccines. A: Edward Jenner is credited for performing the first vaccine experiment in which he demonstrated that inoculation of a boy with purulent material obtained from a cowpox lesion on the hand of a milkmaid protected him against subsequent challenge with variola. This event launched the formal concept of vaccination and established the prototypical approach for developing live attenuated viral vaccines. **B:** The implementation of smallpox vaccination faced many of the same issues of fear and misunderstanding that are prevalent today and impede the deployment of effective vaccines, as illustrated by a political cartoon published in 1804. **C:** The successful eradication of smallpox yielded many lessons about the value of simple, low-cost, local production of vaccine, as illustrated by the collection of vaccine material from the hide of a cow during the initial phases of the World Health Organization–sponsored eradication campaign. There were also lessons on the importance of product stability and simple delivery approaches. **D:** Once vaccinia was lyophilized, it could be reconstituted on site and was not as dependent on maintenance of the cold chain. The bifurcated needle **(D)** was an innovation that provided a simple standardized approach to inoculation without the need for needles or mechanical devices and allowed vaccination to penetrate remote locations. (**A** and **B,** courtesy of the National Library of Medicine; **C,** courtesy of J. Mohr, World Health Organization; **D,** courtesy of James Gathany/Centers for Disease Control and Prevention.)

intentional low-dose infection) to reduce the virulence of subsequent smallpox infection, which was initiated more than 1,000 years ago in India and China. From this arose the concept of vaccination (using an alternative agent to provide immunity against an infectious disease) and the first vaccine used in humans—live cowpox virus. In 1796, Edward Jenner inoculated 8-year old James Phipps with purulent material taken from a cowpox pustule on the hand of milkmaid Sarah Nelmes and introduced it into an incision on the boy's arm. Jenner subsequently proved that the boy was protected from an inoculation of material from a smallpox lesion. He published the work in 1798 and coined the word *vaccine* from the Latin *vacca* for cow, designating the process vaccination. For 80 years, live virus was transferred almost exclusively from human arm to arm by collection of purulent material. Subsequently, vaccine was propagated on the skin of calves using serial inoculation, resulting in vaccinia virus as the distinct vaccine strain.[260] This vaccine was used successfully to eradicate smallpox from the population, and smallpox remains the only human virus infection to be eradicated through a vaccination campaign (Fig. 14.3).

Origin of Inactivated Virus Vaccination

In the 1880s, Louis Pasteur and his colleagues attributed rabies to virus replication to the CNS. Next, they discovered that drying rabies-infected tissue at room temperature attenuated the infectivity of the tissue. The dried rabies-infected tissue was determined to be noninfectious, although serial inoculation of dogs with the tissues provided protection against an otherwise lethal rabies virus challenge. Inoculation of dried rabies-infected CNS tissue was tested in a single human postexposure case in 1885 when Pasteur serially inoculated Joseph Meister, a 9-year-old boy bitten by a rabid dog more than 2 days earlier. The initial inoculations contained highly attenuated virus from rabbit spinal cord dried for 15 days, followed by inoculations with less attenuated virus-infected tissue. In total, the regimen included 13 immunizations over 10 days. The boy was fully protected from disease, representing the beginning of an era in which inactivated vaccines were used for other viral diseases following Pasteur's paradigm of identification, inactivation, and inoculation (Fig. 14.4) and e-Table 14.1.

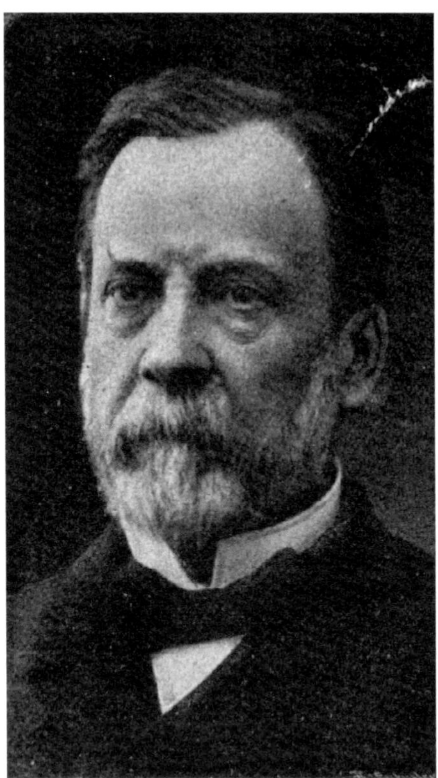

FIGURE 14.4. Origins of inactivated viral vaccines. Louis Pasteur is pictured here as the person responsible for the inactivated viral vaccine concept. His work on the rabies vaccine produced by desiccation of spinal cords from rabid dogs also anticipated the public debates that still occur involving the balance of risk and benefit to the individual and the public from the implementation of vaccines. (Courtesy of the National Library of Medicine.)

Critical Events in the History of Viral Vaccines

Since the introduction of vaccinia virus (Chapters 66 and 67), licensed vaccines have been developed for 15 other viral pathogens (Table 14.1). Notable advances in viral vaccine development over the past century include semieradication of many virus infections; processes for optimization of manufacturing cell lines for next-generation vaccines; utilization of human immune correlates to establish efficacy for licensure; and improvements in vaccine safety monitoring, which is important for public safety but also serves to keep safe and efficacious vaccines from unwarranted negative assessment.

Semieradication Secondary to Effective Vaccine Campaigns

Several vaccines have resulted in regional semieradication of virus disease or dramatic reduction in the incidence or morbidity from infection (polio, measles, mumps, rubella, rabies, and VZV). Other vaccines are highly effective and have been reduced to use only for travelers to endemic areas of the world (yellow fever, Japanese encephalitis). Licensed vaccines for influenza and hepatitis A and B are highly effective, and their impact on frequency of infection has been improved by new strategies for distribution (Table 14.2).

Modernization of Vaccine Manufacturing

The process of manufacturing a vaccine is complex, and the primary cornerstone in overall production is the substrate used for vaccine growth or antigen production. Early-generation vaccines were often grown in animal organ cells, including adenovirus vaccine in monkey kidney cells and Japanese encephalitis virus (JEV) vaccine in mouse brains. During the second half of the 20th century, modernization of vaccine production included the progression to use of cell lines as substrates, including current JEV vaccine in Vero cells and hepatitis B vaccine in yeast. Influenza vaccine researchers continue to develop U.S. marketed vaccines using chicken eggs as the substrate but have developed cell culture–based substrates that are used effectively in some European countries. The transition to cell-based substrates offers a more efficient, more reliable, and more stable manufacturing process.

Surrogate End Points for Vaccine Efficacy

Traditionally, the assessment of vaccine efficacy has been made by determining whether infection or disease has been

TABLE 14.1 Viral Vaccines Licensed in the United States[a]

Virus vaccine	Number of serotypes covered by vaccine	Type of vaccine			Target population	Comments
		Live	Inactivated	VLP		
Adenovirus[b]	2 (types 4 & 7)	+			Military recruits	WT virus in enteric-coated capsules orally to selectively infect the gut; lapse in manufacturing
Hepatitis A	1		+		Travelers, healthcare workers	IM; 2 doses; combined hepatitis A & B vaccine also available
Hepatitis B	1			+	All children	IM or SQ; 3 doses
Human papillomavirus	4 (types 6, 11, 16, & 18)			+	Preteen girls	IM to prevent cervical cancer; 3 doses
Influenza A & B	3 (H1N1, H3N2, & type B)	+	+		Elderly, patients with cardiopulmonary disease, school-age children, others	IM or ID; repeated annually with disrupted virus vaccine, or intranasal delivery of live attenuated vaccine
Japanese encephalitis	1		+		Travelers to endemic region	IM; single dose
Measles	1	+			All children	IM or SQ; single dose; booster recommended at 4–6 y of age
Mumps	1	+			All children	IM or SQ; single dose; booster recommended at 4–6 y of age
Poliovirus	3	+	+		All children	IM or SQ; 3 doses of inactivated vaccine recommended in United States; booster recommended at 4–6 y of age
Rabies	1		+		High-risk or exposed persons	IM; prophylactic 3 doses; therapeutic 4 doses
Rotavirus[b]	4 (G1, G2, G3, & G4)	+			All children	Oral vaccine based on rhesus rotavirus; 3 doses; removed from market because of concerns related to intussusception
	5 (G1, G2, G3, G4, & P[8])	+			All children	Oral vaccine; 3 doses; must start prior to 3 mo of age
	1 (G1P[8])	+			All children	Oral vaccine; 2 doses given at 2 & 4 mo of age
Rubella	1	+			All children	IM or SQ; single dose; booster recommended at 4–6 y of age
Smallpox	1	+			Military & first responder healthcare workers; recommended for laboratory workers using recombinant vaccinia virus	Intradermal vaccine used to eradicate smallpox
Varicella	1	+			All children; the elderly to diminish herpes zoster	IM or SQ; single dose; booster recommended at 4–6 y of age
Yellow fever	1	+	Travelers to endemic region	IM, single dose		
Total number of viruses covered	27	19	9	5		

VLP, virus-like particle; WT, wild-type; IM, intramuscular; SQ, subcutaneous; ID, intradermal.

[a]See individual chapters for specifics on target populations and immunization schedules for individual agents, which may vary or change from this overview. In addition, see the following website for a list of licensed vaccine products, including combination products: http://www.fda.gov/cber/vaccine/licvacc.htm.

[b]RotaShield tetravalent vaccine is no longer available. RotaTeq pentavalent and Rotarix monovalent vaccines are available.

TABLE 14.2 Impact of Licensed Vaccines on Viral Diseases With Well-Defined Surveillance and Estimated Impact on Disease Burden for Other Viral Vaccines

Viral disease	Year of peak U.S. prevalence	Peak number of cases per year in U.S.	Number of annual U.S. cases in modern vaccine era
Impact of licensed vaccines on viral diseases with well-defined surveillance			
Hepatitis A	1971	59,606	1,670[a]
Hepatitis B	1985	26,654	3,374[a]
Measles	1958–1962	503,282	63[a]
Mumps	1967	185,691	2,612[a]
Polio	1951–1954	16,316	0[a]
Rubella	1966–1968	47,745	5[a]
Congenital rubella	1966–1968	823	0[a]
Smallpox	1900–1904	48,164	0[a]
Estimated impact on disease burden for other viral vaccines			
Influenza A & B	Annual epidemics	~50,000 excess deaths per year[b]	Reduces morbidity & mortality; however, effectiveness varies from year to year because of variations in circulating virus strains
Japanese encephalitis	—	—	Only necessary for travel to endemic regions, highly effective
Rabies	<1940	>100 deaths/y	2–3/y[c]
Varicella	<1994	>4 million/y	Vaccine offers 83%–96% efficacy against primary infection[d]
Yellow fever	1905[e]	8,399	Only necessary for travel to endemic regions, highly effective

[a]http://www.cdc.gov/mmwr/preview/mmwrhtml/mm5953a1.htm.

[b]http://www.cdc.gov/mmwr/preview/mmwrhtml/mm5933a1.htm.

[c]http://www.cdc.gov/rabies/location/usa/surveillance/index.html.

[d]http://www.merck.com/product/usa/pi_circulars/v/varivax/varivax_pi.pdf.

[e]Last U.S. epidemic in New Orleans.

prevented. In the process of establishing vaccine efficacy, the use of a human immune correlate of protection is potentially more efficient and has been implemented successfully in the yearly approval process for influenza vaccines. Influenza vaccines typically are approved based on the accepted surrogate of protection, a hemagglutination inhibition (HAI) titer of 1:40 or higher or a fourfold increase over the prevaccination HAI titer. In this case, the immune response serves as a surrogate marker that is predetermined to predict clinical benefit; therefore, the more lengthy process of assessing the presence or absence of influenza infection in a clinical trial is not always needed (http://www.fda.gov/BiologicsBloodVaccines/GuidanceComplianceRegulatoryInformation/Guidances/Vaccines/ucm074794.htm). Similarly, assessing the end result of infection (or absence of) rather than documenting an effect on the virus itself can also be used to assess protective efficacy. HPV vaccines were licensed based on efficacy derived from the prevention of cervical and vulvar cancer, precancerous lesions, and dysplastic lesions (http://www.fda.gov/BiologicsBloodVaccines/Vaccines/ApprovedProducts/ucm111283.htm).

Maintaining Vaccine Availability

Vaccine efficacy, need, utilization, and safety (or perceived safety) all have a significant impact on the success of licensure and sustained availability of a vaccine. Two licensed vaccines that are no longer available are the adenovirus serotypes 4 and 7 and the tetravalent rhesus rotavirus vaccine. Production of the adenovirus vaccine, selectively given to new military recruits, was stopped by the sole manufacturer in 1995 for economic reasons. Since then, morbidity from adenovirus infections has increased among military recruits, and epidemics have occurred in training centers.[169] In addition to economic concerns, safety concerns have also prompted an abrupt end to the use of vaccines. Specifically, RotaShield, a live tetravalent rhesus rotavirus reassortant vaccine against the four major prevalent serotypes (based on VP7, a major outer capsid glycoprotein), was effective but was later withdrawn from market. A postmarketing analysis revealed that the vaccine was associated with an excess rate of intussusception of up to 1 per 2,500 vaccinees that occurred in the immediate postvaccination period, predominantly following the first dose of vaccine.[306] Following withdrawal of RotaShield, subsequent studies led to a significant downward revision of these estimates and have suggested that the early period of increase in intussusception seen after the first dose was followed by a period of compensatory decrease such that there was no net overall increase in the number of cases in vaccinees less than 1 year of age.[306] Furthermore, the excess cases of intussusception occurred mostly when the vaccine was used in children 3 months of age or older to "catch up" rather than in vaccinees who received the ideally recommended schedule of 2, 4, and 6 months of age.[212,403] This case highlights the importance of the analysis of postmarketing data, which needs to be especially thorough and comprehensive because it can dramatically impact the availability of a vaccine that may otherwise have a favorable risk/benefit ratio. Despite the initial conclusions and withdrawal of RotaShield from the market, two newer versions of a rotavirus vaccine have been developed. Pentavalent RotaTeq has been licensed in the United States for infants less than 3 months of age. It consists of a mixture of live attenuated, bovine/human reassortant viruses that express a single VP4 (P1A) as well as VP7 (G) Ag from G1 through G4 strains of rotavirus and VP4 (P1A[8]). P1A is the most common VP4 in G1, G3, and G4 strains and is present in a major portion of G9 viruses that are becoming more prevalent in some regions. The second new vaccine is a monovalent VP7 G1:P1A[8] attenuated human rotavirus strain that was first licensed in Mexico and the Dominican Republic[151] and later in 2008 in the United States. These two vaccines protect against severe gastroenteritis attributable to rotavirus. Large-scale postlicensure evaluations will be essential to more clearly elucidate the overall risks associated with rotavirus vaccines in the general population.

Future Directions in Vaccinology

In recent decades, major advances in viral vaccine development have coincided with the emergence of new technologies (Fig. 14.5). Therefore, selected technologies that are likely to influence future vaccine design are discussed briefly.

Impact of Advances in High-Throughput Sequencing Technology

The Human Genome Project simulated major investments in sequencing technology, resulting in breakthroughs that have increased throughput by orders of magnitude. As a result, it is now feasible to sequence all nucleic acids in samples of interest, such as vaccine preparations. Not surprisingly, such experiments have identified previously unidentified agents or nucleic acids in licensed vaccines, such as porcine circovirus type 1 (PCV1) in the commercial rotavirus vaccine Rotarix.[438] The U.S. Food and Drug Administration (FDA) temporarily suspended use of the vaccine in 2010; however, experts agreed that this highly prevalent nonpathogenic pig virus does not infect humans, and the use of vaccine was reinstituted. Some vaccines are produced in avian or primate cell lines, and thus it was not surprising that RNAs from avian leukosis virus, which is noninfectious for humans, or genetically defective DNAs from simian retrovirus (SRV) were present in products of such cell lines. Another interesting finding of such sequencing efforts is that the vaccine virus populations contain minority variants with polymorphisms or mutations (compared to the known sequence of the vaccine strains). Such variants have been observed for oral polio vaccine (OPV), mumps virus, and VZVs but are not known to affect attenuation.

Advances in Monoclonal Antibody Isolation

The neutralizing determinants on vaccine Ags are *de facto* the epitopes recognized by human Abs that mediate antiviral function. The study of the molecular and structural basis for neutralization has been limited by the difficulty in isolating human mAbs. Recent breakthroughs in this field using enhanced EBV transformation with CpG,[34] human hybridoma formation,[467] plasmablast sorting and cloning,[456] single B-cell sorting and expansion,[440] and other techniques have increased the numbers of human Abs for study by several orders of magnitude. Structural studies of complexes of human Abs with viral Ags have begun to yield fascinating insights into the features of protective Ab epitopes, which often are conformational, quaternary, and otherwise complex.[237]

Advances in Structural Biology

The ability to design optimal antigenic surfaces for induction of neutralizing Abs has long been a dream of vaccine scientists. The goal is to develop synthetic constructs that elicit Abs with predetermined structural specificity. In particular, induction of Abs against epitopes that are hidden in the native viral protein has been a challenge for vaccine design. Investigators working in the areas of structural biology and computational modeling

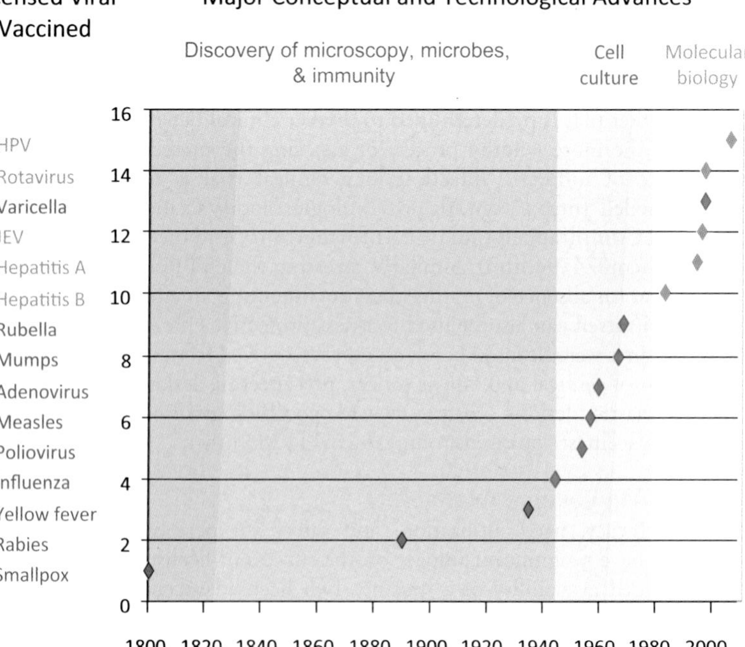

FIGURE 14.5. History of viral vaccines. Viral vaccines can be organized by the major technology that made their development feasible. Licensed viral vaccines are listed on the **left** axis in chronological order. They are color coded, indicating the major development era or technology with which they were associated. Significant advances since the initial age of empiricism have been coincident with the development of cell culture techniques and molecular biology. One can envision that advances in some of the technologies discussed in the text, such as structural biology, advances in sequencing, and gene expression vectors, may facilitate vaccine development for unmet and unanticipated future needs for prevention of viral diseases.

recently have made significant progress in this regard. Computationally designed epitope-scaffolds that are immunogenic have been developed for the HIV-1 gp41 epitopes of the broadly neutralizing mAbs 2F5[326] and 4E10[93] and the RSV F motavizumab epitope.[274] Structural information from HIV gp120 CD4 binding site epitope recognized by the neutralizing Ab b12 has been used to design gp120 reagents to select additional CD4 binding site Abs that have broad neutralizing activity against HIV.[474] Fragments of influenza HA have been expressed to focus the immune response to conserved epitopes in the HA stem region.[41] Computational and structural tools also can be used for design of viral inhibitors—for example, the design of proteins targeting the influenza HA stem that mimic the action of neutralizing Abs. It seems likely that computationally designed Ags will increasingly influence viral vaccine design.

LIVE VIRUS VACCINES

History of Methods for Isolating Attenuated Strains

Varying methods have been used to achieve attenuation for live virus vaccines. Type 2 poliovirus, strain 712, one of the three poliovirus vaccine strains in the live vaccine preparation, is a naturally occurring attenuated human poliovirus that was identified by its lack of virulence for the brain and spinal cord of monkeys.[382] Adenovirus vaccine strains (types 4 and 7) are wild-type human respiratory viruses used in the U.S. military that produced an asymptomatic infection following oral administration that was restricted in replication to the intestinal tract.[68] The remaining attenuated vaccine viruses were derived from wild-type human viruses by serial passage in cell cultures prepared from an unnatural host, leading to the emergence of mutants that were partially restricted in humans at the portal of entry and/or the target organ(s). In this manner, attenuated mutants of rubella virus and types 1 and 3 poliovirus were selected after passage in monkey kidney tissue culture. Vaccine strains of yellow fever virus (17D strain) and measles virus were generated by multiple passage in chick embryo cell culture, whereas mumps virus was attenuated by multiple passages in embryonated eggs.

A critical feature of most successful live vaccine development programs is the identification of preclinical laboratory predictors of attenuation. For the yellow fever virus and poliovirus vaccines, promising vaccine strains were identified by their attenuation for experimental animals. In monkeys, the 17D strain of yellow fever virus exhibited decreased tropism for the liver, suggesting that this mutant might be suitably attenuated for humans[423]—a hypothesis that was confirmed during subsequent clinical trials. Naturally occurring or tissue culture–passaged strains of poliovirus were evaluated for neurovirulence in monkeys by intraspinal inoculation, which was a central innovation that allowed Sabin to identify attenuated strains.[381,382] This testing system was selected because several observations suggested that the spinal cord of monkeys was more permissive than that of humans to the neuronolytic effect of poliovirus.[382] Viruses that caused the least neurovirulence in monkeys were identified, and these strains then were cloned and recloned biologically by the plaque technique to yield progeny with the lowest possible level of monkey neurovirulence. These candidate vaccine strains then were subjected to additional cycles of selection, which led to the identification of mutants that replicated with high efficiency in the intestinal tract without significant increase in neurovirulence for nonhuman primates. These viruses were evaluated in clinical trials and were shown to be satisfactorily attenuated and immunogenic.

Experimental animal systems were not available for evaluating virulence of the other vaccine viruses. Therefore, these viruses were tested for attenuation directly in humans. Initial candidate measles and rubella virus vaccines were insufficiently attenuated, although further passage of rubella virus in monkey kidney cell culture and selection of a cold-adapted, temperature-sensitive mutant of measles virus yielded satisfactory vaccine strains. Attenuation of mumps virus passaged in eggs also was determined in humans. Interestingly, the Jeryl Lynn strain of mumps virus vaccine developed by Maurice Hilleman as a clinical isolate from his daughter was found to be a mixture of two closely related strains of mumps virus.[7] Several other vaccines have been found to be mixtures of virus strains, including the yellow fever virus vaccine and some vaccinia stocks used for smallpox vaccination.

Poliovirus and adenovirus vaccines are administered orally, whereas yellow fever, rubella, measles, and mumps virus vaccines are given parenterally. Each of the currently licensed live virus vaccines is directed against a virus that has a complex pathogenesis of infection in which virus is introduced by inoculation (yellow fever) or by implantation on a mucosal surface (measles, mumps, rubella, and poliovirus) with subsequent spread systemically to the target organ(s). The requirement of such viruses to pass through blood to reach the target organ of disease makes them generally susceptible to serum Abs. It is more difficult to protect against infection by viruses that cause disease at a mucosal portal of entry without the need for viremia.

Advantages of Live Virus Vaccines

The major advantage of live virus vaccines is the activation of all components of the immune system yielding both a balanced systemic and local immune response and a broad humoral and cell-mediated response. This type of comprehensive induction of immune effectors is particularly important for infections in which cell-mediated immunity plays an important role and for mucosal infections in which both local and systemic immunity are required for optimal resistance. As noted, mucosal infection with a live virus vaccine is much more effective in stimulating a local response in the unprimed host than inactivated virus vaccines administered parenterally.[305] Live virus vaccines also can stimulate an immune response to each of the protective Ags of a virus, and this obviates the difficulties that arise from selective destruction of one of the protective Ags that may occur during the inactivation process and can lead to disease potentiation. This advantage is especially important for complex viruses encoding many protective Ags, because it is prohibitively difficult and expensive to immunize with multiple purified proteins or to construct multivalent vectors. Furthermore, immunity induced by live virus vaccines is generally more durable and more effective.[204] There are practical advantages to many live virus vaccines, such as relatively low cost of production and ease of administration. Live viruses contribute to protection in populations because of the induction of herd immunity, sometimes facilitated by transmission of vaccine viruses from a recipient to a contact. The effectiveness of live vaccines in settings of high transmission is illustrated by the use of adenovirus vaccines. Adenovirus vaccines have reduced military respiratory disease morbidity significantly over the past three decades. In 1995, however, the manufacturer of these vaccines ceased production owing to budgetary constraints. Major outbreaks of serious adenovirus infections occurred in military facilities as a consequence.

Disadvantages of Live Virus Vaccines

The major concerns with live virus vaccines are that they (a) can contain adventitious agents; (b) can cause illness directly; (c) can lose their attenuation during manufacture or during replication in vaccinees by reversion or by second-site compensatory mutations; (d) can spread to contacts; and (e) can lose infectivity during storage, transport, or use. The potential for contamination with live adventitious agents always exists as discussed previously. Sources include the original clinical sample from which the virus was isolated, cell culture substrates, laboratory reagents of animal origin (such as serum supplements and trypsin), and contamination from laboratory workers or environments. Cross-contamination of vaccine lots with other viruses in a laboratory facility is possible. Fortunately, contamination of clinical lots of vaccine with major human pathogenic adventitious agents has rarely been a problem in the modern era. Some of the early lots of live poliovirus vaccine were contaminated with live SV40, and the live yellow fever virus vaccine was initially contaminated with an avian leukosis virus. Follow-up of individuals who were given live vaccine contaminated with SV40 or avian leukosis virus has failed to identify any long-term adverse effect, including cancer, associated with exposure to these adventitious viruses.[291,412,446]

Some live virus vaccines, such as the measles virus, rubella virus, and yellow fever virus vaccines, retain a low level of residual virulence. The reactions produced by these vaccines generally are minor and have not interfered with acceptance and widespread use of these products. A more serious problem is that of restoration of a varying degree of virulence during infection by vaccine virus. This occurs with the poliovirus vaccine at an extremely low frequency—that is, about one in 10^6 to 10^7 immunizations.[319] Most vaccine-associated cases of paralysis in vaccinees or their close contacts occur after the first dose and involve the type 3 vaccine strain.[319] A significant proportion of the paralytic illnesses associated with poliovirus vaccine occurs in individuals who are immunocompromised; however, this may not represent a manifestation of genetic alteration of vaccine virus.[319]

The genetic basis for the very rare increase in virulence of the poliovirus vaccine strains during replication *in vivo* is relatively well understood. However, a paradox exists in that mutation toward a higher level of virulence for the CNS occurs rapidly and frequently during replication of poliovirus in the intestinal tract of vaccinees, although vaccine-associated paralytic disease is extremely rare. During manufacture of vaccine, the mutations that are associated with restoration of virulence can be detected at variable low frequency by sequence analysis, and neurovirulence of the final product can be held to a low level by rejecting vaccine lots that exceed the accepted standard for frequency of these mutations.[76] Genetic instability was also a problem with the 17D yellow fever virus vaccine during early field trials. Encephalitis was observed in 1% to 2% of young vaccinees administered virus that had been passaged 20 times beyond the original seed lot.[137]

The problem of genetic instability of live attenuated virus vaccines following replication *in vivo* is an even larger concern for viruses that can cause latent or persistent infection *in vivo* such as herpes viruses or lentiviruses (e.g., HIV). Despite this concern, successful vaccines have been developed for VZV—a herpesvirus that causes chickenpox and zoster—indicating that a successful live attenuated vaccine can be developed for a virus that causes a lifelong infection in humans. This vaccine was licensed first for prevention of childhood chickenpox and has recently been shown to significantly reduce the risk of VZV reactivation or shingles.[333]

Rubella virus can be recovered from the lymphocytes of immunologically normal individuals with arthritis up to 6 years after immunization or natural infection[69]; however, the rubella virus vaccine does not appear to be associated with chronic arthritis.[364] Interestingly, persistence of measles vaccine virus has not been detected, nor has the vaccine virus been implicated in subacute sclerosing panencephalitis.[281] Instead, widespread use of live measles vaccine has almost eradicated this rare but serious sequelae of persistent wild-type measles virus infection.

Several other concerns have been identified for live attenuated virus vaccines. First, there is a theoretical risk that infection of the fetus could occur following vaccination during the first trimester of pregnancy. For rubella vaccine, there is concern that vaccination might lead to development of the congenital rubella syndrome; however, the actual risk appears to be negligible.[339] Second, naturally occurring wild-type viruses may interfere with infection by a live virus vaccine, resulting in a decrease in vaccine efficacy. Such interference has been observed primarily with live poliovirus vaccine strains and is caused by a wide variety of enteric viruses. This phenomenon has also been seen with experimental live attenuated alphavirus vaccines.[270] To overcome this viral–viral interference, multiple doses of polyvalent live virus vaccines are required to assure a protective immune response to each component. Third, defective interfering particles have been identified in preparations of live virus vaccines,[55] and it is likely that they are present in all live virus vaccines to some degree. Fourth, live attenuated measles virus vaccine has been associated with a generalized immunosuppression that was observed to be directly correlated with the level of immune response to the vaccine.[199]

Finally, it should be noted that stability is a serious practical problem with thermolabile vaccine viruses such as measles virus. The need for storage and transport of measles vaccine at low temperature (4°C) has limited its usefulness in some tropical areas where maintenance of a "cold chain" for transport and storage is difficult. Some simple solutions for stabilizing other live virus vaccines have been identified, such as lyophilization of vaccinia virus or using deuterium oxide for water in live poliovirus or influenza vaccine formulations,[200,283] although additional work is needed.

Genetic Basis for Attenuation of Live Viruses

Mutants selected by passage in an unnatural host accumulate many mutations, often making it difficult to define in a precise manner the genetic basis for their attenuation. In some cases, the molecular basis of attenuation has been defined. The genetic basis of this neuroattenuation of each of the three poliovirus vaccine strains has been partially defined.[170] Surprisingly, few mutations are involved. Analyses have identified attenuating nucleotide substitutions in 5′ noncoding sequences and others attenuating in the 3′ noncoding region or in the structural or nonstructural coding regions of type 1, type 2, or type 3 polioviruses.[45,147,367] These mutations can now be monitored during manufacture and following replication *in vivo*. Vaccine lots with an increased frequency of reversion at some residues have been shown to exhibit increased neurovirulence, and such lots can be discarded as unacceptable for human use.[76] Thus, it is now possible to use molecular virological techniques to control the manufacture of vaccines by identifying the presence of the desired attenuating mutations as well as the absence, or low frequency, of unwanted reversions.[76]

The Jennerian approach to the development of live attenuated viruses involves the use of a virus strain of mammalian or avian origin to immunize humans against a human virus that is related antigenically to the animal or avian strain. Mammalian and avian viruses that are well adapted to their natural host often do not replicate efficiently in humans and hence are attenuated. At present, we lack a complete understanding of the genetic basis for this form of host-range restriction. However, those mammalian or avian viral genes that have been identified as being responsible for host-range restriction in humans exhibit significant divergence of nucleotide sequence from that of the corresponding human viral genes. Quadrivalent and pentavalent rotavirus vaccine are examples of the Jennerian approach to vaccine development in which a nonhuman rotavirus strain, the rhesus rotavirus or bovine rotavirus, was found to be attenuated in humans. Because there was a need for a multivalent vaccine that would induce resistance to each of the major human rotavirus serotypes, the Jennerian approach was modified by constructing three reassortant viruses, each of which contained 10 rhesus rotavirus or bovine rotovirus genes plus a single human rotavirus gene encoding one of the major neutralization Ags of the targeted serotypes.

Conventional techniques for attenuation of viruses such as passage of virus at low temperature, mutagenesis followed by selection of mutants with the desired phenotype(s), or passage of virus in heterologous tissues continue to play a significant role in the development of live virus vaccines. These techniques have been used to generate candidate vaccine strains for CMV, ortho- and paramyxoviruses, alphaviruses, flaviviruses, hepatitis A virus, and arenaviruses. Selection for a combination of phenotypes (such as cold adapted and *ts*) is thought to be desirable because the different mutations can have synergistic effects on the stability of the attenuation phenotype *in vivo*.[304] Viruses bearing stable, molecularly defined, identifiable attenuating mutations or attenuating gene constellations represent the vaccine strains of the future, because the genetic basis for attenuation will be known and can be monitored directly during all phases of vaccine development, manufacture, and utilization in humans.

The function of viral proteins can be altered by missense mutations, insertions, or deletions. Classically, attenuated viruses were identified using biologic phenotypes: (a) *ts* mutants; (b) cold-passaged (*cp*) or cold-adapted (*ca*) mutants; (c) small plaque mutants; (d) protease activation (*pa*) mutants (also designated as cleavage mutants); and (e) mutants with altered interaction with host cell receptors. With modern molecular techniques, virulent viruses also can be attenuated by a wide variety of creative approaches including gene deletion, shuffling of gene order, alteration of noncoding regulatory regions contain cis-acting signals required for efficient replication, the use of gene incompatibility in chimeric genomes, and the insertion of genes that encode proteins with known antiviral activities or with known immunoregulatory functions.

INACTIVATED VIRUS VACCINES

Inactivated virus vaccines are available in the United States for the prevention of disease caused by nine separate viral agents (see Table 14.1). The available vaccines are based on either whole inactivated virus or virus-like particles (VLPs) produced from purified protein. The viruses are grown in a variety of cell substrates, including eggs (influenza types A and B), a continuous monkey kidney cell line (poliovirus types 1, 2, and 3), human diploid fibroblasts (rabies, hepatitis A), or mouse brain (JEV vaccine). Virus is then inactivated with a chemical such as formalin or disrupted with a detergent (influenza). The level of efficacy of inactivated viral vaccines differs: Inactivated poliovirus vaccine is highly effective in preventing disease, whereas influenza virus vaccine is only partially protective.

Features of Inactivated Virus Vaccines

Inactivated virus vaccines offer the advantage of immunization with the entire antigenic content of the virus with little or no risk of infection. Only rarely do such vaccines contain a contaminating adventitious agent or residual infectious virus that has resisted inactivation. For example, paralytic disease was produced by some of the early lots of inactivated poliovirus vaccine that contained residual infectious virus.[313,327] Contamination by an infectious adventitious agent was also detected retrospectively in some early lots of inactivated poliovirus. This was of some concern because the contaminating simian virus, SV40, was oncogenic in hamsters.[194] Fortunately, long-term follow-up of individuals who were inoculated with SV40-contaminated vaccine during early infancy failed to show evidence of a vaccine-induced oncogenic effect.[412] Another incident occurred in a research setting where live vaccinia virus was found to be present in a preparation of inactivated vaccinia–HIV recombinant virus being evaluated as a therapeutic vaccine in HIV-infected subjects. Unfortunately, an immunodeficient recipient of this vaccine developed progressive vaccinia caused by residual live virus in the inoculum.[470] Several inactivated whole virus vaccines have potentiated disease rather than prevented it.[143,219] This finding was first observed with formalin-inactivated measles virus vaccine.[143] Initially, this vaccine prevented measles; however, after several years, vaccinees lost their resistance to infection. When subsequently infected with naturally circulating measles virus, the vaccinees developed an atypical illness with accentuated systemic symptoms and pneumonia.[143,310] Retrospective analysis showed that formalin inactivation destroyed the ability of the measles fusion (F) protein to induce hemolysis-inhibiting Abs, although it did not destroy the ability of the H (HA or attachment) protein to induce neutralizing Abs.[320,321] When the H-specific Ab had waned sufficiently to permit extensive infection with measles virus, an altered and sometimes more severe disease was seen at the sites of measles virus replication.[53] This atypical disease is believed to be mediated in part by an altered cell-mediated immune response in which Th2 cells[356] or a delayed-type hypersensitivity reaction[246] were induced preferentially, leading to heightened disease manifestations at the sites of viral replication. Immune complex deposition also plays a role in the pathogenesis of atypical measles.[357]

Potentiation of disease also was observed after parenteral administration of an experimental formalin-inactivated respiratory syncytial virus (FI-RSV) vaccine.[219] In clinical trials conducted in the mid-1960s, an FI-RSV vaccine induced a measurable serum-neutralizing Ab response but did not protect the youngest vaccinees. Unexpectedly, on subsequent natural infection with RSV, the FI-RSV vaccinees developed severe RSV lower respiratory tract disease significantly more often than did infants and young children who had received an inactivated parainfluenza virus vaccine.[219] Speculation on the mechanism of disease potentiation by the inactivated RSV vaccine has centered on several possible aberrations of the immune response to vaccine that involve an imbalance between or within various compartments of the immune system. Most likely, the protective antigenic sites on the F protein were altered by fixation, and the altered Ag induced an aberrant T-cell and cytokine response leading to enhanced disease as recently reviewed.[165] The major lesson learned from the FI-RSV vaccine-enhanced illness is that the chemical treatment and physical purification procedures used for the preparation of each new inactivated vaccine should be evaluated not only for their effect on the magnitude of immune responses but also on the functional characteristics of the response. Typically, the Ab induced should have neutralizing activity, and the T-cell responses should mediate efficient virus clearance.

Potentiation of disease by an inactivated virus vaccine is not limited to vaccines containing measles virus or RSV and has occurred with both human and veterinary vaccines. For example, administration of an inactivated caprine lentivirus vaccine has also been associated with an accelerated, more severe disease in animals subsequently challenged with virus.[273] Vaccine-enhanced pathology is also not limited to inactivated virus vaccines. Immunization with a subunit vaccine of another lentivirus—equine infectious anemia virus (EIAV)—enhanced disease caused by subsequent challenge with a heterologous EIAV strain.[201] A similar phenomenon occurred during the development of a vaccine for feline infectious peritonitis virus (FIPV). FIPV is a CoV that developed more notoriety after the emergence of the severe acute respiratory syndrome (SARS) CoV in 2003. Attempts to develop a vaccine against FIPV have been largely unsuccessful and associated with a vaccine-enhanced illness. A major problem is that Abs are not protective even when given passively for prophylaxis, and they can facilitate virus entry through Fc receptors. Whole virus,[345] recombinant vaccinia expressing the major surface S (spike) glycoprotein,[437] or DNA immunization with IL-12[150] all have led to enhanced disease syndromes. Immunization of ferrets with a recombinant modified vaccinia virus Ankara (MVA) expressing the S glycoprotein has also caused an enhanced disease with hepatitis after SARS CoV immunization. Although the immunological mechanisms responsible for these examples of enhanced disease have not been identified, there are two common features present in these settings to consider. First, there was induction of a memory T-cell response in the absence of prechallenge Ab that could effectively neutralize virus. This is analogous to the conditions associated with measles and RSV vaccine-enhanced disease. Second, these are viruses that have tropism for Fc receptor bearing cells. The presence of binding Ab that does not effectively neutralize virus could thereby facilitate entry and amplify viral replication. Vaccine studies with DNA or recombinant vectors, subunit proteins, or inactivated virus alone or in combination that have induced effective neutralizing Ab responses to the SARS CoV in animal models have not been associated with enhanced illness postchallenge.

Another disadvantage of inactivated virus particle vaccines is that they typically have to be given parenterally because without replication or gene expression, it is difficult for mucosally delivered Ag to elicit a significant inductive event. Parenteral induction of systemic immunity may not fully protect against viruses that infect and cause disease primarily at mucosal surfaces if the gradient of Ab between serum and mucosa is too large or the kinetics of viral entry are too rapid. Therefore, resistance to viral challenge in the upper respiratory tract or in the intestines may be less robust than that conferred by local immunization or infection. This may be the reason inactivated influenza vaccines are only partially protective, and why the inactivated polio vaccine (IPV) can prevent paralytic polio but cannot prevent poliovirus infection and intestinal carriage. There are clear exceptions to this principle, which are best exemplified by the success of parenterally administered HPV vaccine. Although HPV is a purely mucosal pathogen, it has recently been shown that entry into basal epithelial cells is a two-step process that may take several hours.[222] Virus neutralization can be accomplished with much less Ab when given longer access to the viral antigenic sites.

Inactivated virus vaccines are clearly at a disadvantage compared to either live attenuated virus vaccines or vector-based gene delivery with respect to induction of a CTL response. CD8 CTL responses require Ags to be processed through the proteasome so that peptides can be transported into the endoplasmic reticulum and associate with MHC class I molecules. This is best achieved when proteins are synthesized in the host cell cytoplasm and is rarely achieved in primates when Ags enter the APC through the endocytic pathway. For example, inactivated influenza virus is considerably less effective than virus infection in stimulating a primary CTL response in mice. However, inactivated influenza A virus or purified surface glycoproteins derived from it can sometimes stimulate a secondary CTL response in sensitized mice or humans.[5,122] There are new adjuvants and delivery vehicles that have the capacity for moving purified proteins into the MHC class I presentation pathway, and these may be considerations for future vaccine development.

The Guillain-Barré syndrome was associated with widespread use of inactivated influenza A H1N1 (swine) virus vaccine during 1976 and 1977,[240] indicating that unanticipated, delayed, or untoward side effects can be induced by inactivated virus vaccines. This syndrome has been associated only rarely with subsequent influenza virus vaccines and was not reported at all following the rapid introduction of vaccines against the 2009 H1N1 pandemic strain, even though these products were prepared in the same manner as the 1976 vaccine.[240] The basis for this idiosyncratic syndrome associated with the 1976 influenza vaccine is still not defined.

Future Considerations for Inactivated Virus Vaccine Development

Formaldehyde, heat, and oxidation have been shown to produce reactive carbonyl groups on protein Ags that promote

CD4 T-cell responses with Th2 differentiation.[285] Chemical inactivation of poliovirus during vaccine manufacturing can result in modification of a major neutralization epitope. Therefore, inactivating infectivity of nonenveloped and enveloped viruses can adversely affect the antigenicity of the vaccine.[130] It has also been recognized that antigenic changes can occur during selection and amplification of influenza viruses in the allantoic cavity of embryonated eggs—the substrate used to produce virus for the inactivated vaccine.[370] The genetic basis for these mutations involves host cell selection of mutants that replicate more efficiently in eggs. These variants acquire a mutation in or near the receptor binding pocket of the HA that increases their efficiency of replication in eggs but also alters antigenicity and immunogenicity. Nevertheless, influenza viruses that are used to prepare inactivated vaccine for humans are grown in eggs, and such vaccines have been repeatedly shown to be protective. Although this would not be a problem for influenza vaccines produced in mammalian cell culture, vaccine Ags may be modified or processed in ways that compromise antigenicity even in mammalian cell substrates. For example, poliovirus grown in tissue culture contains an uncleaved outer capsid protein, VP1, which is usually cleaved in a natural infection by intestinal proteases. Although tissue culture–grown poliovirus has limited ability to induce Abs that neutralize viruses containing a cleaved VP1,[371] both cleaved and uncleaved VP1 can induce protection from replication of subsequently administered live attenuated poliovirus vaccine.[350] Nevertheless, careful assessment of the substrate-dependent antigenicity and consequences of inactivation is warranted in the development of inactivated virus vaccines.

VIRUS-LIKE PARTICLE VACCINES

There are licensed VLP vaccines for two viral pathogens (HBV and HPV). The VLPs are produced as self-assembling capsid proteins in yeast or insect cells. For the purposes of this section, we will define VLP as self-assembling viral proteins that can mimic the particle structure of virions and present the quaternary structures of oligomeric viral surface proteins but do not package the virus genome. There are other self-assembling nonviral proteins that can be used to display vaccine Ags that are mentioned with nanoparticles in the Delivery Vehicles section.

The initial version of the HBV vaccine was based on surface Ag purified from the blood of persons persistently infected with HBV. The Australia Ag was associated with the disease caused by HBV, and later the Dane particle was found to represent the Australia Ag. Interestingly, electron microscopy revealed not only the Dane particle, which is a 42-nm structure representing the complete infectious virion, but also smaller particles and filaments. The 22-nm particle was found to be comprised of just HBsAg and is noninfectious because it does not contain nucleic acid. This small particle, purified from human plasma, was the first licensed HBV vaccine. An effective second-generation HBsAg vaccine was developed using a recombinant plasmid to express the gene for HBsAg in yeast. Yeast-produced HBsAg self-assembles into uniform 22-nm particles. Although the 22-nm noninfectious particle is smaller in size and technically a defective genomeless subvirion particle, it is considered a VLP because it is made of the same capsid protein (HBsAg) as the full particle. Licensed HBV VLPs are formulated with alum and are now part of the routine pediatric vaccine schedule. This vaccine often is protective against HBV infection and hepatitis even in the absence of detectable Ab response. Immunization against HBV also significantly reduces the frequency of hepatoma and is regarded as the first anticancer vaccine.[67] The immunogenicity of HBV VLP in patients with renal failure, HIV-1 infection, or other immunocompromising conditions is diminished. New adjuvant approaches such as formulation with CpG (TLR-9 agonist), monophosphoryl lipid A (MPL)+alum, or MPL+QS21 are being explored to improve vaccine-induced immunity in those settings.[32,33,91] HBV VLPs are now produced for human use in nine countries using yeast, bacteria, or mammalian cells for manufacturing, and other substrates including transgenic plants are being explored.[375]

HPV particles were first identified by electron microscopy in 1949. In 1983, the association between HPV infection and cervical dysplasia and malignancy was proven.[117] In 1991, it was shown that VLPs lacking genomes could be produced by expression of the L1 and L2[473] or just the L1[224] capsid proteins of papillomaviruses. L1 self-assembles into pentamers, and each VLP is comprised of 72 pentameric capsomeres. If present, one L2 protein is associated with the center of each L1 pentamer on the inner surface of the capsid. These key discoveries led to the development of candidate VLP vaccines. Importantly, the end points for the efficacy trial were chosen carefully. Although prevention of cervical carcinoma was the goal, this target was not an acceptable end point because ablative treatment would be performed if premalignant lesions were detected. Therefore, cervical intraepithelial neoplasia grade 2 or higher was used as the end point for vaccine efficacy trials as a surrogate for cervical carcinoma. Prevention of persistent serotype-specific HPV infection was also a primary end point. Yeast-produced HPV 16 VLP formulated in alum and delivered parenterally was 100% effective in preventing cervical intraepithelial neoplasia.[232] A three-dose regimen of a tetravalent L1-based VLP vaccine based on HPV 16 and 18 (most common causes of cervical intraepithelial neoplasia) and HPV 6 and 11 (most common causes of anogenital warts) is also highly effective.[439] Subsequent studies have shown that HPV VLP immunization can prevent HPV-induced cervical lesions in women[4] and anogenital lesions in both women and men.[146,149] Three doses containing 30 μg of each of the four VLPs formulated with aluminum hydroxyphosphate sulfate (Gardasil) or 20 μg of each of two VLPs formulated with a mixture of aluminum hydroxide and 3-deacylated MPL (AS04) (Cervarix) are sufficient to achieve protective immunity that is durable for more than 5 years.[374] The protection has been correlated with type-specific neutralizing Ab. A nonavalent VLP vaccine including serotypes 6, 11, 16, 18, 31 33, 45, 52, and 58 is being evaluated in efficacy trials in an attempt to extend the coverage against cervical neoplasia from 70% to more than 90%.

Advantages of Virus-Like Particle Vaccines

Capsid proteins from many nonenveloped viruses and the nucleocapsid or matrix proteins together with surface proteins from some enveloped viruses can self-assemble into VLPs and provide a platform technology that may be applicable as vaccines for multiple virus families. VLPs offer several advantages as immunogens. First, the viral nucleic acid is not present in

VLPs, thus there is no concern that viral oncogenes or other pathogenic features of the live virus are present. Second, VLPs present conformational epitopes to the immune system in the same way as native infectious particles so that neutralizing Abs and other protective immune responses are induced efficiently. Some of these epitopes are formed by the juxtaposition of parts of two different capsid proteins. Third, many of the nonenveloped viruses from which immunogenic VLPs have been developed replicate poorly or not at all in tissue culture (e.g., B19 parvovirus, papillomaviruses, and hepatitis E virus), thus precluding the use of purified virus as immunogen. Fourth, because VLPs are noninfectious, chemical inactivation is not required. For this reason, VLPs might prove to be better immunogens than formalin-inactivated whole virus vaccines because the deleterious effects of formalin on structure and immunogenicity can be avoided. Fifth, the immune system responds better to a viral Ag presented as an assembled multimeric particle rather than as an individual monomeric protein. Sixth, the stability of VLPs from nonenveloped viruses may simplify vaccine storage and distribution and also make successful oral delivery feasible in some cases.[318]

Disadvantages of Virus-Like Particle Vaccines

The major disadvantage of VLP vaccines is related to the cost and complexity of manufacture, although costs should become lower with advances and expansion of the options for cell substrates. The biological disadvantage of VLPs compared to replication-competent viruses or vectors is that there is not ongoing production of Ag following vaccination. However, these particles tend to be highly antigenic and stable, and immunogenicity can be enhanced with adjuvants.

Future Considerations for Virus-Like Particle Vaccine Development

VLPs have been engineered successfully for viruses belonging to a wide range of virus families, including both nonenveloped and enveloped viruses. Because of the advantages listed previously and track record of success, they should be considered as a vaccine platform technology for other virus families when possible.

Nonenveloped Virus-Like Particles

The first characterization of synthetic VLPs followed the observation that picornavirus capsid proteins could self-assemble during the *in vitro* translation of viral RNA to yield 75S to 85S particles.[335] Later studies indicated that VLPs could form *in vitro* following translation of picornavirus viral RNA lacking most of the 5′ noncoding region.[80] Next, it was observed that expression of the open reading frames of capsid proteins of nonenveloped viruses by a baculovirus or vaccinia vector in appropriate eukaryotic cells resulted in generation of VLPs.[81,224,473] For picornaviruses, particle assembly requires expression of the entire open reading frame to permit the proteolytic processing of the structural proteins by nonstructural viral-encoded proteases. There are current vaccine development approaches being used for enterovirus 71 that involve VLP technology.[78]

Human parvovirus B19 causes erythema infectiosum, acute and chronic red cell aplasia, and other illnesses. A vaccine candidate consisting of the human parvovirus B19 VP1 and VP2 capsid proteins that form VLPs is being developed.[22] Immunization of humans with this vaccine induces neutralizing Abs that achieve levels equivalent in magnitude and neutralizing activity to those seen following natural infection.[44] Antigenic VLPs can be readily produced for other human (bocavirus)[66] and veterinary parvoviruses,[373] suggesting that VLP-based vaccines may be an appropriate approach for pathogens for this viral family.

Norovirus, the prototypic member of the calicivirus family, also may be a good candidate target for a VLP vaccine. The virus is a 28- to 37-nm nonenveloped particle that is formed by a single major capsid protein (VP1). VP1 is a protein with two domains connected by a short linker. The P domain forms the outer surface of the particle, and the S domain forms an inner shell. The P portion of VP1 can self-assemble 24 protomers to form a 20-nm particle that is immunogenic.[417]

Enveloped Virus-Like Particles

Expression of the nucleoprotein or matrix proteins of some enveloped viruses has also resulted in the production of VLP or virus pseudoparticles. This finding was noted first for the Gag protein of HIV when it was expressed in recombinant vaccinia-infected cells.[178,196] Production of purified HIV pseudovirions is being developed as a vaccine strategy,[127] and the construction of vectors that are competent to produce pseudovirions *in vivo* may improve immunogenicity beyond that of the simple expression of the isolated gene products.[72,182] VLPs have now been produced for several respiratory viral pathogens. Expression of M1, M2, NA, and HA can form influenza VLPs[241]; however, HA is sufficient in the presence of NA.[71] These are potent immunogens that can be constructed to express Ags that can confer broad cross-reactivity[406] or TLR agonists that can provide adjuvant properties.[441] SARS CoV pseudoparticles are formed by transfection of 293 cells with the M (membrane) and N (nucleocapsid) genes.[197] The M protein of Newcastle disease virus (NDV) is sufficient to produce VLPs[337] that can support the incorporation and display of RSV F and G and is immunogenic and protective in animal models.[272] The NDV VLPs appears to be a stable platform for presentation of viral glycoproteins from other viruses as well.[290] Alphaviruses and flaviviruses are also potential viral targets for VLP vaccines. For example, West Nile virus pseudoparticles are formed by co-expression of prM and E.[184] Recently, chikungunya virus VLPs were produced that protected rhesus macaques from lethal challenge.[8]

Novel chimeric particles in which viral Ags are built onto the hepatitis B core VLP[43] are immunogenic in mice. Relatively large structures can be mounted on the recombinant VLPs if inserted covalently into the outer loops or attached through chemical conjugation in the right place and orientation to allow access to the vaccine Ag being displayed. Other chimeric VLPs can be constructed by inserting candidate vaccine Ags into the variable loops that face outward, including norovirus P particles,[418] Chikungunya,[8] or others, and could be selected based on the desired particle size and Ag valency (Fig. 14.6).

OTHER VACCINE APPROACHES

Molecular biology has been an important stimulus for new approaches to make live attenuated virus vaccines. As well, it has provided avenues for production of subunit vaccines and gene delivery vehicles that express viral Ags (e-Fig. 14.9). MAb

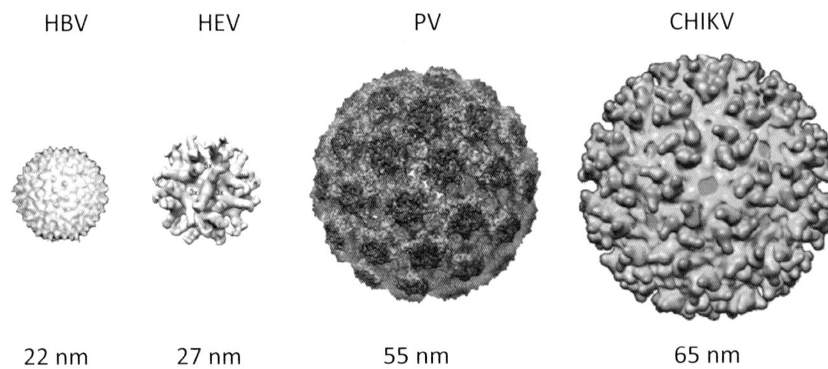

FIGURE 14.6. Variations on VLP size and structure. VLPs assume a wide range of sizes and are shown here as images derived from cryoelectron microscopy. Hepatitis B (HBV),[113] hepatitis E (HEV),[463] bovine papillomavirus (PV) representative of other papillomaviruses,[455] and chikungunya (CHIKV)[9] are shown by order of increasing size. VLP, virus-like particle.

and recombinant DNA technology are now used routinely to produce large quantities of purified viral Ags for use in immunoprophylaxis. MAb immunoaffinity chromatography or lectin chromatography facilitates purification of viral Ags from infected cells, whereas recombinant DNA technology makes it possible to express viral proteins in eukaryotic cells of yeast, insect, or mammalian origin. The use of these techniques has yielded candidate vaccines encompassing a large array of viral proteins that are capable of inducing protective Abs in experimental animals. Immunization by gene delivery is emerging as an important way to mimic certain aspects of live virus infection and can be accomplished by a growing list of delivery methods.

Vaccination With Proteins or Peptides

There are several theoretical advantages to immunizing with selected viral Ags instead of using whole virus particles. Production of recombinant viral proteins or synthetic peptides diminishes the risk of contamination by unrecognized pathogens. In addition, the preparation of vaccines free of nucleic acid eliminates theoretical concerns about recombination or integration of viral nucleic acid. Immunizing with individual Ags or epitopes from the virus might also reduce antigenic competition and focus the response on the most relevant protective antigenic sites.

Production of Viral Proteins in Eukaryotic Cells

Before expression of viral proteins in eukaryotic cells can be used as a method for vaccine production, several obstacles must be overcome. First, it is essential to identify the correct immunogen. Second, it is necessary to produce protein in a highly efficient manner to make this approach economically feasible. Mechanisms to enhance expression of viral proteins that have been pursued focus primarily on identification of strong promoters of gene expression and development of techniques for efficient gene amplification. Third, viral proteins must be separated effectively from host cell protein, DNA, and endogenous adventitious agents. Lastly, the proteins must be produced with the desired structure and activity. This latter requirement is of special concern, as immortalized mammalian cell lines are ideal for producing viral proteins because posttranslational modifications are more likely to be authentic than when these proteins are produced from prokaryotic hosts. Host cell DNA must be greatly reduced in the final vaccine (FDA guidance is <10 ng/dose) to reduce the theoretical potential for oncogenic events. Additionally, removal and inactivation of endogenous viruses must be performed for products made from continuous rodent and other mammalian cell lines. Recombinant DNA techniques to promote secretion of viral glycoproteins into the medium have been developed to facilitate effective separation of viral proteins from host cell proteins. Fourth, the procedures used to produce and purify viral protein must be gentle enough to maintain the protein in its native state, thereby preserving conformationally dependent neutralization epitopes needed to induce protective Abs. Finally, because purified monomeric proteins are typically weak immunogens, they need to be formulated with adjuvants or produced as oligomers or particles to enhance their immunogenicity. The following discussion of these approaches is not intended to be exhaustive in scope but illustrative of current strategies in use or in development.

Recombinant DNA techniques are commonly used to express viral proteins in yeast, insect, or mammalian cells. The usefulness of yeast expression has been described previously for the production of the HBV vaccine and is also used to produce HPV VLPs.[254] Some viral proteins such as the rabies G glycoprotein are more difficult to produce in yeast.[384]

A major advance in viral Ag production has been the development of baculovirus vectors to express foreign genes to high levels in insect cells under control of a strong baculovirus promoter, such as the polyhedrin promoter.[257] Protein can be produced in large quantity (1 mg/10^6 cells) using this system. Viral glycoproteins also can be produced in this system. For example, baculovirus-produced influenza HAs can be produced efficiently and have equivalent or superior immunogenicity to the traditional trivalent split product in adults[27] even though immunogenicity is significantly reduced in more immunologically naive children.[223] The baculovirus system also can be used to express more complicated viral immunogens that require polyprotein processing to generate native immunogenic surface proteins. An example of this is expression of the entire structural protein region (C-E3-E2-6K-E1) of an alphavirus to generate authentic, processed viral proteins capable of inducing an efficient neutralizing Ab response in experimental animals.[193]

Mammalian cells also have been used for the production of viral proteins that can be incorporated in a subunit vaccine. Mammalian cell cultures represent an optimal system for the production of viral proteins because protein folding, transport, and processing closely approximate those that occur in the infected host. Initial approaches were to purify viral proteins from infected cells or from cells transduced with a recombinant virus expression system engineered for high level of expression of the foreign viral Ag[140,141] or by transient transfection with DNA. More recently, cell lines have been developed that can stably produce recombinant proteins or Abs, can be modified for large-scale production, and have achieved regulatory approval for clinical products.

Chinese hamster ovary (CHO) cells have long been a preferred cell line for the production of protein-based therapeutics.[431] These cells have been used to produce viral glycoproteins from HIV and HSV that have been advanced to efficacy trials[135,366,409] and can be modified to improve the manufacturing efficiency and capacity even further. Immortalized human cell lines derived from healthy human embryonic material have also emerged as producer cell lines for protein production such as 293 and PER.C6. Both lines have been used extensively to produce gene delivery vectors, have fully documented passage histories, and have had no adventitious agents or oncogenic or teratogenic potential identified to date. PER.C6 was derived from embryonic retina cells and immortalized with the adenovirus *E1* gene. The 293-ORF6 cell line has a similar development history and contains the adenovirus open reading frame 6 from *E4* as well as the *E1* gene.[54] These fully human cell lines may provide advantages for producing virus glycoproteins that authentically replicate the structures present in human infection, can be adapted to different growth conditions, and can stably produce high levels of recombinant protein without gene amplification.[208] In general, identifying immortalized human cell line platforms for the production of proteins, VLPs, whole virus, or vaccine vectors will be preferable to using primary cell lines that have to be revalidated repeatedly or using less efficient production methods that require transient infection or transfection.

Production of Viral Proteins in Prokaryotic Cells

Production of immunogenic viral proteins in prokaryotic cells is difficult and requires extensive re-engineering of the gene to achieve immunogenic structures because of differences in protein processing and microenvironment. However, there have been some notable successes, especially in the production of VLPs. In particular, a portion of the structural protein from hepatitis E ORF2 produced in *Escherichia coli* self-assembles into particles and was shown to be efficacious in a 100,000-person study.[475] HPV VLPs have also been produced in bacteria, although clinical trials have not yet been reported.[249,311]

Production of Viral Proteins in Plant Cells

Plants have been modified genetically to express virus proteins[63,415] and VLPs,[99] some of which have advanced to clinical trials. Plants can be engineered with selected mammalian glycosidases to provide more authentic posttranslational modifications.[411] The major advantage of this approach is the potential for inexpensive and widely distributed manufacturing capacity.

Protein Purification

Immunoaffinity chromatography, lectin chromatography, and physical separation techniques have been used to purify a variety of viral glycoproteins that have induced partial to complete resistance in animals. When directly compared in animals, resistance induced by immunization is greatest when the purified viral glycoprotein is in its native conformation.[433] In the case of RSV and EBV, purified glycoprotein vaccines induced Abs that were able to bind to glycoprotein in enzyme-linked immunosorbent assays (ELISAs); however, these Abs had a very low level of neutralizing activity.[302,452] In contrast to purified protein immunogens, RSV glycoproteins expressed by a vaccinia virus RSV F or G recombinant induced a titer of neutralizing Abs comparable to that developed by animals infected with the virus.[88] Observations of this type underscore the potential importance of quaternary structures and presentation of proteins in the context of membranes and organized on particles to achieve functional Ab responses.

Synthetic Peptides as Immunogens

During the early 1970s, the use of synthetic peptides as immunogens was studied using a synthetic icosapeptide representing the immunodominant domain of the outer coat protein of bacteriophage MS-2.[239] This peptide, conjugated to a carrier and emulsified in adjuvant, induced Abs in rabbits that neutralized the infectivity of the bacteriophage when goat antirabbit Ig Abs were added to the mixture. Although synthetic peptides were shown subsequently to induce neutralizing Abs that did not depend on the aggregating effect of anti-Ig Abs and to stimulate immunity to certain animal viruses *in vivo*,[38] the immunity induced was less than that achieved when full-length protein, inactivated whole virus, or live virus was used as immunogen. The decreased immunogenicity of synthetic peptides is a consequence of their failure to mimic the conformational epitopes of viral surface proteins. Strategies to augment the immunogenicity of synthetic peptides, such as (a) inclusion of both B-cell and CD4 T-cell epitopes in the peptide, (b) synthesis of oligomeric peptide structures by using polylysine scaffolding,[312] (c) presentation of peptide in a noninfectious viral particle, (d) expression of peptide by infectious virus, or (e) scaffolding of peptide epitopes with constrained conformational structure have not overcome the inherent deficiencies of this approach. Neutralizing epitopes from the membrane proximal region of HIV gp41 and the Synagis epitope from RSV were designed on protein scaffolds to mimic the structure and display the identical contact residues defined by the original peptide-Ab crystal structures. Although these novel Ags were immunogenic and induced Abs that bound HIV gp41 and RSV F, vaccinee sera did not have neutralizing activity.[274,326] Using a much longer peptide may sometimes retain sufficient structural integrity to induce protective Ab responses. For example, a 100-aa peptide from the central region of RSV G can elicit neutralizing Ab to a central conserved region of the protein.[358] Also, a 56-aa peptide from the stem region of the influenza HA can induce Abs to a conserved epitope that has some cross-neutralizing activity.[444]

The fact that CD8 T-cell epitopes are short peptides of 8 to 10 amino acids in length presented in the context of the MHC class I heterodimer suggested that it might be possible to produce peptide vaccines to induce CTL-mediated immunity.[120] CTL induction by peptide vaccines has been achieved in several experimental systems. For example, a peptide in adjuvant induced CTLs and protected mice against Sendai virus infection.[215] Thus far, peptide vaccines have not achieved significant immunogenicity when used in immunologically naive humans unless formulated in preparations with strong adjuvants that are associated with unacceptable reactogenicity. Also, the reductionist approach to vaccine Ags has not been successful when tested in humans. In general, it is better to use a larger antigenic content in vaccines for viruses so that the individual hosts can select the most relevant and effective epitopes for themselves. This principle is also consistent with the concept that vaccination has its largest impact on public health at the population level. Developing tailored, personalized vaccination approaches may be in the distant future for preventive antiviral vaccines, and this type of approach is being explored for therapeutic vaccines against neoplasms and some chronic virus infections. Indeed, immunization with mixtures of long peptides derived from HPV E6 and E7 oncoproteins formulated in incomplete Freund's adjuvant (IFA) has led to remission of HPV16-induced vulvar intraepithelial neoplasia.[217]

Vaccination by Gene Delivery

The age of molecular biology has made it possible to build expression vectors that can serve as a vehicle for gene delivery of vaccine Ags. The development of this technology is attractive because it combines the immunogenicity advantages of live vaccines and the safety advantages of nonliving vaccines. Genes can be modified to be nonfunctional and harmless to the host, improve expression, and yet retain the antigenicity of the expressed protein. Using the host cell for transient protein production provides the opportunity for expression of more native structures than are possible with *in vitro* protein production including glycosylation patterns that may influence antigenicity. Genes can be produced synthetically so that no component of the original virus pathogen is needed in the manufacturing process to avoid the potential complications of infection with live viruses or adventitious agents. Selected immunogenic components of the pathogens can be expressed and combined with molecular adjuvants that enhance and guide the composition of immune responses. In addition, the mechanisms that viruses use to evade or alter immune responses can be removed, or genes can be modified (e.g., by adding ubiquitination sites) to improve processing and Ag presentation.[404] Therefore, it may be possible to improve on the immunity afforded by natural infection by using vector-based expression of viral Ags. New delivery approaches, including vector technology, provide the opportunity to combine Ags from multiple strains or different pathogens to potentially allow broadening of vaccine-induced immunity while simplifying vaccination regimens. They can be categorized by their functional properties (e-Fig. 14.10) and other features that may influence vaccine strategies for a particular virus (e-Table 14.2).

DNA Vaccines

The concept of using bacteria-derived plasmid DNA to deliver vaccine Ags has many attractive features, including ease and flexibility of construction, scalable manufacturing capacity, stability, production of vaccine Ag in host cells, transient expression, no induction of antivector immunity, induction of a balanced CD4 and CD8 T-cell response in addition to an Ab response, and minimal local or systemic reactogenicity.[242]

It was originally found to be possible to express transgenes by direct intramuscular or intradermal inoculation of plasmid DNA in the early 1990s.[419,454] The feasibility of immunization with DNA was demonstrated by the induction of Abs against human growth hormone in mice immunized with a plasmid encoding this foreign protein.[419] The first demonstration of DNA vaccine protection against a virus was in mice challenged with influenza.[288] Subsequently, immunization with DNA that encoded viral Ags, including Ags that can form VLPs, from a wide range of viruses has induced functional (i.e., neutralizing or syncytium-inhibiting) Abs and/or resistance to virus infection.[110] Gene-based immunization promotes host cell synthesis and expression of the vaccine Ag and physiological posttranslational processing and folding in the cell cytoplasm. For these reasons, DNA vaccination can elicit both CD4 and CD8 T-lymphocyte responses with a variety of immunogens in animal models.

Immunization with DNA has several advantages over immunization with purified viral Ags. The most important advantage is that vaccine Ags such as viral glycoproteins can be expressed on the surface of transfected cells and are presented to the immune system in a native state. During the processes of purification of viral proteins, purification and assembly of VLPs, or inactivation of viruses with chemicals, epitopes on viral proteins can be altered that compromise immunogenicity. DNA immunization, which circumvents these problems, more closely resembles immunization with a live virus vaccine than with an inactivated viral Ag. Viral Ags encoded by DNA, whether entire proteins or minimal CTL epitopes, are presented efficiently in the context of MHC class I molecules and are able to induce CD4 T cells and CTLs.[65,243,264,468] In this way, it is possible to induce a balanced immune response more similar to immunity induced by natural infection than to immunity induced by administration of preformed viral Ags. A second advantage of immunization with DNA is its ability to transfect cells without interference by antiviral or antivector Abs. Live attenuated vaccine virus, such as that present in the measles virus vaccine, is effectively rendered noninfectious by Abs. Likewise, Abs to gene-delivery vectors, such as adenovirus serotype 5 (Ad5), can diminish the immunogenicity of this approach, whereas DNA immunization is not affected by pre-existing Abs. Finally, it has been observed that the foreign Ag can be expressed *in vivo* for several months following DNA immunization.[465] Protein expression can also be optimized by modifying the promoter elements (e.g., adding the translation enhancer element from the human T-lymphotropic virus type 1 [HTLV-1] LTR).[26,243] It is thought that the major factor limiting the immunogenicity of DNA vaccines is inefficient transfection of cells. This is partially improved by using delivery devices such as Biojector, and new approaches utilizing electroporation offer the potential for improved potency of DNA vaccines.[388]

The safety profile of DNA vaccines in clinical trials has been excellent to date, without evidence of integration of the vaccine DNA into the human genome or induction of autoimmune reactions, which were some of the early theoretical concerns. Initially, DNA immunization showed limited immunogenicity in humans, despite many examples of vaccine-induced protection in mice and nonhuman primates.[110] The first DNA vaccine demonstrated to be immunogenic in Ag-naive humans expressed the circumsporozoite Ag from *Plasmodium falciparum* and was shown to induce CD8 CTL responses detected by *in vitro* expansion of effectors.[443] Another report described a DNA plasmid expressing the HBsAg that induced Ab as well as vaccine-specific T-cell responses in Ag-naive humans.[378] Through improvements in promoter design, manufacturing process, and delivery, DNA immunization in humans is now showing promise as a platform for inducing significant neutralizing Ab[243,264] and T-cell responses.[163]

Replication-Competent Vectors

The molecular technologies that have made gene delivery possible in general have been applied to the development of stable attenuated virus vaccines, some of which have been used to construct viable recombinants that express the surface proteins of other viruses, thus blurring the distinction between live attenuated viruses and vaccine vectors. Chimeric or live recombinant virus vectors can be designed to deliver the foreign gene from a virulent pathogen in the context of a nonpathogenic expression system, thereby improving safety. The vector design can also take into account manufacturing issues to improve overall production efficiency. The use of a viral vector for immunization has the advantage that the foreign viral Ags are expressed naturally in the context of an infected cell, thereby inducing cellular and humoral immune responses. Vector selection and design can focus vaccine Ag expression to a particular target cell or immunological compartment to tailor the organization of an immune response to a particular pathogen. Delivering the vaccine Ag in a complex structure has the benefit of broadly engaging both the innate and adaptive immune responses to better simulate the immunity to natural infection. Replication-competent vectors have additional immunogenicity advantages over replication-defective vectors, because more prolonged Ag expression and more diverse stimulation of TLR pathways often translate into better Ab production and more durable immune responses.

Chimeric Live Virus Reassortant and Recombinant Vaccines

Two major platforms have emerged to create chimeric viruses. One is based on reassortment of genes that occurs in segmented RNA viruses and is used in two currently licensed vaccines. The other utilizes reverse genetic systems developed to make molecular clones of viruses with nonsegmented RNA genomes. Live attenuated chimeric virus vaccines are distinguished from live viral vectors because the viral vaccine Ag being expressed is derived from the same virus family and replaces the homologous protein from the virus that supplies the coding and noncoding regions constituting the replication-competent particle.

The rhesus and bovine rotavirus vaccines are examples of live attenuated chimeric viruses produced by reassortment. The chimeric viruses contain the attenuating background of the rhesus or bovine rotavirus plus the gene for a human rotavirus VP7 surface protein. Similarly, the live attenuated influenza virus vaccines are chimeric viruses that can be antigenically updated by replacement of the HA and NA genes of the attenuated donor virus with those of a new epidemic or pandemic virus. This process was utilized in the response to the 2009 H1N1 pandemic. While the replication of A/California/7/2009 H1N1-like isolates in eggs was relatively low, the chimeric live virus produced as FluMist had outstanding growth properties that facilitated production.

Construction of recombinant live attenuated chimeric virus vaccines by gene replacement in molecular clones has most commonly utilized flaviviruses and paramyxovirus backgrounds. For flaviviruses, a live attenuated virus vaccine candidate for JEV has been made by the replacement of genes encoding the membrane precursor (prM) and envelope (E) proteins of the attenuated yellow fever virus (YFV) vaccine with those from an attenuated strain of JEV. The resulting JEV-YFV antigenic chimeric recombinant vaccine candidate was attenuated and immunogenic *in vivo.*[173] Both components of this chimeric virus came from attenuated viruses. It has now been evaluated in advanced clinical trials[286] and is being submitted for registration.[175] Chimeric recombinant candidate vaccines have been made between a naturally attenuated tick-borne flavivirus (Langat virus) and a wild-type mosquito-borne dengue type 4 virus (DENV-4), and the resulting recombinant was found to be significantly more attenuated than its tick-borne parent virus for mice.[355] This is an example of an attenuating effect that stems from partial incompatibility between the two components of the chimeric virus. Another strategy is being pursued for the production of a tetravalent dengue virus vaccine in which a DENV-4 background containing an attenuating deletion mutation in the 3′ noncoding region is used to construct antigenic chimeric viruses containing the surface proteins of other dengue serotypes.[278] Alternatively, the 3′ attenuating mutation is reproduced in the other serotypes. Chimeric flavivirus constructs appear to be a stable and effective vaccine platform for these types of viruses. Tetravalent, live attenuated dengue vaccines based on either the attenuated DENV-4 background or the chimeric YFV expressing prM and E from each serotype are immunogenic in humans and are being evaluated in advanced clinical trials.[175,307]

A chimeric virus containing the HN and F surface proteins of parainfluenza virus type 1 (PIV1) substituted for those of an attenuated parainfluenza virus type 3 (PIV3) virus has been constructed and shown to be attenuated and protective in experimental animals.[421] Both bovine and human PIV3 chimeras are being pursued to make vaccines against several other paramyxoviruses including PIV1, -2, and -3, RSV, metapneumovirus, and measles virus. Both human and bovine PIV3 are very amenable to use as a background for chimeric paramyxovirus vaccines; however, other paramyxoviruses are also being developed as vaccine vectors including Sendai virus, NDV, canine distemper virus, and measles virus.[198] Paramyxoviruses have also been constructed as vectors to deliver vaccine Ags from unrelated viruses such as HIV or Ebola.[107]

Poxvirus Vectors

Vaccinia virus is the most commonly used recombinant vector to date.[295] Poxviruses have large genomes into which a variety of foreign viral genes can be inserted and expressed without seriously compromising the capacity of vaccinia virus to replicate. Recombinant vaccinia viruses expressing the surface protein(s) of a large number of viruses have been constructed and are shown to be protective in experimental animals. Polyvalent live vaccinia virus recombinants have been used to successfully immunize experimental animals, even in the presence of immunity to one of the foreign viral Ags,[132] and vaccinia-rabies virus recombinants are being used to control rabies in foxes[342] (e-Table 14.3). Recombinant vaccinia has been evaluated in clinical trials,[158,160,161] although they are not sufficiently attenuated for use in immunocompromised hosts[129,172,365] and are complicated by other idiosyncratic side effects such as myopericarditis.[18] However, new versions of attenuated replication-competent poxvirus vectors such as the Tiantan strain of vaccinia have been constructed as candidate HIV vaccines and are currently being evaluated in clinical trials in China.[103]

Herpesvirus Vectors

Herpesvirus vectors have been developed using HSV-1, EBV, CMV, and some animal alphaherpesviruses. The primary advantages of this vector system are the capacity to package up to 100 kb of foreign DNA and the potential for long-term gene expression from latent episomal DNA that can be present in both neuronal and nonneuronal cells.[52] Herpesviruses have tropism for a wide variety of cells and are efficient at cell binding and attachment even at low particle-to-cell ratios. Vectors can also be pseudotyped to help target delivery into selected host cells. They can be given mucosally as well as parenterally and can be engineered to eliminate immune evasion genes such as the HSV-1 ICP47 that interferes with the transporter associated with antigen processing (TAP) to diminish MHC class I presentation. Live herpesvirus vectors can be attenuated to avoid vector-mediated disease and can also be made replication defective (see later discussion). Because HSV is ubiquitous, a potential disadvantage for this approach is that pre-existing Ab to the vector may diminish immune responses to the transgene product. In a murine model, it was shown that pre-existing HSV immunity did not alter the Ab or proliferative responses to recombinant protein encoded by the HSV vector.[47] Using animal herpesvirus vectors may be an alternative approach to circumvent the potential problem of pre-existing immunity to the vector, although replication is severely restricted when species barriers are crossed.[429] There is a licensed veterinary vaccine for Marek's disease in chickens based on this technology (see e-Table 14.3), and this technology has also been applied in HIV vaccine development. Initially, it was shown that replication-competent HSV vectors expressing Env and Nef showed partial protection against challenge with SIVmac239.[308] Subsequently, rhesus CMV vectors were constructed expressing Env, Gag, Pol, and Rev/Nef/Tat. Animals immunized with either recombinant CMV vectors alone or primed with CMV and boosted with recombinant adenovirus (rAd) vectors had significant protection from a SIVmac239 mucosal challenge. The correlate of protection is thought to be persistence of tissue-resident effector memory CD8 T cells, sustained by the persistence of the vector.[185]

Rhabdovirus Vectors

VSV has been engineered to serve as a vector for recombinant gene delivery. Recombinant VSV can be produced at high titer, is relatively stable, has broad tropism, and can be given mucosally.[220] VSV is a rhabdovirus and is known to have neurovirulence. Therefore, extensive work has been done to attenuate the parent vector by altering the gene order and by truncating the cytoplasmic tail of the major surface glycoprotein.[360] Gene delivery and subsequent immune responses to the recombinant gene product are potent,[179] and rhesus macaques immunized by a VSV vector expressing Env and Gag have been protected from SHIV challenge.[376] Replication-defective VSV vectors have also been developed (see later discussion).

Live Adenovirus Vectors

The live adenovirus vaccine for serotypes 4 and 7 is a licensed and highly effective vaccine that is administered mucosally. Therefore, it has ideal properties for a gene-delivery vehicle and has been developed as a candidate HIV-1 vaccine.[256,347] The advantages are the track record of the vector for both safety and efficacy, as well as the potential for delivery in capsules to the lower intestinal tract.[174,416]

Picornavirus Vectors

Poliovirus vectors have been developed that can express recombinant foreign proteins that are excised by the virus-encoded protease after translation of the recombinant polyprotein.[15] The major advantages of this approach are the long history of successful vaccination with the vector and the capacity for oral delivery and induction of mucosal immunity. The major disadvantage of this system is the relatively small packaging capacity (~200 aa) that requires a library of recombinant viruses in the vaccine to deliver large Ags. There is also the concern of reversion to neurovirulent forms of poliovirus, although there are new design approaches that can probably overcome this problem by manipulating the fidelity of the poliovirus polymerase[19] or substituting the internal ribosomal entry site (IRES) in the 5′ untranslated region with a similar stem-loop structure from rhinovirus.[57] Other issues complicating the use of live poliovirus vectors include pre-existing immunity against the vector in vaccinated persons and the recommendation to only use inactivated poliovirus vaccine in the United States. Although the global eradication campaign seeks to eliminate the need for polio vaccination, as with variola, as long as the virus remains in freezers or the sequence is available in databases, the idea of maintaining immunity to polio in the general population by using poliovirus as a vector for other pathogens has merit. Enteroviruses and rhinovirus vectors have been developed using similar technology and to target different mucosal inductive sites, and new innovations such as removing part of the capsid gene can provide a larger coding region for the vaccine Ag.[108,298]

Bacterial Vectors

Bacterial vectors have also been used to deliver viral Ags. Recombinant bacilli Calmette-Guérin (BCG) has received the most attention. Some advantages of BCG as a vector include (a) its safety record after administration to millions of persons, particularly in developing countries; (b) its persistence and therefore prolonged Ag production that may provide a more durable immune response; (c) its potential for mucosal administration; (d) its innate chemical composition that provides an adjuvant effect through TLR-1, TLR-3, TLR-4, and possibly other pattern recognition receptors; and (e) that immunity against tuberculosis could be a by-product of immune responses to the vector. Advances in mycobacterial genetics have made construction of recombinant vectors feasible,[386] and because of the large capacity for accepting foreign genes, co-expression of cytokines and other immunomodulators is possible.[11,309] In addition, discoveries about how mycobacteria inhibit apoptosis of macrophages to delay immune-mediated clearance have led to the development of attenuated mycobacteria for vaccination against tuberculosis. New promoters, other vector design modifications, and combining with other modalities may further enhance immune responses to the foreign gene products.[375] Other bacterial vectors that have been considered for delivering viral Ags include lactobacilli, salmonella, shigella, and listeria. The salmonella and shigella vectors have also been designed to deliver the gene-based vaccine Ag by plasmid and thereby combine mucosal delivery and adjuvanticity with authentic glycosylation of the gene product.[136] This concept has been tested in early-phase clinical trials to express an HIV-1 envelope protein, although there was poor immunogenicity.

Replication-Defective Vectors

Replication-defective virus vectors have had genes deleted that are essential for replication *in vitro* or *in vivo.* Replication-defective viruses can replicate to high titer in cell lines engineered to express the missing protein that would be encoded by the deleted gene. The viruses produced in such complementing cells can attach and deliver their genetic payload to cells *in vivo* but are unable to replicate. Such vectors undergo an abortive infection *in vivo* but express the foreign protein during this abortive infection and can thereby induce both the humoral and cellular arms of the immune response. Nonreplicating vectors do not retain the virulence of the original agent from which they were derived and would be expected to be safe even in hosts with compromised immune systems, should they encounter the vector. Many vectors retain the antigenicity of structural proteins from the original agent. This raises two issues. The first is reactogenicity. Many vectors can trigger innate immune responses that cause local and systemic reactions in the vaccinee. This is an advantage from the perspective of adjuvanticity but can be limiting at higher doses of the vector. The second is pre-existing immunity to the vector. If the vector is derived from an agent to which the host has had prior exposure, the pre-existing Ab can dampen the immunogenicity of the delivered vaccine Ag. Vector-based vaccines are of particular value when the vaccine target is a virus for which live attenuated or whole inactivated virus vaccines are not considered for safety or other reasons. Vectors have added value when the vaccine strategy is focused on inducing CD8 T-cell responses because they deliver the vaccine Ag to the cytoplasm, allowing access to the MHC class I processing pathway for Ag presentation. Because this characterizes the current strategies for HIV vaccine development, most vector-based vaccine strategies have been evaluated for the induction of protective immunity against lentivirus infection. Therefore, antiviral vaccine vectors will be discussed primarily in the context of HIV vaccine development even though they are also being developed for many other antiviral vaccine programs.

The regulatory approval pathway for vector-based gene delivery will involve scrutiny around issues such as integration, recombination, reversion to replication competence, and reactogenicity. The origins of many vaccine vectors are from the field of gene therapy, and some of the clinical events associated with gene therapy trials still affect the evaluation of vaccine vectors. For example, the 1999 death of a teenager in a gene therapy trial at the University of Pennsylvania prompted extensive reviews of safety data from both human and animal studies of vector-based gene delivery. The 18-year-old patient, who had a rare liver disorder called *ornithine transcarbamylase deficiency,* died after receiving a large dose (3.8×10^{13} particle units [PU]) of E1/E4-deleted serotype 5 adenoviral vector directly into the liver through the right hepatic artery. The death was most likely attributable to an adenovirus-induced cytokine storm with subsequent disseminated intravascular coagulation, acute respiratory distress, and multiorgan failure.[3] This incident compels a cautious approach to dose and route evaluation of any antigenic substance but particularly vector-based products. Another gene therapy incident involved a retrovirus vector used to successfully treat children with X-linked SCID. After 3 years, some of the children developed leukemia associated with the integration of vector DNA into the LMO2 proto-oncogene locus.[176,177]

Adenovirus Vectors

Replication-defective rAds exhibit characteristics that make them ideal vaccine vector candidates, and substantial resources are being invested to develop safe and immunogenic rAd vaccines for infectious agents including HIV, Ebola, plague, anthrax, influenza, tuberculosis, and malaria.[25] These vectors possess desirable qualities for use in vaccination strategies, including efficient transduction of host cells, limited duration of gene expression, vector nonpersistence, the ability to rapidly induce both humoral and cell-mediated immunity, induction of innate immune responses that may provide an adjuvant effect, relatively high stability, and ability to scale up production for manufacturing purposes.[25] Most rAd vaccine candidates are replication-defective owing to a deletion of the E1 region. Some vectors have additional deletions of E3 and E4 to increase capacity for gene insertion and to further reduce the chance of recombination in the packaging cell line to form replication-competent adenovirus. Deletion of E4 also prevents transcription of adenoviral genes encoding structural proteins to reduce antigenic competition with the vaccine Ag. Complementary human embryonic cell lines such as PER.C6[258] or 293-ORF6[48] are used to package the deficient rAd *in vitro* and allow large-scale production. Pre-existing immunity to a given adenovirus serotype has been shown in animal models and in human clinic trials to diminish the immunogenicity of the vaccine Ag. Adenovirus serotype 5 (Ad5) immunity has a high prevalence, particularly in developing countries.[229] Although Ad5 has been commonly used in the initial studies, there are 51 human adenovirus serotypes, and many have now been engineered to express foreign genes. In addition, new vectors have been constructed from adenoviruses derived from chimpanzees and macaques that have favorable properties and will provide options to avoid pre-existing vector-specific immunity. An alternative to using a rare serotype rAd vector is to construct chimeric vectors. For example, adenovirus vectors have been developed in which the shaft and knob portions of the fiber proteins are exchanged.[460] Another novel approach involved making hexon loop chimeras in which the neutralizing targets in hexon are exchanged for those of an uncommon adenovirus serotype.[414] A mucosal route of administration is another potential option for overcoming pre-existing vector immunity, with the added advantage of better induction of immunity in the mucosal compartment. This may be particularly important for inducing immunity against viruses that primarily enter the host through a mucosal surface such as HIV and influenza. Replication-defective rAd has been successfully given mucosally without adverse reactions,[434] even though one study in mice showed that intranasal administration could result in Ag expression in the olfactory bulb.[245] The effects of pre-existing immunity to the vector can also be partially overcome by increasing the dose or by priming with a heterologous vector expressing the vaccine Ag of interest. Finally, one can avoid pre-existing immunity by carefully selecting the target population. For example, children between 6 months and 2 years of age are Ad5 seronegative, which makes recombinant Ad5 vectors a viable choice for immunization of that age group.

The Step study was a phase IIb trial that evaluated E1-deleted recombinant Ad5 vectors expressing HIV-1 Gag, Pol, and Nef in individuals at high-risk of HIV infection. It was stopped prematurely in 2007 because there was a higher frequency of HIV-1 infections among vaccinees than placebo recipients.[49] The increased rate of infection was associated with being uncircumcised and with pre-existing Ad5 Ab. The biological basis for this outcome is not known. HIV-1 vaccine clinical trials utilizing rare serotype rAd vectors and recombinant Ad5 vectors (E1, E3, E4-deleted expressing HIV-1 Env, Gag, and Pol) in heterologous prime-boost combinations with DNA vaccines are still in progress.

Adeno-Associated Virus Vectors

Adeno-associated virus (AAV) vectors are unique because the wild-type virus itself is replication-defective and requires the presence of wild-type adenovirus as a helper virus to propagate. The vector is very simple and contains the promoter, foreign gene, and polyadenylation sequence surrounded by two short noncoding inverted terminal repeats from AAV. No genes from the wild-type AAV are included in the vector. Particles are produced in a packaging cell line that provides the AAV structural proteins. The AAV capsid induces an immune response, and as with other vectors, anti-AAV Ab can diminish immune responses to the foreign gene product expressed by recombinant AAV vectors. Using alternative capsid serotypes and incorporating immune modulators may overcome any limitations posed by pre-existing AAV immunity or allow heterologous boosting and further amplification of immunogenicity induced by primary vaccination. Transduction of muscle cells and APCs is efficient, and expression can be prolonged. A single dose of recombinant AAV has been shown to induce both humoral and cellular immunity sufficient to control SIV infection in macaques.[205] AAV-transduced cells achieve persistent gene expression by delivering concatameric circular episomes that remain transcriptionally active, and there is no evidence for integration.[394] Long-term episomal gene expression has been uniquely demonstrated by delivering neutralizing Ab genes to muscle cells in rhesus macaques and achieving sufficient titers in serum to protect against SIV challenge.[206]

Alphavirus Vectors

Alphaviruses such as Venezuelan equine encephalitis (VEE) virus, Sindbis virus, and Semliki Forest virus (SFV) have been modified to produce three distinct types of immunogens. All take advantage of the alphavirus replicon that is a minimal genome with replication origins and packaging signals. The vectors include the alphavirus nonstructural genes including the replicase and the subgenomic promoter upstream of a foreign gene that replaces the genes encoding alphavirus structural proteins. The replicon itself can be injected as either plasmid DNA or as naked RNA. Alternatively, helper cell lines can be constructed that provide the structural gene products needed for packaging of replicons and particle assembly of nonpropagating vectors.[140] These replication-defective viral particles are extremely efficient in targeting APCs, particularly dendritic cells, and because of the amplification of the RNA, they achieve high-level expression of the foreign protein. They have induced significant humoral and cellular immune responses to a variety of viral proteins in animal models,[192,207,361] and a VEE vector expressing HIV Ags has advanced into clinical trials.[451] The immunogenicity of the VEE vector is in part owing to its tropism for dendritic cells. When minor changes are made in the envelope protein to diminish dendritic cell entry, the induction of immune response is compromised.[259] One unique property of VEE vector-induced immunity is that parenteral immunization has been shown to induce mucosal IgA responses.[186] The mechanism underlying this phenomenon relates to the rapid and dramatic effect that the VEE particles and replicons have on the systemic innate immune response[227]—an effect that occurs in the first 24 hours after inoculation.[424] Because the stimulation of the innate immune system by VEE replicons also appears to enhance adaptive immune responses, replicons that do not express a vaccine Ag can be used as an adjuvant to enhance the protective response to subunit vaccines.[61]

Herpesvirus Vectors

Replication-defective HSVs have been produced in a manner analogous to that of the E1A-deficient adenoviruses—that is, they have had one or more genes deleted that are essential for replication; however, replication *in vitro* is supported in a cell line that constitutively expresses the essential protein needed for replication.[100,289] In contrast to the E1-deficient adenoviruses, the replication-defective HSVs are being developed as vaccines to protect against disease caused by HSV itself, as well as a vector to deliver foreign viral proteins. One potential advantage of herpesvirus vectors is persistent Ag production that may be required for the optimal induction of cellular immune responses. Another approach to vector construction is to package replication-defective HSV amplicons in HSV particles using bacterial artificial chromosome (BAC)-encoded helper viruses with deleted packaging sequences resulting in foreign gene expression without the influence of any residual HSV genes.[154]

Poxvirus Vectors

Attenuated replication-defective poxvirus vectors have been developed to address the known complications of vaccinia virus in immunocompromised persons. The most developed vectors include MVA, avipox (canarypox and fowlpox), and NYVAC (deliberate deletion of 18 genes associated with virulence).[338] MVA was derived by more than 500 passages in chick embryo cells[266,280] and has been evaluated as a vaccine vector for a variety of viral Ags. MVA is a highly attenuated host-range mutant that replicates well in avian cells and has limited replication in BSC-40 and baby hamster kidney (BHK) cells but does not propagate in most mammalian cells.[39,60,113] MVA is nonpathogenic in immunocompromised hosts and has been administered to large numbers of humans without incident.[267,410,449] Attenuation of the MVA recombinant resulted from the loss of nearly 30 kb of genome including genes for immune evasion and host range during its many passages in embryonated eggs.[16] The use of avian poxviruses, referred to as avipox viruses, as vectors represents a second type of host-range restricted poxvirus vector. Avipox viruses are naturally occurring host-range restricted viruses that are replication-deficient in mammalian cells and mammal hosts.[338] Each of these poxvirus vectors has the property of efficient replication *in vitro* in avian cell culture but restricted replication in primates. Avipox vectors have an added advantage because pre-existing immunity to vaccinia does not impact vector delivery. Poxvirus vectors have the following advantages: (a) thermostability, (b) the history of being associated with the extraordinary success of the smallpox eradication campaign, (c) large packaging capacity for foreign genes, and (d) lack of persistence or genomic integration. The major disadvantages are that (a) attenuated vectors are grown in primary cell lines (chicken embryo fibroblasts), and production is difficult to scale up; (b) the foreign gene insert is sometimes unstable; and (c) poxviruses are antigenically complex, and there may be competition between the vector and the inserted gene products for Ag processing and presentation.

After extensive phase I and phase II evaluation,[152,352] a recombinant canarypox vaccine was evaluated in RV144—a controversial phase III efficacy study.[51] This landmark study provides a benchmark as the first demonstration of efficacy for an HIV vaccine.[366] A general population cohort of 16,402 people in Thailand was enrolled in the study and randomized 1:1 vaccine to placebo recipient. Vaccinees received intramuscular injections of a recombinant canarypox vector expressing Env, Gag, and parts of Pol and Nef given at 0, 1, 3, and 6 months and rgp120 formulated in alum given at months 3 and 6. At 18 months, 74 infections had occurred in placebo recipients, and 51 infections had occurred in vaccinees, which was statistically significant. A similar rgp120 did not protect men-who-have-sex-with-men (MSM)[148] or intravenous drug users (IVDU)[353]—populations with much higher incidence. The immune correlate of protection is not yet defined; however, protection appears to be temporally associated with serum Ab titers, even though vaccinee sera does not neutralize commonly transmitted strains using traditional assays.

Limitations of Gene-Based Vectors

It is beyond the scope of this chapter to cover the growing list of potential vectors to deliver genes encoding viral Ags that may be considered for future vaccine development. For example, arenavirus[131] and lentivirus[102] vectors have not been discussed here, and reverse genetic systems have been developed for other virus families[225] that will make recombinant vector development feasible. Each system has a unique set of properties that should be considered when devising a strategy for a particular pathogen. One of the primary considerations is seroprevalence for the vector in the target population. Pre-existing vector-specific immunity can affect both safety and potency of the vaccine. This may be a problem if there is natural immunity to the vector or if competing vaccine programs for other important pathogens converge on the same vector platforms. There are several factors involving safety, Ag selection, immunogenicity, manufacturing, and stability that are important to consider when developing a vector-based vaccine strategy that are pathogen and target population specific (see e-Table 14.2).

Viral Vectors as Vaccines Against the Virus from Which the Vector Was Derived

A practical by-product of the development of gene-based replication-defective viral vaccine vectors is that the vector itself may serve as a novel vaccine platform for the virus from which the vector was derived. The most advanced examples of this are the poxvirus vectors such as MVA or NYVAC. These have been evaluated as candidate smallpox vaccines in clinical trials using replication-competent vaccinia (Dryvax) as a surrogate challenge.[139,341] This type of approach has also been proposed for herpesviruses[116] and adenoviruses. Using the viral vector creates the opportunity to express additional viral Ags[9] or immunomodulatory proteins such as cytokines[70] that could provide adjuvant effects and increase immunogenicity compared to the live attenuated virus platform. Another advantage of this approach is that the vector delivers the antigenic complexity of a live attenuated virus vaccine with a more favorable risk profile because of lack of replication. In addition, the vector provides more options for achieving robust manufacturing capacity, although this is often a challenge for live attenuated viral vaccines.

VACCINE FORMULATION AND DELIVERY

Adjuvants

Adaptive immune responses are controlled by the amount, duration, and formulation of the Ag in conjunction with innate immunity. The Ag sequence and structure determines specificity; however, the adjuvant and context of delivery and Ag presentation determine the composition, location, kinetics, and magnitude of vaccine-induced immune responses (e-Fig. 14.11). Although specificity is a property of the adaptive immune response, many adjuvant effects are mediated by the innate immune system. The most potent and broad-based adaptive immune responses are induced by replication-competent virus vaccines and gene-based viral vectors. These vectors provide efficient Ag presentation and inherently stimulate innate immunity through a variety of signaling pathways, thus limiting a requirement for exogenous adjuvants. By contrast, inactivated virus vaccines, purified viral proteins, or peptide Ags by themselves have relatively weak immunogenicity in a naive host. There are several reasons why replication-competent viral vaccines and gene-based vectors are inherently more immunogenic than inactivated virus or subunit vaccines. First, gene expression provides an ongoing source of the relevant protective Ag that is amplified through replication beyond the dose contained in the original inoculum. Second, Ags produced during transcription in the host cells have native quaternary and multimeric particulate structures and authentic posttranslational modifications. Third, replication-competent viruses and gene-based vectors can broadly engage multiple distinct innate immune and Ag presentation pathways. Indeed, a major advantage of live or attenuated viral vaccines is that expressed antigenic epitopes are processed efficiently through both MHC class I and II pathways. This mechanism contrasts with that of inactivated vaccines where Ag processing is mostly limited to MHC class II presentation, which elicits CD4 T-cell responses but is limited for generating CD8 immunity. Finally, PAMP recognition receptors are engaged on the cell surface, in endocytic vesicles, and in the cytoplasm with live vaccines (e-Fig. 14.12). Therefore, adjuvants are needed to compensate for the diminished immunogenicity of vaccines that are not transcriptionally active in host cells by recruiting additional signaling pathways to activate innate immunity, promoting APC maturation and co-stimulation, and prolonging Ag persistence.

Empirically Derived Adjuvants

Traditionally, adjuvants have been derived from natural products empirically found to have immunostimulating properties. Adjuvants can improve immunogenicity by optimizing the duration of Ag presentation through a "depot" effect and/or through enhancing certain innate stimulatory pathways. It was first discovered that bacterial toxins were more protective when mixed with other substances.[362] A prototypic adjuvant used exclusively in laboratory research is Freund's adjuvant prepared from mycobacterial cell walls. A modern version of IFA

(Montanide ISA-51) is a water-in-oil emulsion composed of mineral oil mixed with the surfactant mannose monooleate in a 1:1 ratio with the aqueous phase. Although vaccines formulated with mineral oil have been administered to more than one million people since 1945, with the emergence of aluminum-based adjuvants, they fell out of favor because of the reactogenicity profile and potential for causing sterile abscesses.[164] They are still frequently used in the context of therapeutic vaccines.

There are two currently licensed adjuvants in the United States for human use in preventive viral vaccines: alum and a combination of alum+MPL. Alum is derived from aluminum hydroxide or aluminum phosphate and is formulated as a gel or used to precipitate protein Ags to create aggregates. It functions as a short-term Ag depot in which Ag that is electrostatically bound to alum is slowly released at the site of inoculation. More recent studies have shown that some of the adjuvant activity conferred by alum is through activation of the "inflammasome" innate signaling pathway.[119] Alum has been the standard adjuvant used in licensed vaccines for several decades. All currently licensed inactivated viral vaccines and hepatitis B VLPs are formulated with alum. Gardasil, the Merck HPV VLP vaccine, is also formulated with alum. More recently, Ab responses can be improved by combining additional immune stimulatory molecules to alum. Indeed, AS04 (Adjuvant System 04, GlaxoSmith-Kline, London, UK) is a combination of alum and a modified synthetic form of MPL, which is a key component of lipopolysaccharide (LPS) that is the ligand for TLR-4. Cervarix, the HPV VLP from GlaxoSmithKline, is formulated with AS04 and is the first adjuvant containing a TLR ligand to be approved for use in humans. The MPL-based adjuvants when combined either with alum (AS04) or with QS21 (AS02) have been shown to have a significant dose-sparing effect and may have additional advantages in terms of the speed and durability of the humoral responses. Formulations that include MPL also stimulate IFN-γ, producing CD4 T-cell responses that may have additional benefit.[316]

After alum, the other most widely used adjuvant in humans is MF59. MF59 is a squalene oil-in-water squalene emulsion that is licensed for human use in Europe. MF59 was designed originally to provide an Ag depot from which Ag would be slowly released as the biodegradable oil was metabolized or removed by macrophages, and as a vehicle for the immunostimulant muramyl tripeptide-phosphatidyl ethanolamine (MTP-PE), a derivative of muramyl dipeptide, the active component of the mycobacterium cell wall fraction in Freund's complete adjuvant. However, clinical studies in humans indicated that MF59 itself was as immunostimulatory as MF59/MTP-PE with less toxicity.[162] Its adjuvant effect is not TLR dependent, but there is evidence that MF59 has some innate immune stimulatory capacity. More than 45 million doses have now been given to humans formulated with seasonal influenza vaccines. MF59 is dose sparing, and clinical studies with H5N1, H1N1, or seasonal trivalent influenza vaccines show that protective levels of immunity can be achieved with as little as 3.75 μg of vaccine Ag.[79] A similar squalene oil-in-water emulsion (AS03) has achieved similar dose-sparing effects when formulated with influenza Ags.[317] MF59-formulated influenza vaccines also result in Abs with greater cross-reactivity and greater avidity to conformational epitopes than alum-formulated vaccines in head-to-head comparisons.[218] As with alum, MF59 tends to promote Th2 responses.[432]

QS21, the active ingredient of immune stimulating complexes (ISCOMs), was discovered in the bark of *Quillaja saponaria,* Molina (soap bark tree). It was named for the tree's scientific name and for being the 21st peak on the high-performance liquid chromatography analysis of the bark extract. The basis for its adjuvant properties is not known.

Rationally Designed Adjuvants

As discoveries were made in the 1980s and early 1990s about the regulation of immune responses by cytokines,[294] chemokines,[7] and co-stimulatory molecules,[392] a more targeted molecular approach was taken to vaccine adjuvants. The trend during the 1990s was to attempt to build the optimal adjuvant effect one cytokine at a time and try to precisely control the processes of cell activation and differentiation.[251,420] This approach may still be possible but has underestimated the complexity of the molecular milieu required to produce a specific effect, and also has underestimated the complexity of effector phenotypes and the importance of timing involved in the successive waves of regulatory events participating in nascent immune responses. For example, in a study evaluating HIV Ags delivering by DNA together with an IL-2-Ig fusion protein also expressed as a plasmid, it was found that the cytokine only provided an adjuvant effect if delivered 48 hours after the vaccine Ag.[20]

More recently, the understanding of how PAMPS[203] are recognized has helped to explain the molecular basis for some traditional adjuvants and has resulted in better characterized products that are now being developed as vaccine adjuvants. PAMPS are recognized by TLRs—a family of type 1 integral membrane proteins—present on plasma membranes or within endosomes.[276] Ligands for any of the 11 currently known human TLRs can produce an integrated set of responses by APCs and other components of the innate immune system to stimulate adaptive immune responses (Chapter 8). Using TLR ligands instead of individual cytokines to adjuvant vaccine-induced immune responses helps to avoid the unanticipated problems that arise when using individual molecular adjuvants in isolation, providing a more authentic stimulus for the host to decide what pattern of cytokines, chemokines, and co-stimulation will be needed for a particular immune response. Empirically developed adjuvant products such as muramyl dipeptide derivatives or MPL are known to stimulate TLR-2 and TLR-4, respectively. Components of live and inactivated virus vaccines such as double-stranded RNA and single-stranded RNA are known to stimulate TLR-3 and TLR-7/8, respectively. Experimental adjuvants such as PolyI:C (TLR-3 agonist) and imidazoquinoline compounds (imiquimod or resiquimod TLR-7/8 agonists) are being explored to mimic these features of live virus infection. Palindromic CpG motifs present in bacterial DNA that are ligands of TLR-9 are also used as experimental adjuvants.

It is beyond the scope of this chapter to review all of the ways that cytokines, chemokines, and activation of TLR signaling pathways are being explored in antiviral vaccine formulations. As described previously, the discovery of PAMP recognition receptors provides an explanation for the activity of some empirically developed adjuvants (e.g., TLR-2 and TLR-4 agonists) and a platform for the rational design of future vaccine adjuvants.

Delivery Vehicles

Delivery of vaccine Ag can determine the immunological compartment that is stimulated and influence the types of APCs that process the vaccine Ag. Many delivery vehicles are formulated with adjuvants or have innate adjuvant properties; however, in this section the term will refer to approaches for transporting Ag to a particular location. A delivery vehicle may allow the mucosal delivery of an Ag that could otherwise only be given parenterally. Alternatively, a delivery vehicle could function as a way of co-delivering a mixture of Ags and adjuvant, produce a depot effect, or otherwise control the timing of release of Ag. More recently, vaccine delivery vehicles have been designed to carry Ag into particular subcellular compartments with the intent of stimulating specific immune responses by accessing distinct Ag processing pathways.

Lipid-Based Carriers

Many virus surface proteins are spatially oriented in lipid envelopes, and that is one rationale to use lipids in the formulation of virus vaccines. Another is that the Ag may be protected by the lipid and allow delivery through harsh environments such as the gastric mucosa or blood, or promote a depot effect when injected. Liposomal vaccine formulations may facilitate DNA transport into target cells and have been used extensively for transfection of cells *in vitro*. Liposomes are vesicles with a roughly spherical lipid bilayer surrounding an aqueous center.[128] If virus-derived proteins are inserted into the membranes (proteoliposomes), they are often referred to as virosomes. Liposomes have been used to deliver peptides, proteins, whole virus, and DNA with and without adjuvants and can be designed to target or co-stimulate selected APCs. The intent is to produce an inert particle that concentrates in the target organ of interest and then releases its payload. Typically, when used for purposes of DNA delivery, cationic lipids are used in the liposome formulation to improve the interaction with the negatively charged nucleic acid. The lipid composition of the liposome can be modified to affect charge, pH sensitivity, thermal stability, and fusogenicity to control release of the products. Virosomes are used in licensed products (non U.S. products) to deliver vaccine Ags for influenza and hepatitis A.[292] More elaborate virosomes in which the proteoliposome is built around a polystyrene bead are being developed as a candidate HIV-1 vaccine, using the scaffolding of the particle to produce more stable conformations of the envelope glycoprotein.[171] As a natural source of liposomes, exosomes are 50- to 90-nm vesicles produced by an endosomal process in which vesicles bud into endosomes (multivesicular bodies) and are then secreted from APCs. Interestingly, these exocytic vesicles contain many of the proteins involved in Ag presentation, including MHC and co-stimulatory molecules.[238] In addition, they have lipid content similar to many enveloped viruses and lipid rafts with high cholesterol content.[157] ISCOMs are another lipid-based vehicle for delivering vaccine Ag. They are 40-nm cage-like structures formed by a complex mixture of lipids and saponins that can be formulated with viral Ags.[6] ISCOMs are able to deliver proteins or peptides to the cytoplasmic compartment, where they can be processed to activate CD8 T cells, and this has also been demonstrated in clinical trials of HPV and HCV vaccine candidates.[387] ISCOMs also have adjuvant properties derived primarily from the saponin component QS21, as described previously.

Synthetic Particles

Synthetic polymers have been used in creative ways to contain or hold vaccine Ags for presentation to the immune system. Microparticles are made from biodegradable polymers complexed with viral Ags.[94] The primary polymer used is poly lactic-co-glycolic acid (PLGA), which can encapsulate DNA by itself or with multiple proteins, adjuvants, or other immunomodulators. PLGA has an extensive history of safety in humans because it is the polymer used in absorbable sutures. Some other advantages of microparticles (1 to 10 μm) include (a) preferential uptake through the phagocytic pathway of dendritic cells; (b) protection of the vaccine product from the environment, resulting in a slow-release depot effect[324]; and (c) a potential payload capacity that is higher than for liposomes or viral vectors. PLGA microparticles coated with cationic surfactants have also been used as a vehicle for DNA delivery by absorption of plasmid DNA to its charged surface.[324] In general, these approaches have not produced the robust gene expression and immunogenicity needed for gene-based vaccination, and the formulations are being empirically modified. One approach has been to produce a hybrid polymer by combining PLGA with other substances such as poly-β amino ester to improve the sensitivity to pH change and more rapidly liberate the DNA.[252] Another approach for DNA delivery has been to use alternative polymers such as poly (ortho esters) (POEs), which had been developed for drug and peptide delivery.[442]

Nanoparticles also have been explored as vehicles to deliver DNA vaccines. Generally sizes of less than 200 nm (close to the size of many viruses) have been used, which are less likely to be forced into the phagolysosome pathway than microparticles. One approach has involved polylysine cationic polymers with imidazole side chains to facilitate escape from endosomes.[253] Another utilizes an oil-in-water microemulsion to produce wax cationic nanoparticles[98] that can be modified to encapsulate DNA.[300] Finally, nonionic block co-polymers have been used to deliver DNA vaccines with promising results in animal models but not in human trials.[400]

Synthetic self-assembling polypeptides can be used to display vaccine Ags on particles to achieve multivalency similar to the use of VLP as Ag scaffolds.[351] Another approach is to use self-assembling proteins from other (nonviral) biological sources such as the yeast protein Ty,[244] although evaluation of these structures in human trials did not induce significant immune responses.[447]

Cell-based Carriers

Dendritic cells are important for Ag presentation, for initiating the innate responses, and for bridging the innate and adaptive immune systems to coordinate a comprehensive response to a virus infection. Therefore, they have been central to several vaccine development efforts. Not surprisingly, dendritic cells themselves have been used as the vehicle for Ag delivery. Autologous dendritic cells have been sorted, expanded *in vitro* with selected cytokines, pulsed with peptide, inactivated whole virus, or vectors and then reinfused into subjects.[255,263,325] Another cell-based vaccine approach utilizes transgenic plants. Potatoes, lettuce, tomatoes, carrots, and corn have all been engineered to produce vaccine Ags that have been evaluated in clinical trials.[415] This technology is also in early stages but has partially overcome some of the initial theoretical concerns that delivery of edible vaccines would result in oral tolerance or possibly result in food allergies to the carrier. A major advantage of transgenic plants is that production does not require an extensive physical infrastructure, and therefore manufacturing is inexpensive and easily distributed.

Conjugates

Vaccines derived by conjugating protein to carbohydrate have been extraordinarily successful for the control of encapsulated bacteria. The protein in this setting helps to redirect the Ag presentation so that alternative Ab isotypes are produced to control the bacteria. Because the carbohydrate structures of viruses are made by the host cell, they are not antigenic targets and often protect the virus from host immune defenses, as exemplified by the "glycan shield" of the HIV-1 gp120. Conjugates for viral Ags have typically been designed to carry the viral Ag into the cytoplasmic compartment of the APC so that processing and MHC class I presentation and CD8 T-cell activation can occur. This objective has been accomplished by using heat shock proteins (HSP70),[64] alpha-2 macroglobulin,[250] and leader sequences that promote membrane translocation to help the protein directly enter the cytoplasm.[189,372] Protein conjugate vaccines with Ab Fc receptors, CpG motifs, and TLR-7/8 agonists[73,450] also have been used to improve the efficiency of uptake of viral Ags to dendritic cells. An additional approach is to target Ag directly to dendritic cells through incorporating the viral Ag into an Ab such as the DEC205 Ab conjugate that delivers Ag directly to dendritic cells.[133,314] This provides an efficient *in vivo* approach for targeting dendritic cells instead of the *ex vivo* approach mentioned earlier, which may be limited to therapeutic vaccines for chronic virus infection and cancer.

Mechanical Devices

Currently licensed vaccines are given orally or by needle and syringe, aerosol, or bifurcated needle in the case of vaccinia. Future vaccines and adjuvants or immunomodulators may utilize more technically sophisticated devices such as microneedles[221] or micromechanical abrasion.[282] Other delivery devices have been adapted or developed in large part to address the need for improving the efficacy of DNA vaccines in humans. Needle-free injection systems such as Biojector or PowderJect have been used to deliver DNA vaccines in clinical trials,[163,378,443] and in both animal models and humans, electroporation has been shown to improve Ag expression and immunogenicity of DNA vaccination.[388,435] In addition, there continue to be new designs for delivery by traditional aerosol or needle and syringe devices that have been designed to improve effectiveness or safety. In particular, there are rapid advances in microneedle (<1 μm) technology in which arrays of needles made from a wide variety of materials (ranging from stainless steel to dissolving crystalline sugars) can effectively deliver vaccines.

Combination Approaches

Co-Delivery or Multivalent Vaccines

Co-delivery of vaccines has become a matter of practicality with more than 13 pathogens being targeted during the childhood immunization series alone. Therefore, combined vaccine formulations such as MMR (measles, mumps, rubella), the tetravalent product that includes varicella vaccine with the MMR combination, IPV (polio serotypes 1, 2, and 3), and influenza (B and A H3N2 and H1N1) are commonly used. Factors such as antigenic competition, interference, and unanticipated adverse reactions need to be considered during the development of combination products.

Co-delivery of different vaccines against the same pathogen can sometimes augment immunogenicity. Simultaneous administration of two different influenza virus vaccines to elderly subjects—namely, an intranasally administered live attenuated[415] influenza A virus candidate vaccine and a parenterally administered licensed inactivated virus vaccine—induced greater resistance to illness than did administration of the inactivated virus vaccine alone.[430] In this situation, the greater immunogenicity of the live virus vaccine in the respiratory tract coupled with the greater efficiency of the inactivated virus vaccine in stimulating systemic immunity appear to act in concert to optimize efficacy. A replication-defective HSV vaccine was found to be most immunogenic when administered by both parenteral and mucosal routes, indicating that the same vaccine preparation can also be given by a combination of routes to augment protection.[289]

Sequential Combination of Vaccines

Sequential combination of different vaccine modalities that focus on inducing immune responses to the same pathogen have recently been referred to as prime-boost strategies.[363] This concept takes advantage of the memory inherent in the adaptive immune response by sequentially amplifying the response to selected Ags. This can be done with combinations of replication-competent or gene-based vectors with inactivated or subunit vaccine approaches or by heterologous vector combinations. Combining vaccine approaches has the potential for eliciting new components of the immune response and for broadening the response to new specificities and immunological compartments. Combining heterologous vectors has the added value of the boost, avoiding pre-existing antivector immunity while amplifying the response to the expressed vaccine Ag.

Combination approaches can be used both for improving the safety of the booster vaccine and for improving immunogenicity beyond either approach alone. Polio vaccination is an example where using combined modalities improved both safety and immunogenicity. It is now recommended that only IPV be used for polio vaccination in the United States. Prior to this, sequential immunization with inactivated poliovirus vaccine followed by live attenuated virus vaccine was used as a safer alternative to OPV, the three-dose live virus vaccine. The combination approach provided immunity against the rare cases of vaccine-associated polio caused by the live virus vaccine and also primed for a booster effect from OPV, which expanded the immune response to the mucosal compartment. Thus, immunogenicity was optimized in the individual and herd immunity was provided to the population by inducing sufficient mucosal immunity in the gastrointestinal tract to prevent the spread of imported strains of poliovirus.[284,350] Sequential immunization with a live attenuated alphavirus vaccine candidate followed with a boost with an inactivated virus vaccine induced higher levels of Ab than live virus alone.[354] In the field of HIV vaccine development, a variety of prime-boost strategies have been evaluated. In some cases, priming has been done with a DNA or gene-based vector followed by subunit protein boost.[82,90,160] This approach led to the first demonstration of efficacy against HIV acquisition using a recombinant canarypox vector expressing Env, Gag, and Pol boosted with recombinant gp120 protein.[366] Other approaches have utilized heterologous vector combinations or DNA priming followed by gene-based vector boosting.[13,183,230,396] These studies have shown that DNA priming followed by recombinant Ad5 boosting can protect against SIV infection in macaques and reduce viral load in vaccinated animals that experience breakthrough infections.[247] This concept is being evaluated in HVTN 505, a phase IIb efficacy trial.

SUMMARY

Vaccine development has occurred primarily through observation and empiricism. In some cases, the emergence of new technologies allowed advances in vaccine development, and occasionally basic research discoveries have led to successful new vaccine approaches. The earliest observations that smallpox did not occur twice in the same individual led to the development of insufflation and variolization. Observing that a relatively innocuous cowpox infection seemed to protect against smallpox led Jenner to vaccinate. When Pasteur observed that an aged bacterial culture did not cause disease in chickens, and subsequently found that those chickens were protected from challenge with fresh cultures, an era of intentional modification and attenuation of microbes began that led to the introduction of many new vaccines. New technologies, such as cell culture, led to a series of new vaccines because viruses such as measles, mumps, rubella, and polio could be cultivated and produced in large quantities. The advent of molecular biology has led to the production of subunit proteins for successful hepatitis B and HPV vaccines and the technical ability to produce reassortant and recombinant viruses. Modern immunology, driven largely by the response to the HIV/acquired immunodeficiency syndrome (AIDS) crisis, has introduced new methods for measuring T-cell function that will help define the role of T cells in vaccine-induced immunity and guide the use of molecular adjuvants. Structural biology is providing an increasingly rapid way to view the atomic structures of viruses and their antigenic determinants bound to Abs and suggesting new approaches for vaccine design. The expanded capacity for nucleic acid sequencing has facilitated the discovery and surveillance of viral threats and has provided new insights to the biology of viruses and immune effectors. Technological advances in engineering and manufacturing have made vaccines safer and have created many new approaches for delivery that will have additional benefits on safety, stability, and ease of administration.

Vaccine development typically has required decades to accomplish and has never been a process that could occur in response to a crisis. However, a better awareness of the inevitability of new emerging infectious diseases and heightened concerns about bioterrorism have challenged traditional processes and compelled the consideration of new approaches. For example, the FDA has created the Two Animal Rule, which is a provision for vaccine licensure based on efficacy data in animal models combined with safety data in humans for diseases that are not conducive to efficacy trials.[415] A test case for the ability to develop vaccines rapidly for emerging infectious diseases occurred during the outbreak of the SARS CoV. This disease was recognized in the winter of 2003; the virus was identified in March 2003; a full-length sequence was obtained in April 2003; and vaccine development of whole inactivated, vector-based, DNA, and subunit vaccines began immediately. Phase I clinical trials of the whole inactivated virus vaccine began in the summer of 2004, and DNA trials started in December 2004. Fortunately, by that time, the epidemic had been contained through classical public health approaches of surveillance and quarantine. In 2009, when the pandemic H1N1/A/California/2009 virus appeared, both commercially licensed approaches and some experimental vaccines were in clinical use or testing within 4 months. It is possible that in the future, platform technologies for classes of viruses will allow even more rapid development time lines. Just as toxoids and polysaccharide conjugates have been successful platform technologies for toxin-producing and encapsulated bacteria, respectively, patterns are emerging for vaccine approaches that have a high likelihood of success against some types of virus. For example, using reassortment to produce live attenuated vaccines for viruses with segmented genomes, or producing VLPs with the capsid proteins of nonenveloped and some enveloped viruses, appear to be viable platforms for those types of viruses. Although this chapter has focused on antiviral vaccines for human pathogens, much can be learned from the development of veterinary vaccines. The list of licensed veterinary antiviral vaccines that are shown in e-Table 14.3 is provided to demonstrate the enormous variety of viruses to which vaccines have been developed, to demonstrate the types of approaches that have had some measure of success against various virus families, and to illustrate that the introduction of gene-based vaccine approaches into veterinary practice is anticipating the evolution of new human vaccines (see e-Table 14.3).

The goal for future vaccine development is to identify preventive strategies for selected pathogens that cause a large disease burden (e.g., HIV-1, RSV, dengue, and HSV) and have the potential for sporadic epidemics or intentional release and high disease severity (e.g., orthopoxviruses, filoviruses, flaviviruses), or emerging pathogens with the potential for causing widespread epidemics (e.g., chikungunya or H5N1 influenza), and at the same time develop platform technologies that can be deployed more rapidly when new virus diseases emerge (e.g., SARS CoV and West Nile virus). The 21st century promises higher capacity for protein production, structure-based Ag design, molecular adjuvants, and delivery devices to direct immune response patterns, a better understanding of the genetics of human immune response polymorphisms and repertoire, and more complete knowledge of immune effector mechanisms. In addition, the safety and efficacy of several classes of gene-based delivery vectors will be determined. These advances will hopefully provide the knowledge and infrastructure needed to develop vaccines for new emerging viruses and for difficult viruses that have eluded vaccine solutions and continue to impact human health.

ACKNOWLEDGMENTS

We acknowledge the extensive work done by Sandra Sitar, done on e-Table 14.1 outlining the history of viral vaccine development. We are grateful to Robert Seder, Richard Schwartz, Rick King, Philip Johnson, and Steve Whitehead for their careful review of selected sections. We also thank our many colleagues who have contributed to our thoughts about viral vaccines, particularly David T. Karzon and Robert M. Chanock, who died since the last edition of this book.[160]

REFERENCES

All cited references are available in the e-book.

1. Reduction of respiratory syncytial virus hospitalization among premature infants and infants with bronchopulmonary dysplasia using respiratory syncytial virus immune globulin prophylaxis. The PREVENT Study Group. *Pediatrics* 1997;99(1):93–99.
2. Palivizumab, a humanized respiratory syncytial virus monoclonal antibody, reduces hospitalization from respiratory syncytial virus infection in high-risk infants. The IMpact-RSV Study Group. *Pediatrics* 1998;102 (3 Pt 1):531–537.
4. Quadrivalent vaccine against human papillomavirus to prevent high-grade cervical lesions. *N Engl J Med* 2007;356(19):1915–1927.
6. Afzal MA, Pickford AR, Forsey T, et al. The Jeryl Lynn vaccine strain of mumps virus is a mixture of two distinct isolates. *J Gen Virol* 1993;74(Pt 5): 917–920.
8. Akahata W, Yang ZY, Andersen H, et al. A virus-like particle vaccine for epidemic Chikungunya virus protects nonhuman primates against infection. *Nat Med* 2010;16(3):334–338.
9. Akhrameyeva NV, Zhang P, Sugiyama N, et al. Development of a glycoprotein D-expressing dominant-negative and replication-defective herpes simplex virus 2 (HSV-2) recombinant viral vaccine against HSV-2 infection in mice. *J Virol* 2011;85(10):5036–5047.
10. Albrecht P, Ennis FA, Saltzman EJ, et al. Persistence of maternal antibody in infants beyond 12 months: mechanism of measles vaccine failure. *J Pediatr* 1977;91(5):715–718.
11. Aldovini A, Young RA. Humoral and cell-mediated immune responses to live recombinant BCG-HIV vaccines. *Nature* 1991;351(6326):479–482.
13. Amara RR, Villinger F, Altman JD, et al. Control of a mucosal challenge and prevention of AIDS by a multiprotein DNA/MVA vaccine. *Science* 2001;292(5514):69–74.
20. Baden LR, Blattner WA, Morgan C, et al. Timing of plasmid cytokine (IL-2/Ig) administration affects HIV-1 vaccine immunogenicity in HIV seronegative subjects. *J Infect Dis* 2011;204(10):1541–1549.
24. Barouch DH, Kunstman J, Kuroda MJ, et al. Eventual AIDS vaccine failure in a rhesus monkey by viral escape from cytotoxic T lymphocytes. *Nature* 2002;415(6869):335–339.
27. Baxter R, Patriarca PA, Ensor K, et al. Evaluation of the safety, reactogenicity and immunogenicity of FluBlok(R) trivalent recombinant baculovirus-expressed hemagglutinin influenza vaccine administered intramuscularly to healthy adults 50–64 years of age. *Vaccine* 2011;29(12):2272–2278.
28. Beasley RP, Hwang LY, Stevens CE, et al. Efficacy of hepatitis B immune globulin for prevention of perinatal transmission of the hepatitis B virus carrier state: final report of a randomized double-blind, placebo-controlled trial. *Hepatology* 1983;3(2):135–141.
32. Beran J. Safety and immunogenicity of a new hepatitis B vaccine for the protection of patients with renal insufficiency including pre-haemodialysis and haemodialysis patients. *Expert Opin Biol Ther* 2008; 8(2): 235–247.
33. Beran J, Hobzova L, Wertzova V, et al. Safety and immunogenicity of an investigational adjuvanted hepatitis B vaccine (HB-AS02V) in healthy adults. *Hum Vaccin* 2010;6(7):578–584.
36. Betts MR, Casazza JP, Koup RA. Monitoring HIV-specific CD8+ T cell responses by intracellular cytokine production. *Immunol Lett* 2001;79(1–2):117–125.
37. Billam P, Bonaparte KL, Liu J, et al. T Cell receptor clonotype influences epitope hierarchy in the CD8+ T cell response to respiratory syncytial virus infection. *J Biol Chem* 2011;286(6):4829–4841.
41. Bommakanti G, Citron MP, Hepler RW, et al. Design of an HA2-based Escherichia coli expressed influenza immunogen that protects mice from pathogenic challenge. *Proc Natl Acad Sci U S A* 2010;107(31):13701–13706.
42. Bomsel M, Tudor D, Drillet AS, et al. Immunization with HIV-1 gp41 subunit virosomes induces mucosal antibodies protecting nonhuman primates against vaginal SHIV challenges. *Immunity* 2011;34(2):269–280.
46. Brecht H, Hammerling U, Rott R. Undisturbed release of influenza virus in the presence of univalent antineuraminidase antibodies. *Virology* 1971;46(2):337–343.
47. Brockman MA, Knipe DM. Herpes simplex virus vectors elicit durable immune responses in the presence of preexisting host immunity. *J Virol* 2002;76(8):3678–3687.
49. Buchbinder SP, Mehrotra DV, Duerr A, et al. Efficacy assessment of a cell-mediated immunity HIV-1 vaccine (the Step Study): a double-blind, randomised, placebo-controlled, test-of-concept trial. *Lancet* 2008;372(9653):1881–1893.
50. Burns JW, Siadat-Pajouh M, Krishnaney AA, et al. Protective effect of rotavirus VP6-specific IgA monoclonal antibodies that lack neutralizing activity. *Science* 1996;272(5258):104–107.
53. Buser F. Side reaction to measles vaccination suggesting the Arthus phenomenon. *N Engl J Med* 1967;277(5):250–251.
58. Cannon MJ, Stott EJ, Taylor G, et al. Clearance of persistent respiratory syncytial virus infections in immunodeficient mice following transfer of primed T cells. *Immunology* 1987;62(1):133–138.
60. Carroll MW, Moss B. Host range and cytopathogenicity of the highly attenuated MVA strain of vaccinia virus: propagation and generation of recombinant viruses in a nonhuman mammalian cell line. *Virology* 1997;238:198–211.
61. Carroll TD, Matzinger SR, Barro M, et al. Alphavirus replicon-based adjuvants enhance the immunogenicity and effectiveness of Fluzone® in rhesus macaques. *Vaccine* 2011;29(5):931–940.
66. Cecchini S, Negrete A, Virag T, et al. Evidence of prior exposure to human bocavirus as determined by a retrospective serological study of 404 serum samples from adults in the United States. *Clin Vaccine Immunol* 2009;16(5):597–604.
67. Chang MH, You SL, Chen CJ, et al. Decreased incidence of hepatocellular carcinoma in hepatitis B vaccinees: a 20-year follow-up study. *J Natl Cancer Inst* 2009;101(19):1348–1355.
68. Chanock RM, Ludwig W, Heubner RJ, et al. Immunization by selective infection with type 4 adenovirus grown in human diploid tissue cultures. I. Safety and lack of oncogenicity and tests for potency in volunteers. *Jama* 1966;195(6):445–452.
69. Chantler JK, Ford DK, Tingle AJ. Persistent rubella infection and rubella-associated arthritis. *Lancet* 1982;1(8285):1323–1325.
71. Chen BJ, Leser GP, Morita E, et al. Influenza virus hemagglutinin and neuraminidase, but not the matrix protein, are required for assembly and budding of plasmid-derived virus-like particles. *J Virol* 2007;81(13):7111–7123.
76. Chumakov KM, Norwood LP, Parker ML, et al. RNA sequence variants in live poliovirus vaccine and their relation to neurovirulence. *J Virol* 1992;66(2):966–970.
78. Chung CY, Chen CY, Lin SY, et al. Enterovirus 71 virus-like particle vaccine: improved production conditions for enhanced yield. *Vaccine* 2010;28(43):6951–6957.
79. Clark TW, Pareek M, Hoschler K, et al. Trial of 2009 influenza A (H1N1) monovalent MF59-adjuvanted vaccine. *N Engl J Med* 2009;361(25):2424–2435.
84. Clements ML, Makhene MK, Karron RA, et al. Effective immunization with live attenuated influenza A virus can be achieved in early infancy. Pediatric Care Center. *J Infect Dis* 1996;173(1):44–51.
91. Cooper CL, Angel JB, Seguin I, et al. CPG 7909 adjuvant plus hepatitis B virus vaccination in HIV-infected adults achieves long-term seroprotection for up to 5 years. *Clin Infect Dis* 2008;46(8):1310–1314.
93. Correia BE, Ban YE, Holmes MA, et al. Computational design of epitope-scaffolds allows induction of antibodies specific for a poorly immunogenic HIV vaccine epitope. *Structure* 2010;18(9): 1116–1126.
95. Crotty S. Follicular helper CD4 T cells (TFH). *Annu Rev Immunol* 2011;29:621–663.
99. D'Aoust MA, Couture MM, Charland N, et al. The production of hemagglutinin-based virus-like particles in plants: a rapid, efficient and safe response to pandemic influenza. *Plant Biotechnol J* 2010; 8(5):607–619.
102. Dai B, Yang L, Yang H, et al. HIV-1 Gag-specific immunity induced by a lentivector-based vaccine directed to dendritic cells. *Proc Natl Acad Sci U S A* 2009;106(48):20382–20387.
103. Dai K, Liu Y, Liu M, et al. Pathogenicity and immunogenicity of recombinant Tiantan Vaccinia Virus with deleted C12L and A53R genes. *Vaccine* 2008;26(39):5062–5071.

104. Day PM, Kines RC, Thompson CD, et al. In vivo mechanisms of vaccine-induced protection against HPV infection. *Cell Host Microbe* 2010;8(3):260–270.
107. DiNapoli JM, Yang L, Samal SK, et al. Respiratory tract immunization of non-human primates with a Newcastle disease virus-vectored vaccine candidate against Ebola virus elicits a neutralizing antibody response. *Vaccine* 2010;29(1):17–25.
108. Doherty PC. The tetramer transformation. *J Immunol* 2011;187(1): 5–6.
111. Doores KJ, Burton DR. Variable loop glycan dependency of the broad and potent HIV-1-neutralizing antibodies PG9 and PG16. *J Virol* 2010;84(20):10510–10521.
112. Dowd KA, Jost CA, Durbin AP, et al. A dynamic landscape for antibody binding modulates antibody-mediated neutralization of west nile virus. *PLoS Pathog* 2011;7(6):e1002111.
114. Dryden KA, Wieland SF, Whitten-Bauer C, et al. Native hepatitis B virions and capsids visualized by electron cryomicroscopy. *Mol Cell* 2006; 22(6):843–850.
116. Dudek T, Knipe DM. Replication-defective viruses as vaccines and vaccine vectors. *Virology* 2006;344(1):230–239.
117. Durst M, Gissmann L, Ikenberg H, et al. A papillomavirus DNA from a cervical carcinoma and its prevalence in cancer biopsy samples from different geographic regions. *Proc Natl Acad Sci U S A* 1983;80(12):3812–3815.
119. Eisenbarth SC, Colegio OR, O'Connor W, et al. Crucial role for the Nalp3 inflammasome in the immunostimulatory properties of aluminium adjuvants. *Nature* 2008;453(7198):1122–1126.
126. Epstein SL. Prior H1N1 influenza infection and susceptibility of Cleveland family study participants during the H2N2 pandemic of 1957: An experiment of nature. *J Infect Dis* 2006;193:49–53.
129. Fenner F, Henderson DA, Arita I, et al. *Smallpox and its eradication* Geneva: World Health Organization; 1988.
131. Flatz L, Hegazy AN, Bergthaler A, et al. Development of replication-defective lymphocytic choriomeningitis virus vectors for the induction of potent CD8+ T cell immunity. *Nat Med* 2010;16(3):339–345.
133. Flynn BJ, Kastenmuller K, Wille-Reece U, et al. Immunization with HIV Gag targeted to dendritic cells followed by recombinant New York vaccinia virus induces robust T-cell immunity in nonhuman primates. *Proc Natl Acad Sci U S A* 2011;108(17):7131–7136.
134. Flynn KJ, Belz GT, Altman JD, et al. Virus-specific CD8+ T cells in primary and secondary influenza pneumonia. *Immunity* 1998;8(6): 683–691.
135. Flynn NM, Forthal DN, Harro CD, et al. Placebo-controlled phase 3 trial of a recombinant glycoprotein 120 vaccine to prevent HIV-1 infection. *J Infect Dis* 2005;191(5):654–665.
137. Fox J, Lennette E, Manso C, et al. Encephalitis in man following vaccination with 17D yellow fever virus. *Am J Hygiene* 1941;36:117–141.
140. Frolov I, Hoffman TA, Pragai BM, et al. Alphavirus-based expression vectors: strategies and applications. *Proc Natl Acad Sci U S A* 1996; 93(21):11371–11377.
143. Fulginiti VA, Eller JJ, Downie AW, et al. Altered reactivity to measles virus. Atypical measles in children previously immunized with inactivated measles virus vaccines. *JAMA* 1967;202(12):1075–1080.
146. Garland SM, Hernandez-Avila M, Wheeler CM, et al. Quadrivalent vaccine against human papillomavirus to prevent anogenital diseases. *N Engl J Med* 2007;356(19):1928–1943.
147. Georgescu MM, Balanant J, Macadam A, et al. Evolution of the Sabin type 1 poliovirus in humans: characterization of strains isolated from patients with vaccine-associated paralytic poliomyelitis. *J Virol* 1997;71(10):7758–7768.
149. Giuliano AR, Palefsky JM, Goldstone S, et al. Efficacy of quadrivalent HPV vaccine against HPV Infection and disease in males. *N Engl J Med* 2011;364(5):401–411.
160. Graham BS, Matthews TJ, Belshe RB, et al. Augmentation of human immunodeficiency virus type 1 neutralizing antibody by priming with gp160 recombinant vaccinia and boosting with rgp160 in vaccinia-naive adults. The NIAID AIDS Vaccine Clinical Trials Network. *J Infect Dis* 1993;167(3):533–537.
164. Graham BS, McElrath MJ, Keefer MC, et al. Immunization with cocktail of HIV-derived peptides in montanide ISA-51 is immunogenic, but causes sterile abscesses and unacceptable reactogenicity. *PLoS One* 2010;5(8):e11995.
165. Graham BS. Biological challenges and technological opportunities for respiratory syncytial virus vaccine development. *Immunol Rev* 2011; 239(1):149–166.
166. Graham BS, Crowe JEJ. Tribute to David T. Karzon, MD and Robert M. Chanock, MD. *Vaccine* 2011;29(21):3725–3727.
167. Graham BS, Walker C. Meeting the challenge of vaccine design to control HIV and other difficult viruses. In: Kaufmann SHE, Rouse BT, Sacks DL, eds. *The Immune Response to Infection* Washington, DC: ASM Press; 2011:559–570.
169. Gray GC, Goswami PR, Malasig MD, et al. Adult adenovirus infections: loss of orphaned vaccines precipitates military respiratory disease epidemics *Clin Infect Dis* 2000;31(3):663–670.
174. Gutekunst RR, White RJ, Edmondson WP, et al. Immunization with live type 4 adenovirus: determination of infectious virus dose and protective effect of enteric infection. *Am J Epidemiol* 1967;86(2):341–349.
175. Guy B, Guirakhoo F, Barban V, et al. Preclinical and clinical development of YFV 17D-based chimeric vaccines against dengue, West Nile and Japanese encephalitis viruses. *Vaccine* 2010;28(3):632–649.
179. Haglund K, Leiner I, Kerksiek K, et al. High-level primary CD8(+) T-cell response to human immunodeficiency virus type 1 gag and env generated by vaccination with recombinant vesicular stomatitis viruses. *J Virol* 2002;76(6):2730–2738.
181. Hammon WM, Coriell LL, Wehrle PF, et al. Evaluation of Red Cross gamma globulin as a prophylactic agent for poliomyelitis. IV. Final report of results based on clinical diagnoses. *J Am Med Assoc* 1953;151(15): 1272–1285.
182. Hammonds J, Chen X, Zhang X, et al. Advances in methods for the production, purification, and characterization of HIV-1 Gag-Env pseudovirion vaccines. *Vaccine* 2007;25(47):8036–8048.
185. Hansen SG, Ford JC, Lewis MS, et al. Profound early control of highly pathogenic SIV by an effector memory T-cell vaccine. *Nature* 2011;473(7348):523–527.
190. Haynes BF, Fleming J, St Clair EW, et al. Cardiolipin polyspecific autoreactivity in two broadly neutralizing HIV-1 antibodies. *Science* 2005;308(5730):1906–1908.
191. Hessell AJ, Hangartner L, Hunter M, et al. Fc receptor but not complement binding is important in antibody protection against HIV. *Nature* 2007;449(7158):101–104.
194. Horvath B, Fornosi F. Excretion of SV40 virus after oral administration of contaminated polio vaccine. *Acta Microbiol Hung* 1964;11:271–275.
198. Hurwitz JL. Development of recombinant Sendai virus vaccines for prevention of human parainfluenza and respiratory syncytial virus infections. *Pediatr Infect Dis J* 2008;27(10 Suppl):S126–128.
202. Janeway CA. Use of concentrated human gamma globulin in the prevention and attenuation of measles. *Bull NY Acad Med* 1945;21:202–202.
204. Johnson PR, Feldman S, Thompson JM, et al. Immunity to influenza A virus infection in young children: a comparison of natural infection, live cold-adapted vaccine, and inactivated vaccine. *J Infect Dis* 1986; 154(1):121–127.
205. Johnson PR, Schnepp BC, Connell MJ, et al. Novel adeno-associated virus vector vaccine restricts replication of simian immunodeficiency virus in macaques. *J Virol* 2005;79(2):955–965.
206. Johnson PR, Schnepp BC, Zhang J, et al. Vector-mediated gene transfer engenders long-lived neutralizing activity and protection against SIV infection in monkeys. *Nat Med* 2009;15(8):901–906.
207. Johnston RE, Johnson PR, Connell MJ, et al. Vaccination of macaques with SIV immunogens delivered by Venezuelan equine encephalitis virus replicon particle vectors followed by a mucosal challenge with SIVsmE660. *Vaccine* 2005;23(42):4969–4979.
209. Kaech SM, Hemby S, Kersh E, et al. Molecular and functional profiling of memory CD8 T cell differentiation. *Cell* 2002;111(6):837–851.
211. Kallewaard NL, McKinney BA, Gu Y, et al. Functional maturation of the human antibody response to rotavirus. *J Immunol* 2008;180(6): 3980–3989.
213. Karron RA, Belshe RB, Wright PF, et al. A live human parainfluenza type 3 virus vaccine is attenuated and immunogenic in young infants. *Pediatr Infect Dis J* 2003;22(5):394–405.

214. Karron RA, Wright PF, Belshe RB, et al. Identification of a recombinant live attenuated respiratory syncytial virus vaccine candidate that is highly attenuated in infants. *J Infect Dis* 2005;191(7):1093–1104.
216. Kaul TN, Welliver RC, Ogra PL. Development of antibody-dependent cell-mediated cytotoxicity in the respiratory tract after natural infection with respiratory syncytial virus. *Infect Immun* 1982;37(2):492–498.
217. Kenter GG, Welters MJ, Valentijn AR, et al. Vaccination against HPV-16 oncoproteins for vulvar intraepithelial neoplasia. *N Engl J Med* 2009;361(19):1838–1847.
218. Khurana S, Verma N, Yewdell JW, et al. MF59 adjuvant enhances diversity and affinity of antibody-mediated immune response to pandemic influenza vaccines. *Sci Transl Med* 2011;3(85):85ra48.
219. Kim HW, Canchola JG, Brandt CD, et al. Respiratory syncytial virus disease in infants despite prior administration of antigenic inactivated vaccine. *Am J Epidemiol* 1969;89(4):422–434.
221. Kim YC, Jarrahian C, Zehrung D, et al. Delivery systems for intradermal vaccination. *Curr Top Microbiol Immunol* 2012;351:77–112.
222. Kines RC, Thompson CD, Lowy DR, et al. The initial steps leading to papillomavirus infection occur on the basement membrane prior to cell surface binding. *Proc Natl Acad Sci U S A* 2009;106(48):20458–20463.
223. King JC, Jr., Cox MM, Reisinger K, et al. Evaluation of the safety, reactogenicity and immunogenicity of FluBlok trivalent recombinant baculovirus-expressed hemagglutinin influenza vaccine administered intramuscularly to healthy children aged 6–59 months. *Vaccine* 2009;27(47):6589–6594.
224. Kirnbauer R, Booy F, Cheng N, et al. Papillomavirus L1 major capsid protein self-assembles into virus-like particles that are highly immunogenic. *Proc Natl Acad Sci U S A* 1992;89(24):12180–12184.
225. Kobayashi T, Antar AA, Boehme KW, et al. A plasmid-based reverse genetics system for animal double-stranded RNA viruses. *Cell Host Microbe* 2007;1(2):147–157.
227. Konopka JL, Thompson JM, Whitmore AC, et al. Acute infection with venezuelan equine encephalitis virus replicon particles catalyzes a systemic antiviral state and protects from lethal virus challenge. *J Virol* 2009;83(23):12432–12442.
230. Koup RA, Roederer M, Lamoreaux L, et al. Priming immunization with DNA augments immunogenicity of recombinant adenoviral vectors for both HIV-1 specific antibody and T-cell responses. *PLoS One* 2010;5(2):e9015.
232. Koutsky LA, Ault KA, Wheeler CM, et al. A controlled trial of a human papillomavirus type 16 vaccine. *N Engl J Med* 2002;347(21):1645–1651.
233. Krause JC, Tumpey TM, Huffman CJ, et al. Naturally occurring human monoclonal antibodies neutralize both 1918 and 2009 pandemic influenza A (H1N1) viruses. *J Virol* 2010;84(6):3127–3130.
235. Kwong PD, Wyatt R, Robinson J, et al. Structure of an HIV gp120 envelope glycoprotein in complex with the CD4 receptor and a neutralizing human antibody. *Nature* 1998;393(6686):648–659.
236. Kwong PD, Doyle ML, Casper DJ, et al. HIV-1 evades antibody-mediated neutralization through conformational masking of receptor-binding sites. *Nature* 2002;420(6916):678–682.
237. Kwong PD, Wilson IA. HIV-1 and influenza antibodies: seeing antigens in new ways. *Nat Immunol* 2009;10(6):573–578.
240. Lasky T, Terracciano GJ, Magder L, et al. The Guillain-Barré syndrome and the 1992–1993 and 1993–1994 influenza vaccines. *N Engl J Med* 1998;339(25):1797–1802.
242. Ledgerwood JE, Graham BS. DNA vaccines: a safe and efficient platform technology for responding to emerging infectious diseases. *Hum Vaccin* 2009;5(9):623–626.
243. Ledgerwood JE, Pierson TC, Hubka SA, et al. A West Nile virus DNA vaccine utilizing a modified promoter induces neutralizing antibody in younger and older healthy adults in a phase I clinical trial. *J Infect Dis* 2011;203(10):1396–1404.
246. Lennon RG, Isacson P. Delayed dermal hypersensitivity following killed measles vaccine. Experience in 9-month-old infants. *J Pediatr* 1967;71(4):525–529.
247. Letvin NL, Rao SS, Montefiori DC, et al. Immune and genetic correlates of vaccine protection against mucosal infection by SIV in monkeys. *Sci Transl Med* 2011;3(81):81ra36.
248. Levine B, Hardwick JM, Trapp BD, et al. Antibody-mediated clearance of alphavirus infection from neurons. *Science* 1991;254(5033):856–860.
256. Lubeck MD, Natuk R, Myagkikh M, et al. Long-term protection of chimpanzees against high-dose HIV-1 challenge induced by immunization. *Nat Med* 1997;3(6):651–658.
264. Martin JE, Pierson TC, Hubka S, et al. A West Nile virus DNA vaccine induces neutralizing antibody in healthy adults during a phase 1 clinical trial. *J Infect Dis* 2007;196(12):1732–1740.
266. Mayr A, Hochstein-Mintzel V, Stickl H. Passage history, properties, and applicability of the attenuated vaccinia virus strain MVA. *Infection* 1975;3:6–14.
269. Mazanec MB, Kaetzel CS, Lamm ME, et al. Intracellular neutralization of Sendai and influenza viruses by IgA monoclonal antibodies. *Adv Exp Med Biol* 1995;371A:651–654.
272. McGinnes LW, Gravel KA, Finberg RW, et al. Assembly and immunological properties of Newcastle disease virus-like particles containing the respiratory syncytial virus F and G proteins. *J Virol* 2011;85(1):366–377.
274. McLellan JS, Correia BE, Chen M, et al. Design and characterization of epitope-scaffold immunogens that present the motavizumab epitope from respiratory syncytial virus. *J Mol Biol* 2011;409(5):853–866.
275. Mease PJ, Ochs HD, Wedgwood RJ. Successful treatment of echovirus meningoencephalitis and myositis-fasciitis with intravenous immune globulin therapy in a patient with X-linked agammaglobulinemia. *N Engl J Med* 1981;304(21):1278–1281.
276. Medzhitov R, Preston-Hurlburt P, Janeway CA, Jr. A human homologue of the Drosophila Toll protein signals activation of adaptive immunity. *Nature* 1997;388(6640):394–397.
280. Meyer H, Sutter G, Mayr A. Mapping of deletions in the genome of the highly attenuated vaccinia virus MVA and their influence on virulence. *J Gen Virol* 1991;72:1031–1038.
281. Meyer HM, Jr., Hopps HE, Parkman PD, et al. Control of measles and rubella through use of attenuated vaccines. *Am J Clin Pathol* 1978;70(1 Suppl):128–135.
283. Milstien JB, Lemon SM, Wright PF. Development of a more thermostable poliovirus vaccine. *J Infect Dis* 1997;175(Suppl 1):S247–S253.
285. Moghaddam A, Olszewska W, Wang B, et al. A potential molecular mechanism for hypersensitivity caused by formalin-inactivated vaccines. *Nat Med* 2006;12(8):905–907.
287. Monsalvo AC, Batalle JP, Lopez MF, et al. Severe pandemic 2009 H1N1 influenza disease due to pathogenic immune complexes. *Nat Med* 2011;17(2):195–199.
290. Morrison TG. Newcastle disease virus-like particles as a platform for the development of vaccines for human and agricultural pathogens. *Future Virol* 2010;5(5):545–554.
291. Mortimer EA, Jr., Lepow ML, Gold E, et al. Long-term follow-up of persons inadvertently inoculated with SV40 as neonates. *N Engl J Med* 1981;305(25):1517–1518.
294. Mosmann TR, Cherwinski H, Bond MW, et al. Two types of murine helper T cell clone. I. Definition according to profiles of lymphokine activities and secreted proteins. *J Immunol* 1986;136(7):2348–2357.
298. Mueller S, Wimmer E. Introducing recombinant picornaviral genomes into cells. *Cold Spring Harb Protoc* 2011;2011(6).
299. Mullbacher A, Ebnet K, Blanden RV, et al. Granzyme A is critical for recovery of mice from infection with the natural cytopathic viral pathogen, ectromelia. *Proc Natl Acad Sci U S A* 1996;93(12):5783–5787.
301. Murphy BR, Prince GA, Walsh EE, et al. Dissociation between serum neutralizing and glycoprotein antibody responses of infants and children who received inactivated respiratory syncytial virus vaccine. *J Clin Microbiol* 1986;24(2):197–202.
307. Murphy BR, Whitehead SS. Immune response to dengue virus and prospects for a vaccine. *Annu Rev Immunol* 2011;29:587–619.
310. Nader P, Horwitz M, Rousseau J. Atypical exanthem following exposure to natural measles. Eleven cases in children previously inoculated with killed vaccine. *J Pediatr* 1968;72:22–28.
313. Nathanson N, Langmuir AD. The Cutter incident. Poliomyelitis following formaldehyde-inactivated poliovirus vaccination in the United States during the Spring of 1955. II. Relationship of poliomyelitis to Cutter vaccine. 1963 [classical article]. *Am J Epidemiol* 1995;142(2):109–140; discussion 107–108.
314. Nchinda G, Kuroiwa J, Oks M, et al. The efficacy of DNA vaccination is enhanced in mice by targeting the encoded protein to dendritic cells. *J Clin Invest* 2008;118(4):1427–1436.

315. Netea MG, Quintin J, van der Meer JW. Trained immunity: a memory for innate host defense. *Cell Host Microbe* 2011;9(5):355–361.
317. Nicholson KG, Abrams KR, Batham S, et al. Immunogenicity and safety of a two-dose schedule of whole-virion and AS03A-adjuvanted 2009 influenza A (H1N1) vaccines: a randomised, multicentre, age-stratified, head-to-head trial. *Lancet Infect Dis* 2011;11(2):91–101.
319. Nkowane BM, Wassilak SG, Orenstein WA, et al. Vaccine-associated paralytic poliomyelitis. United States: 1973 through 1984. *Jama* 1987;257(10):1335–1340.
320. Norrby E, Enders-Ruckle G, Meulen V. Differences in the appearance of antibodies to structural components of measles virus after immunization with inactivated and live virus. *J Infect Dis* 1975;132(3):262–269.
321. Norrby E, Gollmar Y. Identification of measles virus-specific hemolysis-inihibiting antibodies separate from hemagglutination-inhibiting antibodies. *Infect Immun* 1975;11(2):231–239.
326. Ofek G, Guenaga FJ, Schief WR, et al. Elicitation of structure-specific antibodies by epitope scaffolds. *Proc Natl Acad Sci U S A* 2010;107(42):17880–17887.
327. Offit PA. *The Cutter Incident: How America's First Polio Vaccine Led to the Growing Vaccine Crisis.* New Haven, CT: Yale University Press; 2007.
329. Orentas RJ, Hildreth JE, Obah E, et al. Induction of CD4+ human cytolytic T cells specific for HIV-infected cells by a gp160 subunit vaccine. *Science* 1990;248(4960):1234–1237.
333. Oxman MN, Levin MJ, Johnson GR, et al. A vaccine to prevent herpes zoster and postherpetic neuralgia in older adults. *N Engl J Med* 2005;352(22):2271–2284.
342. Pastoret PP, Brochier B. Epidemiology and control of fox rabies in Europe. *Vaccine* 1999;17(13–14):1750–1754.
346. Pejchal R, Walker LM, Stanfield RL, et al. Structure and function of broadly reactive antibody PG16 reveal an H3 subdomain that mediates potent neutralization of HIV-1. *Proc Natl Acad Sci U S A* 2010;107(25):11483–11488.
351. Pimentel TA, Yan Z, Jeffers SA, et al. Peptide nanoparticles as novel immunogens: design and analysis of a prototypic severe acute respiratory syndrome vaccine. *Chem Biol Drug Des* 2009;73(1):53–61.
353. Pitisuttithum P, Gilbert P, Gurwith M, et al. Randomized, double-blind, placebo-controlled efficacy trial of a bivalent recombinant glycoprotein 120 HIV-1 vaccine among injection drug users in Bangkok, Thailand. *J Infect Dis* 2006;194(12):1661–1671.
356. Polack FP, Auwaerter PG, Lee SH, et al. Production of atypical measles in rhesus macaques: evidence for disease mediated by immune complex formation and eosinophils in the presence of fusion-inhibiting antibody. *Nat Med* 1999;5(6):629–634.
357. Polack FP, Hoffman SJ, Crujeiras G, Griffin DE. A role for nonprotective complement-fixing antibodies with low avidity for measles virus in atypical measles. *Nat Med* 2003;9(9):1209–1213.
362. Ramon G. Sur l'augmentation anormale de l'antitoxine chez les chevaux producteurs de serum antidiptherique. *Bull Soc Centr Med Vet* 1925;101:227.
363. Ranasinghe C, Ramshaw IA. Genetic heterologous prime-boost vaccination strategies for improved systemic and mucosal immunity. *Expert Rev Vaccines* 2009;8(9):1171–1181.
364. Ray P, Black S, Shinefield H, et al. Risk of chronic arthropathy among women after rubella vaccination. Vaccine Safety Datalink Team [see comments]. *JAMA* 1997;278(7):551–556.
366. Rerks-Ngarm S, Pitisuttithum P, Nitayaphan S, et al. Vaccination with ALVAC and AIDSVAX to prevent HIV-1 infection in Thailand. *N Engl J Med* 2009;361(23):2209–2220.
368. Richman DD, Wrin T, Little SJ, et al. Rapid evolution of the neutralizing antibody response to HIV type 1 infection. *Proc Natl Acad Sci U S A* 2003;100(7):4144–4149.
373. Roldao A, Mellado MC, Castilho LR, et al. Virus-like particles in vaccine development. *Expert Rev Vaccines* 2010;9(10):1149–1176.
374. Romanowski B. Long term protection against cervical infection with the human papillomavirus: review of currently available vaccines. *Hum Vaccin* 2011;7(2).
375. Rosario M, Hopkins R, Fulkerson J, et al. Novel recombinant Mycobacterium bovis BCG, ovine atadenovirus, and modified vaccinia virus Ankara vaccines combine to induce robust human immunodeficiency virus-specific CD4 and CD8 T-cell responses in rhesus macaques. *J Virol* 2010;84(12):5898–5908.
378. Roy MJ, Wu MS, Barr LJ, et al. Induction of antigen-specific CD8+ T cells, T helper cells, and protective levels of antibody in humans by particle-mediated administration of a hepatitis B virus DNA vaccine. *Vaccine* 2000;19(7–8):764–778.
380. Russell SM, Liew FY. T cells primed by influenza virion internal components can cooperate in the antibody response to haemagglutinin. *Nature* 1979;280(5718):147–148.
381. Sabin A. Properties and behavior of orally administered attenuated poliovirus vaccine. *Jama* 1957;164:1216–1223.
382. Sabin A, Boulger L. History of Sabin attenuated poliovirus oral live vaccine strains. *J Biol Stand* 1973;1:115–118.
383. Sabin AB. Oral poliovirus vaccine: history of its development and use and current challenge to eliminate poliomyelitis from the world. *J Infect Dis* 1985;151(3):420–436.
388. Sardesai NY, Weiner DB. Electroporation delivery of DNA vaccines: prospects for success. *Curr Opin Immunol* 2011;23(3):421–429.
393. Schmitz JE, Kuroda MJ, Santra S, et al. Control of viremia in simian immunodeficiency virus infection by CD8+ lymphocytes. *Science* 1999;283(5403):857–860.
397. Seder RA, Ahmed R. Similarities and differences in CD4+ and CD8+ effector and memory T cell generation. *Nat Immunol* 2003;4(9):835–842.
399. Selin LK, Welsh RM. Plasticity of T cell memory responses to viruses. *Immunity* 2004;20(1):5–16.
401. Sibbet G, Romero-Graillet C, Meneguzzi G, et al. alpha6 integrin is not the obligatory cell receptor for bovine papillomavirus type 4. *J Gen Virol* 2000;81(Pt 2):327–334.
406. Song JM, Van Rooijen N, Bozja J, et al. Vaccination inducing broad and improved cross protection against multiple subtypes of influenza A virus. *Proc Natl Acad Sci U S A* 2011;108(2):757–761.
407. Spear GT, Takefman DM, Sullivan BL, et al. Anti-cellular antibodies in sera from vaccinated macaques can induce complement-mediated virolysis of human immunodeficiency virus and simian immunodeficiency virus. *Virology* 1993;195(2):475–480.
409. Stanberry LR, Spruance SL, Cunningham AL, et al. Glycoprotein-D-adjuvant vaccine to prevent genital herpes. *N Engl J Med* 2002; 347(21):1652–1661.
411. Strasser R, Castilho A, Stadlmann J, et al. Improved virus neutralization by plant-produced anti-HIV antibodies with a homogeneous beta1,4-galactosylated N-glycan profile. *J Biol Chem* 2009;284(31):20479–20485.
412. Strickler HD, Rosenberg PS, Devesa SS, et al. Contamination of poliovirus vaccines with simian virus 40 (1955–1963) and subsequent cancer rates. *JAMA* 1998;279(4):292–295.
413. Sullivan NJ, Martin JE, Graham BS, et al. Correlates of protective immunity for Ebola vaccines: implications for regulatory approval by the animal rule. *Nat Rev Microbiol* 2009;7(5):393–400.
416. Takafuji ET, Gaydos JC, Allen RG, et al. Simultaneous administration of live, enteric-coated adenovirus types 4, 7 and 21 vaccines: safety and immunogenicity. *J Infect Dis* 1979;140(1):48–53.
418. Tan M, Huang P, Xia M, et al. Norovirus P particle, a novel platform for vaccine development and antibody production. *J Virol* 2011;85(2):753–764.
419. Tang DC, DeVit M, Johnston SA. Genetic immunization is a simple method for eliciting an immune response. *Nature* 1992;356(6365):152–154.
423. Theiler M, Smith H. The effect of prolonged cultivation in vitro upon the pathogenicity of yellow fever virus. *J Exp Med* 1939;65:767–787.
424. Tonkin DR, Jorquera P, Todd T, et al. Alphavirus replicon-based enhancement of mucosal and systemic immunity is linked to the innate response generated by primary immunization. *Vaccine* 2010;28(18):3238–3246.
425. Topham DJ, Tripp RA, Doherty PC. CD8+ T cells clear influenza virus by perforin or Fas-dependent processes. *J Immunol* 1997;159(11): 5197–5200.
428. Townsend AR, Gotch FM, Davey J. Cytotoxic T cells recognize fragments of the influenza nucleoprotein. *Cell* 1985;42(2):457–467.
435. Vasan S, Hurley A, Schlesinger SJ, et al. In Vivo Electroporation Enhances the Immunogenicity of an HIV-1 DNA Vaccine Candidate in Healthy Volunteers. *PLoS One* 2011;6(5):e19252.
438. Victoria JG, Wang C, Jones MS, et al. Viral nucleic acids in live-attenuated vaccines: detection of minority variants and an adventitious virus. *J Virol* 2010;84(12):6033–6040.

439. Villa LL, Costa RL, Petta CA, et al. Prophylactic quadrivalent human papillomavirus (types 6, 11, 16, and 18) L1 virus-like particle vaccine in young women: a randomised double-blind placebo-controlled multicentre phase II efficacy trial. *Lancet Oncol* 2005;6(5):271–278.
440. Walker LM, Phogat SK, Chan-Hui PY, et al. Broad and potent neutralizing antibodies from an African donor reveal a new HIV-1 vaccine target. *Science* 2009;326(5950):285–289.
441. Wang BZ, Xu R, Quan FS, et al. Intranasal immunization with influenza VLPs incorporating membrane-anchored flagellin induces strong heterosubtypic protection. *PLoS One* 2010;5(11):e13972.
443. Wang R, Doolan DL, Le TP, et al. Induction of antigen-specific cytotoxic T lymphocytes in humans by a malaria DNA vaccine. *Science* 1998;282(5388):476–480.
444. Wang TT, Tan GS, Hai R, et al. Vaccination with a synthetic peptide from the influenza virus hemagglutinin provides protection against distinct viral subtypes. *Proc Natl Acad Sci U S A* 2010;107(44):18979–18984.
446. Waters TD, Anderson PS, Jr., Beebe GW, et al. Yellow fever vaccination, avian leukosis virus, and cancer risk in man. *Science* 1972;177(43):76–77.
448. Weitkamp JH, Lafleur BJ, Greenberg HB, et al. Natural evolution of a human virus-specific antibody gene repertoire by somatic hypermutation requires both hotspot-directed and randomly-directed processes. *Hum Immunol* 2005;66(6):666–676.
453. Wolf M, Garcea RL, Grigorieff N, et al. Subunit interactions in bovine papillomavirus. *Proc Natl Acad Sci U S A* 2010;107(14):6298–6303.
454. Wolff JA, Malone RW, Williams P, et al. Direct gene transfer into mouse muscle in vivo. *Science* 1990;247(4949 Pt 1):1465–1468.
456. Wrammert J, Smith K, Miller J, et al. Rapid cloning of high-affinity human monoclonal antibodies against influenza virus. *Nature* 2008;453(7195):667–671.
459. Wu X, Yang ZY, Li Y, et al. Rational design of envelope identifies broadly neutralizing human monoclonal antibodies to HIV-1. *Science* 2010;329(5993):856–861.
461. Xing L, Wang JC, Li TC, et al. Spatial configuration of hepatitis E virus antigenic domain. *J Virol* 2011;85(2):1117–1124.
462. Xu R, Ekiert DC, Krause JC, et al. Structural basis of preexisting immunity to the 2009 H1N1 pandemic influenza virus. *Science* 2010; 328(5976):357–360.
465. Yankauckas MA, Morrow JE, Parker SE, et al. Long-term anti-nucleoprotein cellular and humoral immunity is induced by intramuscular injection of plasmid DNA containing NP gene. *DNA Cell Biol* 1993; 12(9):771–776.
467. Yu X, Tsibane T, McGraw PA, et al. Neutralizing antibodies derived from the B cells of 1918 influenza pandemic survivors. *Nature* 2008;455(7212):532–536.
473. Zhou J, Sun XY, Stenzel DJ, et al. Expression of vaccinia recombinant HPV 16 L1 and L2 ORF proteins in epithelial cells is sufficient for assembly of HPV virion-like particles. *Virology* 1991;185(1):251–257.
474. Zhou T, Georgiev I, Wu X, et al. Structural basis for broad and potent neutralization of HIV-1 by antibody VRC01. *Science* 2010;329(5993): 811–817.
475. Zhu FC, Zhang J, Zhang XF, et al. Efficacy and safety of a recombinant hepatitis E vaccine in healthy adults: a large-scale, randomised, double-blind placebo-controlled, phase 3 trial. *Lancet* 2010;376(9744): 895–902.
476. Zhu J, Yamane H, Paul WE. Differentiation of effector CD4 T cell populations. *Annu Rev Immunol* 2010;28:445–489.

CHAPTER 15

Gregory A. Storch • David Wang

Diagnostic Virology

Diagnostic virology continues to evolve rapidly. Viral testing is now essential for the care of a number of patient groups, including hospitalized patients with acute respiratory infections; transplant recipients and other immunocompromised patients; patients infected with human immunodeficiency virus (HIV), hepatitis C virus (HCV), and hepatitis B virus (HBV); and infants with possible congenital infection. Multiple test methods continue to be used, but molecular tests are emerging as the dominant technology. A variety of commercial molecular assays have been or are in the process of being approved or cleared as *in vitro* diagnostic tests by the Food and Drug Administration (FDA). This is an important development because it makes viral diagnostic testing available to more laboratories and it improves the standardization of diagnostic testing. The scope of diagnostic virology has broadened. General categories of viral diagnostic testing and the viruses included in those categories are shown in Table 15.1.

HISTORY OF DIAGNOSTIC VIROLOGY

Modern diagnostic virology dates to the first growth of human viruses in tissue culture reported by Weller and Enders in 1948.[149] This and other landmarks in the history of diagnostic virology are shown in Table 15.2.

SPECIMENS FOR VIRAL DIAGNOSIS

The likelihood of making a specific viral diagnosis depends largely on the quality of the specimen that is received in the laboratory. Important variables include the timing of the specimen in relation to the patient's illness, the type of specimen, the quality and amount of specimen material obtained, and the time and conditions of transport to the laboratory. Although this concept is so basic as to seem trivial, optimizing the variables listed requires knowledge on the part of the physician and attention to logistic considerations that can present substantial barriers to diagnosis.

For the diagnosis of acute viral infections, the best specimens are usually obtained from the site of disease. For example, in the patient with suspected viral meningitis, cerebrospinal fluid (CSF) is the best specimen. In infections involving skin or mucosal surfaces, specimens obtained from those surfaces are usually the only ones required. Viral titers are highest early in the course of an acute illness, so that specimens obtained within the first few days after onset are most likely to be positive.

Viral culture requires more attention to conditions of transport than specimens submitted for detection of viral antigens or nucleic acids, because the viability of the virus must be preserved. A number of clinically important viruses are labile and will not survive prolonged transport. General instructions for transporting specimens for viral culture are shown in Table 15.3. These conditions are usually also suitable for detection of viral antigens and nucleic acids, but consultation with the laboratory performing testing is advised.

For serologic diagnosis, an acute phase serum specimen should be obtained within the first few days of illness and a convalescent phase specimen 2 to 4 weeks later. If a virus-specific immunoglobulin M (IgM) assay is available, the acute phase specimen may be sufficient by itself. Immunoglobulins are stable in serum or plasma. Proper handling of specimens for serologic diagnosis begins with separation of serum or plasma. If testing is performed within several days, the serum or plasma can be stored at 4°C. If a longer delay is involved, the specimen should be frozen at –20°C or –70°C. For certain viral infections, serologic tests can also be performed on saliva or urine.

TABLE 15.1 Categories of Testing Performed in Diagnostic Virology

Category of testing	Specific viruses	Methodology
Respiratory viruses	Influenza A and B, RSV, PIV 1–4, hMPV, rhinoviruses, enteroviruses, coronaviruses, adenoviruses	Rapid antigen tests (influenza A and B, RSV), fluorescent antibody staining (influenza A and B, RSV, PIV 1–3, adenoviruses, hMPV), culture, multiplex NAAT
Gastrointestinal viruses	Rotavirus, norovirus, adenovirus, astrovirus	Rapid antigen tests (rotavirus, norovirus, adenovirus), NAAT
Mucocutaneous viruses	HSV, VZV, HPV	Fluorescent antibody staining (HSV and VZV), culture (HSV and VZV), NAAT
Central nervous system viruses	HSV, VZV, CMV, EBV, HHV-6, JCV, enteroviruses, parechoviruses, West Nile virus, other arboviruses	NAAT, serology (West Nile and other arboviruses)
Opportunistic agents	CMV, EBV, BKV, HHV-6, adenoviruses	NAAT, antigen detection (CMV pp65 assay), cytology (BKV)
Mononucleosis syndrome in nonimmunocompromised individuals	EBV, CMV, HIV	Serology, NAAT
HIV, HCV, HBV viral loads	HIV, HCV, HBV	NAAT
Viral genotyping	HCV, HBV, HPV	Nucleotide sequencing, reverse hybridization, NAAT (Cleavase reaction for HPV)
HIV, HCV, HBV diagnosis	HIV, HCV, HBV	Serology, NAAT
Systemic infections of childhood	Parvovirus B19, measles virus, rubella virus, mumps virus	NAAT, serology
Tropical and emerging infections	Dengue and other flaviviruses; chikungunya and other alphaviruses; hemorrhagic fever viruses including arenaviruses, bunyaviruses, and filoviruses; Hendra and Nipah viruses	Serology, culture, NAAT (hemorrhagic fever testing is done in BSL-4 laboratories)
Unknown virus	Any	Culture, microarray, nucleotide sequencing

BKV, BK virus; CMV, cytomegalovirus; EBV, Epstein-Barr virus; HBV, hepatitis B virus; HCV, hepatitis C virus; HHV-6, human herpesvirus 6; HIV, human immunodeficiency virus; hMPV, human metapneumovirus; HPV, human papillomavirus; HSV, herpes simplex virus; JCV, JC virus; NAAT, nucleic acid amplification testing; PIV, parainfluenza virus; RSV, respiratory syncytial virus; VZV, varicella-zoster virus.

TABLE 15.2 Landmarks in the History of Diagnostic Virology

Year	Landmark
1892	Intranuclear and intracytoplasmic inclusions noted at the base of smallpox lesions[47]
1898	Discovery by Loeffler and Frosch that foot-and-mouth disease of cattle is caused by a filterable agent, referred to as a virus
1929	Complement fixation method described for detection of antibodies to smallpox, vaccinia, and varicella-zoster viruses[6]
1948	First growth of pathogenic human viruses in tissue culture[149]
1956	Detection of influenza virus in respiratory secretions using fluorescent antibody staining[36,80]
1975	Development of monoclonal antibodies as diagnostic reagents[68]
1985	Discovery of PCR[118]
1992	Development of real-time PCR[53]
2002	Beginning of systematic approaches to virus discovery[45,91,148]
2007	Description of multiplex PCR for respiratory viruses[85]

PCR, polymerase chain reaction.

SIGNIFICANCE OF VIRAL DETECTION

As in other areas of microbiology, the detection of a virus in a clinical sample is not proof in and of itself that the detected virus is the cause of the patient's illness. This problem regarding viral causality is exacerbated by polymerase chain reaction (PCR) and other very sensitive detection methods that may reveal very low-level persistent infection or even latent infection, unrelated to the patient's current illness. A determination of whether a causal relationship exists requires consideration of several factors. Two of the most important are (a) the nature of the virus–host interaction and (b) whether the virus is known to cause the disease manifestations that the patient is experiencing. If the virus detected is one known to be associated with persistent or latent infection, its detection may require other supportive evidence before it can be accepted as causal of the patient's current illness. For example, detection of the presence of virus-specific IgM antibodies or of seroconversion, in addition to the presence of the virus, favors acute infection, which, in turn, favors a causal relationship. An alternative approach using molecular methods may be to detect a specific viral RNA that encodes a structural or other protein that is expressed only in active infection. Obviously, detection of a virus known to cause the disease that the patient has is much more likely to be causal than detection of a virus not

TABLE 15.3 Instructions For Obtaining and Transporting Specimens for Viral Testing[a]

Specimen	Instructions[b]
Blood	Volume requirement varies according to the specific test required. Molecular methods generally require lower blood volumes than does culture. The appropriate tube is determined by the test to be performed, the blood component on which the test is performed (whole blood, leukocytes, plasma, or serum), and the preference of the laboratory. Whole blood, leukocytes, and plasma require collection into a tube containing an anticoagulant. The most commonly used anticoagulants are ethylenediaminetetraacetic acid (EDTA) (purple top tube), heparin (green top tube), and acid-citrate-dextrose (yellow top tube). Note: Heparin is inhibitory for some polymerase chain reaction (PCR) procedures, especially those performed on plasma. Some nonculture tests performed on blood may have specific collection tube requirements that can be determined through communication with the laboratory. Most serologic procedures are performed on serum, although some tests can also be performed on plasma. Serum specimens require collection into a tube that does not contain an anticoagulant (red top tube or gold top serum separator tubes). Blood specimens do not have to be placed on ice if transport requires less than 1 day. Note: Prolonged transport can severely compromise the ability to recover cytomegalovirus (CMV) in culture from blood specimens.[114]
Swab	Swabs with Dacron or rayon tips are preferred. If available, swabs designed specifically for collection of viral specimens should be used. Recently, flocked swabs have been shown to be superior to standard swabs.[1,90] Swabs can also be placed in viral transport media. In this case, the shaft of the swab may have to be cut to allow the top of the transport vial to be securely closed. The swab or tube of transport media should be placed on ice if transport will require more than 1 hour.
Fluid	Place in a sterile container.
Tissue	Place in a sterile container with a small amount of viral transport media or sterile saline or phosphate-buffered saline to maintain moisture.
Stool	Obtain at least 4 g of stool. Place in a clean or sterile container.

[a]Specimens other than blood should be transported on ice if more than 1 hour is required for arrival in the laboratory. If a delay of more than 24 hours is anticipated, specimens should be frozen at –70°C and transported on dry ice. Note: Some viruses such as respiratory syncytial virus (RSV) and varicella-zoster virus (VZV) are unlikely to retain viability with freezing. Specimens should not be frozen at –20°C.

[b]Commercial tests may have specific recommendations for collection and transport. These should always be followed to ensure proper assay performance.

known to be associated with that disease. This applies particularly to viruses such as human herpesvirus type 6 (HHV-6) and type 7 (HHV-7), human polyomaviruses such as JC virus, non–high-risk types of human papillomavirus (HPV), and even respiratory or gastrointestinal viruses such as rhinovirus or adenoviruses that may be present in patients who are not ill.

METHODS USED IN DIAGNOSTIC VIROLOGY

Viral Culture

For approximately 50 years, viral culture was the signature method of diagnostic virology laboratories, and it was the method that led to the establishment of virology laboratories as distinct entities apart from other areas of the clinical laboratory. With the advent of immunological and especially of molecular methods, which are more rapid than viral culture and potentially detect a broader range of viruses, cell culture is playing a diminishing role. For this reason, the treatment of cell culture in this chapter will be brief, and the interested reader is referred to other sources.[77,78,125,144]

By their very nature, viruses require living systems for propagation. In the past, inoculation of animals such as suckling mice or of embryonated eggs was used to grow viruses. These methods were largely supplanted by cell culture in the diagnostic laboratory. To grow viruses in cell culture, a clinical sample is prepared and then inoculated onto one or more cell culture types. Typically several cell culture types are inoculated, because no one type supports the growth of all clinically relevant viruses. Cell culture types that are commonly used are shown in Table 15.4. After inoculation, viral growth is detected in one of several ways. Traditionally, the principal method was the appearance of cytopathic effect, which refers to morphologic changes observable by microscopy that occur in virally infected cells (Fig. 15.1). Alternatively, hemadsorption, which refers to the surface binding of erythrocytes by virally infected cells, was used for the detection of influenza, parainfluenza, and mumps viruses. Interference, used to detect rubella virus, refers to the phenomenon that cells infected with certain viruses such as rubella virus become resistant to infection with other viruses that would readily infect the cells if they were uninfected by the first virus. Confirmation of virus growth, suspected based on one of the indicators described previously, can be achieved by immunofluorescence using specific antiviral antibodies. When cytopathic effect is present but immunological stains are negative, electron microscopy of cell culture material can be used to examine the culture. More recently, molecular methods such as VIDISCA (virus discovery based on complementary DNA [cDNA]-amplified fragment length polymorphism) have been used in this situation to detect new viruses growing in cell culture.[107,132]

Presently, most viral culture done in diagnostic virology laboratories is performed using centrifugation cultures, also often referred to as shell-vial cultures (Fig. 15.2). The shell-vial culture method was originally developed for cytomegalovirus (CMV)[42,46] but has subsequently been applied to many other viruses. In this method, viral entry is enhanced by a low-speed centrifugation after inoculation of the clinical sample onto the cell culture, which may be grown on a cover

TABLE 15.4 Cell Culture Types Used to Detect Medically Important Viruses

Primary	Monkey kidney	Influenza viruses, parainfluenza viruses, enteroviruses
	Rabbit kidney	Herpes simplex virus
	Human embryonic kidney	Adenovirus, enteroviruses
Diploid	Fibroblasts (e.g., MRC-5, WI-38)	CMV, VZV, HSV, rhinovirus, enteroviruses (some), adenovirus, RSV
Continuous	HEp-2	RSV, adenovirus, HSV, parainfluenza viruses (some), enteroviruses (some)
	A549	HSV, adenovirus, enteroviruses
	MDCK	Influenza viruses
	LLC-MK2	Parainfluenza viruses, hMPV
	Rhabdosarcoma (RD)	Echoviruses
	Buffalo green monkey	Coxsackieviruses

CMV, cytomegalovirus; hMPV, human metapneumovirus; HSV, herpes simplex virus; RSV, respiratory syncytial virus; VZV, varicella-zoster virus.

slip within a 1-dram vial referred to as a shell vial, but can also be grown within other devices such as 24-well plates that can be conveniently centrifuged. Viral growth is detected by immunofluorescence, typically at 16 and 40 hours after inoculation, allowing detection of viruses much sooner than could be accomplished using conventional tube cultures. It is now possible to purchase cell cultures for centrifugation cultures in which more than one type of cell is present. For example, a commercial system called R-Mix (Diagnostic Hybrids, Inc., Athens, Ohio) combines human adenocarcinoma (A549) and mink lung cell lines for growth of respiratory viruses. After incubation, the R-Mix cells are stained with a mixture of monoclonal antibodies specific for seven respiratory viruses. Similar mixed cell culture systems also exist to detect herpes simplex virus (HSV) and varicella-zoster virus (VZV) and to detect enteroviruses.

Genetically Engineered Cell Lines

Techniques of genetic engineering have been used to modify cell lines either to make them susceptible to viruses to which they are not otherwise susceptible or to create novel means of detecting virus growth. An example is a cell line developed by Stabell and Olivo[126] for the detection of HSV. This cell line, shown in Figure 15.3, consists of baby hamster kidney (BHK) cells that have been transfected with the β-galactosidase gene from *Escherichia coli* under the control of a promoter from the herpes simplex gene *UL39*. The promoter is activated by exposure to HSV proteins ICP0 and VP16. Exposure of the cells to

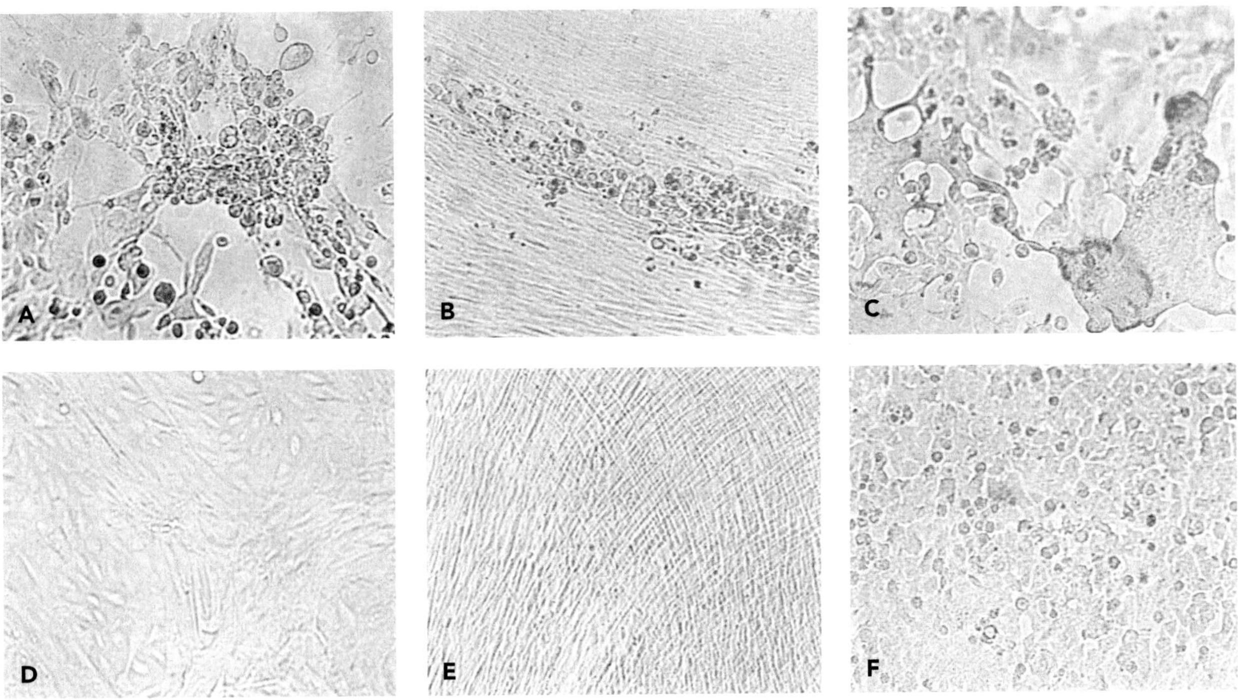

FIGURE 15.1. Cytopathic effect caused by viruses growing in cell culture. Herpes simplex virus growing in primary rabbit kidney cells **(A)**; uninfected primary rabbit kidney cells **(D)**. Cytomegalovirus growing in human embryonic lung fibroblast cells **(B)**; uninfected human embryonic lung fibroblast cells **(E)**. Respiratory syncytial virus growing in HEp-2 cells **(C)**; uninfected HEp-2 cells **(F)**.

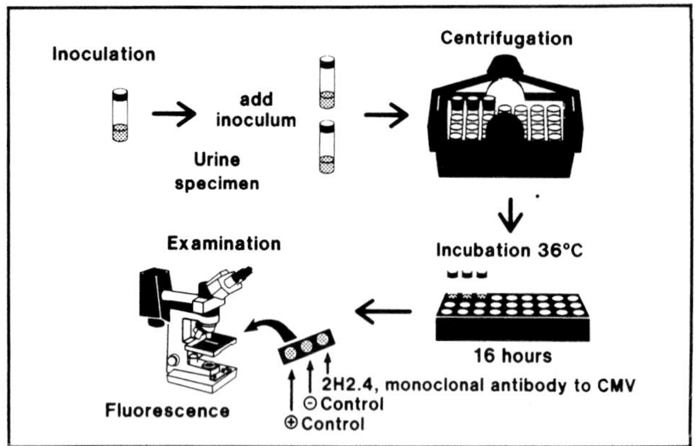

FIGURE 15.2. Shell-vial assay for cytomegalovirus. (From Shuster EA, Beneke JS, Tegtmeier GE, et al. Monoclonal antibody for rapid laboratory detection of cytomegalovirus infections: characterization and diagnostic application. *Mayo Clin Proc* 1985;60:577–585, with permission.)

a specimen containing HSV specifically activates the promoter, causing production of β-galactosidase, which can be detected by a simple histochemical stain of the culture, performed 16 to 24 hours after inoculation. A commercial version of this system, called ELVIS HSV (Diagnostic Hybrids, San Diego, CA), has been shown to have sensitivity comparable to conventional viral culture for detection of HSV in clinical specimens.[127] The system has also been adapted to the performance of HSV antiviral drug susceptibility assays.[133] Another example is the creation of a line of buffalo green monkey (BGM) cells that have been modified to express human decay-accelerating factor, which is a receptor for some enterovirus serotypes.[56] Addition of this molecule increases the ability of unaltered BGM cells to grow enteroviruses. These cells are combined with A549 cells in a commercial product called Super E-Mix (Diagnostic Hybrids).

Electron Microscopy

Viral infections are rarely diagnosed using electron microscopy for the direct visualization of viral particles in specimens. Advantages include speed, lack of requirement for viral viability, and the potential to visualize many different kinds of viral particles. Disadvantages include the cost and complexity of maintaining an electron microscopy, the need for a skilled operator, and limited sensitivity related to the relatively high concentration of viral particles (10^5 to 10^6/L) that is required for visualization.[89] Historically, electron microscopy was used for the evaluation of stool specimens from patients with suspected viral gastroenteritis. Viruses such as rotavirus, astrovirus, and adenovirus could be identified based on their characteristic morphology, but this has been replaced by rapid immunoassays and PCR assays. Electron microscopy can also be used to detect and classify viral particles in fixed tissue obtained by biopsy or at autopsy. Screening of tissue samples by electron microscopy is not useful because of the small area of tissue that can be examined. Thus, electron microscopy is best employed when it is directed by evidence of viral infection detected by routine histology.

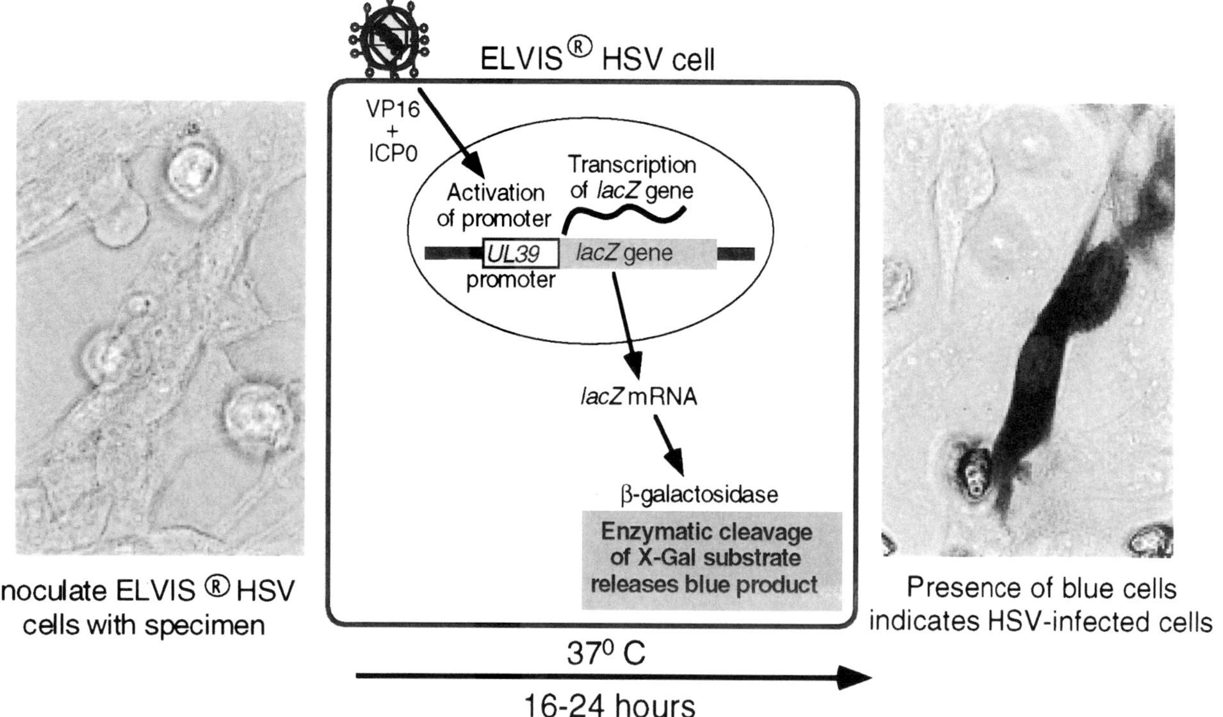

FIGURE 15.3. ELVIS herpes simplex virus (HSV), a genetically engineered cell line for the detection of HSV clinical samples. ELVIS cells are baby hamster kidney (BHK) cells that contain a β-galactosidase gene under the control of the HSV promoter UL39. If HSV is present in the specimen, viral particles enter the cells and the HSV proteins ICP0 and VP16 activate the UL39 promoter, leading to synthesis of β-galactosidase. The presence of β-galactosidase is detected by adding X-gal, a substrate for the enzyme. The activity of β-galactosidase on X-gal results in blue staining of ELVIS cells, visible microscopically.

TABLE 15.5 Viral Inclusions

Virus	Nuclear	Cytoplasmic
Herpes simplex, varicella-zoster	×	
Cytomegalovirus	×	×
Adenovirus	×	
Polyomaviruses (JC and BK)	×	
Parvovirus B19	×	
Poxviruses		×
Measles	×	×
Parainfluenza		×
Rabies		×

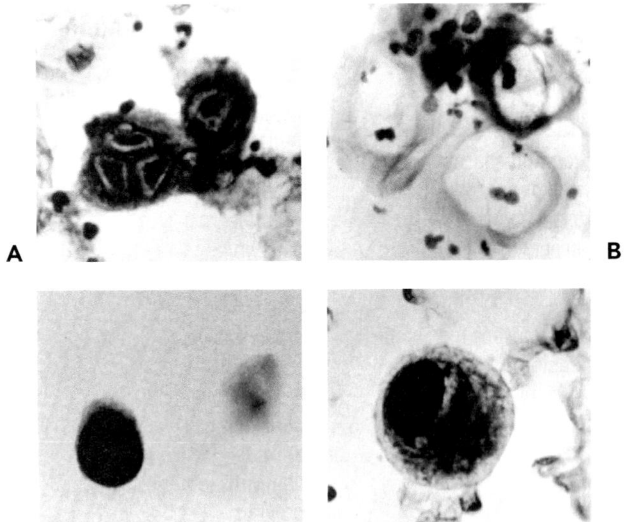

FIGURE 15.4. Cytologic findings suggestive of viral infection. **A:** Cervical smear showing multinucleated cells and the Cowdry type A intranuclear inclusions of herpes simplex infection. **B:** Papanicolaou smear showing binucleate squamous epithelial cells with distinct perinuclear halos. These characteristics, described as *koilocytosis,* are the cellular features associated with human papillomavirus infection. **C:** Urinary epithelial cell containing an enlarged nucleus with smudgy chromatin and a small pale *glassy* intranuclear inclusion indicative of polyomavirus infection. **D:** Cell from bronchoalveolar lavage with a large intranuclear inclusion with a perinuclear clear space (owl's eye cell) indicative of cytomegalovirus infection. (Photographs provided by Dr. Leslie Boucher, Department of Pathology, Washington University, St. Louis, Missouri.)

Light Microscopy

Although viral particles, with the exception of poxviruses, cannot be directly visualized by light microscopy, indirect evidence of viral infection can be detected. The most characteristic signs of viral infection are inclusion bodies (composed of masses of virions), multinucleated cells, and syncytial cells. These findings may be present in cytologic specimens or in tissue examined after histologic staining. Viral inclusions can be found in the nucleus or the cytoplasm of infected cells. The location is characteristic of the responsible virus. The location of viral inclusions is summarized in Table 15.5. Microscopy for detection of the effects of viral infections in clinical specimens is generally carried out in surgical pathology rather than diagnostic virology laboratories.

Cytology and Histology

Cytologic examination for evidence of viral infection can be performed on smears prepared by applying a specimen directly to a microscope slide, on slides prepared by cytocentrifugation of fluids (e.g., bronchoalveolar lavage fluid), and on touch preparations prepared from pieces of unfixed tissue. Viruses that can produce cytologic evidence of infection in respiratory specimens include HSV, CMV, adenoviruses, polyomaviruses, and measles virus (Warthin-Finkeldey cells). Cytologic examination is usually not a sensitive method for detection but provides strong evidence for tissue involvement. Examples of cytologic findings suggestive of viral infection are shown in Figure 15.4. The Tzanck smear is a method sometimes used to detect cytologic evidence of HSV or VZV infection. It is rarely used in diagnostic virology laboratories because techniques such as fluorescent antibody staining and PCR are more sensitive and specific. The Papanicolaou stain (Pap smear) is used to detect evidence of HPV infection in cells obtained from the uterine cervix. HPV infection produces characteristic changes in keratinocytes, including a condensed nucleus with a prominent perinuclear clear zone referred to as *koilocytosis.* More specific evidence of the presence of HPV can be provided by histochemical stains or molecular techniques. Urine cytology may reveal intranuclear inclusions indicative of infection with either CMV or the polyomaviruses, JC and BK. Culture or PCR for CMV and PCR for polyomaviruses, however, are more sensitive and specific techniques. Cytology does not distinguish between JC and BK viruses.

Histologic examination of stained tissue can provide unique information about the role of viral infection in producing tissue inflammation and injury and can be very useful in distinguishing between asymptomatic viral shedding and clinically significant infection. This is particularly useful for CMV infections in which prolonged viral shedding can occur without producing disease. For example, the presence of cytomegalic inclusion cells in tissue obtained by biopsy or at autopsy is often considered to be the gold standard for diagnosing clinically significant CMV infection localized in a specific organ.

Antigen Detection

The detection of viral antigens directly in clinical specimens is widely used to obtain rapid evidence of viral infection. The lack of requirement for virus viability is an important advantage. For some viruses, especially respiratory syncytial virus (RSV) and CMV, the sensitivity of antigen detection may exceed that of viral culture.[111,135] Antigen detection methods can be applied when the following conditions are met: (a) viral antigen is expressed and is present in an accessible specimen, (b) an appropriate antibody (usually but not necessarily monoclonal) is available, (c) antigenic variability does not preclude recognition by immunologic reagents of different strains of the target virus, and (d) the antigen being detected is sufficiently stable that it does not degrade during transport and processing of the specimen. Methods used for viral antigen detection include fluorescent antibody (FA) staining, immunoperoxidase staining, and enzyme immunoassay. The latter can be subdivided

TABLE 15.6 Viral Antigen Detection: Specimens Used and Viruses Detected

Specimen	Viruses detected
Respiratory (nasopharyngeal swab or aspirate, nasopharyngeal wash, tracheal aspirate, bronchoalveolar lavage)	Respiratory syncytial Influenza A, B Parainfluenza 1–3 Adenovirus Human metapneumovirus Measles
Skin or mucous membrane scraping	Herpes simplex Varicella-zoster
Conjunctival or corneal scraping	Herpes simplex Adenovirus
Stool	Rotavirus Adenovirus (enteric serotypes) Norovirus
Blood	Cytomegalovirus (pp65) Hepatitis B (surface antigen) Human immunodeficiency (p24)

into solid phase and lateral flow immunochromatographic assays. The viruses for which antigen detection assays are in widespread use are shown in Table 15.6.

Antigen detection can also be used to detect viral antigens in fixed tissue (immunohistochemistry [IHC]). This method can document the specific viral etiology of a nonspecific finding such as an inclusion body that could be produced by several different viruses. In some cases, IHC also enhances the sensitivity of detection of viruses in tissue compared to standard light microscopy without immunostaining. Immunoperoxidase staining is the most common technique used for viral antigen detection in fixed tissue. IHC can often be performed on formalin-fixed tissue, but for some antigen–antibody combinations, sensitivity is better on fresh frozen tissue.

Fluorescent Antibody Staining

Fluorescent antibody staining is widely used to detect cell-associated viral antigens. In the direct format, a fluorescent label, usually fluorescein isothiocyanate (FITC), is conjugated directly to the antibody that recognizes the viral antigen. In the indirect format, the antiviral antibody is unlabeled and is detected by a second antibody that recognizes immunoglobulins from the animal species of origin of the antiviral antibody. The second antibody carries the fluorescent label. After staining, the specimen is viewed with epi-illumination using ultraviolet (UV) light of the wavelength needed to excite the fluorescent label. The direct method is simpler to use but requires conjugation of each antiviral antibody with the fluorescent label. The indirect method is slightly more sensitive and more versatile, because only the anti-immunoglobulin antibody has to be conjugated with the fluorescent label.

The main applications of FA staining have been to detect respiratory, ocular, cutaneous, and bloodstream pathogens. Many different respiratory specimens can be used, including nasopharyngeal swabs or aspirates, nasal washes, tracheal aspirates, and bronchoalveolar lavage fluid. In each case, the specimen is processed in the laboratory to prepare a pellet of cells, which is spotted onto one or more microscope slides. The cells are air dried, fixed in acetone, and stained with monoclonal antibodies to one or more viruses. For ocular infections, material is scraped from the conjunctiva or cornea, placed on microscope slides, and processed as described for respiratory specimens. Staining is usually directed at detection of HSV and adenovirus antigens. For cutaneous infections, the lesion is scraped with a scalpel blade or swab, and cellular material obtained is placed directly on one or more microscope slides. Alternatively, the base of the lesion can be rubbed vigorously with a swab and the swab submitted to the laboratory, where cellular material is washed from the swab and spotted onto a microscope slide. The use of cytocentrifugation to prepare the slides has been shown to improve the results.[75] Staining is directed at detection of HSV and VZV. In the CMV pp65 antigenemia assay, peripheral blood leukocytes are separated from anticoagulated blood; spotted onto a microscope slide, usually by cytocentrifugation; and stained using a monoclonal antibody specific for the CMV pp65 antigen. The major limitation of FA staining is having an adequate number of cells in the specimen. Immunoperoxidase (IP) staining is similar to FA staining, except that horseradish peroxidase is used in place of a fluorescent label, making it possible to view the stain using light microscopy rather than requiring fluorescence microscopy. It is more often used to detect viral antigens in fixed tissue rather than directly in patient samples.

Enzyme Immunoassay

Enzyme immunoassay (EIA) is a versatile and widely used method that can be applied to the detection of antigens, regardless of whether they are cell associated or in fluid phase. Because intact cells in the specimen are not required, specimen integrity is less important than for FA or IP staining. This may be advantageous when specimen transport time is prolonged. A common assay format for antigen detection is the double antibody sandwich technique, shown in Figure 15.5. In this assay, a *capture* antibody specific for the viral antigen being sought is bound to a reaction surface, for example, the wells of a plastic microtiter tray or the surface of a plastic bead. When the specimen is added, viral antigen present in the specimen binds to the capture antibody. Bound antigen is detected using a different antiviral antibody, the *detector* antibody. The detector antibody can be labeled with an enzyme or can be detected by

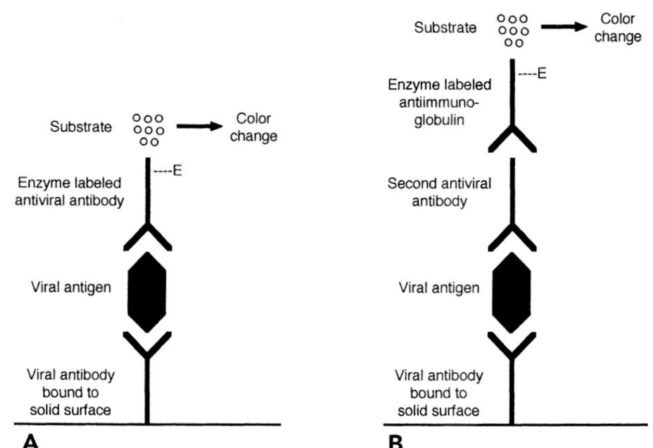

FIGURE 15.5. Enzyme immunoassay (EIA) for antigen detection. **A:** Direct. **B:** Indirect.

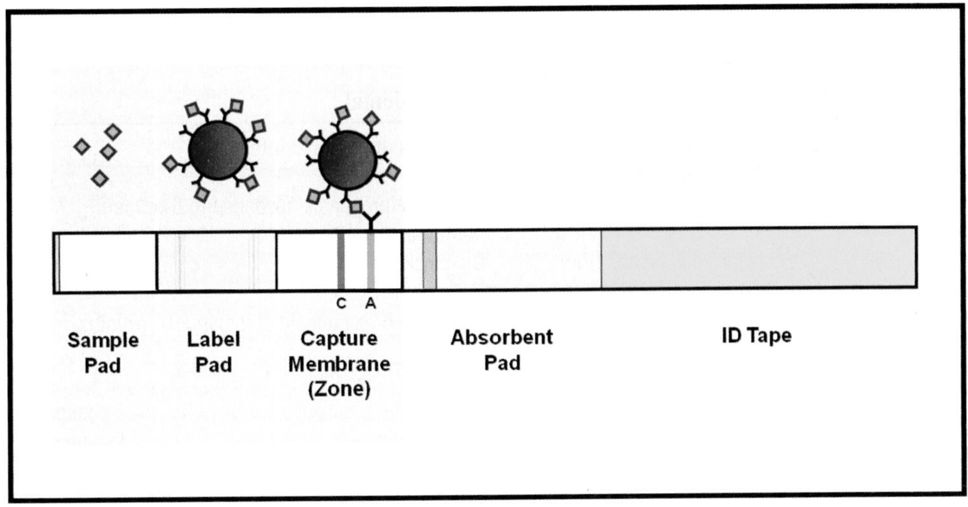

FIGURE 15.6. Lateral flow immunochromatographic assay. The sample is applied to the sample pad. The sample flows across the unit from left to right, drawn by the absorbent pad. Located in the label pad are one or more antibodies, each of which is conjugated to a label such as gold particles. These antibodies bind to antigen present in the sample as it moves across, forming complexes of antigen with conjugated antibody. If present, these complexes are then captured by second antibodies, located in lines in the capture membrane zone. When complexes are captured, the presence of the conjugated label causes the line to become visible. In the figure, antibodies against the target antigen are indicated by "A," and antibodies against a control antigen are indicated by "C." Presence of a colored line corresponding to A is a positive test. Presence of a line corresponding to C in the absence of a line corresponding to A indicates a negative test. Absence of both lines indicates that the test is not valid. (Figure provided by John Tamerius, Quidel Inc.)

the addition of an enzyme-labeled third antibody with specificity for immunoglobulin of the species from which the second antibody was derived. The addition of an enzyme substrate produces a color change or light emission if the enzyme is present. Thus, color change or light emission indicates that viral antigen was present in the specimen being tested. Advantages of EIA include applicability to diverse specimens and potential for automation. Laboratory instruments are now available that can perform EIA to detect either antigens or antibodies. Viruses for which antigen EIA have been widely used are RSV, influenza, rotavirus, enteric adenoviruses, HSV, HBV, and HIV.

Membrane Immunoassay

The lateral flow immunochromatographic assay is a variant of EIA that was first used in home pregnancy tests. A schematic diagram of a lateral flow unit is shown in Figure 15.6. In these tests, a sample is applied directly to a membrane and is drawn across the membrane by capillary action. Antigens in the sample react first with an antibody with specificity for the antigen being detected. This antibody is conjugated to a detector label such as gold particles or fluorescein. If binding occurs, the antigen–antibody complexes sweep across the membrane until they are captured by a second antibody that is bound to the membrane. When the labeled antigen–antibody complexes are captured, a line becomes visible because of the concentration of the label into a limited physical space. Most assays also include a positive control. These assays can be configured as dipsticks or as self-contained cassettes. Standard lateral flow immunochromatographic assays do not require an instrument and are convenient for testing single samples, with results available in 5 to 20 minutes. Multiple commercial versions are now available, mainly for detection of influenza, RSV, and rotavirus. Some of the tests are sufficiently simple to perform that they have been assigned *waived* status under the Clinical Laboratory Improvement Amendments (CLIA), meaning that they can be performed by individuals without specific training who can be working within or outside of a certified clinical laboratory. Unfortunately, sensitivity of these tests has generally been less than that for fluorescent antibody staining, culture, or PCR. This problem was especially true for commercial influenza lateral flow tests in detecting the 2009 H1N1 pandemic.[106] A recent test developed by 3M (3M Rapid Detection RSV or Influenza tests, 3M, St. Paul, MN) achieves increased sensitivity by using fluorescent beads conjugated to a detector antibody and reading the captured antigen–antibody complexes in a fluorescence reader.[41]

Nucleic Acid Detection

Diagnostic virology has been revolutionized by the application of nucleic acid detection techniques, which detect specific DNA or RNA sequences, and can be applied to the detection of virtually any virus. Depending on the target sequence, the assays can be specific for a single virus species or for a group of related viruses. The latter characteristic is particularly advantageous, because it allows nucleic acid detection techniques to be applied to groups of viruses (e.g., the enteroviruses) for which antigenic diversity has precluded successful application of antigen detection techniques. For example, enteroviruses, for which a rapid nonmolecular detection method had not been available, can be detected using reverse-transcription PCR assays that amplify a highly conserved sequence in the 5′ nontranslated region of the genome.[14,115] An overview of applications of nucleic acid testing in diagnostic virology is shown in Table 15.7.

TABLE 15.7 Nucleic Acid Detection for Viral Diagnosis

Target	Specimen(s)	Application(s)
HIV (DNA)	Leukocytes from infant born to HIV-infected mother	Diagnosis of perinatal infection
HIV (quantitative RNA)	Plasma	Viral load (prognosis, response to treatment)
HIV (qualitative RNA)	Plasma	Confirmation of diagnosis
HSV	CSF, ocular fluid, swabs from mucocutaneous lesions	Diagnosis of encephalitis, meningitis, retinitis, mucocutaneous lesions
VZV	CSF, ocular fluid, swabs from mucocutaneous lesions	Diagnosis of encephalitis, meningitis, retinitis, mucocutaneous lesions
CMV	Blood (whole blood, leukocytes, or plasma), CSF, ocular fluid, amniotic fluid	Diagnosis of systemic infection after organ transplantation, encephalitis, radiculomyelitis, retinitis, congenital infection. Quantitative assay performed on blood can be used to assess severity of infection and monitor response to therapy.
EBV	CSF, blood (whole blood, leukocytes, or plasma)	Primary central nervous system lymphoma in AIDS, other EBV infection of the central nervous system, posttransplant lymphoproliferative disorder. Quantitative assay performed on blood can be used to assess the risk of PTLD and the response to therapeutic interventions.
HHV-6, -7	Blood, CSF	Diagnosis of systemic infection and of encephalitis
HHV-8 (Kaposi sarcoma virus)	Blood, pleural or pericardial fluid	Diagnosis of body cavity lymphoma
Adenovirus	Blood, respiratory secretions	Diagnosis and monitoring of disseminated infection in immunocompromised hosts, diagnosis of respiratory tract infection
Parvovirus B19	Serum, amniotic fluid	Diagnosis of acute or chronic parvovirus B19 infection, aplastic crisis, congenital infection
BK virus	Urine, plasma	Assessment of risk of transplant nephropathy in renal transplant recipients and of hemorrhagic cystitis in hematopoietic stem cell transplant recipients
Human papillomavirus	Genital secretions	Detection of viral types associated with cervical carcinoma
Enteroviruses	CSF, blood (whole blood, serum, or plasma)	Diagnosis of meningitis, encephalitis, or systemic infection
Hepatitis C	Plasma	Diagnosis of infection. Quantitative assay is used to assess response to therapy.
Hepatitis B	Serum	Diagnosis of infection when serologic studies are ambiguous. Recognition of virologically active infection. Quantitative assay is used to assess response to therapy and recognize emergence of drug resistance.
Rabies	Saliva, CSF	Diagnosis of rabies
Respiratory viruses	Respiratory samples	Enhanced sensitivity, including detection of noncultivable agents
Gastrointestinal viruses	Feces	Enhanced sensitivity, including detection of noncultivable agents
West Nile and other flavivirus infections	CSF, blood	Rapid diagnosis of CNS infection, especially in immunocompromised hosts, screening of blood units for presymptomatic infection
Dengue	Plasma	Diagnosis of early infection, genotyping
Arenaviruses	Serum or whole blood	Diagnosis of acute infection
Filoviruses	Serum or whole blood	Diagnosis of acute infection
Nipah and Hendra viruses	CSF, throat swabs, urine	Diagnosis of acute infection
Vaccinia and other pox virus infections	Lesion	Diagnosis of acute infection

CMV, cytomegalovirus; CNS, central nervous system; CSF, cerebrospinal fluid; EBV, Ebstein-Barr virus; HHV, human herpesvirus; HIV, human immunodeficiency virus; HSV, herpes simplex virus; PTLD, posttransplant lymphoproliferative disorder.

The earliest attempts at nucleic acid–based diagnosis involved direct hybridization of nucleic acid probes to viral nucleic acids present in clinical specimens. Direct hybridization was never widely adopted because it lacked adequate sensitivity, requiring the presence of 10^4 to 10^5 copies of the target nucleic acid. The development of PCR[118] and other nucleic acid amplification techniques overcame that sensitivity barrier and has led to the development of nucleic acid–based diagnostic tests for many viruses. Nucleic acid amplification tests (NAATs) were originally directed at viruses that were difficult or impossible to cultivate, viruses that grew very slowly in culture, and viruses for which antigen detection could not be applied because of antigenic diversity or because the level of viral antigen in clinical specimens was too low to permit successful detection. NAATs were also very advantageous for specimens such as CSF or ocular fluid for which sample volume could be limiting. Still another advantage of nucleic acid detection as a diagnostic method is the stability of DNA as an analyte, so that detection of viral nucleic acids can be done even when conditions of transport lead to loss of virus viability. Currently NAATs are being applied to all viruses that are of interest in diagnostic virology.

Nucleic Acid Amplification Assays

Target Amplification

Polymerase Chain Reaction. PCR, which is the prototype of target amplification assays, employs short oligonucleotide primers and a thermostable DNA polymerase such as *Taq* polymerase to amplify a segment of target DNA that is typically 100 to 1,000 base pairs (bp) in length. Classic PCR includes repetitive cycles, each consisting of denaturation, primer annealing, and extension steps that take place at different temperatures. Progression through the steps of the cycle is controlled by a thermal cycler that controls the temperature of the reaction. After PCR amplification, the PCR product (also known as the *amplicon*) is detected by gel electrophoresis or by one of several probe-hybridization techniques (e.g., Southern blotting). The analytic sensitivity of PCR can be as low as 1 to 10 copies of target DNA. Because of its simplicity and broad applicability, PCR remains the most widely used NAAT.

Currently, most PCR in diagnostic virology laboratories is carried out using real-time PCR in which reaction products are detected as they are synthesized.[40,52] Numerous specialized instruments for running real-time PCR are now commercially available, including the LightCycler (Roche Diagnostics, Indianapolis, IN), the SmartCycler (Cepheid, Sunnyvale, CA), the ABI TaqMan 7000 series (Applied Biosystems, Foster City, CA), the Rotor Gene (Qiagen, San Diego CA), and many others. Compared with conventional PCR, real-time PCR has several important advantages. Because the accumulation of PCR product is monitored in the reaction tube, no separate detection method (e.g., gel electrophoresis) is required, thus shortening the effective assay time markedly and decreasing the risk of contamination of the laboratory environment by the amplified PCR product. The time from setting up the assay to completion can be less than 1 hour. The use of multiple fluorescent dyes with different emission wavelengths makes it possible to perform multiplex reactions with simultaneous amplification of more than one product. Of great importance, quantification of PCR targets is readily achieved because the generated fluorescence is proportional to the amount of PCR product.

Detection of PCR products in real-time PCR has generally used one of three methods, although other detection methods have also been introduced more recently. The simplest system uses the DNA binding dye SYBR Green, which emits fluorescence when it is bound to double-stranded DNA (dsDNA). When SYBR Green is included in a PCR reaction, the intensity of fluorescence is proportional to the amount of PCR product. Because SYBR Green binds nonspecifically to any dsDNA, signal is generated by undesired amplification products such as primer dimers, as well as by intended amplicons. Discrimination between different amplification products can be achieved through the use of dissociation curves, referred to as *melting point analysis*. Melting point analysis is performed after completion of the amplification reaction by recording fluorescence as the temperature of the reaction mix is gradually increased. When the dissociation temperature (melting point) of the dsDNA reaction product is reached, SYBR Green is released and fluorescence decreases. The melting point is affected by both length and sequence of the PCR product, and thus is precisely defined for a specific PCR product. Unintended amplification products will usually have different melting points, allowing easy discrimination from the intended PCR product.

The other two detection systems are based on the use of oligonucleotide probes that are labeled with fluorescent dyes that interact with one another according to principles of fluorescence resonance energy transfer (FRET). The hybridization probe assay format requires two oligonucleotide probes that are homologous to adjacent portions of one of the strands of the amplified DNA. The probes are chosen so that the 5′ end of one probe is within a few nucleotides of the 3′ end of the other probe. These adjacent ends are each labeled with a fluorescent dye. The dye on the 3′ end is termed the *donor dye* and the dye on the 5′ end is termed the *acceptor dye*. The required property of these dyes is that when they are in close proximity (within a distance of several nucleotides), excitation of the donor dye leads to emission of light by the acceptor dye. When both probes bind to their target sequences, the two dyes are within the proximity required for excitation of the acceptor dye and fluorescence occurs. The fluorescence intensity is proportional to the amount of PCR product.

The other detection system based on interacting fluorescent dyes is the fluorogenic 5′ exonuclease assay (also referred to as the *Taqman assay*). This assay uses a probe that is complementary to a segment of the intended PCR product located between the PCR primers. This probe is labeled with two fluorescent dyes, one called the *reporter* that is linked to the 5′ end of the probe, and the other called the *quencher* that is linked to the 3′ end. When they are in close proximity (i.e., bound to opposite ends of an oligonucleotide probe), the quencher prevents fluorescence by the reporter. During the extension step of PCR, the probe labeled with both dyes binds to the PCR product as it is being synthesized. During extension, the 5′ exonuclease activity of *Taq* polymerase cleaves nucleotides from the 5′ end of the bound probe, releasing the reporter dye away from the quencher, thus allowing it to emit light on excitation. As in the hybridization probe assay, the intensity of fluorescence is proportional to the amount of PCR product.

Because *Taq* polymerase uses only DNA as a template, the use of PCR to detect viral RNA sequences requires the inclusion of a reverse-transcription (RT) step before PCR (RT-PCR). The RT reaction can be performed using a devoted enzyme such as Moloney murine leukemia virus RT or avian myeloblastosis virus RT. Alternatively, heat-stable, multifunctional enzymes such as recombinant *Thermus thermophilus* DNA polymerase are now available that can carry out RT as well as DNA polymerase reactions. Special care must be used in specimen processing because of the susceptibility of RNA to digestion by ribonucleases that may be present in clinical samples. In addition to detecting virion RNA, RT-PCR can also be applied to the detection of viral messenger RNA. This may be particularly useful in the diagnosis of infection caused by viruses that have a latent phase in their life cycle. For these viruses, detection of viral DNA might not distinguish between latent and productive infection, whereas detection of a messenger RNA (mRNA) expressed only in productive infection would be evidence of active viral infection.

RNA Amplification Assays. Several reactions have been developed that are directed at amplification of RNA. *Transcription-based amplification* (Fig. 15.7)[48,73] uses three enzymes, RT, ribonuclease (RNase) H, and T7 RNA polymerase, to amplify a target RNA sequence, employing a series of reactions that mimic the retrovirus replication scheme. An advantage of transcription-based amplification assays is that they are isothermal and do not require complicated instrumentation. The assays begin with synthesis of a DNA strand that is complementary to the RNA target, using a primer that contains a T7 polymerase binding site at its 5′ end. The resulting DNA–RNA hybrid is converted to dsDNA by the action of RNase H and a second primer that also contains a 5′ T7 polymerase binding site. The dsDNA product then serves as a template for transcription driven by T7 RNA polymerase. The newly synthesized RNA transcripts serve as templates for additional cycles of the reaction. Variants of transcription-based amplification include transcription-mediated amplification (TMA),[39] self-sustained sequence replication (3SR),[48] and nucleic acid sequence–based amplification (NASBA).[21] Currently, NASBA assays for HIV, enteroviruses, and CMV pp67 have been approved by the FDA and are marketed by bioMérieux Inc. (Durham, NC) under the trade name NucliSENS. TMA is the basis for the Procleix assays for HIV, HCV, HBV, and West Nile virus marketed by Gen-Probe (San Diego, CA).

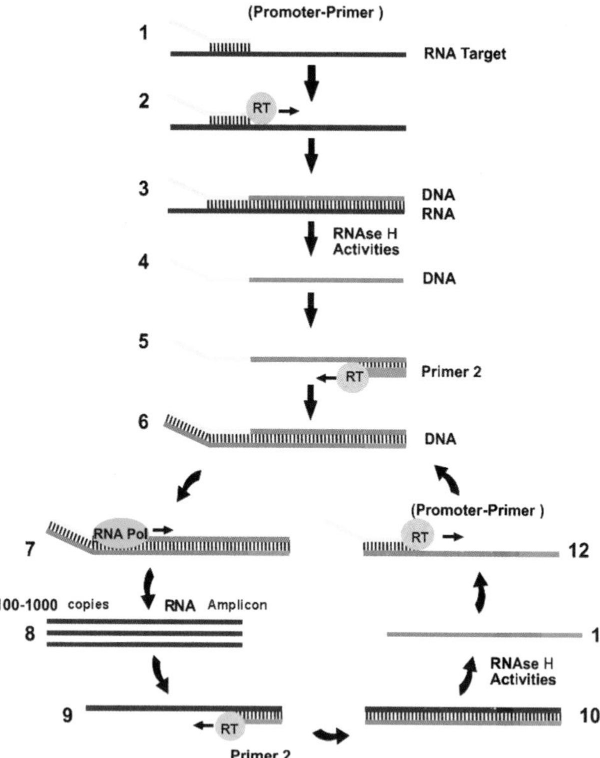

FIGURE 15.7. Transcription-mediated assay, also called 3SR. The 3SR reaction depends on a continuous cycle of reverse transcription and transcription reactions to replicate an RNA target by means of complementary DNA (cDNA) intermediates. Steps 1–6 depict the synthesis of a double-stranded cDNA, which is a transcription template for T7 RNA polymerase. Complete cDNA synthesis is dependent on the digestion of the RNA in the intermediate RNA–DNA hybrid (step 4) by ribonuclease (RNase) H. Transcription-competent cDNAs yield antisense RNA copies of the original target (step 7, right). These transcripts are converted to cDNA containing double-stranded promoters on both ends in an inverted repeat orientation (steps 7–12). These cDNAs can yield either sense or antisense RNA, which can re-enter the cycle.

Signal Amplification

Examples of signal amplification assays include the branched-chain DNA (bDNA) assay,[22] the hybrid capture assay,[51] and the cleavase reaction.[49] The bDNA assay (Fig. 15.8) uses short, branched-chain oligonucleotides to capture the target nucleic acid sequence. Other branched-chain oligonucleotides link multiple molecules of detector enzyme to the captured target. A chemiluminescent substrate allows detection of the target, and measurement of the intensity of emitted light makes it possible to quantify the input target accurately. Because the target itself is not amplified, this reaction is less susceptible than PCR to carryover contamination. Currently, FDA-approved quantitative bDNA assays for HIV and HCV are marketed by Siemens USA (Deerfield, IL) under the trade name Versant.

The hybrid capture assay (Fig. 15.9) is a signal amplification assay that involves a liquid hybridization reaction between the denatured DNA target and RNA probes specific for the viral DNA sequence of interest. If the viral DNA is present, DNA–RNA hybrid molecules are formed and are captured and detected using an antibody specific for DNA–RNA hybrids. This assay can be used as either a qualitative or quantitative assay. Currently, FDA-approved or cleared hybrid capture assays for HPV and CMV are marketed by Qiagen (Valencia, CA).[83,88]

The Invader assay (Fig. 15.10) is an isothermal reaction that makes use of (a) an enzyme referred to as Cleavase that functions as an FEN-1–encoded flap endonuclease,[136] plus (b) two short sequence–specific oligonucleotides termed the probe oligo and the Invader oligo. To initiate the reaction, the two oligos bind to the target DNA with a short region of overlap that is designed to occur at a targeted single nucleotide polymorphism (SNP). The overlap structure occurs only when exact base pairing occurs with the targeted SNP. The resulting structure forms a substrate for the Cleavase enzyme, which cleaves the primary probe oligo at the position of overlap, releasing the 5′ portion, which is termed the *flap oligonucleotide.* The primary probe and the Invader oligos are present in large molar excess, resulting in generation of many cleaved flap oligos if the targeted SNP is present in the template. The flap oligo itself functions as an Invader oligo, binding to a hairpin region of a third oligo, termed a fluorescence resonance energy transfer (FRET) cassette because it contains a fluorophore and a quencher adjacent to one another at one end of the cassette. The sequence of the FRET oligo causes it to assume a hairpin configuration in which the quencher damps fluorescence from the fluorophore. Binding of the flap Invader generates another tertiary DNA structure that also functions as a substrate for the Cleavase enzyme. The resulting cleavage releases the fluorophore away from the quencher, which leads to the generation of a fluorescent signal. Reaction conditions that allow cycling of the probe oligo and the hairpin oligos cycle on and off their

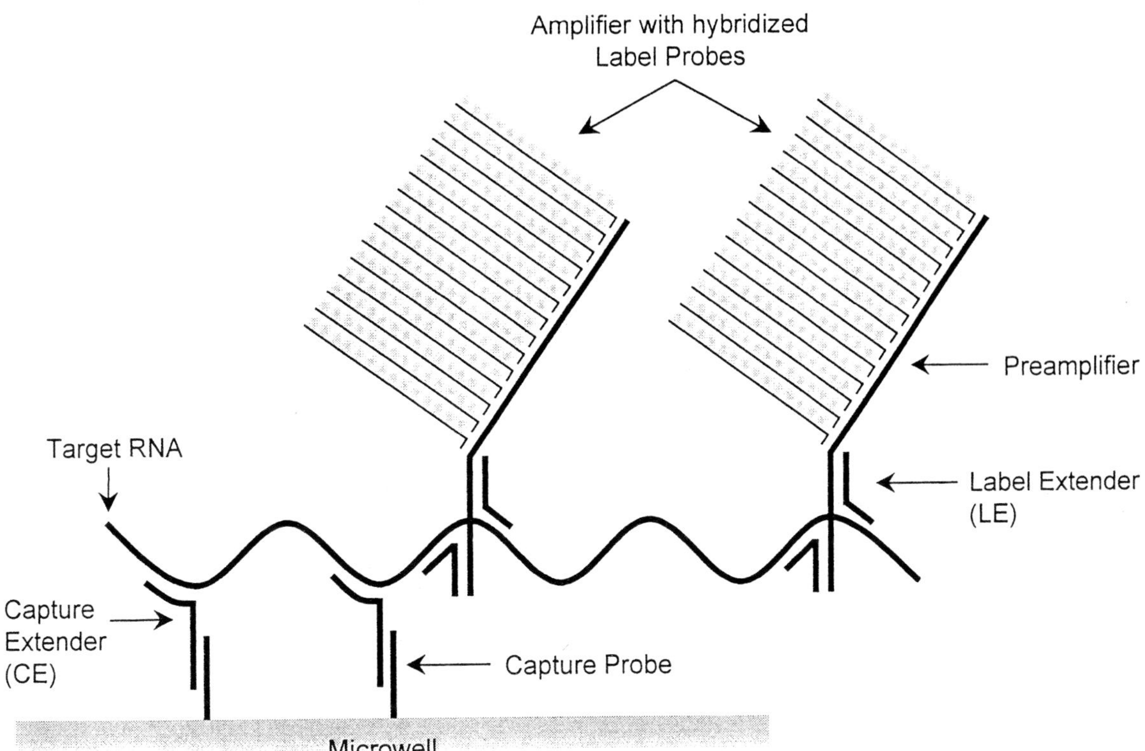

FIGURE 15.8. Branched-chain DNA assay as used for ultrasensitive detection of human immunodeficiency virus (HIV). After liberation of viral nucleic acid from the clinical specimen by a lysis buffer, viral nucleic acid is hybridized with two sets of bifunctional oligonucleotide probes, each of which contains sequences complementary to the target. One set of probes also contains a generic sequence complementary to a capture probe that is bound to the surface of a microtiter tray and serves to bind the target to the solid surface. The other set of probes contains a sequence complementary to *preamplifier* molecules. Additional specificity is achieved because two of the target-specific probes must be juxtaposed in the correct orientation to stabilize the binding of the preamplifier molecule. Each preamplifier molecule binds numerous amplifier molecules, each of which binds many subsequently added alkaline phosphatase–labeled probes. A chemiluminescent substrate is added and generated light is read by a luminometer. The cascade effect results in amplification of the signal generated from initial binding of probes to the target and allows for detection and quantification of nucleic acid present in the specimen. (Courtesy of Bayer Diagnostics, Emeryville, California.)

respective targets result in the generation of 10^6- to 10^7-fold signal amplification per hour. Currently, FDA-approved tests using the Cleavase reaction to detect high-risk HPV types and to genotype HPV types 16 and 18 are marketed by Hologic (Bedford, MA) (formerly Third Wave Technologies) under the trade name Cervista.

The loop-mediated isothermal amplification (LAMP) (Fig. 15.11) is an amplification reaction that employs four primers and a strand-displacing DNA polymerase.[96] It was developed originally by Eiken Chemical Co. (Tokyo, Japan), and additional detailed diagrams of the assay can be viewed on the Eiken web page: http://loopamp.eiken.co.jp/e/lamp/index.html. The inner primers have sense and antisense sequences. When they initiate DNA synthesis, the result is a stem-loop structure, which itself serves as a target for additional amplification. The resulting reaction can produce 10^9 copies of target DNA or RNA in less than 1 hour under isothermal conditions. The reaction can be monitored by measuring turbidity, which results from the accumulation of magnesium pyrophosphate, a by-product of the reaction. Alternatively, the synthesis of dsDNA can be measured using an agent such as SYBR Green, which generates fluorescence when it intercalates between the strands of dsDNA. The reaction has high specificity by virtue of the inclusion of multiple primer sets. The isothermal nature of the reaction, which obviates the requirement for a thermal cycler, makes LAMP attractive for use as a point-of-care test or for use in the developing world.

Contamination

A general concern regarding highly sensitive nucleic acid amplification assays is the occurrence of false-positive findings resulting from contamination of the reaction with exogenous nucleic acids. The source of contaminating nucleic acids can be either amplified products from previous reactions or viral nucleic acids present in a different specimen, especially one containing a high level of the intended target. Prevention of contamination requires fastidious attention to procedural detail within the laboratory. A number of specific preventive techniques are widely used to prevent carryover contamination after PCR, including the use of positive displacement pipettes or plugged pipette tips to block aerosol production, UV irradiation of reaction components (not including *Taq* polymerase and PCR primers that can be inactivated by UV irradiation), use of small working aliquots, and frequent cleaning of equipment and laboratory surfaces with 10% bleach. An important precaution is the physical separation of the laboratory into

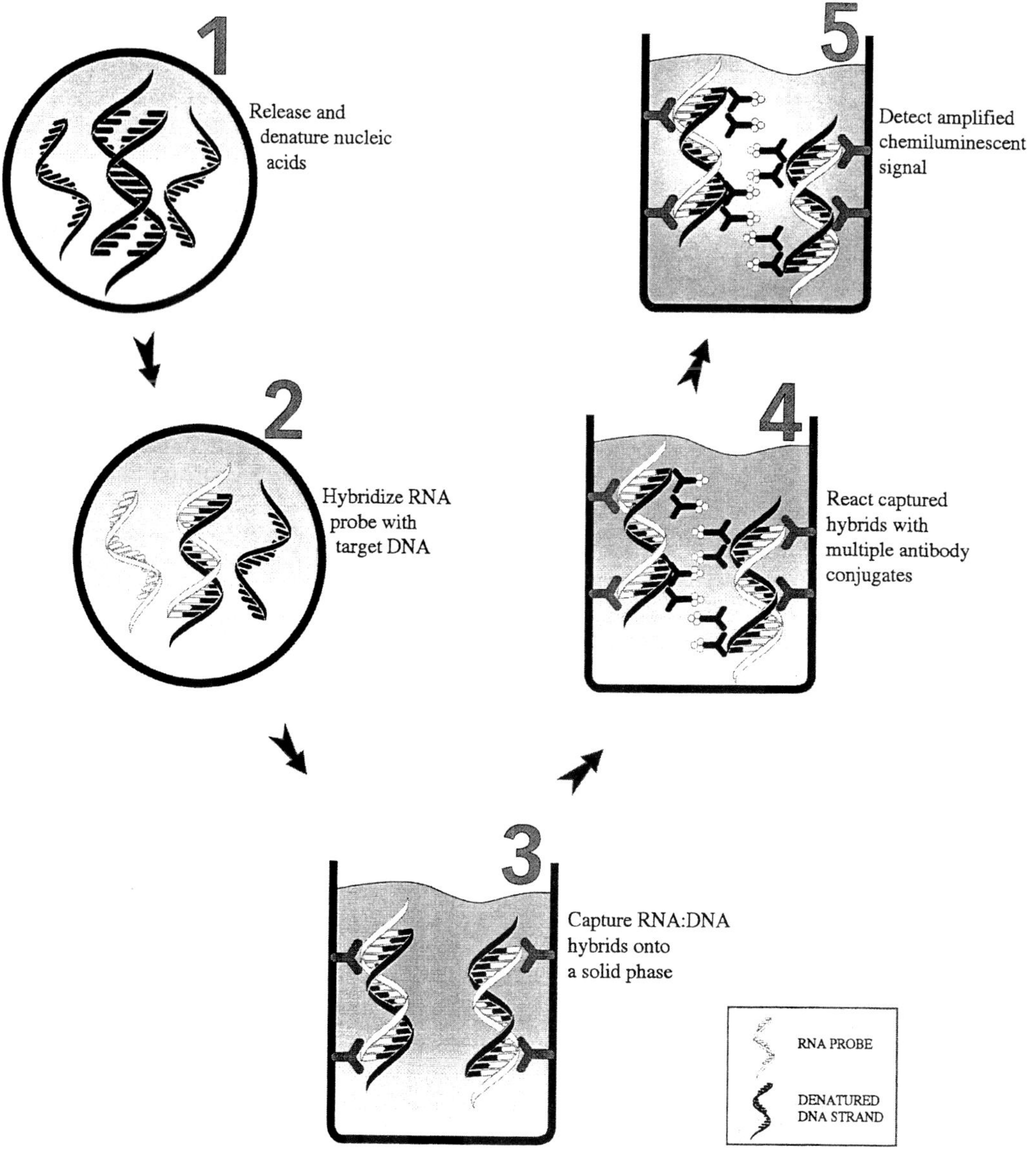

FIGURE 15.9. Hybrid capture assay. In step 1, target DNA is released and denatured. In step 2, RNA probe hybridizes with target DNA. In step 3, RNA–DNA hybrids are captured by an antibody to RNA–DNA hybrids that is bound to the sides of the reaction vessel. In step 4, an enzyme-conjugated antibody that recognizes RNA–DNA hybrids binds to the hybrids. In step 5, a chemiluminescent substrate is added, and light is emitted if hybrids have been formed. (Courtesy of Digene Corporation, Beltsville, Maryland.)

sections where (a) the specimen is prepared, (b) the PCR reaction is set up, (c) the PCR amplification reaction takes place, and (d) the detection of amplification products is carried out. After PCR has taken place, the reaction tube is opened only in the section of the laboratory devoted to product detection. Techniques such as the inclusion of uracil-N-glycosylase or psoralen and isopsoralen derivatives in the reaction mixture were developed to minimize the danger of PCR contamination.[104] Real-time PCR is less susceptible to contamination because product detection does not require manipulating the amplified product. For any form of nucleic acid testing, an additional concern is contamination from one specimen to another, which may occur during specimen handling in the laboratory. Inclusion of negative controls in the reaction setup is important in order to detect this form of contamination.

Nucleotide Sequencing

Sequencing of PCR amplification products can be carried out using the cycle-sequencing reaction[57] or pyrosequencing. Sequence information can be used for several purposes including precise identification of a virus, genotyping, and the presence of mutations associated with antiviral drug resistance or unusual clinical manifestations. Genotypic resistance assays are performed most commonly for HIV, CMV, HBV, and influenza A virus (see section on antiviral susceptibility testing). For HBV, nucleotide sequencing of the nucleocapsid gene

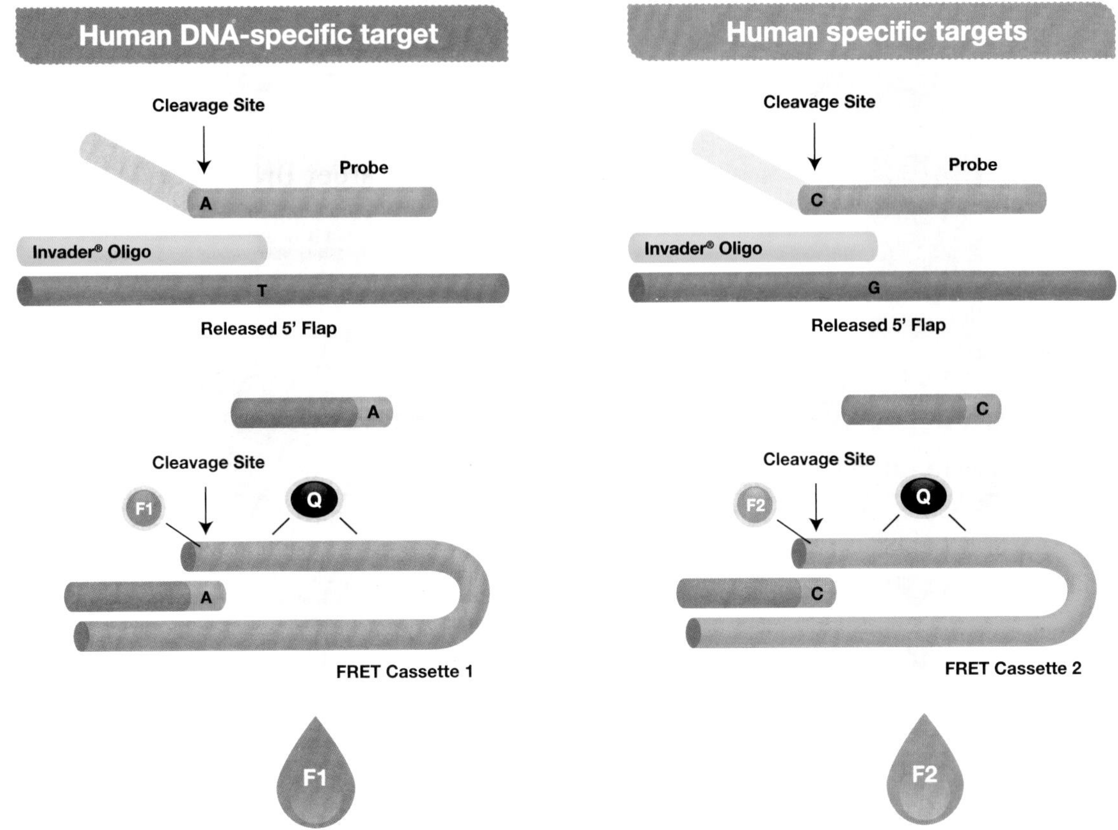

FIGURE 15.10. Invader assay. The **left side** of the figure shows a positive control reaction for human histone 2DNA and the **right side** shows the reaction to detect human papillomavirus (HPV). For each reaction, the probe oligo and the Invader oligo bind to the target, with a short region of overlap occurring at a targeted single nucleotide polymorphism (SNP). This results in a structure that is cleaved by the activity of an enzyme called "Cleavase," releasing the 5′ end of the probe oligo at the position of overlap. The sequence of the released portion is homologous to the 3′ end of a third oligo, which includes a fluorophore (F1 for the human DNA reaction and F2 for the HPV reaction) and a quencher (Q) and is referred to in the figure as the FRET cassette. The hairpin configuration assumed by the FRET cassette brings the quencher sufficiently close to the fluorophore to allow its fluorescence to be quenched. Binding of the released portion of the probe oligo to the FRET cassette results in a region that is another substrate for Cleavase. The activity of Cleavase releases the fluorophore, resulting in generation of a fluorescent signal. (Courtey of Hologic.)

and its associated promoter is also used for detection of core promoter and precore mutations, which have been associated with unusually severe disease and progression to chronic infection.[97] High-throughput ("next-generation") sequencing will probably have important applications in diagnostic virology, including for antiviral susceptibility testing, for identification of viruses growing in cell culture that are not identifiable by conventional means,[130] and for discovery of known[15,154] and novel viruses.[20,99]

Microarray Technology

High-density microarrays consist of hundreds or thousands of oligonucleotide probes bound to a solid phase, usually a small silicon chip. Amplified nucleic acid can be hybridized to the array, and binding to specific probes can be identified. Use of probes representing all possible nucleotide sequence variations within a target sequence allows very rapid determination of nucleotide sequence.[45] Multiple sequence variants present within the specimen can also be detected. Microarray technology has the potential to allow simultaneous detection of multiple infectious disease pathogens, viral and nonviral. An early application in diagnostic virology has been for rapid sequencing to detect HIV mutations associated with resistance to antiretroviral drugs.[70] In another application, sequences representing all sequenced viruses have been selected to create a microarray that can be used to discover unknown viruses. This microarray was successful in categorizing the agent of severe acute respiratory syndrome (SARS) as a new coronavirus.[145] The major application of microarray technology in diagnostic virology to date has been the use of liquid arrays, which are used for the simultaneous detection of multiple respiratory viruses, as exemplified by the xTAG RVP described later. Future uses of liquid arrays and other microarray technology under development include assays to detect multiple viruses (as well as other classes of pathogens) associated with gastroenteritis, sexually transmitted diseases, sepsis, and bioterrorism.

Commercial Nucleic Acid Amplification Platforms and Tests

Government Regulation

In the United States, commercially marketed diagnostic tests and test platforms are regulated by the FDA. Before marketing

LAMP Process

Target DNA

1. Solution temperature at 60°–65° C

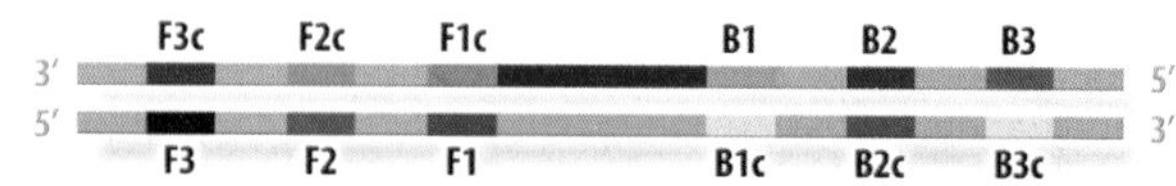

2. Forward Initiating Primer (FIP) anneals to Target Sequence
3. DNA Polymerase initiates synthesis that displaces single strand template DNA
4. Through polymerase activity, a strand complementary to the DNA template is formed

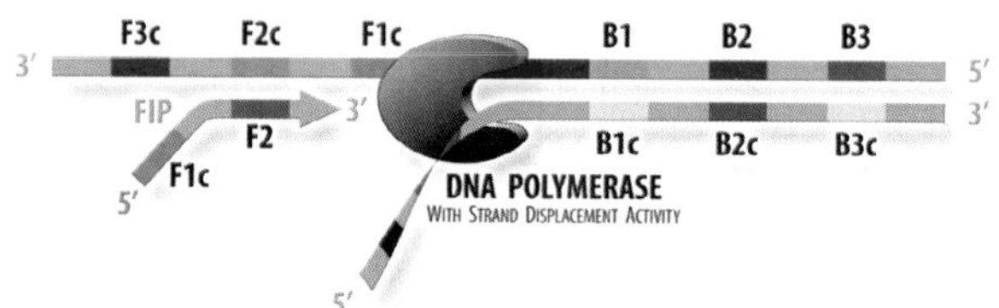

5. The F3 Primer anneals to the F3c Region

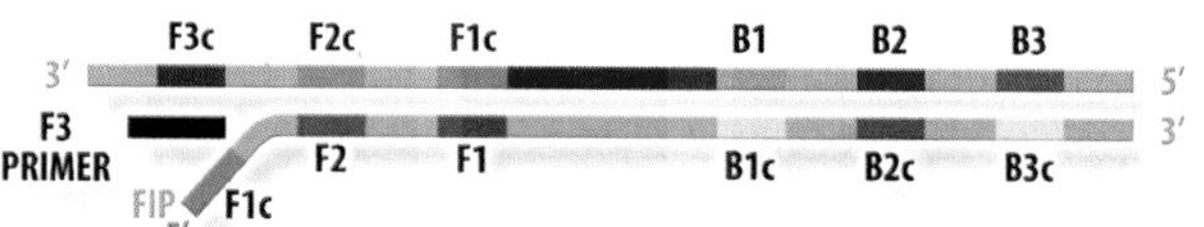

6. DNA Polymerase initiates synthesis and the FIP-linked complementary strand is replaced

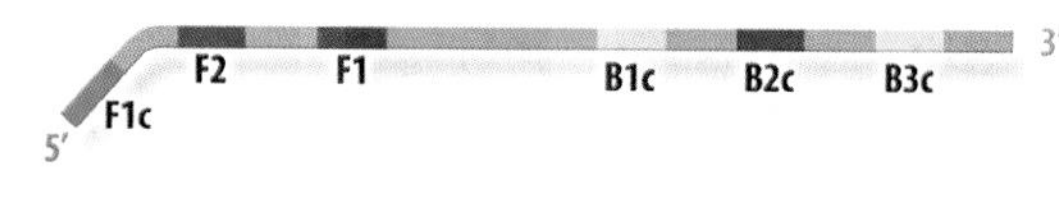

7. This strand forms a "stem loop" at the 5' end due to complementary F1 and F1c regions
8. The BIP anneals to the 3' end of the "stem loop" strand

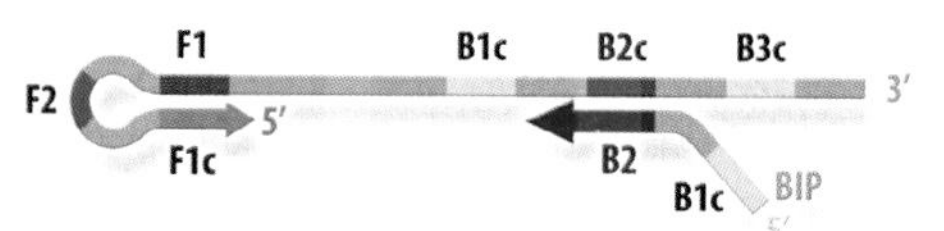

9. The B3 Primer anneals to the B3c target
10. From the 3' end, polymerase synthesizes a complementary DNA strand

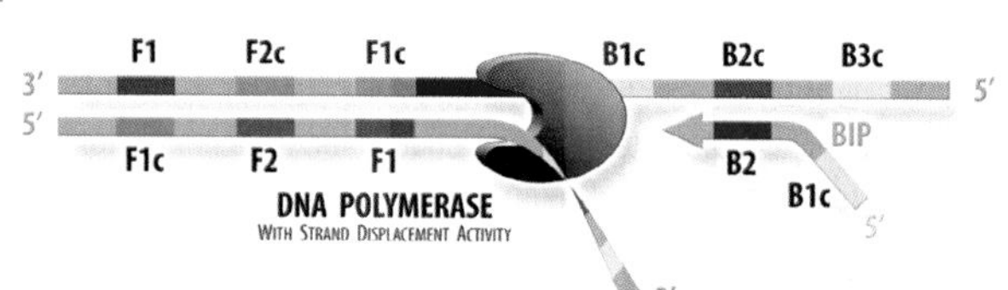

11. DNA reverts from a Loop structure to a linear structure
12. The BIP linked complementary strand is displaced as a single strand

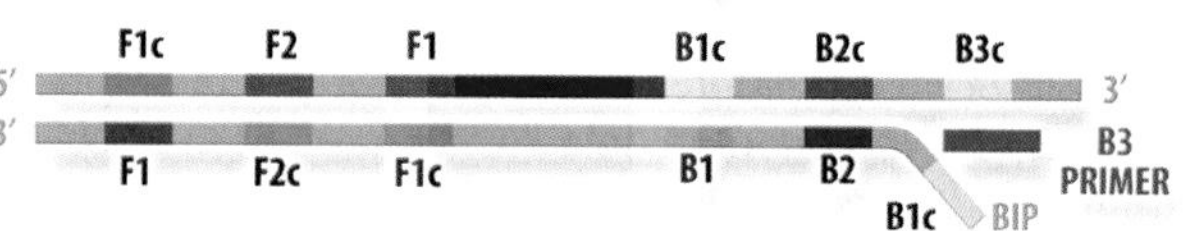

13. This strand forms stem-loops at either end due to the activity of the dual complementary primers

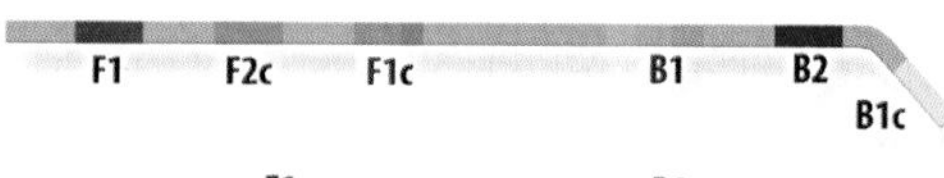

14. This is the starting structure for LAMP Cycling

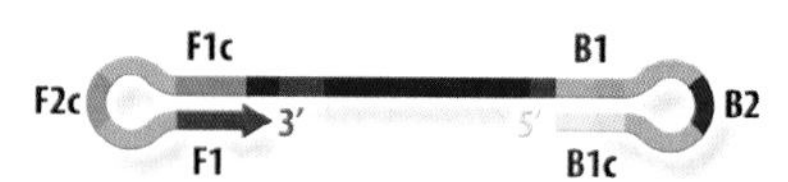

A

FIGURE 15.11. Loop-mediated amplification reaction (LAMP assay). A: Steps leading up to the formation of the "dumbbell" structure. (*continued*)

Cycling Amplification

A dumbbell-like DNA structure is quickly converted into a stem-loop DNA by self-primed DNA synthesis. FIP anneals to the single stranded region in the stem-loop DNA and primes strand displacement DNA synthesis, releasing the previously synthesized strand. This released single strand forms a stem-loop structure at the 3' end because of complementary B1c and B1 regions.

Then, starting from the 3' end of the B1 region, DNA synthesis starts using self-structure as a template, and releases FIP-linked complementary strand (STEP2).

The released single strand then forms a dumbbell-like structure as both ends have complementary F1 - F1c and B1c - B1 regions, respectively (STEP4).

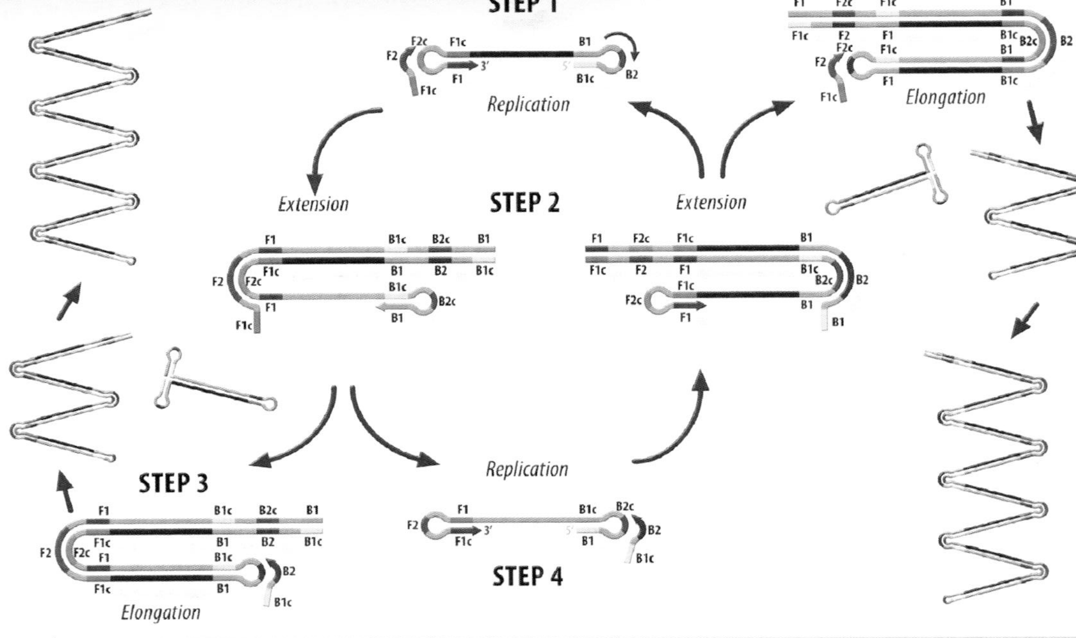

This structure is the 'turn over' structure of the structure formed in STEP1. Similar to the STEPS 1 THROUGH 4, structure in STEP4 leads to self-primed DNA synthesis starting from the 3' end of the B1 region.

Furthermore, BIP anneals to the B2c region and primes strand displacement DNA synthesis, releasing the B1-primed DNA strand. Accordingly, similar structures to STEPS 2 AND 3 as well as the same structure as STEP 1 are produced. With the structure produced in STEP 3, the BIP anneals to the single strand B2c region, and DNA synthesis continues by displacing double stranded DNA sequence. As a result of this process, various sized structures consisting of alternately inverted repeats of the target sequence on the same strand are formed.

B

FIGURE 15.11. (*Continued*) **B:** The cycling steps of the reaction, which lead to extremely rapid amplification. (Courtesy of Meridian Biosciences.)

a test for diagnostic use, a manufacturer must receive authorization from the FDA. This authorization can take one of several forms. If there is no similar test on the market, the manufacturer must apply for premarket approval (PMA). This is a rigorous and expensive process that requires the manufacturer to provide evidence for the accuracy and utility of the proposed test. A test that is "substantially equivalent" to a test that has been previously approved or cleared by the FDA is cleared for use through a mechanism referred to as 510K, after the section of the Federal Food, Drug, and Cosmetic Act that describes the process. Some diagnostic test materials are marketed under the classification "analyte-specific reagent (ASR)." This term is used by the FDA to refer to reagents or materials, including nucleic acid primers and probes, that must meet certain specifications set by the FDA, including being produced utilizing current "good manufacturing practices." In addition, clinical laboratory tests carried out using ASRs must have appropriate labeling appended to the reported results stating that the test was developed and validated by the laboratory and has not undergone FDA clearance or approval. ASRs are intended to be used as components of laboratory-developed tests and can be sold only to laboratories that are qualified under CLIA to perform highly complex testing. ASRs are excluded from the need for premarket approval by the FDA. They cannot be marketed as complete test kits and must be sold without instructions for use or claims regarding performance characteristics.

Individual laboratories may also develop their own assays that are intended for use only in that laboratory. These tests, referred to as "laboratory-developed tests" (sometimes also referred to as "home-brew assays"), are not actively regulated by the FDA, but instead are under the jurisdiction of CLIA passed by the U.S. Congress in 1988. Laboratory-developed tests may use ASRs as components of the test and may also use reagents obtained from diverse sources not specifically labeled as ASRs. The performance of laboratory-developed tests must be verified according to specific criteria established by CLIA.

Overview of Commercial Assays and Platforms

Since the last edition of this book, there has been a dramatic increase in molecular diagnostic tests and test platforms that have been approved or cleared by the FDA for the detection of pathogenic viruses. Tests and platforms approved or cleared by the FDA at the time this chapter was written are shown in Tables 15.8 and 15.9. These tables are adapted from tables that are maintained by the Association for Molecular Pathology (AMP) and are accessible on the AMP website (http://www.amp.org). No single platform permits the detection of all medically important viruses, so laboratories whose mission is broad-based viral diagnosis will need to employ multiple platforms. Currently, laboratories vary widely in the relative proportion of testing that is carried out using commercial platforms versus laboratory-developed tests. Likewise, laboratories that provide different types of service will employ different platforms. For example, hospital-based laboratories may emphasize platforms that provide rapid turnaround time, commercial laboratories may employ platforms that allow high specimen throughput, and government laboratories may employ platforms that allow for testing of viruses of public health significance. The following paragraphs describe several categories of commercial molecular diagnostic tests.

Multiplex Assays

Multiplex PCR refers to PCR reactions in which more than one primer set is incorporated into the reaction mix, allowing the detection of multiple targets. Multiplex assays may be developed either as commercial tests or as laboratory-developed tests. Currently, multiplex assays are being developed for important specimen types to amplify various viral and other microbial agents that are pathogenic at the specific body site. This process is most highly developed for respiratory samples, for which five different multiplex assays are currently cleared by the FDA.

The Proflu+ assay marketed by Prodesse (now Gen-Probe, San Diego, CA), the Simplexa Flu A/B & RSV Test assay marketed by Focus (Cypress, CA), and the Verigene RV+ (Nanosphere, Northbrook, IL) are multiplex real-time assays that use separate primer pairs to simultaneously amplify influenza A and B viruses and RSV plus an internal control. In the Proflu+ and Simplexa assays, unique probes for each virus and the internal control are labeled with separate fluorophores, allowing determination of which virus or viruses have been amplified. The Simplexa assay is run on the 3M Integrated Cycler, an innovative instrument produced by 3M (St. Paul, MN) that has the capability to run 96 assays in 1 hour. Multiple different specimens can be loaded on the instrument and multiple assays can be run simultaneously. The Verigene RV assay uses a very innovative system to detect amplified products in which the amplicons are captured by capture probes that are bound to specific sites on a microarray. Captured amplicons are then detected by binding of silver-coated gold nanospheres that have been tagged with oligonucleotides that are specific for the amplicons and are visualized by light scatter.

The xTAG Respiratory Virus Panel (RVP) marketed by Luminex (Toronto, Ontario, Canada) was the first large multiplex assay to be cleared by the FDA. This assay detects the following viruses in nasopharyngeal swabs: influenza A and B, influenza A subtypes H1 and H3, RSV A and B, parainfluenza 1 through 3, human metapneumovirus (hMPV), enterovirus/rhinovirus, and adenovirus.[85,98] Primers for influenza A hemagglutinin subtype H5, parainfluenza 4, and coronaviruses OC43, 229E, NL63, HKU1, and SARS are also included in the reaction but are not currently cleared for use in the United States. The first step in the reaction is reverse transcription followed by a multiplex PCR reaction that includes primer sets for each target. The resulting amplicons are prepared for detection through a reaction called target-specific primer extension (TSPE). The 3′ end of each of the primers used in TSPE is homologous to one of the amplicons from the multiplex PCR reaction. The 5′ end of the primer consists of a short "tag" sequence that will be used to capture the TSPE product. During the extension reaction that follows annealing of the TSPE primers, biotin-labeled deoxycytidine triphosphate (dCTP) is incorporated into the primer extension product. Detection of the TSPE products uses a set of polystyrene microspheres composed of 100 members. Each member microsphere incorporates two fluorescent dyes in a unique ratio that allows identification by flow cytometry using two lasers, each of which emits light of the appropriate wavelength to excite one of the two fluorescent dyes. Bound to each member of the microsphere set is a short oligonucleotide ("antitag") with sequence homology to one of the tags introduced in the TSPE reaction. These tags are specific for each amplicon amplified by the

TABLE 15.8 Viral Molecular Tests Approved or Cleared by the Food and Drug Administration[a]

Virus	Test Name	Method	Manufacturer
Adenovirus	ProAdeno™+ Assay	Multiplex real-time PCR	Gen-Probe (Prodesse), San Diego, CA
Cytomegalovirus	CMV pp67 mRNA	NASBA	bioMérieux, Durham, NC
Cytomegalovirus	HC1® CMV DNA Test	Hybrid capture	Qiagen, Germantown, MD
Cytomegalovirus (quantification)	COBAS AmpliPrep/COBAS Taqman CMV Test	Real-time PCR	Roche Molecular Diagnostics, Pleasanton, CA
Dengue	CDC DENV 1-4 Real Time RT-PCR Assay	Real-time PCR	Centers for Disease Control and Preventrion, Atlanta, GA
Enteroviruses	NucliSENS EasyQ® Enterovirus	NASBA	bioMérieux, Durham, NC
Enteroviruses	Xpert™ EV	Real-time PCR	Cepheid, Sunnyvale, CA
Hepatitis B virus (quantification)	Abbott Real-time HBV	Real-time PCR	Abbott Molecular, Des Plaines, IL
Hepatitis B virus (quantification)	COABS® TaqMan® HBV Test and COBAS® AmpliPrep/COBAS® TaqMan® HBV Test v 2.0 and COBAS TaqmanHBV Test for use with the HighPure System	Real-time PCR	Roche Molecular Diagnostics, Pleasanton, CA
Hepatitis C virus (quantification)	Abbott Real-Time HCV	Real-time RT-PCR	Abbott Molecular, Des Plaines, IL
Hepatitis C virus (quantification)	VERSANT® HCV RNA 3.0 Assay	bDNA	Siemens Healthcare Diagnostics, Deerfield, IL
Hepatitis C virus (quantification)	COBAS® AmpliPrep/COBAS® TaqMan® HCV Test v 2.0,COBAS® TaqMan® HCV v2.0 for use with the HighPure System, AMPLICOR HCV Test v 2.0, COBAS AMPLIOCOR HCV Test v 2.0	Real-time PCR	Roche Molecular Diagnostics, Pleasanton, CA
HIV (drug resistance)	ViroSeq™ HIV-1 Genotyping System	Sequencing	Celera Diagnostics, Alameda, CA
HIV (drug resistance)	TruGene™ HIV-1 Genotyping and Open Gene DNA Sequencing System	Sequencing	Siemens Healthcare Diagnostics, Deerfield, IL
HIV (quantification)	Abbott Real-Time HIV-1	Real-time RT-PCR	Abbott Molecular, Des Plaines, IL
HIV (quantification)	NucliSENS® HIV-1 QT	NASBA	bioMérieux, Durham, NC
HIV (quantification)	AMPLICOR HIV-1 MONITOR™ Test v1.5, COBAS® AMPLICOR HIV-1 MONITOR™ Test v1.5, COBAS AmpliPrep/COBAS Taqman HIV-1 Test v 2.0, COBAS Taqman HIV-1 Test v 2.0, COBAS® AmpliScreen™ HIV-1 Test, v1.5, COBAS® TaqScreen MPX®	RT-PCR	Roche Molecular Diagnostics, Pleasanton, CA
HIV (quanitification)	VERSANT HIV-1 RNA 3.0 Assay (bDNA)	bDNA	Siemens Healthcare Diagnostics, Deerfield, IL
Herpes simplex virus	BD ProbeTec Herpes Simplex Viruses Qx Amplified DNA Test	SDA	BD Diagnostic Systems, Sparks, MD
Herpes simplex virus	Multicode-RTX Herpes Simplex 1 and 2 kit	Multicode chemistry real-time PCR	Eragen Biosciences, Madison, WI
Herpes simplex virus	IsoAmp HSV Assay	HAD	BioHelix, Beverly, MA
Human metapneumovirus	Pro hMPV+™ Assay	Real time RT-PCR	Gen-Probe (Prodesse), San Diego, CA
Human papilloma- virus	Cervista™ HPV HR and HPV 16/18	Invader® chemistry	Hologic (Third Wave Technologies), Bedford, MA
Human papilloma-virus	HC2® HR and LR, HR, DNA with Pap	Hybrid capture	Qiagen, Germantown, MD
Human papilloma-virus	COBAS® HPV Test	Multiplex real-time PCR and RT-PCR	Roche Molecular Diagnostics, Pleasanton, CA
Human papilloma-virus	Aptima HPV	TMA, HPA	Gen-Probe, San Diego, CA
Influenza virus	Human Influenza Virus Real-Time RT-PCR Detection and Characterization Panel	Real-time RT-PCR	Centers for Disease Control and Prevention, Atlanta, GA
Influenza virus	Xpert™ flu	Real-time PCR	Cepheid, Sunnyvale, CA
Influenza virus	Liat Influenza A/B Assay	Real-Time PCR	IQumm, Marlborough, MA
Influenza virus	Artus Influ A/B RG RT-PCR Jut	Real-Time RT-PCR	Qiagen, Germantown, MD
Influenza virus	Influenza A + B Assay	Real-Time RT-PCR	Quidel, San Diego, CA
Influenza virus	ProFlu Assay	Real-time RT-PCR	Gen-Probe (Prodesse), San Diego, CA
Influenza virus H1N1	Simplexa™ Influenza Test	Real-time RT-PCR	Focus Diagnostics, Cypress, CA

(continued)

TABLE 15.8 Viral Molecular Tests Approved or Cleared by the Food and Drug Administration[a] (*continued*)

Virus	Test Name	Method	Manufacturer
Influenza virus (avian)	Influenza A/H5	Real-time PCR	Centers for Disease Control and Prevention, Atlanta, GA
Parainfluenza viruses 1-3	ProParaFlu+™ Assay	Real-time PCR	Gen-Probe (Prodesse), San Diego, CA
Respiratory viruses (influenza A and B, RSV, parainfluenza 1-3, human metapneumovirus, entero/rhinovirus, adenovirus)	xTAG Respiratory Virus Panel	PCR, RT-PCR, TSPE, Tag sorting	Luminex Molecular Diagnostics, Toronto, CA
Respiratory viruses (influenza A and B, RSV, parainfluenza 1-4, human metapneumovirus, entero/rhinovirus, adenovirus, coronaviruses NL63,HKU1, OC43, 229E)	FilmArray Respiratory Panel	Multiplex, nested PCR and RT-PCR	Biofire Diagnostics, Salt Lake City, UT
Respiratory viruses (influenza A and B, RSV, parainfluenza 1-3, human metapneumovirus, rhinovirus, adenovirus	eSensor Respiratory Virus Panel	PCR, RT-PCR, Probe Hybridization	Gen-Mark Diagnostics, Pasadena, CA
Respiratory viruses (influenza A and B, RSV)	Verigene® Respiratory Virus Plus Nucleic Acid Test	Multiplex gold particle nanoparticle probes	Nanosphere, Northbrook, IL
Respiratory viruses (influenza A and B, RSV)	ProFlu+™ Flu A/B & RSV Test	Multiplex real-time RT-PCR	Focus Diagnostics, Cypress, CA

bDNA, branched chain DNA assay; HAD, helix displacement assay; HPA, hybrid protection assay; SDA, strand displacement assay; TMA, transcription-mediated amplification: TSPE, target-specific primer extension.

[a]Adapted from the web site of the Association for Molecular Pathology (AMP), www.amp.org, accessed November 26, 2012.

TABLE15.9 Molecular Diagnostic Systems Approved/Cleared by the FDA[a]

System	Viruses detected	Manufacturer
NuciSENS EasyQ® System	Enterovirus	bioMérieux, Durham, NC
Procleix® Semi-Automated and TIGRIS Systems	HIV-1, HCV, HBV, WNV	Gen-Probe, San Diego, CA
VERSANT™ 440 Molecular System	HCV	Siemens, Deerfield, IL
Luminex LX 100/200-xTAG Respiratory virus Panel	Respiratory viruses	Luminex, Toronto, Canada
Verigene® System	Influenza A and B, RSV	Nanosphere, Northbrook, IL
Abbott m2000™	HIV-1, HCV	Abbott, Des Plaines, IL
COBAS AmpliPrep/COBAS Taqman, COBAS 4800, COBAS Taqman 48 Analyzer	HIV-1, HBV, HCV, HPV	Roche Diagnostics, Pleasanton, CA
7500 Fast Dx Real-time PCR Instrument	Influenza	Applied Biosystems, Foster City, CA
FilmArray System	Respiratory viruses	Biofire Diagnostics, Salt Lake City, UT
eSensor XT-8 System	Respiratory viruses	GenMark Diagnostics, Pasadena, CA
GeneXpert™ Real-time PCR System	Enteroviruses, Influenza A and B	Cepheid, Sunnyvale, CA
3M Integrated Cycler/Simplexa™ reagent kits and assay protocols	Influenza A and B	Focus Diagnostics, Cypress CA

[a]Adapted from the web site of the Association for Molecular Pathology (AMP), www.amp.org, accessed August 6, 2011.

multiplex reaction. Following the TSPE reaction, the reaction mix is incubated with the microspheres, allowing the microspheres to specifically capture any TSPE products that have been produced. A fluorescent detection signal is generated through the inclusion of streptavidin-phycoerythrin, which binds to the biotin molecules incorporated into the amplicons. As the microspheres pass through the flow cell, they are interrogated by the lasers, allowing identification of the specific microsphere set member and determination of whether or not a TSPE product has been bound. Computer software analyzes the fluorescent events and determines for each virus and internal control whether a threshold of detection has been surpassed. Recently a version that requires less time to complete, called xTAG RVP Fast, was cleared by the FDA for detection of influenza A, influenza A subtype H1, influenza A subtype H3, influenza B, RSV, hMPV, rhinovirus, and adenovirus.

The other large multiplex assay that has been approved by the FDA is the FilmArray Respiratory Panel, which was cleared by the FDA in 2011 for detection in nasopharyngeal swabs of the following viruses: influenza A and B; influenza A subtypes H1, H1 2009, and H3; RSV; hMPV; adenovirus; parainfluenza viruses 1 through 4; rhinovirus/enterovirus; and coronaviruses NL63 and HKU1.[110] Extraction, amplification, and detection are carried out in a self-contained unit referred to as a "pouch." Nucleic acid extraction is accomplished using magnetic beads. The nucleic acid amplification that follows is a multiplex nested PCR assay. The first amplification reaction is a multiplex reaction containing outer primers for each target virus. The reaction mix is then diluted and combined with a new primer-free master mix that contains the fluorescent dye LC Green Plus, which binds to dsDNA. This mix is then moved by microfluidic techniques into an array of individual wells, each of which contains inner primers specific for one target virus. Each target is represented in at least three wells. Production of viral amplicons is confirmed by analyzing melting curves. The entire process from inoculation of sample to availability of results takes approximately 1 hour, with only 2 minutes of hands-on time. The manufacturer also plans to develop a test for gastroenteritis that will include but not be limited to viruses.

Integrated Platforms. The term *integrated platform* refers to test platforms in which nucleic acid extraction, amplification, and product detection are carried out within the same device or instrument. These platforms represent an important advance in diagnostic microbiology because their simplicity allows them to be performed in many laboratories that would not otherwise be able to provide viral diagnostic testing. In fact, they are so simple that they could be performed in a physician's office, although they do not currently have CLIA-waived status, which would permit testing outside of laboratories approved for "high-complexity" testing. To date, two integrated platforms have been approved or cleared by the FDA. The first is the GeneXpert Real-time PCR system, marketed by Cepheid (Sunnyvale, CA). This platform employs test cartridges into which a specimen is inoculated. The cartridge is inserted into the GeneXpert instrument, which performs nucleic acid extraction, amplification, and product detection without any intervention by the user. Tests for enteroviruses[69] and for influenza A and B viruses[105] have currently been cleared by the FDA. The enterovirus assay requires a total of approximately 2½ hours to perform, while the influenza assay requires less than 1 hour. Several GeneXpert bacterial assays have also been cleared by the FDA. The second integrated platform cleared by the FDA is the FilmArray, described previously.

High-Throughput Quantitative Systems

Commercial systems that provide standardized quantitative testing for HIV and HCV RNA and HBV DNA have been approved by the FDA. These systems are the Roche COBAS AmpliPrep/COBAS TaqMan and the Abbott m2000. Both systems include separate automated instruments for nucleic acid extraction and real-time PCR. While these systems are highly automated, they require more hands-on time from laboratory personnel than the truly integrated platforms. Both systems have the capability for moderate to high throughput. Test results are intended for diagnosis, to determine the need for treatment, and to monitor the response to therapy. Tests for quantitative detection of HIV, HCV, and HBV have been approved on both systems. The m2000 system is also FDA approved for detection of *Chlamydia trachomatis* and *Neisseria gonorrhea.* Outside of the United States, additional viral tests are available for the m2000, including HCV genotyping and detection of CMV, Epstein-Barr virus (EBV), HPV, *C. trachomatis,* and *N. gonorrhea.*

Specialized highly automated platforms have also been approved by the FDA for screening donated blood. The Procleix Tigris system has been developed by Gen-Probe in collaboration with Novartis Diagnostics (Emeryville, CA). This is a highly automated instrument that uses FDA-cleared assays (Procleix Ultrio and Ultrio Plus) to test for HIV, HCV, HBV, and West Nile virus (Procleix West Nile Virus Assay). The tests for RNA viruses use the TMA reaction for amplifying RNA. Roche has developed the COBAS s201 system for screening donated blood. This system includes the COBAS AmpliPrep instrument for nucleic acid extraction and the COBAS TaqMan 96 analyzer for performing real-time PCR. The system provides testing for HIV, HCV, HBV, and West Nile virus (TaqScreen MPX Test and TaqScreen West Nile Virus test). Non–real-time PCR assays (COBAS AmpliScreen) have also been approved by the FDA for screening donated blood for HIV, HCV, and HBV.

Serology

Measurement of antiviral antibodies was one of the first methods used for the specific diagnosis of viral infections and it remains an important tool in the diagnostic virology laboratory. The role of serology can be for the diagnosis of acute or current infection or for the determination of immune status to specific viruses. Serologic diagnosis is important for viruses that cannot be cultured readily or for which culture is slow or otherwise impractical. Viruses for which serology is useful in diagnosing acute infection are shown in Table 15.10. Serology is uniquely useful for defining immunity with respect to specific viruses. It is important to use sensitive assays such as EIA for this purpose, because antibody levels indicative of past infection can decline to very low levels years after the infection. The specific assay used must also be selected with care to ensure that it measures antibodies that correlate with immunity. Viruses for which serologic testing is used to determine immune status are shown in Table 15.11.

Kinetics of the Antibody Response

Serologic diagnosis is based on the kinetics of the antibody response to viral infection. Virus-specific antibodies are absent

TABLE 15.10 Serology for Diagnosis of Acute Infection

Epstein-Barr[a]
Cytomegalovirus (mononucleosis syndrome)[a]
Hepatitis viruses (A–E)[b]
Measles[a]
Rubella[a]
Mumps[a]
Parvovirus B19[a]
Encephalitis viruses (e.g., West Nile virus)[a]
Rabies
Hemorrhagic fever viruses[a]
Dengue fever[a]
Human immunodeficiency virus (HIV)
Human T-cell lymphoma or leukemia virus types 1/2 (HTLV-1/2)

[a]Virus-specific immunoglobulin M (IgM) assays are used.

[b]Virus-specific IgM assays are used for hepatitis A, B, and E.

in a susceptible individual but typically become detectable several weeks after the onset of infection. Virus-specific IgM antibodies are often detectable for a short period before virus-specific IgG antibodies. The IgM response tends to decline within approximately 1 to 2 months, although low levels can persist for 1 year or more in some viral infections. IgG antibodies are much more long-lasting and can persist for the life span of the individual. Thus, the absence of virus-specific IgG and IgM antibodies signifies susceptibility to infection; the presence of virus-specific IgM antibodies, with or without virus-specific IgG antibodies, signifies current or very recent infection; and the presence of virus-specific IgG but not IgM antibodies signifies past infection. The latter pattern often, but not always, indicates immunity to subsequent infection.

An alternative serologic approach to the diagnosis of recent infection is based on the concept that the avidity of antigen-specific antibodies increases as the immune response matures.[28] Thus, antibodies produced shortly after infection have low affinity for the causative agent, and antibodies produced late after infection have high affinity. Detection of low-affinity antibodies has been used to diagnose recent infection with CMV,[27] rubella,[116] and HIV.[129]

TABLE 15.11 Serology to Determine Immune Status

Varicella-zoster virus
Herpes simplex virus
Cytomegalovirus
Epstein-Barr virus (immunoglobulin G antibodies to the viral capsid antigen)
Human herpesvirus type 6
Rubella
Measles
Mumps
Parvovirus B19
Hepatitis A virus (total antibodies)
Hepatitis B virus (anti-HBs)
Hepatitis E virus

The relationship between the onset of clinical manifestations of infection and the presence of virus-specific antibodies depends on the incubation period of the infection. In infections with short incubation periods (e.g., acute respiratory infections), antibodies are absent at the onset of symptoms. In viruses with incubation periods of 1 month or longer, however, virus-specific IgG and IgM antibodies are typically present at the onset of symptoms.

Serology in Reinfection and Reactivation

The serologic diagnoses of reinfection and reactivated infection are more complicated than that of initial infection. In both of these cases, the infection occurs in an individual with preexisting, virus-specific IgG antibodies. In reinfection an anamnestic response may occur that results in an increase in the level of virus-specific IgG antibodies with continued absence of virus-specific IgM antibodies. Reactivation of latent infection, for example, in the case of some herpesvirus infections, may result in the appearance of virus-specific IgM as well as IgG antibodies.

Serology in Chronic Infections

The interpretation of serology is unique for viruses that typically cause chronic infection (e.g., HIV) and the related retroviruses human T-cell lymphoma or leukemia virus (HTLV) types 1 and 2. For these agents, the detection of antibodies of any isotype to these viruses (in the absence of artificial immunization) virtually always signifies current infection. In the case of HCV, the confirmed presence of antibodies to the virus corresponds to active infection in approximately 85% of individuals. A recent innovation is the development of tests that simultaneously measure HIV p24 antigen in addition to HIV antibodies. Because p24 antigen may appear some days before the appearance of HIV antibodies, the combined test decreases the "window" during which a recently infected individual is serologically negative but capable of transmitting infection.[100] The Abbott Architect HIV Ag/Ab Combo assay was recently approved by the FDA as an aid in the diagnosis of HIV-1 or -2 infection.

Serologic Assays

Binding Assays

The most widely used assays are those that directly measure binding of antibodies to viral antigens. Examples of binding assays include EIA, radioimmunoassay (RIA), and the indirect immunofluorescent antibody assay (IFA). Binding assays can be used in many different formats. In one common format, a viral antigen, which can consist of virally infected cells, a purified viral preparation, or a recombinant viral protein, is attached to a solid surface such as the inner surface of the well of a microtiter tray, a plastic bead, or a microscope slide in the case of IFA. Serum is added, allowing the binding of antiviral antibodies that might be present in the serum. After an appropriate incubation period, the serum is removed and the well is extensively washed. The next step is the addition of a second antibody (also referred to as a detector antibody) with specificity for human immunoglobulins. The second antibody is typically a mouse monoclonal or a polyclonal antibody from a nonhuman species. It is linked to an enzyme such as horseradish peroxidase. The second antibody binds to any human antibody present (ideally, because of specific binding to the viral antigen). The well is again extensively washed, and the presence of the second antibody is detected based on a colorimetric, radiometric, or fluorescent signal. An important advantage of binding assays is that they can be modified to detect IgM- or IgA-specific antiviral antibodies through the use of isotype-specific detector antibodies.

Immunobinding Assays

The western blot and related recombinant immunobinding assays are binding assays that allow the identification of antibodies to specific viral proteins. In the western blot assay, viral antigens present in infected cells are denatured, separated by gel electrophoresis, transferred to a membrane, and allowed to react with the serum specimen. Binding of antiviral antibodies is detected through the use of labeled detector antibodies. The western blot is cumbersome but provides a very high level of specificity because of the ability to identify binding to individual viral proteins and the production of a characteristic blot fingerprint. Thus, its main application in diagnostic laboratories is the confirmation of screening assays (e.g., EIA) that are less specific. For example, until recently, the western blot was widely used to confirm a positive HIV EIA. Western blot is also considered the gold standard in determining the type specificity of HSV antibodies. The recombinant immunobinding assay differs from the western blot in that specific viral antigens are produced in *in vitro* expression systems and artificially attached to membranes in a predetermined configuration, often in dots or in bands. The membranes are then incubated with serum, and bound antibodies are detected, as in the western blot. Because the antigens used in the immunobinding assay are not denatured as they are in routine western blots, these assays may have advantages in detection of antibodies to conformational epitopes. A recombinant immunobinding assay is used to confirm positive hepatitis C EIA results.

Functional Assays

Functional assays are based on detection of specific activities resulting from the binding of specific antibodies to viral antigens. An important example is the neutralization assay, which measures the ability of antibodies to block viral infectivity. In neutralization assays, serial dilutions of the serum to be tested are incubated with a standardized quantity of infectious virus. After a short incubation period, the serum–virus mixtures are added to cells that support the growth of the virus, in parallel with a similar inoculum of virus that has not been incubated with serum. The neutralizing antibody titer is the highest serum dilution that prevents infection of the cells. The neutralization assay correlates well with protection from infection and is sometimes considered the standard against which other serologic assays should be measured. Because it is cumbersome and expensive, the neutralization assay is now rarely used in routine diagnostic laboratories. Other examples of functional assays are the hemagglutination-inhibition assay, in which the presence of antiviral antibodies is detected by their ability to block virus-induced hemagglutination, and the complement fixation assay, which measures the ability of antiviral antibodies to fix complement, preventing the complement from lysing indicator erythrocytes. Although hemagglutination-inhibition and complement fixation assays have been widely used in the past, they are increasingly being replaced by binding assays.

Agglutination Assays

Viral antigens can be bound to a variety of particles, including fixed erythrocytes and latex particles. Agglutination assays are performed by mixing dilutions of serum with a suspension of antigen-coated particles. The agglutination titer is the highest serum dilution that results in visible agglutination of particles. The advantage of agglutination assays is simplicity; they are rapid and do not require sophisticated equipment. Therefore, they are well suited for *stat* testing and for use under field conditions. For example, a rapid latex agglutination assay for varicella antibodies can be used for rapid determination of the varicella immune status of health care personnel who are exposed to a patient with varicella.

Virus-Specific IgM Assays

Assays for virus-specific IgM antibodies are important because they often allow a specific diagnosis of an acute infection to be made based on analysis of a single serum specimen obtained during the acute phase of illness. These assays are most likely to be useful in diseases with incubation periods that are sufficiently long so that virus-specific IgM levels are present at detectable levels at the onset of illness. Hepatitis A provides an excellent example; because of its incubation period of 2 to 6 weeks, hepatitis A IgM antibodies are virtually always detectable at the time patients seek medical care.

A number of methods are used to measure virus-specific IgM antibodies. Two older methods include (a) separating IgG and IgM fractions before performing the virus-specific antibody assay and (b) performing the virus-specific assay before and after procedures, such as treatment with β-mercaptoethanol, that selectively destroy IgM antibodies. Many modern virus-specific IgM antibody assays use IFA or EIA with a detector antibody that binds only to human IgM. The IgM capture assay is an alternative approach in which IgM antibodies present in the serum sample being tested are first *captured* using an antibody specific for human IgM. A preparation of viral antigen is added, followed by an enzyme-labeled antibody specific for the viral antigen. Binding is detected by the addition of the appropriate enzyme substrate.

Virus-specific IgM assays have several potential pitfalls and must be interpreted in conjunction with clinical findings. False-positive results can occur if the serum being tested contains rheumatoid factor (IgM antibodies to human IgG) plus virus-specific IgG antibodies that form complexes that may be falsely detected by the assay as virus-specific IgM antibodies. This problem can be avoided by pretreatment of the serum to remove either rheumatoid factor or IgG antibodies. One or the other of these pretreatments is included routinely in many commercial virus-specific IgM antibody assays. False-negative results can occur if the serum being tested contains high levels of virus-specific IgG antibodies that may compete with the virus-specific IgM antibodies. The IgM-capture assay configuration avoids this problem, as does serum pretreatment to remove IgG.

Complexities in the nature of the IgM antibody response must also be considered in interpreting virus-specific IgM antibody tests. In some patients, the IgM antibody response is transient or low level, leading to failure to detect virus-specific IgM antibodies, whereas in others, low levels of IgM antibodies may persist for 1 year or longer, decreasing the specificity of the assay as an indicator of very recent infection. In herpesvirus infections, IgM antibodies can sometimes be detected in reactivations as well as in primary infection.

Saliva and Urine Assays

Virus-specific antibodies can often be detected in saliva and urine. These body substances are attractive for use in serologic assays because they avoid the need for phlebotomy. Assays for HIV antibodies in these fluids are commercially available and have performance characteristics similar to assays carried out on serum.[35,138]

Cerebrospinal Fluid Serology

Serologic testing can be applied to CSF for the diagnosis of central nervous system (CNS) infection. For unusual viruses (e.g., rabies), the presence of any virus-specific antibodies within the CSF is diagnostic of active infection. For the diagnosis of encephalitis caused by the alphaviruses, bunyaviruses, or flaviviruses, the presence of virus-specific antibodies in CSF is highly suspicious and the presence of virus-specific IgM antibodies in CSF is diagnostic. For more common viruses (e.g., herpesviruses) or the common respiratory viruses, the mere presence of virus-specific antibodies in CSF is not diagnostic of CNS infection because antibodies produced in the blood are present in the CSF even in the absence of CNS infection. The problem is further complicated by the fact that defects in the blood–brain barrier that can occur during many neurologic diseases can increase the passage of antibodies from blood to CSF. Therefore, for the common viruses, intrathecal synthesis of specific antiviral antibodies must be demonstrated to provide evidence of CNS infection.

Intrathecal synthesis of a specific antiviral antibody is evaluated by determining the quotient of two ratios: (a) the ratio of specific antiviral antibody level in CSF to the level in serum, and (b) the ratio of total IgG in CSF to total IgG in serum ($CSF_{specific\ antibody}$:$serum_{specific\ antibody}$ divided by CSF_{IgG}:$serum_{IgG}$). A quotient greater than 1.5 is evidence of intrathecal antibody synthesis of the specific antibody. The antibody assay used to measure the specific antiviral antibody must have certain special characteristics. First, it must be very sensitive, because CSF antibody levels are usually low (~1,000 times less than serum levels). Second, it must be capable of providing a quantitative result that allows calculation of the CSF-to-serum ratio of specific antibody level. EIA is usually used, but testing of a series of dilutions of CSF and serum is required to obtain linear quantitative estimates of antibody level suitable for calculating the necessary ratio. Because of the complexities involved, accurate determination of intrathecal antibody synthesis of specific antiviral antibodies is performed in only a limited number of reference laboratories.

Measurement of intrathecal antibody synthesis has been used in a variety of CNS infections. The applications for which experience is most extensive are encephalitis caused by HSV and VZV. In HSV encephalitis, the utility of determinations of intrathecal antibody synthesis is limited because intrathecal antibody synthesis may not be detectable until 7 to 10 days after the onset of illness. Interestingly, intrathecal antibody synthesis can persist for years after the acute infection. Therefore, the main application is in cases in which specimens were not available early in the illness to allow a definitive diagnosis based on PCR. A caveat concerning diagnosis by demonstration of intrathecal antibody synthesis is that nonspecific polyclonal intrathecal antibody synthesis can occur in some diseases (e.g., multiple sclerosis).[113] This pitfall can be avoided by evaluating intrathecal synthesis of antibodies to at least one other virus other than the one of primary interest. Serologic diagnosis has been shown to be more sensitive than PCR for diagnosis of VZV vasculopathy.[91] This is explained partly by the fact that CSF samples from some patients in this study were obtained months after the onset of neurologic manifestations.

Antiviral Susceptibility Testing

In recent years, antiviral drugs have been licensed for the treatment of infections caused by HSV, VZV, CMV, influenza A and B, RSV, HIV, HCV, and HBV. Not surprisingly, increasing use of these drugs has been accompanied by the appearance of antiviral drug resistance. Testing for resistance may be required for optimal patient management. Antiviral drug susceptibility testing is performed in some diagnostic virology laboratories and is also available through reference laboratories.

Phenotypic Assays

Antiviral susceptibility testing is divided into phenotypic and genotypic methods. Phenotypic methods analyze the effect of antiviral drugs on the replication of virus, which can be measured by infectivity, viral antigen or nucleic acid production, or effect on the activity of a viral enzyme such as influenza neuraminidase. Phenotypic assays are important because they directly measure the effects of antiviral drugs on viral replication. In addition, they are more universal than genotypic assays because they can be used when the genetic basis for resistance is unknown. In the case of HIV, phenotypic assays are useful in analyzing viruses in which the presence of multiple mutations makes it difficult to predict phenotype from genotypic data. Finally, phenotypic assays must be used to determine the significance of candidate mutations found in drug-resistant isolates. However, from a practical standpoint, phenotypic assays tend to be labor-intensive, slow, and poorly standardized. In addition, there is a theoretical concern that the growth of the virus in cell culture may lead to selection of nonrepresentative viral variants, especially because antiviral resistance may in some instances be associated with decreased viral fitness. For these reasons, phenotypic assays are not performed in most diagnostic virology laboratories. Table 15.12 shows recommended *cut-offs* that define resistance to several drugs used for HSV and CMV infections.

The plaque assay was the traditional method for performing phenotypic susceptibility testing. However, this method is rarely used in diagnostic virology laboratories for the reasons mentioned previously and will not be discussed further here. Assays measuring viral antigen or nucleic acid production are alternatives to infectivity-based assays. A variety of assays have been used in individual laboratories, but they are not commercially available. The ELVIS assay illustrated in Figure 15.3 has also been adapted for the performance of antiviral susceptibility testing.[128,134] For influenza, resistance to neuraminidase inhibitors has been measured using neuraminidase inhibition assays based on either fluorescent or chemiluminescent signal generation.[12,92,93]

Recombinant phenotypic assays have been developed and widely used for HIV. These assays involve insertion of HIV genes that are targets for antiretroviral drugs (polymerase, protease, integrase) from a patient being evaluated into a vector consisting of a rapidly replicating laboratory strain of HIV that also contains a reporter gene (e.g., luciferase) that is used to measure viral growth.[102] These assays allow relatively rapid testing of the susceptibility of HIV to multiple drugs as well as to drug combinations. Commercial tests have been developed by Monogram Biosciences (San Francisco, CA) and Virco

TABLE 15.12 Cut-Offs for Antiviral Susceptibility Testing for Herpes Simplex Virus (HSV) and Cytomegalovirus (CMV) Using the Plaque Reduction Assay

		Cut-off (μM)		
Virus (reference)	**Drug**	**Sensitive**	**Intermediate**	**Resistant**
HSV (117)	Acyclovir	<8		≥8
	Foscarnet	<330		≥330
CMV (18,84)	Ganciclovir	≤6	6–12	>12
	Foscarnet	≤400		>400
	Cidofovir	≤2		>4

(Antwerp, Belgium) and are available in the United States through national reference laboratories. A special case is the HIV drug maraviroc, which blocks HIV entry by binding to the CCR5 receptor. Viruses that use the CXCR4 receptor rather than the CCR5 receptor are resistant to maraviroc. A commercial assay called Trofile (Monogram Biosciences)[150] is used to predict response to maraviroc by determining the receptor tropism of a patient's isolate.

Genotypic Assays

Genotypic assays test for the genetic basis for resistant phenotypes. A variety of methods are used, including detection of restriction fragment length polymorphisms, PCR assays that detect mutations by virtue of differential primer or probe binding, and nucleotide sequencing. With rapid improvements in sequencing technology including the development of pyrosequencing, sequencing-based methods are becoming increasingly used. Genotypic assays are informative only when the genetic basis for resistance is known and are most useful when the resistance being evaluated is accounted for by a limited number of genetic changes.

Genotypic assays have been most widely used for CMV, HIV, HBV, and influenza A, because phenotypic assays for these viruses are slow and expensive or not widely available. Application of genotypic assays requires an extensive body of knowledge concerning the effect of specific mutations on antiviral resistance. Some single mutations may confer high-level resistance, while others may confer only partial resistance, and others are not associated with resistance at all.

For CMV, resistance to the currently FDA-approved drugs ganciclovir, foscarnet, and cidofovir has been related to mutations in the phosphotransferase (*UL97*) and polymerase (*UL54*) genes.[18,84] Most laboratories now use sequencing to detect these mutations. Because ganciclovir-resistance mutations generally arise first in the *UL97* gene, some laboratories sequence this gene first, proceeding to sequencing *UL54* only if no significant mutations are detected in *UL97*, or if the patient is being treated with foscarnet or cidofovir, which exert their antiviral effect by inhibiting this gene. Different mutations within *UL97* or *UL54* are associated with different levels of antiviral resistance.[84]

For HIV, genotypic testing for resistance is commonly used by physicians in the developed world in the management of antiretroviral drug therapy. This testing involves RT-PCR amplification of regions of the polymerase and protease genes and sometimes the integrase gene, followed by nucleotide sequencing of the amplicons. Certain mutations are highly associated with phenotypic resistance and drug failure, whereas the significance of other mutations found in drug-resistant strains is less clear. Interpretation of HIV genotypic testing is most straightforward in patients who are not highly drug experienced and have relatively small numbers of mutations. Patients who have been treated more extensively may have multiple interacting mutations and may also have mutations that lie outside of the segments that are sequenced but nevertheless affect susceptibility to antiretroviral drugs.[43] Several FDA-approved sequencing systems are commercially available to detect HIV drug resistance mutations, including the ViroSeq system marketed by Celera Diagnostics (Alameda, CA) and the TruGene system marketed by Siemens (Deerfield, IL). High-throughput sequencing can be used to detect rare drug-resistant mutants that make up a small percentage of viral genomes.[122] The clinical significance of small minority populations of drug-resistant mutants is still under investigation.[11]

Resistance testing for influenza is related to the two existing classes of influenza antiviral drugs, the adamantanes and the neuroaminidase inhibitors. Resistance to the adamantanes occurs when there are mutations at positions 26, 27, 30, 31, or 34 in the gene encoding the M2 matrix protein, which is the target of the drugs.[11] Resistance to the neuraminidase inhibitors is related to specific mutations in the gene encoding neuraminidase, especially a histidine to tyrosine change at position 274 (N2 numbering), designated H274Y. This mutation became widespread during the 2007–2008 influenza season.[24,50] Pyrosequencing has been effectively used to detect these mutations,[23] as have a variety of PCR-based assays.[19,151]

The presence of resistance of HBV to antiviral agents is detected by sequencing of the DNA polymerase gene. Genotypic testing for HSV is less useful than phenotypic testing because of the diverse genetic loci within the HSV thymidine kinase and polymerase genes that can account for resistance.[37]

SELECTED CLINICAL PROBLEMS

Tables 15.13 through 15.18 provide information related to specific areas of diagnostic virology not covered elsewhere in the chapter.

VIRUS DISCOVERY

Experimental methodologies used for viral discovery have traditionally relied on classic approaches such as electron

TABLE 15.13 Laboratory Diagnosis of Human Herpesvirus Infections

Virus	Clinical problem	Test(s)	Specimen
Herpes simplex	Mucocutaneous lesions	Culture, NAAT, FA stain	Swab of lesion
	Encephalitis or meningitis	NAAT	CSF
Varicella-zoster	Mucocutaneous lesions	Culture, NAAT, FA stain	Swab of lesion
	Encephalitis or meningitis	NAAT	CSF
	CNS vasculopathy	Intrathecal antibody synthesis, NAAT[a]	Serum or plasma plus CSF
Cytomegalovirus	Systemic infection in immunocompromised individual	Quantitative NAAT, pp65 antigenemia assay	Plasma or whole blood
	Mononucleosis syndrome in nonimmunocompromised individual	CMV IgM antibody assay, NAAT	Serum or plasma for antibody assay, plasma or whole blood for NAAT
	Tissue-invasive disease (e.g., involving the gastrointestinal or respiratory tract)	Histology, immunohistochemistry *in situ* hybridization, culture, NAAT	Tissue from involved organ
	Encephalitis	NAAT	CSF
	Retinitis	NAAT	Vitreous or aqueous fluid
Epstein-Barr virus (EBV)	Infectious mononucleosis	Heterophile antibody assay,[b] IgM antibodies to the viral capsid antigen	Serum or plasma
	Posttransplant lymphoproliferative disorder	Quantitative NAAT	Whole blood or plasma
	Primary central nervous system lymphoma	NAAT	CSF
	Encephalitis or meningitis	NAAT[c]	CSF[c]
Human herpesviruses types 6 (HHV-6) and 7 (HHV-7)	Acute infection[d]	NAAT,[e] IgM antibody assay, IgG avidity assay[147]	Plasma (NAAT), plasma or serum for IgM antibody assay or IgG avidity assay[147]
	Systemic infection in immunocompromised individual	NAAT[e]	Whole blood or plasma[e]
	Encephalitis	NAAT[e]	CSF
Human herpesvirus type 8 (HHV-8) (Kaposi sarcoma virus)	Systemic infection[f]	NAAT	Blood or body fluid

CSF, cerebrospinal fluid; FA, fluorescent antibody; Ig, immunoglobulin; NAAT, nucleic acid amplification test.

[a]Intrathecal antibody synthesis has been shown to be more sensitive than NAAT for diagnosis of varicella-zoster virus central nervous system vasculopathy.[91]

[b]Slide tests or other modified heterophile assays are usually used.

[c]Should be performed only in the setting of primary EBV infection. In other clinical settings, specificity and positive predictive values are low.

[d]Some but not all cases have a rash and are diagnosed as roseola.

[e]Approximately 1% of the population has chromosomal integration of HHV-6 and has very high levels of HHV-6 DNA in blood and tissue, which is not indicative of disease attributable to HHV-6. Chromosomal integration in immunocompetent patients can be excluded by testing a follow-up sample (those with chromosomal integration will have persistently high levels of HHV-6 DNA) or a pretransplant sample from the transplant recipient (those with chromosomal integration will have high levels of HHV-6 DNA in the pretransplant sample).

[f]Systemic HHV-8 infection may be associated with body cavity lymphoma or multicentric Castleman disease.

microscopy, cell culture, and antibody-based detection. Despite the success of these approaches, which have resulted in the discovery of many viruses throughout the years, each of these methods suffers from significant limitations. For example, electron microscopy requires high viral titers and may not provide the necessary resolution to unambiguously identify the type of virus even when viral particles are observed. Many viruses cannot be cultured, and those that can often require very specific cell types; crucially, there is no universal cell line capable of broadly supporting growth of all, or even a majority of, known viruses. Antibody-based methods are limited in breadth, require the development of specific reagents for a given viral group, and, most critically, require selection of specific candidates based on prior knowledge in order to be useful in identifying a virus. Due to these limitations, there have been ongoing efforts to develop additional complementary strategies for detecting and discovering novel viruses. In the last decade of the 20th century, various molecular methods were developed in efforts to circumvent limitations of these classic approaches. These molecular methods, including library immunoscreening, degenerate PCR, and representational difference analysis, led to the discovery of many clinically important viruses including

TABLE 15.14 Laboratory Diagnosis of Viral Respiratory and Gastrointestinal Tract Infections

Virus	Test method	Comments
Respiratory tract infections		
Influenza A, B	NAAT	Most sensitive test
	FA stain	Less sensitive than NAAT
	Culture	Less sensitive than NAAT, requires viable virus
	Antigen detection	Low sensitivity, especially for pandemic 2009 H1N1 virus
Respiratory syncytial	NAAT	Most sensitive test
	FA stain	Less sensitive than NAAT
	Culture	Requires viable virus
	Rapid tests	Less sensitive than other methods
Parainfluenza	NAAT	Most sensitive test
	FA stain	Less sensitive than NAAT
	Culture	Requires viable virus
Human metapneumovirus	NAAT	Most sensitive test
	FA stain	Less sensitive than NAAT
Rhinovirus	NAAT	Most sensitive test; primers and probes must be selected carefully to detect all serotypes/genotypes. May be difficult or impossible to distinguish from enteroviruses
	Culture	Requires viable virus; is less sensitive than NAAT. Clade C rhinoviruses have not been successfully cultured as of time of writing
Coronaviruses (OC43, 229E, NL63, HKU1)	NAAT	Most sensitive test
Adenoviruses	NAAT	Most sensitive test
	FA stain	Less sensitive than NAAT or culture
	FA	Less sensitive than culture
Gastrointestinal tract infections		
Rotavirus	Antigen detection	Very sensitive
Norovirus	NAAT	Most sensitive test
	ELISA	Less sensitive than NAAT
Adenoviruses (group F, serotypes 40 and 41)	ELISA	Specific assay for serotypes 40 and 41
	NAAT	Most sensitive test
Astroviruses	NAAT	Most sensitive test

ELISA, enzyme-linked immunosorbent assay; FA, fluorescent antibody; NAAT, nucleic acid amplification test.

HCV, Kaposi sarcoma herpesvirus (KSHV), and others. As these methods have been the subject of other reviews,[65] they will not be discussed in detail here.

The 21st century has witnessed a revolution in the field of virus discovery as evidenced by the dramatic increase in the rate of identification of novel viruses. This increase has been driven largely by the advent of the genomic era, which has created novel sequencing technologies that in turn have geometrically increased the volume of sequencing data that can be generated. The combination of increased sequences in public databases and increased sequencing capacity has enabled the development of new, sophisticated sequence-based approaches for viral detection and discovery. Even existing methods, such as consensus PCR approaches, have benefited from the geometric growth in sequence databases. With the availability of many more viral genome sequences, improved consensus PCR primers can be designed for many viral taxa.

All of the recently developed viral discovery methods are based on detection of viral nucleic acids. Fundamentally, the major challenge in sequence-based viral discovery is identifying the relatively few copies of viral DNA or RNA in specimens that typically contain a vast excess of host genomic DNA and/or RNA. In theory, given unlimited sequencing capacity, there would be no need to be concerned with the host; exhaustive direct sequencing of a given sample should reveal the presence of any viral sequences in the sample no matter how low the abundance of the virus. However, practical limitations on sequencing, either in terms of sheer capacity or cost, have until recently required that additional methods be employed to effectively increase the relative percentage of viral sequence to host sequence. For example, propagation of a virus in cell culture is one means of increasing the relative abundance of viral sequences. Physical purification of virions, by ultracentrifugation or nuclease treatment to eliminate nonencapsidated nucleic acids, is another means of enriching for viral sequences. Subtractive hybridization strategies achieve a similar end point by physically reducing the amount of host sequences. However, we are rapidly approaching a point where sequencing capacity and costs are no longer limiting.

One potential limitation in sequence-based virus discovery is the quantity of nucleic acids available for sequencing. To circumvent this challenge, multiple experimental approaches to increase the total abundance of nucleic acids to levels amenable to further analysis have also been developed. An essential feature

TABLE 15.15 Laboratory Diagnosis of Central Nervous System Infections

Syndrome	Virus	Method[a]
Meningitis	Enterovirus	NAAT
	Herpes simplex virus	NAAT
	Varicella-zoster virus	NAAT
	Human immunodeficiency virus	NAAT on plasma
Encephalitis in nonimmunosuppressed individuals	Herpes simplex	NAAT
	West Nile virus and other arboviruses	IgM antibody assay on serum and CSF[b]
	Varicella-zoster virus	NAAT, intrathecal antibody synthesis[c]
	Epstein-Barr virus	NAAT, IgM antibody assay on serum and plasma
	HHV-6	NAAT
	Rabies	NAAT on CSF and saliva, rabies antibody assay on CSF and serum,[d] FA stain of skin biopsy from nape of neck
	Mumps	NAAT on CSF and saliva, IgM antibody assay on serum
	Lymphocytic choriomeningitis virus	IgG and IgM antibody assays on CSF and serum (acute and convalescent samples), NAAT, culture
Encephalitis in immunosuppressed individuals	Cytomegalovirus	NAAT
	Epstein-Barr virus	NAAT
	Varicella-zoster virus	NAAT, intrathecal antibody synthesis[c]
	JC virus	NAAT

CSF, cerebrospinal fluid; HHV-6, human herpesvirus type 6; Ig, immunoglobulin; NAAT, nucleic acid amplification test.

[a]Indicated test is performed on CSF unless otherwise indicated.

[b]Testing should be performed on CSF and serum. Testing of CSF is more specific for current infection.

[c]Detection of intrathecal antibody synthesis has been shown to be more sensitive than NAAT for the diagnosis of varicella-zoster virus central nervous system vasculopathy.[91]

[d]CSF is preferred if the individual being evaluated has previously received rabies immunization.

TABLE 15.16 Laboratory Diagnosis of Congenital and Neonatal Viral Infections

Virus	Recommended testing
Cytomegalovirus	NAAT or culture of urine and/or saliva during first 2 weeks of life
Herpes simplex	NAAT or culture of a vesicle, CSF, blood (plasma, serum, or whole blood). Conjunctiva, nasopharynx, oropharynx, urine, and rectum/stool may also be tested
Human immunodeficiency virus (HIV)	NAAT for HIV RNA on plasma or DNA on whole blood
Rubella	IgM antibody assay of serum or plasma, NAAT or culture of urine, oropharynx, blood, stool, CSF. Amniotic fluid and products of conception can also be tested
Parvovirus B19	IgM antibody assay of serum or plasma, NAAT of plasma or serum
Hepatitis B	Hepatitis B surface antigen test on serum or plasma
Varicella-zoster virus	NAAT, culture, or FA stain on vesicle, CSF, or blood. NAAT on amniotic fluid
Enteroviruses	NAAT on plasma or serum, CSF, nasopharyngeal or oropharyngeal swab, stool, urine
Hepatitis C	NAAT on plasma or serum on two occasions between 2 and 6 months of age or HCV antibody assay at age ≥15 months of age

CSF, cerebrospinal fluid; FA, fluorescent antibody; Ig, immunoglobulin; NAAT, nucleic acid amplification assay.

TABLE 15.17 Laboratory Diagnosis of Human Immunodeficiency and Other Retrovirus Infections

Indication	Test
Routine diagnosis	ELISA for HIV antibodies[a]
Confirmation of a positive ELISA	Samples that are reactive on the screening HIV antibody or combined HIV antigen–antibody assay should be tested with a confirmatory antibody test that differentiates HIV-1 and HIV-2 antibodies.[b] Patients who are positive with this assay should have a second sample tested for HIV RNA. Rare patients who are reactive on the screening test and the confirmatory HIV-1/HIV-2 antibody assay but negative for HIV RNA should have additional testing performed under the direction of an HIV specialist. This testing might include a repeat of the screening assay, an HIV western blot, or an HIV DNA PCR assay. Patients who are negative with the confirmatory HIV-1/HIV-2 antibody assay should have an HIV RNA assay performed. Patients who are reactive on the screening assay, negative on the confirmatory HIV-1/HIV-2 antibody assay, and positive for HIV RNA are presumed to have recent infection and should be referred immediately to an HIV specialist.[8]
Blood donor screening	ELISA for antibodies to HIV-1 and -2, HIV RNA assay
Infant born to infected mother	HIV RNA or DNA assay at 14–21 days of age, 1–2 months, and 4–6 months[c]
Acute antiretroviral syndrome	HIV RNA assay
Prognosis	Quantitative HIV RNA assay
Response to therapy	Quantitative HIV RNA assay
Resistance to antiretroviral drugs	Genotypic assay based on nucleotide sequencing of the relevant genes, or phenotypic assay based on inserting relevant genes from the patient's HIV strain into a laboratory vector
Diagnosis of HIV-2 infection	ELISA for HIV-2 antibodies[d]
Monitoring of HIV-2 infection	HIV-2 RNA assay[e]
Diagnosis of HTLV-1 or -2 infection	HTLV-1 and 2 antibody ELISA assays
Confirmation of HTLV-1 or -2 infection	HTLV-1 and -2 western blot, line immunoassay or immunofluorescent antibody assay[e]

ELISA, enzyme-linked immunosorbent assay; HIV, human immunodeficiency virus; HTLV, human T-cell lymphoma or leukemia virus; PCR, polymerase chain reaction.

[a]Most FDA licensed tests detect antibodies to both HIV-1 and -2. Third-generation antibody assays are preferred because they detect immunoglobulin M (IgM) as well as IgG antibodies, and thus become positive earlier after infection than assays that detect only IgG antibodies. An alternative approach is to use a fourth-generation test that measures HIV p24 antigen in addition to HIV antibodies.

[b]A licensed rapid HIV antibody test approved by the Food and Drug Administration (FDA) is now available that differentiates HIV-1 and HIV-2 antibodies.

[c]DNA PCR may be preferred while the infant is on prophylactic antiretroviral treatment because of the possibility that antiretroviral therapy may make HIV RNA undetectable.

[d]Most HIV antibody assays currently in use detect antibodies to both HIV-1 and HIV-2, but only one FDA-licensed test differentiates between HIV-1 and HIV-2 antibodies.

[e]Available only in selected reference laboratories.

TABLE 15.18 Laboratory Diagnosis of Tropical and Other Geographically Localized Viral Infections

Virus or syndrome	Location	Preferred tests
Sin nombre virus	Western United States	Virus-specific IgM antibody assay, NAAT
Other hantaviruses	Asia, Europe	Virus-specific IgM antibody assay, NAAT
Colorado tick fever	Western United States	Virus-specific IgM antibody assay, NAAT
Dengue fever	Asia, Central and South America	Virus-specific IgM antibody assay, NAAT
Filoviruses (Ebola and Marburg viruses)	Central Africa	Virus-specific IgM antibody assay, NAAT
Arenaviruses (e.g., Lassa, Junin, many others)	West Africa (Lassa fever), South American (Junin)	Virus-specific IgM antibody assay, NAAT, culture
Hendra and Nipah viruses	Australia, Malaysia, Bangladesh, India	Virus-specific IgM antibody assay, NAAT
Yellow fever	Central Africa, Amazon region	Virus-specific IgM antibody assay, NAAT
Crimean-Congo hemorrhagic fever and other bunyavirus infections	Asia, Africa, Europe	Virus-specific IgM antibody assay, antigen-capture ELISA, culture, NAAT
Rift Valley fever	East Africa	Virus-specific IgM antibody assay, antigen-capture ELISA, culture, NAAT, culture
Chikungunya and other alphavirus infections (O'nyong nyong, sindbis, Mayaro, Ross River)	Africa, India, Central and South America, Europe, Australia (Ross River)	Virus-specific IgM antibody assay, culture, NAAT

ELISA, enzyme-linked immunosorbent assay; IgM, immunoglobulin M; NAAT, nucleic acid amplification test.

of all of these amplification strategies is that no prior knowledge regarding the nature of the sequences to be amplified is required because it is unknown what type of virus may be present.

For sequence-based detection technologies, a key step is the computational analysis required to identify a sequence as viral in nature. In early efforts, only a few sequences were generated and thus analysis could easily be done via commonly used web-interface software. With advances in sequencing capacity, the number of sequences generated from a sample increased initially to hundreds or thousands and now can easily surpass a million sequences or more. In order to efficiently analyze this volume of sequence data, automated high-throughput bioinformatics pipelines had to be developed. Although many variations on this theme exist, most computational pipelines utilize very similar overall strategies. Typically, sequence alignment software, such as BLAST, is used to compare the sequences generated from a sample to established public databases. Sequences with perfect or near-perfect alignments to known sequences (host, viral, bacterial, etc.) can then be categorized based on the identity of the reference sequence to which a given read aligned. Sequences derived from novel viruses are those that have only limited similarity to known viruses in the available databases. For more definitive characterization of the relatedness of these sequences to known viruses, phylogenetic methods are subsequently used.

As mentioned previously, a key driving factor in the advances in virus discovery has been the evolution of sequencing technology. For over 30 years, from its inception in the late 1970s until the late 2000s, Sanger dideoxy sequencing was the dominant sequencing technology in use, and all efforts to identify viruses using sequencing-based strategies relied on this technology. At its highest throughput, automated 96-capillary Sanger sequencing could generate up to approximately 100,000 bp of sequence in a single run. Starting in 2005, the first of the so-called Next Generation (NextGen) sequencing platforms was introduced.[87] These platforms dramatically increased the quantity of sequence that could be produced. For example, the Roche/454 platform in its initial format was capable of generating 100,000 reads of 100 bp length in a single run, or approximately 100-fold greater sequence than a run on the previous instrument standard, the ABI 3730. Over the next few years, this platform rapidly evolved such that by 2009, the Roche/454 platform could readily generate 1,000,000 reads that averaged 400 bp, or 400 megabases (MB) of sequence. Two other major NextGen sequencing platforms, Solexa (Illumina) and SOLiD (ABI), also emerged during this time (reviewed in reference 86). Both of these platforms generate more reads than Roche/454, but of shorter length (up to 125 bp for Illumina, up to 75 for SOLiD). At the current time, these platforms are capable of generating on the order of 100 gigabases (GB) of sequence in a single run. It is the unprecedented growth in sequencing capacity offered by these new platforms that has transformed the process of virus discovery.

Novel Virus Discovery Strategies (2000–2010)

Random Arbitrarily Primed PCR

The 2001 discovery of human metapneumovirus relied on differential display of amplicons generated by a sequence-independent PCR amplification strategy.[139] An unknown virus was passaged in tertiary monkey kidney cells from respiratory secretions of multiple children with respiratory tract infections. From nucleic acids purified from one such culture, a defined set of random, arbitrary primers was hybridized under low stringency to amplify nucleic acids from the culture and an uninfected control. Comparison of the resulting gel electrophoresis patterns yielded unique bands present only in the infected sample. These bands were selectively purified from the gel, sequenced, and found to share only limited sequence identity to avian pneumoviruses. Cultured virus was used to infect cynomolgus macaques, several of which developed mild respiratory symptoms and replicated virus as measured by RT-PCR, thus fulfilling Koch's postulates. Serologic analysis demonstrated that the virus is commonly acquired in childhood, with the majority of adults being seropositive. The human metapneumovirus is now established as one of the leading causes of viral respiratory infection.

DNase-SISPA

In 2001, Allander et al.[2] described DNase-SISPA (sequence-independent single primer amplification), a key virus discovery methodology that would be used to identify numerous novel viruses in the following years. Importantly, specific enrichment for capsid-protected viral nucleic acids in the specimen was carried out prior to nucleic acid extraction, using a combination of ultracentrifugation to pellet virions followed by treatment with DNase to degrade any free nucleic acids, presumably derived primarily from the host. RNA and DNA were independently extracted and analyzed in parallel. RNA was converted to double-stranded cDNA and then treated exactly as the extracted DNA. DNA was digested by restriction enzymes, a common linker was ligated to both ends of the double-stranded DNA fragments, and then the DNA was PCR amplified using a single common linker primer. Amplification products were visualized by gel electrophoresis, and individual bands were recovered from the gel, cloned, and sequenced using standard Sanger sequencing technology. In this proof of principle study, two novel bovine parvoviruses were identified in commercial bovine serum.

Random PCR Amplification-DNA Microarray Hybridization or "Virus Chip"

With the advent of DNA microarrays in the early 1990s, it rapidly became clear that the inherently parallel nature of microarrays could be utilized for massively parallel viral detection. Conceptually, the presence of a virus in a sample could be deduced from the pattern of hybridization to virus-derived oligonucleotide sequences on the microarray or so-called virus chip. The spectrum of viruses that could be detected in a single microarray hybridization was limited in theory only by the availability of viral sequences that could be included in a given microarray. The first broad-range viral detection microarray, which contained ~1,600 oligonucleotides capable of detecting ~140 viruses from all virus families with members known to cause respiratory disease, was described in 2002.[145] Critically, the most highly conserved 70-mer regions from these viruses were incorporated into the microarray to maximize the probability of detecting not only known viruses but also unsequenced or novel viruses by cross-hybridization to these highly conserved elements. The resulting pan-viral microarray is shown in Figure 15.12. The ability of the microarray

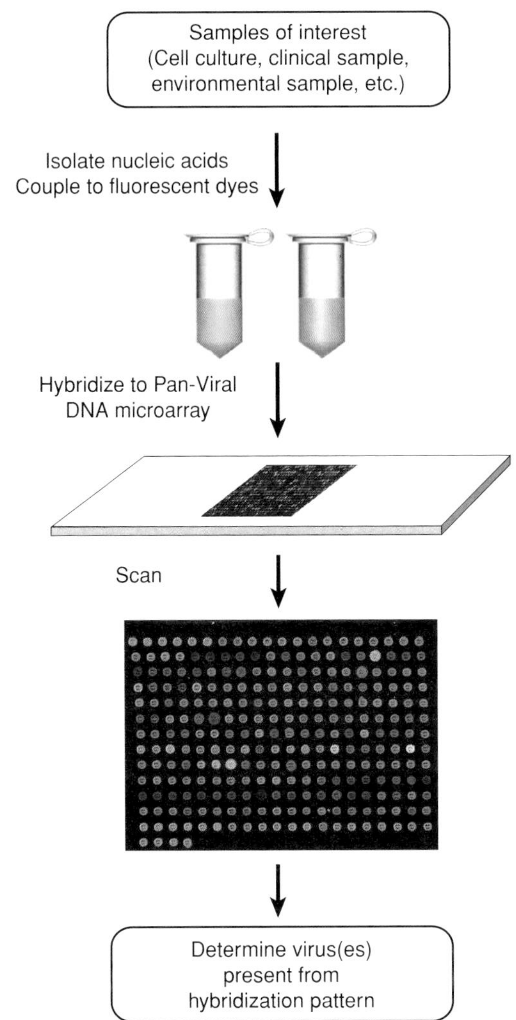

FIGURE 15.12. Pan-viral microarray used for virus discovery. (Wang D, Coscoy L, Zylberberg M, et al. Microarray-based detection and genotyping of viral pathogens. *Proc Natl Acad Sci U S A* 2002;99:15687–15692.)

to detect known viruses was validated using a series of known respiratory viruses grown in cell culture. To demonstrate the feasibility of detecting unknown viruses, multiple unsequenced strains of rhinoviruses grown in culture were hybridized to the microarray. Based on hybridization to many rhinovirus-derived sequences, these viruses could clearly be classified as rhinoviruses. Furthermore, to demonstrate that the method could be applied to human clinical samples and not just to cultured viruses, random PCR amplification of nucleic acids extracted directly from human respiratory specimens was employed. In this strategy, a single primer composed of a fixed linker region at the 5′ end and five or more totally degenerate positions at the 3′ end is the critical reagent.[7,34] The degenerate 3′ end can theoretically hybridize at any position on any DNA template, and when two primers hybridize to complementary strands in close proximity, the subsequent thermocycling generates an amplicon. In this fashion, all nucleic acids in a sample can be amplified at random. Microarray hybridization of randomly amplified nucleic acids extracted from the clinical specimens enabled detection of diverse known human respiratory viruses.

The first application of this approach to identify a novel virus occurred during the SARS outbreak of 2003.[72,146] A second-generation pan-viral DNA microarray that contained ~11,000 70-mers derived from every fully sequenced viral genome in GenBank at the time was used to analyze an unknown virus cultured in Vero cells from the respiratory swab of a SARS patient. Random PCR followed by hybridization to the microarray yielded a hybridization pattern consistent with the presence of a divergent member of the family *Coronaviridae;* only a limited number of coronavirus-derived probes had high signal intensity. In order to rapidly sequence portions of the viral genome, fragments of the unknown virus that were bound to various 70-mers on the microarray were physically recovered, cloned, and sequenced.[146] These sequences shared only 33% identity to murine hepatitis virus, a murine coronavirus, definitively demonstrating that SARS was highly divergent from all previously described viruses.

VIDISCA

The discovery of human coronavirus NL63 in 2004 relied on VIDISCA (*Vi*rus *Dis*covery *c*DNA-*A*FLP [amplified fragment length polymorphism]), a variant of the DNAse-SISPA strategy[140] in combination with classic viral culture. From a 7-month-old child with bronchiolitis, cytopathic effect was detected following culture in tertiary monkey kidney cells. Material from those cultures was further passaged into LLC-MK2 cells. To identify the virus, supernatants from infected and uninfected cells were generated and subjected to VIDISCA. In this protocol, the initial steps were essentially identical to DNAse-SISPA: ultracentrifugation, DNAse treatment, nucleic acid purification, restriction endonuclease digestion, linker ligation, and PCR amplification. At this stage, a second set of PCR reactions was performed using all pairwise combinations of four PCR primers; each primer used contained one additional nucleotide (A, T, G, or C) appended to the 3′ end of the linker primer used in the first round of PCR. Thus, 16 PCR reactions were performed with the goal of identifying specific bands present only in the infected cell culture and absent from the uninfected control. This process reduces the complexity of the banding pattern during gel electrophoresis compared to standard DNase-SISPA as each reaction should contain only one-sixteenth of the amplicons. In this instance, 16 bands unique to the infected sample were cloned, and 13 were determined to have only limited sequence similarity to known coronaviruses. Analysis of the complete genome of coronavirus NL63 determined that it shares 65% nucleotide identity to its closest relative, coronavirus 229E. Follow-up epidemiologic studies have defined an association of coronavirus-NL63 with croup.[141]

Rolling Circle Amplification/Restriction Digest/Gel Electrophoresis

The methods described previously have all utilized sequence-independent PCR amplification. An alternative non–PCR-based, sequence-independent amplification strategy relies on isothermal amplification using phi29 polymerase with random primers. This amplification strategy, also referred to variously as *rolling circle amplification, multiple displacement amplification,* and *whole genome amplification,* takes advantage of the highly processive nature of phi29 polymerase (greater than 70,000 average nucleotide extension) and its strand displacement activity, which can lead to branching and thereby exponential amplification. When incubated with phi29 polymerase and random primers, small circular DNA viruses can be amplified by a factor of 10^4. The products of this amplification, long double-stranded linear concatemers of viral genome monomers, can then be digested by restriction enzymes and visualized by gel electrophoresis. Bands can then be cloned and sequenced. In demonstrating proof of principle, Rector et al.[112] described the detection of a bovine papillomavirus from tissue. Subsequently, this approach would be used to identify the novel human polyomavirus 6.[120]

Random PCR-Sanger High-Throughput Sequencing

The discovery of human bocavirus was the first example where PCR products from randomly amplified clinical material were sequenced en masse[3]; prior examples of sequencing-based discovery described previously relied on gel purification of specific individual target bands. In this study, respiratory secretions from multiple patients with unexplained respiratory illness were pooled, ultracentrifuged to concentrate viral particles, and DNAse-treated to enrich for capsid-protected sequences. Following nucleic acid extraction, random PCR amplification, and size selection of 600- to 1,500-bp amplicons for cloning, 384 clones were sequenced using standard Sanger technology. Sequences with limited amino acid similarity to known parvoviruses were detected. Phylogenetic analysis demonstrated that this novel genome was a previously uncharacterized species of the genus *Bocavirus*. This experimental strategy would be used in many subsequent instances to identify novel viruses. With the evolution of NextGen sequencing platforms, many laboratories subsequently adapted their protocols to utilize NextGen sequencing technologies in place of the traditional Sanger sequencing. Multiple examples of viruses discovered by random PCR-NextGen sequencing will be described in the following sections.

NextGen High-Throughput Sequencing of a cDNA Library

The identification of Merkel cell polyomavirus in Merkel carcinomas was the first instance of the use of a NextGen sequencing platform (Roche/454 FLX platform) to discover a novel virus.[29] The experimental strategy, termed *digital transcriptome subtraction*, entailed sequencing of mRNA isolated from tumor tissue and subsequent computational subtraction of host sequences followed by alignment of the remaining sequences. Proof of concept for this type of strategy was first demonstrated in 2002, wherein an expressed sequence tag (EST) library derived from HeLa cells was subjected to computational subtraction of human sequences.[148] Among the remaining ESTs that did not match to any human sequences were human papillomavirus-18 sequences, which were known to be present in HeLa cells. In the Merkel carcinoma study, a total of four tumor samples were pooled and ~382,000 high-quality sequence reads were generated; from the data, one sequence possessed detectable sequence similarity to the T antigen of known polyomaviruses. The complete genome sequence of the novel virus, designated Merkel polyomavirus, was obtained, and phylogenetic analysis demonstrated that it was a highly divergent polyomavirus. Southern blotting determined that Merkel polyomavirus DNA was clonally integrated in a number of Merkel tumors. Multiple subsequent prevalence studies have determined that ~80% of Merkel carcinoma tissues contain Merkel polyomavirus. This landmark study demonstrated the increased sensitivity achievable by deep sequencing with NextGen platforms as compared to previous efforts, wherein a single sequence of a novel virus (out of >380,000 total sequences sampled) could be detected. Moreover, no steps were taken to enrich the ratio of virus to host.

NextGen High-Throughput Sequencing of Small RNAs

Two studies demonstrated the feasibility of identifying novel viruses by sequencing and assembly of small RNAs.[71,153] Following the discovery of RNA interference (RNAi), it became clear that RNAi has an antiviral function in plants and lower eukaryotic organisms; as a consequence, viral RNA sequences are cleaved to small RNAs ranging in size from ~21 to 25 nt. The presence of these small RNAs could readily be detected by gel-purifying small RNAs, using NextGen platforms to sequence the small RNAs. From these sequences, the application of assembly algorithms to reconstitute larger RNA fragments yielded contigs that could be clearly recognized as viral in nature. In plant experiments designed to analyze the effect of known sweet potato viruses on RNAi, previously undescribed badnaviruses and mastreviruses were detected by assembly of small RNAs.[71] Similarly, analysis of small RNA sequencing data from *Drosophila* cell lines demonstrated that multiple novel viruses, including members of *Nodaviridae, Titiviridae, Birnaviridae,* and *Tetraviridae,* could be identified in this fashion.[153]

Summary of Pathogen Discovery Methods

The methods described for virus discovery in the preceding paragraphs share a common end goal, albeit with multiple variations, namely, to identify nucleic acid sequences derived from viruses present in a sample of interest. The overall process can be dissected into distinct component modules, which in general can be mixed and matched, as illustrated in Figure 15.13. For a given specimen, different methods of processing the initial sample can be applied, different types of nucleic acid can be isolated, different sequence-independent amplification strategies can be used, and, ultimately, a range of technologies can be used as the readout. New combinations of these components continue to evolve.

Representative Novel Human Viruses Discovered (2000–2010)

Parvovirus 4

Screening of human plasma from patients with febrile illness by DNase-SISPA led to the discovery of sequences with only limited identity to known members of the family *Parvoviridae* in 2005.[58] The genome of a novel parvovirus, parvovirus 4, was sequenced. It has been detected to date in blood, bone marrow, and lymphoid tissue from patients with either HCV or HIV/acquired immunodeficiency syndrome (AIDS), in plasma of kidney transplant patients, and in CSF of encephalitis patients. The virus is believed to be parenterally transmitted based on the observation of high detection rates in hemophiliacs and injection drug users, although additional routes of transmission may also exist.

Anelloviruses

TT virus, the prototype anellovirus, was discovered in 1997 using representational difference analysis on human serum[95]

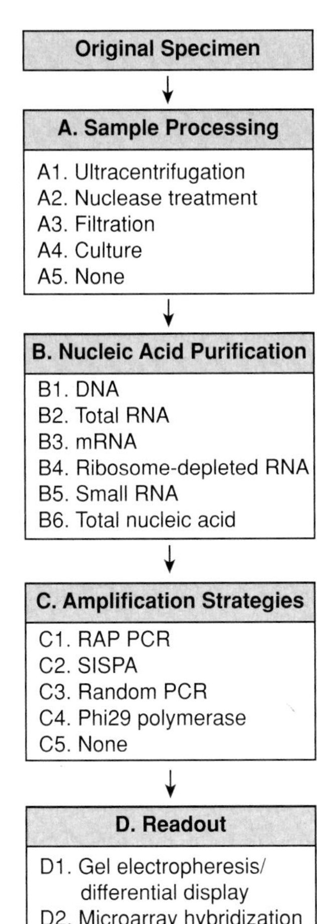

Original Specimen
A. Sample Processing
A1. Ultracentrifugation
A2. Nuclease treatment
A3. Filtration
A4. Culture
A5. None
B. Nucleic Acid Purification
B1. DNA
B2. Total RNA
B3. mRNA
B4. Ribosome-depleted RNA
B5. Small RNA
B6. Total nucleic acid
C. Amplification Strategies
C1. RAP PCR
C2. SISPA
C3. Random PCR
C4. Phi29 polymerase
C5. None
D. Readout
D1. Gel electropheresis/ differential display
D2. Microarray hybridization
D3. Sanger sequencing
D4. NextGen sequencing

FIGURE 15.13. Pathogen discovery methods. Recently developed sequence-based pathogen discovery methods all fundamentally follow a similar overall scheme. A clinical specimen of interest is collected. **A:** If desired, samples can be manipulated to increase the ratio of virus to host by various methods. **B:** Nucleic acid species of interest is isolated. **C:** In cases where the quantity of purified nucleic acid is limiting, random sequencing-independent amplification is applied. **D:** A readout method is selected. For example, the identification of human bocavirus used the sequence of steps A1-A2-B1-C3-D3. The identification of Merkel polyomavirus used the sequence A5-B3-C5-D4.

from a transfusion-associated hepatitis patient. Since its discovery, TT virus and TT-related viruses have been found at high frequencies in a variety of human specimens, including respiratory secretions, stool, and serum. There is currently no known disease association for any of the anelloviruses. Two studies in 2005 described the presence of novel anelloviruses in human blood.[9,58] In one study using DNase-SISPA to analyze serum from patients with febrile illness, two novel anelloviruses, SA1 and SA2, were identified that shared only 32% to 35% similarity to TT virus.[58] In the other study, plasma from healthy donors was enriched for virions by centrifugation through a cesium chloride (CsCl) step gradient. The fractions expected to contain known DNA viruses (1.2 to 1.5 g/mL density) were collected, DNAse treated, and then extracted. Two amplification strategies were then used: (a) shearing followed by linker ligation and sequence-independent PCR (as in DNAse-SISPA) and (b) sequence-independent amplification using phi29 polymerase. In both instances, shotgun libraries were constructed and then sequenced. In this study, seven sequences with limited similarity to anelloviruses were detected. Since these studies, novel anelloviruses have been detected in numerous studies.[30,143]

Novel Bocaviruses

Following the discovery of human bocavirus in respiratory secretions, a second novel bocavirus, named human bocavirus 2, was discovered by two independent groups using similar Sanger sequencing-based screening of stool samples of patients with acute flaccid paralysis[62] and acute gastroenteritis.[5] In the latter study, human bocavirus 2 prevalence of 17% in diarrhea cases was described, as was a statistically significant association between infection with human bocavirus 2 and acute gastroenteritis; however, in another study, no association was detected.[63] During efforts to describe the prevalence of human bocavirus and bocavirus 2 in human stools using consensus PCR, two additional human bocaviruses, human bocavirus 3[5] and human bocavirus 4,[63] were discovered.

KI Polyomavirus

Using Sanger sequencing of pooled respiratory secretions physically enriched for virions, KI polyomavirus (KIV), a novel member of the family *Polyomaviridae,* was discovered in 2007.[4] From the sequences generated, one 363-bp read possessed limited sequence similarity to the simian virus 40 (SV40) VP1 protein. From this one fragment, the complete 5,040-bp circular genome was sequenced. KIV has been detected in respiratory secretions in populations around the world as well as in feces. Seroepidemiologic studies have determined that a high percentage of the general population has been previously infected by KIV.[13,64,94]

WU Polyomavirus

Nearly simultaneously with the discovery of KIV, WU polyomavirus (WUV) was discovered by a similar strategy of high-throughput Sanger sequencing analysis of individual respiratory secretions.[38] From 384 clones that were sequenced from the nasopharyngeal aspirate of a child with pneumonia, six sequence reads that shared 35% to 50% amino acid identity to JC virus and SV40 were detected. The complete genome of 5,229 bp was sequenced, and based on phylogenetic analysis, WUV was found to be most closely related to KIV. To date, WUV has been detected primarily in respiratory secretions, but it has also been detected in a few instances in feces, blood (whole blood, plasma, and serum), CSF, and lymphoid tissue. As with KIV, infection by WUV appears to occur primarily in childhood, with ~90% of adult populations harboring antibodies to WUV.[13,64,94]

Human Polyomaviruses 6 and 7

During efforts to clone genomes of Merkel polyomavirus using rolling circle amplification of DNA collected from skin swab samples, a 1.6-kb BamHI fragment of a novel polyomavirus was detected. Subsequently, the complete genome of a novel virus designated human polyomavirus 6 was sequenced.[120] Based on this sequence, screening of skin swabs using degenerate PCR primers designed from human polyomavirus 6 and WU polyomavirus yielded an additional virus, human polyomavirus 7. Serologic analysis of 95 blood donors using recombinant VP1 capsid protein demonstrated 69% and 35% seropositivity for human polyomavirus 6 and human polyomavirus 7, respectively.[120]

TSV Polyomavirus

Trichodysplasia spinulosa (TSV) is a rare skin disease that occurs exclusively in immunocompromised patients. It is characterized by the development of spicules and follicular papules primarily on the face. Multiple case reports included electron micrographs demonstrating the presence of clusters of ~40-nm viral particles consistent with viruses in the polyomavirus or papillomavirus families. In 2010, DNA from the spicules collected from a heart transplant recipient suffering symptoms of TSV was subjected to rolling circle amplification (RCA). Restriction analysis of the RCA product yielded specific bands, which upon cloning and sequencing yielded a novel polyomavirus genome of 5,232 bp.[142] Quantitative PCR demonstrated that the virus was present at 2×10^5 copies per cell. Prevalence studies performed on plucked eyebrows from 69 immunocompromised renal transplant patients yielded 3 (4%) that were TSV positive. TSV polyomavirus has subsequently been detected in two urine samples from two additional patients.[121]

Human Polyomavirus 9

Human polyomavirus 9 was discovered using a degenerate PCR amplification strategy from the serum of a kidney transplant patient.[121] Sequencing of the compete genome demonstrated that human polyomavirus 9 was most closely related to the African green monkey lymphotropic virus. PCR-based screening of a cohort primarily composed of immunocompromised individuals yielded human polyomavirus 9 in three additional blood samples and one urine sample.

Asfarivirus-Like Virus

Random PCR-Roche/454 high-throughput sequencing was applied to human serum samples collected from patients suffering acute febrile illness and healthy controls in the Middle East. Multiple sequence fragments were detected in a total of four distinct serum samples that shared limited sequence identity (36% to 64% amino acid identity) to African swine fever virus proteins.[81] African swine fever virus is the only known member of the family *Asfarviridae,* and the divergence between the detected sequences and known African swine fever viruses clearly demonstrate that the sequences represent one or more novel members of this family. No human infection with African swine fever virus has been reported. In addition, sequencing of raw sewage collected in Spain also yielded multiple sequence fragments that were most closely related to African swine fever virus. In total, 36 unique fragments were identified, including multiple fragments that shared sequence identity to genes specifically found only in African swine fever virus.

Novel Astroviruses

Astrovirus MLB1 was identified in the first metagenomic analysis of stools from patients with diarrhea.[30] Following filtration of diluted stool supernatant, RNA was extracted and randomly amplified. The amplicons were cloned and 384 clones were sequenced using standard Sanger sequencing. From the stool sample of a 3-year-old child from Australia with acute diarrhea, seven sequences with less than 68% amino acid identity to known astroviruses were detected. The complete genome was sequenced, and phylogenetic analysis demonstrated it was a highly divergent astrovirus. The virus has been detected in stool samples of patients with and without diarrhea from the United States, Mexico, Hong Kong, India, and Nigeria.

Another novel astrovirus, astrovirus VA1, was discovered in stool samples collected from an unexplained outbreak of gastroenteritis in the United States by random PCR high-throughput sequencing. Parallel sequencing efforts using Sanger technology and the Roche/454 platform were used, in combination with conventional rapid amplification of CDNA ends (RACE) protocols, to sequence the entire genome.[32] The robustness of NextGen platforms such as Roche/454 was demonstrated by the fact that the majority of the genome (a contig of 6,581 nt out of the complete genome of 6,586 nt) could be assembled from the initial Roche/454 data. Astrovirus VA1 shared only 61% amino acid identity to its closest relative, mink astrovirus. Real-time RT-PCR screening for astrovirus VA1 demonstrated that astrovirus VA1 was present at high copy number in three out of the six available stool samples from the outbreak. These results raise the possibility that astrovirus VA1 may play a role in causing diarrhea. Viruses very closely related to astrovirus VA1 were subsequently detected in three stool samples from children in Nepal[61] and a patient in the Netherlands with celiac disease.[124] Furthermore, Roche/454 sequencing of encephalitic brain tissue from a child suffering from X-linked agammaglobulinemia yielded a virus closely related to astrovirus VA1.[109] Additional consensus astrovirus RT-PCR screening of stool samples led to the discovery of three additional astroviruses in human stool specimens in two independent studies: astrovirus MLB2, astrovirus VA2/HMO-A, and astrovirus VA3/HMO-B.[31,61]

Saffold Cardiovirus

Saffold virus, a novel member of the *Cardiovirus* genus, was discovered by DNase-SISPA analysis of an unknown virus cultured from a patient stool sample.[59] Saffold-like viruses were subsequently detected directly in a sample of human respiratory secretions using a pan-viral microarray approach[16] as well as in human stool from patients with gastroenteritis by PCR screening.[16,26] Serologic studies using neutralization assays have yielded seropositivity rates of 80% to 90% by adulthood, demonstrating that Saffold infection is a common occurrence.[17,155]

Rhinovirus C

By a consensus PCR strategy, a novel clade of rhinoviruses was identified in patients with influenza-like illness.[74] The many known serotypes of rhinoviruses have traditionally been classified into two clades, rhinovirus A and rhinovirus B. With the discovery in numerous studies of a novel set of related rhinoviruses, a new clade, designated rhinovirus C, has been establis hed.[66–76] These viruses appear to be globally widespread and may contribute to 50% or more of rhinovirus infections. No member of the rhinovirus C clade has been successfully cultivated in the cell lines traditionally used for detection of rhinoviruses.

Cosavirus

Random PCR followed by Sanger sequencing led to the discovery of a novel picornavirus, cosavirus A1, from a stool sample of a child with nonpolio acute flaccid paralysis from Pakistan.[60] Phylogenetic analysis of the complete genome of 7,634 bp determined that it is most closely related to Seneca Valley virus in the genus *Cardiovirus*. In this study, PCR screening identified an additional 34 cosavirus-positive samples in cases and in healthy controls that, based on phylogenetic analysis, were further classified into four distinct genetic groups (A through D). An independent study also using random PCR and Sanger sequencing led to the identification of a proposed genetic group E of cosavirus.[54]

Klassevirus/Salivirus

The identification of the novel picornavirus human klassevirus,[55,144] also known as salivirus,[79] by three independent groups in 2009 relied primarily on Roche/454 sequencing. This virus is most similar to members of the genus *Kobuvirus* and has been detected both in human stool specimens from the United States,[44,55,79] Australia,[55] Nigeria, Tunisia, and Nepal[79] and in raw sewage from Spain.[55] These results demonstrate that klassevirus/salivirus is globally widespread. In one study, 2 of 751 stool samples were positive for klassevirus, with the two positive patients twin siblings.[44] One case-control study in a Nepalese cohort demonstrated a positive association with gastroenteritis ($p = 0.0056$).[79]

Coronavirus HKU1

Degenerate PCR screening of respiratory secretions resulted in the discovery of human coronavirus HKU.[152] This virus has been detected in numerous studies from respiratory samples from patients around the world.

Lymphocytic Choriomeningitis Virus–Like Arenavirus

In one of the earliest applications of Roche/454 high-throughput sequencing to viral detection, an arenavirus was identified in multiple recipients of organs from a common donor.[99] In this case cluster, three organ recipients from the same donor died 4 to 6 weeks after transplantation. RNA was extracted from the CSF, serum, brain, kidney, and liver from two patients, pooled, and sequenced. From a total of 94,043 high-quality sequence reads, 14 had detectable sequence similarity to lymphocytic choriomeningitis virus (LCMV). Following PCR to sequence the complete genome of the virus, RT-PCR testing of multiple specimens from each of the three individuals revealed identical viral sequences in all three patients. Virus was isolated by culture in Vero E6 cells. Using antibodies against LCMV, viral antigen was detected in liver and kidney sections, and seroconversion was observed in one patient.

Lujo Virus

In 2008, a cluster of five cases of undiagnosed hemorrhagic fever was reported in South Africa with four fatalities. Random PCR-Roche/454 high-throughput sequencing was performed on RNA extracted from two postmortem liver biopsies and one serum sample. Analysis of the resulting ~300,000 sequences yielded nine fragments with limited sequence similarity to known arenaviruses.[10] Upon sequencing of the complete genome, phylogenetic analysis demonstrated that the virus, named Lujo virus, was highly divergent from known arenaviruses. Specimens collected from all five patients were positive for Lujo virus by virus isolation using cell culture and by RT-PCR.[103]

Xenotropic Murine Leukemia Virus–Related Virus

In 2006, a novel retrovirus closely related to xenotropic murine leukemia viruses, named xenotropic murine leukemia virus–related virus (XMRV), was first identified by random PCR pan-viral DNA microarray analysis.[137] The samples analyzed were prostate tumor specimens, and presence of the virus was associated with a specific polymorphism of the *RNaseL* gene, a key component of the interferon-induced antiviral defense system. In further studies of prostate cancer specimens, XMRV was also detected in one instance[119] but not in another.[131] Subsequently, one study suggested an association between chronic fatigue syndrome and XMRV.[82] This finding, however, has been contradicted by numerous studies that have failed to detect XMRV in chronic fatigue patients, including a large multicenter blinded study[123] and a study that retested patients previously identified to have the virus in the original study.[67] Furthermore, multiple studies have demonstrated that reagents often used in RT-PCR and other manipulations can be contaminated with XMRV-like sequences, raising the possibility that amplification artifacts and contamination contribute to some of the observations.[131] Finally, one study demonstrated that XMRV likely arose via recombination between two murine retroviruses in the course of prostate tumor xenograft experiments, suggesting that this virus is an artifact of laboratory experimentation.[101] These studies illustrate some of the potential challenges of defining the biological relevance of newly identified agents using primarily molecular approaches.

Prospects and Challenges for the Future

Advances in molecular methods have dramatically increased the rate at which viral genomes can be detected, resulting in our awareness of the existence of many more viral genomes than just a few years ago. For example, following the initial discoveries of BK and JC viruses by culture in 1971, there were no additional polyomaviruses of humans identified until 2007. Since then, a total of seven new polyomaviruses have been identified in humans, all by molecular methods. Parallel situations exist in many viral taxa, wherein geometric increases in the number of known members have been observed. With the continued growth in sequencing capacity, there is little doubt that many more viruses will be identified in the upcoming years. Recently, specific efforts to comprehensively catalog the spectrum of viruses present in humans have begun. One objective of the international Human Microbiome Project is to define the set of viruses present in different anatomic sites in a set of "healthy" adults. These and other similar efforts to define the "viromes" of humans, animals, plants, or environmental niches will undoubtedly uncover a tremendous diversity of new viral genomes. While our ability to identify viral nucleic acids and genomes has grown at an astounding rate, our ability to define the molecular properties and the biological relevance of these new agents has unfortunately lagged behind. In order to effectively study these new viruses, commensurate new developments in traditional virology must occur. For example, novel methods of virus culture must be developed in order to keep pace with the rate of discovery of new viral sequences, as the ability to propagate a virus in culture is, in many instances, the rate-limiting step in our ability to further characterize a virus and to define its pathogenicity. Many of the viruses being discovered today by sequencing-based molecular methods are unlikely to grow in the traditional cell lines utilized by virologists. As an example, the advent of differentiated primary respiratory epithelial cultures has opened new frontiers by enabling the culture of several newly identified respiratory viruses, such as human bocavirus[25] and coronavirus HKU,[108] that have failed to grow previously in traditional respiratory tract–derived cell lines. Another area of great importance is the development of robust animal models for these new agents, which will be a critical part of efforts to define pathogenicity and disease causality. Finally, the criteria used for defining "pathogenicity" must also be revisited. While Koch's postulates, the 100-plus-year-old gold standard for proof of disease causation, have served us well in the past, this era of molecular virus discovery necessitates an enhanced emphasis on the role of epidemiologic and seroepidemiologic approaches in defining disease associations.[33] Furthermore, more nuanced conceptions of microbially induced disease, such as disease as a consequence of imbalance or perturbation of host microbial populations, must also be considered. In summary, technology-driven advances in sequencing have led to a golden era of discovery of new viruses in the first decade of the 21st century. Hopefully, parallel advances in understanding the biology of these new agents will come to fruition in the next decades of the 21st century.

PERSPECTIVE

Diagnostic virology is at a critical point in its history. The field has matured, with detection of a selected group of viral pathogens emerging as an important component of clinical laboratory services at major medical centers. For example, the detection of respiratory viruses; diagnosis and monitoring of viral infections, especially CMV, EBV, and BK virus in immunocompromised patients; viral load and antiviral susceptibility testing for HIV, HCV, and HBV; and testing for HPV have all become mainstream diagnostic procedures. The methodology of diagnostic virology is evolving rapidly, with increasing conversion to molecular methods. The development of standardized commercial molecular tests that have passed through the review processes of the FDA has been relatively slow but is now beginning to gain momentum. At the same time, the process of virus discovery, described earlier, is dramatically expanding the vistas of medical virology. In the coming years, it may become necessary to detect many viruses other than those for which FDA-approved assays are under development. Relatively unbiased methods such as NextGen sequencing, currently being used mainly for virus discovery, will undoubtedly be evaluated in the clinical laboratory setting. In addition, new paradigms, including recognition and diagnosis of diseases that result from multiple microbial interactions as well as diseases that occur uniquely in an individual based on that individual's genetic makeup, may require profound changes in the way in which diagnostic testing is performed. Assays to detect the presence of viruses may need to be combined with assays to evaluate biomarkers that provide information on how the host is reacting to the presence of the virus. Genetic markers may need to be evaluated to help define how an individual patient is likely to respond to viral infection. In addition, there is little doubt that unforeseen technological advances will drive the evolution of the field in directions that are currently impossible to predict.

DISCLOSURES

Dr. Storch serves on the medical advisory board of Roche Molecular Systems and has served as a consultant to Idaho Technology, PrimeraDx, Abbott, and Diagnostic Hybrids. He has received an honorarium from GenProbe and Meridian. He is currently performing research funded by Luminex and Meridian. Dr. Wang has no disclosures.

REFERENCES

1. Abu-Diab A, Azzeh M, Ghneim R, et al. Comparison between pernasal flocked swabs and nasopharyngeal aspirates for detection of common respiratory viruses in samples from children. *J Clin Microbiol* 2008;46:2414–2417.
2. Allander T, Emerson SU, Engle RE, et al. A virus discovery method incorporating DNase treatment and its application to the identification of two bovine parvovirus species. *Proc Natl Acad Sci U S A* 2001;98:11609–11614.
3. Allander T, Tammi MT, Eriksson M, et al. Cloning of a human parvovirus by molecular screening of respiratory tract samples. *Proc Natl Acad Sci U S A* 2005;102:12891–12896.
4. Allander T, Andreasson K, Gupta S, et al. Identification of a third human polyomavirus. *J Virol* 2007;81:4130–4136.
5. Arthur JL, Higgins GD, Davidson GP, et al. A novel bocavirus associated with acute gastroenteritis in Australian children. *PLoS Pathog* 2009;5:e1000391.
6. Bedson S, Bland J. Complement-fixation with filterable viruses and their antisera. *Br J Exp Pathol* 1929;1929:393–404.
7. Bohlander SK, Espinosa R 3rd, Le Beau MM, et al. A method for the rapid sequence-independent amplification of microdissected chromosomal material. *Genomics* 1992;13:1322–1324.
8. Branson BM, Mermin J. Establishing the diagnosis of HIV infection: new tests and a new algorithm for the United States. *J Clin Virol* 2011;52(Suppl 1):S3–S4.
9. Breitbart M, Rohwer F. Method for discovering novel DNA viruses in blood using viral particle selection and shotgun sequencing. *BioTechniques* 2005;39:729–736.
10. Briese T, Paweska JT, McMullan LK, et al. Genetic detection and characterization of Lujo virus, a new hemorrhagic fever-associated arenavirus from southern Africa. *PLoS Pathog* 2009;5:e1000455.
11. Bright RA, Medina MJ, Xu X, et al. Incidence of adamantane resistance among influenza A (H3N2) viruses isolated worldwide from 1994 to 2005: a cause for concern. *Lancet* 2005;366:1175–1181.
12. Buxton RC, Edwards B, Juo RR, et al. Development of a sensitive chemiluminescent neuraminidase assay for the determination of influenza virus susceptibility to zanamivir. *Anal Biochem* 2000;280:291–300.
13. Carter JJ, Paulson KG, Wipf GC, et al. Association of Merkel cell polyomavirus-specific antibodies with Merkel cell carcinoma. *J Natl Cancer Inst* 2009;101:1510–1522.
14. Chapman NM, Tracy S, Gauntt CJ, et al. Molecular detection and identification of enteroviruses using enzymatic amplification and nucleic acid hybridization. *J Clin Microbiol* 1990;28:843–850.
15. Cheval J, Sauvage V, Frangeul L, et al. Evaluation of high-throughput sequencing for identifying known and unknown viruses in biological samples. *J Clin Microbiol* 2011;49:3268–3275.
16. Chiu CY, Greninger AL, Kanada K, et al. Identification of cardioviruses related to Theiler's murine encephalomyelitis virus in human infections. *Proc Natl Acad Sci U S A* 2008;105:14124–14129.
17. Chiu CY, Greninger AL, Chen EC, et al. Cultivation and serological characterization of a human Theiler's-like cardiovirus associated with diarrheal disease. *J Virol* 2010;84:4407–4414.
18. Chou S. Cytomegalovirus UL97 mutations in the era of ganciclovir and maribavir. *Rev Med Virol* 2008;18:233–246.
19. Chutinimitkul S, Suwannakarn K, Chieochansin T, et al. H5N1 Oseltamivir-resistance detection by real-time PCR using two high sensitivity labeled TaqMan probes. *J Virol Methods* 2007;139:44–49.
20. de Vries M, Deijs M, Canuti M, et al. A sensitive assay for virus discovery in respiratory clinical samples. *PLoS One* 2011;6:e16118.
21. Deiman B, van Aarle P, Sillekens P. Characteristics and applications of nucleic acid sequence-based amplification (NASBA). *Mol Biotechnol* 2002;20:163–179.

22. Dewar RL, Highbarger HC, Sarmiento MD, et al. Application of branched DNA signal amplification to monitor human immunodeficiency virus type 1 burden in human plasma. *J Infect Dis* 1994;170: 1172–1179.
23. Deyde VM, Sheu TG, Trujillo AA, et al. Detection of molecular markers of drug resistance in 2009 pandemic influenza A (H1N1) viruses by pyrosequencing. *Antimicrob Agents Chemother* 2010;54:1102–1110.
24. Dharan NJ, Gubareva LV, Meyer JJ, et al. Infections with oseltamivir-resistant influenza A(H1N1) virus in the United States. *JAMA* 2009; 301:1034–1041.
25. Dijkman R, Koekkoek SM, Molenkamp R, et al. Human bocavirus can be cultured in differentiated human airway epithelial cells. *J Virol* 2009; 83:7739–7748.
26. Drexler JF, Luna LK, Stocker A, et al. Circulation of 3 lineages of a novel Saffold cardiovirus in humans. *Emerg Infect Dis* 2008;14:1398–1405.
27. Eggers M, Bader U, Enders G. Combination of microneutralization and avidity assays: improved diagnosis of recent primary human cytomegalovirus infection in single serum sample of second trimester pregnancy. *J Med Virol* 2000;60:324–330.
28. Eisen HN, Siskind GW. Variations in affinities of antibodies during the immune response. *Biochemistry* 1964;3:389–393.
29. Feng H, Shuda M, Chang Y, et al. Clonal integration of a polyomavirus in human Merkel cell carcinoma. *Science* 2008;319:1096–1100.
30. Finkbeiner SR, Allred AF, Tarr PI, et al. Metagenomic analysis of human diarrhea: viral detection and discovery. *PLoS Pathog* 2008;4:e1000011.
31. Finkbeiner SR, Holtz LR, Jiang Y, et al. Human stool contains a previously unrecognized diversity of novel astroviruses. *Virology journal* 2009;6:161.
32. Finkbeiner SR, Li Y, Ruone S, et al. Identification of a novel astrovirus (astrovirus VA1) associated with an outbreak of acute gastroenteritis. *J Virol* 2009;83:10836–10839.
33. Fredericks DN, Relman DA. Sequence-based identification of microbial pathogens: a reconsideration of Koch's postulates. *Clin Microbiol Rev* 1996;9:18–33.
34. Froussard P. A random-PCR method (rPCR) to construct whole cDNA library from low amounts of RNA. *Nucleic Acids Res* 1992;20:2900.
35. Gallo D, George JR, Fitchen JH, et al. Evaluation of a system using oral mucosal transudate for HIV-1 antibody screening and confirmatory testing. OraSure HIV Clinical Trials Group [see comments] [published erratum appears in *JAMA* 1997 Mar 12;227(10):792]. *JAMA* 1997;277: 254–258.
36. Gardner PS, McQuillin J. *Rapid Virus Diagnosis. Application of Immunofluorescence.* 2nd ed. London: Butterworths, 1980.
37. Gaudreau A, Hill E, Balfour HH Jr, et al. Phenotypic and genotypic characterization of acyclovir-resistant herpes simplex viruses from immunocompromised patients. *J Infect Dis* 1998;178:297–303.
38. Gaynor AM, Nissen MD, Whiley DM, et al. Identification of a novel polyomavirus from patients with acute respiratory tract infections. *PLoS Pathog* 2007;3:e64.
39. Giachetti C, Linnen JM, Kolk DP, et al. Highly sensitive multiplex assay for detection of human immunodeficiency virus type 1 and hepatitis C virus RNA. *J Clin Microbiol* 2002;40:2408–2419.
40. Gibson UE, Heid CA, Williams PM. A novel method for real time quantitative RT-PCR. *Genome Res* 1996;6:995–1001.
41. Ginocchio CC, Swierkosz E, McAdam AJ, et al. Multicenter study of clinical performance of the 3M Rapid Detection RSV test. *J Clin Microbiol* 2010;48:2337–2343.
42. Gleaves CA, Smith TF, Shuster EA, et al. Rapid detection of cytomegalovirus in MRC-5 cells inoculated with urine specimens by using low-speed centrifugation and monoclonal antibody to an early antigen. *J Clin Microbiol* 1984;19:917–919.
43. Grant PM, Zolopa AR. The use of resistance testing in the management of HIV-1-infected patients. *Curr Opin HIV AIDS* 2009;4:474–480.
44. Greninger AL, Runckel C, Chiu CY, et al. The complete genome of klassevirus - a novel picornavirus in pediatric stool. *Virol J* 2009;6:82.
45. Gresham D, Curry B, Ward A, et al. Optimized detection of sequence variation in heterozygous genomes using DNA microarrays with isothermal-melting probes. *Proc Natl Acad Sci U S A* 2010;107:1482–1487.
46. Griffiths PD, Panjwani DD, Stirk PR, et al. Rapid diagnosis of cytomegalovirus infection in immunocompromised patients by detection of early antigen fluorescent foci. *Lancet* 1984;2:1242–1245.
47. Guarnieri G. Recherche sulla Pathogenesi ed Etiologia dell'infezione vaccinica e variolosa. *Arch Sci Med* 1892;16:403–423.
48. Guatelli JC, Whitfield KM, Kwoh DY, et al. Isothermal, in vitro amplification of nucleic acids by a multienzyme reaction modeled after retroviral replication [published erratum appears in *Proc Natl Acad Sci U S A* 1990 Oct;87(19):7797]. *Proc Natl Acad Sci U S A* 1990;87:1874–1878.
49. Hall JG, Eis PS, Law SM, et al. Sensitive detection of DNA polymorphisms by the serial invasive signal amplification reaction. *Proc Natl Acad Sci U S A* 2000;97:8272–8277.
50. Hauge SH, Dudman S, Borgen K, et al. Oseltamivir-resistant influenza viruses A (H1N1), Norway, 2007-08. *Emerg Infect Dis* 2009;15:155–162.
51. Hebart H, Gamer D, Loeffler J, et al. Evaluation of Murex CMV DNA hybrid capture assay for detection and quantitation of cytomegalovirus infection in patients following allogeneic stem cell transplantation. *J Clin Microbiol* 1998;36:1333–1337.
52. Heid CA, Stevens J, Livak KJ, et al. Real time quantitative PCR. *Genome Res* 1996;6:986–994.
53. Higuchi R, Dollinger G, Walsh PS, et al. Simultaneous amplification and detection of specific DNA sequences. *Biotechnology (N Y)* 1992;10: 413–417.
54. Holtz LR, Finkbeiner SR, Kirkwood CD, et al. Identification of a novel picornavirus related to cosaviruses in a child with acute diarrhea. *Virol J* 2008;5:159.
55. Holtz LR, Finkbeiner SR, Zhao G, et al. Klassevirus 1, a previously undescribed member of the family Picornaviridae, is globally widespread. *Virol J* 2009;6:86.
56. Huang YT, Yam P, Yan H, et al. Engineered BGMK cells for sensitive and rapid detection of enteroviruses. *J Clin Microbiol* 2002;40:366–371.
57. Innis MA, Myambo KB, Gelfand DH, et al. DNA sequencing with Thermus aquaticus DNA polymerase and direct sequencing of polymerase chain reaction-amplified DNA. *Proc Natl Acad Sci U S A* 1988;85: 9436–9440.
58. Jones MS, Kapoor A, Lukashov VV, et al. New DNA viruses identified in patients with acute viral infection syndrome. *J Virol* 2005;79:8230–8236.
59. Jones MS, Lukashov VV, Ganac RD, et al. Discovery of a novel human picornavirus in a stool sample from a pediatric patient presenting with fever of unknown origin. *J Clin Microbiol* 2007;45:2144–2150.
60. Kapoor A, Victoria J, Simmonds P, et al. A highly prevalent and genetically diversified Picornaviridae genus in South Asian children. *Proc Natl Acad Sci U S A* 2008;105:20482–20487.
61. Kapoor A, Li L, Victoria J, et al. Multiple novel astrovirus species in human stool. *J Gen Virol* 2009;90:2965–2972.
62. Kapoor A, Slikas E, Simmonds P, et al. A newly identified bocavirus species in human stool. *J Infect Dis* 2009;199:196–200.
63. Kapoor A, Simmonds P, Slikas E, et al. Human bocaviruses are highly diverse, dispersed, recombination prone, and prevalent in enteric infections. *J Infect Dis* 2010;201:1633–1643.
64. Kean JM, Rao S, Wang M, et al. Seroepidemiology of human polyomaviruses. *PLoS Pathog* 2009;5:e1000363.
65. Kellam P. Molecular identification of novel viruses. *Trends Microbiol* 1998;6:160–165.
66. Kistler A, Avila PC, Rouskin S, et al. Pan-viral screening of respiratory tract infections in adults with and without asthma reveals unexpected human coronavirus and human rhinovirus diversity. *J Infect Dis* 2007; 196:817–825.
67. Knox K, Carrigan D, Simmons G, et al. No evidence of murine-like gammaretroviruses in CFS patients previously identified as XMRV-infected. *Science* 2011;333:94–97.
68. Kohler G, Milstein C. Continuous cultures of fused cells secreting antibody of predefined specificity. *Nature* 1975;256:495–497.
69. Kost CB, Rogers B, Oberste MS, et al. Multicenter beta trial of the GeneXpert enterovirus assay. *J Clin Microbiol* 2007;45:1081–1086.
70. Kozal MJ, Shah N, Shen N, et al. Extensive polymorphisms observed in HIV-1 clade B protease gene using high-density oligonucleotide arrays. *Nat Med* 1996;2:753–759.
71. Kreuze JF, Perez A, Untiveros M, et al. Complete viral genome sequence and discovery of novel viruses by deep sequencing of small RNAs: a generic method for diagnosis, discovery and sequencing of viruses. *Virology* 2009;388:1–7.

72. Ksiazek TG, Erdman D, Goldsmith CS, et al. A novel coronavirus associated with severe acute respiratory syndrome. *N Engl J Med* 2003; 348:1953–1966.
73. Kwoh DY, Davis GR, Whitfield KM, et al. Transcription-based amplification system and detection of amplified human immunodeficiency virus type 1 with a bead-based sandwich hybridization format. *Proc Natl Acad Sci U S A* 1989;86:1173–1177.
74. Lamson D, Renwick N, Kapoor V, et al. MassTag polymerase-chain-reaction detection of respiratory pathogens, including a new rhinovirus genotype, that caused influenza-like illness in New York State during 2004-2005. *J Infect Dis* 2006;194:1398–1402.
75. Landry ML, Ferguson D, Wlochowski J. Detection of herpes simplex virus in clinical specimens by cytospin-enhanced direct immunofluorescence. *J Clin Microbiol* 1997;35:302–304.
76. Lee WM, Kiesner C, Pappas T, et al. A diverse group of previously unrecognized human rhinoviruses are common causes of respiratory illnesses in infants. *PLoS One* 2007;2:e966.
77. Leland DS. *Clinical Virology.* Philadelphia: W.B. Saunders Company, 1996.
78. Lennette EH, Smith TF, eds. *Laboratory Diagnosis of Viral Infections.* 3rd ed. New York: Marcel Dekker, 1999.
79. Li L, Victoria J, Kapoor A, et al. A novel picornavirus associated with gastroenteritis. *J Virol* 2009;83:12002–12006.
80. Liu C. Rapid diagnosis of human influenza. *Proc Soc Exp Biol Med* 1956;92:883–887.
81. Loh J, Zhao G, Presti RM, et al. Detection of novel sequences related to African Swine Fever virus in human serum and sewage. *J Virol* 2009; 83:13019–13025.
82. Lombardi VC, Ruscetti FW, Das Gupta J, et al. Detection of an infectious retrovirus, XMRV, in blood cells of patients with chronic fatigue syndrome. *Science* 2009;326:585–589.
83. Lorincz AT. Hybrid Capture method for detection of human papillomavirus DNA in clinical specimens: a tool for clinical management of equivocal Pap smears and for population screening. *J Obstet Gynaecol Res* 1996;22:629–636.
84. Lurain NS, Chou S. Antiviral drug resistance of human cytomegalovirus. *Clin Microbiol Rev* 2010;23:689–712.
85. Mahony J, Chong S, Merante F, et al. Development of a respiratory virus panel test for detection of twenty human respiratory viruses by use of multiplex PCR and a fluid microbead-based assay. *J Clin Microbiol* 2007;45:2965–2970.
86. Mardis ER. A decade's perspective on DNA sequencing technology. *Nature* 2011;470:198–203.
87. Margulies M, Egholm M, Altman WE, et al. Genome sequencing in microfabricated high-density picolitre reactors. *Nature* 2005;437:376–380.
88. Mazzulli T, Wood S, Chua R, et al. Evaluation of the Digene Hybrid Capture System for detection and quantitation of human cytomegalovirus viremia in human immunodeficiency virus-infected patients. *J Clin Microbiol* 1996;34:2959–2962.
89. Miller SE. Diagnosis of viral infections by electron microscopy. In: Lennette EH, Lennette DA, Lennette ET, eds. *Diagnostic Procedures for Viral, Rickettsial, and Chlamydial Infections.* 7th ed. Washington, DC: American Public Health Association, 1995:37–78.
90. Munywoki PK, Hamid F, Mutunga M, et al. Improved detection of respiratory viruses in pediatric outpatients with acute respiratory illness by real-time PCR using nasopharyngeal flocked swabs. *J Clin Microbiol* 2011;49:3365–3367.
91. Nagel MA, Cohrs RJ, Mahalingam R, et al. The varicella zoster virus vasculopathies: clinical, CSF, imaging, and virologic features. *Neurology* 2008;70:853–860.
92. Network WGIS. *Manual for the Laboratory Diagnosis and Virological Surveillance of Influenza.* Geneva, Switzerland: WHO Press, 2011.
93. Nguyen HT, Sheu TG, Mishin VP, et al. Assessment of pandemic and seasonal influenza A (H1N1) virus susceptibility to neuraminidase inhibitors in three enzyme activity inhibition assays. *Antimicrob Agents Chemother* 2010;54:3671–3677.
94. Nguyen NL, Le BM, Wang D. Serologic evidence of frequent human infection with WU and KI polyomaviruses. *Emerg Infect Dis* 2009;15: 1199–1205.
95. Nishizawa T, Okamoto H, Konishi K, et al. A novel DNA virus (TTV) associated with elevated transaminase levels in posttransfusion hepatitis of unknown etiology. *Biochem Biophys Res Commun* 1997;241:92–97.
96. Notomi T, Okayama H, Masubuchi H, et al. Loop-mediated isothermal amplification of DNA. *Nucleic Acids Res* 2000;28:E63.
97. Ou JH, Laub O, Rutter WJ. Hepatitis B virus gene function: the precore region targets the core antigen to cellular membranes and causes the secretion of the e antigen. *Proc Natl Acad Sci U S A* 1986;83:1578–1582.
98. Pabbaraju K, Tokaryk KL, Wong S, et al. Comparison of the Luminex xTAG respiratory viral panel with in-house nucleic acid amplification tests for diagnosis of respiratory virus infections. *J Clin Microbiol* 2008; 46:3056–3062.
99. Palacios G, Druce J, Du L, et al. A new arenavirus in a cluster of fatal transplant-associated diseases. *N Engl J Med* 2008;358:991–998.
100. Pandori MW, Hackett J Jr, Louie B, et al. Assessment of the ability of a fourth-generation immunoassay for human immunodeficiency virus (HIV) antibody and p24 antigen to detect both acute and recent HIV infections in a high-risk setting. *J Clin Microbiol* 2009;47:2639–2642.
101. Paprotka T, Delviks-Frankenberry KA, Cingoz O, et al. Recombinant origin of the retrovirus XMRV. *Science* 2011;333:97–101.
102. Parkin NT, Lie YS, Hellmann N, et al. Phenotypic changes in drug susceptibility associated with failure of human immunodeficiency virus type 1 (HIV-1) triple combination therapy. *J Infect Dis* 1999;180:865–870.
103. Paweska JT, Sewlall NH, Ksiazek TG, et al. Nosocomial outbreak of novel arenavirus infection, southern Africa. *Emerg Infect Dis* 2009;15: 1598–1602.
104. Persing DH, Cimino GD. Amplification product inactivation methods. In: Persing DH, Smith TF, Tenover FC, et al., eds. *Diagnostic Molecular Microbiology Principles and Applications.* Washington, DC: American Society for Microbiology, 1993:105–121.
105. Popowitch EB, Rogers E, Miller MB. Retrospective and prospective verification of the Cepheid Xpert influenza virus assay. *J Clin Microbiol* 2011;49:3368–3369.
106. Centers for Disease Control and Prevention. Evaluation of rapid influenza diagnostic tests for detection of novel influenza A (H1N1) virus—United States, 2009. *MMWR* 2009;58:826–829.
107. Pyrc K, Jebbink MF, Berkhout B, et al. Detection of new viruses by VIDISCA. Virus discovery based on cDNA-amplified fragment length polymorphism. *Methods Mol Biol* 2008;454:73–89.
108. Pyrc K, Sims AC, Dijkman R, et al. Culturing the unculturable: human coronavirus HKU1 infects, replicates, and produces progeny virions in human ciliated airway epithelial cell cultures. *J Virol* 2010;84:11255–11263.
109. Quan PL, Wagner TA, Briese T, et al. Astrovirus encephalitis in boy with X-linked agammaglobulinemia. *Emerg Infect Dis* 2010;16:918–925.
110. Rand KH, Rampersaud H, Houck HJ. Comparison of two multiplex methods for detection of respiratory viruses: FilmArray RP and xTAG RVP. *J Clin Microbiol* 2011;49:2449–2453.
111. Ray CG, Minnich LL. Efficiency of immunofluorescence for rapid detection of common respiratory viruses. *J Clin Microbiol* 1987;25:355–357.
112. Rector A, Tachezy R, Van Ranst M. A sequence-independent strategy for detection and cloning of circular DNA virus genomes by using multiply primed rolling-circle amplification. *J Virol* 2004;78:4993–4998.
113. Reiber H, Lange P. Quantitation of virus-specific antibodies in cerebrospinal fluid and serum: sensitive and specific detection of antibody synthesis in the brain. *Clin Chem* 1991;37:1153–1160.
114. Roberts TC, Buller RS, Gaudreault-Keener M, et al. Effects of storage temperature and time on qualitative and quantitative detection of cytomegalovirus in blood specimens by shell vial culture and PCR. *J Clin Microbiol* 1997;35:2224–2228.
115. Rotbart HA. Enzymatic RNA amplification of the enteroviruses. *J Clin Microbiol* 1990;28:438–442.
116. Rousseau S, Hedman K. Rubella infection and reinfection distinguished by avidity of IgG. *Lancet* 1988;1:1108–1109.
117. Safrin S, Elbeik T, Phan L, et al. Correlation between response to acyclovir and foscarnet therapy and in vitro susceptibility result for isolates of herpes simplex virus from human immunodeficiency virus-infected patients. *Antimicrob Agents Chemother* 1994;38:1246–1250.
118. Saiki RK, Scharf S, Faloona F, et al. Enzymatic amplification of beta-globin genomic sequences and restriction site analysis of sickle cell anemia. *Science* 1985;230:1350–1354.
119. Schlaberg R, Choe DJ, Brown KR, et al. XMRV is present in malignant prostatic epithelium and is associated with prostate cancer, especially high-grade tumors. *Proc Natl Acad Sci U S A* 2009;106:16351–16356.

120. Schowalter RM, Pastrana DV, Pumphrey KA, et al. Merkel cell polyomavirus and two previously unknown polyomaviruses are chronically shed from human skin. *Cell Host Microbe* 2010;7:509–515.
121. Scuda N, Hofmann J, Calvignac-Spencer S, et al. A novel human polyomavirus closely related to the African green monkey-derived lymphotropic polyomavirus (LPV). *J Virol* 2011;85:4586–4590.
122. Simen BB, Simons JF, Hullsiek KH, et al. Low-abundance drug-resistant viral variants in chronically HIV-infected, antiretroviral treatment-naive patients significantly impact treatment outcomes. *J Infect Dis* 2009; 199:693–701.
123. Simmons G, Glynn SA, Komaroff AL, et al. Failure to confirm XMRV/MLVs in the blood of patients with chronic fatigue syndrome: a multi-laboratory study. *Science* 2011;334:814–817.
124. Smits SL, van Leeuwen M, van der Eijk AA, et al. Human astrovirus infection in a patient with new onset coeliac disease. *J Clin Microbiol* 2010;48:3416–3418.
125. Specter S, Hodinka RL, Young SA, et al. *Clinical Virology Manual.* 4th ed. Washington, DC: ASM Press, 2009.
126. Stabell EC, Olivo EC. Isolation of a cell line for rapid and sensitive histochemical assay for the detection of herpes simplex virus. *J Virol Methods* 1992;38:195–204.
127. Stabell EC, O'Rourke SR, Storch GA, et al. Evaluation of a genetically engineered cell line and a histochemical beta-galactosidase assay to detect herpes simplex virus in clinical specimens. *J Clin Microbiol* 1993; 31:2796–2798.
128. Stranska R, Schuurman R, Scholl DR, et al. ELVIRA HSV, a yield reduction assay for rapid herpes simplex virus susceptibility testing. *Antimicrob Agents Chemother* 2004;48:2331–2333.
129. Suligoi B, Galli C, Massi M, et al. Precision and accuracy of a procedure for detecting recent human immunodeficiency virus infections by calculating the antibody avidity index by an automated immunoassay-based method. *J Clin Microbiol* 2002;40:4015–4020.
130. Svraka S, Rosario K, Duizer E, et al. Metagenomic sequencing for virus identification in a public-health setting. *J Gen Virol* 2010;91:2846–2856.
131. Switzer WM, Jia H, Hohn O, et al. Absence of evidence of xenotropic murine leukemia virus-related virus infection in persons with chronic fatigue syndrome and healthy controls in the United States. *Retrovirology* 2010;7:57.
132. Tan le V, Van Doorn HR, Van der Hoek L, et al. Random PCR and ultracentrifugation increases sensitivity and throughput of VIDISCA for screening of pathogens in clinical specimens. *J Infect Dev Ctries* 2011; 5:142–148.
133. Tebas P, Stabell EC, Olivo PD. Antiviral susceptibility testing with a cell line which expresses beta-galactosidase after infection with herpes simplex virus. *Antimicrob Agents Chemother* 1995;39:1287–1291.
134. Tebas P, Scholl D, Jollick J, et al. A rapid assay to screen for drug-resistant herpes simplex virus. *J Infect Dis* 1998;177:217–220.
135. The TE, van der Ploeg M, van den Berg AP, et al. Direct detection of cytomegalovirus in peripheral blood leukocytes–a review of the antigenemia assay and polymerase chain reaction. *Transplantation* 1992;54: 193–198.
136. Tsutakawa SE, Classen S, Chapados BR, et al. Human flap endonuclease structures, DNA double-base flipping, and a unified understanding of the FEN1 superfamily. *Cell* 2011;145:198–211.
137. Urisman A, Molinaro RJ, Fischer N, et al. Identification of a novel Gammaretrovirus in prostate tumors of patients homozygous for R462Q RNASEL variant. *PLoS Pathog* 2006;2:e25.
138. Urnovitz HB, Sturge JC, Gottfried TD. Increased sensitivity of HIV-1 antibody detection. *Nat Med* 1997;3:1258.
139. van den Hoogen BG, de Jong JC, Groen J, et al. A newly discovered human pneumovirus isolated from young children with respiratory tract disease. *Nat Med* 2001;7:719–724.
140. van der Hoek L, Pyrc K, Jebbink MF, et al. Identification of a new human coronavirus. *Nat Med* 2004;10:368–373.
141. van der Hoek L, Sure K, Ihorst G, et al. Croup is associated with the novel coronavirus NL63. *PLoS Med* 2005;2:e240.
142. van der Meijden E, Janssens RW, Lauber C, et al. Discovery of a new human polyomavirus associated with trichodysplasia spinulosa in an immunocompromized patient. *PLoS Pathog* 2010;6:e1001024.
143. van Leeuwen M, Williams MM, Koraka P, et al. Human picobirnaviruses identified by molecular screening of diarrhea samples. *J Clin Microbiol* 2010;48:1787–1794.
144. Versalovic J, ed. *Manual of Clinical Microbiology.* 10th ed. Washington, DC: ASM Press, 2011.
145. Wang D, Coscoy L, Zylberberg M, et al. Microarray-based detection and genotyping of viral pathogens. *Proc Natl Acad Sci U S A* 2002;99:15687–15692.
146. Wang D, Urisman A, Liu YT, et al. Viral discovery and sequence recovery using DNA microarrays. *PLoS Biol* 2003;1:E2.
147. Ward KN, Turner DJ, Parada XC, et al. Use of immunoglobulin G antibody avidity for differentiation of primary human herpesvirus 6 and 7 infections. *J Clin Microbiol* 2001;39:959–963.
148. Weber G, Shendure J, Tanenbaum DM, et al. Identification of foreign gene sequences by transcript filtering against the human genome. *Nat Genet* 2002;30:141–142.
149. Weller RH, Enders JF. Production of hemagglutinin by mumps and influenza A viruses in suspended cell tissue cultures. *Proc Soc Exp Biol Med* 1948;69:124–128.
150. Whitcomb JM, Huang W, Fransen S, et al. Development and characterization of a novel single-cycle recombinant-virus assay to determine human immunodeficiency virus type 1 coreceptor tropism. *Antimicrob Agents Chemother* 2007;51:566–575.
151. Wong S, Pabbaraju K, Wong A, et al. Development of a real-time RT-PCR assay for detection of resistance to oseltamivir in influenza A pandemic (H1N1) 2009 virus using single nucleotide polymorphism probes. *J Virol Methods* 2011;173:259–265.
152. Woo PC, Lau SK, Chu CM, et al. Characterization and complete genome sequence of a novel coronavirus, coronavirus HKU1, from patients with pneumonia. *J Virol* 2005;79:884–895.
153. Wu Q, Luo Y, Lu R, et al. Virus discovery by deep sequencing and assembly of virus-derived small silencing RNAs. *Proc Natl Acad Sci U S A* 2010; 107:1606–1611.
154. Yang J, Yang F, Ren L, et al. Unbiased parallel detection of viral pathogens in clinical samples by use of a metagenomic approach. *J Clin Microbiol* 2011;49:3463–3469.
155. Zoll J, Erkens Hulshof S, Lanke K, et al. Saffold virus, a human Theiler's-like cardiovirus, is ubiquitous and causes infection early in life. *PLoS Pathog* 2009;5:e1000416.

Specific Virus Families

SECTION II

CHAPTER 16

Vincent R. Racaniello

Picornaviridae: The Viruses and Their Replication

Viruses in the family *Picornaviridae* have nonenveloped particles with a single-stranded RNA (ssRNA) genome of positive polarity. Among its many members are numerous important human and animal pathogens, such as poliovirus, hepatitis A virus, foot-and-mouth disease virus (FMDV), enterovirus 71, and rhinovirus. The name of the virus family was intended to convey the small size of the viruses (pico, a small unit of measurement [10^{-12}]) and the type of nucleic acid that constitutes the viral genome (RNA).

Picornaviruses have played important roles in the development of modern virology. Foot-and-mouth disease virus was the first animal virus to be discovered, by Loeffler and Frosch in 1898.[305] Poliovirus was isolated 10 years later,[289] a discovery spurred by the emergence of epidemic poliomyelitis at the turn of the 20th century. The discovery in 1949 that poliovirus could be propagated in cultured cells led to studies of viral replication.[135] The plaque assay, an essential method for quantification of viral infectivity, was developed with poliovirus.[130] The first RNA-dependent RNA polymerase identified was that of mengovirus,[29] a picornavirus, and the synthesis of a precursor polyprotein from which viral proteins are derived by proteolytic processing was first identified in poliovirus-infected cells.[477] The first infectious DNA clone of an animal RNA virus was that of poliovirus,[416] and the first three-dimensional structures of animal viruses determined by x-ray crystallography were those of poliovirus[223] and rhinovirus.[435] Poliovirus RNA was the first messenger RNA (mRNA) shown to lack a 5′ cap structure.[215,361] This observation was subsequently explained by the finding that the genome RNA of poliovirus and other picornaviruses is translated by internal ribosome binding,[243,385] a process now known to occur on cellular mRNA.[248,313]

Because they cause serious diseases, poliovirus and FMDV have been the best-studied picornaviruses. Research on poliovirus has produced two effective vaccines; it is likely that poliomyelitis will be eradicated from the globe in the near future. The World Health Organization (WHO) has established a goal of cessation of vaccination, at which time all poliovirus stocks must be destroyed. When this historic event takes place, all research on this virus will cease. Poliovirus is truly a virus with a brilliant past, but with no future.

TABLE 16.1 Members of the Family *Picornaviridae*

Genus	Species
Aphthovirus	*Foot-and-mouth disease virus*
	Equine rhinitis A virus
	Equine rhinitis B virus
Avihepatovirus	*Duck hepatitis A virus*
Cardiovirus	*Encephalomycarditis virus*
	Theilovirus
Enterovirus	*Bovine enterovirus*
	Human enterovirus A (Coxsackievirus, enterovirus)
	Human enterovirus B (Coxsackievirus, echovirus, enterovirus)
	Human enterovirus C (poliovirus, Coxsackievirus, enterovirus)
	Human enterovirus D (enterovirus)
	Porcine enterovirus B
	Simian enterovirus A
	Human rhinovirus A
	Human rhinovirus B
	Human rhinovirus C
Erbovirus	*Equine rhinitis B virus*
Hepatovirus	*Hepatitis A virus*
Kobuvirus	*Aichi virus*
	Bovine kobuvirus
Parechovirus	*Human parechovirus*
	Ljungan virus
Sapelovirus	*Porcine sapelovirus*
	Simian sapelovirus
	Avian sapelovirus
Senecavirus	*Seneca Valley virus*
Tremovirus	*Avian encephalomyelitis virus*
Teschovirus	*Porcine teschovirus*

CLASSIFICATION

The family *Picornaviridae* belongs to the order *Picornavirales* and comprises 12 genera (Table 16.1), which all contain viruses that infect vertebrates.[280] Information on selected viruses is summarized below.

The genus *Aphthovirus* consists of four species: *Foot-and-mouth disease virus* (FMDV), *Bovine rhinitis A* virus, *Bovine rhinitis B virus,* and *Equine rhinitis A virus.* FMDV infects cloven-footed animals (e.g., cattle, goats, pigs, and sheep), primarily via the upper respiratory tract, and has been isolated from at least 70 species of mammals. Seven serotypes of FMDV have been identified; within each serotype are many subtypes. These viruses are highly labile and rapidly lose infectivity at pH values of less than 6.8.

There are two species within the genus *Cardiovirus: Encephalomyocarditis virus* and *Theilovirus.* The encephalomyocarditis viruses (which include strains known as encephalomyocarditis virus, Columbia SK virus, Maus Elberfeld virus, and Mengovirus) are murine viruses, which can also infect many other hosts, including humans, monkeys, pigs, elephants, and squirrels. The second species includes the Theiler's murine encephalomyelitis viruses and human Saffold viruses.

There are 10 species in the *Enterovirus* genus: *Human enterovirus A, B, C, D; Simian enterovirus A, Bovine enterovirus, Porcine enterovirus B,* and *Human rhinovirus A, B, C.* Members of this genus include poliovirus (3 serotypes), Coxsackievirus (25 serotypes), echovirus (28 serotypes), human enterovirus (43 serotypes), and many nonhuman enteric viruses. Enteroviruses such as poliovirus (3 serotypes) and Coxsackievirus (25 serotypes) replicate in the alimentary tract and are resistant to low pH. The acid-labile rhinoviruses (so named because they replicate in the nasopharynx) are important agents of the common cold. There are 100 serotypes of *Human rhinovirus A and B.* Rhinoviruses may also replicate in the lower respiratory tract; the newly discovered *Human rhinovirus C* (49 types) have been associated with severe lower respiratory tract disease.[327]

The genus *Hepatovirus* contains a single species, the human pathogen *Hepatitis A virus* (one serotype). Virions are highly stable and resistant to acid pH and high temperatures (60°C for 10 min). The virus infects epithelial cells of the small intestine and hepatocytes.

The *Parechovirus* genus contains two species, *Human parechovirus* and *Ljungan virus,* a virus of rodents. Parechoviruses are etiologic agents of respiratory and gastrointestinal disease.

Proteins of parechoviruses are substantially diverged from those of other picornaviruses, with no greater than 30% amino acid identity.

The *Erbovirus* genus contains three types of *Equine rhinitis B virus.* These viruses cause upper respiratory tract disease in horses that is associated with viremia and fecal shedding of virus particles. The *Kobuvirus* genus contains two species: *Aichi virus,* which causes gastroenteritis in humans, and *Bovine kobuvirus.* The *Teschovirus* genus consists of 12 serotypes of *Porcine teschovirus.* Some strains can cause polioencephalitis in pigs, also called Teschen/Talfan disease or teschovirus encephalomyelitis. There are three species in the *Sapelovirus* genus: *Porcine sapelovirus, Simian sapelovirus,* and *Avian sapelovirus.* The sole species in the genus *Senecavirus* is *Seneca Valley virus,* found in pigs throughout the United States, but there is no known associated disease. It is currently in clinical trials to assess its value for treating human tumors.[440] *Avian encephalomyelitis virus,* which causes the eponymous disease in young chickens, pheasants, quail, and turkeys, is the sole species in the genus *Tremovirus.*

A number of other related viruses may be members of the *Picornaviridae* but have not been approved as species by the International Committee on Taxonomy of Viruses (ICTV). These include human cosaviruses, identified in the stools of south Asian children,[224,262] human klassevirus/salivirus,[183,225,297] and many others.[280]

VIRION STRUCTURE

Physical Properties

Picornavirus virions are spherical, with a diameter of about 30 nm (Fig. 16.1). The particles are simple, consisting of a protein shell surrounding the naked RNA genome. The virus particles lack a lipid envelope, and their infectivity is insensitive to organic solvents. Cardioviruses, enteroviruses (except rhinoviruses), hepatoviruses, and parechoviruses are acid stable and retain infectivity at pH values of 3.0 and lower. In contrast, rhinoviruses and aphthoviruses are labile at pH values of less than 6.0. Differences in pH stability influence the sites of replication of the virus. For example, rhinoviruses and aphthoviruses replicate in the respiratory tract and need not be acid stable. Because they are acid labile, they cannot replicate in the alimentary tract. Cardioviruses, enteroviruses, hepatoviruses, and parechoviruses pass through the stomach to gain access to the intestine and, therefore, must be resistant to low pH. The structural basis for the acid lability of FMDV is partly understood (see *Entry into Cells*).

The buoyant densities of picornaviruses are quite different (Table 16.2). Cardioviruses and enteroviruses have a buoyant density of 1.34 g/mL, that of FMDV is 1.45 g/mL, and rhinoviruses have an intermediate value (1.40 g/mL). The reason for the difference lies in the permeability of the viral capsid to cesium. The capsid of poliovirus does not allow cesium to reach the RNA interior; thus, the virus bands at an abnormally light buoyant density.[146] In contrast, aphthovirus capsids contain pores that allow cesium to enter.[1] The rhinovirus capsid is permeable to cesium, but the presence of polyamines in the capsid interior limits the amount of cesium that can enter, which provides an explanation for the intermediate buoyant density value of these viruses.[146]

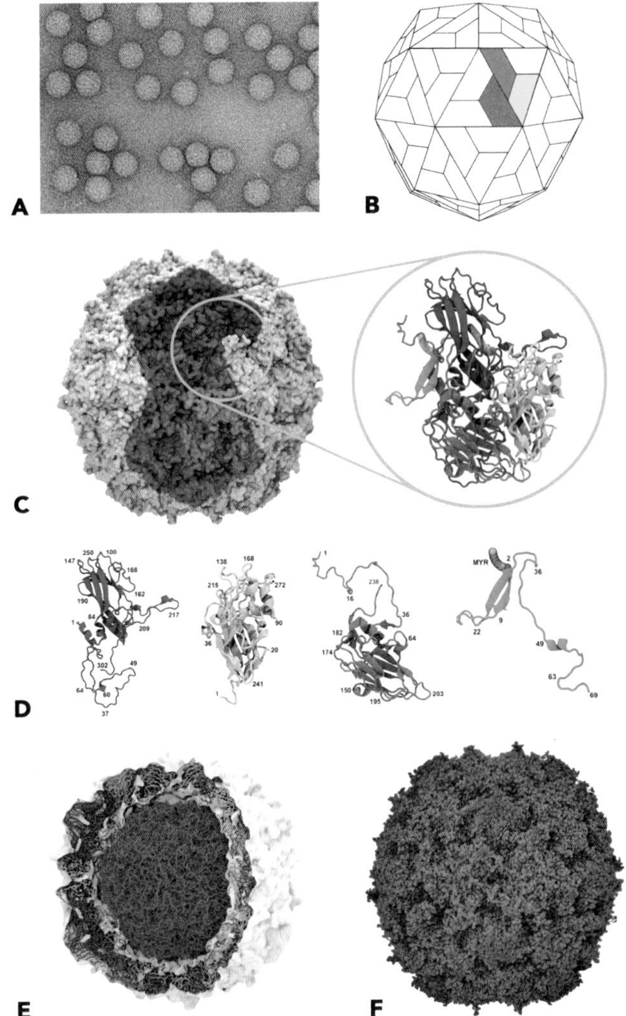

FIGURE 16.1. Structural features of picornaviruses. A: Electron micrograph of negatively stained poliovirus (×270,000 magnification). **B:** Schematic of the picornavirus capsid, showing the pseudoequivalent packing arrangement of VP1 (*blue*), VP2 (*yellow*), and VP3 (*red*). VP4 (*green*) is on the interior of the capsid. A single biologic protomer is colored. **C:** Model of poliovirus type 1, Mahoney, based on x-ray crystallographic structure determined at 2.9 Å. Two adjacent pentamers aligned at the twofold axis of symmetry are shaded dark gray. A single protomer is colored and also expanded at right as a cartoon of the alpha carbon backbone; capsid proteins are color coded according to **B**. **D:** Individual capsid proteins VP1, VP2, VP3, and VP4 are shown as cartoon representations of the alpha carbon backbone. **E:** Virion after 10 nanoseconds of atomistic molecular dynamics simulation. Volumetric (density) map representation is white with protein backbone shown as tubes and colored as in **B**. Lipids are represented as Van der Waals models with coloring by element. RNA is colored purple and associated magnesium ions are colored blue. **F:** All-atom Van der Waals representation of the poliovirus capsid with radial coloring depicting the relative distance from the center of the particle; blue = 133 Å to red = 166 Å. (**A** courtesy of N. Cheng and D. M. Belnap; **C** to **F** courtesy of Jason A. Roberts, WHO Poliomyelitis Regional Reference Laboratory, Victorian Infectious Diseases Reference Laboroatory, North Melbourne, Australia.)

TABLE 16.2 Physical Properties of Some Picornaviruses

Genus	pH stability	Virion buoyant density	Sedimentation coefficient
Aphthovirus	Labile, <6.8	1.43–1.45	142–146S
Cardiovirus	Stable, 3–9	1.33–1.34	160S
Enterovirus			
Enteroviruses	Stable, 3–9	1.34	160S
Rhinoviruses	Labile, <6	1.40	160S
Hepatovirus	Stable	1.32–1.34	160S
Parechovirus	Stable	1.36	160S

Ratio of Particles to Infectious Viruses

The ratio of particles to infectious virus is determined by dividing the number of virus particles in a sample (determined by electron microscopy [EM] or spectrophotometric measurements) by the plaque titer, yielding the particle-to-plaque forming unit (pfu) ratio. This ratio is a measurement of the fraction of virus particles that can complete an infectious cycle. The particle-to-pfu ratio of poliovirus ranges from 30 to 1,000, and that of other picornaviruses is in the same range. The high particle-to-pfu ratio may be caused by the presence of lethal mutations in the viral genome. This explanation, however, probably does not apply to all picornaviruses; it has been shown that the infectivity of aphthovirus RNA approaches one infectious unit per molecule. An alternative explanation is that all viruses do not successfully complete an infectious cycle because they fail at one of several steps that must be completed, including attachment, entry, replication, and assembly.

High-Resolution Structure of the Virion

The capsids of picornaviruses are composed of four structural proteins: VP1, VP2, VP3, and VP4. The results of x-ray diffraction studies, EM observations, and biochemical studies of virus particles and their dissociation products led to the hypothesis that the picornavirus capsid contains 60 structural proteins arranged into an icosahedral lattice.[441] Our understanding of the structure of picornaviruses was substantially advanced in 1985 when the atomic structures of poliovirus type 1[223] and human rhinovirus type 14[435] were determined by x-ray crystallography. Since then, the high-resolution structures of many other picornaviruses have been determined.

The basic building block of the picornavirus capsid is the protomer, which contains one copy each of VP1, VP2, VP3, and VP4. The shell is formed by VP1 to VP3, and VP4 lies on its inner surface (Fig. 16.1). VP1, VP2, and VP3 have no sequence homology, yet all three proteins have the same topology: they form an eight-stranded, antiparallel β-barrel (also called a β-barrel jelly roll or a Swiss-roll β-barrel). This domain is a wedge-shaped structure made up of two antiparallel β-sheets. One β-sheet forms the wall of the wedge, and the second, which has a bend in the center, forms both a wall and the floor. The wedge shape facilitates the packing of structural units to form a dense, rigid protein shell. Packing of the β-barrel domains is strengthened by a network of protein–protein contacts on the interior of the capsid, particularly around the fivefold axes. This network, which is formed by the N-terminal extensions of VP1 to VP3 as well as VP4, is essential for the stability of the virion.

VP4 differs significantly from the other three proteins in that it has an extended conformation. This protein is similar in position and conformation to the NH2-terminal sequences of VP1 and VP3 and functions as a detached NH2-terminal extension of VP2 rather than an independent capsid protein.

The main structural differences among VP1, VP2, and VP3 lie in the loops that connect the β-strands and the N- and C-terminal sequences that extend from the β-barrel domain. These amino acid sequences give each picornavirus its distinct morphology and antigenicity. The C-termini are located on the surface of the virion, and the N-termini are on the interior, indicating that significant rearrangement of the P1 precursor occurs on proteolytic cleavage.

Resolution of the structures of poliovirus and rhinovirus revealed that the β-barrel domains are strikingly similar in structure to those of plant viruses such as southern bean mosaic virus and tomato bushy stunt virus. The capsid proteins of these viruses bear no sequence homology with those of the picornaviruses. It has since become apparent that similar protein topology is found in the capsid proteins of many plant, insect, and vertebrate positive-stranded RNA viruses as well as in the DNA-containing papovaviruses and adenoviruses. These findings suggest that either the polypeptides evolved from a common ancestor or that the β-barrel domain is one of the few ways to allow proteins to pack to form a sphere.

In some viruses, such as the parechoviruses, VP0, the precursor to VP2 + VP4, remains uncleaved, while in hepatitis A virus, VP4 is very small.

Surface of the Virion

Resolution of the structures of poliovirus and human rhinovirus revealed that the surfaces of these viruses have a corrugated topography; a prominent, star-shaped plateau (mesa) is found at the fivefold axis of symmetry, surrounded by a deep depression (canyon) and another protrusion at the threefold axis (Fig. 16.1). It was originally proposed that the canyon is the receptor-binding site—this hypothesis has been proved for a number of enteroviruses. Not all picornaviruses have canyons. The surface of cardioviruses bears a series of depressions, or "pits," which are involved in receptor binding, while that of FMDV is much smoother. As will be discussed later, a flexible loop that projects from the capsid surface binds to the cellular receptor for FMDV.

Interior of the Virion

A network formed by the N-termini on the interior of the capsid contributes significantly to the stability of the virion.

At the fivefold axis of symmetry, the N-termini of five VP3 molecules form a cylindrically parallel β-sheet. This structure is surrounded by five three-stranded β-sheets formed by the N-termini of VP4 and VP1. The myristate group attached to the N-terminus of VP4 mediates the interaction between these two structures.[93] Interactions among pentamers are stabilized by a seven-stranded β-sheet, composed of four β-strands of the VP3 β-barrel and one strand from the N-terminus of VP1 that surround a two-stranded β-sheet made from the N-terminus of VP2 from a neighboring pentamer.[138]

Poliovirus genomes containing an extra 1,500 nucleotides can be successfully packaged, indicating that the interior of the capsid is not fully occupied.[9] It has been suggested that picornaviral capsids are stabilized by interactions with the RNA genome, based on findings with bean pod mottle virus, which is related to picornaviruses. In this virus, ordered RNA can be observed at the threefold axis, and packaging of viral RNA stabilizes subunit interactions.[91,299] Several nucleotides have been tentatively identified in a similar location in the structures of P3/Sabin and rhinovirus type 14.[25,138] In the atomic structure of poliovirus P2/Lansing, RNA bases have been observed stacking with conserved aromatic residues of VP4.[294] The structure of *Seneca Valley virus* revealed the arrangement of the RNA within the capsid.[511] Much of the nucleic acid contacts the inner surface of the capsid, particularly near the twofold axes under VP2. The RNA forms a shell that contacts both VP2 and VP4 and which could serve as a scaffold for capsid assembly or might contribute to virion stability.

Hydrophobic Pocket

Within the core of VP1, just beneath the canyon floor of many picornaviruses, is a hydrophobic tunnel or pocket (Fig. 16.2). Electron density observed in this area has been interpreted to be cell-derived lipids called "pocket factors." In poliovirus types 1 and 3, the pocket is believed to contain sphingosine.[138] An unidentified lipid has been found in human rhinoviruses types 1A and 16, a C16 fatty acid has been modeled in the pocket of coxsackievirus B3,[194,271,348] coxsackievirus A21 is believed to carry myristic acid,[535] and bovine enterovirus contains a mixture of palmitic and myristic acid.[464] In the enterovirus 71 virion, the pocket factor is partly exposed on the floor of the canyon.[403] In contrast, the pocket of human rhinovirus type 14 is empty.[25] The results of introducing amino acid changes in the pocket of rhinovirus 16 suggest that the hydrophobic pocket, and not the pocket factor, is important for maintaining capsid dynamics.[265]

The hydrophobic pocket is also the binding site for anti-picornavirus drugs such as the WIN compounds produced by Sterling-Winthrop[462] as well as similar molecules produced by Janssen Pharmaceuticals (Titusville, NJ)[19,104] (Fig. 16.2). Some of these drugs have been evaluated in clinical trials, such as pleconaril for treatment of common colds caused by rhinoviruses[392] and for enteroviral sepsis syndrome.[356] These hydrophobic, sausage-shaped compounds bind tightly in the hydrophobic tunnel, displacing any lipid that is present, inhibiting either binding or uncoating. Drug-dependent mutants of poliovirus spontaneously lose infectivity at 37°C, probably because they do not contain lipid in the pocket.[347]

Myristate

Myristic acid (*n*-tetradecanoic acid) is covalently linked to glycine at the amino terminus of VP4 of most picornaviruses.[93] This fatty acid is an integral part of the viral capsid. The N-termini of VP3 intertwine around the fivefold axis to form a twisted tube of parallel β-structure.[223] The five myristyl groups extend from the N-termini of VP4 and cradle the twisted tube formed by VP3.[93] The myristyl groups interact with amino acid side chains of VP4 and VP3. Mutagenesis of VP4 has revealed a role for myristic acid modification in virus assembly and in the stability of the capsid.[20,314–316,344]

Neutralizing Antigenic Sites

Viral serotype is determined by the connecting loops and C-termini of the capsid proteins that decorate the outer surface of the virion. These contain the major neutralization antigenic sites of the virus, the amino acid sequences that are recognized by antibodies that block viral infectivity. Such sites are defined by mutations that confer resistance to neutralization with monoclonal antibodies directed against the viral capsid.[334,335,458] Human sera contain antibodies directed against poliovirus antigenic sites identified in mice.[423]

The large area of contact of the poliovirus receptor (PVR) CD155 on the virion surface, compared with other picornavirus–receptor interactions, might provide a clue to why there are many rhinovirus serotypes but only three serotypes of poliovirus.[209] This large interaction area could limit the viability of antibody-escape mutants because they would also compromise their ability to bind CD155.

The capsids of rhinovirus, poliovirus, and other picornaviruses are dynamic, leading to transient display of the buried N-termini of VP1.[246,266,298,411,432,446] Antibodies to this sequence of VP1 neutralize viral infectivity.

GENOME STRUCTURE AND ORGANIZATION

General Features

The genome of picornaviruses is a single positive-stranded RNA molecule (Fig. 16.3). The viral RNA is infectious because it is translated on entry into the cell to produce all the viral proteins required for viral replication. Picornavirus genomic RNA is unique because it is covalently linked at the 5′ end to a protein called VPg (virion protein, genome linked).[142,293] VPg is covalently joined to the 5′-uridylylate moiety of the viral RNA by an O4-(5′-uridylyl)-tyrosine linkage. The tyrosine that is linked to the viral RNA is always the third amino acid from the N-terminus. VPg of different picornaviruses varies in length from 22 to 24 amino acid residues and is encoded by a single viral gene, except in the genome of FMDV, which encodes three VPg genes.[145] VPg is not required for infectivity of poliovirus RNA; if it is removed from viral RNA by treatment with proteinase, the specific infectivity of the viral RNA is not reduced. VPg is not found on viral mRNA that is associated with cellular ribosomes and undergoing translation; these mRNA contain only uridine 5′-phosphate (pU) at their 5′ ends. Poliovirus mRNA differs from virion RNA only by the lack of VPg.[363,389] VPg is removed from virion RNA by a host protein called *unlinking enzyme*.[12] It is not known whether removal of VPg is a prerequisite for association with ribosomes or is a result of that association. Although VPg-linked RNA can be translated in cell-free extracts, it is possible that VPg is rapidly cleaved from the RNA such that only RNA lacking VPg are translated.[169,338,514] VPg is present on nascent RNA

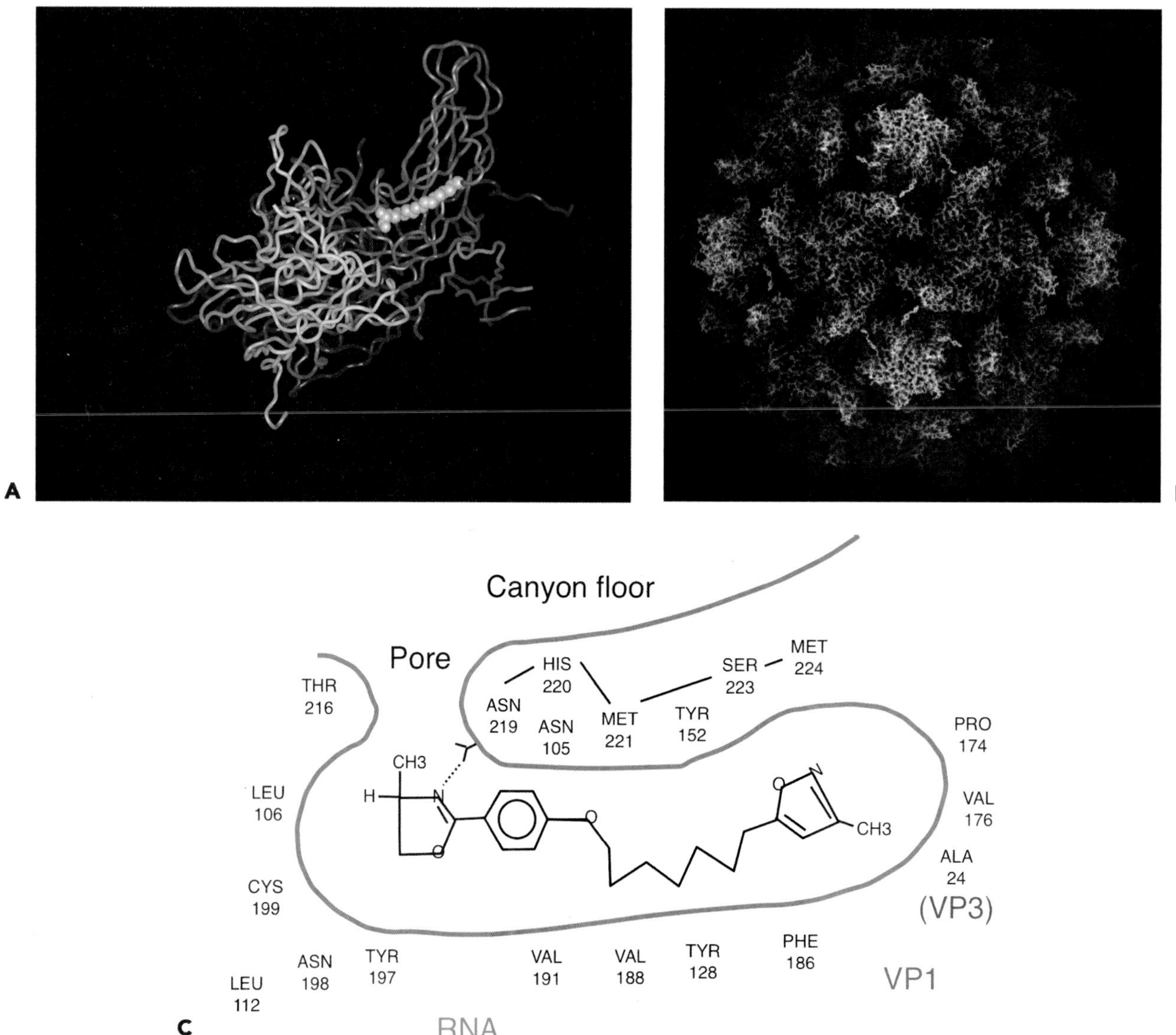

FIGURE 16.2. The hydrophobic pocket in the picornavirus capsid. A: Cellular lipid bound in the hydrophobic pocket of poliovirus type 1. Side view of a protomer, consisting of one copy each of VP1, VP2, VP3, and VP4. RNA is below, and the fivefold axis of symmetry is at the upper right. *Gray spheres* represent what is believed to be a molecule of sphingosine bound in the hydrophobic pocket. The lipid is just below the canyon floor. **B:** Drug bound in the poliovirus pocket. R78206, a WIN-like compound, bound in the poliovirus capsid. The bound drug is the small yellow molecule at the base of the canyon. The drug appears to be exposed on the surface but is actually in the hydrophobic pocket. The capsid model is shown in a radial depth-cued representation, in which atoms are colored according to whether they are near the center of the virus (*blue*) or far from the center (*white*). Residues at the bottom of the canyon are dark because they are at a position of low radius. The bound drug is not depth cued. **C:** WIN52084 bound in the hydrophobic pocket. These drugs displace the lipid from the pocket, thereby blocking infectivity.

chains of the replicative intermediate RNA and on negative-stranded RNA, which has led to the suggestion that VPg is a primer for poliovirus RNA synthesis.[362,389] The role of VPg in viral RNA synthesis is discussed in subsequent sections.

Nucleotide sequence analysis of many picornavirus RNAs has revealed a common organizational pattern (Fig. 16.3). The genomes vary in length from 7 to 8.8 kb. The 5′-noncoding regions of picornaviruses are long (0.5 to 1.5 kb) and highly structured. This region of the genome contains sequences that control genome replication and translation. The 5′-noncoding region contains the internal ribosome entry site (IRES) that directs translation of the mRNA by internal ribosome binding. The 5′-untranslated regions of aphthoviruses, cardioviruses, and erboviruses contain a poly(C) tract that varies in length among different virus strains (80 to 250 nucleotides in cardioviruses, 40 to 400 nucleotides in aphthoviruses). Among cardioviruses, longer poly(C) length is associated with higher virulence in animals.[129,198]

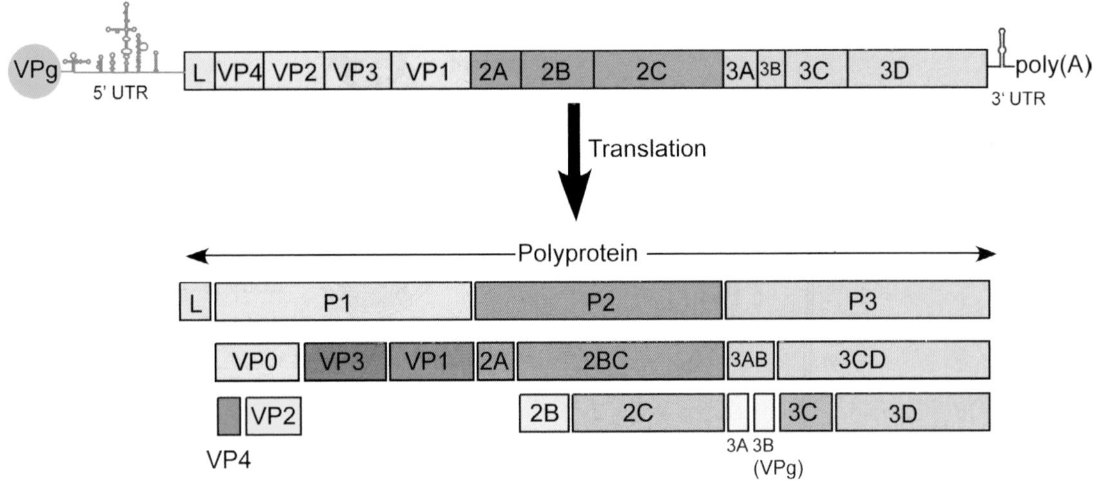

FIGURE 16.3. Organization of a picornavirus genome. Top: Schematic of the viral RNA genome, with the genome-linked protein VPg at the 5′ end, the 5′ untranslated region containing the IRES, the protein coding region, the 3′ untranslated region containing a pseudoknot, and the poly(A) tail. L is a leader protein encoded in the genomes of erboviruses, cardioviruses, and aphthoviruses but not other picornaviruses. Coding regions for the viral proteins are indicated. **Bottom:** Processing pattern of picornavirus polyprotein. Some genomes encode multiple copies of protein coding regions, e.g., there are three VPgs in the FMDV genome, two 2A motifs in Ljungan virus, and three 2A motifs in the duck hepatitis A virus genome.

The 3′-noncoding region of picornaviruses is short, ranging in length from 40 to 330 nucleotides. This region may also contain a secondary structure, a pseudoknot, that has been implicated in controlling viral RNA synthesis.[241] The entire 3′-noncoding region of poliovirus and rhinovirus is not required for infectivity, however.[77,489] Both virion RNA and mRNA contain a 3′ stretch of poly(A).[541] Negative-stranded RNA contains a 5′ stretch of poly(U), which is copied to form poly(A) of the positive strand.[542] The average length of the poly(A) tail varies from 35 nucleotides in encephalomyocarditis virus to 100 nucleotides in aphthoviruses.[5] Viral RNA from which the poly(A) tract is removed is noninfectious.[469]

The results of biochemical studies of poliovirus-infected cells had predicted the presence of a single, long, open reading frame (ORF) on the viral RNA that is processed to form individual viral proteins.[477] This hypothesis was proved when the nucleotide sequence of the poliovirus genome was determined, which revealed that the viral RNA encodes a single ORF.[276,415] A similar strategy for viral gene expression occurs during the replication of all picornaviruses. The polyprotein is cleaved during translation, so that the full-length product is not observed. Cleavage is carried out by virus-encoded proteinases to yield 11 to 15 final cleavage products. Some of the uncleaved precursors also have functions during replication.

To unify the nomenclature of picornavirus proteins, the polyprotein has been divided into three regions: P1, P2, and P3 (Fig. 16.3). The genomes of some picornaviruses encode a leader (L) protein before the P1 region. The P1 region encodes the viral capsid proteins, whereas the P2 and P3 regions encode proteins involved in protein processing ($2A^{pro}$, $3C^{pro}$, $3CD^{pro}$) and genome replication (2B, 2C, 3AB, $3B^{VPg}$, $3CD^{pro}$, $3D^{pol}$). The genome of FMDV encodes three VPg proteins. The genome of Ljungan virus, a parechovirus, may encode two unrelated 2A proteins[249] and that of duck hepatitis A virus in the genus *Avihepatovirus* encodes three 2A motifs.

INFECTIOUS DNA CLONES OF PICORNAVIRUS GENOMES

Recombinant DNA techniques allow the introduction of mutations anywhere in the genome of most animal viruses. An infectious DNA clone—a double-stranded copy of the viral genome carried on a bacterial plasmid—or RNA transcripts derived by *in vitro* transcription, can be introduced into cultured cells by transfection to recover infectious virus. The first infectious DNA clone of an animal RNA virus was that of poliovirus.[416] The infectivity of cloned poliovirus DNA (10^3 pfu/μg) is much lower than that of genomic RNA (10^6 pfu/μg). The development of plasmid vectors incorporating promoters for bacteriophage SP6, T7, or T3 RNA polymerase for the production of RNA transcripts *in vitro* enabled the production of infectious picornavirus RNA from cloned DNA.[503] Such RNA transcripts have an infectivity approaching that of genomic RNA. A similar approach has been adopted for the recovery of many other picornaviruses from cloned DNA copies of the viral genome.

STAGES OF REPLICATION

Replication of picornaviruses occurs in the cell cytoplasm. The first step is attachment to a cell receptor (Fig. 16.4). The RNA genome is then uncoated, a process that involves structural changes in the capsid. Once the positive-stranded viral RNA enters the cytoplasm, it is translated to provide viral proteins essential for genome replication and the production of new virus particles. The viral proteins are synthesized from a polyprotein precursor, which is cleaved nascently. Cleavages are carried out mainly by two viral proteinases, $2A^{pro}$ and $3C^{pro}$ or $3CD^{pro}$. Among the proteins synthesized are the viral

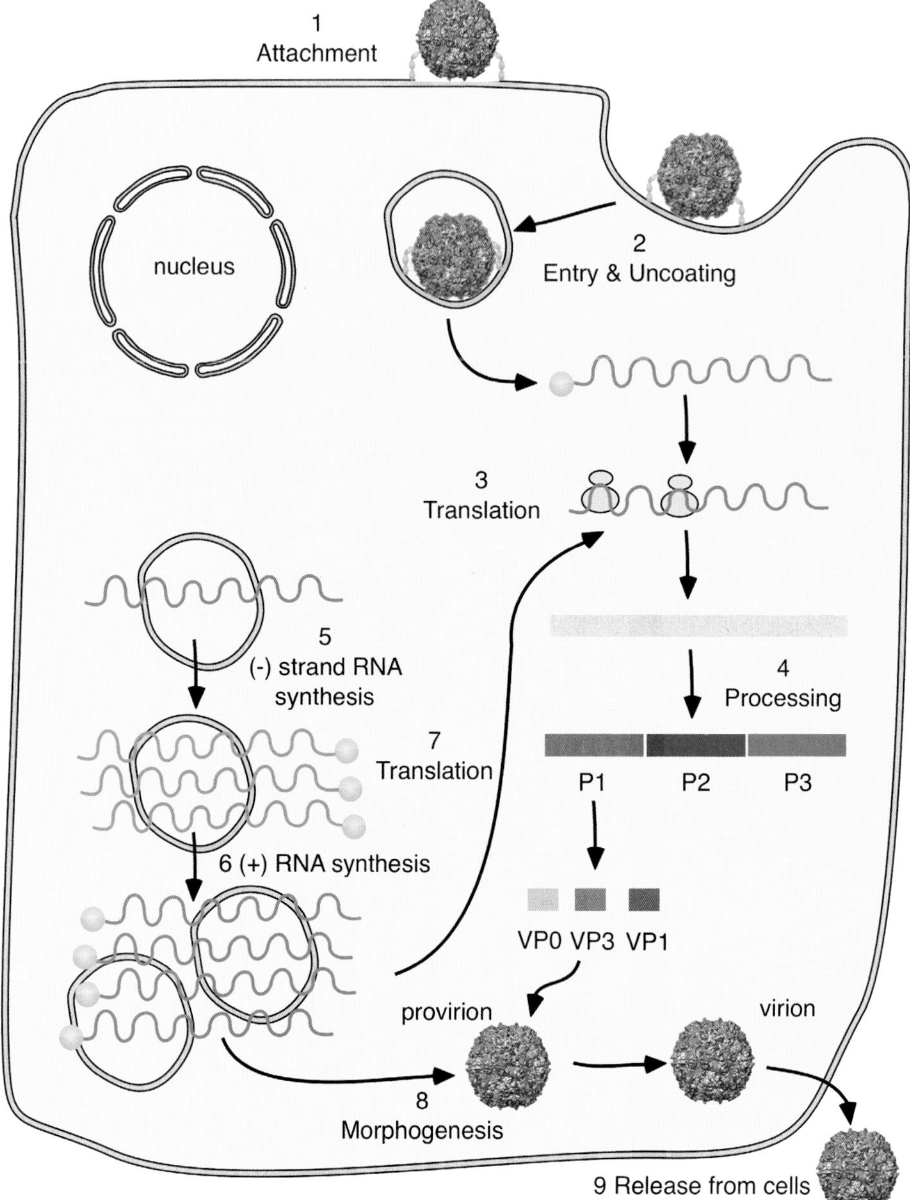

FIGURE 16.4. Overview of the picornavirus replication cycle. Virus binds to a cellular receptor **(1)** and the genome is uncoated **(2)**. VPg (virion protein, genome linked) is removed from the viral RNA, which is then translated **(3)**. The polyprotein is cleaved nascently to produce individual viral proteins **(4)**. RNA synthesis occurs on membrane vesicles induced by viral proteins (not drawn to scale). Viral (+) strand RNA is copied by the viral RNA polymerase to form full-length (–) strand RNAs **(5)**, which are then copied to produce additional (+) strand RNA **(6)**. Early in infection, newly synthesized (+) strand RNA is translated to produce additional viral proteins **(7)**. Later in infection, the (+) strands enter the morphogenetic pathway **(8)**. Newly synthesized virus particles are released from the cell by lysis **(9)**.

RNA–dependent RNA polymerase and accessory proteins required for genome replication and mRNA synthesis. The first step in genome replication is copying of the positive-stranded RNA to form a negative-stranded intermediate; this step is followed by the production of additional positive strands. These events occur on small membranous vesicles that are induced by several virus proteins. Once the pool of capsid proteins is sufficiently large, encapsidation begins. Coat protein precursor P1 is cleaved to produce an immature protomer, which then assembles into pentamers. Newly synthesized, positive-stranded RNA associates with pentamers to form the infectious virus. Empty capsids that are found in infected cells are likely to be a storage form of pentamers.

The entire time required for a single replication cycle ranges from 5 to 10 hours, depending on many variables, including the particular virus, temperature, pH, host cell, and multiplicity of infection. Many picornaviruses are released as the cell loses its integrity and lyses. Other picornaviruses (e.g., hepatitis A virus) are released from cells in the absence of cytopathic effect.

ATTACHMENT

Cellular Receptors and Coreceptors

Like most viruses, picornaviruses initiate infection of cells by first attaching to a receptor on the host cell plasma membrane. The nature of picornavirus receptors remained obscure until 1989, when the receptors for poliovirus and the major group rhinoviruses were identified.[184,332,471] Receptors for many other members of this virus family have since been identified (Table 16.3). Different types of cell surface molecules serve as

TABLE 16.3 Some Cell Receptors for *Picornaviruses*

Virus	Virus receptor	Type of receptor	Coreceptor	References
Aphthovirus				
Foot-and-mouth disease virus (cell culture adapted)	Heparan sulfate	Glycosaminoglycan		(236)
Foot-and-mouth disease virus	$\alpha_v\beta_1$, $\alpha_v\beta_3$, $\alpha_v\beta_6$, $\alpha_v\beta_8$	Integrin		(237,238,351)
Equine rhinitis A virus	Sialic acid	Carbohydrate		(473)
Cardiovirus				
Encephalomyocarditis virus	Vcam-1	Ig-like		(227)
	Sialylated glycophorin A (for hemagglutination only)	Carbohydrate		
Theiler's murine encephalomyelitis virus	Sialic acid	Carbohydrate		(193)
Low neurovirulence strains	Sialic acid	Carbohydrate		(302)
High neurovirulence strains	Heparin sulfate	Proteoglycan		
Enterovirus				
Bovine enterovirus	Sialic acid	Carbohydate		(547)
Coxsackievirus A9	$\alpha_v\beta_3$, $\alpha_v\beta_6$	Integrin	β_2-Microglobulin, GRP78, MHC-1	(431,498,499, 531)
Coxsackieviruses A13, A18, A21	Icam-1 (CD)	Ig-like		(99)
Coxsackievirus A16	P-selectin glycoprotein ligand-1 (PSGL-1), Scavenger receptor class B (SCARB2)	Mucin-like		(360,539)
Coxsackievirus A21	Decay-accelerating factor (CD55)	SCR-like (complement cascade)	Icam-1	(453)
Coxsackievirus A24	Sialic-acid containing, O-linked glycoconjugates	Carbohydrate		(336,359)
Coxsackieviruses B1–B6	Car (coxsackievirus-adenovirus receptor)	Ig-like		(58)
Coxsackievirus B1, B3, B5	Decay-accelerating factor (CD55)	scr-like (complement cascade)	$\alpha_v\beta_6$-Integrin (CVB1) CAR (CVB3)	(4,452,454)
Echovirus 1, 8	$\alpha_2\beta_1$-Integrin (Vla-2)	Integrin	β_2-Microglobulin	(56,521)
Echovirus 3, 6, 7, 11–13, 20, 21, 24, 29, 30, 33	Decay-accelerating factor (CD55)	SCR-like (complement cascade)	β_2-Microglobulin, CD59 (E7)	(57,172,409, 437,520,521)
Echovirus 5	Heparan sulfate	Proteoglycan		(234)
Echovirus 9	$A_v\beta_3$-Integrin	Integrin		(352)
Enterovirus 70	Decay-accelerating factor (CD55) sialic acid	SCR-like (complement cascade) carbohydrate		(8,264)
Enterovirus 71	P-selectin glycoprotein ligand-1 (PSGL-1), Scavenger receptor class B (SCARB2)	Mucin-like		(360,539)
Parechovirus 1	$\alpha_v\beta_3$, $\alpha_v\beta_6$			(497)
Parechovirus 1	$\alpha_v\beta_1$, $\alpha_v\beta_3$ (Vitronectin receptor)	Integrin		(497)
Hepatitis A virus	HAVcr-1	T-cell Ig-like, mucin-like (TIM)		(261)
Polioviruses 1–3	Pvr (CD155)	Ig-like		(332)
Rhinoviruses (major group, 91 serotypes)	Icam-1	Ig-like		(184,471,492)
Rhinoviruses (minor group, 10 serotypes)	Low-density lipoprotein receptor protein family	Signaling receptor		(222)

Ig, Immunoglobulin; SCR, short consensus repeat.

cellular receptors for picornaviruses; some are shared among picornaviruses and members of other virus families. For example, the cell surface protein CD55 is a receptor for certain Coxsackieviruses, echoviruses, and enterovirus 70, and the PVR CD155 is a receptor for alphaherpesviruses. For some picornaviruses (e.g., poliovirus and rhinovirus), a single type of receptor is sufficient for entry of viruses into cells. For other viruses, a second molecule, or coreceptor, is needed for virus entry into cells. For example, Coxsackievirus A21, which attaches to CD55, requires intercellular adhesion molecule 1 (ICAM-1) for entry into cells.[453]

One Type of Receptor Molecule for Virus Binding and Entry

For certain picornaviruses, a single type of receptor molecule is sufficient for virus binding and entry. These include the cell receptors for poliovirus (PVR/CD155), rhinoviruses (ICAM-1, low-density lipoprotein receptor LDLR, LDLR-related protein, very-low-density lipoprotein receptor), EMCV (VCAM-1), hepatitis A virus (TIM-1), and enterovirus 71 (SCBR2, PSGL-1).

The PVR is a type I transmembrane protein and a member of the immunoglobulin (Ig) superfamily of proteins, with three extracellular Ig-like domains: a membrane-distal V-type domain followed by two C2-type domains.[332] Production of PVR in mice is sufficient to overcome the lack of susceptibility of this species to poliovirus infection.[282,421] Because PVR transgenic mice develop poliomyelitis after inoculation with poliovirus by different routes, they have proved to be a valuable model for studying the pathogenesis of poliomyelitis.[417] PVR transgenic mice are not susceptible to infection by the oral route, the natural route of infection in humans, unless the gene encoding type I interferon receptors has been deleted.[370,549] PVR is synthesized in many tissues in transgenic mice, yet the main sites of poliovirus replication are the brain and spinal cord.[282,422] This restricted tropism is regulated by the interferon (IFN)-α/β response, which limits viral replication in extraneural organs.[232]

Expression of PVR on cultured cells derived from different animal species leads to susceptibility to poliovirus infection. Therefore it is likely that PVR is the only molecule required for poliovirus binding and entry. The observation that a monoclonal antibody directed against the lymphocyte homing receptor CD44 blocks poliovirus binding to cells suggests that this protein might be a coreceptor for poliovirus entry.[456,457] It was subsequently shown that CD44 is not a receptor for poliovirus and is not required for poliovirus infection of cells that produce PVR.[72,149] It seems likely that PVR and CD44 are associated in the cell membrane[150] and that anti-CD44 antibodies block poliovirus attachment by blocking the poliovirus-binding sites on PVR.

Orthologs of the *pvr* gene are present in the genomes of a number of mammals, including those not susceptible to poliovirus infection.[231] The amino acid sequence of domain 1 of PVR varies extensively among the nonsusceptible mammals, especially in the regions known to contact poliovirus. The absence of a poliovirus-binding site on these PVR molecules, therefore, explains why poliovirus infection is restricted to simians.

The PVR is an adhesion molecule that participates in the formation of adherens junctions through interaction with nectin-3, a related immunoglobulin-like protein.[349] The PVR is also a recognition molecule for natural killer (NK) cells, and interacts with CD226 and CD96 on NK cells to stimulate their cytotoxic activity.[71,153] It also interacts with T-cell Ig and ITIM domain (TIGIT), regulating T-cell function.[308] The UL141 protein of cytomegalovirus (CMV) blocks surface expression of PVR, leading to evasion of NK cell–mediated killing.[491]

The cell surface receptor for the major group of human rhinoviruses (90 serotypes) was identified by using monoclonal antibodies directed against the cellular binding site to isolate the receptor protein from susceptible cells. Amino acid sequence analysis of the purified protein revealed that it is ICAM-1, a type I transmembrane protein with five immunoglobulin-like domains.[184,471,492] The normal cellular functions of ICAM-1 are to bind its ligand, lymphocyte function–associated antigen 1 (LFA-1) on the surface of lymphocytes and to promote a wide range of immunologic functions.[502] ICAM-1 is expressed on the surfaces of many tissues, including the nasal epithelium, which is the entry site for rhinoviruses.

Three members of the low-density lipoprotein receptor family are receptors for minor group rhinoviruses (10 serotypes). These proteins consist of 7 (LDLR), 8 (VLDLR), or 31 (LRP) ligand-binding repeats, transmembrane and cytoplasmic domains.

Many picornaviruses bind integrins, which are dimeric cell adhesion receptors with α and β subunits. Many integrin receptors recognize the tripeptide Arg-Gly-Asp (RGD) whose presence in the viral capsid suggests interaction with this type of receptor. A number of integrins can serve as entry receptors for FMDV (Table 16.3), although all may not be utilized during infection of animals. Although integrins are sufficient for FMDV infection, their interaction with the viral capsid does not lead to uncoating (see *Entry Into Cells*).

Receptors and Coreceptors Required for Infection

Many enteroviruses bind to decay-accelerating factor (DAF, or CD55), a member of the complement cascade (Table 16.3); it is composed of four extracellular short consensus repeat modules and is attached to the plasma membrane by a glycosylphosphatidyl inositol (GPI) anchor. For most of these viruses, however, interaction with DAF is not sufficient for infection; this molecule is an attachment receptor but does not lead to virion uncoating. For example, Coxsackievirus A21 binds to DAF, but infection does not occur unless ICAM-1 is also bound (Fig. 16.5).[453] In this case, ICAM-1 inserts into the canyon where it triggers capsid uncoating.[534] Coxsackievirus B3 binds DAF but virion uncoating does not occur unless Coxsackievirus-adenovirus receptor (CAR; see below) binds in the canyon.[208]

Echovirus 7, which normally binds DAF, can infect some DAF-negative cells; in these cases CD59 or β_2-microglobulin can serve as coreceptors for entry.[172,521] Some Coxsackie B viruses that bind CD55 may require $\alpha_v\beta_6$-integrin as a coreceptor.[4]

A specific role for coreceptors in virus entry is illustrated by Coxsackievirus B3 entry into polarized epithelial cells.[105] The Coxsackievirus and adenovirus receptor, CAR, mediates cell entry of all Coxsackie B viruses.[58] CAR is not present on the apical surface of epithelial cells that line the intestinal and respiratory tracts, but is a component of the tight junction and is inaccessible to virus entry. Coxsackie B viruses first bind an attachment receptor, DAF, which is present on the apical

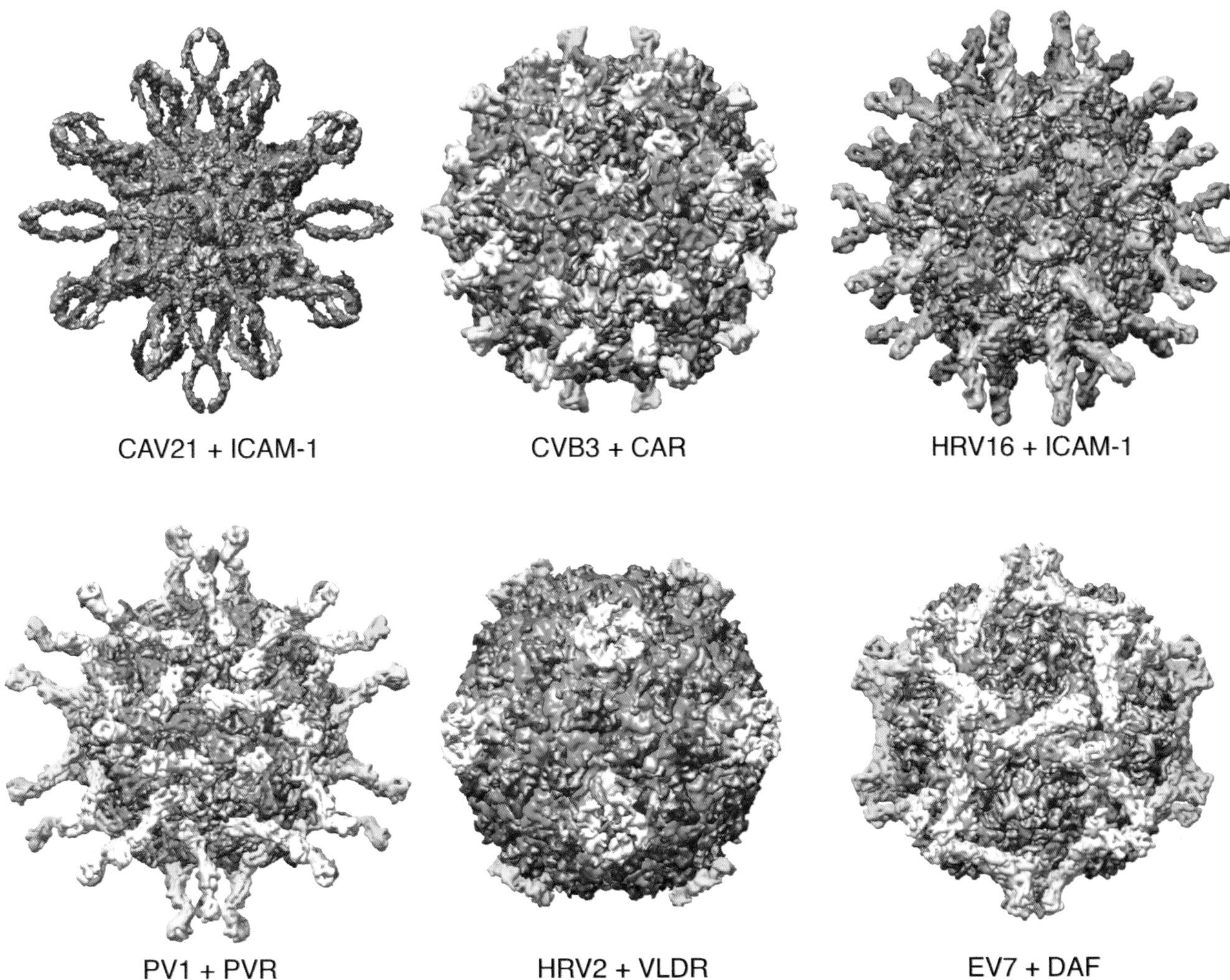

FIGURE 16.5. Interactions of six different picornaviruses with cellular receptors. Immunoglobulin-like cell receptors bind in the canyon, as illustrated for coxsackievirus 21 and ICAM-1, coxsackievirus B3 and CAR, rhinovirus 16 and ICAM-1, and poliovirus type 1 with PVR. A receptor for rhinovirus type 2, very-low-density lipoprotein receptor, binds on the plateau at the fivefold axis, and DAF binds echovirus 7 near the twofold icosahedral axes. Images produced with the Virus Particle Explorer at viberdb.scripps.edu.[83]

surface of epithelial cells. Coxsackievirus B3 binding to DAF activates Abl kinase, which in turn triggers Rac-dependent actin rearrangements, leading to virus movement to the tight junction where it can bind CAR and enter cells.[105]

Enteroviruses that bind integrins typically require a coreceptor for cell entry. For CAV9, it has been suggested that β_2-microglobulin,[499] GRP78, and MHC-1[498] might fulfill this role.

Alternative Receptors

Some viruses bind to different cell surface receptors, depending on the virus isolate or the cell line (Table 16.3). Clinical isolates of FMDV bind to integrin receptors, but passage in cell culture can select for viruses that bind to heparin sulfate, a sulfated glycan.[236,320,443] Cell culture passage may also produce a virus that infects cells independent of heparin sulfate and integrins.[33]

How Picornaviruses Attach to Cell Receptors

Among the picornavirus members, the four capsid proteins are arranged similarly, but the surface architecture varies. These differences account for both the diverse serotypes and the varied modes of interaction with cell receptors. For example, the capsids of enteroviruses have a groove, or canyon, surrounding each fivefold axis of symmetry. In contrast, cardioviruses and aphthoviruses do not have canyons.

The canyons of enteroviruses are the sites of interaction with Ig-like cell receptors. The results of genetic and structural experiments demonstrate that the first Ig-like domain contains the site that binds poliovirus. Cells expressing the first Ig-like domain of PVR, either alone or as a hybrid with other Ig-like proteins, are susceptible to infection with poliovirus.[281,342,450,451] Mutations in the first Ig-like domain of PVR interfere with poliovirus binding.[21,60,343] Mutagenesis of ICAM-1 DNA has revealed that the binding site for rhinovirus is located in the first Ig-like domain.[325,420,472] Models of the interaction of poliovirus, rhinovirus, and Coxsackievirus with their cellular receptors have been produced from cryo-EM and x-ray crystallographic data (Fig. 16.5).[51,53,84,85,207,283,372,536] These models reveal that only domain 1 of PVR or ICAM-1 penetrates the canyon of the respective virus. Mutations that affect receptor binding map to the virion–receptor interface as determined by these structural studies. Mutation of amino acids that line the canyons of poliovirus and rhinovirus can alter the affinity of binding to receptors.[100–102,204,300]

Although the capsids of at least two minor group rhinoviruses possess a canyon around the fivefold axes, it is not the binding site for the minor group receptor, members of the low-density lipoprotein receptor family (Fig. 16.5). Rather, the minor group receptor binds close to the fivefold axis, on the star-shaped plateau that is surrounded by the canyon.[213,413,418,512] In this way multiple low-affinity interactions are combined to yield a high-avidity virus-receptor complex.

Sequence and structural comparisons have revealed why major and minor group rhinoviruses recognize different receptors. A lysine at position 224 of VP1, which is conserved in all minor group rhinoviruses, is the key amino acid that interacts with a negatively charged cluster of LDLR.[512] The electrostatic attraction between Lys1224 and the acidic cluster in LDLR might initiate contact between virus and receptor. Neighboring hydrophobic and basic residues in VP1 could then lead to tight binding between virus and receptor. The conserved lysine is not present in VP1 of major group rhinoviruses, providing an explanation for failure of these viruses to bind LDLR. An exception is rhinovirus 85, a major group serotype that has the conserved lysine; presumably, it does not bind LDLR because of other amino acid differences in neighboring hydrophobic and basic VP1 residues.

It was originally believed that the picornavirus canyons were too deep and narrow to allow penetration by antibody molecules, which contain adjacent immunoglobulin domains.[436] This physical barrier was believed to hide amino acids crucial for receptor binding from the immune system. Structural studies of a rhinovirus–antibody complex, however, revealed that antibody does penetrate deep into the canyon, as does ICAM-1.[463] The shape of the picornavirus canyon, therefore, is not likely to play a role in concealing virus from the immune system.

In contrast to the Ig-like receptors that bind the canyons of enteroviruses, the binding sites for DAF on the virion are diverse. For example, DAF bridges the canyon of Coxsackievirus B3.[196] In contrast, the binding site of DAF on echovirus 7 (Fig. 16.5) and 12 is near the twofold axis.[390,402] These interactions are not sufficient for virion uncoating. Coxsackievirus A21 must also bind ICAM-1, which inserts into the canyon, triggering capsid uncoating.[453,534] Similarly, Coxsackievirus B3 binds DAF but virion uncoating does not occur unless CAR binds in the canyon.[208]

Integrin-binding picornaviruses attach to cell receptors through surface loops. In FMDV, an Arg-Gly-Asp sequence in the flexible, exposed βG-βH loop of the capsid protein VP1 is recognized by integrin receptors on cells.[121,147,306] Arg-Gly-Asp–containing peptides block attachment of FMDV,[44] and alteration of this sequence interferes with virus binding.[322] In Coxsackievirus A9, the Arg-Gly-Asp sequence is present in a 17–amino acid extension of the C-terminus of VP1 and is also the site of attachment to cell receptors.[87,431] Alteration of this sequence does not abolish binding to cells, suggesting that the virus can bind to another cell surface receptor.[228] Echovirus 1 is unusual in that it binds the RGD-independent integrin $\alpha_2\beta_1$ in the canyon.[537]

As discussed, FMDV binds alternative receptors, either integrin or heparan sulfate, depending on the virus isolate. The binding site for heparan sulfate on cell culture–adapted FMDV is a shallow depression on the virion surface, where the three major capsid proteins, VP1, VP2, and VP3, are located.[152] Binding specificity is controlled by two preformed sulfate-binding sites on the capsid. Residue 56 of VP3 is a critical regulator of receptor recognition. In field isolates of the virus, this amino acid is histidine. Adaptation to cell culture selects for viruses with an arginine at this position, which forms the high-affinity, heparan sulfate–binding site.

The interaction of EMCV with its cellular receptor, VCAM-1, has not been studied in detail. The EMCV capsid does not have a canyon, therefore VCAM-1, an Ig-like protein, must interact with the virion in a manner different from the Ig-like receptors of poliovirus and rhinovirus.

Kinetics and Affinity of the Virus–Receptor Interaction

The affinity and kinetics of picornaviruses binding to soluble forms of their receptors have been studied by surface plasmon resonance. Two classes of receptor-binding sites, with distinct binding affinities, exist on the capsids of poliovirus and rhinovirus.[84,326,536] The association rates for the two binding classes are 25 and 13 times higher for the poliovirus–sPVR interaction than for the rhinovirus–sICAM interaction at 20°C. The greater association rate of poliovirus and PVR may be caused, in part, by differences in the extent of contact between virus and receptor. In contrast, whereas two dissociation rate constants exist for the poliovirus–PVR interaction, only one has been reported for the rhinovirus 3–ICAM interaction. The dissociation rates for the poliovirus–sPVR interaction are 1.5 times and 2.0 times faster than for the rhinovirus–sICAM interaction, indicating greater instability of the former complex. The affinity constants for the poliovirus–sPVR interaction are 19 times and 6 times greater than those reported for the rhinovirus–sICAM-1 complex.

In contrast to the observations with poliovirus and rhinovirus, a single class of binding site was found on echovirus 11 for a soluble form of its receptor, CD55.[292] The affinity of this interaction is at least fourfold lower than either of the binding sites on poliovirus for sPVR. The association rate for the interaction between echovirus 11 and CD55 is faster than that of poliovirus–sPVR and rhinovirus–sICAM-1. One explanation for these findings is that the contact between echovirus 11 and CD55 is more extensive than that of the other two virus–receptor complexes. The binding site for CD55 on echovirus 11 may also be more accessible than those of PVR and ICAM-1. The dissociation rate for the echovirus–CD55 interaction is at least 97 times faster than that of either the poliovirus–sPVR or the rhinovirus–sICAM-1 interaction. These findings are consistent with a more accessible binding site for CD55 on echovirus 11, compared with the receptor-binding sites on poliovirus and rhinovirus. Atomic interactions between CD55 and echovirus 11 may be weaker than between the other two viruses and their receptors. The faster dissociation rate of the echovirus 11–CD55 complex may be related to the finding that the interaction does not lead to structural changes of the virus particle,[409] as occurs with poliovirus and rhinovirus. In general, there is a higher affinity for virions of receptors that can uncoat particles ("unzippers"—poliovirus/PVR, HRV/ICAM-1, CVB3/CAR) compared with attachment receptors (E6, 7, 11, 12, CVB3 with DAF). This may reflect the requirement for higher affinity to release the viral RNA.

Why do poliovirus and rhinovirus have two classes of receptor-binding sites? The receptors for both viruses make contacts at two major sites on the virus surface, one in a cleft on the south rim of the canyon, and a second on the side of the mesa on the north rim. These two contact sites may correspond to the two classes of binding sites. Two classes of binding sites may also be a consequence of the structural flexibility exhibited by both viruses, which may cause exposure of different binding sites. Normally internal parts of the poliovirus and rhinovirus capsid proteins have been shown to be transiently displayed on the virion surface, a process called *breathing*.[296,298] As to be discussed later, the interaction of poliovirus and rhinovirus with their cellular receptors leads to irreversible and more extensive structural changes. In contrast to the findings with poliovirus and rhinovirus, binding of echovirus 11 with CD55 can be described by a simple 1:1 binding model. Such behavior, which would be expected for the interaction of two preformed binding sites, is consistent with the fact that the echovirus–CD55 interaction does not result in detectable structural changes in the capsid.[409]

ENTRY INTO CELLS

Once picornaviruses have attached to their cellular receptor, the viral capsid is brought into the cell by the endocytic pathway, followed by genome release into the cytoplasm, the site of picornavirus replication. For some picornaviruses, interaction with a cell receptor serves only to concentrate virus on the cell surface; release of the genome is a consequence of low pH or perhaps the activity of a coreceptor. For other picornaviruses, the cell receptor is also an unzipper and initiates conformational changes in the virus that lead to release of the genome.

Entry by Clathrin-Mediated Endocytosis

Several lines of evidence indicate that FMDVs enter cells by clathrin-mediated endocytosis. Infection is inhibited by sucrose, which eliminates clathrin-coated pits and induces clathrin to polymerize into empty cages, and by expression of a dominant negative form of the clathrin coat assembly protein AP180 that is needed for assembly of clathrin cages.[61] Confocal microscopy also revealed that FMDV enters cells via a clathrin-dependent mechanism.[366] There is also some evidence that entry is dependent on cholesterol in the plasma membrane, a requirement generally observed for lipid rafts[319]; however, cholesterol might be required for clathrin-induced membrane curving.[428] Another aphthovirus, equine rhinitis A virus, binds sialic acid–containing receptors but also enters into cells via clathrin-mediated endocytosis.[185]

LDLR family members that are receptors for minor group HRVs possess C-terminal cytoplasmic domains with tyrosine- and di-leucine–based internalization signals that lead to clustering of the receptors in clathrin-coated pits.[384] Evidence for HRV entry via this pathway includes the inhibition of infection in cells producing dominant negative inhibitors of the clathrin pathway.[47,465] There is some evidence that ICAM-1 binding major group HRVs also enter cells via clathrin-mediated endocytosis, including transmission EM, which shows virions in clathrin-coated pits and vesicles 5 minutes after infection[187] and the fact that dominant negative dynamin inhibits infection.[118] HRV infection also activates signaling pathways with links to the endocytic machinery. The cytoplasmic domain of ICAM-1 binds the adaptor protein ezrin, which links the receptor to Syk, a tyrosine kinase.[519a] When HRV binds ICAM-1, Syk is recruited from the cytoplasm to the plasma membrane together with clathrin. Functional Syk is required for HRV entry via ICAM-1.[291]

When virions enter cells by clathrin-dependent endocytosis they encounter low pH, which triggers release of the viral RNA from the capsid. A role for low pH in infection can be demonstrated by determining the effect on entry of compounds that block acidification, such as weak bases (ammonium chloride, chloroquine, methylamine) ionophores (monensin, nigericin, X537A) or inhibitors of the vacuolar proton ATPase (concanamycin A, bafilomycin A). The pH of early endosomes is 6.5; as these vesicles mature to late endosomes the pH drops to 5.5. Endosomal maturation is dependent not only on vacuolar ATPases but also on microtubules and membrane GTPases of the Rab family. Early to late endosome maturation can be inhibited by drugs that depolymerize microtubules (nocodazole), dominant negative Rabs, or inhibitors of PI3K signaling (wortmannin). In this way it is possible to determine if viral entry occurs from early or late endosomes.

Uncoating by FMDV clearly requires low pH because concanamycin A, monensin, and ammonium chloride all inhibit infection.[43,61,366,517] Entry occurs from the early endosome as determined by experiments with dominant negative Rab proteins.[250] FMDV that bind heparan sulfate enter cells via a caveolae-dependent route, but low pH is still required for infection.[367] Consistent with this mechanism of uncoating, FMDV that has been coated with antibody can bind to, and infect, cells that express Fc receptors, in contrast to poliovirus, which cannot productively infect cells via this pathway.[321] Cell receptors for FMDV are, therefore, *hooks:* they do not induce uncoating-related changes in the virus particle, but rather serve only to tether the virus to the cell and bring it into the endocytic pathway.

Entry of minor group HRVs requires low pH of the late endosome, as infection is inhibited by monensin, bafilomycin A1, nocodazole, and wortmannin.[46,59,74,353,410] ICAM-binding HRVs are also sensitive to bafilomycin and monensin, suggesting that endosome acidification is required for entry.[187,387,483]

Echovirus 7, which binds DAF, enters cells by clathrin-mediated endocytosis, and trafficking into late endosomes is required.[270] However, infection does not appear to require low pH, and therefore the trigger for uncoating and its intracellular location remains in question.

Entry by Caveolin-Mediated Endocytosis

As discussed above, CVB3 binds DAF, a GPI-linked protein localized within lipid rafts on the apical surface of polarized cells. The virus/DAF complex then moves to tight junctions (TJ) where it engages CAR. The virus is then internalized along with the TJ protein occludin by caveolin-1–dependent endocytosis.[107] The role of occludin is not known but it could provide a scaffold for recruiting other molecules. Within 60 minutes, the virus is within caveolin-1–containing vesicles (caveolae and caveosomes). Phosphorylation of caveolin-1 by tyrosine kinases is required for CVB3 entry, but the role of this modification is not known. Dynamin is not required for uptake of this virus, suggesting that other routes of entry are involved. Inhibitors of micropinocytosis (rottlerin and dominant negative Rab34) block infection, indicating a role for this type of uptake.

Echovirus 1, which binds the integrin $\alpha 2\beta 1$, is taken into the cell by the caveolin-mediated endocytic pathway. The receptor is present in raft-like membrane domains that do not contain caveolin. Internalization of the virus does not depend on dynamin, but components of the macropinocytosis pathway, such as PKC, Pak1, and Rac1, are involved. By 30 minutes after infection, the virus appears in vesicular structures that appear to be caveolae.[318] These fuse with caveosomes, delivering the virus and its receptor to the perinuclear region.[397] These may be novel multivesicular bodies; virus transport to them appears to depend on ESCRT proteins.[263]

Caveolin- and Clathrin-Independent Endocytosis

In HeLa cells, poliovirus is taken up into cells by an endocytic pathway that is dependent on actin, ATP, and a tyrosine kinase, but independent of clathrin, caveolin, flotillin, microtubules, and pinocytosis.[76] RNA release from the particle occurs rapidly and within 100 to 200 nm of the cell surface. Entry was different in a highly polarized human brain microvascular endothelial cell line.[106] Poliovirus enters these cells very slowly via dynamin-dependent caveolar endocytosis. Virus binding to PVR induces tyrosine phosphorylation of the receptor cytoplasmic domain, which in turn recruits and activates SHP-2, which is required for infection. These observations emphasize that virus entry pathways are likely to differ substantially according to cell type.

Uncoating

The interaction of enteroviruses and major group rhinoviruses with susceptible cells leads to the conversion of virions to a more slowly sedimenting form (135S versus 160S for native particles).[112,252] The resulting particles, called *altered* (or *A*) *particles,* contain the viral RNA but have lost the internal capsid protein VP4. In addition, the N-terminus of VP1, which is normally on the interior of the capsid, is on the surface of the A particle.[151] This sequence of VP1 is hydrophobic and, as a result, the A particles have an increased affinity for membranes compared with the native virus particle. It is believed that A particles represent a stable intermediate structure in the entry process that terminates with exit of RNA and the production of empty (80S) capsids. In one hypothesis for poliovirus entry, receptor binding leads to these conformational changes; the exposed lipophilic N-terminus of VP1 then inserts into the cell membrane, tethering the A particle to the membrane. A membrane pore is then formed, possibly by both VP4 and VP1, through which the viral RNA can travel to the cytoplasm (Fig. 16.6). The finding that A particles, when added to lipid bilayers, induce the formation of ion channels supports this hypothesis.[493] The trigger for conversion of minor group HRVs is not receptor binding but low pH.[410]

Native poliovirus and rhinovirus particles have been shown to transiently and reversibly expose VP4 and the N-terminus of VP1, a process called "breathing".[296,298] Receptor binding (poliovirus) or low pH (rhinoviruses, cardioviruses, aphthoviruses) lowers the energy barrier for conversion to the A particle, a process that enables genome delivery to the cell. The structure of poliovirus bound to a monoclonal antibody that recognizes the N-terminus of VP1 reveals that this viral protein exits the capsid near the twofold axes, instead of near the propeller tip in 135S particles (see below).

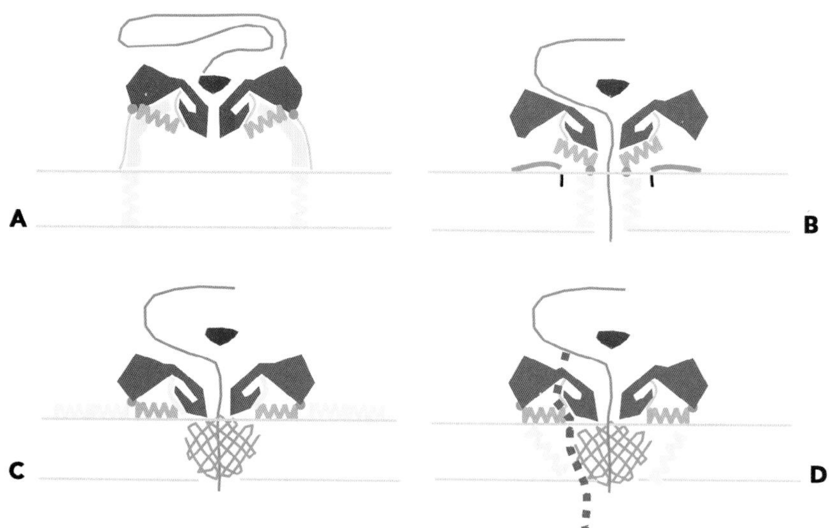

FIGURE 16.6. Hypothetical mechanism for translocation of poliovirus RNA across the cell membrane. A: Cross-section of a virus particle that has just bound poliovirus receptor (PVR) at the cell surface. PVR docks on the capsid in the canyon, above the hydrophobic pocket. The path of VP1 egress would not preclude continued binding to PVR. The viral RNA is in the capsid, and lipid has exited from the hydrophobic pocket. The capsid is colored blue, VP4 is green, and the N-terminus of VP1 is cyan and magenta, PVR is tan, RNA is a green line. At this stage the VP3 β-cylinder (red) blocks a channel at the fivefold axis. **B–D** illustrate alternative models for anchoring of virus particle to the cell membrane by the N-terminus of VP1 and formation of a pore for passage of viral RNA. Upon binding, PVR structural changes occur that move the VP3 β-cylinder out of the way like a float valve and open a channel at the fivefold axis that is contiguous with a pore in the membrane. **(B)** Amphipathic helices at the N-terminus of VP1 form a pore through the membrane. In **C** and **D**, VP4 (*green mesh*) is playing a central role in pore formation. In this case, VP1 may anchor the particle to the membrane. An alternative pathway for release of the genome from the base of the canyon is shown.

Low-resolution, cryo-EM reconstructions of the poliovirus 135S and 80S particles did not reveal openings that could allow for release of the viral genome.[52] Subsequently, higher-resolution structures of the poliovirus A particle and a derivative in which the N-terminal 31 amino acids of VP1 were removed revealed that this sequence of VP1 is likely to exit the virion at the base of the canyon, between the tips of the "stars" at the fivefold axis and the propeller-shaped feature around the threefold axis.[78] It has also been suggested that VP4 exits near the twofold axis, based on the observation that insertion of a cysteine in the N-terminus of VP4 leads to disulfide linking upon breathing.[266]

Cryo-EM reconstructions of 80S particles of HRV2,[213] HRV14, and poliovirus[295] reveal two populations of particles, one with more internal density (presumably RNA) than the other. The poliovirus structures reveal different particle states: some in the process of releasing RNA, others with nucleic acid in the particle, crossing the particle walls, and outside the particle. Analysis of these particles indicates that the viral RNA exits the capsid from openings at the base of the canyon, near where the release of the VP1 N-terminus occurs.[70] The trigger for release of RNA from the capsid is unknown, but may require unfolding of secondary structure.[76]

VP4 is released from the virion during conversion to A particles, but a small amount of this protein might remain and participate with VP1 in membrane channel formation. A virus containing an amino acid change at position 28 of VP4 can bind to cells and be converted to A particles, but these are blocked at a subsequent step in virus entry.[345] Amino acid changes at this position of VP4 reduce the conductance of ion channels and the translocation of viral RNA.[115] These findings suggest that VP4 might play a central role in pore formation. VP4 and VP2 are produced, during virus assembly, from the precursor VP0, which remains uncleaved until RNA encapsidation. Cleavage of VP0, therefore, can be viewed as a way of priming the capsid for uncoating because cleavage separates VP4 from VP2.

While the enterovirus capsid maintains its icosahedral form during uncoating, the acid-labile aphthoviruses dissociate into pentamers at low pH, a process that releases the viral RNA.[510] The mechanism by which low pH causes disassembly of the FMDV capsid has been illuminated by structural and genetic studies. Examination of the atomic structure of the virus revealed a high density of histidine residues lining the pentamer interfaces, which are stabilized by β-sheet interactions.[1] These residues confer stability to the capsid; because the pKa of histidine is 6.8, close to the pH at which the virus dissociates, protonation of the side chains of the histidines might cause electrostatic repulsion, leading to disassembly.[113] To test this hypothesis, a histidine residue at position 142 of VP3 was changed to arginine by mutagenesis. The resulting capsids were more stable at low pH than wild-type capsids,[134] supporting the proposed role of the histidine residue in acid-catalyzed disassembly. Enteroviruses are stable at low pH in part because there are extra β-sheet interactions in VP1.[138] Equine rhinitis A virus is also acid labile; it dissociates into pentamers due to rearrangement of loops in VP2 that disrupt the pentamer interfaces.[501] How aphthoviruses breach the endosome membrane is not known; these viruses do not have a hydrophobic VP1 N-terminus, and A particles are not produced.

If aphthoviruses dissociate into pentamers in the endosome, how is the integrity of viral RNA preserved before it exits to the cytoplasm? A clue is provided by the finding that equine rhinitis A virus capsid dissociation is preceded by the formation of a transient empty particle.[501] It is possible that this protects the viral RNA until it leaves the endosome.

Low pH causes particle expansion of minor group rhinoviruses and the opening of a 10 Å diameter pore at the fivefold axis through which the RNA is presumed to exit.[214]

Regulation of Uncoating by Cellular Molecules

Beneath the canyon floor is a hydrophobic pocket that opens at the base of the canyon and extends toward the fivefold axis of symmetry. The pocket appears to be occupied in many picornaviruses with a fatty acid or related compound (Fig. 16.2). In some picornaviruses (e.g., rhinovirus types 3 and 14), the pockets are apparently empty.[25,550] The hydrophobic pocket appears to be a critical regulator of the receptor-induced structural transitions of enteroviruses. The icosahedral symmetry of the capsid would allow each virion to contain up to 60 lipid molecules. Certain antiviral drugs (e.g., the WIN compounds first identified by Sterling-Winthrop, Inc.) displace the lipid and bind tightly within the pocket.[462] Binding of such drugs to rhinovirus 14 causes conformational changes in the canyon that prevent attachment to cells.[391] In contrast, drug binding to rhinoviruses 1A, 3, and 16 and to poliovirus causes smaller structural changes in the capsid.[182,195,218] Inhibition of rhinovirus 16 binding by these compounds is probably not a consequence of altering the receptor-binding site, but rather the result of preventing conformational changes required for receptor binding. Such compounds do not inhibit binding of poliovirus, but rather uncoating.[330]

The lipids that occupy the hydrophobic pocket were originally believed to contribute to the stability of the native virus particle by locking the capsid in a stable configuration and preventing conformational changes. Removal of the lipid was therefore necessary to provide the capsid with sufficient flexibility to undergo the changes that permit the RNA to leave the shell. This hypothesis comes from the study of antiviral drugs, such as the WIN compounds, that displace the lipid and bind tightly in the hydrophobic pocket. These antiviral compounds block breathing of the rhinovirus capsid, the process by which normally internal parts of the capsid proteins are transiently displayed on the virion surface.[296] Polioviruses containing bound WIN compounds can bind to cells, but the interaction with PVR does not result in the production of A particles.[148,548] WIN compounds appear to inhibit poliovirus infectivity by preventing PVR-mediated conformational alterations that are required for uncoating. Additional support for the role of lipids in uncoating comes from the analysis of poliovirus mutants that cannot replicate unless WIN compounds are present.[347] Such WIN-dependent mutants spontaneously convert to altered particles at 37°C, in the absence of the cell receptor, probably because of the absence of lipid in the hydrophobic pocket. The lipids can be considered to be switches that determine whether the virus is stable (lipid present) or will uncoat (lipid absent). It is not known what causes lipid release from the capsid. PVR docks onto the poliovirus capsid just above the hydrophobic pocket (Fig. 16.6), which suggests that the interaction of the virus with receptor may initiate structural changes in the virion that lead to the release of the lipid.

Incubation of poliovirus with PVR for short periods at low temperatures appears to result in loss of the lipid.[53] The results of computational modeling and kinetic studies suggest that stabilization of virus particles by drugs that replace the lipid is a consequence of increased compressibility rather than increased rigidity.[395,470,500]

TRANSLATION OF THE VIRAL RNA

Internal Ribosome Binding: The Internal Ribosome Entry Site

Once the picornavirus positive-stranded genomic RNA is released into the cell cytoplasm, it must be translated because it cannot be copied by any cellular RNA polymerase and no viral enzymes are brought into the cell within the viral capsid. Several experimental findings led to the belief that translation of the picornavirus genome was accomplished by an unusual mechanism. The positive-stranded RNA genomes lack 5′-terminal cap structures; although virion RNA is linked to the viral protein VPg, this protein is removed by a cellular unlinking enzyme on entry of the RNA into the cell.[13] Furthermore, picornavirus genomes are efficiently translated in infected cells despite inhibition of cellular mRNA translation. Determination of the nucleotide sequence of poliovirus positive-stranded RNA revealed a 741-nucleotide 5′-untranslated region that contains seven AUG codons.[276,415] Similar 5′-noncoding regions were subsequently found in other picornaviruses and shown to contain highly ordered RNA structures.[426,461] These findings led to the suggestion that ribosomes do not scan through picornaviral 5′-untranslated regions, but rather bind to an internal sequence. The 5′-untranslated region of poliovirus positive-stranded RNA was subsequently shown to contain a sequence that promotes internal binding of the 40S ribosomal subunit; it was called the *internal ribosome entry site* (IRES) (Fig. 16.7).

All picornavirus RNA contain an IRES, as do other viral and some cellular mRNAs.[313] Viral IRES have been placed in four groups based on a variety of criteria, including primary

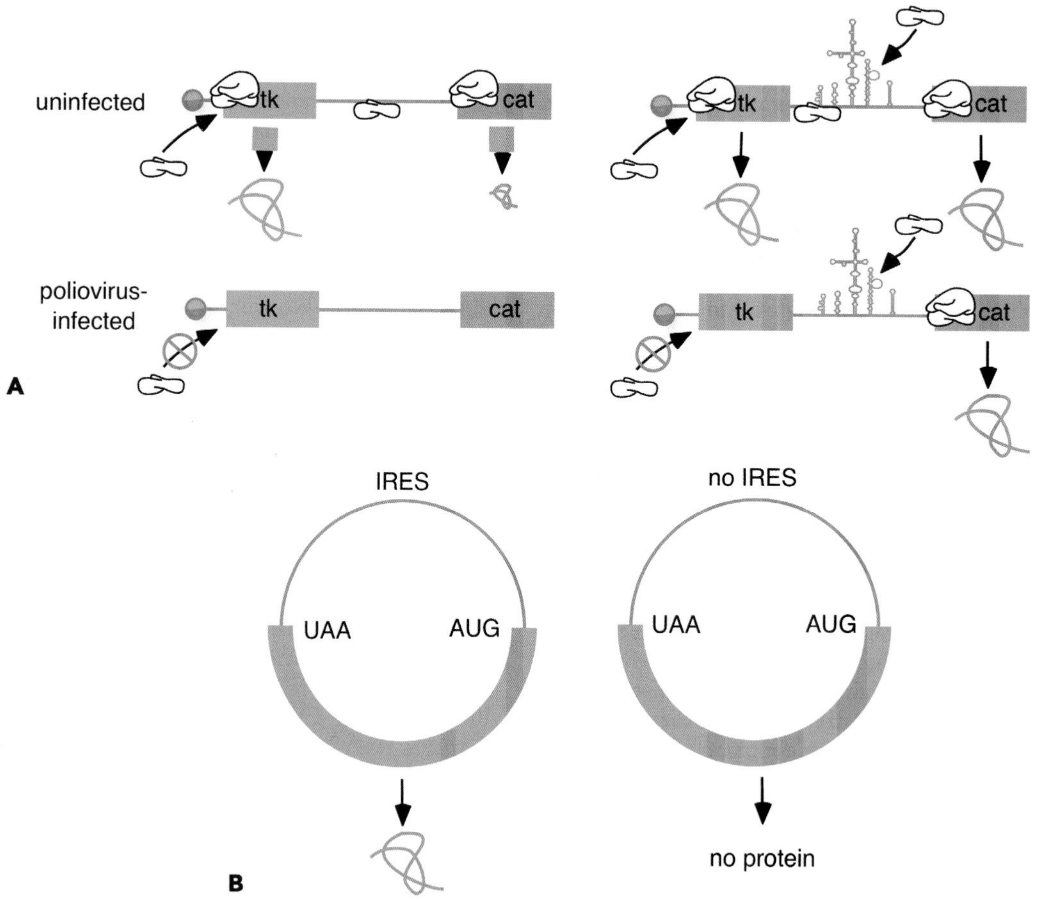

FIGURE 16.7. Discovery of the internal ribosome entry site (IRES). A: Bicistronic messenger RNA (mRNA) assay used to discover the IRES. Plasmids were constructed that encode two reporter molecules, thymidine kinase (tk) and chloramphenicol acetyl transferase (cat), separated by an IRES or a spacer. After introduction into mammalian cells, the plasmids give rise to mRNA of the structure shown in the figure. In uninfected cells (*top line*), both reporter molecules can be detected, although cat synthesis is inefficient without an IRES and is probably caused by reinitiation. In poliovirus-infected cells, 5′ end–dependent initiation is inhibited, and no proteins are detected without an IRES, demonstrating internal ribosome binding. **B:** Circular mRNA assay for an IRES. Circular mRNA were constructed and translated *in vitro* in cell extracts. In the absence of an IRES, no protein is observed because 5′-end initiation requires a free 5′ end. Inclusion of an IRES allows protein translation from the circular mRNA, demonstrating internal ribosome binding.

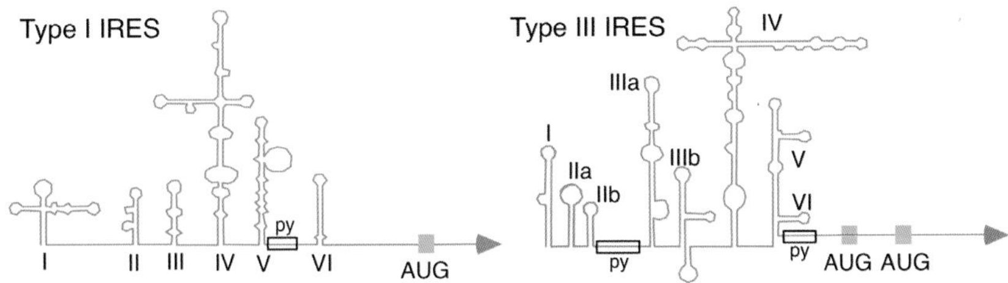

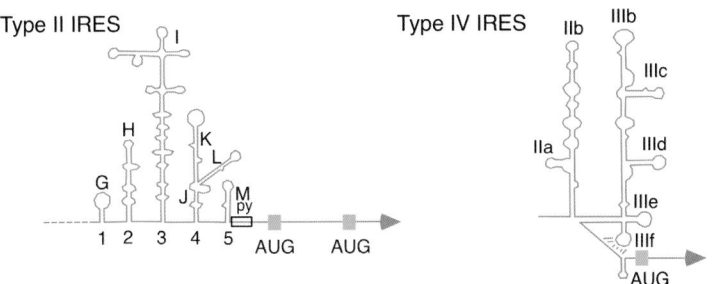

FIGURE 16.8. Four major types of picornaviral internal ribosome entry sites (IRES). The type I IRES is found in the genomes of enteroviruses. The genomes of cardioviruses and aphthoviruses contain a type II IRES. The IRES of hepatitis A virus is type III, and the type IV IRES is represented by porcine teschovirus 1; other picornaviruses with this type of IRES include simian virus 2, porcine enterovirus 8, simian picornavirus type 9, avian encephalomyelitis virus, and Seneca Valley virus.

sequence, secondary structure, location of the initiation codon, and activity in different cell types (Fig. 16.8). In the type I IRES (found in the genomes of enteroviruses and rhinoviruses), and the type III IRES (hepatitis A virus), the initiation codon is located 50 to 100 nucleotides beyond the 3′-end of the IRES, whereas it is located at the 3′-end of a type II IRES (cardioviruses and aphthoviruses). The IRES of porcine teschovirus, avian encephalomyelitis virus, and hepatitis C virus (a member of the *Flaviviridae*) are classified as a type IV IRES.

There is little nucleotide sequence conservation among different IRES elements. The picornavirus IRES contains extensive regions of RNA secondary structure (Fig. 16.7) that is not strictly conserved but is crucial for ribosome binding. One sequence motif that is conserved among picornavirus IRES is a GNRA sequence (G, guanine; N, any nucleotide; R, purine; A, adenine) in stem-loop IV of the type I IRES and in stem-loop I of the type II IRES. Another conserved element is an Yn-Xm-AUG motif, in which Yn is a pyrimidine-rich region and Xm is a 15- to 25-nucleotide spacer followed by an AUG codon. Translation initiation mediated by a type I IRES involves binding of the 40S ribosomal subunit to the IRES and scanning of the subunit to the AUG initiation codon. The 40S subunit probably binds at the AUG initiation codon of a type II IRES.

The type III IRES has little homology with type I and type II IRES except for the Yn-Xm-AUG motif. It is structurally distinct, consisting of two major domains, and in addition requires intact eIF4F complex.[11] The type IV IRES functions in a prokaryotic-like manner. The secondary structures of these RNA elements facilitate direct interaction with the small 40S ribosome.[143,144,242,468] These interactions place a portion of the RNA within the P site of the 40S ribosomal subunit as observed by *in vitro* toeprinting and structural analyses of RNA–protein complexes. Initiation of translation mediated by the type IV IRES is therefore independent of all canonical translation proteins including the ternary complex of eIF2α-GTP-met-tRNAi. The only initiation protein required is DHX29, necessary to unwind secondary structure surrounding the initiation codon.[401,546] No met-tRNAi is required, as the first amino acid of this polyprotein is glycine.[242]

The IRES of Aichi virus is distinct from types I, II, and III IRES and may represent a distinct class.[546] Domain I is not related to elements found in any other IRES. Domain J consists of a long, interrupted basal helix and an apical four-way helical junction, similar to but smaller than domain IV in type I IRES. Its apical subdomain (Jb) also includes a GNRA tetraloop, which is essential for the function of type I and type II IRES. The apex of AV domain K contains an element identical to an apical motif in domain J of type II IRES that is essential for specific interaction with eIF4G.[42,95] These domains are otherwise unrelated. An equivalent of domain K of type 2 IRES is also absent. Finally, the initiation codon is preceded by an Yn motif as in the type I/II IRES, but in contrast, it is sequestered in a long, stable hairpin, explaining why this IRES requires the DExH-box protein DHX29.

Mechanism of Internal Ribosome Binding

Different sets of translation initiation proteins are needed for internal initiation mediated by various IRES. Internal ribosome binding via the type III IRES requires all of the initiation proteins, including eIF4E. A subset of translation initiation proteins is required for the activity of most picornavirus IRES.

Translation initiation via a type I IRES involves binding of the 40S ribosomal subunit to the IRES, followed by scanning of the subunit to the initiation codon. The 40S subunit may bind directly to the RNA, or might be recruited to the IRES by interacting with translation initiation proteins. In cells infected with some picornaviruses, eIF4G is cleaved, inactivating the translation of most cellular mRNA. This observation led to the belief that eIF4G is not required for function of the IRES of poliovirus and other picornaviruses. The C-terminal fragment of eIF4G, which contains binding sites for eIF3 and eIF4A (Fig. 16.9), however, stimulates IRES-mediated translation.[79,371] These findings have led to a model in which the 40S ribosomal subunit is recruited to the IRES through interaction with eIF3 bound to the C-terminal domain of eIF4G, which

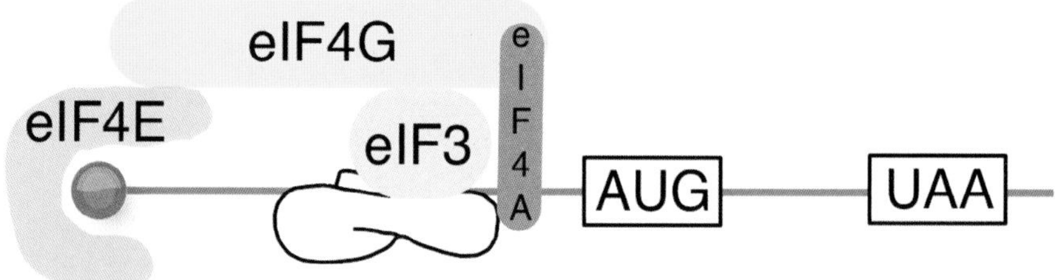

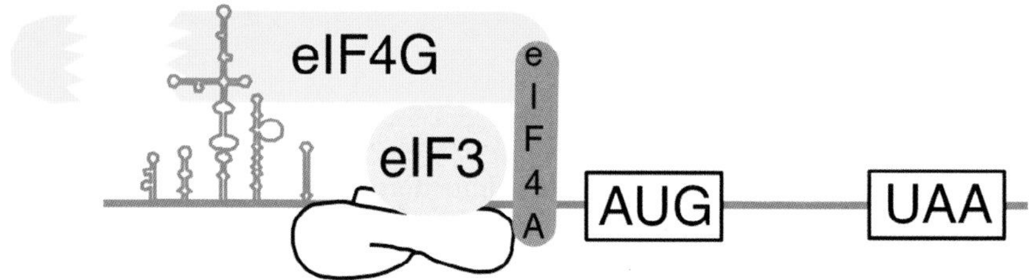

FIGURE 16.9. Models for translation initiation complex formation. In 5′ end–dependent initiation, the 40S subunit is recruited to the messenger RNA (mRNA) through its interaction with eIF3, which binds eIF4G. The latter initiation factor is part of eIF4F, which also contains eIF4A, a helicase to unwind RNA secondary structure, and eIF4E, the cap-binding protein. Binding of eIF4E to the cap thus positions eIF4E at the 5′ end and positions the 40S subunit on the mRNA. In IRES-dependent translation, a 5′ end is not required. The eIF3–40S complex is believed to be recruited to the RNA by the interaction of eIF4G with the IRES.

binds directly to the IRES. Stimulation of IRES function by the C-terminal proteolytic fragment of eIF4G may explain the observation that IRES activity is enhanced in cells in which the poliovirus protease $2A^{pro}$ is expressed.[200] Protease $2A^{pro}$ is one of the picornaviral proteinases responsible for cleavage of eIF4G. Although the IRES of most picornaviruses function with cleaved eIF4G, that of hepatitis A virus requires intact eIF4G.[69] The 40S ribosomal subunit binds at or near the AUG initiation codon of the type II IRES, and no scanning occurs.

The poliovirus IRES functions poorly in reticulocyte lysates, in which capped mRNA can be translated efficiently. Addition of a cytoplasmic extract to reticulocyte lysates restores efficient translation from this IRES. These observations led to the suggestion that ribosome binding to the IRES requires cell proteins other than the canonical translation proteins. Such proteins have been identified by their ability to bind the IRES and restore internal initiation in reticulocyte lysates (reviewed in[139]). One host protein identified by this approach is the La protein, which binds to the 3′-end of the poliovirus IRES.[331] This protein is associated with the 3′-termini of newly synthesized small RNA, including transcripts of cellular RNA polymerase III. La protein is present in low amounts in reticulocyte lysates; addition of the protein to such lysates stimulates the activity of the poliovirus IRES.[331] La is a nuclear protein that is relocalized to the cytoplasm in poliovirus-infected cells.[459] La protein is also required for efficient function of the encephalomyocarditis virus IRES.[272]

Polypyrimidine tract-binding protein (PTB) is composed of four RNA binding domains and functions as a regulator of pre-mRNA splicing. It binds the poliovirus IRES[211] and is required by all type I IRES.[230] Removal of this protein from a cell extract with an RNA affinity column inhibits the function of the FMDV IRES[358,398] and that of encephalomyocarditis virus, but does not affect translation by 5′ end–dependent initiation.[258] The deficiency in the function of these IRES is restored by adding the purified protein back to the lysate. The depleted lysate, however, still supports the function of the IRES from Theiler's murine encephalomyocarditis virus, another picornavirus. It was subsequently shown that the requirement for polypyrimidine tract-binding protein by the encephalomyocarditis virus IRES depends on the nature of the reporter and the size of an A-rich bulge in the IRES.[259] It is thought that PTB protein facilitates initiation via the type I IRES by modulating binding of eIF4G to the viral RNA through the interaction between the RNA-binding motifs 1 and 2 of PTB protein, the bottom of domain V of the type I IRES, and the RNA-binding motifs 3 and 4 within the single-stranded region of the viral RNA surrounding domain V of the IRES.[257] Unlike the type I IRES, multiple copies of PTB protein are required to bind the FMDV, EMCV, and other type II IRES. RNA-binding domains 1 and 2 of one PTB molecule binds domain F of the IRES, and RNA-binding domains 3 and 4 bind domains D and E of the IRES. RNA-binding domains 1 and 2 of a second molecule of PTB bind domain K of the IRES, and RNA-binding domains 3 and 4 interact with IRES domains H, I, and L, all with lower affinity.[256]

HeLa cell extracts also contain unr, an RNA-binding protein with five cold-shock domains that is required for IRES function.[229] Recombinant unr stimulates the function of the rhinovirus IRES in the reticulocyte lysate and acts synergistically with recombinant PTB protein to stimulate translation mediated by the rhinovirus IRES *in vitro.* However, the poliovirus IRES inefficiently mediates translation initiation in $unr^{-/-}$ cells even though PTB is present.[73]

Ribosome-associated poly r(C)-binding proteins bind at multiple sites within the poliovirus IRES.[65,155] One binding site for these proteins has been identified within stem loop IV of the poliovirus IRES.[65] Mutations in this region that abolish binding of poly r(C)-binding proteins cause decreased translation *in vitro.* Furthermore, depletion of poly r(C)-binding proteins from HeLa cell translation extracts results in inhibition of poliovirus IRES function.[66] When this assay was used to survey a wide range of picornaviral IRES elements, it was found that poly r(C)-binding proteins are required for function of the type I, but not the type II, IRES.[518] A second binding site for poly r(C)-binding proteins has been identified within a cloverleaf RNA structure that forms within the first 108 nucleotides of the positive-stranded poliovirus RNA genome.[155,377] The interaction of poly r(C)-binding proteins with this part of the RNA has been proposed to regulate whether a positive-stranded RNA molecule is translated or replicated.

The nuclear-cytoplasmic protein SRp20 functions with poly r(C)-binding protein 2 to promote initiation on poliovirus mRNA.[50] SRp20 binds to the KH3 domain of poly r(C)-binding protein 2. Depletion of SRp20 from cellular lysates by monoclonal antibodies or from cells by short interfering RNAs reduced IRES-mediated translation by 50%. Polysome analysis of infected cells by sucrose gradient fractionation demonstrated that both SRp20 and poly r(C)-binding protein 2 are at least partly associated with translation initiation complexes bound to stem loop V of the poliovirus 5′-UTR.[140]

Murine proliferation–associated protein 1 (Mpp-1) is required for the function of the foot-and-mouth disease virus IRES. This protein binds to a central domain of the viral IRES and acts synergistically with polypyrimidine tract-binding protein to increase the binding of eIF4F. It has been suggested that Mpp-1 may determine the tissues in which the IRES functions. To test this hypothesis, a recombinant virus was constructed by replacing the IRES of Theiler's virus with that of FMDV. Theiler's virus replicates in the mouse brain, but the recombinant virus cannot, possibly because of the absence of Mpp-1 in this organ.[398]

The DExH-box helicase DHX29 is necessary for the activity of the Aichi virus IRES.[546] Initially this protein was identified because it enabled efficient 48S complex formation on cellular mRNAs possessing highly structured 5′UTRs.[401] It is believed to be required for proper placement of the ribosome on RNAs possessing prokaryotic-like IRES elements, such as those of classic swine fever virus and the intergenic IRES of CrPV.[401]

No single cellular protein has been identified that is essential for the function of all viral IRES. A common property of cellular proteins needed for IRES activity is that they are RNA-binding proteins that can form multimers with the potential to contact the IRES at multiple points. This observation has led to the hypothesis that such proteins may act as RNA chaperones, maintaining the IRES in a structure that permits it to bind directly to the translational machinery.[235] IRES that do not require such chaperones may fold properly without the need for cellular proteins.

Processing of the Viral Polyprotein

Picornavirus proteins are synthesized by the translation of a single, long, ORF encoded by the viral positive-stranded RNA genome, followed by cleavage of the polyprotein by virus-encoded proteinases (Figs. 16.3 and 16.10). This strategy allows the synthesis of multiple protein products from a single RNA genome. The polyprotein is not observed in infected cells because it is processed as soon as the protease coding sequences have been translated. The polyprotein precursor is processed cotranslationally by intramolecular reactions (in *cis*) in what are called *primary cleavages,* followed by secondary processing in *cis* or in *trans* (intermolecular). All picornavirus genomes encode at least one proteinase, $3C^{pro}/3CD^{pro}$, and some encode L^{pro} or $2A^{pro}$.

The first protein encoded in the genome of aphthoviruses, cardioviruses, and erboviruses is the L protein (Figs. 16.3 and 16.10). The L protein of aphthoviruses and erboviruses is a proteinase that releases itself from the polyprotein by cleaving between its C-terminus and the N-terminus of VP4.[217,475] Based on sequence analysis, it was suggested that FMDV L^{pro} is related to thiol proteases.[178] This prediction was supported by the results of site-directed mutagenesis, which showed that Cys-51 and His-148 are the active-site amino acids.[396,427] The atomic structure of L^{pro} reveals that it consists of two domains, with a topology related to that of papain, a thiol proteinase[189] (Fig. 16.11). The active-site His is located at the top of the central α-helix, and substrate binds in the groove between the two domains. Besides releasing itself from the polyprotein, L^{pro} also cleaves the translation initiation factor eIF4G, causing inhibition of cellular translation.[119] The cardiovirus L protein, which does not have proteolytic activity, is released from the P1 precursor by $3C^{pro}$.[374]

In cells infected with enteroviruses (and possibly sapeloviruses), the primary cleavage between P1 and P2 is mediated by $2A^{pro}$. Cellular proteins are also cleaved by $2A^{pro}$, including eIF4GI, eIF4GII, Pabp, heart muscle dystrophin, and nucleoporins.[27,86,180,181,191,192,247,268,286,375] In the protein precursor of rhinovirus, poliovirus, and some other enteroviruses, the cleavage site for $2A^{pro}$ is between tyrosine and glycine. Other sites cleaved by $2A^{pro}$ include threonine-glycine and phenylalanine-glycine in certain Coxsackieviruses and echoviruses. Based on sequence alignments, it was suggested that the structure of $2A^{pro}$ would resemble that of small bacterial chymotrypsin-like proteinases (e.g., *Streptomyces griseus* proteinase A) and would possess a catalytic triad consisting of His-20, Asp-38, and an active-site nucleophile of Cys-109 rather than serine.[48] The results of site-directed mutagenesis and the resolution of the atomic structure of rhinovirus and Coxsackievirus B4 $2A^{pro}$ confirm that these residues comprise the active site and that the fold of $2A^{pro}$ is very similar to that of *Streptomyces griseus* proteinase A[45,388,467,545] (Fig. 16.11). However, $2A^{pro}$ differs from all known chymotrypsin-like proteinases in that the N-terminal domain is not a β-barrel, but rather a four-stranded antiparallel β-sheet. The larger C-terminal domain contains a six-stranded antiparallel β-barrel. The active-site catalytic triad is located in a cleft between the two domains. Another unusual feature of $2A^{pro}$ is a tightly bound zinc ion located at the beginning of the C-terminal domain. Biochemical and structural studies indicate that zinc is essential for the structure of the enzyme.[388,466,516]

The 2A/2B junction of aphthoviruses, avihepatoviruses, cardioviruses, erboviruses, senecaviruses, teschoviruses, Ljungan virus and duck hepatitis virus is cleaved not by proteolysis but by an unusual mechanism called ribosomal skipping.[126] Changes within the conserved amino acid sequence Asn-Pro-Gly-Pro,

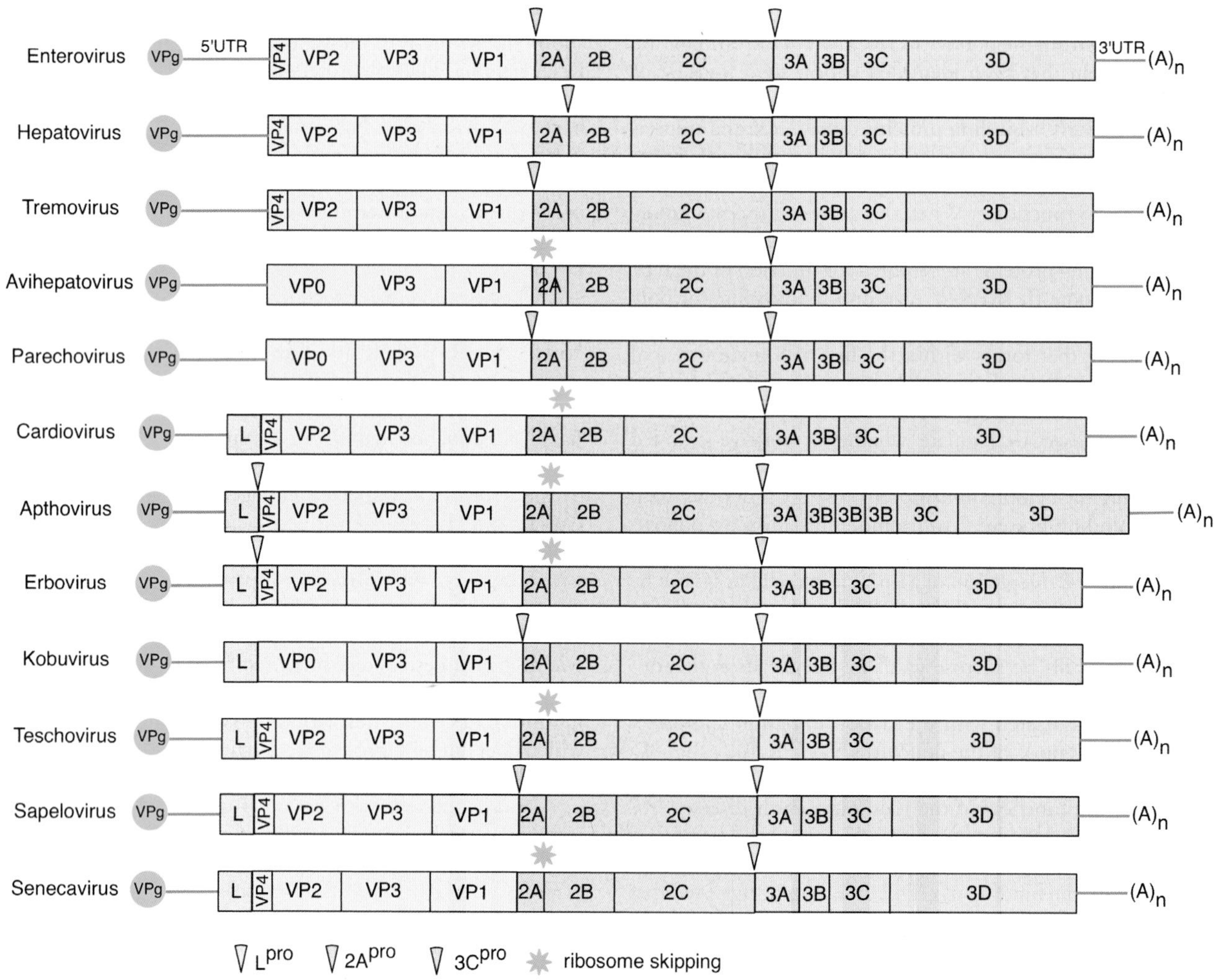

Enterovirus VPg 5'UTR VP4 VP2 VP3 VP1 2A 2B 2C 3A 3B 3C 3D 3'UTR (A)n
Hepatovirus VPg VP4 VP2 VP3 VP1 2A 2B 2C 3A 3B 3C 3D (A)n
Tremovirus VPg VP4 VP2 VP3 VP1 2A 2B 2C 3A 3B 3C 3D (A)n
Avihepatovirus VPg VP0 VP3 VP1 2A 2B 2C 3A 3B 3C 3D (A)n
Parechovirus VPg VP0 VP3 VP1 2A 2B 2C 3A 3B 3C 3D (A)n
Cardiovirus VPg L VP4 VP2 VP3 VP1 2A 2B 2C 3A 3B 3C 3D (A)n
Apthovirus VPg L VP4 VP2 VP3 VP1 2A 2B 2C 3A 3B 3B 3B 3C 3D (A)n
Erbovirus VPg L VP4 VP2 VP3 VP1 2A 2B 2C 3A 3B 3C 3D (A)n
Kobuvirus VPg L VP0 VP3 VP1 2A 2B 2C 3A 3B 3C 3D (A)n
Teschovirus VPg L VP4 VP2 VP3 VP1 2A 2B 2C 3A 3B 3C 3D (A)n
Sapelovirus VPg L VP4 VP2 VP3 VP1 2A 2B 2C 3A 3B 3C 3D (A)n
Senecavirus VPg L VP4 VP2 VP3 VP1 2A 2B 2C 3A 3B 3C 3D (A)n

L^pro 2A^pro 3C^pro ribosome skipping

FIGURE 16.10. Primary cleavages of picornavirus polyprotein. In all viruses shown, the P2–P3 cleavage is carried out by 3C^pro (*green triangle*). In some picornaviruses, the P1-P2 cleavage is carried out by 2A^pro (*magenta triangle*) or 3C^pro; in others, the 2A/2B bond is separated by ribosome skipping (*orange asterisk*). The L^pro proteinase (*blue triangle*) of aphthoviruses and erboviruses catalyzes its release from VP4.

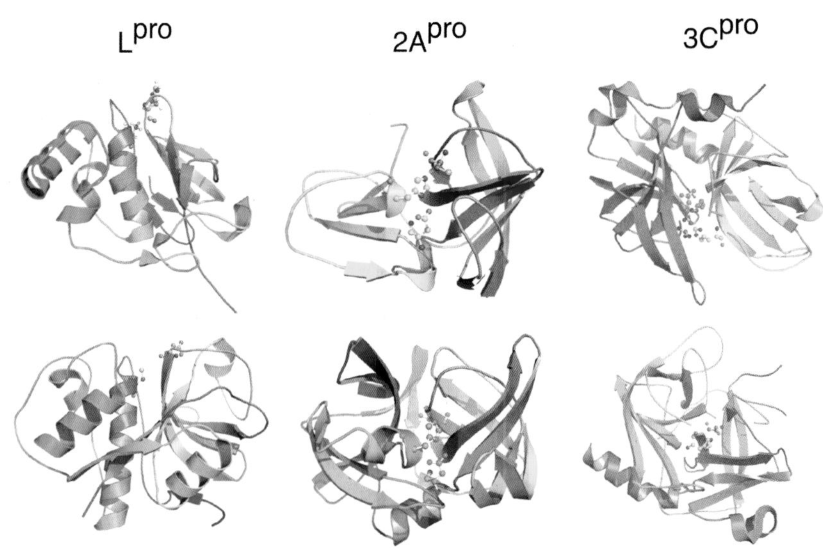

FIGURE 16.11. Three-dimensional structures of L^pro of foot-and-mouth disease virus, rhinovirus 2A^pro, and hepatitis A virus 3C^pro. Below each is the cellular proteinase that is structurally similar to each viral enzyme. Catalytic residues are drawn as *balls* and *sticks*. Images drawn with MacPymol using the following pdb files: 2sga, 2hrv, 2jqg, 1pip, 1hav, 5cha.

which contains the cleavage site Gly-Pro, disrupt cleavage.[374] The mechanism of NPG/P-mediated cleavage is not understood. It has been suggested that aphthovirus and cardiovirus 2A might modify the ribosome, causing the translational machinery to skip the synthesis of a glycyl-prolyl peptide bond at the C-terminus of 2A.[127] If this model is correct, it would represent a novel mechanism for the release of proteins from a polyprotein precursor without enzymatic cleavage. Similar 2A-like sequences have been found in other viral genomes and trypanosome non-LTR retrotransposons.[310] The ability of the 2A sequence to yield two proteins from a single open reading frame, without proteinase activity, has led to its use in many research and biomedical applications.[438]

Because only enteroviruses and possibly sapeloviruses have proteolytically active $2A^{pro}$, in cells infected with other picornaviruses, the VP1–2A cleavage is either carried out by $3C^{pro}$[245,374,448,449] or in Ljungan virus by an NPG/P sequence following the VP1 protein[249] (Fig. 16.10).

The polyprotein of Aichi virus, a member of the *Kobuvirus* genus, is unusual because the L and 2A proteins are not proteinases and there is no NPG/P motif at the 2A/2B junction. The only active proteinase encoded in the genome of this virus is $3C^{pro}$ and $3CD^{pro}$, which can process all cleavage sites in the polyprotein, including the VP1/2A site.[445] Efficient cleavage of the VP1/2A site requires tight binding of 3CD to the 2A region of the substrate.

All picornaviruses encode $3C^{pro}$, which carries out a primary cleavage between 2C and 3A (Fig. 16.10). Unlike the other picornavirus proteinases, $3C^{pro}$ also carries out secondary cleavages of the P1 and P2 precursors. Poliovirus $3C^{pro}$ cleaves only at the Gln-Gly dipeptide; however, $3C^{pro}$ of other picornaviruses has less strict cleavage specificities and cleaves at other sites, including Gln-Ser, Gln-Ile, Gln-Asn, Gln-Ala, Gln-Thr, and Gln-Val. Clearly, other determinants of cleavage exist because not all such dipeptides in picornavirus polyproteins are cleaved by $3C^{pro}$. Additional determinants include accessibility of the cleavage site to the enzyme, recognition of secondary and tertiary structures in the substrate by the enzyme, and amino acid sequences surrounding the cleavage site. For example, efficient cleavage of poliovirus Gln-Gly pairs requires an Ala at the P4 position (Gln is residue P1, numbering is toward the N-terminus).[64]

Sequence comparisons with cellular proteinases led to the prediction that $3C^{pro}$ folds similarly to the chymotrypsin-like serine proteinases, in particular *Staphylococcus aureus* proteinase.[48,174–177] The putative catalytic triad was believed to consist of His-40, Asp-71 (aphthoviruses and cardioviruses) or Glu-71 (enteroviruses and rhinoviruses), and Cys-147 as the nucleophilic residue, in contrast to serine in cellular serine proteinases. These predictions have been confirmed by site-directed mutagenesis and by resolution of the atomic structures of rhinovirus, hepatitis A virus, poliovirus, FMDV, and enterovirus 71 $3C^{pro}$.[89,186,201,267,323,346,388,519] The viral enzyme folds into two equivalent β-barrels like chymotrypsin (Fig. 16.11), but differs in some of the connecting loops, the orientation of the catalytic residues, and in areas needed for transition-state stabilization. The acidic member of the catalytic triad, Glu or Asp, points away from the active-site His and, therefore, is not believed to assist in catalysis. However, $3C^{pro}$ also binds viral RNA (see discussion of genome replication and mRNA synthesis), and this binding site is distal from the active site of the enzyme. The presence of this RNA-binding site imposes evolutionary constraints on $3C^{pro}$ that are not found in other proteinases.

Both $3C^{pro}$ and $2A^{pro}$ are active in the nascent polypeptide and release themselves from the polyprotein by self-cleavage. After the proteinases have been released, they cleave the polyprotein in *trans*. The cascade of processing events varies for different picornaviruses. In cells infected with rhinovirus and enteroviruses, the initial event in the processing cascade is the release of the P1 precursor from the nascent P2–P3 protein by $2A^{pro}$. The activity of $2A^{pro}$ does not depend on whether it is cleaved from the precursor,[210] but further processing of P1 by $3CD^{pro}$ does not occur unless $2A^{pro}$ is released from P1.[357,543] Next, $3CD^{pro}$ is released from the P3 precursor by autocatalytic cleavage. This proteinase, which contains the entire sequence of the viral RNA polymerase, carries out secondary cleavage of glutamine-glycine dipeptides in poliovirus P1 far more efficiently than $3C^{pro}$.[253,544] Both $3C^{pro}$ and $3CD^{pro}$ process proteins of the P2 and P3 regions with similar efficiency. The $3D^{pol}$ sequence within $3CD^{pro}$ may be required to recognize structural motifs in properly folded P1, allowing efficient processing by the $3C^{pro}$ part of the enzyme. The presence of multiple activities in a single protein is not found among eukaryotic proteinases and is an example of how the coding capacity of small viral genomes can be maximized. Not all picornaviruses require $3CD^{pro}$ to process P1; aphthoviruses, cardioviruses, and hepatoviruses produce $3C^{pro}$ that can cleave P1 without additional viral protein sequence.

An advantage of the polyprotein strategy is that expression can be controlled by the rate and extent of proteolytic processing. Alternative use of cleavage sites can also produce proteins with different activities. For example, because $3CD^{pro}$ is required for processing of the poliovirus capsid protein precursor P1, the extent of capsid protein processing can be controlled by regulating the amount of $3CD^{pro}$ that is produced. Because $3CD^{pro}$ does not possess RNA polymerase activity, some of it must be cleaved to allow RNA replication.

A final processing step occurs during maturation, when VP0 is cleaved to form VP4 and VP2. This event is discussed later.

VIRAL RNA SYNTHESIS

In the 1950s, it was believed that the genome of RNA viruses was replicated by the cellular DNA-dependent RNA polymerase, through an intermediate DNA strand. The replication of RNA viruses, therefore, was thought to occur entirely in the cell nucleus. In the early 1960s, studies of mengovirus showed that virus infection results in the induction of a cytoplasmic enzyme that can synthesize viral RNA in the presence of actinomycin D.[30] This observation suggested that viral genome replication occurred through a virus-specific, RNA-dependent RNA polymerase because cellular RNA synthesis is DNA dependent; it occurs in the nucleus and is sensitive to actinomycin D. A similar cytoplasmic, actinomycin D–resistant genome replication system was discovered in poliovirus-infected cells.[28]

In poliovirus-infected cells, the positive-stranded genome is amplified to about 50,000 copies per cell through a negative-stranded intermediate. Three forms of viral RNA have been identified in the cell; single-stranded RNA, replicative intermediate (RI), and replicative form (RF). Single-stranded RNA, the most abundant form, is exclusively positive stranded; free negative strands have never been detected in infected cells. RI is full-length RNA from which six to eight nascent strands are attached. RI is largely of positive polarity with nascent negative strands, although the opposite configuration has been detected. RF is a double-stranded structure, consisting of one full-length copy of the positive and negative strands. Viral RNA synthesis is asymmetric; the synthesis of positive strands is 30 to 70 times greater than the synthesis of negative strands.[162,364]

Viral RNA-Dependent RNA Polymerase, 3D^{pol}

The first evidence for a viral RNA-dependent RNA polymerase activity came from experiments in which lysates from cells infected with mengovirus or poliovirus were assayed for viral RNA polymerase activity by the incorporation of a radioactive nucleotide into viral RNA.[29] Initial experiments demonstrated that the viral RNA polymerase is associated with a cellular membrane fraction, subsequently shown to be comprised of smooth membranes, which was called the *RNA replication complex.*[166] A major component of the replication complex was a viral protein that migrated at 63,000 d on polyacrylamide gels (therefore, called p63), which was suggested to be the viral RNA-dependent RNA polymerase. Other viral and host proteins, including 2BC, 2C, 3AB, and 3C^{pro}, however, were detected in the RNA replication complexes.

A limitation of this early work was that replication complexes only copied viral RNA already present in the complex, and did not respond to added RNA. Attempts were made, therefore, to purify a template-dependent enzyme from membrane fractions of infected cells, using a poly(A) template and an oligo(U) primer. A poly(U) polymerase activity was purified from poliovirus-infected cells, which could also copy poliovirus RNA in the presence of an oligo(U) primer. Highly purified preparations contained only p63, the major viral protein found in membranous replication complexes.[141,504] This protein is the poliovirus RNA polymerase, now known as 3D^{pol}. In the absence of an oligo(U) primer, 3D^{pol} cannot copy poliovirus RNA. Recombinant 3D^{pol} purified from bacteria or insect cells also requires the presence of an oligo(U) primer to copy poliovirus RNA.[354,404] 3D^{pol}, therefore, is a template- and primer-dependent enzyme that can copy poliovirus RNA. Its molecular weight predicted from the amino acid sequence is 53 kd.

The structures of three of the four types of polymerases—DNA-dependent DNA polymerase, DNA-dependent RNA polymerase, and RNA-dependent DNA polymerase (reverse transcriptase)—are characterized by analogy with a right hand, consisting of a palm, fingers, and thumb. The palm domain contains the active site of the enzyme. The first structure of an RNA-dependent RNA polymerase is that of poliovirus 3D^{pol}, first determined at 2.6 Å resolution by x-ray crystallography.[202] Additional structures of 3D^{pol} from poliovirus, three rhinovirus serotypes, and coxsackievirus B3 provide resolution of virtually all amino acids in the protein, offering a complete picture of the enzyme.[22,81,307,488] The enzyme has the same overall shape as other polymerases, although the fingers and thumb differ (Fig. 16.12). The fingers and thumb domains interact, resulting in an encircled active site. The palm domain contains four conserved amino acid motifs (B, C, D, E) that are found in other RNA-dependent polymerases. Amino acids 1 to 68 (forming the ring finger) cross the active site under the index finger and extend to the enzyme surface. The ring finger, which is the top of the channel through which nucleoside triphosphates enter, includes conserved motif F that is important for interacting with the triphosphates. Template and primer molecules that contact the front face of 3D^{pol} probably use the opening for nucleotide exchange, as do other polymerases. A template RNA channel in the fingers domain of all the picornavirus polymerases is lined with basic amino acids that are predicted to interact with viral template as it enters the active site. Alteration of amino acids in this channel identifies key residues for template binding or elongation.[284]

The RNA polymerase 3D^{pol} is produced by cleavage of a precursor protein, 3CD^{pro}, which is highly active as a proteinase, binds *cre* (see below), but has no polymerase activity. It was suggested that processing of 3CD affected the location of the N-terminus of 3D^{pol}, which is buried in a surface pocket in 3D^{pol}. There it makes hydrogen bonds that position Asp238, an essential residue that selects for the 2′ OH group of substrate rNTP (ribonucleoside triphosphate), in the active site. On proteolysis, the N-terminal Gly was believed to push Asp-238 a distance of 1.4 Å into the catalytic site. However, a comparison of structures of 3D^{pol} and 3CD^{pro} did not show a significant difference in the position of Asp238.[317,488] Resolution of the structure of the coxsackievirus B3 3D^{pol} reveals an unusual conformation for residue 5, which is located at a distortion within a β-strand that is conserved in all known 3D^{pol} structures.[81] Substitution of more hydrophobic residues at this position results in higher enzymatic activity. It has been proposed that this residue becomes buried during the repositioning of the nucleotide that takes place before phosphoryl transfer, which cannot occur if the N-terminus has not been properly generated by proteolytic processing.

The first poliovirus 3D^{pol} structure revealed that the polymerase molecules interacted in a head-to-tail manner and formed fibers; subsequently, the protein was shown to form a lattice.[311] The implication was that RNA would be replicated as it moved along the lattice, rather than the polymerase moving on the template. The head-to-tail fibers were formed by interface I, which involves more than 23 amino acid side chains between the thumb of one polymerase and the back of the palm of another (Fig. 16.13). Amino acid changes in the back of the thumb that disrupt this interface impaired replication.[120,221] Repetition of this interaction in a head-to-tail fashion results in long fibers of polymerase molecules 50 Å in diameter. A similar interface was observed in crystals of 3D^{pol} of rhinovirus 14 but not rhinoviruses 16 or 1b.[307] Interface II is formed by N-terminal polypeptide segments, which may lead to a network of polymerase fibers in combination with interactions at interface I. These N-terminal polypeptide segments may originate from different polymerase molecules. The N-terminus of 3D^{pol} is required for enzyme activity, which would support the idea that interface II interactions are of functional consequence. Furthermore, intermolecular cross-linking has been observed between cysteines engineered at Ala-29 and Ile-441 of poliovirus 3D^{pol}[221] and disruption of these interactions led to lethality.[486] Polymerase-containing oligomeric structures resembling those seen with purified 3D^{pol} were observed on the surface of vesicles isolated from poliovirus-infected cells.[311] Because picornavirus RNA synthesis occurs on membranous vesicles, the concept of a flat, catalytic lattice is mechanistically attractive.

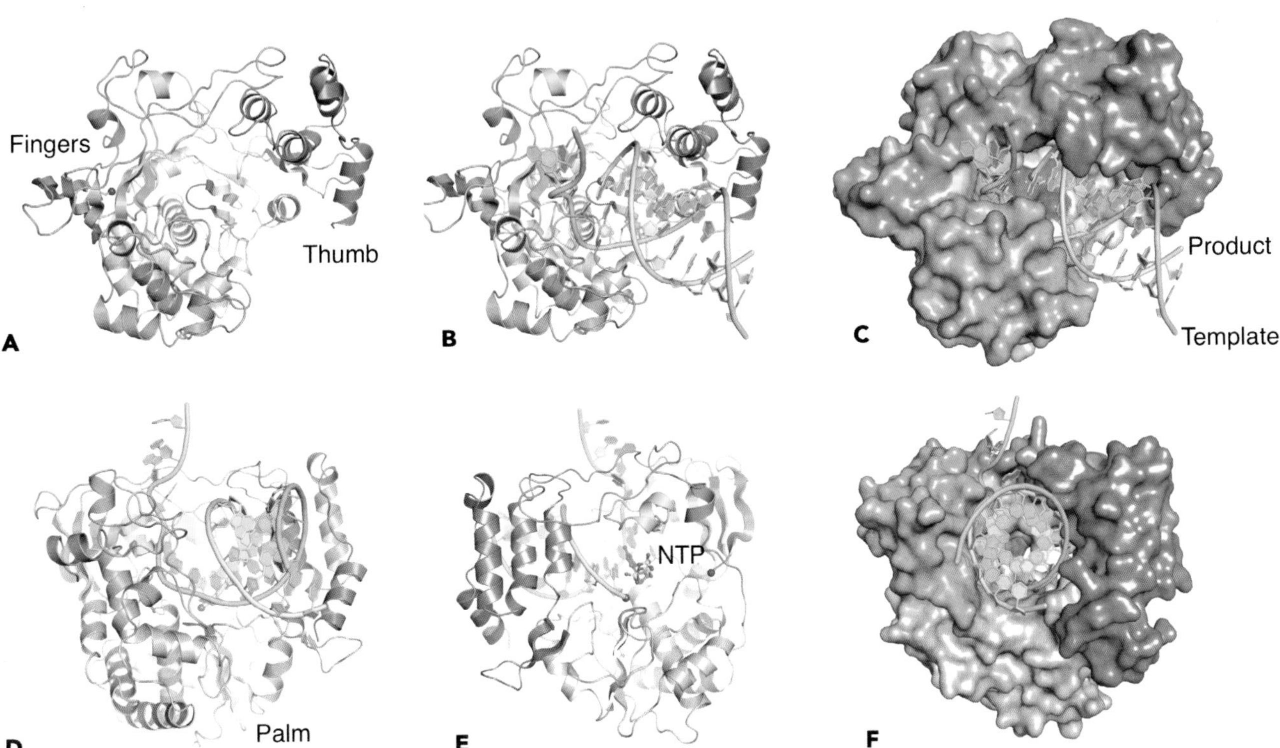

FIGURE 16.12. Three-dimensional structure of poliovirus 3D^{pol}. Structure of poliovirus 3D^{pol} polymerase and its elongation complex with primer-template RNA. The polymerase structure can be described by analogy to a cupped right hand, consisting of palm (*gray*) and thumb (*blue*) domains and a fingers domains with four discrete structural elements known as the index (*green*), middle (*orange*), ring (*yellow*), and pinky (*red*) fingers. The structure of the elongation complex shows the path of the RNA as the template strand (*cyan*) enters the polymerase from the top and of the template-product (*gold*) duplex as it exits the polymerase between the pinky finger and thumb structures.[220] **A-C:** Views from the top of the polymerase looking down into the active site (*magenta*) of 3D^{pol} in the absence of RNA **(A)**, the 3D^{pol} elongation complex with bound RNA **(B)**, and the elongation complex with a surface representation of the polymerase to show how the product RNA duplex is clamped in place between the pinky finger and thumb structures **(C)**. **D:** Front view of the elongation complex showing the path template and product RNA strands. **E:** Back view of the elongation complex showing the NTP entry channel with the priming 3′ OH (*red sphere*) positioned above the active site and a bound di-deoxy-CTP (*green ball-and-stick with phosphate groups in red and yellow*). **F:** Surface representation of the elongation complex looking down the axis of the exiting RNA duplex. 3D^{pol} from poliovirus and closely related picornaviruses is activated upon cleavage from the viral polyprotein, resulting in a newly created N-terminus that becomes buried in a pocket at the base of the finger domain that is ≈15 Å away from the active site itself (*blue sphere* in **A** and **E**). (Courtesy of Olve Peersen, Colorado State University.)

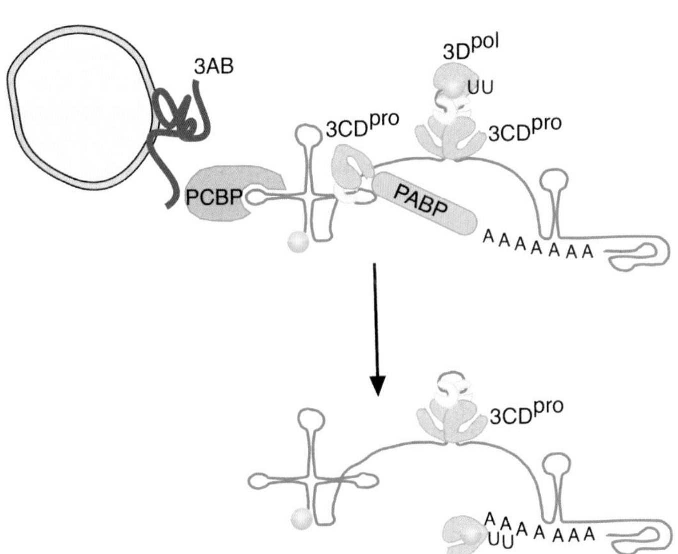

FIGURE 16.13. Model for the synthesis of poliovirus (–) strand RNA. The (+) strand template is shown in green with the 5′-cloverleaf structure, the internal *cre* sequence, and the 3′ pseudoknot. A ribonucleoprotein complex is formed when poly r(C)-binding protein (PCBP) and 3CD^{pro} bind the cloverleaf structure. The ribonucleoprotein complex interacts with PABP1, which is bound to the 3′-poly(A) sequence, producing a circular template. Protease 3CD^{pro} cleaves membrane-bound 3AB to produce VPg and 3A. The *cre* sequence binds 3D^{pol}, 3CD^{pro}, and VPg. VPg-pUpU is synthesized by 3D^{pol} using the sequence AAACA of *cre* as template. The complex is transferred to the 3′ end of the genome, and 3D^{pol} uses VPg-pUpU to prime RNA synthesis.

Viral Accessory Proteins

The poliovirus capsid proteins are not required for viral RNA synthesis; the region of the viral genome that encodes these proteins can be deleted without affecting the ability of viral RNA to replicate in cells.[260] The capsid coding regions of rhinovirus, Theiler's virus, and Mengovirus, however, contain a *cis*-acting RNA sequence required for genome replication.[304,328,329] A *cis*-acting RNA sequence required for RNA replication has also been identified in the poliovirus protein 2C coding region.[171] Genetic and biochemical studies implicate most proteins of the P2 and P3 regions of the genome in RNA synthesis.

2A Protein

As discussed above, 2A^{pro} protein is necessary for proteolytic cleavage of the polyprotein. The protein also appears to have a role in RNA replication. A deletion within the 2A^{pro} coding sequence severely inhibits replication of subgenomic replicons, which lack the capsid region and are not dependent on proteolytic activity of 2A^{pro} to release the P1 region.[98] In another approach, a second IRES element was placed in the poliovirus genome before the 2A^{pro} coding region, effectively alleviating the need for the processing activity of the enzyme. Such viruses are viable.[339] Deletion of part of the coding region for 2A^{pro} is lethal, however. These results suggest that 2A^{pro} also plays a role in viral RNA replication. By using a cell-free replication system, it was possible to determine the effect of 2A^{pro} on each step of the replication cycle.[255] The results show that 2A^{pro} stimulates the initiation of negative-strand synthesis, but has no effect on positive-strand synthesis. How 2A^{pro} achieves this affect is not known, but it has been suggested that the proteinase might modify a cellular protein required for negative-strand RNA synthesis.[255]

2B Protein

The 2B protein is a small, hydrophobic, membrane-associated protein that is involved at an early step of viral RNA synthesis. Alterations of the 2B protein of poliovirus and coxsackievirus lead to viruses with defects in RNA synthesis.[251,505] Adaptation of rhinoviruses to mouse cells is mediated in part by amino acid changes in 2B, which allow viral RNA synthesis in this host cell.[206] The C-terminus of 2B contains a hydrophobic region and a conserved putative amphipathic α-helix that appear to be crucial to the function of the protein and its association with membranes.[506] Protein 2B has been called a *viroporin,* a protein that oligomerizes and inserts into membranes to create channels.[2,170] The exact role of 2B in RNA synthesis, however, is not known. Synthesis of protein 2B leads to an inhibition of protein secretion from the Golgi apparatus[35,123] and permeabilization of membranes,[2,7,444,508,509] which may play a role in release of virus from cells. Protein 2B is also partly responsible for the proliferation of membranous vesicles in infected cells, which are the sites of viral RNA replication. Because protein 3A has the same effect, it is not clear whether altered membrane proliferation is responsible for the RNA-defective phenotype in 2B mutants.

2C Protein

Protein 2C is a highly conserved protein with membrane-, RNA-, and NTP-binding regions.[131,429,430,508,509] The structure of 2C suggests that it contains three domains, with amphipathic α-helices at both the N- and C-termini that mediate peripheral association with membranes[285,487] and a central region with NTP-binding domains. Mutations responsible for resistance of poliovirus and echovirus to guanidine hydrochloride, which blocks viral RNA replication, are located in the 2C protein.[278,399] This compound has been shown to inhibit specifically the initiation of negative-stranded RNA synthesis and has no effect on initiation of positive-stranded RNA synthesis or on elongation on either strand.[40] The nucleoside triphosphatase (NTPase) activity of protein 2C is inhibited by guanidine.[394] Protein 2C shares amino acid homology with known RNA helicases, proteins encoded by most positive-stranded RNA viruses with large genomes. These enzymes are believed to be necessary to unwind double-stranded RNA structures that form during RNA replication. Purified protein 2C, however, does not have RNA helicase activity.[429] Alteration of conserved amino acids within the NTPase domain of 2C results in loss of viral infectivity; 2C, therefore, may have two functions during viral RNA synthesis: as an NTPase and directing replication complexes to cell membranes. Synthesis of 2C causes disassembly of the Golgi apparatus and endoplasmic reticulum (ER), and formation of vesicular structures similar, but not identical to, those that constitute the replication complex.[6,92]

2BC Protein

Much of protein 2BC, the precursor to 2B and 2C, remains uncleaved during infection, and its presence is critical to viral replication.[92] Synthesis of 2BC causes membrane permeabilization to a greater degree than 2B synthesis alone,[7] and leads to the formation of vesicles that are more similar to those formed during viral infection than does protein 2C.[6,92] The C-terminus of 2B and the N-terminus of 2C may interact intramolecularly in 2BC, and protein cleavage may cause a conformational change that alters the properties of 2B and 2C individually.[35,507] Larger 2BC-containing precursors are also required for certain steps of replication,[254] although an intact 2C–3A junction is not strictly required.[380]

3AB Protein

A strongly hydrophobic region in the C-terminus of 3A mediates the association of 3A and its precursor, 3AB, with membranes.[124,474,495] Amino acid changes in the hydrophobic region of 3A yield replication-defective viruses.[163,287] Changes in viral host range have been mapped to changes in 3A protein.[49,206,287,365] The solution structure of 3A demonstrates that it is a homodimer, with the dimer interface located in the central region of the protein.[474] The requirement for 3A dimerization during infection has not been explored. Protein 3B, also known as VPg, plays an indispensable role in viral replication by acting as a protein primer for viral RNA synthesis (see below). Protein 3AB is believed to anchor VPg in membranes for the priming step of RNA synthesis. The purified protein greatly stimulates 3D^{pol} activity *in vitro*[379,405,424] as well as the proteolytic activity of 3CD^{pro}.[340] 3AB interacts with 3D^{pol} and 3CD^{pro} in infected cells and with 3D^{pol} in the yeast two-hybrid system.[226] Amino acid changes in 3D^{pol} that disrupt its interaction with 3AB result in viruses with defects in protein processing and viral RNA synthesis.[161,163] A complex of 3AB and 3CD^{pro} also binds the 3′-terminal sequence of poliovirus RNA.

Cellular Accessory Proteins

Early studies of poliovirus replication using purified components suggested that a host cell protein is required for copying the viral RNA by 3D^{pol} in the absence of an oligo(U) primer.[116] Although this protein was never identified, the concept of a host factor required for poliovirus replication endured, largely because an ample precedent was seen for the participation of host cell components in a viral RNA replicase. The best-studied example is the RNA replicase of the bacteriophage Qβ, which is a multisubunit enzyme consisting of a 65-kd virus-encoded protein and three host proteins: ribosomal protein S1 and translation factors EF-Tu and EF-Ts.[203] The 65-kd viral protein has no RNA polymerase activity in the absence of the host factors but has sequence similarity with known RNA-dependent RNA polymerases. A subunit of the translation initiation factor eIF-3 is part of the polymerase from brome mosaic virus.[412] Two different experimental systems have been used to provide additional evidence that poliovirus RNA synthesis requires host cell components.

When purified poliovirus RNA is incubated *in vitro* with a cytoplasmic extract prepared from cultured, permissive cells, the viral RNA is translated, the resulting protein is proteolytically processed, and the genome is replicated and assembled into new infectious virus particles.[338] When guanidine, an inhibitor of poliovirus RNA synthesis, is included in the reaction, complexes are formed, but elongation cannot occur.[38] The preinitiation complexes can be isolated free of guanidine and, when added to new cytoplasmic extracts, RNA synthesis occurs. In the absence of cytoplasmic extract, preinitiation complexes do not synthesize viral RNA.[37] These results indicate that one or more soluble cellular components are required for the initiation of viral RNA replication. A similar conclusion comes from studies in which poliovirus RNA is injected into oocytes derived from the African clawed toad, *Xenopus laevis.* Poliovirus RNA cannot replicate in *Xenopus* oocytes unless it is coinjected with a cytoplasmic extract from human cells.[154]

Cellular poly r(C)-binding proteins are required for poliovirus RNA synthesis. These proteins bind to a cloverleaf-like secondary structure, also called a stem-loop I, that forms in the first 108 nucleotides of positive-stranded RNA (Fig. 16.13). Binding of poly r(C)-binding protein to the cloverleaf is necessary for the binding of viral protein 3CD^{pro} to the opposite side of the same cloverleaf.[16,18,155,377] Formation of a ribonucleoprotein complex composed of the 5′ cloverleaf, 3CD^{pro}, and a cellular protein is essential for the initiation of viral RNA synthesis.[18] The human cell protein required for replication of poliovirus RNA in *Xenopus* oocytes has also been identified as poly r(C)-binding protein.[155] A model of how these interactions lead to viral RNA synthesis is shown in Figure 16.14. The ternary complex with stem-loop I may also function during positive-strand RNA synthesis.[515]

Another candidate for a host protein that is essential for poliovirus RNA synthesis is poly(A)-binding protein 1. This protein interacts with poly r(C)-binding protein, 3CD^{pro}, and the 3′-poly(A) tail of poliovirus RNA, circularizing the genome[40,212] (Fig. 16.13). Formation of this circular ribonucleoprotein complex is required for negative-strand RNA synthesis.

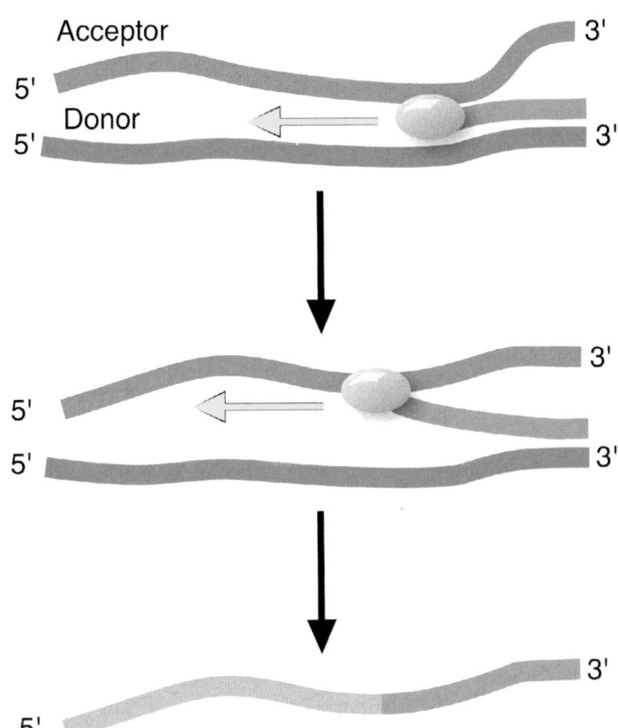

FIGURE 16.14. Schematic diagram of RNA recombination in picornavirus-infected cells by template switching, or copy choice. Two parental genomes, the acceptor and donor, are shown. The RNA polymerase (*blue*) is shown copying the 3′ end of donor RNA and switching to the acceptor genome **(middle)**. As a result of this template switch, the recombinant RNA shown is formed **(bottom)**.

Protein-Primed RNA Synthesis

As discussed, poliovirus 3D^{pol} is a primer-dependent enzyme that will not copy poliovirus RNA *in vitro* without an oligo(U) primer. The discovery of VPg linked to poliovirus genome RNA, as well as to the 5′ end of newly synthesized positive- and negative-stranded RNA, suggested that VPg might be involved in the initiation of RNA synthesis. This hypothesis was supported by the finding that both VPg and a uridylylated form of the protein, VPg-pUpU, can be found in infected cells.[110] Furthermore, VPg-pUpU can be synthesized *in vitro* in a membrane fraction from poliovirus-infected cells.[481] It was also argued that a precursor of VPg, known as *3AB,* is likely to participate in the initiation reaction. 3AB is a membrane-bound polypeptide and, therefore, an ideal candidate to act as a VPg donor in membranous replication complexes. Viruses containing a mutation in 3AB that decreases its hydrophobicity are defective in initiation of RNA synthesis, *in vitro* uridylylation of VPg, and *in vivo* synthesis of positive-stranded viral RNA.[161,163] Because no protein larger than VPg has been detected linked to nascent RNA strands, it is likely that 3AB is rapidly cleaved by the proteinase 3C^{pro} to form VPg-linked RNA. Additional evidence that VPg can serve as a primer for poliovirus RNA synthesis comes from experiments in which synthetic VPg is first uridylylated *in vitro,* then added to an *in vitro* polymerase reaction containing a poly(A) template and 3D^{pol}.[381] The labeled, uridylylated VPg is extended to form poly(U). Poliovirus RNA replication is primed by a genome-linked protein, a mechanism also involved in adenovirus DNA replication. A model for VPg priming of poliovirus RNA synthesis is shown in Figure 16.13.

The template for uridylylation of VPg is an RNA hairpin, the *cis*-acting replication element, *cre,* located in the coding region of picornaviruses.[382,425,540] The cre functions independent of position in the genome, and its location differs among viruses. Protein 3C is a major determinant of RNA binding activity, but 3AB may also be involved in cre recognition.[378,533] Whether cre-dependent VPg uridylylation is involved only in (+) strand RNA synthesis, or also during synthesis of the (–) strand, is controversial.[173,341,350,425]

The results of genetic analyses indicate that the binding site for VPg (as part of 3AB) on 3D^{pol} is on the surface of the enzyme near conserved motif E, on the back side of the palm near the base of the thumb, which is distant from the catalytic center.[312] Because uridylylation of VPg takes place at the same polymerase active site used for chain elongation, it must occur through the opposite side of the nucleotide channel used for chain elongation. How the uridylated VPg is transferred to the front side of the polymerase for use in priming RNA synthesis is not known. The primer might be transferred through the nucleotide channel, or, as suggested by experimental results, to another polymerase molecule.[485] Resolution of the structure of rhinovirus 3D^{pol} suggested that VPg could bind via the front face of the polymerase.[22] However, structure of the FMDV 3D^{pol} bound to VPg revealed that the protein does not bind to the active site, consistent with the results of genetic analyses. Whether there are virus-specific mechanisms of VPg priming remains to be determined.

Cellular Site of RNA Synthesis

Picornaviral RNA synthesis, like that of most RNA viruses, occurs in the cytoplasm of the cell. Picornavirus infection leads to the proliferation and rearrangement of intracellular membranes in infected cells. The ER and Golgi apparatus are destroyed in this process, and the cytoplasm fills with double-membraned vesicles.[115,447] Viral RNA replication occurs on the cytoplasmic surfaces of these vesicles.[63,92,133] Membrane localization of viral RNA replication proteins may ensure high local concentrations of replication components, increasing the rates or efficiencies of replication reactions. It has also been suggested that membrane localization of viral RNA replication proteins could promote their oligomerization.[311]

Poliovirus proteins 3A and 2BC are sufficient to induce the formation of vesicles that are biochemically and ultrastructurally similar to those observed in virus-infected cells.[476] Because viral proteins 2A and 2BC are known to localize to the ER, a plausible hypothesis is that they promote vesicle formation from this site.[124] One source of virus-induced vesicles may be those that participate in ER-to-Golgi trafficking. Budding of vesicles from the ER is initiated by COPII coats; these fuse to create the ER-Golgi intermediate compartment (ERGIC). COPI coats initiate budding of vesicles from the ERGIC that move to the Golgi. It has been suggested that poliovirus-induced vesicles are morphologically similar to COPII vesicles, which are involved in anterograde transport.[442] The COPII proteins Sec13/31 were shown to colocalize with the viral 2B protein on the surface of the vesicles. The inhibition of poliovirus and rhinovirus RNA replication by brefeldin A, however, apparently contradicts this hypothesis.[158,233,324] Brefeldin A interferes with formation of COPI, but not COPII or autophagic vesicles, by inhibiting the exchange of guanosine triphosphate (GDP) for guanosine triphosphate (GTP) by the adenosine diphosphate (ADP) ribosylation factor, Arf. Brefeldin prevents COPI coat assembly by targeting the Arf1 guanine exchange factors GBF1, BIG1 and BIG2. A brefeldin-resistant form of GBF1 was found to allow poliovirus replication in the presence of the drug.[54] Viral protein 3A binds GBF1, recruiting it to replication complexes, and this interaction, which BFA functionally interferes with, is required for replication.[54,290] When poliovirus proteins are synthesized in cells in the absence of viral RNA replication, membrane remodeling is insensitive to brefeldin A, indicating that the drug inhibits viral replication (by interfering with GBF1), not remodeling of cellular membranes.[54]

The binding of 3A to GBF1 diverts the protein from its normal function in the secretory pathway, and explains inhibition of protein secretion by viral infection.[123] The result is an inhibition of COPI vesicle formation; these may be diverted to form viral replication complexes. In support of this hypothesis, components of COPI coats have been found in association with echovirus replication complexes.[158]

The vesicles induced during poliovirus and rhinovirus infection may also be derived from the cellular autophagosomal pathway. In response to a variety of stimuli, including cellular starvation, cells break down cytoplasmic proteins and organelles within autophagosomes, double-membraned structures that mature and become degradative. The poliovirus-induced vesicles bear several hallmarks of autophagosomes, including their double-membraned structure, the presence of cytoplasmic content within the vesicles,[447] and colocalization with autophagosomal markers latency-associated membrane protein 1 (LAMP1) and LC3.[239] In support of the autophagosomal origin of virus-induced vesicles, stimulation of autophagy increased virus yield, whereas inhibition of the autophagosomal pathway by drugs or small interfering RNA (siRNA) reduced virus yield.[239] These findings indicate that components of the cellular autophagosomal pathway are subverted to provide membranous supports for viral RNA replication complexes. Autophagosomes are induced during infection with other picornaviruses, including FMDV, enterovirus 71, EMCV, rhinoviruses, and coxsackieviruses (reviewed in[277]). They are not present in rhinovirus 1A–infected cells,[414] however, and it is not clear if they are needed for replication of rhinovirus 2.[75] Replication membranes in rhinovirus 1A–infected cells appear to be derived from the Golgi apparatus, whose fragmentation correlates with the presence of the viral 3A protein.[414]

A recent study on the three-dimensional architecture of the poliovirus-induced replication complexes revealed that membrane remodeling begins with the formation, often in association with a Golgi antigen, of a network of irregularly shaped, single-membrane, branching tubular structures.[55] Later in infection these become double-membraned structures, but the highest rates of viral RNA synthesis occur when the mainly single-membraned convoluted tubules are present.

At least two viral proteins, 2C and 3AB, bring the replication complex to membranous vesicles. As discussed, 3AB is a hydrophobic protein that anchors the protein primer VPg in the membrane for RNA synthesis. Protein 3AB binds 3D^{pol} and 3CD^{pro}, thereby recruiting the replication complex to membranes. Protein 2C has an RNA-binding domain, which could also anchor viral RNA to membranes in the replication complexes.[132]

Translation and Replication of the Same RNA Molecule

The genomic RNA of picornaviruses is not only mRNA but also the template for synthesis of negative-stranded RNA. How does the viral polymerase, traveling in a 3′ to 5′ direction on the positive strand, avoid collisions with ribosomes translating in the opposite direction? It is believed that a mechanism exists to avoid the two processes occurring simultaneously. *In vitro* experiments using inhibitors of protein synthesis demonstrate that, when ribosomes are frozen on the viral RNA, replication of the RNA is inhibited. In contrast, when ribosomes are released from the viral RNA, its replication is increased.[39] These results suggest that replication and translation cannot occur on the same template simultaneously.

A mechanism for regulating viral RNA translation and replication involves cleavage of poly r(C)-binding protein. This protein functions in IRES-dependent translation by binding stem-loop IV[65,155] (Fig. 16.15), and in viral RNA synthesis by binding stem-loop I.[157,377] Poly r(C)-binding protein is cleaved by viral $3C^{pro}$; the cleaved protein can no longer stimulate IRES-dependent protein synthesis but is competent to participate in the initiation of viral RNA synthesis.[386] Another mechanism involves binding of 3CD to stem-loop I, which increases the binding affinity of poly r(C)-binding protein for stem-loop I and decreases it for stem-loop IV.[156] Cleavage of PTB by $3C^{pro}$ also leads to reduced viral translation.[26] The consequence of these modifications is that viral IRES-dependent translation is down-regulated, and ribosomes are cleared from the viral mRNA, allowing unimpeded transit of RNA polymerase.

Whether there exist mechanisms to regulate translation and replication of RNA, experimental evidence indicates that some ribosome and RNA polymerase collisions do occur. This conclusion is based on the isolation of a poliovirus variant whose genome contains an insertion of a 15 nucleotide sequence from 28S ribosomal RNA (rRNA).[88] Apparently, the RNA polymerase collided with a ribosome, copied 15 nucleotides of rRNA, and then returned to the viral RNA template.

Discrimination of Viral and Cellular RNA

The RNA-dependent RNA polymerases of picornaviruses are template-specific enzymes. Poliovirus $3D^{pol}$ copies only viral RNA, not cellular mRNA, in infected cells. The purified enzyme, however, will copy any polyadenylated RNA if provided with an oligo(U) primer. This observation has led to the suggestion that template specificity probably resides in the interaction of replication proteins with sequence elements in the viral RNA. The *cis*-acting RNA elements located within the coding region of picornaviruses, which direct the uridylylation of VPg, are binding sites for $3CD^{pro}$ (Fig. 16.13). The 3′-noncoding region of the viral positive-stranded RNA contains an RNA pseudoknot conserved among picornaviruses that is believed to play a role in the specificity of copying by $3D^{pol}$.[241] Disruption of the pseudoknot by mutagenesis produces viruses that have impaired RNA synthesis, indicating the importance of the structure in the synthesis of negative-stranded RNA. $3D^{pol}$ or $3CD^{pro}$ cannot bind to the 3′ end of poliovirus RNA unless 3AB is present. The interaction of 3AB–$3D^{pol}$ may determine the specificity of binding to the 3′ pseudoknot.

Despite experimental results that underscore the importance of the pseudoknot in RNA synthesis, polioviruses from which the entire 3′-noncoding region of the viral RNA has been removed are able to replicate.[77,489] This finding has led to the suggestion that template specificity imparted by terminal structures of RNA might be of greater importance early in infection. During the initiation phases of replication, the 3′ pseudoknot structure might facilitate template selection when few viral polymerase molecules are available and membrane association has not yet provided high concentrations of replication components. Later, determinants of template selection by the polymerase might include the membrane association of the RNA polymerase. Template specificity may also be conferred

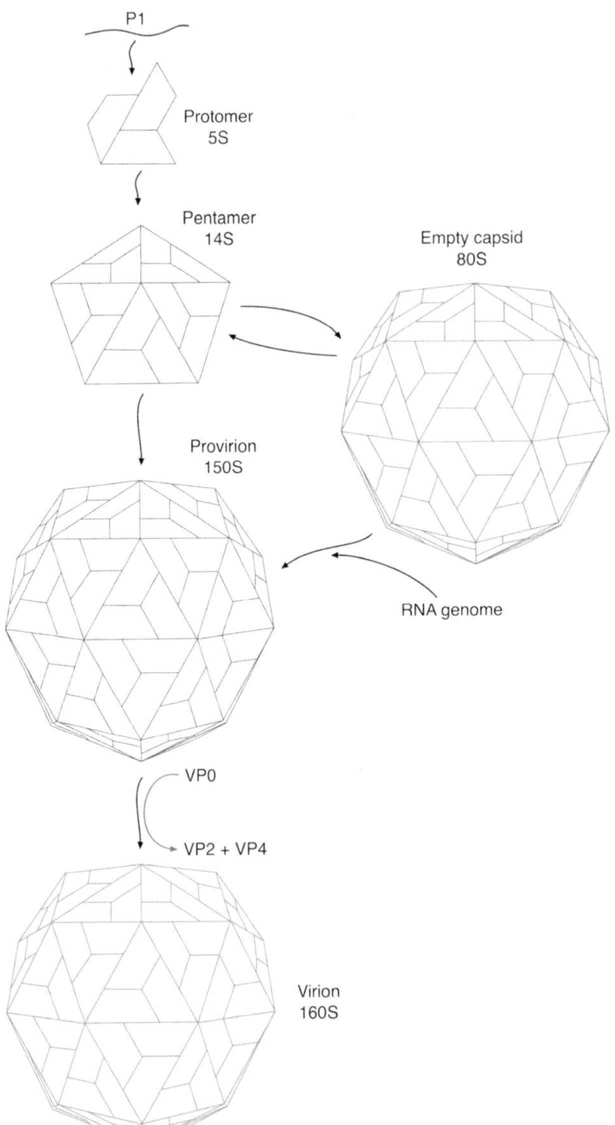

FIGURE 16.15. Morphogenesis of picornaviruses. The capsid protein precursor, P1, folds nascently, is cleaved from P2, and then is further cleaved to VP0 + VP3 + VP1 by $3CD^{pro}$. Protomers (5S) self-assemble into 14S pentamers, and pentamers assemble into 80S empty capsids. In one model of encapsidation, RNA is threaded into the empty capsid, producing a 150S provirion in which VP0 is uncleaved. Another possibility is that pentamers assemble around the RNA genome and that empty capsids are storage depots for pentamers. Cleavage of VP0 is the final morphogenetic step that produces the infectious 160S virion. The proteinase responsible for the cleavage of VP0 is unknown.

by the position of the 3D^{pol} gene at the very 3′ end of the viral RNA; translation places the polymerase at the 3′ end of the genome, ready for initiation.

A cloverleaf-like structure that forms in the 5′-noncoding region also plays an important role in template specificity. The finding that a mutation in a cloverleaf-like structure in the 5′-noncoding region that affects RNA synthesis could be complemented by a suppressor mutation in 3C^{pro} led to the suggestion that 3C^{pro} might bind the cloverleaf and play a role in viral RNA replication.[17] It was subsequently found that 3CD^{pro} binds the cloverleaf structure in the positive strand, together with a cellular protein, now known to be poly r(C)-binding protein, that is required for complex formation.[16,18,377] The RNA-binding domain of 3CD^{pro} is contained within the 3C^{pro} portion of the protein, on the opposite face of the molecule from the site involved in proteolysis. Mutations within this domain abolish complex formation and RNA replication without affecting viral protein processing. 3CD^{pro}, therefore, plays an important role in viral RNA synthesis by participating in formation of a ribonucleoprotein complex at the 5′ end of the positive-stranded RNA. A structural model of rhinovirus 3C^{pro} bound to stem-loop I shows that RNA binding induces changes in the proteinase active site, although their effect on catalytic activity is not known.[94] A role for these interactions in viral RNA replication is suggested in the model in Figure 16.13.

ORIGINS OF DIVERSITY

Misincorporation of Nucleotides

As with all other RNA viruses, the picornaviruses have very high error rates, because of misincorporation during chain elongation and the lack of proofreading ability in RNA polymerases. With error frequencies as high as one misincorporation per 10^3 to 10^4 nucleotides, RNA virus populations exist as *quasispecies*, or mixtures of many different genome sequences.[125]

It has been suggested that RNA viruses exist on the threshold of error catastrophe, to maximize diversity and adaptability.[125] A moderate increase in error frequency would be expected to destroy the virus population. In one study, it was estimated that each poliovirus genome synthesized after multiple rounds of replication in an infected cell contains two point mutations.[111] In the presence of the antiviral drug ribavirin, each poliovirus genome contained 15 point mutations, and yields of poliovirus in infected cells were 0.00001% of untreated cells. Similar observations have been made with FMDV[188] and Coxsackievirus B3.[179] These findings demonstrate that RNA viruses do exist at the error threshold, and that ribavirin is an RNA virus mutagen that inhibits virus replication by increasing the RNA polymerase error rate beyond the threshold.

High RNA virus error rates are believed to be necessary to enable survival of the virus population under selective pressure. Consequently, viruses with less error-prone RNA polymerases should be at a competitive disadvantage in complex environments such as an infected animal. To test this hypothesis, a poliovirus mutant resistant to the antiviral effects of ribavirin was isolated.[393,513] Resistance to ribavirin was conferred by a single amino acid change in 3D^{pol} that reduces errors during replication. The high-fidelity mutant virus replicated and spread poorly in mice, and was unable to compete with a low-fidelity virus. The results indicate that mutations, and the formation of a diverse quasispecies, benefits viral populations, particularly in an infected animal. Analysis of a ribavirin-resistant mutant of FMDV reveals no restriction of the viral quasispecies.[23] This apparent paradox is explained by the observation that the RNA polymerase mutation increased the frequency of misincorporation of natural nucleotides while decreasing the frequency of the incorporation of ribavirin nucleotide.

Recombination

Recombination, the exchange of nucleotide sequences among different genome RNA molecules, was first discovered in cells infected with poliovirus, and was subsequently found to occur during infection with other positive- and negative-stranded RNA viruses. The frequency of recombination, which is calculated by dividing the yield of recombinant virus by the sum of the yields of parental viruses, can be relatively high. In one study of poliovirus and FMDV, the recombination frequency was 0.9%, leading to the estimation that 10% to 20% of the viral genomes recombine in one growth cycle. When poliovirus recombination is studied by quantitative polymerase chain reaction, obviating the necessity to select for viable viruses, the recombination frequency for marker loci 600 nucleotides apart is 2×10^{-3}, similar to estimates obtained using selectable markers.[244] RNA recombination also occurs in natural infections. For example, intertypic recombinants among the three serotypes of Sabin poliovirus vaccine strains are readily isolated from the intestines of vaccinees; some recombinants contain sequences from all three serotypes.[80] The significance of these recombinants is unknown, but it has been suggested that such viruses are selected for their improved ability to replicate in the human alimentary tract compared with the parental viruses. Recombination in nature has also been demonstrated among nonpolio enteroviruses[460] (reviewed in[309]).

Poliovirus recombination, which mainly occurs between nucleotide sequences of the two parental genome RNA strands that have a high percentage of nucleotide identity, is called *base pairing dependent* (Fig. 16.14). RNA recombination is believed to be coupled with the process of genome RNA replication: it occurs by template switching during negative-strand synthesis, as first demonstrated in poliovirus-infected cells[275] and subsequently in cell-free extracts.[482] The RNA polymerase first copies the 3′ end of one parental positive strand, then switches templates and continues synthesis at the corresponding position on a second parental positive strand. Template switching in poliovirus-infected cells occurs predominantly during negative-strand synthesis because the concentration of positive-strand acceptors for template switching is 30 to 70 times higher than that of negative-strand acceptors. This template-switching mechanism of recombination is also known as *copy-choice.* A prediction of the copy-choice mechanism is that recombination frequencies should be lower between different poliovirus serotypes, a prediction that has been verified experimentally. For example, recombination between poliovirus types 1 and 2 occurs about 100 times less frequently than among type 1 polioviruses (the different poliovirus serotypes differ by about 15% in their nucleotide sequences).[273] The cause of template switching is not known, but it might be triggered by pausing of the polymerase during chain elongation.

ASSEMBLY OF VIRUS PARTICLES

Morphogenesis of picornaviruses has been studied extensively because the 60-subunit capsid is relatively simple and the assembly intermediates can be readily detected in infected cells (Fig. 16.15). During the synthesis of the P1 protein, the capsid protein precursor, the central β-barrel domains form, and intramolecular interactions among the surfaces of these domains lead to formation of the structural units. Once P1 is released from the 2A protein, the VP0–VP3 and VP3–VP1 bonds are cleaved by proteinase 3CD^{pro}. These cleavage sites are located in flexible regions between the β-barrels; considerable movement of the aminotermini and carboxyltermini occurs after cleavage, but the contacts between β-barrels are not disturbed.[223] In the mature capsid, the carboxyltermini of VP1, VP2, and VP3 are on the outer surface of the capsid, whereas the aminotermini are on the interior, where they participate in an extensive network of interactions among protomers. This process produces the first assembly intermediate in the poliovirus pathway, the 5S protomer, the immature structural unit consisting of one copy each of VP0, VP3, and VP1. Five protomers then assemble to form a pentamer, which sediments at 14S. Cleavage of P1 is probably required for assembly of the pentamer.[373] This conclusion is supported by examination of the virion structure. The β-cylinder at the fivefold axis of symmetry is formed from the N-termini of neighboring VP3 molecules; the cylinder is surrounded by a bundle composed of the aminotermini of VP0 and VP1. For these interactions to occur, proteolytic cleavage of the capsid proteins must occur to allow movement of the aminotermini.

Pentamers are important intermediates in the assembly of all picornaviruses.[67,433] They can self-assemble *in vitro* or *in vivo* into 80S empty capsids; in one model of assembly, newly synthesized viral RNA is inserted into these particles to form the provirion,[240] in which the capsid protein VP0 remains uncleaved. This assembly model would seemingly require an opening in the empty capsid through which the RNA can enter. Examination of the high-resolution x-ray crystallographic structure of these particles does not provide evidence for such an opening.[41] This finding does not exclude this morphogenetic pathway because the pore might be dynamic and not observed in the crystals. In an alternative morphogenesis pathway, 4S pentamers assemble with virion RNA to form provirions. In this model, for which there is some experimental support,[365] the empty capsids found in infected cells serve as storage depots for 14S pentamers.

The final morphogenetic step involves cleavage of most of the VP0 molecules to VP4 + VP2. The proteinase that carries out this final maturation cleavage has not been identified. The VP0 scissile bond is located on the interior of empty capsids and mature virions and is inaccessible to viral or cellular proteinases. The presence of a conserved serine in VP2 near one of the cleaved termini of VP2 led to a model that cleavage occurs by a novel autocatalytic serine protease-like mechanism in which basic viral RNA groups serve as proton abstracters during the cleavage reaction.[24] Replacement of ser-10, however, does not impair VP0 cleavage.[205] In another hypothesis, a conserved histidine in VP2 is involved in catalysis, together with the viral RNA.[41,114] Replacement of this histidine with different amino acids leads to lack of infectivity or highly unstable particles, supporting the involvement of VP2 histidine 195 in mediating VP0 cleavage during assembly.[216]

The structure of the 80S particle reveals differences in the network formed by the N-terminal extensions of the capsid proteins on the inner surface of the shell, compared with the native virion.[41] In empty capsids, VP4 and the entire N-terminal extensions of VP1 and VP2 are disordered, and many stabilizing interactions that are present in the mature virion are not present. Thus, cleavage of VP0 establishes the ordered N-terminal network, an interlocking seven-stranded β-sheet formed by residues from adjacent pentamers. This network results in an increase in particle stability and the acquisition of infectivity.

The picornavirus encapsidation process is highly specific, resulting in packaging of only positive-stranded RNA, and not viral mRNA, negative-stranded viral RNA, or any cellular RNA.[363,364] VPg is probably not an encapsidation signal because VPg-containing negative-stranded RNA is not packaged. The coupling of encapsidation to viral RNA synthesis may explain the selective packaging of viral positive-stranded RNA. In infected cells, newly synthesized RNA is packaged into virions within 5 minutes, whereas incorporation of capsid proteins in virions requires at least 20 minutes.[31] The pool of viral RNA available for packaging, therefore, is small, and the pool of capsid proteins is large. If capsid formation is inhibited with *p*-fluorophenylalanine, the accumulated RNA cannot be packaged after removal of the inhibitor.[199] These results suggest that packaging of the viral genome is linked to RNA synthesis, and would explain why only RNA containing VPg are encapsidated. This conclusion is questioned by more recent findings showing that inhibition of virion assembly by hydantoin, which targets the 2C protein, does not effect genome replication. Furthermore, when hydantoin from infected cells after RNA synthesis is complete, and in the presence of an inhibitor of replication, normal levels of virions are produced.[369]

During its synthesis, the P1 capsid protein precursor is linked to myristic acid at the aminoterminal glycine residue of VP4 that is exposed after removal of the initiation Met residue.[93] The myristate groups, which form part of a network of interactions between subunits that form when protomers assemble into pentamers, cluster around the fivefold axis of symmetry and stabilize the β-cylinder that is made by the aminotermini of five copies of VP3. Mutagenesis indicates that the myristate group plays a role in stabilizing pentamers and, therefore, virions.[20,314–316,344]

EFFECTS OF VIRAL MULTIPLICATION ON THE HOST CELL

Inhibition of 5′ End–Dependent mRNA Translation

Cleavage of eIF4G

In cultured mammalian cells, poliovirus infection results in inhibition of cellular protein synthesis. By 2 hours after infection, polyribosomes are disrupted and translation of nearly all cellular mRNA stops, replaced by viral mRNA translation (Fig. 16.16). Poliovirus mRNA, but not capped mRNA, can be translated in extracts from infected cells. In such extracts, the eIF4GI/II component of the translation initiation factor eIF4F has been cleaved.[136,434,496] Cleavage of eIF4G separates the N-terminal eIF4E-binding domain of eIF4G from the C-terminal fragment

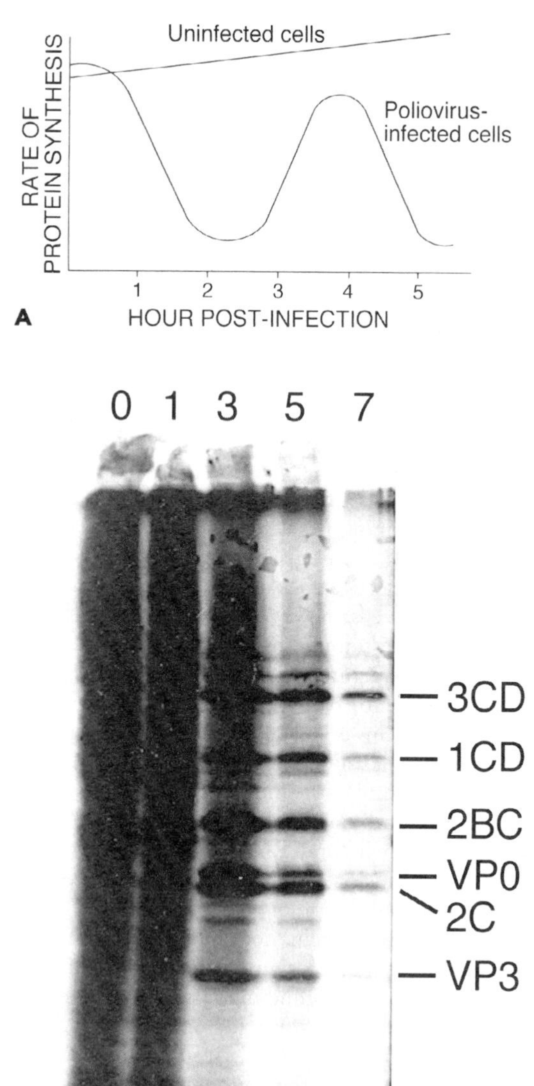

FIGURE 16.16. Inhibition of cellular translation in cells infected with poliovirus. A: Protein synthesis in poliovirus-infected and uninfected cells at different times after infection. Poliovirus infection results in inhibition of host cell translation beginning about 1 hour after infection. The increase in translation beginning 3 hours after infection is caused by the synthesis of viral proteins. **B:** Polyacrylamide gel showing inhibition of cellular translation. At different times after infection (top of each lane), cells were incubated with ^{35}S-methionine for 15 minutes; the cell extracts were then fractionated on an SDS-polyacrylamide gel. By 5 hours after infection, host translation is markedly inhibited and replaced by the synthesis of viral proteins, identified at the **right**.

(Fig. 16.17). The assumption that the C-terminal fragment of eIF4G cannot support the translation of capped mRNA has been proved incorrect.[10] It is now believed that picornavirus-induced translational inhibition is not caused by inability of p100 to support capped mRNA translation, but to the viral RNA outcompeting host cell mRNA for the limiting concentration of p100. Optimal function of the IRES does require the C-terminal fragment of eIF4G, which, as discussed previously, is necessary to anchor 40S ribosomal subunits to the IRES. Although both eIF4GI and eIF4GII are cleaved in poliovirus- and rhinovirus-infected cells, the kinetics of shutoff of host translation correlates with cleavage of eIF4GII and not eIF4GI.[180,478]

Both forms of eIF4G are cleaved by protease 2A^{pro} of poliovirus and rhinovirus.[180,478] *In vitro* cleavage of eIF4G by purified 2A^{pro} of rhinovirus is inefficient unless eIF4G is bound to eIF4E.[197] This finding indicates that eIF4G is not cleaved as an individual polypeptide, but rather as part of the eIF4F complex. Binding of eIF4E to eIF4G may induce conformational changes in eIF4G that make it a more efficient substrate for the protease. Poliovirus 2A^{pro} efficiently cleaves eIF4GI, but not eIF4GII, consistent with the differential cleavage of these proteins during virus infection.[180] The L^{pro} protein cleaves eIF4GI in cells infected with FMDV. The cleavage sites in eIF4GI for the two proteinases are different: L^{pro} cleaves between Gly-479 and Arg-480, whereas 2A^{pro} cleaves between Arg-486, and Gly-487.[274,288]

Modulation of eIF4F Activity

Two related low-molecular-weight cell proteins, 4E-BP1 and 4E-BP2, bind to eIF4E and inhibit translation by 5′ end–dependent scanning, but not by internal ribosome entry (Fig. 16.17).[383] 4E-BP1 is identical to a protein called PHAS-I (phosphorylated heat- and acid-stable protein regulated by insulin), which was previously known to be an important phosphorylation substrate in cells treated with insulin and growth factors.[301] Phosphorylation of 4E-BP1 *in vitro* blocks its association with eIF4E. Binding of either 4E-BP1 or 4E-BP2 to eIF4E does not prevent it from interacting with the 5′ cap but does inhibit binding to eIF4G. Consequently, active eIF4F is not formed. eIF4G and the 4E-BP have a common sequence motif that binds eIF4E. Treatment of cells with hormones and growth factors leads to the phosphorylation of 4E-BP1 and its release from eIF4E. Those mRNAs with extensive secondary structure in the 5′-untranslated region, which are translated poorly, are preferentially sensitive to the phosphorylation state of 4E-BP1. As expected, translation by internal ribosome binding is not affected when 4E-BP1 is dephosphorylated. Binding of extracellular ligands leads to phosphorylation of 4E-BP through a signaling pathway that includes the target of rapamycin.[532]

Infection with several picornaviruses causes alteration of the phosphorylation state of 4E-BP1 and 4E-BP2 (Fig. 16.17). Infection of cells with encephalomyocarditis virus causes inhibition of cellular translation, but in contrast to the shutoff that occurs in poliovirus-infected cells, shutoff of cellular protein synthesis occurs late in infection and is not mediated by cleavage of eIF4G. Infection with encephalomyocarditis virus induces dephosphorylation of 4E-BP1, which then binds eIF4E to prevent it from forming eIF4F.[132] Translation of cellular mRNA is inhibited, but that of the viral RNA is not inhibited because it contains an IRES. Dephosphorylation of 4E-BP1 also occurs late in cells infected with poliovirus, but this event does not coincide with inhibition of cellular translation, which occurs earlier in infection.[165] Inhibition of translation by dephosphorylation of 4E-BP also influences the ability of the cell to productively combat viral infection by reducing production of type I interferons.[97]

Efficient translation initiation requires the formation of a closed loop on mRNA. Circularization of the RNA is mediated

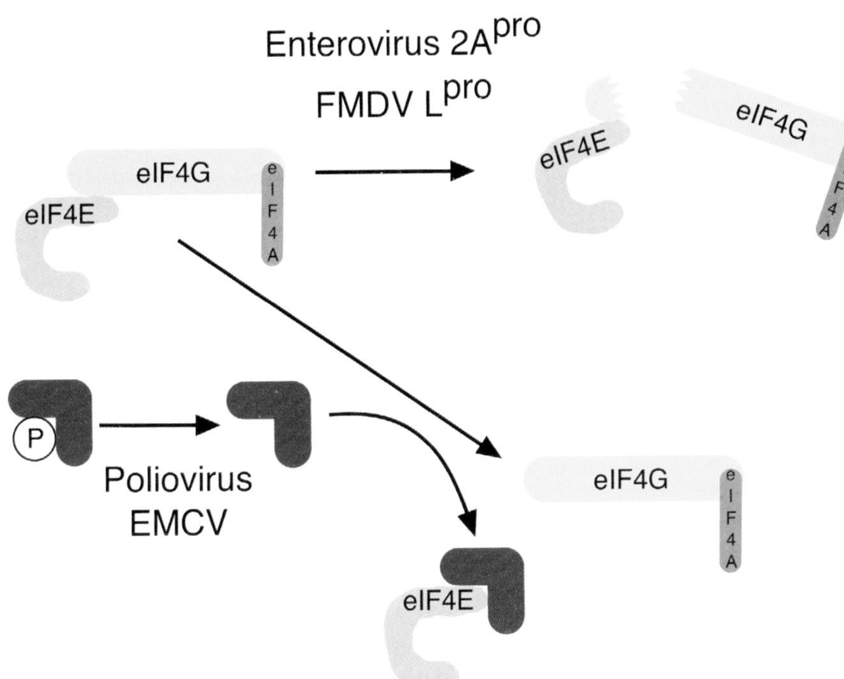

FIGURE 16.17. Two mechanisms for regulating eIF4F activity in picornavirus-infected cells. The proteins 4E-BP1 and 4E-BP1 bind eIF4E and prevent it from interacting with eIF4G. 4E-BP1 binds eIF4E when it is dephosphorylated, an event that occurs in cells infected with poliovirus and encephalomyocarditis virus. Cleavage of eIF4G takes place in cells infected with poliovirus, rhinovirus, and foot-and-mouth disease virus, among others. Cleavage reduces the efficiency of translation of capped messenger RNA (mRNA). 5′ end–dependent initiation is inhibited because capped mRNA cannot compete with viral mRNA for the translation machinery.

by the interaction of eIF4G bound at the 5′ end of the RNA and poly(A) binding protein bound to the poly(A) tail at the 3′ end. The initial synthesis of picornavirus specific proteins is stimulated by the interaction of eIF4G with poly(A) binding protein.[333,479] Like eIF4G, poly(A) binding protein is cleaved during enterovirus infection by viral proteinases $2A^{pro}$ and $3C^{pro}$; however, the kinetics of poly (A) binding protein cleavage are slower than those of eIF4G.[247] Cleavage of poly(A) binding protein is necessary but not sufficient for efficient inhibition of cellular translation; instead, cleavage of this protein is believed to participate in the switch from RNA translation to replication (see "Translation and Replication of the Same RNA molecule").[68] The effect of poly(A) binding protein cleavage during this switch is controversial, as depletion of poly(A) binding protein from cell lysates did not reduce virus production.[480] The cellular polyadenylation factor CstF-64 is cleaved by enterovirus 71 $3C^{pro}$ proteinase, impairing the addition of poly(A) to host cell mRNAs.[524]

Formation of the eIF4F complex can also be regulated by miRNAs. During enterovirus infection, transcription of miR-141 is enhanced. Because multiple binding sites for this miRNA are found within the 3′-UTR of the eIF4E mRNA, levels of eIF4E—and consequently the eIF4F complex—are reduced, and cellular protein synthesis is impaired.[219] Viral translation is unaffected as it does not require eIF4E.

The production of double-stranded RNA during infection with many viruses leads to activation of Pkr, phosphorylation of eIF2α, and inhibition of translation. It occurs very late in the replication cycle of poliovirus.[368] Like most cellular mRNAs, the polyprotein encoded by picornaviral mRNA begins with an AUG, and early in infection initiation of protein synthesis requires the ternary complex of eIF2-GTP-met-tRNA$_i$. Late in infection, phosphorylation of serine 52 of the alpha subunit of eIF2 prevents the recycling of the ternary complex after initiation. However, poliovirus specific protein synthesis continues throughout infection. It is believed that initiation of translation late during infection occurs independently of eIF2.[523,530] The exact mechanism for this mode of initiation is not well understood but is thought to be dependent on the generation of a fragment of eIF5 that functions in a similar manner as eIF2 in recruiting the initiating tRNA to the small 40S ribosomal subunit while bound to the mRNA.[530] The proteolytic activity of $2A^{pro}$ is believed to be required to enable poliovirus mRNA translation in the absence of eIF2.[419]

Stress-Associated RNA Granules

Sequestering of mRNA away from the translation apparatus in processing (P) bodies and stress granules is a another mechanism by which cellular mRNA translation can be impaired.[15] P bodies and stress granules are two nonmembranous cytoplasmic aggregates composed of RNA and protein, including many proteins involved in mRNA translation. These granules are believed to form when translation is inhibited in the presence of intracellular and extracellular stresses, including viral infection. When stress conditions are alleviated, the mRNAs found in these aggregates can either be deadenylated and degraded or returned to the pool of actively translated RNAs.

Stress granules are thought to be nucleated on two cellular proteins, T-cell–restricted intracellular antigen-1 (TIA-1) and the RasGAP SH3-domain binding protein 1 (G3BP). Reduction of either protein impairs formation of stress granules, and overproduction of either component stimulates formation of these aggregates.[164,494] Stalled translation complexes consisting of mRNA, eIF4E, eIF4G, eIF4A, eIF3, poly(A) binding protein, and phosphorylated eIF2α are found within these granules. The presence of phosphorylated eIF2α is a hallmark of stress granules. Formation of stress granules is enhanced during early picornavirus infection, and correlates with the inhibition of cellular translation but is independent of eIF2α phosphorylation. Late in viral infection, the viral proteinase $3C^{pro}$ cleaves

RasGAP SH3-domain binding protein 1a, dissembling stress granules, an event required for efficient viral replication. The presence of an altered form of cleaved RasGAP SH3-domain binding protein 1^{Q326E} prevents the disassembly of stress granules and impairs viral replication.[528] Instead, a noncanonical form of stress granules remains, an aggregate containing only TIA-1.[400,529] The opposite is observed during infection with members of the *Discistroviridae:* cricket paralysis virus infection prohibits stress granule formation as defined by foci of the *Drosophila* homologs of TIA-1 and RasGAP SH3-domain binding protein 1, Rox8 and Rin. Addition of potent inducers of stress granules such as arsenite and patemine A to the culture medium is unable to overcome viral inhibition.[269]

Processing (P-) bodies are a second type of nonmembrane bound aggregate found in the cytoplasm. These aggregates, which are the sites of RNA deadenylation and mRNA repression, are composed of proteins such as the decapping enzymes Dcp1a, Dcp2, and proteins that mediate mRNA deadenylation including Pan3, the CCR4/Not 1 complex, Xrn-1, a 5′-3′ RNA exonuclease, and the DEAD-box helicase p54/Rck. In uninfected cells, P-bodies are the consequence of micro RNA (miRNA)–mediated repression.[137] Ultrastructural analysis of these granules suggests that there is an anchoring core composed of proteins required for repression with proteins mediating decay on the periphery. The protein that bridges between the two regions of the aggregate is p54/Rck.[103] P-bodies are found in proximity to both the ribosome and mitochondria. Although cellular mRNA translation is inhibited during picornavirus infection, the RNA is not degraded, possibly due to inhibition of P-body formation. The $3C^{pro}$ proteinase of poliovirus cleaves several P-body components including Xrn1, Dcp1a, and Pan 3, disrupting P-body formation.[128]

Inhibition of Cellular RNA Synthesis

Infection of cells with picornaviruses leads to a rapid inhibition of host cell RNA synthesis catalyzed by all three classes of DNA-dependent RNA polymerase. RNA polymerases I, II, and III from poliovirus-infected cells are enzymatically active, suggesting that accessory proteins may be the target of transcriptional inhibition. Studies of *in vitro* systems have demonstrated the inhibition of specific transcription factors required by each of the three RNA polymerases. The RNA polymerase factor TFIID, which is a multiprotein complex, is inactivated in poliovirus-infected cells.[279] This inactivation appears to be caused, at least in part, by cleavage of a subunit of TFIID, the TATA-binding protein, by protease $3C^{pro}$.[79] A pol III DNA-binding transcription factor, TFIIC, is also cleaved and inactivated by $3C^{pro}$.[96] The target of $3C^{pro}$ is a subunit of TFIIIC, which contacts the pol III promoter. The pol I transcription factors SL-1 (selectivity factor) and UBF (upstream binding factor) are inactivated in poliovirus-infected cells by $3C^{pro}$, resulting in inhibition of pol I transcription.[32,439]

Because poliovirus replication occurs in the cytoplasm, cleavage of RNA polymerase transcription factors requires that the viral proteinase $3C^{pro}$ enter the nucleus. $3C^{pro}$ lacks a nuclear localization signal (NLS), but the precursor $3CD^{pro}$ enters the nucleus by virtue of an NLS in protein $3D^{pol}$. Transcription factors in the nucleus are then cleaved by either $3CD^{pro}$ or $3C^{pro}$ that is released by autocatalysis.[455] Rhinovirus 16 $3CD^{pro}$ has also been shown to enter the nucleus.[14]

Inhibition of Nucleocytoplasmic Trafficking

Infection of cells with picornaviruses leads to the disruption of nucleocytoplasmic trafficking. One mechanism by which this is achieved is the proteolysis of nucleoporins, proteins that constitute the nuclear pore complex. In cells infected with poliovirus, two protein components of the nuclear pore complex are cleaved, Nup153 and Nup62.[191,192] The proteinase responsible for cleavage of Nup62 in rhinovirus-infected cells is $2A^{pro}$.[376] This cleavage results in the cytoplasmic accumulation of nuclear proteins, some of which, such as La protein[459] and SRp20,[140] are required for viral replication. The rates and processing profiles of Nup by $2A^{pro}$ proteinases of different rhinoviruses vary widely.[522] The rhinovirus $3C^{pro}$ and its precursor $3CD^{pro}$ are imported into the nucleus, leading to the degradation of nuclear pore components.[160]

Another mechanism of disruption of nucleocytoplasmic trafficking involves the L protein of cardioviruses (the 2A protein of these viruses is not a proteinase). The L protein binds directly to the Ran-GTPase, a key regulator of nucleocytoplasmic transport.[406] Infection also leads to phosphorylation of nucleoporins Nup62, Nup153, and Nup214.[407] Staurosporine, a broad-spectrum protein kinase inhibitor, and ERK and p38 MAP kinase inhibitors block Nup phosphorylation and restore normal nuclear trafficking.[408] Inhibition of Nup activity is therefore achieved by phosphorylation in cardiovirus-infected cells and by proteolysis in cells infected with enteroviruses.

The disruption of nucleocytoplasmic trafficking by picornaviruses not only provides cytoplasmic access to nuclear proteins needed for viral replication, but blocks the export of cell mRNAs with antiviral activity produced as part of the innate immune response.

Inhibition of Protein Secretion

Transport of both secretory and plasma membrane proteins is blocked in picornavirus-infected cells.[123] The 2B and 2BC proteins block protein secretion from the Golgi apparatus, and the 3A protein blocks vesicular traffic from the ERGIC to the Golgi complex.[34,62,124,444] Inhibition of protein secretion by poliovirus protein 3A is not required for viral growth in cell culture.[122] Protein 3A inhibits protein transport by binding to and inhibiting GBF1, a guanine exchange factor that is needed for activity of Arf1 and is required for the transport through the secretory pathway.[54] Cells infected with the poliovirus mutant 3A-2, which has a single amino acid change in the protein, have reduced inhibition of protein transport.[124] This amino acid change abrogates binding of 3A to GBF1 and therefore does not inhibit activity of the protein.[525,527] Because the 3A protein prevents secretion of cytokines[122] and major histocompatibility complex I (MHC-I)–dependent antigen presentation,[117] it is likely to modulate the innate and adaptive immune responses of the host and, therefore, the outcome of infection. Consistent with this hypothesis, when the 3A mutation is introduced into the genome of Coxsackievirus B3, the mutant is less pathogenic in mice, although the mechanism of attenuation is not known.[526] Inhibition of protein secretion in cells infected by FMDV is caused not by protein 3A but by protein 2BC.[337]

Cell Death and Virus Release

When cells are productively infected with poliovirus, they develop the characteristic morphologic changes known as *cytopathic effects.* These include condensation of chromatin, nuclear blebbing, proliferation of membranous vesicles, changes in membrane permeability, leakage of intracellular components, and shriveling of the entire cell. The cause of cytopathic effects is unknown. One hypothesis is that leakage of lysosomal contents is partly responsible.[190] Although cellular RNA, protein, and DNA synthesis are inhibited during the first few hours of infection, they cannot account for cytopathic effects.

When poliovirus reproduction is hindered by certain drugs or other restrictive conditions, cell death occurs through induction of apoptosis.[490] Although certain manifestations of cytopathic effects and apoptosis are similar (e.g., chromatin condensation and nuclear deformation), the pathways leading to their induction differ.[3] During productive infections of cultured cells with poliovirus, apoptosis is blocked by a virus-encoded inhibitor.[490] Viral replication and central nervous system injury in mice infected with poliovirus, however, are associated with apoptosis.[167] Viral inducers of apoptosis include proteins 2C, $2A^{pro}$, and $3C^{pro}$,[36,168,303] and inhibitors of apoptosis include L^{pro}, 2B, and 3A.[82,122,159,355,538] The ability of different strains of Theiler's murine encephalomyelitis virus to induce apoptosis may be a determinant of disease. The TO strain of Theiler's virus, which causes a persistent demyelinating disease in mice, encodes an additional protein, L*.[90] This protein is produced by initiation from an AUG that is 13 nucleotides downstream from the initiator AUG of the polyprotein, in a different reading frame. In contrast, nondemyelinating strains of the virus (e.g., GDVII) do not encode L*. It was subsequently found that L* has antiapoptotic properties in macrophages, is critical for virus persistence,[159] and prevents antiviral cytotoxic T-cell activation.[538] The ability of L* to inhibit apoptosis may be a key factor in determining whether infection of mice results in acute disease or persistence and demyelination.

The autophagosomes that form in cells infected with some picornaviruses (see "Cellular Site of Viral RNA Synthesis") may also play a role in virus release from the cell. Suppressing proteins in the autophagic pathway reduces viral release, suggesting a mechanism for nonlytic exit of newly synthesized virus from the infected cell.[484]

PERSPECTIVES

Since the identification in 1908 of poliovirus as the etiologic agent of poliomyelitis, research on the virus has waxed and waned. With each lull in activity, questions were raised about whether it was productive to continue research on the virus. Each time, new technologies emerged that allowed the field to advance and become active once again. Today, research on poliovirus is as vibrant as ever. The difficulties encountered in the effort to globally eradicate this virus have allowed research to continue. Nevertheless, work on other picornaviruses has become highly productive, and research on a wide range of cardioviruses, aphthoviruses, enteroviruses, and members of many other genera flourishes. Many questions remain about nearly every stage of the replicative cycle, and an unprecedented array of experimental techniques and reagents are available to address them. Genome-wide RNA interference screens are being applied to picornaviruses, and have already identified hundreds of cell genes that not only are required for picornavirus infection but regulate replication.[108,109] It can be anticipated that cellular genes will be involved in all aspects of the picornaviral replication cycle, from receptor binding and entry to macromolecular synthesis, assembly of new virus particles, and release. Studies of these processes will contribute to understanding questions about how the viral RNA is released from the capsid, whether RNA synthesis proceeds in infected cells as has been learned from *in vitro* systems, how replication complexes are produced in infected cells, and how the viral RNA enters the virion and becomes folded to fit in a very small space. Because poliovirus is a model system, its study provides a unique opportunity to address fundamental questions in virology. The polio eradication program has made impressive gains—as of this writing in April 2012 there have been fewer than 47 cases of paralytic disease, and remarkably, India has been polio free for over 1 year. When the time comes for research on poliovirus to cease, the picornavirus field will be ready to move on to other fascinating subjects. As viral discovery in general has greatly accelerated in the past 5 years, the size of the *Picornaviridae* has grown remarkably. With this growth come new opportunities to study fascinating new viral systems, one of which might some day become the next model system for this virus family.

REFERENCES

All cited references are available in the e-book.

1. Acharya R, Fry E, Stuart D, et al. The three-dimensional structure of foot-and-mouth disease virus at 2.9 Å resolution. *Nature* 1989;337:709–716.
3. Agol VI, Belov GA, Bienz K, et al. Two types of death of poliovirus-infected cells: caspase involvement in the apoptosis but not cytopathic effect. *Virology* 1998;252(2):343–353.
11. Ali IK, McKendrick L, Morley SJ, et al. Activity of the hepatitis A virus IRES requires association between the cap-binding translation initiation factor (eIF4E) and eIF4G. *J Virol* 2001;75(17):7854–7863.
12. Ambros V, Pettersson RF, Baltimore D. An enzymatic activity in uninfected cells that cleaves the linkage between poliovirion RNA and the 5′ terminal protein. *Cell* 1978;15(4):1439–1446.
13. Ambros V, Baltimore D. Purification and properties of a HeLa cell enzyme able to remove the 5′-terminal protein from poliovirus RNA. *J Biol Chem* 1980;255(14):6739–6744.
18. Andino R, Rieckhof GE, Achacoso PL, et al. Poliovirus RNA synthesis utilizes an RNP complex formed around the 5′-end of viral RNA. *EMBO J* 1993;12(9):3587–3598.
20. Ansardi DC, Luo M, Morrow CD. Mutations in the poliovirus P1 capsid precursor at arginine residues VP4-ARG34, VP3-ARG223, and VP1-ARG129 affect virus assembly and encapsidation of genomic RNA. *Virology* 1994;199(1):20–34.
22. Appleby TC, Luecke H, Shim JH, et al. Crystal structure of complete rhinovirus RNA polymerase suggests front loading of protein primer. *J Virol* 2005;79(1):277–288.
25. Arnold E, Rossmann MG. Analysis of the structure of a common cold virus, human rhinovirus 14, refined at a resolution of 3.0 Å. *J Mol Biol* 1990;211(4):763–801.
29. Baltimore D, Franklin RM. A new ribonucleic acid polymerase appearing after mengovirus infection of L-cells. *J Biol Chem* 1963;238:3395–3400.
32. Banerjee R, Weidman MK, Navarro S, et al. Modifications of both selectivity factor and upstream binding factor contribute to poliovirus-mediated inhibition of RNA polymerase I transcription. *J Gen Virol* 2005;86(Pt 8):2315–2322.
33. Baranowski E, Ruiz-Jarabo CM, Sevilla N, et al. Cell recognition by foot-and-mouth disease virus that lacks the RGD integrin-binding motif: flexibility in aphthovirus receptor usage. *J Virol* 2000;74(4):1641–1647.

37. Barton DJ, Black EP, Flanegan JB. Complete replication of poliovirus in vitro: preinitiation RNA replication complexes require soluble cellular factors for the synthesis of VPg-linked RNA. *J Virol* 1995;69(9):5516–5527.
39. Barton DJ, Morasco BJ, Flanegan JB. Translating ribosomes inhibit poliovirus negative-strand RNA synthesis. *J Virol* 1999;73(12):10104–10112.
40. Barton DJ, O'Donnell BJ, Flanegan JB. 5′ cloverleaf in poliovirus RNA is a *cis*-acting replication element required for negative-strand synthesis. *EMBO J* 2001;20(6):1439–1448.
41. Basavappa R, Syed R, Flore O, et al. Role and mechanism of the maturation cleavage of VP0 in poliovirus assembly: structure of the empty capsid assembly intermediate at 2.9 Å resolution. *Protein Sci* 1994;3(10):1651–1669.
46. Bayer N, Schober D, Prchla E, et al. Effect of bafilomycin A1 and nocodazole on endocytic transport in HeLa cells: implications for viral uncoating and infection. *J Virol* 1998;72(12):9645–9655.
50. Bedard KM, Daijogo S, Semler BL. A nucleo-cytoplasmic SR protein functions in viral IRES-mediated translation initiation. *EMBO J* 2007;26(2):459–467.
53. Belnap DM, McDermott BM Jr, Filman DJ, et al. Three-dimensional structure of poliovirus receptor bound to poliovirus. *Proc Natl Acad Sci U S A* 2000;97(1):73–78.
54. Belov GA, Feng Q, Nikovics K, et al. A critical role of a cellular membrane traffic protein in poliovirus RNA replication. *PLoS Pathog* 2008;4(11):e1000216.
55. Belov GA, Nair V, Hansen BT, et al. Complex dynamic development of poliovirus membranous replication complexes. *J Virol* 2012;86(1):302–312.
58. Bergelson JM, Cunningham JA, Droguett G, et al. Isolation of a common receptor for Coxsackie B viruses and adenoviruses 2 and 5. *Science* 1997;275(5304):1320–1323.
62. Beske O, Reichelt M, Taylor MP, et al. Poliovirus infection blocks ERGIC-to-Golgi trafficking and induces microtubule-dependent disruption of the Golgi complex. *J Cell Sci* 2007;120(Pt 18):3207–3218.
66. Blyn LB, Towner JS, Semler BL, et al. Requirement of poly(rC) binding protein 2 for translation of poliovirus RNA. *J Virol* 1997;71(8):6243–6246.
68. Bonderoff JM, Larey JL, Lloyd RE. Cleavage of poly(A)-binding protein by poliovirus 3C proteinase inhibits viral internal ribosome entry site-mediated translation. *J Virol* 2008;82(19):9389–9399.
70. Bostina M, Levy H, Filman DJ, et al. Poliovirus RNA is released from the capsid near a twofold symmetry axis. *J Virol* 2011;85(2):776–783.
74. Brabec M, Blaas D, Fuchs R. Wortmannin delays transfer of human rhinovirus serotype 2 to late endocytic compartments. *Biochem Biophys Res Commun* 2006;348(2):741–749.
76. Brandenburg B, Lee LY, Lakadamyali M, et al. Imaging poliovirus entry in live cells. *PLoS Biol* 2007;5(7):e183.
77. Brown DM, Cornell CT, Tran GP, et al. An authentic 3′ noncoding region is necessary for efficient poliovirus replication. *J Virol* 2005;79(18):11962–11973.
78. Bubeck D, Filman DJ, Cheng N, et al. The structure of the poliovirus 135S cell entry intermediate at 10-angstrom resolution reveals the location of an externalized polypeptide that binds to membranes. *J Virol* 2005;79(12):7745–7755.
81. Campagnola G, Weygandt M, Scoggin K, et al. Crystal structure of coxsackievirus B3 3D^{pol} highlights the functional importance of residue 5 in picornavirus polymerases. *J Virol* 2008;82(19):9458–9464.
84. Casasnovas JM, Springer TA. Kinetics and thermodynamics of virus binding to receptor. Studies with rhinovirus, intercellular adhesion molecule-1 (ICAM-1), and surface plasmon resonance. *J Biol Chem* 1995;270(22):13216–13224.
87. Chang KH, Day C, Walker J, et al. The nucleotide sequences of wild-type coxsackievirus A9 strains imply that an RGD motif in VP1 is functionally significant. *J Gen Virol* 1992;73(Pt 3):621–626.
91. Chen ZG, Stauffacher C, Li Y, et al. Protein-RNA interactions in an icosahedral virus at 3.0 Å resolution. *Science* 1989;245(4914):154–159.
93. Chow M, Newman JF, Filman D, et al. Myristylation of picornavirus capsid protein VP4 and its structural significance. *Nature* 1987;327(6122):482–486.
94. Claridge JK, Headey SJ, Chow JY, et al. A picornaviral loop-to-loop replication complex. *J Struct Biol* 2009;166(3):251–262.
104. Cox S, Buontempo PJ, Wright-Minogue J, et al. Antipicornavirus activity of SCH 47802 and analogs: in vitro and in vivo studies. *Antiviral Res* 1996;32(2):71–79.
105. Coyne CB, Bergelson JM. Virus-induced Abl and Fyn kinase signals permit coxsackievirus entry through epithelial tight junctions. *Cell* 2006;124(1):119–131.
106. Coyne CB, Kim KS, Bergelson JM. Poliovirus entry into human brain microvascular cells requires receptor-induced activation of SHP-2. *EMBO J* 2007;26(17):4016–4028.
107. Coyne CB, Shen L, Turner JR, et al. Coxsackievirus entry across epithelial tight junctions requires occludin and the small GTPases Rab34 and Rab5. *Cell Host Microbe* 2007;2(3):181–192.
108. Coyne CB, Bozym R, Morosky SA, et al. Comparative RNAi screening reveals host factors involved in enterovirus infection of polarized endothelial monolayers. *Cell Host Microbe* 2011;9(1):70–82.
109. Coyne CB, Cherry S. RNAi screening in mammalian cells to identify novel host cell molecules involved in the regulation of viral infections. *Methods Mol Biol* 2011;721:397–405.
111. Crotty S, Maag D, Arnold JJ, et al. The broad-spectrum antiviral ribonucleoside ribavirin is an RNA virus mutagen. *Nat Med* 2000;6(12):1375–1379.
118. DeTulleo L, Kirchhausen T. The clathrin endocytic pathway in viral infection. *EMBO J* 1998;17(16):4585–4593.
122. Dodd DA, Giddings TH Jr, Kirkegaard K. Poliovirus 3A protein limits interleukin-6 (IL-6), IL-8, and beta interferon secretion during viral infection. *J Virol* 2001;75(17):8158–8165.
123. Doedens JR, Kirkegaard K. Inhibition of cellular protein secretion by poliovirus proteins 2B and 3A. *EMBO J* 1995;14(5):894–907.
124. Doedens JR, Giddings TH Jr, Kirkegaard K. Inhibition of endoplasmic reticulum-to-Golgi traffic by poliovirus protein 3A: genetic and ultrastructural analysis. *J Virol* 1997;71(12):9054–9064.
127. Donnelly ML, Luke G, Mehrotra A, et al. Analysis of the aphthovirus 2A/2B polyprotein 'cleavage' mechanism indicates not a proteolytic reaction, but a novel translational effect: a putative ribosomal 'skip'. *J Gen Virol* 2001;82(Pt 5):1013–1025.
128. Dougherty JD, White JP, Lloyd RE. Poliovirus-mediated disruption of cytoplasmic processing bodies. *J Virol* 2011;85(1):64–75.
138. Filman DJ, Syed R, Chow M, et al. Structural factors that control conformational transitions and serotype specificity in type 3 poliovirus. *EMBO J* 1989;8(5):1567–1579.
139. Fitzgerald KD, Semler BL. Bridging IRES elements in mRNAs to the eukaryotic translation apparatus. *Biochim Biophys Acta* 2009;1789(9–10):518–528.
140. Fitzgerald KD, Semler BL. Re-localization of cellular protein SRp20 during poliovirus infection: bridging a viral IRES to the host cell translation apparatus. *PLoS Pathog* 2011;7(7):e1002127.
142. Flanegan JB, Petterson RF, Ambros V, et al. Covalent linkage of a protein to a defined nucleotide sequence at the 5′-terminus of virion and replicative intermediate RNAs of poliovirus. *Proc Natl Acad Sci U S A* 1977;74(3):961–965.
145. Forss S, Schaller H. A tandem repeat gene in a picornavirus. *Nucleic Acids Res* 1982;10(20):6441–6450.
151. Fricks CE, Hogle JM. Cell-induced conformational change in poliovirus: externalization of the amino terminus of VP1 is responsible for liposome binding. *J Virol* 1990;64(5):1934–1945.
152. Fry EE, Lea SM, Jackson T, et al. The structure and function of a foot-and-mouth disease virus-oligosaccharide receptor complex. *EMBO J* 1999;18(3):543–554.
155. Gamarnik AV, Andino R. Two functional complexes formed by KH domain containing proteins with the 5′ noncoding region of poliovirus RNA. *RNA* 1997;3(8):882–892.
160. Ghildyal R, Jordan B, Li D, et al. Rhinovirus 3C protease can localize in the nucleus and alter active and passive nucleocytoplasmic transport. *J Virol* 2009;83(14):7349–7352.
164. Gilks N, Kedersha N, Ayodele M, et al. Stress granule assembly is mediated by prion-like aggregation of TIA-1. *Mol Biol Cell* 2004;15(12):5383–5398.
165. Gingras AC, Svitkin Y, Belsham GJ, et al. Activation of the translational suppressor 4E-BP1 following infection with encephalomyocarditis virus and poliovirus. *Proc Natl Acad Sci U S A* 1996;93(11):5578–5583.
171. Goodfellow I, Chaudhry Y, Richardson A, et al. Identification of a *cis*-acting replication element within the poliovirus coding region. *J Virol* 2000;74(10):4590–4600.

176. Gorbalenya AE, Donchenko AP, Blinov VM, et al. Cysteine proteases of positive strand RNA viruses and chymotrypsin-like serine proteases. A distinct protein superfamily with a common structural fold [see comments]. *FEBS Lett* 1989;243(2):103–114.
179. Graci JD, Gnadig NF, Galarraga JE, et al.. Mutational robustness of an RNA virus influences sensitivity to lethal mutagenesis. *J Virol* 2012; 86(5):2869–2873.
180. Gradi A, Svitkin YV, Imataka H, et al. Proteolysis of human eukaryotic translation initiation factor eIF4GII, but not eIF4GI, coincides with the shutoff of host protein synthesis after poliovirus infection. *Proc Natl Acad Sci U S A* 1998;95(19):11089–11094.
183. Greninger AL, Runckel C, Chiu CY, et al. The complete genome of klassevirus—a novel picornavirus in pediatric stool. *Virol J* 2009;6:82.
184. Greve JM, Davis G, Meyer AM, et al. The major human rhinovirus receptor is ICAM-1. *Cell* 1989;56:839–847.
185. Groppelli E, Tuthill TJ, Rowlands DJ. Cell entry of the aphthovirus equine rhinitis A virus is dependent on endosome acidification. *J Virol* 2010;84(12):6235–6240.
191. Gustin KE, Sarnow P. Effects of poliovirus infection on nucleo-cytoplasmic trafficking and nuclear pore complex composition. *EMBO J* 2001; 20(1–2):240–249.
194. Hadfield AT, Lee W, Zhao R, et al. The refined structure of human rhinovirus 16 at 2.15 A resolution: implications for the viral life cycle. *Structure* 1997;5(3):427–441.
196. Hafenstein S, Bowman VD, Chipman PR, et al. Interaction of decay-accelerating factor with coxsackievirus B3. *J Virol* 2007;81(23):12927–12935.
198. Hahn H, Palmenberg AC. Encephalomyocarditis viruses with short poly(C) tracts are more virulent than their mengovirus counterparts. *J Virol* 1995;69(4):2697–2699.
208. He Y, Chipman PR, Howitt J, et al. Interaction of coxsackievirus B3 with the full length coxsackievirus-adenovirus receptor. *Nat Struct Biol* 2001; 8(10):874–878.
209. He Y, Mueller S, Chipman PR, et al. Complexes of poliovirus serotypes with their common cellular receptor, CD155. *J Virol* 2003;77(8):4827–4835.
212. Herold J, Andino R. Poliovirus RNA replication requires genome circularization through a protein-protein bridge. *Mol Cell* 2001;7(3): 581–591.
213. Hewat EA, Neumann E, Blaas D. The concerted conformational changes during human rhinovirus 2 uncoating. *Mol Cell* 2002;10(2):317–326.
216. Hindiyeh M, Li QH, Basavappa R, et al. Poliovirus mutants at histidine 195 of VP2 do not cleave VP0 into VP2 and VP4. *J Virol* 1999;73(11): 9072–9079.
220. Hobdey SE, Kempf BJ, Steil BP, et al. Poliovirus polymerase residue 5 plays a critical role in elongation complex stability. *J Virol* 2010;84(16): 8072–8084.
223. Hogle JM, Chow M, Filman DJ. Three-dimensional structure of poliovirus at 2.9 Å resolution. *Science* 1985;229:1358–1365.
224. Holtz LR, Finkbeiner SR, Kirkwood CD, et al. Identification of a novel picornavirus related to cosaviruses in a child with acute diarrhea. *Virol J* 2008;5:159.
225. Holtz LR, Finkbeiner SR, Zhao G, et al. Klassevirus 1, a previously undescribed member of the family *Picornaviridae,* is globally widespread. *Virol J* 2009;6:86.
226. Hope DA, Diamond SE, Kirkegaard K. Genetic dissection of interaction between poliovirus 3D polymerase and viral protein 3AB. *J Virol* 1997;71(12):9490–9498.
232. Ida-Hosonuma M, Iwasaki T, Yoshikawa T, et al. The alpha/beta interferon response controls tissue tropism and pathogenicity of poliovirus. *J Virol* 2005;79(7):4460–4469.
236. Jackson T, Ellard FM, Ghazaleh RA, et al. Efficient infection of cells in culture by type O foot-and-mouth disease virus requires binding to cell surface heparan sulfate. *J Virol* 1996;70(8):5282–5287.
239. Jackson WT, Giddings TH Jr, Taylor MP, et al. Subversion of cellular autophagosomal machinery by RNA viruses. *PLoS Biol* 2005;3(5):e156.
241. Jacobson SJ, Konings DA, Sarnow P. Biochemical and genetic evidence for a pseudoknot structure at the 3′ terminus of the poliovirus RNA genome and its role in viral RNA amplification. *J Virol* 1993;67(6):2961–2971.
243. Jang SK, Krausslich H-G, Nicklin MJH, et al. A segment of the 5′ nontranslated region of encephalomyocarditis virus RNA directs internal entry of ribosomes during in vitro translation. *J Virol* 1988;62:2636–2643.
244. Jarvis TC, Kirkegaard K. Poliovirus RNA recombination: mechanistic studies in the absence of selection. *EMBO J* 1992;11(8):3135–3145.
249. Johansson S, Niklasson B, Maizel J, et al. Molecular analysis of three Ljungan virus isolates reveals a new, close-to-root lineage of the Picornaviridae with a cluster of two unrelated 2A proteins. *J Virol* 2002;76(17): 8920–8930.
250. Johns HL, Berryman S, Monaghan P, et al. A dominant-negative mutant of rab5 inhibits infection of cells by foot-and-mouth disease virus: implications for virus entry. *J Virol* 2009;83(12):6247–6256.
253. Jore J, De Geus B, Jackson RJ, et al. Poliovirus protein 3CD is the active protease for processing of the precursor protein P1 in vitro. *J Gen Virol* 1988;69(Pt 7):1627–1636.
255. Jurgens CK, Barton DJ, Sharma N, et al. $2A^{pro}$ is a multifunctional protein that regulates the stability, translation and replication of poliovirus RNA. *Virology* 2006;345(2):346–357.
262. Kapoor A, Victoria J, Simmonds P, et al. A highly prevalent and genetically diversified Picornaviridae genus in South Asian children. *Proc Natl Acad Sci U S A* 2008;105(51):20482–20487.
265. Katpally U, Smith TJ. Pocket factors are unlikely to play a major role in the life cycle of human rhinovirus. *J Virol* 2007;81(12):6307–6315.
266. Katpally U, Fu TM, Freed DC, et al. Antibodies to the buried N terminus of rhinovirus VP4 exhibit cross-serotypic neutralization. *J Virol* 2009;83(14):7040–7048.
269. Khong A, Jan E. Modulation of stress granules and P bodies during dicistrovirus infection. *J Virol* 2011;85(4):1439–1451.
270. Kim C, Bergelson JM. Echovirus 7 entry into polarized intestinal epithelial cells requires clathrin and rab7. *MBio* 2012;3(2):e00304–e00311.
271. Kim SS, Smith TJ, Chapman MS, et al. Crystal structure of human rhinovirus serotype 1A (HRV1A). *J Mol Biol* 1989;210(1):91–111.
275. Kirkegaard K, Baltimore D. The mechanism of RNA recombination in poliovirus. *Cell* 1986;47(3):433–443.
277. Klein KA, Jackson WT. Picornavirus subversion of the autophagy pathway. *Viruses* 2011;3(9):1549–1561.
282. Koike S, Taya C, Kurata T, et al. Transgenic mice susceptible to poliovirus. *Proc Natl Acad Sci U S A* 1991;88:951–955.
283. Kolatkar PR, Bella J, Olson NH, et al. Structural studies of two rhinovirus serotypes complexed with fragments of their cellular receptor. *EMBO J* 1999;18(22):6249–6259.
284. Kortus MG, Kempf BJ, Haworth KG, et al. A template RNA entry channel in the fingers domain of the poliovirus polymerase. *J Mol Biol* 2012;417(4):263–278.
290. Lanke KH, van der Schaar HM, Belov GA, et al. GBF1, a guanine nucleotide exchange factor for Arf, is crucial for coxsackievirus B3 RNA replication. *J Virol* 2009;83(22):11940–11949.
291. Lau C, Wang X, Song L, et al. Syk associates with clathrin and mediates phosphatidylinositol 3-kinase activation during human rhinovirus internalization. *J Immunol* 2008;180(2):870–880.
293. Lee YF, Nomoto A, Detjen BM, et al. A protein covalently linked to poliovirus genome RNA. *Proc Natl Acad Sci U S A* 1977;74(1):59–63.
294. Lentz KN, Smith AD, Geisler SC, et al. Structure of poliovirus type 2 Lansing complexed with antiviral agent SCH48973: comparison of the structural and biological properties of three poliovirus serotypes. *Structure* 1997;5(7):961–978.
295. Levy HC, Bostina M, Filman DJ, et al. Catching a virus in the act of RNA release: a novel poliovirus uncoating intermediate characterized by cryo-electron microscopy. *J Virol* 2010;84(9):4426–4441.
296. Lewis JK, Bothner B, Smith TJ, et al. Antiviral agent blocks breathing of the common cold virus. *Proc Natl Acad Sci U S A* 1998;95(12): 6774–6778.
297. Li L, Victoria J, Kapoor A, et al. A novel picornavirus associated with gastroenteritis. *J Virol* 2009;83(22):12002–12006.
298. Li Q, Yafal AG, Lee YM, et al. Poliovirus neutralization by antibodies to internal epitopes of VP4 and VP1 results from reversible exposure of these sequences at physiological temperature. *J Virol* 1994;68(6): 3965–3970.
307. Love RA, Maegley KA, Yu X, et al. The crystal structure of the RNA-dependent RNA polymerase from human rhinovirus: a dual function target for common cold antiviral therapy. *Structure* 2004;12(8): 1533–1544.

311. Lyle JM, Bullitt E, Bienz K, et al. Visualization and functional analysis of RNA-dependent RNA polymerase lattices. *Science* 2002;296(5576): 2218–2222.
314. Marc D, Drugeon G, Haenni AL, et al. Role of myristoylation of poliovirus capsid protein VP4 as determined by site-directed mutagenesis of its N-terminal sequence. *EMBO J* 1989;8(9):2661–2668.
315. Marc D, Masson G, Girard M, et al. Lack of myristoylation of poliovirus capsid polypeptide VP0 prevents the formation of virions or results in the assembly of noninfectious virus particles. *J Virol* 1990;64(9): 4099–4107.
316. Marc D, Girard M, van der Werf S. A Gly1 to Ala substitution in poliovirus capsid protein VP0 blocks its myristoylation and prevents viral assembly. *J Gen Virol* 1991;72(Pt 5):1151–1157.
317. Marcotte LL, Wass AB, Gohara DW, et al. Crystal structure of poliovirus 3CD protein: virally encoded protease and precursor to the RNA-dependent RNA polymerase. *J Virol* 2007;81(7):3583–3596.
318. Marjomaki V, Pietiainen V, Matilainen H, et al. Internalization of echovirus 1 in caveolae. *J Virol* 2002;76(4):1856–1865.
319. Martin-Acebes MA, Gonzalez-Magaldi M, Sandvig K, et al. Productive entry of type C foot-and-mouth disease virus into susceptible cultured cells requires clathrin and is dependent on the presence of plasma membrane cholesterol. *Virology* 2007;369(1):105–118.
320. Martinez MA, Verdaguer N, Mateu MG, et al. Evolution subverting essentiality: dispensability of the cell attachment Arg-Gly-Asp motif in multiply passaged foot-and-mouth disease virus. *Proc Natl Acad Sci U S A* 1997; 94(13):6798–6802.
321. Mason PW, Baxt B, Brown F, et al. Antibody-complexed foot-and-mouth disease virus, but not poliovirus, can infect normally insusceptible cells via the Fc receptor. *Virology* 1993;192:568–577.
323. Matthews DA, Smith WW, Ferre RA, et al. Structure of human rhinovirus 3C protease reveals a trypsin-like polypeptide fold, RNA-binding site, and means for cleaving precursor polyprotein. *Cell* 1994;77(5): 761–771.
327. McErlean P, Shackelton LA, Andrews E, et al. Distinguishing molecular features and clinical characteristics of a putative new rhinovirus species, human rhinovirus C (HRV C). *PLoS One* 2008;3(4):e1847.
328. McKnight KL, Lemon SM. Capsid coding sequence is required for efficient replication of human rhinovirus 14 RNA. *J Virol* 1996;70(3): 1941–1952.
332. Mendelsohn CL, Wimmer E, Racaniello VR. Cellular receptor for poliovirus: molecular cloning, nucleotide sequence, and expression of a new member of the immunoglobulin superfamily. *Cell* 1989;56(5):855–865.
334. Minor PD, Schild GC, Bootman J, et al. Location and primary structure of a major antigenic site for poliovirus neutralization. *Nature* 1983;301(5902):674–679.
335. Minor PD, Ferguson M, Evans DM, et al. Antigenic structure of polioviruses of serotypes 1, 2 and 3. *J Gen Virol* 1986;67(Pt 7):1283–1291.
337. Moffat K, Howell G, Knox C, et al. Effects of foot-and-mouth disease virus nonstructural proteins on the structure and function of the early secretory pathway: 2BC but not 3A blocks endoplasmic reticulum-to-Golgi transport. *J Virol* 2005;79(7):4382–4395.
338. Molla A, Paul AV, Wimmer E. Cell-free, de novo synthesis of poliovirus. *Science* 1991;254:1647–1651.
339. Molla A, Paul AV, Schmid M, et al. Studies on dicistronic polioviruses implicate viral proteinase $2A^{pro}$ in RNA replication. *Virology* 1993; 196(2):739–747.
341. Morasco BJ, Sharma N, Parilla J, et al. Poliovirus cre(2C)-dependent synthesis of VPgpUpU is required for positive- but not negative-strand RNA synthesis. *J Virol* 2003;77(9):5136–5144.
344. Moscufo N, Chow M. Myristate-protein interactions in poliovirus: interactions of VP4 threonine 28 contribute to the structural conformation of assembly intermediates and the stability of assembled virions. *J Virol* 1992;66(12):6849–6857.
347. Mosser AG, Rueckert RR. WIN 51711-dependent mutants of poliovirus type 3: evidence that virions decay after release from cells unless drug is present. *J Virol* 1993;67(3):1246–1254.
348. Muckelbauer JK, Kremer M, Minor I, et al. The structure of coxsackievirus B3 at 3.5 A resolution. *Structure* 1995;3(7):653–667.
350. Murray KE, Barton DJ. Poliovirus CRE-dependent VPg uridylylation is required for positive-strand RNA synthesis but not for negative-strand RNA synthesis. *J Virol* 2003;77(8):4739–4750.
362. Nomoto A, Detjen B, Pozzatti R, et al. The location of the polio genome protein in viral RNAs and its implication for RNA synthesis. *Nature* 1977;268(5617):208–213.
363. Nomoto A, Kitamura N, Golini F, et al. The 5′-terminal structures of poliovirion RNA and poliovirus mRNA differ only in the genome-linked protein VPg. *Proc Natl Acad Sci U S A* 1977;74(12):5345–5349.
364. Novak JE, Kirkegaard K. Improved method for detecting poliovirus negative strands used to demonstrate specificity of positive-strand encapsidation and the ratio of positive to negative strands in infected cells. *J Virol* 1991;65:3384–3387.
370. Ohka S, Igarashi H, Nagata N, et al. Establishment of a poliovirus oral infection system in human poliovirus receptor-expressing transgenic mice that are deficient in alpha/beta interferon receptor. *J Virol* 2007;81(15):7902–7912.
371. Ohlmann T, Rau M, Morley SJ, et al. Proteolytic cleavage of initiation factor eIF-4 gamma in the reticulocyte lysate inhibits translation of capped mRNAs but enhances that of uncapped mRNAs. *Nucleic Acids Res* 1995;23(3):334–340.
372. Olson NH, Kolatkar PR, Oliveira MA, et al. Structure of a human rhinovirus complexed with its receptor molecule. *Proc Natl Acad Sci U S A* 1993;90:507–511.
376. Park N, Skern T, Gustin KE. Specific cleavage of the nuclear pore complex protein Nup62 by a viral protease. *J Biol Chem* 2010;285(37):28796–28805.
377. Parsley TB, Towner JS, Blyn LB, et al. Poly (rC) binding protein 2 forms a ternary complex with the 5′-terminal sequences of poliovirus RNA and the viral 3CD proteinase. *RNA* 1997;3(10):1124–1134.
381. Paul AV, van Boom JH, Filippov D, et al. Protein-primed RNA synthesis by purified poliovirus RNA polymerase. *Nature* 1998;393(6682): 280–284.
382. Paul AV, Rieder E, Kim DW, et al. Identification of an RNA hairpin in poliovirus RNA that serves as the primary template in the in vitro uridylylation of VPg. *J Virol* 2000;74(22):10359–10370.
385. Pelletier J, Sonenberg N. Internal initiation of translation of eukaryotic mRNA directed by a sequence derived from poliovirus RNA. *Nature* 1988;334:320–325.
386. Perera R, Daijogo S, Walter BL, et al. Cellular protein modification by poliovirus: the two faces of poly(rC)-binding protein. *J Virol* 2007;81(17): 8919–8932.
387. Perez L, Carrasco L. Entry of poliovirus into cells does not require a low-pH step. *J Virol* 1993;67(8):4543–4548.
388. Petersen JF, Cherney MM, Liebig HD, et al. The structure of the 2A proteinase from a common cold virus: a proteinase responsible for the shut-off of host-cell protein synthesis. *EMBO J* 1999;18(20):5463–5475.
389. Pettersson RF, Ambros V, Baltimore D. Identification of a protein linked to nascent poliovirus RNA and to the polyuridylic acid of negative-strand RNA. *J Virol* 1978;27(2):357–365.
393. Pfeiffer JK, Kirkegaard K. Increased fidelity reduces poliovirus fitness and virulence under selective pressure in mice. *PLoS Pathog* 2005;1(2):e11.
394. Pfister T, Wimmer E. Characterization of the nucleoside triphosphatase activity of poliovirus protein 2C reveals a mechanism by which guanidine inhibits poliovirus replication. *J Biol Chem* 1999;274(11):6992–7001.
396. Piccone ME, Zellner M, Kumosinski TF, et al. Identification of the active-site residues of the L proteinase of foot-and-mouth disease virus. *J Virol* 1995;69(8):4950–4956.
397. Pietiainen V, Marjomaki V, Upla P, et al. Echovirus 1 endocytosis into caveosomes requires lipid rafts, dynamin II, and signaling events. *Mol Biol Cell* 2004;15(11):4911–4925.
398. Pilipenko EV, Pestova TV, Kolupaeva VG, et al. A cell cycle-dependent protein serves as a template-specific translation initiation factor. *Genes Dev* 2000;14(16):2028–2045.
401. Pisareva VP, Pisarev AV, Komar AA, et al. Translation initiation on mammalian mRNAs with structured 5′UTRs requires DExH-box protein DHX29. *Cell* 2008;135(7):1237–1250.
402. Plevka P, Hafenstein S, Harris KG, et al. Interaction of decay-accelerating factor with echovirus 7. *J Virol* 2010;84(24):12665–12674.
403. Plevka P, Perera R, Cardosa J, et al. Crystal structure of human enterovirus 71. *Science* 2012;336(6086):1274.
406. Porter FW, Bochkov YA, Albee AJ, et al. A picornavirus protein interacts with Ran-GTPase and disrupts nucleocytoplasmic transport. *Proc Natl Acad Sci U S A* 2006;103(33):12417–12422.

407. Porter FW, Palmenberg AC. Leader-induced phosphorylation of nucleoporins correlates with nuclear trafficking inhibition by cardioviruses. *J Virol* 2009;83(4):1941–1951.
408. Porter FW, Brown B, Palmenberg AC. Nucleoporin phosphorylation triggered by the encephalomyocarditis virus leader protein is mediated by mitogen-activated protein kinases. *J Virol* 2010;84(24):12538–12548.
410. Prchla E, Kuechler E, Blaas D, et al. Uncoating of human rhinovirus serotype 2 from late endosomes. *J Virol* 1994;68(6):3713–3723.
414. Quiner CA, Jackson WT. Fragmentation of the Golgi apparatus provides replication membranes for human rhinovirus 1A. *Virology* 2010;407(2): 185–195.
416. Racaniello VR, Baltimore D. Cloned poliovirus complementary DNA is infectious in mammalian cells. *Science* 1981;214:916–919.
421. Ren R, Costantini FC, Gorgacz EJ, et al. Transgenic mice expressing a human poliovirus receptor: A new model for poliomyelitis. *Cell* 1990;63: 353–362.
422. Ren R, Racaniello V. Human poliovirus receptor gene expression and poliovirus tissue tropism in transgenic mice. *J Virol* 1992;66:296–304.
423. Rezapkin G, Neverov A, Cherkasova E, et al. Repertoire of antibodies against type 1 poliovirus in human sera. *J Virol Methods* 2010;169(2):322–331.
429. Rodriguez PL, Carrasco L. Poliovirus protein 2C has ATPase and GTPase activities. *J Biol Chem* 1993;268(11):8105–8110.
432. Roivainen M, Piirainen L, Rysa T, et al. An immunodominant N-terminal region of VP1 protein of poliovirion that is buried in crystal structure can be exposed in solution. *Virology* 1993;195(2):762–765.
435. Rossmann MG, Arnold E, Erickson JW, et al. Structure of a human common cold virus and functional relationship to other picornaviruses. *Nature* 1985;317:145–153.
440. Rudin CM, Poirier JT, Senzer NN, et al. Phase I clinical study of Seneca Valley Virus (SVV-001), a replication-competent picornavirus, in advanced solid tumors with neuroendocrine features. *Clin Cancer Res* 2011;17(4):888–895.
442. Rust RC, Landmann L, Gosert R, et al. Cellular COPII proteins are involved in production of the vesicles that form the poliovirus replication complex. *J Virol* 2001;75(20):9808–9818.
443. Sa-Carvalho D, Rieder E, Baxt B, et al. Tissue culture adaptation of foot-and-mouth disease virus selects viruses that bind to heparin and are attenuated in cattle. *J Virol* 1997;71(7):5115–5123.
450. Selinka H-C, Zibert A, Wimmer E. Poliovirus can enter and infect mammalian cells by way of an intercellular adhesion molecule 1 pathway. *Proc Natl Acad Sci U S A* 1991;88:3598–3602.
453. Shafren DR, Dorahy DJ, Ingham RA, et al. Coxsackievirus A21 binds to decay-accelerating factor but requires intercellular adhesion molecule 1 for cell entry. *J Virol* 1997;71(6):4736–4743.
458. Sherry B, Mosser AG, Colonno RJ, et al. Use of monoclonal antibodies to identify four neutralization immunogens on a common cold picornavirus, human rhinovirus 14. *J Virol* 1986;57(1):246–257.
462. Smith TJ, Kremer MJ, Luo M, et al. The site of attachment in human rhinovirus 14 for antiviral agents that inhibit uncoating. *Science* 1986;233(4770):1286–1293.
464. Smyth M, Pettitt T, Symonds A, et al. Identification of the pocket factors in a picornavirus. *Arch Virol* 2003;148(6):1225–1233.
471. Staunton DE, Merluzzi VJ, Rothlein R, et al. A cell adhesion molecule, ICAM-1, is the major surface receptor for rhinoviruses. *Cell* 1989;56:849–853.
477. Summers DF, Maizel JV. Evidence for large precursor proteins in poliovirus synthesis. *Proc Natl Acad Sci U S A* 1968;59:966–971.
478. Svitkin YV, Gradi A, Imataka H, et al. Eukaryotic initiation factor 4GII (eIF4GII), but not eIF4GI, cleavage correlates with inhibition of host cell protein synthesis after human rhinovirus infection. *J Virol* 1999;73(4):3467–3472.
484. Taylor MP, Kirkegaard K. Potential subversion of autophagosomal pathway by picornaviruses. *Autophagy* 2008;4(3):286–289.
485. Tellez AB, Crowder S, Spagnolo JF, et al. Nucleotide channel of RNA-dependent RNA polymerase used for intermolecular uridylylation of protein primer. *J Mol Biol* 2006;357(2):665–675.
486. Tellez AB, Wang J, Tanner EJ, et al. Interstitial contacts in an RNA-dependent RNA polymerase lattice. *J Mol Biol* 2011;412(4):737–750.
488. Thompson AA, Peersen OB. Structural basis for proteolysis-dependent activation of the poliovirus RNA-dependent RNA polymerase. *EMBO J* 2004;23(17):3462–3471.
489. Todd S, Towner JS, Brown DM, et al. Replication-competent picornaviruses with complete genomic RNA 3′ noncoding region deletions. *J Virol* 1997;71(11):8868–8874.
490. Tolskaya EA, Romanova LI, Kolesnikova MS, et al. Apoptosis-inducing and apoptosis-preventing functions of poliovirus. *J Virol* 1995;69(2): 1181–1189.
492. Tomassini JE, Graham D, DeWitt CM, et al. cDNA cloning reveals that the major group rhinovirus receptor on HeLa cells is intercellular adhesion molecule 1. *Proc Natl Acad Sci U S A* 1989;86:4907–4911.
493. Tosteson MT, Chow M. Characterization of the ion channels formed by poliovirus in planar lipid membranes. *J Virol* 1997;71(1):507–511.
501. Tuthill TJ, Harlos K, Walter TS, et al. Equine rhinitis A virus and its low pH empty particle: clues towards an aphthovirus entry mechanism? *PLoS Pathog* 2009;5(10):e1000620.
504. Van Dyke TA, Flanegan JB. Identification of poliovirus polypeptide p63 as a soluble RNA-dependent RNA polymerase. *J Virol* 1980;35: 732–740.
511. Venkataraman S, Reddy SP, Loo J, et al. Structure of Seneca Valley Virus-001: an oncolytic picornavirus representing a new genus. *Structure* 2008;16(10):1555–1561.
512. Verdaguer N, Fita I, Reithmayer M, et al. X-ray structure of a minor group human rhinovirus bound to a fragment of its cellular receptor protein. *Nat Struct Mol Biol* 2004;11(5):429–434.
513. Vignuzzi M, Stone JK, Arnold JJ, et al. Quasispecies diversity determines pathogenesis through cooperative interactions in a viral population. *Nature* 2006;439(7074):344–348.
515. Vogt DA, Andino R. An RNA element at the 5′-end of the poliovirus genome functions as a general promoter for RNA synthesis. *PLoS Pathog* 2010;6(6):e1000936.
519. Wang J, Fan T, Yao X, et al. Crystal structures of enterovirus 71 3C protease complexed with rupintrivir reveal the roles of catalytically important residues. *J Virol* 2011;85(19):10021–10030.
519a. Wang X, Lau C, Wiehler S, et al. Syk is downstream of intercellular adhesion molecule-1 and mediates human rhinovirus activation of p38 MAPK in airway epithelial cells. *J Immunol* 2006;177:6859–6870.
524. Weng KF, Li ML, Hung CT, et al. Enterovirus 71 3C protease cleaves a novel target CstF-64 and inhibits cellular polyadenylation. *PLoS Pathog* 2009;5(9):e1000593.
526. Wessels E, Duijsings D, Niu TK, et al. A viral protein that blocks Arf1-mediated COP-I assembly by inhibiting the guanine nucleotide exchange factor GBF1. *Dev Cell* 2006;11(2):191–201.
527. Wessels E, Duijsings D, Lanke KH, et al. Molecular determinants of the interaction between coxsackievirus protein 3A and guanine nucleotide exchange factor GBF1. *J Virol* 2007;81(10):5238–5245.
528. White JP, Cardenas AM, Marissen WE, et al. Inhibition of cytoplasmic mRNA stress granule formation by a viral proteinase. *Cell Host Microbe* 2007;2(5):295–305.
529. White JP, Lloyd RE. Poliovirus unlinks TIA1 aggregation and mRNA stress granule formation. *J Virol* 2011;85(23):12442–12454.
530. White JP, Reineke LC, Lloyd RE. Poliovirus switches to an eIF2-independent mode of translation during infection. *J Virol* 2011;85(17): 8884–8893.
534. Xiao C, Bator CM, Bowman VD, et al. Interaction of coxsackievirus A21 with its cellular receptor, ICAM-1. *J Virol* 2001;75(5):2444–2451.
535. Xiao C, Bator-Kelly CM, Rieder E, et al. The crystal structure of coxsackievirus A21 and its interaction with ICAM-1. *Structure* 2005;13(7):1019–1033.
541. Yogo Y, Wimmer E. Polyadenylic acid at the 3′-terminus of poliovirus RNA. *Proc Natl Acad Sci U S A* 1972;69(7):1877–1882.
542. Yogo Y, Teng MH, Wimmer E. Poly(U) in poliovirus minus RNA is 5′-terminal. *Biochem Biophys Res Commun* 1974;61(4):1101–1109.
544. Ypma-Wong MF, Dewalt PG, Johnson VH, et al. Protein 3CD is the major poliovirus proteinase responsible for cleavage of the P1 capsid precursor. *Virology* 1988;166(1):265–270.
546. Yu Y, Sweeney TR, Kafasla P, et al. The mechanism of translation initiation on Aichivirus RNA mediated by a novel type of picornavirus IRES. *EMBO J* 2011;30(21):4423–4436.
549. Zhang S, Racaniello VR. Expression of PVR in intestinal epithelial cells is not sufficient to permit poliovirus replication in the mouse gut. *J Virol* 1997;71:4915–4920.

CHAPTER 17

Mark A. Pallansch • M. Steven Oberste • J. Lindsay Whitton

Enteroviruses: Polioviruses, Coxsackieviruses, Echoviruses, and Newer Enteroviruses

HISTORY

The history of enteroviruses (EVs) is very much the history of poliovirus (PV). In fact, many of the PV milestones are landmarks in the study of EV and, in fact, all of virology.

Poliomyelitis is believed to be an ancient disease. It has been suggested that the depiction of a young man with an atrophic limb on an Egyptian stele from the second millennium bc represents a sequela of poliomyelitis.[197] The first clinical descriptions of poliomyelitis were made in the 1800s, with reports of cases of paralysis with fever. In 1840, von Heine[153] published a monograph more specifically describing the affliction. His contributions and those published later by Medin[271] from Sweden led to paralytic poliomyelitis being referred to as *Heine-Medin disease.* Another early report, by Charcot and Joffroy,[65] described the pathologic changes in the anterior horn motor neurons of the spinal cord in poliomyelitis.

The 1900s began a new era in poliomyelitis investigations and the beginning of an understanding of the infectious nature of this disease. Wickman[418] and others recognized the communicable nature of poliomyelitis, the importance of asymptomatic infected individuals in transmission of PV, and the role of enteric infection in disease pathogenesis. The role of the gastrointestinal tract in the initiation and spread of PV infection was later confirmed by Trask et al.[396] In a classic study, Viennese investigators Landsteiner and Popper[241] proved the infectious nature of poliomyelitis by successfully transmitting the clinical disease and its pathology to monkeys following inoculation of central nervous system (CNS) tissue homogenates from human cases.

Despite this progress, a number of unfortunate misconceptions emerged about poliomyelitis that initially confused scientists and misdirected efforts for control. These misconceptions included a belief that the virus was exclusively neurotropic, that the nasopharynx was a major site for virus entry into the CNS, and that the virus spread to the nervous system before viremia and by way of the olfactory nerve. As a result of these misconceptions and the failure of several poorly conceived immunization attempts, some with rather disastrous results,[328] an atmosphere of pessimism existed by the middle of the 20th century concerning the eventual control of poliomyelitis, even among scientists working in the field. In 1945, Burnet[49] wrote, "The practical problem of preventing infantile paralysis has not been solved. It is even doubtful whether it ever will be solved." The eventual realization that virus entered via the oral–gastrointestinal route and that CNS disease followed a viremia did much to boost hopes for effective immunization.[36]

Building on studies of others, Enders et al.[105] performed a landmark study showing that PV could be propagated in non-neural tissue culture. These investigations had implications for all of virology because they indicated, first, that PV grew in various tissue culture cells that did not correspond to the tissues infected during the human disease, and second, that PV destroyed cells with a specific cytopathic effect. Neutralization tests showed that PV has three serotypes,[39] and serologic tests[25] confirmed that most infected individuals do not manifest clinical disease. These investigations laid a critical framework for the development of a vaccine, and they clarified a host of confusing data, such as the apparent presence of second attacks of poliomyelitis.

A variety of vaccines were subsequently produced, with the most well known being the Salk inactivated polio vaccine (IPV) delivered via the intramuscular route (licensed in 1955 in the United States) and the Sabin live, attenuated vaccine (oral polio vaccine [OPV]) delivered via the oral route (licensed in 1961–1962). The importance of these vaccines and the individuals who produced them can begin to be realized by noting that more Americans knew the name of Jonas Salk than the president of the United States. The real impact of these vaccines will ultimately be felt with the complete global eradication of poliomyelitis. The eradication will undoubtedly provide a fitting dramatic finale to the compelling story of poliomyelitis.

Poliovirus work has had a continuing significant impact on the field of molecular virology. PV was the first animal virus completely cloned and sequenced,[227,337] the first RNA animal virus for which an infectious clone was constructed,[336] and the first human virus that had its three-dimensional structure solved by x-ray crystallography.[164] In 1989, Mendelsohn et al.[279] identified the PV receptor, CD155, a finding that was followed by the generation of mice carrying CD155 as a transgene.[234,344]

Coxsackieviruses (group A) were first isolated during poliomyelitis outbreaks in 1947 from the feces of paralyzed children in Coxsackie, New York.[89] These isolates were obtained by inoculation of suckling mice, the pathogenicity in mice clearly differentiating these viruses from PV. In the following year, the first coxsackievirus (CV) group B was isolated from cases of aseptic meningitis.[276] The original CV group A (CVA) isolates produced myositis with flaccid hind limb paralysis in newborn mice, whereas the coxsackieviruses group B (CVB) produced a spastic paralysis and generalized infection in newborn mice, with myositis and involvement of the brain, pancreas, heart, and brown fat.

In 1951, echoviruses were first isolated from the stool of asymptomatic individuals.[349] Echoviruses received their name because they were *e*nteric isolates, *c*ytopathogenic in tissue culture, isolated from *h*umans, and *o*rphans (i.e., unassociated with a known clinical disease). Subsequent studies have shown that echoviruses, in fact, do cause a variety of human diseases. After this period of rapid growth in the number of enteroviruses, there were several decades where new enteroviruses were uncommonly identified. This changed with the introduction of molecular detection methods, and the last 15 years have seen a rapid expansion in the number of recognized enteroviruses. This period of discovery is still in progress.

INFECTIOUS AGENTS

Physical and Chemical Properties

Enteroviruses are distinguished from other picornaviruses on the basis of physical properties, such as buoyant density in cesium chloride and stability in weak acid. Many aspects of enteroviral pathology, transmission, and general epidemiology are directly related to the biophysical properties and their cytolytic life cycle. The infectious virus is relatively resistant to many common laboratory disinfectants, including 70% ethanol, isopropanol, dilute Lysol, and quaternary ammonium compounds. The virus is insensitive to lipid solvents, including ether and chloroform, and it is stable in many detergents at ambient temperature. Formaldehyde, glutaraldehyde, strong acid, sodium hypochlorite, and free residual chlorine inactivate enteroviruses. Concentration, pH, extraneous organic materials, and contact time affect the degree of inactivation by these compounds. Similar inactivation is achieved when virus is present on fomites, although conditions may not be exactly comparable.[1] In general, most reagents that inactivate EV depend on active chemical modification of the virion, whereas most extractive solvents have no effect.

Enteroviruses are relatively thermostable, but less so than hepatitis A virus. Most enteroviruses are readily inactivated at 42°C, although some sulfhydryl reducing agents and magnesium cations can stabilize viruses so that they are relatively stable at 50°C.[8,99] The relative sensitivity to modest elevations in temperature makes it possible to use pasteurization to inactivate EV in many biologically active preparations.[160]

As with other infectious agents, ultraviolet light can be used to inactivate EV, particularly on surfaces. In addition, the process of drying on surfaces significantly reduces virus titers. The degree of virus loss by drying is related to porosity of the surfaces and the presence of organic material.[2] Many studies of EV inactivation have been conducted using PV as a model enterovirus. A report describing strain-specific differences for glutaraldehyde inactivation among echovirus 25 isolates implies, however, that the assumption that PV is representative of all EV may not be valid.[62] The inactivation of infectivity may not be directly related to the destruction of the viral genome, because the polymerase chain reaction (PCR) can be used to amplify viral RNA, even after inactivation of virus has occurred.[259] This would suggest that reactivation of infectivity may be possible in some circumstances. In fact, some examples of recovered infectivity have been reported through increased multiplicity of infection in cell culture,[372,443] but the practical significance of these observations is not clear.

Antigenic Characteristics and Taxonomy

As described in Chapter 16, the picornaviruses are among the simplest RNA viruses, having a highly structured capsid with little place for elaboration. Yet, despite the limited genetic material and structural constraints, evolution within the picornaviruses has resulted in a large number of readily distinguishable members. This variability has been categorized antigenically as serotype.

Each of the serotypes correlates with the immunologic response of the human host, protection from disease, receptor usage, and, to a lesser extent, the spectrum of clinical disease. These correlations, however, have only a partial relationship with the original classification of enteroviruses into polioviruses, coxsackie A or B viruses, and echoviruses, based on biological activity and disease: human CNS disease with flaccid paralysis (poliomyelitis); flaccid paralysis in newborn mice, human CNS disease, and herpangina (coxsackie A viruses); spastic paralysis in newborn mice and human CNS and cardiac disease (coxsackie B viruses); and no disease in mice and (originally) no human disease (echoviruses). Within each of these groups, isolates can be readily distinguished on the basis of antigenicity as measured with antisera raised in animals. The original classification scheme broke down with the identification of viruses serologically identical to known echoviruses that were found to cause disease in mice and humans. This and other inconsistencies led to a numbering of new EV serotypes starting with EV68. These antigenic groupings, which define the serotypes, became increasingly more complicated as the number of different viruses grew. Despite these limitations, the serotype remains the single most important physical and immunologic property that distinguishes the different EVs. Most of the prototype EV strains are maintained in the American Type Culture Collection, Manassas, Virginia, and in many of the World Health Organization (WHO) collaborating reference laboratories.

Despite the importance of the antigenic properties, the introduction of molecular typing methods and a reassessment of the limitations of the old classification scheme led to the development of the current classification system that divides the members of the EV genus into species on the basis of genome organization and sequence similarity as well as biological properties (Table 17.1).

The human enteroviruses are now classified into four species: *Enterovirus A* (EV-A), EV-B, EV-C, and EV-D. In this system, members within an EV species:

> share greater than 70% aa [amino acid] identity in the polyprotein, share greater than 60% aa identity in P1, share greater than 70% aa identity in the nonstructural proteins 2C + 3CD, share a limited range of host cell receptors, share a limited natural host range, have a genome base composition (G + C) which varies by no more than 2.5%, share a significant degree of compatibility in proteolytic processing, replication, encapsidation, and genetic recombination.[230]

Coding for the capsid proteins, the P1 region provides a reliable correlation between sequence relatedness and the traditional definition of serotype. This also appears to be true for the various individual capsid protein regions, with the exception of VP4; the VP4 sequence does not always correlate with serotype and, therefore, is not reliable for serotype identification.

The molecular studies have also provided a framework in which the EV antigenic relationships can be better understood. These studies suggest that the nucleotide sequence of VP1 can function as an excellent surrogate for the reference antigenic typing methods that use neutralization tests in order to distinguish EV serotypes. VP1 nucleotide sequence identity of at least 75% (85% aa identity) between an isolate and a serotype prototype strain suggests that the isolate is serotypically identical to the prototype (assuming that the next highest identity with other prototype strains is less than 70%). For example, a capsid sequence identity of 85.4% aa between CVA3 and A8 compared with a mean sequence identity among prototype strains of 71.5% confirmed the antigenic relationships that had previously been described and suggested that these two viruses probably derived relatively recently from a common ancestor.[318] Similarly, capsid sequences with more than 96% identity confirmed the antigenic relationships between CVA11 and A15 and between A13 and A18;[46] as a result, CVA15 and A18 have been reclassified as A11 and A15, respectively. In this way, the use of VP1 sequencing studies has supported and clarified early serologic data and also led to proposals regarding the classification of isolates into new EV serotypes.[312,316]

No general correlation is found, however, between sequence similarities with serotype in genome segments outside of the capsid region because of frequent recombination in the noncapsid regions. For example, sequencing studies have shown that phylogenetic trees constructed from sequences from varying genome regions of members of EV-C and *Poliovirus* have incongruities between the capsid region and noncapsid regions,[46] suggesting that viruses with a PV capsid may recombine with these CV nonstructural protein coding regions to acquire different nonstructural protein sequences and, similarly, viruses with a CV capsid protein sequence may recombine to acquire different nonstructural protein sequences.[255] These findings imply that recombination occurs between PV and other EV-C viruses within the nonstructural protein coding regions, and this shuffling of different nonstructural protein coding regions may lead to serotypes with selective advantages that become dominant. The frequency of recombination in the noncapsid region supports the idea that serotype is defined by the capsid region and that limited correlations likely exist between the serotype of isolates and other phenotypic characteristics not associated with the capsid proteins. The findings also demonstrated that the phylogenetic clustering of prototype strains changes, depending on the nonstructural region that is analyzed.

Recombination within the nonstructural proteins was also found among EV-A and EV-B prototype members with other members of the same species, consistent with their classification into two separate species.[314,318] An analysis of multiple isolates within several EV-B serotypes[319] found relatively frequent interserotypic recombination of the noncoding regions, which appeared to occur at least once every 6 years for the isolates that were analyzed. Although no evidence was found of interserotypic recombination within the capsid (perhaps because of structural constraints specific for a particular serotype), intraserotypic recombination within this region appeared to occur.

Additional sequencing studies showed that the 5′ untranslated region (UTR) of enteroviruses forms two clusters: the viruses of EV-C and EV-D compose cluster I, whereas EV-A and EV-B compose cluster II.[46,188]

Sequencing studies have also demonstrated significant similarities between human rhinoviruses and the human enteroviruses, resulting in a reclassification of the human rhinoviruses as members of three different species within the genus *Enterovirus*.[230] Despite the reclassification, the rhinoviruses have several unique properties and are covered separately in this volume (see Chapter 18).

TABLE 17.1 Picornavirus Genera, Species,[a] and (Sero)Types

Genera and species	No. of types	Comments
Genus *Enterovirus*	**269**	
Human enterovirus A[b]	22	Five have been found only in nonhuman primates
Human enterovirus B[b]	60	Two have been found only in nonhuman primates
Human enterovirus C[b]	21	
Human enterovirus D[b]	4	
Human rhinovirus A[b]	77	
Human rhinovirus B[b]	25	
Human rhinovirus C[b]	49	
Simian enterovirus A	1	
Bovine enterovirus	2	Possible third type detected in sheep
Porcine enterovirus B	3	
Unclassified	5	Detected in nonhuman primates
Genus *Hepatovirus*[b]	**1**	
Genus *Cardiovirus*	**12**	
Encephalomyocarditis virus[b]	1	
Theilovirus[b]	11	
Genus *Kobuvirus*	**3**	
Aichi virus[b]	1	
Bovine kobuvirus	1	Also found in sheep and pigs
Porcine kobuvirus	1	
Unclassified	2	One virus detected in rodents and one in dogs
Genus *Teschovirus*	**11**	
Genus *Erbovirus*	**3**	
Genus *Aphthovirus*	**11**	
Foot-and-mouth disease virus	7	
Bovine rhinitis A virus	1	
Bovine rhinitis B virus	2	
Equine rhinitis A virus	1	
Genus *Parechovirus*	**20**	
Human parechovirus[b]	16	Types 1 and 2 formerly classified in genus *Enterovirus*
Ljungan virus	4	
Genus *Sapelovirus*	**8**	
Simian sapelovirus	3	
Porcine sapelovirus	1	Formerly porcine enterovirus A in genus *Enterovirus*
Avian sapelovirus	1	
Unclassified	3	One virus detected in rodents and two in sea lions
Genus *Senecavirus*	**1**	
Genus *Tremovirus*	**1**	
Genus *Avihepatovirus*	**3**	
Proposed genus Aquamavirus	**1**	
Proposed genus Cosavirus[b]	**4**	
Proposed genus Megrivirus	**1**	
Proposed genus Salivirus[b]	**1**	
Unclassified picornaviruses	**18**	Viruses detected in bats, cats, rodents, sheep, birds, fish, and reptiles

[a]The classification scheme shown is from the Picornavirus Study Group of the International Committee on the Taxonomy of Viruses (Knowles NJ, Hovi T, Hyypiä T, et al. Picornaviridae. In: King AMQ, Adams MJ, Carstens EB, et al., eds. *Virus Taxonomy: Classification and Nomenclature of Viruses: Ninth Report of the International Committee on Taxonomy of Viruses*. San Diego: Elsevier, 2011:855–880; and http://www.picornaviridae.com). The types that compose the human enterovirus species are listed in Tables 17.4 through 17.7.

[b]At least one virus in the genus or species has been detected in humans.

In addition to the genetic relatedness, many different EV serotypes share some antigenicity. For example, PV1 and 2 share a common antigen, and antigenic relationships also exist between coxsackieviruses A3 and A8, A16 and EV71, and A24 and EV70, and between echoviruses 6 and 30, and 12 and 29. When virions are disrupted by heating, particularly in the presence of detergent, nonsurface antigens are exposed that are shared broadly among many EVs.[280]

Despite this lack of understanding of molecular variation in virus structure as measured by polyclonal antibodies, high-resolution studies of the virion surface have been particularly useful in identifying the targets of neutralization of EV by monoclonal antibodies.[165,327] Other less investigated antigenic sites elicit immune responses that are not neutralizing but nevertheless contribute to serotype identity. The observed structure of some antigenic sites has been shown to span noncontinuous polypeptide chains, providing an explanation for why antigenicity of the virus is destroyed by disruption of the virion structure.

Antisera raised in animals to each of the enteroviruses are largely type specific and are used to determine serotype in a neutralization assay. The PV neutralizing antibody response is serotype specific, with the exception of some minor cross-reaction between PV1 and 2. A monoclonal antibody has been described that reacts with this shared site that is not found on PV3.[403] As noted, heat-disrupted virions, particularly those heated in the presence of detergent, induce antibodies that react with many EVs.[280] These broadly reacting antibodies are generally not neutralizing, and at least one of these epitopes has been mapped to the amino-terminal region of capsid protein VP1.[362] Although measurable *in vitro* differences are found in antigenic properties among strains within a serotype, the significance of these differences during natural infection has not been determined. Several PVs isolated during outbreaks have demonstrated different antigenic properties when compared with the reference vaccine strains.[140,186] In all cases, immunity derived from vaccination has been sufficient to provide protection and control of these strains.[43] In addition, even in the face of massive immunization campaigns, no antigenic *escape mutants* resistant to neutralization have ever been observed, and successive genotypes of PV have been eliminated. Natural antigenic variants have also been identified with panels of monoclonal antibodies for several nonpolio EVs.[148,329]

Propagation and Assay in Cell Culture

One of the prominent characteristics of enteroviruses is the cytolytic nature of growth in cell culture. For many years, PV was the prototype of a lytic viral infection. At the microscopic level, infection is usually manifest within 1 to 7 days by the appearance of a characteristic cytopathic effect, which features visible rounding, shrinking, nuclear pyknosis, refractility, and cell degeneration (Fig. 17.1). The earliest effects can be seen in less than 24 hours if the inoculum contains many infectious particles. With fewer virions, however, visible changes are not recognizable for several days, although a sufficient number of cells are infected. In addition, some EVs either do not cause cytopathic effect at all or do so only after several passages. In general, once focal cytopathic effect is detected, infection spreads rapidly throughout the cell sheet with total destruction of the monolayer, sometimes in a matter of hours.

All known EVs can be propagated in either cell culture or in suckling mice. Most of the serotypes can be grown in at least one human or primate continuous cell culture. No cell line, however, can support the growth of all cultivable EVs. Even after many years of experimentation, a few serotypes (e.g., CVA19) can be propagated only in suckling mice. The typical host range of human EV in cell cultures or animals is shown in a broad, generalized way in Table 17.2 and is not clearly associated specifically with a given virus species.[275] Infection of target cells depends on viruses binding to specific receptors on the cell surface. Collectively, the EVs use many different receptors. A practical adaptation resulting from the identification and genetic cloning of EV receptors is the introduction of the receptor into animals and cells that do not normally permit virus infection. This approach has resulted in advances in understanding both the pathogenesis of PV infection in a nonprimate animal model system and its practical application in the diagnostic laboratory. The L20B cells, which are murine cells that express CD155, are now used routinely to selectively isolate PV (see Diagnosis) as part of the global PV laboratory network supporting the poliomyelitis eradication initiative.[333]

Infection in Experimental Animals: Host Range

The natural host for all human enteroviruses is the human. Although serologically distinct picornaviruses with the same physical properties as human EV have been found in many animals, human beings do not usually have recognizable infections with these animal EV. On the other hand, some animals are susceptible to experimental infection with human EV. These include nonhuman primates and CD155 transgenic mice for polioviruses, mice and some monkeys for coxsackieviruses A and B, and monkeys for echoviruses. Human EV can infect nonhuman primates, perhaps related to the homology that several simian EVs share with human viruses, but the infections appear to be largely subclinical.[313,334] Among higher primates, chimpanzees and gorillas appear to be able to acquire PV infection and develop disease from humans through natural exposure.[100] CVB5 is closely related antigenically to the porcine EV causing swine vesicular disease, with about 50% genetic homology over the entire genome. Genetic studies of a number of strains of swine vesicular disease virus, as well as epidemiologic information gleaned from outbreaks, strongly suggest that a human CVB5 was specifically introduced into swine decades ago and led to establishment in this new host.[448]

Although most coxsackie A viruses have been successfully grown in various cell culture systems, isolation from clinical specimens is sometimes unsuccessful, necessitating the inoculation of suckling mice. Inoculation of suckling mice and subsequent virus identification is a process analogous to that of cell culture inoculation. A blind passage in mice may be necessary if the inoculum is of very low titer or, possibly, because passage of the virus is needed for it to adapt to growth in mice. The two groups of coxsackieviruses can be distinguished by the distinct pathology that they cause in mice (Figs. 17.2 and 17.3). With CVA infection, newborn mice develop flaccid paralysis and severe, extensive degeneration of skeletal muscle (sparing the tongue, heart, and CNS), and they may have renal lesions. Death usually occurs within a week. CVB infection proceeds more slowly and is characterized by spastic paralysis and tremors associated with encephalomyelitis, focal myositis, necrosis of brown fat pads, myocarditis, hepatitis, and acinar cell

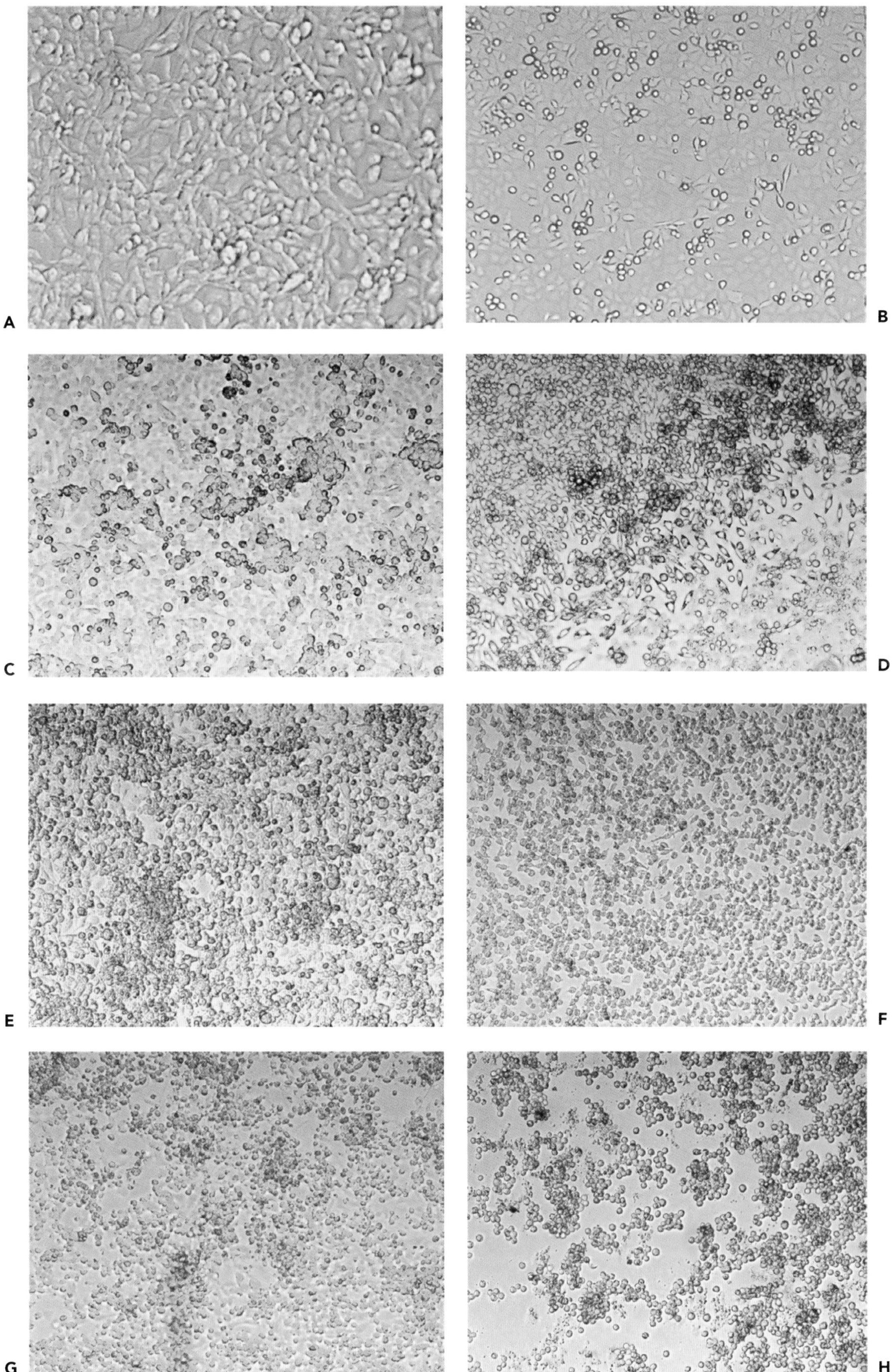

FIGURE 17.1. Normal and poliovirus (PV)-infected rhabdomyosarcoma (RD) cells and CD155 transgenic mouse L cells (L20B) in culture. **A:** Monolayer of normal RD cells in culture. **B:** RD cell culture showing early stage of cytopathic effect typical of PV infection. Approximately 25% of the cells in the culture show cytopathic effect (especially rounding) indicative of virus multiplication (1+ cytopathic effect score). **C:** RD cell culture illustrating more advanced cytopathic effect (3+ to 4+ cytopathic effect). **D:** Almost 100% of the cells are affected, and most of the cell sheet has come loose from the wall of the culture tube. **E–H:** Similar stages of cytopathic effect are shown as in **A–D,** but in this case L20B cells are infected with PV.

TABLE 17.2 Usual Host Range of Human Enteroviruses: Animal and Tissue Culture Spectrum[a]

		Cytopathic effect		Illness and pathology	
Virus	Antigenic types[b]	Monkey kidney tissue culture	Human tissue culture	Suckling mouse	Monkey
Polioviruses	1–3	+	+	–	+
Coxsackieviruses, group A	1–22, 24	±	±	+	–
Coxsackieviruses, group B	1–6	+	+	+	–
Echoviruses	1–33	+	±	–	–
Enteroviruses	68–116	+	+	–	–

[a] Many enteroviral strains have been isolated that do not conform to these categories.

[b] New types, beginning with type 68, are now assigned enterovirus type numbers instead of coxsackievirus or echovirus numbers. Types 68–116 have been identified.
Adapted from Melnick JL. Enteroviruses: polioviruses, coxsackieviruses, echoviruses, and newer enteroviruses. In: Fields BN, Knipe DM, Howley PM, eds. *Fields Virology*. 3rd ed. Philadelphia: Lippincott-Raven, 1996:655–712.

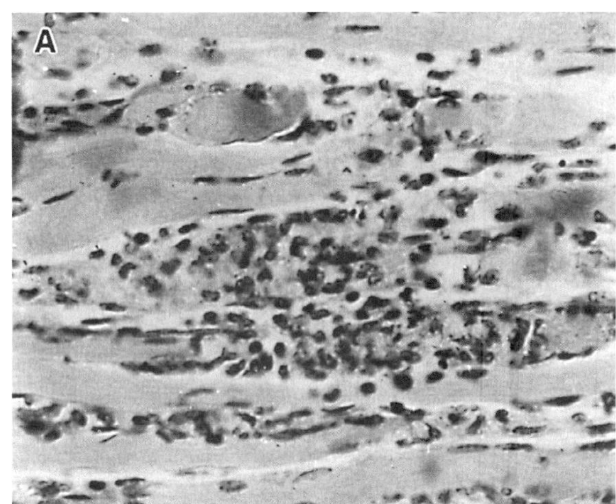

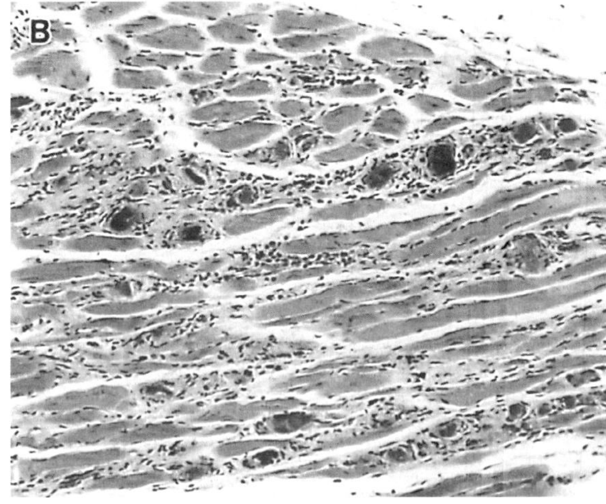

FIGURE 17.2. **Photomicrographs of lesions of striated muscle in suckling mice infected with coxsackieviruses. A:** Two sarcolemmic tubes with numerous mononuclear phagocytes and remnants of hyaline material within the sarcolemmic sheaths. Acute stage of infection with Conn-5 strain, prototype of coxsackievirus B1 (CVB1) (×450). **B:** Partly mineralized residual masses surrounded by fibrous capsules, and sometimes by giant cells. The remainder of the muscle is completely restored. Texas-1 strain of CVA4, 11 days after onset of paralysis (×180). (From Melnick JL. Current status of poliovirus infections. *Clin Microbiol Rev* 1996;9[3]:293–300, with permission.)

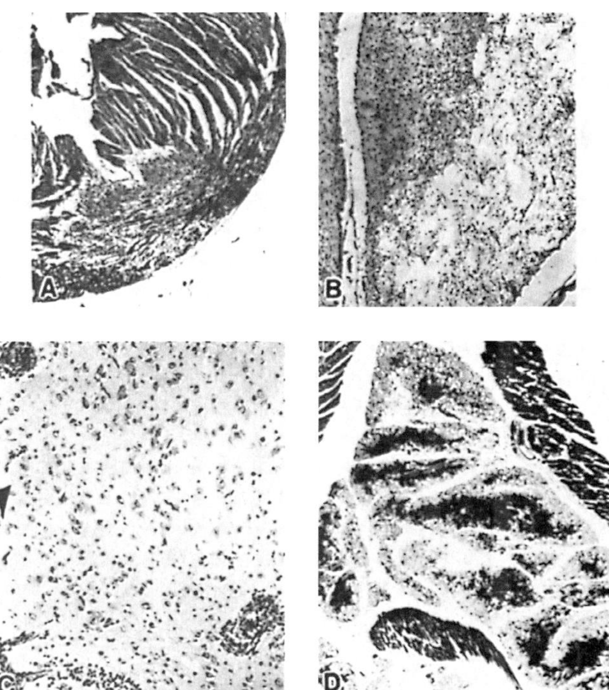

FIGURE 17.3. **Photomicrographs of lesions in heart, brain, and fat lobules of suckling mice in acute stage of infection with Conn-5 strain of coxsackievirus B1 (CVB1) (90). A:** Heart. Large zone of myocardial necrosis at apex of left ventricle (×170). **B:** Brain. Rarefaction after necrosis in cerebrum (×140). **C:** Brain. Encephalitis showing marked perivascular cuffing and leptomeningitis (×190). **D:** Fat lobes. Interlobular edema and acute necrotizing steatitis, illustrating the selective destruction of the peripheral parts of the lobules, which are shown as pale margins, with preservation of the central parts, which are shown as dark fuchsinophilic areas (×72). (From Melnick JL. Current status of poliovirus infections. *Clin Microbiol Rev* 1996;9[3]:293–300, with permission.)

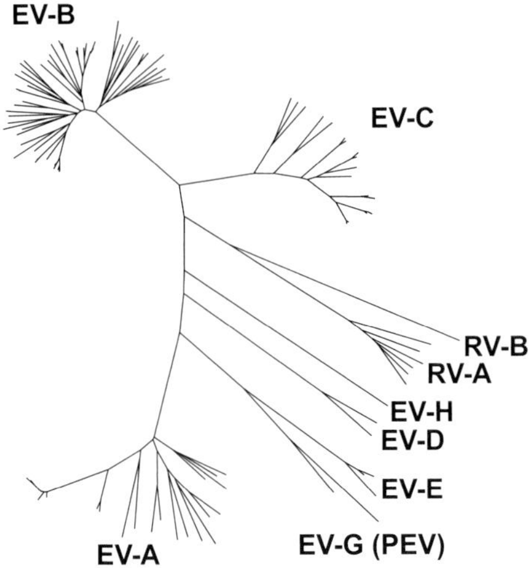

FIGURE 17.4. Dendrogram of genus *Enterovirus*. The figure illustrates the phylogenetic relationship among the prototype strains (see Tables 17.4 through 17.7) within the genus *Enterovirus* and the distinct grouping of isolates into each of the species of viruses that affects humans and other related animal enteroviruses based on the amino acid sequence of the P1 (capsid) coding region of the genomes. Species: EV-A (formerly *Human enterovirus A*); EV-B (formerly *Human enterovirus B*); EV-C (formerly *Human enterovirus C*); EV-D (formerly *Human enterovirus D*); RV-A (formerly *Human rhinovirus A*); RV-B (formerly *Human rhinovirus B*); EV-E (formerly *Bovine enterovirus*); EV-G (formerly *Porcine enterovirus B*); EV-H (formerly *Simian enterovirus B*). Not shown: EV-F (*Bovine enterovirus 2*), EV-J (*Simian virus 6* and related viruses), and RV-C. (Data from M. S. Oberste.)

pancreatitis. Echoviruses, except for some isolates of echovirus type 9, do not generally cause disease in mice.

Other Human Picornaviruses

In addition to the enteroviruses, rhinoviruses (Chapter 18), and hepatitis A (Chapter 19), other picornaviruses that infect humans have been recently discovered or previously considered to be enteroviruses and reclassified as a separate genus (Table 17.1). These genera are genetically distinct from the EV genus (Fig. 17.4) but share some physical and structural similarity with EV. On the basis of a very low genetic relationship, differences in viral proteins and processing, and a novel 2A protease, echoviruses 22 and 23 were reclassified as a new genus, *Parechovirus*. Additional members of this genus exist, including additional serotypes of human parechovirus,[192] as well as a separate species first isolated in Swedish bank voles, Ljungan virus; Ljungan virus has been associated with diabetes in its natural host and may have a possible role in human disease.[302] The human parechoviruses (HPeVs) cause a similar spectrum of illnesses as the EVs and can often be detected in cerebrospinal fluid (CSF) from meningitis cases at a frequency similar to that of the EVs.[409,422] Serologic studies suggest that HPeV infection occurs at an early age, as most children were seropositive by the age of 2 years.[3,198,385] HPeV3 has been associated with sepsis-like illness and CNS disease in infants.[32,41]

Another distinct picornavirus genus associated with human infection is *Kobuvirus*.[434] Although little information is currently available about this virus, it appears that it is often associated with gastroenteritis in young children and infection is common. Members of the genus *Cardiovirus* have also been associated with disease in humans, but they do not appear to be a major cause of human illness.[301,309] Viruses in the proposed genus Salivirus are related to kobuviruses and have also been associated with gastroenteritis in humans.[167,250] Another proposed genus, Cosavirus, has been detected at a relatively high frequency in stool, but there is no known association with disease. What is notable about all of these newer genera is that the currently available molecular reagents for the detection of EV do not detect these viruses (see Diagnosis).

PATHOGENESIS AND PATHOLOGY

Entry into the Host

Virus infection normally requires that the virion can attach to the cell surface, and it was long imagined that each virus would have a single receptor. For poliovirus, at least, this may be the case: the virus binds to the poliovirus receptor (PVR,[279] now named CD155), a transmembrane glycoprotein in the immunoglobulin superfamily that mediates adhesion of natural killer (NK) cells, and triggers their effector functions. PVR (human CD155) appears to be the major factor regulating the virus's natural host range, which is limited to humans and Old World primates. CD155 homologs/orthologs have been identified and characterized in mice[289] and in New World monkeys; the extracellular domains share ~70% amino acid homology with hCD155, and these homologs do not support efficient PV binding or infection. Several laboratories have generated transgenic mice that express PVR, and in many of the resulting models, PV was shown to induce neurologic disease and paralysis following parenteral administration.[82,117,189,233,279,295,342–344,449] However, oral administration did not cause disease even when the PVR transgene was regulated by a promoter that drove protein expression in enterocytes and microfold (M) cells; PV appeared to bind to the intestinal cells, but productive infection was not observed following oral inoculation of greater than 10^8 plaque-forming units/mL (pfu) of virus.[449] These findings are consistent with studies of humans and susceptible primates, in which hCD155 expression has been identified in many tissues, but productive infection is limited largely to the CNS. Thus, factors other than PVR expression play a key role in determining *in vivo* tropism.

It is now generally accepted that some viruses, or viral strains, may have more than one receptor, perhaps expanding their potential host range. EV71, most frequently associated with hand-foot-and-mouth disease in children but capable of causing devastating neurologic pathology,[381] has at least two receptors: scavenger receptor B2[435] and P-selectin glycoprotein ligand-1.[303] Indeed, some viruses appear to interact with two different surface molecules on a single cell, perhaps in series, with one protein acting as the binding moiety, before "handing over" the virus to a second protein that facilitates its entry into the cell. This is thought to occur for some CVBs that bind to decay accelerating factor (DAF, CD55) but then must interact with another protein, the *c*oxsackievirus and *a*denovirus *r*eceptor (CAR), in order to enter the cell.

Site of Primary Replication

Human enteroviruses are spread by the fecal–oral route and respiratory droplets, so systemic infection requires the virus to cross the gastrointestinal wall, most of which is lined with epithelial cells that form a barrier to invasion. Perhaps surprisingly, given the many years of study, the primary site of PV infection and replication in the intestine remain unknown. PV has been identified in lymphoid tissues, such as the tonsils,[36] and in lymphoid aggregates, commonly termed Peyer's patches (PPs), that are present in the ileum of the small intestine. PPs are overlaid with a specialized follicle-associated epithelium (FAE) that contains M cells, which can transport certain molecules from the gastrointestinal lumen, across the epithelial layer, and into cells in the PP. Some studies suggest that PV may replicate within these epithelial cells and lymphoid cells,[204] while others suggest that the virus may be transcytosed through the M cell, subsequently establishing infection in an unidentified cell in the PP.[375] The cells in which CVB initially replicates are also uncertain; this issue is further clouded by the predominant use, in mouse models, of the intraperitoneal route of infection. Human rhinovirus (HRV) infects epithelial cells of the airways. Infection of the nasal epithelium causes few detectable pathologic changes, even if rhinitis is quite severe, and—as is true for many virus-induced diseases—many of the symptoms appear to be caused by the host response rather than by direct virus-mediated tissue damage.[420,421]

Spread in the Host

Following replication in the alimentary tract, PV enters the blood, thereby potentially gaining access to all tissues; however, in normal hosts, viral replication is highly restricted, being readily detected mainly in the CNS.[36] PV can enter the CNS in two ways: first, from the blood—the virus is thought to be able to cross the blood brain barrier (BBB), perhaps independently of the PVR,[437] thereby accessing the CNS parenchyma; and second, by retrograde axonal transport, in which the virus (apparently in the form of an intact virion) ascends the neuronal axon, perhaps in endosomes, and uncoating begins when PV reaches the cell body.[320–322] This may underpin provocation poliomyelitis, a phenomenon in which a traumatized limb is more susceptible to paralytic polio. The trauma may be directly associated with the virus, as reported in 1935, when it was noted that paralysis first appeared in (or was most severe in) the limb that had received an intramuscular inoculation of "pre-Salk" polio vaccine.[244] Such inoculation poliomyelitis also was observed in the "Cutter incident," when an incompletely inactivated Salk vaccine was administered.[297] However, provocation poliomyelitis does not require that trauma and virus be administered to the same limb; when PV was administered intravascularly to monkeys that had received innocuous injections into one limb, paralysis was more likely to develop in the injected muscles.[38] Provocation poliomyelitis also has been reproduced in a mouse model.[139] Mechanisms other than retrograde axonal transport may contribute. For example, the peripheral trauma may increase the permeability of the BBB locally, in the region that innervates the injured muscle; this could explain why provocation poliomyelitis still occurs in traumatized limbs despite scission of the ipsilateral peroneal muscle.[296] Dissemination of CVB and other enteroviruses appears to occur largely by the hematogenous route. Viremia is frequently found, when sought; this is true even in rhinovirus infection of normal or asthmatic children,[432] in which spread to the lower respiratory tract was thought to occur by more direct means.

Cell and Tissue Tropism

It has been proposed that the observed *in vivo* tropism of PV for the CNS may result from differing efficiencies of viral internal ribosome entry site (IRES) utilization by the various cell types. However, this explanation appears to be incorrect; the PV IRES is equally functional in many cell types *in vivo*, including those that do not support virus replication in the living animal.[211] Rather, the explanation may lie in the ability of an infected cell (or tissue) to respond to type I interferons (T1IFNs). Following PV infection, PVR transgenic mice lacking the receptor for these key antiviral cytokines developed severe lesions not only in the CNS but also in the liver, spleen, and pancreas.[190] Thus, in immunocompetent PVR transgenic mice (and, by extension, in the natural hosts), the absence of apparent PV infection in most hCD155+ peripheral tissues may result from these cells' being able to mount rapid and strong T1IFN responses; and the apparent neurotropism of the virus in immunocompetent hosts may reflect a reduced or delayed T1IFN response within the CNS.[190]

CVB3 can cause pancreatitis, myocarditis, and meningoencephalitis. Enteroviruses, and especially CVB, have been implicated in up to one-third of human pancreatitis cases.[22,326,404] In the mouse model, the pancreas appears to be the first major site of abundant CVB3 replication, with virus titers reaching ~10^4 pfu/gram after only 12 hours, and ~10^{10} pfu/gram at 24 hours postinfection.[277,278] As shown in Figure 17.5A, there is a large inflammatory infiltrate and widespread destruction of the exocrine pancreas, but the islets of Langerhans remain apparently unaffected. Transmission electron microscopy (Fig. 17.5B and C) reveals, in infected acinar cells, nuclear pyknosis and the accumulation of small double-membraned autophagy-like vesicles, also termed compound membrane vesicles, which are characteristic of enterovirus-infected cells. CVB4 also causes pancreatitis,[339,340,406] the severity of which depends on the virus isolate that is used; a single amino acid change in VP1 appears to be largely responsible for switching the phenotype from mild pancreatitis to a more severe form.[51,142] CVB has been found in acinar cells but not in islets of Langerhans[356,407,410] by immunohistochemistry[23,406] and by *in situ* hybridization.[23,407,410] CAR expression correlates with the observed pathology: the receptor messenger RNA (mRNA) is expressed at very high levels in acinar cells but not in the pancreatic ducts or the islets of Langerhans (204), consistent with the observation that CVB-infected mice do not develop hyperglycemia.[277,338] Cre recombinase-mediated deletion of CAR from the pancreas confers substantial, albeit incomplete, protection against organ damage during CVB infection.[203]

A role for EV-B, and in particular CVB, also has been suggested in type 1 diabetes (T1D), and evidence is available to support this notion.[40,75,341] Several studies have implicated antibody or T-cell cross-reactivity between CVB and host proteins to explain the observed correlations.[107,179,180,299,300,353] The innate immune system, too, may be involved; a human genome-wide scan for nonsynonymous single nucleotide polymorphisms, comparing healthy individuals to diabetic patients, identified MDA5 as a T1D susceptibility locus.[379] However, despite many years of study, a causal role for CVB (or any enterovirus) in T1D has not been convincingly demonstrated in humans, and the issue remains controversial. It is possible that, as has been proposed for pancreatitis, enteroviruses are a co-factor in T1D, very rarely initiating disease in healthy islets but tipping

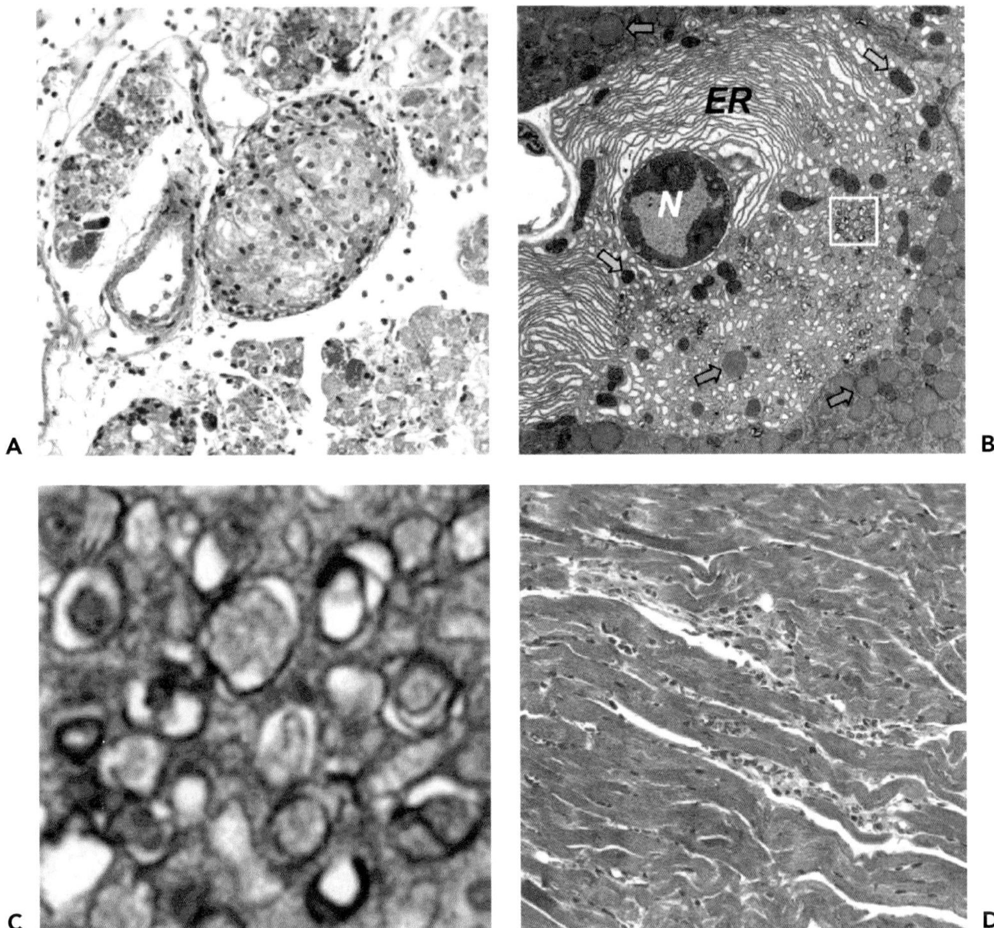

FIGURE 17.5. Histopathology and electron microscopy of coxsackievirus B3 (CVB3)-infected mice. **A:** Inflammatory infiltrate of pancreas with destruction of the exocrine pancreas but sparing of the islets of Langerhans. **B:** Transmission electron microscopy of infected acinar cells showing nuclear pyknosis. **C:** Further magnification of **B** showing accumulation of small double-membraned autophagy-like vesicles. **D:** Infected heart myocardium showing inflammatory infiltrate that contains predominantly macrophages, T cells, and natural killer cells.

the balance in individuals who—unbeknownst to them—have ongoing islet inflammation and are in prediabetic status.

CVB has long been considered one of the principal causes of viral myocarditis,[81] and this view has been confirmed in several recent reports.[16,106,262,264,266] The inflammatory infiltrate (Fig. 17.5D) contains predominantly macrophages, T cells, and natural killer cells. Several mechanisms have been proposed to explain CVB-mediated cardiomyocyte destruction. The first is direct, virus-mediated damage. Cardiomyocytes can be infected *in vitro*,[152,206] and infected cells are rapidly lysed.[158] These *in vitro* findings are corroborated by *in vivo* ultrastructural studies of myocardial tissue, which show clear evidence of virus infection of cardiac muscle cells and cell death.[131,163,228] The second proposed mechanism is immunopathologic damage. The inflammatory infiltrate contains CD8+ T cells, natural killer cells, and macrophages,[67,129,156,370] and other studies have implicated $\gamma\delta$ T cells in CVB pathogenesis.[174–176,178] Finally, studies have implicated autoimmunity in CVB-triggered myocarditis.[176,299,353–355] One potential means by which this could occur is via molecular mimicry (i.e., immunologic cross-reactivity between viral and heart proteins), and there is evidence that this occurs at both the antibody[121,122] and T-cell[176,177,181] levels. However, recent studies in mice that lack CAR expression only on cardiomyocytes casts doubt on the importance of molecular mimicry in CVB-induced myocarditis. Thus, virus replication in the heart is a prerequisite for myocardial destruction, and this is difficult to reconcile with molecular mimicry; these data do not, of course, exclude a role for autoimmunity induced by other means, for example, by virus-driven exposure of sequestered cardiac antigens.

Immune Response

Innate Immunity

The innate immune response plays a central role in regulating virus infection, as illustrated earlier by the important role played by T1IFNs in regulating PV tissue tropism and pathogenesis. RNA viruses may trigger one (or more) of at least three sensor groups:[208] Toll-like receptors (TLRs), retinoic acid–inducible gene I (RIG-I)-like receptors (RLRs), and NOD-like receptors (NLRs, some of which assemble into larger structures termed inflammasomes). The interactions between enteroviruses and NLRs have not been reported, so

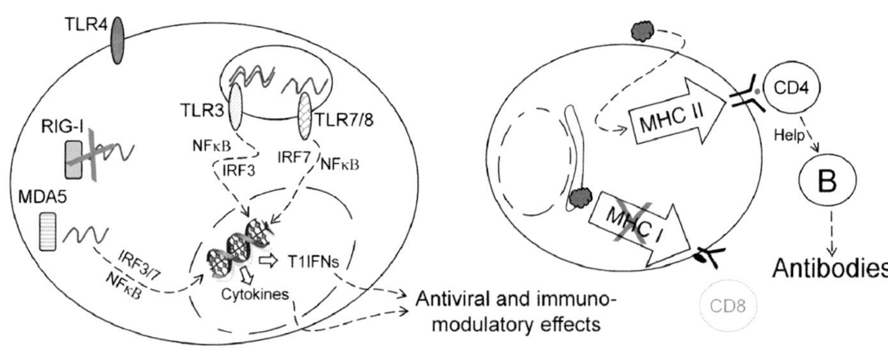

FIGURE 17.6. Signaling through Toll-like receptors (TLRs) during enterovirus infections. TLR4 on human pancreatic cells is triggered by infection. TLR3 senses double-stranded RNA (dsRNA) molecules and a strong TLR3-triggered response may protect against enteroviral myocarditis. Other internal TLRs also can contribute to the control of coxsackievirus B (CVB) infections.

herein we focus on the first two sensor groups. Triggering of TLRs and RLRs alters the expression of hundreds of genes including a variety of cytokines, chemokines, and other proteins, some of which can directly counter virus infection (e.g., *p*rotein *k*inase regulated by *R*NA [PKR, discussed later] and type I interferons), while others may regulate the development of the adaptive antiviral immune response. The roles of cell surface and internal TLRs during enterovirus infections have been evaluated in the CVB model (Fig. 17.6). TLR4 on human pancreatic cells is triggered by CVB4,[398] and TLR4 knockout (KO) mice infected with CVB3 show reduced virus titers and myocarditis.[109] A comparison of male and female mice confirmed that TLR4 signaling was correlated with the severity of myocarditis.[118] However, the administration of TLR4 stimulants such as lipopolysaccharides (LPSs) greatly increased the severity of CVB-induced myocarditis, suggesting that CVB-mediated triggering of TLR4 *in vivo* is likely to be submaximal.[242,346] TLR3 senses double-stranded RNA (dsRNA) molecules, which are commonly produced during the replication of RNA viruses.[13] One study of CVB4 infection of TLR3-deficient mice suggested that TLR3 was almost indispensable for the innate response to this virus[347] and, when compared to wild-type (wt) mice, TLR3KO mice showed increased mortality and developed more severe myocarditis following CVB3 infection.[298,416] Genomic screening of patients diagnosed with enteroviral myocarditis or dilated cardiomyopathy (DCM) revealed two TLR3 sequence variants, both of which showed reduced responsiveness to ligand;[120] this suggests that a strong TLR3-triggered response may protect against enteroviral myocarditis. Other internal TLRs also can contribute to the control of CVB infections. For example, human cardiac inflammatory responses to CVB are reported to be dependent largely on TLR7 and TLR8,[397] both of which recognize single-stranded RNA (ssRNA) and other small molecules.[151] Contrary to the reported beneficial effects of a strong TLR3 response to enteroviruses, a strong TLR8 response may be associated with adverse outcomes in patients with enterovirus-associated DCM.[365] Autophagy is up-regulated by TLRs, and the most potent pro-autophagic effects are mediated by ssRNA/TLR7 signaling.[91] Electron microscopic (EM) studies of poliovirus-infected cells revealed an association between PV and double-membraned intracellular vesicles,[88] subsequently shown to be autophagy related.[368] Extensive membrane remodeling occurs in a poliovirus-infected cell, mediated by the viral 2BC and 3A proteins,[383] and the resulting vesicles carry several autophagosome-related proteins.[391,392] A similar relationship between CVB and autophagic vesicles has been reported,[134] and there is a marked increase in double-membraned structures within CVB-infected cells, both in tissue culture[424,441] and *in vivo.*[214] Although autophagy is generally thought to support the replication of these viruses, to date, the effects have been determined only in tissue culture cells and are extremely modest; inhibiting autophagy in cells infected with PV,[193] CVB3,[424] CVB4,[441] or EV71[173] reduces production of each of these viruses by only 1.5- to 4-fold. To date, few studies have evaluated autophagy during enteroviral replication *in vivo.*

Three RLRs have been identified: RIG-I, MDA5 (melanoma differentiation–associated gene 5), and LGP2 (laboratory of genetics and physiology 2). Unlike TLRs, these proteins are expressed in most cell types. All are activated by nucleic acids, and all are cytosolic, although it has been reported that RIG-I co-localizes with F-actin, and thus is associated with the cytoskeleton.[293] Many RNA viruses produce abundant dsRNA and ssRNA with 5′ triphosphate and, therefore, strongly activate RIG-I. In the absence of RIG-I, the innate response to several RNA virus families is abrogated.[257] The 5′ terminus of an enteroviral RNA lacks the 5′ triphosphate moiety, instead bearing a modified protein (VPg), and, for this reason, these viruses do not stimulate RIG-I. Infected cells appear to rely largely on MDA5 to alert them to the presence of picornaviral RNA. This sensor is tripped by the cardiovirus encephalomyocarditis virus (EMCV),[127,210] and two recent publications using MDA5 knockout mice suggest that enteroviruses, too, trigger MDA5 signaling.[183,414] MDA5, like RIG-I, is degraded in poliovirus-infected HeLa cells, providing one possible mechanism by which enteroviruses might paralyze the innate immune response.[28] However, the observation that MDA5 deficiency has a marked effect during CVB3 infection suggests that, if MDA5 degradation occurs in CVB-infected cells, the process does not prevent MDA5-mediated triggering of the innate response.

At least two observations have been made that may be relevant to both TLR- and RLR-mediated responses to CVB (and, possibly, other enteroviruses). First, many cells—exemplified by macrophages and dendritic cells—are phagocytic and engulf dead or dying cells. Thus, although human dendritic cells (DCs) cannot be productively infected by CVB,[239] these cells can consume debris from CVB-infected cells, thereby potentially introducing viral materials to the cytosolic and intravesicular sensors, potentially inducing an antiviral state in the DCs.[238] Second, as well as degrading the sensors themselves, some enteroviruses can interrupt the downstream signaling upon which the innate response depends. Signaling via TLR3 and the RLRs rely, respectively, on proteins named TRIF and MAVS, both of which are degraded in CVB-infected cells, apparently by the viral 3C protease.[292]

NK cells, which are part of the innate response to many infections, are important in protecting against CVB-induced pancreatitis in the mouse model.[408] The importance of NK cells in combating human enteroviral infections is unknown, but human NK cells can produce interferon-γ (IFN-γ) in response to CVB-infected cells.[182]

Adaptive Immunity

Antibodies and CD8+ T cells together provide a strong antigen-specific barrier against virus infections. Under normal circumstances, these two arms of the adaptive response complement each other. However, members of the *Enterovirus* species appear to be an exception to this general rule. Patients with X-linked agammaglobulinemia are highly susceptible to enteroviral infections,[282] and after receiving live poliovirus vaccine, such individuals may continue to shed virulent poliovirus for up to ~20 years.[219,267] The near-absolute requirement for antibodies in protecting against enteroviruses has been confirmed in an animal model of CVB3 infection, using B-cell knockout (BcKO) mice; these mice cannot eradicate the virus, and high titers are present in many organs.[278] These observations suggest that, for agammaglobulinemic hosts infected with an enterovirus, there may be some deficit in the backup system that, for most viruses, is provided by CD8+ T-cell responses. This may, in part, explain why most studies of enteroviral infections, in mouse and man, have identified strong antibody responses, while CD8+ T-cell responses—so easily detected in most virus infections—are weak (if detected at all). The enterovirus genus is large, and the adaptive responses to only a select few enteroviral species will be discussed later.

HUMAN ENTEROVIRUS A

The best-studied pathogen in this species is EV71. The virus triggers an immunoglobulin M (IgM) response that is detectable as early as 2 days postinfection,[399] as well as a strong neutralizing IgG response that recognizes epitopes in the N-terminal segment of VP1.[387] Neutralizing antibodies, when transferred to uninfected neonatal recipient mice, are able to protect against a lethal challenge infection.[445] Studies of knockout mice showed that B cells, in particular, were important for survival following EV71 infection, and B-cell–deficient mice treated with virus-specific antibody either before or during EV71 infection had lower virus titers, less severe disease, and lower mortality.[253] Memory T-helper 1 (Th1) CD4+ T-cell responses specific for three epitopes in VP1 have been identified in EV71-positive individuals,[116] but no CD8+ T-cell epitopes have been reported.

HUMAN ENTEROVIRUS B

CVBs are the best-studied pathogens in this species and, as described earlier, can trigger severe acute and chronic diseases including myocarditis, DCM, pancreatitis, and aseptic meningitis. Infection by these viruses triggers a rapid and strong neutralizing antibody response. Virus-specific IgM appears during the first week of infection, followed by a strong neutralizing IgG response. The CVB3-specific IgM titer wanes over time, but IgG antibodies persist.[256] Work in T-cell–deficient (nude) mice indicates that at least some of the CVB-specific antibody response is T-cell independent,[150,364,426] although some studies suggest that CD4+ T-cell help may be important for the induction of strong neutralizing antibody responses.[246] B cells appear to be targeted by CVB[278] and may provide a reservoir for the virus during persistent CVB infection. Viral RNA-positive cells, most probably B cells, can be found in the splenic follicles and germinal centers;[14,195,207,229,278] approximately 1% of B cells are infected with CVB3 *in vivo,* and these cells may accelerate the systemic distribution of virus.[278] T cells can help control CVB infection, although much less effectively than antibodies. *In vivo* analyses of CVB-specific T cells has been challenging because these viruses, despite replicating to high titers in mice, induce remarkably weak CD8+ T-cell responses.[378,213a] Nevertheless, some responses can be identified, exemplified by CD4+ T-cell responses against epitopes expressed by CVB4.[143,144] CD8+ T-cell responses are particularly meager. Epitopes in several viral proteins have been identified in human studies, but their detection required ~2 weeks of *in vitro* peptide antigen restimulation.[416]

HUMAN ENTEROVIRUS C

This species contains a number of coxsackie A viruses, but the most important pathogen is PV, which induces a strong neutralizing antibody response that is necessary to control the infection. Virus infection and vaccination induce strong and long-lasting humoral responses,[79] but the immunity is not sterilizing and secondary infections of the gut can occur. Susceptibility to such reinfections, and subsequent shedding of PV, may be controlled by IgA.[48] PV-driven T-cell proliferation has been observed in infant vaccinees, and the responses appear to be cross-reactive across different enteroviruses.[202] However, PV-specific T-cell responses in OPV-vaccinated infants may be weaker than those in adults.[405] OPV induces major histocompatibility complex (MHC) class II–restricted memory CD4+ T-cell responses targeted to epitopes in all four capsid proteins.[377] CD8+ T-cell responses to PV vaccination are long-lived but, as is true for most CVB-specific responses, they became detectable only after several rounds of *in vitro* restimulation, suggesting that T-cell numbers *in vivo* were low.[413] Mice are not naturally infected by PV, but PVR-transgenic (PVR-Tg) animals have allowed the analysis of T- and B-cell responses and their roles in antiviral protection. Adoptive transfer of PV-primed B cells together with a VP4-specific CD4+ T-cell clone protected PVR-Tg mice against a lethal challenge of PV, but neither cell population alone was protective, indicating that the virus-specific B cells required T-cell help.[265]

Release from Host

Virion assembly and RNA packaging of enteroviruses remain very poorly understood. Although enteroviruses are generally considered to be highly lytic—and, therefore, released from cells upon their lysis—there is some evidence from cell culture studies consistent with PV release by nonlytic means.[330,401] It has been proposed that autophagy-mediated release of PV may occur, permitting the virus to exit a cell in a noncytolytic manner;[193] this proposed mechanism has, memorably, been termed AWOL (*a*utophagy-mediated exit *w*ith*o*ut *l*ysis).[390]

Virulence

Viral virulence is a complex interplay between virus and host, and some of the contributing elements, such as receptor distribution and host responses, have been discussed earlier. Here, we will focus on selected enteroviral sequences and proteins and their contributions to a virulent phenotype. Wild-type PV is more neurovirulent than the attenuated viruses that constitute the oral vaccine, and studies have identified, in all three PV serotypes, changes in the 5′ noncoding region that can alter neurovirulence. For example, sequence comparison between the attenuated Sabin 3 virus and revertants from cases of vaccine-associated poliomyelitis showed that a single U-C change in the viral IRES, at position 472, conferred a growth advantage in the human intestine and resulted in increased neurovirulence, although, on its own, the change was insufficient to confer full neurovirulence;[108] a second change, leading to an amino acid substitution in VP3, almost completely restored virulence.[417] Mutations in the IRES of PV types 1 and 2 also modulate the neurovirulent phenotype.[212,260,261] The *in vivo* neuroattenuating phenotype imposed by changes in the IRES, together with tissue culture studies showing apparent cell-specific effects of the IRES mutations,[146] led to the proposal that neuroattenuation might be explained by a neuron-specific reduction in usage of the mutated IRES. However, *in vivo* analyses have demonstrated that, while the Sabin 3 IRES sequence is indeed less effectively utilized in neurons, this defect also is observed in other cells and tissues.[212] Thus, another explanation was sought. The importance of T1IFNs in modulating PV neurovirulence *in vivo* has been described earlier. Cardiovirulence in CVB3 also has been mapped to various locations in the 5′ nontranslated region (NTR), ~80 to 240 bases from the 5′ end of the genome,[64,104,400] although the capsid region, too, plays a part.[395] In contrast to the extensive mapping of the limits of, and functional domains within, the PV IRES, analysis of the CVB IRES has been limited.

Persistence

Although both PV and CVB are rapidly cytolytic in many of the cell types that they infect, both viruses can establish persistent or chronic infection in tissue culture.[78,119,269,331] In neuroblastoma cells, PV persistence is associated with accrual of mutations in the capsid region,[330] and for both PV and CVB, moving from a cytolytic to persistent phenotype in cell culture may be inversely related to the capacity of the virus to adsorb to the receptor and/or to the level of receptor expression.[53,240] It recently has been reported that, during persistent infection of cultured cells that express low levels of CAR, CVB accumulated changes in the capsid that allow the variant virus to bind to novel (non-DAF, non-CAR) molecules, and this more promiscuous activity conferred a replicative advantage upon the variant.[52] Cellular factors contribute to the establishment of PV persistence.[126] Cell cycle status may play a role in the case of CVB, which does not replicate efficiently in tissue culture cells rendered quiescent by drugs or by serum starvation but undergoes productive and cytolytic replication when the cell cycle is triggered.[112,113]

Enteroviral persistent infections can take place under two general scenarios. First, a chronic productive enterovirus infection can occur in immunocompromised hosts. As noted earlier, agammaglobulinemic individuals who receive oral polio vaccine may retain, and excrete, the virus for many years. One study of individuals with primary immunodeficiency who had developed vaccine-associated paralytic poliomyelitis found that approximately one in five secreted vaccine-derived PV at 6 months after their last OPV dose, but this frequency declined to 0% when the interval was 10 years.[222] The low prevalence of the underlying condition means that such persons are rare; only ~40 such individuals have been identified.[429] Fortunately, a more common potential cause of immunosuppression, human immunodeficiency virus (HIV) infection, seems not to correlate with PV persistence/shedding.[24,157] Second, immunocompetent hosts may carry virus (or at least viral RNA) for many years. Given the frequency of enteroviral infections, it is reasonable to suppose that this is the more common of the two types of enterovirus persistence. In the vast majority of cases in which enteroviral persistence *in vivo* has been reported in immunocompetent hosts, infectious virus was not identified; rather, viral materials (most commonly RNA) were reported and infectious particles, if sought, were not found. CVB RNA has frequently been detected by PCR in many analyses of cardiac biopsies from individuals with DCM[20,21,45,232] or inflammatory peripheral myopathy.[44] From results obtained in a murine model of polymyositis, the authors concluded that the RNA was maintained in double-stranded form, with little indication of virus mutation/evolution.[386] However, recent analyses of CVB3 genomes isolated from the hearts of persistently infected mice suggest that CVB persistence *in vivo* may be dependent upon the deletion of nucleotides at the 5′ end of the genome.[226] Several deletions were reported, some extending to nucleotide 49, and all affecting the 5′ cloverleaf structure that is considered vital for RNA replication. Importantly, the materials were infectious; although replicating very slowly, they could be maintained in culture and did not require a helper virus. The VPg protein was present on several of the deletion mutant genomes and, notably, ~25% of RNA encapsidated into virions was negative sense. The authors proposed that the encapsidation of negative strands might occur because the terminal deletions, by altering RNA replication, markedly reduced the ratio of positive to negative strands. Similar 5′ terminal deletion variants subsequently were identified in CVB3 that had been passed in primary tissue culture cells[225] and, critically, in a CVB2 genome isolated from the heart of a human who had succumbed to enteroviral myocarditis.[63] The poor infectivity of these mutated viruses may explain why infectious virus was not identified in the vast majority of previous studies in which enterovirus RNA was found. To date, there is no evidence to suggest that these terminally deleted variants can be transmitted under normal circumstances.

EPIDEMIOLOGY

Demographics

Despite the nearly ubiquitous nature of EV infections and the wide variety of clinical presentations, the demographics of the various infections and diseases have some consistent characteristics. In particular, several factors, including age, sex, and socioeconomic status, have largely predictable effects.

One of the most important determinants of EV infection outcome is age. Different age groups have different susceptibilities to infection, severity of illness, clinical manifestations, and prognoses following EV infection. Understanding these age effects on outcome of infection is complicated by the widely divergent prior history of infection and resulting immunity. Nevertheless, it is possible to make certain generalizations.

The largest amount and duration of virus shedding occurs on primary infection with a given EV serotype. Because infection is so common, most primary infections occur during childhood. For these reasons, young children are probably the most important transmitters of EV, particularly within households. The greater exposure of children to virus during infection may make them more likely to have significant clinical symptoms. For example, in outbreaks of meningitis, children typically have higher rates of disease than adults.[134,191] Most studies, however, do not separately determine age-specific infection rates and disease rates, and the relative rates at which adults are infected are not generally known.

The incidence of poliomyelitis is relatively low for the first 4 to 6 months of life in countries in which control through vaccination has not yet been achieved, because of the frequent presence of protective maternal antibody. In these countries, an increased incidence is seen of paralytic disease in children older than 6 months compared with children in wealthier developed countries, presumably related to an earlier exposure to virus as a result of poor sanitary conditions. Ironically, areas with improved hygiene may have a decrease in infant exposure, leaving an older (unexposed) population susceptible to epidemic disease, with high rates of paralytic disease during an outbreak.[335] Adults are more likely to be severely affected in both developing and developed countries, tending to acquire paralytic poliomyelitis rather than nonparalytic CNS disease (i.e., aseptic meningitis), abortive illness, or asymptomatic infection.[56,57,170] The reason for the increase in severity later in life is unknown. A possible reason relates to the finding that fast axonal flow, which appears important in the spread of PV within the CNS,[200] increases with age. In addition, it may be that CD155 expression or host factors important in replication change with age.

Severity of a number of enteroviral diseases besides poliomyelitis may be strikingly age related. An indirect indication is that a delay in first infection with a number of EVs increases risk of more severe disease. For example, exanthema associated with CVA and echoviruses are for the most part milder in children than in adults. On the other hand, some EVs cause more severe disease in newborns than in older children and adults, possibly inducing a fulminant *viral sepsis* with myocarditis, encephalitis, and sometimes death (see Clinical Features: Neonate and Infant Disease).[68,194] In addition, recent outbreaks of hand-foot-and-mouth disease caused by EV71 have been associated with a significant CNS complication, fatal brainstem encephalitis, that was restricted largely to young children (Table 17.3) (see Clinical Features: Meningitis and Encephalitis).[235,258,428]

In general, encephalitis and aseptic meningitis caused by EV appear to be most frequent among those 5 to 14 years of age rather than those older or younger. In a 10-year surveillance summary from the United States,[286] adults tended to be overrepresented among cases of severe disease (paralysis, encephalitis, meningitis, carditis) when compared with the age distribution of the EV-infected population as a whole. In another study, the mean age among patients with CVB meningitis (7.7 years) or pericarditis (9.9 years) was greater than the mean age of patients with CVB gastroenteritis (1.3 years).[96]

Enterovirus infections are more prevalent among persons of lower socioeconomic status and those living in urban areas.[145,196] In a study utilizing active surveillance of healthy children for EV infections in West Virginia during 1951–1953, the rate of isolations among children in a lower socioeconomic setting was two- to sevenfold higher than among children in a higher socioeconomic setting.[168] A similar study in Ghana during 1971–1973 further indicated that EV isolations were significantly more frequent among children in areas with poorer sanitation and in urban areas during both rainy and dry seasons.[325]

TABLE 17.3 Some Enterovirus 71 Outbreaks, 1969–2009

Year	Location	Clinical findings
1969–1973	California	Aseptic meningitis, encephalitis
1972	New York	Aseptic meningitis, encephalitis, hand-foot-and-mouth disease
1972	Australia	Aseptic meningitis, rash, polyneuritis, acute respiratory infection
1973	Sweden	Aseptic meningitis, hand-foot-and-mouth disease
1973	Japan	Hand-foot-and-mouth disease, aseptic meningitis
1975	Bulgaria	Aseptic meningitis, encephalitis, acute myocarditis, acute flaccid paralysis
1978[a]	Hungary	Aseptic meningitis, encephalitis, acute flaccid paralysis
1985	Hong Kong	Monoplegia
1986	Australia	Central nervous system involvement
1987	United States	Acute flaccid paralysis, meningitis, encephalitis
1989	China	Hand-foot-and-mouth disease
1997	Malaysia	Fatal encephalitis, acute flaccid paralysis, hand-foot-and-mouth disease
1998	Taiwan	Fatal encephalitis, hand-foot-and-mouth disease
2000–2001	Australia	Severe neurologic disease, pulmonary edema
2005–2009	Viet Nam	Severe neurologic disease, hand-foot-and-mouth disease
2006	Brunei Darussalam	Severe neurologic disease, hand-foot-and-mouth disease, herpangina
2007–2009	China	Fatal encephalitis, hand-foot-and-mouth disease

[a]A mixed epidemic of tick-borne encephalitis (chiefly in adults) and enterovirus 71 disease (chiefly in children).

Adapted from Melnick JL. Enteroviruses: polioviruses, coxsackieviruses, echoviruses, and newer enteroviruses. In: Fields BN, Knipe DM, Howley PM, eds. *Fields Virology*. 3rd ed. Philadelphia: Lippincott-Raven, 1996:655–712; with additional data from World Health Organization. *A Guide to Clinical Management and Public Health Response for Hand, Foot and Mouth Disease (HFMD)*. Geneva: World Health Organization, 2011.

Paradoxically, poliomyelitis and possibly other EV diseases tend to be *diseases of development*. In the case of poliomyelitis, improvement in a country's hygienic and socioeconomic conditions (before vaccination programs) successfully reduces the incidence of paralysis caused by PV and leads to a transitional period in which there is a delay in age of first infection with a subsequent temporary increase in the paralysis-to-infection ratio. Before the introduction of the PV vaccine in the United States and other developed countries, paralytic poliomyelitis was disproportionately a disease of the middle and upper socioeconomic classes; this disease distribution was a result of infection at an older age, when paralysis was a more frequent complication. Ironically, the delay was a result of improved hygiene. The infant mortality rate, a general indicator of a country's level of health development, may be inversely correlated with the age-specific incidence of poliomyelitis.[274]

Enterovirus diseases, and possibly also EV infections, occur more frequently in males than in females,[132,287] although some exceptions have been described.[94] In numerous reports, the male-to-female ratio appears generally to range between about 1.2 and 2.5:1; that is, approximately 55% to 70% of such diseases occur in males. Male predominance tends to be greater for the more severe diseases (e.g., CNS disease or carditis) than for less-severe disease (e.g., pleurodynia, hand-foot-and-mouth disease, respiratory disease, acute hemorrhagic conjunctivitis, rash, or undifferentiated febrile illness).

The apparent predominance of enteroviral infections among males may have both sociologic and biological explanations. Population-based measurements of infection (e.g., serosurveys), which should be gender neutral, have not consistently demonstrated a higher infection rate for males. Several additional explanations for the male predominance have been proposed on the basis of studies of infections in healthy children:[123] a longer duration of virus excretion occurs in males than in females (leading to increased chance of identifying infected males); and a higher virus titer occurs in the feces of males (leading to a similar increase in diagnosis). Another possibility is that, indeed, more frequent infections occur in males because of a greater exposure to the pathogen, perhaps because of differences in the parental treatment and play habits of younger boys and greater activity among older boys. An additional possibility is that males are more likely to develop a serious illness from a given EV infection than females. For example, the reason that human myopericarditis is more common in adolescent and adult males than in females (except in pregnant and postpartum women)[423] could be caused by sex-related endocrine effects leading to differences in disease susceptibility.

Transmission

Enteroviruses can be isolated from both the lower and upper alimentary tract and can be transmitted by both fecal–oral and respiratory routes. Fecal–oral transmission may predominate in areas with poor sanitary conditions, whereas respiratory transmission may be important in more developed areas.[169] The relative importance of the different modes of transmission probably varies with the particular EV and environmental setting. It is believed that almost all EVs, except possibly EV70, can be transmitted by the fecal–oral route; however, it is not known whether most can also be transmitted by the respiratory route. EV70 and CVA24 variant, the agents that cause acute hemorrhagic conjunctivitis, are seldom isolated from the respiratory tract or stool specimens and are probably primarily spread by direct or indirect contact with eye secretions.[236] Enteroviruses that cause a vesicular exanthem presumably can be spread by direct or indirect contact with vesicular fluid, which contains infectious virus.

It is likely that EVs are transmitted in the same manner as are other viruses causing the common cold—that is, by hand contact with secretions (e.g., on the hand of another person) and autoinoculation to the mouth, nose, or eyes. Direct bloodstream inoculation, usually by laboratory accidents (e.g., needlesticks) can result in EV infection; however, neither blood transfusion nor mosquito or other insect bite appears to be a significant route of transmission. The isolation of EV from flies has led to a suspicion that houseflies (*Musca domestica*) and various filth flies may be vehicles of mechanical transmission. No evidence indicates that venereal transmission is important.

Transmission within households has been well studied for both PV and nonpolio EV. Small children generally introduce EV into the family, although young adults make up the majority of index cases in some outbreaks of acute hemorrhagic conjunctivitis.[366] Intrafamily transmission can be rapid and relatively complete, depending on duration of virus excretion, household size, number of siblings, socioeconomic status, immune status of household members, and other risk factors.[145] Transmission has been generally found to be greatest in large families of lower socioeconomic status with a greater number of children 5 to 9 years of age and with no evidence of serologic immunity to the virus type. Not surprisingly, infections in different family members can result in different clinical manifestations.

Observations of household transmission of various EVs have documented that many infected contacts do not become ill and that the extent of secondary transmission varies with different EVs. Household secondary attack rates in susceptible members may be greatest for the agents of acute hemorrhagic conjunctivitis (EV70 and CVA24 variant) and for PV, and of lesser magnitude for the coxsackieviruses and echoviruses. In some studies, secondary attack rates may be 90% or greater, although they are typically lower. New York Virus Watch data indicate that EV infections were more frequent among children 2 to 9 years of age and that secondary CV infections were more frequent in mothers (78%) than in fathers (47%).[231] In the same study, coxsackieviruses spread to 76% of exposed susceptible persons versus 25% of exposed persons who had detectable antibody to the infecting type; echoviruses infected 43% of those who were susceptible and only one person with antibody. The greater spread of polioviruses and coxsackieviruses may derive from longer periods of virus excretion.

Transmission occurs within the neighborhood and community, particularly where people congregate. In addition, as with many other viruses, EV can be rapidly transmitted within institutions when circumstances permit (e.g., crowding, poor hygiene, or contaminated water). School teams or activity groups and institutionalized ambulatory retarded children or adults may be at special risk.[11] Despite crowding, EV transmission is not usually accelerated to a noticeable degree in institutions where good sanitation is found.

As a result of widespread but incomplete PV immunization, rare PV-susceptible enclaves have arisen. These usually consist of unvaccinated religious groups in countries with an otherwise high prevalence of PV immunity. Despite the barrier of millions of immune persons, PV outbreaks have occurred in some of these enclaves.[324] The frequency and ease of international travel may result in the continuous introduction of wild-type PV in all regions of the world, indicating that a large proportion of the population must be vaccinated if poliomyelitis epidemics are to be prevented. This suggests that herd immunity may be of only limited value in protecting groups of susceptible persons who have regular contact with outside populations, and it raises questions about the risks that such groups may pose to the community at large.

Nosocomial transmission of various CVA and B and the echoviruses has also been well documented, typically in newborn nurseries. Hospital staff may have been involved in mediating transmission in some of these outbreaks. EV70, as well as CVA24 variant, is highly transmissible and can cause outbreaks in ophthalmology clinics when instruments are inadequately cleaned between patients. An apparent outbreak of CVA1, which included some fatal cases, has been reported in bone marrow transplant recipients.[394]

Although human EVs have been isolated from various environmental sources, humans are thought to make up the only important natural reservoir.[101,110] Survival beyond a few weeks does not generally occur, although EV can survive for months in favorable environmental conditions; these favorable conditions include neutral pH, moisture, and low temperatures, especially in the presence of organic matter, which protects against inactivation. Simian enteroviruses have been identified that are closely related to a number of human viruses,[149,305,307,315,334] and human enteroviruses have been detected in free-living nonhuman primates,[308] but it is not known whether primates can serve as a reservoir for human infection.

Although little evidence suggests that EVs found in the environment are of public health importance, concern has been expressed about possible dangers of contaminated sources of water (Fig. 17.7). Recreational swimming water has been investigated in several studies, and EVs have been isolated from swimming and wading pools in the absence of fecal coliforms and in the presence of *recommended* levels of free residual chlorine. CVB5 was isolated from an unchlorinated lake swimming area during an outbreak at a boys' camp in Vermont, although the outbreak itself was explained by person-to-person transmission. In one study, the relative risk of EV infection among children was found to be significantly higher for beach swimmers, especially for those younger than 4 years of age.[84] These reports suggest that swallowing of contaminated pool or lake water may theoretically account for transmission, but no proof exists that this type of transmission is significant in recreational settings.

Enteroviruses have been found in surface and ground waters throughout the world. In the tropics, virus survival is more prolonged in ground water because it is cooler than surface water. As in the case with swimming pools, EV can be found in these waters even after chlorination and even in the absence of fecal coliforms. In industrialized countries, EV transmission from potable water is apparently uncommon but is a constant source of concern for public health investigators, because the usual conditions under which city drinking water is chlorinated may be insufficient to completely inactivate enteroviruses.

Enteroviruses have been isolated from raw or partly cooked mollusks and crustacea and their overlying waters.[134] Shellfish rapidly concentrate many viruses, including EV. These viruses can survive in oysters for 3 weeks at temperatures of 1°C to 21°C. To date, no outbreak of EV disease has been attributed to consumption of shellfish. Other food-borne transmission

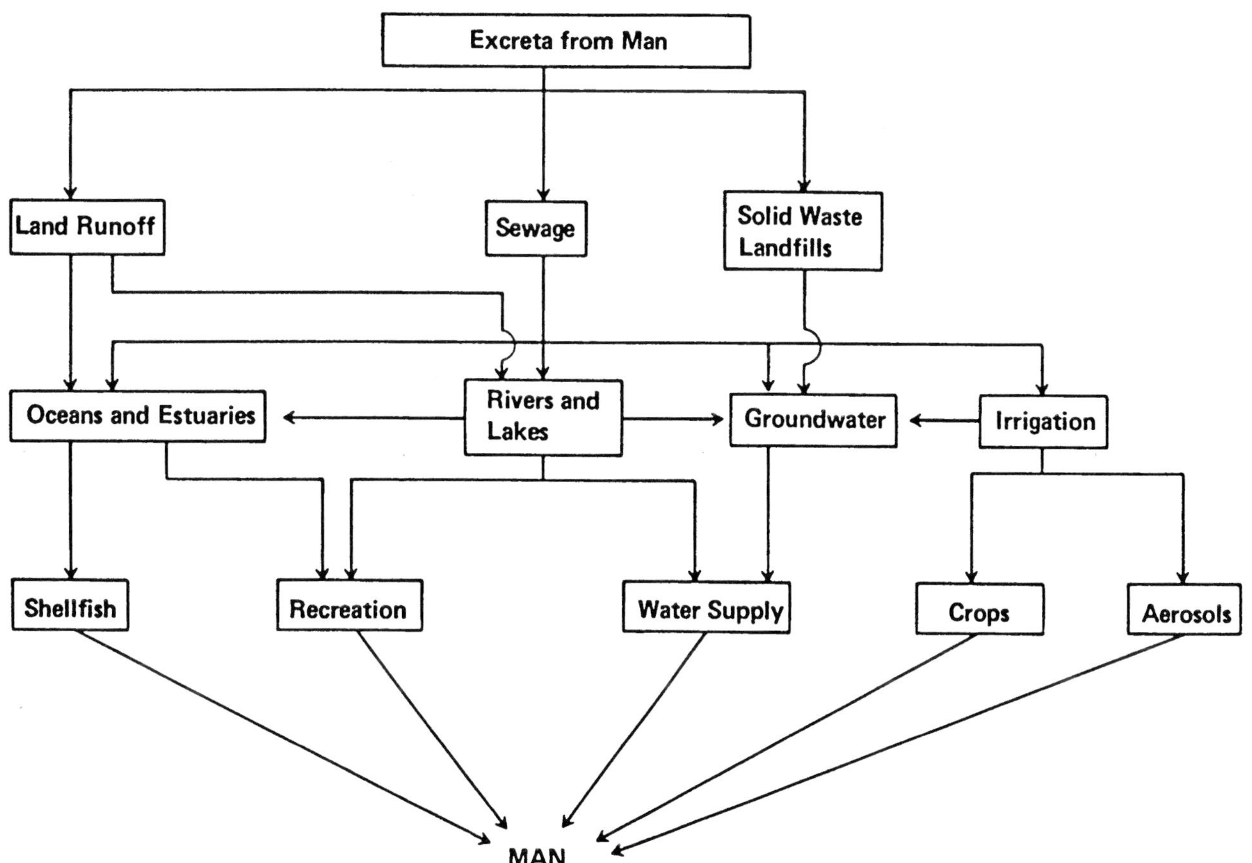

FIGURE 17.7. Routes of potential enteric virus transmission in the environment. (From Melnick JL. Current status of poliovirus infections. *Clin Microbiol Rev* 1996;9[3]:293–300, with permission.)

has been documented but is thought to be uncommon. A 1976 outbreak of aseptic meningitis attributed to echovirus type 4 was apparently caused by consumption of contaminated coleslaw at a large picnic (Centers for Disease Control and Prevention, unpublished data, 1976).

Enteroviruses, especially polioviruses, are regularly found in sewage. Enteroviruses are more prevalent in sewage from areas with low socioeconomic conditions or with large proportions of young children. In addition, sewage workers have been shown to have a higher prevalence of serum antibodies to EV than highway maintenance workers, which is consistent with an occupational risk.[74]

Soil and crops also provide conditions favorable to EV. Enteroviruses survive well in sludge and remain on the surface of sludge-treated soil and even on crops. Air samples from aerosolized spray irrigants using contaminated effluents have also been found to contain EV.[285] Survival of EV on vegetable food crops exposed to contaminated water or fertilizer has not been proved to be associated with virus transmission.

Prevalence and Disease Incidence

Incidence data about diseases caused by particular EV types can be derived from prospective longitudinal surveillance of a defined population or from a sample of the population in which the occurrence of disease or infection can be reliably determined. The Virus Watch program in the 1960s in U.S. cities exemplifies this type of surveillance study, in which specimens from subject children were obtained every 2 weeks for virologic evaluation.[80,231,382] Although difficult and extremely expensive, such prospective cohort studies avoid many of the pitfalls of passive surveillance, and they allow interpretations about both infection and disease incidence.

Less-useful information is based on passive case finding. Ascertainment may be incomplete because the surveillance system is likely to identify a case only if it is easily recognizable and diagnosed by someone who decides to report it. Because such data indicate neither how many ill persons were not reported nor how many ill persons had negative laboratory tests, the information is mostly of qualitative value; however, it may be useful in indicating trends. Despite these limitations, occasional reports do appear.[29,221]

In the United States, EV surveillance data are collected and analyzed by the Centers for Disease Control and Prevention (CDC). The data have been reported irregularly since the beginning of the program in 1961.[221,286,288] In the United States, the only notifiable enteroviral diseases are poliomyelitis and encephalitis. These are reportable by diagnosis only (e.g., encephalitis) and not etiology (e.g., echovirus encephalitis). Such disease-based surveillance is the most accessible but least representative of all surveillance data.

Enterovirus excretion does not necessarily imply association with disease, because most such excretion is asymptomatic. This applies particularly to developing countries where EVs are ubiquitous and childhood infections commonplace and characteristically silent.

Enterovirus activity in populations can be either sporadic or epidemic, and certain EV types are associated with both sporadic and epidemic disease occurrences. The reported incidence or prevalence of a given EV disease may actually or artifactually be increased in an outbreak situation when sudden focus of attention improves diagnosis and reporting of cases, but this may also increase reporting of *noncases*. In addition, there may be a tendency for other strains to be excluded when a particular strain is predominant in a community; however, large communities with summer enteroviral disease typically support co-circulation of several different types simultaneously and in no particular pattern.

An important concept in understanding the epidemiology of the EVs is variation: by serotype, by time, by geographic location, and by disease. This concept is illustrated in surveillance studies of nonpolio EV infections. For example, Figure 17.8 summarizes the data for the years 1970–1998 for CVB3, echovirus 11, and echovirus 30 isolates in the United States collected and analyzed by the CDC. These data illustrate endemic and epidemic patterns of EV prevalence. The epidemic pattern, as typified by E11 and E30, is characterized by peaks in numbers of isolations followed by periods with few

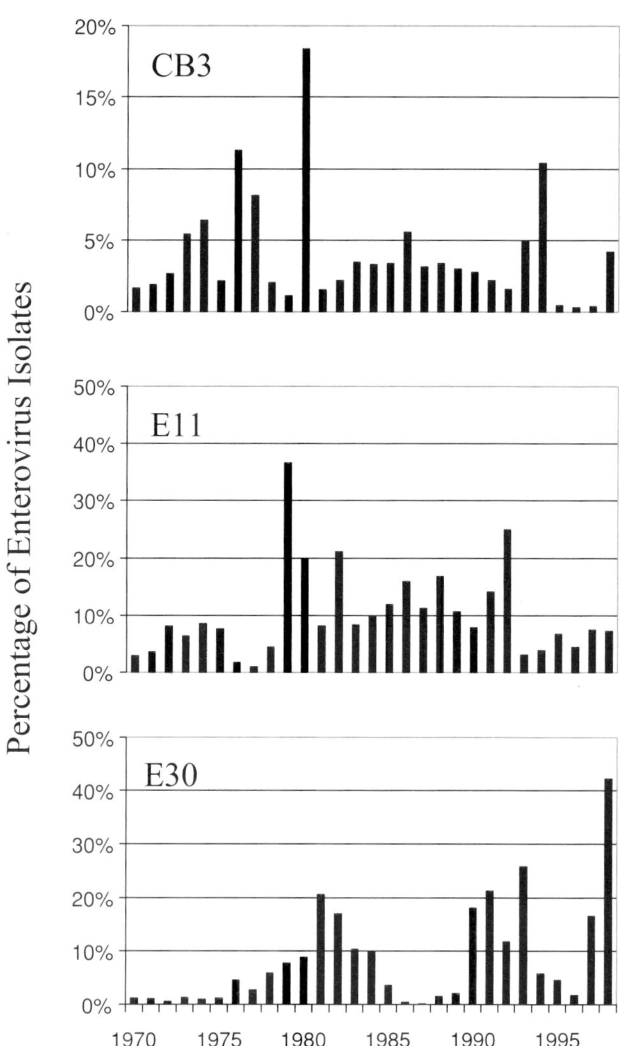

FIGURE 17.8. Reported enterovirus isolations in the United States, 1970–1998. The graphs represent the percentage of total enterovirus isolations in a given year for each of three common serotypes, coxsackievirus B3 (CB3), echovirus 11 (E11), and echovirus 30 (E30). Note that full scale for the coxsackievirus B3 panel is 20%, whereas it is 50% for both of the echoviruses.

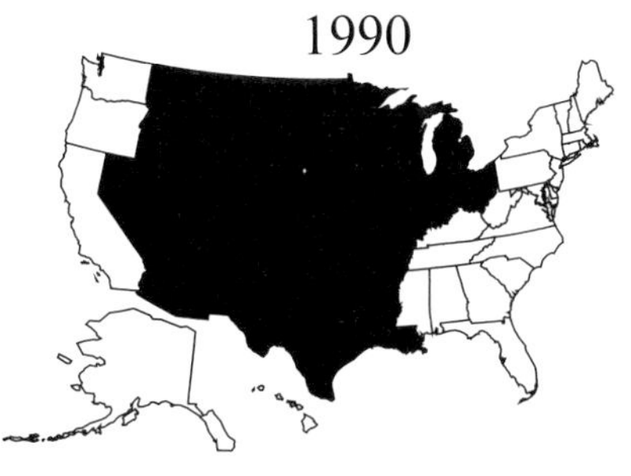

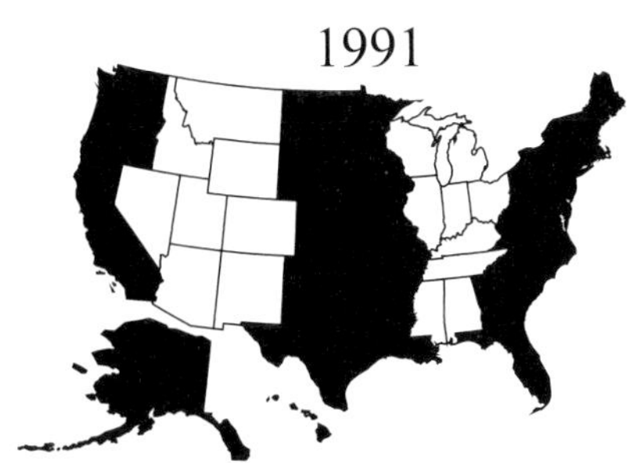

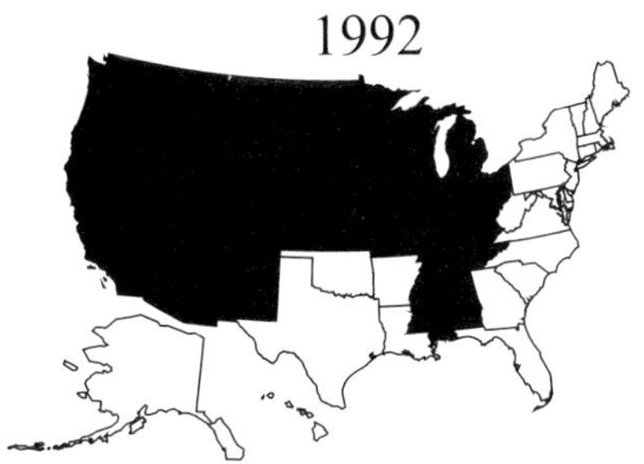

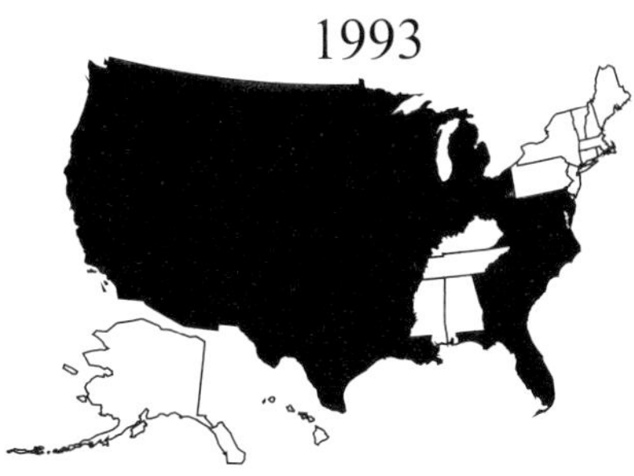

FIGURE 17.9. Geographic distribution of echovirus 30 isolates in the United States, 1990–1993. Maps represent regions of the United States where echovirus 30 was one of the three most common enterovirus isolates for the given year. States are shaded on a regional basis, because not all states report enterovirus isolation data.

isolations.[221] These peaks may be sharp (1- or 2-year) or broad (multiyear) periods of increased virus isolations. For example, during the study period, several major epidemics occurred of echovirus 30 in the United States: outbreaks from 1981 to 1982, 1990 to 1994, and 1997 to 1998. By contrast, endemic viruses (e.g., CVB3) are isolated nearly every year and in similar numbers each year. Even with endemic viruses, larger outbreaks do occasionally occur, as with CVB3 in 1980. Similar endemic and epidemic patterns are seen for the other echoviruses and coxsackie A viruses.

Variation by location is also a major characteristic of EV. Outbreaks can be restricted to small groups (e.g., schools and day care centers) or to select communities, or they may become widespread at the regional, national, or even international level. Outbreaks in small groups can sometimes be linked epidemiologically to a breakdown in hygiene practices. Even during national outbreaks of a specific serotype, the location of virus activity may not be uniform. During the period 1990–1993, echovirus 30 was the most commonly isolated EV in the United States (Fig. 17.9). As can be seen in the figure, not all parts of the country had echovirus 30 isolates during the entire period. Some areas, such as the New England states, had extensive circulation in only 1 year, whereas other areas, such as the entire western United States, had extensive virus circulation for 3 or more of the 4 years. It is important to note, therefore, that aggregate national data can obscure significant regional and local variation in viral prevalence.

In temperate climates, EVs are characteristically found during the summer and early autumn, although outbreaks can continue into the winter. In fact, naturally occurring EVs have a distinct seasonal pattern of circulation that varies by geographic area; in contrast, live attenuated PV (mostly vaccine strains) are isolated year round, reflecting the routine administration of poliomyelitis vaccine to children. In tropical and semitropical areas, circulation tends to be year-round or associated with the rainy season. In the United States, 23 years of surveillance indicated that 78% of EV isolations were made during the five summer or fall months of June to October.[221] In a 6-year study of viral CNS disease, 85% of enteroviral disease, compared with 12% to 26% of diseases caused by other viral agents, occurred between June and November.[286]

Many studies have examined the prevalence of antibodies to the EVs in specific populations, as has been reviewed elsewhere,[273,284] with several important conclusions. First, the number of persons who have neutralizing antibody to any given EV is large, indicating a high incidence of past infection. A high incidence of recent infection is also suggested by surveys of IgM antibodies to EV, which typically show 4% to 6% positivity. Second, infections with one serotype of EV can boost antibody titers to other EV serotypes as measured by either IgM or neutralization. The pattern of the heterotypic response varies by serotype and among individuals. The nature of this heterotypic response has been explored through the identification of specific epitopes using monoclonal antibodies and peptide antisera.[141,362,433] Third, the pattern of antibody prevalence by serotype varies by geographic location, time, and age. Thus, prevalence data from different years and locations are not directly comparable. These three points must be considered when interpreting the findings of serologic studies of associations between EV infection and disease.

Molecular Epidemiology

Study of the molecular variation of viral proteins or nucleic acid may contribute significant epidemiologic information on viral diseases (see Diagnosis). Molecular epidemiologic studies have helped in our understanding of EVs including the following: providing the opportunity for unequivocal strain identification, providing insights into EV classification and taxonomy, clarifying the origins of outbreaks, and allowing identification of strains transmitted between outbreaks. For the EVs, and in particular PV, the primary method used to generate epidemiologic information is direct analysis of genomic variation using nucleic acid sequencing. Previously, both monoclonal antibodies and oligonucleotide fingerprinting were also used to study variation in PV and EV; however, these approaches are limited by their ability to show similarities and small differences only among relatively closely related viruses. Neither technique, however, is able to readily detect any patterns among seemingly unrelated virus isolates. The introduction of the technique of genomic nucleic acid sequencing and its application to the study of wild PV isolates from different parts of the world has significantly extended the epidemiologic power of molecular studies.[348] By analyzing the random mutations that occur in the genome of different PVs, closely related viruses were easily detected, and, in addition, more distantly related viruses were clustered into distinct geographic groupings of endemic circulation. This approach allowed epidemiologic links to be extended beyond those identified with other techniques.

Nucleic acid sequencing technology has been most comprehensively applied to studies of PV, where the information has proved valuable for supporting the global PV eradication program.[215–217] From these studies, it is possible to determine (a) if an isolated PV is related to vaccine virus, (b) similarities among isolates in an epidemic, and (c) differences among isolates from different geographic areas. By comparing the changes that are observed between virus strains, the geographic and temporal origin of a virus can be determined. Building on a nucleic acid sequence database of PV strains worldwide, it has been possible to develop rapid approaches to tracking wild PV strains.[9,254,294,348,450]

Studies on the molecular epidemiology of nonpolio EV have focused on the evolutionary inference derived from the comparison of virus isolates within a serotype over time, as well as the comparison of isolates from different serotypes and even between different genera within the *Picornaviridae*. Molecular epidemiologic studies using sequencing have been reported for CVB1, CVB5, echovirus 30, and EV71.[47,102,237,310,452] One of the studies of CVB5 isolates examined the pattern of genetic changes over three separate outbreaks in the United States. The nucleotide sequence from multiple isolates from the epidemics showed that each of the epidemics was caused by a single genotype. The genotype of CVB5 observed in the 1967 epidemic showed more similarity to the virus observed in the 1983 epidemic than to viruses isolated during the intervening years,[237] suggesting discontinuous transmission of epidemic CVB5 in the United States during this time. In an analogous manner, echovirus 30 genotypes have demonstrated an overlapping succession among the isolates characterized in the United States.[310] More than one genotype may be found in certain periods, and the displaced genotype can be found in other parts of the world after isolations have ceased in the United States for many years. In studies of EV71 isolates, three distinct genotypes have been characterized.[47] Unlike the situation with echovirus 30 and more similar to the CVB5 example, the transition from one genotype to another occurred during a single year, 1987, and the older genotype has not been isolated since in the United States despite isolation in other parts of the world.

CLINICAL FEATURES

Most EV infections are asymptomatic. On the other hand, these viruses can cause a spectrum of clinically distinct syndromes when they lead to disease. Tables 17.4 through 17.7 list the prototype EV strains and the illness, if any, in the person from whom the prototype virus was isolated. Individual serotypes generally lead to varied symptomatology and disease processes. Similarly, individual clinical disorders can generally be caused by a number of different EVs. On occasion, however, particular syndromes are associated with specific EVs

TABLE 17.4 Enterovirus Species A (EV-A)

Type	Prototype strain	Geographic origin	Illness or source prototype virus	Accession number
CVA2	Fleetwood	Delaware	Poliomyelitis	AY421760
CVA3	Olson	New York	Meningitis	AY421761
CVA4	High Point	North Carolina	Sewage of community with polio	AY421762
CVA5	Swartz	New York	Poliomyelitis	AY421763
CVA6	Gdula	New York	Meningitis	AY421764
CVA7	Parker	New York	Meningitis	AY421765
CVA8	Donovan	New York	Poliomyelitis	AY421766
CVA10	Kowalik	New York	Meningitis	AY421767
CVA12	Texas-12	Texas	Flies in community with polio	AY421768
CVA14	G-14	South Africa	None	AY421769
CVA16	G-10	South Africa	None	U05876
EV71	BrCr	California	Meningitis[a]	U22521
EV76	10226	France	Gastroenteritis	AY697458
EV89	10359	Bangladesh	Acute flaccid paralysis	AY697459
EV90	10399	Bangladesh	Acute flaccid paralysis	AY697460
EV91	10406	Bangladesh	Acute flaccid paralysis	AY697461
EV114	11610	Bangladesh	Acute flaccid paralysis	NA

NA, information not available.

[a]An identical strain was isolated from the brain of a fatal encephalitis case in the same local outbreak of central nervous system disease.

TABLE 17.5 Enterovirus Species B (EV-B)[a]

Type	Prototype strain	Geographic origin	Illness yielding prototype virus	Accession number
CVA9	Bozek	New York	Meningitis	D00627
CVB1	Conn-5	Connecticut	Meningitis	M16560
CVB2	Ohio-1	Ohio	Summer grippe	AF085363
CVB3	Nancy	Connecticut	Minor febrile illness	M16572
CVB4	JVB	New York	Chest and abdominal pain	X05690
CVB5	Faulkner	Kentucky	Mild paralytic disease with atrophy	AF114383
CVB6	Schmidt	Philippine Islands	None	AF105342
E1	Farouk	Egypt	None	AF029859
E2	Cornelis	Connecticut	Meningitis	AY302545
E3	Morrisey	Connecticut	Meningitis	AY302553
E4	Pesascek	Connecticut	Meningitis	AY302557
E5	Noyce	Maine	Meningitis	AF083069
E6	D'Amori	Rhode Island	Meningitis	AY302558
E7	Wallace	Ohio	None	AY302559
E9	Hill	Ohio	None	X84981
E11	Gregory	Ohio	None	X80059
E12	Travis	Philippine Islands	None	X79047
E13	Del Carmen	Philippine Islands	None	AY302539
E14	Tow	Rhode Island	Meningitis	AY302540
E15	CH 96-51	West Virginia	None	AY302541
E16	Harrington	Massachusetts	Meningitis	AY302542
E17	CHHE-29	Mexico City	None	AY302543
E18	Metcalf	Ohio	Diarrhea	AF317694
E19	Burke	Ohio	Diarrhea	AY302544
E20	JV-1	Washington, DC	Fever	AY302546
E21	Farina	Massachusetts	Meningitis	AY302547
E24	DeCamp	Ohio	Diarrhea	AY302548
E25	JV-4	Washington, DC	Diarrhea	AY302549
E26	Coronel	Philippine Islands	None	AY302550
E27	Bacon	Philippine Islands	None	AY302551
E29	JV-10	Washington, DC	None	AY302552
E30	Bastianni	New York	Meningitis	AF162711
E31	Caldwell	Kansas	Meningitis	AY302554
E32	PR-10	Puerto Rico	Meningitis	AY302555
E33	Toluca-3	Mexico	None	AY302556
EV69	Toluca-1	Mexico	None	AY302560
EV73	CA55-1988	California	Unknown	AF241359
EV74	10213	California	Unknown	AY556057
EV75	10219	Oklahoma	Unknown	AY556070
EV77	CF496-99	France	Unknown	AJ493062
EV78	W137-126/99	France	Unknown	AY208120
EV79	10384	California	Unknown	AY843297
EV80	10387	California	Unknown	AY843298
EV81	10389	California	Unknown	AY843299
EV82	10390	California	Unknown	AY843300
EV83	10392	California	Unknown	AY843301
EV84	10603	Côte d'Ivoire	None	DQ902712
EV85	10353	Bangladesh	Acute flaccid paralysis	AY843303
EV86	10354	Bangladesh	Acute flaccid paralysis	AY843304
EV87	10396	Bangladesh	Acute flaccid paralysis	AY843305
EV88	10398	Bangladesh	Acute flaccid paralysis	AY843306
EV97	10355	Bangladesh	Acute flaccid paralysis	AY843307
EV100	10500	Bangladesh	Acute flaccid paralysis	DQ902713
EV101	10361	Côte d'Ivoire	None	AY843308
EV106	10634	Bangladesh	Acute flaccid paralysis	NA
EV107	TN94-0349	Thailand	None	AB266609

NA, information not available.

[a]Echovirus types 1 and 8 share antigens, type 1 having the broader spectrum. Type 10 was soon excluded from this group: it turned out to be a larger RNA virus and was reclassified as a prototypic reovirus. Type 28 was reclassified as rhinovirus type 1. Types 22 and 23 have been reclassified as members of the genus *Parechovirus* and are named parechovirus 1 and 2; these viruses along with Ljungan virus represent the only members of this new genus. Type 34, DN-19, is now considered a prime strain of CV A24, rather than a distinct echovirus. Additional newer serotypes (EV73 and higher) are proposed new types defined on the basis of genetic sequence information.

TABLE 17.6 Enterovirus Species C (EV-C)

Type	Prototype strain	Geographic origin	Illness in person with prototype	Accession number
CVA1	Tompkins	Coxsackie, NY	Poliomyelitis	AF499635
CVA11	Belgium-1	Belgium	Epidemic myalgia	AF499636
CVA13	Flores	Mexico	None	AF499637
CVA17	G-12	South Africa	None	AF499639
CVA19	NIH-8663	Japan	Guillain-Barré syndrome	AF499641
CVA20	IH-35	New York	Infectious hepatitis	AF499642
CVA21	Kuykendall; Coe	California	Poliomyelitis, mild respiratory disease	AF546702
CVA22	Chulman	New York	Vomiting and diarrhea	AF499643
CVA24	Joseph	South Africa	None	D90457
PV1	Brunhilde	Maryland	Paralytic poliomyelitis	AY560657
PV2	Lansing	Michigan	Fatal paralytic poliomyelitis	AY082680
PV3	Leon	California	Fatal paralytic poliomyelitis	K01392
EV96	10358	Bangladesh	Acute flaccid paralysis	EF015886
EV99	10461	Bangladesh	Acute flaccid paralysis	EF555644
EV102	10424	Bangladesh	Acute flaccid paralysis	EF555645
EV104	CL-1231094	Switzerland	Acute respiratory illness	EU840733
EV105	TW/NTU07	NA	NA	NA
EV109	NICA08–4327	Nicaragua	Acute respiratory illness	GQ865517
EV116	126	Russia	NA	JX514942
EV117	LIT22	NA	Pneumonia	JQ446368
EV118	ISR10	NA	Pneumonia	JQ768163

NA, information not available.

(Table 17.8). For example, acute hemorrhagic conjunctivitis is usually caused by the CVA24 variant or EV70. Acute flaccid paralysis is usually caused by PV or EV71. The occasional isolates from cases of diabetes are usually CVB serotypes.

Poliomyelitis

As is true for nonpolio EV, infection of most patients with PV does not result in disease or lead to any symptomatology. The most common symptomatic disease caused by PV, known as *abortive poliomyelitis,* is a mild febrile illness with or without gastrointestinal signs that occurs in 4% to 8% of individuals. The incubation period from infection to the onset of abortive poliomyelitis is usually 1 to 3 days, although symptoms can be seen as late as 5 days after infection. Less frequently, PV infection results in aseptic meningitis. This nonparalytic illness has the typical features of viral meningitis, with fever, headache, and meningeal signs but an absence of signs of CNS parenchymal involvement. The meningitis has a self-limited course and lasts for a few days to 2 weeks.

On average, only about 1 in 200 PV infections in a fully susceptible population results in the paralytic disease known as *poliomyelitis.* The incubation period from infection to the onset of paralysis is usually 4 to 10 days, although it can be as short as 3 days or longer than a month. The paralysis generally occurs 2 to 5 days after headaches occur and peaks within a few days. Usually, a prodrome occurs with sensory complaints and shooting or aching pains in muscle. The muscle pains may reflect growth of the virus in this tissue, which is known to occur.[270] In children can be seen a biphasic or *dromedary* course of neurologic involvement, and paralysis can occur as the initial symptom.

Paralysis is classified as either spinal or bulbar, depending on whether the spinal cord or brainstem, respectively, is involved. Not infrequently, the spinal form becomes associated with the bulbar form during the course of the disease, resulting in so-called *bulbospinal polio.* Spinal polio is usually asymmetric, flaccid, and limited to the extremities and trunk and varies from mild weakness to quadriplegia. Only about 10% to 15%

TABLE 17.7 Enterovirus Species D (EV-D)

Type	Prototype strain	Geographic origin	Illness in person with prototype	Accession number
EV68	Fermon	California	Lower respiratory illness	AY426531
EV70	J670/71	Japan and Singapore	Acute hemorrhagic conjunctivitis	D00820
EV94	E210	Egypt	Detected in sewage	DQ916376
EV111	KK2640	Cameroon	None[a]	JF416935

[a]The prototype strain was detected in a chimpanzee, but another strain of EV111 was detected in a human with acute flaccid paralysis in the Democratic Republic of the Congo.

TABLE 17.8 Clinical Syndromes Associated with Infections by Enteroviruses

Polioviruses, types 1–3
- Paralysis (complete to slight muscle weakness)
- Aseptic meningitis
- Undifferentiated febrile illness, particularly during the summer

Coxsackieviruses, group A, types 1–24
- Herpangina
- Acute lymphatic or nodular pharyngitis
- Aseptic meningitis
- Paralysis
- Exanthema
- Hand-foot-and-mouth disease (A10, A16)
- Pneumonitis of infants
- "Common cold"
- Hepatitis
- Infantile diarrhea
- Acute hemorrhagic conjunctivitis (type A24 variant)

Coxsackieviruses, group B, types 1–6
- Pleurodynia
- Aseptic meningitis
- Paralysis (infrequently)
- Severe systemic infection in infants, meningoencephalitis, and myocarditis
- Pericarditis, myocarditis
- Upper respiratory illness and pneumonia
- Rash
- Hepatitis
- Undifferentiated febrile illness

Echoviruses, types 1–33
- Aseptic meningitis
- Paralysis
- Encephalitis, ataxia, or Guillain-Barré syndrome
- Exanthema
- Respiratory disease
- Others: Diarrhea
- Pericarditis and myocarditis
- Hepatic disturbance

Enterovirus, types 68–116[a]
- Pneumonia and bronchiolitis
- Acute hemorrhagic conjunctivitis (type 70)
- Paralysis (types 70, 71)[b]
- Meningoencephalitis (types 70, 71)
- Hand-foot-and-mouth disease (type 71)

[a]Since 1969, new enterovirus types have been assigned enterovirus type numbers rather than being subclassified as coxsackieviruses or echoviruses. The vernacular names of the previously identified enteroviruses have been retained.

[b]Numerous additional types have been identified in stool from acute flaccid paralysis cases, but an etiologic link has not been confirmed.

Adapted from Melnick JL. Enteroviruses: polioviruses, coxsackieviruses, echoviruses, and newer enteroviruses. In: Fields BN, Knipe DM, Howley PM, eds. *Fields Virology*. 3rd ed. Philadelphia: Lippincott-Raven, 1996:655–712.

of poliomyelitis cases are bulbar, a term indicating involvement of the motor cranial nerves or medullary centers controlling respiration and the vasomotor system. Cranial nerves IX and X, those most affected, lead to paralysis of the pharyngeal and laryngeal muscles with resultant difficulty swallowing and talking. Involvement of other cranial nerves can lead to weakness of the face (VII) and tongue (XII). Most dreaded is involvement of the brainstem reticular formation, resulting in respiratory compromise, potentially requiring ventilatory support. Also seen is autonomic involvement, which manifests as abnormalities of sweating, urination, defecation, and blood pressure control. Recovery can be delayed significantly. Not infrequently, one extremity is left severely weak and atrophic, with a relatively normal contralateral limb.

The pathology of poliomyelitis is one of inflammation and destruction of the gray matter of the CNS, especially of the spinal cord. Motor neurons up and down the neuraxis can be infected, including upper motor neurons located rostrally in the brainstem and cerebral hemispheres in addition to the anterior horn lower motor neurons in the spinal cord. The widespread nature of the gray matter infection demonstrates that the disease is frequently a polioencephalomyelitis (i.e., inflammation of the gray matter of the brain and spinal cord) rather than merely a poliomyelitis (inflammation of the gray matter of the spinal cord). Interestingly, perivascular mononuclear inflammatory cells can persist for months, although virus is difficult to culture from the spinal cord after a week.[37] Although the focus of pathology in the spinal cord is in the anterior horn, abnormalities also occur outside the motor system in the posterior horn and intermediolateral column. Similarly, the brainstem shows involvement of a number of sensory cranial nerve nuclei and of the reticular formation in addition to the motor cranial nerve nuclei. Neurons die with evidence of chromatolysis followed by neuronophagia. Recent investigations of CD155 transgenic mice have reported that spinal cord neurons die by apoptosis.[125]

Poliomyelitis or acute flaccid paralysis can occur as a result of infection with other EVs besides PV. EV71 is emerging as the most important virulent neurotropic EV during the poliomyelitis eradication period. This virus causes epidemics of poliomyelitis-type disease, including bulbar disease.[72] In an EV71 epidemic in Bulgaria in 1975, a paralytic disease occurred in as many as 21% of approximately 700 patients, with a case fatality rate approaching 30%.[373] EV71 is also associated with epidemic encephalitis and meningitis (see Clinical Features: Meningitis and Encephalitis). EV70, a cause of epidemics of acute hemorrhagic conjunctivitis, can lead to a severe and acute paralytic disease.[411] The incidence of paralysis is probably 1 of 10,000 infections.[197] These patients can also have cranial nerve palsies, autonomic abnormalities, and sensory signs. Sometimes, EV70 infections cause isolated cranial nerve palsies, most commonly involving the facial nerve. The eye disease is usually spread by direct or indirect contamination of the eye rather than the fecal–oral route. Some echoviruses and coxsackieviruses have also been associated with acute flaccid paralysis (e.g., CVA7 virus).[137]

Postpolio Syndrome and Amyotrophic Lateral Sclerosis

Patients with postpolio syndrome complain of new weakness, fatigue, and pain decades after paralytic poliomyelitis. One subgroup of this syndrome, called *postpoliomyelitis progressive muscular atrophy*, is an uncommon primary neurologic disorder manifested by slowly progressive atrophy of muscles with evidence of ongoing motor nerve damage.[54] Some investigators have reported a persistent PV infection in the spinal fluid or

CNS tissue from patients with postpoliomyelitis progressive muscular atrophy,[248,249,290,333,371] but others have failed to confirm these findings.[201,272,361] One of the groups that originally reported EV genome in patients with postpolio syndrome later claimed that both patients and controls had evidence of enteroviral genome in the CNS.[291] Although the PV genome of a mouse-adapted mutant PV has been reported to persist at low levels following experimental infection of mice,[97] the only consistent evidence for persistent PV infection in humans has been found in individuals who are immunocompromised. We await more convincing data demonstrating that a persistent infection underlies the postpolio syndrome.

The issue of whether PV can persist in postpoliomyelitis progressive muscular atrophy has raised questions about whether PV or another EV is involved in amyotrophic lateral sclerosis, a chronic progressive weakening disease of unknown cause associated with death of motor neurons. A possible role for EV in amyotrophic lateral sclerosis seems unlikely given the immunocompetence of these patients and the noninflammatory pathology of the disease. Although some studies have reported enteroviral genomic sequences in tissues of patients with amyotrophic lateral sclerosis and motor neuron diseases, a recent investigation failed to find evidence to support this.[304]

Meningitis and Encephalitis

Aseptic meningitis is a nonbacterial inflammation of the meninges associated with fever, headache, photophobia, and meningeal signs in the absence of signs of brain parenchymal involvement.[358] The syndrome is the most common CNS infection, with 7,000 cases of aseptic meningitis reported per year in the United States and an actual incidence believed to be 10-fold higher.[357]

Enteroviruses are the main recognized cause of aseptic meningitis in both children and adults in developed countries. Enteroviruses were identified in 85% to 95% of cases in which a specific pathogen was cultured.[358] In one study, 62% of infants younger than 3 months of age with aseptic meningitis had CVB as the etiologic agent.[209] Of note, aseptic meningitis is the most common clinical syndrome caused by EV that results in medical attention.

Enteroviruses should be suspected as the causative agent for aseptic meningitis occurring in the summer and fall in temperate zones. The seasonal increase in incidence of enteroviral aseptic meningitis may result because the fecal–oral route of transmission is facilitated in warm periods when less clothing is worn.[197] Fever is common in patients with EV-induced aseptic meningitis, as with most cases of aseptic meningitis. At times, the fever has a biphasic pattern, initially associated with constitutional symptoms and then returning with meningeal signs. One may see nonneurologic abnormalities associated with enteroviral meningitis (e.g., rash), which may be helpful in the diagnosis and identification of the particular enteroviral serotype.[197] For example, rashes have been associated with CNS disease caused by CVA5, A9, and A16 and echoviruses 4, 6, 9, and 16. The rash associated with echovirus 9 meningitis can be petechial, resembling that seen with meningococcemia.

Encephalitis signifies that the brain parenchyma is infected and is not infrequently associated with a disturbed state of consciousness, focal neurologic signs, and seizures. The distinction between aseptic meningitis and encephalitis is important because the absence of parenchymal involvement in aseptic meningitis suggests a more benign condition and more favorable prognosis. Encephalitis is usually associated with aseptic meningitis, usually resulting in a meningoencephalitis.

Although a specific virus is not usually identified in most cases of encephalitis, and although the number of cases in which an EV has been identified as the cause of encephalitis is low, EVs nevertheless rank second to herpes simplex virus and comparable to arboviruses as a recognized cause of encephalitis in the United States. The New York State Department of Health found evidence of EV genome by PCR in the spinal fluid of 3 of 41 cases of encephalitis over the period from July 1997 to November 1998;[172] herpes simplex virus genome and arbovirus genome were each found in 5 cases.

Patients with EV encephalitis usually have a global neurologic depression in function, although occasionally seen are focal neurologic signs, resembling herpes simplex virus encephalitis.[283] Cases associated with an acute cerebellar ataxia have been reported in children infected with various EVs, including PV, echoviruses 6 and 9, and coxsackieviruses A2 and A9.[197] Other uncommon clinical manifestations reported include acute hemiplegia, opsoclonus-myoclonus, movement disorders, and Guillain-Barré syndrome.[197]

The meningeal syndrome is usually self-limited and benign, with evidence of improvement in days to a week. Deaths have been reported, however, following infection with a number of enteroviruses, including CVB1 and echoviruses 9, 17, and 21.[197] Morbidity and mortality are also increased in the neonate. The neonate's disease tends to be especially severe when the disease appears soon after birth, perhaps reflecting perinatal spread of virus to the fetus from the mother. Mortality is increased in the neonate partly because the aseptic meningitis can be associated with systemic disease (e.g., hepatitis and myocarditis) as well as encephalitis. The largest study of recovered patients failed to find any neurodevelopmental abnormalities above levels seen in controls.[352]

Isolation of EV may be unsuccessful because a particular EV may grow poorly in cell culture or because inhibitory factors (e.g., neutralizing antibody) may be present in the spinal fluid. With the use of reverse transcriptase (RT)-PCR, EV genome may be found in a significant number of culture-negative spinal fluid samples from cases of aseptic meningitis. The potential usefulness of RT-PCR can be seen in a report of a Swiss epidemic of aseptic meningitis caused by echovirus 30, when the EV genome was identified using this technique in 42 of 50 spinal fluid cultures (84%) that were negative for virus isolation.[133] On the other hand, the use of RT-PCR may be unsuccessful because some so-called generic RT-PCR primers may fail to hybridize well to particular EVs because of a difference in target sequence.

In some areas of the world, epidemics of EV71[72,373] have been associated with a high incidence of aseptic meningitis as well as CNS parenchymal involvement; the CNS infection has caused acute flaccid paralysis as well as a more varied clinical symptomatology.[274] As noted, EV71 is emerging as the most significant neurotropic EV in some areas of the world. This virus circulates in the United States, and 26% of adults tested in a seroepidemiologic study in New York in 1972 had antibody.[95] An epidemic of EV71 infection in 1998 in Taiwan caused frequent CNS disease and more than 100,000 reports of hand-foot-and-mouth disease or herpangina (see Respiratory Infections, Herpangina, and Hand-Foot-and-Mouth

Disease), which may correspond to 1 million actual cases of EV infection.[161] The patients with hand-foot-and-mouth disease had vesicular lesions on their hands, feet, mouth, and, at times, buttocks, whereas the patients with herpangina had vesicular lesions of the palate and pharynx. Of special concern was the finding of 405 severe cases with associated complications, 78 of which were fatal. Among the more severe cases, the case fatality rate in different areas ranged from 7.7% to 31.0%. Most of the hospitalized cases (80%) and the deaths (91%) were in children younger than 5 years of age. The most frequent complication was encephalitis. Other serious complications, which were associated at times with encephalitis, included aseptic meningitis, myocarditis, and pulmonary edema and hemorrhage. It is unclear whether the pulmonary signs were related to viral invasion of the lungs or to brain injury from the viral encephalitis.

A review[172] of 41 hospitalized children with neurologic complications and culture-confirmed EV71 infection during the Taiwan epidemic in 1998 demonstrated an unusual and rather distinctive neurologic manifestation, brainstem encephalitis or rhombencephalitis. The mean age of the 41 children was 2.5 years (with a range from 3 months to 8.2 years). There was frequently an associated condition: hand-foot-and-mouth disease in 68%, or herpangina in 15%. The neurologic disease usually followed the initial illness of fever and skin or mucosal lesions, and it was manifested as rhombencephalitis (37 patients), aseptic meningitis (3 patients), and acute flaccid paralysis (associated with the disease in 4 patients, and following rhombencephalitis in 3 of the 4). At times, breathing difficulties and coma were seen in the patients with rhombencephalitis, progressing to death in five. The brainstem and spinal cord pathology was presumably related to direct viral injury, because virus was cultured from the spinal cord and brainstem of the one patient who underwent autopsy. Five of the patients who survived had neurologic sequelae. EV71 brainstem involvement was also seen during an epidemic in Malaysia in 1997, but not in earlier epidemics. In contrast, hand-foot-and-mouth disease and herpangina did not occur during the previous epidemics in Bulgaria and Hungary. It is not clear whether the changes in EV71 disease phenotype represent the emergence (or re-emergence) of a more virulent strain or whether it is related to the serologic status of the at-risk populations.

The presence of immunodeficiency predisposes to a syndrome of EV-induced aseptic meningitis or meningoencephalitis, at times producing a persistent CNS infection. McKinney et al.[270] reviewed more than 40 cases of chronic enteroviral meningoencephalitis in patients with congenital immunodeficiencies, most commonly X-linked agammaglobulinemia. Clinical features were remarkably varied and included headaches, seizures, ataxia, a disturbed state of consciousness, motor deficits, personality changes with cognitive decline, and sensory disturbances. At times, patients had other associated abnormalities, such as a dermatomyositis syndrome (in 21 of 41 patients; see Clinical Features: Muscle Disease), rashes (16 of 35 cases), edema (20 of 40 cases), and hepatitis (15 of 32 patients). Although some cases started abruptly, most tended to be slowly progressive, at times lasting years, and with a frequent fatal outcome. Most patients had a spinal fluid mononuclear cell pleocytosis with an increase in protein. Some cases at autopsy had evidence of inflammatory infiltrates in the heart, lungs, kidneys, adrenal glands, thyroid, and pancreas, in addition to the CNS.

Cardiac Disease

Myocarditis is an inflammation of the myocardium associated with damage that is unrelated to an ischemic injury. Myocarditis is frequently self-limited and subclinical, with few if any sequelae. On the other hand, the acute disease can lead to significant morbidity and even death. On the basis of well-established criteria, one study found evidence of myocarditis in approximately 1% of autopsies.[136]

In some cases, myocardial inflammation may persist, producing a chronic myocarditis that can progress to dilated cardiomyopathy.[61,205,354] In dilated cardiomyopathy, the heart is large, with impaired function and evidence of heart failure but with little or no inflammation. The incidence of dilated cardiomyopathy in the United States has been reported to be 6 per 100,000 cases,[77] with approximately 100,000 new cases each year. Because of the high mortality of dilated cardiomyopathy, patients are frequent recipients of heart transplants, making up perhaps 50% of all cardiac transplant patients. Of note is the observation that nonpolio EVs, especially CVB3, cause acute and chronic myocarditis in experimental animals, and that a contribution from the immune system to the chronic disease has been proposed (see Pathogenesis earlier).

Acute Cardiac Disease

CVB has long been considered one of the principal causes of viral myocarditis,[81] and this view has been confirmed in several recent reports.[16,106,262,264,266] Epidemiologic and other studies suggest that 70% of the general public will be exposed to cardiotropic viruses, and half of these individuals will develop acute viral myocarditis.[306] It is believed that 1.5% of enteroviral infections, including 3.2% of CVB infections, result in overt cardiac signs or symptoms.[137] Myocarditis is a frequent autopsy finding in children who die of overwhelming CV infection.[209] The peak age group in which myocarditis caused by CVB occurs is young adults, primarily between the ages of 20 and 39 years, with a higher prevalence among men.[425]

However, even the larger group of symptom-free individuals is at risk; collapse and death of young and vigorous individuals, especially during exertion, can result from catastrophic dysfunction of the electrical pathways in the heart, as a consequence of unsuspected acute viral myocarditis.[31,415] A remarkably high prevalence of asymptomatic myocarditis has been shown by necropsy studies of victims of violent or accidental deaths; in this relatively random human population, approximately 1% had active myocarditis.[136]

A summary of data from varied sources shows that the prevalence of enteroviral infection in acute myocarditis on the basis of serologic studies is 34% (214 positives in 636 patients) compared with 4% (44 of 1,139) of controls (199). However, these serologic studies demonstrating seroconversion with an EV do not prove that EV caused the cardiomyopathy, as they may result merely from an unrelated EV infection. In addition, evidence suggests that multiple EVs can circulate at the time of an epidemic, so that isolation of an EV does not prove its role in a disease; for example, more than 10 EVs were recovered from the community during an echovirus 9 epidemic.[197]

A meta-analysis of data obtained from molecular studies (slot blot hybridization, *in situ* hybridization, and RT-PCR) published in 12 reports found 23% of cases (68 of 289) and 6% of controls (14 of 216) had evidence of EV genome in heart tissue, giving an odds ratio of 4.4 with a 95% confidence interval of 2.4 to 8.2.[27] These data, coupled with reports of positive virus isolations from the heart, indicate that EV may represent a common cause of acute myocarditis. The surprisingly large number of positive findings in controls is presumed to result from difficulties in obtaining appropriately controlled heart tissue.

Chronic Cardiac Disease

Human DCM has multiple causes, both inherited and sporadic. A prior history of enteroviral infection of the heart, especially with CVB, has been implicated in sporadic human dilated cardiomyopathy.[26,382] Although the majority of patients with symptoms recover well from acute myocarditis, the disease can have serious long-term sequelae; some 10% to 20% of people with symptoms (i.e., ~20,000 to 40,000 patients per year in the United States) will develop chronic disease, progressing over time to DCM.[306,380] A summary of serologic data from multiple sources found that the prevalence of EV in dilated cardiomyopathy was 25% (64 of 260) compared to 10% of controls (26 of 255).[268] These serologic data suffer from the same drawbacks that are noted earlier.

In contrast to acute myocarditis, no reports are found of isolation of EV from chronic dilated cardiomyopathy, suggesting that the virus may have a restricted expression or disappear following the acute infection; however, some reports exist of EV VP1 antigen in the heart of patients with dilated cardiomyopathy and chronic coronary disease.[15]

The difficulty in isolating infectious virus led to studies probing affected tissues for persistent enteroviral genome. A meta-analysis of data from molecular studies described in 17 published reports found 23% of the patients and 7% of controls had evidence of enteroviral genome, giving an odds ratio of 3.8 with a 95% confidence interval of 2.1 to 4.6.[27] The meta-analysis data are supportive of an association between EV infection and chronic cardiac disease; however, it remains a possibility that RNA from other laboratory-based enteroviral studies contaminated test samples in the highly sensitive PCR studies. Most of the hybridization and PCR studies did not include sequencing of the viral genome and, therefore, failed to prove more directly that an EV was involved. In a few cases, however, partial sequencing was done of the RNA found in clinical samples; for example, Archard et al.[20] identified the amplified sequence as CVB.

Not all the viral genomic studies have been positive. One investigation involving a nested PCR failed to find evidence of EV RNA in 287 heart biopsy specimens from 38 patients with dilated cardiomyopathy and 39 patients with heart failure of unknown cause.[92] At least two other studies have also resulted in negative findings.[251,369] The lack of consistent reproducible results regarding the presence of enteroviral genome in tissue from patients with cardiomyopathy indicates that further studies are needed under careful, blinded conditions.

Muscle Disease Including Pleurodynia

The relationship of EV to inflammatory muscle diseases was initially recognized because of the myotropism of coxsackieviruses in suckling mice. This observation was fueled by the association of these viruses with epidemic pleurodynia on the Danish island of Bornholm. The latter disease, called *Bornholm disease,* is an acute febrile illness with myalgia, especially involving the chest and abdomen, but without muscle weakness. It has occurred as an epidemic and also sporadically in various locales. Relapses can occur. CVB3 and B5 are the most frequently recognized causative agents, although other EVs have also been isolated.[446] The limited information from muscle biopsy findings suggests that the inflammation in this disease may be confined to the endomysial part of the muscle and, therefore, is not a true myositis.[87]

Enteroviruses have been implicated in acute and chronic inflammatory muscle disease. The acute diseases, which are usually called *acute polymyositis* or *myositis,* are characterized by fever with myalgia, elevated muscle enzymes, and, at times, myoglobinuria. Chronic inflammatory muscle diseases, which are generally classified as polymyositis, dermatomyositis, or inclusion body myositis, have a subacute to chronic progressive weakness with a distinctive pathology on muscle biopsy. Dermatomyositis is distinguished from the other two inflammatory myopathies because it is associated with a characteristic rash.

The causes of chronic inflammatory myopathy are generally unknown. Hypotheses concerning the etiology of polymyositis and dermatomyositis include a direct virus infection, especially an EV infection, or an autoimmune process in which the virus infection triggers a reaction against muscle (see Pathogenesis earlier). That coxsackieviruses cause acute and chronic inflammatory myopathy in experimental animals provides additional support for their involvement in human inflammatory muscle diseases. Investigations of these model systems may help clarify the pathogenesis of these diseases in humans.

Enteroviruses have been isolated from cases of inflammatory myopathies, but these isolations have generally been rare and from single cases with acute[33] or atypical clinical pictures.[389] The inability to isolate virus from cases of chronic inflammatory myopathy has raised the possibility of a restricted expression of the virus with little infectious virus present. For this reason, investigators have probed muscle tissue from patients with inflammatory myopathy for picornaviral genome. Some reports involving slot blot or *in situ* hybridization studies of muscle tissues from patients with inflammatory myopathies have shown positive results using EV-specific probes.[444] In some cases, the product amplified in an RT-PCR has been identified as CVB sequence.[21] In contrast, other studies using RT-PCR and nucleic acid hybridization have found negative results.[245,247,328] It remains a possibility that an EV could trigger an autoimmune inflammatory muscle disease and then disappear. Studies regarding the possible role of EV in chronic fatigue syndrome have similarly failed to find reproducible evidence of EV involvement.[87]

Of special interest with respect to the issue of EV involvement in inflammatory muscle disease is the observation that patients with immunodeficient states can manifest a disease similar to dermatomyositis with an accompanying persistent echovirus infection.[412,419] It should be noted, however, that questions have been raised whether these patients had a true myositis (i.e., inflammation of the muscle) or a fasciitis with interstitial inflammation in the endomysium.[87] The inflammatory muscle disease is associated with a chronic encephalomyelitis as well as a more disseminated disease in which EV, especially echoviruses, can be cultured from the spinal fluid (see Clinical Features: Meningitis and Encephalitis earlier).[451] Although virus has occasionally been isolated from affected muscle, it remains unclear whether the dermatomyositis syndrome in patients who are immunodeficient is a result of direct virus invasion of the muscle or an immune-mediated disease associated with virus persistence. The existence of this syndrome similar to dermatomyositis demonstrates that echoviruses, and perhaps other EVs, can produce a chronic myositis in humans that is associated with persistent infection and chronic inflammation.

Diabetes

Both genetic and environmental factors, including EV infection, have been implicated in the cause of insulin-dependent diabetes. A number of epidemiologic and serologic studies have demonstrated a relationship between EV infection and the development of diabetes. D'Alessio[84] found that 15 of 84 cases (17.8%) of newly diagnosed insulin-dependent diabetes had evidence of IgM antibody against CVB, compared with 5 of 71 controls (7.0%). The individuals with IgM antibody were especially common in association with human leukocyte antigen (HLA)-DR3 positivity. A prospective study in Finland found a greater incidence of serologic conversion of EV antibodies among children who developed insulin-dependent diabetes than among those who did not.[187] The antibody present in the prediabetic period was directed against a number of different EV serotypes, including CVA9, B1, B2, B3, and B5.[351] At times, the EV antibodies are associated with autoantibodies to GAD_{65} and other important targets.

Rare, but well-documented, isolations of CVB4 have come from the pancreases of patients with acute-onset as well as fatal cases of insulin-dependent diabetes.[341,345] Some of the isolates have been demonstrated to be diabetogenic when inoculated into certain mouse strains[441] and nonhuman primates.[442] Patients dying from coxsackieviral myocarditis can have an associated pancreatitis, including islitis. More recent investigations have involved probing tissues from patients for evidence of EV genome. An *in situ* hybridization study showed evidence of EV genome in the islets of autopsy pancreases from 7 of 12 newborn infants who died of fulminant CV infection (and 6 of the 7 had islitis), in the islets of autopsy pancreases of 4 of 65 adults with type 1 diabetes, and in one of the pancreatic control tissues from 40 nondiabetic patients.[440]

Although it is likely that EVs are capable of causing diabetes mellitus in animals and humans, it remains unclear how often this occurs in humans and what if any immune mechanisms are involved.

Eye Infections

Acute hemorrhagic conjunctivitis is characterized by a short incubation period of 24 to 48 hours preceding a rapid onset of uniocular or binocular symptoms and signs. Patients manifest excessive lacrimation, pain, periorbital swelling, and redness of the conjunctiva (from subconjunctival petechiae to frank hemorrhages).[438] Keratitis with accompanying pain and possible visual impairment as well as anterior uveitis may be seen. The epidemic disease can also be associated with nonophthalmic symptoms and signs, such as neurologic dysfunction (see Clinical Features earlier) and respiratory and gastrointestinal disturbances. The disease usually resolves without sequelae in 1 to 2 weeks.

The first pandemic of acute hemorrhagic conjunctivitis was recognized in 1969 in Africa. Within 2 years, two EVs, a new antigenic variant of CVA24 and a previously unknown EV serotype designated EV70, were implicated as causative agents responsible for the epidemics of this disease.[252] During the first pandemic from 1969 to 1971, hundreds of millions of people were likely to have been infected. Subsequent epidemics of acute hemorrhagic conjunctivitis have continued in various locations throughout the world. Other EVs have also been recognized as causes of acute hemorrhagic conjunctivitis (e.g., echovirus type 7)[363] and as causes of sporadic conjunctivitis and keratoconjunctivitis.[213] The ocular disease caused by EV is often indistinguishable from acute hemorrhagic conjunctivitis caused by various adenovirus serotypes.

Respiratory Infections, Herpangina, and Hand-Foot-and-Mouth Disease

Enteroviruses are a common cause of respiratory illnesses. Enteroviruses were isolated in 1.7% of 3,119 respiratory specimens submitted for viral culture from 1983 to 1994[70] and in 6.4% of all the viruses that were isolated from these specimens (54 of 838). Respiratory illness occurred in 15% of EV infections collected by the WHO from 1967 to 1974[137] and 21% of cases from the CDC obtained from 1970 to 1979.[18] The EVs implicated in these respiratory infections included CVA (12.4%), CVB (20.3%), and echoviruses (12.6%).[137]

Enteroviral respiratory infections are more frequently associated with upper respiratory infections (e.g., the common cold, croup, and epiglottitis) than with lower respiratory infections (e.g., pneumonia). The infections are frequently subclinical, but if they cause clinical disease it tends to be self-limited and mild, with a short incubation period of 1 to 3 days. More severe lower respiratory infections may be related to a higher dose of virus in the inoculum. In a series of infants with CVB infections, 30 of 77 patients had marked abnormalities (e.g., interstitial inflammation and hemorrhage), and 12 had virus isolated from the lung.[209]

Herpangina is a febrile illness of relatively sudden onset with complaints of fever and sore throat. Characteristic lesions are found on the anterior tonsillar pillars, soft palate, uvula, and tonsils, and on the posterior pharynx. The illness, which has a predilection for the young, is usually self-limited and disappears within a few days. At times, the disease is associated with more significant clinical abnormalities (e.g., meningitis). Hand-foot-and-mouth disease is an illness associated with vesicular lesions of the hands, feet, mouth, and, at times, buttocks.

A number of EVs have been identified as causes for herpangina, including CVA and B serotypes; echovirus types 6, 9, 11, 16, 17, 22, and 25;[70] and EV71. The main causes of hand-foot-and-mouth disease are CVA10 and A16 and EV71.[137] The pathogenesis of the lesions seen in herpangina is not clear; however, experimental infection of rhesus monkeys with CVA4 may provide a model system for the study of the pathogenesis of herpangina. In this system, ingestion of the virus by the oral route leads to multiplication in the lower gastrointestinal tract, followed by viremia, and then multiplication in the oropharynx.[376]

Neonate and Infant Disease

Neonates are at increased risk from enteroviral infections. This increased susceptibility is present in humans as well as experimental animals infected with varied EVs.[71]

The increased risk of neonates to EV infection was apparent in the prevaccine era with respect to PV. Although the incidence of paralytic disease among neonates approached 40%

born to mothers with poliomyelitis at the time of delivery, the overall incidence of neonatal poliomyelitis was an infrequent occurrence, perhaps related to the protective effect of maternal antibody.[431] Neonatal poliomyelitis generally had a shorter incubation period and a higher case fatality rate than found with disease later in life, demonstrating the increased susceptibility of immature hosts to EV infection. Infection of the mother early in gestation was associated with an increased risk of abortion, stillbirth, and prematurity.[71]

Nonpolio EVs are a not infrequent cause of infection in neonates and infants. In a series from the CDC, EV isolates from patients younger than 2 months of age included echoviruses (51%), CVB (45%), and CVA (4%).[288] Echovirus serotypes included 4, 9, 11, 17 to 20, 22 (now classified as human parechovirus 1), and 31.

The most frequent presentation in the neonate with nonpolio EV is asymptomatic infection.[196] Symptomatic cases most commonly manifest a self-contained febrile illness, at times associated with irritability and nonspecific signs of infection, making EV infection a leading cause of fever in the infant. A rash of variable character is seen in more than 30% of cases.[4] More serious infections can be seen, with the peak of symptoms correlating with viremia.[86] Nonpolio EVs are the most frequently identified cause of aseptic meningitis in infants younger than 1 month of age and are believed responsible for more than one-third of these cases.[301] An increased susceptibility of the neonatal CNS to CV infection may be related to the virus's predilection for neonatal stem cells.[111] In a small series of patients with pneumonia in the first month of life, EVs were implicated in 15% of cases (6 of 40).[5] Usually, the mother has a history of fever or respiratory symptoms a week before the delivery, although mothers can be asymptomatic or have a more severe disease.

One of the serious infections caused by EVs is a sepsis-like disease. In one series, EVs were implicated in 65% of infants younger than 3 months of age admitted to the hospital for suspected sepsis.[85] In another series, evidence was seen of enteroviral genome in 80 of 345 infants younger than 90 days of age admitted to a medical center with suspected sepsis.[50] A number of other studies have yielded similar results, emphasizing the importance of EV as a cause for a sepsis-like syndrome among neonates and infants.[86] In fact, EVs tend to be a more common cause of this syndrome than bacteria in the summer and fall.[50] There may be extensive multiorgan involvement in severely affected cases, especially ones that go on to a fatal outcome; the organs affected include liver, lung, heart, pancreas, and brain.

The incidence and severity of EV infections among infants can be better appreciated by reviewing a study conducted in Nassau County, New York, from 1970 to 1979.[209] Of 153,250 live births, 77 infants younger than 3 months required hospitalization for CVB infection. These 77 cases were from a pool of 602 infants who tested positive for CVB, demonstrating the high frequency of CVB infection in infants. The attack rate might have been even higher than was found, because the positive samples from this study were from only a limited number of infants hospitalized in the community. A total of 24 mothers had evidence of a viral-like infection occurring within a period from 10 days before delivery to 5 days after delivery. The most common syndrome that was seen was aseptic meningitis. Some of the infections in the infants were very serious, as evidenced by the finding that eight children died from overwhelming CVB infection. All but one of these eight had evidence of myocarditis.

Severe EV disease in the young is associated with an early age of illness, prematurity, a more severe illness in the mother, multiorgan disease, low socioeconomic status, bottle-feeding, specific EV types, and an absence of neutralizing antibody to the pathogen.[4] The level of maternal neutralizing antibody appears to be important both for determining the risk of developing infection and for modulating disease severity.[7] Long-term sequelae following neonatal myocarditis or CNS infection appear infrequent.[4,357]

Nonpolio enteroviral infection can affect the fetus, inducing clinical abnormalities and causing overt disease in the neonate. Reports exist of abortion and stillbirth associated with maternal enteroviral infections, although these are infrequent.[4] The relationship between maternal EV infection and congenital anomalies in the newborn remains unclear.

A number of routes exist by which EV can cause neonatal disease. Studies have found evidence of placentitis and viral infection in fetal tissues.[4] Virus can enter the placenta or fetus from contaminated maternal blood, feces, or vaginal secretions, which can occur during pregnancy, with virus penetrating the fetal membranes, or at the time of the delivery. In addition, infection of the neonate can result from a viremia, because EVs have been cultured from cord blood,[199] but it is unclear how often this route of transmission occurs. Infection can also occur from virus shed by other neonates or hospital staff in the nursery. In cases involving nursery outbreaks, implementation of infection controls (e.g., strict hand washing and the isolation of affected patients) has a role in prevention of new cases.

DIAGNOSIS

Differential and Presumptive Diagnosis

The process of diagnosing an EV infection or establishing that an EV infection produced a particular clinical syndrome can be complicated and challenging. This problem results from the biology and epidemiology of EV infections, as well as from limitations in current diagnostic methodologies. Although it is possible to demonstrate that a person is infected with an enterovirus, this association does not necessarily prove likely disease causation. On the other hand, a presumptive diagnosis in certain epidemiologic and clinical situations can be possible with a high degree of certainty on clinical grounds alone.

Several related biological properties complicate the diagnosis of EV-induced disease. The first is that most virus replication and infection typically occur in the respiratory and gastrointestinal tract. These infections are often asymptomatic, with few if any systemic clinical signs. Because these infections are extremely common, even random sampling of healthy individuals can demonstrate EV infections at substantial rates. For this reason, the simple recovery or detection of virus from certain nonsterile sites does not establish a firm linkage to disease, and it may be merely coincidental.

A second difficulty is that even when illness results from the EV infection, most of the signs and symptoms are relatively generic and usually lack specificity. The collection of appropriate clinical specimens for virus isolation or detection is critical to laboratory confirmation of EV infection. For example, the exclusive use of CNS or cardiac specimens to diagnose

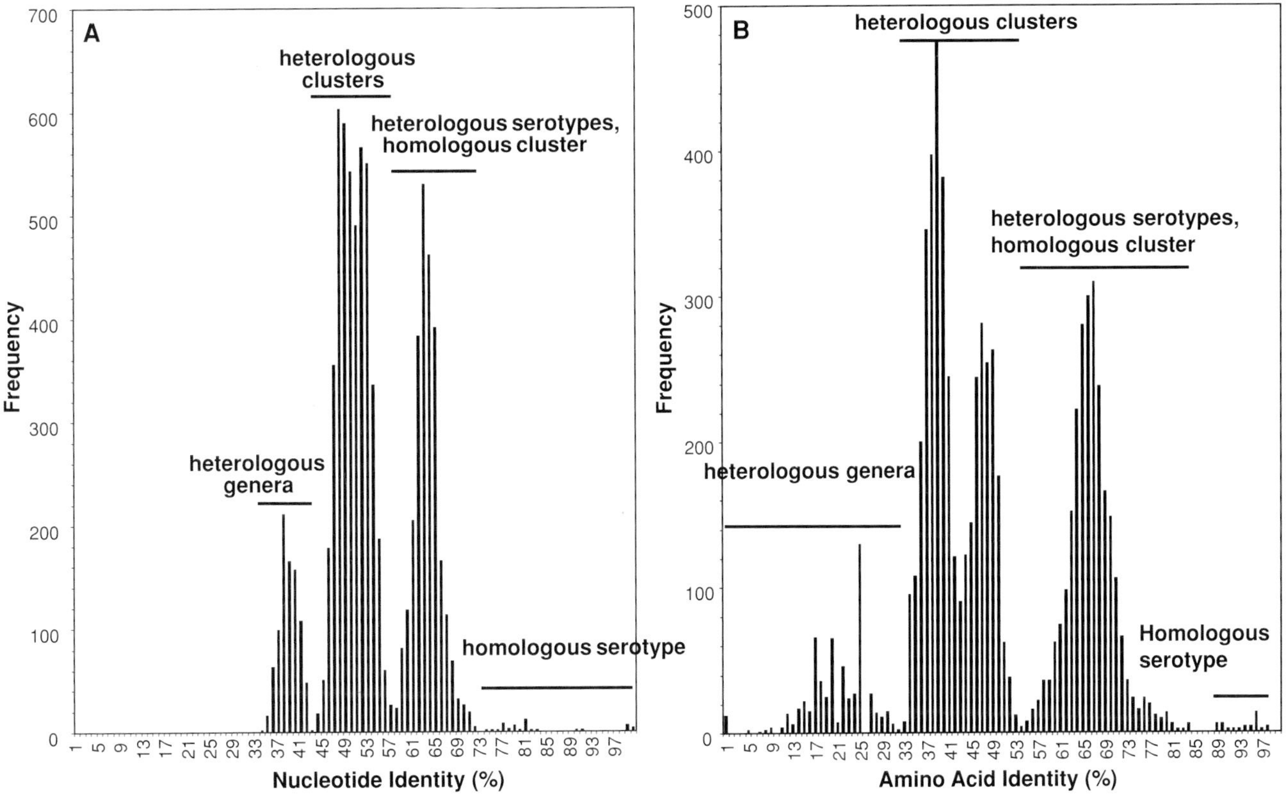

FIGURE 17.11. Serotype identification using sequence data. Frequency distribution of pairwise identity scores for comparison of VP1 nucleotide and deduced amino acid sequences. Serotype identification of an isolate can be achieved by comparing the sequence of the isolate with known sequences in VP1 for all serotypes and looking for identities of greater than 75% in nucleotide sequence or greater than 88% in amino acid. **A:** Nucleotide sequence distribution. **B:** Amino acid sequence distribution. (From: Oberste MS, Maher K, Kilpatrick DR, Flemister MR, Brown BA, Pallansch MA. Typing of human enteroviruses by partial sequencing of VP1. *J Clin Microbiol.* 1999;37:1288–1293.)

VP1 sequence with a database containing VP1 sequences for the prototype and variant strains of all human EV serotypes. The following guidelines have been suggested:

> (i) a partial or complete VP1 nucleotide sequence identity of ≥75% (>85% amino acid identity) between a clinical EV isolate and serotype prototype strain may be used to establish the serotype of the isolate, on the provision that the second highest score is <70%; (ii) a best-match nucleotide sequence identity of <70% may indicate that the isolate represents an unknown (that is, new) serotype; and (iii) a sequence identity between 70% and 75% indicates that further characterization is required before the isolate can be identified firmly.[316]

Using these guidelines, strains of homologous serotypes can be easily discriminated from heterologous serotypes and new serotypes can be identified (Fig. 17.11). This method can greatly reduce the time required to type an EV isolate and can be used to type isolates that are difficult or impossible to type using standard immunologic reagents. The technique is also useful to rapidly determine whether viruses isolated during an outbreak are epidemiologically related.

FIGURE 17.10. Enterovirus nucleotide and amino acid sequence variation, and location of primers used for virus detection and identification. A: Sequence conservation at sites in the enterovirus (EV) 5′ nontranslated region (NTR) that are targeted by published real-time reverse transcriptase-polymerase chain reaction (RT-PCR) primers. The consensus sequence at each site and the sequences of the widely used Rotbart primers and probe are indicated for comparison. Mismatches between a primer and the human enterovirus consensus are underlined. Numbers indicate nucleotide positions relative to the genome of poliovirus 1, Mahoney strain (GenBank J02281). **B:** Sequence conservation at sites in the EV 5′ NTR that are targeted by the published nucleic acid sequence–based amplification (NASBA) methods, as in panel **A**. **C:** Nucleotide sequence variation across the enterovirus genome. Complete genome sequences for reference strains of all human enterovirus serotypes were aligned, the sequence identity within each window of 18 residues was plotted versus the nucleotide position, and the window was advanced in one-residue increments across the genome. An expanded view of the 5′ NTR analysis is shown in the **upper plot**. Peaks labeled 1–5 are sites commonly targeted by enterovirus molecular detection assays. **D:** Enterovirus genome map. Boundaries of mature protein products are approximate. **E:** Amino acid sequence variation across the enterovirus genome. Deduced polyprotein amino acid sequences for reference strains of all human enterovirus serotypes were aligned; the sequence identity within each window of six residues was plotted versus the amino acid position and the window was advanced in one-residue increments across the genome. **F:** Locations of RT-PCR products used for molecular serotyping.

Virus Isolation

Many of the detailed procedures for the established laboratory diagnosis of EV infections using virus isolation have been described.[135] The traditional techniques for detecting and characterizing EV rely on the time-consuming and labor-intensive procedures of viral isolation in cell culture and neutralization by reference antisera. Isolation of EV from specimens using appropriate cultured cell lines is often possible within 2 or 3 days and remains a very sensitive method for detecting these viruses. The best specimens for isolation of virus are, in order of preference, stool specimens or rectal swabs, throat swabs or washings, and CSF. Throat swabs or washings and CSF are most likely to yield virus isolates if they are obtained early in the acute phase of the illness. For cases of acute hemorrhagic conjunctivitis, the best specimens are conjunctival swabs,[438] although occasionally virus can be isolated from tears.[439] Since the major pandemic in 1981, however, isolation of EV70 from patients with acute hemorrhagic conjunctivitis has been very difficult, and molecular methods provide the only sensitive method to detect this agent.[374]

The procedure for virus isolation involves inoculation of appropriate specimens onto susceptible cultured cells. No single cell line exists that is capable of growing all human enteroviruses. It is common practice to use several types of human and primate cells to increase the spectrum of viruses that can be detected.[69] Even with a variety of cells, however, several CVA serotypes fail to propagate in culture. The coxsackieviruses, including those that do not grow in cell culture, can be isolated and propagated in suckling mice.

As a consequence of current PV eradication activities and the importance of PV as a public health problem, specific diagnostic procedures have been developed to detect this virus. In general, PV grows well on a variety of primate and human cell culture lines, but it cannot be distinguished from other EVs solely on the basis of cytopathic effect. Polioviruses are unique in the use of CD155, which is distinct from receptors used by all other EVs to infect cells. This receptor has been transfected and expressed in a murine cell line that normally cannot be infected by most EVs but is permissive to viral replication when the viral genome is present within the cell. One of these transfected murine cells, L20B, can grow PV and has been exploited selectively to isolate PV, even in the presence of other EVs.[171] When a specimen is inoculated onto these cells and a characteristic EV cytopathic effect is seen, the virus can be presumptively identified as a PV. A few strains of certain nonpolio EV serotypes are able to grow on the parent murine cells, however, and therefore growth on L20B cells is not a definitive identification of PV, and confirmatory testing is required.

In routine diagnostic testing, all EV growth in cell culture is detected by its cytopathic effect, and the isolate is typically confirmed as a specific EV by neutralization with type-specific antisera, by immunofluorescence with type-specific monoclonal antibodies, or by PCR coupled with sequencing. For clinical management of routine cases, it is seldom critical to identify the specific nonpolio EV type. A high index of suspicion for an EV infection can be developed by reflecting on the clinical picture, the virus isolate's cytopathic effect and cell culture systems utilized, and knowledge of basic EV epidemiology.

Antibody Tests

Serologic diagnosis of EV infection can be made by comparing titers in acute and convalescent phase (*paired*) serum specimens. In general, however, EV serodiagnosis is more relevant to epidemiologic studies than to clinical diagnosis (see Epidemiology earlier). The most basic serologic test is that of neutralization in cell culture. Many serologic studies rely on the detection of IgM antibody as evidence for recent EV infection, and this is now widely used as an alternative to the neutralization and complement fixation test. Several groups have developed an enzyme-linked immunosorbent assay (ELISA) for EV-specific IgM.[30,263] These tests have been found positive for nearly 90% of culture-confirmed CVB infections and can be performed rapidly. The ELISA has been successfully applied for epidemiologic investigations of outbreaks,[130] as well as for specific diagnostic use.[90]

In most cases, the IgM ELISA test is not serotype specific. Depending on the configuration and sensitivity of the test, from 10% to nearly 70% of serum samples show a heterotypic response caused by other EV infections. This heterotypic response has been exploited to measure broadly reactive antibody, and the assay used to detect EV infection generically.[42,384] In attempting to characterize the exact nature of the response using different antigens, it is clear that the human immune response to EV infection includes antibodies that react with both serotype-specific epitopes and shared epitopes.[120] Despite this problem, which is inherently biological, a fairly high concordance of results remains between assays of different configurations.[162] In summary, the IgM assays that are generally used in epidemiologic studies have very good sensitivity and appear to be very specific for EV infection; however, these assays detect heterotypic antibodies resulting from other EV infections and, therefore, cannot be considered strictly serotype specific.

PREVENTION AND CONTROL

Treatment

Although no currently available drug treatment for enteroviral infections is in clinical use, the effectiveness of a variety of drugs *in vitro,* as well as in animal models, has been documented. In addition, varied new directions for future therapeutic intervention are being pursued.

Several potential therapies (e.g., IFN and antiviral antibody) target early stages in the virus life cycle, such as spread. IFN-α and IFN-β have been found to be effective in CVA24 *in vitro* infections.[243] Pilot studies have been conducted administering intravenous immunoglobulin in neonates suspected of having enteroviral infection.[7] Pooled immunoglobulin delivered intravenously or via a shunt into the spinal fluid has also been used in patients who are agammaglobulinemic with chronic encephalitis and meningitis associated with nonpolio enteroviruses. Patients who are immunodeficient with persistent EV infections, including PV infections, represent a particular challenge to effective treatment. Although intravenous immunoglobulin may protect these patients from poliomyelitis and may appear to stabilize and improve some of the infections, the disease may progress; most of these infections, however, spontaneously cease. In some cases, efficacy may be limited by inadequate amounts of the relevant antibody in the immunoglobulin pool (e.g., if the infection involves an unusual and rare EV serotype), as well as problems in the delivery of adequate levels of antibody to the infected cells. One report documented the failure to clear persistent PV excretion despite treatment with intravenous immunoglobulin, breast milk, and ribavirin.[261a] Interestingly, a successful clearance of PV may apparently follow intercurrent diarrheal infections caused by other pathogens, perhaps because of damage to gut lymphoid tissue, which acts as a main site of PV replication.[222]

A number of specific antiviral compounds have been developed to target enteroviral proteins and steps in the virus's life cycle. The *WIN compounds* and related derivatives, which were originally shown to be effective against rhinovirus, have shown the most consistent results and have been those most studied mechanistically. These drugs bind a hydrophobic site near the surface of the virion called the *pocket*,[447] which lies in the floor of the *canyon* where the virion binds to the cellular receptor. By binding to the pocket, these compounds are believed to interfere with viral attachment and uncoating. Variations in activity of WIN compounds against different picornaviruses are presumably related to the particular fit of the drug into the pocket of a specific EV strain. Oral administration of WIN 54954 significantly decreased the number of upper respiratory infections following challenge with CVA21 (i.e., 3 of 27 patients in the treated group had an upper respiratory infection versus 15 of 23 in the placebo group) with decreased associated symptoms and viral titers.[367] Adverse reactions, however, curtailed further investigations with this drug. Pleconaril or VP 63843 is a more recently developed pocket-binding compound with a broad *in vitro* inhibitory activity against 95% of the 215 nonpolio EVs that were tested.[332] Significant activity was noted against some serotypes, such as echovirus 11. A randomized, double-blind study involving the administration of pleconaril following a challenge with CVA21 showed statistically significant decreases in viral shedding in nasal secretions, nasal mucous production, and total respiratory illness symptom scores in patients treated with pleconaril compared with subjects treated with placebo.[367] Another phase II trial of the same drug against enteroviral meningitis showed a statistically significant decrease in disease duration (9.5 days in the placebo group versus 4.0 days in the controls).[359] A subsequent study, however, failed to have the statistical power to show efficacy in infants with enteroviral meningitis.[6] A problem with all of these antiviral compounds is that mutant viruses resistant to the drug can arise. In the case of resistance to rhinovirus, the mutant viruses tend to have bulky amino acid substitutions that sterically block entry of the drug into the pocket.[154] These mutant viruses may not be as significant a problem as expected, because drug-resistant CVB3 mutants that appeared in tissue culture following exposure to the WIN compounds tended to be attenuated when inoculated into mice.[138]

Enviroxime is an antiviral drug that targets nonstructural protein 3A, leading to a block in the synthesis of plus-strand viral RNA. Although this compound inhibits EV and rhinovirus *in vitro* infections, it is toxic and not effective in humans.[98] Resistance to enviroxime is determined by changes in the amino acid at position 30 in protein 3A.[155]

An antiviral strategy promoted recently involves the use of drug-sensitive dominantly inhibitory viruses, generated as a result of a targeted drug treatment, which interfere with growth of drug-resistant viruses.[83] Regions of the virus that can serve as targets for drugs that lead to the generation of these dominant defective viruses include (a) the capsid and polymerase coding region, because of the proteins' oligomeric properties (i.e., there is interference during interactions with the respective wild-type protein); (b) cre and VPg (genome-linked virus protein), perhaps because their malfunction leads to inhibitory intermediates; and (c) 2A, perhaps because the uncleaved intramolecular cleavage of VP1–2A is inhibitory during assembly of the virus capsids. The 2A proteinase seemed to be an especially attractive target because of its inability to be rescued in *trans* and the dominant inhibition of the uncleaved product on virus growth.

The administration of small interfering RNA (siRNA) has also been examined as a possible strategy for control of EV infections. This approach has been used to inhibit *in vitro* infections of PV as well as CVB3.[10,128] The use of a pool of siRNA to target multiple sites throughout the virus genome may be able to limit the emergence of resistant viruses arising from mutations. The possibility of designing an siRNA that is effective against many closely related EV makes this an especially attractive approach for human infections. As with all siRNA approaches, further testing in varied EV infections of animals and then humans is necessary, including the development of an efficient and appropriate delivery system.

Vaccines

Efforts have been initiated to develop a vaccine against EV71, and several approaches have been evaluated in animal models. Mice immunized with a DNA vaccine encoding VP1,[402,430] or with synthetic peptides encoding B-cell epitopes from VP1,[115] mount a neutralizing VP1-specific IgG response; passive transfer of vaccine-induced antibodies to neonatal mice conferred substantial protection against a normally lethal EV71 challenge.[114] A virus-like particle (VLP) vaccine induced a strong and sustained neutralizing IgG response.[73] Finally, transgenic mice have been developed in which VP1 is expressed in the milk of nursing mothers; EV71-specific antibodies were induced in the suckling pups.[73] In both of the latter studies, the antibody responses protected neonatal mice against a normally lethal EV71 challenge.[66,73]

Poliovirus Vaccine and Eradication

The PV field was fortunate to have more than one excellent vaccine, because both the killed intramuscular vaccine of Salk and the oral attenuated vaccine of Sabin were available. Both of these vaccines result in production of anti-PV antibody (Fig. 17.12) with subsequent protection from disease.[300] Although there has been a continuing advocacy for one or the other vaccine over the years, it is clear that each has advantages and disadvantages (Tables 17.9 and 17.10) and that appropriate circumstances exist for the use of each. With the incidence of PV declining dramatically, the United States has switched from OPV to the exclusive use of IPV in 2000 (at 2 months, 4 months, 6 to 18 months, and 4 to 6 years of age). The main benefit for this change was the elimination of vaccine-associated paralytic poliomyelitis (VAPP), and subsequent studies have shown that this was accomplished.[12]

In 1988, in part based on the rapid progress of eradication activities in the Americas, the World Health Assembly unanimously adopted a resolution calling for the global eradication of PV before the end of the 20th century. This resolution was reaffirmed in May of 1999, 2004, and 2011, and an acceleration of activities was urged with particular focus on the

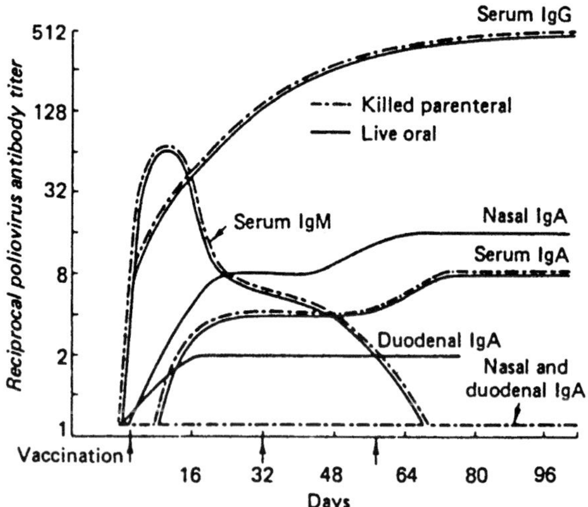

FIGURE 17.12. Serum and secretory antibody responses to oral administration of live attenuated polio vaccine and to intramuscular inoculation of killed poliovirus (PV) vaccine. (From: Ogra PL, Karzon DT. Formation and function of poliovirus antibody on different tissues. *Prog Med Virol.* 1971;13:156–193.)

remaining endemic areas. These accelerated activities include additional rounds of National Immunization Days, intensified surveillance in high-risk communities, and mopping up in focal reservoirs.

A progress report on the global efforts to eradicate PV is provided on a website of the WHO.[427] Four fundamental components compose the strategy to eradicate PV.[185] First is the achievement and maintenance of high levels of routine immunization. With the accelerated activities resulting from the Expanded Program on Immunization of the WHO, routine coverage with three doses of OPV in children younger than 1 year of age reached nearly 90% of the world's children by 1990; however, maintenance of these levels has not been completely successful, and some erosion of routine immunization has occurred. Because of the inability of routine immunization to control PV circulation in many developing countries, the second element of the strategy is the use of National Immunization Days for the delivery of vaccine to all children younger than 5 years of age in a very short period of time, usually from 1 to a few days.[34] The mass immunization interferes with the spread of wild PV through a rapid increase in population

TABLE 17.9 Killed Poliovirus Vaccine: Advantages and Disadvantages

Advantages
- Safe because inactivation ensures no infectious virus exists
- Can be used in immunodeficient and immunosuppressed individuals
- Provides excellent systemic immunity

Disadvantages
- Requires intramuscular injection with repeated doses
- More expensive than live vaccine
- Potential hazards because of the use of wild seed virus in production
- Reduced intestinal immunity compared with natural infection

TABLE 17.10 Live Poliovirus Vaccine: Advantages and Disadvantages

Advantages
- Confers strong systemic and intestinal immunity
- Relatively inexpensive
- Provides herd immunity because the virus is excreted into the environment, expanding immunity
- Oral delivery
- Relatively safe

Disadvantages
- Can mutate to neurovirulent form, causing vaccine-associated paralytic poliomyelitis
- Contraindicated in immunodeficient and immunosuppressed individuals
- Requires monkeys for safety testing
- Can lead to circulating vaccine-derived polioviruses causing outbreaks of poliomyelitis

immunity and abruptly decreases the *chains of transmission* in a country. This strategy was used in many early immunization efforts in the 1960s and was applied successfully in Cuba to achieve and maintain the elimination of PV from that country following 3 successive years of annual campaigns.[350] Multiple rounds in a given year are now routinely carried out for all endemic countries, and the National Immunization Days have grown in an extraordinary way as more countries have adopted this strategy. Some campaigns now represent the largest public health activities on record and often represent the largest multinational health events as well.

The third basic element is the use of surveillance based on cases of acute flaccid paralysis.[35] One of the major differences between the smallpox eradication program and the efforts to eradicate PV is the low rate of clinical disease following PV infection. Because less than 1% of infected susceptible individuals will develop paralytic illness, most infections are not clinically recognized. Therefore, unlike smallpox, where almost all infections were symptomatic, PV is difficult to detect; this is certainly a challenge to eradication efforts. To improve the sensitivity of detecting PV infection and yet achieve a practical system, surveillance was developed around the unique clinical presentation of paralytic poliomyelitis. To avoid the requirement for extensive neurologic examinations, which are not feasible in many developing countries, the surveillance was simplified to include any case of acute flaccid paralysis. This system reports many other diseases in addition to poliomyelitis, such as Guillain-Barré syndrome, transverse myelitis, and traumatic neuropathy. This loss of specificity, however, is compensated for by a gain in sensitivity, because most cases of true poliomyelitis are reported. The incidence of non–PV-induced flaccid paralysis is also used as an indicator of surveillance sensitivity (>2 cases per 100,000 population younger than 15 years of age is considered an operational indicator of adequate quality), although it is not clear if the expected rate is the same in different countries or would be expected to be constant over time. Regardless, acute flaccid paralysis surveillance has proved to be remarkably efficient for detection of wild PV circulation.

The remaining part of surveillance is focused on detection of the virus. Two stool specimens are collected from all cases of acute flaccid paralysis and tested in a global network of laboratories to attempt isolation of PV.[184] The major advantages of this surveillance system are simplicity, practicality, and reasonable sensitivity for detection of PV. The major disadvantages are the requirements to (a) rapidly collect, transport, and test a large number of specimens from all areas of the world and (b) have high-quality laboratory testing. Despite these challenges, the global network of 146 laboratories was able to process more than 200,000 specimens in 2011 and provide this information in a timely manner to the Eradication Program.[59]

The last element of the eradication strategy is the use of *mopping-up* activities.[93] This strategy focuses on an area or country where the previous three parts of the program have successfully reduced the number of PV cases to a small number, and where surveillance has localized the remaining reservoirs of transmission. It is then possible to intensify immunization activities in those targeted communities that contain the remaining circulating virus, or the last *chains of transmission.* These intensified activities usually involve active searches in communities for children, including house-to-house or boat-to-boat immunization.[19] Teams visit all residences in the area and ensure that children are not missed. With further reduction of poliovirus circulation to only parts of a limited number of countries, a further increase in vaccine coverage was achieved by more focused Supplemental Immunization Activities. These immunization campaigns were focused on the remaining reservoirs of polio circulation within the endemic countries and conducted many times nearly year round. As a result of this intensified effort, by the end of 2011, only four countries continued to maintain polio circulation.

These elements of PV eradication strategy have proved successful in large parts of the world. Since the program began, almost all countries are now free of indigenous PV circulation. This can be seen in Figure 17.13, where in 1988 PV was found on all the continents (except Australia), with estimates of more than 350,000 cases of PV each year. In 2011, the number of countries with PV was only 16, and all of the Americas, Europe, and the Far East have been certified to be free of PV.[58] The only countries with endemic PV cases were in south Asia (Pakistan and Afghanistan) and Sub-Saharan Africa (Nigeria).

Numerous unknowns and potential obstacles remain to be faced in the eradication efforts. Because of the inherent insensitivity of detecting PV infection, it is important that surveillance quality be achieved and maintained for a period of time.

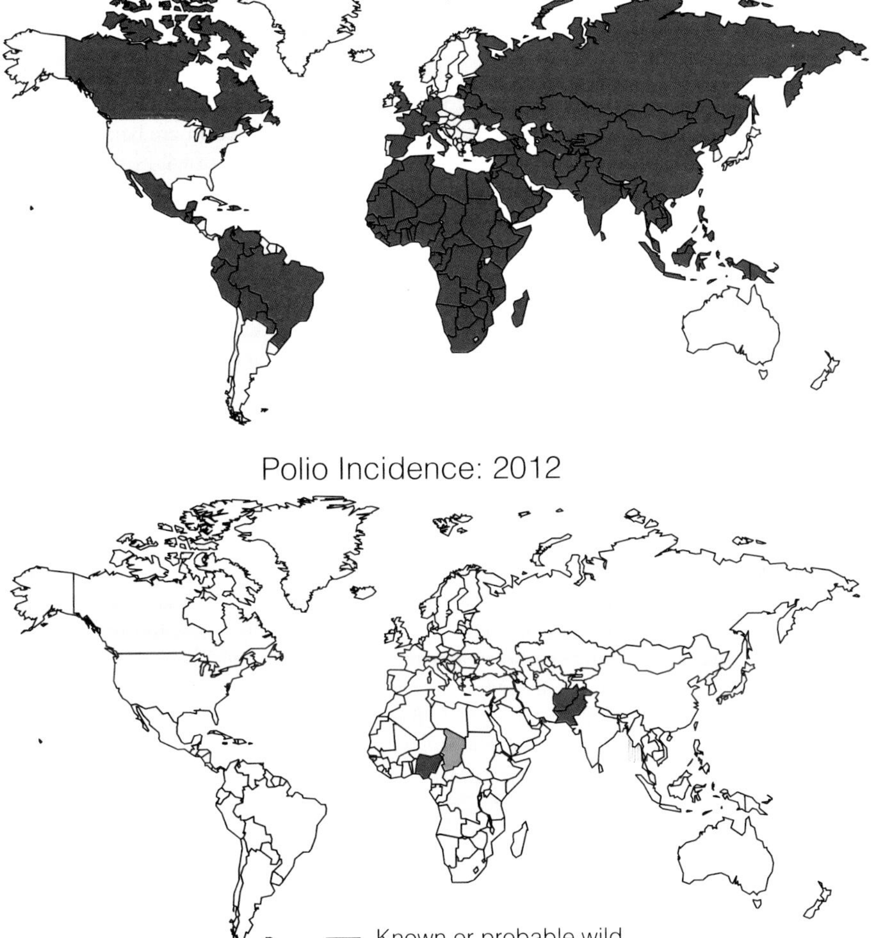

FIGURE 17.13. World map depicting the circulation of wild poliovirus (PV) for 1988 and 2012 as reported to the World Health Organization. In 2012, intermediate shaded country had eliminated indigenous transmission but following importation re-established transmission in the country for a period exceeding 12 months. (Adapted from Centers for Disease Control and Prevention, unpublished data.)

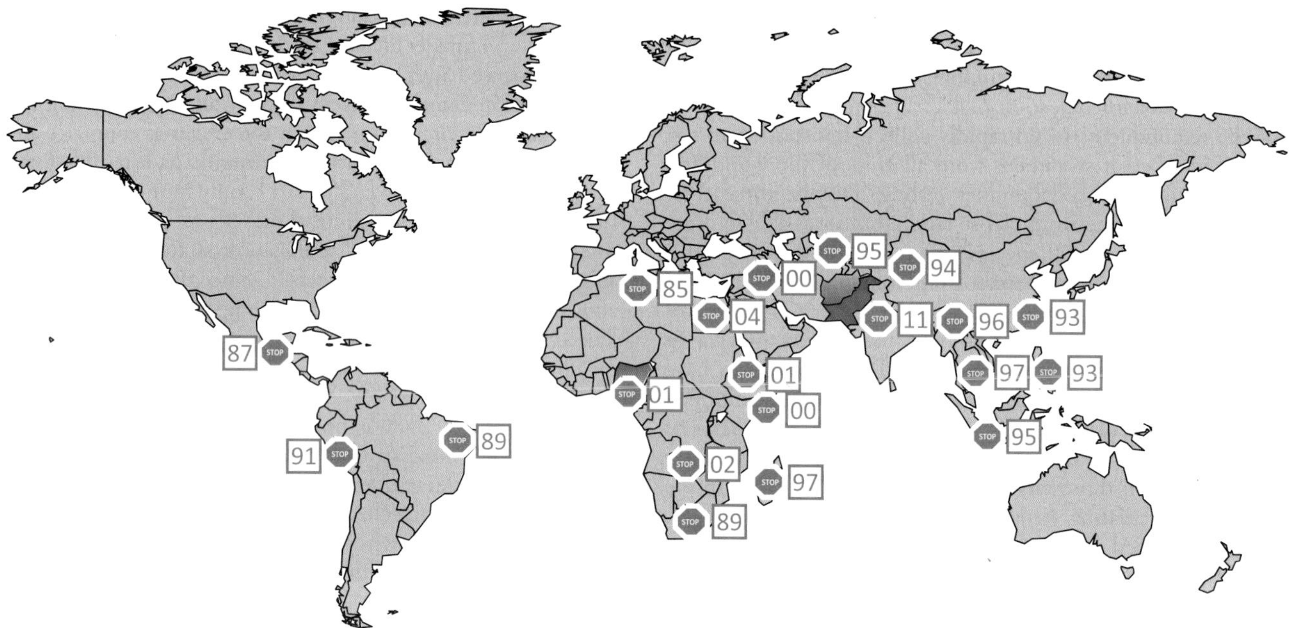

FIGURE 17.14. World map depicting type 1 poliovirus (PV) genotypes in different regions from 1985/2011 and the years in which the eradication occurred. Shaded countries represent remaining endemic circulation for the two remaining type 1 genotypes. Each symbol represents a distinct genotype that has been eradicated and the year when that occurred. (Adapted from Centers for Disease Control and Prevention, unpublished data.)

Although the exact length of time required to be assured of success is not known in all circumstances, the minimal requirement for certification is 3 years. Previous experience indicates that if excellent surveillance is achieved and maintained, PV genotypes that have not been detected for a period of 1 year will not be detected ever again. This has been true for more than three dozen genotypes that have been eliminated from circulation (Fig. 17.14).

After wild virus circulation is interrupted, the accidental release of viruses from laboratories or vaccine-manufacturing facilities will represent a significant risk to the PV-free world. Therefore, it will be necessary to institute proper containment of the virus. A plan for these steps of containment has been drafted and will be implemented in phases as eradication proceeds. In the first pre-eradication phase, preparation for later phases is to be undertaken by conducting an inventory of all institutions and laboratories that have wild PV or potentially infectious materials. This survey for wild PV and potentially infectious materials has been completed in the polio-free regions of the world and has been completed in more than 100 countries, including the United States.[55] Wherever possible, use of vaccine strains of PV in the laboratory should be substituted for wild strains. In the second phase, after the last wild PV has been isolated anywhere in the world, all work with wild PV will be done at a higher biosafety level of containment (BSL-3/polio). Once all countries and regions have been certified as being free of circulating PV, and once all laboratories have properly contained, referred, or destroyed their PV stocks and potentially infectious materials, the Global Certification Commission will declare wild PV eradicated. The last phase of containment will occur sometime in the future when the decision is made to stop vaccination with OPV. At that time, all infectious PV will need to be in containment. The containment requirements for this last phase are being developed. In addition, the special containment needs associated with IPV production are being assessed. Of particular concern are the current use of wild strains and the associated risk of an accidental release of virus during vaccine production. One way to limit this danger that is under consideration and active development is to prepare the IPV from the live Sabin attenuated vaccine strains.[76]

Once eradication of wild PV is achieved, the only disease caused by PV in the world will be as a result of the use of live OPV. In most parts of the world, the disease burden caused by VAPP already exceeds that of wild PV. In addition, the continued use of OPV poses a risk for outbreaks from vaccine-derived polioviruses (VDPVs). VDPVs are derived from OPV but differ from the OPV strains and from the frequent PV isolates seen soon after vaccination with OPV by having more than 1% nucleotide changes in the coding region for VP1. The demarcation of more than 1% is somewhat arbitrary but is consistent with the approximate 1 year of circulation of the virus. More recently, this definition has been modified for PV type 2 to be greater than 0.6% difference from the parent vaccine strain. Most OPV-like isolates and most PV excreted from patients with VAPP have less than 1% nucleotide change in the VP1 coding region and, therefore, are not classified as VDPVs because the duration of infection is short and because random mutations do not accumulate as observed with VDPVs. VDPVs fall into three groups: (a) circulating VDPVs (cVDPVs), (b) VDPVs isolated from individuals with immune deficiencies (iVDPVs), and (c) ambiguous VDVPs (aVDPVs) in which the source of infection is unknown.

Although recognized as a potential problem associated with OPV for more than 40 years, the occurrence of multiple episodes involving cVDPVs within the last 12 years has explicitly demonstrated this risk. The first documented cVDPV outbreak of poliomyelitis occurred on the island of Hispaniola in 2000–2001, with 21 virologically confirmed cases in Haiti and the Dominican Republic, and with many more apparent cases from which no specimens were collected.[218,220] Since this outbreak in Hispaniola, cVDPV outbreaks have occurred in numerous countries, including the large multiyear outbreak of type 2 cVDPV in Nigeria (http://www.polioeradication.org/Dataandmonitoring/Poliothisweek/Circulatingvaccine-derivedpoliovirus.aspx). In addition, cVDPVs have been recognized retrospectively in other countries, particularly Egypt, where the type 2 cVDPV was endemic for possibly 10 years.[436] cVDPVs circulate in regions that have inadequate vaccine coverage along with an absence of natural infection from circulating wild PV of the same serotype. The strains are of particular concern because they have caused paralytic disease and have a capacity for sustained person-to-person spread similar to wild-type PV.[106a] The presence of cVDPVs underscores the importance of maintaining excellent surveillance, the need to maintain high vaccine coverage, and the continued risk from suboptimal use of OPV, even in polio-free areas of the world.

Although not as great a concern as cVDPVs, an issue that complicates PV eradication is the demonstrated excretion of iVDPVs, at times for periods of more than a decade. The occurrence of iVDPVs is rare, however, even in immunosuppressed patients. Although both iVDPVs and cVDPVs can occur in the absence of any recombination, recombination has only been observed in the case of iVDPVs with other vaccine PV strains and not with other members of EV-C. This is presumably because of the absence of EV-C co-infections in the tissue supporting the chronic PV infection, in contrast to the frequent recombination observed between vaccine strains that occurs in normal vaccinees. Interestingly, prolonged excretion with PV occurs with viruses derived from OPV, and not with wild PV,[222] perhaps because the greater neurovirulence of wild PV would be expected to lead to a uniformly fatal outcome in immunosuppressed individuals or because individuals with severe immune deficiencies are likely to live in PV-free countries and, therefore, are only exposed to vaccine strains. Currently no evidence indicates that patients with cell-mediated deficiencies are at increased risk for chronic PV infections. Prolonged excretion of PV has not been observed in studies undertaken specifically to look at HIV-infected children and adults.[147,157]

Included in the VDPV group are ambiguous VDPVs (aVDPVs), in which the source of infection is unknown (e.g., VDPV isolates from environmental sources), no known immunodeficiency is found in the patient, or the isolate is not associated with a PV outbreak. For example, in more than 10,000 vaccine-related isolates studied in WHO Network laboratories in 2011, there were 67 cVDPVs (from 6 recent outbreaks).[60,427]

Because of the risks evident from VAPP and VDPVs, the WHO has concluded that continued use of OPV following wild PV eradication is incompatible with the ultimate goal of polio eradication. Therefore, sometime after the eradication of wild PV, all use of OPV for routine immunization will stop. This has significant implications for immunization policy decisions and raises two very important basic questions regarding the management of risks: What vaccination policies will be recommended for PV? How will future PV outbreaks or cases be controlled after OPV use has stopped? With regard to the first question, one option that countries could elect would be to completely stop vaccination for PV. In the absence of wild PV and competing health priorities, this option may be very attractive to many countries, particularly those with limited access to resources. In contrast, concerns about the potential use of PV as a bioterrorism agent means that some countries will continue to vaccinate indefinitely with IPV, as they are doing now. For some countries, particularly middle-income countries, however, the decision about which option to choose may not be simple.

Ideally, it should be possible to describe accurately all of the advantages and disadvantages of choices related to future vaccination policy. It is difficult, however, to estimate and quantitate risks for all populations associated with the cessation of OPV use because of inadequate knowledge about reversion of vaccine strains and viral genetic determinants for neurovirulence and transmissibility. It is also not clear what protective benefits are possible in the absence of high levels of routine IPV use. An attempt to use elements of decision analysis and disease modeling has been made to try to provide better information regarding risk assessments.[103,393]

Regardless of decisions made about immunization policies, future generations will have an increasing susceptibility to PV as immunization becomes the only source of immunity. For this reason, another key component of activities related to posteradication risk management is the establishment of a global stockpile of vaccine to respond to any outbreak in the future. In most developed countries in temperate climates, IPV has proved very effective in preventing outbreaks in the general population and may remain the vaccine of choice for small outbreaks in the countries. Much remains unknown about the potential for IPV to control PV circulation in developing countries because IPV induces a lower level of mucosal immunity than OPV.[124] Because OPV is the only vaccine that has ever been demonstrated to stop circulation of PV in developing countries, it will likely remain the vaccine of choice for the global stockpile. If an outbreak does occur, it is reasonable to expect that it will be caused by a single serotype in a specific place or time, prompting the maintenance of monovalent OPV strains in the stockpile. Monovalent OPV strains of all three types are already licensed, and types 1 and 3 are being used for the last stages of polio eradication.[76] The use of monovalent OPV strains will eliminate the need to introduce undesirable additional strains into the population. Details remain, however, about the response plans and the use of the stockpile that need to be completed. In addition, issues remain about what should be done at the boundaries of the response population. It may be that the process of eliminating OPV may be as complicated and difficult as the process of eradicating the wild virus.

When the eradication program began, it was assumed that the vaccines available at the time were sufficient for the successful achievement of the goal. With the growing knowledge of the risks associated with OPV and the possible difficulties associated with either continuing or stopping its use in the future, hindsight indicates that the availability of additional options would be highly desirable. In the intervening years many new approaches to vaccinology have been developed, raising the possibility of developing new PV vaccines (e.g., genetically engineered PV, noninfectious DNA, or immunogenic peptides). Although some or all of these vaccines might allow protection with greater safety than the present vaccines, no easy way exists to assess the effectiveness of an untested vaccine against poliomyelitis, given the licensing requirements and demonstration of efficacy. The testing would be expensive and extensive, and passing the test may not ensure universal acceptance of a new intervention. Despite the significant difficulties involving testing these new interventions, it seems appropriate to continue active investigations in this area.[159]

The world has endured the crippling effects of PV for millennia, yet the end of these particular viruses is approaching. It is possible that the next edition of this chapter will treat PV quite differently, possibly even as a historic footnote rather than a major focus of public health activities.

PERSPECTIVES

For 25 to 50 years before the identification of acquired immunodeficiency syndrome, much of human virology was focused on PV. With the eradication of poliomyelitis imminent, the picornavirology field is changing and will never be the same again. It is somewhat ironic to realize that, despite the incredible advances in our understanding of the molecular aspects of PV and the availability of extraordinarily powerful molecular tools for studying PV, the eradication of poliomyelitis will become a reality as a result of the use of the Salk and Sabin vaccines, vaccines that were generated empirically in the middle of the last century before the breakthroughs in our understanding of the molecular biology of PV.

But perhaps it is unfair to belittle the achievements of modern techniques in the eradication of PV. Certainly, the tools of molecular biology were and will continue to be important in monitoring and tracking PV and identifying strains; it also may be that new technology and knowledge will make a better PV vaccine. Novel diagnostic methods developed to assist in surveillance of poliomyelitis are likely to aid in the identification of new enteroviruses, provide better and more accurate descriptions of the epidemiology of EV infections, and lead to new anti-EV drugs, nonpolio EV vaccines, and a better understanding of the relationship of EV to acute and chronic human disease.

What new directions will drive the field of picornavirology? Pressure exists to develop new antiviral treatments and vaccines. New antiviral approaches will take advantage of knowledge of virus receptors, structures of capsid and nonstructural proteins, and immunologic features of the disease. New vaccines will be pursued and developed. The ability of EV71 to mount large epidemics and to be a major cause of neurologic disease, especially acute flaccid paralysis, is likely to have already generated special interest with respect to vaccine development. The many diseases that the coxsackieviruses cause also makes this group of viruses of great interest from the point of view of vaccine development. In addition, investigations of coxsackieviral diseases may clarify the pathogenesis of virus-induced autoimmune diseases.

Despite the development of new treatments and vaccines, enteroviruses will still be very much with us, even after the eradication of PV.

ACKNOWLEDGMENTS

We thank Drs. Olen Kew, Tapani Hovi, and Konstantin Chumakov for providing unpublished data.

REFERENCES

All cited references are available in the e-book.

1. Abad FX, Pinto RM, Bosch A. Disinfection of human enteric viruses on fomites. *FEMS Microbiol Lett* 1997;156(1):107–111.
2. Abad FX, Pinto RM, Bosch A. Survival of enteric viruses on environmental fomites. *Appl Environ Microbiol* 1994;60(10):3704–3710.
3. Abed Y, Wolf D, Dagan R, et al. Development of a serological assay based on a synthetic peptide selected from the VP0 capsid protein for detection of human parechoviruses. *J Clin Microbiol* 2007;45(6):2037–2039.
4. Abzug M. Perinatal enterovirus infections. In: Rotbart HA, ed. *Human enterovirus infections.* Washington, DC: ASM Press, 1995:221–238.
5. Abzug MJ, Beam AC, Gyorkos EA, Levin MJ. Viral pneumonia in the first month of life. *Pediatr Infect Dis J.* 1990;9(12):881–885.
6. Abzug MJ, Cloud G, Bradley J, et al. Double blind placebo-controlled trial of pleconaril in infants with enterovirus meningitis. *Pediatr Infect Dis J.* Apr 2003;22(4):335–341.
7. Abzug MJ, Keyserling HL, Lee ML, Levin MJ, Rotbart HA. Neonatal enterovirus infection: virology, serology, and effects of intravenous immune globulin. *Clin Infect Dis.* 1995;20(5):1201–1206.
8. Ackermann WW, Fujioka RS, Kurtz HB. Cationic modulation of the inactivation of poliovirus by heat. *Arch Environ Health.* 1970;21(3): 377–381.
9. Afif H, Sutter RW, Kew OM, et al. Outbreak of poliomyelitis in Gizan, Saudi Arabia: cocirculation of wild type 1 polioviruses from three separate origins. *J Infect Dis.* 1997;175(Suppl 1):S71–S75.
10. Ahn J, Jun ES, Lee HS, et al. A small interfering RNA targeting coxsackievirus B3 protects permissive HeLa cells from viral challenge. *J Virol.* Jul 2005;79(13):8620–8624.
11. Alexander JP Jr, Chapman LE, Pallansch MA, Stephenson WT, Torok TJ, Anderson LJ. Coxsackievirus B2 infection and aseptic meningitis: a focal outbreak among members of a high school football team. *J Infect Dis.* 1993;167(5):1201–1205.
12. Alexander LN, Seward JF, Santibanez TA, et al. Vaccine policy changes and epidemiology of poliomyelitis in the United States. *JAMA.* 2004; 292(14):1696–1701.
13. Alexopoulou L, Holt AC, Medzhitov R, Flavell RA. Recognition of double-stranded RNA and activation of NF-k B by Toll-like receptor 3. *Nature.* 2001;413(6857):732–738.
14. Anderson DR, Wilson JE, Carthy CM, Yang D, Kandolf R, McManus BM. Direct interactions of coxsackievirus B3 with immune cells in the splenic compartment of mice susceptible or resistant to myocarditis. *J Virol.* 1996;70:4632–4645.
15. Andreoletti L, Bourlet T, Moukassa D, et al. Enteroviruses can persist with or without active viral replication in cardiac tissue of patients with end-stage ischemic or dilated cardiomyopathy. *J Infect Dis.* 2000;182(4): 1222–1227.
16. Andreoletti L, Leveque N, Boulagnon C, Brasselet C, Fornes P. Viral causes of human myocarditis. *Arch Cardiovasc Dis* 2009;102(6–7):559–568.
17. Anonymous. Deaths among children during an outbreak of hand, foot, and mouth disease–Taiwan, Republic of China, April-July 1998. *MMWR Morbid Mortal Wkly Rep* 1998;47(30):629–632.
18. Anonymous. *Enterovirus Surveillance Report, 1970–1979.* Atlanta: Centers for Disease Control, 1981.
19. Anonymous. From the Centers for Disease Control and Prevention. Final stages of poliomyelitis eradication–Western Pacific Region, 1997–1998. *JAMA.* 1999;281(18):1690–1691.
20. Archard LC, Khan MA, Soteriou BA, et al. Characterization of Coxsackie B virus RNA in myocardium from patients with dilated cardiomyopathy by nucleotide sequencing of reverse transcription-nested polymerase chain reaction products. *Hum Pathol.* 1998;29(6):578–584.
21. Archard LC, Richardson PJ, Olsen EG, Dubowitz V, Sewry C, Bowles NE. The role of Coxsackie B viruses in the pathogenesis of myocarditis, dilated cardiomyopathy and inflammatory muscle disease. *Biochem Soc Symp.* 1987;53:51–62.
22. Arnesjo B, Eden T, Ihse I, Nordenfelt E, Ursing B. Enterovirus infections in acute pancreatitis. *Scand J Gastroenterol* 1976;11(7):645–649.
23. Arola A, Kalimo H, Ruuskanen O, Hyypia T. Experimental myocarditis induced by two different coxsackievirus B3 variants: aspects of pathogenesis and comparison of diagnostic methods. *J Med Virol.* 1995;47:251–259.

24. Asturias EJ, Grazioso CF, Luna-Fineman S, Torres O, Halsey NA. Poliovirus excretion in Guatemalan adults and children with HIV infection and children with cancer. *Biologicals.* Jun 2006;34(2):109–112.
25. Aycock WL. The significance of the age distribution of poliomyelitis: evidence of transmission through contact. *Am J Hyg.* 1928;8:35–54.
26. Baboonian C, Davies MJ, Booth JC, McKenna WJ. Coxsackie B viruses and human heart disease. *Curr Top Microbiol Immunol.* 1997;223:31–52.
27. Baboonian C, Treasure T. Meta-analysis of the association of enteroviruses with human heart disease. *Heart.* 1997;78(6):539–543.
28. Barral PM, Morrison JM, Drahos J, et al. MDA-5 is cleaved in poliovirus-infected cells. *J Virol.* 2007;81(8):3677–3684.
29. Bell EJ, McCartney RA. A study of Coxsackie B virus infections, 1972–1983. *J Hyg.* 1984;93(2):197–203.
30. Bell EJ, McCartney RA, Basquill D, Chaudhuri AK. Mu-antibody capture ELISA for the rapid diagnosis of enterovirus infections in patients with aseptic meningitis. *J Med Virol.* 1986;19(3):213–217.
31. Bendig JWA, O'Brien PS, Muir P, Porter HJ, Caul EO. Enterovirus sequences resembling coxsackievirus A2 detected in stool and spleen from a girl with fatal myocarditis. *J.Med.Virol.* 2001;64:482–486.
32. Benschop KSM, Schinkel J, Minnaar RP, et al. Human parechovirus infections in Dutch children and the association between serotype and disease severity. *Clin Infect Dis.* 2006;42:204–210.
33. Berlin BS, Simon NM, Bovner RN. Myoglobinuria precipitated by viral infection. *JAMA.* 1974;227(12):1414–1415.
34. Birmingham ME, Aylward RB, Cochi SL, Hull HF. National immunization days: state of the art. *J Infect Dis.* 1997;175(Suppl 1):S183–188.
35. Birmingham ME, Linkins RW, Hull BP, Hull HF. Poliomyelitis surveillance: the compass for eradication. *J Infect Dis.* 1997;175(Suppl 1): S146–S150.
36. Bodian D. Emerging concept of poliomyelitis infection. *Science.* 1955; 122(3159):105–108.
37. Bodian D. Histopathologic basis of clinical findings in poliomyelitis. *Am J Med.* May 1949;6(5):563–578.
38. Bodian D. Viremia in experimental poliomyelitis. II. Viremia and the mechanism of the provoking effect of injections or trauma. *Am J Hyg.* 1954;60(3):358–370.
39. Bodian D, Morgan IM, Howe HA. Differentiation of types of poliomyelitis viruses. III. The grouping of fourteen strains into three basic immunological types. *Am J Hyg.* 1949;49:234–245.
40. Boettler T, von HM. Protection against or triggering of Type 1 diabetes? Different roles for viral infections. *Expert Rev Clin Immunol.* 2011; 7(1):45–53.
41. Boivin G, Abed Y, Boucher FD. Human parechovirus 3 and neonatal infections. *Emerg Infect Dis.* Jan 2005;11(1):103–105.
42. Boman J, Nilsson B, Juto P. Serum IgA, IgG, and IgM responses to different enteroviruses as measured by a coxsackie B5-based indirect ELISA. *J Med Virol.* 1992;38(1):32–35.
43. Bothig B, Danes L, Dittmann S. Immunogenicity of oral poliomyelitis vaccine (OPV) against variants of wild poliovirus type 3. *Bull World Health Organ* 1990;68(5):597–600.
44. Bowles NE, Dubowitz V, Sewry CA, Archard LC. Dermatomyositis, polymyositis, and Coxsackie-B-virus infection. *Lancet.* 1987;1(8540): 1004–1007.
45. Bowles NE, Richardson PJ, Olsen EG, Archard LC. Detection of Coxsackie-B-virus-specific RNA sequences in myocardial biopsy samples from patients with myocarditis and dilated cardiomyopathy. *Lancet.* 1986;1:1120–1123.
46. Brown B, Oberste MS, Maher K, Pallansch MA. Complete genomic sequencing shows that polioviruses and members of human enterovirus species C are closely related in the noncapsid coding region. *J Virol.* Aug 2003;77(16):8973–8984.
47. Brown BA, Oberste MS, Alexander JP Jr, Kennett ML, Pallansch MA. Molecular epidemiology and evolution of enterovirus 71 strains isolated from 1970 to 1998. *J Virol.* 1999;73(12):9969–9975.
48. Buisman AM, Abbink F, Schepp RM, Sonsma JA, Herremans T, Kimman TG. Preexisting poliovirus-specific IgA in the circulation correlates with protection against virus excretion in the elderly. *J. Infect. Dis.* 2008;197(5):698–706.
49. Burnet FM. Poliomyelitis in the light of recent experimental work. *Health Bull* 1945;(81–82):2173–2177.
50. Byington CL, Taggart EW, Carroll KC, Hillyard DR. A polymerase chain reaction-based epidemiologic investigation of the incidence of nonpolio enteroviral infections in febrile and afebrile infants 90 days and younger. *Pediatrics.* 1999;103(3):E27.
51. Caggana M, Chan P, Ramsingh A. Identification of a single amino acid residue in the capsid protein VP1 of coxsackievirus B4 that determines the virulent phenotype. *J Virol.* 1993;67(8):4797–4803.
52. Carson SD, Chapman NM, Hafenstein S, et al. Variation of coxsackievirus B3 capsid primary structure, ligands, and stability are selected in a coxsackievirus and adenovirus receptor-limited environment. *J Virol* 2011; 85:3306–3314.
53. Carson SD, Kim KS, Pirruccello SJ, Tracy S, Chapman NM. Endogenous low-level expression of the coxsackievirus and adenovirus receptor enables coxsackievirus B3 infection of RD cells. *Journal of General Virology.* 2007;88(Pt 11):3031–3038.
54. Cashman NR, Maselli R, Wollmann RL, Roos R, Simon R, Antel JP. Late denervation in patients with antecedent paralytic poliomyelitis. *New England Journal of Medicine.* 1987;317(1):7–12.
55. Centers for Disease Control and Prevention. National laboratory inventory for global poliovirus containment—United States, November 2003. *MMWR - Morbidity & Mortality Weekly Report.* 2004;53(21): 457–459.
56. Centers for Disease Control and Prevention. Notes from the field: poliomyelitis outbreak—Republic of the Congo, September 2010–February 2011. *MMWR Morb Mortal Wkly Rep.* 2011;60(10):312–313.
57. Centers for Disease Control and Prevention. Outbreak of polio in adults–Namibia, 2006. *MMWR Morb Mortal Wkly Rep.* Nov 10 2006; 55(44):1198–1201.
58. Centers for Disease Control and Prevention. Progress toward interruption of wild poliovirus transmission - worldwide, January 2011-March 2012. *Morbidity & Mortality Weekly Report.* 2012;61(19):353–357.
59. Centers for Disease Control and Prevention. Tracking progress toward global polio eradication, 2010–2011. *Morbidity & Mortality Weekly Report.* 2012;61:265–269.
60. Centers for Disease Control and Prevention. Update on vaccine-derived polioviruses–worldwide, July 2009-March 2011. *Morbidity & Mortality Weekly Report.* 2011;60(25):846–850.
61. Cetta F, Michels VV. The autoimmune basis of dilated cardiomyopathy. *Ann Med.* Apr 1995;27(2):169–173.
62. Chambon M, Bailly JL, Peigue-Lafeuille H. Comparative sensitivity of the echovirus type 25 JV-4 prototype strain and two recent isolates to glutaraldehyde at low concentrations. *Appl Environ Microbiol.* 1994; 60(2):387–392.
63. Chapman NM, Kim KS, Drescher KM, Oka K, Tracy S. 5′ terminal deletions in the genome of a coxsackievirus B2 strain occurred naturally in human heart. *Virology.* 2008;375(2):480–491.
64. Chapman NM, Romero JR, Pallansch MA, Tracy S. Sites other than nucleotide 234 determine cardiovirulence in natural isolates of coxsackievirus B3. *J.Med.Virol.* 1997;52(3):258–261.
65. Charcot JM, Joffroy A. Cas de paralysie infantile spinale avec lesins des cornes anterieures de la substance grise de la moelle epiniere. *Arch Physiol Norm Pathol.* 1870;3:134–152.
66. Chen HL, Huang JY, Chu TW, et al. Expression of VP1 protein in the milk of transgenic mice: a potential oral vaccine protects against enterovirus 71 infection. *Vaccine.* 2008;26(23):2882–2889.
67. Chen SX, Mei SW, Bao SH, et al. Immunological status and pathology of coxsackie B viral myocarditis and dilated cardiomyopathy. *Chin Med J (Engl).* 1993;106:659–664.
68. Chiou CC, Liu WT, Chen SJ, et al. Coxsackievirus B1 infection in infants less than 2 months of age. *American Journal of Perinatology.* 1998;15(3): 155–159.
69. Chonmaitree T, Ford C, Sanders C, Lucia HL. Comparison of cell cultures for rapid isolation of enteroviruses. *J Clin Microbiol.* 1988;26(12): 2576–2580.
70. Chonmaitree T, Mann L. Respiratory infections. In: Rotbart HA, ed. *Human enterovirus infections.* Washington, DC: ASM Press; 1995: 255–270.
71. Chow LH, Beisel KW, McManus BM. Enteroviral infection of mice with severe combined immunodeficiency. Evidence for direct viral pathogenesis of myocardial injury. *Laboratory Investigation.* 1992;66(1):24–31.

72. Chumakov M, Voroshilova M, Shindarov L, et al. Enterovirus 71 isolated from cases of epidemic poliomyelitis-like disease in Bulgaria. *Arch Virol.* 1979;60(3–4):329–340.
73. Chung YC, Ho MS, Wu JC, et al. Immunization with virus-like particles of enterovirus 71 elicits potent immune responses and protects mice against lethal challenge. *Vaccine.* 2008;26(15):1855–1862.
74. Clark CS, Bjornson AB, Schiff GM, Phair JP, Van Meer GL, Gartside PS. Sewage worker's syndrome [letter]. *Lancet.* 1977;1(8019):1009.
75. Clements GB, Galbraith DN, Taylor KW. Coxsackie B virus infection and onset of childhood diabetes. *Lancet.* 1995;346(8969):221–223.
76. Cochi SL, Sutter RW, Aylward RB. Possible global strategies for stopping polio vaccination and how they could be harmonized. *Dev Biol (Basel).* 2001;105:153–158; discussion 159.
77. Codd MB, Sugrue DD, Gersh BJ, Melton LJ, 3rd. Epidemiology of idiopathic dilated and hypertrophic cardiomyopathy. A population-based study in Olmsted County, Minnesota, 1975–1984. *Circulation.* Sep 1989; 80(3):564–572.
78. Colbere-Garapin F, Duncan G, Pavio N, Pelletier I, Petit I. An approach to understanding the mechanisms of poliovirus persistence in infected cells of neural or non-neural origin. *Clin Diagn Virol.* 1998;9(2–3): 107–113.
79. Conyn-Van Spaendonck MA, de Melker HE, Abbink F, Elzinga-Gholizadea N, Kimman TG, van Loon T. Immunity to poliomyelitis in the Netherlands. *American Journal of Epidemiology.* Feb 1 2001;153(3):207–214.
80. Cooney MK, Hall CE, Fox JP. The Seattle virus watch. 3. Evaluation of isolation methods and summary of infections detected by virus isolations. *American Journal of Epidemiology.* 1972;96(4):286–305.
81. Crainic R, Couillin P, Blondel B, Cabau N, Boue A, Horodniceanu F. Natural variation of poliovirus neutralization epitopes. *Infection & Immunity.* 1983;41(3):1217–1225.
82. Crotty S, Hix L, Sigal LJ, Andino R. Poliovirus pathogenesis in a new poliovirus receptor transgenic mouse model: age-dependent paralysis and a mucosal route of infection. *Journal of General Virology.* 2002;83(Pt 7):1707–1720.
83. Crowder S, Kirkegaard K. Trans-dominant inhibition of RNA viral replication can slow growth of drug-resistant viruses. *Nat Genet.* Jul 2005; 37(7):701–709.
84. D'Alessio DJ. A case-control study of group B Coxsackievirus immunoglobulin M antibody prevalence and HLA-DR antigens in newly diagnosed cases of insulin-dependent diabetes mellitus. *American Journal of Epidemiology.* 1992;135(12):1331–1338.
85. Dagan R, Hall CB, Powell KR, Menegus MA. Epidemiology and laboratory diagnosis of infection with viral and bacterial pathogens in infants hospitalized for suspected sepsis. *J Pediatr.* 1989;115(3):351–356.
86. Dagan R, Menegus M. Nonpolio enteroviruses and the febrile infant. In: Rotbart HA, ed. *Human enterovirus infections.* Washington, DC: ASM Press; 1995:239–254.
87. Dalakas MC. Enteroviruses and human neuromuscular diseases. In: Rotbart HA, ed. *Human enterovirus infections.* Washington, DC: ASM Press; 1995:387–398.
88. Dales S, Eggers HJ, Tamm I, Palade GE. Electron microscopic study of the formation of poliovirus. *Virology.* 1965;26:379–389.
89. Dalldorf G, Sickles GM. An unidentified, filtrible agent isolated from the feces of children with paralysis. *Science.* 1948;108:61–62.
90. Day C, Cumming H, Walker J. Enterovirus-specific IgM in the diagnosis of meningitis. *Journal of Infection.* 1989;19(3):219–228.
91. de Jong AS, de Mattia F, van Dommelen MM, et al. Functional analysis of picornavirus 2B proteins: effects on calcium homeostasis and intracellular protein trafficking. *Journal of Virology.* 2008;82(7):3782–3790.
92. de Leeuw N, Melchers WJ, Balk AH, de Jonge N, Galama JM. No evidence for persistent enterovirus infection in patients with end-stage idiopathic dilated cardiomyopathy. *J Infect Dis.* 1998;178(1): 256–259.
93. de Quadros CA, Andrus JK, Olive JM, Carrasco P. Strategies for poliomyelitis eradication in developing countries. *Public Health Reviews.* 1993; 21(1–2):65–81.
94. Dechkum N, Pangsawan Y, Jayavasu C, Saguanwongse S. Coxsackie B virus infection and myopericarditis in Thailand, 1987–1989. *Southeast Asian Journal of Tropical Medicine & Public Health.* 1998;29(2): 273–276.
95. Deibel R, Gross LL, Collins DN. Isolation of a new enterovirus (38506). *Proceedings of the Society for Experimental Biology & Medicine.* 1975;148(1):203–207.
96. Dery P, Marks MI, Shapera R. Clinical manifestations of coxsackievirus infections in children. *American Journal of Diseases of Children.* 1974; 128(4):464–468.
97. Destombes J, Couderc T, Thiesson D, Girard S, Wilt SG, Blondel B. Persistent poliovirus infection in mouse motoneurons. *J Virol.* Feb 1997;71(2):1621–1628.
98. Diana GD, Pevear DC. Antipicornavirus drugs: current status. *Antiviral Chemistry & Chemotherapy.* 1997;8:401–408.
99. Dorval BL, Chow M, Klibanov AM. Stabilization of poliovirus against heat inactivation. *Biochemical & Biophysical Research Communications.* 1989;159(3):1177–1183.
100. Douglas JD, Soike KF, Raynor J. The incidence of poliovirus in chimpanzees (Pan troglodytes). *Laboratory Animal Care.* 1970;20(2):265–268.
101. Dowdle WR, Birmingham ME. The biologic principles of poliovirus eradication. *J Infect Dis.* 1997;175(Suppl 1):S286-S292.
102. Drebot MA, Campbell JJ, Lee SH. A genotypic characterization of enteroviral antigenic variants isolated in eastern Canada. *Virus Res.* 1999;59(2):131–140.
103. Duintjer Tebbens RJ, Pallansch MA, Kew OM, et al. Uncertainty and sensitivity analyses of a decision analytic model for posteradication polio risk management. *Risk Analysis.* 2008;28:855–876.
104. Dunn JJ, Bradrick SS, Chapman NM, Tracy SM, Romero JR. The stem loop II within the 5′ nontranslated region of clinical coxsackievirus B3 genomes determines cardiovirulence phenotype in a murine model. *J. Infect. Dis.* 2003;187(10):1552–1561.
105. Enders JF, Weller TH, Robbins FC. Cultivation of the Lansing strain of poliomyelitis virus in cultures of various human embryonic tissues. *Science.* 1949;109:85–87.
106. Esfandiarei M, McManus BM. Molecular biology and pathogenesis of viral myocarditis. *Annu Rev Pathol.* 2008;3:127–155.
106a. Estívariz CF, Watkins MA, Handoko D, et al. A large vaccine-derived poliovirus outbreak on Madura Island–Indonesia, 2005. *J Infect Dis.* 2008; 197(3):347–354.
107. Estrin M, Smith C, Huber SA. Coxsackievirus B-3 myocarditis. T-cell autoimmunity to heart antigens is resistant to cyclosporin-A treatment. *American Journal of Pathology.* 1986;125:244–251.
108. Evans DM, Dunn G, Minor PD, et al. Increased neurovirulence associated with a single nucleotide change in a noncoding region of the Sabin type 3 poliovaccine genome. *Nature.* 1985;314:548–550.
109. Fairweather D, Yusung S, Frisancho S, et al. IL-12 receptor á1 and Toll-like receptor 4 increase IL-1á- and IL-18-associated myocarditis and coxsackievirus replication. *Journal of Immunology.* 2003;170(9):4731–4737.
110. Feachem R, Garelick H, Slade J. Enteroviruses in the environment. *Tropical Diseases Bulletin.* 1981;78(3):185–230.
111. Feuer R, Mena I, Pagarigan RR, Harkins S, Hassett DE, Whitton JL. Coxsackievirus B3 and the neonatal CNS: the roles of stem cells, developing neurons, and apoptosis in infection, viral dissemination, and disease. *Am J Pathol.* Oct 2003;163(4):1379–1393.
112. Feuer R, Mena I, Pagarigan RR, Hassett DE, Whitton JL. Coxsackievirus replication and the cell cycle: a potential regulatory mechanism for viral persistence / latency. *Medical Microbiology and Immunology (Berlin).* 2004;193(2/3):83–90.
113. Feuer R, Mena I, Pagarigan RR, Slifka MK, Whitton JL. Cell cycle status affects coxsackievirus replication, persistence, and reactivation in vitro *Journal of Virology.* 2002;76(9):4430–4440.
114. Foo DG, Alonso S, Chow VT, Poh CL. Passive protection against lethal enterovirus 71 infection in newborn mice by neutralizing antibodies elicited by a synthetic peptide. *Microbes Infect.* Sep 2007;9(11):1299–1306.
115. Foo DG, Alonso S, Phoon MC, Ramachandran NP, Chow VT, Poh CL. Identification of neutralizing linear epitopes from the VP1 capsid protein of Enterovirus 71 using synthetic peptides. *Virus Res.* Apr 2007;125(1):61–68.
116. Foo DG, MacAry PA, Alonso S, Poh CL. Identification of human CD4 T-cell epitopes on the VP1 capsid protein of enterovirus 71. *Viral Immunology.* 2008;21(2):215–224.
117. Freistadt MS, Kaplan G, Racaniello VR. Heterogeneous expression of poliovirus receptor-related proteins in human cells and tissues. *Mol. Cell Biol.* 1990;10(11):5700–5706.

118. Frisancho-Kiss S, Davis SE, Nyland JF, et al. Cutting edge: cross-regulation by TLR4 and T cell Ig mucin-3 determines sex differences in inflammatory heart disease. *Journal of Immunology.* 2007;178(11): 6710–6714.
119. Frisk G, Lindberg MA, Diderholm H. Persistence of coxsackievirus B4 infection in rhabdomyosarcoma cells for 30 months. Brief report. *Archives of Virology.* 1999;144(11):2239–2245.
120. Frisk G, Nilsson E, Ehrnst A, Diderholm H. Enterovirus IgM detection: specificity of mu-antibody-capture radioimmunoassays using virions and procapsids of Coxsackie B virus. *J Virol Meth.* 1989;24(1–2): 191–202.
121. Gauntt CJ, Arizpe HM, Higdon AL, et al. Molecular mimicry, anti-coxsackievirus B3 neutralizing monoclonal antibodies, and myocarditis. *Journal of Immunology.* 1995;154:2983–2995.
122. Gauntt CJ, Higdon AL, Arizpe HM, et al. Epitopes shared between coxsackievirus B3 (CVB3) and normal heart tissue contribute to CVB3-induced murine myocarditis. *Clin Immunol Immunopathol.* 1993;68: 129–134.
123. Gelfand HM, Holguin AH, Marchetti GE, Feorino PM. A continuing surveillance of enterovirus infections in healthy children in six United States cities. I. Viruses isolated during 1960 and 1961. *Am J Hyg.* Nov 1963;78:358–375.
124. Ghendon Y, Robertson SE. Interrupting the transmission of wild polioviruses with vaccines: immunological considerations. *Bulletin of the World Health Organization.* 1994;72(6):973–983.
125. Girard S, Couderc T, Destombes J, Thiesson D, Delpeyroux F, Blondel B. Poliovirus induces apoptosis in the mouse central nervous system. *J Virol.* Jul 1999;73(7):6066–6072.
126. Girard S, Gosselin AS, Pelletier I, Colbere-Garapin F, Couderc T, Blondel B. Restriction of poliovirus RNA replication in persistently infected nerve cells. *Journal of General Virology.* 2002;83(Pt 5):1087–1093.
127. Gitlin L, Barchet W, Gilfillan S, et al. Essential role of mda-5 in type I IFN responses to polyriboinosinic:polyribocytidylic acid and encephalomyocarditis picornavirus. *Proceedings of the National Academy of Sciences, U.S.A.* 2006;103(22):8459–8464.
128. Gitlin L, Stone JK, Andino R. Poliovirus escape from RNA interference: short interfering RNA-target recognition and implications for therapeutic approaches. *J Virol.* Jan 2005;79(2):1027–1035.
129. Godeny EK, Gauntt CJ. In situ immune autoradiographic identification of cells in heart tissues of mice with coxsackievirus B3-induced myocarditis. *American Journal of Pathology.* 1987;129:267–276.
130. Goldwater PN. Immunoglobulin M capture immunoassay in investigation of coxsackievirus B5 and B6 outbreaks in South Australia. *J Clin Microbiol.* 1995;33(6):1628–1631.
131. Gomez RM, Lopez Costa JJ, Pecci Saavedra G, Berria MI. Ultrastructural study of cell injury induced by coxsackievirus B3 in pancreatic and cardiac tissues. *Medicina.(B.Aires).* 1993;53:300–306.
132. Gondo K, Kusuhara K, Take H, Ueda K. Echovirus type 9 epidemic in Kagoshima, southern Japan: seroepidemiology and clinical observation of aseptic meningitis. *Pediatr Infect Dis J.* 1995;14(9):787–791.
133. Gorgievski-Hrisoho M, Schumacher JD, Vilimonovic N, Germann D, Matter L. Detection by PCR of enteroviruses in cerebrospinal fluid during a summer outbreak of aseptic meningitis in Switzerland. *J Clin Microbiol.* 1998;36(9):2408–2412.
134. Goyal SM, Gerba CP. Comparative adsorption of human enteroviruses, simian rotavirus, and selected bacteriophages to soils. *Appl Environ Microbiol.* 1979;38(2):241–247.
135. Grandien M, Forsgren M, Ehrnst A. Enteroviruses and Reoviruses. In: Lennette EH, Schmidt NJ, eds. *Diagnostic procedures for viral, rickettsial, and chlamydial infections.* 6th ed. Washington, DC: American Public Health Association; 1989:513–569.
136. Gravanis MB, Sternby NH. Incidence of myocarditis. A 10-year autopsy study from Malmo, Sweden. *Arch Pathol Lab Med.* Apr 1991;115(4): 390–392.
137. Grist NR, Bell EJ, Assaad F. Enteroviruses in human disease. *Prog Med Virol.* 1978;24:114–157.
138. Groarke JM, Pevear DC. Attenuated virulence of pleconaril-resistant coxsackievirus B3 variants. *J Infect Dis.* Jun 1999;179(6):1538–1541.
139. Gromeier M, Wimmer E. Mechanism of injury-provoked poliomyelitis. *J Virol.* 1998;72(6):5056–5060.
140. Guo R, Tang EH, Wang H, et al. Preliminary studies on antigenic variation of poliovirus using neutralizing monoclonal antibodies. *J Gen Virol.* 1987;68(Pt 4):989–994.
141. Haarmann CM, Schwimmbeck PL, Mertens T, Schultheiss HP, Strauer BE. Identification of serotype-specific and nonserotype-specific B-cell epitopes of coxsackie B virus using synthetic peptides. *Virology* May 1 1994; 200(2):381–389.
142. Halim S, Ramsingh AI. A point mutation in VP1 of coxsackievirus B4 alters antigenicity. *Virology.* 2000;269(1):86–94.
143. Halim SS, Collins DN, Ramsingh AI. A therapeutic HIV vaccine using coxsackie-HIV recombinants: a possible new strategy. *AIDS Res Hum Retroviruses.* 2000;16(15):1551–1558.
144. Halim SS, Ostrowski SE, Lee WT, Ramsingh AI. Immunogenicity of a foreign peptide expressed within a capsid protein of an attenuated coxsackievirus. *Vaccine.* 2001;19(7–8):958–965.
145. Hall CE, Cooney MK, Fox JP. The Seattle virus watch program. I. Infection and illness experience of virus watch families during a community-wide epidemic of echovirus type 30 aseptic meningitis. *American Journal of Public Health & the Nations Health.* 1970;60(8):1456–1465.
146. Haller AA, Stewart SR, Semler BL. Attenuation stem-loop lesions in the 5′ noncoding region of poliovirus RNA: neuronal cell-specific translation defects. *J Virol.* 1996;70(3):1467–1474.
147. Halsey NA, Pinto J, Rosales F, et al. Search for poliovirus carriers in persons with primary immune deficiency diseases in the United States, Mexico and Brazil. *Bull World Health Organ* 2004;82:3–8.
148. Hartig PC, Webb SR. Coxsackievirus B4 heterogeneity: effect of passage on neutralization and mortality. *Acta Virologica.* 1986;30(6):475–486.
149. Harvala H, Sharp CP, Ngole EM, Delaporte E, Peeters M, Simmonds P. Detection and genetic characterization of enteroviruses circulating among wild populations of chimpanzees in Cameroon; relationship with human and simian enteroviruses. *J Virol.* 2011;85:4480–4486.
150. Hashimoto I, Komatsu T. Myocardial changes after infection with Coxsackie virus B3 in nude mice. *Br J Exp Pathol.* 1978;59(1):13–20.
151. Heck CF, Shumway SJ, Kaye MP. The Registry of the International Society for Heart Transplantation: sixth official report–1989. *J Heart Transplant.* 1989;8:271–276.
152. Heim A, Canu A, Kirschner P, et al. Synergistic interaction of interferon-á and interferon-g in coxsackievirus B3-infected carrier cultures of human myocardial fibroblasts. *J Infect Dis.* 1992;166:958–965.
153. von Heine J. *Beobachtungen uber Lahmungszustande der untern Extermitaten und deren Behandlung.* Stuttgart: Kohler; 1840.
154. Heinz BA, Rueckert RR, Shepard DA, et al. Genetic and molecular analyses of spontaneous mutants of human rhinovirus 14 that are resistant to an antiviral compound. *J Virol.* 1989;63(6):2476–2485.
155. Heinz BA, Vance LM. Sequence determinants of 3A-mediated resistance to enviroxime in rhinoviruses and enteroviruses. *J Virol.* 1996; 70(7):4854–4857.
156. Henke A, Huber SA, Stelzner A, Whitton JL. The role of CD8 + T lymphocytes in coxsackievirus B3-induced myocarditis. *Journal of Virology.* 1995;69(11):6720–6728.
157. Hennessey KA, Lago H, Diomande F, et al. Poliovirus vaccine shedding among persons with HIV in Abidjan, Cote d'Ivoire. *J Infect Dis.* Dec 15 2005;192(12):2124–2128.
158. Herzum M, Huber SA, Weller R, Grebe R, Maisch B. Treatment of experimental murine Coxsackie B3 myocarditis. *Eur Heart J.* 1991;12 (Suppl D):200–202.
159. Heymann DL, Sutter RW, Aylward RB. A global call for new polio vaccines. *Nature.* Apr 7 2005;434(7034):699–700.
160. Hilfenhaus J, Nowak T. Inactivation of hepatitis A virus by pasteurization and elimination of picornaviruses during manufacture of factor VIII concentrate. *Vox Sanguinis.* 1994;67(Suppl 1):62–66.
161. Ho M, Chen ER, Hsu KH, et al. An epidemic of enterovirus 71 infection in Taiwan. Taiwan Enterovirus Epidemic Working Group. *New England Journal of Medicine.* 1999;341(13):929–935.
162. Hodgson J, Bendig J, Keeling P, Booth JC. Comparison of two immunoassay procedures for detecting enterovirus IgM. *J Med Virol.* 1995; 47(1):29–34.
163. Hofschneider PH, Klingel K, Kandolf R. Toward understanding the pathogenesis of enterovirus-induced cardiomyopathy: molecular and ultrastructural approaches. *J Struct Biol.* 1990;104:32–37.

164. Hogle JM, Chow M, Filman DJ. Three-dimensional structure of poliovirus at 2.9 A resolution. *Science.* 1985;229(4720):1358–1365.
165. Hogle JM, Filman DJ. The antigenic structure of poliovirus. *Philosophical Transactions of the Royal Society of London - Series B: Biological Sciences.* 1989;323(1217):467–478.
166. Hohenadl C, Klingel K, Mertsching J, Hofschneider PH, Kandolf R. Strand-specific detection of enteroviral RNA in myocardial tissue by in situ hybridization. *Molecular & Cellular Probes.* 1991;5(1):11–20.
167. Holtz LR, Finkbeiner SR, Zhao G, et al. Klassevirus 1, a previously undescribed member of the family Picornaviridae, is globally widespread. *Virol J.* 2009;6:86.
168. Honig EI, Melnick JL, Isacson P, Parr R, Myers IL, Walton M. An endemiological study of enteric virus infections: poliomyelitis, coxsackie, and orphan (ECHO) viruses isolated from normal children in two socioeconomic groups. *J Exp Med.* Feb 1 1956;103(2):247–262.
169. Horstmann DM. Enterovirus infections of the central nervous system. The present and future of poliomyelitis. *Medical Clinics of North America.* 1967;51(3):681–692.
170. Horstmann DM. Poliomyelitis: severity and type of disease in different age groups. *Ann NY Acad Sci.* 1955;61:956–967.
171. Hovi T, Stenvik M. Selective isolation of poliovirus in recombinant murine cell line expressing the human poliovirus receptor gene. *J Clin Microbiol.* 1994;32(5):1366–1368.
172. Huang CC, Liu CC, Chang YC, Chen CY, Wang ST, Yeh TF. Neurologic complications in children with enterovirus 71 infection. *New England Journal of Medicine.* 1999;341(13):936–942.
173. Huang SC, Chang CL, Wang PS, Tsai Y, Liu HS. Enterovirus 71-induced autophagy detected in vitro and in vivo promotes viral replication. *J. Med. Virol.* 2009;81(7):1241–1252.
174. Huber S, Sartini D. T cells expressing the V g 1 T-cell receptor enhance virus-neutralizing antibody response during coxsackievirus B3 infection of BALB/c mice: differences in male and female mice. *Viral Immunology.* 2005;18(4):730–739.
175. Huber S, Song WC, Sartini D. Decay-accelerating factor (CD55) promotes CD1d expression and Vgamma4+ T-cell activation in coxsackievirus B3-induced myocarditis. *Viral Immunology.* 2006;19(2):156–166.
176. Huber SA. Autoimmunity in coxsackievirus B3 induced myocarditis. *Autoimmunity.* Feb 2006;39(1):55–61.
177. Huber SA. Autoimmunity in myocarditis: relevance of animal models. *Clin Immunol Immunopathol.* 1997;83(2):93–102.
178. Huber SA, Born W, O'Brien R. Dual functions of murine gammadelta cells in inflammation and autoimmunity in coxsackievirus B3-induced myocarditis: role of Vgamma1+ and Vgamma4+ cells. *Microbes Infect.* 2005;7(3):537–543.
179. Huber SA, Lodge PA. Coxsackievirus B-3 myocarditis in Balb/c mice. Evidence for autoimmunity to myocyte antigens. *American Journal of Pathology.* 1984;116:21–29.
180. Huber SA, Lyden DC, Lodge PA. Immunopathogenesis of experimental Coxsackievirus induced myocarditis: role of autoimmunity. *Herz.* 1985; 10:1–7.
181. Huber SA, Moraska A, Cunningham M. Alterations in major histocompatibility complex association of myocarditis induced by coxsackievirus B3 mutants selected with monoclonal antibodies to group A streptococci. *Proc Natl Acad Sci U.S.A.* 1994;91(12):5543–5547.
182. Huhn MH, Hultcrantz M, Lind K, Ljunggren HG, Malmberg KJ, Flodstrom-Tullberg M. IFN-g production dominates the early human natural killer cell response to Coxsackievirus infection. *Cellular Microbiology.* 2008;10(2):426–436.
183. Huhn MH, McCartney SA, Lind K, Svedin E, Colonna M, Flodstrom-Tullberg M. Melanoma differentiation-associated protein-5 (MDA-5) limits early viral replication but is not essential for the induction of type 1 interferons after Coxsackievirus infection. *Virology.* 2010;401(1):42–48.
184. Hull BP, Dowdle WR. Poliovirus surveillance: building the global Polio Laboratory Network. *J Infect Dis.* 1997;175(Suppl 1):S113–S116.
185. Hull HF, Ward NA, Hull BP, Milstien JB, de Quadros C. Paralytic poliomyelitis: seasoned strategies, disappearing disease. *Lancet.* 1994; 343(8909):1331–1337.
186. Huovilainen A, Kinnunen L, Ferguson M, Hovi T. Antigenic variation among 173 strains of type 3 poliovirus isolated in Finland during the 1984 to 1985 outbreak. *J Gen Virol.* 1988;69(Pt 8):1941–1948.
187. Hyöty H, Hiltunen M, Lonnrot M. Enterovirus infections and insulin dependent diabetes mellitus–evidence for causality. *Clinical & Diagnostic Virology.* 1998;9(2–3):77–84.
188. Hyypiä T, Hovi T, Knowles NJ, Stanway G. Classification of enteroviruses based on molecular and biological properties. *J Gen Virol.* 1997; 78(Pt 1):1–11.
189. Ida-Hosonuma M, Iwasaki T, Taya C, et al. Comparison of neuropathogenicity of poliovirus in two transgenic mouse strains expressing human poliovirus receptor with different distribution patterns. *Journal of General Virology.* 2002;83(Pt 5):1095–1105.
190. Ida-Hosonuma M, Iwasaki T, Yoshikawa T, et al. The alpha/beta interferon response controls tissue tropism and pathogenicity of poliovirus. *Journal of Virology.* 2005;79(7):4460–4469.
191. Irvine DH, Irvine AB, Gardner PS. Outbreak of E.C.H.O. virus type 30 in a general practice. *Brit Med J.* 1967;4(582):774–776.
192. Ito M, Yamashita T, Tsuzuki H, Takeda N, Sakae K. Isolation and identification of a novel human parechovirus. *J Gen Virol.* 2004;85:391–398.
193. Jackson WT, Giddings TH Jr, Taylor MP, et al. Subversion of cellular autophagosomal machinery by RNA viruses. *PLoS Biology.* 2005;3(5): e156.
194. Jankovic B, Pasic S, Kanjuh B, et al. Severe neonatal echovirus 17 infection during a nursery outbreak. *Pediatr Infect Dis J.* 1999;18(4): 393–394.
195. Jarasch N, Martin U, Zell R, Wutzler P, Henke A. Influence of pan-caspase inhibitors on coxsackievirus B3-infected CD19 + B lymphocytes. *Apoptosis.* 2007;12(9):1633–1643.
196. Jenista JA, Powell KR, Menegus MA. Epidemiology of neonatal enterovirus infection. *J Pediatr.* 1984;104(5):685–690.
197. Johnson R. *Viral Infections of the Nervous System.* 2nd ed. Philadelphia: JB Lippincott-Raven; 1998.
198. Joki-Korpela P, Hyypia T. Diagnosis and epidemiology of echovirus 22 infections. *Clin Infect Dis.* 1998;27(1):129–136.
199. Jones MJU, Kolb M, Votava HJ, Johnson RL, Smith TF. Case reports. Intrauterine echovirus type II infection. *Mayo Clinic Proceedings.* 1980;55(8): 509–512.
200. Jubelt B, Gallez-Hawkins G, Narayan O, Johnson RT. Pathogenesis of human poliovirus infection in mice. I. Clinical and pathological studies. *Journal of Neuropathology & Experimental Neurology.* 1980;39(2):138–148.

CHAPTER 18

James E. Gern • Ann C. Palmenberg

Rhinoviruses

HISTORY

The common cold has been recognized for millennia, and both the illness and prescribed remedies have been influenced by and engendered a broad body of folklore. In fact, the name of the illness stems from the belief that being chilled causes the illness, a concept that studies using experimental inoculation techniques have been unable to verify.[53] In Chinese traditional medicine, colds were considered an illness of wind and cold, and the Roman physician Galen wrote "The white-colored substance (the phlegma) collects mostly…in those who have been chilled in some way".[14] Through the ages, ideas about pathogenesis have varied widely, and suggestions for common cold cures were creative and occasionally bizarre, but seldom helpful. Enthusiasm for a cure for the common cold remains quite high today; a web-based search yielded 4,120,000 hits in response to the terms "common cold cure."

In modern times, Kruse in 1914[139] demonstrated that cell-free filtrates of nasal secretions from affected individuals could transmit colds. In 1930, Dochez et al.[50] confirmed these findings by transmitting colds to volunteers and apes using filtered nasal secretions that were free of bacteria, indicating a viral etiology. Progress in finding the cause for common colds was accelerated by the establishment of the Common Cold Unit (CCU) by the UK Medical Research Council in 1946.[237] The building was originally a hospital established by Harvard University and the American Red Cross to support Great Britain in World War II, and after the war the building was donated to the British government. At the time one virus was presumed to cause colds, and another to cause influenza.[237] The goals of the CCU, led by Christopher Andrewes and later David Tyrrell, were to identify the common cold virus, its means of transmission, and host characteristics that promoted more severe illness. From 1946 until the unit closed in 1989, more than 20,000 volunteers participated in these studies.

Rhinoviruses were discovered beginning in 1956 by two groups working independently.[190,198] It was not long before researchers realized that several families of viruses caused common cold illnesses, and that human rhinovirus (HRV) serotypes were numerous. In 1967, a collaborative program classified the known rhinoviruses into 55 different serotypes,[1] serotypes 56 through 89 were added in 1971,[2] and the remainder of the classical serotypes were added in 1987.[88]

The development of molecular techniques for detecting HRV in a variety of clinical specimens led to a renewed period of discovery related to HRV classification and epidemiology. Recent findings include the discovery of the genetically distinct HRV-C species viruses that do not grow in standard tissue culture, and additional insights into the role of HRV not only in common colds, but also otitis, sinusitis, lower respiratory infections, asthma, and acute exacerbations of chronic respiratory diseases such as asthma.

Infectious Agent

Classification

The human rhinoviruses comprise the HRV-A, HRV-B, and HRV-C species of the *Enterovirus* genus in the *Picornaviridae* family. Classification is based on overt similarities in genome organization, capsid properties, and primary sequence conservation.[185] Viruses are assigned to these species classifications if they share greater than 70% amino acid identity in the P1, 2C, and 3CD regions with other members. Within species, isolates are subdivided into numeric genotypes (Fig. 18.1). For the HRV-A and HRV-B, several historic clinical panels archived by the American Type Culture Collection, were combined and indexed into 101 original HRV types after assessment of antigenic crossreactivity or serotyping in rabbits. HRV-A87 was subsequently reassigned to the *Enterovirus D* (HEV-D68) after reevaluation of genetic, immunogenic, and receptor use (decay-accelerating factor as a receptor) properties.[210] New HRV isolates, especially for the HRV-C, are now rarely tested for immunogenicity. Type assignments still respect the historic naming system, but rely more heavily on sequence comparisons, primarily of the VP1 protein or VP4/VP2. Strains within a common genotype generally share greater than 12% to 15% aligned amino acid identity in either or both of these regions. Full genome sequencing indicated that some historic types are more closely related than this (e.g., A09 and A95, or A29 and A44), and others such as A45 and A95 defining "clade D" may be sufficiently different as to warrant eventual designation as a fourth species (Fig. 18.1). Because many HRV-C's are not yet fully sequenced, genotype assignments in this species still rely on comparative VP1 data. Nomenclature conventions for all HRVs cite both the species letter and genotype assignment (e.g., A16, B14, C01) to prevent ambiguity among assigned HRV-A (77 types), HRV-B (25 types), and HRV-C (49 types).

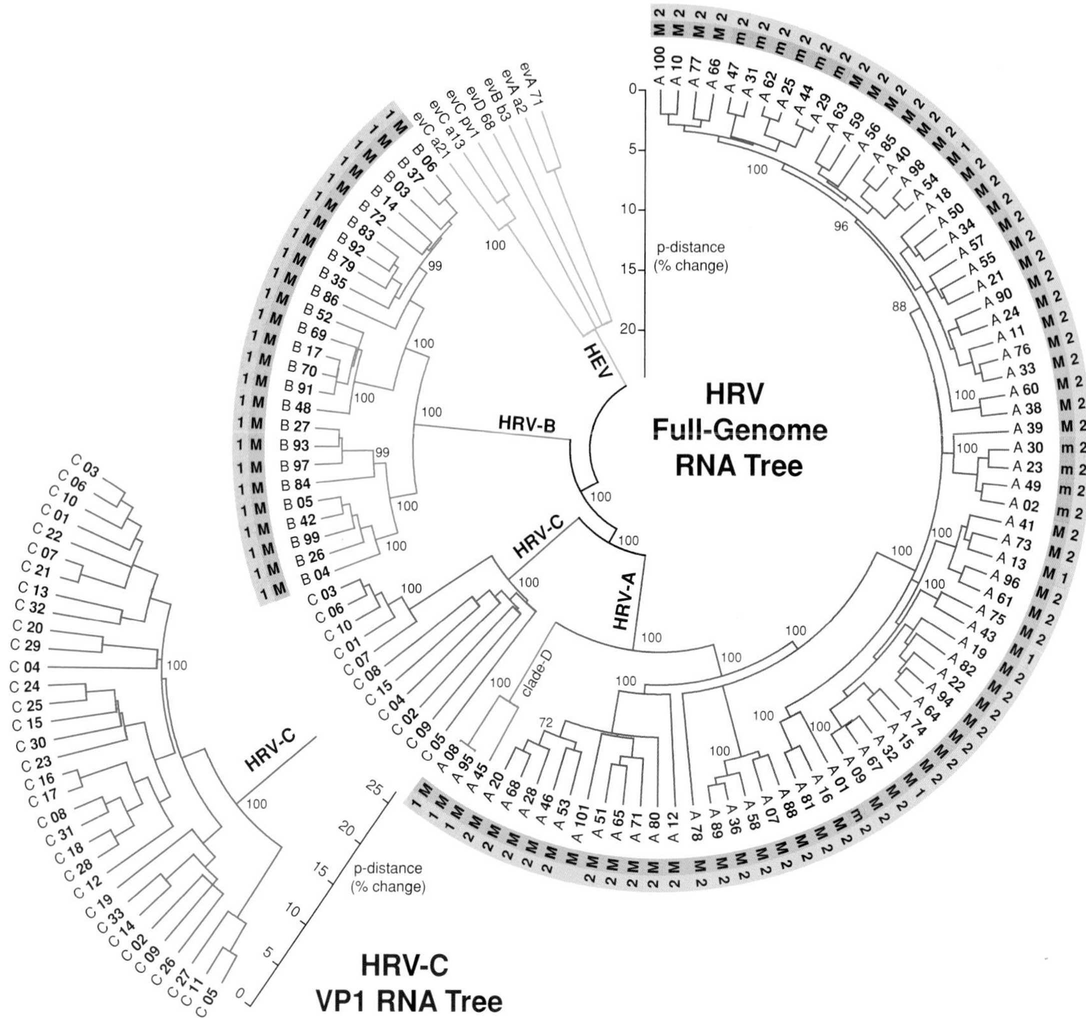

FIGURE 18.1. Circle phylogram relationships for known genotypes of human rhinovirus (HRV)-A, HRV-B, and HRV-C. The tree was calculated with neighbor-joining methods from aligned, full-genome RNA sequences, and rooted with data from human enterovirus (HEV)-A, HEV-B, and HEV-C species (similar to 186). The outer ring ("1" or "2") indicates anticapsid drug group types, if known.[7] The inner ring shows members of the Major ("M," intercellular adhesion molecule 1 [ICAM-1]) and minor ("m," low-density lipoprotein receptor [LDL-R]) receptor groups. The HRV-C receptor is unknown. Because few HRV-C are fully sequenced, relationships among these genotypes rely on partial VP1 RNA data (lower left). Bootstrap values (percent of 2,000 replicates) are indicated at key nodes.

Physical Characteristics

As enteroviruses, the HRV have genome organizations (Fig. 18.2) and capsid structures (Fig. 18.3) similar to those of polioviruses, coxsackie viruses, and enteric cytopathic human orphan (ECHO) viruses. But unlike other enteroviruses that remain viable at pH 3.0, HRV particles are unstable at pH below 5 to 6. The icosahedral capsid (~30 nm diameter) has 60 copies each, of proteins VP1, VP2, VP3, and VP4, named in order of descending electrophoretic mobility. The protein shell surrounds a densely packed, single-stranded, positive-sense RNA genome of 7079 (C01) to 7233 (B92) bases, a count that does not include the variable length 3′ poly(A) tail. Several HRV capsids have been resolved at the atomic level resolution, including A01 (*1r1a*), A02 (*1fpn*), A16 (*1ayn*), B03 (*1rhi*), and B14 (*4hrv*), with multiple structure variants showing receptor interactions (e.g., A16 with intercellular adhesion molecule 1 [ICAM-1], *1d3e*) or antiviral drug interactions (e.g., A16 with pleconaril, *1c8m*). Like poliovirus, the surfaces of HRV-A&B capsids are dominated by the three largest proteins (Fig. 18.3). VP4 is internal to the structure, centered near the fivefold axis. Around the exterior fivefold plateau, a symmetrical "canyon" provides receptor binding sites and immunogenic surfaces. There are no current structures for an HRV-C, but available sequences indicate significant deletions in the VP1 regions contributing to the fivefold plateau, so it is likely the HRV-C have unique topologies.[161] Common to all HRV, the VP1 cores surround a hydrophobic "pocket" or cavity, which can uptake and bind antiviral drugs like pleconaril or other capsid-binding agents. Type-1 long (e.g., B14) or type-2 short (e.g., A16) pocket shapes are defined for most

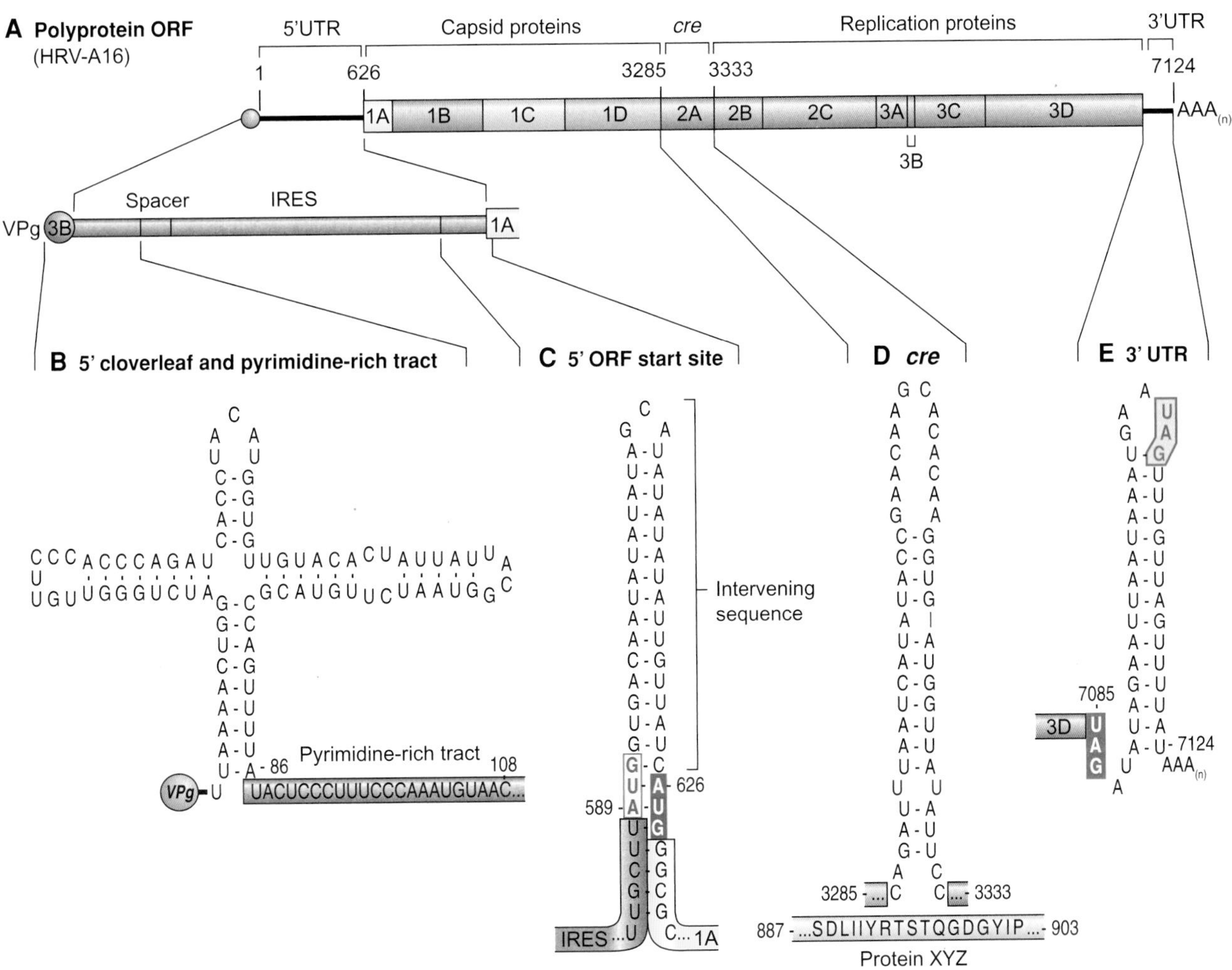

FIGURE 18.2. The genome of an HRV encodes a single polyprotein open reading frame (ORF) **(A)**. Important RNA structural motifs include a 5′ cloverleaf **(B)**, ORF start-site stem **(C)**, a *cre* element **(D)**, and 3′ stem motif **(E)**.

HRV-A&B and determine whether a virus is susceptible to particular drugs aimed at inhibiting the uncoating process.[7]

The HRV genome is messenger-sense, encoding the polyprotein open reading frame (ORF) and multiple important RNA structural motifs (Fig. 18.2). Adjacent to the 5′ cloverleaf, a regulatory feature for translation and replication, each HRV encodes a strain-specific pyrimidine-rich tract that may be involved in suppressing innate immunity triggers.[186] The type-1 internal ribosome entry site (IRES) 3′ to this tract, includes a variable-length stem structure pairing the ORF start site (AUG) with an upstream AUG. Unlike poliovirus, intervening sequences between these AUGs are probably not scanned by initiating ribosomes.[114] The picornavirus VPg uridylylation reaction, required for RNA synthesis, is templated by a special structure called the *cre* (*cis*-acting replication element) whose location varies in every species of picornavirus. For the HRV-A, the *cre* is in the 2A gene.[225] For the HRV-B, the *cre* is in the 2C gene.[225] The HRV-C *cre* has been proposed as one of two sites in the 1B gene.[37,186,225] Neither has been confirmed experimentally. The short, 3′ untranslated sequences (untranslated regions, UTRs) are of highly variable sequence. Invariably, they configure as an inclusive stem motif displaying at least one bogus termination codon in the terminal loop. This codon may be in-frame or out-of-frame with the authentic ORF stop site, and has been proposed to play a role in the recruitment of translation termination factors.[186]

Pathogenesis and Pathology

Entry into the Host

The primary portal of entry for HRV infections is through inoculation of either the eyes or nose. Studies of seronegative infected volunteers have shown that very low doses of HRV, substantially less than the amount needed to infect cells *in vitro* (one tissue culture infectious dose$_{50}$ [TCID$_{50}$]), can cause infection when introduced via the conjunctiva or nasal mucosa.[41] In contrast, approximately 10,000 times as much virus is needed to cause productive infection when the inoculation site is the tongue or external nares.[41]

Site of Primary Replication

The primary site of infection is the airway epithelium. In studies of airway tissues from either natural or experimentally induced colds, detection of viral protein or RNA is largely confined to the epithelial layer, along with an occasional cell in

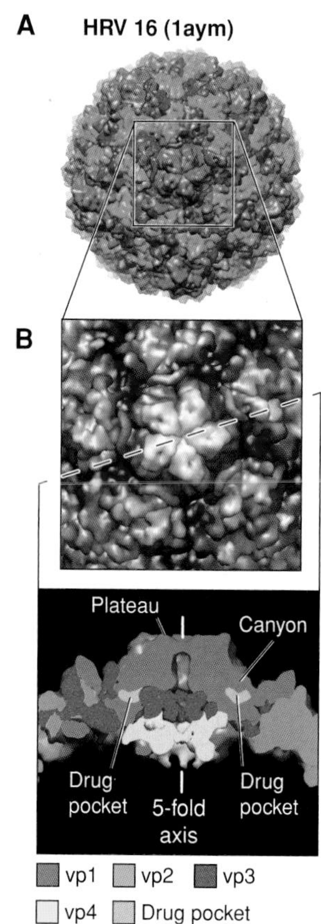

FIGURE 18.3. Capsid structure of a human rhinovirus (HRV) **(A)**, illustrates the icosahedral surface topography of VP1, VP2 and VP3 proteins. The VP4 is internal to the capsid **(B)**. Type 1 and type 2 antiviral capsid drugs bind in a pocket, internal to VP1.

the subepithelial layer (Fig. 18.4).[11,23,175] Highly differentiated epithelial cells grown at air–liquid interface are more resistant to HRV infection compared to undifferentiated monolayers of cells.[154] In addition, mechanical damage to well-differentiated cells significantly enhances viral replication *in vitro*.[116] These findings suggest that the epithelial barrier function is an important contributor to the resistance against HRV infections. In addition, differentiation of epithelial cells in tissue culture in the presence of interleukin-13 (IL-13) *in vitro* causes increased numbers of goblet cells and greater HRV replication *in vitro*, suggesting that HRV replication is increased in goblet cells.[143]

Spread

For years it was assumed that HRV infection was confined to the upper airway and did not affect the chest except under unusual circumstances. In fact, one of the breakthroughs that led to successful propagation of HRV in cell culture was the discovery that this virus replicated best at 33°C to 35°C. It was assumed that the lower airways were at core temperature (37°C), and this characteristic was thought to limit HRV replication to the cooler upper airways. Contrary to these initial assumptions, direct measurements in the lower airways have shown that large- and medium-sized airways are at the ideal temperature for HRV replication (Fig. 18.5).[163] In addition, cultured lower airway epithelial cells support HRV replication *in vitro* at least as well, and perhaps even better, than cells derived from the upper airways.[155,174]

Following experimental inoculation of the upper airway, HRV has been detected in the lower airways of individuals with a variety of techniques. Secretions from the lower airways sampled by bronchoscopy and bronchial lavage were analyzed by reverse transcriptase–polymerase chain reaction (RT-PCR), and more than half of the lower airway specimens tested positive for HRV.[73,214] These findings were extended by subsequent

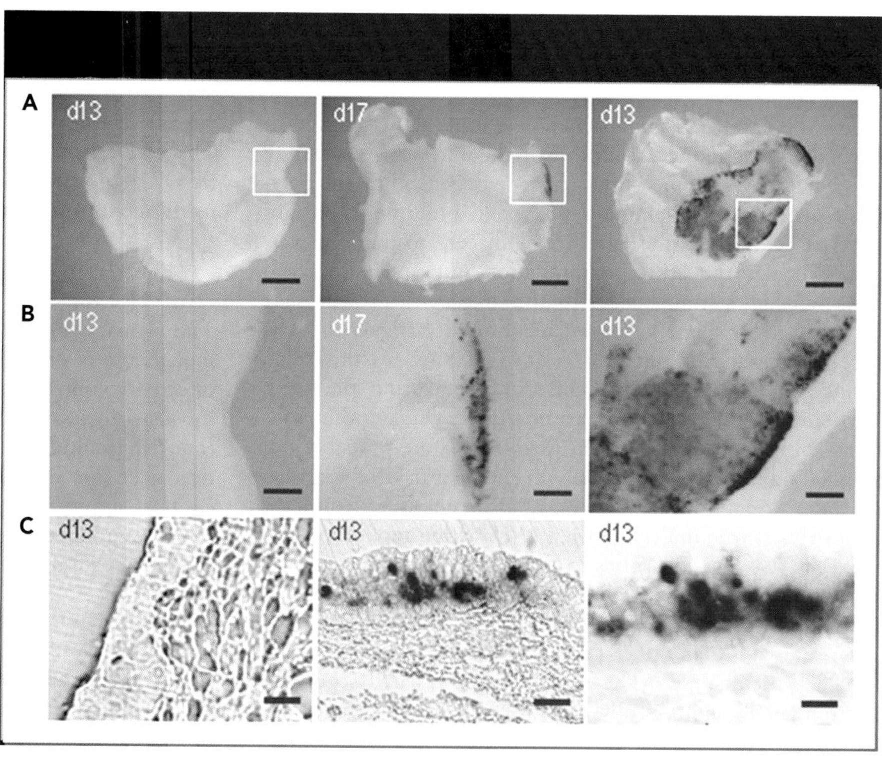

FIGURE 18.4. Human rhinovirus (HRV)-C15 replication within epithelial cells in sinus organ culture. A: Sinus tissue in organ culture was inoculated with HRV-C15 **(center and right)** or medium alone **(left)**, and whole mounts of the tissue were analyzed for HRV-C15 RNA by *in situ* hybridization (purple stain). Scale bars, 1 mm. **B:** Higher magnification view of the areas boxed in panel **a**, showing uninfected cells **(left)** or cells containing viral RNA **(center and right)**. Scale bars, 0.15 mm. C: Sections of mock **(left)** or HRV-C infected **(center and right)** sinus tissue. Right panel is counterstained with eosin (pink). Scale bars, 15 μm. (From Bochkov YA, Palmenberg AC, Lee WM, et al. Molecular modeling, organ culture and reverse genetics for the emerging respiratory pathogen human rhinovirus C. *Nat Med* 2011;17:627–632; with permission.)

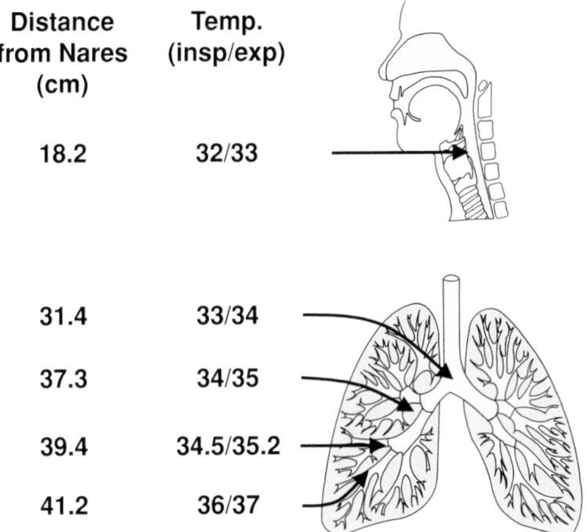

FIGURE 18.5. Temperatures in the lower airways are ideal for human rhinovirus (HRV) replication. Direct measurements of temperature in lower airways have been recorded at measured distances from the nares using a bronchoscope equipped with a small thermistor.[163] Even when the inspired air is at room temperature (26.7°C), airway temperatures in the medium and large airways are in the range of 33°C to 35°C. In contrast, small airway temperatures approach core temperature (37°C). insp, inspiration; exp, expiration.

studies demonstrating the presence of intracellular HRV RNA and protein using in situ hybridization and immunohistochemistry, respectively.[175,187] Analysis of sputum has been used to provide an estimate of the quantity and kinetics of viral shedding from the large lower airways. After experimental inoculation of seronegative volunteers, viral shedding from the upper airway peaks 2 to 4 days later. Analysis of sputum specimens 3, 7, and 14 days after inoculation revealed that peak levels of virus in the sputum occurred 3 to 7 days after inoculation.[175] In addition, about half of the volunteers had viral shedding in the sputum that was equal to or exceeded that found in the nasal secretions. Notably, only small amounts of virus were detected in bronchial lavage specimens, which originate from distal airways and alveoli.[175] These findings suggest that HRV replication is greatest in the upper airway in most individuals, and that high-level replication can also occur in the large- and medium-sized airways.

Data from natural cold studies also provide evidence of lower airway infections with HRV. Viral recovery from sputum during colds can exceed that obtained from upper airway samples.[106] In epidemiologic studies, HRV is frequently detected in children who are hospitalized with wheezing illnesses and in infants with pneumonia.[166,167,193] In wheezing infants, HRV has been detected in lower airway biopsies, and HRV detection was associated with reduced lung function in these infants.[158] In children with tracheostomies, samples of nasal mucus can be obtained directly from the lower airway without contamination from nasal secretions, and HRV detection rates from upper versus lower airway specimens are similar.[217]

In addition to infecting the nasopharynx, conjunctiva, and lower airways, HRV has also been recovered in specimens obtained from the middle ear and sinuses.[29,117,194,196] The respiratory epithelium in each of these two locations is contiguous with that of the nasopharynx, and the virus presumably spreads via local extension. Rhinovirus viremia has been detected in infected children by PCR but not by recovery of infectious virus,[260] and a study of experimentally infected adults showed no evidence of circulating HRV RNA.[45] Therefore, systemic infections do not occur in immune competent individuals. HRV are inactivated at pH less than 6, thus preventing swallowed virus from replicating in the gastrointestinal tract.

Cell and Tissue Tropism

Biopsies of the upper airway from infected volunteers show a patchy pattern of infection with small foci of infected cells.[10,195,256] Point cultures of the airway have demonstrated high levels of HRV shedding in the nasopharynx and especially in the adenoidal region. Examination of biopsies obtained during experimentally induced colds suggest that a specific type of nonciliated adenoidal epithelial cell, resembling the intestinal M cell, expresses high levels of ICAM-1 and supports high-level viral replication.[255] It is possible that these cells play a sentinel role in the detection of viral respiratory infections.

The receptors for HRV are also expressed by airway cells other than epithelial cells. Besides epithelial cells, HRV can bind to macrophages, monocytes, eosinophils, and fibroblasts.[72,75,90] Macrophages and monocytes are good sources of type I and type III interferons,[131,136] which may explain why there is little or no HRV replication in these cells. Airway fibroblasts[75] and possibly smooth muscle cells[140] support HRV replication in tissue culture, but it has not been established whether these cells, which are located several cell layers under the epithelial surface, are infected *in vivo.*

Receptors

All HRV-A&B use ICAM-1 (88 "major" types) or alternatively, low-density lipoprotein receptor (LDL-R, 11 "minor" types) for recognition and attachment to cells.[78,243] In addition, the major group virus HRV-A89 binds to heparan sulfate in the absence of ICAM-1.[242] The external cellular receptor(s) used by the HRV-C are most certainly different but yet to be identified.[23,161] Studies utilizing atopic force spectroscopy indicate that after initial HRV binding, multiple receptors are rapidly recruited (within 200 ms).[205]

Species Tropism

Rhinoviruses primarily infect humans. Chimpanzees can be infected, but although viral shedding can be detected, there are few or no signs or symptoms of illness.[108] HRV replication in rabbit smooth muscle cells has been reported by a single group.[86] HRV do not bind to murine ICAM-1, but can bind to murine LDL-R.[261] Accordingly, minor group viruses can replicate in murine epithelial cells,[24,236] and strains have been selected for this property by serial passage in murine cell lines.[17,91] In addition, epithelial cells from transgenic mice engineered to express human ICAM-1 support replication of major group viruses.[17]

The demonstration that HRV can grow in murine epithelial cells has led to the development of murine models of HRV infection.[17,24,178,180,236] Several features of these models resemble infection of the human, including replication in the respiratory epithelium, induction of type I interferons and neutrophil chemokines, and neutrophilic airway inflammation.[17,180] In addition, HRV infection of mice increases inflammation in response to allergen exposure, suggesting that these models could be informative for asthma.[17] Limitations of the models include the requirement of a large inoculating dose, and short duration (<24 hours) of significant viral replication and shedding. A second rodent model of picornavirus respiratory infection was developed using a genetically altered strain of Mengovirus, a natural mouse pathogen that causes a polio-like syndrome.[206] Intranasal inoculation of rats with attenuated Mengovirus causes infection of the airway epithelium with similarities to HRV infections in humans. The ability to investigate HRV host–cell interactions *in vivo* using the genetic tools available in rodent models should yield important new insights into the pathogenesis of infection in humans.

Immune Response

Immunohistochemistry

HRV infections produce relatively little cytopathology. Findings on biopsy during the peak of the illness include tissue edema and a sparse infiltration of neutrophils and mononuclear cells.[253,254] The relative lack of pathology together with the small number of infected cells suggests that the immune response to HRV rather than direct virus-induced injury contributes most to respiratory symptoms.[97]

Mediators of Inflammation

HRV infection induced a variety of proinflammatory cytokines and mediators (Table 18.1). Most of these factors are present in peak concentrations during the acute cold, and correlate with illness severity and viral shedding.[16] There is only circumstantial evidence that these immune mediators contribute to the pathogenesis of cold signs and symptoms, and the specific roles for most of these factors have yet to be defined. Kinins, leukotrienes, and histamine are of special interest due to their effects on vasodilation and edema, which are prominent findings during acute colds.[110,262] HRV infection of volunteers with asthma induced increased mRNA and activity of human kallikrein, a critical enzyme for the release of kinins, in the lower airways.[33] These mediators can also cause smooth muscle contraction as well as edema, and thus could promote airway obstruction in patients with asthma. Notably, common colds have little effect on concentrations of histamine in the nose,[61] and second-generation antihistamines (which are specific H1-receptor antagonists), have no effect on cold symptoms.[176] Leukotrienes (LTs) are overproduced during viral respiratory infections,[70] but the cystinyl leukotriene receptor antagonist montelukast did not affect cold symptoms in experimentally infected volunteers.[134] In addition, administration of LTB4 to the nose before experimental inoculation had no significant effects on either viral replication or symptoms.[251] Kinins are increased early in the course of a cold,[200] but testing of their role in pathogenesis awaits the development of safe and effective kinin inhibitors. HRV-induced cytokines may also promote vascular permeability; experiments conducted *in vitro* demonstrate that tumor necrosis factor α (TNF-α), IL-1β, and IFN-γ can each increase vascular permeability.[212] Analysis of nasal secretions after experimental inoculation demonstrates that the thin rhinorrhea during the early stages of a cold contains serum proteins (e.g., immunoglobulin [IgG], albumin), and as the cold progresses the composition shifts to mucin proteins.[110,262] This progression suggests that the pathophysiology of rhinorrhea is time-dependent, and shifts from vascular leakage initially to local secretion of mucus during the mid to latter stages of a cold.

Epithelium

The airway epithelium is the first line of defense against HRV infections. Mucins, antimicrobial peptides, and surfactant proteins in the mucous layer nonspecifically deter infection.[103] In addition, well-differentiated epithelial cells are relatively

TABLE 18.1 HRV-Induced Mediators and Cytokines

Category	Examples	Comments	References
Mediators	Kinins	Vasodilation and edema	(110,200,262)
	Leukotrienes	↑Vascular permeability and bronchoconstriction	(70)
	Nitric oxide	Vasodilation, bronchoconstriction	(43,64,208)
Antivirals	IFN-α	Low concentrations in nasal secretions[a]	(131,137)
	IFN-β	Possibly deficient in asthma	(131,247)
	IFN-λ (IL-28, IL-29)	Possibly deficient in asthma	(36,131)
	β-Defensins	Activity against bacteria and enveloped viruses	(58,201)
Chemokines	CXCL10	Attracts Th1 cells	(137,223,246)
	CXCL8	Attracts neutrophils	(74,230,235)
	CCL2	Attracts monocytes, T cells, and dendritic cells	(87)
Cytokines	IL-1	Proinflammatory	(199)
	IL-6	Proinflammatory	(154)
Growth factors and tissue repair	G-CSF	↑Production of neutrophils in bone marrow	(118)
	TGF-β	↑Collagen synthesis, immunoregulation	(52)
	VEGF	Angiogenesis and airway remodeling	(44)

[a]True for all interferons.

IFN, interferon; IL, interleukin; G-CSF, granulocyte-colony stimulating factor; TGF, transforming grown factor; VEGF, vascular endothelial growth factor.

resistant to HRV infection.[154] The epithelium may serve as a barrier against HRV infection; HRV replication is enhanced when apical cells of well-differentiated epithelial cell cultures are either damaged or stripped away.[116] This property may help to explain how exposure to factors such as pollutants and allergic inflammation that can damage epithelium also increase the risk and/or severity of HRV illnesses. HRV infection itself can disrupt the barrier function of the epithelium,[207] which may contribute to synergistic effects with bacteria, allergens, or irritants.

In addition to being the principal host cells for HRV infections, airway epithelial cells initiate antiviral and proinflammatory immune responses (Fig. 18.6). Attachment of HRV to ICAM-1 activates signaling cascades that lead to the activation of chemokine genes such as *CXCL10*.[69,136] Once HRV particles uncoat in the endosome, the release of single-stranded RNA activates additional innate immune sensors. These include toll-like receptors (TLRs) (e.g., TLR-3, TLR-7) that are expressed on endosomal membranes, and the double-stranded RNA-dependent protein kinase (PKR) and RNA helicases (retinoic acid-induced gene I [RIG-I] and melanoma-differentiation-associated gene-5 [MDA-5]). MDA-5 binds to double-stranded RNA that is formed during the replication process, and appears to be an important contributor to anti-HRV IFN responses.[220,244] The role of RIG-I, which binds to the 5′ triphosphate motif and longer stretches of double-stranded RNA,[19] is more controversial. One recent *in vitro* study found that TLR-3 was constitutively expressed on airway

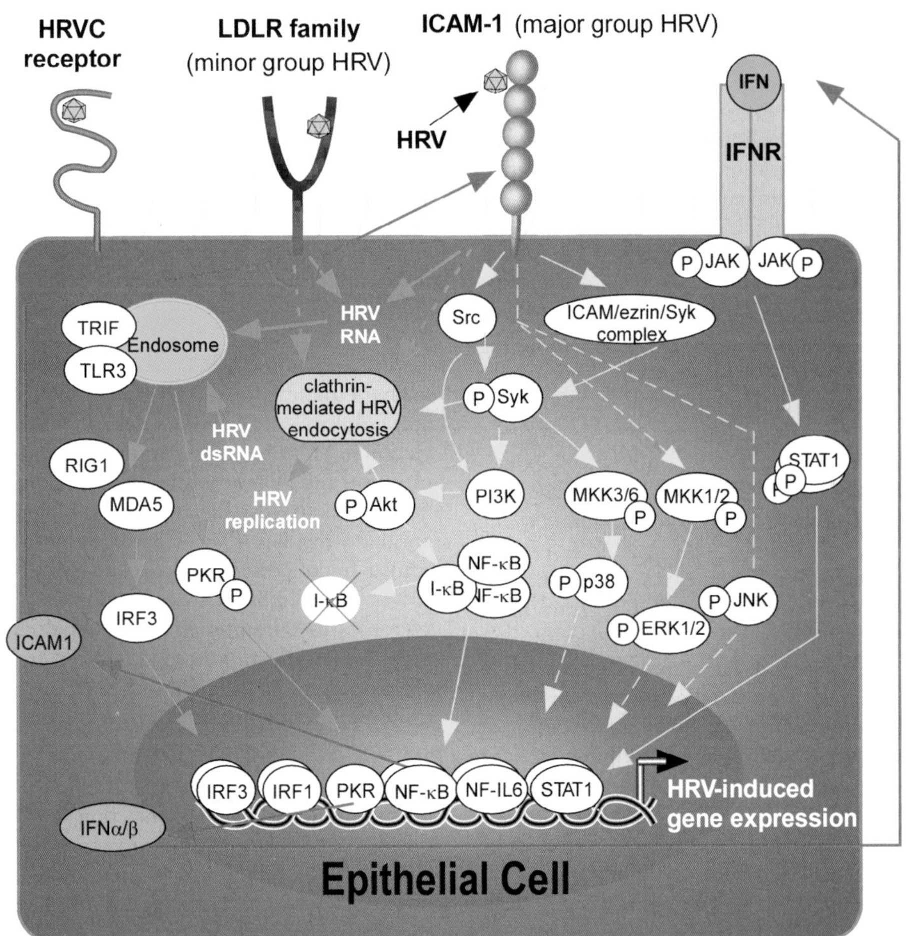

FIGURE 18.6. Airway epithelial cells initiate the immune response to human rhinovirus (HRV). Major group HRV binds to intercellular adhesion molecule 1 (ICAM-1) and minor group HRV binds to low-density lipoprotein receptors (LDL-Rs) on the surface of cells, such as epithelial cells and leukocytes, that would be abundant in the airway, to induce downstream signaling. The receptor and signaling pathways induced by HRV-C types has yet to be elucidated. Upon ligation of HRV to surface receptors on epithelial cells, direct uncoating of viral RNA or clathrin-mediated endocytosis leads to the release/replication of HRV RNA into the cytoplasm. This viral RNA is detected by endosomal receptors, such as toll-like receptor 3 (TLR-3), to propagate downstream signaling and induction of gene expression, including the production of interferons (IFNs) that can exert an autocrine/paracrine effect by binding to IFN receptors and triggering a janus kinase (JAK)-signal transducers and activators of transcription (STAT) signaling cascade. Replication-independent signaling is also induced upon HRV infection, and includes the activation of Src, Syk, and mitogen-activated protein kinase (MAPK) signaling cascades. Yellow solid lines, data to support link; dashed lines, indirectly connected (may have signaling molecules in between); red lines, signaling induced by product of HRV-induced gene transcription; green lines, replication-dependent signaling. (From Gavala ML, Bertics PJ, Gern JE. Rhinoviruses, allergic inflammation, and asthma. *Immunol Rev* 2011;242:69–90, with permission.)

epithelial cells, and activation of TLR-3 led to induction of RIG-I and MDA-5.[220] Subsequently, all three of these molecules contributed to upregulation of innate IFN responses to HRV infection.

Engagement of cell surface receptors and RNA-sensing molecules leads to activation of several signaling cascades, including nuclear factor kappa B (NFκB), janus kinase (JAK)-signal transducers and activators of transcription (STAT) pathways, and mitogen-activated protein kinases (MAPKs).[60,87,99,132,136,144,146,179,180,245,263] Viral proteases can also contribute to cell activation; the 3C protease cleaves the transcription factor organic cation transporter-1 (OCT-1),[6] which negatively regulates CXCL8 (interleukin-8) transcription. The net result of these actions is activation of viral sensing and antiviral effector pathways, IFNs, and a variety of proinflammatory cytokines and chemokines.[22,31,202] Type I IFNs inhibit HRV replication by inducing multiple antiviral pathways, and also prime epithelial cells to synthesize chemokines such as CXCL10.[6,137] IFN-γ has several effects on viral replication and inflammatory responses. It is a potent inducer of ICAM-1[135] and soluble ICAM-1,[250] and effects on viral replication in cultured epithelial cells depend on experimental conditions. In addition to affecting viral receptor expression, IFN-γ also enhances the HRV-induced secretion of chemokines such as CCL5.[135] HRV-induced chemokines from epithelial cells and other sources attract a variety of cells into the airway, including dendritic cells, monocytes, macrophages, epithelial cells, and lymphocytes (Table 18.1). The ensuing cellular response promotes antiviral effects and killing of infected cells, but also increases inflammation that contributes to the pathophysiology of illness.

Cellular Immune Responses

Macrophages are the principal cells in lower airway secretions, and it is likely that these cells are important contributors to the innate antiviral response. Considering that little to no replication of HRV has been observed in airway macrophages or blood monocytes,[72,146] the signaling pathways could differ from those in epithelial cells, in which viral replication processes provide potent innate immune stimulation. As in epithelial cells, HRV activate NF-κB and STAT-1-dependent pathways. For example, HRV-induced secretion of CCL2 involves activation of NF-κB and phosphorylation of activating transcription factor-2 (ATF-2).[87] Furthermore, HRV-A16 induces STAT-1 tyrosine phosphorylation and IFN-α release in monocytes.[136] NF-κB activation, but not the p38 MAPK, has been reported to be involved in HRV-mediated TNF-α release by monocytes.[146]

Macrophages are important sources of cytokines (e.g., TNF-α), chemokines (e.g., CXCL8 [IL-8], CXCL10 [IP-10], CCL2 [MCP-1]), and type I and type III IFNs during HRV infections.[87,127,131,146] Although epithelial cells and macrophages in isolation can both respond to HRV infection, co-culture of these cells leads to synergistic enhancement of selected chemokines such as CXCL10, and this synergy has been linked to macrophage secretion of IFN-α.[137] Airway dendritic cells are interdigitated into the epithelium, and as major producers of type I IFNs[215] they are likely to be important in orchestrating the early innate response to HRV infection.

Neutrophils are the most numerous cells in airway secretions during an HRV cold.[118,231,254] Experiments conducted after experimental HRV inoculation demonstrate that granulocyte-colony stimulating factor (G-CSF) is secreted into the nasal secretions within 24 hours, followed closely by increased in circulating G-CSF that can boost the production of neutrophil precursors in the bone marrow.[118] Neutrophils increase in the blood 1 to 2 days after inoculation, and are then recruited to upper and lower airway secretions. Neutrophilic inflammation correlates with respiratory symptoms, and it is suspected that these cells have both antiviral and proinflammatory effects during the cold.[16,79,118,230,231] The $P2X_7$ receptor is a cation channel expressed on epithelial cells and leukocytes that is activated after binding ATP, and can therefore initiate inflammatory responses secondary to virus-induced cellular damage and other stimuli that release ATP. In volunteers who were experimentally inoculated with HRV, $P2X_7$ pore activity measured in blood cells correlated with the influx of neutrophils into upper airway secretions during the acute cold.[46]

Lymphocyte numbers dip briefly in the blood during an acute cold, and rise in nasal secretions, but to a lesser extent than neutrophils.[151,152] T-cell responses are critical for resolution of HRV infections, as indicated by reports of prolonged and sometimes severe symptoms in immunosuppressed individuals or those with primary immune deficiencies.[68,112] T-cell responses can be directed at either serotype-specific or shared antigens.[71] Vigorous HRV-specific proliferative responses in seronegative volunteers at baseline were associated with milder clinical symptoms, suggesting a potential role for lymphocytes in the initial antiviral response.[188]

Role of Antibody

Antibody responses can be detected as early as 7 to 14 days following experimental inoculation, and it is likely that both IgG and IgA responses to HRV contribute to protection from reinfection.[41,66,192] Preexisting antibody reduces the rates of HRV infection and illness. Studies of natural infections among families found that the infection rate for individuals with serum antibody was half that of antibody-negative subjects,[41,66] and similar findings were reported in trials of experimental inoculation.[4,28] In addition to protection associated with antibody responses to a homotypic virus, serial challenges with heterotypic virus also produced a reduced frequency of infection, suggesting either the presence of cross-reacting antibodies or protective mechanisms not involving antibody.[65]

Release from Host and Mode of Transmission

The transmission of HRV infections has been the subject of a number of creative and innovative studies. Dick and colleagues[49] compared the HRV transmission rates from experimentally infected donors to seronegative recipients under controlled conditions. Some volunteers wore arm restraints or plastic collars designed to prevent hand to face contact; rates of transmission were similar for these volunteers compared to those with no restraints. These results are in agreement with observations that a related virus (coxsackievirus A21) could be spread by aerosol droplets.[40] On the other hand, Dr. Jack Gwaltney and colleagues[81] found that contact with coffee cups or plastic tiles contaminated with wet secretions could transmit HRV infections to volunteers who handled the fomites and then rubbed their eyes and nares with their fingertips. In addition, transmission of HRV can be inhibited by cleaning the hands with virucidal solutions, or by the use of virucidal tissues when blowing the nose.[48] Notably, items with dried secretions contain little virus and were not able to transmit colds. Collectively, these findings indicate that HRV can be transmitted by either aerosol or fomites, and that the predominant mode of transmission may depend on age, personal hygiene, and degree of viral shedding.

Virulence

With the very large number of HRV serotypes and genotypes, it is likely that some are more or less virulent. Early studies relying on tissue culture documented that at least 20 different HRV serotypes could cause wheezing illnesses. Larger studies using molecular diagnostics indicate that HRV-C infections appear to be overrepresented in more severe illnesses, including wheezing in infants and young children,[8] and acute exacerbations of childhood asthma.[20] There is also a single report of HRV-C recovery from pericardial fluid in a child with signs and symptoms of systemic infection.[228] Given that prevailing HRV strains change almost completely, additional studies include community surveillance over multiple seasons to definitively establish whether HRV-C are more virulent, and whether there are selected types of HRV-A and HRV-B with the same properties.

Persistence

Several studies have observed that following acute HRV infections, virus can sometimes be detected for weeks,[120,259] and this has led to speculation that HRV might cause chronic infection. In fact, studies that have performed HRV typing following either natural or experimentally induced infections provide definitive evidence that most HRV infections are cleared after 1 to 2 weeks.[45,184] Prolonged detection of HRV is usually explained by serial infections with different HRV types, and shedding of a singly viruses for four weeks or longer is a rare event in immunocompetent individuals.[119] In contrast, immunodeficient or immunocompromised patients can shed the same HRV type for prolonged periods, and can have more severe illnesses.[68,112,130]

Detection of HRV in the absence of respiratory symptoms is common, and rates of asymptomatic infection in infants are especially high (25% to 44%).[141,150,240] This could be a reflection of the age-related increased susceptibility to all HRV infections (symptomatic or not), but it is also true that mild symptoms (e.g., sore throat) may not be recognized in infants. In surveillance studies of infants, 10% to 20% of these "asymptomatic infections" reflect viral shedding following recovery from a cold, or a prodromal period just before the onset of respiratory illness.[109,120,240,257] Studies that have performed serial sampling of respiratory secretions have found no evidence that HRV establishes a "carrier state" characterized by persistent low-level viral shedding.[119,184,191] The quantity of viral shedding is not a good differentiator of symptomatic versus asymptomatic infection.[191] Notably, both symptomatic and asymptomatic infections can elicit immune responses.[123] When considered together, these findings indicate that detection of HRV shedding by culture or PCR is indicative of infection, and that asymptomatic infections are common and need to be considered in epidemiologic studies linking infection to illness outcomes.

Epidemiology

Age

HRV infections are most common in infants and young children. There is evidence that infection rates are somewhat lower in the first 6 months of life, and then rates are relatively high throughout infancy and early childhood.[18,47,66,105,113,238] Among young adults, infections rates are greater in mothers and women of similar age compared to men. In older adults, this relationship is reversed and illness rates are higher in men.[82]

Morbidity

HRV cause a broad spectrum of illness including asymptomatic infections, common colds, and other upper respiratory illnesses, bronchitis and wheezing illnesses, and lower respiratory tract infections including bronchiolitis, bronchitis, wheezing, and pneumonia (Fig. 18.7). The wide range of illness suggests that there are a number of factors related to the virus, the host, and the environment that contribute to the severity of illness. With 100 traditional serotypes and more than 40 HRV-C types, it is likely that there are species or strain-specific patterns of virulence. The C viruses appear to be overrepresented in studies of hospitalized children[51,89,145,148,153,156,162,166] and acute exacerbations of asthma,[20] but longitudinal data including large numbers of HRV illnesses of varying severity are needed to confirm these findings.

Most of the morbidity associated with HRV infections is in high-risk groups: infants, the elderly, immunocompromised individuals, and patients with chronic respiratory diseases such as asthma,[39,129,182] chronic obstructive lung disease,[258] and cystic

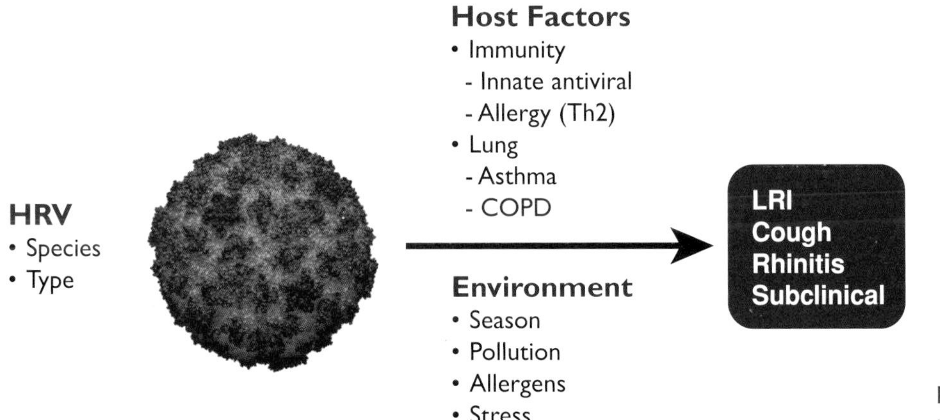

FIGURE 18.7. The spectrum of human rhinovirus (HRV) illness (see text).

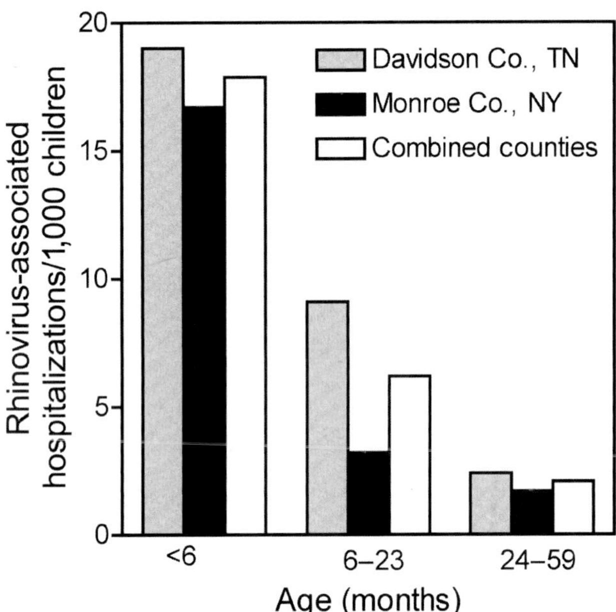

FIGURE 18.8. Age-related hospitalization rates for rhinovirus lower respiratory infection. (From Miller EK, Lu X, Erdman DD, et al. Rhinovirus-associated hospitalizations in young children. *J Infect Dis* 2007;195:773–781, with permission.)

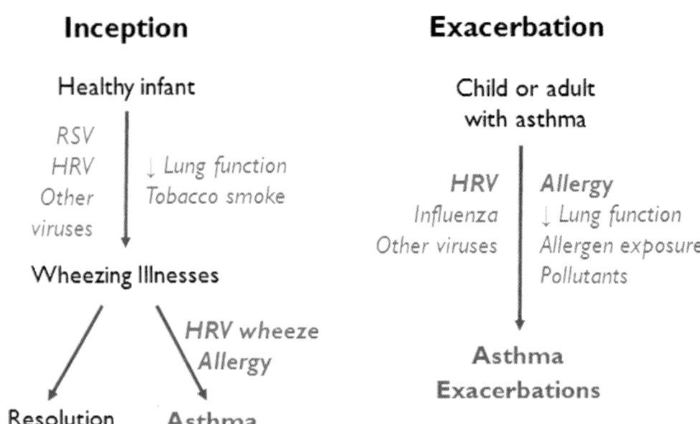

FIGURE 18.9. Human rhinovirus (HRV) infections and asthma (see text).

fibrosis.[35,222,249] Risk factors for HRV wheezing illnesses in early life include maternal atopy, a history of previous wheezing episodes, and increased airway resistance on infant lung function tests.[122,168,224,239] Population-based hospitalization rates were calculated for children hospitalized in Rochester, New York, and Nashville, Tennessee (Fig. 18.8); one major children's hospital serves the population in each of these communities.[167] Young age and a history of previous asthma or wheezing were two risk factors for HRV lower respiratory illness. Finally, several studies indicate that allergic children are especially likely to develop acute wheezing illnesses with HRV infections.[100,184,204]

Environmental factors that contribute to the severity of HRV illness include tobacco smoke and other pollutants.[57,181,241] Several studies have provided evidence that stress increases the severity of natural and experimentally induced colds.[34,226] Seasonal influences have been linked to cold prevalence, and likely also affect severity of illness. Notably, vitamin D status has been shown to be associated with the prevalence of upper respiratory illnesses, although specific links to HRV infections have not been established.[76]

HRV infections have been closely linked to the inception and exacerbation of asthma (Fig. 18.9). Many respiratory viruses can cause wheezing episodes in infancy, and low lung function and environmental exposures such as tobacco smoke increase the risk for wheeze. Most children recover fully, but a subset subsequently develop recurrent wheezing illnesses and asthma. Wheezing with HRV infections during infancy and early childhood is one of the strongest indicators of risk for subsequent childhood asthma, especially in those individuals who develop allergen-specific IgE (allergic sensitization) at an early age.[113,138,142] The causality of this relationship is uncertain. Once asthma has become established, viral respiratory illnesses (most commonly caused by HRV) are the most common trigger for acute exacerbations of asthma. The relationship between HRV infections and acute asthma is especially close in childhood; HRV infection is detected in up to 85% of asthma exacerbations in children compared to about half of exacerbations in adults.[13,100,101,129,182,184] There is a remarkable similarity in the seasonal patterns of HRV infections and exacerbations of asthma, especially in school-aged children in whom hospitalizations due to asthma have a strong fall and spring preponderance year after year.[125,126,128] Even so, the use of routine monitoring of respiratory secretions for HRV in children with asthma demonstrates that only a subset of HRV infections cause exacerbations.[184] Children with respiratory allergies are at greatest risk for virus-induced wheezing, and other risk factors include exposure to allergens or pollutants, obstructive changes on lung function testing, and failure to use asthma-control medications.[30,57,77,125,177,241]

Origin and Spread of HRV Infections

In general, transmission of HRV infections is relatively inefficient. Children have the highest rates of HRV illnesses, and also appear to transmit infections most effectively. In family surveillance studies, transmission from children to other children and adults was much more common than transmission from adult to children or other adults.[98,191] Epidemics with HRV are uncommon, although they have been reported to occur associated with "flu-like" illnesses in nursing homes.[62,102] Secondary attack rates within families vary between 30% and 70%.

Conditions that affect transmission of HRV infections were identified in studies of experimentally inoculated HRV "donors" and seronegative adult "recipients". Short-term (15 minute to 3 hours) contact led to transmission rates of less than 10%, even in the presence of loud vocalization, card playing, and kissing.[41,83] Higher rates of transmission were observed among donor and recipient married couples (38% transmission rate),[42] and in a crowded research hut in Antarctica (88% to 100% transmission rate).[104] Transmission of natural colds in a more spacious Antarctic hut occurred at a relatively low rate (~1% per day among 200 inhabitants), and it was notable that transmission rates were similar among long-term residents and recent arrivals to the research station.[248] In clinical studies that reproduced the close contact of the studies in Antarctica, the best predictor of transmission of a cold from a donor to a seronegative recipient, was the duration of exposure

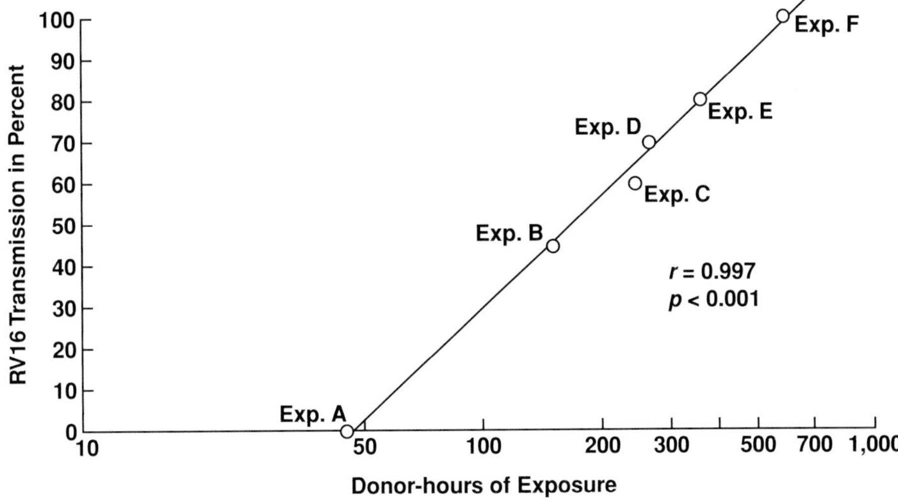

FIGURE 18.10. Relationship between the exposure and transmission of human rhinovirus (HRV)-A16. A series of experiments (A–F) was conducted in which donors with severe experimentally induced colds (HRV-A16) were housed with seronegative recipients for varying lengths of time. The groups were housed in a clinical research unit from 5 to 79 hours, and samples of nasal lavage fluid were obtained for 10 days and analyzed for viral shedding. One donor-hour of exposure (DHE) was defined as exposure to one infected donor for 1 hour. There was a straight-line relationship between the logarithm of DHE and the risk of HRV transmission. (From Meschievitz CK, Schultz SB, Dick EC. A model for obtaining predictable natural transmission of rhinoviruses in human volunteers. *J Infect Dis* 1984;150:195–201, with permission.)

(Fig. 18.10).[165] In general, factors that promote transmission include young age, symptomatic illness, crowding, high-level viral shedding from the index case, and seronegativity of the recipient.[124,172]

Prevalence and Seroepidemiology

HRV infections occur year round, with increased prevalence in the fall and spring (Fig. 18.11).[66,157,171,257] The increased prevalence in the fall has led to speculation that school-based transmission among children may drive this trend.[126] HRV infections continue during the wintertime, but account for less than 50% of infections during this period of time due to the plethora of other respiratory viruses found at this time of year. The prevalence of HRV infections increases again in the spring, and is lowest in the summertime. Overall, HRV infections account for about half of common cold infections over the entire year, and more than 80% of infections during peak seasons in the spring and fall HRV.

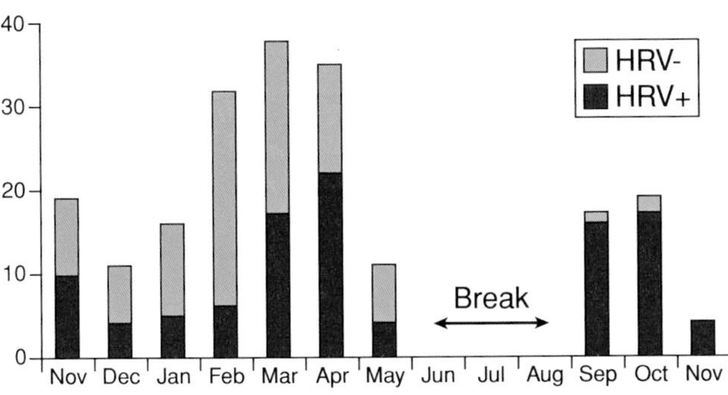

FIGURE 18.11. Seasonality of human rhinovirus (HRV) infections. Between October 1994 and November 1995, 200 young adults (mean age 24 years, mostly university students) were followed for the occurrence of common cold symptoms. Nasopharyngeal aspirates obtained during periods of illness were analyzed by polymerase chain reaction (PCR) for rhinoviruses and other respiratory viruses. The graph depicts the monthly occurrence of upper respiratory illnesses, and illnesses that were positive for HRV by PCR-based diagnostics are indicated by the blue bars. Data from.[157]

More than 20 types of HRV can circulate within a community at any given period of time, and the composition of HRV types in a single community changes almost completely from season to season and year to year.[170,184] Some studies have reported species-specific patterns of HRV prevalence,[166,184] but because the range of viruses differs markedly with season and location, several years of data will be necessary to confirm these patterns.

Serologic responses to the various rhinovirus types can be detected in infants, and the number of serotypes to which antibodies are present increased throughout childhood and adolescence.[80,172] The prevalence of serotype-specific antibodies peaks in young adults (mean percent positive = 60%), and remains at 40% to 50% throughout adulthood. Type-specific antibody in the same individual can persist at relatively stable levels for years.[229]

Epidemiologic studies of HRV prevalence are best conducted with molecular diagnostics because of difficulties in culturing these viruses (especially the C species viruses). Serologic tests can be performed for culturable viruses, but due to the large number of serotypes, antibody responses are measured mainly in experimental inoculation studies performed with a single serotype.[84,234]

Genetic Diversity of Virus

As might be predicted from the original HRV typing system, a large degree of sequence diversity among the HRVs manifests as amino acid changes in capsid surface regions mapped as neutralizing immunogenic epitopes (Nims). Completion of the full cohort of HRV-A&B sequences identified extensive evidence for historic recombination among species clades (Fig. 18.12). Surprisingly, these recombinants had not exchanged capsid regions. The most common trades included the 5′ UTR, primarily upstream of the IRES, or less frequently, fragments from P2-P3 regions. Recent HRV sequencing from multiple field isolates confirmed this idea, showing clearly

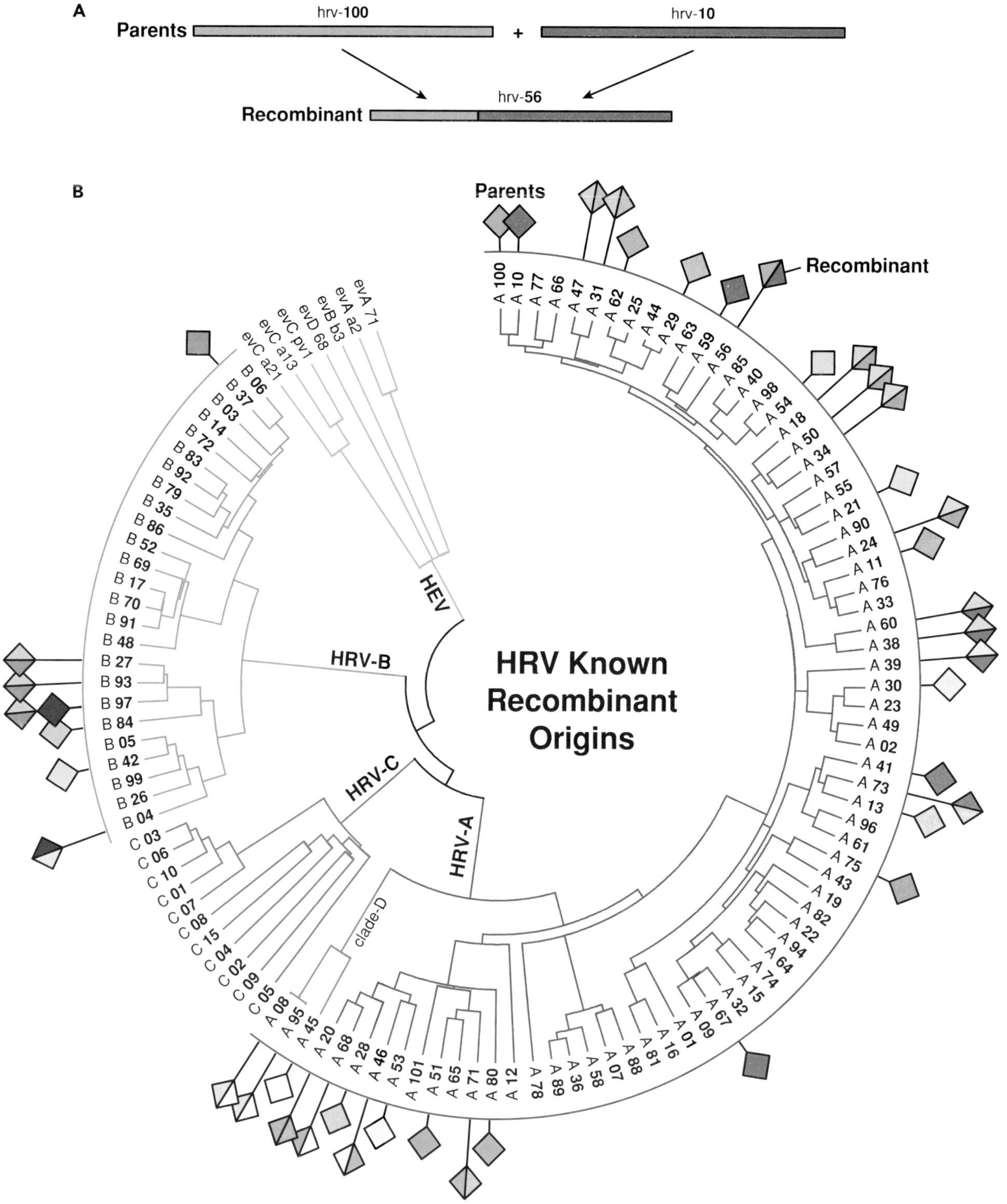

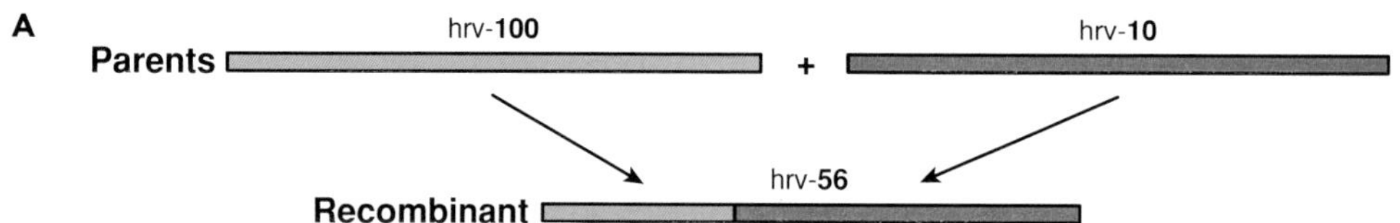

FIGURE 18.12. Recombinant origins for many human rhinovirus (HRV). A&B were uncovered by genome sequencing.[186] Parents (solid boxes) or progeny (two-color boxes) are founders of many clades.

that the HRV-A and HRV-C frequently recombine, and when they do, they exchange not the expected capsid Nims, but 5′ UTR regions, including the pyrimidine-rich tracts, and their respective 2A protease genes.[107,164] Comparative 2A work is underway to document why evolution apparently favors these particular recombinants. Possibly, divergent protease specificities may help these viruses regulate the overall cell response to infection.

Picornavirus polymerases have a high error rate, estimated at 10^{-3} to 10^{-4} errors/nucleotide/cycle of replication. As a result, HRV types exist as quasispecies populations. Analysis of 34 full HRV sequences of prototype strains demonstrated that the HRV genome as a whole is under purifying selective pressure, with focal areas of diversifying pressure at antigenic sites in the structural genes, and in the 3C protease and 3D polymerase.[133] Mutation rates have also been determined for HRV-A39 after experimental inoculation.[38] The calculated mutation rate after 5 days of replication *in vivo* was 3.4×10^{-4} mutations/nucleotides over the whole ORF, and specific hypervariable mutation sites were located within VP1, VP2, VP3, 2C, and 3C sequences.[38]

Clinical Features

Experimental inoculation studies have enabled detailed observations of the time course of clinical manifestations of HRV infection.[21,42,49,54,56,104,165] Following inoculation with virus, the first signs of illness are usually sore or scratchy throat with an onset as soon as 16 hours postinoculation, followed by malaise and rhinitis. The first nasal symptoms are rhinorrhea, which usually begins with a watery discharge. During the peak of the cold, the discharge becomes mucoid or purulent, and is accompanied by nasal congestion, cough, and headache. Low grade fevers can occur in infected children, and are uncommon among adults with HRV infections. The latent period after infection is generally 1 to 2 days, and peak symptoms generally occur between 2 and 4 days following inoculation. Most colds are either over or are clearly subsiding within one week; cough and nasal symptoms that persist for two weeks or longer suggest either secondary bacterial sinusitis,[221] or else a second infection with a different virus.[119] There are few symptoms to differentiate HRV illnesses from those caused from other viruses. Studies of adults indicate that HRV may be more likely to present with sore throat, have prominent nasal symptoms in most individuals, and are less likely to be associated with fever.[12]

HRV can also cause infections of the middle ear, sinuses, and lower airways. Eustation tube dysfunction occurs in about half of experimentally induced or naturally occurring HRV infections.[25,160,173] Studies of natural colds also link detection of HRVs in the nasal secretions or middle ear fluid to otitis media (OM).[9,29,32,196,211,227,252] A prospective one-year study of the role of viral URI in OM enrolled 294 children between the ages of 6 months and 3 years, and the viruses most often detected were HRV and adenoviruses (27% of OM for each virus).[32] Approximately one third of HRV infections were complicated by acute OM, and another 20% of cases had asymptomatic middle ear effusions. Another recent longitudinal study prospectively sampled nasal secretions of 1- to 5-year-old children and siblings at the onset of either cold or otologic symptoms.[5] HRV infection was detected at least once in 70% of the children, and 44% of these infections were associated with either OM with effusion or acute OM.

To investigate effects of HRV on the paranasal sinuses, Gwaltney and colleagues[85] performed sinus computerized tomography (CT) scans during the peak symptom period following experimental HRV inoculation of 31 adults, and during the acute cold 27 subjects (87%) had swelling and or mucosal thickening and fluid collection in one or both of the maxillary sinuses (Fig. 18.13). A subset of the study subjects had repeat scans two weeks later, and these abnormalities had spontaneously subsided in 79%. Likewise, Puhakka et al.[203] tracked findings on serial plain radiographs in individuals with naturally acquired common colds, and found that 38% developed mucosal thickening and either air fluid levels or opacification of the sinuses on day 7 of the cold. These abnormalities resolved without treatment on follow-up films obtained on day 21. Together, these findings provide evidence that HRV infections can cause acute sinusitis. Whether the illness is caused by HRV or a combination or HRV plus bacteria has not been resolved, but an important clinical point is that the illness subsided without antibiotic treatment.

In infants, HRV can cause bronchiolitis, which is a syndrome consisting of upper airway symptoms that progress to severe cough, wheezing, and tachypnea. In severe cases, significant air trapping and hypoventilation can lead to hypoxia

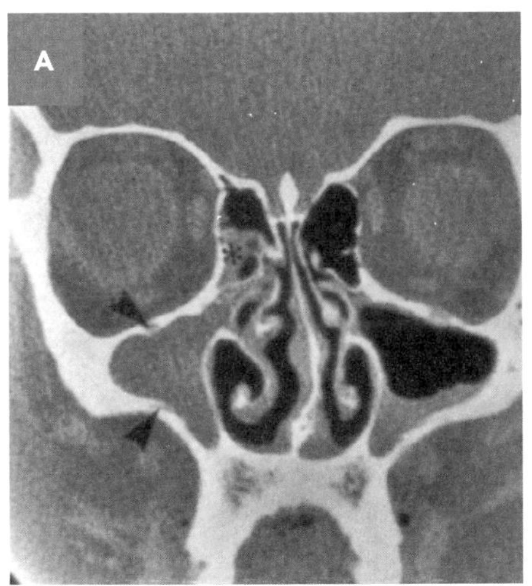

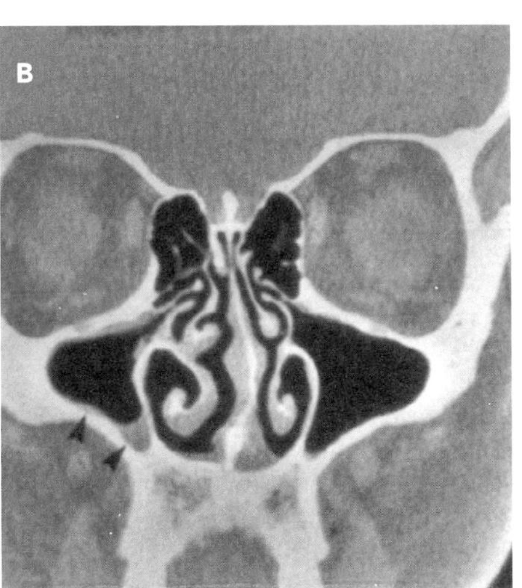

FIGURE 18.13. Computerized tomography (CT) scans during an experimentally induced human rhinovirus (HRV) infection. The initial scan obtained on day 4 postinoculation **(A)** shows bilateral effusions in the maxillary sinuses (*arrows*) and abnormalities in the right ethmoid sinuses (*asterisk*). The follow-up scan on day 13 of the illness **(B)** shows some residual abnormality of the right maxillary sinus (*arrows*). (From Gwaltney JM, Jr, Phillips CD, Miller RD, et al. Computed tomographic study of the common cold. *N Engl J Med* 1994;330:25–30, with permission © Massachusetts Medical Society.)

and need for hospitalization for supportive care. HRV is second only to respiratory syncytial virus as a cause for bronchiolitis in infants.[26,115,121,122,149,169,218] In patients with chronic asthma, HRV infections often begin with typical cold symptoms and then progress to asthma exacerbations that include severe cough, wheezing, shortness of breath, and in severe cases, hypoxia. Similar exacerbations of chronic respiratory symptoms also occur in patients with cystic fibrosis or chronic obstructive pulmonary disease (COPD).[35,222,249,258]

Diagnosis

Differential

HRV infections cause respiratory symptoms that are quite similar to those caused by other respiratory viruses. Compared to influenza, HRV is less likely to cause fever, myalgia, and headache. In general, signs and symptoms of rhinitis are prominent, but there are few true differentiating features. The spring and fall peaks in HRV epidemiology follow the same general pattern as hay fever in many geographic locations. Differentiation of common cold and allergy symptoms can be difficult, but there are some differences in symptom profiles. Compared to respiratory allergies, HRV infections are of shorter duration, are more likely to cause sore throat, and are less likely to cause nasal and ocular pruritus.

Laboratory

Virus Isolation and Identification

Tissue culture is a relatively insensitive method for HRV detection. Fetal lung fibroblast cells (WI-38, MRC-5, and Wis.L cells) or HRV-sensitive lines of HeLa cells are commonly used for HRV detection. Notably, HRV-C viruses cannot be cultured in standard cell lines, which lack the receptor to bind C species viruses, but have been propagated in organ cultures of sinus epithelium.[23] Typing of HRV-A and HRV-B species isolates is possible using specific antisera.

HRV detection is greatly improved through the use of RT-PCR[67,111,147] or other molecular techniques,[51,133] which are available mainly through research laboratories. The 5′ untranslated region contains several highly conserved regions that are usually targeted for primer design (Fig. 18.14). Because HRV-C's do not grow in standard tissue culture conditions, partial genomic sequencing has been used to classify these viruses into "types".[216] The regions usually targeted for genotyping are the 5′ UTR, VP2-4, or VP1. Sequences in the capsid protein coding region are more variable, which helps to distinguish genotypes but also complicates the design of broadly applicable primers. Higher rates of success (close to 100%) have been achieved by targeting the 5′ UTR.[148] Classification based on partial sequences must be considered as tentative, since recombination among HRV can occur.[186]

Nasopharyngeal lavage specimens or swabs are the best specimens for HRV detection, and yields are lower from throat swabs.[165,224] A "nose-blow" technique has been used to obtain nasal secretions for clinical research protocols using PCR-based diagnostics with good recovery rates.[95,184,197] Viral transport medium containing a protein source such as gelatin or albumin helps to stabilize the viral capsid for best results with tissue culture or molecular techniques. Nasal swabs obtained at home and mailed to the laboratory also provide specimens suitable for analysis by molecular techniques.[191]

Prevention and Control

The cure for the common cold remains enigmatic. Many approaches have been explored, including nutritional supplements, immune modulators, antiviral agents, and mediator antagonists to block specific common cold symptoms.[232] Vitamin C has long been touted for common cold treatment; however, a meta-analysis of common cold treatment studies found no significant effects on either prevention or treatment.[55] A Cochrane review of clinical studies found evidence that zinc lozenges reduce common cold duration, but have significant side effects including bad taste and nausea.[219] Topical zinc was marketed as a homeopathic treatment for colds, but was taken off the market due to association with anosmia.[3] Large-scale trials of Echinacea have provided no evidence of efficacy.[15,233] There is evidence that warm drinks, as recommended for generations, can provide symptomatic relief from malaise and nasal symptoms without troublesome side effects.[209]

Improved knowledge of HRV molecular virology has led to several attempts to develop antivirals. IFN-α has antiviral effects *in vitro* and shortens the duration and severity of colds, but topical application led to nasal irritation and bleeding.[63,92,94] Anti-ICAM-1 and soluble ICAM-1 were developed to prevent binding of major group viruses to their receptor.[27,159,183] Capsid

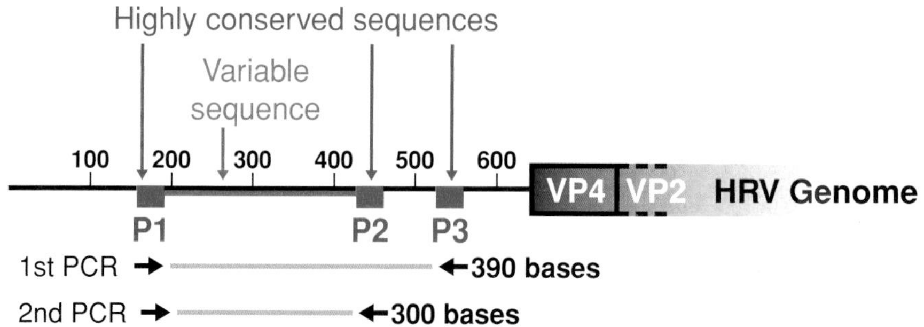

FIGURE 18.14. Selection of primers for polymerase chain reaction (PCR)–based diagnostic tests for human rhinovirus (HRV) infection. The most conserved sites in the HRV genome are in the 5′ untranslated region in the area of stem loop structures that bind ribosomal proteins. These sites are targeted for primer design (P1, P2, P3) that can be used for single or nested reverse-transcriptase PCR. (Figure courtesy of Wai Ming Lee, PhD, University of Wisconsin-Madison.)

binding agents that bind to the VP1 pocket and inhibit viral binding and/or uncoating[7,213,234] have shown modest antiviral effects and efficacy in clinical trials.[93,95] An inhibitor to the 3C protease (rupintrivir) also showed broad anti-HRV activity *in vitro* and efficacy in clinical trials.[96] Unfortunately, these antiviral approaches have not so far led to development of a clinically useful medication. The molecules tested to date have been limited by combinations of modest efficacy, side effects, and/or drug interactions.[232]

Medications targeting specific symptoms can be helpful in relieving some aspects of the common cold. Examples include use of decongestants and topical ipratropium for relief of congestion and rhinorrhea, respectively.[59] Cough syrups are ineffective. Notably, marketing of combination cough and cold medications to children has been stopped by the U.S. Food and Drug Administration (FDA) due to reports of toxicity with overdoses, and even a small number of children receiving standard doses of these medications. A recent study suggests that vapor rub (petroleum jelly with aromatic oils) may relieve common cold symptoms, perhaps by stimulation of ion channels.[189]

Perspective

The development of molecular diagnostic tests for HRV has led to a better appreciation of their role in respiratory illnesses, especially with respect to lower respiratory illness in young children and patients with chronic lung diseases. Findings from recent studies underscore the ubiquitous nature of HRV infections, and at the same time have led to some caution in interpretation of viral detection due to high rates of asymptomatic illness. That HRV is linked to a full spectrum of respiratory illness also raises questions about the nature of factors that modify illness severity. Identification of environmental and personal determinants of illness severity could provide new preventive strategies, and this is especially important for high risk populations.

Another revelation for common cold researchers was the discovery of the HRV-C species in 2006. After a hiatus of almost 20 years following the cataloguing of what most virologists considered to be the final HRV serotypes, clinical studies utilizing molecular diagnostics led to the discovery of another estimated 50 to 60 HRV types. There is growing evidence that HRV-C viruses may be more likely than other species to cause lower respiratory illness in infants and children, and acute exacerbations of asthma.

Finally, the cure for the common cold remains elusive. After some initial failures took the wind out of the sails of these efforts, the recognition that HRV infections are an important cause of lower respiratory illnesses has generated renewed interest in this effort. Recent advances in understanding the molecular pathogenesis of HRV illnesses, including HRV-C, provide reason for renewed optimism that this goal will be achieved.

REFERENCES

All cited references are available in the e-book.

4. Alper CM, Doyle WJ, Skoner DP, et al. Prechallenge antibodies: moderators of infection rate, signs, and symptoms in adults experimentally challenged with rhinovirus type 39. *Laryngoscope* 1996;106:1298–1305.
5. Alper CM, Winther B, Mandel EM, et al. Rate of concurrent otitis media in upper respiratory tract infections with specific viruses. *Arch Otolaryngol Head Neck Surg* 2009;135:17–21.
6. Amineva SP, Aminev AG, Palmenberg AC, et al. Rhinovirus 3C protease precursors 3CD and 3CD′ localize to the nuclei of infected cells. *J Gen Virol* 2004;85:2969–2979.
7. Andries K, Dewindt B, Snoeks J, et al. Two groups of rhinoviruses revealed by a panel of antiviral compounds present sequence divergence and differential pathogenicity. *J Virol* 1990;64:1117–1123.
8. Arden KE, Mackay IM. Newly identified human rhinoviruses: molecular methods heat up the cold viruses. *Rev Med Virol* 2010;20:156–176.
9. Arola M, Ruuskanen O, Ziegler T, et al. Clinical role of respiratory virus infection in acute otitis media. *Pediatr* 1990;86:848–855.
10. Arruda E, Boyle TR, Winther B, et al. Localization of human rhinovirus replication in the upper respiratory tract by in situ hybridization. *J Infect Dis* 1995;171:1329–1333.
12. Arruda E, Pitkaranta A, Witek TJJ, et al. Frequency and natural history of rhinovirus infections in adults during autumn. *J Clin Microbiol* 1997;35:2864–2868.
13. Atmar RL, Guy E, Guntupalli KK, et al. Respiratory tract viral infections in inner-city asthmatic adults. *Arch Int Med* 1998;158:2453–2459.
14. Atzl I, Helms R. A short history of the common cold. In: Eccles R, ed. *Common Cold*. Birkhauser Verlag: Basel, Switzerland; 2009:1–21.
15. Barrett B, Brown R, Rakel D, et al. Echinacea for treating the common cold: a randomized trial. *Ann Intern Med* 2010;153:769–777.
16. Barrett B, Brown R, Voland R, et al. Relations among questionnaire and laboratory measures of rhinovirus infection. *Eur Respir J* 2006;28:358–363.
17. Bartlett NW, Walton RP, Edwards MR, et al. Mouse models of rhinovirus-induced disease and exacerbation of allergic airway inflammation. *Nat Med* 2008;14:199–204.
18. Beem M. Rhinovirus infections in nursery school children. *J Pediatr* 1969;74:818.
19. Binder M, Eberle F, Seitz S, et al. Molecular mechanism of signal perception and integration by the innate immune sensor retinoic acid-inducible gene-I (RIG-I). *J Biol Chem* 2011;286:27278–27287.
20. Bizzintino J, Lee WM, Laing IA, et al. Association between human rhinovirus C and severity of acute asthma in children. *Eur Respir J* 2011;37(5) 1037–1042.
22. Bochkov YA, Hanson KM, Keles S, et al. Rhinovirus-induced modulation of gene expression in bronchial epithelial cells from subjects with asthma. *Mucosal Immunol* 2010;3:69–80.
23. Bochkov YA, Palmenberg AC, Lee WM, et al. Molecular modeling, organ culture and reverse genetics for the emerging respiratory pathogen human rhinovirus C. *Nat Med* 2011;17:627–632.
24. Brockman-Schneider RA, Amineva SP, Bulat MV, et al. Serial culture of murine primary airway epithelial cells and ex vivo replication of human rhinoviruses. *J Immunol Methods* 2008;339:264–269.
26. Calvo C, Pozo F, Garcia-Garcia M, et al. Detection of new respiratory viruses in hospitalized infants with bronchiolitis: a three-year prospective study. *Acta Paediatr* 2010;99(6):883–887.
29. Chantzi FM, Papadopoulos NG, Bairamis T, et al. Human rhinoviruses in otitis media with effusion. *Pediatr Allergy Immunol* 2006;17:514–518.
30. Chauhan AJ, Inskip HM, Linaker CH, et al. Personal exposure to nitrogen dioxide (NO2) and the severity of virus-induced asthma in children. *Lancet* 2003;361:1939–1944.
31. Chen Y, Hamati E, Lee PK, et al. Rhinovirus induces airway epithelial gene expression through double-stranded RNA and IFN-dependent pathways. *Am J Respir Cell Mol Biol* 2006;34:192–203.
32. Chonmaitree T, Revai K, Grady JJ, et al. Viral upper respiratory tract infection and otitis media complication in young children. *Clin Infect Dis* 2008;46:815–823.
33. Christiansen SC, Eddleston J, Bengtson SH, et al. Experimental Rhinovirus Infection Increases Human Tissue Kallikrein Activation in Allergic Subjects. *Int Arch Allergy Immunol* 2008;147:299–304.
34. Cohen S. Psychological stress and susceptibility to upper respiratory infections. *Am J Respir Crit Care Med* 1995;152:S53–S58.
36. Contoli M, Message SD, Laza-Stanca V, et al. Role of deficient type III interferon-lambda production in asthma exacerbations. *Nat Med* 2006;12:1023–1026.
37. Cordey S, Gerlach D, Junier T, et al. The cis-acting replication elements define human enterovirus and rhinovirus species. *RNA* 2008;14:1568–1578.
38. Cordey S, Junier T, Gerlach D, et al. Rhinovirus genome evolution during experimental human infection. *PLoS One* 2010;5:e10588.

39. Corne JM, Marshall C, Smith S, et al. Frequency, severity, and duration of rhinovirus infections in asthmatic and non-asthmatic individuals: a longitudinal cohort study. *Lancet* 2002;359:831–834.
41. D'Alessio DJ, Meschievitz CK, Peterson JA, et al. Short-duration exposure and the transmission of rhinoviral colds. *J Infect Dis* 1984;150:189–194.
42. D'Alessio DJ, Peterson JA, Dick CR, et al. Transmission of experimental rhinovirus colds in volunteer married couples. *J Infect Dis* 1976;133:28–36.
43. de Gouw HW, Grünberg K, Schot R, et al. Relationship between exhaled nitric oxide and airway hyperresponsiveness following experimental rhinovirus infection in asthmatic subjects. *Eur Respir J* 1998;11:126–132.
44. De SD, Dagher H, Ghildyal R, et al. Vascular endothelial growth factor induction by rhinovirus infection. *J Med Virol* 2006;78:666–672.
45. DeMore JP, Weisshaar EH, Vrtis RF, et al. Similar colds in subjects with allergic asthma and nonatopic subjects after inoculation with rhinovirus-16. *J Allergy Clin Immunol* 2009;124:245–252.
46. Denlinger LC, Shi L, Guadarrama A, et al. Attenuated P2×7 pore function as a risk factor for virus-induced loss of asthma control. *Am J Respir Crit Care Med* 2009;179:265–270.
49. Dick EC, Jennings LC, Mink KA, et al. Aerosol transmission of rhinovirus colds. *J Infect Dis* 1987;156:442–448.
51. Dominguez SR, Briese T, Palacios G, et al. Multiplex MassTag-PCR for respiratory pathogens in pediatric nasopharyngeal washes negative by conventional diagnostic testing shows a high prevalence of viruses belonging to a newly recognized rhinovirus clade. *J Clin Virol* 2008;43: 219–222.
52. Dosanjh A. Transforming growth factor-beta expression induced by rhinovirus infection in respiratory epithelial cells. *Acta Biochim Biophys Sin (Shanghai)* 2006;38:911–914.
53. Douglas RC Jr, Couch RB, Lindgren KM. Cold doesn't affect the "common cold" in study of rhinovirus infections. *JAMA* 1967;199:29–30.
55. Douglas RM, Hemila H, Chalker E, et al. Vitamin C for preventing and treating the common cold. *Cochrane Database Syst Rev* 2007:CD000980.
56. Doyle WJ, Skoner DP, Fireman P, et al. Rhinovirus 39 infection in allergic and nonallergic subjects. *J Allergy Clin Immunol* 1992;89:968–978.
59. Eccles R, Eriksson M, Garreffa S, et al. The nasal decongestant effect of xylometazoline in the common cold. *Am J Rhinol* 2008;22:491–496.
60. Edwards MR, Hewson CA, Laza-Stanca V, et al. Protein kinase R, IkappaB kinase-beta and NF-kappaB are required for human rhinovirus induced pro-inflammatory cytokine production in bronchial epithelial cells. *Mol Immunol* 2007;44:1587–1597.
65. Fleet WF, Couch RB, Cate TR, et al. Homologous and heterologous resistance to rhinovirus common cold. *Am J Epidemiol* 1965;82:185–196.
66. Fox JP, Cooney MK, Hall CE, et al. Rhinoviruses in Seattle families, 1975–1979. *Am J Epidemiol* 1985;122:830–846.
67. Gama RE, Horsnell PR, Hughes PJ, et al. Amplification of rhinovirus specific nucleic acids from clinical samples using the polymerase chain reaction. *J Med Virol* 1989;28:73–77.
68. Garbino J, Soccal PM, Aubert JD, et al. Respiratory viruses in bronchoalveolar lavage: a hospital-based cohort study in adults. *Thorax* 2009;64: 399–404.
69. Gavala ML, Bertics PJ, Gern JE. Rhinoviruses, allergic inflammation, and asthma. *Immunol Rev* 2011;242:69–90.
70. Gentile DA, Fireman P, Skoner DP. Elevations of local leukotriene C4 levels during viral upper respiratory tract infections. *Ann Allergy Asthma Immunol* 2003;91:270–274.
72. Gern JE, Dick EC, Lee WM, et al. Rhinovirus enters but does not replicate inside monocytes and airway macrophages. *J Immunol* 1996;156: 621–627.
73. Gern JE, Galagan DM, Jarjour NN, et al. Detection of rhinovirus RNA in lower airway cells during experimentally-induced infection. *Am J Respir Crit Care Med* 1997;155:1159–1161.
74. Gern JE, Vrtis R, Grindle KA, et al. Relationship of upper and lower airway cytokines to outcome of experimental rhinovirus infection. *Am J Respir Crit Care Med* 2000;162:2226–2231.
75. Ghildyal R, Dagher H, Donninger H, et al. Rhinovirus infects primary human airway fibroblasts and induces a neutrophil chemokine and a permeability factor. *J Med Virol* 2005;75:608–615.
76. Ginde AA, Mansbach JM, Camargo CA Jr. Association between serum 25-hydroxyvitamin D level and upper respiratory tract infection in the Third National Health and Nutrition Examination Survey. *Arch Intern Med* 2009;169:384–390.
77. Green RM, Cusotvic A, Sanderson G, et al. Synergism between allergens and viruses and risk of hospital admission with asthma: case-control study. *Br Med J* 2002;324:763–766A.
79. Grünberg K, Smits HH, Timmers MC, et al. Experimental rhinovirus 16 infection. Effects on cell differentials and soluble markers in sputum in asthmatic subjects. *Am J Respir Crit Care Med* 1997;156:609–616.
81. Gwaltney JM Jr, Hendley JO. Transmission of experimental rhinovirus infection by contaminated surfaces. *Am J Epidemiol* 1982;116: 828–833.
83. Gwaltney JM Jr, Moskalski PB, Hendley JO. Hand-to-hand transmission of rhinovirus colds. *Ann Intern Med* 1978;88:463–467.
85. Gwaltney JM Jr, Phillips CD, Miller RD, et al. Computed tomographic study of the common cold. *N Engl J Med* 1994;330:25–30.
87. Hall DJ, Bates ME, Guar L, et al. The role of p38 MAPK in rhinovirus-induced monocyte chemoattractant protein-1 production by monocytic-lineage cells. *J Immunol* 2005;174:8056–8063.
89. Han TH, Chung JY, Hwang ES, et al. Detection of human rhinovirus C in children with acute lower respiratory tract infections in South Korea. *Arch Virol* 2009;154:987–991.
91. Harris JR, Racaniello VR. Changes in rhinovirus protein 2C allow efficient replication in mouse cells. *J Virol* 2003;77:4773–4780.
92. Hayden FG, Albrecht JK, Kaiser DL, et al. Prevention of natural colds by contact prophylaxis with intranasal alpha$_2$-interferon. *N Engl J Med* 1986;314:71–75.
93. Hayden FG, Coats T, Kim K, et al. Oral pleconaril treatment of picornavirus-associated viral respiratory illness in adults: efficacy and tolerability in phase II clinical trials. *Antivir Ther* 2002;7:53–65.
95. Hayden FG, Herrington DT, Coats TL, et al. Efficacy and safety of oral pleconaril for treatment of colds due to picornaviruses in adults: results of 2 double-blind, randomized, placebo-controlled trials. *Clin Infect Dis* 2003;36:1523–1532.
96. Hayden FG, Turner RB, Gwaltney JM, et al. Phase II, randomized, double-blind, placebo-controlled studies of ruprintrivir nasal spray 2-percent suspension for prevention and treatment of experimentally induced rhinovirus colds in healthy volunteers. *Antimicrob Agents Chemother* 2003;47: 3907–3916.
97. Hendley JO. The host response, not the virus, causes the symptoms of the common cold. *Clin Infect Dis* 1998;26:847–848.
99. Hewson CA, Haas JJ, Bartlett NW, et al. Rhinovirus induces MUC5AC in a human infection model and in vitro via NF-kappaB and EGFR pathways. *Eur Respir J* 2010;36:1425–1435.
100. Heymann PW, Carper HT, Murphy DD, et al. Viral infections in relation to age, atopy, and season of admission among children hospitalized for wheezing. *J Allergy Clin Immunol* 2004;114:239–247.
102. Hicks LA, Shepard CW, Britz PH, et al. Two outbreaks of severe respiratory disease in nursing homes associated with rhinovirus. *J Am Geriatr Soc* 2006;54:284–289.
104. Holmes MJ, Reed SE, Stott EJ, et al. Studies of experimental rhinovirus type 2 infections in polar isolation and in England. *J Hyg (Lond)* 1976;76: 379–393.
106. Horn MEC, Reed SE, Taylor P. Role of viruses and bacteria in acute wheezy bronchitis in childhood: a study of sputum. *Arch Dis Child* 1979; 54:587–592.
107. Huang T, Wang W, Bessaud M, et al. Evidence of recombination and genetic diversity in human rhinoviruses in children with acute respiratory infection. *PLoS One* 2009;4:e6355.
110. Igarashi Y, Skoner DP, Doyle WJ, et al. Analysis of nasal secretions during experimental rhinovirus upper respiratory infections. *J Allergy Clin Immunol* 1993;92:722–731.
111. Ireland DC, Kent J, Nicholson KG. Improved detection of rhinoviruses in nasal and throat swabs by seminested RT-PCR. *J Med Virol* 1993;40: 96–101.
112. Ison MG, Hayden FG, Kaiser L, et al. Rhinovirus infections in hematopoietic stem cell transplant recipients with pneumonia. *Clin Infect Dis* 2003;36:1139–1143.
113. Jackson DJ, Gangnon RE, Evans MD, et al. Wheezing rhinovirus illnesses in early life predict asthma development in high-risk children. *Am J Respir Crit Care Med* 2008;178:667–672.
115. Jacques J, Bouscambert-Duchamp M, Moret H, et al. Association of respiratory picornaviruses with acute bronchiolitis in French infants. *J Clin Virol* 2006;35:463–466.

116. Jakiela B, Brockman-Schneider R, Amineva S, et al. Basal cells of differentiated bronchial epithelium are more susceptible to rhinovirus infection. *Am J Respir Cell Mol Biol* 2008;38:517–523.
117. Jang YJ, Kwon HJ, Park HW, et al. Detection of rhinovirus in turbinate epithelial cells of chronic sinusitis. *Am J Rhinol* 2006;20: 634–636.
118. Jarjour NN, Gern JE, Kelly EA, et al. The effect of an experimental rhinovirus 16 infection on bronchial lavage neutrophils. *J Allergy Clin Immunol* 2000;105:1169–1177.
119. Jartti T, Lee WM, Pappas T, et al. Serial viral infections in infants with recurrent respiratory illnesses. *Eur Respir J* 2008;32:314–320.
120. Jartti T, Lehtinen P, Vuorinen T, et al. Persistence of rhinovirus and enterovirus RNA after acute respiratory illness in children. *J Med Virol* 2004; 72:695–699.
121. Jartti T, Lehtinen P, Vuorinen T, et al. Respiratory picornaviruses and respiratory syncytial virus as causative agents of acute expiratory wheezing in children. *Emerg Infect Dis* 2004;10:1095–1101.
122. Jartti T, Lehtinen P, Vuorinen T, et al. Bronchiolitis: age and previous wheezing episodes are linked to viral etiology and atopic characteristics. *Pediatr Infect Dis J* 2009;28:311–317.
123. Jartti T, Paul-Anttila M, Lehtinen P, et al. Systemic T-helper and T-regulatory cell type cytokine responses in rhinovirus vs. respiratory syncytial virus induced early wheezing: an observational study. *Respir Res* 2009; 10:85.
125. Johnston NW, Johnston SL, Duncan JM, et al. The September epidemic of asthma exacerbations in children: a search for etiology. *J Allergy Clin Immunol* 2005;115:132–138.
126. Johnston NW, Johnston SL, Norman GR, et al. The September epidemic of asthma hospitalization: school children as disease vectors. *J Allergy Clin Immunol* 2006;117:557–562.
128. Johnston SL, Pattemore PK, Sanderson G, et al. The relationship between upper respiratory infections and hospital admissions for asthma: a time trend analysis. *Am J Respir Crit Care Med* 1996;154: 654–660.
129. Johnston SL, Pattemore PK, Sanderson G, et al. Community study of role of viral infections in exacerbations of asthma in 9–11 year old children. *BMJ* 1995;310:1225–1229.
130. Kainulainen L, Vuorinen T, Rantakokko-Jalava K, et al. Recurrent and persistent respiratory tract viral infections in patients with primary hypogammaglobulinemia. *J Allergy Clin Immunol* 2010;126:120–126.
131. Khaitov MR, Laza-Stanca V, Edwards MR, et al. Respiratory virus induction of alpha-, beta- and lambda-interferons in bronchial epithelial cells and peripheral blood mononuclear cells. *Allergy* 2009;64: 375–386.
132. Kim J, Sanders SP, Siekierski ES, et al. Role of NF-kappa B in cytokine production induced from human airway epithelial cells by rhinovirus infection. *J Immunol* 2000;165:3384–3392.
133. Kistler AL, Webster DR, Rouskin S, et al. Genome-wide diversity and selective pressure in the human rhinovirus. *Virol J* 2007;4:40.
134. Kloepfer KM, DeMore JP, Vrtis RF, et al. Effects of montelukast on patients with asthma after experimental inoculation with human rhinovirus 16. *Ann Allergy Asthma Immunol* 2011;106:252–257.
135. Konno S, Grindle KA, Lee WM, et al. Interferon-γ enhances rhinovirus-induced RANTES secretion in human airway epithelial cells. *Am J Respir Cell Mol Biol* 2002;26:594–601.
136. Korpi-Steiner NL, Bates ME, Lee WM, et al. Human rhinovirus induces robust IP-10 release by monocytic cells, which is independent of viral replication but linked to type I interferon receptor ligation and STAT1 activation. *J Leukoc Biol* 2006;80:1364–1374.
137. Korpi-Steiner NL, Valkenaar SM, Bates ME, et al. Human monocytic cells direct the robust release of CXCL10 by bronchial epithelial cells during rhinovirus infection. *Clin Exp Allergy* 2010;40:1203–1213.
138. Kotaniemi-Syrjanen A, Vainionpaa R, Reijonen TM, et al. Rhinovirus-induced wheezing in infancy–the first sign of childhood asthma? *J Allergy Clin Immunol* 2003;111:66–71.
140. Kuo C, Lim S, King NJ, et al. Rhinovirus infection induces expression of airway remodelling factors in vitro and in vivo. *Respirology* 2011;16: 367–377.
141. Kusel MM, de Klerk NH, Holt PG, et al. Role of respiratory viruses in acute upper and lower respiratory tract illness in the first year of life: a birth cohort study. *Pediatr Infect Dis J* 2006;25:680–686.
142. Kusel MM, de Klerk NH, Kebadze T, et al. Early-life respiratory viral infections, atopic sensitization, and risk of subsequent development of persistent asthma. *J Allergy Clin Immunol* 2007;119:1105–1110.
143. Lachowicz-Scroggins ME, Boushey HA, Finkbeiner WE, et al. Interleukin-13 induced mucous metaplasia increases susceptibility of human airway epithelium to rhinovirus infection. *Am J Respir Cell Mol Biol* 2010; 43:652–661.
144. Lau C, Wang X, Song L, et al. Syk associates with clathrin and mediates phosphatidylinositol 3-kinase activation during human rhinovirus internalization. *J Immunol* 2008;180:870–880.
145. Lau SK, Yip CC, Tsoi HW, et al. Clinical features and complete genome characterization of a distinct human rhinovirus (HRV) genetic cluster, probably representing a previously undetected HRV species, HRV-C, associated with acute respiratory illness in children. *J Clin Microbiol* 2007;45:3655–3664.
146. Laza-Stanca V, Stanciu LA, Message SD, et al. Rhinovirus replication in human macrophages induces NF-kappaB-dependent tumor necrosis factor alpha production. *J Virol* 2006;80:8248–8258.
147. Lee WM, Grindle KA, Pappas TE, et al. A high-throughput, sensitive and accurate multiplex PCR-microsphere flow cytometry system for large-scale comprehensive detection of respiratory viruses. *J Clin Microbiol* 2007;45:2626–2634.
148. Lee WM, Kiesner C, Pappas T, et al. A diverse group of previously unrecognized human rhinoviruses are common causes of respiratory illnesses in infants. *PLoS One* 2007;2:e966.
149. Legg JP, Warner JA, Johnston SL, et al. Frequency of detection of picornaviruses and seven other respiratory pathogens in infants. *Pediatr Infect Dis J* 2005;24:611–616.
150. Lemanske RF Jr, Jackson DJ, Gangnon RE, et al. Rhinovirus illnesses during infancy predict subsequent childhood wheezing. *J Allergy Clin Immunol* 2005;116:571–577.
153. Linsuwanon P, Payungporn S, Samransamruajkit R, et al. High prevalence of human rhinovirus C infection in Thai children with acute lower respiratory tract disease. *J Infect* 2009;59:115–121
154. Lopez-Souza N, Dolganov G, Dubin R, et al. Resistance of differentiated human airway epithelium to infection by rhinovirus. *Am J Physiol Lung Cell Mol Physiol* 2004;286:L373–L381.
155. Lopez-Souza N, Favoreto S, Wong H, et al. In vitro susceptibility to rhinovirus infection is greater for bronchial than for nasal airway epithelial cells in human subjects. *J Allergy Clin Immunol* 2009;123: 1384–1390.
156. Mackay IM. Human rhinoviruses: the cold wars resume. *J Clin Virol* 2008;42:297–320.
157. Makela MJ, Puhakka T, Ruuskanen O, et al. Viruses and bacteria in the etiology of the common cold. *J Clin Microbiol* 1998;36: 539–542.
158. Malmstrom K, Pitkaranta A, Carpen O, et al. Human rhinovirus in bronchial epithelium of infants with recurrent respiratory symptoms. *J Allergy Clin Immunol* 2006;118:591–596.
161. McErlean P, Shackelton LA, Andrews E, et al. Distinguishing molecular features and clinical characteristics of a putative new rhinovirus species, human rhinovirus C (HRV C). *PLoS One* 2008;3:e1847.
162. McErlean P, Shackelton LA, Lambert SB, et al. Characterisation of a newly identified human rhinovirus, HRV-QPM, discovered in infants with bronchiolitis. *J Clin Virol* 2007;39:67–75.
163. McFadden ER Jr, Pichurko BM, Bowman HF, et al. Thermal mapping of the airways in humans. *J Appl Physiol* 1985;58:564–570.
164. McIntyre CL, William Leitch EC, Savolainen-Kopra C, et al. Analysis of genetic diversity and sites of recombination in human rhinovirus species C. *J Virol* 2010;84:10297–10310.
165. Meschievitz CK, Schultz SB, Dick EC. A model for obtaining predictable natural transmission of rhinoviruses in human volunteers. *J Infect Dis* 1984;150:195–201.
166. Miller EK, Edwards KM, Weinberg GA, et al. A novel group of rhinoviruses is associated with asthma hospitalizations. *J Allergy Clin Immunol* 2009;123:98–104.
167. Miller EK, Lu X, Erdman DD, et al. Rhinovirus-associated hospitalizations in young children. *J Infect Dis* 2007;195:773–781.
168. Miller EK, Williams JV, Gebretsadik T, et al. Host and viral factors associated with severity of human rhinovirus-associated infant respiratory tract illness. *J Allergy Clin Immunol* 2011;127:883–891.

169. Miron D, Srugo I, Kra-Oz Z, et al. Sole pathogen in acute bronchiolitis: is there a role for other organisms apart from respiratory syncytial virus? *Pediatr Infect Dis J* 2010;29:e7–e10.
170. Monto AS, Bryan ER, Ohmit S. Rhinovirus infections in Tecumseh, Michigan: Frequency of illness and number of serotypes. *J Infect Dis* 1987;156:43–49.
173. Moody SA, Alper CM, Doyle WJ. Daily tympanometry in children during the cold season: association of otitis media with upper respiratory tract infections. *Int J Pediatr Otorhinolaryngol* 1998;45:143–150.
174. Mosser AG, Brockman-Schneider RA, Amineva SP, et al. Similar frequency of rhinovirus-infectable cells in upper and lower airway epithelium. *J Infect Dis* 2002;185:734–743.
175. Mosser AG, Vrtis R, Burchell L, et al. Quantitative and qualitative analysis of rhinovirus infection in bronchial tissues. *Am J Respir Crit Care Med* 2005;171:645–651.
176. Muether PS, Gwaltney JM Jr. Variant effect of first- and second-generation antihistamines as clues to their mechanism of action on the sneeze reflex in the common cold. *Clin Infect Dis* 2001;33:1483–1488.
177. Murray CS, Poletti G, Kebadze T, et al. Study of modifiable risk factors for asthma exacerbations: virus infection and allergen exposure increase the risk of asthma hospital admissions in children. *Thorax* 2006;61:376–382.
178. Nagarkar DR, Bowman ER, Schneider D, et al. Rhinovirus infection of allergen-sensitized and -challenged mice induces eotaxin release from functionally polarized macrophages. *J Immunol* 2010;185:2525–2535.
179. Newcomb DC, Sajjan U, Nanua S, et al. PI 3-kinase is required for rhinovirus-induced airway epithelial cell IL-8 expression. *J Biol Chem* 2005;280(44):36952–36961.
180. Newcomb DC, Sajjan US, Nagarkar DR, et al. Human rhinovirus 1B exposure induces phosphatidylinositol 3-kinase-dependent airway inflammation in mice. *Am J Respir Crit Care Med* 2008;177:1111–1121.
182. Nicholson KG, Kent J, Ireland DC. Respiratory viruses and exacerbations of asthma in adults. *BMJ* 1993;307:982–986.
184. Olenec JP, Kim WK, Lee WM, et al. Weekly monitoring of children with asthma for infections and illness during common cold seasons. *J Allergy Clin Immunol* 2010;125:1001–1006.
185. Palmenberg AC, Rathe JA, Liggett SB. Analysis of the complete genome sequences of human rhinovirus. *J Allergy Clin Immunol* 2010;125:1190–1199.
186. Palmenberg AC, Spiro D, Kuzmickas R, et al. Sequencing and analyses of all known human rhinovirus genomes reveals structure and evolution. *Science* 2009;324:55–59.
187. Papadopoulos NG, Bates PJ, Bardin PG, et al. Rhinoviruses infect the lower airways. *J Infect Dis* 2000;181:1875–1884.
188. Parry DE, Busse WW, Sukow KA, et al. Rhinovirus-induced peripheral blood mononuclear cell responses and outcome of experimental infection in allergic subjects. *J Allergy Clin Immunol* 2000;105:692–698.
189. Paul IM, Beiler JS, King TS, et al. Vapor rub, petrolatum, and no treatment for children with nocturnal cough and cold symptoms. *Pediatr* 2010;126:1092–1099.
191. Peltola V, Waris M, Osterback R, et al. Rhinovirus transmission within families with children: incidence of symptomatic and asymptomatic infections. *J Infect Dis* 2008;197:382–389.
193. Piralla A, Rovida F, Campanini G, et al. Clinical severity and molecular typing of human rhinovirus C strains during a fall outbreak affecting hospitalized patients. *J Clin Virol* 2009;45:311–317.
194. Pitkaranta A, Arruda E, Malmberg H, et al. Detection of rhinovirus in sinus brushings of patients with acute community-acquired sinusitis by reverse transcription-PCR. *J Clin Microbiol* 1997;35:1791–1793.
195. Pitkaranta A, Puhakka T, Makela MJ, et al. Detection of rhinovirus RNA in middle turbinate of patients with common colds by in situ hybridization. *J Med Virol* 2003;70:319–323.
197. Powell KR, Shorr R, Cherry JD, et al. Improved method for collection of nasal mucus. *J Infect Dis* 1977;136:109–111.
200. Proud D, Naclerio RM, Gwaltney JM, et al. Kinins are generated in nasal secretions during natural rhinovirus colds. *J Infect Dis* 1990;161:120–123.
201. Proud D, Sanders SP, Wiehler S. Human rhinovirus infection induces airway epithelial cell production of human beta-defensin 2 both in vitro and in vivo. *J Immunol* 2004;172:4637–4645.
202. Proud D, Turner RB, Winther B, et al. Gene expression profiles during in vivo human rhinovirus infection: insights into the host response. *Am J Respir Crit Care Med* 2008;178:962–968.
203. Puhakka T, Makela MJ, Alanen A, et al. Sinusitis in the common cold. *J Allergy Clin Immunol* 1998;102:403–408.
204. Rakes GP, Arruda E, Ingram JM, et al. Rhinovirus and respiratory syncytial virus in wheezing children requiring emergency care. IgE and eosinophil analyses. *Am J Respir Crit Care Med* 1999;159:785–790.
205. Rankl C, Kienberger F, Wildling L, et al. Multiple receptors involved in human rhinovirus attachment to live cells. *Proc Natl Acad Sci U S A* 2008;105:17778–17783.
206. Rosenthal LA, Amineva SP, Szakaly RJ, et al. A rat model of picornavirus-induced airway infection and inflammation. *Virol J* 2009;6:122.
207. Sajjan U, Wang Q, Zhao Y, et al. Rhinovirus disrupts the barrier function of polarized airway epithelial cells. *Am J Respir Crit Care Med* 2008;178:1271–1281.
208. Sanders SP, Siekierski ES, Porter JD, et al. Nitric oxide inhibits rhinovirus-induced cytokine production and viral replication in a human respiratory epithelial cell line. *J Virol* 1998;72:934–942.
209. Sanu A, Eccles R. The effects of a hot drink on nasal airflow and symptoms of common cold and flu. *Rhinology* 2008;46:271–275.
211. Savolainen-Kopra C, Blomqvist S, Kilpi T, et al. Novel species of human rhinoviruses in acute otitis media. *Pediatr Infect Dis J* 2009;28:59–61.
213. Shepard DA, Heinz BA, Rueckert RR. WIN 52035–2 inhibits both attachment and eclipse of human rhinovirus 14. *J Virol* 1993;67:2245–2254.
216. Simmonds P, McIntyre C, Savolainen-Kopra C, et al. Proposals for the classification of human rhinovirus species C into genotypically assigned types. *J Gen Virol* 2010;91:2409–2419.
217. Simons E, Schroth MK, Gern JE. Analysis of tracheal secretions for rhinovirus during natural colds. *Pediatr Allergy Immunol* 2005;16:276–278.
218. Singh AM, Moore PE, Gern JE, et al. Bronchiolitis to asthma: a review and call for studies of gene-virus interactions in asthma causation. *Am J Respir Crit Care Med* 2007;175:108–119.
219. Singh M, Das RR. Zinc for the common cold. *Cochrane Database Syst Rev* 2011:CD001364.
220. Slater L, Bartlett NW, Haas JJ, et al. Co-ordinated role of TLR3, RIG-I and MDA5 in the innate response to rhinovirus in bronchial epithelium. *PLoS Pathog* 2010;6:e1001178.
222. Smyth AR, Smyth RL, Tong CYW, et al. Effect of respiratory virus infections including rhinovirus on clinical status in cystic fibrosis. *Arch Dis Child* 1995;73:117–120.
223. Spurrell JC, Wiehler S, Zaheer RS, et al. Human airway epithelial cells produce IP-10 (CXCL10) in vitro and in vivo upon rhinovirus infection. *Am J Physiol Lung Cell Mol Physiol* 2005;289:L85–L95.
224. Spyridaki IS, Christodoulou I, de BL, et al. Comparison of four nasal sampling methods for the detection of viral pathogens by RT-PCR-A GA(2)LEN project. *J Virol Methods* 2009;156:102–106.
225. Steil BP, Barton DJ. Cis-active RNA elements (CREs) and picornavirus RNA replication. *Virus Res* 2009;139:240–252.
226. Stone AA, Bovbjerg DH, Neale JM, et al. Development of common cold symptoms following experimental rhinovirus infection is related to prior stressful life events. *Behav Med* 1992;18:115–120.
228. Tapparel C, L'Huillier AG, Rougemont AL, et al. Pneumonia and pericarditis in a child with HRV-C infection: a case report. *J Clin Virol* 2009;45:157–160.
230. Teran LM, Johnston SL, Schroder JM, et al. Role of nasal interleukin-8 in neutrophil recruitment and activation in children with virus-induced asthma. *Am J Respir Crit Care Med* 1997;155:1362–1366.
232. Turner RB. New considerations in the treatment and prevention of rhinovirus infections. *Pediatr Ann* 2005;34:53–57.
233. Turner RB, Bauer R, Woelkart K, et al. An evaluation of *Echinacea angustifolia* in experimental rhinovirus infections. *N Engl J Med* 2005;353:341–348.
234. Turner RB, Dutko FJ, Goldstein NH, et al. Efficacy of oral WIN 54954 for prophylaxis of experimental rhinovirus infection. *Antimicrob Agents Chemother* 1993;37:297–300.
235. Turner RB, Weingand KW, Yeh CH, et al. Association between interleukin-8 concentration in nasal secretions and severity of symptoms of experimental rhinovirus colds. *Clin Infect Dis* 1998;26:840–846.
236. Tuthill TJ, Papadopoulos NG, Jourdan P, et al. Mouse respiratory epithelial cells support efficient replication of human rhinovirus. *J Gen Virol* 2003;84:2829–2836.

238. van der Zalm MM, Uiterwaal CS, Wilbrink B, et al. Respiratory pathogens in respiratory tract illnesses during the first year of life: a birth cohort study. *Pediatr Infect Dis J* 2009;28:472–476.
239. van der Zalm MM, Uiterwaal CS, Wilbrink B, et al. The influence of neonatal lung function on rhinovirus-associated wheeze. *Am J Respir Crit Care Med* 2011;183:262–267.
240. van der Zalm MM, van Ewijk BE, Wilbrink B, et al. Respiratory pathogens in children with and without respiratory symptoms. *J Pediatr* 2009; 154:396–400.
241. Venarske DL, Busse WW, Griffin MR, et al. The relationship of rhinovirus-associated asthma hospitalizations with inhaled corticosteroids and smoking. *J Infect Dis* 2006;193:1536–1543.
242. Vlasak M, Goesler I, Blaas D. Human rhinovirus type 89 variants use heparan sulfate proteoglycan for cell attachment. *J Virol* 2005;79: 5963–5970.
243. Vlasak M, Roivainen M, Reithmayer M, et al. The minor receptor group of human rhinovirus (HRV) includes HRV23 and HRV25, but the presence of a lysine in the VP1 HI loop is not sufficient for receptor binding. *J Virol* 2005;79:7389–7395.
244. Wang Q, Nagarkar DR, Bowman ER, et al. Role of double-stranded RNA pattern recognition receptors in rhinovirus-induced airway epithelial cell responses. *J Immunol* 2009;183:6989–6997.
245. Wang X, Lau C, Wiehler S, et al. Syk is downstream of intercellular adhesion molecule-1 and mediates human rhinovirus activation of p38 MAPK in airway epithelial cells. *J Immunol* 2006;177:6859–6870.
246. Wark PA, Bucchieri F, Johnston SL, et al. IFN-gamma-induced protein 10 is a novel biomarker of rhinovirus-induced asthma exacerbations. *J Allergy Clin Immunol* 2007;120:586–593.
247. Wark PA, Johnston SL, Bucchieri F, et al. Asthmatic bronchial epithelial cells have a deficient innate immune response to infection with rhinovirus. *J Exp Med* 2005;201:937–947.
248. Warshauer DM, Dick EC, Mandel AD, et al. Rhinovirus infections in an isolated Antarctic station: Transmission of the viruses and susceptibility of the population. *Am J Epidemiol* 1989;129:319–340.
249. Wat D, Gelder C, Hibbitts S, et al. The role of respiratory viruses in cystic fibrosis. *J Cyst Fibros* 2008;7:320–328.
250. Whiteman SC, Spiteri MA. IFN-gamma regulation of ICAM-1 receptors in bronchial epithelial cells: soluble ICAM-1 release inhibits human rhinovirus infection. *J Inflamm (Lond)* 2008;5:8.
251. Widegren H, Andersson M, Borgeat P, et al. LTB4 increases nasal neutrophil activity and conditions neutrophils to exert antiviral effects. *Respir Med* 2011;105:997–1006.
252. Winther B, Alper CM, Mandel EM, et al. Temporal relationships between colds, upper respiratory viruses detected by polymerase chain reaction, and otitis media in young children followed through a typical cold season. *Pediatr* 2007;119:1069–1075.
254. Winther B, Farr B, Thoner RB, et al. Histopathologic examination and enumeration of polymorphonuclear leukocytes in the nasal mucosa during experimental rhinovirus colds. *Acta Otolaryngol* 1984;413(suppl):19–24.
255. Winther B, Greve JM, Gwaltney JMJ, et al. Surface expression of intercellular adhesion molecule 1 on epithelial cells in the human adenoid. *J Infect Dis* 1997;176:523–525.
256. Winther B, Gwaltney JM Jr, Mygind M, et al. Sites of rhinovirus recovery after point inoculation of the upper airway. *JAMA* 1986;256:1763–1767.
257. Winther B, Hayden FG, Hendley JO. Picornavirus infections in children diagnosed by RT-PCR during longitudinal surveillance with weekly sampling: Association with symptomatic illness and effect of season. *J Med Virol* 2006;78:644–650.
258. Wiselka MJ, Kent J, Cookson JB, et al. Impact of respiratory virus infection in patients with chronic chest disease. *Epidemiol Infect* 1993;111: 337–346.
259. Wood LG, Powell H, Grissell TV, et al. Persistence of rhinovirus RNA and IP-10 gene expression after acute asthma. *Respirology* 2011;16:291–299.
260. Xatzipsalti M, Kyrana S, Tsolia M, et al. Rhinovirus viremia in children with respiratory infections. *Am J Respir Crit Care Med* 2005;172(8): 1037–1040.
262. Yuta A, Doyle WJ, Gaumond E, et al. Rhinovirus infection induces mucus hypersecretion. *Am J Physiol Lung Cell Mol Physiol* 1998;274: L1017–L1023.
263. Zaheer RS, Proud D. Human rhinovirus-induced epithelial production of CXCL10 is dependent upon IFN regulatory factor-1. *Am J Respir Cell Mol Biol* 2010;43:413–421.

CHAPTER 19

F. Blaine Hollinger • Annette Martin

Hepatitis A Virus

HISTORY

Reports of icteric disease in ancient Chinese literature, as reviewed by Zuckerman,[419] and a letter from Pope Zacharias to Archbishop St. Boniface of Mainz during the 8th century AD describing an outbreak of jaundice may refer to hepatitis A; however, it cannot be distinguished from jaundice attributable to other causes. It was not until the 17th, 18th, and 19th centuries that scattered epidemics of jaundice affecting diverse populations were recorded more frequently. The disease, which was common in military troops, was called *campaign jaundice*. In time, an infectious cause was suspected by several clinicians, especially for the milder, more contagious forms called *epidemic catarrhal jaundice*.[143] In 1912, Cockayne[54] used the term *infectious hepatitis* to describe this epidemic form of the disease, and support for a viral cause gained favor from that point forward.[260]

Epidemiologic studies and human volunteer experiments performed during and after World War II confirmed the viral cause of hepatitis A and defined its relatively short incubation period and its fecal–oral mode of transmission. These studies also demonstrated the uniqueness of this disease from *homologous serum jaundice*, another form of hepatitis having a longer incubation period.[30,153,154,205] In 1947, MacCallum[235] introduced the terms *hepatitis A* and *hepatitis B* to categorize these diseases, terms that were adopted in 1973 by the World Health Organization (WHO) Expert Committee on Viral Hepatitis.[401] Between the mid-1950s and early 1970s, the studies of Murray[270] and of Krugman et al[205,207] at the Willowbrook State School for the mentally handicapped were instrumental in further defining the seroepidemiologic relationships between hepatitis A and B that eventually led to the evaluation of new methods for the immunoprophylaxis of these diseases. One of the hepatitis viruses, designated MS-1, was transmitted primarily by the fecal–oral route. The disease was highly infectious, had a relatively short incubation period of 4 ± 2 weeks, and defined classic viral hepatitis type A. The MS-1 strain of hepatitis A virus (HAV) was later used to infect adult volunteers,[30] leading to the identification of the virus in their feces by immune electron microscopy, as reported by Feinstone et al[101] in 1973. Highly sensitive immunoassays were subsequently developed for the detection of HAV antigens and specific antibodies,[162] culminating in the development of immunoglobulin M (IgM)-specific anti-HAV tests to distinguish recent HAV infection from a previous infection.[223] In 1967, Deinhardt et al[79] provided the first evidence for propagation of HAV in small primates, leading to the subsequent recovery of the CR326 strain of human HAV from an experimentally infected *Saguinus mystax*.[252] In 1979, Provost and Hilleman[304] were successful in cultivating and serially passaging this HAV strain in cell culture—an important step that ultimately contributed to the development of a vaccine.

VIRUS CLASSIFICATION

HAV is a nonenveloped, positive-sense, single-stranded RNA virus classified within the family *Picornaviridae* that otherwise include many medically and veterinary important pathogens subclassified into 12 genera based on genotypic and serologic characterization (Fig. 19.1). HAV differs from other picornaviruses by several attributes, as reviewed by Martin and Lemon[249]: (a) HAV is resistant to high temperatures, low pH, and drugs that inactivate many picornaviruses; (b) HAV replicates very slowly and generally without cytopathic effect in cell culture; (c) nucleotide and amino acid sequences, as well as predicted sizes of several HAV proteins are dissimilar; and (d) only one serotype of HAV has been identified, and one antigenic neutralization site is immunodominant. Therefore, HAV has been classified as the type species of a separate genus—*Hepatovirus*—and is still the only identified member of this genus. One other distinct species of picornavirus found in chickens and other birds, avian encephalomyelitis virus,[251] was tentatively classified within the *Hepatovirus* genus on the basis of a close phylogenetic relationship to HAV.[351] However, based on substantial molecular divergence in several proteins and its polyprotein translation mechanism, this virus has been assigned recently to a separate new genus within the *Picornaviridae* family—the *Tremovirus* genus.

VIRUS HOST RANGE AND EXPERIMENTAL MODEL SYSTEMS

HAV infects humans and nonhuman primates. Serologic and experimental infectivity studies in nonhuman primates using acute-phase sera from HAV-infected patients have revealed that HAV can be transmitted to chimpanzees (*Pan troglodytes*)[78,82,256] and other Old World primates, such as vervet (*Chlorocebus* sp.), African green monkeys (*Cercopithecus aethiops*), rhesus and cynomolgus macaques (*Macaca mulatta* and *M. fascicularis*), as well as several species of New World primates, such as tamarins (*Saguinus* sp.), marmosets (*Callithrix* sp.), squirrel (*Saimiri* sp.), and owl monkeys (*Aotus* sp.).[18,79,165,307] Disease in nonhuman primates resembles that in humans but is usually milder.[307] There are several reports of isolation of HAV-related viruses from Old World monkeys in the wild, several of which have significant sequence variation and minor

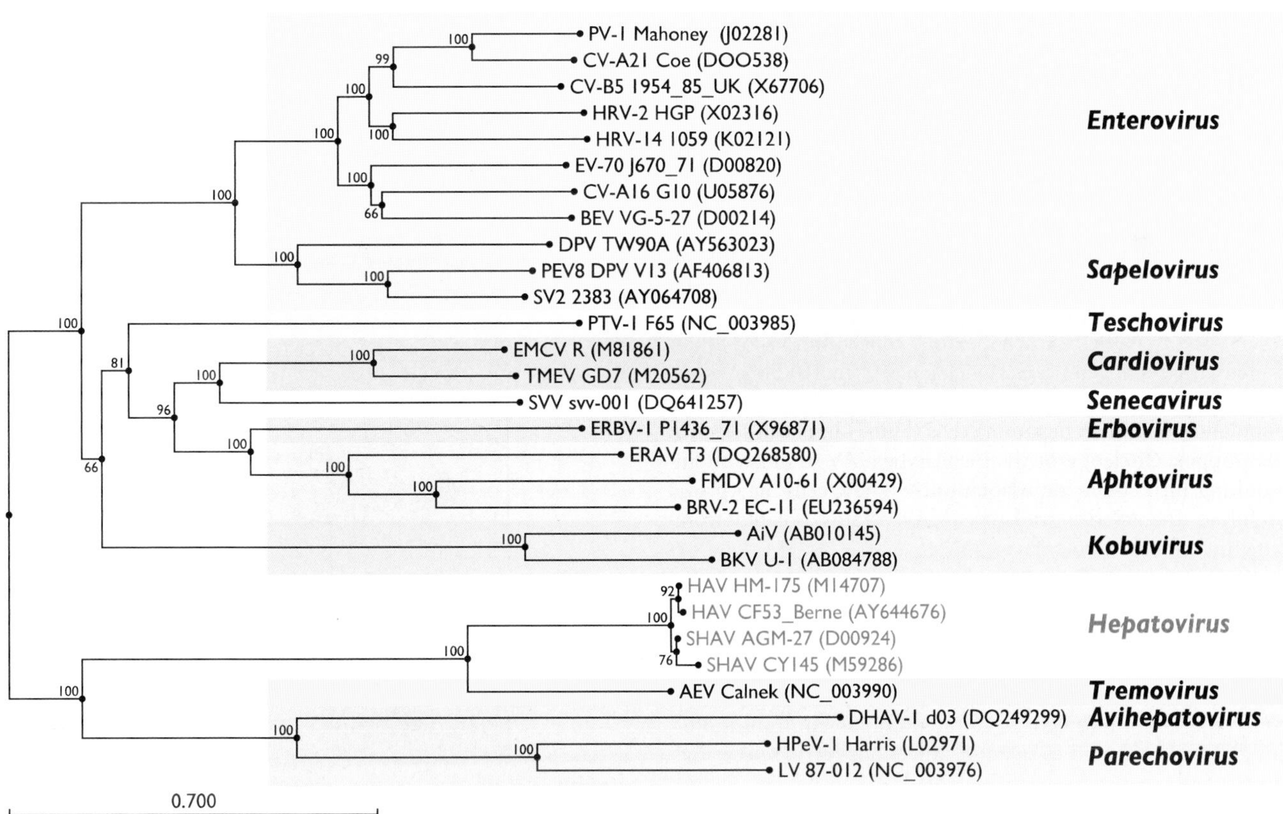

FIGURE 19.1. Phylogenetic relationship of hepatitis A virus (HAV) and simian HAV (SHAV) to representative species of other *Picornaviridae* genera. The relationship was examined by mid-pointed rooted neighbor-joining tree based on P1 (capsid) amino acid similarities using Clustal alignments (accession numbers for sequences of selected picornavirus strains are indicated in parentheses). Bootstrap values (%) are illustrated at nodes, and the genetic distance per amino acid per site is shown by the *horizontal bar*. The grouping in 12 genera is marked by *colored boxes*. HAV appears most closely related to tremoviruses (avian encephalomyelitis virus, AEV).

antigenic differences with human HAV[45,94,274,376] (see the Diversity of the Infectious Agent section). The simian virus isolated from an African green monkey caused severe hepatitis in African green monkeys, rhesus macaques, and tamarins but not in chimpanzees (although the virus replicated and the animals seroconverted).[94] Correspondingly, after 20 passages in marmosets, human HAV MS-1 was more virulent for marmosets but was attenuated for chimpanzees.[40] This suggests that host, species-specific variants may have been selected. To date, no rodent animal model has been shown to be susceptible to HAV, although experimental infection in guinea pigs resulted in virus replication in the absence of clinical disease.[166] Chimpanzees, tamarins, and marmosets have been most extensively used as animal models of HAV infection.

HAV is usually difficult to adapt and grow *in vitro.* The virus was first isolated *ex vivo* in marmoset liver explant cultures and was subsequently propagated in continuous fetal rhesus monkey kidney cells[304] and in a variety of different types of mammalian cells. Primary African green monkey kidney (AGMK) cells, primary human fibroblast cells, and continuous human diploid lung (MRC5) cells often have been used because of their suitability as potential vaccine substrates. Cell lines derived from AGMK (e.g., BS-C-1, Vero), fetal rhesus kidney (FRhK4), or human hepatoma (PLC/PRF/5) tissue also have been useful for studying virus replication and for propagating large amounts of virus.[71,106,308] Surprisingly, HAV also replicates in cells of guinea pig, porcine, or dolphin origin.[87]

Wild-type HAV strains collected from infected patients usually replicate very slowly and to relatively low titers in cultured cells, often requiring weeks or even months and blind passages to reach maximal titers. With continued *in vitro* passage, however, the virus becomes progressively adapted to growth in cell culture, replicating more rapidly and achieving higher titers.[57,59,71] During this process, the viral genome accumulates several mutations (see the Molecular Determinants of Hepatitis A Virus Adaptation to Cell Culture and Attenuation *In Vivo* section). Even when well adapted, HAV usually takes several days to weeks to reach maximal concentrations of propagated virus, achieving typical yields of 10^6 to 10^8 50% tissue culture infectious doses ($TCID_{50}$)/mL of virus. Recently, a subpopulation of human hepatoma cells (Huh7) has been selected that support efficient growth of wild-type HAV strains without requiring further genetic adaptation.[202] These cells may prove useful to characterize wild-type HAV strains isolated from patients and environmental samples.

In contrast to many other picornaviruses, HAV usually has few or no visible effects on the host cell. Thus, detection of HAV multiplication has usually required indirect methods: immunologic assays for viral antigens and hybridization or real-time polymerase chain reaction (RT-PCR) assays for HAV RNA. Radioimmunofocus or infrared fluorescent immunofocus assays can be used to quantify infectious HAV, select viral clones, and measure neutralizing anti-HAV antibodies.[66,222]

As with other positive-strand viruses, purified genomic RNA, whether extracted from virions or produced synthetically from cloned complementary DNA (cDNA) of cell culture-adapted HAV, is replication competent when transfected into permissive cultured cells.[58] Accordingly, using synthetic RNA in cell culture and also applying findings from other picornaviruses, it has been possible to elucidate several features of the HAV replication strategy.

MORPHOLOGY AND PROPERTIES OF HEPATITIS A VIRIONS

Virion Structure and Physicochemical Properties

HAV is a nonenveloped, approximately 27-nm spherical virus particle as first determined by Feinstone et al,[101] who used immune-electron microscopy and negative staining techniques on stool specimens collected from acute-phase hepatitis A patients (Fig. 19.2). Mature HAV virions purified from feces collected from infected humans or chimpanzees band at 1.32 to 1.34 g/cm^3 in cesium chloride (CsCl) and sediment at approximately 156S to 160S in neutral sucrose solutions.[342] Additional populations of viral particles with different sedimentation characteristics have been isolated from human feces and cell culture. Particles with lower density that band at about 1.27 g/cm^3 in CsCl and sediment at 70S to 80S are abundant in feces collected during early infection and probably represent empty capsids devoid of genomic RNA (also called *procapsids*) (see Fig. 19.2). Other premature or defective particles, including particles harboring capsid protein precursors, also can be observed.[26,224,342] These alternative structures are

A

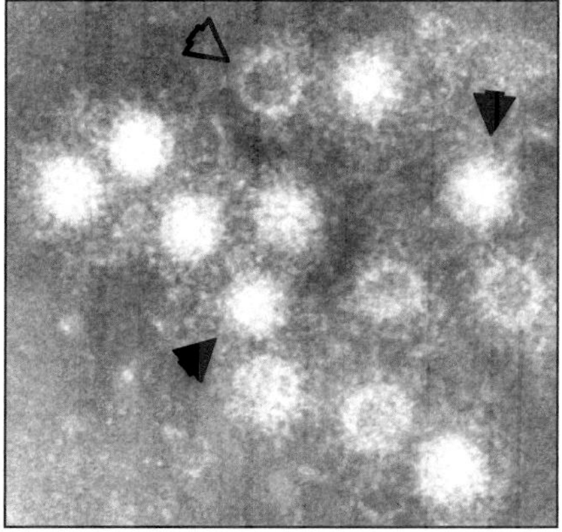

B

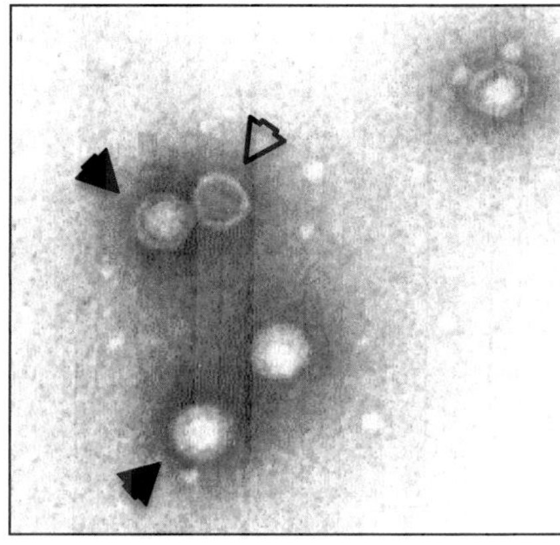

FIGURE 19.2. Hepatitis A virus (HAV) particles observed by electron microscopy. A: Immune electron micrograph of HAV particles from human stool heavily coated with and aggregated by human convalescent antibody. **B:** Negative staining showing 27- to 28-nm HAV particles with cubical symmetry purified from human stool. Both virions (*closed arrowheads*) and procapsids devoid of genomic material (*open arrowheads*) can be found. (Courtesy of Dr. Stephen M. Feinstone, Food and Drug Administration, Bethesda, MD.)

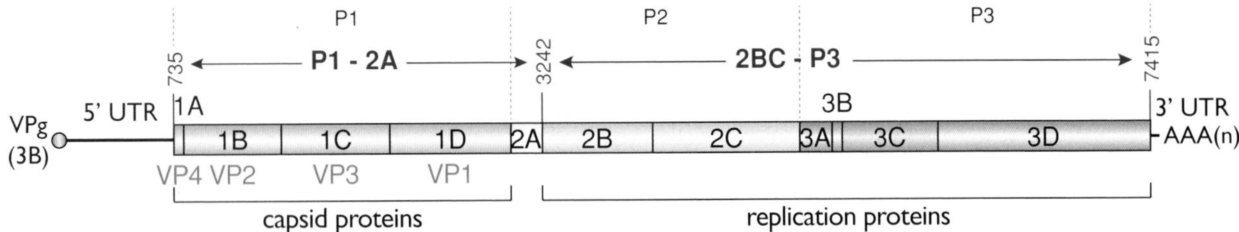

FIGURE 19.3. Hepatitis A virus (HAV) genome organization. The positive-strand RNA genome contains a single open reading frame (ORF), 5′ and 3′ untranslated regions (UTRs), is linked at its 5′ terminus to the virus-encoded protein 3B (also referred to as VPg), and is polyadenylated [AAA(n)] at its 3′ terminus. The ORF encodes capsid proteins 1A-D (also referred to as VP1-4 in the order indicated below the genome scheme; 1AB or VP4-VP2 precursor also is known as VP0), protein 2A that is involved in particle assembly as 1D-2A (VP1-2A) precursor, and proteins 2B-C and 3A-D involved in genome replication. *Dotted lines* delineate commonly termed P1, P2, and P3 coding segments in picornaviruses, whereas primary cleavage of HAV polyprotein generates P1-2A and 2BC-P3 polypeptides (which sequences are indicated by *double-headed arrows*). Numbering above the genome indicates nucleotide positions within the wild-type HM175 strain of HAV (GenBank accession number M14707).

morphologically indistinguishable from typical HAV and have the same major surface antigens.

The HAV capsid encloses the viral genome, which is a linear, single-stranded, 33S RNA molecule of positive polarity approximately 7.5 kilobases (kb) in length.[59,65,342] The viral genome encodes a single polyprotein that is subsequently cleaved primarily by the unique virus-encoded protease 3C to generate four capsid proteins (VP1-VP4) at its N-terminus and the nonstructural proteins involved in genome replication at its C-terminus (Fig. 19.3).

The HAV capsid contains 60 copies of the three major capsid proteins VP1, VP2, and VP3.[120,342] Attempts to determine the atomic structure of HAV by X-ray crystallography have not been successful, although such studies have provided high-resolution images of virus particles from several other picornaviral genera. Medium-resolution images of the HAV particle, obtained by cryo-electron microscopy (Fig. 19.4) and generated by R. H. Cheng and collaborators (personal communication, 2011), suggest that there are prominent features at the icosahedral surface of the particle around fivefold and threefold axes of symmetry but no marked depression around the fivefold axes in contrast to the canyon found in enteroviruses.[250]

Hepatitis A Virus Resistance to Physical and Chemical Agents

In common with the enteroviruses, HAV is stable at low pH.[327] It retains most of its infectivity when subjected to pH 1.0 for 2 hours at room temperature and is still infectious after 5 hours. The thermal stability of HAV, however, is considerably greater than that of other picornaviruses.[344] Incubation of the virus for at least 4 weeks at room temperature (25°C) results in only a 100-fold decrease in infectivity.[259,350] Significant loss of infectivity starts to occur with exposure at 60°C for short periods, and infectivity is destroyed almost instantaneously by heating above 85°C at neutral pH.[285,305,344]

HAV has been found to survive for days to months in experimentally contaminated fresh water, seawater, wastewater, soils, marine sediment, live oysters, and cream-filled cookies.[350] Outbreaks of hepatitis A have been reported following ingestion of partially cooked bivalve mollusks, suggesting that even steaming may be insufficient to destroy the virus in this food source. In addition, HAV infectivity is highly resistant to drying, and infectious virus has been recovered from acetone-fixed cell sheets. The virus is also highly resistant to detergents, surviving a 1% concentration of sodium dodecyl sulfate, as well as to organic solvents such as diethyl ether, chloroform, or trichlorotrifluoroethane.[294,344] Thus, solvent-detergent inactivation procedures do not reduce the infectivity of HAV, explaining why hepatitis A transmission has occasionally been associated with the administration of high purity, solvent-

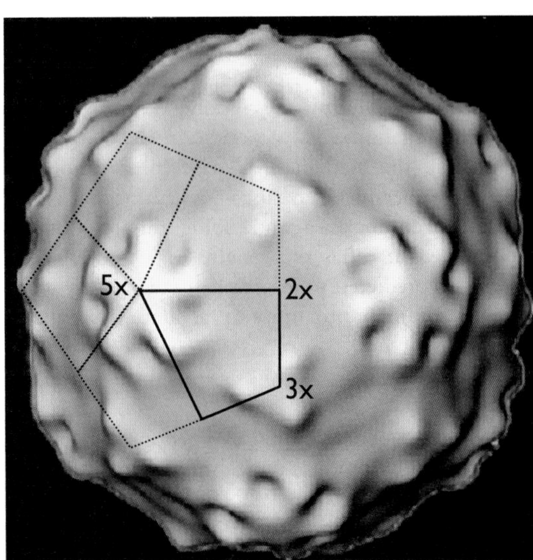

FIGURE 19.4. Medium-resolution image of the structure of the hepatitis A virus (HAV) particle as revealed by cryo-electron microscopy. The solid kite defines a protomer that is likely occupied by single copies of each capsid protein VP1, VP2, and VP3. Five copies of such a protomer are linked at the fivefold (5×) axis of symmetry to form a pentamer assembly subunit. The mature particle contains 12 pentamers arranged on an icosahedral surface or 60 copies of each individual capsid protein. Threefold (3×) and twofold (2×) axes also are indicated. Coloring is based on the distance from the center of the particle, with *yellow* depicting exposed regions at the surface of the particle. (Courtesy of Profs. R. Holland Cheng, University of California at Davis, Davis, CA, and Tatsuo Miyamura, National Institute of Infectious Diseases, Tokyo, Japan.)

detergent–treated clotting factor concentrates.[227] These properties of the virus are likely to contribute significantly to its ability to spread through the environment and to cause common-source outbreaks of hepatitis.

Inactivation of HAV was reviewed by Coulepis et al.[63] Appropriate measures rely on autoclaving (121°C for 20 minutes), exposure to chlorine-containing compounds (sodium hypochlorite, 3–10 mg/L at 20°C for 5–15 minutes or free residual chlorine concentrations of 2.0–2.5 mg/L for 15 minutes),[294] or to a quaternary ammonium formulation containing 23% hydrogen chloride (HCl). HAV also is inactivated by incubation in 3% formaldehyde for 5 minutes, or in 70% ethanol for 60 minutes, and by β-propiolactone or ultraviolet irradiation.[258]

GENOME STRUCTURE

Genomic Organization

Similar to all picornaviral genomes, the HAV genome is a single-stranded RNA molecule of positive polarity that can be divided into three parts (see Fig. 19.3): (a) a relatively lengthy 5′ untranslated region (UTR) that does not have a cap structure at its 5′ end but instead has a 2.5 kDa, covalently bound, virus-encoded protein—VPg (also known as 3B)[389]; (b) a single, large open reading frame (ORF) encoding a polyprotein of approximately 2,227 amino acids in length that is proteolytically processed into structural (P1-2A) and nonstructural (2B-C and P3 or 3A-D) viral polypeptides; and (c) a short 3′ UTR of 63 nucleotides that is followed by a poly(A) tail of varying lengths (40–80 nucleotides) typical of picornavirus genomes. Complete sequence lengths range from 7,470 to 7,487 nucleotides excluding the 3′ poly(A) tail.

The HAV genome is very rich in A+U bases (62%) as compared to the median A+U base composition of 54% found among other picornaviruses—a feature that is likely to affect base-pair composition and biologically relevant folds of the genome. As in other picornaviruses, however, the HAV genome also is predicted to exist as a circular entity with both 5′ and 3′ ends in close proximity to facilitate RNA translation to replication switches.[284]

Untranslated Regions

The nucleotide sequence of the HAV genome begins at the 5′ end with two uridyl residues typical of picornaviruses. The 5′ UTR is approximately 729 to 749 nucleotides long and has a high level of secondary RNA structure comprising several complex stem-loop structures (Fig. 19.5). RNA secondary structure and tertiary interactions (pseudoknots) within this segment of the genome have been established by a combination of (a) phylogenetic comparative sequence analyses to predict thermodynamically stable base pairing, (b) functional genetic studies, and (c) direct biophysical and nuclease mapping techniques with single- or double-strand–specific ribonucleases (RNases).[41,215,336] Among HAV strains, the 5′ UTR appears to be the most conserved region of the genome (≥89% nucleotide identity among strains representing genotypes I, II, and III).[41] All picornavirus genomes have secondary structural elements at their extreme 5′ end that differ in length and folding.[284] In the case of HAV, the 5′ UTR has an unbranched terminal stem of very low free energy comprising the 41 5′ terminal nucleotides. This element (stem-loop I; see Fig. 19.5) is likely to be important for RNA replication.

As in all picornaviruses, the most dominant structural unit in the HAV 5′ UTR is the internal ribosome entry site (IRES), which determines the initiation of viral translation in a 5′ cap-independent fashion (see Fig. 19.5). Depending on structural similarities at the secondary and tertiary levels, and the nature of cellular translation factors required to initiate translation, picornaviral IRESs are divided into four groups.[284] The HAV IRES makes up a group on its own, designated type III IRES, which is distinct from all other known IRESs.[20,284] The boundaries of the HAV IRES were mapped by using bicistronic messenger RNAs (mRNAs) comprised of a first reporter gene followed by various segments of the HAV 5′ UTR that controlled translation of a second, downstream reporter gene. Characterization of their translation activities in reticulocyte lysates or in cell culture revealed that the IRES is located between nucleotides 154 and 735.[43,125]

Between the 5′ terminal stem-loop I and the IRES lies a sequence of approximately 110 nucleotides (nucleotides 42–154) that includes (a) two pseudoknots (IIa and IIb, nucleotides 42–94),[336] the sequence of which is highly conserved among HAV strains, and (b) a partially ordered polypyrimidine tract and a single-stranded region (nucleotides 95–154),[149] which are susceptible to naturally occurring mutations, particularly deletions.[41] This 5′ spacer domain corresponds to the most variable segment in length and sequence among all picornaviruses.[284] These sequences may function as replication elements and/or contribute essential virus–host interactions.

The 3′ UTR of HAV RNA shows a high proportion of differences between HAV strains (up to 20%). It has been less extensively studied than the 5′ UTR but also has a high propensity to form higher-order structures. Hypothetical structural models of the HAV 3′ UTR have been proposed based on probing with specific RNases and computer-aided predictions, suggesting that a pseudoknot structure is favored[85] (e-Fig. 19.1).

Structural Proteins and Replication Proteins

Uniquely among *Picornaviridae* genera, the primary cleavage of the HAV polyprotein occurs between the P1-2A and 2BC-P3 segments of the polyprotein under the direction of the only protease encoded by the virus—the 3C protein[184,248] (see Fig. 19.3). The P1-2A segment comprises four structural polypeptides (in order): VP4 (1A), VP2 (1B), VP3 (1C), and VP1 (1D), named according to their homologs in the poliovirus capsid based on relative molecular masses, with VP1 being the largest. These proteins are approximately 23, 222, 246, and 274 amino acids in length, respectively (Table 19.1).[59,138,247] VP1, however, has a heterogeneous carboxy terminus,[138] reflecting a unique maturation mechanism. Whereas VP2, VP3, and VP1 comprise the viral capsid, VP4 is substantially smaller than its homologs in other picornaviruses and has never been experimentally determined to be part of the HAV capsid. The 2A protein of HAV does not encode a primary cleavage function as found in the 2A proteins of most other picornaviruses, neither is it involved in genome replication.[250] HAV 2A functions in capsid assembly as a fusion precursor with VP1[60] and remains attached to some otherwise fully formed virions.[9] In-frame insertions within the HAV genome of exogenous protein coding sequences, flanked by 3C cleavage sites at the 2A/2B junction, has resulted in replication-competent virus, further

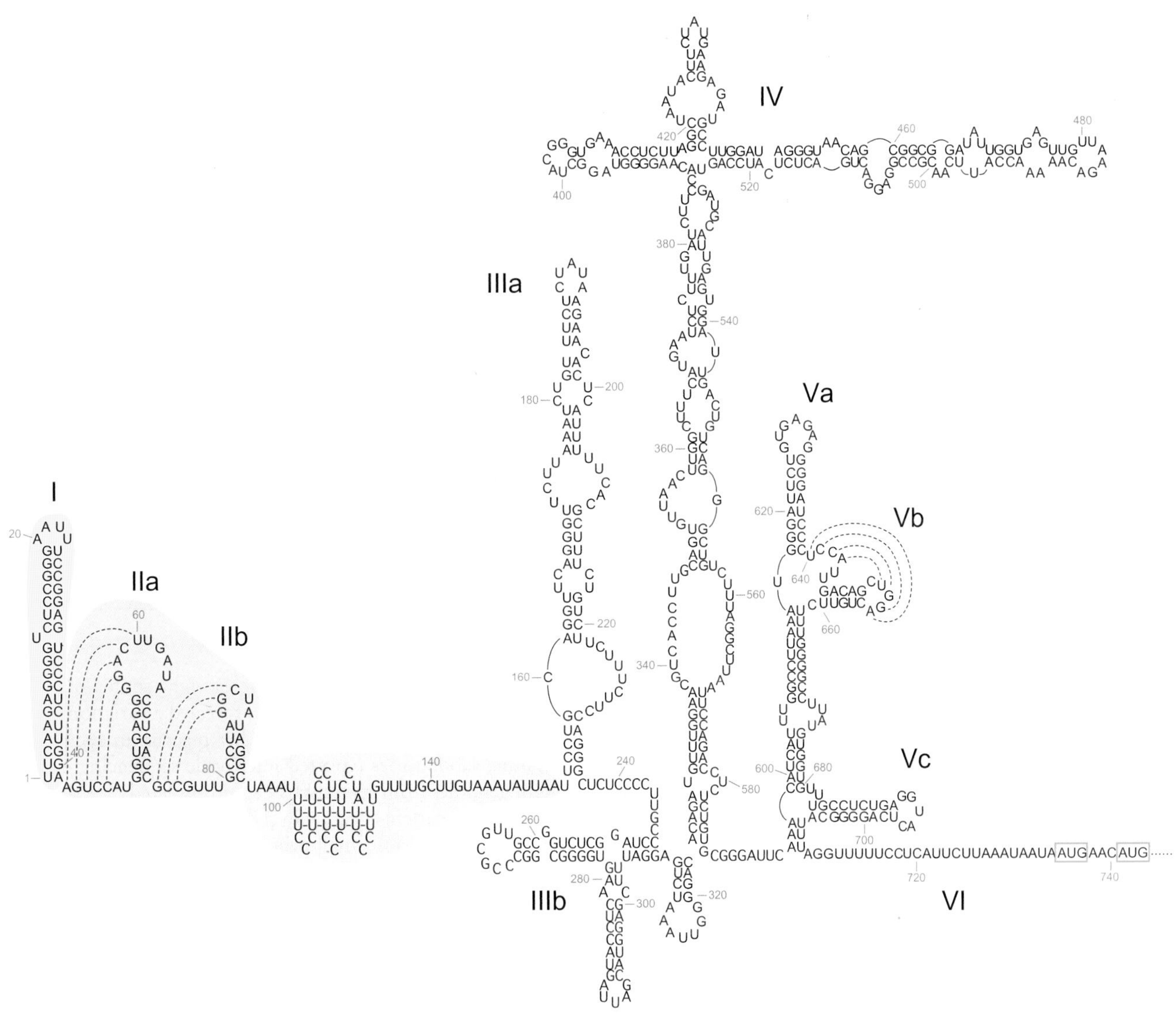

FIGURE 19.5. Proposed RNA structure of the 5′ untranslated region (5′ UTR) of hepatitis A virus (HAV; wild-type HM175 strain, accession number M14707). Nucleotides (in *blue*) are numbered according to their positions within the HAV genome. Subdomains comprised of stem-loop structures are numbered sequentially (Roman numerals). Putative tertiary pseudoknots are represented by *dotted lines* to indicate possible interactions between nucleotides. The 5′ terminal stem-loop structure (I), pseudoknot elements (IIa-b), and polypyrimidine tract/single-stranded region (see text) are represented by *yellow, pink,* and *gray-shaded areas,* respectively. The internal ribosome entry site (IRES) is delineated by the *blue-shaded area* and comprises RNA structures IIIa to VI (nucleotides 154–735). The two in-frame AUG initiator codons of the viral polyprotein are boxed. (Modified from Martin A, Lemon S. The molecular biology of hepatitis A virus. In: Ou J-H, ed. *Hepatitis Viruses.* Norwell, MA: Kluwer Academic Publishers; 2002:23–50, with kind permission from Springer Science+Business Media B.V.)

confirming that 2A has no function in *cis* with the remainder of the nonstructural proteins.[21]

Nonstructural proteins derived from the 2BC-P3 segment of the polyprotein probably all contribute directly to the assembly of the membrane-bound viral replicase complex (see Table 19.1). Proteins 2B and 2C, and probably also the precursor 2BC, are involved in directing the rearrangements of cellular membranes required for replicase assembly.[130,369] It has been suggested that 2B, containing hydrophobic sequences, anchors the replicase complexes to altered intracellular membranes.[130] 2C has NTPase activity[126] and contains an RNA helicase sequence motif.[84]

Among the P3 nonstructural proteins, 3D is assumed to be the viral RNA-dependent RNA polymerase, although no direct data exist. 3C has been crystallized and is a chymotrypsin-like cysteine protease[3,23,409] (Fig. 19.6). It appears to be the only virus-encoded protease of HAV, which is responsible for all co- or posttranslational cleavage events within the HAV polyprotein except for those at VP4/VP2 and VP1/2A junctions.[151,242] In addition, HAV 3C protease and/or its precursors 3ABC and 3CD also appear to cleave cellular IRES-transacting factors and adaptor molecules acting in interferon signaling pathways (see the Infectious Viral Life Cycle and the Pathogenesis and

TABLE 19.1 Hepatitis A Virus Structural and Nonstructural Proteins

Viral Protein	Number of amino acids	Function	Properties
1A = VP4	21–23	Capsid protein?	Found as 1AB precursor in immature particles Presence not demonstrated in virions
1B = VP2	222	Capsid protein	
1C = VP3	246	Capsid protein	Contributes to the major neutralization antigenic site
1D = VP1	272–274	Capsid protein	Heterogeneous C-terminus Also found as 1D-2A precursor in immature particles Contributes to the major neutralization antigenic site
2A	71	Essential for capsid assembly	Only characterized as P1-2A and 1D-2A precursors
2B	251	Probable membrane anchoring for the virus replication complex	Also found as 2BC precursor
2C	335	NTPase and helicase activities	Also found as 2BC precursor
3A	74	Probable membrane anchoring for 3B	3ABC precursor associates with mitochondrial membranes
3B = VPg	23	Initiation of RNA replication?	Covalently linked to the 5′ end of the genome
3C	219	Chymotrypsin-like cysteine protease	Cleaves all protein junctions except for 1D/2A and 1A/1B 3ABC and 3CD precursors cleave adaptor proteins of the host interferon signaling pathways
3D	489	RNA-dependent RNA polymerase	

Host Immune Responses sections). P3 also generates protein 3B (also referred to as VPg), which is attached to the 5′ end of both positive- and negative-strand RNAs,[389] and protein 3A, which comprises a hydrophobic 21 amino acid stretch that is believed to anchor the 3AB precursor of VPg (3B) to cellular membranes and to target the 3ABC precursor to mitochondrial membranes.[404]

DIVERSITY OF THE INFECTIOUS AGENT

Genetic Diversity

HAV identification and initial characterization were done with strain MS-1 isolated in 1964 from the blood and stools of a patient in New York.[101,204] In the mid-1980s, the first comparative study of the nucleotide sequences of HAV performed by RNase T1 oligonucleotide mapping of eight strains originating from diverse geographic sources revealed a variation in the order of magnitude reported for other picornaviruses.[390] Several other laboratories reported nucleotide sequencing of full-length genomes from several HAV strains isolated directly from the stools of patients (e.g., HM175; Australia, 1976),[59,71] or after a few passages in small primates or cell culture (e.g., LA; USA, 1976),[275] MBB (North Africa, 1978),[286] and GBM (Germany, 1976).[136] Wild-type strain HM175 has been adapted to yield the widest range of mutants in cell culture, including attenuated, persistently infecting, cytopathic and neutralization-resistant variants (see the Molecular Determinants of Hepatitis A Virus Adaptation to Cell Culture section). Attenuated mutants of HM175,[193] CR326 (Costa Rica, 1960),[231] H2 (China, 1982),[244] and variants of strains GBM[384] and MBB[167] are the best characterized candidates for live attenuated vaccines,

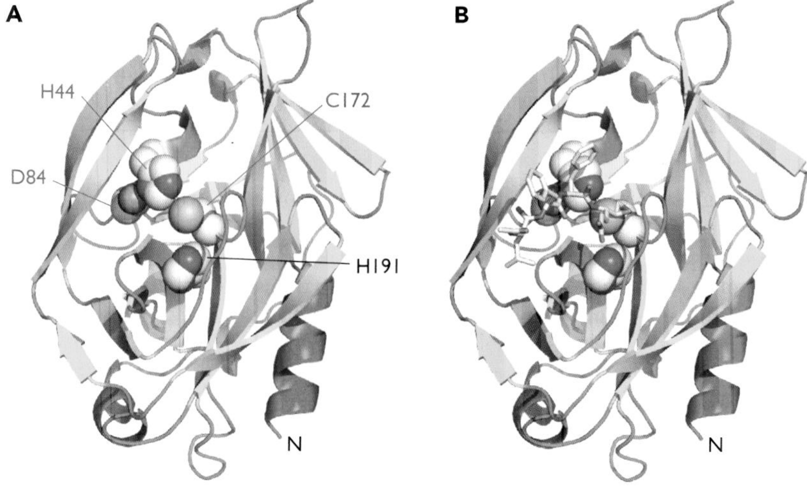

FIGURE 19.6. **Ribbon representation of the crystal structure of hepatitis A virus (HAV) 3C protease** (PDB accession 2HAL).[409] **A:** Ribbon is colored by secondary structure with *red,* helix; *yellow,* sheet; *green,* loop. Side chains of the catalytic triad (D84, H44, C172) are shown as spheres across the top of the active site. The side chain of H191, the primary residue responsible for the glutamine specificity in P1, is also shown as spheres. **B:** A stick representation of the LFFE-FMK inhibitor, which mimics substrate residues P1-P4, is shown bound in the active site. Spheres and sticks are colored by atom type. (Courtesy of Dr. Bruce A. Malcolm, Johnson and Johnson Infectious Diseases and Vaccines, Beerse, Belgium.)

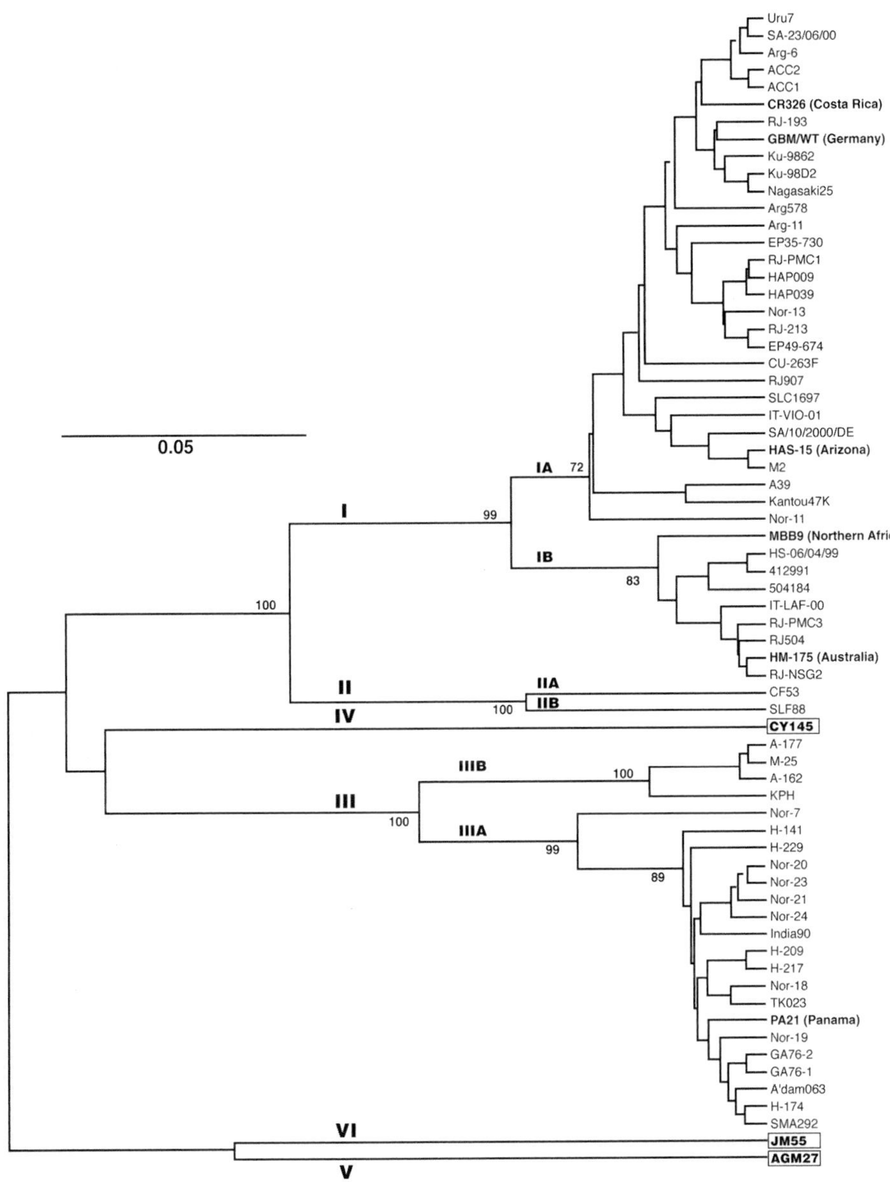

FIGURE 19.7. Phylogenetic tree based on hepatitis A virus (HAV) sequences (168 nucleotides) in the 2A region. Statistically significant bootstrap values (%) are given at the nodes, and genetic distance per nucleotide per site is shown by the *horizontal bar.* Genotypes are indicated by *Roman numerals,* whereas subgenotypes are indicated by *A* and *B.* The country of origin is indicated for best characterized strains of genotypes I, II, and III. The prototype MS-1 strain of HAV (not shown) belongs to subgenotype IA. The only known representatives of genotypes IV, V, and VI were collected from Old World monkeys. (Modified from Lu L, Ching KZ, de Paula VS, et al. Characterization of the complete genomic sequence of genotype II hepatitis A virus (CF53/Berne isolate). *J Gen Virol* 2004;85:2943–2952, with permission.)

as reviewed by Flehmig et al,[107] Hu et al,[168] and Provost et al[303] (see the Hepatitis A Vaccines section).

The genetic diversity of HAV has further been investigated by determining the partial genomic nucleotide sequences of 152 HAV strains recovered from various human or simian sources and geographical areas[234] (Fig. 19.7). Following virus purification by capture with an HAV monoclonal antibody, reverse transcription of viral RNA, and amplification by RT-PCR,[181] genotypic analysis was based on the nucleotide sequence of a short genomic segment (168 nucleotides) that encompassed the relatively variable 2A coding sequence (originally thought to span the VP1/2A junction).

Additional phylogenetic studies were more recently carried out using a wider range of HAV isolates that were under-represented in the initial genotyping studies. This included HAV strains from South America, North and Central Africa, and India. In addition, full-length VP1 sequences (900 nucleotides) were chosen to establish nucleotide comparisons, considering that several residues of VP1 contribute to the major immunodominant site of HAV. Overall strain variation in the complete VP1 gene was found to be higher than 20% at the nucleotide level and around 10% at the amino acid level.[62]

The current view is that HAV circulates worldwide as a total of six genotypes (≤85% identity) with three genotypes (I, II and III) subdivided into subtypes A and B (86%–92.5% identity within subtypes)[234] (see Fig. 19.7). Genotypes I, II, and III comprise all human strains, among which subgenotype IA and genotype III are the most prevalent worldwide (e-Fig. 19.2). Each of the three simian HAV genotypes are defined by a single strain isolated from naturally infected Old World monkeys, cynomolgus macaques (genotypes IV and VI),[274,318] and African green monkeys (genotype V).[376] All simian HAV strains have a typical signature sequence at the VP3/VP1 junction that distinguishes them from human strains.[42,318,376]

Clusters within genotypes predominate in certain geographic regions (see e-Fig. 19.2), such as a group of subgenotype

IA strains with more than 97% identity that represent nearly all of the viruses from the United States, suggesting endemic spread. Other regions, such as Europe and Japan, have a greater genetic mixture of viruses, suggesting regular introduction of strains by travelers returning from endemic regions. A higher degree of heterogeneity than reported previously has been found in strains isolated in South America.[67]

To better define the HAV mode of evolution in populations, full-length VP1 sequences of a collection of genotype IA HAV strains isolated in France from 1984 to 2001 were analyzed. This revealed a mean rate of 9.76×10^{-4} nucleotide substitutions per site per year, and an estimation of a synonymous substitution rate around 5×10^{-3} substitutions per site per year. The latter is clearly lower than that observed for other representative members of the family *Picornaviridae* and may be related to the slower replication cycle of HAV, its particular tropism, or its transmission mode.[265]

Virion Antigenic Structure and Diversity

Comparisons of the nucleotide sequences of various human HAV strains from widely separated geographic regions have demonstrated high amino acid conservation in the sequences of the viral capsid proteins (>70%). Likewise, viruses belonging to distinct genotypes elicit antibodies with substantial cross-neutralizing activity, suggesting that there is only one HAV serotype among human strains.[353] A primate HAV strain recovered from a captive New World monkey (owl monkey) was considered to be a human (genotype IIIA) rather than a simian strain following biological characterization and sequence analysis[42,318] (see e-Fig. 19.2). Conversely, in strains of HAV isolated from naturally infected Old World monkeys (cynomolgus and African green monkeys), some monoclonal antibodies are capable of distinguishing unique epitopes, indicating some degree of antigenic singularity in simian strains.[274,376] However, whereas African green monkey virus from genotype V caused no disease in chimpanzees, it elicited an anti-HAV response that protected the chimpanzees against disease after challenge with the virulent human-derived HM175 strain.[94] These observations suggest that even simian and human strains of HAV demonstrate substantial antigenic cross-reactivity.

Neutralization epitopes of HAV are conformational and generally are not displayed on isolated HAV proteins. Correspondingly, neutralizing murine monoclonal antibodies do not recognize denatured capsid proteins, and antisera raised against proteins expressed by recombinant DNA techniques show only weak reactivity with native capsids and have very limited virus neutralization activity.[170] Most murine monoclonal antibodies to HAV compete with each other and are able to substantially block the binding of polyclonal human antibodies to virus in solid-phase competition immunoassays.[171,354] Similarly, human and chimpanzee neutralizing monoclonal anti-HAV antibodies recovered by phage display have been shown to compete with murine monoclonal antibodies.[199,326] This suggests that there may be only a limited number of antigenic epitopes that are closely clustered on the surface of the virus.

Antigenic variants of HAV that resist neutralization by murine monoclonal antibodies have been selected in cell culture by continued passage of HM175 virus in the presence of these antibodies.[354] Sequencing of the genomic regions encoding their capsid proteins revealed single amino acid changes in each mutant with a limited number of changes confined to VP3 (two mutations) and VP1 (four mutations).[296,297] Similarly, in strain HAS-15 (Arizona, 1979), a small number of mutations that confer resistance to neutralizing antibodies also were selected in VP3 and VP1.[273] Competition studies with these mutants confirmed the existence of an immunodominant site composed of residues of VP1 (at positions 102, 171, and 176) and VP3 (at positions 70 and 74) that are likely to be closely positioned on the surface of the HAV particle and reside on exposed loops that connect β strands of the capsid proteins. This feature is likely to distinguish HAV from enteroviruses, for which equivalent residues do not lie in close vicinity at the surface of the capsid.[160] A crystallographic structure of the HAV capsid would shed light on the conformational nature of the immunodominant antigenic site. An apparently distinct site involving C-terminal residues of VP1 has been identified from HM175 neutralization escape mutants.[297] In addition, two continuous epitopes near the N-terminus of VP1 (residues 11–25) and within VP3 (residues 110–121), which elicit weak neutralizing activity as peptides also may represent secondary neutralization sites.[34,95] In the case of poliovirus, the VP1 N-terminus is internally located in the virion capsid but is exposed during virus attachment to cells.[44]

The finding of limited amino acid changes among multiple neutralization escape mutants suggests that there are important constraints to the antigenic or structural variations of HAV. Recently, however, several HAV variants bearing substitutions or deletions at or around the immunodominant neutralization site or secondary neutralization sites were isolated in sporadic cases or during outbreaks of hepatitis A. These strains showed at least partial resistance to antiserum generated against HAV vaccine or to murine monoclonal anti-HAV antibodies, suggesting a potential for the emergence of HAV antigenic variants or new serotypes in the population.[62,119,123,292,323]

INFECTIOUS VIRAL LIFE CYCLE

Attachment and Entry

HAV has been shown to bind to a wide range of cultured animal cells, including nonpermissive cells. Although nothing is known about viral determinants involved in HAV cell attachment, it has been observed that mature virions attach relatively rapidly and in a calcium-dependent way[25,352,394,412] but undergo comparatively slow uncoating with release of viral RNA into the cytoplasm about 4 hours postinfection.[27]

A candidate cellular receptor (HAVcr1), a mucin-like class 1 integral membrane glycoprotein of 451 amino acids[370] (Fig. 19.8A), was first identified in HAV-susceptible AGMK cells using an expression cloning strategy and a monoclonal antibody that blocked binding of HAV to the cell surface.[191] A molecule with 95% amino acid similarity was concomitantly identified in an HAV-susceptible hybrid marmoset-Vero cell line.[14] A human homolog of HAVcr1 (with 79% identity) was later shown to interact with cell culture–adapted HAV.[100] The N-terminal cysteine-rich immunoglobulin-like region of the HAVcr1 ectodomain is sufficient for binding HAV, but both this region and the mucin-like region are required for viral particle conformational changes leading to HAV uncoating[346] (Fig. 19.8A,B). A soluble form of HAVcr1 also is able to neutralize wild-type HAV,[345] providing additional evidence for the role of this molecule as the HAV receptor *in vivo*. Recent

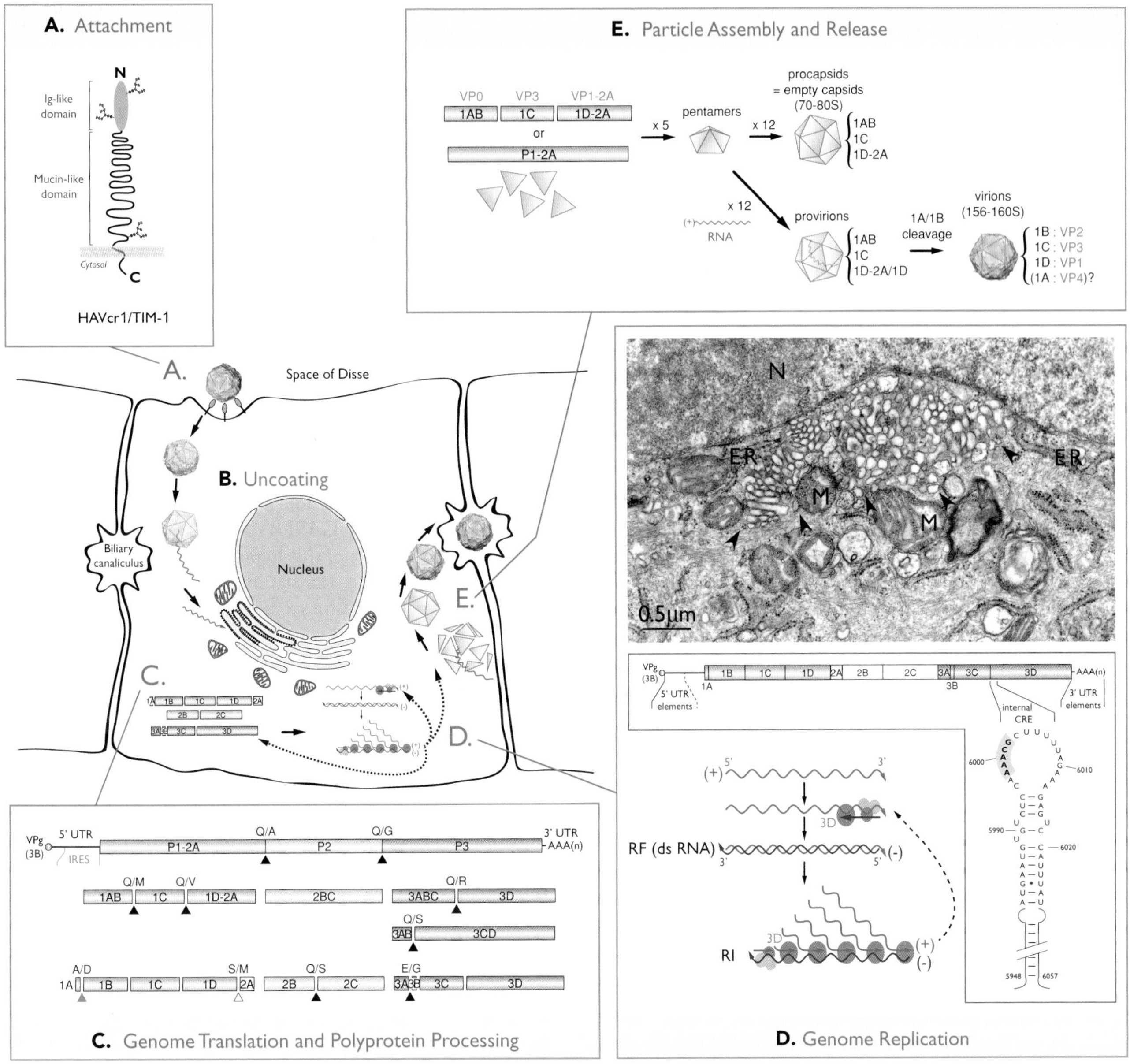

FIGURE 19.8. Hepatitis A virus (HAV) infectious life cycle. A: HAV enters hepatocytes by attachment to a cellular receptor, likely HAVcr1/TIM-1. This receptor, as schematically represented, comprises an N-terminal immunoglobulin-like domain and a mucin-like domain with three N-glycosylated sites (branched elements).[370] **B:** Details of HAV uncoating remain largely unknown. **C:** Once released within the cell cytoplasm, virion RNA serves as a template for translation of the viral polyprotein, which is subsequently cleaved as depicted. Cleavages are carried out by HAV protease 3C at most junctions (*black triangles*), likely by a cellular protease at the 1D/2A junction (*open triangle*), or upon RNA encapsidation at the 1A/1B junction (*gray triangle*). Dipeptides representing cleavage sites between stable polypeptide precursors or mature proteins are indicated above corresponding boxes. **D:** Genome replication subsequently takes place within the virus-induced tubular vesicular network. The electron micrograph of FRhK-4 cells infected with cell culture–adapted HAV demonstrates rearrangement of cytosolic membranes into a network of tubular-vesicular structures (delineated by *arrowheads*), which appear closely associated with membranes of the endoplasmic reticulum (ER) and mitochondria (M) in the vicinity of the nucleus (N).[130] The positive-strand RNA is used as a template by the viral replicase complex comprised of polymerase 3D and other nonstructural proteins for minus-strand RNA synthesis, thereby generating replicating forms (RF). The minus-strand RNA serves in turn as a template for the synthesis of multiple positive-strand RNAs (replication intermediates, RI). *Cis*-active RNA elements (CRE) located at the 5′ and 3′ terminal regions of the genome, as well as within the 3D coding sequence are required for RNA replication. The stem-loop structure of the internal CRE, as depicted below the genome, includes a relatively lengthy stem (nucleotide numbering from HAV full-length genome) and a large loop that contains a motif boxed in *orange*, typical of all picornaviral CREs and necessary for their function.[405] Newly synthesized positive-strand RNAs can be either engaged in translation, replication, or encapsidation, as represented by *dashed arrows* within the cell. (Electron micrograph courtesy of Dr. Rainer Gosert, Institute for Medical Microbiology, Basel, Switzerland.) **E:** Virion assembly is likely to proceed through indicated assembly intermediates, ultimately leading to the production of infectious virions, which are subsequently released into biliary canaliculi.

studies have identified *TIM-1,* an atopy susceptibility gene, as the gene that encodes HAVcr1.[261] The T-cell immunoglobulin mucin (TIM) gene family, particularly TIM-1, are cell surface receptors that are important in T-cell regulation and Th-cell differentiation (see the Clinical Features section). HAVcr1 is widely distributed in different tissues[100]; thus, the tropism of HAV for the liver remains an enigma waiting to be resolved.

A surrogate entry mechanism of HAV has been proposed via immunocomplexes with HAV-specific immunoglobulin A (IgA), which are present in significant amounts during acute infection. This was based on the observation that HAV/IgA complexes can be endocytosed in hepatocyte cultures via the hepatocellular asialoglycoprotein receptor (ASGPR), which mediates uptake of IgA.[88] IgA-mediated transcytosis of HAV via polymeric immunoglobulin receptor also was observed *in vitro* and proposed as a mechanism for HAV to overcome the epithelial barrier of the intestinal tract.[86]

Genome Translation, Polyprotein Processing, and Replication

The entire HAV life cycle occurs in the cytoplasm of the cell (Fig. 19.8). HAV genome translation and replication appear to take place in association with a tubular-vesicular membranous network specifically rearranged from cytosolic membranes by proteins 2B, 2C, or 2BC in HAV-infected cells,[130,369] as is the case for other picornaviruses (Fig. 19.8D). The HAV 2B protein is localized predominantly in the endoplasmic reticulum (ER),[76] suggesting that the tubular vesicular structures may be derived from the ER.[197] Unlike enterovirus homologous proteins, HAV 2B has little, if any, effect on ER and Golgi calcium homeostasis, or on protein trafficking through the secretory pathway,[76] which is consistent with the hypothesis that hepatitis A virions may use the secretory pathway to exit the cell.[28]

Translation

Uncoated RNA is translated via an IRES-dependent mechanism that involves cellular factors so that 40S ribosomal subunits bind and begin translation at the correct initiation codon and not at multiple AUG codons scattered throughout the 5′ UTR. This mechanism contrasts with typical eukaryotic translation, in which 40S subunits recognize an m7G-cap at the 5′ mRNA terminus (not present in the HAV genome) and then scan for the nearest AUG within an appropriate sequence motif.[203] Initiation of HAV translation may start at either of two in-frame AUG codons at positions 735 through 737 and 741 through 743[366] (see Fig. 19.5). Although either codon could function independently, selective deletion experiments have demonstrated that the second of these codons is preferentially used *in vitro* and in cells.[366]

The HAV IRES is far less efficient for directing translation in acellular systems and in various cell lines than are encephalomyocarditis virus (EMCV) and foot-and-mouth disease virus (FMDV) IRES, for example.[32,43,125,396] Inefficient translation is likely owing to the fact that the HAV IRES uniquely requires intact cellular initiation factor eIF-4G to function, unlike other picornavirus IRESs that utilize a cleaved fragment of this factor,[31] and that it probably competes poorly for this and other necessary cellular factors. HAV translation and replication are thus likely to depend on continued synthesis of host factors. Consistent with this hypothesis is the fact that HAV generally does not shut off host protein synthesis, unlike other picornaviruses. In the context of virus/cell competition, HAV appears to have adopted a naturally biased, deoptimized codon usage with respect to that of its cellular host.[12,322] It has been hypothesized that this finely tuned strategy, observed specifically in the capsid coding region, might avoid competition between HAV and the host cell for cellular transfer RNAs (tRNAs), modulate translation kinetics, and allow proper protein folding to reach the highest viral fitness.[12]

HAV IRES activity appears to be modulated by several cellular proteins, including polypyrimidine tract-binding protein (PTB),[51,129] glyceraldehyde 3-phosphate dehydrogenase (GAPDH),[51,331,408] poly(rC) binding protein 2 (PCBP2),[133] and lupus autoantigen (La).[61] GAPDH and PTB compete for binding to overlapping sites in the IRES (stem-loop III at the 5′ end of the IRES)[331] (see Fig. 19.5). Although the mechanisms by which these cellular proteins modulate the translational activities of HAV IRES are unknown, it has been speculated that GAPDH may have a destabilization effect on RNA secondary structure, leading to translation suppression,[408] whereas PTB may have a stabilizing action on higher-ordered RNA structures, thereby reversing GAPDH action and stimulating translation.[129,408] In support of this hypothesis, a naturally occurring mutation that enhances translation in AGMK cells[332] decreases the affinity of GAPDH for stem-loop III in the IRES.[408]

Polyprotein Processing

Hepatoviruses follow a unique cleavage cascade distinct from all other picornavirus genera, as reviewed in Martin and Lemon.[249] The primary, co-translational cleavage during HAV polyprotein translation is mediated by the unique virus-encoded protease (3C) at the 2A/2B junction, thus releasing a P1-2A precursor of 836 amino acids from the downstream nonstructural proteins[128,248] (Fig. 19.8C). In most picornavirus genera, the primary polyprotein cleavage also occurs at the 2A/2B junction, although by a different mechanism; a unique sequence of amino acids (Asn-Pro-Gly-Pro) located at the 2A/2B junction possesses an inherent propensity to induce ribosome skipping, resulting in "cleavage" of the nascent polyprotein between Gly and Pro residues. Enteroviruses encode a second protease (2A) that autocatalytically cleaves its own N-terminus at the P1/2A junction.[284]

The key protease 3C carries out most other cleavages in the HAV polyprotein,[151,182,242,330,368] as in other picornaviruses. The 3C-specific cleavage sites are formed by at least six residues surrounding the scissile bonds (amino acids at positions P4-P1 upstream, and P′1-P′2 downstream, of the cleavage site). HAV 3C is in general less discriminating than other picornaviral 3C proteases and recognizes Gln or Glu residues at position P1, any small residue or even charged residues with large side chains at position P′1 (e.g., Gln/Arg at the 3C/3D site), virtually any amino acid at position P′2, and residues with large side chains at position P4[241] (see Figs. 19.6 and 19.8C). The 3C-mediated cleavages occur according to preferential site order and also release stable intermediate precursors, such as 2BC, 3ABC, 3CD that appear to contribute specific functions in the HAV life cycle (see Table 19.1).[210,301,310,404]

Cleavage at two junctions, VP1(1D)/2A and VP4(1A)/VP2(1B), is not carried out by the 3C protease. Uniquely among picornaviruses, VP1 is apparently released from 2A by cellular proteases.[138,247] The C-terminus of VP1 is heterogeneous,[138] with a predominant form releasing a 2A protein of

71 amino acids. It has been proposed that, as for Mengovirus, cellular proteases may trim 2A sequences from VP1-2A to generate VP1 intermediate forms, as well as mature VP1 protein.[138,247] The maturation cleavage at the VP4 (1A)/VP2 (1B) junction, similar to other picornaviruses, takes place in late stages of virion morphogenesis (see Fig. 19.8E) and occurs by an unknown, perhaps autocatalytic, mechanism to yield capsid proteins VP4 and VP2.

RNA Replication

Within the membrane-bound replicase complex, the virion RNA serves as a template for negative-strand RNA synthesis by the RNA-dependent, RNA polymerase 3D, generating double-stranded replicative forms (dsRNA) (Fig. 19.8D). This negative-strand intermediate then acts in turn as a template for the synthesis of multiple positive-strand RNA molecules, yielding replication intermediates (RIs). This asymmetric process suggests that mechanisms of replication of positive and negative strands may show some differences. Newly synthesized positive-strand RNAs can be translated into proteins, replicated, or packaged into new virions.

There are several genomic *cis*-active RNA elements (CREs) required for the initiation of viral RNA replication. Terminal sequences and/or structures present at the 5′ and 3′ ends of the genome, as well as the poly(A) 3′ terminal tail are likely to contain important replication elements. Consistent with this hypothesis, HAV genome-length RNAs that lacked the two 5′ terminal nucleotides (UU) or nucleotides 2 and 3 (UC), which are thought to be involved in a stem-loop structure (see Fig. 19.5), were not infectious.[150] One study suggested that elements required for RNA replication may extend downstream of nucleotide 151 of the 5′ UTR (i.e., beyond the polypyrimidine tract), because a genome containing only the 5′ terminal 151 nucleotides of the 5′ UTR followed by the EMCV IRES was noninfectious, in contrast to chimeric genomes containing the first 237 HAV nucleotides fused to EMCV IRES.[185] Likewise, whereas deletion of the pyrimidine-rich tract (nucleotides 96–139) did not alter viral replication in cell culture, deletions that also included nucleotides 140 through 144 immediately downstream of it (in a predicted single-stranded region (see Fig. 19.5) yielded a temperature-sensitive virus[336] with defective RNA synthesis.[338] The importance of the poly(A) 3′ terminal tail has been corroborated by observations that viral replication is delayed in cells transfected with genomes lacking part or all of the poly(A) sequence, and the poly(A) tail is concomitantly regenerated in progeny virus.[212]

In addition, other internal CREs first identified in a rhinovirus genome[262] have been subsequently identified in several other picornavirus genera and are often located within genomic coding sequences. These elements comprise stem-loop structures of variable lengths with a common apical loop containing an "AAAC" motif.[356] In poliovirus, the CRE was shown to template the uridylylation of 3B (VPg)—the small genome-linked protein—generating VPg-pUpU that functions as a protein primer for viral RNA synthesis.[287] It is still debated whether both negative- and positive-strand RNA synthesis require CRE-dependent VPg uridylylation or whether negative-strand synthesis can be primed by VPg.[356] For HAV, a CRE has been identified in the 3D coding sequence by combined phylogenetic and thermodynamic predictive strategies, as well as mutational analyses.[405] HAV CRE comprises a larger stem loop with lower free-folding energy than CREs of other picornaviruses (see Fig. 19.8D), suggesting that there are likely to be important differences in the details of the VPg uridylylation templated process for HAV. This is further supported by the apparent targeting of HAV 3A (and likely also the 3AB precursor of VPg) to mitochondrial rather than ER membranes.[389,404] Evidence suggests that internal CREs function coordinately with the other *cis*-active RNA sequences and structures at the 5′ and 3′ termini of picornavirus RNAs to mediate RNA replication, presumably via ribonucleoprotein interactions that might be facilitated by the NTPase activity of 2C.[356] Along these lines, interactions between HAV proteins 3C and 3AB with structures formed at both termini of the HAV genome have been documented *in vitro*.[22,211,213,293]

Translation to Replication Switches

Interestingly, several cellular proteins may be involved in the finely tuned regulation of HAV RNA translation to replication switches, given that the same genomic molecule may be engaged in either process and that viral polysomes must be cleared of ribosomes before RNA replication can occur. Several sites for binding of GAPDH in the HAV 3′ UTR have been described.[85] Therefore, binding of GAPDH to both 5′[51,331,408] (see earlier discussion) and 3′ termini of the HAV genome might promote the establishment of their close spatial proximity and have a role in RNA translation-replication switches. Viral protein and RNA syntheses also might be coordinated by the binding of full-length PCBP2 to the polypyrimidine tract of the 5′ UTR, whereas a truncated form of this cellular protein, which is cleaved by HAV 3C protease, has lesser affinity for HAV RNA, thus possibly facilitating the switch toward replication.[414] Similarly, another IRES *trans*-acting factor—PTB[129]—is cleaved upon overexpression of HAV 3C protease, resulting in translation inhibition and hypothetically replication turn on.[189] However, the biological relevance of these observations is uncertain, because cleavage of these cellular factors has not been confirmed in HAV-infected cells, maybe as the result of low 3C quantities being present owing to protracted virus growth. HAV IRES was shown to be stimulated by polyadenylation in an acellular system, in contrast to FMDV IRES, suggesting a possible role for the 3′ terminal poly(A) residues of the genome in regulating HAV translation.[290] More recently, poly(A)-binding protein (PABP) was shown to interact with polyadenylated HAV 3′ UTR.[413] This could hypothetically allow the bridging of HAV IRES via PABP-eIF4G interaction, resulting in the circularization of the RNA, such as in poliovirus and cellular mRNAs.[158] PABP also is targeted by HAV 3C protease in HAV-infected cells yielding a C-terminally truncated polypeptide that is able to bind to the polypyrimidine tract of HAV 5′ UTR. This might result in the curtailment of translation and the promotion of RNA replication.[413]

Particle Assembly and Release

The mechanisms of HAV particle assembly are likely to differ significantly from those of other picornaviruses, consistent with detection of immature particle intermediates in HAV-infected cells.[26,33] Recombinant vaccinia virus–mediated expression of HAV polyprotein or of capsid protein precursor P1-2A, on the one hand, and nonstructural protein precursor 2BC-P3, on the other hand, results in the assembly of capsid-like structures.[60,400] Using this system and C-terminally truncated P1-2A polypeptides, the presence of nonstructural protein 2A as a C-terminal extension of P1 was shown to be essential for both efficient 3C-mediated internal processing of P1-2A and the first step in virion morphogenesis.[60] The N-terminal domain of 2A is actually instrumental for assembling five copies of 1AB (VP4-VP2 or VP0), 1C (VP3), and 1D-2A (VP1-2A) polypeptides into pentamers, as a direct primary signal and/or as a consequence of its critical role in 3C-mediated processing of P1-2A, notably at the VP0/VP3 junction. However, whether pentamers are first assembled with five copies of uncleaved P1-2A precursors or cleaved VP0, VP3, VP1-2A polypeptides remains uncertain[33,60,300] (Fig. 19.8E). In other picornaviruses, the assembly of pentamers is initiated by N-terminally myristoylated VP4 protein.[284] VP4 of HAV, however, is considerably smaller than VP4 proteins of other picornaviruses (at most 23 amino acids) and is not myristoylated, despite the presence of an internal consensus myristoylation signal.[367] Twelve pentamers subsequently assemble into complete procapsids (empty capsids) or incorporate virion RNA to form provirions. N-terminal fusion of heterologous sequences to VP0 did not prevent the assembly of procapsids,[416] further suggesting that VP4 is not a critical determinant of HAV capsid assembly. The presence of the 3ABC precursor of 3C appears to improve P1-2A cleavage and particle assembly.[210] Cleavage at the VP1/2A junction begins after assembly of complete capsids and releases the mature VP1 capsid protein as well as larger VP1 polypeptides of intermediate lengths that, along with uncleaved VP1-2A, can still be detected in low amounts in procapsids and provirions.[33,60,300] C-terminal residues of 2A are important for efficient cleavage at the VP1/2A junction,[60] which is likely carried out by a cellular protease that remains to be identified. Maturation cleavage of VP0 to release VP2 depends on RNA encapsidation, occurs by an as yet undetermined mechanism, and is associated with a conformational change to generate mature virions.[26] Cleavage of VP1-2A and VP0 into corresponding mature capsid proteins is accompanied by an increase in the specific infectivity of viral particles.[26,60] The fate of 2A and VP4 in this process is unknown, and efforts to detect them in infected cells or virions have been unsuccessful.

Although a large proportion of the newly synthesized particles remains cell associated, there is extensive release of progeny virus into cell culture supernatant fluids by an as yet unknown mechanism. In polarized, human colonic epithelial cell cultures (Caco-2), release of virus occurs almost exclusively into apical supernatant fluids, mimicking the secretion of HAV across the apical canalicular membrane of the hepatocyte into the biliary system.[28] Interestingly, this process is largely blocked by an inhibitor of the cellular secretory pathway (Brefeldin A), suggesting that virus release may involve vectorial vesicular transport mechanisms.[28]

MOLECULAR DETERMINANTS OF HEPATITIS A VIRUS ADAPTATION TO CELL CULTURE AND ATTENUATION *IN VIVO*

In contrast to the invariably transient nature of HAV infections in humans, infection of cultured cells, such as FRhK4, BS-C-1, or MRC5, is typically not associated with any dramatic cellular injury and commonly leads to long-term persistence of the virus in cells. In addition, the HAV replication cycle in cell culture is typically slow. Most cell culture–adapted HAV variants attain maximal accumulation within 3 to 13 days but are not cytolytic. However, highly adapted variants of HAV that replicate rapidly (2–3 days) and cause cytopathic effects in cultured cells have been described.[38,68,226,264] The development of a cytopathic effect depends on the interaction between particular HAV strains and cells at certain passage levels. In most cases, rapid cytolytic growth was selected by passaging HAV HM175 from persistently infected cells at intervals of 3 to 7 days.[38] Some strains of HAV, however, were cytopathic within several passages after direct isolation from human feces.[264] Cellular injury appears to arise from the induction of apoptotic pathways leading to programmed cell death.[38,130,131] Continuous passage of the virus in cell culture frequently results in a reduction in the ability of the virus to replicate in primates, resulting in attenuation of HAV virulence *in vivo*.[302]

Infectious cloned cDNAs of both wild-type and cell culture–adapted HAV strains are available and have made it possible to study the effects of mutations on the growth of HAV in cell culture and on its virulence for primates, as reviewed by Purcell and Emerson.[308] The development of reporter subgenomic replicons lacking structural protein sequences that are capable of autonomous replication also have contributed to a better understanding of whether cell culture–adaptive mutations acted at the level of genome replication.[407] Several concepts have emerged about mutations selected during adaptation or passage in cultured cells (Fig. 19.9): (a) mutations in gene 2B or 2C appear to be essential for the adaptation and efficient genome replication of HM175[56,91,93,407] and probably other strains[135]; (b) mutations in the 5′ UTR (especially in the variable region around nucleotide 200) are not essential but enhance growth in a cell-type–restricted fas hion[75,115,116,117,137]—a cluster of mutations in the IRES appear to act by modulating translation efficiency in certain cells, perhaps through cell-type–specific interactions with accessory cellular proteins[75,117,332]; and (c) other mutations or deletions throughout the genome, notably in 3A and 3D coding sequences, also contribute to enhanced growth of various HAV strains.[135,136,201,264,308,415]

The effect of several cell culture–adapting mutations on HAV virulence has been evaluated following inoculation of tamarins (or occasionally chimpanzees) with virus or genomic RNA corresponding to wild-type HAV carrying cell culture–adapting mutations, or chimeras comprised of an attenuated HM175 variant and a virulent African green monkey strain. These experiments revealed that neither the 2B gene nor the 5′ UTR (including the polypyrimidine tract and IRES) are implicated in HAV virulence,[56,92,116,134,337] whereas the 2C gene (in particular, nucleotide 4563) plays a major role in virulence of HM175 in tamarins[92,312] (see Fig. 19.9). The VP1-2A region also is an important determinant for HAV virulence, although not for adaptation to cultured cells.[92] Genetic analysis of clinical viral isolates collected in patients experiencing self-limited acute, severe acute, or fulminant hepatitis failed to demonstrate clear associations of particular viral genome polymorphisms in the 5′ UTR/IRES, 2B, or 2C sequences with disease phenotypes.[111,113,237]

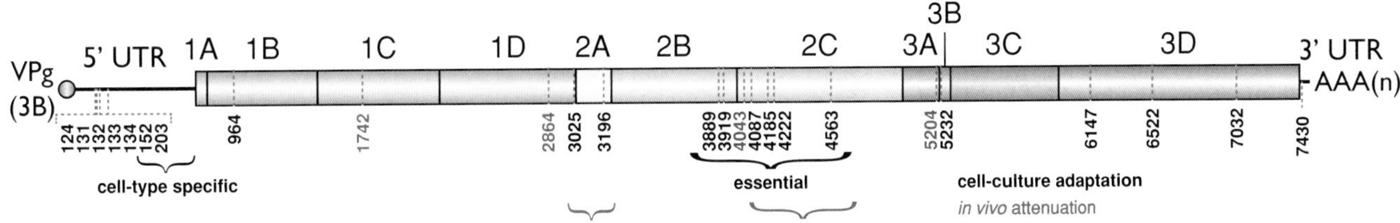

FIGURE 19.9. Substitutions existing between the cell culture–adapted HM175/p35 strain, used to produce inactivated hepatitis A virus (HAV) vaccines (GenBank accession number M16632), and its wild-type HM175 counterpart (GenBank accession number M14707) are represented by *dotted red lines* with their nucleotide position within the HAV full-length genome indicated below. Substitutions in the untranslated regions and those that result in amino acid changes are shown in *black font*, whereas silent changes are shown in *gray font*. Substitutions that are essential to cell culture adaptation and/or *in vivo* attenuation, or involved in cell-type modulation of HAV translation or replication (see text), are indicated by *curly braces*.

PATHOGENESIS AND HOST IMMUNE RESPONSES

Virus Replication *In Vivo*

Natural infection with HAV usually follows ingestion of virus from material contaminated with feces containing HAV. The sequence of events that begins with entry via the gastrointestinal tract and ultimately results in hepatitis has not been completely resolved. Consistent with the hypothesis that some cells of the gastrointestinal tract may be susceptible to HAV are studies in orally infected owl monkeys in which virus has been isolated from various levels of the gastrointestinal tract 3 to 35 days postinfection, and viral antigen has been identified by immunofluorescence in the epithelial cells of the intestinal crypts and in cells of the lamina propria from the duodenum, jejunum, and ileum.[13] Recognition that a transient rebound in fecal HAV RNA shedding has been observed in HAV-infected chimpanzees in the absence of a concomitant relapsing rise of virus-specific RNA in the serum or liver also suggests the possibility of an independent gastrointestinal replication compartment.[214] Whether this represents a *bona fide* site of replication of HAV remains to be clarified, however, because previous studies could not identify HAV antigen or genomic material in the intestinal mucosa of experimentally infected tamarins.[204,253,254]

The primary site of replication for HAV is the liver, as demonstrated by virus detection in hepatocytes within days and even hours after infection.[204,219,254,298] HAV is then released from

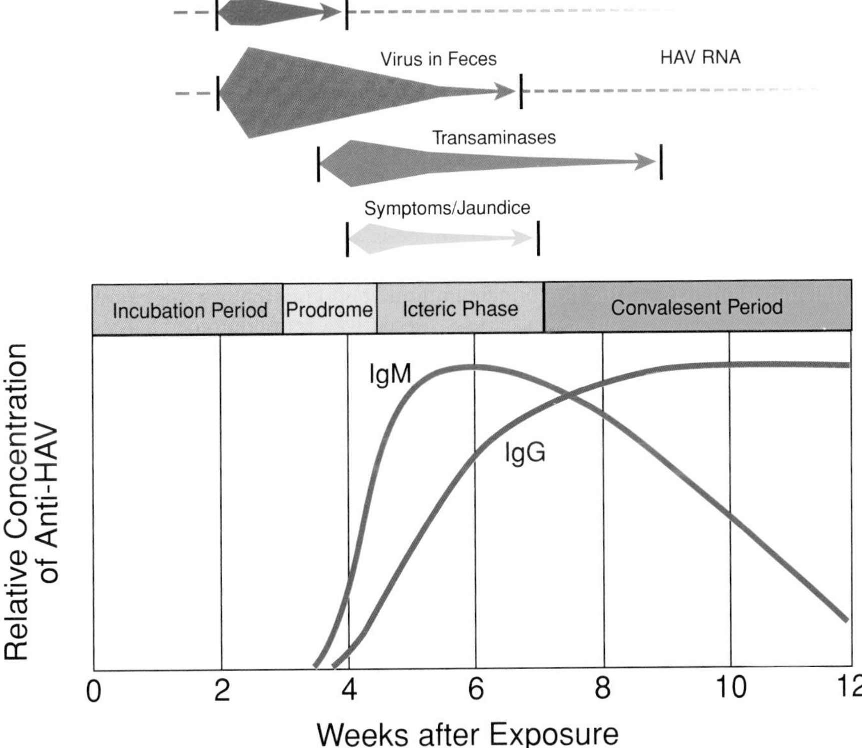

FIGURE 19.10. Clinically relevant immunologic and biologic events associated with hepatitis A virus (HAV) infection in humans divided into the four clinical stages. Following a period when virus in blood and feces has been shown to be transmissible, HAV RNA genomic material continues to be detected over a finite period of time (*dotted lines*) in some samples in the absence of documented infectivity (see text).

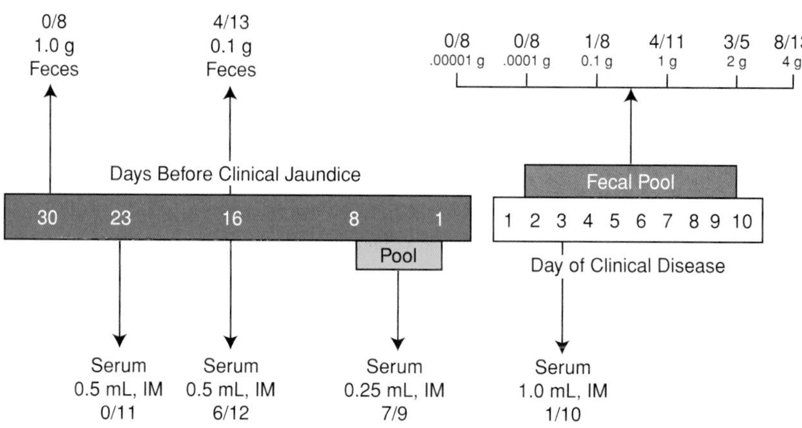

FIGURE 19.11. Relative levels of hepatitis A virus (HAV) infectivity observed for fecal and serum samples collected during the incubation period before clinical jaundice and the early stages of acute icteric hepatitis A. The number of subjects tested preceded by the number developing clinical hepatitis A is provided for each quantity of sample evaluated. In the absence of a diagnostic HAV assay in the 1960s to determine susceptibility, the number tested is not necessarily equivalent to the number of susceptible subjects; thus, the infectivity rate may be underestimated.[205] IM, intramuscular.

infected hepatocytes into the bile canaliculi and passes into the intestine, after which it is detected in stools.[308,328] According to this virus replication sequence, relatively high concentrations of HAV (up to 10^9 infectious virions per gram of stool)[309,371] are shed in the feces before the alanine aminotransferase (ALT) level initially becomes elevated and before the onset of clinical symptoms or jaundice[64,109,145,162,311] (Fig. 19.10). Communicability is highest during this interval.[169,186,206,311] Early human studies have documented excretion of infectious HAV in stool specimens collected as early as 2 to 3 weeks before and up to 8 days after the onset of jaundice[152,206] (Fig. 19.11). By contrast, transmission is severely curtailed during the acute and early convalescent stages of the disease, requiring increasingly larger quantities of fecal material to elicit an infection.[206,207,233,386] In adults, viral particles are more often detected in the stools of jaundiced patients in contrast to patients who develop clinical symptoms without jaundice or who display no clinical disease.[83,109] It is noteworthy that fecal shedding of presumably encapsidated HAV RNA can occur for several weeks after hepatitis develops, notably in infants,[316,319,364] whereas recurrent shedding of HAV RNA has been observed in patients who have relapsing illness.[347] In one study,[319] HAV RNA was detected in fecal samples from three preterm infants up to 4 to 5 months after they had developed acute hepatitis A. In addition to these observations, viral RNA and HAV antigen persist in the liver of infected chimpanzees more than 30 weeks after ALT levels have returned to normal and hepatic inflammation has resolved.[214]

Virus is observed in blood (viremia) at about the same time extensive shedding of the virus in feces is occurring (see Fig. 19.10), although at levels generally 2 to 4 $\log_{10}$ units lower than those in stool.[35,55,219] Viremia precedes the appearance of clinical and laboratory evidence of hepatitis by at least 2 weeks, and its level tends to diminish dramatically during the period of liver enzyme elevation. In some situations, HAV appears to circulate in the blood enclosed in lipid-associated membrane fragments that may transiently protect the virus from neutralizing antibody.[221] In parallel with what has been observed in stool samples, HAV genomic material has been detected in the blood of infected patients and chimpanzees for much longer periods after onset of the disease than originally assumed (>10 weeks), although at concentrations several orders of magnitude lower than in acute-phase samples and always accompanied by virus-specific antibody.[35,112,219,280,410] The clinical significance of these observations has not been determined, because transmission or infectivity of blood components or fecal material containing HAV genomic material at these later time intervals has never been documented.

Evidence has been obtained for the replication of HAV in the oropharynx and salivary glands in orally inoculated chimpanzees and marmosets shortly after the appearance of virus in the blood; this could represent an early replicative event for the virus.[55,298] Correspondingly, the presence of low titers of infectious virus in saliva collected from patients during the acute phase of the disease[5,238,309] and in macaques infected by the intravenous route[4] supports this conclusion. It is also possible, however, that the saliva may be contaminated by HAV entering the mouth during mastication through crevicular fluid that originates at the root–capillary interface, is released at the gingival surface, and contains serous material.[163] Finally, HAV antigen and/or genomic material has been observed in the kidney and spleen of infected owl monkeys, the biological relevance of which remains unknown.[13]

Immune Responses and Liver Disease

Early clinical studies in patients with acute hepatitis A reported either the absence of type I interferon[395] or only transient increases in serum levels of interferons and type I interferon-induced human MxA protein[180,228,411]—key components of the host innate immune responses that exert an antiviral effect on several viruses. Recently, a transcriptome analysis in HAV-infected chimpanzees revealed that the first evidence of an interferon response occurred at week 1 postinfection, as indicated by low-level increases of intrahepatic interferon-stimulated gene (ISG)-15 transcripts.[214] However, unlike many other genes, most ISG transcripts were up-regulated to a minimal degree and for only a few weeks in these HAV-infected animals. This paucity of type I interferon-induced ISG expression contrasts sharply with early and high-level induction of such genes in acute-resolving hepatitis C virus (HCV) infection. This is despite similar levels of viremia and 100-fold higher levels and much longer persistence of HAV RNA in the liver, and despite the presence of dsRNA in up to 10% of hepatocytes. The dsRNA corresponds to HAV replicative intermediates and forms (see Fig. 19.8D) and represents a potent pathogen-associated molecular pattern (PAMP) recognized by innate immune sensors.[214]

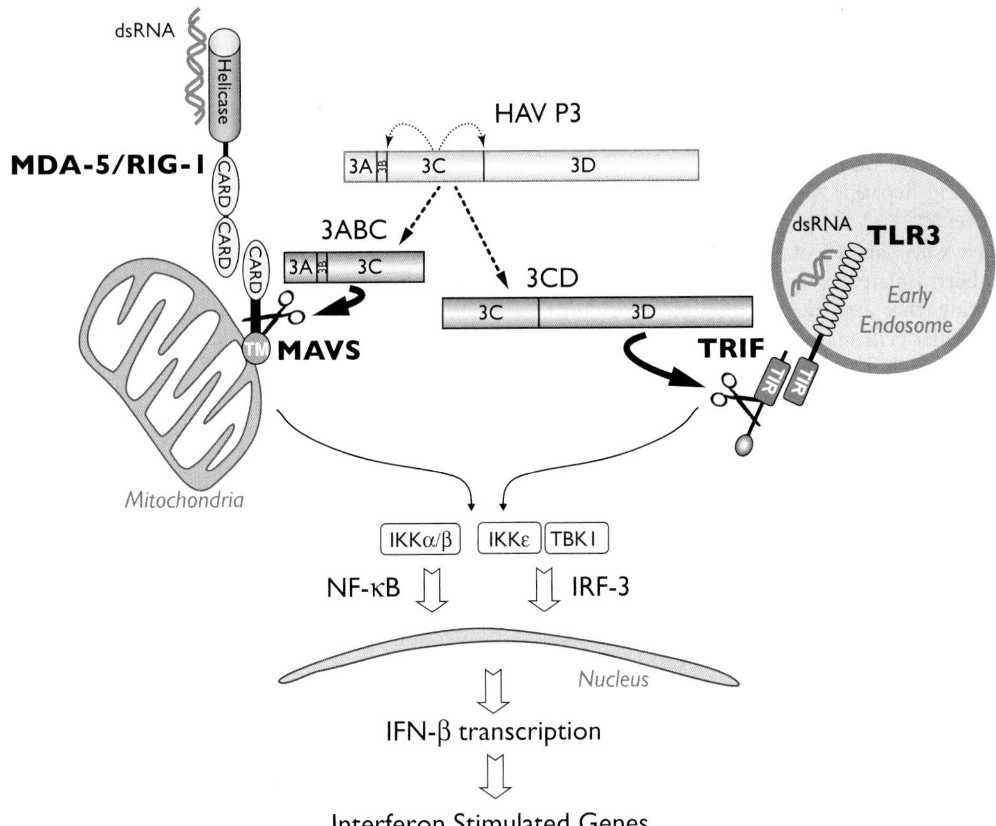

FIGURE 19.12. Interferon-activating pathways disrupted by hepatitis A virus (HAV) 3C protease precursors. Cytosolic HAV RNA (double-stranded RNA [dsRNA]) is most likely sensed by the cellular RNA helicase MDA-5, which interacts through caspase-recruitment domains (CARD) with the adaptor protein MAVS localized on the mitochondrial outer membrane. This induces the activation of kinases (IKKα/β, TBK-1, IKKε) of the IκB complex and subsequent activation of latent cytoplasmic transcription factors IRF-3 and NF-κB that results in the synthesis of interferon (IFN)-β as well as interferon-stimulated genes (ISG). Within an endosomal compartment, sensing of dsRNA by toll-like receptor 3 (TLR3) induces the dimerization of TLR3 and subsequent recruitment of the adaptor protein TRIF through shared toll/interleukin-1 receptor (TIR) domains. This also results in the signalization of IFN-β and ISG synthesis. Two different 3C protease processing intermediates derived from HAV P3 polypeptide block these signaling pathways by directing cleavage of the adaptor proteins: polypeptide 3ABC cleaves MAVS[404] and polypeptide 3CD possesses altered substrate specificity compared to mature 3C that allows cleavage of TRIF.[310] (Modified from a scheme courtesy of Prof. Stanley M. Lemon, University of North Carolina, Chapel Hill, NC, USA)

Altogether, these observations suggest that HAV has evolved strategies to evade protective host innate immune responses induced by dsRNA that can be summarized as follows (Fig. 19.12). Initial studies revealed that HAV infection blocked interferon-β expression in cell culture by inhibiting interferon regulatory factor 3 (IRF3) activation mediated by retinoic acid–inducible gene I (RIG-I) or melanoma differentiation–associated gene 5 (MDA5); signal transduction appeared disrupted between RIG-I/MDA5 and downstream kinases.[37,102] It was further shown that this disruption operated through cleavage of the adaptor molecule (MAVS) of the MDA-5/RIG-I–mediated signaling pathway by HAV 3ABC polypeptide. A stable and proteolytically active 3C protease precursor, 3ABC is directed to the mitochondrial membrane where MAVS localizes, owing to the presence of a mitochondrial targeting transmembrane domain in 3A.[404] In addition, evidence indicates that the 3CD protease-polymerase precursor processing intermediate disrupts toll-like receptor 3 (TLR3) interferon signaling by directing the cleavage of the corresponding adaptor molecule TRIF at two noncanonical 3C cleavage sites.[310] Thus, HAV proteins interfere with the two major cellular antiviral response pathways (RIG-I/MDA5/MAVS and TLR3/TRIF), possibly facilitating HAV replication during the clinically silent early weeks of infection.

The mechanisms responsible for hepatocellular injury and virus clearance in hepatitis A are incompletely characterized. The presence of large quantities of virus in the liver and stools prior to the onset of hepatic inflammation argues against a major direct cytopathic effect of HAV. Furthermore, in the absence of extensive adaptation of HAV to cell culture, HAV infections *in vitro* are noncytopathic and cell metabolism is relatively unaffected. Clinical hepatitis coincides with the appearance of robust humoral[183] and cellular (see below) immune responses. Because of this, the possibility of humoral immunopathogenesis has been examined, although no complement-dependent, antibody-mediated cytolytic activity has been demonstrated against HAV-infected cells.[118] Circulating immune complexes containing HAV and HAV-specific antibodies (primarily immunoglobulin M [IgM]) have been found during infection.[17,39,246] However, although immune complexes may be present in the kidney,[164] immunoglobulin and complement deposits were not found at the sites of liver cell damage, and resolution of disease occurred at a time when antibody levels were rising and hepatitis A antigen could still be easily detected in the liver.[245]

Natural killer cells capable of lysing HAV-infected cultured cells have been isolated from patients with acute hepatitis A,[16] suggesting that nonspecific immune mechanisms involving natural killer cells may play a role in hepatocellular damage. Clinical studies have revealed that lymphocytes recovered from the liver and blood of patients with acute hepatitis A contain human leukocyte antigen (HLA)-restricted, HAV-specific, CD8+ cytotoxic T cells that produce interferon-γ in response to HAV-infected cultured cells.[108,209,239,379,380] This is consistent with the pathology of hepatitis A being largely the result of cell-mediated immune responses to the infection, as reviewed by Vallbracht and Fleischer[378] and Siegl and Weitz.[343] Highly conserved HAV-specific epitopes restricted by HLA-A2 and other alleles were recognized by CD8+ T cells collected from patients with acute, postacute, and resolved HAV infections.[329] Most patients showed a multispecific T-cell response against at least two epitopes located within HAV VP1, VP2, VP3, 2B, 2C, and 3D regions of the HAV polyprotein, with the response directed against the 3D epitope being reproducibly immunodominant in HLA-A2 patients. These results and the existence of a single serotype suggest that immune escape in HAV infection does not appear to play a major role in the pathogenesis of this infection.

Although a dominant role for CD8+ T cells in both liver injury and control of HAV infections in humans has been postulated, a recent study in HAV-infected chimpanzees pointed to a potentially significant role for CD4+ T cells in HAV clearance. CD4+ T cells produced multiple cytokines when viremia first declined, rebounded with a transient relapse of HAV fecal shedding, and remained detectable for many weeks until the HAV genome was cleared from the liver, whereas CD8+ T-cell frequency and effector functions did not appear to be as closely associated with virus control, at least in chimpanzees.[417] It is noteworthy that viremia declines rapidly following the appearance of the humoral response, suggesting that neutralizing antibodies also play a major role in clearing viremia.[225] Correspondingly, a transcriptome analysis in HAV-infected chimpanzees revealed a remarkable activation of genes involved in B-cell development at 3 to 4 weeks postinfection.[214]

EPIDEMIOLOGY

Hepatitis A is one of the most common causes of infectious jaundice in the world today and is frequently associated with recurrent epidemics. Humans and other primates are the only natural reservoirs for HAV. Based on incidence rates from confirmed acute HAV cases, the geographic distribution of HAV infection appears to be changing as countries improve their level of sanitation and personal hygiene (D. Shouval, personal communication, 2011)[178] (Fig. 19.13). In populations in which living conditions are crowded and sanitation is nonexistent or inadequate, prevalence studies reveal that infections occur at an early age and that close to 100% of children acquire immunity during the first decade of life[110,141,179,257,361] (Fig. 19.14). In contrast, in modern urban societies or in developing nations where improvements in sanitation and personal hygiene have delayed infection, a reduction in anti-HAV prevalence among younger persons has been found.[142,177,179,257,324,360] Thus, large segments of the population remain susceptible, and epidemics can occur after chance introduction of the virus to such an area. This has resulted in a paradoxical increase in the number

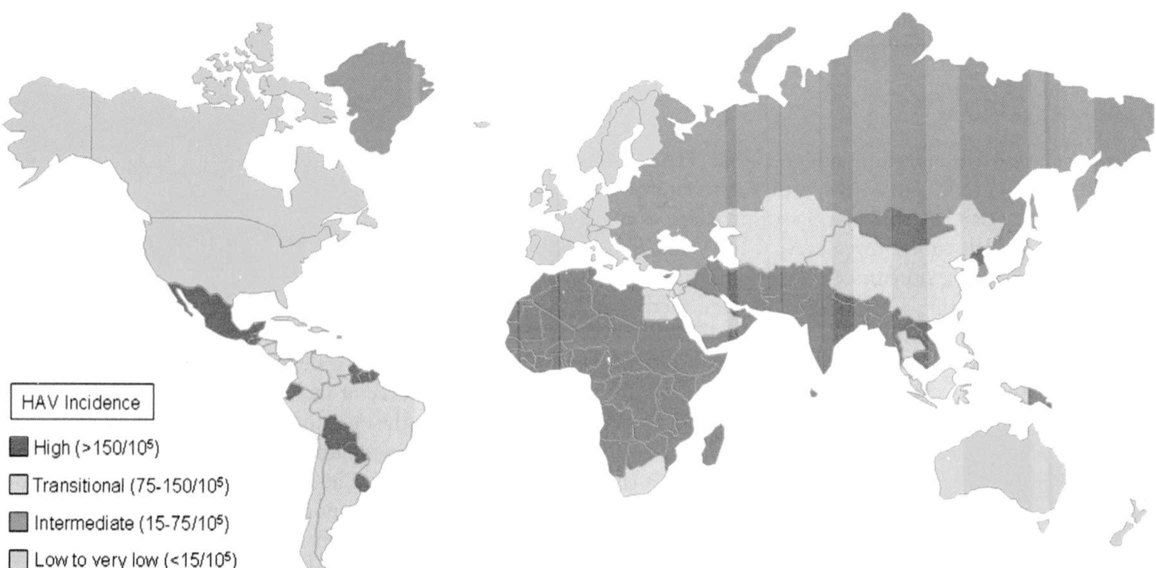

FIGURE 19.13. Estimated global hepatitis A virus incidence levels based on age-seroprevalence rates by country or region from samples that are representative of the general population, 2005. (Courtesy of Prof. Daniel Shouval, Hadassah-Hebrew University Hospital, Jerusalem, Israel.)

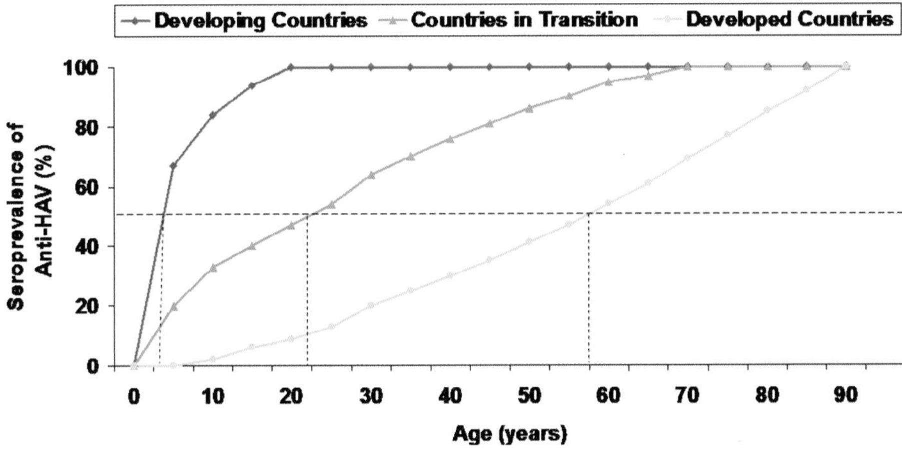

FIGURE 19.14. Age-specific hepatitis A virus seroprevalence curves in developed and developing countries and those in transition demonstrating age at which 50% of the people have immunity.[179]

of cases observed in adults as they escape early childhood infection where disease manifestations are mild, and transition to adulthood where clinical disease is more overt and severe. An example of this changing epidemiology was the large epidemic that occurred in Shanghai in 1988 with more than 300,000 cases recorded.[406]

In the United States, the incidence of acute, symptomatic cases of HAV declined from 12.8 cases/100,000 population in 1980 to 0.9 cases/100,000 in 2008[49] (Fig. 19.15). At least a part of this decline is attributable to implementation of vaccine programs in high-risk populations (see the Prevention and Control section). The actual incidence of disease throughout the United States is estimated to be much higher because (a) many persons contract such a mild form of hepatitis that they do not seek treatment, and (b) physicians underreport hospitalized cases, although deaths are usually reported.

The incubation period for hepatitis A ranges from 10 to 50 days, with a mode of approximately 1 month, regardless of the route of infection.[276,288,289] Higher doses of virus, however, lead to a shorter incubation period.[289,309] When two cases occur less than 14 days apart during a point source epidemic, they are more likely to be coprimary, rather than secondary, cases. Correspondingly, cases occurring more than 60 days apart presumably result from secondary spread of the infection.[207,386] Although the median incubation periods for viral hepatitis A through E are distinctly different, there is considerable overlap; thus, knowledge of the incubation period is rarely useful in determining etiology. In addition, the patient may not know the time of exposure.

Of those with overt hepatitis A, from 21% to 53% are hospitalized, with the lowest being among children and the highest among persons 60 years of age or older. More than 70% of the adult clinical cases are jaundiced. In the United States, an estimated 100 persons die of fulminant hepatitis annually. Table 19.2 provides mortality data by age group for hospitalized patients with icteric hepatitis A increasing from 0.23% for those younger than 30 years to 1.8% to 2.1% for those older than 49 years. An overall case fatality rate of less than 0.015%

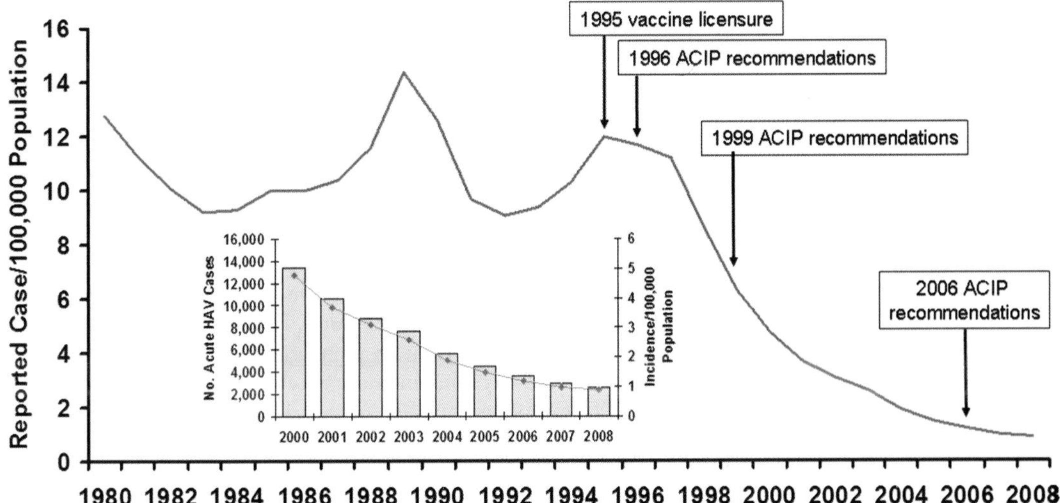

FIGURE 19.15. Incidence of acute hepatitis A per 100,000 population, United States, by year and Advisory Committee on Immunization Practices (ACIP) recommendations.[49] The inset covers the years 2000 to 2008 and shows the number of acute hepatitis A virus cases and the incidence/100,000 population in more detail.

TABLE 19.2 Predicted Outcome After an Infection With Hepatitis A Virus[a]

	Predicted outcome	
Parameter	**Children (<5 y) (%)**	**Adults (%)**
Inapparent infection	80–95	10–25
Anicteric or icteric disease	5–20	75–90
Complete recovery	≥99	≥98
Chronic disease	None	
Mortality rate (hospitalized cases)		
<30 y	0.23	
30–49 y	0.3–0.6	
>49 y	1.8–2.1	

[a]Refer to the text regarding atypical manifestations of hepatitis A.

was recorded among 310,746 cases of hepatitis A that occurred in Shanghai in 1988.[406] This translated to a mortality rate of 0.3% to 0.6% for the 8,647 patients who were hospitalized, of whom 90.8% were between the ages of 20 and 40 years. Some of these patients had an underlying hepatitis B infection.

As expected, the presence of HAV in feces facilitates virus dissemination and accounts for the person-to-person mode of spread of hepatitis A. In the United States, the epidemiologic characteristics of acute hepatitis A cases reported to the Centers for Disease Control and Prevention (CDC) from 2001 to 2007 changed annually[47] to include household or sexual contacts with a person who had hepatitis A, international travel, men who had sex with other men, illicit drug users, and children and employees associated with daycare centers or with contacts of these individuals (e-Fig. 19.3). No risk factor was disclosed in more than 50% of the cases, although HAV-contaminated food was often suspected. Percentages are found to vary each year; however, a trend exists toward proportionally more cases being attributed to international travel, especially to Mexico and Central/South America, although sexual or household contact also is frequently implicated.

In contrast to this person-to-person mode of spread, sudden, explosive epidemics of hepatitis A within communities or confined populations usually result from fecal contamination from a single source,[63] such as drinking water,[266] milk, or food.[104] Contamination of food can occur during cultivation, harvesting, processing, distribution, or preparation. Most food handlers with hepatitis A do not transmit HAV to patrons; when this occurs, however, the incriminated food is usually an item that is served uncooked or without further cooking (e.g., sandwiches, salads, pastries). Recent sources of large outbreaks have implicated frozen raspberries and strawberries, as well as iceberg lettuce.[104] An example of foodborne outbreaks in three states of the United States following the consumption of contaminated green onions[393] is illustrated by an increase in the number of cases reported in 2003 (see e-Fig. 19.3). Several other foodborne outbreaks of hepatitis A have resulted from the consumption of raw or inadequately cooked oysters and clams obtained from water polluted with sewage.[147,321,406] The role of mollusks has been that of virus concentrators of water polluted by sewage and not as a source for virus replication. During feeding, physiologically active bivalves (e.g., oysters or mussels) can filter up to 10 gallons of water per hour over a short period during which HAV can be concentrated at least 100 times and persist for about 7 days.[96] As expected, nonbivalve shellfish (e.g., lobsters, shrimp) do not impart the same risk.

Hepatitis A molecular epidemiology is being widely and successfully used to characterize sources of infection and transmission patterns.[272] These molecular studies can provide strong epidemiologic links of disease transmission between persons who travel to an endemic area[316,318,372] or during investigations of foodborne outbreaks.[8] Such analyses are facilitated by the use of nucleic acid sequencing and phylogenetic evaluations to identify unique strains and determine genetic relatedness. Current phylogenetic analyses generally use a 315-bp nucleotide fragment from the 1D-2AB region of the genome because of its high degree of variability.[272] Population-based studies provide evidence that HAV is often transmitted by networks of persons who display similar risk factors for infection.[372]

As discussed previously, HAV communicability is apparently highest during the clinically silent incubation period when virus replication reaches a peak[169,186,206,311] (see Fig. 19.11). By the time the patient seeks medical attention or the transaminases reach a peak and the patient becomes jaundiced, clinically relevant viremia also has significantly diminished. In one study, an acute-phase serum sample from a human with clinical disease was a million-fold less infectious when inoculated into chimpanzees than a stool sample collected on the same day,[309] and serum samples from three other strains of HAV were at least 1,000 times less infectious. Despite these observations, HAV transmission through blood remains a rare but potential cause of posttransfusion hepatitis.[19,148,164,219] In the past, the problem was amplified in neonatal intensive care units where infants developed a covert infection after receiving blood components from an infected donor. They subsequently transmitted the virus to healthcare workers and family members, presumably by the fecal–oral route.[15,200,279,319] The rarity of transfusion-associated hepatitis A in adults probably can be attributed to several closely associated factors. First, the viremic stage is short, and the concentration of HAV in the blood is relatively low, as previously reviewed. The absence of an HAV carrier state[207] also contributes to the rarity of HAV transmission through blood. Thus, for transmission to occur, an infected donor would have to donate blood to a susceptible recipient during a very restricted interval. In addition, because most recipients are given more than 1 unit of blood, an anti–HAV-positive unit may be transfused concurrently with the HAV-positive unit, thereby neutralizing the virus. Several of these scenarios often do not apply to neonates, which is why the risk is greater in this group. Current blood bank practices do not include specific screening of prospective donors for evidence of active HAV infection. However, nucleic acid testing for HAV is being done by the plasma industry, and whereas there is a wide variation in pool sizes and sensitivities, the general conclusion is that the HAV nucleic acid–reactive yield is relatively low with a range of 1 positive donation in 120,000 to 1,805,500 donations (S. Stramer, personal communication, 2011).

From 1989 to 1995, several outbreaks of hepatitis A occurred among hemophiliacs in Europe, South Africa, and the United States who received solvent- and detergent-treated factor VIII.[243,315] Implicated lots were devoid of appreciable amounts of neutralizing anti-HAV and contained HAV genomic material whose genetic sequence was identical to that obtained from infected patients. The solvent or detergent treatment had no effect on infectivity of this nonenveloped virus (see the Morphology and Properties of Hepatitis A Virions section) but could have been responsible for dispersing HAV in the product by releasing the virus from a nonneutralizable, lipid-associated environment. Effective heat-inactivation procedures, a preference for recombinant factor VIII, and vaccination have significantly reduced this risk.

Little evidence is found for transmission of HAV by exposure to urine or the nasopharyngeal secretions of infected patients.[1,124,154,187,236,277] Other identified potential sources of exposure to HAV are nonhuman primates, usually chimpanzees, that have infected caretakers and other zoo personnel in close contact with them.[74,81,159] In these situations, vaccination has been highly effective.

CLINICAL FEATURES

The outcome of hepatitis A can be extremely variable depending on the age when acquired (see Table 19.2). Patients with inapparent or subclinical hepatitis have neither symptoms nor jaundice. These asymptomatic cases previously went unrecognized but now can be identified by detecting biochemical or serologic alterations in the blood. Other patients can develop anicteric hepatitis or icteric hepatitis. Symptoms ranging from mild and transient to severe and prolonged can accompany anicteric or icteric hepatitis. Most patients recover completely; however, some develop fulminant hepatitis and die. As noted in Table 19.2, the disease is milder in children than in adults, complete recovery is the rule, and chronic disease has not been observed.[216] Hospitalization for and death caused by fulminant hepatic failure is age dependent. Whereas two-thirds of the clinical cases occur in children and young adults, more than 70% of the deaths are observed in patients older than 50 years. The mortality rate is considerably higher among patients with chronic hepatitis B or C who are superinfected with HAV,[144,196,382,406] primarily when the underlying liver disease is advanced.

Symptoms and Signs

A typical course of acute hepatitis A can be divided into four clinical phases: (a) incubation or preclinical period (time between exposure and the first day of symptoms), (b) prodromal or preicteric stage, (c) icteric phase, and (d) convalescent period (see Fig. 19.10).

During the incubation phase, the patient remains asymptomatic despite active replication of the virus. A short prodromal or preicteric phase, varying from a few days to more than a week, precedes the onset of jaundice. In more than half of patients, the prodromal state typically is characterized by anorexia, fever, fatigue, malaise, myalgia, nausea, and vomiting. In hepatitis A, the transition from well-being to acutely ill occurs abruptly (within a period of 24 hours) in more than 60% of the cases, whereas the onset is more insidious in hepatitis B. Fever higher than 100.5°F is more common in acute hepatitis A than in acute hepatitis B.[386] Diarrhea, nausea, and vomiting are more frequent in children than in adults.[220] Weight loss of 2 to 10 pounds is common as a result of the anorexia that accompanies disorders of taste and smell.[157,349] Older children and adults often complain of right upper quadrant pain or discomfort as a consequence of hepatomegaly.[386]

The icteric phase of acute viral hepatitis is ushered in by the appearance of golden-brown urine caused by bilirubinuria, followed one to several days later by pale stools and yellowish discoloration of the mucous membranes, conjunctivae, sclerae, and skin. This icteric phase begins within 10 days of the initial symptoms in more than 85% of HAV cases,[420] prompting patients to seek medical attention. Fever, if present, usually subsides after the first few days of jaundice.

Physical examination of the patient with a typical case of acute disease reveals the presence of jaundice accompanied by tenderness to palpation or percussion of the liver, which may be enlarged. Measurement by percussion is essential, because a reduction in size in a patient whose condition is deteriorating often heralds massive necrosis. Approximately 5% to 15% of patients have splenomegaly; however, generalized adenopathy is not a component of the disease and should trigger further investigation. Palmar erythema and spider angiomata may be observed.

Several atypical manifestations of hepatitis A have been reported, including the development of cholestasis, the possible induction of type 1 autoimmune hepatitis, extrahepatic manifestations, and relapsing hepatitis.[188,325] HAV-infected patients who present with cholestatic hepatitis A initially have pruritus, fever, diarrhea, and weight loss. The serum bilirubin usually remains above 10 mg/dL for more than 12 weeks, whereas the ALT level is often less than 500 IU/L. Resolution of the disease is slow; however, recovery is complete within 2 to 8 months.[127,334] HAV also has been associated with acute acalculous cholecystitis with jaundice on rare occasions[268,283] and to trigger the onset of autoimmune hepatitis. Extrahepatic manifestations of hepatitis A are unusual,[69] although transient rashes are observed infrequently, as are arthralgia, arthritis, hemolysis, leukocytoclastic vasculitis, membranoproliferative glomerulonephritis, and pancreatitis.[164,174,399] Finally, relapsing hepatitis occurs in 3% to 20% of the cases of acute hepatitis A. Recrudescence of the disease, usually less severe than the original episode, occurs 4 to 15 weeks after the initial symptoms have resolved. In some patients, only biochemical changes are observed. IgM anti-HAV either reappears or increases in titer, and HAV genomic material is detected in feces and serum. More than one relapse can occur, and enzyme elevations can persist for 5 to 12 months, although chronic sequelae are not observed.

Occasionally, more extensive necrosis of the liver occurs during acute viral hepatitis A, leading to severe impairment of hepatic synthetic processes, excretory functions, and detoxifying mechanisms. This entity, designated *fulminant hepatitis* if hepatic encephalopathy occurs during the first 6 to 8 weeks of illness or within 1 to 4 weeks after jaundice, is characterized by the sudden onset of high fever, marked abdominal pain, vomiting, and jaundice followed by the development of encephalopathy associated with deep coma and seizures.[282] A jaundice-to-encephalopathy time >7 days is an important prognostic indicator when determining the need for a liver transplant. This, however, is only one of several factors that are employed to determine survival in cases of fulminant hepatitis A. Other variables include coagulopathy (international normalized ratio [INR] >3.85), age (<10 or >40 years), elevated serum bilirubin and creatinine levels, intubation, and the use of pressors.[281,365] Although ascites, a bleeding diathesis, and decerebrate rigidity can lead to death in 70% to 90% of patients, in at least one study,[365] the overall survival rate in fulminant hepatitis A among those spontaneously recovering and not requiring a liver transplant was 55%. Fortunately, fulminant liver failure is rare, occurring in less than 1.0% of the icteric patients hospitalized for acute viral hepatitis A.

Host factors that might influence the severity of hepatitis A infection are not well known. Viremia in patients with fulminant hepatitis A was found to be significantly lower than in classical forms of the disease, raising the hypothesis that fulminant hepatitis A might be associated with a strong immunological response.[314] A recent study found a relationship between HAV-induced severe liver disease and a six amino acid insertion in HAVcr1/TIM-1, a potential functional receptor for HAV[52,198] (see the Infectious Viral Life Cycle section). This gene polymorphism appeared to offer protection against the development of atopic diseases while predisposing the individual to severe HAV-induced disease. A possible explanation for this may stem from observations that the long form of TIM-1 binds HAV more efficiently and that natural killer T cells expressing the long form of TIM-1 are more cytotoxic for HAV-infected hepatocytes.[198] In addition, it was found that the association of IgA with HAVcr1/TIM-1 enhances the interaction of HAVcr1/TIM-1 with HAV, suggesting a potential role for IgA/HAVcr1 interaction in the pathogenesis of HAV by enhancing viral entry in cells expressing low levels of HAVcr1/TIM-1.[362]

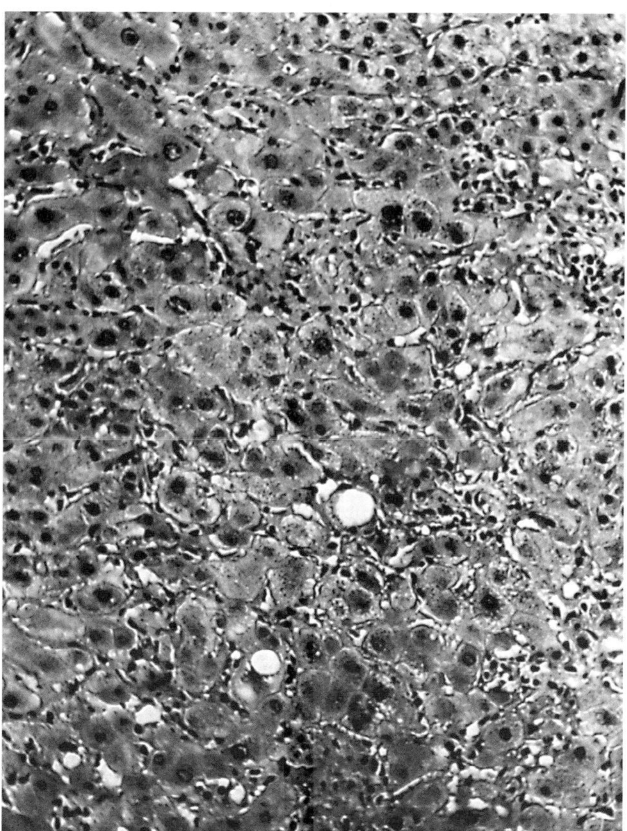

FIGURE 19.16. Classic acute viral hepatitis. Lobular disarray characterized by anisocytosis, anisonucleosis, ballooning, and Kupffer cell hypertrophy (H&E, ×190). (From Ishak KG. Light microscopic morphology of viral hepatitis. *Am J Clin Pathol* 1976;65(Suppl 5):787–827, with permission.)

Laboratory Features

The initial laboratory evaluation of the patient with acute hepatitis should include a biochemical liver panel, complete blood count (CBC), and INR. Serum ALT and aspartate aminotransferase (AST) concentrations are highly sensitive indicators of hepatocellular injury. They provide a quantitative assessment of acute damage sustained by the liver, although the eventual outcome cannot be predicted from the level attained. Within hepatocytes, AST is found in mitochondria (80%) and the cytosol (20%), whereas ALT is limited to the cytosol, which may partially explain the aminotransferase patterns seen in acute hepatitis (i.e., ALT > AST). Damage to the plasma membrane leading to ionic and water shifts[375] is followed by ballooning degeneration of hepatocytes (Fig. 19.16) and leakage of ALT from the cytosol. Consequently, high ALT:AST ratios (>1.4) are observed in uncomplicated acute viral hepatitis cases. Exceptions include those situations in which severe tissue necrosis develops, resulting in the release of mitochondrial AST into the blood. In these situations, the lactic dehydrogenase (LDH) enzyme also is significantly elevated. For the jaundiced patient, total serum bilirubin usually remains below 10 mg/dL, although levels of 20 mg/dL are occasionally observed. After reaching a peak in 1 to 2 weeks, the rate of decline is more gradual, with resolution occurring within 6 weeks of onset in most patients.[320] As liver injury improves, discordant findings between serum and urine bilirubin can occur when elevated levels of serum bilirubin may not be accompanied by bilirubinuria owing to the *de novo* synthesis of a conjugated form of bilirubin (delta bilirubin) that is irreversibly (covalently) bound to albumin,[388] thereby impairing its excretion in the urine.

Certain serum proteins (e.g., albumin, prothrombin, and fibrinogen) are synthesized exclusively or predominantly by the liver and can be affected by HAV injury. However, because the intravascular half-lives of the various plasma-clotting factors are relatively short (hours to days), measurement of both the INR and partial thromboplastin time may more accurately reflect early and potentially serious derangements in liver function than does measurement of serum albumin, which has a half-life of 3 weeks.

Generally, the patient with typical acute viral hepatitis has a normal or slightly reduced number of neutrophils and a relative lymphocytosis.[155] When the white blood count is more than 12,000/mm^3, a more serious form of the disease should be anticipated. Although mild to moderate reduction in red blood cell survival is frequent in acute viral hepatitis,[195] the hematocrit and hemoglobin remain within normal limits. Occasionally, however, hemolytic anemia occurs, often in association with glucose-6-phosphate dehydrogenase deficiency.[132,173,240] Rarely does agranulocytosis, thrombocytopenia, red cell aplasia, or aplastic anemia accompany acute viral hepatitis.[69,97,271]

Histologic Findings

In acute hepatitis A, both degenerative and regenerative parenchymal changes coexist with a diffusely distributed accumulation of mononuclear inflammatory cells.[176] Lobular disarray (see Fig. 19.16) is accompanied by swollen hepatocytes (ballooning degeneration) with indistinct plasma membranes, enlarged nuclei, and a featureless cytoplasm except for some cytoplasmic remnants condensed around the nuclei (e-Fig. 19.4). Acidophilic degeneration (apoptosis) also occurs with cells becoming shriveled and angulated while displaying increased eosinophilia. Both types of degeneration result in the migration of affected cells or cellular debris into the spaces of Disse and eventually into the sinusoids, where they are surrounded by Kupffer cells and undergo phagocytosis and digestion. Activation of Kupffer cells in the sinusoids and macrophages in the portal tracts results in marked hypertrophy and hyperplasia of these cells. The portal tracts are enlarged as a result of edema accompanied by a moderate to heavy infiltration of lymphocytes, although neutrophils and eosinophils can be present. Plasma cells are uncommon. Inflammatory cells can spill over into the adjacent parenchyma, a process called *interface hepatitis;* however, less than 25% of the limiting plate is involved. During the recovery stage, regeneration is prominent, as manifested by anisonucleosis, the presence of numerous bi- and trinucleated cells, and mitosis. The inflammatory response diminishes, although Kupffer cell hypertrophy persists for a few weeks. The damaged hepatic tissue is usually restored within 8 to 12 weeks.

In 5% to 10% of patients, focal necrosis gives way to zones of necrosis that bridge portal tracts or join portal areas to terminal hepatic veins.[36,103] When this process involves entire lobules or adjacent lobules, the terms *submassive* (involving the central and middle zones of lobules) or *massive* (involving entire lobules) are applied. The latter is characterized further by the proliferation of cholangioles in the periportal areas infiltrated by neutrophils (Fig. 19.17). Confluent hepatic necrosis is potentially a progressive lesion that can lead to fulminant hepatitis and death, which appears to be inevitable when necrosis involves more than 65% to 80% of the total hepatocyte fraction.[121,335] Conversely, complete regeneration of the liver is observed in survivors.[53,194]

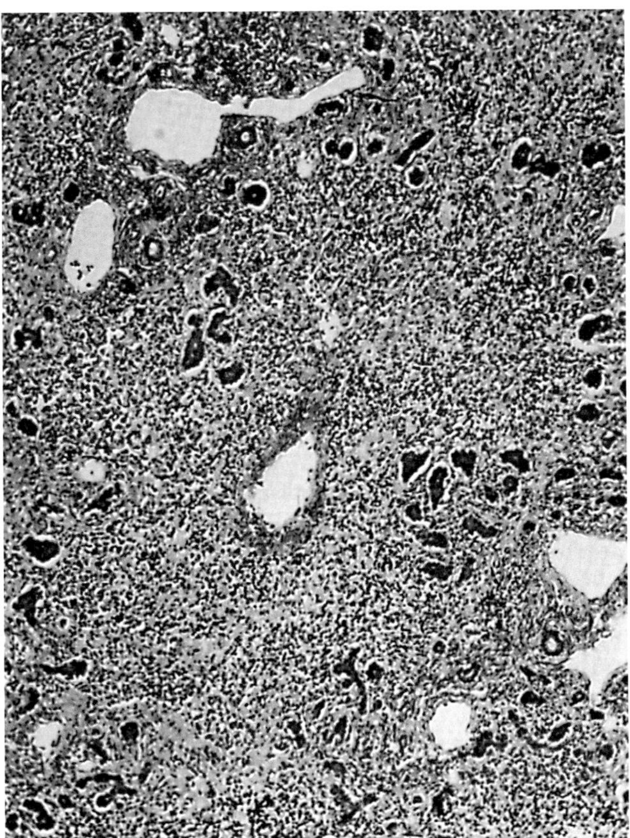

FIGURE 19.17. Acute viral hepatitis with massive necrosis. All liver cells have "dropped out." Note proliferating periportal cholangioles and infiltration of stroma and portal areas with inflammatory cells (H&E, × 73). (From Ishak KG. Light microscopic morphology of viral hepatitis. *Am J Clin Pathol* 1976;65 (Suppl 5):787–827, with permission.)

In rare cases of acute viral hepatitis A accompanied by jaundice, severe centrilobular cholestasis associated with disruption of bile canaliculi and periportal inflammation is observed that sometimes resembles chronic hepatitis, which never occurs in hepatitis A. This appears to be more common in hepatitis A than in hepatitis B or C but is less common than in acute hepatitis E.[139,334] Plasma cells are often prominent in this condition.

Just as it is difficult to determine the cause of acute hepatitis without serologic data, the pathologic changes in acute-phase liver tissue obtained from humans with different forms of viral hepatitis are qualitatively similar.[103,176] In general, liver tissue from patients with acute hepatitis A has less conspicuous parenchymal changes (including focal necrosis, Kupffer cell proliferation, acidophilic bodies, and ballooning degeneration) and less occurrence of steatosis than does tissue from patients with acute hepatitis C; however, necrosis and mononuclear cell inflammation of the periportal region are more evident than in biopsies from patients with acute hepatitis B.[2,103,208] In addition, the limiting plate is more likely to be disrupted in hepatitis A.

DIAGNOSIS

Because the agents of viral hepatitis often cannot be distinguished clinically and HAV superinfection of hepatitis B and C carriers can occur, serologic means are required for identification. The most favored acute viral hepatitis profile includes assays for IgM anti-HAV, hepatitis B surface antigen (HBsAg), IgM antibodies to the hepatitis B core antigen (IgM anti-HBc), and antibodies to HCV (anti-HCV). Idiosyncrasies of the assays, however, often make it desirable to perform ancillary tests that will confirm a positive response. Figure 19.18 is the approach used to diagnose acute hepatitis A, determine immunity, and assess the need for vaccination.

Amplification and sequencing of HAV RNA is being used to determine the genetic relatedness of isolates to identify infection sources and transmission patterns during epidemiologic case investigations[80,172,315,316,318,372] (see the Epidemiology section). Immunocytochemical staining and physicochemical studies have been used to identify HAV and viral antigen in liver tissue from infected primates obtained early in the course of the disease.[169,197,214,254,269,339] None of these methods, however, is practical in a clinical setting; they are not necessary unless incontrovertible proof for the presence of infectious virus or its source is needed.

To establish the diagnosis of acute or recent hepatitis A, blood samples are examined for the presence of acute-phase IgM-specific anti-HAV[39,77,232] (see Figs. 19.10 and 19.18). Rarely, this test may be nonreactive when the patient first seeks medical assistance but will invariably become positive within the next 7 to 10 days.[230] Conceptually, the *total* anti-HAV test also will be positive when the IgM anti-HAV assay is positive,

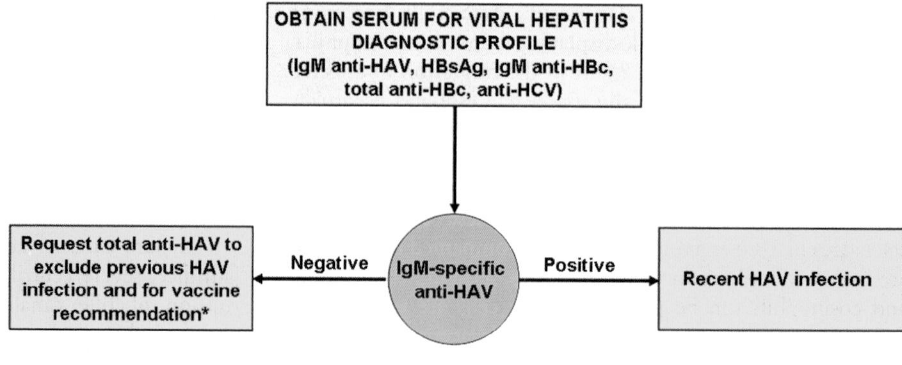

FIGURE 19.18. Serologic diagnosis of acute hepatitis A and immunity. IgM anti-HAV (immunoglobulin M antibodies to the hepatitis A virus); HBsAg (hepatitis B surface antigen); IgM anti-HBc (immunoglobulin M antibodies to the hepatitis B core antigen); total anti-HBc (immunoglobulin G [IgG] and IgM antibodies to the hepatitis B core antigen); anti-HCV (antibodies to the hepatitis C virus); total anti-HAV (IgG and IgM antibodies to the hepatitis A virus).

because it detects both immunoglobulin G (IgG) and IgM antibodies. Should it be negative, a false-positive IgM anti-HAV result should be entertained. The IgM anti-HAV antibody rapidly increases in titer over a period of 4 to 6 weeks and then declines to nondetectable levels within 3 to 6 months in most patients (range of <30 to >420 days), with persistence for more than 200 days in 13.5% of cases.[190] In more than 85% of patients, the liver enzymes will be normal before or at the time of disappearance of IgM anti-HAV. IgG anti-HAV eventually replaces the IgM antibody, persists for years after infection, and appears to confer lifelong immunity[348] (see Fig. 19.10).

The total anti-HAV assay is used primarily to determine the immune status of an individual after vaccination or to assess risk in a person traveling to an endemic region or working in a high-risk area. In the absence of either IgM anti-HAV or an abnormal ALT level, clinicians can assume that the antibody being detected by this assay is of the IgG type, indicating previous infection with HAV—or successful vaccination—and protection against future infection. These conclusions are valid only if passively acquired antibody from blood components, maternal antibodies crossing the placenta, or immune globulin immunoprophylaxis can be excluded.

MANAGEMENT OF ACUTE VIRAL HEPATITIS

No specific treatment for acute viral hepatitis exists, and hospitalization is not ordinarily indicated. Therapy should be supportive and aimed at maintaining comfort and adequate nutritional balance. For most jaundiced patients, strict bed rest and prolonged confinement are probably not indicated.[50] In one study, for example, strenuous activity did not appear to have any adverse effect on the clinical course of acute viral hepatitis.[313]

The diet should conform to the patient's appetite and wishes; it must, however, supply adequate protein and calories. As a general rule, modest consumption of alcohol (<30 g/day for men and <15 g/day for women) during convalescence (6–24 weeks after symptoms develop) does not seem to be harmful when the ALT level has decreased to less than 1.5 times the upper limit of normal.[373] Nevertheless, because of the direct hepatotoxic effect of ethanol, abstinence from alcoholic beverages during the acute phase of hepatitis seems prudent. Finally, women who are taking oral contraceptives need not discontinue their use during the course of hepatitis.[333]

No indication exists for corticosteroids in the treatment of acute, uncomplicated hepatitis A. They have no effect on the rate of resolution of the underlying disease process and may increase the rate of relapse or result in death from fulminant hepatitis, especially if administered during the incubation or prodromal stage of infection.[29,98,99] Conversely, a 4-week course of prednisone with tapering doses can hasten resolution in some patients who have developed prolonged, moderate to severe cholestasis, although complete recovery without therapy will eventually occur in all.[325] Abruptly stopping prednisone or shortening the interval of therapy can result in a relapse.

Specific antiviral therapy is not yet available for HAV, partly because chronicity is not an issue and outcome of the disease is generally favorable. However, amantadine and interferon-alpha have been reported to interfere with HAV replication in cell culture.[397,403] Amantadine was shown to inhibit HAV IRES-mediated translation in hepatoma cells. However, whether effective treatment doses could be transposed to the clinical setting remains to be demonstrated.

Treatment of fulminant hepatitis A is based on a thorough understanding of the pathophysiology of this disorder, which has been reviewed.[299,359] Although mortality rates are relatively high, the immediate transfer of the patient to a liver transplant facility and the aggressive management of complications have been responsible for much of the improvement in survival rates. Orthotopic liver transplantation (OLT) or auxiliary partial OLT remain the only therapeutic modalities available for achieving a nonfatal outcome in the most severely affected patients with fulminant hepatitis A, leading to 1-year survival rates of 80% or more. The use of artificial or bioartificial liver support systems to perform all of the functions of the liver remains elusive and cannot currently be recommended outside of clinical trials.

PREVENTION AND CONTROL

Decisions concerning the prevention of hepatitis A must consider the immunobiology of the disease and the principal routes of transmission.[161] The most effective control measures must prevent fecal contamination by infected individuals before their clinical disease becomes apparent. Thus, the most critical control measure is proper hand washing and the avoidance of work practices that facilitate contamination of hands when taking care of children younger than 2 years, especially infected neonates where nosocomial transmission has occurred in relatives, family, staff, and physicians having direct contact with these individuals.[15,90,200,279,319] Because the personal hygiene of young children is often difficult to control, they should be restrained from close contact with their susceptible playmates during the first 2 weeks of illness or for at least 2 weeks after the onset of jaundice.

Considering the low order of infectivity that is present during the icteric stage of disease in adults (see Fig. 19.11), many authorities have suggested that strict enteric precautions within the hospital are not necessary.[255,267] In general, universal precautions should be adequate. Thus, isolation of patients in private rooms and the use of gowns or masks are unnecessary unless direct and excessive exposure to feces or fecally contaminated items is anticipated.

Immune Globulin Immunoprophylaxis

Prevention of clinical manifestations of hepatitis A through the administration of conventional intramuscular immune globulin (IGIM) was documented initially by Stokes and Neefe[358] in 1944 during a common-source outbreak at a summer camp in which they observed an 87% reduction in the attack rate among those receiving IGIM. Similar immunoprophylaxis studies were carried out simultaneously in military personnel and institutionalized children.[122,156] In each instance, IGIM was capable of preventing anicteric or icteric hepatitis A in 80% to 90% of the participants when given up to 6 days before the expected onset of illness, and doses as low as 0.01 to 0.02 mL/kg were found to be protective.

IGIM collected from any geographic region should be protective against HAV infection because only a single human HAV serotype exists. Current lots of IGIM are sterile preparations of concentrated antibodies that have tested negative for HBsAg, human immunodeficiency virus (HIV), and HCV. Although the U.S. Food and Drug Administration (FDA) has not yet set minimal concentration requirements for IGIM, the level of anti-HAV in the 16.5% formulation has ranged from about 33 IU/mL to 63 IU/mL in lots assayed between 2005 and 2007 (M-Y Yu, CBER, FDA, personal communication, 2011). Peak levels of antibody are achieved approximately 2 days after intramuscular administration, and the half-life of IgG is 23 days.

Studies performed in institutions and those conducted during community outbreaks indicate that IGIM can either completely suppress or modify the infection in HAV-susceptible persons, depending on the concentration of anti-HAV administered and the interval from exposure to treatment[89,146,357] (e-Fig. 19.5). Larger doses of IGIM may provide protection lasting a few more weeks; however, more importantly, passive-active responses are curtailed, leaving a larger percentage of susceptibles available for infection following another exposure. IGIM is unlikely to be effective if given more than 3 weeks after exposure. The theoretical concern—that individuals might acquire HAV from persons who develop subclinical hepatitis after IGIM treatment—has not been borne out by epidemiologic investigations.[357] Once the occupants of a household have received adequate prophylactic treatment, rigid isolation or compulsive cleanliness is not necessary. Commercial enzyme-linked immunosorbent (EIA) assays for anti-HAV following IGIM administration are usually unable to detect anti-HAV in the blood unless the procedure is optimized.[7] When sera were evaluated with a sensitive neutralization assay, however, low-level neutralizing antibody was found to persist for at least 14 weeks, depending on dose and concentration of antibody.[114,353] Based on these observations, it can be assumed that very low levels of anti-HAV are sufficient to prevent infection.

Although IGIM may not interfere with the immune response to inactivated vaccines or to oral poliovirus or yellow fever vaccine,[192] it may interfere with the response to other live attenuated vaccines such as measles, mumps, rubella, and varicella. Therefore, IGIM should be delayed at least 2 weeks after such immunizations, or, if IGIM is administered initially for hepatitis A prophylaxis, at least 3 months should pass before these other vaccines are administered.[48]

Hepatitis A Vaccines

As nations improve their level of sanitation and hygiene, the age at which individuals will become infected is being delayed until adulthood, at which time the likelihood of developing symptomatic or serious illness is considerably higher (see Fig. 19.14 and Table 19.2). With the development, evaluation, and subsequent licensure of cell culture–derived hepatitis A vaccines in Europe in 1991 and the United States in 1995,[11,218] the potential for long-term immunity has become a reality.

Two types of hepatitis A vaccines have been developed: either alum- or influenza virosome-adjuvanted, formaldehyde-inactivated vaccines that are available worldwide (Havrix, Vaqta, Avaxim, and Epaxal) (e-Table 19.1), or freeze-dried, live attenuated vaccines that have been used primarily in China and recently introduced into India.[340] In general, these vaccines were initially evaluated in nonhuman primates, then their safety and efficacy were confirmed in clinical trials in humans. Both types use cell culture–derived HAV grown in human diploid cell cultures. In addition to these monovalent vaccines, the HAV-specific antigen has been combined with other vaccines such as the hepatitis B vaccine (Twinrix, Twinrix Junior, and Ambirix from GlaxoSmithKline [GSK]) or typhoid vaccines (ViATIM or Vivaxim from Sanofi Pasteur and Hepatyrix from GSK). None of the HAV vaccines induce antigenic competition with other vaccines or increase the frequency of adverse events.[6,24] Except for Epaxal, all other inactivated vaccines are free of thimerosal as a preservative.

All inactivated vaccines have similar immunogenicity and require two injections given 6 to 12 months apart, although this interval can be extended to 36 months. The vaccines should be administered by the intramuscular route, because suboptimal responses can result if the vaccine is administered in the gluteal region, especially in obese adults. Accelerated stability tests at 37°C for up to 3 weeks and after 15 months at 2°C to 8°C have revealed no loss of immunogenicity. In contrast, freezing may be deleterious to the product.

To prepare the alum-adsorbed Havrix hepatitis A vaccine, SmithKline Beecham (now GSK) extracted the cell culture–adapted HM175 strain of HAV from MRC5 cells[140] by freezing and thawing. This crude harvest is tested for the absence of extraneous agents, microbiologic sterility, and antigen identity[291] and then treated with formalin to ensure viral inactivation. Residual MRC5 cellular protein and traces of formalin and neomycin remain in the vaccine. No serious adverse events caused by this inactivated vaccine have been recorded in either outbreak settings or in field trials involving approximately 24,000 individuals.[10,278] Postmarketing experience of unsolicited events from a population of uncertain size precludes establishing reliable estimates of frequency of adverse events or their causal relationship to the vaccine.

The formalin-inactivated, alum-adsorbed, hepatitis A vaccine Vaqta, distributed by Merck & Co. Inc. is prepared from MRC5 cell monolayers infected with the attenuated strain of HAV CR326F.[229,303] Antigen is extracted by lysis of infected cells and then concentrated, purified, and treated with formalin. The purified preparation is free from detectable MRC5 protein and contains only trace amounts of nonviral protein, DNA, bovine albumin, formaldehyde, and neomycin. The antigen is composed of monodispersed, full and empty, HAV particles. As with Havrix, undesirable side effects (e.g., injection-site pain/tenderness, fever, and headache) were mild in nature and of short duration. In a postmarketing surveillance study, no adverse events were identified among more than 42,000 individuals.[278]

Immunogenicity in adults, adolescents, and children 1 year of age or older is excellent, with protective levels of antibody (≥20 mIU/mL) being achieved in virtually all subjects after the primary injection. Two large efficacy trials involving more than 19,000 children have been conducted with the Havrix and Vaqta vaccines.[175,391] The only cases that were observed in the Vaqta group occurred during the first 16 days, presumably among persons who had been infected before or shortly after the initial injection. The two cases that occurred in the Havrix group were relatively mild when compared with the cases in the control group.[175] Adverse events in these trials were mild and self-limited, and vaccine efficacy ranged from 95% to 100% (Fig. 19.19). During a 9-year follow-up period

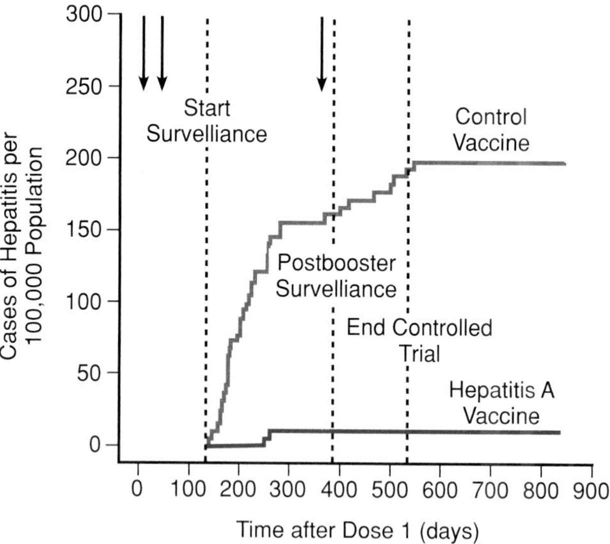

FIGURE 19.19. Cumulative rates of symptomatic infection with hepatitis A virus in healthy children receiving hepatitis B surface antigen vaccine (control group) and hepatitis A vaccine (Havrix, GlaxoSmithKline, Research Triangle Park, NC). Timing of vaccine administrations is represented (*arrows*) with doses being given at 0, 1, and 12 months. *Dashed lines* indicate when surveillance was started, when postbooster surveillance was begun, and when the controlled trial was terminated at crossover. (Modified from Innis BL, Snitbhan R, Kunasol P, et al. Protection against hepatitis A by an inactivated vaccine. *JAMA* 1994;271:1328–1334, with permission.)

in a community-wide Vaqta study, no vaccine recipient developed hepatitis A despite continuing community exposure.[392]

Estimates using kinetic models suggest that protective levels of neutralizing antibody could persist in most vaccinees for 20 years or more.[381,398] Development of IgM anti-HAV after vaccination is rare,[341] and the ALT level remains normal, so confusion with recent viral hepatitis should not be an issue. Immunogenicity data for infants are limited; however, initial studies have indicated excellent responses in seronegative infants. In contrast, responses in infants with pre-existing maternal antibody have resulted in a suboptimal response, especially in those under 6 months of age.[72,105,295,374,377] A subsequent booster dose of vaccine, however, results in an anamnestic response in most, indicating that priming of the immune response had occurred despite the lower anti-HAV concentrations observed initially.[72,105] Currently, the vaccine is only recommended for children 1 year of age and older. Other factors associated with reduced immunogenicity include immunosuppression from disease or drugs and advanced age.

The bivalent Twinrix vaccine contains a pooled formulation of the inactivated HAV and a purified recombinant HBsAg hepatitis B vaccine. It is indicated for susceptible individuals 18 years of age and older who are, or will be, at risk for exposure to both viruses. This risk includes (a) travelers to endemic areas of high or intermediate endemicity for both HAV and hepatitis B virus (HBV) who are at increased risk because of behavioral or occupational factors; (b) patients with chronic liver disease; (c) persons at risk through their work, such as emergency medical assistance teams; (d) men who have sex with men; (e) military recruits; (f) illicit drug users, injecting or noninjecting; and (g) persons with clotting factor disorders. In patients with chronic liver disease, baseline serology suggests that fewer than 40% may qualify for the bivalent vaccine because of natural immunity to one or the other virus. Primary immunization with the Twinrix vaccine includes three doses given on a 0-, 1-, and 6-month schedule, although a four-dose regimen (0, 7, and 21–30 days with a booster at 12 months) may be used if time is of the essence. Seroconversion and protective levels of anti-HAV were observed after one dose in 93.8% of healthy adult volunteers, although the anti-HBs response was unexceptional until after the third dose, as it is with the conventional hepatitis B vaccine. In contrast, responsiveness is reduced for both vaccines, but especially HBV, in patients with chronic liver disease with bridging fibrosis or cirrhosis. For the HBsAg nonresponders, booster injections with high concentrations of HBsAg (e.g., the Merck dialysis formulation) are sometimes required to achieve immunity. Adverse reactions have been rare and include hypersensitivity reactions and anaphylaxis.

At least two live attenuated hepatitis A vaccines used in China over the past decade have been reported to be safe and immunogenic and to achieve comparable seroprotection levels for more than 10 years following a single-dose immunization schedule.[244,402,418] These vaccines contain the H2 and LA-1 strains of HAV that were adapted for growth in human diploid cell cultures at lower temperature (32°C). In a recent clinical trial comparing these two vaccines, a 95% protective efficacy to prevent clinical infection was observed in more than 450,000 children.[402] Herd immunity in the nonvaccinated population also was observed. Although subclinical infection may not be averted in all recipients, there is no evidence to indicate that the vaccine virus is shed in the feces or that it

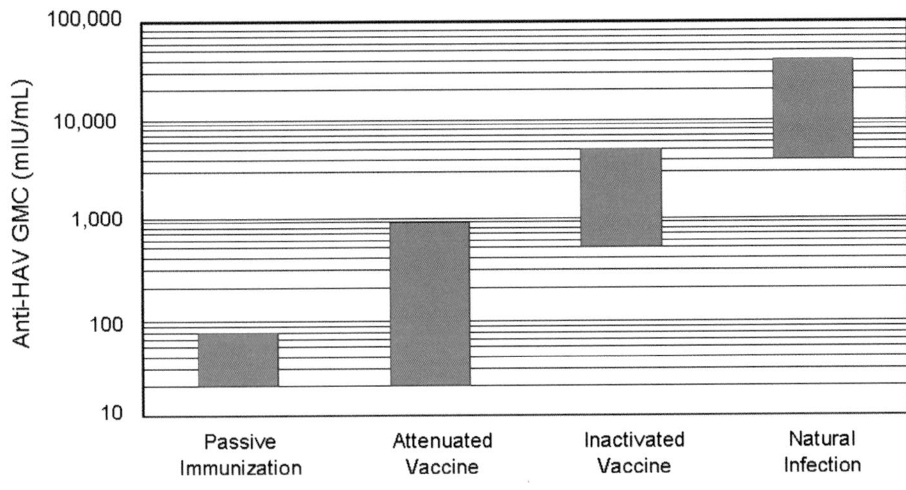

FIGURE 19.20. Anti–hepatitis A virus (HAV) geometric mean concentration (GMC; mIU/mL) observed in persons after passive and active immunization and after natural HAV infection. (Modified from Lemon S. Hepatitis A virus: current concepts of the molecular virology, immunobiology and approaches to vaccine development. *Rev Med Virol* 1992;73–87, with permission.)

causes vaccine-associated infections. Accordingly, reversion to a more virulent strain has not occurred. Oral inoculation has been unsuccessful, however, even when higher doses of vaccine were administered.

Strategies for the Use of Hepatitis A Virus Vaccine and Immune Globulin

Anti-HAV Responses After Passive and Active Immunization

Qualitative differences in protective antibody responses are observed following active and passive immunization probably because of differences in the affinity of antibodies.[225] Figure 19.20 compares anti-HAV responses in the following situations[217]: (a) at 3 to 5 days after receiving 5 mL of IGIM (passive immunization), (b) at 6 to 12 months after one injection of live attenuated HAV vaccine, (c) at 6 to 12 months after two injections of inactivated hepatitis A vaccine, and (d) at 10 to 20 years after a natural infection. Despite these disparities, protection against disease is comparable, implying that very low and even nondetectable levels of anti-HAV may confer protection.

Pre-Exposure Prophylaxis

Although universal childhood immunization for hepatitis A is a worthy goal, it is unlikely that such a recommendation will be issued by policy makers in developing countries or regions with transitional economies, given the economic and political realities of global immunization programs. Even in developed countries, the integration of hepatitis A vaccination into routine childhood immunization schedules has been slow to materialize. Within the United States, however, several recommendations were formulated by the Advisory Committee on Immunization Practices (ACIP) beginning shortly after the vaccine was introduced in 1995, even though the annual number of prevaccination deaths from hepatitis A placed it at the bottom of the list of other infectious diseases for which vaccination was subsequently recommended. At first the focus was on vaccinating high- and intermediate-risk groups and children living in communities with the highest disease rates. In 1999, this was expanded to include children residing in states, counties, or communities that had consistently elevated rates of hepatitis A (≥10 cases/100,000 population or twice the national average).[48] The final step in this strategy came in 2006, when routine hepatitis A vaccination of children was recommended nationwide. Administration of IGIM was relegated to more specific indications (see later discussion).

A recent assessment of the impact of this novel immunization strategy revealed that the incidence of hepatitis A in 2003, when compared with a prevaccination baseline period (1990–1997), declined 76% to 2.6 cases/100,000 population[387] (see Fig. 19.15). Although this decline was seen throughout the United States regardless of vaccination policy, it was more pronounced in those states where vaccination was implemented (88% vs. 53% decline in rate). A decline in the incidence rates also was seen in all age groups. A similar reduction in disease incidence in the vaccinated and older nonvaccinated population also was observed following universal immunization of toddlers 18 to 24 months of age in Israel, suggesting marked herd protection and the possibility that catch-up vaccination programs may not be necessary[73] (e-Fig. 19.6).

As shown in Table 19.3, immunization should be offered to persons traveling from industrialized countries to regions of the world where HAV is endemic and where the risk of acquiring hepatitis A is enhanced because of living conditions and the length of stay (e.g., Asia [except Japan]; Africa, Latin America and the Caribbean, eastern Europe, the Middle East, and the Commonwealth of Independent States). Routine immunization for U.S. military personnel could be reserved for those who regularly travel to endemic areas or those in rapid-deployment

TABLE 19.3 Risk Groups Potentially Targeted for Pre-Exposure Prophylaxis

- Travelers to or workers in foreign countries (including the military) where the risk of acquiring hepatitis A is enhanced
- American Indians/Alaskan natives
- Persons who work with HAV or with nonhuman primates
- Persons with chronic liver disease
- Men who have sex with men
- Persons who have clotting factor disorders
- Persons residing in areas where extended community outbreaks exist
- Refugees residing in temporary camps after catastrophes

units. For other soldiers, typical reassignment or deployment times of several weeks would be sufficient for generating a protective response to vaccination.

It has been reported that the incidence of symptomatic hepatitis A for a 1-month trip to a developing country is 3 to 6 cases/1,000 susceptible travelers.[355] In contrast, the incidence rate is sixfold higher (20 cases/1,000) in persons whose travel arrangements or personal hygiene place them in jeopardy of acquiring an infection. In making a recommendation for vaccination, it is important to recognize that hepatitis A is contracted at least 100 times more frequently than is typhoid fever or cholera.[355] For most travelers, vaccine alone will suffice if the first dose is administered at least 2 weeks prior to expected exposure to HAV. For both immediate and long-term protection of older adults (>40 years), immunocompromised persons and persons with chronic liver disease or other chronic medical conditions where the immune response may be muted, and who are planning to depart for an endemic area in 2 weeks or less, the simultaneous administration of inactivated hepatitis A vaccine with IGIM (0.02–0.06 mL/kg) should provide optimal protection with the stipulation that separate syringes and injection sites are used.[46,385] The anti-HAV titers, however, are about twofold lower when compared with those observed when vaccine alone is administered but more than 100 times higher than levels considered to be protective.

At-risk individuals who are allergic to components in the vaccine or who do not elect to receive the vaccine can be given small doses of IGIM (0.02–0.04 mL/kg or 2.0 mL for adults) if the anticipated period of exposure is 2 to 3 months. Larger doses (0.05–0.06 mL/kg or 5.0 mL for adults) should be administered every 4 to 6 months for more prolonged exposure.

Vaccine also should be offered to staff and residents of institutions for the mentally disabled or to members of other relatively closed communities who are at high risk for acquiring hepatitis A. It also should be offered to preschool children attending daycare centers, including the staff, parents and siblings, and to any other group whose occupation, lifestyle, or behavior places them in the high-risk category (e.g., illicit drug users, injecting or noninjecting, and men who have sex with other men). Other groups that have been targeted for possible immunization for hepatitis A are listed in Table 19.3.

One of the more contentious recommendations concerns the administration of hepatitis A vaccine to patients with chronic liver disease, especially those with hepatitis B or C. Several reports have suggested that the occurrence of hepatitis A in these patients is associated with a higher frequency of severe illness or fulminant hepatic failure, leading to substantially higher case fatality rates.[196,382] Other investigators, however, have reported conflicting data on the clinical course and outcome of hepatitis A in chronic liver disease.[263,363] In the interim, it seems prudent to offer vaccination to all patients with chronic liver disease as recommended by the ACIP. Physicians should recognize, however, that no data indicate that a concurrent hepatitis A infection will place patients with chronic liver disease at increased risk for a life-threatening outcome unless they have advanced liver disease (e.g., cirrhosis).

Postexposure Prophylaxis

There has been considerable movement to revamp the strategy on postexposure prophylaxis favoring the use of hepatitis A vaccine over IGIM following exposure to HAV. Advantages include long-term protection, ease of administration, higher acceptability and availability, and comparable cost. Initial data was limited to experiments in marmosets and chimpanzees.[70,306,317] Primates were vaccinated 1 to 3 days after being challenged orally or parenterally and were protected against hepatitis A disease or had an attenuated infection without virus shedding. A randomized, double-blind, active-control, noninferiority trial conducted in Kazakhstan and supported by the CDC, was designed to compare the efficacy of hepatitis A vaccine (n = 568) to IGIM (n = 522) in preventing laboratory-confirmed, symptomatic HAV infection when given to at-risk subjects within 14 days after exposure.[383] This study found that HAV occurred infrequently in either treatment group, meeting a prespecified criterion for noninferiority for these prophylactic measures. Rates of infection, however, were higher in the vaccine group (8.6%) than in the IGIM group (6.7% overall) and for all HAV study points examined (clinical and subclinical), suggesting that the IGIM performed modestly better than the vaccine in these per-protocol populations (e-Fig. 19.7). Regardless, the ACIP in 2007 updated their recommendations for postexposure prophylaxis to include either hepatitis A vaccine alone or IGIM alone in most exposure circumstances (Table 19.4). The only situation where both vaccine and IGIM were recommended was in a person who shared illicit drugs with a case, and even in this situation, vaccine alone also was an option.

TABLE 19.4 Advisory Committee on Immunization Practices Recommendations for Postexposure Prophylaxis Using Vaccine or Immunoglobulin M Alone

- Close personal contact (household and sexual contacts)[a]
- Outbreak in childcare centers (staff and attendees; consider household members of diapered attendees)
- Common-source exposure (food handlers of index worker and patrons if identified and treated within 2 weeks of exposure)
- Outbreak confirmed in schools, hospitals, and work settings

[a]Consider vaccine alone or both vaccine and immunoglobulin M if the contact shared illicit drugs with case.

PERSPECTIVES

Detailed studies of early innate and adaptive immune responses to HAV that have been undertaken recently are likely to provide a better understanding of critical responses that lead to the elimination of virus from the host. In addition, through comparative analyses with host responses to another hepatotropic virus—HCV—such studies may help understand why HCV may establish persistent infections in humans whereas HAV never does. A better understanding of HAV virulence mechanisms could lead to the development of novel therapies designed to subvert severe outcomes. As developing countries transition from high endemicity to low endemicity, the need for universal vaccination of the population will become more compelling. The development of an oral vaccine would be of great benefit in this situation.

ACKNOWLEDGMENTS

This work was supported in part by the Eugene B. Casey Foundation and the William and Sonya Carpenter Fund, Baylor College of Medicine (F.B.H.), and the Institut Pasteur, the Centre National de la Recherche Scientifique (CNRS), and the Agence Nationale de Recherche sur le Sida et les Hépatites Virales (ANRS), France (A.M.). We gratefully acknowledge colleagues who provided data prior to publication and support for illustrations, and the Service Image of Institut Pasteur for help with generation of figures.

REFERENCES

All cited references are available in the e-book.

2. Abe H, Beninger PR, Ikejiri N, et al. Light microscopic findings of liver biopsy specimens from patients with hepatitis type A and comparison with type B. *Gastroenterology* 1982;82:938–947.
3. Allaire M, Chernaia MM, Malcolm BA, et al. Picornaviral 3C cysteine proteinases have a fold similar to chymotrypsin-like serine proteinases. *Nature* 1994;369:72–76.
5. Amado LA, Villar LM, de Paula VS, et al. Exposure to multiple subgenotypes of hepatitis A virus during an outbreak using matched serum and saliva specimens. *J Med Virol* 2011;83:768–775.
7. Ambrosch F, Wiedermann G, Andre FE, et al. Comparison of HAV antibodies induced by vaccination, passive immunization, and natural infection. In: Hollinger FB, Lemon SM, Margolis HS, eds. *Viral Hepatitis and Liver Disease.* Baltimore: Williams & Wilkins; 1991:98–100.
8. Amon JJ, Devasia R, Xia G, et al. Molecular epidemiology of foodborne hepatitis A outbreaks in the United States, 2003. *J Infect Dis* 2005; 192:1323–1330.
9. Anderson DA, Ross BC. Morphogenesis of hepatitis A virus: isolation and characterization of subviral particles. *J Virol* 1990;64: 5284–5289.
10. Andre FE, D'Hondt E, Delem A, et al. Clinical assessment of the safety and efficacy of an inactivated hepatitis A vaccine: rationale and summary of findings. *Vaccine* 1992;10(Suppl 1):S160–S168.
11. Andre FE, Hepburn A, D'Hondt E. Inactivated candidate vaccines for hepatitis A. *Prog Med Virol* 1990;37:72–95.
12. Aragones L, Guix S, Ribes E, et al. Fine-tuning translation kinetics selection as the driving force of codon usage bias in the hepatitis A virus capsid. *PLoS Pathog* 2010;6:e1000797.
13. Asher LV, Binn LN, Mensing TL, et al. Pathogenesis of hepatitis A in orally inoculated owl monkeys (*Aotus trivirgatus*). *J Med Virol* 1995;47:260–268.
19. Barbara JA, Howell DR, Briggs M, et al. Post-transfusion hepatitis A. *Lancet* 1982;1:738.
20. Beales LP, Holzenburg A, Rowlands DJ. Viral internal ribosome entry site structures segregate into two distinct morphologies. *J Virol* 2003;77: 6574–6579.
21. Beard MR, Cohen L, Lemon SM, et al. Characterization of recombinant hepatitis A virus genomes containing exogenous sequences at the 2A/2B junction. *J Virol* 2001;75:1414–1426.
24. Bienzle U, Bock HL, Kruppenbacher JP, et al. Immunogenicity of an inactivated hepatitis A vaccine administered according to two different schedules and the interference of other "travellers" vaccines with the immune response. *Vaccine* 1996;14:501–505.
26. Bishop NE, Anderson DA. RNA-dependent cleavage of VP0 capsid protein in provirions of hepatitis A virus. *Virology* 1993;197:616–623.
27. Bishop NE, Anderson DA. Uncoating kinetics of hepatitis A virus virions and provirions. *J Virol* 2000;74:3423–3426.
28. Blank CA, Anderson DA, Beard M, et al. Infection of polarized cultures of human intestinal epithelial cells with hepatitis A virus: vectorial release of progeny virions through apical cellular membranes. *J Virol* 2000;74:6476–6484.
31. Borman AM, Kean KM. Intact eukaryotic initiation factor 4G is required for hepatitis A virus internal initiation of translation. *Virology* 1997;237:129–136.
33. Borovec SV, Anderson DA. Synthesis and assembly of hepatitis A virus-specific proteins in BS-C-1 cells. *J Virol* 1993;67:3095–3102.
35. Bower WA, Nainan OV, Han X, et al. Duration of viremia in hepatitis A virus infection. *J Infect Dis* 2000;182:12–17.
36. Boyer JL, Klatskin G. Pattern of necrosis in acute viral hepatitis—prognostic value of bridging (subacute hepatic necrosis). *N Engl J Med* 1970;283:1063–1071.
38. Brack K, Frings W, Dotzauer A, et al. A cytopathogenic, apoptosis-inducing variant of hepatitis A virus. *J Virol* 1998;72:3370–3376.
41. Brown EA, Day SP, Jansen RW, et al. The 5′ nontranslated region of hepatitis A virus RNA: secondary structure and elements required for translation in vitro. *J Virol* 1991;65:5828–5838.
43. Brown EA, Zajac AJ, Lemon SM. In vitro characterization of an internal ribosomal entry site (IRES) present within the 5′ nontranslated region of hepatitis A virus RNA: comparison with the IRES of encephalomyocarditis virus. *J Virol* 1994;68:1066–1074.
46. Centers for Disease Control and Prevention. Update: Prevention of hepatitis A after exposure to hepatitis A virus and in international travelers. Updated recommendations of the Advisory Committee on Immunization Practices (ACIP). *MMWR* 2007;56:1080–1084.
49. Centers for Disease Control and Prevention. Viral hepatitis statistics and surveillance—surveillance data for acute viral hepatitis—United States, 2008. Atlanta: Centers for Disease Control and Prevention; 2010.
50. Chalmers TC, Eckhardt RD, Reynolds WE, et al. The treatment of acute infectious hepatitis. Controlled studies of the effects of diet, rest, and physical reconditioning on the acute course of the disease and on the incidence of relapses and residual abnormalities. *J Clin Invest* 1955;34:1163–1235.
52. Chatenoud L, Bach JF. Genetic control of hepatitis A severity and susceptibility to allergy. *J Clin Invest* 2011;121:848–850.
53. Chenard-Neu MP, Boudjema K, Bernuau J, et al. Auxiliary liver transplantation: regeneration of the native liver and outcome in 30 patients with fulminant hepatic failure—a multicenter European study. *Hepatology* 1996;23:1119–1127.
55. Cohen JI, Feinstone S, Purcell RH. Hepatitis A virus infection in a chimpanzee: duration of viremia and detection of virus in saliva and throat swabs. *J Infect Dis* 1989;160:887–890.
58. Cohen JI, Ticehurst JR, Feinstone SM, et al. Hepatitis A virus cDNA and its RNA transcripts are infectious in cell culture. *J Virol* 1987;61:3035–3039.
59. Cohen JI, Ticehurst JR, Purcell RH, et al. Complete nucleotide sequence of wild-type hepatitis A virus: comparison with different strains of hepatitis A virus and other picornaviruses. *J Virol* 1987;61:50–59.
60. Cohen L, Benichou D, Martin A. Analysis of deletion mutants indicates that the 2A polypeptide of hepatitis A virus participates in virion morphogenesis. *J Virol* 2002;76:7495–7505.
62. Costa-Mattioli M, Cristina J, Romero H, et al. Molecular evolution of hepatitis A virus: a new classification based on the complete VP1 protein. *J Virol* 2002;76:9516–9525.
63. Coulepis AG, Anderson BN, Gust ID. Hepatitis A. *Adv Virus Res* 1987; 32:129–169.
67. Cristina J, Costa-Mattioli M. Genetic variability and molecular evolution of hepatitis A virus. *Virus Res* 2007;127:151–157.
69. Cuthbert JA. Hepatitis A: old and new. *Clin Microbiol Rev* 2001;14:38–58.
71. Daemer RJ, Feinstone SM, Gust ID, et al. Propagation of human hepatitis A virus in African green monkey kidney cell culture: primary isolation and serial passage. *Infect Immun* 1981;32:388–393.
72. Dagan R, Amir J, Mijalovsky A, et al. Immunization against hepatitis A in the first year of life: priming despite the presence of maternal antibody. *Pediatr Infect Dis J* 2000;19:1045–1052.
73. Dagan R, Leventhal A, Anis E, et al. Incidence of hepatitis A in Israel following universal immunization of toddlers. *JAMA* 2005;294:202–210.
76. De Jong AS, de Mattia F, Van Dommelen MM, et al. Functional analysis of picornavirus 2B proteins: effects on calcium homeostasis and intracellular protein trafficking. *J Virol* 2008;82:3782–3790.
77. Decker RH, Kosakowski SM, Vanderbilt AS, et al. Diagnosis of acute hepatitis A by HAVAB-M, a direct radioimmunoassay for IgM anti-HAV. *Am J Clin Pathol* 1981;76:140–147.
79. Deinhardt F, Holmes AW, Capps RB, et al. Studies on the transmission of human viral hepatitis to marmoset monkeys. I. Transmission of disease, serial passages, and description of liver lesions. *J Exp Med* 1967; 125:673–688.

80. Dentinger CM, Bower WA, Nainan OV, et al. An outbreak of hepatitis A associated with green onions. *J Infect Dis* 2001;183:1273–1276.
82. Dienstag JL, Feinstone SM, Purcell RH, et al. Experimental infection of chimpanzees with hepatitis A virus. *J Infect Dis* 1975;132:532–545.
85. Dollenmaier G, Weitz M. Interaction of glyceraldehyde-3-phosphate dehydrogenase with secondary and tertiary RNA structural elements of the hepatitis A virus 3′ translated and non-translated regions. *J Gen Virol* 2003;84:403–414.
86. Dotzauer A, Brenner M, Gebhardt U, et al. IgA-coated particles of hepatitis A virus are translocalized antivectorially from the apical to the basolateral site of polarized epithelial cells via the polymeric immunoglobulin receptor. *J Gen Virol* 2005;86:2747–2751.
88. Dotzauer A, Gebhardt U, Bieback K, et al. Hepatitis A virus-specific immunoglobulin A mediates infection of hepatocytes with hepatitis A virus via the asialoglycoprotein receptor. *J Virol* 2000;74:10950–10957.
89. Drake ME, Ming C. Gamma globulin in epidemic hepatitis: comparative value of two dosage levels, apparently near the minimal effective level. *J Am Med Assoc* 1954;155:1302–1305.
92. Emerson SU, Huang YK, Nguyen H, et al. Identification of VP1/2A and 2C as virulence genes of hepatitis A virus and demonstration of genetic instability of 2C. *J Virol* 2002;76:8551–8559.
93. Emerson SU, Huang YK, Purcell RH. 2B and 2C mutations are essential but mutations throughout the genome of HAV contribute to adaptation to cell culture. *Virology* 1993;194:475–480.
94. Emerson SU, Tsarev SA, Govindarajan S, et al. A simian strain of hepatitis A virus, AGM-27, functions as an attenuated vaccine for chimpanzees. *J Infect Dis* 1996;173:592–597.
100. Feigelstock D, Thompson P, Mattoo P, et al. The human homolog of HAVcr-1 codes for a hepatitis A virus cellular receptor. *J Virol* 1998;72: 6621–6628.
101. Feinstone SM, Kapikian AZ, Purcell RH. Hepatitis A: detection by immune electron microscopy of a viruslike antigen associated with acute illness. *Science* 1973;182:1026–1028.
102. Fensterl V, Grotheer D, Berk I, et al. Hepatitis A virus suppresses RIG-I-mediated IRF-3 activation to block induction of beta interferon. *J Virol* 2005;79:10968–10977.
104. Fiore AE. Hepatitis A transmitted by food. *Clin Infect Dis* 2004;38: 705–715.
105. Fiore AE, Shapiro CN, Sabin K, et al. Hepatitis A vaccination of infants: effect of maternal antibody status on antibody persistence and response to a booster dose. *Pediatr Infect Dis J* 2003;22:354–359.
106. Flehmig B. Hepatitis A-virus in cell culture: I. propagation of different hepatitis A-virus isolates in a fetal rhesus monkey kidney cell line (Frhk-4). *Med Microbiol Immunol* 1980;168:239–248.
108. Fleischer B, Fleischer S, Maier K, et al. Clonal analysis of infiltrating T lymphocytes in liver tissue in viral hepatitis A. *Immunology* 1990;69: 14–19.
113. Fujiwara K, Yokosuka O, Imazeki F, et al. Analysis of hepatitis A virus protein 2B in sera of hepatitis A of various severities. *J Gastroenterol* 2007; 42:560–566.
114. Fujiyama S, Iino S, Odoh K, et al. Time course of hepatitis A virus antibody titer after active and passive immunization. *Hepatology* 1992; 15:983–988.
116. Funkhouser AW, Raychaudhuri G, Purcell RH, et al. Progress toward the development of a genetically engineered attenuated hepatitis A virus vaccine. *J Virol* 1996;70:7948–7957.
117. Funkhouser AW, Schultz DE, Lemon SM, et al. Hepatitis A virus translation is rate-limiting for virus replication in MRC-5 cells. *Virology* 1999; 254:268–278.
121. Gazzard BG, Portmann B, Murray-Lyon IM, et al. Causes of death in fulminant hepatic failure and relationship to quantitative histological assessment of parenchymal damage. *Q J Med* 1975;44:615–626.
122. Gellis SS, Stokes JJ, Brother GM, et al. The use of human immune serum globulin (gamma globulin) in infectious (epidemic) hepatitis in the Mediterranean theater of operations. I. Studies on prophylaxis in two epidemics of infectious hepatitis. *JAMA* 2011;128:1062–1063.
125. Glass MJ, Jia XY, Summers DF. Identification of the hepatitis A virus internal ribosome entry site: in vivo and in vitro analysis of bicistronic RNAs containing the HAV 5′ noncoding region. *Virology* 1993;193: 842–852.
127. Gordon SC, Reddy KR, Schiff L, et al. Prolonged intrahepatic cholestasis secondary to acute hepatitis A. *Ann Intern Med* 1984;101:635–637.
129. Gosert R, Chang KH, Rijnbrand R, et al. Transient expression of cellular polypyrimidine-tract binding protein stimulates cap-independent translation directed by both picornaviral and flaviviral internal ribosome entry sites in vivo. *Mol Cell Biol* 2000;20:1583–1595.
130. Gosert R, Egger D, Bienz K. A cytopathic and a cell culture adapted hepatitis A virus strain differ in cell killing but not in intracellular membrane rearrangements. *Virology* 2000;266:157–169.
131. Goswami BB, Kulka M, Ngo D, et al. Apoptosis induced by a cytopathic hepatitis A virus is dependent on caspase activation following ribosomal RNA degradation but occurs in the absence of 2′-5′ oligoadenylate synthetase. *Antiviral Res* 2004;63:153–166.
132. Gotsman I, Muszkat M. Glucose-6-phosphate dehydrogenase deficiency is associated with increased initial clinical severity of acute viral hepatitis A. *J Gastroenterol Hepatol* 2001;16:1239–1243.
133. Graff J, Cha J, Blyn LB, et al. Interaction of poly(rC) binding protein 2 with the 5′ noncoding region of hepatitis A virus RNA and its effects on translation. *J Virol* 1998;72:9668–9675.
134. Graff J, Emerson SU. Importance of amino acid 216 in nonstructural protein 2B for replication of hepatitis A virus in cell culture and in vivo. *J Med Virol* 2003;71:7–17.
136. Graff J, Normann A, Feinstone SM, et al. Nucleotide sequence of wild-type hepatitis A virus GBM in comparison with two cell culture-adapted variants. *J Virol* 1994;68:548–554.
137. Graff J, Normann A, Flehmig B. Influence of the 5′ noncoding region of hepatitis A virus strain GBM on its growth in different cell lines. *J Gen Virol* 1997;78(Pt 8):1841–1849.
138. Graff J, Richards OC, Swiderek KM, et al. Hepatitis A virus capsid protein VP1 has a heterogeneous C terminus. *J Virol* 1999;73:6015–6023.
144. Hadler SC. Global impact of hepatitis A virus infection: changing patterns. In: Hollinger FB, Lemon SM, Margolis HS, eds. *Viral Hepatitis and Liver Disease.* Baltimore: Williams & Wilkins; 1991:14–20.
146. Hall WT, Madden DL, Mundon FK, et al. Protective effect of immune serum globulin (ISG) against hepatitis A infection in a natural epidemic. *Am J Epidemiol* 1977;106:72–75.
156. Havens WP, Jr., Paul JR. Prevention of infectious hepatitis with gama globulin. *JAMA* 1945;129:272.
159. Hillis WD. An outbreak of infectious hepatitis among chimpanzee handlers at a United States Air Force Base. *Am J Hyg* 1961;73:316–328.
161. Hollinger FB. International symposium on active immunization against hepatitis A. *Vaccine* 1992;10(Suppl 1):S6–S7.
162. Hollinger FB, Bradley DW, Dreesman GR, et al. Detection of viral hepatitis type A. *Am J Clin Pathol* 1976;65:854–865.
173. Ibe M, Rude B, Gerken G, et al. Coombs-negative severe hemolysis associated with hepatitis A. *Z Gastroenterol* 1997;35:567–569.
174. Inman RD, Hodge M, Johnston ME, et al. Arthritis, vasculitis, and cryoglobulinemia associated with relapsing hepatitis A virus infection. *Ann Intern Med* 1986;105:700–703.
175. Innis BL, Snitbhan R, Kunasol P, et al. Protection against hepatitis A by an inactivated vaccine. *JAMA* 1994;271:1328–1334.
176. Ishak KG. Light microscopic morphology of viral hepatitis. *Am J Clin Pathol* 1976;65 Suppl 5:787–827.
179. Jacobsen KH, Wiersma ST. Hepatitis A virus seroprevalence by age and world region, 1990 and 2005. *Vaccine* 2010;28:6653–6657.
182. Jewell DA, Swietnicki W, Dunn BM, et al. Hepatitis A virus 3C proteinase substrate specificity. *Biochemistry* 1992;31:7862–7869.
184. Jia XY, Summers DF, Ehrenfeld E. Primary cleavage of the HAV capsid protein precursor in the middle of the proposed 2A coding region. *Virology* 1993;193:515–519.
188. Jung YM, Park SJ, Kim JS, et al. Atypical manifestations of hepatitis A infection: a prospective, multicenter study in Korea. *J Med Virol* 2010;82:1318–1326.
190. Kao HW, Ashcavai M, Redeker AG. The persistence of hepatitis A IgM antibody after acute clinical hepatitis A. *Hepatology* 1984;4:933–936.
191. Kaplan G, Totsuka A, Thompson P, et al. Identification of a surface glycoprotein on African green monkey kidney cells as a receptor for hepatitis A virus. *Embo J* 1996;15:4282–4296.
194. Karvountzis GG, Redeker AG, Peters RL. Long term follow-up studies of patients surviving fulminant viral hepatitis. *Gastroenterology* 1974; 67:870–877.

196. Keeffe EB. Is hepatitis A more severe in patients with chronic hepatitis B and other chronic liver diseases? *Am J Gastroenterol* 1995;90:201–205.
197. Khan NC, Hollinger FB, Melnick JL. Localization of hepatitis A virus antigen to specific subcellular fractions of hepatitis-A-infected chimpanzee liver cells. *Intervirology* 1984;21:187–194.
198. Kim HY, Eyheramonho MB, Pichavant M, et al. A polymorphism in TIM1 is associated with susceptibility to severe hepatitis A virus infection in humans. *J Clin Invest* 2011;121:1111–1118.
199. Kim SJ, Jang MH, Stapleton JT, et al. Neutralizing human monoclonal antibodies to hepatitis A virus recovered by phage display. *Virology* 2004;318:598–607.
201. Konduru K, Kaplan GG. Determinants in $3D^{pol}$ modulate the rate of growth of hepatitis A virus. *J Virol* 2010;84:8342–8347.
202. Konduru K, Kaplan GG. Stable growth of wild-type hepatitis A virus in cell culture. *J Virol* 2006;80:1352–1360.
204. Krawczynski KK, Bradley DW, Murphy BL, et al. Pathogenetic aspects of hepatitis A virus infection in enterally inoculated marmosets. *Am J Clin Pathol* 1981;76:698–706.
205. Krugman S, Giles JP, Hammond J. Infectious hepatitis. Evidence for two distinctive clinical, epidemiological, and immunological types of infection. *JAMA* 1967;200:365–373.
206. Krugman S, Ward R, Giles JP, et al. Infectious hepatitis: detection of virus during the incubation period and in clinically inapparent infection. *N Engl J Med* 1959;261:729–734.
207. Krugman S, Ward R, Giles JP. The natural history of infectious hepatitis. *Am J Med* 1962;32:717–728.
208. Kryger P, Christoffersen P. Liver histopathology of the hepatitis A virus infection: a comparison with hepatitis type B and non-A, non-B. *J Clin Pathol* 1983;36:650–654.
210. Kusov Y, Gauss-Muller V. Improving proteolytic cleavage at the 3A/3B site of the hepatitis A virus polyprotein impairs processing and particle formation, and the impairment can be complemented in trans by 3AB and 3ABC. *J Virol* 1999;73:9867–9878.
212. Kusov YY, Gosert R, Gauss-Muller V. Replication and in vivo repair of the hepatitis A virus genome lacking the poly(A) tail. *J Gen Virol* 2005; 86:1363–1368.
214. Lanford RE, Feng Z, Chavez D, et al. Acute hepatitis A virus infection is associated with a limited type I interferon response and persistence of intrahepatic viral RNA. *Proc Natl Acad Sci U S A* 2011;108:11223–11228.
216. Lednar WM, Lemon SM, Kirkpatrick JW, et al. Frequency of illness associated with epidemic hepatitis A virus infections in adults. *Am J Epidemiol* 1985;122:226–233.
217. Lemon S. Hepatitis A virus: current concepts of the molecular virology, immunobiology and approaches to vaccine development. *Rev Med Virol* 1992;73–87.
218. Lemon SM. Inactivated hepatitis A vaccines. *JAMA* 1994;271:1363–1364.
219. Lemon SM. The natural history of hepatitis A: the potential for transmission by transfusion of blood or blood products. *Vox Sang* 1994;67(Suppl 4):19–23.
223. Lemon SM, Brown CD, Brooks DS, et al. Specific immunoglobulin M response to hepatitis A virus determined by solid-phase radioimmunoassay. *Infect Immun* 1980;28:927–936.
225. Lemon SM, Murphy PC, Provost PJ, et al. Immunoprecipitation and virus neutralization assays demonstrate qualitative differences between protective antibody responses to inactivated hepatitis A vaccine and passive immunization with immune globulin. *J Infect Dis* 1997;176:9–19.
226. Lemon SM, Murphy PC, Shields PA, et al. Antigenic and genetic variation in cytopathic hepatitis A virus variants arising during persistent infection: evidence for genetic recombination. *J Virol* 1991;65:2056–2065.
229. Lewis JA, Armstrong ME, Larson VM, et al. Use of a live, attenuated hepatitis A vaccine to prepare a highly purified, formalin-inactivated hepatitis A vaccine. In: Hollinger FB, Lemon SM, Margolis HS, eds. *Viral Hepatitis and Liver Disease.* Baltimore: Williams & Wilkins; 1991:94–97.
232. Locarnini SA, Ferris AA, Lehmann NI, et al. The antibody response following hepatitis A infection. *Intervirology* 1977;8:309–318.
234. Lu L, Ching KZ, de Paula VS, et al. Characterization of the complete genomic sequence of genotype II hepatitis A virus (CF53/Berne isolate). *J Gen Virol* 2004;85:2943–2952.
236. MacCallum FO, Bradley WH. Transmission of infective hepatitis to human volunteers. *Lancet* 1944;2:228.
237. Mackiewicz V, Cammas A, Desbois D, et al. Nucleotide variability and translation efficiency of the 5′ untranslated region of hepatitis A virus: update from clinical isolates associated with mild and severe hepatitis. *J Virol* 2010;84:10139–10147.
238. Mackiewicz V, Dussaix E, Le Petitcorps MF, et al. Detection of hepatitis A virus RNA in saliva. *J Clin Microbiol* 2004;42:4329–4331.
243. Mannucci PM, Gdovin S, Gringeri A, et al. Transmission of hepatitis A to patients with hemophilia by factor VIII concentrates treated with organic solvent and detergent to inactivate viruses. The Italian Collaborative Group. *Ann Intern Med* 1994;120:1–7.
246. Margolis HS, Nainan OV, Krawczynski K, et al. Appearance of immune complexes during experimental hepatitis A infection in chimpanzees. *J Med Virol* 1988;26:315–326.
247. Martin A, Benichou D, Chao SF, et al. Maturation of the hepatitis A virus capsid protein VP1 is not dependent on processing by the 3Cpro proteinase. *J Virol* 1999;73:6220–6227.
248. Martin A, Escriou N, Chao SF, et al. Identification and site-directed mutagenesis of the primary (2A/2B) cleavage site of the hepatitis A virus polyprotein: functional impact on the infectivity of HAV RNA transcripts. *Virology* 1995;213:213–222.
249. Martin A, Lemon S. The molecular biology of hepatitis A virus. In: Ou J-H, ed. *Hepatitis Viruses.* Norwell, MA: Kluwer Academic Publishers; 2002:23–50.
250. Martin A, Lemon SM. Hepatitis A virus: from discovery to vaccines. *Hepatology* 2006;43(Suppl 1):S164–S172.
261. McIntire JJ, Umetsu SE, Macaubas C, et al. Immunology: hepatitis A virus link to atopic disease. *Nature* 2003;425:576.
263. Mele A, Tosti ME, Stroffolini T. Hepatitis associated with hepatitis A superinfection in patients with chronic hepatitis C. *N Engl J Med* 1998; 338:1771–1773.
264. Morace G, Pisani G, Beneduce F, et al. Mutations in the 3A genomic region of two cytopathic strains of hepatitis A virus isolated in Italy. *Virus Res* 1993;28:187–194.
265. Moratorio G, Costa-Mattioli M, Piovani R, et al. Bayesian coalescent inference of hepatitis A virus populations: evolutionary rates and patterns. *J Gen Virol* 2007;88:3039–3042.
266. Morse LJ, Bryan JA, Hurley JP, et al. The Holy Cross college football team hepatitis outbreak. *JAMA* 1972;219:706–708.
270. Murray R. Viral hepatitis. *Bull N Y Acad Med* 1955;31:341–358.
272. Nainan OV, Armstrong GL, Han XH, et al. Hepatitis A molecular epidemiology in the United States, 1996–1997: sources of infection and implications of vaccination policy. *J Infect Dis* 2005;191:957–963.
273. Nainan OV, Brinton MA, Margolis HS. Identification of amino acids located in the antibody binding sites of human hepatitis A virus. *Virology* 1992;191:984–987.
276. Neefe J, Gellis S, Stokes JJ. Homologous serum hepatitis and infectious (epidemic) hepatitis: studies in volunteers bearing on immunological and other characteristics of the biological agents. *Am J Med* 1946;1:3–22.
278. Niu MT, Salive M, Krueger C, et al. Two-year review of hepatitis A vaccine safety: data from the Vaccine Adverse Event Reporting System (VAERS). *Clin Infect Dis* 1998;26:1475–1476.
280. Normann A, Jung C, Vallbracht A, et al. Time course of hepatitis A viremia and viral load in the blood of human hepatitis A patients. *J Med Virol* 2004;72:10–16.
281. O'Grady JG, Alexander GJ, Hayllar KM, et al. Early indicators of prognosis in fulminant hepatic failure. *Gastroenterology* 1989;97:439–445.
284. Palmenberg AC, Neubauer D, Skern T. Genome organization and encoded proteins. In: Ehrenfeld E, Domingo E, Roos RP, eds. *The Picornaviruses.* Washington, DC: ASM Press; 2010:3–17.
291. Peetermans J. Production, quality control and characterization of an inactivated hepatitis A vaccine. *Vaccine* 1992;10(Suppl 1):S99–S101.
292. Perez-Sautu U, Costafreda MI, Cayla J, et al. Hepatitis A virus vaccine escape variants and potential new serotype emergence. *Emerg Infect Dis* 2011;17:734–737.
297. Ping LH, Lemon SM. Antigenic structure of human hepatitis A virus defined by analysis of escape mutants selected against murine monoclonal antibodies. *J Virol* 1992;66:2208–2216.
298. Pinto MA, Marchevsky RS, Baptista ML, et al. Experimental hepatitis A virus (HAV) infection in *Callithrix jacchus:* early detection of HAV antigen and viral fate. *Exp Toxicol Pathol* 2002;53:413–420.

299. Polson J, Lee WM. AASLD position paper: the management of acute liver failure. *Hepatology* 2005;41:1179–1197.
301. Probst C, Jecht M, Gauss-Muller V. Processing of proteinase precursors and their effect on hepatitis A virus particle formation. *J Virol* 1998;72:8013–8020.
304. Provost PJ, Hilleman MR. Propagation of human hepatitis A virus in cell culture in vitro. *Proc Soc Exp Biol Med* 1979;160:213–221.
306. Purcell RH, D'Hondt E, Bradbury R, et al. Inactivated hepatitis A vaccine: active and passive immunoprophylaxis in chimpanzees. *Vaccine* 1992;10(Suppl 1):S148–S151.
307. Purcell RH, Emerson SU. Animal models of hepatitis A and E. *ILAR J* 2001;42:161–177.
309. Purcell RH, Feinstone SM, Ticehurst JR, et al. Hepatitis A virus. In: Vyas GN, Dienstag JL, Hoofnagle JH, eds. *Viral Hepatitis and Liver Disease.* Orlando, FL: Grune & Stratton; 1984:9–22.
310. Qu L, Feng Z, Yamane DY, et al. Disruption of TLR3 signaling due to cleavage of TRIF by the hepatitis A virus protease-polymerase processing intermediate, 3CD. *PLoS Pathog* 2011;7:e1002169.
312. Raychaudhuri G, Govindarajan S, Shapiro M, et al. Utilization of chimeras between human (HM-175) and simian (AGM-27) strains of hepatitis A virus to study the molecular basis of virulence. *J Virol* 1998;72: 7467–7475.
314. Rezende G, Roque-Afonso AM, Samuel D, et al. Viral and clinical factors associated with the fulminant course of hepatitis A infection. *Hepatology* 2003;38:613–618.
317. Robertson BH, D'Hondt EH, Spelbring J, et al. Effect of postexposure vaccination in a chimpanzee model of hepatitis A virus infection. *J Med Virol* 1994;43:249–251.
318. Robertson BH, Jansen RW, Khanna B, et al. Genetic relatedness of hepatitis A virus strains recovered from different geographical regions. *J Gen Virol* 1992;73(Pt 6):1365–1377.
319. Rosenblum LS, Villarino ME, Nainan OV, et al. Hepatitis A outbreak in a neonatal intensive care unit: risk factors for transmission and evidence of prolonged viral excretion among preterm infants. *J Infect Dis* 1991;164:476–482.
324. Schenzle D, Dietz K, Frosner GG. Antibody against hepatitis A in seven European countries. II. Statistical analysis of cross-sectional surveys. *Am J Epidemiol* 1979;110:70–76.
325. Schiff ER. Atypical clinical manifestations of hepatitis A. *Vaccine* 1992; 10(Suppl 1):S18–S20.
326. Schofield DJ, Satterfield W, Emerson SU, et al. Four chimpanzee monoclonal antibodies isolated by phage display neutralize hepatitis a virus. *Virology* 2002;292:127–136.
329. Schulte I, Hitziger T, Giugliano S, et al. Characterization of CD8+ T-cell response in acute and resolved hepatitis A virus infection. *J Hepatol* 2011;54:201–208.
332. Schultz DE, Honda M, Whetter LE, et al. Mutations within the 5′ nontranslated RNA of cell culture-adapted hepatitis A virus which enhance cap-independent translation in cultured African green monkey kidney cells. *J Virol* 1996;70:1041–1049.
334. Sciot R, Van Damme B, Desmet VJ. Cholestatic features in hepatitis A. *J Hepatol* 1986;3:172–181.
336. Shaffer DR, Brown EA, Lemon SM. Large deletion mutations involving the first pyrimidine-rich tract of the 5′ nontranslated RNA of human hepatitis A virus define two adjacent domains associated with distinct replication phenotypes. *J Virol* 1994;68:5568–5578.
337. Shaffer DR, Emerson SU, Murphy PC, et al. A hepatitis A virus deletion mutant which lacks the first pyrimidine-rich tract of the 5′ nontranslated RNA remains virulent in primates after direct intrahepatic nucleic acid transfection. *J Virol* 1995;69:6600–6604.
339. Shimizu YK, Mathiesen LR, Lorenz D, et al. Localization of hepatitis A antigen in liver tissue by peroxidase-conjugated antibody method: light and electron microscopic studies. *J Immunol* 1978;121:1671–1679.
340. Shouval D. Module 18: hepatitis A. In: *The immunological basis for immunization series.* Geneva, Switzerland, World Health Organization; 2011:1–39.
342. Siegl G, Frosner GG, Gauss-Muller V, et al. The physicochemical properties of infectious hepatitis A virions. *J Gen Virol* 1981;57:331–341.
344. Siegl G, Weitz M, Kronauer G. Stability of hepatitis A virus. *Intervirology* 1984;22:218–226.
346. Silberstein E, Xing L, van de Beek W, et al. Alteration of hepatitis A virus (HAV) particles by a soluble form of HAV cellular receptor 1 containing the immunoglobin- and mucin-like regions. *J Virol* 2003;77:8765–8774.
347. Sjogren MH, Tanno H, Fay O, et al. Hepatitis A virus in stool during clinical relapse. *Ann Intern Med* 1987;106:221–226.
348. Skinhoj P, Mikkelsen F, Hollinger FB. Hepatitis A in Greenland: importance of specific antibody testing in epidemiologic surveillance. *Am J Epidemiol* 1977;105:140–147.
350. Sobsey MD, Shields PA, Hauchman FS, et al. Survival and persistence of hepatitis A virus in environmental samples. In: Zuckerman AJ, ed. *Viral Hepatitis and Liver Disease.* New York: Alan R. Liss; 1988:121–124.
353. Stapleton JT, Jansen R, Lemon SM. Neutralizing antibody to hepatitis A virus in immune serum globulin and in the sera of human recipients of immune serum globulin. *Gastroenterology* 1985;89:637–642.
355. Steffen R. Risk of hepatitis A in travellers. *Vaccine* 1992;10(Suppl 1): S69–S72.
356. Steil BP, Barton DJ. Cis-active RNA elements (CREs) and picornavirus RNA replication. *Virus Res* 2009;139:240–252.
357. Stokes J, Jr., Farquhar JA, Drake ME, et al. Infectious hepatitis; length of protection by immune serum globulin (gamma globulin) during epidemics. *J Am Med Assoc* 1951;147:714–719.
358. Stokes JJ, Neefe J. The prevention and attenuation of infectious hepatitis by gamma globulin. *JAMA* 1945;127:144–145.
360. Szmuness W, Dienstag JL, Purcell RH, et al. Distribution of antibody to hepatitis A antigen in urban adult populations. *N Engl J Med* 1976;295:755–759.
361. Szmuness W, Dienstag JL, Purcell RH, et al. The prevalence of antibody to hepatitis A antigen in various parts of the world: a pilot study. *Am J Epidemiol* 1977;106:392–398.
362. Tami C, Silberstein E, Manangeeswaran M, et al. Immunoglobulin A (IgA) is a natural ligand of hepatitis A virus cellular receptor 1 (HAVCR1), and the association of IgA with HAVCR1 enhances virus-receptor interactions. *J Virol* 2007;81:3437–3446.
363. Tassopoulos N, Papaevangelou G, Roumeliotou-Karayannis A, et al. Double infections with hepatitis A and B viruses. *Liver* 1985;5:348–353.
365. Taylor RM, Davern T, Munoz S, et al. Fulminant hepatitis A virus infection in the United States: incidence, prognosis, and outcomes. *Hepatology* 2006;44:1589–1597.
367. Tesar M, Jia XY, Summers DF, et al. Analysis of a potential myristoylation site in hepatitis A virus capsid protein VP4. *Virology* 1993;194: 616–626.
369. Teterina NL, Bienz K, Egger D, et al. Induction of intracellular membrane rearrangements by HAV proteins 2C and 2BC. *Virology* 1997;237:66–77.
371. Tjon GM, Coutinho RA, van den Hoek A, et al. High and persistent excretion of hepatitis A virus in immunocompetent patients. *J Med Virol* 2006;78:1398–1405.
372. Tjon GM, Wijkmans CJ, Coutinho RA, et al. Molecular epidemiology of hepatitis A in Noord-Brabant, The Netherlands. *J Clin Virol* 2005; 32:128–136.
373. Tozun N, Forbes A, Anderson MG, et al. Safety of alcohol after viral hepatitis. *Lancet* 1991;337:1079–1080.
374. Troisi CL, Hollinger FB, Krause DS, et al. Immunization of seronegative infants with hepatitis A vaccine (HAVRIX; SKB): a comparative study of two dosing schedules. *Vaccine* 1997;15:1613–1617.
380. Vallbracht A, Maier K, Stierhof YD, et al. Liver-derived cytotoxic T cells in hepatitis A virus infection. *J Infect Dis* 1989;160:209–217.
381. Van Damme P, Thoelen S, Cramm M, et al. Inactivated hepatitis A vaccine: reactogenicity, immunogenicity, and long-term antibody persistence. *J Med Virol* 1994;44:446–451.
382. Vento S, Garofano T, Renzini C, et al. Fulminant hepatitis associated with hepatitis A virus superinfection in patients with chronic hepatitis C. *N Engl J Med* 1998;338:286–290.
383. Victor JC, Monto AS, Surdina TY, et al. Hepatitis A vaccine versus immune globulin for postexposure prophylaxis. *N Engl J Med* 2007; 357:1685–1694.
386. Ward R, Krugman S, Giles JP, et al. Infectious hepatitis; studies of its natural history and prevention. *N Engl J Med* 1958;258:407–416.
387. Wasley A, Samandari T, Bell BP. Incidence of hepatitis A in the United States in the era of vaccination. *JAMA* 2005;294:194–201.

391. Werzberger A, Mensch B, Kuter B, et al. A controlled trial of a formalin-inactivated hepatitis A vaccine in healthy children. *N Engl J Med* 1992;327:453–457.
392. Werzberger A, Mensch B, Nalin DR, et al. Effectiveness of hepatitis A vaccine in a former frequently affected community: 9 years' followup after the Monroe field trial of VAQTA. *Vaccine* 2002;20:1699–1701.
397. Widell A, Hansson BG, Oberg B, et al. Influence of twenty potentially antiviral substances on in vitro multiplication of hepatitis A virus. *Antiviral Res* 1986;6:103–112.
398. Wiens BL, Bohidar NR, Pigeon JG, et al. Duration of protection from clinical hepatitis A disease after vaccination with VAQTA. *J Med Virol* 1996;49:235–241.
404. Yang Y, Liang Y, Qu L, et al. Disruption of innate immunity due to mitochondrial targeting of a picornaviral protease precursor. *Proc Natl Acad Sci U S A* 2007;104:7253–7258.
405. Yang Y, Yi M, Evans DJ, et al. Identification of a conserved RNA replication element (cre) within the $3D^{pol}$-coding sequence of hepatoviruses. *J Virol* 2008;82:10118–10128.
406. Yao G. Clinical spectrum and natural history of viral hepatitis A in a 1988 Shanghai epidemic. In: Hollinger FB, Lemon SM, Margolis HS, eds. *Viral Hepatitis and Liver Disease.* Baltimore: Williams & Wilkins; 1991: 76–78.
407. Yi M, Lemon SM. Replication of subgenomic hepatitis A virus RNAs expressing firefly luciferase is enhanced by mutations associated with adaptation of virus to growth in cultured cells. *J Virol* 2002;76:1171–1180.
408. Yi M, Schultz DE, Lemon SM. Functional significance of the interaction of hepatitis A virus RNA with glyceraldehyde 3-phosphate dehydrogenase (GAPDH): opposing effects of GAPDH and polypyrimidine tract binding protein on internal ribosome entry site function. *J Virol* 2000;74:6459–6468.
409. Yin J, Cherney MM, Bergmann EM, et al. An episulfide cation (thiiranium ring) trapped in the active site of HAV 3C proteinase inactivated by peptide-based ketone inhibitors. *J Mol Biol* 2006;361:673–686.
413. Zhang B, Morace G, Gauss-Muller V, et al. Poly(A) binding protein, C-terminally truncated by the hepatitis A virus proteinase 3C, inhibits viral translation. *Nucleic Acids Res* 2007;35:5975–5984.
417. Zhou Y, Callendret B, Xu D, et al. Dominance of the CD4+ T helper cell response during acute resolving hepatitis A virus infection. *J Exp Med* 2012;209:1481–1492.
418. Zhuang FC, Qian W, Mao ZA, et al. Persistent efficacy of live attenuated hepatitis A vaccine (H2-strain) after a mass vaccination program. *Chin Med J (Engl)* 2005;118:1851–1856.

CHAPTER 20

Kim Y. Green

Caliciviridae: The Noroviruses

The family *Caliciviridae* is composed of small (27 to 40 nm), nonenveloped, icosahedral viruses that possess a linear, positive-sense, single-stranded RNA (ssRNA) genome. The five genera of the family are *Norovirus, Sapovirus, Nebovirus, Lagovirus,* and *Vesivirus.* The major human pathogens in the family are the noroviruses and sapoviruses, which cause acute gastroenteritis. Important veterinary pathogens include vesiviruses such as feline calicivirus (FCV), which causes a respiratory disease in cats, and lagoviruses such as rabbit hemorrhagic disease virus (RHDV), which causes an often fatal hemorrhagic disease in rabbits. This chapter provides a description of the family *Caliciviridae,* with major emphasis on the noroviruses because of their prominent role in sporadic and epidemic gastroenteritis.[147]

HISTORY

The establishment of a viral etiology for gastroenteritis in humans was a decades-long process that was hampered by the fastidious nature of many of these viruses for growth in cell culture.[213] Volunteer studies carried out in the 1940s and 1950s in the United States and Japan played a major role in establishing that filterable, nonbacterial infectious agents can cause enteric disease.[213] An important advance occurred in 1972 with the discovery of Norwalk virus (NV) by Kapikian et al.[214] Stool material from a rectal swab obtained from an ill individual involved in a gastroenteritis outbreak that had occurred at an elementary school in Norwalk, Ohio, in October 1968 was administered to adult volunteers as a bacteria-free filtrate and serially passaged to other volunteers, inducing acute gastroenteritis in certain individuals.[112,113] Stool material from these volunteers was then examined for the presence of viruses by the technique of immune electron microscopy (IEM), which involves the direct observation of antigen–antibody complexes by EM.[11,13,18,214] The fecal filtrate was incubated with prechallenge or convalescent-phase serum from a volunteer who had become ill following ingestion of the filtrate. Figure 20.1 shows the striking difference between the appearance of the small, round virus particles (described as 27 to 30 nm in diameter with a hint of surface structure) after incubation with the prechallenge serum (part A and B) and after incubation with convalescent-phase serum (parts C and D). The increase in visible virus-specific antibodies in the convalescent serum from individuals involved in the original Norwalk outbreak, as well as in volunteers challenged with the virus derived from the outbreak, led to the conclusion that NV was the etiologic agent.[214] Norwalk virus would become the prototype strain for a large group of related *Norwalk-like viruses* or *small round structured viruses,* known now as the noroviruses.

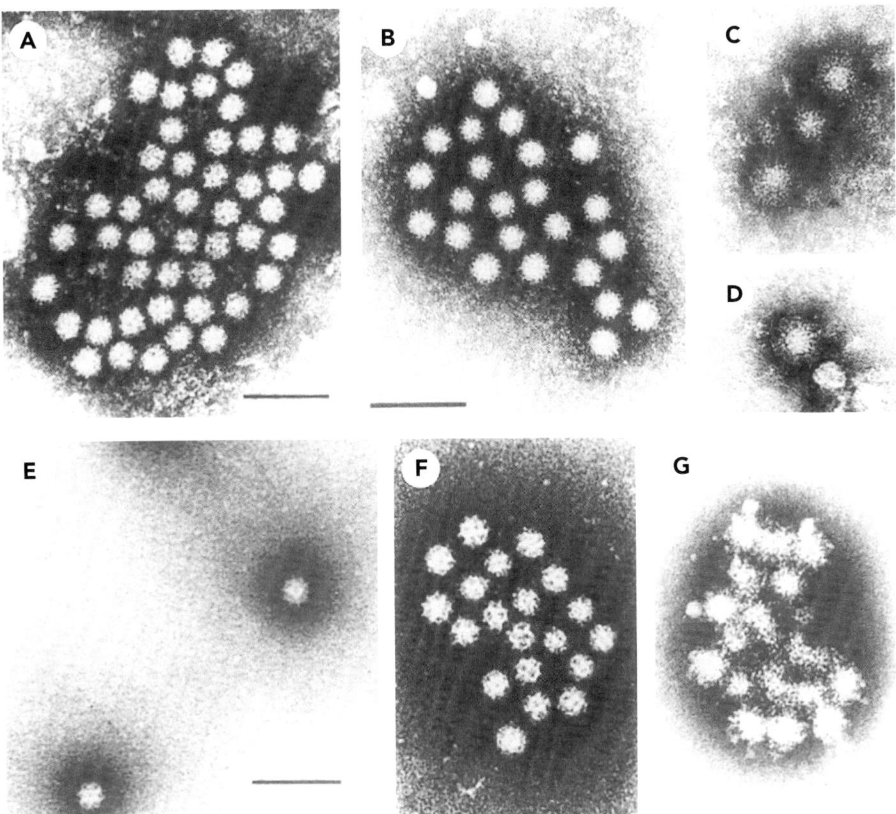

FIGURE 20.1. Norwalk virus (NV) (genus *Norovirus*) and Sapporo virus (genus *Sapovirus*) in stool material. A: NV particles in a stool filtrate visualized by immune electron microscopy (IEM). **B:** An aggregate observed after incubation of NV stool filtrate with a 1:5 dilution of volunteer's prechallenge serum. Particles have a light coating of antibody molecules. The amount of antibody present on this aggregate was given a rating of 1 to 2 to 2+ and the serum was given an overall rating of 1 to 2+ on a scale of 1 to 4. **C, D:** Three single particles **(C)** and one individual particle **(D)** observed after incubation of the NV stool filtrate with a 1:5 dilution of the same volunteer's postchallenge convalescent serum. Particles are heavily coated with antibody molecules. At high antibody levels (antibody excess), large aggregates may not be seen. The amount of antibody was given a rating of 4+ and the serum was given an overall rating of 4+ on a scale of 1 to 4. **E:** Sapporo virus particles in stool material visualized by direct electron microscopy (EM). The distinct, hollow cup-like structures are apparent. **F:** Sapporo virus particles after incubation with guinea pig hyperimmune serum. The amount of antibody was given a 1+ rating. **G:** An aggregate observed after incubation of Sapporo virus stool filtrate with guinea pig hyperimmune serum. The amount of antibody was given a rating of 4+ on a scale of 1 to 4. (**A–D** from Kapikian AZ, Wyatt RG, Dolin R, et al. Visualization by immune electron microscopy of a 27-nm particle associated with acute infectious nonbacterial gastroenteritis. *J Virol* 1972;10:1075–1081, with permission. **E–G** from Nakata S, Kogawa K, Numata K, et al. The epidemiology of human calicivirus/Sapporo/82/Japan. *Arch Virol Suppl* 1996;12:263–270, with permission.)

The techniques used in the discovery of the NV proved instrumental in the subsequent characterization of other fastidious enteric viruses (including human rotaviruses, astroviruses, parvoviruses, enteroviruses, and hepatitis A virus) by an approach that became known as *particle* or *direct* virology.[213] Norovirus reference strains such as Hawaii virus (from a family outbreak of gastroenteritis that occurred in Honolulu in 1971) and Snow Mountain virus (from an outbreak in a Colorado resort camp in 1976) were discovered in 1977 and 1982, respectively.[116,468] In 1976, Madeley and Cosgrove[296] reported the presence of "typical" caliciviruses in the stools of infants and young children (2 to 18 months of age), and these viruses showed a striking morphologic similarity to previously characterized animal caliciviruses that were known to exhibit "classical" distinct cup-like depressions on the surface of the virion. That same year, Flewett and Davies[130] observed similar calicivirus particles in a sample from the intestinal lumen of a child at autopsy and in the feces of a child with gastroenteritis. Chiba et al[90] described a "classical" calicivirus, associated with gastroenteritis, in infants and young children living in an infant home in Sapporo, Japan, in 1977. Another virus (later designated Sapporo/82/Japan) that exhibited classical calicivirus morphology was subsequently detected from this same infant home (Fig. 20.1E).[340] Hyperimmune serum was raised in guinea pigs against Sapporo/82/Japan virus particles purified from stool material, and IEM was used to establish its antigenic characteristics (Fig. 20.1F and 20.1G, respectively). The Sapporo virus would become the prototype strain for the *Sapporo-like viruses* or *classical caliciviruses,* known now as the sapoviruses.

In the late 1980s, the stool filtrate derived from the Norwalk, Ohio, outbreak was again fed to adults in volunteer studies to obtain adequate quantities of virus particles to

TABLE 20.1 Taxonomic Structure of the *Caliciviridae*

Genus	Species	Representative strain
Norovirus (NoV)	*Norwalk virus* (NV)	Hu/NoV/GI.1/Norwalk/1968/US
Sapovirus (SaV)	*Sapporo virus* (SV)	Hu/SaV/GI.1/Sapporo/1982/JP
Lagovirus (LaV)	*Rabbit hemorrhagic disease virus* (RHDV)	Ra/LaV/RHDV/GH/1988/DE
	European brown hare syndrome virus (EBHSV)	Ha/LaV/EBHSV/GD/1989/FR
Nebovirus (NeV)	*Newbury-1 virus* (NBV)	Bo/NeV/NBV/Newbury-1/1976/UK
Vesivirus (VeV)	*Vesicular exanthema of swine virus* (VESV)	Po/VeV/VESV/VESV-A48/1948/US
	Feline calicivirus (FCV)	Fe/VeV/FCV/F9/1958/US

The cryptograms are organized as follows: host species from which the virus was obtained/genus/species (or genogroup)/strain name/year of occurrence/country of origin. Abbreviations for the host species are Fe, feline; Ha, Hare; Hu, Human; Po, Porcine; Ra, Rabbit. Country abbreviations are DE, Germany; FR, France; JP, Japan; US, United States.

GenBank Accession numbers and references for description of representative viruses: Norwalk virus, M87661[202,214]; Sapporo virus, U65427[89,352]; RHDV, M67473[325]; EBHSV, Z69620[258]; VESV, AF181082[345,490]; FCV, M86379[64]; Newbury-1 virus, DQ013304.[53,361]

Adapted from Virus taxonomy: 2011 release. International Committee on the Taxonomy of Viruses web page. http://ictvonline.org/virusTaxonomy.asp?version=2011

characterize the viral genome, a major advance by Jiang et al[199] that established the classification of Norwalk virus as a member of the *Caliciviridae.* The complete RNA genome sequences of Norwalk virus and the closely related Southampton virus were determined and found to be organized into three major open reading frames (ORF1, -2, and -3) with a polyadenylated 3′ end[176,202,253,254] (see Genome Structure and Organization). The ORF1 was shown to encode a large polyprotein that was proteolytically processed into the mature nonstructural proteins.[273,276] The ORF2 encoded the major capsid protein, VP1, and ORF3 encoded a minor structural protein, VP2. The human noroviruses initially segregated into two major phylogenetic groups within what would become the genus *Norovirus* of the *Caliciviridae* that were designated as genogroups I (GI) and II (GII), with NV belonging to GI and the Hawaii and Snow Mountain viruses belonging to GII.[266,487] In addition, sequence analysis of the "classical" caliciviruses confirmed that they were distinct from the noroviruses, ultimately forming a separate genus, *Sapovirus,* within the *Caliciviridae.*[252,274,309]

CLASSIFICATION

Members of the virus family *Caliciviridae* have a virion protein, genome (VPg)-linked, positive-sense RNA genome that is polyadenylated and surrounded by a nonenveloped, icosahedral capsid of 27 to 40 nm in diameter. The capsid is constructed predominantly from a major structural protein, VP1, of approximately 60,000 D. The five genera of the family *Caliciviridae—Norovirus, Sapovirus, Lagovirus, Nebovirus,* and *Vesivirus*—each represent a distinct phylogenetic clade in the family[92,152] (e-Fig. 20.1). Within each genus, one or more species has been defined based primarily on genetic relatedness, and the current taxonomic structure of the *Caliciviridae* is shown in Table 20.1. It is possible that additional genera will be established, following characterization of the unique genomes of Tulane virus (simian),[128] St. Valérian virus (porcine),[251] and Bayern virus (avian)[509] (e-Fig. 20.1). Below the level of species in certain genera (*Norovirus* and *Sapovirus*), provisional genetic typing systems (consisting of genogroups subdivided into genetic clusters or genotypes) have proven useful in epidemiologic studies (see Molecular Epidemiology).

VIRION STRUCTURE

Calicivirus virions exhibit T = 3 icosahedral symmetry. The capsid contains 90 dimers of the VP1 capsid protein that form a shell from which 90 arch-like capsomeres protrude at the local and strict twofold axes.[86,381,382,384] These arches are arranged in such a way that 32 large hollows are seen at the icosahedral five- and threefold positions, and these hollows are seen as cup-like structures on the surface of caliciviruses (*calici* is derived from the Latin word *calyx,* or "cup"). Electron cryomicroscopy and computer image processing studies of representative caliciviruses show subtle variation in the capsid structures that are consistent with their differences in appearance by negative-stain EM, which can range from a feathery appearance (many noroviruses, such as Norwalk virus in Fig. 20.1A) to the presence of sharply defined "cups" (many sapoviruses, such as Sapporo virus in Fig. 20.1E and the vesiviruses).[86,383]

Self-assembly of the norovirus VP1 into virus-like particles (VLPs) is an efficient process and does not require RNA[201] or the minor capsid protein, VP2.[256,263] This feature has been especially useful in the study of the fastidious caliciviruses, because recombinant (r) VLPs expressed in the baculovirus system have served as a surrogate for native virions.[154,201,203] The NV rVP1 (180 copies) characteristically self-assembles into 38-nm particles with T = 3 symmetry, but it can form smaller VLPs (23 nm) with T = 1 symmetry composed of 60 copies of VP1.[498]

The atomic structure of the Norwalk rVLP has been determined by x-ray crystallography.[382] These structural studies

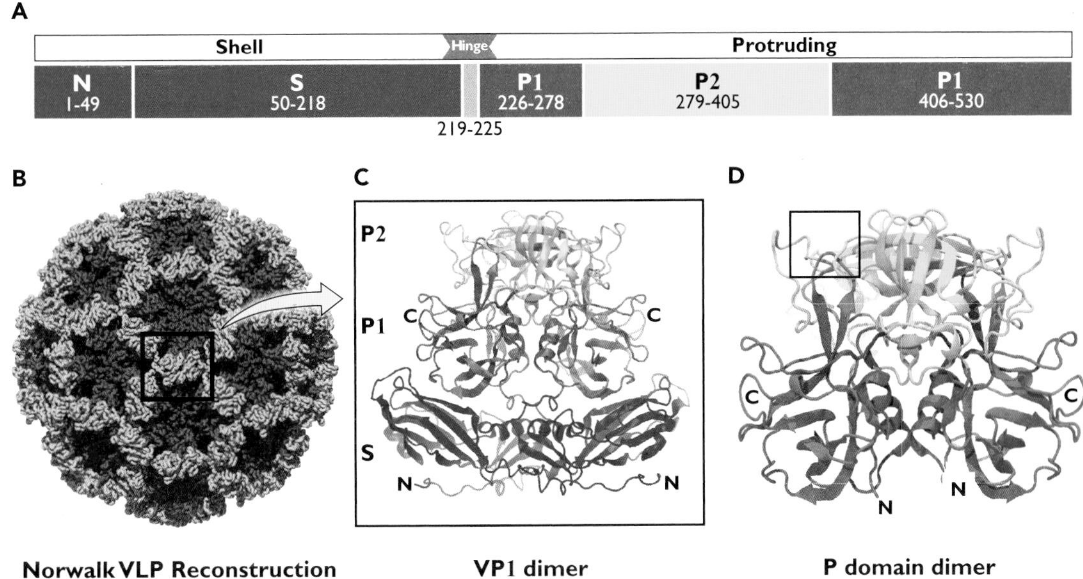

FIGURE 20.2. Organization of the norovirus major capsid protein, VP1. A: The Norwalk virus major capsid protein VP1 is 539 amino acids (aa) in length and is organized into two major parts, shell (S) and protruding (P), connected by a hinge (H) region. The aa borders of the defined domains are N-terminal (N) arm, 1 to 49; S, 50 to 218; hinge, 219 to 225; P1, 226 to 278 and 406 to 530; and P2, 279 to 405. (Adapted from Prasad BV, Hardy ME, Dokland T, et al. X-ray crystallographic structure of the Norwalk virus capsid. *Science* 1999;286:287–290.) **B:** Model of the T = 3 Norwalk virus whole capsid, determined at 3.4-Å resolution.[382] The capsid is composed of 90 dimers of VP1, with the S, P1, and P2 domains shown in blue, red, and yellow, respectively. The box highlights the arrangement of a VP1 dimer as it is displayed on the surface of the virion. **C:** Three-dimensional ribbon representation of a VP1 dimer derived from x-ray crystallography studies of Norwalk virus recombinant virus-like particles (rVLPs) at 3.4 Å, showing the presentation of the P2 domain at the top of an arch supported by two P1 domain "arms".[382] The S domain forms the internal scaffold of the virion that surrounds the RNA genome and positions the arch to the virion surface. The N-terminus (N) and C-terminus (C) of the VP1 are indicated. **D:** Three-dimensional ribbon representation of a P domain–only dimer, determined at 1.4-Å resolution.[91] The box highlights the location of a histo-blood group antigen (HBGA) carbohydrate binding site mapped within the P2 domain (see Fig. 20.7). (Images provided by B. V. V. Prasad.)

have defined two major domains in the VP1—the shell (S) and the protruding (P) arm (Fig. 20.2). The S domain forms the inner part of the capsid that surrounds the RNA genome and maintains the icosahedral contacts of the T = 3 structure, and the P domain forms the arch-like protrusions that emanate from the shell and contain the dimeric contacts.[382] The amino acid residues that correspond to the S and P subdomains in the NV VP1 (530 amino acids in length) are diagrammed in Figure 20.2A. A ribbon model of the VP1 dimeric subunit derived from the crystallographic structure of the capsid shows a more detailed view of these domains and their interactions (Fig. 20.2B, C). The NH_2-terminal (N) arm, located within the S domain, consists of residues 1 to 49 and faces the interior of the capsid. The part of the S domain that forms a classic eight-stranded antiparallel β-sandwich fold consists of amino acids (aa) 50 to 225 (which includes a flexible hinge). The entire S domain (aa 1 to 225) corresponds to the N-terminal region of the capsid protein that is relatively conserved among noroviruses in sequence comparisons. The P domain, which is linked to the S domain through a flexible hinge (aa 219 to 225), corresponds to the C-terminal half of the VP1, which is more variable in amino acid sequence. The P domain is divided into the P1 subdomain, encompassing aa 226 to 278 and 406 to 520, and the P2 subdomain, encompassing aa 279 to 405. The P1 subdomains form the sides of the arch of the capsomeres and position the highly variable P2 subdomain at the top of the arch. In the dimeric form of the capsid protein, two P2 subdomains form what appears to be a bilobed structure at the surface of the virion. The exposure of the variable P2 region on the surface is consistent with its role in the formation of a major antigenic site and in receptor binding.[10,47,85,86,107,110,172,178,185,221,271,281,348,382,398,459,497] It has been proposed that the highly conserved S domain may function as an icosahedral scaffold with the N-terminal arm providing a switch to facilitate the appropriate curvature, and that the P domain may be a replaceable module for conferring strain differences and antigenic specificity.[85,86,382] Structural studies of other caliciviruses have shown a similar organization, with an internal shell domain serving as the scaffold for the more variable protruding domain.[85,220]

Knowledge of the capsid structure has informed study of capsid assembly and facilitated the expression of subviral forms of the capsid that have proven useful in several areas of research (e-Fig. 20.2).[460] The extreme N-terminus of the NV VP1 protein (first 20 aa) was not required for the assembly of native-sized 38-nm VLPs with T = 3 symmetry.[36] Expression of the NV VP1 S region alone (beginning with the extreme N-terminus of the VP1 and including amino acid residues 1 to 227) resulted in the formation of smooth particles (designated "S" particles in e-Fig. 20.2) of approximately 30 nm in diameter.[36]

Although initial expression of the NV P region alone did not yield VLPs in baculovirus or bacterial systems,[36,458] the native P domain from NV and other noroviruses formed *P dimers* that were recognized by antibodies and carbohydrates similarly to intact VLPs.[458] The ability to produce rapidly P dimers (and mutagenized forms) accelerated structure and function studies of the norovirus capsid protein.[61,463,464,465] Further genetic engineering to include a four to seven arginine-rich sequence at the C-terminus of the P domain resulted in the generation of small, subviral particles termed *P particles* that were assembled from 12 dimers of the P domain and that showed T = 1 symmetry[460,463] (e-Fig. 20.2). Recently, expression of the P domain with a further modified terminus allowed the production of *small P particles.*[457]

GENOME STRUCTURE AND ORGANIZATION

Caliciviruses have a linear, single-stranded, positive-sense RNA genome (ranging from approximately 7.3 to 8.5 kb [kilobases] in length) (Fig. 20.3A). Genomes characteristically begin with a 5′ end terminal pGpU sequence that is covalently linked to a small protein, VPg. A short conserved region (CR) at the 5′ end is repeated internally in the genome near the beginning of a subgenomic-sized RNA transcript that is co-terminal with the 3′ end of the genome.[179,254,324,331,344] The nonstructural proteins are encoded beginning near the 5′ end of the genome, and the structural proteins (VP1 and VP2) are encoded toward the 3′ end of the genome in the region corresponding to a subgenomic RNA. Calicivirus genomes are organized into two or more major ORFs, depending on the genus. The noroviruses and vesiviruses encode the VP1 structural protein in a separate ORF (ORF2), whereas sapoviruses, lagoviruses, and neboviruses encode a VP1 that is contiguous with the large nonstructural polyprotein in ORF1 (Fig. 20.3B). All caliciviruses have a relatively small ORF near the 3′ end that encodes the minor structural protein, VP2. The VP2 is variable in size (12,000 to 29,000 D) and sequence identity among the caliciviruses.[65,418] Murine norovirus genomes analyzed thus far contain a unique conserved ORF (ORF4),[467] with an encoded protein of 23,800 D

A Genome Organization

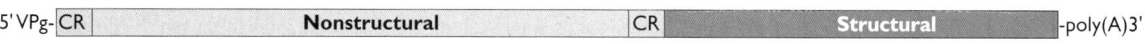

B Reading Frame Usage

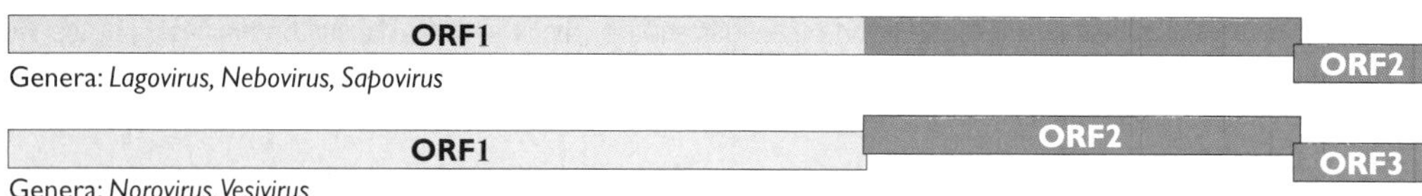

C Gene Order and Cleavage Sites

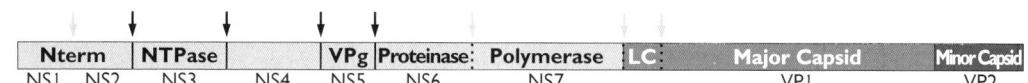

FIGURE 20.3. Comparative features of calicivirus genomes. A: The positive-sense RNA genome is covalently linked to a virion protein genome (VPg) at the 5′ end and polyadenylated at the 3′ end. Nonstructural proteins are encoded beginning from the 5′ end of the genome and the structural proteins are encoded toward the 3′ end. A conserved region (CR) of nucleotide sequence is shared between the 5′ end of the viral genome and the 5′ end of an abundant subgenomic RNA species produced during replication that serves as a template for translation of the viral structural proteins. **B:** Calicivirus genome organization. Calicivirus genomes are organized so that the major capsid protein coding sequence is either in frame or not with the upstream nonstructural protein sequence. The genomic organization and reading frame usage are shown for representative strains in the genera *Lagovirus* (Ra/LaV/RHDV/GH/1988/DE, GenBank Accession Number M67473), *Nebovirus* (Bo/NeV/NBV/Newbury-1/1976/UK, GenBank Accession Number DQ013304), *Sapovirus* (Hu/SaV/Manchester/1993/UK, GenBank Accession Number X86560), *Norovirus* (Hu/NoV/Norwalk/1968/US, GenBank Accession Number M87661), and *Vesivirus* (Fe/VeV/FCV/F9/1958/US, GenBank Accession Number M86379). **C:** A large polyprotein (encoded in open reading frame 1 [ORF1]) is translated from the viral RNA genome, and it is processed into precursors and final products by a virus-encoded protease. The proteolytic processing strategy varies among the caliciviruses, but all viruses encode domains for at least seven protein functions indicated here as nonstructural (NS) proteins NS1 through NS7.[434] An extra cleavage site is present in the ORF1 of caliciviruses in which the capsid protein sequence is in frame with the nonstructural polyprotein encoded in ORF1. Cleavage at this site is thought to release the VP1 from the polyprotein so that the RNA-dependent RNA polymerase (NS7) can adopt an active conformation early in the replicative cycle. A cleavage site unique to the vesiviruses is present to release the leader of the capsid protein (LC) from a capsid precursor encoded in ORF2.[438] Mapped cleavage sites conserved and utilized among all calicivirus genera are indicated with a dark arrow; cleavage sites that vary in utilization among the family are indicated with a light arrow.[238,273,276,358,359,434,435,438,506]

(designated VF-1) that has been implicated in modulation of the host innate immune response *in vivo.*[318]

Viral Proteins

Structural Proteins

Three proteins are found in mature calicivirus virions: VP1, VP2, and VPg.[436] The VP1 (~60,000 D), which is the major structural protein of the virus, is present in 180 copies (90 dimers) per virion.[383] The predominance of VP1 in the formation of the viral capsid structure (see Virion Structure) is consistent with its critical role in determining the antigenic phenotype of the virus and its interactions with host cells.

The VP2 (12,000 to 29,000 D) is considered a minor structural protein because it is present in only one to two copies per virion, and its function is unknown.[145,146,436] The ablation of VP2 expression in an infectious FCV complementary DNA (cDNA) clone by the introduction of a stop codon in its reading frame did not abolish RNA replication; however, infectious virions could not be recovered without an intact VP2.[433] Although VP1 can self-assemble into rVLPs independently of the presence of VP2,[256,263] the presence of VP2 may increase the efficiency of VP1 expression and enhance the stability of rVLPs generated in the baculovirus expression system.[35] Evidence for a direct interaction between the VP1 and VP2 capsid proteins has been reported for both NV[74,145,146] and FCV,[108,211] further suggesting a role in particle maturation or stability.

The VPg is covalently linked to the genomic and subgenomic RNA in infected cells,[120,180] and is a minor component in virions at an estimated one or two copies per particle.[410,436] Although the VPg is present in virions, it likely functions primarily as a nonstructural protein during replication (see Nonstructural Proteins).

Nonstructural Proteins

Caliciviruses derive their mature nonstructural proteins (designated here as NS1 through NS7) by proteolytic cleavage of a large polyprotein encoded in ORF1 (Fig. 20.3C). The length of the noncleaved polyprotein precursor is approximately 200,000 D (excluding the in-frame VP1 capsid protein sequences of the lagoviruses, neboviruses, and sapoviruses). This large precursor has never been observed, most likely because proteolytic processing is rapid and co-translational.[273,276,439] The proteolytic cleavages are mediated by a virus-encoded cysteine proteinase (NS6^{Pro}).[50] The location of the cleavage sites in the ORF1 polyprotein that define the borders of the final nonstructural protein cleavage products has been determined for calicivirus strains representing the genera *Norovirus,*[34,273,276,434] *Vesivirus,*[435] *Lagovirus,*[238,506] and *Sapovirus.*[359] Some variation is seen among the proteolytic processing strategies, but the overall gene order of the calicivirus nonstructural proteins is conserved. The lagoviruses, represented by RHDV, have the highest number (six) of mapped cleavage sites. The polyprotein of RHDV is cleaved at these six sites to release seven final products (designated as NS1 through NS7 in Fig. 20.3C and Table 20.2). Five cleavage sites for the norovirus ORF1 polyprotein (represented by Southampton virus) have been mapped that would release six mature products.[273,276] The noroviruses differ from the lagoviruses in that a protease cleavage site has not been directly mapped in the extreme N-terminal protein, although evidence suggests that additional processing (or modification) of the protein can occur in cells.[419,434] The vesivirus cleavage map (represented by FCV) contains five mapped cleavage sites to release six mature nonstructural proteins, and each cleavage event is essential in the virus replication cycle.[435] The vesiviruses show yet another variation in processing, in that no evidence exists for efficient viral protease-mediated cleavage between the Pro and polymerase (Pol) proteins, even in virus-infected cells.[306,357,435,439] In addition, vesiviruses bear a unique cleavage site in a capsid protein precursor protein that is processed by NS6^{Pro} to release the leader of the capsid (LC) and the major capsid protein, VP1[438,470] (Fig. 20.3C). The predicted nonstructural protein cleavage map of human sapovirus strain, Mc10, shows an overall similarity with that of the vesiviruses.[359] Sapoviruses (and other caliciviruses in which the capsid region is in frame with the nonstructural polyprotein) bear an additional protease cleavage site in the ORF1 polyprotein between the polymerase and capsid coding regions. A number of stable precursor proteins have been described also for the caliciviruses, and it is likely that these proteins have defined functions in replication.[34,39,93,238,325,326,434,435]

The calicivirus dipeptide cleavage recognition sites are consistent with those described for the picornavirus 3C cysteine proteinase.[174] The calicivirus cleavage sites identified thus far have either a negatively charged glutamic acid (E) or polar glutamine (Q) in the first position (designated P1). More variation exists within the second position of the dipeptide cleavage site (designated P1′). Studies of the calicivirus proteinase substrate specificity have shown some tolerance in the P1′ position at certain cleavage sites.[174,438,505] The conformation of the protein surrounding the dipeptide recognition site is also important for efficient cleavage by the proteinase.[174,439]

The availability of proteolytic cleavage maps for the calicivirus nonstructural polyproteins has enabled studies that elucidate the functions and structures of individual proteins.[175] Biochemical studies first confirmed enzymatic activities in calicivirus proteins corresponding to an NTPase (NTPase or NS3^{NTPase}),[300] a chymotrypsin-like cysteine proteinase (Pro or NS6^{Pro}),[50] and an RNA-dependent RNA polymerase (Pol or NS7^{Pol}).[479] The three-dimensional structures for the latter two enzymes have been reported. The norovirus Pro shares structural similarities with classical chymotrypsin-like serine proteases[188,189,339,518] (Fig. 20.4A). A cleft containing the active site catalytic residues (His 30, Glu 54, and Cys 139 for Norwalk virus) involved in substrate cleavage is located between two domains. The N-terminal domain (blue) starts with an α-helix followed by a five-stranded twisted antiparallel β-sheet. The structure of this domain contains features of both the simpler four-stranded β-sheet found in the N-terminal domain of picornaviral 2A proteinases and the more commonly found complete β-barrels observed in the N-terminal domains of most chymotrypsin-like proteinases. The C-terminal domain (red) adopts the structure of a classical six-stranded β-barrel found in a wide range of viral and nonviral chymotrypsin-like proteinases. Co-crystallization of the protease with an active site-directed peptide inhibitor (acetyl-Glu-Phe-Gln-Leu-Gln-propenyl ethyl ester) has given detailed insight into the interaction of substrate with the catalytic residues such as Cys 139 (the active site nucleophile) within the cleft[189] (Fig. 20.4B). The norovirus RNA-dependent RNA polymerase has a classical "right hand" (finger, thumb, and palm) organization,[346,347,517] with the C-terminus of the protein positioned in the active site cleft (Fig. 20.5A). Modeling of the

TABLE 20.2 Calicivirus Nonstructural Proteins

Calicivirus nonstructural protein (NS)	Picornavirus counterpart	Function	Reported properties (genus)	References
NS1	2A	Unknown	Cleavage and release essential for replication (VeV)	(435)
NS2	2B	Unknown	Binding partner with host cell VAP-A (NoV)	(125)
			Golgi co-localization and disassembly (NoV)	(129)
			C-terminal hydrophobic region (NoV)	(125,129)
			Present in membranous replication complexes (VeV)	(155)
			Interacts with NS3, NS4, NS6–7 (VeV)	(211)
NS3	2C	NTPase	NTP binding, hydrolysis of NTP (LaV, NoV)	(300,375)
			Present in membranous replication complexes (VeV)	(155)
NS4	3A	Unknown	Forms stable precursor with VPg: proposed VPg anchor (VeV)	(435)
			Present in membranous replication complexes (VeV)	(155)
			Inhibits actin cytoskeleton remodeling (NoV)	(182)
			ER/Golgi trafficking antagonist (NoV)	(422)
NS5	3B	VPg	Present in virions, covalently linked to RNA (VeV)	(58,180)
			Binding partner with eIF3 (NoV)	(103)
			Binding partner with eIF4E (VeV)	(148)
			Nucleotidylated by RdRP at conserved tyrosine (LaV)	(295)
			Functions in protein-primed RNA synthesis (NoV)	(399)
			Conserved tyrosine essential for replication of virus (VeV, NoV)	(327,446)
			Sequence homology with eIF1A (NoV, VeV)	(439)
			Present in membranous replication complexes (VeV)	(155)
			Linked to cellular trans-Golgi network protein 2 RNA in cells (NoV)	(446)
NS6	3C	Proteinase (Pro)	Proteinase activity, cysteine in active site (NoV, VeV, LaV, SaV)	(50,276,359,439)
			Mediates cleavage and release of ORF1-encoded proteins (LaV, NoV, VeV, SaV)	(276,359,439,506)
			Mediates cleavage of capsid precursor protein, PreVP1 (VeV)	(438)
			Cleaves cellular proteins (VeV, NoV)	(250,503)
			Structural analysis shows chymotrypsin-like folding (NoV)	(339)
NS7	3D	RNA-dependent RNA polymerase (Pol)	Contains Pol motif hYGDDhhY/V (VeV, NoV, LaV, SaV)	(199,309,325,342)
			In vitro activity is primer independent (LaV, NoV, VeV)	(134,479,493)
			Transcription activity on negative-strand template (LaV)	(331)
			Enzymatically active as ProPol (NS6–7) precursor form (VeV, NoV)	(33,493)
			Interacts with VPg, PreVP1, VP2 (VeV)	(211)
			Present in membranous replication complexes (VeV)	(155)
			Structural analysis reveals carboxyl-terminus in active site cleft (NoV)	(347)

ER, endoplasmic reticulum; LaV, Lagovirus; NoV, Norovirus; NTP, nucleotide triphosphate; NTPase, nucleotide triphosphatase; ORF1, open reading frame 1; RdRP, RNA-dependent RNA polymerase; SaV, Sapovirus; VeV, Vesivirus; VPg, virion protein, genome.

interaction of Pol with an RNA template in the presence of manganese and cytidine triphosphate (CTP) shows that the initiation of RNA synthesis occurs within the active site cleft (Fig. 20.5B–D). Binding of the primer/template RNA duplex displaces the C-terminal tail away from the active site, allowing the central helix of the thumb domain to position itself for interaction with the primer strand and minor groove of the primer–template duplex.[517] Two divalent metal ions (likely Mg^{2+} in cells) help mediate catalysis by forming coordination bonds with three highly conserved aspartic acid residues and the nucleoside triphosphate (NTP). After nucleotidyl transfer has occurred, the pyrophosphate is released from the enzyme. The primer–template duplex is predicted to translocate in a manner that places the newly incorporated nucleotide into the same position as that of the 3′ end of the primer strand immediately prior to nucleotidyl transfer. This translocation process

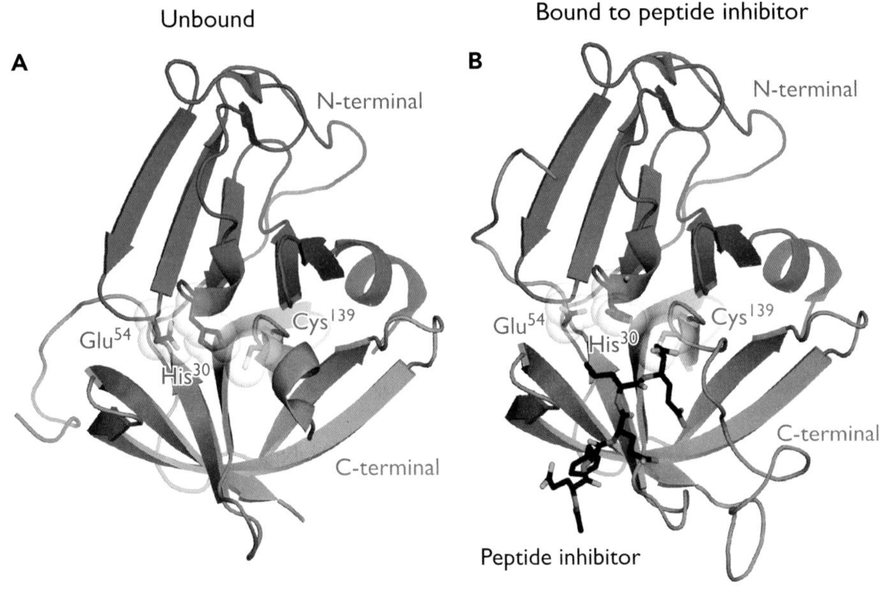

FIGURE 20.4. Structure of the norovirus proteinase. A: Three-dimensional ribbon representation of the Norwalk virus protease structure resolved at 1.5 Å shows that it adopts the conformation of a classical serine protease, in which a cleft containing the enzymatic active site is located between two β-barrel domains. The active site is positioned at the opening of the cleft and composed of residues His 30, Glu 54, and Cys 139 (the *catalytic triad*). The conformation of the loops and β-strands are thought to play a role in positioning the active site residues for proteolysis. **B:** Modeled interaction of Norwalk virus protease with an inhibitor that blocks proteolysis.[188,189,339,518] (Images provided by K. Ng.)

provides the space needed to form the binding site for the next incoming nucleoside triphosphate.

Although the gene order of the nonstructural proteins and strong structural and functional homology in the Pro and Pol enzymes suggest a common ancestor for the caliciviruses and picornaviruses,[342] it is striking that several proteins encoded in the calicivirus ORF1 share little or no detectable sequence relatedness with the picornaviruses. These include the extreme N-terminal proteins NS1 and NS2 (corresponding in gene order to the picornavirus 2A and 2B proteins), the NS4 (corresponding to the picornavirus 3A protein), and the NS5 (corresponding to the VPg). Although the roles of these proteins in replication require further investigation, evidence for some functional homology with the picornaviruses has been

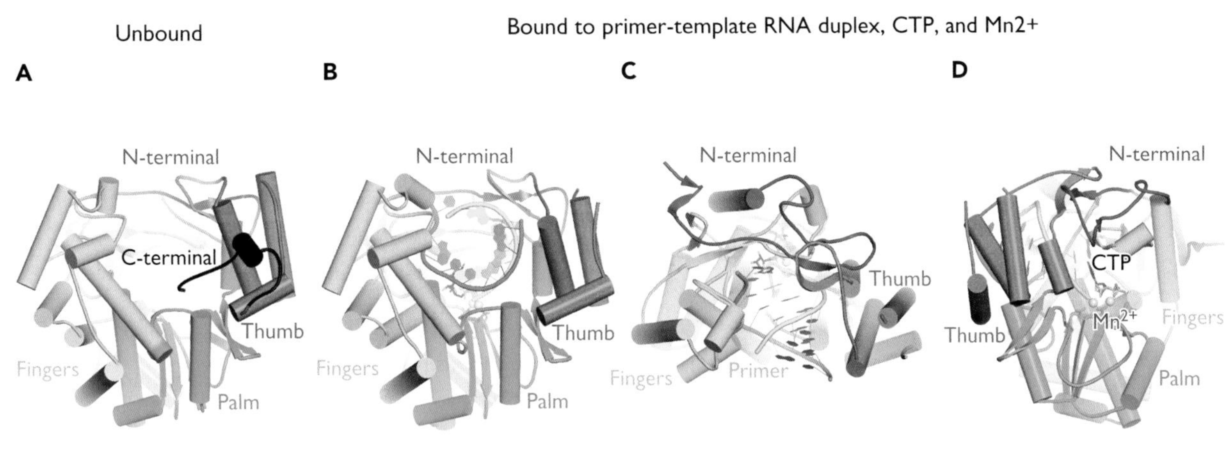

FIGURE 20.5. Structure of the norovirus RNA-dependent RNA polymerase. A: The norovirus RNA-dependent RNA polymerase adopts the classic "right hand" structure characteristic of polynucleotide polymerases as shown in this stick model. The fingers (blue) and palm (green) domains form a rigid unit, while the thumb (red) domain is flexible and can assume either a "closed" or "open" conformation. An N-terminal domain bridges the fingers and thumb domains. When the polymerase is unbound to template, the C-terminal end of the protein appears to lie within the active site cleft.[347] **B–D:** The front, top, and side views, respectively, of the Norwalk RNA polymerase bound to a primer–RNA duplex, cytidine triphosphate (CTP), and metal divalent cation, Mn^{2+}.[346,347,517] (Images provided by K. Ng.)

proposed.[25,129,422] A summary of the calicivirus nonstructural proteins and their known properties is shown in Table 20.2.

STAGES OF REPLICATION

Replication Strategy

The replication strategy elucidated thus far for the caliciviruses shares many features with those of other positive-strand RNA viruses (Fig. 20.6). Caliciviruses attach and enter the cell, the RNA genome is released, and translation of the genome occurs via the host cell machinery. Certain newly translated viral proteins interact with the host cell to establish defined sites of virus replication (characteristically involving reorganized intracellular membranes), while other proteins function as replicative enzymes. Newly synthesized positive-strand RNA genomes are covalently linked to VPg and packaged into virions that are released from lysed cells. The replication cycle of a calicivirus is rapid: new viral progeny can be detected within hours after infection.

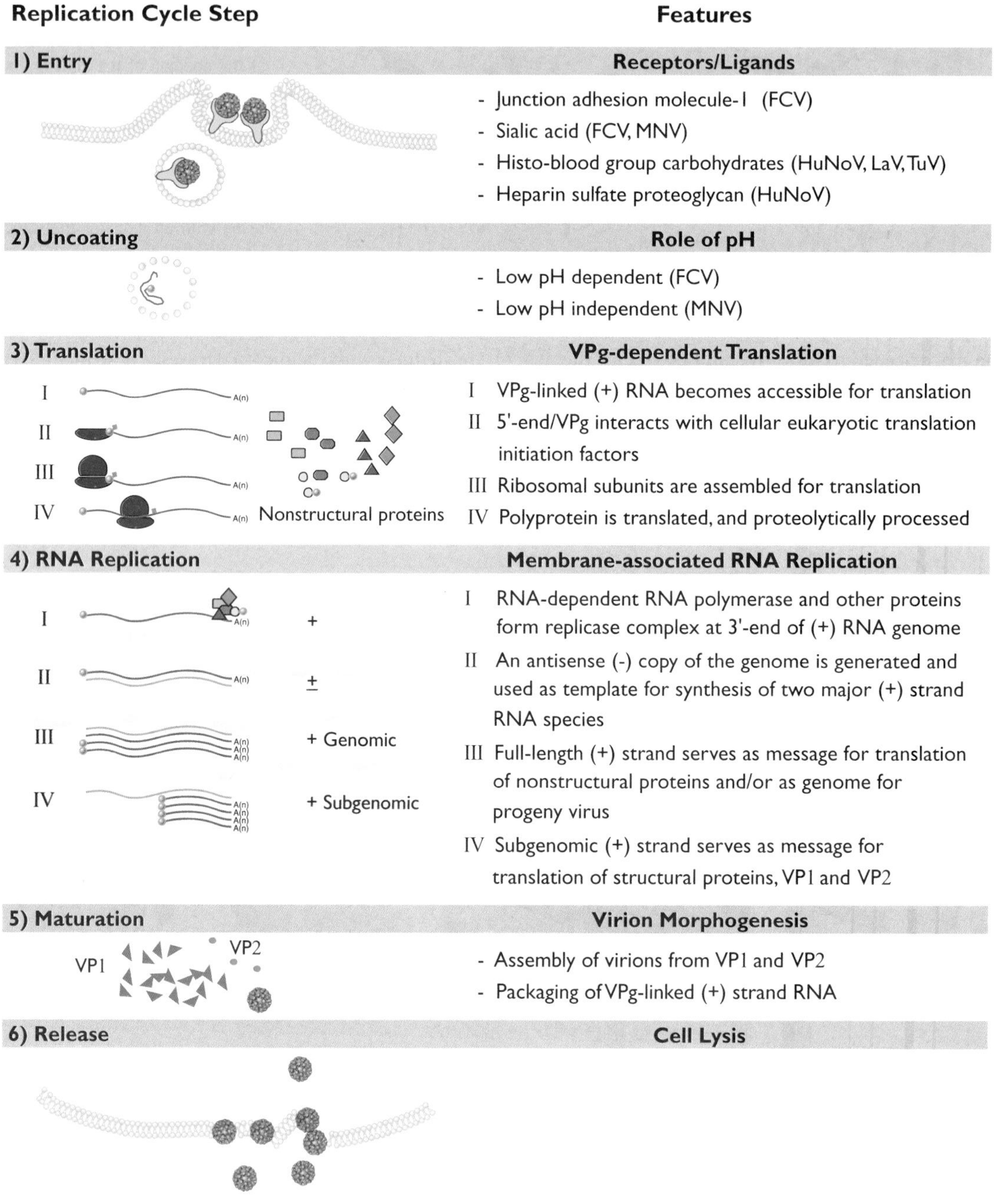

Replication Cycle Step | Features

1) Entry — Receptors/Ligands
- Junction adhesion molecule-1 (FCV)
- Sialic acid (FCV, MNV)
- Histo-blood group carbohydrates (HuNoV, LaV, TuV)
- Heparin sulfate proteoglycan (HuNoV)

2) Uncoating — Role of pH
- Low pH dependent (FCV)
- Low pH independent (MNV)

3) Translation — VPg-dependent Translation

Nonstructural proteins

I VPg-linked (+) RNA becomes accessible for translation
II 5'-end/VPg interacts with cellular eukaryotic translation initiation factors
III Ribosomal subunits are assembled for translation
IV Polyprotein is translated, and proteolytically processed

4) RNA Replication — Membrane-associated RNA Replication

I +
II ±
III + Genomic
IV + Subgenomic

I RNA-dependent RNA polymerase and other proteins form replicase complex at 3'-end of (+) RNA genome
II An antisense (-) copy of the genome is generated and used as template for synthesis of two major (+) strand RNA species
III Full-length (+) strand serves as message for translation of nonstructural proteins and/or as genome for progeny virus
IV Subgenomic (+) strand serves as message for translation of structural proteins, VP1 and VP2

5) Maturation — Virion Morphogenesis

VP1 VP2

- Assembly of virions from VP1 and VP2
- Packaging of VPg-linked (+) strand RNA

6) Release — Cell Lysis

FIGURE 20.6. Schematic diagram of the proposed replication strategy of the caliciviruses. Consistent with other positive-strand RNA viruses, the replication cycle of a calicivirus involves the following stages: **(1)** entry, **(2)** uncoating, **(3)** translation, **(4)** RNA replication, **(5)** maturation, and **(6)** release, as reviewed in the text. FCV, feline calicivirus; LaV, lagovirus; MNV, murine norovirus; HuNoV, human norovirus; TuV, Tulane virus.

Reverse genetics systems have been developed for several caliciviruses, including FCV,[432] porcine enteric calicivirus,[77] Tulane virus,[492] RHDV,[277] and murine norovirus,[83,489,515] based on the construction of infectious full-length cDNA clones of the viral genome. Murine norovirus is presently the only norovirus that grows efficiently in cell culture,[507] making this virus an important model.[508] Human norovirus infectious cDNA clones have remained elusive in the absence of a fully permissive cell culture system to verify recovery of virus, but replication in cells can be studied following expression of proteins from full-length cDNA clones[21,219] or in stable RNA replicon-bearing cell lines.[79]

Mechanism of Attachment

Calicivirus virions must first interact with the host cell. Carbohydrates, including those present on various histo-blood group antigens (HBGAs), have been implicated in the binding of a number of calicivirus strains to cells[245,301,403,443,455,462,516] (Fig. 20.6). Structural studies have verified that the norovirus VP1 interacts with HBGA carbohydrates[61,91] (Fig. 20.7). Receptor recognition is essential for the caliciviruses, as transfection of infectious calicivirus RNA into nonpermissive cells (i.e., those that cannot be infected with virions) allows replication and recovery of infectious progeny virus.[162,245,298] The junction adhesion molecule-1 (JAM-1), an immunoglobulin-like cellular membrane protein, has been identified as a functional receptor for FCV,[299] making this the first experimentally verified cellular receptor in the family. Structural and modeling studies have shown that FCV interacts with feline (f) JAM-1 through binding of the P2 domain of the capsid to the distal membrane domain (D1) of fJAM-1[37,38,363] (e-Fig. 20.3).

Nearly all norovirus VLPs bind to one or more HBGA carbohydrates, and as noted earlier, structural studies have defined interactions with certain HBGA saccharides at the amino acid level[61] (Fig. 20.7). A correlation was found between susceptibility to Norwalk virus infection in adult volunteers and HBGA secretor status, which is linked to the *FUT2* gene[269] (see Cell and Tissue Tropism). A similar pattern of genetic susceptibility to RHDV (lagovirus) infection in rabbits was associated with genes involved in the modification of HBGAs, indicating a role for blood group carbohydrates in host cell recognition by lagoviruses.[161] Experiments to verify that HBGAs can serve as a functional receptor for the noroviruses have been unsuccessful, hampered in part by the unavailability of a permissive cell culture system. Expression of the human *FUT2* gene product (fucosyltransferase-2) in nonpermissive cells enhanced binding of Norwalk virus VLPs to cells *in vitro* but did not render them permissive for the virus.[162]

Mechanism of Entry and Intracellular Trafficking

Variation has been noted among caliciviruses in their requirements for entry into cells and subsequent infection. Feline calicivirus replication was inhibited by chloroquine, a reagent that raises lysosomal pH, indicating dependence on a low pH step during entry.[244,444] In contrast, murine norovirus (strain MNV-1) was not dependent on the acidification of endosomes for infectivity.[143,373] Feline caliciviruses use clathrin-mediated endocytosis for entry into mammalian cells,[444] whereas MNV-1 apparently does not enter via clathrin- or caveolin-mediated pathways.[143,373] An endocytic pathway was proposed for MNV-1 entry that likely involves cholesterol-sensitive lipid rafts and dynamin II (at least in RAW264.7 cells).[143,373,374]

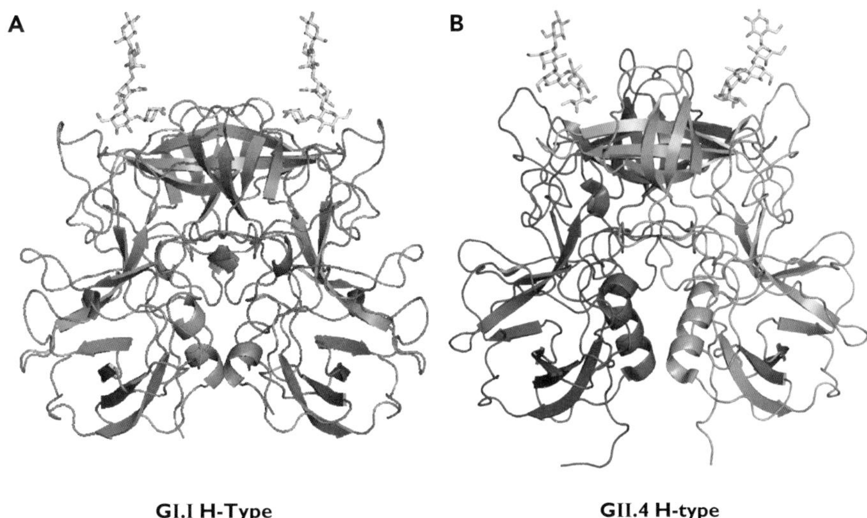

FIGURE 20.7. Interaction of representative norovirus VP1 dimers with H carbohydrates from histo-blood group antigens (HBGAs). For both GI.1 and GII.4 noroviruses, HBGA carbohydrates interact with the distal surface of the capsid, but differences in these interactions have been noted. The Norwalk virus (GI.1) carbohydrate binding site contains residues that project from a well-structured antiparallel β-sheet near the P domain dimeric interface and favors a precise and limited recognition of a terminal Gal-Fuc or Gal-acetamido combination. In contrast, the VA387 (GII.4) binding site is formed by residues located in two surface-exposed loops near the P domain dimeric interface that broadly recognize a terminal fucosyl moiety. (Courtesy of B. V. V. Prasad with data adapted from Cao S, Lou Z, Tan M, et al. Structural basis for the recognition of blood group trisaccharides by norovirus. *J Virol* 2007;81:5949–5957; and Choi JM, Hutson AM, Estes MK, et al. Atomic resolution structural characterization of recognition of histo-blood group antigens by Norwalk virus. *Proc Natl Acad Sci U S A* 2008;105:9175–9180.)

Uncoating

The uncoating events that allow the calicivirus positive-sense RNA genome to become accessible to the cellular translational machinery have not been defined. Uncoating is a rapid process: MNV genome was released within 1 hour after infection.[374] Binding to the cellular receptor induces a conformational change in the capsid of FCV, suggesting that uncoating may, in part, be receptor binding mediated.[37] FCV infection is associated with an increase in permeability of the host cell membrane soon after virus entry via clathrin-coated endosomes and exposure to low pH.[444] It was proposed that this acidification process might change the conformation of the FCV virion structure to facilitate release of the viral RNA.[444] Analysis of norovirus (Norwalk) VLPs by mass spectrometry has shown that they are stable under acidic conditions; a disassembly model has been proposed in which T = 3 particles (containing 180 copies of VP1) disassociate into predominantly dimers in the presence of alkaline conditions.[426]

Translation

Calicivirus genomic RNA in virions requires the presence of the covalently linked VPg protein in order to establish an infection after release (or transfection) into cells.[58] The initiation of translation of the incoming positive-strand genome is likely mediated through interactions of the VPg protein with the cellular translation machinery.[82,103,148,165] Calicivirus replication is associated with an inhibition of host cell translation, and the viral proteinase ($NS6^{Pro}$) has been shown to cleave certain cellular proteins involved in translation, which may, in part, give the viral RNA a competitive advantage.[250] The ORF1 of the virus is translated first to produce a large polyprotein, which is processed rapidly into precursors and products by $NS6^{Pro}$ at several essential cleavage sites.[435] Some of these nonstructural proteins and their precursors function to set up replication sites within the host cell,[25,194] while others (such as the RNA-dependent RNA polymerase, $NS7^{Pol}$) play a role in replication of the viral RNA (Table 20.2).

An abundant VPg-linked subgenomic positive-strand RNA serves as a bicistronic message for translation of the structural proteins VP1 and VP2,[179,344] and the regulation of translation of VP2 from the subgenomic RNA (translated at approximately 20% of the levels of VP1) was mapped to an upstream RNA sequence element in the VP1 coding region of approximately 70 nucleotides designated as the termination upstream ribosomal binding site (TURBS).[322,323] The TURBS site contains two motifs, one of which mediates base pairing between the viral subgenomic messenger RNA and the cellular 18S ribosomal subunit.[322] This interaction may function as a "tether," positioning the ribosome for immediate reinitiation of translation following termination of translation of the VP1 gene.[291,292]

Replication of Genomic Nucleic Acid

As with all other positive-strand RNA viruses, the replication of calicivirus RNA is associated with host cell membranes.[155] A marked rearrangement of intracellular membranes occurs, and evidence exists for the initiation of RNA replication in a perinuclear site that contains membranes associated with endoplasmic reticulum, trans-Golgi network, and endosomal membrane markers.[25,194] The initiation of synthesis of an antisense (negative)-strand RNA from the genomic RNA template occurs beginning at the 3′ end of the genomic positive-strand RNA and likely involves interactions with cellular proteins.[166] The negative-strand RNA, in turn, serves as a template for transcription of two major positive-strand RNA species corresponding to the full-length genome (genomic RNA) and the approximately terminal one-third of the genome toward the 3′ end (subgenomic RNA).[344]

The calicivirus RNA genome bears conserved regions of secondary structure,[292,378,429] and functional RNA regulatory elements have been mapped both internally and near the ends of the genome.[26] Transcription from the start site for the subgenomic RNA species on the negative-strand template (nt 5,296 of RHDV) was found to require an upstream sequence of 50 nt for full polymerase activity in *in vitro* studies,[331] consistent with its role in the formation of a subgenomic promoter. The corresponding region of MNV was mapped also as bearing a promoter for subgenomic RNA synthesis from the negative-strand template.[429]

Assembly

A two-stage process has been proposed for the maturation of calicivirus (FCV) particles.[237] The first stage involves the rapid aggregation and assembly of capsid precursor proteins into 5S subunits, which then pass through several intermediate forms (with varying stability) to form stable 15S subunits. The second stage involves the association of 15S subunits with newly synthesized RNA genomes to form infectious particles (that sediment at 170S). Protein–protein interactions have been detected between the FCV VPg (covalently linked to the RNA genome) and the capsid precursor as well as between the RNA-dependent RNA polymerase $NS7^{Pol}$ and the capsid precursor, suggesting that these interactions may be related to packaging of the newly synthesized RNA into the viral capsid.[211] In addition, successful assembly of the infectious FCV virions was linked to an efficient expression of the virus minor capsid protein, VP2.[433]

The VPg-linked genomic and subgenomic positive-strand RNA species are found in FCV and RHDV particles of distinct densities, indicating that they are not packaged together in the same virion.[324,343] The incorporation of subgenomic RNA into the lower-density (LD) particles suggests that a packaging signal is located within the 3′ terminal 2,400 nucleotides of the genome. It has been suggested that LD particles (which would not be infectious) may be associated with FCV strains of higher virulence, but their function, if any, in the virus life cycle is unknown.[343]

Release

Calicivirus-infected cells undergo lysis, and it is presumed that the majority of progeny viruses are released during this process. The triggering of apoptosis has been associated with calicivirus infection both *in vitro*[7,49,135,341,437] and *in vivo,*[12,84,208,223,334,337,386,472] and apoptotic changes in cellular membranes may be one of the mechanisms by which cells lyse and release viral particles.

PATHOGENESIS AND PATHOLOGY

Caliciviruses cause a broad range of diseases in many different animal hosts (Table 20.3). This section will focus on the noroviruses, but there are important common themes in pathogenesis shared by all caliciviruses. Illnesses range from

TABLE 20.3 Pathogenesis and Disease Manifestations of Representative Calicivirus Strains

Calicivirus strain	Genus	Host	Site of replication[a]	Clinical disease[b]
Norwalk virus	Norovirus	Human	Enteric	Gastroenteritis
Jena virus	*Norovirus*	Cattle	Enteric	Gastroenteritis
Murine norovirus-1 (MNV-1)	*Norovirus*	Mouse	Enteric, lymphoid cells	Fulminant organ dysfunction[c]
Pistoia virus	*Norovirus*	Lion	Enteric	Hemorrhagic enteritis[d]
Canine norovirus	*Norovirus*	Dog	Enteric	Gastroenteritis
Swine 43	*Norovirus*	Pig	Enteric	Not established
Sapporo virus	*Sapovirus*	Human	Enteric	Gastroenteritis
Porcine enteric calicivirus (Cowden)	*Sapovirus*	Pig	Enteric	Gastroenteritis
Mink enteric calicivirus	*Sapovirus*	Mink	Enteric	Gastroenteritis
Rabbit hemorrhagic disease virus	*Lagovirus*	Rabbit	Liver, systemic	Organ dysfunction, pulmonary hemorrhage[e]
European brown hare syndrome virus	*Lagovirus*	Hare	Liver, systemic	Organ dysfunction, pulmonary hemorrhage
Bovine enteric calicivirus (Newbury-1 virus)	*Nebovirus*	Cattle	Enteric	Gastroenteritis
Bovine enteric calicivirus (Nebraska virus)	*Nebovirus*	Cattle	Enteric	Gastroenteritis
Feline calicivirus	*Vesivirus*	Cat	Mouth, upper respiratory	Stomatitis, pneumonia
Feline calicivirus-VS	*Vesivirus*	Cat	Systemic	Fulminant organ dysfunction[f]
San Miguel sea lion virus	*Vesivirus*	Sea lion	Mucosal, systemic	Skin (flipper) lesions, pneumonia
Canine calicivirus (No. 48)	*Vesivirus*	Dog	Enteric	Gastroenteritis
Vesivirus isolate 2117	*Vesivirus*	Unknown	Unknown	Unknown[g]
Tulane virus	Unclassified	Monkey	Enteric	Gastroenteritis
St. Valérian virus (AB90)	Unclassified	Pig	Enteric	Not established
Bayern virus	Unclassified	Chicken	Enteric	Not established

[a]Site of replication is based on observed pathologic effects in tissue and in some cases, confirmed by immunohistochemistry. For many caliciviruses, the primary site of replication in the host has not been fully established.

[b]The characteristic clinical disease associated with each representative calicivirus strain is shown. Swine norovirus,[448] St.Valérian virus,[251] and Bayern virus[509] were detected in screening surveys of nonselected stool specimens: the clinical disease outcome has not been established. Norwalk virus, representative of the human noroviruses associated with acute gastroenteritis, is generally associated with self-limiting vomiting and diarrhea of 24 to 48 hours' duration. However, the illness can be severe and life-threatening in certain individuals (see text). Sapporo virus, representative of the human sapoviruses associated with acute gastroenteritis, has most often been associated with self-limiting gastroenteritis in younger age groups.[89] In general, infection outcome in the family *Caliciviridae* can range from asymptomatic (subclinical) to lethal.

[c]Most variants of the MNV-1 strain of murine norovirus are lethal only in certain mice that lack an innate immune system, but evidence exists for varying pathogenicity among MNV strains and variants.[26,217,467,507]

[d]First case report described illness in one lion cub,[304] natural history not established.

[e]Rabbit hemorrhagic disease virus emerged as a highly lethal disease in rabbits in China in 1984,[290] but was likely endemic in rabbits worldwide prior to 1984[224]

[f]Feline calicivirus strains have emerged in recent years designated as "virulent systemic" (VS) that are associated with high morbidity and mortality in cats. In addition, the virus can cause a persistent, asymptomatic infection in cats.[385]

[g]Vesivirus 2117 was discovered as a contaminant in cultured Chinese hamster ovary cells.[357]

mild to life-threatening, and evidence exists for the emergence of calicivirus strains with increased virulence. Asymptomatic infection occurs in susceptible populations,[106,377] and shedding of virus can extend days to weeks after resolution of acute symptoms.[24,140]

Adult volunteer studies have been successful in defining important features of norovirus gastroenteritis, pathogenesis, and immunity.[213] Presently, there is no animal model that directly recapitulates the full range of disease symptoms observed in humans (see Clinical Features), but animals in which evidence for infection has been reported following challenge with human noroviruses include gnotobiotic piglets[84] and calves,[440] monkeys,[394,447] and chimpanzees.[48,158,512]

Noroviruses have been detected in the feces of mice (e.g., strain MNV-1),[210,217,337] pigs (strain SW418),[448] cattle (strain Jena virus),[275] and dogs (strain 170/07),[305] leading to the investigation of these viruses as model systems for the human noroviruses. Bovine norovirus (strain Jena) caused diarrhea and severe blunting of the small intestinal villi in newborn calves similar to that observed in human norovirus infection, and virus antigen-positive cells were observed in epithelial cells of the villi and the lamina propria.[364]

Entry into the Host

Noroviruses enter the body predominantly via the oral route. Virions are acid stable, consistent with an ability to survive passage through the stomach. Indirect evidence from epidemiologic studies suggests that viruses can enter also via aerosols, such as in those generated from the explosive vomiting that often occurs during illness.[66,70,302,303,372]

Based on volunteer studies with NV, the incubation period is short, ranging from 10 to 51 hours, with a mean of 24 hours.[24,43,112,113,442,511] Acute illness usually lasts about 24 to 48 hours. The incubation period recorded in 22 naturally occurring outbreaks of norovirus gastroenteritis was between 24 and 48 hours in 20 of the outbreaks, and the range was from 4 to 77 hours.[216] The incubation period of experimentally induced Snow Mountain virus illness ranged from 19 to 41 hours, with a mean of 27 hours.[116]

Studies in volunteers demonstrated that the Norwalk, Hawaii, Montgomery County, and Snow Mountain viruses induced gastroenteritis when administered by the oral route.[112,113,206,265,332,442,511] Transmission via the respiratory route has not been established for this group of agents, although it has been suggested from epidemiologic observations in selected settings.[66,71,302,408] The virus was detected in vomitus obtained from infected volunteers[157]; vomitus has been considered to be a source of transmission in certain settings.[70] Oral-to-oral transmission has been suggested: norovirus RNA was detected in washings from the mouths of individuals with norovirus infection (in one case, up to 2 weeks postillness) and in 10/17 (59%) of patients hospitalized with norovirus gastroenteritis who had vomited within 24 hours prior to sample collection.[231] Nasopharyngeal washings from a volunteer with experimentally induced Norwalk gastroenteritis did not induce illness in three volunteers.[112]

Site of Primary Replication

The site of primary replication for the noroviruses has not been established, but it is assumed that they replicate in the upper intestinal tract. Biopsies of the jejunum of volunteers who develop gastrointestinal illness following oral administration of the Norwalk or Hawaii virus exhibit histopathologic lesions.[3,114,413,414] A broadening and blunting of the villi of the proximal small intestine occurs, although the mucosa itself remains histologically intact (Fig. 20.8). Infiltration with mononuclear cells and cytoplasmic vacuolization is also observed. Biopsies obtained during the convalescent phase of illness are normal. Blunting and atrophy of the villi was observed also in the small intestine of pigs infected with porcine enteric calicivirus (PEC), a sapovirus,[132] and in newborn calves infected with Jena virus, a bovine norovirus.[364] When viewed by transmission EM, the epithelial cells are intact, but there is shortening of the microvilli. Virus has not been observed in epithelial cells of the mucosa by EM. Of interest is that the characteristic jejunal lesion has also been observed in volunteers who were fed NV or Hawaii virus but who did not become ill.[320,413,414] Histologic lesions are not observed in the gastric fundus, antrum, or rectal mucosa of volunteers with NV-induced illness.[502] The examination of intestinal biopsies from pediatric patients infected with norovirus who had undergone small intestinal transplantation showed increased mononuclear infiltrates in the lamina propria and villous blunting when compared with uninfected controls.[334] Duodenal biopsies from immunocompetent individuals with acute norovirus gastroenteritis showed evidence of shortened villus height (which decreased the overall villus surface area by approximately 47%) and noted also the infiltration of a dense population of intraepithelial CD8 lymphocytes.[472]

A transient malabsorption of fat, d-xylose, and lactose is observed during experimentally induced NV illness.[43,413] Levels

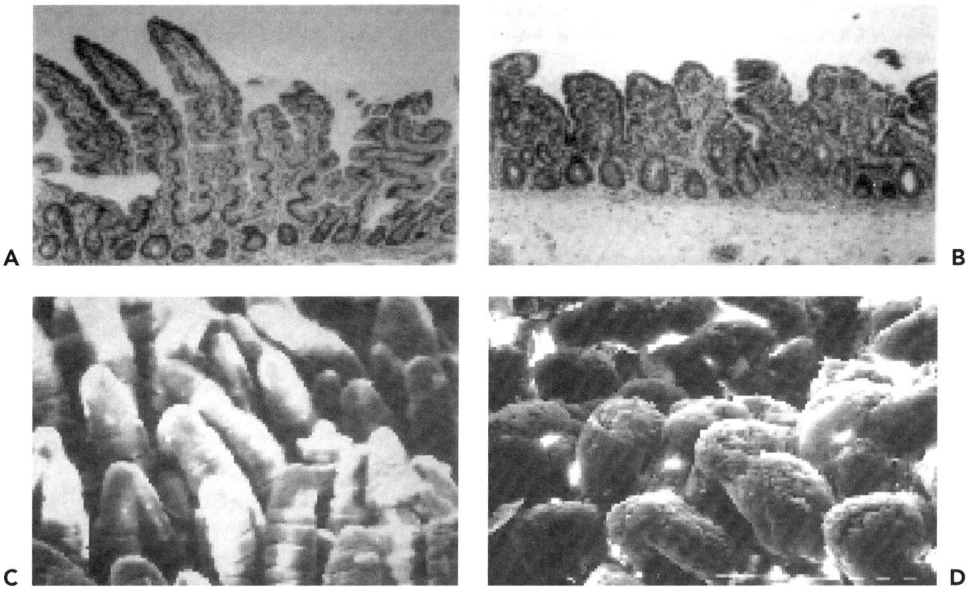

FIGURE 20.8. Pathology of norovirus and sapovirus infection in the jejunum. A: Normal-appearing jejunal tissue from biopsy of a volunteer prior to challenge with Norwalk virus (NV). Hematoxylin and eosin (H&E), 390. **B:** Broadened and flattened villi in jejunal biopsy tissue from same volunteer during illness with Norwalk-induced gastroenteritis. H&E, 390. **C:** Scanning electron microscopy (EM) showing normal-appearing jejunal tissue from biopsy of pig prior to challenge with porcine enteric calicivirus. **D:** Scanning EM showing shortening, blunting, fusion, or absence of villi in jejunal biopsy from same pig following challenge with porcine enteric calicivirus. (**A,B** from Agus SG, Dolin R, Wyatt RG, et al. Acute infectious nonbacterial gastroenteritis: intestinal histopathology. Histologic and enzymatic alterations during illness produced by the Norwalk agent in man. *Ann Intern Med* 1973;79:18–25, with permission. **C,D** from Flynn WT, Saif LJ, Moorhead PD. Pathogenesis of porcine enteric calicivirus-like virus in four-day-old gnotobiotic pigs. *Am J Vet Res* 1988;49:819–825, with permission.)

of small intestinal brush-border enzymes (trehalase and alkaline phosphatase) were significantly decreased when compared with baseline and convalescent-phase values, whereas adenylate cyclase activity in the jejunum was not elevated following NV- or Hawaii virus—induced illness.[3,265] Gastric secretion of hydrochloric acid, pepsin, and intrinsic factor did not appear to be altered during NV illness.[320] Elevation of serum transaminase levels was reported in four pediatric patients at approximately two 2 weeks following acute illness.[474]

A marked delay in gastric emptying was observed in infected volunteers who became ill and developed the typical jejunal mucosal lesion.[320] It has been proposed that abnormal gastric motor function is responsible for the nausea and vomiting associated with these viral agents.[320] An analysis of epithelial barrier and secretion function in norovirus-positive human duodenal biopsy tissue showed that the tight junction proteins occludin, claudin-4, and claudin-5 were reduced, and anion secretion was stimulated.[472] It was proposed that norovirus diarrhea could result from both epithelial barrier and secretory pathway dysfunction.

Spread in the Host

The major site of norovirus replication is presumably the upper small intestinal tract (duodenum and upper jejunum), but there is evidence that extraintestinal spread of the virus can occur. Viral RNA has been detected in serum and cerebrospinal fluid of a 23-month-old patient with encephalopathy.[196] In an analysis of 39 patients with acute norovirus gastroenteritis (confirmed by the detection of viral RNA in stool), norovirus RNA was detected in the serum of 6 (15%) patients by real-time PCR.[453] Human noroviruses can establish an enteric infection in gnotobiotic piglets[84] and chimpanzees[48] when administered by the intravenous route.

Cell and Tissue Tropism

Human noroviruses are presumed to target cells in the small intestine due to the observed pathologic lesion (blunted villi), but the specificity of this interaction has been difficult to establish. Radiolabeled Norwalk rVLPs bind to a variety of cultured cell types, and in certain cells, they are apparently internalized with a low efficiency.[497] Norwalk VLPs bind to the surface of human intestinal epithelial cells bearing H1 or H2/3 HBGAs present in fixed tissue sections from secretor-positive (but not secretor-negative) individuals,[301] but the expression of these antigens on the surface of Huh-7 cells (a human liver cell line) does not confer full susceptibility to a productive Norwalk virus infection.[162] It was speculated that human noroviruses might bind nonepithelial cells in the gut: Sakai virus (a GII norovirus) was shown to bind to cells within the lamina propria and Brunner gland of human duodenum,[73] and chimpanzees infected with Norwalk virus displayed Norwalk virus antigen-positive cells within the lamina propria of the upper small intestine.[48] The murine norovirus infects macrophage and dendritic cells of the mouse immune system,[507] but this cell tropism has not been confirmed for human noroviruses in *in vitro* studies.[257] Gnotobiotic piglets challenged with a GII.4 norovirus strain displayed virus-positive enterocytes in the duodenum and jejunum.[84]

For years speculation was that a genetically determined variation in virus receptors in the intestinal tract might be responsible for long-term resistance to NV.[30,41,98,239,369] Recent studies have found evidence for such a mechanism that involves the ABH and Lewis carbohydrate antigens present on gut epithelial cells,[301] which is reviewed elsewhere.[117,191,261,262,461] Expression of these carbohydrate antigens on cells is controlled by enzymes that are products of alleles at the ABO, FUT2, and FUT3 loci. Individuals with two mutated FUT2 alleles, and therefore devoid of H-type antigens on their gut (and other mucosal) epithelial cells, are called *nonsecretors*. It was first observed that RHDV (lagovirus) virions and RHDV rVLPs were able to bind to ABH histo-blood group antigens (present also on human blood cells) that were expressed on epithelial cells of the respiratory and digestive tracts of rabbits.[403] Furthermore, the binding of RHDV to human blood cells was blocked by saliva from human individuals who were secretor positive for H carbohydrates, but not from individuals who were nonsecretors. The subsequent discovery that Norwalk VLPs could bind to HBGAs expressed on human intestinal epithelial cells[301] suggested that genetically determined host factors relating to histo-blood group antigens might play a role in mediating susceptibility to infection. This hypothesis was confirmed in human volunteers, in which the secretor status of the individual was a major correlate in susceptibility to infection with NV.[269] On oral challenge with NV, only secretor individuals with H type 1 antigens were susceptible to infection, whereas nonsecretors were resistant. In a retrospective analysis of volunteers in earlier NV challenge studies, the secretor status was again identified as a major correlate of susceptibility to infection.[190] Furthermore, the ABO blood group antigens have also been linked to susceptibility to Norwalk infection, with B blood group antigen individuals rarely showing evidence of infection and illness with NV.[192,269] Variation likely exists among the noroviruses in their recognition of host cell carbohydrates.[61,91,186,461] Infection in volunteers challenged with GII Snow Mountain virus (unlike those challenged with NV) showed no correlation between ABH secretor status and susceptibility,[268] suggesting that the link to protection in type B individuals might be limited to GI noroviruses.[395] Attempts to correlate susceptibility with ABH secretor status or blood type in naturally occurring disease have yielded variable results.[170,255,351,441]

The role of HBGA recognition by noroviruses has been the subject of intense study from the perspective of structure,[242] evolution,[47,105,272] and host restriction.[63,262] It is not yet clear whether these molecules serve only as attachment ligands on host cells or are functional receptors that enable the entry of virus (see Mechanism of Attachment).

Immune Response

Immunity to noroviruses in humans is poorly understood.[310] Adults consistently demonstrate a high degree of susceptibility to both naturally occurring and experimentally induced NV illness. In some norovirus outbreaks, more than 80% of adults became ill.[216] In addition, approximately 50% of unselected adult volunteers consistently developed illness following challenge with NV.[43,112,442,511] Resistance to norovirus illness likely involves a complex interplay between the genetic and immunological susceptibility of the host and exposure to evolving norovirus strains.

Adaptive Immunity

Because serum or intestinal secretory neutralizing antibodies to the noroviruses cannot yet be measured in tissue culture, most of the information about immunity comes from early volunteer studies. Although the use of high doses of challenge virus in these early studies has been noted,[147] they established that there are two forms of immunity to NV: one is short term and the other is long term.[112,369,511] Short-term immunity, which follows the traditional pattern, is apparently virus (possibly serotype) specific. Thus, volunteers who become ill following NV (GI.1) challenge are usually resistant to rechallenge with this virus 6 to 14 weeks later. Challenge of such volunteers with the heterotypic Hawaii virus (GII.1), however, induces illness. Similarly, volunteers who recently became ill following infection with Hawaii virus are susceptible to challenge with NV.[511] Long-term immunity, however, deviates from the traditional pattern. Twelve volunteers who were challenged with the NV on two occasions, 27 to 42 months apart, exhibited two different patterns of resistance to sequential challenge.[369] Six volunteers developed gastrointestinal illness following the initial challenge, and they developed it again following rechallenge 27 to 42 months later. In contrast, the other six individuals failed to become ill following the initial challenge and were also resistant after rechallenge 31 to 34 months later. Serologic studies in which prechallenge serum antibodies to NV were measured by IEM and radioimmunoassay (RIA) failed to provide an explanation for the difference in susceptibility.[99,156,369] Paradoxically, volunteers who did not become ill had little, if any, antibody to NV measurable by IEM in either prechallenge serum specimen.[369] Also, they failed to develop a significant serologic response following each challenge. Volunteers who became ill following each challenge, and who were evaluated serologically, developed a serologic response after each challenge, however. The observation that serum antibody to NV does not correlate with resistance to illness has been reproduced in more recent volunteer studies.[149,206,269] It was found also that the levels of local jejunal antibodies did not correlate with resistance to illness in volunteer studies and during natural outbreaks of disease.[30,42,156,205,206,297] Naturally acquired immunity, however, may play some role in protection at the mucosal level. A recent volunteer study showed that the development of a rapid mucosal IgA response (indicating prior exposure to NV or a related norovirus) was associated with resistance to illness following challenge with NV.[269] Furthermore, antibody was shown to be critical for the clearance of MNV in the mouse model.[68]

The discovery that NV and other human noroviruses recognize HBGAs has led to the development of assays that measured HBGA carbohydrate-blocking activity (or "blockade") of serum antibodies.[279] The presence of antibodies that blocked binding of Norwalk VLPs to H type 1 or H type 3 glycans at the time of Norwalk virus challenge was shown to correlate with protection from illness in adult volunteers, leading to the proposal that HBGA blocking assays might serve as a surrogate test for neutralization in the absence of traditional cell culture–based virus neutralization assays.[387] Consistent with this, chimpanzees vaccinated with a Norwalk VLP immunogen and resistant to Norwalk virus infection when subsequently challenged were shown also to develop serum antibodies that block binding of Norwalk VLPs to synthetic HBGA carbohydrates.[48] Application of this technique in the first efficacy study of norovirus vaccines in adult volunteers showed a correlation between levels of prechallenge HBGA-blocking titers and protection from illness.[22] A hemagglutination inhibition assay (HAI) to measure serum antibodies was shown also to correlate with protection from illness in volunteers challenged with Norwalk virus.[101,193]

Cell-Mediated Immunity

Cell-mediated immune responses were studied in volunteers following oral immunization with Norwalk rVLPs.[452] The VLPs elicited a cell-mediated immune response that included virus-specific proliferative responses. There was an increase in γ-interferon (IFN) in the absence of IL-4 production, suggesting a dominant T-helper type 1 (Th-1) pattern of cytokine production. In a study of 15 volunteers infected with Snow Mountain virus, significant increases in serum γ-IFN and IL-2, but not IL-6 or IL-10, were detected on day 2 after challenge, again showing a dominant Th-1 response.[268] Depletion of CD4+ cells prior to stimulation of peripheral blood mononuclear cells with norovirus antigen led to a decrease in γ-IFN, again consistent with a Th-1 dominant response that is characteristic of cell-mediated immunity.[268]

Both CD4 and CD8 T cells are required for virus clearance from the intestine following challenge with MNV.[67] Evidence for cross-reactive T-cell epitopes shared among different norovirus genogroups and genotypes was found in mice immunized with VLPs representing human and murine noroviruses.[280]

Innate Immunity

The innate immune response was found to be important in the control of murine norovirus (strain MNV-1) in mice: certain mouse strains deficient in components of the innate immune system (such as STAT1 or receptors for interferon) developed a disseminated, lethal infection when challenged with MNV-1.[217] It has been reported that MDA-5, an intracellular sensor of double-stranded RNA, may be involved in the recognition and control of MNV.[315] Caliciviruses have been shown to be sensitive to various types of interferon *in vitro*.[76,78,79,80,229,328]

Release from Host and Transmission

Noroviruses are released from the enteric tract of the host in feces and have been detected also in vomitus.[151,157,227,317] Viral RNA can be detected in feces before the onset of symptoms and shedding in stool can last several days to weeks in immunocompetent individuals[24,141,149,360] and even longer in immunocompromised patients.[136,222,223,289,406,450] In a study of 13 elderly patients (60 to 98 years of age), the average duration of norovirus shedding was 14.3 days, with some individuals shedding up to 32 days.[16] In pediatric patients (3 months to 7 years of age), the average length of shedding was 16 days, with three patients younger than 6 months of age shedding for more than 40 days.[338] Studies of the natural history of norovirus in a community found that 26% of 99 patients examined shed virus (detected by reverse transcriptase [RT]-PCR) up to 3 weeks after the onset of illness, with the highest rate (38%) of prolonged shedding in children younger than 1 year of age.[393] This observation indicates that infected individuals recovering from norovirus illness can continue shedding beyond the symptomatic period, a finding that has implications in the management of outbreaks.[100,329,367,388,477,496] Norovirus RNA has been detected in washings from the mouths of individuals who experienced norovirus infection for several days after symptoms subsided, suggesting that oral-to-oral transmission of norovirus might occur.[231] The detection of norovirus RNA in the sera of children with gastroenteritis has been reported, but it is not known whether this RNA corresponds to that of circulating infectious virus (viremia) or noninfectious (inactivated) virus present in circulating immune cells.[453]

Noroviruses are spread by several modes of transmission (see Fig. 20.9B for a summary of the reported modes of transmission in 5,036 norovirus outbreaks that occurred in Europe between 2000 and 2011). The predominant modes of transmission for the noroviruses are person-to-person contact and food- or water-borne spread.[248] Contamination of surfaces and objects by infected individuals can lead to inadvertent exposure.[184,283,477] Several epidemiologic investigations have linked exposure to noroviruses in air or in aerosolized vomitus with infection.[31,66,142,302,303,408]

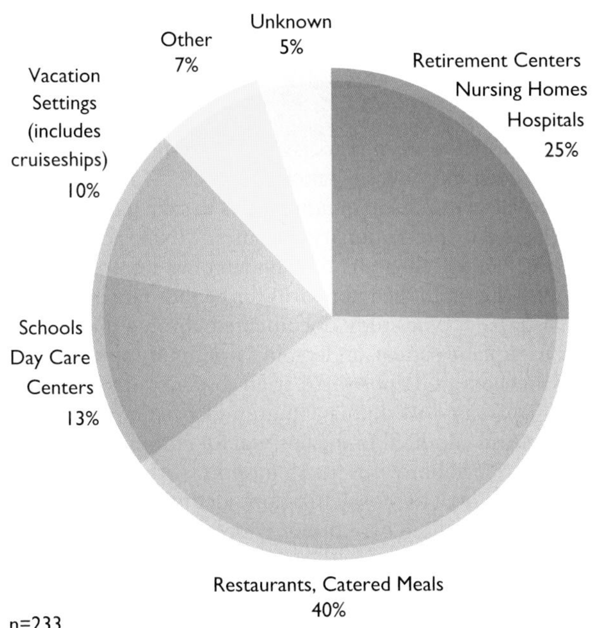

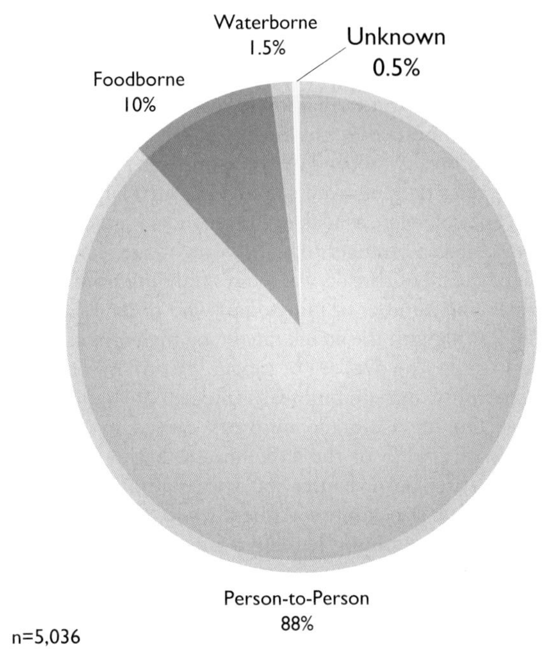

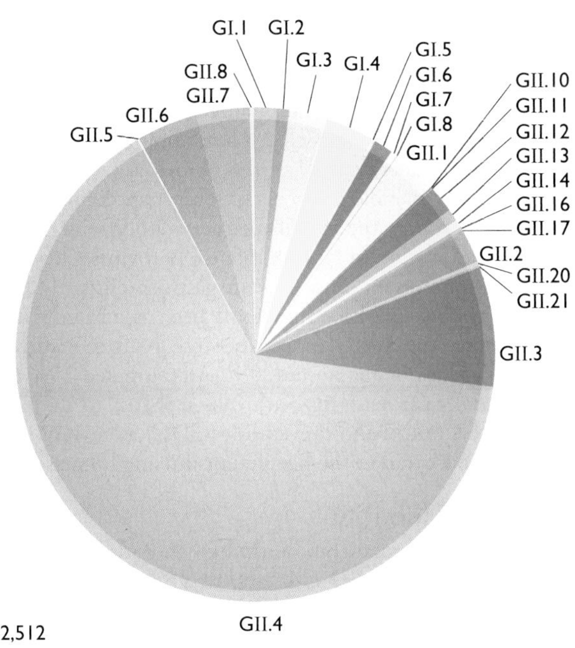

FIGURE 20.9. Features of norovirus epidemiology. A: Settings of transmission for 233 outbreaks of nonbacterial gastroenteritis in the United States from July 1997 to June 2000. Noroviruses were detected in stool samples from individuals in 93% of these outbreaks by reverse transcriptase-polymerase chain reaction (RT-PCR). (Data adapted from Fankhauser RL, Monroe SS, Noel JS, et al. Epidemiologic and molecular trends of "Norwalk-like viruses" associated with outbreaks of gastroenteritis in the United States. *J Infect Dis* 2002;186:1–7; and http://www.cdc.gov/ncidod/dvrd/revb/gastro/norovirus.htm.) **B:** Reported modes of transmission for 5,036 norovirus outbreaks that occurred over a 5-year period (2001–2006) in Europe. (Data adapted from Kroneman A, Verhoef L, Harris J, et al. Analysis of integrated virological and epidemiological reports of norovirus outbreaks collected within the Foodborne Viruses in Europe network from 1 July 2001 to 30 June 2006. *J Clin Microbiol* 2008;46:2959–2965; and www.rivm.nl/en/aboutrivm/projects/index.) **C:** Norovirus genotypes associated with gastroenteritis outbreaks that occurred over an 11-year period (2000–2011) in Europe. The Genogroup II noroviruses were detected in 2,256 (90%) of the 2,512 samples analyzed, with the GII.4 genotype detected in 1,627 (65%) of the total number tested. (Data from the Foodborne Viruses in Europe Network, http://www.noronet.nl. Personal communication, A. Kroneman and M. Koopmans.)

The explosive nature of some NV outbreaks, in which a large number of persons become ill within 24 to 48 hours, indicates that infection is often acquired from a common source. This was suggested in the original NV outbreak, but a common-source exposure could not be identified.[2] Later, a review of 38 NV-associated outbreaks suggested that a common source of infection was likely in 31 (82%).[215] The vehicle of transmission could be identified in 17 of the 31 outbreaks, including water in 13 instances and food in four others. Water-borne infection was attributed to a municipal water system (twice), semipublic water supply (seven times), stored water on a cruise ship (twice), and recreational swimming (twice). The food-borne outbreaks were associated with the ingestion of oysters or salad. Primary person-to-person transmission occurred in 7 of the 38 outbreaks.[216] Sufficient data were available from 26 of the outbreaks to permit estimation of secondary attack rates.[216] In 20 of 23 common-source outbreaks and in each of 3 person-to-person outbreaks, secondary transmission was observed, with attack rates ranging from 4% to 32%. In a large outbreak for which age data were available, the secondary attack rate was highest in children younger than 10 years of age. The median duration of the 38 outbreaks was 7 days (ranging from 1 day to 3 months). The number of individuals who became ill ranged from 2 to 2,000, with the attack rate being higher in common-source outbreaks (median 60%, range 23% to 93%) than in primary person-to-person outbreaks (median 39%, range 31% to 42%).[216] In the Colorado outbreak caused by the Snow Mountain virus, 61% of the 418 illnesses began on a single day.[116,332] A water-borne source was suggested as the etiologic agent because the attack rate was directly related to the amount of water- or ice-containing beverages consumed. In addition, the water supply was contaminated by a leaking septic tank and was inadequately chlorinated. The efficient transmission of human caliciviruses by contaminated food and water vehicles has raised concerns about public safety in a global market economy.[147,379,411,482,491]

The infectious dose for noroviruses is low, with an estimated median infectious dose of 18 viruses.[466] Exposure to higher levels of virus likely increases the risk of illness.[288] In a study that examined norovirus fecal load, higher numbers (greater than 100-fold) of norovirus genome copies were detected in individuals shedding GII (median, 3.0×10^8 genome copies per gram feces) strains compared to GI (median, 8.4×10^5 genome copies per gram feces).[75] It was proposed that the higher levels of GII shedding might account for a higher transmissibility of these viruses through the fecal–oral route.[75] However, high levels of GI shedding have been reported: the median peak of GI Norwalk virus shed in the stool of 16 volunteers was 9.5×10^{10} genome copies per gram feces.[24]

Noroviruses are remarkably stable. The NV retains infectivity for volunteers following (a) exposure of the stool filtrate to pH 2.7 for 3 hours at room temperature, (b) treatment with 20% ether at 4°C for 18 hours, or (c) incubation at 60°C for 30 minutes.[112] Norwalk virions remain infectious when stored in ground water at room temperature in the dark for as long as 61 days, and RNA could be detected in such samples after storage at room temperature for 3 years.[420] NV is resistant to inactivation following treatment with 3.75 to 6.25 mg/L of chlorine (free residual chlorine of 0.5 to 1.0 mg/L), a chlorine concentration consistent with that found in a drinking water distribution system.[225] NV, however, is inactivated following treatment with 10 mg/L of chlorine, a concentration that is used to treat water supply systems after contamination has been detected. NV is more resistant to inactivation by chlorine than poliovirus type 1, human rotavirus (Wa), simian rotavirus (SA11), or f2 bacteriophage.[225]

Virulence

Virulence determinants have not been defined for the human noroviruses, but differences in clinical outcome, ranging from asymptomatic infection to life-threatening diarrhea, suggest that strain differences exist,[187] as shown for other caliciviruses (Table 20.3). A compelling feature of norovirus epidemiology that supports strain differences (especially in the GII.4 genotype) is the striking variation in disease prevalence in certain years, with sharp increases in global outbreaks and disease burden.[123,147]

Persistence

Noroviruses have been associated with prolonged infection in immunocompromised patients,[139,223,348,396] and, therefore, nosocomial transmission of noroviruses to such patients should be prevented by precautionary measures.[430] Nine adult patients receiving kidney allografts and undergoing immunosuppression were shown to shed norovirus for periods ranging from 97 to 898 days.[412] One study documented chronic diarrhea in a heart transplant patient undergoing immunosuppressive therapy who shed a GII norovirus strain over 2 years.[348] A 36-yr year-old patient with human immunodeficiency virus (HIV) infection and admitted to the hospital for chronic diarrhea was reported to shed norovirus for 15 months (with stools collected 5 months prior to hospitalization identified as norovirus-positive).[504] Deaths in two chronic lymphocytic leukemia (CLL) patients were associated with prolonged norovirus diarrhea.[62] Immunocompromised patients with norovirus infection were reported to be at increased risk for the development of pneumatosis intestinalis.[228]

EPIDEMIOLOGY

Age

Noroviruses have been associated with infection and disease in all age groups. The estimated overall prevalence of norovirus in infants and young children hospitalized for the treatment of gastroenteritis is approximately 12% according to a recent review of published studies.[371] making the noroviruses second only to the rotaviruses as etiologic agents of severe gastroenteritis in this young age group. In the surveillance period following efficacious rotavirus vaccination in Finnish infants, noroviruses became the single most important cause of acute gastroenteritis.[519]

The noroviruses have frequently been associated with gastroenteritis in the elderly, especially those living in institutional settings such as nursing homes.[126,153] An estimated 25% of 233 nonbacterial gastroenteritis outbreaks reported to the Centers for Disease Control and Prevention (CDC) from July 1997 to June 2000 occurred in the hospital or nursing home setting.[126]

Morbidity/Mortality

Although precise data on morbidity and mortality are not available, several studies estimate a significant burden from norovirus-associated disease.[169,409] In the United States, an estimated 71,000 hospitalizations are associated with norovirus gastroenteritis each year, at a cost of $493 million per year.[286] In a review of published studies, noroviruses were consistently reported as the second most important cause (after rotavirus) of severe gastroenteritis in infants and young children worldwide, with an estimated 200,000 deaths per year in children younger than 5 years of age in developing countries.[371] Noroviruses have been linked to gastrointestinal illness in neonates.[321] Norovirus infection and disease in preterm infants receiving intensive care in a hospital nursery unit have been reported,[19] and in one such setting necrotizing enterocolitis occurred more frequently in preterm infants with norovirus infection.[445] In an analysis of medical registrations (such as doctor visits, hospitalizations, and deaths) associated with gastroenteritis of unspecified cause during periods of high norovirus outbreak activity in the Netherlands, it was estimated that elderly individuals (65 years of age and older) were at increased risk for serious illness requiring medical intervention and death.[478] In Sweden, an overall excess mortality rate was found in elderly patients hospitalized for the treatment of severe norovirus gastroenteritis that was acquired in the community,[164] and a case-fatality rate of 2% was reported in a large norovirus outbreak that occurred in six nursing homes in Israel.[60] An analysis of the role of various enteric pathogens in hospitalized patients in Canada (from 2001 to 2004) estimated that noroviruses were responsible for a mean hospitalization incidence rate of 1.6 cases per 100,000 and that the average age of hospitalized patients was 59 years old.[404] Over the 4-year period, 43 deaths were attributed to noroviruses, making it a leading cause of mortality among the enteric pathogens studied.[404] Noroviruses have been associated with increased morbidity and mortality in patients with an underlying illness such as cardiovascular disease or who are immunosuppressed or receiving chemotherapy.[62,216,223,232,312,400,417,430]

Origin and Spread of Epidemics

Noroviruses are the single most important cause of nonbacterial gastroenteritis outbreaks. In an analysis of 233 nonbacterial gastroenteritis outbreaks reported to the CDC between July 1997 and June 2000, 217 (93%) were associated with noroviruses.[126] In a larger survey of 3,714 nonbacterial gastroenteritis outbreaks that occurred in Europe between 1995 and 2000, 85% were associated with noroviruses.[287] Outbreaks often occur in hospitals, long-term care facilities, camps, recreational areas, elementary schools, daycare centers, cruise ships, retirement centers, colleges, restaurants, social events with catered meals, families, the military, prisons, and community settings (see Fig. 20.9A for predominant settings of outbreaks in the United States between 1997 and 2000). Outbreaks can vary in size, involving small family groups to hundreds of individuals.[195,311,513]

Especially noteworthy is the predominant role of the noroviruses in food-related outbreaks of gastroenteritis. Noroviruses are the leading cause of food-borne illness in the United States (followed by *Salmonella* [nontyphoidal], *Clostridium perfringens, Campylobacter* spp., and *Staphylococcus aureus*), accounting for approximately 26% of all reported outbreaks.[409] An analysis of 8,271 food-borne outbreaks reported to the CDC (1991–2000) showed that norovirus outbreaks were often larger than bacterial outbreaks (median persons affected: 25 vs. 15), with 10% of the affected individuals seeking medical care and 1% being hospitalized.[501] In a study of water-borne outbreaks in Finland, 18 (64%) of 28 outbreaks evaluated were associated with norovirus.[313] Bivalve mollusks (such as oysters and mussels) are an important cause of food-borne norovirus outbreaks.[9,234,285,316,335,495]

Noroviruses have also been documented as important agents of gastroenteritis in military populations in several different areas of the world.[4,20,104,314] Among U.S. military personnel deployed to South America or West Africa, NV infection was detected in 10% of ill personnel, second in importance to enterotoxigenic *Escherichia coli,* which was the most frequently encountered pathogen (17%).[52] In addition, large-scale outbreaks of gastroenteritis have been attributed to the noroviruses on ships such as aircraft carriers on which hundreds of crew members became ill.[45,94,365,423]

Although the majority of traveler's diarrhea has been attributed to enterotoxigenic *E. coli,*[40] an increasing number of reports have linked noroviruses to such illness.[5,6,17,81,121,405] Norovirus transmission during airplane travel, in addition to that on recreational cruise ships, has been reported, illustrating the potential ease with which strains can be spread globally.[233,469,481,500]

Prevalence and Seroepidemiology

Noroviruses have a worldwide distribution. Most individuals in both developed and developing countries show evidence of infection with norovirus before adulthood, reflecting the global distribution and endemic nature of these viruses.[203] A study of Finnish infants and children, aged 0 to 14 years, found that antibody prevalence against GII.4 noroviruses reached 91.2% in children older than 5 years of age.[353] The prevalence of antibody to the GII viruses (Mexico, Hawaii, or Lordsdale) appears to be greater than that of the GI viruses in most[97,204,355,431] but not all[102,109] studies, which likely reflects the predominance of circulating GII strains. The prevalence of norovirus antibodies characteristically increased more gradually by age in developed than in developing countries.[203]

The incidence of norovirus gastroenteritis has been estimated in several community-based studies. In the United States, an enhanced surveillance study of acute gastroenteritis (that included pathogen identification with diagnostic assays) in a single state (Georgia) estimated that norovirus was the predominant cause of acute gastroenteritis, accounting for 6,500 (16%) and 640 (12%) per 100,000 person-years of community and outpatient acute gastroenteritis episodes, respectively.[169] In the Netherlands, 18% of the community cases of gastroenteritis over a single winter season and at least 5% of gastroenteritis cases that resulted in a visit to a physician were associated with norovirus infection.[241] Furthermore, a 1-year prospective population-based cohort study showed that noroviruses were the single most important cause of gastroenteritis overall in nearly all age groups in the Netherlands.[106] In Germany, the incidence of norovirus gastroenteritis in the community requiring medical attention was reported as 626 cases/per 100,000 person-years, making it the predominant known cause of acute gastroenteritis in that country.[218] In England, the community incidence of norovirus gastroenteritis was 4.5 cases/per 100 person-years, corresponding to approximately 2 million episodes per/year.[376]

Genetic Diversity of Virus

Molecular epidemiologic studies have demonstrated a marked genetic diversity among circulating noroviruses. Genetic typing of circulating strains has proven to be a useful tool in elucidating the source and spread of outbreaks,[247,482,483] and regional data-sharing networks have been established in several areas of the world.[133,246,336,480] Genetic typing systems for the noroviruses have been proposed based on relatedness in the complete VP1 capsid protein, which presumably would correlate with the antigenic specificity.[247,520] One such system (Table 20.4) shows the division of the genus Norovirus into six major phylogenetic clades, or genogroups, designated GI through GV. Genogroups I, II, and III are further subdivided into 9, 21, and 3 genotypes, respectively.

Large-scale molecular epidemiologic studies have given insight into important genetic features of the noroviruses. An analysis of the genetic typing data from 2,512 noroviruses associated with outbreaks in Europe from 2000 to 2011 shows the marked genetic variation in the genotypes of circulating

TABLE 20.4 Norovirus Genogroups and Genotypes as Determined by VP1 Relatedness

Reference virus	Genogroup	Genotype	GenBank accession number
Hu/NoV/GI.1/Norwalk/1968/US	I	1	M87661
Hu/NoV/GI.2/Southampton/1991/UK	I	2	L07418
Hu/NoV/GI.3/Desert Shield 395/1990/SA	I	3	U04469
Hu/NoV/GI.4/Chiba 407/1987/JP	I	4	AB022679
Hu/NoV/GI.5/Musgrove/1989/UK	I	5	AJ277614
Hu/NoV/GI.6/BS5(Hesse3)/1997/DE	I	6	AF093797
Hu/NoV/GI.7/Winchester/1994/UK	I	7	AJ277609
Hu/NoV/GI.8/Boxer/2001/US	I	8	AF538679
Hu/NoV/GI.9/Vancouver730/2004/CA	I	9	HQ637267
Hu/NoV/GII.1/Hawaii/1971/US	II	1	U07611
Hu/NoV/GII.2/Melksham/1994/UK	II	2	X81879
Hu/NoV/GII.3/Toronto 24/1991/CA	II	3	U02030
Hu/NoV/GII.4/Bristol/1993/UK	II	4	X76716
Hu/NoV/GII.5/Hillingdon/1990/UK	II	5	AJ277607
Hu/NoV/GII.6/Seacroft/1990/UK	II	6	AJ277620
Hu/NoV/GII.7/Leeds/1990/UK	II	7	AJ277608
Hu/NoV/GII.8/Amsterdam/1998/NL	II	8	AF195848
Hu/NoV/GII.9/VA97207/1996/US	II	9	AY038599
Hu/NoV/GII.10/Erfurt546/2000/DE	II	10	AF427118
Po/NoV/GII.11/Sw918/1997/JP	II	11	AB074893
Hu/NoV/GII.12/Wortley/1990/UK	II	12	AJ277618
Hu/NoV/GII.13/Fayetteville/1998/US	II	13	AY113106
Hu/NoV/GII.14/M7/1999/US	II	14	AY130761
Hu/NoV/GII.15/J23/1999/US	II	15	AY130762
Hu/NoV/GII.16/Tiffin/1999/US	II	16	AY502010
Hu/NoV/GII.17/CS-E1/2002/US	II	17	AY502009
Po/NoV/GII.18/OH-QW101/2003/US	II	18	AY823304
Po/NoV/GII.19/OH-QW170/2003/US	II	19	AY823306
Hu/NoV/GII.20/Luckenwalde591/2002/DE	II	20	EU373815
Hu/NoV/GII.21/IF1998/2003/IR	II	21	AY675554
Hu/NoV/GII.22/Yuri/2002/JP	II	22	AB083780
Bo/NoV/GIII.1/Jena/1980/DE	III	1	AJ011099
Bo/NoV/GIII.2/Newbury-2/1976/UK	III	2	AF097917
Ov/NoV/GIII.3/Norsewood30/2007/NZ	III	3	EU193658
Hu/NoV/GIV.1/Alphatron 98–2/1998/NL	IV	1	AF195847
Lion/NoV/GIV.2/Pistoia/387/2006/IT	IV	2	EF450827
Mu/NoV/GV.1/MNV-1/2002/US	V	1	AY228235
Ca/NoV/GVI/Bari/91/2007/IT	VI	1	FJ875027
Ca/NoV/GVI/Viseu/2007/PT	VI	2	GQ443611

Country abbreviations are CA, Canada; DE, Germany; IR, Iraq; IT, Italy; JP, Japan; NL, Netherlands; NZ, New Zealand; PT, Portugal; SA, Saudi Arabia; UK, United Kingdom; US, United States. Species abbreviations are Bo, bovine; Ca, canine; Hu, human; Mu, murine; Po, porcine; Ov, ovine

Note: According to classification system of the online norovirus typing tool at http://www.rivm.nl/mpf/norovirus/typingtool. Kroneman A, Vennema H, Deforche K, et al. An automated genotyping tool for enteroviruses and noroviruses. *J Clin Virol* 2011;51:121–125.

strains (Fig. 20.9C). The GII noroviruses, particularly those of the GII.4 cluster, were the predominant viruses detected, and this distribution reflects the epidemiologic pattern observed in most other parts of the world. In an analysis of 773 norovirus outbreaks reported to the CDC from 1994 to 2006, 629 (81.4%) were caused by GII viruses and 342 (44.2%) of these were caused by GII.4 strains.[521] Major shifts in the predominant circulating strain can occur,[56,127,138,284,350,389,485,499,521] and the factors (host or viral) responsible for the emergence of an epidemic norovirus strain are under investigation. Sequence analysis of the GII.4 noroviruses that emerged on a global level in the early 2000s identified the presence of an amino acid insertion in the VP1 P2 domain, suggesting a possible change in the antigenic or receptor recognition phenotype.[110] Further evolution in the GII.4 cluster was described,[56] and several studies have examined the possibly unique propensity of this genotype to undergo genetic (and antigenic) drift.[10,47,51,57,118,271,272,336,421,428] Genetic variation has been detected in other regions of the genome such as the emergence of the "GGIIb-pol" polymerase type that was found in norovirus strains in combination with several different VP1 genotypes.[389,390] Additional reports of unique polymerase sequences have led to the conclusion that recombination is a driving mechanism of norovirus evolution.[55,144]

Evidence for mixed norovirus infections within the same individual or within the same outbreak has been reported in many epidemiologic studies.[14,54,150,167,282,449] In addition, a marked genetic diversity among norovirus strains has been documented in pediatric patients.[137,173,235,307,522] Such diverse and mixed infections may allow recombination between RNA genomes, a possibility suggested from sequence analyses of naturally occurring noroviruses in several species.[55,124,171,177,198,362,398,488] The presence of diverse norovirus sequences in shellfish samples is common,[87,95,260] suggesting another potential source for mixed infection. Infection of feline kidney cells with two distinct recombinant FCV strains bearing different fluorescent markers has demonstrated that co-infection of the same cell can readily occur, further supporting the potential for recombination of RNA genomes during replication.[1]

CLINICAL FEATURES

Viral gastroenteritis is generally considered to be mild and self-limiting, although the illness can be incapacitating during the symptomatic phase that usually lasts 24 to 48 hours (Fig. 20.10). Illness induced by the noroviruses can be sufficiently severe to require medical intervention, with an increased risk for life-threatening dehydration at both ends of the age spectrum.[20,104,216,232,366,400,423] Immunocompromised patients with norovirus infection are at increased risk for morbidity and mortality, and an increasing number of reports have linked norovirus to chronic gastroenteritis in patients undergoing transplantation or chemotherapy[46,131,312,401,406,417,430,450,494] (see Treatment).

Clinical manifestations observed in 31 volunteers experimentally infected with noroviruses who became ill included the following: fever above 99.4°F (45%), diarrhea (81%), vomiting (65%), abdominal discomfort (68%), anorexia (90%), headache (81%), and myalgias (58%).[511] The illnesses were characteristically mild and usually lasted 24 to 48 hours; however, one volunteer was given parenteral fluid because he vomited 20 times within a 24-hour period. The number of clinical signs and symptoms can vary among volunteers receiving the same inoculum.[113] Illnesses induced by the Hawaii, Montgomery County, and Snow Mountain viruses in volunteers cannot be distinguished clinically from those caused by Norwalk virus.[116,511] Subclinical infections with Norwalk or Hawaii virus have been observed under experimental as well as natural conditions.

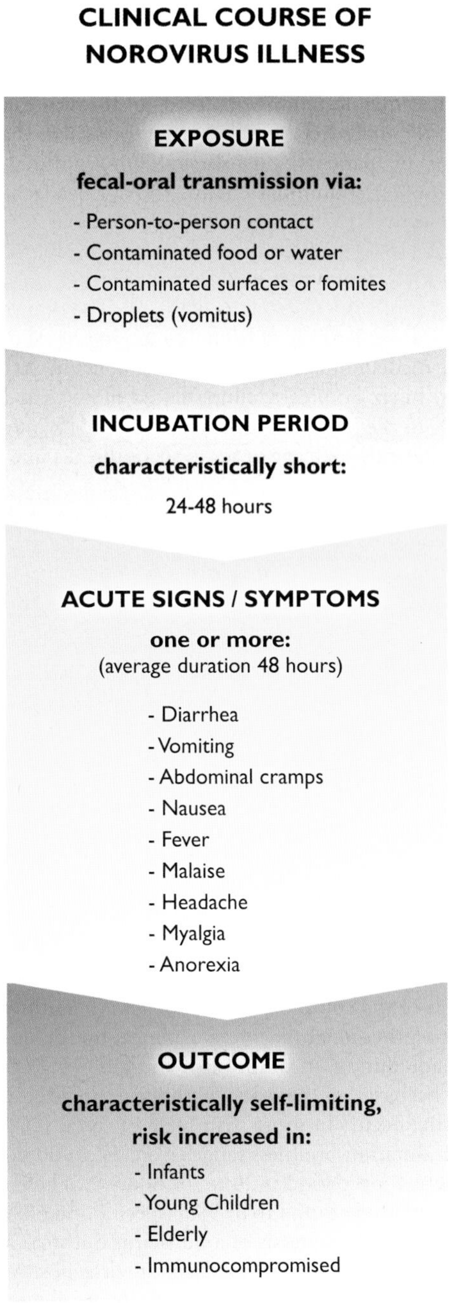

Of 16 volunteers who developed illness following Norwalk or Hawaii virus infection, 14 developed transient lymphopenia.[115] This was attributed to a redistribution of circulating lymphocytes to the site of viral infection in the small intestine.

CLINICAL COURSE OF NOROVIRUS ILLNESS

EXPOSURE

fecal-oral transmission via:

- Person-to-person contact
- Contaminated food or water
- Contaminated surfaces or fomites
- Droplets (vomitus)

INCUBATION PERIOD

characteristically short:

24-48 hours

ACUTE SIGNS / SYMPTOMS

one or more:

(average duration 48 hours)

- Diarrhea
- Vomiting
- Abdominal cramps
- Nausea
- Fever
- Malaise
- Headache
- Myalgia
- Anorexia

OUTCOME

characteristically self-limiting, risk increased in:

- Infants
- Young Children
- Elderly
- Immunocompromised

FIGURE 20.10. Clinical course of norovirus disease.

The lymphocytes remaining in the circulation responded normally or exhibited an exaggerated response to mitogenic stimuli.

Clinical manifestations observed in 38 outbreaks associated with NV included the following (expressed as the median percentage of patients): nausea (79%), vomiting (69%), diarrhea (66%), abdominal cramps (30%), headache (22%), fever (subjective) (37%), chills (32%), myalgias (26%), and sore throat (18%).[216] Bloody stools were not reported. Vomiting occurred more frequently than diarrhea in children, whereas in adults the reverse was observed. The duration of illness in 28 outbreaks ranged from 2 hours to several days, with a mean or median of between 12 and 60 hours in 26 of the 28 outbreaks. In six outbreaks, illness lasted more than 3 days in up to 15% of the affected individuals. The attack rates did not differ significantly with age or sex in six outbreaks in which this was analyzed.[216]

A 2-year study in children (5 years of age or younger) compared the severity of acute diarrheal episodes caused by noroviruses with rotaviruses in hospital emergency and outpatient settings; most cases for both viruses ranged from moderate to severe, although illness was overall less severe for norovirus-infected individuals.[354] The clinical course of norovirus illness in preterm infants has been reported to include a distended abdomen and symptoms such as apnea or a sepsis-like appearance: vomiting was not a predominant symptom in these patients.[19] Noroviruses have been reported as associated with the following rare conditions or sequelae: convulsions,[72,319] encephalopathy,[196,356] and necrotizing enterocolitis.[445]

DIAGNOSIS

Differential

An analysis of the common features of 38 NV outbreaks indicates that a provisional diagnosis of illness by the noroviruses can be made during an outbreak if the following criteria are met: (a) bacterial or parasitic pathogens are not detected, (b) vomiting occurs in more than 50% of cases, (c) the mean or median duration of illness ranges from 12 to 60 hours, and (d) the incubation period is 24 to 48 hours.[215] These so-called Kaplan criteria were found to be 99% specific and 68% specific for the provisional diagnosis of a norovirus outbreak when re-evaluated with samples confirmed as norovirus positive.[476]

Differential diagnosis of sporadic norovirus illness in individual patients is difficult, due to shared clinical features (see Clinical Features) with a wide range of enteric pathogens and disease syndromes.

Laboratory

Reverse Transcriptase-Polymerase Chain Reaction

Currently, RT-PCR is the most widely used technique for detection of noroviruses.[23] With this method, noroviruses can be detected in clinical specimens (feces or vomitus) and contaminated food, water, or fomites. The application of real-time quantitative (q) RT-PCR has gained widespread use because it allows rapid detection as well as comparison of viral RNA levels.[209,473] There are several considerations for optimal performance of RT-PCR techniques.[23] First, the viral RNA extraction procedure should allow the purification of an RNA template that is nondegraded and free of inhibitors of the RT-PCR reaction. Internal RNA controls can be used in the assay of clinical and environmental samples to avoid false-negative results.[370,415] Second, the choice of primers is important, because considerable genetic diversity exists among circulating strains. Several primer pairs have been described that were deduced from highly conserved regions of the RNA genome (usually the polymerase region).[484] RT-PCR, coupled with sequence analysis of the amplicons, has been used extensively to detect and characterize noroviruses in various outbreaks (see Molecular Epidemiology). Norovirus identification is increasingly included in multiplex assays that detect a wide array of enteric pathogens, facilitated by an accumulating norovirus database that has allowed the design of broadly reactive primers and probes.[160,197,278,424,510]

Immunoassays

Immunoassays for the detection of noroviruses have been developed that employ hyperimmune antisera prepared against rVLPs.[201,203] Although sensitive, these assays are often highly specific for the immunizing VLP.[149,200,203,212] Progress has been made in the development of norovirus-specific and cross-reactive monoclonal antibodies[168,178,181,236,267,270,368,425,514] for use in enzyme-linked immunosorbent assays (ELISAs) that can detect viral antigen in clinical specimens; commercial diagnostic ELISA kits are now available.

The ELISAs that use rVLPs as antigen are specific, sensitive, and efficient for detecting infection with the human caliciviruses and have been used in several large-scale seroepidemiologic studies (see Prevalence and Seroepidemiology). The Norwalk rVLP ELISA has been shown to detect broadly reactive antibody responses in volunteers given NV, Hawaii virus, or Snow Mountain virus, although the maximal response was observed in volunteers challenged with NV.[149,154,330,471] Thus, it is impossible to identify the antigenic type of an infecting norovirus strain by serologic analysis because of the cross-reactive antibodies detected by ELISA.[32,349] The demonstration of an antibody response in 50% or more of the individuals involved (or examined) in an outbreak to a calicivirus antigen is strong evidence linking the virus with the outbreak.[216]

PREVENTION AND CONTROL

Treatment

The noroviruses characteristically induce a mild, self-limited gastroenteritis that normally resolves without complications.[43,111,112,113,206,442,511] As noted, hospitalization for severe dehydration, although rare, can occur with norovirus gastroenteritis. Oral fluid and electrolyte replacement therapy is usually sufficient to replace fluid loss.[96,380,477] Oral rehydration therapy should not be administered to patients with depressed consciousness because of the possibility of fluid aspiration. Parenteral administration of fluids may be necessary, however, if severe vomiting or diarrhea occurs.

Oral administration of bismuth subsalicylate after onset of symptoms significantly reduced the severity and duration of abdominal cramps during experimentally induced norovirus illness in adults.[442] In addition, the median duration of gastrointestinal symptoms was reduced from 20 to 14 hours. The number, weight, and water content of stools, as well as the extent of virus excretion, were not significantly affected by

TABLE 20.5 Various Treatment Protocols Tested in Normal and Immunocompromised Patients with Norovirus Gastroenteritis

Patient status at time of norovirus illness	Age	Norovirus treatment	Dose or modification of Immunosuppressive therapy (IST)	Reported outcome[b]	Reference
Normal	Adult	Bismuth subsalicylate	420 mg	Reduced abdominal cramping	(442)
Normal	12–60 years	Nitazoxanide	Oral, 500 mg, 2× x daily	Shorter duration of illness	(402)
AML	43 years	Nitazoxanide	Oral, 500 mg, 2× daily	Improvement	(427)
Immunocompromised	All[a]	Immunoglobulin	Oral, 25 mg/kg, 4× x daily	Decreased stool output	(131)
HIV	36 years	Immunoglobulin	IV, 400 mg/kg, 1× daily	Minimal 2-day improvement	(504)
Stem cell/lung transplant	56 years	Modify IST	Drug switch	Improvement	(46)
Intestinal transplant	<2 years	Modify IST	Dose reduction	Improvement	(223)
Renal transplant	Adult	Modify IST	Dose reduction	Improvement	(401)
Renal transplant	Adult	Modify IST	Dose reduction	Improvement	(412)

AML, acute myelogenous leukemia; HIV, human immunodeficiency virus; IST, immunosuppressive therapy.

[a]Two study groups: one with average age of 2 years old, the other with male adults.

[b]Long term follow-up information unavailable for most patients.

treatment. The use of various medications for symptomatic treatment of acute diarrhea in infants and young children (aged 1 month to 5 years) was reviewed: bismuth subsalicylate, loperamide, anticholinergic agents, adsorbents, or Lactobacillus-containing compounds were not recommended by the American Academy of Pediatrics and, in addition, the use of opiates as well as opiate and atropine combination drugs was contraindicated.[380]

Although direct-acting antivirals for the treatment of norovirus gastroenteritis are not yet available, treatment protocols implemented for other pathogens have been evaluated in a small number of individuals with norovirus disease, with varying success (Table 20.5). Improvement in chronic norovirus diarrhea has been reported in immunocompromised patients following reduction in immunosuppressive therapy (IST) drugs; however, careful monitoring of these patients is required (Table 20.5). Efforts are in progress to develop antiviral drugs to target specific stages of the norovirus life cycle, but their safety and clinical efficacy have not been established.[188,229,392,397]

Vaccines

A vaccine for the control of norovirus gastroenteritis is not yet available, but a promising efficacy study in adult volunteers has shown recently that administration of Norwalk virus rVLPs as vaccine provided protection against illness when vaccinees were challenged with Norwalk virus.[22] Additional work will be needed to determine the number of antigenic components required to provide protection against a broad range of norovirus antigenic types and variants. Various routes of administration, formulations, and expression systems for rVLPs (or subunit forms) are under investigation.[27,28,48,122,163,451,452,454,456,460] A safe and effective vaccine could reduce the incidence of epidemic viral gastroenteritis. A vaccine would be of special importance to college students, military personnel, nursing home residents, and individuals in various institutional settings. In addition, it might reduce the number of episodes of severe gastroenteritis in infants and children. Although norovirus gastroenteritis tends to be a mild illness, a reduction in diarrheal episodes may be especially important in the debilitated, malnourished infant, because it has been suggested that repeated diarrheal episodes may be a precipitating factor in the development of malnutrition through sequential damage to the intestinal mucosa.[308] The impact of norovirus infection on normal gastrointestinal microflora or underlying disease conditions,[59] when elucidated, may provide additional data to support norovirus immunoprophylaxis.

Infection Control

Specific methods are not available for the prevention of human calicivirus infection or illness. Outbreak management generally focuses on containment by the prevention of spread to other areas by ill or exposed individuals, frequent handwashing, and effective environmental decontamination.[8,69,88,226,249,293,469,477] The noroviruses are generally resistant to detergent or ethanol-based cleaning of environmental surfaces and fomites and require additional chemical disinfection.[29,119,477] Reliance on the use of alcohol-based hand sanitizers over handwashing has been reported to actually increase the risk of norovirus transmission and infection in patient care settings.[44,486] Effective disinfectants have been reported to include hypochlorite at 5,000 ppm (domestic bleach is approximately 5% sodium hypochlorite and can be used as a 10% solution), hydrogen peroxide–based cleaners, and phenolic-based cleaners.[29,477]

Special care must be given to the hygienic processing of food in view of the frequent occurrence of food-borne outbreaks.[240,475] Depuration of oysters does not adequately clear tissues of NV,[15,159,416] and recent studies have shown that NV binds to oyster tissues via carbohydrate structures similar to those of human histo-blood group antigens.[259,294] Precaution must be taken to prevent contamination of oyster beds with feces, vomitus, or sewage treatment plant effluent. Measures that increase the purity of drinking water or swimming pool water should also decrease the frequency of outbreaks.[282] Various technological processes are under development to inactivate noroviruses in agricultural food products and shellfish prior to market[183,230,243,264,333]; human volunteer studies remain important in establishing their efficacy in the absence of an *in vitro* infectivity assay for the human strains.[391]

PERSPECTIVE

Caliciviruses are a highly diverse and evolving family of single-stranded RNA viruses. Because these viruses have a proven ability to persist silently in nature, next-generation pathogen discovery techniques, such as deep sequencing, are sure to uncover many new host species for these viruses. Rabbit hemorrhagic disease virus remained undetected as a pathogen until its sudden emergence as the etiologic agent of a deadly rabbit hemorrhagic disease three decades ago. Murine norovirus, likely present in laboratory mice for decades, was discovered only when genetically engineered laboratory mice lacking a functional innate immune system developed unexplained illness and died, thus prompting investigation. Even recognized calicivirus pathogens may shift suddenly in virulence, as shown by the recent emergence of lethal "virulent systemic" FCV strains. Human GII.4 noroviruses, currently the predominant genotype, periodically undergo genetic drift to cause sharp increases in the number of global gastroenteritis outbreaks, affecting millions.

The diversity and rapid evolution of viruses in the *Caliciviridae* present a constant challenge in the management of disease and in the development of vaccines, and noroviruses are no exception. Human norovirus research is complicated even further by the continued absence of a fully permissive cell culture system, thus hindering the ability to determine serotypic diversity. Despite this stubborn, lingering technical obstacle, important strides have been made in the last few years, and more are on the horizon. Norovirus vaccines containing antigens from the major capsid protein, VP1, have advanced in clinical trials, and the first demonstration of vaccine efficacy has been achieved. The serious nature of prolonged norovirus shedding and illness in immunocompromised patients has become apparent, and intense efforts are in progress to identify an effective antiviral drug. Drug development for human noroviruses is facilitated by the availability of molecular biology–driven tools such as recombinant enzymes expressed from cDNA clones and a human norovirus replicon–bearing cell line. These tools, coupled with the investigation of caliciviruses that grow in cell culture such as feline calicivirus and murine norovirus, each with powerful reverse genetics systems, are bringing the field closer to the realization of effective approaches for norovirus control. The next few years should be remarkable.

REFERENCES

All cited references are available in the e-book.

1. Abente EJ, Sosnovtsev SV, Bok K, et al. Visualization of feline calicivirus replication in real-time with recombinant viruses engineered to express fluorescent reporter proteins. *Virology* 2010;400:18–31.
7. Al-Molawi N, Beardmore VA, Carter MJ, et al. Caspase-mediated cleavage of the feline calicivirus capsid protein. *J Gen Virol* 2003;84: 1237–1244.
16. Aoki Y, Suto A, Mizuta K, et al. Duration of norovirus excretion and the longitudinal course of viral load in norovirus-infected elderly patients. *J Hosp Infect* 2010;75:42–46.
19. Armbrust S, Kramer A, Olbertz D, et al. Norovirus infections in preterm infants: wide variety of clinical courses. *BMC Res Notes* 2009;2:96.
21. Asanaka M, Atmar RL, Ruvolo V, et al. Replication and packaging of Norwalk virus RNA in cultured mammalian cells. *Proc Natl Acad Sci U S A* 2005;102:10327–10332.
22. Atmar RL, Bernstein DI, Harro CD, et al. Norovirus vaccine against experimental human Norwalk virus illness. *N Engl J Med* 2011;365:2178–2187.
23. Atmar RL, Neill FH, Le Guyader FS. Detection of human caliciviruses in fecal samples by rt-PCR. *Methods Mol Biol* 2011;665:39–50.
24. Atmar RL, Opekun AR, Gilger MA, et al. Norwalk virus shedding after experimental human infection. *Emerg Infect Dis* 2008;14:1553–1557.
25. Bailey D, Kaiser WJ, Hollinshead M, et al. Feline calicivirus p32, p39 and p30 proteins localize to the endoplasmic reticulum to initiate replication complex formation. *J Gen Virol* 2010;91:739–749.
32. Belliot G, Noel JS, Li JF, et al. Characterization of capsid genes, expressed in the baculovirus system, of three new genetically distinct strains of "Norwalk-like viruses". *J Clin Microbiol* 2001;39:4288–4295.
33. Belliot G, Sosnovtsev SV, Chang KO, et al. Norovirus proteinase-polymerase and polymerase are both active forms of RNA-dependent RNA polymerase. *J Virol* 2005;79:2393–2403.
34. Belliot G, Sosnovtsev SV, Mitra T, et al. In vitro proteolytic processing of the MD145 norovirus ORF1 nonstructural polyprotein yields stable precursors and products similar to those detected in calicivirus-infected cells. *J Virol* 2003;77:10957–10974.
35. Bertolotti-Ciarlet A, Crawford SE, Hutson AM, et al. The 3′ end of Norwalk virus mRNA contains determinants that regulate the expression and stability of the viral capsid protein VP1: a novel function for the VP2 protein. *J Virol* 2003;77:11603–11615.
36. Bertolotti-Ciarlet A, White LJ, Chen R, et al. Structural requirements for the assembly of Norwalk virus-like particles. *J Virol* 2002;76:4044–4055.
37. Bhella D, Gatherer D, Chaudhry Y, et al. Structural insights into calicivirus attachment and uncoating. *J Virol* 2008;82:8051–8058.
38. Bhella D, Goodfellow IG. The cryo-electron microscopy structure of feline calicivirus bound to junctional adhesion molecule A at 9-angstrom resolution reveals receptor-induced flexibility and two distinct conformational changes in the capsid protein VP1. *J Virol* 2011;85:11381–11390.
46. Boillat Blanco N, Kuonen R, Bellini C, et al. Chronic norovirus gastroenteritis in a double hematopoietic stem cell and lung transplant recipient. *Transpl Infect Dis* 2011;13:213–215.
48. Bok K, Parra GI, Mitra T, et al. Chimpanzees as an animal model for human norovirus infection and vaccine development. *Proc Natl Acad Sci U S A* 2011;108:325–330.
50. Boniotti B, Wirblich C, Sibilia M, et al. Identification and characterization of a 3C-like protease from rabbit hemorrhagic disease virus, a calicivirus. *J Virol* 1994;68:6487–6495.
52. Bourgeois AL, Gardiner CH, Thornton SA, et al. Etiology of acute diarrhea among United States military personnel deployed to South America and west Africa. *Am J Trop Med Hyg* 1993;48:243–248.
55. Bull RA, Hansman GS, Clancy LE, et al. Norovirus recombination in ORF1/ORF2 overlap. *Emerg Infect Dis* 2005;11:1079–1085.
56. Bull RA, Tu ET, McIver CJ, et al. Emergence of a new norovirus genotype II.4 variant associated with global outbreaks of gastroenteritis. *J Clin Microbiol* 2006;44:327–333.
58. Burroughs JN, Brown F. Presence of a covalently linked protein on calicivirus RNA. *J Gen Virol* 1978;41:443–446.
60. Calderon-Margalit R, Sheffer R, Halperin T, et al. A large-scale gastroenteritis outbreak associated with norovirus in nursing homes. *Epidemiol Infect* 2005;133:35–40.
61. Cao S, Lou Z, Tan M, et al. Structural basis for the recognition of blood group trisaccharides by norovirus. *J Virol* 2007;81:5949–5957.
62. Capizzi T, Makari-Judson G, Steingart R, et al. Chronic diarrhea associated with persistent norovirus excretion in patients with chronic lymphocytic leukemia: report of two cases. *BMC Infect Dis* 2011;11:131.
64. Carter MJ, Milton ID, Meanger J, et al. The complete nucleotide sequence of a feline calicivirus. *Virology* 1992;190:443–448.
66. Caul EO. Small round structured viruses: airborne transmission and hospital control [see comments]. *Lancet* 1994;343:1240–1242.
67. Chachu KA, LoBue AD, Strong DW, et al. Immune mechanisms responsible for vaccination against and clearance of mucosal and lymphatic norovirus infection. *PLoS Pathog* 2008;4:e1000236.
73. Chan MC, Ho WS, Sung JJ. In vitro whole-virus binding of a norovirus genogroup II genotype 4 strain to cells of the lamina propria and Brunner's glands in the human duodenum. *J Virol* 2011;85:8427–8430.
75. Chan MC, Sung JJ, Lam RK, et al. Fecal viral load and norovirus-associated gastroenteritis. *Emerg Infect Dis* 2006;12:1278–1280.

77. Chang KO, Sosnovtsev SS, Belliot G, et al. Reverse genetics system for porcine enteric calicivirus, a prototype sapovirus in the Caliciviridae. *J Virol* 2005;79:1409–1416.
79. Chang KO, Sosnovtsev SV, Belliot G, et al. Stable expression of a Norwalk virus RNA replicon in a human hepatoma cell line. *Virology* 2006; 353:463–473.
84. Cheetham S, Souza M, Meulia T, et al. Pathogenesis of a genogroup II human norovirus in gnotobiotic pigs. *J Virol* 2006;80:10372–10381.
86. Chen R, Neill JD, Noel JS, et al. Inter- and intragenus structural variations in caliciviruses and their functional implications. *J Virol* 2004; 78:6469–6479.
89. Chiba S, Nakata S, Numata-Kinoshita K, et al. Sapporo virus: history and recent findings. *J Infect Dis* 2000;181:S303–S308.
90. Chiba S, Sakuma Y, Kogasaka R, et al. An outbreak of gastroenteritis associated with calicivirus in an infant home. *J Med Virol* 1979;4:249–254.
91. Choi JM, Hutson AM, Estes MK, et al. Atomic resolution structural characterization of recognition of histo-blood group antigens by Norwalk virus. *Proc Natl Acad Sci U S A* 2008;105:9175–9180.
101. Czako R, Atmar RL, Opekun AR, et al. Serum hemagglutination inhibition activity correlates with protection from gastroenteritis in persons infected with Norwalk virus. *Clin Vaccine Immunol* 2012;19:284–287.
103. Daughenbaugh KF, Fraser CS, Hershey JW, et al. The genome-linked protein VPg of the Norwalk virus binds eIF3, suggesting its role in translation initiation complex recruitment. *EMBO J* 2003;22:2852–2859.
106. de Wit MA, Koopmans MP, Kortbeek LM, et al. Sensor, a population-based cohort study on gastroenteritis in the Netherlands: incidence and etiology. *Am J Epidemiol* 2001;154:666–674.
110. Dingle KE. Mutation in a Lordsdale norovirus epidemic strain as a potential indicator of transmission routes. *J Clin Microbiol* 2004;42:3950–3957.
112. Dolin R, Blacklow NR, DuPont H, et al. Biological properties of Norwalk agent of acute infectious nonbacterial gastroenteritis. *Proc Soc Exp Biol Med* 1972;140:578–583.
113. Dolin R, Blacklow NR, DuPont H, et al. Transmission of acute infectious nonbacterial gastroenteritis to volunteers by oral administration of stool filtrates. *J Infect Dis* 1971;123:307–312.
115. Dolin R, Reichman RC, Fauci AS. Lymphocyte populations in acute viral gastroenteritis. *Infect Immun* 1976;14:422–428.
116. Dolin R, Reichman RC, Roessner KD, et al. Detection by immune electron microscopy of the Snow Mountain agent of acute viral gastroenteritis. *J Infect Dis* 1982;146:184–189.
125. Ettayebi K, Hardy ME. Norwalk virus nonstructural protein p48 forms a complex with the SNARE regulator VAP-A and prevents cell surface expression of vesicular stomatitis virus G protein. *J Virol* 2003;77:11790–11797.
126. Fankhauser RL, Monroe SS, Noel JS, et al. Epidemiologic and molecular trends of "Norwalk-like viruses" associated with outbreaks of gastroenteritis in the United States. *J Infect Dis* 2002;186:1–7.
129. Fernandez-Vega V, Sosnovtsev SV, Belliot G, et al. Norwalk virus N-terminal nonstructural protein is associated with disassembly of the Golgi complex in transfected cells. *J Virol* 2004;78:4827–4837.
130. Flewett TH, Davies H. Letter: Caliciviruses in man. *Lancet* 1976;1:311.
131. Florescu DF, Hermsen ED, Kwon JY, et al. Is there a role for oral human immunoglobulin in the treatment for norovirus enteritis in immunocompromised patients? *Pediatr Transplant* 2011;15:718–721.
134. Fukushi S, Kojima S, Takai R, et al. Poly(A)- and primer-independent RNA polymerase of Norovirus. *J Virol* 2004;78:3889–3896.
143. Gerondopoulos A, Jackson T, Monaghan P, et al. Murine norovirus-1 cell entry is mediated through a non-clathrin-, non-caveolae-, dynamin- and cholesterol-dependent pathway. *J Gen Virol* 2010;91:1428–1438.
145. Glass PJ, White LJ, Ball JM, et al. Norwalk virus open reading frame 3 encodes a minor structural protein. *J Virol* 2000;74:6581–6591.
147. Glass RI, Parashar UD, Estes MK. Norovirus gastroenteritis. *N Engl J Med* 2009;361:1776–1785.
148. Goodfellow I, Chaudhry Y, Gioldasi I, et al. Calicivirus translation initiation requires an interaction between VPg and eIF 4 E. *EMBO Rep* 2005; 6:968–972.
149. Graham DY, Jiang X, Tanaka T, et al. Norwalk virus infection of volunteers: new insights based on improved assays. *J Infect Dis* 1994;170:34–43.
155. Green KY, Mory A, Fogg MH, et al. Isolation of enzymatically active replication complexes from feline calicivirus-infected cells. *J Virol* 2002;76:8582–8595.
157. Greenberg HB, Wyatt RG, Kapikian AZ. Norwalk virus in vomitus [letter]. *Lancet* 1979;1:55.
161. Guillon P, Ruvoen-Clouet N, Le Moullac-Vaidye B, et al. Association between expression of the H histo-blood group antigen, alpha1, 2fucosyltransferases polymorphism of wild rabbits, and sensitivity to rabbit hemorrhagic disease virus. *Glycobiology* 2009;19:21–28.
162. Guix S, Asanaka M, Katayama K, et al. Norwalk virus RNA is infectious in mammalian cells. *J Virol* 2007;81:12238–12248.
164. Gustavsson L, Andersson LM, Lindh M, et al. Excess mortality following community-onset norovirus enteritis in the elderly. *J Hosp Infect* 2011;79:27–31.
165. Gutierrez-Escolano AL, Brito ZU, del Angel RM, et al. Interaction of cellular proteins with the 5′ end of Norwalk virus genomic RNA. *J Virol* 2000;74:8558–8562.
166. Gutierrez-Escolano AL, Vazquez-Ochoa M, Escobar-Herrera J, et al. La, PTB, and PAB proteins bind to the 3(′) untranslated region of Norwalk virus genomic RNA. *Biochem Biophys Res Commun* 2003;311:759–766.
169. Hall AJ, Rosenthal M, Gregoricus N, et al. Incidence of acute gastroenteritis and role of norovirus, Georgia, USA, 2004–2005. *Emerg Infect Dis* 2011;17:1381–1388.
174. Hardy M, Crone T, Brower J, et al. Substrate specificity of the Norwalk virus 3C-like proteinase. *Virus Res* 2002;89:29.
179. Herbert TP, Brierley I, Brown TD. Detection of the ORF3 polypeptide of feline calicivirus in infected cells and evidence for its expression from a single, functionally bicistronic, subgenomic mRNA. *J Gen Virol* 1996;77:123–127.
180. Herbert TP, Brierley I, Brown TD. Identification of a protein linked to the genomic and subgenomic mRNAs of feline calicivirus and its role in translation. *J Gen Virol* 1997;78:1033–1040.
182. Hillenbrand B, Gunzel D, Richter JF, et al. Norovirus non-structural protein p20 leads to impaired restitution of epithelial defects by inhibition of actin cytoskeleton remodelling. *Scand J Gastroenterol* 2010;45: 1307–1319.
188. Hussey RJ, Coates L, Gill RS, et al. A structural study of norovirus 3C protease specificity: binding of a designed active site-directed peptide inhibitor. *Biochemistry* 2011;50:240–249.
189. Hussey RJ, Coates L, Gill RS, et al. Crystallization and preliminary X-ray diffraction analysis of the protease from Southampton norovirus complexed with a Michael acceptor inhibitor. *Acta Crystallogr Sect F Struct Biol Cryst Commun* 2010;66:1544–1548.
190. Hutson AM, Airaud F, LePendu J, et al. Norwalk virus infection associates with secretor status genotyped from sera. *J Med Virol* 2005; 77:116–120.
194. Hyde JL, Sosnovtsev SV, Green KY, et al. Mouse norovirus replication is associated with virus-induced vesicle clusters originating from membranes derived from the secretory pathway. *J Virol* 2009;83:9709–9719.
196. Ito S, Takeshita S, Nezu A, et al. Norovirus-associated encephalopathy. *Pediatr Infect Dis J* 2006;25:651–652.
199. Jiang X, Graham DY, Wang K, et al. Norwalk virus genome cloning and characterization. *Science* 1990;250:1580–1583.
201. Jiang X, Wang M, Graham DY, et al. Expression, self-assembly, and antigenicity of the Norwalk virus capsid protein. *J Virol* 1992;66:6527–6532.
202. Jiang X, Wang M, Wang K, et al. Sequence and genomic organization of Norwalk virus. *Virology* 1993;195:51–61.
203. Jiang X, Wilton N, Zhong WM, et al. Diagnosis of human caliciviruses by use of enzyme immunoassays. *J Infect Dis* 2000;181(Suppl 2): S349–S359.
209. Kageyama T, Kojima S, Shinohara M, et al. Broadly reactive and highly sensitive assay for Norwalk-like viruses based on real-time quantitative reverse transcription-PCR. *J Clin Microbiol* 2003;41:1548–1557.
211. Kaiser WJ, Chaudhry Y, Sosnovtsev SV, et al. Analysis of protein-protein interactions in the feline calicivirus replication complex. *J Gen Virol* 2006;87:363–368.
213. Kapikian AZ. The discovery of the 27-nm Norwalk virus: an historic perspective. *J Infect Dis* 2000;181:S295–S302.
214. Kapikian AZ, Wyatt RG, Dolin R, et al. Visualization by immune electron microscopy of a 27-nm particle associated with acute infectious nonbacterial gastroenteritis. *J Virol* 1972;10:1075–1081.
215. Kaplan JE, Feldman R, Campbell DS, et al. The frequency of a Norwalk-like pattern of illness in outbreaks of acute gastroenteritis. *Am J Public Health* 1982;72:1329–1332.

216. Kaplan JE, Gary GW, Baron RC, et al. Epidemiology of Norwalk gastroenteritis and the role of Norwalk virus in outbreaks of acute nonbacterial gastroenteritis. *Ann Intern Med* 1982;96:756–761.
217. Karst SM, Wobus CE, Lay M, et al. STAT1-dependent innate immunity to a Norwalk-like virus. *Science* 2003;299:1575–1578.
218. Karsten C, Baumgarte S, Friedrich AW, et al. Incidence and risk factors for community-acquired acute gastroenteritis in north-west Germany in 2004. *Eur J Clin Microbiol Infect Dis* 2009;28:935–943.
223. Kaufman SS, Chatterjee NK, Fuschino ME, et al. Characteristics of human calicivirus enteritis in intestinal transplant recipients. *J Pediatr Gastroenterol Nutr* 2005;40:328–333.
225. Keswick BH, Satterwhite TK, Johnson PC, et al. Inactivation of Norwalk virus in drinking water by chlorine. *Appl Environ Microbiol* 1985; 50:261–264.
228. Kim MJ, Kim YJ, Lee JH, et al. Norovirus: a possible cause of pneumatosis intestinalis. *J Pediatr Gastroenterol Nutr* 2011;52:314–318.
231. Kirby A, Dove W, Ashton L, et al. Detection of norovirus in mouthwash samples from patients with acute gastroenteritis. *J Clin Virol* 2010; 48:285–287.
237. Komolafe OO, Jarrett O. A possible maturation pathway of calicivirus particles. *Microbios* 1986;46:103–111.
241. Koopmans M, Vinje J, de Wit M, et al. Molecular epidemiology of human enteric caliciviruses in The Netherlands. *J Infect Dis* 2000;181:S262–S269.
245. Kreutz LC, Seal BS, Mengeling WL. Early interaction of feline calicivirus with cells in culture. *Arch Virol* 1994;136:19–34.
246. Kroneman A, Harris J, Vennema H, et al. Data quality of 5 years of central norovirus outbreak reporting in the European Network for food-borne viruses. *J Public Health (Oxf)* 2008;30:82–90.
247. Kroneman A, Vennema H, Deforche K, et al. An automated genotyping tool for enteroviruses and noroviruses. *J Clin Virol* 2011;51:121–125.
250. Kuyumcu-Martinez M, Belliot G, Sosnovtsev SV, et al. Calicivirus 3C-like proteinase inhibits cellular translation by cleavage of poly(A)-binding protein. *J Virol* 2004;78:8172–8182.
252. Lambden PR, Caul EO, Ashley CR, et al. Human enteric caliciviruses are genetically distinct from small round structured viruses [letter]. *Lancet* 1994;343:666–667.
253. Lambden PR, Caul EO, Ashley CR, et al. Sequence and genome organization of a human small round-structured (Norwalk-like) virus. *Science* 1993;259:516–519.
258. Le Gall G, Huguet S, Vende P, et al. European brown hare syndrome virus: molecular cloning and sequencing of the genome. *J Gen Virol* 1996; 77:1693–1697.
260. Le Guyader FS, Bon F, DeMedici D, et al. Detection of multiple noroviruses associated with an international gastroenteritis outbreak linked to oyster consumption. *J Clin Microbiol* 2006;44:3878–3882.
265. Levy AG, Widerlite L, Schwartz CJ, et al. Jejunal adenylate cyclase activity in human subjects during viral gastroenteritis. *Gastroenterology* 1976;70:321–325.
268. Lindesmith L, Moe C, Lependu J, et al. Cellular and humoral immunity following Snow Mountain virus challenge. *J Virol* 2005;79:2900–2909.
269. Lindesmith L, Moe C, Marionneau S, et al. Human susceptibility and resistance to Norwalk virus infection. *Nat Med* 2003;9:548–553.
270. Lindesmith LC, Beltramello M, Donaldson EF, et al. Immunogenetic mechanisms driving norovirus GII.4 antigenic variation. *PLoS Pathog* 2012;8:e1002705.
273. Liu B, Clarke IN, Lambden PR. Polyprotein processing in Southampton virus: identification of 3C-like protease cleavage sites by in vitro mutagenesis. *J Virol* 1996;70:2605–2610.
276. Liu BL, Viljoen GJ, Clarke IN, et al. Identification of further proteolytic cleavage sites in the Southampton calicivirus polyprotein by expression of the viral protease in E. coli. *J Gen Virol* 1999;80:291–296.
277. Liu G, Ni Z, Yun T, et al. A DNA-launched reverse genetics system for rabbit hemorrhagic disease virus reveals that the VP2 protein is not essential for virus infectivity. *J Gen Virol* 2008;89:3080–3085.
279. LoBue AD, Lindesmith L, Yount B, et al. Multivalent norovirus vaccines induce strong mucosal and systemic blocking antibodies against multiple strains. *Vaccine* 2006;24:5220–5234.
280. LoBue AD, Lindesmith LC, Baric RS. Identification of cross-reactive norovirus CD4+ T cell epitopes. *J Virol* 2010;84:8530–8538.
286. Lopman BA, Hall AJ, Curns AT, et al. Increasing rates of gastroenteritis hospital discharges in US adults and the contribution of norovirus, 1996–2007. *Clin Infect Dis* 2011;52:466–474.
287. Lopman BA, Reacher MH, Van Duijnhoven Y, et al. Viral gastroenteritis outbreaks in Europe, 1995–2000. *Emerg Infect Dis* 2003;9:90–96.
291. Luttermann C, Meyers G. A bipartite sequence motif induces translation reinitiation in feline calicivirus RNA. *J Biol Chem* 2007;282:7056–7065.
294. Maalouf H, Schaeffer J, Parnaudeau S, et al. Strain-dependent norovirus bioaccumulation in oysters. *Appl Environ Microbiol* 2011;77:3189–3196.
295. Machin A, Martin Alonso JM, Parra F. Identification of the amino acid residue involved in rabbit hemorrhagic disease virus VPg uridylylation. *J Biol Chem* 2001;276:27787–27792.
296. Madeley CR, Cosgrove BP. Letter: Caliciviruses in man. *Lancet* 1976; 1:199–200.
299. Makino A, Shimojima M, Miyazawa T, et al. Junctional adhesion molecule 1 is a functional receptor for feline calicivirus. *J Virol* 2006; 80:4482–4490.
300. Marin MS, Casais R, Alonso JM, et al. ATP binding and ATPase activities associated with recombinant rabbit hemorrhagic disease virus 2C-like polypeptide. *J Virol* 2000;74:10846–10851.
301. Marionneau S, Ruvoen N, Le Moullac-Vaidye B, et al. Norwalk virus binds to histo-blood group antigens present on gastroduodenal epithelial cells of secretor individuals. *Gastroenterology* 2002;122:1967–1977.
308. Mata LJ, Urrutia JJ, Gordon JE. Diseases and disabilities. In: Mata LJ, ed. *The Children of Santa Maria Cauque: a Prospective Field Study of Health and Growth.* Cambridge, Massachusetts: MIT Press; 1978:254–292.
309. Matson DO, Zhong WM, Nakata S, et al. Molecular characterization of a human calicivirus with sequence relationships closer to animal caliciviruses than other known human caliciviruses. *J Med Virol* 1995;45:215–222.
313. Maunula L, Miettinen IT, von Bonsdorff CH. Norovirus outbreaks from drinking water. *Emerg Infect Dis* 2005;11:1716–1721.
314. McCarthy M, Estes MK, Hyams KC. Norwalk-like virus infection in military forces: epidemic potential, sporadic disease, and the future direction of prevention and control efforts. *J Infect Dis* 2000;181:S387–S391.
315. McCartney SA, Thackray LB, Gitlin L, et al. MDA-5 recognition of a murine norovirus. *PLoS Pathog* 2008;4:e1000108.
318. McFadden N, Bailey D, Carrara G, et al. Norovirus regulation of the innate immune response and apoptosis occurs via the product of the alternative open reading frame 4. *PLoS Pathog* 2011;7:e1002413.
319. Medici MC, Abelli LA, Dodi I, et al. Norovirus RNA in the blood of a child with gastroenteritis and convulsions–a case report. *J Clin Virol* 2010; 48:147–149.
320. Meeroff JC, Schreiber DS, Trier JS, et al. Abnormal gastric motor function in viral gastroenteritis. *Ann Intern Med* 1980;92:370–373.
322. Meyers G. Characterization of the sequence element directing translation reinitiation in RNA of the calicivirus rabbit hemorrhagic disease virus. *J Virol* 2007;81:9623–9632.
324. Meyers G, Wirblich C, Thiel HJ. Genomic and subgenomic RNAs of rabbit hemorrhagic disease virus are both protein-linked and packaged into particles. *Virology* 1991;184:677–686.
325. Meyers G, Wirblich C, Thiel HJ. Rabbit hemorrhagic disease virus–molecular cloning and nucleotide sequencing of a calicivirus genome. *Virology* 1991;184:664–676.
327. Mitra T, Sosnovtsev SV, Green KY. Mutagenesis of tyrosine 24 in the VPg protein is lethal for feline calicivirus. *J Virol* 2004;78:4931–4935.
331. Morales M, Barcena J, Ramirez MA, et al. Synthesis in vitro of rabbit hemorrhagic disease virus subgenomic RNA by internal initiation on (-) sense genomic RNA: mapping of a subgenomic promoter. *J Biol Chem* 2004;279:17013–17018.
334. Morotti RA, Kaufman SS, Fishbein TM, et al. Calicivirus infection in pediatric small intestine transplant recipients: pathological considerations. *Hum Pathol* 2004;35:1236–1240.
338. Murata T, Katsushima N, Mizuta K, et al. Prolonged norovirus shedding in infants <or=6 months of age with gastroenteritis. *Pediatr Infect Dis J* 2007; 26:46–49.
339. Nakamura K, Someya Y, Kumasaka T, et al. A norovirus protease structure provides insights into active and substrate binding site integrity. *J Virol* 2005;79:13685–13693.
340. Nakata S, Kogawa K, Numata K, et al. The epidemiology of human calicivirus/Sapporo/82/Japan. *Arch Virol Suppl* 1996;12:263–270.

342. Neill JD. Nucleotide sequence of a region of the feline calicivirus genome which encodes picornavirus-like RNA-dependent RNA polymerase, cysteine protease and 2C polypeptides. *Virus Res* 1990;17:145–160.
343. Neill JD. The subgenomic RNA of feline calicivirus is packaged into viral particles during infection. *Virus Res* 2002;87:89–93.
344. Neill JD, Mengeling WL. Further characterization of the virus-specific RNAs in feline calicivirus infected cells. *Virus Res* 1988;11:59–72.
345. Neill JD, Meyer RF, Seal BS. The capsid protein of vesicular exanthema of swine virus serotype A48: relationship to the capsid protein of other animal caliciviruses. *Virus Res* 1998;54:39–50.
346. Ng KK, Cherney MM, Vazquez AL, et al. Crystal structures of active and inactive conformations of a caliciviral RNA-dependent RNA polymerase. *J Biol Chem* 2002;277:1381–1387.
347. Ng KK, Pendas-Franco N, Rojo J, et al. Crystal structure of Norwalk virus polymerase reveals the carboxyl terminus in the active site cleft. *J Biol Chem* 2004;279:16638–16645.
348. Nilsson M, Hedlund KO, Thorhagen M, et al. Evolution of human calicivirus RNA in vivo: accumulation of mutations in the protruding P2 domain of the capsid leads to structural changes and possibly a new phenotype. *J Virol* 2003;77:13117–13124.
353. Nurminen K, Blazevic V, Huhti L, et al. Prevalence of norovirus GII-4 antibodies in Finnish children. *J Med Virol* 2011;83:525–531.
354. O'Ryan ML, Pena A, Vergara R, et al. Prospective characterization of norovirus compared with rotavirus acute diarrhea episodes in Chilean children. *Pediatr Infect Dis J* 2010;29:855–859.
357. Oehmig A, Buttner M, Weiland F, et al. Identification of a calicivirus isolate of unknown origin. *J Gen Virol* 2003;84:2837–2845.
359. Oka T, Yamamoto M, Katayama K, et al. Identification of the cleavage sites of sapovirus open reading frame 1 polyprotein. *J Gen Virol* 2006;87:3329–3338.
361. Oliver SL, Asobayire E, Dastjerdi AM, et al. Genomic characterization of the unclassified bovine enteric virus Newbury agent-1 (Newbury1) endorses a new genus in the family Caliciviridae. *Virology* 2006;350:240–250.
364. Otto PH, Clarke IN, Lambden PR, et al. Infection of calves with bovine norovirus GIII.1 strain Jena virus: an experimental model to study the pathogenesis of norovirus infection. *J Virol* 2011;85:12013–12021.
369. Parrino TA, Schreiber DS, Trier JS, et al. Clinical immunity in acute gastroenteritis caused by Norwalk agent. *N Engl J Med* 1977;297:86–89.
371. Patel MM, Widdowson MA, Glass RI, et al. Systematic literature review of role of noroviruses in sporadic gastroenteritis. *Emerg Infect Dis* 2008;14:1224–1231.
373. Perry JW, Taube S, Wobus CE. Murine norovirus-1 entry into permissive macrophages and dendritic cells is pH-independent. *Virus Res* 2009;143:125–129.
374. Perry JW, Wobus CE. Endocytosis of murine norovirus 1 into murine macrophages is dependent on dynamin II and cholesterol. *J Virol* 2010;84: 6163–6176.
375. Pfister T, Wimmer E. Polypeptide p41 of a Norwalk-like virus is a nucleic acid-independent nucleoside triphosphatase. *J Virol* 2001;75:1611–1619.
376. Phillips G, Tam CC, Conti S, et al. Community incidence of norovirus-associated infectious intestinal disease in England: improved estimates using viral load for norovirus diagnosis. *Am J Epidemiol* 2010;171:1014–1022.
377. Phillips G, Tam CC, Rodrigues LC, et al. Prevalence and characteristics of asymptomatic norovirus infection in the community in England. *Epidemiol Infect* 2010;138(10):1454–1458.
380. Practice parameter: the management of acute gastroenteritis in young children. American Academy of Pediatrics, Provisional Committee on Quality Improvement, Subcommittee on Acute Gastroenteritis [see comments]. *Pediatrics* 1996;97:424–435.
382. Prasad BV, Hardy ME, Dokland T, et al. X-ray crystallographic structure of the Norwalk virus capsid. *Science* 1999;286:287–290.
383. Prasad BV, Matson DO, Smith AW. Three-dimensional structure of calicivirus. *J Mol Biol* 1994;240:256–264.
385. Radford AD, Addie D, Belak S, et al. Feline calicivirus infection. ABCD guidelines on prevention and management. *J Feline Med Surg* 2009;11:556–564.
387. Reeck A, Kavanagh O, Estes MK, et al. Serological correlate of protection against norovirus-induced gastroenteritis. *J Infect Dis* 2010;202:1212–1218.
389. Reuter G, Krisztalovics K, Vennema H, et al. Evidence of the etiological predominance of norovirus in gastroenteritis outbreaks–emerging new-variant and recombinant noroviruses in Hungary. *J Med Virol* 2005;76:598–607.
393. Rockx B, De Wit M, Vennema H, et al. Natural history of human calicivirus infection: a prospective cohort study. *Clin Infect Dis* 2002;35:246–253.
394. Rockx BH, Bogers WM, Heeney JL, et al. Experimental norovirus infections in non-human primates. *J Med Virol* 2005;75:313–320.
395. Rockx BH, Vennema H, Hoebe CJ, et al. Association of histo-blood group antigens and susceptibility to norovirus infections. *J Infect Dis* 2005; 191:749–754.
399. Rohayem J, Robel I, Jager K, et al. Protein-primed and de novo initiation of RNA synthesis by norovirus 3Dpol. *J Virol* 2006;80:7060–7069.
401. Roos-Weil D, Ambert-Balay K, Lanternier F, et al. Impact of norovirus/sapovirus-related diarrhea in renal transplant recipients hospitalized for diarrhea. *Transplantation* 2011;92:61–69.
402. Rossignol JF, El-Gohary YM. Nitazoxanide in the treatment of viral gastroenteritis: a randomized double-blind placebo-controlled clinical trial. *Aliment Pharmacol Ther* 2006;24:1423–1430.
403. Ruvoen-Clouet N, Ganiere JP, Andre-Fontaine G, et al. Binding of rabbit hemorrhagic disease virus to antigens of the ABH histo-blood group family. *J Virol* 2000;74:11950–11954.
404. Ruzante JM, Majowicz SE, Fazil A, et al. Hospitalization and deaths for select enteric illnesses and associated sequelae in Canada, 2001–2004. *Epidemiol Infect* 2011;139:937–945.
409. Scallan E, Hoekstra RM, Angulo FJ, et al. Foodborne illness acquired in the United States–major pathogens. *Emerg Infect Dis* 2011;17:7–15.
412. Schorn R, Hohne M, Meerbach A, et al. Chronic norovirus infection after kidney transplantation: molecular evidence for immune-driven viral evolution. *Clin Infect Dis* 2010;51:307–314.
413. Schreiber DS, Blacklow NR, Trier JS. The mucosal lesion of the proximal small intestine in acute infectious nonbacterial gastroenteritis. *N Engl J Med* 1973;288:1318–1323.
420. Seitz SR, Leon JS, Schwab KJ, et al. Norovirus infectivity in humans and persistence in water. *Appl Environ Microbiol* 2011;77:6884–6888.
422. Sharp TM, Guix S, Katayama K, et al. Inhibition of cellular protein secretion by norwalk virus nonstructural protein p22 requires a mimic of an endoplasmic reticulum export signal. *PLoS One* 2010;5:e13130.
426. Shoemaker GK, van Duijn E, Crawford SE, et al. Norwalk virus assembly and stability monitored by mass spectrometry. *Mol Cell Proteomics* 2010;9:1742–1751.
427. Siddiq DM, Koo HL, Adachi JA, et al. Norovirus gastroenteritis successfully treated with nitazoxanide. *J Infect* 2011;63:394–397.
429. Simmonds P, Karakasiliotis I, Bailey D, et al. Bioinformatic and functional analysis of RNA secondary structure elements among different genera of human and animal caliciviruses. *Nucleic Acids Res* 2008;36:2530–2546.
432. Sosnovtsev S, Green KY. RNA transcripts derived from a cloned full-length copy of the feline calicivirus genome do not require VPg for infectivity. *Virology* 1995;210:383–390.
433. Sosnovtsev SV, Belliot G, Chang KO, et al. Feline calicivirus VP2 Is essential for the production of infectious virions. *J Virol* 2005;79:4012–4024.
434. Sosnovtsev SV, Belliot G, Chang KO, et al. Cleavage map and proteolytic processing of the murine norovirus nonstructural polyprotein in infected cells. *J Virol* 2006;80:7816–7831.
435. Sosnovtsev SV, Garfield M, Green KY. Processing map and essential cleavage sites of the nonstructural polyprotein encoded by ORF1 of the feline calicivirus genome. *J Virol* 2002;76:7060–7072.
436. Sosnovtsev SV, Green KY. Identification and genomic mapping of the ORF3 and VPg proteins in feline calicivirus virions. *Virology* 2000;277:193–203.
438. Sosnovtsev SV, Sosnovtseva SA, Green KY. Cleavage of the feline calicivirus capsid precursor is mediated by a virus-encoded proteinase. *J Virol* 1998;72:3051–3059.
439. Sosnovtseva SA, Sosnovtsev SV, Green KY. Mapping of the feline calicivirus proteinase responsible for autocatalytic processing of the nonstructural polyprotein and identification of a stable proteinase-polymerase precursor protein. *J Virol* 1999;73:6626–6633.
440. Souza M, Azevedo MS, Jung K, et al. Pathogenesis and immune responses in gnotobiotic calves after infection with the genogroup II.4-HS66 strain of human norovirus. *J Virol* 2008;82:1777–1786.
442. Steinhoff MC, Douglas RG Jr, Greenberg HB, et al. Bismuth subsalicylate therapy of viral gastroenteritis. *Gastroenterology* 1980;78:1495–1499.
443. Stuart AD, Brown TD. {alpha}2,6-Linked sialic acid acts as a receptor for feline calicivirus. *J Gen Virol* 2007;88:177–186.

444. Stuart AD, Brown TD. Entry of feline calicivirus is dependent on clathrin-mediated endocytosis and acidification in endosomes. *J Virol* 2006;80:7500–7509.
445. Stuart RL, Tan K, Mahar JE, et al. An outbreak of necrotizing enterocolitis associated with norovirus genotype GII.3. *Pediatr Infect Dis J* 2010;29:644–647.
446. Subba-Reddy CV, Goodfellow I, Kao CC. VPg-primed RNA synthesis of norovirus RNA-dependent RNA polymerases by using a novel cell-based assay. *J Virol* 2011;85:13027–13037.
448. Sugieda M, Nagaoka H, Kakishima Y, et al. Detection of Norwalk-like virus genes in the caecum contents of pigs. *Arch Virol* 1998;143:1215–1221.
452. Tacket CO, Sztein MB, Losonsky GA, et al. Humoral, mucosal, and cellular immune responses to oral Norwalk virus-like particles in volunteers. *Clin Immunol* 2003;108:241–247.
453. Takanashi S, Hashira S, Matsunaga T, et al. Detection, genetic characterization, and quantification of norovirus RNA from sera of children with gastroenteritis. *J Clin Virol* 2009;44:161–163.
455. Tamura M, Natori K, Kobayashi M, et al. Genogroup II noroviruses efficiently bind to heparan sulfate proteoglycan associated with the cellular membrane. *J Virol* 2004;78:3817–3826.
457. Tan M, Fang PA, Xia M, et al. Terminal modifications of norovirus P domain resulted in a new type of subviral particles, the small P particles. *Virology* 2011;410:345–352.
458. Tan M, Hegde RS, Jiang X. The P domain of norovirus capsid protein forms dimer and binds to histo-blood group antigen receptors. *J Virol* 2004;78:6233–6242.
459. Tan M, Huang P, Meller J, et al. Mutations within the P2 domain of norovirus capsid affect binding to human histo-blood group antigens: evidence for a binding pocket. *J Virol* 2003;77:12562–12571.
460. Tan M, Huang P, Xia M, et al. Norovirus P particle, a novel platform for vaccine development and antibody production. *J Virol* 2011;85: 753–764.
464. Tan M, Xia M, Cao S, et al. Elucidation of strain-specific interaction of a GII-4 norovirus with HBGA receptors by site-directed mutagenesis study. *Virology* 2008;379:324–334.
466. Teunis PF, Moe CL, Liu P, et al. Norwalk virus: how infectious is it? *J Med Virol* 2008;80:1468–1476.
468. Thornhill TS, Wyatt RG, Kalica AR, et al. Detection by immune electron microscopy of 26- to 27-nm viruslike particles associated with two family outbreaks of gastroenteritis. *J Infect Dis* 1977;135:20–27.
472. Troeger H, Loddenkemper C, Schneider T, et al. Structural and functional changes of the duodenum in human norovirus infection. *Gut* 2009;58:1070–1077.
474. Tsuge M, Goto S, Kato F, et al. Elevation of serum transaminases with norovirus infection. *Clin Pediatr (Phila)* 2010;49:574–578.
476. Turcios RM, Widdowson MA, Sulka AC, et al. Reevaluation of epidemiological criteria for identifying outbreaks of acute gastroenteritis due to norovirus: United States, 1998–2000. *Clin Infect Dis* 2006;42:964–969.
477. Updated norovirus outbreak management and disease prevention guidelines. *MMWR Recomm Rep* 2011;60:1–20.
478. van Asten L, Siebenga J, van den Wijngaard C, et al. Unspecified gastroenteritis illness and deaths in the elderly associated with norovirus epidemics. *Epidemiology* 2011;22:336–343.
479. Vazquez AL, Martin Alonso JM, Casais R, et al. Expression of enzymatically active rabbit hemorrhagic disease virus RNA- dependent RNA polymerase in Escherichia coli. *J Virol* 1998;72:2999–3004.
484. Vinje J, Vennema H, Maunula L, et al. International collaborative study to compare reverse transcriptase PCR assays for detection and genotyping of noroviruses. *J Clin Microbiol* 2003;41:1423–1433.
486. Vogel L. Hand sanitizers may increase norovirus risk. *CMAJ* 2011; 183:E799–E800.
487. Wang J, Jiang X, Madore HP, et al. Sequence diversity of small, round-structured viruses in the Norwalk virus group. *J Virol* 1994;68: 5982–5990.
489. Ward VK, McCormick CJ, Clarke IN, et al. Recovery of infectious murine norovirus using pol II-driven expression of full-length cDNA. *Proc Natl Acad Sci U S A* 2007;104:11050–11055.
492. Wei C, Farkas T, Sestak K, et al. Recovery of infectious virus by transfection of in vitro-generated RNA from tulane calicivirus cDNA. *J Virol* 2008;82:11429–11436.
493. Wei L, Huhn JS, Mory A, et al. Proteinase-polymerase precursor as the active form of feline calicivirus RNA-dependent RNA polymerase. *J Virol* 2001;75:1211–1219.
497. White LJ, Ball JM, Hardy ME, et al. Attachment and entry of recombinant Norwalk virus capsids to cultured human and animal cell lines. *J Virol* 1996;70:6589–6597.
498. White LJ, Hardy ME, Estes MK. Biochemical characterization of a smaller form of recombinant Norwalk virus capsids assembled in insect cells. *J Virol* 1997;71:8066–8072.
501. Widdowson MA, Sulka A, Bulens SN, et al. Norovirus and foodborne disease, United States, 1991–2000. *Emerg Infect Dis* 2005;11:95–102.
502. Widerlite L, Trier JS, Blacklow NR, et al. Structure of the gastric mucosa in acute infectious bacterial gastroenteritis. *Gastroenterology* 1975; 68:425–430.
503. Willcocks MM, Carter MJ, Roberts LO. Cleavage of eukaryotic initiation factor eIF4G and inhibition of host-cell protein synthesis during feline calicivirus infection. *J Gen Virol* 2004;85:1125–1130.
504. Wingfield T, Gallimore CI, Xerry J, et al. Chronic norovirus infection in an HIV-positive patient with persistent diarrhoea: a novel cause. *J Clin Virol* 2010;49:219–222.
506. Wirblich C, Thiel HJ, Meyers G. Genetic map of the calicivirus rabbit hemorrhagic disease virus as deduced from in vitro translation studies. *J Virol* 1996;70:7974–7983.
507. Wobus CE, Karst SM, Thackray LB, et al. Replication of Norovirus in cell culture reveals a tropism for dendritic cells and macrophages. *PLoS Biol* 2004;2:e432.
511. Wyatt RG, Dolin R, Blacklow NR, et al. Comparison of three agents of acute infectious nonbacterial gastroenteritis by cross-challenge in volunteers. *J Infect Dis* 1974;129:709–714.
517. Zamyatkin DF, Parra F, Alonso JM, et al. Structural insights into mechanisms of catalysis and inhibition in Norwalk virus polymerase. *J Biol Chem* 2008;283:7705–7712.
518. Zeitler CE, Estes MK, Venkataram Prasad BV. X-ray crystallographic structure of the Norwalk virus protease at 1.5-A resolution. *J Virol* 2006; 80:5050–5058.
521. Zheng DP, Widdowson MA, Glass RI, et al. Molecular epidemiology of genogroup II-genotype 4 noroviruses in the United States between 1994 and 2006. *J Clin Microbiol* 2010;48:168–177.
522. Zintz C, Bok K, Parada E, et al. Prevalence and genetic characterization of caliciviruses among children hospitalized for acute gastroenteritis in the United States. *Infect Genet Evol* 2005;5:281–290.

CHAPTER 21

Ernesto Méndez* • Carlos F. Arias

Astroviruses

The family *Astroviridae* includes human and animal astroviruses that show icosahedral morphology; they are nonenveloped and their genome is composed of plus-sense, single-stranded RNA (ssRNA), with three open-reading frames, whose organization distinguishes them from other virus families.

Astroviruses (AstV) have been isolated from a variety of animal species. In most mammals, astrovirus infections are associated with gastroenteritis. In particular, human astroviruses (HAstV) have been found to be the second or third most common cause of viral diarrhea in young children and cause of sporadic gastroenteritis outbreaks. Avian AstV, on the other hand, have been linked with more severe intestinal and extraintestinal manifestations of disease.

*Deceased.

HISTORY

The term *astrovirus* was coined by Madeley and Cosgrove in 1975 to describe small, round viruses with a distinctive five- or six-pointed, star-like appearance (astron, *star* in Greek) of about 28 to 30 nm in diameter.[86] They were observed by direct electron microscopy (EM) in the stools of infants hospitalized with diarrhea and in outbreaks of gastroenteritis in newborn nurseries (Fig. 21.1). Subsequently, viral particles of similar size and morphology were identified by EM in association with gastroenteritis in a wide variety of young mammals and birds.

An important milestone was achieved in 1981 when Lee and Kurtz reported the isolation and passage of HAstV in primary cell cultures.[82] This achievement led to the recognition of five HAstV serotypes in 1984,[79] development of an enzyme immunoassay (EIA) to detect viral antigen in the late 1980s,[60] and confirmation of its medical importance.[61] The molecular characterization of astrovirus isolates subsequently permitted the recognition of 8 serotypes of HAstV and the design of molecular probes for use as diagnostic tools. Metagenomic approaches have allowed the identification of novel AstV from humans and animal species in recent years.[16,33,35,115] The efficient propagation of HAstV in cell lines[147] and of turkey isolates in animal models.[72] has further advanced our knowledge of the molecular and structural biology, as well as of pathogenesis of these viruses.

CLASSIFICATION

The general organization of the astrovirus genome places the open reading frames (ORF) encoding the nonstructural proteins at the 5′ end, and the ORF encoding the structural proteins at the 3′ end. Distinctive features of this family include the morphology of viruses,[116] the lack of an RNA-helicase domain encoded in the genome, and the usage of a ribosomal frameshifting mechanism to translate the RNA-dependent RNA polymerase (RdRp).[65]

Astroviruses were originally classified into genera and species based only on the host of origin; however, recent characterization of novel AstV has shown that isolates from different animal species can be genetically similar, while genetically

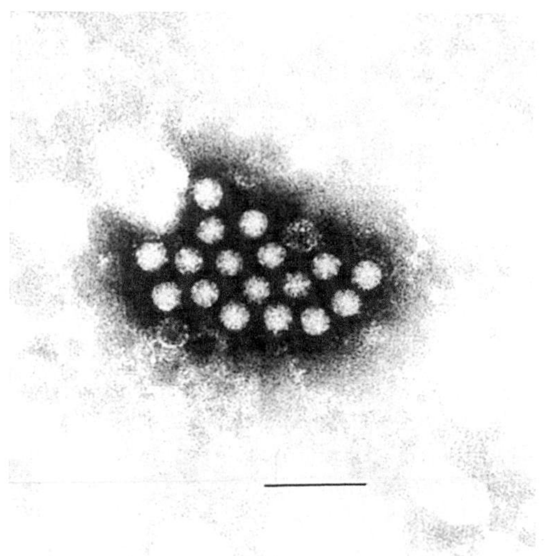

FIGURE 21.1. Electron micrograph of human astrovirus in a fecal specimen. Bar = 100 nm. (Courtesy of T. W. Lee and J. B. Kurtz.)

diverse viruses can be isolated from the same animal species.[69,85,152] These findings have led to a proposed new classification scheme based on the amino acid sequence of ORF2 (Astroviruses Study Group, 9th Report ICTV, 2010),[17] which encodes the capsid polyprotein and represents the most variable region of the genome (see below). Two genera are distinguished within the *Astroviridae* family: *Mamastrovirus* and *Avastrovirus* (Fig. 21.2). Viruses belonging to the genus *Mamastrovirus* include isolates from a number of mammals, including humans, pigs (PAstV), cats (FeAstV), minks (MAstV), sheep (OAstV), calfs (BoAstV), dogs (CaAstV), bats (BAstV), rats (RAstV), deer (CcAstV), and marine mammals, such as sea lions (CSlAstV) and bottlenose dolphins (BdAstV), among others. This genus includes two genogroups, GI and GII, with 10 and 9 genotype species, respectively. Both genogroups comprise viruses from human and animal origin. Of note, recently identified human viruses are very similar to animal isolates, such as mink and sheep,[69] among others. HAstV previously classified within one species that comprised serotypes 1 to 8 (based on their reactivity to hyperimmune sera; HAstV-1 to -8) are now included in the proposed genotype G1 of genogroup I. The genetic diversity found among pig,[85] bat,[152] and human[69] isolates places them into highly divergent groups, suggesting that they have different ancestors that probably emerged during interspecies transmission.[85]

Viruses from the genus *Avastrovirus* include isolates from turkeys (TAstV), ducks (DAstV), chicken (CAstV), and guinea fowl. This genus includes two proposed species in genogroup GI (GIA, GIB) and one in genogroup II (GIIA). Similarly to canonical HAstV, members of some of these species can be distinguished by serology, indicating the existence of viral serotypes in some, such as in TAstV-2 and ANV.[132,134] In general, avastroviruses show higher diversity than mamastroviruses.

VIRION STRUCTURE AND COMPOSITION

Virion Structure

Ultrastructural analysis by EM of human viruses propagated in cell culture in the presence of trypsin revealed icosahedral particles of 41 nm, with spikes protruding from the surface.[116] The star-like form of the particles was observed only after alkaline treatment. Recent studies by cryo-EM and image processing of trypsin-treated and untreated HAstV particles confirmed the spiked icosahedral structure of virions (Fig. 21.3) (K. Dryden et al.,

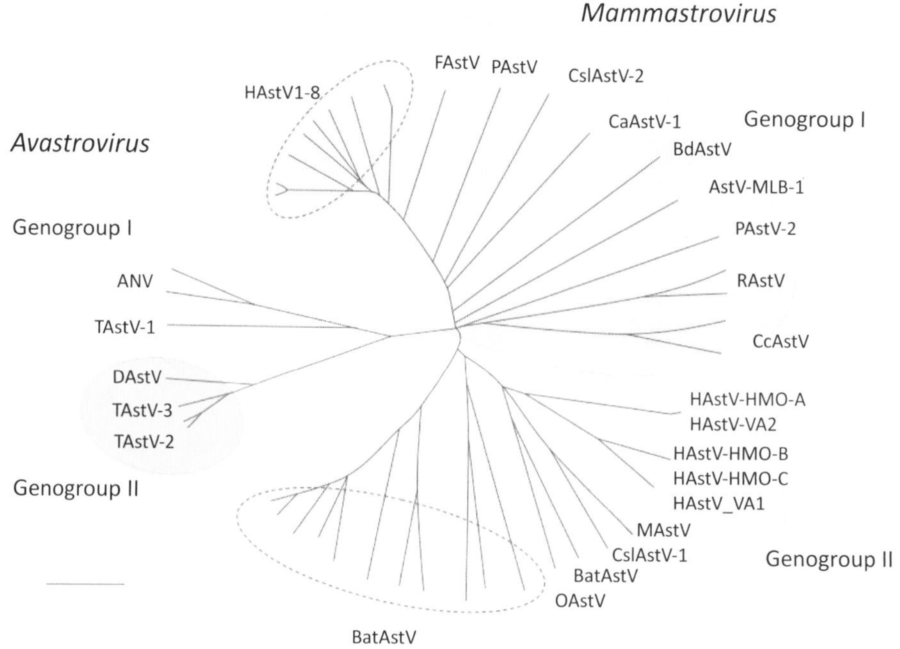

FIGURE 21.2. The *Astroviridae* family includes two genera with two genogroups each. Virus species are classified based on the ORF2 amino acid sequence distances. (Classification proposed by the Astroviruses Study Group, 9th Report ICTV, 2010.[17])

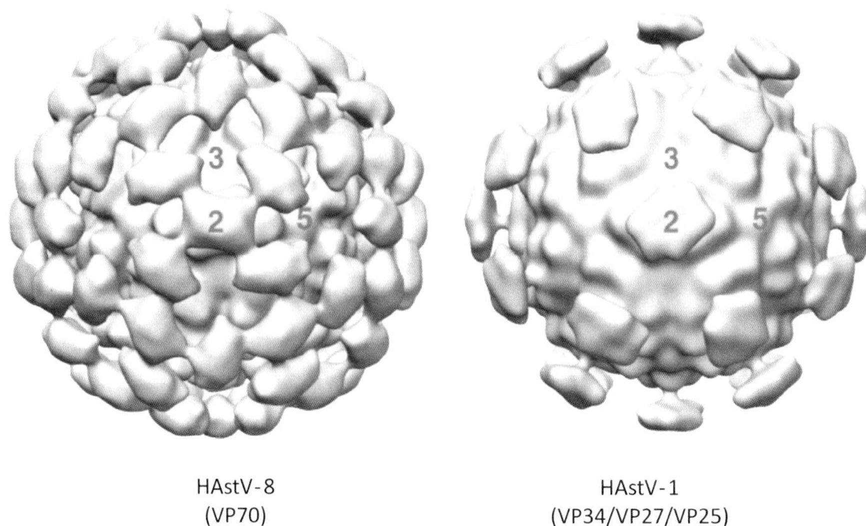

FIGURE 21.3. Three-dimensional reconstruction of HAstV obtained by cryo-electron microscopy. Purified particles of HAstV-8 and HAstV-1 by cesium chloride gradients, untreated or treated with trypsin, respectively. Protein composition is indicated. Images were obtained at 23–25 Å of resolution. (Courtesy of K. Dryden, University of Virginia.)

unpublished results). Remarkable differences are observed between the two types of particles. The untreated virus, 46 nm in diameter, contains 180 copies of a single protein of 70 kd arranged in a T = 3 icosahedral symmetry. Two kinds of spikes, localized at two- and fivefold vertices, can be observed in these particles. Two protein layers can be distinguished. The internal layer forms the capsid core and is almost identical to that of treated particles, at the highest resolution reached (23–25 Å); however, the distal layer that forms the spikes shows dramatic changes after trypsin treatment. This treatment results in the cleavage of the 70-kd protein into three polypeptides that is required for virus infectivity (see below). The main difference between the two types of particles is the number of spikes observed, more likely due to disordering of the projections located around the fivefold vertices in the trypsin-treated virions (K. Dryden et al., personal communication).

Virion Composition

Astrovirus particles are formed by the viral genome surrounded by an icosahedral capsid formed by a single protein of 70 to 90 kd, or by at least three proteins in the range of 25 to 34 kd, depending on the extent of proteolytic processing of the virion.[12,93,119] Extracellular particles, released from HAstV-8 infected cells, are formed by protein VP70, which results from the intracellular processing of VP90, the full-length primary protein product encoded in ORF2[94] (see below). Fully infectious particles obtained by exhaustive treatment of the virus with trypsin are constituted by three proteins, in the range of 32–34, 27–29, and 25–26 kd, depending on the virus strain, with the last two proteins overlapping in sequence.[93,119] Thus, proteins of different size (between 24 and 90 kd), probably representing final and intermediate cleavage products, can be found in particles of HAstV.[12] The size of some of the proteins identified in animal viruses is similar to that of proteins found in human strains; thus, PAstV contains proteins of 31, 30, and 36 kd,[125] and OAstV contains two proteins of approximately 33 kd[58]; however, PAstV also contains proteins of 39 and 13 kd,[125] not usually detected in mature HAstV particles. An isolated report indicates that HAstV particles may contain a small protein of 5.2 kd, but its nature was not established.[78]

In addition to proteins derived from ORF2, proteins coded by ORF1a have been suggested to be present in viral particles, since antibodies to purified HAstV-1 virions recognize a recombinant protein containing amino acids 757 to 899 of nsp1a.[89]

GENOME STRUCTURE AND ORGANIZATION

Astroviruses have an ssRNA genome of positive polarity [ssRNA(+)] (Fig. 21.4) that varies in length from 6.17 kb for the human strain MLB-1[33] to 7.72 kb for DAstV-2,[37]

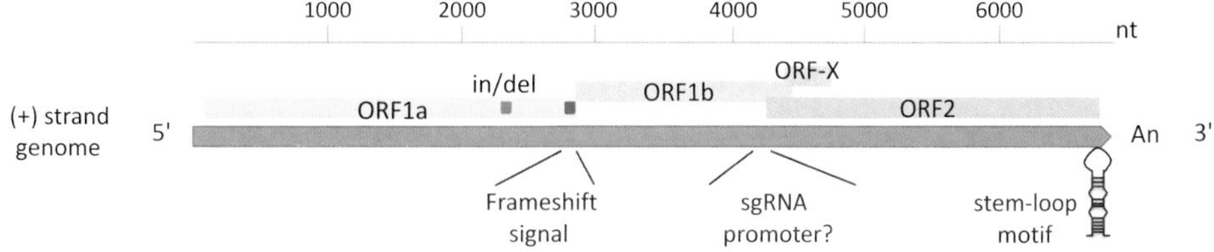

FIGURE 21.4. Genome organization of human astrovirus. The genomic RNA, approximately 6.8 kb, contains three recognized open reading frames (ORF1a, ORF1b, and ORF2). ORF-X has been proposed as functional, given its conservation among AstVs. The genome contains three elements conserved among all members of the family: the frameshift signal (*blue square*), the sequence upstream of ORF2 that putatively acts as promoter for synthesis of the subgenomic (sg) RNA, and the stem-loop at the ORF2 3′ end. Also shown are the insertion/deletion (In/del) region (*red square*) and the presence of a poly(A) tail at the 3′ end.

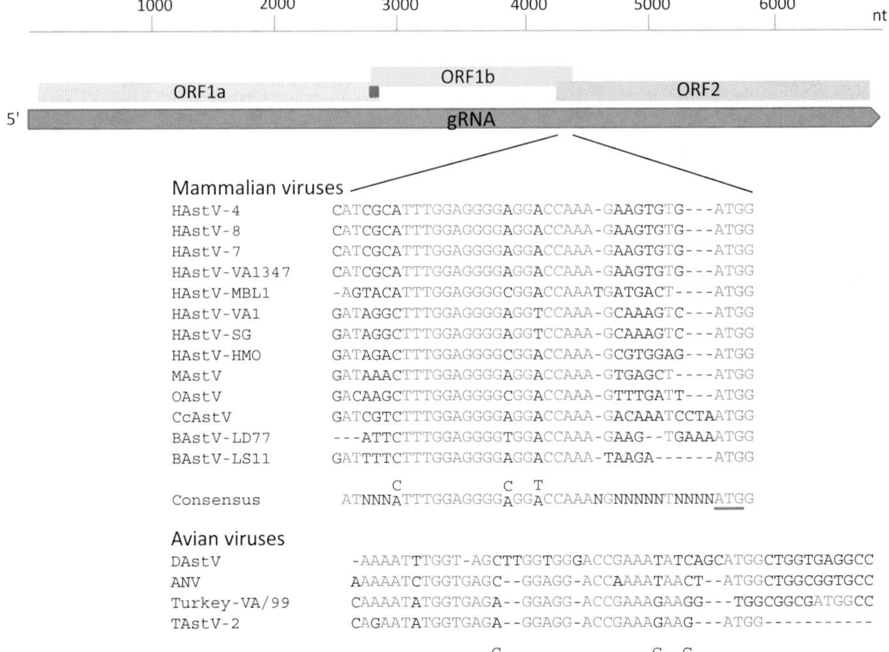

FIGURE 21.5. Conserved sequences upstream of the ORF2 initiation codon that might represent the promoter for sgRNA synthesis. Red letters indicate those completely conserved among viruses of the same genus; the ORF2 initiation codon is underlined. Viruses within each genus have a different consensus sequence.

excluding the poly(A) tail at the 3 end (e-Table 21.1 and e-Fig. 21.1). The RNA extracted from AstV particles, as well as RNA transcribed from a full-length genomic copy of complementary DNA (cDNA) clone, are able to initiate a productive infection in cultured cells,[42] although with different efficiencies. The viral genome includes 5′ and 3′ untranslated regions (UTRs), and three ORFs of variable length in different isolates (e-Table 21.1). The two ORFs located towards the 5′ end of the genome, designated ORF1a and ORF1b, encode nonstructural proteins that are presumed to be involved in transcription and replication of the virus genome, based on the sequence motifs they contain (see below). Variation of the ORF1a length in HAstV is mainly due to insertions or deletions (in/del regions) present near the 3′ end of ORF1a.[55,144] The third ORF, found at the 3′ end of the genome and designated ORF2, encodes the capsid polyprotein. ORF1a and ORF1b overlap in 10 to 148 nucleotides (nt) in the genome of mammalian viruses, and between 10 and 45 nt in avian viruses. The overlapping region contains an essential signal for translation of the viral RNA polymerase (encoded in ORF1b) through a frameshift mechanism[65] (see below).

Two positive-sense RNA species have been identified in astrovirus-infected cells: the full-length genomic RNA (gRNA), and a subgenomic RNA (sgRNA) of ~2.4 kb[104] (see below, Transcription/Replication section). Based on the transcription initiation site determined for the sgRNA in HAstV-1 and HAstV-2,[103,146] ORF1b and ORF2 overlap in 8 nt; however, the length of this overlapping may vary, and it is not present in DAstV; rather, it is 24 nt apart in this virus.[37] The highly conserved sequence around the ORF2 start codon has been suggested to be part of the promoter for synthesis of the sgRNA,[68] as described for alphaviruses; however, this region differs in length and sequence between mammalian and avian viruses (Fig. 21.5). This conserved sequence shows partial identity with the 5′ end of the gRNA,[68] suggesting that it has an important role for the synthesis of both gRNA and sgRNA. Analysis of recombinant AstV isolated from different species has identified this region as a hot spot for recombination.[132,140,148] Of note, the terminal 19 nt of ORF2 and the adjacent 3′ -UTR are highly conserved among most

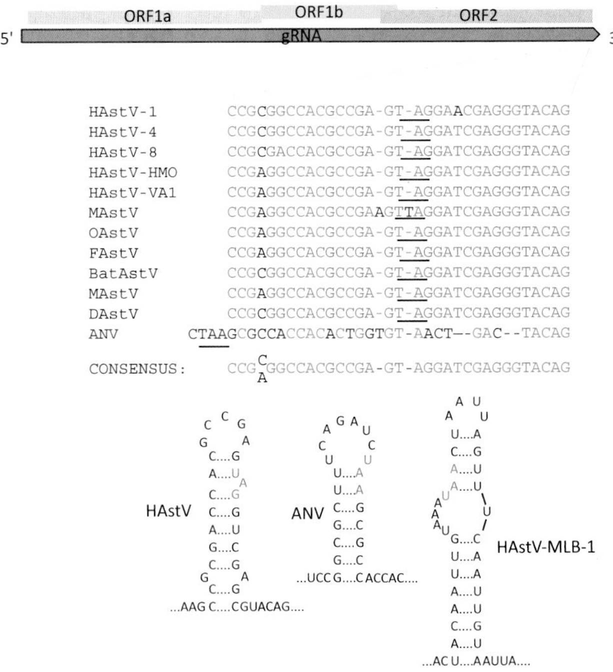

FIGURE 21.6. Conserved sequence and secondary structure at the 3′ end of the ORF2 sequence. The relative position of these sequences is indicated in the upper diagram. Red letters on the sequence comparison indicate conserved nucleotides. The stop codon is underlined in the sequence and in red letters in the stem-loop structures. Although some strains lack this sequence conservation, such as ANV and HAstV-MLB1, a stem-loop structure in this region is also predicted.

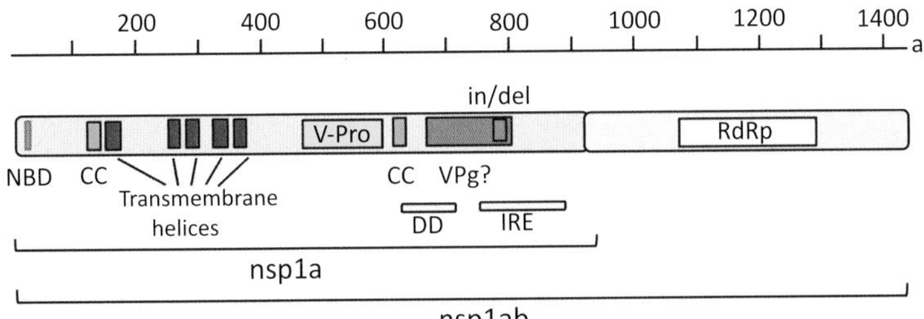

FIGURE 21.7. Nonstructural proteins predicted from the nucleotide sequence of ORF1a and ORF1b. NBM, nucleotide binding motif; CC, coiled-coil; v-Pro, viral protease; VPg, viral protein attached to the genome; in/del, insertion/deletion; DD, putative death domain; IRE, immune reactive epitope; RdRp, RNA-dependent RNA polymerase.

AstV, and similarities have been observed in the sequence and folding of the 3′ -UTR of viruses from other families, such as avian infectious bronchitis virus (a coronavirus), a dog norovirus, and equine rhinovirus serotype 2 (a picornavirus),[85,101] suggesting that it is relevant for astrovirus genome replication (Fig. 21.6).

ORF1a and ORF1b

The polypeptide encoded by ORF1a (nsp1a) is 874 to 936 amino acids (aa) in length in most mammalian viruses, although it can be as short as 787 in a human isolate and can reach 1,240 in avian viruses (e-Table 21.1). Five to six helical transmembrane motifs followed by a viral serine protease motif (v-Pro) are predicted in nsp1a[68] (Fig. 21.7). The v-Pro has features consistent with trypsin-like proteases, with a serine at the third catalytic amino acid residue.[131] A viral protein genome-linked (VPg) encoded downstream of the protease motif has also been predicted based on its similarity with the VPg of calicivirus[3]; however, its synthesis in astrovirus-infected cells has not been investigated. Two predicted coiled-coil structures are present in nsp1a, one just upstream of the first helical transmembrane motif, and the second one downstream of the protease motif, suggesting that some protein products of nsp1a might form oligomers.[68] One region containing insertion/deletions (in/del), located downstream of the VPg motif, was related to the efficiency of HAstV to synthesize viral RNA species and to adaptation to cultured cells[55,144]; however, it is not known whether the RNA sequence or the encoded protein is involved in modulating those events. ORF1b encodes a polypeptide of 515 to 539 aa that contains motifs of an RdRp, which are similar to RdRp of picornaviruses, caliciviruses, and certain plant viruses.[3,65]

Regions that could potentially encode an RNA helicase and a methyltransferase have not been identified in the astrovirus genome.[65] Given the putative existence of a VPg, the absence of a methyltransferase could be understandable; however, the absence of an RNA helicase domain is unusual for a plus-strand RNA virus with a genome length of more than 6,000 nt, like astrovirus.[65] The amino terminus of nsp1a shows similarity with an NTP binding motif of some helicases,[3] but lacks other motifs, such as the substrate binding and NTP hydrolysis domains present in these enzymes.[135]

ORF2

The largest sequence variability in the astrovirus genome is found in ORF2, which codes for the virus structural polyprotein. This polypeptide varies from 672 to 851 aa in length in TastV-1 and a porcine strain, respectively. In general, the ORF2 of avian viruses codes for shorter polyproteins (e-Table 21.1). The N-terminal half of the polyprotein is more conserved than the C-terminal domain, encompasses a region of basic character that is conserved among astroviruses,[67,142] and is thought to interact with the genomic RNA in the virion.[43] On the other hand, the C-terminal half of the protein shows considerable sequence variability among astroviruses isolated from different species, even among different isolates from the same animal species; the sequence of this region defines the serotypes in HAstV (Fig. 21.8). A delimited region with abundant insertion or deletions among different astroviruses is also present in the carboxy half of the capsid protein.[142] The acidic character of a small portion of the protein, located close to the carboxy terminus (residues 649 to 702 for HAstV-8), is highly conserved among all members of the *Astroviridae* family.[92] The last five amino acid residues at the C-terminal end

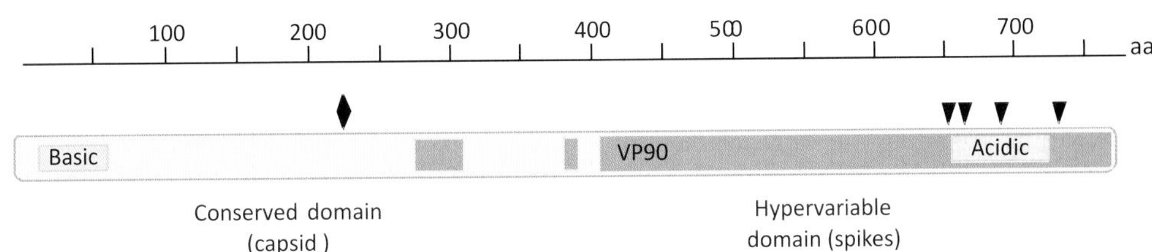

FIGURE 21.8. Features of the structural protein. The primary ORF2 product (named VP90 in HAstV-8), contains two domains that can be distinguished by their degree of conservation: the N-terminal domain is highly conserved and forms the core of the capsid, while the hypervariable C-terminal domain forms the spikes of the virus particle. VP90 contains basic and acidic regions that are highly conserved among all AstVs characterized. The diamond in the conserved domain indicates a lethal mutation identified in HAstV-1 and the black arrows indicate motifs recognized by caspases, important for virus maturation and cell egress.

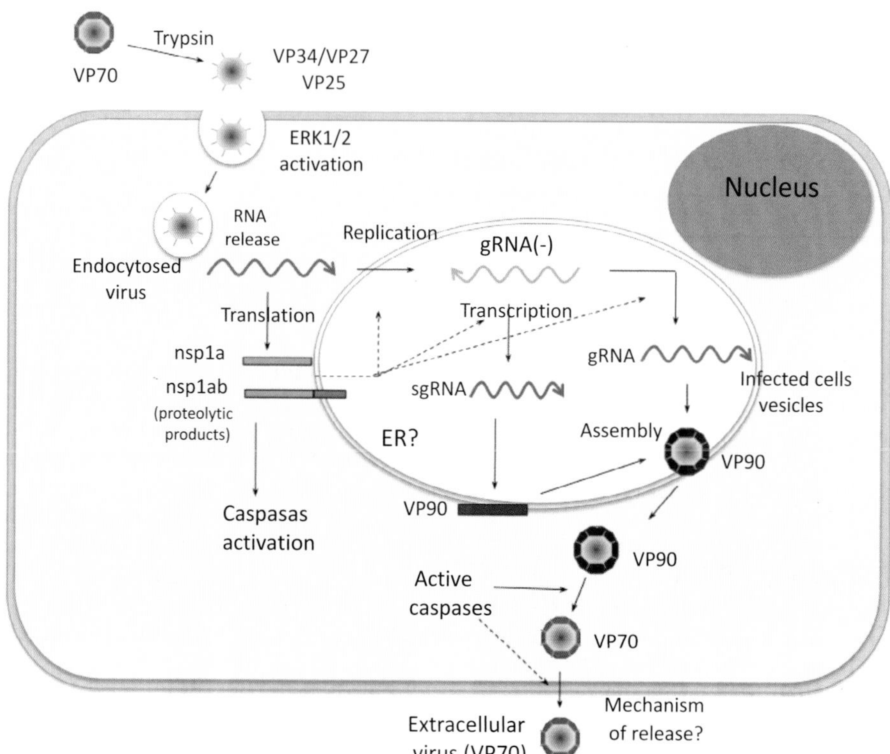

FIGURE 21.9. Replication cycle of HAstV. See details in the text.

are conserved, particularly among human and some other mammalian strains.

The conserved domain of the structural protein forms the capsid core of the particle, whereas the hypervariable C-terminal domain forms the spikes of the virion; thus, this last domain is predicted to participate in the early interactions of the virus with the host cell.[76]

An alternative ORF (named ORF-X) of 91 to 122 codons overlapping ORF2 in a +1 reading frame has been described in all HAstV and some other mammalian viruses[36] (Fig. 21.4). Its initiation codon, usually located 41–50 nt downstream of the ORF2 AUG, is placed in a better Kozak's consensus sequence than that of ORF2, and might be translated through a leaky scanning mechanism. It remains to be determined whether ORF-X is actually translated and, if it is, its significance for virus replication.

STAGES OF REPLICATION

Attachment and Entry

Studies directed toward understanding the early interactions of astroviruses with their host cells have been limited; however, a general view of the replication cycle can be depicted (Fig. 21.9). Cell receptor molecules for these viruses have not been identified. Different HAstV strains show different tropism in cultured cells[19]; thus, it is likely that their initial interactions with the host cells might be different.

The infectivity of human astroviruses is greatly enhanced (3 to 5 logs) by, and probably requires, the treatment of the virus particles with trypsin.[8,93,119] Although the proteolytic pathway of VP70 processing present in the virion has been elucidated for HAstV-8,[93] the mechanism by which this treatment enhances virus infectivity is still unknown. Trypsin cleavage of the precursor polyprotein induces drastic structural changes in the particles[8] (Fig. 21.3) and the generation in HAstV-8 of three final products: VP34, VP25, and VP27 (see details in the Protein Synthesis and Processing section). VP34 represents the conserved domain and forms the capsid core, while both VP25 and VP27 form the spikes on the virion surface. In spite of its high variability, VP25 contains two conserved structural motifs that have been suggested to be involved in the interaction of the virus with the host cell, one of which includes residues Lys455, Ser554, Thr575, and Glu610, predicted to interact with oligosaccharide moieties that could act as cell receptors or co-receptors (Fig. 21.10) (Dr. Y.J. Tao, unpublished data). Antibodies that recognize the spike proteins VP25 and VP27 neutralize virus infectivity,[9,119] probably by blocking virus binding.

Early studies on HAstV entry in HEK-293 Graham cells using endocytosis-blocking agents (ammonium chloride, methylamine, and dansylcadaverine), as well as ultrastructural analysis, indicated that an endocytic, coated pit–dependent pathway is used by the virus to enter cells.[30] Recently, a clathrin-dependent endocytosis was confirmed to be a functional pathway for the entry of HAstV-8 into Caco-2 cells (unpublished results).

The interaction of HAstV with the host cell provokes activation of the ERK1/2 signaling pathway within the first 15 minutes after virus attachment.[107] Although the mechanism for this activation is unknown, it was independent of virus replication, suggesting that this pathway is triggered during virus binding or entry into the cell. Accordingly, ERK1/2 seems to be required at early times to establish a productive infection,

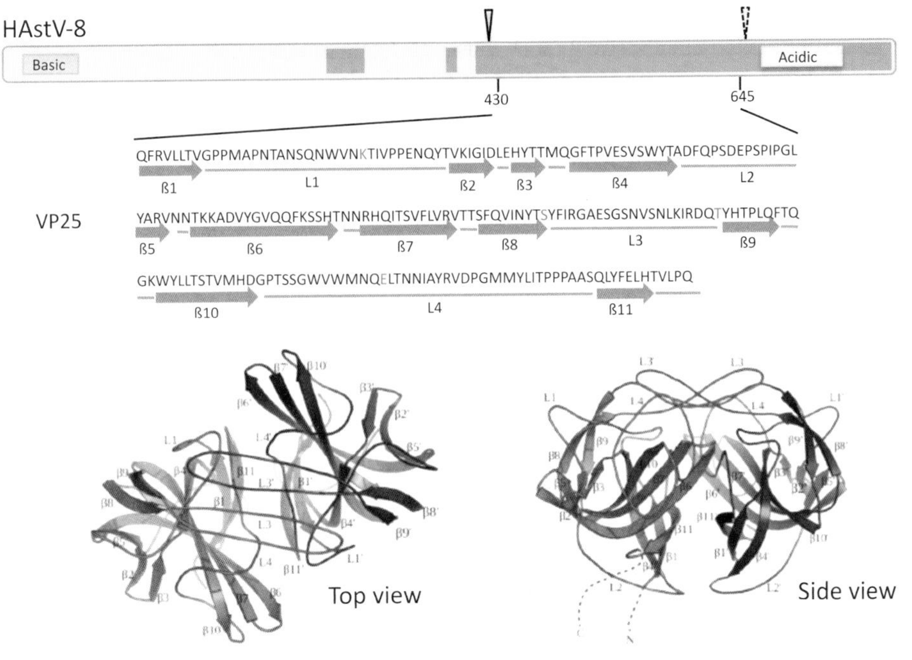

FIGURE 21.10. Three-dimensional structure of the spike protein VP25. The hypervariable region of HAstV-8 VP90, including residues 430 to 645, crystalized to 1.8 Å resolution as a dimer. The upper diagram shows the relative position of the crystalized protein; the cleavage carried out by trypsin is indicated (*arrowheads*, as in Fig. 21.15). Amino acid residues Lys455, Ser554, Thr575, and Glu610 (red in the sequence) are strictly conserved in all eight HAstV serotypes, and have been proposed as potentially interacting with cell surface carbohydrate motifs during the early virus–cell interactions. Top and side views of the spike are shown. (Courtesy of Dr. Y. J. Tao, Rice University.)

since inhibitors of this kinase blocked synthesis of viral proteins and RNA and, consequently, reduced virus yield. HAstV also induce an increase in the epithelial barrier permeability that is independent of virus replication, apparently due to an interaction between the capsid protein and the cell surface.[105] It has been suggested that HAstV could trigger tight junction instability to reach putative receptors present in the basolateral membrane; however, the fact that the increase in permeability is observed after at least 16 hours of addition of the virus suggests that more than a requirement for infection, it is a consequence of the cellular transduction signal pathways induced by the virus.

Uncoating

The mechanism through which the viral genomic RNA is released from the infecting virus particle into the cytoplasm for translation, the cell site where it occurs, and the cellular and viral factors involved in this event are unknown.

Translation

No detectable changes in cellular protein synthesis are observed upon HAstV infection. As do most cellular mRNAs, astroviral RNA contains a polyA tail at the 3′ end, but the presence of a cap structure at its 5′ end has not been described. Since a VPg has been suggested to be encoded in astrovirus ORF1a,[3] this protein could modulate the translation of viral mRNAs by interacting with translation initiation factors, as has been described for other viruses, such as calicivirus.[23,29]

Nonstructural Polyproteins Synthesis and Processing

After uncoating, the gRNA is translated into nonstructural proteins that are produced as polyprotein precursors and subsequently proteolytically processed into smaller proteins. ORF1a directs the synthesis of protein nsp1a (of about 100 kd), whereas protein nsp1ab (160 kd) is derived from both ORF1a and ORF1b, through a frameshift mechanism of translation (see below). Proteins nsp1a and nsp1ab are apparently processed co-translationally at their amino terminus, so that the expected full-length proteins are not, or very rarely, observed in HAstV-infected cells (Fig. 21.11). Information regarding processing of the nonstructural polyproteins has been obtained by *in vitro* translation, transient expression of cDNA clones, and analysis of HAstV-infected cells, using antibodies to different regions of nsp1a and nsp1ab.[41,45,95,145] No specific processing of nsp1a and nsp1ab were observed by *in vitro* translation of cDNA-derived transcripts,[45] suggesting a requirement for cellular factors.

In HAstV-1-infected Caco-2 cells, Willcocks et al.[145] detected proteins of 74, 34, 20, 6.5, and 5.5 kd with antibodies raised to the predicted C-terminal 298 aa of nsp1a. Proteins of 20 and 74 kd—in addition to products of 88, 27, and 19 kd—were also detected in Caco-2 cells infected with an HAstV-8 strain using antibodies to several regions of nsp1a.[95] The 19- and 20-kd proteins likely represent the most N-terminal products of nsp1a, apparently cleaved out by a cellular protease, probably a signalase, because it is produced by *in vitro* translation experiments only in the presence of microsomes,[91] it occurs co-translationally,[41,95] and it is independent of the v-Pro activity.[41] The 27-kd protein represents the v-Pro and probably spans from around amino acid residue 410 to 654 of nsp1a.[41] Proteins of 160, 75, and 38 to 40 kd, and phosphorylated forms of 21 to 27 kd were also detected with antibodies to a synthetic peptide that comprises aa residues 778 to 792 of nsp1a.[54]

Translation of the RdRp occurs through a ribosomal-1 frameshift mechanism in the overlapping region between ORF1a and ORF1b. The signal that modulates this event has two key features, conserved among all astroviruses: a heptameric sequence (AAAAAAC) and the potential to form a downstream stem-loop structure[18] (Fig. 21.12). Translation of heterologous proteins, with the HAstV frameshift signal included, revealed that its efficiency varies between

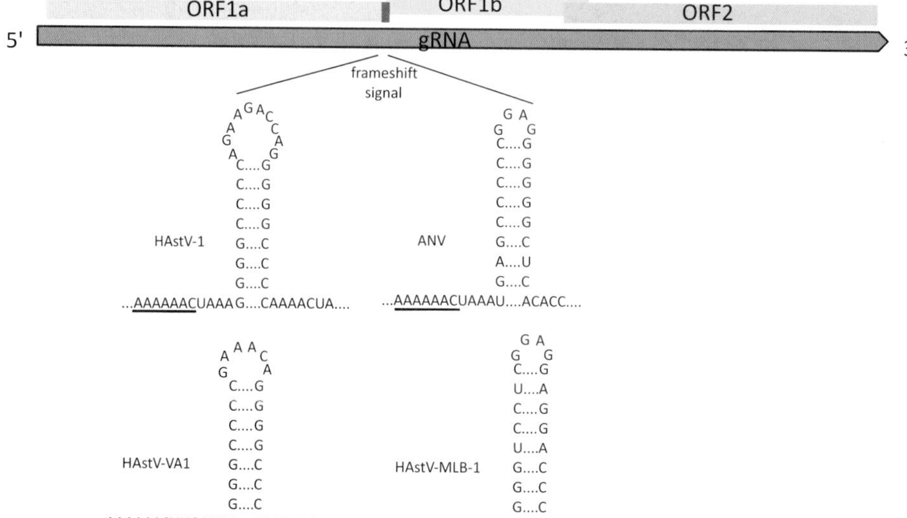

FIGURE 21.11. The frameshift signal (fss) of astroviruses is composed by a slippery sequence (*underlined*) and a stem-loop structure. The length and sequence of the loop and of the region between the slippery motif and stem-loop structure are not important for its function,[18] as seen for the viruses shown.

7% and 28%, depending on the system in which it was evaluated[84]; however, the efficiency of the frameshift has not been determined in HAstV-infected cells. Antibodies raised to recombinant proteins containing the RdRp motif identified a protein of 57 kd as the final product in Caco-2 cells infected with an HAstV-8 strain.[95]

In summary, proteins of 27, 20, 19, 6.5, and 5.5 kd, as well as the phosphorylated 21 to 27 kd polypeptides, seem to represent the final processing products of polyprotein nsp1a, whereas a 57 to 59 kd protein represents the mature protein derived from ORF1b. The proteins observed of 145, 88, 85, 75, and 34 kd most likely represent intermediate products of the nonstructural protein processing (Fig. 21.11). With exception of the cleavage that releases the 20 kd most amino-terminal polypeptide, all other cleavages at nsp1a and nsp1ab polyproteins are believed to depend on the v-Pro activity, although only those identified at around amino acid residues 410 and 655 of nsp1a have been confirmed.[41] Crystal analysis of the v-Pro domain (Fig. 21.13) showed that the enzyme contains a basic S1 pocket that recognizes and cleaves acidic residues (Glu and Asp) at position P1.[131] Thus, Asp-413, but not Ala-409, and Glu-654 seem to be the actual residues cleaved by v-Pro on nsp1a. The C-terminal region of nsp1a contains many acidic residues that prevent the prediction of cleavage sites downstream of Glu-654 recognized by the viral enzyme to generate the 6.5 and 5.5 kd products observed.

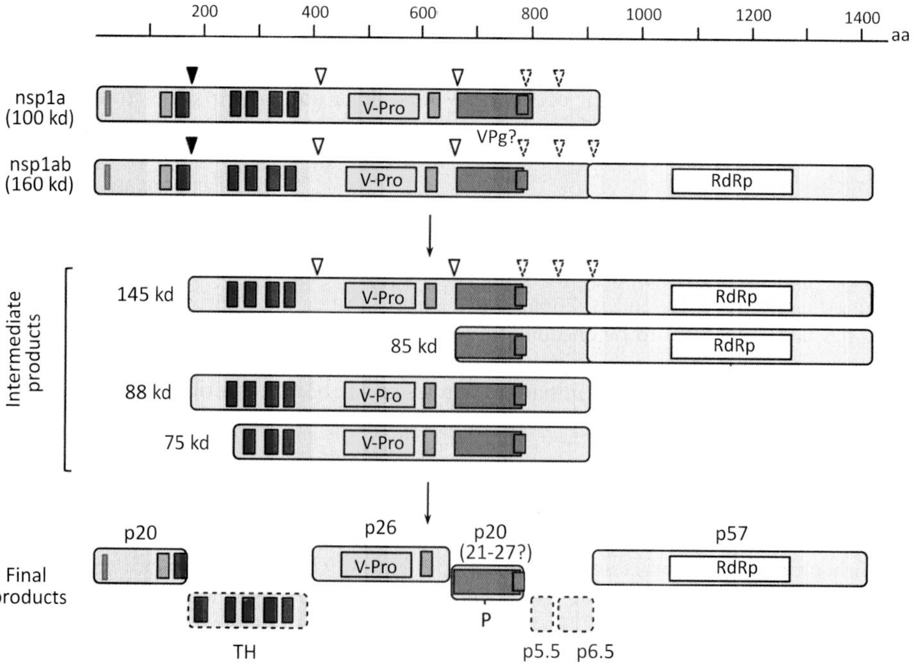

FIGURE 21.12. Processing of the nonstructural proteins. Nsp1a and nsp1ab are processed by cellular (*closed triangle*) and viral (*open triangles*) proteases. Although only the cleavages around amino acid residues 410 and 654 have been confirmed to be due to v-Pro, indirect evidence that would explain the protein processing products observed suggests that the downstream cleavages (*dashed triangles*) are also due to viral protease. No products from the hydrophobic region have been identified and the smaller products of 5.5 and 6.5 kd have not been mapped into nsp1a (*dotted boxes*).

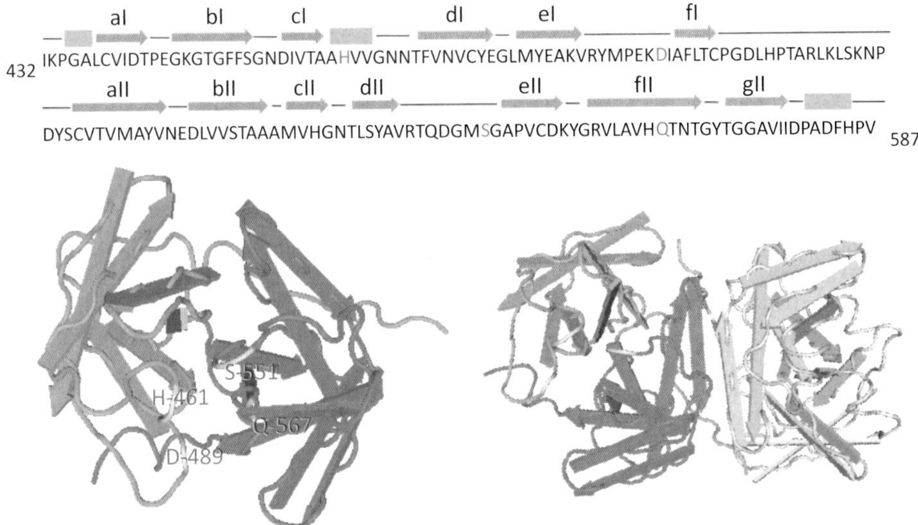

FIGURE 21.13. Diagram representing the structure of the HAstV-1 viral protease. Residues 432 to 587 of HAstV-1 nsp1a **(upper sequence)** were crystalized to 2.0 Å resolution. Monomer **(left)** with the two domains in blue and pink, and the catalytic residues in *yellow* and *red letters* is shown on the left. In the dimer **(right)**, two domains of a monomer are colored and the other monomer is in grey. Structure was obtained from Protein Data Bank (ID code 2w5e).

Structural Polyprotein Synthesis and Processing

The structural proteins of HAstV, encoded in ORF2, are synthesized from the sgRNA as a polyprotein precursor of 87 to 90 kd. Studies with HAstV-8 have revealed that the 90-kd primary translation product is intracellularly cleaved at Asp-657 to yield a product of 70 kd (named VP70)[7] through intermediates of 75 to 85 kd,[94] whose biological relevance, if any, is unknown (Fig. 21.14). Processing of VP90 to VP70 is carried out by cellular enzymes (caspases) that are involved in apoptotic processes,[7] and whose activity is triggered during viral infection by an unknown mechanism.[7,53] The pan-caspases inhibitor Z-VAD-fmk strongly inhibits this processing, whereas specific inhibitors of caspase activity partially block it. On the contrary, some proapoptotic factors—such as TNF-related apoptosis-inducing ligand (TRAIL) and staurosporine, which triggers different apoptotic pathways—enhance the cleavage of VP90 to VP70.[94] It is believed that caspases are important for processing the structural polyprotein precursor in most, if not all, astroviruses since the caspase-recognition motifs present at the carboxy-terminal region of VP90 are highly conserved among different strains. For HAstV-8, caspase-3 and caspase-9 seem particularly important for processing VP90; however, other caspases might also be involved, since VP90 is substrate of caspase-8 and caspase-4 *in vitro*.[7] Also, it cannot be excluded that different caspases are responsible for cleavage of VP90 from different astrovirus strains, since the motifs recognized by caspases in this precursor protein vary among viruses. Of interest, the VP90 to VP70 processing is not required for VP90 to assemble as viral particles, but it is important for the egress of the virus from infected cells[7,91] (see below).

Extracellular particles of HAstV-8 formed by VP70 are weakly infectious, but its infectivity is strongly enhanced by treatment of the viral particles with trypsin,[8,93] which is present in the intestinal lumen. Protein VP70 present in the extracellular virion is initially cleaved to yield 41 kd (VP41, the N-terminal product) and 28 kd (VP28, the C-terminal product) polypeptides. VP41 is subsequently cleaved at its carboxy terminus to yield a mature protein of 34 kd (VP34), whereas

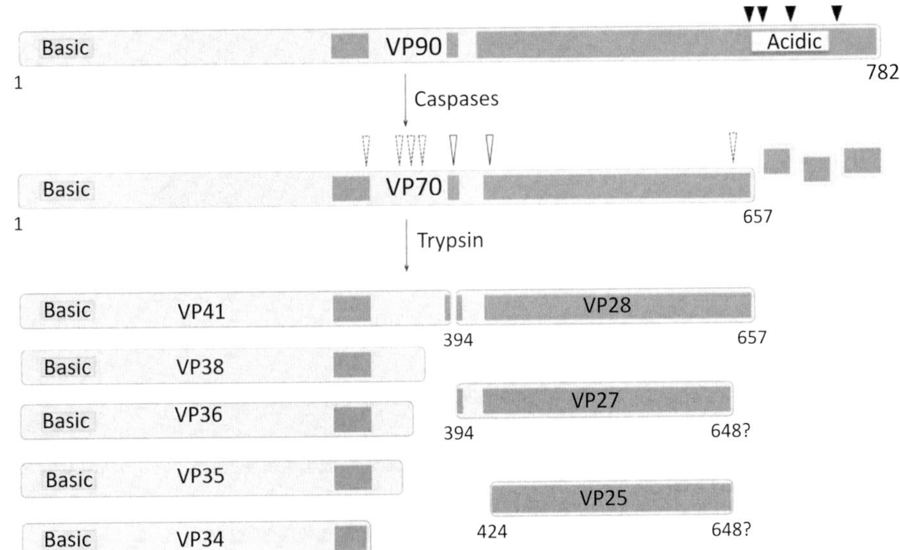

FIGURE 21.14. Processing of the structural protein VP90. The primary product of ORF2 is sequentially processed at its carboxy terminus by caspases to generate VP70, the protein present in the extracellular particles. These particles are processed by trypsin to generate protein intermediates of variable size, and the final products VP34, VP27, and VP25. Closed arrowheads represent cleavages carried out by caspases; open, long arrowheads represent cleavages by trypsin. The cleavage sites indicated by dashed arrowheads have not been precisely determined, therefore the carboxy-terminus of the intermediate and final products is unknown.

VP28 is cleaved to final products of 27 and 25 kd (VP27 and VP25, respectively) that share their carboxy terminus.[93] Thus, the full infectious virus is constituted by VP34, VP27, and VP25.

The C-terminal products VP25 and VP27 (or VP26 and VP29 in HAstV-2) are recognized by neutralizing antibodies,[9,119] whereas VP34 (VP32 in HAstV-2) contain cross-reaction epitopes that have been used for diagnosis.[59] Although not tested, the infectivity of other astroviruses may also depend on trypsin treatment, since sites susceptible to trypsin cleavage are conserved in the capsid protein from avian and mammalian viruses.

Transcription/Replication

Astrovirus RNA synthesis has been poorly studied. Given the structure and organization of the astrovirus genome, it is believed that these viruses follow a strategy similar to that of alphaviruses to replicate and transcribe their genome.[44] Based on this assumption, the gRNA would be used as a template to synthesize a full-length negative-sense RNA, gRNA(-), which in turn would be used as a template to produce both the full-length gRNA and the sgRNA. These positive-strand RNA molecules are initially observed in HAstV-8–infected Caco-2 cells at 8 hours postinfection (hpi) (Fig. 21.15), indicating that at this time gRNA(-) is already synthesized, although at undetectable levels. In a different study gRNA(-) was detected starting at 9 hpi and it accumulated to 0.7% to 4% of gRNA.[64] Similarly to alphavirus, it is believed that the viral transcriptase recognizes a *cis*-element that acts as a promoter on gRNA(-) to synthesize the sgRNA, which in the case of HAstV can reach five- to tenfold higher molar abundance than the full length gRNA.[104] A sequence located around the ORF2 initiation codon that is highly conserved among most known astroviruses might represent that promoter (see above, Fig. 21.5).

Synthesis of gRNA(-) and accumulation of gRNA require cell protein synthesis, but not cellular DNA transcription.[64] v-Pro, RdRp, VP90, gRNA(-), and viral particles have all been found to be associated with internal cell membranes.[91] This suggests that RNA replication and the first steps of morphogenesis are carried out associated with the observed membranous structures that probably derive from the ER, since viral phosphoproteins of 21 to 27 kd, which interact with the RdRp,[38] and are likely involved in RNA replication, localize to this organelle.[54]

Besides v-Pro and RdRp, no specific function has been assigned to the rest of the ORF1a and ORF1b products. Since the 20-kd N-terminal product of nsp1a is cleaved co-translationally, it is likely that the cleavage is carried out by a signalase.[95] This protein thus might target the replication complexes to membranes, although the predicted region containing highly hydrophobic transmembrane helixes (amino acid residues 178 to 409) could also contribute to association of the replication complexes to membranes. A potential VPg has been suggested as possible product of nsp1a,[3] just downstream of the protease, opening the possibility that AstV RNA synthesis would be primer dependent. Further studies are required to confirm this hypothesis.

Assembly and Release

The expression of ORF2 in cultured cells using recombinant vaccinia virus[28] or baculovirus[22] as vectors leads to the assembly of virus-like particles, indicating that the encoded protein is able to assemble in the absence of viral RNA; however, these particles were unstable and showed atypical morphology when purified, indicating a defective assembly.[22,105]

Virus assembly tolerates some deletion or changes in the 70 N-terminal basic amino acids of VP90/VP70, which are thought to interact with the gRNA in the particles.[43] The infectivity of a recombinant virus in which aa residues 11 to 30 were replaced by 8 or 9 amino acids of a foreign sequence reduced to about 50%. In contrast, viruses carrying the same foreign sequence in place of aa residues 31 to 50 of the capsid protein showed a drastic reduction to 0.1% of infectivity. Substituting the 5 C-terminal aa of ORF2 was also very deleterious to virus infectivity.[43] A single-point lethal mutation was described in HAstV-1 VP34 (Thr-227 to Ala or Ser),[88] however, whether the defect on infectivity was due to a defective assembly was not studied.

The ORF2 primary product of HAstV-8, VP90, forms intracellular particles that can be found associated with membranes or in the cytosol.[91] Apparently, VP90 assembles into particles associated with membranous structures, where viral nonstructural proteins and the sense and antisense genomic RNA are also present[91]; therefore RNA replication is also thought to occur associated with these structures (Fig. 21.16).

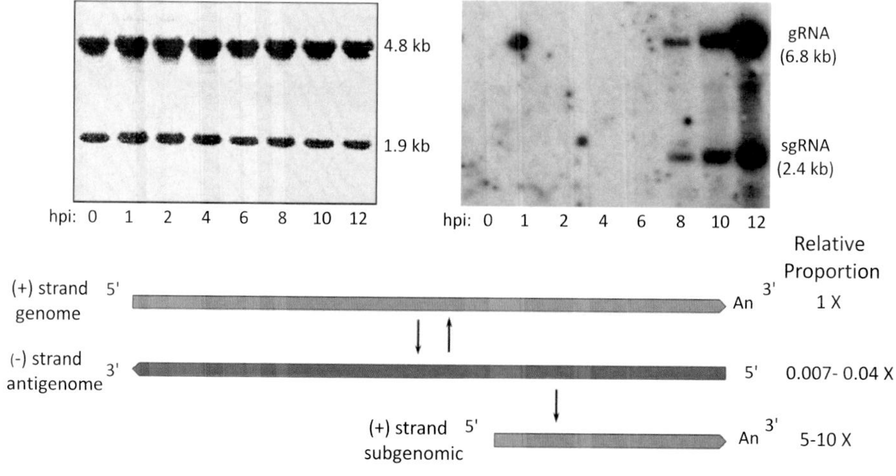

FIGURE 21.15. Astrovirus RNA species and their relative proportion produced during infection of HAstV. Total RNA from HAstV-8-infected cells at a multiplicity of infection of 2 were separated by gel electrophoresis. Ribosomal RNA was detected by staining with ethidium bromide **(upper left)**, and viral RNAs by Northern blot with a negative-polarity RNA probe that is able to detect both gRNA and sgRNA **(upper right)**. The hours postinfection (hpi) at which each sample was taken is shown. The lower scheme depicts the astrovirus RNA species and their relative amounts in infected cells.[64,104]

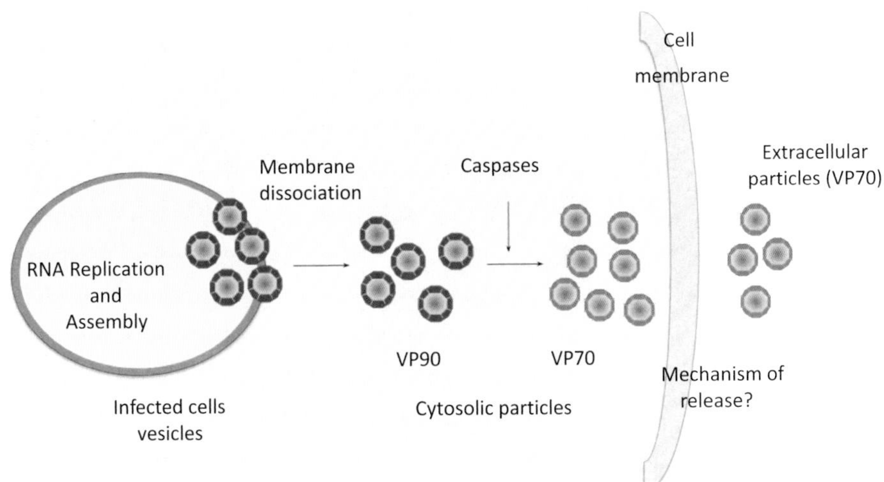

FIGURE 21.16. Model of VP90 processing and virus maturation. See details in the text.

It is believed that rearrangement of internal membranes is induced by AstV infection, since it is observed in intestinal epithelial cells of lambs infected with OAstV but not in uninfected cells.[48]

HAstV infection induces the activation of caspases in Caco-2 cells through an unknown mechanism. Activity of initiator (caspase-8, -9, and -4), and executioner (caspase-3 and -7) caspases is clearly detected at 12 hpi. Apoptotic markers, such as lamin A and poly (ADP-ribose)-polymerase (PARP) cleavage, are also detected at 12 hpi, although cell death is not observed up to 48 hpi, even at high moi.[7] A putative death domain (pDD), localized downstream of the v-Pro domain (aa residues 620 to 714 of nsp1a), was suggested as responsible for activation of caspases[53]; however, given that cleavage at Glu-654 by v-Pro would split this putative domain, its role in caspase activation requires further investigation. Recent findings that v-Pro may cleave Asp residues[131] open the possibility that this enzyme might cleave and activate pro-caspases.

Proteolytic processing by caspases of the VP90 assembled into particles, to yield VP70, is required for cell egress of the virus, since inhibitors of these proteases prevents it, while it is promoted by pro-apoptotic factors, such as TRAIL.[94] It is believed that after their initial assembly associated with membranes, the viral particles formed by VP90 separate from these structures, exposing its carboxy terminus, such that it is now available to caspase cleavage.[91] In addition to its role in cleaving VP90 to VP70, the activity of Cap-3 seems to be required by the virus to exit the cell.[7] Although the cellular process mediated by this caspase to allow virus egress is not known, the cell death induced by this protease seems not to be necessary; thus, a nonlytic mechanism seems to be involved in the release of HAstV. On the other hand, since a cytopathic effect was observed upon infection with porcine.[125] and chicken[10] astrovirus strains, these viruses could use more than one mechanism to exit the cell.

PATHOGENESIS AND PATHOLOGY

As a gastrointestinal pathogen, HAstV can be transmitted to a host through the fecal–oral route, as shown by human volunteer studies, but also person to person, as it was found in an outbreak of gastroenteritis in California.[97] Illness in adults can also be due to exposure to a larger dose of astrovirus or through fomites, and contaminated food or water.[2,13] In the case of avian viruses transmission is also through a fecal–oral route, facilitated by the large amount of viruses secreted in feces and the usual contact of animals with them, although it has also been proposed to occur by vertical transmission from parents to their offspring.[137]

Mammalian astroviruses affect mainly epithelial cells of the intestinal tract. Histopathologic studies of an immunocompromised child persistently infected, having a pronounced diarrhea, showed that astrovirus infection was limited to the small intestine. Infection involves the mature epithelial cells near the microvilli tips; it was more extensive in the jejune than in the duodenum, but not in the stomach (Fig. 21.17).[122] Morphologic abnormalities in the intestine suggested that, despite severe diarrhea, an inflammatory response does not occur. Studies with other mamastroviruses indicate that AstV can infect epithelial cells (OAstV and BoAstV) as well as subepithelial macrophages (OAstV) and M cells (BoAstV) of the small intestine.[130,150] OAstV particles were observed in vacuoles of the enterocytes, very similar to those found during infection of HAstV in cultured cells. OAstV infection resulted in diarrhea on days 2 to 4 postinfection and a transient villus atrophy and crypt hypertrophy.[48] Although BoAstV was considered as nonpathogenic because it was unable to induce diarrhea in gnotobiotic animals, inflammatory mononuclear cells above the dome villi were observed on infection with this virus. In addition, the lamina propria was infiltrated with neutrophils and contained cells with degenerate nuclei. Lymphoid-cell depletion was noted in the central region of germinal centers beneath infected dome villi.[150]

Astrovirus was recently found as the only pathogen in the central nervous system (CNS) of an immunodeficient patient who died of encephalitis.[115] Expression of structural proteins was specifically localized in astrocytes, but not in macrophages or neurons. Infiltration of macrophages and inflammation were found in the CNS of the patient, although evidence of astrovirus infection was not found in gastrointestinal postmortem samples. Of note, the human strain associated with encephalitis

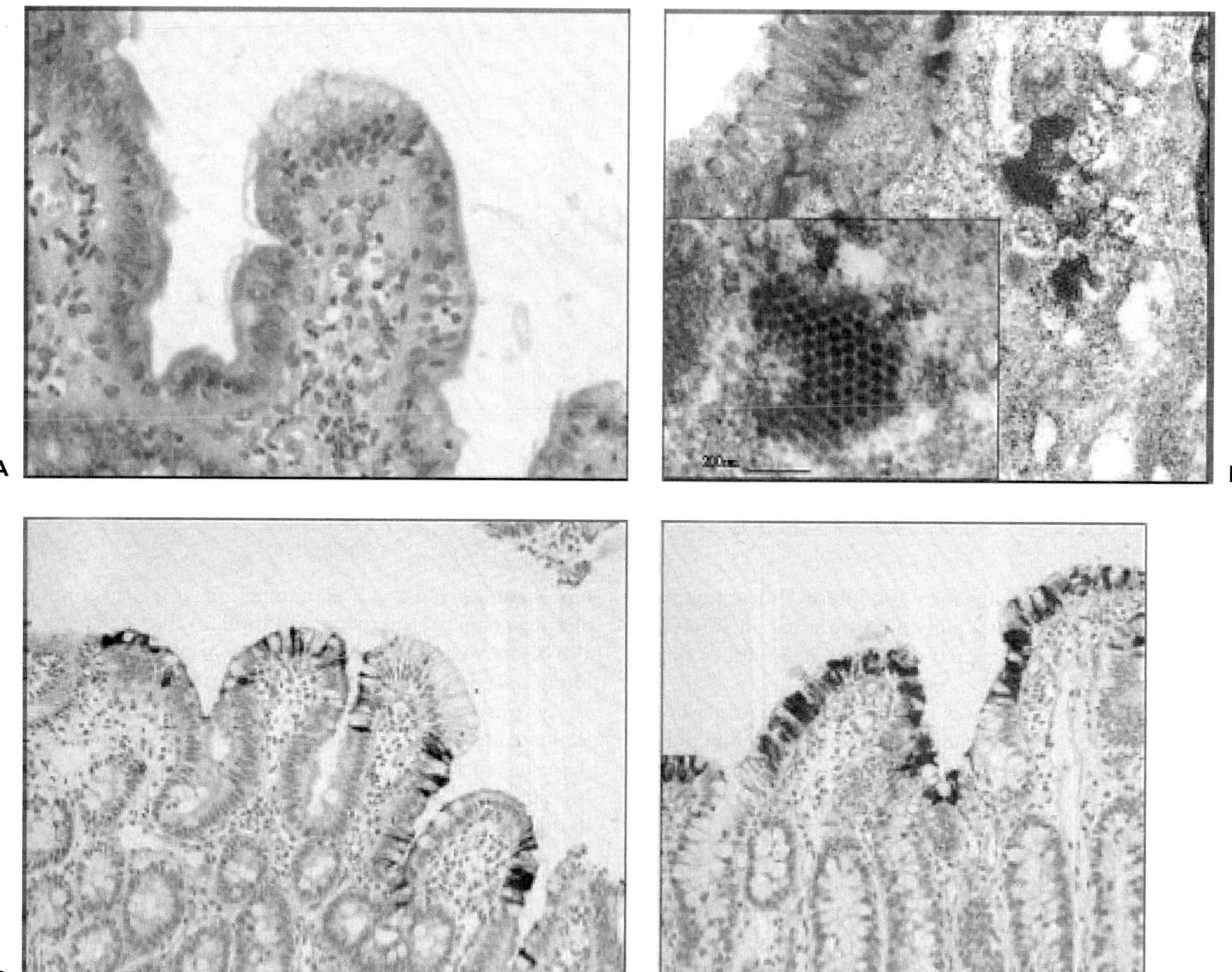

FIGURE 21.17. A: Photomicrograph of a jejunal biopsy specimen from a bone marrow transplant recipient with astrovirus infection demonstrating villus blunting, nonspecific alterations in surface epithelial cells and a mixed lamina propria inflammatory infiltrate, but without the presence of viral inclusion bodies (original magnification, x 100). Photomicrographs of **(B)** duodenal and **(C)** jejunal biopsies from a bone marrow transplant recipient with astrovirus infection immunostained with anti-astrovirus antibody and demonstrating progressively more extensive staining of surface epithelial cells, most commonly near the villus tips (original magnifications, ×40 and ×100, respectively). **D:** Electron micrographs of a jejunal enterocyte demonstrating cytoplasmic paracrystalline viral arrays of astrovirus [original magnifications, ×32,000 and ×100,000 (inset)]. (From Sebire NJ, Malone M, Shah N, et al. Pathology of astrovirus associated diarrhoea in a paediatric bone marrow transplant recipient. *J Clin Pathol* 2004;57:1001–1003, with permission.)

was genetically related to a novel human astrovirus associated with an outbreak of gastroenteritis (strain VA1)[35] and with celiac disease.[127] It was also found in feces of five children with nonpoliovirus acute flaccid paralysis,[69] although it was also present in one healthy child. In addition, an astrovirus strain was found in the CNS of minks suffering from a neurologic disease (shaking mink syndrome) by metagenomics.[16] In this last case, the syndrome was transmitted from infected to healthy animals by inoculation of brain homogenates. These findings suggest that AstV might cause neurologic diseases in mammals; however, the mechanism by which astrovirus could reach the CNS after infecting the gastrointestinal tract is unknown.

Lack of inflammation after intestinal astrovirus infection in humans[122] and turkeys[72] and the ability of HAstV to induce apoptosis in cultured cells[53,94] suggest that this form of programmed cell death, in which inflammation is not frequently observed, could contribute to gastrointestinal disease. However, more than one mechanism could participate in the disease produced by these viruses since, for instance, inflammation was observed in the CNS upon AstV infection.[115] Inflammation was also observed in premature children with necrotizing enterocolitis associated with HAstV, although in this case it was unclear whether inflammation was due to bacteria or HAstV spread.[5,6]

Structural proteins may also be involved in pathogenesis, since the capsid protein is able to increase the permeability of monolayers of epithelium cells in culture.[105] Apparently, no virus replication is needed for the capsid protein to have this effect, but transduction signals are likely involved since barrier permeability was clearly increased at 20 hours after treatment with inactivated virus or the purified protein, but not earlier.

The HAstV-1 capsid protein binds C1q and mannose-binding lectin, blocking the complement activation through the classical and lectin pathways, respectively. Interaction of the virion with C1q is likely conserved among astroviruses, given the high conservation of the complement system in animals as well as of the region through which the capsid protein interacts with C1q (aa residues 79 to 108).

TAstV-2, isolated from birds with poult enteritis mortality syndrome (characterized by enteritis, growth depression, lymphoid atrophy, immunosuppression, and high mortality rates), has been used as a model to study astrovirus pathogenesis in young turkeys.[72] Experimental infection of turkeys with TAstV-2 has shown that infectious virus can be recovered from many tissues, including blood, indicating the occurrence of viremia. The intestine, however, appears to be the only organ in which astrovirus replicates in this disease model.[11] Turkeys developed diarrhea on days 1 through 3 that persisted through 4 more days. In the intestines, no drastic morphologic changes or apoptosis were observed by light microscopy in infected animals; however, the F-actin distribution pattern changed at the apical region of jejunum tight junctions, which correlated with zones of infected cells. It has been suggested that these changes, together with defects in Na^+ absorption probably due to modifications of expression and cell distribution of sodium/hydrogen exchangers, might provoke osmotic diarrhea.[110] Intracytoplasmic aggregates of astrovirus were found in enterocytes on the sides and base of villi in the ileum and distal jejunum on day 3.

Avian astroviruses may spread to other tissues besides intestine, such as kidney, pancreas, lymphoid organs and liver, causing more severe diseases; however, this effect might depend on many factors, such as animal age and route of infection (vertical or horizontal), maternal antibody levels, size of the infecting dose, virus strain, and the presence of co-infecting pathogens.[66,128,133,136]

Immunity

Determinants of immunity to astrovirus are not well understood. Symptomatic astrovirus infection is found primarily in two age groups: young children and elderly, institutionalized patients. Indirect evidence suggests that astrovirus-specific antibodies could play a role in limiting infection in the host. The existence of astrovirus serotypes in different animal species, classified mainly on the basis of neutralizing antibody reactivity against the carboxy region of the capsid protein, suggests that antibodies exert immune pressure on the virus.[70] The biphasic age distribution of symptomatic infection suggests that antibody acquired early in life provides some kind of protection from illness through most of adult life and that immunity to astrovirus wanes late in life. Immunoglobulin therapy of immunocompromised patients with persistent astrovirus infection resulted in virus clearance and diarrhea elimination.[15] However, the role of astrovirus-specific antibodies to clear the virus was not defined because no neutralizing antibodies were measured in the immunoglobulin preparation utilized. On the other hand, bone marrow transplant patients with chronic diarrhea did not respond to the immunoglobulin treatment, although this preparation was demonstrated to have antibodies to the homologous infecting astrovirus serotype.[27] Thus, the response of patients to immunoglobulin treatment for virus clearance could be caused by additional unspecific factors more than to astrovirus-specific antibodies.

The normal mucosal immune system could be important in protecting individuals from repeated infections with human astrovirus.[100] T cells that recognize astrovirus antigens in a human leukocyte antigen (HLA)–restricted manner were found to reside in the intestinal lamina propria of healthy adults. These human astrovirus–specific CD4+ T cells produced helper T-cell subtype 1 (T_H1)-type cytokines, interferon gamma, and tumor necrosis factor, when activated.

The complement system is one of the initial host responses to pathogens, important in both innate and adaptive immunity. By blocking the complement system,[51,57] as mentioned earlier, HAstV could alter an effective immune response of the host. However, on the other hand, binding of C1q to the capsid protein already assembled in the virion, if it occurs, could facilitate phagocytosis and elimination of the virus by C1q acting as opsonin.

In animals, the role of the humoral immune response to limit astrovirus infection is also not clear. Koci et al.[71] found that virus replication in small turkeys infected with TAstV was limited, even though the infection did not induce a significant adaptive immune response, evaluated through measurement of a specific increase in the population of CD4+ and CD8+ T cells. Because there was no protection against TAstV upon secondary challenge, the limitation of virus replication was attributed to an innate response, mediated by production of nitric oxide. In chickens, protective immunity can be conferred by the capsid protein, since inoculation of this protein partially protected animals from disease,[123] although the role of humoral and cellular immunity in this partial protection is still unknown.

EPIDEMIOLOGY

HAstV infections have been found worldwide primarily, but not exclusively, in young children with diarrhea. Several studies associate astroviruses with diarrhea in immunocompromised patients, including adults,[15,25,27,40,50,149] and with necrotizing enterocolitis (NEC) in premature children.[5,6] Sporadic outbreaks of gastroenteritis caused by astrovirus have been reported among elderly patients[83] and military recruits.[13] Large, food-borne outbreaks, affecting thousands of individuals in Japan, have occurred among school-aged children and adults as well.[112] In children, studies in different populations[26,113] have revealed HAstV as the second most important cause of gastroenteritis, after rotavirus, with incidences varying between 4.2% and 7.3%, although incidences lower than 1% have also been reported. Higher incidences of HAstV have been rarely reported in children with diarrhea, such as in native populations of Brazil and southeast Mexico, with incidences of 56%[39] and 28%,[87] respectively. The age distribution of HAstV can vary depending on several factors; however, in a study carried out in Spain, approximately 80% of the astrovirus infections occurred in children under 3 years of age.[56] The age-specific HAstV incidences (episodes per year) found in an Egyptian study (0.38 for infants <6 months, 0.40 for infants 6 to 11 months, and 0.16 for children between 12 and 23 months) were similar to those found for rotavirus.[109]

Most astrovirus infections in humans are detected in the winter months in temperate regions and in the rainy season in more tropical climates.[26,141] Both community-acquired and

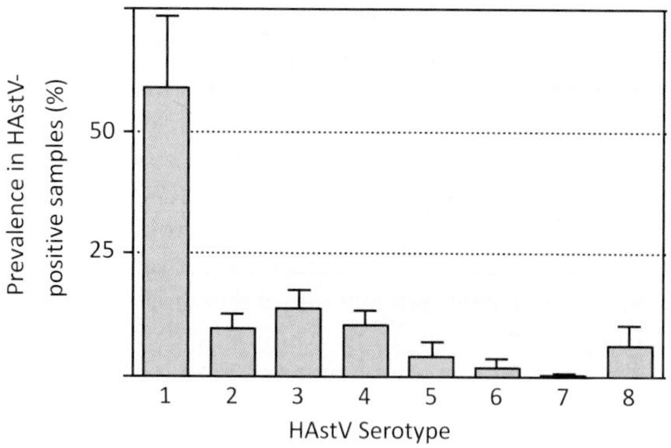

FIGURE 21.18. Prevalence of HAstV serotypes in children with diarrhea. This graph compiles data from eight studies in different countries with 461 astrovirus-positive samples. (Adapted from Monroe, SS. Molecular epidemiology of human astroviruses, In: Desselberger U, Gray JJ, eds. *Perspectives in Medical Virology. Viral Gastroenteritis.* Vol. 9. Amsterdam: Elsevier, 2003:607–616.)

nosocomial infections, particularly among immunocompromised patients[25,40] and premature children, have been observed.

Eight serotypes have been mainly described among viruses that circulate in the human population. In general, serotype 1 of HAstV is the most common type found in children[102] (Fig. 21.18), but the predominant serotype can vary with time and location. Thus, in a study in the United Kingdom, 72% of the community-acquired astroviruses encountered between 1975 and 1987 were serotype 1[78]; while in Australia serotypes 1, 3, and 4 were regularly found in a period of 18 years.[120] In contrast, a longitudinal study of diarrhea in a cohort of Mexican children found that astrovirus serotype 2 was the most common (35%).[52] In a different study with samples from different geographic regions in Mexico, all eight serotypes, except serotype 5, were found, with serotype 8 being as frequent as serotype 1 in one of the studied regions.[96] Analyzing AstV from different regions of India, putative recombinant viruses were found to be the most prevalent in children under 24 months of age.[138] Recombinant viruses containing RdRp and the capsid protein from different canonical HAstV have also been identified in different populations of Kenya.[148]

Epidemiologic studies of AstV in the human population have been limited so far to the canonical HAstV serotypes 1 to 8. However, the recent identification of novel AstV in humans[33–35,69] by highly sensitive methods highlights the necessity to analyze the prevalence of these novel viruses to determine their actual impact in public health, especially because they were found to be genetically related to animal viruses and some were isolated from patients with more severe diseases, such as encephalitis. Limited studies suggest that these viruses, similarly to the canonical HAstV, may be distributed worldwide in the human population.[32,69] Given their genetic relationship with animal viruses and the potential for interspecies transmission, it would be possible that wild animals may become part of the epidemiologic equation.

Morbidity and Mortality

Although the gastroenteritis caused by HAstV is usually a mild, self-limiting illness that does not require hospitalization, more severe gastroenterologic disease that may result in death has also been reported.[112] Astrovirus infection has been associated with intestinal diseases other than gastroenteritis, such as celiac disease[127] and intussusception,[4,63] and it was found as the only pathogen in the CNS of a child with encephalitis.[115] In a population of Mayan infants, astrovirus was the most common enteric pathogen identified in stool samples collected during a prospective study of oral poliovirus immunogenicity.[87] In 61% of the infants, astrovirus was detected by EIA in at least one stool sample over the 18-week period each infant was followed. Of 305 diarrheal episodes reported at study visits, 26% were associated with astrovirus. The enzyme immuno assay (EIA) results were confirmed by reverse transcription-polymerase chain reaction (RT-PCR) in a subset of EIA-positive and -negative samples. The reason for the high prevalence of astrovirus infection and the low rate of rotavirus infection (4%) in this semiclosed community is not known, but it may be related to temperature, rainfall, humidity, or other environmental factors.

HAstV were shown to be an important cause of outbreaks of diarrhea in the childcare setting. Children up to 36 months of age attending childcare centers were at greatest risk of developing diarrhea.[99] An investigation of eight outbreaks of astrovirus diarrhea in six childcare centers showed that 20% of the children with diarrhea shed astrovirus.[98]

Origin and Transmission

Epidemiologic data indicate that contaminated food is the main source for HAstV infection. HAstV has been found in bivalve mollusks, indicating that seafood may contribute to gastroenteritis caused by HAstV.[139] HAstV has also been detected in water from different origins, including drinking water, rivers, dams, wastewater, and effluents from water treatment plants.[81,90,108,114] Sequence analysis of HAstV strains recovered from water and clinical samples from hospitalized patients showed that virus strains from both origins were identical,[108] confirming that water supplies are an important source of HAstV contamination. In ground water, the infectivity of astrovirus can be maintained for months; besides, it is partially resistant to chlorination,[31] which is widely used for wastewater treatment in many countries.

The identification of astroviruses in the human population—different from canonical HAstV but genetically related to AstV isolated from rats,[24] minks,[69] marine mammals,[117] and pigs[85]—suggested that wild mammals might act as reservoirs for human AstV, and that interspecies transmission occurs. The identification of a recombinant virus containing sequences derived from HAstV-4 and CslAstV in sea lions supports this hypothesis.[117] A high diversity of AstV has been found in mammals, such as bats[152] and pigs,[85] suggesting that the emergence of novel viruses in humans is possible.

Seroprevalence

Antibodies to canonical HAstV tend to be acquired in early childhood, which is consistent with the age at which children are primarily infected. An early survey of 87 children less than 10 years of age in the Oxford region of the United Kingdom revealed that antibody prevalence rises rapidly from 7% in 6- to 12-month-old infants to 70% by school age.[77] This study was focused on detecting HAstV antibodies by immunofluorescence of astrovirus-infected cells; therefore, the prevalence of antibodies to astrovirus in this population could be underestimated.

The presence of high titers of antibodies to HAstV, particularly to HAstV-1 capsid protein,[27] in gammaglobulin pools from the United States indicates that HAstV infection with this serotype is very common. As expected, based on the most frequent HAstV serotype found to cause infection in different studies, one study of seroprevalence among children treated at a hospital in the United Kingdom found rates of 86% for serotype 1, 1% for serotype 2, 8% for serotype 3, and 6% for serotype 4.[111] In an age-stratified sample from The Netherlands, seroprevalence of neutralizing antibodies was again higher for serotype 1 (91%), but it was different for the other serotypes.[75] Studies to determine the seroprevalence of antibodies to the recently identified human isolates—such as HAstV-HMO, -MLB, and -VA1—are still pending, although limited studies with the HAstV-MLB-like virus strain indicate that they are also widely distributed in the human population.[34,69]

CLINICAL FEATURES

Characteristics of Human Illness

Gastroenteritis caused by astrovirus infection primarily affects young children throughout the world. Table 21.1 summarizes the clinical features associated with this disease; however, these features can vary depending on the population studied. For instance, 12.4% of outpatients under 36 months of age infected with HAstV in Argentina got diarrhea, 41.6% had fever, and 16.6% of the patients required hospitalization[46]; in Egypt, diarrhea caused by HAstV in children under the age of 3 years was similar to that caused by rotavirus, and severe dehydration was present in 17% of these patients.[109] Complications such as dehydration can develop in patients with underlying gastrointestinal disease, poor nutritional status, and mixed infection.[26]

TABLE 21.1 Clinical Symptoms of Human Astrovirus Infection

Diarrhea	72%–100%
Duration of diarrhea (days, average)	2–3
Maximum number of stools/24 h	4
Bloody diarrhea	0%
Abdominal pain	50%
Vomiting	20%–70%
Duration of vomiting (days, average)	1
Maximum number of vomiting episodes/24 h	1
Fever	20%–25%
Maximum fever (Celsius)	37.9
Dehydration to some degree	24%–30%
Severe dehydration	0%–5%
Hospitalization	6%
Duration of hospitalization (days, average)	6
Severity score[a] (1–20) (average)	5
Otitis	13%
Bronchiolitis	33%
Admission diagnosis of gastroenteritis	18.7%–48%

[a]Twenty point scoring system (Ruuska T, Vesikari T. Rotavirus disease in Finnish children: use of numerical scores for clinical severity of diarrhoeal episodes. *Scand J Infect Dis.* 1990;22:259–267.).

Adapted from Walter JE, Mitchell DK. Astrovirus infection in children. *Curr Opin Infect Dis* 2003;16:247–253.

Adult human volunteer studies established the incubation period to be 3 to 4 days and the highest viral shedding at day 6, which appeared to be proportional to the severity of the illness; seroconversion was confirmed at day 28.[97] Development of disease in these patients was limited and dependent on the size of the inoculum. A shorter incubation period of 24 to 36 hours was calculated from the secondary spread characteristics during an outbreak of gastroenteritis in a Japanese kindergarten.[74] In general, astrovirus diarrhea is milder than that caused by rotavirus and does not lead to significant dehydration or hospitalization.[141] Persistent gastroenteritis caused by astrovirus has been associated with strains belonging to serotype 3.[21] Deaths associated with gastrointestinal astrovirus infection are extremely rare but have been reported.[126]

Additional gastrointestinal diseases associated with canonical HAstV include intussusception[4,63] and necrotizing enterocolitis,[5,6] while the recently described HAstV-VA1 was found in celiac disease.[127] HAstV was found in 3 out of 6 pediatric patients (between 4 and 7 months) with ileocolic intussusception; in two, HAstV was the only pathogen found and one died.[4] In premature children, HAstV was the most frequently associated viral pathogen with necrotizing enterocolitis.[6]

HAstV has been found to be the cause of chronic diarrhea among immunocompromised patients, children, and adults, and of outbreaks in pediatric patients undergoing bone marrow transplantation[27] and pediatric primary immunodeficiency units.[40] Among gastrointestinal viruses, HAstV have been found more frequently in patients with a number of immune diseases, such as human immunodeficiency (HIV positives), combined immunodeficiency, congenital T-cell immunodeficiency, chronic lymphocytic leukemia, Waldenström's macroglobulinemia, and immunodeficiency polyendocrinopathy.[15,40,50,149] Patients treated with fludarabine, which is known to deplete CD4+ T cells, developed persistent diarrhea caused by HAstV.[15]

Astroviruses have been identified in feces of children with nonpoliovirus flaccid paralysis[69] and in frontal cortex biopsy of a patient with X-linked agammaglobulinemia who developed encephalitis.[115]

Clinical Features in Avian Species

Intestinal and extraintestinal illness has been noted in avian species infected with astroviruses. Avian nephritis virus (ANV) infects chickens, and the viral antigen can be found in different organs (e.g., liver, spleen, pancreas, kidney, jejunum, and ileum) of this animal. This virus has been associated with growth retardation and acute interstitial nephritis.[62] Antigenically ANV-unrelated astrovirus (confirmed to be different by sequence analysis of a specific region of the nonstructural polyprotein) isolated from chickens were found in the small intestine, but rarely in other organs; these viruses were associated with mild diarrhea.[10] In ducks, astrovirus infection is associated with fatal hepatitis, with mortality rates of up to 50%.[47] Subcutaneous injection of a 20% (w/v) suspension of astrovirus-infected livers into 2- to 3-day-old ducklings recapitulated the hepatitis with all of the histologic features of the original animals and caused death within 2 to 4 days in 25% of the ducklings. Serial passage of this agent in ducks resulted in mortality rates of 25% to 55%. However, asymptomatic DAstV infections seem to be present at high frequency since a significant seroprevalence on healthy animals can be found; a high seroprevalence to DAstV was also found in flocks that present a very low mortality rate.[137] Turkey astrovirus has been associated with diarrhea and the high mortality disease poult enteritis mortality syndrome (PEMS). TAstV was isolated from the thymus of an infected animal with PEMS,[73] but it could be detected in different tissues (e.g., bursa, thymus, spleen, kidney, pancreas, and skeletal muscle).[106] The small intestine, however, seems to be the main tissue where virus replication occurs.[11] Asymptomatic infections have been also found in turkeys as well as in chickens infected with AstV.[137]

DIAGNOSIS

Electron Microscopy

Astroviruses have been detected by direct EM examination of negative-stained fecal specimens. The sensitivity of this methodology has been estimated to be 10^6 to 10^7 virus particles per gram of stool. Usually, patients with diarrhea caused by astrovirus shed large numbers of viral particles (equivalent to approximately 10^{10} or 10^{11} of virus genomes per gram of feces).[55] However, in those patients who may be excreting fewer viral particles, usage of antiviral antibodies for immunoelectron microscopy facilitates identification of the virus.

Enzyme Immunoassays

Herrmann et al. developed an EIA that relies on a group-reactive monoclonal antibody (8E7) that maps to the conserved domain of the capsid protein of HAstV serotypes 1 to 8 (amino acid residues 71 to 260) to capture viral antigen, and a polyclonal antiserum as the detector antibody.[60] This EIA had a comparable sensitivity (91%) and specificity (98%) to immune EM. EIA has been useful for rapid detection of astrovirus antigen in studies in which a large number of human samples have been assayed. However, antibodies developed by Herrmann do not recognize the recently described novel HAstV strains.

The high antigenic divergence of avian viruses has not allowed the obtention of antibodies to common epitopes to be used in immunoassays to detect all AstV that infect flocks; the DAstV capsid carboxy-terminal region has been successfully used to detect prevalence of antibodies to this virus in ducks.[143]

Molecular Techniques

As more information regarding the sequence of astrovirus genomes became available, detection techniques that employ molecular probes and RT-PCR were developed. At present, the complete genome sequence of several human and animal AstV strains, as well as the ORF2 sequences from a high number of isolates, have been determined. The high sequence variability that exists among these viruses does not allow the use of universal primers for all members of the *Astroviridae* family. However, based on these sequences, oligonucleotides from selected regions of the genome have been used as primers to diagnose closely related viruses by RT-PCR and sequencing of the amplicon. Particularly, primers derived from different regions along the genome have been successfully used for RT-PCR to detect typical HAstV and animal viruses. The sensitivity of this methodology increased when it was coupled to a cell-culture system in clinical and environmental water samples.[49] Given that different pathogens are associated with enteric infections in humans and animals, methods based in RT-PCR have been developed recently for diagnosis of multiple human or animal viruses, including astroviruses, in a single tube.[14,118,124,151]

Diagnosis by RT-PCR has also been used to detect the presence of astrovirus in animals; however, in the case of avian astroviruses, as mentioned, common oligonucleotides cannot be used due to the high genome diversity, which is even higher than among mammastroviruses. In spite of this, quantitative RT-PCR assays for ANV and CAstV, able to detect 180 and 105 RNA copies, respectively, have been used to specifically demonstrate the presence of these viruses in the gut and kidney of field and experimental infected animals.[129] Sensitivity for ANV detection increased (detecting up to 18 RNA copies) when oligonucleotides that amplify the 3 -UTR conserved region were used.[136]

Metagenomic analysis has revealed the existence of novel astroviruses in samples from patients with diseases that had not been previously associated with these viruses,[69,115] contributing to changing the virologist community's view of their behavior and relevance. This powerful technology can help to identify emerging astroviruses, as well as many other novel pathogens, and will provide the basis to design biological reagents for specific diagnosis.

Oligonucleotide microarrays have also been used as a powerful technology to identify previously unknown viruses belonging to different families. This methodology has been evaluated to detect and type HAstV using viral cDNA or RNA from reference strains adapted to cultured cells or wild-type strains from feces.[20] More studies are needed to determine the usefulness and sensitivity of this methodology with clinical samples.

PREVENTION AND CONTROL

Gastroenteritis caused by astrovirus is generally a mild, self-limiting illness that can disrupt an individual's activities for a few days but does not require specific therapy. In the young child or adult patient who becomes dehydrated, oral or intravenous fluid resuscitation may be necessary. Intravenous immunoglobulin may be a useful adjunct in severely immunodeficient patients who fail to respond to conservative measures,[15] but larger studies are needed to determine efficacy and establish indications. Of note, immunoglobulin treatment has been suggested as a possible cause of encephalitis in an immunodeficient patient,[115] although this was not confirmed.

Interruption of transmission is the key factor in preventing astrovirus infection. This is especially important in hospitals and other institutions, daycare centers, and families, where person-to-person transmission is likely to occur. Astrovirus is resistant to a number of treatments, including normal disinfectants,[80,121] and it can survive in water after chlorination.[1,81] Therefore, universal hygienic procedures must be enforced in these settings. No vaccines have been developed for astrovirus infections in any host animal; however, inoculation of the recombinant, baculovirus-expressed capsid protein to hens partially protected the offspring for the presence of gut lesions and weight depression after virus challenge.[123] Thus, this kind of antigen eventually could be useful in evaluating vaccine candidates in other animal species, including humans.

PERSPECTIVES

The perception of the relevance of AstV in public health is changing given the discovery in recent years of novel viruses isolated from humans that show genetic similarities with animal strains, some of which have been associated with diseases other than gastroenteritis. Further characterization of HAstV genetically related to animal strains will help to better understand the public health importance of astroviruses. The available evidence indicates that interspecies transmission might be common in astroviruses. Epidemiologic studies designed to search for AstV in nongastrointestinal diseases, such as those related to the CNS, will be useful in understanding the spectrum of pathology these viruses may be associated with, and could change the current knowledge we have about the epidemiology and pathology of astrovirus-associated disease. Although animal models have been established for avian viruses, models for mammalian viruses are required to study the determinants of protective immunity in these viruses and the pathogenesis of the diseases they cause. The structural analysis of AstV proteins that has already started with viral protease, and spike protein should continue to help in the understanding of the molecular determinants of infection as well as the role specific viral proteins play in the virus replication cycle. So far, neither cellular receptors nor the virus capsid protein domains involved in virus entry and cell egress have been identified for AstV. It is expected that further structural characterization of viral capsid proteins will allow us to undertake new approaches targeted to understand these processes, and also probably to control infection. Significant gaps exist in our understanding of astrovirus genome replication, especially since it occurs in the absence of a viral encoded RNA-helicase, a peculiar feature of AstV; therefore, the identification of viral and cellular proteins that participate in this process will be useful in elucidating its mechanism. The cell response to HAstV infection has proven to be partially beneficial for virus cell entry and egress; however, the cell factors and mechanisms involved in these processes are only beginning to be characterized. Further studies are required to advance our understanding of these stages of the virus lifecycle. Although infectious clones for HAstV and ANV have been available for some time, reverse genetics in AstV has been poorly exploited. The systems for reverse genetics should be improved and used to identify the virus molecular determinants involved in the virus replication cycle.

ACKNOWLEDGMENTS

We apologize to our colleagues whose work has not been cited due to space constraints. We thank Dr. K. Dryden and Dr. Y. J. Tao for providing unpublished data. Our laboratory acknowledges the financial support from DGAPA–National University of Mexico (UNAM) and the National Council for Science and Technology (CONACYT).

REFERENCES

1. Abad FX, Pinto RM, Villena C, et al. Astrovirus survival in drinking water. *Appl Environ Microbiol* 1997;63:3119–3122.
2. Abad FX, Villena C, Guix S, et al. Potential role of fomites in the vehicular transmission of human astroviruses. *Appl Environ Microbiol* 2001;67:3904–3907.
3. Al-Mutairy B, Walter JE, Pothen A, et al. Genome Prediction of Putative Genome-Linked Viral Protein (VPg) of Astroviruses. *Virus Genes* 2005; 31:21–30.
4. Aminu M, Ameh EA, Geyer A, et al. Role of astrovirus in intussusception in Nigerian infants. *J Trop Pediatr* 2009;55:192–194.
5. Bagci S, Eis-Hubinger AM, Franz AR, et al. Detection of astrovirus in premature infants with necrotizing enterocolitis. *Pediatr Infect Dis J* 2008; 27:347–350.
6. Bagci S, Eis-Hubinger AM, Yassin AF, et al. Clinical characteristics of viral intestinal infection in preterm and term neonates. *Eur J Clin Microbiol Infect Dis* 2010;29:1079–1084.
7. Banos-Lara MR, Mendez E. Role of individual caspases induced by astrovirus on the processing of its structural protein and its release from the cell through a non-lytic mechanism. *Virology* 2010;401:322–332.
8. Bass DM, Qiu S. Proteolytic processing of the astrovirus capsid. *J Virol* 2000;74:1810–1814.
9. Bass DM, Upadhyayula U. Characterization of human serotype 1 astrovirus-neutralizing epitopes. *J Virol* 1997;71:8666–8671.
10. Baxendale W, Mebatsion T. The isolation and characterisation of astroviruses from chickens. *Avian Pathol* 2004;33:364–370.
11. Behling-Kelly E, Schultz-Cherry S, Koci M, et al. Localization of astrovirus in experimentally infected turkeys as determined by in situ hybridization. *Vet Pathol* 2002;39:595–598.
12. Belliot G, Laveran H, Monroe SS. Capsid protein composition of reference strains and wild isolates of human astroviruses. *Virus Res* 1997; 49:49–57.
13. Belliot G, Laveran H, Monroe SS. Outbreak of gastroenteritis in military recruits associated with serotype 3 astrovirus infection. *J Med Virol* 1997;51:101–106.
14. Beuret C. Simultaneous detection of enteric viruses by multiplex real-time RT-PCR. *J Virol Methods* 2004;115:1–8.
15. Bjorkholm M, Celsing F, Runarsson G, et al. Successful intravenous immunoglobulin therapy for severe and persistent astrovirus gastroenteritis after fludarabine treatment in a patient with Waldenstrom's macroglobulinemia. *Int J Hematol* 1995;62:117–120.
16. Blomstrom AL, Widen F, Hammer AS, et al. Detection of a novel astrovirus in brain tissue of mink suffering from shaking mink syndrome by use of viral metagenomics. *J Clin Microbiol* 2010;48:4392–4396.
17. Bosch A, Guix S, Krishna NK, et al. Astroviruses. In: King AMQ, Adams MJ, Carstens EB, Lefkowitz EJ, eds. *Virus Taxonomy: Classification and Nomenclature of Viruses: Ninth Report of the International Committee on Taxonomy of Viruses.* San Diego: Elsevier; 2012.
18. Brierley I, Vidakovic M. Ribosomal frameshifting in astroviruses. In: Desselberger U, Gray JJ, eds. *Perspectives in Medical Virology. Viral Gastroenteritis, vol. 9.* Amsterdam: Elsevier; 2003:587–606.
19. Brinker JP, Blacklow NR, Herrmann JE. Human astrovirus isolation and propagation in multiple cell lines. *Arch Virol* 2000;145:1847–1856.
20. Brown DW, Gunning KB, Henry DM, et al. A DNA oligonucleotide microarray for detecting human astrovirus serotypes. *J Virol Methods* 2008; 147:86–92.
21. Caballero S, Guix S, El-Senousy WM, et al. Persistent gastroenteritis in children infected with astrovirus: association with serotype-3 strains. *J Med Virol* 2003;71:245–250.
22. Caballero S, Guix S, Ribes E, et al. Structural requirements of astrovirus virus-like particles assembled in insect cells. *J Virol* 2004;78:13285–13292.
23. Chaudhry Y, Nayak A, Bordeleau ME, et al. Caliciviruses differ in their functional requirements for eIF4F components. *J Biol Chem* 2006;281: 25315–25325.
24. Chu DK, Chin AW, Smith GJ, et al. Detection of novel astroviruses in urban brown rats and previously known astroviruses in humans. *J Gen Virol* 2010;91:2457–2462.
25. Cox GJ, Matsui SM, Lo RS, et al. Etiology and outcome of diarrhea after marrow transplantation: a prospective study. *Gastroenterology* 1994;107:1398–1407.
26. Cruz JR, Bartlett AV, Herrmann JE, et al. Astrovirus-associated diarrhea among Guatemalan ambulatory rural children. *J Clin Microbiol* 1992; 30:1140–1144.
27. Cubitt WD, Mitchell DK, Carter MJ, et al. Application of electronmicroscopy, enzyme immunoassay, and RT-PCR to monitor an outbreak of astrovirus type 1 in a paediatric bone marrow transplant unit. *J Med Virol* 1999;57:313–321.

28. Dalton RM, Pastrana EP, Sanchez-Fauquier A. Vaccinia virus recombinant expressing an 87-kilodalton polyprotein that is sufficient to form astrovirus-like particles. *J Virol* 2003;77:9094–9098.
29. Daughenbaugh KF, Wobus CE, Hardy ME. VPg of murine norovirus binds translation initiation factors in infected cells. *Virol J* 2006;3:33.
30. Donelli G, Superti F, Tinari A, et al. Mechanism of astrovirus entry into Graham 293 cells. *J Med Virol* 1992;38:271–277.
31. Espinosa AC, Mazari-Hiriart M, Espinosa R, et al. Infectivity and genome persistence of rotavirus and astrovirus in groundwater and surface water. *Water Res* 2008;42:2618–2628.
32. Finkbeiner SR, Holtz LR, Jiang Y, et al. Human stool contains a previously unrecognized diversity of novel astroviruses. *Virol J* 2009;6:161.
33. Finkbeiner SR, Kirkwood CD, Wang D. Complete genome sequence of a highly divergent astrovirus isolated from a child with acute diarrhea. *Virol J* 2008;5:117.
34. Finkbeiner SR, Le BM, Holtz LR, et al. Detection of newly described astrovirus MLB1 in stool samples from children. *Emerg Infect Dis* 2009; 15:441–444.
35. Finkbeiner SR, Li Y, Ruone S, et al. Identification of a novel astrovirus (astrovirus VA1) associated with an outbreak of acute gastroenteritis. *J Virol* 2009;83:10836–10839.
36. Firth AE, Atkins JF. Candidates in Astroviruses, Seadornaviruses, Cytorhabdoviruses and Coronaviruses for +1 frame overlapping genes accessed by leaky scanning. *Virol J* 2010;7:17.
37. Fu Y, Pan M, Wang X, et al. Complete sequence of a duck astrovirus associated with fatal hepatitis in ducklings. *J Gen Virol* 2009;90:1104–1108.
38. Fuentes C, Guix S, Bosch A, et al. The C-Terminal nsP1a protein of human astrovirus is a phosphoprotein that interacts with the viral polymerase. *J Virol* 2011;85:4470–4479.
39. Gabbay YB, Chamone CB, Nakamura LS, et al. Characterization of an astrovirus genotype 2 strain causing an extensive outbreak of gastroenteritis among Maxakali Indians, Southeast Brazil. *J Clin Virol* 2006; 37:287–292.
40. Gallimore CI, Taylor C, Gennery AR, et al. Use of a heminested reverse transcriptase PCR assay for detection of astrovirus in environmental swabs from an outbreak of gastroenteritis in a pediatric primary immunodeficiency unit. *J Clin Microbiol* 2005;43:3890–3894.
41. Geigenmuller U, Chew T, Ginzton N, et al. Processing of nonstructural protein 1a of human astrovirus. *J Virol* 2002;76:2003–2008.
42. Geigenmuller U, Ginzton NH, Matsui SM. Construction of a genome-length cDNA clone for human astrovirus serotype 1 and synthesis of infectious RNA transcripts. *J Virol* 1997;71:1713–1717.
43. Geigenmuller U, Ginzton NH, Matsui SM. Studies on intracellular processing of the capsid protein of human astrovirus serotype 1 in infected cells. *J Gen Virol* 2002;83:1691–1695.
44. Geigenmuller U, Mendez E, Matsui M. Studies on the molecular biology of human astrovirus. In: Desselberger U, Gray JJ, eds. *Perspectives in Medical Virology. Viral Gastroenteritis, vol. 9.* Amsterdam: Elsevier; 2003:573–586.
45. Gibson CA, Chen J, Monroe SA, et al. Expression and processing of nonstructural proteins of the human astroviruses. *Adv Exp Med Biol* 1998; 440:387–391.
46. Giordano MO, Martinez LC, Isa MB, et al. Childhood astrovirus-associated diarrhea in the ambulatory setting in a Public Hospital in Cordoba city, Argentina. *Rev Inst Med Trop Sao Paulo* 2004;46:93–96.
47. Gough RE, Collins MS, Borland E, et al. Astrovirus-like particles associated with hepatitis in ducklings. *Vet Rec* 1984;114:279.
48. Gray EW, Angus KW, Snodgrass DR. Ultrastructure of the small intestine in astrovirus-infected lambs. *J Gen Virol* 1980;49:71–82.
49. Grimm AC, Cashdollar JL, Williams FP, et al. Development of an astrovirus RT-PCR detection assay for use with conventional, real-time, and integrated cell culture/RT-PCR. *Can J Microbiol* 2004;50:269–278.
50. Grohmann GS, Glass RI, Pereira HG, et al. Enteric viruses and diarrhea in HIV-infected patients. Enteric Opportunistic Infections Working Group. *N Engl J Med* 1993;329:14–20.
51. Gronemus JQ, Hair PS, Crawford KB, et al. Potent inhibition of the classical pathway of complement by a novel C1q-binding peptide derived from the human astrovirus coat protein. *Mol Immunol* 2010;48:305–313.
52. Guerrero ML, Noel JS, Mitchell DK, et al. A prospective study of astrovirus diarrhea of infancy in Mexico City. *Pediatr Infect Dis J* 1998;17: 723–727.
53. Guix S, Bosch A, Ribes E, et al. Apoptosis in astrovirus-infected CaCo-2 cells. *Virology* 2004;319:249–261.
54. Guix S, Caballero S, Bosch A, et al. C-terminal nsP1a protein of human astrovirus colocalizes with the endoplasmic reticulum and viral RNA. *J Virol* 2004;78:13627–13636.
55. Guix S, Caballero S, Bosch A, et al. Human astrovirus C-terminal nsP1a protein is involved in RNA replication. *Virology* 2005;333: 124–131.
56. Guix S, Caballero S, Villena C, et al. Molecular epidemiology of astrovirus infection in Barcelona, Spain. *J Clin Microbiol* 2002;40: 133–139.
57. Hair PS, Gronemus JQ, Crawford KB, et al. Human astrovirus coat protein binds C1q and MBL and inhibits the classical and lectin pathways of complement activation. *Mol Immunol* 2010;47:792–798.
58. Herring AJ, Gray EW, Snodgrass DR. Purification and characterization of ovine astrovirus. *J Gen Virol* 1981;53:47–55.
59. Herrmann JE, Cubitt WD, Hudson RW, et al. Immunological characterization of the Marin County strain of astrovirus. *Arch Virol* 1990; 110:213–220.
60. Herrmann JE, Nowak NA, Perron-Henry DM, et al. Diagnosis of astrovirus gastroenteritis by antigen detection with monoclonal antibodies. *J Infect Dis* 1990;161:226–229.
61. Herrmann JE, Taylor DN, Echeverria P, et al. Astroviruses as a cause of gastroenteritis in children. *N Engl J Med* 1991;324:1757–1760.
62. Imada T, Yamaguchi S, Mase M, et al. Avian nephritis virus (ANV) as a new member of the family Astroviridae and construction of infectious ANV cDNA. *J Virol* 2000;74:8487–8493.
63. Jakab F, Peterfai J, Verebely T, et al. Human astrovirus infection associated with childhood intussusception. *Pediatr Int* 2007;49:103–105.
64. Jang SY, Jeong WH, Kim MS, et al. Detection of replicating negative-sense RNAs in CaCo-2 cells infected with human astrovirus. *Arch Virol* 2010;155:1383–1389.
65. Jiang B, Monroe SS, Koonin EV, et al. RNA sequence of astrovirus: distinctive genomic organization and a putative retrovirus-like ribosomal frameshifting signal that directs the viral replicase synthesis. *Proc Natl Acad Sci U S A* 1993;90:10539–10543.
66. Jindal N, Patnayak DP, Chander Y, et al. Comparison of capsid gene sequences of turkey astrovirus-2 from poult-enteritis-syndrome-affected and apparently healthy turkeys. *Arch Virol* 2011;156(6):969–977.
67. Jonassen CM, Jonassen TO, Saif YM, et al. Comparison of capsid sequences from human and animal astroviruses. *J Gen Virol* 2001;82: 1061–1067.
68. Jonassen CM, Jonassen TT, Sveen TM, et al. Complete genomic sequences of astroviruses from sheep and turkey: comparison with related viruses. *Virus Res* 2003;91:195–201.
69. Kapoor A, Li L, Victoria J, et al. Multiple novel astrovirus species in human stool. *J Gen Virol* 2009;90:2965–2972.
70. Koci MD. Immunity and resistance to astrovirus infection. *Viral Immunol* 2005;18:11–16.
71. Koci MD, Kelley LA, Larsen D, et al. Astrovirus-induced synthesis of nitric oxide contributes to virus control during infection. *J Virol* 2004; 78:1564–1574.
72. Koci MD, Moser LA, Kelley LA, et al. Astrovirus induces diarrhea in the absence of inflammation and cell death. *J Virol* 2003;77:11798–11808.
73. Koci MD, Seal BS, Schultz-Cherry S. Molecular characterization of an avian astrovirus. *J Virol* 2000;74:6173–6177.
74. Konno T, Suzuki H, Ishida N, et al. Astrovirus-associated epidemic gastroenteritis in Japan. *J Med Virol* 1982;9:11–17.
75. Koopmans MP, Bijen MH, Monroe SS, et al. Age-stratified seroprevalence of neutralizing antibodies to astrovirus types 1 to 7 in humans in The Netherlands. *Clin Diagn Lab Immunol* 1998;5:33–37.
76. Krishna NK. Identification of structural domains involved in astrovirus capsid biology. *Viral Immunol* 2005;18:17–26.
77. Kurtz J, Lee T. Astrovirus gastroenteritis age distribution of antibody. *Med Microbiol Immunol (Berl)* 1978;166:227–230.
78. Kurtz JB, Lee TW. Astroviruses: human and animal. *Ciba Found Symp* 1987;128:92–107.
79. Kurtz JB, Lee TW. Human astrovirus serotypes. *Lancet* 1984;2:1405.
80. Kurtz JB, Lee TW, Parsons AJ. The action of alcohols on rotavirus, astrovirus and enterovirus. *J Hosp Infect* 1980;1:321–325.

81. Le Cann P, Ranarijaona S, Monpoeho S, et al. Quantification of human astroviruses in sewage using real-time RT-PCR. *Res Microbiol* 2004; 155:11–15.
82. Lee TW, Kurtz JB. Serial propagation of astrovirus in tissue culture with the aid of trypsin. *J Gen Virol* 1981;57:421–424.
83. Lewis DC, Lightfoot NF, Cubitt WD, et al. Outbreaks of astrovirus type 1 and rotavirus gastroenteritis in a geriatric in-patient population. *J Hosp Infect* 1989;14:9–14.
84. Lewis TL, Matsui SM. Studies of the astrovirus signal that induces (−1) ribosomal frameshifting. *Adv Exp Med Biol* 1997;412:323–330.
85. Luo Z, Roi S, Dastor M, et al. Multiple novel and prevalent astroviruses in pigs. *Vet Microbiol* 2011;149:316–323.
86. Madeley CR, Cosgrove BP. Letter: Viruses in infantile gastroenteritis. *Lancet* 1975;2:124.
87. Maldonado Y, Cantwell M, Old M, et al. Population-based prevalence of symptomatic and asymptomatic astrovirus infection in rural Mayan infants. *J Infect Dis* 1998;178:334–339.
88. Matsui SM, Kiang D, Ginzton N, et al. Molecular biology of astroviruses: selected highlights. *Novartis Found Symp* 2001;238:219–233; discussion 233–236.
89. Matsui SM, Kim JP, Greenberg HB, et al. Cloning and characterization of human astrovirus immunoreactive epitopes. *J Virol* 1993;67:1712–1715.
90. Maunula L, Kalso S, Von Bonsdorff CH, et al. Wading pool water contaminated with both noroviruses and astroviruses as the source of a gastroenteritis outbreak. *Epidemiol Infect* 2004;132:737–743.
91. Mendez E, Aguirre-Crespo G, Zavala G, et al. Association of the astrovirus structural protein VP90 with membranes plays a role in virus morphogenesis. *J Virol* 2007;81(19):10649–10658.
92. Mendez E, Arias CF. Astroviruses. In: Knipe DM, Howley PM, eds. *Fields Virology*, 5th ed. Philadelphia: Lippincott Williams & Willkins; 2007: 981–1000.
93. Mendez E, Fernandez-Luna T, Lopez S, et al. Proteolytic processing of a serotype 8 human astrovirus ORF2 polyprotein. *J Virol* 2002;76:7996–8002.
94. Mendez E, Salas-Ocampo E, Arias CF. Caspases mediate processing of the capsid precursor and cell release of human astroviruses. *J Virol* 2004;78: 8601–8608.
95. Mendez E, Salas-Ocampo MP, Munguia ME, et al. Protein products of the open reading frames encoding nonstructural proteins of human astrovirus serotype 8. *J Virol* 2003;77:11378–11384.
96. Mendez-Toss M, Griffin DD, Calva J, et al. Prevalence and genetic diversity of human astroviruses in Mexican children with symptomatic and asymptomatic infections. *J Clin Microbiol* 2004;42:151–157.
97. Midthun K, Greenberg HB, Kurtz JB, et al. Characterization and seroepidemiology of a type 5 astrovirus associated with an outbreak of gastroenteritis in Marin County, California. *J Clin Microbiol* 1993;31: 955–962.
98. Mitchell DK, Matson DO, Jiang X, et al. Molecular epidemiology of childhood astrovirus infection in child care centers. *J Infect Dis* 1999; 180:514–517.
99. Mitchell DK, Van R, Morrow AL, et al. Outbreaks of astrovirus gastroenteritis in day care centers. *J Pediatr* 1993;123:725–732.
100. Molberg O, Nilsen EM, Sollid LM, et al. CD4+ T cells with specific reactivity against astrovirus isolated from normal human small intestine. *Gastroenterology* 1998;114:115–122.
101. Monceyron C, Grinde B, Jonassen TO. Molecular characterisation of the 3′-end of the astrovirus genome. *Arch Virol* 1997;142:699–706.
102. Monroe SS. Molecular epidemiology of human astroviruses. In: Desselberger U, Gray JJ, eds. *Perspectives in Medical Virology. Viral Gastroenteritis, vol. 9.* Amsterdam: Elsevier; 2003:607–616.
103. Monroe SS, Jiang B, Stine SE, et al. Subgenomic RNA sequence of human astrovirus supports classification of Astroviridae as a new family of RNA viruses. *J Virol* 1993;67:3611–3614.
104. Monroe SS, Stine SE, Gorelkin L, et al. Temporal synthesis of proteins and RNAs during human astrovirus infection of cultured cells. *J Virol* 1991;65:641–648.
105. Moser LA, Carter M, Schultz-Cherry S. Astrovirus increases epithelial barrier permeability independently of viral replication. *J Virol* 2007; 81:11937–11945.
106. Moser LA, Schultz-Cherry S. Pathogenesis of astrovirus infection. *Viral Immunol* 2005;18:4–10.
107. Moser LA, Schultz-Cherry S. Suppression of astrovirus replication by an ERK1/2 inhibitor. *J Virol* 2008;82:7475–7482.
108. Nadan S, Walter JE, Grabow WO, et al. Molecular characterization of astroviruses by reverse transcriptase PCR and sequence analysis: comparison of clinical and environmental isolates from South Africa. *Appl Environ Microbiol* 2003;69:747–753.
109. Naficy AB, Rao MR, Holmes JL, et al. Astrovirus diarrhea in Egyptian children. *J Infect Dis* 2000;182:685–690.
110. Nighot PK, Moeser A, Ali RA, et al. Astrovirus infection induces sodium malabsorption and redistributes sodium hydrogen exchanger expression. *Virology* 2010;401:146–154.
111. Noel J, Cubitt D. Identification of astrovirus serotypes from children treated at the Hospitals for Sick Children, London 1981–93. *Epidemiol Infect* 1994;113:153–159.
112. Oishi I, Yamazaki K, Kimoto T, et al. A large outbreak of acute gastroenteritis associated with astrovirus among students and teachers in Osaka, Japan. *J Infect Dis* 1994;170:439–443.
113. Palombo EA, Bishop RF. Annual incidence, serotype distribution, and genetic diversity of human astrovirus isolates from hospitalized children in Melbourne, Australia. *J Clin Microbiol* 1996;34:1750–1753.
114. Pusch D, Oh DY, Wolf S, et al. Detection of enteric viruses and bacterial indicators in German environmental waters. *Arch Virol* 2005;150(5):929–947.
115. Quan PL, Wagner TA, Briese T, et al. Astrovirus encephalitis in boy with X-linked agammaglobulinemia. *Emerg Infect Dis* 2010;16:918–925.
116. Risco C, Carrascosa JL, Pedregosa AM, et al. Ultrastructure of human astrovirus serotype 2. *J Gen Virol* 1995;76(Pt 8):2075–2080.
117. Rivera R, Nollens HH, Venn-Watson S, et al. Characterization of phylogenetically diverse astroviruses of marine mammals. *J Gen Virol* 2010; 91:166–173.
118. Rohayem J, Berger S, Juretzek T, et al. A simple and rapid single-step multiplex RT-PCR to detect Norovirus, Astrovirus and Adenovirus in clinical stool samples. *J Virol Methods* 2004;118:49–59.
119. Sanchez-Fauquier A, Carrascosa AL, Carrascosa JL, et al. Characterization of a human astrovirus serotype 2 structural protein (VP26) that contains an epitope involved in virus neutralization. *Virology* 1994;201: 312–320.
120. Schnagl RD, Belfrage K, Farrington R, et al. Incidence of human astrovirus in central Australia (1995 to 1998) and comparison of deduced serotypes detected from 1981 to 1998. *J Clin Microbiol* 2002;40:4114–4120.
121. Schultz-Cherry S, King DJ, Koci MD. Inactivation of an astrovirus associated with poult enteritis mortality syndrome. *Avian Dis* 2001;45:76–82.
122. Sebire NJ, Malone M, Shah N, et al. Pathology of astrovirus associated diarrhoea in a paediatric bone marrow transplant recipient. *J Clin Pathol* 2004;57:1001–1003.
123. Sellers H, Linneman E, Icard AH, et al. A purified recombinant baculovirus expressed capsid protein of a new astrovirus provides partial protection to runting-stunting syndrome in chickens. *Vaccine* 2010;28: 1253–1263.
124. Sellers HS, Koci MD, Linnemann E, et al. Development of a multiplex reverse transcription-polymerase chain reaction diagnostic test specific for turkey astrovirus and coronavirus. *Avian Dis* 2004;48:531–539.
125. Shimizu M, Shirai J, Narita M, et al. Cytopathic astrovirus isolated from porcine acute gastroenteritis in an established cell line derived from porcine embryonic kidney. *J Clin Microbiol* 1990;28:201–206.
126. Singh PB, Sreenivasan MA, Pavri KM. Viruses in acute gastroenteritis in children in Pune, India. *Epidemiol Infect* 1989;102:345–353.
127. Smits SL, van Leeuwen M, van der Eijk AA, et al. Human astrovirus infection in a patient with new-onset celiac disease. *J Clin Microbiol* 2010; 48:3416–3418.
128. Smyth JA, Connor TJ, McNeilly F, et al. Studies on the pathogenicity of enterovirus-like viruses in chickens. *Avian Pathol* 2007;36:119–126.
129. Smyth VJ, Jewhurst HL, Wilkinson DS, et al. Development and evaluation of real-time TaqMan(R) RT-PCR assays for the detection of avian nephritis virus and chicken astrovirus in chickens. *Avian Pathol* 2010; 39:467–474.
130. Snodgrass DR, Angus KW, Gray EW, et al. Pathogenesis of diarrhoea caused by astrovirus infections in lambs. *Arch Virol* 1979;60:217–226.
131. Speroni S, Rohayem J, Nenci S, et al. Structural and biochemical analysis of human pathogenic astrovirus serine protease at 2.0 A resolution. *J Mol Biol* 2009;387:1137–1152.

132. Strain E, Kelley LA, Schultz-Cherry S, et al. Genomic analysis of closely related astroviruses. *J Virol* 2008;82:5099–5103.
133. Tang Y, Murgia MV, Ward L, et al. Pathogenicity of turkey astroviruses in turkey embryos and poults. *Avian Dis* 2006;50:526–531.
134. Tang Y, Saif YM. Antigenicity of two turkey astrovirus isolates. *Avian Dis* 2004;48:896–901.
135. Tanner NK, Linder P. DExD/H box RNA helicases: from generic motors to specific dissociation functions. *Mol Cell* 2001;8:251–262.
136. Todd D, Trudgett J, McNeilly F, et al. Development and application of an RT-PCR test for detecting avian nephritis virus. *Avian Pathol* 2010;39: 207–213.
137. Todd D, Wilkinson DS, Jewhurst HL, et al. A seroprevalence investigation of chicken astrovirus infections. *Avian Pathol* 2009;38:301–309.
138. Verma H, Chitambar SD, Gopalkrishna V. Astrovirus associated acute gastroenteritis in western India: predominance of dual serotype strains. *Infect Genet Evol* 2010;10:575–579.
139. Vilarino ML, Le Guyader FS, Polo D, et al. Assessment of human enteric viruses in cultured and wild bivalve molluscs. *Int Microbiol* 2009; 12:145–151.
140. Walter JE, Briggs J, Guerrero ML, et al. Molecular characterization of a novel recombinant strain of human astrovirus associated with gastroenteritis in children. *Arch Virol* 2001;146:2357–2367.
141. Walter JE, Mitchell DK. Astrovirus infection in children. *Curr Opin Infect Dis* 2003;16:247–253.
142. Wang QH, Kakizawa J, Wen LY, et al. Genetic analysis of the capsid region of astroviruses. *J Med Virol* 2001;64:245–255.
143. Wang X, Wang Y, Xie X, et al. Expression of the C-terminal ORF2 protein of duck astrovirus for application in a serological test. *J Virol Methods* 2011;171:8–12.
144. Willcocks MM, Ashton N, Kurtz JB, et al. Cell culture adaptation of astrovirus involves a deletion. *J Virol* 1994;68:6057–6058.
145. Willcocks MM, Boxall AS, Carter MJ. Processing and intracellular location of human astrovirus non-structural proteins. *J Gen Virol* 1999;80 (Pt 10):2607–2611.
146. Willcocks MM, Carter MJ. Identification and sequence determination of the capsid protein gene of human astrovirus serotype 1. *FEMS Microbiol Lett* 1993;114:1–7.
147. Willcocks MM, Carter MJ, Laidler FR, et al. Growth and characterisation of human faecal astrovirus in a continuous cell line. *Arch Virol* 1990;113:73–81.
148. Wolfaardt M, Kiulia NM, Mwenda JM, et al. Evidence of a recombinant wild-type human astrovirus strain from a Kenyan child with gastroenteritis. *J Clin Microbiol* 2011;49:728–731.
149. Wood DJ, David TJ, Chrystie IL, et al. Chronic enteric virus infection in two T-cell immunodeficient children. *J Med Virol* 1988;24:435–444.
150. Woode GN, Pohlenz JF, Gourley NE, et al. Astrovirus and Breda virus infections of dome cell epithelium of bovine ileum. *J Clin Microbiol* 1984; 19:623–630.
151. Yan H, Yagyu F, Okitsu S, et al. Detection of norovirus (GI, GII), Sapovirus and astrovirus in fecal samples using reverse transcription single-round multiplex PCR. *J Virol Methods* 2003;114:37–44.
152. Zhu HC, Chu DK, Liu W, et al. Detection of diverse astroviruses from bats in China. *J Gen Virol* 2009;90:883–887.

CHAPTER 22

Richard J. Kuhn

Togaviridae

The togaviruses are simple enveloped plus-strand RNA viruses that are spherical in appearance and contribute significantly to human disease. Although they were originally classified together with several groups of viruses that are transmitted predominantly by insects, more recent analyses have categorized them into a distinct family with two genera: *Alphavirus* and the *Rubivirus*.[167,208] The *Alphavirus* genus is by far the larger of the two, with about 30 recognized members, whereas the *Rubivirus* genus is composed of a single member, rubella virus. Virus classification into each group is determined by genome organization and nucleotide homologies. The alphaviruses are responsible for a variety of human and animal diseases, involving encephalitis, arthritis, fever, and rash, and are transmitted primarily by arthropod vectors. Viruses such as Chikungunya (CHIKV) and Venezuelan equine encephalitis virus (VEEV) have been responsible for recent human outbreaks and have raised awareness of the significance and potential threat of alphaviruses to human health. Rubella virus is a common childhood illness for which an effective vaccine is available. However, in the absence of immunity, the virus can induce severe congenital defects in the fetuses of infected women.

Sindbis virus (SINV), the type-member of the alphavirus genus, has been studied extensively, in large part due to its facile growth in cell culture and its ability to cause mild or inapparent illness in humans. The virus has an 11.7-kb RNA genome that is capped at its 5′ end and contains a poly A tract at its 3′ terminus.[265] Virions have a spherical icosahedral arrangement of proteins that has facilitated their structural analysis. The detailed knowledge of the viral life cycle, which is the focus of this chapter, has been exploited for the development of alphavirus gene expression vectors. Many members of this virus group have been studied for their role in pathogenesis. Rubella virus, as expected from its classification, shares a number of properties with the alphaviruses, yet has several important distinctions that are highlighted throughout the chapter.

CLASSIFICATION OF VIRUSES WITHIN THE *TOGAVIRIDAE* FAMILY

Viruses transmitted by arthropods have been referred to as arboviruses.[208] It was originally noted that many arboviruses had a similar morphologic structure, as observed by electron microscopy, that resembled a Roman cloak (in Latin, *toga*), hence the name togaviruses. Originally, the family *Togaviridae* consisted of group A (alphaviruses) and group B (flaviviruses); however, the genera *Rubivirus* and *Pestivirus* were later added based on their similar physical properties but despite their lack of arthropod transmission. With the development of sequencing, it became apparent that the original joint classification for these viruses was in error. The *togaviruses* have nonstructural or replication proteins encoded at the 5′ end of their genome RNA, whereas the 3′ end encodes the proteins that comprise the virus particle, or virion. In the togaviruses, these structural proteins are translated from a subgenomic messenger RNA (mRNA) that derives from, and is co-terminal with, the 3′ end of the genome.[219,265]

The larger of the two genera within togaviruses, the *Alphaviruses,* has been classified into seven antigenically related complexes.[209] Most phylogenetic analyses support this classification, but several recent additions add complexity to the organization. The alphaviruses have a worldwide geographic distribution, including the continent of Antarctica. The alphaviruses have classically been described as either Old World or New World viruses, depending on their distribution, and it is likely that several transoceanic exchanges have occurred.[209] Most alphaviruses are transmitted by arthropod vectors that probably control their geographic dispersal. However, the recent identification of the salmonid viruses, salmon pancreas disease virus, and sleeping disease virus (infecting rainbow trout), present examples of alphaviruses for which arthropod transmission is unlikely.[293,309] These salmonid viruses appear to have diverged from the Old World–New World lineages early in alphavirus evolution, with no present-day close relatives. Another identified alphavirus, southern elephant seal virus, has been isolated from the louse *Lepidophthirus macrorhini*.[151] This isolation demonstrates not only that alphaviruses are transmitted by lice, but that they can also infect marine mammals, and a recent report suggests a marine origin for the alphaviruses.[51] Given this wide host range, it seems probable that amphibian- and reptile-specific alphaviruses also await future identification.

Although the alphaviruses and rubella virus have been classified within the same family, the evolutionary relationship between them is obscure.[54] They have a similar genome organization, and their virions share physical similarities, yet their replication and assembly strategies are sufficiently diverse to question whether they arose from a direct ancestor.

VIRION STRUCTURE

Structure of Mature Virion

The structure of the alphavirus virion has been extensively studied, and numerous high-resolution structural studies now provide a near-atomic view of the virion. Although a variety of biophysical methods were used to elaborate the alphavirus structure, work that has advanced the field the most has come from cryo-electron microscopy (cryo-EM) and image reconstruction techniques.[93,94,287,288] The virion is 70 nm in diameter, with a molecular mass of 52×10^6 D and a density of 1.22 g per cc. It is composed of repeating units of the E1 and E2 transmembrane glycoproteins, the capsid or nucleocapsid protein (C), a host-derived lipid bilayer, and a single molecule of genome RNA. The protein components of the virion are arranged as a T = 4 icosahedral lattice, with 240 copies of each subunit.[27,198,201] These subunits interact with one another to form a rigid structure across the membrane in a one-to-one relationship between glycoprotein E2 and the capsid protein. Smaller amounts of another membrane-associated protein, 6K, are also found in the virus particle.[64,162] More recently it has been discovered that another small protein, the TransFrame (TF) protein, is found in substoichiometric amounts in the virion.[47] The lipid bilayer is derived from the host plasma membrane and is enriched in cholesterol and sphingolipid, molecules that are required for entry and budding.[114] Inside the bilayer, the C surrounds the genome RNA and forms an icosahedral shell. Thus, the alphaviruses are composed of multiple organized shells of molecules that effectively protect and deliver the viral RNA to susceptible host cells.

Cryo-EM has been used extensively to study the structure of alphaviruses, including SINV,[198] Semliki Forest virus (SFV),[283] Ross River virus (RRV),[27] VEEV,[197,315] Western equine encephalitis virus (WEEV),[247] Aura virus,[316] CHIKV,[298a] and Barmah Forest virus (BFV).[122] The most recent studies with VEEV, BFV, and SINV are the most advanced, with a resolution between 4.4 and 7.0 Å reported for these viruses.[122,315] The surface view of the virion, seen in Figure 22.1 for SINV, reveals a spherical particle with spike protrusions rising 100 Å from the surface. The icosahedral nature of the particle results in an ordered distribution of the petal-like spikes. The asymmetric unit, which is shaded in green in Figure 22.1A, contains four E1–E2 heterodimers. Each spike consists of three heterodimers of E1 and E2 glycoproteins. A total of 80 spikes reside on icosahedral threefold (solid black triangle in Fig. 22.1A) and quasi-threefold axes (open white triangles in Fig. 22.1A). Earlier biochemical studies established the nature of the heterodimer, and this relationship has been confirmed

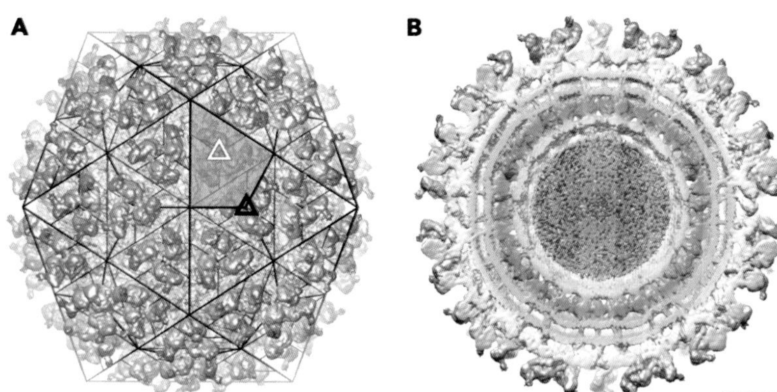

FIGURE 22.1. Structure of alphaviruses determined using cryo-EM. A: Surface-shaded view of Sindbis virus as determined by cryo-electron microscopy (cryo-EM) at 7.0 Å. The trimeric petal-shaped spikes are visible, with solid triangles representing the threefold axes, and white triangles representing quasi-threefold axes. One of the asymmetric units is highlighted by green shading. **B:** The same view as shown in A but with the front half of the reconstructed structure removed. The outer layer containing spikes is shown in blue, whereas the underlying skirt density is in magenta. Crossing the lipid bilayer (cyan) reveals the ordered capsid protein (green; residues 114–264), a disordered region containing a mix of protein and RNA (yellow), and a region containing the remainder of the RNA genome (red). The transmembrane densities of E1 and E2 are seen spanning the outer and inner leaflets of the lipid bilayer (cyan). (Reproduced from Tang J, Jose J, Chipman P, et al. Molecular links between the E2 envelope glycoprotein and nucleocapsid core in Sindbis virus. *J Mol Biol* 2011;414:442–459; copyright 2011, with permission from Elsevier.)

by cryo-EM reconstructions[218,321] and by x-ray crystallography.[145,289] Although the protein lattice occupies a substantial surface area, small openings are present in the virion that reveal the underlying lipid bilayer. These openings are most pronounced at the twofold axes, but can also be found at the fivefold axes and around the base of each spike.

The transmembrane components of the two glycoproteins are clearly seen in the cryo-EM reconstructions (Fig. 22.1B). The shape of density suggests that each transmembrane segment traverses the bilayer as a helix, although the E1 transmembrane domain is better represented by two alpha helices separated by a two amino acid kink.[315] For SINV the E1 glycoprotein has five amino acid residues that penetrate across to the inner side of the membrane (cdE1), whereas E2 has 33 amino acids (cdE2) that interact with the nucleocapsid core.[14,148,153,271] This interaction is observed in cryo-EM reconstructions and demonstrates that each E2 molecule makes specific contacts with each capsid protein. The nucleocapsid core has a T = 4 arrangement of capsid protein, with the C-terminal protease domain forming pentameric and hexameric projections that appear as capsomeres on the surface of nucleocapsid cores (shown in green in Fig. 22.1B). The genome RNA does not appear to assume regular symmetry within the nucleocapsid core and is not ordered in the reconstructions (red in Fig. 22.1B).

Structure of Immature Virion

The structure of the immature virus containing an uncleaved precursor to E2, called PE2 or p62, has also been solved using cryo-EM.[46,200] Mutant versions of both SINV and SFV were used for independent structure determinations resulting in similar structures. The extra density corresponding to the small protein E3 was found predominantly between the petals of the spike resulting in a dual-lobed petal. At a resolution of 25 Å, no apparent differences were found in the skirt or other regions of the spike and suggest that following cleavage of PE2 and release of E3, no significant conformational changes occur in the virus structure. The immature form of the virus that contains PE2 has been proposed to stabilize the fusion protein as it transits the mildly acidic environment of the Golgi.[155,157,291]

Structural Proteins of the Virion

The proteins that comprise the alphavirus virion are synthesized as a polyprotein from a subgenomic RNA and are shown in Figure 22.2. The structures of the three major virion proteins have been determined by x-ray crystallography to high resolution. The capsid protein functions to encapsidate the genome RNA and forms a T = 4 icosahedron prior to release from the cell. The 264 amino acid capsid protein of SINV was crystallized, although the N-terminal 105 residues have been absent in all of the final structures.[29] It was suggested that the highly basic N-terminal domain was susceptible to proteases and degraded during crystal growth. A similar observation was made for the SFV capsid protein.[28] The C-terminal residues 114 to 264 of the SINV capsid protein form a chymotrypsin-like fold with the ultimate residue tryptophan 264 bound in the active-site protease pocket. The fold contains two Greek key *β*–barrel domains that bring the catalytic triad of Ser215, His141, and Asp163 into juxtaposition for activity.[86] This structure substantiated biochemical and genetic data that proposed that the capsid protein had an autocatalytic serine protease activity.[10,85,168] The atomic structure of the capsid protein was used to generate a "pseudoatomic" resolution structure of the alphavirus nucleocapsid core (Figure 22.3) by fitting its coordinates into the cryo-EM density.[27,179,228] This was accomplished and it was suggested that the missing residues of the N-terminus would point inward from the core surface and interact with the negatively charged viral RNA. The recent 4.4 Å cryo-EM structure of VEEV provides support for the earlier fitted structures, but the N-terminal basic domain residues (1–110). Remains obscure as ordered density within the nucleocapsid core has not been observed.[315]

The E1 protein functions as a class II fusion machine to promote the joining of viral and cellular membranes under conditions of low pH. The structure of the E1 molecule from SFV was solved using x-ray crystallography.[138] The starting material for crystallization was the SFV spike cleaved with subtilisin, which released the ectodomains of the E1 and E2 glycoproteins.[307] Unfortunately, the crystals contained only the E1 polypeptide, and it was assumed that E2 was proteolyzed.

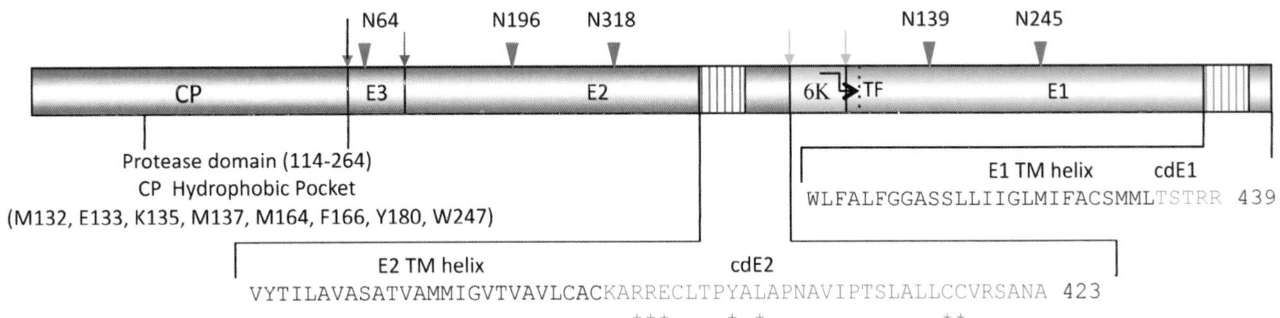

FIGURE 22.2. A schematic of the Sindbis virus structural polyprotein. The individual proteins are color coded, with protease cleavage sites indicated by an *arrow*. N-linked glycosylation sites are shown by green arrowheads. The amino acids that comprise the transmembrane and cytoplasmic domains of both E1 and E2 are shown. *Asterisks* indicate residues of cdE2 that interact with the capsid protein. The TransFrame (TF) protein is identified by the *bent arrow* followed by the *dotted line* crossing E1.

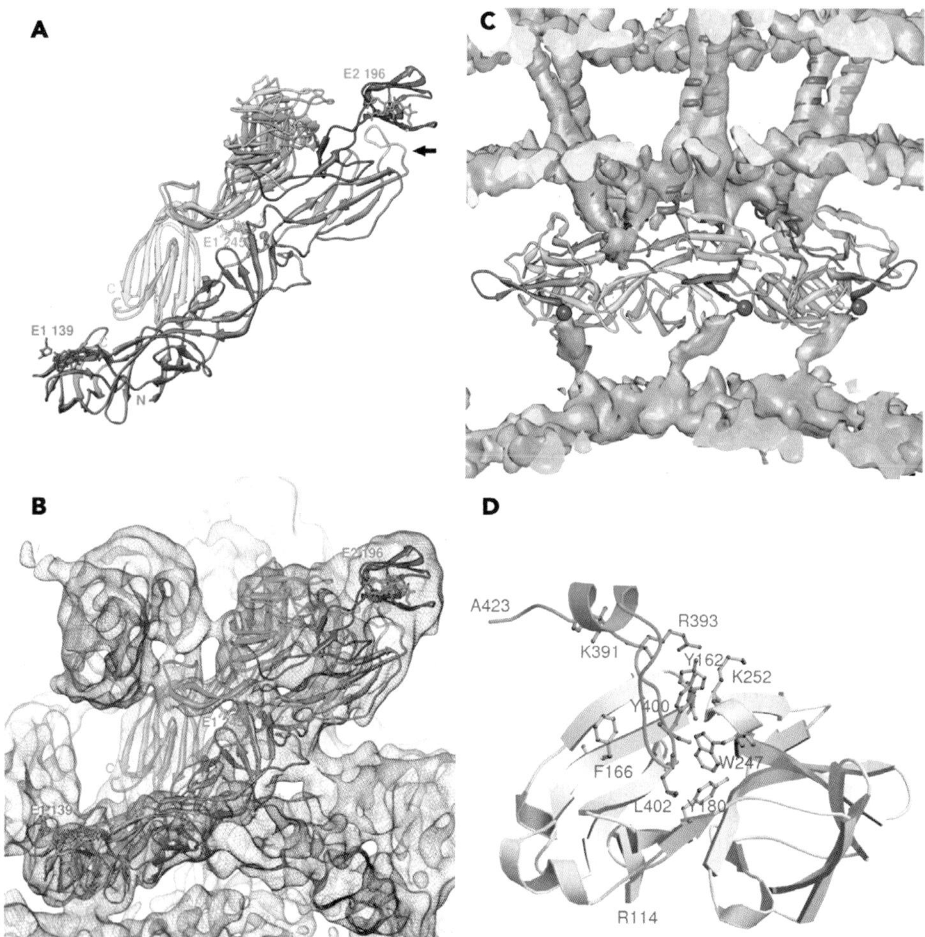

FIGURE 22.3. Pseudoatomic representation of the Sindbis virus structural proteins based on the 7.0 Å cryo-electron microscopy (cryo-EM) reconstruction. A: The structure of E1 and E2 of Sindbis virus. E1 is shown in red. The A and C domains of E2 are shown in two colors, with one representing the structure from the crystal structure (cyan) and the other obtained by fitting the crystal structure into the cryo-EM map (green). The B domain of E2 (blue) is a homology-modeled structure derived from the Chikungunya crystal structure. The arrow points to the E1 fusion peptide (yellow). **B:** Same as in **A** but fitted into the cryo-EM density (grey mesh). **C:** Cross-section of the fitted cryo-EM structure showing the transmembrane helices of E1 (red) and E2 (green) and the underlying N-terminal protease domain of the capsid protein (residues 114–264). Below capsid residue 114 (blue ball), the remaining N-terminal residues of the capsid are not identified but must interact with the underlying genome RNA. Additional EM density is shown in gray. **D:** Interactions between the capsid protein and the cdE2. The residues that comprise cdE2 (amino acids 391–423) were modeled according to the cryo-EM density and are shown as they interact with the hydrophobic pocket of the capsid protein. Residues of the capsid that have been shown as important in this interaction—F166, Y180, and W247—are highlighted. (Reproduced from Tang J, Jose J, Chipman P, et al. Molecular links between the E2 envelope glycoprotein and nucleocapsid core in Sindbis virus. *J Mol Biol* 2011;414:442–459; copyright 2011, with permission from Elsevier.)

The structure of the E1 ectodomain (residues 1–383) is shown in Figure 22.3 and contains three β–barrel domains. Domain I, the so-called central domain, links domains II and III. The extended domain II contains at its distal end the fusion peptide, a short loop of hydrophobic amino acids that promotes insertion of the protein into the target membrane. Domain III has an immunoglobulin (Ig)-like fold and connects at its C-terminus with the transmembrane domain of the protein.

The structure of E1 is remarkably similar to that of the flavivirus E protein.[217,269] Unlike the alphaviruses, the flavivirus E protein functions both in receptor attachment and in membrane fusion. In the alphaviruses, these two activities are carried out by proteins E2 and E1, respectively. In the flaviviruses, the E protein is oriented roughly parallel to the lipid membrane, and it was anticipated that E1 might assume a similar orientation in the alphavirus virion.[124] This was essentially verified once the E1 atomic structure was fitted into the cryo-EM density. This fitting was accomplished for both SFV and SINV, and most recently for CHIKV.[138,145,207,289] Furthermore, for SINV, the two sites of E1 glycosylation were mapped onto the cryo-EM structure, and these sites at Asn139 and Asn245 were used as positional markers to fix the position of E1 in the virion.[207] E1 lies at an angle of ~50 degrees relative to the surface of the membrane (Figure 22.3B), and it forms an icosahedral lattice comprising the region that has been referred to as the skirt.[138,207] The crystallographic E1 dimer, which is a back-to-back dimer as opposed to a face-to-face dimer seen in the flaviviruses, is essentially preserved in the arrangement of E1 in the virion. The interface residues that make contact in the crystallographic dimer are presumably those that are important for forming the icosahedral lattice in the virion.

Although E1 comprises the skirt region of the alphavirus surface, the majority of the protruding spike is comprised of the E2 molecule. E2 constitutes the petals that make up the spike, and covers the distal end of the E1 molecule that points outward. E2 serves to engage cell surface receptor molecules required for entry of the virion into the cell. The crystal structure of E2 together with both E1 and E3 for CHIKV was solved and reveals a three-immunoglobulin domain protein.[289] Domain B is located at the outermost point of the spike and contains the residues that have been implicated in receptor binding and as well as those involved in binding neutralizing antibodies. Domain B exhibits mobility in the context of the spike and was absent from the intact SINV E1–E2 trimer structure done at low pH.[145] At the other end of the protein, located closest to the viral membrane, is the C-terminal domain C. The N-terminal domain A (residues 1–132 in SINV) is the central bridge of E2, and connections are made to the B domain by β–ribbon connectors. The β–ribbon connector is flanked by a pair of well-conserved histidine residues that might function as an acid switch to release the connector and B domain under acidic conditions. Although E3 does not directly contact E1, its contact with the β–ribbon connector holds it in place to prevent movement of the B domain while the virus is in the process of egress from the cell in an immature state. The furin cleavage of the p62 to release E3, therefore, releases the clamp holding the B domain and activating the complex for pH-triggered fusion. E1 and E2 have extensive contacts with each other, promoting the spike architecture (Fig. 22.3).

In addition to the three major structural proteins identified by cryo-EM in the virion, two small transmembrane proteins are present in sub-stoichiometric amounts and can be identified using purified virus and mass spectrometry. The existence of the 6K protein in the virion has been well established, but more recently the TF protein (~8 kD) has also been found within SFV particles.[47] Given the low abundance and presumably random distribution of these small transmembrane proteins, they have not been detected using high-resolution cryo-EM, and their membrane architecture has to date prevented x-ray crystal structures. Whether the TF and 6K proteins exist as oligomers is also unknown.

GENOME STRUCTURE AND ORGANIZATION

The togavirus genome resides on a positive-strand RNA that contains a 5′ terminal 7-methylguanosine and a 3′ terminus that is polyadenylated. The alphavirus genome, represented in Figure 22.4 by the type virus SINV, is approximately 11.7 kb in length, whereas rubella virus is nearly 2 kb shorter, at 9.8 kb.[40,265] The genomes segregate their replication and virion protein coding regions into two segments, with the replication region mapping to the 5′ two-thirds and the structural region mapping to the 3′ one-third. Limited nucleotide homology exists between genomes in the two genera, although there are several sequences in both translated and nontranslated regions that do have homology; however, most evidence suggests that their replication and assembly strategies are quite different.[40]

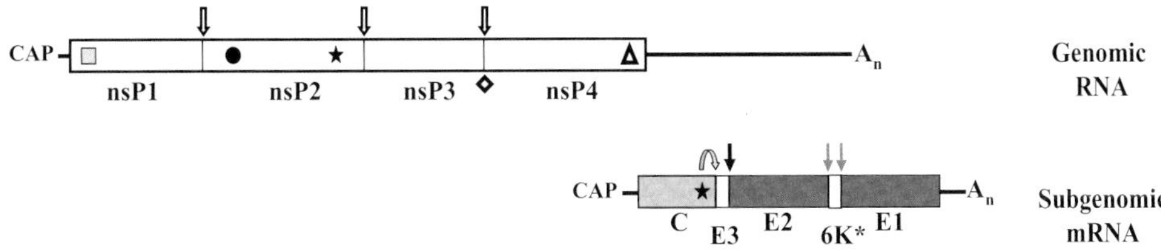

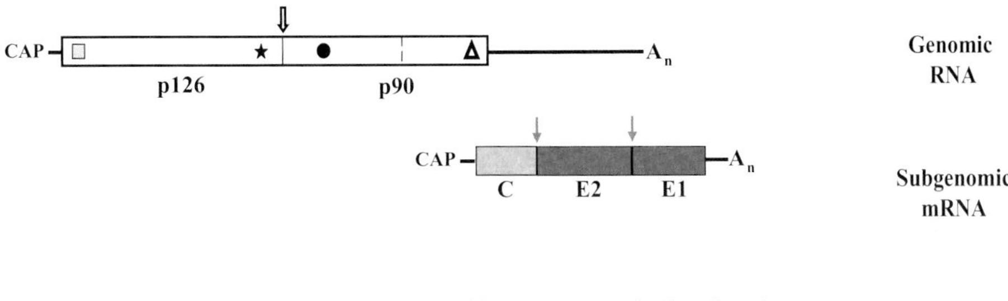

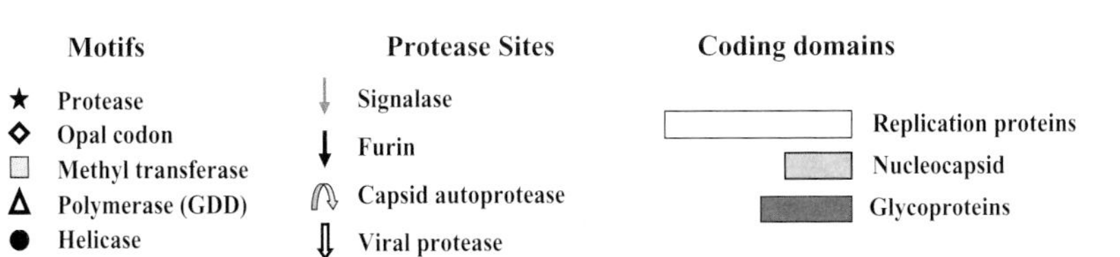

FIGURE 22.4. The genomes of Sinbis virus and rubella virus. Nontranslated regions are shown by the *solid line* and translated regions are shown in *boxes*. *Open boxes* indicate replication proteins and *shaded boxes* represent structural or virion proteins. Motifs and cleavage sites are indicated according to the scheme. The subgenomic mRNAs are not shown to scale with the genomic RNAs.

The nonstructural or replication proteins are translated from the genome RNA, whereas the structural or virion proteins are translated from a subgenomic mRNA.[191,251] In SINV, the 5′ nontranslated region (NTR) is 59 nucleotides, about average for the alphaviruses, whereas the 3′ NTR is also close to the average in length at 322 nucleotides.

Using comparative genome analyses and functional genetic studies of defective interfering particles and viruses, four conserved regions (conserved sequence element [CSE]) of the alphavirus genome were identified as *cis*-acting elements important for replication.[184,185–186] Two conserved regions are found near the 5′ end of the genome, one is found in the junction region between nonstructural and structural genes, and one is found at the 3′ end immediately preceding the poly (A). Three presumably similar functioning CSEs can also be found in the rubella genome.[40] In the alphaviruses, each CSE has been shown to interact in a host-dependent manner, suggesting that host factors may play a role in their function.[44,97,98,123,187,188] It has been shown that a U-rich region in the 3′ NTR of SINV contains elements responsible for viral RNA stability and that the cellular HuR protein binds this region, thus decreasing the rate of cell-mediated decay of the genome RNA.[260] In addition, studies have shown that host proteins bind to the 3′ end of the minus-strand RNA of SINV, and in one case the protein was identified as the mosquito homolog to the La protein.[193,194–195]

ALPHAVIRUS REPLICATION

Mechanism of Attachment and Receptors

Alphaviruses display an extremely broad host range, both in terms of susceptible animal species and in terms of cells in culture. This broad host range has prompted speculation as to the nature of the receptor, with two hypotheses proposed to explain this phenomenon.[266] In the first, the virus E2 glycoprotein contains multiple receptor-binding sites so that distinct cellular receptors can bind the viral surface protein. The second hypothesis proposes that the virus uses a ubiquitous receptor that is highly conserved across species, including both mammals and mosquitoes. Data exist to support each model, and it is likely that a combination of the two is the true strategy for alphavirus attachment to the cell.

The variety of molecules that have been implicated in SINV argues for multiple distinct receptor-binding sites on E2.[266] The use of the laminin receptor with its high conservation across species suggests that it might serve as a receptor in multiple cell types and multiple host species.[295] However, the picture remains obscure for SINV because laminin receptor functions in baby hamster kidney cells but not in chicken embryo fibroblasts, where a 63-kD protein has been implicated.[296] In mouse neuroblastoma cells, proteins of 74 and 110 kD have been reported as possible SINV cellular receptors.[278] DC-SIGN and L-SIGN, C-type lectins that bind mannose-enriched carbohydrates, have also been implicated as receptors of alphaviruses that have been produced in mosquito cells.[118] Very recent studies using a genome-wide RNA interference (RNAi) screen in *Drosophila* cells identified the natural resistance-associated macrophage protein (NRAMP) as a cellular receptor functioning to permit SINV infection.[226] Likewise, NRAMP2, the vertebrate homolog, allowed for SINV, but not RRV, entry into mammalian cells. This new approach and finding raises the possibility that a family of related conserved multipass membrane proteins may serve as receptors for other alphaviruses.

Natural isolates of EEEV utilize cell surface heparan sulfate as an attachment receptor.[65] This use of heparan sulfate may direct tropism of EEEV and promote enhanced neurovirulence. In contrast, passage of several other alphaviruses in culture leads to the accumulation of adaptive mutations, some of which introduce basic amino acids in their E2 glycoprotein.[18,20,21,119] This increase in positively charged amino acids in E2 leads to high efficiency attachment to cells through heparan sulfate molecules. The importance of this interaction was demonstrated genetically by the generation of a Chinese hamster ovary cell line using retroviral insertional mutagenesis that was deficient in the expression of heparan sulfate and chondroitin sulfate.[108] These cells were resistant to SINV infection and defective in binding virus. The substitution of a single residue on the E2 glycoprotein of RRV was sufficient to permit heparan sulfate binding, and this attachment was mapped using cryo-EM to the distal tip of the spike.[97,317] The binding of heparan sulfate does not result in conformational changes in the virion, nor does it enhance the fusion process.[257,317] Therefore, it likely serves simply as a mechanism to attach the particle to the cell surface with high affinity so an efficient interaction with the entry receptor can occur. In contrast to what is observed in cell culture with SINV, infection of mice results in the development of large-plaque viral mutants with a reduced affinity for heparan sulfate and a greater viremia.[21] However, given these diverse observations, the utilization of heparan sulfate and its role in pathogenesis among the different alphaviruses requires further investigation.

Mechanisms of Entry, Membrane Fusion, and Uncoating

Following attachment to cells and engagement with an entry receptor, alphaviruses proceed via the endocytic pathway to gain access to the cell interior (Fig. 22.5).[38,98,166] Structural and biochemical experiments demonstrate that binding of RRV to heparan sulfate does not induce conformational changes in the virion.[257,317] However, other receptors may induce conformational changes in the particle that might mediate entry such as the reduction of disulfide bonds to disrupt protein–protein interactions.[1,11,199,237] Despite these suggestions that disulfide exchange may play a role in alphavirus entry, the use of thiol-blocking reagents failed to show a significant inhibition of infection.[77] However, it is clear that the attachment of SINV to cells results in the exposure of new epitopes defined by monoclonal antibodies and suggests that protein rearrangements occur following receptor engagement.[48,172] Similar observations have been made using purified virus and treatment with heat, pH, and reducing agents.[171] In addition, the recent observations on the role of virion and protein dynamics in the flavivirus life cycle, suggest that other structurally related viruses might employ particle dynamics to sense their environment as they search for an entry receptor.[40a] In addition to the role of thiol exchange reactions that have been proposed to play a role in alphavirus entry, there has even been a suggestion that cell penetration may occur at the cell surface in the absence of fusion by conformational rearrangements in the envelope glycoproteins.[1,199] However, it has been fairly well established that membrane fusion triggered by an exposure to acidic conditions

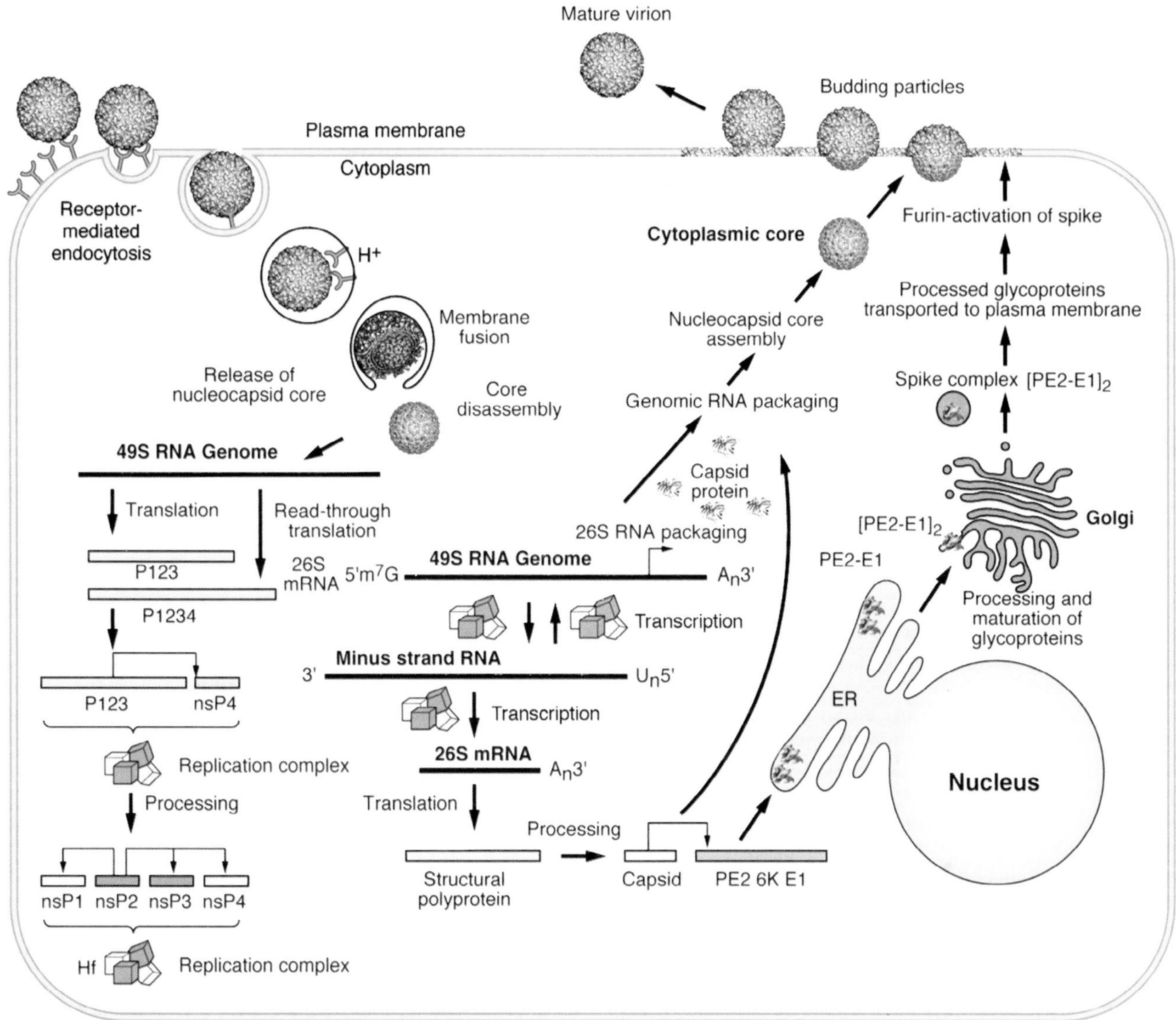

FIGURE 22.5. Life cycle of an alphavirus. The start of the life cycle is shown on the **left** with the attachment of a virion to the cellular receptor. Following fusion of the viral envelope, disassembly of the core, and release of the genome RNA, replication proteins are translated and processed **(bottom left)**. These proteins enable the replication of the input genome RNA **(bottom center)**, and translation of the subgenomic mRNA into structural proteins. Cytoplasmic assembly of genome RNA and capsid produces the nucleocapsid core that associates with processed glycoproteins **(right)** at the plasma membrane resulting in budding. (Scale varies.)

is the gateway for the release of genome RNA into the cytoplasm (Fig. 22.6).

Receptor-bound viruses undergo endocytosis into coated vesicles using a clathrin-dependent pathway. This pathway was demonstrated by DeTulleo and Kirchhausen[38] using dominant-negative mutants of dynamin to block the formation of clathrin-coated pits and prevent entry of SFV and SINV. The vesicles are subsequently acidified, providing the trigger for fusion between viral and cellular membranes. Acid-induced fusion is supported by numerous studies, but most convincingly by the use of lysosomotropic weak bases that raise the pH of endocytic vesicles and prevent entry of alphaviruses.[77,99,310] Although it has been argued that viral RNA replication might also be affected by the acidification, pseudotyped viruses containing alphavirus envelope proteins are also inhibited in entry by this treatment.[42,100,246]

The role of the alphavirus E1 and E2 glycoproteins in the entry process has been firmly established (Figs. 22.6 and 22.7). In the presence of acidic pH, the E1–E2 heterodimer is destabilized and the two proteins dissociate.[291,293] The dissociation of the proteins results in the exposure of the fusion peptide that is found on the distal tip of E1.[4,74,88,138] The fusion peptide of E1 inserts into the target membrane in a cholesterol-dependent manner followed by the trimerization of E1.[3,73,116,189,206,292] A large conformational change in E1 results in domain III and the stem-anchor region of the protein packing against domain II, resulting in the viral and target membranes being brought into close opposition (Fig. 22.6).[76] A set of E1 trimers, possibly

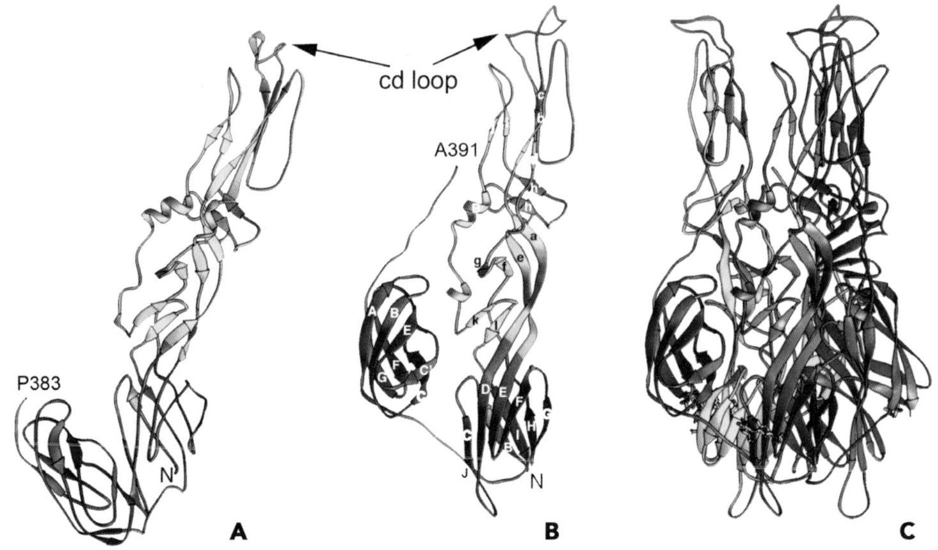

FIGURE 22.6. Postfusion structure of the Semliki Forest virus E1 protein. **A** and **B:** Neutral and low pH forms of the soluble E1 ectodomain lacking amino acid residues 392–438, respectively. The orientation of the protein presents the fusion loop (cd loop) toward the target membrane **(top)**. **C:** This rearrangement would occur after E1 has undergone trimerization as shown here. (Modified from an image provided by Dr. Felix Rey; 76.)

resembling what has been seen in liposomes, results in membrane deformation and promotes membrane mixing.[74] Finally, a fusion pore will form as the two membranes complete the process, and the nucleocapsid core will be released into the cytoplasm (Fig. 22.7).

Rey et al.[138] recognized that the structural features of the alphavirus E1 and flavivirus E proteins were distinct from the structures of other previously identified fusion proteins such as hemagglutinin (HA) from influenza, and proposed that they represented a novel class of fusion machines. They termed these class II membrane fusion proteins and elaborated several distinguishing features that separated the two classes. Class II fusion proteins are composed predominantly of β-strands, contain an internal fusion peptide, and have a companion protein that stabilizes the structure; this companion protein forms an activated metastable structure following proteolytic processing of a precursor protein. In the alphaviruses, PE2 is proteolytically activated by cleavage to generate E3 and E2, with E2 and E1 forming a stable heterodimer.[155,156] Mutagenesis experiments have provided insight into the fusion process and the residues that play regulatory and supporting roles in this process. As predicted, a pH-sensitive histidine residue in E1 (SFV H3) appears to regulate the low pH-dependent folding of E1 that is required for fusion.[215] Several other well-conserved histidines in E1 were evaluated and found unable to influence the activity. In addition, Kielian and colleagues[152] found that a salt bridge is formed within domain II of the E1 trimer core, which appears critical for stabilizing the homotrimer fusion intermediate.

Biochemical experiments with SFV have defined the requirements and steps in the alphavirus fusion process. Kielian et al.[116,159,206] demonstrated a strict dependence on cholesterol for fusion. This requirement has been narrowed down to the sterol 3β hydroxyl group in cholesterol.[31,176,290,312] A mutant was isolated (named *srf-3* for sterol requirement in function) that was cholesterol independent and had an amino acid substitution of a proline to serine at E1 residue 226. This mutation did not affect fusion with normal membranes but significantly enhanced fusion to cholesterol-free membranes.[24,280] In mosquito cells, the *srf-3* mutant grew better than wild-type virus.[5] The importance of this region of E1, which lies in the ij loop, for alphavirus fusion was further demonstrated by mutation of a conserved histidine at position 230 to alanine with the resulting virus particles being noninfectious, but capable of proceeding through E1 homotrimer formation under low pH conditions and suggesting a late step in fusion.[23] However, the exact role of cholesterol to promote fusion is not known. The structure of the postfusion form of E1 has been determined using x-ray crystallography.[74,75,76] This was accomplished using a soluble form of the E1 ectodomain known as E1* following exposure to low pH in the presence of liposomes, and solubilization with detergents. The structure of this homotrimer reveals the movement of domain III by 37 Å toward the fusion peptide and target membrane (Fig. 22.6)[76] and is similar to changes that are induced by class I fusion protein activation.[115] It is important to note that the addition of exogenous domain III can inhibit fusion by binding to E1 and preventing fold-back of the endogenous domain III.[146] This fold-back process appears to be reversible and is mediated by a series of interactions between the domain I and domain III linker region.[320] A complete picture of the virion during the fusion process is not available, despite several attempts using cryo-EM to examine these steps.[46,62,84,199]

Following the fusion of the viral and cellular membranes, the nucleocapsid core is released into the cytoplasm. The stability of that core is not known, but uncoating has been suggested to require the interaction of the core with ribosomes. This is based on several reports that suggest that ribosomal RNA competes for a site on the capsid protein and that displacement of this site results in disassembly.[253,254,305] This site has been identified in SINV capsid protein between residues 94 and 105 and coincides with a predicted site for genome RNA binding.[308] It has also been suggested that the core might be primed for uncoating by exposure to low pH, which causes the core to become unstable.[303,306] This exposure to low pH could occur in the endosome because both E1 and 6K have been proposed to have ion channel properties.[158,169,304] However, studies using pre-formed cores microinjected into naïve cells demonstrated that these cores do uncoat presumably devoid of conditions of low pH.[258] Whether these cores interact with ribosomes to promote disassembly and release of genome RNA remains to be shown.

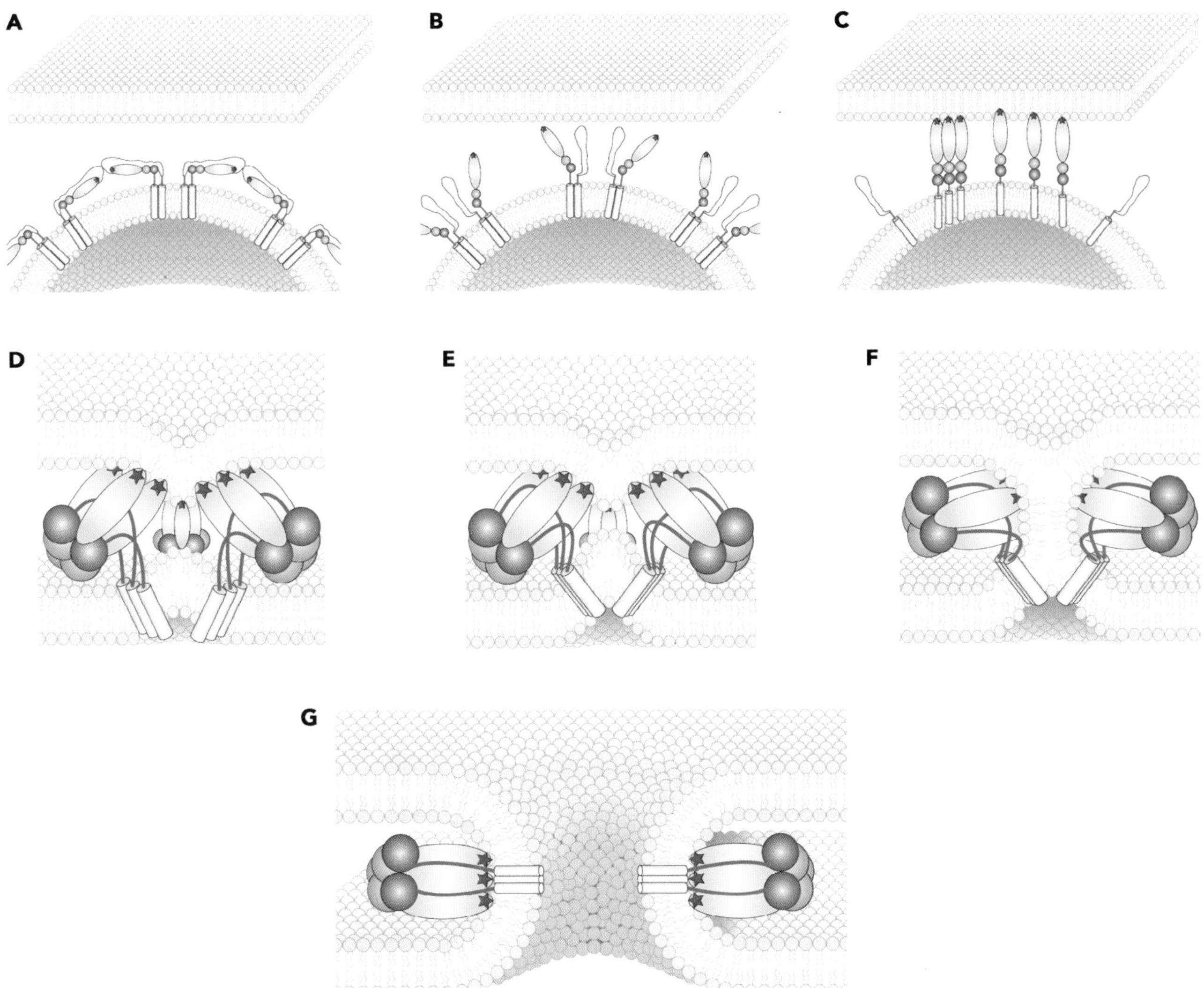

FIGURE 22.7. Model of alphavirus fusion. A: Native virions with E1 represented by two circles (domains I and III) and an extended oval (domain II), and E2 in the background and covering the E1 fusion peptide (*star*). **B:** Low pH triggers dissociation of E1 and E2 and fusion peptide exposure. **C:** Low pH and cholesterol-dependent insertion of the fusion loop into the target membrane, aligning E1 and promoting trimerization. **D:** Fold-back process by which domain III and the stem region move toward the fusion loop. **E:** Folding of domain III and the stem region against domain II of the trimer pulls the transmembrane domains toward one another distorting the viral membrane. **F:** Opposing dome-like deformations in the two membranes leads to mixing of the outer leaflets (termed hemifusion). **G:** Close opposition of the fusion peptides and transmembrane domains resolve into the fusion pore. (Courtesy of Dr. Margaret Kielian. Reprinted from Kielian M, Rey FA. Virus membrane-fusion proteins: more than one way to make a hairpin. *Nat Rev Microbiol* 2006;4:67–76, with permission from Macmillan Publishers Ltd: Nature Review Microbiology, © 2006.)

Translation and the Role of Viral-Encoded Replication Proteins

The genome RNA serves as an mRNA for the synthesis of the nonstructural or replication proteins (Fig. 22.4). These are produced by two polyproteins that originate translation at nucleotide 60 in SINV.[268] The smaller but more abundant polyprotein P123 terminates translation at an opal codon following 1,897 amino acids. Readthrough of the opal codon occurs with a low frequency (~10% to 20%) and results in the production of the larger P1234 polyprotein. Not all alphaviruses have a termination codon to control the production of the two polyproteins, but mutagenesis of the opal codon in SINV adversely affects replication.[144] Processing of the polyproteins occurs through the action of a virus-encoded protease located within the nonstructural protein 2 (nsP2).[39,91,92] The processing of the polyprotein to generate precursor and end-product nsP's is believed to regulate the synthesis of viral RNAs.[35,137,250] Translation of the structural polyprotein proceeds through a subgenomic mRNA that is initiated near the coding region for the C-terminus of P1234. The subgenomic mRNA is 3′ co-terminal with the genome RNA and is produced later in the infection.[268]

Initial studies of the replication proteins used temperature-sensitive mutants that were conditional lethal for viral

TABLE 22.1 Translation Products of Alphaviruses (Sindbis Virus)

Protein	Size (aa)	Function
Nonstructural Proteins		
nsP1	540	Methyltransferase and guanylyltransferase; anchors replicase complex to membranes
nsP2	807	NTPase, helicase, RNA triphosphatase, protease responsible for processing of non-structural polyprotein
nsP3	556	Phosphoprotein with unknown function(s) but important for minus-strand synthesis; contains macro domain and SH3-binding regions
nsP4	610	RNA-dependent RNA polymerase (RdRp), terminal transferase
Structural Proteins		
Capsid	264	Encapsidates genomic RNA to form nucleocapsid core; carboxyl domain is an autocatalytic serine protease
E3	64	N-terminal domain is uncleaved leader peptide for E2; E3 + E2 = pE2.
E2	423	Presents the major neutralizing epitopes and is responsible for receptor binding
6K	55	Leader peptide for E1, enhances particle release, putative ion channel
TF	70	TransFrame (TF) protein, putative ion channel, enhances particle infectivity, expression prevents synthesis of E1
E1	439	Responsible for membrane fusion activity

replication. These studies established complementation groups and identified specific functions of the replication proteins.[264] Four complementation groups were identified, and these correlated with the four nsP's. Once sequence information was available, motifs were identified that verified function and permitted phylogenetic relationships between other virus families to be established. This resulted in the suggestion of an alphavirus-like superfamily that contained RNA virus members from several plant families and argued for an evolutionary relationship between them.[2,267]

The nsP's are multifunctional proteins with their known activities shown in Table 22.1. However, it is likely that additional unknown activities exist. Guanine-7-methyltransferase and guanylyltransferase activities necessary for mRNA and genome RNA capping have been shown to reside within nsP1.[127,173,174] This capping activity is distinct from cellular capping enzymes in substrate preference.[6] Several genetic studies have confirmed the identity of amino acids critical for the methyltransferase function, but the domain required for guanylyltransferase activity has not be identified and may flank the conserved methyltransferase domain.[8,227] A *ts* mutant that mapped to Ala348 of nsP1 in SINV demonstrated a role of the protein in minus-strand RNA synthesis.[87] A defect in minus-strand synthesis has also been seen with mutations in nsP4, and some of these have been complemented with changes in nsP1 at residues 349 and 374, suggesting sites for nsP1 and nsP4 interaction.[43] nsP1 is the only alphavirus nonstructural protein that has been shown to be membrane associated.[128,203] The membrane association has been suggested to occur by a palmitoylated cysteine at residue 420 (in SINV).[7,127] Mutations that disrupt palmitoylation did not alter the distribution of replication complexes and show only modest reductions in growth. However, nsP1 can still bind to membranes through a patch of positively charged and hydrophobic amino acids between residues 245 and 264.[9] Nuclear magnetic resonance spectroscopy of a corresponding peptide suggests that this sequence can form an amphipathic α-helix that can interact with liposomes.[129] This membrane anchoring of the replication complex associated with nsP1 is probably required for efficient replicase activity.

The largest of the replication proteins is nsP2, with a length of about 800 amino acids. The N-terminal half of the protein has helicase, nucleoside triphosphatase, and RNA triphosphatase activities,[78,79,221,281] whereas the C-terminal half contains a novel cysteine protease domain and a nonfunctional methyltransferase domain.[263,282] The structure for the C-terminal two domains of the VEEV nsP2 was solved by Watowich and colleagues using x-ray crystallography (Fig. 22.8).[234] The structure shows that the active site of the protease is positioned close to the interface between the two domains. Although related to proteases papain and cathepsin X, the fold of the nsP2 protease domain appears to be unique and a new

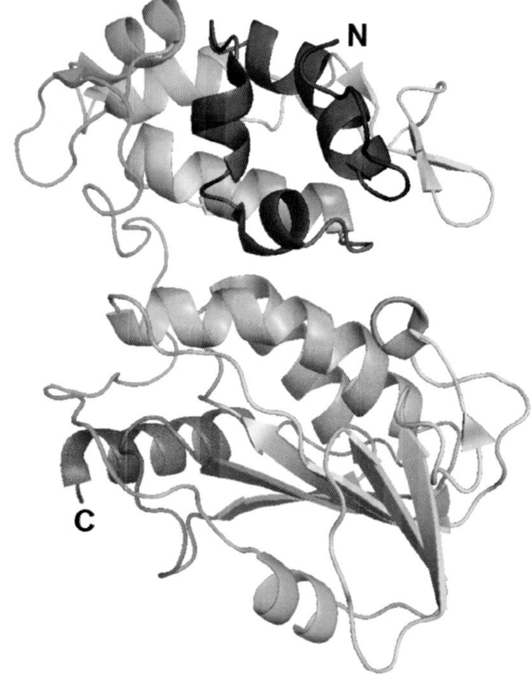

FIGURE 22.8. Structure of the Venezuelan equine encephalitis virus nsP2 protease. A ribbon diagram showing the protease colored from blue (N-terminus) through red (C-terminus) representing residues N468 to S787. The catalytic dyad residues, C477 and H546, are found in the N-terminal protease domain **(top)**, whereas the methyltransferase-like domain **(bottom)** comprises the C-terminal domain. (Courtesy of Dr. Joyce Jose; generated in PyMole using the PDB coordinates 2HWK from Russo AT, White MA, Watowich SJ. The crystal structure of the Venezuelan equine encephalitis alphavirus nsP2 protease. *Structure* 2006;14:1449–1458.)

form of cysteine protease structure. Although having a similar tertiary structure with known methyltransferases such as FtsJ, the S-adenosylmethionine (SAM) substrate binding site is very different in backbone alignment and sequence, arguing against any methyltransferase activity. However, by mapping several previously identified *ts* mutants affected in RNA synthesis onto the C-terminal domain, it was suggested that the domain functions as an RNA-binding scaffold that regulates protease activity and RNA synthesis.[233,234]

The nsP2 protein has a nuclear localization sequence that results in 50% of the protein reaching the nucleus,[222,223] and it has been reported that nsP2 of VEEV undergoes both nuclear import as well as export.[177] Abrogation of the signal results in a slightly defective virus, but at least in SFV the mutant has lost neuropathogenesis, arguing for a role of nsP2 in host interactions.[220] Studies have identified a role for nsP2 from the Old World alphaviruses in the induction of cytopathic effects and the establishment of persistent infections, and is discussed later in the chapter.[41,55] In addition, experiments have provided a link between nsP2 and the host response, resulting in shutoff of minus-strand RNA synthesis.[240] Genetic studies identified conditional lethal mutations demonstrating RNA-defective phenotypes that implicated nsP2 in the regulation of minus-strand synthesis and in the initiation of subgenomic RNA synthesis.[37,87,241] Furthermore, the role of the protease activity to regulate the temporal control of RNA synthesis has been well established and is described later.[35,137]

The function of the nsP3 protein remains obscure, although genetic analyses indicate that it plays a role in RNA synthesis and neurovirulence.[131,276,297] The protein is highly conserved among alphaviruses at its N-terminus, whereas the C-terminal 200 amino acids are rich in serine and threonine residues. The protein is phosphorylated on serines and threonine; however, this modification is not required for replication, and its function in the virus life cycle is not known.[130,143,204,284,285] The protein has a weak affinity for membranes and will associate with them when expressed in the absence of the other nsPs.[202,284] A crystal structure of both the CHIKV and VEEV N-terminal 160 residues of nsP3 confirmed previous suggestions that this region contains a macro domain (the VEEV structure is shown in Fig. 22.9).[80,163] These domains function as ADP-ribose binding modules and have also been shown capable of single-strand RNA binding. The exact function(s) of the macro domain awaits additional studies. Although the C-terminal end of nsP3 is not well conserved, a proline-rich sequence found in most alphaviruses was identified as a target site for Src-homology 3 domain containing proteins amphiphysin-1 and amphiphysin-2.[185] Disruption of the binding sequence by mutation or reduction of amphiphysin-2 by RNAi reduced replication in both SINV and SFV. It is unclear how this interaction influences RNA replication; however, the amphiphysins have been implicated as membrane-binding proteins, involved in endocytosis, and membrane trafficking, and the virus may usurp these functions to facilitate RNA synthesis.

The core of the virus replication complex is the RNA-dependent RNA polymerase (RdRp) that maps to nsP4.[87,121] Interestingly, because of the opal codon in SINV, synthesis of P123 is significantly greater than the level of P1234 and thus nsP4 levels are lower than that of the other nsP's. Furthermore, modifications that increase the synthesis of nsP4, such as the removal of the opal termination codon, result in reduced virus replication.[144] The majority of the protein from the C-terminus constitutes the RdRp domain based on homology with other polymerases and predicted secondary structures.[111] A short region exists at the N-terminus that lacks a counterpart in other viral polymerases, and it has been suggested that it might be a binding domain for the other nsP's.[87,249] The N-terminus of nsP4 also contains a conserved tyrosine residue, and this serves to make the protein unstable in infected cells.[36,248,252] deGroot et al.[36] examined the degradation of nsP4 and showed that it was degraded by the N-end rule pathway. It has been suggested that free nsP4 is rapidly degraded, whereas nsP4 that is a component of replicase complexes is protected and relatively stable. Therefore, it was not a surprise that attempts to express the full-length nsP4 in heterologous systems were initially unsuccessful. However, expression of nsP4 lacking the first 97 amino acids was successful, and this truncated nsP4 displayed a terminal adenylyltransferase activity.[275] This terminal transferase activity was suggested to play a role in the maintenance of the poly (A) tract at the 3′ end of positive-strand RNAs. The nsP4 protein was subsequently expressed as an N-terminal small ubiquitin-like modifier (SUMO) fusion protein that was cleaved after purification, and nsP4 was shown to possess de novo minus-strand synthesis activity that was dependent on the correct 3′ end of positive-strand template.[229] Proteomic studies have been used to identify host proteins that might interact with nsP4 during virus infection.[33] In this study the authors demonstrated that a total of 29 host proteins were associated with nsP4 in a temporally regulated pattern. Among the proteins identified, two proteins known as GTPase-activating protein SH3-domain binding protein 1 and 2 (G3BP1 and G3BP2) were

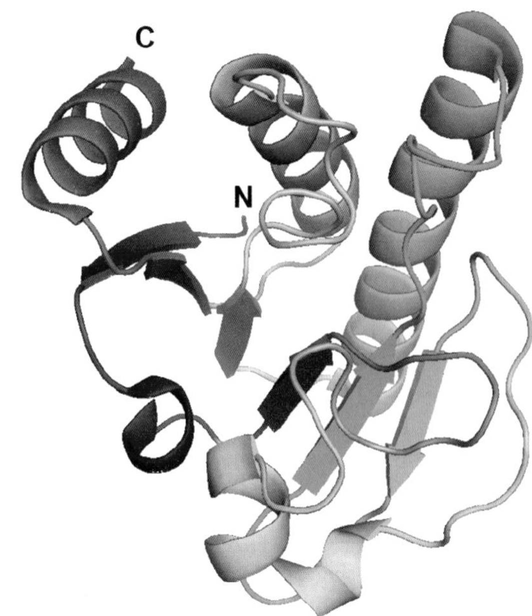

FIGURE 22.9. Structure of the Venezuelan equine encephalitis virus nsP3 macro domain. A ribbon diagram showing the nsP3 macro domain colored from blue (N-terminus) through red (C-terminus) representing residues A1 to E160. The structure consists of a six-stranded β-sheet ringed by three α-helices. (Courtesy of Dr. Joyce Jose; generated in PyMole using the PDB coordinates 3GQE from Malet H, Coutard B, Jamel S, et al. The crystal structures of Chikungunya and Venezuelan equine encephalitis virus nsP3 macro domains define a conserved adenosine binding pocket. *J Virol* 2009;83:6534–6545.)

also shown to interact with nsP2 and nsP3.[32] However, the role of these proteins is unclear; they may function to reduce the pool of RNAs available for translation by recruiting the viral RNA to the stress granule pathway.

Transcription and Replication of Genomic Nucleic Acid

Alphavirus-infected cells produce three species of RNAs: genome plus-strand RNA, complementary minus-strand RNA, and subgenomic mRNA. The synthesis of these three species is tightly regulated by the availability of specific nsP's (Fig. 22.10).[35,136,137] Replication is initiated on the cytoplasmic surface of endosomes and lysosomes on structures termed cytopathic vacuoles.[61] All four nsP's can be found associated with each other and within these vacuoles.[126] In elegant studies by Strauss et al.[35] it was shown that proteolytic site selection controlled the processing of the nsP's and determined the components of the replicase complex. This was accomplished by assessing cleavage-site preferences and determining which enzymes (nsP2 or its precursors) could affect processing. Additional studies by the Sawicki laboratory using temperature-sensitive mutants established the biochemical nature of the replicase complex.[15,37,239,242] In complementary work, the Rice laboratory carried out *in vivo* replication studies using nsP's expressed in a vaccinia vector to discern the functional complexes.[135–137] Despite earlier problems, they were successful in developing a system for template-dependent initiation of SINV.[134]

RNA replication begins with the initiation of minus-strand synthesis. This event requires the 3′ CSE and host proteins/factors.[56,72,90,123] *In vitro* studies using polymerase extracts suggest the poly (A) tract may not serve as template for the initiation of minus-strand synthesis, although the details of this initiation event are not known.[89] Minus-strand synthesis requires P123 or P23 and nsP4, but a cleavage-defective P1234 is not functional.[135–137,250] Similarly, in the vaccinia system, expression of the individual nsPs was not sufficient for complex formation and minus-strand synthesis.[135,136] As minus-strand synthesis continues, nsPs continue to be translated and concentrations of the protease precursors increase. Cleavage at the nsP1–nsP2 and nsP2–nsP3 junctions results in the switch over to plus-strand synthesis, presumably by a change in the conformation and composition of the replicase complex (Fig. 22.10). Synthesis of minus strands by the replicase requires continuous protein synthesis, and it has been suggested that nsP2 engages the host response by using the RNase L-dependent pathway to inhibit host cell translation.[82,240] As

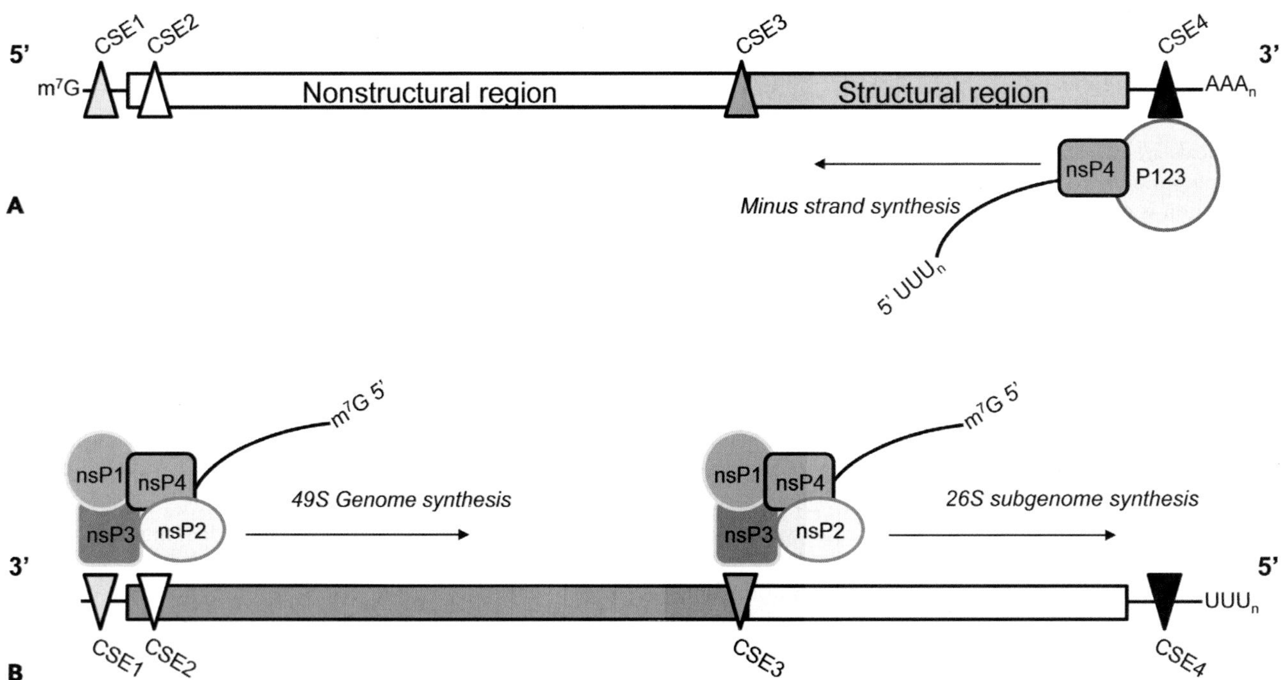

FIGURE 22.10. The conserved sequence elements (CSEs) and nonstructural proteins involved in alphavirus genome replication. A: A schematic of minus-strand synthesis from a plus-strand template. A protein complex composed of P123 and nsP4, and presumably host proteins (not shown), initiate synthesis of the minus strand from the 3′ end of the genome. CSE4, a 19nt element, is found just upstream of the polyA tract. CSE4 is thought to act as a promoter for minus-strand synthesis, perhaps via a cyclization event with CSE2, a 51nt element located within the nsP1 coding region (not shown). **B:** A schematic of full-length 49S genomic and 26S subgenomic RNA syntheses from a minus-strand template. An accumulation of P123 allows processing of P123 polyproteins in *trans* into the individual nonstructural proteins. Presumably, the altered conformation of the replicase complex shifts template preference to the minus strand. CSE1, comprising the first 44nt of the 5′ genome, acts as a promoter for synthesis of full-length 49S genomic RNA from a minus-strand template, perhaps in conjunction with CSE2. Fully processed replicase complexes also associate on the CSE3 element, which span the 3′ end of the nsP4 coding sequence and the junction region between the nonstructural and structural genes. These CSE3-associated replicase complexes efficiently transcribe the 26S subgenomic message. Note that a replicase complex composed of nsP1, P23, and nsP4 may also be capable of plus-strand synthesis (not shown). (Courtesy of Jonathan Snyder.)

with most plus-strand RNA viruses, synthesis is asymmetric with minus-strand synthesis about 2% to 5% the level of plus-strand genome RNA.[298]

Although the viral protein composition of the minus- and plus-strand replicases is known, the role of host proteins in the complex is not. From studies with the CSEs, host cell–dependent effects were observed and several host proteins were shown to bind to the conserved RNA elements.[56,193,194,195] Furthermore, Fayzulin and Frolov[44] showed that although the 51 nt CSE is dispensable in mammalian cells, in mosquito cells mutations have a deleterious effect. Interestingly, adaptive mutations occur in the 5′ NTR, as well as in nsP2 and nsP3, suggesting their involvement in CSE function. Frolov et al.,[56] using chimeric templates and *trans*-competition experiments, showed that the 5′ NTR is a component of the promoter for not only plus-strand synthesis, but also for minus-strand synthesis. From these data, they proposed a model for the initiation of minus-strand RNA synthesis that requires the 5′ and 3′ ends of the genome RNA to be brought together. This would be accomplished using components of the host translational machinery, which is involved in cap and poly (A) binding. Despite the attractiveness of the model, the lack of a purified reconstituted system for RNA synthesis has hampered progress in understanding alphavirus RNA replication.

The synthesis of the subgenomic mRNA is controlled by a minimal promoter element that spans from −19 to +5 relative to the start of mRNA synthesis. A larger fragment from −98 to +14 provides three- to sixfold more activity and constitutes the fully active promoter.[214] As with the 5′ and 3′ CSEs, the subgenomic promoter appears to interact with host factors, as mutations in the promoter have differential effects, depending on replication in vertebrate versus invertebrate hosts.[101,102,311] This promoter has been extensively employed in gene expression and replicon studies using alphaviruses, including the use of multiple tandem promoters.[19,57,59]

Perhaps the most informative studies on alphavirus replication in recent years have emerged using advanced imaging techniques. These approaches have shed light on the spatial and temporal assembly of replication complexes. Most intriguing is the observation that membrane-derived structures competent for RNA synthesis appear to form initially at the plasma membrane (Fig. 22.11). Studies from both SFV and SINV demonstrate that the membrane invaginations referred to as spherules first accumulate on the plasma membrane and are

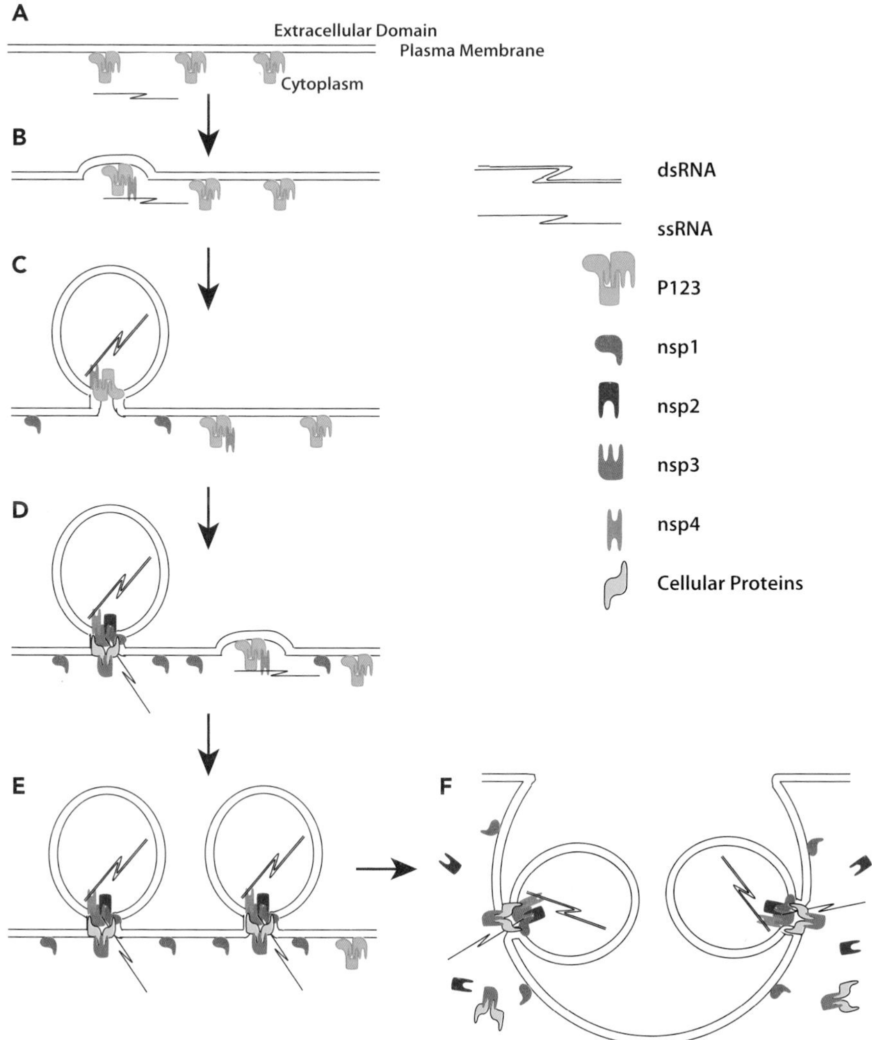

FIGURE 22.11. Assembly of alphavirus replication complexes. A: Replication complexes consisting of P123 and genome RNA are found at the plasma membrane. With the addition of nsP4 **(B)**, the RNA-dependent RNA synthesis (RdRp), synthesis of double-stranded DNA (dsRNA) occurs **(C)** along with the formation of membrane spherules. Upon processing of P123 **(D)**, replication complexes switch to the synthesis of genomic and subgenomic RNA. As replication continues **(E** and **F)** free nsP1, nsP2, and nsP3 are found, with the latter protein associating with specific host proteins and nsP1 remaining membrane associated. At later stages, multiple spherules coalesce into cytopathic vacuoles type 1 (CPV-1) within the cytoplasm. (Adapted by Thomas Edwards and R.J.K. with permission from Drs. Elena Frolova and Ilya Frolov.[60])

later internalized using the actin–myosin network.[60,262] These structures appear to contain all of the nonstructural proteins as well as double-stranded RNA but are devoid of any structural proteins. Structures known as cytopathic vacuoles type 1 and type 2 (CPVI and CPVII) were described previously as containing the replication proteins and viral glycoproteins, respectively.[61,202] The role of CPV2 appears to guide the glycoproteins to the site of budding; however, the role of CPV1 for RNA synthesis is not as clear. CPV1 structures form later in RNA replication, probably as a result of spherule recruitment from the plasma membrane, but it has been suggested that they may not be the major site for viral RNA synthesis at least in mammalian cells.[60]

Assembly of Nucleocapsid Core, Glycoprotein Synthesis, and Processing

The subgenomic RNA, which is made at approximately three times the level of the genomic RNA, is translated to produce the structural or virion proteins.[216] The order of translation is capsid-PE2(E3+E2)-6K-E1 (Fig. 22.2). Translation of the structural polyprotein is enhanced due to the presence of a hairpin secondary structure in the subgenomic mRNA between residues 77 and 139.[59] The polyprotein is processed by host and viral proteases to generate the authentic structural proteins that will end up in the virion, and the membrane topology of the glycoproteins is shown in Figure 22.12. The capsid protein is translated first and is released by proteolysis immediately after the ribosome clears the junction between it and PE2. The capsid functions as an autoprotease, and sequence and mutational analyses suggested that the C-terminal domain of the capsid contained a serine-like protease.[10,86] This hypothesis was confirmed by the x-ray crystal structure of the C-terminal domain from SINV.[29] The protein has a chymotrypsin-like fold, with His141, Asp163, and Ser215 forming the catalytic triad. Interestingly, the C-terminal residue, Trp264, remains in the active site pocket and presumably prevents transcleavage by the protease. With the self-cleavage of the capsid protein, the new N-terminus of the polyprotein now contains a signal sequence for translocation of the PE2 sequence across the endoplasmic reticulum (ER) membrane.[69] Additional signal sequences are present at the C-terminus of E2, permitting translocation of 6K, and at the C-terminus of 6K, permitting translocation of E1 (Fig. 22.12). The expression of TF protein, which contains the first 43 amino acids of 6K, and then shifts to the -1 reading frame that prevents the synthesis of E1.[47] Proteins E1, E2, 6K, and TF are transmembrane proteins, whereas E3 is released from most alphavirus particles following cleavage of its PE2 precursor.[95,210,211,232,236] SFV retains the cleaved E3 with the virion; however, it is unclear whether it has a postcleavage function.[321]

Following autoproteolysis, the capsid protein transiently associates with the ribosome, and assembly into a core particle appears to be both rapid and efficient, with no observed intermediates.[259,279] A specific "packaging sequence" has been identified in the genome RNA in SINV that promotes encapsidation of RNA into the assembling core.[300] In SINV, this sequence has been identified as nucleotides 945 to 1076, and attempts to identify the nature of the recognition element have met with limited success.[150] However, there is conservation of structural and functional components of packaging signal across diverse alphaviruses.[117] The packaging sequence on the genome RNA is recognized by residues 81 to 113 in the capsid protein.[71,299] A deletion of residues 97 to 106 results in a failure to efficiently package genome RNA, although cores still form with heterologous RNA incorporated.[192] Although most alphaviruses package their genomes with high efficiency, Aura virus has been described as an alphavirus that packages its subgenomic mRNA as well.[230,231] The development of alphaviruses as gene expression vectors has prompted much investigation into the packaging requirements, and in VEEV, packaging has been shown to

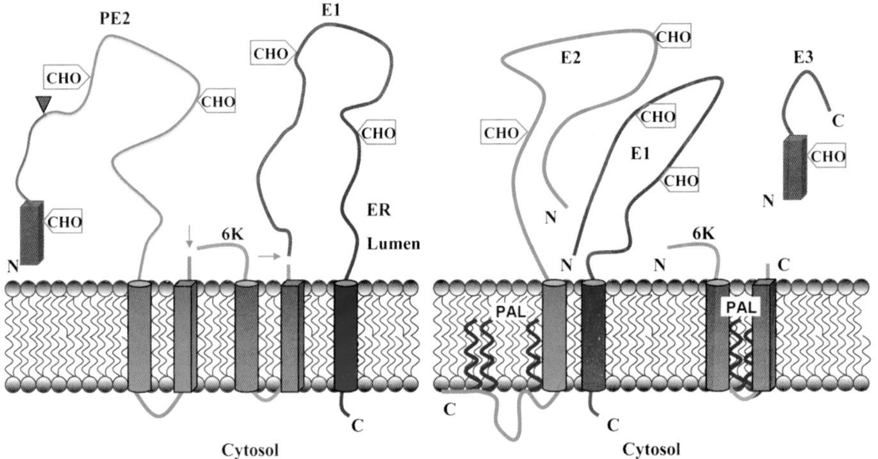

FIGURE 22.12. Schematic model for the configuration of the E1 and E2 glycoproteins in the membrane. Left: Configuration of the glycoproteins after signalase cleavage of 6K and E1, but before cleavage of PE2. **Right:** Configuration of glycoproteins after the maturation cleavage of PE2 into E3 and E2. Note the *dark red jagged lines* on the cytoplasmic side of E2 and 6K that represent palmitoylation sites (PALs). Glycosylation sites are indicated by CHO. Signal sequences are indicated as *colored rectangular blocks*. Stop-transfer sequences are indicated as *colored cylinders*. The shapes of the polypeptides do not imply their native configuration. (Courtesy of Dr. Joyce Jose.)

require expression of nsP123, although the mechanism and the generality of this requirement have not been shown.[286]

Although *in vitro* systems for core assembly have been described, the stepwise assembly process has not been clearly elaborated.[272–274,301,302] The capsid protein requires the addition of nucleic acid to initiate the assembly process, and in the presence of full-length wild-type protein, assembly proceeds rapidly. Using a truncated capsid protein, the initial step appears to involve a protein dimer complexed with RNA.[273,274] Cores are found in the cytoplasm and attached to membranes, probably through their interaction with E2 (reviewed in[68,110]). Cytoplasmic cores have a well-defined size and T = 4 icosahedral symmetry, similar to *in vitro* assembled cores, but not identical to the well-ordered T = 4 symmetry in cores found within virus particles.[178,196] However, the symmetry of the core does not necessarily dictate the symmetry of the virion, and it is likely that the icosahedral architecture of the glycoprotein scaffold is the driving force behind the strict T = 4 organization of alphavirus.[52,138,207] This is supported by the observation from Forsell et al.,[53] who produced a SFV capsid protein with a deletion in residues 40 to 118. This mutant was unable to assemble cores, but virus particles were produced that had the expected T = 4 symmetry.

In parallel with the formation of the nucleocapsid in the cytoplasm, the envelope proteins that were translocated into the ER are processed and undergo posttranslational modifications (Fig. 22.5). High mannose chains are added to all potential N-linked glycosylation sites, and the oligosaccharide chains are trimmed depending on the availability of the site.[243,245] Palmitoylation occurs at several sites in E2 and 6K/TF.[17,64] In a set of elegant studies, Brown et al. showed that E1 and PE2 undergo a complex series of folding intermediates.[22,120,180,181] These intermediates require chaperones and disulfide bond formation and exchange. The E1 and E2 glycoproteins form a heterodimer in the ER, but it is not known whether higher-order oligomerization takes place here.[218,321] Oligomerization of PE2 and E1 is also a requirement for the transport of the glycoproteins, but the presence of the capsid (CP) is not required.[70,105,157] It has been shown that PE2 oligomerizes with a partially folded intermediate of E1 and that this oligomerization is sufficient for the proteins to exit the ER. After the heterodimer reaches the trans-Golgi network, but prior to arrival at the plasma membrane, PE2 is cleaved by furin.[34] This cleavage is required for virion entry and fusion activation in new cells, although revertants can be readily isolated that suppress the requirement for cleavage.[96,211]

Virion Budding

The final stage of the virus life cycle is the effective interaction between the capsid protein and the glycoproteins to promote virus budding. Thin-section electron microscopy of infected cells has shown a clustering of nucleocapsid cores at the plasma membrane at sites of budding but it is likely that the interaction occurs earlier, perhaps in the vicinity of CPVII.[261] All evidence suggests that a proper interaction between the cores and glycoprotein spikes is required for budding.[109] When the glycoproteins have been expressed in the absence of the capsid protein, virus-like particles have not been observed. In SFV, virions have been shown to bud from specific sites in polarized cells,[225] and virus has been reported to bud intracellularly in insect cells.[175] There also appears to be a requirement for cholesterol in the membrane to support budding,[159,164] and host cell lipid metabolism has also been implicated.[186] Several systems have been reported that show the exogenously produced capsid cores can be introduced into naïve cells expressing the viral glycoproteins and particles can be released, suggesting that RNA synthesis is not required for budding.[26,258]

The interaction between the capsid protein and the envelope glycoproteins has been investigated extensively, with most of the available data coming from molecular genetic and structural studies.[109,271] X-ray crystallography of the capsid protein identified a hydrophobic pocket that was occupied by the amino-terminal arm of a neighboring capsid protein. The nature of the arm residues bound in the hydrophobic pocket suggested that a tyr-ala-leu motif found in the cytoplasmic domain of the E2 glycoprotein might function in a similar manner and bind into the capsid protein pocket.[133,256] An extensive number of mutagenesis experiments involving SFV and SINV have established residues of the E2 cytoplasmic domain that were important for the interaction with the tyrosine, which is conserved in the alphaviruses, as an important one.[64,109,270,319] E2 peptides have also been used to inhibit budding, suggesting residues involved in process and similar peptides were shown to bind to capsids.[30,170] In addition, cryo-EM studies have shown that the cytoplasmic domain of E2 clearly extends down into the core to the site of the hydrophobic pocket.[271,179,271,318] As was mentioned previously, deletions that disrupt the accumulation of nucleocapsid cores do not prevent budding because lateral interaction between the glycoproteins appear to be the driving force as long as capsid interactions do occur.[287]

The 6K protein, which has been estimated at 5 to 10 molecules per virion, has been implicated in the budding process and in the formation of virions.[63,64] Removal of 6K from the genome of SFV did not influence the formation of the E1–E2 heterodimer or its transport to the cell surface, but it did reduce budding.[149] Other studies have shown that mutations in 6K can influence glycoprotein trafficking and virion assembly.[238] E2 and 6K appear to interact, as mutations in 6K can be suppressed by mutations in E2,[107] and chimeric viruses containing an SINV glycoprotein and an RRV 6K are highly defective for virus formation.[314] Recently, it has been shown that a frameshift occurs at a low frequency during translation of the region encoding 6K resulting in the production of the TF protein shown in Figure 22.13.[47] The TF protein shares 47 amino acids with 6K and contains the transmembrane domain that has been implicated in channel formation. The remaining 23 residues are unique to TF and since there is a –1 frameshift followed by a termination codon, no E1 is produced from this polyprotein. Preliminary data suggest that TF also has a role in virus replication and is incorporated into the virion but whether its function(s) overlaps with 6K is not yet known.

Effects on the Host Cell

Alphaviruses have a wide host range and must interact with a variety of cellular receptors, either ubiquitous or unrelated molecules. Because the nature of these receptors is largely unknown, equally unknown is the signaling that such molecules might engage in following virion attachment and early steps in entry. Clearly, the response of most vertebrate cells to viral infection is distinct from the response of invertebrate cells. However, in both cases there appears to be a balance between the needs of the virus to effectively propagate and the needs of the host to control virus infection and dissemination. Host

```
SINV    CUGCCUGCCUUUUUUAGUGGUUGCC (10022)
WEEV    CUGCAUGCCUUUUUUAUUGGUUGCA (9821)
EEEV    UGGGCCGGCUUUUUUACUUGUCUGC (9955)
CHIKV   AACGUUGGCUUUUUUAGCCGUAAUG (9951)
RRV     GCCAUUUUCUUUUUUAGUGUUACUG (9973)
SFV     GAGCCUUUCUUUUUUAGUGCUACUG (9825)
```
A

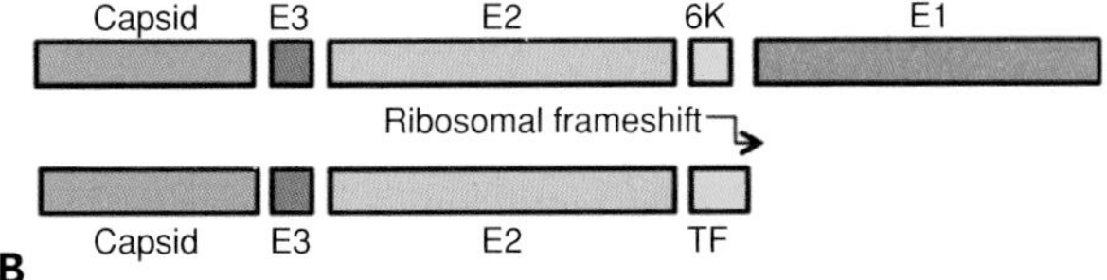

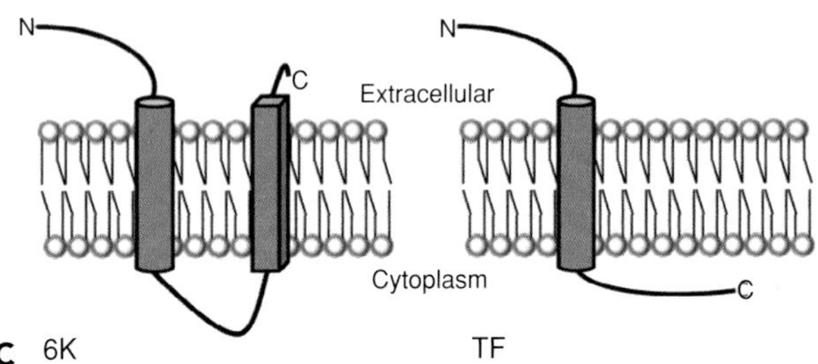

FIGURE 22.13. Ribosomal frameshifting during translation of the 26S subgenomic RNA yields a newly described protein, TransFrame (TF). A: Sequence alignment of various alphaviruses demonstrates the conservation of a putative slippery site motif within the 6K gene (underlined for Sindbus virus). The coordinate of the first nucleotide of the slippery site is indicated in parentheses for each virus. **B:** The typical protein products obtained from normal translation of the 26S subgenomic RNA **(top)**, and the protein products obtained in the case of a frameshift event **(bottom)**. Note that the amino terminal regions of the 6K and TF proteins share the same sequence. **C:** A model of the putative membrane topology of the mature 6K and TF proteins. The N- and C-termini are denoted. 6K **(left)** contains both a transmembrane anchor (cylindrical), and a membrane spanning region that acts as the signal sequence for E1 (rectangular). TF **(right)** contains only the transmembrane anchor (cylindrical); the frameshift event prevents production of the E1 signal sequence. (Courtesy of Jonathan Snyder.)

macromolecular synthesis is inhibited in vertebrate cells shortly after infection (reviewed in 268). Host protein synthesis is shut off at 3 hours after infection, although virus protein translation continues unabated. This has been an intensive area of investigation, and four mechanisms for shutoff have been proposed: (a) an altered intracellular environment such as K^+ concentration that would favor viral translation, (b) direct competition for translational machinery, (c) inhibition of cellular translation by the capsid protein, and (d) inhibition of translation by one of the nonstructural proteins. The development and use of replicon systems that contain only the *cis*-acting replication signals and the coding region for replication proteins suggested that the structural proteins were not responsible for translational shutoff.[58] Furthermore, studies investigating the establishment of persistence identified changes in SINV nsP2, at Pro726 to serine, which reduced cytopathic effects of the virus.[55] A variety of studies suggest that alphavirus infection promotes the double-stranded RNA-activated protein kinase (PKR)-dependent and PKR-independent pathways to reduce host cell translation.[66,235] Mutations in nsP2 suggest that the shutoff of host cell transcription and translation are distinct events and strongly influence the decreased production of a α/β interferon.[81] However, the role of nsP2 in host cell shutoff appears to function only in the Old World alphaviruses. It has been shown that in VEEV and other New World alphaviruses that a region of the capsid protein encompassing residues 33-68 and not nsP2 is responsible for transcriptional shutoff and cytopathogenicity.[67] This region of the VEEV capsid protein has also been shown to be responsible for nuclear trafficking of the protein to the nucleus.[12]

Most infections by alphaviruses of vertebrate cells in culture lead to the induction of apoptosis.[139] Apoptosis of infected neurons is a major determinant of neurovirulence, as demonstrated for SINV.[142] In contrast, mosquito cells can undergo a variety of effects from persistent infections to cell death caused by necrosis.[112] It has also been possible to establish persistent infection of vertebrate cells using defective interfering particles, followed by genetic changes to the helper virus in nsP2.[41] An alternative method was used by selecting for replicons that were noncytopathic to BHK cells, and again, amino acids substitutions were detected in the coding region for nsP2,[55] suggesting a major role for this protein in modulating the virus–host interaction.

A number of antiviral proteins produced in infected cells have been described for the alphaviruses. A small hydrophobic peptide of 3,200 D was shown to be produced in persistently infected mosquito cells, and this peptide could activate an antiviral state.[161] This peptide induced the synthesis of a 55-kD protein and inhibited the replication of alphavirus RNA.[160] The rat zinc-finger antiviral protein (ZAP), originally identified as a retrovirus resistance protein, was shown to inhibit multiple alphaviruses.[16] This protein inhibited viral translation by binding to viral mRNA, although its exact mechanism of action is not known.[83] It is likely that many additional proteins, such as interferon-stimulated genes, will demonstrate direct antiviral activity and might be exploited to control alphavirus infection.

Defective Interfering Genomes and Replicon Systems

Defective interfering (DI) genomes replicate and are packaged in the presence of helper virus, and retain all *cis*-acting sequences necessary for RNA replication. Several alphavirus DI genomes have been molecularly characterized, and all retain the 3′ CSE that was previously described. The 5′ end of the DI genomes was found to be more heterogenous, with the 5′ CSE, cellular transfer RNA (tRNA) sequences, or the 5′ 142 nucleotides from the subgenomic mRNA located at the 5′ end of the DI RNA. The study of DI genomes provided a powerful genetic tool to identify the location and function of required cis-acting sequence elements.[141] The development of DI genomes for genetic purposes gave way to the construction of replicons, which supported RNA replication but were incapable of infection of new cells because they lacked the structural proteins.[140,244,313] The structural proteins could be supplied by additional helper RNAs so that the replicons could be packaged and used to efficiently infect target cells.[19]

The alphavirus replicon has become a standard gene expression system. The system has proven useful for examining protein expression in heterogenous systems and the development of vaccines.[244] SINV, SFV, and VEEV replicons have been widely used and can allow for targeting to specific cells.[148,214,244] By introducing a mutation in nsP2 that renders the replicon noncytopathic, continuous replication in the absence of cell death can occur for SINV.[55] For VEEV, mutations in the 5′ nontranslated region and nsP3 were also required for persistent infection by the replicon.[205] Multiple subgenomic promoters can be employed for the expression of several proteins of interest in a regulated fashion. To further reduce the chance of recombination between replicon and helper RNAs to generate an infectious genome, tricomponent replicon systems have been developed that can produce at least 1,000 packaged replicons per cell.[45]

RUBIVIRUS REPLICATION

Virion Structure and Entry

Although once considered a close cousin of the alphaviruses, molecular analyses of rubella virus have revealed significant differences.[54] Whereas rubella virions are similar to alphaviruses in protein composition and morphology, the particles have yet to yield to high-resolution structural analysis, and it is unlikely that the particles share the property of icosahedral symmetry with the alphaviruses. The rubella virion is composed of three structural proteins that share the same name as alphaviruses, yet differ in amino acid sequence.[40] The virions are pleomorphic in shape and are around 60 to 70 nm in diameter.[182] The two type I envelope glycoproteins, E1 and E2, form heterodimers, and have 13 and 7 amino acids on their inner cytoplasmic face. All three structural proteins are membrane associated with the C-terminus of the capsid containing the signal sequence for E2.[190] The structural proteins are cleaved by signal peptidase, with the signal sequence for E1 present at the C-terminus of E2.[103] The capsid protein is a phosphoprotein of 293 or 300 amino acids, depending on which AUG codon is used to initiate the polyprotein.[165]

Rubella virus is restricted to growth in humans and is not transmitted by insects, as are the alphaviruses. However, the virus can replicate in a wide range of mammalian cell types and can infect experimental animals producing subclinical results. Thus, like alphaviruses, a ubiquitous cellular receptor may function in entry, although none has yet been identified. The virus also appears to enter through a receptor-mediated endocytosis pathway with membrane fusion promoted by an acidified endosome,[113] and a class II fusion mechanism is expected.

Transcription, Translation, and Genome Replication

The placement of rubella virus in the family *Togaviridae* implies a common genome structure and replication strategy. Complete nucleotide sequences are available for several strains of rubella virus.[40,212] The 9,762 nucleotide genome RNA contains a 5′ terminal 7-methylguanosine and a 3′ terminus that is polyadenylated.[191,294] The genomes of rubiviruses and alphaviruses are compared in Figure 22.4, and a more complete discussion of rubella replication is provided in Chapter 24. The replication proteins P150 and P90 are encoded by the genome RNA, whereas the structural proteins are derived from the subgenomic mRNA. Although there is no amino acid sequence homology among the structural proteins, limited homologies do exist within the replication proteins.[40] The construction of a rubella virus complementary DNA (cDNA) clone from which infectious RNA could be generated permitted molecular genetic studies on the virus that were, up until then, quite limited.[213,294]

Three species of RNA are synthesized in infected cells: complementary minus-strand RNA, genome RNA, and subgenomic mRNA. On infection, the genome RNA is translated into a 200-kD polyprotein that is cleaved by a virus-encoded protease.[50] Unlike its alphavirus counterpart, the rubella enzyme is a metalloprotease that contains zinc-binding domains, and it cleaves P200 in trans.[295] Virus replication complexes can be found in association with cellular membranes. Virus-specific vacuoles have been identified and colocalize with lysosomal markers, similar to those found for alphaviruses.[125] There is a close association between these replication complexes, identified with antibodies to P150, and ER and Golgi membranes, presumably to facilitate translation and packaging of genome RNAs.[224]

Attempts to identify cellular proteins that might participate in RNA replication have focused on proteins that bind to the 5′ and 3′ NTRs. A 5′ stem-loop structure predicted to form on the plus-strand RNA was shown to bind to the La autoantigen. Several cellular proteins were shown to bind to the 3′ NTR.[183,184] One of these proteins was identified as calreticulin, although decreased binding of calreticulin did not correlate with reduced virus replication.[255] The nonstructural protein P90 has been shown to bind to the retinoblastoma protein Rb through an Rb-binding motif.[13] Mutation of this motif reduces virus replication, but it is unclear whether the defect is related to a reduction in binding.[49]

The capsid protein has also been implicated in RNA replication. It has been shown to complement a replication defect resulting from a deletion of 169 amino acids from P150.[277] Exactly how this might function is not known, but the amino terminal 88 residues of the capsid were sufficient for complementation, and these might function by binding to RNA. In addition, the capsid protein has been shown to influence the replication of rubella replicons,[25] although once again the mechanism is not known. The capsid protein has also been shown to bind to mitochondrial matrix protein p32 and the proapoptotic protein Bax.[106] The function of capsid in binding these proteins is to prevent apoptosis and enhance RNA replication.

Virus Assembly

A packaging signal has been located between nucleotides 347 and 375 of the genome RNA, and it interacts with capsid residues 28 to 56.[154] Phosphorylation of the capsid protein occurs and has been suggested to act as a regulatory mechanism to prevent binding of nonviral RNAs to the capsid.[132] With the retention of the capsid protein signal sequence at its C-terminus, the capsid remains associated with the ER membrane. This association may be important for ensuring close connectivity with the envelope glycoproteins through their transmembrane domains. Glycoproteins E1 and E2 are believed to have functions similar to their alphavirus counterparts, although rubella virions bud into the Golgi.[104] Virions undergo a maturation step after Golgi budding that may release the capsid signal sequence because morphologic changes occur in the core of the virion.[224] The structures of the mature and immature rubella virions await structural techniques but will probably require electron tomography, as they lack the icosahedral symmetry present in the alphaviruses.

PERSPECTIVES

Our knowledge of togaviruses has grown dramatically thanks in large part to the ability to genetically manipulate these relatively "simple" plus-strand RNA viruses. Insights into alphaviruses have been obtained more quickly than for rubella virus due to their greater replication efficiency in cultured cells and their well-organized virions. Structural studies of the alphaviruses have progressed rapidly, leveraging the icosahedral nature of the virus particles and the ability to obtain large quantities of homogeneous preparations. The ability to express capsid proteins in heterologous systems has facilitated both structural and biochemical studies of capsid structure and its assembly pathway. The structure determinations of the native and postfusion forms of the E1 protein have provided exceptional insights into the entry process and the structure of the virion. The atomic structures of the E1 and E2 heterodimer, in both low pH and neutral forms, have provided insight into the sequential entry process employed by these viruses.

Significant gaps still persist in understanding the replication process of the togaviruses. Although the protease domain of nsP2 and the macro domain of nsP3 have been determined, the full-length proteins have proven difficult to express in large quantities, to purify to homogeneity, and to crystallize. Furthermore, it is expected that the functional entities will be complexes of viral and probably cellular proteins that will further complicate structural analyses. The ability to reconstitute purified and functional replication complexes will be an important milestone to decipher RNA replication. In contrast, significant progress has been made in understanding the cellular response to viral infection and the recruitment of cellular proteins to promote or inhibit the virus replication complex. Systems-level studies to evaluate the total cellular environment altered in virus infection are beginning to yield a comprehensive picture of how the virus perturbs and subjugates the cell. The use of advanced and real-time optical imaging as well as electron tomography promises to provide a temporal and spatial view of virus infection. However, most studies continue to rely on standard cell culture systems and it will be important to verify what occurs in more natural target cells such as neurons.

With the growing knowledge of togaviruses, their utility in gene expression and gene therapy continues to be exploited and expanded. Future directions that will further benefit this system will be in understanding the nature of the cellular receptors and the structure of the E2 protein that is involved in binding these receptors. With this knowledge, newly designed alphavirus vectors will be engineered to specifically and efficiently target the replicon to cells and tissues of interest.

REFERENCES

All cited references are available in the e-book.

1. Abell BA, Brown DT. Sindbis virus membrane fusion is mediated by reduction of glycoprotein disulfide bridges at the cell surface. *J Virol* 1993;67:5496–5501.
2. Ahlquist P, Strauss EG, Rice CM, et al. Sindbis virus proteins nsP1 and nsP2 contain homology to nonstructural proteins from several RNA plant viruses. *J Virol* 1985;53:536–542.
3. Ahn A, Gibbons DL, Kielian M. The fusion peptide of Semliki Forest virus associates with sterol-rich membrane domains. *J Virol* 2002;76:3267–3275.
5. Ahn A, Schoepp RJ, Sternberg D, et al. Growth and stability of a cholesterol-independent Semliki Forest virus mutant in mosquitoes. *Virology* 1999;262:452–456.
8. Ahola T, Laakkonen P, Vihinen H, et al. Critical residues of Semliki Forest virus RNA capping enzyme involved in methyltransferase and guanylyltransferase-like activities. *J Virol* 1997;71:392–397.
9. Ahola T, Lampio A, Auvinen P, et al. Semliki Forest virus mRNA capping enzyme requires association with anionic membrane phospholipids for activity. *EMBO J* 1999;18:3164–3172.
10. Aliperti G, Schlesinger MJ. Evidence for an autoprotease activity of Sindbis virus capsid protein. *Virology* 1978;90:366–369.
11. Anthony RP, Pardes AM, Brown DT. Disulfide bonds are essential for the stability of the Sindbis virus envelope. *Virology* 1993;190:330–336.
12. Atasheva S, Gorchakov R, English R, et al. Development of Sindbis viruses encoding nsP2/GFP chimeric proteins and their application for studying nsP2 functioning. *J Virol* 2007;81:5046–5057.
16. Bick MJ, Carroll JW, Gao G, et al. Expression of the zinc-finger antiviral protein inhibits alphavirus replication. *J Virol* 2003;77:11555–11562.
20. Byrnes AP, Griffin DE. Binding of Sindbis virus to cell surface heparan sulfate. *J Virol* 1998;72:7349–7356.
21. Byrnes AP, Griffin DE. Large-plaque mutants of Sindbis virus show reduced binding to heparan sulfate, heightened viremia, and slower clearance from the circulation. *J Virol* 2000;74:644–651.
22. Carleton M, Brown DT. Disulfide bridge-mediated folding of Sindbis virus glycoproteins. *J Virol* 1996;70:5541–5547.
23. Chanel-Vos C, Kielian M. A conserved histidine in the ij loop of the Semliki Forest virus E1 protein plays an important role in membrane fusion. *J Virol* 2004;78:13543–13552.
25. Chen MH, Icenogle JP. Rubella virus capsid protein modulates viral genome replication and virus infectivity. *J Virol* 2004;78:4314–4322.
27. Cheng RH, Kuhn RJ, Olson NH, et al. Nucleocapsid and glycoprotein organization in an enveloped virus. *Cell* 1995;80:621–630.
29. Choi HK, Tong L, Minor W, et al. Structure of Sindbis virus core protein reveals a chymotrypsin-like serine proteinase and the organization of the virion. *Nature (London)* 1991;354:37–43.
32. Cristea IM, Carroll JW, Rout MP, et al. Tracking and elucidating alphavirus-host protein interactions. *J Biol Chem* 2006;281:30269–30278.
33. Cristea IM, Rozjabek H, Molloy KR, et al. Host factors associated with the Sindbis virus RNA-dependent RNA polymerase: role for G3BP1 and G3BP2 in virus replication. *J Virol* 2010;84:6720–6732.
35. de Groot RJ, Hardy RH, Shirako Y, et al. Cleavage-site preferences of Sindbis virus polyproteins containing the nonstructural proteinase: Evidence for temporal regulation of polyprotein processing in vivo. *EMBO J* 1990;9:2631–2638.
36. de Groot RJ, Rümenapf T, Kuhn RJ, et al. Sindbis virus RNA polymerase is degraded by the N-end rule pathway. *Proc Natl Acad Sci U S A* 1991;88:8967–8971.
37. De I, Sawicki SG, Sawicki DL. Sindbis virus RNA-negative mutants that fail to convert from minus-strand to plus-strand synthesis: role of the nsP2 protein. *J Virol* 1996;70:2706–2719.
38. DeTulleo L, Kirchhausen T. The clathrin endocytic pathway in viral infection. *EMBO J* 1998;17:4585–4593.
39. Ding M, Schlesinger MJ. Evidence that Sindbis virus nsP2 is an autoprotease which processes the virus nonstructural polyprotein. *Virology* 1989;171:280–284.
40. Dominguez G, Wang C-Y, Frey TK. Sequence of the genome RNA of rubella virus: Evidence for genetic rearrangement during togavirus evolution. *Virology* 1990;177:225–238.
42. Edwards J, Brown DT. Sindbis virus infection of a Chinese hamster ovary cell mutant defective in the acidification of endosomes. *Virology* 1991;182:28–33.
44. Fayzulin R, Frolov I. Changes of the secondary structure of the 5′ end of the Sindbis virus genome inhibit virus growth in mosquito cells and lead to accumulation of adaptive mutations. *J Virol* 2004;78:4953–4964.
47. Firth AE, Chung BY, Fleeton MN, et al. Discovery of frameshifting in Alphavirus 6K resolves a 20-year enigma. *Virol J* 2008;5:108.

50. Forng RY, Frey TK. Identification of the rubella virus nonstructural proteins. *Virology* 1995;206:843–853.
51. Forrester NL, Palacios G, Tesh RB, et al. Genome-scale phylogeny of the alphavirus genus suggests a marine origin. *J Virol* 2012;86:2729–2738.
52. Forsell K, Griffiths G, Garoff H. Preformed cytoplasmic nucleocapsids are not necessary for alphavirus budding. *EMBO J* 1996;15:6495–6505.
53. Forsell K, Xing L, Kozlovska T, et al. Membrane proteins organize a symmetrical virus. *EMBO J* 2000;19:5081–5091.
54. Frey TK. Molecular biology of rubella virus. *Adv Virus Res* 1994;44:69–160.
55. Frolov I, Agapov E, Hoffman TA Jr, et al. Selection of RNA replicons capable of persistent noncytopathic replication in mammalian cells. *J Virol* 1999;73:3854–3865.
56. Frolov I, Hardy R, Rice CM. Cis-acting RNA elements at the 5′ end of Sindbis virus genome RNA regulate minus- and plus-strand RNA synthesis. *RNA* 2001;7:1638–1651.
57. Frolov I, Hoffman TA, Pragai BM, et al. Alphavirus-based expression vectors: strategies and applications. *Proc Natl Acad Sci U S A* 1996;93:11371–11377.
58. Frolov I, Schlesinger S. Comparison of the effects of Sindbis virus and Sindbis virus replicons on host cell protein synthesis and cytopathogenicity in BHK cells. *J Virol* 1994;68:1721–1727.
60. Frolova EI, Gorchakov R, Pereboeva L, et al. Functional Sindbis virus replicative complexes are formed at the plasma membrane. *J Virol* 2010;84:11679–11695.
61. Froshauer S, Kartenbeck J, Helenius A. Alphavirus RNA replicase is located on the cytoplasmic surface of endosomes and lysosomes. *J Cell Biol* 1988;107:2075–2086.
63. Gaedigk-Nitschko K, Ding M, Schlesinger MJ. Site-directed mutations in the Sindbis virus 6K protein reveal sites for fatty acylation and the underacylated protein affects virus release and virion structure. *Virology* 1990;175:282–291.
65. Gardner CL, Ebel GD, Ryman KD, et al. Heparan sulfate binding by natural eastern equine encephalitis viruses promotes neurovirulence. *Proc Natl Acad Sci U S A* 2011;108:16026–16031.
66. Garmashova N, Gorchakov R, Frolova E, et al. Sindbis virus nonstructural protein nsP2 is cytotoxic and inhibits cellular transcription. *J Virol* 2006;80:5686–5696.
71. Geigenmüller-Gnirke U, Nitschko H, Schlesinger S. Deletion analysis of the capsid protein of Sindbis virus: Identification of the RNA binding region. *J Virol* 1993;67:1620–1626.
73. Gibbons DL, Ahn A, Chatterjee PK, et al. Formation and characterization of the trimeric form of the fusion protein of Semliki Forest Virus. *J Virol* 2000;74:7772–7780.
74. Gibbons DL, Erk I, Reilly B, et al. Visualization of the target-membrane-inserted fusion protein of Semliki Forest virus by combined electron microscopy and crystallography. *Cell* 2003;114:573–583.
76. Gibbons DL, Vaney M-C, Roussel A, et al. Conformational change and protein-protein interactions of the fusion protein of Semliki Forest virus. *Nature* 2004;427:322–325.
77. Glomb-Reinmund S, Kielian M. The role of low pH and disulfide shuffling in the entry and fusion of Semliki Forest virus and Sindbis virus. *Virology* 1998;248:372–381.
79. Gorbalenya AE, Koonin EV, Donchenko AP, et al. A novel superfamily of nucleoside triphosphate-binding motif containing proteins which are probably involved in duplex unwinding in DNA and RNA replication and recombination. *FEBS Lett* 1988;235:16–24.
80. Gorbalenya AE, Koonin EV, Lai MMC. Putative papain-related thiol proteases of positive-strand RNA viruses. *FEBS Lett* 1991;288:201–205.
81. Gorchakov R, Frolova E, Frolov I. Inhibition of transcription and translation in Sindbis virus-infected cells. *J Virol* 2005;79:9397–9409.
82. Gorchakov R, Frolova E, Sawicki S, et al. A new role for ns polyprotein cleavage in Sindbis virus replication. *J Virol* 2008;82:6218–6231.
83. Guo X, Carroll JW, Macdonald MR, et al. The zinc finger antiviral protein directly binds to specific viral mRNAs through the CCCH zinc finger motifs. *J Virol* 2004;78:12781–12787.
84. Haag L, Garoff H, Xing L, et al. Acid-induced movements in the glycoprotein shell of an alphavirus turn the spikes into membrane fusion mode. *EMBO J* 2002;21:4402–4410.
86. Hahn CS, Strauss JH. Site-directed mutagenesis of the proposed catalytic amino acids of the Sindbis virus capsid protein autoprotease. *J Virol* 1990;64:3069–3073.
88. Hammar L, Markarian S, Haag L, et al. Prefusion rearrangements resulting in fusion Peptide exposure in Semliki forest virus. *J Biol Chem* 2003;278:7189–7198.
89. Hardy RW. The role of the 3′ terminus of the Sindbis virus genome in minus-strand initiation site selection. *Virology* 2006;345:520–531.
91. Hardy WR, Strauss JH. Processing of the nonstructural polyproteins of Sindbis virus: Study of the kinetics in vivo using monospecific antibodies. *J Virol* 1988;62:998–1007.
92. Hardy WR, Strauss JH. Processing the nonstructural proteins of Sindbis virus: Nonstructural proteinase is in the C-terminal half of nsP2 and functions both in *cis* and *trans*. *J Virol* 1989;63:4653–4664.
96. Heidner HW, McKnight KL, Davis NL, et al. Lethality of PE2 incorporation into Sindbis virus can be suppressed by second-site mutations in E3 and E2. *J Virol* 1994;68:2683–2692.
97. Heil ML, Albee A, Strauss JH, et al. An amino acid substitution in the coding region of the E2 glycoprotein adapts Ross River Virus to utilize heparan sulfate as an attachment moiety. *J Virol* 2001;7:6303–6309.
100. Hernandez R, Luo TC, Brown DT. Exposure to low pH is not required for penetration of mosquito cells by Sindbis virus. *J Virol* 2001;75:2010–2013.
101. Hertz JM, Huang HV. Evolution of the Sindbis virus subgenomic mRNA promoter in cultured cells. *J Virol* 1995;69:7768–7774.
103. Hobman TC, Lundstrom ML, Mauracher CA, et al. Assembly of rubella virus structural proteins into virus-like particles in transfected cells. *Virology* 1994;202:574–585.
104. Hobman TC, Woodward L, Farquhar MG. Targeting of a heterodimeric membrane protein complex to the Golgi: rubella virus E2 glycoprotein contains a transmembrane Golgi retention signal. *Mol Biol Cell* 1995;6:7–20.
106. Ilkow CS, Goping IS, Hobman TC. The Rubella virus capsid is an anti-apoptotic protein that attenuates the pore-forming ability of Bax. *PLoS Pathog* 2011;7:e1001291.
109. Jose J, Przybyla L, Edwards TJ, et al. Interactions of the cytoplasmic domain of Sindbis virus E2 with nucleocapsid cores promote alphavirus budding. *J Virol* 2012;86:2585–2599.
110. Jose J, Snyder JE, Kuhn RJ. A structural and functional perspective of alphavirus replication and assembly. *Future Microbiol* 2009;4:837–856.
113. Katow S, Sugiura A. Low pH-induced conformational change of rubella virus envelope proteins. *J Gen Virol* 1988;69(Pt 11):2797–2807.
116. Kielian MC, Helenius A. Role of cholesterol in fusion of Semliki Forest virus with membranes. *J Virol* 1984;52:281–283.
117. Kim DY, Firth AE, Atasheva S, et al. Conservation of a packaging signal and the viral genome RNA packaging mechanism in alphavirus evolution. *J Virol* 2011;85:8022–8036.
118. Klimstra WB, Nangle EM, Smith MS, et al. DC-SIGN and L-SIGN can act as attachment receptors for alphaviruses and distinguish between mosquito cell- and mammalian cell-derived viruses. *J Virol* 2003;77:12022–12032.
119. Klimstra WB, Ryman KD, Johnston RE. Adaptation of Sindbis virus to BHK cells selects for use of heparan sulfate as an attachment receptor. *J Virol* 1998;72:7357–7366.
121. Koonin EV, Dolja VV. Evolution and taxonomy of positive-strand RNA viruses: implications of comparative analysis of amino acid sequences. *Crit Rev Biochem Mol Biol* 1993;28:375–430.
122. Kostyuchenko VA, Jakana J, Liu X, et al. The structure of barmah forest virus as revealed by cryo-electron microscopy at a 6-angstrom resolution has detailed transmembrane protein architecture and interactions. *J Virol* 2011;85:9327–9333.
123. Kuhn RJ, Hong Z, Strauss JH. Mutagenesis of the 3′ nontranslated region of Sindbis virus RNA. *J Virol* 1990;64:1465–1476.
124. Kuhn RJ, Zhang W, Rossmann MG, et al. Structure of dengue virus: implications for flavivirus organization, maturation, and fusion. *Cell* 2002;108:717–725.
125. Kujala P, Ahola T, Ehsani N, et al. Intracellular distribution of rubella virus nonstructural protein P150. *J Virol* 1999;73:7805–7811.
126. Kujala P, Ikaheimonen A, Ehsani N, et al. Biogenesis of the Semliki Forest virus RNA replication complex. *J Virol* 2001;75:3873–3884.

131. LaStarza MW, Lemm JA, Rice CM. Genetic analysis of the nsP3 region of Sindbis virus: evidence for roles in minus-strand and subgenomic RNA synthesis. *J Virol* 1994;68:5781–5791.
132. Law LM, Everitt JC, Beatch MD, et al. Phosphorylation of rubella virus capsid regulates its RNA binding activity and virus replication. *J Virol* 2003;77:1764–1771.
133. Lee S, Owen KE, Choi HK, et al. Identification of a protein binding site on the surface of the alphavirus nucleocapsid and its implication in virus assembly. *Structure* 1996;4:531–541.
135. Lemm JA, Rice CM. Assembly of functional Sindbis virus RNA replication complexes: requirement for coexpression of P123 and P34. *J Virol* 1993;67:1905–1915.
136. Lemm JA, Rice CM. Roles of nonstructural polyproteins and cleavage products in regulating Sindbis virus RNA replication and transcription. *J Virol* 1993;67:1916–1926.
137. Lemm JA, Rumenapf T, Strauss EG, et al. Polypeptide requirements for assembly of functional Sindbis virus replication complexes: a model for the temporal regulation of minus- and plus-strand RNA synthesis. *EMBO J* 1994;13:2925–2934.
138. Lescar J, Roussel A, Wein MW, et al. The fusion glycoprotein shell of Semliki Forest virus: an icosahedral assembly primed for fusogenic activation at endosomal pH. *Cell* 2001;105:137–148.
139. Levine B, Huang Q, Isaacs JT, et al. Conversion of lytic to persistent alphavirus infection by the bcl-2 cellular oncogene. *Nature* 1993; 361:739–742.
140. Levis R, Huang H, Schlesinger S. Engineered defective interfering RNAs of Sindbis virus express bacterial chloramphenicol acetyltransferase in avian cells. *Proc Natl Acad Sci U S A* 1987;84:4811–4815.
141. Levis R, Weiss BG, Tsiang M, et al. Deletion mapping of Sindbis virus DI RNAs derived from cDNAs defines the sequences essential for replication and packaging. *Cell* 1986;44:137–145.
142. Lewis J, Wesselingh SL, Griffin DE, et al. Alphavirus-induced apoptosis in mouse brains correlates with neurovirulence. *J Virol* 1996;70: 1828–1835.
143. Li G, LaStarza MW, Hardy WR, et al. Phosphorylation of Sindbis virus nsP3 *in vivo* and *in vitro*. *Virology* 1990;179:416–427.
144. Li G, Rice CM. Mutagenesis of the in-frame opal termination codon preceding nsP4 of Sindbis virus: Studies of translational readthrough and its effect on virus replication. *J Virol* 1989;63:1326–1337.
145. Li L, Jose J, Xiang Y, et al. Structural changes of envelope proteins during alphavirus fusion. *Nature* 2010;468:705–708.
146. Liao M, Kielian M. Domain III from class II fusion proteins functions as a dominant-negative inhibitor of virus membrane fusion. *J Cell Biol* 2005;171:111–120.
148. Liljeström P, Garoff H. Internally located cleavable signal sequences direct the formation of Semliki Forest virus membrane proteins from a polyprotein precursor. *J Virol* 1991;65:147–154.
149. Liljeström P, Lusa S, Huylebroeck D, et al. In vitro mutagenesis of a full-length cDNA clone of Semliki Forest virus: the small 6000-molecular-weight membrane protein modulates virus release. *J Virol* 1991;65: 4107–4113.
151. Linn ML, Gardner J, Warrilow D, et al. Arbovirus of marine mammals: a new alphavirus isolated from the elephant seal louse, Lepidophthirus macrorhini. *J Virol* 2001;75:4103–4109.
152. Liu CY, Kielian M. E1 mutants identify a critical region in the trimer interface of the Semliki forest virus fusion protein. *J Virol* 2009;83:11298–11306.
153. Liu N, Brown DT. Transient translocation of the cytoplasmic (Endo) domain of a type I membrane glycoprotein into cellular membranes. *J Cell Biol* 1993;120:877–883.
154. Liu Z, Yang D, Qiu Z, et al. Identification of domains in rubella virus genomic RNA and capsid protein necessary for specific interaction. *J Virol* 1996;70:2184–2190.
155. Lobigs M, Garoff H. Fusion function of the Semliki Forest virus spike is activated by proteolytic cleavage of the envelope glycoprotein precursor p62. *J Virol* 1990;64:1233–1240.
156. Lobigs M, Wahlberg JM, Garoff H. Spike protein oligomerization control of Semliki Forest virus fusion. *J Virol* 1990;64:5214–5218.
158. Loewy A, Smyth J, von Bonsdorff CH, et al. The 6-kilodalton membrane protein of Semliki Forest virus is involved in the budding process. *J Virol* 1995;69:469–475.
161. Luo T, Brown DT. Purification and characterization of a Sindbis virus-induced peptide which stimulates its own production and blocks virus RNA synthesis. *Virology* 1993;194:44–49.
163. Malet H, Coutard B, Jamal S, et al. The crystal structures of Chikungunya and Venezuelan equine encephalitis virus nsP3 macro domains define a conserved adenosine binding pocket. *J Virol* 2009;83:6534–6545.
164. Marquardt MT, Phalen T, Kielian M. Cholesterol is required in the exit pathway of Semliki Forest virus. *J Cell Biol* 1993;123:57–65.
165. Marr LD, Sanchez A, Frey TK. Efficient in vitro translation and processing of the rubella virus structural proteins in the presence of microsomes. *Virology* 1991;180:400–405.
168. Melancon P, Garoff H. Processing of the Semliki Forest virus structural polyprotein: role of the capsid protease. *J Virol* 1987;61:1301–1309.
169. Melton JV, Ewart GD, Weir RC, et al. Alphavirus 6K proteins form ion channels. *J Biol Chem* 2002;277:46923–46931.
170. Metsikkö K, Garoff H. Oligomers of the cytoplasmic domain of the p62/E2 membrane protein of Semliki Forest virus bind to the nucleocapsid in vitro. *J Virol* 1990;64:4678–4683.
171. Meyer WJ, Gidwitz S, Ayers VK, et al. Conformational alteration of Sindbis virion glycoproteins induced by heat, reducing agents, or low pH. *J Virol* 1992;66:3504–3513.
173. Mi S, Durbin R, Huang HV, et al. Association of the Sindbis virus RNA methytransferase activity with the nonstructural protein nsP1. *Virology* 1989;170:385–391.
174. Mi S, Stollar V. Expression of Sindbis virus nsP1 and methyltransferase activity in Escherichia coli. *Virology* 1991;184:423–427.
177. Montgomery SA, Johnston RE. Nuclear import and export of Venezuelan equine encephalitis virus nonstructural protein 2. *J Virol* 2007; 81:10268–10279.
178. Mukhopadhyay S, Chipman PR, Hong EM, et al. In vitro-assembled alphavirus core-like particles maintain a structure similar to that of nucleocapsid cores in mature virus. *J Virol* 2002;76:11128–11132.
179. Mukhopadhyay S, Zhang W, Gabler S, et al. Mapping the structure and function of the E1 and E2 glycoproteins in alphaviruses. *Structure* 2006;14:63–73.
180. Mulvey M, Brown DT. Assembly of the Sindbis virus spike protein complex. *Virology* 1996;219:125–132.
181. Mulvey M, Brown DT. Formation and rearrangement of disulfide bonds during maturation of the Sindbis virus E1 glycoprotein. *J Virol* 1994;68: 805–812.
182. Murphy FA. Togavirus morphology and morphogenesis. In: Schlesinger RW, ed. *The Togaviruses*. New York: Academic Press; 1980:241–316.
183. Nakhasi HL, Cao X-Q, Rouault TA, et al. Specific binding of host cell proteins to the 3′-terminal stem-loop structure of rubella virus negative-strand RNA. *J Virol* 1991;65:5961–5967.
185. Neuvonen M, Kazlauskas A, Martikainen M, et al. SH3 domain-mediated recruitment of host cell amphiphysins by alphavirus nsP3 promotes viral RNA replication. *PLoS Pathog* 2011;7:e1002383.
186. Ng CG, Coppens I, Govindarajan D, et al. Effect of host cell lipid metabolism on alphavirus replication, virion morphogenesis, and infectivity. *Proc Natl Acad Sci U S A* 2008;105:16326–16331.
187. Niesters HGM, Strauss JH. Defined mutations in the 5′ nontranslated sequence of Sindbis virus RNA. *J Virol* 1990;64:4162–4168.
192. Owen KE, Kuhn RJ. Identification of a region in the Sindbis virus nucleocapsid protein that is involved in specificity of RNA encapsidation. *J Virol* 1996;70:2757–2763.
194. Pardigon N, Strauss JH. Cellular proteins bind to the 3′ end of Sindbis virus minus strand RNA. *J Virol* 1992;66:1007–1015.
195. Pardigon N, Strauss JH. Mosquito homolog of the La autoantigen binds to Sindbis virus RNA. *J Virol* 1996;70:1173–1181.
197. Paredes A, Alwell-Warda K, Weaver SC, et al. Venezuelan equine encephalomyelitis virus structure and its divergence from Old World alphaviruses. *J Virol* 2001;75:9532–9537.
198. Paredes AM, Brown DT, Rothnagel R, et al. Three-dimensional structure of a membrane-containing virus. *Proc Natl Acad Sci U S A* 1993;90: 9095–9099.
199. Paredes AM, Ferreira D, Horton M, et al. Conformational changes in Sindbis virions resulting from exposure to low pH and interactions with cells suggest that cell penetration may occur at the cell surface in the absence of membrane fusion. *Virology* 2004;324:373–386.

200. Paredes AM, Heidner H, Thuman-Commike P, et al. Structural localization of the E3 glycoprotein in attenuated Sindbis virus mutants. *J Virol* 1998;72:1534–1541.
201. Paredes AM, Simon ML, Brown DT. The mass of the Sindbis virus nucleocapsid suggests it has T = 4 icosahedral symmetry. *Virology* 1993; 187:329–332.
202. Peranen J, Kaariainen L. Biogenesis of type I cytopathic vacuoles in Semliki Forest virus-infected BHK cells. *J Virol* 1991;65:1623–1627.
205. Petrakova O, Volkova E, Gorchakov R, et al. Noncytopathic replication of Venezuelan equine encephalitis virus and eastern equine encephalitis virus replicons in Mammalian cells. *J Virol* 2005;79:7597–7608.
206. Phalen T, Kielian M. Cholesterol is required for infection by Semliki Forest virus. *J Cell Biol* 1991;112:615–623.
207. Pletnev SV, Zhang W, Mukhopadhyay S, et al. Locations of carbohydrate sites on alphavirus glycoproteins show that E1 forms an icosahedral scaffold. *Cell* 2001;105:127–136.
208. Porterfield JS. Comparative and historical aspects of the Togaviridae and Flaviviridae. In: Schlesinger S, Schlesinger MJ, eds. *The Togaviridae and Flaviviridae.* New York: Plenum Press; 1986:1–19.
209. Powers AM, Brault AC, Shirako Y, et al. Evolutionary relationships and systematics of the alphaviruses. *J Virol* 2001;75:10118–10131.
211. Presley JF, Polo JM, Johnston RE, et al. Proteolytic processing of the Sindbis virus membrane protein precursor PE2 is nonessential for growth in vertebrate cells but is required for efficient growth in invertebrate cells. *J Virol* 1991;65:1905–1909.
213. Pugachev KV, Abernathy ES, Frey TK. Improvement of the specific infectivity of the rubella virus (RUB) infectious clone: determinants of cytopathogenicity induced by RUB map to the nonstructural proteins. *J Virol* 1997;71:562–568.
215. Qin ZL, Zheng Y, Kielian M. Role of conserved histidine residues in the low-pH dependence of the Semliki Forest virus fusion protein. *J Virol* 2009;83:4670–4677.
217. Rey FA, Heinz FX, Mandl C, et al. The envelope glycoprotein from tick-borne encephalitis virus at 2 Å resolution. *Nature (London)* 1995; 375:291–298.
218. Rice CM, Strauss JH. Association of Sindbis virion glycoproteins and their precursors. *J Mol Biol* 1982;154:325–348.
219. Rice CM, Strauss JH. Nucleotide sequence of the 26S mRNA of Sindbis virus and deduced sequence of the encoded virus structural proteins. *Proc Natl Acad Sci U S A* 1981;78:2062–2066.
220. Rikkonen M. Functional significance of the nuclear-targeting and NTP-binding motifs of Semliki Forest virus nonstructural protein nsP2. *Virology* 1996;218:352–361.
221. Rikkonen M, Peranen J, Kaariainen L. ATPase and GTPase activities associated with Semliki Forest virus nonstructural protein nsP2. *J Virol* 1994;68:5804–5810.
224. Risco C, Carrascosa JL, Frey TK. Structural maturation of rubella virus in the Golgi complex. *Virology* 2003;312:261–269.
226. Rose PP, Hanna SL, Spiridigliozzi A, et al. Natural resistance-associated macrophage protein is a cellular receptor for sindbis virus in both insect and mammalian hosts. *Cell Host Microbe* 2011;10:97–104.
228. Roussel A, Lescar J, Vaney M-C, et al. Structure and interactions at the viral surface of the envelope protein E1 of Semliki Forest virus. *Structure* 2006;14:75–86.
229. Rubach JK, Wasik BR, Rupp JC, et al. Characterization of purified Sindbis virus nsP4 RNA-dependent RNA polymerase activity in vitro. *Virology* 2009;384:201–208.
231. Rümenapf T, Strauss EG, Strauss JH. Subgenomic mRNA of Aura alphavirus is packaged into virions. *J Virol* 1994;68:56–62.
233. Russo AT, Malmstrom RD, White MA, et al. Structural basis for substrate specificity of alphavirus nsP2 proteases. *J Mol Graph Model* 2010; 29:46–53.
234. Russo AT, White MA, Watowich SJ. The crystal structure of the Venezuelan equine encephalitis alphavirus nsP2 protease. *Structure* 2006;14: 1449–1458.
235. Ryman KD, Meier KC, Nangle EM, et al. Sindbis virus translation is inhibited by a PKR/RNase L-independent effector induced by alpha/beta interferon priming of dendritic cells. *J Virol* 2005;79:1487–1499.
236. Salminen A, Wahlberg JM, Lobigs M, et al. Membrane fusion process of Semliki Forest virus II: Cleavage-dependent reorganization of the spike protein complex controls virus entry. *J Cell Biol* 1992;116:349–357.
238. Sanz MA, Carrasco L. Sindbis virus variant with a deletion in the 6K gene shows defects in glycoprotein processing and trafficking: lack of complementation by a wild-type 6K gene in trans. *J Virol* 2001;75:7778–7784.
239. Sawicki D, Barkhimer DB, Sawicki SG, et al. Temperature sensitive shut-off of alphavirus minus strand RNA synthesis maps to a nonstructural protein, nsP4. *Virology* 1990;174:43–52.
240. Sawicki DL, Perri S, Polo JM, et al. Role for nsP2 proteins in the cessation of alphavirus minus-strand synthesis by host cells. *J Virol* 2006; 80:360–371.
242. Sawicki SG, Sawicki DL, Kääriäinen L, et al. A Sindbis virus mutant temperature-sensitive in the regulation of minus-strand RNA synthesis. *Virology* 1981;115:161–172.
244. Schlesinger S. Alphavirus expression vectors. *Adv Virus Res* 2000;55: 565–577.
247. Sherman MB, Weaver SC. Structure of the recombinant alphavirus Western equine encephalitis virus revealed by cryoelectron microscopy. *J Virol* 2010;84:9775–9782.
248. Shirako Y, Strauss EG, Strauss JH. Modification of the 5′ terminus of Sindbis virus genomic RNA allows nsP4 RNA polymerases with nonaromatic amino acids at the N terminus to function in RNA replication. *J Virol* 2003;77:2301–2309.
250. Shirako Y, Strauss JH. Regulation of Sindbis virus RNA replication: uncleaved P123 and nsP4 function in minus-strand RNA synthesis, whereas cleaved products from P123 are required for efficient plus-strand RNA synthesis. *J Virol* 1994;68:1874–1885.
253. Singh I, Helenius A. Role of ribosomes in Semliki Forest virus nucleocapsid uncoating. *J Virol* 1992;66:7049–7058.
255. Singh NK, Atreya CD, Nakhasi HL. Identification of calreticulin as a rubella virus RNA binding protein. *Proc Natl Acad Sci U S A* 1994; 91:12770–12774.
256. Skoging U, Vihinen M, Nilsson L, et al. Aromatic interactions define the binding of the alphavirus spike to its nucleocapsid. *Structure* 1996; 4:519–529.
257. Smit JM, Waarts B-L, Kimata K, et al. Adaptation of alphaviruses to heparan sulfate: Interaction of Sindbis and Semliki Forest virus with liposomes containing lipid-conjugated heparin. *J Virol* 2002;76:10128–10137.
258. Snyder JE, Azizgolshani O, Wu B, et al. Rescue of infectious particles from preassembled alphavirus nucleocapsid cores. *J Virol* 2011; 85:5773–5781.
260. Sokoloski KJ, Dickson AM, Chaskey EL, et al. Sindbis virus usurps the cellular HuR protein to stabilize its transcripts and promote productive infections in mammalian and mosquito cells. *Cell Host Microbe* 2010; 8:196–207.
261. Soonsawad P, Xing L, Milla E, et al. Structural evidence of glycoprotein assembly in cellular membrane compartments prior to Alphavirus budding. *J Virol* 2010;84:11145–11151.
262. Spuul P, Balistreri G, Kaariainen L, et al. Phosphatidylinositol 3-kinase-, actin-, and microtubule-dependent transport of Semliki Forest Virus replication complexes from the plasma membrane to modified lysosomes. *J Virol* 2010;84:7543–7557.
264. Strauss EG, Lenches EM, Strauss JH. Mutants of Sindbis virus. I. Isolation and partial characterization of 89 new temperature-sensitive mutants. *Virology* 1976;74:154–168.
265. Strauss EG, Rice CM, Strauss JH. Complete nucleotide sequence of the genomic RNA of Sindbis virus. *Virology* 1984;133:92–110.
268. Strauss JH, Strauss EG. The alphaviruses: gene expression, replication, and evolution. *Microbiol Rev* 1994;58:491–562.
270. Suomalainen M, Liljestrom P, Garoff H. Spike protein-nucleocapsid interactions drive the budding of alphaviruses. *J Virol* 1992;66:4737–4747.
271. Tang J, Jose J, Chipman P, et al. Molecular links between the E2 envelope glycoprotein and nucleocapsid core in Sindbis virus. *J Mol Biol* 2011;414:442–459.
272. Tellinghuisen TL, Hamburger AE, Fisher BR, et al. In vitro assembly of alphavirus cores by using nucleocapsid protein expressed in Escherichia coli. *J Virol* 1999;73:5309–5319.
274. Tellinghuisen TL, Perera R, Kuhn RJ. In vitro assembly of Sindbis virus core-like particles from cross-linked dimers of truncated and mutant capsid proteins. *J Virol* 2001;75:2810–2817.
275. Tomar S, Hardy RW, Smith JL, et al. Catalytic core of alphavirus nonstructural protein nsP4 possesses terminal adenylyltransferase activity. *J Virol* 2006;80:9962–9969.

277. Tzeng WP, Frey TK. Complementation of a deletion in the rubella virus p150 nonstructural protein by the viral capsid protein. *J Virol* 2003; 77:9502–9510.
278. Ubol S, Griffin DE. Identification of a putative alphavirus receptor on mouse neural cells. *J Virol* 1991;65:6913–6921.
281. Vasiljeva L, Merits A, Auvinen P, et al. Identification of a novel function of the alphavirus capping apparatus. RNA 5′-triphosphatase activity of Nsp2. *J Biol Chem* 2000;275:17281–17287.
284. Vihinen H, Ahola T, Tuittila M, et al. Elimination of phosphorylation sites of Semliki Forest virus replicase protein nsP3. *J Biol Chem* 2001; 276:5745–5752.
286. Volkova E, Gorchakov R, Frolov I. The efficient packaging of Venezuelan equine encephalitis virus-specific RNAs into viral particles is determined by nsP1–3 synthesis. *Virology* 2006;344:315–327.
289. Voss JE, Vaney MC, Duquerroy S, et al. Glycoprotein organization of Chikungunya virus particles revealed by X-ray crystallography. *Nature* 2010;468:709–712.
290. Waarts B-L, Bittman R, Wilschut J. Sphingolipid and cholesterol dependence of alphavirus membrane fusion. *J Biol Chem* 2002;277:38141–38147.
292. Wahlberg JM, Bron R, Wilschut J, et al. Membrane fusion of Semliki Forest virus involves homotrimers of the fusion protein. *J Virol* 1992; 66:7309–7318.
294. Wang CY, Dominguez G, Frey TK. Construction of rubella virus genome-length cDNA clones and synthesis of infectious RNA transcripts. *J Virol* 1994;68:3550–3557.
295. Wang KS, Kuhn RJ, Strauss EG, et al. High-affinity laminin receptor is a receptor for Sindbis virus in mammalian cells. *J Virol* 1992;66:4992–5001.
297. Wang Y-F, Sawicki SG, Sawicki D. Alphavirus nsP3 functions to form replication complexes transcribing negative-strand RNA. *J Virol* 1994; 68:6466–6475.
299. Weiss B, Geigenmüller-Gnirke U, Schlesinger S. Interactions between Sindbis virus RNAs and a 68 amino acid derivative of the viral capsid protein further defines the capsid binding site. *Nucleic Acids Res* 1994; 22:780–786.
300. Weiss B, Nitschko H, Ghattas I, et al. Evidence for specificity in the encapsidation of Sindbis virus RNAs. *J Virol* 1989;63:5310–5318.
302. Wengler G, Boege U, Wengler G, et al. The core protein of the alphavirus Sindbis virus assembles into core-like nucleoproteins with the viral genome RNA and with other single-stranded nucleic acids *in vitro*. *Virology* 1982;118:401–410.
305. Wengler G, Wengler G. Identification of a transfer of viral core protein to cellular ribosomes during the early stages of alphavirus infection. *Virology* 1984;134:435.
306. Wengler G, Wengler G. In vitro analysis of factors involved in the disassembly of Sindbis virus cores by 60S ribosomal subunits identifies a possible role of low pH. *J Gen Virol* 2002;83:2417–2426.
310. White J, Kartenbeck J, Helenius A. Fusion of Semliki Forest virus with the plasma membrane can be induced by low pH. *J Cell Biol* 1980; 87:264–272.
311. Wielgosz MM, Raju R, Huang HV. Sequence requirements for Sindbis virus subgenomic mRNA promoter function in cultured cells. *J Virol* 2001;75:3509–3519.
313. Xiong C, Levis R, Shen P, et al. Sindbis virus: an efficient, broad host range vector for gene expression in animal cells. *Science* 1989;243:1188–1191.
315. Zhang R, Hryc CF, Cong Y, et al. 4.4 Å cryo-EM structure of an enveloped alphavirus Venezuelan equine encephalitis virus. *EMBO J* 2011; 30:3854–3863.
317. Zhang W, Heil M, Kuhn RJ, et al. Heparin binding sites on Ross River virus revealed by electron cryo-microscopy. *Virology* 2005;332:511–518.
318. Zhang W, Mukhopadhyay S, Pletnev SV, et al. Placement of the structural proteins in Sindbis virus. *J Virol* 2002;76:11645–11658.
319. Zhao H, Lindqvist B, Garoff H, et al. A tyrosine-based motif in the cytoplasmic domain of the alphavirus envelope protein is essential for budding. *EMBO J* 1994;13:4204–4211.
320. Zheng Y, Sanchez-San Martin C, Qin ZL, et al. The domain I-domain III linker plays an important role in the fusogenic conformational change of the alphavirus membrane fusion protein. *J Virol* 2011;85:6334–6342.

CHAPTER 23

Diane E. Griffin

Alphaviruses

The genus *Alphavirus* includes 29 species that can be classified antigenically into at least eight complexes (Table 23.1). Alphaviruses are geographically restricted in their distributions and have been found on all continents and on many islands. In nature, alphaviruses cycle between invertebrate insect vectors and vertebrate hosts. For most alphaviruses, the insect vectors are mosquitoes; however, other hematophagous arthropods, such as lice or mites, are vectors for a few. The vertebrate hosts are generally mammals or birds, although fish are hosts for the aquatic alphaviruses. In general, the pathogenic alphaviruses are divided into the viruses that cause human disease characterized by rash and arthritis, primarily found in the Old World, and viruses that cause encephalitis, primarily found in the New World. For many alphaviruses, no human or veterinary disease has been recognized. Larger mammals, such as humans and horses, that tend to develop severe or fatal disease are often dead-end hosts unimportant to the endemic virus transmission cycles but can be important for sustaining epidemics.

HISTORY

Records of diseases almost certainly attributable to alphaviruses date to the 18th and 19th centuries, when epidemics of fatal encephalitis in horses in the northeastern United States and outbreaks of arthritis in Southeast Asia were recognized and recorded.[111,300,788] The first clear report of epidemic encephalitis comes from the summer of 1831, when 75 horses died in Massachusetts.[300] Over the next 100 years, several local outbreaks of encephalitis in horses were noted along the Atlantic seaboard of the United States and in the Pampas region of South America.[683] However, the first alphavirus to be cultured was western equine encephalitis virus (WEEV). This virus was isolated in 1930 from the central nervous system (CNS) tissues of 2 horses involved in an epidemic of equine encephalitis in the San Joaquin Valley of California.[522] Eastern equine encephalitis virus (EEEV) was isolated from the brains of affected horses in New Jersey and Virginia in 1933.[786] Both diseases occurred in summertime epidemics, suggesting an arthropod vector, and

TABLE 23.1 Alphaviruses, Abbreviations, Biological Features, and Association with Disease

Virus (abbreviation)	Antigenic complex	Principal vertebrate reservoir host	Geographic distribution	Human disease	Animal disease
Aura (AURA)	WEE	?	South America		
Barmah Forest (BF)	BF	Birds	Australia	Fever, arthritis, rash	
Bebaru (BEB)	SF	?	Asia		
Cabassou (CAB)	VEE	?	French Guiana		
Chikungunya (CHIK)	SF	Primates	Africa, Southeast Asia, Philippines, Indonesia	Fever, arthritis, rash	
Eastern equine encephalitis (EEE)	EEE	Birds	North America, South America, Caribbean	Fever, encephalitis	Horse, pheasant, emu, pigeon, turkey
Everglades (EVE)	VEE	Mammals	Florida	Fever, encephalitis	
Fort Morgan (FM)	WEE	Birds	Colorado		
Getah (GET)	SF	Mammals	Asia	Fever	Horse
Highlands J (HJ)	WEE	Birds	North America		Horse, turkey, emu, pheasant, duck, crane
Mayaro (MAY)	SF	Mammals	South America	Fever, arthritis, rash	
Middelburg (MID)	MID	?	Africa		
Mosso das Pedras/78V3531	VEE	?	South America		
Mucambo (MUC)	VEE	?	South America, Caribbean		
Ndumu (NDU)	NDU	?	Africa		
O'nyong-nyong (ONN)	SF	?	East Africa	Fever, arthritis, rash	
Pixuna (PIX)	VEE	Mammals	Brazil		
Rio Negro/AG80 (RN)	VEE	Mammals	Argentina		
Ross River (RR)	SF	Mammals	Australia, South Pacific	Fever, arthritis, rash	
Salmonid alphavirus (SAV)	?	Fish	North Atlantic		Trout, salmon
Semliki Forest (SF)	SF	?	Africa	Fever, encephalitis	Horse
Sindbis (SIN)	WEE	Birds	Australia, Africa, Northern Europe, Middle East	Fever, arthritis, rash	
Southern elephant seal (SES)	?	Seals	Antarctica		
Tonate (TON)	VEE	?	South America	Fever, encephalitis	
Trocara (TRO)	WEE	?	South America		
Una (UNA)	SF	?	South America, Trinidad		Horse
Venezuelan equine encephalitis (VEE)	VEE	Mammals	South America, North America	Fever, encephalitis	Horse
Western equine encephalitis (WEE)	WEE	Birds, mammals	North America, South America	Fever, encephalitis	Horse, emu
Whataroa (WHA)	WEE	Birds	New Zealand, Australia		

in 1933, Kelser showed WEEV transmission by mosquitoes.[388] In 1936, an epizootic of equine encephalitis occurred in the Guajira region of Venezuela; the virus isolated was not neutralized by antisera against EEEV or WEEV and was designated Venezuelan equine encephalitis virus (VEEV).[420]

Summertime epidemics of polyarthritis were recognized in Australia and New Guinea in 1928,[183,572] and subsequent outbreaks were reported in Northern Europe, Africa, and Southeast Asia.[727] It is likely, of course, that the alphavirus-induced arthritic diseases are much older than these dates but were not clearly described or differentiated from more prevalent infections in these regions, such as dengue. This is considered to be particularly true of outbreaks of chikungunya virus (CHIKV) that have occurred in India and Southeast Asia over the past 200 years.[111,788] Viruses associated with epidemic polyarthritis were eventually isolated, both from mosquitoes collected in the areas of human disease and later from humans. The first of these viruses was isolated in 1952 from a pool of *Culex* spp.

mosquitoes collected near Sindbis, Egypt.[782] However, it was many years before Sindbis virus (SINV) was linked to human disease.[493]

The first clear association of an alphavirus with arthritic disease came in 1953, when CHIKV was isolated in Tanzania from the blood of people with severe arthritis.[668] During the next several years, several viruses that cause arthritis, often accompanied by a rash, were isolated in Africa, Australia, and South America.[122,537,884] These viruses were added to the growing list of arthropod-borne (arbo) viruses, defined by the World Health Organization in 1967 as "viruses which are maintained in nature principally, or to an important extent, through biological transmission between susceptible vertebrate hosts by haematophagous arthropods; they multiply and produce viremia in the vertebrates, multiply in the tissues of arthropods, and are passed on to new vertebrates by the bites of arthropods after a period of extrinsic incubation".[621]

In 1954, arboviruses were divided by Casals and Brown into three serologic groups—A, B, and C—based on cross-reactivity in hemagglutination inhibition (HI) tests.[556,621] EEEV, WEEV, and VEEV constituted the group A arboviruses. A second cross-reacting set, including dengue, St. Louis encephalitis, and yellow fever viruses, constituted the group B arboviruses, and the nonreactive viruses were designated group C. As viruses became classified on the fundamental properties of the virion and the genome, the group A viruses became the *Alphavirus* genus within the *Togaviridae* family of enveloped RNA viruses.

INFECTIOUS AGENTS

Alphaviruses are enveloped plus-strand RNA viruses with icosahedral symmetry (Fig. 23.1). The virions are 60 to 70 nm in diameter and sensitive to ether and detergent. Cryo-electron microscopy structures are available for many.[18,418,496,549,618,722,901–903] The RNA is contained within a capsid formed by a single protein arranged as an icosahedron with T = 4 symmetry. The nucleocapsid is enclosed in a lipid envelope derived from the host cell plasma membrane that contains the viral-encoded glycoproteins E1 and E2. These proteins form heterodimers that are grouped as trimers to form 80 knobs on the virion surface. Glycoproteins are arranged such that 240 copies of each interact with 240 copies of capsid protein.

The 49S genome is composed of a single-strand, nonsegmented, capped, and polyadenylated message sense RNA that is infectious. Complete sequence information is available for representatives of all currently known *Alphavirus* species.[129,161,206,219,297,402,431,434,437,518,764] The genomes are 11 to 12 kb in size and are organized with the nonstructural proteins (nsPs) at the 5′ end and the structural proteins at the 3′ end. The nsPs are translated from genomic RNA and the structural proteins from a subgenomic RNA.[765] Four nsPs function to replicate the viral RNA and produce the subgenomic RNA (see Chapter 22).

Five potential structural proteins (C, E3, E2, 6K, and E1) are encoded in the subgenomic RNA as a polyprotein, and an additional transframe protein (TF) is produced by −1 ribosomal frameshifting within the 6K coding region.[141,215] The N-terminal portion of C is basic and is presumed to bind the viral genomic RNA, whereas the more conserved C-terminal portion interacts with other copies of the C protein to form the nucleocapsid and also interacts with the cytoplasmic tail of E2.[765,901]

E3 is a small, cysteine-rich glycoprotein that serves as a signal sequence for pE2 (the precursor containing E3 and E2), mediates proper folding of E2, and is necessary for pE2 to

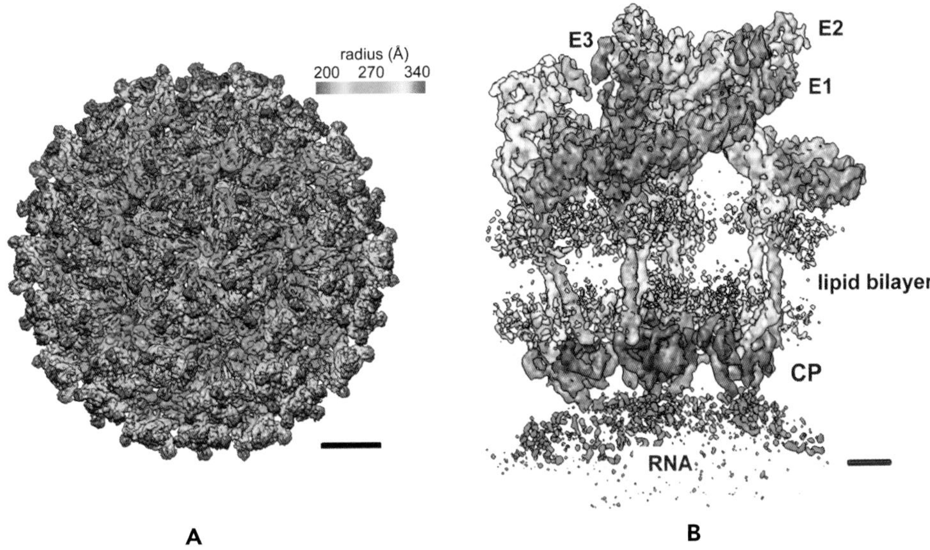

FIGURE 23.1. Three-dimensional (3D) reconstruction of the Venezuelan equine encephalitis virus (VEEV) virion. A: Radially colored 3D reconstruction of VEEV showing the E1 basal triangle (*green*) and E2 central protrusion (*blue*) for each spike. Scale bar: 10 nm. **B:** One asymmetric unit of the virus containing four unique copies of E1 (*magenta*), E2 (*cyan*), E3 (*orange*), and capsid (CP, *blue*). The cryo-electron microscopy densities for the viral membrane (*yellow*) and genomic RNA (*green*) are also displayed at slightly lower isosurface threshold. (Courtesy of Wah Chiu; reproduced with permission from Zhang R, Hryc CF, Cong Y, et al. 4.4A cryo-EM structure of an enveloped alphavirus Venezuelan equine encephalitis virus. *EMBO J* 2011;30:3854–3863.)

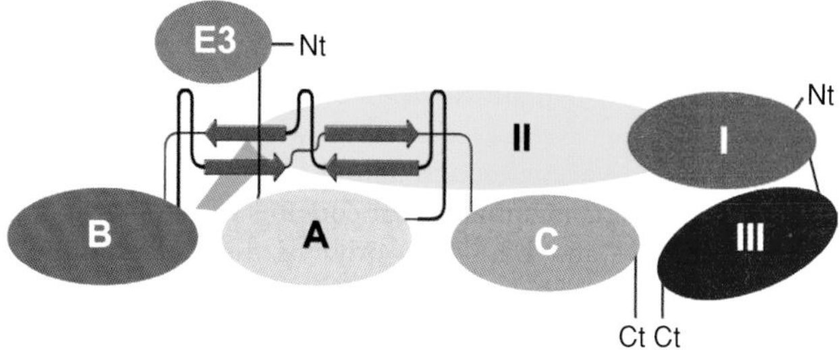

FIGURE 23.2. Domain structure of the glycoprotein spike. Schematic diagram of the E1pE2 heterodimer drawn "untwisted" to show the domains positioned with respect to one another and their connectivity. Domains of E1 (I, red; II, yellow; III, blue; fusion loop, orange) and pE2 (A, cyan; B, dark green; C, pink; E3, gray) are shown. Ct, C-terminus; Nt, N-terminus. (Courtesy of Felix Rey; reproduced with permission from Voss JE, Vaney MC, Duquerroy S, et al. Glycoprotein organization of chikungunya virus particles revealed by x-ray crystallography. *Nature* 2011;468:709–712.)

heterodimerize with E1 for transport to the cell surface.[468,599] As part of the pE2-E1 heterodimer, E3 prevents premature activation of E1.[362,840,844] E3 is cleaved from E2 by furin in the trans-Golgi, remains associated with the spike under acidic conditions, and is usually shed when virions bud from the cell surface.[737,904]

The E2 glycoprotein is a transmembrane protein that has two or three N-linked carbohydrates and contains the most important epitopes for neutralizing antibody. E2 is organized into three immunoglobulin domains (A, B, and C) (Fig. 23.2). Domain A (residues 1–132) is at the center and top of the heterotrimer and has receptor and neutralizing antibody-binding sites. Domain B is at the spike tip, and C is toward the viral membrane.[455,840] The intracytoplasmic portion interacts with the capsid and has a second stretch of hydrophobic amino acids and myristoylation sites that tether it to the inner surface of the membrane.

The 6K protein serves as a signal peptide for E1, is cleaved from E1 and E2 by signal peptidase, and is important for budding, and small amounts are incorporated into the virion.[238,461] The E1 protein has one or two N-linked carbohydrates, a short (one or two residue) intracytoplasmic tail, and a positionally conserved internal hydrophobic stretch of amino acids in the N-terminal portion that serves as the fusion peptide for virion entry into the cell. E1 is organized into three β-sheet-rich domains (I, II, and III) similar to the flavivirus E protein with the internal fusion loop at the tip of domain II[253,443] (see Fig. 23.2). The function of TF has not yet been defined but can be incorporated into virions.[215]

Propagation and Assay in Tissue Culture

Initial isolations of alphaviruses were accomplished by intracerebral inoculation into suckling mice—a host very susceptible to infection with most alphaviruses.[335,668,689,781,782,867,884] Many alphaviruses can also be isolated and propagated efficiently in primary chick embryo fibroblasts (CEFs) and in various continuous mammalian cell lines such as human epithelial (HeLa, MRC5) cells, baby hamster kidney (BHK) cells, monkey kidney (Vero) cells, and mouse fibroblast and neuroblastoma cells[108,581] (Fig. 23.3).

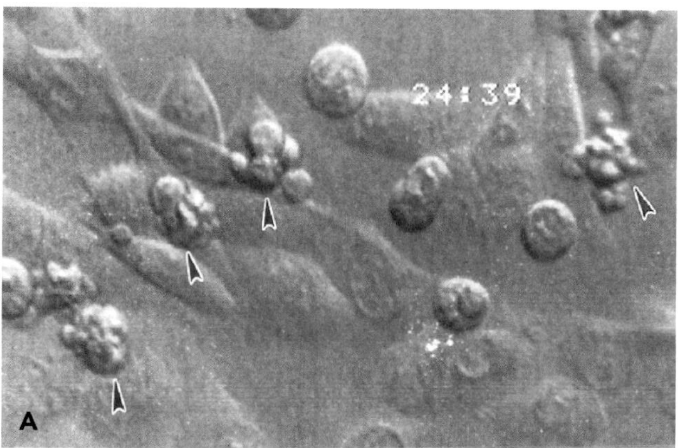

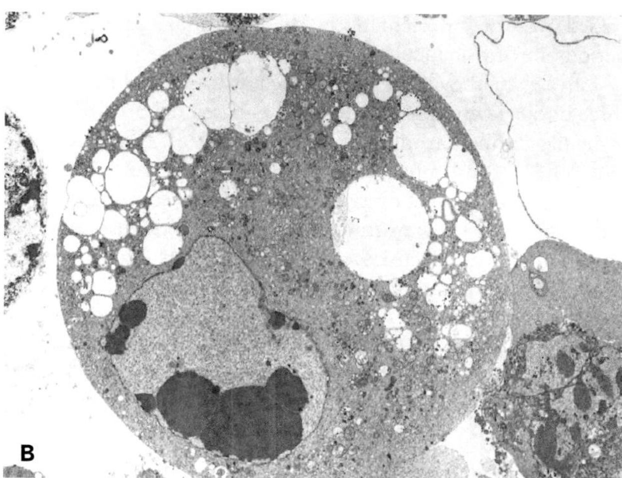

FIGURE 23.3. Effects of Sindbis virus infection on vertebrate cells. A: Cytopathic effects (*CPE*) of rounding, shrinkage, and cytoplasmic blebbing in baby hamster kidney (BHK) cells infected at a low multiplicity. **B:** Electron micrograph of an infected BHK cell showing chromosomal condensation and cytopathic vacuoles.

Most alphaviruses will form plaques on susceptible mammalian or avian cells under an agar overlay. Mosquito cell lines also support replication, although often without cytopathic effect (CPE).[635,761,763,803] The first plaque assay of an animal virus was performed using WEEV on CEF cells,[190] and plaque assay remains a convenient and sensitive way to quantify infectious virus. Plaque size has been used to differentiate strains and is determined by the type of overlay used, by relative virus binding to negatively charged sulfated polysaccharides present in the overlay, and by replication efficiency.[87,96,775]

Biological Characteristics

Hemagglutination

Alphaviruses can hemagglutinate avian (e.g., goose, chicken) erythrocytes,[581,684] and hemagglutination has been used as a method for quantifying virus and HI for measuring antiviral antibody.[144] Hemagglutination requires prior exposure of the virus to acidic pH, depends primarily on the E1 glycoprotein, and reflects binding of the fusion domain of the E1 glycoprotein to lipids in the erythrocyte membrane.[130,144,829,873] E2 also participates in hemagglutination because some monoclonal antibodies (MAbs) specific for E2 also have HI activity.[67,640] The HI test has been useful for determining antigenic relationships among alphaviruses.[107]

Cellular Receptors

Binding of virus to the cell surface and entry into the cell is a multistep process that depends on virus glycoproteins E1 and E2, cell surface molecules, low pH in the endosome, and fusion of membrane lipids. Variations in any of these components will affect the efficiency of infection and the likelihood that any particular cell will become infected *in vivo*. Virus-specific attachment to cells is primarily a function of the E2 glycoprotein. The important role for E2 in initiating virus–cell interaction is evidenced by the ability of anti-E2 MAbs to inhibit binding to cells,[96,474] of anti-idiotypic antibodies to E2-specific MAbs to recognize putative virus receptors on cells,[823,852] and of amino acid changes in E2 to alter virus binding to cells of different types.[189,438]

Identification of specific alphavirus receptors has been difficult and may be complicated by experimental use of virus strains that are adapted to replicate in tissue culture.[411] Because each alphavirus infects a wide range of hosts, often including birds, mammals, and mosquitoes, they must either use an evolutionarily well-conserved cell surface molecule or multiple molecules as receptors. None of the alphavirus receptors identified to date appears to be used exclusively, suggesting the possibility of several receptors. Alternatively, alphaviruses may use receptor-coreceptor combinations to achieve wide host range and the specific tropisms observed *in vivo*.

The first alphavirus receptor to be identified was the major histocompatibility complex (MHC) class I molecule receptor for Semliki Forest virus (SFV) on mouse and human cells.[315] This molecule is not absolutely required because cells lacking MHC molecules can still be infected with SFV.[583] The high-affinity laminin receptor is a receptor for SINV on BHK cells and a potential receptor for SINV and VEEV on C6/36 mosquito cells.[474,850] Again, this molecule appears to account for only a portion of the total virus interaction with the cells studied and does not contribute to SINV binding to avian cells.[850] Ross River virus (RRV) uses the $\alpha_1\beta_1$ integrin on HeLa cells for binding.[426] SINV and VEEV can use natural resistance–associated macrophage protein (NRAMP) for binding to insect and mammalian cells.[664] The type of cell in which the virus is grown can also influence initial virus–receptor interactions. For instance, SINV grown in mosquito cells is enriched in high-mannose carbohydrates that bind the C-type lectins DC-SIGN and L-SIGN on the surface of dendritic cells (DCs).[410]

Heparan sulfate (HS), a ubiquitously expressed glycosaminoglycan is an important initial binding molecule for certain strains of many alphaviruses. The use of HS is selected for by virus passage in vertebrate cells. However, wild-type strains of EEEV bind HS, so this property is not exclusively determined by passage in tissue culture.[242] For these viruses, addition of heparin or lactoferrin, treatment of cells with heparinase, or the use of cells deficient in HS decreases binding to cells and plaque formation.[59,96,242,312,409,411,426,740,843] Interaction with HS—a highly sulfated, negatively charged molecule—probably explains the effects of ionic strength and charge on the attachment of virus to cells.[499,501,611] The heparin-binding domain of the E2 glycoprotein is on domain A and overlaps a neutralizing epitope (see Fig. 23.2). Changes toward more positively charged amino acids in the region around E2–70 increase the efficiency of attachment to cells in tissue culture.[59,97,242,411]

Entry requires endocytosis followed by a conformational change in the trimer of E1-E2 heterodimers induced by exposure to low pH.[313,729,739,879] The E1 fusion peptide is protected in the virion heterotrimer by the B domain of E2, and this association is stabilized by E3.[455,840] When exposed to acidic pH, E1 dissociates from E2 and forms stable E1 homotrimers in the presence of cholesterol-containing membranes. During this conformational change, the fusion peptide is exposed and inserted into the outer leaflet of the lipid bilayer.[83,252,253] Fusion with the cell membrane to initiate infection depends on the presence of a membrane potential and sphingolipid.[314,570,899]

Effects on Vertebrate Cells

Alphaviruses replicate rapidly in most vertebrate cell lines with the release of progeny virus typically within 4 to 6 hours after infection. At the time of virus entry, there is an increase in permeability perhaps owing to pore formation by the E1, 6K, and/or TF proteins.[492,871,872] Insertion of newly synthesized glycoproteins into the plasma membrane renders infected cells capable of adenosine triphosphatase (ATP)-dependent polykaryocyte formation on exposure to acid pH.[389] Infection causes extensive CPE characterized by cell rounding, shrinkage, and cytoplasmic blebbing (see Fig. 23.3A), with the death of infected cells within 24 to 48 hours.[449,635] Alphavirus-induced CPE has been linked to shut off of host cell transcription and translation,[246] endoplasmic reticulum (ER) stress,[574] and induction of apoptosis.[20,26,257,270,351,449,656,699] The ability of alphaviruses to induce cell death, combined with the ability to express heterologous genes and activate natural killer (NK) cells, has led to their development as potential oncolytic agents.[344,454,552,633,634,808,809,830]

Shut off of host cell functions in Old World viruses (e.g., SINV, SFV) has been linked to the effects of nuclear nsP2 and in New World viruses (e.g., VEEV, EEEV) to the effects of C.[14,32,247] Activation of protein kinase R (PKR) results in phosphorylation of eIF2α, which shuts down host protein synthesis without affecting translation of viral 26S subgenomic RNA.[834] Alphavirus escape from eIF2α phosphorylation is owing to the presence of a hairpin loop structure in the subgenomic messenger RNA (mRNA) downstream of the initiation codon that allows the 40S ribosome to initiate translation in the absence of eIF2.[185,804,834] This initiation process utilizes host cell factors ligatin and MCT-1/DFNR[738] and does not depend on mTOR signaling.[530] Alphavirus-induced inhibition of host protein synthesis can also be PKR-independent perhaps through late suppression of mTOR.[265,530]

The apoptotic process is associated with blebbing of the plasma membrane, condensation of nuclear chromatin, and formation of apoptotic bodies (see Fig. 23.3B). Viral proteins are concentrated in the surface blebs from which budding continues to occur.[665] This process does not hamper, and may enhance, virus replication because inhibition of apoptosis usually decreases virus yield.[445,458,699]

The mechanism(s) by which alphaviruses induce apoptosis is not completely understood and likely differs with virus and type of target cell. Apoptosis of cultured cells can be initiated at the endosomal membrane during SINV fusion.[364] Membrane-bound sphingomyelinases are activated releasing ceramide, an efficient inducer of cellular apoptosis.[363,366] SFV-induced apoptosis requires RNA synthesis and accumulation[777,828] and is independent of p53.[258,828] Other events in alphavirus-induced cell death often include early activation of poly(adenosine diphosphate [ADP] ribose) polymerase,[564,596] activation of proapoptotic Bcl-2 family member proteins Bad or Bak,[539] loss of mitochondrial membrane integrity, and release of cytochrome c.[50,828] Cellular caspases are activated with cleavage of caspase-3 substrates and fragmentation of chromosomal DNA.[825]

Apoptotic death is accelerated by glycoprotein-induced ER stress,[50,234,574] sphingomyelinase deficiency,[567] low levels of extracellular Ca^{++},[825] expression of Bax,[574] and activation of Bid.[828] Alphavirus-induced apoptosis can be slowed or prevented by expression of ceramidase,[363] altered Ras signaling,[365,413] expression of $p21^{WAF1/CIP1}$,[338] expression of Bcl-2 family member and interacting proteins,[270,449,451,458,539,552,574,699,826,828] expression of the ER stress protective protein Parkin,[574] mutation of nsP2,[246,574] phosphorylation of PKCδ,[910] inhibition of constitutive expression of NFκB,[462] and caspase inhibition.[565,695,828]

Alphavirus-induced vertebrate cell death can also occur by caspase-independent, nonapoptotic mechanisms. Alphaviruses efficiently shut down protein, ribosomal RNA (rRNA) and mRNA synthesis in infected cells,[246,264,510,556] deplete nicotinamide adenine dinucleotide (NAD) and energy stores,[199,825] and induce dysfunction of $Na^{+}K^{+}$ adenosine triphosphatase (ATPase) causing loss of membrane potential and changes in intracellular cation concentrations.[51,827] Genome replication without structural protein synthesis can induce cell death.[828] For Old World viruses, expression of nsP2 alone is cytotoxic, and this property is independent of its protease activity and can be separated from the effects of nsP2 on host transcription.[187,233,246,247,264,507,605,777] Although immature neurons die by apoptosis, mature neurons are more resistant to apoptotic cell death.[257,307] This resistance is attributable to an intrinsic ability to suppress virus replication.[120,835] Mature motor neurons, infected by virulent strains of virus, die by a necrotic process and are not protected from death by Bcl-2 family member proteins.[307,393] Autophagic clearance of viral proteins may promote neuronal survival.[588]

Persistent infection can occasionally be established in mammalian cell cultures *in vitro.* Mouse fibroblasts producing interferon (IFN), or BHK cells with a high concentration of defective interfering particles, can establish SINV persistent infection.[345,869] Infection with SINV or SINV replicons that have mutations in the C-terminal methyl transferase–like domain of nsP2 results in reduced viral RNA synthesis, decreased CPE, and persistent infection in some vertebrate cell lines.[7,187,233,235,507,605] Persistent infection can also be established if the cell infected is resistant to virus-induced apoptosis.[90,449,824,835]

Effects on Invertebrate Cells

Studies of alphavirus infection of cell lines derived from *Aedes albopictus* (e.g., C6/36, U4.4) and *Aedes aegypti* (e.g., Aag2) larvae demonstrate differences in alphavirus replication between vertebrate and invertebrate cells. The time course of virus replication is similar; however, frequently, virus matures within vesicular structures and virions are released by exocytosis rather than at the plasma membrane.[523,763] Virions are relatively deficient in cholesterol and have detectable differences in structure.[296,310,754] There is only a modest effect on host gene expression,[225,696] and persistent noncytopathic infection, or death by a nonapoptotic process,[383] is more likely than in vertebrate cells.

The uncloned lines derived from *Ae. albopictus* larvae contain many types of cells with properties representative of different mosquito tissues. Lytic infection occurs in clones that support high levels of virus replication,[523,803] whereas persistent infection is associated with a short period of relatively high virus replication followed by a decrease in virus production and often in the numbers of cells in the culture that are producing virus.[164,547,548] The decrease in virus production is not associated with activation of the signal transducer and activator of transcription (STAT), immune deficiency (IMD), or toll insect innate response pathways but is associated with decreased processing of the nonstructural polyprotein and expression of the protease inhibitor TEPII.[225,547] Lytic infection can also be induced by viruses engineered to express death-inducing insect proteins such as reaper or michelob_x.[849] Transcriptional analysis of persistently infected cells shows an increase in mRNAs associated with vesicle formation and the Notch signaling pathway.[547]

RNA interference (RNAi) is an important insect defense mechanism, and SFV infection of U4.4 or Aag2 cells leads to production of virus-derived small interfering RNAs (viRNAs) derived from replicative double-stranded (dsRNA) that are unevenly distributed across the genome and variable in efficiency for mediating antiviral RNAi.[736] This RNAi signal can spread from cell to cell and inhibit replication.[37] The RNAi pathway is defective in C6/36 cells[74]; however, the IMD, and not the toll innate response pathway, can suppress SINV replication in these cells.[41]

Superinfection Exclusion

Vertebrate and invertebrate cells infected with one alphavirus cannot be productively infected with the same, or a closely related, alphavirus at a later time. Exclusion is established after translation of the nsP genes of the first virus to enter. The superinfecting genome can be translated but not replicated,[762] probably owing to the presence of the transacting nsP2 protease that prematurely cleaves the replicase polyprotein required for minus-strand synthesis.[384]

Antigenic Composition

All alphaviruses are related and share common antigenic sites, as revealed by HI and complement fixation (CF) tests with polyclonal immune sera[107] and by cytotoxic T-cell lysis of infected cells.[465,550] Antigenic cross-reactivities may confer some cross protection and interfere with sequential alphavirus immunizations.[106,181,277,465,508] These cross-reactivities formed the basis for the original classification into the group A arboviruses and continue to be a valuable means for initial identification and classification of alphaviruses.[107] Closely related viruses within a serogroup form a complex. Seven broad antigenic complexes have been identified within the alphavirus serogroup: Barmah Forest, eastern equine encephalitis (EEE), Middelburg (MID), Ndumu (NDU), Semliki Forest, Venezuelan equine encephalitis (VEE), and western equine encephalitis (WEE).[427,626,806] A few viruses remain unclassified and will probably form one or more additional complexes (see Table 23.1). The Barmah Forest, EEE, MID, and NDU complexes each contain only a single virus, whereas the Semliki Forest, VEE, and WEE complexes include several viruses. Viruses within each complex can be subtyped using reactivity with MAbs, kinetic HI, or neutralization assays.[98]

Antibodies to E1 are more likely to cross-react with other alphaviruses than are antibodies to E2.[67,343,892] This is

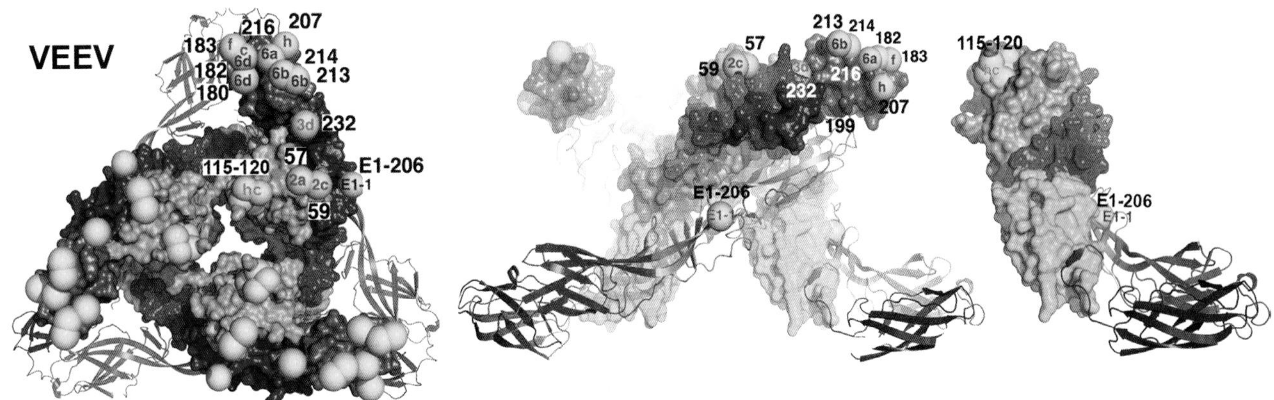

FIGURE 23.4. Neutralization escape mutations and positions affecting host range and tissue tropism mapped on the Venezuelan equine encephalitis virus spike. Neutralizing antibody escape mutations are displayed as yellow spheres on the spike with epitope written in the spheres. E1 is shown in ribbons and E2 in surface rendering using the colors defined in Figure 23.2. The **left panel** shows a top-down view of the spike, the **middle panel** shows the spike from the side, and the **right panel** shows the far right dimer from the middle panel. (Courtesy of Felix Rey; reproduced with permission from Voss JE, Vaney MC, Duquerroy S, et al. Glycoprotein organization of chikungunya virus particles revealed by x-ray crystallography. *Nature* 2011;468:709–712.)

consistent with the documented sequence conservation in the E1 protein. Competitive binding assays using MAbs have identified approximately seven epitopes on the E1 glycoproteins of SINV, SFV, WEEV, and VEEV.[67,343,519,662,703] Most E1 epitopes are not exposed on the virion surface but are present on the surface of infected cells or on acid-exposed virions.[15,282,320,519,703] These transitional epitopes map to domain III in a region buried at the spike interfaces[840] (Fig. 23.4). The *in vitro* biological activities of antibodies to E1 include HI, neutralization of virus infectivity, and inhibition of fusion.[15,67,282,343,703] Neutralizing epitopes map to domains I, II, and III.[282,455]

Antibodies to E2 are usually alphavirus specific. Competitive binding assays using MAbs identify four to five epitopes on the E2 glycoproteins of SINV, SFV, RRV, and VEEV.[67,394,519,586,662] *In vitro* biological activities of antibodies to E2 include HI, neutralization of virus infectivity, and blocking of virus binding to the cell surface.[662] Many anti-E2 MAbs have both neutralizing and HI activity, suggesting that these functions overlap.[282] Neutralization escape mutants, naturally occurring variants, λgt11 expression libraries, site-directed mutagenesis, and recombinant viruses have been used to identify amino acids contributing to the various epitopes on E2 and have identified two major neutralizing sites[704,758,851] that have been mapped onto the crystal structure of the E1-E2 heterodimer and trimerized spike and are in domain B[8,282,367,455,840] (see Fig. 23.4). This is an exposed hydrophilic region that often includes an N-linked carbohydrate. There are linear, as well as conformational, determinants in this region because these MAbs frequently react in Western blots and recognize λ fusion proteins, and antibodies to peptides from this region are protective against challenge.[851]

The second neutralizing epitope on E2 appears to be primarily conformational and is in domain A. This region is responsible for binding to HS and is obscured if pE2 is not cleaved.[96,675,840] Visualization by cryo-electron microscopy of the binding of HS and MAbs to this epitope on SINV and RRV identifies the domain A knob on the glycoprotein spike.[742,902]

Evolution and Phylogeny

Alphaviruses, which replicate in arthropods, birds, reptiles, fish, and mammals, derive from a single unknown protoalphavirus and are part of the alphavirus superfamily of viruses. Viruses in this superfamily, including many RNA plant viruses, have a similar genetic organization and replicase proteins but diverse coat proteins.[417,766] Among alphaviruses, amino acids important in secondary structure (e.g., cysteines and those close to one another in adjacent β sheets and α helices) have been conserved for the glycoproteins E1, E2, and E3, consistent with a similar three-dimensional structure of the virion for all.[219] The most variable regions of the genome are in the C-terminus of nsP3 and the N-terminus of C.[219] Highly conserved regions in the nsP1 and nsP4 genes have allowed development of primers to detect a broad range of alphaviruses by reverse transcription polymerase chain reaction (RT-PCR).[201,290] Sequence information from the entire genome generally groups the viruses similarly to that derived by antigenic analysis (Fig. 23.5) and has detected at least one recombination event.[297] Criteria for species demarcation of alphaviruses combine genetic, ecological, and antigenic information. Species generally have distinct transmission cycles and differ by more than 23% at the nucleotide level and 10% in amino acid sequence when E1 genes are compared.

The origin of the alphaviruses is unclear. Partial genome sequencing has suggested origins both in the Americas and in the Old World.[107,267,434,626,859] Recently, comparison of whole genome sequences from all known alphaviruses has suggested an origin from the louse-borne aquatic alphaviruses[219] (see Fig. 23.5). All of these scenarios require repeated movement across the globe to explain the current virus distributions.

Like other RNA viruses, alphaviruses undergo genetic change primarily by accumulation of point mutations in the genomic RNA; however, deletions and duplications also occur.[1,217] Mutation occurs at a rate that is slower ($1–7 \times 10^{-4}$ substitutions/nucleotide/year) than is estimated for other RNA viruses,[93,146] presumably because fitness must be maintained in both insect vectors and vertebrate hosts.[147] Recombination

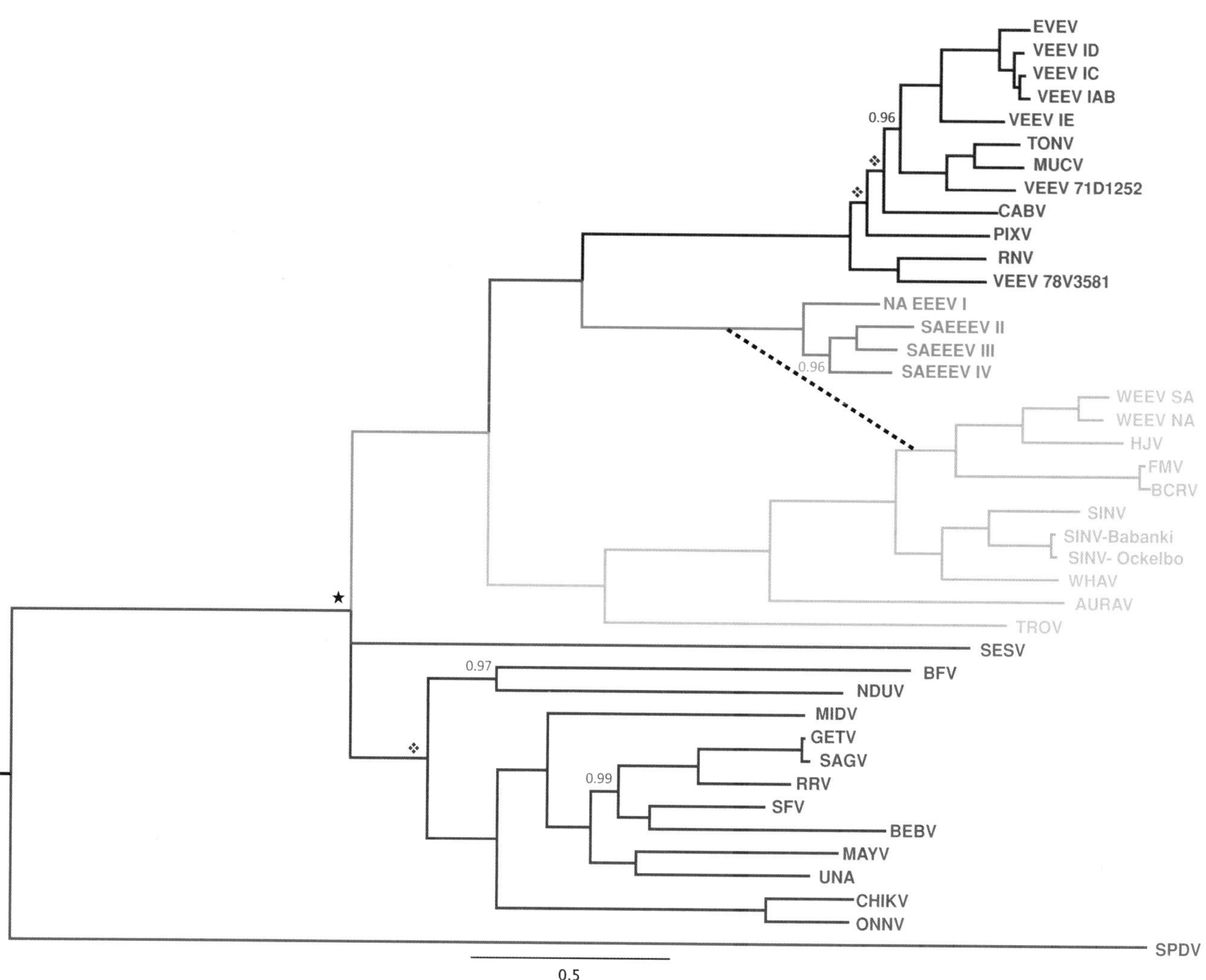

FIGURE 23.5. Alphavirus phylogenetic tree produced using the E2, 6K, and E1 structural protein genes and Bayesian methods with midpoint rooting. The tree includes representatives from all alphavirus species, and the *dashed line* indicates the recombination between ancestors of Sindbis and eastern equine encephalitis viruses that led to the western equine encephalitis virus (WEEV) group. Roman numerals indicate major subtypes of some species, and scale indicates 50% nucleotide sequence divergence. All posterior probabilities were 1 except as indicated; nodes with a diamond had posterior probabilities less than 0.9, and nodes with a star had no posterior support. A similar tree utilizing full-length sequences without the WEEV recombinant group showed a similar topology except Middelburg virus was basal to chikungunya and o'nyong-nyong viruses, and Una, Mayaro, Semliki Forest, and Bebaru viruses were grouped separately together with Getah, Sagiyama, and Ross River viruses.[219] (Courtesy of Scott Weaver; from Forrester NL, Palacios G, Tesh RB, et al. 2012. Genome-scale phylogeny of the alphavirus genus suggests a marine origin. *J Virol* 2012;86(5):2729–2738.)

between alphaviruses can be demonstrated *in vitro* but is infrequent and usually puts the chimeric virus at a replicative disadvantage.[93,146] However, successful recombination has occurred at least occasionally in nature because WEEV resulted from recombination between EEE- and Sindbis-like viruses (see Fig. 23.5) at the junction of E3 and E2, an event that is estimated to have occurred thousands of years ago.[219,421,766]

Alphaviruses replicate in and are transmitted horizontally by a wide range of invertebrate, primarily mosquito, species. However, each virus usually has a principal or preferred vector for the enzootic cycle. Most alphaviruses can infect various vertebrates but have birds, mammals, or fish as their primary amplifying and reservoir hosts (see Table 23.1). The specific invertebrate vector and vertebrate host used by an alphavirus will contribute significantly to determining the geographic distribution of that virus. Experiments modeling evolution *in vitro* show that fewer mutations accumulate if replication alternates between vertebrate and invertebrate cells, although diversity, fitness, and adaptability are greater with serial passage.[149,150,153,276,856] Experiments employing *in vivo* passage show that serial passage in mosquitoes increases mosquito infection and that passage in vertebrates produces higher viremias; however, alternately passaged viruses do not change fitness.[149] It is hypothesized that short transmission seasons and host mobility influence alphavirus genetic diversity and evolution in a geographic region.[146,858] Viruses using avian enzootic hosts (e.g., EEEV, WEEV, SINV) extend over wide geographic regions and evolve as a few highly conserved genotypes, whereas viruses using mammalian enzootic hosts with a more limited range of dispersal (e.g., RRV, VEEV) evolve within multiple geographically restricted genotypes.[490,688]

Some strains of alphaviruses associated with epidemics or epizootics are antigenically and biologically distinguishable from enzootic strains. Phylogenetic evidence indicates that, at least for VEEV and WEEV, the virulent epizootic strains evolve by mutation from avirulent viruses being maintained in the enzootic cycle.[23,61,629,657]

PATHOGENESIS AND PATHOLOGY IN VERTEBRATES

Excellent and well-studied model systems exist for several alphaviruses, and much of our detailed knowledge about alphavirus pathogenesis comes from investigations in mice. Information from these models will be combined where appropriate with information from studies of humans with alphavirus-induced disease to deduce the pathogenesis of infection. Specifics will be covered in sections on the individual viruses.

Entry

The primary mode of alphavirus transmission to vertebrates is through the bite of an infected insect, most often a mosquito. Mosquitoes salivate during feeding and deposit virus-infected saliva extravascularly.[819] Saliva virus titers are highest early after the mosquito is infected and decline, along with transmission rates, after 1 to 2 weeks; however, mosquitoes remain infected for life.[525,833] The high-mannose glycans on virus from mosquitoes inhibits induction of IFN by myeloid DCs,[718] and proteins in saliva further facilitate transmission by skewing the host cellular immune response toward Th2 cytokines.[794]

Sites of Primary Replication

The initial sites of virus replication vary with the virus and host. Mice have received the most extensive study. After subcutaneous inoculation, viruses may infect skeletal muscle or fibroblasts at the local site (e.g., EEEV, WEEV, SFV, RRV, SINV, and Getah virus) or be taken up by and infect Langerhans cells in the skin (e.g., VEEV)[287,325,466,553] (Fig. 23.6). Langerhans cells and DCs transport virus to lymph nodes draining the site of inoculation that also may become infected.[242,487] *In vitro,* human DCs are susceptible to infection with VEEV but not to infection with CHIKV or EEEV[241,573,702,707,753]; thus, the importance of DC infection after mosquito inoculation is likely to differ with the infecting virus.

Spread

Alphaviruses induce a substantial plasma viremia in their amplifying hosts and in hosts susceptible to disease (Fig. 23.7). The ability to mount and sustain a viremia depends on the continued efficient production of virus, delivery of virus into the vascular system, and slow clearance from the blood. Animal studies have shown that small plaque viruses are generally less virulent because they are cleared more rapidly from the circulation than are large plaque viruses.[354,360,623] This phenomenon is related to the ability of small plaque viruses to bind HS and thus to be rapidly removed from the circulation by the highly sulfated glycosaminoglycans in the liver.[97] Ability to invade target organs depends in part on the duration and height of the viremia but also on other characteristics of the virus important for tissue invasion.[484]

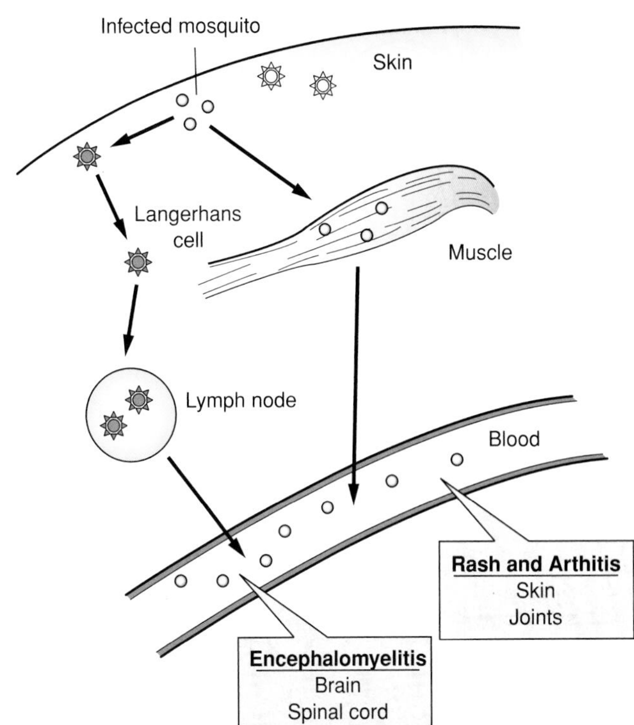

FIGURE 23.6. Basic steps in alphavirus infection of vertebrates. Virus is delivered extravascularly by an infected mosquito and infects local muscle cells or Langerhans cells in the skin. Langerhans cells can carry virus to local lymph nodes, where further replication may occur. Virus is delivered to the blood and spreads to target tissues such as skin, joints, and the central nervous system, in addition to distant muscle and lymphatic tissue.

Cell and Tissue Tropism

Viruses that replicate initially in skeletal muscle and lymph nodes near the site of inoculation often spread through the bloodstream to more distant skeletal muscles and other lymphatic tissues. In addition, cardiac myocytes, osteoblasts, brain and spinal cord neurons, and brown fat cells are secondary sites of replication for many alphaviruses in mice[9,466,535,554] (see Fig. 23.6). Getah virus causes polymyositis.[325,554,713] EEEV, WEEV, SFV, and SINV cause encephalitis[44,242,350,466,838]; RRV and CHIKV cause myositis and arthritis[244,543,907]; and VEEV causes lymphoid depletion and encephalitis.[260,359,845]

In humans, the skin is a target for alphaviruses that cause a rash,[230,493] the joints for alphaviruses that cause arthritis,[229,328,543,772] muscle for alphaviruses that cause myalgia,[543,590,907] and the nervous system for alphaviruses that cause encephalitis.[245,760] RRV and SINV have been recovered from skin biopsies.[423,424,493] RRV replicates in skin basal epidermal and eccrine duct epithelial cells.[230] CHIKV is found in fibroblasts and macrophages.[328,428] Human synovial cells support RRV infection *in vitro,*[373] and RRV RNA is detected in synovial biopsy specimens.[747] Joint fluid taken from humans with acute arthritis has

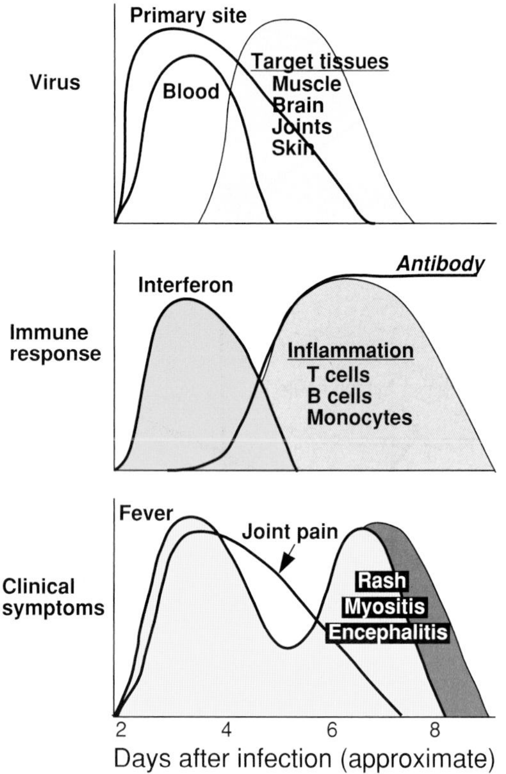

FIGURE 23.7. Schematic diagram of the pathogenesis of alphavirus-induced disease. Viremia may be accompanied by production of interferon, other proinflammatory cytokines, and fever. Virus then spreads through the blood to other target tissues. As the immune response is induced, the viremia is terminated; however, fever is renewed with appearance of a mononuclear inflammatory response in the infected tissue. In infections that lead to rash and arthritis, joint pain usually appears early after infection and prior to the appearance of the rash.

not yielded infectious virus; however, viral antigen and RNA can be detected in macrophages, and these cells support RRV and CHIKV replication *in vitro*.[328,373,854]

The mechanism by which encephalitic alphaviruses enter the CNS is not entirely clear. Neuroinvasiveness is a component of virulence that varies between viruses and virus strains.[188] Murine studies have shown infection or transport by cerebrovascular endothelial cells,[396,602,748] infection of choroid plexus epithelial cells,[466] infection of olfactory neurons,[133,670,792,837] and transport by peripheral nerves.[152] Once within the CNS, virus can spread cell to cell or through the cerebrospinal fluid (CSF).[349,584,792] For most encephalitic alphaviruses, the targeted cell within the CNS is the neuron,[350,466,584] where cellular protein synthesis is suppressed[804] and damage can be severe and irreversible. In mice that recover from neuronal infection, infectious virus is cleared but viral RNA persists.[223,446,521,821] SFV, RRV, and VEEV can cause persistent infection of microglial and oligodendroglial cells leading to demyelination.[94,160,226,715]

Immune Responses

Innate Responses

Early responses to alphavirus infection include production of cytokines and chemokines and activation of NK cells.[271]

Type I (α/β) IFN is induced *in vivo* after many, but not all, alphavirus infections of experimental animals[242,255,358,721,807] and humans[328,677,702,853] (see Fig. 23.7). The amount of IFN produced by infected tissues is usually linked to the level of virus replication, and IFN production continues if virus is not cleared.[91,224,294,328,358,702] IFN rapidly appears in serum, and levels are diminished by splenectomy, suggesting that lymphoid tissue is one important source.[358,415,416]

Several different cell systems have been used to determine the mechanisms by which alphaviruses induce and control synthesis of IFN in response to infection. Viruses vary in their ability to induce IFN production by different types of cells,[623,702,721] and the cellular sources of IFN probably differ with time after infection. In tissue culture cell lines, IFN production, shutoff of host protein synthesis, and CPE are controlled either by nsP2 (SINV, SFV) or C (VEEV, EEEV).[14,81,235,246,247] In these cells, shutoff of host gene expression suppresses antiviral responses.[14,81,247,894]

The primary source of early IFN *in vivo* may be plasmacytoid DCs for some alphaviruses[730] but not for others.[702] SFV induction of IFN by myeloid DCs requires fusion but not replication, and it is independent of MyD88.[322] For SINV and RRV, N-linked glycans on E2 are important determinants of IFN production by DCs.[719]

Induction of IFN requires viral entry and RNA synthesis.[57,322,881] Data from *ts* mutants suggest that formation of dsRNA is the necessary step in replication for IFN induction. Viruses with mutations in the protease domain of nsP2, which cannot process the nonstructural polyprotein and thus cannot initiate plus-strand RNA synthesis, do not induce IFN.[298,497] In infected fibroblasts and epithelial cells, dsRNA and higher-ordered RNA structures activate MDA5 and PKR, which are important intracellular sensors of alphavirus infection,[49] and stimulate phosphorylation of interferon regulatory factor (IRF) 3[610,706] and formation of the IRF3/CBP/p300 transcriptional activation complex for immediate early IFNs.[57] This process is independent of mTOR pathway activation.[175] NsP1/nsP2 cleavage affects IRF3 activation and IFN induction by SINV without affecting shutoff of host transcription or translation.[158] Virulent strains of EEEV do not induce IFN after fibroblast infection, whereas attenuated strains do, which is potentially associated with decreased binding to HS and increased infection of lymphoid tissue.[242,243]

Production of IFN follows the initial release of virus from infected cells by 2 to 3 hours[327] and for some, but not all, alphavirus strains is regulated by nuclear importation of nsP2 and by whether host protein synthesis is shut off before IFN can be synthesized.[81,92,881] The ability of CHIKV to induce IFN mRNA and protein is cell type dependent.[702] Primary human monocytes infected by CHIKV produce IFN-α, interleukin (IL)-6, and IL-12[319]; however, similarly infected primary human fibroblasts produce IFN-β mRNA but no protein, because the mRNA is not translated.[881]

IFN is an important part of the host response to alphavirus infection, and virus replication is sensitive to its effects.[12,155,172,441,680,718,753,787,905] Animals can be protected from lethal infection if treated with IFN or IFN inducers before or soon after infection.[12,358,375,477,714] Animals unable to respond to IFN owing to deletions of the IFN receptor or crucial IFN signaling molecules develop more severe disease than wild-type mice.[12,95,155,157,210,224,279,679,702,756,880] Furthermore, absence of an IFN response allows virus replication in cells previously resistant to infection.[224,678,679,810] IFN appears to act primarily to limit virus replication early, during the time the specific immune response is being induced (see Fig. 23.7). Treatment of cells with IFN inhibits alphavirus replication[90,172,358,540,551,681]; however, the mechanism by which this occurs, and therefore the IFN-induced host responses important for control of replication, are not known. Attachment and entry are not affected,[172,641] although later replication steps, including formation of replication complexes, structural protein synthesis, and morphogenesis, are inhibited.[551,641,787]

In addition to inhibiting host cell protein synthesis, alphaviruses can also interfere with IFN signaling by decreasing Janus kinase (JAK) activation and STAT phosphorylation and nuclear translocation.[236,733,894] This is a property of either nsP1 or nsP2.[236,734]

Antiviral proteins PKR and RNase L have a limited role in the IFN-induced antiviral response *in vitro* and *in vivo.*[681] However, activation of PKR improves the stability of IFN mRNA.[49,706] Interestingly, infected ribonuclease (RNase) L–deficient fibroblasts fail to shut off minus-strand RNA synthesis or form stable replication complexes and establish persistent infection, suggesting a role for RNase L in virus replication.[698]

IFN-induced proteins that can inhibit alphavirus replication include human MxA,[432] zinc-finger antiviral protein (ZAP),[63,292,392,435,488,905] viperin,[905] the large form of 2′,5′-oligoadenylate synthetase,[82] interferon-stimulated gene (ISG) 20,[905] and ISG15.[440,441] Transgenic expression of MxA, a large cytoplasmic guanosine triphosphatase (GTPase), in IFN-α/β receptor-deficient mice results in decreased SFV replication by preventing accumulation of genomic and subgenomic RNA and provides some protection against fatal disease.[311] ZAP is an RNA-binding protein that prevents accumulation of viral RNA by blocking translation of incoming viral genomic RNA.[63,291] This is accomplished by binding to specific viral mRNA sequences and interaction with the host DEAD box helicase p72 and RNA-processing exosome.[135,292] ISG15 is an ubiquitin-like molecule that exerts its antiviral effect by conjugating proteins, although the mechanism for suppression of virus replication remains unknown.[251]

Viruses and virus strains vary in their sensitivity to the antiviral activities of IFN, and this may or may not correlate with virulence.[24,68,174,756,894] Mutations associated with altered sensitivity to IFN have been mapped to the 5′ nontranslated region (NTR), nsP1, and nsP2.[235,667,756,880]

IFN may also contribute to alphavirus-induced disease. Fever during the viremic phase of infection, as is seen with CHIKV and RRV, is probably a response to the IFN induced early after infection (see Fig. 23.7). It has been postulated that the rapidly fatal disease induced by alphaviruses in newborn mice may be owing to the production of large amounts of IFN and pro-inflammatory cytokines.[807] Acute-phase responses induced by alphaviruses prior to the virus-specific immune response include up-regulation of toll-like receptor expression and increases in tumor necrosis factor (TNF), IL-1, and IL-6, and levels generally correlate with the extent of virus replication.[278,512,702,807,874] Adult mice deficient in IL-1β have reduced mortality after CNS infection with a neurovirulent strain of SINV, again suggesting that cytokine effects may contribute to mortality.[457]

Virus-Specific Adaptive Responses

Both cellular and humoral immune responses are induced by infection (see Fig. 23.7). In experimentally infected adult mice, antiviral antibody is usually detected in serum within 3 to 4 days after infection.[280,592,713] The cellular immune response, manifested by the presence of virus-reactive lymphocytes in draining lymph nodes and blood and the infiltration of mononuclear cells into infected tissues, also appears within 3 to 4 days after infection.[283,509] These responses appear later (7–10 days after infection) in neonatal mice.[721] Both appear to play a role in recovery from infection and protection against reinfection.

Humoral Immunity

Virus-specific immunoglobulin M (IgM) antibody is detectable very early in human disease, often provides a means for rapid diagnosis of infection, and can persist for many months after recovery.[69,99,103,112,115,288,424,495,571] Virus-specific immunoglobulin A (IgA) also appears early in infection but declines rapidly.[114] Immunoglobulin G (IgG) antibody is present in serum after 7 to 14 days and is maintained at relatively high levels for years.[101,183,396] Many lines of evidence support the hypothesis that recovery from alphavirus infection depends in large part on the antibody response.[91,284,906] Rapidity of antibody synthesis is predictive of outcome from encephalitis because patients without evidence of antibody at the time of illness onset are most likely to die.[99] Antibody can neutralize virus infectivity and promote virus clearance by the reticuloendothelial system in conjunction with complement.[356] Appearance of antibody correlates with cessation of viremia (see Fig. 23.7).

The most extensive experimental studies to define the antibody specificity and the mechanisms of antibody-mediated recovery and protection have been done using VEEV, SFV, and SINV infection of mice. Passive transfer of antibody before or after infection is protective. Both neutralizing and nonneutralizing MAbs against multiple epitopes on the E1, E2, and E3 glycoproteins can protect against alphavirus challenge and promote recovery.[65,66,289,343,502,519,597,757,892] There is a correlation of protection with the ability of the MAb to bind to the surface of infected cells, although this is not absolute.[757] Protection requires intact bivalent antibody but does not require complement.[323,503] However, virus clearance from blood is delayed in complement-deficient mice.[324]

Treatment of immune deficient mice persistently infected with SINV or SFV with antiviral antibody clears infectious virus from the CNS without causing neurologic damage.[21,448] Clearance of infectious virus is rapid, whereas the decline in viral RNA occurs more slowly.[448,521] E2-specific MAbs can down-regulate intracellular virus replication *in vivo* and *in vitro* by a nonlytic mechanism.[448] Antibody against an N-terminal peptide of VEEV E2 that is not neutralizing can limit virus replication *in vivo,*[342] and a nonneutralizing MAb to SFV E2 can limit virus replication *in vitro.*[66] Anti-E3 MAbs inhibit production of VEEV.[597] Anti-E1 MAbs may also be able to alter intracellular virus replication.[128]

In vitro studies show that the process by which antibody alters intracellular virus replication requires bivalent antibody but does not require the Fc portion of the MAb, complement, or other cells[448,824]; however, the effects of antibody are amplified by treatment of infected cells with IFN-α.[172] Soon after antibody binding, virion budding from the plasma membrane is inhibited.[173] *In vivo* studies also show that IFN and antibody act synergistically to promote recovery, although the mechanisms by which these systems interact have not been identified.[95,154]

After recovery from encephalitis, viral RNA remains detectable in the CNS for life. Therefore, one consequence of a nonlytic mechanism for clearance of virus from tissue is that the virus genome is not completely eliminated if the originally infected cells survive.[446,447] This leads to a need for long-term control of virus replication that is accomplished in part by infiltration of antibody-producing B cells into the CNS.[281,286,521,821]

Antibody also is important for protection from infection.[538] Inactivated vaccines protect against EEE, VEE, and WEE.[636,638] Delivered before or shortly after infection, passive transfer of antibody can protect from acute fatal disease but may predispose to late disease.[284,399,712]

Cellular Immunity

Alphavirus infection induces virus-specific lymphoproliferative, cytokine, and cytotoxic T-cell responses.[4,283,385,498,531] Cytokines increased in plasma during acute disease include IL-4, IL-6, IL-10, IL-12, IL-13, and IFN-γ.[328,853] After epidermal virus inoculation, Langerhans cells increase expression of MHC class II antigens and accessory and costimulatory molecules that enhance activation of naive T cells.[370] The mononuclear inflammatory process in alphavirus encephalitis is immunologically specific[509] and includes infiltration of NK cells, $CD4^+$ and $CD8^+$ T lymphocytes, B cells, and macrophages.[346,521,529,541] Relative proportions of these mononuclear cells vary with the time after infection.[346,521,529] T cells play a role in virus clearance and in protection from challenge.[200,897] Viral RNA levels in the CNS of SINV-infected mice decrease more rapidly when $CD8^+$ T cells are present.[400] Mice lacking the ability to produce antibody can clear infectious virus from some populations of neurons through production of IFN-γ,[64,84] and IFN-γ downregulates SINV replication in mature neurons *in vitro* through a JAK/STAT-dependent mechanism.[89,90] In animals infected with virulent strains of virus, cellular immune responses contribute to tissue damage and fatal disease.[273,399,563,669]

Pathologic Changes

Encephalomyelitis

Pathologic changes in the CNS of humans with fatal neurologic disease and mice with experimentally induced encephalomyelitis begin with perivascular infiltration of mononuclear and polymorphonuclear inflammatory cells.[509,529,577] Adhesion molecules (e.g., ICAM-1, VCAM-1) are up-regulated on endothelial cells and integrins LFA-1 and VLA-4 are important mediators of mononuclear cell entry.[347,741,750] This phase of infection may include extravasation of red blood cells and endothelial cell swelling and hyperplasia.[577] Lymphocytes and monocytes move from the perivascular regions to areas of the parenchyma with virus-infected neurons. This inflammatory process is accompanied by gliosis and evidence of inflammatory and glial cell apoptosis.[245]

Neonatal mice and human infants may die with widespread virus-induced neuronal cell death before the inflammatory process—a manifestation of the cellular immune response—can be initiated.[555] Immature neurons die by an apoptotic process,[452] whereas death of mature neurons may be characterized by cytoplasmic swelling, vacuolation, membrane breakdown, and cellular degeneration suggesting necrosis.[245,307,555] Demyelination has been described as a consequence of EEEV and WEEV infection in humans[52,576,577] and of WEEV, RRV, and SFV infection of mice, probably as a result of infection of oligodendrocytes.[94,532,715]

Reticuloendothelial Infection

The pathology of VEE in horses includes cellular depletion of bone marrow, spleen, and lymph node tissue, and pancreatic necrosis.[405] Small mammals also develop widespread infection of reticuloendothelial system tissues and may develop ileal necrosis.[40,266,845] Leukopenia is commonly observed during human infection.[534]

Arthritis

In CHIKV- and RRV-induced arthritis, there is hyperplasia of the synovial lining, vascular proliferation, and mononuclear cell infiltration.[328,747] Synovial fluid contains increased protein, $CD4^+$ T lymphocytes, activated NK cells and macrophages, and increased levels of monocyte chemotactic protein (MCP)-1/CCL2, IL-6, and IL-8.[145,229,328] Persistent infection is suggested by the presence of RRV RNA 5 weeks after onset of symptoms[747] and CHIKV antigen and RNA in synovial macrophages 18 months after acute disease in a patient with chronic arthritis.[328]

Rash

Skin biopsies taken from patients with RRV-induced rash show perivascular infiltration of lymphocytes (primarily $CD8^+$ T cells) and monocytes without evidence of immune complex deposition.[230]

Release and Transmission

A common feature of alphaviruses is their transmission by insects and maintenance in a natural cycle of replication in vertebrate and invertebrate hosts. Arthropod vectors become infected by feeding on a viremic host, are able to transmit the virus 4 to 10 days later (external incubation), and remain persistently infected. Maintenance of this cycle requires an amplifying host that develops a viremia of sufficient magnitude to infect feeding mosquitoes. For many alphaviruses, humans are dead-end hosts unable to infect mosquitoes efficiently. However, human-mosquito-human transmission has been important in epidemics of RRV, o'nyong nyong virus (ONNV), and CHIKV-induced polyarthritis,[478,689,790] and horse-mosquito-horse transmission is important in epizootics of VEE.[659,771]

Other modes of transmission are occasionally important. Horses infected with VEEV may shed virus in nasal, eye, and mouth secretions, as well as in urine and milk, resulting in the potential for transmission by the respiratory route.[118,405] Aerosol transmission of VEEV, CHIKV, and Mayaro virus has occurred in laboratory settings,[118,378,439,788,799] and aerosolized VEEV has been developed as an agent of biological warfare.[728] EEEV persists in the feather follicles of infected pheasants, and transmission among penned pheasants can occur through feather picking and cannibalism.[697] Person-to-person transmission has not been documented.[439,659]

Veterinary Correlates and Animal Models

WEEV, EEEV, and VEEV—the first alphaviruses to be cultured—came to the attention of virologists because they caused fatal disease in horses; these viruses remain important equine pathogens.[182,522,786] EEEV and WEEV cause encephalitis in horses, whereas VEEV causes severe respiratory disease associated with leukopenia; encephalitis may or may not be present. Getah virus causes an urticarial rash and hind leg edema in horses.[717] WEEV, EEEV, and Highlands J virus (HJV) cause disease in domesticated birds such as chickens, pigeons, pheasants, turkeys, and emus.[42,167,213,221,476,822,868] The alphaviruses associated with arthritis in humans have not been recognized as important causes of disease in domestic animals.

Good small animal models exist for the encephalitogenic alphaviruses but are less satisfactory for study of the arthritogenic alphaviruses. In mice, alphaviruses generally infect lymphatic tissue, muscle, brown fat, brain, and spinal cord; however, the extent and relative importance of infection at these sites differs among these viruses. For instance, RRV and Getah virus cause primarily myositis, VEEV causes reticuloendothelial infection, and WEEV and EEEV cause encephalitis with neurons as the main target cells.[9,526,554] In mice infected with relatively avirulent strains of SFV, RRV, and VEEV, the acute encephalitic phase is accompanied by infection of oligodendroglial cells and demyelination.[94,715] For all alphaviruses, fatal disease in mice is usually associated with CNS infection even if encephalitis is not a manifestation of the human infection. For instance, SINV infection of mice is studied as a model for acute viral encephalitis, although SINV causes arthritis and rash, not encephalitis, in humans.[349,489,820] Specifics of these animal model systems are discussed with the individual viruses.

Virulence

Virulence is a measure of the ability of the virus to cause fatal disease; for alphaviruses, this usually reflects the severity of neurologic disease. Outcome is influenced by characteristics of both the host and the virus. An early virus determinant of virulence is induction of IFN and susceptibility to IFN-mediated inhibition of replication. Viruses that induce IFN and are susceptible to IFN are generally attenuated.[12,92,158,235,243,734,756,880] Most alphaviruses show an age-dependent susceptibility to disease.[9,75,294,554,584,713] Resistance increases with maturation and is associated with decreased virus replication in tissues at the site of virus inoculation and in target tissues (e.g., brain), not with changes in induction of IFN or the ability of infected mice to mount a virus-specific immune response.[280,287,554] The ability of a virus strain to cause fatal disease or a particular complication of infection also often depends on the genetic background of the host[186,759,792,814]; however, the specific genetic determinants of susceptibility are just beginning to be identified.[793] Avirulent alphavirus strains may replicate poorly even in newborn animals, whereas virulent strains can usually replicate well and cause disease in adult and newborn animals. The role of the response to IFN is unclear, although older mice increase ISG12 whereas young mice do not.[429]

For encephalitic alphaviruses, another viral determinant of virulence is their ability to enter the CNS efficiently (neuroinvasiveness). Many alphavirus strains can cause fatal disease after intracerebral or intranasal inoculation but not after subcutaneous or intraperitoneal inoculation. The duration of viremia often correlates with virulence with virulent strains sustaining longer viremias than avirulent strains.[355,357,360] Peripheral replication, viremia, neuroinvasiveness, and neurotropism (ability to replicate in CNS cells) all contribute to virulence.

The viral determinants of virulence have been most extensively studied in murine models for SINV, SFV, RRV, and VEEV infections. Viruses with altered virulence have been selected after chemical mutagenesis,[48,85] by passage in tissue culture,[58,166,395,783] by passage in mice,[284,517,783] by isolation of MAb escape mutants[842] or plaque variants,[354] and by manipulation of complementary DNA (cDNA) virus clones.[166,485,779,815] Nucleotide and amino acid changes affecting virulence have been mapped to the 5′ NTR, nsP1, nsP2, nsP3, E1, and E2. Virulence determinants in the glycoproteins map to receptor-binding regions of the E2 A and B domains[840] (see Fig. 23.4). Specifics are covered in the sections dealing with each of these viruses.

Persistence

There is substantial evidence that alphaviruses can persist after appearance of an immune response and clearance of infectious virus from the circulation and from tissue.[447] Pathologic examination of CNS tissue from human cases of progressive WEEV months to years after resolution of acute encephalitis has shown an active inflammatory process.[575,577] Viral RNA and proteins can be detected in the nervous system long after recovery of mice from SINV or SFV-induced encephalitis and for several weeks in the joints of humans with RRV-induced arthritis.[186,285,396,447,521,747,821] It is postulated that this persistence of RNA is attributable to failure of the virus or the immune system to eliminate the infected cells. Interestingly, passive antibody protection predisposes to persistent infection and the late onset of progressive disease.[399,712]

Congenital Infection

Alphaviruses can be transmitted transplacentally. This has been documented in mice for RRV, SFV, VEEV, and Getah virus[3,30,35,524,755] and in humans for RRV, WEEV, VEEV, and CHIKV.[6,231,380,723] In mice, the virus infects the placenta, where it is able to persist and spread to the fetus despite the development of maternal antibody. The outcome of fetal infection depends on the timing of infection relative to transfer of maternal antiviral IgG to the fetus. Fetuses are protected if transfer occurs prior to infection; however, transfer of antibody after fetal infection does not mediate recovery.[524] In monkeys, congenital infection with VEEV induces malformations of the brain and eye.[471] In humans, no abnormalities were observed in infants infected with RRV at 11 to 19 weeks gestation; however, earlier infection may lead to fetal death.[6] Epidemics of VEE are associated with increases in spontaneous abortion.[659,862] No effect on pregnancy outcome was identified during the CHIKV outbreak on Reunion Island.[231]

PATHOGENESIS AND PATHOLOGY IN MOSQUITOES

The ability of alphaviruses to infect mosquitoes efficiently with spread to and replication in the salivary glands is essential for maintaining the natural cycle of transmission. Not all mosquitoes taking a blood meal from a viremic host will become infected, and not all infected mosquitoes develop the ability to transmit virus. Many alphaviruses preferentially infect a narrow range of mosquito species, and this host specificity plays an important role in determining the geographic distribution of the virus. Even within a species, strains of mosquitoes may vary in susceptibility to infection. *Ae. albopictus* collected from different geographic regions show differences in susceptibility to infection with CHIKV and in the amount of virus produced after infection.[789] Field and laboratory populations of *Culex tarsalis* differ in susceptibility to WEEV.[334] Strains of virus also differ in their abilities to infect mosquitoes, and laboratory-adapted strains may establish infection relatively inefficiently.[557,710,711,831,833]

The extrinsic incubation period—or the time between taking an infected blood meal and ability to transmit infection—depends on the rapidity of virus replication and dissemination to the salivary glands. This period is relatively short (2–7 days) for alphaviruses compared to other arboviruses.[710]

Entry and Sites of Primary Replication

Posterior midgut epithelial cells are the initial sites of infection,[77,558,612,708,864] and infection is facilitated when virus in the serum is concentrated next to these cells as the blood meal clots[866] (Fig. 23.8). Susceptibility of mosquitoes to alphavirus infection is determined in large part by the ability of the virus to infect midgut epithelial cells.[334,397,710] Changes both in the virus and vector can affect this interaction.[889] WEEV rapidly fuses with microvillar membrane preparations from *Cx. tarsalis* mosquitoes, and both WEEV and CHIKV bind better to membranes from susceptible mosquitoes than to membranes from refractory mosquitoes,[334,546] which is consistent with a role for viral structural proteins as determinants of vector specificity, midgut infection, and dissemination.[612,813,832,833] The high-affinity laminin receptor A is a receptor for VEEV and SINV on the surface of C6/36 larval *Ae. albopictus* cells,[474,850] and proteins of 60 and 38 kDa have been identified as putative receptors for CHIKV on brush-border membranes from *Ae. aegypti*.[546]

Host cell membrane cholesterol levels affect the efficiency of alphavirus entry.[473] Mosquitoes, like other insects, do not synthesize cholesterol and obtain sterols needed for reproduction and development from dietary blood. Cholesterol-independent mutants of SFV replicate better than parental SFV in cholesterol-depleted C6/36 cells and in adult *Ae. albopictus* mosquitoes.[16]

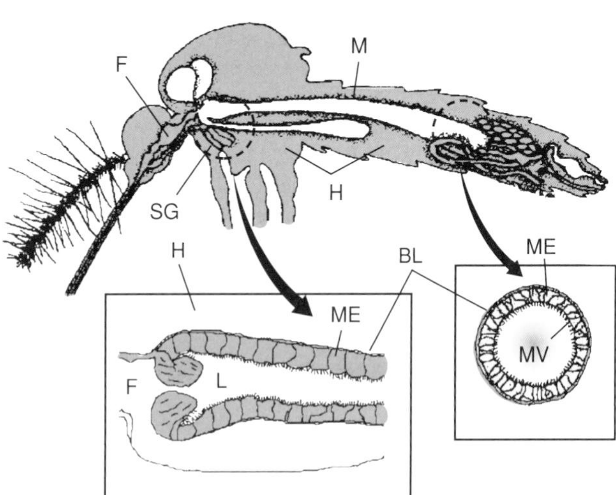

FIGURE 23.8. Diagram of mosquito internal anatomy showing the essential sites for alphavirus infection. BL, basal lamina; L, lumen; F, foregut; M, midgut; ME, midgut epithelium; MV, microvilli or brush border; SG, salivary gland. (Adapted from Weaver SC, Scott TW, Lorenz LH, et al. Togavirus-associated pathologic changes in the midgut of a natural mosquito vector. *J Virol* 1988;62:2083–2090.)

Replication in midgut epithelial cells is regulated by the RNAi innate antiviral response that is triggered by virus-derived dsRNA and small interfering RNAs.[109,387,397,559] RNAi affects infection rate of the midgut, intensity of infection, and virus dissemination to secondary tissues and is probably an important determinant of vector competence.[387,397]

Spread

For the mosquito to become capable of transmission, virus must reach the salivary glands and replicate there (see Fig. 23.8). For most alphaviruses, spread beyond the midgut to other tissues is through the hemolymph.[710] Virus buds primarily from the basolateral surface of the infected midgut epithelial cells and accumulates next to the basal lamina,[710] which is a layered structure composed of mucopolysaccharide that acts as a barrier to hemocoel entry. Dissemination of SINV from the midgut of *Ae. aegypti* mosquitoes depends on expression of endosomal proteins UNC93A and synaptic vesicle-2.[110] Replication of ONNV in *Anopheles gambiae* is controlled by expression of heat shock protein cognate 70B.[731,732] Infected midgut epithelial cells often degenerate and slough 36 to 48 hours after infection; this process may facilitate penetration of the virus into the hemocoel.[710,865]

Infection of salivary gland acinar cells from the hemolymph requires that the virus again traverse a basal lamina—a process that may depend primarily on hemolymph titer. The fat body is an important site for virus amplification.[855,864] EEEV infects the midgut, fat body, muscle, and salivary glands without involving the nervous system or the ovarioles,[708,864] whereas VEEV infects the nervous system[855] and SINV infects respiratory tissue.[73]

Once salivary gland infection is established, virus matures by budding into apical cavities or randomly into vesicles basolaterally and apically. This process may be associated with cytopathic changes in the salivary glands.[525] The rapidity of virus growth and dissemination to the salivary glands depend on the ambient temperature. Higher temperatures accelerate the transmission cycle in warm months.[650,816] This can be as short as 2 to 3 days.[710] In general, virus content of an individual mosquito reaches a peak within 4 to 7 days after infection.[525,710] Some tissues (e.g., fat bodies) produce large amounts of virus, and some (e.g., head ganglia) produce small amounts; others (e.g., ovarioles and Malpighian tubules) remain virus negative.[523]

For transovarial transmission to occur, virus must be able to infect oocytes early in development. Failure to infect ovarioles precludes efficient transovarial transmission of most alphaviruses.[73,176,708,855] However, the presence of RRV and CHIKV in field-caught male mosquitoes suggests that vertical transmission can occur.[463,639,795] Eggs can also be infected after they have been fertilized. Low levels of vertical transmission have been documented in the laboratory for RRV in *Aedes vigilax*, for SINV in *Aedes australis*, and for CHIKV in *Ae. aegypti*.[506,589] Vertical transmission in nature has been reported for RRV, SINV, and WEEV.[176,237,463]

Pathology, Persistence, and Host Response

Although generally considered to be benign for the invertebrate vector, infection may reduce survival and reproductive capacity.[709,710] The IMD pathway of innate immunity can be activated by infection to decrease virus replication.[41] Suppression of the RNAi response increases virus replication and mosquito mortality after infection.[143,387] Mosquitoes remain infected and infectious for life.[525,710] In the fat body and salivary glands, infection is persistent, although titers decline after the acute phase of infection, decreasing efficiency of transmission.[708]

ALPHAVIRUSES ASSOCIATED PRIMARILY WITH ENCEPHALITIS

Eastern Equine Encephalitis

EEE was first recognized as a disease of horses in the northeastern United States. In the summer of 1831, more than 75 horses died in three coastal counties of Massachusetts.[300] Between 1845 and 1912, epizootics were recorded on Long Island and in North Carolina, New Jersey, Florida, Maryland, and Virginia.[300,710] The virus responsible for EEE was first isolated in 1933 from the brains of affected horses in New Jersey and Virginia during a widespread outbreak that also involved coastal areas of Delaware and Maryland.[786] South American eastern equine encephalitis virus (SA-EEEV) was first isolated in 1936 from a horse in Argentina.[683] Although human cases were suspected earlier, it was not demonstrated until 1938 when an outbreak in the northeastern United States resulted in 30 cases of fatal encephalitis in children living in the same areas as equine cases. At that time, EEEV was isolated from the CNS of humans,[867] as well as from pigeons[221] and pheasants.[868]

Based on seasonality, location of cases near salt marsh areas, lack of evidence of transmission from horse to horse through contact, short period of equine viremia, and geographic distribution of cases, Ten Broeck et al.[785] postulated that insects transmitted infection and that birds were likely to be the reservoir host. The first arthropod isolates were actually from chicken mites and lice, which can transmit infection only inefficiently.[193,710] Transmission of EEEV by *Aedes sollicitans* in the laboratory was accomplished in 1934[520]; subsequently, multiple *Aedes* species were shown to be competent vectors, although recovery of EEEV from naturally infected mosquitoes did not occur until 1949 with isolates from *Mansonia perturbans* in Georgia[337] and *Culiseta melanura* in Louisiana.[127] Subsequent work showing the competence of *Cs. melanura* and a consistent association between infected birds and the isolation of virus from this vector has led to the current understanding that *Cs. melanura* is the primary enzootic vector for North American eastern equine encephalitis virus (NA-EEEV) strains.[27,162,436,710]

Epidemiology

NA-EEEV causes localized outbreaks of equine, pheasant, and human encephalitis in the summer. The virus is enzootic in North America from Maine southward along the Atlantic seaboard and Gulf Coast to Texas, in the Caribbean, and in Central America[254] (Fig. 23.9). Inland foci exist in the Great Lakes Region and have extended to South Dakota and Quebec.[136] The primary enzootic cycle is maintained in shaded swamps where the vector is the ornithophilic mosquito *Cs. melanura*[27,159,710] (Fig. 23.10). Birds are the primary reservoir host, and many species are susceptible to infection.[406] The amplifying species for NA-EEEV are wading birds, migratory passerine songbirds, and starlings.[162,204,414,514] Young birds are probably important for virus amplification because they are more susceptible to infection, have a prolonged viremia, and are less defensive toward mosquitoes.[162] Multiple mosquito species, such as *Coquillettidia perturbans, Ochlerotatus canadensis,* and various *Aedes* species, may serve as bridge vectors for transmission to susceptible mammals.[27,159,528,710] In temperate areas, the virus is most likely periodically reintroduced by migratory viremic birds or windborne infected mosquitoes from subtropical areas of year-round transmission.[716,861,878,895] Reptiles with viremias that are prolonged and persist through hibernation may maintain the virus focally.[877] There is no convincing evidence for overwintering in mosquitoes, and ovarioles are not involved after experimental infection of *Cs. melanura* with NA-EEEV.[708]

SA-EEEV is enzootic along the northern and eastern coasts of South America and in the Amazon Basin[123] (see Fig. 23.9). In South and Central America, the enzootic cycle is maintained in moist forests where *Culex (Melanoconion)* spp. appear to be the primary vectors.[710,818] Forest-dwelling rodents, bats, and marsupials are frequently infected and may provide a reservoir; however, these transmission cycles are not well characterized.[28,710] Infection of reptiles and amphibians is also likely.[159]

Morbidity and Mortality

NA-EEEV is the most virulent of the encephalitic alphaviruses, with a high mortality owing to encephalitis. Most cases are associated with exposure to wooded areas adjacent to swamps and marshes,[98] and approximately equal numbers occur in females and males.[211] Children under 10 years of age are most susceptible,[211] with 1 in 8 infections resulting in encephalitis; in adults, 1 in 23 infections result in encephalitis.[261] The case fatality rate was 60% to 70% in earlier studies and 30% to 50% in more recent studies, with the highest rates in children and the elderly.[98,125,171,207,211,632] SA-EEEV is much less virulent and causes little human disease despite evidence of human infection in areas of endemic transmission.[13,123,180,682]

Origin and Spread of Epidemics

In the northern part of the North American region, human and equine cases of EEE occur between July and October; in the southern region, cases can occur throughout the year.[125,632] In the Caribbean, outbreaks appear to be linked to virus introduction by southbound migratory songbirds.[710] In North America, human and equine cases usually occur near swamps maintaining enzootic transmission. Outbreaks are initiated when the virus spreads from the enzootic cycle involving ornithophilic mosquitoes into mosquito populations that feed on various hosts (see Fig. 23.10). Multiple species of mosquitoes with catholic feeding habits have been implicated as potential bridge vectors in different regions.[27,159,528,694,710]

Cases of equine encephalitis are usually the first indication of an outbreak. In the absence of immunization, epizootics appear approximately every 5 to 10 years and are associated with heavy rainfall and warmer water temperatures that increase the populations of enzootic and epizootic mosquito vectors.[444] Most of the epidemics have occurred in Massachusetts and surrounding states[211]; however, the largest recorded outbreak occurred in 1947 in Louisiana and Texas, with 14,344 cases of equine encephalitis and 11,722 horse deaths.[129] Since 1955, an average of eight cases of EEE have been diagnosed in humans in the United States each year[125,126] (Fig. 23.11).

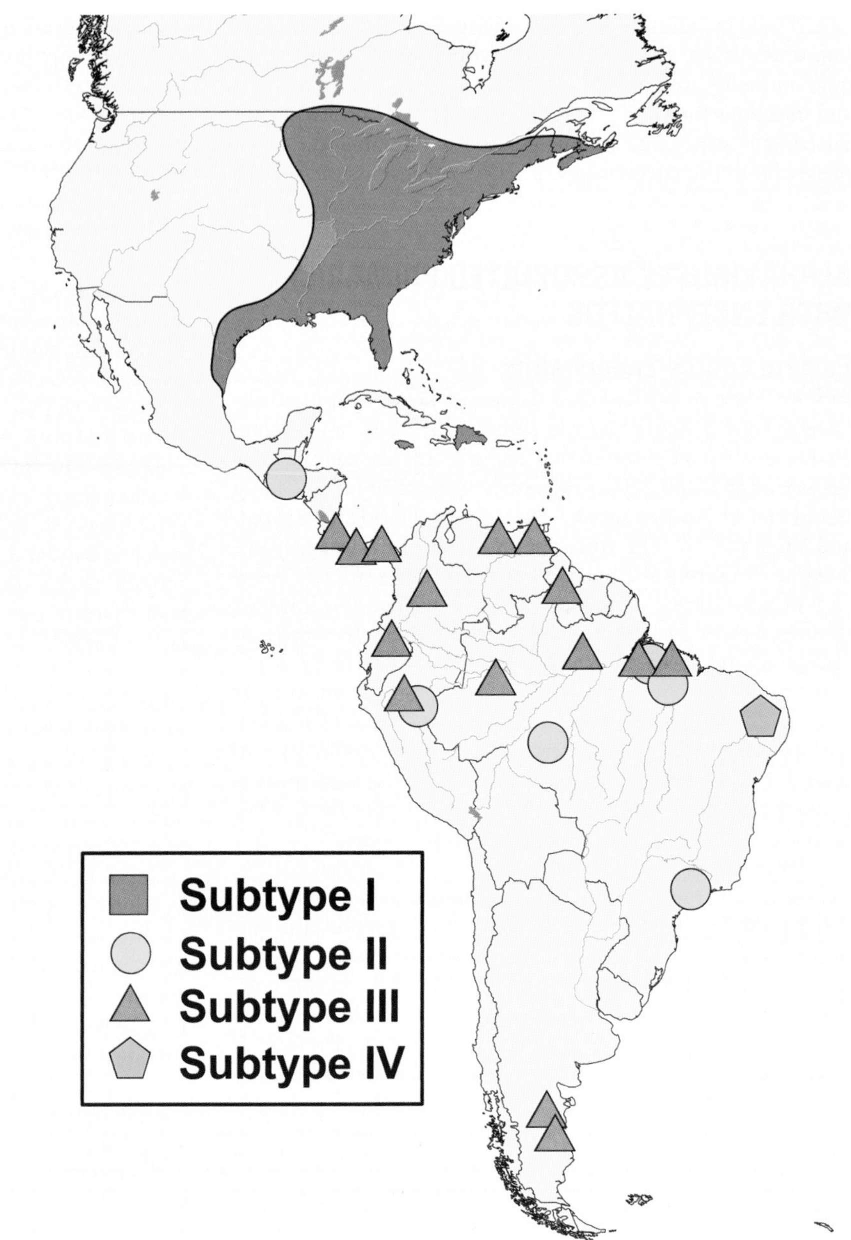

FIGURE 23.9. Geographic distribution of eastern equine encephalitis virus. The map shows the locations for isolation of North American eastern equine encephalitis virus (subtype I) and the three South American eastern equine encephalitis virus lineages (subtypes I, II, and III).[861] (Courtesy of Scott Weaver; from Weaver SC, Powers AM, Brault AC, et al. Molecular epidemiologic studies of veterinary arboviral encephalitides. *Vet J* 1999; 157:123–138.)

Molecular Epidemiology

Antigenic differences between North and South American strains of EEEV have long been recognized,[117] and the strains can be distinguished by reactivity with MAbs to the E1 glycoprotein.[663] Sequence comparisons indicate that EEEV has evolved independently in North and South America over the past 1,000 years, with 23% to 24% nucleotide and 9% to 11% amino acid sequence divergence.[29] There is one lineage of NA-EEEV (lineage I) and three lineages of SA-EEEV: on the coasts of South and Central America (lineage II), in the Amazon basin (lineage III), and in Brazil (lineage IV)[78,861] (see Fig. 23.9). Isolates of NA-EEEV are highly conserved, differing over a large geographic range by less than 3% in nucleotide sequence consistent with birds as the vertebrate reservoir hosts. The calculated yearly nucleotide substitution rate is 2.7×10^{-4}.[78,861] The two main lineages of SA-EEEV (II and III) exhibit 17% to 21% nucleotide divergence and 3% to 5% amino acid divergence and are evolving at a slower rate (1.2×10^{-4} substitutions/nucleotide/year).[29] The South American groups are estimated to have diverged 1,000 to 2,000 years ago and appear to be evolving locally, which is consistent with small mammals as the reservoir hosts.[29,858,861]

Clinical Features and Pathology

Illness caused by infection with NA-EEEV may consist of 1 to 2 weeks of fever, chills, malaise, and myalgias followed by recovery. In cases of encephalitis, these prodromal symptoms are followed by the fulminant onset of increased headache, vomiting, restlessness, irritability, seizures, obtundation, and coma.[171,207,211] Meningismus is frequent, and focal signs including cranial nerve palsies and hemipareses are not uncommon.[171,632] Hyponatremia owing to inappropriate secretion of

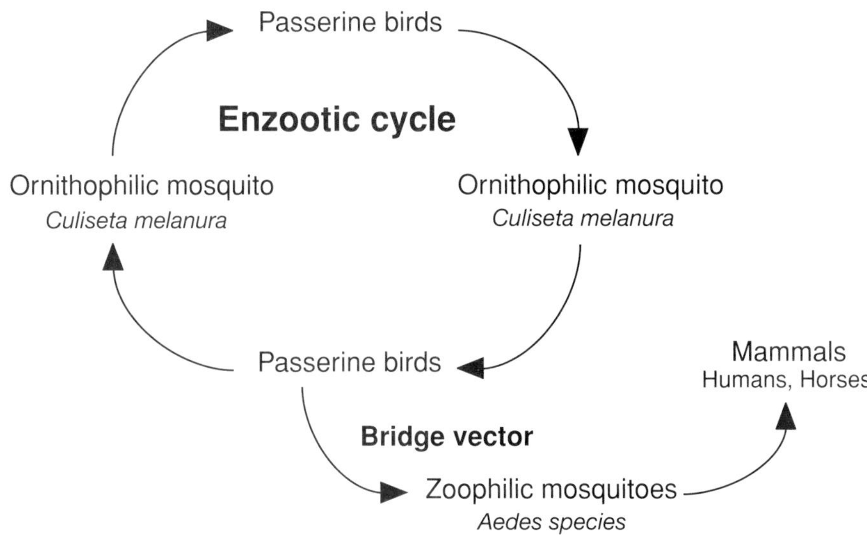

FIGURE 23.10. Enzootic and epidemic/epizootic cycles of eastern equine encephalitis virus as an example of an alphavirus that uses a species of mosquito with different host feeding preferences to bridge from the enzootic avian-ornithophilic mosquito cycle to infect mammals such as humans and horses. Similar mechanisms are operative in transmission of Sindbis virus to humans.

antidiuretic hormone is a common complication, and edema of the face and extremities has been noted.[171,207] Death typically occurs within 2 to 10 days after onset of encephalitis.

CSF examination shows increased pressure and white cell counts ranging from 10 to 2,000/μL. Polymorphonuclear leukocytes are often abundant early in disease, with a shift to mononuclear cells over the first few days of illness.[171] The presence of red blood cells or xanthochromia is not uncommon.[632] CSF protein levels are increased, whereas glucose is low to normal.[207,632] Electroencephalographic (EEG) findings are relatively nonspecific, usually showing slowing.[171] Computed tomography (CT) scans may be normal or show only edema.[171,632] Magnetic resonance imaging (MRI) scans are more often abnormal, with focal lesions most commonly observed in the thalamus, basal ganglia, and brain stem.[171]

Poor outcome is predicted by high CSF white cell count or severe hyponatremia but not by the size of the radiographic lesions.[171] Recovery is more likely in individuals who have a long (5–7 day) prodrome and do not develop coma.[632] Sequelae, including paralysis, seizures, and mental retardation, are common, with 35% to 80% of survivors, particularly children, having significant long-term neurological impairment.[171,207,211]

Histopathology on fatal cases demonstrates a diffuse meningoencephalitis with widespread neuronal destruction; perivascular cuffing with polymorphonuclear, as well as mononuclear, leukocytes; and vasculitis with vessel occlusion in the cortex, basal ganglia, and brain stem. The spinal cord is frequently spared.[207,222,760] Virus antigen is localized to neurons, and neuronal death is marked by cytoplasmic swelling and

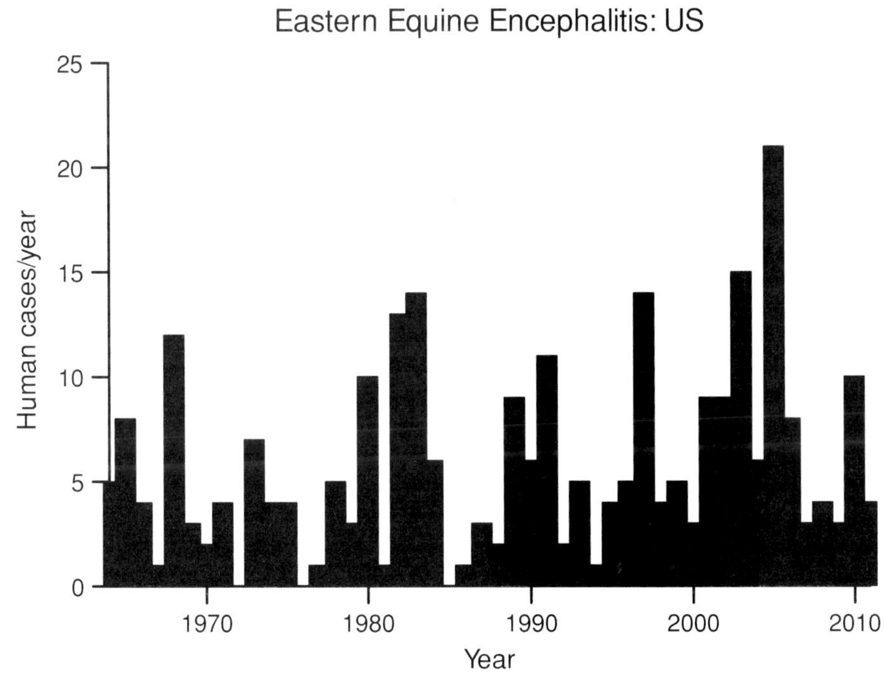

FIGURE 23.11. Numbers of human cases of eastern equine encephalitis reported annually in the United States since 1964. (Based on data from the Centers for Disease Control and Prevention.)

nuclear pyknosis.[245] Apoptotic glial and inflammatory cells are frequently found in the regions of affected neurons.[207,245]

Veterinary Correlates, Host Range, and Animal Models

NA-EEEV is an important cause of disease in horses, pheasants, emus, and turkeys and can also cause encephalitis in penguins, sheep, deer, dogs, and pigs.[53,167,221,293,476,697,780] Horses develop signs of depression, progressive incoordination, seizures, and prostration. The case fatality rate is 80% to 90%. Most survivors are left with neurologic sequelae.[710] Birds vary in their susceptibility—some species develop disease, whereas many others show no morbidity or mortality despite a prolonged viremia.[406,476] Chickens, turkeys, emus, and whooping cranes often develop fatal viscerotropic disease with multifocal necrosis in the heart, kidney, and pancreas and lymphoid depletion in thymus, spleen, and bursa.[167,293,822] Pheasants develop encephalitis with 50% to 70% mortality, whereas penguins develop nonfatal encephalitis.[476,697]

Laboratory studies of macaques, marmosets, mice, guinea pigs, and hamsters generally confirm the neurovirulence of NA-EEEV for mammals.[222,466,592,670,760,786,838,893] NA-EEEV can initiate CNS infection in experimental animals by infecting choroid plexus epithelial cells or olfactory neurons.[466,670] Peripheral replication is in fibroblasts, skeletal muscle, and osteoblasts.[838] Macaques and marmosets develop encephalitis, whereas New World *Aotus* monkeys develop viremia without evidence of disease.[202] Young mice show extensive neuronal damage and rapid death.[838] Older mice are relatively resistant to peripheral inoculation; however, after intracerebral inoculation, they develop seizures and die rapidly.[242,466] Guinea pigs develop encephalitis after aerosol exposure to NA-EEEV with neuronal death, inflammation, and vasculitis.[670] Hamsters develop a biphasic fatal illness with hepatitis and lymphatic organ infection followed by encephalitis characterized by extensive vasculitis and microhemorrhages.[592]

Virulence

NA-EEEV is more virulent than SA-EEEV in humans and experimental animals.[12,123,710] Construction and testing of chimeric viruses in mice indicate that both structural and nsPs contribute to virulence.[10] Viruses with a temperature-sensitive, small plaque phenotype, and decreased virulence for mice and hamsters have been selected after chemical mutagenesis.[85] One determinant of the neurovirulence of NA-EEEV is the ability to bind HS. Increased HS binding is associated with decreased tropism for lymphoid tissue, decreased production of IFN, and increased replication in the CNS.[242]

Diagnosis, Treatment, and Prevention

Diagnosis is based on virus isolation or detection of RNA or antibody. Virus can be isolated from CSF, blood, or CNS tissue by inoculation into newborn mice or onto various tissue culture cells. Detection and identification of virus in field and clinical samples can also be accomplished through various nucleic acid amplification assays.[430] Antibody is usually measured by enzyme immunoassay (EIA), with detection of IgM in serum and CSF particularly useful.[99,100] No specific therapies have been developed for treatment of EEE; thus, treatment is supportive.[645]

Infection in mosquito populations can be monitored by virus isolation, by nucleic acid amplification, or by seroconversion of sentinel pheasants or chickens. This information can be used to guide insecticide spraying to reduce adult and larval mosquito populations and prevent human cases. A formalin-inactivated vaccine based on an NA-EEEV strain (PE-6) is available for horses and emus and for investigational use in humans to protect laboratory workers. This vaccine does not induce significant neutralizing or anti-E2 antibody to SA-EEEV.[767]

Western Equine Encephalitis

Epizootics of viral encephalitis in horses were described in 1908 in Argentina. In 1912, 25,000 horses were estimated to have died in the central plains of the United States.[683] In the summer of 1930, a similar epizootic occurred in the San Joaquin Valley of California, causing an estimated 6,000 cases of equine encephalitis. During this outbreak, WEEV was isolated from the brains of two affected horses by intraocular inoculation of another horse, and this virus was subsequently used to infect other animals.[522] WEEV was suspected at that time to be a cause of human encephalitis. In 1938, WEEV was recovered from the brain of a child with fatal encephalitis.[335]

Mosquitoes were implicated in disease transmission when it was demonstrated that horses developed a viremia[336] and that experimentally infected *Ae. aegypti* mosquitoes were capable of transmitting the virus to horses.[388] However, it was not until the summer of 1941 during a widespread epidemic in the northern plains of the United States and Canada that the virus was isolated from naturally infected *Cx. tarsalis* mosquitoes.[299] Subsequently, WEEV was isolated from *Cx. tarsalis* in other epizootic sites and recognized to be the principal vector.

Other New World Western Equine Encephalitis Complex Viruses

The WEE complex in the New World includes three viruses in addition to WEEV: Highlands J (HJ), Buggy Creek, and Aura viruses.[102] These viruses have different ecological niches and vary in virulence. Only WEEV is recognized to cause human disease.[98] Viruses in the WEE complex found in the Old World (e.g., SINV and Whataroa virus) are discussed in the later Sindbis section. WEEV, HJV, and Fort Morgan virus all belong to the lineage that diverged since recombination between a Sindbis-like virus and an EEE-like virus.[297] Aura virus is a "pre-recombinant" virus (see Fig. 23.5).

Highlands J

WEEV-like viruses were first isolated in the eastern part of the United States in 1952. In 1960, the prototype HJV was isolated from a blue jay in Florida.[317] HJV is enzootic on the U.S. East Coast and is maintained in a cycle similar to that of EEEV, with *Cs. melanura* the primary vector and migrating birds the primary reservoir. All alphaviruses in the WEEV complex isolated in the eastern United States are strains of HJV.[309] Rates of divergence of WEEV and HJV of 0.1% to 0.2% per year have been estimated.[146] HJV can occasionally cause encephalitis in horses[381] and is a recognized pathogen for various avian species, including turkeys, pheasants, partridges, ducks, emus, hawks, and whooping cranes.[19,213,293,861]

Fort Morgan, Buggy Creek, and Stone Lakes

Fort Morgan virus and its close relative Buggy Creek virus were originally isolated from swallows and sparrows in eastern Colorado[105] and Oklahoma.[332] These viruses exist as two lineages found primarily in the western plains of North America[591,607] and are transmitted to cliff swallows and sparrows by cimicid swallow nest bugs (*Oeciacus vicarius*).[86] Neither virus is recognized as a pathogen for humans; however, the viruses cause encephalitis in nestling house sparrows.[578] Recently, a third related virus, Stone Lakes virus, was isolated from swallow bugs in California.[76]

AURA

Aura virus was isolated in 1959 in Brazil from *Culex (Melanoconion)* spp. collected near the Aura River and later from *Aedes serratus* in Brazil and Argentina.[121] This virus is likely to be related to the "Sindbis-like" virus that recombined with EEEV to produce WEEV.[674] It has not been linked to human disease and is relatively nonpathogenic for mice.

Epidemiology

WEEV is widely distributed in the western plains and valleys of the United States and Canada and in South America. In North America, WEEV is maintained in an endemic cycle involving domestic and passerine birds (particularly finches and sparrows) and *Cx. tarsalis,* a mosquito well adapted to irrigated agricultural areas.[98] Occasional isolations have been made from *Aedes melanimon* and *Aedes dorsalis,* which also are competent vectors. There is evidence for a transmission cycle involving *Ae. melanimon* and the black-tailed jackrabbit[98,302] in addition to the *Cx. tarsalis*–avian cycle. Increased transmission is associated with greater abundance of *Cx. tarsalis.*[46] Serosurveys and virus isolations provide evidence of natural infection in chickens, pheasants, rodents, rabbits, ungulates, tortoises, and snakes. In some areas of South America, most mosquitoes from which WEEV has been isolated feed primarily on mammals and antibodies are common in small mammals including rats and rabbits, whereas in other areas, antibodies are found primarily in birds.[726,861] A recent survey of horses in the Pantanal region of Brazil found 36% seropositivity for WEEV.[603] Interseasonal persistence can occur in saltwater marshes, perhaps by overwintering in adults.[648,649]

MORBIDITY AND MORTALITY

WEEV in the western United States has caused epidemics of encephalitis in humans, horses, and emus; however, the case fatality rate of 10% for humans, 20% to 40% for horses, and 10% for emus is lower than for NA-EEEV. In older children and adults, males are two to three times more likely to develop disease than females.[472] The estimated case to infection ratio is 1:58 in children younger than 5 years and 1:1150 in adults.[98] Clinically apparent disease is most common in the very young and those older than 50 years.[472] Severe disease, seizures, fatal encephalitis, and significant sequelae are more likely to occur in infants and in young children.[194,412] The overall case fatality rate is 3% but rises to 8% in those older than 50 years.[472] Accidental infections involving aerosolized virus in the laboratory have been reported[222] and have led WEEV to be regarded as a potential bioterroist threat.[728]

The rare occurrence of significant human disease during equine outbreaks of WEE in South America may be related to the feeding habits of the vector or to a lower virulence of South American strains for humans and horses.[169,683]

ORIGIN AND SPREAD OF EPIDEMICS

There have been large, often widespread epidemics of equine encephalitis occurring from mid June to late September in North America with significant spillover into the human population. These outbreaks correlated with regional increases in the population densities of *Cx. tarsalis.*[587] Major epizootics occurred every 2 to 3 years in the United States from 1931 to 1952. In 1941, more than 3,400 human WEE cases were reported in the plains of the western United States and Canada, with attack rates of up to 167 cases/100,000 population.[98] During the 1952 epidemic in California's Central Valley, attack rates were 36 cases/100,000 humans and 1120/100,000 equids.[98] Seroprevalence in humans was 34% in rural areas of California endemic for WEEV in 1960[232] but only 1.3% to 2.6% in similar areas from 1993 to 1995.[646] Human cases of WEE have steadily declined to fewer than one to two human cases/year over the past 20 years (Fig. 23.12). This decline is

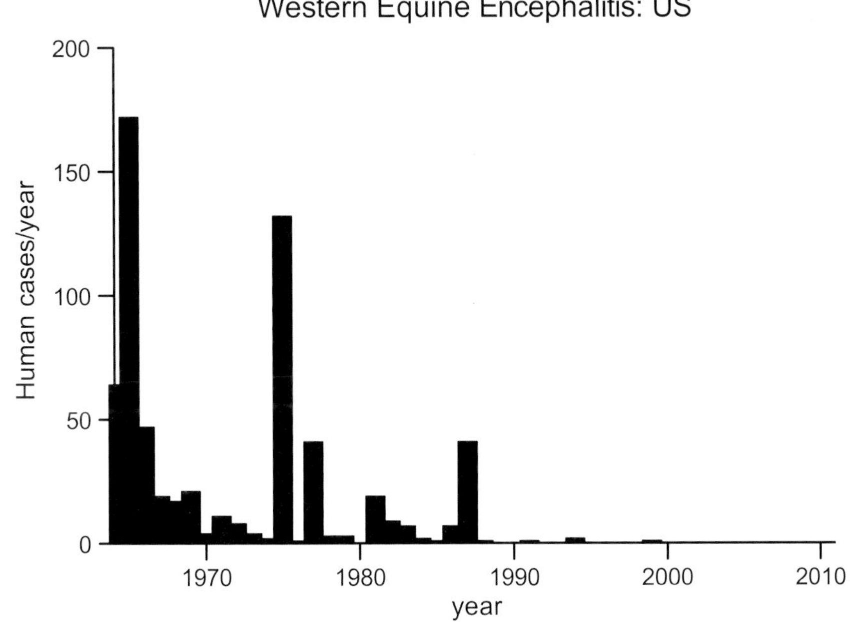

FIGURE 23.12. Numbers of human cases of western equine encephalitis reported annually in the United States since 1964. (Based on data from the Centers for Disease Control and Prevention.)

not understood but does not appear to be owing to a decrease in virus virulence or change in vector competence.[218,647,900]

Studies of differential virulence of epizootic and enzootic strains in South America first suggested that epizootic strains arise from nonpathogenic enzootic strains.[61] Sequence analysis of the viruses found at the initial focus of the 1982 WEE epizootic in Argentina indicated that the enzootic virus was the source of a virulent variant, which emerged by mutation or selection to cause the epizootic. The epizootic vector in South America is *Aedes albifasciatus,* and rabbits may serve as an amplifying host.[861]

Molecular Epidemiology

WEEV has four major lineages—two in South America and two widely distributed in North and South America and the Caribbean.[859,861] One was isolated during the 1982–1983 epizootic in Argentina, a second is related to the McMillan strain found in North and South America and Cuba from 1930 to 1972, a third was found in the same regions from 1964 to 1993, and a fourth was found in Brazil and Argentina. Within California, separately evolving lineages have been identified in the Central Valley and the southern part of the state.[419]

Clinical Features and Pathology

WEEV causes encephalitis with signs and symptoms similar to those of EEE. Transmission can occur by aerosols as well as by mosquitoes.[642] There is a 3- to 5-day prodrome of fever and headache that may progress to restlessness, tremor, irritability, nuchal rigidity, photophobia, altered mental status, and paralysis.[214,412,516] Infants often present with rigidity, seizures, and a bulging fontanel.[214,516] Transplacental transmission results in perinatal infection manifesting within the first week of life as fever, failure to feed, and seizures.[516,723] CSF pleocytosis is typical with 100 to 1,500 cells/μL. Neutrophils are present early in disease and mononuclear cells later.[516] In infants less than 1 year of age, approximately 60% of survivors have brain damage, and in some the disease is progressive.[516,576] Common problems are cognitive disabilities associated with quadriplegia, spasticity, recurring seizures, cortical atrophy, ventricular dilation, and intracranial calcification.[194,214,576,751] In older individuals, recovery is typically rapid, with remission of signs and symptoms within 5 to 10 days, and sequelae are less common (5%).[214] Age-dependent susceptibility is likely related to the maturation-dependent ability of neurons to respond to IFN and limit virus replication.[120]

Pathology of acute cases of WEE shows leptomeningitis and perivascular cuffing with neutrophils in the earliest cases and lymphocytes, plasma cells, and macrophages at later times. In areas of neuronal degeneration, there is inflammation accompanied by endothelial hyperplasia, petechial hemorrhages, and glial nodules. Lesions are found primarily in the basal ganglia, brain stem, cerebellum, cerebral cortex, and spinal cord, with areas of focal necrosis and demyelination in the subcortical white matter and basal ganglia.[214,576,577]

Occasionally in infants and children, there is pathologic evidence of progressive disease consistent with persistent infection.[516,576,577] Individuals surviving months to years after onset of encephalitis (often with progressive disease) may have cystic lesions, gliosis, and demyelination with areas of active mononuclear inflammation.[576,577]

Veterinary Correlates, Host Range, and Animal Models

WEE was first recognized as a neurologic disease of equids characterized by fever, incoordination, drowsiness, and anorexia leading to prostration, coma, and death in approximately 40% of affected animals.[182] Emus also develop symptomatic, often fatal disease characterized by ataxia, paralysis, and tremors.[42] As a part of its enzootic cycle, WEEV infects sparrows, finches, blackbirds, mourning doves, pheasants, cowbirds, swallows, and chickens. The virus can cause fatal disease in sparrows, whereas chickens, which are often used as sentinels, develop asymptomatic infection.[651]

Experimentally infected newborn mice die within 48 hours after infection with involvement of skeletal muscle, cartilage, and bone marrow. In weanling mice, the brain, heart, lung, and brown fat appear to be the primary target tissues.[9] After intracerebral inoculation, there is infection of the choroid plexus and ependyma with spread to neurons and glial cells in the brain, cerebellum, and brain stem and to motor neurons in the spinal cord.[466] After peripheral inoculation, WEEV replicates in skeletal and cardiac muscle cells, causes a necrotizing myocarditis, and occasionally spreads to the CNS.[466,535] Hamsters are more susceptible to WEEV-induced disease than mice, with high mortality owing to encephalitis after intranasal or intraperitoneal inoculation.[375] Neurons are infected, and neuropathologic changes include perivascular inflammation, microcavitation, and astrocytic hypertrophy.[909] Cynomolgus and rhesus macaques are susceptible to intranasal, aerosol, and intracerebral infection and develop dose-dependent signs of encephalitis with fever, tremors, and altered consciousness. Pathology shows encephalitis with infection of neurons accompanied by mononuclear inflammation.[642,893]

Virulence

Variants of WEEV with decreased pathogenicity for mice and hamsters (e.g., B628 clone 15) have been selected by passage on CEF cells.[909] Large plaque strains tend to be more virulent than small plaque strains.[354] Epizootic strains appear to be optimized for viremia and neuroinvasiveness and are generally more virulent for mice and guinea pigs than are enzootic strains.[61,62,303] North American isolates vary substantially in their virulence for mice but are generally more virulent than South American strains.[218,469,561] The molecular bases for any of these differences have not been defined; however, preliminary sequencing suggests that structural region genes are important determinants of virulence.[561]

Diagnosis, Treatment, and Prevention

Diagnosis can be made by detection of WEEV-specific IgM in serum, by isolation of virus in mice or cultured cells, or by nucleic acid amplification.[99,430] Small molecule screening has identified potential lead compounds that inhibit WEEV replication and are partially protective in mice.[377,604] An inactivated vaccine is available for horses and as an experimental preparation for laboratory workers.[638] Preclinical studies of approaches to protection include activation of innate immunity,[470] DNA virus vectors expressing IFN or viral proteins, and chimeric alphaviruses.[33,45,248,560,774,890,891]

Venezuelan Equine Encephalitis

Equine disease was recognized in South America in the 1920s. In 1936, a virus (VEEV) was isolated from the brains of encephalitic horses during an outbreak of equine encephalitis that spread from the central river valleys of Colombia into the Guajira region of Venezuela. This virus was antigenically distinct from the viruses causing equine encephalitis in the eastern and western portions of North America (EEEV and WEEV) and became the third encephalitic alphavirus identified in the Americas.[56,420] Between 1943 and 1963, many VEEV-related viruses, including the prototypic Trinidad donkey (TrD) strain,[637] were isolated in South America, Central America, and southern regions of the United States.[11] The first reported human cases of VEE were in laboratory workers[118,439]; subsequently, human disease was documented in the general population during equine outbreaks, and virus was isolated from ill humans.[637,692,857]

Studies in Central America during this period indicated an enzootic cycle involving *Culex (Melanoconion)* spp. mosquitoes and rodents.[239] In 1969, an epizootic/epidemic of VEE appeared and spread from Peru through Central America and into Texas, causing human disease and a high mortality in horses.[11] Virus isolations during the epizootic were primarily from *Psorophora confinnis* and *Ae. sollicitans* mosquitoes and from horses, suggesting that the epizootic and enzootic transmission cycles differed.[404,771]

Venezuelan Equine Encephalitis Complex Viruses

Using a short incubation HI test, isolates of viruses related to VEEV were originally classified into subtypes I through IV: VEE (I), Everglades (EVE, II), Mucambo (MUC, III), and Pixuna (PIX, IV).[896] When Cabassou (CAB) and AG80–663 (Rio Negro [RN]) viruses were isolated and shown to be within the VEEV antigenic complex, they became subtypes V and VI.[104,181] The VEE subtype I viruses have been further subdivided serologically into IAB, IC, ID, IE, and IF (Mosso das Pedras)[104,857,896] and the MUC subtype III viruses into IIIA, IIIB (Tonate [TON]/Bijou Bridge), IIIC, and IIID.[403,857] Analysis of the phylogenetic relationships of the VEE complex viruses gained from sequencing has led to a recognition of eight species within the VEEV complex[402,518,629] (Fig. 23.13; see Table 23.1).

Everglades

EVE virus (serotype II) was first recognized in southern Florida in the 1960s in persons living near Everglades National Park. Transmission is widespread in Florida with *Culex (Melanoconion) cedecei* as the primary vector and cotton rats (*Sigmodon hispidus*) the main vertebrate reservoir.[148,863] Disease in humans is usually mild.[198]

Mucambo

MUC virus (serotype IIIA) was first isolated (BeAn 8) from a Brazilian monkey in 1954.[123] Three clades have been identified, with temporally defined clades 1 and 2 from Trinidad and clade 3 from Brazil.[38,39] The virus causes fatal disease in newborn mice and in adult mice after intracerebral, but not peripheral, inoculation. Experimentally inoculated guinea pigs and horses survive infection.[725]

Tonate

TON virus (serotype IIIB) was first isolated in 1973 from a bird (*Psarocolius decumanus*) captured in French Guiana[181] and

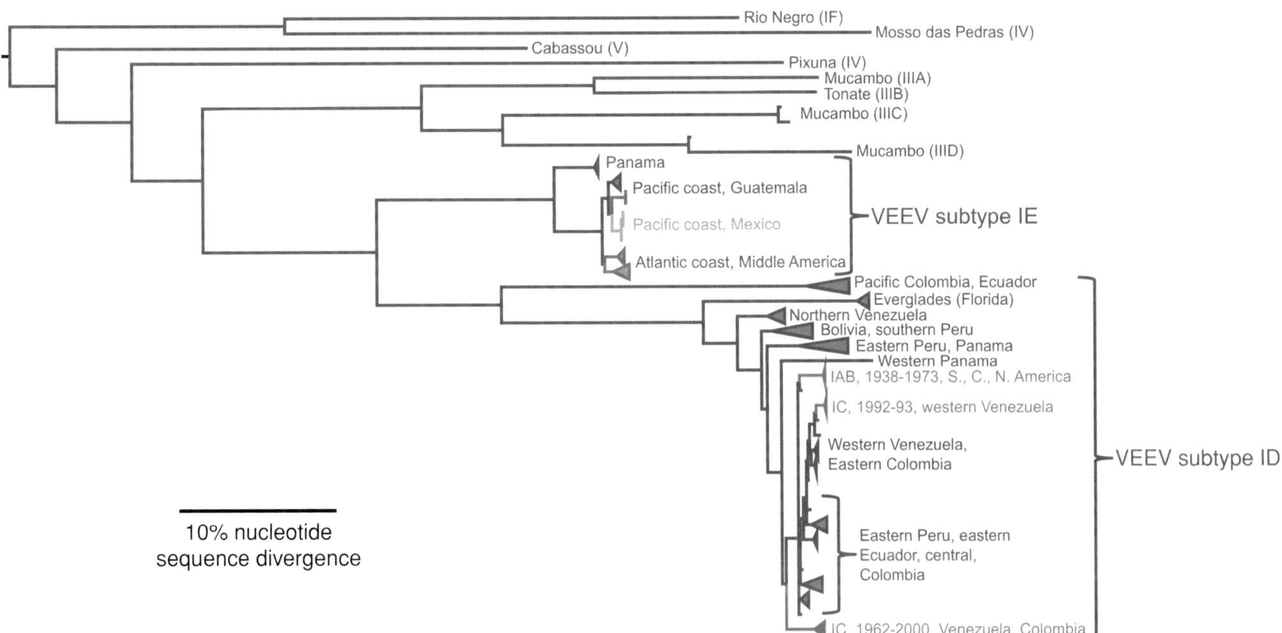

FIGURE 23.13. Venezuelan equine encephalitis virus phylogenetic tree showing relationships of epizootic (colored *red* and *orange*) and enzootic/endemic strains (colored *green*). Strains are abbreviated with country followed by year of collection. The tree was generated using 817 nucleotide sequences from the PE2 envelope glycoprotein gene using maximum likelihood methods. (Courtesy of Scott Weaver.)

subsequently from *Culex portesi*.[595] TON virus (Bijou Bridge) has also been recovered from cliff swallow bugs and birds in North America.[536] Human seropositivity is 11.9% in French Guiana, with the highest rates in savannah areas.[776] Infection is most often associated with a mild dengue-like illness but has caused fatal encephalitis in a young child.[331]

Pixuna

PIX virus (serotype IV) was first isolated (BeAr 35645) from *Anopheles (Stethomyia) nimbus* mosquitoes in Belem, Brazil, in 1961[725] and has also been identified in Argentina.[613,614] There is no evidence that it causes disease in humans or horses.

Cabassou

CAB virus (serotype V) was first isolated (CaAr 508) from mosquitoes in French Guiana in 1974.[181] This virus is not neurovirulent for adult mice or guinea pigs.

Rio Negro

RN virus (serotype VI) was first isolated (AG80–663) from *Culex (Melanoconion) delpontei* near the Rio Negro in Argentina in 1980.[104] The virus circulates in neotropical regions of Argentina,[527,613,614] where it has caused outbreaks of acute febrile illness.[151] Suckling mice die within 2 to 3 days; however, adult mice and guinea pigs survive infection.[104]

Epidemiology

Enzootic VEE complex viruses are involved in perennially active transmission cycles in subtropical and tropical areas of the Americas (e.g., EVE in Florida; VEE ID and IE in Central America; Mosso das Pedras, MUC, PIX, CAB, and RN in South America). In enzootic areas, mosquito isolates are primarily from *Culex (Melanoconion)* spp. mosquitoes that live in tropical and subtropical swamps throughout the Americas, breed near aquatic plants, and feed at dawn and dusk on various rodents, birds, and other vertebrates.[11,212,239,272] Wild birds are susceptible to infection; however, mammals, such as cotton rats, spiny rats, bats, and opossums, are the most likely reservoir hosts, as determined by virus isolation, levels of viremia, serology, and resistance to disease.[47,113,205,272,857]

Morbidity and Mortality

Clinically evident human infection can occur with enzootic, as well as epizootic, VEE complex viruses.[11,198,331,776,857] Humans living in areas of enzootic transmission have a high prevalence of antibody owing to infection associated mostly with undiagnosed mild febrile illnesses, often assumed to be dengue.[11,205,272,701,776] During epizootics, human attack rates vary widely.[659] The apparent to inapparent infection ratio is estimated at 1:11.[72] All ages and both sexes are equally susceptible to infection; however, disease manifestations vary with age.[659] Individuals younger than 15 years are more likely to develop fulminant disease with reticuloendothelial infection, lymphoid depletion, and encephalitis. In older children and young adults, a relatively benign influenza-like illness is most common.[198] Individuals older than 50 years are prone to develop encephalitis, although most recover.[198] The incidence of encephalitis in clinically ill humans is generally less than 5% and the mortality less than 1%.[659] Essentially all deaths occur in children.

Origin and Spread of Epidemics

VEE epizootics/epidemics have occurred at approximately 10- to 20-year intervals in cattle ranching areas of Venezuela, Colombia, Peru, and Ecuador when heavy rainfall leads to increased populations of epizootic mosquito vectors and herd immunity decreases.[659] Formalinized vaccines containing residual live virus were probably responsible for initiating the IAB outbreaks in South America that spread to Central America and Texas between 1969 and 1972[404] and in Peru in 1973.[629,860] Viruses causing epizootics are subtype IAB, IC, or IE, whereas enzootic viruses are ID, IE, or IF. During 1995, a major VEE IC outbreak occurred in coastal areas of Venezuela and Colombia that caused disease in 75,000 to 100,000 people. This region had experienced a similar outbreak in 1962–1964. A ID virus obtained from a mosquito pool collected in Venezuela in 1983, when there was no epidemic activity, was similar in sequence and indicated that the epizootic IC virus was not maintained in a separate cycle but rather evolved by mutation from an enzootic ID virus[629,657,862] (Figs. 23.13 and 23.14). A similar process accounted for the emergence of a IC virus in 1992–1993 from a ID virus.[23] Epizootic potential is correlated with positive-charge mutations in E2 that increase the level of viremia in equines and may also increase infectivity for the mosquito vector *Ochlerotatus taeniorhynchus*.[23,80,275] During epizootics, horses are an important amplifying species, and susceptible equines provide a means for virus spread.[771]

Detailed phylogenetic studies have delineated six major lineages of enzootic VEEV, including five subtype ID strains and the subtype IE lineage (see Fig. 23.13). All epizootic strains from major outbreaks fall into a clade nested within one of these lineages.[857] Enzootic IE viruses were the source of epizootic IE strains in two recent equine epizootics in Mexico.[579] Interestingly, these epizootic IE strains cause encephalitis in horses with little viremia.[262,685]

During outbreaks, virus has been isolated from several species of mosquitoes. Those most incriminated as VEEV vectors include *Ochlerotatus sollicitans, Oc. taeniorhynchus, Psorophora columbiae,* and *P. confinnis*.[771,857] After an epizootic, IC viruses may persist in a natural cycle and serve as a source for subsequent smaller outbreaks.[566]

Molecular Epidemiology

Sequence analysis of the VEE complex viruses shows the greatest divergence for the E2 glycoprotein and the C-terminal region of nsP3.[518,629] Five enzootic subtype ID lineages have been identified: Colombia and coastal Ecuador, Panama, Colombia, western Venezuela, and northern Peru (see Fig. 23.13). All epizootic IAB and IC strains are related to ID strains from Colombia, Venezuela, and Peru.[629,857] Three distinct geographically separate IE lineages have also been recognized: northwestern Panama, Pacific coast (Mexico and Guatemala), and Gulf/Caribbean coast (Mexico and Belize).[580]

Clinical Features and Pathology

Infection with enzootic, as well as epizootic, strains of VEEV can cause significant human disease, with the most common signs and symptoms being fever, headache, tremors, prostration, nausea, and vomiting that last from 3 to 4 days.[11] Accidental laboratory aerosol infections of young adults with epizootic strains of VEEV caused a febrile illness with the abrupt onset of chills, headache, myalgia, somnolence, vomiting, diarrhea, and pharyngitis 2 to 5 days after exposure without evidence of encephalitis.[118,198,439] Natural epidemic human infection was first described in 1952 in Colombia and subsequently

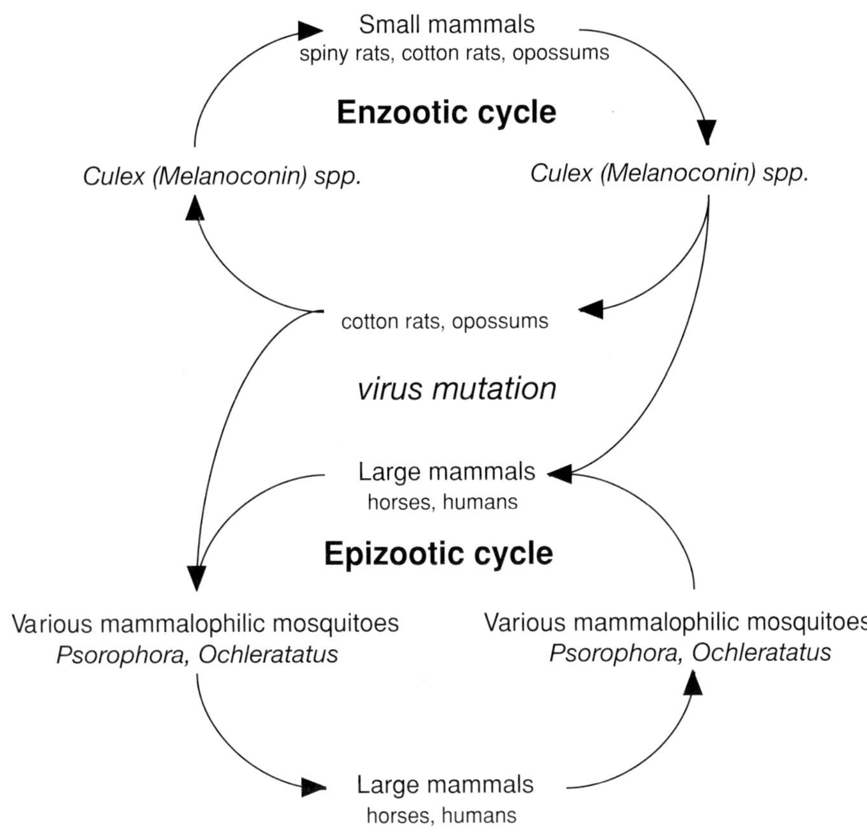

FIGURE 23.14. Enzootic and epidemic/epizootic cycles of Venezuelan equine encephalitis virus as an example of an alphavirus for which the epizootic strain arises by mutation from the enzootic virus. Similar mechanisms may be operative in transmission of epidemic western equine encephalitis virus.

in Venezuela and Panama during the 1962–1964 outbreak that resulted in 32,000 human cases and 190 deaths.[198,368] The 1995 outbreak in Colombia caused an estimated 75,000 human cases—3,000 with neurologic complications and 300 deaths.[659,862] The case fatality rate is 0.7% to 1%. Neurologic disease tends to appear 4 to 10 days after onset of illness, with headache and vomiting the most common initial symptoms. Specific neurologic signs include focal or generalized seizures, paresis, behavioral changes, and stupor or coma.[659,862] Children recovering from encephalitis may be left with neurological deficits, particularly seizure disorders.[442] Fetal abnormalities, spontaneous abortions, and stillbirths may occur with infection during pregnancy.[659,862]

Laboratory studies often show lymphopenia. Pathology on fatal cases has shown myocarditis, focal centrilobular hepatic necrosis and inflammation, generalized lymphoid depletion, cerebral edema, and vasculitis.[368] Congenitally infected infants show severe neurologic damage with widespread necrosis, hemorrhage, and hypoplasia resulting—in the most severe cases—in hydranencephaly.[870]

Veterinary Correlates, Host Range, and Animal Models

Enzootic strains of the VEE complex can infect horses, although these infections are asymptomatic or cause short-term fever, low-level viremia, and little clinical illness and may immunize horses against infection with epizootic strains (IAB, IC, and IE).[316,857] Equine disease induced by epizootic strains is characterized by fever, depression, and diarrhea leading to death 6 to 8 days after infection. Viremia persists until death, with titers up to 10^8 infectious units/mL blood. Virus can also be recovered from eye washings, nasal washings, and urine. Leukopenia coincides with the viremia and is progressive in fatal cases. In animals that recover, antibody appears approximately 7 days after infection.[405] Pathology on fatal cases shows pancreatic necrosis and cellular depletion in bone marrow, lymph nodes, and spleen. The brains of horses with signs of neurologic disease show swollen cerebrovascular endothelial cells, edema, extravasation of blood, and leukocytic infiltration into the perivenular spaces.[260,405]

Infection of macaques by aerosol or subcutaneous inoculation with enzootic and epizootic strains of virus elicits a biphasic febrile response—the first phase is coincident with the viremia and the second phase with termination of viremia—that is, the appearance of the immune response[260,534,644] (see Fig. 23.7). Leukopenia is common. Symptoms are usually mild, consisting of anorexia, loose stools, and irritability, and occasionally loss of balance, tremor, or myoclonus.[534,760] Examination of tissues shows lymphocyte depletion early, mild hepatitis, myocarditis, and encephalitis. Lesions in the brain are found primarily in the olfactory cortex and basal ganglia and consist of lymphocytic perivascular cuffing and glial nodules.[260]

Experimental infection of small laboratory animals with VEEV produces various disease patterns. After subcutaneous inoculation of guinea pigs, rabbits, or hamsters with virulent strains of VEEV, there is a viremia. Virus replicates in bone marrow, lymph nodes, spleen, and brain, with rapid destruction of myeloid and lymphoid cells in lymph nodes, spleen, thymus, intestinal and conjunctival lymphoid tissue, liver, and bone marrow; damage to the intestinal wall and pancreas; cerebral hemorrhage; and neuronal cell death.[260,359,845] Death occurs 2 to 4 days after infection and may be associated with ileal necrosis, bacteremia, and endotoxemia.[266] EVE, MUC, and PIX viruses are progressively less virulent.[359]

In addition to myeloid and lymphoid necrosis, susceptible strains of mice develop encephalomyelitis leading to death in 6 to 9 days after infection with the TC-83 vaccine strain, as well as wild-type strains of VEEV.[260,376,475] After subcutaneous inoculation, virus replicates first in DCs or Langerhans cells, which migrate to the draining lymph node where virus is amplified[487] (see Fig. 23.6). Virus enters the CNS by the olfactory route after respiratory or peripheral inoculation. Initial infection is of olfactory epithelium, with spread to olfactory neurons and then caudally to all regions of the brain, causing encephalitis and neuronal apoptosis.[133,351,759,760,837] Virus also infects the pancreas, liver, and teeth. Fatal disease has an immunopathologic component that depends on the strain of mouse infected.[132,475,760] There can also be transplacental transmission of infection.[755]

Virulence

Comparative studies of the virulent TrD and avirulent TC-83 strains of the IAB serotype and construction of recombinant viruses have led to identification of the 5′ NTR (nt 3) and the E2 glycoprotein (residue 120) as important determinants of VEEV virulence for mice.[166,401] Attenuated viruses infect DCs less efficiently and replicate less well in lymphoid tissue and in the CNS than virulent viruses.[487,759] Virulence for guinea pigs is determined by both envelope and nonenvelope genes.[274,625] Determinants of equine virulence are different from determinants of murine virulence but also lie largely within the E2 glycoprotein.[79,275,629] Changes most frequently associated with acquisition of equine virulence for ID strains are a Thr to Met change at position 360 of nsP3 and replacement of uncharged residues with Arg at positions 193 and 213 of the E2 glycoprotein.[23,846] Acquisition of surface charge changes in E2 are also associated with emergence of epizootic IE strains.[79]

Diagnosis, Treatment, and Prevention

Diagnosis can be made by virus isolation from blood or pharynx[118,439,862] or by documenting the presence of anti-VEEV IgM or a rise in IgG antibody. HI, CF, neutralization, or EIA tests can be used for serologic diagnosis and nucleic acid amplification for detection of viral RNA. Antibody responses to enzootic versus epizootic strains can be differentiated with an epitope-blocking EIA.[848]

Treatment is generally supportive; however, passive transfer of antibody can protect mice before, or up to 24 hours after, challenge.[263,340,341] The D-(-) enantiomer of carbodine, an inhibitor of cellular cytidine triphosphate synthetase, and antisense morpholino oligomers suppress VEEV replication *in vitro* and improve the outcome of infected mice.[374,593]

The earliest vaccines developed for horses and laboratory workers were formalin-inactivated preparations.[636,638] These vaccines had repeated problems with residual live virus producing disease and with poor immunogenicity and are no longer in use.[404,629,860] A live attenuated vaccine (TC-83), developed by serial passage of the virulent TrD strain in guinea pig heart tissue culture cells,[58] is protective for horses and laboratory workers; however, 15% to 30% of recipients develop fever and pharyngeal viral shedding.[616] Therefore, a formalin-inactivated TC-83 vaccine (C-84) was produced.[196] Both the live and inactivated vaccines are immunogenic, although live TC-83 provides better protection against aerosol challenge in hamsters than C-84 and is therefore preferred despite the reactogenicity.[361] To produce a more optimal vaccine, several experimental DNA, inactivated, and attenuated live virus vaccines are under development.[131,191,192,500,594,643]

Several measures are effective in controlling outbreaks. These include immunizing equines, limiting equine movements from regions of infection, applying larvacides to mosquito breeding sites, and spraying insecticides to control adult mosquitoes.[659,771,857] Protection of human populations relies primarily on personal protection from mosquito bites.

ALPHAVIRUSES ASSOCIATED PRIMARILY WITH POLYARTHRITIS AND RASH

Chikungunya

An outbreak of a crippling arthritic disease of sudden onset was first recorded in the Newala District of Tanzania in 1952.[661] Retrospective case reviews have suggested that CHIKV epidemics in Africa occurred as early as 1779 but were confused with dengue.[111] Because of the severe arthritic symptoms, the disease was given the name *chikungunya,* meaning "to walk bent over" in the Kimakonde language of Mozambique.[328,661] The virus, isolated in 1953 from serum and from *Aedes* spp. and *Culex* spp. mosquitoes, was related to the group A arboviruses[668] (see Fig. 23.5). Subsequent epidemics were recognized in the Transvaal of South Africa, Zambia, India, Southeast Asia, and the Philippines. From 2004 to 2007, a large epidemic affected islands in the Indian Ocean and India, with spread to Southeast Asia and Europe.[628,654]

Epidemiology

CHIKV causes epidemics of rash and arthritis in India, Southeast Asia, Indonesia, the Philippines, most of sub-Saharan Africa, and Indian Ocean islands with recent extension into southern Europe[269,390,433,655,788] (Fig. 23.15). In Africa, the virus

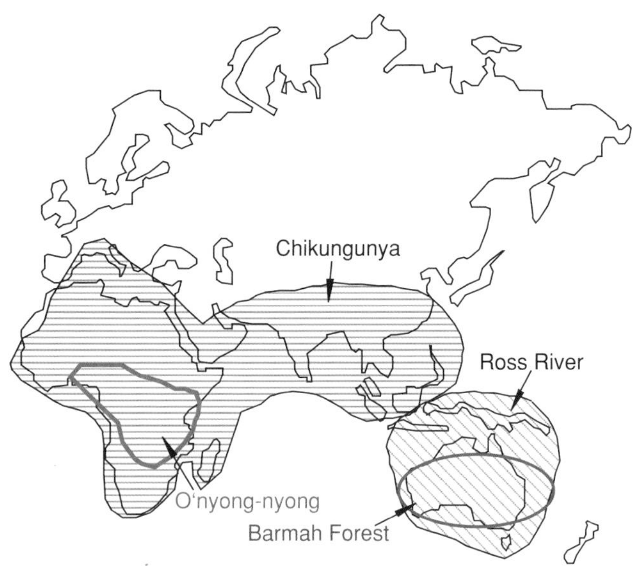

FIGURE 23.15. Geographic distributions of several alphaviruses that cause epidemic polyarthritis and rash: chikungunya, o'nyong-nyong, Barmah Forest, and Ross River viruses.

is maintained in cycles similar to that of yellow fever virus. There is a rural cycle involving *Aedes africanus, Aedes furcifer,* nonhuman primates, and other mammals and an urban cycle involving *Ae. aegypti* or *Ae. albopictus* and humans.[137,177,812] In rural areas, the disease is endemic with small numbers of cases occurring most years.[177] In urban areas, outbreaks are sporadic and explosive, with infection of a large proportion of the susceptible population within a few weeks.[250,601,654,661] In Asia, there is no evidence for a sylvatic cycle; rather, urban transmission is by *Ae. aegypti* and rural transmission is by *Ae. albopictus* in a human-mosquito-human cycle.[326,568,627] Laboratory-acquired infections have also been reported.[799]

Morbidity and Mortality

All ages and both sexes are susceptible to chikungunya, and disease is usually self-limiting and rarely life threatening. However, approximately 0.3% of cases are atypical or severe with nephritis, hepatitis, meningoencephalitis, thrombocytopenia, or encephalopathy. The case fatality rate has been estimated at 1 in 1,000, with most of the deaths either in neonates infected peripartum, adults with underlying conditions, or the elderly.[119,195,654,660,707] The epidemic on Reunion Island affected almost 40% of the population (estimated 300,000 cases) and led to an excess of 254 deaths.[250,318,653] Infants infected at birth are susceptible to CNS complications including cerebral edema and hemorrhage resulting in long-term disabilities.[249] Musculoskeletal symptoms are recurrent or persistent in approximately 40% of adults and are more likely to affect females than males.[752,887]

Origin and Spread of Epidemics

Outbreaks typically occur during the rainy season and are associated with increased population densities of mosquitoes.[112,390,433,478] After an epidemic, the disease usually vanishes from an affected region for years, possibly because large portions of the population have become immune. The recent epidemics that began in Kenya in 2004 and spread to Comoros, Reunion Island, the Seychelles, Mauritius, and Mayotte in 2005 were associated with the emergence of a new strain that arose from the East African lineage[382,705] (Fig. 23.16). Related outbreaks have been reported in India, Sri Lanka, Thailand, Malaysia, Singapore, France, and Italy, with imported cases recognized in many countries.[318,598] Many of the recent outbreaks have been associated with a strain of virus that can be efficiently transmitted by *Ae. albopictus.*[326,833] Because susceptible mosquitoes are widely distributed, travelers provide a source of CHIKV introduction into many other geographic regions.[318,598,652,796]

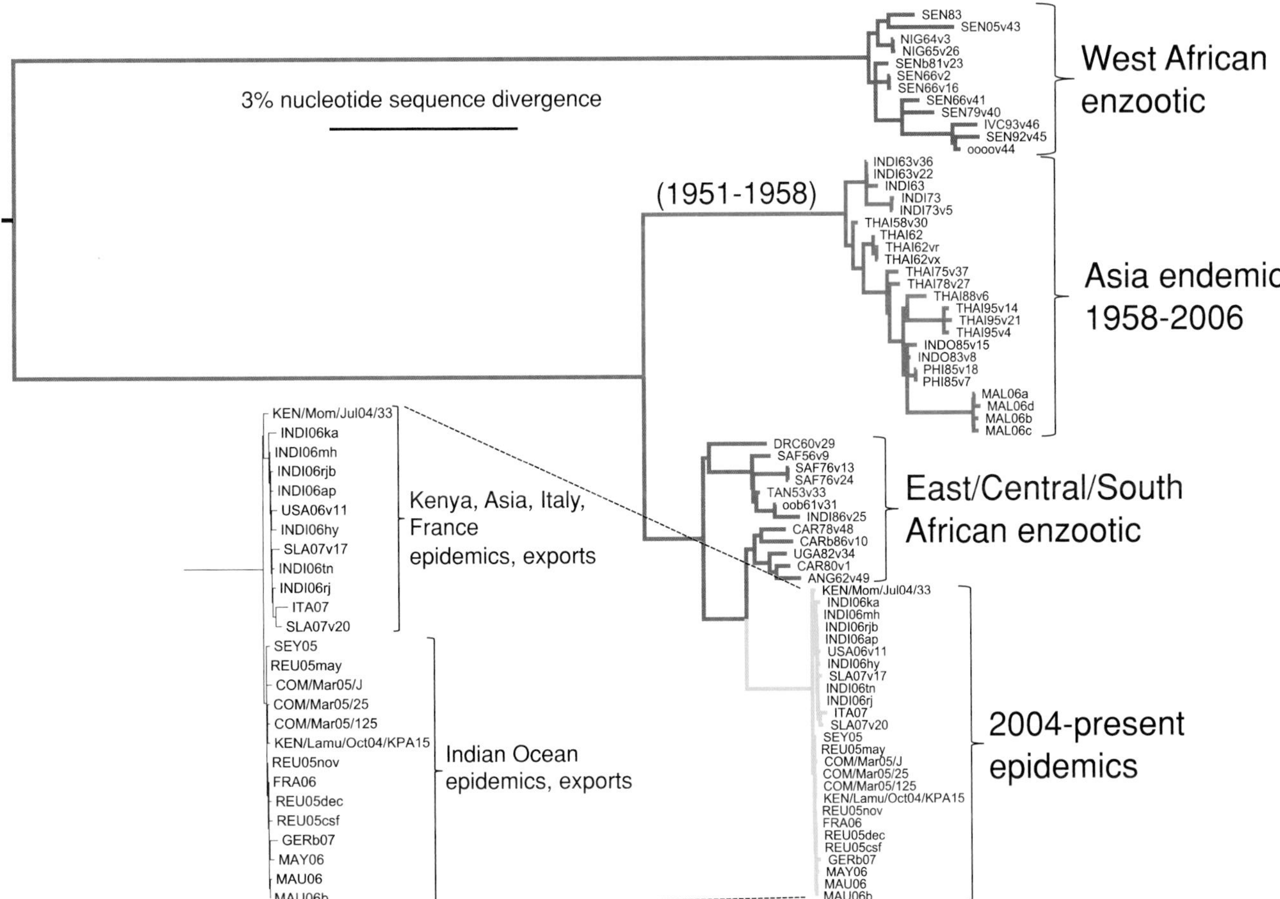

FIGURE 23.16. Chikungunya virus phylogenetic tree derived from genomic nucleotide sequences and Bayesian methods. Strains are abbreviated with country followed by year of collection. All posterior probability values were 1.0 except for some within the 2004 to present epidemic clade shown in *yellow*. Estimated time frame for emergence of the 1958–2006 Asian endemic clade is indicated in *parentheses*. (Courtesy of Scott Weaver.)

There is some evidence that virus can be maintained within mosquito populations by low rates of transovarial or venereal transmission.[506,639,795]

Molecular Epidemiology

CHIKV is a member of the SFV complex, evolved from an ancestor in Africa, and was probably introduced into Asia 70 to 90 years ago.[839] Two distinct lineages exist—one in western Africa and another in southern and eastern Africa and Asia[627,628,705] (see Fig. 23.16). In the latter lineage, the Asian strains group as a genotype distinct from the African strains, and analysis of isolates from recent outbreaks suggest that the Indian Ocean strains originated in Kenya and evolved separately from the viruses that spread to Sri Lanka, Singapore, and the Maldives.[301,382,705,839] Analysis of genetic changes over time suggests positive selection driven by cellular immune responses to the virus and enhanced transmissibility by *Ae. albopictus,* an important vector for outbreaks, particularly in rural areas.[301,568,705,800,813,833] Adaptation of endemic Asian strains to *Ae. albopictus* was restricted by interaction between threonine at E1–98 and the adaptive E1–226 alanine to valine substitution. This allowed African strains that had adapted to this vector to replace the endemic strains in many countries[326,568,811,812–813] and possibly increase virulence.[628]

Clinical Features and Pathology

Chikungunya is of sudden onset with an incubation period estimated at 3 to 12 days.[661] No prodrome is recognized.[112] Fever rises rapidly to 103°F to 104°F and may be accompanied by a rigor. The onset of fever corresponds to the period of viremia and may be related to the ability of this virus to induce large amounts of type I IFN[140,255,328,853] (see Fig. 23.7). Monocytes are infected and are a source of IFN during infection.[319] Virus titers in blood can reach greater than 10^6 plaque-forming units (pfu)/mL, and viral load correlates with disease severity and IFN production.[112,140,328,702] Joint pain appears suddenly and can be incapacitating. Essentially any joint can be involved, and pain may be accompanied by swelling and paresthesias.[69,391,569] Headache, conjunctivitis, and gastrointestinal symptoms are common; in 80%, a maculopapular rash appears 4 to 8 days after the initial illness. The rash may be associated with a second rise in fever (see Fig. 23.7), lasts approximately 2 days, and is described as "irritating" or "itchy".[70,661] Atypical cases with severe disease and increased mortality can develop bullous dermatosis, encephalitis, myelopathy, pneumonia, and diabetes.[142,195,778] Fibroblasts in skin and joints and satellite cells in muscle are targets for infection.[155,590] Leukopenia is frequent.[70,140,328,887] Plasma levels of TNF, IFN-γ, and MCP-1 are increased.[672]

Joint pains and myalgias may continue in a milder form for many months after the original illness.[168,668,752] Chronic pain is more likely in females and those older than 60 years with a high viral load during the acute illness.[328,887] Synovial tissue harbors persistently infected perivascular macrophages, fibroblast hyperplasia, activated NK cells, and $CD4^+$ T cells but few $CD8^+$ T cells.[328] Cytokines are increased during the response to infection, and persistent arthralgia is associated with elevated plasma levels of IL-6 and granulocyte macrophage colony-stimulating factor.[139,140,569] Joint x-rays are usually normal or show soft tissue swelling without evidence of bone or joint damage, although erosive arthritis has been reported.[391,495] In India, but not Africa, inguinal lymphadenopathy and red swollen ears are also observed as part of the clinical picture.[112]

Animal Models and Host Range

Mice and nonhuman primates can be infected with CHIKV. In wild-type mice, disease severity is age dependent.[155] Neonatal mice develop fatal disease.[784] Two-week-old mice survive infection but develop weight loss, difficulty walking, myositis, foot swelling, tenosynovitis, and vasculitis.[543,907] Local inoculation of adult mice causes foot swelling associated with macrophage infiltration and production of inflammatory cytokines, particularly TNF, IFN-γ, and MCP-1.[244,672]

Fibroblasts are target cells for CHIKV infection and a major source of IFN-α/β.[702] Adult interferon α/β receptor (IFNAR)- and STAT1-deficient mice develop fatal disease with replication in the liver, muscle, joint, and skin fibroblasts and occasional dissemination to the choroid plexus, leptomeninges, and ependyma of the CNS.[155,157,702] Infection of pregnant mice does not result in fetal infection.[157]

Adult cynomolgus macaques infected intravenously or intradermally develop a dose-dependent viremia, fever, rash, liver enzyme elevation, arthritis, and meningoencephalitis.[428] Peak production of IFN-α/β coincides with peak viremia. Pathology shows persistent mononuclear cell infiltration into lymphatic tissue, joints, muscle, and liver associated with prolonged presence of CHIKV RNA in macrophages at these sites.[428] Pregnant rhesus macaques infected with enzootic West African and epidemic Indian strains of CHIKV develop viremia, rash, joint swelling, leucopenia, and cytokine increases after infection; however, fetuses did not become infected, providing further evidence that transplacental transmission is infrequent.[134]

Diagnosis, Treatment, and Prevention

The primary differential diagnoses for chikungunya fever are dengue and o'nyong-nyong (ONN) fevers. Dengue overlaps the chikungunya geographic distribution extensively but is characterized more by myalgia than arthralgia.[391] ONN is clinically similar but has geographic overlap only in Africa[112] (see Fig. 23.15). Laboratory parameters are variable and not particularly helpful in the diagnosis.[628] CHIKV can be isolated from plasma or detected by nucleic acid amplification during the initial fever.[288,600,668,784] Detection of IgM antibody provides a means of early diagnosis and can persist for months, particularly in those with persistent symptoms.[69,100,288]

Treatment is generally symptomatic with anti-inflammatory agents. Drugs that inhibit MCP-1 synthesis decrease muscle and joint inflammation in mice.[672] Passive transfer of immunoglobulin containing antibody to CHIKV can protect neonatal wild-type mice and IFNAR-/- mice from fatal infection.[156] IFN-α is protective in mice, although only if given prior to infection.[244]

A live attenuated vaccine (TSI-GSD-218) has been developed by passage of a CHIKV isolate from Thailand in MRC-5 cells.[197] This vaccine induces long-term production of neutralizing antibody, can be used to protect laboratory workers from infection,[508] and is undergoing further development.[628] A formalin-inactivated vaccine can elicit protective immune responses in mice.[244,797] Additional approaches to vaccination include DNA, chimeric engineered viruses, and virus-like particles.[18,398,494,617,796,847]

O'nyong-nyong

In 1959, an outbreak of a new disease, originally mistaken for dengue, was reported from northwestern Uganda.[727] It is likely that a similar epidemic occurred in the same region in 1904–1906.[727] The name *o'nyong-nyong* originated from one of the first tribes to be affected—the Acholi—and refers to the painful joints that are characteristic of the disease.[295] During the 1959 outbreak, ONNV was isolated from the serum of a patient with acute arthritis[884] and from anopheline mosquitoes.[886] ONNV is a member of the SFV complex and antigenically is most closely related to CHIKV, from which it is estimated to have diverged thousands of years ago.[627,884] The virus re-emerged in southern Uganda in 1996–1997, suggesting a 30- to 50-year epidemic cycle.[431] In 1967, Igbo Ora, now recognized to be a strain of ONNV,[431,627] was isolated from humans in western Nigeria.[537]

Epidemiology

ONNV causes sporadic, widespread outbreaks of fever, rash, and arthritis with high attack rates. The first epidemic recognized originated in northwestern Uganda in 1959 and spread south and east to Kenya, Tanzania, Zaire, Malawi, Mozambique, and Zambia to affect more than two million people.[885] More recent outbreaks of ONNV/Igbo Ora infection have been documented in West and Central Africa.[60,422,453,622]

The enzootic vector and vertebrate reservoir host for ONNV are unknown. Interepidemic seroconversions and mosquito isolations indicate continuous sporadic transmission in East Africa, and it is possible that humans or nonhuman primates are the primary reservoir.[431] ONNV is transmitted principally by *Anopheles funestus* and *An. gambiae* and is the only alphavirus known to be transmitted by anopheline mosquitoes.[486,886] Human-mosquito-human transmission occurs during epidemics, and spread from one region to another occurs through the movement of viremic humans.[689] The most recent outbreak began near swamps and lakes in the rural Rakai District of south-central Uganda. Serosurveys showed infection rates of 45% to 96% in areas of epidemic transmission, with the ratio of apparent to inapparent infection ranging from 1:4 to 1:24.[453,537,689] All ages and both sexes are equally susceptible.[407] Among domestic animals in the same region, cattle have the highest seroprevalence (40%),[582] although the enzootic reservoir for this virus is not known.

Clinical Features and Pathology

The onset of fever associated with ONNV is sudden and often accompanied by a rigor. The characteristic syndrome includes joint pains, rash, lymphadenitis, and conjunctivitis. Fever is typically moderate (100°F–101°F) and lasts approximately 5 days. Joint pain most often occurs in the knees, although ankles, elbows, wrists, and fingers can also be affected. The pain usually lasts 6 to 7 days and is severe enough to be immobilizing in 80% to 90% of patients but can persist for up to 3 months. The generalized morbilliform maculopapular rash erupts 4 to 7 days after the onset of symptoms and is similar to that of chikungunya. It begins on the face and extends to the trunk and extremities, occasionally affecting the palms. Cervical lymphadenopathy distinguishes the disease from chikungunya, occurs in approximately half of patients, and most frequently involves posterior cervical lymph nodes. Leukopenia is common. Fatalities have not been described; however, morbidity is substantial.[407,453,537,727]

Diagnosis

ONNV is often clinically confused with malaria, measles, dengue, and rubella[622,727] but also resembles chikungunya. Virus can be isolated, or nucleic acid amplified, from blood early in the illness.[60,622,885] Diagnostic serology includes a positive IgM EIA or neutralizing antibody to ONNV that is more than two-fold greater than that to CHIKV.[689] IgM persists for about 60 days after infection.[407]

Ross River

Epidemics of polyarthritis in Australia probably date from at least 1886 but were first clearly described in towns on the Murrumbidgee River in New South Wales in 1928 and then in troops stationed in the Northern Territory and Queensland during World War II.[306,353,489] Serologic studies suggested an alphavirus as the causative agent, and RRV (strain T48) was first isolated from *Ae. vigilax* mosquitoes trapped near the Ross River in Queensland in 1959.[306,489] The first human isolate was made in 1971 from the blood of a child with fever.[184] In 1979, RRV spread from Australia to Fiji, Samoa, and the Cook Islands, causing an explosive outbreak of tens of thousands of cases of polyarthritis on these Pacific islands.[306] Virus was first isolated from the serum of patients with polyarthritis during this epidemic.

Epidemiology

RRV is endemic throughout the coastal regions of much of northern and central Australia and epidemic in the rest of Australia, Papua New Guinea, and the Solomon Islands.[666,790] In general, the Wallace and Weber hypothetical lines in the Indo-Australian archipelago that separate the fauna of the Oriental and Australian regions appear also to separate the geographic distributions of CHIKV and RRV[489] (see Fig. 23.15). RRV is the most common mosquito-borne pathogen in Australia, with approximately 5,000 cases reported each year, an annual incidence of 14 to 50/100,000 population, and 10-year seroconversion rates of 24% in some areas.[676] Cases are most common in the north and occur primarily in late summer and early autumn with some evidence of an increasing incidence.[306,489,676] Two salt marsh–breeding mosquitoes—*Aedes camptorhynchus* and *Ae. vigilax*—are probably the major vectors in coastal regions of Australia.[676] In inland areas, the freshwater-breeding mosquito *Culex annulirostris* is the major vector; in urban areas, *Aedes notoscriptus* appears to be involved in transmission.[676] Various mammals, primarily macropods such as kangaroos and wallabies, and potentially pteropid bats, appear to serve as vertebrate hosts for the enzootic cycle.[116,306,676] In urban areas, horses and brushtail possums are likely involved in transmission.[386]

Morbidity and Mortality

Infection rates can be as high as 1:30 during outbreaks.[489] Estimates of apparent to inapparent infections range from 1:3 to 1:1.[306,772] Seroprevalence and disease incidence are similar in males and females. Clinically apparent infections are rare in children, and the highest incidence of disease is in the 25- to 40-year age group.[306,353]

Origin and Spread of Epidemics

In Australia, outbreaks are seasonal and have been associated with prolonged inundation of salt marshes owing to increased tidal heights or heavy rains during the summer[339,353,489,801,883] and with a loss of herd immunity in reservoir populations.[116] In arid regions, outbreaks often occur within 2 or 3 weeks of heavy rains, suggesting that RRV survives in desiccation-resistant mosquito eggs with vertical transmission.[463] This is further suggested by isolation of RRV from field-caught immature and male *Ae. vigilax* and *Aedes tremulus* mosquitoes.[463] Both urban and rural cycles of transmission occur. Epidemic polyarthritis, initiated by a viremic traveler from Australia to Fiji, spread to several South Pacific Islands between 1979 and 1980 in explosive outbreaks similar to urban chikungunya, with a man-mosquito-man transmission cycle and *Aedes polynesiensis* as the vector.[666,790] Human viremias of more than 10^6 mosquito infectious dose 50 (ID_{50})/mL have been documented.[790] Cases in travelers suggest that RRV has been reintroduced to Fiji.[408]

Molecular Epidemiology

Strains of RRV originally isolated from the northeastern (Queensland), southeastern (New South Wales), and western regions of Australia are antigenically and genetically distinguishable.[371,687,888] However, the northeastern lineage has not been recovered since 1977 and, along with the western lineage, has been replaced by the southeastern lineage.[1,371] This replacement accompanied the appearance of duplication in the C-terminal domain of nsP3 first identified in a virus recovered in 1979 from a patient in Fiji.[1,5] The data suggest genetic divergence and independent evolution of RRV within geographically isolated enzootic foci consistent with mammals as a vertebrate reservoir.[687] However, overall diversity is low, perhaps owing to purifying selection.[371] Sequencing of intrahost populations of RRV reveal substantial diversity and evidence of mixed infections.[467]

Clinical Features and Pathology

RRV infection most often induces fever, arthralgia, and rash (see Fig. 23.6), although not all patients develop all three symptoms.[308,788] Usually the illness has a sudden onset. Fever is the initial symptom, which is low grade, and is typically followed by the onset of pain, swelling, and tenderness in multiple joints. Joint involvement is usually symmetrical, and both small and large joints can be affected. Characteristically, the rash appears on the third or fourth day of illness; is maculopapular, nonpruritic, and present on the face, trunk, and extremities with occasional involvement of the palms and soles; and generally lasts 3 to 4 days.[228] Frequent accompanying signs and symptoms include lymphadenopathy, lethargy, headache, myalgias, and photophobia. The average period of incapacity is 6 weeks, and symptoms gradually resolve in most affected individuals over 3 to 6 months.[304,308]

Examination of synovial fluid shows increased protein; the presence of $CD4^+$ T lymphocytes, monocytes, and activated macrophages; and increased levels of TNF, IFN-γ, and MCP-1.[145,229,460] Cell counts are moderately increased, ranging from 1,500 to 15,000 cells/mm^3,[229] and RRV RNA is present.[747] RRV replicates in, and can cause persistent infection of, synovial macrophages *in vitro.*[854] It is postulated that infection of these cells leads to cytokine production and inflammatory arthritis *in vivo.*[772]

The skin lesions show mononuclear perivascular inflammation without evidence of immune complex deposition. Most of the infiltrating cells are $CD8^+$ T lymphocytes. RRV antigen is present in the basal epidermal and eccrine duct epithelial cells.[230]

Animal Models and Host Range

Despite its extensive host range, RRV induces clinically evident disease only in humans, mice, and horses.[43,783] The prototype T48 strain has been extensively passaged in mice, and virulence is age dependent.[526,554] In newborn mice, T48 infects cardiac muscle, causing myocardial necrosis and death 3 to 4 days after infection.[554,715] One-week-old mice survive, and infection of the CNS leads to demyelination and destruction of the internal granule cell layer of the cerebellum.[715] In 2- to 3-week-old mice, RRV causes myositis, arthritis, and weakness, with virus replication in muscle, perichondrium, periosteum, and skin.[545,554] Macrophages are prominent components of the disease-inducing inflammatory process.[460,673] Soluble mediators that contribute to disease severity include complement, TNF, IFN-α/β, IFN-γ, MCP-1, and macrophage inhibitory factor (MIF).[321,459,460,542,544] Adult mice develop an asymptomatic viremia that persists for 5 to 9 days.[720] In pregnant mice, virus can replicate in the placenta and spread to the fetus.[524]

The less virulent NB5092 strain induces severe myositis and muscle cell death in newborn mice after subcutaneous inoculation.[554] Mice become stiff and unable to move and then gradually regenerate muscle and recover function after virus is cleared.[554] CNS disease is minimal, with patchy infection of ependymal cells and ependymitis leading to hydrocephalus. Neurons are only occasionally infected.[526] Brown fat is another important site of virus replication.[554] By 1 week of age, mice no longer develop signs of disease.[554]

Virulence

To identify determinants of virulence for mice, virulent T48 has been compared to the less virulent NB5092 and DC5692 strains with different passage histories.[206,240] Virulence has been associated primarily with amino acid differences in nsP1 and E2.[379,395,517,783,841,842] Changes in nsP1 affect disease without affecting virus replication, whereas changes in E2 usually affect replication. Induction and susceptibility to IFN also influence disease development.[459] Of unproven but possible significance is the fact that the epidemic strain of RRV in the Pacific differed from the parent Australian strain by a change from Thr to Ala at E2–219 and duplication in nsP3.[1,93]

Diagnosis, Treatment, and Prevention

Diagnosis is aided by geographic location and travel history. The differential diagnosis includes rubella, other alphavirus-induced arthritidies, and Henoch-Schönlein syndrome.[228] Virus can be recovered from blood early in disease[666,790]; however, most diagnoses are made using serology. The most sensitive and commonly used serologic test is an IgM capture EIA that can remain positive for 1 to 2 years after the onset of disease.[115]

In mice, treatment with sulfasalazine to block NFκB or with bindarit to inhibit MCP-1 synthesis decreases inflammation and tissue damage.[460,671] In contrast, treatment with etanercept to block TNF enhances virus replication, inflammation, and tissue damage.[898]

Vector control and personal protection against mosquito bites remain the primary means of prevention.[305,798] An aluminum hydroxide adjuvanted inactivated whole virus vaccine that protects mice from infection and disease induces neutralizing antibody in humans at levels predicted to be protective and is in clinical development.[2,17,330]

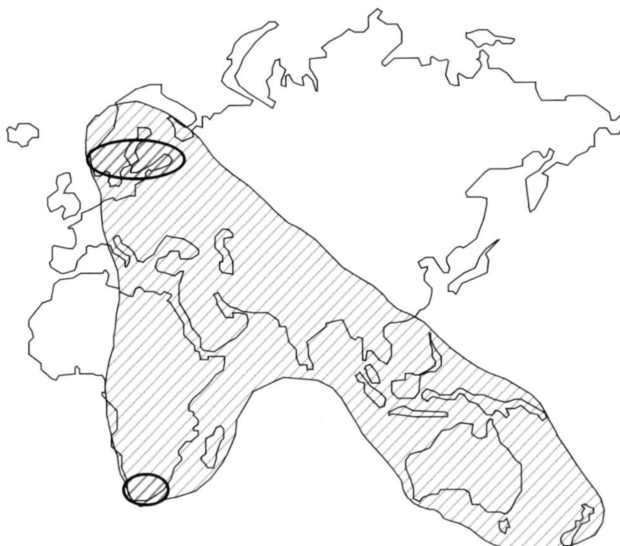

FIGURE 23.17. Geographic distribution of Sindbis virus. Northern Europe and South Africa, regions with significant outbreaks of arthritis, and rash disease in humans are designated in *blue.*

Sindbis

The prototype strain of SINV—AR339—was initially isolated from *Culex univittatus* mosquitoes collected near Sindbis, Egypt, in 1952.[782] Humans living in the Nile Delta at that time had a seroprevalence of 27%, although no disease was associated with infection.[782] Over the next 25 years, SINV was isolated in Europe, the Middle East, Africa, India, Asia, Australia, and the Philippines from various mosquito and vertebrate species. SINV was first isolated from the blood of febrile humans in Uganda in 1961 and recognized in South Africa as a cause of rash and arthritis in 1963.[493]

Epidemiology

SINV is the most widely distributed of the alphaviruses causing arthritis in man (Fig. 23.17). The primary sites of recognized SINV-mediated human disease are in northern Europe (Ockelbo in Sweden, Pogosta fever in Finland, and Karelian fever in Russia)[203] and South Africa.[380] In the many other regions where the virus exists, human infection occurs but results only in subclinical disease, fever, or mild arthralgias. The basic maintenance cycle of SINV is between *Culex* spp. or *Culiseta* spp. mosquitoes and wild birds.[489] In Sweden, the enzootic cycle involves *Culex torrentium, Culiseta morsitans,* and passerine birds.[227,480,482] In Finland, grouse are an important vertebrate host.[425] Vertical transmission in mosquitoes can occur.[176]

Morbidity and Mortality

The age-adjusted prevalence for SINV is 2% to 8% in endemic regions of northern Europe and 0.1% to 0.2% in neighboring nonendemic areas. Risk is highest between the 60th and 64th parallels and is associated with spending time in the woods or marshland and exposure to mosquito bites.[88,203,425,479,691] The ratio of symptomatic to asymptomatic cases is 1:17, with 45- to 65-year-old women most likely to develop disease.[88]

Origin and Spread of Epidemics

Spread of SINV from its enzootic cycle between birds and ornithophilic mosquitoes to humans involves bridge vectors with less specialized feeding habits[817] (see Fig. 23.10). In northern Europe, the primary bridge vector is *Aedes cinereus,* and availability of this species may determine the frequency of human infection. Cases begin to appear in late July and continue into the fall. Large outbreaks occur approximately every 7 years, perhaps in association with fluctuating grouse populations.[479,690]

Molecular Epidemiology

Antigenic and genetic analyses of strains from different locations indicate the presence of five geographically distributed distinct genotypes: Africa and Europe (I), Australia (II), East Asia (III), Azerbaijan and China (IV), and New Zealand (V, Whataroa).[481,482,686,688] Strains isolated in northern Europe and South Africa, where most SINV-induced disease occurs, are more closely related to each other than to strains isolated in south and central Europe and the Middle East, where disease is rare.[372,724] The phylogeographic distribution is consistent with migratory birds as the major vertebrate host.[481,688]

Clinical Features

The primary clinical manifestations are itching rash, arthritis, fever, and muscle pain.[203,424,820] The rash is distributed diffusely over the trunk and limbs and can affect the palms and soles. Skin lesions have a macular base with central vesicle formation and are occasionally hemorrhagic.[203,493] Joint pain preferentially affects large joints and may be severe enough to be immobilizing. Macrophages infected with SINV become activated; release MIF, TNF, IL-1β, and IL-6; and express matrix metalloproteinases.[31] Most patients recover within 14 days; however, joint pain and stiffness may persist for months to years.[203,424,820] In Australia, SINV-induced arthritis and rash is milder and less frequent than RRV-induced disease or SINV-induced disease in northern Europe and Africa.[489]

Animal Models and Host Range

SINV can infect various vertebrates and has been extensively studied in mice as a model for acute encephalitis. In mice, there is an age-dependent susceptibility to fatal encephalitis.[369] In young mice, virus replicates to high titer and spreads rapidly, causing death in 3 to 5 days. In older mice, virus replication is more restricted, and they often recover. After peripheral inoculation, virus replicates in muscle, produces a viremia, and then spreads to the brain and spinal cord, where the primary target cells are neurons.[349] Ability of SINV to spread to the CNS and cause fatal disease depends on the strain of virus and the genetic background of the mouse.[350,483,484,721,792,814] C57BL/6 mice are most susceptible to fatal encephalomyelitis after infection with neurovirulent strains, and this is determined in part by a gene on chromosome 2.[792,793,814] Neuronal death requires contributions of the host, such as glutamate excitotoxicity and immunopathology.[163,273,563,669] Deficiencies of IFN signaling or acid sphingomyelinase increase susceptibility to fatal encephalitis.[95,567]

In nonfatal encephalitis, neutralizing antibody and an SINV-specific perivascular mononuclear inflammatory response consisting of T cells and monocytes appears within 3 to 4 days after infection.[529] Spread of infection is limited initially by IFN-α/β,[95] and infectious virus is cleared within 7 to 8 days after infection, primarily through the effects of antiviral antibody and IFN-γ.[64,89–91,286,448] Viral RNA persists in the CNS after clearance of infectious virus, and reactivation of infection appears to be prevented by continued presence of T lymphocytes and antibody-secreting B cells within the CNS.[285,447,521,821]

Virulence

Strains of SINV differing in virulence have been derived from independent isolates from Egypt (AR339), South Africa (SR86), and Israel (SV-Peleg). Variants of AR339 and SV-Peleg differing in virulence have been derived by passage in mice and in tissue culture.[284,483] Virulence is determined primarily by the 5′ NTR and the E2 glycoprotein but can be influenced by changes in E1 and the nsPs.[165,485,513,773] Changes in nucleotide 5 or 8 from A to G increase neurovirulence by unknown mechanisms.[188,513] Several amino acid changes in the E2 glycoprotein affect virulence by altering efficiency of virus entry into the CNS or by enhancing neuronal infection.[54,165,438,815] Neuroinvasion is affected by changes at residues 55 and 190 of E2.[188] A Gln to His change at E2-55 increases efficiency of infection of neurons and is a major determinant of increased virulence in older mice.[438,815]

Diagnosis, Treatment, and Prevention

The major differential in SINV is with other causes of acute rash and arthritis, such as parvovirus B19 and rubella. The virus can be recovered from skin lesions and from blood[423,424,493]; however, the diagnosis is most often made by serology. SINV-specific IgM increases during the acute phase of the disease and then tends to decrease slowly for 3 to 4 years, independent of persistent symptoms.[571]

Mice can be protected from fatal encephalitis by treatment with drugs that inhibit inflammation and glutamate excitotoxicity.[273,348,631] Mice can also be passively protected with antibody but develop progressive destruction of infected regions of the brain.[399]

Barmah Forest

Barmah Forest virus (BFV) was first isolated in 1974 from *Cx. annulirostris* mosquitoes collected in the Barmah Forest in the Murray River Valley region of southeastern Australia and soon thereafter in southwest Queensland.[25] It is the only recognized member of the BFV complex and has a unique E2 protein without N-linked glycosylation.[418,437] Human disease was first reported in 1986 with an epidemic of polyarthritis in New South Wales,[71] and BFV was first isolated from the blood of a patient in 1988.[609] The geographic range of BFV is expanding.[802] In 1989, BFV—previously restricted to eastern portions of Australia—was isolated in western Australia with subsequent outbreaks of human disease.[464]

The vertebrate reservoir host is unknown; however, serosurveys suggest that horses and marsupials, particularly brushtail possums, may play a role.[386,464] On the other hand, sequence analysis shows a high degree of homology over the geographic distribution consistent with an avian vertebrate host.[620] The main mosquito vectors are not well established but appear to include *Cx. annulirostris, Ae. vigilax, Ae. notoscriptus,* and *Ae. camptorhynchus.*[352,464] Transmission in coastal areas is influenced by temperature, tides, and socioeconomic factors.[562]

Disease is most common in the 30- to 50-year age group, with men and women equally affected.[55] The most common clinical features are fever, lethargy, polyarthritis, and myalgia accompanied by a vesicular rash.[25,55,609] Diagnosis may not be made because the illness is frequently mild and overlaps the clinical spectrum and geographic distribution of RRV and SINV infections (see Figs. 23.15 and 23.17). Rash is more prominent in BFV, whereas arthritis is more prominent in RRV[216] and the serology is distinct.[609] In over half of infected individuals, recovery takes several weeks, with lethargy the most prominent persisting symptom.[55]

Mayaro and Una

Mayaro virus was first isolated in 1954 from febrile forest workers in Trinidad and then from several individuals with fever and frontal headache in the Guama River area of Brazil.[22,122] The virus is widely distributed in South America.[220,505,791] Human cases are sporadic and occur primarily in persons with recent contact with humid tropical forests.[805] There are two distinct genotypes. Genotype D contains isolates from Trinidad and north central South America, and genotype L contains isolates from Brazil.[624] The principal mosquito vectors are in the forest-dwelling genus *Haemagogus,* and the vertebrate hosts are mammals, mainly nonhuman primates. Airborne transmission to laboratory personnel has also occurred.[378] Symptoms include fever, headache, arthralgia, myalgia, vomiting, diarrhea, and rash that last from 3 to 5 days.[505] The diagnosis can be made by isolation of virus from blood or by serology using an IgM capture EIA.[100] Una virus is closely related to Mayaro virus and was first isolated from *Psoraphora ferox* mosquitoes in the Amazonian region of Brazil in 1959.[121] It is widely distributed in Central and South America.[121,178,179] Vertebrate hosts include nonhuman primates.[178] This virus is pathogenic for mice but is not recognized to cause human disease.

OTHER ALPHAVIRUSES

Semliki Forest

SFV was first isolated in 1942 from *Aedes abnormalis* collected in the Semliki Forest of western Uganda.[743] It is widely distributed in Africa with mosquito (e.g., *Ae. africanus, Aedes argenteopunctatus*) isolates documented from Mozambique, Nigeria, and the Central African Republic.[491,504,511] Although SFV is one of the most extensively studied of the alphaviruses and serosurveys indicate that human infection is relatively common,[333,504,743] SFV has been linked to human disease on only two occasions. In the first case, reported in 1979, a 26-year-old laboratory worker in Germany with a 1-year history of "purulent bronchitis" working with the Osterrieth strain of SFV developed fever and headache followed by seizures, coma, and death from encephalitis. SFV was isolated from CSF and from brain. No antiviral antibody was detectable at the time the CNS symptoms began, although it was detected at the time of death 1 week later.[882] The history of chronic pulmonary infections and failure to produce antiviral antibody rapidly suggest that this individual had an immunodeficiency disorder involving antibody production. In 1987, SFV was isolated from serum samples of individuals in the Central African Republic with fever, persistent headache, myalgias, and arthralgias.[504]

Animal Models

SFV can cause encephalitis in horses, mice, rats, hamsters, rabbits, and guinea pigs.[36,75,743,908] Severity and type of disease depend on the age of the animal at the time of infection, the route of inoculation, and the virulence of the strain of SFV used for infection.[75,287] Mice have been most extensively studied, and the strain of inbred mouse infected can also influence outcome.[769]

In newborn and suckling mice inoculated peripherally, virulent and avirulent strains of SFV replicate rapidly and extensively in muscle, elicit a high-titered viremia, spread to the CNS, and cause death within 2 to 4 days.[208,287,553] Evidence suggests that SFV enters the brain across cerebrovascular endothelial cells.[208,396,748] Once within the CNS, the virus replicates primarily in neurons and spreads rapidly along neural pathways, producing neuronal cell death.[584]

In weanling (3- to 5-week-old) mice, SFV replicates rapidly but reaches lower peak titers in muscle, blood, and brain than in younger animals.[287] Virus enters perivascular regions of the brain and initiates foci of infection within the CNS. After intranasal inoculation, virus infects olfactory neurons first and then spreads within the CNS.[584] The primary target cells in the brain are neurons, although oligodendrocytes are also infected.[36,208,396] Neurons control virus replication more effectively than oligodendrocytes.[226] A mononuclear inflammatory response consisting of T lymphocytes, B lymphocytes, and monocytes is apparent 3 to 4 days after infection, peaks at 2 to 3 weeks, and is mostly resolved by 6 weeks.[541]

Mice infected with virulent strains can be passively protected from fatal encephalitis with immune serum but then develop a delayed disease associated with persistent infection, inflammation, and neuronal degeneration.[712] Mice that survive infection develop demyelination, which is accompanied by mild paralysis, 2 to 4 weeks after infection.[138,770] Clearance of infectious virus is complete 7 to 10 days after infection, and this clearance is mediated by antibody.[208] Viral RNA and protein persist for months.[186,396] Focal areas of demyelination are found 14 to 21 days after SFV infection and are characterized initially by swelling and vacuolation of oligodendrocytes and loss of myelin sheaths followed by remyelination.[94] Demyelination is macrophage mediated and appears to be the result of oligodendrocyte infection, the immune response to infection, and induction of an autoimmune response to myelin.[209,532,768] SJL mice have prolonged inflammatory responses and demyelination after infection compared with other strains of mice.[186,744]

SFV infection of the CNS can also increase the susceptibility of mice to induction of experimental autoimmune encephalomyelitis,[533] apparently by damaging the blood–brain barrier, increasing adhesion molecule expression on endothelial cells, and facilitating entry of autoimmune T lymphocytes into the CNS.[748,749]

Virulence

Isolates from mosquitoes collected in 1942 in Bwamba, Uganda,[743] in 1948 in Kumba, Nigeria,[491] and in 1959 in Namacurra, Mozambique[511] have given rise to various laboratory strains of SFV with differing levels of virulence. The most commonly studied are virulent strains V12, V13, and L10 (Uganda strain independently passaged in mice in Bethesda [V] and London [L]) and avirulent strain A7 (Mozambique strain AR2066 passaged in mice) and its less virulent derivative A7-74.[75] In addition, avirulent strains of L10 have been derived by chemical mutagenesis (e.g., m9).[48] Virulent and avirulent strains differ in their ability to invade and replicate in the CNS of weanling mice and rats after peripheral inoculation, although all strains cause fatal disease in newborn or suckling mice.[36,208,287,553] In 3- to 4-week-old mice, avirulent SFV is restricted in replication and spread in the CNS compared to virulent strains of virus and compared to avirulent strains in younger mice.[585] This difference in replication is associated with decreased budding of infectious virus and is independent of the host immune response.[208] Mature neurons and pancreatic and myocardial cells can be made more susceptible to avirulent virus by treatment with aurothiomalate compounds that induce intracellular membrane proliferation.[208,700] In general, reduced virulence correlates with reduced replication in neurons.[44]

In vitro studies of the differences between virulent and avirulent strains of SFV have shown differential replication in neuronal cells[34] and differences in susceptibility to IFN.[174] Efforts to identify specific nucleotide and amino acid changes important for virulence have utilized comparative sequence analysis and an infectious SFV cDNA clone pSP6-SFV4 derived from the prototype virulent L10 strain. Construction of SFV4/A7 chimeric viruses has shown that determinants of virulence reside in both the structural and nonstructural regions of the genome.[779] E2, nsP2, and nsP3 are important determinants of virulence.[208,256,259,658,693]

Other Semliki Forest–Related Viruses

The SFV complex includes eight viruses and has representatives in both the Old World (Bebaru virus, chikungunya, Getah, ONN, Ross River, and Simliki Forest) and the New World (Mayaro and Una) (see Table 23.1 and Fig. 23.5). Recently identified southern elephant seal virus is phylogenetically, but not antigenically, related to SFV. Human disease, when present, is generally characterized by fever that may be accompanied by arthritis and rash. CHIKV, ONNV, RRV, and SFV have been discussed previously.

Getah

Getah virus was first isolated from *Culex* spp. mosquitoes collected in Malaysia in 1955 and causes myositis when inoculated into mice.[325] It is maintained in a cycle similar to Japanese encephalitis virus with transmission by *Culex tritaeniorhynchus* and amplification in domestic pigs.[735] Getah virus is widespread and ranges from Eurasia to Southeast and Far East Asia, the Pacific Islands, and Australasia. Disease in humans is limited to fever,[456] although it causes abortion in pigs and is an important pathogen of horses.[717] The equine disease is characterized by fever, an urticarial rash, and hind leg edema but is not life threatening.[717]

Southern Elephant Seal

Southern elephant seal virus was isolated from lice residing on southern elephant seals on Macquarie Island, Australia. It is phylogenetically related to SFV but does not cross-react serologically. No disease has been recognized in infected seals.[427]

Salmonid Alphavirus

Salmonid alphavirus (SAV) causes sleeping disease in rainbow trout and pancreas disease in farmed Atlantic salmon.[329,836,875,876] SAV has unusually large E1 and E2 structural glycoproteins and relatively low (30%–34%) homology to other alphaviruses.[836,876] Six subtypes have been identified.[745] Subtypes 1, 4, and 5 are closely related and have been isolated from farms in Britain with pancreas disease. Subtype 2 causes sleeping disease in Europe, and subtype 3 causes disease on salmon farms in Norway. Subtype 6 is represented by a single isolate from Ireland. SAV causes significant disease on fish farms, which is characterized by abnormal swimming behavior and lack of appetite. Histopathology shows degeneration of the pancreas and of cardiac and skeletal muscles.[515] SAV is shed in feces and mucus and can be horizontally transmitted.[268] Sea lice can be infected; however, their role in transmission is unclear.[606] Subtype 5 SAV RNA sequences have been detected in wild marine fish, suggesting that marine reservoirs exist.[746]

DIAGNOSIS

The differential diagnosis of alphavirus-induced diseases often includes more than one alphavirus in addition to other mosquito-borne viral diseases such as dengue and West Nile fevers, other rash diseases such as rubella and parvovirus B19, and other causes of encephalitis. IgM capture EIAs can be used for diagnosis early in disease.[99,100,103] The IgM response is relatively specific for each antigenic complex and is useful even at later times, because IgM persists for at least 2 to 3 weeks after onset of disease.[100] Virus isolation and identification remain useful; however, nucleic acid amplification tests have simplified virus identification in clinical samples.[630] RT-PCR primers have been designed that can amplify the conserved region of all alphaviruses,[201,290,608] as well as alphavirus-specific regions,[430] and should be useful for rapid diagnosis.

PREVENTION AND CONTROL

Treatment

At this time, there is no available specific antiviral treatment for any alphavirus-induced disease, although compound screening has identified potential antiviral therapies for evaluation in animals.[170,374,377,593,604,619,645] Therapeutic MAbs and immune system activators are being evaluated in animal models.[341,470] Several neuroprotective drugs protect mice from fatal encephalitis.[163,273,348,563,631] Supportive treatment for those with encephalitis can be lifesaving because individuals may make remarkable recoveries from coma. Symptomatic treatment for arthritis with anti-inflammatory drugs and immune modulators can be beneficial.

Vaccines

Formalin-inactivated vaccines against EEE, WEE, and VEE are available for horses and against EEE for birds. Experimental inactivated vaccines against EEE, WEE, and VEE are also available for laboratory workers exposed to these agents, with yearly booster doses required for EEE and WEE.[196] PE-6—the investigational inactivated EEE vaccine for humans—induces good immunoreactivity against the NA-EEEV but not SA-EEEV.[767] An inactivated VEE vaccine that uses the V3526 strain is under evaluation,[500] and an inactivated RRV vaccine is in human trials.[17]

Live attenuated vaccines have been developed for VEEV (TC-83) and CHIKV.[450] Substantial side effects are common after immunization with TC-83,[196,616] and new attenuated strains are under investigation.[594,643] Alternative approaches in preclinical development include MAbs, DNA vaccines, chimeric alphaviruses, alphavirus replicons, and adenovirus-vectored vaccines.[191,192,263,340,594,774] In both horses and humans, prior vaccination against one alphavirus can interfere with development of neutralizing antibody to subsequent alphavirus vaccines.[106,181,508,615]

Other

Prevention of infection with most alphaviruses relies primarily on efforts to control mosquito populations by spraying and reducing breeding places. Various means can be used for assessing the need for mosquito abatement. These include monitoring mosquito population densities, seroconversion of sentinel animals, and presence of virus in populations of mosquitoes capable of transmitting virus to humans or domestic animals. Individual use of protective measures, such as mosquito repellents and protective clothing, are important.

PERSPECTIVE

The ability to construct full-length cDNA alphavirus clones that can be transcribed into infectious RNA has advanced understanding of the functions of various genes and their importance for replication and virulence in the multiple hosts necessary for maintenance of these viruses in their natural cycles. An understanding of the three-dimensional structures of proteins in the virion has greatly aided interpretation of much of the sequence and virulence data previously acquired. Further sequence information on virulent and avirulent strains, functional and structural analysis of the nsPs, and assessment of host–cell interactions is likely to provide the next level of understanding of virus–host relationships.

In addition, there is a need for improved approaches to prevention and treatment. There is a particular need for understanding the components of the immune response necessary for noncytolytic virus clearance, protection from reinfection, and immune modulation of disease. New and improved vaccines are needed for protection during outbreaks and for laboratory workers. In addition, there is a need for effective anti-alphaviral drugs, and an understanding of the structure of viral proteins may offer new approaches to therapeutics. Both of these areas have implications for biological defense purposes, because many alphaviruses can be transmitted by aerosol and VEEV, EEEV, and WEEV are on the U.S. Centers for Disease Control and Prevention category B list of critical biological agents.[124]

REFERENCES

All cited references are available in the e-book.

1. Aaskov J, Jones A, Choi W, et al. Lineage replacement accompanying duplication and rapid fixation of an RNA element in the nsP3 gene in a species of alphavirus. *Virology* 2011;410:353–359.
5. Aaskov JG, Mataika JU, Lawrence GW, et al. An epidemic of Ross River virus infection in Fiji, 1979. *Am J Trop Med Hyg* 1981;30:1053–1059.

7. Agapov EV, Frolov I, Lindenbach BD, et al. Noncytopathic Sindbis virus RNA vectors for heterologous gene expression. *Proc Natl Acad Sci U S A* 1998;95:12989–12994.
11. Aguilar PV, Estrada-Franco JG, Navarro-Lopez R, et al. Endemic Venezuelan equine encephalitis in the Americas: hidden under the dengue umbrella. *Future Virol* 2011;6:721–740.
14. Aguilar PV, Weaver SC, Basler CF. Capsid protein of eastern equine encephalitis virus inhibits host cell gene expression. *J Virol* 2007;81:3866–3876.
15. Ahn A, Klimjack MR, Chatterjee PK, et al. An epitope of the Semliki Forest virus fusion protein exposed during virus-membrane fusion. *J Virol* 1999;73:10029–10039.
17. Aichinger G, Ehrlich HJ, Aaskov JG, et al. Safety and immunogenicity of an inactivated whole virus Vero cell-derived Ross River virus vaccine: A randomized trial. *Vaccine* 2011;29:9376–9384.
22. Anderson CR, Downs WG, Wattley GH, et al. Mayaro virus: a new human disease agent. II. Isolation from blood of patients in Trinidad, B.W.I. *Am J Trop Med Hyg* 1957;6:1012–1016.
23. Anishchenko M, Bowen RA, Paessler S, et al. Venezuelan encephalitis emergence mediated by a phylogenetically predicted viral mutation. *Proc Natl Acad Sci U S A* 2006;103:4994–4999.
27. Armstrong PM, Andreadis TG. Eastern equine encephalitis virus in mosquitoes and their role as bridge vectors. *Emerg Infect Dis* 2010;16:1869–1874.
29. Arrigo NC, Adams AP, Weaver SC. Evolutionary patterns of eastern equine encephalitis virus in North versus South America suggest ecological differences and taxonomic revision. *J Virol* 2010;84:1014–1025.
37. Attarzadeh-Yazdi G, Fragkoudis R, Chi Y, et al. Cell-to-cell spread of the RNA interference response suppresses Semliki Forest virus (SFV) infection of mosquito cell cultures and cannot be antagonized by SFV. *J Virol* 2009;83:5735–5748.
49. Barry G, Breakwell L, Fragkoudis R, et al. PKR acts early in infection to suppress Semliki Forest virus production and strongly enhances the type I interferon response. *J Gen Virol* 2009;90:1382–1391.
50. Barry G, Fragkoudis R, Ferguson MC, et al. Semliki Forest virus-induced endoplasmic reticulum stress accelerates apoptotic death of mammalian cells. *J Virol* 2010;84:7369–7377.
54. Bear JS, Byrnes AP, Griffin DE. Heparin-binding and patterns of virulence for two recombinant strains of Sindbis virus. *Virology* 2006;347:183–190.
56. Beck CE, Wyckoff RWG. Venezuelan equine encephalomyelitis. *Science* 1938;88:530.
58. Berge TO, Banks IS, Tigertt WD. Attenuation of Venezuelan equine encephalomyelitis virus by in vitro cultivation in guinea-pig heart cells. *Am J Hyg* 1961;73:209–218.
63. Bick MJ, Carroll JW, Gao G, et al. Expression of the zinc-finger antiviral protein inhibits alphavirus replication. *J Virol* 2003;77:11555–11562.
64. Binder G, Griffin DE. Interferon-γ–mediated site specific clearance of alphavirus from CNS neurons. *Science* 2001;293:303–306.
65. Boere WAM, Benaissa-Trouw BJ, Harmsen M, et al. Neutralizing and nonneutralizing monoclonal antibodies to the E2 glycoprotein of Semliki Forest virus can protect mice from lethal encephalitis. *J Gen Virol* 1983;64:1405–1408.
69. Borgherini G, Poubeau P, Jossaume A, et al. Persistent arthralgia associated with chikungunya virus: a study of 88 adult patients on reunion island. *Clin Infect Dis* 2008;47:469–475.
76. Brault AC, Armijos MV, Wheeler S, et al. Stone Lakes virus (family Togaviridae, genus Alphavirus), a variant of Fort Morgan virus isolated from swallow bugs (Hemiptera: Cimicidae) west of the Continental Divide. *J Med Entomol* 2009;46:1203–1209.
79. Brault AC, Powers AM, Holmes EC, et al. Positively charged amino acid substitutions in the E2 envelope glycoprotein are associated with the emergence of Venezuelan equine encephalitis virus. *J Virol* 2002;76:1718–1730.
80. Brault AC, Powers AM, Ortiz D, et al. Venezuelan equine encephalitis emergence: enhanced vector infection from a single amino acid substitution in the envelope glycoprotein. *Proc Natl Acad Sci U S A* 2004;101:11344–11349.
81. Breakwell L, Dosenovic P, Karlsson Hedestam GB, et al. Semliki Forest virus nonstructural protein 2 is involved in suppression of the type I interferon response. *J Virol* 2007;81:8677–8684.
84. Brooke CB, Deming DJ, Whitmore AC, et al. T cells facilitate recovery from Venezuelan equine encephalitis virus-induced encephalomyelitis in the absence of antibody. *J Virol* 2010;84:4556–4568.
89. Burdeinick-Kerr R, Govindarajan D, Griffin DE. Noncytolytic clearance of Sindbis virus infection from neurons by gamma interferon is dependent on Jak/STAT signaling. *J Virol* 2009;83:3429–3435.
91. Burdeinick-Kerr R, Wind J, Griffin D. The synergistic roles of antibody and interferon in noncytolytic clearance of Sindbis virus from different regions of the central nervous system. *J Virol* 2007;81:5628–5636.
96. Byrnes AP, Griffin DE. Binding of Sindbis virus to cell-surface heparan sulfate. *J Virol* 1998;72:7349–7356.
97. Byrnes AP, Griffin DE. Large-plaque mutants of Sindbis virus show reduced binding to heparan sulfate, heightened viremia and slower clearance from the circulation. *J Virol* 2000;74:644–651.
98. Calisher CH. Medically important arboviruses of the United States and Canada. *Clin Microbiol Rev* 1994;7:89–116.
100. Calisher CH, El-Kafrawi AO, Al-Deen Mahmud MI, et al. Complex-specific immunoglobulin M antibody patterns in humans infected with alphaviruses. *J Clin Microbiol* 1986;23:155–159.
105. Calisher CH, Monath TP, Muth DJ, et al. Characterization of Fort Morgan virus, an alphavirus of the western equine encephalitis virus complex in an unusual ecosystem. *Am J Trop Med Hyg* 1980;29:1428–1440.
109. Campbell CL, Keene KM, Brackney DE, et al. *Aedes aegypti* uses RNA interference in defense against Sindbis virus infection. *BMC Microbiol* 2008;8:47.
121. Causey OR, Casals J, Shope RE, et al. Aura and Una, two new group A arthropod-borne viruses. *Am J Trop Med Hyg* 1963;12:777–781.
127. Chamberlain RW, Rubin H, Kissling RE, et al. Recovery of virus of eastern equine encephalomyelitis from a mosquito, *Culiseta melanura* (Coquillett). *Proc Soc Exp Biol Med* 1951;77:396–397.
133. Charles PC, Walters E, Margolis F, et al. Mechanism of neuroinvasion of Venezuelan equine encephalitis virus in the mouse. *Virology* 1995;208:662–671.
135. Chen G, Guo X, Lv F, et al. p72 DEAD box RNA helicase is required for optimal function of the zinc-finger antiviral protein. *Proc Natl Acad Sci U S A* 2008;105:4352–4357.
137. Chevillon C, Briant L, Renaud F, et al. The chikungunya threat: an ecological and evolutionary perspective. *Trends Microbiol* 2008;16:80–88.
138. Chew-Lim M, Suckling AJ, Webb HE. Demyelination in mice after two or three infections with avirulent Semliki Forest virus. *Vet Pathol* 1977;14:67–72.
140. Chow A, Her Z, Ong EK, et al. Persistent arthralgia induced by Chikungunya virus infection is associated with interleukin-6 and granulocyte macrophage colony-stimulating factor. *J Infect Dis* 2011;203:149–157.
141. Chung BY, Firth AE, Atkins JF. Frameshifting in alphaviruses: a diversity of 3′ stimulatory structures. *J Mol Biol* 2010;397:448–456.
143. Cirimotich CM, Scott JC, Phillips AT, et al. Suppression of RNA interference increases alphavirus replication and virus-associated mortality in Aedes aegypti mosquitoes. *BMC Microbiol* 2009;9:49.
147. Coffey LL, Beeharry Y, Borderia AV, et al. Arbovirus high fidelity variant loses fitness in mosquitoes and mice. *Proc Natl Acad Sci U S A* 2011;108:16038–16043.
149. Coffey LL, Vasilakis N, Brault AC, et al. Arbovirus evolution in vivo is constrained by host alternation. *Proc Natl Acad Sci U S A* 2008;105:6970–6975.
162. Dalrymple JM, Young OP, Eldridge BF, et al. Ecology of arboviruses in a Maryland freshwater swamp. III.Vertebrate hosts. *Am J Epidemiol* 1972;96:129–140.
164. Davey MW, Dalgarno L. Semliki Forest virus replication in cultured *Aedes albopictus* cells: studies on the establishment of persistence. *J Gen Virol* 1974;24:453–463.
173. Despres P, Griffin JW, Griffin DE. Effects of anti-E2 monoclonal antibody on Sindbis virus replication in AT3 cells expressing bcl-2. *J Virol* 1995;69:7006–7014.
184. Doherty RL, Carley JG, Best JC. Isolation of Ross River virus from man. *Med J Aust* 1972;1:1083–1084.
187. Dryga SA, Dryga OA, Schlesinger S. Identification of mutations in a Sindbis virus variant able to establish persistent infection in BHK cells: the importance of a mutation in the nsP2 gene. *Virology* 1997;228:74–83.
190. Dulbecco R. Production of plaques in monolayer tissue cultures by single particles of an animal virus. *Pathology* 1952;38:747–752.

195. Economopoulou A, Dominguez M, Helynck B, et al. Atypical Chikungunya virus infections: clinical manifestations, mortality and risk factors for severe disease during the 2005–2006 outbreak on Reunion. *Epidemiol Infect* 2009;137:534–541.
196. Edelman R, Ascher MS, Oster CN, et al. Evaluation in humans of a new, inactivated vaccine for Venezuelan equine encephalitis virus (C-84). *J Infect Dis* 1979;140:708–715.
197. Edelman R, Tacket CO, Wasserman SS, et al. Phase II safety and immunogenicity study of live chikungunya virus vaccine TSI-GSD-218. *Am J Trop Med Hyg* 2000;62:681–685.
198. Ehrenkranz NJ, Ventura AK. Venezuelan equine encephalitis virus infection in man. *Ann Rev Med* 1974;25:9–14.
203. Espmark A, Niklasson B. Ockelbo disease in Sweden: Epidemiological, clinical and virological data from the 1982 outbreak. *Am J Trop Med Hyg* 1984;33:1203–1211.
207. Farber S, Hill A, Connerly ML, et al. Encephalitis in infants and children caused by the virus of the eastern variety of equine encephalitis. *J Am Med Assoc* 1940;114:1725–1731.
215. Firth AE, Chung BY, Fleeton MN, et al. Discovery of frameshifting in Alphavirus 6K resolves a 20-year enigma. *Virol J* 2008;5:108.
217. Forrester NL, Guerbois M, Adams AP, et al. Analysis of intrahost variation in Venezuelan equine encephalitis virus reveals repeated deletions in the 6-kilodalton protein gene. *J Virol* 2011;85:8709–8717.
218. Forrester NL, Kenney JL, Deardorff E, et al. Western equine encephalitis submergence: lack of evidence for a decline in virus virulence. *Virology* 2008;380:170–172.
219. Forrester NL, Palacios G, Tesh RB, et al. Genome-scale phylogeny of the alphavirus genus suggests a marine origin. *J Virol* 2012;86(5):2729–2738.
222. Fothergill LRD, Dingle JH, Farber S, et al. Human encephalitis caused by the virus of the eastern variety of equine encephalomyelitis. *N Engl J Med* 1939;219:411–422.
223. Fragkoudis R, Ballany CM, Boyd A, et al. In Semliki Forest virus encephalitis, antibody rapidly clears infectious virus and is required to eliminate viral material from the brain, but is not required to generate lesions of demyelination. *J Gen Virol* 2008;89:2565–2568.
234. Frolov I, Schlesinger S. Comparison of the effects of Sindbis virus and Sindbis virus replicons on host cell protein synthesis and cytopathogenicity in BHK cells. *J Virol* 1994;68:1721–1727.
236. Fros JJ, Liu WJ, Prow NA, et al. Chikungunya virus nonstructural protein 2 inhibits type I/II interferon-stimulated JAK-STAT signaling. *J Virol* 2010;84:10877–10887.
242. Gardner CL, Ebel GD, Ryman KD, et al. Heparan sulfate binding by natural eastern equine encephalitis viruses promotes neurovirulence. *Proc Natl Acad Sci U S A* 2011;108:16026–16031.
251. Giannakopoulos NV, Arutyunova E, Lai C, et al. ISG15 Arg151 and the ISG15-conjugating enzyme UbE1L are important for innate immune control of Sindbis virus. *J Virol* 2009;83:1602–1610.
265. Gorchakov R, Frolova E, Williams BR, et al. PKR-dependent and -independent mechanisms are involved in translational shutoff during Sindbis virus infection. *J Virol* 2004;78:8455–8467.
273. Greene IP, Lee E-Y, Prow NA, et al. Protection from fatal viral encephalomyelitis: AMPA receptor antagonists have a direct effect on the inflammatory response to infection. *Proc Natl Acad Sci U S A* 2008;105:3575–3580.
275. Greene IP, Paessler S, Austgen L, et al. Envelope glycoprotein mutations mediate equine amplification and virulence of epizootic Venezuelan equine encephalitis virus. *J Virol* 2005;79:9128–9133.
280. Griffin DE. Role of the immune response in age-dependent resistance of mice to encephalitis due to Sindbis virus. *J Infect Dis* 1976;133:456–464.
284. Griffin DE, Johnson RT. Role of the immune response in recovery from Sindbis virus encephalitis in mice. *J Immunol* 1977;118:1070–1075.
285. Griffin DE, Metcalf T. Clearance of virus infection from the CNS. *Curr Opin Virol* 2011;1:216–221.
290. Grywna K, Kupfer B, Panning M, et al. Detection of all species of the genus Alphavirus by reverse transcription-PCR with diagnostic sensitivity. *J Clin Microbiol* 2010;48:3386–3387.
292. Guo X, Ma J, Sun J, et al. The zinc-finger antiviral protein recruits the RNA processing exosome to degrade the target mRNA. *Proc Natl Acad Sci U S A* 2007;104:151–156.
295. Haddow AJ, Davies CW, Walker AJ. O'nyong-nyong fever: An epidemic virus disease in East Africa. I. Introduction. *Trans R Soc Trop Med Hyg* 1960;54:517–522.
297. Hahn CS, Lustig S, Strauss EG, et al. Western equine encephalitis virus is a recombinant virus. *Proc Natl Acad Sci U S A* 1988;85:5997–6001.
306. Harley D, Sleigh A, Ritchie S. Ross River virus transmission, infection, and disease: a cross-disciplinary review. *Clin Microbiol Rev* 2001;14: 909–932.
307. Havert MB, Schofield B, Griffin DE, et al. Activation of divergent neuronal cell death pathways in different target cell populations during neuroadapted Sindbis virus infection of mice. *J Virol* 2000;74:5352–5356.
321. Herrero LJ, Nelson M, Srikiatkhachorn A, et al. Critical role for macrophage migration inhibitory factor (MIF) in Ross River virus-induced arthritis and myositis. *Proc Natl Acad Sci U S A* 2011;108:12048–12053.
328. Hoarau JJ, Jaffar Bandjee MC, Krejbich TP, et al. Persistent chronic inflammation and infection by chikungunya arthritogenic alphavirus in spite of a robust host immune response. *J Immunol* 2010;184:5914–5927.
331. Hommel D, Heraud JM, Hulin A, et al. Association of Tonate virus (subtype IIIB of the Venezuelan equine encephalitis complex) with encephalitis in a human. *Clin Infect Dis* 2000;30:188–190.
333. Horling J, Vene S, Franzen C, et al. Detection of Ockelbo virus RNA in skin biopsies by polymerase chain reaction. *J Clin Microbiol* 1993;31: 2004–2009.
335. Howitt B. Recovery of the virus of equine encephalomyelitis from the brain of a child. *Science* 1938;88:455–456.
336. Howitt BF. Equine encephalitis. *J Infect Dis* 1932;51:493–510.
337. Howitt BF, Dodge HR, Bishop LK, et al. Recovery of the virus of eastern equine encephalomyelitis from mosquitoes (*Mansonia perturbans*) collected in Georgia. *Science* 1949;110:141–142.
347. Irani DN, Griffin DE. Regulation of lymphocyte homing into the brain during viral encephalitis at various states of infection. *J Immunol* 1996;156:3850–3857.
349. Jackson AC, Moench TR, Griffin DE. The pathogenesis of spinal cord involvement in the encephalomyelitis of mice caused by neuroadapted Sindbis virus infection. *Lab Invest* 1987;56:418–423.
350. Jackson AC, Moench TR, Trapp BD, et al. Basis of neurovirulence in Sindbis virus encephalomyelitis of mice. *Lab Invest* 1988;58:503–509.
352. Jacups SP, Whelan PI, Currie BJ. Ross River virus and Barmah Forest virus infections: a review of history, ecology, and predictive models, with implications for tropical northern Australia. *Vector Borne Zoonotic Dis* 2008;8:283–297.
355. Jahrling PB, Gorelkin L. Selective clearance of a benign clone of Venezuelan equine encephalitis virus from hamster plasma by hepatic reticuloendothelial cells. *J Infect Dis* 1975;132:667–676.
361. Jahrling PB, Stephenson EH. Protective efficacies of live attenuated and formaldehyde-inactivated Venezuelan equine encephalitis virus vaccines against aerosol challenge in hamsters. *J Clin Microbiol* 1984;19 :429–431.
366. Joe AK, Foo H, Kleeman L, et al. The transmembrane domains of Sindbis virus envelope glycoproteins induce cell death. *J Virol* 1998;72: 3935–3943.
369. Johnson RT, McFarland HF, Levy SE. Age-dependent resistance to viral encephalitis: Studies of infections due to Sindbis virus in mice. *J Infect Dis* 1972;125:257–262.
379. Jupille HJ, Oko L, Stoermer KA, et al. Mutations in nsP1 and PE2 are critical determinants of Ross River virus-induced musculoskeletal inflammatory disease in a mouse model. *Virology* 2011;410:216–227.
380. Jupp PG, Blackburn NK, Thompson DL, et al. Sindbis and West Nile virus infections in the Witwatersrand-Pretoria region. *S Afr Med J* 1986; 70:218–220.
383. Karpf AR, Brown DT. Comparison of Sindbis virus-induced pathology in mosquito and vertebrate cell cultures. *Virology* 1998;240:193–201.
387. Keene KM, Foy BD, Sanchez-Vargas I, et al. RNA interference acts as a natural antiviral response to o'nyong-nyong virus (Alphavirus; Togaviridae) infection of *Anopheles gambiae*. *Proc Natl Acad Sci U S A* 2004;101: 17240–17245.
388. Kelser RA. Mosquitoes as vectors of the virus of equine encephalomyelitis. *J Am Vet Med Assoc* 1933;82:767–771.
397. Khoo CC, Piper J, Sanchez-Vargas I, et al. The RNA interference pathway affects midgut infection- and escape barriers for Sindbis virus in Aedes aegypti. *BMC Microbiol* 2010;10:130.
402. Kinney RM, Pfeffer M, Tsuchiya KR, et al. Nucleotide sequences of the 26S mRNAs of the viruses defining the Venezuelan equine encephalitis antigenic complex. *Am J Trop Med Hyg* 1998;59:952–964.

404. Kinney RM, Tsuchiya KR, Sneider JM, et al. Molecular evidence for the origin of the widespread Venezuelan equine encephalitis epizootic of 1969 to 1972. *J Gen Virol* 1992;73:3301–3305.
410. Klimstra WB, Nangle EM, Smith M, et al. DC-SIGN and L-SIGN can act as attachment receptors for alphaviruses and distinguish between mosquito cell- and mammalian cell-derived viruses. *J Virol* 2003;77: 12022–12032.
411. Klimstra WB, Ryman KD, Johnston RE. Adaptation of Sindbis virus to BHK cells selects for use of heparan sulfate as an attachment receptor. *J Virol* 1998;72:7357–7366.
418. Kostyuchenko VA, Jakana J, Liu X, et al. The structure of Barmah Forest virus as revealed by cryo-electron microscopy at a 6-angstrom resolution has detailed transmembrane protein architecture and interactions. *J Virol* 2011;85:9327–9333.
420. Kubes V, Rios FA. The causative agent of infectious equine encephalomyelitis in Venezuela. *Science* 1939;90:20–21.
424. Kurkela S, Manni T, Myllynen J, et al. Clinical and laboratory manifestations of Sindbis virus infection: prospective study, Finland, 2002–2003. *J Infect Dis* 2005;191:1820–1829.
427. La Linn M, Gardner J, Warrilow D, et al. Arbovirus of marine mammals: a new alphavirus isolated from the elephant seal louse, *Lepidophthirus macrorhini*. *J Virol* 2001;75:4103–4109.
436. LeDuc JW, Suyemoto W, Eldridge BF, et al. Ecology of arboviruses in a Maryland freshwater swamp. II. Blood feeding patterns of potential mosquito vectors. *Am J Epidemiol* 1972;96:123–128.
439. Lennette EH, Koprowski H. Human infection with Venezuelan equine encephalomyelitis virus: A report on eight cases of infection acquired in the laboratory. *J Am Med Assoc* 1943;13:1088–1095.
441. Lenschow DJ, Lai C, Frias-Staheli N, et al. IFN-stimulated gene 15 functions as a critical antiviral molecule against influenza, herpes, and Sindbis viruses. *Proc Natl Acad Sci U S A* 2007;104:1371–1376.
445. Levine B, Goldman JE, Jiang HH, et al. Bcl-2 protects mice against fatal alphavirus encephalitis. *Proc Natl Acad Sci U S A* 1996;93:4810–4815.
446. Levine B, Griffin DE. Persistence of viral RNA in mouse brains after recovery from acute alphavirus encephalitis. *J Virol* 1992;66:6429–6435.
448. Levine B, Hardwick JM, Trapp BD, et al. Antibody-mediated clearance of alphavirus infection from neurons. *Science* 1991;254:856–860.
449. Levine B, Huang Q, Isaacs JT, et al. Conversion of lytic to persistent alphavirus infection by the Bcl-2 cellular oncogene. *Nature* 1993;361: 739–742.
452. Lewis J, Wesselingh SL, Griffin DE, et al. Alphavirus-induced apoptosis in mouse brains correlates with neurovirulence. *J Virol* 1996;70:1828–1835.
455. Li L, Jose J, Xiang Y, et al. Structural changes of envelope proteins during alphavirus fusion. *Nature* 2010;468:705–708.
457. Liang X-H, Goldman JE, Jiang HH, et al. Resistance of interleukin-1β-deficient mice to fatal Sindbis virus encephalitis. *J Virol* 1999;73: 2563–2567.
460. Lidbury BA, Rulli NE, Suhrbier A, et al. Macrophage-derived proinflammatory factors contribute to the development of arthritis and myositis after infection with an arthrogenic alphavirus. *J Infect Dis* 2008; 197:1585–1593.
464. Lindsay MDA, Johansen CA, Broom AK, et al. Emergence of Barmah Forest virus in Western Australia. *Emerg Infec Dis* 1995;1:22–25.
465. Linn ML, Mateo L, Gardner J, et al. Alphavirus-specific cytotoxic T lymphocytes recognize a cross-reactive epitope from the capsid protein and can eliminate virus from persistently infected macrophages. *J Virol* 1998;72:5146–5153.
467. Liu WJ, Rourke MF, Holmes EC, et al. Persistence of multiple genetic lineages within intrahost populations of Ross River virus. *J Virol* 2011; 85:5674–5678.
478. Lumsden WH. An epidemic of virus disease in Southern Province, Tanganyika territory, in 1952–53. *Trans R Soc Trop Med Hyg* 1955;49:33–57.
485. Lustig S, Jackson AC, Hahn CS, et al. The molecular basis of Sindbis virus neurovirulence in mice. *J Virol* 1988;62:2329–2336.
487. MacDonald GH, Johnston RE. Role of dendritic cell targeting in Venezuelan equine encephalitis virus pathogenesis. *J Virol* 2000;74: 914–922.
493. Malherbe H, Strickland-Cholmley M, Jackson AL. Sindbis virus infection in man: Report of a case with recovery of virus from skin lesions. *S Afr Med J* 1963;37:547–552.
504. Mathiot CC, Grimaud G, Garry P, et al. An outbreak of human Semliki Forest virus infections in Central African Republic. *Am J Trop Med Hyg* 1990;42:386–393.
507. Mayuri, Geders TW, Smith JL, et al. Role for conserved residues of Sindbis virus nonstructural protein 2 methyltransferase-like domain in regulation of minus-strand synthesis and development of cytopathic infection. *J Virol* 2008;82:7284–7297.
509. McFarland HF, Griffin DE, Johnson RT. Specificity of the inflammatory response in viral encephalitis. I. Adoptive immunization of immunosuppressed mice infected with Sindbis virus. *J Exp Med* 1972;136:216–226.
515. McLoughlin MF, Graham DA. Alphavirus infections in salmonids–a review. *J Fish Dis* 2007;30:511–531.
520. Merrill MH, Lacaillade CW, Ten Broeck C. Mosquito transmission of equine encephalomyelitis. *Science* 1934;80:251–252.
521. Metcalf TU, Griffin DE. Alphavirus-induced encephalomyelitis: Antibody-secreting cells and viral clearance from the nervious system. *J Virol* 2011;85:11490–11501.
522. Meyer KF, Haring CM, Howitt B. The etiology of epizootic encephalomyelitis of horses in the San Joaquin Valley. *Science* 1931;74:227–228.
529. Moench TR, Griffin DE. Immunocytochemical identification and quantitation of mononuclear cells in cerebrospinal fluid, meninges, and brain during acute viral encephalitis. *J Exp Med* 1984;159:77–88.
536. Monath TP, Lazuick JS, Cropp CB, et al. Recovery of Tonate virus ("Bijou Bridge" strain), a member of the Venezuelan equine encephalomyelitis virus complex, from cliff swallow nest bugs (*Oeciacus vicarius*) and nestling birds in North America. *Am J Trop Med Hyg* 1980;29:969–983.
544. Morrison TE, Simmons JD, Heise MT. Complement receptor 3 promotes severe Ross River virus-induced disease. *J Virol* 2008;82:11263–11272.
559. Myles KM, Wiley MR, Morazzani EM, et al. Alphavirus-derived small RNAs modulate pathogenesis in disease vector mosquitoes. *Proc Natl Acad Sci U S A* 2008;105:19938–19943.
566. Navarro JC, Medina G, Vasquez C, et al. Postepizootic persistence of Venezuelan equine encephalitis virus, Venezuela. *Emerg Infect Dis* 2005; 11:1907–1915.
571. Niklasson B, Espmark A, Lundstrom J. Occurrence of arthralgia and specific IgM antibodies three to four years after Ockelbo disease. *J Infect Dis* 1988;157:832–835.
575. Noran HH. Chronic equine encephalitis. *Am J Pathol* 1944;20: 259–267.
584. Oliver KR, Fazakerley JK. Transneuronal spread of Semliki Forest virus in the developing mouse olfactory system is determined by neuronal maturity. *Neuroscience* 1998;82:867–877.
588. Orvedahl A, MacPherson S, Sumpter R Jr, et al. Autophagy protects against Sindbis virus infection of the central nervous system. *Cell Host Microbe* 2010;7:115–127.
590. Ozden S, Huerre M, Riviere JP, et al. Human muscle satellite cells as targets of chikungunya virus infection. *PLoS One* 2007;2:e527.
594. Paessler S, Weaver SC. Vaccines for Venezuelan equine encephalitis. *Vaccine* 2009;27 Suppl 4:D80–D85.
609. Phillips DA, Murray JR, Aaskov JG, et al. Clinical and subclinical Barmah Forest virus infection in Queensland. *Med J Aust* 1990;152:463–466.
610. Pichlmair A, Schulz O, Tan CP, et al. Activation of MDA5 requires higher-order RNA structures generated during virus infection. *J Virol* 2009;83:10761–10769.
626. Powers AM, Brault AC, Shirako Y, et al. Evolutionary relationships and systematics of the alphaviruses. *J Virol* 2001;75:10118–10131.
628. Powers AM, Logue CH. Changing patterns of chikungunya virus: re-emergence of a zoonotic arbovirus. *J Gen Virol* 2007;88:2363–2377.
636. Randall R, Maurer FD, Smadel JE. Immunization of laboratory workers with purified Venezuelan equine encephalomyelitis vaccine. *J Immunol* 1949;63:313–318.
637. Randall R, Mills JW. Fatal encephalitis in man due to the Venezuelan virus of equine encephalomyelitis in Trinidad. *Science* 1944;99: 225–226.
647. Reisen WK, Fang Y, Brault AC. Limited interdecadal variation in mosquito (Diptera: Culicidae) and avian host competence for western equine encephalomyelitis virus (Togaviridae: Alphavirus). *Am J Trop Med Hyg* 2008;78:681–686.
652. Reiter P, Fontenille D, Paupy C. *Aedes albopictus* as an epidemic vector of chikungunya virus: another emerging problem? *Lancet Infect Dis* 2006; 6:463–464.

654. Renault P, Solet JL, Sissoko D, et al. A major epidemic of chikungunya virus infection on Reunion Island, France, 2005–2006. *Am J Trop Med Hyg* 2007;77:727–731.
668. Ross RW. The Newala epidemic - The virus: isolation, pathogenic properties and relationship to the epidemic. *J Hyg* 1956;54:177–191.
672. Rulli NE, Rolph MS, Srikiatkhachorn A, et al. Protection from arthritis and myositis in a mouse model of acute chikungunya virus disease by bindarit, an inhibitor of monocyte chemotactic protein-1 synthesis. *J Infect Dis* 2011;204:1026–1030.
674. Rumenapf T, Strauss EG, Strauss JH. Aura virus is a new world representative of Sindbis-like viruses. *Virology* 1995;208:621–633.
676. Russell RC. Ross River virus: ecology and distribution. *Annu Rev Entomol* 2002;47:1–31.
677. Ryman KD, Klimstra WB. Host responses to alphavirus infection. *Immunol Rev* 2008;225:27–45.
692. Sanmartin-Barberi C, Groot H, Osorno-Mesa E. Human epidemic in Colombia caused by the Venezuelan equine encephalomyelitis virus. *Am J Trop Med Hyg* 1954;3:283–293.
700. Scallan MF, Fazakerley JK. Aurothiolates enhance the replication of Semliki Forest virus in the CNS and the exocrine pancreas. *J Neurovirol* 1999;5:392–4002.
703. Schmaljohn AL. Protective monoclonal antibodies define maturational and pH-dependent antigenic changes in Sindbis virus E1 glycoprotein. *Virology* 1983;130:144–154.
705. Schuffenecker I, Iteman I, Michault A, et al. Genome microevolution of chikungunya viruses causing the Indian Ocean outbreak. *PLoS Med* 2006;3:e263.
708. Scott TW, Hildreth SW, Beaty BJ. The distribution and development of eastern equine encephalitis virus in its enzootic mosquito vector, *Culiseta melanura*. *Am J Trop Med Hyg* 1984;33:300–310.
717. Sentsui H, Kono Y. An epidemic of Getah virus infection among racehorses: Isolation of the virus. *Res Vet Sci* 1980;29:157–161.
719. Shabman RS, Rogers KM, Heise MT. Ross River virus envelope glycans contribute to type I interferon production in myeloid dendritic cells. *J Virol* 2008;82:12374–12383.
725. Shope RE, Causey OR, de Andrade AH. TheVenezuelan equine encephalomyelitis complex of group A arthropod-borne viruses, including Mucambo and Pixuna from the Amazon region of Brazil. *Am J Trop Med Hyg* 1964;13:723–727.
736. Siu RW, Fragkoudis R, Simmonds P, et al. Antiviral RNA interference responses induced by Semliki Forest virus infection of mosquito cells: characterization, origin, and frequency-dependent functions of virus-derived small interfering RNAs. *J Virol* 2011;85:2907–2917.
743. Smithburn KC, Haddow AJ. Semliki Forest virus. I. Isolation and pathogenic properties. *J Immunol* 1944;49:141–173.
746. Snow M, Black J, Matejusova I, et al. Detection of salmonid alphavirus RNA in wild marine fish: implications for the origins of salmon pancreas disease in aquaculture. *Dis Aquat Organ* 2010;91:177–188.
750. Soilu-Hanninen M, Roytta M, Salmi AA, et al. Semliki Forest virus infection leads to increased expression of adhesion molecules on splenic T-cells and on brain vascular endothelium. *J Neurovirol* 1997;3:350–360.
756. Spotts DR, Reichert RA, Kalkhan MA, et al. Resistance to alpha/beta interferons correlates with the epizootic and virulence potential of Venezuelan equine encephalitis viruses and is determined by the 5′ noncoding region and glycoproteins. *J Virol* 1998;72:10286–10291.
760. Steele KE, Twenhafel NA. Pathology of animal models of alphavirus encephalitis. *Vet Pathol* 2010;47:790–805.
765. Strauss JH, Strauss EG. The alphaviruses: Gene expression, replication and evolution. *Microbiol Rev* 1994;58:491–562.
766. Strauss JH, Strauss EG. Recombination in alphaviruses. *Semin Virol* 1997;8:85–94.
781. Taylor RM, Hurlbut HS. The isolation of Coxsackie-like viruses from mosquitoes. *J Egypt Med Assoc* 1953;36:489–494.
785. Ten Broeck C, Hurst EW, Traub E. Epidemiology of equine encephalomyelitis in the eastern United States. *J Exp Med* 1935;62:677–685.
788. Tesh RB. Arthritides caused by mosquito-borne viruses. *Ann Rev Med* 1982;33:31–40.
791. Tesh RB, Watts DM, Russell KL, et al. Mayaro virus disease: An emerging mosquito-borne zoonosis in tropical South America. *Clin Infect Dis* 1999;28:67–73.
793. Thach DC, Kleeberger SR, Tucker PC, et al. Genetic control of neuroadapted Sindbis virus replication in female mice maps to chromosome 2 and associates with paralysis and mortality. *J Virol* 2001;75:8674–8680.
794. Thangamani S, Higgs S, Ziegler S, et al. Host immune response to mosquito-transmitted chikungunya virus differs from that elicited by needle inoculated virus. *PLoS One* 2010;5:e12137.
804. Toribio R, Ventoso I. Inhibition of host translation by virus infection in vivo. *Proc Natl Acad Sci U S A* 2010;107:9837–9842.
812. Tsetsarkin KA, Chen R, Sherman MB, et al. Chikungunya virus: evolution and genetic determinants of emergence. *Curr Opin Virol* 2011;1:310–317.
813. Tsetsarkin KA, McGee CE, Volk SM, et al. Epistatic roles of E2 glycoprotein mutations in adaption of chikungunya virus to *Aedes albopictus* and *Ae. aegypti* mosquitoes. *PLoS One* 2009;4:e6835.
815. Tucker PC, Strauss EG, Kuhn RJ, et al. Viral determinants of age-dependent virulence of Sindbis virus in mice. *J Virol* 1993;67:4605–4610.
824. Ubol S, Levine B, Lee S-H, et al. Roles of immunoglobulin valency and the heavy-chain constant domain in antibody-mediated downregulation of Sindbis virus replication in persistently infected neurons. *J Virol* 1995;69:1990–1993.
826. Ubol S, Tucker PC, Griffin DE, et al. Neurovirulent strains of alphavirus induce apoptosis in Bcl-2-expressing cells; role of a single amino acid change in the E2 glycoprotein. *Proc Natl Acad Sci U S A* 1994;91:5202–5206.
828. Urban C, Rheme C, Maerz S, et al. Apoptosis induced by Semliki Forest virus is RNA replication dependent and mediated via Bak. *Cell Death Differ* 2008;15:1396–1407.
833. Vazeille M, Moutailler S, Coudrier D, et al. Two chikungunya isolates from the outbreak of La Reunion (Indian Ocean) exhibit different patterns of infection in the mosquito, *Aedes albopictus*. *PLoS One* 2007;2:e1168.
834. Ventoso I, Sanz MA, Molina S, et al. Translational resistance of late alphavirus mRNA to eIF2alpha phosphorylation: a strategy to overcome the antiviral effect of protein kinase PKR. *Genes Dev* 2006;20:87–100.
836. Villoing S, Bearzotti M, Chilmonczyk S, et al. Rainbow trout sleeping disease virus is an atypical alphavirus. *J Virol* 2000;74:173–183.
840. Voss JE, Vaney MC, Duquerroy S, et al. Glycoprotein organization of chikungunya virus particles revealed by X-ray crystallography. *Nature* 2010;468:709–712.
853. Wauquier N, Becquart P, Nkoghe D, et al. The acute phase of Chikungunya virus infection in humans is associated with strong innate immunity and T CD8 cell activation. *J Infect Dis* 2011;204:115–123.
859. Weaver SC, Kang W, Shirako Y, et al. Recombinational history and molecular evolution of western equine encephalomyelitis complex alphaviruses. *J Virol* 1997;71:613–623.
865. Weaver SC, Scott TW, Lorenz LH, et al. Togavirus-associated pathologic changes in the midgut of a natural mosquito vector. *J Virol* 1988;62:2083–2090.
866. Weaver SC, Scott TW, Lorenz LH, et al. Detection of eastern equine encephalomyelitis virus deposition in *Culiseta melanura* following ingestion of radiolabeled virus in blood meals. *Am J Trop Med Hyg* 1991;44:250–259.
867. Webster LT, Wright FH. Recovery of eastern equine encephalomyelitis virus from brain tissue of human cases of encephalitis in Massachusetts. *Science* 1938;88:305–306.
877. White G, Ottendorfer C, Graham S, et al. Competency of reptiles and amphibians for eastern equine encephalitis virus. *Am J Trop Med Hyg* 2011;85:421–425.
882. Willems WR, Kaluza G, Boschek B, et al. Semliki Forest virus: Cause of a fatal case of human encephalitis. *Science* 1979;203:1127–1129.
884. Williams MC, Woodall JP. O'nyong-nyong fever: An epidemic virus disease in East Africa. II. Isolation and some properties of the virus. *Trans R Soc Trop Med Hyg* 1961;55:135–141.
886. Williams MC, Woodall JP, Corbet PS, et al. O'nyong-nyong fever: An epidemic virus disease in East Africa VIII. Virus isolations from Anopheles mosquitoes. *Trans R Soc Trop Med Hyg* 1965;59:300–306.

CHAPTER 24

Tom C. Hobman

Rubella Virus

Rubella virus (RV) is the etiologic agent of *rubella,* a mild exanthematous disease associated with low-grade fever, lymphadenopathy, and a short-lived morbilliform rash. Rubella was first described as a distinct disease in the early 1800s.[143] Prior to acquiring its more common name, the disease was named *Rötheln* by the German physician de Bergen,[65] leading to the common name of German measles, a milder form of the much more serious exanthem caused by the paramyxovirus, measles virus. Subsequently, in 1866 the disease name was anglicized to *rubella* by the British physician Veale.[243]

Predominantly a childhood disease, RV is endemic in many parts of the world. The introduction of comprehensive vaccination programs in most industrialized regions including the Americas, Western Europe, Japan, and Australia has drastically reduced the incidence of disease in these areas. Indeed, the indigenous circulation of rubella was officially declared eliminated in the United States in 2005. However, developed nations are still very much at risk for rubella outbreaks due to immigration from areas where RV vaccination is lacking. For example, in Africa and Southeast Asia, scheduled infant immunization against rubella is 0.1% and 4%, respectively.[258] Because a very large proportion of the world's population is still susceptible to RV (Fig. 24.1), we can expect that epidemics of rubella will still occur on a regular basis.

Until the keen observations of the ophthalmologist Norman Gregg, rubella was considered a relatively benign infection, associated with considerably less morbidity than measles. In 1941, Gregg encountered a large number of children with cataracts, many of whom had additional serious congenital defects. He noted that an apparent epidemic of congenital cataracts was directly preceded by a large rubella outbreak. Gregg proposed that the cataracts and the often associated congenital cardiac abnormalities were the consequence of maternal infection during pregnancy.[83] Further studies by other investigators confirmed that the virus could have devastating effects on a developing fetus when acquired by the mother in early pregnancy.[254] The realization that viruses can act as teratogenic agents spurred the efforts to develop an attenuated vaccine.

A key step in vaccine development was isolation and growth of RV in cultured cells.[182,253] In 1969, the first rubella vaccine was licensed in the United States, 5 years after the last major epidemic in that country and shortly before the next significant outbreak was predicted to occur. Fortunately, no other major rubella epidemics occurred, largely in part because of the adoption of universal vaccination in infancy, which has been remarkably successful in controlling natural rubella and its devastating teratogenic effects.[213]

INFECTIOUS AGENT

RV is an enveloped positive-strand RNA virus in the family *Togaviridae.* There are two genera that compose the *Togaviridae: Alphavirus,* which includes Sindbis and Semliki Forest viruses, and *Rubivirus,* whose sole member is RV. Togaviruses share a common genome organization and replication strategy (Fig. 24.2). Whereas alphaviruses employ animal reservoirs and arthropod vectors for transmission, humans appear to be the only natural host and reservoir for RV. Although only one serotype exists, there are at least 10 genotypes of RV (Fig. 24.3), which can be grouped into two clades.[264] Circulation of clade 2 viruses, which contain three genotypes, is limited to Eurasia, while clade 1 viruses are more widely distributed. The genome of RV is a 5′ capped positive-sense RNA molecule of approximately 10 kilobases (kb) with a poly (A) tail. There is no serologic cross-reactivity between the alphaviruses and RV, and only limited genome sequence similarity, predominantly within the nonstructural genes in regions that encode functional domains such as the polymerase and protease activities.

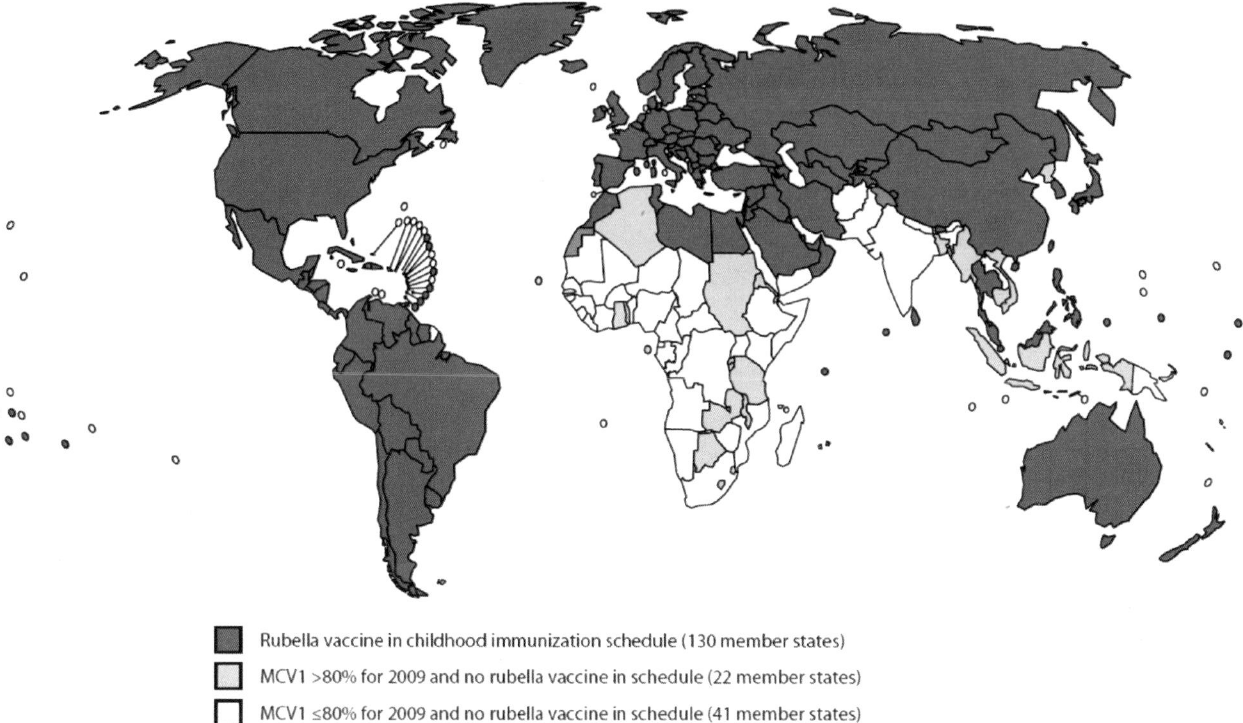

FIGURE 24.1. World map showing countries that have comprehensive rubella vaccination strategies. (From Progress toward control of rubella and prevention of congenital rubella syndrome—worldwide, 2009. *MMWR Morb Mortal Wkly Rep* 2010;59[40]: 1307–1310.)

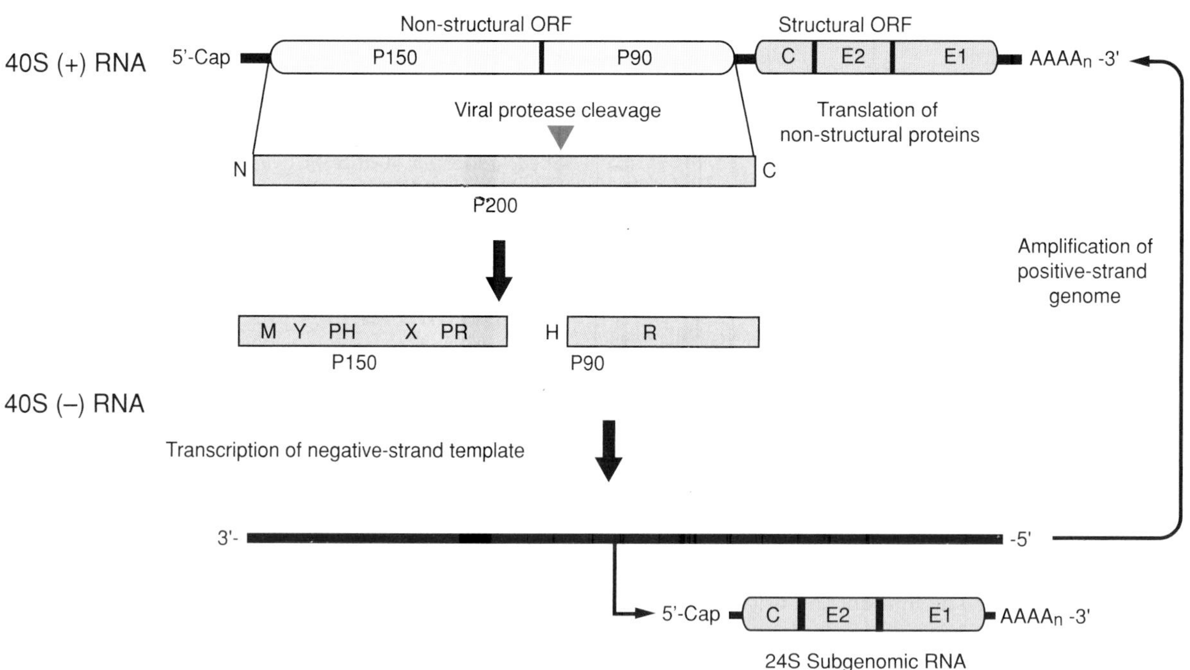

FIGURE 24.2. Organization and expression of the rubella virus (RV) genome. The genome is a single-stranded 40S RNA containing two open reading frames (ORFs). The 5′ proximal ORF encodes the nonstructural proteins p150 and p90. The 40S genome serves as a messenger RNA (mRNA) for translation of the nonstructural protein precursor p200, which is cleaved by a virus-encoded protease to produce p150 and p90. The relative positions of methyltransferase (M), Y, proline hinge (PH), X, protease (PR), helicase (H), and RNA-dependent polymerase (R) domains within p150 and p90 proteins are shown. These two proteins form the viral replicase that synthesizes a negative-sense 40S RNA, which then serves as a template for synthesis of more genomic RNA and the 24S subgenomic RNA. Both the 40S and 24S positive-sense RNAs are capped and polyadenylated.

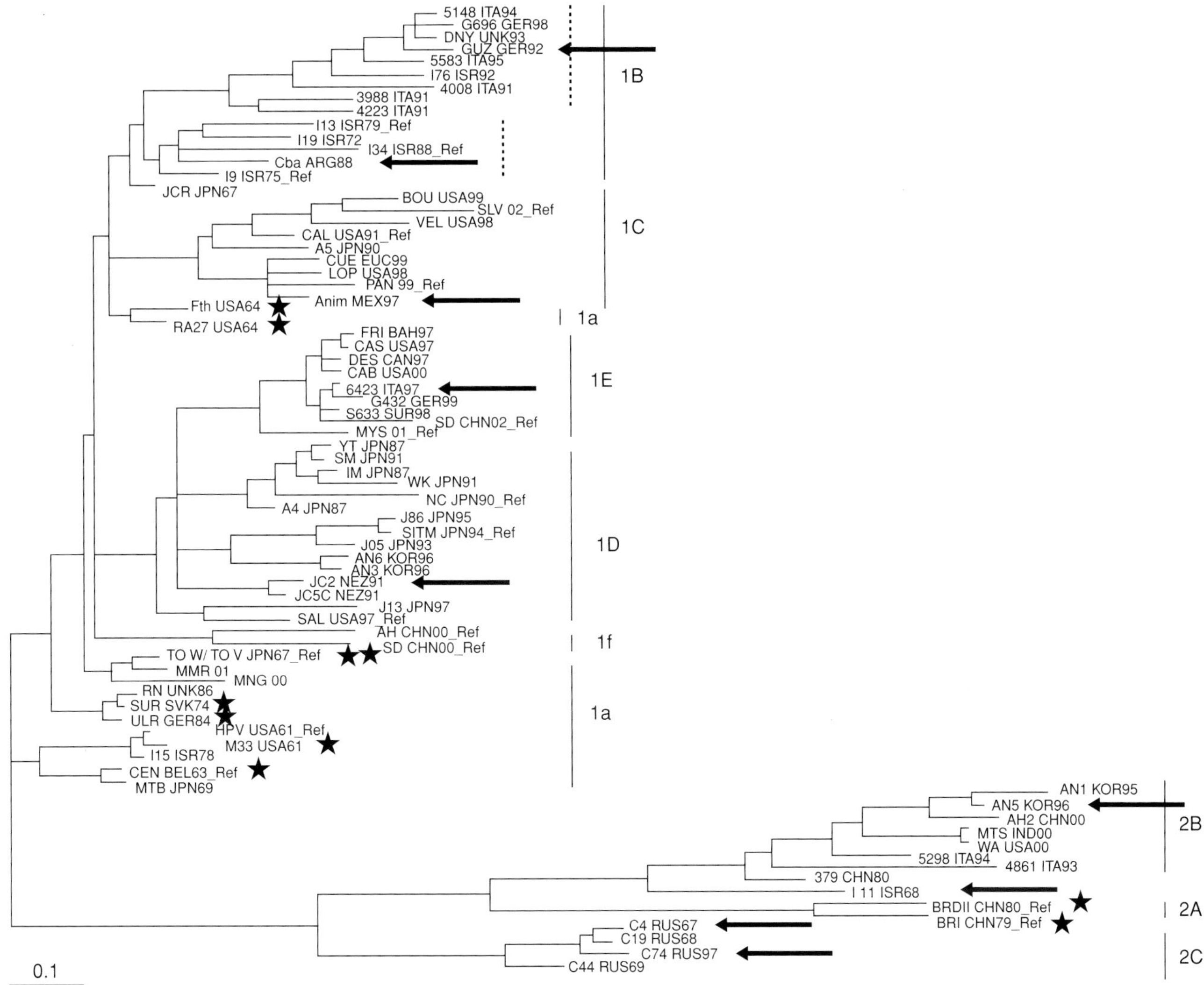

FIGURE 24.3. Phylogenetic tree of rubella virus (RV) genotypes based on analyses of *E1* gene nucleotide sequences. Based on the analyses, there are two main clades 1 and 2, which are composed of seven and three genotypes, respectively. Reference strains for each genotype are indicated by "Ref." Strains whose genomic sequence have been reported previously are indicated by stars, whereas those strains whose genomic sequences were determined by Zhou et al are indicated by arrows. Two sub-branches within genotype 1B are indicated by dashed lines. (From Zhou Y, Ushijima H, Frey TK. Genomic analysis of diverse rubella virus genotypes. *J Gen Virol* 2007;88[Pt 3]:932–941, with permission.)

Morphology and Physicochemical Properties of the Virion

By transmission electron microscopy, RV virions appear as spherical particles with a mean diameter of 61 nm.[160] Virus particles can often be observed budding into the Golgi complex of infected cells (Fig. 24.4). They have an electron-dense nucleocapsid core surrounded by a host-derived envelope.[159] The nucleocapsid (30 to 40 nm in diameter) is composed of a single molecule of genomic RNA and multiple copies of capsid protein. Between the core and the envelope is an electron-lucent region giving the virions the appearance of having a ring or "toga" surrounding the nucleocapsid, from which the name is derived. Virus-encoded glycoprotein spikes project 6 to 8 nm outward from the lipid envelope[236] and denote the virion surface. Early electron microscopic studies suggest that the RV nucleocapsids exhibit a T = 3 icosahedral symmetry,[144] distinguishing them from those of alphaviruses that are arranged with a T = 4 symmetry; however, this has not been confirmed by subsequent high-resolution analyses.

The buoyant density of rubella virions in sucrose gradients is 1.18 to 1.19 g/mL.[104] In comparison, the buoyant density of alphavirus virions is 1.20 g/mL, a difference that may be attributable to a wider electron-lucent zone between the core and envelope in rubella virions. The reported sedimentation coefficient of RV virions ranges from 240S and 350S.[9] The reason for this heterogeneity is not known but may be due in part to contamination of the virus preparations by host cell–derived membranous material. The difficulty in obtaining highly purified homogenous preparations of RV virions is one of the numerous technical reasons that has impeded the progress of structural analysis.

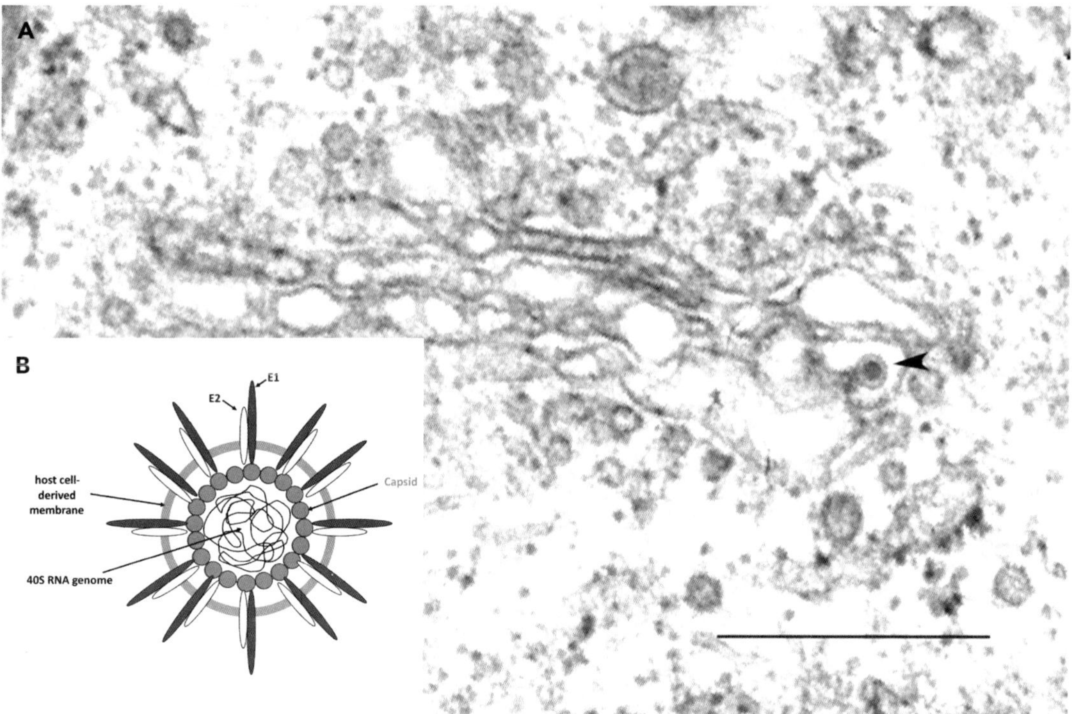

FIGURE 24.4. A: Electron micrograph of a rubella virion budding into the lumen of a Golgi cisterna in an infected Vero cell. Note the electron-lucent halo that surrounds the electron-dense nucleocapsid. Bar = 0.5 μm. (Courtesy of Dr. John Law and Ms. Honey Chan). **B:** Schematic of a rubella virus (RV) virion.

The infectivity of RV virions is rapidly lost following exposure to protein denaturing agents (formaldehyde, ethylene oxide, and β-propiolactone) or treatments/reagents that cause lesions in nucleic acids (ultraviolet light or photodynamic dyes). Moreover, because it is an enveloped virus, exposure of RV preparations to nonionic or ionic detergents and lipid solvents abrogates the infectivity of virions.[181] Virions are rapidly inactivated by incubation at 56°C for less than 20 minutes, and even at much lower temperatures such as 37°C, RV loses activity slowly ($t_{1/2}$ = 48 hours).[152] When stored at temperatures less than –60°C in the presence of protein stabilizers, RV preparations maintain their infectivity for many years. Fortunately, with respect to vaccine distribution, lyophilized RV preparations are stable for years at 4°C and for months at ambient temperatures.[184]

Biological Characteristics

RV has a restricted host range (only humans) *in vivo* but replicates in a wide variety of cultured mammalian cell lines, including primary African green monkey kidney cells, BHK21, RK13, and Vero cell lines. All strains of the virus (including wt+ strains) are slightly temperature sensitive, with higher yields of virus obtained when infected cells are cultured at 35°C rather than at 37°C. The vaccine strains RA27/3 and Cendehill are completely growth restricted at 39°C, while some wt+ isolates are still able to replicate at 41°C, albeit at lower levels.[36]

In comparison to the rapid lytic infection of mammalian cells by the alphaviruses, RV replicates more slowly, with an eclipse phase of 10 to 12 hours (c.f. 4 hours for Sindbis or Semliki Forest viruses), and peak titers of secreted virus are not observed until 36 to 48 hours.[87,242] By comparison, peak viral titers for alphaviruses are observed within 8 hours. As well as exhibiting relatively slow replication kinetics, the amount of infectious virus progeny released per cell is estimated to be 1,000-fold less than for alphaviruses. Under optimal conditions, RV-infected BHK-21 and Vero cells can produce titers of 10^7 and 10^8 plaque-forming units (pfu) per mL, respectively.[10,241] The relatively feeble replication of RV may be due to a number of factors including low uptake of virus and/or inefficiencies associated with the replicase/transcriptase complex or limitations of the assembly process. For example, RV buds into the Golgi complex, which is a much smaller membrane compartment than the endoplasmic reticulum or the plasma membrane. Another factor that may play a role is the high G + C content of the viral genome (69.5%), which is predicted to form stable secondary and tertiary structures that may impede replication/transcription or translation.[68] Also related to the G + C content, the codon usage by RV is different from that of mammalian cells, requiring utilization of transfer RNAs (tRNAs) that may be of low abundance, a factor that has been suggested to limit the rate of protein synthesis.[225]

Effects on Host Cell

Although RV can have devastating effects on the developing human fetus, infection of most cultured primate or rodent cell lines does not result in major cytopathology. However, in some cell lines (Vero, BHK-21, and RK13), when high multiplicities of infection (MOIs) are employed, the virus causes rounding and detachment of cells commencing at 24 hours postinfection and increasing over the next 72 hours. Much of the RV-induced cytopathic effect is likely the result of apoptosis.[61,149,195] Virions that are first inactivated by ultraviolet light do not induce apoptosis, indicating that viral replication is required to cause cell death.[61,100] The cytopathic determinants of RV have been mapped to the nonstructural genes,[193] and in agreement with this, expression of RV structural proteins alone in Vero cells does not induce apoptosis.[100] Paradoxically, primary human embryonic fibroblasts seem to be particularly immune to RV-induced apoptosis.[3]

At low (less than 1) or moderate (1 to 3) MOIs, little virus cytopathic effect is observed in most cultured cells[61,116] and chronic infections can readily be established (see Replication Strategy section). Induction of apoptosis in response to RV infection is undoubtedly an important antiviral defense mechanism that is employed by cells against many RNA viruses. Because viruses are obligate parasites, they require a living cell for replication. Depending on the apoptotic stimuli, cells can be killed in a matter of hours, a situation that would be seemingly problematic for RV, which has a long eclipse period and whose replication peak occurs between 2 and 4 days postinfection.[87] However, the maximum RV-induced apoptosis does not occur until after 5 days postinfection,[149] which is consistent with a scenario where the virus actively blocks apoptosis early in infection. Indeed, a recent study revealed that RV-infected cells are highly resistant to apoptotic stimuli.[107] Mapping studies showed that the capsid protein is responsible for this process, which presumably provides a window of opportunity for the virus to replicate before apoptosis is initiated.

In most cell types, cellular macromolecular synthesis on a global level does not appear to be significantly affected, even following high-multiplicity infections (5 to 10 pfu per cell). For example, host cell RNA synthesis continues normally and protein synthesis is only slightly reduced at 72 hours postinfection in several highly permissive cell lines.[87] However, in mitogen-stimulated peripheral blood mononuclear cells (PBMCs), host cell protein synthesis was reportedly inhibited by more than 90% at 48 hours postinfection.[38] The capsid protein has been shown to block translation *in vitro,*[108] but it has yet to be determined whether this viral protein is responsible for inhibition of protein synthesis in PBMCs or other cell types.

A number of characteristic morphologic changes occur in RV-infected cells. Similar to other togaviruses, RV infection is accompanied by drastic rearrangement of cellular membranes. For example, the endoplasmic reticulum (ER), Golgi complex, and mitochondria are often closely arranged around the virus replication complexes (Fig. 24.5), which are derived from endosomes and/or lysosomes.[125,127] This arrangement of organelles could in theory facilitate the efficient transfer of virus genome from the site of RNA replication (endosomes) to the area of virus assembly (Golgi complex). Whereas organelle rearrangement is common in togavirus-infected cells, the formation of electron-dense plaques (22 to 25 nm in thickness) between organelles is unique to RV infection.[123] The plaques (Fig. 24.6) and associated organelles have been termed confronting membranes or confronting cisternae and commonly involve outer membranes of mitochondria and rough ER, adjacent mitochondria, and adjacent ER membranes, respectively. Expression of capsid protein in the absence of other viral proteins induces mitochondrial clustering and formation of plaques,[15] and immunoelectron microscopy revealed that capsid protein is a major component of the plaques.[109] It has been known for years that a large pool of capsid protein is targeted to the surface

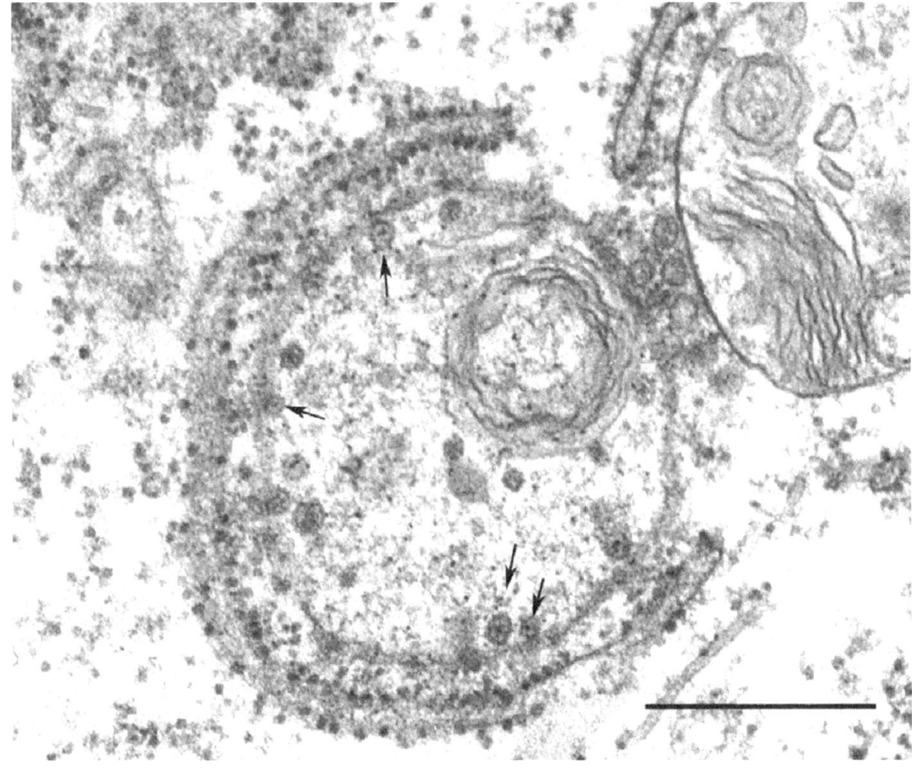

FIGURE 24.5. Electron micrograph of viral replication complex is associated with rough endoplasmic reticulum. Spherules are indicated by arrows. Bar = 0.5 μm. (Courtesy of Dr. John Law and Ms. Honey Chan.)

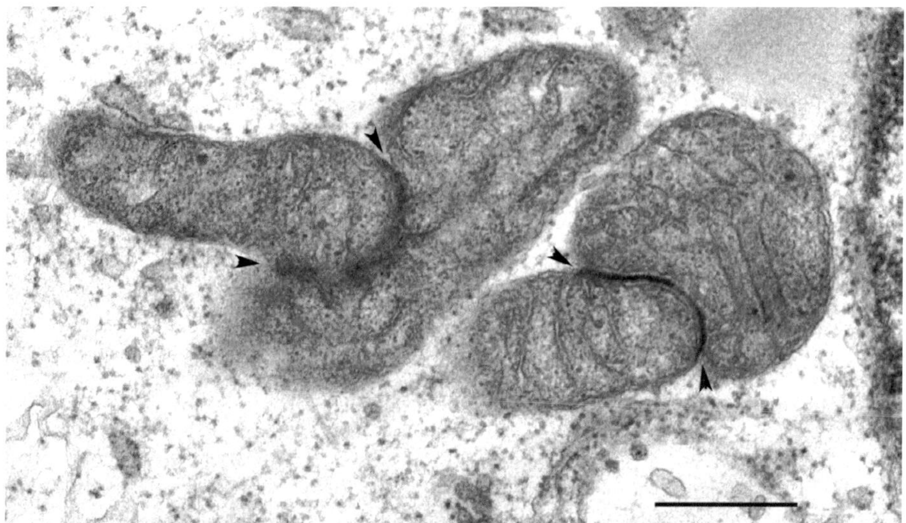

FIGURE 24.6. Aggregation of mitochondria and formation of electron-dense intermitochondrial plaques in rubella virus (RV)-infected cells. Bar = 0.5 μm. (Courtesy of Dr. John Law and Ms. Honey Chan.)

of mitochondria,[16,126] and recently it was discovered that capsid affects mitochondrial import.[109] The latter may explain the loss of cristae and dysmorphic (club-shaped) mitochondria in RV-infected cells.[122] Together, these observations reflect the close link between RV replication and mitochondrial physiology.

Phenotypic Variation

Although there are now recognized to be at least 10 genotypes of RV (Fig. 24.3), there is only one serotype, and infection with one strain provides protection against all others recognized to date. However, the limited genetic differences seen (0.8% to 2.1% at the amino acid level[221,263]) are associated with differences in hemagglutination,[133] plaque morphology,[116] temperature sensitivity, virus yield, and cell tropism.[36] Compared to natural RV infection, administration of vaccine strains is associated with milder acute symptoms and a lower incidence of complications such as joint and neurological symptoms,[21,66,229] as well as teratogenic effects.[13]

The major neutralization epitopes appear to be highly conserved among RV strains,[22,69] although differences have been noted in the kinetics of neutralization[81] and in reactivity to certain monoclonal antibodies.[36] However, both infection and immunization are believed to provide protection against all other strains for the duration of the immune response elicited, except in cases where incomplete immunity is induced.[230]

The vaccine strains RA27/3 and Cendehill display different tissue tropisms from wt+ strains, including growth restriction in both PBMCs and the B-cell lines, Raji and Cess cells.[36] These two strains also show limited replication in cells derived from human joint tissue,[152] with the Cendehill strain completely inhibited in synovial organ cultures and chondrocytes. In comparison, wt+ strains replicate to high titer (10^6 to 10^7 pfu/mL) in joint cells. The determinants that govern growth in joint tissue have been mapped to the 5′ end of the genome, which encodes the nonstructural proteins, and as such, it is likely that replication rather than binding and entry events determine tropism.[135]

Structure and Organization of the Genome

The genome of RV is a single molecule of positive-strand RNA of approximately 10 kb with a GC content of 69.5%, by far the highest of any RNA virus sequenced to date.[6] The 5′ end of the RNA has a 7-methyl-guanosine cap,[166] while at the 3′ end there is a poly (A) tract with a mean length of 53 nucleotides.[246] The genome consists of two nonoverlapping polycistronic open reading frames (ORFs) separated by a nontranslated region of 123 nucleotides (Fig. 24.2).[192] The 5′ proximal ORF (approximately 6,385 nucleotides) encodes the nonstructural proteins, while the 3′ proximal ORF (3,189 nucleotides) encodes the three structural proteins, capsid, E2, and E1. The structural proteins are translated from a 5′ capped and polyadenylated subgenomic RNA that is collinear with the 3′ one-third of the 40S genome.[166] The complete nucleotide sequences have been determined for the genomes of several wild-type and vaccine strains of RV[68] and are available in GenBank. In addition, infectious complementary DNA (cDNA) clones of several strains have been produced and used to map genetic elements involved in viral replication and attenuation.[135,196,246,259]

Cis-Acting Elements

The availability of infectious RV cDNA clones[135,196,259] and replicons[237] has enabled the application of reverse genetics to study the roles of *cis*-acting elements in genome replication. Both the 5′ and 3′ untranslated regions (UTRs) of the RV genome are believed to form secondary structures that influence transcription and translation events. For example, the predicted 5′ stem-loop (5′SL), which encompasses nucleotides 15 to 65, has a terminal loop as well as a bulge in the stem and a hinge region (Fig. 24.7). It is believed to form a pseudoknot,[194] a structure that has been shown in a number of plant and animal viruses to enhance binding of proteins that function in RNA replication.[57,110] Within the single-stranded leader sequence (nucleotides 1 to 14) and the stem-loop, there are three AUG codons starting at nucleotides 3, 41, and 57. Translation of the long ORF encoding the nonstructural genes is initiated at AUG_{41}, while the first and third AUGs are in a different reading frame and are terminated at nucleotides 54 and 90, respectively. Indeed, site-specific mutagenesis studies suggest that AUG_3 is not essential for viral replication,[194] nor is it known whether short peptides that originate from either AUG_3 or AUG_{57} play any role in virus biology. However, it is notable that the

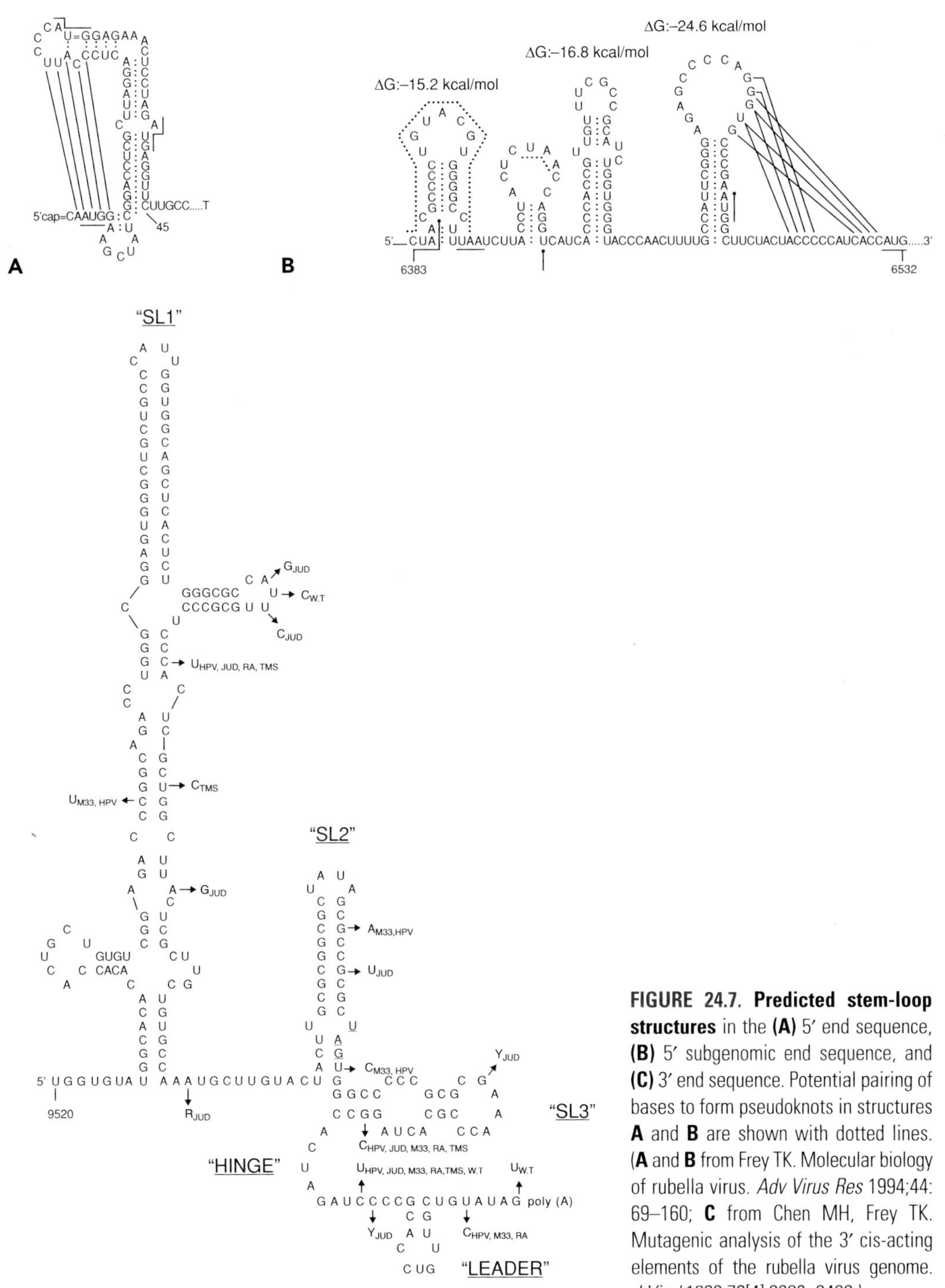

FIGURE 24.7. Predicted stem-loop structures in the **(A)** 5′ end sequence, **(B)** 5′ subgenomic end sequence, and **(C)** 3′ end sequence. Potential pairing of bases to form pseudoknots in structures **A** and **B** are shown with dotted lines. (**A** and **B** from Frey TK. Molecular biology of rubella virus. *Adv Virus Res* 1994;44:69–160; **C** from Chen MH, Frey TK. Mutagenic analysis of the 3′ cis-acting elements of the rubella virus genome. *J Virol* 1999;73[4]:3386–3403.)

three AUG codons are conserved in all strains sequenced to date.[135,194] Analysis of the 5′ end sequences of a number of RV strains revealed that the stem-loop is largely conserved and that polymorphisms are restricted to the terminal loop or the hinge region.[110,194] Mutations in the 5′SL are associated with differences in viral yield and plaque morphology,[194] as well as tropism for joint tissue.[135]

Between the nonstructural and structural genes is a 123-bp region that is predicted to form a series of stem-loops (Fig. 24.7). This region shares 58% identity with the equivalent region in the Sindbis virus genome and may be important for regulating synthesis of the subgenomic RNA. In addition, translation of the structural genes is affected by mutations in this region, which forms the 5′ end of the subgenomic RNA.[180] In the 3′ UTR, there is a stretch of 59 nucleotides following the stop codon at nucleotide 9701. A complex secondary structure involving three major stem-loop structures[43] has been predicted for the 3′ terminal 240 nucleotides (Fig. 24.7).

These 3′ UTR sequences function in *cis* to regulate transcription, specifically, synthesis of plus-strand viral RNAs but not negative-sense RNA.[44]

Encapsidation Signal

Mapping studies revealed that capsid protein binds with relatively high affinity to a 29-nucleotide segment located in the 5′ nonstructural gene region between nucleotides 347 and 375.[132]

Nonstructural ORF and Protein Products

The nonstructural (NS) genes are located in the 5′ end of the viral genome within a long ORF commencing at AUG_{41}. The NS ORF is translated as a single polyprotein greater than 200 kD that is cleaved into two products, p150 and p90,[140] that function in replication and transcription of viral RNAs (Fig. 24.2). The gene order of the 5′ ORF is NH_2-p150-p90-COOH. The two nonstructural proteins have several enzymatic activities including RNA polymerase, protease, and helicase and together form the viral replicase. Proteolytic processing of the p200 polyprotein marks the switch from synthesis of negative-strand genomic RNA to synthesis of plus-strand RNA.[128]

p150 contains several domains that are conserved among other RNA virus-encoded proteins. A protease domain located in the carboxyl portion of p150 (Fig. 24.2) is responsible for cleavage of the nonstructural precursor protein p200 and is critical for virus replication.[42,260] Mutagenesis studies have shown that the RV protease is a metalloprotease that requires divalent cations for activity[130,131] and functions in both *cis* and *trans* modes.[129] A putative methyltransferase domain in the amino terminus is believed to have a role in capping the viral RNA.[211] p150 also contains an X domain that has homology to the nonstructural proteins of alphaviruses, coronaviruses, and hepatitis E virus.[80] The function of the X domain is not well characterized, but it is required for *trans* cleavage by the RV protease and in alphaviruses at least is important for replication.[86] Interestingly, the X domain is the region that is most highly conserved between RV and alphaviruses.[60] Two other domains of unknown function, Y and a proline hinge, are also present in p150. The order of these domains in p150 is NH_2–methyltransferase–Y domain–proline hinge domain–X domain–protease–COOH. The second nonstructural protein, p90, comprises 905 amino acid residues and contains the replicase and helicase motifs. Based on comparison with global RNA-dependent RNA polymerase consensus sequences,[111] the GDD tripeptide at amino acids 1965 to 1967 of p90 is the active site of the RV replicase. An RNA-stimulated nucleoside triphosphatase (NTPase) that promotes unwinding of the template during RNA replication is associated with the helicase motif.[85]

The localization of RV nonstructural proteins, p150 and p90, is less well studied than that of the structural proteins. This is because the nonstructural proteins are present at relatively low concentrations in infected cells, and furthermore, attempts to produce useful antibodies against these antigens has met with limited success. However, it has been reported that p150 associates with long tubular structures that correspond to sites of viral RNA synthesis.[118] p90 has been detected in discrete cytoplasmic puncta that form linear chains.[5] The identity of the p90-associated structures was not determined, but it is likely that they are replication complexes derived from endocytic vacuoles. Presumably, a large pool of p150 is also localized to the p90-positive foci. No information regarding sequences that target the nonstructural proteins to endocytic membranes has been reported.

Structural ORF and Protein Products

The structural genes are contained within the 3′ ORF of the 40S genomic RNA; however, they are actually translated from a subgenomic 24S RNA that is produced in infected cells. There are two in-frame AUG initiation codons in the subgenomic RNA separated by 21 nucleotides. The downstream AUG is in the more favorable context for translation initiation, but *in vitro* mutagenesis experiments indicate that both codons can be used.[47] The 24S subgenomic RNA encodes three structural proteins, which are translated in the order NH2-C-E2-E1-COOH.[165] Unlike alphavirus structural proteins, which require both host cell signal peptidase and a capsid-associated protease for complete processing,[150] processing of the RV structural polyprotein (Fig. 24.8) into C, E2, and E1 only requires signal peptidase, which is encoded by the host cell.[139,224]

In the absence of genomic RNA, coordinated expression of the RV structural proteins in mammalian cells results in the assembly and secretion of rubella virus-like particles (VLPs).[94,199] The VLPs, which resemble native virions in terms of morphology and antigenicity, have served as a useful tool for studying virus assembly, and as a consequence, the roles of RV structural proteins and their domains in the assembly process are relatively well understood. The fact that rubella VLPs are efficiently assembled and secreted in the absence of genomic RNA indicates that virus budding is not tightly linked to nucleocapsid assembly.

Capsid

The capsid protein is a phosphoprotein with an apparent molecular mass of 33 to 35 kD.[139] The protein contains 300 amino acid residues and is rich in arginine and proline residues, particularly at its amino terminus, which gives it a net positive charge[46] and facilitates its interaction with genomic RNA during nucleocapsid formation. Capsid protein often migrates as a doublet on SDS-PAGE gels. The reason for this remains unknown, but it is not due to the use of an alternate translation start site.[47,139] Virion-associated capsid protein can be isolated as disulfide-linked dimers, but intermolecular disulfide bonding is not necessary for formation of virus particles.[12,124]

Cleavage of the RV capsid protein from the polyprotein precursor is distinct from that of alphavirus capsid proteins, which contains an autoprotease that separates the capsid protein from the polyprotein.[150] As a consequence, alphavirus capsids are free in the cytoplasm of infected cells. RV capsid protein, in contrast, lacks autoprotease activity, and separation from E2 is carried out by host cell signal peptidase.[46] The E2 signal peptide is therefore retained as the carboxyl terminus of capsid protein (Fig. 24.8), where it serves to confer membrane association of the protein.[91,139,224] The membrane association of RV capsid protein is unique among togaviruses and may account for some of the unusual morphogenetic features of the virus. For example, retention of the E2 signal peptide on capsid protein is necessary for assembly of VLPs and presumably infectious virions.[120]

Role of the Capsid Protein in Virus Assembly. The primary function of capsid protein during virus assembly is to homo-oligomerize and bind viral genomic RNA to form

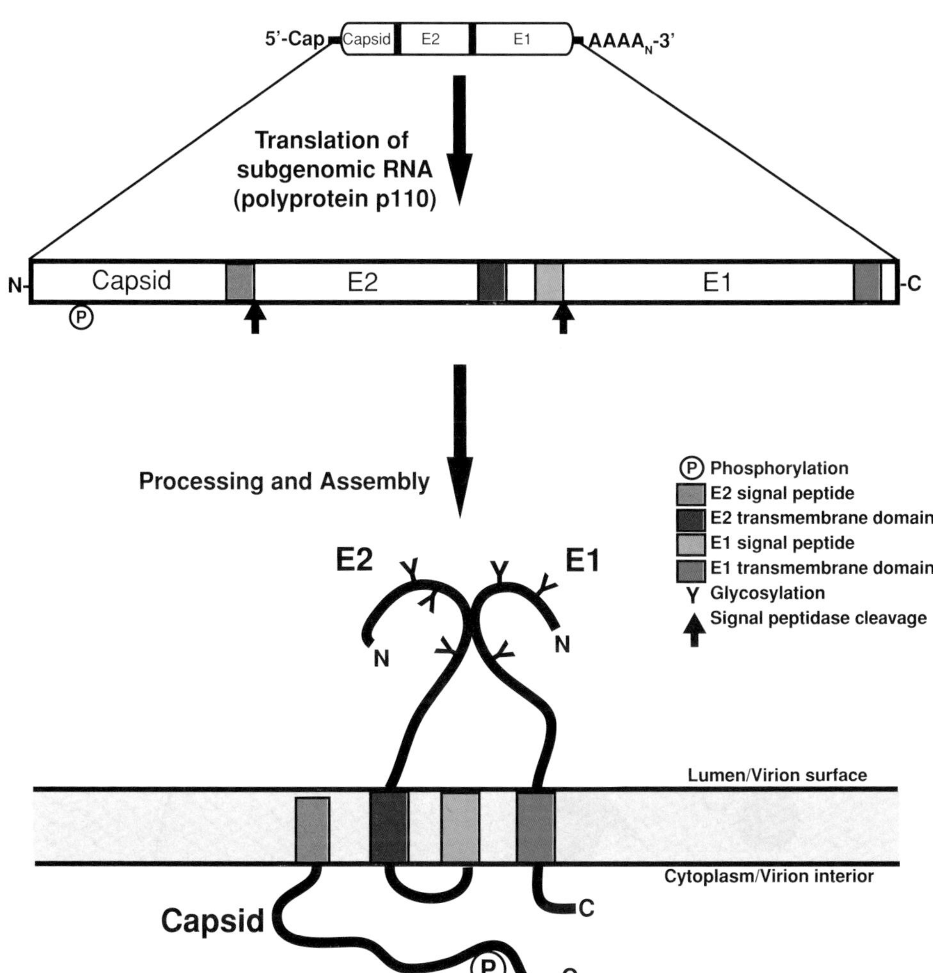

FIGURE 24.8. Processing of rubella virus (RV) structural proteins. The 24S RNA serves as the messenger RNA (mRNA) for translation of a structural polyprotein precursor, which is then cleaved by host signal peptidase to produce capsid, E2 and E1. The relative membrane orientations of the structural proteins immediately following translocation into the endoplasmic reticulum (ER) are shown. The amino (N) and carboxyl (C) termini of the proteins are indicated.

the nucleocapsid. The RNA-binding domain of capsid protein resides within amino acid residues 28 to 56 and binds to a packaging signal (nucleotides 347 to 375) in the genomic RNA.[132] Posttranslational modification of capsid protein may play an important role in regulating the formation of nucleocapsids because phosphorylation of serine 46 within the RNA-binding domain negatively regulates RNA binding.[119,121] This is believed to prevent nonspecific binding of cellular RNAs to capsid protein and to delay binding of genomic RNA until the virion components are targeted to the budding site. *In vitro,* capsid protein is a substrate for protein phosphatase IA, an enzyme that has been implicated in Golgi-associated functions.[121] Accordingly, targeting of capsid protein to the Golgi complex, followed by dephosphorylation at this site, could explain how nucleocapsid assembly is synchronized with virus assembly (Fig. 24.9). Supporting this scenario is the observation that virion-associated capsid protein has a higher affinity for viral RNA and contains significantly less phosphate than cell-associated capsid protein.[119,121] Similar to alphaviruses,[223] it is thought that capsid protein drives budding of RV through interactions with the envelope glycoproteins; however, direct binding between RV capsid protein and E2 and/or E1 has yet to be demonstrated.

Nonstructural Roles of the Capsid Protein. In addition to nucleocapsid assembly, the RV capsid protein plays a role in regulating viral transcription and replication. The first indication of this nonstructural function came from the observation that expression of capsid protein rescues the replication of an RV replicon containing an in-frame deletion of p150.[238] Further analyses indicated that the capsid protein is involved in modulating viral genomic and subgenomic RNA synthesis.[239] In the absence of capsid protein expression, the ratio of genomic RNA to subgenomic RNA is substantially lower. It is believed that a pool of capsid protein that associates with the replication complexes is responsible for regulating synthesis of viral RNAs. Interestingly, the effects of capsid protein on transcription depend on the levels of replicon RNA.[45] At low levels of RNA, capsid protein expression enhances replication of viral RNA, but with higher levels of RNA, capsid protein is inhibitory for this process.

Given its multiple roles, it is not surprising that the RV capsid protein is associated with multiple organelles. Consistent with its function in virus assembly, pools of capsid protein are localized to the Golgi.[11,94] Transport of capsid to the Golgi region from the site of its synthesis, the ER, depends on E1 and E2.[74,120] Capsid also localizes to mitochondria and to virus

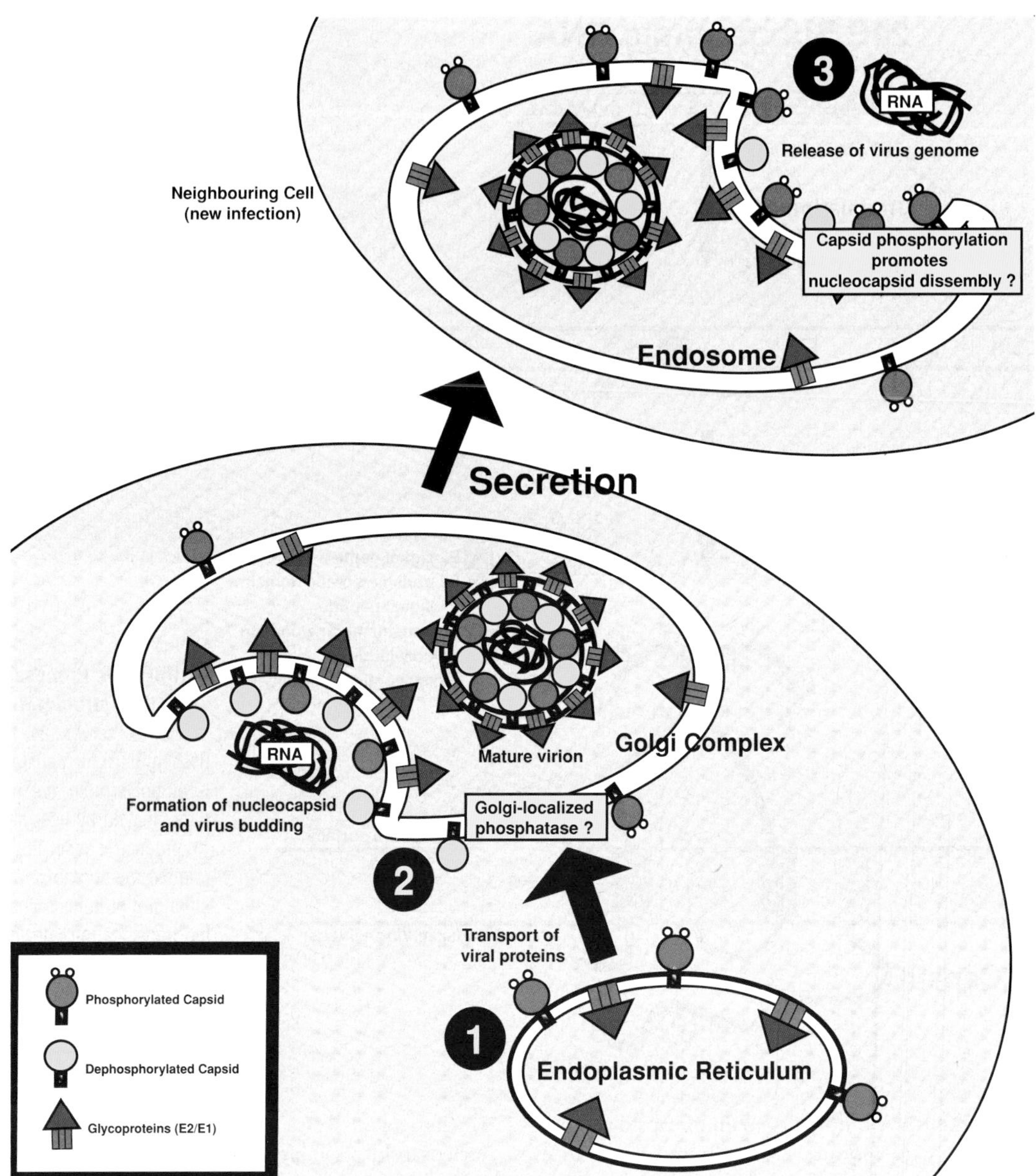

FIGURE 24.9. Model to illustrate the putative roles of dynamic phosphorylation of capsid protein in virus replication. 1: Phosphorylation of newly synthesized capsid protein prevents nonspecific binding of RNA and premature formation of nucleocapsid at the early stages of virus assembly. **2:** Capsid protein is subsequently targeted to the Golgi complex and dephosphorylation of the protein at this stage allows interaction with the genomic RNA, formation of the nucleocapsid, and subsequent virus budding. **3:** Timely rephosphorylation of capsid protein before or during virus entry promotes the disassembly of nucleocapsid.

replication complexes.[16,123] In contrast, the glycoproteins E1 and E2 are targeted only to the virus budding site (Golgi), suggesting that they do not have major nonstructural roles. Together with p150, replication complex–localized capsid protein[118] is thought to modulate replication of viral RNA, whereas the mitochondrial pool of capsid plays one or more critical roles in virus–host interactions (Fig. 24.10). For example, it potently blocks apoptosis by sequestering the proapoptotic host protein Bax into nonfunctional complexes.[107] RV capsid also interferes with mitochondrial import,[109] a critical process that is linked to apoptosis in mammalian cells.[183] Finally, it has been known for more than a decade that capsid interacts with the mitochondrial matrix protein p32.[16] The precise function of this interaction is not clear, but several lines of evidence suggest that it is important for virus replication. First, ablation of the p32-binding site in capsid protein reduces the replication efficiency of RV by 1,000-fold.[15] Second, depletion of cellular p32 pools by RNA interference results in a 10-fold reduction in virus replication.[49] Capsid protein–p32 interactions may also be important for synthesis of subgenomic RNA and/or translation of structural proteins. Finally, loss of stable binding between capsid protein and p32 is correlated with reduced mitochondrial clustering in

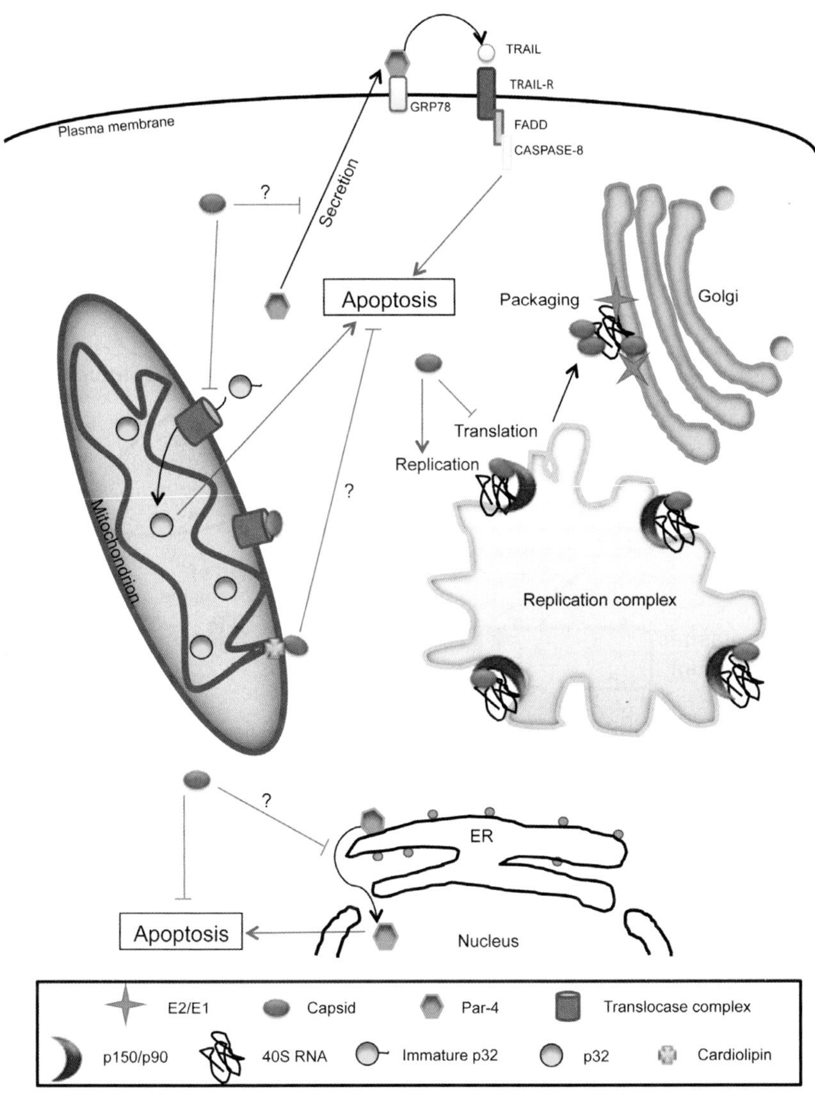

FIGURE 24.10. Integrated model of rubella virus (RV) capsid nonstructural functions. At the replication complex, capsid associates with nonstructural proteins (p150 and p90) and regulates transcription and replication of viral RNA. Late in the infection cycle, local sequestration of translation initiation factors such as poly(A) binding protein (PABP) may modulate the switch from translation to packaging of the genomic RNA, a mechanism that would leave the viral RNA available for packaging into nucleocapsids at the Golgi complex. Capsid prevents apoptosis by binding to Bax and inducing the formation of hetero-oligomers that are incompetent for pore formation at the mitochondria and potentially at the endoplasmic reticulum (ER) membranes. Capsid may also inhibit apoptosis by preventing translocation of pro-apoptotic proteins such as p32 into the mitochondria or by engaging in complexes with the mitochondrial lipid, cardiolipin. (Modified from Ilkow CS, Willows SD, Hobman TC. Rubella virus capsid protein: a small protein with big functions. *Future Microbiol* 2010;5[4]:571–584.)

the perinuclear region. Together, these results suggest that interactions between capsid protein and p32 are important for RV-induced rearrangement of mitochondria, a phenomenon that is associated with optimal replication.

Envelope Proteins

E1 and E2 are type I membrane proteins that dimerize to form the spike complexes on the surface of the virion (Fig. 24.8). The major functions of these spikes are to bind receptors on the host cell and to mediate fusion with cell membranes.[114] The envelope proteins, E1 in particular, are the major antigenic determinants against which neutralizing antibodies are directed.[249]

E1 is 481 amino acid residues in length and exhibits an apparent molecular mass of 58 kD when analyzed by SDS-PAGE. The mature protein contains three asparagine-linked oligosaccharide moieties.[95] An amino terminal signal peptide facilitates translocation of E1 into the ER and a 22–amino acid hydrophobic sequence at its carboxyl terminus mediates membrane association.[96] E1 also contains a carboxyl terminal tail of 13 amino acid residues that is exposed to the cytoplasm. E2 (282 amino acids residues) contains two stretches of hydrophobic amino acid residues near its carboxy terminus, an 18–amino acid residue transmembrane domain, and the E1 signal peptide.[11,46] These two hydrophobic domains are separated by a 7–amino acid residue loop that is rich in basic amino acid residues. Similar to E1, translocation of E2 into ER membranes is mediated by an amino terminal signal peptide.[91] E2 is heavily glycosylated and contains both asparagine-linked and O-linked carbohydrates.[96,136] Finally, both glycoproteins are modified by the addition of palmitate prior to virus assembly.[93,249] The role of this modification in spike protein function has not been investigated, but it is possible that acylation may serve to further stabilize and/or orientate E2 and E1 in the membrane. The membrane orientations of the RV structural proteins are shown in Figure 28.8.

Replication Strategy

The replication strategy of RV is similar to that of alphaviruses in many respects, but there are several quantitative and qualitative differences. As discussed previously, RV replication is less robust and much slower than that of alphaviruses.[87] In addition, it is not possible to obtain a uniformly infected population of cells within 24 hours, even at high multiplicities of infection.[214] The reason for this phenomenon is not clear, but

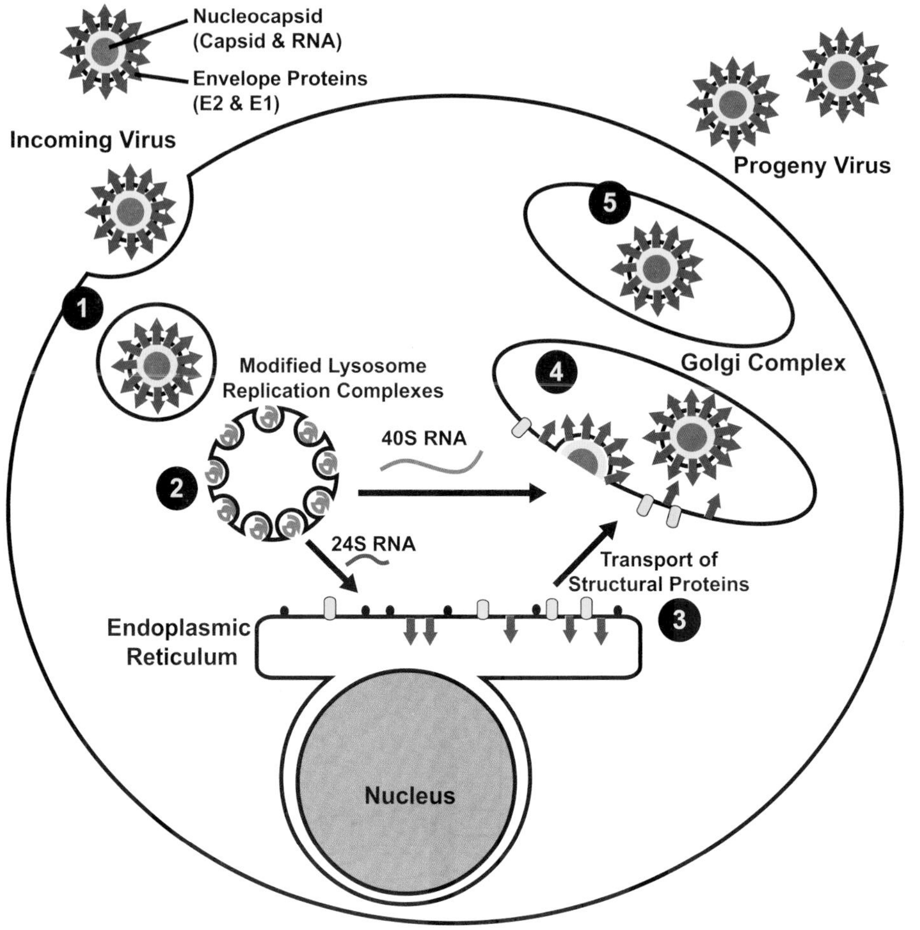

FIGURE 24.11. Entry and exit strategy of rubella virus (RV). 1: Uptake of RV is dependent upon receptor-mediated endocytosis. The low pH of the endosome/lysosome induces virus uncoating. **2:** RNA replication occurs at the cytopathic vacuoles that originate from endosomes/lysosomes. Genome amplification and synthesis of the 24S subgenomic RNA also occurs at these sites. **3:** Synthesis of structural proteins takes place at the endoplasmic reticulum and processing by the host cell signal peptidase separates the polyprotein into individual structural proteins. Subsequently, the structural proteins assemble and are transported to the Golgi complex. **4:** Nucleocapsid assembly and virus budding occur at the Golgi complex. **5:** Rubella virions undergo a series of maturation events before exocytosis.

given the fact that eventually all cells within a permissive culture become infected, it is possible that a cell cycle–dependent factor is required for RV entry or early viral replication events. Another major difference from the alphaviruses is that a large pool of the nascent RV capsid protein remains membrane associated.[120,224] This may be one of the reasons that RV nucleocapsid assembly differs from that of alphaviruses, which are not membrane associated. Free nucleocapsids are rarely observed in RV-infected cells but rather assembly is coincident with virus budding at the Golgi complex, a process that is hypothesized to be regulated by reversible phosphorylation of the capsid protein.[121] A schematic diagram of how RV enters, replicates, and exits from host cells is shown in Figure 24.11.

Virus Entry

Host cell–encoded proteins and lipids are important for virion binding,[50,142] after which the virus is internalized by receptor-mediated endocytosis.[186] At low pH, the envelope glycoproteins become fusogenic, and capsid undergoes a conformational change and becomes hydrophobic,[114,145] indicating that the acidic environment within endosomes induces fusion of the viral envelope with cellular membranes followed by release of genomic RNA from the nucleocapsid. The type I membrane protein myelin oligodendrocyte glycoprotein binds to the E1 glycoprotein and was recently identified as a host receptor for RV.[50] This protein is most highly expressed in the central nervous system, but in epithelial and lymphoid cells, which serve as the portals of entry and initial sites of replication, myelin oligodendrocyte glycoprotein levels are much lower. As such, it cannot be ruled out that the virus uses different receptors in different cell types.

Replication Complexes

Similar to all other plus-strand RNA viruses that infect mammalian cells, replication of RV RNA occurs in association with cellular membranes. Cytoplasmic vacuoles (Fig. 24.5) with regularly shaped invaginations or spherules (60 nm in diameter) are observed in RV-infected cells.[127] The spherules are connected to the vacuolar membranes by thin membranous necks and can be stained with antibodies against p150 and double-stranded RNA, suggesting that they are the sites of viral RNA synthesis.[118,125] These vacuoles also co-localize with lysosomal markers, indicating that they are derived from endosomes and/or possibly lysosomes.[138]

Recently, replication complexes in RV-infected cells have been analyzed using electron microscopy and freeze fracture techniques.[64] Replication of viral RNA occurs within protected membranous pockets of the cytopathic vacuoles. The vacuoles are surrounded by rough ER, an arrangement that may facilitate binding between RNA and the capsid protein (which is synthesized on the surface of the ER) to promote nucleocapsid formation. In a number of fundamental aspects, RV replication complexes are similar to those found in alphavirus-infected cells.[71] However, there are several important distinctions between them. First, assembled nucleocapsids are rarely observed near replication complexes in RV-infected cells. In contrast, nucleocapsids are regularly observed surrounding the replication complexes of alphavirus-infected cells. In RV-infected cells, formation of the replication complexes coincides with the rearrangement of other cellular structures. Specifically, rough ER and Golgi are in close proximity to the virus-modified endocytic organelles, and mitochondria cluster to regions of the cell containing replication complexes.[123,127] Although mitochondrial aggregation in the vicinity of replication complexes also occurs in alphavirus-infected cells, the close association of the rough ER and Golgi with replication complexes is unique to RV-infected cells. Recruitment of ER and Golgi membranes to the replication complexes may be necessary to coordinate translation of the structural proteins and packaging of the genomic RNA. Mitochondria are also recruited to the replication complexes, but the reason for this is not clear. It has been suggested that this arrangement of organelles would increase the availability of adenosine triphosphate (ATP) for virus replication, but solid evidence to support this theory is lacking.

Targeting of Structural Proteins to the Budding Site

Following synthesis of the subgenomic RNA, the RV structural proteins are translated in association with ER membranes. The structural polyprotein precursor is cleaved by signal peptidase at two sites (Fig. 24.8) to generate the three structural proteins.[91,96] The structural proteins are then posttranslationally modified and transported to the Golgi complex, which is the primary site of virus budding. Processing and transport of the RV structural proteins have been extensively studied using transfection experiments. When co-expressed, E2 and E1 heterodimerize, form intramolecular disulfide bonds in the ER, and are transported to and retained in the Golgi.[11,99] Targeting of the virus glycoproteins to the Golgi complex is independent of capsid, indicating that accumulation of E2 and E1 in this organelle is the major factor in determining the budding site. In the absence of E2, E1 does not target to the Golgi but rather is retained in a smooth ER compartment.[98] The membrane proximal regions of the structural proteins have important roles in regulating the localization and transport of these proteins. For example, within the transmembrane and the cytoplasmic domains of E1 resides an ER retention signal that prevents or delays transport of nascent viral glycoproteins from the ER.[92] Co-expression of E2 appears to mask the ER retention signal in E1, thereby allowing transport of the E2-E1 heterocomplex from the ER to the Golgi after a maturation period. The transmembrane domain of E2, in turn, contains a retention signal that mediates retention of the E2-E1 heterodimer in the Golgi.[97]

The highly regulated transport of RV glycoproteins may serve as a quality control mechanism to ensure only properly assembled subunits reach the virus budding site. The half-life for transport of the RV glycoproteins to the Golgi is 60 to 90 minutes (whereas for alphavirus glycoproteins it is approximately 25 minutes).[90] Dimerization of E1 and E2 in the ER is not rate limiting as evidenced by the fact that these two proteins associate rapidly following synthesis. E2 achieves its mature conformation shortly after synthesis and has been proposed to function as a scaffold for E1. Accordingly, the rate-limiting step for transport of the glycoproteins is the relatively slow maturation and folding of E1 in the ER.[99] The mature ectodomain of E1 contains 20 cysteine residues that participate in the formation of intramolecular disulfide bonds.[84] It is hypothesized that the ER retention signal in E1 is required to retain nascent E1 in the ER until it has achieved the proper conformation, which includes the formation of intramolecular disulfide bonds. Indeed, replacing the E1 transmembrane domain with analogous domains from other membrane glycoproteins actually increases the rate of ER-to-Golgi transport for E1 and E2.[74] The E2 transmembrane and cytoplasmic domains are required for assembly of E2-E1 heterodimers and therefore have an indirect role in regulating transport of the RV glycoproteins from the ER to the Golgi. Finally, mutagenesis studies have shown that N-linked glycosylation is important for maturation and intracellular transport of both E1 and E2 glycoproteins.[95,198]

As well as regulating targeting of E1 to the Golgi complex, E2 is required for transport of the capsid protein to the intracellular budding site.[11,94] The carboxyl terminus of E2, which includes the transmembrane and cytoplasmic domains, is essential for this process[74] and formation of VLPs[120] and likely infectious virions. Lateral interactions between the E2 signal peptide and the transmembrane regions of E2 and/or E1 may facilitate transport of capsid from the ER to the Golgi by incorporation into ER-derived transport vesicles. In contrast, the analogous regions of E1 are not required for localization of capsid to the juxtanuclear region. Together, these results indicate that the E2 carboxyl terminus governs the targeting of all three RV structural proteins to the virus budding site.

Virus Assembly and Secretion

RV budding has been reported to occur at both the Golgi complex and the plasma membrane, depending on cell type and the time postinfection.[10,244] However, several lines of evidence suggest that the primary site for virus budding is the Golgi complex. First, the presence of a signal in E2 mediates retention of the structural proteins in the Golgi complex, and consequently, only a small fraction of the RV structural proteins reaches the plasma membrane.[97,99] Second, budding at the plasma membrane reportedly occurs late in infection, suggesting that this is not the principal budding site. Furthermore, virion membrane composition is more similar to that of intracellular membranes rather than the plasma membrane.[8]

Unlike alphavirus nucleocapsids, which are formed in the cytoplasm of infected cells prior to budding, RV nucleocapsids form in association with cellular membranes coincident with budding and are rarely observed in the cytoplasm of infected cells.[126] It has also been hypothesized that RV employs a mechanism to prevent premature assembly of nucleocapsids (Fig. 24.9). Specifically, reversible phosphorylation of the RNA-binding region of capsid may regulate assembly and disassembly of RV nucleocapsids.[119,121] Whether phosphorylation of capsid proteins has any role in assembly of alphavirus nucleocapsids has not been investigated.

The mechanisms that regulate interactions between the nucleocapsid and spike glycoproteins during virus budding are largely unknown. With respect to the budding reaction, it is tempting to speculate that electrostatic interactions between the cytoplasmic domain of E2, which is rich in basic amino acid residues, and clusters of acidic amino acid residues in the capsid are involved. Indeed, nonconservative mutations in this E2 domain drastically affect the assembly of VLPs.[74] It is also well established that the transmembrane domains of the structural proteins are important for targeting to the budding site. In this respect, lateral interactions between the transmembrane domains of E1, E2, and capsid protein may be important for the budding reaction. Finally, it is important to consider that interactions between RV structural proteins and host cell proteins contribute to efficient budding of virus particles.

A morphologic study that employed freeze-substitution electron microscopy revealed that rubella virions undergo a maturation process following budding into the Golgi.[206] Specifically, at early time points, intra-Golgi virions exhibited homogenous interiors with fine contacts between the core and the particle membrane. At later time points the virion cores appeared denser and were smaller in diameter such that they were clearly delineated from the virion membrane. These results indicate that the virion maturation process involves compaction of the nucleocapsid. Several lines of evidence suggest that the E1 transmembrane and cytoplasmic domains also function in virion maturation and/or secretion. Replacement of the E1 transmembrane domain does not affect budding of VLPs in the Golgi, but secretion of the particles into the extracellular space is blocked.[73] Similarly, introduction of point mutations into the E1 transmembrane and/or cytoplasmic domains drastically reduces virus secretion without affecting the assembly process at the Golgi.[200,259] These rather surprising data indicate that virus assembly at the Golgi complex is not coupled to secretion and that E1 is involved in a late-stage maturation event that is necessary for virus secretion.

There is limited information regarding the interactions between RV virions and polarized cells. Because it causes a systemic infection, the virus must cross one or more epithelial layers, including the upper respiratory epithelium. Cultured epithelial cells can be infected from the apical and basal membranes, indicating that RV receptors are not confined to one surface.[73] The secretion of virus particles varies according to cell type. In two of the three polarized cell lines examined, virions were released primarily from the apical surface, but significant quantities were also secreted from the basolateral membrane. Presumably, secretion of rubella virions from the apical surface facilitates virus spread from person to person, whereas basolateral secretion could be important for establishing a systemic infection and/or crossing the placenta prior to fetal infection.

RV Persistence

Although cell death by apoptosis occurs in highly susceptible cell lines infected at high MOIs, infection of a wide variety of cells *in vitro* with low MOIs results in little cytopathology and viral persistence.[1,3,70,255] In fact, a recent study has shown that RV-infected cells are quite resistant to a variety of apoptotic stimuli as a result of interaction between the capsid protein and the host protein Bax.[107] These findings are consistent with earlier observations that while temperature-sensitive mutants and defective interfering (DI) particles develop in and may play a role in controlling replication in persistently infected cells, neither is required to establish persistent infection.[70,255] During long-term persistence in RV-infected Vero cells, DI RNAs become the dominant species of viral RNA, with genomic RNA decreasing to low levels. Persistence in cultured cells is thus a chronic infection, with the majority of cells expressing viral antigen and RNA, much of which is DI RNA. These cultures release low levels of temperature-sensitive progeny virus and DI particles. Finally, while it cannot be ruled out that interferons play a role in viral persistence, they are clearly not essential because persistent RV infections can be established in interferon-deficient cell lines such as Vero and BHK-/21 cells.[222] Moreover, exogenous interferon was not found to have an effect on RV persistence in these cell lines.

The virus can persist for many months in congenitally infected human fetuses, and multiple organ systems are affected (see Mechanisms of Teratogenesis section). Following postnatal infection, PBMCs are an established site of RV persistence *in vivo,* particularly in adults who develop rubella-associated arthritis following natural infection or immunization.[35] Viral persistence *in vivo* occurs in the presence of high levels of neutralizing antibody, which not only may limit viral spread but also has been suggested to actually promote viral persistence. To date, however, this theory has yet to be substantiated. Another site of persistence *in vivo* is joint tissue,[39,67] which has led to speculation that RV plays a role in development of degenerative joint disease (see Complications section).

In vitro, both wt+ and vaccine strains of RV can infect and persist in chondrocyte-derived cell lines[36] and in primary cultures of human joint tissue.[152] Except for the Cendehill vaccine strain, all other RV strains can replicate and persist in joint tissue for more than 3 months. Interestingly, virus derived from these chronically infected cultures was temperature sensitive, but no DI particles were detected.

Animal Models of Rubella Virus Infection

There are no reliable animal models for the study of clinically symptomatic rubella infection. However, a variety of laboratory animals (including nonhuman primates) can be asymptomatically infected with RV. For example, rhesus and African green monkeys develop viremia, shed virus in respiratory secretions, and produce humoral immune responses in a manner that is similar to acute rubella in humans.[101] However, attempts to model the teratogenic effects of rubella in various animals, including baboons, cynomolgus monkeys, marmosets, and rats, have produced inconsistent results with, at best, low incidence of defects such as cataracts or stillbirths.[248,251] Infection of the central nervous system (CNS) has been shown to occur in immunosuppressed BALB/c mice, and as such, it is possible that this system could work as a small animal model to understand the effects of RV on the brain.[141] Unfortunately, none of the animal systems has proven sufficiently reliable to study details of the pathogenesis of either acquired or congenital rubella.

Antigenic Composition and Determinants

Complement-Fixing and Hemagglutinating Antigens

Early serologic tests for rubella used crude complement fixation antigens extracted from virus-infected cells and purified on sucrose gradients. A more slowly sedimenting fraction from the gradients with a density of 1.08 to 1.10 in sucrose (as compared to a density of 1.18 to 1.20 for intact virions) was shown to have hemagglutinating (HA) activity.[236] HA activity is also associated with cell-free virus preparations[105] and can be extracted from infected cells or supernatant virus using Tween 80 and ether, resulting in a 26S particle that retains biological activity. By electron microscopy, it appears as a 15-nm rosette with a hollow core.[235]

B-Cell Epitopes

The E1 glycoprotein is the immunodominant surface molecule of the virus particle as evidenced by the fact that it is the major target for the host's humoral immune system.[256] Antibodies to both E2 and capsid are also found in humans, although at lower levels and of lower avidity. Mapping of antigenic domains on the viral proteins was first carried out using monoclonal antibodies.[256] Later, detailed studies on the fine antigenic structure of each viral protein were carried out using recombinant proteins, proteolytic peptide fragments, and synthetic peptides to deduce antigenic sites.[40,147,154] At least five distinct nonoverlapping immunoreactive regions were identified in the E1 protein ($E1_{11-39}$, $E1_{154-179}$, $E1_{199-239}$, $E1_{226-277}$, and $E1_{389-412}$). Cellular proliferative responses to these peptides were found in 29% to 83% of the subjects tested,[154] including one peptide ($E1_{208-239}$) that contained a previously identified neutralization domain.[257] Reactivity with this peptide in an enzyme-linked immunoassay (ELISA) correlates well with assays that measure hemagglutination inhibition (HAI) and virus neutralization.[54,157] To date, two B-cell epitopes have been identified on the capsid protein, C_{1-30} and C_{96-123}, and one ($E2_{31-105}$) on the E2 glycoprotein.[40,147,173]

T-Cell Epitopes

There are at least 17 RV-specific T-cell epitopes, but the precise limit of each epitope is not known.[147,154,172] A minimum of four immunodominant sites are located on E1, and these display reactivity to T cells from several donors with different HLA haplotype backgrounds.[178] Subsequently, minimal T-helper-cell epitopes were identified at $E1_{280-287}$, $E1_{385-393}$, and $E1_{410-420}$ using T-cell lines from seropositive healthy donors, with variation in responsiveness found between individuals.[141] Interestingly, binding of the peptide $E1_{272-285}$ to HLA-DR and its recognition by RV-specific clones is influenced by DRβ polymorphisms.[177]

At least three T-cell epitopes have been found on the E2 protein.[154,172] One of these peptides ($E2_{54-65}$) is present in approximately 50% of T-cell lines derived from donors with the HLA-DR7 phenotype.[170] With respect to the capsid protein, a peptide ($C_{265-273}$) is recognized by T-cell clones derived from donors expressing the DRB1*0403 and DRB1*0901 alleles.[171] However, this peptide is recognized promiscuously by HLA-DR molecules that have common residues in pocket 4 of the peptide-binding groove and therefore likely defines a DR supertype.[176]

EPIDEMIOLOGY

Incidence

Prior to the introduction of immunization programs, rubella was endemic worldwide, with regular seasonal peaks occurring in the spring months in temperate climates. In addition, epidemics of rubella occurred at intervals of 6 to 9 years as the pool of susceptible individuals reached a threshold. Epidemics still occur in developing and tropical countries, but the lack of effective monitoring programs, together with the absence of serious clinical symptoms in affected children, has made them difficult to assess.[209] Regional variations in the age of onset of rubella, the incidence of the disease, and the appearance and spread of epidemics are determined by population densities, socioeconomic factors, and levels of medical sophistication in a given community. When these rubella outbreaks occur, they are accompanied by birth defects associated with congenital rubella syndrome (CRS). The teratogenic effects of rubella were a significant factor that spurred vaccine development following the rubella pandemic between 1962 and 1965. In this epidemic, an estimated 12.5 million cases of rubella occurred in the United States alone, resulting in up to 20,000 children born with congenital abnormalities.[28] Today, CRS has been reduced to a handful of cases in both Europe and North America, with a declaration by the Centers for Disease Control and Prevention (CDC) in 2005 that endemic CRS had been eliminated from the United States.[2] However, residual cases are seen in immigrants who may not have been immunized in their country of origin.[18] Despite an increase in rubella vaccination worldwide, less than 40% of the global birth cohort was covered as of 2009.[258] Indeed, most of Africa and India and parts of Asia are not vaccinated against rubella (Fig. 24.1). It has been estimated that even in nonepidemic years, there are more than 100,000 infants born with CRS annually.

Age

Prior to the introduction of universal rubella immunization, peak infection occurred in the 5- to 9-year-old age group.[102] After vaccine implementation, the disease shifted from children to young adults until its virtual elimination from Europe and North America in recent years.[30] In countries that have not implemented vaccination programs, infection at an early age is still the norm, with high seroconversion rates found in both preschool populations and in the 5- to 9-year-old age group.[79] In many developing countries, women of childbearing age are susceptible to rubella and the incidence of CRS during rubella outbreaks is 1 to 2 per 1,000 live births.[58]

Origin and Spread of Epidemics

The are no animal reservoirs for RV, and therefore, continued cycling of the virus within the human population is required for perpetuation of the disease between seasons of maximal endemic occurrence. In countries where rubella immunization is not carried out and congenital infection is still common, the surviving infants shed high levels of virus for many months, forming a potential source for maintenance of the virus for relatively long periods. Enhanced vaccination programs have been very effective in disrupting virus circulation in much of the developed world. However, localized outbreaks of rubella still occur with regular frequency in countries where vaccination is practiced. Often, vaccine refusal on the basis of religious grounds is the major factor in such outbreaks. For example, in 2005, 214 cases of rubella occurred in an Amish community in Canada.[14] Similar outbreaks have been reported in the United States among religious communities and Hispanic populations.[28] More recently, between 2009 and 2010, an outbreak of 1,900 cases of rubella was reported in Bosnia and Herzegovina, a situation that resulted from decreased vaccine uptake during the 1992–1995 war.[106] Together, these studies demonstrate the importance of maintaining high levels of herd immunity in developed countries, because rubella can be reintroduced into the population by foreign travel or from recent immigrants travelling from endemic areas. To prevent outbreaks, it has been estimated that at least 85% of the population must be immune to RV,[4] whereas to maintain elimination, a 90% level of immunity among children is required.[88]

Molecular Epidemiology

Based on sequence comparison of the *E1* gene, at least 10 genotypes of RV representing two clades (RG1 and 2) have been identified[264] (Fig. 24.3). The RG1 clade comprises viral isolates from North America, Europe, and Japan, whereas RG2 was

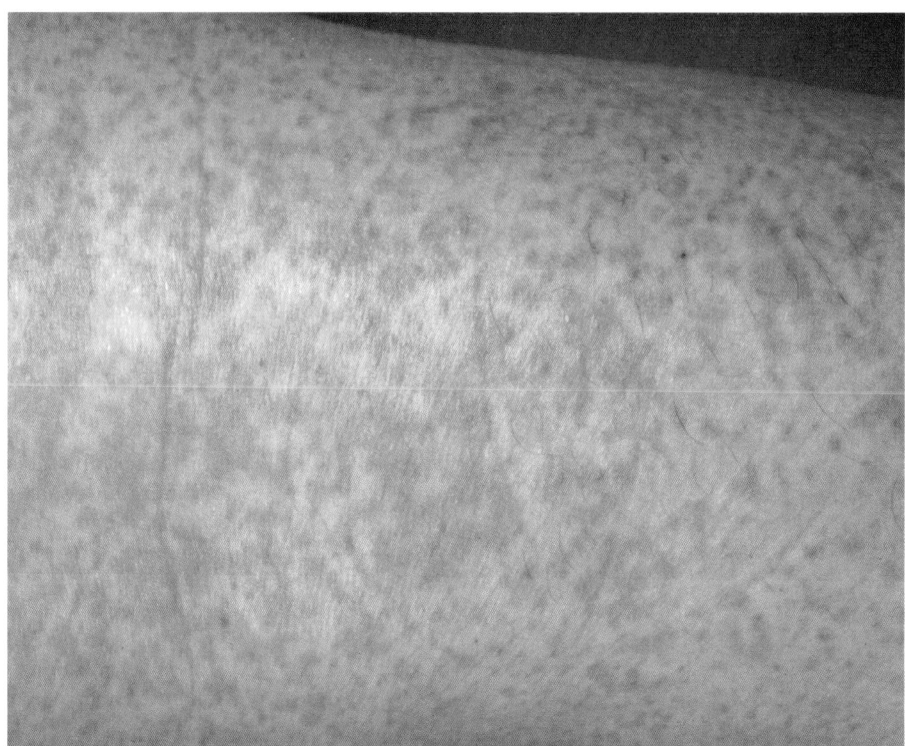

FIGURE 24.12. Characteristic skin rash on patient with acute rubella. (Reproduced with permission from Logical Images, Inc.)

identified using isolates from China and India. RG1 and RG2 differ by 8% to 10% at the nucleotide level, as opposed to less than 5% among genotypes within each clade. RG2 has more genetic diversity than RG1 and may in fact consist of multiple clades. These genetic differences have been useful in tracking RV spread around the world and changes in endemic strains over time. Nevertheless, the differences in *E1* genes result in only 1% to 3% substitutions at the amino acid level, attesting to a high degree of genetic conservation between rubella strains. Finally, only one strain from clade 2 contained a mutation in one of the known epitopes defined by monoclonal antibodies, the first indication of a serotype variant.

CLINICAL FEATURES

Acute Rubella

Postnatal infection with RV is usually mild and frequently subclinical.[7,62] Symptoms, when present, typically include sore throat and low-grade fever, a maculopapular rash, lymphadenopathy, and, in some cases, conjunctivitis and/or arthralgia. The rash (Fig. 24.12) is first seen on the face and spreads in centripetal fashion. The lesions appear as distinct pink maculopapules that fade rapidly over several days. A pronounced posterior cervical and suboccipital adenopathy is often present. In the majority of cases, the clinical syndrome clears in days and is seldom attended by more significant symptoms, but arthropathy, thrombocytopenia, and encephalopathy can occur.[19] However, these serious sequelae and death as a result of RV infection are rare. The course of the acquired infection and the accompanying immune response are shown in Figure 24.13.

The virus is spread through respiratory secretions, and the mucosa of the upper respiratory tract and the nasopharyngeal lymphoid tissue serve as portals of virus entry as well as the initial sites for viral replication. Spread of virus via lymphatics or a transient viremia then seeds regional lymph nodes. Local replication of virus in these nodes accounts for the posterior cervical and occipital nodal enlargement that typically appears 5 to 9 days before the onset of the rash. The incubation period (approximately 14 days) is followed by the appearance of virus in serum and the onset of viral shedding into the nasopharynx and stool, providing a source of spread to susceptible individuals. High levels of virus can be found in nasopharyngeal

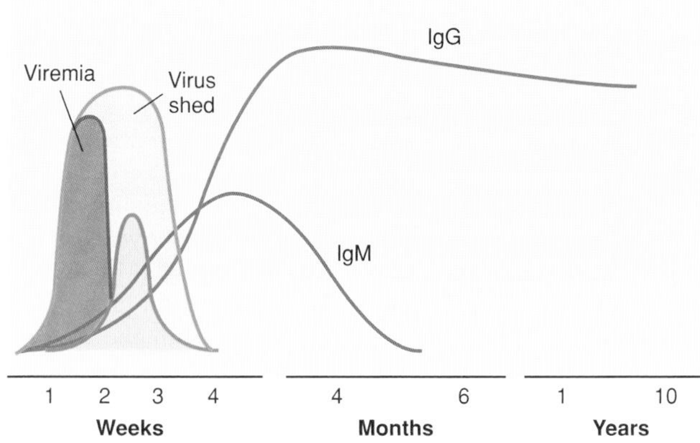

FIGURE 24.13. Time course showing viremic phase, rash, and immunoglobulin M (IgM) and IgG development during acute rubella infection from the time of infection initiation by droplet spray. Patients are infectious and shed virus from the time of infection until 1 to 2 weeks after the appearance of rash. IgM is present by day 10 and peaks around 4 weeks postinfection, by which time low-avidity IgG is also present.

secretions, exceeding 10^5 tissue culture infectious dose 50 ($TCID_{50}$) per 0.1 mL even in vaccinated individuals.[7] The viremic phase may be marked by mild prodromal symptoms and malaise. The maculopapular rash appears at 14 to 21 days after natural exposure but somewhat earlier following experimental infection or vaccination. The presence of virus in serum ceases shortly after the rash appears, coincident with the onset of detectable circulating antibodies.

Immune Response

A serologic response can be detected at the onset of rash and continues to evolve over the next few weeks (Fig. 24.13). Generally, immunoglobulin M (IgM) antibody is first detected at 10 days postinfection, after which peak levels occur at 4 weeks postinfection but can persist for more than 7 months after acute infection.[212,228] By 3 weeks, RV-specific antibodies are present in all immunoglobulin classes, including IgG, IgA, IgD, and IgE. At early stages of primary infection, IgG is of low avidity, maturing gradually during the next 3 months.[25]

When measured by immunoprecipitation or immunoblot techniques, the majority of the immunoglobulin response appears to be directed at the E1 glycoprotein, with proportionally lesser amounts of the response against E2 or capsid.[41] Interestingly, males have a more rapid and robust antibody response than females, although females have a higher anti-E2 response.[158] Whether there are pathologic consequences of these differences is not known.

Transient depression of lymphocyte responsiveness to mitogenic stimulation follows natural or vaccine infections in children and adults.[26] Despite this generalized immune suppression, RV-specific cell-mediated immune responses develop and can be measured *in vitro* within 1 or 2 weeks of onset of clinical illness. The cellular responses wane over the next few years but persist at low levels indefinitely after natural rubella. In contrast, they are difficult to detect following vaccination. More detailed studies have defined the epitope specificity of defined CD4+ and CD8+ T-cell clones[134,172,175] (see Antigenic Composition and Determinants section).

Complications

Joint Symptoms

The most common complications of natural rubella are acute arthralgia and/or arthritis, particularly in adolescent and adult women.[219] Incidence rates for joint involvement range between 30% and 60% during outbreaks. For example, in one report, 52% of adult females and 9% of adult males developed arthropathy, with symptoms being more severe among women.[229] The joint symptoms usually begin within a week of the appearance of the rash and may involve any joint, with the fingers and knees being most commonly affected. Although these symptoms usually resolve within several weeks, they can persist for months or even years, in which case they are episodic. Rarely, chronic severe arthropathy that is significantly disabling has been reported.[35] A similar range of less severe symptoms occurs 9 to 27 days following vaccination but is less common than after natural rubella.[229] A report on rubella vaccine–associated arthritis, based on analysis of the Vaccine Adverse Events Reporting System (VAERS) database, has confirmed that rubella vaccine in adult women is associated with chronic arthritis that can persist for at least 1 year.[76]

Factors that affect the incidence of joint symptoms include age and gender,[229] as well as major histocompatibility complex (MHC) type of the infected individual.[155] Hormonal influences also affect the incidence of joint symptoms, with adult females being most susceptible. The underlying pathogenesis of rubella arthritis is unknown, but the mechanism may involve local viral replication. Several groups have reported the isolation of RV from synovial fluids of symptomatic joints for up to a month following acute infection.[67,162] Virus has also been isolated from PBMCs of symptomatic individuals[35] and can be detected in women with chronic arthropathy postvaccination by reverse transcriptase-polymerase chain reaction (RT-PCR) amplification of PBMC RNA using RV-specific primers.[156] Replication and persistence of virus in extra-articular sites and deposition of immune complexes on articular surfaces may therefore play a role in the acute stage.

RV can also infect and persist in joint tissue for prolonged periods *in vitro,* forming foci of infection that are positive for viral antigen.[152] Overall, the body of evidence indicates that RV is a highly arthrotropic virus and a plausible candidate as one of several viral triggers (including human parvovirus, hepatitis C, and human T-cell lymphotropic virus type 1 [HTLV-1]) of chronic degenerative forms of arthritis.

Thrombocytopenia

A number of different viral infections result in reduced platelets either by inhibiting their production or by causing their lysis.[202] For example, binding of viral immune complexes to Fc receptors on the platelet surface triggers immune-mediated clearing of both the complex and its associated platelet.[115] This causes a transient asymptomatic depression of thrombocyte counts and is quite common with rubella.[52] Thrombocytopenic purpura is seen following rubella infection; however, this condition is relatively rare (1 in 1,500 cases)[240] and is usually self-limiting. However, it may even occur in the absence of rash. Accordingly, undiagnosed RV infections are likely the cause of some cases of idiopathic thrombocytopenic purpura. Very rarely is epidemic rubella associated with hemolytic anemia.

Encephalopathy

The most serious complication of postnatal rubella is postinfectious encephalopathy or encephalomyelitis.[17] Estimated to occur in 1 in 6,000 cases of natural infection, rubella encephalitis is rarely reported in countries with comprehensive vaccination policies. However, occasionally, case reports indicate that this disorder can appear during rubella outbreaks. The symptoms of rubella encephalopathy appear abruptly 1 to 6 days following the onset of rash in an otherwise typical case of rubella. The most frequently encountered symptoms include headache, vomiting, stiff neck, lethargy, and generalized convulsions.[250] In rare cases, RV antigens have been detected within brain tissue,[51] and virus has been isolated from cerebrospinal fluid (CSF), indicating that it has the capacity to invade the mature CNS.[220]

Postnatal rubella encephalopathy usually requires only supportive treatment, and the disease course is generally concluded within a few days; the survival rate approximates 80%. Among the 20% of patients who do not survive, the disease course typically includes coma, respiratory distress, apnea, and then death, usually within a few days of onset of symptoms.

Congenital Rubella Syndrome

Although postnatal rubella is rarely associated with severe complications, infection *in utero* following transplacental transmission of virus from the mother has dire consequences for the developing fetus. These are reflected in a constellation of symptoms collectively called congenital rubella syndrome.[52,251]

Pathogenesis of Congenital Rubella Syndrome

In general, maternal infection shortly before conception does not lead to intrauterine infection.[63] However, when infection occurs after conception, the virus is present in placental villi approximately 10 days after the onset of rash in the mother and can be detected in the fetus after 20 to 30 days.[113] Transplacental transmission occurs in up to 90% of cases during the first 8 weeks of gestation, falling to a low of 25% to 35% during the second trimester and rising again near term.[7,75,251] This fluctuating incidence of fetal infection is likely related to changes in the placenta during pregnancy. In early gestation, infection of the placenta causes scattered foci of necrotic syncytiotrophoblast and cytotrophoblast cells, as well as damage to the vascular endothelium, resulting in placental hypoplasia.[75] Infection at later stages is associated with multifocal mononuclear cell infiltrates in the placental membranes, cord, and decidua, along with vasculitis.[251] In cases where fetal infection occurs, the virus can spread widely and almost any organ may be infected. A chronic and generally nonlytic infection is then established in the fetus.[187]

Clinical Consequences

The effects of RV invasion of fetal tissue are quite varied, and early infection may result in resorption of the embryo. Whether placental infection alone can lead to spontaneous abortion or abnormalities of fetal development is not established. In the majority of cases, the infected fetus will survive and the pregnancy continues to term, with premature delivery or stillbirths being rare outcomes.[153] In many countries, clinically recognized maternal rubella during the first 8 weeks of gestation is an indication for therapeutic abortion due to the high incidence of congenital defects. Although these are not universal, some degree of neurologic deficit including sensorineural deafness is found in most cases. The current rubella vaccine RA27/3 has extremely low teratogenicity, and inadvertent vaccination in early pregnancy is not considered an indication for therapeutic abortion, although immunization at this time should be avoided.[31,191]

The most common clinical manifestations of congenital rubella are listed in Table 24.1. In addition to the high incidence of sensorineural deafness (~80%), cataracts are detected in 50% to 60% of neonates infected in the first 8 weeks of pregnancy.[7] Congenital heart disease is also found in more than half of CRS babies, usually manifested as patent ductus arteriosus or pulmonary artery or valvular stenosis. Other common defects include glaucoma, retinopathy, psychomotor retardation, neonatal thrombocytopenia purpura, hepatomegaly and/or splenomegaly, and intrauterine growth retardation.[52] Less frequent features (present in 5% to 10%) include adenopathy, bony radiolucencies, hepatitis, and hemolytic anemia. Many of the clinical manifestations of congenital rubella are evident at birth or shortly thereafter. This includes a reddish-blue (purpuric) maculopapular rash termed the *blueberry muffin* rash (Fig. 24.14). Other clinical signs, including hepatosplenomegaly and jaundice, usually resolve within weeks. In addition, there are defects that are not recognized at birth but may be manifest in childhood (e.g., mental or physical retardation) or in adolescence (type 1 diabetes).

TABLE 24.1 Manifestations of Congenital Rubella Syndrome

Group A	Group B
Eye manifestations • Cataracts • Congenital glaucoma • Retinitis Congenital heart defects • Patent ductus arteriosus • Pulmonary artery stenosis Sensorineural hearing loss Pigmentary neuropathy	Purpura Hepatosplenomegaly Jaundice Microcephaly Meningoencephalitis Radiolucent bone disease Progressive or late-onset manifestations • Mental retardation • Diabetes mellitus • Progressive panencephalitis

At birth, CRS is accompanied by clinical signs that include bulging anterior fontanel, microcephaly, lethargy, irritability, and motor tone abnormalities.[251] RV can be isolated from almost any organ at birth and from selected tissues for up to 1 year or more in surviving infants.[151] More than 80% of congenitally infected newborns contain substantial amounts of RV in their nasopharyngeal secretions and urine, and 3% will continue to shed virus for as long as 20 months. This chronic shedding of RV by neonates is an indicator of early gestational infection[56] and a major source of virus for dissemination to others.

Mechanisms of Teratogenesis

Most of our information on rubella embryopathy comes from careful pathologic analyses conducted following the major

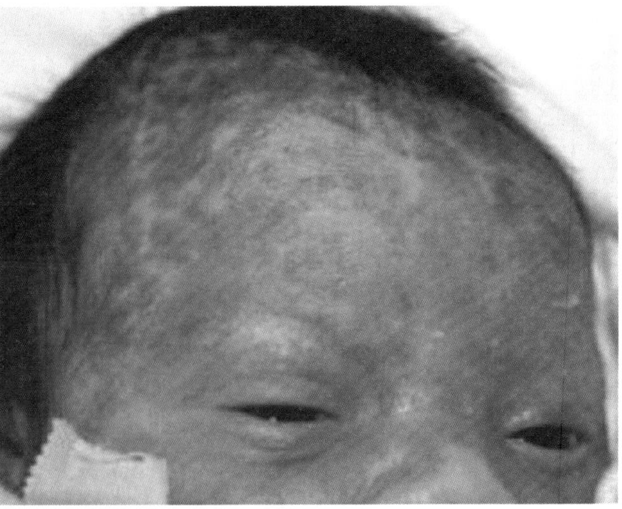

FIGURE 24.14. Infant with congenital rubella showing characteristic "blueberry muffin" maculopapular rash. (From Dermatology Online Journal, dermatology.cdlib.org.)

rubella pandemic of the 1960s. Data from these studies led to the idea that direct cytolytic effects of RV to cells in the retinal epithelium, myocardium, skeletal muscle, and neural tissue underlie much of the observed damage in CRS.[117,210,233] The widespread nature of the tissue damage indicates that RV infects most fetal organ systems. Infection of focal clones of cells and their progeny during critical stages of the ontogeny of fetal organs was believed to give rise to the wide range of abnormalities that together compose CRS.

Because there are no animal models that recapitulate the teratogenic effects of RV infection, direct effects on human fetal cells *in situ* can only be extrapolated from studies in cell culture. Multiple studies reporting that cultured cells infected with RV exhibited signs of apoptosis[61,100,122,149,195] and that human embryonic cells persistently infected with RV produce lower levels of collagen and are less responsive to epidermal growth factor[261] led to the hypothesis that altered cell physiology and induction of programmed cell death were integral to the teratogenic activity of the virus. However, a later study reported that RV infection does not induce apoptosis in human embryonic fibroblasts, but rather induces expression of multiple of antiapoptotic genes.[3] These findings are consistent with a more recent report showing that the capsid protein blocks apoptosis in human embryonic and adult cultured cell lines.[107] Accordingly, it is quite possible that a predominantly noncytopathic RV infection of selected embryonic cell types *in utero* upsets the normal delicate balance of cellular growth and differentiation and has profound effects on organogenesis. These effects, alone or in concert, could explain the observation that the small but otherwise apparently normal organs of congenital rubella infants contain reduced numbers of cells.[161] In addition to these direct effects of RV replication in host tissue, it is possible that immune-mediated damage occurs in CRS.

Fetal Immune Response in CRS

The persistence of RV in fetal tissue throughout gestation, and in infants with CRS for prolonged periods after birth, raises the question of how the virus avoids immune elimination. Clearly, neither transferred maternal IgG nor fetal IgM (detected at around 15 weeks' gestation[251]) can eliminate virus *in utero*, although both have neutralizing capacity *in vitro*.[53] It has been suggested that antibody may in fact promote persistence; however, this phenomenon has only been observed *in vitro*[1,34] and it is not at all clear whether it can occur in the absence of the complement system and phagocytic cells. Two recent studies[3,107] suggest that the ability of RV to block apoptosis may also play a role in establishment and/or maintenance of persistence by thwarting innate antiviral defenses. Moreover, because the thymus does not mature until 15 weeks, the fetus is highly vulnerable to viral infection prior to this time. Interferon-α is present early in gestation and therefore may limit viral spread, a scenario that could explain why only 0.1% to 0.001% of cells from fetal organs contain detectable virus.[203]

Postnatal infection induces IgG class antibodies against each of the three structural proteins of the virus; however, CRS infants often lack antibodies to the capsid protein and demonstrate weak humoral reactivity to the E2 protein.[59,197] Perhaps more telling, these children show selective tolerance to the E1 protein[146] and, more specifically, possess little or no antibody to the putative E1 neutralization domain.[157,197]

Infants with CRS also demonstrate prolonged impairment of RV-specific cell-mediated immune responses, including cytotoxicity, and lymphokine secretion *in vitro*.[26,59] T-cell lines derived from several congenital rubella children and adults failed to respond to RV peptides that stimulate lymphocyte proliferative responses in normal immune adult donor cells.[172] These data suggest that early fetal infection results in selective immune tolerance to a limited but critical number of RV epitopes that must be recognized to clear the virus.

Late-Onset Sequelae

Although many of the effects of fetal rubella that manifest at birth are transient, some defects such as retinopathy, mental retardation, hearing loss, and endocrine abnormalities may not become clinically apparent for several years.[148,215] Psychomotor retardation (62%), cardiac abnormalities (58%), and mental retardation (42%) are also associated with CRS, and multiorgan disease is found in 88% of patients.[78]

Delayed Endocrine Disease

Congenital RV infection is associated with a variety of delayed endocrine abnormalities, including type 1 diabetes, thyroid disease, and polyglandular autoimmunity.[201,215] Early reports suggested that type 1 diabetes occurs in as many as 10% to 40% of CRS patients. However, while more recent analyses from a diabetes-focused perspective confirmed that *in utero* RV infection undoubtedly predisposes to diabetes, the proportion is probably less than 10%.[72] Conversely, postnatal rubella does not have a clear association with type 1 diabetes.[23]

The mechanism by which RV causes diabetes is not understood, and certainly the lack of a suitable animal model has limited progress in this area. However, a number of older studies in hamsters have provided some intriguing results. For example, Syrian hamster pups infected with an adapted rubella RA 27/3 vaccine virus exhibited hypoinsulinemia and hyperglycemia.[204] In these animals, cell-free RV was recoverable from pancreas, viral antigens were present in islet cells, and a mononuclear infiltration of the islets occurred over the first 3 weeks of the infection. Moreover, islet cell antibodies developed in 40% of the infected pups.

RV-induced damage to the pancreas may therefore be a combination of viral replication in islets, compounded by the triggering of an autoimmune reaction that perpetuates beta-cell damage. Evidence in favor of this theory includes the identification of a monoclonal antibody to RV capsid protein that reacts with pancreatic islet cell Ia2 protein.[112] In addition, CD4 and CD8 T-cell clones isolated from CRS patients recognize peptides of the diabetes-associated autoantigen GAD65 in an HLA-restricted manner.[174,179] Also, 20% to 40% of sera from CRS patients in a selected series were found to contain antibodies that react with thyroid tissue.[48,77,216] Finally, CRS is also associated with growth hormone deficiency, and therefore, pituitary involvement is another complication. Relatedly, hamsters immunized with recombinant RV E1 or E2 develop pituitary autoantibodies.[262] In summary, these observations suggest that viral-induced autoimmunity may partially account for the late appearance of polyendocrine diseases that frequently complicate congenital rubella.

Delayed Neurologic Disease

A rare late-onset encephalitis following rubella has been described, referred to as progressive rubella panencephalitis

(PRP).[234,252] Like other slow viral diseases of the CNS, PRP is characterized by a prolonged asymptomatic period, followed by the onset of symptoms of neural deterioration during the second decade of life. The pathogenesis of PRP is unclear; however, immune complexes are consistently identified, suggesting ongoing viral replication.[55] The near-complete destruction of Purkinje cells indicates either some degree of selective tropism of RV for these cells within the CNS or a negative effect on their metabolism. This could also account for the selective loss of myelin and oligodendroglia, although immunopathologic mechanisms could also be active.

DIAGNOSIS

Differential

The most common symptoms of rubella (lymphadenopathy, erythematous rash, and low-grade fever) can be readily confused with similar illnesses associated with maculopapular rash caused by other common viral and nonviral pathogens or even some drug treatments. The differential diagnosis includes parvovirus, measles, human herpesvirus 6 (roseola), and rash-associated enteroviruses, such as echovirus 9 and coxsackievirus A9.[7] In particular, parvovirus infections can be confused with rubella because their clinical presentations are so similar and both can be associated with arthritis or arthralgia.[217] Moreover, in endemic areas, dengue, West Nile, Sindbis, chikungunya, and Ross River virus infections should be considered.[7] Therefore, a definitive diagnosis of rubella can only be made using specific laboratory tests.

Similarly, confirmation of a diagnosis of CRS cannot be established solely on the basis of clinical findings. It requires either the direct isolation of RV or serologic evidence of acute infection in the infant. In the absence of confirmatory laboratory data, a clinical diagnosis compatible with CRS requires the presence of any two of the following: cataracts and/or congenital glaucoma, congenital heart disease, hearing loss, or pigmentary retinopathy. In the presence of only one of the preceding manifestations, the additional finding of purpura, hepatosplenomegaly, jaundice, microcephaly, mental retardation, meningoencephalitis, or radiolucent bone disease is indicative of CRS (Table 24.1).[33] In countries in which rubella vaccination is not carried out (or is in the process of being implemented), surveillance for CRS is important to monitor for prevalence or effectiveness of the vaccination policy. A combination of eye and congenital heart anomalies has been proposed as a sensitive and specific sentinel for CRS to identify infants for further laboratory investigation.[207]

Laboratory

Diagnosis of postnatal rubella and congenital infection (following birth) is normally carried out by detection of rubella-specific IgM by enzyme immunoassay (EIA) using commercial assays.[232] The capture assay is preferred over indirect assays, which have been shown to give false-positive results with other acute viral infections such as parvovirus, Epstein-Barr virus, or cytomegalovirus,[226] or when rheumatoid factor is present.[82] IgM is usually detectable for 6 to 8 weeks after acute rubella[7] but can be detected for longer in some patients and is present for up to a year in congenitally infected infants.[227]

Virus isolation may occasionally be warranted, particularly to confirm infection during pregnancy. In acute infection, RV is readily isolated from throat swabs or nasopharyngeal secretions for approximately 1 week before and up to 2 weeks after the appearance of rash.[265] Virus can also be isolated from circulating lymphocytes for up to 1 month postinfection,[37] but this is too expensive for routine clinical diagnostic purposes. Cord blood or placental tissue may be used to confirm congenital infection at the time of birth. In addition, virus can readily be isolated from throat swabs or urine of the neonate.[56]

Over the last 10 to 15 years, a variety of nucleic acid amplification–based techniques have been developed to detect RV genomic RNA in clinical samples. Reverse transcription of RNA isolated from patient tissue/cells or fluid is required prior to amplification of the cDNA by PCR using primers specific for a selected region of the RV genome (usually the *E1* gene). PCR-based detection of RV RNA has been used to detect virus in cases of suspected congenital infection using samples obtained by amniocentesis, cordocentesis, and chorionic villus sampling for *in utero* diagnosis.[24,205] A comparison of nested RT-PCR on amniotic fluid with measurement of rubella IgM in fetal blood has confirmed both the specificity and the sensitivity of the genome amplification technique.[137] Finally, adaption of multiplexed real time–based PCR assays allows molecular genotyping as well as exquisitely accurate and sensitive detection of as little as one plaque-forming unit of RV in clinical samples.[163,164]

PREVENTION AND CONTROL

Vaccines

Development

Following isolation of RV in cell culture in 1962,[182] attenuation of the virus was carried out by serial passage in a variety of cell lines, giving rise to several vaccine strains that came into use around 1970. These included the original vaccine used widely in North America, HPV77/DE5[27]; the Cendehill strain, used more extensively in Europe[185]; and several Japanese strains.[218] The HPV77/DE5 strain was the predominant strain used in North America until 1979, when it was replaced by the RA27/3 vaccine due to concerns of waning immunity in HPV77/DE5 vaccine recipients.[103] The RA27/3 strain was derived from an isolate from the kidney of a RV-infected fetus and was attenuated by passaging 4 times in human embryonic kidney cells followed by passage 17 to 25 times in WI-38 fibroblasts.[188] This strain of virus induces a more vigorous immune response than HPV77/DE5 and has the added advantage that it was attenuated in human cells and is therefore not subject to possible side effects associated with vaccines grown in nonhuman cells. RA27/3 was licensed in 1979 and is now the only rubella vaccine available in North America. It is also widely used in other countries, including the majority of those in Europe, in Australia and New Zealand, and in South America. However, in parts of Asia, locally produced rubella vaccine strains are used. In Japan, five vaccine strains (KRT, TO-336, Matsuura, TCRB19, and Matsuba) have been developed,[169] whereas in China, BRD-2 has been compared in clinical studies to RA27/3.[247] The most recent reporting indicates that 130 of the 193 World Health Organization (WHO) member states (Fig. 24.1) now employ RV vaccine in their national immunization programs.[29] Yet, this does not include most of Africa and India and large areas of Asia, and as such, it represents less than 50% of the global birth cohort. The WHO initiated a campaign to eliminate rubella and CRS from the Americas by 2010 and the European region by 2015.

Vaccine Administration

Rubella vaccine is usually given in combination with measles and mumps as the measles-mumps-rubella (MMR) vaccine between 12 and 15 months of age, with a subsequent booster dose prior to school entry or in adolescence. Subcutaneous administration induces an antibody response in approximately 95% of recipients older than 12 months of age, detectable at 4 weeks postimmunization. The majority of vaccinated children report only mild symptoms, and transmission to susceptible bystanders seems not to occur. Although the antibody titers are lower than those following natural infection, protection is believed to endure for more than 21 years in the majority of those immunized.[168] However, in 10% of women tested in the United States, titers had dropped to low or undetectable levels in 5 years, although they responded rapidly to challenge with high-titer RA27/3.[167] In view of this, rubella vaccination should be given to all women of childbearing age found to have low or undetectable antibody titers, preferably 1 month before conception or postpartum. Immunization during pregnancy should be avoided (see Risk in Pregnancy section).

Adverse Reactions

The current RA27/3 vaccine is well tolerated but not problem free. Certainly, the incidence of acute adverse reactions is lower than after natural rubella[229] but still higher than that reported for some other vaccine strains.[21] Symptoms include fever, lymphadenopathy, arthralgia/arthritis, paresthesia, and carpal tunnel syndrome. Between 10% and 30% of adult rubella seronegative women vaccinated with the RA27/3 vaccine develop acute, usually transient, arthritis or arthralgia.[189,229,231] The joint reactions can be recurrent or persistent, similar to symptoms following natural rubella, and viral persistence may be associated with ongoing symptoms.[35] Subsequent studies have questioned the link between RV vaccination and joint manifestations, and it is probably prudent to conclude that the incidence of vaccine-induced chronic arthritis is lower than previously reported.[229] However, the finding of an association of certain HLA-DR haplotypes with a higher incidence of joint symptoms following RA27/3 rubella vaccination[155] suggests that the virus may cause joint symptoms in small numbers of genetically predisposed individuals. This factor should be taken into account in any future studies based on analysis of populations.

Vaccine side effects and complications are a serious challenge to maintaining herd immunity, and the higher incidence of arthralgia and arthritis particularly in female vaccines has most certainly had negative consequences. However, by far the most damage to effective uptake of MMR vaccine stems from a report by Wakefield et al[245] that ultimately led to the belief among a significant number of people that this vaccine was linked to autism. Numerous larger and much better controlled studies failed to confirm a causal relationship between the MMR vaccine and autism, but unfortunately the damage was done and the rate of vaccine uptake dropped dramatically. Predictably, this led to an increase in the number of cases of measles and, to a lesser extent, rubella. Fortunately, the journal that published the Wakefield et al paper, the *Lancet,* retracted the paper from the published record in 2010. However, it will still be some time before we have fully recovered from the effects of this fraudulent report.

Risk in Pregnancy

A serious concern of rubella vaccination programs has been the potential risk to the developing fetus in mothers who are immunized during early pregnancy. In such instances, the placenta and fetus may become infected, although the isolation rate is only 3%.[208] Moreover, one survey of 515 children born of mothers inadvertently immunized within 3 months of conception showed that none had malformations compatible with CRS.[20] This included cases of vaccination with the earlier Cendehill and HPV-77 vaccines, as well as with the current RA27/3 vaccine. Vaccine strains of RV therefore appear to be far less teratogenic than wt+ RV, and even in one case where the fetus was infected no signs of CRS were detected at birth. Because a potential risk to the fetus still exists (estimated at 1.3% when the mother is vaccinated 1 to 2 weeks before to 4 to 6 weeks after conception[32]), pregnancy remains a contraindication to rubella vaccination. However, inadvertent vaccination of a seronegative pregnant woman is not sufficient reason for termination of pregnancy.

New Vaccine Strategies

Because the current rubella vaccines are considered highly effective, there is limited interest in developing a subunit vaccine. Nevertheless, live attenuated vaccines are not recommended for children with immunodeficiency diseases or for women in the early stages of pregnancy who might be living or working in a situation where they risk exposure. For these situations, a subunit vaccine that provides some protection, even if only for a limited time, may be appropriate. Use of the E1 protein, which contains the major neutralizing epitopes, has been proposed,[257] but such vaccine platforms have not been developed further. In addition, DNA vaccines incorporating genes for all three structural proteins, or just E1 and E2, have been constructed and have shown some promise in mice.[190] However, for general use, a live attenuated vaccine that promotes the strongest and most enduring immune response is still advisable. With current knowledge on the genetic determinants of virulence and joint tropism, the potential exists for development of a recombinant vaccine designed to be highly immunogenic but not associated with unwanted side effects. Nevertheless, the overall success of current vaccines likely precludes further development of next-generation recombinant vaccines.

PERSPECTIVE

With the availability of relatively inexpensive and safe vaccines, rubella is most certainly a preventable disease. Indeed, much of the industrialized world has adopted comprehensive immunization policies that have curtailed virus circulation and CRS; however, more than 50% of the global birth cohort is still susceptible to rubella.[29] The cost of medical care for children with CRS easily justifies implementation of comprehensive immunization programs on economic grounds alone.[89] Yet RV is still endemic in many developing countries, and sadly, these are the least well-equipped nations to deal with the very high costs of caring for CRS children.

Compounding matters is the fact that to prevent RV transmission, herd immunity needs to exceed 85%[4] and the cost of proper surveillance for RV can be prohibitive. As a result of inadequate surveillance, the actual numbers of rubella and CRS are vastly underreported. For example, based on seroprevalence data and statistical modeling for the Southeast Asia region, it is estimated that more than 46,000 infants are born with CRS each year, yet only 13 cases of CRS were reported between 2000 and 2009.[29] Accordingly, RV is still a significant human pathogen that takes an enormous toll on the health of the world's population through the widespread manifestations of CRS, most notably in relation to blindness and hearing defects.

On the positive side, significant progress has been made with respect to understanding virus–host interactions at the molecular level, and the complete sequences of multiple wild-type and vaccine strains of RV are known. By pooling the knowledge from these studies through further investigation, we will be in a better position to understand the underlying mechanisms of teratogenicity and virus-induced autoimmune diseases such as diabetes and arthritis.

REFERENCES

All cited references are available in the e-book.

1. Abernathy ES, Wang CY, Frey TK. Effect of antiviral antibody on maintenance of long-term rubella virus persistent infection in Vero cells. *J Virol* 1990;64:5183–5187.
2. Achievements in public health: elimination of rubella and congenital rubella syndrome-US, 1969–2004. *Ann Pharmacother* 2005;39:1151–1152.
3. Adamo P, Asis L, Silveyra P, et al. Rubella virus does not induce apoptosis in primary human embryo fibroblast cultures: a possible way of viral persistence in congenital infection. *Viral Immunol* 2004;17:87–100.
4. Anderson RM, May RM. Immunisation and herd immunity. *Lancet* 1990;335:641–645.
6. Auewarakul P. Composition bias and genome polarity of RNA viruses. *Virus Res* 2005;109:33–37.
7. Banatvala JE, Brown DW. Rubella. *Lancet* 2004;363:1127–1137.
8. Bardeletti G, Gautheron DC. Phospholipid and cholesterol composition of rubella virus and its host cell BHK 21 grown in suspension cultures. *Arch Virol* 1976;52:19–27.
10. Bardeletti G, Tektoff J, Gautheron D. Rubella virus maturation and production in two host cell systems. *Intervirology* 1979;11:97–103.
11. Baron MD, Ebel T, Suomalainen M. Intracellular transport of rubella virus structural proteins expressed from cloned cDNA. *J Gen Virol* 1992;73:1073–1086.
12. Baron MD, Forsell K. Oligomerization of the structural proteins of rubella virus. *Virology* 1991;185:811–819.
15. Beatch MD, Everitt JC, Law LJ, et al. Interactions between rubella virus capsid and host protein p32 are important for virus replication. *J Virol* 2005;79:10807–10820.
16. Beatch MD, Hobman TC. Rubella virus capsid associates with host cell protein p32 and localizes to mitochondria. *J Virol* 2000;74:5569–5576.
17. Bechar M, Davidovich S, Goldhammer G, et al. Neurological complications following rubella infection. *J Neurol* 1982;226:283–287.
18. Berger BE, Omer SB. Could the United States experience rubella outbreaks as a result of vaccine refusal and disease importation? *Hum Vaccin* 2010;6:1016–1020.
24. Bosma TJ, Corbett KM, O'Shea S, et al. PCR for detection of rubella virus RNA in clinical samples. *J Clin Microbiol* 1995;33:1075–1079.
25. Bottiger B, Jensen IP. Maturation of rubella IgG avidity over time after acute rubella infection. *Clin Diagn Virol* 1997;8:105–111.
26. Buimovici-Klein E, Cooper LZ. Cell-mediated immune response in rubella infections. *Rev Infect Dis* 1985;7(Suppl 1):S123–S128.
27. Buynak EB, Hilleman MR, Weibel RE, et al. Live attenuated rubella virus vaccines prepared in duck embryo cell culture. I. Development and clinical testing. *JAMA* 1968;204:195–200.
28. Centers for Disease Control and Prevention (CDC). Elimination of rubella and congenital rubella syndrome–United States, 1969–2004. *Morb Mortal Wkly Rep* 2005;54:279–282.
29. Centers for Disease Control and Prevention (CDC). Progress toward control of rubella and prevention of congenital rubella syndrome—worldwide, 2009. *Morb Mortal Wkly Rep* 2010;59:1307–1310.
30. Centers for Disease Control and Prevention (CDC). Progress toward elimination of measles and prevention of congenital rubella infection–European region, 1990–2004. *Morb Mortal Wkly Rep* 2005;54:175–178.
34. Chantler JK, Davies MA. The effect of antibody on rubella virus infection in human lymphoid cells. *J Gen Virol* 1987;68(Pt 5):1277–1288.
35. Chantler JK, Ford DK, Tingle AJ. Persistent rubella infection and rubella-associated arthritis. *Lancet* 1982;1:1323–1325.
36. Chantler JK, Lund KD, Miki NP, et al. Characterization of rubella virus strain differences associated with attenuation. *Intervirology* 1993;36:225–236.
37. Chantler JK, Tingle AJ. Isolation of rubella virus from human lymphocytes after acute natural infection. *J Infect Dis* 1982;145:673–677.
38. Chantler JK, Tingle AJ. Replication and expression of rubella virus in human lymphocyte populations. *J Gen Virol* 1980;50:317–328.
39. Chantler JK, Tingle AJ, Petty RE. Persistent rubella virus infection associated with chronic arthritis in children. *N Engl J Med* 1985;313:1117–1123.
40. Chaye H, Ou D, Chong P, et al. Human T- and B-cell epitopes of E1 glycoprotein of rubella virus. *J Clin Immunol* 1993;13:93–100.
41. Chaye HH, Mauracher CA, Tingle AJ, et al. Cellular and humoral immune responses to rubella virus structural proteins E1, E2, and C. *J Clin Microbiol* 1992;30:2323–2329.
42. Chen JP, Strauss JH, Strauss EG, et al. Characterization of the rubella virus nonstructural protease domain and its cleavage site. *J Virol* 1996;70:4707–4713.
43. Chen MH, Frey TK. Mutagenic analysis of the 3′ cis-acting elements of the rubella virus genome. *J Virol* 1999;73:3386–3403.
44. Chen MH, Frolov I, Icenogle J, et al. Analysis of the 3′ cis-acting elements of rubella virus by using replicons expressing a puromycin resistance gene. *J Virol* 2004;78:2553–2561.
45. Chen MH, Icenogle JP. Rubella virus capsid protein modulates viral genome replication and virus infectivity. *J Virol* 2004;78:4314–4322.
46. Clarke DM, Loo TW, Hui I, et al. Nucleotide sequence and in vitro expression of rubella virus 24S subgenomic messenger RNA encoding the structural proteins E1, E2 and C. *Nucleic Acids Res* 1987;15:3041–3057.
47. Clarke DM, Loo TW, McDonald H, et al. Expression of rubella virus cDNA coding for the structural proteins. *Gene* 1988;65:23–30.
49. Claus C, Chey S, Heinrich S, et al. Involvement of p32 and microtubules in alteration of mitochondrial functions by rubella virus. *J Virol* 2011;85:3881–3892.
50. Cong H, Jiang Y, Tien P. Identification of the myelin oligodendrocyte glycoprotein as a cellular receptor for rubella virus. *J Virol* 2011;85:11038–11047.
54. Cordoba P, Lanoel A, Grutadauria S, et al. Evaluation of antibodies against a rubella virus neutralizing domain for determination of immune status. *Clin Diagn Lab Immunol* 2000;7:964–966.
56. Cradock-Watson JE, Miller E, Ridehalgh MK, et al. Detection of rubella virus in fetal and placental tissues and in the throats of neonates after serologically confirmed rubella in pregnancy. *Prenat Diagn* 1989;9:91–96.
57. Cui T, Porter AG. Localization of binding site for encephalomyocarditis virus RNA polymerase in the 3′-noncoding region of the viral RNA. *Nucleic Acids Res* 1995;23:377–382.
58. Cutts FT, Robertson SE, Diaz-Ortega JL, et al. Control of rubella and congenital rubella syndrome (CRS) in developing countries, Part 1: Burden of disease from CRS. *Bull World Health Organ* 1997;75:55–68.
59. de Mazancourt A, Waxham MN, Nicolas JC, et al. Antibody response to the rubella virus structural proteins in infants with the congenital rubella syndrome. *J Med Virol* 1986;19:111–122.
61. Duncan R, Muller J, Lee N, et al. Rubella virus-induced apoptosis varies among cell lines and is modulated by Bcl-XL and caspase inhibitors. *Virology* 1999;255:117–128.

62. Dwyer DE, Robertson PW, Field PR. Broadsheet: clinical and laboratory features of rubella. *Pathology* 2001;33:322–328.
63. Enders G, Nickerl-Pacher U, Miller E, et al. Outcome of confirmed periconceptional maternal rubella. *Lancet* 1988;1:1445–1447.
64. Fontana J, Lopez-Iglesias C, Tzeng WP, et al. Three-dimensional structure of Rubella virus factories. *Virology* 2010;405:579–591.
65. Forbes JA. Rubella: historical aspects. *Am J Dis Child* 1969;118:5–11.
68. Frey TK. Molecular biology of rubella virus. *Adv Virus Res* 1994;44: 69–160.
69. Frey TK, Abernathy ES, Bosma TJ, et al. Molecular analysis of rubella virus epidemiology across three continents, North America, Europe, and Asia, 1961–1997. *J Infect Dis* 1998;178:642–650.
70. Frey TK, Hemphill ML. Generation of defective-interfering particles by Rubella virus in vero cells. *Virology* 1988;164:22–29.
71. Froshauer S, Kartenbeck J, Helenius A. Alphavirus RNA replicase is located on the cytoplasmic surface of endosomes and lysosomes. *J Cell Biol* 1988;107:2075–2086.
72. Gale EA. Congenital rubella: citation virus or viral cause of type 1 diabetes? *Diabetologia* 2008;51:1559–1566.
73. Garbutt M, Chan H, Hobman TC. Secretion of rubella virions and virus-like particles in cultured epithelial cells. *Virology* 1999;261: 340–346.
74. Garbutt M, Law LM, Chan H, et al. Role of rubella virus glycoprotein domains in assembly of virus-like particles. *J Virol* 1999;73:3524–3533.
75. Garcia AG, Marques RL, Lobato YY, et al. Placental pathology in congenital rubella. *Placenta* 1985;6:281–295.
76. Geier DA, Geier MR. Rubella vaccine and arthritic adverse reactions: an analysis of the Vaccine Adverse Events Reporting System (VAERS) database from 1991 through 1998. *Clin Exp Rheumatol* 2001;19:724–726.
80. Gorbalenya AE, Koonin EV, Lai MM. Putative papain-related thiol proteases of positive-strand RNA viruses. Identification of rubi- and aphthovirus proteases and delineation of a novel conserved domain associated with proteases of rubi-, alpha- and coronaviruses. *FEBS Lett* 1991; 288:201–205.
83. Gregg NM. Congenital cataract following German measles in the mother. *Trans Ophthalmol Soc Aust* 1941:35–46.
84. Gros C, Linder M, Wengler G, et al. Analyses of disulfides present in the rubella virus E1 glycoprotein. *Virology* 1997;230:179–186.
85. Gros C, Wengler G. Identification of an RNA-stimulated NTPase in the predicted helicase sequence of the Rubella virus nonstructural polyprotein. *Virology* 1996;217:367–372.
87. Hemphill ML, Forng RY, Abernathy ES, et al. Time course of virus-specific macromolecular synthesis during rubella virus infection in Vero cells. *Virology* 1988;162:65–75.
91. Hobman TC, Gillam S. In vitro and in vivo expression of rubella virus glycoprotein E2: the signal peptide is contained in the C-terminal region of capsid protein. *Virology* 1989;173:241–250.
92. Hobman TC, Lemon HF, Jewell K. Characterization of an endoplasmic reticulum retention signal in the rubella virus E1 glycoprotein. *J Virol* 1997;71:7670–7680.
93. Hobman TC, Lundstrom ML, Gillam S. Processing and intracellular transport of rubella virus structural proteins in COS cells. *Virology* 1990;178:122–133.
94. Hobman TC, Lundstrom ML, Mauracher CA, et al. Assembly of rubella virus structural proteins into virus-like particles in transfected cells. *Virology* 1994;202:574–585.
95. Hobman TC, Qiu ZY, Chaye H, et al. Analysis of rubella virus E1 glycosylation mutants expressed in COS cells. *Virology* 1991;181:768–772.
96. Hobman TC, Shukin R, Gillam S. Translocation of rubella virus glycoprotein E1 into the endoplasmic reticulum. *J Virol* 1988;62:4259–4264.
97. Hobman TC, Woodward L, Farquhar MG. Targeting of a heterodimeric membrane protein complex to the Golgi: rubella virus E2 glycoprotein contains a transmembrane Golgi retention signal. *Mol Biol Cell* 1995;6:7–20.
98. Hobman TC, Woodward L, Farquhar MG. The rubella virus E1 glycoprotein is arrested in a novel post-ER, pre-Golgi compartment. *J Cell Biol* 1992;118:795–811.
99. Hobman TC, Woodward L, Farquhar MG. The rubella virus E2 and E1 spike glycoproteins are targeted to the Golgi complex. *J Cell Biol* 1993; 121:269–281.
100. Hofmann J, Pletz MW, Liebert UG. Rubella virus-induced cytopathic effect in vitro is caused by apoptosis. *J Gen Virol* 1999;80(Pt 7):1657–1664.
101. Horstmann DM. Discussion paper: the use of primates in experimental viral infections–rubella and the rubella syndrome. *Ann N Y Acad Sci* 1969;162:594–597.
103. Horstmann DM, Schluederberg A, Emmons JE, et al. Persistence of vaccine-induced immune responses to rubella: comparison with natural infection. *Rev Infect Dis* 1985;7(Suppl 1):S80–S85.
107. Ilkow CS, Goping IS, Hobman TC. The rubella virus capsid is an anti-apoptotic protein that attenuates the pore-forming ability of Bax. *PLoS Pathog* 2011;7:e1001291.
108. Ilkow CS, Mancinelli V, Beatch MD, et al. Rubella virus capsid protein interacts with poly(A)-binding protein and inhibits translation. *J Virol* 2008;82:4284–4294.
109. Ilkow CS, Weckbecker D, Cho WJ, et al. The rubella virus capsid protein inhibits mitochondrial import. *J Virol* 2010;84:119–130.
110. Johnstone P, Whitby JE, Bosma T, et al. Sequence variation in 5′ termini of rubella virus genomes: changes affecting structure of the 5′ proximal stem-loop. *Arch Virol* 1996;141:2471–2477.
111. Kamer G, Argos P. Primary structural comparison of RNA-dependent polymerases from plant, animal and bacterial viruses. *Nucleic Acids Res* 1984;12:7269–7282.
112. Karounos DG, Wolinsky JS, Thomas JW. Monoclonal antibody to rubella virus capsid protein recognizes a beta-cell antigen. *J Immunol* 1993;150:3080–3085.
114. Katow S, Sugiura A. Low pH-induced conformational change of rubella virus envelope proteins. *J Gen Virol* 1988;69:2797–2807.
118. Kujala P, Ahola T, Ehsani N, et al. Intracellular distribution of rubella virus nonstructural protein P150. *J Virol* 1999;73:7805–7811.
119. Law LJ, Ilkow CS, Tzeng WP, et al. Analyses of phosphorylation events in the rubella virus capsid protein: role in early replication events. *J Virol* 2006;80:6917–6925.
120. Law LM, Duncan R, Esmaili A, et al. Rubella virus E2 signal peptide is required for perinuclear localization of capsid protein and virus assembly. *J Virol* 2001;75:1978–1983.
121. Law LM, Everitt JC, Beatch MD, et al. Phosphorylation of rubella virus capsid regulates its RNA binding activity and virus replication. *J Virol* 2003;77:1764–1771.
122. Lee JY, Bowden DS. Rubella virus replication and links to teratogenicity. *Clin Microbiol Rev* 2000;13:571–587.
123. Lee JY, Bowden DS, Marshall JA. Membrane junctions associated with rubella virus infected cells. *J Submicrosc Cytol Pathol* 1996;28:101–108.
125. Lee JY, Marshall JA, Bowden DS. Characterization of rubella virus replication complexes using antibodies to double-stranded RNA. *Virology* 1994; 200:307–312.
126. Lee JY, Marshall JA, Bowden DS. Localization of rubella virus core particles in vero cells. *Virology* 1999;265:110–119.
127. Lee JY, Marshall JA, Bowden DS. Replication complexes associated with the morphogenesis of rubella virus. *Arch Virol* 1992;122:95–106.
128. Liang Y, Gillam S. Mutational analysis of the rubella virus nonstructural polyprotein and its cleavage products in virus replication and RNA synthesis. *J Virol* 2000;74:5133–5141.
129. Liang Y, Yao J, Gillam S. Rubella virus nonstructural protein protease domains involved in trans- and cis-cleavage activities. *J Virol* 2000;74: 5412–5423.
130. Liu X, Ropp SL, Jackson RJ, et al. The rubella virus nonstructural protease requires divalent cations for activity and functions in trans. *J Virol* 1998;72:4463–4466.
131. Liu X, Yang J, Ghazi AM, et al. Characterization of the zinc binding activity of the rubella virus nonstructural protease. *J Virol* 2000;74:5949–5956.
132. Liu Z, Yang D, Qiu Z, et al. Identification of domains in rubella virus genomic RNA and capsid protein necessary for specific interaction. *J Virol* 1996;70:2184–2190.
134. Lovett AE, McCarthy M, Wolinsky JS. Mapping cell-mediated immunodominant domains of the rubella virus structural proteins using recombinant proteins and synthetic peptides. *J Gen Virol* 1993;74:445–452.
135. Lund KD, Chantler JK. Mapping of genetic determinants of rubella virus associated with growth in joint tissue. *J Virol* 2000;74:796–804.

136. Lundstrom ML, Mauracher CA, Tingle AJ. Characterization of carbohydrates linked to rubella virus glycoprotein E2. *J Gen Virol* 1991;72:843–850.
137. Mace M, Cointe D, Six C, et al. Diagnostic value of reverse transcription-PCR of amniotic fluid for prenatal diagnosis of congenital rubella infection in pregnant women with confirmed primary rubella infection. *J Clin Microbiol* 2004;42:4818–4820.
138. Magliano D, Marshall JA, Bowden DS, et al. Rubella virus replication complexes are virus-modified lysosomes. *Virology* 1998;240:57–63.
139. Marr LD, Sanchez A, Frey TK. Efficient in vitro translation and processing of the rubella virus structural proteins in the presence of microsomes. *Virology* 1991;180:400–405.
140. Marr LD, Wang CY, Frey TK. Expression of the rubella virus nonstructural protein ORF and demonstration of proteolytic processing. *Virology* 1994;198:586–592.
143. Maton W. Some account of a rash liable to be mistaken for scarlatina. *Med Trans Coll Physicians (London)* 1815;5:149–165.
144. Matsumoto A, Higashi M. Electron microscopic studies on the morphology and morphogenesis of togaviruses. *Ann Rep Inst Virus Res Kyoto Univ* 1974;17:11–12.
145. Mauracher CA, Gillam S, Shukin R, et al. pH-dependent solubility shift of rubella virus capsid protein. *Virology* 1991;181:773–777.
146. Mauracher CA, Mitchell LA, Tingle AJ. Differential IgG avidity to rubella virus structural proteins. *J Med Virol* 1992;36:202–208.
147. McCarthy M, Lovett A, Kerman RH, et al. Immunodominant T-cell epitopes of rubella virus structural proteins defined by synthetic peptides. *J Virol* 1993;67:673–681.
149. Megyeri K, Berencsi K, Halazonetis TD, et al. Involvement of a p53-dependent pathway in rubella virus-induced apoptosis. *Virology* 1999;259:74–84.
150. Melancon P, Garoff H. Processing of the Semliki Forest virus structural polyprotein: role of the capsid protease. *J Virol* 1987;61:1301–1309.
152. Miki NP, Chantler JK. Differential ability of wild-type and vaccine strains of rubella virus to replicate and persist in human joint tissue. *Clin Exp Rheumatol* 1992;10:3–12.
153. Miller E, Cradock-Watson JE, Pollock TM. Consequences of confirmed maternal rubella at successive stages of pregnancy. *Lancet* 1982;2:781–784.
154. Mitchell LA, Decarie D, Tingle AJ, et al. Identification of immunoreactive regions of rubella virus E1 and E2 envelope proteins by using synthetic peptides. *Virus Res* 1993;29:33–57.
155. Mitchell LA, Tingle AJ, MacWilliam L, et al. HLA-DR class II associations with rubella vaccine-induced joint manifestations. *J Infect Dis* 1998;177:5–12.
156. Mitchell LA, Tingle AJ, Shukin R, et al. Chronic rubella vaccine-associated arthropathy. *Arch Intern Med* 1993;153:2268–2274.
158. Mitchell LA, Zhang T, Tingle AJ. Differential antibody responses to rubella virus infection in males and females. *J Infect Dis* 1992;166:1258–1265.
160. Murphy FA, Halonen PE, Harrison AK. Electron microscopy of the development of rubella virus in BHK-21 cells. *J Virol* 1968;2:1223–1227.
161. Naeye RL, Blanc W. Pathogenesis of congenital rubella. *JAMA* 1965;194:1277–1283.
164. Okamoto K, Fujii K, Komase K. Development of a novel TaqMan real-time PCR assay for detecting rubella virus RNA. *J Virol Methods* 2010;168:267–271.
165. Oker-Blom C. The gene order for rubella virus structural proteins is NH_2-C-E2-E1-COOH. *J Virol* 1984;51:354–358.
166. Oker-Blom C, Ulmanen I, Kaariainen L, et al. Rubella virus 40S genome RNA specifies a 24S subgenomic mRNA that codes for a precursor to structural proteins. *J Virol* 1984;49:403–408.
167. O'Shea S, Best JM, Banatvala JE. Viremia, virus excretion, and antibody responses after challenge in volunteers with low levels of antibody to rubella virus. *J Infect Dis* 1983;148:639–647.
168. O'Shea S, Woodward S, Best JM, et al. Rubella vaccination: persistence of antibodies for 10–21 years. *Lancet* 1988;2:909.
169. Otsuki N, Abo H, Kubota T, et al. Elucidation of the full genetic information of Japanese rubella vaccines and the genetic changes associated with in vitro and in vivo vaccine virus phenotypes. *Vaccine* 2011;29:1863–1873.
170. Ou D, Chong P, Choi Y, et al. Identification of T-cell epitopes on E2 protein of rubella virus, as recognized by human T-cell lines and clones. *J Virol* 1992;66:6788–6793.
171. Ou D, Chong P, McVeish P, et al. Characterization of the specificity and genetic restriction of human CD4+ cytotoxic T cell clones reactive to capsid antigen of rubella virus. *Virology* 1992;191:680–686.
172. Ou D, Chong P, Tingle AJ, et al. Mapping T-cell epitopes of rubella virus structural proteins E1, E2, and C recognized by T-cell lines and clones derived from infected and immunized populations. *J Med Virol* 1993;40:175–183.
175. Ou D, Mitchell LA, Decarie D, et al. Characterization of an overlapping CD8+ and CD4+ T-cell epitope on rubella capsid protein. *Virology* 1997;235:286–292.
176. Ou D, Mitchell LA, Decarie D, et al. Promiscuous T-cell recognition of a rubella capsid protein epitope restricted by DRB1*0403 and DRB1*0901 molecules sharing an HLA DR supertype. *Hum Immunol* 1998;59:149–157.
177. Ou D, Mitchell LA, Domeier ME, et al. Characterization of the HLA-restrictive elements of a rubella virus-specific cytotoxic T cell clone: influence of HLA-DR4 beta chain residue 74 polymorphism on antigenic peptide-T cell interaction. *Int Immunol* 1996;8:1577–1586.
178. Ou D, Mitchell LA, Ho M, et al. Analysis of overlapping T- and B-cell antigenic sites on rubella virus E1 envelope protein. Influence of HLA-DR4 polymorphism on T-cell clonal recognition. *Hum Immunol* 1994;39:177–187.
179. Ou D, Mitchell LA, Metzger DL, et al. Cross-reactive rubella virus and glutamic acid decarboxylase (65 and 67) protein determinants recognised by T cells of patients with type I diabetes mellitus. *Diabetologia* 2000;43:750–762.
180. Pappas CL, Tzeng WP, Frey TK. Evaluation of cis-acting elements in the rubella virus subgenomic RNA that play a role in its translation. *Arch Virol* 2006;151:327–346.
182. Parkman PD, Buescher EL, Artenstein MS. Recovery of rubella virus from army recruits. *Proc Soc Exp Biol Med* 1962;111:225–230.
183. Paschen SA, Weber A, Hacker G. Mitochondrial protein import: a matter of death? *Cell Cycle* 2007;6:2434–2439.
185. Peetermans J, Huygelen C. Attenuation ob rubella virus by serial passage in primary rabbit kidney cell cultures. I. Growth characteristics in vitro and production of experimental vaccines at different passage levels. *Arch Gesamte Virusforsch* 1967;21:133–143.
186. Petruzziello R, Orsi N, Macchia S, et al. Pathway of rubella virus infectious entry into Vero cells. *J Gen Virol* 1996;77:303–308.
188. Plotkin SA, Farquhar J, Katz M, et al. A new attenuated rubella virus grown in human fibroblasts: evidence for reduced nasopharyngeal excretion. *Am J Epidemiol* 1967;86:468–477.
189. Polk BF, Modlin JF, White JA, et al. A controlled comparison of joint reactions among women receiving one of two rubella vaccines. *Am J Epidemiol* 1982;115:19–25.
190. Pougatcheva SO, Abernathy ES, Vzorov AN, et al. Development of a rubella virus DNA vaccine. *Vaccine* 1999;17:2104–2112.
193. Pugachev KV, Abernathy ES, Frey TK. Improvement of the specific infectivity of the rubella virus (RUB) infectious clone: determinants of cytopathogenicity induced by RUB map to the nonstructural proteins. *J Virol* 1997;71:562–568.
194. Pugachev KV, Frey TK. Effects of defined mutations in the 5′ nontranslated region of rubella virus genomic RNA on virus viability and macromolecule synthesis. *J Virol* 1998;72:641–650.
195. Pugachev KV, Frey TK. Rubella virus induces apoptosis in culture cells. *Virology* 1998;250:359–370.
196. Pugachev KV, Galinski MS, Frey TK. Infectious cDNA clone of the RA27/3 vaccine strain of Rubella virus. *Virology* 2000;273:189–197.
197. Pustowoit B, Liebert UG. Predictive value of serological tests in rubella virus infection during pregnancy. *Intervirology* 1998;41:170–177.
199. Qiu Z, Ou D, Hobman TC, et al. Expression and characterization of virus-like particles containing rubella virus structural proteins. *J Virol* 1994;68:4086–4091.
204. Rayfield EJ, Kelly KJ, Yoon JW. Rubella virus-induced diabetes in the hamster. *Diabetes* 1986;35:1278–1281.
205. Revello MG, Baldanti F, Sarasini A, et al. Prenatal diagnosis of rubella virus infection by direct detection and semiquantitation of viral RNA

in clinical samples by reverse transcription-PCR. *J Clin Microbiol* 1997; 35:708–713.
206. Risco C, Carrascosa JL, Frey TK. Structural maturation of rubella virus in the Golgi complex. *Virology* 2003;312:261–269.
207. Rittler M, Lopez-Camelo J, Castilla EE. Monitoring congenital rubella embryopathy. *Birth Defects Res A Clin Mol Teratol* 2004;70:939–943.
208. Robertson SE, Cutts FT, Samuel R, et al. Control of rubella and congenital rubella syndrome (CRS) in developing countries, Part 2: Vaccination against rubella. *Bull World Health Organ* 1997;75:69–80.
211. Rozanov MN, Koonin EV, Gorbalenya AE. Conservation of the putative methyltransferase domain: a hallmark of the 'Sindbis-like' supergroup of positive-strand RNA viruses. *J Gen Virol* 1992;73:2129–2134.
212. Sarnesto A, Ranta S, Vaananen P, et al. Proportions of Ig classes and subclasses in rubella antibodies. *Scand J Immunol* 1985;21:275–282.
215. Sever JL, South MA, Shaver KA. Delayed manifestations of congenital rubella. *Rev Infect Dis* 1985;7(Suppl 1):S164–S169.
217. Shirley JA, Revill S, Cohen BJ, et al. Serological study of rubella-like illnesses. *J Med Virol* 1987;21:369–379.
219. Smith CA, Petty RE, Tingle AJ. Rubella virus and arthritis. *Rheum Dis Clin North Am* 1987;13:265–274.
222. Stanwick TL, Hallum JV. Role of interferon in six cell lines persistently infected with rubella virus. *Infect Immun* 1974;10:810–815.
225. Takkinen K, Vidgren G, Ekstrand J, et al. Nucleotide sequence of the rubella virus capsid protein gene reveals an unusually high G/C content. *J Gen Virol* 1988;69:603–612.
226. Thomas HI, Barrett E, Hesketh LM, et al. Simultaneous IgM reactivity by EIA against more than one virus in measles, parvovirus B19 and rubella infection. *J Clin Virol* 1999;14:107–118.
227. Thomas HI, Morgan-Capner P, Cradock-Watson JE, et al. Slow maturation of IgG1 avidity and persistence of specific IgM in congenital rubella: implications for diagnosis and immunopathology. *J Med Virol* 1993;41:196–200.
228. Thomas HI, Morgan-Capner P, Enders G, et al. Persistence of specific IgM and low avidity specific IgG1 following primary rubella. *J Virol Methods* 1992;39:149–155.
229. Tingle AJ, Allen M, Petty RE, et al. Rubella-associated arthritis. I. Comparative study of joint manifestations associated with natural rubella infection and RA 27/3 rubella immunisation. *Ann Rheum Dis* 1986;45:110–114.
230. Tingle AJ, Chantler JK, Kettyls GD, et al. Failed rubella immunization in adults: association with immunologic and virological abnormalities. *J Infect Dis* 1985;151:330–336.
231. Tingle AJ, Mitchell LA, Grace M, et al. Randomised double-blind placebo-controlled study on adverse effects of rubella immunisation in seronegative women. *Lancet* 1997;349:1277–1281.
232. Tipples G, Hiebert J. Detection of measles, mumps, and rubella viruses. *Methods Mol Biol* 2011;665:183–193.
234. Townsend JJ, Baringer JR, Wolinsky JS, et al. Progressive rubella panencephalitis. Late onset after congenital rubella. *N Engl J Med* 1975;292: 990–993.
235. Trudel M, Marchessault F, Payment P. Characterisation of rubella virus hemagglutinin rosettes. *J Virol Methods* 1981;2:195–201.
236. Trudel M, Ravaoarinoro M, Payment P. Reconstitution of rubella hemagglutinin on liposomes. *Can J Microbiol* 1980;26:899–904.
237. Tzeng WP, Chen MH, Derdeyn CA, et al. Rubella virus DI RNAs and replicons: requirement for nonstructural proteins acting in cis for amplification by helper virus. *Virology* 2001;289:63–73.
238. Tzeng WP, Frey TK. Complementation of a deletion in the rubella virus p150 nonstructural protein by the viral capsid protein. *J Virol* 2003;77: 9502–9510.
239. Tzeng WP, Frey TK. Rubella virus capsid protein modulation of viral genomic and subgenomic RNA synthesis. *Virology* 2005;337: 327–334.
242. Vaheri A, Sedwick WD, Plotkin SA, et al. Cytopathic effect of rubella virus in RHK21 cells and growth to high titers in suspension culture. *Virology* 1965;27:239–241.
243. Veale H. History of an epidemic of Rötheln with observations on its pathology. *Edinburgh Med J* 1866;12:404–414.
244. von Bonsdorff C-H, Vaheri A. Growth of rubella virus in BHK-21 cells: electron microscopy of morphogenesis. *J Gen Virol* 1969;5:47–51.
245. Wakefield AJ, Murch SH, Anthony A, et al. Ileal-lymphoid-nodular hyperplasia, non-specific colitis, and pervasive developmental disorder in children. *Lancet* 1998;351:637–641.
246. Wang C-Y, Dominguez G, Frey TK. Construction of rubella virus genome-length cDNA clones and synthesis of infectious RNA transcripts. *J Virol* 1994;68:3550–3557.
247. Wang SS, Han YR, Su WN, et al. Studies on the reactogenicity and immunogenicity of the BRD-2 and RA27/3 live attenuated rubella vaccines. *Vaccine* 1984;2:277–280.
248. Wang Z, Yao P, Song Y, et al. Characteristics and mechanisms of isolated rubella virus, strain JR23: infection of the central nervous system of BALB/c mice. *Intervirology* 2003;46:79–85.
249. Waxham MN, Wolinsky JS. Detailed immunologic analysis of the structural polypeptides of rubella virus using monoclonal antibodies. *Virology* 1985;143:153–165.
250. Waxham MN, Wolinsky JS. Rubella virus and its effects on the central nervous system. *Neurol Clin* 1984;2:367–385.
251. Webster WS. Teratogen update: congenital rubella. *Teratology* 1998;58: 13–23.
252. Weil ML, Itabashi H, Cremer NE, et al. Chronic progressive panencephalitis due to rubella virus simulating subacute sclerosing panencephalitis. *N Engl J Med* 1975;292:994–998.
253. Weller TH, Neva FA. Propagation in tissue culture of cytopathic agents from patients with rubella-like illness. *Proc Soc Exp Biol Med* 1962;111: 215–225.
256. Wolinsky JS, McCarthy M, Allen-Cannady O, et al. Monoclonal antibody-defined epitope map of expressed rubella virus protein domains. *J Virol* 1991;65:3986–3994.
257. Wolinsky JS, Sukholutsky E, Moore WT, et al. An antibody- and synthetic peptide-defined rubella virus E1 glycoprotein neutralization domain. *J Virol* 1993;67:961–968.
258. World Health Organization. *WHO vaccine-preventable diseases monitoring system, 2009 global summary.* Geneva: World Health Organization, 2009.
259. Yao J, Gillam S. Mutational analysis, using a full-length rubella virus cDNA clone, of rubella virus E1 transmembrane and cytoplasmic domains required for virus release. *J Virol* 1999;73:4622–4630.
260. Yao J, Yang D, Chong P, et al. Proteolytic processing of rubella virus nonstructural proteins. *Virology* 1998;246:74–82.
261. Yoneda T, Urade M, Sakuda M, et al. Altered growth, differentiation, and responsiveness to epidermal growth factor of human embryonic mesenchymal cells of palate by persistent rubella virus infection. *J Clin Invest* 1986;77:1613–1621.
262. Yoon JW, Choi DS, Liang HC, et al. Induction of an organ-specific autoimmune disease, lymphocytic hypophysitis, in hamsters by recombinant rubella virus glycoprotein and prevention of disease by neonatal thymectomy. *J Virol* 1992;66:1210–1214.
263. Zheng DP, Frey TK, Icenogle J, et al. Global distribution of rubella virus genotypes. *Emerg Infect Dis* 2003;9:1523–1530.

CHAPTER 25

Brett D. Lindenbach • Catherine L. Murray • Heinz-Jürgen Thiel • Charles M. Rice

Flaviviridae

INTRODUCTION

The first human virus was discovered over one century ago when Walter Reed demonstrated that yellow fever could be experimentally transferred via the filtered serum of an infected individual, and that this infectious agent was transmitted to humans by mosquitoes.[817] It is now appreciated that yellow fever virus (YFV) is but one representative of a large family of related positive-strand RNA viruses, the *Flaviviridae* (from the Latin *flavus,* "yellow"). This family currently consists of three genera: *Flavivirus, Pestivirus* (from the Latin *pestis,* "plague"), and *Hepacivirus* (from the Greek *hepar, hepatos,* "liver")[851] (Table 25.1). A fourth genus, *Pegivirus* (*pe*rsistent *G*B virus), has recently been proposed to encompass the previously unclassified GB virus A (GBV-A), GBV-C, and GBV-D.[805] As detailed later, the *Flaviviridae* share similarities in virion morphology, genome organization, and replication strategy but exhibit diverse biological properties and lack serologic cross-reactivity. The phylogenetic relationships of the *Flaviviridae* are shown in Figure 25.1. The increasing significance of *Flaviviridae* as human and animal pathogens emphasizes that their study remains no less pertinent than in Reed's time.

Family Classification

Positive-stranded RNA viruses are classified into three superfamilies based on the evolutionary relatedness of their RNA-dependent RNA polymerases (RdRPs). The *Flaviviridae* are members of superfamily 2, bearing distant similarity to coliphages and the plant-infecting carmo-, tombus-, diantho-, and subgroup I luteoviruses.[418] Before the era of molecular biology, some members of the family *Flaviviridae* were classified as *Togaviridae.*

Family Characteristics and Replication Cycle

This chapter is organized around common features of the family *Flaviviridae* life cycle (Fig. 25.2). The enveloped virions are composed of a lipid bilayer with two or more species of envelope (E) glycoprotein surrounding a nucleocapsid, which consists of a single-stranded, positive-sense RNA genome complexed with multiple copies of a small, basic capsid (C) protein. Binding and uptake are believed to involve receptor-mediated endocytosis. The low pH of the endosome induces fusion of the virion envelope with cellular membranes. Following uncoating of the nucleocapsid, the RNA genome is released into the cytoplasm. The genome serves three discrete roles within the life cycle: as the messenger RNA (mRNA) for translation of all viral proteins, a template during RNA replication, and the genetic material packaged within new virus particles. The organization

TABLE 25.1 Members of the *Flaviviridae*

Taxonomic unit	Representative examples
Genus *Flavivirus*[54]	
Mosquito-borne viruses	*Yellow fever virus* (YFV)
	Dengue virus, types 1 to 4 (DENV-1 to DENV-4)
	Japanese encephalitis virus (JEV)
	Kokobera virus (KOKV)
	West Nile virus (WNV)
Tick-borne viruses	*Tick-borne encephalitis virus,* European subtype (TBEV-Eu)
	Tick-borne encephalitis virus, Far Eastern subtype (TBEV-FE)
	Omsk hemorrhagic fever virus (OHFV)
	Tyuleniy virus (TYEV)
Viruses with no known vector	*Modoc virus* (MODV)
	Rio Bravo virus (RBV)
Unclassified	*Cell fusing agent virus* (CFAV)
Genus *Hepacivirus*[1]	*Hepatitis C virus* (HCV), seven genotypes
	GB virus B (GBV-B; unclassified)
	Canine hepacivirus (CHV; unclassified)
Genus *Pestivirus*[4]	*Bovine viral diarrhea virus 1* (BVDV-1)
	Bovine viral diarrhea virus 2 (BVDV-2)
	Border disease virus (BDV)
	Classical swine fever virus (CSFV)[a]
	Giraffe-1 pestivirus (unclassified)
Genus *Pegivirus* (proposed)	*GB virus A* (GBV-A)
	GB virus C (GBV-C), "*Hepatitis G virus* (HGV)"
	GB virus D (GBV-D)

Numbers in superscript indicate the current number of virus species recognized within each group.

[a]CSFV was formerly called *hog cholera virus* (HCV). The name was changed to avoid confusion with *hepatitis C virus*.

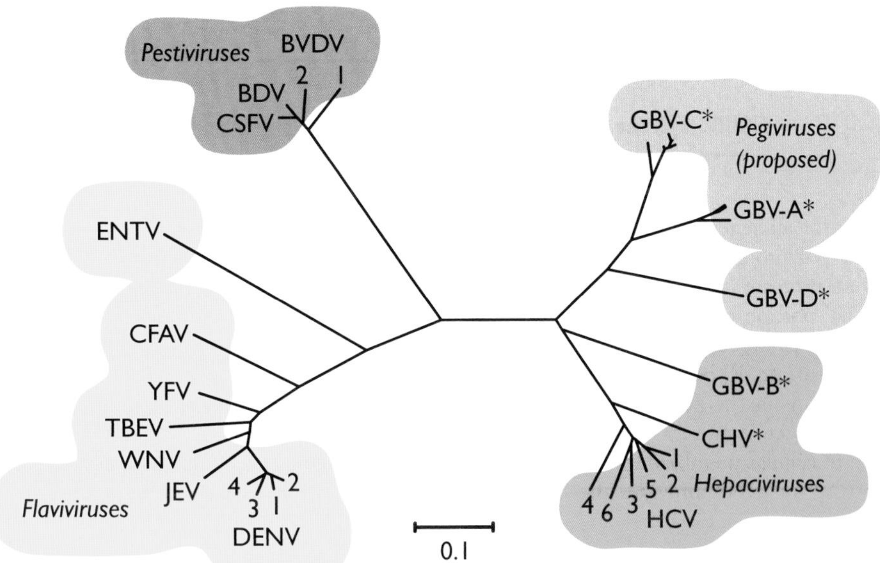

FIGURE 25.1. The family *Flaviviridae*. Phylogenetic tree based on neighbor-joining analysis of the viral RNA-dependent RNA polymerases (RdRPs). Shown are members of the *Flavivirus* genus: yellow fever virus (YFV), dengue virus (DENV) serotypes 1 through 4, West Nile virus (WNV), Japanese encephalitis virus (JEV), tick-borne encephalitis virus (TBEV), cell-fusing agent virus (CFAV), and Entebbe bat virus (ENTV); the *Pestivirus* genus: bovine viral diarrhea virus (BVDV) types 1 and 2, classical swine fever virus (CSFV), and border disease virus (BDV); the *Hepacivirus* genus: hepatitis C virus (HCV) genotypes 1 through 6, GB virus B (GBV-B, proposed assignment), and canine hepacivirus (CHV, proposed assignment); and the proposed *Pegivirus* genus: GB virus A (GBV-A), GB virus C (GBV-C), and GB virus D (GBV-D). The scale bar indicates amino acid substitutions per position.

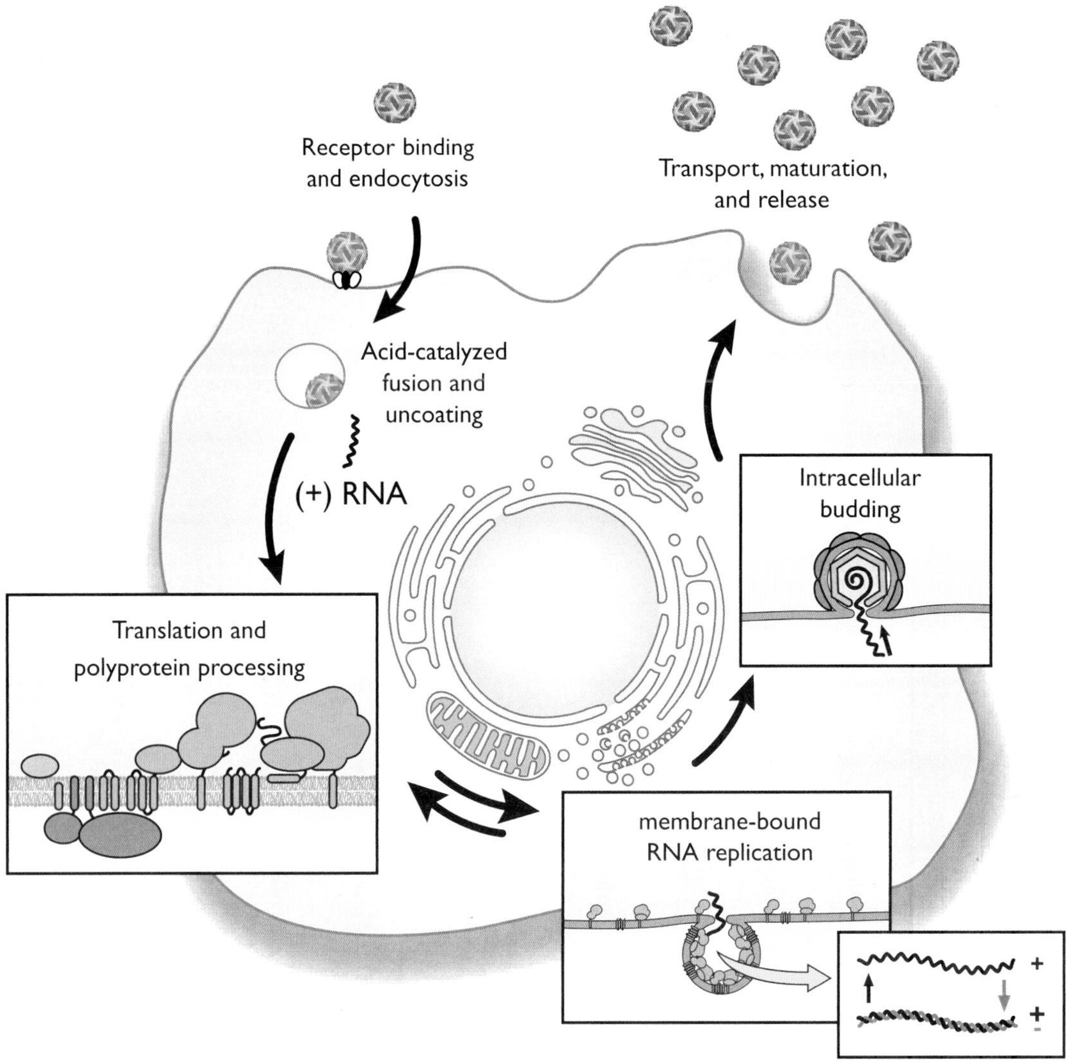

FIGURE 25.2. The life cycle of the *Flaviviridae*. See text for further details.

of the genome is similar for all genera. Viral proteins are produced as part of a single polyprotein that is cleaved by a combination of host and viral proteases. The structural proteins are located in the N-terminal portion of the polyprotein with the nonstructural (NS) proteins in the remainder. Sequence motifs characteristic of a serine protease, RNA helicase, and an RdRP are found in similar locations in the polyproteins of all three genera.[585] RNA replication occurs entirely in the cytoplasm in close association with intracellular membranes; the synthesis of a genome-length minus-strand RNA provides the intermediate. Progeny virions assemble by budding into an intracellular membrane compartment, most likely the endoplasmic reticulum (ER), then transit through the host secretory pathway and are released at the cell surface.

FLAVIVIRUSES

Background and Classification

The *Flavivirus* genus consists of more than 50 species, many of which are arthropod-borne human pathogens. Flaviviruses cause a variety of diseases, including fever, encephalitis, and hemorrhagic fevers. Entities of major global concern include dengue virus (DENV)—with its associated dengue hemorrhagic fever (DHF) and dengue shock syndrome (DSS)—Japanese encephalitis virus (JEV), West Nile virus (WNV), and YFV (reviewed in[537]). Other flaviviruses with regional or endemic distribution include Murray Valley encephalitis virus (MVEV) and St. Louis encephalitis virus (SLEV). *Tick-borne encephalitis virus* (TBEV) is a name commonly applied to either central European encephalitis virus or Far Eastern encephalitis virus, although these are clearly distinct species.[208] Decreases in mosquito control efforts during the latter part of the 20th century, coupled with societal factors (e.g., increased transportation and dense urbanization), have contributed to the re-emergence of flaviviruses such as DENV in South and Central America. Following an outbreak in New York City in 1999, WNV has spread throughout much of North America and Central America.

Flavivirus species are further categorized into antigenic complexes and subcomplexes based on serologic criteria or into clusters, clades, and species, according to molecular phylogenetics.[117] Mosquito-borne and tick-borne flaviviruses, although distinct, appear to have evolved via a common ancestral line that diverged from viruses with no known arthropod vector. DENV circulates as four distinct serotypes, which show significant sequence diversity (reviewed in[337]). Some reports have documented intertypic recombination among DENV isolates, although the taxonomic status of these isolates is currently unclear.

The development of the first live-attenuated flavivirus vaccine, YFV strain 17D,[849] led to Max Theiler's recognition by the Nobel Prize committee in 1951. Only a limited number of flavivirus vaccines are available, including inactivated TBEV and JEV for use in humans and inactivated WNV for use in animals.[694] Development of effective DENV vaccines that exhibit cross-protection between serotypes is proving to be particularly challenging. The ability to genetically manipulate flaviviruses has led to novel approaches, including live attenuated chimeric vaccines based on the YFV-17D backbone.

Structure and Physical Properties of the Virion

Infectious flavivirus particles are roughly spherical, approximately 50 nm in diameter, and surrounded by a lipid envelope[615] (Fig. 25.3). Viruses sediment between 170 and 210S and have buoyant densities of 1.19 to 1.23 g/cm^3 depending on the lipid composition, which can vary by host.[745] The outer shell of the particle is made up of two viral proteins, envelope (E) and membrane (M). The E glycoprotein is the major antigenic determinant of the virion and mediates binding and fusion during virus entry. The M protein is a small proteolytic fragment of the precursor (pr)M protein and is produced during viral maturation within the secretory pathway. Removal of the lipid envelope with nonionic detergents reveals discrete nucleocapsids (120 to 140S; 1.30 to 1.31 g/cm^3), which consist of capsid (C) protein and genomic RNA (reviewed in[745]). Isolated nucleocapsids become unstable under high salt conditions, disassembling into C protein dimers.[399]

Cryoelectron microscopy and image reconstruction have provided a wealth of information on flavivirus structure. Mature infectious particles of DENV[430] and WNV[610] display a relatively smooth outer surface. Fitting the E protein crystal structure[722] into the electron density maps showed that glycoprotein dimers lie flat across the surface of the virion. Interestingly, the 180 copies of E are tightly packed in an unusual herringbone array that completely covers the lipid bilayer. Beneath the protein shell, the M protein associates closely with the membrane. Notably, the nucleocapsid lacks discernible symmetry, and neither E nor M sequences extend through the membrane to make contacts with the nucleocapsid.[956]

Immature flavivirus particles adopt various appearances as they egress through the secretory pathway.[667] Soon after they are formed, immature virions are larger (60 nm in diameter) than mature virions and display 60 prominent spikes on their surface.[957] Each protrusion is composed of three E-prM heterodimers, with the prM molecule capping the E fusion peptide. As immature particles pass through the low pH environment of the *trans*-Golgi network, a dramatic rearrangement of the glycoproteins occurs. The immature virions now adopt a smooth appearance almost indistinguishable from mature particles, with the exception that prM remains attached.[946] This conformational change is followed by cleavage of prM by the host cell enzyme furin[802] and the release of the protective fragment upon exit from the cell, revealing the mature virions.[946] This process is not always efficient, and immature or partially mature particles can be released in significant quantities. Although immature particles are deemed noninfectious because they cannot undergo fusion,[303] they have recently been shown to initiate infection when internalized in complex with anti-prM antibodies by cells bearing the Fc receptor.[735] The mechanism of this is not well understood, but it may invoke prM cleavage in the endosome and could be especially relevant during secondary infection when antibody levels are high. In addition, partially matured particles that retain only some prM have been visualized in flavivirus populations and can undergo attachment and fusion to initiate infection similar to fully mature particles.[137]

Small, noninfectious subviral particles (SVPs) are the final class of particles released from flavivirus-infected cells. SVPs

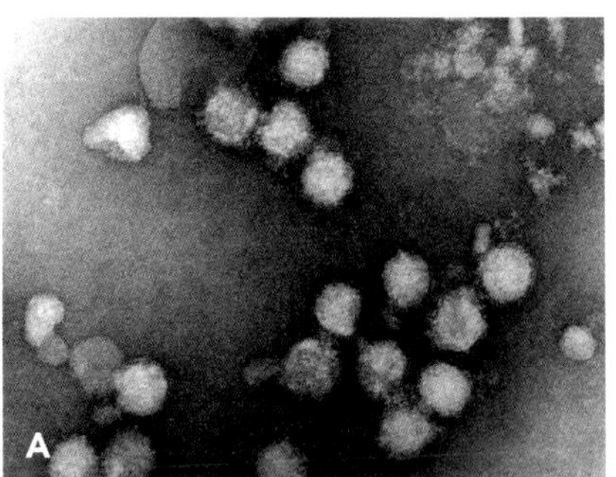

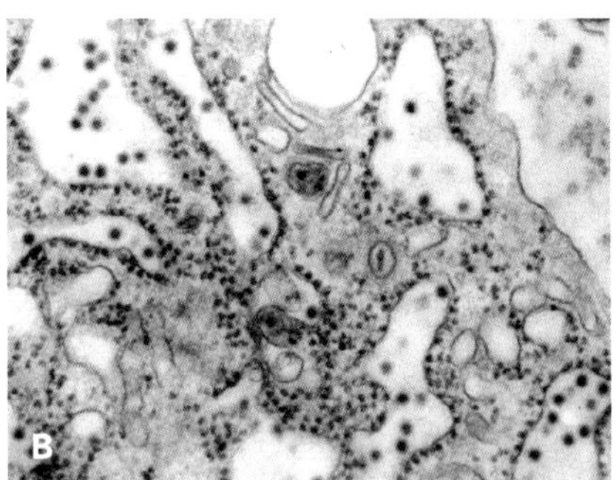

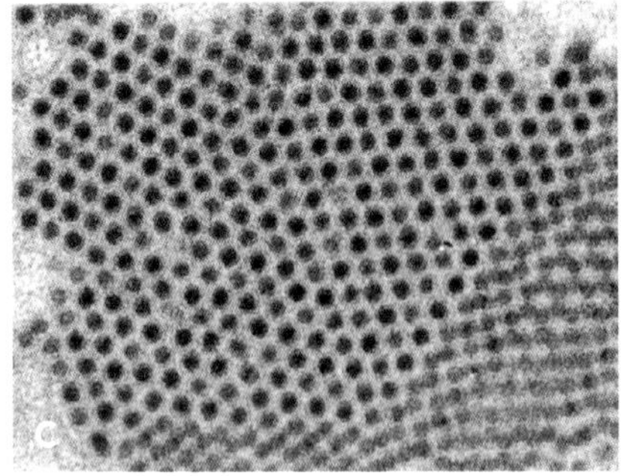

FIGURE 25.3. Electron micrographs of flavivirus particles and virus-infected cells. A: Purified St. Louis encephalitis virus (SLEV) negatively stained with ammonium molybdate (Murphy FA. Togavirus morphology and morphogenesis. In: Schlesinger RW. *The Togaviruses: Biology, Structure, Replication.* Academic Press: New York; 1980:241–316). Surface projections appear as a very thin, indistinct layer. (Courtesy of Dr. Frederick A. Murphy.) **B:** Thin section of a baby hamster kidney (BHK)-21 cell at 48 hours after infection showing SLEV particles in the cisternae of the endoplasmic reticulum (Whitfield SG, Murphy FA, Sudia WD. St. Louis encephalitis virus: an ultrastructural study of infection in a mosquito vector. *Virology* 1973;56:70–87). (Courtesy of Drs. Frederick A. Murphy, Sylvia G. Whitfield, and A. K. Harrison.) **C:** Paracrystalline array of SLEV particles in the salivary gland of a *Culex pipiens* mosquito 25 days after blood meal feeding on an infected suckling mouse. (Courtesy of Sylvia G. Whitfield, Frederick A. Murphy, and W. Daniel Sudia.)

contain E and M proteins but lack C and RNA.[797] They complete the same maturation process as whole virions and can undergo fusion with a target cell[760]; due to lack of a genome, however, they are not infectious. Recombinant subviral particles (RSPs) form in cells experimentally transfected with only prM and E, indicating that interactions between these envelope proteins are sufficient to drive budding.[14,512,760] RSPs are generally about 30 nm in diameter and slightly less dense than infectious virus (1.14 g/cm^3),[760] although virion-sized particles have also been observed in these expression systems.[16,512] Cryo-electron microscopy and image reconstruction of TBEV RSPs suggests a markedly different arrangement of the E proteins compared to infectious virions. Thirty E dimers lie flat against the surface in a $T = 1$ icosahedral shell[232] rather than a herringbone array.[430] It is hypothesized that this arrangement may resemble a fusion intermediate that is adopted as E dimers rearrange to trimers upon virus entry.[611]

Binding and Entry (see Video in e-Book)

Flaviviruses infect a variety of target cells through receptor-mediated endocytosis, followed by intracellular membrane fusion. Flavivirus receptors are not well characterized, perhaps because these viruses use a range of entry factors for different cell types and employ more than one host molecule to enter a target cell. Highly sulphated glycosaminoglycans, such as heparin sulphate, are ubiquitously expressed molecules used as initial attachment factors by many viruses. These factors have also been shown to play a role in binding and entry of flaviviruses, such as DENV,[132] YFV,[269] TBE,[426] and JEV.[130] However, high affinity for glycosaminoglycans in tissue culture–adapted strains is associated with *in vivo* attenuation.[458] C-type lectins are cellular proteins that bind mannose-rich glycans and are involved in flavivirus infection of dendritic cells (DCs). Intradermal DCs are often the primary targets encountered by the arthropod-delivered pathogens and can transport the virus to draining lymph nodes where a second round of replication initiates viremia. C-type lectin Dendritic cell-specific intercellular adhesion molecule 3-grabbing nonintegrin (DC-SIGN) is thought to function as an attachment receptor for DENV infection of DCs.[516,624,833] WNV preferentially uses DC-SIGN-related (DC-SIGNR),[182] while YFV-17D, which lacks glycan modifications on E, can infect DC cells in a lectin-independent manner.[39] The mannose receptor is a C-type lectin that is constitutively internalized by clathrin-mediated endocytosis and has been suggested to play a role in endocytosis of DENV, JEV, and TBEV.[584] Interestingly, C-type lectin domain family 5, member A (CLEC5) interacts with DENV but does not mediate its entry; instead, CLEC5 binding triggers the release of inflammatory cytokines, leading to DHF/DSS-like symptoms in mice.[131]

Additional receptors that have been implicated in flavivirus entry include the glycosphingolipid neolactotetraosylceramide,[26] low-density lipoprotein receptor (LDL-R),[138] laminin receptor 1,[850,857] $\alpha v\beta 3$ integrins,[144] and a CD14-containing complex.[134] Heat shock proteins have also been suggested as entry factors. GRP78 (BIP) plays a role in liver cell uptake of DENV,[112,368] and Hsp90/Hsp70 acts in DENV and JEV entry into human monocytes/macrophages, neuroblastoma cell lines, and mosquito cells.[180,720,723] Finally, virus particles opsonized with subneutralizing concentrations of immunoglobulins show enhanced binding and infection of cells expressing Fc receptors.[661,764] It is widely speculated that antibody-enhanced infection is relevant to the pathogenesis of DSS and DHF, which occur more frequently in people previously exposed to other DENV serotypes.

After capture by the appropriate receptor(s), flaviviruses are internalized by endocytosis. Single particle tracking of fluorescently labeled DENV particles has shown that virions diffuse across the surface of the cell until they encounter a preformed clathrin-coated pit.[871] Following internalization, DENV particles are delivered to early or intermediate endosomes, which then mature into late endosomes.[871] Fusion of the viral and host membranes occurs during endosomal trafficking, although the exact compartment that triggers this event seems to differ between strains and flavivirus species, perhaps indicating an optimal pH.[871] In the acidic environment, E protein dimers dissociate and undergo an irreversible conformational change to become fusogenic trimers.[13,810] The fusion peptide, previously buried at the E homodimer interface, is exposed and inserts into the endosomal membrane (Video 25.1). The efficiency of fusion is influenced by the lipid composition of target membranes: cholesterol, oleic acid, and anionic lipids such as bis(monoacylglycero)phosphate and phosphatidylserine enhance fusion, whereas lyophosphatidylcholine inhibits the process.[812,813,950] Lipid composition can also influence the pH threshold of fusion.[420] Following fusion, viral genomes are immediately accessible for translation.[420]

Genome Structure

As for other positive-strand RNA viruses, the genomes of flaviviruses are infectious.[662] Full-length infectious complementary DNA (cDNA) clones have been constructed for several species, allowing flavivirus biology to be dissected by reverse genetics.[491,725,742] Flavivirus genomes consist of a single, positive-strand RNA of approximately 11 kilobases (kb) in length (sedimentation, 42S) with a 5′ type 1 cap, m^{7}GpppAmN[151,901] (Fig. 25.4). The cap structure serves to stabilize the viral RNA, initiate translation, and subvert innate antiviral defenses.[178,253] Unlike cellular mRNAs, flavivirus genomes lack a 3′ polyadenylate tail.[901] Genomes encode a single long open reading frame (ORF, ~3,400 codons) flanked by 5′ and 3′ noncoding regions (NCRs) of ~100 nucleotides (nt) and 400 to 700 nt, respectively[544] (Fig. 25.4).

The sequence of the 5′ NCR is not well conserved between flaviviruses, although common secondary structural elements have been identified, including a bifurcating 5′ stem-loop (5′ SL). These structures influence viral genome translation, as antisense oligonucleotides complementary to the 5′ SL abolish DENV translation and replication, and second-site mutations in this region compensate for replication defects caused by reduced viral cap methylation. In addition, 5′ SL likely acts as a promoter to initiate RNA replication by binding the viral NS5 polymerase/methyltransferase protein.[196,236,237,506] Consistent with this, deletions within the 5′ NCR cause severe defects in DENV-4 replication, but not viral translation.[113] Interestingly, one of the viable mutants exhibited a limited host-range growth phenotype, suggesting that host-specific factors interact with either the 5′ NCR or the complementary 3′ end of the negative strand. Indeed, several human proteins, including La and TIAR, can bind to the 3′ end of negative-strand RNA.[472,778,938] WNV replication is inhibited in a TIAR-knockout cell line,[472] and mutagenesis of the TIA-1/TIAR binding sites suggests a role in initiating positive-strand RNA synthesis.[217]

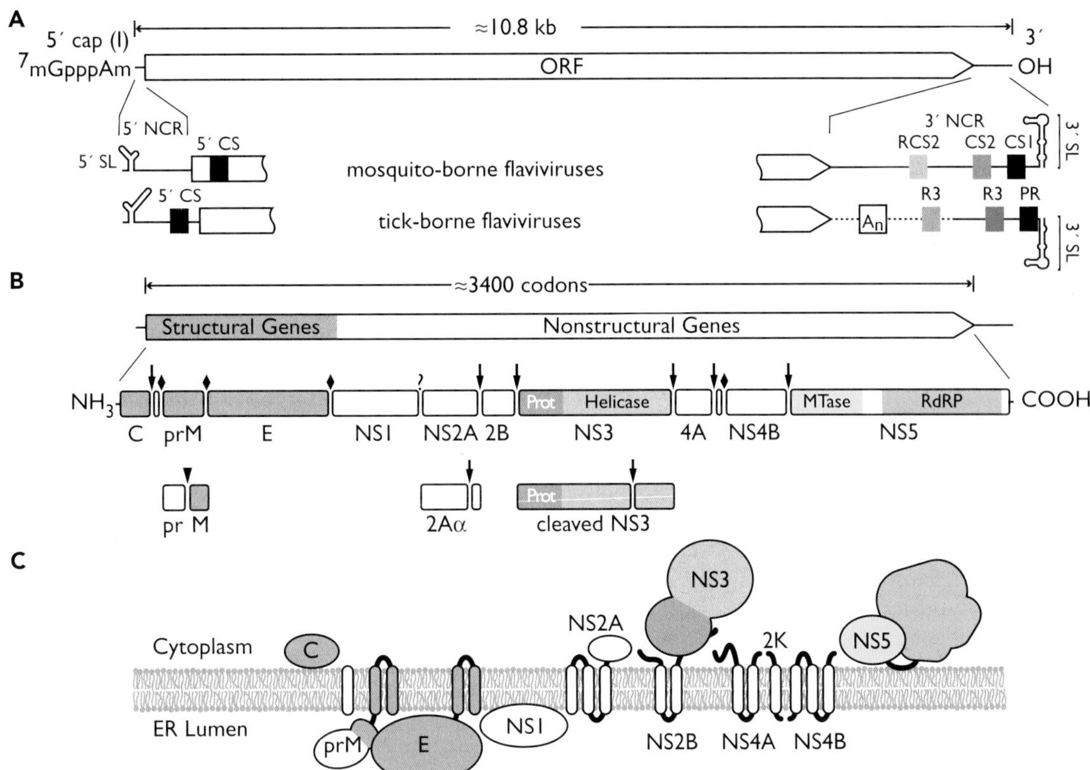

FIGURE 25.4. Flavivirus genome structure and protein expression. A: Genome structure and RNA elements. The viral genome is depicted with the open reading frame (ORF), the 5′ cap, and the 5′ and 3′ noncoding regions (NCR) indicated. Functionally significant RNA structures within the viral genome are indicated. (See the text for further details.) **B:** Polyprotein processing and cleavage products. Boxes below the genome indicate precursors and mature proteins generated by the proteolytic processing cascade. Structural proteins are colored purple, while nonstructural (NS) proteins are white or shaded according to their enzymatic subunits, as indicated. Cleavage sites for host signalase (♦), the viral serine protease (downward arrow), furin or related protease (triangle), or unknown proteases (?) are indicated. **C:** Polyprotein membrane topology. The proposed membrane orientation of the flavivirus proteins is shown. The proteins are approximately to scale (areas are proportional to the number of amino acids) and arranged in order (left to right) of their appearance in the polyprotein.

The organization of the 3′ NCR differs between mosquito-borne viruses, tick-borne viruses, and viruses with no known vector. Nevertheless, conserved regions, sequence duplications, and predicted RNA secondary structures are shared among the groups (Fig. 25.4). The greatest structural similarity is a long (90 to 120 nt) 3′ stem-loop (3′ SL) that differs in primary sequence between mosquito-borne and tick-borne flaviviruses.[296] Mutational analysis of DENV-2 and WNV revealed essential virus-specific and host-specific functional regions within the 3′ SL.[216,856,947,953] The 3′ SL enhances translation of reporter mRNAs containing the DENV 3′ NCR,[140,335] while DENV-2 translation and replication were inhibited by a corresponding antisense oligonucleotide.[336] The 3′ SL also interacts with several important proteins, including the viral NS2A, NS3, and NS5 proteins[129,175,535] and translation elongation factor 1A (EF1A).[75,183,185] These results are intriguing, because EF1A, and its prokaryotic homolog EF-Tu, contribute to the replication of other positive-strand RNA viruses.[81,314,379,951] In addition, the human La autoantigen,[185,262,875] polypyrimidine tract binding (PTB) protein,[185] and murine Mov34 protein[822] were found to bind 3′ SL of DENV-4 and JEV, although the functional relevance of these interactions is presently unknown.

Upstream of the 3′ SL lie conserved sequence repeats (CS1, CS2, CS3, RCS2, and RCS3), secondary structures, and putative pseudoknots.[296] Some of these structures confer resistance to the cellular 5′-3′ exoribonuclease Xrn-1,[252,785] suggesting that this region of the genome forms a compact structure.

Flavivirus genomes can be circularized through long-distance base pairing between elements located near the 5′ and 3′ ends. In mosquito-borne flaviviruses, these interactions are mediated by the 5′ UAR (upstream of AUG region), 5′ DAR (downstream of AUG region), and 5′ CS (conserved sequence), which base-pair with the 3′ UAR, 3′ DAR, and 3′ CS1 regions, respectively, located more than 10 kb downstream at the base of the 3′ SL.[354] A distinct set of long-distance interactions circularizes the genomes of tick-borne flaviviruses.[394,410] These long-range base pairs are important for RNA replication, presumably by bringing the 5′ SL–bound NS5 protein in proximity to the 3′ site of minus-strand initiation.[18,96,167,196,236,237,248,354,394,410,940] It should be noted that genome circularization requires the melting of local secondary structures within the 5′ and 3′ ends and leads to the occlusion of the translation start site. Thus, large-scale conformation changes within the flavivirus genome may regulate the switch from translation to RNA replication.

Translation and Proteolytic Processing

The efficiency of genome translation is a primary determinant of flavivirus infectivity.[209] The viruses therefore use several mechanisms to ensure translational competence, including specialized structures within the 5′ and 3′ NCRs. Translation is cap dependent, and 2′-O methylation of the 5′ cap helps to overcome innate antiviral defenses that down-regulate translation in infected cells.[178] While translation initiates via ribosomal scanning, many mosquito-borne flaviviruses lack a canonical Kozak initiation motif and contain several AUG codons near the correct start site. To help ensure proper AUG selection, DENV uses a small RNA stem-loop embedded within the C gene to induce ribosomal pausing over the authentic initiation codon.[155]

Translation of the single, long ORF produces a large polyprotein that is co- and posttranslationally cleaved into at least 10 proteins (Fig. 25.4B). The N-terminal region of the polyprotein encodes the structural proteins (C-prM-E), which are followed by the NS proteins (NS1-NS2A-NS2B-NS3-NS4A-2K-NS4B-NS5).[119,120,726] Host signal peptidase is responsible for cleavages between C/prM, prM/E, E/NS1, and 2K-NS4B. A virus-encoded serine protease, NS2B-3, processes at the NS2A/NS2B, NS2B/NS3, NS3/NS4A, NS4A/2K, and NS4B/NS5 junctions. The enzyme responsible for NS1–2A cleavage is presently unknown. The expected topology of the flavivirus polyprotein is depicted in Figure 25.4C.

Features of the Structural Proteins

C Protein

Capsid (C) protein is a highly basic protein of ~11 kD. The nascent protein contains a C-terminal hydrophobic tail that serves as a signal peptide for ER translocation of prM. This anchor is cleaved in two steps, first by the viral NS2B-3 protease and then by signal peptidase.[503] Mature C protein folds into a compact dimer with each monomer containing four α-helices[193,372,529] (Fig. 25.5). The N-terminal region of the protein remains unstructured and, along with charged residues at the C-terminus, is thought to be involved in RNA binding.[398] An internal hydrophobic region mediates membrane association of C.[529]

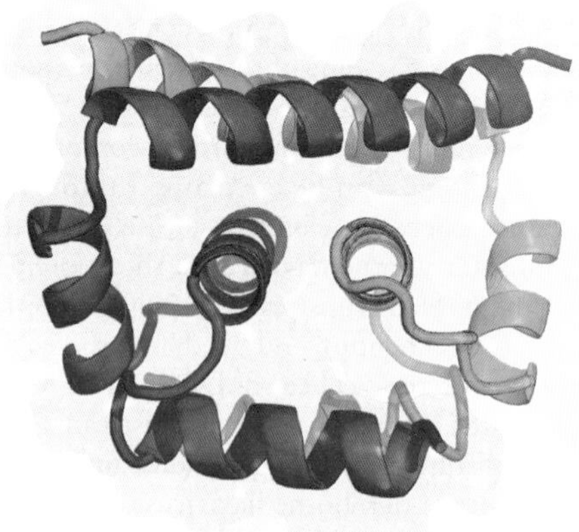

FIGURE 25.5. Flavivirus C protein structure. The WNV-KUN C protein is shown as a ribbon diagram with the protein surface rendered transparent, from PDB accession number 1SFK.[193] One monomer of the dimer is colored blue, the other green.

Overall, flavivirus C proteins demonstrate remarkable functional flexibility, with tolerance for large deletions. YFV C retains its ability to package RNA even after deletion of nearly 40 residues from the N-terminus or 27 residues of the C-terminus; internal deletions of the hydrophobic sequence are less tolerated.[654] The TBEV C protein can accept deletions of up to 16 amino acids from the central hydrophobic helix, albeit with increased production of empty particles.[409] Mutants containing larger deletions are not viable but can be rescued by second-site changes that increase the hydrophobicity of downstream sequences.[411] WNV tolerates small deletions in hydrophobic helix $\alpha 2$ to various degrees. Remarkably, infectivity of the deleted genomes was improved by even larger deletions—up to one-third of the C protein sequence—encompassing all of helix $\alpha 3$.[765] This results in the loss of a hydrophilic stretch, again suggesting the importance of hydrophobicity. It is not yet clear how C protein dimers are organized within the apparently disordered nucleocapsids, but interaction with RNA or DNA can induce isolated C protein dimers to assemble into nucleocapsid-like particles *in vitro*.[399]

Membrane Glycoprotein prM

The glycoprotein precursor of M, prM (~26 kD), is translocated into the ER via a signal sequence provided by the hydrophobic tail of C. Signal peptidase cleavage is delayed, however, until the viral serine protease cleaves on the cytosolic side of the membrane to generate the mature form of C.[19,503,924] This delay seems to result from the combination of a fairly short (14 to 22 amino acids) signal sequence, suboptimal residues at the signalase cleavage site, and residues in downstream regions of prM[504,815] and E protein.[511] Interestingly, uncoupling signal peptidase cleavage from NS2B-3 processing leads to increased production of empty virus particles.[459,504,505] Coordinated cleavage therefore serves to delay structural protein processing until the viral serine protease has accumulated and replication is under way, which may limit the release of immunogenic but noninfectious SVPs early in infection.

The N-terminal region of prM contains one to three N-linked glycosylation sites[122] and six conserved cysteine residues, all of which are disulfide linked.[633] The prM protein folds rapidly and assists in the proper folding of E.[415,511] The C-terminal transmembrane (TM) domains of prM and E act as ER retention signals and may assist in their heterodimerization.[486,641,643] A major function of prM is to prevent E from undergoing acid-catalyzed rearrangement and fusion during transit of the virions through the secretory pathway.[302,322] The crystal structure of DENV prM in complex with E has recently been solved and demonstrates how this function is performed.[471] The pr domain is a unique fold consisting of seven β strands, with the previously identified disulfide bonds stabilizing the structure. In immature particles, the pr region sits at the tip of the E protein, forming the pr-E spike and shielding the fusion peptide from the cellular environment (Fig. 25.6A). prM is not accessible to furin cleavage in these particles due to steric hindrance.[471] The acidity of the *trans*-Golgi compartment induces a global rearrangement that exposes the furin cleavage site.[946] After cleavage, the pr peptide does not immediately

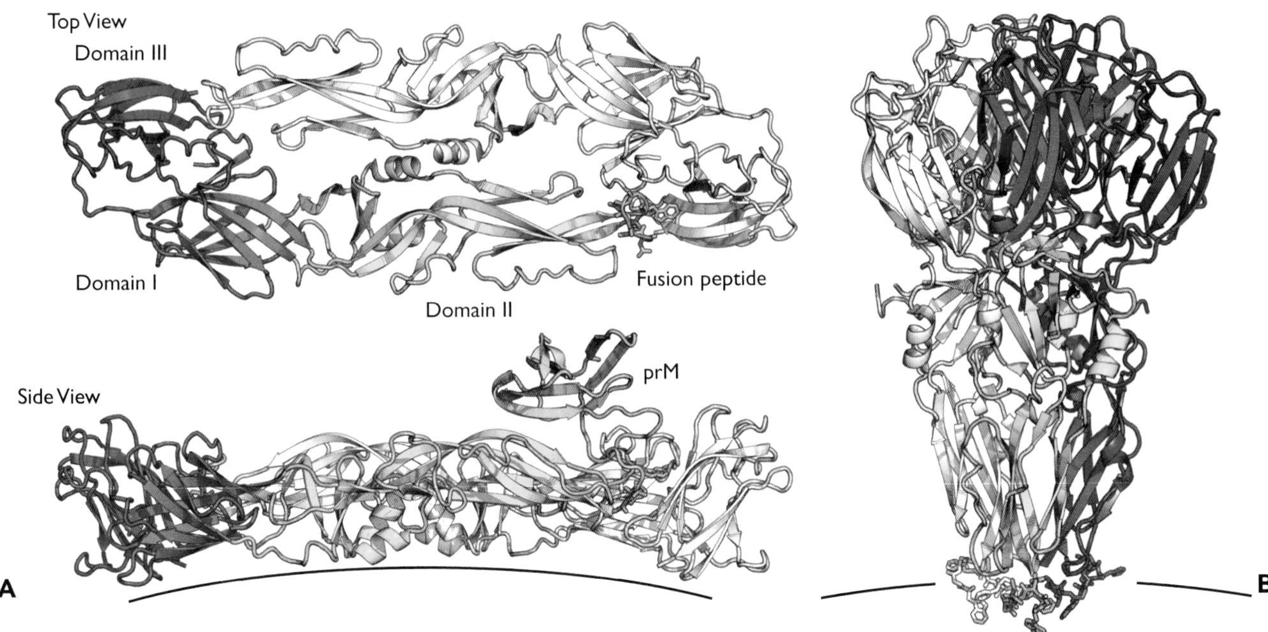

FIGURE 25.6. Flavivirus glycoprotein structures. A: The structure of a dengue virus 2 (DENV-2) E glycoprotein dimer is represented in this ribbon diagram, as viewed perpendicular **(top)** or laterally **(bottom)** with respect to the lipid bilayer. One E monomer is colored red (domain I), yellow (domain II), and blue gray (domain III). The amino acid side chains of the fusion peptide are shown (orange). Rendered from PDB 1OAN.[591] In the **bottom panel**, the low pH conformation of the DENV-2 pr protein from PDB 3C5X[471] was modeled onto the structure of 1OAN. **B:** tick-borne encephalitis virus (TBEV) E protein trimers in their postfusion form, colored as in **A**. Rendered from PDB 1URZ.[98]

disassociate from the virus particle.[802] Exposure to the neutral pH of the extracellular space is required to release pr and reveal the fusion-competent mature virion. This delay prevents the cleaved particles from undergoing premature membrane fusion within the Golgi.

Envelope Glycoprotein

E protein (~53 kD) is the major protein on the surface of flavivirus virions. E is synthesized as a type I membrane protein containing 12 conserved cysteines that form disulfide bonds[634]; in some viral species E is N-glycosylated.[123,909] Proper folding, stabilization in low pH, and secretion of E depends on co-expression with prM.[415,511] E is a class II fusion protein that mediates both receptor binding and membrane fusion.

Atomic resolution structures of E proteins from several flaviviruses have been solved in pre- and postfusion conformations.[98,382,591–592,593,625,635,722,958] In its prefusion form, E folds into an elongated structure rich in β-sheets and forming head-to-tail homodimers that lie parallel to the virus envelope.[591,722] Each E protein is composed of three domains: DI, which forms an eight-stranded β-barrel; DII, a long, finger-like domain that projects along the virus surface; and DIII, which maintains an immunoglobulin-like fold (Fig. 25.6A). The fusion peptide[12] is located at the tip of DII and remains covered by the pr peptide or buried in a hydrophobic pocket formed by DI and DIII of the partner monomer until triggered to insert into the target cell membrane.[722] DIII projects slightly from the virion surface and is thought to be involved in receptor binding; it is a major target of neutralizing antibodies.[145] Between the ectodomain of E and the membrane is a short but functionally important stem region composed of two α-helices that lie parallel to the plane of the membrane.[15,956]

On exposure to low pH, E protein dimers dissociate into monomeric subunits, which then form fusogenic trimers.[13,810,811] Interestingly, the WNV E protein crystal structure shows an array of perpendicular monomers, suggesting a mechanism for E protein rotation without exposing the fusion loop.[635,814] Crystal structures of postfusion E show the protein folded back onto itself, bringing the N-terminal fusion peptide, with its associated cellular membrane, into proximity with C-terminal TM domain, which is still integrated in the viral membrane[98,592] (Fig. 25.6B). To accomplish this, DIII must rotate and fold back more than 30 Å in relation to DI. Indeed, neutralizing antibodies against DIII can inhibit a postattachment step of viral entry,[636] and a soluble, recombinant form of DIII is a potent dominant-negative inhibitor of fusion.[478] In addition, DII rotates relative to DI,[98,592] with similar displacement of DII seen in crystals of native E protein grown in the presence of the detergent β-octylglucoside.[591,958] Residues that influence the pH threshold for membrane fusion surround the DI/DII pocket.[591] Protonation of conserved histidines at the interface of DI and DIII also contribute to E domain rearrangements in TBEV RSPs.[249] Mutagenesis studies of WNV, however, failed to identify histidine residues that entirely control the switch.[629]

Features of the Nonstructural Proteins

NS1 Glycoprotein

The NS1 glycoprotein (~46 kD) is translocated into the ER during synthesis and processed at its N-terminus by host signal peptidase. The C-terminus of NS1 arises through NS1–2A cleavage by an unknown ER-resident host enzyme, which requires the eight C-terminal residues of NS1 and greater than 140 amino acids of NS2A.[227,228,340] In addition, JEV expresses an elongated form of NS1, termed NS1′, which arises through a ribosomal −1 frameshifting event.[80,238,547,565]

NS1 contains two or three N-linked glycosylation sites and 12 conserved cysteines that form disulfide bonds.[79,461,547,797,884] Around 30 minutes after synthesis, NS1 simultaneously forms highly stable homodimers and acquires an affinity for membranes.[910,911] As NS1 lacks a known membrane interaction domain, the nature of its membrane association remains unclear. One possibility is that dimerization creates a hydrophobic surface for peripheral membrane binding. Alternatively, it has been reported that DENV-2 NS1 exhibits properties of a glycosylphosphatidylinositol (GPI)-anchored protein, although this mechanism seems inconsistent with the C-terminal peptide sequence of this protein.[902]

NS1 is retained within a secretory-derived compartment, expressed on the surface of infected cells, and efficiently secreted from mammalian, but not insect, cells.[491,816] The relative distribution of NS1 within these compartments is regulated through an unknown mechanism involving a short, N-terminal region of the protein.[942] The secreted form of NS1 accumulates to high levels in human sera and tissues and can be used to diagnose flavivirus infections at an early stage.[8,147,531] Secreted NS1 forms soluble, hexameric lipoprotein particles of ~10 nm that appear as three dimers held together in a barrel configuration.[172,239,304] The secreted form of NS1 can bind to uninfected cells by interaction with sulfated glycosaminoglycans[33] and can be internalized and trafficked to late endosomes, where it accumulates.[9] The function of endocytosed NS1 is not yet clear, but it may enhance subsequent infection with the homologous virus.[9]

The intracellular form of NS1 localizes to sites of viral RNA synthesis and plays an essential role in genome replication.[533,904] Mutations in NS1 can lead to dramatic defects in RNA replication and infectious virus production.[170,619,620] *trans*-Complementation studies revealed that NS1 functions at an early stage in RNA replication through a genetic interaction with NS4A.[395,396,490,492]

The extracellular forms of NS1 are highly antigenic and induce a strong humoral response. Secreted NS1 was originally characterized as a soluble, complement-fixing antigen present in the serum and tissues of DENV-infected animals. Antibodies that recognize cell surface–bound NS1 can direct complement-mediated lysis of infected cells and protect animals from lethal disease; other NS1-specific antibodies are protective in a complement-independent manner.[148,149] Antibody-mediated cross-linking of cell surface NS1 can also induce signaling cascades in DENV-2–infected cells, and it has been proposed that NS1 may contribute to pathogenesis by inducing antibodies that cross-react with human proteins. Despite the strong link between NS1-specific humoral responses and complement fixation, recent evidence indicates that WNV NS1 can inhibit the alternative pathway of complement activation by binding to and inhibiting the serum protein factor H. Furthermore, DENV, WNV, and YFV NS1 inhibit the classical pathway of complement fixation by binding to and increasing the turnover of complement factor C4. NS1 clearly plays an important role in flavivirus-specific humoral responses.

NS2A and NS2B Proteins

NS2A is a relatively small (~22 kD) hydrophobic protein. Its N-terminus is generated by an unidentified ER-resident host enzyme,[228] whereas the C-terminus is generated by NS2B-3 cleavage in the cytoplasm. Thus, NS2A is membrane spanning, although the precise topology of the protein is unknown. In addition, the YFV serine protease can cleave at an internal site in NS2A to generate a C-terminally truncated form, NS2Aα.[123,630] Interestingly, mutations at the YFV NS2Aα cleavage site block virus particle production and can be suppressed by a second mutation on the surface of the NS3 helicase domain.[434] Mutations in KUNV NS2A similarly block virus assembly, while the protein also localizes to subcellular sites of RNA replication and interacts with replicase components NS3, NS5, and the 3′ NCR of genome RNA. The involvement of NS proteins, in particular the NS2–3 region, in replication and infectious virus assembly appears to be an emerging theme for all three genera of the family *Flaviviridae.*

DENV-2 and WNV NS2A can also inhibit interferon (IFN) signaling, as evidenced by specific mutations in the protein that diminish this inhibitory activity and attenuate virulence in mice.[498,500,613] Interestingly, these mutations are cell culture adaptive and enhance the ability of KUNV replicons to establish persistence in IFN-competent cell lines. Remarkably, NS2A of the tick-borne flavivirus Langat does not share this property, which appears to be carried out instead by NS5.[66]

NS2B is also a small (~14 kD) membrane-associated protein.[154] NS2B forms a stable complex with NS3, serves to anchor this complex to cellular membranes, and acts as an essential co-factor for the NS2B-3 serine protease.[229] The co-factor activity lies in a central peptide that intercalates within the fold of the serine protease domain.[31,125,221]

NS3 Protein

NS3 is a large (~70 kD) multifunctional protein, encoding enzymatic activities required for polyprotein processing and RNA replication. The N-terminal third of the protein is the catalytic domain of the NS2B-3 serine protease,[50,124,279] which has specificity for substrates containing adjacent basic residues at the NS2A/NS2B, NS2B/NS3, NS3/NS4A, and NS4B/NS5 junctions.[122] In addition, this protease generates the C-termini of mature capsid protein[19,924] and NS4A[481] and can cleave at internal sites within NS2A and NS3.

Soluble, recombinant forms of the NS2B-3 serine protease domain have been purified and crystallized for x-ray diffraction.[125,221,733] These structures show that the co-factor region of NS2B contributes a β-strand to complete the chymotrypsin-like fold of the protease (Fig. 25.7A), similar to hepatitis C virus (HCV) NS3-4A. The C-terminal region of the NS2B co-factor can adopt multiple conformations that may alternately help to form the substrate-binding pocket or project outward from the protease fold; it is not yet clear whether these structural rearrangements are biologically significant.

As for other members of the *Flaviviridae,* the C-terminal region of NS3 encodes a supergroup 2 RNA helicase–nucleoside triphosphatase (NTPase).[280] NS3 demonstrates RNA-stimulated NTPase and RNA unwinding activities[890,899] and mutagenesis of the active site residues confirmed that these activities are essential for viral replication.[549] This region of NS3 also exhibits RNA triphosphatase (RTPase) activity, proposed to dephosphorylate the 5′ end of the genome before cap addition.[900] Recent

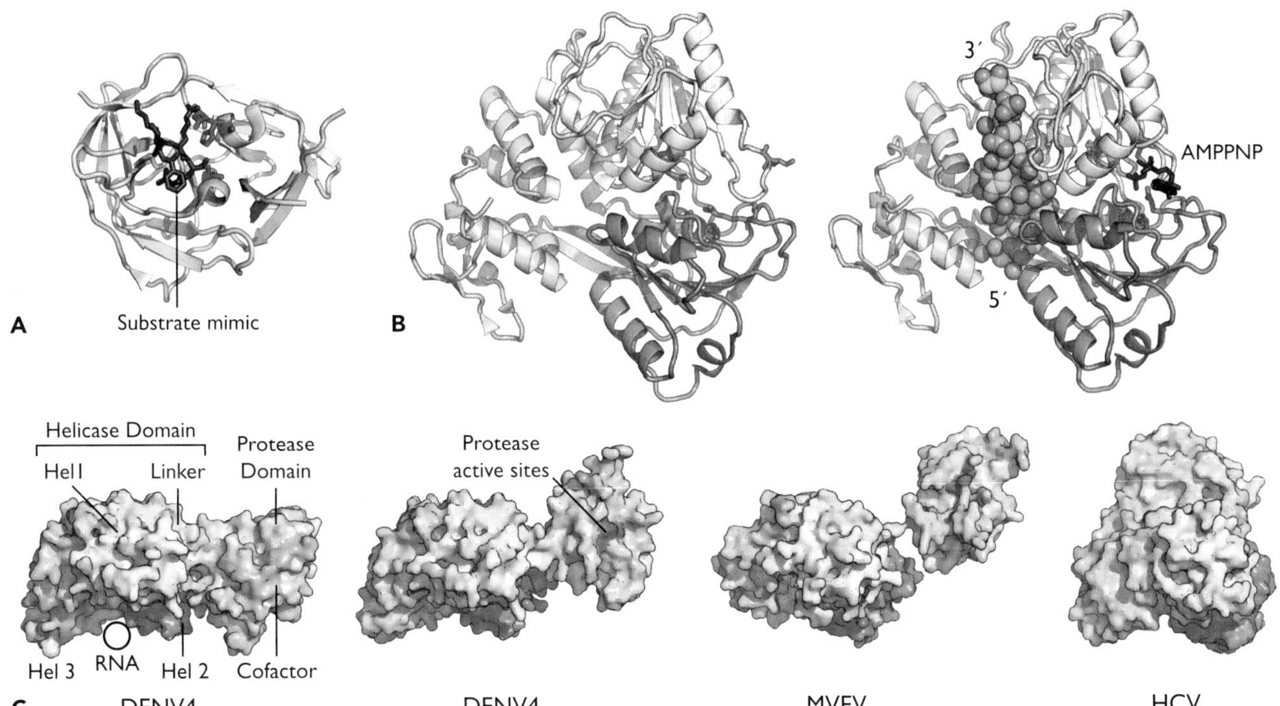

FIGURE 25.7. Viral NS3 proteins. A: The structure of the West Nile virus (WNV) NS2B-3 serine protease domain, with NS2B co-factor peptide (green), NS3 protease domain (pink), and a substrate-based inhibitor (black). Active-site residues are shown in red. Rendered from PDB number 2FP7.[221] **B:** Structure of the dengue fever 4 (DENV-4) NS3 helicase domain with **(left)** or without **(right)** bound RNA substrate (colored spheres) and adenosine triphosphate (ATP) analog (black). Note the adenosine triphosphatase (ATPase) active site (red) becomes structured at the interface of domain I (cyan) and domain II (purple) upon RNA binding. The RNA is bound within a cleft formed by the first two domains and domain III (gold). Rendered from PDB numbers 2JLQ and 2JLV.[523] **C:** Structural interdomain flexibility within full-length NS3. Shown are two conformations of full-length DENV-4 NS3 (PDBs 2VBC[522] and 2WHX,[521] respectively), Murray Valley encephalitis virus (MVEV) (PDB 2WV9[31]), and hepatitis C virus (HCV) (PDB 1CU1[930]). Shown is a structural alignment of the helicases, with molecular surfaces colored as in **A** and **B** and the protease-helicase linker in yellow.

studies show that RTPase is dependent on the Walker B motif in the helicase–NTPase catalytic core for phosphodiester bond hydrolysis.[41,58] Thus, all three nucleic acid–modifying activities of NS3 rely on a common active center. In addition to its roles in RNA replication, the helicase domain of NS3 has been implicated in virus assembly,[434,655] a role that is separable from the known enzymatic activities and can function *in trans*.[655]

Crystal structures of isolated DENV and YFV NS3 helicase domains show three subdomains, two structurally conserved RecA-like domains that are involved in NTP hydrolysis, and a unique C-terminal domain that may be involved in virus-specific RNA and protein recognition.[523,916,921] Co-crystallization of the DENV helicase with or without RNA substrates and nucleoside analogs revealed the structural basis for RNA-stimulated adenosine triphosphatase (ATPase) activity and substrate unwinding[523] (Fig. 25.7B). The structures of full-length DENV and MVEV NS3 have recently been solved in complex with their corresponding NS2B co-factors.[31,521,522] In these structures, the serine protease and helicase regions largely retain their domain folds, forming an elongated binary complex. However, the relative orientation of the domains differ, and greatly differ from the orientation of the related domains in HCV NS3, implying that the flexible linker region may play an important role in coordinating enzyme activities (Fig. 25.7C). The DENV structure also revealed that the serine protease domain can contribute to RNA helicase activity.[522]

Truncated forms of NS3, which result from alternative serine protease cleavage events in the helicase domain, have been observed *in vitro* and *in vivo*. The role of these cleavages is unclear, although it is possible that the products could have a distinct function. In this regard, replication defects caused by deletions in the KUNV helicase domain can be complemented *in trans*, while deletions in the serine protease domain cannot be complemented.[374,396,499]

Finally, the NS3 proteins of Langat, DENV-2, and WNV have been shown to induce apoptosis, in some cases through activation of caspase-8.[691,704,776] Flaviviruses are often cytopathic in mammalian cells, although whether this is the normal pathway for cell killing requires further study. The DENV NS2B-3 serine protease can also down-regulate the activation of type I IFN in human dendritic cells, although the relevant protease substrate(s) have not been identified.[736]

The NS4A and NS4B Proteins

NS4A and NS4B are small (16 kD and 27 kD, respectively) hydrophobic proteins. NS4A has been implicated in RNA replication through a genetic interaction with NS1[490] and co-localization with replication complexes.[535] Similar to the coordinated processing of C protein, signal peptidase cleavage at the 2K/NS4B junction requires prior cleavage by the NS2B-3 serine protease at a site just upstream of the 2K internal signal peptide.[481,690] Overexpression studies showed that NS4A can induce membrane rearrangements and/or formation of autophagosomes, and that regulated NS4A/2K/4B cleavage is necessary for this activity.[560,586,738] Mutations in NS4A and 2K have been found to confer resistance to a potent inhibitor of flavivirus RNA replication and to overcome superinfection exclusion, further implicating this region in RNA replication.[966,967]

NS4B is a polytopic membrane protein that co-localizes with NS3 at the presumed sites of RNA replication.[481,587] NS4B is posttranslationally modified to a form that migrates faster on sodium dodecyl sulfate-polyacrylamide gel electrophoresis (SDS-PAGE),[123,690] although the identity and function of this modification remain to be determined. Similar to NS2A, DENV NS4A and NS4B can block type I IFN signaling.[613] NS4B has the strongest antagonistic effect, which requires either proper processing of the NS4A–NS4B polyprotein or expression of NS4B with an N-terminal signal peptide.[612] Similarly, WNV NS4A and NS4B block IFN signaling by inducing an unfolded protein response in the ER, which can down-regulate Jak-STAT signaling.[20]

NS5 Protein

NS5 is a large (103 kD), highly conserved, multifunctional phosphoprotein with RNA capping and RdRP activities encoded within its N- and C-terminal regions, respectively.[181] Formation of a type 1 RNA cap involves multiple steps, including (a) removal of one phosphate from a 5′ triphosphorylated RNA substrate by an RTPase, (b) addition of a 5′-5′ guanosine cap (from guanosine triphosphate [GTP]) by a guanylyltransferase, (c) N7-methylation of the guanylyl cap by a methyltransferase (MTase), and (d) 2′-O methylation of the second residue by the same or another MTase. As mentioned earlier, the NS3 helicase–NTPase exhibits RTPase activity, which suggests that NS3 and NS5 function together during RNA capping.[41,900] The flavivirus guanylyltransferase proved to be elusive for many years, although recent evidence indicates that the N-terminal domain of NS5 is capable of performing this reaction.[361] Finally, the N-terminal region of NS5 encodes conserved MTase motifs and is capable of performing both N7 and 2′-O methylation in a coordinated fashion.[211,417,713] The structure of the NS5 capping domain has been solved by x-ray crystallography under a variety of conditions, revealing high-resolution structures of these reaction pathways[181,211,266,931] (Fig. 25.8A). Mutagenesis of the NS5 capping domain showed that the methylation events are separable and that N7 methylation is required for viral translation and replication, while 2′-O methylation allows the virus to avoid innate antiviral defenses.[178,195,427,964] Interestingly, cellular casein kinase 1 can phosphorylate YFV NS5 *in vitro* at a serine residue near the methyltransferase active site, which inhibits 2′-O methylation.[67,68] While inhibitors of this kinase affect YFV replication, it is not known if this site is phosphorylated *in vivo.*

The C-terminal domain of NS5 contains conserved RdRP motifs[417,726] and structurally resembles other RNA polymerases, forming a "right hand" structure with palm, fingers, and thumb subdomains[181,543,932] (Fig. 25.8B). NS5 RNA polymerase activity has been confirmed with purified, recombinant protein[1,181,305,826]; mutagenesis of the polymerase active site; and supplying the activity *in trans* from a KUNV replicon. The major product of *in vitro* RdRP reactions is often a self-primed copy-back RNA. However, NS5 is capable of initiating RNA synthesis *de novo,*[1,632,948] which likely reflects the authentic mechanism in infected cells. NS5 forms a complex with NS3[371,389] and stimulates NS3 NTPase and RTPase activities.[175,939] Cross-linking studies have shown that both proteins bind to the 3′ SL of the viral genome.[129] Along with genome circularization, this may serve to initiate minus-strand synthesis by 5′ SL–bound NS5.[196,237,354,940]

WNV and DENV-2 NS5 have been shown to localize at sites of viral RNA synthesis,[534,898] although this has been

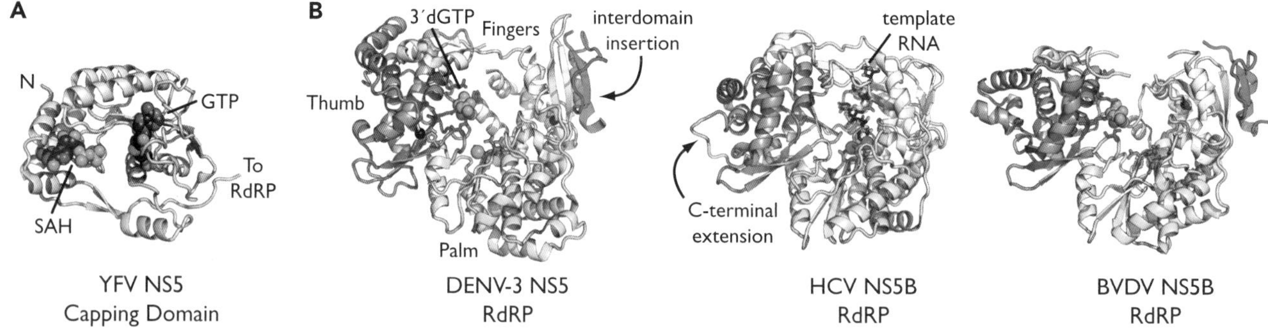

FIGURE 25.8. Viral NS5 and NS5B proteins. A: The yellow fever virus (YFV) capping domain is shown, with bound methyl donor S-adenosyl-L-homocysteine (SAH) and guanosine triphosphate (GTP). Rendered from PDB number 3EVC.[266] **B:** A structural comparison of RNA-dependent RNA polymerases (RdRP) domains across the *Flaviviridae.* The dengue virus 3 (DENV-3) RdRP domain is shown, with the canonical finger (cyan), palm (pink), and thumb (purple) domains indicated. A flavivirus-specific interdomain insertion is shown in green. This structure shows the binding site of a GTP analog, which is important for activating *de novo* RNA synthesis. GTP-binding residues are blue, RdRP active-site residues are red, and a catalytic Mg^{2+} ion is shown as a green sphere. Structural Zn^{2+} ions are shown in black. This model is a composite structure, rendered from PDB numbers 2J7U and 2J7W.[932] The hepatitis C virus (HCV) NS5B RdRP is shown with bound template RNA; the HCV-specific C-terminal extension is shown in yellow. Rendered from PDB number 1NB7.[637] The bovine viral diarrhea virus 1 (BVDV-1) NS5B RdRP is shown modeled in the GTP-bound state by rendering PDB number 2JCQ and the GTP analog from 2J7W. The pestivirus-specific N-terminal extension is shown in green.

difficult to show for other viruses. Biochemical studies indicate that only a small fraction of NS5 co-fractionates with replicase activity,[298,868] and the protein is frequently localized to the nucleus of flavivirus-infected cells.[181,389] These results suggest that NS5 may play additional roles, other than in RNA replication, in the virus life cycle. In this regard, DENV-2 NS5 induces interleukin-8 (IL-8) transcription and secretion, which may enhance viral spread or disease by recruiting inflammatory cells to the site of infection.[562] In addition, NS5 has been shown to block the Jak-STAT pathway of IFN signaling.[66,181]

RNA Replication

The flavivirus NS proteins presumably recruit the viral genome out of translation and into a replication complex. Replication begins with the synthesis of a genome-length minus-strand RNA, which then serves as a template for new plus-strand genomes. Minus-strand RNA has been detected as early as 3 hours after infection.[492] Viral RNA synthesis is asymmetric, with approximately 10-fold more positive strands accumulating compared to minus strands.[152,620] Flavivirus replication can be followed by metabolic labeling of virus-specific RNA in the presence of actinomycin D, an inhibitor of DNA-dependent RNA polymerases. Three major species of labeled flavivirus RNA have been described, including the plus-strand genome, a double-stranded replicative form (RF), and a heterogeneous population of replicative intermediates (RIs) that most likely represent duplex regions and recently synthesized RNAs displaced by nascent strands undergoing elongation.[146,152] Pulse-chase analyses indicate that RF and RI are precursors to genome RNA,[146,152] indicating semiconservative and asymmetric replication.[146]

In addition to genome-length plus- and minus-strand products of RNA replication, 0.2- to 0.6-kb subgenomic flavivirus RNAs (sfRNAs) are produced in infected cells.[485,762,869] sfRNAs are co-linear with the 3′ end of the genome and are produced through incomplete degradation of the genome by the cellular 5′-3′ exoribonuclease Xrn1.[678,785] The Xrn1 resistance of this region is due to conserved secondary structures and pseudoknots located within the 3′ NCR.[252,785] While controversy exists over whether sfRNAs are needed for efficient RNA replication, a WNV mutant that does not produce sfRNAs is less cytopathic in cell culture and less pathogenic in mice.[252,678,785] Interestingly, supplying sfRNA *in trans* restored WNV cytopathic effect in cell culture, suggesting that these small RNAs may have a specific but as yet unknown target.[678]

Membrane Reorganization and the Compartmentalization of Flavivirus Replication

Biochemical studies of flavivirus-infected cells show that replicase activity is concentrated in dense membrane fractions that are enriched for most viral NS proteins. Treatment with nonionic detergents increases sensitivity to nucleases and proteases, indicating that the active replicase resides within a membrane-bound compartment. Consistent with this, ultrastructural changes in perinuclear membranes can be detected in flavivirus-infected cells.[898] In general, the earliest event is the proliferation of ER membranes, followed by the appearance of smooth vesicular structures around the time of early logarithmic virus production. These structures, sometimes referred to as double-membrane vesicles or vesicle packets, are small clusters of ~90-nm vesicles within the lumen of the ER.[898,904] They are frequently adjacent to ER-derived convoluted membranes, which can appear as randomly folded membranes or highly ordered "paracrystalline arrays".[454,616,898] Electron tomography revealed that these vesicles are invaginations of the ER and retain connectivity to the cytosol through a neck-like pore, sometimes apposed to sites of virus assembly[898] (Fig. 25.9).

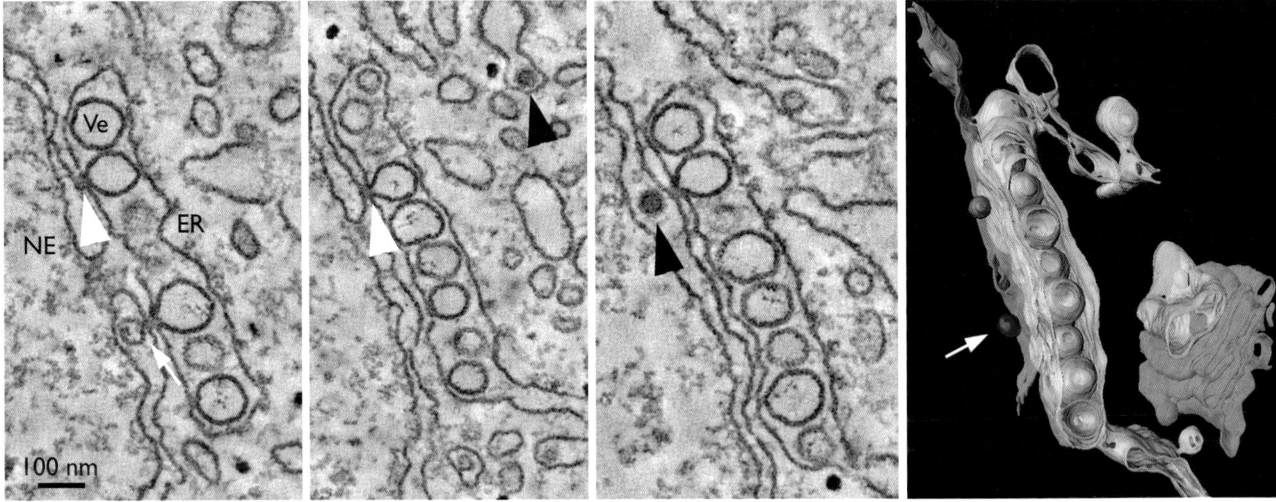

FIGURE 25.9. Sites of dengue virus (DENV) RNA replication and virus particle assembly. The three tomographic slices, each ~2 nm thick, show DENV-induced vesicles (Ve) associated with the endoplasmic reticulum (ER) and nuclear envelope (NE). White arrowheads indicate necked connections between the Ve and ER membranes; black arrowheads indicate virus particles. To the right is a three-dimensional reconstruction of the membrane surfaces (tan) and virus particles (red). The white arrow indicates a putative site of virus budding. (Courtesy of Drs. Sonja Welsch and Ralf Bartenschlager. Adapted from Welsch S, Miller S, Romero-Brey I, et al. Composition and three-dimensional architecture of the dengue virus replication and assembly sites. *Cell Host Microbe* 2009;5:365–375, with permission from Elsevier.)

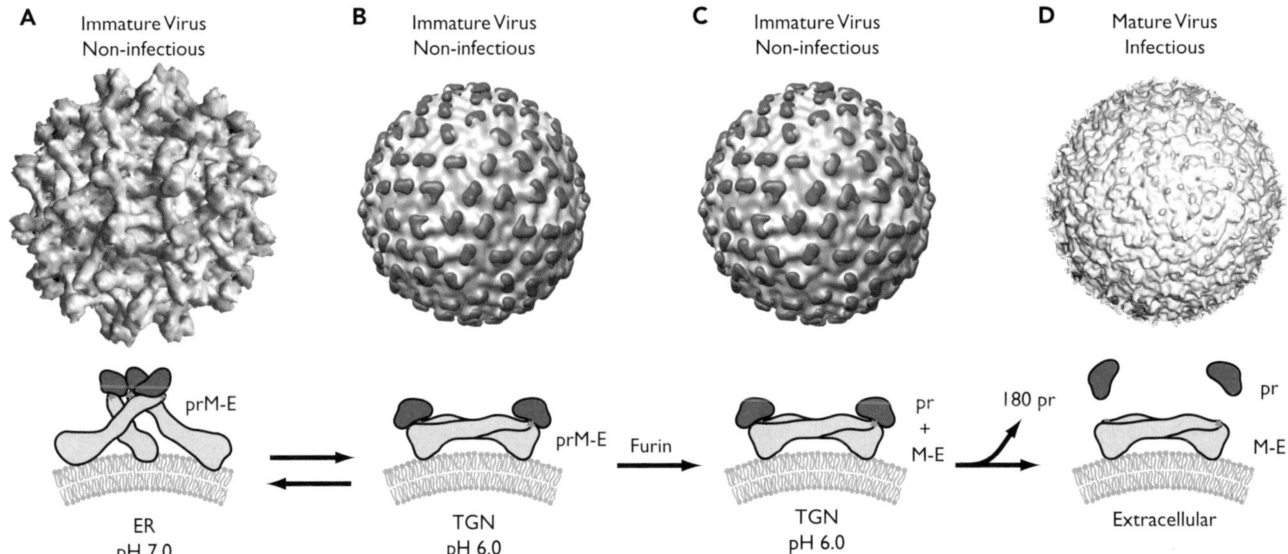

FIGURE 25.10. Flavivirus particle maturation. Nascent, noninfectious, immature particles undergo a pH-dependent conformational rearrangement of the viral glycoproteins E (gray) and precursor M (prM) (blue). Mature, infectious particles form upon furin cleavage of prM and release of the pr fragment. (Adapted from Perera R, Kuhn RJ. Structural proteomics of dengue virus. *Curr Opin Microbiol* 2008;11:369–377, with permission from Elsevier.)

Perinuclear vesicle packets have been confirmed as the sites of viral RNA synthesis by metabolic labeling of nascent RNA, *in situ* hybridization, and immunodetection of double-stranded RNA (dsRNA) (presumably RF and RI).

The pathways of flavivirus-induced membrane reorganization are currently being worked out. One important clue comes from the ability of DENV-2 NS3 to recruit the cellular fatty acid synthase to sites of replication, at least by late times of infection.[319] In addition, DENV induces autophagosome formation in infected cells,[393,463,560,651] leading to turnover of triglycerides into free fatty acids, β-oxidation of lipids, and increased adenosine triphosphate (ATP) levels that promote virus replication.[320]

Assembly and Release of Particles from Flavivirus-Infected Cells

Similar to replication, early ultrastructural studies indicated that flavivirus morphogenesis occurs in close association with intracellular membranes.[615] The assembly process is thought to commence by association of C protein dimers with genomic RNA, followed by budding into ER membranes containing the E–prM glycoprotein complex. Recent electron tomography studies of DENV-infected cells have shown that replicase-containing vesicle packets and ER-associated sites of virus budding are part of one continuous network. Pores within the replication vesicles appear to release newly synthesized viral RNA directly adjacent to budding DENV particles.[898] These findings suggest a potential mechanism for coupling of flavivirus replication and assembly.[397] Interdependence of these processes is a common theme among RNA viruses and might serve to reduce the propagation of defective genomes. Coupling flavivirus replication and assembly may also explain the roles of NS2A and NS3 proteins in infectious virus assembly.[434,465,497,655]

Following assembly, nascent virions are transported through the secretory pathway and released at the cell surface.[536] It is during secretion that immature particles undergo acid-induced E–prM rearrangement and prM cleavage (Fig. 25.10). Additional virion maturation steps occur during egress, including glycan modification of prM and E (for some viruses) by trimming and terminal addition.[123,169,309,547] This implies that virions move through an exocytosis pathway similar to that used for host cell surface glycoproteins. In addition to the secretory pathway machinery, other host factors have been implicated in flavivirus morphogenesis. Inhibitor and RNA interference studies implicate the Src family kinase c-Yes in WNV egress from the ER.[333] A serine/threonine protein phosphatase inhibitor, I(2)(PP2A), has also been found to bind the WNV C protein, although its importance for infectivity was minimal.[350]

HEPATITIS C VIRUSES

Background and Classification

HCV was identified in 1989 through expression cloning of immunoreactive cDNA from the plasma of a chimpanzee infected with an etiologic agent known to cause non-A non-B viral hepatitis.[143] The virus currently infects more than 130 million people worldwide and remains a significant public health concern. HCV typically causes chronic hepatotropic infections, which can progress over decades to fibrosis, cirrhosis, and liver cancer. Based on difficulties in detecting HCV *in vivo,* the virus was originally thought to replicate poorly. Yet mathematical models of HCV dynamics indicate that a chronically infected patient produces approximately 10^{12} virions per day, with a virion half-life of only a few hours.[666]

Based on its evolutionary history, HCV is classified into seven genotypes, which differ from each other by more than 30% at the nucleotide level.[614,788] Each genotype is further divided into numerous subtypes. HCV genotypes show differences in worldwide distribution, disease progression, and susceptibility to treatment. In addition, intergenotypic and intersubtype recombinant HCV genomes have been described.[788]

While no HCV vaccine exists, advances in treatment have been made. Pegylated IFN-α and ribavirin—the standard of care for over a decade—have burdensome side effects and do not cure many of the patients treated. The most common HCV genotype, genotype 1, is also the most difficult to treat with this therapy.[334] Recently, however, HCV-specific antiviral drugs—such as protease inhibitors—have begun to reach the clinic. While the new drugs must still be used in combination with IFN and ribavirin, first-generation protease inhibitors have almost doubled the chances of treatment success.

In addition to HCV, the genus *Hepacivirus* may contain a few related viruses that are awaiting taxonomic classification. An HCV-like virus was recently identified in domestic dogs with respiratory illness.[388] This virus appears to be closely related to HCV and has been tentatively designated canine hepacivirus (CHV), although it has not been formally classified within this genus. In addition, GB virus B (see later) appears to be closely related to the hepaciviruses.

Experimental Systems

HCV research was limited for years by the lack of convenient laboratory culture systems and small animal models. However, many of these technical hurdles have been overcome in the past decade.

Shortly after the sequence of the HCV genome was fully elucidated, the first consensus cDNA clones were constructed. RNA transcripts from these cDNAs were shown to be infectious by direct intrahepatic inoculation into chimpanzees.[412,925] Chimpanzee infectious clones have been used to show that all viral enzymes, the *p7* gene, and 3′ NCR are essential for HCV replication *in vivo.*[414,750,926] Furthermore, the ability to use genetically defined inocula to initiate clonal infections provided a useful tool to study virus evolution and immune responses.[106] Despite their demonstrated utility *in vivo,* however, these infectious transcripts failed to replicate after transfection into cultured cells.

Subgenomic HCV replicons were developed in 1999 and proved to be the first broadly useful system for studying HCV RNA replication in cell culture.[509] Subgenomic replicons are bicistronic constructs in which the HCV internal ribosome entry site (IRES) drives expression of the neomycin resistance gene and the encephalomyocarditis virus (EMCV) IRES drives expression of the HCV NS proteins. Following RNA transfection into a human hepatoma line, Huh-7, the original genotype 1b (Con1 strain) replicon replicated to low levels.[509] Cell culture–adaptive mutations were later found to increase RNA replication efficiency up to 10,000 times.[77] These mutations, many of which cluster in NS5A, are thought to increase RNA accumulation at the expense of infectious virus production, although their mechanisms of action are not well understood (reviewed in[43]). In addition to Con1, subgenomic replicons have now been constructed for additional genotype 1b strains, as well as genotype 1a and 2a isolates.

Full-length genotype 1a and 1b genomes bearing adaptive mutations were shown to replicate in cell culture but did not produce infectious virus particles.[78,355,676] The HCV pseudoparticle (HCVpp) system was therefore developed to examine the role of the viral glycoproteins in entry. HCVpp are defective retrovirus particles expressing a reporter gene and displaying the HCV envelope proteins on their surface.[46,201,343] Pseudoparticles undergo low-pH–mediated entry by using the known HCV entry factors and continue to be a valuable system to study entry in isolation from RNA replication. HCVpp differ from authentic particles, however, in their acid susceptibility[343] and their assembly in a post-Golgi compartment rather than in the ER.[751]

In 2005, production of authentic HCV in cell culture (HCVcc) was achieved for the first time. An HCV isolate from an unusual case of acute fulminant hepatitis in Japan (JFH-1) was found to replicate in culture without the need for adaptive mutations.[392] Remarkably, full-length JFH-1 also produced low levels of infectious virus.[883,959] Infectious titers could be increased with passage or by engineering chimeric genomes based on a related genotype 2a strain, J6.[487,675] A cell culture–adapted genotype 1a genome that produces infectious HCVcc has also been developed, albeit with lower infectivity.[937]

The chimpanzee remains the only animal model that reproduces clinical aspects of HCV infection, including a high rate of viral persistence and the development of HCV-specific innate and adaptive immune responses. Advances have been made, however, in generating small animal models for HCV infection. Immunodeficient mouse strains with liver injury can be repopulated with human hepatocytes and infected with HCV. Two commonly used liver injury models are the toxic urokinase plasminogen activator transgene (Alb-uPA mice)[568,570] and a conditionally lethal fumaryl acetoacytate hydrolase deficiency ($FAH^{-/-}$ mice).[73] Recently, immunocompetent mice that express human HCV entry factors have been developed as a model for the early steps of infection.[198]

Structure and Physical Properties of the Virion

HCV particles are enveloped and contain the viral proteins core (C), E1, and E2, as well as the genomic RNA. Virions are between 30 and 80 nm in diameter.[88,317,949] For a virus of this size, HCV exhibits an unusually low and heterogeneous buoyant density. In highly infectious acute-phase chimpanzee serum, HCV-specific RNA is detected in fractions with densities ranging from 1.03 to 1.10 g/mL.[87,331] The particle density is inversely correlated with infectivity, with low-density virions being more infectious than high-density particles. Similar to serum-derived virus, the peak of HCVcc RNA has a buoyant density of approximately 1.15 g/mL,[116,487,883,937,959] whereas the peak infectivity is near 1.10 g/mL.[116,487,959] Passage of cell culture–grown virus in animals[488] or primary hepatocyte cultures[682] increases the proportion of low-density, high-infectivity virus, highlighting the impact of host cell environment on virion composition.

The high density observed for noninfectious particles may come from immunoglobulin binding to the virus and/or represent nonenveloped nucleocapsids.[23] The low buoyant density of infectious HCV appears to reflect the ability of the virus to interact with serum lipoproteins.[22,631,692,855] The lipidome of HCV particles is very similar to low-density lipoproteins (LDLs) and very-low-density lipoproteins (VLDLs), including an enrichment of cholesteryl esters.[569] Immunoprecipitation and immunogold-electron microscopy (EM) studies have detected apolipoprotein (Apo) AI,[416] ApoB,[416,631,855] ApoC1,[572] and ApoE[631] in association with serum-derived HCV. Apolipoprotein E and ApoC1 are also associated with HCVcc,[126,569,572] but ApoB is generally lacking, leading to controversy about

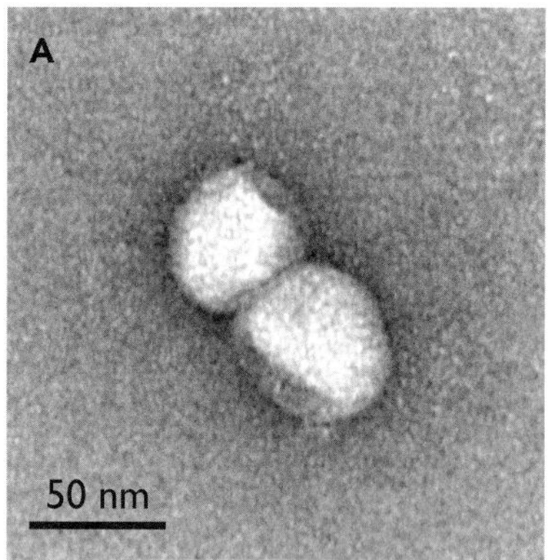

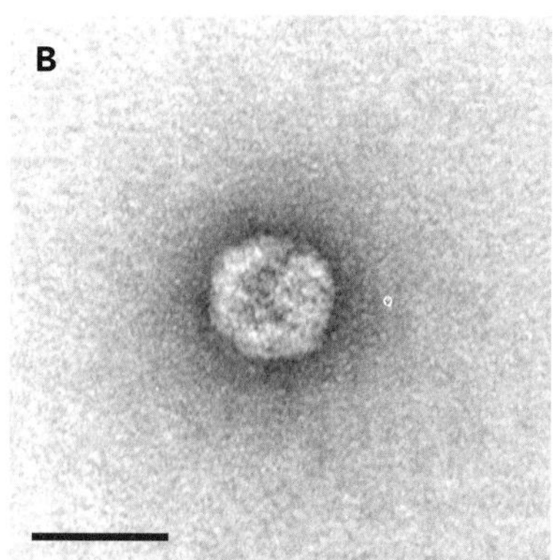

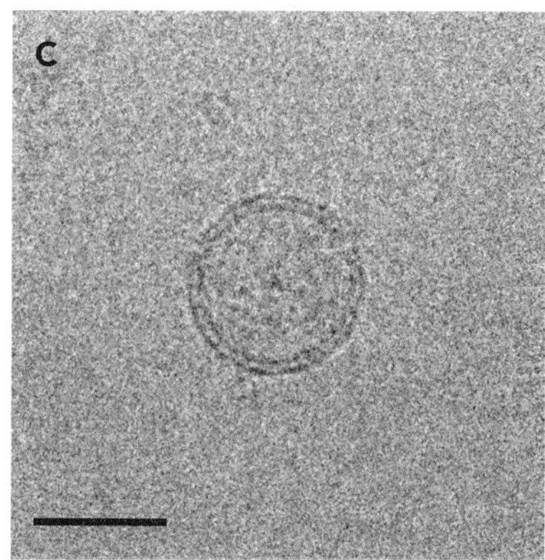

FIGURE 25.11. Hepatitis C virus (HCV) particles produced in cell culture. A: Virus particles were purified and negative stained with uranyl acetate. **B:** A representative virus particle after extraction with 0.2% NP-40 and negative staining. **C:** A representative enveloped virus particle as imaged through cryoelectron microscopy. (Adapted from Gastaminza P, Dryden KA, Boyd B, et al. Ultrastructural and biophysical characterization of hepatitis C virus particles produced in cell culture. *J Virol* 2010;84:10999–11009, with permission of the American Society for Microbiology Press.)

its functional importance (reviewed in[44]). The propensity of HCV to interact closely with lipids has led to the hypothesis that at least a portion of circulating virus is internalized in host lipoproteins to form a "lipoviral" particle,[22] which may provide camouflage for the virus to escape neutralizing antibodies.

Although unambiguous visualization of HCV from patient samples remains a challenge, negative stain and cryoelectron microscopy studies have started to reveal structural features of HCV grown in cell culture[264,569,883] (Fig. 25.11). One recent study detected two predominant classes of HCV particles, each making up approximately half of the preparation. The first were spherical, pleomorphic particles, ~55 nm in diameter, containing a lipid bilayer and an electron-dense core (Fig. 25.11C). These particles, which are presumably infectious HCV, were enriched in low-density fractions and had a relatively smooth, featureless surface that reacted with E2- and ApoE-specific antibodies. The second class of particles, electron-dense structures ~45 nm in diameter, is presumed to be naked nucleocapsids. This class was enriched in high-density, low-infectivity fractions and lacked a membrane or visible surface projections. Similar particles were seen after detergent treatment of infectious virus, which is expected to remove the viral envelope.[264] Unfortunately, the reconstruction of high-resolution models of the virus particle is currently limited by particle heterogeneity, relatively low yields, and lack of symmetry in both classes of HCV particles.

Binding and Entry

HCV infects target hepatocytes through a multistep process that involves several cell surface molecules. Virus particles initially attach to glycosaminoglycans[45,268] and possibly the LDL receptor (LDL-R),[4,598] which may interact with virion-associated ApoB and ApoE. Following attachment, virus particles employ four specific entry factors to mediate uptake: scavenger receptor class B type I (SR-BI, aka SCARBI),[758] CD81,[679] claudin 1 (CLDN1),[224] and occludin (OCLN).[681]

SR-BI, which is highly expressed on hepatocytes, plays important physiologic roles in the selective uptake of cholesterol and cholesteryl esters from lipoproteins. SR-BI can interact with the E2 hypervariable region 1 (HVR1),[758] and its overexpression enhances virion binding to CHO cells,[224] suggesting a role for SR-BI in primary attachment. Blocking antibody studies have both supported a role for SR-BI in binding,[121] as well as shown the importance of SR-B1 at a postbinding step that is closely linked to CD81.[386,952] Antibodies directed at E2 HVR1 similarly block a postattachment step of HCV entry.[878] The physiologic SR-BI binding partner, PDZK1, is also important for entry.[225] Perhaps because the lipoviral particle shares commonalities with the natural ligands of SR-BI, various lipoproteins modulate HCV infectivity. Specifically, high-density lipoproteins (HDLs) can enhance HCV fusion in a manner dependent on SR-BI lipid transfer, ApoCI, and the E2 HVR1.[47,199,571,880] In contrast, oxidized LDL,[882] VLDL,[542] and serum amyloid A[114,453] inhibit HCV entry.

The tetraspanin CD81 binds tightly to the glycoprotein E2 via residues in the CD81 large extracellular loop.[328,670,679] Antibodies targeting CD81 do not affect HCVpp binding to hepatocytes[166] but inhibit HCV infection after virus attachment.[421] Because HVR1 masks the CD81 binding site, a conformational change may be required to prime E2 for binding to this co-receptor.[37] CD81 interacts with another HCV entry factor, CLDN1,[313,929] forming a complex that is essential for HCV infection.[312] Receptor tyrosine kinases, such as epidermal growth factor receptor (EGFR), appear to regulate CD81–CLDN1 interactions and to promote HCV membrane fusion.[527] Interaction of CD81 with another host factor, EWI-2wint, inhibits virus uptake.[734] In addition to its role in entry, interaction of HCV with lymphocyte-expressed CD81 may contribute to the immune dysregulation seen in some patients with chronic infection.[173,739,865]

Two tight junction proteins, CLDN1[224] and OCLN,[59,496,681] are essential for postbinding steps of HCV uptake. In addition, CLDN family members-6 and -9 can also mediate entry.[563] The involvement of tight junction proteins suggests that HCV could traffic across the surface of the hepatocyte in order to engage all of its entry factors. Indeed, binding to CD81 activates a Rho guanosine triphosphatase (GTPase), which may mediate cytoskeleton rearrangements. Furthermore, recombinant E2 promotes relocalization of CD81 to tight junctions.[94] In conflict with this hypothesis, however, is the finding that CLDN1 can form complexes with CD81 on the basolateral surface of hepatocytes.[312] In addition, single particle tracking has visualized HCV internalization outside tight junctions—although this may represent the nonpolarized nature of the cultured hepatoma cells.[159]

Following attachment, HCV is taken up via clathrin-mediated endocytosis.[76,564] Internalized virions co-localize with clathrin light chain and the E3 ubiquitin ligase c-Cbl prior to uncoating.[159] Intracellular HCV is delivered to Rab5a-positive early endosomes,[159] which likely provide the acidic environment necessary to induce rearrangement of the HCV glycoproteins into their fusogenic form.[343,864] Surprisingly, extracellular HCVcc particles are resistant to inactivation by low pH, suggesting that interactions at or near the cell surface prime the virus for fusion.[864] This is functionally similar to pestiviruses[425] but in contrast to flavivirus particles, which are primed during maturation,[946] and to HCVpp,[343,644] which have structural and compositional differences from authentic HCV particles.

Genome Structure

The HCV genome is an uncapped, 9.6-kb RNA containing highly structured 5′ and 3′ ends (Fig. 25.12A). The 5′ NCR is a well-conserved, 341-nt sequence element that folds into a complex structure consisting of four major domains and a pseudoknot.[324] The first 120 nt serves as a minimal replication element, although compelling genetic evidence shows that the entire 5′ NCR (or its complement in the negative strand) plays an important role in efficient positive-strand RNA synthesis.[70,247,282,290,404,525,721] The 5′ NCR also contains an IRES, which directs the cap-independent translation of the single large ORF.

Interestingly, the liver-specific micro-RNA (miR)-122 binds to two sites within the HCV 5′ NCR, and these interactions are required for efficient viral replication.[377,469] While miR-122 can stimulate IRES-mediated translation in an Argonaute 2-dependent manner,[325,366,732,907] elegant genetic experiments revealed that a major function of miR-122 is to sequester the 5′ end of the genome, perhaps protecting it from RNA degradation or from activation of innate antiviral responses.[532] Nuclease-resistant oligonucleotides that antagonize miR-122 function *in vivo* profoundly decrease HCV replication in experimentally infected chimpanzees and show promise for future therapeutics,[447] although viral escape can occur in cell culture.[474]

A number of functionally important RNA structures have been identified within the HCV ORF.[867] Genetic analysis indicated that an RNA stem-loop within the C gene is important for viral fitness.[561,876] An RNA structure in NS5B, termed 5BSL3.2, forms a long-distance base-pairing interaction with upstream RNA sequences with the 3′ NCR.[246] This "kissing" interaction is essential for replication, although its function remains to be determined. In addition, the HCV ORF contains fewer UA and UU dinucleotides than expected

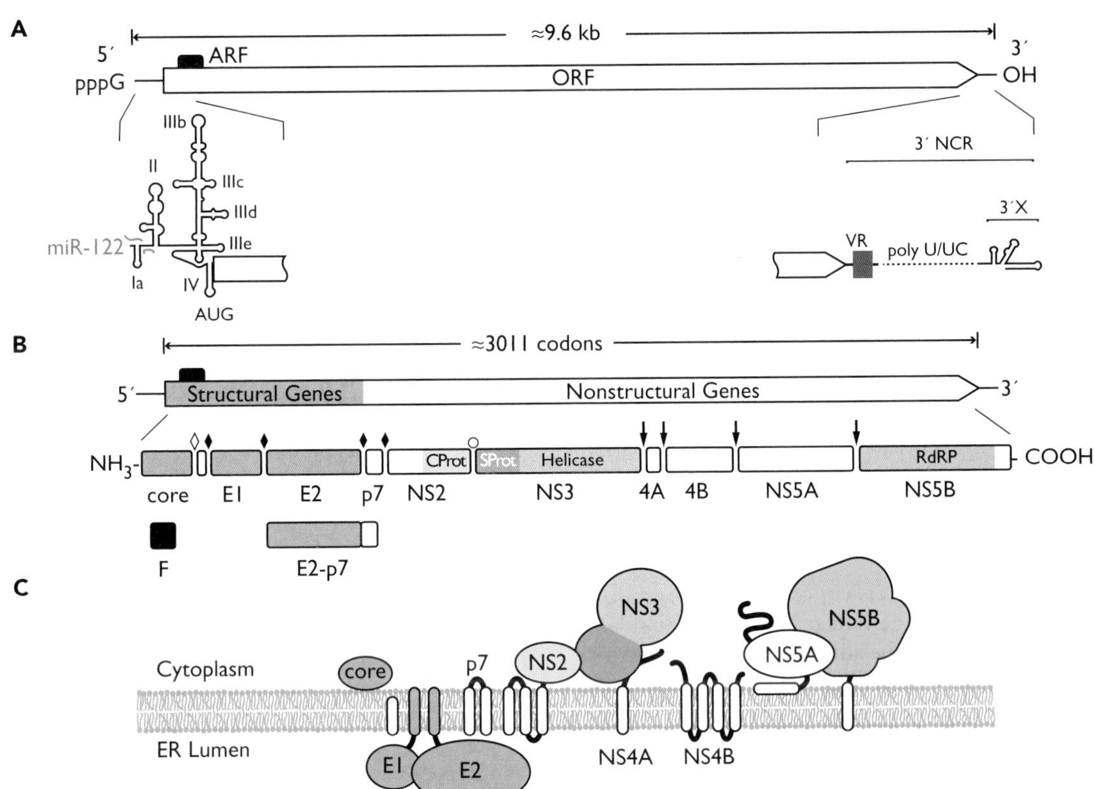

FIGURE 25.12. Hepacivirus genome structure and protein expression. A: Hepatitis C virus (HCV) genome structure and RNA elements. Important RNA elements are indicated as in Figure 25.4. The binding sites of micro-RNA (miR)-122 are indicated in red; the alternative reading frame (ARF) is indicated by a black box. **B:** Polyprotein processing and cleavage products. Cleavage sites are indicated as in Figure 25.4 except the NS2/3 cleavage, which is mediated by the NS2 cysteine autoprotease (open bullet). **C:** Polyprotein membrane topology. See the legend of Figure 25.4 for symbol definitions and the text for further details.

by chance.[308] This is significant because these dinucleotides are the preferred cleavage sites of the IFN-stimulated RNase L. Based on the large-scale computerized folding of numerous positive-strand RNA viral genomes, the HCV ORF is also predicted to contain an unusually high rate of internal base pairing.[789] Intriguingly, this feature is common among viruses that cause persistent infections. Thus, the observed bias in nucleotide composition and propensity for internal base pairing within the HCV ORF may reflect adaptation to evolutionary pressure exerted by innate antiviral pathways.

The 3′ NCR was originally thought to terminate in polyadenosine or polyuridine. Improved methods for producing 3′ terminal cDNAs later revealed, however, that the HCV 3′ NCR actually consists of a short (~40 nt) variable domain and a polyuridine/polypyrimidine (polyU/UC) tract, followed by a highly conserved 98-nt 3′ X domain.[413,827] Mutagenesis studies revealed that the 3′X domain is essential for RNA replication and that the polyU/UC tract must be at least 26 nt in length.[245,926,935,941] A number of cellular factors have been found to bind to the HCV 3′ NCR, including RNA-binding proteins polypyrimidine-tract binding (PTB) protein,[278,363,866] heterogeneous ribonuclear protein C,[150,277] glyceraldehyde-3-phosphate dehydrogenase,[671] HuR,[801] and La autoantigen.[799]

Translation and Proteolytic Processing

In addition to its roles in replication, the HCV 5′ NCR acts as an IRES to direct cap-independent translation of the viral genome. The IRES is encoded by 5′ NCR domains II through IV (Fig. 25.12A), although flanking sequences can influence activity. In the current model of HCV IRES function, free 40S ribosomal subunits directly bind to the 5′ NCR domains IIId through f and adopt an mRNA-bound conformation.[645,669,798] The IRES–40S complex then binds eIF3 and the ternary complex eIF2–GTP–Met-$tRNA_i$ to form a 48S intermediate complex, in which the initiating AUG codon at nt 342 is positioned within the ribosomal P site.[367,645] The HCV IRES directly interacts with eIF3 via determinants in domain IIIb[164] and thereby functionally mimics the 5′ cap-binding complex eIF4F.[793] Following GTP hydrolysis and release of eIF2, the 60S ribosomal subunit is recruited to form a translationally active 80S complex.[367,645,669] Under some conditions the HCV IRES does not require eIF3 or ternary complex and is also capable of directing translation from non-AUG initiation sites.[444,846] This mechanism, which utilizes eIF5B to recruit Met-$tRNA_i$, may allow the virus to initiate translation despite cellular eIF2 phosphorylation by the viral RNA sensor protein kinase R (PKR).

A number of cellular factors have been reported to contribute to HCV IRES activity. The human La protein stimulates translation by binding near the initiator AUG and recruiting the 40S ribosomal subunit[168,693]; inhibiting La strongly decreases HCV gene expression and replication.[168,194] Other host factors that stimulate HCV IRES activity include proteosome α-subunit PSMA7[428] and nucleolin.[365] In addition, polycytidine binding proteins 1 and 2 and PTB were shown to bind the 5′ NCR, although their functions in the virus life cycle remain to be defined.[43] IRES-mediated translation can be inhibited by long-distance base pairing of 5′ NCR nt 24 to 38 to a stem-loop region (nt 428 to 442) within the C gene region.[405] Interestingly, this part of the 5′ NCR overlaps with one of the miR-122 binding sites.[377]

Translation of the HCV genome produces a large polyprotein (~3,000 amino acids) that is proteolytically cleaved to produce 10 viral proteins (Fig. 25.12B): the virion structural components core (C) and glycoproteins E1 and E2, and the presumed NS proteins p7, NS2, NS3, NS4A, NS4B, NS5A, and NS5B. Mature forms of the HCV proteins arise via co- and posttranslational cleavage mediated by cellular and host-encoded proteases. During structural region processing, cleavages between C/E1, E1/E2, and E2/p7 are mediated by signal peptidase; mature C protein is released from the E1 signal peptide via signal peptide peptidase (SPP). Within the NS region, signal peptidase mediates cleavage of p7/NS2. The remainder of the NS region is processed by two virus-encoded proteases: the NS2 cysteine autoprotease mediates cleavage at the NS2/3 junction, whereas the NS3-4A serine protease cleaves at all downstream junctions (Fig. 25.12C).

In addition to proteins encoded by the large ORF, it appears that small protein products can be produced from the +1 reading frame of the C gene. At least three different forms of alternative reading frame protein (ARFP) have been described: ARFP/F (frameshift), ARFP/DF (double frameshift), or ARFP/S (short form). Although it is thought that these products are produced via ribosomal frameshifting, alternate translational initiation sites may also be involved.[89] It is equally unclear what role, if any, ARFP expression plays in the virus life cycle. Mutant genomes with a disrupted +1 reading frame are highly attenuated *in vivo,*[561,876] although this may be due to disruption of conserved RNA secondary structures within the C gene.

Features of the Structural Proteins

C Protein

Core (C) is the first protein encoded by the HCV genome. It is among the most conserved of the viral proteins and is thought to multimerize and bind RNA to form the viral nucleocapsid. Proteolytic processing of the C protein occurs in two steps. First, the C/E1 junction is cleaved by host signal peptidase to yield a 191–amino acid, membrane-anchored form of C and the N-terminus of E1.[329] Subsequent cleavage within the C-terminal membrane anchor by SPP liberates the mature form of C[559,640,752,933] and is essential for infectivity.[832] The authentic SPP cleavage site has not yet been determined but likely occurs somewhere between residues 173 and 182[351]; recent genetic evidence suggests that the C-terminus is at position 177.[419] In addition, N-terminally truncated forms of C have been described, but their mechanism of production is unknown.[218]

Following removal of the membrane anchor, the mature C protein consists of two domains.[86] The N-terminal domain I (DI, ~120 amino acids) is hydrophilic and can bind RNA nonspecifically,[752] associate with the 5′ NCR,[783,828] and mediate dimerization of the RNA 3′X region.[171] *In vitro,* interaction of DI with structured RNA can induce the assembly of nucleocapsid-like particles.[431] C protein likely dimerizes through homotypic binding elements in domains I and II,[86,406,518,548] as well as a potential disulfide bond at Cys 128.[432] C protein has also been shown to associate with E1 and E2.[49,502,623] Domain I may also be the target of phosphorylation by protein kinases A and C.[517]

Domain II (~50 amino acids) contains primarily hydrophobic residues. *In vitro,* this domain is important for folding of truncated recombinant protein (residues 1 to 169) into an

α-helix–rich dimer.[86] DII is also important for localizing C to ER-associated lipid droplets,[38,85,604] which play an important but unclear role in virus particle assembly.[588,777] Lipid droplet association requires prior cleavage with SPP[559] and is enhanced by the actions of diacylglycerol acyltransferase-1 (DGAT-1), an ER-resident enzyme that catalyzes a final step in triglyceride synthesis.[326] It has been proposed that trafficking of C to lipid droplets increases the risk of liver steatosis in patients with chronic HCV, as well as promotes the development of steatosis in certain transgenic mice that overexpress the protein. Indeed, C binding to lipid droplets displaces adipocyte differentiation–related protein (ADRP) and leads to redistribution, clustering, and increased synthesis of these organelles in cell culture.[84,190]

The HCV C protein has been implicated in numerous cellular pathways, including altered signaling, transcriptional control, apoptosis, and cellular transformation.[558,845]

Envelope Glycoproteins

The HCV glycoproteins E1 (~30 kD) and E2 (~70 kD) form a noncovalent heterodimer that mediates viral attachment and membrane fusion. Both E1 and E2 are type I TM glycoproteins that contain a large extracellular domain and a single C-terminal TM domain. To generate this topology, the E1 and E2 TM segments, which each contain two short (<20 amino acids) hydrophobic stretches separated by charged residues, adopt an intramembrane hairpin structure during translocation. Following signal peptidase cleavage, the luminal C-termini reorient to face the cytoplasm, yielding tandem proteins each with a single membrane anchor.[156] Following biogenesis, the glycoproteins are retained in the ER.[203,207,740]

Structural information regarding E1 is not available. Recently, however, biophysical characterization of the E2 ectodomain has produced a structural model that can be compared to flavivirus protein E.[422,905] E2 is a three-domain protein with a high proportion of β-sheet, as well as random coil, β-turns and other natively unfolded regions; the overall structure of E2 is the same at both acidic and neutral pH.[422,905] Three variable regions, including HVR1, can be deleted without affecting CD81 binding.[554] HVR1 is followed by domain I (DI), which likely contains eight β-strands and includes the determinants of CD81 interaction. Several glycosylation sites cluster on DI and may shield the CD81 binding site from antibody neutralization. The highly conserved domain II (DII) is largely unstructured and includes the candidate fusion loop at residues 502 to 520; it also encompasses HVR2. The fusion peptide may be buried by contacts with E1 prior to fusion. Domain III (DIII) is connected to DII by an extendable linker encompassing the intergenotypic variable region (IgVR) and contains residues that may assist DI in CD81 binding. DIII is followed by a flexible stem that connects it to the TM domain.[422]

E1 and E2 likely associate as a class II fusion protein complex.[922] Formation of E1-E2 heterodimers is a slow process, with folding of each glycoprotein dependent on the other[95,582,653] and on the chaperone calnexin.[204] Residues within the E1 and E2 TM domains are important for heterodimerization,[642] as are interactions of the ectodomains.[936] The membrane proximal linker in E2 is also important for heterodimerization and HCVpp entry.[202] Construction of HCVpp bearing E1 and E2 from different genotypes indicates regions of intergenotypic incompatibility in DI and HVRII and additional sequences in DII, IgVR, and the stem region of E2, confirming functionally important determinants.[7] Although E1 and E2 interactions in the ER membrane are noncovalent, recent studies of infectious virions suggest that the assembled glycoproteins form large covalent complexes stabilized by disulfide bonds.[879] These bridges may block acid-induced conformational changes until a trigger initiates entry, explaining the pH resistance of HCV particles.[864]

The HCV glycoproteins are important humoral antigens that can lead to virus neutralization and therefore employ strategies to evade the immune response. HVR1 is a major target of neutralizing antibodies.[391,895] HVR1-specific antibodies can protect chimpanzees from infection with homologous HCV strains,[231] and early induction of HVR1-specific antibodies correlates with viral clearance in humans.[11,965] To avoid neutralization, HVR1 exhibits a high level of sequence variability even within a single patient, largely driven by immunogenic selection.[230,553,599,896] In addition, protein glycosylation likely also contributes to immune evasion by the envelope proteins. The E1 and E2 ectodomains are heavily N-glycosylated (generally 4 and 11 sites, respectively). Certain glycosylation site mutants are highly sensitive to neutralizing antibodies, suggesting the glycans mask conserved epitopes from the immune response.[323] Glycosylation is also important for the proper folding and secretion of E2,[795] as well as for the assembly and infectivity of HCVpp[274] and HCVcc.[323]

Features of the Nonstructural Proteins

p7 Protein

p7 is a small (~7 kD) hydrophobic protein that spans the membrane twice, with ER-luminal N- and C-termini and a short, basic, cytoplasmic loop (Fig. 25.13A). Incomplete or delayed processing by host signal peptidase between E2, p7, and NS2 can lead to the production of E2-p7 and E2-p7-NS2.[482,590,676,773] In model membrane systems, p7 multimerizes to form hexameric, cation-conductive membrane channels that are inhibited by amantadine and hexamethylene amiloride[294,519,600,659,689] (Fig. 25.13B).

HCV p7 is essential for virus assembly and infectivity *in vitro* and *in vivo*.[373,750,809] In virus-producing cells, p7 was found to equilibrate pH gradients, reducing the number of acidic vesicles and raising the pH of lysosomes.[915] Interestingly, a p7 mutant that lacks channel activity could be complemented by the influenza M2 protein or by treatment with bafilomycin A1, demonstrating that p7 acts as a viroporin to modulate intracellular pH during virus production.[915] However, a p7 deletion mutant was not complemented by these treatments, suggesting that the protein plays an additional role during virus assembly. In this regard, p7 appears to interact with NS2 at a very early stage of virus morphogenesis.[83,370,530]

NS2 Protein

NS2 (~23 kD) is a membrane-spanning protein with cysteine protease activity.[287,330,513,770] The membrane topology of NS2 has not been fully elucidated but likely incorporates three N-terminal TM segments[369,370] (Fig. 25.13C). The C-terminal region of NS2 contains the protease active site residues, His-952, Glu-972, and Cys-993.[287,330,513] The only known function of this enzyme is to cleave the NS2/3 junction. Optimal autoprotease activity requires co-expression of NS2

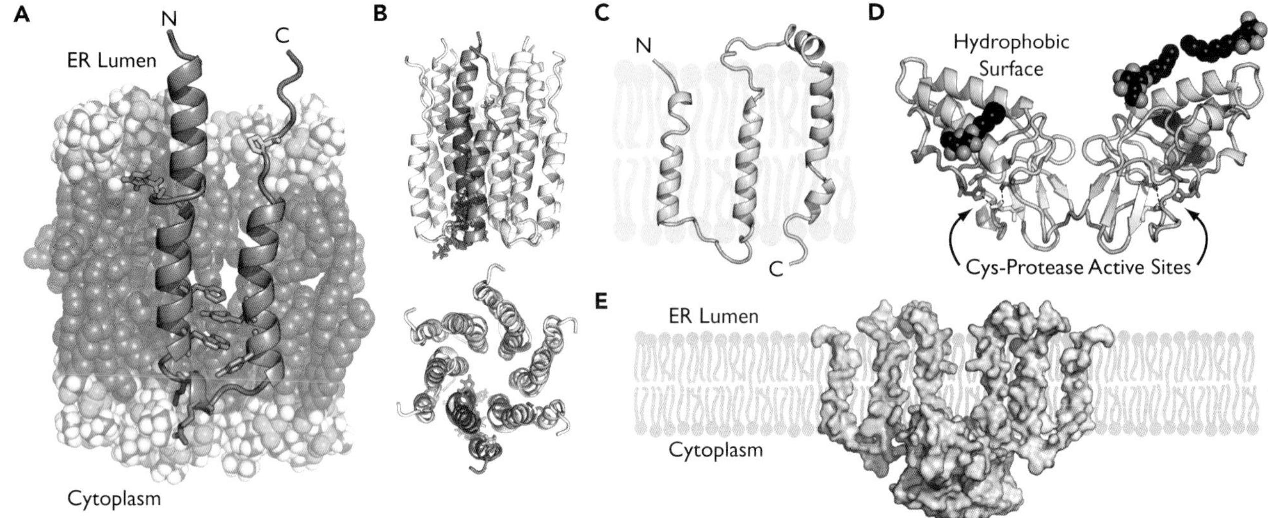

FIGURE 25.13. Structure of the hepatitis C virus (HCV) p7 and NS2 proteins. A: Model of the p7 monomer in a lipid bilayer.[600] Functionally important, conserved residues His-17 (green); Lys-33 and Arg-35 (magenta); Pro-58 (yellow); and Phe-26, Trp-30, Tyr-42, and Tyr-45 (slate) are shown. (Nuclear magnetic resonance [NMR] coordinates and membrane modeling kindly provided by C. Chipot and F. Penin.) **B:** Model of a p7 hexamer as viewed from the side or from the endoplasmic reticulum (ER) lumen. (Modeling coordinates kindly provided by C. Chipot and F. Penin.) **C:** Model of NS2 transmembrane (TM) domains, based on NMR data.[370] **D:** The dimeric NS2 cysteine protease domain. Monomeric subunits are colored green and blue; active-site residues, red; C-terminal residues, yellow; co-crystallized detergent molecules are shown as spheres. Rendered from PDB number 2HD0.[513] **E:** A model of the full-length NS2, based on the models presented in **C** and **D**.

with the N-terminal zinc-binding domain of NS3, although the mechanism of enhancement is not clear.[287,330,770] Notably, NS2/3 cleavage is inhibited by NS4A, the co-factor that promotes NS3 folding into a compact serine protease structure.[179]

The x-ray crystal structure of the NS2 C-terminal domain demonstrated a cysteine protease with the active-site geometry of a serine protease.[513] The C-terminus of NS2 is bound in the substrate-binding pocket, suggesting that further protease activity is blocked following NS2/3 cleavage (Fig. 25.13D). Interestingly, the protease domain homodimerizes, leading to the formation of two composite active sites at the dimer interface. This architecture reveals a mechanism that can control polyprotein processing and explains the ability of some NS2-3 mutants bearing distinct defects to reform an active autoprotease *in trans*.[287,716]

NS2 has an important albeit unclear role in virus particle assembly. Genetic experiments suggested that the N-terminal region of NS2 interacts with the structural proteins and/or p7, whereas downstream regions of NS2 interact with other NS proteins.[675] Indeed, further genetic and biochemical studies confirm NS2 interactions with E1, E2, p7, NS3, and NS4A, indicating that NS2 contributes to virus particle assembly by bringing together viral structural and NS proteins.[83,370,400,530,672,688,803]

NS3 Protein

HCV NS3 (~70 kD) is a multifunctional protein, containing an N-terminal serine protease domain and a C-terminal RNA helicase/NTPase domain.[605] Both enzyme activities are critical for viral replication and have been characterized biochemically and structurally.

The serine protease domain of NS3 requires interaction with NS4A, as well as coordination of a structural Zn^{2+} ion, for complete folding and enzyme activity.[42,226,483] The NS3-4A protease is responsible for cleavage at the NS3/4A, NS4A/4B, NS4B/5A, and NS5A/5B sites.[606] The protease first cleaves the NS3/4A site *in cis,* whereas subsequent cleavages occur *in trans,* with the preferred order NS5A/B > NS4A/B > NS4B/5A. Cleavage sites are well conserved and conform to the sequence (Asp/Glu)XXXX(Cys/Thr)/(Ser/Ala). In addition, NS3 has been shown to mediate internal cleavages within NS3, NS4B, and NS5A, although the functional relevance of these events is not yet known.[43]

NS3-4A is structurally similar to other chymotrypsin-like proteases, with active site residues His-57, Asp-81, and Ser-139, and a substrate-binding surface located in a cleft between two β-barrel subdomains.[606] The first subdomain includes an intercalated β-strand from the central region of NS4A. In the absence of the NS4A co-factor, the N-terminal 28 residues of NS3 remain flexible[557] and the protein is rapidly degraded.[914] NS3 interacts with cellular membranes through two N-terminal amphipathic helices and through its interaction with NS4A.[90,914] Interestingly, the structure of a single-chain, full-length NS3 shows the C-terminus coordinated by the serine protease, as would be expected from the *cis*-cleavage reaction[930] (Fig. 25.7C).

The mechanism of protease activity initiates through deprotonation of Ser-139 by His-57; Ser-139 in turn acts as a nucleophile to attack the carbonyl carbon of the scissile peptide bond, forming a transient covalent link between the catalytic serine and C-terminal substrate. Dissociation of the N-terminal product allows hydrolysis of the tetrahedral intermediate to occur, regenerating the active site and C-terminal product. NS3-4A has an unusually shallow and hydrophobic substrate-binding surface that accommodates six amino acids.

However, the recognition of *trans*-cleaved substrates (NS4A/B, NS4B/5A, and NS5A/B) involves a relatively stable interaction between Cys residues at the substrate P1 position and a conserved Phe residue within NS3.[680] This interaction slows the release of N-terminal products, which can inhibit subsequent catalysis.[501,808] The discovery of this product-based inhibition led to the development of peptidomimetic compounds that potently inhibit NS3-4A serine protease activity and HCV replication *in vivo*.[442,606] Interestingly, the preference for threonine at the P1 position of the NS3/4A cleavage site appears to reflect the selection of a substrate that is easily released following autocleavage.[887,930]

In addition to its essential role in HCV polyprotein processing, NS3-4A serine protease manipulates the host cellular environment by cleaving the human mitochondrial antiviral-signaling (MAVS), TIR-domain-containing adapter-inducing interferon-β (TRIF), and tyrosine-protein phosphatase non-receptor type 2 (PTPN2) proteins (reviewed in[606]). MAVS is a key molecule involved in transducing signals from retinoic acid-inducible gene I (RIG-I) and melanoma differentiation-associated 5 (MDA5) proteins, which are cytoplasmic sensors of viral RNA that activate interferon regulatory factor-3 (IRF-3). TRIF is involved in the Toll-like receptor 3 pathway, which senses dsRNA in the extracellular and endolysosomal compartments. Thus, cleavage of MAVS and TRIF serves to subvert innate antiviral defenses.[470,473,581] PTPN2 is a protein tyrosine phosphatase that resets the epithelial growth factor (EGF) receptor and other growth factor signals. Cleavage of PTPN2 may therefore contribute to altered cell growth and the development of liver cancer.[97]

Similar to other *Flaviviridae*, the C-terminal domain of HCV NS3 encodes a superfamily 2 RNA helicase/NTPase. These enzymes utilize the energy derived from NTP hydrolysis to translocate along and unwind double-stranded nucleic acids.[697] NS3 has been shown to unwind RNA and DNA homo- and heteroduplexes by binding to an unpaired region of a template strand and translocating in a 3′ to 5′ direction.[43,306,339]

Like other RNA helicases, HCV NS3 contains two RecA-like subdomains with ATPase active site residues at their interface. *Flaviviridae* helicases also contain an α-helix–rich, third subdomain of unclear function. Co-crystallization studies revealed that nucleic acids are bound with a cleft formed between the first two subdomains and subdomain 3.[402,538] The mechanism of NS3-4A helicase activity has recently been revealed through elegant structural biology, traditional ensemble enzymology, and single-molecule biophysical studies.[29,205,301,467,468,774,775] NS3 sequentially translocates in the 3′ to 5′ direction along the tracking strand's phosphodiester backbone, unwinding one base pair for each ATP hydrolyzed.[301] Other studies have suggested a spring-loaded mechanism can lead to larger apparent step sizes of up to 3 nt.[29] Dimerization of NS3 helicase domains appears to facilitate cooperative unwinding of long templates. Helicase activity and substrate recognition are also stimulated by the NS3 serine protease domain and NS4A, and the helicase in turn stimulates NS3-4A serine protease activity.[62,63,300,342,429,648] The helicase function of full-length NS3 can also be up-regulated by NS5B, presumably through interactions with the serine protease domain.[954] Likewise, the NS3 helicase activity facilitates NS5B-mediated RNA synthesis.[674] Helicase activity can be down-regulated by the cellular enzyme protein arginine N-methyltransferase 1 (PRMT1), which methylates one or more arginines within the NTP-coordinating motif VI.[206,724] In addition, many cell culture–adaptive mutations map to the surface of the helicase and to the region linking the protease and helicase,[43] suggesting that these are critical sites of protein interaction and/or conformational changes.

Although the precise roles of the NS3 helicase are not fully understood, the NTPase and helicase activities are essential for HCV replication and viral infectivity,[414,441] and the helicase domain has been implicated in virus particle assembly.[617]

NS4A and NS4B Proteins

NS4A is the smallest (~8 kD) NS protein, yet it has multiple functions in the virus life cycle. The central region of the protein acts as a co-factor for the serine protease and facilitates recognition of RNA substrates by the full-length NS3 protease/helicase.[61] The hydrophobic N-terminal TM region of NS4A anchors NS3-4A to cellular membranes. NS4A also physically interacts with NS4B, NS5A, and uncleaved NS4B-5A.[30,484] The acidic C-terminal region of NS4A contributes to HCV helicase activity,[61] NS5A phosphorylation,[383,407] RNA replication,[489] and virus particle assembly.[673]

NS4B (~27 kD) is an integral membrane protein containing four central TM domains separating cytoplasmic N- and C-terminal regions.[284] The N-terminal region of NS4B encodes two amphipathic helices, the second of which can alter its topology to insert in the membrane, and thereby invert the orientation of the first helix.[284,520] The C-terminus of NS4B also encodes two α-helices, the second of which is membrane associated[283] and can be palmitoylated.[943] In addition, the central region of NS4B encodes a partially conserved nucleotide-binding motif and exhibits NTPase and adenylate kinase activities.[212,854] NS4B can also bind RNA, with an affinity for the 3′ terminus of the minus strand, and a small-molecule inhibitor of this activity decreases HCV replication.[213]

NS4B forms oligomers and plays a critical role in organizing the membrane-bound replication complex.[285,657,943] Expression of NS4B is sufficient to induce membrane alterations resembling the *membranous web,* where HCV RNA replication occurs.[210,281] Consistent with an important role in RNA replication, a number of cell culture–adaptive mutations have been mapped to NS4B (reviewed in[43]). NS4B has also been genetically linked to virus particle assembly, although its function in this process is not yet clear.[375]

NS5A Protein

NS5A (~56 to 58 kD) is a proline-rich, homodimeric, RNA-binding phosphoprotein that plays multiple roles in the viral life cycle. NS5A is a multidomain protein that contains an N-terminal Zn^{2+}-binding domain I (DI), a central conserved domain II (DII), and a C-terminal variable domain III (DIII); these domains are separated by two short linkers of low complexity sequence (LCS).[842] DI includes an N-terminal amphipathic helix that mediates membrane association.[91,214,665] X-ray crystallography revealed that DI adopts a novel protein fold and contains a unique Zn^{2+}-binding motif[843] (Fig. 25.14A, B). Interestingly, the same DI structure has been crystallized in two distinct homodimeric conformations: in one case DI formed a homodimeric claw with a basic groove postulated to bind RNA[843]; in the other case DI dimers formed a barrel-shaped structure[514] (Fig. 25.14B, C). Both dimer forms contain well-conserved residues at their interface, suggesting that these

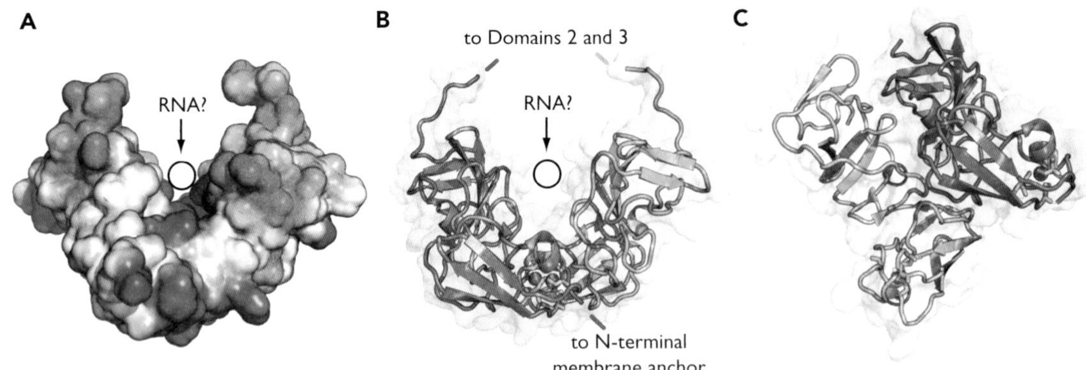

FIGURE 25.14. Structures of hepatis C virus (HCV) NS5A protein. A: Surface electrostatic potential of the dimeric NS5A zinc-binding domain, as rendered from PDB 1ZH1.[843] Negative charges in red and positive charges in blue. **B:** The NS5A zinc-binding domain (PDB 1ZH1), with individual monomeric subunits colored purple and green. Zn^{2+} ions are shown in red, and coordinating residues are shown in yellow. **C:** An alternative structure of the NS5A zinc-binding domain, as rendered from PDB 3FQM.[514] The purple subunit is structurally aligned the same as the purple subunit in **B**.

alternate conformations may be functionally important—perhaps representing a molecular switch or a mechanism of higher-order oligomerization. NS5A homodimers have been observed in cell culture, although the dimer form was not resolved.[352] DII and DIII appear to contain natively unfolded regions, although NMR spectroscopy supports α-helical content within DIII.[477,877] In line with this flexibility, DIII is tolerant of large deletions and insertions.[27,345,495,556,605,841] One unusual feature of NS5A is a central region (amino acids 227 to 277), which overlaps the first LCS and part of DII, termed the IFN sensitivity-determining region (ISDR). Sequence variation within the ISDR was originally thought to correlate with IFN responsiveness in chronically infected patients, although the predictive value of this variation was later discredited.[219,660] Nevertheless, the ISDR likely has other important functions, described later.

NS5A is phosphorylated by multiple cellular serine kinases and can be found in basally phosphorylated (56 kD) and hyperphosphorylated (58 kD) forms. The relevant cellular kinases and phosphoacceptor sites in NS5A are not fully characterized. Basal phosphorylation involves two regions of NS5A: a central region that encompasses the ISDR and a large C-terminal region of DIII.[830] Basal phosphorylation likely involves casein kinase II or a related member of the CMCG kinase family, although other kinases have been implicated.[158,346,347,353,401,717] Hyperphosphorylation involves residues in the first LCS, Ser-224, Ser-228, and Ser-231,[830] although it is not clear whether these are the sites of hypophosphorylation or whether they are required for downstream phosphorylation events. NS5A hyperphosphorylation appears to be mediated by casein kinase Iα,[702,703] although Polo-like kinase 1 has also been implicated in this process.[133] Furthermore, NS5A hyperphosphorylation requires the co-expression of NS3–5A *in cis*[407,626] and interaction between NS5A and NS4A.[30,383]

NS5A plays multiple key roles in RNA replication. The first line of evidence came from the identification of cell culture–adaptive mutations that enhance the replication efficiency of genotype 1a and 1b replicons, many of which mapped to hyperphosphorylation determinants within NS5A.[43,77] Several adaptive mutations (including those in other NS proteins) are associated with decreased NS5A hyperphosphorylation, suggesting that hyperphosphorylation negatively regulates replication.[43,77] However small molecules that block NS5A hyperphosphorylation can either inhibit or enhance HCV replication depending on the viral genetic background,[627] indicating that replication in cell culture may require a balance between different NS5A phosphoforms. Furthermore, cell culture–adaptive mutations associated with low hyperphosphorylation strongly inhibit HCV replication in chimpanzees.[110] While the consequences of NS5A hyperphosphorylation are not fully understood, adaptive mutations associated with decreased hyperphosphorylation correlate with increased interaction between NS5A and hVAP-A,[223] a cellular vesicle trafficking protein and putative HCV replication factor.[260] Furthermore, an important function of NS5A is to bind to and activate PI4KIIIα, a cellular lipid kinase that is essential for HCV replication complex formation.[719,823] Consistent with this, NS5A localizes to sites of viral RNA synthesis.[281] NS5A also interacts with NS5B and can inhibit its RdRP activity *in vitro*,[784] and NS5A mutations that block these interactions are detrimental for replication in cell culture.[781] Furthermore, NS5A binds G/U-rich RNA and exhibits a high affinity for the polypyrimidine tract of the HCV 3′ NCR.[345] The minimal RNA-binding domain of NS5A consists of DI and the first LCS,[352] although DII and DIII may contribute to RNA binding as well.[242] Finally, the RNA-binding ability of NS5A can be regulated by cyclophilin A (CypA), a cellular proline *cis-trans* isomerase that is essential for HCV replication.[128,157,233,234,243,622,646,696,877,891,927]

NS5A also plays an important role in virus particle assembly, primarily through determinants in DIII.[28,840] Specifically, virus assembly requires phosphorylation of NS5A residue Ser-457 by casein kinase IIα.[840] Interestingly, mutation of this residue resulted in decreased hyperphosphorylation, suggesting a possible switch between genome replication and virion assembly. Furthermore, virus morphogenesis is dependent on recruitment of NS5A to lipid droplets through its interaction with the C protein.[28,546,588] NS5A also interacts with ApoE, an essential host factor for HCV particle assembly, and recruits annexin A2, a cellular phospholipid-binding protein that enhances virus production.[34]

In addition to replication and assembly factors, NS5A has been reported to interact with numerous cellular partners in pathways such as signal transduction, transcriptional control, cell death regulation, and cell cycle control.[318] While the molecular details for many of these observations have not yet been elucidated, NS5A has been found to interact with p53, a tumor suppressor protein; Grb-2, an adaptor protein involved in mitogen signaling; phosphatidylinositol 3 kinase (PI3K), a lipid kinase involved in cell survival through the AKT pathway; FBL-2, a geranylgeranylated F-box protein that is required for the replication of genotype 1b replicons; SRCAP, an ATPase that activates cellular transcription; karyopherin β3, a protein involved in nuclear trafficking; Cdk1/2, cyclin-dependent kinases that regulate cell cycle control; and Fyn, Hck, Lck, and Lyn, Src-family kinases.[43,318] In addition, although the molecular consequences of the ISDR have not been explained, NS5A does appear to manipulate innate antiviral defenses. NS5A can bind to and antagonize PKR, a cytoplasmic sensor of dsRNA, as well as induce IL-8 expression, which can antagonize type I IFN responses.[254–256,684–686]

Because of its important roles in the virus life cycle, NS5A is a promising target for antiviral drug design. Based on the requirement for interaction with CypA, HCV replication is potently inhibited by cyclosporin A and derivates.[622,891] One promising candidate is DEBIO-025, which inhibits HCV replication but lacks cyclosporin's immunosuppressive effects.[157,646] A new class of NS5A inhibitors was recently identified in a replicon-based screen, leading to compounds that appear to target DI and inhibit HCV replication at picomolar concentrations.[261,464] Interestingly, the most potent compounds are symmetric, suggesting that they may bind to NS5A dimers.

NS5B Protein

NS5B (~68 kD) is the major enzyme of HCV RNA replication, the RdRP. Similar to other polymerases, NS5B has a right-hand structure, with distinct finger, palm, and thumb domains[5,99,100] (Fig. 25.8B). HCV NS5B was the first RdRP to be structurally solved in a closed, active conformation, demonstrating extensive contacts between the finger and thumb domains surrounding a preformed active site. Subsequent studies showed that the active structure opens into an inactive form via movement of the thumb domain.[74] Conserved RdRP motifs and catalytic residues are primarily located in the palm domain and serve to properly align the RNA template, NTP substrates, and two divalent cations that catalyze nucleotide transfer (reviewed in[872]). Structures of NS5B in complex with divalent cations and NTP revealed an active-site geometry remarkably similar to human immunodeficiency virus (HIV) reverse transcriptase (an RNA-dependent DNA polymerase [RdDP]) and the RdRP of the dsRNA bacteriophage ϕ6.[99,637] In addition, a low-affinity GTP-binding pocket was identified at the interface of the thumb and finger domains.[99] Mutation of this GTP binding site has shown that it is dispensable for RdRP activity *in vitro* but critical for RNA replication in cell culture.[115,707] The finger domain also contains a polar groove, which holds the template RNA; correct positioning of the template 3′ end is ensured by a β-hairpin that protrudes from the thumb into the active-site cavity.[338,637,707] This structure may act as a flap that is displaced during RNA synthesis to allow the dsRNA product to exit the polymerase core. The polymerase also contains a C-terminal regulatory loop that wraps around the thumb and inserts into the active site, decreasing RNA binding and RdRP activity.[466,707] In addition to the core RdRP structure, NS5B contains a 21–amino acid C-terminal hydrophobic tail that posttranslationally inserts into the ER membrane.[364,766] Mutations that interfere with membrane association destroy RNA replication.[462,603] Although the tail anchor can be functionally replaced with a heterologous membrane anchor,[460] other evidence suggests that it contains important determinants for intramembrane protein–protein interaction.[92] Nevertheless, tail anchor deletion mutants retain RdRP activity and permit the efficient expression and purification of soluble, active, recombinant NS5B for biochemical and structural studies.[923]

In vitro, NS5B has been shown to elongate annealed primers or self-priming copy-back templates.[56] RNA synthesis utilizes the divalent cations Mg^{2+} or Mn^{2+} to catalyze nucleotide incorporation at a rate of 150 to 200 nt/minute.[508,638,708] NTP analogs containing 2′C-methyl groups are potent chain-terminating RdRP inhibitors of HCV and other *Flaviviridae.*[184] As the purine 2′ position is not involved in catalysis, these compounds may impose steric constraints within the catalytic core. Resistance to these inhibitors is easily acquired in HCV by mutation of Ser-282-Thr in the NTP binding pocket, although this mutation has adverse effects on RNA replication.[583]

During authentic genome replication, NS5B is thought to initiate RNA synthesis *de novo* (i.e., without a primer).[524,708,710,963] Comparative enzymatic studies showed that the efficiency of *de novo* initiation correlates with the efficiency of replication in cell culture, and that residue 405 on the thumb domain is an important determinant of initiation.[767,786] As for other RNA polymerases, NS5B initiates with a purine nucleotide, which can be mono-, di-, or triphosphorylated.[706,707,780] *De novo* initiation is destroyed by NS5B mutations that affect GTP binding but do not disrupt NTP incorporation.[712] The β-hairpin and C-terminal regulatory loop of NS5B, which limit dsRNA binding, also control *de novo* initiation versus primed synthesis.[136,466,707] High GTP concentrations may serve to structurally rearrange these elements, thereby favoring *de novo* initiation.[315] RNA templates that are efficiently used for *de novo* initiation, at least *in vitro,* contain limited secondary structure and an unpaired 3′ end.[385] NS5B can also utilize circular RNA templates, suggesting that a free 3′ end is not absolutely required and that RNA is loaded when NS5B is in the open conformation.[709] Nevertheless, the aforementioned template requirements are notably different from the natural site of HCV minus-strand initiation, the 3′ NCR, which terminates with a uridylate base paired in a stable stem-loop. When the HCV 3′ NCR is used as a template in *de novo* initiation reactions, only internally initiated minus strands are produced.[385,403,639,820] Addition of a few unpaired 3′ nt, however, leads to the production of template-length minus-strand products.[639] Thus, authentic initiation of HCV minus-strand synthesis may depend on the local unwinding of 3′ secondary structures, perhaps by the NS3-4A helicase.

NS5B RdRP activity depends on higher-order interactions. Important contacts between NS5B domains were revealed through structural studies with nonnucleoside RdRP inhibitors (NNIs), which can allosterically block polymerase activity.[74,139,153,191,299,515,859,860,885] In addition to intramolecular interactions, oligomerization of NS5B leads to cooperative stimulation of polymerase activity,[699,886] and the NS3-4A helicase can enhance primed RNA synthesis.[674] Although both NS4B and NS5A mutations inhibit RNA synthesis,[674,784] mutations in NS5A that inhibit interaction with NS5B are detrimental for RNA replication.[781] Genetic studies indicate that NS5B binds NS5A primarily via residues on the back of the thumb and inner surface of the fingers.[699]

In addition to template-directed RNA synthesis, NS5B may have terminal nucleotide transferase (TnTase) activity, adding one or a few untemplated nt to the 3′ end of an RNA substrate.[56,705,780] It should be noted that several reports did not detect this TnTase activity or showed that a cellular TnTase copurified with NS5B.[390,508,638,923] Nevertheless, the TnTase activity of a highly purified NS5B preparation was shown to depend on RdRP active-site residues.[705,712] Moreover, NS5B TnTase activity can convert an RNA lacking a 3′ initiation site into a useful template for *de novo* initiation,[705] suggesting that TnTase activity may contribute to maintaining genome integrity.

RNA Replication

Because many copies of the structural proteins are needed to package each nascent genome, *Flaviviridae* genomes must be translated more frequently than they are replicated. Indeed, HCV subgenomic replicon-bearing cells produce a ~1,000-to-1 molar ratio of viral proteins to viral RNA.[701] One way to achieve this is by cross-talk between the determinants that control translation and genome replication. For instance, the cellular PTB protein binds to the HCV 5′ NCR and C coding region where it may modulate IRES activity,[25,362,858] and to the 3′ NCR where it may repress replication.[362,866] Similarly, La protein was shown to bind to both HCV NCRs. For the related pestiviruses, several NF/NFAR proteins bind the 5′ and 3′ NCRs and regulate genome circularization, and might also be involved in regulating HCV translation versus replication.[359,360] HCV translation may also be autoregulated through product inhibition: low levels of C protein can enhance IRES-mediated translation, whereas high concentrations inhibit it.[82,955] Finally, it is interesting to note that polycytidine-binding protein 2 (PCBP-2) binds to the HCV 5′ NCR.[251,800] PCBP-2 also interacts with the 5′ NCR and RdRP of another positive-strand RNA virus, poliovirus, to control the switch between translation and replication.[259]

HCV RNA replication takes place in a dense perinuclear matrix of ~85-nm vesicles termed the membranous web[210,281] (Fig. 25.15). Several studies have shown that the membranous web is likely to be derived from the rough ER,[43] although these structures can be insoluble in nonionic detergents, suggesting that they are sphingomyelin rich.[6,779] Formation of the membranous web is mediated by both NS4B[210] and NS5A[719] and may utilize autophagic pathways[200] and activate ER stress.[831] The process of HCV replication also induces the expression of genes involved in lipid metabolism.[192,387,818] Furthermore, replication is stimulated by increased availability of saturated and monounsaturated fatty acids and inhibited by polyunsaturated fatty acids or inhibitors of fatty acid synthesis,[387] suggesting that specific lipids and/or membrane fluidity are important for the function of the membranous web. In addition, altering cholesterol metabolism pharmacologically can lead to the disassembly of the replicase and inhibit RNA replication due to reduced geranylgeranylation.[387,934]

The HCV replicase can be accessed biochemically by using permeabilized cells, cell lysates, or membrane preparations isolated from HCV replicon-bearing cells.[6,10,311,439,589,701,928] These *in vitro* systems allow the elongation of endogenous RNA templates to be studied, but they do not accept exogenous RNA. Nevertheless, the sensitivity of RNA synthesis to heparin[311] and the pulse-chase metabolic labeling of single-stranded RNA (ssRNA) into dsRNA[439] suggest that at least a limited amount of *de novo* synthesis occurs *in vitro*. Furthermore, *in vitro* RdRP activity is protected from nuclease and protease degradation by a detergent-sensitive membrane,[589,701] suggesting that RNA synthesis is enclosed within the membranous web. These data support the hypothesis that active replicase is bound by a limiting membrane and demonstrate that a vast excess of NS proteins are produced. This enclosed replicase presumably includes a channel for the exchange of NTPs with nascent RNA and pyrophosphate, similar to the spherule structures proposed for other positive-strand RNA viruses.

Similar to other *Flaviviridae*, HCV RNA replication initiates with the synthesis of genome-length, negative-strand RNAs, which exist as partially double-stranded replicative intermediates or fully double-stranded replicative forms.[10] Negative-strand RNA then serves as a template for multiple rounds of positive-strand synthesis, leading to the asymmetric

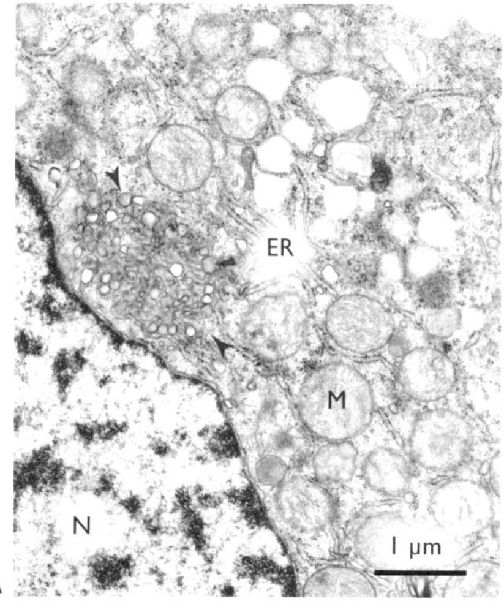

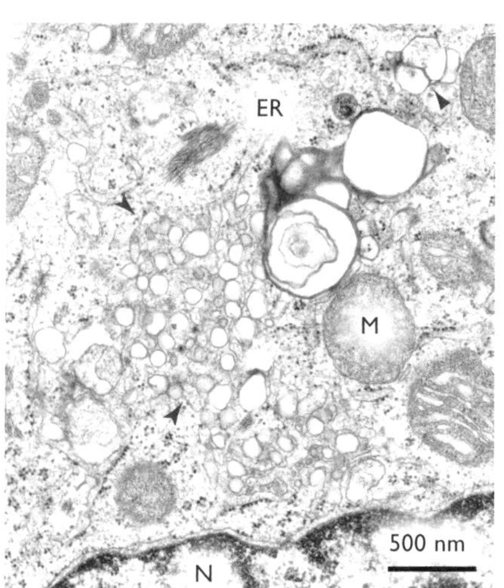

FIGURE 25.15. Membranous webs, the site of hepatitis C virus (HCV) RNA replication. A: Membrane alterations in Huh-7 cells harboring an HCV subgenomic replicon. **B:** Higher magnification of the membranous web (arrows). M, mitochondria; N, nucleus. (Courtesy of R. Gosert and D. Moradpour. Adapted from Gosert R, Egger D, Lohmann V, et al. Identification of the hepatitis C virus RNA replication complex in Huh-7 cells harboring subgenomic replicons. *J Virol* 2003;77(9):5487–5492. Used with permission of the American Society for Microbiology Press.)

accumulation of nearly 10 positive strands for every negative strand.[6,445,509,589,701] At least for cell culture–adapted genotype 1b replicons that do not make infectious virus, each cell contains approximately 100 negative strands, 1,000 positive-strands, and 1,000,000 copies of each viral protein.[701] A number of factors, however, influence the rate of HCV RNA replication. In Huh-7 cells, genotype 1b replication is robust in exponentially growing cells and repressed in growth-arrested cells.[628,677,769] Interestingly, this block may be caused by a reduced pool of pyrimidine nucleotides, because replication can be restored in confluent cells by supplementing media with uridine and cytosine.[628] In addition, co-transfected replicons interfere with each other, suggesting that they compete for limiting cellular factors.[222,507] Given that replication-defective genomes also compete but that translation-defective genomes do not, one of these limiting cellular factors may interact with an NS protein.[507]

Virus Assembly

Similar to the related *Flaviviridae,* HCV particles bud directly into the ER, transit the secretory pathway, and are released through exocytosis. A model of HCV particle assembly has recently emerged, tying this process to the unique lipid metabolism of hepatocytes. Infectious virus production begins when SPP-processed core protein migrates to ER-associated cytoplasmic lipid droplets.[559] Core is thought to recruit the membrane-associated replication complex through its interaction with NS5A,[546,588,28] while the p7–NS2 complex recruits viral structural and NS proteins to the sites of virus assembly.[83,370,530,672,688,803]

HCV particle formation is associated with VLDL assembly, which also takes place in the secretory pathway of hepatocytes. Consistent with this, inhibitors of serum lipoprotein assembly strongly inhibit HCV particle production,[263,344] and NS5A has been shown to interact with apolipoproteins.[60,176,223] During budding, nascent HCV particles may become associated with ER-luminal lipid droplets displaying ApoE. Lipid droplets are the triglyceride source for maturing VLDL particles and, *in vivo,* a large proportion may fuse with nascent ApoB-positive lipoproteins (reviewed in[44]). HCV egresses through the secretory pathway, where the ion channel activity of p7 may protect nascent virions from premature fusion induced by the low pH of the secretory compartment.[915] While intracellular HCV particles are infectious, their buoyant density becomes lower as they egress in a maturation process that parallels VLDL.[265] Like VLDL, blocking secretion of HCV leads to degradation of the high-density particles in a post-ER compartment.[263]

In addition to the VLDL secretory pathway, a number of other host factors have been implicated in HCV assembly, including the NS5A-associated factor annexin A2,[34] autophagy proteins Atg7 and beclin-1,[829] and heat shock protein HSC70.[652]

PESTIVIRUSES

Background and Classification

Pestiviruses are animal pathogens of major economic importance for the livestock industry. They include the type member, bovine viral diarrhea virus (BVDV), as well as classical swine fever virus (CSFV) and border disease virus (BDV) of sheep.[851] New pestiviruses are frequently being isolated from animals, bovine serum, or cell cultures. The International Committee on the Taxonomy of Viruses currently recognizes four pestivirus species (BVDV-1, BVDV-2, CSFV, and BDV) and four tentative species (atypical pestivirus, Bungowannah virus, giraffe-1 pestivirus, and pronghorn antelope pestivirus).[271,494] Within the family *Flaviviridae,* pestiviruses show greater similarity in genome structure and mechanism of initiating translation to the hepaciviruses than to the flaviviruses.

Pestivirus infections can be subclinical or produce a range of symptoms, including acute diarrhea, hemorrhagic syndrome, acute fatal disease, and wasting disease (reviewed in[852]). CSFV, typically transmitted oronasally, leads to acute or chronic hemorrhagic syndromes with significant mortality. In contrast, ruminant pestiviruses usually result in subclinical infection or cause mild symptoms in adult animals. A notable exception is BVDV-2, which has been associated with a severe, acute hemorrhagic condition in cattle.[165,664,714] In addition, diaplacental transmission of pestiviruses can cause fetal death, malformation, or persistent infection of the fetus; for cattle this can lead to the development of mucosal disease. Two biotypes of pestiviruses, cytopathic (cp) and noncytopathic (ncp) viruses, are distinguished by their ability to cause cytopathic effects in cell culture.

Live attenuated strains, inactivated virus preparations, and subunit vaccines are available for immunization against pestivirus-induced diseases.[594] Such vaccines should prevent diaplacental infection. Early attempts at vaccination with an attenuated cpBVDV strain resulted in genome recombination and the emergence of fatal mucosal disease in persistently infected cattle.[53] While improved vaccines have been developed by combining multiple attenuating mutations,[574] genetic recombination remains a concern.

Structure and Physical Properties of the Virion

Pestiviruses have been difficult to purify because of modest growth in cell culture, inefficient release from infected cells, and association with serum components and cellular debris.[452] Virus particles visualized by electron microscopy[594,894] are spherical and 40 to 60 nm in diameter[341] (Fig. 25.16). Structure and symmetry of the core have not been characterized. In addition to the genome RNA and lipid envelope, the particles are composed of four structural proteins: the core protein (C) and three envelope glycoproteins, E^{rns} (for ribonuclease, secreted), E1, and E2.[749,853] E^{rns} and E2 have been detected on the surface of CSFV and BVDV particles by immunogold labeling,[894] and disulfide bonds connect the envelope proteins on the virion surface.[853] Pestivirus virions have a buoyant density of 1.134 g/mL and are inactivated by heat, organic solvents, and detergents.[746] Similar to HCV, virion infectivity is stable over a relatively broad range of pH.[480]

Binding and Entry

Binding and entry of pestiviruses involves initial attachment, interaction with specific receptor(s), internalization, and membrane fusion. Pestiviruses can be detected in a variety of tissue types *in vivo,* including epithelial cells, endothelial cells, PBMCs, the gastrointestinal tract, and neurons. Highly permissive cell lines for the propagation of pestiviruses and infectious cDNA clones have allowed the study of viral entry in culture. Bovine CD46 has been identified as a cellular receptor for

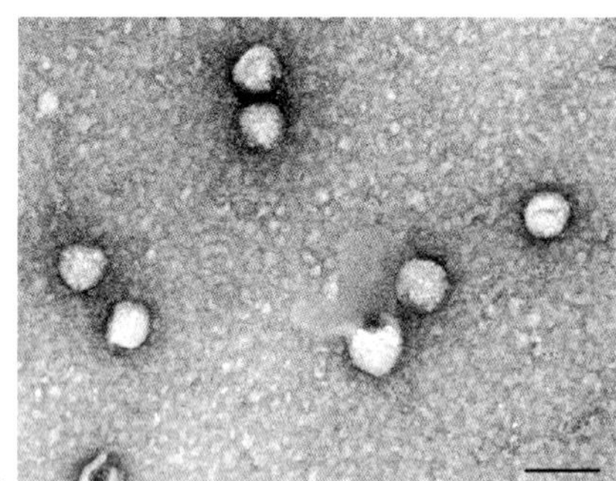

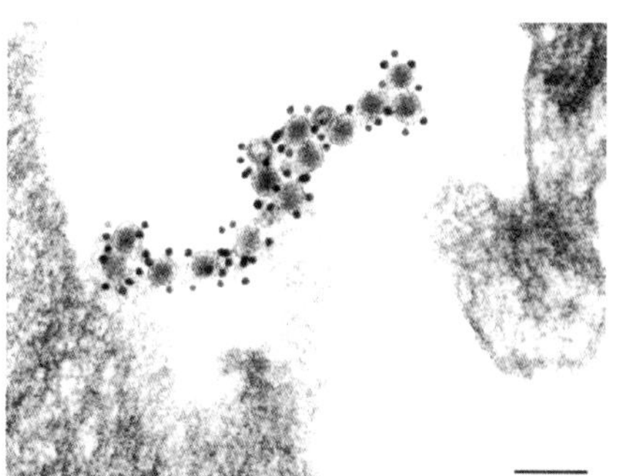

FIGURE 25.16. Pestivirus particles. A: Classical swine fever virus (CSFV) virions negatively stained with uranyl acetate **B:** Ultrathin section of swine testicular epitheloid cells infected with CSFV and immunostained with E^{rns}-specific monoclonal antibody (mAb) 24/16 and colloidal gold. Bar = 100 nm. (Courtesy of F. Weiland. Adapted from Weiland F, Weiland E, Unger G et al. Localization of pestiviral envelope proteins E^{rns} and E2 at the cell surface and on isolated particles. *J Gen Virol* 1999; 80[5]:1157–1165. Used with permission of Society for General Microbiology).

BVDV-1 and BVDV-2, including primary clinical isolates.[551] Experiments using chimeric CD46 molecules identified a discrete subregion within complement control protein repeat 1 as essential for BVDV binding and uptake.[423] The viral ligand for CD46 is probably E2, which is also the major determinant of cell culture tropism, at least for ruminant pestiviruses.[476,718] The LDL receptor was also suggested to assist in BVDV entry,[4] although later evidence found no role for this molecule in bovine cell infection.[424] In addition, E^{rns} of cell culture–adapted viruses binds cell surface glycosaminoglycans, which may act as an initial attachment factor.[356,357] Finally, ectopically expressed E2 ectodomain inhibits BVDV entry at a step downstream of viral interaction with CD46, suggesting the involvement of an as-yet-unidentified entry factor.[862]

After binding, BVDV enters target cells via clathrin-dependent endocytosis followed by acid-dependent fusion in the endosome.[297,425,457] Similar to HCV, BVDV must be primed to respond to low pH. Breakage of disulfide bonds between the glycoproteins during endocytosis may contribute to destabilizing the virion.[425]

Interestingly, E1 and E2 are sufficient for entry of CSFV or BVDV glycoprotein-pseudotyped particles; E^{rns} is nonessential in this system.[737,888] Charged residues in the TM domains of E1 and E2 play a critical role in protein heterodimer formation and pseudoparticle entry.[737]

Genome Structure

Pestivirus genomes are approximately 12.3 kb in length.[162,601] Similar to HCV, pestivirus genomes lack a 5′ cap and 3′ poly(A) tract[102,601] (Fig. 25.17A). A long ORF of approximately 4,000 codons is flanked by a 5′ NCR of 372 to 385 nt and a 3′ NCR of 185 to 273 nt.[32,102,160] Two 5′ terminal stem-loop structures in the BVDV genome (domains Ia and Ib in Fig. 25.17A) are important for efficient RNA replication.[250,945] A 5′ terminal GUAU sequence is essential for BVDV replication, as its complement may be a promoter for plus-strand synthesis.[250] Provided that this tetranucleotide sequence is retained, substitutions and deletions of hairpin Ia and part of Ib do not abolish replication.[52] Thus, the 5′ signals essential for pestivirus genome replication are significantly shorter than for the hepaciviruses. Following the ORF, the 3′ NCR consists of a variable region, a single-stranded region, and a conserved 3′ terminal stem-loop.[189,944] Mutational analyses indicate that the terminal stem-loop and the upstream single-stranded region harbor important primary and secondary structural elements that probably function *in cis* to direct minus-strand initiation. In contrast, deletions in the variable region are well tolerated.[360,650,944]

Translation and Polyprotein Processing

Cap-independent translation initiation of the pestivirus genome is mediated by an IRES that bears structural and functional similarity to that of HCV (compare Figs. 25.12A and 25.17A).[103,189,687,729] The minimal pestivirus IRES includes 5′ NCR domains II and III and can be influenced by structured sequences downstream from the initiator AUG.[142,621,687,729] As for HCV, the pestivirus IRES binds ribosomal 40S subunits without the need for translation initiation factors eIF4A, eIF4B, and eIF4F.[668,669,794] The pestivirus genome encodes a large polyprotein that is processed into individual viral proteins: N^{pro}-C-E^{rns}-E1-E2-p7-NS2-NS3-NS4A-NS4B-NS5A-NS5B (Fig. 25.17B).[161,163,578,602,695]

Unlike other *Flaviviridae,* the first pestivirus protein is an NS protein, N^{pro}. This is an autoprotease responsible for cleavage at the N^{pro}/C site.[806,912] Processing of the pestivirus structural region appears to be mediated by at least three additional proteases. Host signal peptidase is believed to cleave at the C/E^{rns}, E1/E2, E2/p7, and p7/NS2 sites, with incomplete cleavage at the E2/p7 site leading to accumulation of an uncleaved product.[215,310,749] SPP mediates further processing of the pestivirus C protein in the TM region.[321] The E^{rns}-E1 polyprotein (gp62) is processed slowly at a novel type of signal peptidase cleavage site.[71,749] The NS region is processed by the NS2 autoprotease,[437] which performs an incomplete cleavage at the NS2/3 junction,[3] and the NS3-4A serine protease, which cleaves the remainder of the polyprotein.[834,913,920] As detailed later, certain cytopathic pestiviruses generate the authentic N-terminus of NS3 via several different mechanisms.

N^{pro} Autoprotease

N^{pro} is an NS autoprotease that cleaves at a conserved site between Cys-168 and Ser-169 of the polyprotein.[806,912] The active-site residues involved in this activity include Glu-22,

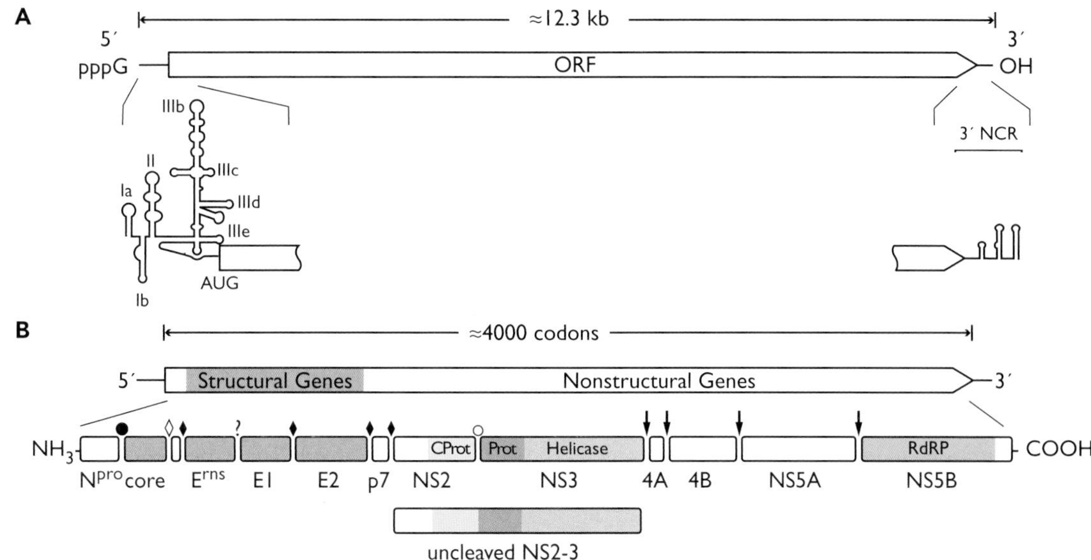

FIGURE 25.17. Pestivirus genome structure and protein expression. A: Genome structure and RNA elements. Important RNA elements are indicated as in Figure 25.4. **B:** Polyprotein processing and cleavage products. Symbols identifying proteolytic cleavages for the cpBVDV NADL strain are the same as those described in Figure 25.4 except for the proposed autocatalytic cleavage releasing the N-terminal nonstructural protein Npro from the pestivirus polyprotein, which is indicated by a closed bullet. See text for details.

His-49, and Cys-69, leading to the suggestion that N^{pro} may be an unusual subtilisin-like cysteine protease.[747] N^{pro} is dispensable for pestivirus replication in cell culture but is required for virulence in animals.[55,552,607,835,861] N^{pro} inhibits IFN production[135,272,435,741,744] by targeting the cellular transcription factor IRF-3 for degradation.[48,135,332,771] However, CSFV mutants that lack this activity remain virulent in animals.[743]

Pestivirus Structural Proteins

The capsid (C) protein is a 14-kD, highly basic, RNA-binding protein.[618] The N-terminus of C is generated by the autocleavage of N^{pro}.[912] The nascent C protein encodes a C-terminal signal peptide that leads to translocation of E^{rns} into the ER. Similar to HCV, pestivirus C protein undergoes sequential maturational cleavages by signal peptidase and SPP.[321] Mature C is a natively unfolded protein that nonspecifically binds RNA with low affinity.[618] Remarkably, functional C protein can tolerate sizeable deletions, duplications, and insertions; for one of these mutants, severe defects in virus assembly were suppressed by a second site mutation in the NS3 helicase domain.[727] These data suggest that C protein does not form an icosahedral nucleocapsid but may function like a histone protein to condense nucleic acids.

The E^{rns} glycoprotein (44 to 48 kD, formerly known as E0 or gp44/48) is heavily glycosylated on seven to nine asparagine residues and forms disulfide-linked homodimers.[449,853] E^{rns} associates with membranes and virus particles via a C-terminal amphipathic helix[235,847] but is also secreted from infected cells in soluble form.[749,892,894] The most unusual feature of E^{rns} is that it encodes a ribonuclease (RNase) activity with specificity for uridine residues.[316,768] This RNase activity contributes to the ability of pestiviruses to inhibit the induction of type I IFN by exogenous dsRNA.[358,526,540,550,574] Antibodies that inhibit RNase activity tend to neutralize virus infectivity,[908] and mutations in E^{rns} that destroy enzymatic activity give rise to viruses that are attenuated *in vivo*.[573,574,881] While homodimerization is dispensable for RNase activity,[908] viral mutants that are unable to form E^{rns} complexes are less virulent,[848] suggesting that the glycoprotein may have additional functions *in vivo*. Recombinant E^{rns} is toxic to lymphocytes *in vitro*,[104] which may contribute to the leukopenia seen in natural infections.[821] Although cytotoxicity is a feature of other soluble RNases,[761] it is not yet clear whether the enzymatic activity of E^{rns} is related to its toxicity. The C-terminal domain of E^{rns} can promote its translocation across cellular membranes, suggesting that it may have an intracellular target or function.[448] Recombinant E^{rns}, however, can also bind strongly to the surface of cells, probably via interaction with glycosaminoglycans, and inhibit viral infection.[356,894]

E1 and E2 are integral membrane glycoproteins that contain two to three and four to six N-linked glycosylation motifs, respectively.[893] E2 forms homodimers,[853,893] as well as disulfide-linked heterodimers with E1.[749] Heterodimer formation is essential for viral entry and involves the interaction of charged residues within the TM domains of E1 and E2. Recombinant CSFV E2 can bind to cells and block infection of CSFV and BVDV, suggesting a common receptor or co-receptor for binding and entry of these pestiviruses.[348] In addition, E2 expression inhibits BVDV superinfection at the level of viral entry.[862,863] Infectious pestivirus particles are neutralized by monoclonal antibodies that recognize E^{rns} or E2,[197,656,873,892,893,903] and these antigens can elicit protective immunity.[349,748,874]

p7 Protein

The p7 protein consists of a central charged region separating hydrophobic termini. Similar to the HCV protein, pestivirus p7 is dispensable for RNA replication[55] but required for the production of infectious virus particles.[310,475] Another similarity is that E2–p7 cleavage, most likely by host signal peptidase, is inefficient.[215] Uncleaved E2–p7 is not required for replication in cell culture and both E2–p7 and p7 appear to remain cell associated.[310] Furthermore, pestivirus p7 protein may form ion channels *in vitro* and *in vivo*.[295,528]

Pestivirus Nonstructural Proteins

The NS2 protein (~54 kD) is a cysteine autoprotease, distantly related to the NS2-3 autoprotease of HCV and GB viruses, which is responsible for processing NS2-3 (~125 kD).[436,438] Remarkably, a cellular chaperone protein, DNAJC14 (originally identified as Jiv for J-domain protein interacting with viral protein), is an essential co-factor for NS2-mediated proteolysis. DNAJC14, a member of the heat shock protein (HSP) 40 family of chaperones, interacts irreversibly with NS2 and facilitates interaction of the catalytic and substrate residues.[436] As discussed later, NS2-3 cleavage is essential for pestivirus RNA replication, and the efficiency of processing is a key regulator of RNA accumulation and cytopathogenicity. Interestingly, pestivirus NS2-3 cleavage is incomplete, and the unprocessed form of the protein is essential for infectious virus production.[3,608]

As for other *Flaviviridae,* the pestivirus NS3 protein (~80 kD) contains an N-terminal serine protease domain[50,279,913] and a C-terminal RNA helicase.[280] The NS3 serine protease, along with its NS4A co-factor,[836,920] cleaves between leucine and small uncharged amino acids: L↓(S/A/N).[834,920] Substitutions that eliminate serine protease activity abolish viral RNA replication, confirming its essential role in virus viability.[288,920] Interestingly, protease activity is retained when threonine is substituted for the serine nucleophile.[836] The NS3 protein of BVDV has been purified and shown to possess RNA helicase[889] and RNA-stimulated NTPase[825] activities. Site-directed mutagenesis of the conserved helicase and NTPase motifs abolished viral replication.

The pestivirus NS4A (~10 kD) and NS4B (~38 kD) proteins share similar size, organization, and function with their HCV analogs, although sequence homology between the genera is negligible. NS4A is an essential co-factor for the NS3 serine protease activity.[836,920] NS4B is a multispanning membrane protein that associates with rearranged cellular membranes involved in RNA replication.[897] Similar to HCV, the pestivirus NS4B protein encodes an NTPase activity of unclear function.[273] While a ~45 kD NS4A-4B precursor is transiently produced in pestivirus-infected cells, genetic analysis revealed that it is not essential for BVDV replication in cell culture.[257]

The remaining two proteins, NS5A (~58 kD) and NS5B (~75 kD), are present as mature cleavage products, as well as an uncleaved NS5A-5B precursor.[161,163,443] NS5A is essential for RNA replication, although its precise functions have not been fully elucidated.[289,844] Similar to HCV, pestivirus NS5A proteins contain an N-terminal amphipathic helix and a zinc-coordinating motif.[93,753,844] Furthermore, NS5A is phosphorylated by a cellular serine or threonine kinase with properties similar to enzyme(s) that modify flavivirus NS5 and hepacivirus NS5A.[715] Genetic analysis revealed that defects in the *NS5A* gene can be efficiently complemented *in trans,* whereas mutations in other pestivirus NS genes cannot.[289]

NS5B contains motifs characteristic of RdRP.[160] The RNA polymerase activity of recombinant NS5B has been characterized *in vitro* and found to extend template-primed RNA into double-stranded copy-back products[440,510,807,960] or to catalyze *de novo* initiation from short, synthetic RNA or DNA templates.[384,440] The structure of BVDV NS5B is similar to the HCV polymerase and to other RdRPs, containing a palm subdomain surrounded by finger and thumb subdomains.[141] The pestivirus NS5B structure reveals a unique N-terminal region, which suggests a role for GTP in *de novo* initiation, and provides a framework for understanding the molecular mechanisms of small-molecule inhibitors of BVDV replication.[35,177,647,819]

RNA Replication

The basic mechanisms of pestivirus RNA replication appear to be similar to those described for HCV. RNA accumulation is associated with cytoplasmic membranes and requires NS3 through NS5B. Cellular components are also involved; for example, NFAR proteins associate specifically with the 5′ and 3′ termini of the BVDV genome.[359] The 3′ NCR also contains determinants that ensure efficient termination of translation, which is essential for efficient pestivirus RNA replication.[360] Negative- and positive-strand RNAs have been detected from 4 to 6 hours after pestivirus infection, followed by the asymmetric synthesis of additional minus- and excess plus-strand RNA.[275] Double-stranded RF RNA and partial duplex RI RNA have been tentatively identified.[275,276,695]

Insights into the regulation of BVDV RNA replication and virus assembly have emerged from the study of ncp and cpBVDV. In addition to displaying differences in cytopathogenicity, both biotypes show altered NS2-3 processing. cpBVDV produces both NS3 and uncleaved NS2-3 in large amounts, whereas ncpBVDV was thought to express only the uncleaved protein. This suggested that uncleaved NS2-3 could serve as a functional RNA replicase component. It has been shown, however, that NS2/3 cleavage is absolutely required for RNA replication and that the efficiency of this process is regulated by the NS2 co-factor, DNAJC14.[436] Early after ncpBVDV infection, NS2/3 cleavage is nearly complete, allowing efficient NS3 production and the initiation of RNA replication. At later time points, when uncomplexed DNAJC14 levels are limiting, autoprocessing becomes inefficient and viral RNA synthesis rates decline.[437] cpBVDV viruses overcome the decline of endogenous DNAJC14 and promote continuous NS2-3 cleavage through a variety of genetic variations, as described later.

During replication, nonhomologous recombination can occur within pestivirus genomes and between pestivirus RNA and host cellular mRNA (reviewed in[580]). One likely mechanism is copy-choice template recruitment during minus-strand synthesis, which is consistent with the coding orientation of cellular inserts. An alternative mechanism of RNA recombination has been demonstrated by using a cell culture–based system in which homologous and nonhomologous recombination occurred between two overlapping transcripts that each lacked different essential parts of the viral RdRP.[258] Statistical analysis of recombination sites also supports the hypothesis that homologous recombination contributes to pestivirus diversity in nature.[376]

Assembly and Release of Virus Particles

Other than the features of the virion structural proteins described previously, little information is available on the assembly and release of pestiviruses. Electron microscopic examination of infected cells suggests that pestiviruses mature in intracellular vesicles and are released by exocytosis.[69,291] Consistent with intracellular budding, pestivirus envelope proteins are retained within the secretory pathway[292,894] and brefeldin A, a potent inhibitor of ER–Golgi transport, inhibits the secretion of viral particles but does not block their assembly.[539] Interestingly, E^{rns} and E2 have been immunolocalized on isolated virus particles by electron microscopy, but E2 was not detected in particles undergoing secretion (or perhaps reattachment) at the cell surface.[894] This suggests that E2 may be conformationally inaccessible to antibodies before maturation. As with other members of the *Flaviviridae,* NS proteins play an important role in pestivirus virion assembly or release, including p7, NS2-3, NS3-4A, and NS5B.[3,24,475,608,617]

Pathogenesis of Mucosal Disease and the Generation of Cytopathic Pestiviruses

Mucosal disease, the most severe outcome of BVDV infection, is usually fatal.[580] This disease occurs only after *in utero* infection with an ncpBVDV strain between 40 and 125 days of gestation, leading to the birth of immunotolerant animals that remain persistently infected for life. In the case of an animal exhibiting mucosal disease, both cp and ncp biotypes of BVDV can be found.[555] The close serologic relatedness of isolated ncp–cp pairs led to the suggestion that cpBVDV might arise from ncpBVDV by a rare mutational event. Genetic characterization of a number of these ncp–cp pairs has verified this hypothesis and led to the remarkable discovery that most cpBVDV strains are generated via RNA recombination,[54] although a few cpBVDV strains lack obvious genome rearrangements.[580,663] The presence of these genome rearrangements strongly correlates with increased NS3 expression, enhanced RNA replication, and cytopathic effects in cell culture. Figure 25.18 illustrates a few of the remarkable cpBVDV genome alterations that have been discovered.

Common features of some cpBVDV variants include genome rearrangements or mutations that activate NS2-3 autoprotease activity, leading to increased production of NS3 and augmented RNA replication. For instance, strain NADL (Fig. 25.18A) contains a fragment of the cellular *DNAJC14* gene (also known as Jiv) inserted within NS2.[731] As described earlier, DNAJC14 is an essential co-factor of the NS2 protease, and overexpression of a critical 90–amino acid DNAJC14 subdomain enhances NS2-3 cleavage, regardless of whether the fragment is provided *in cis* or *in trans.*[437] Interestingly, a much smaller insertion is found in the *NS2* gene of cpBVDV strain CP7, which contains a 27-nt duplication from an upstream region of the *NS2* gene in an alternate reading frame.[837] As with the DNAJC14 fragment, this insertion leads to increased NS2-3 processing and a virus that is cytopathic in culture.[567,576] Other viral insertions at or very close to the same site have been described.[36] For other cpBVDV isolates, increased NS2-3 autoprotease activity appears to result from point mutations that have accumulated within the *NS2* gene.[433]

Another common rearrangement in cpBVDV isolates is the insertion of ubiquitin or ubiquitin-like genes immediately upstream of NS3,[40,577,698,838] leading to NS2/3 processing by ubiquitin C-terminal hydrolase or related enzymes (e.g., strain

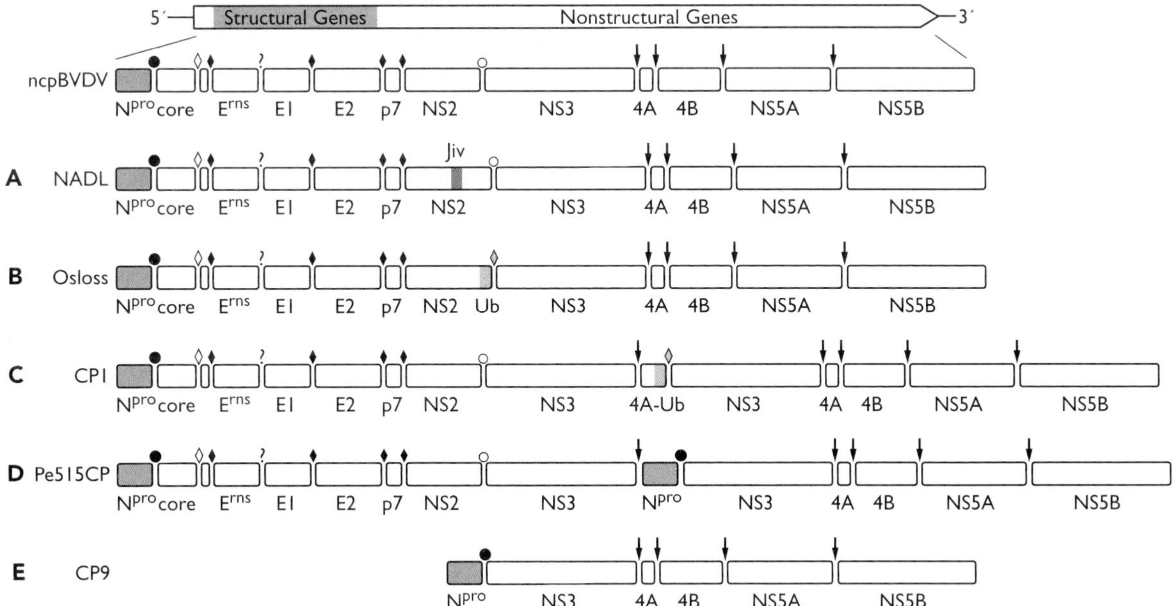

FIGURE 25.18. Genome rearrangements associated with cytopathic bovine viral diarrhea virus (cpBVDV). The **top diagram** indicates the polyprotein of a typical noncytopathic BVDV (ncpBVDV) isolate. Below, the polyproteins encoded by five different cpBVDV isolates generated by RNA recombination are shown. **A:** The genome of BVDV1 strain NADL. **B:** The genome of BVDV1 strain Osloss. **C:** The genome of BVDV1 strain CP1. **D:** The genome of BVDV1 strain Pe515CP. **E:** The genome of BVDV1 strain CP9. As discussed in the text, these cpBVDV polyprotein structures allow the production of both NS2-3 and NS3. In-frame insertions of host sequences (colored boxes) are present in NADL, Osloss, and CP1. The NS2 autoprotease is responsible for NS3 production in the NADL strain, but the inserted ubiquitin sequences in Osloss and CP1 provide sites for processing by host ubiquitin C-terminal hydrolase (orange diamond). For Pe515CP and the CP9 DI RNA, the N^{pro} autoprotease (maroon box) mediates the cleavage producing the NS3 N terminus. The nomenclature and organization of the cleavage products and the symbols for the normal processing enzymes are defined in Figure 25.17.

Osloss) (Fig. 25.18B). In strains such as CP1, this may be accompanied by additional genome rearrangements, such as duplication of the *NS3* and *NS4A* genes[578] (Fig. 25.18C). All the strains described previously also express uncleaved NS2-3, which is important for infectious virion production.[3] Another type of insertion includes the light chain 3 gene of cellular microtubule-associated proteins, which is targeted for cleavage by a cellular protease.[244,575]

A third type of cpBVDV genome configuration repositions the N^{pro} autoprotease immediately upstream of NS3. In strain Pe515CP, N^{pro} is duplicated together with the *NS3* and *NS4A* genes[578] (Fig. 25.18D). Other cpBVDV isolates, such as CP9, contain a precise deletion of the C-E^{rns}-E1-E2-p7-NS2 coding region, resulting in an in-frame fusion of N^{pro} and NS3[839] (Fig. 25.18E). Such subgenomic RNAs replicate autonomously but require ncpBVDV helper viruses to provide packaging functions *in trans*.[55] For CSFV, cp subgenomic RNAs have been isolated in which the entire coding sequence upstream of NS3 has been deleted.[579]

cpBVDV genome rearrangements strongly correlate with increased NS3 expression and enhanced RNA replication. These phenotypes, however, can be uncoupled from cytopathogenicity in cell culture. For instance, a temperature-sensitive mutant of CP7 containing a point mutation in NS2 is ncp at 39.5°C but retains high NS3 expression, although RNA replication is reduced.[649] Selection for variants of cpBVDV in cell culture resulted in an ncpBVDV strain that still produces NS3 and viral RNA at levels comparable to the cp parent but encodes a point mutation in NS4B that attenuates the cytopathic effect.[700] Other ncpBVDV strains also show changes in NS4B.[257] Given that cpBVDV can cause ER stress[378] and NS4B is involved in membrane reorganization,[897] it seems plausible that cytopathic effects may result from overcommitment of cellular membranes to viral replication. Proteome analysis of infected cell cultures showed that cp or ncp viruses differentially regulate host signal transduction pathways, although these studies were not conducted with an isotype-matched cp–ncp pair of viruses.[21] In infected animals, increased cell death may be sufficient to induce widespread tissue injury and inflammation. Animals with mucosal disease also show increased numbers of infected cells, suggesting that differences in cpBVDV tropism may also contribute to the disease.[479]

GB VIRUSES

Discovery and Classification

In the early 1990s, a residual number of hepatitis cases were still not attributable to hepatitis A through E viruses. Efforts aimed at identifying additional hepatitis agents revealed three novel viruses that have been tentatively assigned to the family *Flaviviridae*. Two of these viruses, GBV-A and GBV-B, were cloned via representational difference analysis from the sera of tamarins experimentally infected with the GB hepatitis agent.[792] The GB agent was originally derived from the serum of a 34-year-old surgeon, "GB," who had acute hepatitis, by serial passage in tamarins.[188] Both viruses are similar to HCV yet genetically quite distinct.[609] Although originally derived from a human hepatitis case, subsequent work showed that GBV-A is an indigenous monkey virus that was likely acquired during passage in tamarins.[107,456] Some human cases that are not A through E hepatitis show serologic reactivity to both GBV-A and GBV-B, but reverse transcription-polymerase chain reaction (RT-PCR) has failed to detect either virus in human samples. Rather, a third related virus, GBV-C, was subsequently identified in humans.[791] Working independently, another group that was immunoscreening cDNA libraries from non-A, non-B hepatitis cases identified an agent, initially termed hepatitis G virus (HGV), which later turned out to be an independent isolate of GBV-C.[493] Because this virus has not been convincingly shown to cause human disease, including hepatitis, we will refer to it by its original designation, GBV-C.

A virus distantly related to GBV-A and GBV-C was recently discovered in Old World frugivorous bats in Bangladesh.[220] This virus has been designated GBV-D.

Based on sequence relatedness and overall genome structure, GBVs have been classified as members of the family *Flaviviridae*. GBV-B is considered to be a member of the genus *Hepacivirus*.[851] It has recently been proposed that GBV-A, GBV-C, and GBV-D be classified as a separate genus, *Pegivirus*, although this awaits formal ratification by taxonomists.[805] According to the proposed classification strategy, GBV-B would be renamed GBV and other GBVs would be renamed as pegiviruses according to their host of origin.

The inability to detect GBV-A or GBV-B in human samples led to investigation into their origins. Interestingly, GBV-A has been detected in several species of New World monkeys in the absence of experimental infection or overt disease.[107,455] Viral sequences isolated from a single primate species are highly related, whereas sequences derived from separate species show greater divergence, indicating that GBV-A has adapted to its primate hosts over extended periods of time.[107,127,455] The distribution of GBV-B in nature is unknown because the only source of this virus is the original tamarin-passaged GB serum. Despite intensive efforts, it has not been reisolated from natural sources.

Since its initial discovery, GBV-C infection has been found to be surprisingly common in the human population. Approximately 15% of healthy volunteer blood donors have markers of previous or ongoing infection with this virus,[804] and GBV-C has also been found in chimpanzees.[2,72,595] Phylogenetic analysis of GBV-C sequences has been complicated by an apparent bias against synonymous substitutions in some parts of the genome, leading to differences in inferred evolutionary relationships.[787] The molecular basis for this bias is unclear but may involve evolutionary constraints imposed by RNA structures[789] or cryptic ORFs.[658,796] Nevertheless, GBV-C has been classified into four or five genotypes.[787] Remarkably, variation among GBV-C isolates reflects the geographic distribution of human migration, suggesting the long-term co-evolution of this virus and its host. Given the rate at which RNA viruses typically evolve, this finding suggests that GBV-C is subject to unusual evolutionary constraints.

Clinical Perspective

Although GBV-A and GBV-B were originally derived from a case of human hepatitis, it is unclear whether either virus was the cause of the disease. It is now clear that GBV-A is not associated with any known disease and is likely to have been acquired during tamarin passage. GBV-B can infect and cause hepatitis in New World monkeys such as tamarins, marmosets, and owl monkeys, but it does not infect chimpanzees.[101,108,446] Because of this preference for lower primates, GBV-B is unlikely to be a human virus. Attempts to identify GBVs in the original GB clinical sample have failed, possibly because of degradation over prolonged storage.[2,763]

Human infection with GBV-C is well documented, although direct association of this virus with any human disease has proved to be elusive.[804] While the virus is usually cleared within 2 years,[64] persistent infections can last for years without clinical effects.[17] Clearance usually correlates with the appearance of antibodies against the viral E2 glycoprotein.[804] GBV-C appears to be primarily lymphotropic *in vivo*,[450,451] although evidence also exists for hepatotropic isolates.[240] GBV-C is transmitted parenterally or sexually, and a vertical transmission route is also likely.[65,804] Because these routes also transmit many other human viruses, GBV-C co-infections with HBV, HCV, or HIV are not uncommon. Needless to say, co-infection with human hepatitis viruses has likely contributed to the confusing association of GBV-C with disease.

Intriguingly, there is a possible interaction between GBV-C and HIV. It has been noted that patients co-infected with the two viruses tend to have higher CD4+ T-cell counts, lower HIV titers, and slower HIV disease progression.[804] Based on these observations, as well as *in vitro* experiments, it has been proposed that GBV-C may interfere with HIV replication by altering expression of cytokines, chemokines, and chemokine receptors,[683,918] decreasing T-cell activation,[541] directly inhibiting HIV-1 entry,[327,381,408,596] or eliciting cross-reactive antibodies that neutralize HIV particles.[597] It has also been argued, however, that as a lymphotropic virus, the presence of GBV-C viremia may simply reflect the higher CD4+ counts in HIV nonprogressors.[870] Thus, the underlying reasons for the correlation between GBV-C infection and slower HIV progression are not yet clear.

Experimental Systems

Little work has been done on GBV-A because it is an indigenous monkey virus that is not associated with disease. On the other hand, GBV-B is the closest relative of HCV and has been extensively studied as a surrogate model system. GBV-B can be readily cultured in primary tamarin or marmoset hepatocytes[51,101,446] but replicates poorly (if at all) in many immortalized cell lines.[105] Full-length GBV-B cDNAs have been assembled and shown to be infectious and cause hepatitis in tamarins.[109,545,757] Based on these functional clones, subgenomic GBV-B replicons have been constructed and can replicate in the human hepatoma lines Huh-7 and Hep3B, albeit with low efficiency.[186,187]

GBV-C has been reportedly cultured in human hepatoma lines,[772] primary human lymphocytes,[267] peripheral blood mononuclear cells,[241] and a derivative of the Daudi Burkitt lymphoma line.[782] Reminiscent of HCV, replication levels are low in these cell culture systems. Nevertheless, a GBV-C cDNA clone was constructed and shown to be infectious in primary human CD4+ T-cells.[919] GBV-C subgenomic replicons can persistently replicate in Huh-7 cells.[118]

Virion Structure and Entry

Particles of GBV-A and GBV-B have not been characterized. Similar to HCV, GBV-C particles exhibit unusually low and heterogeneous buoyant density, with peaks near 1.07 to 1.09 g/mL and 1.17 g/mL[566,754,917] due to interaction with lipoproteins. Treatment with detergents or organic solvents removes the viral envelope and shifts the peak of viral RNA to a higher-density form that may represent nucleocapsids,[566,754,917] although, paradoxically, GBV-A and GBV-C do not encode an obvious capsid gene. Little is known about the entry mechanism of GBV, although it has been proposed that GBV-C utilizes the LDL receptor.[4]

Genome Structure and Expression

As with other *Flaviviridae,* the GBVs encode a single long ORF containing structural genes followed by NS genes, flanked by 5′ and 3′ NCRs.[456,609] As for HCV and the pestiviruses, GBVs utilize an IRES to direct cap-independent translation.[286,790] Compared to other *Flaviviridae,* however, the GBV-A and GBV-C 5′ NCRs are much longer (>500 nt) and appear to fold into a similar structure that differs from other family members. The GBV-B 5′ NCR is also much longer than the corresponding HCV sequence, but the two regions share significant similarities in primary, secondary, and tertiary structure. In fact, critical regions of the GBV-B and HCV IRESs can be functionally exchanged.[380,728,730]

The GBV-A and GBV-C 3′ NCRs lack a poly(U/UC) tract and are highly conserved only within these virus groups, with the exception of more broadly conserved terminal stem-loop structures.[174,919] The GBV-B 3′ NCR is 361 nt long, containing a short poly(U) stretch 30 nt downstream of the stop codon, followed by a unique 309-nt sequence.[109,756] Although this region of the GBV-B genome does not display homology to HCV, the terminal 82 nt of the sequence can fold into a structure reminiscent of the HCV 3′ X region.

As with HCV, GBV-B contains a basic capsid protein followed by two envelope glycoproteins, E1 and E2. The genomes for GBV-A and GBV-C also contain E1 and E2 glycoproteins, but they lack any obvious capsid-like sequence.[493,609] The initiation codons used by these viruses have not been firmly mapped but appear to be conserved AUG codons immediately upstream of the E1 gene.[790] It has been observed, however, that individuals infected with GBV-C generate antibodies against a small basic peptide that can be translated from an in-frame upstream AUG, suggesting that such a protein is expressed *in vivo*.[917] Alternative explanations for the lack of a capsid-like protein include the possibilities that GBV-A and GBV-C might usurp a capsid-like protein from the host cell or a co-infecting virus, or that additional GBV proteins may be involved. In this regard, a region of the GBV-C *NS5A* gene exhibiting a bias against synonymous mutation has been noted to potentially encode a small basic protein (10 kD, pI 11.5) in an alternate reading frame.[658] Further characterization of GBV-A and GBV-C particles will be needed to demonstrate the nature of their nucleocapsid.

GBV-B encodes a 13-kD protein that shows partial homology to HCV p7.[270] This protein is predicted to span the membrane four times and can be processed by signal peptidase into two tandem p7-like proteins.[270,824] Remarkably, only the second half of p13, which has greater similarity to the HCV *p7* gene, is needed for infectivity in tamarins.[824] Furthermore, the GBV-B *p13* gene can be functionally replaced by HCV p7.[293]

The NS proteins of GBVs show the greatest similarity to HCV, and the boundaries of cognate NS2, NS3, NS4A, NS4B, NS5A, and NS5B proteins have been proposed.[456,609] Catalytic residues of the HCV NS2/3 autoprotease are conserved among GBV NS2 proteins, and this enzymatic activity has been demonstrated for GBV-C.[57] Similarly, the GBV NS3 proteins encode an N-terminal serine protease and C-terminal RNA helicases.[456,609] The GBV-B serine protease activity shares substrate specificity with the HCV enzyme and requires the virus-specific NS4A co-factor.[111,755,759] Consistent with this high degree of similarity, inhibitors of the HCV serine protease also inhibit the GBV-B protease.[101] NTP-dependent RNA helicase activity has also been demonstrated for NS3 proteins of GBV-B and GBV-C.[307,961] The GBV-B NS5B has been shown to possess primer-dependent and *de novo* initiation RdRP and terminal transferase activities, albeit with different cation selectivity.[711,962] The tail anchor of GBV-B NS5B can functionally substitute for the tail anchor of HCV NS5B.[92]

PERSPECTIVES

Our understanding of the *Flaviviridae* has increased tremendously in the recent years, although significant gaps remain. The recent identification of new members of the *Flaviviridae* such as the GBVs and CHV has deep implications for understanding the origins and diversity of these viruses. For a few viruses in the family, viral and host proteins required for genome replication have been identified and some of them have been characterized in molecular detail. A major remaining task is to understand how these components come together to form a functional replicase. Similarly, the processes of virus entry and particle assembly are only incompletely understood. It is very curious that flaviviruses and pestiviruses can tolerate large deletions and insertions within their C genes, and that some GBVs lack recognizable nucleocapsid genes altogether. These observations suggest that alternative mechanisms must allow viral genomes to condense into small virus particles. It is also curious that HCV assembly has been tied to VLDL assembly, although the molecular basis for this association remains unclear. Finally, a major overarching goal is to translate our knowledge of these viruses into improvements in human and animal health. The recent development of HCV-specific antivirals demonstrates the feasibility of this approach, although major challenges remain to develop broadly acting antiviral strategies. Similarly, vaccine development remains an important priority, particularly for dengue and HCV, with no clear solutions in sight. Clearly, we have only just begun to understand the *Flaviviridae*.

REFERENCES

All cited references are available in the e-book.

3. Agapov EV, Murray CL, Frolov I, et al. Uncleaved NS2-3 is required for production of infectious bovine viral diarrhea virus. *J Virol* 2004; 78(5):2414–2425.
10. Ali N, Tardif KD, Siddiqui A. Cell-free replication of the hepatitis C virus subgenomic replicon. *J Virol* 2002;76(23):12001–12007.
21. Ammari M, McCarthy FM, Nanduri B, et al. Analysis of Bovine Viral Diarrhea Viruses-infected monocytes: identification of cytopathic and non-cytopathic biotype differences. *BMC Bioinformatics* 2010;11(Suppl 6): S9.
24. Ansari IH, Chen LM, Liang D, et al. Involvement of a bovine viral diarrhea virus NS5B locus in virion assembly. *J Virol* 2004;78(18):9612–9623.
27. Appel N, Pietschmann T, Bartenschlager R. Mutational analysis of hepatitis C virus nonstructural protein 5A: potential role of differential phosphorylation in RNA replication and identification of a genetically flexible domain. *J Virol* 2005;79(5):3187–3194.
28. Appel N, Zayas M, Miller S, et al. Essential role of domain III of nonstructural protein 5A for hepatitis C virus infectious particle assembly. *PLoS Pathog* 2008;4(3):e1000035.
29. Appleby TC, Anderson R, Fedorova O, et al. Visualizing ATP-dependent RNA translocation by the NS3 helicase from HCV. *J Mol Biol* 2011; 405(5):1139–1153.
42. Bartenschlager R, Ahlborn-Laake L, Mous J, et al. Kinetic and structural analyses of hepatitis C virus polyprotein processing. *J Virol* 1994; 68(8):5045–5055.
43. Bartenschlager R, Frese M, Pietschmann T. Novel insights into hepatitis C virus replication and persistence. *Adv Virus Res* 2004;63:71–180.
44. Bartenschlager R, Penin F, Lohmann V, et al. Assembly of infectious hepatitis C virus particles. *Trends Microbiol* 2011;19(2):95–103.
46. Bartosch B, Dubuisson J, Cosset FL. Infectious hepatitis C virus pseudo-particles containing functional E1-E2 envelope protein complexes. *J Exp Med* 2003;197(5):633–642.
54. Becher P, Tautz N. RNA recombination in pestiviruses: cellular RNA sequences in viral genomes highlight the role of host factors for viral persistence and lethal disease. *RNA Biol* 2011;8(2):216–224.
55. Behrens SE, Grassmann CW, Thiel HJ, et al. Characterization of an autonomous subgenomic pestivirus RNA replicon. *J Virol* 1998;72(3):2364–2372.
56. Behrens SE, Tomei L, De Francesco R. Identification and properties of the RNA-dependent RNA polymerase of hepatitis C virus. *EMBO J* 1996; 15(1):12–22.
73. Bissig KD, Wieland SF, Tran P, et al. Human liver chimeric mice provide a model for hepatitis B and C virus infection and treatment. *J Clin Invest* 2010;120(3):924–930.
76. Blanchard E, Belouzard S, Goueslain L, et al. Hepatitis C virus entry depends on clathrin-mediated endocytosis. *J Virol* 2006;80(14):6964–6972.
77. Blight KJ, Kolykhalov AA, Rice CM. Efficient initiation of HCV RNA replication in cell culture. *Science* 2000;290(5498):1972–1974.
83. Boson B, Granio O, Bartenschlager R, et al. A concerted action of hepatitis C virus p7 and nonstructural protein 2 regulates core localization at the endoplasmic reticulum and virus assembly. *PLoS Pathog* 2011; 7(7):e1002144.
91. Brass V, Bieck E, Montserret R, et al. An amino-terminal amphipathic alpha-helix mediates membrane association of the hepatitis C virus nonstructural protein 5A. *J Biol Chem* 2002;277(10):8130–8139.
98. Bressanelli S, Stiasny K, Allison SL, et al. Structure of a flavivirus envelope glycoprotein in its low-pH-induced membrane fusion conformation. *EMBO J* 2004;23(4):728–738.
109. Bukh J, Apgar CL, Yanagi M. Toward a surrogate model for hepatitis C virus: an infectious molecular clone of the GB virus-B hepatitis agent. *Virology* 1999;262(2):470–478.
110. Bukh J, Pietschmann T, Lohmann V, et al. Mutations that permit efficient replication of hepatitis C virus RNA in Huh-7 cells prevent productive replication in chimpanzees. *Proc Natl Acad Sci U S A* 2002; 99(22):14416–14421.
126. Chang KS, Jiang J, Cai Z, et al. Human apolipoprotein E is required for infectivity and production of hepatitis C virus in cell culture. *J Virol* 2007;81(24):13783–13793.
131. Chen ST, Lin YL, Huang MT, et al. CLEC5A is critical for dengue-virus-induced lethal disease. *Nature* 2008;453(7195):672–676.
141. Choi KH, Groarke JM, Young DC, et al. The structure of the RNA-dependent RNA polymerase from bovine viral diarrhea virus establishes the role of GTP in de novo initiation. *Proc Natl Acad Sci U S A* 2004;101(13):4425–4430.
143. Choo Q-L, Kuo G, Weiner AJ, et al. Isolation of a cDNA clone derived from a blood-borne non-A, non-B viral hepatitis genome. *Science* 1989; 244(4902):359–362.
159. Coller KE, Berger KL, Heaton NS, et al. RNA interference and single particle tracking analysis of hepatitis C virus endocytosis. *PLoS Pathog* 2009;5(12):e1000702.

171. Cristofari G, Ivanyi-Nagy R, Gabus C, et al. The hepatitis C virus core protein is a potent nucleic acid chaperone that directs dimerization of the viral (+) strand RNA in vitro. *Nucleic Acids Res* 2004;32(8):2623–2631.
178. Daffis S, Szretter KJ, Schriewer J, et al. 2′-O methylation of the viral mRNA cap evades host restriction by IFIT family members. *Nature* 2010;468(7322):452–456.
181. Davidson AD. Chapter 2. New insights into flavivirus nonstructural protein 5. *Adv Virus Res* 2009;74:41–101.
188. Deinhardt F, Holmes AW, Capps RB, et al. Studies on the transmission of human viral hepatitis to marmoset monkeys. I. Transmission of disease, serial passage, and description of liver disease. *J Exp Med* 1967; 125(4):673–688.
198. Dorner M, Horwitz JA, Robbins JB, et al. A genetically humanized mouse model for hepatitis C virus infection. *Nature* 2011;474(7350):208–211.
201. Drummer HE, Maerz A, Poumbourios P. Cell surface expression of functional hepatitis C virus E1 and E2 glycoproteins. *FEBS Lett* 2003; 546(2–3):385–390.
211. Egloff MP, Benarroch D, Selisko B, et al. An RNA cap (nucleoside-2′-O-)-methyltransferase in the flavivirus RNA polymerase NS5: crystal structure and functional characterization. *EMBO J* 2002;21(11):2757–2768.
220. Epstein JH, Quan PL, Briese T, et al. Identification of GBV-D, a novel GB-like flavivirus from old world frugivorous bats (Pteropus giganteus) in Bangladesh. *PLoS Pathog* 2010;6:e1000972.
221. Erbel P, Schiering N, D'Arcy A, et al. Structural basis for the activation of flaviviral NS3 proteases from dengue and West Nile virus. *Nat Struct Mol Biol* 2006;13(4):372–373.
224. Evans MJ, von Hahn T, Tscherne DM, et al. Claudin-1 is a hepatitis C virus co-receptor required for a late step in entry. *Nature* 2007;446(7137): 801–805.
226. Failla C, Tomei L, De Francesco R. Both NS3 and NS4A are required for proteolytic processing of hepatitis C virus nonstructural proteins. *J Virol* 1994;68(6):3753–3760.
240. Fogeda M, López-Alcorocho JM, Bartolomé J, et al. Existence of distinct GB virus C/hepatitis G virus variants with different tropism. *J Virol* 2000;74(17):7936–7942.
246. Friebe P, Boudet J, Simorre JP, et al. Kissing-loop interaction in the 3′ end of the hepatitis C virus genome essential for RNA replication. *J Virol* 2005;79(1):380–392.
247. Friebe P, Lohmann V, Krieger N, et al. Sequences in the 5′ nontranslated region of hepatitis C virus required for RNA replication. *J Virol* 2001;75(24):12047–12057.
257. Gallei A, Orlich M, Thiel HJ, et al. Noncytopathogenic pestivirus strains generated by nonhomologous RNA recombination: alterations in the NS4A/NS4B coding region. *J Virol* 2005;79(22):14261–14270.
258. Gallei A, Pankraz A, Thiel HJ, et al. RNA recombination in vivo in the absence of viral replication. *J Virol* 2004;78(12):6271–6281.
264. Gastaminza P, Dryden KA, Boyd B, et al. Ultrastructural and biophysical characterization of hepatitis C virus particles produced in cell culture. *J Virol* 2010;84(21):10999–11009.
265. Gastaminza P, Kapadia SB, Chisari FV. Differential biophysical properties of infectious intracellular and secreted hepatitis C virus particles. *J Virol* 2006;80(22):11074–11081.
270. Ghibaudo D, Cohen L, Penin F, et al. Characterization of GB virus B polyprotein processing reveals the existence of a novel 13-kDa protein with partial homology to hepatitis C virus p7 protein. *J Biol Chem* 2004; 279(24):24965–24975.
273. Gladue DP, Gavrilov BK, Holinka LG, et al. Identification of an NTPase motif in classical swine fever virus NS4B protein. *Virology* 2011;411 (1):41–49.
284. Gouttenoire J, Penin F, Moradpour D. Hepatitis C virus nonstructural protein 4B: a journey into unexplored territory. *Rev Med Virol* 2010; 20(2):117–129.
286. Grace K, Gartland M, Karayiannis P, et al. The 5′ untranslated region of GB virus B shows functional similarity to the internal ribosome entry site of hepatitis C virus. *J Gen Virol* 1999;80(Pt 9):2337–2341.
287. Grakoui A, McCourt DW, Wychowski C, et al. A second hepatitis C virus-encoded proteinase. *Proc Natl Acad Sci U S A* 1993;90(22):10583–10587.
293. Griffin S, Trowbridge R, Thommes P, et al. Chimeric GB virus B genomes containing hepatitis C virus p7 are infectious in vivo. *J Hepatol* 2008;49(6):908–915.
294. Griffin SD, Beales LP, Clarke DS, et al. The p7 protein of hepatitis C virus forms an ion channel that is blocked by the antiviral drug, Amantadine. *FEBS Lett* 2003;535(1–3):34–38.
295. Griffin SD, Harvey R, Clarke DS, et al. A conserved basic loop in hepatitis C virus p7 protein is required for amantadine-sensitive ion channel activity in mammalian cells but is dispensable for localization to mitochondria. *J Gen Virol* 2004;85(Pt 2):451–461.
301. Gu M, Rice CM. Three conformational snapshots of the hepatitis C virus NS3 helicase reveal a ratchet translocation mechanism. *Proc Natl Acad Sci U S A* 2010;107(2):521–528.
310. Harada T, Tautz N, Thiel HJ. E2-p7 region of the bovine viral diarrhea virus polyprotein: processing and functional studies. *J Virol* 2000;74(20):9498–9506.
312. Harris HJ, Davis C, Mullins JG, et al. Claudin association with CD81 defines hepatitis C virus entry. *J Biol Chem* 2010;285(27):21092–21102.
316. Hausmann Y, Roman-Sosa G, Thiel HJ, et al. Classical swine fever virus glycoprotein E rns is an endoribonuclease with an unusual base specificity. *J Virol* 2004;78(10):5507–5512.
321. Heimann M, Roman-Sosa, G, Martoglio B, et al. Core protein of pestiviruses is processed at the C terminus by signal peptide peptidase. *J Virol* 2006;80(4):1915–1921.
326. Herker E, Harris C, Hernandez C, et al. Efficient hepatitis C virus particle formation requires diacylglycerol acyltransferase-1. *Nat Med* 2010; 16(11):1295–1298.
330. Hijikata M, Mizushima H, Akagi T, et al. Two distinct proteinase activities required for the processing of a putative nonstructural precursor protein of hepatitis C virus. *J Virol* 1993;67(8):4665–4675.
343. Hsu M, Zhang J, Flint M, et al. Hepatitis C virus glycoproteins mediate pH-dependent cell entry of pseudotyped retroviral particles. *Proc Natl Acad Sci U S A* 2003;100(12):7271–7276.
346. Huang L, Sineva EV, Hargittai MR, et al. Purification and characterization of hepatitis C virus non-structural protein 5A expressed in Escherichia coli. *Protein Expr Purif* 2004;37(1):144–153.
347. Huang Y, Staschke K, De Francesco R, et al. Phosphorylation of hepatitis C virus NS5A nonstructural protein: a new paradigm for phosphorylation-dependent viral RNA replication? *Virology* 2007;364(1):1–9.
354. Iglesias NG, Gamarnik AV. Dynamic RNA structures in the dengue virus genome. *RNA Biol* 2011;8(2):249–257.
370. Jirasko V, Montserret R, Lee JY, et al. Structural and functional studies of nonstructural protein 2 of the hepatitis C virus reveal its key role as organizer of virion assembly. *PLoS Pathog* 2010;6(12):e1001233.
377. Jopling CL, Yi M, Lancaster AM, et al. Modulation of hepatitis C virus RNA abundance by a liver-specific MicroRNA. *Science* 2005; 309(5740):1577–1581.
384. Kao CC, Del Vecchio AM, Zhong W. De novo initiation of RNA synthesis by a recombinant Flaviviridae RNA-dependent RNA polymerase. *Virology* 1999;253(1):1–7.
388. Kapoor A, Simmonds P, Gerold G, et al. Characterization of a canine homolog of hepatitis C virus. *Proc Natl Acad Sci U S A* 2011;108(28): 11608–11623.
412. Kolykhalov AA, Agapov EV, Blight KJ, et al. Transmission of hepatitis C by intrahepatic inoculation with transcribed RNA. *Science* 1997;277(5325):570–574.
413. Kolykhalov AA, Feinstone SM, Rice CM. Identification of a highly conserved sequence element at the 3′ terminus of hepatitis C virus genome RNA. *J Virol* 1996;70(6):3363–3371.
414. Kolykhalov AA, Mihalik K, Feinstone SM, et al. Hepatitis C virus-encoded enzymatic activities and conserved RNA elements in the 3′ nontranslated region are essential for virus replication in vivo. *J Virol* 2000;74(4):2046–2051.
430. Kuhn RJ, Zhang W, Rossmann MG, et al. Structure of dengue virus: implications for flavivirus organization, maturation, and fusion. *Cell* 2002;108(5):717–725.
433. Kümmerer BM, Meyers G. Correlation between point mutations in NS2 and the viability and cytopathogenicity of Bovine viral diarrhea virus strain Oregon analyzed with an infectious cDNA clone. *J Virol* 2000;74(1):390–400.
434. Kümmerer BM, Rice CM. Mutations in the yellow fever virus nonstructural protein NS2A selectively block production of infectious particles. *J Virol* 2002;76(10):4773–4784.

436. Lackner T, Müller A, König M, et al. Persistence of bovine viral diarrhea virus is determined by a cellular cofactor of a viral autoprotease. *J Virol* 2005;79(15):9746–9755.
437. Lackner T, Müller A, Pankraz A, et al. Temporal modulation of an autoprotease is crucial for replication and pathogenicity of an RNA virus. *J Virol* 2004;78(19):10765–10775.
438. Lackner T, Thiel HJ, Tautz N. Dissection of a viral autoprotease elucidates a function of a cellular chaperone in proteolysis. *Proc Natl Acad Sci U S A* 2006;103(5):1510–1515.
440. Lai VC, Kao CC, Ferrari E, et al. Mutational analysis of bovine viral diarrhea virus RNA-dependent RNA polymerase. *J Virol* 1999;73(12):10129–10136.
442. Lamarre D, Anderson PC, Bailey M, et al. An NS3 protease inhibitor with antiviral effects in humans infected with hepatitis C virus. *Nature* 2003;426(6963):186–189.
447. Lanford RE, Hildebrandt-Eriksen ES, Petri A, et al. Therapeutic silencing of microRNA-122 in primates with chronic hepatitis C virus infection. *Science* 2010;327(5962):198–201.
450. Laskus T, Radkowski M, Wang LF, et al. Detection of hepatitis G virus replication sites by using highly strand-specific Tth-based reverse transcriptase PCR. *J Virol* 1998;72(4):3072–3075.
451. Laskus T, Radkowski M, Wang LF, et al. Lack of evidence for hepatitis G virus replication in the livers of patients coinfected with hepatitis C and G viruses. *J Virol* 1997;71(10):7804–7806.
467. Levin MK, Gurjar M, Patel SS. A Brownian motor mechanism of translocation and strand separation by hepatitis C virus helicase. *Nat Struct Mol Biol* 2005;12(5)429–435.
471. Li L, Lok SM, Yu IM, et al. The flavivirus precursor membrane-envelope protein complex: structure and maturation. *Science* 2008;319(5871):1830–1834.
487. Lindenbach BD, Evans MJ, Syder AJ, et al. Complete replication of hepatitis C virus in cell culture. *Science* 2005;309(5734):623–626.
491. Lindenbach BD, Rice CM. Molecular biology of flaviviruses. *Adv Virus Res* 2003;59:23–61.
492. Lindenbach BD, Rice CM. trans-Complementation of yellow fever virus NS1 reveals a role in early RNA replication. *J Virol* 1997;71(12):9608–9617.
493. Linnen J, Wages J Jr, Zhang-Keck ZY, et al. Molecular cloning and disease association of hepatitis G virus: a transfusion-transmissible agent. *Science* 1996;271(5248):505–508.
508. Lohmann V, Körner F, Herian U, et al. Biochemical properties of hepatitis C virus NS5B RNA-dependent RNA polymerase and identification of amino acid sequence motifs essential for enzymatic activity. *J Virol* 1997;71(11):8416–8428.
509. Lohmann V, Körner F, Koch JO, et al. Replication of subgenomic hepatitis C virus RNAs in a hepatoma cell line. *Science* 1999;285(5424):110–113.
510. Lohmann V, Overton H, Bartenschlager R. Selective stimulation of hepatitis C virus and pestivirus NS5B RNA polymerase activity by GTP. *J Biol Chem* 1999;274(16):10807–10815.
513. Lorenz IC, Marcotrigiano J, Dentzer TG, et al. Structure of the catalytic domain of the hepatitis C virus NS2-3 protease. *Nature* 2006;442(7104):831–835.
514. Love RA, Brodsky O, Hickey MJ, et al. Crystal structure of a novel dimeric form of NS5A domain I protein from hepatitis C virus. *J Virol* 2009;83(9):4395–4403.
519. Luik P, Chew C, Aittoniemi J, et al. The 3-dimensional structure of a hepatitis C virus p7 ion channel by electron microscopy. *Proc Natl Acad Sci U S A* 2009;106(31):12712–12716.
524. Luo G, Hamatake RK, Mathis DM, et al. De novo initiation of RNA synthesis by the RNA-dependent RNA polymerase (NS5B) of hepatitis C virus. *J Virol* 2000;74(2):851–863.
527. Lupberger J, Zeisel MB, Xiao F, et al. EGFR and EphA2 are host factors for hepatitis C virus entry and possible targets for antiviral therapy. *Nat Med* 2011;17(5):589–595.
528. Luscombe CA, Huang Z, Murray MG, et al. A novel hepatitis C virus p7 ion channel inhibitor, BIT225, inhibits bovine viral diarrhea virus in vitro and shows synergism with recombinant interferon-alpha-2b and nucleoside analogues. *Antiviral Res* 2010;86(2):144–153.
529. Ma L, Jones CT, Groesch TD, et al. Solution structure of dengue virus capsid protein reveals another fold. *Proc Natl Acad Sci U S A* 2004;101(10):3414–3419.
530. Ma Y, Anantpadma M, Timpe JM, et al. Hepatitis C virus NS2 protein serves as a scaffold for virus assembly by interacting with both structural and nonstructural proteins. *J Virol* 2011;85(1):86–97.
532. Machlin ES, Sarnow P, Sagan SM. Masking the 5′ terminal nucleotides of the hepatitis C virus genome by an unconventional microRNA-target RNA complex. *Proc Natl Acad Sci U S A* 2011;108(8):3193–3198.
533. Mackenzie JM, Jones MK, Young PR. Immunolocalization of the dengue virus nonstructural glycoprotein NS1 suggests a role in viral RNA replication. *Virology* 1996;221(1):232–240.
551. Maurer K, Krey T, Moennig V, et al. CD46 is a cellular receptor for bovine viral diarrhea virus. *J Virol* 2004;78(4):1792–1799.
558. McLauchlan J. Properties of the hepatitis C virus core protein: a structural protein that modulates cellular processes. *J Viral Hepat* 2000;7(1):2–14.
559. McLauchlan J, Lemberg MK, Hope G, et al. Intramembrane proteolysis promotes trafficking of hepatitis C virus core protein to lipid droplets. *EMBO J* 2002;21(15):3980–3988.
561. McMullan LK, Grakoui A, Evans MJ, et al. Evidence for a functional RNA element in the hepatitis C virus core gene. *Proc Natl Acad Sci U S A* 2007;104(8):2879–2884.
565. Melian EB, Hinzman E, Nagasaki T, et al. NS1′ of flaviviruses in the Japanese encephalitis virus serogroup is a product of ribosomal frameshifting and plays a role in viral neuroinvasiveness. *J Virol* 2010;84(3):1641–1647.
568. Mercer DF, Schiller DE, Elliott JF, et al. Hepatitis C virus replication in mice with chimeric human livers. *Nat Med* 2001;7(8):927–933.
569. Merz A, Long G, Hiet MS, et al. Biochemical and morphological properties of hepatitis C virus particles and determination of their lipidome. *J Biol Chem* 2011;286(4):3018–3032.
570. Meuleman P, Libbrecht L, De Vos R, et al. Morphological and biochemical characterization of a human liver in a uPA-SCID mouse chimera. *Hepatology* 2005;41(4):847–856.
572. Meunier JC, Russell RS, Engle RH, et al. Apolipoprotein C1 association with hepatitis C virus. *J Virol* 2008;82(19):9647–9656.
574. Meyers G, Ege A, Fetzer C, et al. Bovine viral diarrhea virus: prevention of persistent fetal infection by a combination of two mutations affecting Erns RNase and Npro protease. *J Virol* 2007;81(7):3327–3338.
579. Meyers G, Thiel HJ. Cytopathogenicity of classical swine fever virus caused by defective interfering particles. *J Virol* 1995;69(6):3683–3689.
580. Meyers G, Thiel HJ. Molecular characterization of pestiviruses. *Adv Virus Res* 1996;47:53–118.
588. Miyanari Y, Atsuzawa K, Usuda N, et al. The lipid droplet is an important organelle for hepatitis C virus production. *Nat Cell Biol* 2007;9(9):1089–1097.
589. Miyanari Y, Hijikata M, Yamaji M, et al. Hepatitis C virus non-structural proteins in the probable membranous compartment function in viral genome replication. *J Biol Chem* 2003;278(50):50301–50308.
591. Modis Y, Ogata S, Clements D, et al. A ligand-binding pocket in the dengue virus envelope glycoprotein. *Proc Natl Acad Sci U S A* 2003;100(12):6986–6991.
592. Modis Y, Ogata S, Clements D, et al. Structure of the dengue virus envelope protein after membrane fusion. *Nature* 2004;427(6972):313–319.
605. Moradpour D, Evans MJ, Gosert R, et al. Insertion of green fluorescent protein into nonstructural protein 5A allows direct visualization of functional hepatitis C virus replication complexes. *J Virol* 2004;78(14):7400–7409.
606. Morikawa K, Lange CM, Gouttenoire J, et al. Nonstructural protein 3-4A: the Swiss army knife of hepatitis C virus. *J Viral Hepat* 2011;18(5):305–315.
608. Moulin HR, Seuberlich T, Bauhofer O, et al. Nonstructural proteins NS2-3 and NS4A of classical swine fever virus: essential features for infectious particle formation. *Virology* 2007;365(2):376–389.
609. Muerhoff AS, Leary TP, Simons JN, et al. Genomic organization of GB viruses A and B: two new members of the Flaviviridae associated with GB agent hepatitis. *J Virol* 1995;69(9):5621–5630.
610. Mukhopadhyay S, Kim BS, Chipman PR, et al. Structure of West Nile virus. *Science* 2003;302(5643):248.

611. Mukhopadhyay S, Kuhn RJ, Rossmann MG. A structural perspective of the flavivirus life cycle. *Nat Rev Microbiol* 2005;3(1):13–22.
617. Murray CL, Jones CT, Rice CM. Architects of assembly: roles of *Flaviviridae* non-structural proteins in virion morphogenesis. *Nat Rev Microbiol* 2008;6(9):699–708.
618. Murray CL, Marcotrigiano J, Rice CM. Bovine viral diarrhea virus core is an intrinsically disordered protein that binds RNA. *J Virol* 2008; 82(3):1294–1304.
627. Neddermann P, Quintavalle M, Di Pietro C, et al. Reduction of hepatitis C virus NS5A hyperphosphorylation by selective inhibition of cellular kinases activates viral RNA replication in cell culture. *J Virol* 2004;78(23):13306–13314.
649. Pankraz A, Preis S, Thiel HJ, et al. A single point mutation in nonstructural protein NS2 of bovine viral diarrhea virus results in temperature-sensitive attenuation of viral cytopathogenicity. *J Virol* 2009; 83(23):12415–12423.
655. Patkar CG, Kuhn RJ. Yellow fever virus NS3 plays an essential role in virus assembly independent of its known enzymatic functions. *J Virol* 2008;82(7):3342–3352.
665. Penin F, Brass V, Appel N, et al. Structure and function of the membrane anchor domain of hepatitis C virus nonstructural protein 5A. *J Biol Chem* 2004;279(39):40835–40843.
666. Perelson AS, Herrmann E, Micol F, et al. New kinetic models for the hepatitis C virus. *Hepatology* 2005;42(4):749–754.
667. Perera R, Kuhn RJ. Structural proteomics of dengue virus. *Curr Opin Microbiol* 2008;11(4):369–377.
672. Phan T, Beran RK, Peters C, et al. Hepatitis C virus NS2 protein contributes to virus particle assembly via opposing epistatic interactions with the E1-E2 glycoprotein and NS3-NS4A enzyme complexes. *J Virol* 2009;83(17):8379–8395.
675. Pietschmann T, Kaul A, Koutsoudakis G, et al. Construction and characterization of infectious intragenotypic and intergenotypic hepatitis C virus chimeras. *Proc Natl Acad Sci U S A* 2006;103(19):7408–7413.
679. Pileri P, Uematsu Y, Campagnoli S, et al. Binding of hepatitis C virus to CD81. *Science* 1998;282(5390):938–941.
681. Ploss A, Evans MJ, Gaysinskaya VA, et al. Human occludin is a hepatitis C virus entry factor required for infection of mouse cells. *Nature* 2009;457(7231):882–886.
700. Qu L, McMullan LK, Rice CM. Isolation and characterization of noncytopathic pestivirus mutants reveals a role for nonstructural protein NS4B in viral cytopathogenicity. *J Virol* 2001;75(22):10651–10662.
702. Quintavalle M, Sambucini S, Di Pietro C, et al. The alpha isoform of protein kinase CKI is responsible for hepatitis C virus NS5A hyperphosphorylation. *J Virol* 2006;80(22):11305–11312.
708. Ranjith-Kumar CT, Kao CC. Biochemical activities of the HCV NS5B RNA-dependent RNA polymerase. In: Tan SL, ed. *Hepatitis C Viruses: Genomes and Molecular Biology.* Norfolk, UK: Horizon Bioscience; 2006: Chapter 10.
713. Ray D, Shah A, Tilgner M, et al. West Nile virus 5′-cap structure is formed by sequential guanine N-7 and ribose 2′-O methylations by nonstructural protein 5. *J Virol* 2006;80(17):8362–8370.
717. Reed KE, Xu J, Rice CM. Phosphorylation of the hepatitis C virus NS5A protein in vitro and in vivo: properties of the NS5A-associated kinase. *J Virol* 1997;71(10):7187–7197.
719. Reiss S, Rebhan I, Backes P, et al. Recruitment and activation of a lipid kinase by hepatitis C virus NS5A is essential for integrity of the membranous replication compartment. *Cell Host Microbe* 2011;9(1):32–45.
722. Rey FA, Heinz FX, Mandl C, et al. The envelope glycoprotein from tick-borne encephalitis virus at 2 Å resolution. *Nature* 1995;375(6529):291–298.
725. Rice CM, Grakoui A, Galler R, et al. Transcription of infectious yellow fever virus RNA from full-length cDNA templates produced by in vitro ligation. *New Biol* 1989;1(3):285–296.
727. Riedel C, Lamp B, Heimann M, et al. Characterization of essential domains and plasticity of the classical swine fever virus Core protein. *J Virol* 2010;84(21):11523–11531.
731. Rinck G, Birghan C, Harada T, et al. A cellular J-domain protein modulates polyprotein processing and cytopathogenicity of a pestivirus. *J Virol* 2001;75(19):9470–9482.
749. Rümenapf T, Unger G, Strauss JH, et al. Processing of the envelope glycoproteins of pestiviruses. *J Virol* 1993;67(6):3288–3294.
750. Sakai A, Claire MS, Faulk K, et al. The p7 polypeptide of hepatitis C virus is critical for infectivity and contains functionally important genotype-specific sequences. *Proc Natl Acad Sci U S A* 2003;100(20):11646–11651.
756. Sbardellati A, Scarselli E, Tomei L, et al. Identification of a novel sequence at the 3′ end of the GB virus B genome. *J Virol* 1999;73(12): 10546–10550.
758. Scarselli E, Ansuini H, Cerino R, et al. The human scavenger receptor class B type I is a novel candidate receptor for the hepatitis C virus. *EMBO J* 2002;21(19):5017–5025.
765. Schlick P, Taucher C, Schittl B, et al. Helices alpha2 and alpha3 of West Nile virus capsid protein are dispensable for assembly of infectious virions. *J Virol* 2009;83(11):5581–5591.
768. Schneider R, Unger G, Stark R, et al. Identification of a structural glycoprotein of an RNA virus as a ribonuclease. *Science* 1993;261(5125): 1169–1171.
770. Schregel V, Jacobi S, Penin F, et al. Hepatitis C virus NS2 is a protease stimulated by cofactor domains in NS3. *Proc Natl Acad Sci U S A* 2009;106(13):5342–5347.
775. Serebrov V, Pyle AM. Periodic cycles of RNA unwinding and pausing by hepatitis C virus NS3 helicase. *Nature* 2004;430(6998):476–480.
788. Simmonds P, Bukh J, Combet C, et al. Consensus proposals for a unified system of nomenclature of hepatitis C virus genotypes. *Hepatology* 2005;42(4):962–973.
790. Simons JN, Desai SM, Schultz DE, et al. Translation initiation in GB viruses A and C: evidence for internal ribosome entry and implications for genome organization. *J Virol* 1996;70(9):6126–6135.
791. Simons JN, Leary TP, Dawson GJ, et al. Isolation of novel virus-like sequences associated with human hepatitis. *Nat Med* 1995;1(6):564–569.
792. Simons JN, Pilot-Matias TJ, Leary TP, et al. Identification of two flavivirus-like genomes in the GB hepatitis agent. *Proc Natl Acad Sci U S A* 1995;92(8):3401–3405.
803. Stapleford KA, Lindenbach BD. Hepatitis C virus NS2 coordinates virus particle assembly through physical interactions with the E1-E2 glycoprotein and NS3-NS4A enzyme complexes. *J Virol* 2011;85(4):1706–1717.
804. Stapleton JT. GB virus type C/Hepatitis G virus. *Semin Liver Dis* 2003;23(2):137–148.
805. Stapleton JT, Foung S, Muerhoff AS, et al. The GB viruses: a review and proposed classification of GBV-A, GBV-C (HGV), and GBV-D in genus Pegivirus within the family *Flaviviridae*. *J Gen Virol* 2011;92(Pt 2): 233–246.
807. Steffens S, Thiel HJ, Behrens SE. The RNA-dependent RNA polymerases of different members of the family Flaviviridae exhibit similar properties in vitro. *J Gen Virol* 1999;80(Pt 10):2583–2590.
809. Steinmann E, Penin F, Kallis S, et al. Hepatitis C virus p7 protein is crucial for assembly and release of infectious virions. *PLoS Pathog* 2007; 3(7):e103.
823. Tai AW, Benita Y, Peng LF, et al. A functional genomic screen identifies cellular cofactors of hepatitis C virus replication. *Cell Host Microbe* 2009;5(3):298–307.
824. Takikawa S, Engle RE, Emerson SU, et al. Functional analyses of GB virus B p13 protein: development of a recombinant GB virus B hepatitis virus with a p7 protein. *Proc Natl Acad Sci U S A* 2006;103(9):3345–3350.
825. Tamura JK, Warrener P, Collett MS. RNA-stimulated NTPase activity associated with the p80 protein of the pestivirus bovine viral diarrhea virus. *Virology* 1993;193(1):1–10.
827. Tanaka T, Kato N, Cho MJ, et al. Structure of the 3′ terminus of the hepatitis C virus genome. *J Virol* 1996;70(5):3307–3312.
836. Tautz N, Kaiser A, Thiel HJ. NS3 serine protease of bovine viral diarrhea virus: characterization of active site residues, NS4A cofactor domain, and protease-cofactor interactions. *Virology* 2000;273(2):351–363.
837. Tautz N, Meyers G, Stark R, et al. Cytopathogenicity of a pestivirus correlates with a 27-nucleotide insertion. *J Virol* 1996;70(11):7851–7858.
840. Tellinghuisen TL, Foss KL, Treadaway J. Regulation of hepatitis C virion production via phosphorylation of the NS5A protein. *PLoS Pathog* 2008;4(3):e1000032.
843. Tellinghuisen TL, Marcotrigiano J, Rice CM. Structure of the zinc-binding domain of an essential component of the hepatitis C virus replicase. *Nature* 2005;435(7040):374–379.

852. Thiel, H-J, Plagemann PGW, Moennig V. Pestiviruses. In: Fields BN, Knipe DM, Howley PM, eds. *Fields Virology*, 3rd ed. New York: Raven Press; 1986;1:1059–1073.
853. Thiel HJ, Stark R, Weiland E, et al. Hog cholera virus: molecular composition of virions from a pestivirus. *J Virol* 1991;65(9):4705–4712.
861. Tratschin JD, Moser C, Ruggli N, et al. Classical swine fever virus leader proteinase N^{pro} is not required for viral replication in cell culture. *J Virol* 1998;72(9):7681–7684.
862. Tscherne DM, Evans MJ, Macdonald MR, et al. Transdominant inhibition of bovine viral diarrhea virus entry. *J Virol* 2008;82(5):2427–2436.
864. Tscherne DM, Jones CT, Evans MJ, et al. Time- and temperature-dependent activation of hepatitis C virus for low-pH-triggered entry. *J Virol* 2006;80(4):1734–1741.
869. Urosevic N, van Maanen M, Mansfield JP, et al. Molecular characterization of virus-specific RNA produced in the brains of flavivirus-susceptible and -resistant mice after challenge with Murray Valley encephalitis virus. *J Gen Virol* 1997;78(Pt 1):23–29.
871. van der Schaar HM, Rust MJ, Chen C, et al. Dissecting the cell entry pathway of dengue virus by single-particle tracking in living cells. *PLoS Pathog* 2008;4(12):e1000244.
879. Vieyres G, Thomas X, Descamps V, et al. Characterization of the envelope glycoproteins associated with infectious hepatitis C virus. *J Virol* 2010;84(19):10159–10168.
883. Wakita T, Pietschmann T, Kato T, et al. Production of infectious hepatitis C virus in tissue culture from a cloned viral genome. *Nat Med* 2005; 11(7):791–796.
889. Warrener P, Collett MS. Pestivirus NS3 (p80) protein possesses RNA helicase activity. *J Virol* 1995;69(3):1720–1726.
894. Weiland F, Weiland E, Unger G, et al. Localization of pestiviral envelope proteins E(rns) and E2 at the cell surface and on isolated particles. *J Gen Virol* 1999;80(Pt 5):1157–1165.
897. Weiskircher E, Aligo J, Ning G, et al. Bovine viral diarrhea virus NS4B protein is an integral membrane protein associated with Golgi markers and rearranged host membranes. *Virol J* 2009;6:185.
898. Welsch S, Miller S, Romero-Brey I, et al. Composition and three-dimensional architecture of the dengue virus replication and assembly sites. *Cell Host Microbe* 2009;5(4):365–375.
905. Whidby J, Mateu G, Scarborough H, et al. Blocking hepatitis C virus infection with recombinant form of envelope protein 2 ectodomain. *J Virol* 2009;83(21):11078–11089.
912. Wiskerchen M, Belzer SK, Collett MS. Pestivirus gene expression: the first protein product of the bovine viral diarrhea virus large open reading frame, p20, possesses proteolytic activity. *J Virol* 1991;65(8): 4508–4514.
913. Wiskerchen M, Collett MS. Pestivirus gene expression: protein p80 of bovine viral diarrhea virus is a proteinase involved in polyprotein processing. *Virology* 1991;184(1):341–350.
915. Wozniak AL, Griffin S, Rowlands D, et al. Intracellular proton conductance of the hepatitis C virus p7 protein and its contribution to infectious virus production. *PLoS Pathog* 2010;6(9):e1001087.
920. Xu J, Mendez E, Caron PR, et al. Bovine viral diarrhea virus NS3 serine proteinase: polyprotein cleavage sites, cofactor requirements, and molecular model of an enzyme essential for pestivirus replication. *J Virol* 1997;71(7):5312–5322.
925. Yanagi M, Purcell RH, Emerson SU, et al. Transcripts from a single full-length cDNA clone of hepatitis C virus are infectious when directly transfected into the liver of a chimpanzee. *Proc Natl Acad Sci U S A* 1997; 94(16):8738–8743.
926. Yanagi M, St Claire M, Emerson SU, et al. In vivo analysis of the 3′ untranslated region of the hepatitis C virus after in vitro mutagenesis of an infectious cDNA clone. *Proc Natl Acad Sci U S A* 1999;96(5): 2291–2295.
937. Yi M, Villanueva RA, Thomas DL, et al. Production of infectious genotype 1a hepatitis C virus (Hutchinson strain) in cultured human hepatoma cells. *Proc Natl Acad Sci U S A* 2006;103(7):2310–2315.
940. You S, Padmanabhan R. A novel in vitro replication system for Dengue virus. Initiation of RNA synthesis at the 3′-end of exogenous viral RNA templates requires 5′- and 3′-terminal complementary sequence motifs of the viral RNA. *J Biol Chem* 1999;274(47):33714–33722.
946. Yu IM, Zhang W, Holdaway HA, et al. Structure of the immature dengue virus at low pH primes proteolytic maturation. *Science* 2008;319(5871): 1834–1837.
956. Zhang W, Chipman PR, Corver J, et al. Visualization of membrane protein domains by cryo-electron microscopy of dengue virus. *Nat Struct Biol* 2003;10(11):907–912.
957. Zhang Y, Corver J, Chipman PR, et al. Structures of immature flavivirus particles. *EMBO J* 2003;22(11):2604–2613.
959. Zhong J, Gastaminza P, Cheng G, et al. Robust hepatitis C virus infection in vitro. *Proc Natl Acad Sci U S A* 2005;102(26):9294–9299.
960. Zhong W, Gutshall LL, Del Vecchio AM. Identification and characterization of an RNA-dependent RNA polymerase activity within the nonstructural protein 5B region of bovine viral diarrhea virus. *J Virol* 1998;72(11):9365–9369.

CHAPTER 26

Theodore C. Pierson • Michael S. Diamond

Flaviviruses

Flaviviruses acquired their name from the jaundice associated with the liver dysfunction caused by yellow fever virus (YFV) infections. YFV played an important historical role in defining the nature of viruses in general. Seminal studies by Walter Reed and colleagues[780] demonstrated that the etiology of yellow fever was a filterable agent that could be transmitted through the bite of a mosquito, confirming the postulates of Carlos Finlay. YFV was the first flavivirus isolated (in 1927) and the first to be propagated *in vitro*.[790,820] These advances led remarkably rapidly to the development of an effective YFV vaccine that remains in use today.[569] Experiments with the louping ill virus (LIV) in 1931 established that ticks also were capable of transmitting viruses associated with human disease.[119] The discovery that antisera raised against some, but not all, viruses that caused similar diseases (e.g., encephalitis) cross-reacted with heterologous viruses provided a method to investigate the relatedness of flaviviruses.[126–128,876] This was refined further with the development of a standardized hemagglutination inhibition test that allowed classification of 10 different flaviviruses and distinguished them from alphaviruses.[127] These two groups of viruses were referred to thereafter as group A and B arboviruses, respectively. The first full-length flavivirus genome (YFV) were sequenced in 1985 by Charles Rice and colleagues.[680] Subsequent advances in the molecular genetics of flaviviruses have increased our understanding of the relationships between viruses that was originally revealed by serology (described below). Seventy-three viruses of the *Flavivirus* genus (classified as 53 distinct species) have since been defined (http://www.ICTVonline.org/index.asp).

FLAVIVIRUS DIVERSITY, EVOLUTION, AND DISTRIBUTION

Molecular Phylogeny

Phylogenic relationships among members of the flavivirus genus have been established through the analysis of individual genes, and, more recently, the entire open reading frame of the genome.[73,160,248,274,275,402,435,910] Analysis of the phylogenic tree of flaviviruses with respect to key features of the biology and ecology of these viruses has proven insightful.[248,271] Three groups of viruses are defined based on their mode of transmission: tick-borne flaviviruses (TBFVs), mosquito-borne flaviviruses viruses (MBFVs), and those flaviviruses with no known vector (NKV). The earliest divergence from a monophyletic origin separates flaviviruses based on their mode of transmission.[435,528] One lineage arising from the earliest branch of the phylogenic tree contains viruses transmitted by ticks and two groups of NKV viruses (Fig. 26.1). The second includes the mosquito-borne viruses and the Entebbe bat virus (ENTV) group of NKV viruses.[402] The MBFVs are grouped further as a function of their association with mosquitoes of the *Aedes* and *Culex* genera. Viruses in these two clades cause hemorrhagic disease and encephalitis in humans and livestock, respectively. Although many of the viruses in the *Culex* clade infect avian hosts, *Aedes* viruses generally do not. Conversely, *Culex* viruses are not maintained in nature in infection cycles involving primates.

The tick-borne flaviviruses include 12 species divided into three groups[274,402] (Fig. 26.1). The largest group of TBFVs is associated with mammalian hosts (typically rodents), and includes viruses that cause encephalitis (e.g., tick-borne encephalitis viruses [TBEVs]) and hemorrhagic fever (Omsk hemorrhagic fever virus [OHFV] and Kyasanur Forest disease virus [KFDV]) in humans. In addition, three species of mammalian TBFVs have not been associated with disease (Royal Farm virus [RFV], Karshi virus [KSIV], and Gadgets Gully virus [GGYV]). Viruses of the TBEV serocomplex are thought to represent a continuous evolutionary cline (a genetic gradient) that originated in Africa and moved from east to west across the Northern Hemisphere; the genetic distance between viruses in the mammalian tick-borne group correlates with increases in geographic distance.[274,910] This is reflected by the asymmetric branching pattern of the phylogenic tree of the mammalian viruses[911] (Fig. 26.1). The evolution of RFV, KSIV, and GGYV is not associated with this TBEV serocomplex cline, nor understood. This second group of TBFVs replicates within seabirds and ornithophilic ticks but does not cause disease in humans. These viruses have a broad geographic range that presumably reflects the migratory patterns of their avian hosts.[271,274] The sole member of the final group of TBFVs is the Kadam virus (KADV). KADV is found in Africa and is typically associated with livestock.[271] An understanding of the relationship between KADV and other members of the TBFVs has evolved. Although these viruses have been assigned to both the mammalian or sea bird groups of flaviviruses, a more recent analysis of the complete coding sequence of TBFVs places this virus in its own group, which is supported by unique features of its envelope protein and the fact that it encodes a polyprotein that is smaller than the rest of the TBFVs.[274]

MBFVs diverged early into two lineages; viruses within each of these lineages are subdivided based on their association with mosquitoes of the *Aedes* genus or *Culex* genus[275,402] (Fig. 26.1). Viruses of the *Aedes* clade are a paraphyletic group thought to predate and give rise to the *Culex* viruses.[271] One branch of the MBFV portion of the phylogenic tree includes viruses of the YFV group, the recently proposed Edge Hill virus (EHV) group, and two NKV viruses, discussed below. The YFV group includes Wesselsbron virus (WESSV), Sepik virus (SEPV), and YFV. WESSV is a veterinary pathogen transmitted by *Aedes* mosquitoes that causes a nonfatal febrile illness in humans. Very little is known about the clinical significance and vector biology of SEPV infection. Both SEPV and WESSV are found in Africa and Asia.[275] The seven viruses of the EHV group are transmitted predominantly by *Aedes* mosquitoes, are found primarily in Africa (except for EHV, which is present in Australia), and share the unique property of encoding five (instead of six) disulfide bridges in the envelope glycoprotein. Human cases have been associated only with Banzi virus infection (BANV).[275] The second branch of the MBFV phylogenic tree contains dengue viruses (DENVs), which are transmitted by *Aedes* mosquitoes, a large group of viruses vectored by *Culex* mosquitoes (e.g., Japanese encephalitis virus [JEV], West Nile virus [WNV]), and a group of *Aedes*-vectored viruses closes related to the *Culex* flaviviruses (e.g., Spondweni virus, SPOV).[402] The diversity of viruses in the JEV serocomplex and DENV is described in detail below.

FIGURE 26.1. Phylogenetic tree of viruses in the genus *Flavivirus* reveals the evolutionary relationships among viruses transmitted by different vectors. A maximum-likelihood tree was generated using the complete polyprotein sequence of the indicated flaviviruses as detailed by Kitchen and colleagues.[402] The viral taxa are abbreviated and colored according to their mode of transmission. The host reservoir for each virus is indicated in *gray*. Viruses that frequently cause disease in humans are indicated with *red asterisks*. APOIV, Apoi virus; MODV, Modoc virus; MMLV, Montana myotis leukoencephalitis virus; RBV, Rio Bravo virus; TYUV, Tyuleniy virus; MEAV, Meaban virus; SREV, Saumaurez Reef virus; KADV, Kadam virus; GGYV, Gadgets Gully virus; KSIV, Karshi virus; RFV, Royal Farm virus; DTV, Deer tick virus; POWV, Powassan virus; AHFV, Alkhurma hemorrhagic fever virus; KFDV, Kyasanur Forest disease virus; LGTV, Langat virus (LGTV); OHFV, Omsk hemorrhagic fever virus; TBEV-FE, Tick-borne encephalitis virus-far eastern subtype; TBEV-S, Tick-borne encephalitis virus-Siberian subtype; GGEV, Greek goat encephalomyelitis virus; TSEV, Turkish sheep encephalitis virus; TBEV-E, Tick-borne encephalitis virus-European subtype; LIV, Louping ill virus; SSEV, Spanish sheep encephalomyelitis virus; ENTV, Entebbe bat virus; YOKV, Yokose virus; YFV, Yellow fever virus; SEPV, Sepik virus; WESSV, Wesselsbron virus; EHV, Edge Hill virus; BOUV, Bouboui virus; BANV, Banzi virus; UGSV, Uganda S virus; JUGV, Jugra virus; POTV, Potiskum virus; SABV, Saboya virus; DENV-4, Dengue virus serotype 4; DENV-2, Dengue virus serotype 2; DENV-1, Dengue virus serotype 1; DENV-3, Dengue virus serotype 3; KEDV, Kedougu virus; SPOV, Spondweni virus; ZIKV, Zika virus; IGUV, Iguape virus; KOKV, Kokobera virus; AROAV, Aroa virus; BSQV, Bussuquara virus; ILHV, Ilheus virus; ROCV, Rocio virus; BAGV, Bagaza virus; SLEV, St. Louis encephalitis virus; KUNV, Kunjin virus; WNV, West Nile virus; JEV, Japanese encephalitis virus; MVEV, Murray Valley encephalitis virus; and USUV, Usutu virus. The tree was kindly provided by Dr. Edward Holmes and modified with permission.

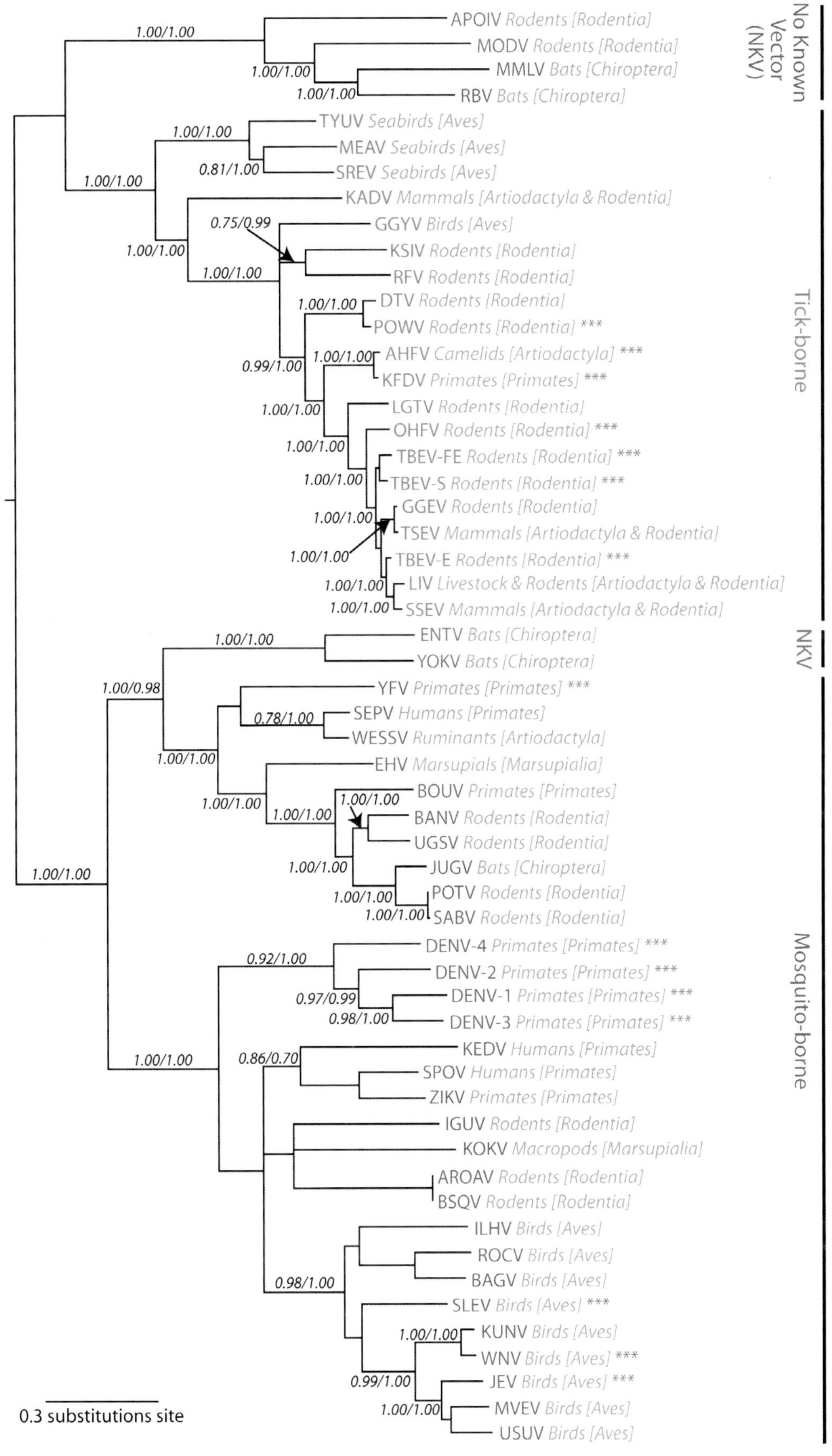
No Known Vector (NKV)
APOIV Rodents [Rodentia]
MODV Rodents [Rodentia]
MMLV Bats [Chiroptera]
RBV Bats [Chiroptera]
TYUV Seabirds [Aves]
MEAV Seabirds [Aves]
SREV Seabirds [Aves]
KADV Mammals [Artiodactyla & Rodentia]
GGYV Birds [Aves]
KSIV Rodents [Rodentia]
RFV Rodents [Rodentia]
DTV Rodents [Rodentia]
POWV Rodents [Rodentia] ***
AHFV Camelids [Artiodactyla] ***
KFDV Primates [Primates] ***
LGTV Rodents [Rodentia]
OHFV Rodents [Rodentia] ***
TBEV-FE Rodents [Rodentia] ***
TBEV-S Rodents [Rodentia] ***
GGEV Rodents [Rodentia]
TSEV Mammals [Artiodactyla & Rodentia]
TBEV-E Rodents [Rodentia] ***
LIV Livestock & Rodents [Artiodactyla & Rodentia]
SSEV Mammals [Artiodactyla & Rodentia]
Tick-borne
ENTV Bats [Chiroptera]
YOKV Bats [Chiroptera]
NKV
YFV Primates [Primates] ***
SEPV Humans [Primates]
WESSV Ruminants [Artiodactyla]
EHV Marsupials [Marsupialia]
BOUV Primates [Primates]
BANV Rodents [Rodentia]
UGSV Rodents [Rodentia]
JUGV Bats [Chiroptera]
POTV Rodents [Rodentia]
SABV Rodents [Rodentia]
DENV-4 Primates [Primates] ***
DENV-2 Primates [Primates] ***
DENV-1 Primates [Primates] ***
DENV-3 Primates [Primates] ***
KEDV Humans [Primates]
SPOV Humans [Primates]
ZIKV Primates [Primates]
IGUV Rodents [Rodentia]
KOKV Macropods [Marsupialia]
AROAV Rodents [Rodentia]
BSQV Rodents [Rodentia]
ILHV Birds [Aves]
ROCV Birds [Aves]
BAGV Birds [Aves]
SLEV Birds [Aves] ***
KUNV Birds [Aves]
WNV Birds [Aves] ***
JEV Birds [Aves] ***
MVEV Birds [Aves]
USUV Birds [Aves]
Mosquito-borne
1.00/1.00
0.81/1.00
0.75/0.99
0.99/1.00
0.78/1.00
1.00/0.98
0.92/1.00
0.97/0.99
0.98/1.00
0.86/0.70
0.99/1.00
0.3 substitutions site

By comparison to the vector-borne flaviviruses, relatively little is known about the NKV viruses. These viruses are most commonly found in rodents or bats, in which they do not appear to cause disease or a high viremia. NKV viruses of rodents are found only in the New World, whereas those capable of infecting bats are found in both the Old and New Worlds.[270] Although the majority of NKV viruses (12 species) diverged with the TBFVs, two species of bat-associated viruses appear to have evolved from a lineage transmitted by mosquitoes and then lost this trait secondarily (Yokose virus [YOKV] and ENTV)[270,434,806] (Fig. 26.1). These viruses are most similar to the *Aedes* species–vectored viruses of the YFV group. Of interest, studies with chimeric YFV and DENV engineered to express the envelope genes of Modoc virus (MODV) suggest that the host-restriction of NKV viruses may be at a postentry step of the virus life cycle.[138]

Evolution

Many flaviviruses are transmitted by insect vectors, which is a unique feature of the genus not shared by the pestiviruses and hepaciviruses of the *Flaviviridae* family. One hypothesis is that flaviviruses evolved from an ancestral virus that was not vectored. Phylogenic analysis of NS5 sequences supports this notion[271,435]; these studies indicate that the majority of NKV viruses diverged from a lineage that gave rise to vector-borne viruses early in the evolution of flaviviruses. In this context, MBFVs arose from the TBFV lineage. An alternative hypothesis, supported by the analysis of NS3 and complete genome sequences, is that MBFVs diverged first and then gave rise to TBFVs and the majority of NVK viruses[73,275,274,402] (Fig. 26.1). Flaviviruses likely originated in the Old World during the last 10,000 years since the last ice age.[160,270] All of the TBFVs, with the exception of Powassan virus (POWV), are found in the Old World.[271] POWV is found in far eastern Russia and Canada. Deer tick virus (DTV) is a subtype of POWV isolated in New England.[813] That significant speciation of POWV in the New World has not yet occurred suggests a relatively recent introduction. The most divergent MBFVs are found in the Old World.[271] The earliest lineages of the *Aedes* clade viruses are thought to originate in Africa; only DENV and YFV are now found in the New World.[271] Finally, the distribution of the NKV viruses also appears consistent with an Old World origin. Viruses that infect bats are found in either the Old or New World, whereas those associated with rodents occupy restricted niches in the New World. It is possible that bats played an important role in the introduction of these viruses into the New World.[248]

Inspection of the phylogenic trees for MBFV and TBFVs revealed striking differences that may reflect distinct biology of the vectors that transmit them. The portion of the tree that includes the TBEV group is highly asymmetric, with a step-wise branching pattern associated with the evolutionary cline of these

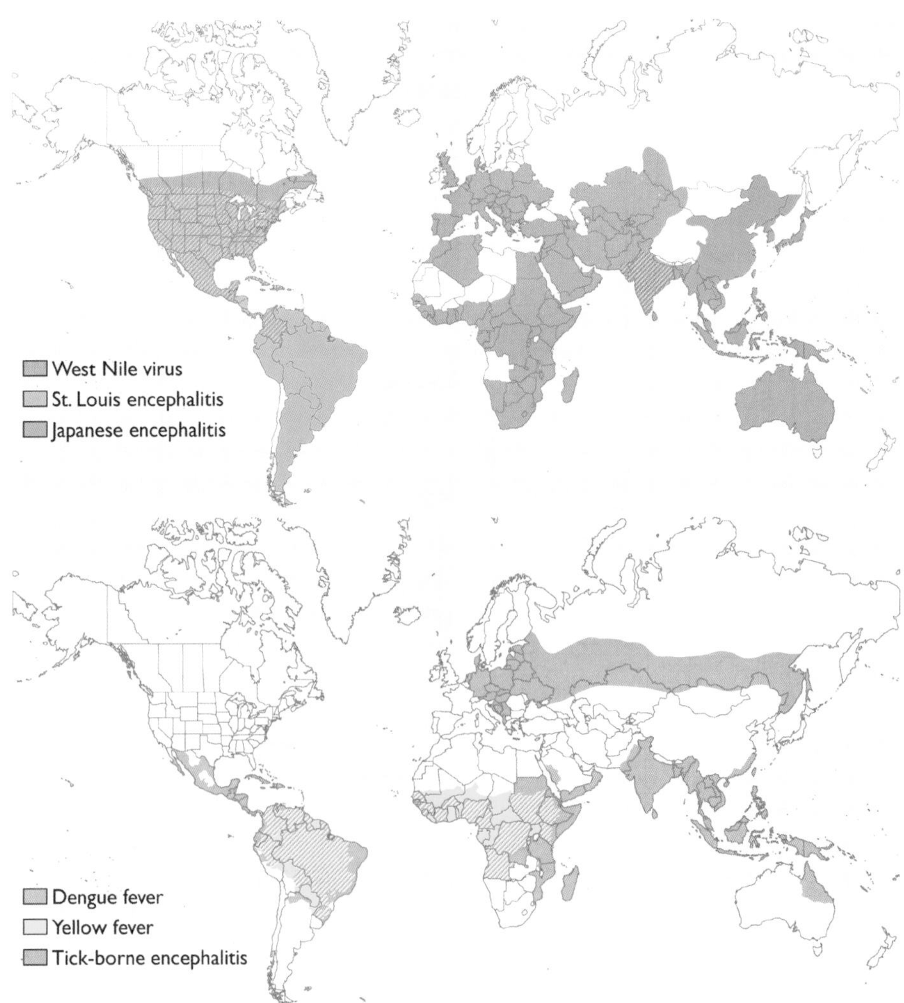

FIGURE 26.2. Global distribution of flaviviruses. The global distribution of flaviviruses with significant impact on global health.

viruses.[910,911] In contrast, the phylogenic tree for MBFVs is more balanced and does not result in a greater number of branches than predicted by chance. MBFVs evolution appears to involve slow phases punctuated by periods of rapid change and diversification. The last two centuries have been characterized by extensive cladogenesis (change that results in new branches on the phylogenetic tree) for the DENV and JEV complexes.

Overall, TBFVs appear to have evolved more slowly than the MBFVs (0.56 times the rate of mosquito-borne viruses).[911] Several aspects of tick biology may limit the number of replication cycles and dispersal of TBFVs in nature that contribute to clinal pattern and modest rate of evolution: (a) ticks live for relatively long periods (2 to 7 years), (b) ticks feed only three times during their lifespan, (c) ticks may transmit viruses to other ticks during co-feeding, minimizing the importance of the vertebrate host for increasing replication cycles, and (d) ticks are relatively immobile unless carried by a vertebrate host. By comparison, MBFVs are transmitted by vectors with the capacity for wider distributions and are quickly replicated through many cycles in the mosquito vector and vertebrate hosts. MBFVs are found in overlapping distributions (e.g., the four serotypes of DENV), whereas TBFVs characteristically occupy defined and nonoverlapping niches.[270]

Global Distribution

Flaviviruses are found on six different continents where they are responsible for endemic and epidemic disease each year (Fig. 26.2). The geographic distribution of flaviviruses has proven quite dynamic, enabling emergence in new geographic areas and increased disease incidence.[514] For example, since its introduction into the Western Hemisphere in 1999, it took only 4 years for the WNV to spread across the United States, where it is now an endemic pathogen. The contribution of human activity toward the spread of flaviviruses is significant.[271] Prior to the development of rapid intercontinental transportation, the movement of flaviviruses between the Old World and New World was uncommon. YFV (and potentially the *Aedes aegypti* mosquito) were introduced into the Americas during the slave trade 300–400 years ago. Importation of YFV by travelers into nonendemic areas, and DENV and WNV into the New World, has been described.[110]

FLAVIVIRUS COMPOSITION AND ANTIGENIC STRUCTURE

Structure

Flaviviruses are small spherical particles composed of three structural proteins, an ~11 kb positive-sense genomic RNA, and a lipid envelope. The envelope (E) protein is a ~53 kD structural protein that functions in multiple steps of the virus life cycle including assembly, budding, attachment to target cells, and viral membrane fusion (reviewed by[591]). The E protein is also the major target of neutralizing antibodies (reviewed by[647,688]). The structure of the ectodomain of the E protein has been determined at the atomic level for several flaviviruses.[557,559,591,623,647,679,918] Flavivirus E protein is an elongated, type II viral fusion protein composed of three distinct domains connected by short flexible hinges (Fig. 26.3AB). Domain I (E-DI) is an eight-stranded β-barrel located in the center of the E protein molecule. This central domain contains two of the six disulfide bonds present in the E protein structure, as well as a site for the addition of an asparagine-linked (N-linked) carbohydrate. Domain II (E-DII) is an elongated structure that mediates dimerization of E proteins on the mature virion. A highly conserved glycine-rich loop composed of 13 amino acids located at the tip of E-DII is thought to insert into the membranes of target cells.[10,98,558] In the context of the dimer, the E-DII fusion loop (E-DII-FL) sits in a hydrophobic pocket formed at the interface of E-DI and domain III (E-DIII). The introduction of mutations into the fusion loop blocks fusion between virions and the membranes of synthetic liposomes.[162] For some flaviviruses, E-DII contains a second N-linked glycosylation site. E-DIII adopts an immunoglobulin-like fold at the carboxy-terminus (C-terminus) of the E protein ectodomain and is stabilized by a single disulfide bridge. E-DIII is the portion of the E protein that projects farthest from the surface of the mature virion and is speculated to contain binding sites for cellular factors involved in virus attachment and entry.[71,153,455,520,679] Many of the most potent neutralizing antibodies characterized to date recognize epitopes on E-DIII (discussed below). The E protein is tethered to the viral membrane by a helical stem (the stem anchor) and two transmembrane domains.[11,591,915]

The precursor to membrane protein (prM) is a ~20 kD protein that facilitates E protein folding and trafficking.[501] In addition, interactions with the E protein prevent the adventitious fusion of the virus during egress.[321] Virion maturation is regulated by the proteolytic cleavage of prM, which results in the formation of a "pr" protein that is ultimately released from the virion and an ~8 kD membrane-associated M peptide. The structure of the "pr" peptide has been determined at the atomic level and is composed of seven β strands held together by three disulfide bonds (Fig. 26.4A).[466] prM interacts with the E protein near at the tip of E-DII adjacent to the fusion loop.[916,917] prM is anchored into the viral membrane via two transmembrane domains.[591,915] Recent studies suggest that antibodies specific for prM are commonly produced *in vivo*.[61,191]

Flaviviruses assemble on virus-induced membranes derived from the endoplasmic reticulum (ER).[353,502,513,861] Virus particles bud into the lumen of these membrane structures as immature virions on which E and prM proteins form heterotrimeric spikes that project from the surface of the virion. Within each spike, the prM protein is located at the tip of the trimer. Immature virions incorporate 60 trimers arranged with icosahedral symmetry (Fig. 26.4B).[907,916,917] Transit of the immature virion through the mildly acidic compartments of the trans-Golgi network (TGN) triggers an extensive rearrangement of E proteins on the immature virion; the lower pH induces a structural transition such that E proteins lie flat as antiparallel dimers on the surface of the virion, analogous to the structure of the mature virion discussed below.[907] Under acidic conditions, prM remains associated with the fusion loop on this structure and protrudes from the surface of an otherwise smooth virus particle. This pH-dependent conformational change increases the susceptibility of prM for a furin-like serine protease.[777] Cleavage of prM is the hallmark of the virion maturation process, and is a required step in the virus life cycle.[223] Release of the virion into the neutral conditions of the extracellular milieu results in the dissociation of the pr peptide.[466,907] Mature virions are relatively smooth virus particles that incorporate 180 copies of the E protein arranged with an unusual herringbone pseudo-T = 3 icosahedral symmetry[425,590,591] (Fig. 26.5A).

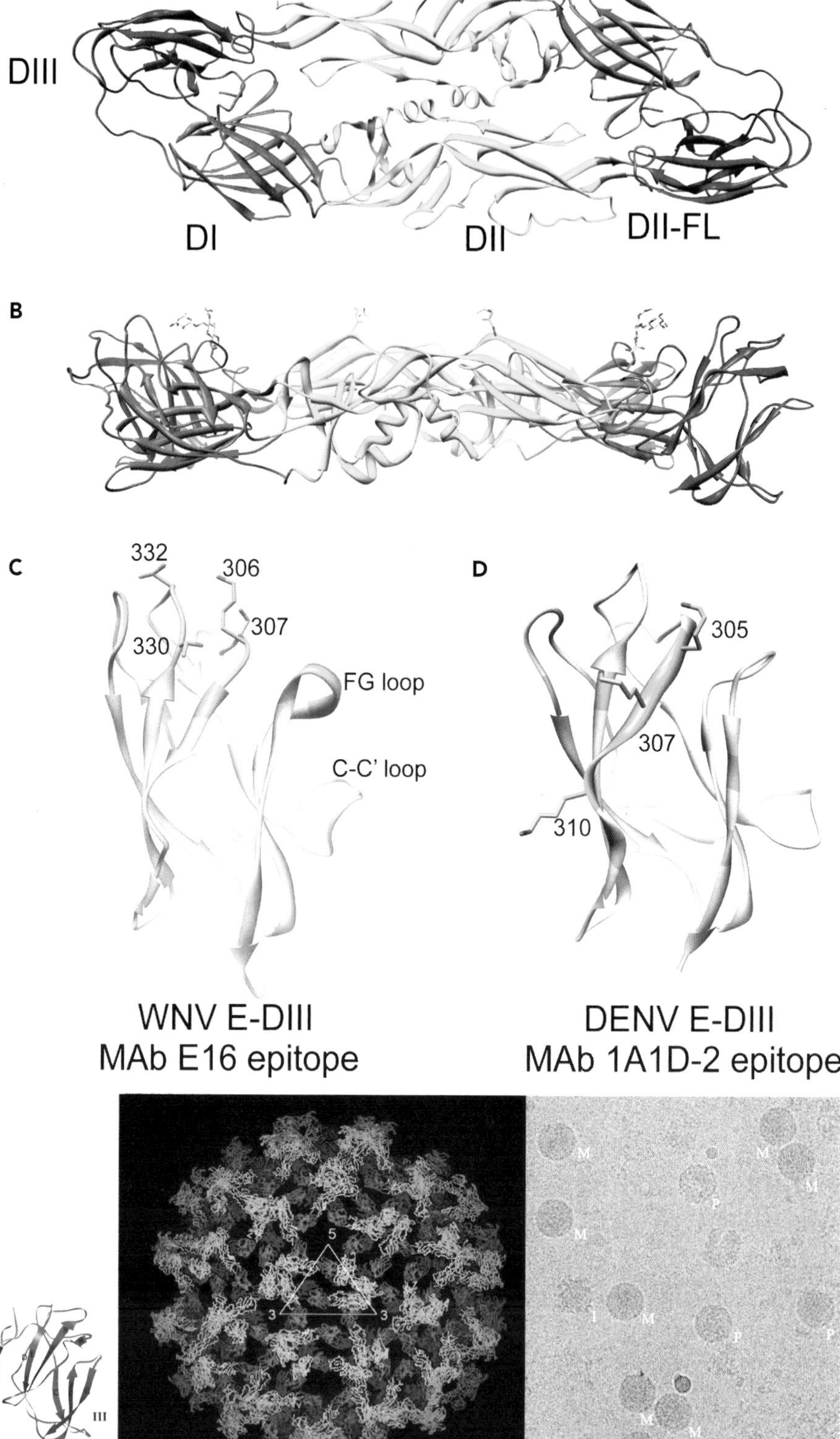

FIGURE 26.3. Structure of the flavivirus E protein. The envelope (E) proteins of flaviviruses are elongated class II viral fusion proteins composed of three structurally distinct domains. **A:** Ribbon diagram of the Dengue virus (DENV) E protein dimer as seen from the top; individual domains of each E protein monomer are indicated (domain I, E-DI, *red;* domain II, E-DII, *yellow;* and domain III, E-DIII, *blue*). The fusion loop at the tip of E-DII is shown in *green.* **B:** DENV E protein as viewed from the side. The stem anchor connecting the E protein to the viral membrane is not shown. The two N-linked carbohydrate modifications at positions Asn67 and Asn154 are shown. **C:** Structure of the West Nile virus (WNV) E-DIII highlighting amino acids that form the epitope recognized by the type-specific neutralizing mAb E16. Residues identified in structural studies as antibody contacts are shown in *brown*; the side chains of residues demonstrated to be critical for antibody binding are shown and labeled. **D:** Structure of the DENV E-DIII highlighting the epitope recognized by the group-reactive mAb 1A1D-2. Residues identified in structural studies as antibody contacts are shown in *brown*; the side chains of residues demonstrated to be critical for antibody binding are shown and labeled. We thank Mr. Phong Lee (National Institute of Allergy and Infectious Diseases [NIAID], National Institutes of Health [NIH]) for preparation of the figure.

FIGURE 26.4. The immature flavivirus virion. The structure of prM and the immature flavivirus virion. **A:** Ribbon representation of the Dengue virus (DENV) pr peptide complexed with the DENV E protein. The pr peptide is shown in *cyan.* Domains I, II, and III of the E protein are shown in *red, yellow,* and *blue,* respectively. **B:** Surface-shaded representation of the immature DENV virion at neutral pH. **C:** Cryo-electron microscopy visualization of extracellular DENV reveals the heterogeneity of virions released from mosquito cell cultures. Immature (I) and mature (M) virions are indicated. Partially mature virions (P) characterized by the appearance of smooth and spiky features on the same virion comprise a significant fraction of the virions released from cells.

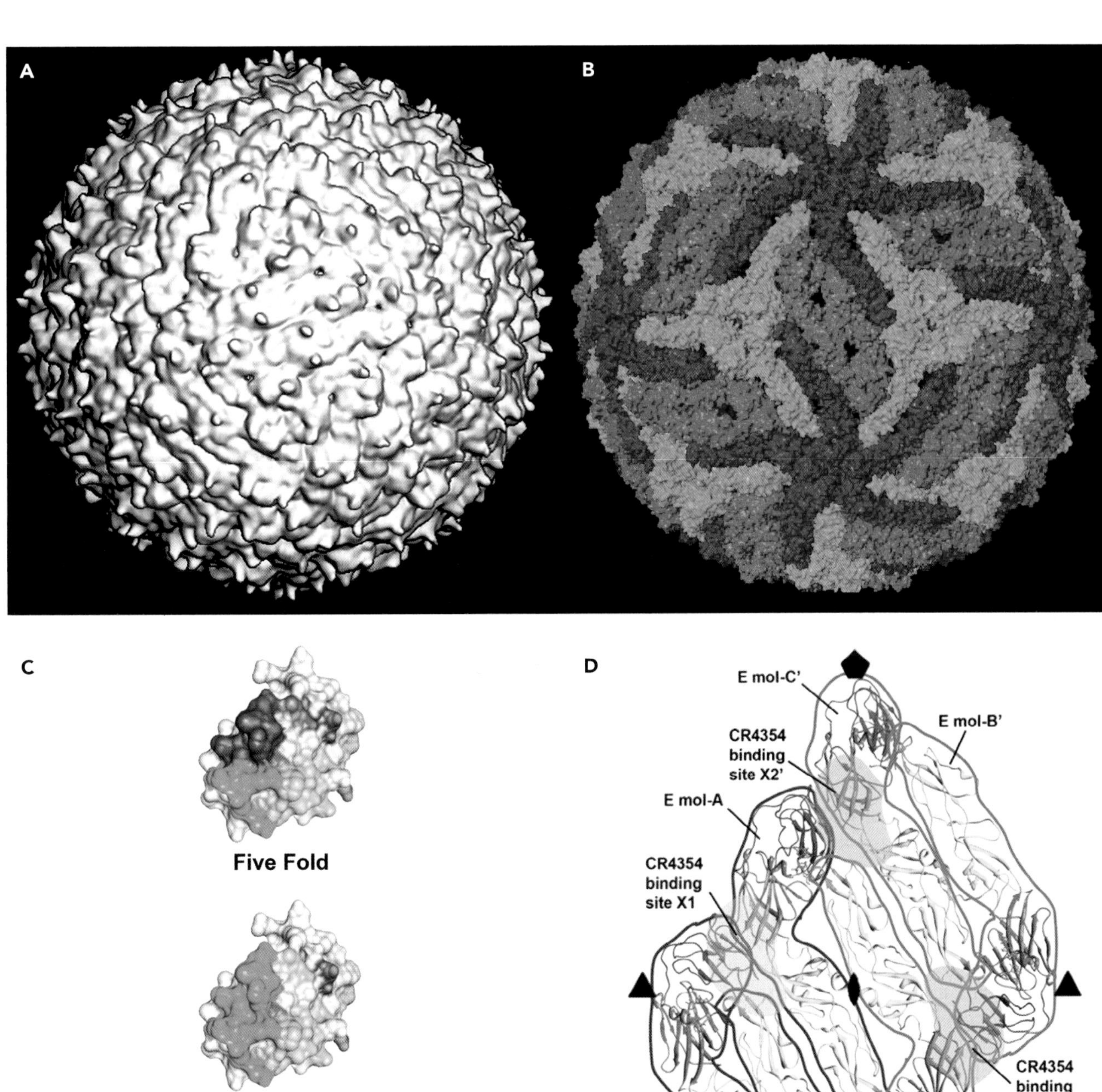

FIGURE 26.5. The arrangement of E proteins on the mature flavivirus increases the complexity of the antigenic surface of the virus particle. **A:** Structure of the mature DENV virion. **B:** Structure of the mature virion highlighting the association of E proteins proximal to the two-, three-, and five-fold symmetry axis of the virion, shown in *red, green,* and *blue,* respectively. **C:** Epitope accessibility varies as a function of the location of a particular E protein on the surface of the pseudo-icosahedral mature virion. Residues important for the binding of mAb E16 are highlighted in *green* for E proteins of each symmetry environment. The steric conflicts that prevent binding of E16 to E proteins proximal to the fivefold symmetry axis are shown in *dark green.* Accessibility of amino acids involved in 1A1D-2 binding are shown in *pink*; steric conflicts that prevent binding to E proteins on the mature virion are shown in *red.* **D:** The complex epitope of mAb 4354 composed of multiple E proteins is shown. Individual domains of each E protein monomer are indicated (domain I, E-DI, *red*; domain II, E-DII, *yellow*; and domain III, E-DIII, *blue*).

Each virion is composed of 30 sets of three antiparallel dimers. In this configuration, E proteins exist in one of three chemically distinct dimer environments defined by their proximity to the two-, three-, or fivefold symmetry axis (Fig. 26.5B).

The Antigenic Surface

Flaviviruses were first classified according to serologic reactivity.[127,188] These early studies generally agreed with approaches that group viruses as a function of genetic relatedness (discussed above, Fig. 26.1).[522] Flavivirus-reactive antibodies are classified as a function of their capacity to discriminate between the antigens of viruses within and between related serologic groups of viruses.[829] For example, monoclonal antibodies that react with DENV may be type-specific (a single DENV serotype), subcomplex-specific (more than one DENV serotype), complex reactive (all DENV viruses), or flavivirus-group reactive (multiple flaviviruses).[322] Type-specific mAbs provided a rapid and specific method for distinguishing between antigenically related viruses.[324,572] Furthermore, recent studies indicate that antibodies differentially recognize different genotypes within a given serotype.[99,751,852]

E Protein Epitopes Recognized by Neutralizing Antibodies

The majority of neutralizing antibodies bind epitopes on the E protein (reviewed in[688]). Early studies distinguished epitopes on the E protein based on the biochemical and functional properties of mAbs including a capacity to bind and compete for viral antigens, neutralize virus, and inhibit hemagglutination of red blood cells.[251,319,322,394,395,411,642,690] An early model of the antigenic structure of the E protein was proposed by Heinz and colleagues that featured three nonoverlapping antigenic domains (A, B, and C); more refined clusters of epitopes within each domain were based on functional differences.[286,318] These studies also identified a small number of antibodies that bound the E protein outside of these domains. This advance not only provided a framework to classify antibodies based on their epitope, but also provided context to consider relationships between epitope location and the functional properties of mAbs.[689] Antigenic domain A epitopes were recognized by cross- and group-reactive antibodies, domain B epitopes were typically type specific, and domain C epitopes were recognized by subtype-specific mAbs.[286,521] These epitopes were subsequently shown to correspond to E-DII, E-DIII, and E-DI, respectively.[679]

All three domains of the E protein are recognized by neutralizing antibodies, albeit with widely varying potency. Epitopes of some of the most well-characterized antibodies to date are described below, although it should be anticipated that this list will expand as greater insight to the complexity of the antigenic surface of the virion is obtained:

E-DIII-LR

Many of the most potent neutralizing antibodies characterized to date bind epitopes on E-DIII. Potently neutralizing antibodies that bind an epitope on the domain III lateral ridge (E-DIII-LR) of several flaviviruses have been identified.[52,150,170,279,627,647,689,708,751] mAb E16 is a type-specific WNV-reactive mAb that neutralizes at picomolar concentrations *in vitro* and protects mice from lethal challenge when administered 5 days after infection.[581,582,627,648] The structure of E16 bound to E-DIII has been determined and revealed a binding footprint composed of four discontinuous loops centered on amino acids of the BC loop and amino-terminal region (positions 306, 307, 330, and 332)[624] (see Fig. 26.3C). Type-specific neutralizing antibodies against DENV-2 have been mapped to an epitope composed of multiple regions of the upper lateral surface of E-DIII, including the FG loop.[279,360,380,794,795] The binding of many of these antibodies to DIII is also sensitive to amino acid substitutions on the BC loop, C-C′ loop, the amino-terminal region (residue 301), or the A-strand (e.g., residue 304); the latter structure is also recognized by antibodies that neutralize DENV with subcomplex specificity, as discussed below. For example, the highly characterized mAb 3H5 recognizes an epitope composed of residues on both the FG loops and the A strand.[795] Mapping experiments with type-specific DENV-1,[751] DENV-3,[99,852] JEV,[891] and TBEV[786] antibodies have identified similar epitopes.

E-DIII A-Strand

Antibodies with a pattern of complex and subcomplex reactivity have been mapped to the A-strand of E-DIII.[497,671,795,824] mAb 1A1D-2 potently neutralizes DENV-1, DENV-2, and DENV-3, but fails to bind DENV-4 viruses. The structure of mAb 1A1D-2 bound to E-DIII was solved and revealed that this antibody binds an epitope on the A strand and is sensitive to mutation of DENV residues 305, 307, and 310 (see Fig. 26.3D).[497] In addition, these studies identified residues in the G strand that play a role in antibody binding, consistent with mapping studies of other complex- and group-reactive antibodies.[280,489,751,824]

E-DII-FL

Antibodies that bind the fusion loop of E-DII are highly cross-reactive.[168,171,629,787] Although mutation of conserved fusion loop residues reduces antibody binding, other adjacent structures also may contribute to the fine specificity of antibody binding and the functional properties of these antibodies.[266,629] The structure of the WNV fusion loop-reactive antibody mAb E53 bound to soluble E proteins has been determined.[149] Residues shown to be important antibody contacts include those of the fusion loop (residues 104–107, and 109–110) as well as residues of the BC-loop of E-DII.[629] The fusion loop epitope is also poorly accessible on the mature virion, as discussed in detail below.[629,787]

E-DI

Antibodies that bind E-DI have also been characterized. mAb 5H2 is a type-specific antibody that neutralizes DENV-4. Neutralization escape studies mapped 5H2 binding to an epitope that includes residue 174 of E-DI.[445] DI-reactive antibodies that bind WNV (E121; residues 175, 191, 193, and 194), DENV2 (mAb DV2–48, residue 177), and TBEV (IC3 and i2, residues D181 and K171, respectively) also have been characterized.[338,521,629,794] The recently described WNV mAb CR4354 that binds a complex epitope that includes the linker between E-DI and E-DII will be described in detail below.[384]

Antibodies That Bind the prM Protein

Antibodies that react with the prM protein have been described.[61,121,191,229,844] Generally, these antibodies are characterized by low neutralizing activity *in vitro.* Recent studies suggest that anti-prM antibodies are elicited frequently *in vivo,* and may contribute to the pathogenesis of DENV infection as discussed below.[191,685] Human monoclonal antibodies to WNV prM protein have been isolated and mapped to residues V19, T20, T24, and L33.[121]

Complexities of Antibody Recognition of the Virion

The complex and dynamic arrangement of the E proteins on the surface of flaviviruses complicates an understanding of how antibodies interact with flaviviruses. E proteins exist on the mature virus particle in different chemical environments (Fig. 26.5B; defined in relation to the two-, three-. and five-fold symmetry axes of the pseudo-icosahedral particle), which impacts antibody recognition. Amino acids involved in antibody recognition may be differentially accessible for antibody binding depending on their location on the virus particle.[624,629,787] As mentioned above, the WNV mAb E16 binds a cluster of residues on the upper lateral surface of E-DIII.[624] However, this epitope is not uniformly accessible for antibody binding on all E proteins on the mature virus; steric constraints imposed by the tight packing of E-DIII on E proteins at the fivefold axis of symmetry prevent antibody binding to these molecules (Fig. 26.5C).[383,624] Therefore, although the mature virion incorporates 180 copies of the E protein, a maximum of 120 antibodies physically can bind the virus particle. This is not an unusual feature of this antibody as none of the antibodies studied to date using structural methods appear capable of binding all E proteins on the intact mature virus particle. In fact, the molecular basis for recognition by many antibodies cannot be explained using static models of virion structure.

Epitopes Can Be Composed of More Than One Protein on the Surface of the Virion

Virions contain 180 individual E proteins. To date, most of the well-characterized antibodies are capable of binding monomeric E proteins, indicating their epitopes are composed of residues contained within a single E protein molecule. However, complex epitopes composed of contact residues from adjacent E proteins have been described.[168,384,521] mAb CR4354 is a human antibody that binds the hinge between E-DI and E-DII. Mapping studies using recombinant forms of the E protein failed to identify the CR4354 epitope because this antibody was unable to bind soluble forms of the E protein. A loss-of-function substitution at position K136 was defined by neutralization escape studies.[850] Cryoelectron microscopic reconstructions of CR4354 Fab fragments bound to the mature virion revealed a complex epitope composed of residues on neighboring E proteins (Fig. 26.5D).[384]

Incomplete Virion Maturation Impacts Antibody-Mediated Neutralization

Cleavage of prM is a required step in the flavivirus life cycle; mutation of the RRXR/S motif in prM recognized by furin-like proteases renders TBEV noninfectious.[223] However, biochemical analysis of preparations of flaviviruses released from cells indicated that a substantial amount of prM may remain uncleaved. Recent studies demonstrate that more than 90% of DENV virions could be precipitated with anti-prM antibodies.[368] Electron microscopy studies identified virus particles with structural features of both mature and immature virions (hereafter referred to as "partially mature virions") (Fig. 26.4C).[653] Several lines of evidence suggest that partially mature virions are infectious. Virions produced in the presence of ammonium chloride display a reduced sensitivity to inactivation when exposed to acid, presumably because pH-mediated changes in the conformation of E protein are reversible when complexed with prM.[285] In addition, the carbohydrate on prM can mediate attachment of the lineage II 956 strain of WNV (which lacks an N-linked carbohydrate on the E protein) onto cells expressing the c-type lectin CD209L.[183] Although these studies demonstrate that virions containing prM may be infectious, the stoichiometric requirements of prM cleavage have not yet been determined.

The presence of partially mature secreted virions impacts antibody recognition in at least two ways. Increasing the efficiency of virion maturation resulted in a marked reduction in the sensitivity of WNV to neutralization by antibodies that bind several structurally distinct epitopes, including the DI-LR and DII-FL epitopes recognized by mAbs E121 and E53, respectively.[607] Conversely, decreasing the extent of virion maturation enhanced neutralization by these mAbs. An analysis of the sensitivity of polyclonal antibody elicited by vaccination with two distinct candidate WNV vaccines revealed maturation state-dependent changes in neutralization potency in roughly half the volunteers.[607] The structural basis for this pattern of recognition has been investigated.[149] mAb E53 does not efficiently bind the E protein on mature virions due to poor accessibility of the fusion loop epitope on the mature virus particle. In addition to modulating the potency of neutralizing antibodies, uncleaved prM on infectious virus particles may interact directly with antibodies, resulting in enhanced infection of Fcγ-receptor bearing cells *in vitro* and *in vivo* as discussed below.[61,191,347,685,912]

Impact of Structural Dynamics of the Virus Particle

Flaviviruses present a complex and dynamic antigenic surface to the immune system that is not fully captured by the static models of virion structure. It has long been appreciated that proteins are in constant motion and sample an ensemble of conformations at equilibrium.[84] Proteins incorporated into virus particles also are structurally dynamic.[361,888] Virus "breathing" has been demonstrated for several unrelated classes of viruses,[88,459] and may affect antibody recognition.[467,905] As an example, the accessibility of the A-strand epitope on the mature virion is limited by steric constraints arising from the arrangement of E proteins on the virus particle. The binding of Fab fragments of the subcomplex-reactive A-strand–specific mAb 1A1D-2 to mature DENV virions was shown to be temperature dependent; significant Fab binding was observed only after incubation at 37°C.[497] Cryoelectron microscopic reconstruction of mature DENV bound by the 1A1D-2 FAb revealed significant changes in the arrangement and orientation of E proteins on the surface of the virus particle. These results suggested that the binding of 1A1D-2 stabilized the E proteins in a state distinct from the herringbone arrangement found on mature virions. More recent studies suggest the impact of viral dynamics on antibody-mediated neutralization is widespread among antibodies of differing specificity. Analysis of the neutralizing activity of a panel of mAbs specific for structurally distinct epitopes revealed a time- and temperature-dependent aspect of neutralization of WNV and DENV attributed to changes in epitope accessibility arising from the dynamic motion of E proteins on the virion.[210] Given sufficient time, even epitopes that are poorly accessible in all three symmetry axes of the mature virion may support some level of neutralization. The scope of the structural conformations sampled by flaviviruses at equilibrium is not yet understood. Changes in the configuration of E proteins on dynamic virions have the potential to affect several aspects of antibody binding (functional affinity, bivalency, antibody binding orientation), and thus, complicates our understanding of the antigenic surface of the flavivirus virion.

Antibodies to NS1 Can Protect In vivo

NS1, a protein that is absent from the virion, is secreted at high levels into the extracellular environment during flavivirus infection, predominantly as a hexamer,[238] with significant accumulation (up to 50 μg/ml) in the sera of DENV-infected patients.[6,28,470,906] In addition, soluble NS1 can bind back to the plasma membrane of cells through an interaction with specific sulfated glycosaminoglycans.[29] Furthermore, NS1 is expressed directly on the surface of infected cells, possibly via glycosyl phosphatidyl inositol (GPI) linkage,[354] lipid raft association,[621] or through an as-yet undefined mechanism. Several groups also have generated nonneutralizing, yet protective mAbs against NS1.[155,156,194,230,323,665,720,721,723–725] Therefore, protection against flavivirus infections *in vivo* does not always correlate with neutralizing activity *in vitro.*[93,690,722] Beyond direct virus neutralization, antibody binding to virions or virus-infected cells can trigger protective Fc-dependent antiviral activities through complement activation or Fc-γ receptor–mediated immune complex clearance mechanisms. Fc-γ receptors can activate or inhibit immune responses depending on their cytoplasmic domain and association with specific signaling molecules.[617] A requirement for Fc effector function has been established for protective anti-NS1 mAbs. NS1 is expressed on the cell surface or secreted into the extracellular space and antagonizes complement control of flavivirus infection by binding the negative regulator factor H or by promoting C4 degradation.[24,154] Passive transfer of mAbs against NS1 can protect mice against lethal infection by WNV and YFV,[155,722] and this requires an intact Fc moiety.[725] Mechanistic studies using immunodeficient mice demonstrate that protective anti-NS1 mAbs recognize cell surface–associated NS1 and trigger Fc-γ receptor–dependent phagocytosis and clearance of WNV-infected cells.[156]

CLINICAL AND PATHOLOGIC SYNDROMES OF THE FLAVIVIRUSES

DENGUE VIRUS

History, Global Distribution, and Epidemic Cycle

The natural cycle of epidemic Dengue virus (DENV) infection is between the mosquito vector (*Aedes albopictus* or *Aedes aegypti)* and humans (Fig. 26.6). After mosquito inoculation, DENV infection causes a spectrum of clinical disease ranging from self-limited Dengue fever (DF) to a life-threatening hemorrhagic and capillary leak syndrome (Dengue hemorrhagic fever [DHF]/Dengue shock syndrome [DSS]). Globally, there is significant diversity among DENV strains, including four distinct serotypes (DENV-1, DENV-2, DENV-3, and DENV-4) that differ at the amino acid level in the viral envelope proteins by 25% to 40%. DENV causes an estimated 25 to 100 million infections and 250,000 cases of DHF/DSS per year worldwide, with 2.5 billion people at risk.[298,562]

Although a dengue-like syndrome may have occurred in China several times during the first millennium AD, the initial description of a DENV epidemic is attributed to Benjamin Rush, a physician in Philadelphia, in his article reporting a febrile outbreak in 1780.[694] Primary DENV infection and epidemics were common in North America, the Caribbean, Asia, and Australia during the 18th and 19th centuries, presumably due to the widespread ecology of the mosquito vectors. During World War II, DENV spread to and through Southeast Asia. Troop movement and the destruction of the environment and human settlements are believed to have promoted the spread of DENV and their mosquito vectors throughout Southeast Asia and the Western Pacific.[433] Since 1950, the number of people infected has risen steadily, such that today DENV is the leading arthropod-borne viral disease in the world. With the spread and co-circulation of multiple DENV serotypes, secondary infection with heterologous serotypes and epidemic DHF/DSS emerged 50 years ago in Southeast Asia,[310] and more recently in the Americas in 1981[420] and South Asia in 1989.[551] Since the 1950s, epidemics involving thousands of people with multiple DENV serotypes and strains occur annually in multiple parts of the world, including the Americas, Asia, Africa, and Australia, in essence wherever the primary mosquito vector *Aedes aegypti* is present. Indeed, after a recent outbreak of DENV

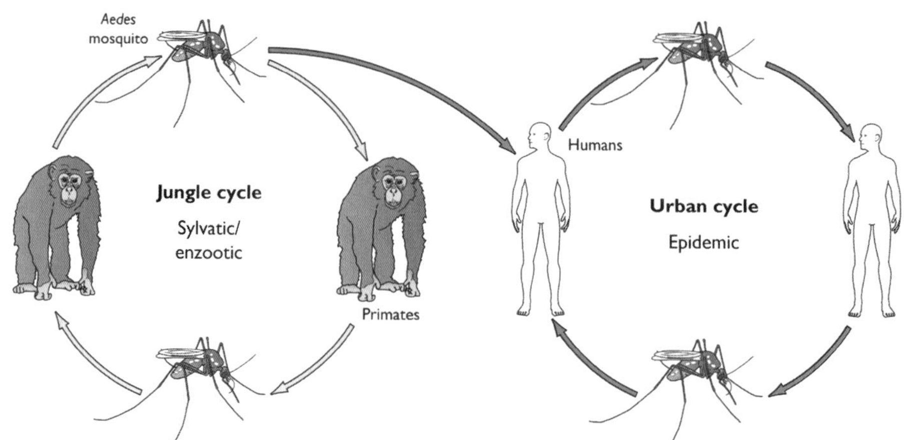

FIGURE 26.6. Life cycle of Dengue virus (DENV). DENV circulates in nature in two relatively distinct transmission cycles vectored by *Aedes* sp. mosquitoes. DENV infection of humans results in a sufficiently high viremia to support infection of feeding mosquitoes; transmission cycles of DENV do not require an enzootic amplifying host. DENV may also replicate in a sylvatic cycle. Although incompletely understood, the contribution of sylvatic strains of DENV to human infections appears minimal.

in Key West Florida in 2009, a serosurvey conducted by the Centers for Disease Control and Prevention (CDC) reported that 5.4% of households had evidence of recent DENV infection.[1] As a reflection of this, the global incidence of DHF/DSS has increased more than 500-fold, with more than 100 countries affected by outbreaks of dengue.[442]

DENV Diversity

Globally, there is significant diversity among DENV strains. The four serotypes of DENV (DENV-1, DENV-2, DENV-3, and DENV-4) are genetically distinct but cause similar diseases and share epidemiologic features. All DENV strains are members of the Dengue antigenic complex; inclusion of a strain as DENV is based on antigen cross-reactivity, sequence homology, and genome organization.[120] The four serotypes of DENV were historically distinguished by limited cross-neutralization or hemagglutination inhibition using serum from infected individuals. Subsequent sequencing analysis revealed that individual serotypes of DENV can differ from one another at the amino acid level significantly, with 30% to 40% variation in the viral envelope proteins. However, within a given serotype, amino acid homology is much greater, with conservation levels at approximately 90% or higher. Therefore, individual DENV serotypes (e.g., DENV-1 versus DENV-4) vary far more than distinct viruses in Japanese encephalitis serocomplex (e.g., WNVs and JEVs vary by 10% to 15% at the amino acid level), which has led some to consider DENV as a group of four different viruses that are linked by serology, epidemiology, and disease pathogenesis. Differences in severity associated with individual serotypes or particular sequences of serotypes in sequential infection have been observed, and it still is unclear whether some serotypes are inherently more pathogenic than others. DENV-2 viruses have been commonly associated with DHF/DSS,[36,112,821] as are DENV-1 and DENV-3 viruses.[273,314,551] In comparison, DENV-4 appears more commonly to be clinically mild, although it can cause severe disease.[619]

Genetic variation of DENV, however, is not limited to serotype. Geographic variants within a serotype were initially identified by RNase fingerprint assays.[678,847] Subsequently, nucleic acid sequencing confirmed differences within each serotype, allowing for classification of genotypes that vary further by up to approximately 6% and 3% at the nucleotide and amino acid levels, respectively.[337,681] DENV genotype classification was originally defined by sequence variation within a given genomic region (e.g., *E* and *NS1* genes). More recent analysis has used high-throughput full genome sequencing technologies to assign phylogenetic classification. Although there remains some dissonance among investigators, most classification schemes include five DENV-1 genotypes, four or five DENV-2 genotypes, four DENV-3 genotypes, and two or three DENV-4 genotypes.[682,874] Beyond serotype and genotype, two further types of DENV complexity should be mentioned: strain variation and quasispecies. DENV strain variation refers to the limited change that occurs among individual isolates; this was classically described as within a serotype, although as DENV continues to emerge and evolve, variation now occurs within a genotype. Strain variation within a genotype may be functionally important, as it can affect antibody neutralization, presumably due to changes at key sites within exposed epitopes.[99,794,852,925]

In addition to serotype, genotype, and strain variation, DENV has the capacity to accumulate variation rapidly within an individual host. Viral quasispecies comprises a cloud of variants that are genetically linked through mutation. It is observed during infection by many RNA viruses (e.g., hepatitis C virus [HCV], human immunodeficiency virus [HIV], and influenza) and creates diversity that allows a viral population to adapt rapidly to dynamic environments and evolve resistance to immune responses, vaccines, and antiviral drugs.[450,848] DENV exists as a collection of highly similar variants forming a quasispecies[869] by virtue of its error-prone NS5 polymerase, which has an estimated mutation rate of 10^3 to 10^5 substitutions per nucleotide copied per round of replication.[137,836] Preliminary studies suggest that genetic diversity is greater in the structural proteins, which may have less constraint to maintain integral functions. The study of genetic and intrahost diversity for DENV is still in its relative infancy, and thus more analysis is warranted to define how mutation and variation impact fitness, tropism, and resistance.

Clinical Features of Acute DF: Primary DENV Infection

DENV infection of humans after mosquito inoculation causes a spectrum of clinical disease ranging from inapparent disease (~50% of infections[37,112,224]), self-limited dengue fever (DF) to severe DHF and DSS. A classical presentation of DF is an abrupt onset of a debilitating febrile illness characterized by headache, retroorbital pain, myalgias, arthralgias, and a maculopapular rash that occurs after a 2- to 7-day incubation period after mosquito inoculation.[700] Some individuals experience severe bone and joint pain ("break-bone fever") and develop petechial hemorrhages that are associated with mild to severe thrombocytopenia. There is no specific constellation of signs or symptoms to differentiate DF from other acute flu-like viral syndromes, so a health care provider must have a high index of suspicion for diagnosis in the setting of the appropriate epidemiology. DF also may present in a less classical form as an undifferentiated febrile illness with rash along with mild upper respiratory symptoms (cough, pharyngitis, rhinitis), particularly in children. DF is usually self-limited, lasting 1 to 2 weeks, although some (up to 25% of hospitalized patients) experience a prolonged postinfectious fatigue and depression syndrome that can persist for weeks, akin to that seen after Epstein-Barr virus (EBV) infection and mononucleosis.[739] Because of the debilitating fever and musculoskeletal symptoms, the morbidity toll is high in clinically apparent DF, whereas the mortality rate is exceedingly low. Primary DF usually occurs during the initial DENV infection of an individual, with the exception of infants from immune mothers that have acquired antibodies transplacentally.

Clinical Features of DHF/DSS: Secondary and Infant DENV Infection

The incidence of the most severe form of DENV disease, DHF/DSS, varies considerably between primary and secondary infections. A secondary DENV infection results when a person previously infected with one serotype is exposed to a different serotype, and is the single most important risk factor for severe dengue disease.[112,224,294,305] Epidemiologic data in Thailand has shown greater than 10-fold higher rates of DHF/DSS during secondary compared to primary infection of children.[843] It should be pointed out that even during secondary infection, DHF/DSS is quite rare, with only 0.5% of secondary infections progressing to the most severe forms of dengue disease. DHF/DSS is characterized by rapid onset of capillary leakage accompanied by thrombocytopenia and mild to moderate liver damage, reflected by increases in serum levels of hepatic enzyme (e.g., aspartate aminotransferase [AST] and alanine aminotransferase [ALT]).[301] DHF/DSS usually occurs as a second phase of the illness, after a short period of defervescence from the initial fever. Hemorrhagic manifestations are observed in a subset of DHF/DSS cases and include petechiae, epistaxis, gastrointestinal bleeding (hematemesis or melena), menorrhagia, and a positive tourniquet test. Use of the term hemorrhagic fever instead of dengue capillary-leak syndrome has led many to anticipate that bleeding is the greatest threat. Rather, fluid loss into tissue spaces with hemoconcentration and hypotension can result in shock, which carries the highest risk of mortality.[612] From a diagnostic standpoint, an elevated hematocrit and upper abdominal ultrasonogram showing a thickened gall bladder wall, hepatomegaly, ascites, or pleural effusions are evidence of fluid shifts associated with a capillary leak syndrome.

Whereas DHF/DSS occur largely after secondary infection by a different DENV serotyope in children and adults,[273] in infants younger than age one born to dengue-immune mothers, primary infection can cause severe DHF/DSS.[305,356,764] In clinical studies, maternal anti-DENV neutralization antibody titers and age of the infant correlated with disease. The actual age at which DHF/DSS occur in infants (peak at 7 months) corresponds to the age at which maximum enhancing activity for DENV infection in primary monocytes is observed in vitro.[405] Severe clinical manifestations of DHF/DSS are more prevalent in infants[311] and there is an approximately fourfold higher mortality rate compared to other age groups.[373] Infants represent approximately 5% of children hospitalized with DHF/DSS in many parts of Southeast Asia.[140,273,303] The more prevalent or severe clinical manifestations associated with infant DHF/DSS include seizures, hepatic dysfunction, thrombocytopenia, high-grade fever, diffuse rash, peripheral edema, ascites, and frank shock.[356]

Although it is not fully accepted by the field, some clinical studies have suggested that severe DENV infection also can have neurologic manifestations including transverse myelitis, Guillain-Barre syndrome, encephalitis, and encephalopathy,[769,841] occurring in as many as 1% to 6% of DHF/DSS cases.[122,325] In contrast to other encephalitic flaviviruses (e.g., JEV, WNV, or tick-borne encephalitis viruses), DENV historically has not been considered as neurotropic. However, the discovery of DENV and anti-DENV immunoglobulin M (IgM) in the cerebrospinal fluid of patients with encephalopathy suggests that it may be capable of causing central nervous system (CNS) infection as part of a severe DHF/DSS syndrome, at least in a subset of individuals.[507,769] In support of this, focal imaging abnormalities have been detected in brain MRI scans of DENV-infected patients.[122,872] Although these results are suggestive, bona fide DENV encephalitis and CNS disease may not be fully accepted until its antigens are reliably detected in the brains of encephalopathic patients and a more complete understanding of the molecular determinants for neurotropism is acquired.

Pathologic Features of DHF/DSS

Although DENV is the leading mosquito-borne transmitted viral infection in the world, there are few detailed autopsy series of patients who succumbed to DHF/DSS, and fewer performed with newer molecular techniques and markers. Detailed histopathologic studies that might inform a basic understanding of DENV pathogenesis are rare because much of the lethal disease occurs in regions lacking sophisticated laboratory infrastructure, highly trained personnel, and repositories for long-term tissue storage. Forensic studies also are complicated by lack of standardization of histologic procedures and variation in the quality of specimen preparation and storage.

A recent summary of the autopsy literature from a total of 160 fatal DHF/DSS cases occurring primarily in children and adolescents was published.[531] Pathologic findings in the liver of DHF/DSS cases include centrilobular necrosis, changes in fatty tissue, inflammatory leukocyte infiltration, and Kupffer cell hyperplasia.[70,113] Gross macroscopic examination revealed multiple hemorrhagic foci. Microscopic analysis has shown increased inflammatory infiltrates around the portal vessels, sinusoidal congestion, small hemorrhages, midzonal hepatocyte necrosis, and microvesicular steatosis.[228,293] In other tissues (spleen or lung) hemorrhage, tissue edema, and plasma leakage have been observed.[50]

A key to understanding the pathogenesis of severe DENV infection is defining cellular tropism of infection, which could influence the host inflammatory response that results in the capillary leakage syndrome. Autopsy series have shown the presence of DENV antigen or nucleic acid in cells of the skin, liver, spleen, lymph nodes, kidney, lung, thymus, or brain.[38,50,165,293,377,392,553,692] However, several of these studies used in situ hybridization or reverse transcriptase polymerase chain reaction (RT-PCR) based assays, and thus have not definitively shown that infectious virus is produced in a given cell of a target tissue. In severe DENV cases, infectious virus can be reliably isolated from blood, lymphoid tissues, and the liver, although the cellular source of the virus remains controversial. Studies in humans, nonhuman primates, and small animal models support a role for infection of myeloid cells (blood monocytes, tissue macrophages, Kupffer cells), and possibly other cells including hepatocytes[296] and endothelial cells.[50,912]

YELLOW FEVER VIRUS

History, Global Distribution, and Epidemic Cycle

Several recent excellent reviews have described the epidemiology and historical details of yellow fever virus (YFV) infection.[41,222,246] YFV, the causative agent of yellow fever virus (YFV), was first isolated (strain Asibi) in 1927 after inoculation of a rhesus monkey with the blood of a patient from Ghana.[789] YFV originated in Africa, was imported into the Americas during the slave trade, and had the first reported epidemic in the Yucatan in 1648.[45] Historically, large epidemics of YF disease occurred beyond these regions and were described in the 17th through 20th centuries as far north in the Americas as Canada, as well as in parts of Europe including Spain, Italy, France, and England.[566] Despite the presence of an effective vaccine (17D strain) that was developed in 1937 by Max Theiler and colleagues,[820] with more than 500 million doses administered to humans,[246] YFV infection has remained a public health threat in restricted parts of the world. Currently, YFV is endemic in the tropical regions of Africa and the Americas, infects humans and nonhuman primates, and is transmitted by mosquitoes including *Aedes aegypti*. The World Health Organization (WHO) estimates an incidence of 200,000 cases per year, leading to about 30,000 deaths, with the majority occurring in sub-Saharan Africa.[890] Overall, 44 countries in Africa and the Americas are considered within the modern YFV endemic zone, with almost 900 million people at risk of infection.[222,246]

The sylvatic or jungle cycle of YFV in which transmission occurs between mosquitoes and wild monkeys explains why extensive vaccination campaigns have reduced but not eradicated infection. In East Africa, YFV infection is maintained enzootically in monkey transmission cycles in the jungle with the *Aedes africanus* mosquito vector. Periodically, infection may cross into humans during an intermediate savannah cycle, with transmission by several different *Aedes* mosquito species (e.g., *Aedes bromeliae*). Indeed, in the Americas, most cases appear to be a result of humans intruding on the jungle cycle of YFV.[47] Epidemic YFV infection (human–mosquito–human cycle) ensues in urban or domestic areas with *Aedes aegypti* as the principal mosquito vector. Rapid urbanization in Africa and the Americas with population shifts from rural to urban settings combined with the collapse of mosquito eradication programs has allowed the *A. aegypti* vector to repopulate many parts of the world, and caused YFV to be classified as a reemerging threat for humans.[246]

YFV Diversity

YFV does not belong to an antigenic subgroup based on plaque reduction neutralization assays,[120] but shows greater genetic relationship to other African flaviviruses including Banzi, Zika, Wesselsbron, and Bouboui viruses. Indeed, cross-protection against YFV infection in monkeys has been shown after immunization with some of these related viruses.[326] Although there is only one serotype of YFV, there is significant diversity within the genus. Seven genotypes have been proposed including two West African genotypes, a single Central/South African genotype, two East African genotypes, and two South American genotypes.[222] These genotypes of YFV were originally defined based on nucleotide variation of greater than 9% in the prM, E, and 3′ UTR gene regions[601,858] and have been confirmed with full-genome sequencing of YFV isolates.[851] Phylogenic studies suggest that YFV originated in East or Central Africa and was introduced subsequently into West Africa and South America.[600,601] Beyond genotypes, sequence analysis of 79 YFV strains isolated from 1935 to 2001 in Brazil revealed further strain divergence into clades that differ at the nucleotide and amino acid level by up to 7% and 5%, respectively.[842] The physiologic basis for genotype-specific amino acid variation between YFV isolates remains uncertain, although it is likely that selection confers a phenotypic advantage in a given host.

Clinical Features of YFV Infection

In humans, YFV infection causes a variable clinical syndrome ranging from no symptoms, to mild febrile flu-like illness, to fulminate and possibly fatal disease. Approximately 15% of people who become infected develop severe visceral disease, and in this group there is a 20% to 50% case fatality rate.[564] Symptoms occur within 3 to 6 days of mosquito inoculation and include an abrupt onset of fever, chills, myalgia, back pain, and headache or the first "period of infection," which usually lasts 3 days and corresponds to peak viremia. During this phase, individuals are infectious to mosquitoes. In some, this stage may be followed by a short "period of remission," with defervescence and improvement of clinical signs and symptoms. Shortly after, in a subset (20%) of patients, fever and symptoms worsen ("period of intoxication") with vomiting, epigastric pain, and jaundice (which gives yellow fever its name); this is associated with YFV replication in the liver, an absence of viremia, and measurable anti-YFV antibodies in serum. As time progresses, severe YFV infection evolves into a hemorrhagic fever characterized by severe hepatitis, renal failure, hemorrhage, shock, and multiorgan failure. A bleeding diathesis manifests with melena, hematemesis, epistaxis, ecchymosis, menorrhagia, petechial hemorrhages, and blood oozing from mucous membranes. Renal failure is associated with an abrupt decrease in urine output and with albuminuria. Laboratory tests show leukopenia, thrombocytopenia, and a coagulopathy. Death occurs on the 7th to 10th day of illness and is preceded by hemodynamic and cardiovascular instability, acute liver failure, hypothermia, hypoglycemia, and coma. For those individuals surviving severe YFV infection, convalescence is prolonged with hepatitis and associated constitutional symptoms persisting sometimes for months.

Pathologic Features of YFV Infection

Macroscopic gross pathology of tissues from YFV infection autopsy studies show an enlarged and icteric liver and edematous and enlarged kidneys and heart. Microscopic pathologic analyses of the liver reveal six major features,[246,408,567] which occur primarily during the last "period of intoxication": (a) eosinophilic degeneration of hepatocytes and Kupffer cells; (b) midzonal hepatocellular swelling and necrosis, with sparing of the cells in the portal area; (c) the presence of Councilman bodies coincident with hepatocyte cell death; (d) absence of leukocyte inflammatory infiltrates; (e) microvesicular fatty changes and lipid accumulation, likely secondary to decreased apoprotein synthesis by hepatocytes; and (f) retention of the reticulin structure. YFV antigen and RNA are demonstrable in hepatocytes by immunohistochemistry or in situ hybridization,[187] and this coupled with the absence of inflammation, suggests that the cell death is mediated directly by virus infection, likely via apoptotic mechanisms.[567,666]

In the kidney, severe eosinophilic degeneration and a microvesicular fatty change of renal tubular epithelium are observed, analogous to that seen in the liver. Viral antigen can be detected by immunohistochemistry in renal tubular cells.[187] Glomerular damage and albuminuria with changes in the basement membrane and degeneration of cells lining Bowman's capsule may be due to direct viral injury[567] or secondary to decreased blood flow during the sepsis syndrome.[246] The spleen shows an overall loss of lymphocytes, hyperplasia of the follicle, appearance of large mononuclear tissue histiocytes, and significant degeneration of cells with accumulation of fragmented nuclei.[409] In monkeys, necrosis of B-cell follicular areas of the spleen is more apparent.[568] In the heart, myocardial cells also undergo apoptotic changes as in other organs, in the absence of a significant cellular inflammatory response. Patchy lesions have been described in sinoatrial (SA) node and bundle of His,[495] which could explain the paradoxical bradycardia (Faget's sign) and late cardiac death, observed in some severe YFV cases.

Hemorrhagic manifestations and damage to and plasma leakage from capillaries are characteristic findings of severe

YFV infection.[567] The bleeding manifestations are attributed to decreased synthesis of vitamin K–dependent coagulation factors by the injured liver, disseminated intravascular coagulation, and reduced platelet numbers and function. Beyond direct bleeding, there is additional vascular dysfunction, with pleural and peritoneal effusions, and edema of several other organs, including the brain. At present, the precise pathogenesis of the vascular leakage syndrome associated with YFV remains unknown, although highly elevated levels of proinflammatory and vasoactive cytokines are observed.[814]

WEST NILE VIRUS

History, Global Distribution, and Epidemic Cycle

West Nile virus (WNV) was first isolated in 1937 in the West Nile district of Uganda from a woman with an undiagnosed febrile illness.[766] Historically, WNV caused sporadic outbreaks of a mild febrile illness in regions of Africa, the Middle East, Asia, and Australia. Indeed, in the 1950s, detailed studies of WNV showed recurrent outbreaks in Israel[66,260] and high levels of seroconversion in adults from Egypt[352,549]; these outbreaks and others in Africa generally were not associated with severe human disease. However, in the 1990s, the epidemiology of infection changed. New outbreaks in Eastern Europe were associated with higher rates of neurologic disease.[348] In 1999, WNV entered North America, and caused seven human fatalities in the New York area as well a large number of avian and equine deaths. Over the last decade, WNV has spread to all 48 of the lower United States as well as to parts of Canada, Mexico, the Caribbean, and South America. Because of the increased range, the number of human cases has continued to rise: in the United States between 1999 and 2012, 36,500 cases were confirmed and associated with 1,500 deaths (http://www.cdc.gov/ncidod/dvbid/westnile/surv&control.htm).

WNV cycles in nature between *Culex* mosquitoes and birds, but also infects and causes disease in humans, horses, and other vertebrate species. (Fig. 26.7) Ticks also have been implicated as having a minor role in transmission in some parts of the world,[510] although few isolates have been obtained. Although its enzootic cycle is overwhelmingly between mosquitoes and birds, with vertebrate species serving as "dead-end" hosts because of low-level and transient viremia, nonviremic transmission of WNV between co-feeding mosquitoes[330] suggests that vertebrates could act as reservoirs for mosquito infection. Most (~85%) human infections in the Northern Hemisphere occur in the late summer, with a peak number of cases in August and September. This reflects the seasonal activity of *Culex* mosquito vectors and a requirement for virus amplification in the late spring and early summer in avian hosts. In warmer parts of the world, virtually year-round transmission has been observed. Although more than 100 avian species are susceptible to WNV infection, in the United States, some are particularly vulnerable, with a large number of deaths in crows, blue jays, and hawks. The magnitude of dying birds in a community in the early summer often predicts the severity of human or equine disease weeks later.[415] Ecologic studies suggest that *Culex pipiens*, the dominant enzootic (bird-to-bird) and bridge (bird-to-human) vector of WNV in urbanized areas in the northeast and north-central United States, shifts its feeding preferences from birds to humans during the late summer and early fall, coincident with the dispersal of its preferred host, the American robin (*Turdus migratorius*).[393]

WNV Diversity

Sequencing and phylogenic analysis of full-length genomes has resulted in a division of WNV strains into four distinct lineages,[67,358,447,510] with lineage 1 strains further separated into three clades (1a, 1b, and 1c). This topic has been analyzed in great detail in a recent study.[537] Clade 1a comprises isolates from Europe, the Middle East, Russia, and the Americas, and includes all strains from the recent epoch in the United States and Canada. Clade 1b contains the naturally attenuated Australian variant, Kunjin virus, which forms a tight cluster with approximately 2% to 3% difference at the amino acid level from North American WNV strains.[719] Clade 1c comprises isolates from India only. Historically, lineage 2 isolates were isolated from sub-Saharan Africa and Madagascar, and generally showed less ability to cause disease in humans and animals[54,348]; a more recent study suggests that lineage 2 isolates now circulate in parts of Eastern Europe, some of which cause severe disease.[226] There are fewer sequenced strains from lineage 3 and 4 WNV, with only one lineage 3 isolate from Austria in 1997[33] and several lineage 4 isolates[510] from Russia between 2002 and 2006. Within a given ecological niche, possibly because of the enzootic cycle, WNV has remarkable genetic stability despite its error-prone RNA-dependent RNA polymerase; full-length sequencing analysis of North American isolates over the past decade

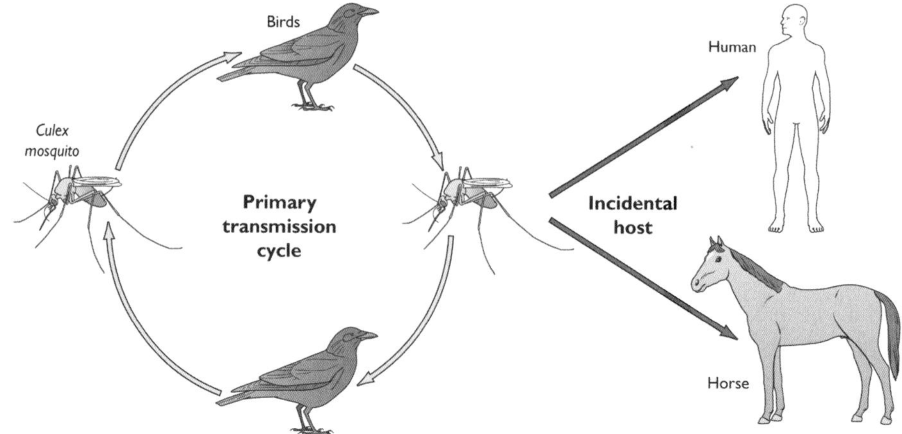

FIGURE 26.7. Transmission cycle of West Nile virus (WNV). WNV is maintained in nature in an enzootic transmission cycle between mosquitoes and birds. Many vertebrate species, including humans, may also be infected as "dead-end" hosts for WNV. The resulting transient low-level viremia in mammalian hosts does not support sufficient infection of the mosquito vector to continue the transmission cycle.

has revealed a rate of approximately five nucleotide and fewer than one amino acid mutation per genome per year, with little geographic subdivision.[181,810]

Clinical Features of WNV Infection

Seroprevalence studies suggest that most (~80%) cases are subclinical, without significant symptoms. Among clinical cases, many develop a self-limiting illness that is termed WNV fever. This syndrome begins after a 2- to 14-day incubation period and is characterized by fever accompanied by myalgias, arthralgias, headache, fatigue, gastrointestinal complaints, maculopapular rash, or lymphadenopathy. This nonneuroinvasive form of WNV infection can be severe, as 38% of patients with WNV fever were hospitalized with a mean length of stay of 5.4 days.[350] A subset of the symptomatic cases progress to the neuroinvasive forms of WNV infection, including acute flaccid paralysis, meningitis, encephalitis, and ocular manifestations[34,742]; in many instances, a combination of these syndromes is present. Overall, about 1 in 150 WNV infections result in the most severe and potentially lethal form of the disease. During an epidemic, on a human population scale, the seroconversion rate is approximately 3%[588,832] and the attack rate for severe disease during an epidemic is about 7 per 100,000.[350] The risk of severe WNV infection is greatest in the elderly.[151,603,832] At least two studies have estimated a 20-fold increased risk of neuroinvasive disease and death in those older than 50 years of age.[350,603] Persistent movement disorders, cognitive complaints, and functional disability may occur after West Nile neuroinvasive disease. West Nile poliomyelitis-like disease may result in limb weakness and long-term morbidity. Moreover, even patients with apparently mild cases of acute disease have sustained subjective and somatic sequelae following WNV infection. Therefore, the neurologic and functional disability associated with WNV infection represents a considerable source of morbidity in patients long after their recovery from acute illness.[740,741,742,743]

Although most human WNV infections occur after the bite of an infected *Culex* mosquito, other routes including transfusion, organ transplantation, and placental and breast milk transmission. In 2002, 23 cases of WNV infection were identified after transfusion of blood products.[639] These cases led to the development and implementation of nucleic acid amplification tests, which have been used to identify infected pools or individual blood product samples[115,644] and largely prevent transmission by transfusion. Nucleic acid screening of blood donors have not completely eliminated transfusion-transmitted WNV infections, as "breakthrough" infections have occurred, and were attributed to units that had levels of viremia below the sensitivity of the screening assay.[116] In addition to transfusion-associated WNV infection, several cases by organ transplantation have been reported.[427,428] Because of the relatively low incidence of WNV infection in organ transplantation and risk of false-positives that can occur with wide scale testing, screening is not mandated.

Pathologic Features of WNV Infection

WNV causes encephalitis in several vertebrate species including humans, horses, and birds, by virtue of its ability to infect and cause injury to neurons through direct (viral-induced) and indirect (immune response induced) mechanisms.[129] Pathologic observations in humans, however, is limited by the small number of autopsy studies on individuals succumbing to WNV infection. Gross macroscopic examination of organs (brain, lung, kidney, and spleen) tends to be unremarkable.[630] Microscopic examination of the brain in humans and other animals reveals histologic changes that are consistent with the clinical disease.[221,630] This includes neuronal cell death, activation of resident microglia and infiltrating macrophages, perivascular and parenchymal accumulation of $CD4^+$ and $CD8^+$ lymphocytes and $CD138^+$ plasma cells, and formation of microglial nodules. These lesions, which tend to be patchy in distribution, occur in the brainstem, cerebral cortex, hippocampus, thalamus, and cerebellum.[630] In addition, overt meningitis with cellular infiltrates in the meninges can be readily apparent. In some cases, destruction of vascular structures with focal hemorrhage is present, suggestive of a vasculitis; this may be associated with local compromise of the blood–brain barrier.[200,868] Immunohistochemical analysis confirms that WNV antigen is present in neurons from multiple regions of the brain, although other cells (e.g., astrocytes or $CD11b^+$ myeloid cells) may be infected to lesser degrees.[176,208]

In addition, WNV infection can cause a poliomyelitis-like syndrome of acute flaccid paralysis.[257,458] Patients show markedly decreased motor responses in the paretic limbs, preserved sensory responses, and widespread asymmetric muscle denervation without evidence of demyelination or myopathy.[458] Microscopically, in the spinal cord, an intense inflammatory infiltrate around large and small blood vessels is observed with large numbers of microglia in the ventral horn. Anterior horn motor neurons are targeted by WNV,[458,754] and studies suggest that axonal transport from peripheral neurons can mediate WNV entry into the spinal cord and induce acute flaccid paralysis.[705]

Although most mammalian WNV infections are cleared by the adaptive immune response, persistence in the kidney has been described, albeit infrequently. Hamsters experimentally infected with WNV developed chronic renal infection and viruria for up to 8 months, despite clearance from blood and the appearance of neutralizing antibodies. Although minimal histopathology was reported, WNV antigen staining was detected in the renal epithelium, interstitial cells, and tubules.[816] Of interest, these persistent viruses evolved genetically and no longer caused neuroinvasive disease on challenge of naïve animals.[895] Analogous to the studies in hamsters, WNV RNA was demonstrated in 5 of 25 urine samples from convalescent humans 1.6 to 6.7 years after the initial infection, although infectious virus was not successfully isolated.[599] However, a separate larger study did not detect viral RNA in urine, and thus analysis of additional patient cohorts may be required to better define renal persistence and its significance in humans.[254]

Persistent WNV infection in the CNS also has been suggested by experimental infection studies in monkeys, hamsters, and mice. In monkeys, WNV persisted at least 5.5 months after initial infection and was isolated in the cerebellum and cerebral subcortical ganglia but had lost its neurovirulence and cytopathic properties.[655] In hamsters, persistent WNV RNA and foci of WNV antigen-positive cells were identified in the CNS of hamsters between 28 to 86 days after infection,[758] and this was associated with long-term neurologic sequelae. In mice, infectious WNV persisted in the brains of wild-type animals up to 4 months, and viral RNA could be detected at 6 months in up 12% of mice, even in animals with subclinical infection.[16] Consistent with this, virus-specific B- and

T-cell immune responses persisted in the CNS of mice up to 4 months after infection.[785]

JAPANESE ENCEPHALITIS VIRUS

History, Global Distribution, and Epidemic Cycle

Japanese encephalitis virus (JEV) is a mosquito-transmitted flavivirus and the prototype virus of the JEV antigenic serocomplex. JEV causes severe neurologic disease, primarily in Asia, where it accounts for about 35,000 to 50,000 cases and 10,000 to 15,000 deaths annually.[831] JEV epidemics were originally described in Japan in the 1870s, and the virus was initially recovered in 1935 from the brain of an infected human in Tokyo; this isolate was established as the prototype Nakayama JEV strain.[460] Although most human infections are asymptomatic or result in mild symptoms, greater than 50% of the severe clinical cases are fatal or result in devastating long-term neurologic sequelae.[736] Moreover, as JEV-induced disease largely occurs in children living in rural areas, it is likely vastly underreported in most regions of Asia.[736,768]

The enzootic cycle of JEV is between waterbirds (e.g., egrets and herons) and mosquitoes, with pigs also serving as an amplifying host. JEV is transmitted primarily by *Culex* mosquitoes (principally *Culex tritaeniorhynchus*) that breed in rice fields and stagnant water. Humans and other vertebrate animals are considered incidental targets and dead-end hosts, as they do not produce a viremia sufficient to infect mosquitoes. Two epidemiologic patterns are observed: in northern temperate areas JEV infections occur during the summer months, whereas as in tropical climates, year-round transmission of JEV has been described.[267]

Globally, despite the introduction of several inactivated and live-attenuated vaccines (see Vaccine section below), JEV remains the most important cause of arthropod-transmitted viral encephalitis. Disease caused by JEV is widely distributed in Asia, with outbreaks historically occurring in Japan, China, Taiwan, Korea, the Philippines, India, parts of Southeast Asia, and the far-eastern region of Russia. Although cases in China appear to be declining, possibly due to large-scale vaccination campaigns, epidemic activity in India, Nepal, and other parts of Southeast Asia appears to be escalating. More recently, JEV has been described in Pakistan, Papua New Guinea, and Australia, suggesting that its geographic range may be expanding.[312,313]

JEV Diversity

Phylogenic analysis suggests that JEV evolved from an ancestral flavivirus in Africa within the last few centuries.[268] Based on sequence analysis primarily of the viral structural genes, JEV was initially classified into one single serotype with four distinct genotypes (I–IV),[145,146,835] with as much as 12% variation at the nucleotide level. These divisions have been confirmed by full-length genome sequencing on a subset of isolates. Genotype I includes isolates from Thailand, Cambodia, Korea, China, Japan, Vietnam, Taiwan, and Australia from 1967 to the present. Genotype II includes strains from Thailand, Malaysia, Indonesia, Papua New Guinea, and Australia from 1951 to 1999. Genotype III includes isolates recovered from mostly temperate areas of Asia including Japan, China, Taiwan, the Philippines, and the Asian subcontinent between 1935 and the present. Finally, genotype IV includes strains from Indonesia that were isolated only in 1980 and 1981. More recently, a fifth, more divergent genotype (V) has been proposed based on full-genome sequencing of a 1952 isolate from a patient in the Muar region Malaysia.[560] This strain has approximately 20% and 9% nucleotide and amino acid divergence, respectively, and shows significant variation with respect to neutralization by JEV-specific monoclonal antibodies.[315]

Because genotypes I and III largely occurred in epidemic regions and genotypes II and IV were associated with endemic transmission, differences in strain virulence were hypothesized to explain the epidemiologic patterns of JEV.[146] However, as the geographic range of JEV has expanded, there are now several examples in which strains of individual genotypes cause either epidemic or endemic disease depending on the region or country.[772]

Clinical Features of JEV Infection

In humans, the JEV infection can be asymptomatic or produce a range of clinical syndromes including a mild nonspecific febrile illness, aseptic meningitis, seizures, encephalitis, and poliomyelitis-like flaccid paralysis. Disease onset usually begins with a 1- to 2-week period of flu-like symptoms including headache, fever, cough, and upper respiratory symptoms, as well as gastrointestinal complaints such as nausea, vomiting, and diarrhea. In infants and young children the disease can progress rapidly as the virus invades the CNS and infects and injures neurons. CNS invasion is heralded by nuchal rigidity, photophobia, and altered mental status. JEV infection in the CNS can share features with Parkinson's disease including mask-like facies, hypertonia, tremor, and cogwheel rigidity. Other CNS symptoms include seizures (more common in children than adults), ataxia, involuntary movements (e.g., choreoathetosis, facial grimacing, and lip-smacking), and cranial nerve palsies. Associated with this are elevated white blood cell counts and pressure in the cerebrospinal fluid (CSF) and abnormal electroencephalography (EEG) examinations. Imaging studies in the brain have revealed thalamic and basal ganglia abnormalities during the acute phase of disease.[768] Upper rather than lower extremity paralysis is more common, and lower motor neuron disease of the spinal cord can develop. Death can occur, especially in children, within 3 to 5 days of CNS symptoms, or much later due to complications associated with hospitalization or cardiopulmonary status. A recent prospective study evaluated the clinical features and long-term prognosis of 118 children with encephalitis due to JEV in Malaysia.[633] Only 44% of patients had full recovery, with 8% dying during the acute phase of the illness and 31% having persistent and severe neurologic sequelae. These included chronic seizures, motor dysfunction, and neuropsychiatric symptoms such as mental retardation and psychiatric disorders.

Pathologic Features of JEV Infection

JEV infection in the brain results in neuronal degeneration, necrosis, microglial nodule formation, and perivascular and parenchymal leukocyte infiltrates as well as focal hemorrhage. Parenchymal damage in the CNS is attributed to both direct cytopathic effect of the virus in nonrenewing populations of neurons and the resultant inflammatory state induced by activated microglia and infiltrating leukocytes. Although these histologic findings can occur throughout the brain, they usually are more restricted to the gray matter in the cortex, midbrain, and brainstem, providing anatomic correlates for the tremor and dystonias associated with CNS infection. Focal lesions are seen predominantly in the thalamus and cerebral peduncles but also are commonly observed in the substantia nigra, cerebral and cerebellar cortices, and the anterior horn of the spinal cord,[768] the latter of which is associated with a poliomyelitis-like acute flaccid paralysis.[771] In patients who die rapidly, there may be little histologic evidence of inflammation, but instead, high levels of JEV antigen can be detected in morphologically intact neurons.[362]

ST. LOUIS ENCEPHALITIS VIRUS

History, Global Distribution, and Epidemic Cycle

St. Louis encephalitis virus (SLEV) is a mosquito-borne member of the JEV serocomplex capable of causing severe neurologic disease in humans. SLEV was first discovered in 1933 following a large epidemic of encephalitis in St. Louis, Missouri (1,095 cases and 225 deaths).[185,508,675] More than 10,000 cases of severe illness and 1,000 deaths have since been attributed to SLEV infection, reflecting annual endemic transmission (~50 cases/year) punctuated by epidemic periods that occur every 5 to 15 years.[563] At least 41 epidemics of SLEV have occurred in the United States since 1933,[185] the largest of these in 1975.[167] During this epidemic, SLEV cases were reported in 29 states and the District of Columbia; the greatest number of illnesses occurred in Ohio, Mississippi, Indiana, and Illinois. Roughly 1,500 confirmed cases were reported, resulting in 171 fatalities. The most recent large outbreak of SLEV occurred in central Florida during 1990, resulting in 222 laboratory-confirmed cases and 14 deaths.[543]

SLEV is found in much of the New World; distribution ranges from Canada to Argentina, and across North America.[675] SLEV is maintained in nature in enzootic cycles between *Culex* mosquitoes and passeriform and columbiform birds. Of interest, the transmission cycle of this virus varies by region due to differences in the biology of the primary vector mosquitoes.[675] In the eastern and central United States, the principal vectors of SLEV are *Culex pipiens* and *Culex quinquefasciatus* mosquitoes. *Culex tarsalis* is the primary vector for SLEV in Western states, whereas *Culex nigripalpus* transmits SLEV in Florida. The avian hosts of SLEV in these transmission cycles include house finches, house sparrows, and mourning doves. The mechanism of virus transmission and amplification in South and Central America is less clear. SLEV has been isolated from 11 different mosquito genera, many of which feed primarily on mammals.

Both WNV and SLEV are antigenically related members of the JEV serogroup that share a similar transmission cycle between *Culex* mosquitoes and birds. How the introduction of WNV in North America has impacted the epidemiology of SLEV is of significant interest. Analysis of the number of neuroinvasive cases attributed to SLEV reported to the CDC between 1999 and 2007 revealed a threefold reduction by comparison with data in the pre-WNV era.[674] Interpretation of this finding is complicated by changes in the intensity of surveillance and local testing for arboviral diseases in the years after the introduction of WNV. Because major epidemics of SLEV have occurred infrequently in the past, the modest number of clinical cases may simply reflect a nadir in the natural cycle of this virus. Alternatively, the existence of cross-reactive antibodies in WNV-immune avian reservoirs may disrupt the transmission cycle of SLEV via competition for avian hosts. Although the infection of house finches with WNV has been shown to confer protection from subsequent infection by SLEV, the reciprocal is not true. Prior exposure of finches to SLEV prevents mortality following WNV infection but not the low-level of viremia that is sufficient for transmission of WNV.[232] Similar findings were reported in a golden hamster model of infection.[817] The disappearance of SLEV from regions of California following introduction of WNV is consistent with the notion that competition may allow for the local displacement of the virus from historically endemic areas.[676] Additional study and surveillance are required to clarify the dynamics and interactions between these two related pathogens in North America.

SLEV Diversity

Phylogenic studies grouped SLEV isolates into seven genetic lineages (I–VII), many of which were divided further into clades of related genotypes.[421,538] These groups correspond roughly to the geographic distribution of each lineage of SLEV.[830] For example, lineage I include viruses isolated in the western United States, whereas lineage V contains South American strains and an isolate from Trinidad. However, the relationship between phylogenic relatedness and geographic region is imperfect. SLEV strains vary considerably with respect to virulence in avian and mammalian hosts; these differences correlate roughly with geographic distribution.[90,571] In addition to regional persistence, sequence analysis reveals that SLEV may be transported between regions.[421]

Clinical and Pathologic Features of SLEV Infection

As is the case for both WNV and JEV, the majority of SLEV infections of humans are clinically asymptomatic. The ratio of apparent to inapparent infections has been reported to range from 1:16 to 1:425.[563] Increasing age is a significant factor influencing susceptibility to severe illness. Symptomatic illness is noted after an incubation period of 5 to 15 days and is characterized by mild malaise, fever, headache, nausea, myalgia, sore throat, and cough.[103] Severe neurologic manifestations including encephalitis and aseptic meningitis may occur and can be fatal. Case fatality rates for SLEV range from 5% to 20%, with fatalities increasing in the elderly.[675] Although most SLEV cases resolve spontaneously and without sequelae, many patients (30% to 50%) experience an extended convalescence lasting up to 3 years. This phase is characterized by headache, depression, memory loss, and weakness.[103,675]

TICK-BORNE ENCEPHALITIS VIRUSES

History, Global Distribution, and Epidemic Cycle

Tick-borne encephalitis virus (TBEV) causes a fatal neurologic syndrome that primarily affects individuals ranging from northern China and Japan, through Russia, to parts of Northern Europe.[525] TBEV infection was first described in 1931 after a pattern of seasonal meningoencephalitis cases in Austria was observed.[732] In 1939, experiments confirmed that this seasonal encephalitis in humans was caused by a virus transmission by the tick, *Ixodes persulcatus.*[923] Although a highly effective

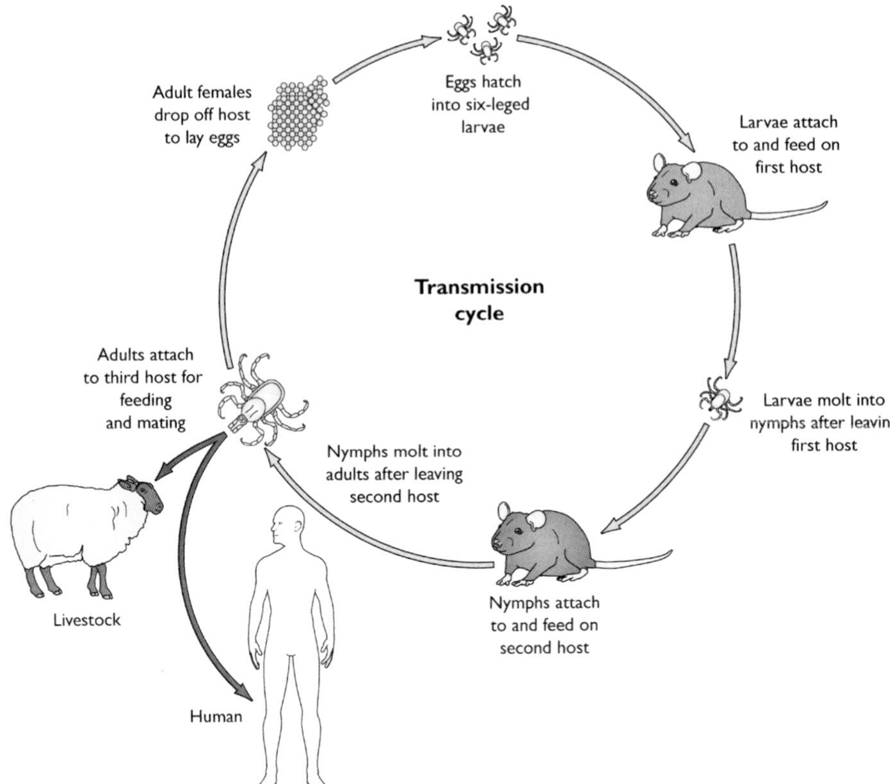

FIGURE 26.8. Life cycle of tick-borne encephalitis virus (TBEV). The transmission of tick-borne flaviviruses is connected to the life cycle of the vector due to a requirement for the tick to feed prior to transition through each of its developmental stage. Ticks are infected during this blood meal, molt, and then may infect a mammalian host. Nonviremic transmission between co-feeding ticks has also been shown to be an important mechanism of transmission and is not pictured.

formalin-inactivated vaccine has been implemented in some European countries (e.g., Austria) with marked reductions in case numbers,[320] TBEV-induced morbidity and mortality continue to rise.[799] Between 1990 and 2007, about 9,000 cases per year were reported in Europe and Russia[799]; currently, TBEV is believed to cause approximately 14,000 human cases per year, the majority of which occur in parts of Russia.[277] This increase is thought to be due to changes in climate, population dynamics and range of permissive ticks, and shifts in land usage. Within Russia, Siberia has the highest number of TBEV cases, whereas the Czech Republic has the greatest incidence.[525] The relative virulence of TBEV decreases with its westward spread, with the far-eastern subtype having a case-fatality rate of almost 40%.

In the enzootic cycle, TBEV is maintained between ticks and different vertebrate hosts, with humans as incidental hosts (Fig. 26.8). TBEV is transmitted primarily by the hard tick *Ixodes ricinus,* although in Eastern Europe and Russia the principal vector is *Ixodes persulcatus.* Infection is seasonal, usually occurring between March and November,[371] and coincides with seasonal peaks of feeding activity of the particular tick involved in transmission. TBEV is endemic from central Europe to Far East Asia, with cases reported in 34 countries.[798] Ticks can become chronically infected after sampling viremic blood, or by transstadial or transovarial transmission. In addition, infected ticks can transmit virus to uninfected ticks during co-feeding on rodents.[277,444] This is because the local skin environment supports TBEV replication, and migratory infected cells transport virus within the skin allowing for transmission in the absence of viremia.[443]

One exception to TBEV transmission by tick inoculation is the syndrome of biphasic milk fever, which results from oral infection and was first identified in Russia between 1947 and 1951. During milk fever epidemics, whole families contracted TBEV infection, and this was associated with the consumption of goat milk. Goats develop subclinical TBEV infection after tick bite and become the source of infectious virus after secretion into milk. Analogously, TBEV transmission to humans has been reported after consumption of unpasteurized cow or sheep milk or dairy products.[277] These findings are supported by experiments in mice in which TBEV infection was established after oral feeding.[654]

TBEV Diversity

Based on sequence similarity, three main subtypes of TBEV exist: the Far Eastern genotype 1 (previously Russian Spring and Summer encephalitis), European genotype 2 (previously Central European encephalitis), and Siberian genotype 3 (previously west-Siberian). These TBEV genotypes are closely related[218,339] and transmitted by the ticks *Ixodes ricinus* (European subtypes) and *Ixodes persulcatus* (Asian subtypes).[277] Within these three genotypes, there is an approximately 1.2% to 1.7% difference at the amino acid level. The Far Eastern, European, and Siberian genotypes 1, 2, and 3 differ from each other by approximately 5% to 7% at the amino acid level. In addition to these three TBEV genotypes, two additional genotypes (4 and 5) have been described based on nucleotide and amino acid differences.[193] Other viruses that are antigenically related across Europe, Asia, and North America are classified as part of the TBEV serocomplex,[118] also termed the mammalian group of tick-borne flaviviruses. In addition to TBEV, this group includes Omsk hemorrhagic fever virus (OHFV), Louping ill virus (LIV), Langat virus (LGTV), Powassan virus (POWV), Kyasanur Forest disease virus (KFDV), Kadam virus (KADV), Royal Farm virus (RFV), Gadgets Gully virus (GGYV), Alkhurma hemorrhagic fever virus (AHFV), and Karshi virus (KSIV). Of these viruses, TBEV, LIV, and POWV cause encephalitis in humans and animals, whereas OHFV, KFDV, and AHFV cause hemorrhagic fever.[278,695] LGTV is a naturally occurring avirulent virus (analogous to Kunjin virus among WNV strains), and no clinical disease has been reported for KSIV, RFV, or GGYV.

Clinical Features of TBEV Infection

About one-third of patients after inoculation with an infected tick will become symptomatic,[371] with men affected twice as frequently as women, although this could reflect exposure bias. The incubation period for TBEV infection in humans varies, but for most individuals is approximately 1 to 2 weeks. A prodrome of fatigue, musculoskeletal pain, and headache lasts a few days, and is followed by an abrupt onset of fever, nausea, vomiting, and myalgias; this phase is associated with thrombocytopenia, leukopenia, and mildly elevated levels of liver enzymes in the serum. Subsequent to this, several clinical syndromes of TBEV infection develop, as reviewed previously[277,371]:

1. *Febrile syndrome.* This illness is characterized by high fever (39°C) with no evidence of neuroinvasion. It lasts from 1 to 5 days, and upon defervescence, patients recover completely.
2. *Meningitis.* This is the most common form of clinically apparent TBEV infection occurring in approximately 50% of individuals. After the onset of fever, symptoms worsen with progressive headache, nausea, vomiting, and photophobia. All patients exhibit a CSF leukocyte pleocytosis after lumbar puncture. Fever lasts 1 to 2 weeks, with gradual recovery.
3. *Meningoencephalitis.* This form occurs in approximately 10% of cases, is more severe, and is associated with damage to the CNS. Individuals become weak, lethargic, and develop focal signs of disease including hemiparesis, hemiplegia, seizures, and autonomic instability. Up to 30% of these cases are fatal, and survivors have long-term neurologic sequelae with slow convalescence.
4. *Poliomyelitis-like disease.* This is characterized by a prodrome of limb weakness or numbness that progresses to paralysis. Paralysis occurs more frequently in the upper limbs, with the proximal segments affected more often. Recovery is slow, partial, and occurs in only one-half of patients, with the remainder showing progressive deterioration.
5. *Polyradiculitis.* This syndrome has a biphasic course with fever, headache, and myalgia followed by defervescence. Approximately one week later the second phase starts and is characterized by pain and damage in peripheral nerves, sometimes coupled with meningitis. Recovery from this form of TBEV infection is usually complete.
6. *Chronic or persistent infection.* This form has been described in Siberia and Far East Russia, although not in Europe, and is believed to associate uniquely with the Siberian subtype of TBEV. Chronic or persistent infection is characterized by a late phase (months or even years later) deterioration of the neurologic sequelae that developed during the acute illness. Alternatively, chronic TBEV infection can begin with the acute phase of disease, such that neurologic symptoms occur years after a tick bite. Clinical symptoms can include epilepsy, Parkinsonian movement and cognitive disorders, and progressive muscle atrophy, ultimately with dementia and death ensuing. Although infectious virus has not been routinely recovered in autopsy studies, a TBEV strain was isolated from a patient who died of a progressive (2-year) form of tick-borne encephalitis 10 years after experiencing a tick bite.[276]
7. *Postencephalitic syndrome.* Both retrospective and prospective clinical trials have shown that TBEV infection is associated with a slow recovery period that has considerable long-term morbidity.[289,370,554] This postencephalitic syndrome occurs in approximately 40% to 60% of patients, and includes memory disturbances, headache, and affective and gait disorders. The frequency of these symptoms was proportionately higher in more severe cases.

Pathologic Features of TBEV Infection

Gross pathologic analysis of the brain of humans who succumb to lethal TBEV infection shows edema and hyperemia. Microscopic lesions occur in a patchy distribution throughout the CNS but are most prominent in the brainstem, basal ganglia, thalamus, cerebellum, and spinal cord. The cerebral and spinal meninges show a diffuse leukocyte infiltration, predominantly with lymphocytes. In the parenchyma of the brain and spinal cord, perivascular infiltrates, microglial nodules, and necrosis of neurons is observed. Notably, Purkinje cell neurons in the cerebellum and anterior horn motor neurons in the spinal cord are preferentially targeted and injured by TBEV.[371] Immunohistochemical analysis of brains from 28 autopsy cases[250] showed prominent TBEV antigen staining in Purkinje cells, neurons of the dentate gyrus, the brainstem, and basal ganglia, with T lymphocytes detected in direct apposition to TBEV-infected neurons.

PATHOGENESIS AND IMMUNITY

Virus Entry and Tropism

Flavivirus entry into cells is mediated by the envelope proteins and can be considered in three relatively discrete steps (Fig. 26.9). The first step involves the attachment of the virus particle to the cell. Collisions between virions and target cells are not always productive. "Attachment factors" promote infection by increasing the duration of contact between the virion and cell surface, and thereby increase the likelihood that subsequent steps in the virus entry pathway will occur. Attachment factors are not strictly required for infection. In contrast, interactions with viral "receptors" promote required events during virus entry. Although the distinction between these two types of cellular factors is clear for some viruses (e.g., HIV), the cell biology of flavivirus entry remains poorly understood.

Several cellular factors have been suggested to function as attachment factors or receptors during the flavivirus entry (reviewed by Lindenbach, Murray, Thiel, and Rice in Chapter 25 of this volume). The interaction between flaviviruses and glycosaminoglycans (GAGs) have been documented.[147,332,455,523] The binding site for these sulfated polysaccharides on the virion has been mapped to positively charged surfaces of the E protein.[147,523] Passage of virus in cell culture selects for variants that bind more efficiently to GAGs, although this adaptation appears to be associated with reduced fitness *in vivo*.[454,456,523] Treatment

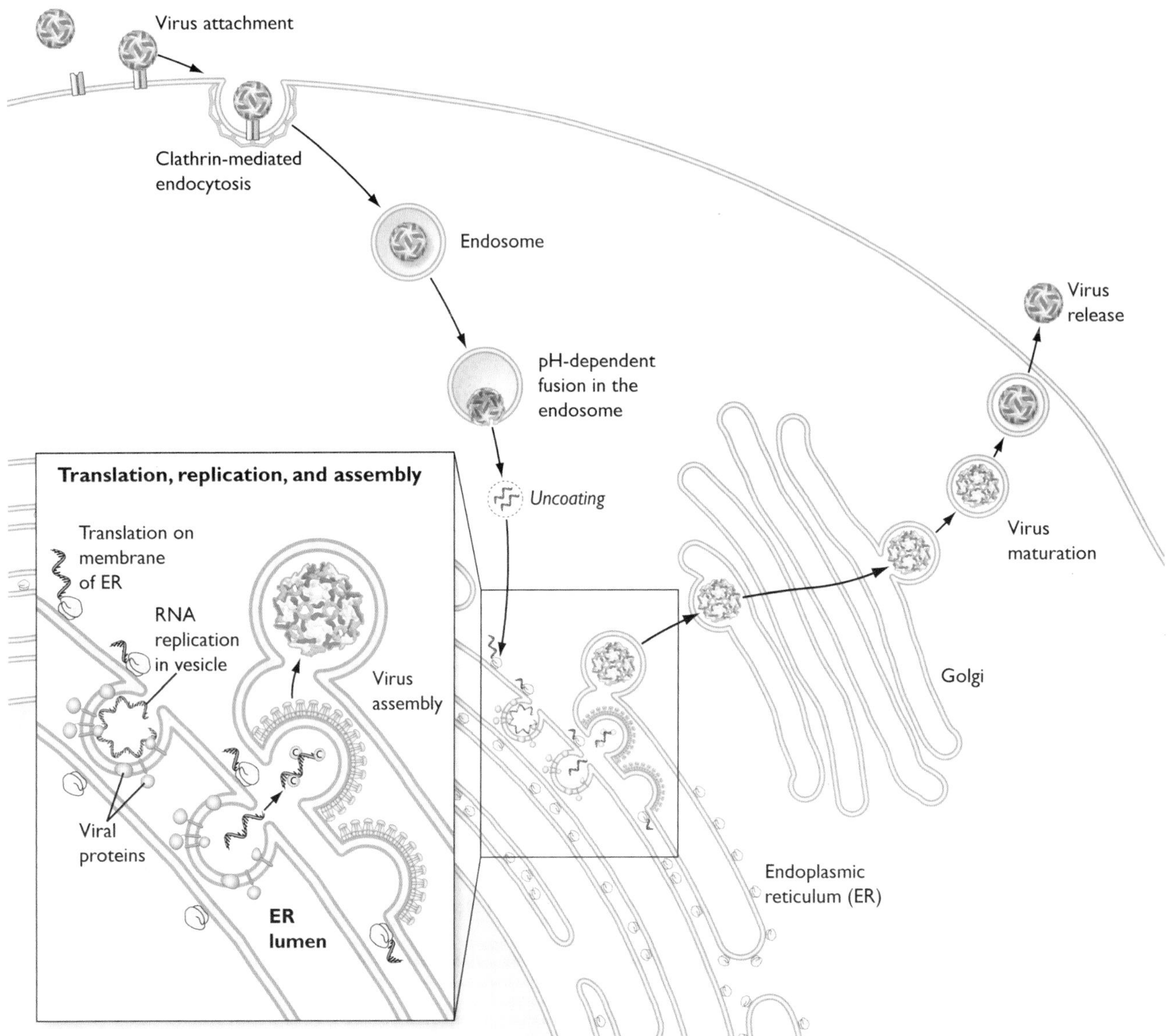

FIGURE 26.9. The replication cycle of flaviviruses. Flaviviruses bind cells of the host through poorly defined interactions with one or more molecules on target cells. Viruses are internalized via clathrin-mediated endocytosis and fuse with membranes of the late endosome in a pH-dependent manner. Viral RNA replication begins shortly thereafter in association with membranes of the host cell. Cells actively replicating flaviviruses reveal striking host membrane rearrangements thought to coordinate the processes of genomic RNA replication and virus assembly. Virus particles assemble at and bud into the endoplasmic reticulum and are secreted from the cell. During egress, virion maturation occurs in the acidic compartments of the Golgi and is characterized by cleavage of the prM protein by a furin-like protease.

of cells with heparan sulfate can inhibit infection.[147,457,485] GAGs are thought to promote more efficient attachment to cells via electrostatic interactions with the virus particle.

Cellular lectins also increase the efficiency of flavivirus attachment. CD209 Dendritic Cell-Specific Intercellular Adhesion Molecule-3-Grabbing Non-integrin (DC-SIGN) is a calcium-dependent c-type lectin that serves as an attachment factor for several classes of viruses (reviewed in[839]), including some flaviviruses.[183,605,811] These interactions are mediated by N-linked sugars on the prM and E proteins of the virion.[182,406,480,504] CD209 is expressed *in vivo* on a subset of dendritic cells (DCs) and macrophages.[839] The infectivity of DCs by DENV correlates with CD209 expression; immature DCs express CD209 and are more permissive to infection than mature DCs expressing lower levels of CD209.[811,893] Antibodies against CD209 or soluble forms of this lectin are capable of blocking DENV infection of DCs.[605,811] Experiments with truncated forms of CD209 suggest that internalization of CD209 is not required to increase the efficiency of virus attachment to selected cell types.[503] CD209L Dendritic Cell-Specific Intercellular Adhesion Molecule-3-Grabbing Non-integrin-Related protein (DC-SIGNR)[183,811] and the mannose receptor (MR)[556] have also been identified as attachment factors for flaviviruses.

Recent studies have identified members of the TIM and TAM families of phosphatidylserine receptors that function as attachment and potentially signaling factors for flaviviruses. These cellular protein directly (in the case of TIM1) or indirectly (in the case of TAM proteins) bind lipids incorporated into the membrane of the virus particle. The expression pattern of this family of molecules may explain, in part, the broad cellular tropism of these viruses in vitro. Furthermore, the interaction of cellular proteins with the lipid envelope of the virion, thought to be buried by the dense icosahedral array of E proteins described above), raises questions about the structure(s) of infectious flaviviruses.[543a]

Flavivirus enter cells via clathrin-mediated endocytosis.[2,152,262,424,838] Elegant single-particle tracking studies of DENV suggest that virions move across the surface of cells until they encounter preformed clathrin-coated pits. Virus particles are then internalized and traffic into late Rab7-positive endosomal compartments where viral fusion occurs.[838] Fusion between viral and cellular membranes is triggered by the acidic environment of endosomes. How viruses sense the low-pH environment is not completely understood, but may involve the protonation of key histidine residues on the E protein.[241,375,608] Fusion may also be governed by the lipid composition of the endosome.[909] That flaviviruses have the ability to fuse with synthetic liposomes devoid of proteins indicates that this process does not require interactions with a cellular receptor.[162,264]

The molecular basis for the tropism of flaviviruses is unknown. A wide variety of cell lines representing different lineages and species may be infected *in vitro.* This suggests cellular factors involved in virus entry are either highly conserved (from mosquitoes to man) or redundant. Targets for flavivirus infection *in vivo* appear more restricted and include monocytes, macrophages, hepatocytes, neurons, endothelial cells, and DCs.[38,704] Tropism may be regulated at a postentry level through the activities of interferon and interferon-stimulated genes.[704,859]

Mechanisms of Dissemination

Blood-Borne Viruses

For both viscerotropic (e.g., DENV and YFV) and encephalitic (e.g., WNV, JEV, and TBEV) flaviviruses, the skin is the likely initial infection site after insect inoculation, with resident dendritic cells[117,529] or epidermal keratinocytes[478] believed to be the primary target cells. The dose of virus inoculated by the mosquito under conditions of natural infection is not known precisely, but likely ranges from 10^3 to 10^5 plaque-forming units (PFU),[731,791] depending on the flavivirus and insect vector. Active WNV replication can be detected at the subcutaneous site of infection within one day of infection,[107] and virus spread to the lymph node occurs in animals infected by mosquitoes or with mosquito salivary extracts.[731,792] Proteins in mosquito saliva alter cytokine levels and other components of innate immunity, leading to local immunosuppression or dysregulation,[729] and enhanced spread and replication.

Flaviviruses disseminate to local lymph nodes either associated with migratory infected dendritic cells[663] or as free virus that transudates directly into lymphatic fluid.[369] Macrophages on the floor of the subcapsular sinus and in the medulla of lymph nodes capture viral particles efficiently, serving as possible targets of virus amplification infection and initiators of innate and adaptive immune responses.[369] Virus produced in the draining lymph nodes likely spreads to intravascular venous compartments via efferent lymphatic drainage. Virus in the bloodstream can directly infect blood cells or visceral tissues, which can result in further dissemination and secondary viremia.

The infectivity of flaviviruses in plasma, the fluid component of blood, appears remarkably short, with a half-life in mice ranging from 2 to 10 minutes for DENV and WNV, respectively.[242] The loss of infectivity is due in part, to complement (C3 and C4 components) opsonization via mannose-binding lectin recognition of N-linked glycans on the surface of virions.[242] The short half-life of infectious flavivirus in plasma may also reflect sequestration and removal by different visceral organs.[355] Alternatively, flaviviruses may transit rapidly into the cellular compartment of blood. One study of patients with DENV infections of different disease severity showed DENV antigen (prM and NS3) predominantly in cells of monocyte ($CD14^+$, $CD32^+$) lineage, with up to 80% to 90% of cells of expressing viral antigen.[216] This finding of DENV in blood monocytes is consistent with prior literature[526] but contrasts with newer studies in rhesus macaques, suggesting that platelets become positive for dengue antigen during the course of infection.[632] Finally, another explanation for the rapid drop of plasma infectivity is that flaviviruses adhere readily to erythrocytes in whole blood.[683]

Neurotropic Viruses

Flavivirus neuropathogenesis requires neuroinvasiveness, the capacity to enter the CNS, and neurovirulence, the ability to propagate efficiently within cells of the CNS. In classical studies, phenotypic distinctions were made among different arthropod-borne viruses on the basis of replication efficiency and pathogenic potential in peripheral versus CNS tissues.[5] A main principle was the relationship between peripheral virus burden and the propensity to cause neuroinvasion. Viruses with a low capacity to replicate in the periphery generally had less neuroinvasive potential, regardless of their intrinsic neurovirulence. Aerosol-acquired and, perhaps, mucosal infections are possible exceptions, as these may use alternate routes of CNS entry.

Data from several studies indicate that the time of onset, magnitude, and duration of viremia, as well as the integrity of the host immune system influences the risk of entry into the CNS. Therefore, the neuropathogenic potential of most flaviviruses is a balance between the replication efficiency and the effectiveness of early host defenses in clearing viremia. Neuroinvasiveness is affected by both viral and host factors. Based on genetic analysis of virulent and attenuated strains of JEV, TBEV, YFV, and WNV, viral determinants of neuroinvasiveness map primarily to the E protein.[54,56,130,541,615,616] The mechanisms associated with these genetic determinants have not been determined, but are believed to relate to increased viral infectivity of key target cells through enhanced binding and penetration.

Animal models of infection of encephalitic flaviviruses have begun to define factors that govern virus entry into the brain and spinal cord. Crossing of the blood–brain barrier (BBB) likely occurs through a hematogenous route, as increased viral burden in the serum correlates with earlier and enhanced viral entry into the brain.[204] Accordingly, changes in endothelial cell permeability may facilitate CNS entry; these may be triggered by vasoactive cytokines[509,868] or activation of matrix metalloproteinases that degrade the BBB extracellular matrix.[845,864] Additional possible mechanisms may contribute to CNS infection of flaviviruses, including the following: (a) direct infection or passive transport through the endothelium,[212,488,846] and (b) infection of olfactory neurons and rostral spread from the olfactory bulb.[107] Access through the olfactory bulb is believed to occur either after infection by the aerosol or intranasal route[602,618,669] or in the context of hematogenous dissemination of virus.[542] The olfactory bulb is vulnerable to direct infection because of the exposure of its nerve terminals within the olfactory mucosa; (c) a "Trojan horse" mechanism in which virus is transported by infected immune cells that traffic to the CNS[865]; (d) access to the CNS after breakdown of BBB integrity[139,412]; and (e) direct axonal retrograde transport from infected peripheral neurons.[351,584,705,860] Although much has been learned from infection studies in mice and hamsters, the precise mechanisms of CNS entry of encephalitic flaviviruses in humans and other animals requires additional study.

Mechanisms of Immune Control: Innate Immunity

Cellular Innate Immunity

Macrophages

Although only limited studies have directly addressed the function of cellular innate immunity in flavivirus infection, emerging data suggest that macrophages play key roles in orchestrating control of infection. Macrophages can limit infection though direct viral clearance, enhanced antigen presentation to B and T cells, and production of proinflammatory or antiviral cytokines and chemokines.[426,527] The protective role of macrophages is highlighted by studies in mice, which demonstrated exacerbated WNV, TBEV, DENV, or YFV disease after selective macrophage depletion.[63,234,390,663,924] Macrophages may control flaviviruses through the production of nitric oxide (NO) and other reactive oxygen intermediates after stimulation of inducible nitric oxide synthetase (NOS-2).[422,484,712,713] Activation of macrophages in response to flavivirus infection also promotes release of type I interferon (IFN), tumor necrosis factor (TNF)-α, interleukin (IL)-1β, IL-8, and other cytokines, some of which have antiviral activity and reduce viral replication, at least in culture.[757] Despite their protective role in innate defense, macrophages also are targets of infection by some flaviviruses[416,441,684] and have the potential to contribute to pathogenesis through antibody-dependent enhancement of infection mediated by Fc-γ and complement receptors.[123,261,641] The macrophage cell surface receptor CLEC5a independently has been reported to interact with DENV directly, resulting in DAP12 phosphorylation and the release of proinflammatory cytokines.[144] Therefore, in some circumstances macrophages can contribute to flavivirus-induced disease, although the contribution to clearance versus pathogenesis may vary depending on the specific virus, the presence of preexisting nonneutralizing antibodies, and the specific proinflammatory molecules that are produced.

Neutrophils

Although polymorphonuclear leukocytes (neutrophils) are among the first circulating leukocytes to respond to infection or inflammatory stimuli, their function in flavivirus infection remains uncertain. Some studies suggest a protective function; however, others indicate that neutrophils can contribute to flavivirus pathogenesis. A protective role was reported in the context of WNV infection as macrophages produced neutrophil chemoattractive chemokines (CXCL1 and CXCL2), neutrophils rapidly migrated to the site of infection, and mice depleted of neutrophils 1 or 2 days after virus infection developed higher viremia and experienced earlier death.[30] Paradoxically, if neutrophils were depleted prior to infection, viremia was reduced and survival was enhanced.[30] Analogously, depletion of neutrophils resulted in prolonged survival and decreased mortality in Murray Valley encephalitis virus-infected mice, and neutrophil infiltration and disease correlated with NOS-2 expression within the CNS.[14] Finally, transcriptional gene signatures from whole blood showed a greater abundance of neutrophil transcripts in patients who progressed to DSS, a finding supported by higher plasma levels of proteins associated with neutrophil degranulation.[334] Although further studies are warranted, neutrophils may prevent or promote flavivirus disease, depending on the specific virus and immunologic context.

Dendritic Cells

Human peripheral blood contains two types of dendritic cells (DCs), plasmacytoid DCs (pDCs) and myeloid DCs (mDCs), which can be distinguished based on function and distinctive surface markers. pDCs lack phagocytic capacity and are less efficient in capturing and presenting antigens to T cells, but they produce extraordinarily high levels of type I IFN in the presence of viruses or bacteria,[759] and are thus considered to play a crucial role in antiviral immunity.[802,803] Low levels of DENV replication were observed in pDCs, but proinflammatory cytokines were produced rapidly and could accumulate to high levels. This cytokine response was not dependent on viral replication, but dependent on endosomal toll-like receptor 7 (TLR7), and could be induced by purified DENV RNA.[797,862] In prospective clinical studies, the absolute number of circulating pDCs remained stable early in moderately ill children with dengue fever or other nondengue, febrile illnesses. However, there was an early decrease in circulating pDCs in children who subsequently developed DHF, as a blunted blood pDC response was associated with an altered innate immune response, higher viremia levels, and severe disease.[646] Of interest, the host origin of the flavivirus influences the response that is generated by pDCs, as WNV grown in mammalian cells was a potent inducer of IFN-α secretion in pDCs, whereas pDCs failed to produce IFN-α when exposed to WNV grown in mosquito cells.[762]

mDCs reside and circulate throughout the body, enabling them to transport antigens from the periphery to lymphoid tissues. They are professional antigen-presenting cells that transmit incoming infectious signals to B and T cells to orchestrate rapid and efficient adaptive immune responses.[783] mDCs are more readily infected by flaviviruses *ex vivo,* and are thought to contribute to viral spread and early immune system priming depending on the particular virus. For example, WNV efficiently infects mouse mDCs and induces a type I IFN and proinflammatory cytokine response through RIG-I-like pattern recognition receptors and IPS-1-dependent signaling cascade.[178,800] In comparison, also in mice, JEV induced impaired responses through MyD88-dependent and -independent pathways, with blunted co-stimulatory molecule expression and production of the antiinflammatory cytokine IL-10, which resulted in poor T-cell priming.[7] DENV productively infects human mDCs and induces release of high levels of chemokines and proinflammatory cytokines, with the notable exception of type I IFN,[686,687] although this latter finding has not been observed with all strains of DENV.[35,469] Moreover, mature mDCs were capable of supporting antibody-dependent enhancement (ADE) of DENV, whereas immature DCs, due to expression of higher levels of DC-SIGN, did not promote ADE.[87]

Despite an accumulating wealth of data on purified mDC *ex vivo,* few studies have assessed their direct function *in vivo* in the context of flavivirus infection. A recent report showed that selective genetic deletion of $CD8\alpha^+$ mDCs resulted in defective cross-presentation and virus-specific $CD8^+$ T-cell responses to WNV.[331] The generation of diphtheria toxin receptor transgenic mice that selectively deplete DC subsets may allow further dissection of the net function of mDCs in flavivirus infection.

Natural Killer Cells

Natural killer (NK) cells are innate immune lymphocytes that serve as a first line of defense against a variety of infections.[75] NK cells mediate protection through the recognition and killing of target cells and the production of immunomodulatory cytokines, particularly IFN-γ, which enhances innate immunity and shapes the subsequent adaptive immune response.[161] Unlike adaptive T and B lymphocytes, NK cells do not rearrange their receptor genes somatically, but rely on a fixed number of inhibitory and activating cell receptors that recognize major histocompatibility complex (MHC) class I and class I–like molecules, as well as other ligands.[111] The function of NK cells in flavivirus infection remains uncertain. Some *in vitro* studies suggest that human NK cells can expand and inhibit WNV infection of cells through both cytolytic (antibody-dependent cell-mediated cytotoxicity [ADCC]) and non-cytolytic (IFN-γ) activities.[914] The activating human NK-cell receptor, NKp44 has been reported to directly bind to domain III of DENV and WNV E proteins. This interaction induced IFN-γ secretion and lysis of WNV-infected targets by NK cells.[328] However, flavivirus infection may inhibit NK-cell killing by increasing the cell surface expression of class I MHC molecules,[209,329,400] which sends a negative signal to NK cells.[363] *In vivo,* the function of NK cells in flavivirus infection also remains unclear. Although NK cells expand and become activated in YFV- and DENV-infected humans and mice,[140,610,747] antibody depletion of NK cells in mice did not alter morbidity or mortality after WNV infection.[755]

$\gamma\delta$ T Cells

$\gamma\delta$ T cells contribute to the innate defense against several viruses by virtue of their relative frequency in blood and epithelial sites and ability to respond rapidly to nonpeptide antigens and secrete proinflammatory cytokines and chemokines. Because they lack classical MHC restriction, $\gamma\delta$ T cells can react with viral antigens in the absence of conventional antigen processing.[781] $\gamma\delta$ T cells are divided into functionally distinct subsets, which have disparate effects on host immunity to pathogen infection. Splenic $V\gamma1^+$ $\gamma\delta$ T cells contribute to eliminating *Listeria* infection by virtue of their IFN-γ activity.[536] In comparison, $V\gamma4^+$ $\gamma\delta$ T cells enhance Th1-cell activation through IFN-γ– and CD1-dependent mechanisms.[349] To date, much of the initial analysis of $\gamma\delta$ T cell function during flavivirus infection has focused on studies with WNV in mice, although recent studies confirm that human and monkey $\gamma\delta$ T cells also are activated rapidly after YFV infection.[196,611] Mice deficient in $\gamma\delta$ T cells were more susceptible to WNV infection,[867] and this was in part due to their ability to produce IFN-γ, which has direct antiviral effects.[756] Moreover, mice depleted of $V\gamma1^+$ $\gamma\delta$ T cells have enhanced viremia and higher WNV mortality, whereas the opposite is observed with depletion of $V\gamma4^+$ $\gamma\delta$ T cells.[877] Subsequent work showed that $\gamma\delta$ T cells also contribute to the development of a protective $CD8^+$ T-cell response against WNV, as $TCR\delta^{-/-}$ mice were more susceptible than wild type mice to secondary WNV challenge.[866] This priming effect may reflect DC maturation (increased expression of surface co-stimulatory and class II MHC molecules and secretion of IL-12) that is promoted by $\gamma\delta$ T cells after activation by WNV.[231]

Mast Cells

Mast cells contribute to a variety of inflammatory reactions and host defense against pathogens[519] by secreting chemokines, cytokines, and inflammatory lipid mediators and granule-associated products. Mast cells express several Fc receptors, reside primarily in tissues, and associate closely with vascular beds.[744] Recent studies suggest that infection or activation of mast cells in tissues by DENV can promote viral clearance[776] or have immunopathologic consequences that contribute to the vasculopathy associated with secondary infection. DENV infection of mast cells *ex vivo* resulted in increased secretion of chemokines, including CCL5 without inducing degranulation,[398] and production of vasoactive cytokines was enhanced in the presence of subneutralizing concentrations of antibody that promotes ADE.[399] Antibody-enhanced DENV infection of mast cells in culture also resulted in significant production of TNF-α, which can stimulate endothelial cells,[108] as well as massive mast cell apoptosis that occurs via global caspase activation.[109] Although more investigation is needed, DENV-infected mast cells may contribute to endothelial cell activation and permeability via local production of cytokines.

Cell-Intrinsic Immunity

Recognition and Control of Flaviviruses by Host Sensors

Interferon (IFN) responses are an essential host defense program against many viruses, including flaviviruses. IFNs are produced during the earliest stages of viral infection after recognition of pathogen-associated molecular patterns (PAMPs) by specific pathogen recognition receptors (PRRs). In mammalian cells, the host detects and responds to infection by flaviviruses by primarily recognizing viral RNA through several distinct PRRs including the cell surface and endosomal RNA sensors TLR3 and TLR7, and the cytoplasmic RNA sensors retinoic acid–inducible gene I (RIG-I) and melanoma-differentiation–associated gene 5 (MDA5) (Fig. 26.10). Binding of single- and/or double-stranded (ds) viral RNA to these PRR results in downstream activation of transcription factors, such as IFN regulatory factors 3 and 7 (IRF-3 and IRF-7) and NF-κB, and induction of IFN-α and IFN-β. Secretion of IFNs followed by engagement of the IFN-$\alpha\beta$ receptor (IFNAR) in an autocrine and paracrine fashion activates janus kinase (JAK)-signal transducer and activator of transcription (STAT) pathway–dependent and independent signal transduction cascades[465] that induce the expression of hundreds of IFN-stimulated genes (ISGs), a subset of which likely have antiviral activity against flaviviruses (Fig. 26.11).[733]

Recent studies suggest that RIG-I and MDA5 contribute to the induction of host IFN and antiviral response to flaviviruses (Fig. 26.10). Murine embryonic fibroblasts (MEFs) deficient in RIG-I and MDA5 showed decreased IRF-3 activation, delayed induction of host interferon and ISG responses, and augmented WNV and DENV replication.[239,240,500,604] RIG-I

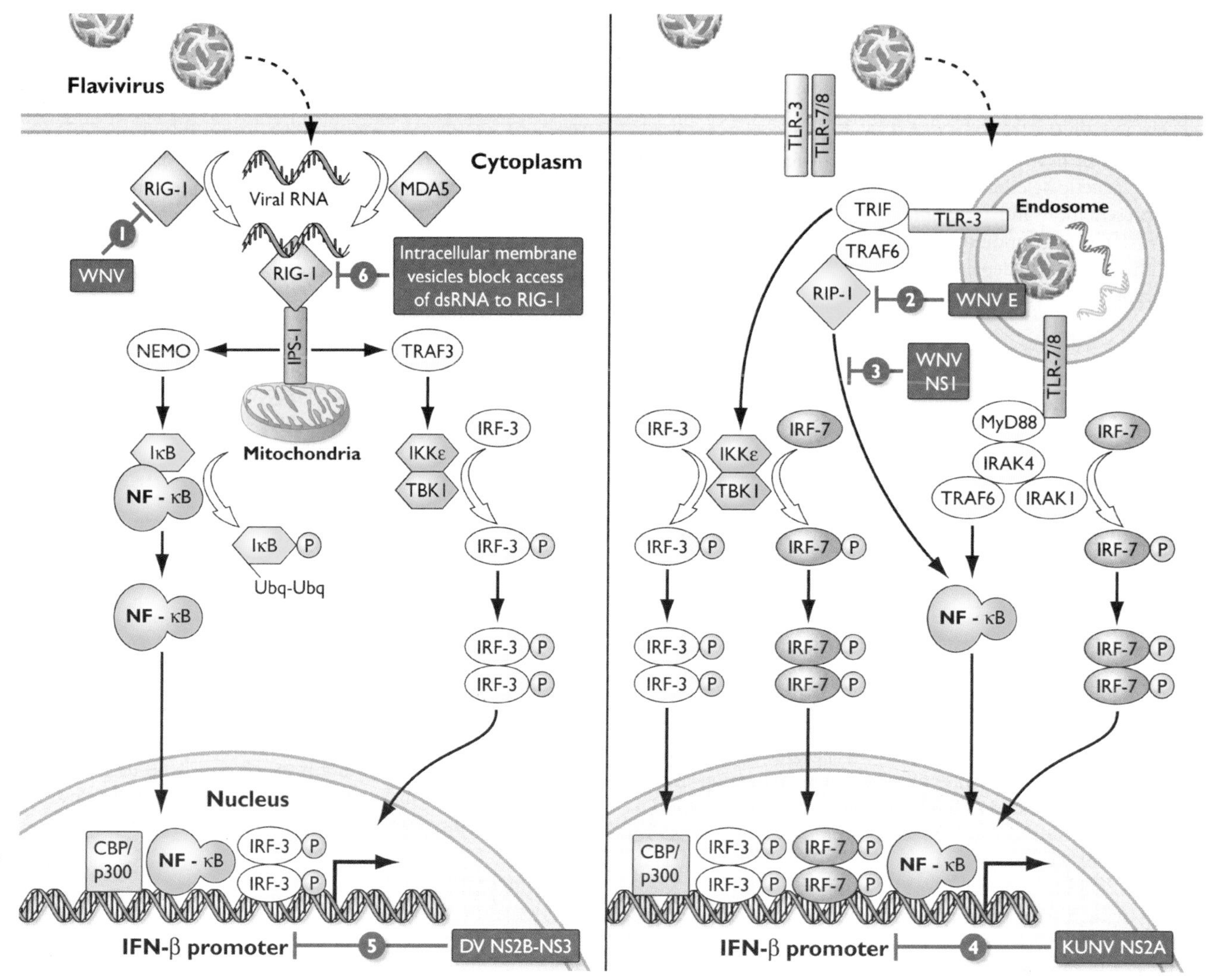

FIGURE 26.10. Detection of flavivirus RNA by pathogen recognition receptors (PRRs) and mechanisms of viral evasion. (Left) Cytoplasmic PRR and signaling cascade. Infection by flaviviruses produces double-stranded RNA (dsRNA) replication intermediates that display motifs recognized by retinoic acid–inducible protein I (RIG-I) and possibly, the melanoma disassociation-associated 5 (MDA5) helicase. Binding of viral RNA promotes an interaction with IPS-1 that results in recruitment of signaling proteins (NEMO and TRAF3) that activate interferon regulatory factor 3 (IRF-3) and nuclear factor kappa B (NF-κB). These transcription factors translocate to the nucleus and bind to the promoter region of the IFN-*β* gene leading to transcription and translation. **(Right)** Toll-like receptor (TLR) signaling cascade. In some cells, the transmembrane PRRs TLR3 and TLR7/8 in endosomes recognize double-stranded RNA (dsRNA) and single-stranded RNA (ssRNA) motifs leading to recruitment of cytoplasmic adaptor molecules (TIR-domain-containing adapter-inducing interferon-*β* [TRIF] and Mmeloid differentiation primary response gene (88) [MYD88], respectively), which initiate signaling cascades (via I kappaB kinase [IKK] TANK-binding kinase 1 [TBK1] Receptor-Interacting Protein 1 [RIP-1] and interleukin-1 receptor-associated kinase 4 [IRAK-4]) that activate IRF-3, IRF-7, and NF-κB, resulting in IFN-*β* gene transcription. Mechanisms of evasion by flaviviruses are believed to include the following: (1) a delay in recognition of West Nile virus (WNV) RNA by RIG-I; (2) impairment of RIP-1 signaling by high mannose carbohydrates on the structural E protein; (3) attenuation of TLR3 signaling by the NS1 protein; (4) reduction in IFN-*β* gene transcription by the Kunjin virus (KUNV) NS2A protein; (5) reduction of type I IFN production by catalytically active dengue virus (DENV) NS2B-NS3 protein; and (6) viral dsRNA intermediates localized to specialized membrane vesicles, which prevent rapid detection by intracellular sensors such as RIG-I.

appears to prime the early type I IFN response, whereas MDA5 has a more apparent role in a second phase of IFN-dependent gene expression that occurs later in the course of infection. A genetic deficiency of IPS-1 (also known as Cardif, mitochondrial antiviral signaling protein [MAVS], or virus-induced signaling adaptor [VISA]), an essential RIG-I and MDA5 adaptor molecule that is anchored to the outer leaflet of mitochondria, completely disabled the innate IFN response[178,240] and was associated with enhanced WNV lethality in mice with dysregulated immune responses.[800] RIG-I–dependent signaling appears dominant in mice, as animals deficient in RIG-I were more vulnerable to JEV infection,[379] and a deficiency of proteins that regulate the Tripartite motif-containing protein 25 (TRIM25)-mediated ubiquination and activation of RIG-I resulted in enhanced WNV replication and mortality.[863] Consistent with this, JEV and DENV induce the host type I IFN response

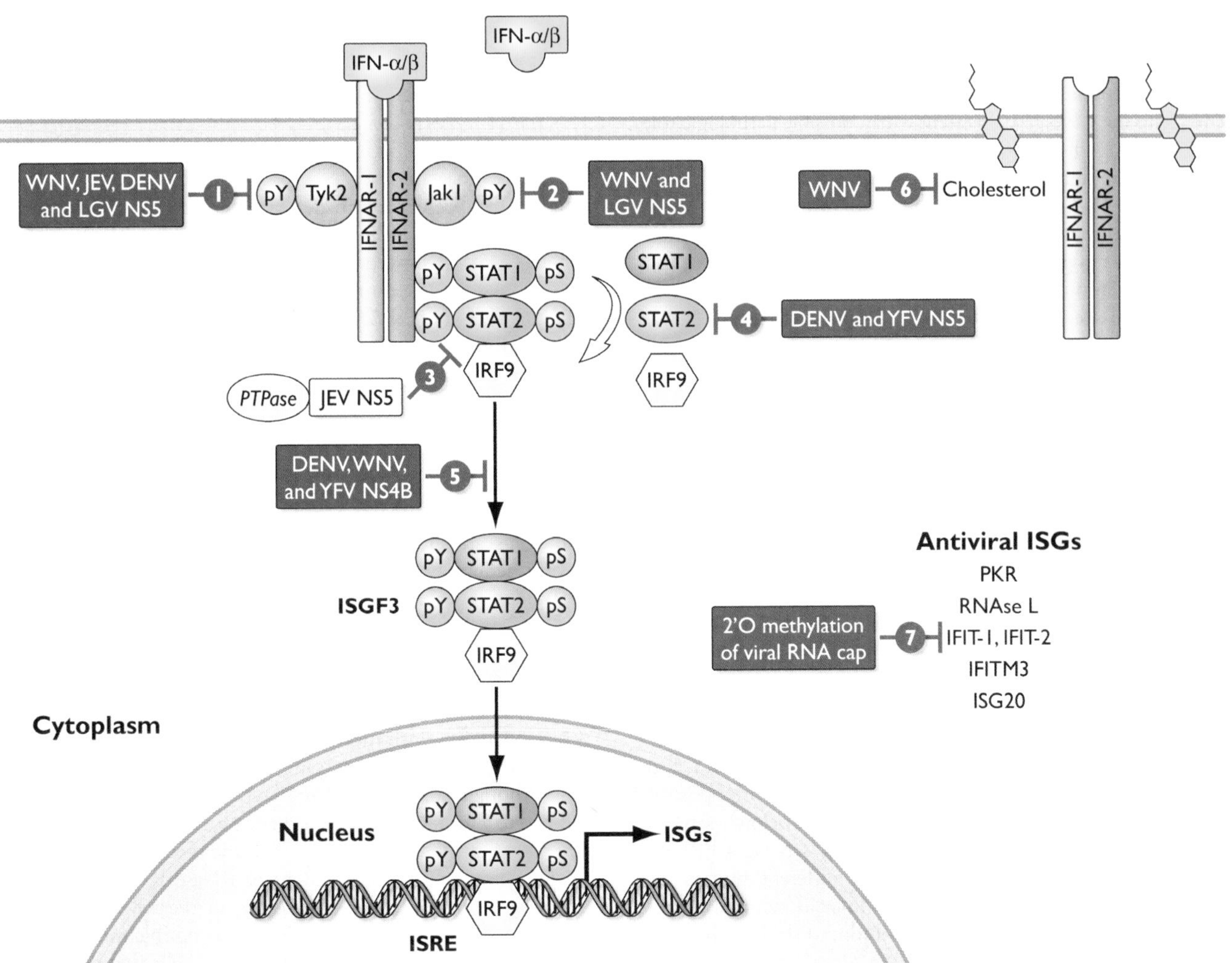

FIGURE 26.11. Type I interferon (IFN) signaling and mechanisms of disruption by flaviviruses. Secretion of IFN by a flavivirus-infected cell results in autocrine and paracrine signaling through the heterodimeric IFN-$\alpha\beta$ receptor (IFNAR). Binding by IFN results in activation and tyrosine phosphorylation of Janus kinase (JAK) family members (JAK1 and Tyk2) and the cytoplasmic tail of the IFNAR. This promotes recruitment of the signal transducers and activators of transcription (STAT1) and STAT2, which themselves become phosphorylated by the JAKs. Phosphorylated STAT1 and STAT2 proteins heterodimerize, associate with IRF-9, and translocate to the nucleus, where they bind interferon-sensitive response element (ISRE) sequences to induce expression of hundreds of interferon-stimulated genes (ISGs). Mechanisms of evasion by flaviviruses are believed to include the following: blockade of phosphorylation of (1) Tyk2 and (2) JAK1 by flavivirus NS5; (3) activation of a phosphotyrosine phosphatase by JEV NS5; (4) reduction in STAT2 gene and protein expression by Dengue virus (DENV) and Yellow fever virus (YFV) NS5; (5) attenuation of STAT signaling by flavivirus NS4B; (6) downregulation of the IFNAR through virus-induced redistribution of cellular cholesterol; and (7) antagonism of interferon-induced protein with tetratricopeptide repeats (IFIT) family genes effector functions by 2′O methylation of flavivirus RNA.

through a mechanism involving RIG-I/IRF-3 and NF-κB.[136] MDA5 may be less important for flavivirus recognition, as IFN production by MDA5$^{-/-}$ myeloid dendritic cells remains largely intact after WNV infection,[256] and a deficiency of MDA5 in mice did not affect survival after JEV,[379] although higher mortality rates are observed after WNV infection (H. Lazear and M. Diamond, unpublished results). Despite data from murine embryonic fibroblasts (MEF) suggesting that RIG-I and likely MDA5 recognize WNV RNA and induce type I IFN responses, IFN-α and β production in mice appears independent of IPS-1[800] or the downstream transcription factor IRF-3.[89,174] Therefore, individual cell types (myeloid, fibroblast, and neuronal) use distinct PRR responses to protect against flavivirus infection through both IFN-dependent and IFN-independent pathways.[177]

TLR3, which is expressed on the surface of fibroblasts and in the endosomes of myeloid cells, promotes IRF-3 phosphorylation after binding ds viral RNA through a complex signaling cascade that includes recruitment of TIR-domain-containing adapter-inducing interferon-β (TRIF) and activation of the kinases TANK-binding kinase 1 (TBK1) and I kappaB kinase (IKKε).[535,735] Initial studies with TRIF-deficient MEF suggested that TLR3 may be dispensable for recognition of flaviviruses in cells,[239] although subsequent cell culture studies showed a proinflammatory and protective effect of TLR3 after DENV infection.[604,834] Experiments in TLR3$^{-/-}$ mice have had conflicting results. TLR3$^{-/-}$ mice injected by an intraperitoneal route paradoxically showed decreased WNV lethality despite higher peripheral viral titers, presumably because of blunted cytokine responses (e.g., TNF-α) that normally facilitate virus entry into the CNS.[868] Consistent with a possible pathologic role, preliminary studies suggest a functional TLR3 allele is a risk factor for severe human TBEV infection.[397] In comparison, other studies with TLR3$^{-/-}$ mice and a different North American WNV strain showed increased viral burden in the brain and enhanced lethality,[176] as might be anticipated for a PRR that triggers a protective host immune response. *Ex vivo* and *in vivo* experiments suggest a cell-specific role for TLR3, as it protected against WNV largely by restricting replication in neurons.

TLR7 is an endosomal PRR that detects guanosine and uridine-rich single-stranded RNA[207] and activates IRF-7 via the Myeloid differentiation primary response gene (88) (MYD88) adaptor molecule. IRF-7 was identified as a primary regulator of antiviral gene induction after YFV infection,[247] with some of this activation occurring through TLR7 recognition of viral RNA.[667,668,797,862] Similarly, DENV stimulates IFN production in pDCs in a TLR7-dependent manner after virus uncoating.[862] The antiviral IFN-α response against WNV is mediated primarily by IRF-7,[175] and at least some of this signal is attributed to recognition of viral RNA by TLR7. Indeed, both TLR7$^{-/-}$ and MyD88$^{-/-}$ mice show increased susceptibility to WNV infection, and this was associated with increased local infection and decreased production of IL-1β, IL-6, IL-12, IL-23, and several chemokines, which altered leukocyte trafficking and virus control in several tissues.[572a,805,828,878] In addition to its possible antiviral effects as an IFN effector molecule (see below), dsRNA-dependent protein kinase R (PKR) also may serve as a PRR for inducing interferon responses. In three different human cell lines, small interfering RNA (siRNA) knockdown and chemical inhibition of PKR blocked WNV-induced IFN synthesis.[255]

Type I IFN Signaling Pathway

Type I IFNs induce an antiviral state by upregulating genes with both direct and indirect inhibitory functions.[651] In mice, for example, there are at least 14 IFN-α and one IFN–β isoforms, in addition to multiple other subtypes.[840] IFN-α and IFN-β are considered the dominant functional type I IFN in humans and are secreted by many cell types following virus infection. Type I IFN primes adaptive immune responses through stimulation of DCs, activation of B and T cells, and by preventing death of recently activated T cells.[451,452,784] Pretreatment of cells with IFN-α or IFN-β inhibits flavivirus replication *in vitro,*[68,203,482,505,849] but treatment after infection is less effective.[13,166,203,704,778] Although flaviviruses can antagonize IFN-induced responses after infection, IFN still restricts replication and spread *in vivo.* Mice lacking the type I IFN receptor (IFNAR$^{-/-}$) or downstream signaling components (e.g., STAT1) show enhanced lethality and replication after infection with WNV,[385,704] DENV,[748] YFV,[548] or MVEV.[496] Increased infection occurred in normally resistant cell populations and tissues after flavivirus infection of IFNAR$^{-/-}$ mice, suggesting that IFN acts, in part, to restrict viral tropism. The importance of type I IFN in controlling flavivirus infection has been confirmed in therapeutic disease models. Pretreatment of animals with IFN-α or inducers of IFN-α attenuates infection by SLEV, WNV, YFV, and Modoc viruses.[106,366,463,464,650,812] The relevance of these pathways has been confirmed in vivo as several recent microarray analyses have shown that animals or primary cells infected with flaviviruses produce a potent innate antiviral transcriptional gene signature characterized by genes downstream of type I IFN signaling.[35,334,668,710]

Type I IFN-Induced Genes that Control Flavivirus Infection

Progress has been made in defining the specific IFN-induced antiviral genes that limit flavivirus infection (Fig. 26.11). Initial studies showed that dsRNA-dependent PKR and 2′-5′-oligoadenylate synthase (Oas) proteins mediated intrinsic cell resistance to WNV.[706] PKR is activated by binding dsRNA and phosphorylates the eukaryotic translation initiation factor 2 (eIF2-α) resulting in attenuation of protein synthesis.[552] PKR also may have independent antiviral effects by activating signaling pathways that augment type I IFN production[48,255] and directly regulating IFN-β mRNA stability.[738] RNase L is activated by 2′-5′-linked oligoadenylates that are synthesized by Oas enzymes. RNase L inhibits viral infections by functioning as an endoribonuclease that cleaves viral RNA[920,921] and by generating small self-RNA PAMPs that amplify antiviral immunity through a RIG-I and MDA5-dependent pathway.[517,518] RNase L$^{-/-}$ MEF and macrophages supported increased WNV replication in *vitro,*[706,717] and knockdown of RNase L enhanced infectivity in human cells.[483] Moreover, mice deficient in RNase L showed increased lethality following WNV infection, with higher viral loads in peripheral tissues at early time points after infection.[706]

Although susceptibility to flaviviruses in mice has been mapped to a mutation in the *Oas* gene 1b, resulting in the expression of a truncated Oas isoform,[532,643] the mechanism of control by this gene appears independent of RNase L[717] and the type I IFN signaling pathway.[104] Knock-in of the wild-type Oas1b allele into a flavivirus-induced disease susceptible mouse generated a resistant phenotype,[716] and murine cells that ectopically expressed Oas1b resisted WNV infection by preventing viral RNA accumulation inside infected cells.[372] Although biochemical studies have shown that Oas1b itself is an inactive 2′-5′ Oas, recent experiments suggest that Oas1b inhibits Oas1a activity, resulting in reduced 2′-5′ oligoA production in response to poly(I:C).[220] Negative regulation of 2′-5′ Oas by inactive Oas1b proteins may tune the RNase L response that could cause significant damage in cells, if it were not tightly controlled.

More recent studies have used ectopic expression and siRNA or short hairpin RNA (shRNA) knockdown strategies to identify key and novel ISGs that restrict infection of different flaviviruses. A large-scale ectopic lentivirus screen identified several regulatory and effector ISGs that inhibit infection of WNV and YFV in human cells.[733] Ectopic expression of ISG15, a ubiquitin-like protein that conjugates to key proteins of the cellular innate immune response,[253] inhibited replication of the JEV in human medulloblastoma cells,[343] although ISG15$^{-/-}$ mice or neurons are not more susceptible to WNV infection (M. Samuel, D. Lenschow, and M. Diamond, unpublished observations). Members of the Interferon-inducible transmembrane (IFITM) proteins were recently shown to inhibit an early entry step in infection of DENV and WNV in cells.[94] This observation was confirmed by ectopic expression studies in HEK293 cells.[359] Other studies have suggested that viperin[359,804] and ISG20[359,922] also may inhibit infection by flaviviruses. Although the field is rapidly advancing with respect to identifying antiviral ISG against flaviviruses, definitive studies in genetically deficient animals may be required to establish the cell- and tissue-specific nonredundant effects of individual ISG in controlling flavivirus infection in the context of a robust type I IFN response.

Chemokines

Depending on the specific flavivirus infection, individual chemokines and cytokines can either protect or contribute to pathogenesis. For encephalitic flaviviruses, production of inflammatory chemokines in the brain by neuronal and non-neuronal cells coordinates recruitment of lymphocytes for clearance of viral infection. Chemokines that have been detected in the brain or CSF after WNV, JEV, or TBEV infection of mice include CXCL9 (MIG), CXCL10 (IP-10), CXCL11 (I-TAC), CCL2, (MCP-1), CCL3 (MIP-1a), CCL4 (MIP-1b), and CCL5 (RANTES).[245,291,404,746,825] WNV infection in the brain is associated with the early expression of the T-cell chemoattractant CXCL10 by virally infected neurons[404]; this expression proceeds in a caudal to rostral direction with higher levels detected in the cerebellum. This regional heterogeneity in CXCL10 expression is due to differential regulation by WNV-infected cortical versus cerebellar granule cell neurons and leads to enhanced trafficking of WNV-specific T cells that express the CXCL10 receptor CXCR3 into the cerebellum.[913] Loss of CXCL10 or CXCR3 via targeted deletion or neutralizing antibody administration leads to decreased recruitment of WNV-specific $CD8^+$ T cells into the CNS, especially within the cerebellum, increased viral loads, and enhanced mortality.[404,913] In contrast, antagonism of polarized CXCR4–CXCL12 interactions along the BBB improved survival from lethal WNV infection through enhanced intraparenchymal migration of WNV-specific $CD8^+$ T cells within the brain, leading to reduced viral loads and decreased immunopathology.[540]

A genetic deficiency in CCR2, a chemokine receptor on inflammatory monocytes and other leukocyte subtypes, resulted in markedly increased WNV-induced mortality in C57BL/6 mice,[477] and was associated with a selective reduction of monocyte accumulation in the brain. Subsequent experiments showed that CCR2 mediates selective peripheral blood monocytosis in the context of WNV infection, and this is critical for accumulation of protective monocytes in the brain. Although a protective role for CCL2–CCR2 interactions was observed with a virulent WNV isolate, an opposing phenotype was seen after infection with an attenuated strain; neutralization of CCL2 reduced the number of microglia in the brain during WNV infection but prolonged the life of infected animals.[252] Therefore, depending on the virulence of the strain, CCL2–CCR2-dependent monocyte accumulation and migration may differentially affect disease outcome after WNV infection.

Additional studies have established that the chemokines CCL3, CCL4, and CCL5, all of which bind to the chemokine receptor CCR5, are strongly induced within the brain after WNV infection.[258,404,746] Moreover, targeted deletion of CCR5 is associated with depressed leukocyte trafficking, increased viral burden, and enhanced mortality.[258] An analysis of WNV infection in humans with CCR5Δ32, a defective *CCR5* allele, showed that homozygosity for the allele correlated with an increased risk of symptomatic disease.[259,475,476] Because the mouse studies examined the entire brain with regard to expression and leukocyte trafficking, and the human studies did not report on specific neurologic symptoms, it remains unclear whether CCR5-expressing leukocytes also exhibit regional specificity during CNS recruitment. Finally, a case of YFV vaccine-associated viscerotropic disease was associated with genetic polymorphisms in both *CCR5* and *CCL5* genes.[662]

For viscerotropic flaviviruses such as DENV, the function of chemokine interaction with their receptors remains less certain. Although DENV-infected wild-type mice produce high levels of chemokines CCL2, CCL3, and CCL5 in their spleen and liver, $CCR1^{-/-}$ mice had a phenotype similar to wild-type mice, whereas infection of $CCR2^{-/-}$ or $CCR4^{-/-}$ mice showed attenuated lethality, liver damage, leukocyte activation, and levels of IL-6 and IFN-γ without significant differences in viral load.[283] Therefore, chemokine–chemokine receptor interactions in the context of DENV infection appear to contribute to the development of disease. Nevertheless, in an encephalitic mouse model of DENV infection, CXCL10 interaction with CXCR3 was required for clearance and resistance to infection.[344]

Complement Activation and Flaviviruses

The complement system is a family of serum and cell surface proteins that recognize PAMPs, altered-self ligands, and immune complexes. Although complement activation inhibits infection of many viruses (reviewed in[27,788]), it has both protective and pathogenic roles in flavivirus infection depending on the specific virus, phase of the infection, and immune status of the host. Activation of the complement cascade triggers several antiviral functions, including pathogen opsonization and/or lysis, and priming of adaptive immune responses. Complement is activated through the classical, lectin, and alternative pathways depending on specific recognition molecules.[855,856] Classical pathway activity is triggered by C1q binding to antigen–antibody complexes on the surface of pathogens. The lectin pathway is initiated by mannose binding lectin (MBL) or ficolin recognition of carbohydrate structures on the surface of microbes or apoptotic cells. The alternative pathway is constitutively active at low levels through the spontaneous hydrolysis of C3 and also amplifies activation of the classical and lectin pathways. The classical, lectin, and alternative pathways generate convertase enzymes (C4bC2a for classical and lectin, and C3bBb for the alternative), which cleave C3, the central component of the complement system, and expose a reactive internal thioester bond on C3b necessary for covalent attachment to target surfaces. The binding of C3b back to C4b2a and C3bBb C3 convertases forms the classical and alternative pathway C5 convertases, respectively. These enzymes cleave C5 and promote assembly of C5b-9 membrane attack complex (MAC), which lyses pathogens or infected cells. Sublytic amounts of C5b-9 on a cell surface can activate granulocytes and endothelial cells, whereas soluble C5b-9 independently induces inflammation through cytokine induction. The release of anaphylatoxins (C3a and C5a) by the C3 and C5 convertases also promotes chemotaxis of immune cells via the interaction with specific G-protein coupled transmembrane receptors (C3aR and C5aR). Deposition of C3 and C4 fragments (C3b and C4b) on a pathogen facilitates binding and phagocytosis by complement receptors (CR1, CR3, CR4, and CRIg), a process called opsonization, which helps to clear microbial infections.[125]

Protective Activity of Complement on Flavivirus Infection

Complement can limit flavivirus infection by stimulating adaptive immune responses or by directly neutralizing infection. In support of an immune priming role for complement, $C3^{-/-}$ mice are more susceptible to lethal WNV infection and show greater viral burden and reduced antiviral antibody titers.[547] Infection studies with mice lacking C1q, MBL, C4, or factor B establish that all complement activation pathways protect against WNV infection.[243,545] However, each activation pathway appears to exert distinct effects in response to WNV infection. Humoral IgM responses to WNV depend upon activation of C3 by the lectin recognition pathway. In contrast, both the lectin and alternative pathways appear necessary for efficient T-cell priming, as $C4^{-/-}$, factor $B^{-/-}$, and factor $D^{-/-}$ mice exhibited reduced WNV-specific $CD8^{+}$ T-cell responses.[545] The T-cell defects in $C4^{-/-}$ mice may be indirect as depressed IgM responses could affect viral opsonization and antigen presentation. The terminal lytic complement components (C5–C9) do not appear to serve a major function in protection, as C5 neither contributed to protection against WNV pathogenesis nor augmented the neutralizing efficacy of complement-fixing anti-WNV neutralizing antibodies in mice.[546]

Flaviviruses directly trigger complement activation, which can inhibit infectivity. Increasing concentrations of serum complement neutralize WNV or DENV in cell culture and *in vivo* in the absence of antibody, and this depends on recognition of N-linked glycans on the surface of the virion by MBL.[242] Complement activation by flaviviruses occurs *in vivo,* as C3 and C4 consumption occur prior to the induction of a specific antibody response.[545]

Complement augments antibody-mediated neutralization of flaviviruses, including YFV, DENV, and WNV.[192,547,775] The C1q component of complement is sufficient to enhance the potency of antibody neutralization as it reduces the number of antibodies that must bind the virion to neutralize infectivity.[546] The protective efficacy of flavivirus neutralizing antibodies *in vivo* correlates with IgG subclasses that efficiently fix complement.[546,724]

Pathologic Effects of Complement on Flavivirus Infection

In myeloid cells that express complement receptors, antibody-dependent complement activation paradoxically may enhance viral infection.[123,124] Blockade of complement receptor-3 (CD11b/CD18) abrogated the complement-dependent enhancement of WNV infection in this model system. Therefore, under certain circumstances, antibody and complement-dependent opsonization of flaviviruses may increase infection in myeloid cells.

During severe secondary DENV infection, a vascular leakage syndrome occurs with fluid transudation into serosal spaces. Although the pathogenesis of DENV infection remains incompletely understood, a pathologic role for complement activation has been proposed.[28,85] In early clinical studies, reduced levels of C3 and C4 and factor B and increased catabolic rates of C3 and C1q were observed, particularly in patients with severe DENV disease.[85] In addition, C3 breakdown products and anaphylatoxins accumulated in the circulation of severely ill patients and peaked at the day of maximum vascular leakage.[157,516] Circulating immune complexes formed by virions and DENV-specific antibodies have been hypothesized to cause the pathologic complement activation.[85] One alternative hypothesis is that infected cells express sufficient amounts of DENV antigens (E or NS1 proteins) on their surface, thereby facilitating immune complex formation and complement deposition.[69] Indeed, DENV-infected endothelial cells activate human complement in the presence of antibodies resulting in C5b-9 deposition.[26,28]

Humoral Immunity

Humoral immunity contributes significantly to the host response to flavivirus infection. Virus challenge experiments using inbred strains of mice identified the importance of B cells during a protective response.[204,205] The importance of antiviral antibody has been established directly. Passive administration of virus-reactive mAbs, purified polyclonal γ-globulin, and immune sera confers significant protection in small animal models of flavivirus infection.[202] For example, transfer of heat-inactivated WNV-immune serum into wild-type mice completely protects from lethal infection with WNV; administration of antibody into *uMT* or *RAG1* KO mouse strains prior to virus challenge delays mortality but does not protect from death.[204] Antibodies may also protect from disease when administered therapeutically after infection.[202] Although neutralizing antibody titers correlate with protection by several flavivirus vaccines,[60,320,533,575] the relationship may be imperfect.[81] Antibodies also may exert protective effects via effector functions mediated by the Fc portion of the antibody molecule, including complement fixation, antibody-mediated cellular cytotoxicity, and facilitating virus and clearance.[546,724,725] Protective antibodies that bind epitopes on the prM and E structural proteins incorporated into virions, as well as the nonstructural protein NS1, have been characterized.[211,381]

Stoichiometric Requirements for Neutralization

Antibody-mediated neutralization of flaviviruses requires engagement by antibodies with a stoichiometry that exceeds a particular threshold (reviewed by[211]). From this perspective, the number of antibodies bound to the virion is controlled by the functional avidity of the antibody for viral antigens on the virion, and the number of times an epitope is displayed on the virion in a context in which it is accessible for antibody binding. Complexities that modulate the accessibility of viral epitopes include the dense arrangement of E proteins on the surface of the mature virion,[497,624,629,787] the extent of virion maturation,[607] and the structural dynamics of the virus particle.[210,497] Antibody avidity determines the fraction of accessible antibody epitopes bound by antibody molecules at any concentration of antibody.[211,403] The mAb E16 binds a relatively accessible epitope on the E-DIII-LR and supports neutralization at a low occupancy.[648] Similar findings were reported for neutralizing anti-DENV antibodies that bind a similar epitope.[279] By comparison, antibodies that bind poorly accessible "cryptic" epitopes may neutralize only at saturation.[280,607,648,787] It is notable that some epitopes are not displayed with a frequency that allows engagement of the virion with a stoichiometry that allows for neutralization, even when fully occupied. Therefore, antibodies that bind cryptic epitopes may be incapable of neutralization regardless of their functional affinity for the virion.[607,648] The limited neutralizing activity of prM-specific antibodies may simply reflect an inability to bind the virion enough times (Fig. 26.12).

The stoichiometric requirements for neutralization of WNV have been estimated.[648] Experiments with E-DIII-LR-specific mAbs demonstrate that neutralization requires occupancy of 20% to 25% of accessible epitopes on the mature virion. Because only 120 epitopes on the mature virion are accessible for antibody binding, this translates into a requirement for engagement of the virion by roughly 30 antibody molecules. The functional significance of this number is not yet clear. Of potential interest, it does agree with predictions of the "coating

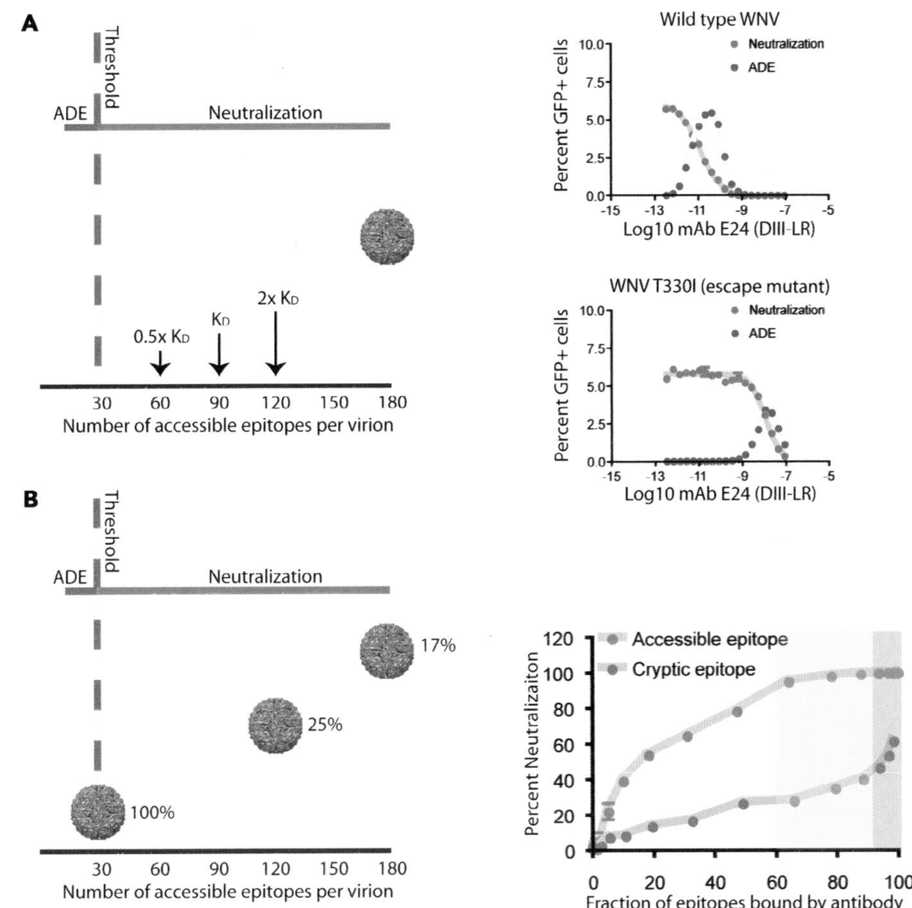

FIGURE 26.12. Antibody affinity and epitope accessibility govern the neutralization potency of anti-flavivirus antibodies. Neutralization of flaviviruses is a multiple-hit phenomenon that requires engagement of the virion by antibody with a stoichiometry that exceeds a threshold estimated at approximately 30 antibody molecules. The number of antibody molecules bound to the virion at any given antibody concentration is determined in part by the strength of the antibody–virion interaction and epitope accessibility. **A:** The affinity of antibody–virion interactions determines the fraction of epitopes displayed on the virion bound by antibody at given concentration. **(Right)** Therefore, changes in antibody affinity (conferred in this example via mutation of the antibody epitope) results in a change in the number of antibodies bound to the virus particle at each antibody dilution and a shift in the neutralization profile toward higher concentrations of antibody. **B:** Epitope accessibility, which may vary considerably depending on its location on the virion and the maturation state of the virion, governs the occupancy requirements for neutralization. For a theoretical flavivirus displaying 180 epitopes, an epitope occupancy of 17% is required to exceed a stoichiometric threshold of 30 antibody molecules. A reduction in epitope accessibility translates into increases in the fraction of epitopes that must be engaged to support virus neutralization. **(Right)** Antibodies that bind highly accessible determinants may completely neutralize infection at relatively modest occupancy (60%, *green shading*), whereas antibodies that bind poorly accessible structures neutralize infection only at full occupancy (*red shading*). (Reproduced from Dowd KA, Pierson TC. Antibody-mediated neutralization of flaviviruses: a reductionist view. *Virology.* 2011;411(2):306–315, with permission.)

theory" model that suggest the number of antibodies required to neutralize a virion is determined by surface area of the virus particle.[114] It will be important to determine the stoichiometric requirements for neutralization by antibodies that bind other epitopes; this is complicated experimentally as antibody-mediated neutralization of many other epitopes is modulated by the extent of maturation and structural dynamics of the virion.

Mechanisms of Neutralization

Antibodies have the capacity to neutralize directly the infectivity of viruses via several mechanisms that act at distinct steps in the virus life cycle. Anti-flavivirus antibodies can block virus attachment to host cells.[170,317,624] At present, it is unknown whether antibodies that block attachment to cells do so by interfering with specific interactions with receptor on the target cells or via a general steric hindrance mechanism. Flavivirus-reactive antibodies also may block infection to virions after the attachment step. Studies by Gollins and Porterfield demonstrated that antibodies could block the uncoating and infectivity of WNV, even when added after virions attached to cells. Furthermore, they demonstrated that antibodies could directly block fusion of virions to synthetic liposomes.[263] These observations have been expanded to include other flaviviruses and antibodies.[689,822] Analysis of the ability of a large panel of TBEV-reactive antibodies to block liposomal fusion reveal mAbs capable of blocking fusion completely (25% of antibodies tested), partially (58% of antibodies tested), or not at all (17% of antibodies tested).[786] These results suggest that an ability to block fusion is a relatively common functional property of neutralizing antibodies. Two recent atomic structures illustrate different ways antibodies that decorate the virus particle may block fusion. Experiments with Fab fragments of mAb E16 suggest this antibody blocks the radial expansion of the virus particle and traps it in an intermediate step of the fusion process following exposure of the virus to acidic conditions.[382] In contrast, the complex epitope recognized by the mAb CR4354, which was composed of multiple E proteins, suggests a mechanism of inhibition by which E proteins on the surface are cross-linked together, preventing the rearrangements that propel fusion.[384]

How an antibody neutralizes flavivirus infection may depend on context, as an individual antibody may block virus infection at more than one step of the virus entry pathway. For example, mAb E16 partially blocks attachment at relatively high antibody concentration. Virus binding is not significantly inhibited at lower concentrations of antibody at which significant virus neutralization is observed.[210,624] This observation suggests that the stoichiometric requirements for neutralization may differ depending on the mechanism of inhibition.

Antibody-Dependent Enhancement of Infection

Antibody-dependent enhancement (ADE) of infection describes a phenomenon in which a significant increase in the efficiency of virus infection is observed in the presence of virus-reactive antibody.[306,307] Although ADE has been demonstrated for several families of viruses *in vitro,* a role for enhancing antibodies *in vivo* has been suggested in only a few contexts, including secondary DENV infection.[300] Passive transfer of DENV-reactive antibodies increases viral burden and exacerbates disease in an IFN-$\alpha\beta\gamma$ receptor-deficient murine model (AG129 mice) of infection and pathogenesis[39,912] and increases viremia in primates.[265,297] The mechanism of ADE has been studied extensively, but remains incompletely understood. ADE is most commonly, although not exclusively, observed on cells that express Fc-γ or complement receptors.[300] Antibodies enhance infection by increasing the efficiency of virus attachment to target cells and thus, is of significantly reduced magnitude on cells with the capacity to bind viruses via other attachment factors.[648] For example, Fc-γ-receptor expressing immature dendritic cells do not support ADE due to the expression of CD209. By comparison, ADE occurs with mature dendritic cells that lack expression of CD209.[811] ADE can be inhibited by antibodies that block Fc-γ-receptor interactions,[640] enzymatic removal of the heavy chain of the antibody molecule,[912] and removal of the N-linked sugar on IgG molecules.[39,265,648]

What are the properties of antibodies that enhance infection? Virus neutralization and the phenomenon of ADE are related by the number of antibody molecules bound to the virion; antibodies that neutralize flaviviruses also have the potential to enhance infection at subneutralizing concentrations.[211] Antibodies that bind the virion with low affinity will enhance infection at higher concentrations relative to molecules that engage the virion via high affinity interactions. Furthermore, antibodies that recognize poorly accessible epitopes support ADE at higher concentrations than antibodies that bind readily accessible determinants. Estimates of the stoichiometric requirements for ADE identified a requirement for more than a single antibody molecule; enhancement of Fc-γ-RII-expressing cells required engagement of at least 15 DIII-LR-specific mAbs.[648] Presumably this is the minimal number of antibodies required for stable attachment of the virion–antibody complex to cells. Whether the requirements for ADE differ on cells expressing other Fc-γ-receptor molecules has not been investigated.

Recent studies indicate that complement can restrict ADE. Complement minimized ADE of WNV and DENV infection in Fc-γR-expressing cells.[544,899] Experiments with mouse sera deficient in individual complement components indicate that C1q is sufficient to restrict ADE of WNV infection *in vitro.* This effect was IgG subclass-dependent, as C1q restricted ADE by a human IgG_3 isotype-switch variant, but had little effect on IgG_2 and IgG_4 subclass variants; these results correlate with the known affinity of human IgG subclasses for C1q.[74] The addition of complement reduces the stoichiometry of neutralization by antibodies such that for IgG subclasses that bind C1q avidly, the reduced threshold of neutralization falls below the minimal number of antibodies required for ADE of infection.[647,648]

The Repertoire of Antibodies Elicited *In vivo*

The composition of the polyclonal antibody response elicited by infection is incompletely understood. Recent studies suggest that the humoral immune response of humans is directed against the highly conserved fusion loop of E-DII.[61,191,823] In agreement, biochemical studies with recombinant proteins and virus particles incorporating mutations in the fusion loop suggest a significant portion of the reactivity maps to this conserved structure.[168,169,628] Functional approaches to measure the relative contribution of epitopes on the E protein toward the neutralizing and protective activity of sera are being developed.[186,607,628,853]

T-Cell–Mediated Control

CD8+ T Cells

CD8+ T cells, by virtue of their ability to lyse infected target cells and produce inflammatory cytokines (e.g., IFN-γ and TNF-α), can have either protective or pathologic effects depending on the context. Indeed, depending on the flavivirus strain and experimental system, beneficial or adverse functions of CD8+ T cells have been reported. Experiments in small animal models and *in vitro* demonstrate that T lymphocytes can be an essential component of protection against infection by several different flaviviruses, including WNV, DENV, YFV, and JEV.[77,100,101–102,490,595,596,664,752,765,901,903] Consistent with this, individuals with hematologic malignancies and impaired T-cell function have an increased risk of neuroinvasive WNV infection.[598,658] Upon recognition of a flavivirus-infected cell that expresses class I MHC molecules, antigen-restricted cytotoxic T lymphocytes (CTLs) proliferate, release proinflammatory cytokines,[101,209,388,426,664] and lyse cells directly through the delivery of perforin and granzymes A and B, or via Fas-Fas ligand interactions. After WNV infection, mice deficient in CD8+ T cells had higher and sustained WNV burdens in the spleen and CNS and increased mortality.[752,870] CD8+ T cells require perforin and Fas ligand interactions to control infection of virulent North American WNV strains, as mice deficient in these molecules had increased CNS viral burdens and lethality.[753,755] Moreover, adoptive transfer of wild-type but not perforin or Fas-ligand–deficient CD8+ T cells decreased CNS viral burden and enhanced survival. In comparison, granzymes appear important for the control of the lineage II isolate Sarafend, with perforin, Fas, and Fas ligand having a more limited role in modulating infection.[871] The net function of CD8$^+$ T cells in infection by other encephalitic flaviviruses (e.g., JEV or MVEV) also varies. Initial reports showed that JEV-specific cytotoxic CD8$^+$ T cells could reduce production of infectious virus from infected macrophage and neuronal-like cells *in vitro.*[595] Moreover, adoptive transfer of anti-JEV CD8$^+$ T cells by an intracerebral route protected adult but not newborn or suckling BALB/c mice against lethal JEV challenge.[596] However, in vaccine immunization studies, challenge experiments in CD8 T cell$^{-/-}$ mice, indicate that CD8$^+$ T cells are dispensable and that antibody was the most critical component of protection.[637] CD8$^+$ T cells may have a lesser role *in vivo* in JEV infection because of active subversion of the antigen-presentation pathway by the virus; recent reports suggest that JEV infection leads to active depletion and impairment of CD8α^+CD11c$^+$ dendritic cells,[7,8] which are the cells that predominantly mediate cross-presentation of antigen and priming of CD8$^+$ T-cell responses in vivo.[331] With MVEV infection, effector CD8$^+$ T cells in the brain appear pathologic, as mice deficient in granule exocytosis (perforin or granzyme B) or Fas-mediated cytotoxicity showed delayed and reduced mortality.[471]

For DENV, which generally does not cause encephalitis, the protective or pathologic function of CD8$^+$ T cells depends on whether the response is primary or memory. During primary infection of mice, depletion of CD8$^+$ T cells before infection resulted in significantly higher viral loads. DENV-specific CD8$^+$ T cells produced IFN-γ and TNF-α, and exhibited cytotoxic activity *in vivo.*[903] In comparison, a pathogenic role of CD8$^+$ T cells has been described during secondary DENV infection. Due to the significant amino acid sequence homology among the four serotypes, there is a high potential for T-cell cross-reactivity during secondary heterologous DENV infection. Serotype cross-reactive CD8$^+$ T cells are preferentially activated during secondary infection in humans in a phenomenon termed "original antigenic sin".[577] These cross-reactive CD8$^+$ T cells exhibit altered cytokine production and reduced cytolytic activity.[49,57,524,578] Aberrant cytokine production by T cells could contribute to severe DENV disease, as higher levels of proinflammatory mediators may contribute to endothelial cell dysfunction or damage, leading to plasma leakage.[534]

CD4$^+$ T Cells

CD4$^+$ T cells can restrict or contribute to pathogenesis depending on the flavivirus, and whether the response is primary or anamnestic. Studies in mice have shown that CD4$^+$ T cells restrict pathogenesis of primary WNV infection. A genetic or acquired deficiency of CD4$^+$ T-cell function resulted in protracted WNV infection in the CNS that culminated in uniform lethality by 50 days after infection. CD4$^+$ T cells protect against primary WNV infection by providing help for antibody responses, sustaining WNV-specific CD8$^+$ T-cell responses in the CNS that enable viral clearance, producing antiviral cytokines, and killing cells.[102,765] A protective role for CD4$^+$ T cells against lethal JEV infection in mice was observed as depletion reduced and adoptive transfer promoted survival.[77] Moreover, in humans, impaired JEV-specific CD4$^+$ T-cell function (e.g., IFN-γ secretion) was seen preferentially in patients with encephalitis and neurologic sequelae.[430] Consistent with this, CD4$^{-/-}$ mice also showed greater susceptibility to CNS infection by a neuroadapted strain of YFV.[490] In comparison, depletion of CD4$^+$ T cells prior to DENV infection in mice had no effect on tissue viral burden, DENV-specific antibody titers or neutralizing activity, or CD8$^+$ T-cell responses.[901]

Memory CD4$^+$ T cells can have protective or pathologic consequences, depending on the context. For DENV, immunization schemes that elicit antigen-specific CD4$^+$ T cells prior to infection of mice resulted in significantly lower viral burden after challenge with homologous DENV.[901] Therefore, induction of CD4$^+$ T cells by immunization can contribute to viral clearance. However, during heterologous secondary DENV infection, cross-reactive CD4$^+$ memory T cells may be stimulated by antigen from the secondary infection. These CD4$^+$ T cells then augment the response of memory CD8$^+$ T cells, which can result in an overexuberant production of inflammatory cytokines and an increased risk for severe DENV disease.[57]

CD4$^+$CD25$^+$FoxP3$^+$ Regulatory T Cells

Regulatory CD4$^+$ T cells (Tregs) are a subset of CD4$^+$ T cells that can suppress effector T cells to control reactivity to self-antigens and pathogens.[702,801] These cells function to blunt inflammation and to maintain antigen-specific T-cell homeostasis.[432,625] A recent study showed that Tregs control the development of symptomatic WNV infection in humans and mice.[449] Symptomatic WNV-infected mice and humans had lower Treg frequencies compared with asymptomatic cohorts, and Treg-deficient mice developed lethal WNV infection at a higher rate than controls. Of interest, in severe DENV infection in humans, although Tregs expand and function normally, their relative frequencies are insufficient to control the immunopathology of severe disease.[506] Given their relatively recent identification, future studies will undoubtedly clarify the role of Tregs in preventing or promoting flavivirus pathogenesis.

Flavivirus Immune Evasion

Evasion of the Type I IFN Pathway. Flaviviruses have evolved several strategies to avoid and/or attenuate induction of type I IFN and its effector responses. In cell culture, flaviviruses are largely resistant to the antiviral effects of IFN once infection is established.[203] This may explain in part, the relatively modest therapeutic window for IFN-α administration that has been observed clinically in animal models or humans infected with JEV, SLEV, and WNV.[132,374,670,770] Experiments by several groups have demonstrated that individual flaviviruses attenuate IFN signaling at distinct steps in the cascade.

Inhibition of IFN-β Gene Induction. Three mechanisms have been described by which flaviviruses minimize the induction of IFN-β (Fig. 12.10).

1. IFN-β gene transcription. Studies with KUNV have identified the nonstructural protein NS2A as an inhibitor of *IFN-β* gene transcription.[491,492] Incorporation of an *A30P* mutation of *NS2A* into a KUNV genome resulted in a virus that elicits more rapid and sustained synthesis of type I IFN; infection of this mutant virus *in vitro* and *in vivo* was highly attenuated. The exact cellular target of NS2A and its mechanism of inhibition remain unknown.
2. PRR detection. Highly pathogenic WNV strains evade IRF-3-dependent recognition pathways without actively antagonizing the host defense signaling pathways.[239] Virulent WNV strains delay activation of PRR, such as RIG-I,

through mechanisms that are not clear to provide the virus with a kinetic advantage in the infected cell to elude host detection during replication at early times after infection.[386] In contrast, less pathogenic strains of WNV induce greater levels of IFN at early time points.[385]

3. PRR signaling. Studies in human mDCs suggest that DENV infection interferes with the type I IFN production[797] prior to *IFN-β* gene induction as IRF-3 phosphorylation is not induced.[686,687] Although the precise mechanism remains uncertain, ectopic expression studies show that a catalytically active NS2B–NS3 complex is sufficient for IFN antagonism. Activation of IRF-3 in response to dsRNA (poly (I:C)) also was inhibited in HeLa cells infected with WNV or stably propagating a subgenomic replicon.[734] Although initial experiments suggested that NS1 might mediate this inhibitory effect,[886] more recent work has questioned these results.[42] Alternatively, the high mannose carbohydrates on the E protein may independently block the production of IFN-*β*, IL-6, and TNF-*α* that is induced by dsRNA in macrophages. This effect was not directly dependent on TLR3 but instead occurred downstream at the level of the signaling intermediate and NF-*κ*B activator, receptor-interacting protein (RIP)-1.[17] Based on studies with macrophages from different age cohorts, this E protein–dependent inhibitory pathway may be dysregulated in elderly humans, leading to a pathogenic cytokine response.[416] Although the mechanistic basis for how specific forms of the E protein alter antiviral signaling programs remains uncertain, glycosylated E proteins can potentially signal through multiple cell surface lectins including the mannose receptor[556] and CLEC5a.[144]

Impaired IFNAR Pathway Signaling. In addition to antagonizing induction of *IFN-β* gene responses, several flaviviruses target the JAK-STAT signaling pathway for evasion to prevent the induction of antiviral ISG with possible antiviral activity (Fig 26.11). Therefore, even when type I IFN is produced, it may not achieve its inhibitory effect because of attenuated signaling capacity. Because the nonstructural proteins NS2A, NS3, NS4A, NS4B, and NS5 mediate many of the viral evasion mechanisms described below, these countermeasures are largely intrinsic to infected cells.

1. Phosphorylation of JAKs. Studies with LGV and WNV have shown interference with phosphorylation of both JAK1 and Tyk2.[68,290] A variation on this was observed with JEV, which showed complete inhibition of phosphorylation of Tyk2 with little effect on JAK1 phosphorylation.[482] Expression of a subgenomic replicon or infection of cells with DENV also inhibited Tyk2 phosphorylation and had no effect on IFNAR expression.[333] However, there may be cell- or virus-specific effects as JEV also inhibits STAT1 and STAT2 activation in the setting of normal levels of Tyk2 phosphorylation.[479]
2. STAT2 gene expression. DENV antagonizes IFN function by reducing STAT2 expression.[364] Cell lines that stably propagated subgenomic DENV replicons were resistant to the antiviral effects of IFN-*α*, had reduced levels of STAT2, and blunted ISG responses. DENV NS5 protein mediates binding and degradation of human but not mouse STAT2 via a ubiquitin and proteasome-dependent process,[20] and this species-specific effect in part explains the restriction of DENV infection in wild-type mice.[21]
3. Cholesterol redistribution. Flavivirus infection can actively promote re-localization of cholesterol to intracellular membranous sites of replication. This redistribution diminishes the formation of cholesterol-rich lipid rafts in the plasma membrane and attenuates the IFN antiviral signaling response.[512]
4. NS proteins as specific IFN antagonists. Several groups have begun to define the viral determinants and mechanisms that mediate IFN attenuation. Ectopic expression studies in A549 cells with DENV showed that NS2A, NS4A, or NS4B enhanced replication of an IFN-sensitive virus by blocking nuclear localization of STAT1.[594] Subsequent experiments showed that NS4B of DENV, WNV, and YFV partially block STAT1 activation and ISG induction.[593] Mutagenesis studies have identified a sequence determinant on WNV NS4B (E22/K24) that controls IFN resistance in cells that express subgenomic replicons.[227]

Although NS5 attenuates JAK-STAT signaling after LGV, JEV, and TBEV infection, the mechanism of NS5 inhibition appears to have virus-specific characteristics. For TBEV, a sequence in the methyltransferase domain of NS5 binds the PDZ protein scribble to inhibit JAK-STAT signaling.[879] For JEV, the N-terminal 83 residues of NS5 inhibit JAK-STAT signaling through a protein-tyrosine phosphatase-dependent mechanism.[481] Finally, for LGV, the JAK-STAT inhibitory domain was mapped to sites within the RNA-dependent RNA polymerase domain.[638]

Impaired IFN Effector Functions. Although flaviviruses devote a significant segment of their genome to inhibiting JAK-STAT signaling, they also target individual downstream antiviral effector molecules. Viperin is a candidate antiviral ISG with inhibitory activity against HCV, influenza virus, HIV, and Sindbis virus, possibly because of its ability to alter lipid raft formation. JEV, however, counteracts viperin by promoting rapid proteasome-dependent degradation.[131] The mechanism of this inhibition remains unclear, as transfection of individual JEV proteins failed to explain the phenotype, suggesting that a combined effect of viral proteins or replication is required.

More recent studies have shown that 2′O methylation modification of flavivirus RNA encoded by the methyltransferase activity of NS5 can antagonize the antiviral effects of the IFN-induced genes, IFIT-1 and IFIT-2.[179] A WNV mutant in NS5 (E218A) that specifically lost 2′O methylation activity replicated poorly in primary macrophages and mice, but showed restored virulence in cells and animals lacking IFN*αβ*R or IFIT-1.

Evasion of the Complement Pathway by NS1. To minimize recognition and/or destruction by complement, viruses have evolved strategies to evade or exploit complement to establish infection.[27,788] Flavivirus NS1 is expressed on cell surfaces, secreted from infected cells, and accumulates in the serum of infected individuals, with high circulating levels correlating with severe DENV disease.[28,468] WNV NS1 attenuates complement activation of the alternative pathway by enhancing the cofactor activity of factor H for factor I–mediated cleavage of C3b to iC3b, which decreases deposition of C3b and the C5b–C9 membrane attack complex on cell surfaces.[154] As an additional mechanism by which flaviviruses can evade complement, NS1 also binds to C4 and C1s, which enhanced the cleavage of C4 to C4b and reduced C4b and C3b deposition on cell surfaces.[24] Soluble NS1 has also been reported to bind the complement regulatory factors

C4bp[25] and clusterin, the latter of which normally inhibits the formation of the C5b–C9 membrane attack complex.[439]

Class I MHC and NK Cell Evasion. Because of their capacity to directly kill virally infected cells or produce inflammatory cytokines that control early stages of infection, NK cells are an important initial defense against many viruses. NK cells lyse infected cells by releasing cytotoxic granules that contain perforin and granzymes, or by binding to apoptosis-inducing receptors on target cells. NK cell activation is finely regulated through a balance of activating (Ly49D, Ly49H, and NKG2D) and inhibitory cell surface receptors (killer-cell immunoglobulin-like receptors (KIRs), immunoglobulin-like inhibitory receptors (ILTR), and CD94-NKG2A). To control the consequences of untoward activation of NK cells, inhibitory receptors are expressed constitutively, some of which bind to host MHC class I molecules on opposing cells and transmit inhibitory signals through intracellular tyrosine-based inhibitory motifs in their cytoplasmic domains. A decrease in expression of class I MHC molecules on a cell may prompt NK cell activation by attenuating the inhibitory signals. Therefore, NK-cell target recognition occurs after ligation of activating receptors and repression of inhibitory receptors on the cell surface.

Although many viruses attempt to avoid NK responses by expressing MHC class I homologs, flaviviruses may evade NK cell cytotoxicity by increasing surface expression of class I MHC molecules.[400,493,494] Expression of class I MHC molecules is stimulated by increasing the transport activity of transporter associated with antigen processing (TAP)[561,592] and by NF-kB–dependent transcriptional activation of MHC class I genes.[389] The rapid increase in expression of MHC class I suggests that early in the course of infection, flaviviruses may overcome susceptibility to NK cell–mediated lysis, even if it is at the expense of later recognition by an adaptive CD8$^+$ T-cell response. Consistent with this, splenocytes from WNV-immunized mice had poor NK-cell lytic activity[561] and mice with acquired deficiencies in NK cells demonstrated no increased morbidity or mortality compared to wild type controls.[755]

Intrinsic ADE. The ligation of monocyte or macrophage Fc-γ receptors by IgG immune complexes, rather than aiding host defenses, have been hypothesized to suppress innate immunity, increase production of IL-10, and bias T-helper cell responses, leading to increased infectious output by infected cells.[304,587] Initial studies with the unrelated Ross River alphavirus in RAW 264.7 macrophage-like cells showed that infection by ADE suppressed expression of CXCL10, NOS-2, IRF-1, TNF-α, and IFN-γ.[472,515] Subsequent experiments with DENV in the THP-1 monocytic cell line confirmed that ADE attenuated innate immune responses by downregulating the RIG-I/MDA5 signaling pathway and decreasing production of type I IFN and ISGs.[837] However, more recent experiments with DENV infection of primary human monocytes[86,419] did not demonstrate suppressed production of inhibitory or immunomodulatory cytokines in the context of ADE. One caveat to the concept of intrinsic ADE is that enhanced viral entry and infectivity (via DENV immune complex interaction with Fc-γ receptor) yields higher levels of viral nonstructural proteins in a cell, which themselves independently suppress innate immunity[197,198] irrespective of Fc-γ receptor signaling. Although the idea that intrinsic ADE of infection suppresses innate immunity and modulates disease severity of DENV infection is appealing,[304] it remains to be distinguished from the enhanced infectivity *per se* and confirmed in a physiologically relevant setting.

ANIMAL MODELS OF FLAVIVIRUS PATHOGENESIS AND DISEASE

Animal models of viral infections are used to address fundamental questions that are difficult to answer in human studies. These investigations are often directed toward defining basic mechanisms of viral pathogenesis (tropism, dissemination, and virulence) and host immune responses (protective and pathologic), but also are important for determining relative efficacy of candidate vaccines and antiviral agents. Although what constitutes a good animal model varies among investigators, in general, the most useful surrogate models mimic features of human disease, are reproducible, and have the capacity for high-throughput experimentation. The weakness of many animal models is they often do not fully recapitulate human disease with respect to kinetics, viral replication and spread, or disease phenotype, and thus restraint is required in applying these results to the human condition. Animal models of flavivirus infection are varied in their fidelity to human disease, and thus in their utility in providing basic insight into pathogenesis, immune control, and likely efficacy of vaccines or antiviral agents. This section reviews the strengths and weaknesses of key animal models, and what investigators in the field have learned by using them.

Dengue Virus

One of the major limitations in identifying and working with animal models of DENV infection is that humans are the only known host to develop disease after infection. A second consideration is that severe DENV infection and its plasma leakage syndrome is associated with preexisting maternal antibody in infants and secondary infection in children and adults, suggesting an immunopathogenesis mechanism, which has been difficult to recapitulate in animals. Although each of the animal models described below has been informative for understanding DENV infection, their inability to mimic human disease has limited the insight on human DENV infection.

Non-Human Primate Model of DENV Infection

Although humans are the natural host for DENV, serologic data support the existence of a sylvatic cycle between mosquitoes and nonhuman primates (NHPs).[857] Several species of monkeys (e.g., chimpanzees and rhesus macaques) have been infected experimentally with DENV and develop viremia and adaptive immune responses,[308,309,718] although in most cases, there is limited evidence of the severe disease seen in humans. One study in macaques showed thrombocytopenia, transiently reduced complement levels, and enhanced peak viremia after secondary infection with heterologous DENV serotype, although only 1 of 44 animals developed a syndrome that shared features of severe human disease.[309] A more recent study observed features of DHF in six rhesus macaques after high-dose (10^7 PFU per animal) intravenous infection with a DENV-2 strain,[632] including neutropenia, thrombocytopenia, clotting abnormalities, and petechial hemorrhage.

In addition, NHPs have been used as a model to study ADE and its consequences *in vivo*. *In vivo* enhancement of viremia was observed in juvenile rhesus monkeys after passive transfer of antibody and heterologous DENV challenge.[297] Analogously, an approximately 100-fold increase of DENV-4 viremia was demonstrated in juvenile rhesus monkeys that received a cross-reactive mAb recognizing the fusion loop in DII.[265] In neither model, however, was evidence of severe vascular leak observed despite the increase in DENV replication. NHPs also have been used to evaluate adaptive immune response and protection of live-attenuated or subunit-based DENV vaccine candidates.[158,213,418]

Mouse Models

A recent review describes the utility and clinical features of individual mouse models of DENV infection in great detail (see Table 1 in Yauch and Shresta[902]). Below, we describe some features of the more commonly used models in the field. In general, there have been several hurdles to establishing mouse models of DENV disease pathogenesis: (a) the majority of models are not ideal because most mice do not develop the same clinical disease as humans; (b) it has been difficult to infect mice reliably and reproducibly with low passage clinical and mosquito isolates (hence, many studies are performed with laboratory- or mouse-adapted strains that have uncertain relevance to the strains that cause human disease); and (c) DENV is virulent in humans because it has evolved specific countermeasures to evade the human immune response.[198] In mice, these evasion mechanisms may not function, resulting in rapid control. One example is the recent finding that DENV NS5 promotes degradation of human but not mouse STAT2, a key protein in the type I IFN signaling cascade.[21]

IFN-Signaling Deficient Mice

Because of the importance of STAT2 and the IFN response in restricting DENV infection, mice (AG129) lacking receptors for both type I (IFN-α/β) and type II (IFN-γ) were tested and shown vulnerable to intraperitoneal (i.p.) infection with a mouse-adapted (New Guinea C) DENV-2 strain[360] or intravenous (i.v.) infection with a laboratory-adapted (PL046) DENV-2 strain.[748] In these studies, however, mice succumbed to DENV infection because of rapid spread to the CNS, resulting in encephalitis and paralysis, which are not common features of human disease. Similar results were observed in STAT1$^{-/-}$ mice,[749] although in some cases hemorrhage was observed after inoculation at multiple sites.[144] Subsequent investigation identified mouse adapted (DENV-2 D2S10) and nonadapted strains (DENV-2 Y98P) that cause rapid death of AG129 mice associated with some characteristics of human disease, including cytokine storm, vascular leakage, and high TNF-α levels[750,808] after i.v. or i.p. infection.

AG129 mice have been used as a model to test antiviral candidates[148,737,782] or to explore the role of ADE in disease severity. Two groups showed that preexisting cross-reactive monoclonal or polyclonal antibody facilitate ADE *in vivo* and promote more severe DENV disease including vascular leakage.[39,912] Importantly, when the Fc fragment of the antibody was eliminated by proteolysis or modified genetically, enhanced replication and disease were no longer observed, thus confirming the longstanding hypothesis that ADE can cause severe disease in an animal.[299] Cellular and tissue tropism have been examined in the ADE model in AG129 mice[39,912]; the virus targets appear similar to that described in human autopsy studies, with antigen present in the lymph node, spleen, and bone marrow, with significant infection in myeloid cells, and possibly sinusoidal endothelial cells in the liver. Although the comparative data are intriguing, the absence of IFN in mice independently broadens cellular and tissue tropism of flaviviruses,[704] and thus some caution in interpretation is warranted.

Immunocompetent Mice

The successful infection of immunocompetent mice with DENV strains would allow more detailed analysis of the kinetics and function of protective immune responses. Although most DENV strains replicate poorly in wild-type laboratory strains of mice, recent reports suggest that infection may be possible, with the development of a spectrum of disease. Subcutaneous and systemic hemorrhage was induced in wild-type C57BL/6 mice after intradermal (i.d.) infection with a laboratory passaged DENV-2 16681 strain.[141] With this strain, C57BL/6 and BALB/c mice also developed thrombocytopenia, elevated levels of systemic TNF-α, and liver damage.[142,635] However, none of these experiments showed evidence of vascular leakage, the hallmark of severe DENV disease in humans. Studies with a mouse-adapted DENV-2 strain (P23085) that was injected i.p. in 4 week-old BALB/c or C57BL/6 mice showed thrombocytopenia, liver injury, and the development of a vascular permeability and shock-like syndrome.[23,774] This promising mouse model, which has not yet been validated extensively, recently was used to assess the function of platelet-activating factor, macrophage migration inhibitory factor, and chemokine receptors in the pathogenesis of DENV.[22,283,774]

Mouse–Human Chimeras

Because most mouse strains do not sustain DENV replication after infection, mouse-human chimeras have been developed. Early studies using severe combined immunodeficient (SCID) mice engrafted with human peripheral blood lymphocytes showed marginal infection with a DENV-1 strain.[894] Subsequent studies engrafted human tumor cells (K562, HepG2, Huh-7),[12,80,486] which supported DENV replication but caused CNS disease and not a vascular leakage syndrome. Nonobese diabetic (NOD)/SCID or NOD/SCID IL2R$\gamma^{-/-}$ have been engrafted with CD34^{+} human cord blood hematopoietic progenitor cells. After infection with DENV-2, these chimeric mice developed some of the signs of severe human disease including fever, rash, and thrombocytopenia.[65,357,589] In an analogous model, RAG2$^{-/-}$ x γ chain$^{-/-}$ mice engrafted with CD34^{+} human fetal liver stem cells and infected with DENV-2, developed viremia and fever and produced human-specific anti-DENV antibody responses.[440] Although engraftment of human cells is advantageous as the response of human cells, pathogenesis, and possibly tropism can be analyzed, the chimeric models have limitations: (a) the disease phenotype generated to date recapitulates only some of the features of severe DENV; (b) technically, the mouse-to-mouse level of chimerism is variable, making phenotypic analysis challenging; (c) the throughput of experiments is low, making these models less practical for vaccine or antiviral testing; and (d) the immune cross-talk between human and mouse cells within an animal may be altered, limiting interpretation of effects on immunity.

Yellow Fever Virus

Despite the fact that YFV was isolated in 1927 and that a vaccine was developed 10 years later, our understanding of the mechanisms underlying the virulence and pathogenesis of virulent YFV remains surprisingly limited. Analogous to DENV, part of this stems from the lack of a small animal model that recapitulates the viscerotropism of human infection. Given the reemergence of YFV, an improved understanding of its pathogenesis and a vehicle for testing novel vaccines and antiviral agents through the use of existing and new animal models of disease is now a research priority.

Human Vaccine Model

Vaccination with the attenuated 17D strain of YFV has conferred protection to hundreds of millions of humans worldwide. Recent prospective analyses have examined the interaction of 17D YFV with the innate immune system and how this might be important for triggering long-term protective adaptive immunity.[661] A systems biology approach defined early gene signatures that predicted immune responses in humans vaccinated with yellow fever vaccine YF-17D. Computational analyses identified induction of genes (e.g., complement protein C1qB, TNFRS17, and eukaryotic translation initiation factor 2 alpha kinase 4) that correlated with and predicted protective B- and T-cell responses with high accuracy in an independent, blinded trial.[668]

Nonhuman Primate Model of Severe YFV Infection

YFV cycles in nature as part of a sylvatic cycle between *Aedes* mosquitoes and wild monkeys. Rhesus and cynomolgus monkeys develop viscerotropic disease, analogous to humans, ranging from mild to fulminate hepatitis, whereas African and New World NHPs have milder or silent infections.[567] The pathogenesis of YFV infection in rhesus monkeys resembles severe human disease with the development of jaundice, acute renal failure, coagulopathy, and shock,[568] although the course is more severe, not biphasic, produces markedly higher viral burden, and is also associated with severe necrosis of lymphoid tissue.[409,568] The coagulopathy in monkeys is associated with a global decrease in synthesis of clotting factors secondary to direct hepatic damage and impaired hemostasis associated with abnormalities of platelet function.[567]

In contrast to that described for DENV, preexisting immunity to heterologous flaviviruses results in protection rather than enhanced pathogenesis in NHPs. Rhesus monkeys that were infected previously with DENV were protected against YFV challenge, and recipients of anti-DENV antibodies by passive transfer showed no evidence of enhanced disease.[567,818] Monkeys immunized with other flaviviruses,[326] similar to humans with prior exposure to flaviviruses,[570] manifest a lower incidence of severe YFV disease.

Rodent Models of YFV Infection

Historical infection studies in mice and hamsters with nonadapted YFV did not cause viscerotropic disease. Syrian golden hamsters, however, did develop disease that more closely resembled human YFV infection (hepatitis, hepatic necrosis, splenic necrosis), but this phenotype requires serial passage of YFV *in vivo,* and renal disease was not observed.[539,897] In comparison, peripheral infection of wild-type mice does not cause viscerotropic disease. However, YFV-induced encephalitis can be induced in suckling mice after i.p. or intracranial (i.c.) inoculation, in adult mice if the blood-brain barrier is disturbed, or if mouse-adapted strains are used.[44,236,237,567,711] Because these models do not cause viscerotropism, they are of limited relevance to understanding the pathophysiology of human YFV infection, and have been largely restricted to vaccine and antiviral testing. More recent subcutaneous infection studies of mice that are deficient in IFN-signaling revealed viscerotropic YFV infection and disease (liver and spleen necrosis) without a requirement for virus adaptation.[548] This study suggests that nonadapted YFV has little ability to evade the antiviral activity of IFN-α/β in mice, whereas species-specific antagonism of IFN-α/β antiviral activity in primate hosts may contribute to infection outcome.

West Nile Virus

WNV and other encephalitic flaviviruses are generally more promiscuous in their ability to infect and cause disease in different species of animals. Beyond its endemic cycle in multiple species of birds, WNV causes severe disease in horses, and can periodically infect other mammals sometimes with severe consequences.[91] Although the molecular basis for its broad animal tropism remains uncharacterized, as a result of this, it has been easier to develop animal models of infection that recapitulate features of human disease using low-passage field isolates. However, the frequency of neuroinvasive disease may vary significantly among animal strains, making some models preferred for studying pathogenesis and disease outcome.

Non-Human Primate Model of WNV Infection

NHP models of WNV infection are important because of their potential for use in evaluating vaccine and therapeutic candidates. In one study of five intradermally infected rhesus macaques, the clinical course, level and duration of viremia, and antibody response were similar to that occurring in uncomplicated human WNV infection, although it was unclear whether virus entered the brain in these animals.[672] This model of sustained viremia and measurable immune responses has been used to evaluate the efficacy of WNV vaccine candidates.[884] Analogously, in baboons, after intradermal infection, WNV accumulated to high levels in blood and was associated with a transient macular rash, but failed to cause encephalitis or other severe clinical signs.[889] Although these NHP models do not develop WNV encephalitis, it remains possible that the frequency of neuroinvasive disease parallels human infection (1:150), and thus would require much larger studies to identify severe cases. In contrast to infection via a peripheral route, i.c. inoculation of rhesus monkeys with different African and Asian WNV strains results in persistent viral infection in the CNS and other organs.[655] These animals sustained a prolonged infection course and showed evidence of fatal encephalitis with diffuse neuronal degeneration and necrosis and inflammation. Similar severe clinical manifestations (fever, tremors, and spasticity) were observed in rhesus macaques challenged via a frontal lobe injection with the New York 1999 strain of WNV.[19]

Hamster Model

Syrian golden hamsters are an excellent small animal model for studying WNV pathogenesis, vaccine efficacy, and antiviral screening. Intraperitoneal or even oral infection of a New York isolate of WNV results in viremia of 5 to 6 days in duration, followed by the development of virus-specific antibodies.[714,896] Clinical signs of encephalitis (weakness, tremor, ataxia, and paralysis) were apparent within 6 to 7 days of infection with an approximately 50% mortality rate. WNV disease correlated with the detection of viral antigen and neuronal degeneration in several regions of the brain including the cerebral cortex, basal ganglia, hippocampus, cerebellum, and brainstem. Because of their larger size relative to mice, hamsters have been used to elucidate particular aspects of neuropathogenesis. WNV spread to the CNS can occur through a retrograde axonal transport mechanism as the virus moves from peripheral motor neurons into the spinal cord.[705,860] Electrophysiology studies have shown that respiratory distress associated with WNV infection is caused by diaphragmatic suppression through lesions in the brainstem and cervical spinal cord, or altered vagal afferent function.[583]

In the hamster model, infectious WNV can be cultured from the brains of hamsters up to 53 days after initial infection,[896] suggesting that persistent replication occurs. Persistent WNV infection or protein production in the spinal cord causes continued neuronal dysfunction, chronic neuropathologic lesions, and poliomyelitis-like disease, and can be measured using electrophysiologic approaches.[758] Consistent with persistent infection in the brain, hamsters also develop persistent viruria, as infectious WNV can be cultured from urine for several weeks.[826]

The hamster model has been used to evaluate candidate therapeutics or vaccines against WNV disease. Studies with small molecule inhibitors,[586] antiviral cytokines,[580] synthetic oligonucleotides,[827] and humanized monoclonal antibodies[581] have been performed with varying efficacy, especially when administered as postexposure therapy.[199] Analogously, immunization with single-cycle,[885] recombinant subunit,[761] or live-attenuated[815] vaccines have elicited durable protective immunity, and thus has provided a robust preclinical small animal model for assessment and comparison of the surrogate markers of protection.

Mouse Models

Infection studies in several inbred laboratory strains of mice have provided insight into the fundamental mechanisms of WNV dissemination, pathogenesis, and immune system control. Over the last decade, most studies have been performed with North American WNV strains and wild-type and immunodeficient strains of C57BL/6 mice. The strengths of this particular model include the following: (a) depending on the dose of virus and age of mice, a subset of wild-type mice develop neuroinvasive disease, whereas the remainder are infected with minimal or limited spread to the CNS. Therefore, the mechanisms by which the immune system restricts viral entry or facilitates viral clearance can be studied; (b) many features of pathogenesis and neuropathology appear remarkably similar to that observed in humans; (c) nonadapted low-passage WNV isolates cause disease in wild-type mice. Therefore, this model can be used to define the genetics of virus attenuation; (d) there are a large number of transgenic, knockout, and conditional knock-out mice available from academic laboratories and public consortia to study the role of specific genes or cells in pathogenesis; and (e) genes (e.g., CCR5 and OAS-1b) that predict susceptibility in mice have been corroborated as risk factors for human WNV disease.[201] Nonetheless, there are limitations to the model including the compressed disease time course, the difficulty in obtaining CSF samples in live animals because of size, and a rather flat virus dose–response curve after peripheral infection. Moreover, the mouse anti-WNV antibody response appears directed at a distinct dominant neutralizing epitope than the human response.[628]

Following peripheral inoculation of mice, initial WNV replication is thought to occur in keratinocytes and skin Langerhans dendritic cells,[117] with mosquito saliva modulating the local proinflammatory cytokine response.[730] Dendritic cells migrate to and seed draining lymph nodes, resulting in a primary viremia and subsequent infection of peripheral tissues such as the spleen and occasionally, the kidney. By the end of the first week, WNV is largely cleared from the serum and peripheral organs, and infection in the CNS is observed in a subset of immunocompetent animals. Mice that succumb to infection develop CNS pathology similar to that observed in human WNV cases, including infection and injury of brainstem, hippocampal, and spinal cord neurons.[754] WNV infection is detected at much lower levels in nonneuronal CNS cell populations, such as $CD11b^+$ cells[176,828] or astrocytes.[208] In most surviving wild-type mice, WNV is cleared from all tissue compartments within 2 to 3 weeks after infection. However, persistent WNV infection in the brains of class II MHC,[765] $CD8^+$ T-cell[752] or perforin deficient mice[755] was routinely observed. Analogously, a small subset of wild-type mice sustained WNV persistence in the CNS, even in the setting of a robust antibody response and inflammation.[16] Remarkably, WNV persistence in the CNS was observed even in mice with subclinical infections, as treatment with the immunosuppressive drug cyclophosphamide resulted in active viral replication.

PREVENTION AND CONTROL

Flavivirus Vaccines

Successful vaccination programs have dramatically reduced the global health burden of flavivirus infections. More than 500 million doses of vaccine to prevent YFV infection have been administered since its development in 1937, and effective vaccines have blunted the impact of JEV and TBEV as discussed below. Nonetheless, safe and effective vaccines for several clinically significant flaviviruses still remain elusive. As an example, up to 100 million DENV infections occur each year, and severe disease manifestations are occurring with an increased frequency.[882] New flavivirus vaccines and improvement on safety of existing vaccines is urgently needed. The development of molecular clone technology, more sophisticated animal models of infection, and insights from structural biology have aided recent efforts in these areas.

Yellow Fever Virus

The live-attenuated YFV 17D vaccine is considered among the most safe and effective ever developed, an achievement for which Max Theiler was awarded the Nobel Prize in 1951. An excellent historical account of the development of this vaccine has been written by Monath.[569] The current YFV vaccine was derived from a virus (the Asibi strain) isolated in 1927 from a West African man with a mild febrile illness.[789] The Asibi strain was passaged 176 times in the embryonic tissue of mice and chickens to yield the YF-17D virus with considerably reduced neurotropic and viscerotropic properties.[565,819] Vaccines currently in use are substrains of YF-17D; strain YF-17DD is used in vaccines produced for South America (passage 287–289), whereas the YF-17D-204 strain (passages 235–240) is distributed elsewhere, including the United States.[46,779] The consensus sequence of the vaccine strains differs from the parent Asibi strain by approximately 20 amino acids as well as by 4 nucleotide changes in the 3′ UTR.[565] Vaccine is produced in chicken embryos, lyophilized, and administered by subcutaneous injection following reconstitution in saline. A single dose of YFV vaccine contains roughly 10^4 to 10^6 PFU.[46]

The Immune Response to YF-17 Infection

The host response to YF-17D infection involves both the adaptive and innate arms of the immune system.[569] Recent studies highlight the significance of the innate response to YF-17D in shaping the adaptive immune response to vaccination.[247,661,667] YF-17D activates mDCs and pDCs through multiple TLR proteins, including TLR2, TLR7, TLR8, and TLR9, resulting in the induction of proinflammatory cytokines and IFN-α.[667,668] Of interest, a capacity to interact with multiple TLR pathways does not appear functionally redundant; these interactions tune the adaptive response by influencing the balance of Th1 and Th2 cytokines and the quality of the anti-YFV T cell response.[667] Indeed, YF-17D infection induces a mixture of Th1 and Th2 cytokines *in vivo*,[247,709] and YF-17D infected DCs present viral antigen to T cells despite inefficient replication in these cells.[40,636]

YF-17D vaccination induces a low-grade and transient viremia that peaks on day 5.[565] Defervescence is coincident with a reduction in viremia and the detection of cellular and humoral responses. YF-17D infection induces a polyfunctional $CD8^+$ T-cell response of considerable magnitude (2% to 13% of $CD8^+$ T cells) that peaks roughly 2 weeks postimmunization.[3] Analysis of the breadth of this response demonstrates that all 10 viral proteins contain epitopes recognized by $CD8^+$ T cells; reactivity with epitopes in E, NS3, and NS5 proteins were most common.[4,247] The virus-specific $CD8^+$ T-cell response contracts at approximately day 30 postinfection to a size that corresponds to approximately 5% to 10% of the magnitude of the original response, with memory $CD8^+$ T cells persisting for years.[4,555]

Vaccination with YF-17D also elicits a rapid neutralizing antibody response in virtually all recipients.[60,645] Kinetic analysis of vaccinated adults revealed that approximately 87% have neutralizing antibodies at 2 weeks postvaccination, with virtually 100% of subjects developing neutralizing antibody by day 28.[448] YFV-reactive IgM can be detected by day 9, peaks between days 14 and 17, and persists for more than one year. YFV-specific IgG is detected between days 10 and 17 and peaks approximately 1 month postvaccination.[569] Neutralizing antibodies persist for decades. More than 90% of vaccinated subjects had neutralizing antibody when examined 16 to 19 years postimmunization.[693] Indeed, neutralizing antibody was detected in 80% of vaccinated U.S. military personnel when assayed 30 to 35 years after receiving YF-17D.[656] Despite the impressive longevity of the antibody response, booster immunizations are still recommended every 10 years.[779]

The neutralizing antibody response correlates with protection from infection.[60,533,569,575] Roughly 94% of primates with a neutralizing antibody titer greater or equal to 0.7 logs (1/5 dilution of serum) were protected from a lethal challenge with YF-Asibi.[533] As a comparison, the mean neutralizing antibody titer of recipients of the YF-17D vaccine at 28 days postimmunization is 2.2 logs (1/160 serum dilution).[575]

Adverse Events Arising from YF-17D Vaccination

More than 500 million doses of YF-17D have been administered to humans with a high track record of safety.[246] The most common side effects from YF-17D vaccination are transient headache, myalgia, and low-grade fever.[779] Severe adverse events (SAEs) following vaccination have been reported, albeit at a very low frequency. The risk of SAEs following vaccination increases with age; the incidence of SAEs in vaccine recipients greater than 70 years of age is roughly 10-fold higher than that for individuals aged 19 to 29.[391] Three main classes of SAEs have been reported:

1. Anaphylactic reactions are infrequent (1 in 135,000) and likely a result of allergic responses to components of the vaccine including egg and chicken proteins, gelatin, and latex.[387,779] Hypersensitivity to eggs is a contraindication for vaccination.[569]
2. Vaccine-associated neurologic disease (YEL-AND) is associated with invasion of the CNS by the vaccine strain. This SAE was most commonly reported prior to the establishment of the vaccine seed system (in 1945) and in infants prior to changes in the recommendations for vaccination of children less than 6 months old (in 1960).[565] The mechanism underlying the increased risk of YEL-AND in infants remains uncertain, but may reflect differences in the level or duration of viremia, the integrity of the BBB, or a failure to mount an effective immune response.[569] Twenty-nine cases of YEL-AND have been reported since 1990 with a case fatality ratio of 6.9%[569] with an incidence of 0.4 to 0.8 per 100,000 doses.[487,779]
3. Vaccine-associated viscerotropic disease (YEL-AVD) is a recently reported SAE that mimics many aspects of naturally acquired YFV infection. YEL-AVD is characterized by the rapid onset of high fever (within 2 to 5 days of vaccination), malaise, and myalgia that is followed by jaundice, oliguria, cardiovascular instability, and hemorrhage. Analysis of the sequence of viruses recovered from vaccine recipients with YEL-AVD failed to identity mutations associated with this SAE.[46] Risk factors for YEL-AVD include advanced age and a history of thymus disease or thymectomy. As of 2010, 57 cases of YEL-AVD have been reported with a case fatality rate of 64%. In the United States, the incidence is estimated as 0.3 to 0.5 per 100,000 doses.[779]

New Vaccine Approaches

Despite the demonstrable success of the live-attenuated YF-17D vaccine, the potential for SAE has prompted efforts to develop new vaccines with improved safety. Perspectives supporting a need for new vaccine approaches have been given.[316] A new inactivated whole virus vaccine candidate, XRX-001, is being developed to complement the existing YF-17D vaccine, particularly for contraindicated populations. XRX-001 is a β-propiolactone inactivated YF-17D virus that is produced in Vero cells and adsorbed to aluminum hydroxide.[573] Two doses of vaccine in the presence or absence of adjuvant was sufficient to elicit a neutralizing antibody response in mice. The neutralizing antibody titers achieved following XRX-001 vaccination were equivalent or better than those with live-attenuated YF-17D vaccination experiments performed in parallel. Experiments in hamsters and NHPs confirmed that vaccination protected against lethal challenge with YFV.[573] Evaluation of this candidate vaccine in human clinical trials is underway (clinical trials.gov identified NCT00995865).

Dengue Virus

Four antigenically related serotypes of DENV circulate in nature. Although natural infection by DENV is thought to confer protection from re-infection by a homologous DENV serotype,[700] an increased risk of severe clinical manifestations following secondary infection by a heterologous DENV has been demonstrated.[112,224,294,305] Therefore, the potential for an exacerbated clinical outcome in a DENV sensitized–individual complicates the development of a safe and effective vaccine. A perceived requirement of candidate DENV vaccines is that administration confers simultaneous, durable protection against all four different DENV serotypes. Given the considerable effort and resources required to bring a safe and effective vaccine against a single pathogen to market, a tetravalent DENV vaccine is among the most ambitious vaccine development efforts undertaken. DENV vaccine research traces its roots to the 1940s[701] and has advanced from empirical administration of passaged strains to rational design that exploits the advances of molecular and structural virology.[217]

Live Attenuated Dengue Vaccines Derived from Extensive Passaging

The earliest efforts to produce a vaccine against DENV were undertaken by Sabin and colleagues.[701] DENV-1 (Hawaii strain) was passaged in mice via intracranial inoculation, isolated as a brain homogenate, and used to challenge human volunteers. Although the first six passages of DENV in mice did not sufficiently attenuate the virus and caused fever in human subjects, experiments with virus passaged seven or more times conferred protection following challenge with DENV-infected mosquitoes.[700,701] Similar experiments were performed using the DENV-1 Mochizuki strain.[340,341] A more extensively passaged mouse brain–derived DENV-1 isolate was the first DENV vaccine candidate evaluated in the field during an outbreak of DENV-3 in Puerto Rico; this heterologous protection experiment suggested an efficacy of about 40%.[59,703]

Extensive passage in tissue culture also has been used to attenuate DENV for use in vaccines. Investigators in Thailand developed vaccine candidates for all four serotypes of DENV via serial passages in primary dog kidney (PDK) or primary green monkey kidney (PGMK) cells.[882] Aventis Pasteur/Sanofi Pasteur licensed these strains for clinical vaccine development. The safety and immunogenicity of tetravalent formulations was investigated in clinical trials in adults[376,696] and in children.[697] Although these vaccines were generally well tolerated, reactogenicity was noted, particularly after the first dose of vaccine. Furthermore, the DENV-3 component of the vaccine replicated more robustly in vaccinated subjects and was immunodominant. Although changes in the relative doses of each component strain of the vaccine were tested to reduce the dominance of DENV-3 and reactogenicity, development of this tetravalent candidate was halted. These studies highlight the complexity and challenge of eliciting a balanced immune response against four different viruses representing all DENV serotypes.

Investigators at the Walter Reed Army Institute of Research (WRAIR) developed a tetravalent vaccine composed of four highly passaged DENV. These viruses were produced by serial passage of clinical isolates of DENV in PDK cells, and the formulation of candidate tetravalent vaccines were studied in several monovalent and tetravalent clinical trials.[217] A phase I clinical evaluation of two doses of vaccine administered 6 months apart demonstrated that the vaccine was well-tolerated and elicited a tetravalent neutralizing antibody response in all subjects.[763] Concerns as to the durability of the tetravalent humoral response in humans has prompted the commercial partner (GlaxoSmithKline) to suspend clinical trials (J Toussaint, personal communication) with this vaccine candidate.

Live-Attenuated Dengue Vaccines: Rational Design using Molecular Biology

The development of molecular infectious clones of flaviviruses has enabled the construction and characterization of variants with attenuating mutations. The 3′ UTR of flaviviruses folds into RNA structures that function to regulate genomic RNA replication, translation, and cytopathicity.[159,649] The introduction of a 30 nucleotide deletion in the 3′ UTR of DENV-4 (strain 814669) yielded a markedly attenuated virus *in vivo,* which still elicited a robust humoral response in monkeys and humans.[213,550] Vaccination with DENV-4Δ30 resulted in low-level viremia (~1.6 logs) in 70% of recipients,[213] which is not sufficient for blood-meal transmission of the vaccine to mosquito vectors. Similar results were reported with a DENV-1Δ30 virus constructed from the Western Pacific 1974 strain.[214] In contrast, DENV-2 and DENV-3 viruses incorporating the Δ30 deletion were not attenuated sufficiently to warrant further study as vaccine candidates.[78,79] A second DENV-3 virus, however, encoding two deletions in the 3′ UTR (DENV-3Δ30/31) appears more promising; monkeys immunized with this variant were not viremic, mounted a robust neutralizing antibody response, and were protected from challenge by wild-type virus.[82]

The development of chimeric flaviviruses encoding the structural genes of heterologous viruses is a second attenuation approach that has yielded several promising vaccine candidates. The first chimeric viruses were constructed by introducing the C, prM, and E genes of DENV-1 or DENV-2 into the genetic background of DENV-4.[95] These viruses were immunogenic and attenuated as immunization of monkeys elicited neutralizing antibodies and reduced viremia following challenge with a homologous wild-type strain.[96] These early studies established that the structural proteins conferred the serologic specificity of chimeric DENV. Chimeric vaccine candidates encoding the heterologous C-prM-E and prM-E cassettes have been characterized; viruses constructed using the latter replicated more efficiently than those encoding all three structural genes, perhaps due to a requirement for interaction between RNA elements in the capsid gene and the 3′ UTR.[96] Several tetravalent chimeric flavivirus vaccine candidates using molecular backbones of DENV4Δ30, YF-17D, and DENV-2 viruses are in advanced stages of clinical development.[446,597]

A tetravalent DENV vaccine using chimeras constructed with the DENV-4Δ30 backbone is being developed by the National Institute of Allergy and Infectious Disease (NIAID),

National Institutes of Health (NIH). Because the DENV-4 backbone of these viruses is already attenuated by the Δ30 deletion, viruses were constructed using the structural genes from wild-type strains. A chimeric DENV-2/DENV-4Δ30 virus encoding the prM-E of the New Guinea C DENV-2 strain has been evaluated in phase I clinical studies.[215,883] Although chimeric DENV4Δ30 encoding the structural proteins of DENV-3 could be recovered, these viruses were overattenuated *in vivo.*[78] A second chimeric virus strategy involved replacing the 3′ UTR of a DENV-3 virus with the DENV-4Δ30 UTR described above is being evaluated.[82] Tetravalent formations of the NIAID vaccine candidates are in phase I clinical trials and include both chimeric viruses and those encoding a Δ30 deletion.

Because of the extensive safety profile of the YF-17D vaccine, several chimeric viruses also have been constructed by replacing genes encoding the structural proteins of YF-17D with those of heterologous flaviviruses.[292] This platform, called ChimeriVax™ (licensed by Sanofi Pasteur), has been used to create chimeric viruses expressing the prM-E proteins of all four serotypes of DENV.[284] The structural genes of these chimeric viruses were obtained from low-passage primary isolates of human dengue cases. Preclinical and clinical studies demonstrate that ChimeriVax-DENV is safe, with minimal and nonsevere adverse reactions (reviewed by[292]). Studies in suckling mice infected via the intracranial route demonstrated that chimeric DENV-YF-17D has lost the neurovirulent phenotype associated with the YF-17D backbone. Vaccination of monkeys and humans results in a low and transient viremia of reduced magnitude compared to the parental viruses. Preclinical studies in monkeys immunized with a single dose of a tetravalent formulation showed excellent immunogenicity, and 92% percent of immunized animals remained aviremic after challenge with wild-type DENV.[287] A randomized phase IIb study of this vaccine candidate in dengue-experienced subjects (clinicaltrials.gov identifier NCT00842530) revealed only modest efficacy (30.2%) that was not uniform among serotypes; no protection against infection by DENV2 viruses.[697a]

A third chimeric tetravalent DENV vaccine formulation has been generated using the Thai DENV-2 PDK-53 vaccine strain as the backbone.[345,346] Although these vectors are immunogenic and protective in mouse models, they have only recently entered phase I clinical trials in humans (clinical trials.gov identifier NCT01110551).

Alternative Vaccine Strategies

DNA Vaccines. DNA-based DENV vaccines offer several advantages including ease of production, transport, and storage. Furthermore, administration of multiple DNA constructs encoding different flavivirus antigens avoids viral interference.[726] The first DNA vaccine for DENV encoded the prM and a secreted form of the E protein lacking the transmembrane domains of the DENV-2 New Guinea C strain.[413] Plasmids that express prM and E proteins may be particularly immunogenic, as they can produce secreted subviral particles *in vivo,* which display the E protein in a highly ordered array analogous to that present on infectious virions.[233] Two vaccinations with four plasmids encoding the envelope proteins of each DENV serotype were sufficiently immunogenic in mice to confer protection from heterologous challenge with any of the four dengue viruses.[417] However, a phase I clinical evaluation of three doses of a monovalent DENV-1 DNA vaccine revealed only modest immunogenicity.[58]

Recombinant Subunit Vaccines. DENV vaccines composed of recombinant E proteins also have been studied. Analogous to DNA vaccines, this approach may simplify the task of eliciting a balance tetravalent response.[217] High-level expression of soluble forms of the E protein has been achieved using insect cell gene expression technologies. Whether the antigens in subunit vaccines are capable of eliciting the full spectrum of antibody specificities required for a maximally protective response, particularly those spanning multiple E protein oligomers on the intact virion, remains uncertain.

Other/Modified Viral Vectors. Several viral expression vectors have been studied in mice and primates as possible DENV vaccine platforms including vaccinia virus,[97,195] alphavirus,[143,881] adenovirus,[673] and measles virus.[92]

Japanese Encephalitis Virus

JEV is a principal cause of pediatric encephalitis in Asia and has been a focus of vaccine development efforts since before World War II.[302] Inactivated suspensions of JEV-infected mouse brains were administered to military personnel in response to an outbreak of Japanese B virus (now recognized as JEV) on Okinawa in 1945.[699] Although circumstances did not permit a complete evaluation of efficacy, this vaccine elicited neutralizing antibodies in a subset of vaccinated subjects at titers that protected mice from lethal infection.[698] Since that time, considerable progress has been made toward developing a safe and effective JEV vaccine. Three vaccination approaches have reduced the incidence of JEV in countries with the means to utilize them. However, ~35,000 to 50,000 cases of JEV disease annually are still seen; as such, efforts to develop effective and economical vaccines with improved safety profiles continue.[53]

Mouse-Brain Derived JEV Vaccines

Vaccines produced from JEV-infected mouse brains have been effective at controlling JEV in many parts of Asia, including Japan, South Korea, Taiwan, and Thailand.[235] The Research Foundation for Microbial Diseases of Osaka University (BIKEN) produced the majority of mouse-brain derived JEV vaccine licensed for international use between 1954 and 2005. This vaccine platform uses genotype III Nakayama or Beijing-1 strains for different markets.[53] Brain tissue from intracranially infected mice is homogenized, and virus is purified by ultracentrifugation and filtration steps. The materials are inactivated by formalin during this process.[335] These vaccines were used primarily in Japan, Korea, Thailand, Malaysia, Sri Lanka, and Vietnam to protect against endemic JEV.[53] The BIKEN vaccine was licensed for travelers in the United States and elsewhere and marketed as JE-VAX™.[235]

Efficacy studies of mouse brain–derived JEV vaccines suggest that they are modestly immunogenic, and thus require multiple boosts. A placebo-controlled double-blind evaluation of monovalent (Nakayama strain) or bivalent (Nakayama and Beijing strains) formulations of JE-VAX conducted in Thailand revealed an efficacy of 91% in children receiving two doses of vaccine 7 days apart.[335] However, interpretation of these studies is complicated by the prevalence of individuals with prior flavivirus experience in JEV-endemic regions. Studies of the immunogenicity of two doses of JE-VAX in flavivirus-naïve subjects revealed only 33% seroconversion at 26 weeks postvaccination; in subsequent studies, near complete seroconversion was achieved using a third dose.[657,707] Attempts to measure the durability of antibody responses elicited by mouse brain–derived vaccine in endemic regions have been complicated by the potential boosting by naturally acquired flavivirus infection. Studies of military vaccine recipients suggest that neutralizing antibodies may persist for at least 3 years.[244] Vaccine is typically administered in two doses separated by 1 to 4 weeks, followed by a booster 1 to 2 years later. Travelers require a rapid three-dose vaccination regimen (days 0, 7, and 30).[235]

Although mouse brain–derived JEV vaccines have shown efficacy in humans, they are reactogenic and raise concerns about vaccine safety. Roughly 20% of JE-VAX recipients experience local adverse events including swelling, redness, and tenderness at the vaccination site, and mild systemic symptoms are also relatively common. Severe allergic and neurologic (acute disseminated encephalomyelitis [ADEM]) complications of vaccination have been observed (10 to 260 and 0.1 to 2 per 100,000 vaccinees, respectively).[53,235] Fatalities from ADEM resulted in cessation of production of JE-VAX in 2005 in favor of newer vaccines with more favorable safety profiles.

Live Attenuated JEV Vaccines

SA14-14-2 is a live-attenuated JEV vaccine that has been administered to more than 300 million individuals.[302] The parental SA14 strain was isolated from the larvae of *Culex pipiens* mosquitoes collected in China in 1954, and causes lethal neurologic disease when inoculated into weanling mice via the intracranial route. The attenuated strain was developed after extensive passaging of the SA14 strain in cell culture, and in hamsters and suckling mice.[613,898] The SA12-1-7 strain was isolated by passage of SA14 in newborn mice 10 times and 100 passages in primary hamster kidney cells.[614] Although this virus was considerably less virulent than SA14, it was not genetically stable and reverted to a neurovirulent phenotype following a single passage in mice, or several passages in primary cell cultures.[908] Derivatives of this virus with greater genetic stability were subsequently developed and evaluated. SA14-5-3 was derived from SA12-1-7 by additional passages in cell culture and plaque purification steps. Clinical studies demonstrated vaccine safety in humans but only modest immunogenicity, with seroconversion rates of 85% and 61% in endemic and nonendemic regions, respectively.[302] SA14-5-3 was licensed for use in China; altogether about 5 million children were vaccinated.[908] To improve immunogenicity, additional passages of SA14-5-2 in suckling mice yielded the SA14-14-2 strain. A single dose of SA14-14-2 induced a neutralizing antibody response in 85 to 100% of non-immune recipients.[767,833,898] Case-controlled studies demonstrated that a single dose of SA14-14-2 vaccine provided considerable protection (80% to 99%),[76,327,431,626] which was durable even after 5 years.[809] SA-14-14-2 was licensed for use in China in 1988, and subsequently distributed in Nepal, South Korea, Sri Lanka, Thailand, and India.

Inactivated JEV Vaccines Produced in Cell Culture

The IC51 (or IXIARO) vaccine is a formalin-inactivated vaccine produced in certified Vero cells under serum free conditions and adjuvanted with aluminum hydroxide.[235] IC51 uses the SA14-14-2 JEV strain,[414] and is administered in two doses 28 days apart, each containing ~6 μg of purified virus. Licensure was granted based on a noninferiority immunogenicity study comparing the response of recipients receiving IC51 to those vaccinated with a three-dose regimen of JE-VAX. Although a single dose of IC51 was poorly immunogenic (41% seroconversion), 4 weeks after the last of three doses, 96% of recipients had detectable neutralizing antibodies, and these persisted in most subjects 6 months after vaccination.[414] No significant local or systemic adverse events were associated with vaccination; rare events await a more detailed analysis of larger populations of vaccine recipients. IC51 was licensed for use in the United States as a traveler's vaccine in 2009 for individuals older than 17 years of age. An inactivated JEV vaccine derived from the genotype III P3 strain and produced in hamster cell cultures also has been used extensively in China, with as many as 70 million doses of this vaccine administered each year.[302]

New Vaccination Approaches

ChimeriVax-JE, or IMOJEV, is a promising live attenuated vaccine constructed using the attenuated YF17D backbone described above (reviewed by[55]). ChimeriVax-JE was constructed by inserting the prM-E genes of YF-17D, with genes encoding the envelope proteins of SA-14-14-2. Vaccination with ChimeriVax-JE elicits a protective response in mice and primate studies.[55,288,576] Clinical studies in humans reveal the vaccine is well tolerated and immunogenic (reviewed by[292]).

Tick-Borne Encephalitis Virus

Two inactivated TBEV vaccines are used to prevent infection in Europe, but are not licensed in the United States.[677] Kunz and colleagues[436,437] developed the first licensed vaccine in 1973 using the Austrian Neudörfl strain of TBEV grown in chick embryo fibroblasts, after inactivation with formalin and adjuvanting with aluminum hydroxide. Today, this vaccine is distributed as FSME-IMMUN by Baxter Biosciences. A second vaccine, produced by Novartis and marketed as Encepur,[83,407] was licensed in 1991. It is produced using similar methods, except the German K23 strain of TBEV is substituted. Both inactivated TBEV vaccines are administered in three doses and require boosting. The conventional schedule requires three vaccinations at 0, 1–3 months, and 9–12 months, and a booster at 3 years, followed by additional booster vaccinations every 5 years. These vaccines are highly immunogenic; virtually 100% of vaccinated subjects develop significant neutralizing antibody titers following their third dose,[436] and antibodies persist for at least 5 years.[652,887] The effectiveness of current TBEV vaccines in the field has been estimated at about 99%.[320] Despite the availability of effective vaccine, TBEV incidence in parts of Europe recently has increased, coincident with poor vaccine coverage.[438]

West Nile Virus

Several strategies for vaccination against WNV have been developed and evaluated in clinical studies (reviewed in[51]). Live-attenuated flavivirus chimeras have been developed for WNV using the strategies described above for DENV and JEV. ChimeriVax WNV was constructed by replacing the genes encoding the prM-E proteins of YF-17D with those of WNV.[292] Two vaccines were developed using this approach. ChimeriVax-WN01 encodes the unmodified sequence of the NY99 strain, and was developed as a veterinary vaccine that has been in use in horses since roughly 2006.[498,499] ChimeriVax-

WN02 differs from the veterinary vaccine by three amino acid substitutions in the E protein introduced to reduce neurovirulence, and a fourth adventitious substitution that arose during adaption of the vaccine lot to growth on Vero cells.[292] ChimeriVax-WN02 has been shown to be safe and immunogenic in phase I and phase II clinical trials in humans.[72,574] Chimeric flavivirus vaccine candidates have also been constructed using the DENV4Δ30 backbone described earlier (see DENV section) and have proven to be safe and immunogenic in preclinical[606] and clinical studies (A. Durbin, S. Whitehead, and colleagues, unpublished data; ClinicalTrials.gov identifier: NCT00094718).

Despite their effectiveness, concerns about the potential hazards associated with the use of live-attenuated viral vaccines provide a strong rationale for the development of other approaches. DNA vaccination has also shown promise for WNV vaccination. DNA vaccine constructs typically express genes encoding the prM and E structural proteins. Expression of prM-E *in vitro* is sufficient for the production of small virus-like subviral particles on which the E proteins are arrayed with icosahedral symmetry[233]; DNA vaccines are thought to produce subviral particles upon administration *in vivo.* Two phase I clinical studies of a WNV nucleic acid vaccine have been performed.[180,453,530] These trials demonstrated that three doses of vaccine were well-tolerated and capable of eliciting both a T-cell and neutralizing antibody response. A similar construct has proven to be efficacious at reducing WNV incidence in horses and a variety of birds.[51]

An adjuvanted subunit vaccine containing a soluble fragment of the WNV E protein has been developed[473,474,873] and studied in humans (ClinicalTrials.gov identifier: NCT00707642). A truncated form of the E protein lacking the transmembrane domains (referred to as 80% E) was produced in *Drosophila* S2 cells and purified using immunoaffinity chromatography. Preclinical studies demonstrate that administration of a single dose of adjuvanted protein was immunogenic and capable of eliciting a neutralizing antibody response.[473,474,873] To date, the results of a phase I clinical study of this vaccine have not been published.

Replivax-WN is a truncated form of the WNV genome encoding a large deletion in the gene encoding the capsid protein. This construct can be complemented *in vitro* using cell lines that express the capsid protein to yield pseudoinfectious virus particles. Infection of cells with these virus particles is not productive, yet it results in the production of subviral particles composed of prM and E. Immunization with RepliVax particles has been shown to be safe in preclinical studies and stimulates a robust adaptive response.[606,884,885] A similar modification of the Kunjin virus genome has been evaluated as a candidate WNV vaccine.[133]

Altogether four veterinary vaccines have been licensed for use including a formalin-inactivated adjuvanted whole virus vaccine (WN-Innovator, Fort Dodge Animal Health), a canarypox vector expressing prM and E (Recombitek equine WNV vaccine),[219,378,760] ChimeriVax-WN01 (PreveNile),[292] and a DNA vaccine construct that served as the basis for the human vaccine described above (WN-Innovator DNA, Fort Dodge Animal Health).[180]

Therapeutics

At present, no specific therapy has been approved for use in humans with any flavivirus infection, as all current treatments are supportive. For example, treatment of severe DHF/DSS currently consists of careful patient monitoring and aggressive fluid management. Although tissue culture and animal model studies have applied multiple screening strategies to generate novel therapies against flaviviruses, development has remained challenging. Among the impediments are the rapid development of resistance for monotherapy, a need to efficiently cross the BBB for inhibitors of the encephalitic flaviviruses, and regulatory hurdles for the design and implementation of multicenter trials, given the sporadic temporal and spatial occurrence of many flavivirus infections.

Existing Antiviral Agents: Ribavirin, Mycophenolic Acid and Human IFN-α

Ribavirin is a broad-spectrum antiviral agent and has been used clinically to treat respiratory syncytial, hepatitis C, Lassa fever, and Crimean-Congo hemorrhagic fever viruses. It acts as a guanosine analog and competitively inhibits inosine monophosphate dehydrogenase (IMP), resulting in depleted intracellular guanosine pools.[462] This activity has been proposed to interfere with the guanylylation step of RNA capping, inhibit viral polymerases, or compromise the integrity of the viral genome by being incorporated directly into the nascent RNA strand and serving as a template for both cytidine and uridine.[172,173,184] Ribavirin has inhibitory activity against flaviviruses infection in cell culture,[166,365,807] albeit at relatively high micromolar concentrations. Limited animal studies have been performed with varying results. Although a beneficial therapeutic effect of ribavirin was observed in YFV-infected hamsters,[366,715] treatment of YFV-infected NHP had minimal positive effect,[564] and increased mortality was observed in WNV-infected hamsters.[580] A combination of ribavirin with IFN-α_{2b} also failed to improve outcome of flavivirus-induced encephalitis in mice.[463] Finally, during a WNV outbreak in Israel in 2000, in an uncontrolled study, 37 patients received ribavirin and had a higher mortality rate.[151]

Mycophenolic acid (MPA) is a nonnucleoside inhibitor of IMP dehydrogenase that is used clinically to prevent rejection of transplanted organs. The immunosuppressive properties of MPA are attributed to its antiproliferative effect on lymphocytes *in vitro.* MPA inhibits to varying degrees the replication of a number of DNA, RNA, and retroviruses. Several studies have demonstrated that MPA inhibits flavivirus infection in cells by limiting viral RNA replication.[206,585,807] Although MPA blocks flavivirus infection in cell culture, its immunosuppressive properties *in vivo* likely overshadow its direct antiviral effects, as no study has reported therapeutic benefit in animals.

Type I IFN induces an antiviral state within cells through the induction of antiviral proteins and by modulating adaptive immune responses. Despite the ability of flaviviruses to antagonize its signaling pathways, pretreatment of cells with type I IFN potently inhibits infection by many flaviviruses. Nonetheless, IFN may still have therapeutic potential. Pretreatment of rodents with IFN-α inhibited SLEV infection and resulted in decreased WNV viral loads and mortality.[106,580] Analogously, treatment of before or after YFV infection also improved survival rates.[366] Administration of IFN-α reduced complications in human SLEV cases and has been used in an uncontrolled manner to treat small numbers of human cases of WNV encephalitis.[374,461,670] However, in Vietnam, a double-blinded, randomized placebo-controlled clinical trial was performed in

1,112 children with suspected or documented encephalitis virus infection; treatment with IFN-α_{2a} failed to improve outcome.[770]

Passive Antibody Therapy

Through experiments in a variety of experimental systems, it is well established that antibodies can neutralize flavivirus infection *in vitro* and *in vivo,* and prophylaxis or immunization can provide sterilizing immunity and prevent infection. The ability to cure animals with established flavivirus infection by passive transfer of antibodies, however, is more challenging and depends on the dosage, time of administration, and individual flavivirus.[691] For some flaviviruses, there are concerns that treatment could promote ADE and paradoxically exacerbate disease. In both monkeys and mice, subneutralizing concentrations of antibody enhanced DENV infectivity[39,265,309,912] and thus could complicate the antibody therapy. Apart from or perhaps related to ADE, an "early-death" phenomenon[579] has been reported that could also limit the utility of antibody therapy. According to this model, animals that have preexisting humoral immunity but do not respond well to viral challenge may succumb to infection more rapidly than animals without preexisting immunity. Although it has been described after passive acquisition of antibodies against YFV and Langat encephalitis viruses,[43,269,875] this phenomenon was not observed after transfer of monoclonal or polyclonal antibodies against WNV,[64,225,627] JEV,[396] or TBEV.[423]

Although preexposure passive transfer of neutralizing antibodies protects successfully against infection by many flaviviruses[199,691] postexposure therapeutic studies have been performed in a more limited fashion, primarily with antibodies against WNV, TBEV, and DENV. In therapeutic trials, immune human γ-globulin protected mice and hamsters against WNV-induced mortality.[62,64,225,367] Therapeutic intervention even 5 days after WNV infection reduced mortality; this time point is significant because in rodents WNV spreads to the brain and spinal cord by day 4. Therefore, passive transfer of immune antibody improved clinical outcome even after WNV had disseminated into the CNS. Analogously, postexposure treatment with polyclonal immune immunoglobulin decreased TBEV lethality in mice, with the degree of protection correlating with the amount of antibody administered and the time interval between infection and treatment.[423]

Humans have received passive therapy with immune γ-globulin against flavivirus infection. The largest experience is with commercial anti-TBEV antibody preparations (Encegam® and FSME-Bulin®). These products were available beginning in the 1970s, and recommended for treatment within a few days of a tick bite at risk for TBEV infection,[105] with between 70,000 and 200,000 doses administered.[18] However, worsened illness after treatment was reported in three children,[410,854] although no definitive clinical trial was ever conducted. Subsequently, immune γ-globulin production was suspended in the European Union, and Latvia remains the only European country where TBEV-specific immunoglobulin is still given.[105] In comparison, case reports have described improvement in humans with neuroinvasive WNV infection after receiving immune γ-globulin.[295,745] Although promising, γ-globulin immunotherapy against WNV infection in humans has limitations: (a) batch variability may affect the quantitative titer and functional activity; (b) it is purified from human plasma and has a theoretical risk of transmitting infectious agents; and (c) it requires a large volume of administration, which can increase adverse events in patients with cardiac or renal comorbidities.

More recently, humanized or human monoclonal antibodies or antibody derivatives with therapeutic activity against WNV infection[272,627,823,850] have been developed. These human or humanized antibody fragments have high neutralizing activity *in vitro* and provide excellent protection in rodents. When some humanized mAbs were given as a single dose 5 or 6 days after infection, 90% of mice or hamsters were protected.[581,627] Acute flaccid paralysis in hamsters also was blocked by treatment several days after infection using one anti-WNV neutralizing antibody.[705] A phase II randomized, double-blinded clinical trial to evaluate safety and efficacy of this humanized antibody (E16, also termed MGAWN1) against severe WNV infection was recently completed (ClinicalTrials.gov identifier: NCT00515385). Neutralizing antibody therapeutics show promise, as they directly inhibit transneuronal spread of WNV infection and prevent the development of paralysis *in vivo.* Future use of a combination of monoclonal antibodies that bind distinct epitopes and neutralize by independent mechanisms could diminish the potential risk of selecting escape variants *in vivo,* especially in immunocompromised individuals who generate high-grade viremia and tissue viral burden.

Antibody-based therapeutics more recently have been proposed as a possible treatment for DENV infection. Although somewhat counterintuitive, because of the theoretical risk of ADE and immune-enhanced disease *in vivo,* genetically engineered antibody variants (E60-N297Q, 82.11-LALA, and 87.11-LALA) that recognize conserved epitopes in domain II or domain III and cannot bind FcγR exhibited prophylactic and therapeutic efficacy against ADE-induced lethal challenge of DENV-2 in mice.[39,61] These observations suggest a novel strategy for the design of antibody-based therapeutics against DENV.

Nucleic Acid Inhibitors

RNA Interference

RNA interference (RNAi) is a cellular process that specifically degrades RNA within the cytoplasm of cells in a sequence-specific manner. RNAi occurs in plants, nematodes, parasites, insects, and mammalian cells and functions as a regulator of cellular gene expression and an innate defense against RNA viruses. RNAi uses dsRNA to target and degrade sequence-specific single-stranded RNA (ssRNA). The cytoplasmic ribonuclease Dicer recognizes and cleaves long dsRNA molecules into approximately 21 to 25 base pair small interfering RNA (siRNA) molecules; these associate with the RNA-induced silencing complex (RISC) to target and degrade complementary ssRNA molecules.[773] The viral targets of RNAi have included double-stranded replicative-intermediate RNA or highly structured hairpin regions in single-stranded viral genomic RNA. In addition, any single-stranded viral RNA may be targeted and converted first to dsRNA by a cellular RNA-dependent RNA polymerase before recognition by Dicer.[9]

Many mammalian viruses appear susceptible to treatment with exogenous siRNA. Cells that express virus-specific siRNA or shRNA are resistant to infection by WNV,[15,249,631,900] DENV,[793] YFV,[634] SLEV,[904] and JEV.[429] The sequence-specific activity of siRNA against viruses has led to great interest in its potential as antiviral therapy. Administration of siRNA to mice reduces flavivirus infection and affords partial protection against lethal challenge.[32,429,634,904] WNV-specific siRNA could act efficiently as a therapeutic after viral challenge, although administration within 6 hours of infection was required.[429] No significant protection was observed when siRNA was delivered 24 hours after infection.[32] Although promising, RNAi-based therapeutics against viruses may await the development of delivery systems that allow more effective activity against actively replicating viruses.

Antisense Technology

Antisense oligomers have been used to modulate gene expression of pathogenic viruses, and several are in various stages of clinical development.[511] These compounds inhibit flaviviruses by binding RNA in a sequence-specific manner, effectively blocking access to a particular region of the viral genome. The development of phosphorodiamidate morpholino oligomers (PMOs) has enhanced water solubility and nuclease resistance,[796] and the conjugation of arginine-rich peptides to PMOs has facilitated cellular uptake and inhibitory activity.[609] Sequence-specific antisense oligomers have inhibitory activity in cell culture against several flaviviruses, including WNV[189,190] and DENV.[336,401] Low micromolar concentrations of arginine-rich peptide-conjugated PMOs that target the 5′ untranslated or 3′ cyclization sequences inhibited flavivirus infection by 5 to 6 $\log_{10}$ PFU/ml[190,401] when administered as pretreatment. However, when given either 2 or 4 days after infection, peptide-conjugated PMOs had little or no antiviral effect. PMO directed against the 5′ and 3′ conserved sequences partially protected mice from WNV or DENV infection and disease without causing appreciable toxicity,[189,782] although selection of resistant mutants was observed.[189] Some clinical improvement was observed when PPO was administered to mice at day 5 after infection, although statistically significant differences were not achieved. AVI Biopharma initiated a phase I human clinical trial for treatment of WNV infection (ClinicalTrials.gov identifier: NCT00091845) with AVI-4020, but the study was terminated prematurely due to a limited pool of eligible subjects.

Flavivirus Antiviral Peptides

Fuzeon™ is a peptide-based fusion inhibitor approved for clinical use in HIV-infected patients. Although structurally distinct, the flavivirus E proteins undergo an analogous series of pH-dependent conformational changes that permit entry, fusion, and nucleocapsid escape into the cytoplasm (see section on Virus Entry and Tropism). Exogenous administration of peptides corresponding to prM protein[919] or the stem anchor domains[342,727,728] of WNV and DENV E proteins inhibit infectivity in cell culture, likely during a late stage of the fusion process. Peptides corresponding to sites in domain II and the domain I–II hinge interface also inhibited DENV infection in cell culture at the level of virus–cell attachment.[163] Finally, another group identified two E protein peptides that could inhibit WNV infection with half maximal effective concentration (EC50) values as low as about 3 mM. Mice challenged with WNV that had been administered these inhibitory peptides showed reduced viremia and lethality.[31] Although this is an emerging area of therapeutic development for flaviviruses with multiple possible targets, clinical studies have not yet been initiated.

Iminosugars

In flavivirus-infected mammalian cells, a 14-residue oligosaccharide $(Glc)_3(Man)_9(GlcNAc)_2$ is added in the ER to specific asparagine residues on the prM and E virion proteins. This high-mannose carbohydrate is sequentially modified in the ER and Golgi by resident glucosidases to generate N-linked glycans that lack the terminal $\alpha(1,2)$ and $\alpha(1,3)$ glucose residues. Trimming of N-linked glycans in the ER is required for efficient assembly and secretion of flaviviruses in mammalian cells.[164,892] Iminosugar derivatives, such as deoxynojirimycin or castanospermine, inhibit endoplasmic reticulum α-glucosidases I and II. This prevents processing of high-mannose N-linked glycans from nascent glycoproteins, a step that is required for interaction with the ER chaperones, calnexin, and calreticulin. Several flaviviruses are strongly inhibited by α-glucosidase inhibitors *in vitro*[135,164,281,737,880,892] and *in vivo.*[134,880] One possible advantage of α-glucosidase inhibitors is that they target a host enzyme that is an essential step in virus secretion rather than the virus directly, and are thus less likely to select for resistant variants.

High-Throughput Screens with Small Molecule Inhibitors

Over the last decade, high-throughput screens (HTS) with small molecule libraries have identified classes of "druggable" compounds that inhibit flavivirus infection. Several strategies have been utilized in high-throughput platforms including approaches that target viral enzymes, host proteins, key viral protein structures, and viral replication.[620] HTS screens that directly or indirectly assess flavivirus replication have measured inhibition of cytopathic effect of viral infection, reporter gene expression in the context of a flavivirus replicon, or viral antigen expression by immunofluorescence and automated microscopy.[282,622,659,660] Among viral targets, inhibitors that attenuate NS2B-NS3 protease activity, NS5 methyltransferase activity, and NS5 RNA-dependent RNA polymerase activity of different flaviviruses have been identified. Possible host targets for HTS include furin-like enzymes or signal peptidases that promote virion maturation, c-Src and c-Yes kinases that are required for assembly and maturation, cholesterol and lipid biosynthesis, and immune response genes. High-resolution x-ray crystal structures of key viral proteins (e.g., C, prM, E, NS3, and NS5) have informed structure-based design and *in silico* screening of inhibitors to augment the potency of lead antiviral compounds. Co-crystallization of lead candidate inhibitors with protein targets can determine the topology and consequences of binding, so that structure-activity related variants with augmented efficacy can be designed.

More limited studies have been performed with small molecule inhibitors in animals to assess therapeutic potential. One oral pyrazine derivative with broad-spectrum antiviral activity, T-705 (6-fluoro-3-hydroxy-2-pyrazinecarboxamide) was protective in rodents when administered twice daily beginning 2 days after WNV infection.[586] However, administration of T-705 at days 3 or 4 after infection showed little apparent efficacy. A small molecule nucleoside analog (e.g., NITD203) that targets flavivirus RNA synthesis showed efficacy against DENV in mouse models,[148] although its significance as a possible therapeutic agents appears limited by *in vivo* toxicity.

Given their continued global emergence and expansion, the development of antiviral agents against flaviviruses as a complement to intensive vaccine design strategies is essential. At present, several candidate therapies that act through distinct mechanisms are moving through various stages of preclinical and clinical development. Based on the pathogenesis of infection by different flaviviruses, therapeutic agents may pair potent and direct antivirals with drugs that mitigate immune system–mediated inflammation and damage. For the encephalitic flaviviruses, inhibitors may need to cross the BBB efficiently to allow for control of local replication within neurons. For some flaviviruses where disease is sporadic and less predictable on an annual basis, regulatory hurdles will be encountered in implementing multicenter trials. Because of this, extensive preclinical experiments in small animals and NHPs may be useful to define whether a candidate therapeutic should reach human clinical trials. Ongoing pathogenesis and infection studies will inform novel drug design strategies that target individual viral proteins. Experiments in animals should continue to define the essential components of the protective immune response, and the immunologic risk factors that predispose to severe neurologic disease. Ultimately, a combination drug strategy that blocks viral infection, minimizes tissue injury, and limits the development of resistant variants will likely be more effective than single agents.

ACKNOWLEDGMENTS

We thank Mr. Ethan Tyler (OD, NIH) for preparation Figures 2, 6 to 8, 10, and 11; Dr. Richard Kuhn (Purdue University) for preparation of Figures 4 and 5; and Dr. Jiraphan Junjhon (Purdue University) for providing the unpublished image of DENV used in Figure 26.4C.

REFERENCES

All cited references are available in the e-book.

10. Allison SL, Schalich J, Stiasny K, et al. Mutational evidence for an internal fusion peptide in flavivirus envelope protein E. *J Virol* 2001;75(9): 4268–4275.
11. Allison SL, Stiasny K, Stadler K, et al. Mapping of functional elements in the stem-anchor region of tick-borne encephalitis virus envelope protein E. *J Virol* 1999;73(7):5605–5612.
17. Arjona A, Ledizet M, Anthony K, et al. West Nile virus envelope protein inhibits dsRNA-induced innate immune responses. *J Immunol* 2007; 179(12):8403–8409.
20. Ashour J, Laurent-Rolle M, Shi PY, et al. NS5 of dengue virus mediates STAT2 binding and degradation. *J Virol* 2009;83(11):5408–5418.
21. Ashour J, Morrison J, Laurent-Rolle M, et al. Mouse STAT2 restricts early dengue virus replication. *Cell Host Microbe* 2010;8(5):410–421.
24. Avirutnan P, Fuchs A, Hauhart RE, et al. Antagonism of the complement component C4 by flavivirus nonstructural protein NS1. *J Exp Med* 2010;207(4):793–806.
27. Avirutnan P, Mehlhop E, Diamond MS. Complement and its role in protection and pathogenesis of flavivirus infections. *Vaccine* 2008;26 (Suppl 8):I100–I107.
28. Avirutnan P, Punyadee N, Noisakran S, et al. Vascular leakage in severe dengue virus infections: a potential role for the nonstructural viral protein NS1 and complement. *J Infect Dis* 2006;193(8):1078–1088.
32. Bai F, Wang T, Pal U, et al. Use of RNA interference to prevent lethal murine West Nile virus infection. *J Infect Dis* 2005;191(7):1148–1154.
39. Balsitis SJ, Williams KL, Lachica R, et al. Lethal antibody enhancement of dengue disease in mice is prevented by Fc modification. *PLoS Pathog* 2010;6(2):e1000790.
41. Barnett ED. Yellow fever: epidemiology and prevention. *Clin Infect Dis* 2007;44(6):850–856.
46. Barrett AD, Teuwen DE. Yellow fever vaccine - how does it work and why do rare cases of serious adverse events take place? *Curr Opin Immunol* 2009;21(3):308–313.
52. Beasley DW, Barrett AD. Identification of neutralizing epitopes within structural domain III of the West Nile virus envelope protein. *J Virol* 2002;76(24):13097–13100.
53. Beasley DW, Lewthwaite P, Solomon T. Current use and development of vaccines for Japanese encephalitis. *Expert Opin Biol Ther* 2008;8(1): 95–106.
54. Beasley DW, Li L, Suderman MT, et al. Mouse neuroinvasive phenotype of West Nile virus strains varies depending upon virus genotype. *Virology* 2002;296(1):17–23.
56. Beasley DW, Whiteman MC, Zhang S, et al. Envelope protein glycosylation status influences mouse neuroinvasion phenotype of genetic lineage 1 West Nile virus strains. *J Virol* 2005;79(13):8339–8347.
61. Beltramello M, Williams KL, Simmons CP, et al. The human immune response to Dengue virus is dominated by highly cross-reactive antibodies endowed with neutralizing and enhancing activity. *Cell Host Microbe* 2010;8(3):271–283.
63. Ben-Nathan D, Huitinga I, Lustig S, et al. West Nile virus neuroinvasion and encephalitis induced by macrophage depletion in mice. *Arch Virol* 1996;141(3–4):459–469.
64. Ben-Nathan D, Lustig S, Tam G, et al. Prophylactic and therapeutic efficacy of human intravenous immunoglobulin in treating West Nile virus infection in mice. *J Infect Dis* 2003;188(1):5–12.
70. Bhamarapravati N, Tuchinda P, Boonyapaknavik V. Pathology of Thailand haemorrhagic fever: a study of 100 autopsy cases. *Ann Trop Med Parasitol* 1967;61(4):500–510.
81. Blaney JE Jr, Matro JM, Murphy BR, et al. Recombinant, live-attenuated tetravalent dengue virus vaccine formulations induce a balanced, broad, and protective neutralizing antibody response against each of the four serotypes in rhesus monkeys. *J Virol* 2005;79(9):5516–5528.
85. Bokisch VA, Top FH Jr, Russell PK, et al. The potential pathogenic role of complement in dengue hemorrhagic shock syndrome. *N Engl J Med* 1973;289(19):996–1000.
87. Boonnak K, Slike BM, Burgess TH, et al. Role of dendritic cells in antibody-dependent enhancement of dengue virus infection. *J Virol* 2008;82(8):3939–3951.
94. Brass AL, Huang IC, Benita Y, et al. The IFITM proteins mediate cellular resistance to influenza A H1N1 virus, West Nile virus, and dengue virus. *Cell* 2009;139(7):1243–1254.
95. Bray M, Lai CJ. Construction of intertypic chimeric dengue viruses by substitution of structural protein genes. *Proc Natl Acad Sci U S A* 1991; 88(22):10342–10346.
96. Bray M, Men R, Lai CJ. Monkeys immunized with intertypic chimeric dengue viruses are protected against wild-type virus challenge. *J Virol* 1996;70(6):4162–4166.
98. Bressanelli S, Stiasny K, Allison SL, et al. Structure of a flavivirus envelope glycoprotein in its low-pH-induced membrane fusion conformation. *EMBO J* 2004;23(4):728–738.
100. Brien JD, Uhrlaub JL, Hirsch A, et al. Key role of T cell defects in age-related vulnerability to West Nile virus. *J Exp Med* 2009;206(12):2735–2745.
104. Brinton MA. Characterization of West Nile virus persistent infections in genetically resistant and susceptible mouse cells. I. Generation of defective nonplaquing virus particles. *Virology* 1982;116(1):84–98.
105. Broker M, Kollaritsch H. After a tick bite in a tick-borne encephalitis virus endemic area: current positions about post-exposure treatment. *Vaccine* 2008;26(7):863–868.
110. Bryant JE, Holmes EC, Barrett AD. Out of Africa: a molecular perspective on the introduction of yellow fever virus into the Americas. *PLoS Pathog* 2007;3(5):e75.
112. Burke DS, Nisalak A, Johnson DE, et al. A prospective study of dengue infections in Bangkok. *Am J Trop Med Hyg* 1988;38(1):172–180.
113. Burke T. Dengue haemorrhagic fever: a pathological study. *Trans R Soc Trop Med Hyg* 1968;62(5):682–692.
115. Busch MP, Caglioti S, Robertson EF, et al. Screening the blood supply for West Nile virus RNA by nucleic acid amplification testing. *N Engl J Med* 2005;353(5):460–467.
119. Calisher CH, Gould EA. Taxonomy of the virus family Flaviviridae. *Adv Virus Res* 2003;59:1–19.
120. Calisher CH, Karabatsos N, Dalrymple JM, et al. Antigenic relationships between flaviviruses as determined by cross-neutralization tests with polyclonal antisera. *J Gen Virol* 1989;70(Pt 1):37–43.

121. Calvert AE, Kalantarov GF, Chang GJ, et al. Human monoclonal antibodies to West Nile virus identify epitopes on the prM protein. *Virology* 2011;410(1):30–37.
123. Cardosa MJ, Gordon S, Hirsch S, et al. Interaction of West Nile virus with primary murine macrophages: role of cell activation and receptors for antibody and complement. *J Virol* 1986;57(3):952–959.
124. Cardosa MJ, Porterfield JS, Gordon S. Complement receptor mediates enhanced flavivirus replication in macrophages. *J Exp Med* 1983; 158(1):258–263.
135. Chang J, Wang L, Ma D, et al. Novel imino sugar derivatives demonstrate potent antiviral activity against flaviviruses. *Antimicrob Agents Chemother* 2009;53(4):1501–1508.
140. Chau TN, Quyen NT, Thuy TT, et al. Dengue in Vietnamese infants–results of infection-enhancement assays correlate with age-related disease epidemiology, and cellular immune responses correlate with disease severity. *J Infect Dis* 2008;198(4):516–524.
144. Chen ST, Lin YL, Huang MT, et al. CLEC5A is critical for dengue-virus-induced lethal disease. *Nature* 2008;453(7195):672–676.
147. Chen Y, Maguire T, Hileman RE, et al. Dengue virus infectivity depends on envelope protein binding to target cell heparan sulfate. *Nat Med* 1997; 3(8):866–871.
149. Cherrier MV, Kaufmann B, Nybakken GE, et al. Structural basis for the preferential recognition of immature flaviviruses by a fusion-loop antibody. *EMBO J* 2009;28(20):3269–3276.
154. Chung KM, Liszewski MK, Nybakken G, et al. West Nile virus non-structural protein NS1 inhibits complement activation by binding the regulatory protein factor H. *Proc Natl Acad Sci U S A* 2006;103(50):19111–19116.
164. Courageot MP, Frenkiel MP, Dos Santos CD, et al. Alpha-glucosidase inhibitors reduce dengue virus production by affecting the initial steps of virion morphogenesis in the endoplasmic reticulum. *J Virol* 2000; 74(1):564–572.
168. Crill WD, Chang GJ. Localization and characterization of flavivirus envelope glycoprotein cross-reactive epitopes. *J Virol* 2004;78(24):13975–13986.
175. Daffis S, Samuel MA, Suthar MS, et al. Interferon regulatory factor IRF-7 induces the antiviral alpha interferon response and protects against lethal West Nile virus infection. *J Virol* 2008;82(17):8465–8475.
179. Daffis S, Szretter KJ, Schriewer J, et al. 2′-O methylation of the viral mRNA cap evades host restriction by IFIT family members. *Nature* 2010;468:452–456.
182. Davis CW, Mattei LM, Nguyen HY, et al. The location of asparagine-linked glycans on West Nile virions controls their interactions with CD209 (dendritic cell-specific ICAM-3 grabbing nonintegrin). *J Biol Chem* 2006;281(48):37183–37194.
191. Dejnirattisai W, Jumnainsong A, Onsirisakul N, et al. Cross-reacting antibodies enhance dengue virus infection in humans. *Science* 2010; 328(5979):745–748.
198. Diamond MS. Mechanisms of evasion of the type I interferon antiviral response by flaviviruses. *J Interferon Cytokine Res* 2009;29(9):521–530.
204. Diamond MS, Shrestha B, Marri A, et al. B cells and antibody play critical roles in the immediate defense of disseminated infection by West Nile encephalitis virus. *J Virol* 2003;77:2578–2586.
210. Dowd KA, Jost CA, Durbin AP, et al. A dynamic landscape for antibody binding modulates antibody-mediated neutralization of west nile virus. *PLoS Pathog* 2011;7(6):e1002111.
211. Dowd KA, Pierson TC. Antibody-mediated neutralization of flaviviruses: a reductionist view. *Virology* 2011;411(2):306–315.
213. Durbin AP, Karron RA, Sun W, et al. Attenuation and immunogenicity in humans of a live dengue virus type-4 vaccine candidate with a 30 nucleotide deletion in its 3′-untranslated region. *Am J Trop Med Hyg* 2001;65(5):405–413.
217. Durbin AP, Whitehead SS. Dengue vaccine candidates in development. *Curr Top Microbiol Immunol* 2010;338:129–143.
221. Eldadah AH, Nathanson N. Pathogenesis of West Nile Virus encepahlitis in mice and rats. II. Virus multiplication, evolution of immunofluorescence, and development of histological lesions in the brain. *Am J Epidemiol* 1967;86(3):776–790.
225. Engle M, Diamond MS. Antibody prophylaxis and therapy against West Nile Virus infection in wild type and immunodeficient mice. *J Virol* 2003;77:12941–12949.
235. Fischer M, Lindsey N, Staples JE, et al. Japanese encephalitis vaccines: recommendations of the Advisory Committee on Immunization Practices (ACIP). *MMWR Recomm Rep* 2010;59(RR-1):1–27.
239. Fredericksen BL, Gale M Jr. West Nile virus evades activation of interferon regulatory factor 3 through RIG-I-dependent and -independent pathways without antagonizing host defense signaling. *J Virol* 2006; 80(6):2913–2923.
246. Gardner CL, Ryman KD. Yellow fever: a reemerging threat. *Clin Lab Med* 2010;30(1):237–260.
258. Glass WG, Lim JK, Cholera R, et al. Chemokine receptor CCR5 promotes leukocyte trafficking to the brain and survival in West Nile virus infection. *J Exp Med* 2005;202(8):1087–1098.
259. Glass WG, McDermott DH, Lim JK, et al. CCR5 deficiency increases risk of symptomatic West Nile virus infection. *J Exp Med* 2006;203(1): 35–40.
260. Goldblum N, Sterk VV, Paderski B. West Nile fever; the clinical features of the disease and the isolation of West Nile virus from the blood of nine human cases. *Am J Hyg* 1954;59(1):89–103.
261. Gollins S, Porterfield J. Flavivirus infection enhancement in macrophages: radioactive and biological studies on the effect of antibody and viral fate. *J Gen Virol* 1984;65:1261–1272.
262. Gollins SW, Porterfield JS. Flavivirus infection enhancement in macrophages: an electron microscopic study of viral cellular entry. *J Gen Virol* 1985;66(Pt 9):1969–1982.
264. Gollins SW, Porterfield JS. pH-dependent fusion between the flavivirus West Nile and liposomal model membranes. *J Gen Virol* 1986;67: 157–166.
265. Goncalvez AP, Engle RE, St Claire M, et al. Monoclonal antibody-mediated enhancement of dengue virus infection in vitro and in vivo and strategies for prevention. *Proc Natl Acad Sci U S A* 2007;104(22): 9422–9427.
266. Goncalvez AP, Purcell RH, Lai CJ. Epitope determinants of a chimpanzee Fab antibody that efficiently cross-neutralizes dengue type 1 and type 2 viruses map to inside and in close proximity to fusion loop of the dengue type 2 virus envelope glycoprotein. *J Virol* 2004;78(23):12919–12928.
271. Gould EA, de Lamballerie X, Zanotto PM, et al. Origins, evolution, and vector/host coadaptations within the genus Flavivirus. *Adv Virus Res* 2003;59:277–314.
274. Grard G, Moureau G, Charrel RN, et al. Genetic characterization of tick-borne flaviviruses: new insights into evolution, pathogenetic determinants and taxonomy. *Virology* 2007;361(1):80–92.
275. Grard G, Moureau G, Charrel RN, et al. Genomics and evolution of Aedes-borne flaviviruses. *J Gen Virol* 2010;91(Pt 1):87–94.
277. Gritsun TS, Lashkevich VA, Gould EA. Tick-borne encephalitis. *Antiviral Res* 2003;57(1-2):129–146.
280. Gromowski GD, Barrett ND, Barrett AD. Characterization of dengue virus complex-specific neutralizing epitopes on envelope protein domain III of dengue 2 virus. *J Virol* 2008;82(17):8828–8837.
292. Guy B, Guirakhoo F, Barban V, et al. Preclinical and clinical development of YFV 17D-based chimeric vaccines against dengue, West Nile and Japanese encephalitis viruses. *Vaccine* 2010;28(3):632–649.
293. Guzman MG, Alvarez M, Rodriguez R, et al. Fatal dengue hemorrhagic fever in Cuba, 1997. *Int J Infect Dis* 1999;3(3):130–135.
297. Halstead SB. In vivo enhancement of dengue virus infection in rhesus monkeys by passively transferred antibody. *J Infect Dis* 1979;140(4): 527–533.
298. Halstead SB. Pathogenesis of dengue: challenges to molecular biology. *Science* 1988;239(4839):476–481.
302. Halstead SB, Jacobson J. Japanese encephalitis vaccines. In: Plotkin SA, Orenstein WA, Offit PA, eds. *Vaccines.* 5th ed. Philadelphia: Saunders Elsevier; 2008:311–352.
305. Halstead SB, Nimmannitya S, Cohen SN. Observations related to pathogenesis of dengue hemorrhagic fever. IV. Relation of disease severity to antibody response and virus recovered. *Yale J Biol Med* 1970;42(5): 311–328.
306. Halstead SB, O'Rourke EJ. Antibody-enhanced dengue virus infection in primate leukocytes. *Nature* 1977;265(5596):739–741.
307. Halstead SB, O'Rourke EJ. Dengue viruses and mononuclear phagocytes. I. Infection enhancement by non-neutralizing antibody. *J Exp Med* 1977;146(1):201–217.

308. Halstead SB, Shotwell H, Casals J. Studies on the pathogenesis of dengue infection in monkeys. I. Clinical laboratory responses to primary infection. *J Infect Dis* 1973;128(1):7–14.
318. Heinz FX, Berger R, Tuma W, et al. A topological and functional model of epitopes on the structural glycoprotein of tick-borne encephalitis virus defined by monoclonal antibodies. *Virology* 1983;126(2):525–537.
320. Heinz FX, Holzmann H, Essl A, et al. Field effectiveness of vaccination against tick-borne encephalitis. *Vaccine* 2007;25(43):7559–7567.
321. Heinz FX, Stiasny K, Puschner-Auer G, et al. Structural changes and functional control of the tick-borne encephalitis virus glycoprotein E by the heterodimeric association with protein prM. *Virology* 1994;198(1):109–117.
322. Henchal EA, Gentry MK, McCown JM, et al. Dengue virus-specific and flavivirus group determinants identified with monoclonal antibodies by indirect immunofluorescence. *Am J Trop Med Hyg* 1982;31(4):830–836.
327. Hennessy S, Liu Z, Tsai TF, et al. Effectiveness of live-attenuated Japanese encephalitis vaccine (SA14-14-2): a case-control study. *Lancet* 1996;347(9015):1583–1586.
348. Hubalek Z, Halouzka J. West Nile fever - a reemerging mosquito-borne viral disease in Europe. *Emerg Inf Dis* 1999;5(5):643–650.
359. Jiang D, Weidner JM, Qing M, et al. Identification of five interferon-induced cellular proteins that inhibit west nile virus and dengue virus infections. *J Virol* 2010;84(16):8332–8341.
360. Johnson AJ, Roehrig JT. New mouse model for dengue virus vaccine testing. *J Virol* 1999;73(1):783–786.
364. Jones M, Davidson A, Hibbert L, et al. Dengue virus inhibits alpha interferon signaling by reducing STAT2 expression. *J Virol* 2005;79(9):5414–5420.
383. Kaufmann B, Nybakken GE, Chipman PR, et al. West Nile virus in complex with the Fab fragment of a neutralizing monoclonal antibody. *Proc Natl Acad Sci U S A* 2006;103(33):12400–12404.
384. Kaufmann B, Vogt MR, Goudsmit J, et al. Neutralization of West Nile virus by cross-linking of its surface proteins with Fab fragments of the human monoclonal antibody CR4354. *Proc Natl Acad Sci U S A* 2010;107(44):18950–18955.
393. Kilpatrick AM, Kramer LD, Jones MJ, et al. West Nile virus epidemics in North America are driven by shifts in mosquito feeding behavior. *PLoS Biol* 2006;4(4):e82.
400. King NJ, Kesson AM. Interferon-independent increases in class I major histocompatibility complex antigen expression follow flavivirus infection. *J Gen Virol* 1988;69(Pt 10):2535–2543.
402. Kitchen A, Shackelton LA, Holmes EC. Family level phylogenies reveal modes of macroevolution in RNA viruses. *Proc Natl Acad Sci U S A* 2011;108(1):238–243.
404. Klein RS, Lin E, Zhang B, et al. Neuronal CXCL10 directs CD8+ T cell recruitment and control of West Nile virus encephalitis. *J Virol* 2005;79(17):11457–11466.
405. Kliks SC, Nimmanitya S, Nisalak A, et al. Evidence that maternal dengue antibodies are important in the development of dengue hemorrhagic fever in infants. *Am J Trop Med Hyg* 1988;38(2):411–419.
425. Kuhn RJ, Zhang W, Rossmann MG, et al. Structure of dengue virus: implications for flavivirus organization, maturation, and fusion. *Cell* 2002;108(5):717–725.
429. Kumar P, Lee SK, Shankar P, et al. A single siRNA suppresses fatal encephalitis induced by two different flaviviruses. *PLoS Med* 2006;3(4):e96.
431. Kumar R, Tripathi P, Rizvi A. Effectiveness of one dose of SA 14-14-2 vaccine against Japanese encephalitis. *N Engl J Med* 2009;360(14):1465–1466.
436. Kunz C. TBE vaccination and the Austrian experience. *Vaccine* 2003;21(Suppl 1):S50–S55.
442. Kyle JL, Harris E. Global spread and persistence of dengue. *Annu Rev Microbiol* 2008;62:71–92.
455. Lee E, Lobigs M. Substitutions at the putative receptor-binding site of an encephalitic flavivirus alter virulence and host cell tropism and reveal a role for glycosaminoglycans in entry. *J Virol* 2000;74(19):8867–8875.
466. Li L, Lok SM, Yu IM, et al. The flavivirus precursor membrane-envelope protein complex: structure and maturation. *Science* 2008;319(5871):1830–1834.
469. Libraty DH, Pichyangkul S, Ajariyakhajorn C, et al. Human dendritic cells are activated by dengue virus infection: enhancement by gamma interferon and implications for disease pathogenesis. *J Virol* 2001;75(8):3501–3508.
476. Lim JK, McDermott DH, Lisco A, et al. CCR5 deficiency is a risk factor for early clinical manifestations of West Nile virus infection but not for viral transmission. *J Infect Dis* 2010;201(2):178–185.
484. Lin YL, Huang YL, Ma SH, et al. Inhibition of Japanese encephalitis virus infection by nitric oxide: antiviral effect of nitric oxide on RNA virus replication. *J Virol* 1997;71(7):5227–5235.
492. Liu WJ, Wang XJ, Clark DC, et al. A single amino acid substitution in the West Nile virus nonstructural protein NS2A disables its ability to inhibit alpha/beta interferon induction and attenuates virus virulence in mice. *J Virol* 2006;80(5):2396–2404.
497. Lok SM, Kostyuchenko V, Nybakken GE, et al. Binding of a neutralizing antibody to dengue virus alters the arrangement of surface glycoproteins. *Nat Struct Mol Biol* 2008;15(3):312–317.
503. Lozach PY, Burleigh L, Staropoli I, et al. Dendritic cell-specific intercellular adhesion molecule 3-grabbing non-integrin (DC-SIGN)-mediated enhancement of dengue virus infection is independent of DC-SIGN internalization signals. *J Biol Chem* 2005;280(25):23698–23708.
513. Mackenzie JM, Westaway EG. Assembly and maturation of the flavivirus Kunjin virus appear to occur in the rough endoplasmic reticulum and along the secretory pathway, respectively. *J Virol* 2001;75(22):10787–10799.
514. Mackenzie JS, Gubler DJ, Petersen LR. Emerging flaviviruses: the spread and resurgence of Japanese encephalitis, West Nile and dengue viruses. *Nat Med* 2004;10(12 Suppl):S98–S109.
516. Malasit P. Complement and dengue haemorrhagic fever/shock syndrome. *Southeast Asian J Trop Med Public Health* 1987;18(3):316–320.
523. Mandl CW, Kroschewski H, Allison SL, et al. Adaptation of tick-borne encephalitis virus to BHK-21 cells results in the formation of multiple heparan sulfate binding sites in the envelope protein and attenuation in vivo. *J Virol* 2001;75(12):5627–5637.
527. Marianneau P, Steffan AM, Royer C, et al. Infection of primary cultures of human Kupffer cells by Dengue virus: no viral progeny synthesis, but cytokine production is evident. *J Virol* 1999;73(6):5201–5206.
529. Marovich M, Grouard-Vogel G, Louder M, et al. Human dendritic cells as targets of dengue virus infection. *J Investig Dermatol Symp Proc* 2001;6(3):219–224.
532. Mashimo T, Lucas M, Simon-Chazottes D, et al. A nonsense mutation in the gene encoding 2′-5′-oligoadenylate synthetase/L1 isoform is associated with West Nile virus susceptibility in laboratory mice. *Proc Natl Acad Sci U S A* 2002;99(17):11311–11316.
533. Mason RA, Tauraso NM, Spertzel RO, et al. Yellow fever vaccine: direct challenge of monkeys given graded doses of 17D vaccine. *Appl Microbiol* 1973;25(4):539–544.
534. Mathew A, Rothman AL. Understanding the contribution of cellular immunity to dengue disease pathogenesis. *Immunol Rev* 2008;225:300–313.
543a. Meertens L, Carnec X, Lecoin MP, et al. The TIM and TAM families of phosphatidylserine receptors mediate dengue virus entry. *Cell Host Microbe* 2012;12:544–557.
544. Mehlhop E, Ansarah-Sobrinho C, Johnson S, et al. Complement protein C1q inhibits antibody-dependent enhancement of flavivirus infection in an IgG subclass-specific manner. *Cell Host Microbe* 2007;2(6):417–426.
545. Mehlhop E, Diamond MS. Protective immune responses against West Nile virus are primed by distinct complement activation pathways. *J Exp Med* 2006;203(5):1371–1381.
548. Meier KC, Gardner CL, Khoretonenko MV, et al. A mouse model for studying viscerotropic disease caused by yellow fever virus infection. *PLoS Pathog* 2009;5(10):e1000614.
550. Men R, Bray M, Clark D, et al. Dengue type 4 virus mutants containing deletions in the 3′ noncoding region of the RNA genome: analysis of growth restriction in cell culture and altered viremia pattern and immunogenicity in rhesus monkeys. *J Virol* 1996;70(6):3930–3937.
553. Miagostovich MP, Ramos RG, Nicol AF, et al. Retrospective study on dengue fatal cases. *Clin Neuropathol* 1997;16(4):204–208.
558. Modis Y, Ogata S, Clements D, et al. Structure of the dengue virus envelope protein after membrane fusion. *Nature* 2004;427(6972):313–319.
564. Monath TP. Treatment of yellow fever. *Antiviral Res* 2008;78(1):116–124.
565. Monath TP. Yellow fever vaccine. *Expert Rev Vaccines* 2005;4(4):553–574.

566. Monath TP. Yellow fever: Victor, Victoria? Conqueror, conquest? Epidemics and research in the last forty years and prospects for the future. *Am J Trop Med Hyg* 1991;45(1):1–43.
567. Monath TP, Barrett AD. Pathogenesis and pathophysiology of yellow fever. *Adv Virus Res* 2003;60:343–395.
569. Monath TP, Cetron MS, Teuwen DE. Yellow fever vaccine. In: Plotkin SA, Orenstein WA, Offit PA, eds. *Vaccines*. 5th ed. Philadelphia: Saunders Elsevier; 2008:959–1055.
577. Mongkolsapaya J, Dejnirattisai W, Xu XN, et al. Original antigenic sin and apoptosis in the pathogenesis of dengue hemorrhagic fever. *Nat Med* 2003;9(7):921–927.
578. Mongkolsapaya J, Duangchinda T, Dejnirattisai W, et al. T cell responses in dengue hemorrhagic fever: are cross-reactive T cells suboptimal? *J Immunol* 2006;176(6):3821–3829.
589. Mota J, Rico-Hesse R. Humanized mice show clinical signs of dengue fever according to infecting virus genotype. *J Virol* 2009;83(17):8638–8645.
591. Mukhopadhyay S, Kuhn RJ, Rossmann MG. A structural perspective of the flavivirus life cycle. *Nat Rev Microbiol* 2005;3(1):13–22.
594. Munoz-Jordan JL, Sanchez-Burgos GG, Laurent-Rolle M, et al. Inhibition of interferon signaling by dengue virus. *Proc Natl Acad Sci U S A* 2003;100:14333–14338.
597. Murphy BR, Whitehead SS. Immune response to dengue virus and prospects for a vaccine. *Annu Rev Immunol* 2011;29:587–619.
599. Murray K, Walker C, Herrington E, et al. Persistent infection with West Nile virus years after initial infection. *J Infect Dis* 2010;201(1):2–4.
603. Nash D, Mostashari F, Fine A, et al. The outbreak of West Nile virus infection in the New York City area in 1999. *N Engl J Med* 2001;344(24): 1807–1814.
605. Navarro-Sanchez E, Altmeyer R, Amara A, et al. Dendritic-cell-specific ICAM3-grabbing non-integrin is essential for the productive infection of human dendritic cells by mosquito-cell-derived dengue viruses. *EMBO Rep* 2003;4(7):723–728.
607. Nelson S, Jost CA, Xu Q, et al. Maturation of West Nile virus modulates sensitivity to antibody-mediated neutralization. *PLoS Pathog* 2008; 4(5):e1000060.
612. Ngo NT, Cao XT, Kneen R, et al. Acute management of dengue shock syndrome: a randomized double-blind comparison of 4 intravenous fluid regimens in the first hour. *Clin Infect Dis* 2001;32(2):204–213.
620. Noble CG, Chen YL, Dong H, et al. Strategies for development of Dengue virus inhibitors. *Antiviral Res* 2010;85(3):450–462.
624. Nybakken GE, Oliphant T, Johnson S, et al. Structural basis of West Nile virus neutralization by a therapeutic antibody. *Nature* 2005;437 (7059):764–769.
627. Oliphant T, Engle M, Nybakken G, et al. Development of a humanized monoclonal antibody with therapeutic potential against West Nile virus. *Nat Med* 2005;11(5):522–530.
628. Oliphant T, Nybakken GE, Austin SK, et al. The induction of epitope-specific neutralizing antibodies against West Nile virus. *J Virol* 2007;81: 11828–11839.
629. Oliphant T, Nybakken GE, Engle M, et al. Antibody recognition and neutralization determinants on domains I and II of West Nile Virus envelope protein. *J Virol* 2006;80(24):12149–12159.
638. Park GS, Morris KL, Hallett RG, et al. Identification of residues critical for the interferon antagonist function of Langat virus NS5 reveals a role for the RNA-dependent RNA polymerase domain. *J Virol* 2007; 81(13):6936–6946.
639. Pealer LN, Marfin AA, Petersen LR, et al. Transmission of West Nile virus through blood transfusion in the United States in 2002. *N Engl J Med* 2003;349(13):1236–1245.
640. Peiris JS, Gordon S, Unkeless JC, et al. Monoclonal anti-Fc receptor IgG blocks antibody enhancement of viral replication in macrophages. *Nature* 1981;289(5794):189–191.
641. Peiris JS, Porterfield JS. Antibody-mediated enhancement of Flavivirus replication in macrophage- like cell lines. *Nature* 1979;282(5738):509–511.
643. Perelygin AA, Scherbik SV, Zhulin IB, et al. Positional cloning of the murine flavivirus resistance gene. *Proc Natl Acad Sci U S A* 2002; 99(14):9322–9327.
645. Pfister M, Kursteiner O, Hilfiker H, et al. Immunogenicity and safety of BERNA-YF compared with two other 17D yellow fever vaccines in a phase 3 clinical trial. *Am J Trop Med Hyg* 2005;72(3):339–346.
647. Pierson TC, Fremont DH, Kuhn RJ, et al. Structural insights into the mechanisms of antibody-mediated neutralization of flavivirus infection: implications for vaccine development. *Cell Host Microbe* 2008;4(3): 229–238.
648. Pierson TC, Xu Q, Nelson S, et al. The stoichiometry of antibody-mediated neutralization and enhancement of West Nile virus infection. *Cell Host Microbe* 2007;1:135–145.
661. Pulendran B. Learning immunology from the yellow fever vaccine: innate immunity to systems vaccinology. *Nat Rev Immunol* 2009;9(10):741–747.
667. Querec T, Bennouna S, Alkan S, et al. Yellow fever vaccine YF-17D activates multiple dendritic cell subsets via TLR2, 7, 8, and 9 to stimulate polyvalent immunity. *J Exp Med* 2006;203(2):413–424.
668. Querec TD, Akondy RS, Lee EK, et al. Systems biology approach predicts immunogenicity of the yellow fever vaccine in humans. *Nat Immunol* 2009;10(1):116–125.
679. Rey FA, Heinz FX, Mandl C, et al. The envelope glycoprotein from tick-borne encephalitis virus at 2 A resolution. *Nature* 1995;375(6529): 291–298.
684. Rios M, Zhang MJ, Grinev A, et al. Monocytes-macrophages are a potential target in human infection with West Nile virus through blood transfusion. *Transfusion* 2006;46(4):659–667.
685. Rodenhuis-Zybert IA, van der Schaar HM, da Silva Voorham JM, et al. Immature dengue virus: a veiled pathogen? *PLoS Pathog* 2010;6(1): e1000718.
686. Rodriguez-Madoz JR, Belicha-Villanueva A, Bernal-Rubio D, et al. Inhibition of the type I interferon response in human dendritic cells by dengue virus infection requires a catalytically active NS2B3 complex. *J Virol* 2010;84(19):9760–9774.
687. Rodriguez-Madoz JR, Bernal-Rubio D, Kaminski D, et al. Dengue virus inhibits the production of type I interferon in primary human dendritic cells. *J Virol* 2010;84(9):4845–4850.
690. Roehrig JT, Mathews JH, Trent DW. Identification of epitopes on the E glycoprotein of Saint Louis encephalitis virus using monoclonal antibodies. *Virology* 1983;128(1):118–126.
691. Roehrig JT, Staudinger LA, Hunt AR, et al. Antibody prophylaxis and therapy for flaviviral encephalitis infections. *Ann N Y Acad Sci* 2001: 286–297.
693. Rosenzweig EC, Babione RW, Wisseman CL Jr. Immunological studies with group B arthropod-borne viruses. IV. Persistence of yellow fever antibodies following vaccination with 17D strain yellow fever vaccine. *Am J Trop Med Hyg* 1963;12:230–235.
694. Rush AB. An account of the bilious remitting fever, as it appeared in Philadelphia in the summer and autumn of the year 1780. *Medical Enquiries Observations* 1789:104–117.
697a. Sabchareon A, Wallace D, Sirivichayakul C, et al. Protective efficacy of the recombinant, live-attenuated, CYD tetravalent dengue vaccine in Thai schoolchildren: a randomised, controlled phase 2b trial. *Lancet* 2012;380:1559–1567.
700. Sabin AB. Research on dengue during World War II. *Am J Trop Med Hyg* 1952;1(1):30–50.
701. Sabin AB, Schlesinger RW. Production of Immunity to Dengue with Virus Modified by Propagation in Mice. *Science* 1945;101(2634): 640–642.
704. Samuel MA, Diamond MS. Type I IFN protects against lethal West Nile virus infection by restricting cellular tropism and enhancing neuronal survival. *J Virol* 2005;79:13350–13361.
705. Samuel MA, Wang H, Siddharthan V, et al. Axonal transport mediates West Nile virus entry into the central nervous system and induces acute flaccid paralysis. *Proc Natl Acad Sci U S A* 2007;104(43):17140–17145.
706. Samuel MA, Whitby K, Keller BC, et al. PKR and RNAse L contribute to protection against lethal West Nile virus infection by controlling early viral spread in the periphery and replication in neurons. *J Virol* 2006;80(14):7009–7019.
711. Sawyer WA, Lloyd W. The Use of Mice in Tests of Immunity against Yellow Fever. *J Exp Med* 1931;54(4):533–555.
717. Scherbik SV, Paranjape JM, Stockman BM, et al. RNase L plays a role in the antiviral response to West Nile virus. *J Virol* 2006;80(6):2987–2999.
721. Schlesinger JJ, Brandriss MW, Putnak JR, et al. Cell surface expression of yellow fever virus non-structural glycoprotein NS1: consequences of interaction with antibody. *J Gen Virol* 1990;71(Pt 3):593–599.

727. Schmidt AG, Yang PL, Harrison SC. Peptide inhibitors of dengue-virus entry target a late-stage fusion intermediate. *PLoS Pathog* 2010; 6(4):e1000851.
732a. Schoggins JW, Dorner M, Feulner M, et al. Dengue reporter viruses reveal viral dynamics in interferon receptor-deficient mice and sensitivity to interferon effectors in vitro. *Proc Natl Acad Sci U S A* 2012;109:14610–14615.
733. Schoggins JW, Wilson SJ, Panis M, et al. A diverse range of gene products are effectors of the type I interferon antiviral response. *Nature* 2011; 472(7344):481–485.
736. Schuh AJ, Tesh RB, Barrett AD. Genetic characterization of Japanese encephalitis virus genotype II strains isolated from 1951 to 1978. *J Gen Virol* 2011;92(Pt 3):516–527.
740. Sejvar JJ. The long-term outcomes of human West Nile virus infection. *Clin Infect Dis* 2007;44(12):1617–1624.
742. Sejvar JJ, Haddad MB, Tierney BC, et al. Neurologic manifestations and outcome of West Nile virus infection. *JAMA* 2003;290(4): 511–515.
745. Shimoni Z, Niven MJ, Pitlick S, et al. Treatment of West Nile virus encephalitis with intravenous immunoglobulin. *Emerg Infect Dis* 2001; 7(4):759.
748. Shresta S, Kyle JL, Snider HM, et al. Interferon-dependent immunity is essential for resistance to primary dengue virus infection in mice, whereas T- and B-cell-dependent immunity are less critical. *J Virol* 2004; 78(6):2701–2710.
750. Shresta S, Sharar KL, Prigozhin DM, et al. Murine model for dengue virus-induced lethal disease with increased vascular permeability. *J Virol* 2006;80(20):10208–10217.
751. Shrestha B, Brien JD, Sukupolvi-Petty S, et al. The development of therapeutic antibodies that neutralize homologous and heterologous genotypes of dengue virus type 1. *PLoS Pathog* 2010;6(4):e1000823.
752. Shrestha B, Diamond MS. The role of CD8+ T cells in the control of West Nile virus infection. *J Virol* 2004;78(15):8312–8321.
756. Shrestha B, Wang T, Samuel MA, et al. Gamma interferon plays a crucial early antiviral role in protection against West Nile virus infection. *J Virol* 2006;80(11):5338–5348.
764. Simmons CP, Chau TN, Thuy TT, et al. Maternal antibody and viral factors in the pathogenesis of dengue virus in infants. *J Infect Dis* 2007; 196(3):416–424.
765. Sitati E, Diamond MS. CD4+ T Cell responses are required for clearance of West Nile virus from the central nervous system. *J Virol* 2006; 80(24):12060–12069.
766. Smithburn KC, Hughes TP, Burke AW, et al. A neurotropic virus isolated from the blood of a native of Uganda. *Am J Trop Med Hyg* 1940;20:471–492.
769. Solomon T, Dung NM, Vaughn DW, et al. Neurological manifestations of dengue infection. *Lancet* 2000;355(9209):1053–1059.
770. Solomon T, Dung NM, Wills B, et al. Interferon alfa-2a in Japanese encephalitis: a randomised double-blind placebo-controlled trial. *Lancet* 2003;361(9360):821–826.
779. Staples JE, Gershman M, Fischer M. Yellow fever vaccine: recommendations of the Advisory Committee on Immunization Practices (ACIP). *MMWR Recomm Rep* 2010;59(RR-7):1–27.
780. Staples JE, Monath TP. Yellow fever: 100 years of discovery. *JAMA* 2008; 300(8):960–962.
786. Stiasny K, Brandler S, Kossl C, et al. Probing the flavivirus membrane fusion mechanism by using monoclonal antibodies. *J Virol* 2007;81(20): 11526–11531.
787. Stiasny K, Kiermayr S, Holzmann H, et al. Cryptic properties of a cluster of dominant flavivirus cross-reactive antigenic sites. *J Virol* 2006; 80(19):9557–9568.
788. Stoermer KA, Morrison TE. Complement and viral pathogenesis. *Virology* 2011;411(2):362–373.
792. Styer LM, Lim PY, Louie KL, et al. Mosquito saliva causes enhancement of West Nile virus infection in mice. *J Virol* 2011;85(4):1517–1527.
795. Sukupolvi-Petty S, Austin SK, Purtha WE, et al. Type- and subcomplex-specific neutralizing antibodies against domain III of dengue virus type 2 envelope protein recognize adjacent epitopes. *J Virol* 2007; 81(23):12816–12826.
811. Tassaneetrithep B, Burgess TH, Granelli-Piperno A, et al. DC-SIGN (CD209) mediates dengue virus infection of human dendritic cells. *J Exp Med* 2003;197(7):823–829.
814. ter Meulen J, Sakho M, Koulemou K, et al. Activation of the cytokine network and unfavorable outcome in patients with yellow fever. *J Infect Dis* 2004;190(10):1821–1827.
816. Tesh RB, Siirin M, Guzman H, et al. Persistent West Nile virus infection in the golden hamster: studies on its mechanism and possible implications for other flavivirus infections. *J Infect Dis* 2005;192(2): 287–295.
818. Theiler M, Anderson CR. The relative resistance of dengue-immune monkeys to yellow fever virus. *Am J Trop Med Hyg* 1975;24(1):115–117.
828. Town T, Bai F, Wang T, et al. Toll-like receptor 7 mitigates lethal West Nile encephalitis via interleukin 23-dependent immune cell infiltration and homing. *Immunity* 2009;30(2):242–253.
838. van der Schaar HM, Rust MJ, Chen C, et al. Dissecting the cell entry pathway of dengue virus by single-particle tracking in living cells. *PLoS Pathog* 2008;4(12):e1000244.
843. Vaughn DW, Green S, Kalayanarooj S, et al. Dengue viremia titer, antibody response pattern, and virus serotype correlate with disease severity. *J Infect Dis* 2000;181(1):2–9.
846. Verma S, Lo Y, Chapagain M, et al. West Nile virus infection modulates human brain microvascular endothelial cells tight junction proteins and cell adhesion molecules: Transmigration across the in vitro blood-brain barrier. *Virology* 2009;385(2):425–433.
852. Wahala WM, Donaldson EF, de Alwis R, et al. Natural strain variation and antibody neutralization of Dengue serotype 3 viruses. *PLoS Pathog* 2010;6(3):e1000821.
853. Wahala WM, Kraus AA, Haymore LB, et al. Dengue virus neutralization by human immune sera: role of envelope protein domain III-reactive antibody. *Virology* 2009;392(1):103–113.
860. Wang H, Siddharthan V, Hall JO, et al. West Nile virus preferentially transports along motor neuron axons after sciatic nerve injection of hamsters. *J Neurovirol* 2009;15(4):293–299.
864. Wang P, Dai J, Bai F, et al. Matrix metalloproteinase 9 facilitates West Nile virus entry into the brain. *J Virol* 2008;82(18):8978–8985.
867. Wang T, Scully E, Yin Z, et al. IFN-γ-producing $\gamma\delta$ T cells help control murine West Nile virus infection. *J Immunol* 2003;171:2524–2531.
870. Wang Y, Lobigs M, Lee E, et al. CD8+ T cells mediate recovery and immunopathology in West Nile virus encephalitis. *J Virol* 2003;77(24): 13323–13334.
893. Wu SJ, Grouard-Vogel G, Sun W, et al. Human skin Langerhans cells are targets of dengue virus infection. *Nat Med* 2000;6(7):816–820.
896. Xiao SY, Guzman H, Zhang H, et al. West Nile virus infection in the golden hamster (Mesocricetus auratus): a model for West Nile encephalitis. *Emerg Infect Dis* 2001;7(4):714–721.
901. Yauch LE, Prestwood TR, May MM, et al. CD4+ T cells are not required for the induction of dengue virus-specific CD8+ T cell or antibody responses but contribute to protection after vaccination. *J Immunol* 2010;185(9): 5405–5416.
902. Yauch LE, Shresta S. Mouse models of dengue virus infection and disease. *Antiviral Res* 2008;80(2):87–93.
907. Yu IM, Zhang W, Holdaway HA, et al. Structure of the immature dengue virus at low pH primes proteolytic maturation. *Science* 2008; 319(5871):1834–1837.
912. Zellweger RM, Prestwood TR, Shresta S. Enhanced infection of liver sinusoidal endothelial cells in a mouse model of antibody-induced severe dengue disease. *Cell Host Microbe* 2010;7(2):128–139.
915. Zhang W, Chipman PR, Corver J, et al. Visualization of membrane protein domains by cryo-electron microscopy of dengue virus. *Nat Struct Biol* 2003;10(11):907–912.
916. Zhang Y, Corver J, Chipman PR, et al. Structures of immature flavivirus particles. *EMBO J* 2003;22(11):2604–2613.
919. Zheng A, Umashankar M, Kielian M. In vitro and in vivo studies identify important features of dengue virus pr-E protein interactions. *PLoS Pathog* 2010;6(10):e1001157.

CHAPTER 27

Stuart C. Ray • Justin R. Bailey • David L. Thomas

Hepatitis C Virus

HISTORY

By the mid-1970s, it was apparent that at least one viral hepatitis agent other than hepatitis A virus (HAV) or hepatitis B virus (HBV) was the primary agent of posttransfusion hepatitis, a syndrome termed "non-A, non-B" hepatitis (NANBH).[197,335] Studies of transfusion recipients revealed that NANBH tended to be milder in its acute form than HBV but could cause severe complications including cirrhosis and liver failure.[16] Inoculation of chimpanzees with blood components from humans having both acute and chronic NANBH resulted in characteristic elevations of hepatic transaminases, providing a valuable animal model for NANBH and establishing the chronic nature of NANBH.[17] By the mid-1980s, physicochemical studies of infectious inocula had revealed that the NANBH agent was a small (less than 80 nm), enveloped virus; however, the agent defied efforts directed at conventional viral cultivation and immunological detection.[76,159]

Serial passage of NANBH in chimpanzees provided key pathologic, physiologic, and biochemical insights, as well as a well-characterized pool of specimens in which the agent was known to be present. A team led by Michael Houghton assembled a lambda phage library of complementary DNA (cDNA) derived from one such high-titer chimpanzee plasma specimen and then screened more than 1 million expression clones using serum from a chronic NANBH patient to find a single positive cDNA clone called 5-1-1.[116] This discovery led to initial assays for detection of antibodies to the newly named hepatitis C virus (HCV),[18,116,352] and the 5-1-1 antigen continues to be a component of anti-HCV serologic tests.

The first cDNA clone enabled further characterization of the genome as a positive-strand RNA molecule of almost 10,000 nucleotides containing a single open reading frame with an organization consistent with the *Flaviviridae*.[117] Discovery of the authentic 5′ and 3′ untranslated regions (UTRs) led to a full-length cDNA clone of the HCV genome that, when transcribed, was infectious by direct intrahepatic injection in chimpanzees.[337] The development of *in vitro* model systems was relatively intractable until the development of subgenomic RNA replicons[387] and then successful passage in cell culture of a clone from one strain.[670]

HCV continues to present unresolved scientific and clinical challenges. Questions persist regarding fundamental aspects of the HCV life cycle, replication dynamics *in vivo*, mechanisms of persistence, and pathogenesis. Screening of blood products using antibody- and then nucleic acid–based testing, combined with other blood banking practices, provides a sound basis for the virtual elimination of transfusion-transmitted HCV infection; nonetheless, new infections continue to occur via other routes. Nearly 3% of humans remain chronically infected with

HCV, and although treatment continues to improve in efficacy and availability, HCV infection remains a major cause of death and disability worldwide.

PATHOGENESIS AND PATHOLOGY

Entry into the Host

As discussed in the Transmission section later (under Epidemiology), the primary route of HCV entry is percutaneous, although permucosal infection has also been described. Experimentally, HCV infection can be achieved by intravenous injection of HCV virions or intrahepatic injection of HCV genomic RNA.[337,694]

Cell and Tissue Tropism

As depicted in Figure 27.1, HCV replication *in vivo* occurs primarily or exclusively in hepatocytes, the major parenchymal cell of the liver.[505] The basis for this tropism is likely to be multifactorial, including entry facilitated by proteins expressed at particularly high levels on hepatocytes (e.g., low-density lipoprotein receptor [LDL-R][446] and scavenger receptor class B type I [SR-BI][185,248,557]), dependence on liver-specific miR-122 for efficient replication,[299] and utilization of the liver's lipoprotein assembly pathway for virion production.[280] Tissue-specific subcellular localization and dynamic interaction between viral components and more broadly expressed proteins on which HCV replication depends (such as CD81,[195,248,270,320,499] claudins [CLDNs],[183,267,270,422] occludin [OCLN],[500] epidermal growth factor receptor,[392] and cyclophilins[257]) may also contribute to liver-specific tropism. HCV entry is discussed in detail in Chapter 25.

Extrahepatic Replication

Productive infection of other cell types is controversial,[70,362] but there is evidence for extrahepatic detection of HCV negative-strand replicative intermediates,[106,375,701] sequence variant compartmentalization,[459,562] and *in vitro* replication in a variety of cell types.[602,608] Viral dynamic modeling of data from the anhepatic phase of liver transplantation suggested that in a subset of patients with end-stage liver disease, an extrahepatic compartment exists that contributes no more than 3% to 4% of plasma viremia.[142,505]

Model Systems *In Vitro*

During the first decade after HCV was discovered, the only robust model was the chimpanzee infected with primary or chimpanzee-passaged HCV isolates. Efforts to culture HCV from human and chimpanzee serum using primary hepatocytes or hepatoma cell lines were limited by relatively insensitive tools for measuring and visualizing infection, inconsistent cell lines, and the inherent variability of HCV isolates (see Genetic Diversity, later).[284,290,313,444,445,454,570,697] Without an efficient culture system, screening of candidate antivirals was hampered.

The First Infectious Clone

In 1997, two groups separately reported chimpanzee infection with infectious clones of HCV,[337,694] generated from acute phase isolate H77[17] by using overlapping sequences spanning the genome (Fig. 27.2) to identify low-frequency polymorphisms

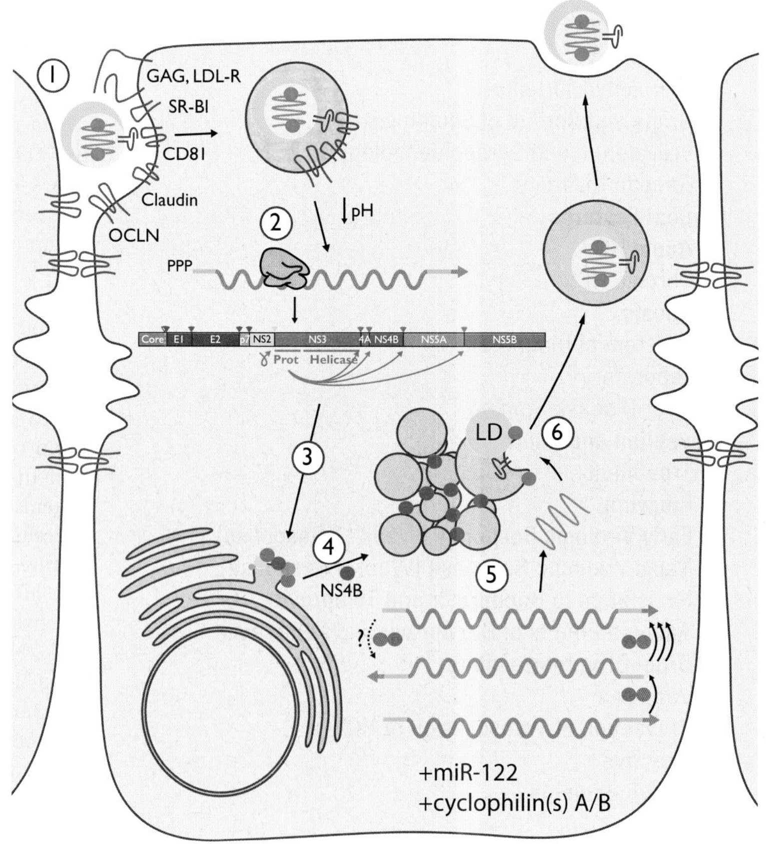

FIGURE 27.1. Life cycle of hepatitis C virus (HCV). Initial binding and internalization **(1)** probably involve glycosaminoglycans (GAGs) and low-density lipoprotein receptor (LDL-R), which may interact with viral envelope proteins or with virion-associated lipoproteins. Entry depends directly on binding of E2 with the tetraspanin CD81, as well as interactions with scavenger receptor BI (SR-BI) and tight junction proteins claudin-1 and occludin (OCLN). The viral genome is released from late endosomes **(2)** in a pH-dependent manner, followed by internal ribosome entry site (IRES)-dependent polyprotein synthesis **(3)** with initial cleavages among the structural proteins mediated by signalase and signal peptide peptidase followed by cleavage of the NS2–NS3 junction by NS2-NS3 cysteine protease; the remaining junctions are cleaved by the NS3-NS4A serine protease. NS4B recruits and rearranges endoplasmic reticulum (ER) membranes **(4)** to form a *membranous web,* the principal site of viral replication. Minus-strand and subsequent plus-strand RNA syntheses are affected by the NS5B RNA-dependent RNA polymerase (RdRp) **(5)** and depend on miR-122 and cyclophilin B, as well as conserved structural elements at the 5′ and 3′ ends of the genome. Core protein associates with lipid droplets (LDs) in the lipoprotein assembly pathway **(6)**, linked to NS5A and other members of the replication complex by interaction with NS2. Viroporin p7 is necessary for production of stable viral particles coated with E1 and E2, which fold in a cooperative manner and are glycosylated in a manner consistent with ER but not Golgi processing.

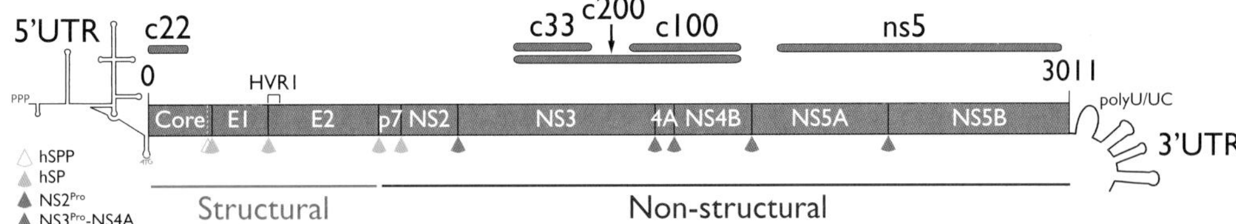

FIGURE 27.2. Map of the hepatitis C virus (HCV) genome, depicting the 5′ untranslated region (5′UTR), capsid core, envelope genes *E1* and *E2*, viroporin p7, membrane-anchored cysteine protease NS2, serine protease-helicase NS3, NS3 protease co-factor NS4A, membrane remodeling protein NS4B, phosphoprotein NS5A, RNA-dependent RNA polymerase NS5B, and the 3′UTR. Depicted as green bars are protein segments used as antigens in HCV enzyme immune assay (EIA) and recombinant immunoblot assay (RIBA) (c22,[268,609] c100-3[352]). Cleavages of the polyprotein are due to the action of signal peptidase (solid orange), signal peptide peptidase (open orange), NS2 cysteine autoprotease (green), and NS3-NS4A serine protease (blue).

that were likely to be either artifactual (generated during cDNA cloning) or biologically genuine but less infectious. By removing such minor sequence variations, they constructed consensus sequences that were infectious, paving the way for the generation of consensus sequences from other isolates in search of clones that would replicate efficiently *in vitro.*[51]

HCV Replicons

In 1999, the efficient replication of subgenomic replicons in hepatoma cell line Huh-7 was reported, representing the first culture system that depended on HCV enzymes for propagation of a selectable marker (driven in a 2-internal ribosome entry site [IRES bicistronic construct) and permitting more direct study of the viral life cycle.[387] Highly replicative subtype subgenomic replicons were developed and were shown to depend on intact viral enzymatic sequences and negative-strand subgenome intermediates, inhibited by interferon-α.[64,386] This latter characteristic opened the door to "curing" of cultures with interferon, resulting in Huh-7–derived cell lines like Huh-7.5[65] that were more permissive for HCV replication, an important tool for subsequent achievements including authentic culture of HCV *in vitro.*

Although cell culture adaptation of replicons permitted greater dynamic range of replication sufficient for screening inhibitors and studying viral protein interactions, the adaptive changes[64,343,386] were often found to impair infectivity *in vivo,*[85] and when they included the structural and *p7* genes, these replicons did not produce structural proteins or viral RNA in the supernatant. Strains that were assembled from human isolates as consensus clones but required no adaptive changes as replicons were identified, including subtype 1b strain HCV-N, which was also infectious in chimpanzees,[285] and subtype 2a strain JFH-1.[315,316] When these were assembled as full-genome replicons, JFH-1 was found to produce infectious viral particles.

HCV Cell Culture

In 2005, the complete replication cycle of HCV in culture was described, using the subtype 2a strain JFH-1 in Huh-7–derived cells that had been made more permissive by eradication of HCV subgenomic replicon infection with interferon.[670,706] Subsequently, the HCV cell culture (HCVcc) platform was broadened to include subtype 1a strain H77-S.[696] As discussed in Chapter 25, this system and derivatives such as chimeric structural and nonstructural regions[248] and reporter constructs[328] provide new avenues for investigation of HCV biology and immunity.

HCV Pseudoparticles

Prior to the advent of HCVcc, HCV pseudoparticles (HCVpp) were developed to study HCV entry, which was found to be similar to other members of the *Flaviviridae,* and CD81 was found to be necessary but not sufficient for E1E2-mediated entry.[46,279] HCVpp expressing a variety of *E1E2* genes have facilitated study of cross-subtype and cross-genotype neutralization[436,478] and have been used to demonstrate that neutralizing antibodies drive the rapid evolution of E2 during acute HCV infection.[170,382]

Virion Production without HCV Replication

There are many uses for high-titer stocks of HCV, but these can be difficult to generate and achievable titers are dependent on genomic characteristics (e.g., culture adaptive mutations) that may interfere with intended uses. A novel system for generating virions was recently developed to address these challenges, using cells conditioned by replication of a West Nile virus replicon.[638] Because this system does not depend on HCV replication, it is potentially HCV sequence (i.e., genotype) independent.

Model Systems *In Vivo*

The initial model for HCV infection was the chimpanzee, essential to the discovery of this virus and to key experiments described herein (e.g., Transmission, Immune Response, and Genetic Diversity sections). The chimpanzee remains the only model for studying the full range of host–HCV interactions, from acute to chronic infection.[84] The availability and use of chimpanzees is very limited,[22] and other models are available that are relevant to specific areas.

Mice with Implanted Ectopic Human Liver Grafts

The Trimera severe combined immunodeficiency (SCID) mouse model, in which liver fragments remain viable for weeks after ectopic implantation (e.g., under the kidney capsule), can be used for studying HCV infection. The level of replication is modest ($10^{4.8}$ IU/mL) but high enough for testing antiviral regimens.[286] The liver tissue in this model does not maintain normal architecture.

Mice with Liver Injury and Human Hepatocyte Xenografts

SCID mice transgenic for urokinase plasminogen activator (uPA) driven by the albumin promoter develop severe neonatal liver injury that is rescued by infused hepatocytes that engraft and occupy the space of the involuting liver.[431] Similarly, RAG$^{-/-}$/interleukin-2 receptor-γ–deficient (IL2R$\gamma^{-/-}$) mice bred for fumaryl acetoacetate hydrolase deficiency (FAH$^{-/-}$) develop hepatic toxicity but can be rescued pharmacologically with NTBC (2-[2-nitro-4-trifluoromethylbenzoyl]-1,3-cyclohexanedione) or by transfer of the *FAH* gene. These FRG mice (FAH$^{-/-}$, RAG$^{-/-}$, IL2R$\gamma^{-/-}$) will accept infusions of human hepatocytes after infection with a uPA-expressing adenovirus (presumably to proteolytically damage the liver stroma).[35] These mice can achieve physiologic levels of human albumin and lipoprotein levels, and after infection with HCV they can develop high levels of HCV RNA (10^6 IU/mL) and maintain these levels for months. The mice are difficult to breed and remain immunodeficient, and hepatocyte engraftment is highly variable; however, they are a useful model for HCV replication and have enabled mechanistic study of phenomena such as HCV neutralization *in vivo*.[434]

Humanized Mouse

A different approach from those described earlier was the recent development of a genetically humanized mouse model of HCV infection that partially addresses host restriction factors that block HCV infection of mouse hepatocytes.[168] Using adenovirus gene delivery to induce expression of potential restriction factors for entry, CD81,[499] SR-BI,[557] CLDN-1,[183] and OCLN,[500] they found that human CD81 and OCLN were required for entry in the mouse. Mouse SR-BI knockout and human SR-BI complementation confirmed the necessity of SR-BI for HCV entry and that mouse SR-BI could substitute for human SR-BI in HCV entry. The remaining host restrictions for HCV infection of mice are unknown, but the use of adenovirus gene delivery may have enhanced innate antiviral responses, and the stable expression of CD81 and OCLN in the mouse will facilitate further study. At present, the genetically humanized mouse model supports entry but not replication of HCV.

Spread

The mode of spread of HCV throughout the liver is poorly understood. High-level viremia achieved by HCV provides ample opportunity for virions to interact with hepatocytes, yet it appears that only about 10% to 20% of hepatocytes are infected during chronic infection.[378] Lack of uniform infection may be explained by innate responses that could render cells refractory and adaptive immunity that could interfere with entry of free virions.[588] Cell-to-cell spread[449] within the liver could circumvent antibody responses, and data from *in vitro* culture on human hepatoma cell lines support this mode of spread,[630] suggesting that virus spread *in vivo* is relatively resistant to neutralizing antibody compared with infection with free virions, yet is dependent on the same key entry factors (HCV envelope, CD81, SR-BI, OCLN, and CLDN family members).[79] These data are supported by the observation of foci of infection during *in vitro* culture, suggesting that this is a potential mode of local spread; however, it is clear that humoral immune pressure drives HCV evolution during chronic infection,[382] suggesting that a major component of spread during chronic HCV infection remains subject to antibody-mediated neutralization.

Immune Response

Each component of the host immune response to HCV is balanced in some way by viral components. As a result, multiple viral proteins (depicted in Figs. 27.1 and 27.2, with a detailed functional discussion in Chapter 25) have immune-evasive roles in addition to more direct functions in the viral life cycle. These include Core (capsid), E1 and E2 (envelope), NS3-NS4A (serine protease), NS5A (polyfunctional phosphoprotein), and NS5B (RNA-dependent RNA polymerase).

Innate Immune Response

The innate immune response is of great importance in control of HCV infection,[214] and the virus has evolved a variety of mechanisms to evade this response (Fig. 27.3). Interferon signaling is a key component of the innate responses against HCV. Type I, II, and III interferons (IFN-α and IFN-β; IFN-γ; and IFN-λ, respectively) have all been shown to be important, early intrahepatic responses in HCV infection.[60,363,374,626] Type I and II interferons are induced by overlapping signaling pathways. IFN-regulatory factor 3 (IRF3), a latent cytoplasmic transcription factor, can be activated by viral infection and translocated to the nucleus where it induces the transcription of IFN-β. In autocrine and paracrine fashion, IFN-β stimulates activation of the Janus-activated kinase and signal transducer and activators of transcription (JAK-STAT) signaling pathway and synthesis of IFN-α, as well as multiple other antiviral cytokines and chemokines, inhibiting viral replication and orchestrating the subsequent adaptive immune response.[221] HCV NS3-NS4A blocks IRF3 activation by proteolytically cleaving TIR domain–containing adapter-inducing interferon-β (TRIF) and mitochondrial antiviral signaling protein (MAVS). TRIF is an adapter protein for the double-stranded RNA (dsRNA) sensing molecule Toll-like receptor 3,[377] and MAVS is an adapter protein in the retinoic-acid-inducible gene I (RIG-I) signaling cascade.[439] These cleavages underscore the importance of these pathways for antiviral immunity, and impairment of interferon stimulated gene (ISG) expression was reversed by treatment with small-molecule inhibitors of the NS3-NS4A protease.[377,389,439]

Defects in JAK-STAT signaling have also been described in HCV transgenic mice.[66] In HCV transgenic mouse and human liver biopsies, impairment of JAK-STAT signaling is linked to hypomethylation of STAT1 and increased expression of protein phosphatase 2A (PP2A).[175] There is also evidence that NS5A protein can stimulate IL-8, inhibit dsRNA-activated protein kinase (PKR), and interfere with 2′,5′-oligoadenylate synthetase (2,5-OAS), antagonizing type 1 interferon signaling.[223,305,344,501] Overexpression of HCV core protein also interferes with IFN signaling, likely through direct interaction with STAT1.[67,381] Other studies suggest that ubiquitin-specific peptidase 18 (USP18) may be up-regulated by long-term interferon stimulation, blocking activation of ISG15 and suppressing JAK-STAT signaling, and leading to refractoriness to type 1 IFN stimulation.[401,553] The inhibitory effect of HCV proteins on the interferon activation cascade is incomplete, as gene expression microarray studies have shown type 1 interferon responses in the livers of acutely and chronically HCV-infected chimpanzees.[60,592] Hepatic levels of ISG expression in chronically infected humans vary significantly for unclear reasons.[109,552]

Natural killer (NK) cells are also likely to play a very important role in control of HCV infection. NK and natural killer T-lymphocyte (NKT) cells are abundant in the liver and prime cellular immune responses through production of IFN-γ and other cytokines.[138,639] Binding of the E2 protein to CD81 has been associated with inhibition of NK cell activity.[138,639] HLA Cw*04 and related haplotypes, which bind inhibitory

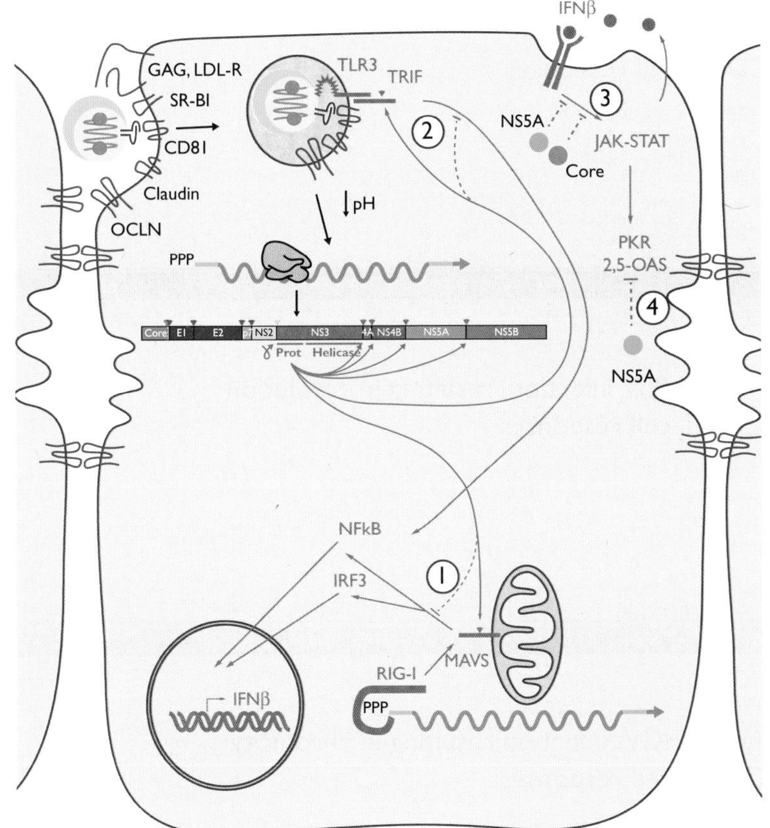

FIGURE 27.3. Innate responses to hepatitis C virus (HCV) and their evasion by the virus. Cytoplasmic HCV double-stranded RNA (dsRNA) can be sensed by RIG-I **(1)**, resulting in signaling through mitochondrial antiviral signaling protein (MAVS) and subsequent nuclear translocation of nuclear factor (NF)-κB and phosphorylated IRF3 that activate an antiviral program including secretion of interferon-β (IFN-β), which has autocrine and paracrine activity; HCV NS3-NS4A protease cleaves MAVS, blocking this signaling.[213,389,439] Viral dsRNA may be sensed in endosomes by Toll-like receptor 3 (TLR3) **(2)**, which signals via the adapter molecule TIR domain–containing adapter-inducing interferon-β (TRIF), resulting in nuclear translocation of NF-κB and expression of IFN-β; NS3-NS4A protease cleaves TRIF, interfering with this response.[377] IFN-β effects depend on the JAK-STAT signaling pathway, which is inhibited **(3)** by HCV core and NS5A proteins. Inflammatory responses including type I interferons activate host antiviral molecules including protein kinase (PKR) and 2′,5′-oligoadenylate synthetase (2,5-OAS), which are antagonized **(4)** by NS5A. Further details and additional innate responses and evasive mechanisms are described in the text and Table 27.1.

killer immunoglobulin-like receptors (KIR) on NK cells, have been associated with viral persistence.[325] The least inhibitory human leukocyte antigen (HLA)-C-KIR haplotypes are most strongly associated with recovery.

Dendritic cells are critical for orchestration of both innate and adaptive immune responses. Toll-like receptor 7 (TLR7) is expressed by plasmacytoid dendritic cells (pDCs), and pDCs produce type I interferon when co-cultured with Huh-7 cells containing replicating HCV RNA[606]; however, data regarding the effect of HCV infection on pDCs *in vivo* are less clear.[153,306] HCV may interfere with NK cell activation of dendritic cells,[297] and there is some evidence that HCV infection may be associated with impaired peripheral dendritic cell function.[40,307] This impairment may explain the collapse of the cellular immune response during the transition from acute to chronic infection.[133,564]

Cellular Immune Response

There is strong evidence that both CD4 and CD8 T-cell responses are critical for control of HCV infection, but there is limited understanding of failure of these responses leading to chronicity. HCV-specific T cells develop rapidly during acute infection and are then detectable for years in blood and liver in individuals after clearance of infection. During chronic infection, stronger polyclonal CD8 T-cell responses in the liver and circulation have been associated with lower circulating HCV loads,[465,525] though CD8 T-cell responses to HCV epitopes are only detectable *ex vivo* in half of human immunodeficiency virus (HIV)-negative individuals chronically infected with HCV, whether obtained from peripheral blood or liver.[327,340]

Induction of T-Cell Responses

HCV-specific T cells typically become detectable in the blood 5 to 10 weeks after infection.[127,371,573,615,643] In experimentally infected chimpanzees, intrahepatic T-cell responses appear another 4 to 8 weeks later.[127,615] In intravenous drug users, there is significant overlap in the number of T-cell epitopes targeted during acute infection in individuals with subsequent resolving versus persistent infection outcomes.[133,564] Even at the height of the response, HCV-specific CD8 T cells rarely target more than 10 epitopes, regardless of outcome, with little evidence of immunodominance.[133,340] While acute phase CD4 and CD8 T-cell responses are usually detectable regardless of outcome, in individuals who progress to chronic infection, they disappear rapidly and may be less vigorous.[133,160,259,308,441,564,616,644] HCV-specific T cells produce IL-2 and IFN-γ in individuals who go on to clear infection, and acquisition of full effector function may be a key factor leading to viral control in individuals with spontaneous clearance. In individuals who clear infection, functional effector CD8 T cells peak in the blood just after the initial drop in viremia, usually about 8 to 12 weeks after infection.[127,251,368,371,615,616]

Anti-HCV T-cell responses are not focused on one viral protein or genomic region, and there is little evidence of immunodominance in general[133,340,564] when compared with responses to HIV and influenza.[10,379] Comprehensive analyses of CD4 and CD8 T-cell responses in persons with acute infection, using overlapping peptides composing the HCV polyprotein, have revealed widely dispersed epitopes (Fig. 27.4).[133,368,564] In persons with certain uncommon alleles, such as HLA-B*27 and HLA-B*57, immunodominant responses to functionally

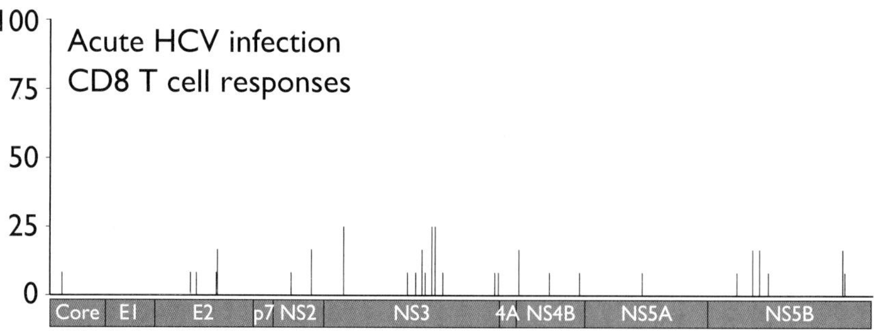

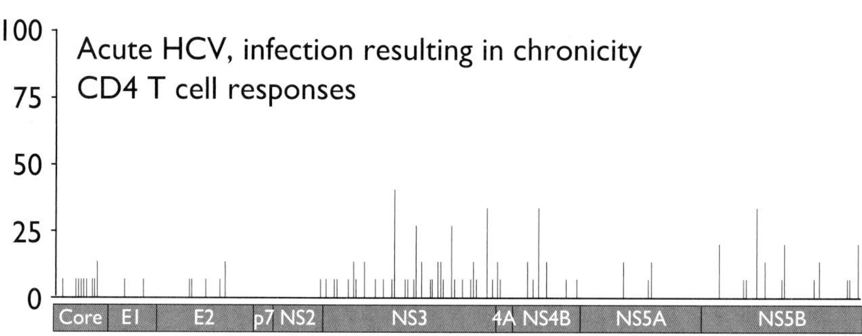

FIGURE 27.4. Anti–hepatitis C virus (HCV) T-cell epitopes are widely dispersed across the polyprotein during acute infection. The per-person frequency at which responses were detected using ELISpot is indicated for epitopes centered at positions indicated along the polyprotein. CD8 T-cell responses in 12 persons with acute HCV infection are indicated in the upper panel (adapted from two reports, with many outcomes unknown due to early interferon treatment[133,368]), while the middle and lower panels depict CD4 T-cell responses from 18 subjects with resolving acute HCV and 13 subjects who progressed to chronicity, respectively.[564] (Middle and lower panels © 2012, Schulze zur Wiesch et al. Originally published in *The Journal of Experimental Medicine.* 209:61–75.)

constrained epitopes have been described,[469,470,477,549] whereas each person with the more common allele HLA-A*02 targets a few of the dozens of epitopes restricted by that allele.[673]

Role of T Cells in Clearance of HCV

A central role for T cells in clearance of HCV was illustrated by studies in which T cells (CD4 or CD8) were depleted in chimpanzees in the context of acute HCV infection.[251,573] Depletion of CD8 T cells, from an animal that had rapidly and spontaneously cleared HCV infection twice, led to prolonged viremia after reinfection, with control occurring when CD8 T cells returned.[573] Depletion of CD4 T cells had a somewhat different effect, with widely fluctuating levels of viremia associated with progressive escape mutations at epitopes targeted by previously primed CD8 T-cell epitope responses.[251,573]

In humans, spontaneous clearance of HCV has been associated with expression of certain major histocompatibility complex (MHC) class I molecules, with various studies showing association with the presence of HLA-B*57, HLA-B*27, HLA-A*11, HLA-A*03, or HLA-Cw*01, and the absence of HLA-Cw*04.[326,349,420,617] Some of the differences in observed associations may be due to variation in predominant circulating HCV genotypes. The mechanism by which these particular alleles favor clearance of viremia is generally unknown, though there is evidence that some protective alleles bind and present to T cells epitopes that are particularly immunogenic and/or functionally conserved,[470] whereas risk alleles may be ligands for inhibitory receptors of NK cells.[617] The latter mechanism is supported by evidence that polymorphisms in NK receptors may also play an important role in HCV clearance.[325]

HCV clearance has also been associated with MHC class II genes, particularly DQB1*0301 and HLA-DRB1*1101.[269,617] In a study using peptides spanning the HCV polyprotein, individuals with resolved infections targeted an average of 10 MHC class II epitopes (range 3 to 28), whereas individuals with chronic infection targeted an average of 1 epitope (range 0 to 8). Epitopes most frequently recognized were in core and nonstructural proteins, which may reflect differences in protein processing or mismatch in other regions between the circulating virus and library peptides.[150,235,489,560,565] In chimpanzees, a subset of dominant CD4 T-cell epitopes were targeted prior to clearance of infection, and subdominant populations were detected only after clearance.[269]

Memory Responses

Anti-HCV CD8 T-cell responses have been detected in individuals who have been exposed to HCV but have not seroconverted.[81,340] Studies in chimpanzees have also shown that CD4 and CD8 memory T-cell responses are important for protection against reinfection with HCV.[48,189,251,400,458,507,573,681] Control of a second infection is associated with rapid expansion of memory CD4 and CD8 cells.[363] Expansion of HCV-specific T cells was observed 2 to 3 weeks after reinfection compared to 10 to 12 weeks after initial exposure to virus. Depletion of CD8 T cells led to prolonged viremia after reinfection, and depletion of CD4 T cells also led to impaired control, despite the presence of previously primed HCV-specific CD8 T cells.[251,573] Even more importantly, a recent study demonstrated that reinfected humans tend to develop broader T-cell responses and lower peak viremia and are more likely to spontaneously clear their second HCV infection.[478]

T-Cell Responses During Chronic Viremia

Despite T-cell responses, most HCV-infected individuals remain persistently infected. In individuals who progress to chronic infection, HCV-specific CD8 T cells become dysfunctional, possibly due to CD4 T-cell dysfunction.[29,258,390,564,675] HCV-specific CD8 T cells obtained from peripheral blood during chronic infection show poor *ex vivo* proliferation and IFN-gamma production, low intracellular stores of perforin, and decreased ability to lyse target cells.[29,258,390,675] These functions are not consistently restored after successful treatment.[442]

Anti-HCV T-cell responses have been studied primarily in peripheral blood; due to compartmentalization of the T-cell response, such studies are likely to underestimate the breadth and magnitude of intrahepatic responses. Approximately a third of chronically infected individuals have intrahepatic anti-HCV T-cell responses that can be expanded *ex vivo.*[339,687] Intrahepatic anti-HCV T-cell responses may be associated with lower serum HCV RNA levels, higher degrees of hepatic inflammation, and higher rates of response to interferon-based treatment[465,466]; thus, responses that contribute to clearance may, if unsuccessful, contribute to injury.[102] In spite of quantitative differences in number and breadth and some differences in phenotype[53] of T-cell responses, there are many similarities.[585] Such inferences from PBMCs have been supported by indirect correlations such as viral escape substitutions in epitopes that were detected in assays of PBMCs.[134,629]

Many HCV-specific CD8 T cells express the counterregulatory molecule PD-1.[104,258,541,675] Studies in murine models have shown that PD-1 binds to programmed death ligands 1 and 2 (PD-L1 and PD-L2), and ligation leads to dephosphorylation of signaling molecules downstream of the T-cell receptor (TCR), decreasing T-cell sensitivity to stimulation.[108,366,476] Blockade by anti–PD-L1 antibodies leads to increased proliferation of both CD8 and CD4 T cells directed against HCV.[312,455,495,511,524,637] Interestingly, levels of PD-1 expression in acute infection do not appear to correlate with outcome of infection. In model systems, direct activation of CD8 T cells by hepatic parenchymal cells, without help from CD4 T cells, may result in impaired CD8 T cells that express high levels of PD-1.[692] Some recent studies have suggested that high levels of PD-1 may indicate a high level of immune activation, but not necessarily T-cell exhaustion.[176]

T-cell immunoglobulin and mucin domain–containing molecule-3 (TIM-3) may also play a role in modulation of HCV-specific T-cell responses. Expression of both TIM-3 and PD-1 on CD8 cells during acute infection was associated with persistence, and like PD-1, blockade of TIM-3 increased proliferation of HCV-specific CD8 T cells.[421] Recent studies have suggested that 2B4 (CD244), another inhibitory molecule on exhausted T cells in the lymphocytic choriomeningitis virus model of chronic infection, may also play a role in modulating HCV-specific CD8 T cells. HCV-specific CD8 T cells show increased expression of 2B4, and 2B4 stimulation reduced the increase in proliferation of HCV-specific T cells usually seen after PD-1 blockade.[561]

Interaction with other immune cells likely also modulates antiviral T-cell activity. Liver-infiltrating CD8 T cells may have decreased expression of the co-stimulatory molecule CD86.[301,355] Regulatory T cells (T_{reg})[298,376] may modulate HCV-specific T-cell activity, and increased early IL-10 production during chronic HCV infection may drive CD4 T cells to become T_{reg}.[209] These CD4CD25^{high} T cells are enriched in peripheral blood during chronic HCV infection and may infiltrate the chronically infected liver, potentially protecting it from injury.[69,71,92,590,678]

HCV Evasion of T-Cell Response

In addition to innate and adaptive host responses that are functionally inadequate for clearing infection, there appears to be selection for HCV mutations that enable response evasion while maintaining adequate replicative fitness to sustain infection. T-cell recognition of HCV is reduced by amino acid replacements that occur *in vivo,*[103,134,628] and such changes have been correlated with persistence.[134,181] Multiple cross-sectional studies have shown enrichment of amino acid changes in predicted or confirmed cytotoxic T-lymphocyte (CTL) epitopes among chronically infected individuals with corresponding HLA types.[207,232,365,521,540,629] Observed mechanisms of reduced recognition during HCV infection (Fig. 27.5) include changes adjacent to epitopes that result in impaired processing for MHC class I presentation,[329,566] changes in anchor residues that reduce binding affinity for MHC class I,[134,628] and mutations that affect TCR contact residues.[686]

Amino acid replacements have potential fitness costs that may balance the fitness gain associated with escaping a T-cell response. These substitutions could disrupt functions of HCV proteins or RNA genomic elements[299,642] or create neoantigen. Loss of protein function in this context has been observed, as have compensatory changes that appear to restore function[470,477,539,549]; such compensatory changes must be considered when analyzing HCV evolution in the context of an immune response and may be detected in searches for long-range interactions across the genome.[165] Neoantigen could be recognized by other T cells, as has been observed for HIV[15]; however, this does not appear to be common in HCV. Lack of recognition of the neoantigen produced by escape substitutions could be due to repertoire fixation,[686] analogous to the phenomenon of original antigenic sin observed in repeated infections.[334] A novel additional mechanism, the exploitation by HCV of a hole in the human T-cell repertoire[686] such that the mutant form is not recognized at all, may not be surprising for a virus that has been adapting to humans for a very long time.[576] Consistent with that mechanism, CD8 T cells specific for epitopes that have escape substitutions, though low in frequency, may express high levels of the memory marker CD127 similar to those found in persons with spontaneous clearance.[53,311] Escape mutations are not generally observed in epitopes targeted by CD4 T cells[220,564]; this is not surprising given the indirect role of CD4 T cells in antiviral responses, because a viral variant with an escape substitution in a CD4

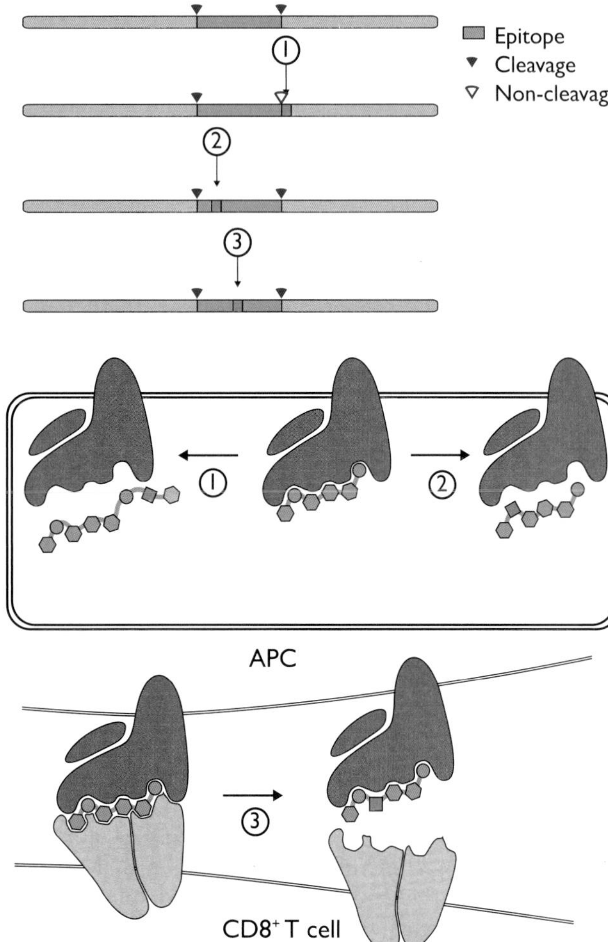

FIGURE 27.5. Evolutionary escape from CD8 T-cell response. Mechanisms for escape from recognition from CD8 T cells that have been demonstrated for hepatitis C virus (HCV) include **(1)** change in a residue affecting proteasomal processing, resulting in C-terminal extensions that cannot be trimmed in the endoplasmic reticulum (ER); **(2)** change in an anchor residue, resulting in loss of affinity for major histocompatibility complex (MHC) class I; and **(3)** change in a T-cell receptor (TCR) contact residue.

T-cell epitope might not have a survival advantage relative to nearby variants lacking such a substitution.

Humoral Immune Response

There is increasing evidence for the importance of the humoral immune response in control and clearance of HCV infection. Antibodies against HCV are not absolutely required for clearance of infection, as demonstrated in individuals with congenital agammaglobulinemia.[4] In individuals with normal humoral immunity, however, binding antibody responses against structural and nonstructural HCV proteins are detectable within weeks to months of infection.[110,467] Using autologous virus, neutralizing antibodies can sometimes be detected within this same time period.[170,494]

Envelope proteins E1 and E2 are type I transmembrane proteins that exist on infectious virions as a cross-linked heterodimer.[660] The structure of E1 is unknown, but recent mutational and computational analysis has produced a draft structure of E2[342] that is supported by functional and antibody mapping studies.[11,321] HCV envelope binds directly to CD81, and mutational analysis suggests that this binding involves E2 residues in domain I (Fig. 27.6). Although anti-E1 and anti-E2 antibodies can be detected in persons with acute and chronic HCV infection,[467] almost all neutralizing antibodies target E2 and inhibit entry at a postattachment step.[272,544,659]

There are numerous direct and indirect lines of evidence to suggest that antibodies against HCV decrease the risk of infection after exposure (see also Passive Immunization section, later). First, there were fewer HCV infections in liver transplant recipients who received immune globulin prior to 1990, the first year that immune globulin preparations were screened for HCV seroreactivity.[199] Second, immune globulin in a randomized controlled study reduced the incidence of sexual HCV transmission.[497] In addition, inoculum-specific neutralizing antibodies directed at the hypervariable region 1 (HVR-1) reduced infection in chimpanzees; however, HVR-1 variability resulted in breakthrough infection.[192,194,680] More recently, prophylactic treatment with a broadly neutralizing monoclonal antibody protected against HCV challenge in a human liver chimeric mouse model.[369]

Neutralizing antibodies may also play a role in modulating ongoing HCV infection. Individuals with primary hypogammaglobulinemia had more rapid progression of disease and poorer response to interferon treatment,[63] and individuals with humoral immune defects have fewer amino acid changes in E2.[73,231]

Evasion of the Neutralizing Antibody Response

The development of pseudotyped lentiviruses for measuring neutralizing antibodies to HCV[46,385,532] has revealed that chronic infection is associated with significant titers of neutralizing antibodies,[385] and a case report of a chronically infected individual showed continuous rounds of escape from neutralizing antibody.[666] During acute infection, neutralizing antibodies drive sequence evolution, suggesting that they have an impact on fitness *in vivo,* and early appearance of HVR-1–specific and/or neutralizing antibodies is associated with an increased likelihood of spontaneous viral clearance.[13,170,494,708,709] Individuals reinfected after clearance of infection have lower second peak viremia, increased likelihood of clearance of the second infection, and a more broadly neutralizing antibody response.[424,478]

The enormous diversity of the virus and tolerance of amino acid changes in E1E2 contribute to escape from this host response (Table 27.1). As with HIV-1, heavy glycosylation of E1 and E2 may provide a "glycan shield" that obscures conserved, functionally important domains (Fig. 27.6).[272] During the transition from acute to chronic infection, acceleration of evolution in HCV envelope genes is likely to be due to the appearance of neutralizing antibodies.[382] Because they are immunodominant targets of humoral immunity while also tolerating extensive nonsynonymous variation, HVR-1 and, to a lesser degree, HVR-2 and the intergenotypic variable region (igVR) contribute to neutralizing antibody escape (Fig. 27.6, marker 2).[42,47,193,523,659] Antibodies targeting the HVR-1 are common *in vivo,* but, given the variability of the region, they tend to be strain specific. In a study of neutralizing antibody development in acute HCV infection, neutralizing antibody escape mutations were mapped to the HVR-1.[170] Most broadly neutralizing antibodies bind to the E2-CD81-binding site.[80,320,369,479,544,659] Some of these epitopes are linear, while others are conformational in nature. While the

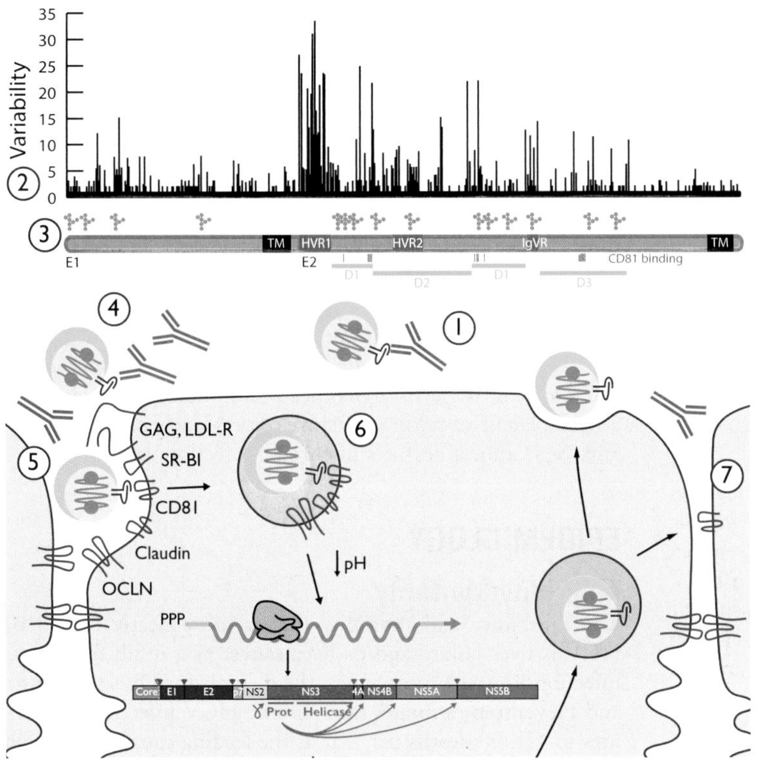

FIGURE 27.6. Evasion of anti–hepatitis C virus (HCV) antibody-mediated responses. Neutralization of HCV by antibodies can block infection of the cell **(1)**. Binding of neutralizing antibodies (red) can be evaded by variability in the envelope proteins **(2)** illustrated here in a plot of Wu-Kabat amino acid variability[691] and by dense glycosylation at approximately 15 positions **(3)**. Nonneutralizing antibodies **(4**, green) and lipoproteins **(5)** may hinder neutralizing antibody binding to HCV envelope glycoproteins, and delayed exposure of conserved domains until late in the entry process may prevent their recognition on free virions **(6)**. Cell-to-cell transfer of virions is resistant to neutralizing antibodies *in vitro,* suggesting an additional mode of escape for local spread of infection **(7)**. Along the envelope gene map are indicated transmembrane regions (TMs), hypervariable regions (HVRs), intergenotypic variable regions (IgVRs), putative tertiary domains (D1–D3), and CD81-binding residues (vertical lines).

CD81-binding site is highly conserved, many of these broadly neutralizing antibodies can induce escape mutations in HCV cell culture, suggesting that replication-competent escape variants may also exist *in vivo.*[320]

Several other mechanisms in addition to antigenic variability may contribute to HCV resistance to antibody-mediated neutralization. It appears that the CD81-binding site may be partially shielded from neutralizing antibodies by the HVR-1 and by N-linked glycosylation (Fig. 27.6, marker 3).[42,187,272] Lipid shielding of the virion may also play a role, because studies have suggested that some neutralization epitopes are less accessible in particles associated with very low-density lipoproteins (VLDLs) or high-density lipoproteins (HDLs) (Fig. 27.6, marker 5).[90,665] Additional mechanisms of evasion of neutralizing antibodies may include nonneutralizing antibodies that bind E1E2 in a manner that interferes with binding of neutralizing antibodies, and postendocytic conformational changes in E1E2 revealing conserved determinants of entry (Figure 27.6, markers 4 and 6, respectively).[545,705] *In vitro* demonstration of direct cell-to-cell spread of HCV, resistant to most neutralizing antibodies, suggests an additional potential mechanism for immune evasion (Fig. 27.6, marker 7)[79,630,685]; however, strong evidence for antibody-driven HCV evolution[170,382] suggests that neutralizing antibodies apply significant selection pressure *in vivo.*

Release from Host and Transmission

HCV RNA has been detected in small amounts in a variety of secreted body fluids including saliva, tears, and urine,[111,204,430] but transmission primarily results from percutaneous exposure

TABLE 27.1 HCV Proteins Contributing to Persistence

Protein	Immune function	Evasion mechanism	References
Core	TNF-α and lymphotoxin signaling	Interference with intracellular signaling	(107,414,707)
E1, E2	Antibody binding, neutralization	Glycan shield	(272)
		Cell-to-cell spread	(79,630,685)
		Evolution/escape	(170,187,318–320,382,545,568,666,680)
NS3-NS4A	TLR3 signaling	TRIF cleavage	(377)
	RIG-I signaling	MAVS cleavage	(389,439)
NS5A	PKR, 2,5-OAS responses	Direct interaction	(222,223)
		IL-8 stimulation	(501)
Any	MHC epitope recognition by T cells	Evolution/escape (see Fig. 27.5)	(134,351,521,614,628)

MAVS, mitochondrial antiviral signaling protein; MHC, major histocompatibility complex; 2,5-OAS, 2′,5′-oligoadenylate synthetase; PKR, protein kinase RNA-activated; RIG-I; TLR, Toll-like receptor; TNF, tumor necrosis factor; TRIF, TIR domain–containing adapter-inducing interferon-β.

to blood or rarely from mucosal exposure to genital secretions, as discussed in the section on Transmission later.

Virulence

In spite of their extreme heterogeneity, genetic variants of HCV (genotypes and subtypes) have remarkably similar clinical manifestations; for example, there have been no reported outbreaks of acute fulminant hepatitis, and persons infected in common-source outbreaks have displayed a wide range of outcomes.[151,322] Moreover, efforts to identify viral determinants of fibrosis progression have not revealed consistent associations. Response to treatment is strongly affected by viral genotype, with genotype 1 being relatively refractory to interferon-based therapy as discussed in the Treatment section.

HCV subverts hepatic lipoprotein metabolism (see Virus Assembly section for HCV in Chapter 25), so it is not surprising that steatosis and insulin resistance are common features in HCV infection (see Clinical Features, later).[281] Multiple studies have found a significantly stronger association between genotype 3 HCV infection and steatosis[151] than for other HCV genotypes; this association may be related to genotype-specific disruption of lipid biosynthesis pathways.[118] Steatosis is also strongly associated with visceral obesity.[5] Geographic variation in host factors as well as viral genetic types (see Genetic Diversity, later) could confound association of viral genotype with some manifestations.

During initial HCV infection, the peak of hepatic injury (illustrated by the peak in alanine aminotransferase [ALT] in Fig. 27.7) follows, rather than coinciding with, the peak of viremia.[102] This consistent observation, combined with observations of liver pathology and cell culture, suggests that lysis of HCV-infected cells results primarily from the host antiviral immune response.[102,115] The association of chronic infection with progressive liver disease and hepatocellular carcinoma is discussed in the Clinical Features section later.

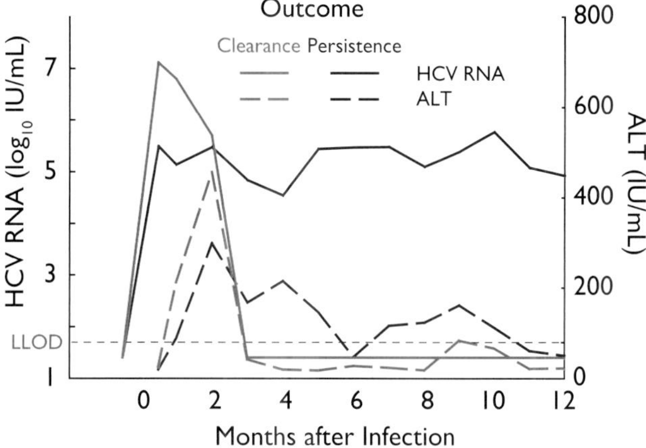

FIGURE 27.7. Patterns of acute hepatitis C virus (HCV) infection, resulting in spontaneous resolution or chronicity. The initial peak of viremia is followed by a peak in alanine aminotransferase (ALT) indicating cytolysis, temporally associated with the detection of cell-mediated responses to HCV that do not differ qualitatively by outcome when measured *ex vivo*.[133] Initial level of viremia is higher in those who clear compared with those who later progress to chronic infection.[383]

Persistence

When untreated, acute infection with HCV may spontaneously resolve or persist as chronic HCV infection (Fig. 27.7, discussed further in Clinical Features, later). Spontaneous clearance of HCV occurs in approximately one-third of untreated infections. This resolution occurs in the first 2 years and is generally complete, with no residual viral RNA in serum or liver.[135,424] Persistent HCV infection occurs in two-thirds of infected persons, is attributable to the evasion mechanisms discussed earlier, and is associated with persistent viremia at a level of 5 to 7 log_{10} IU/mL in 90% of individuals.[627] Spontaneous resolution during chronicity is rare.[9] Because persistence is marked by high-level viremia and constant evolution in immunocompetent hosts, HCV appears to persist dynamically and there is no evidence of a stable, latent reservoir or archive of previously dominant variants. See Clinical Features of chronic infection, later.

EPIDEMIOLOGY

Morbidity/Mortality

The morbidity and mortality that is most clearly caused by HCV is liver failure and/or liver cancer as a result of chronic infection. In the Unites States, the Centers for Disease Control and Prevention estimates that chronic HCV infection contributes to 15,000 deaths per year, is the leading cause of liver failure leading to transplantation, and in 2007 superseded HIV as a cause of death (Fig. 27.8).[184,394,684] HCV-related liver morbidity and mortality increase with older age and greater duration of HCV infection and are expected to rise in the coming decades. Using multistate disease models, one group recently estimated that HCV-related liver failure and cancer will continue to increase until 2020–2023 without widespread treatment.[147] Liver-related mortality is predicted to rise from 146,667 cases in 2000–2009 to 254,550 cases in 2010–2019 and 283,378 in 2020–2029. Reliable worldwide estimates of HCV-related mortality are not available.

HCV-infected persons are at increased risk of more than liver failure. In one study, 10,259 HCV antibody–positive blood donors were compared to donors matched by year of donation, age, gender, and zip code and followed for a mean of 7.7 years.[261] Compared to the HCV-uninfected donors, the risk of death was 3.13-fold higher in HCV-infected donors, who were more likely to die of not just liver-related but also drug/alcohol-related events, trauma/suicide, and cardiovascular causes. Persons with HCV infection are also at much higher risk of some medical conditions such as mixed cryoglobulinemic vasculitis and porphyria cutanea tarda (see Clinical Features later).[6,154] The degree to which HCV infection contributes to less specific medical syndromes such as chronic fatigue/arthritis or mental illness is more difficult to establish.

Origin and Spread of Epidemics

HCV infection spread during the 20th century, strongly correlated with expanded production of syringes and their worldwide use for both conventional medicine and illicit drugs.[172,215,397] Drucker and co-workers[172] estimated that global syringe production rose from 100,000 per year in 1920 to 7.5 million per year by 1952. Widespread use of percutaneous injections for medicinal (and then illicit) drug use antedated appreciation of blood-borne transmission of infection

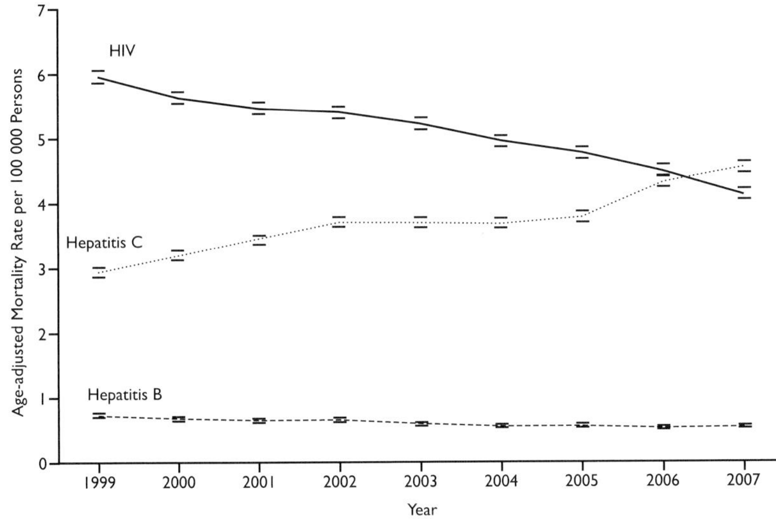

FIGURE 27.8. Annual age-adjusted mortality rates from hepatitis B and hepatitis C virus and human immunodeficiency virus (HIV) infections listed as causes of death in the United States between 1999 and 2007. Because a decedent can have multiple causes of death, a record listing more than one type of infection was counted for each type of infection. (From Ly KN, Xing J, Klevens RM, et al. The increasing burden of mortality from viral hepatitis in the United States between 1999 and 2007. *Ann Intern Med* 2012;156:271–278.)

and spread HCV throughout the world. This trend explains the 5- to 20-fold increased HCV prevalence rates in certain regions where unsafe injections were widespread and among injection drug users (IDUs) (see Global Burden, Incidence, and Prevalence).[215] Transfusions of blood products also contributed to HCV infection, especially when donors were paid and no measures were in place to screen blood for infection.[399]

Prior to the 20th century, HCV infection was probably sustained by percutaneous practices such as scarification rituals and circumcision. This conjecture is supported by evidence of transmission by such practices where they still occur and by molecular clock estimates derived from analyses of worldwide HCV RNA sequences (see Genetic Diversity).[332,509]

Prevalence and Seroepidemiology

Transmission

HCV can be transmitted by percutaneous exposure to contaminated blood, from a mother to her infant, and by sexual intercourse. There is no evidence HCV can penetrate intact skin, but permucosal transmission has occurred when blood was splashed into eyes.

The likelihood that HCV transmission will occur is directly related to the inoculum and the exposure type. Blood is the usual inoculum, typically contains 5 to 7 $\log_{10}$ copies of HCV RNA per mL, and rarely transmits HCV when viremia is not detected.[166,627] Although HCV RNA has been amplified from most other body fluids, it is not clear to what extent other body fluids harbor infectious virions.[204,430,671]

Percutaneous exposures such as unsafe medical procedures and injection drug use are the usual routes of HCV transmission worldwide. HCV transmission almost always occurs following very large percutaneous inocula, such as transfusion of a contaminated unit of blood.[182,669] However, even very small (less than 10 μL) blood inocula may contain infectious virions to establish infection in a recipient if injected percutaneously, and nosocomial exposure may occur if strict universal precautions are not observed.[14,293] Blood spiked with an HCV reporter virus was loaded into syringes and viability was recovered from 71% of tuberculin syringes kept at 22°C for 7 days.[480] This finding correlates with studies of health care personnel with accidental needlestick exposures in whom transmission occurs in 1% to 2% overall and more often from hollow-bore needles, which contain a larger inoculum than a solid-bore needle.[330,528] Repeated small-volume exposures to HCV explain the high rates of HCV among injection drug users (see later).

Nonmedical percutaneous exposures such as body piercing and tattooing are plausible risks and epidemiologically linked to HCV prevalence in many countries, though they are likely to be confounded by other risky behaviors in some populations.[276,336,395,411,426,438,462,506,601]

The frequency by which HCV is transmitted sexually is controversial. On the one hand, long-term monogamous partners of individuals with HCV infection almost never acquire HCV.[30] In one study, 895 monogamous sexual partners of persons with chronic HCV infection were followed for over 8,000 person-years, and there were no instances of sexual HCV transmission, despite unprotected intercourse occurring an average of 1.8 times per week.[654] On the other hand, HCV infection occurs in persons acknowledging high-risk sexual practices (and no other exposure),[650] and there are multiple outbreaks among HIV-infected men who have high-risk sexual exposures with other men.[145,648] One speculation is that, as with HIV, the risk of sexual HCV transmission is greater during the acute phase of infection when viremia peaks and prior to formation of neutralizing antibodies. In addition, anal intercourse may cause mucosal tears that promote HCV transmission. Permucosal spread of HCV may also explain the association of HCV infection with intranasal use of cocaine.[125]

HCV transmission from a mother to her infant occurs infrequently (2% to 10%).[413,527,700] How and when infection occurs in this setting is not known, but risk is increased by maternal HIV infection and/or high HCV RNA levels, prolonged rupture of membranes, and internal fetal monitoring.[413,624]

Global Burden, Incidence, and Prevalence

There are an estimated 185 million HCV-infected persons in the world, or 2.2% of the human population.[688,689] There are marked differences in HCV prevalence between regions (Fig. 27.9) and, even within countries, between age and risk groups. Egypt appears to have the highest HCV prevalence, which is as high as 50% in persons born before 1960.[215] The history of HCV infection in Egypt is exemplary of global

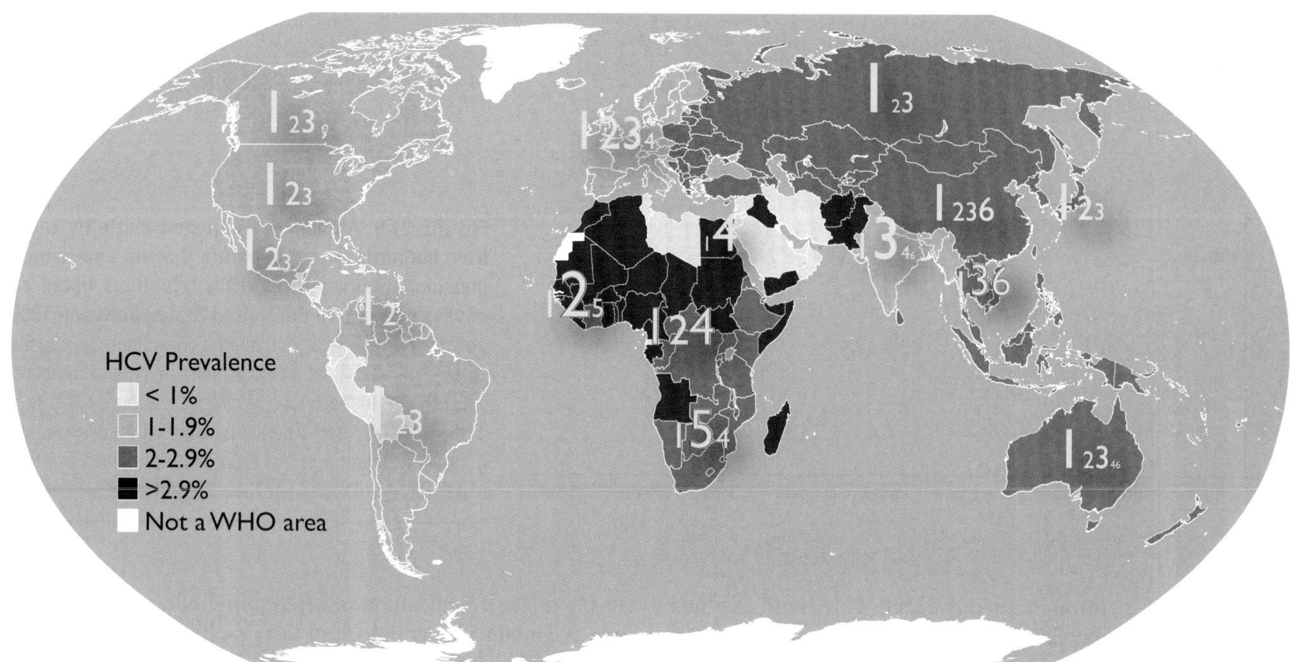

FIGURE 27.9. Map depicting geographic variation in the relative prevalence of hepatitis C virus (HCV) infection and genotypes. Shading of country indicates prevalence. Yellow numerals indicate prevalent HCV genotypes in different regions, with font size corresponding to relative genotype prevalence within each region; red outlining indicates genotypes with greatest intraregional diversity. HCV prevalence is highest, and genetically most diverse, in Africa. Genotype 1 is prevalent worldwide, whereas genotypes 4 and 5 are almost exclusively found in north-central and southern Africa, respectively. Genotype 7 (provisionally assigned and not depicted) has been reported very rarely in persons with epidemiologic links to central Africa. (HCV prevalence estimates adapted from World Health Organization. Global burden of disease [GBD] for hepatitis C. *J Clin Pharmacol* 2004;44:20–29, with permission. Relative genotype prevalence within each region based on sources cited in the text.)

transmission patterns. From the 1950s to the 1980s, the Egyptian Ministry of Health embarked on a campaign to eradicate schistosomiasis infection by intravenously administering tartar emetic to millions of citizens.[589] The effort, commended at the time as a public health model, occurred before there was widespread appreciation for blood-borne transmission of infectious agents. HCV was transmitted extensively because of the widespread reuse of insufficiently cleaned injection equipment.[215] Consequently, the prevalence of HCV infection can exceed 50% in persons alive during that campaign while being 1% to 2% in those born after. In addition, more than 90% of HCV infections in Egypt are genotype 4, which make up less than 10% of genotypes in most other regions of the world.[520]

There is molecular and epidemiologic evidence of similar transmission patterns elsewhere. In studies modeling HCV sequences, Tanaka and co-workers[610] estimated rapid expansion of HCV-1b in Japan in the 1920s, in Europe in the 1940s, and in the United States (HCV-1a) in the 1960s.[610] Population data from southern Italy show that the HCV prevalence is 1.3% in subjects younger than 30 years and 33% in those older than 60 years of age; the odds of infection were doubled in those who recalled reusable glass syringe use.[260] Thus, as mentioned earlier (in Origin and Spread), it appears HCV was widely transmitted worldwide during the 1900s due to stepped-up production of syringes and their worldwide use both for conventional and illicit drugs.[172,397,509]

The overall prevalence of HCV infection in Europe is 1% to 2%. However, country-specific rates vary considerably, with the lowest HCV prevalence (less than 0.5%) reported from Sweden, Germany, and the Netherlands while prevalence rates of 2% to 3% have been reported in some Mediterranean countries.[271] There is less information on incident HCV infection. Although HCV surveillance is required in European countries, new infection information is restricted to symptomatic events (which are the minority of HCV infections) and thus data on trends and comparisons across regions are crude. Overall, because procedures to screen blood donations were implemented, most new infections in Europe are linked to injection drug use or recent health care exposure.[408]

United States Prevalence and Incidence

In the United States, an estimated 3 million persons have chronic HCV infection. Several key epidemiologic trends explain the incidence and prevalence of HCV infection. As in other parts of the world, unsafe medical injections probably contributed to an early expansion of HCV prevalence following World War II. Transfusion of blood and blood products caused new HCV infections until 1992, when the most effective screening measures were adopted. However, it was the epidemic of injection drug use from the 1950s to the 1980s that caused most HCV infections in the United States. Whereas there were probably fewer than 500,000 persons with chronic HCV infection in the early 1950s, by the mid-1990s there were an estimated 3.5 million persons with chronic HCV infection and another 1 million to 1.5 million who had recovered.[31] Much of that epidemic spread was due to injection drug use.

Not only does injection drug use cause most HCV infections in the United States, but also most injection drug users have been HCV infected. HCV infection generally occurs within the first years of initiating the illicit use of injected drugs with annual incidence rates of 10% to 30%.[135,228,266] In one cohort, 80% of subjects acknowledging 2 or more years of injection use were infected with the virus, a prevalence that was higher than that of HIV or HBV infection.[229,625] Early acquisition of HCV is probably related to the practice of older (infected) IDUs teaching new (uninfected) initiates by demonstrating first on themselves and then on the new initiate.[228] Although sharing of needles and syringes causes some HCV transmission, Hagan and co-workers[265] estimated that 37% of new cases were due to sharing of other equipment.

After peaking in the 1980s, HCV incidence has dropped markedly in the United States.[98] Elimination of transfusion-related transmission contributed to the reduction in incidence. However, most of the decline is attributed to a reduction of HCV due to injection drug use that is not fully explained.[19] However, because HCV serology remains positive in most instances even when viremia is cleared, the 20-year surge in HCV incidence among persons born between 1945 and 1964 remains serologically evident.

The best data on HCV prevalence in the Unites States come from the serial National Health and Nutrition Examination Surveys (NHANES).[32] By testing blood collected from a subset of persons representing households in the United States around 1990, it was estimated that 4.1 million individuals had been infected with HCV, or 1.6% of the general population. Approximately two-thirds of those infected were born between 1945 and 1965. The survey was repeated 10 years later and showed the same number of HCV-infected individuals in the same age cohort that was 10 years older. Omitted from this survey were nearly 2 million incarcerated persons in the United States, who probably represent another 250,000 to 500,000 HCV-infected persons.[39] The prevalence of HCV infection in the United States is also higher among racial minorities than in Caucasian Americans, and greater in African Americans than in Mexican Americans. In non-Hispanic Blacks 40 to 49 years of age, the HCV prevalence was 14% compared to a general population prevalence of 1.6%. HCV infection was detected in only 1% of those 20 to 29 years of age.

Genetic Diversity

Genetic variability is one of the most remarkable features of HCV, contributing to evasion of host immune responses and complicating development of diagnostics, therapeutics, and effective vaccines. HCV genomic sequences can be clustered phylogenetically into related groups (genotypes and subtypes), are distinct between individuals, and are highly variable within each infected individual at any given point in time (i.e., quasispecies diversity[314,406]) and over time (i.e., quasispecies divergence).

Global Diversity of HCV

Soon after HCV was discovered, it was apparent that genetically distinct strains were prevalent in different geographic areas. International standards for nomenclature established six major genotypes that are phylogenetically distinct, and subsequent reports have resulted in the proposal of a seventh genotype (Fig. 27.10).[248,346,451,530,577] Within genotypes, phylogenetically

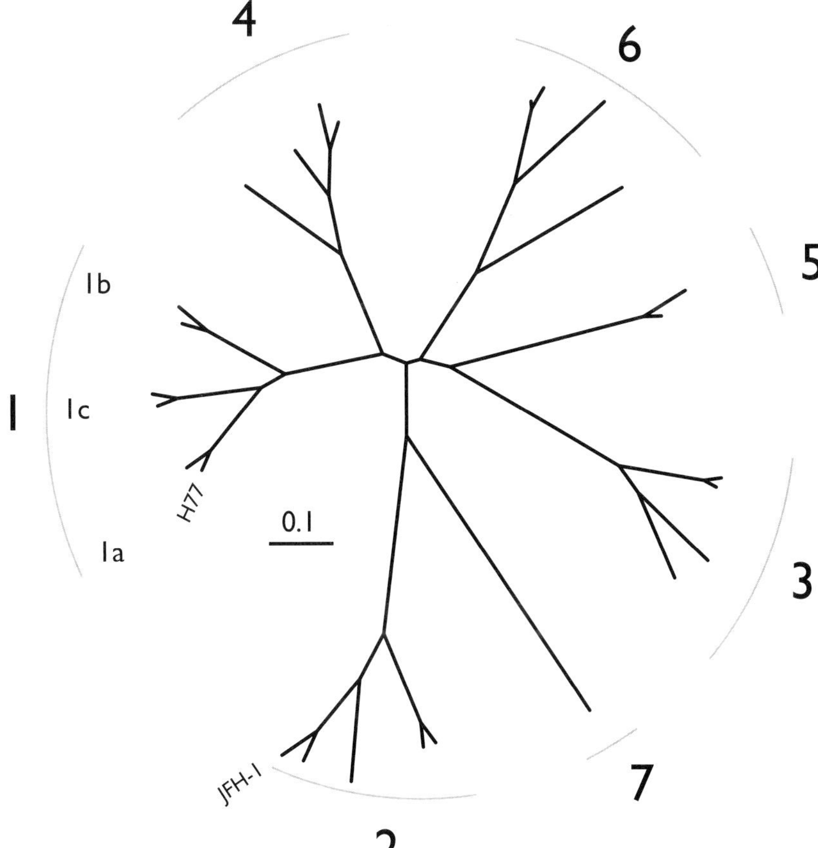

FIGURE 27.10. Phylogenetic tree of representative sequence from the seven proposed genotypes of hepatitis C virus (HCV). Full-genome nucleotide sequences were aligned and analyzed using a maximum likelihood model with estimation of invariant sites and modeling of variable rates using the gamma distribution, with bootstrap resampling to confirm support for each genotype cluster. Reference isolates H77 (AF009606) and JFH-1 (AB047639) are indicated. Subtypes of genotype 1 (1a, 1b, 1c) are indicated for illustration.

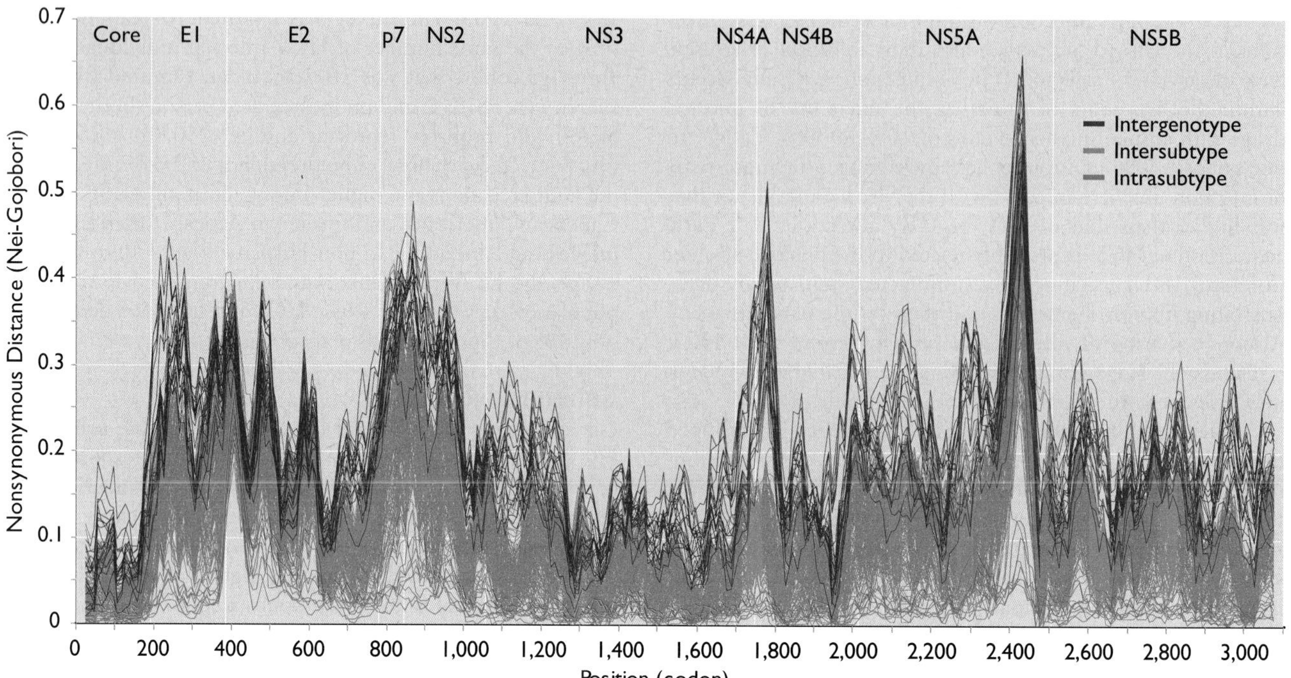

FIGURE 27.11. Genetic variability of hepatitis C virus (HCV) by genomic region. Using an alignment of full-genome sequences from all seven proposed genotypes, the polyprotein open reading frame (ORF) was analyzed using VarPlot (described in[523]) to calculate mean pairwise nonsynonymous distance in a sliding window of 50 codons at intervals of 10 codons. For intergenotype comparisons (blue), there are 21 curves representing each pairwise comparison among the seven genotypes. For genotypes having at least two subtype representatives, there is a curve for each pair of subtypes (red). There is one curve representing mean intrasubtype distance for each subtype having at least four available sequences (green), including subtypes of genotypes 1, 2, 3, 4, and 6; for subtypes having many full-genome sequences, 10 were identified randomly.

distinct clusters may be found that are called subtypes. Clinically, HCV genotypes and subtypes are very similar (see Virulence), though they vary in responsiveness to interferons (genotypes 1 and 4 are less responsive) and, in more complex ways, in susceptibility to direct-acting antiviral agents (see Treatment).

The pairwise distance between genotypes ranges from 29% to 34% for genomic nucleotide sequences and 24% to 33% for amino acid sequences spanning the polyprotein. The protein-coding differences between genotypes are not uniformly distributed across the genome; rather, they are greatest in the E1, E2, p7, NS2, N-terminus of NS4B, and V3 region[287] of NS5A, and most conserved in core (blue curves in Fig. 27.11). As that figure illustrates, the contours of pairwise distance are remarkably consistent between genotypes, reflecting neutral evolution as a dominant force in the divergence of genotypes.[576] Even in the most variable regions (e.g., HVR-1, positions 384 to 410 in the polyprotein using standard genome numbering[345]), there are severe constraints on amino acids with regard to specific amino acids[415] and biophysical properties.[488]

Variation within genotype (i.e., genetic distance between pairs of subtypes) is about half of the intergenotype diversity, with similar regions of divergence and conservation (red curves in Fig. 27.11); a notable exception is the N-terminus of NS4B, the significance of which is unclear. Variation within subtype (green curves in Fig. 27.11) is more restricted, yet remarkably consistent considering that each tracing represents one subtype from widely divergent genotypes (1, 2, 3, 4, and 6, which sufficient representatives). Hypervariable region locations that differ among genotypes suggest different selection pressures.[282]

Potentially confounding genotype assignment and diagnostics is recombination, which is a dominant mode of evolution in HBV and HIV.[531,579] Intergenotype recombination has been reported in HCV sequences,[59,300,302,373,474] and standards for confirmation and nomenclature of recombinant forms are available.[346] While recombination among HCV subtypes has clearly occurred *in vivo* and hybrid genomes can be generated *in vitro*,[248,498,559] this appears to be a rare occurrence given how often distinct HCV genomes simultaneously infect the same host.[56,580,658] HCV recombination may be limited by superinfection exclusion, which has been demonstrated for HCV *in vitro*.[558]

Because intergenotypic recombination is rare, phylogenetic trees obtained from any segment of the genome will reflect genotypic clustering seen on the full-genome tree, on a scale determined by the variability in that segment of the genome.[530] By international consensus,[346] the reference genomic regions for HCV genotype/subtype assignment are core/E1[86,128] and NS5B[591] (see Diagnosis section).

Global Molecular Epidemiology of HCV

Accurate estimation of the relative prevalence of HCV genotypes in a region depends on population-based sampling,[33,452,520] which is rarely performed. Nonetheless, it is clear that HCV genotypes are nonuniformly distributed among geographic regions, with dominant features depicted in Figure 27.9.[131,323,347,464,575]

Genotype 1 is the most widely dispersed worldwide, and phylodynamic analyses are consistent with global expansion in the population and dispersion from 1940 to 1980 and suggest that subtype 1b may have disseminated, possibly in blood products, earlier than subtype 1a.[397,509] These trends are corroborated by other studies,[354,536] and subtype 1a is often associated with recent or ongoing drug use in North America and northern Europe.[55,135,241,452]

Independent analyses of sequence data from other countries in the western hemisphere are consistent with expansion of epidemics during the second half of the 20th century but involving a wider variety of subtypes.[25,360] Taken together, these studies do not suggest that HCV subtypes differ significantly in terms of transmissibility or association with specific routes of transmission; rather, specific HCV subtypes appear to dominate epidemics as a result of founder effects, and the presence of highly diverse variants of one genotype in a region suggests a local origin.[576]

The epidemic in Egypt[215] is dominated by subtype 4a but includes diverse subtypes of genotypes 1 and 4,[514,520] perhaps reflecting its proximity to Central Africa where genotypes 1 and 4 appear to be endemic[216,338,427,460,473,482,672] and may share a common origin.[461,547] Genotype 2 is highly diverse in West Africa, where subtype boundaries can be indistinct, suggesting a local origin of this subtype.[96,295,538] In Southeast Asia, genotypes 3 and 6 appear to be epidemic, including among IDUs, with subtypes 1b and 2a associated with older infections[428,506,578,631–634] (note that in 2005, sequences that had been assigned to subtypes 7a, 8a, 9a, 10a, and 11a were reclassified as subtypes 6d, 6k, 6h, 3k, and 6g, respectively[577]). Genotype 5 is found in southern Africa, with limited dispersal.[26]

Origins of HCV

Available evidence summarized in the previous section suggests that HCV is endemic in widely separated regions of the globe. While nonprimate hepaciviruses have been discovered recently in dogs and horses,[89,309] those isolates are very distinct from HCV, and their origin, prevalence, and tropism are not known.

HCV genotypes appear to have arisen hundreds or perhaps thousands of years ago.[397,509,583] Without sequence data older than 50 years to "calibrate" such molecular clock analyses, phylogenetic saturation at the HCV genotype level may preclude accurate estimation of the age of HCV.[576]

Quasispecies Variability: Mechanisms

HCV exists in each infected host as a swarm of genetically related but distinct variants, collectively called a quasispecies.[162,163,177,314,406] This characteristically diverse set of viruses in an individual arises from one or more "founder" sequences from the predictably diverse quasispecies present in the donor(s), selected randomly or based on phenotypic characteristics by a transmission bottleneck that is poorly understood.[88]

Diversity is generated by mutations introduced by the NS5B RNA-dependent RNA polymerase, which lacks a proofreading function and has an estimated error rate of 10^{-3} to 10^{-5} per nucleotide per replication cycle.[45,174] Enhancing this diversity is the high rate of viral replication, with 10^{10} to 10^{12} virions produced per day.[468] This dynamic, error-prone replication is likely to generate a vast array of mutants every day.[535] Because each HCV genome is produced by the error-prone NS5B polymerase and the number of intracellular replication events (from positive to negative, and negative to positive strand) is at least two but could be larger, each infected cell can generate a diverse population of viral genomes. In contrast, HIV undergoes a single round of error-prone cDNA synthesis per infected cell, with subsequent proviral replication (during cell division) and RNA genome synthesis by host DNA and RNA polymerases, respectively.[38]

Due to neutral drift and sequential selection events (addressed in the next section), HCV quasispecies sequences have motifs that gradually change over time and during passage among individuals, making sequence analysis suitable for forensic and epidemiologic linkage studies.[243,273,322,484]

Assessment of a complex quasispecies can be confounded by methodologic artifacts. Nucleic acid contamination of specimens and analytical intermediates is a common problem, which can be reduced (if not completely eliminated) by taking appropriate precautions.[357] Amplification in multiple cycles, as with the polymerase chain reaction, can introduce sequence artifacts and distort the frequency distribution of sequence variants. These phenomena can inflate or suppress estimates of diversity and evolutionary change and must be considered at all stages from specimen selection and processing through analysis and interpretation.[384,582,664] The biological site of specimen selection may also affect the results due to compartmentalization,[91,396,459,562,569] though the limitations of quasispecies sampling may confound such analyses, and the biological implications of compartmentalization remain controversial.

Quasispecies Evolution During Acute HCV Infection

A diverse viral population, under influence from a variety of selection pressures in a complex host environment, is an ideal situation for viral adaptation in a Darwinian manner.[680] The quasispecies is shaped by positive selection pressure from the host (see Immune Response) and negative selection pressure due to functional constraints imposed by requirements of the viral life cycle (see Chapter 25 for discussion of essential protein motifs and constrained RNA structures at both ends of the genome); therefore, each host's HCV quasispecies directly reflects dynamic aspects of both the host and pathogen.

During acute HCV infection, the diverse quasispecies may be targeted by cellular and humoral immune responses (see Immune Response), which have the potential to reduce the fitness of variants carrying epitopes they recognize and therefore apply positive selection pressure. In people studied during the first months of acute HCV viremia, this selection pressure has been observed in individual epitopes,[628] and more broadly as an excess of amino acid replacements in CD8 T-cell epitopes (studied in nonenvelope genes, to avoid confounding by antibody responses).[134,614] Detailed analysis spanning the HCV polyprotein at multiple time points in four subjects displayed the same phenomena and also demonstrated that nontargeted substitutions represented reversions to the subtype consensus sequence at a rate that was directly related to the conservation of that site in reference sequences.[351] In that study, the rate of mutation in nonenvelope genes declined during the transition to chronicity, consistent with progressive T-cell dysfunction.[133,541,564] Some escape mutations require compensatory changes to restore fitness,[470,539] possibly accounting for additional changes observed during acute HCV infection that do not fall within targeted epitopes.[134,351] In comparison with HIV, HCV evolution during acute infection is relatively limited, reflecting CD8 T-cell dysfunction, HCV genomic inflexibility, or both.[496]

The envelope (E1E2) region of the HCV genome is highly variable (as noted earlier) and has a much higher rate of evolution within hosts than other regions of the genome.[252] Humoral immune responses directed against envelope genes *E1* and *E2* have the potential to neutralize HCV, and the HCVpp and HCVcc systems provide the means to correlate E1E2 evolution with neutralizing antibody responses (see section on the Humoral Immune Response). HCV escape from neutralizing antibodies[666] drives the evolution of envelope sequences during acute infection.[170] This is contrasted with relative stasis of HCV

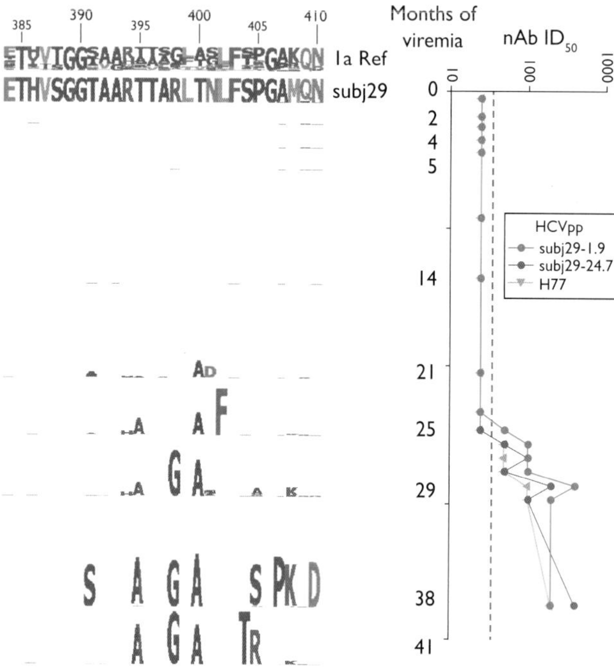

FIGURE 27.12. Evolution of hypervariable region 1 (HVR-1) during the transition from acute to chronic infection. HVR-1 evolution **(left panel)** correlated with neutralizing antibody (nAb) responses **(right panel)** in subject 29 (subj29) from the BBAASH cohort[136] studied from initial viremia (month 0) to chronicity. Type 1 sequence logos[247] were used to demonstrate the variability among 388 reference sequences (1aRef) as well as the initial viral quasispecies (subj29, month 0). Amino acid sequence positions are indicated according to H77.[345] For months 2 through 41, type 2 logos[247] were used to compare amino acid sequences to month 0 sequence, with the height of each amino acid determined by the $\log_2$ unlikelihood of an amino acid at a given position relative to the initial sequence. To determine nAb infectious dose 50 (ID_{50}) titers, autologous HCV pseudoparticles (HCVpp) expressing E1E2 from month 2 and month 25 visits, as well as HCVpp-H77, were incubated with serial twofold dilutions of autologous plasma. When 50% neutralization was not detected at the starting plasma dilution of 1:50 (dashed line), the result was recorded as one-half this value, a titer of 1:25. (From Liu L, Fisher BE, Dowd KA, et al. Acceleration of hepatitis C virus envelope evolution in humans is consistent with progressive humoral immune selection during the transition from acute to chronic infection. *J Virol* 2010;84:5067–5077. Copyright © 2010, American Society for Microbiology.)

envelope sequences in persons with severely impaired humoral immunity[73,231,348] and in chimpanzees with poor anti-E2 responses[49] even during 8 to 10 years of chronic viremia.[522] Both stasis and driven evolution are illustrated by HVR-1 evolution in a subject with acute HCV infection progressing to chronicity (Fig. 27.12) in whom neutralizing antibody responses were not detected in the first 2 years of high-level viremia, during which there was no evolution of HVR-1, whereas there was rapid evolution following the detection of neutralizing antibodies.[382] Delayed onset of neutralizing antibody responses is typical in those developing persistent HCV infection[13,170,494,708,709] and appears to explain the acceleration of envelope evolution during the transition from acute to chronic infection.[382]

Common-source outbreaks (like the one illustrated in Fig. 27.13) facilitate examination of HCV evolution with respect to host–pathogen interactions and provide strong evidence for nonrandom evolution.[521,614] HLA allele-specific adaptations of HCV subtype 1b in the Irish outbreak (due to HCV contamination of anti-D immunoglobulin, which occurred in 1977–1978) were distinct from previously identified adaptations in other populations with HCV subtype 1a and 3a infections, suggesting HCV subtype-specific pathways for evolution.[420] Study of this cohort revealed a protective effect (associated with spontaneous clearance) of HLA-A*03, and the "footprints" of this response have been observed in HLA-A*03$^+$ members of the anti-D immunoglobulin HCV infection cohort; additional study demonstrated that escape mutation was associated with impaired viral replication *in vitro.*[207]

Implications for Virologic Inference *In Vitro*

In vitro HCV replication systems have provided important insights regarding the viral life cycle, but these observations depend primarily on a very limited set of isolates growing in cell lines with impaired innate immunity[324]; most human isolates of HCV do not propagate in cell culture, for reasons that are not clear. *In vivo* models that support replication of more diverse isolates in hepatocytes (rather than hepatoma cell lines) are described in Chapter 25 (HCV Experimental Systems section) and may enable investigation of a more representative variety of HCV strains.

CLINICAL FEATURES

Acute HCV

Acute HCV infection is usually asymptomatic,[135,448] though a minority of persons will present with more typical symptoms of acute viral hepatitis (malaise, fatigue, anorexia, nausea, abdominal pain, jaundice, dark urine, and sometimes pale stool). While HCV can cause fulminant hepatitis, this presentation is rare.[190,246,304,398,690,693,698] In general, the latent period (from exposure to symptoms or laboratory abnormalities) is approximately 7 weeks (range 1 to 16 weeks).[448] In many cases, the only sign of acute infection may be elevation of "hepatic transaminases"[1,135,661] (ALT and aspartate aminotransferase [AST] from damaged or dead hepatocytes; these enzymes may also be released from nonhepatic cells, particularly AST from cardiac or skeletal myocytes, in association with other conditions).

Most exposures that result in HCV infection are percutaneous (see Transmission), after which hematogenous infection of the liver is presumed to occur. Viremia is detectable within days[448]

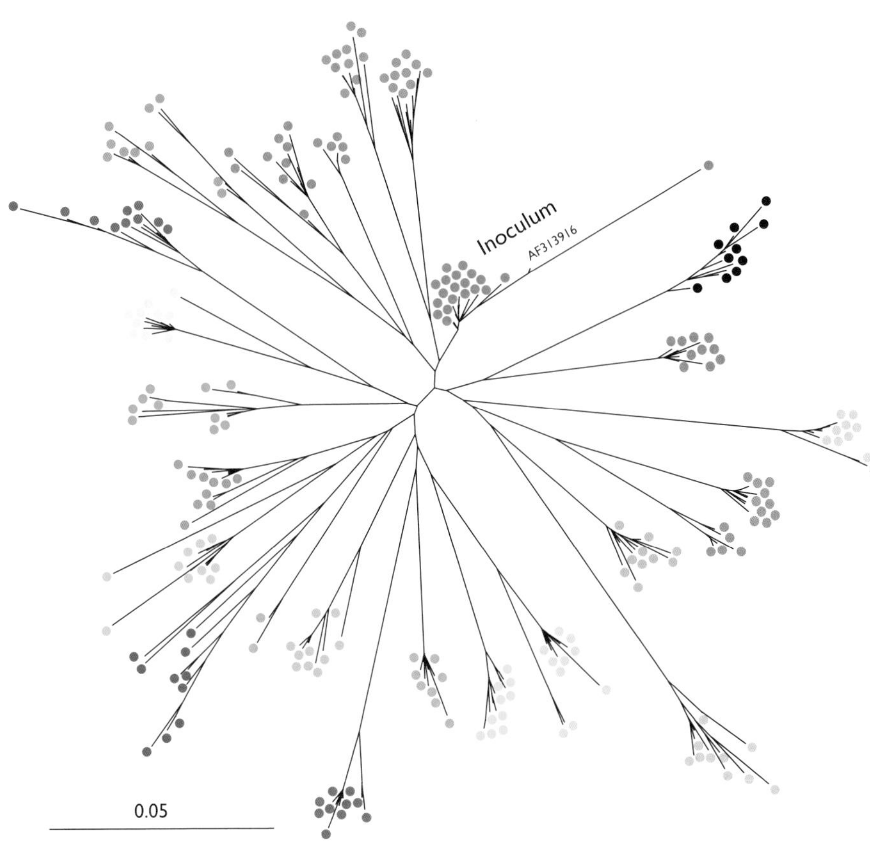

FIGURE 27.13. Phylogenetic analysis of hepatitis C virus (HCV) 18 to 22 years after common-source outbreak, using 10 complementary DNA (cDNA) clones from each study subject to obtain the sequence of a 698-nt region spanning the E1/E2 junction. "Inoculum" indicates 20 clones from inoculum source plasma (10 each from 2 specimens) and a full-length clone (AF313916) obtained in an independent study of this material using smaller amplicons. (From Ray SC, Fanning L, Wang XH, et al. Divergent and convergent evolution after a common-source outbreak of hepatitis C virus. *J Exp Med* 2005;201:1753–1759. Copyright © Ray SC et al, 2005.)

and reaches levels of 10^5 to 10^7 IU/mL within weeks. A decrease in viremia, 1 to 2 weeks later, is associated with a sharp rise in hepatic transaminase levels in blood. This sharp rise is thought to result from immune-mediated cytolysis as adaptive responses to HCV develop (Fig. 27.7),[2,48,135,191,448,571] with more severe hepatitis and higher initial viremia being associated with higher rates of spontaneous clearance of viremia.[234,383,661] When treatment is not instituted and spontaneous clearance does not occur within 12 months, late spontaneous resolution is rare.

Predictors of Spontaneous Clearance

Spontaneous clearance of HCV RNA usually occurs within 6 months of infection and is associated with having overt symptoms of hepatitis, non-African descent, and lack of HIV infection.[234,661] The recognition that a linked set of alleles surrounding the IL28B gene (encoding IFN-λ3) was strongly associated with success of interferon-based therapy[233] (see Treatment, later) was echoed by the discovery that the same protective genotype was associated with spontaneous recovery from acute HCV,[623] apparently independent of viral genotype.[353,515,623] The protective IL28B genotype is more frequently found in Asians and least frequently among persons with African ancestry, in keeping with the clinically observed effect of race.[623] The mechanistic basis of these observations remains unknown.[41]

Chronic HCV

For the 60% to 85% in whom spontaneous resolution does not occur, chronic HCV infection is a heterogeneous condition, with highly individual manifestations and rates of progression (Fig. 27.14).[245] Associated morbidity and mortality occur almost exclusively when the disease progresses to cirrhosis and end-stage liver disease that may manifest as hepatocellular carcinoma (see subsection later). Chronic HCV infection is characterized by high-level viremia and fluctuating hepatic inflammation and transaminase levels,[331,492,683] yet chronically infected people typically have few symptoms that are directly attributable to HCV infection. It is difficult to establish a causal

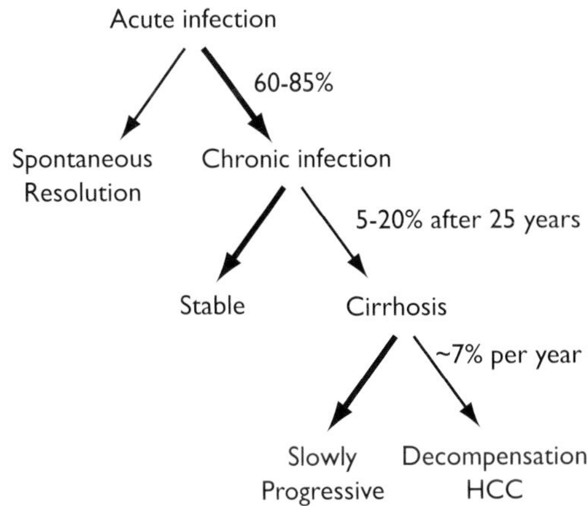

FIGURE 27.14. Progression of hepatitis C virus (HCV) infection. Most HCV infections are persistent and stable, but a minority will progress to cirrhosis within 20 to 30 years. Of those with cirrhosis, most are slowly progressive, but 7% per year will develop either hepatocellular carcinoma (HCC) or decompensated liver disease.[291,550]

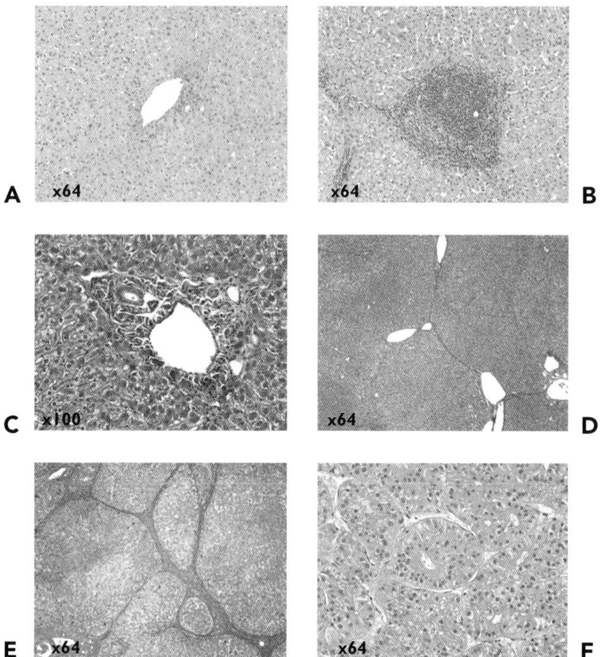

FIGURE 27.15. Histology illustrating progression of hepatitis C virus (HCV)-related liver disease. A: Normal portal tract (hematoxylin and eosin [H&E] stain). **B:** Portal inflammation (H&E stain). **C:** No fibrosis (trichrome stain). **D:** Bridging fibrosis (trichrome stain). **E:** Cirrhosis (trichrome stain). **F:** Hepatocellular carcinoma (HCC) (H&E stain). (Courtesy of Michael Torbenson, MD.)

relation between HCV and nonspecific symptoms, though they do tend to improve after successful therapy.[58,212,586]

The level of HCV RNA in the blood tends to be stable over long periods of time within 1 $\log_{10}$ of 10^6 IU/mL in 90% of individuals. Conditions associated with modest increases include HIV infection, male gender, and increasing age and body mass index, whereas lower levels may be found in those with ongoing HBV infection and more advanced stage of liver disease.[21,125,288,621,627,635] Although the HCV RNA level in the blood is correlated with the level in the liver,[668] there is not a strong correlation between HCV RNA level and fibrosis progression.

Chronic HCV infection is associated with varying degrees of chronic inflammation and steatosis. Lymphocytic infiltrates are typically found in periportal regions of the liver (Fig. 27.15), though these do not correlate strongly with liver disease progression.[567] For reasons that are not clear, many individuals will not develop significant fibrosis despite decades of high-level viral infection, while others have more production than resorption of collagen, also initially in the periportal region. This process may be stable or progress to formation of septae that expand to form bridges between lobules, and further expansion may result in the severe scarring and regeneration that characterize cirrhosis. Increasing portal venous pressure may lead to portal hypertension and neoplastic transformation may lead to hepatocellular carcinoma, hallmarks of end-stage liver disease.

Although people of African descent are more likely to develop chronic HCV than Caucasians, they appear to have a milder course, with less inflammation and progression to fibrosis.[137,613] One potential explanation for this is differences in frequencies of alleles near certain genes such as *IL28B* that are known to affect clearance and may modulate inflammation, though the mechanisms remain poorly understood.

Alcohol consumption is frequent in persons with chronic HCV and is strongly associated with liver disease progression.[12,493] Along with its well-known hepatotoxicity, alcohol use is associated with reduced access to and early discontinuation of HCV treatment.[23] Elimination of alcohol consumption should be attempted to reduce complications in all persons with chronic HCV.[24,237,443,584,695]

Chronic HCV infection is also associated with metabolic dysfunction including insulin resistance, type 2 diabetes, lipid derangement, and steatosis that may be more common in (but not exclusive to) persons infected with HCV genotype 3 (see Virulence, earlier).[129,281,412,423,463] This association is stronger for HCV than for HBV, suggesting that the mechanism may be specific to HCV.[572,682] Potential contributing mechanisms to metabolic dysfunction in HCV include down-regulation of hepatocyte insulin receptor substrate 1[75] and glucose transporter 2[310] and up-regulation of PP2A (see Innate Immune Response, earlier).[57,175]

Flares of hepatitis (with elevated serum transaminases and/or bilirubin), common in HBV infection,[491] are rare in chronic HCV and should prompt a search for other causes. For example, acute HAV infection during chronic HCV infection may be associated with severe acute hepatitis, including liver failure[656]; for this reason, persons with chronic HCV infection should be vaccinated for HAV and HBV if susceptible.[24]

Hepatocellular Carcinoma

Hepatocellular carcinoma (HCC) is a growing problem in countries like the United States with relatively recent HCV epidemics and is a major established problem in countries like Japan and Egypt where the epidemic of HCV infection occurred 10 to 20 years earlier.[610] Because cirrhosis is often unrecognized, and HCC causes few symptoms until advanced, screening for cirrhosis and HCC is an important aspect of HCV management. Unfortunately, there are few effective, inexpensive screening tools. Serum testing for α-fetoprotein (AFP) has limited diagnostic utility.[82]

Unlike HBV, which is associated with a substantially elevated risk of HCC at all stages of infection, the association of HCC with HCV primarily arises after a person develops cirrhosis.[83,146,550,581] While a direct pathogenetic role of HCV in HCC cannot be dismissed,[101,196,225] and studies in which the core protein was overexpressed under control of a strong promoter have suggested potential for induction of proto-oncogenes and suppression of apoptosis,[105,107,112,414,517–519,551,574,604,707] the data are conflicting,[483] and chronic inflammation may be sufficient to trigger HCC in those cases that precede cirrhosis.[456]

Extrahepatic Manifestations

Although the liver is the principal site of HCV replication, chronic infection is associated with a wide variety of extrahepatic manifestations.[262] A common feature of these conditions is chronic inflammation.

Essential mixed cryoglobulinemia, a condition in which cold-precipitating immune complexes are deposited in multiple organ systems, is strongly associated with HCV infection, though other inflammatory conditions may be implicated. Manifestations often include purpuric rash, weakness, and joint pain but may also include Raynaud syndrome and vasculitis complicated by membranoproliferative glomerulonephritis and neuropathy.[94,404,440] HCV tests are positive for anti-HCV antibodies and HCV RNA in a large proportion of affected individuals,[6] HCV treatment can result in remission,[93,201] and rituximab-mediated B-cell depletion may augment therapeutic response.[542] The chronic stimulation of B cells implicated in HCV-related cryoglobulinemia[543] may also explain the elevated risk (approximately 2.5-fold) of non-Hodgkin lymphoma[144]; mechanistically, the potential for HCV E2 to cross-link the B-cell receptor with the co-stimulatory CD19/CD21/CD81 receptor complex may play a role in development of lymphoma (reviewed in[662]).

Porphyria cutanea tarda (PCT), characterized primarily by disorders of the skin (blistering, hyperpigmentation) and nails (onycholysis) worsened by sun exposure and complicated by scarring, is associated with liver disease and is caused by reduced activity of uroporphyrinogen decarboxylase. It is a multifactorial disease, potentiated by mutations in the *HFE* gene (associated with hereditary hemochromatosis and found in 15% of persons with PCT), as well as HCV infection, alcohol, and estrogen use—all of which should be evaluated in persons presenting with PCT.[72]

Other conditions that may be observed at increased frequency include detection of antithyroid antibodies and, in some studies, increased prevalence of thyroiditis even before interferon therapy (see also Adverse Effects of Peginterferon and Ribavirin Therapy, later).[121,140,157,173,636] The association between chronic HCV infection and thyroiditis has been supported by a meta-analysis, though the mechanism remains unclear.[27,28]

DIAGNOSIS

Clinically, HCV is suspected in persons with otherwise unexplained liver disease. In asymptomatic persons, this infection should be suspected in any person reporting risk factors for infection (see Epidemiology, earlier) or having elevated hepatic transaminases even in the absence of known risk factors, because the infection is highly prevalent. Because of shared risk factors and increased severity of disease, the U.S. Public Health Service recommends HCV testing for all HIV-infected persons upon entry into health care. Because more than two-thirds of persons with HCV infection in the United States were born between 1945 and 1965, the U.S. Public Health Service has recommended that everyone in that "birth cohort" be tested once for HCV infection. The cost-effectiveness of birth cohort testing has already been demonstrated.[526]

Differential Diagnosis

Other viral causes of acute hepatitis (described in Clinical Features, earlier) include the named hepatitis viruses (HAV, HBV with or without the delta hepatitis agent, or hepatitis E virus [HEV]), yellow fever virus, and a wide range of viruses with broader tropism including Epstein-Barr virus (EBV) and cytomegalovirus (CMV). In immunocompromised hosts, adenovirus and other agents with broad tropism can also cause hepatitis. Nonviral causes of acute hepatitis include leptospirosis, tuberculosis, rickettsia and rickettsia-like organisms, numerous toxins (alcohol, acetaminophen, isoniazid, and *Amanita phalloides* toxin being prominent), anoxia/hypoperfusion, and autoimmune disease.

Chronic hepatitis may be caused by HBV and occasionally HEV (in immunocompromised hosts), as well as toxoplasmosis, autoimmune hepatitis, and nonalcoholic steatohepatitis.

Laboratory

The recommended approach for diagnosis of HCV infection is testing for HCV antibodies by enzyme immune assay (EIA). When the screening EIA is positive, the next step is usually to test for HCV RNA to establish that there is ongoing infection.[237]

Serologic Testing

The standard screen for HCV infection is anti-HCV EIA,[24] which detects antibodies to recombinant HCV proteins core, NS3, NS4, and NS5 (see Fig. 27.2).[113,417,457] Additional antibody testing can also be performed using recombinant immunoblot assay (RIBA),[653] which indicates separately the reactivity to antigens that are tested together in the EIA. RIBA is not an independent confirmatory test. Instead, the results indicate whether the antibodies detected on EIA are to HCV or due to nonspecific cross-reactivity.[255] In the situation with a positive HCV EIA and negative HCV RNA result, a positive RIBA indicates that there was indeed prior HCV infection, which may have resolved spontaneously (or from treatment). In that setting a negative RIBA would imply the EIA was falsely positive. The signal strength of EIA may also provide an indication of the specificity of the result,[20,486] though there is no clear cutoff value[563] and current versions of the EIA interpreted according to manufacturer specifications have a specificity of greater than 99%.[122]

Current versions of HCV EIA have increased sensitivity to about 97%[132,647] and become positive within 4 to 8 weeks of infection.[44,135,255] Because specificity is not 100%, positive tests in low-risk individuals may be false-positives, and additional testing such as HCV RNA may be needed.[237,255] Clearance of HCV viremia (spontaneously or after successful treatment) is associated with decreasing antibody levels, sometimes below the level of what would be considered positive on EIA (seroreversion),[372,607] which can complicate inference of past events.

Early reports of false-negative EIA tests in immunocompromised individuals[100] have been addressed in third-generation immunoassays, resulting in a very low rate of false-negatives even in HIV infection and dialysis settings[512,618]; nevertheless, RNA testing should be used if suspected on the basis of elevated risk or hepatic transaminases.[512,598]

Viral Nucleic Acid Detection and Quantitation

Direct viral testing currently depends on detection of the viral genome in plasma or serum, with concentrations expressed in terms of international units (IU).[546] HCV RNA detection methods use reverse transcriptase-polymerase chain reaction (RT-PCR) (qualitative and quantitative), transcription-mediated amplification (TMA), and branched DNA (bDNA) for signal amplification. Approved RT-PCR assays have linear ranges from 1.7 to 7 $\log_{10}$ IU/mL, while bDNA has somewhat lower sensitivity but greater reproducibility.[95] Although TMA has been shown to detect low-level viremia in some specimens that are negative by RT-PCR, TMA and RT-PCR assays appear to have equivalent utility in detecting HCV RNA during or at the end of treatment to predict sustained virologic response (SVR).[74,447] Though most assays have targeted the 5′ UTR due to its relatively high conservation, it is feasible to detect or quantitate HCV RNA by targeting the extremely conserved 3′ terminus of the genome.[171]

HCV Genotype Determination

HCV genotype is the strongest single biological predictor of HCV treatment success.[24] Commercially available assays depend on amplification of targets near the 5′ end of the genome and use sequencing or reverse hybridization to determine genotype (and, in some cases, subtype). Mixed infections occur but are uncommon. The gold standard for genotype determination is phylogenetic analysis of nucleotide sequences obtained from a phylogenetically informative genomic region; by international consensus, either the E1 or NS5B region may be used for definitive assignment.[128,577,591]

Liver Disease Staging

Because the progression of HCV-related liver disease is highly variable, staging is important for informing treatment decisions, lifestyle modification, and prognosis. Although the liver biopsy remains the reference standard for staging and provides a wealth of information beyond fibrosis stage, it is invasive and expensive, and other modalities are gaining prominence as they are validated.

Liver biopsy is the standard reference tool for assessing liver fibrosis grade (inflammation) and stage (fibrosis). Tissue examination may detect other causes of liver disease, as well as conditions such as iron overload and steatosis that are important contributors to HCV-related liver disease and may help guide therapy. Histologic stage is assigned on a standard scale, with widely used examples including Batts-Ludwig,[50] International Association for the Study of the Liver (IASL),[156] Metavir, and Ishak.[51a,289] Scores range from no fibrosis to cirrhosis, staged as 0 to 4 (for Batts-Ludwig, IASL, and Metavir) or 0 to 6 (for Ishak). In addition to cost and discomfort, the value of a liver biopsy is limited by sampling error and imprecision[120]; its value is being reassessed and noninvasive alternatives are being evaluated.

Noninvasive markers of fibrosis offer the potential for more frequent assessment than the standard liver biopsy interval of 4 to 5 years. Serum markers (only some of which are approved by the Food and Drug Administration [FDA]) and sonographic elastography (a measure of liver stiffness, not yet evaluated by the FDA, but widely available in Europe) are most informative at the extremes, whereas intermediate values may not discriminate well between mild and severe fibrosis.[237,533]

PREVENTION AND CONTROL

Treatment

All currently approved regimens for treating HCV infection include type I interferon, with the highest response rates associated with pegylated interferon (peginterferon) alfa plus ribavirin, with or without a protease inhibitor (reviewed in[554]). While effective in most participants in clinical trials, HCV treatment remains expensive and is associated with significant side effects. When liver transplantation is necessary, HCV infection of the graft is inevitable without treatment.[188,505,513]

TABLE 27.2 Hepatitis C Virus Direct-Acting Antivirals in Current Phase III Studies

Agent	Drug Class
Asunaprevir (BMS-650032)	NS3-NS4A protease inhibitor
Faldaprevir (BI201335)	NS3-NS4A protease inhibitor
Simeprevir (TMC435)	NS3-NS4A protease inhibitor
Vaniprevir (MK-7009)	NS3-NS4A protease inhibitor
Daclatasvir (BMS-790052)	NS5A inhibitor
Sofosbuvir (GS-7977)	NS5B polymerase inhibitor
Silymarin	NS5B Polymerase inhibitor

The only direct-acting antivirals (DAAs) currently approved in the United States or Europe for HCV treatment are the protease inhibitors boceprevir[356] and telaprevir,[275,418] which are reversibly covalent inhibitors of the NS3-NS4A serine protease. Additional DAAs are in advanced (phase III) development (Table 27.2), including noncovalent NS3-NS4A protease inhibitors (asunaprevir/BMS-650032, faldaprevir/BI201335, simeprevir/TMC435, and vaniprevir/MK-7009), an NS5A inhibitor (daclatasvir), and NS5B polymerase inhibitors (sofosbuvir/GS-7977 and silymarin).

Goals of Treatment

The principal goal of antiviral therapy is the amelioration or prevention of disease. Because not all patients are affected by HCV in the same way and because there can be serious adverse events, treatment is individualized. In 2009, guidelines for use of peginterferon and ribavirin suggested the benefits of treatment would outweigh the risks for persons most likely to respond (e.g., genotype 2 infection) and those most in need (e.g., significant fibrosis) and those with the fewest complicating medical problems (e.g., no depression). However, because there are so many factors to consider, treatment decisions were often individualized.[237] Recent therapeutic advances have added even more variables, and selection of the patient for treatment remains a highly individualized practice.

The primary goal of therapy is SVR, defined as undetectable HCV RNA 24 weeks after the end of a treatment regimen (Fig. 27.16); SVR appears to represent a cure of infection. This outcome is associated with loss of intrahepatic RNA and histologic improvement.[62,367,403] The durability of SVR was assessed in a study of 1,343 people from nine randomized multicenter trials who had SVR after interferon-based treatment,[605] demonstrating that 99.1% remained HCV RNA negative after an average follow-up of 4 years. Whether the 0.9% of persons with recurrent viremia had relapse or were reinfected was not known.

In contrast to SVR, other outcomes are often described as follows (Fig. 27.16): null nonresponse, consistently detectable HCV RNA with less than 2 $\log_{10}$ reduction by week 24; partial response, consistently detectable HCV RNA with reduction by more than 2 $\log_{10}$ at week 24; breakthrough, suppression to undetectable HCV RNA level that becomes detectable again during therapy; and relapse, suppression of HCV RNA to undetectable levels through the completion of treatment

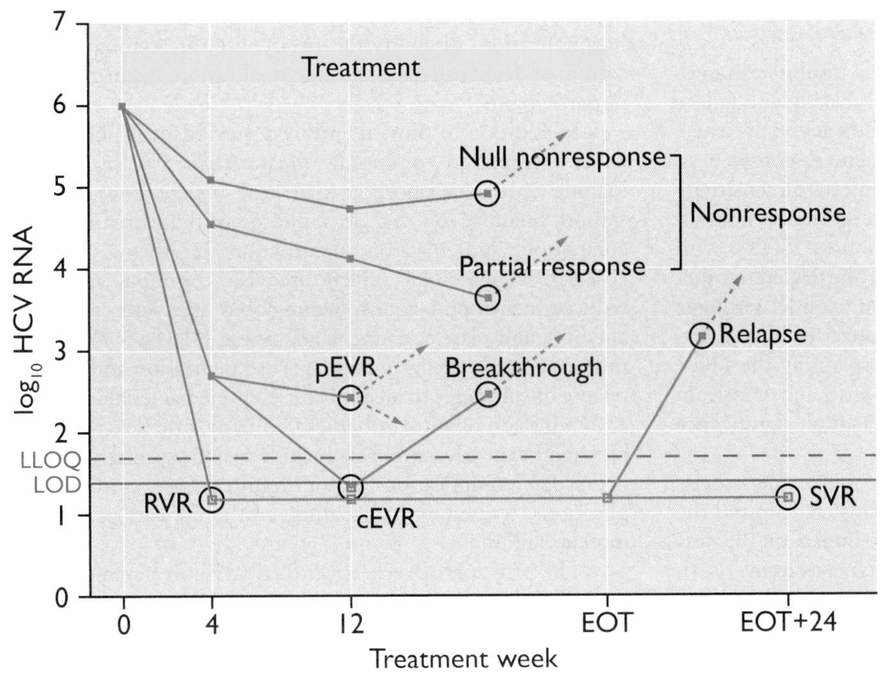

FIGURE 27.16. Outcomes and patterns of treatment response at times during treatment and at end of treatment (EOT). Outcomes (sustained virologic response [SVR], relapse, breakthrough, and nonresponse) are predicted by early patterns of viral response: rapid, complete early, and partial early virologic response (RVR, cEVR, and pEVR, respectively). Dashed arrows indicate subsequent trajectory of viremia. LLOQ, lower limit of quantitation; LOD, limit of detection.

followed by viremia during subsequent follow-up. Nonresponse can be used to describe collectively the null response and incomplete response patterns (i.e., to distinguish from those who achieve viral suppression), though these terms are not used uniformly (nonresponse is sometimes used to refer specifically to null response).

Mechanisms of Action

Interferon-α

Type I interferons are antiviral and regulate proliferation and immunity. Encoded by more than 10 IFN-α genes and one IFN-β gene, these proteins bind the type I interferon receptor, a heterodimer of IFNAR1 and IFNAR2[114] that signals through the JAK-STAT pathway to induce hundreds of interferon-stimulated genes (ISGs).[317] Among these ISGs are PKR, 2,5-OAS, and MxA. These ISGs and others are typically up-regulated during acute HCV infection.[60] Antiviral effects of activated PKR include phosphorylation and inactivation of eukaryotic translation initiation factor 2A (EIF2A) and nuclear localization of nuclear factor (NF)-κB; in addition, HCV NS5A can bind and interfere with PKR function.[224] Type I interferons also up-regulate MHC class I expression and NK cell killing functions.[61] Currently recommended therapy is based on peginterferon α due to greater efficacy than other interferon preparations currently available.[237] These are derivatives of IFN-α (2a or 2b) to which polyethylene glycol has been added for improved pharmacokinetics and efficacy.[219,264,402]

Ribavirin

Like type I interferons, ribavirin is broadly antiviral and is effective as a component of HCV therapy; however, its principal mode of anti-HCV action is unclear.[485] As an inhibitor of inosine monophosphate dehydrogenase and via direct interaction with RNA polymerases, ribavirin may increase the error rate of the HCV RNA-directed RNA polymerase to a level that induces lethal mutagenesis,[139] an effect that may be inapparent at high replication levels but may be unmasked in combination therapy.[161,361] Alternatively, ribavirin may have immunomodulatory effects.[529] In clinical trials, the most pronounced effect of ribavirin is reduction of viremia relapse after completion of therapy.[219]

Efficacy of Combination Therapy with Pegylated Interferon and Ribavirin

The standard regimen for treatment of chronic HCV infection is subcutaneous injection of peginterferon α (180 μg of 2a, or 1.5 μg/kg of 2b) weekly. Patients take ribavirin orally with half the daily dose each morning and night; those with genotypes 2 and 3 receive 800 mg daily and those with genotype 1 receive 800–1,400 mg based on body weight.[237]

Outcomes with the two peginterferon α formulations (2a or 2b) in combination with ribavirin are comparable, with approximately 40% and 80% of previously untreated patients with chronic HCV genotype 1 versus genotype 2 or 3 achieving a sustained virologic response, respectively.[219,402] The optimal duration of therapy varies by genotype, with genotype 1 requiring 48 weeks of therapy and persons without HIV infection who have HCV genotype 2 or 3 achieving high rates of SVR with 24 weeks of therapy.[264]

Predictors of Treatment Success During Interferon-Based Therapy

Well-established determinants of clinical response to these drugs include HCV genotype (genotypes 2, 3, 5, and 6 most responsive, genotype 1 least responsive), HIV infection (coinfection less responsive), stage of liver disease (early stage more responsive than cirrhosis), race (Asians more responsive than Caucasians, who are more responsive than persons with African ancestry), age (<40 years more responsive), sex (females more responsive than males), baseline HCV RNA level (lower levels more responsive), and body weight (lower weight more responsive).[26,36,52,148,158,167,202,303,409,410,487,640,641,667,702,703,710] Though not uniformly measured, insulin resistance (see Clinical Features, earlier) is strongly associated with failure of interferon-based therapy.[124,155,646] Within genotype, there appear to be viral determinants of treatment responsiveness, particularly in the NS5A (specifically, the interferon sensitivity determining region, or ISDR[180]) and core proteins, summarized in Tavis et al[611]; inconsistent detection of ISDRs, with differences among distinct populations, may be related to other differences among those populations,[481] with subtler virologic determinants unmasked only when the impact of host genetics is minimized. Long-range correlations spanning the HCV genome[34,165] might affect treatment response and constrain evolution of resistance,[164] but their biological significance remains to be demonstrated.

It was recently discovered through a genome-wide association study that a series of polymorphisms clustered around the IL28B gene (encoding IFN-λ3) has a major impact on the outcome of HCV treatment[233] (as well as spontaneous recovery[623]), summarized in.[41] The protective haplotype is enriched in Asian populations, uncommon in African populations, and intermediate in Caucasians; this genotype correlates well with overall success rates of interferon-based therapy, explains about half of the effect of race on treatment success, and may explain divergent findings from different races regarding the importance of HCV polymorphisms in ISDR and core noted earlier. Clinical testing for *IL28B* polymorphisms became available within a year of that discovery, ostensibly to assist in prediction of treatment response, yet the mechanism of this effect remains poorly understood. The presence of the protective *IL28B* haplotype is also associated prior to the start of therapy with lower intrahepatic ISG expression,[277] which in turn was previously shown to predict treatment success.[109,552] Taken together, these results suggest that *IL28B* genotype is one of multiple factors contributing to the phenotype associated with treatment response.[41]

Uncommonly, HCV infection is detected during the acute phase.[398] Compared to chronic infection, acute HCV infection is more responsive to interferon-based treatment with overall SVR rates greater than 80%, and the response is significantly less genotype dependent than during chronic infection.[294] A recent meta-analysis supports monitoring for up to 12 weeks after presentation with acute HCV and in those with persistent viremia using interferon-based therapy[130] such as peginterferon with ribavirin.[68] Rates of SVR in HIV-infected individuals with acute HCV may be lower.[358]

Adverse Effects of Pegylated Interferon and Ribavirin Therapy

Most recipients of the combination of peginterferon α and ribavirin experience adverse medication effects. Patients receiving standard doses of peginterferon α-2a or -2b in a large trial (more than 1,000 participants receiving each drug),[419] the following adverse effects were reported: fatigue (63% to 66%), headache (42% to 50%), nausea (36% to 42%), insomnia (39% to 41%), pyrexia (23% to 35%), anemia (34%), myalgia (22% to 27%), neutropenia (26% to 31%), depression (21% to 25%), irritability (25%), or rash (22% to 28%).

Adverse events resulted in early discontinuation of treatment in 13% of those participants and dose reduction in 43%. Serious adverse events (resulting in new or prolonged hospitalization, disability/incapacity, life-threatening complication, or death) attributed to the medications occurred in 4% of participants.

In addition to those mentioned previously, major adverse effects[278] reported commonly (greater than 5%) by patients include arthralgia, anorexia, diarrhea, anxiety, poor concentration, memory loss, hair loss, photosensitivity, itching, nasal congestion, and injection site reactions (erythema, pain, or abscess). Hematologic effects are also common, including reduced neutrophil count, hemoglobin (see later regarding anemia), and platelet count. Uncommon (1% to 5%) but significant adverse effects include marked depression and anxiety, relapse of substance or alcohol abuse, severe bacterial infection, and induction of autoantibodies. Similarly, rare (less than 1%) but significant adverse effects include major psychiatric events, neurologic complications, autoimmune disease, cardiac complications, worsening of hepatitis, and renal, cardiac, or pulmonary failure.

The principal adverse effect of ribavirin is hemolytic anemia. The degree of anemia is highly variable, in part due to polymorphisms in the gene for inosine triphosphatase (ITPA); the protective alleles are associated with reduced ITPA activity and intraerythrocyte accumulation of inosine triphosphate, providing potential for pharmacologic intervention that would make ribavirin less toxic.[198] In combination with peginterferon (which contributes to anemia), ribavirin dose reduction is required in 25% of patients treated for genotype 1 infection and must be discontinued in less than 5%.[419]

Viral Dynamics

As increasingly potent therapy approaches an abrupt halt in virus production, mathematical modeling has provided increasingly precise estimates of viral dynamics because at steady state (just prior to initiation of therapy) the rate of virion clearance must equal the rate of virion production.[405,468,490] The implications of viral dynamic modeling include providing testable hypotheses regarding therapeutic mechanisms, evaluating the contributions of immunologic control to therapeutic efficacy, and predicting clinical outcomes including drug resistance.[535]

Initiation of antiviral treatment is followed by a delay that varies among drug regimens and then a decline in viremia that fits a biphasic decay model.[468] Current models provide estimates of an HCV half-life as short as 45 minutes (reviewed in[143]). The 7- to 10-hour delay observed following treatment initiation of interferon-based therapy may be due to interferon signaling[143] and is shortened to 2 hours with DAA-based therapy.[227] The subsequent first phase of decline, lasting 1 to 2 days, is rapid and attributed primarily to viral clearance unmasked by reduced production. A second, slower phase of decline may be attributed to clearance of infected cells (either through cell death or termination of productive HCV infection). Because early viral dynamics are linked to drug efficacy, it is reasonable to expect that they would be predictive of outcome.

In clinical trials, early viral dynamics have been found to predict outcome with sufficient accuracy so that they are now used to guide early therapeutic decisions from stopping rules to adjustments in treatment duration. Increasingly potent regimens have required enhanced precision of these definitions, and such changes are likely to continue.

Early Virologic Response (Week 12 Response)

Lack of HCV RNA suppression at week 12 (lack of early virologic response [EVR]) consistently predicts failure of treatment. When defined as reduction of HCV by at least 2 $\log_{10}$, the proportion of treatment-naïve individuals who went on to achieve SVR in the context of treatment with peginterferon α-2a or -2b was 0% to 3%,[149,219] and EVR was generally adopted as a "stopping rule" due to futility. The positive predictive value of EVR in those studies was low, with 65% to 72% achieving SVR. When EVR was subdivided into complete EVR (cEVR, lack of detectable HCV RNA at week 12, Fig. 27.16) versus partial EVR (pEVR, EVR with detectable HCV RNA at week 12), the proportion going on to SVR was 74% to 83% versus 21% to 38%, but cEVR was achieved in only 64% to 65% of those treated with combination therapy[149,219] for mixed genotype cohorts, and in only 40% to 45% of persons with genotype 1.[419]

Rapid Virologic Response (Week 4 Response)

Just as slow response is highly predictive of treatment failure, rapid response is highly predictive of treatment success. In treatment-naïve persons with chronic HCV genotype 1, 80% to 92% of patients treated with peginterferon α-2a or -2b and ribavirin who achieved a rapid virologic response (RVR, undetectable viremia at week 4) went on to achieve SVR,[200,419] though only 11% to 12% of treatment-naïve patients with HCV genotype 1 achieved RVR when treated with peginterferon α-2a or -2b.

RVR is also associated with comparable success rates with shorter durations of therapy. For genotype 1–infected individuals, shortening the duration of peginterferon α-2a therapy from 48 to 24 weeks is associated with higher failure rates overall, but in the subset with RVR the outcomes are comparable.[264,296] For genotype 2– and 3–infected individuals with early-stage fibrosis and low baseline HCV RNA levels, shortening the treatment duration from 24 to 12 or 16 weeks in those with RVR may be appropriate.[237]

Less than 1 $\log_{10}$ reduction in HCV RNA at week 4 (which occurred in 10% to 11% of patients) also had strong negative predictive value in genotype 1–infected patients treated with peginterferon and ribavirin, with less than 5% of these individuals achieving SVR.[419] In contrast, lack of RVR in this setting has a poor negative predictive value.

Boceprevir and Telaprevir

In May 2011, the NS3-NS4A serine protease inhibitors boceprevir (formerly SCH503034) and telaprevir (formerly VX-950) were approved by the FDA for use in combination with peginterferon and ribavirin for treatment of chronic HCV genotype 1 infection.[537] These linear tetrapeptide analogs bind to the NS3 protease active site with a ketoamide center that functions as a covalent serine trap.[380,472]

Short-term monotherapy with these agents demonstrated significant but incomplete reductions in HCV RNA level, and more detailed study of specimens from the telaprevir trial showed rapid emergence of resistance.[555,556] Clinical trials of boceprevir (recommended dose 800 mg with food every 7 to 9 hours) or telaprevir (recommended dose 750 mg with fat-containing food every 7 to 9 hours), in combination with peginterferon and ribavirin at standard doses, resulted in approximately 70% SVR, compared with 40% SVR in those treated with the prior standard of care.[275,356,418]

Boceprevir therapy includes a 4-week lead-in phase of peginterferon and ribavirin, followed by addition of boceprevir. The total duration can be fixed at 48 weeks (4-week lead-in plus 44 weeks of triple therapy). Alternatively, treatment-naïve patients without cirrhosis may be treated using response-guided therapy (RGT) during which early HCV RNA dynamics determine treatment duration: if HCV RNA is undetectable at week 8 (week 4 of boceprevir), the duration of triple therapy is 28 weeks (24 weeks of boceprevir); if HCV RNA is detectable at any visit after week 8 but negative at week 24 and subsequent visits, boceprevir is discontinued at week 36 and peginterferon and ribavirin are continued for an additional 12 weeks. RGT is recommended only for treatment-naïve patients without cirrhosis, and all treatment should be discontinued if the HCV RNA level is greater than 100 IU/mL at treatment week 12, or detectable at week 24.[236]

Telaprevir is initiated as part of triple therapy and continued for 12 weeks, after which peginterferon and ribavirin are continued to the end of treatment. For treatment-naïve patients without cirrhosis that have an *extended RVR,* defined as HCV RNA undetected at weeks 4 and 12, duration of therapy can be abbreviated at 24 weeks; for others (with cirrhosis and/or slower response dynamics), peginterferon and ribavirin are continued to complete an overall treatment duration of 48 weeks. All treatment should be discontinued if the HCV RNA level is greater than 1,000 IU/mL at week 4 or week 12 or detectable at week 24.[236]

In treatment-experienced patients with HCV genotype 1, boceprevir- or telaprevir-containing triple therapy resulted in overall rates of SVR that were much higher than for peginterferon plus ribavirin, 64% to 66% versus 17% to 21%.[37,704] Not surprisingly, these rates varied depending on the dynamics of the prior treatment response, with 75% to 83% of prior relapsed patients achieving SVR and only 52% to 59% of prior partial responders achieving SVR after triple therapy. Prior null responders (Fig. 27.16) were excluded from the boceprevir trial,[37] but in the telaprevir trial 29% of prior null responders achieved an SVR; most prior null responders who did not achieve SVR had detectable treatment-emergent resistance mutations.[704]

Resistance to Boceprevir and Telaprevir

Boceprevir and telaprevir select for characteristic changes at NS3 codons 36 (V to M, A, or L), 54 (T to A or S), 155 (R to K or T), 156 (A to S, T, or V), and 168 (D to N) both *in vitro* and *in vivo.*[432,612] Based on *in vitro* models of single substitutions, V36A/M is expected to have a modest impact both on resistance (4-fold increased IC_{50}) and replication capacity (less than 10% reduction), A156V/T the greatest impact on resistance (greater than 50-fold increased IC_{50}) and replication capacity (>50% reduction), and the other substitutions are expected to be intermediate between those extremes.[555] Combined substitutions at codons 36+155 or codons 36+156 have enhanced resistance and fitness relative to the 155 and 156 single substitutions. Changes at other NS3 codons, including 43 and 55, are less consistently observed and may have less-pronounced impact on resistance.

In the pivotal phase 3 trials in which boceprevir was combined with peginterferon and ribavirin, baseline viral sequence data were available for 980 patients treated with boceprevir. Analysis of these NS3 sequences revealed 43 patients (4%)

with pretreatment resistance-associated variants V36M, T54A/S, V55A, and/or R155K.[432] The SVR rate in this population was 65% (28/43). Among the 36 patients in this subgroup who were interferon responsive (greater than or equal to 1 log_{10} reduction in HCV RNA during 4-week peginterferon/ribavirin lead-in therapy), the SVR rate was 78% (28/36), comparable to the 73% to 81% SVR rate observed in the overall population of interferon-responsive patients. Therefore, in this small subpopulation, the response did not appear to be hampered by the presence of high-level resistance mutations at baseline as long as patients were responsive to lead-in peginterferon/ribavirin. In the seven patients with high-level resistance mutations at baseline who were nonresponsive to interferon as defined by a less than 1 log_{10} reduction in HCV RNA during the 4-week peginterferon/ribavirin lead-in therapy, SVR was not observed. By contrast, in the overall population, 28% to 38% of patients who were nonresponsive to interferon during the 4-week lead-in period achieved SVR. Currently, there is no clinical indication for baseline resistance testing.[236]

In agreement with the aforementioned baseline data, the R155K substitution has been observed in untreated individuals with chronic HCV[350] and may represent an escape mutant for an HLA-A*68–restricted T-cell epitope.[548] At baseline and after unsuccessful treatment, R155K resistance substitutions are observed more frequently in persons with HCV subtype 1a infection than those with subtype 1b infection, reflecting a lower genetic barrier for subtype 1a.[555] Specifically, for subtype 1a codon R155 is AGG, requiring only one nucleotide substitution to become AAG (K), whereas for subtype 1b the same R155 is encoded by CGG and requires two changes to become AAG.

Following termination of unsuccessful treatment with boceprevir or telaprevir, the frequency of resistant variants tends to decay and wild-type variants predominate in peripheral blood.[603] Whether the frequency of resistant variants returns to pretreatment baseline or will have an impact on future treatment success is not known. Current understanding of viral dynamics and resistance supports discontinuation of failing DAA-based therapy as early as possible to avoid an increase in the frequency and fitness (through compensatory mutation) of resistant variants, to preserve future treatment options.[236]

Adverse Effects of Boceprevir and Telaprevir

Both boceprevir and telaprevir are associated with increased frequency and severity of anemia relative to peginterferon and ribavirin.[292,504] Management of anemia by reducing ribavirin dose was not associated with a reduced rate of SVR in these trials.[236]

Rash is the most prominent adverse effect associated with telaprevir, with rash noted in 56% versus 32% of those receiving telaprevir, peginterferon, and ribavirin versus those receiving only peginterferon and ribavirin, respectively.[292] In 4% of cases the rash was severe (involving at least 50% of the body surface area), in 6% of cases telaprevir was discontinued due to rash, and in 1% of cases the entire regimen was discontinued due to rash.

Drug–Drug Interactions

In a manner analogous to (but distinct from) HIV protease inhibitors, preliminary studies reveal that boceprevir and telaprevir have significant interactions with other drugs as a result of metabolism by and inhibition of hepatic cytochromes. The range of drugs potentially affected is large and likely to change frequently; clinicians must consult authoritative references for specific information about concomitant medications.

Investigational Agents

Discoveries revealing key steps in the life cycle of HCV have provided promising targets for antiviral development, including HCV p7,[393] NS3-NS4A protease, NS3 helicase, NS4B,[178,179] NS5A,[370] NS5B polymerase,[429] NS5A–cyclophilin interaction,[119,208,257,453] and miR122.[364,657] Drugs discussed here have completed or are currently in phase 3 trials (Table 27.2). A notable challenge for drug design is the NS3 helicase, which has been difficult to target selectively.[218]

NS3 protease inhibitor classes include linear covalent (FDA-approved agents boceprevir and telaprevir), linear noncovalent, and macrocyclic compounds. The pharmacokinetics, potency, and resistance profiles of NS3 protease inhibitors vary. NS3 protease inhibitors currently in FDA phase 3 development (Table 27.2) include two noncovalent linear inhibitors (asunaprevir/BMS-650032 and BI 201335) and two macrocyclic inhibitors (TMC435350 and vaniprevir/MK-7009).

Daclatasvir/BMC-790052 is a potent inhibitor of NS5A that was used, in combination with asunaprevir, in the first interferon-sparing regimen with a significant rate of SVR (36% in prior nonresponders to peginterferon and ribavirin).[388] In this small phase 2a study of patients with chronic HCV genotype 1, 4 of 11 patients who received the interferon-sparing regimen had SVR, and 9 of 10 patients who received peginterferon alfa-2a and ribavirin in addition to asunaprevir and daclatasvir had an SVR. Mild to moderate diarrhea affected most patients in both groups but did not require dose modification.

Small-molecule NS5B polymerase inhibitors include active site nucleoside/nucleotide analogs (competitors and chain terminators) and drugs that bind outside the active site. The latter have multiple potential binding sites in the thumb and palm domains of the NS5B crystal structure. GS-7977 (previously PSI-7977), a chain terminator nucleotide analog prodrug,[450] which has *in vitro* activity against genotypes 1, 2, and 3,[359] was recently reported to achieve SVR in some subjects with HCV genotypes 2 and 3 who received an interferon-free regimen.[226]

Silymarin, an extract of milk thistle, has been shown to have anti-inflammatory properties,[502,503] but it has been difficult to assess such studies due to the fact that silymarin is a mixture of many compounds and standardization has been difficult. Silibinin, which is a component of silymarin, directly inhibits NS5B polymerase.[7]

Vaccines

There is no licensed vaccine for HCV, in spite of substantial interest given the high burden of disease worldwide,[688,689] ongoing community and nosocomial transmission,[97,358,484] limited access to treatment in populations at highest risk,[211,425] evidence for protection from passive immunization (see later), and evidence for protective immunity against chronic infection after primary infection in humans[424,478] and chimpanzees.[363] The two major vaccine categories, prophylactic (preventive) and therapeutic, may share mechanistic features but have different goals and rationales. It is important to note that unlike most viral infections, a prophylactic vaccine for HCV might include a vaccine that allows (typically mild) acute infection but prevents chronic infection.

Passive Immunization

Passive immunization can be highly protective for some viral infections (e.g., hepatitis B virus, varicella-zoster virus), though its role in HCV infection has not been established and no FDA-licensed anti-HCV immune globulin preparation is available. Unlike HBV, HCV viremia was delayed but not prevented in chimpanzees treated with anti-HCV immune globulin postexposure.[341] Indirect evidence for protection by passive immunization was gleaned from HCV infections that occurred after anti-HCV–positive donations were excluded from commercial immunoglobulin preparations prior to the implementation of nucleic acid testing for HCV.[78] More recent studies, augmented by pseudoparticle-based neutralization assays (see Humoral Immune Response, earlier)[46] and use of the chimpanzee model, revealed evidence for passive protection by neutralizing antibodies *in vitro* and *in vivo*.[699]

Investigations of passive immunization have been facilitated by the development of humanized mouse models of HCV entry and infection (see Model Systems In Vivo, earlier). A genetically humanized mouse model demonstrated protection by passive immunization, using entry (without replication) as a surrogate for infection.[168] Similarly, use of the Alb-uPA SCID mouse model with engrafted human liver has demonstrated neutralization *in vivo* by polyclonal serum,[655] though neutralization may be less efficient *in vivo* than *in vitro*.[434] These systems also support identification and evaluation of broadly neutralizing monoclonal antibodies.[80,238,369] Studies of maternal–infant transmission of HCV, a setting in which passive immunization might be anticipated, has not revealed correlation between protection and the presence of neutralizing antibodies in the serum of mother or child.[169,435]

Prophylactic Vaccine Development

Natural infection with HCV generates an immune response that is initially robust and is largely maintained in those who spontaneously clear viremia (see Immune Response, earlier). Prior infection does not prevent reinfection in humans[8,253,478] or chimpanzees,[87,189] but chronicity is greatly reduced in secondary infections[254,424,478] even with heterologous challenge.[363] Although a portion of this apparent protection may be due to host differences,[41,325,617,623] known genetic markers explain only a minority of the clearance phenotype.

A meta-analysis of vaccine studies in chimpanzees (including 63 naïve, 53 vaccinated, and 36 rechallenged animals),[141] most of which were challenged with homologous virus, revealed that HCV-specific immune responses were generated and reduced the rate of chronic infection ($p < .001$) in vaccinated animals (28%) relative to naïve animals (62%) and similarly to rechallenged animals (17%). Peak RNA levels and duration of viremia were also reduced by vaccination. Assays for T-cell responses by IFN-γ ELISpot, performed in only a small number of animals, did not predict efficacy; however, vaccine antigens based on structural proteins were significantly ($p = .01$) more protective (14% chronicity) than those containing nonstructural proteins (46% chronicity). This latter finding is at odds with the highly protective effect of prior cleared HCV infection (i.e., rechallenge after exposure to the full genome) and the consistent importance of HLA class I alleles[469] and CD8 T cells[573] in spontaneous resolution. Therefore, past vaccines have not achieved the protection afforded by natural infection, and further optimization of antigen, adjuvant, vector, route, and/or schedule is needed.

The protective role of antibody responses in HCV infection remains controversial, in part due to data demonstrating an essential role for CD8 T cells in spontaneous clearance[573] in association with a strong CD4 T-cell response[251] and evidence that individuals with congenital agammaglobulinemia can clear infection without treatment.[4] Additionally, hyperimmune serum appeared to be only partially protective in the chimpanzee model[194] due to breakthrough of minor sequence variants, and the extreme variability of the HCV envelope gene (see Genetic Diversity) may limit the breadth of protection provided by an antibody-based vaccine or passive immunization. Nonetheless, antibodies generated by chimpanzees after two vaccinations with recombinant E1 + E2 from the HCV-1 strain (subtype 1a) neutralized HCVpp and HCVcc constructs with envelope proteins derived from genotypes 1, 4, 5, and 6.[437] Similarly, vaccination of mice and macaques with HCVpp displaying E1 and/or E2 from subtype 1a stimulated production of antibodies that neutralized HCV genotypes 1, 2, 4, and 5.[230] E1E2 subunit vaccination of a small number of healthy human volunteers elicited antibody responses that neutralized heterologous isolates.[217,516,587]

Vaccines that elicit robust T-cell responses without neutralizing antibodies may not prevent new HCV infections, but they may prevent chronic infection[210] and associated serious complications. As noted previously (see Immune Response), spontaneous resolution is associated with broadly targeted, polyfunctional CD4 and CD8 T-cell responses. Adenovirus serotypes rarely or never found in humans (addressing the problem of pre-existing immunity[123]) and expressing HCV NS3-NS5B proteins were recently used to vaccinate healthy volunteers, resulting in sustained T-cell responses targeting multiple viral proteins.[43] It is not known whether such a vaccine will prevent chronic HCV infection in humans.

Therapeutic Vaccine Development

A therapeutic vaccine, to be used during chronic infection to augment pharmacologic therapy, modulate chronic disease outcome, or clear chronic infection, is an attractive goal for improving the health of many millions of people with limited treatment options. As an adjunct to conventional antiviral therapy, a therapeutic vaccine would have the potential to reduce duration and/or dose of antivirals, thereby reducing toxicity, cost, and failure rate. Evidence of low-level viremia at end of treatment in persons who subsequently experience relapse underscores the potential value of this approach; in addition, suppression of viremia during therapy may optimize the immune system's ability to augment responses that were previously suppressed by the tolerizing effects of chronic viremia.

Therapeutic vaccines have demonstrated modest efficacy in pilot studies, illustrating the challenge of stimulating immune responses to a chronic infection. Humans injected with E1 protein subunit developed anti-E1 responses but no significant change in viremia or inflammation.[471,676] IC41, a multiepitope peptide-based vaccine, stimulated peptide-specific CD4 and CD8 responses in healthy volunteers,[205,206] had inconsistent effects on the level of viremia in chronic infection,[333] and induced HCV-specific T-cell responses near the end of interferon-based treatment without preventing relapse.[677] TG4040, a modified vaccinia Ankara (MVA) vaccine using an attenuated poxvirus to express NS3-NS5B proteins, stimulated measurable T-cell responses in a minority of recipients, some of whom had transient reductions in viremia.[263]

Prevention of Transmission of HCV

Because the transmission routes of HCV are well defined (see Transmission, earlier), behavioral measures for prevention can be effective if applied consistently. HCV transmission by medical procedures can be stopped by strict observance of infection control protocols.[239,293,512] Although blood transfusions were once an important route of HCV transmission, transfusion transmission has virtually been eliminated by testing donors for HCV antibodies and RNA.[399] Nonetheless, even in some economically developed nations, HCV transmission still occurs in hospitals and traditional medical centers. In one report from Spain, 67% of acute HCV infections were linked to receipt of medical care.[408] The World Health Organization estimates that unsafe injections continue to cause 2.3 million to 4.7 million new HCV infections each year.[283]

HIV Co-Infection with HCV

The complications of HCV are more frequent and severe in persons with HIV, leading to HCV's designation in 1999 as an opportunistic infection,[99,595] and liver disease related to viral hepatitis continues to be a major cause of death among persons with HIV worldwide.[674] For these reasons, people with HIV should be screened for HCV upon entry into care, for any unexplained elevation of hepatic transaminases, and periodically in the setting of risky behavior.

Due primarily to shared routes of transmission, approximately one-quarter of persons with HIV infection also have HCV infection.[619] HIV infection increases the likelihood of transmission of HCV from mother to child[274,624,700] and among men who have sex with men.[240,249,645,648,649,651,652] After exposure to HCV infection, the likelihood of becoming chronically infected is higher in persons with HIV infection,[391,424,433,620] and in those with chronic infection, progression to end-stage liver disease is more frequent and rapid in those with HIV.[242,250,596] HCV RNA levels in persons with HIV are higher than in those without HIV.[186,621,622,627] There has been concern about evidence of fibrosis progression in the first 1 to 2 years of HCV infection in some cohorts,[203] though pre-existing liver disease could not be excluded, fibrosis has not previously been assessed during acute infection, and longer follow-up is needed to clarify this issue.[663]

Whether chronic HCV infection alters the course of HIV or the response to antiretroviral therapy is not clear. Greub and co-workers[256] suggested that even among the subset of HIV/HCV co-infected persons in whom HIV was fully suppressed by antiretroviral therapy, CD4 lymphocyte responses were reduced compared to HIV-infected controls without HCV. Sulkowski and co-workers[597] failed to detect an association once the strong interaction of HCV and injection drug use was considered. What is clear is that adherence to antiretroviral therapy is the dominant determinant of clinical outcomes in HIV/HCV co-infected persons.

Even though treatment of HIV in persons with HIV may be complicated by hepatotoxicity[3,126,152,244,256,416,475,508,534,593,598,599–600,619] significant complications are rare, therapy can be monitored and adjusted, and antiretroviral therapy appears to reduce liver disease progression.[54,77,510] Treatment of HCV in those co-infected with HIV is more complicated due to cytopenias and other toxicities, and concomitant therapies increase the potential for drug–drug interactions, particularly with direct-acting antiviral agents for HCV.[594] These challenges, and the lower likelihood of SVR in persons with HIV infection (discussed in the Treatment section earlier), underscore the need for safer and more effective antiviral agents for HCV.

PERSPECTIVE

A more detailed understanding of the HCV life cycle remains a high priority; we have limited understanding of the trade-offs between replication and virion production, their basis in the viral sequence, and how these are modulated. Current model systems are incompatible with "wild" isolates, and a robust immunocompetent small-animal model is sorely needed. Our nascent understanding of the systems biology of antiviral immunity is underscored by the puzzle of *IL28B* polymorphisms and HCV: intense study has failed to identify the key genetic determinant and its mechanism, with potentially broad implications for innate and adaptive antiviral immunity; this is made more interesting by the relative lack of effect of *IL28B* polymorphisms on HBV or HIV pathogenesis.[407] Epidemiology of HCV, including genotype distribution, is rarely obtained on a population basis; more accurate assessment would have a broad impact on treatment and prevention efforts. Although the safety and efficacy of treatment are likely to improve, worldwide eradication of HCV will depend on a multifaceted approach; therefore, development of a vaccine that prevents chronic infection continues to be an important goal.

ACKNOWLEDGMENTS

We acknowledge Michael Torbenson for providing histology images, John Ticehurst for helpful suggestions, and support from NIH R01 DA024565 (S.C.R.) and R01 DA016078 (D.L.T.).

REFERENCES

All cited references are available in the e-book.

6. Agnello V, Chung RT, Kaplan LM. A role for hepatitis C virus infection in Type II cryoglobulinemia. *N Engl J Med* 1992;327:1490–1495.
24. Anonymous. National Institutes of Health Consensus Development Conference Statement: management of hepatitis C: 2002–June 10–12, 2002. *Hepatology* 2002;36:S3–S20.
37. Bacon BR, Gordon SC, Lawitz E, et al. Boceprevir for previously treated chronic HCV genotype 1 infection. *N Engl J Med* 2011;364:1207–1217.
41. Balagopal A, Thomas DL, Thio CL. IL28B and the control of hepatitis C virus infection. *Gastroenterology* 2010;139:1865–1876.
43. Barnes E, Folgori A, Capone S, et al. Novel adenovirus-based vaccines induce broad and sustained T cell responses to HCV in man. *Sci Transl Med* 2012;4:115ra1.
45. Bartenschlager R, Lohmann V. Replication of hepatitis C virus. *J Gen Virol* 2000;81:1631–1648.
46. Bartosch B, Dubuisson J, Cosset FL. Infectious hepatitis C virus pseudo-particles containing functional E1- E2 envelope protein complexes. *J Exp Med* 2003;197:633–642.
47. Bartosch B, Vitelli A, Granier C, et al. Cell entry of hepatitis C virus requires a set of co-receptors that include the CD81 tetraspanin and the SR-B1 scavenger receptor. *J Biol Chem* 2003;278:41624–41630.

64. Blight KJ, Kolykhalov AA, Rice CM. Efficient initiation of HCV RNA replication in cell culture. *Science* 2000;290:1972–1974.
65. Blight KJ, McKeating JA, Rice CM. Highly permissive cell lines for subgenomic and genomic hepatitis C virus RNA replication. *J Virol* 2002; 76:13001–13014.
73. Booth JC, Kumar U, Webster D, et al. Comparison of the rate of sequence variation in the hypervariable region of E2/NS1 region of hepatitis C virus in normal and hypogammaglobulinemic patients. *Hepatology* 1998;27:223–227.
85. Bukh J, Pietschmann T, Lohmann V, et al. Mutations that permit efficient replication of hepatitis C virus RNA in Huh-7 cells prevent productive replication in chimpanzees. *Proc Natl Acad Sci U S A* 2002;99: 14416–14421.
86. Bukh J, Purcell RH, Miller RH. At least 12 genotypes of hepatitis C virus predicted by sequence analysis of the putative E1 gene of isolates collected worldwide. *Proc Natl Acad Sci USA* 1993;90:8234–8238.
88. Bull RA, Luciani F, McElroy K, et al. Sequential bottlenecks drive viral evolution in early acute hepatitis C virus infection. *PLoS Pathog* 2011; 7:e1002243.
89. Burbelo PD, Dubovi EJ, Simmonds P, et al. Serology enabled discovery of genetically diverse hepaciviruses in a new host. *J Virol* 2012;86:6171–6178.
96. Candotti D, Temple J, Sarkodie F, et al. Frequent recovery and broad genotype 2 diversity characterize hepatitis C virus infection in Ghana, West Africa. *J Virol* 2003;77:7914–7923.
102. Chang KM, Rehermann B, Chisari FV. Immunopathology of hepatitis C. *Springer Semin Immunopathol* 1997;19:57–68.
103. Chang KM, Rehermann B, McHutchison JG, et al. Immunological significance of cytotoxic T lymphocyte epitope variants in patients chronically infected by the hepatitis C virus. *J Clin Invest* 1997;100:2376–2385.
109. Chen L, Borozan I, Feld J, et al. Hepatic gene expression discriminates responders and nonresponders in treatment of chronic hepatitis C viral infection. *Gastroenterology* 2005;128:1437–1444.
116. Choo Q-L, Kuo G, Weiner AJ, et al. Isolation of a cDNA clone derived from a blood-borne non-A, non-B viral hepatitis genome. *Science* 1989; 244:359–362.
120. Cohen EB, Afdhal NH. Ultrasound-based hepatic elastography: origins, limitations, and applications. *J Clin Gastroenterol* 2010;44:637–645.
125. Conry-Cantilena C, Vanraden MT, Gibble J, et al. Routes of infection, viremia, and liver disease in blood donors found to have hepatitis C virus infection. *N Engl J Med* 1996;334:1691–1696.
128. Corbet S, Bukh J, Heinsen A, et al. Hepatitis C virus subtyping by a core-envelope 1-based reverse transcriptase PCR assay with sequencing and its use in determining subtype distribution among Danish patients. *J Clin Microbiol* 2003;41:1091–1100.
133. Cox AL, Mosbruger T, Lauer GM, et al. Comprehensive analyses of CD8+ T cell responses during longitudinal study of acute human hepatitis C. *Hepatology* 2005;42:104–112.
134. Cox AL, Mosbruger T, Mao Q, et al. Cellular immune selection with hepatitis C virus persistence in humans. *J Exp Med* 2005;201:1741–1752.
135. Cox AL, Netski DM, Mosbruger T, et al. Prospective evaluation of community-acquired acute-phase hepatitis C virus infection. *Clin Infect Dis* 2005;40:951–958.
141. Dahari H, Feinstone SM, Major ME. Meta-analysis of hepatitis C virus vaccine efficacy in chimpanzees indicates an importance for structural proteins. *Gastroenterology* 2010;139:965–974.
143. Dahari H, Guedj J, Perelson AS, et al. Hepatitis C viral kinetics in the era of direct acting antiviral agents and IL28B. *Curr Hepat Rep* 2011;10: 214–227.
144. Dal ML, Franceschi S. Hepatitis C virus and risk of lymphoma and other lymphoid neoplasms: a meta-analysis of epidemiologic studies. *Cancer Epidemiol Biomarkers Prev* 2006;15:2078–2085.
146. Davila JA, Morgan RO, Shaib Y, et al. Hepatitis C infection and the increasing incidence of hepatocellular carcinoma: a population-based study. *Gastroenterology* 2004;127:1372–1380.
149. Davis GL, Wong JB, McHutchison JG, et al. Early virologic response to treatment with peginterferon alfa-2b plus ribavirin in patients with chronic hepatitis C. *Hepatology* 2003;38:645–652.
161. Dixit NM, Layden-Almer JE, Layden TJ, et al. Modelling how ribavirin improves interferon response rates in hepatitis C virus infection. *Nature* 2004;432:922–924.
162. Domingo E, Martinez-Salas E, Sobrino F, et al. The quasispecies (extremely heterogeneous) nature of viral RNA genome populations: biological relevance–a review. *Gene* 1985;40:1–8.
168. Dorner M, Horwitz JA, Robbins JB, et al. A genetically humanized mouse model for hepatitis C virus infection. *Nature* 2011;474:208–211.
170. Dowd KA, Netski DM, Wang XH, et al. Selection pressure from neutralizing antibodies drives sequence evolution during acute infection with hepatitis C virus. *Gastroenterology* 2009;136:2377–2386.
171. Drexler JF, Kupfer B, Petersen N, et al. A novel diagnostic target in the hepatitis C virus genome. *PLoS Med* 2009;6:e31.
180. Enomoto N, Sakuma I, Asahina Y, et al. Mutations in the nonstructural protein 5A gene and response to interferon in patients with chronic hepatitis C virus 1b infection. *N Engl J Med* 1996;334:77–81.
181. Erickson AL, Kimura Y, Igarashi S, et al. The outcome of hepatitis C virus infection is predicted by escape mutations in epitopes targeted by cytotoxic T lymphocytes. *Immunity* 2001;15:883–895.
182. Esteban JI, Lopez-Talavera JC, Genesca J, et al. High rate of infectivity and liver disease in blood donors with antibodies to hepatitis C virus. *Ann Intern Med* 1991;115:443–449.
183. Evans MJ, von Hahn T, Tscherne DM, et al. Claudin-1 is a hepatitis C virus co-receptor required for a late step in entry. *Nature* 2007;446: 801–805.
188. Fan X, Lang DM, Xu Y, et al. Liver transplantation with hepatitis C virus-infected graft: interaction between donor and recipient viral strains. *Hepatology* 2003;38:25–33.
193. Farci P, Shimoda A, Coiana A, et al. The outcome of acute hepatitis C predicted by the evolution of the viral quasispecies. *Science* 2000;288: 339–344.
194. Farci P, Shimoda A, Wong D, et al. Prevention of hepatitis C virus infection in chimpanzees by hyperimmune serum against the hypervariable region 1 of the envelope 2 protein. *Proc Natl Acad Sci U S A* 1996;93: 15394–15399.
210. Folgori A, Capone S, Ruggeri L, et al. A T-cell HCV vaccine eliciting effective immunity against heterologous virus challenge in chimpanzees. *Nat Med* 2006;12:190–197.
213. Foy E, Li K, Sumpter R, et al. Control of antiviral defenses through hepatitis C virus disruption of retinoic acid-inducible gene-I signaling. *Proc Natl Acad Sci U S A* 2005;102:2986–2991.
214. Foy E, Li K, Wang C, et al. Regulation of interferon regulatory factor-3 by the hepatitis C virus serine protease. *Science* 2003;300:1145–1148.
215. Frank C, Mohamed MK, Strickland GT, et al. The role of parenteral antischistosomal therapy in the spread of hepatitis C virus in Egypt. *Lancet* 2000;355:887–891.
219. Fried MW, Shiffman ML, Reddy KR, et al. Peginterferon alfa-2a plus ribavirin for chronic hepatitis C virus infection. *N Engl J Med* 2002;347: 975–982.
221. Gale M, Foy EM. Evasion of intracellular host defence by hepatitis C virus. *Nature* 2005;436:939–945.
223. Gale MJJ, Korth MJ, Tang NM, et al. Evidence that hepatitis C virus resistance to interferon is mediated through repression of the PKR protein kinase by the nonstructural 5A protein. *Virology* 1997;230:217–227.
229. Garfein RS, Vlahov D, Galai N, et al. Viral infections in short-term injection drug users: the prevalence of the hepatitis C, hepatitis B, human immunodeficiency, and human T-lymphotropic viruses. *Am J Public Health* 1996;86:655–661.
233. Ge D, Fellay J, Thompson AJ, et al. Genetic variation in IL28B predicts hepatitis C treatment-induced viral clearance. *Nature* 2009;461: 399–401.
234. Gerlach JT, Diepolder HM, Zachoval R, et al. Acute hepatitis C: high rate of both spontaneous and treatment-induced viral clearance. *Gastroenterology* 2003;125:80–88.
236. Ghany MG, Nelson DR, Strader DB, et al. An update on treatment of genotype 1 chronic hepatitis C virus infection: 2011 practice guideline by the American Association for the Study of Liver Diseases. *Hepatology* 2011;54:1433–1444.
237. Ghany MG, Strader DB, Thomas DL, et al. Diagnosis, management, and treatment of hepatitis C: an update. *Hepatology* 2009;49:1335–1374.
250. Graham CS, Baden LR, Yu E, et al. Influence of human immunodeficiency virus infection on the course of hepatitis C virus infection: a meta-analysis. *Clin Infect Dis* 2001;33:562–569.

251. Grakoui A, Shoukry NH, Woollard DJ, et al. HCV persistence and immune evasion in the absence of memory T cell help. *Science* 2003; 302:659–662.
252. Gray RR, Parker J, Lemey P, et al. The mode and tempo of hepatitis C virus evolution within and among hosts. *BMC Evol Biol* 2011;11:131.
255. Gretch DR. Diagnostic tests for hepatitis C. *Hepatology* 1997;26:43S–47S.
256. Greub G, Ledergerber B, Battegay M, et al. Clinical progression, survival, and immune recovery during antiretroviral therapy in patients with HIV-1 and hepatitis C virus coinfection: the Swiss HIV Cohort Study. *Lancet* 2000;356:1800–1805.
263. Habersetzer F, Honnet G, Bain C, et al. A poxvirus vaccine is safe, induces T-cell responses, and decreases viral load in patients with chronic hepatitis C. *Gastroenterology* 2011;141:890–899.
264. Hadziyannis SJ, Sette H Jr, Morgan TR, et al. Peginterferon-alpha2a and ribavirin combination therapy in chronic hepatitis C: a randomized study of treatment duration and ribavirin dose. *Ann Intern Med* 2004;140:346–355.
272. Helle F, Duverlie G, Dubuisson J. The hepatitis C virus glycan shield and evasion of the humoral immune response. *Viruses* 2011;3:1909–1932.
273. Hellinger WC, Bacalis LP, Kay RS, et al. Health care-associated hepatitis C virus infections attributed to narcotic diversion. *Ann Intern Med* 2012;156:477–482.
275. Hezode C, Forestier N, Dusheiko G, et al. Telaprevir and peginterferon with or without ribavirin for chronic HCV infection. *N Engl J Med* 2009; 360:1839–1850.
277. Honda M, Sakai A, Yamashita T, et al. Hepatic interferon-stimulated genes expression is associated with genetic variation in interleukin 28B and the outcome of interferon therapy for chronic hepatitis C. *Gastroenterology* 2010;139:499–509.
279. Hsu M, Zhang J, Flint M, et al. Hepatitis C virus glycoproteins mediate pH-dependent cell entry of pseudotyped retroviral particles. *Proc Natl Acad Sci U S A* 2003;100:7271–7276.
289. Ishak K, Baptista A, Bianchi L, et al. Histological grading and staging of chronic hepatitis. *J Hepatol* 1995;22:696–699.
292. Jacobson IM, McHutchison JG, Dusheiko G, et al. Telaprevir for previously untreated chronic hepatitis C virus infection. *N Engl J Med* 2011; 364:2405–2416.
294. Jaeckel E, Cornberg M, Wedemeyer H, et al. Treatment of acute hepatitis C with interferon alfa-2b. *N Engl J Med* 2001;345:1452–1457.
295. Jeannel D, Fretz C, Traore Y, et al. Evidence for high genetic diversity and long-term endemicity of hepatitis C virus genotypes 1 and 2 in West Africa. *J Med Virol* 1998;55:92–97.
296. Jensen DM, Morgan TR, Marcellin P, et al. Early identification of HCV genotype 1 patients responding to 24 weeks peginterferon alpha-2a (40 kd)/ribavirin therapy. *Hepatology* 2006;43:954–960.
299. Jopling CL, Schutz S, Sarnow P. Position-dependent function for a tandem microRNA miR-122-binding site located in the hepatitis C virus RNA genome. *Cell Host Microbe* 2008;4:77–85.
302. Kalinina O, Norder H, Mukomolov S, et al. A natural intergenotypic recombinant of hepatitis C virus identified in St. Petersburg. *J Virol* 2002; 76:4034–4043.
303. Kanai K, Kako M, Okamoto H. HCV genotypes in chronic hepatitis C and response to interferon. *Lancet* 1992;339:1543.
309. Kapoor A, Simmonds P, Gerold G, et al. Characterization of a canine homolog of hepatitis C virus. *Proc Natl Acad Sci U S A* 2011;108:11608–11613.
315. Kato T, Date T, Miyamoto M, et al. Efficient replication of the genotype 2a hepatitis C virus subgenomic replicon. *Gastroenterology* 2003;125: 1808–1817.
317. Katze MG, He Y, Gale M Jr. Viruses and interferon: a fight for supremacy. *Nat Rev Immunol* 2002;2:675–687.
318. Keck ZY, Li SH, Xia J, et al. Mutations in hepatitis C virus E2 located outside the CD81 binding sites lead to escape from broadly neutralizing antibodies but compromise virus infectivity. *J Virol* 2009;83:6149–6160.
322. Kenny-Walsh E. Clinical outcomes after hepatitis C infection from contaminated anti-D immune globulin. Irish Hepatology Research Group. *N Engl J Med* 1999;340:1228–1233.
327. Kim AY, Lauer GM, Ouchi K, et al. The magnitude and breadth of hepatitis C virus-specific CD8+ T cells depend on absolute CD4+ T-cell count in individuals coinfected with HIV-1. *Blood* 2005;105:1170–1178.
337. Kolykhalov AA, Agapov EV, Blight KJ, et al. Transmission of hepatitis C by intrahepatic inoculation with transcribed RNA. *Science* 1997; 277:570–574.
342. Krey T, d'Alayer J, Kikuti CM, et al. The disulfide bonds in glycoprotein E2 of hepatitis C virus reveal the tertiary organization of the molecule. *PLoS Pathog* 2010;6:e1000762.
346. Kuiken C, Simmonds P. Nomenclature and numbering of the hepatitis C virus. *Methods Mol Biol* 2009;510:33–53.
350. Kuntzen T, Timm J, Berical A, et al. Naturally occurring dominant resistance mutations to hepatitis C virus protease and polymerase inhibitors in treatment-naive patients. *Hepatology* 2008;48:1769–1778.
351. Kuntzen T, Timm J, Berical A, et al. Viral sequence evolution in acute hepatitis C virus infection. *J Virol* 2007;81:11658–11668.
356. Kwo PY, Lawitz EJ, McCone J, et al. Efficacy of boceprevir, an NS3 protease inhibitor, in combination with peginterferon alfa-2b and ribavirin in treatment-naive patients with genotype 1 hepatitis C infection (SPRINT-1): an open-label, randomised, multicentre phase 2 trial. *Lancet* 2010;376:705–716.
361. Lanford RE, Chavez D, Guerra B, et al. Ribavirin induces error-prone replication of GB virus B in primary tamarin hepatocytes. *J Virol* 2001; 75:8074–8081.
362. Lanford RE, Chavez D, Von Chisari F, et al. Lack of detection of negative-strand hepatitis C virus RNA in peripheral blood mononuclear cells and other extrahepatic tissues by the highly strand-specific rTth reverse transcriptase PCR. *J Virol* 1995;69:8079–8083.
364. Lanford RE, Hildebrandt-Eriksen ES, Petri A, et al. Therapeutic silencing of microRNA-122 in primates with chronic hepatitis C virus infection. *Science* 2010;327:198–201.
367. Lau DT, Kleiner DE, Ghany MG, et al. 10-year follow-up after interferon-a therapy for chronic hepatitis C. *Hepatology* 1998;28:1121–1127.
368. Lauer GM, Lucas M, Timm J, et al. Full-breadth analysis of CD8(+) T-cell responses in acute hepatitis C virus infection and early therapy. *J Virol* 2005;79:12979–12988.
369. Law M, Maruyama T, Lewis J, et al. Broadly neutralizing antibodies protect against hepatitis C virus quasispecies challenge. *Nat Med* 2008; 14:25–27.
371. Lechner F, Wong DK, Dunbar PR, et al. Analysis of successful immune responses in persons infected with hepatitis C virus. *J Exp Med* 2000;191: 1499–1512.
377. Li K, Foy E, Ferreon JC, et al. Immune evasion by hepatitis C virus NS3/4A protease-mediated cleavage of the Toll-like receptor 3 adaptor protein TRIF. *Proc Natl Acad Sci USA* 2005;102:2992–2997.
383. Liu L, Fisher BE, Thomas DL, et al. Spontaneous clearance of primary acute hepatitis C virus infection correlated with high initial viral RNA level and rapid HVR1 evolution. *Hepatology* 2012;55:1684–1691.
384. Liu SL, Rodrigo AG, Shankarappa R, et al. HIV quasispecies and resampling. *Science* 1996;273:415–416.
385. Logvinoff C, Major ME, Oldach D, et al. Neutralizing antibody response during acute and chronic hepatitis C virus infection. *Proc Natl Acad Sci U S A* 2004;101:10149–10154.
386. Lohmann V, Korner F, Dobierzewska A, et al. Mutations in hepatitis C virus RNAs conferring cell culture adaptation. *J Virol* 2001;75: 1437–1449.
387. Lohmann V, Korner F, Koch J, et al. Replication of subgenomic hepatitis C virus RNAs in a hepatoma cell line. *Science* 1999;285:110–113.
388. Lok AS, Gardiner DF, Lawitz E, et al. Preliminary study of two antiviral agents for hepatitis C genotype 1. *N Engl J Med* 2012;366:216–224.
389. Loo YM, Owen DM, Li K, et al. Viral and therapeutic control of IFN-beta promoter stimulator 1 during hepatitis C virus infection. *Proc Natl Acad Sci USA* 2006;103:6001–6006.
394. Ly KN, Xing J, Klevens RM, et al. The increasing burden of mortality from viral hepatitis in the United States between 1999 and 2007. *Ann Intern Med* 2012;156:271–278.
398. Maheshwari A, Ray S, Thuluvath PJ. Acute hepatitis C. *Lancet* 2008; 372:321–332.
402. Manns MP, McHutchison JG, Gordon SC, et al. Peginterferon alfa-2b plus ribavirin compared with interferon alfa-2b plus ribavirin for initial treatment of chronic hepatitis C: a randomised trial. *Lancet* 2001;358:958–965.
403. Marcellin P, Boyer N, Gervais A, et al. Long-term histologic improvement and loss of detectable intrahepatic HCV RNA in patients with

chronic hepatitis C and sustained response to interferon-α therapy. *Ann Intern Med* 1997;127:875–881.

404. Marcellin P, Descamps V, Martinot Peignoux M, et al. Cryoglobulinemia with vasculitis associated with hepatitis C virus infection. *Gastroenterology* 1993;104:272–277.
406. Martell M, Esteban JI, Quer J, et al. Hepatitis C virus (HCV) circulates as a population of different but closely related genomes: quasispecies nature of HCV genome distribution. *J Virol* 1992;66:3225–3229.
408. Martinez-Bauer E, Forns X, Armelles M, et al. Hospital admission is a relevant source of hepatitis C virus acquisition in Spain. *J Hepatol* 2008; 48:20–27.
410. Martinot-Peignoux M, Marcellin P, Pouteau M, et al. Pretreatment serum hepatitis C virus RNA levels and hepatitis C virus genotype are the main and independent prognostic factors of sustained response to interferon alfa therapy in chronic hepatitis C. *Hepatology* 1995;22:1050–1056.
413. Mast EE, Hwang LY, Seto DS, et al. Risk factors for perinatal transmission of hepatitis C virus (HCV) and the natural history of HCV infection acquired in infancy. *J Infect Dis* 2005;192:1880–1889.
415. McAllister J, Casino C, Davidson F, et al. Long-term evolution of the hypervariable region of hepatitis C virus in a common-source-infected cohort. *J Virol* 1998;72:4893–4905.
418. McHutchison JG, Everson GT, Gordon SC, et al. Telaprevir with peginterferon and ribavirin for chronic HCV genotype 1 infection. *N Engl J Med* 2009;360:1827–1838.
419. McHutchison JG, Lawitz EJ, Shiffman ML, et al. Peginterferon alfa-2b or alfa-2a with ribavirin for treatment of hepatitis C infection. *N Engl J Med* 2009;361:580–593.
423. Mehta SH, Brancati FL, Strathdee SA, et al. Hepatitis C virus infection and incident type 2 diabetes. *Hepatology* 2003;38:50–56.
424. Mehta SH, Cox A, Hoover DR, et al. Protection against persistence of hepatitis C. *Lancet* 2002;359:1478–1483.
425. Mehta SH, Genberg BL, Astemborski J, et al. Limited uptake of hepatitis C treatment among injection drug users. *J Community Health* 2008; 33:126–133.
431. Mercer DF, Schiller DE, Elliott JF, et al. Hepatitis C virus replication in mice with chimeric human livers. *Nat Med* 2001;7:927–933.
436. Meunier JC, Engle RE, Faulk K, et al. Evidence for cross-genotype neutralization of hepatitis C virus pseudo-particles and enhancement of infectivity by apolipoprotein C1. *Proc Natl Acad Sci U S A* 2005;102: 4560–4565.
439. Meylan E, Curran J, Hofmann K, et al. Cardif is an adaptor protein in the RIG-I antiviral pathway and is targeted by hepatitis C virus. *Nature* 2005;437:1167–1172.
443. Mitchell AE, Colvin HM, Palmer BR. Institute of Medicine recommendations for the prevention and control of hepatitis B and C. *Hepatology* 2010;51:729–733.
448. Mosley JW, Operskalski EA, Tobler LH, et al. Viral and host factors in early hepatitis C virus infection. *Hepatology* 2005;42:86–92.
452. Nainan OV, Alter MJ, Kruszon-Moran D, et al. Hepatitis C virus genotypes and viral concentrations in participants of a general population survey in the United States. *Gastroenterology* 2006;131:478–484.
453. Nakagawa M, Sakamoto N, Tanabe Y, et al. Suppression of hepatitis C virus replication by cyclosporin A is mediated by blockade of cyclophilins. *Gastroenterology* 2005;129:1031–1041.
467. Netski DM, Mosbruger T, Depla E, et al. Humoral immune response in acute hepatitis C virus infection. *Clin Infect Dis* 2005;41:667–675.
468. Neumann AU, Lam NP, Dahari H, et al. Hepatitis C viral dynamics in vivo and the antiviral efficacy of interferon-alpha therapy. *Science* 1998;282: 103–107.
470. Neumann-Haefelin C, Oniangue-Ndza C, Kuntzen T, et al. Human leukocyte antigen B27 selects for rare escape mutations that significantly impair hepatitis C virus replication and require compensatory mutations. *Hepatology* 2011;54:1157–1166.
477. Oniangue-Ndza C, Kuntzen T, Kemper M, et al. Compensatory mutations restore the replication defects caused by cytotoxic T lymphocyte escape mutations in hepatitis C virus polymerase. *J Virol* 2011;85:11883–11890.
478. Osburn WO, Fisher BE, Dowd KA, et al. Spontaneous control of primary hepatitis C virus infection and immunity against persistent reinfection. *Gastroenterology* 2010;138:315–324.
481. Pascu M, Martus P, Hohne M, et al. Sustained virological response in hepatitis C virus type 1b infected patients is predicted by the number of mutations within the NS5A-ISDR: a meta-analysis focused on geographical differences. *Gut* 2004;53:1345–1351.
484. Patel PR, Larson AK, Castel AD, et al. Hepatitis C virus infections from a contaminated radiopharmaceutical used in myocardial perfusion studies. *JAMA* 2006;296:2005–2011.
494. Pestka JM, Zeisel MB, Blaser E, et al. Rapid induction of virus-neutralizing antibodies and viral clearance in a single-source outbreak of hepatitis C. *Proc Natl Acad Sci U S A* 2007;104:6025–6030.
499. Pileri P, Uematsu Y, Campagnoli S, et al. Binding of hepatitis C virus to CD81. *Science* 1998;282:938–941.
500. Ploss A, Evans MJ, Gaysinskaya VA, et al. Human occludin is a hepatitis C virus entry factor required for infection of mouse cells. *Nature* 2009; 457:882–886.
501. Polyak SJ, Khabar KS, Paschal DM, et al. Hepatitis C virus nonstructural 5A protein induces interleukin-8, leading to partial inhibition of the interferon-induced antiviral response. *J Virol* 2001;75:6095–6106.
504. Poordad F, McCone J, Bacon BR, et al. Boceprevir for untreated chronic HCV genotype 1 infection. *N Engl J Med* 2011;364:1195–1206.
509. Pybus OG, Charleston MA, Gupta S, et al. The epidemic behavior of the hepatitis C virus. *Science* 2001;292:2323–2325.
511. Radziewicz H, Ibegbu CC, Fernandez ML, et al. Liver-infiltrating lymphocytes in chronic human hepatitis C virus infection display an exhausted phenotype with high levels of PD-1 and low levels of CD127 expression. *J Virol* 2007;81:2545–2553.
515. Rauch A, Kutalik Z, Descombes P, et al. Genetic variation in IL28B is associated with chronic hepatitis C and treatment failure: a genome-wide association study. *Gastroenterology* 2010;138:1338–1345.
520. Ray SC, Arthur RR, Carella A, et al. Genetic epidemiology of hepatitis C virus throughout Egypt. *J Infect Dis* 2000;182:698–707.
521. Ray SC, Fanning L, Wang XH, et al. Divergent and convergent evolution after a common-source outbreak of hepatitis C virus. *J Exp Med* 2005;201: 1753–1759.
522. Ray SC, Mao Q, Lanford RE, et al. Hypervariable region 1 sequence stability during hepatitis C virus replication in chimpanzees. *J Virol* 2000; 74:3058–3066.
523. Ray SC, Wang YM, Laeyendecker O, et al. Acute hepatitis C virus structural gene sequences as predictors of persistent viremia: hypervariable region 1 as a decoy. *J Virol* 1999;73:2938–2946.
525. Rehermann B, Chang KM, McHutchison JG, et al. Quantitative analysis of the peripheral blood cytotoxic T lymphocyte response in patients with chronic hepatitis C virus infection. *J Clin Invest* 1996;98:1432–1440.
533. Rockey DC, Bissell DM. Noninvasive measures of liver fibrosis. *Hepatology* 2006;43:S113–S120.
535. Rong L, Dahari H, Ribeiro RM, et al. Rapid emergence of protease inhibitor resistance in hepatitis C virus. *Sci Transl Med* 2010;2:30ra32.
546. Saldanha J, Lelie N, Heath A. Establishment of the first international standard for nucleic acid amplification technology (NAT) assays for HCV RNA. WHO Collaborative Study Group. *Vox Sang* 1999;76:149–158.
547. Salemi M, Vandamme AM. Hepatitis C virus evolutionary patterns studied through analysis of full-genome sequences. *J Mol Evol* 2002;54: 62–70.
550. Sangiovanni A, Prati GM, Fasani P, et al. The natural history of compensated cirrhosis due to hepatitis C virus: A 17-year cohort study of 214 patients. *Hepatology* 2006;43:1303–1310.
555. Sarrazin C, Kieffer TL, Bartels D, et al. Dynamic hepatitis C virus genotypic and phenotypic changes in patients treated with the protease inhibitor telaprevir. *Gastroenterology* 2007;132:1767–1777.
564. Schulze zur Wiesch J, Ciuffreda D, Lewis-Ximenez L, et al. Broadly directed virus-specific CD4+ T cell responses are primed during acute hepatitis C infection, but rapidly disappear from human blood with viral persistence. *J Exp Med* 2012;209:61–75.
566. Seifert U, Liermann H, Racanelli V, et al. Hepatitis C virus mutation affects proteasomal epitope processing. *J Clin Invest* 2004;114:250–259.
573. Shoukry NH, Grakoui A, Houghton M, et al. Memory CD8+ T cells are required for protection from persistent hepatitis C virus infection. *J Exp Med* 2003;197:1645–1655.
576. Simmonds P. Genetic diversity and evolution of hepatitis C virus - 15 years on. *J Gen Virol* 2004;85:3173–3188.

577. Simmonds P, Bukh J, Combet C, et al. Consensus proposals for a unified system of nomenclature of hepatitis C virus genotypes. *Hepatology* 2005;42:962–973.
580. Simmonds P, Smith DB, McOmish F, et al. Identification of genotypes of hepatitis C virus by sequence comparisons in the core, E1 and NS-5 regions. *J Gen Virol* 1994;75:1053–1061.
582. Smith DB, McAllister J, Casino C, et al. Virus 'quasispecies': making a mountain out of a molehill? *J Gen Virol* 1997;78:1511–1519.
583. Smith DB, Pathirana S, Davidson F, et al. The origin of hepatitis C virus genotypes. *J Gen Virol* 1997;78:321–328.
584. Soriano V, Puoti M, Sulkowski M, et al. Care of patients coinfected with HIV and hepatitis C virus: 2007 updated recommendations from the HCV-HIV International Panel. *AIDS* 2007;21:1073–1089.
587. Stamataki Z, Coates S, Abrignani S, et al. Immunization of human volunteers with hepatitis C virus envelope glycoproteins elicits antibodies that cross-neutralize heterologous virus strains. *J Infect Dis* 2011;204: 811–813.
589. Strickland GT. Liver disease in Egypt: hepatitis C superseded schistosomiasis as a result of iatrogenic and biological factors. *Hepatology* 2006; 43:915–922.
591. Stuyver L, Van Arnhem W, Wyseur A, et al. Classification of hepatitis C viruses based on phylogenetic analysis of the envelope 1 and nonstructural 5B regions and identification of five additional subtypes. *Proc Natl Acad Sci U S A* 1994;91:10134–10138.
595. Sulkowski MS, Mast EE, Seeff LB, et al. Hepatitis C virus infection as an opportunistic disease in persons infected with human immunodeficiency virus. *Clin Infect Dis* 2000;30(Suppl 1):S77–S84.
596. Sulkowski MS, Mehta SH, Torbenson MS, et al. Rapid fibrosis progression among HIV/hepatitis C virus-co-infected adults. *AIDS* 2007;21: 2209–2216.
597. Sulkowski MS, Moore RD, Mehta SH, et al. Hepatitis C and progression of HIV disease. *JAMA* 2002;288:199–206.
598. Sulkowski MS, Thomas DL. Hepatitis C in the HIV-infected patient. *Clin Liver Dis* 2003;7:179–194.
605. Swain MG, Lai MY, Shiffman ML, et al. A sustained virologic response is durable in patients with chronic hepatitis C treated with peginterferon alfa-2a and ribavirin. *Gastroenterology* 2010;139:1593–1601.
607. Takaki A, Wiese M, Maertens G, et al. Cellular immune responses persist and humoral responses decrease two decades after recovery from a single-source outbreak of hepatitis C. *Nat Med* 2000;6:578–582.
613. Terrault NA, Im K, Boylan R, et al. Fibrosis progression in African Americans and Caucasian Americans with chronic hepatitis C. *Clin Gastroenterol Hepatol* 2008;6:1403–1411.
614. Tester I, Smyk-Pearson S, Wang P, et al. Immune evasion versus recovery after acute hepatitis C virus infection from a shared source. *J Exp Med* 2005;201:1725–1731.
618. Thio CL, Nolt KR, Astemborski J, et al. Screening for hepatitis C virus in human immunodeficiency virus-infected individuals. *J Clin Microbiol* 2000;38:575–577.
619. Thomas DL. The challenge of hepatitis C in the HIV-infected person. *Annu Rev Med* 2008;59:473–485.
620. Thomas DL, Astemborski J, Rai RM, et al. The natural history of hepatitis C virus infection: host, viral, and environmental factors. *JAMA* 2000; 284:450–456.
621. Thomas DL, Astemborski J, Vlahov D, et al. Determinants of the quantity of hepatitis C virus RNA. *J Infect Dis* 2000;181:844–851.
623. Thomas DL, Thio CL, Martin MP, et al. Genetic variation in IL28B and spontaneous clearance of hepatitis C virus. *Nature* 2009;461:798–801.
624. Thomas DL, Villano SA, Riester KA, et al. Perinatal transmission of hepatitis C virus from human immunodeficiency virus type 1-infected mothers. *J Infect Dis* 1998;177:1480–1488.
628. Timm J, Lauer GM, Kavanagh DG, et al. CD8 epitope escape and reversion in acute HCV infection. *J Exp Med* 2004;200:1593–1604.
629. Timm J, Li B, Daniels MG, et al. Human leukocyte antigen-associated sequence polymorphisms in hepatitis C virus reveal reproducible immune responses and constraints on viral evolution. *Hepatology* 2007;46:339–349.
630. Timpe JM, Stamataki Z, Jennings A, et al. Hepatitis C virus cell-cell transmission in hepatoma cells in the presence of neutralizing antibodies. *Hepatology* 2008;47:17–24.
642. Tuplin A, Wood J, Evans DJ, et al. Thermodynamic and phylogenetic prediction of RNA secondary structures in the coding region of hepatitis C virus. *RNA* 2002;8:824–841.
648. van de Laar T, Pybus O, Bruisten S, et al. Evidence of a large, international network of HCV transmission in HIV-positive men who have sex with men. *Gastroenterology* 2009;136:1609–1617.
652. van der Helm JJ, Prins M, del Amo J, et al. The hepatitis C epidemic among HIV-positive MSM: incidence estimates from 1990 to 2007. *AIDS* 2011;25:1083–1091.
654. Vandelli C, Renzo F, Romano L, et al. Lack of evidence of sexual transmission of hepatitis C among monogamous couples: results of a 10-year prospective follow-up study. *Am J Gastroenterol* 2004;99:855–859.
656. Vento S, Garofano T, Renzini C, et al. Fulminant hepatitis associated with hepatitis A virus superinfection in patients with chronic hepatitis C. *N Engl J Med* 1998;338:286–290.
658. Viazov S, Ross SS, Kyuregyan KK, et al. Hepatitis C virus recombinants are rare even among intravenous drug users. *J Med Virol* 2010;82: 232–238.
660. Vieyres G, Thomas X, Descamps V, et al. Characterization of the envelope glycoproteins associated with infectious hepatitis C virus. *J Virol* 2010;84:10159–10168.
661. Villano SA, Vlahov D, Nelson KE, et al. Persistence of viremia and the importance of long-term follow-up after acute hepatitis C infection. *Hepatology* 1999;29:908–914.
666. von Hahn T, Yoon JC, Alter H, et al. Hepatitis C virus continuously escapes from neutralizing antibody and T-cell responses during chronic infection in vivo. *Gastroenterology* 2007;132:667–678.
670. Wakita T, Pietschmann T, Kato T, et al. Production of infectious hepatitis C virus in tissue culture from a cloned viral genome. *Nat Med* 2005; 11:791–796.
674. Weber R, Sabin CA, Friis-Moller N, et al. Liver-related deaths in persons infected with the human immunodeficiency virus: the D:A:D study. *Arch Intern Med* 2006;166:1632–1641.
675. Wedemeyer H, He XS, Nascimbeni M, et al. Impaired effector function of hepatitis C virus-specific CD8+ T cells in chronic hepatitis C virus infection. *J Immunol* 2002;169:3447–3458.
680. Weiner AJ, Geysen HM, Christopherson C, et al. Evidence for immune selection of hepatitis C virus (HCV) putative envelope glycoprotein variants: potential role in chronic HCV infections. *Proc Natl Acad Sci U S A* 1992;89:3468–3472.
683. Wilson LE, Torbenson M, Astemborski J, et al. Progression of liver fibrosis among injection drug users with chronic hepatitis C. *Hepatology* 2006;43:788–795.
688. World Health Organization. Global burden of disease (GBD) for hepatitis C. *J Clin Pharmacol* 2004;44:20–29.
694. Yanagi M, Purcell RH, Emerson SU, et al. Transcripts from a single full-length cDNA clone of hepatitis C virus are infectious when directly transfected into the liver of a chimpanzee. *Proc Natl Acad Sci U S A* 1997;94:8738–8743.
697. Yoo BJ, Selby MJ, Choe J, et al. Transfection of a differentiated human hepatoma cell line (Huh7) with in vitro-transcribed hepatitis C virus (HCV) RNA and establishment of a long-term culture persistently infected with HCV. *J Virol* 1995;69:32–38.
699. Yu MYW, Bartosch B, Zhang P, et al. Neutralizing antibodies to hepatitis C virus (HCV) in immune globulins derived from anti-HCV-positive plasma. *Proc Natl Acad Sci USA* 2004;101:7705–7710.
702. Zein NN, Rakela J, Krawitt EL, et al. Hepatitis C virus genotypes in the United States: epidemiology, pathogenicity, and response to interferon therapy. *Ann Intern Med* 1996;125:634–639.
704. Zeuzem S, Andreone P, Pol S, et al. Telaprevir for retreatment of HCV infection. *N Engl J Med* 2011;364:2417–2428.
706. Zhong J, Gastaminza P, Cheng G, et al. Robust hepatitis C virus infection in vitro. *Proc Natl Acad Sci U S A* 2005;102:9294–9299.

CHAPTER 28

Paul S. Masters • Stanley Perlman

Coronaviridae

HISTORY

Coronaviruses are enveloped RNA viruses that are broadly distributed among humans, other mammals, and birds, causing acute and persistent infections. Members of this family were isolated as early as the 1930s as the causative agents of infectious bronchitis in chickens,[25] transmissible gastroenteritis in pigs,[142] and severe hepatitis and neurologic diseases in mice.[75,186] It was not until the 1960s, however, that these viruses,[27,32] as well as certain human respiratory viruses,[8,391] were recognized to share characteristics that merited their being grouped together. Their most notable common feature, revealed by electron microscopy, was a fringe of widely spaced, club-shaped spikes that projected from the virion surface; these spikes were morphologically distinct from the surface projections of ortho- and paramyxoviruses. The halo of spikes was described as giving the viral particle the appearance of the solar corona, which prompted the name that was adopted for this new virus group.[7]

Over the next 40 years, coronaviruses were studied mainly because they cause economically significant respiratory and gastrointestinal diseases in domestic animals and because they provide unique models for viral pathogenesis. In humans, two coronaviruses were known to be responsible for a substantial fraction of common colds, particularly those that circulate in winter months. This situation changed dramatically with the emergence in 2002 of a devastating new human disease, severe acute respiratory syndrome (SARS), which was caused by a previously unknown coronavirus.[143,288,440] Research stimulated by the SARS outbreak has led to great strides in our understanding of coronaviruses; by 2005, two additional, widespread human respiratory coronaviruses had been discovered.[573,615] Moreover, the search for animal virus reservoirs has nearly tripled the total number of identified coronaviruses,[255,394,616] although most of the recently discovered species are known only as genomic sequences and have yet to be isolated or propagated experimentally.

CLASSIFICATION

The coronaviruses are the largest group within the *Nidovirales* (Fig. 28.1), an order that comprises the families *Coronaviridae, Arteriviridae,*[524] and *Roniviridae.*[102] The arteriviruses, a small group of mammalian pathogens, are discussed in Chapter 29. The roniviruses, which infect shrimp, and a very recently isolated mosquito-borne virus,[416,663] which is not yet classified, are currently the only members of the order having invertebrate hosts. Nidoviruses are membrane-enveloped, nonsegmented positive-strand RNA viruses that are set apart from other RNA viruses by certain distinctive characteristics.[194] Their most significant common features are (a) an invariant general genomic organization, with a very large replicase gene upstream of the structural protein genes; (b) the expression of the replicase-transcriptase polyprotein by means of ribosomal frame shifting; (c) a collection of unique enzymatic activities contained within the replicase-transcriptase protein products; and (d) the expression of downstream genes via transcription of multiple

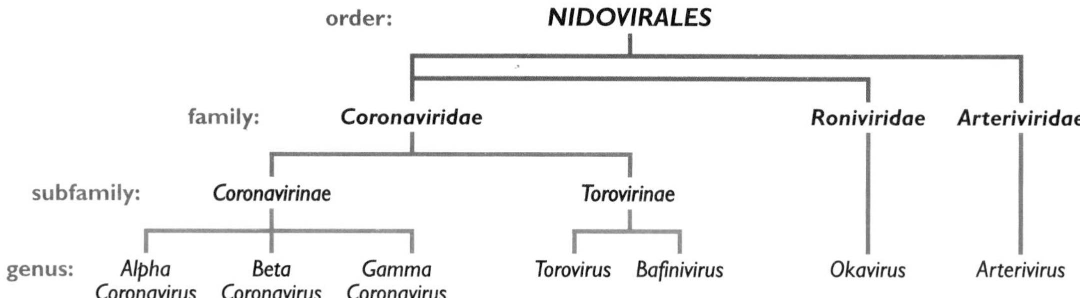

FIGURE 28.1. Taxonomy of the order *Nidovirales*.

3′-nested subgenomic messenger RNAs (mRNAs). This last property has provided the name for the order, which comes from the Latin *nido,* for "nest".[157] It should be noted that the replicative similarities among the three nidovirus families are offset by marked differences in the numbers, types, and sizes of their structural proteins and great variation among the morphologies of their virions and nucleocapsids.

Coronaviruses are now classified as one of two subfamilies (*Coronavirinae*) in the family *Coronaviridae* (see Fig. 28.1). The other subfamily, *Torovirinae,* includes the toroviruses, which are pathogens of cattle, horses, and swine,[523] and the bafiniviruses, whose sole member is the only nidovirus currently known to infect fish.[505] This chapter will concentrate almost exclusively on the *Coronavirinae.*

Coronaviruses have long been sorted into three groups, originally on the basis of serologic relationships and, subsequently, on the basis of phylogenetic clustering.[193,195] Following proposals that were recently ratified by the International Committee on Taxonomy of Viruses (ICTV),[57] these groups—the alpha-, beta-, and gammacoronaviruses—have now been accorded the taxonomic status of genera (see Fig. 28.1). The ICTV classifications have also established rigorous criteria for coronavirus species definitions, in a manner consistent with those used for other viral families. As a consequence, some viruses previously considered to be separate species are currently recognized as a single species—for example, the viruses now grouped within alphacoronavirus 1 or betacoronavirus 1 (Table 28.1). Additionally, the new classification criteria resolve any previous uncertainty about the taxonomic assignment of the virus that caused SARS (severe acute respiratory syndrome coronavirus [SARS-CoV]) as a betacoronavirus.[153,197,374,473,483,521,534,535]

Almost all alpha- and betacoronaviruses have mammalian hosts. In contrast, the gammacoronaviruses, with a single exception, have been isolated from avian hosts. Several of the viruses listed in Table 28.1 have been studied for decades, specifically those included in the species alphacoronavirus 1, betacoronavirus 1, murine coronavirus, and avian coronavirus. The focus on these viruses came about largely because they were amenable to isolation and growth in tissue culture. However, since 2004, molecular surveillance and genomics efforts initiated in the wake of the SARS epidemic have led to the discovery of a multitude of previously unknown coronaviruses that now constitute most members of this subfamily.[616] Notably, most of the newly recognized species were identified in bats, which constitute one of the largest orders within the mammals. Diverse coronaviruses have been described from bats, principally in Asia but also in Africa, Europe, and North and South America. These viruses include likely predecessors of SARS-CoV[308,332] but also four unique species of alphacoronaviruses and three species of betacoronaviruses. Birds have also proven to be a rich source of new viruses. Novel avian coronaviruses have been found to infect geese, pigeons, and ducks,[255] and highly divergent coronaviruses recently identified in bulbuls, thrushes, and munias[617] have the potential to define a fourth genus in the *Coronavirinae.* It has been proposed that bats and birds are ideally suited as reservoirs for the incubation and evolution of coronaviruses, owing to their common ability to fly and their propensity to roost and flock.[616]

Five of the viruses in Table 28.1 are associated with human disease. The most categorically harmful of these, SARS-CoV, which is discussed at length later in this chapter, does not currently infect the human population. The remaining four human coronaviruses (HCoVs), the alphacoronaviruses HCoV-229E and HCoV-NL63, and the betacoronaviruses HCoV-OC43 and HCoV-HKU1, typically cause common colds. Remarkably, HCoV-NL63 and HCoV-HKU1 were only discovered recently, in the post-SARS era,[573,615] despite the fact that each has a worldwide prevalence and has been in circulation for a long time.[461,618] Although generally associated with upper respiratory tract infections, the extant HCoVs can also cause lower respiratory tract infections and have more serious consequences in the young, the elderly, and immunocompromised individuals. In particular, HCoV-NL63 is strongly associated with childhood croup,[574] and the most severe HCoV-HKU1, -OC43, and -229E infections are manifest in patients with other underlying illnesses.[460]

VIRION STRUCTURE

Virus and Nucleocapsid

Virions of coronaviruses are roughly spherical and exhibit a moderate degree of pleomorphism. In the earlier literature, viral particles were reported to have average diameters of 80 to 120 nm but were far from uniform, with extreme sizes from 50 to 200 nm.[389] The spikes of coronaviruses, typically described as club-like or petal-shaped, emerge from the virion surface as stalks with bulb-like distal termini. Some of the variation in particle size and shape was likely attributable to stresses exerted by virion purification or distortions introduced by negative staining of samples for electron microscopy. More recent studies, employing cryo-electron microscopy and cryo-electron tomography,[21,30,413,415] have produced images (e.g., Fig. 28.2A) in which virion size and shape are far more regular, although still

TABLE 28.1 Classification of Coronaviruses

Species[a]	GenBank accession[b]	Previous names for viruses included in newly defined species
Genus *Alphacoronavirus*		
Alphacoronavirus 1	EU186072	Feline coronavirus type I (FeCoV I)
	AY994055	Feline coronavirus type II (FeCoV II), Feline infectious peritonitis virus (FIPV)
	GQ477367	Canine coronavirus (CCoV)
	AJ271965	Transmissible gastroenteritis virus (TGEV)
Human coronavirus 229E (HCoV-229E)	AF304460	
Human coronavirus NL63 (HCoV-NL63)	AY567487	
Porcine epidemic diarrhea virus (PEDV)	AF353511	
Rhinolophus bat coronavirus HKU2 (*Rh*-BatCoV HKU2)	EF203067	
Scotophilus bat coronavirus 512 (*Sc*-BatCoV 512)	DQ648858	
Miniopterus bat coronavirus 1 (*Mi*-BatCoV 1)	EU420138	
Miniopterus bat coronavirus HKU8 (*Mi*-BatCoV HKU8)	EU420139	
Genus *Betacoronavirus*		
Betacoronavirus 1[c]	U00735	Bovine coronavirus (BCoV)
	EF446615	Equine coronavirus (EqCoV)
	AY903460	Human coronavirus OC43 (HCoV-OC43)
	DQ011855	Porcine hemagglutinating encephalomyelitis virus (PHEV)
Murine coronavirus[d]	AY700211	Mouse hepatitis virus (MHV)
	FJ938068	Rat coronavirus (RCoV)
Human coronavirus HKU1 (HCoV-HKU1)	AY597011	
Severe acute respiratory syndrome–related coronavirus (SARSr-CoV)	AY278741	Human severe acute respiratory syndrome coronavirus (SARS-CoV)
	DQ022305	Severe acute respiratory syndrome–related *Rhinolophus* bat coronavirus HKU3 (SARSr-*Rh*-BatCoV HKU3)
	DQ071615	Severe acute respiratory syndrome–related *Rhinolophus* bat coronavirus Rp3 (SARSr-*Rh*-BatCoV Rp3)
Tylonycteris bat coronavirus HKU4 (*Ty*-BatCoV HKU4)	EF065505	
Pipistrellus bat coronavirus HKU5 (*Pi*-BatCoV HKU5)	EF065509	
Rousettus bat coronavirus HKU9 (*Ro*-BatCoV HKU9)	EF065513	
Genus *Gammacoronavirus*		
Avian coronavirus[e]	AJ311317	Infectious bronchitis virus (IBV)
	EU022526	Turkey coronavirus (TuCoV)
Beluga whale coronavirus SW1	EU111742	

[a]Listed viruses are those for which complete genome sequences are available. Novel viruses that have not yet been formally classified include Bulbul coronavirus HKU11,[617] Thrush coronavirus HKU12,[617] Munia coronavirus HKU13,[617] Asian leopard cat coronavirus,[139] and Mink coronavirus.[592]

[b]Representative GenBank accession numbers are given for viruses in each species; in many cases, multiple genomic sequences for a given virus are available.

[c]Other viruses included in the species Betacoronavirus 1 are Human enteric coronavirus (HECoV) and Canine respiratory coronavirus (CRCoV), for which only partial genomic sequences are available.

[d]Other viruses included in the species Murine coronavirus are Puffinosis virus (PCoV) and Sialodacryoadenitis virus (SDAV), for which only partial genomic sequences are available.

[e]Other viruses included in the species Avian coronavirus are Pheasant coronavirus (PhCoV), Goose coronavirus (GCoV), Pigeon coronavirus (PCoV), and Duck coronavirus (DCoV), for which only partial genomic sequences are available.[255]

pleomorphic. These studies, which examined a number of alpha- and betacoronaviruses, converge on mean particle diameters of 118 to 136 nm, including the contributions of the spikes, which project some 16 to 21 nm from the virion envelope.

Enclosed within the virion envelope is the nucleocapsid—a ribonucleoprotein that contains the viral genome. The structure of this component is relatively obscure in images of whole virions; however, its makeup has been partially displayed by electron micrographs of spontaneously disrupted virions or of virions solubilized with nonionic detergents.[59,109,183,269,366] Such studies revealed another distinguishing characteristic of coronaviruses: They have helically symmetric nucleocapsids.

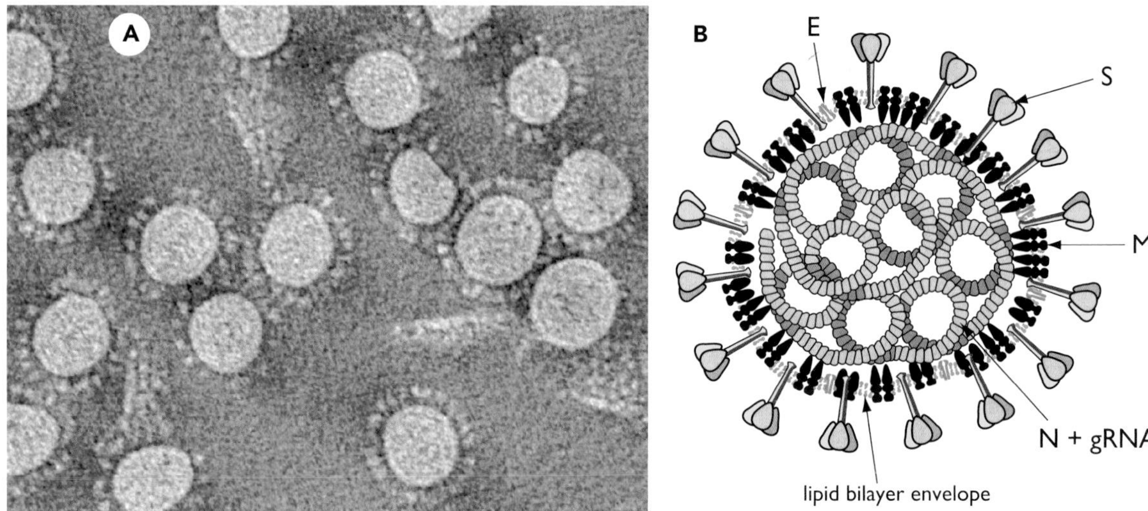

FIGURE 28.2. Coronavirus structure. A: Cryo-electron tomographic image of purified virions of mouse hepatitis virus (MHV), reconstructed as described in reference 415. (Courtesy of Benjamin Neuman, David Bhella, and Stanley Sawicki.) **B:** Schematic showing the major structural proteins of the coronavirus virion: S, spike protein; M, membrane protein; E, envelope protein; and N, nucleocapsid protein.

Helical symmetry is common for negative-strand RNA virus nucleocapsids, although it is highly unusual for positive-strand RNA animal viruses, almost all of which have icosahedral capsids. The best-resolved images of the coronavirus nucleocapsid, which were obtained with HCoV-229E, showed filamentous structures 9 to 13 nm in diameter, with 3- to 4-nm-wide central canals[59]; these filaments were thinner and less sharply segmented than paramyxovirus nucleocapsids. However, widely ranging and sometimes discrepant parameters have been reported for the nucleocapsids of other coronaviruses,[378] varying with both the viral species and the method of preparation.[109,183,269,366,476] Thus, further work is needed to clearly define the diameter, symmetry, length, and protein: RNA stoichiometry of this virion component in isolation. More recent coronavirus ultrastructural studies suggest that when packaged within the virion envelope, the helical nucleocapsid is quite flexible, forming coils and other structures that fold back on themselves.[21,413]

Virion Structural Proteins

Coronaviruses contain a canonical set of four major structural proteins: the spike (S), membrane (M), and envelope (E) proteins, all of which are located in the membrane envelope, and the nucleocapsid (N) protein, which is found in the ribonucleoprotein core (see Fig. 28.2B).

The distinctive surface spikes of coronaviruses are composed of trimers of S molecules.[30,129,529] S is a class I viral fusion protein[41] that binds to host cell receptors and mediates the earliest steps of infection.[95] In some cases, S protein can also induce cell–cell fusion late in infection. The S monomer is a transmembrane protein of 128 to 160 kDa, composed of a very large N-terminal ectodomain and a tiny C-terminal endodomain (Fig. 28.3). This protein is inserted, via a cleaved signal peptide,[62] into the endoplasmic reticulum (ER), where it obtains N-linked glycosylation increasing its mass by some 40 kDa.[224,487] Comprehensive mapping of glycosylation sites has not been carried out for any S protein; however, an analysis of the SARS-CoV S protein showed that at least half of its 23 candidate sites are glycosylated.[287] The early steps of glycosylation occur co-translationally, and this modification assists monomer folding and proper oligomerization; terminal glycosylation is then completed subsequent to trimerization.[129] S protein monomer folding is also accompanied by the formation of intramolecular disulfide bonds among a subset of the numerous cysteine residues of the ectodomain.[425] The positions of S protein cysteines are well conserved in each coronavirus genus[2,153]; disulfide linkages have yet to be mapped.

In many beta- and gammacoronaviruses (e.g., mouse hepatitis virus [MHV], bovine coronavirus [BCoV], and infectious bronchitis virus [IBV]), the S protein is partially or completely cleaved by a furin-like host cell protease into two polypeptides, denoted S1 and S2, which are roughly equal in size. Correspondingly, in coronaviruses that do not have detectably cleaved mature S proteins, the N-terminal and C-terminal halves of the molecule are also designated S1 and S2, respectively. S protein cleavage occurs immediately downstream of a highly basic pentapeptide motif,[2,62,361] and the extent of proteolysis correlates with the number of positively charged residues in the motif.[36] The S1 domain is extremely variable, exhibiting very low homology across the three genera and often diverging extensively among different isolates of a single coronavirus.[181,430,597] By contrast, the S2 domain is highly conserved.[111] For those coronaviruses in which it occurs, S1-S2 cleavage is a late event in virion assembly and release from infected cells. For many other coronaviruses, an alternative type of S protein cleavage (S2′) takes place during the initiation of infection, activating the molecule for fusion.[28] The differing functions of S1 and S2 and the role of proteolysis are discussed later (see the Viral Entry and Uncoating section).

A complete high-resolution structure has not yet been determined for any coronavirus S protein, although a cryo-electron microscopic reconstruction of the SARS-CoV S protein is available,[30] and partial crystal structures have been solved for particular S protein domains.[144,208,323,325,624,630,655]

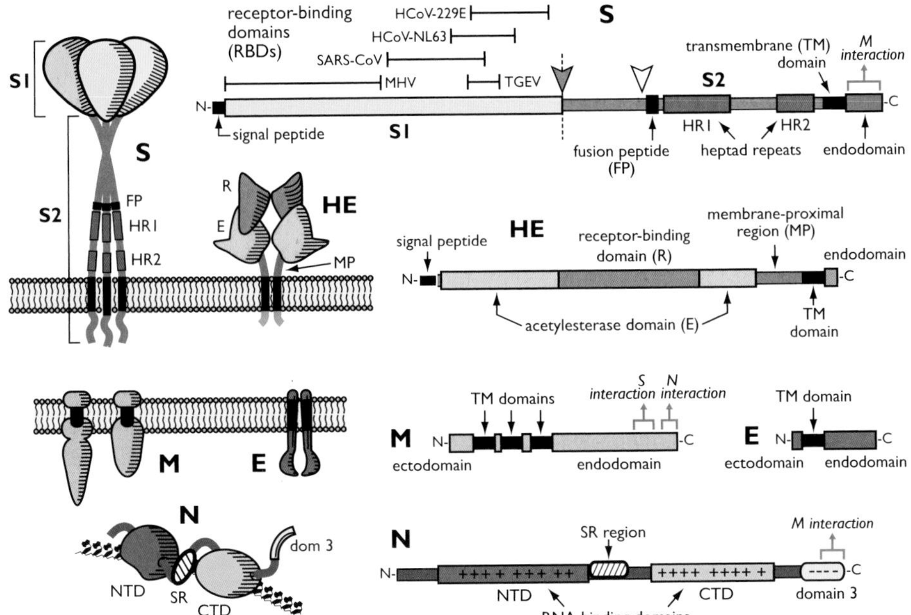

FIGURE 28.3. Virion structural proteins. Folded and linear representations of the spike (S), hemagglutinin-esterase (HE), membrane (M), envelope (E), and nucleocapsid (N) proteins. The size scale for the linear diagram of S is half of that for the other proteins. In the linear diagram of S, *solid* and *open arrowheads* indicate the S1-S2 and alternative (S2′) cleavage sites, respectively. In the linear diagrams of S, M, and N, *red brackets* indicate mapped regions involved in assembly interactions (see the Assembly and Release of Virions section).

Nevertheless, all currently available structural and biochemical evidence accords well with an early proposal that S is functionally analogous to the influenza HA protein.[111] In this model, the S1 domains of the S protein oligomer make up the bulbous, receptor-binding portion of the spike. The narrow stalk of the spike, distancing the bulb from the membrane, is a coiled-coil structure formed by association of heptad repeat regions (HR1 and HR2) of the S2 domains of monomers (see Fig. 28.3).

The most abundant structural protein in coronaviruses—the M protein[544,546]—gives the virion envelope its shape. The M monomer, which ranges from 25 to 30 kDa, is a polytopic membrane protein that is embedded in the envelope by three transmembrane domains.[14,486] At its amino terminus is a very small ectodomain; the C-terminal endodomain of M accounts for the major part of the molecule and is situated in the interior of the virion or on the cytoplasmic face of intracellular membranes (see Fig. 28.3). Although it is inserted co-translationally into the ER membrane, the M protein generally does not bear an amino-terminal signal peptide.[62,486] For IBV and MHV, either the first or the third transmembrane domain of M alone suffices as a signal for insertion and anchoring of the protein in its native membrane orientation.[350,363,384] Anomalously, M proteins of the alphacoronavirus 1 species do contain cleavable N-terminal signal peptides, although it is not clear whether these are necessary for membrane insertion.[263,584] The ectodomain of M is modified by glycosylation, which is usually N linked.[60,251,402,536,632] However, a subset of betacoronavirus M proteins exhibit O-linked glycosylation, and the MHV M protein has served as a model for study of this type of post-translational modification.[116,349,419] Glycosylation of M influences both organ tropism and the interferon (IFN)-inducing capacity of some coronaviruses.[72,113,311]

M proteins are moderately well conserved within each coronavirus genus but diverge considerably across genera. The most variable part of the molecule is the ectodomain. By contrast, a short segment, overlapping the third transmembrane domain and the start of the endodomain, exhibits a high degree of sequence conservation that is seen even in torovirus M proteins.[132] Like most multispanning membrane proteins, the M protein has been refractory to crystallization; however, recent cryo-electron microscopic and tomographic reconstructions have provided a glimpse of the structure of this protein within the virion envelope.[21,413,415] These studies reveal that the large carboxy terminus of M extends some 6 to 8 nm into the viral particle and is compressed into a globular domain, consistent with early work showing that the endodomain is very resistant to proteases.[61,384,486,490] The observed M structures are likely to be dimers, the monomers of which are associated through multiple interacting regions. M dimers appear to adopt two different conformations: a compact form that promotes greater membrane curvature and a more elongated form that contacts the nucleocapsid.[415]

The E protein is a small polypeptide of 8 to 12 kDa that is found in limited amounts in the virion envelope.[189,344,647] Despite its minor presence, no wild-type coronavirus has been discovered to lack this protein. Engineered knockout or deletion of the *E* gene has effects ranging from moderate[124] to severe[293,296] to lethal.[105,428] Thus, although E is not always essential, it is critical for coronavirus infectivity (see the Assembly and Release of Virions section). E protein sequences are widely divergent, even among closely related coronaviruses.[293] However, all E proteins share a common architecture: a short hydrophilic amino terminus, followed by a large hydrophobic region, and, lastly, a large hydrophilic C-terminal tail (see Fig. 28.3). E is an integral membrane protein,[100,335,582] but it does not have a cleavable signal peptide[465] and is not glycosylated. Beta- and gammacoronavirus E proteins are palmitoylated on cysteine residues downstream and adjacent to the hydrophobic region[38,101,335,354,647]; this modification remains to be found in an alphacoronavirus E protein.[189] The membrane topology of E is not completely resolved. Most evidence indicates that this polypeptide transits the membrane once, with an N-terminal exodomain and a C-terminal endodomain.[101,420,465,564,582] Contrary to this are reports that E has a hairpin conformation, placing both of its termini on the cytoplasmic face of membranes,[12,368] or that E can have multiple membrane topologies.[648] Also unresolved is the oligomeric state of E protein. The hydrophobic region of the SARS-CoV E protein forms multimers, from dimers through pentamers.[564,610] A pentameric alpha-helical bundle structure has been solved for this domain,[449] although it is not yet clear whether this reflects the organization of the native protein.

Residing in the interior of the virion, the N protein is the sole protein constituent of the helical nucleocapsid.[222] Monomers of this 43- to 50-kDa protein bind along the RNA genome in a beads-on-a-string configuration common to other helical viral nucleocapsids (see Fig. 28.2B). However, unlike the nucleoproteins of rhabdo- and paramyxoviruses, the coronavirus N protein provides little or no protection for its genome against the action of ribonucleases.[366,408] The bulk of the N protein monomer is made up of two independently folding domains—designated the N-terminal domain (NTD) and the C-terminal domain (CTD)—although neither includes its respective terminus of the N molecule (see Fig. 28.3). Crystal or solution structures have been determined for NTDs and CTDs of SARS-CoV, IBV, and MHV.[76,164,200,234,253,493,555,646] Flanking the NTD and CTD are three spacer segments, the central one of which contains a serine- and arginine-rich tract (the SR region), which was noted to resemble the SR domains of RNA-splicing factors.[442] Another functionally distinct region of N, the carboxy-terminal domain 3, has been defined genetically.[236,279,441,442] The spacer segments and domain 3 are each likely to be intrinsically disordered polypeptides.[66,67] Most of the N molecule, including the NTD and CTD, is highly basic; by contrast, domain 3 is acidic. There is only a moderate degree of sequence homology among N proteins across the three genera, with the exception of a stretch of 30 amino acids within the NTD that is highly conserved among all coronaviruses.[380]

The N protein is a phosphoprotein,[272,352,515,542] modified at a limited number of serine and threonine residues. Phosphorylation sites have been mapped for a representative coronavirus from each genus, and targeted sites, collectively, fall in every domain and spacer region of the N molecule.[55,77,604,619] Thus, a general pattern for N protein phosphorylation cannot yet be discerned, nor have all responsible kinases been identified, although there is evidence linking glycogen synthase kinase-3 to phosphorylation of the SR region.[619] The role of phosphorylation is also not known but is thought to have regulatory impact. Phosphorylation has been suggested to trigger a conformational change in N protein,[541] and it may enhance the affinity of N for viral versus nonviral RNA.[77]

The most conspicuous function of the N protein is to bind to viral RNA. Nucleocapsid formation must involve both sequence-specific and nonspecific modes of RNA binding. Specific RNA substrates that have been identified for N protein include the transcription-regulating sequence (TRS)[200,412,539] (see the Viral RNA Synthesis section) and the genomic RNA packaging signal[96,396] (see the Assembly and Release of Virions section). The NTD and the CTD are each separately capable of binding to RNA ligands *in vitro,* and the structures of these domains offer some clues as to how this is accomplished. The NTD consists of a U-shaped β-platform with an extruding β-hairpin, which presents a putative RNA-binding groove rich in basic and aromatic amino acid residues.[164,200,493] The CTD forms a tightly interconnected dimer, which exhibits a potential RNA-binding groove lined by basic α-helixes.[253,555] Some work suggests that in the intact N protein, optimal RNA binding requires concerted contributions from both the NTD and the CTD.[67,235] A significant fraction of nucleocapsid stability also results from interactions among N monomers.[408] This level of association is generally attributed to the CTD[67,164,253,646]; however, additional regions of N–N interaction have been mapped to the NTD and to domain 3.[164,235,253] Another crucial function of N protein is to bind to M protein.[162,546] This capability is provided by domain 3 of N.[236,295,585]

A fifth prominent structural protein—the hemagglutinin-esterase (HE) protein—is found in only a subset of the betacoronaviruses, including murine coronavirus, betacoronavirus 1, and HCoV-HKU1. In virions of these species, HE forms a secondary set of short projections of 5 to 10 nm arrayed beneath the canopy of S protein spikes.[204,435,550] The 48-kDa HE monomer is composed almost entirely of an N-terminal ectodomain; this is followed by a transmembrane anchor and a very short C-terminal endodomain (see Fig. 28.3). HE is inserted into the ER by means of a cleaved signal peptide and acquires an additional 17 kDa of N-linked glycosylation at multiple sites.[221,271,640] The assembled protein is a homodimer, the subunits of which are connected by disulfide bonds.[221] As its name indicates, the HE protein contains a pair of associated activities. First, it is a hemagglutinin—that is, it has the capability to bind to sialic acid moieties found on cell surface glycoproteins and glycolipids.[54,272] Second, HE exhibits acetylesterase activity with specificity for either 9-*O*- or 4-*O*-acetylated sialic acids.[274,472,520,590,591] These characteristics are thought to allow HE to act as a cofactor for S protein, assisting attachment of virus to host cells, as well as expediting the travel of virus through the extracellular mucosa.[99] Consistent with this notion, the presence of HE in MHV dramatically enhances neurovirulence in the mouse host.[265] Conversely, the HE protein is a burden to the virus in tissue culture, where its expression is rapidly counterselected.[343] The two activities of the HE protein are strikingly similar to the receptor-binding and receptor-destroying activities found in influenza C virus,[590,591] and, remarkably, the coronavirus *HE* gene is clearly related to the influenza C virus *HEF* gene.[359] Moreover, toroviruses also possess a homolog of the *HE* gene,[99,305] raising the possibility that all three of these virus groups evolved from a common ancestor.[359,522] This kinship is further corroborated by the crystal structure of the BCoV HE protein, which reveals separate receptor-binding and acetylesterase domains perched atop a truncated membrane-proximal region.[650] The HE protein thus resembles a squat version of its influenza virus counterpart, shortened because it lacks the fusion domain stalk of the HEF protein.

GENOME STRUCTURE AND ORGANIZATION

Basic and Accessory Genes

The coronavirus genome, which ranges from 26 to 32 kb, is the largest among all RNA viruses, including RNA viruses that have segmented genomes. This exceptional RNA molecule acts in at least three capacities[50,194]: as the initial mRNA of the infectious cycle (see the Expression of the Replicase-Transcriptase Complex section), as the template for RNA replication and transcription (see the Viral RNA Synthesis section), and as the substrate for packaging into progeny viruses (see

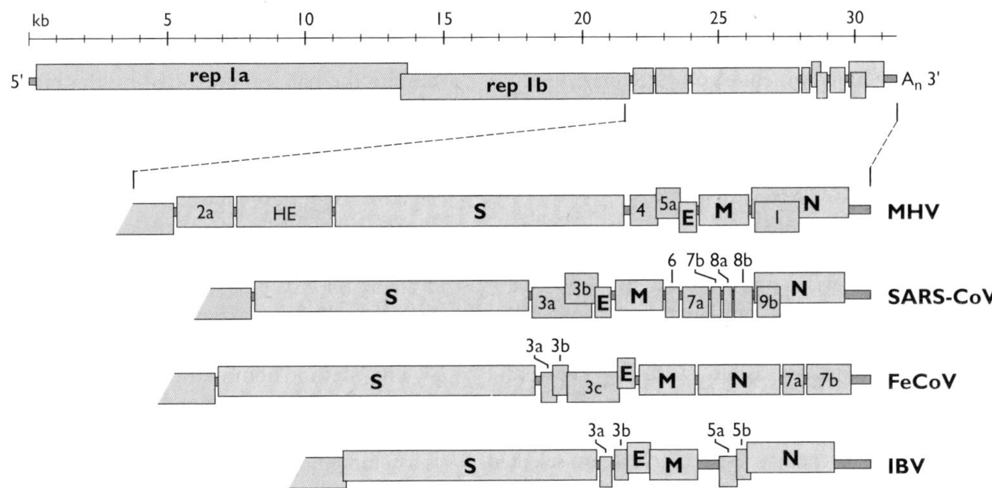

FIGURE 28.4. Coronavirus genome organization. A schematic of the complete genome of MHV is shown at the top. The replicase gene constitutes two ORFs, rep 1a and rep 1b, which are expressed by a ribosomal frameshifting mechanism (see the Expression of the Replicase-Transcriptase Complex section). The expanded region shows the downstream portion of the genomes of two betacoronaviruses (MHV and SARS-CoV), an alphacoronavirus (FeCoV), and a gammacoronavirus (IBV). The sizes and positions of accessory genes are indicated, relative to the basic genes *S, E, M*, and *N*. MHV, mouse hepatitis virus; ORFs, open reading frames; SARS-CoV, severe acute respiratory syndrome coronavirus; FeCoV, feline coronavirus; IBV, infectious bronchitis virus.

the Assembly and Release of Virions section). Consistent with its role as an mRNA, the coronavirus genome has a standard eukaryotic 5′-terminal cap structure[301] and a 3′ polyadenylate tail.[302,351,503,599] The genome comprises a basic set of genes in the invariant order *5′-replicase-S-E-M-N-3′*, with the huge *replicase* gene occupying two-thirds of the available coding capacity (Fig. 28.4). The replicase-transcriptase is the only protein translated from the genome; the products of all downstream open reading frames (ORFs) are derived from subgenomic mRNAs. The 5′-most position of the *replicase* gene is dictated by the requirement for expression of the replicase to set in motion all subsequent events of infection. The organization of the other basic genes, however, does not seem to reflect any underlying principle, because engineered rearrangement of the downstream gene order is completely tolerated.[121]

Dispersed among the basic genes in the 3′-most third of the genome, there are from one to as many as eight additional ORFs, which are designated accessory genes[378,407] (see Fig. 28.4). These can fall in any of the intergenic intervals downstream of the *replicase* gene,[616] except, curiously, never between the *E* and *M* genes. In some cases, an accessory gene can be partially or entirely embedded as an alternate reading frame within another gene—for example, the internal (*I*) gene of MHV or the *3b* gene of SARS-CoV. Accessory genes are generally numbered according to the smallest transcript in which they fall. Consequently, there is usually no relatedness among identically named accessory genes in coronaviruses of different genera, such as the *3a* genes of SARS-CoV, feline coronavirus (FeCoV), and IBV (see Fig. 28.4). Some of these extra ORFs are thought to have been acquired through ancestral recombination with RNA from cellular or heterologous viral sources. The *HE* gene is the best-supported example of this type of horizontal genetic transfer.[359] Two other such candidates are the *2a* gene found in murine coronavirus and betacoronavirus 1, which encodes a putative 2′,3′-cyclic phosphodiesterase,[385,485] and gene *10* of beluga whale coronavirus, which encodes a putative uridine-cytidine kinase.[394] Notably, the *2a* gene has a homolog embedded as a module within the *replicase* gene of the toroviruses,[522] which is a situation also consistent with horizontal transfer. The origin of most accessory genes, however, remains an open question. It is plausible that some of them evolved through intragenomic recombination, resulting in gene duplication and subsequent divergence, as suggested for several of the accessory genes of SARS-CoV.[241]

Almost all accessory genes that have been examined are expressed during infection, although their functions are incompletely understood. The protein products of most accessory genes are nonstructural; however, this rule is not without exception. The HE protein, the MHV I protein,[165] and the products of SARS-CoV ORFs 3a, 6, 7a, 7b, and 9b[231,407,502,627] are all components of virions. Mutational knockout or deletion of accessory genes has revealed that none are essential for viral replication in tissue culture. Conversely, accessory gene ablation,[103,115,206] or transfer to another virus,[452,559] can have profound effects on viral pathogenesis. In some cases, the basis for this is understood to result from interactions with host innate immunity (see the Immune Response and Viral Evasion of the Immune Response section). For other accessory genes, though, potential *in vivo* functions have not yet been elucidated.[125,165,645]

Coronavirus Genetics

Classical coronavirus genetics focused principally on two types of mutants.[299] The first were naturally arising viral variants, particularly deletion mutants, which offered clues to genetic changes responsible for different pathogenic traits.[430,583,603] The second were temperature-sensitive (*ts*) mutants isolated from MHV following chemical mutagenesis.[282,477,501,545] Some of these proved to be valuable in analyses of the functions of structural proteins.[279,360,380,474] However, owing to the large target size of the *replicase* gene, most of such randomly generated mutants had conditional-lethal, RNA-negative phenotypes. Complementation analyses of these latter mutants yielded early insights into the multiplicity of functions entailed by coronavirus RNA synthesis.[22,176,177,501] There has been a recent resurgence of interest in classical replicase *ts* mutants, which are currently sorted into five complementation groups, because they can now be fully examined by the tools of reverse genetics.[138,499,543]

The development of coronavirus reverse genetics proceeded in two phases.[130] Initially, a method called *targeted RNA recombination* was devised at a time when it was uncertain whether the construction of full-length infectious complementary DNA (cDNA) clones of coronavirus genomes would ever become technically feasible. With this method, a synthetic donor RNA bearing mutations of interest is transfected into cells that have been infected with a recipient parent virus possessing some characteristic that can be selected against.[279,377,380] In its current form, for manipulation of MHV, the technique uses a chimeric recipient parent virus designated fMHV (Fig. 28.5A). The fMHV chimera is a mutant of MHV that contains the S protein ectodomain from the FeCoV feline infectious peritonitis virus (FIPV) and can therefore only grow in feline cells (see the Virion Attachment to Host Cells section). The restoration of its ability to grow in murine cells, via recombination with donor RNA containing the MHV *S* gene, enables a strong selection for viruses bearing site-specific mutations[292,381]; unwanted secondary crossover events distal to the *S* gene are eliminated owing to the rearrangement of downstream genes in fMHV.[190] Targeted RNA recombination remains a powerful method to recover structural or accessory protein or 3′ untranslated region (UTR) mutants.

To obtain access to the major part of the coronavirus genome, however, it was necessary to create full-length cDNAs, despite the barriers presented by the huge size of the *replicase* gene and the high instability of various regions when propagated in bacterial clones. Three innovative strategies were developed to overcome these inherent difficulties.[130] In the first (see Fig. 28.5B), a full-length cDNA copy of a coronavirus genome is assembled downstream of a cytomegalovirus (CMV) promoter in a bacterial artificial chromosome (BAC) vector, which is stable by virtue of its low copy number.[5,6] The infection is then launched from transfected BAC DNA through transcription of infectious coronavirus RNA by host RNA polymerase II. This method of initiating infection obviates potential limitations of *in vitro* capping and synthesis of genomic RNA. In the second strategy (see Fig. 28.5C), a full-length genomic cDNA is assembled by *in vitro* ligation of smaller cloned cDNA fragments, some of the boundaries of which have been chosen so as to interrupt regions of instability.[642,643] The ligation occurs in a directed order that is dictated by the use of asymmetric restriction sites. Infectious genomic RNA is then transcribed *in vitro* and used to transfect susceptible host cells. An extension of this method has demonstrated the construction of a coronavirus genome entirely from synthetic cDNAs.[26] In the third strategy (see Fig. 28.5D), the genome of vaccinia virus is used as the cloning vector for a full-length coronavirus cDNA that is generated by long-range reverse transcription polymerase chain reaction (RT-PCR).[94,561] The cDNA is then amenable to manipulation by the repertoire of techniques available for poxvirus reverse genetics.[51,94] Infections are launched from *in vitro*–synthesized RNA or else from transfected cDNA

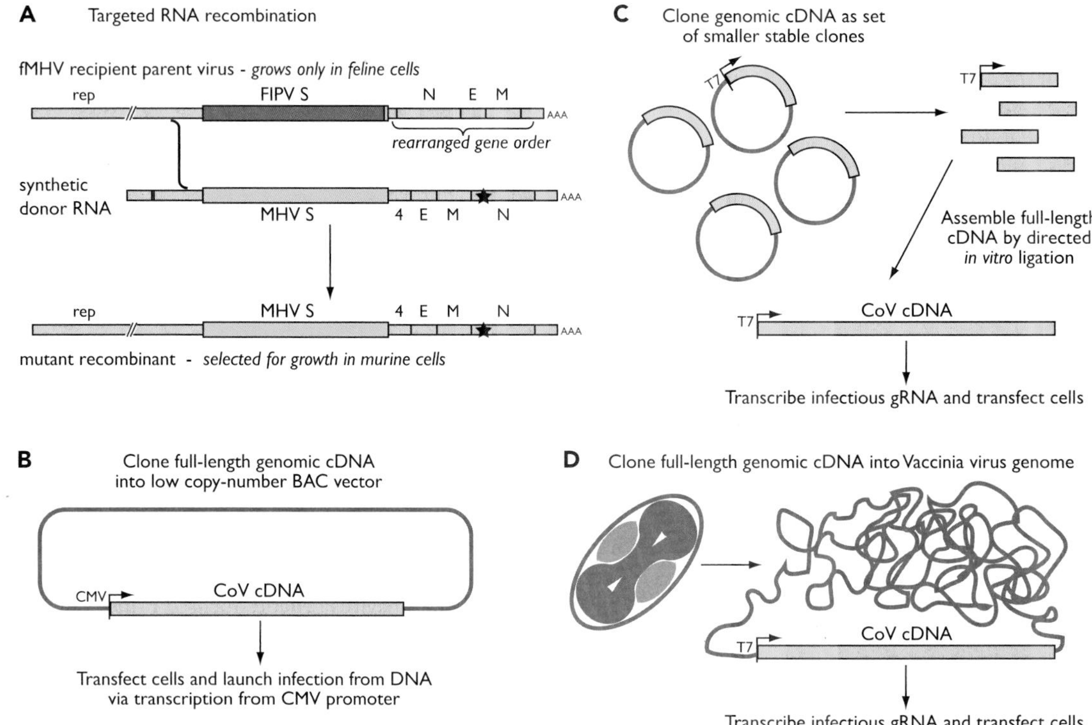

FIGURE 28.5. Methods for coronavirus reverse genetics. A: Targeted RNA recombination, which is applicable to the downstream third of the genome, shown here for transduction of a mutation (*star*) into the mouse hepatitis virus *N* gene. **B–D:** Three schemes developed for complete reverse genetics, based on stable production of full-length genomic complementary DNAs.

transcribed *in vivo* by fowlpox-encoded T7 RNA polymerase.[58] Collectively, these systems developed for complete reverse genetics provide an important pathway toward unraveling the complexities of the coronavirus replicase.

CORONAVIRUS REPLICATION

Virion Attachment to Host Cells

Coronavirus infections are initiated by the binding of virions to cellular receptors (Fig. 28.6). There then follows a series of events culminating in the delivery of the nucleocapsid to the cytoplasm, where the viral genome becomes available for translation. Individual coronaviruses usually infect only one or a few closely related hosts. The interaction between the viral S protein and its cognate receptor constitutes the principal determinant governing coronavirus host species range and tissue tropism. This has been most convincingly shown in two ways. First, the expression of a particular receptor in nonpermissive cells of a heterologous species renders those cells permissive for the corresponding coronavirus.[127,146,330,331,399,567,639] Second, the engineered replacement of the S protein ectodomain changes the host cell species specificity or tissue tropism of a coronavirus in a predictable fashion.[207,292,410,453,495] The amino-terminal, more variable half of the spike protein, S1, is the part that binds to receptor. Binding leads to conformational changes that result in fusion between virion and cell membranes, mediated by the more conserved half of the spike protein, S2. The region of S1 that contacts the receptor—the receptor-binding domain (RBD)—varies among different coronaviruses (see Fig. 28.3). For MHV, the RBD maps to the N-terminal section of S1.[290,554] By contrast, RBDs for SARS-CoV,[614,625] HCoV-NL63,[337] transmissible gastroenteritis virus (TGEV),[188] and HCoV-229E[34] fall in the middle or C-terminal sections of S1.

The known cellular receptors for alpha- and betacoronaviruses are listed in Table 28.2; to date, no receptors have been identified for gammacoronaviruses. The MHV receptor mCEACAM1 was the first discovered coronavirus receptor (as well as one of the first receptors defined for *any* virus).[606,607] That this molecule is the only biologically relevant receptor for MHV was made clear by the demonstration that homozygous *Ceacam1*$^{-/-}$ knockout mice are totally resistant to infection by high doses of MHV.[215] CEACAM1 is a member of the carcinoembryonic antigen (CEA) family within the immunoglobulin (Ig) superfamily and, in its full-length form, contains four Ig-like domains.[146] A diversity of two- and four-Ig domain isoforms is generated by multiple alleles and alternative splicing variants of *Ceacam1*.[97,145,147,422,423,641] The wide range of pathogenicity of MHV in mice is thought to be strongly affected by the interactions of S proteins of different virus strains with the array of receptor isoforms that are expressed in mice of different genetic backgrounds. Although their S proteins are phylogenetically very close to that of MHV, the betacoronaviruses BCoV and HCoV-OC43 do not use CEACAMs to infect their

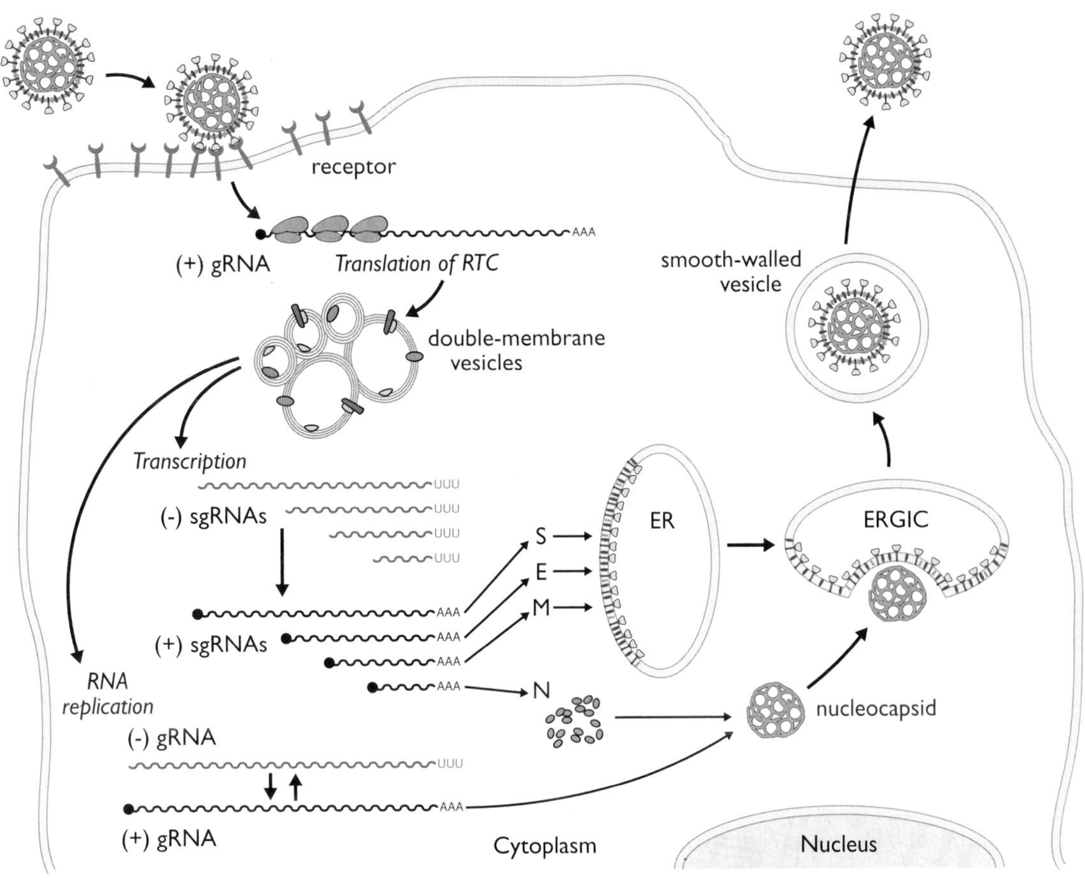

FIGURE 28.6. Overview of coronavirus replication (see text for details).

TABLE 28.2 Coronavirus Receptors

Virus	Receptor	References
Alphacoronaviruses		
TGEV	pAPN[a]	127
PRCoV	pAPN	128
PEDV	pAPN	322
FeCoV II, FIPV	fAPN[b]	567
FeCoV I	Unknown, but *not* fAPN[b]	148,223
CCoV	cAPN	29
HCoV-229E	hAPN	639
HCoV-NL63	ACE2	219
Betacoronaviruses		
MHV	mCEACAM1[c]	411,606
BCoV	N-acetyl-9-*O*-acetylneuraminic acid	504
HCoV-OC43	N-acetyl-9-*O*-acetylneuraminic acid	291
SARS-CoV	ACE2[d]	331

TGEV, transmissible gastroenteritis virus; pAPN, porcine aminopeptidase N; PRCoV, porcine respiratory coronavirus; PEDV, porcine epidemic diarrhea virus; FeCoV, feline coronavirus; fAPN, feline aminopeptidase N; FIPV, feline infectious peritonitis virus; CCoV, canine coronavirus; cAPN, canine aminopeptidase N; HCoV, human coronavirus; hAPN, human aminopeptidase N; ACE2, angiotensin-converting enzyme 2; MHV, mouse hepatitis virus; mCEACAM1, murine carcinoembryonic antigen–related adhesion molecule 1; BCoV, bovine coronavirus; SARS-CoV, severe acute respiratory syndrome coronavirus.

[a]Mammalian aminopeptidase N is also known as CD13.

[b]Although the receptor for FeCoV I remains to be identified, the lectin fDC-SIGN serves as a coreceptor for both FeCoV I and FeCoV II.[471]

[c]The related molecule mCEACAM2 functions weakly as an MHV receptor in tissue culture; however, it is not an alternate receptor in the mouse host *in vivo*.[215]

[d]Human CD209L (L-SIGN), a lectin family member, can also act as a receptor for SARS-CoV but with much lower efficiency than ACE2[254]; a related lectin, DC-SIGN, can serve as a coreceptor.[376,635]

hosts; rather, the only currently known attachment factor for these viruses is N-acetyl-9-*O*-acetylneuraminic acid.[291,504] The recently solved structure of the MHV RBD complexed with mCEACAM1 has allowed the identification of key residues at the S protein–receptor interface.[443] Coupled with mutational analysis, this structure reveals why the S proteins of BCoV and HCoV-OC43 cannot bind the MHV receptor and, conversely, why MHV does not bind to bovine or human CEACAMs.

Many alphacoronaviruses use aminopeptidase N (APN) of their respective host species as a receptor (see Table 28.2).[127,567,639] APN (also called CD13) is a cell-surface, zinc-binding protease that is resident in respiratory and enteric epithelia and in neural tissue. The APN molecule is a heavily glycosylated homodimer. Mutational and inhibitor studies have shown that its enzymatic activity is not required for viral attachment and entry.[126] In general, the receptor activities of APN homologs are not interchangeable among species[126,281]; however, feline aminopeptidase N (fAPN) can serve as a receptor not only for FIPV but also for canine coronavirus (CCoV), TGEV, and HCoV-229E.[567] This circumstance has been exploited for the construction of chimeric APN molecules to map the basis for receptor recognition. Such studies have found three small, linearly discontinuous determinants in APN that govern the species specificity of this subgroup of alphacoronaviruses.[29,214,280,569]

The receptor for SARS-CoV—angiotensin-converting enzyme 2 (ACE2)—was discovered with notable rapidity following the isolation of the virus.[331] ACE2 is a cell-surface, zinc-binding carboxypeptidase involved in regulation of cardiac function and blood pressure. It is expressed in epithelial cells of the lung and the small intestine, which are the primary targets of SARS-CoV, as well as in heart, kidney, and other tissues.[209] As with APN, the receptor role of ACE2 appears to be independent of its enzymatic activity. Although the SARS-CoV S protein binds to the catalytic domain of ACE2, active-site mutation or chemical inhibition does not detectably affect the ability of ACE2 to associate with S protein or to promote syncytia formation.[331,333,398] The crystal structure of the SARS-CoV S protein RBD in complex with ACE2 shows the RBD cradling one lobe of the claw-like catalytic domain of its receptor.[325] Remarkably, ACE2 also serves as the receptor for the alphacoronavirus HCoV-NL63,[219] and the corresponding structural complex for that virus reveals that the HCoV-NL63 RBD and the SARS-CoV RBD bind to the same motifs.[624] Because the SARS-CoV and HCoV-NL63 RBDs have neither sequence nor structural homology, this finding strongly supports the notion that they have independently evolved to bind to the same hotspot on the ACE2 surface.[623,624] Analyses of the SARS-CoV RBD–ACE2 interface have additionally demonstrated the structural basis for the final jump of SARS-CoV from palm civets to human hosts (see the Epidemiology section). These studies found that merely four critical residues constitute the major species barrier between the civet and human ACE2 molecules, and that mutation of only two key RBD residues was sufficient for civet SARS-CoV S protein to gain the ability to productively bind human ACE2.[323,333]

Viral Entry and Uncoating

The entry of virions into cells results from large-scale rearrangements of the S protein that lead to the fusion of viral and cellular membranes.[41] These rearrangements are triggered by some combination of receptor binding, proteolytic cleavage of S, and exposure to acidic pH. The S proteins of many coronaviruses are uncleaved in mature virions and require an encounter with a protease at the entry step of infection to separate the receptor-binding and fusion components of the spike. The details of proteolytic activation are still incompletely understood but have been best studied for SARS-CoV. In the cell types in which this virus is most commonly grown in tissue culture, viral entry depends on cathepsins, which are acid-activated endosomal proteases. The infectivity of SARS-CoV is thus suppressed by cathepsin inhibitors or by lysosomotropic agents.[517] However, cell-bound SARS-CoV can alternatively be activated by treatment with extracellular proteases, such as trypsin or elastase. This route of activation greatly enhances the infectivity of SARS-CoV and allows the virus to enter from the cell surface, thereby rendering the infection insensitive to lysosomotropic agents.[383] The same pattern of proteolytic activation—cathepsin-dependence and its circumvention by exogenously added protease—is observed with a particular strain of MHV (MHV-2) that is unique in having an uncleaved S protein.[464]

The site of cleavage of receptor-bound SARS-CoV S protein by cathepsin or by exogenous trypsin differs from that of the S1-S2 cleavage, which occurs in other coronaviruses upon exit from cells. Cleavage at entry takes place at a locus (S2′) within the S2 half of the molecule, immediately upstream of the putative fusion peptide[28] (see Fig. 28.3). It is not yet clear if cleavage at analogous S2′ sites is the pattern for all coronavirus S proteins; however, the emerging pattern is that proteolytic activation of S protein is required for infectivity and that coronaviruses have evolved in different ways to ensure that this occurs.[41] Recent studies provide evidence that for the SARS-CoV S protein, the most biologically relevant protease may be TMPRSS2.[187,382,514] This transmembrane serine protease, which is expressed in pneumocytes, co-localizes with and binds to ACE2. In cells expressing TMPRSS2, SARS-CoV enters at the cell surface and is insensitive to cathepsin inhibitors and lysosomotropic agents.

Just as the mechanism of S protein proteolytic activation is variable, so too is its location. Some coronaviruses, such as most strains of MHV, fuse with the plasma membrane,[547,601] whereas others, such as TGEV,[212] HCoV-229E,[421] and SARS-CoV,[517] can enter cells through receptor-mediated endocytosis and then fuse with the membranes of acidified endosomes. The boundary between these two modes of entry may easily shift. For one strain of MHV (MHV-4), as few as three amino acid changes in the heptad repeat region of S2 switches the virus from plasma membrane fusion to acid pH-dependent fusion.[180] It remains unresolved whether acidic pH, *per se,* is required for S protein conformational changes[90,154,324] or whether this reflects the requirements for activation of endosomal proteases during infection of some types of cells.[517]

The coronavirus S protein is a class I viral fusion protein with domains functionally similar to those of the fusion proteins of phylogenetically distant RNA viruses, such as influenza virus, human immunodeficiency virus (HIV), and Ebola virus, but on a much larger scale.[41,42] As in those other viral fusion proteins, the coronavirus S2 moiety contains two separated heptad repeats—HR1 and HR2—with a fusion peptide upstream of HR1 and the transmembrane domain immediately downstream of HR2 (see Fig. 28.3). The exact assignment of the fusion peptide is not agreed upon, however.[41,367,450] Receptor-mediated conformational changes in S1, and the dissociation of S1 from S2, are thought to initiate major rearrangements in the remaining S2 trimer that proceed through multiple intermediate states.[133,324] These rearrangements ultimately expose the fusion peptide, which interacts with the host cellular membrane, and the two heptad repeats in each monomer are brought together to form an antiparallel, six-helix bundle. The six-helix bundle is an extremely stable, rod-like complex, the biophysical properties of which have been extensively studied.[40,42,242,348,568] Highly similar crystallographic structures have been solved for the six-helix complexes from both the MHV S protein[629] and the SARS-CoV S protein.[144,552,630] These show the three HR1 helices forming a central, coiled-coil core some two to three times larger than its counterparts in other viruses. Arrayed around this, the three shorter HR2 helices, in an antiparallel orientation, pack into the grooves between the HR1 monomers via hydrophobic interactions. The outcome of the formation of the six-helix bundle is the juxtaposition of the viral and cellular membranes in sufficient proximity to allow mixing of their lipid bilayers and the deposition of the contents of the virion into the cytoplasm.

Expression of the Replicase-Transcriptase Complex

Following delivery of the viral nucleocapsid to the cytoplasm, the next event is the translation of the *replicase* gene from the genomic RNA. This gene consists of two large ORFs—rep 1a and rep 1b—that share a small region of overlap (see Fig. 28.4). Translation of the entire replicase depends on a mechanism called *ribosomal frameshifting,* whereby, with a fixed probability, a translating ribosome shifts one nucleotide in the −1 direction, from the rep 1a reading frame into the rep 1b reading frame.[378] This repositioning is programmed by two RNA elements (Fig. 28.7A), embedded near the region of overlap, that were discovered in studies of IBV.[46,47] The first element is the 5′-UUUAAAC-3′ heptanucleotide slippery sequence, which is identical for all known coronaviruses and has apparently been selected as optimal for its role.[48,457] The second element, located a short distance downstream of the slippery sequence, is an extensively characterized RNA pseudoknot structure.[49,405] This latter component was initially thought to be a classic two-stem (H-type) pseudoknot; however, recent analyses of SARS-CoV frameshifting support a more elaborate structure that includes a third stem loop within pseudoknot loop 2.[20,141,456]

The two elements act together to produce the coterminal polyprotein products pp1a and pp1ab. During most rounds of translation, the elongating ribosome unwinds the pseudoknot and translation terminates at the rep 1a stop codon, yielding the smaller product, pp1a. Some fraction of the time, however, the pseudoknot blocks the mRNA entrance channel of the ribosome.[213,403,528] The consequent pause required for the ribosome to melt out the mRNA structure allows the simultaneous slippage of the P and A site transfer RNAs (tRNAs) into the rep 1b reading frame. This results in the synthesis of pp1ab when elongation resumes.[20,47] Studies of reporter gene expression suggest that the incidence of coronaviral ribosomal frameshifting is as high as 25% to 30%; however, the *in vivo* frequency in infected cells remains to be quantitated. It is thought that the role of programmed frameshifting is to provide a fixed ratio of translation products for assembly into a macromolecular complex.[457] It is also possible that frameshifting forestalls expression of the enzymatic products of rep 1b until the products of rep 1a have prepared a suitable environment for RNA synthesis.

Polyproteins pp1a (440–500 kDa) and pp1ab (740–810 kDa) are autoproteolytically processed into mature products that are designated nsp1 to nsp16 (except for the gammacoronaviruses, which do not have a counterpart of nsp1). From work begun with early studies of MHV,[134,135,525] complete processing schemes have now been solved for replicases of multiple coronaviruses representing all three genera[659,661] (see Fig. 28.7B). Processing also generates many long-lived partial proteolytic products, which may have functional importance. There are two types of polyprotein cleavage activity.[17,358] One or two papain-like proteases (PL^{pro}), which are situated in nsp3, carry out the relatively specialized separation of nsp1, nsp2, and nsp3. The main protease (M^{pro})—nsp5—performs the remaining 11 cleavage events. M^{pro} is often designated the 3C-like protease ($3CL^{pro}$) to point out its distant relationship to the 3C proteins of picornaviruses. Several crystal structures have been determined for PL^{pro} and M^{pro} of SARS-CoV and other

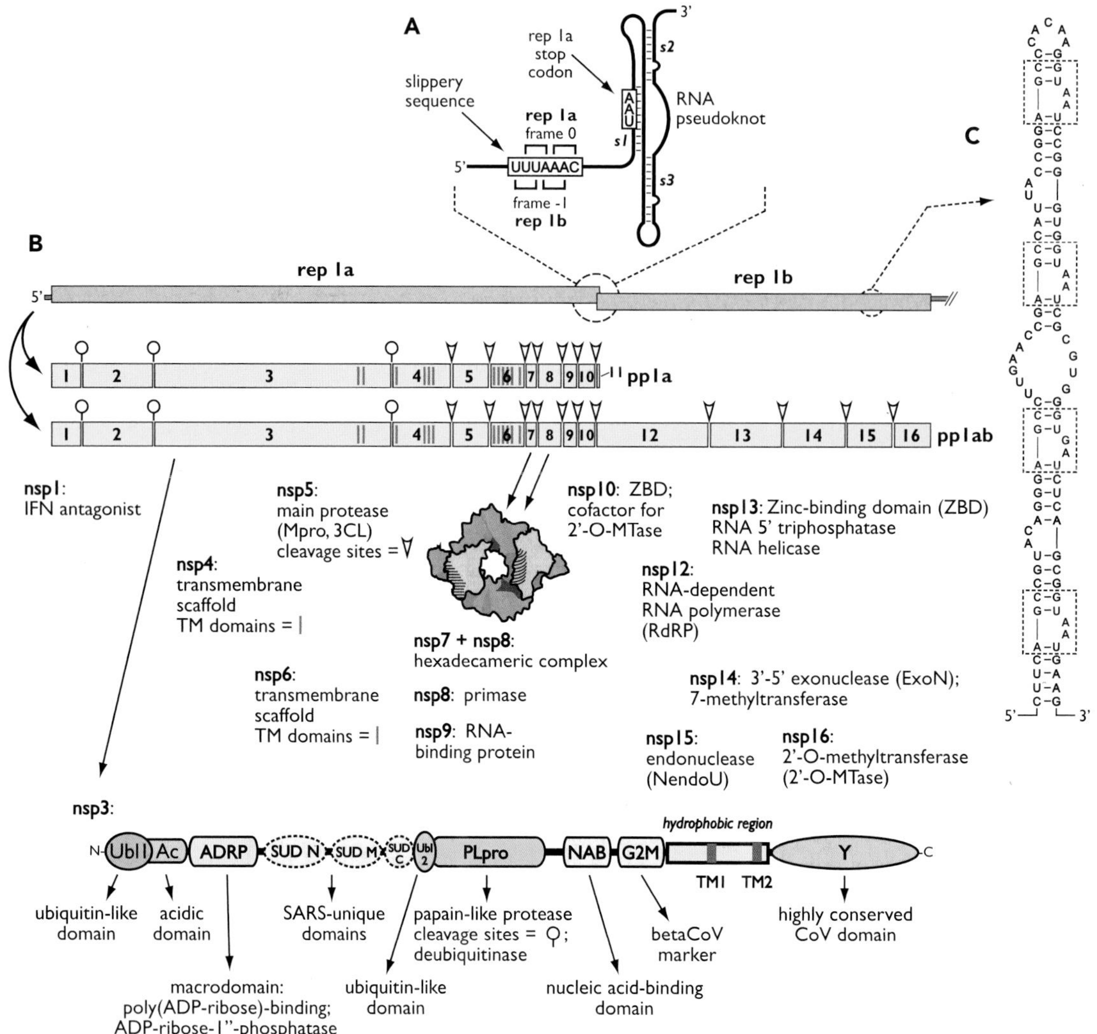

FIGURE 28.7. Coronavirus replicase gene and protein products. A: Ribosomal frameshifting elements of the SARS-CoV *replicase* gene. Pseudoknot stems are indicated as s1, s2, and s3. **B:** Polyprotein pp1a and pp1ab processing scheme for alpha- and betacoronaviruses. The gammacoronavirus processing scheme is identical, except for the absence of nsp1. Known functions and properties of nsp1 through nsp16 are listed; nsp11 is an oligopeptide generated when ribosomal frameshifting does not occur. Transmembrane domains in nsp3, nsp4, and nsp6 are indicated by *red vertical lines*. The nsp3 schematic shown is for SARS-CoV[414]; some modules differ in other coronaviruses. **C:** The RNA packaging signal located in the nsp15-encoding region of the MHV genome.[81] This element is found only in a subset of the betacoronaviruses (MHV, betacoronavirus 1, and HCoV-HKU1); repeat units are boxed. SARS-CoV, severe acute respiratory syndrome coronavirus; MHV, mouse hepatitis virus; HCoV, human coronavirus.

coronaviruses,[9,469,612,631] and these enzymes present attractive targets for antiviral drug design.[468,633,634]

The processed nsps assemble to form the coronavirus replicase, which is also referred to as the replicase-transcriptase complex (RTC).[660] The challenge of defining the roles of the many nsp components of the RTC was initially addressed by foundational studies in bioinformatics,[196,317] which is a discipline that continues to inform the analysis of this intricate molecular machinery.[414,521] Besides PL^{pro} and M^{pro}, the products of rep 1a contain several activities that establish cellular conditions favorable for infection. Some of these are directly linked to RNA synthesis. Others are nonessential for viral replication in tissue culture; however, they can have major effects on virus–host interactions (see the Immune Response and Viral Evasion of the Immune Response section). The very first polyprotein product—nsp1—exhibits a broad repertoire of antagonistic activities that selectively inhibit host protein synthesis and IFN signaling.[230,258,259] By contrast, nsp2 is completely expendable and, as yet, has no demonstrated function.[199]

Nsp3 is by far the largest of the RTC proteins. It consists of a concatenation of individual structural modules that are arranged as globular domains separated by flexibly disordered linkers[414] (see Fig. 28.7B). At the amino terminus of nsp3 are ubiquitin-like (Ubl1) and acidic (Ac) domains[506] that interact with the SR region of the N protein.[237] It is proposed that this interaction tethers the genome to the assembling RTC to allow formation of the initiation complex for RNA synthesis. As mentioned earlier, located within nsp3 are one (in SARS-CoV and gammacoronaviruses) or two PL^{pro} modules (in most other coronaviruses). In addition to protease activity, PL^{pro} domains possess deubiquitinase activity,[341,469,612] which forms another part of the viral arsenal that counters host innate immunity.[136,174] A highly conserved domain of nsp3 has adenosine diphosphate-ribose-1″-phosphatase (ADRP) and poly(adenosine diphosphate [ADP]-ribose)-binding activities,[152,494] which, although nonessential for replication, help confer resistance to host defenses.[158,297] At the C-terminus of nsp3 is a conserved region, designated the Y domain, containing three metal-binding clusters of cysteine and histidine residues.[414,662] The potential functions of other domains of nsp3 (NAB, G2M, SUD),[73,414,507,521] which appear only in various subsets of coronaviruses, remain to be elucidated.

Notably, the rep 1a products nsp3, nsp4, and nsp6 each contain multiple transmembrane helices that anchor the RTC to intracellular membranes.[262,424] These proteins also appear to be responsible for remodeling cellular membranes to form structures that are dedicated to viral RNA synthesis.[92,178] Recent cryo-electron tomographic imaging has revealed an extensive network of convoluted membranes, double-membrane vesicles (DMVs), and vesicle packets, all continuous with the ER, induced by coronavirus infection[277] (Fig. 28.8). Anchorage and compartmentalization of the RTC are thought to provide a scaffold for recruitment of soluble nsps, to offer protection from ribonucleases, and to sequester double-stranded viral

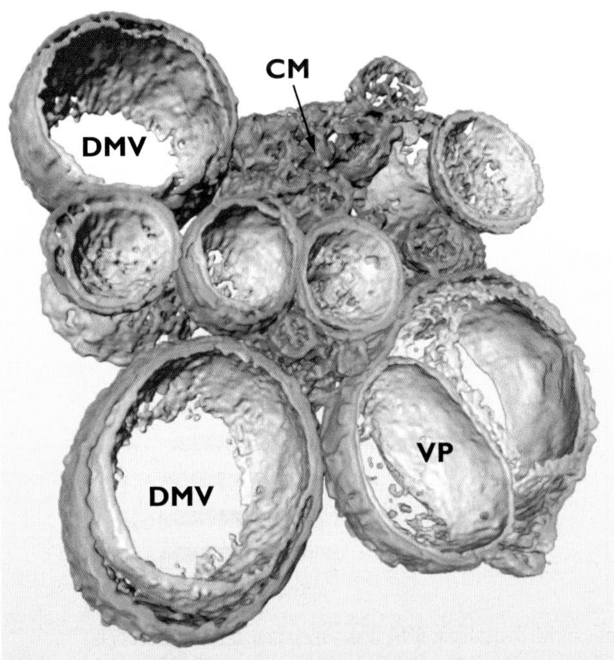

FIGURE 28.8. Membranous compartments for RNA replication and transcription induced by coronavirus infection. Shown is a cryo-electron tomographic reconstruction of the network of intracellular membrane rearrangements found in SARS-CoV-infected Vero cells. There are three types of structures: convoluted membranes (*CM*), which are the major sites of nsp accumulation; double-membrane vesicles (*DMV*), which appear to be the sites of active RNA synthesis; and vesicle packets (*VP*), which are formed by the merger of DMV. (From Knoops K, Kikkert M, Worm SH, et al. SARS-coronavirus replication is supported by a reticulovesicular network of modified endoplasmic reticulum. *PLoS Biol* 2008;6:e226.)

RNA intermediates that might activate host innate immunity (see the Immune Response and Viral Evasion of the Immune Response section).

The most C-terminal rep 1a products are nsp7 through nsp10, a cluster of essential small proteins.[131] Structural studies have revealed that two of these—nsp7 and nsp8—form a hexadecameric supercomplex with a central channel large enough to accommodate double-stranded RNA.[651] This formidable assembly has thus been proposed to act as a processivity clamp for the RNA polymerase. Nsp9 is a single-stranded RNA-binding protein,[151,553] and nsp10 defines a novel structural class of zinc finger proteins.[257,548]

The processed products encoded by rep 1b contain several well-studied enzymatic activities, including many that are common to all positive-strand RNA viruses. Most prominent in this latter class is the coronavirus RNA-dependent RNA polymerase (RdRp), which is contained in nsp12. Sequence alignment and homology modeling indicate that nsp12 has the fingers, palm, and thumb domains characteristic of several viral RdRps and reverse transcriptases[628]; however, to date, this protein has proven refractory to structural determination. Additionally, nsp12 has an unusually large NTD, at least part of which mediates targeting to the RTC.[52] Coronavirus RdRp activity, *in vitro,* is primer dependent.[83,560] Remarkably, a second RdRp activity resides in nsp8 and is capable of synthesizing short RNA oligomers.[240] Nsp8 is thus the optimal candidate for the requisite primase. Another enzyme crucial to RNA synthesis is the helicase of nsp13. This activity unwinds RNA duplexes with a 5′ to 3′ polarity, suggesting that its role is to prepare the template ahead of the RdRp.[247,248] The nsp13 helicase has an amino-terminal zinc finger domain that is found only in nidoviruses.[510]

Like many RNA viruses, coronaviruses contain machinery capable of catalyzing multiple steps of the pathway for synthesis of the 5′-terminal cap structure of mRNA. An RNA 5′-triphosphatase, which would be required for the first step, is yet another property of nsp13.[247,248] Intriguingly, a guanylyltransferase has thus far not been identified among the nsps. The nsp14 C-terminus and nsp16, respectively, harbor N7-methyltransferase and 2′-*O*-methyltransferase activities.[82,123] These enzymes operate in an obligatory sequential manner, with guanosine-N7 methylation preceding ribose-2′-*O* methylation. Activation of the nsp16 methyltransferase requires nsp10 as a cofactor, and the crystal structure of a heterodimer of these two proteins suggests that nsp10 serves as a platform to stabilize nsp16.[43,122] Genetic evidence also implicates nsp10 as a regulator of polyprotein processing by the nsp5 M^{pro}.[138]

Finally, there are two rep 1b–encoded activities that are not found outside the order *Nidovirales*[194,521]; surprisingly, both are ribonucleases. The first is an endonuclease, designated NendoU, which resides in nsp15. NendoU hydrolyzes both single- and double-stranded RNA and specifically cleaves downstream of uridylate residues, producing 2′-3′ cyclic phosphates.[33,246] Although it bears homology to XendoU, an enzyme involved in small nucleolar RNA (snoRNA) processing, the potential role of NendoU in coronavirus RNA synthesis is not clear. It is also unresolved whether NendoU is essential or if lethal mutations constructed in nsp15 affect some other function of that protein.[246,260] The second activity is ExoN, a 3′-5′ exonuclease that is associated with the amino-terminal portion of nsp14.[395] This enzyme is not essential for viral replication; however, nsp14 mutants have a greatly enhanced mutation rate, supporting the notion that ExoN provides a proofreading function for the coronavirus RdRp.[149,150] Such a corrective activity may be critical for maintenance of the stability of the exceptionally large coronavirus genome.

Viral RNA Synthesis

Expression and assembly of the RTC sets the stage for viral RNA synthesis (see Fig. 28.6), a process resulting in the replication of genomic RNA and the transcription of multiple subgenomic RNAs (sgRNAs).[299,433,577] The latter species serve as mRNAs for the genes downstream of the *replicase* gene. Each sgRNA consists of a leader RNA of 70 to 100 nucleotides, which is identical to the 5′ end of the genome, joined to a body RNA, which is identical to a segment of the 3′ end of the genome. The fusion of the leader RNA to body RNAs occurs at short motifs—TRSs—examples of which are listed in Figure 28.9. Like the genome, the sgRNAs have 5′ caps and 3′ polyadenylate tails. Together, these transcripts form a 3′-nested set—the single most distinctive feature of the order *Nidovirales*.[157,194] Synthesis of both genomic RNA and sgRNAs proceeds through negative-strand intermediates.[24,509] The negative sense RNAs, which possess 5′ oligouridylate tracts[220] and 3′ antileaders,[508] are roughly a tenth to a hundredth as abundant as their positive sense counterparts.

At their 5′ and 3′ termini, coronavirus genomes contain *cis*-acting RNA elements that allow their selective recognition as templates for the RTC and play essential roles in RNA synthesis (see Fig. 28.9). The initial localization of these elements was carried out in studies of defective interfering (DI) RNAs, which are extensively deleted genomic variants that propagate by competing for the viral RNA synthesis machinery.[69,371,393,445,575] Manipulations of natural and artificially constructed DI RNAs, evaluated by transfection into helper-virus–infected cells, made possible the mapping of sequences

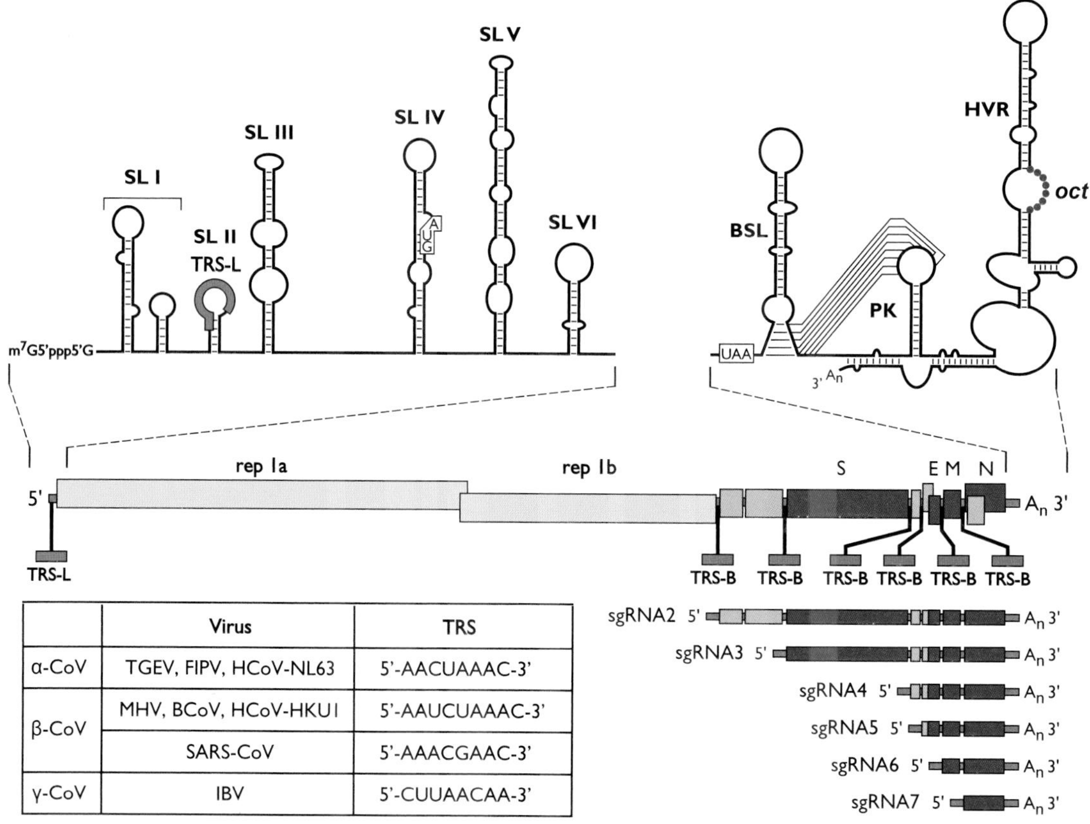

	Virus	TRS
α-CoV	TGEV, FIPV, HCoV-NL63	5'-AACUAAAC-3'
β-CoV	MHV, BCoV, HCoV-HKU1	5'-AAUCUAAAC-3'
	SARS-CoV	5'-AAACGAAC-3'
γ-CoV	IBV	5'-CUUAACAA-3'

FIGURE 28.9. Coronavirus RNA synthesis. Shown are a schematic of MHV genomic RNA and the nested set of transcribed subgenomic RNA species that are a defining feature of the order *Nidovirales*. The leader and body copies of the TRS (TRS-L and TRS-B, respectively) are denoted by *green boxes*. At the **left** are listed examples of consensus TRSs that have been experimentally confirmed[462,463,531,562]; the inferred TRSs of other coronaviruses are identical or highly similar to these. Expanded regions above the genome depict *cis*-acting RNA structures at the genome termini. The structures shown are those characterized for MHV.[190,202,346,667] Homologous structures exist in the BCoV[53,622] and SARS-CoV genomes,[192,261] and counterparts of some of these elements appear in other coronaviruses.[80,107,605] The 5′ expanded region represents the 210-nt 5′ UTR and the first 140 nt of the *rep 1a* gene; the elements shown are SLs I through VI, numbered as originally described for BCoV.[53,202] TRS-L is denoted in *green* in SL II; the start codon of rep 1a is *boxed* in SL IV. The 3′ expanded region represents the 301-nt 3′ UTR. The elements shown are the bulged stem loop (*BSL*), the pseudoknot (*PK*), the hypervariable region (*HVR*), and the conserved coronavirus octanucleotide motif (*oct*); the stop codon for the upstream *N* gene is *boxed*. MHV, mouse hepatitis virus; TRS, transcription-regulating sequence; BCoV, bovine coronavirus; SARS-CoV, severe acute respiratory syndrome coronavirus; UTR, untranslated region; nt, nucleotide; SL, stem loop.

that are critical for the replication and transcription of DI RNA and, presumably, also for genomic RNA.[45,379] More recently, *cis*-acting RNA elements have been dissected through reverse genetics of the intact viral genome, complemented by *in vitro* biochemical and structural analyses. The most completely characterized structures and sequences are those of the betacoronaviruses MHV, BCoV, and SARS-CoV (see Fig. 28.9).

At the 5′ end of the genome, the elements that participate in viral RNA synthesis extend well beyond the 5′ UTR into the replicase coding region, making up a set of seven stem loops.[53,202,346,467] One of these displays the leader copy of the TRS (TRS-L) in its loop, and another sequesters the start codon of the *rep 1a* gene within its stem. Many, but not all, of these defined structures can be exchanged among the genomes of different betacoronaviruses.[202,261] Significantly, functional analyses have shown that either the stability[202,346] or the instability[329] of a given RNA stem can be critical for viral fitness, suggesting that these structures operate in a dynamic manner during RNA synthesis.

At the 3′ end of the genome, *cis*-acting RNA elements are confined entirely to the 3′ UTR[190] and are functionally interchangeable among the betacoronaviruses.[192,228,622] These elements consist of a bulged stem loop[228] and an adjacent pseudoknot[605] that have each been demonstrated to be essential for viral replication. Further downstream is a hypervariable region, which is completely dispensable for viral replication but yet harbors 5′-GGAAGAGC-3′, an octanucleotide motif that is universally conserved in the coronaviruses.[191,347] Notably, the bulged stem loop and the pseudoknot partially overlap, and they therefore can not fold up simultaneously. The two structures are thus thought to constitute a molecular switch between different steps of RNA synthesis.[190,227] In addition, the first loop of the pseudoknot forms a duplex with the extreme 3′ end of the genome and genetically interacts with the RTC subunits nsp8 and nsp9.[667] On this basis, a mechanism has been proposed in which alternate RNA conformations of the 3′ UTR facilitate the transition between initiation of negative-strand RNA synthesis by the nsp8 primase and elongation by the nsp12 RdRp. However, this scheme does not yet incorporate potential cross talk between the 5′ and 3′ ends of the genome,[329] and much remains to be learned about how *cis*-acting RNA elements are recognized by, and cooperate with, the RTC.

A central issue in coronavirus RNA synthesis is how the leader RNA becomes attached to the body segments of the sgRNAs. It became clear from early work that transcription involves a discontinuous process. Ultraviolet (UV) transcriptional mapping demonstrated that sgRNAs are not processed from a genome-length precursor,[250,537] and mixed infections with two different strains of MHV showed that leader RNAs could reassort between separate sgRNA body segments.[372] It was also clearly established by DI RNA studies, and later confirmed by genomic reverse genetics,[527,664] that the TRSs play key roles in sgRNA formation. The efficiency of fusion at an individual body TRS (TRS-B) is, in part, governed by how closely it conforms to the leader TRS (TRS-L).[217,369,576] Nonetheless, factors such as the local sequence context of the TRS and the position of the TRS relative to the 3′ end of the genome also profoundly influence transcription levels.[286,429,580]

Originally, the leader-to-body fusion event was envisioned to occur by a leader-primed mechanism during positive-strand RNA synthesis.[298,300,652] However, there is now broad, although not universal, agreement that fusion takes place through discontinuous extension of negative-strand RNA synthesis.[433,496,498,664] In this model, both genomic and subgenomic negative-strand RNAs are initiated by the RTC at the 3′ end of the (positive-strand) genome template (Fig. 28.10). A pause in RNA synthesis occurs when the RdRp crosses a TRS-B. At this point, the RdRp may continue to elongate the growing negative strand. Alternatively, it may switch to the leader at the 5′ end of the genome template, guided by the complementarity between the 3′ end of the nascent negative strand and the TRS-L of the genome. The resulting negative-strand sgRNA, in partial duplex with positive-strand gRNA, then serves as the template for synthesis of multiple copies of the corresponding positive-strand sgRNA.

Leader-to-body fusion during negative-strand synthesis is amply supported by accumulated experimental results with coronaviruses and the closely related arteriviruses. First, as necessitated by the model, negative-strand sgRNAs contain antileaders at their 3′ ends.[508] Second, in infected cells, there exist transcription intermediates containing negative-strand sgRNAs in association with the genome. These complexes actively participate in transcription[24,497] and can be biochemically separated from replication intermediates containing genome-length negative-strand RNAs.[500] Finally, as would be predicted for discontinuous negative-strand synthesis, engineered (or naturally occurring) variant nucleotides incorporated into the TRS-B, rather than the TRS-L, end up in the leader–body junction of the resulting sgRNA.[238,434,579,664] There remains, however, considerable further work to be done to elucidate the details of the model.[433,498] It is not clear how the transcribing RdRp might continuously monitor the ability of its nascent product to base pair to the TRS-L. Additionally, the synthesis of genome-length negative strands would require the RdRp to bypass all of the TRS-B sites in the genome template. This may come about through a stochastic process, or it may be actively promoted by some RTC component under certain conditions. These and other questions will need to be addressed, possibly with the aid of a robust *in vitro* viral RNA synthesizing system.[578] Such a system may also be decisive in assessing the potential roles of host factors in transcription and replication. Several cellular proteins, including hnRNP A1,[327,512,513] polypyrimidine tract-binding protein,[326,526] mitochondrial aconitase,[404] and polyadenylate-binding protein,[532] have been proposed to take part in coronavirus RNA synthesis, mainly based on their ability to bind *in vitro* to genomic RNA segments. Because many putative host factors also play critical or essential roles in normal cellular functions, it has been difficult to convincingly demonstrate their specific involvement in viral processes. As yet, only a single candidate host factor has been shown to be required for *in vitro* viral RNA synthesis.[578]

In addition to its central role in sgRNA formation, template switching is also at the heart of RNA recombination—another prominent feature of coronavirus RNA synthesis. Significant rates of both homologous and nonhomologous RNA recombination have been found among selected and unselected markers during the course of infection.[266,267,268,370] It is presumed, but remains to be formally demonstrated, that coronavirus RNA recombination results from a copy-choice mechanism, as originally established for poliovirus.[273] In MHV, recombination takes place at an estimated frequency of 1% per 1.3 kb (almost 25% over the entire genome)—the

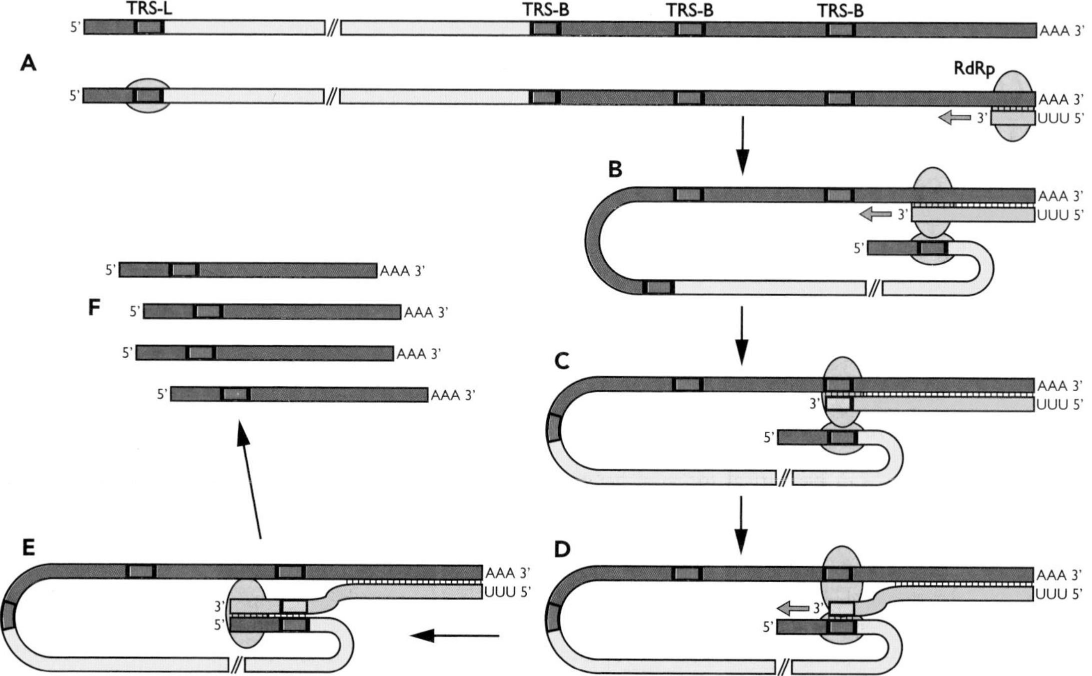

FIGURE 28.10. Coronavirus transcription through discontinuous extension of negative-strand RNA synthesis.[496,498,664] **A, B:** Negative-strand sgRNA synthesis initiates at the 3′ end of the positive-strand genomic RNA template. In the version of the model shown here, the genomic template loops out in such a way as to allow a component of the RTC to constantly monitor the potential complementarity of the 3′ end of the nascent negative-strand RNA with the TRS-L. **C:** Transcription pauses at a TRS-B. At this point, elongation may resume, thereby bypassing the TRS-B. **D:** Alternatively, the nascent negative strand may switch templates, binding to the TRS-L. **E:** Resumption of elongation results in completion of synthesis of an antileader-containing negative-strand sgRNA. **F:** The resulting complex of genome and negative-strand sgRNA acts as template for the synthesis of multiple copies of the corresponding positive-strand sgRNA. sgRNA, subgenomic RNA; RTC, replicase-transcriptase complex; TRS, transcription-regulating sequence. (Adapted from Zúñiga S, Sola I, Alonso S, et al. Sequence motifs involved in the regulation of discontinuous coronavirus subgenomic RNA synthesis. *J Virol* 2004;78:980–994.)

highest rate observed for any RNA virus.[22] On a fine scale, the sites of crossover are random,[19] although selective pressures can generate the appearance of local clustering of recombinational hot spots.[18] This facility for RdRp strand switching may make a major contribution to the ability of the huge coronavirus genome to evolve and to circumvent the accumulation of deleterious mutations. It also serves as the basis for targeted RNA recombination (see the Coronavirus Genetics section).

Assembly and Release of Virions

The immediate outcome of transcription is to enable translation of the proteins that build progeny viruses. The membrane-bound proteins M, S, and E are initially inserted into the ER; from there, they transit to the site of virion assembly, the endoplasmic reticulum–Golgi intermediate compartment (ERGIC).[275,285,563] Here, nucleocapsids composed of progeny genomes encapsidated by N protein coalesce with the envelope components to form virions, which bud into the ERGIC[117,222,378] (see Fig. 28.6).

Coronavirus assembly occurs through a network of cooperative interactions, most of which involve M protein. However, despite its central role, M is not assembly competent by itself. Expression of M protein alone does not result in virion-like structures, and M traverses the secretory pathway beyond the budding site, as far as the *trans*-Golgi.[275,362,363,489] The first virus-like particle (VLP) systems developed for coronaviruses led to the key finding that co-expression of E protein with M protein is sufficient to yield the formation of particles that are released from cells and appear morphologically identical to coronavirus envelopes.[37,582] More recently, it has been shown that the additional co-expression of N protein substantially increases the efficiency of VLP formation[38,519] and can even compensate for mutational defects in M.[15] Other viral structural proteins, in particular S protein, are gathered into virions but are not specifically required for the assembly process. Because virions and VLPs contain very little E protein, this indicates that lateral interactions between M molecules provide the driving force for envelope morphogenesis. Investigations of the ability of M protein mutants to support VLP assembly concluded that M–M interactions occur via multiple contacts throughout the molecule, especially between the transmembrane domains.[114,120] Recent cryo-electron tomographic reconstructions of whole virions suggest that the M protein forms dimers that are maintained through multiple monomer–monomer contacts, while dimer–dimer interactions occur among the globular endodomains.[415]

It remains enigmatic how E protein critically assists M in envelope formation. Like M, E protein by itself moves to a compartment past the ERGIC[93,100]; however, co-expression or infection somehow secures localization of M and E at the budding site. Some evidence suggests that E protein promotes assembly by inducing membrane curvature.[100,166,465] Other work indicates a role for E in maintaining M protein in an assembly-competent state by preventing its nonproductive aggregation—a function that crucially depends on palmitoylation of E.[38] Such a chaperone-like role would be consistent with demonstrations that diverse heterologous E proteins, and even truncated versions of M protein, can functionally replace E protein in MHV.[293,294] Finally, there are reports that point to a need for E protein to facilitate the release of assembled virions from infected cells.[364,427] These roles are not mutually exclusive, and some recent studies have begun to assign individual functions to various regions of the E molecule. The C-terminal endodomain of the IBV E protein governs Golgi localization[100,101] and when linked to a heterologous transmembrane domain can support VLP and virion assembly.[364,491] Conversely, the transmembrane domain of E alters the host secretory pathway in a way that promotes virus release.[491] This latter effect is potentially a consequence of the putative ion channel properties of the E transmembrane domain[449,609,610,638]; however, it is unresolved whether native E protein acts as an ion channel at intracellular membranes *in vivo.*[420]

The dispensability of S protein for VLP formation is consistent with earlier observations that spikeless (noninfectious) virions were formed by infected cells treated with the glycosylation inhibitor tunicamycin[224,487] or by cells infected with particular S mutants.[360,474] S protein thus appears to play a passive role in assembly; however, during its passage through the secretory pathway, it is captured by M protein for virion incorporation.[387,426] For some S proteins, localization at or near the budding compartment is abetted by targeting signals contained in the endodomain.[353,386,611] The S endodomain is also the region of the protein that interacts with M during assembly.[39,636] Conversely, the ability of M protein to interact with S maps to a locus close to the C-terminus of the M endodomain[118] (see Fig. 28.3).

Virion assembly is completed by condensation of the nucleocapsid with the envelope components. This is brought about principally by N and M protein interactions, which have been mapped to domain 3 of N[236,585] and the extreme C-terminus of the M endodomain[162,295] (see Fig. 28.3). These interacting regions likely account for the thread-like connections that have been visualized between the M protein endodomain and the nucleocapsid in virion reconstructions.[21,415] Nucleocapsid formation is presumed to be concomitant with genome replication; however, the details of how the nucleocapsid traffics to the budding compartment are not known. It is also not well understood how coronaviruses selectively package genomic RNA from among the many positive- and negative-strand viral RNA species that are synthesized during infection. DI RNA analyses have mapped the genomic packaging signal of MHV to a small span of RNA sequence embedded in the region of the *replicase* gene that encodes nsp15[169,373,575] (see Fig. 28.7C). Highly homologous structures exist in the genomes of BCoV and HCoV-HKU1.[81,96] However, for most coronaviruses, including SARS-CoV,[256] packaging signals are clearly not found at the same locus, and the relevant structures for these viruses may occur at a large distance, near the 5′ ends of their respective genomes.[80,161] The mechanism by which the MHV packaging signal operates is undetermined. Some studies have shown that it is specifically bound by N protein,[96,396] although other work demonstrates that M protein, in the absence of N, acts as the discriminatory factor for packaging signal recognition.[406,409]

Following assembly and budding, progeny virions are exported from infected cells by transport to the plasma membrane in smooth-walled vesicles and are released by exocytosis. It remains to be more clearly defined whether coronaviruses follow the constitutive pathway for post-Golgi transport of large cargo or, alternatively, if specialized cellular machinery must be diverted for their exit.[222] For some coronaviruses, but not others, a fraction of S protein that has not been assembled into virions transits to the plasma membrane, where it can mediate fusion between infected cells and adjacent, uninfected cells. This leads to the formation of large, multinucleate syncytia, enabling the spread of infection by a means not subject to neutralization by antibody. For MHV, cell–cell fusion depends on S1-S2 cleavage carried out by a furin-like protease late in infection.[119] However, this form of proteolytic activation of S does not appear to affect virus–cell fusion that occurs at the initiation of infection. Similarly, the SARS-CoV S protein has different proteolytic requirements for cell–cell and virus–cell fusion.[168,516] On the opposite side of the membrane from the cleaved ectodomain, the cysteine-rich region of the S protein endodomain also plays a critical role in cell–cell fusion[36,68,636]; specifically, this has been shown to depend on the palmitoylation of a subset of endodomain cysteine residues.[388]

PATHOGENESIS AND PATHOLOGY OF CORONAVIRUS INFECTIONS

General Principles

Most coronaviruses spread to susceptible hosts by respiratory or fecal–oral routes of infection, with replication first occurring in epithelial cells (Table 28.3). Some, including HCoV-OC43, HCoV-229E, and porcine respiratory coronavirus (PRCoV), replicate principally in respiratory epithelial cells, where they produce virus and cause local respiratory symptoms. Other coronaviruses, including TGEV, BCoV, porcine hemagglutinating encephalomyelitis virus (PHEV), CCoV, FeCoV, and enteric strains of MHV, infect epithelial cells of the enteric tract. Some of these viruses, such as TGEV, cause diarrhea that is particularly severe, and sometimes fatal, in young animals.[492] Inapparent enteric infection of adult animals maintains the virus in the population.[98] In addition to local infection of the respiratory or enteric tracts, several coronaviruses cause severe disease. For example, SARS-CoV spreads from the upper airway to cause a severe lower respiratory tract infection, whereas FIPV spreads systemically to cause a generalized wasting disease in felines.[439,448] Rat coronavirus strains cause respiratory infection or sialodacryoadenitis owing to infection of the salivary and lacrimal glands[446] but can also interfere with reproduction by infecting the female urogenital tract.[571] PHEV of swine predominantly causes enteric infection but is also neurotropic.[389] Infection spreads to nerves that innervate the stomach of infected piglets and prevents gastric emptying, resulting in vomiting and wasting disease. The ability to cause localized versus systemic disease is mirrored in polarized tissue culture cells. Thus, coronaviruses such as MHV, which can cause systemic disease, enter the apical side of cells and exit the basolateral side, whereas others, such as HCoV-229E, which causes only a localized infection, enter and

TABLE 28.3 Representative Coronaviruses and Associated Diseases

Virus	Host species	Sites of infection	Clinical disease
Alphacoronaviruses			
CCoV	Canine	GI tract	Gastroenteritis
FeCoV	Felidae	GI tract, respiratory	Gastroenteritis
FIPV	Felidae	Systemic disease	Peritonitis, wasting disease
HCoV-229E	Human	Respiratory	Upper respiratory tract infection
HCoV-NL63	Human	Respiratory	Upper respiratory tract infection, croup
PEDV	Pig	GI tract	Gastroenteritis
TGEV	Pig	GI tract, respiratory	Gastroenteritis
BatCoV	Bat	GI tract, respiratory	Unknown
Rabbit CoV	Rabbit	Heart, GI tract, respiratory	Enteritis, myocarditis
Betacoronaviruses			
BCoV	Bovine, ruminants	GI tract, respiratory	Enteritis, upper and lower respiratory tract infection
HCoV-OC43	Human	Respiratory	Upper respiratory tract infection
HCoV-HKU1	Human	Respiratory	Upper and lower respiratory tract infection
MHV	Mouse, rat	GI tract, liver, brain, lungs	Gastroenteritis, hepatitis, encephalitis, chronic demyelination
PHEV	Pig	Respiratory, brain	Vomiting, wasting, encephalomyelitis
RCoV	Rat	Respiratory, salivary and lachrymal glands, urogenital tract	Respiratory tract infection, metritis, sialodacryoadenitis
SARS-CoV	Human	Respiratory, GI tract	Pneumonia (SARS)
BatCoV	Bat	GI tract, respiratory	Unknown
Gammacoronaviruses			
IBV	Chicken	Respiratory, kidney	Bronchitis, nephritis
TuCoV	Turkey	GI tract	Gastroenteritis

CCoV, canine coronavirus; GI, gastrointestinal; FeCoV, feline coronavirus; FIPV, feline infectious peritonitis virus; HCoV, human coronavirus; PEDV, porcine epidemic diarrhea virus; TGEV, transmissible gastroenteritis virus; BatCoV, bat coronavirus; CoV, coronavirus; BCoV, bovine coronavirus; MHV, mouse hepatitis virus; PHEV, porcine hemagglutinating encephalomyelitis virus; RCoV, rat coronavirus; SARS-CoV, severe acute respiratory syndrome coronavirus; SARS, severe acute respiratory syndrome; IBV, infectious bronchitis virus; TuCoV, turkey coronavirus.

exit the cell apically.[481,482,595] Specific examples are described in more detail later.

Animal Coronavirus Infections

Several coronavirus infections have been extensively studied in their natural hosts. Here, we will focus on murine and feline coronavirus infections.

Mouse Hepatitis Virus

MHV, which until the advent of SARS was the most widely studied coronavirus, causes enteric, hepatic, and neurologic infections of susceptible strains of rodents. Remarkably, closely related strains of MHV, all of which use the same host cell receptor for entry,[606] infect different organs. Enteric strains, such as MHV-Y and MHV-RI, are a major problem in animal research facilities.[98] These viruses spread within infected colonies to young, uninfected animals. They do not generally cause symptomatic disease but may subtly impair the host immune response to other pathogens and immunological stimuli.[98,540] Studies of MHV pathogenesis predominantly use the neurotropic JHM and A59 strains of virus (JHM virus [JHMV] and MHV-A59), in part because they cause a demyelinating encephalomyelitis with similarities to the human disease multiple sclerosis (MS). Originally isolated from a mouse with hindlimb paralysis, JHMV became progressively more virulent on passage in mice.[16,75] The most virulent strains of JHMV cause rapidly fatal acute encephalitis with widespread neuronal infection.[600] Subsequently, most studies have used either attenuated JHMV variants or the mildly neurovirulent MHV-A59 strain for studies of demyelination. Infection with these viruses results in minimal infection of neurons, with oligodendrocytes, microglia, and astrocytes commonly infected.[167,276,313] Myelin destruction occurs during the process of virus clearance from infected glia.[594] Initial studies suggested that demyelination resulted from virus-mediated lysis of oligodendrocytes.[304,600] However, more recent studies show that demyelination is largely immune mediated. In support of this, irradiated mice or congenitally immunodeficient mice (mice with severe combined immunodeficiency [SCID]) or with a disrupted recombination activation gene [$RAG^{-/-}$]) do not develop demyelination after infection with JHMV. When these mice, which lack T and B cells, are reconstituted with virus-specific T cells, demyelination rapidly develops[593,620] (Fig. 28.11). Demyelination is accompanied by infiltration of macrophages and activated microglia into the white matter of the spinal cord.[621] Little is known, however, about how macrophages and microglia are actually attracted to the spinal cord or about the nature of the signals that cause these cells to phagocytose infected myelin. Both CD4 and CD8 T cells are required for virus clearance from the central nervous system (CNS), with CD8 T cells considered most important in

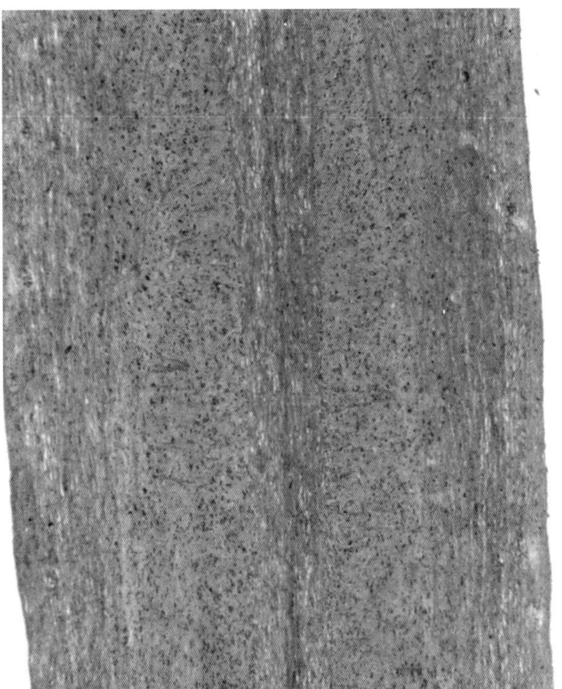

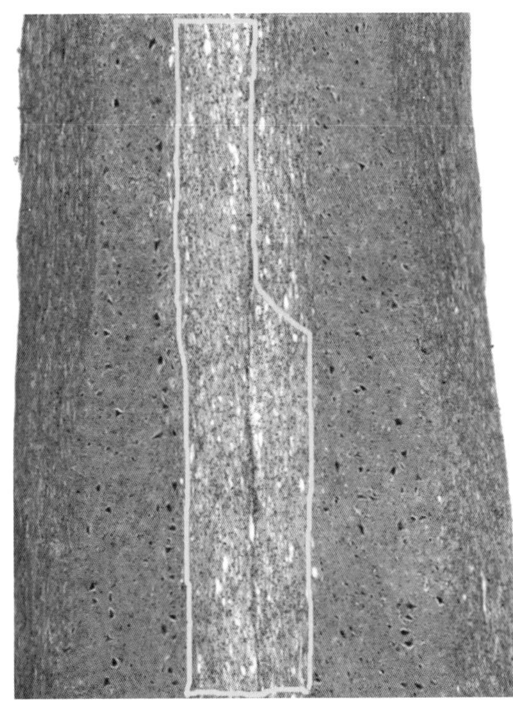

FIGURE 28.11. Immune-mediated demyelination in mice infected with a neurotropic MHV. RAG1$^{-/-}$ mice, lacking T and B cells, were infected with a neurotropic coronavirus as described.[620] Four days later, some mice received adoptively transferred spleen cells from a wild-type C57Bl/6 mouse that was previously immunized intraperitoneally with MHV **(B)**. All mice were sacrificed 8 days later and analyzed for demyelination (marked with a *yellow line* in **B**). Demyelination was observed only in mice that received adoptively transferred MHV-immune cells **(B)** and not in those that did not **(A)**, showing that myelin destruction is largely mediated by T cells during the process of virus clearance. MHV, mouse hepatitis virus.

this process.[608] CD8 T cells eliminate virus from infected astrocytes and microglia by perforin-dependent pathways, whereas clearance from oligodendrocytes is IFN-γ dependent.[340,432] However, T-cell–mediated virus clearance is not complete, and antivirus antibody is required to prevent virus recrudescence.[338] Virus persistence in neonatal mice occurs, in part, because virus variants mutated in an immunodominant CD8 T-cell epitope are selected in specific strains of mice, with subsequent evasion of the cytototoxic T-cell immune response.[451] However, this mechanism of immune evasion has not been detected in older mice that are persistently infected with JHMV. The antivirus CD4 T-cell response, while critical for virus clearance, is also pathogenic. Partial diminution of this response decreases morbidity and mortality, whereas enhancement of the antivirus CD4 T-cell response increases disease severity.[11]

Other strains of MHV, including MHV-A59, MHV-2, and MHV-3, infect both the liver and the CNS. Most notably, MHV-3 causes a fulminant hepatitis in susceptible strains of mice and chronic neurologic infections in semisusceptible strains.[649] In susceptible strains, MHV-3 infects macrophages, resulting in up-regulation of several proinflammatory cytokines, including fibrinogen-like protein 2 (FGL2), a transmembrane procoagulant molecule.[431] FGL2 is also expressed by Foxp3^{+} regulatory T cells.[511] Expression of this molecule results in prothrombin cleavage, with consequent disseminated intravascular coagulation (DIC), hepatic hypoperfusion, and necrosis.[375] Levels of FGL2 are better predictors of a fatal outcome than virus titers. It is known that the propensity to develop severe disease occurs at a postentry step because the MHV-3 receptor, CEACAM1, is expressed in both resistant and susceptible strains of mice. Like JHMV, MHV-3 also infects the CNS; however, infection of this organ occurs only in strains that do not develop a fulminant hepatitis. MHV-3 does not cause a demyelinating disease but rather ependymitis, hydrocephalus, encephalitis, and thrombotic vasculitis.[315,589] The pathogenesis of these entities is not well studied but appears to be immune mediated. Unlike most other strains of MHV, MHV-3 directly infects T and B cells, resulting in lymphocyte apoptosis and lymphopenia.[303] Lymphopenia, with consequent immunosuppression, facilitates virus persistence and its immunopathologic consequences.

Feline Enteric Coronavirus and Feline Infectious Peritonitis Virus

Feline enteric coronavirus (FeCoV) commonly causes mild or asymptomatic infection in domestic cats and other felines. Two serotypes of FeCoV are recognized, with serotype II strains arising by recombination of serotype I FeCoV with CCoV in dually infected animals.[216] In some cats infected persistently with FeCoV, mutations in the virus occur, resulting in the development of a lethal disease called *feline infectious peritonitis* (FIP); FIPV is the virulent strain of FeCoV. Virulence correlates with the ability of the virus to replicate in macrophages.[110] The nature of the mutations required for transition from FeCoV to FIPV is not well understood, although, at least for serotype II viruses, virulence maps in part to the surface glycoprotein.[488] This was shown using reverse genetics, in which S proteins from virulent and avirulent strains were swapped and tested for their ability to cause severe disease in cats. FIPV causes a multiphasic

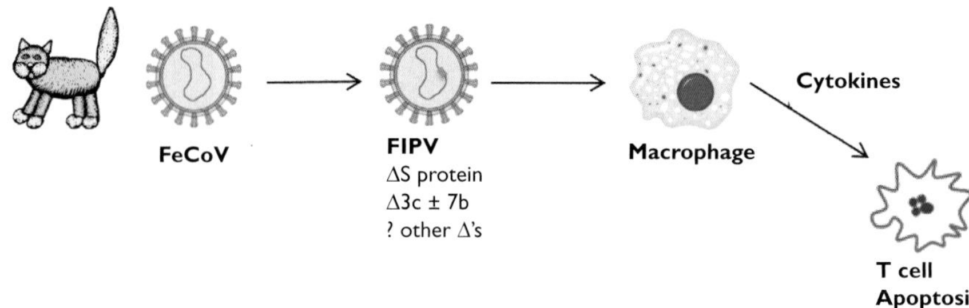

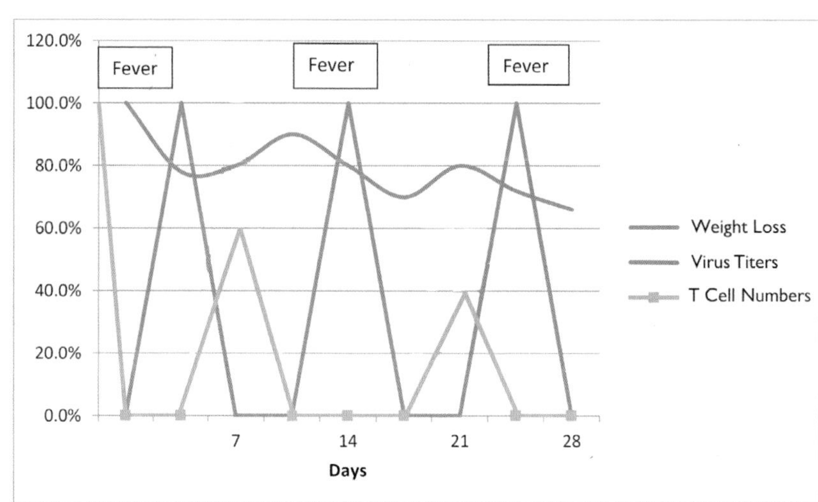

FIGURE 28.12. Recurrent feline infectious peritonitis (FIP). FIP virus—the etiologic agent of FIP—occurs in felines persistently infected with feline coronaviruses. **Upper panels:** Mutations in the S glycoprotein and the ORF3b and 7b proteins occur as virus gains the ability to replicate in macrophages. Infected macrophages serve to transport the virus to sites in the host distant from the initial infection. These infected cells also express several cytokines that are believed to contribute to T-cell apoptosis. **Lower panel:** Clinical disease is characterized by recurrent bouts of virus replication accompanied by fever and clinical disease. Lymphopenia subsequently occurs as disease progresses. The pattern of disease shown in the figure is representative of progressive disease; however, the rate and extent of recurrence of virus replication, as well as the rate of weight loss and of development of lymphopenia, are variable from animal to animal. (Based on De Groot-Mijnes JD, van Dun JM, van der Most RG, et al. Natural history of a recurrent feline coronavirus infection and the role of cellular immunity in survival and disease. *J Virol* 2005;79:1036–1044.)

disease with relapses that result, ultimately, in immunosuppression, weight loss, and death (Fig. 28.12). Each episode is characterized by increased virus replication, fever, and lymphopenia.[112] FIPV does not directly infect lymphocytes. Rather, lymphopenia is believed to be a consequence of infection and activation of macrophages and dendritic cells. Subsequent lymphocyte depletion occurs when cells are exposed to high levels of proinflammatory cytokines, such as tumor necrosis factor, released by these infected cells.[205] Virus dissemination occurs when infected macrophages traffic throughout the body and are deposited in the vasculature. Infected macrophages provoke a pyogranulamatous reaction, which is responsible for many disease manifestations of FIP, such as peritonitis and serositis. Another consequence of immune dysregulation is hypergammaglobulinemia. Antibody-antigen complex formation commonly occurs in FIPV-infected cats and may contribute to vascular injury.[252] However, its precise role in pathogenesis remains uncertain because it is a late manifestation of disease and may make only a minor contribution to disease progression. Neutralizing antibody against the S glycoprotein enhances FIPV infection of macrophages. Enhanced macrophage infection is mediated by virus entry through Fcγ receptors, although virus binding to fAPN—the specific FIPV host cell receptor—is also likely required.[110] This phenomenon has been demonstrated *in vitro* using isolated macrophages and also occurs in cats that have been previously immunized with vectors that express the S glycoprotein.[581] FIPV, but not FeCoV, uptake is augmented by neutralizing antibody that contributes to the propensity of FIPV strains to replicate in macrophages. Although the potential occurrence of antibody-enhanced disease has hindered vaccine development and was raised as a potential difficulty in development of a live attenuated SARS-CoV vaccine, it has never been demonstrated in the natural infection. In fact, cats infected with FeCoV often develop only low antivirus neutralizing antibody titers.[226]

Human Coronavirus Infections

Human Coronaviruses, Other Than Severe Acute Respiratory Syndrome Coronavirus, Associated with Respiratory and Enteric Disease

Prior to 2003, HCoVs were primarily considered to be agents of upper respiratory tract disease and to cause little mortality. In general, whereas coronaviruses were readily isolated from infected birds and other animal species, and serially propagated in continuous cell lines, isolation of HCoVs from infected individuals was only rarely achieved.[389] HCoV-229E and HCoV-OC43 were isolated from patients with upper respiratory tract infections in the 1960s.[210,390,570] There are striking differences in extent of genetic variability when isolates of HCoV-OC43 and HCoV-229E are compared. HCoV-229E isolated at geographically distinct locations show little evidence of variability.[87] In contrast, isolates of HCoV-OC43 isolated from the United States and from France differ in sequence, and virus from the same geographic area but isolated in different years show considerable sequence variations.[587] The ability of HCoV-OC43 to tolerate mutations probably accounts for its ability to grow in mouse cells and infect the mouse brain[389] as well as its ability to cross species (see the Epidemiology section). In contrast, HCoV-229E does not readily cross species

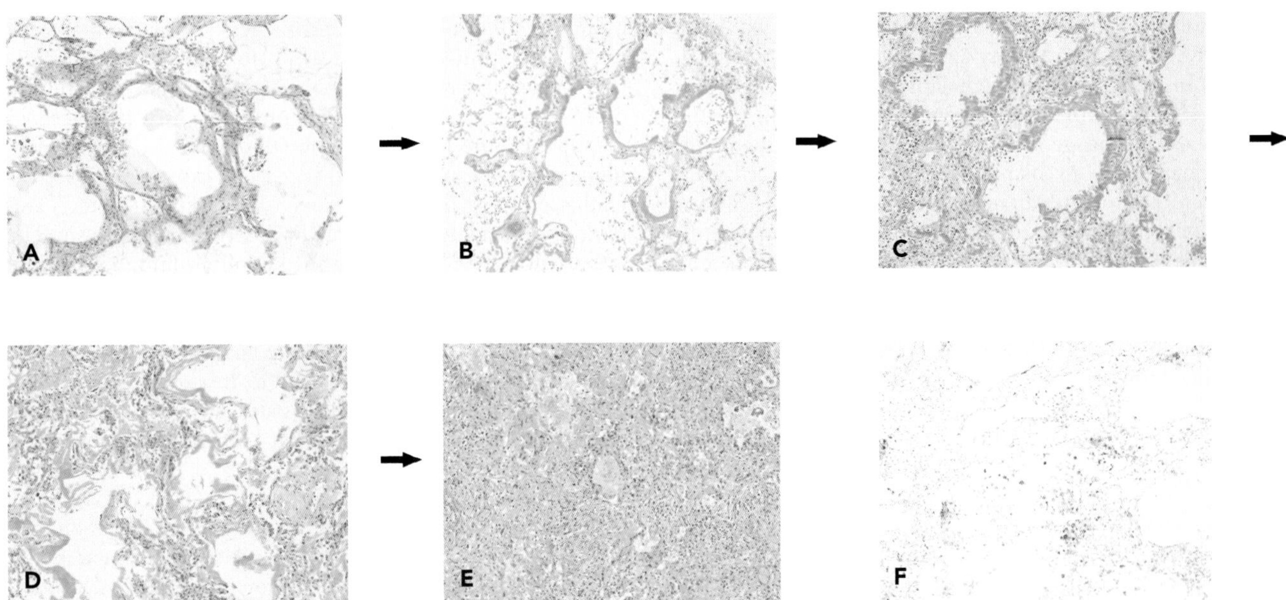

FIGURE 28.13. Pathologic changes in lungs of patients with SARS. Lung samples obtained on autopsy were examined for pathologic changes following SARS-CoV infection. **A–E:** Hematoxylin and eosin stain showing the progression of SARS pneumonia. Early stages of the SARS infection show edema and early hyaline membrane formation **(A)**, hyaline membrane formation **(B)**, and increased inflammatory cell infiltration and pneumocyte hyperplasia **(C)**. As the disease progresses, fibrotic changes become apparent **(D)**. Late manifestations include obliteration of the alveolar volume by fibrous tissue, reactive pneumocytes, and inflammatory cells **(E)**. **F:** Viral antigen is detected most prominently during early stages of the infection in macrophages and alveolar pneumocytes. Magnification, ×100. SARS, severe acute respiratory syndrome; SARS-CoV, severe acute respiratory syndrome coronavirus. (Courtesy of Dr. John Nicholls, University of Hong Kong.)

and does not infect mice. Even in mice that are transgenic for expression of the HCoV-229E host cell receptor (human aminopeptidase N [hAPN]), the virus does not grow unless mice are also rendered immunodeficient by genetic disruption of the *STAT1* gene.[306]

Several new HCoVs were isolated from the respiratory tracts of patients in the post-SARS era. HCoV-NL63, which causes mild respiratory disease, displays homology with HCoV-229E.[460] Phylogenetic analyses suggest that HCoV-NL63 and HCoV-229E diverged approximately 1,000 years ago.[461] A novel feature of HCoV-NL63 is that unlike HCoV-229E, HCoV-NL63 does not use hAPN as a receptor. Rather, infection of cells is mediated by ACE2, the same molecule that is used by SARS-CoV, an unrelated betacoronavirus.[219,331] However, unlike SARS-CoV, HCoV-NL63 does not use cathepsin L or require endosomal acidification to infect ACE2-expressing cells[232] and does not cause severe respiratory disease. HCoV-HKU1, isolated from an adult patient in Hong Kong with pneumonia,[615] also generally causes mild respiratory disease.

A role for HCoVs in the etiology of the human disease MS was postulated based on the ability of murine coronaviruses to cause chronic demyelinating diseases. Coronavirus-like particles have occasionally been detected in the CNS of patients with MS and have also been isolated from the brains of patients after passage in mice or murine cell lines. HCoV-229E RNA was detected in about 44% (40 of 90) of human brains tested, with similar frequencies in brains from MS patients and patients who died from other neurologic diseases or normal control subjects.[13] HCoV-OC43 sequences were detected in 23% (21 of 90) of brains tested, with 36% incidence in brains from MS patients and 14% in that of controls. Although these results are suggestive, the role of non-SARS-CoV HCoVs in diseases outside the respiratory tract, especially in those involving the CNS, is not proven and requires further investigation.

Severe Acute Respiratory Syndrome Coronavirus Infections

SARS-CoV causes the most severe disease of any HCoV.[79,310,439,448,602] The virus infects both upper airway and alveolar epithelial cells, resulting in mild to severe lung injury. Virus or viral products are also detected in other organs, such as the kidney, liver, and small intestine, and in stool. Although the lung is recognized as the organ most severely affected by SARS-CoV, the exact mechanism of lung injury is controversial. Levels of infectious virus appear to diminish as clinical disease worsens, consistent with an immunopathologic mechanism.[437] However, this conclusion must be tempered because patient samples were obtained from nasopharyngeal aspirates, not from the lungs or other organs. Thus, it is not known whether virus titers in the lung also decrease as virus is cleared. Furthermore, virus titers obtained from patients at autopsy do not provide longitudinal information about the relationship between viral load and disease. The SARS-CoV spike protein may also contribute to disease severity. Administration of the SARS-CoV S protein to mice with pre-existing lung injury enhanced disease severity.[239,289] ACE2 appears to have a protective role in animals with lung injury, and S protein may exacerbate disease by causing its down-regulation.[289]

Pathologic findings are nonspecific in patients who died from SARS. Cells in the upper airway were initially infected, resulting in cell sloughing but relatively little epithelial cell damage. However, virus rapidly spread to the alveoli, causing diffuse alveolar damage. This was characterized by pneumocyte desquamation, alveolar edema, inflammatory cell infiltration, and hyaline membrane formation (Fig. 28.13). Over time, alveolar damage progressed, eventually resulting in pathologic signs of acute lung injury (ALI) and, in the most severe cases, acute respiratory distress syndrome (ARDS). Most notably, multinucleated giant cells, originating either from macrophages or respiratory epithelial cells, were detected in autopsy specimens. Although virus could be cultured from infected patients for several weeks, viral antigen was rarely detected in lung autopsy samples after 10 days postinfection.[137,172,318,417]

Like other coronaviruses, such as MHV and FIPV, SARS-CoV infects macrophages and dendritic cells; however, unlike these two animal coronaviruses, it causes an abortive infection in these cells.[314,436,533] Several proinflammatory cytokines and chemokines, such as interferon-inducible protein (IP)-10 (CXCL10), monocyte chemoattractant protein (MCP)-1 (CCL2), macrophage inflammatory protein (MIP)-1α (CCL3), RANTES (regulated on activation normal T cell expressed and secreted) (CCL5), MCP-2 (CCL8), tumor necrosis factor (TNF), and interleukin (IL)-6, are expressed by infected dendritic cells; many of these molecules are also elevated in the serum of SARS-CoV–infected patients.[310] Lymphopenia and neutrophilia were detected in infected patients and were likely to be primarily cytokine driven.[613] A potentially confounding factor is that many patients with SARS in the 2003 epidemic were treated with corticosteroids,[538] and steroid treatment is a well-known cause of lymphopenia.

An important unresolved issue is how SARS-CoV causes severe respiratory disease in humans. This question is virtually impossible to address in patients, because SARS has not recurred in humans since 2004. SARS-CoV infects several species of animals, including mice, ferrets, hamsters, cats, and monkeys,[549] although most of these animals develop either mild or no clinical disease, making them not useful for studies of lethal SARS. However, serial passage of SARS-CoV in mice or rats resulted in the isolation of several rodent-adapted strains that cause severe disease in some strains of young mice and rats.[400,401,478] Most importantly, these strains cause a fatal disease in all aged rodents, paralleling the age-dependent severity observed in infected patients.[140] An age-dependent increase in disease severity is also observed in aged animals experimentally infected with the original human isolates, although disease severity is less than that observed with the mouse-adapted strains.[479] Animals with severe disease, whether infected with human isolates of SARS-CoV or rodent-adapted strains, show pathologic signs of ALI, increased levels of proinflammatory chemokines and cytokines, and diminished T-cell responses. These observations suggest that immune dysregulation contributes to severe disease in these animals, paralleling pathologic changes observed in infected humans.

Immune Response and Viral Evasion of the Immune Response

As in most viral infections, both the innate and adaptive arms of the immune response are required for successful virus clearance and must be appropriately controlled to minimize bystander immunopathologic damage. One of the first steps in the host immune response to a coronavirus infection is the production of type I IFN (IFN-α/β). Plasmacytoid dendritic cells (pDCs) are the source for most IFN-α/β produced in coronavirus-infected hosts, although other cells, such as macrophages, also express IFN.[63,484,657] pDC expression of IFN is mediated by signaling through a toll-like receptor (TLR) 7- and interferon regulatory factor (IRF) 7-dependent pathway. The importance of IFN signaling in the initial immune response to coronaviruses was shown using mice that are defective in expression of the IFN-α/β receptor (IFNAR$^{-/-}$).[63,244] Infection of IFNAR$^{-/-}$ mice with mildly virulent strains of MHV results in rapid and uniformly fatal diseases. Additionally, the importance of the IFN response is also evidenced by the multiple IFN evasive mechanisms that coronaviruses employ, as described later. Although the importance of the IFN response is well established, little is known about which specific IFN-induced proteins are most critical for protection. Ribonuclease L (RNase L) appears to have a role in the immune response to neurotropic strains of MHV[243]; however, whether this molecule is also important in the immune response to nonneurotropic strains of coronavirus remains to be determined.

Once the initial IFN response is induced, virus clearance requires expression of proinflammatory cytokines and chemokines and their receptors, such as CCL2, CXCL9, CXCL10, CCL3, to mediate T-cell and macrophage trafficking to sites of infection.[31] Infection of the CNS also requires breakdown of the blood–brain barrier, which is partially neutrophil dependent. In the absence of neutrophils or of neutrophil chemoattractants, such as CXCL1 and CXCL2, breakdown does not occur, resulting in more severe disease.[658] A robust T-cell response is required for destruction of infected cells and clearance of infectious virus. T-cell responses are poor in felines with progressive FIP (see Fig. 28.12) and in some strains of mice with severe SARS-CoV infections[112,653] Virus is not cleared in MHV- or SARS-CoV–infected mice that lack T cells, again demonstrating the importance of the response in clearance.[621] Both CD4 and CD8 T-cell epitopes have been identified in mice infected with MHV or SARS-CoV and in patients with SARS. Most epitopes are located on the N, M, and S proteins.[78,345,444,447] Once virus has been cleared, the proinflammatory response must be controlled to prevent immunopathology. In MHV-infected mice, regulatory CD4 T cells, characterized by Foxp3 expression, are important for dampening a potentially pathogenic immune response.[565] IL-10, another anti-inflammatory factor important for minimizing immunopathologic changes in MHV-infected mice, is expressed predominantly by virus-specific CD4 and CD8 T cells in the infected brain.[339,566] As described earlier for MHV-infected mice, T cells are responsible for initial virus clearance; however, an effective antivirus antibody response is required to prevent virus recrudescence.[338] Similarly, a robust neutralizing antibody response was detected in survivors during the 2002–2003 SARS outbreak.[56]

Coronaviruses use several approaches, both active and passive, to evade the host IFN response and thereby establish a productive infection (Table 28.4). Coronaviruses replicate in DMVs (see Fig. 28.8), which may shield viral RNA from recognition by intracellular sensor molecules, such as RIG-I, MDA5, and TLR3. Thus, in fibroblasts or conventional DCs infected with MHV or SARS-CoV, no IFN is induced.[173,586,656] However,

TABLE 28.4 Coronavirus Proteins with Immunoevasive Properties

Protein	Virus source	Function	References
nsp1	MHV, SARS-CoV, SARSr-BatCoV Rp3, BatCoV HKU4, BatCoV HKU9, TGEV	a. Suppresses host protein expression through direct inhibition of translation or by promoting degradation of host mRNA, including IFN mRNA	230,258,259
		b. Inhibits IFN induction and signaling	598,666
nsp3 (PL^{pro})	SARS-CoV, HCoV-NL63, MHV	Blocks IRF3 activation and NF-κB signaling	91,136,174,654
nsp3 (ADRP)	SARS-CoV, HCoV-229E, MHV	a. Interferes with IFN-induced antiviral activity	158,297
		b. Enhances host proinflammatory cytokine expression	
nsp16	MHV	Evades MDA5 activation, evades IFIT recognition	106,665
ORF 3b protein	SARS-CoV	Inhibits IFN synthesis and signaling	283
ORF 5a protein	MHV	Interferes with IFN-induced antiviral activity	278
ORF 6 protein	SARS-CoV	Inhibits STAT1 nuclear translocation	175
ORF 7 protein	TGEV	Interferes with PKR and 2′–5′ OAS/RNase L activities	103
N protein	MHV, SARS-CoV	Inhibits IFN induction; interferes with 2′–5′ OAS/RNase L activity	283,637
M protein	SARS-CoV	Inhibits IRF3 activation	518

nsp, nonstructural protein; MHV, mouse hepatitis virus; SARS-CoV, severe acute respiratory syndrome coronavirus; SARSr, severe acute respiratory syndrome–related; BatCoV, bat coronavirus; TGEV, transmissible gastroenteritis virus; mRNA, messenger RNA; IFN, interferon; PL^{pro}, papain-like protease; HCoV, human coronavirus; IRF, interferon regulatory factor; NF-κB, nuclear factor-kappaB; ADRP, adenosine diphosphate-ribose-1″-phosphatase; MDA5, melanoma differentiation-associated gene 5; IFIT, IFN-induced proteins with tetratricopeptide repeats; ORF, open reading frame; STAT, signal transducers and activators of transcription; PKR, double stranded RNA-dependent protein kinase; OAS/RNase L, oligoadenylate synthetase/ribonuclease L.

the IFN response does not appear to be actively blocked in these cells, because infection with Sendai virus or exposure to poly I-C induces IFN. In some cells, such as macrophages, microglia, and oligodendrocytes, coronaviruses induce an IFN response by signaling through MDA5, and in oligodendrocytes, RIG-I.[328,484] To counter IFN induction through activation of MDA5, all coronaviruses express a 2′-*O*-methyltransferase (nsp16; see the Expression of the Replicase-Transcriptase Complex section). In the absence of 2′-*O*-methylation, viral RNA induces a potent MDA5-dependent IFN response, which limits replication in wild-type animals but not in those deficient in IFNAR expression[665] (see Table 28.4). Additionally, SARS-CoV, but not MHV nsp3, inhibits IFN induction by antagonizing IRF3 and NF-κB function.[136,174]

Once IFNs are expressed, they bind to IFNAR, resulting in the up-regulation of a large number of interferon-stimulated genes (ISGs). Several coronaviral proteins inhibit either IFN signaling or specific ISGs (see Table 28.4). In addition to inhibiting IFN induction, the nsp16 2′-*O*-methyltransferase counters the ability of IFN-induced proteins IFIT1 and IFIT2 (also referred to as ISG56 and ISG54) to inhibit translation of viral mRNA.[106] N protein inhibits IFN signaling, as do SARS-CoV, MHV and TGEV nsp1, and SARS-CoV ORF3b and ORF6 proteins.[173] The mechanism of action of some of these proteins has been elucidated. The N protein interferes with 2′,5′-oligoadenylate synthase-associated RNase L activity.[637] Nsp1 appears to enhance host cell mRNA degradation and inhibit host cell protein synthesis, with specific effects on IFN signaling.[259,598,666] The karyopherin complex is required for nuclear import of STAT1, a critical component of the IFN signaling pathway, as well as the import of many other host proteins. SARS-CoV ORF6, by binding karyopherin α2, sequesters karyopherin β1 in the cytoplasm, indirectly inhibiting nuclear translocation of STAT1.[175]

EPIDEMIOLOGY

Human Coronaviruses Other Than Severe Acute Respiratory Syndrome Coronavirus

Four known coronaviruses—HCoV-OC43, HCoV-229E, HCoV-NL63, and HCoV-HKU1—are endemic in human populations. HCoV-OC43 and HCoV-229E cause up to 30% of all upper respiratory tract infections, based on several prospective studies.[245,389] The variable range of detection reflects year-to-year variability, detection methods, season, and age of subjects. These studies also suggest that peak activity occurs every 2 to 4 years.[184,264,397] In temperate climates, infections occur predominantly in the winter and early spring. HCoV-OC43 and HCoV-229E have also been associated with severe pneumonia in neonates and aged populations, especially those with underlying illnesses, such as chronic obstructive pulmonary disease, or those requiring intensive care.[163,198] The high rate of HCoV infections early in life and the pattern of infections during outbreaks demonstrate that HCoVs are efficiently transmitted in human populations, most likely via large and, to a lesser extent, small droplets. Serologic studies suggest that infection with HCoV-229E and HCoV-OC43 frequently occurs in young children and then repeatedly throughout life.[245,264,556,557] Neutralizing antibodies against HCoV-OC43 or HCoV-229E have been detected in about 50% of school-age children and up to 80% of adults.[264,389,458]

HCoV-NL63 and HCoV-HKU1 also have worldwide distributions, causing up to 10% of respiratory tract infections.[1,460] Initial reports suggested that HCoV-NL63 was associated with severe respiratory disease; however, subsequent population-based studies showed that most patients developed mild disease, similar to those infected with HCoV-229E or HCoV-OC43. HCoV-NL63 is also an important etiologic agent of acute laryngotracheitis (croup).[1] HCoV-HKU1 was initially identified in an elderly patient with severe pneumonia,

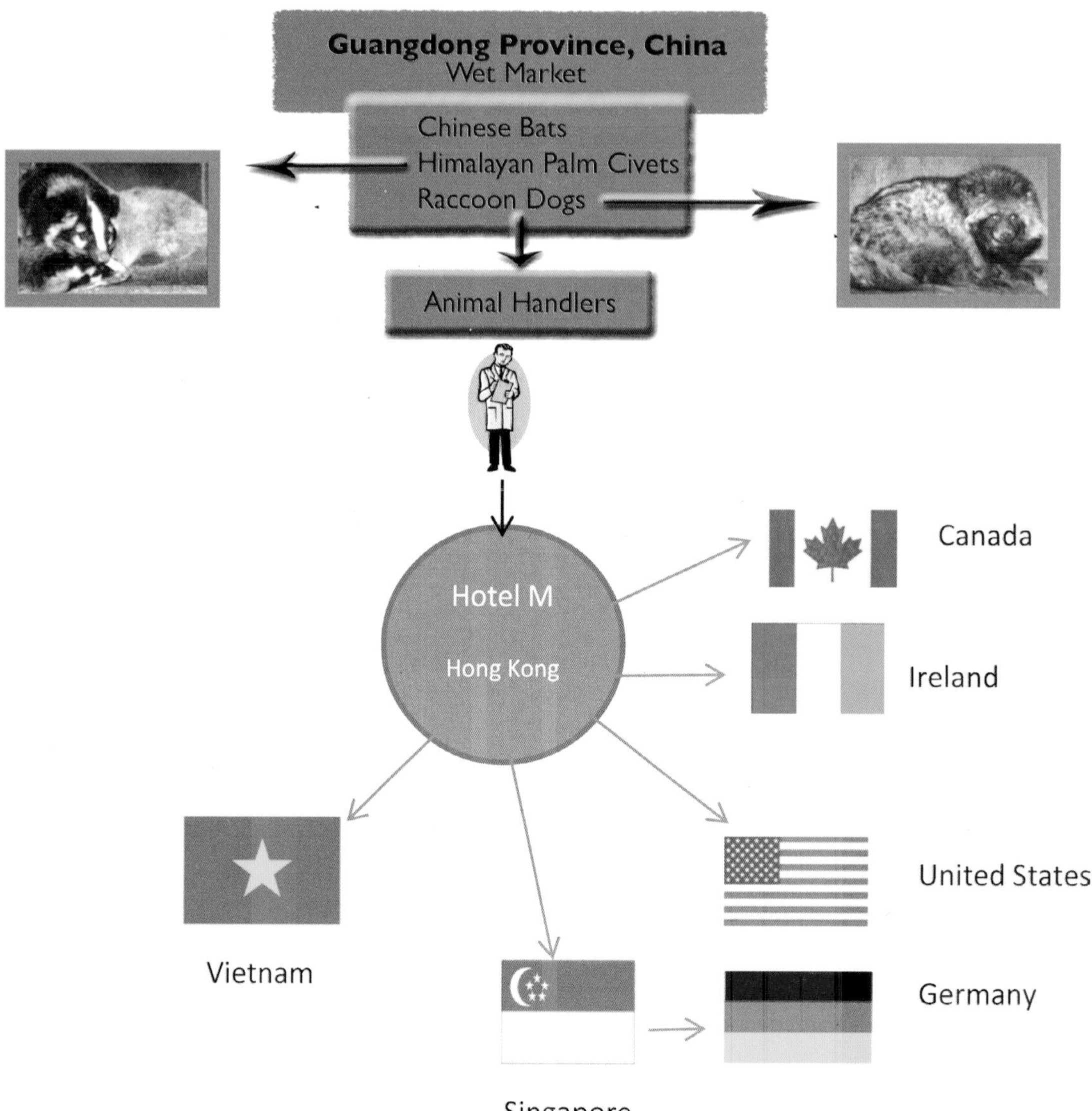

FIGURE 28.14. SARS-CoV spread from infected bats to infect humans in wet markets in Guangdong Province, China. SARS-related coronaviruses were detected in Chinese horseshoe bats and other bat species in China. The virus spread to human populations, likely animal handlers, in wet markets in Guangdong Province. Spread occurred either indirectly, via infection of exotic animals such as Himalayan palm civets, or directly, with subsequent human transmission to Himalayan palm civets and other exotic animals. This transmission occurred more than once, because a fraction of the animal handlers were positive for anti–SARS-CoV antibody.[203] In one episode, a physician taking care of an animal handler became infected. He then flew to Hong Kong and stayed at Hotel M, where he inadvertently infected several other people staying at the hotel, probably via superspreading events. These infected individuals then flew to other countries, resulting in the international outbreak. SARS-CoV, severe acute respiratory syndrome coronavirus; SARS, severe acute respiratory syndrome.

although more recent studies suggest that it is associated with both mild and severe respiratory infections.[460,615]

Severe Acute Respiratory Syndrome

During the 2002–2003 epidemic, SARS-CoV was isolated from several exotic animals, including Himalyan palm civets (*Paguma larvata*) and raccoon dogs (*Nyctereutes procyonoides*), in wet markets in Guangdong Province in China[203] (Fig. 28.14). Subsequent investigations showed that SARS-CoV could not be detected in these animals in the wild but that severe acute respiratory syndrome–related coronaviruses (SARSr-CoV) could be isolated from wild bats in China[308,332] (see Table 28.1). Bats are now considered to be the ultimate source for SARS-CoV, with probable infection of human populations occurring after initial adaptation to animals in Chinese wet markets. Sequences from several distinct SARSr-CoVs have been amplified from Chinese horseshoe bats from Hong Kong and several provinces in China, and 30% to 85% of bats of this genus (*Rhinolophus*) had serologic evidence of infection with a SARSr-CoV. *N* gene sequences for three SARSr bat coronaviruses (BatCoVs) differed by 3% to 6%, similar to the level of difference between the N proteins

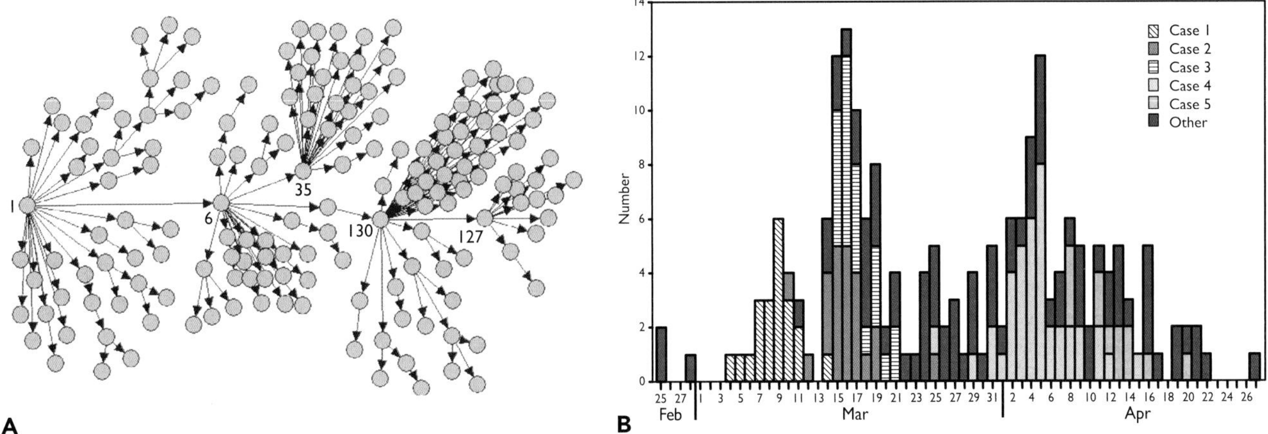

FIGURE 28.15. Role of superspreading events in SARS-CoV epidemics. SARS-CoV spread in Singapore in 2003, illustrated here, via superspreading and non-superspreading events. Most infected persons transmitted virus to fewer than five susceptible contacts. However, in a few instances, infected individuals were highly contagious, resulting in infection of larger numbers of contacts. The basis for superspreading events is not known but likely is a manifestation of larger virus burdens in a few infected patients. **A:** Probable cases of SARS by reported source of infection. **B:** Number of probable cases of SARS, by date of onset of fever and probable source of infection. SARS-CoV, severe acute respiratory syndrome coronavirus; SARS, severe acute respiratory syndrome. (From Leo YS, Chen M, Heng BH, et al. Severe Acute Respiratory Syndrome — Singapore, 2003. *Morb Mortal Wkly Rep* 2003;52:405–411.)

of each of these viruses and that of SARS-CoV. This degree of difference between SARS-CoV and the various SARSr-BatCoVs indicates that the precise source of the 2002–2003 SARS outbreak viruses remains unknown. Neither SARS-CoV nor reconstructed BatCoVs can use the Chinese horseshoe bat ACE2 protein to enter target cells, raising the possibility that the bat host receptor is unrelated to ACE2[26]; alternatively, the virus that was the actual progenitor for SARS-CoV may have originated from a BatCoV distantly related to the SARSr-CoVs identified thus far.[225]

Serologic studies demonstrated that SARS-CoV had not circulated to a significant extent in humans prior to the outbreak in 2002–2003.[64,320] However, some persons working in wild animal wet markets in China had serologic evidence of a SARS-CoV–like infection acquired before the 2003 outbreak but reported no SARS-like respiratory illness.[203] Thus, virus may have circulated in these wild animal markets for a few years, with the SARS outbreak occurring only when a confluence of factors facilitated spread into larger populations. Although animals were the original source of SARS, its global spread occurred by human-to-human transmission. Transmission appeared to occur through close contact—that is, direct person-to-person contact, fomites, or infectious droplets and probably aerosols in some instances.[438] Because transmission usually only occurred after onset of illness and most efficiently after the patient was sufficiently ill to be hospitalized, most spread occurred in household and healthcare settings but infrequently in other settings.[440] There was also substantial patient-to-patient variation in efficiency of transmission, which, in part, was associated with the degree of illness severity. Many susceptible persons were infected in superspreading events; however, fortunately, only a minority of infected individuals were involved in this type of spread[342,475] (Fig. 28.15). Superspreading events, which occurred when a single individual infected multiple susceptible contacts, may have resulted from high virus burdens or a tendency for these individuals to aerosolize virus more efficiently than most infected persons. Most infected individuals spread the virus to only one or a few susceptible persons, suggesting that virus spread was relatively inefficient.[342,475] The outbreak was partly controlled using quarantining, and the lack of efficient spread contributed to the success of this approach. Because the SARS outbreak was controlled in June 2003, only 17 cases of SARS were subsequently confirmed, and none of these occurred after June 2004. Thirteen of these 17 cases resulted from laboratory exposures, including 7 secondary cases associated with one of the cases.[336] The other 4 cases occurred in southern China and resulted from exposure in the community, presumably to SARS-CoV–infected animals from wild animal markets.[334]

Genetic Diversity of Coronaviruses

The SARS outbreak demonstrated the ability of coronaviruses to cross species, as the virus, naturally a bat virus, was able to infect small mammals, such as the Himalayan palm civet, and humans. Initially predicted from studies of coronavirus-infected cultured cells,[23] the ability of coronaviruses to cross species was also demonstrated when the betacoronaviruses HCoV-OC43, PHEV, and BCoV were analyzed[588] (Fig. 28.16). It is estimated that PHEV diverged from HCoV-OC43 and BCoV 100 to 200 years ago, whereas HCoV-OC43 and BCoV diverged about 100 years ago. Whether the common ancestor of HCoV-OC43 and BCoV was a human or bovine virus is not known. More recently, BCoV has crossed species to infect many ruminants, including elk, giraffe, and antelope,[4] and also canines.[159,160] Other phylogenetic studies suggest that the porcine alphacoronavirus TGEV resulted from cross-species transmission of a CCoV.[355]

In addition to their ability to cross species, coronaviruses readily undergo recombination (see the Viral RNA Synthesis section). Recombination events between canine (CCoV-I) and feline (FeCoV-I) coronaviruses and an unknown coronavirus resulted in the appearance of two novel viruses (CCoV-II and FeCoV-II).[355] In another illustration, new strains of IBV

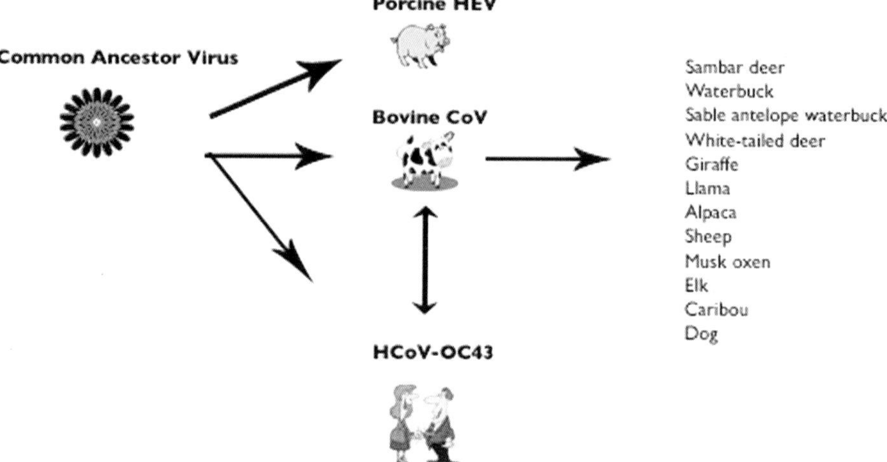

FIGURE 28.16. Coronaviruses mutate and recombine to cross species barriers. Phylogenetic analyses indicate that HCoV-OC43, BCoV, and PHEV shared a common ancestor and diverged about 200 years ago. More recently (100–130 years ago), HCoV-OC43 and BCoV diverged; however, it is not known whether BCoV infected human populations or HCoV-OC43 crossed species barriers to infect bovids. BCoV then spread to many ruminants and to dogs, probably via contact with infected domesticated cows. HCoV, human coronavirus; BCoV, bovine coronavirus; PHEV, porcine hemagglutinating encephalomyelitis virus.

have been detected in chicken populations and appear to have resulted from recombination between circulating vaccine and wild-type IBV strains.[284] This propensity for recombination has raised concerns about the use of live attenuated coronavirus vaccines (see the Prevention section).

CLINICAL FEATURES

Human Coronaviruses Other Than Severe Acute Respiratory Syndrome Coronavirus

In humans, coronaviruses have been clearly shown to cause respiratory disease, including its most severe manifestation—SARS. HCoVs have occasionally been implicated in enteric disease, particularly in newborns, using electron microscopy.[185,270,365] Electron microscopy has been used in these studies, because efforts to propagate human enteric coronaviruses in tissue culture cells have thus far been unsuccessful, hindering further studies. Because other particles in stool specimens (e.g., cellular membranes) can have similar morphology to coronaviruses, electron microscopic detection of coronavirus particles in stools is not considered diagnostic of infection. However, polymerase chain reaction (PCR) assays designed to detect coronavirus RNA sequences in pathologic specimens will now make it possible to determine whether these viruses play a role in enteric diseases. It seems likely that coronaviruses will be the etiologic agent in a fraction of patients with gastroenteritis, given the ability of these viruses to cause enteritis in a variety of domestic and companion animals.

Clinical features of infections in humans follow two distinct patterns: one for the non–SARS-CoV coronaviruses (i.e., HCoV-229E, -NL63, -OC43, -HKU1), and one for the zoonotic coronavirus SARS-CoV. Among the HCoVs, HCoV-229E and HCoV-OC43 were extensively characterized in volunteer studies in the 1960s.[389] Human volunteers inoculated intranasally with respiratory coronaviruses developed symptoms that included fever, headache, malaise, chills, rhinorrhea, sore throat, and cough, with peak infection observed 3 to 4 days following infection. About half of the volunteers challenged with virus developed illness, and approximately 30% were asymptomatically infected, as indicated by detection of virus in the upper respiratory tract. Symptoms lasted for a mean of 7 days, with a range of 3 to 18 days. Natural infection in both adults and children is also usually associated with a common cold–like illness.[44,389] Natural infection is probably acquired in a fashion similar to that for many other respiratory viruses (i.e., inoculation of infectious secretions from infected persons or fomites onto mucous membranes of the upper respiratory tract or inhalation of infectious droplets), with primary infection of ciliated epithelial cells in the nasopharynx.[3] Destruction of these cells, combined with exuberant production of chemokines and cytokines by resident and infiltrating cells, results in signs and symptoms of clinical illness.

HCoV infections are also occasionally associated with lower respiratory tract disease in children and adults. Coronaviruses have been detected in children hospitalized with lower respiratory tract disease at varying rates, although usually less than 8% of patients.[88,155,179,556,557,572] One caveat is that coronaviruses are also sometimes detected in well, control patients; thus, the presence of virus may not be etiologically related to the illness.[108] Coronavirus infection has also been detected in adults with acute respiratory tract illness, including about 5% of those hospitalized with lower respiratory tract disease.[108,155,163,182,198] Studies using PCR to detect viral RNA in middle ear fluids suggest that coronaviruses, like other respiratory viruses, can cause otitis media.[454,455] In addition, HCoVs have been associated with wheezing and exacerbations of asthma.[245,556] HCoV-NL63 and HCoV-HKU1 have also been detected in persons with acute upper and lower respiratory tract illness,[1,108,182,556,557] and as described earlier, HCoV-NL63 is associated with croup in children younger than 3 years.[574] Studies of natural infection and volunteer studies have shown that reinfection with coronaviruses is common, demonstrating that infection does not induce stable protective immunity.[245,264,389] For example, previously infected volunteers developed symptomatic disease if infected 1 year later with the same strain of HCoV-229E.[470]

Severe Acute Respiratory Syndrome Coronavirus Infections

In contrast to the mild illness usually associated with HCoV infections, SARS-CoV have nearly always resulted in a serious lower respiratory tract illness that required hospitalization, often in an intensive care unit (up to 20% of infections)[438] (Fig. 28.17). In the 2002–2003 epidemic, approximately 8,000 individuals were infected, with an overall mortality rate of 10%. Disease severity increased proportionally with age. Thus, no mortality occurred in patients younger than

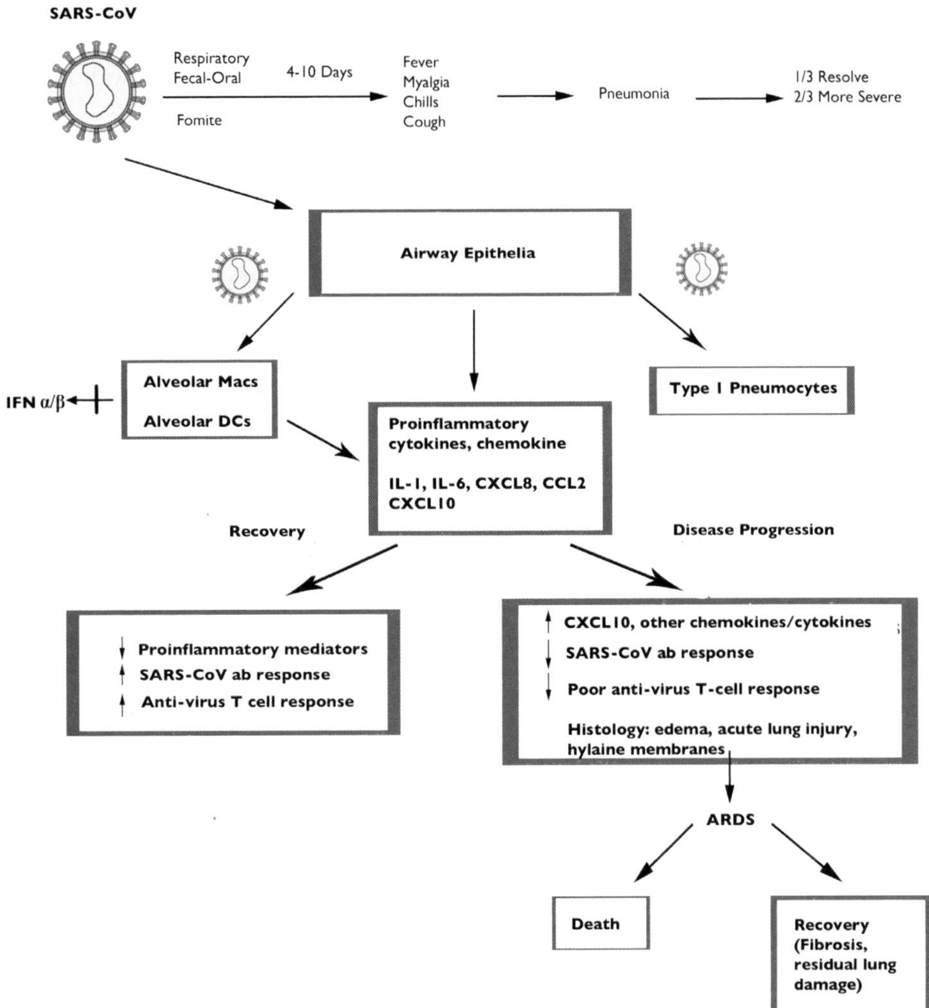

FIGURE 28.17. Clinical disease in patients infected with SARS-CoV. SARS-CoV spread to susceptible individuals via respiratory and fecal–oral routes and, less commonly, if at all, via fomites. Virus replication was initiated in the upper airway epithelial cells, based primarily on animal studies and *in vitro* studies using primary cultures of airway epithelial cells. Virus subsequently spread to the lower respiratory tract, with infection of type 1 pneumocytes and macrophages and dendritic cells most prominent. The infection of the latter two cell types was abortive, resulting in production of proinflammatory cytokines and chemokines such as CXCL10 and CXCL8 but not type 1 IFN. In patients who recovered, expression of proinflammatory cytokines diminished, and robust antivirus antibody responses were detected. In patients who developed progressively more severe disease, cytokine production continued and patients remained lymphopenic without developing an effective anti-SARS-CoV antibody response. Some of these patients died, and significant long-term morbidity was found in many of the survivors. SARS-CoV, severe acute respiratory syndrome coronavirus; IFN, interferon.

24 years, although about 50% of infected individuals older than 60 years succumbed to the infection. Mortality was also greater in patients with underlying disease. Clinical disease in patients with SARS was not diagnostic; however, some features were more common in SARS patients compared to those infected with other pathogens.[35,318,437,438] Illness usually had an onset of 4 to 7 days, although occasionally an incubation period of as little as 2 days or as long as 10 to 14 days was observed. Disease was characterized by systemic symptoms such as fever, malaise, and myalgias. Unlike many other respiratory tract infections, upper respiratory tract signs and symptoms such as rhinorrhea, sore throat, and nasal congestion were not common, although they still occurred in a minority of patients. The first lower respiratory tract symptoms (usually a nonproductive cough and shortness of breath) developed several days after onset of systemic symptoms. Respiratory symptoms were often accompanied by evidence of involvement of other organ systems. Thus, whereas diarrhea occurred at disease onset in fewer than 25% of patients, up to 70% developed gastrointestinal disease during the course of the illness. Most patients developed abnormal liver function tests (70%–90%) and lymphopenia (70%–95%), with a substantial drop in both CD4 and CD8 T-cell numbers.[104,438] Patients who failed to resolve their illness often had progressive respiratory failure leading to ARDS and death weeks to months

after illness onset.[56,171,321] In these patients, lymphocyte and platelet counts remained abnormally low, whereas neutrophilia and elevated titers of virus or viral RNA in clinical specimens for prolonged periods of time were common features. Asymptomatic or mild illness was uncommon, as illustrated by studies of exposed healthcare workers. In these studies, fewer than 1% of those without a SARS-like illness had serologic evidence of infection.[70,218,466] Most survivors of SARS-CoV infection achieved full recovery, although pulmonary function abnormalities sometimes took months to subside.[86,626] Some, however, had persistently abnormal pulmonary function. Curiously, a fraction of survivors showed more evidence of neurologic or psychiatric disease than expected based on the degree of respiratory illness or steroid use. Although brains were not commonly studied during the 2002–2003 epidemic, a few studies did demonstrate SARS-CoV infection of the brain, suggesting that CNS infection may have occurred in some cases.[84,201,307,316]

DIAGNOSIS

Most HCoV infections, other than SARS-CoV, are not diagnosed because they cause mild, self-limited upper respiratory disease, and no specific therapy is available. Diagnosis is laboratory-based because coronavirus infections cannot be distinguished clinically from other causes of upper respiratory tract infections, such as rhinoviruses. However, in some clinical settings, such as in hospitalized patients with pneumonia and in epidemiologic studies, specific diagnosis is important. Coronavirus infections in animals and humans were initially diagnosed by isolation of infectious virus, by electron microscopy, and in serologic assays, with the caveat that some coronaviruses, especially those in the stool, are not easily cultured. HCoV-229E and related alphacoronaviruses have sometimes been isolated in human diploid cell lines. Other HCoVs, most notably HCoV-OC43, initially required cell organ culture systems for isolation,[389] although this virus can now be grown in tissue culture cells. HCoV-NL63 can infect monkey kidney LLC-MK2 cells or Vero cells,[170,460,573] whereas HCoV-HKU1 has been grown only in primary human airway epithelial cells.[463] RT-PCR–based methods and immunofluorescence assays (IFA) for virus antigen have largely replaced these other methods for the diagnosis of respiratory coronavirus infections.[108,156,163,198,392] PCR primers can be designed to be broadly reactive or strain specific, based on primer location and design. With a sensitive system to detect the PCR amplicon (e.g., a real-time assay), fewer than five RNA copies in the reaction mixture can be consistently detected.[156] A multiplex real-time RT-PCR assay has also been described that is able to detect all four respiratory coronaviruses and may become the diagnostic method of choice.[184]

Electron microscopic examination of clinical material, although laborious, contributed to the identification and characterization of many coronaviruses, including SARS-CoV.[143,288,389,439] At present, electron microscopy is used most commonly to identify coronaviruses in patients with enteritis,[270] because none of these coronaviruses have been cultured; however, because other particles in clinical specimens can resemble coronaviruses and coronaviruses may be present without causing disease, identification of such particles does not confirm infection.

Various serologic assays have been used to detect coronavirus infections, including complement fixation, hemagglutination inhibition (HI) for viruses with an HE protein (i.e., some betacoronaviruses), neutralization, IFAs, and enzyme-linked immunoassays (EIAs). Initially, these assays used virus lysates or inactivated whole virus; more recently, cloned expressed proteins, synthesized peptides, and pseudoviruses have been used as antigens for serologic assays.[319,357,389,418,458,558]

SARS or another coronavirus infection of equivalent severity presents a different diagnostic situation. A specific diagnosis is critical because a positive result will guide clinical management and have public health implications. However, testing should only be considered when, based on the likelihood of an exposure and clinical features of the illness, infection is plausible. SARS-CoV was initially isolated in fetal rhesus kidney cells and Vero cells; however, during the 2002–2003 epidemic, a combination of serologic and RT-PCR assays, not virus culture, were used to detect and confirm SARS-CoV infection.[440] With very sensitive PCR assays (e.g., a nested or real-time PCR assay) and RNA extraction procedures that increased the amount of specimen available for the assay, the positivity rate in respiratory specimens obtained during the second and third days of illness increased from less than 40% to more than 80% as the epidemic progressed.[459] SARS N protein EIA was positive in 50% to 80% of serum specimens collected during the first week of illness[74] and in more than 50% of respiratory and stool specimens collected during the second and third weeks of illness.[309] SARS-CoV–specific antibodies were usually detected by 14 days into the illness, although sometimes not until 4 weeks after infection.[229,233] Whereas RT-PCR provided the best way to make an early diagnosis, serologic assays were important in confirming or ruling out SARS-CoV as the cause of infection. Because serum specimens from persons not infected with SARS during the 2002–2003 outbreak have rarely tested positive for SARS-CoV antibodies,[320] a single serum specimen positive for SARS-CoV antibodies was usually considered diagnostic; a negative test on a serum specimen collected late in the illness (28 days or later after onset of illness) could be used to rule out SARS-CoV infection.

TREATMENT

At present, there are no antiviral drugs for HCoV infections, and therapy is supportive. During the major part of the SARS epidemic, most patients were treated with ribavirin or high-dose steroids, based on the idea that the virus would be susceptible to ribavirin and steroids might diminish immune-mediated bystander damage.[538] Late in the outbreak, based on their ability to inhibit SARS-CoV replication *in vitro* and/or in experimental animals, IFN-α, SARS convalescent-phase immune globulin, and lopinavir plus ritonavir (two protease inhibitors licensed for the treatment of HIV) were used to treat patients.[65,85,89,356,530] However, a large-scale review of all of these therapies concluded that whereas some showed efficacy in inhibiting SARS-CoV replication in tissue culture cells, none showed a beneficial effect in patients.[538] The molecular biology of coronavirus infection suggests several potential targets for antiviral drugs, including the viral RdRp, virus-encoded proteases, host cell receptors used by the virus for entry, and the viral S glycoprotein. Subsequent to the outbreak, several antiviral drugs targeting these viral proteins or processes have been developed and evaluated for their ability to inhibit SARS-CoV replication *in vitro.* These include specific coronavirus protease inhibitors,[468] monoclonal antibodies that inhibit SARS-CoV binding to cells,[551] peptides from the heptad repeat regions of the S protein or from ACE2 that inhibit receptor binding or fusion,[40,211] and small interfering RNAs.[71] If SARS or another severe coronavirus-mediated disease emerges, *in vitro* and animal model studies of antiviral drugs will be used to guide treatment.

PREVENTION

No vaccines are available to prevent HCoV infection; however, vaccines against common veterinary coronaviruses, such as IBV and CCoV, are routinely used to prevent serious disease in young animals. Efforts are ongoing to improve these vaccines and to enhance safety and efficacy while minimizing the likelihood of reversion to a virulent strain.[492] In addition, various SARS-CoV vaccines have been developed, including inactivated whole virus, live virus vectors expressing single viral proteins and recombinant proteins, and DNA vaccines.[10,480] Nearly all of these vaccines express the surface glycoprotein and are designed to induce SARS-CoV neutralizing antibodies. For some of these vaccines, efficacy has been demonstrated in animal models. Large stocks of anti–SARS-CoV neutralizing antibody have been prepared and will be used for passive immunization of healthcare workers and other high-risk personnel if SARS recurs.

In general, live attenuated vaccines are likely to be most effective in inducing protective immune responses against coronaviruses. This has been illustrated elegantly in the case of TGEV—an important cause of neonatal diarrhea and death in swine. In the mid-1980s, a naturally occurring, attenuated variant of TGEV—PRCoV—was identified in pig populations. This virus, which causes mild disease and no enteritis, induces an immune response in pigs that is protective against TGEV and largely eliminated it from dually infected populations.[312] Live attenuated vaccines induce not only neutralizing antibodies but also antivirus T-cell responses, which are required for virus clearance from infected cells in SARS and other coronavirus infections. However, the development of live coronavirus vaccines is challenging.[492] First, in many instances, natural infection does not prevent either subsequent infection or disease, therefore an effective vaccine would need to be superior to immunity induced naturally. Second, the genetic and antigenic variability of coronaviruses and their ability to readily recombine hinder vaccine development. Thus, a vaccine may not provide equal protection from all antigenic variants, and subsequent recombination with vaccine strains could increase the number of different strains circulating in the wild. As an example, recombinants of IBV vaccine strains with virulent wild-type strains have caused disease outbreaks in chicken flocks.[249,596] In addition, the finding that immunization with an S protein–expressing FIPV vaccine led to more severe disease after subsequent natural infection raises the concern that other coronavirus vaccines might also enhance, rather than protect, from disease.[581] Several strategies to minimize the likelihood of recombination and to attenuate candidate vaccines without compromising efficacy have been recently described. These include engineering viruses with deletions in nsp1, important for the anti-IFN response,[666] or in E protein, important for virus assembly.[124] In other approaches to minimizing the likelihood of recombination of vaccine viruses, the coronavirus genome has been reconstructed, changing the order of structural genes at the 3′ end[121] or modifying the leader and body TRSs (see the Viral RNA Synthesis section) to eliminate homology with natural virus sequences.[644]

In the absence of effective vaccines and antiviral drugs, the most important ways to prevent coronavirus infections are a highly active public health surveillance system and good infection control practices. This was demonstrated unequivocally during the SARS outbreak in 2002–2003, in which sharing of information by national public health agencies and governments and involvement of international agencies such as the World Health Organization resulted in the rapid identification of a coronavirus as the cause of SARS and implementation of measures that minimized spread. At the local level, strict attention to good isolation and infection control practices and identification and management of exposed persons (contacts) minimized human-to-human spread of the virus within a few months of its global spread. The low risk of SARS-CoV transmission before hospitalization and the low rate of asymptomatic infection facilitated the efficacy of these public health measures.[70,218,466] The identification of cases of laboratory-acquired SARS-CoV, with subsequent transmission to others after one of these cases,[334,336] reinforces the importance of strict attention to safe laboratory practices. These practices include handling the virus in the appropriate type of facility, using standardized operating procedures, and providing appropriate training and medical surveillance programs for staff.

PERSPECTIVES

Many important problems remain to be resolved by future studies of coronaviruses. One critical task will be to broaden our picture of how coronaviruses jump between species. We need to know whether cross-species viral trafficking events, both abortive and successful, are rare or common. Although there has been a recent expansion of our knowledge of spike protein interactions with receptors and associated proteases, we cannot yet fully gauge the height of the barrier preventing productive adaptation by a spike protein to new receptors and proteases. Such information will be directly relevant to forestalling or coping with the re-emergence of a SARS-related (or other) coronavirus from ubiquitous bat reservoirs. Related to this is the challenge of developing *in vitro* culture systems for virus species that are currently only known through their genomic sequences. A second area of crucial importance will be to further develop our understanding of the immunopathogenesis of the more severe human and animal coronaviruses and to more precisely delineate the correlates of immune protection. This will better inform the effective design and evaluation of vaccines for control of these agents. Finally, one of the most exciting areas of future research will be to address the many gaps in our basic knowledge of the intricacies of the coronavirus RTC—the largest and most complicated machinery of RNA synthesis found in any RNA virus. The past few years have seen tremendous advances in this field, particularly in structural and biochemical studies, and it is likely that progress will continue apace. A long-term goal will be the total *in vitro* reconstitution of coronavirus RNA synthesis, which would definitively demonstrate the roles of the many viral replicase subunits as well as those of putative host factors. It can be expected that studies of this type will reveal fundamental principles common to all RNA-dependent RNA synthesis, in addition to mechanisms unique to the order *Nidovirales*. Knowledge derived from this enterprise will be critical for the design of antiviral drugs to combat diseases caused by existing and emerging coronaviruses.

REFERENCES

All cited references are available in the e-book.

4. Alekseev KP, Vlasova AN, Jung K, et al. Bovine-like coronaviruses isolated from four species of captive wild ruminants are homologous to bovine coronaviruses, based on complete genomic sequences. *J Virol* 2008;82:12422–12431.
6. Almazán F, González JM, Pénzes Z, et al. Engineering the largest RNA virus genome as an infectious bacterial artificial chromosome. *Proc Natl Acad Sci U S A* 2000;97:5516–5521.
7. Almeida JD, Berry DM, Cunningham CH, et al. Coronaviruses. *Nature* 1968;220:650.
11. Anghelina D, Pewe L, Perlman S. Pathogenic role for virus-specific CD4 T cells in mice with coronavirus-induced acute encephalitis. *Am J Pathol* 2006;169:209–222.
13. Arbour N, Day R, Newcombe J, et al. Neuroinvasion by human respiratory coronaviruses. *J Virol* 2000;74:8913–8921.
19. Banner LR, Lai MM. Random nature of coronavirus RNA recombination in the absence of selection pressure. *Virology* 1991;185:441–445.
21. Bárcena M, Oostergetel GT, Bartelink W, et al. Cryo-electron tomography of mouse hepatitis virus: insights into the structure of the coronavirion. *Proc Natl Acad Sci U S A* 2009;106:582–587.
22. Baric RS, Fu K, Schaad MC, et al. Establishing a genetic recombination map for murine coronavirus strain A59 complementation groups. *Virology* 1990;177:646–656.
23. Baric RS, Sullivan E, Hensley L, et al. Persistent infection promotes cross-species transmissibility of mouse hepatitis virus. *J Virol* 1999;73:638–649.
26. Becker MM, Graham RL, Donaldson EF, et al. Synthetic recombinant bat SARS-like coronavirus is infectious in cultured cells and in mice. *Proc Natl Acad Sci U S A* 2008;105:19944–19949.
28. Belouzard S, Chu VC, Whittaker GR. Activation of the SARS coronavirus spike protein via sequential proteolytic cleavage at two distinct sites. *Proc Natl Acad Sci U S A* 2009;106:5871–5876.
30. Beniac DR, Andonov A, Grudeski E, et al. Architecture of the SARS coronavirus prefusion spike. *Nat Struct Mol Biol* 2006;13:751–752.
31. Bergmann CC, Lane TE, Stohlman SA. Coronavirus infection of the central nervous system: host-virus stand-off. *Nat Rev Microbiol* 2006;4:121–132.
37. Bos EC, Luytjes W, van der Meulen HV, et al. The production of recombinant infectious DI-particles of a murine coronavirus in the absence of helper virus. *Virology* 1996;218:52–60.
38. Boscarino JA, Logan HL, Lacny JJ, et al. Envelope protein palmitoylations are crucial for murine coronavirus assembly. *J Virol* 2008;82:2989–2999.
40. Bosch BJ, Martina BE, van der Zee R, et al. Severe acute respiratory syndrome coronavirus (SARS-CoV) infection inhibition using spike protein heptad repeat-derived peptides. *Proc Natl Acad Sci U S A* 2004;101:8455–8460.
41. Bosch BJ, Rottier PJM. Nidovirus entry into cells. In: Perlman S, Gallagher T, Snijder EJ, eds. *Nidoviruses*. Washington, DC: ASM Press; 2008:361–377.
43. Bouvet M, Debarnot C, Imbert I, et al. In vitro reconstitution of SARS-coronavirus mRNA cap methylation. *PLoS Pathog* 2010;6:e1000863.
47. Brierley I, Digard P, Inglis SC. Characterization of an efficient coronavirus ribosomal frameshifting signal: requirement for an RNA pseudoknot. *Cell* 1989;57:537–547.
53. Brown CG, Nixon KS, Senanayake SD, et al. An RNA stem-loop within the bovine coronavirus nsp1 coding region is a cis-acting element in defective interfering RNA replication. *J Virol* 2007;81:7716–7724.
56. Cameron MJ, Ran L, Xu L, et al. Interferon-mediated immunopathological events are associated with atypical innate and adaptive immune responses in patients with severe acute respiratory syndrome. *J Virol* 2007;81:8692–8706.
57. Carstens EB. Ratification vote on taxonomic proposals to the International Committee on Taxonomy of Viruses (2009). *Arch Virol* 2010;155:133–146.
59. Caul EO, Ashley CR, Ferguson M, et al. Preliminary studies on the isolation of coronavirus 229E nucleocapsids. *FEMS Microbiol Lett* 1979;5:101–105.
63. Cervantes-Barragan L, Züst R, Weber F, et al. Control of coronavirus infection through plasmacytoid dendritic-cell-derived type I interferon. *Blood* 2007;109:1131–1137.
70. Chang WT, Kao CL, Chung MY, et al. SARS exposure and emergency department workers. *Emerg Infect Dis* 2004;10:1117–1119.
75. Cheever FS, Daniels JB, Pappenheimer AM, et al. A murine virus (JHM) causing disseminated encephalomyelitis with extensive destruction of myelin. *J Exp Med* 1949;90:181–194.
78. Chen H, Hou J, Jiang X, et al. Response of memory CD8+ T cells to severe acute respiratory syndrome (SARS) coronavirus in recovered SARS patients and healthy individuals. *J Immunol* 2005;175:591–598.
79. Chen J, Subbarao K. The immunobiology of SARS. *Annu Rev Immunol* 2007;25:443–472.
81. Chen SC, van den Born E, van den Worm SH, et al. New structure model for the packaging signal in the genome of group IIa coronaviruses. *J Virol* 2007;81:6771–6774.
82. Chen Y, Cai H, Pan J, et al. Functional screen reveals SARS coronavirus nonstructural protein nsp14 as a novel cap N7 methyltransferase. *Proc Natl Acad Sci U S A* 2009;106:3484–3489.
86. Chiang CH, Shih JF, Su WJ, et al. Eight-month prospective study of 14 patients with hospital-acquired severe acute respiratory syndrome. *Mayo Clin Proc* 2004;79:1372–1379.
93. Cohen JR, Lin LD, Machamer CE. Identification of a Golgi complex-targeting signal in the cytoplasmic tail of the severe acute respiratory syndrome coronavirus envelope protein. *J Virol* 2011;85:5794–5803.
101. Corse E, Machamer CE. The cytoplasmic tail of infectious bronchitis virus E protein directs Golgi targeting. *J Virol* 2002;76:1273–1284.
106. Daffis S, Szretter KJ, Schriewer J, et al. 2′-O methylation of the viral mRNA cap evades host restriction by IFIT family members. *Nature* 2010;468:452–456.
112. De Groot-Mijnes JD, van Dun JM, van der Most RG, et al. Natural history of a recurrent feline coronavirus infection and the role of cellular immunity in survival and disease. *J Virol* 2005;79:1036–1044.
115. De Haan CA, Masters PS, Shen X, et al. The group-specific murine coronavirus genes are not essential, but their deletion, by reverse genetics, is attenuating in the natural host. *Virology* 2002;296:177–189.
117. De Haan CA, Rottier PJ. Molecular interactions in the assembly of coronaviruses. *Adv Virus Res* 2005;64:165–230.
121. De Haan CA, Volders H, Koetzner CA, et al. Coronaviruses maintain viability despite dramatic rearrangements of the strictly conserved genome organization. *J Virol* 2002;76:12491–12502.
123. Decroly E, Imbert I, Coutard B, et al. Coronavirus nonstructural protein 16 is a cap-0 binding enzyme possessing (nucleoside-2′O)-methyltransferase activity. *J Virol* 2008;82:8071–8084.
124. DeDiego ML, Alvarez E, Almazán F, et al. A severe acute respiratory syndrome coronavirus that lacks the E gene is attenuated in vitro and in vivo. *J Virol* 2007;81:1701–1713.
127. Delmas B, Gelfi J, L'Haridon R, et al. Aminopeptidase N is a major receptor for the entero-pathogenic coronavirus TGEV. *Nature* 1992;357:417–420.
130. Deming DJ, Baric RS. Genetics and reverse genetics of nidoviruses. In: Perlman S, Gallagher T, Snijder EJ, eds. *Nidoviruses*. Washington, DC: ASM Press; 2008:47–64.
136. Devaraj SG, Wang N, Chen Z, et al. Regulation of IRF-3-dependent innate immunity by the papain-like protease domain of the severe acute respiratory syndrome coronavirus. *J Biol Chem* 2007;282:32208.
143. Drosten C, Günther S, Preiser W, et al. Identification of a novel coronavirus in patients with severe acute respiratory syndrome. *N Engl J Med* 2003;348:1967–1976.
144. Duquerroy S, Vigouroux A, Rottier PJ, et al. Central ions and lateral asparagine/glutamine zippers stabilize the post-fusion hairpin

conformation of the SARS coronavirus spike glycoprotein. *Virology* 2005;335:276–285.

150. Eckerle LD, Lu X, Sperry SM, et al. High fidelity of murine hepatitis virus replication is decreased in nsp14 exoribonuclease mutants. *J Virol* 2007;81:12135–12144.
162. Escors D, Ortego J, Laude H, et al. The membrane M protein carboxy terminus binds to transmissible gastroenteritis coronavirus core and contributes to core stability. *J Virol* 2001;75:1312–1324.
164. Fan H, Ooi A, Tan YW, et al. The nucleocapsid protein of coronavirus infectious bronchitis virus: crystal structure of its N-terminal domain and multimerization properties. *Structure* 2005;13:1859–1868.
169. Fosmire JA, Hwang K, Makino S. Identification and characterization of a coronavirus packaging signal. *J Virol* 1992;66:3522–3530.
170. Fouchier RA, Hartwig NG, Bestebroer TM, et al. A previously undescribed coronavirus associated with respiratory disease in humans. *Proc Natl Acad Sci U S A* 2004;101:6212–6216.
171. Fowler RA, Lapinsky SE, Hallett D, et al. Critically ill patients with severe acute respiratory syndrome. *JAMA* 2003;290:367–373.
173. Frieman M, Heise M, Baric R. SARS coronavirus and innate immunity. *Virus Res* 2008;133:101–112.
174. Frieman M, Ratia K, Johnston RE, et al. Severe acute respiratory syndrome coronavirus papain-like protease ubiquitin-like domain and catalytic domain regulate antagonism of IRF3 and NF-kappaB signaling. *J Virol* 2009;83:6689–6705.
175. Frieman M, Yount B, Heise M, et al. Severe acute respiratory syndrome coronavirus ORF6 antagonizes STAT1 function by sequestering nuclear import factors on the rough endoplasmic reticulum/Golgi membrane. *J Virol* 2007;81:9812–9824.
180. Gallagher TM, Escarmis C, Buchmeier MJ. Alteration of the pH dependence of coronavirus-induced cell fusion: effect of mutations in the spike glycoprotein. *J Virol* 1991;65:1916–1928.
182. Garbino J, Crespo S, Aubert JD, et al. A prospective hospital-based study of the clinical impact of non-severe acute respiratory syndrome (Non-SARS)-related human coronavirus infection. *Clin Infect Dis* 2006; 43:1009–1015.
187. Glowacka I, Bertram S, Müller MA, et al. Evidence that TMPRSS2 activates the severe acute respiratory syndrome coronavirus spike protein for membrane fusion and reduces viral control by the humoral immune response. *J Virol* 2011;85:4122–4134.
190. Goebel SJ, Hsue B, Dombrowski TF, et al. Characterization of the RNA components of a putative molecular switch in the 3′ untranslated region of the murine coronavirus genome. *J Virol* 2004;78:669–682.
192. Goebel SJ, Taylor J, Masters PS. The 3′ cis-acting genomic replication element of the severe acute respiratory syndrome coronavirus can function in the murine coronavirus genome. *J Virol* 2004;78:7846–7851.
194. Gorbalenya AE. Genomics and evolution of the Nidovirales. In: Perlman S, Gallagher T, Snijder EJ, eds. *Nidoviruses.* Washington, DC: ASM Press; 2008:15–28.
195. Gorbalenya AE, Enjuanes L, Ziebuhr J, et al. Nidovirales: evolving the largest RNA virus genome. *Virus Res* 2006;117:17–37.
196. Gorbalenya AE, Koonin EV, Donchenko AP, et al. Coronavirus genome: prediction of putative functional domains in the non-structural polyprotein by comparative amino acid sequence analysis. *Nucleic Acids Res* 1989;17:4847–4861.
197. Gorbalenya AE, Snijder EJ, Spaan WJ. Severe acute respiratory syndrome coronavirus phylogeny: toward consensus. *J Virol* 2004;78:7863–7866.
200. Grossoehme NE, Li L, Keane SC, et al. Coronavirus N protein N-terminal domain (NTD) specifically binds the transcriptional regulatory sequence (TRS) and melts TRS-cTRS RNA duplexes. *J Mol Biol* 2009; 394:544–557.
201. Gu J, Gong E, Zhang B, et al. Multiple organ infection and the pathogenesis of SARS. *J Exp Med* 2005;202:415–424.
202. Guan BJ, Wu HY, Brian DA. An optimal cis-replication stem-loop IV in the 5′ untranslated region of the mouse coronavirus genome extends 16 nucleotides into open reading frame 1. *J Virol* 2011;85:5593–5605.
203. Guan Y, Zheng BJ, He YQ, et al. Isolation and characterization of viruses related to the SARS coronavirus from animals in southern China. *Science* 2003;302:276–278.
216. Herrewegh AA, Smeenk I, Horzinek MC, et al. Feline coronavirus type II strains 79-1683 and 79-1146 originate from a double recombination between feline coronavirus type I and canine coronavirus. *J Virol* 1998;72:4508–4514.
218. Ho KY, Singh KS, Habib AG, et al. Mild illness associated with severe acute respiratory syndrome coronavirus infection: lessons from a prospective seroepidemiologic study of health-care workers in a teaching hospital in Singapore. *J Infect Dis* 2004;189:642–647.
219. Hofmann H, Pyrc K, van der Hoek L, et al. Human coronavirus NL63 employs the severe acute respiratory syndrome coronavirus receptor for cellular entry. *Proc Natl Acad Sci U S A* 2005;102:7988–7993.
222. Hogue BG, Machamer CE. Coronavirus structural proteins and virus assembly. In: Perlman S, Gallagher T, Snijder EJ, eds. *Nidoviruses.* Washington, DC: ASM Press; 2008:179–200.
225. Hon CC, Lam TY, Shi ZL, et al. Evidence of the recombinant origin of a bat severe acute respiratory syndrome (SARS)-like coronavirus and its implications on the direct ancestor of SARS coronavirus. *J Virol* 2008; 82:1819–1826.
232. Huang IC, Bosch BJ, Li F, et al. SARS coronavirus, but not human coronavirus NL63, utilizes cathepsin L to infect ACE2-expressing cells. *J Biol Chem* 2006;281:3198–3203.
236. Hurst KR, Kuo L, Koetzner CA, et al. A major determinant for membrane protein interaction localizes to the carboxy-terminal domain of the mouse coronavirus nucleocapsid protein. *J Virol* 2005;79:13285–13297.
237. Hurst KR, Ye R, Goebel SJ, et al. An interaction between the nucleocapsid protein and a component of the replicase-transcriptase complex is crucial for the infectivity of coronavirus genomic RNA. *J Virol* 2010; 84:10276–10288.
239. Imai Y, Kuba K, Rao S, et al. Angiotensin-converting enzyme 2 protects from severe acute lung failure. *Nature* 2005;436:112–116.
240. Imbert I, Guillemot JC, Bourhis JM, et al. A second, non-canonical RNA-dependent RNA polymerase in SARS coronavirus. *EMBO J* 2006; 25:4933–4942.
243. Ireland DD, Stohlman SA, Hinton DR, et al. RNase L mediated protection from virus induced demyelination. *PLoS Pathog* 2009;5:e1000602.
244. Ireland DD, Stohlman SA, Hinton DR, et al. Type I interferons are essential in controlling neurotropic coronavirus infection irrespective of functional CD8 T cells. *J Virol* 2008;82:300–310.
246. Ivanov KA, Hertzig T, Rozanov M, et al. Major genetic marker of nidoviruses encodes a replicative endoribonuclease. *Proc Natl Acad Sci U S A* 2004;101:12694–12699.
253. Jayaram H, Fan H, Bowman BR, et al. X-ray structures of the N- and C-terminal domains of a coronavirus nucleocapsid protein: implications for nucleocapsid formation. *J Virol* 2006;80:6612–6620.
258. Kamitani W, Huang C, Narayanan K, et al. A two-pronged strategy to suppress host protein synthesis by SARS coronavirus Nsp1 protein. *Nat Struct Mol Biol* 2009;16:1134–1140.
259. Kamitani W, Narayanan K, Huang C, et al. Severe acute respiratory syndrome coronavirus nsp1 protein suppresses host gene expression by promoting host mRNA degradation. *Proc Natl Acad Sci U S A* 2006;103: 12885–12890.
277. Knoops K, Kikkert M, Worm SH, et al. SARS-coronavirus replication is supported by a reticulovesicular network of modified endoplasmic reticulum. *PLoS Biol* 2008;6:e226.
278. Koetzner CA, Kuo L, Goebel SJ, et al. Accessory protein 5a is a major antagonist of the antiviral action of interferon against murine coronavirus. *J Virol* 2010;84:8262–8274.
279. Koetzner CA, Parker MM, Ricard CS, et al. Repair and mutagenesis of the genome of a deletion mutant of the coronavirus mouse hepatitis virus by targeted RNA recombination. *J Virol* 1992;66:1841–1848.
283. Kopecky-Bromberg SA, Martínez-Sobrido L, Frieman M, et al. Severe acute respiratory syndrome coronavirus open reading frame (ORF) 3b, ORF 6, and nucleocapsid proteins function as interferon antagonists. *J Virol* 2007;81:548–557.
284. Kottier SA, Cavanagh D, Britton P. Experimental evidence of recombination in coronavirus infectious bronchitis virus. *Virology* 1995;213:569–580.
288. Ksiazek TG, Erdman D, Goldsmith CS, et al. A novel coronavirus associated with severe acute respiratory syndrome. *N Engl J Med* 2003; 348:1953–1966.
289. Kuba K, Imai Y, Rao S, et al. A crucial role of angiotensin converting enzyme 2 (ACE2) in SARS coronavirus-induced lung injury. *Nat Med* 2005;11:875–879.

292. Kuo L, Godeke GJ, Raamsman MJ, et al. Retargeting of coronavirus by substitution of the spike glycoprotein ectodomain: crossing the host cell species barrier. *J Virol* 2000;74:1393–1406.
293. Kuo L, Hurst KR, Masters PS. Exceptional flexibility in the sequence requirements for coronavirus small envelope protein function. *J Virol* 2007;81:2249–2262.
295. Kuo L, Masters PS. Genetic evidence for a structural interaction between the carboxy termini of the membrane and nucleocapsid proteins of mouse hepatitis virus. *J Virol* 2002;76:4987–4999.
296. Kuo L, Masters PS. The small envelope protein E is not essential for murine coronavirus replication. *J Virol* 2003;77:4597–4608.
306. Lassnig C, Sanchez CM, Egerbacher M, et al. Development of a transgenic mouse model susceptible to human coronavirus 229E. *Proc Natl Acad Sci U S A* 2005;102:8275–8280.
308. Lau SKP, Woo PCY, Li KSM, et al. Severe acute respiratory syndrome coronavirus-like virus in Chinese horseshoe bats. *Proc Natl Acad Sci U S A* 2005;102:14040–14045.
310. Lau YL, Peiris JSM. Pathogenesis of severe acute respiratory syndrome. *Curr Op Immunol* 2005;17:404–410.
314. Law HK, Cheung CY, Ng HY, et al. Chemokine upregulation in SARS coronavirus infected human monocyte derived dendritic cells. *Blood* 2005;106:2366–2376.
318. Lee N, Hui D, Wu A, et al. A major outbreak of severe acute respiratory syndrome in Hong Kong. *N Engl J Med* 2003;348:1986–1994.
320. Leung DT, van Maren WW, Chan FK, et al. Extremely low exposure of a community to severe acute respiratory syndrome coronavirus: false seropositivity due to use of bacterially derived antigens. *J Virol* 2006;80:8920–8928.
321. Lew TW, Kwek TK, Tai D, et al. Acute respiratory distress syndrome in critically ill patients with severe acute respiratory syndrome. *JAMA* 2003;290:374–380.
323. Li F. Structural analysis of major species barriers between humans and palm civets for severe acute respiratory syndrome coronavirus infections. *J Virol* 2008;82:6984–6991.
325. Li F, Li W, Farzan M, et al. Structure of SARS coronavirus spike receptor-binding domain complexed with receptor. *Science* 2005;309:1864–1868.
328. Li J, Liu Y, Zhang X. Murine coronavirus induces type I interferon in oligodendrocytes through recognition by RIG-I and MDA5. *J Virol* 2010;84:6472–6482.
329. Li L, Kang H, Liu P, et al. Structural lability in stem-loop 1 drives a 5′ UTR-3′ UTR interaction in coronavirus replication. *J Mol Biol* 2008;377:790–803.
331. Li W, Moore MJ, Vasilieva N, et al. Angiotensin-converting enzyme 2 is a functional receptor for the SARS coronavirus. *Nature* 2003;426:450–454.
332. Li W, Shi Z, Yu M, et al. Bats are natural reservoirs of SARS-like coronaviruses. *Science* 2005;310:676–679.
333. Li W, Zhang C, Sui J, et al. Receptor and viral determinants of SARS-coronavirus adaptation to human ACE2. *EMBO J* 2005;24:1634–1643.
336. Lim PL, Kurup A, Gopalakrishna G, et al. Laboratory-acquired severe acute respiratory syndrome. *N Engl J Med* 2004;350:1740–1745.
338. Lin MT, Hinton DR, Marten NW, et al. Antibody prevents virus reactivation within the central nervous system. *J Immunol* 1999;162:7358–7368.
340. Lin MT, Stohlman SA, Hinton DR. Mouse hepatitis virus is cleared from the central nervous systems of mice lacking perforin-mediated cytolysis. *J Virol* 1997;71:383–391.
342. Lipsitch MT, Cohen T, Cooper B, et al. Transmission dynamics and control of severe acute respiratory syndrome. *Science* 2003;300:1966–1970.
346. Liu P, Li L, Keane SC, et al. Mouse hepatitis virus stem-loop 2 adopts a uYNMG(U)a-like tetraloop structure that is highly functionally tolerant of base substitutions. *J Virol* 2009;83:12084–12093.
359. Luytjes W, Bredenbeek PJ, Noten AF, et al. Sequence of mouse hepatitis virus A59 mRNA 2: indications for RNA recombination between coronaviruses and influenza C virus. *Virology* 1988;166:415–422.
370. Makino S, Keck JG, Stohlman SA, et al. High-frequency RNA recombination of murine coronaviruses. *J Virol* 1986;57:729–737.
375. Marsden PA, Ning Q, Fung LS, et al. The Fgl2/fibroleukin prothrombinase contributes to immunologically mediated thrombosis in experimental and human viral hepatitis. *J Clin Invest* 2003;112:58–66.
378. Masters PS. The molecular biology of coronaviruses. *Adv Virus Res* 2006;66:193–292.
381. Masters PS, Rottier PJ. Coronavirus reverse genetics by targeted RNA recombination. *Curr Top Microbiol Immunol* 2005;287:133–159.
382. Matsuyama S, Nagata N, Shirato K, et al. Efficient activation of the severe acute respiratory syndrome coronavirus spike protein by the transmembrane protease TMPRSS2. *J Virol* 2010;84:12658–12664.
383. Matsuyama S, Ujike M, Morikawa S, et al. Protease-mediated enhancement of severe acute respiratory syndrome coronavirus infection. *Proc Natl Acad Sci U S A* 2005;102:12543–12547.
389. McIntosh K. Coronaviruses: a comparative review. *Curr Top Microbiol Immunol* 1974;63:85–129.
400. Nagata N, Iwata N, Hasegawa H, et al. Mouse-passaged severe acute respiratory syndrome-associated coronavirus leads to lethal pulmonary edema and diffuse alveolar damage in adult but not young mice. *Am J Pathol* 2008;172:1625–1637.
406. Narayanan K, Chen CJ, Maeda J, et al. Nucleocapsid-independent specific viral RNA packaging via viral envelope protein and viral RNA signal. *J Virol* 2003;77:2922–2927.
407. Narayanan K, Huang C, Makino S. Coronavirus accessory proteins. In: Perlman S, Gallagher T, Snijder EJ, eds. *Nidoviruses.* Washington, DC: ASM Press; 2008:235–244.
413. Neuman BW, Adair BD, Yoshioka C, et al. Supramolecular architecture of severe acute respiratory syndrome coronavirus revealed by electron cryomicroscopy. *J Virol* 2006;80:7918–7928.
414. Neuman BW, Joseph JS, Saikatendu KS, et al. Proteomics analysis unravels the functional repertoire of coronavirus nonstructural protein 3. *J Virol* 2008;82:5279–5294.
415. Neuman BW, Kiss G, Kunding AH, et al. A structural analysis of M protein in coronavirus assembly and morphology. *J Struct Biol* 2011;174:11–22.
417. Nicholls JM, Butany J, Poon LL, et al. Time course and cellular localization of SARS-CoV nucleoprotein and RNA in lungs from fatal cases of SARS. *PLoS Med* 2006;3:e27.
426. Opstelten DJ, Raamsman MJ, Wolfs K, et al. Envelope glycoprotein interactions in coronavirus assembly. *J Cell Biol* 1995;131:339–349.
432. Parra B, Hinton D, Marten N, et al. IFN-gamma is required for viral clearance from central nervous system oligodendroglia. *J Immunol* 1999;162:1641–1647.
434. Pasternak AO, van den Born E, Spaan WJ, et al. Sequence requirements for RNA strand transfer during nidovirus discontinuous subgenomic RNA synthesis. *EMBO J* 2001;20:7220–7228.
437. Peiris JS, Chu CM, Cheng VC, et al. Clinical progression and viral load in a community outbreak of coronavirus-associated SARS pneumonia: a prospective study. *Lancet* 2003;361:1767–1772.
438. Peiris JS, Guan Y, Yuen KY. Severe acute respiratory syndrome. *Nat Med* 2004;10:S88–S97.
439. Peiris JS, Lai ST, Poon LL, et al. Coronavirus as a possible cause of severe acute respiratory syndrome. *Lancet* 2003;361:1319–1325.
440. Peiris JS, Yuen KY, Osterhaus AD, et al. The severe acute respiratory syndrome. *N Engl J Med* 2003;349:2431–2441.
443. Peng G, Sun D, Rajashankar KR, et al. Crystal structure of mouse coronavirus receptor-binding domain complexed with its murine receptor. *Proc Natl Acad Sci U S A* 2011;108:10696–10701.
448. Perlman S, Dandekar AA. Immunopathogenesis of coronavirus infections: implications for SARS. *Nat Rev Immunol* 2005;5:917–927.
451. Pewe L, Wu G, Barnett EM, et al. Cytotoxic T cell-resistant variants are selected in a virus-induced demyelinating disease. *Immunity* 1996;5:253–262.
453. Phillips JJ, Chua MM, Lavi E, et al. Pathogenesis of chimeric MHV4/MHV-A59 recombinant viruses: the murine coronavirus spike protein is a major determinant of neurovirulence. *J Virol* 1999;73:7752–7760.
456. Plant EP, Pérez-Alvarado GC, Jacobs JL, et al. A three-stemmed mRNA pseudoknot in the SARS coronavirus frameshift signal. *PLoS Biol* 2005;3:e172.
460. Pyrc K, Berkhout B, van der Hoek L. The novel human coronaviruses NL63 and HKU1. *J Virol* 2007;81:3051–3057.
461. Pyrc K, Dijkman R, Deng L, et al. Mosaic structure of human coronavirus NL63, one thousand years of evolution. *J Mol Biol* 2006;364:964–973.

463. Pyrc K, Sims AC, Dijkman R, et al. Culturing the unculturable: human coronavirus HKU1 infects, replicates, and produces progeny virions in human ciliated airway epithelial cell cultures. *J Virol* 2010;84:11255–11263.
468. Ratia K, Pegan S, Takayama J, et al. A noncovalent class of papain-like protease/deubiquitinase inhibitors blocks SARS virus replication. *Proc Natl Acad Sci U S A* 2008;105:16119–16124.
475. Riley S, Fraser C, Donnelly CA, et al. Transmission dynamics of the etiological agent of SARS in Hong Kong: impact of public health interventions. *Science* 2003;300:1961–1966.
478. Roberts A, Deming D, Paddock CD, et al. A mouse-adapted SARS-coronavirus causes disease and mortality in BALB/c mice. *PLoS Pathog* 2007;3:e5.
484. Roth-Cross JK, Bender SJ, Weiss SR. Murine coronavirus mouse hepatitis virus is recognized by MDA5 and induces type I interferon in brain macrophages/microglia. *J Virol* 2008;82:9829–9838.
488. Rottier PJ, Nakamura K, Schellen P, et al. Acquisition of macrophage tropism during the pathogenesis of feline infectious peritonitis is determined by mutations in the feline coronavirus spike protein. *J Virol* 2005;79:14122–14130.
490. Rottier PJ, Welling GW, Welling-Wester S, et al. Predicted membrane topology of the coronavirus protein E1. *Biochemistry* 1986;25:1335–1339.
491. Ruch TR, Machamer CE. The hydrophobic domain of infectious bronchitis virus E protein alters the host secretory pathway and is important for release of infectious virus. *J Virol* 2011;85:675–685.
492. Saif LJ. Animal coronavirus vaccines: lessons for SARS. *Dev Biol (Basel)* 2004;119:129–140.
497. Sawicki SG, Sawicki DL. Coronavirus transcription: subgenomic mouse hepatitis virus replicative intermediates function in RNA synthesis. *J Virol* 1990;64:1050–1056.
498. Sawicki SG, Sawicki DL, Siddell SG. A contemporary view of coronavirus transcription. *J Virol* 2007;81:20–29.
499. Sawicki SG, Sawicki DL, Younker D, et al. Functional and genetic analysis of coronavirus replicase-transcriptase proteins. *PLoS Pathog* 2005; 1(4):e39.
505. Schütze H, Ulferts R, Schelle B, et al. Characterization of white bream virus reveals a novel genetic cluster of nidoviruses. *J Virol* 2006;80: 11598–11609.
509. Sethna PB, Hung SL, Brian DA. Coronavirus subgenomic minus-strand RNAs and the potential for mRNA replicons. *Proc Natl Acad Sci U S A* 1989;86:5626–5630.
514. Shulla A, Heald-Sargent T, Subramanya G, et al. A transmembrane serine protease is linked to the severe acute respiratory syndrome coronavirus receptor and activates virus entry. *J Virol* 2011;85:873–882.
518. Siu KL, Kok KH, Ng MH, et al. Severe acute respiratory syndrome coronavirus M protein inhibits type I interferon production by impeding the formation of TRAF3.TANK.TBK1/IKKepsilon complex. *J Biol Chem* 2009;284:16202–16209.
519. Siu YL, Teoh KT, Lo J, et al. The M, E, and N structural proteins of the severe acute respiratory syndrome coronavirus are required for efficient assembly, trafficking, and release of virus-like particles. *J Virol* 2008;82: 11318–11330.
521. Snijder EJ, Bredenbeek PJ, Dobbe JC, et al. Unique and conserved features of genome and proteome of SARS-coronavirus, an early split-off from the coronavirus group 2 lineage. *J Mol Biol* 2003;331:991–1004.
523. Snijder EJ, Horzinek MC. Toroviruses: replication, evolution and comparison with other members of the coronavirus-like superfamily. *J Gen Virol* 1993;74:2305–2316.
533. Spiegel M, Schneider K, Weber F, et al. Interaction of severe acute respiratory syndrome-associated coronavirus with dendritic cells. *J Gen Virol* 2006;87:1953–1960.
538. Stockman LJ, Bellamy R, Garner P. SARS: systematic review of treatment effects. *PLoS Med* 2006;3:e343.
546. Sturman LS, Holmes KV, Behnke J. Isolation of coronavirus envelope glycoproteins and interaction with the viral nucleocapsid. *J Virol* 1980; 33:449–462.
549. Subbarao K, Roberts A. Is there an ideal animal model for SARS? *Trends Microbiol* 2006;14:299–303.
561. Thiel V, Herold J, Schelle B, et al. Infectious RNA transcribed in vitro from a cDNA copy of the human coronavirus genome cloned in vaccinia virus. *J Gen Virol* 2001;82:1273–1281.
565. Trandem K, Anghelina D, Zhao J, et al. Regulatory T cells inhibit T cell proliferation and decrease demyelination in mice chronically infected with a coronavirus. *J Immunol* 2010;184:4391–4400.
566. Trandem K, Zhao J, Fleming E, et al. Highly activated cytotoxic CD8 T cells express protective IL-10 at the peak of coronavirus-induced encephalitis. *J Immunol* 2011;186:3642–3652.
573. Van der Hoek L, Pyrc K, Jebbink MF, et al. Identification of a new human coronavirus. *Nat Med* 2004;10:368–373.
574. Van der Hoek L, Sure K, Ihorst G, et al. Croup is associated with the novel coronavirus NL63. *PLoS Med* 2005;2:e240.
578. Van Hemert MJ, van den Worm SH, Knoops K, et al. SARS-coronavirus replication/transcription complexes are membrane-protected and need a host factor for activity in vitro. *PLoS Pathog* 2008;4:e1000054.
581. Vennema H, de Groot RJ, Harbour DA, et al. Early death after feline infectious peritonitis virus challenge due to recombinant vaccinia virus immunization. *J Virol* 1990;64:1407–1409.
582. Vennema H, Godeke GJ, Rossen JW, et al. Nucleocapsid-independent assembly of coronavirus-like particles by co-expression of viral envelope protein genes. *EMBO J* 1996;15:2020–2028.
586. Versteeg GA, Bredenbeek PJ, van den Worm SH, et al. Group 2 coronaviruses prevent immediate early interferon induction by protection of viral RNA from host cell recognition. *Virology* 2007;361:18–26.
588. Vijgen L, Keyaerts E, Lemey P, et al. Evolutionary history of the closely related group 2 coronaviruses: porcine hemagglutinating encephalomyelitis virus, bovine coronavirus, and human coronavirus OC43. *J Virol* 2006;80:7270–7274.
591. Vlasak R, Luytjes W, Spaan W, et al. Human and bovine coronaviruses recognize sialic acid-containing receptors similar to those of influenza C viruses. *Proc Natl Acad Sci U S A* 1988;85:4526–4529.
594. Wang F-I, Hinton D, Gilmore D, et al. Sequential infection of glial cells by the murine hepatitis virus JHM strain (MHV-4) leads to a characteristic distribution of demyelination. *Lab Invest* 1992;66:744–754.
598. Wathelet MG, Orr M, Frieman MB, et al. Severe acute respiratory syndrome coronavirus evades antiviral signaling: role of nsp1 and rational design of an attenuated strain. *J Virol* 2007;81:11620–11633.
600. Weiner LP. Pathogenesis of demyelination induced by a mouse hepatitis virus (JHM virus). *Arch Neurol* 1973;28:298–303.
602. Weiss SR, Navas-Martin S. Coronavirus pathogenesis and the emerging pathogen severe acute respiratory syndrome coronavirus. *Microbiol Mol Biol Rev* 2005;69:635–664.
605. Williams GD, Chang RY, Brian DA. A phylogenetically conserved hairpin-type 3′ untranslated region pseudoknot functions in coronavirus RNA replication. *J Virol* 1999;73:8349–8355.
606. Williams RK, Jiang G, Holmes KV. Receptor for mouse hepatitis virus is a member of the carcinoembryonic antigen family of glycoproteins. *Proc Natl Acad Sci U S A* 1991;88:5533–5536.
615. Woo PCW, Lau SKP, Chu C-M, et al. Characterization and complete genome sequence of a novel coronavirus, coronavirus HKU1, from patients with pneumonia. *J Virol* 2005;79:884–895.
616. Woo PCW, Lau SKP, Huang Y, et al. Coronavirus diversity, phylogeny and interspecies jumping. *Exp Biol Med* 2009;234:1117–1127.
620. Wu GF, Dandekar AA, Pewe L, et al. CD4 and CD8 T cells have redundant but not identical roles in virus-induced demyelination. *J Immunol* 2000;165:2278–2286.
624. Wu K, Li W, Peng G, et al. Crystal structure of NL63 respiratory coronavirus receptor-binding domain complexed with its human receptor. *Proc Natl Acad Sci U S A* 2009;106:19970–19974.
639. Yeager CL, Ashmun RA, Williams RK, et al. Human aminopeptidase N is a receptor for human coronavirus 229E. *Nature* 1992;357: 420–422.
642. Yount B, Curtis KM, Baric RS. Strategy for systematic assembly of large RNA and DNA genomes: transmissible gastroenteritis virus model. *J Virol* 2000;74:10600–10611.
643. Yount B, Curtis KM, Fritz EA, et al. Reverse genetics with a full-length infectious cDNA of severe acute respiratory syndrome coronavirus. *Proc Natl Acad Sci U S A* 2003;100:12995–13000.
644. Yount B, Roberts RS, Lindesmith L, et al. Rewiring the severe acute respiratory syndrome coronavirus (SARS-CoV) transcription circuit: engineering a recombination-resistant genome. *Proc Natl Acad Sci U S A* 2006;103:12546–12551.

650. Zeng Q, Langereis MA, van Vliet AL, et al. Structure of coronavirus hemagglutinin-esterase offers insight into corona and influenza virus evolution. *Proc Natl Acad Sci U S A* 2008;105:9065–9069.
651. Zhai Y, Sun F, Li X, et al. Insights into SARS-CoV transcription and replication from the structure of the nsp7-nsp8 hexadecamer. *Nat Struct Mol Biol* 2005;12:980–986.
653. Zhao J, Zhao J, Van Rooijen N, et al. Evasion by stealth: inefficient immune activation underlies poor T cell response and severe disease in SARS-CoV-infected mice. *PLoS Pathog* 2009;5:e1000636.
656. Zhou H, Perlman S. Mouse hepatitis virus does not induce Beta interferon synthesis and does not inhibit its induction by double-stranded RNA. *J Virol* 2007;81:568–574.
660. Ziebuhr J. Coronavirus replicative proteins. In: Perlman S, Gallagher T, Snijder EJ, eds. *Nidoviruses.* Washington, DC: ASM Press; 2008:65–81.
661. Ziebuhr J, Snijder EJ, Gorbalenya AE. Virus-encoded proteinases and proteolytic processing in the Nidovirales. *J Gen Virol* 2000;81:853–879.
664. Zúñiga S, Sola I, Alonso S, et al. Sequence motifs involved in the regulation of discontinuous coronavirus subgenomic RNA synthesis. *J Virol* 2004;78:980–994.
665. Züst RL, Cervantes-Barragan L, Habjan M, et al. Ribose 2′-O-methylation provides a molecular signature for the distinction of self and non-self mRNA dependent on the RNA sensor Mda5. *Nat Immunol* 2011;12:137–143.
666. Züst RL, Cervantes-Barragan L, Kuri T, et al. Coronavirus non-structural protein 1 is a major pathogenicity factor: implications for the rational design of coronavirus vaccines. *PLoS Pathog* 2007;3:e109.
667. Züst R, Miller TB, Goebel SJ, et al. Genetic interactions between an essential 3′ cis-acting RNA pseudoknot, replicase gene products, and the extreme 3′ end of the mouse coronavirus genome. *J Virol* 2008;82:1214–1228.

CHAPTER 29

Eric J. Snijder • Marjolein Kikkert

Arteriviruses

HISTORY AND CLASSIFICATION OF ARTERIVIRUSES

The family *Arteriviridae*[68] was established in 1996 and currently comprises the following four enveloped, plus-stranded RNA viruses: equine arteritis virus (EAV), lactate dehydrogenase-elevating virus (LDV) of mice, porcine reproductive and respiratory syndrome virus (PRRSV), and simian hemorrhagic fever virus (SHFV). Three of these (EAV, LDV, and SHFV) were first isolated and characterized about 50 years ago.[62,161,189] The porcine arterivirus PRRSV emerged only about 20 years ago,[36,227] causing vast epidemics of a previously unknown reproductive and respiratory disease in swine in both Europe (genotype I) and North America (genotype II). Remarkably, the subsequent molecular characterization of PRRSV strains from both continents revealed considerable genetic differences, suggesting that the two PRRSV genotypes evolved separately and are only distantly related to a common ancestor.[152,170] PRRSV infection can cause high-mortality disease outbreaks and has developed into the most prevalent disease of swine worldwide. Recently, a large outbreak of highly virulent PRRSV affected the Asian pig industry, causing enormous economic losses.[194,246]

In general, the consequences of arterivirus infection can range from an asymptomatic, persistent or acute infection to abortion or lethal hemorrhagic fever.[199,226] EAV is capable of inducing a variety of symptoms, including necrosis of the small muscular arteries from which the name of the family prototype EAV was derived. The name of the mouse arterivirus LDV is derived from the increase in the level of lactate dehydrogenase (LDH) caused by LDV infection.[161] The virus, which has been used extensively as an *in vivo* research model, is able to escape immune surveillance and establish a largely asymptomatic persistent infection.[22,155] SHFV was isolated from outbreaks of fatal hemorrhagic fever in macaque colonies[189] that were probably caused by inadvertent transmission by humans from African monkeys to macaques.

The unification of the previously unclassified arteriviruses was the direct result of the sequence analysis of their genomes, which revealed an intriguing relationship with coronaviruses and toroviruses (discussed in Chapter 28). Despite striking differences in genome size and virion structure, the genome organization and expression strategy of these viruses were found to be comparable and their replicase genes were postulated to share common ancestry[54] (e-Fig. 29.1). One of the most prominent features of their genome expression strategy, the generation of a nested set of subgenomic (sg) messenger RNAs (mRNAs), provided the basis for the name *Nidovirales*

(L. *nidus* = nest) that was given to the novel virus order comprising the arterivirus and coronavirus families in 1996. Subsequently, the order was further expanded with the invertebrate virus family *Roniviridae* and the genus *Bafinivirus*, which contains fish nidoviruses.[83] Most recently, the isolation of the first insect nidoviruses (proposed family name *Mesoniviridae*) was reported,[140,249] yet again expanding the exceptional host range of the order *Nidovirales*. Furthermore, on the basis of its partial genome sequence, a novel nidovirus isolated from Australian possums (wobbly possum disease virus) appears to represent yet another nidovirus lineage, which is relatively closely related to the *Arteriviridae*.[66a]

Nidoviruses represent a distinct lineage among plus-strand RNA viruses (e-Fig. 29.1). The complex evolutionary relationship between arteriviruses and nidoviruses with a much larger genome has been reviewed extensively elsewhere.[83] Related replicase genes and replication strategies have been combined with seemingly unrelated sets of structural protein genes. RNA recombination likely was an important factor in these evolutionary events and was also invoked to explain some internal rearrangements of arterivirus genomes.[52,81,103]

VIRION STRUCTURE

Arteriviruses have been observed as spherical particles, 50 to 60 nm in diameter, and possess a relatively smooth, mostly featureless surface, which is likely explained by the small ectodomains of the two major envelope proteins (Fig. 29.1; see[20,68,175,182] and references therein). The nucleocapsid structure has long been assumed to be isometric, but recent cryo-electron tomography studies of PRRSV revealed a rather pleomorphic and "disorganized" core structure (average diameter 39 nm). These findings are clearly incompatible with an icosahedral core and suggest a resemblance to the nucleocapsid structure proposed for coronaviruses, a helical coil, or an even more loosely organized filamentous structure[61,182]

The buoyant density of arteriviruses is 1.13 to 1.17 g/cm^3 in sucrose, and their sedimentation coefficient ranges from 214S to 230S. Virions are highly unstable in solutions containing low concentrations of nonionic detergents or at a pH other than 6.0 to 7.5, and quickly lose their infectivity when stored at temperatures higher than 4°C.

The arterivirus nucleocapsid structure (Fig. 29.2, e-Fig. 29.2) is composed of the 12.7 to 15.7 kb RNA genome and the nucleocapsid protein (N). The crystal structure for the capsid-forming C-terminal domain of PRRSV N[59]; e-Fig. 29.2B) suggested that it represents a new class of viral capsid–forming domains, a hypothesis further supported by cryo-EM studies.

Based on studies with EAV and PRRSV, the lipid bilayer that surrounds the nucleocapsid is now presumed to contain seven envelope proteins (Table 29.1, Fig. 29.2), an unusually large number compared to other plus-stranded RNA viruses. In this chapter, we refer to the glycoproteins as "GPx", where x indicates the number of the corresponding open reading frame

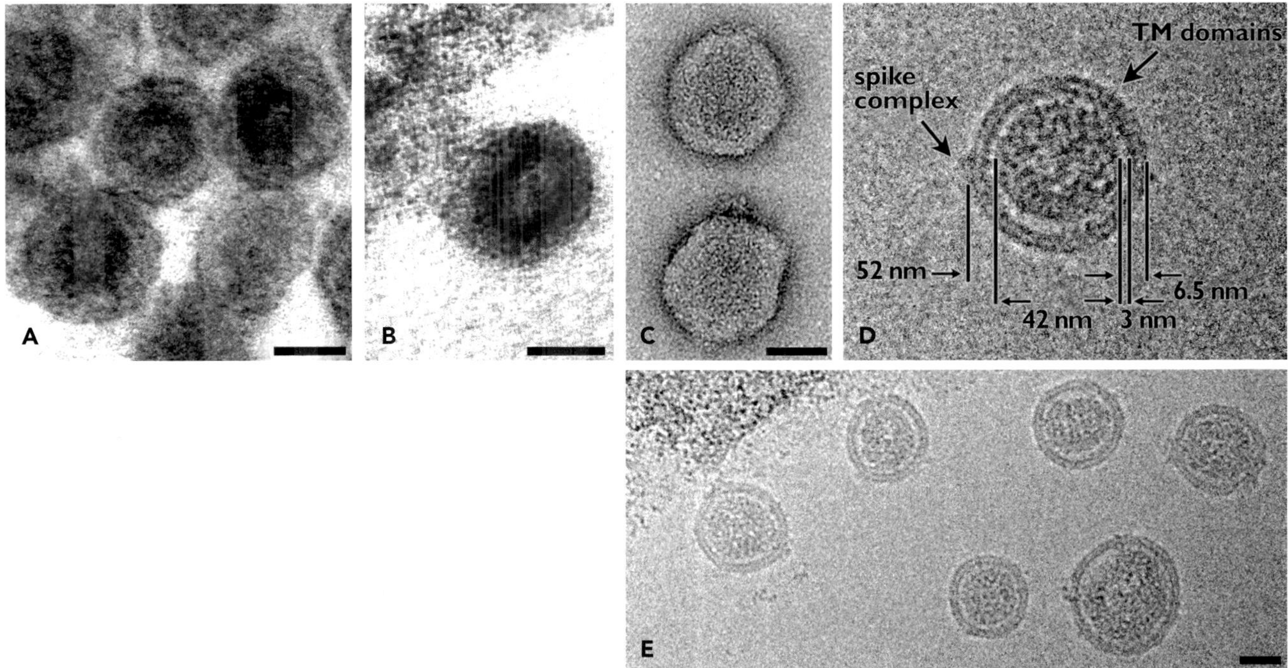

FIGURE 29.1. Electron micrographs of arterivirus particles. A: Transmission electron microscopic (EM) image of extracellular porcine reproductive and respiratory system virus (PRRSV) particles. **B:** Transmission EM image of an equine arteritis virus (EAV) particle budding from smooth intracellular membranes. **C:** Negatively stained, purified PRRSV particles. **D–E:** Cryo-EM of PRRSV particles in vitreous ice. **Panel D** shows a typical PRRSV particle with dimensions indicated. A possible spike protein complex and the striated appearance that most likely corresponds to the transmembrane domains of envelope proteins are visible. All bars are 25 nm. (A and B from Snijder EJ, Meulenberg JJM. The molecular biology of arteriviruses. *J GenVirol* 1998;79:961–979 with permission; **C–E** from Spilman MS, Welbon C, Nelson E, et al. Cryo-electron tomography of porcine reproductive and respiratory syndrome virus: organization of the nucleocapsid. *J GenVirol* 2009;90:527–535, with permission.)

TABLE 29.1 Molecular Properties of Arteriviruses

			Replicase proteins			Structural proteins[c]		
Virus[a]	**Host**	**Genome size (kb)**	**ORF**	**Size (aa)**	**Nsps**[b]	**ORF**	**Protein name**[d]	**Size (aa)**
EAV	Horse	12.7	1a	1,727	9	2a	E	67
	Donkey		1ab	3,175	13	2b	GP2 (GP2b/G_S)	227
						3	GP3	163
						4	GP4	152
						5	GP5 (G_L)	255
						5a	ORF5a protein	59
						6	M	162
						7	N	110
LDV	Mouse	14.1	1a	2,206	10	2a	E	70
			1ab	3,616	14	2b	GP2 (VP3-M)	227
						3	GP3	191
						4	GP4	175
						5	GP5 (VP3-P)	199
						5a	ORF5a protein	47
						6	M (VP2)	171
						7	N (VP1)	115
PRRSV	Pig	15.1	1a	2,397	10	2a	GP2 (GP2a)	249
			1ab	3,854	14	2b	E	70
						3	GP3	265
						4	GP4	183
						5	GP5	201
						5a	ORF5a protein	43
						6	M	173
						7	N	128
SHFV	Monkey	15.7	1a	2,105	10?	2a′	ORF2a′ protein	281
			1ab	3,594	14?	2b′	ORF2b′ protein	94
						3′	ORF3′ protein	204
						4′	ORF4′ protein	205
						2a	E	80
						2b	GP2 (GP2b)	214
						3	GP3	179
						4	GP4	182
						5	GP5	278
						5a	ORF5a protein	64
						6	M	162
						7	N	111

ORF, open reading frame; EAV, equine arteritis virus; aa, amino acid; GP, glycoprotein; nsp, nonstructural protein; LDV, lactate dehydrogenase-elevating virus; PRRSV, porcine reproductive and respiratory syndrome virus; SHFV, simian hemorrhagic fever virus.

[a]Molecular characteristics were based on the sequences of the EAV-Bucyrus (European Molecular Biology Laboratory (EMBL) database accession number NC_002532), PRRSV-Lelystad (accession number M96262), LDV-P (accession number U15146), and the SHFV-LVR (accession number NC_003092).

[b]Numbers of nsps are based on the known (EAV) or predicted (LDV/PRRSV/SHFV) replicase processing schemes as depicted in Figure 29.3 and e-Figure 29.6. Nsp8 is identical to the N-terminal domain of nsp9.

[c]Not all proteins listed here have been identified in all four arterivirus particles.

[d]Alternative names used in other (older) publications are indicated in brackets; SHFV protein nomenclature has been adapted with the most recent recommendations of the *Arteriviridae* study group of the International Committee on Taxonomy of Viruses (ICTV).[68]

(ORF) in the genome (Table 29.1, Figs. 29.2 and 29.3). For simplicity, the GP encoded by ORF2a (PRRSV) or ORF2b (EAV/LDV) will be called GP2. Among arterivirus envelope proteins two major and five minor species are discriminated. The two major species, the nonglycosylated triple-spanning membrane protein M and GP5, form a disulfide-linked hetero dimer[57,69,174] (Fig. 29.2). By separately knocking out the expression of each of the structural proteins, it was established that all major and minor structural proteins are required for the production of infectious progeny,[131,232] with the possible exception of the recently discovered ORF5a protein.[75,94]

Studies of GP2, GP3, and GP4, which form a heterotrimer in the virion[230,232] (Fig. 29.2), have further highlighted their importance. Knockout mutants for minor structural protein genes produced noninfectious subviral particles consisting of GP5, M, N, and the genome RNA.[231,232,243] When one of the

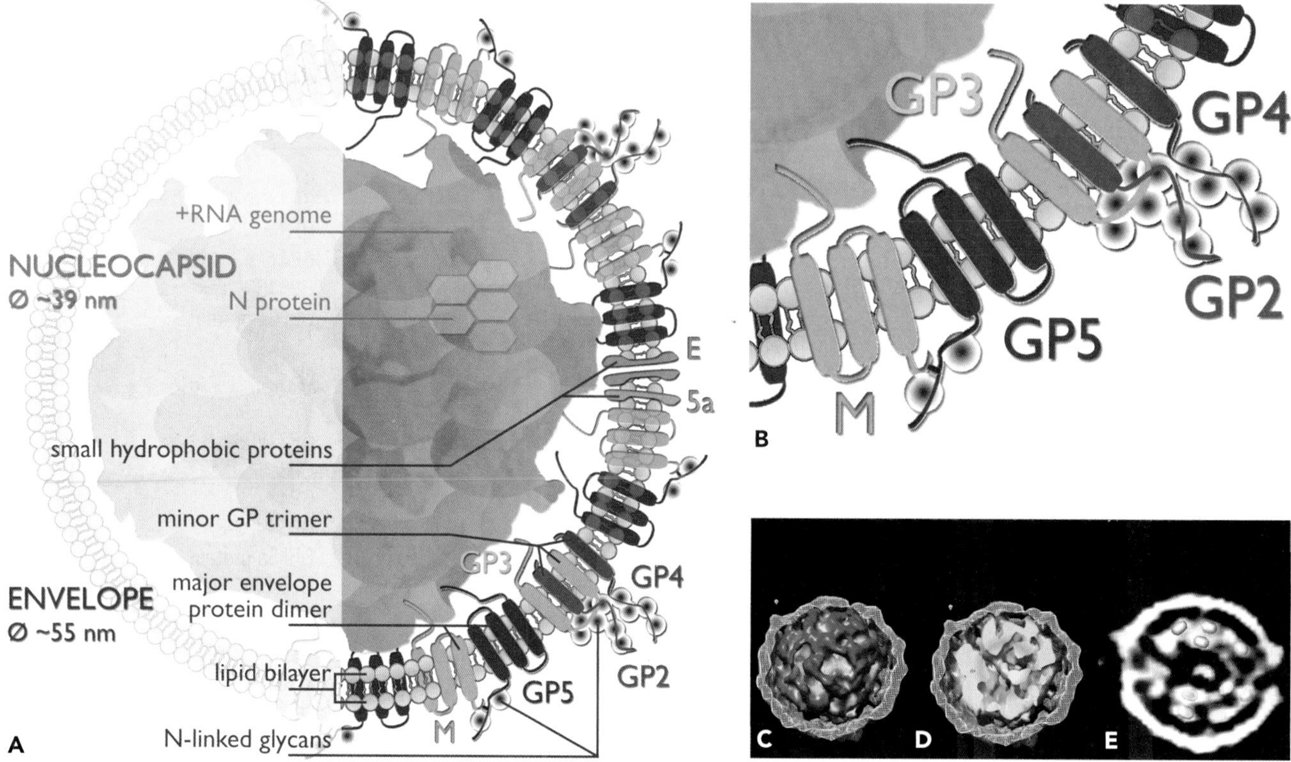

FIGURE 29.2. Arterivirus structure. A: The presumed location and topology of the envelope proteins GP2 to GP5, E, and M, the recently identified open reading frame (ORF)5a protein, and the N protein are shown (see also Table 29.1 and Fig. 29.3). The major envelope proteins GP5 and M form a disulfide-linked heterodimer. The minor glycoproteins GP2, GP3, and GP4 form a disulfide-linked heterotrimer. Seen **Panel B** for a close-up. In addition, also GP_2-GP_4 dimers (not depicted) have been identified in equine arteritis virus (EAV) particles. It should be noticed that not all proteins depicted here have been identified in all four arterivirus particles. **C–E:** Cryo-electron microscopy–based tomographic reconstruction of a porcine reproductive and respiratory syndrome virus (PRRSV) particle,[182] revealing that the virion core is not solid, but consists of a two-layered shell that surrounds a hollow central cavity. **C:** Cutaway view of the internal core, obtained by peeling away the envelope (shown in mesh representation). The core, which is separated from the envelope by a 3-nm gap, appears disorganized and to consist of density strands that are bundled together into a ball. The data suggest a model for the core in which two layers of N dimers form a linked chain (see also **Panel E**). The core is shown as an isosurface, colored by the radius from the center of the particle (from red to blue). **D:** The core has been cut open to show the internal structure, including the central density (red-orange) typically seen in the tomograms. **E:** A 6.3-nm thick slab through the center of one PRRSV particle tomogram, with several copies of the crystal structure of the dimeric C-terminal domain of N, rendered at a comparable resolution and superimposed on the oblong densities in the core. (See also e-Fig. 29.2). (**C–E** from Spilman MS, Welbon C, Nelson E, et al. Cryo-electron tomography of porcine reproductive and respiratory syndrome virus: organization of the nucleocapsid. *J GenVirol* 2009;90:527–535, with permission.)

components of the GP2-GP3-GP4 trimer or the small non-glycosylated envelope protein (E)[176] was lacking, the incorporation of the three minor GPs into virions was blocked.[231] Taken together, these data indicate that the basic protein scaffold of the arterivirus particle consists of the three major structural polypeptides, N, M, and GP5. Whether the incorporation of (genome) RNA is essential for the formation of the nucleocapsid structure, and which RNA sequences/structures specifically interact with N, remains to be established.

GENOME STRUCTURE AND ORGANIZATION

The arterivirus genome is a plus-stranded, 3′-polyadenylated RNA molecule, likely containing a cap structure at its 5′ end.[165] Full-length genomic sequences (see also Table 29.1) have been obtained for European and North American isolates of EAV, a large number of European, North American, and Asian PRRSV isolates, two LDV strains, and three SHFV isolates. The arterivirus replicase gene consists of the large ORFs 1a and 1b and roughly occupies the 5′ three-fourths of the polycistronic genome (Fig. 29.3). In contrast to the more conserved ORF1b region, the size of ORF1a is variable (encoding between 1,727 [EAV] and about 2,500 amino acids [PRRSV]), which largely explains the genome size differences encountered among arteriviruses. The region downstream of the replicase gene contains 8 to 11 relatively small genes, most of which have both 5′- and 3′-terminal sequences that overlap with neighboring genes. These genes encode mostly (or exclusively) structural proteins and are translated from sg mRNAs (see below). Their organization is

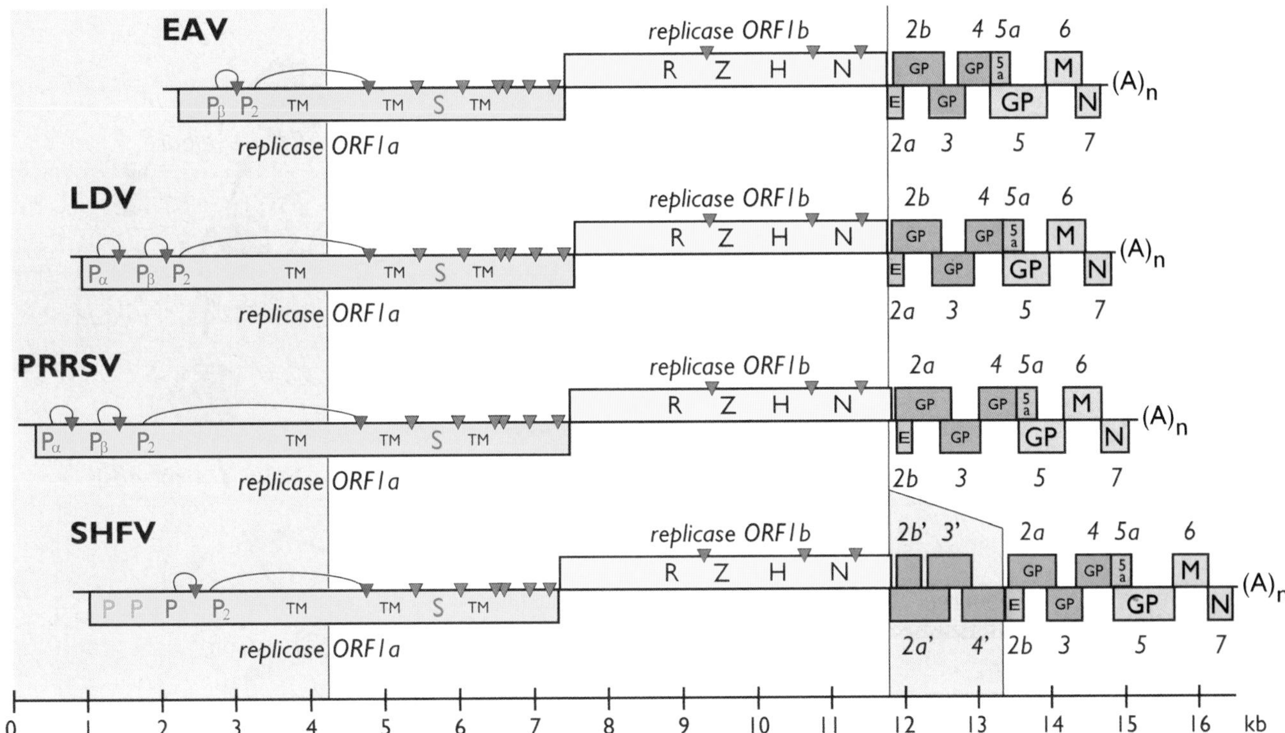

FIGURE 29.3. Arterivirus genome organization. The family prototype equine arteritis virus (EAV) is shown at the **top**. The replicase open reading frames (ORFs) 1a and 1b are followed by the gene encoding the E protein, three genes (ORFs 2a/b-4) encoding minor glycoproteins, the recently discovered ORF5a (presumably encoding a minor envelope protein), and the genes for the three major structural proteins GP5, M, and N (blue). The 3′-proximal region of the simian hemorrhagic fever virus (SHFV) genome carries a large insertion (highlighted in grey), containing four ORFs that may encode additional virion proteins. In the replicase ORFs, the positions corresponding to known or predicted cleavage sites in the encoded polyproteins is depicted. *Red arrowheads* represent sites cleaved by the nsp4 serine proteinase (S), the viral main protease. The papain-like proteinase domains (P) in the quite variable nsp1-nsp2 region and their (predicted) cleavage sites (*blue*) are also shown. The processing scheme of the SHFV nsp1 region remains to be elucidated. The three (putative) transmembrane domains (TM) in the ORF1a-encoded polyprotein are indicated (residing in nsp2, nsp3, nsp5). In ORF1b, the domains encoding the four most conserved nidovirus replicase domains are depicted: the RNA-dependent RNA polymerase (R), (putative) multinuclear zinc-binding domain (Z), RNA helicase (H), and the NendoU endoribonuclease domain (N).

generally well conserved in the arterivirus genome. An exception is the region downstream of the SHFV replicase gene, which contains four additional ORFs, comprising about 1.6 kb, which may have arisen from the duplication of ORFs 2a to 4.[68,81]

THE ARTERIVIRUS REPLICATION CYCLE

Attachment and Entry

The entry of PRRSV and EAV requires a low pH, suggesting that it occurs via the standard endocytic route[101,137,141] (Fig. 29.4). Clathrin heavy-chain knockdown suppressed EAV infection[141] and electron microscopy revealed arterivirus particles contained in relatively small vesicles that appeared to be clathrin coated.[100,101]

The host factors required for arterivirus entry have been studied in detail only for PRRSV (e-Fig. 29.3). Several viral and cellular players have been implicated in binding, entry, and uncoating, although their exact roles remain to be defined in more detail (for recent reviews see 203,224). Sialoadhesin (or sialic acid-binding immunoglobulin [Ig]-like lectin 1 [CD169]; 216), a macrophage-restricted membrane protein, mediates the internalization of the virus by porcine alveolar macrophages (PAMs), the primary target cells of PRRSV.[64,66] In addition, glycosaminoglycans (heparan sulfate) on the cell surface[51] and sialic acids on the virion surface[50] were implicated in the initial binding step. It is believed that the virus initially binds heparin-like molecules on the cell surface and that subsequently internalization via clathrin-mediated endocytosis is triggered by the interaction of CD169 with sialic acids on the ectodomains of the GP5/M dimer.[204] Expression of porcine CD169 in nonsusceptible cell lines can mediate PRRSV internalization, but not disassembly and productive infection,[216] indicating that additional factors must be required for successful infection. This notion is further supported by the fact that MARC-145 cells, which are commonly used to grow PRRSV, do not express CD169 on their surface.[64] In particular CD163, a member of the scavenger receptor cysteine-rich (SRCR) family, was implicated in the early stages of PRRSV infection.[26] Although normally a macrophage-specific antigen, CD163 is aberrantly expressed on MARC-145 cells, possibly explaining their unique susceptibility to PRRSV infection among nonengineered cell lines. Expression of CD163 from various species rendered a variety of nonpermissive cell lines susceptible to PRRSV infection, in the

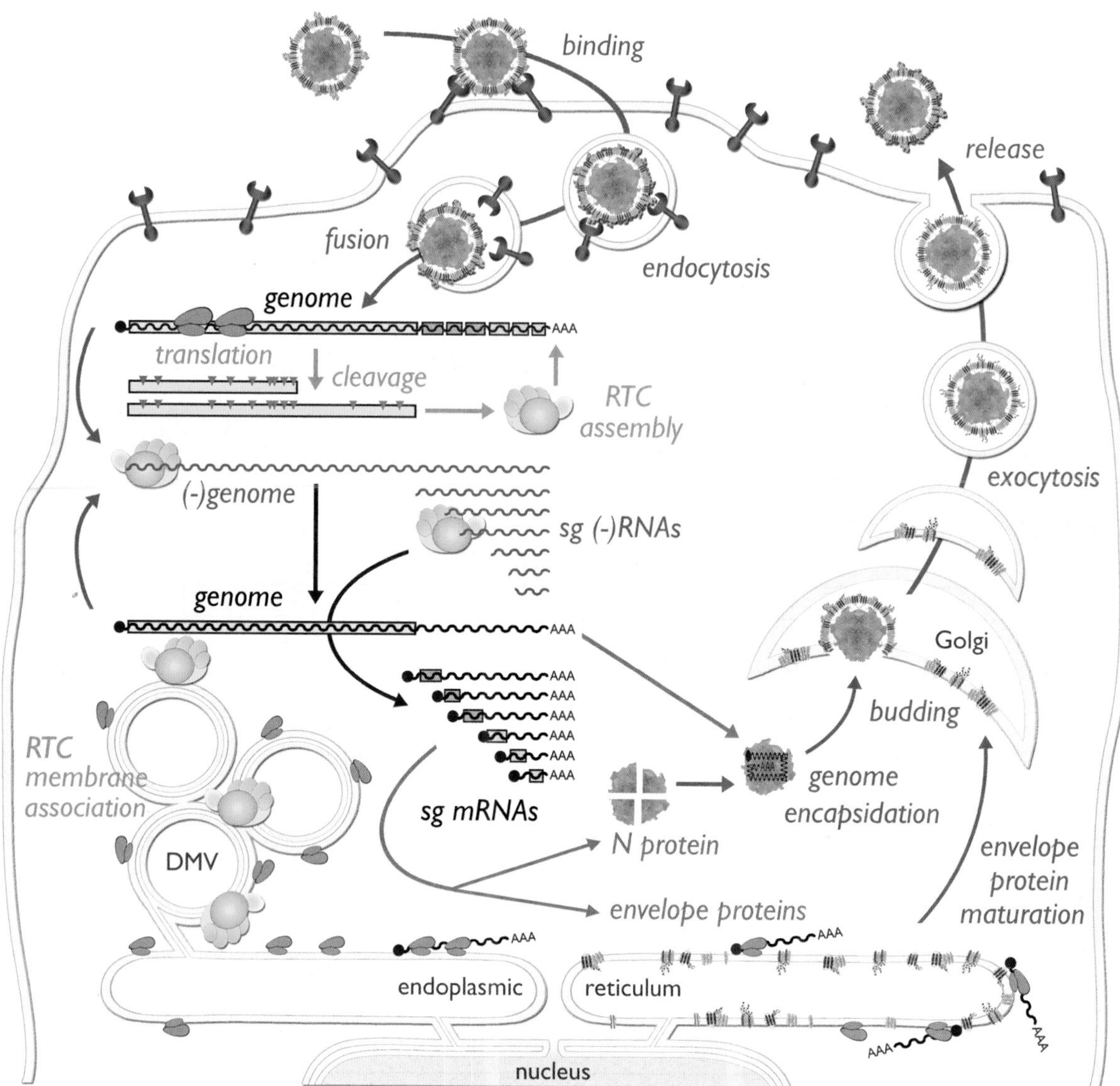

FIGURE 29.4. Overview of arterivirus replication. Following entry by receptor-mediated endocytosis and release of the genome into the cytosol, genome translation yields the pp1a and pp1ab replicase polyproteins (shown as *yellow bars*). Following polyprotein cleavage by multiple internal proteases, the viral nonstructural proteins assemble into a replication and transcription complex (RTC) that engages in minus-strand RNA synthesis. Both full-length and subgenome-length minus strands are produced, with the latter templating the synthesis of subgenomic messenger RNAs (mRNAs) required to express the structural protein genes in the 3′-proximal quarter of the genome. Ultimately, novel genomes are packaged into nucleocapsids that become enveloped by budding from smooth intracellular membranes, after which the new virions leave the cell by following the exocytic pathway. (See text for more details.)

absence of detectable CD169 expression. It was postulated that in PAM, CD169 and CD163 work together, with the former serving as receptor for internalization and the latter playing a key role in virus uncoating and genome release, which are thought to occur in association with the early endosome, following its acidification[211] (e-Fig. 29.3).

Which virion proteins direct the fusion between viral envelope and endosomal membrane remains one of the key questions to be addressed. A role for the minor glycoproteins in arterivirus receptor recognition and tropism has not been rigorously excluded.[44] In fact, recent data show that a chimeric PRRSV carrying E, GP2, GP3, and GP4 of EAV acquired the broad tropism for cultured cells that is typical of the latter virus.[193] These findings are in line with the previously observed phenotypes of recombinant viruses in which the GP5 or M ectodomain was replaced, which did not result in an altered tropism in cell culture.[60,219] These studies, together with the identification of several other host factors as potential “PRRSV entry mediators”,[203,224] illustrate that several questions and controversies regarding arterivirus entry remain to be addressed.

Genome Translation and Replication

The arterivirus replication cycle (Fig. 29.4) is presumed to be entirely cytoplasmic, despite the fact that at least two viral proteins are (in part) targeted to the nucleus (see below). The incoming genome is translated into the two large replicase polyproteins pp1a (1,727 to 2,502 amino acids) and pp1ab (3,175 to 3,959 amino acids), which comprise all functions required for viral RNA synthesis.[131] Despite the relatively large 5′ nontranslated region (NTR), translation presumably initiates following "conventional" ribosomal scanning of the genomic 5′ NTR.[206] ORF1b translation requires a -1 ribosomal frame shift (estimated efficiency of 15% to 20%) just before ORF1a translation is terminated[54] (Fig. 29.3). The ORF1a/1b overlap region contains two signals that are assumed to promote this event: a so-called "slippery" sequence, which is the actual ribosomal frame shift site, and a downstream RNA pseudoknot structure.

Following proteolytic processing of the replicase polyproteins, a complex for viral RNA synthesis is formed that generates a genome-length minus strand (or "anti-genome"), the template for genome replication. In addition, a complex transcription mechanism operates to produce complementary nested sets of sg-length minus-strand RNAs and sg mRNAs[55] (see below and Fig. 29.5). The RNA signals involved in arterivirus genome replication remain to be studied in detail. The coding regions of the genomes are flanked by 5′ and 3′ NTRs of 156 to 221 and 59 to 117 nucleotides, respectively. However, natural and synthetic defective interfering RNAs of EAV invariably require at least 300 nucleotides from both genome termini for efficient replication, indicating that replication signals extend into the coding sequences.[130,198] Likewise, in the case of PRRSV, a so-called "kissing interaction" between the loop sequences of RNA hairpin structures in the 3′ NTR and the N protein gene was found to be crucial for viral RNA synthesis.[218]

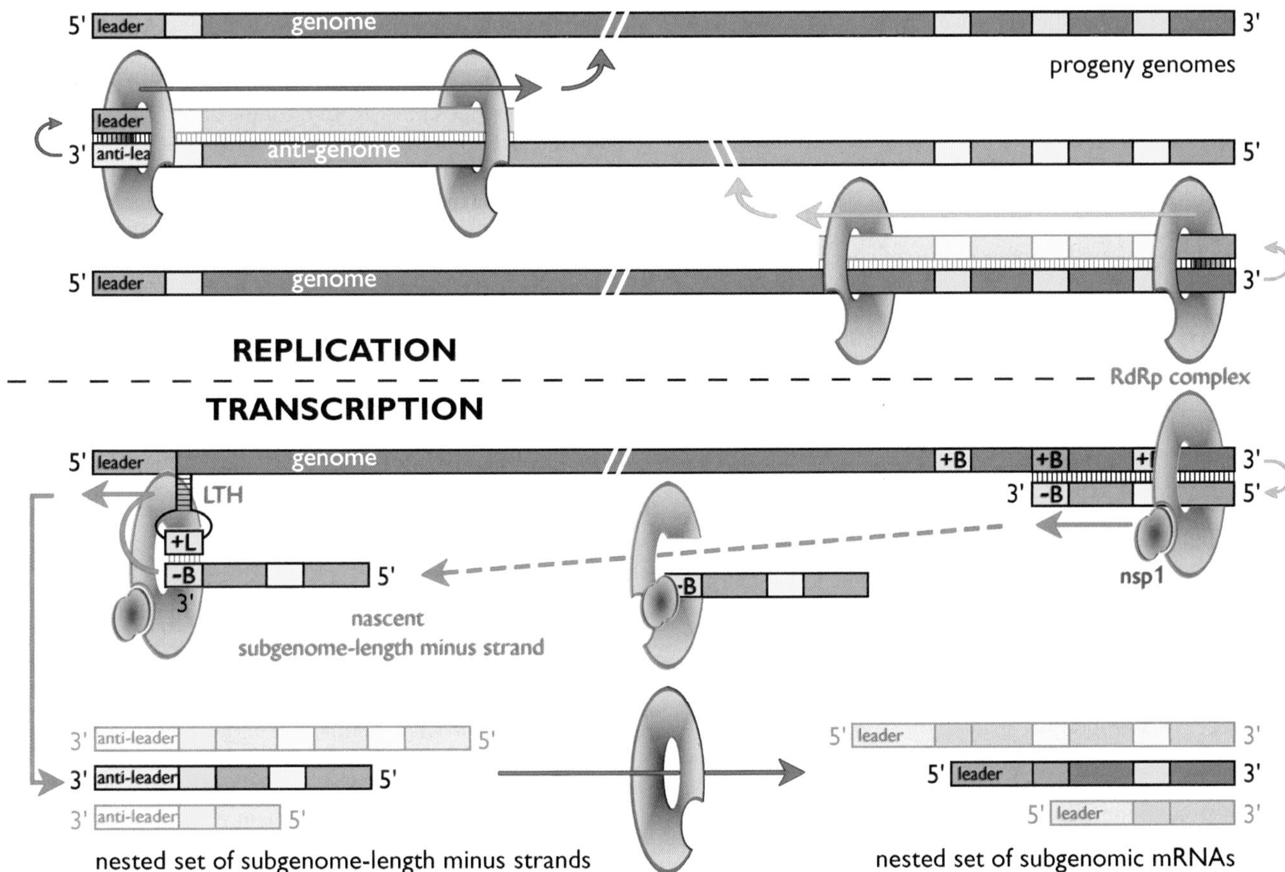

FIGURE 29.5. Arterivirus RNA synthesis. Model for arterivirus (and coronavirus) replication and transcription[146,166–167,168] using a hypothetical arterivirus genome encoding three subgenomic messenger RNAs (mRNAs). The top half of the scheme depicts the replication of the genome by the viral RNA-dependent RNA polymerase (RdRp) complex, which requires a full-length minus-strand intermediate (anti-genome). The bottom half illustrates how minus-strand RNA synthesis can be interrupted at a body transcription-regulating sequence (TRS) (+B), after which the nascent minus strand, having a body TRS complement (-B) at its 3′ end, is redirected to the leader TRS (+L) near the 5′-end of the genome. This +L sequence is thought to be "presented" for base pairing by a viral RNA structure, the leader TRS hairpin (LTH), that is critical for subgenomic RNA synthesis. Guided by a base-pairing interaction between the complementary –B and +L sequences, RNA synthesis is resumed to add the complement of the genomic leader sequence (anti-leader) to each nascent subgenome-length minus strand. Subsequently, the subgenome-length minus strand RNAs each serve as template to produce one of the subgenomic mRNAs. The RdRp complexes engaged in replication and transcription may be (partially) different. For example, in the equine arteritis virus (EAV) model, nsp1 has been identified as a regulatory factor that is dispensable for replication but required to regulate the accumulation levels of the different subgenomic RNAs, most likely by controlling a step during minus strand RNA synthesis. See text for more details.

Using a combination of approaches, detailed RNA secondary structure models were developed for the EAV 5′ and 3′ NTRs. In the 5′ NTR, a region involved in translation, replication, and transcription,[205] (e-Fig. 29.4B), one domain in particular was found to be crucial for sg RNA production (see below). This so-called "leader TRS [transcription-regulating sequence] hairpin" (LTH) is potentially conserved in the 5′ NTR of all arteriviruses (e-Fig 29.4C). The importance of the other structural features of the EAV 5′ NTR and, for example, their involvement in RNA–protein interactions, remains to be investigated because few of these elements are conserved in other arteriviruses.[205] A possible exception is EAV hairpin C (termed SL2 in PRRSV; 115) that was reported to be crucial for PRRSV replication and subgenomic RNA synthesis in particular (e-Fig. 29.4C).

The 3′ NTR of the arterivirus genome does not contain obviously conserved primary sequences. For EAV, the 3′-terminal CC motif immediately upstream of the poly(A) tail plays a critical role in viral RNA synthesis.[15] Furthermore, a stem-loop structure near the 3′-terminus of the EAV genome is also required for RNA synthesis[14] (e-Fig. 29.5A) and its loop was implicated in an essential pseudoknot interaction with an upstream stem-loop structure residing in the N protein gene.[15] This conformation was predicted to be conserved in all arteriviruses and proposed to constitute a molecular switch that could regulate the specificity or timing of viral (minus strand) RNA synthesis (e-Fig. 29.5B).

Various proteins from MA-104 cells bind to arterivirus-derived RNA sequences.[90,122] and the *in vitro* RNA-synthesizing activity of semi-purified EAV replication and transcription complexes depends on the presence of a soluble host protein of 59 to 70 kD, which remains to be identified.[212]

Synthesis and Translation of Subgenomic mRNAs

One of the hallmarks of the replication cycle of arteriviruses (and other nidoviruses) is the synthesis of a 3′-co-terminal nested set of sg mRNAs (Fig. 29.5) from which the genes in the 3′ end of the genome are expressed. In the case of arteriviruses, all these genes encode structural proteins. Arterivirus sg mRNAs also have a common 5′ end, the so-called "leader sequence," which is derived from the 5′ end of the genome.[55] This property is shared with coronaviruses, but—remarkably—not with some other nidoviruses (toroviruses and roniviruses; for reviews, see 83,146,168). Supported by the presumed common ancestry of the arterivirus and coronavirus replicase genes, leader-to-body fusion during arterivirus sg RNA synthesis was proposed to rely on a mechanism of discontinuous RNA synthesis similar to that previously proposed for coronaviruses. In both virus groups, short conserved TRSs are present at the 3′ end of the leader sequence ("leader TRS") and at the 5′ end of each of the transcription units specifying a sg mRNA "body" ("body TRS"; reviewed in 146,168,175). The observation that arterivirus-infected cells contain a nested set of sg-length minus-strand RNAs, complementary to the sg mRNAs, is another important parallel with coronaviruses.[30,53]

With the exception of the smallest species, the arterivirus sg mRNAs are structurally polycistronic, but most of them are assumed to be functionally monocistronic. Notable exceptions are mRNAs 2 and 5 (in EAV, LDV, and PRRSV; Fig. 29.3), which are functionally bicistronic transcripts from which the partially overlapping gene sets E/GP2 and ORF5a/GP5 are expressed.[75,94,176] The mRNAs tentatively numbered 4 and 6 are thought to be used to translate the corresponding SHFV gene sets, and also mRNA2 of this virus was proposed to be functionally bicistronic.[81]

A substantial number of models for coronavirus and arterivirus sg mRNA synthesis have been proposed and reviewed extensively (see also Chapter 28; 146,168,175, and references therein). The detection of sg-length minus strands indicated that the discontinuous step in sg RNA synthesis likely occurs during minus-strand RNA synthesis. This concept was subsequently supported by data from biochemical and genetic studies with coronaviruses and arteriviruses and resulted in a model (Fig. 29.5; e-Fig. 29.4) in which discontinuous extension of minus-strand RNA synthesis yields sg-length minus-strand templates for sg mRNA synthesis.[166,168]

Direct proof for base-pairing between leader TRS and anti-body TRS was obtained from reverse genetics studies using an EAV infectious complementary DNA (cDNA) clone.[147,214] The mechanism by which the transcriptase is translocated between the body and leader TRS in the genomic template, a step that may resemble copy-choice RNA recombination,[19,147,214] remains to be elucidated. Arterivirus sg RNAs are produced in nonequimolar, but relatively constant amounts, thus providing a mechanism to regulate the expression of the various structural protein genes. EAV reverse genetics studies have rigorously demonstrated that transcription depends on duplex formation between leader TRS and anti-body TRS and that—in general—the relative amount of sg mRNA correlates with the calculated stability of this duplex.[147,148,214] Sequences flanking the body TRS, the relative order and/or location of body TRSs in the genome, and possibly also higher order RNA structure were also shown or postulated to influence transcription.[145] Structural studies on the 5′-proximal part of the EAV genome[205] placed the leader TRS in a single-stranded loop of the structure referred to as the "leader TRS hairpin" (or LTH; e-Fig. 29.4B,C), which was characterized as a critical player in transcription.[206]

At the protein level, transcription-specific functions have been attributed to several replicase subunits, in particular nonstructural protein 1 (nsp1) and nsp10, for which mutations were described that resulted in the (near) complete inactivation of sg mRNA synthesis.[138,196,198,208] EAV nsp1 controls the accumulation levels of viral genome and individual sg mRNAs in the infected cell by determining the levels at which the minus-strand templates for each of these molecules are produced.[138] An N-terminal zinc finger (ZF) domain was implicated in this function, but also other nsp1 domains appear to be important. Mutagenesis of nsp1 triggered the evolution of numerous nsp1 pseudorevertants with compensatory mutations that invariably rescued both balanced EAV mRNA accumulation and efficient virus production.[138] In the case of PRRSV, where nsp1 is internally cleaved into nsp1α and nsp1β, the ZF-containing nsp1α subunit is presumed to fulfill a similar role in transcription regulation.[102]

Arterivirus Proteinases and Posttranslational Processing of the Replicase

The proteolytic maturation of the arterivirus pp1a and pp1ab replicase polyproteins involves the rapid autoproteolytic release of three or two N-terminal nsps and the subsequent cleavage of the remaining part of both polyproteins by the viral nsp4 "main protease." The posttranslational processing of the replicase polyproteins has been studied most extensively for EAV (see 202,248, and references therein; e-Fig. 29.6A,B) for which pp1a and pp1ab are cleaved 8 and 11 times, respectively, by three ORF1a-encoded proteinases (see below). In combination with the ORF1a/1b ribosomal frame shift, this yields 13 processing end products (named nonstructural protein [nsp] 1 to 12, including nsp7α and nsp7β; Fig. 29.3; e-Fig. 29.6E). Of these, nsp1-8 are generated from ORF1a, whereas nsp10-12 are entirely ORF1b-encoded and nsp9, due to the ribosomal frame shift consisting of a small, ORF1a-encoded N-terminal domain (identical to nsp8) and a large C-terminal part that is encoded by ORF1b and includes the viral RNA-dependent RNA polymerase (RdRp) domain. EAV reverse genetics studies with cleavage site mutants underscored the critical importance of replicase polyprotein processing for virus replication.[202,209] The nsp3-8 region of pp1a (and likely also pp1ab) is subject to two alternative processing cascades, with the "major pathway" requiring an interaction with nsp2 as a cofactor, to mediate cleavage of the nsp4/5 site[222] (e-Fig. 29.6D).

The three EAV proteinase domains in nsp1, nsp2, and nsp4[74,175,248] (e-Fig. 29.6) and their corresponding cleavage sites are well conserved in the other arteriviruses (Fig. 29.3). EAV nsp1 and nsp2 both contain a papain-like proteinase domain (PLP; formerly referred to as PCP or CP for [papain-like] cysteine protease) that mediates their rapid release from the polyprotein,[178] whereas nsp4 includes a chymotrypsin-like serine proteinase (SP), the arterivirus main proteinase.[180] PRRSV and LDV, in addition to having homologs of these three EAV proteinases, possess a fourth nonstructural proteinase,[52] which mediates the rapid release of an additional N-terminal cleavage product. This PLPα possibly is a duplication of the proteinase (PLPβ) present in the C-terminal domain of EAV nsp1 and appears to have become inactivated in EAV.[52] The sequence analysis of the SHFV nsp1 region revealed an even more complex situation, with an array of three potential PLP domains present in the 480-residue region upstream of the (predicted) nsp1/nsp2 junction. The nsp4 SP combines the His-Asp-Ser catalytic triad of classical chymotrypsin-like proteinases with the substrate specificity of the so-called 3C-like cysteine proteinases, a subgroup of chymotrypsin-like enzymes named after the picornavirus 3C proteinases. Specific residues in the substrate-binding region of the SP are assumed to determine its specificity for cleavage sites containing Glu (or sometimes Gln) as the P1 residue and mainly Gly, Ala, or Ser at the P1′ position. Nine such sites were identified in EAV pp1a/pp1ab, and they were all found to be conserved in the other family members.[175,202,248]

Nsp4 structures have been obtained by x-ray crystallography for both EAV and PRRSV[11,195] (e-Fig. 29.7). The protein consists of three domains, with domains I and II forming the typical chymotrypsin-like two-β-barrel fold of the SP. The C-terminal domain III is dispensable for proteolytic activity and may be involved in fine-tuning replicase polyprotein cleavage.[200,201] Recent structural studies also elucidated the structures of PRRSV nsp1α[186] and nsp1β,[238] including their respective PLP domains (e-Fig. 29.7), which—in line with previous studies—were both confirmed to employ a Cys-His tandem as active site residues. Both PLPα and PLPβ appear to act exclusively *in cis* and the two structures indeed revealed the presence of the C-terminal region of the proteins in the PLP substrate-binding pocket, suggesting an intramolecular cleavage mechanism that would preclude further proteolytic reactions. Both nsp1α and nsp1β of PRRSV have also been implicated in evasion of the host's immune response (see below), but this was most directly demonstrated for the PLP that resides in the N-terminal domain of the highly variable nsp2 subunit. This PLP2, which possesses both *cis* and *trans* cleavage activities,[86,179] not only directs the critical cleavage of the nsp2/3 site in pp1a and pp1ab, but is also able to remove ubiquitin (Ub) and Ub-like modifiers like ISG15 from yet-to-be-identified substrates in the infected cell.[213] The protein is distantly related to the ovarian tumor domain (OTU) family of deubiquitinating enzymes.[76,123,187]

Replicase Proteins and the Replication Complex

Although accelerated by research efforts following the emergence of severe acute respiratory syndrome (SARS)-coronavirus, the functional dissection of the complex array of nidovirus nonstructural protein functions is still in its infancy. Even the arterivirus replicase polyproteins are of extraordinary size and complexity, despite their twofold smaller size compared to nidoviruses with larger genomes like coronaviruses and roniviruses. Therefore, future studies will undoubtedly reveal both novel similarities and differences between these two groups. In arteriviruses, with the notable exception of the role of nsp1 in sg mRNA synthesis (see above), the ORF1a-encoded functions mainly appear important for the regulation of replicase gene expression (by proteolytic processing; see above) and formation of the membrane-anchored "scaffold" for the replication/transcription complex. The ORF1b-encoded proteins, on the other hand, appear to be more directly involved in viral RNA synthesis.

Except for the proteins from the nsp1 region,[31,197] all replicase subunits localize to the perinuclear region of the infected cell (e-Fig. 29.8A–D; 207), where they are associated with intracellular membranes that are derived from the endoplasmic reticulum (ER). Upon arterivirus infection, these host cell membranes are modified into vesicular double-membrane structures that presumably carry the viral replication complex (e-Fig. 29.9A–F).[149,177,212] The formation of closely paired membranes and double membrane vesicles (DMVs) is a typical feature of arterivirus-infected cells described many years ago.[18,184,234] Recent electron tomography studies of EAV-infected cells revealed that these structures are in fact interconnected and form a network of modified ER[99] (e-Fig. 29.9E). Biochemical and electron microscopy studies have implicated ORF1a-encoded subunits that contain hydrophobic, probable trans-membrane domains (in particular nsp2, nsp3, and nsp5; e-Fig. 29.6C) in the formation of these membrane structures.[71,149,158,177,207]

Replicase ORF1b is the most conserved part of the arterivirus genome and encodes the core enzymes for viral RNA synthesis—RdRp (nsp9) and helicase (nsp10).[54,83,140] Recombinant EAV nsp9 is able to initiate RNA synthesis *de novo* in the absence of other viral or cellular proteins, but could not utilize sequences derived from the 3′ end of the viral genome as a template,[13] suggesting additional requirements for its activity *in vivo*. The predicted NTP binding and superfamily 1 helicase activities of arterivirus nsp10 were corroborated by *in vitro* assays with recombinant nsp10. These also revealed the 5′-to-3′ polarity of the unwinding reaction, a property shared with coronaviruses,[12,169] although it has not been reconciled with the protein's presumed role in unwinding local double-stranded

RNA structures that might hinder the RdRp during viral RNA synthesis, which proceeds in the opposite direction. As in all nidoviruses, the helicase is linked to an N-terminal zinc-binding domain that might assist the proper folding of nsp10 and/or mediate interactions of the protein with its substrate RNAs. This domain was also implicated in a remarkable transcription-specific defect.[208,210]

Advanced bioinformatics studies provided the first evidence to suggest that nsp11, and its coronavirus homolog nsp15, contain a nidovirus-specific endoribonuclease activity (NendoU; 173). Subsequently, this prediction was experimentally verified in biochemical assays for recombinant coronavirus nsp15[91] and EAV nsp11.[139] In the meantime, the site-directed mutagenesis of key NendoU residues had been found to exert pleiotropic effects on EAV RNA synthesis, including a complete block in some of the mutants and more moderate effects in others.[157] The exact function of the NendoU domain, a genetic marker of vertebrate nidoviruses,[140] remains to be elucidated, and in particular its substrate specificity in the infected cell is an enigma. Recombinant NendoU-containing proteins exhibit broad substrate specificity *in vitro,* processing both single-stranded and double-stranded RNA substrates 3′ of pyrimidines.[139] However, in the context of the infected cell, NendoU activity or substrate specificity may be controlled via specific protein–protein interactions or compartmentalization of the enzyme as part of the membrane-associated replication and transcription complex.

The final ORF1b-encoded replicase subunit of arteriviruses, nsp12, has not been the subject of experimental studies, and sequence comparisons did not suggest a function or a relationship to any other known protein family.

Assembly and Release

EAV N partially co-localizes with the complex for viral RNA synthesis (197; e-Fig. 29.8D). Because N is not required for replication or transcription,[131,208,232] this suggests that genome encapsidation may occur (or begin) at the site of viral RNA synthesis. Recent electron tomography studies of EAV-infected cells revealed a network of N-containing sheets and tubules in close vicinity of the membrane structures where viral RNA synthesis is thought to occur, but the functional significance of these N structures remains to be studied in more detail.[99]

Arteriviruses acquire their envelope by budding of preformed nucleocapsids into the lumen of the smooth endoplasmic reticulum and/or the Golgi complex[121,184,234] (e-Fig. 29.8E–F and e-Fig. 29.9G–H). Most arterivirus envelope proteins are retained in intracellular membranes (e-Fig. 29.8E–F), and the formation of the GP5-M heterodimer is a primary determinant of virus budding.[231,232,243] The transport of GP5 and M to the Golgi complex appears to depend on complex formation and correlates with the production of infectious virus.[60,174,219] After budding, virions accumulate in intracellular vesicles, which are transported to the plasma membrane and release the progeny virus.

Major Structural Proteins

The three major structural proteins GP5, M, and N are encoded—in this order—by the three most 3′-proximal ORFs in the arterivirus genome (Fig. 29.3 and Table 29.1). N is small (12 to 15 kD) and contains many basic residues, in particular in its presumably disordered N-terminal domain, which is thought to interact with the genomic RNA during nucleocapsid assembly.[59,61] The C-terminal "capsid-forming" half of N forms dimers in solution and is the basis for a proposed "nidovirus nucleocapsid fold" that is also encountered in the much larger coronavirus N protein.[61] The EAV and PRRSV N proteins are phosphorylated.[56,235] In the case of PRRSV N, phosphoserines mapped to both the RNA binding domain and the capsid-forming domain where they may modulate nucleic acid binding activity or protein–protein interactions.[235]

The nonglycosylated M protein (16 to 20 kD) resembles the coronavirus M protein in that its N-terminal half presumably traverses the membrane three times,[56,70,127] resulting in an N_{exo}-C_{endo} configuration with a short ectodomain of only 10 to 18 residues exposed at the virion surface. One of the membrane-spanning fragments is thought to function as an internal signal sequence. The arterivirus M protein forms disulfide-linked heterodimers with the 24 to 54 kD GP5, a step probably driven by the formation of a disulfide bridge between a conserved Cys residue in the M ectodomain and a Cys residue in the GP5 ectodomain.[57,69,174] EAV GP5-M heterodimers are thought to be essential for virus assembly, possibly by inducing the membrane curvature required for virus budding.[57,60,174]

Despite considerable differences in primary structure, the major GPs of arteriviruses (GP5) share common structural features. They contain an N-terminal signal sequence that is assumed to be cleaved from a short ectodomain. The central hydrophobic region probably spans the membrane three times and is followed by a cytoplasmic domain of 50 to 75 amino acids. In the case of LDV and PRRSV, the ectodomain is only about 30 residues long and contains one to three N-linked glycans.[70,127] The ectodomain of EAV GP5 is 95 residues long and usually possesses a single N-linked polylactosamine side chain,[56] although in some strains an additional N-linked glycan is present. In addition, in the case of LDV, GP5 glycosylation occurs by the addition of variable numbers of lactosamine repeats.[110] Nonneuropathogenic and neuropathogenic strains typically contain three and one polylactosaminoglycan chain(s), respectively (see below).

Minor Structural Proteins

The minor arterivirus GP encoded by ORF2a (PRRSV) or ORF2b (EAV/LDV) is a conventional class I integral membrane protein with an N-terminal signal peptide, a C-terminal transmembrane segment, and 1 to 4 potential N-glycosylation sites in its ectodomain. GP2 occurs in EAV-infected cells in a variety of monomeric conformations and in complex with other minor GPs.[228,231] Complex formation is a prerequisite for incorporation into virions.[231,232] Cysteine residues in the EAV GP2 ectodomain form both intramolecular and intermolecular cysteine bridges, the latter involving a cysteine in the ectodomain of GP4, which also is a typical class I integral membrane protein.[228]

GP3 is a heavily glycosylated integral membrane protein with an uncleaved N-terminal signal sequence and a hydrophobic C-terminal domain, suggesting the protein is anchored in the membrane with both termini.[87,229] Like GP2 and GP4, EAV GP3 localizes to the endoplasmic reticulum, both in infected cells and in expression systems.[229] Following initial conflicting reports, PRRSV GP3 is now firmly believed to be present in virions,[48,232] which is also in line with the data obtained for EAV. Following virus release, GP3 becomes disulfide-linked to the GP2-GP4 heterodimers, and this postassembly maturation event yields a complex of three covalently bound minor GPs. As a result, EAV particles contain both GP2-GP4 heterodimers and GP2-GP3-GP4 heterotrimers.[230,231]

Like GP2, GP4 is a predicted class I membrane protein with a cleaved signal sequence and multiple N-glycosylation sites in its ectodomain.[129,215,229] Little is known about the properties or function of GP4, apart from the oligomerization described above and the finding that GP4 may be responsible for an interaction of the GP2-GP3-GP4 trimer with GP5.[44] Recent reverse genetics studies with PRRSV mutants lacking specific glycans in GP2, GP3, and GP4 documented the general importance of these posttranslational modifications for virus viability and interactions with CD163.[45]

The higher order structure of the small E protein is unknown, but this protein is essential for virus infectivity[176] and may in fact be associated with trimer of minor GPs.[231] The protein has been proposed to oligomerize and form an ion channel that could play a role during viral entry.[106] Furthermore, its N-terminus contains a myristoylation signal that is conserved across arteriviruses and is functional in EAV and PRRSV. A block of the fatty acid addition was not lethal, but knockout mutants were crippled and displayed a small-plaque phenotype.[63,190]

Finally, another gene encoding a small generally hydrophobic protein was recently identified in EAV[75] and PRRSV.[94] Bioinformatics analyses revealed a potential open reading frame (ORF5a) overlapping the 5′ end of ORF5, and the ORF5a protein was identified in purified PRRSV virions. EAV reverse genetics revealed that the protein is not essential, but knockout mutants showed a significant reduction of progeny titers.

Replication in Cultured Cells and Host Cell Interactions

With the exception of EAV, arteriviruses have a very restricted host specificity (for reviews, see 155, 175 and references therein). LDV grows in primary cultures of mouse macrophages, but not in macrophage or other cell lines. In addition to primary macrophages from their respective hosts, SHFV and PRRSV also replicate in cell lines of African green monkey kidney cells (MA-104 and derivatives thereof, like the MARC-145 cell line discussed above). EAV replicates efficiently in primary cultures of horse macrophages and kidney cells, and— remarkably—also in a variety of cell lines such as baby hamster kidney, rabbit kidney, and African green monkey kidney and mouse C2C12 cells.[245]

One-step growth experiments have shown that maximum progeny virus titers are generally released by 10 to 15 h postinfection. The maximum titers obtained in cell culture are 10^6 to 10^7 tissue culture infectious dose $(TCID)_{50}$/ml for PRRSV, but may exceed 10^8 PFU/ml for EAV and SHFV.[155,175] In general, arterivirus infection of macrophages and cell lines is highly cytocidal, resulting in rounding of the cells and detachment from the culture plate surface, although recently a model for persistent noncytopathic infection with EAV in human HeLa cells was established.[245]

Arteriviruses interact with a variety of host factors and mechanisms. For example, arteriviruses were claimed to induce or modulate apoptosis in cell lines and/or cultured macrophages.[3,39,185,251] PRRSV also induces apoptosis in germ cells *in vivo.*[188] In both macrophages and MARC-145 cells, PRRSV stimulated antiapoptotic pathways early in infection, but late in infection cells died from caspase-dependent apoptosis, culminating in secondary necrosis.[39]

Despite the cytoplasmic replication cycle of arteriviruses, some viral proteins are directed (in part) to the nucleus of infected cells (e-Fig. 29.8), specifically nsp1 (see above) and the N protein. A nuclear localization signal, for interaction with the nuclear transporters importin α and β, was identified at positions 41-47 of PRRSV N,[164] which—like its EAV counterpart–accumulates in the nucleoli of infected cells.[164,197] Remarkably, a block of CRM1-mediated nuclear export with the drug leptomycin B resulted in the nuclear accumulation of EAV N, indicating that the protein apparently shuttles between cytoplasm and nucleus before playing its role in cytoplasmic virus assembly.[197] Various nuclear host proteins interact with PRRSV N (reviewed by 240), including fibrillarin, nucleolin, and poly(A)-binding protein, but the functional implications of these findings remain to be unraveled. Using reverse genetics, a knockout mutation for the nuclear localization signal of PRRSV N was engineered and yielded a viable, although seriously attenuated, mutant virus.[105] Compared to the wild-type control, pigs infected with this mutant virus showed reduced viremia and significantly higher neutralizing antibody titers.

PATHOGENESIS AND PATHOLOGY OF ARTERIVIRUS INFECTIONS

The natural host range of arteriviruses is restricted to horses and donkeys (EAV), pigs (PRRSV), mice (LDV), and several genera of African and Asian monkeys (SHFV). Recent outbreaks of equine viral arteritis in New Mexico, United States (2006) and Normandy, France (2007) increased the interest of horse owners and veterinarians in EAV treatment and vaccines. Highly virulent PRRSV variants, causing the so-called "porcine high fever disease," emerged in China in 2006 and still continue to cause problems in this and surrounding countries.[107,194,246]

Site of Primary Replication, Spread, and Cell and Tissue Tropism

Macrophages appear to be the primary target cell for all arteriviruses.[155] Cell surface molecules mediating entry into these cells are only known for PRRSV and have been discussed above. Following respiratory transmission, EAV initially replicates in lung macrophages and endothelial cells.[5,88] The virus then spreads to draining lymph nodes, from where it becomes disseminated throughout the body via the circulation. By the third day of infection, a viremia has developed and virus can be isolated from practically all tissues.

Reported primary target cells for PRRSV replication are fully differentiated porcine lung alveolar macrophages and other cells of the monocyte/macrophage lineage including pulmonary intravascular macrophages, subsets of macrophages in lymph nodes and spleen, and intravascular macrophages of the placenta and umbilical cord.[65,104,191] After spreading through the circulation, PRRSV replicates persistently in tonsils, lungs, and lymphoid organs (reviewed in 192).

IMMUNE RESPONSES

Several arteriviruses cause persistent infections despite the presence of an adaptive immune response. Neither neutralizing antibodies nor effective helper and cytolytic T lymphocytes are able to control virus replication in these persistently infected animals. Therefore, arteriviruses must have developed strategies to evade immune responses, underpinning the importance of studying immunity in natural and experimental infections in order to enhance our understanding of the underlying mechanisms. For a more detailed overview of the immune response to arterivirus infection, the reader is also referred to a variety of other review articles,[5,43,114,125,134] and references therein.

Innate Immune Response

It is rather unclear at present which pattern-recognition receptors (PRRs) of the innate immune system recognize arteriviruses during infection of different cell types. Several reports have suggested or speculated on the involvement of toll-like receptor 3 (TLR3) during infection of PRRSV in macrophages and lymphoid tissue (see 43 and references therein). A study with EAV in knockout mouse embryonic fibroblasts suggested that of the cytosolic retinoic acid inducible I–like receptors (RLRs), melanoma differentiation–associated gene (MDA5) is predominantly involved in the recognition of this virus.[213] Experimental infection of $TLR7^{-/-}$ mice with LDV revealed the importance of this TLR expressed by plasmacytoid dendritic cells (pDCs) for the induction of type I interferon (IFN) and the activation of lymphocytes during LDV infection.[1]

In vitro studies using alveolar and blood-derived macrophages demonstrated that tumor necrosis factor (TNF)-α and other proinflammatory cytokines are induced following infection with virulent EAV strains.[5,132] In the case of PRRSV, it is generally believed that a rather weak innate immune response is induced (see 5,43,132,134, and references therein). Induction of TNF-α as well as IFN-α by PRRSV and also the sensitivity to these innate cytokines, seems to depend on the isolate. Chen et al.[33] suggested that this may at least in part relate to variability in nsp2, in which abundant changes and deletions were found among different isolates, which seem to influence host immune responses. Multiple studies reported that PRRSV induces interleukin 8 (Il-8), whereas the induction of Il-6 as well as that of Il-10 is debated (see also below; 43, and references therein).

LDV induced natural killer (NK) cells in infected mice and as a consequence a large increase in serum IFN-γ was observed, but these responses were unable to control LDV replication.[124] LDV also elicits IFN-α induction through TLR7 activation in plasmacytoid dendritic cells, but the virus is not sensitive to a systemic IFN-α response in mice.[1]

Humoral Immune Response

Antigenic cross-reactivity between different arterivirus species has not been demonstrated, with the exception of antibodies directed against the single linear neutralization site of LDV GP5, which do not only neutralize LDV, but also PRRSV.[156] Sera from EAV-infected horses recognize N, M, GP5, and GP2.[34,118] In addition, antibodies against the nonstructural proteins nsp2, nsp4, nsp5, and nsp12 were found in experimentally or persistently infected horses, whereas animals vaccinated with a modified live virus (MLV) vaccine against EAV produced antibodies against nsp2 and nsp12, and much less against nsp4 and nsp5.[79] PRRSV-infected pigs produce antibodies directed against the structural proteins GP2 to GP5, M, and N, with the antibodies recognizing N being detected earliest and most abundantly.[43,112,128] The early humoral response against PRRSV also includes antibodies against nsp1 and particularly nsp2, which develop to titers as high as those of the anti-N antibodies.[95]

It has been proposed that LDV- and PRRSV-specific antibodies contribute to antibody-dependent enhancement (ADE) of infection.[25,241,242] For PRRSV, certain nonneutralizing epitopes in the N and GP5 proteins induce antibodies that seem responsible for ADE through opsonization, leading to enhanced internalization of the virus into macrophages.[27,43,125]

Neutralizing antibodies (NAs) in arterivirus-infected animals are predominantly directed to the major glycoprotein GP5.[6,24,34,82,143,153,154] The neutralization site in EAV, PRRSV, and LDV GP5 was mapped to the ectodomain of the protein.[8,34,110,154] For EAV, its four major neutralization sites are conformation-dependent, and interaction of GP5 with M is critical for neutralization.[8] For LDV and PRRSV, the primary neutralization site was mapped close to the GP5 N-terminus and exhibits 77% amino acid identity, probably explaining the observation that LDV neutralizing antibodies to GP5 also neutralize PRRSV.[154,156] For PRRSV, a second NA-binding domain was identified in the GP4 ectodomain[129]; however, neutralization by monoclonal antibodies directed against this region is less effective than neutralization by GP5 antibodies.[223] The GP4 region is subject to immune selection, and it is therefore highly heterogeneous among different PRRSV strains.[40,41]

The production of NA in EAV-infected horses coincides with virus clearance, suggesting that the humoral immune response plays an important role in recovery.[77] In contrast, NA against LDV and PRRSV are detected only very late, 1 to 2 months after infection, are produced at low levels, and are believed to not or hardly reduce viremia.[24,58,112,241] One of the most common hypotheses for the delayed or absent NA production in PRRSV infection, or after vaccination, is the presence of an immuno-dominant decoy epitope, just upstream of the GP5 neutralization epitope, which induces a strong nonneutralizing antibody response.[143] Insertion of another epitope in between the neutralizing and decoy epitopes increased the neutralizing response, suggesting that the juxtapositioning of the two original epitopes indeed plays a role.[72] In addition, the glycosylation state of the GP5 ectodomain in the vicinity of the neutralizing epitope and glycosylation of GP3 may influence the efficiency of NA production.[220] Similarly, in the case of nonneuropathogenic strains of LDV, the GP5 ectodomain contains three polylactosaminoglycan chains, as opposed to a single polylactosaminoglycan in the ectodomain of neuropathogenic strains. It was postulated that the nonneuropathogenic strains can establish persistent infections because neutralizing antibodies bind less efficiently to the highly glycosylated ectodomain of their GP5. In contrast, neuropathogenic strains are not able to persist.[32,110,155] Yet another explanation for inefficient neutralization was inspired by the observation that PRRSV infection in piglets manipulates the development of the B-cell repertoire.[21] Together with the general idea that PRRSV suppresses (innate) immune responses (see below), this may explain the delayed and aberrant antibody production that is observed (reviewed in 43,89,97,114).

The humoral immune response against SHFV varies with the species of monkey and the virus isolate that is tested.[84,85] The rapid death of macaques after SHFV infection precludes an effective host immune response. Virulent SHFV strains, which cause acute disease in patas monkeys, induced neutralizing antibodies at 7 days postinfection. The production of neutralizing antibodies correlated with the complete clearance of the virus from the circulation by 21 days postinfection.

On the other hand, SHFV strains that cause a persistent infection in these monkeys induce very low antibody titers.

Cell-Mediated Immune Response

Cell-mediated immunity (CMI) to arterivirus infection has not yet been characterized in great detail. Studies in ponies experimentally infected with EAV have shown that cytotoxicity induced by EAV-stimulated peripheral blood mononuclear cells (PBMC) was virus-specific, genetically restricted, mediated by CD8+ T cells, and that the precursors persist for at least 1 year after infection.[5,28]

Cell-mediated responses in PRRSV-infected animals include CD4+, CD8+, and double positive T cells, which appear transiently between 2 and 8 weeks after experimental infection (reviewed in 43,134,237) or become more pronounced at later stages.[126] The abundance of PRRSV-specific T cells and IFN-gamma–producing cells in both acute and persistently infected animals is highly variable and does not correlate to the level of virus in lymphoid tissue.[58,126,237] Several studies indicate that the strongest CMI inducers of PRRSV are proteins M, N, and GP4.[43]

Cytotoxic and helper T-cell responses were detected in LDV-infected mice, but did not reduce LDV replication.[67] Additional studies are required to determine whether there is a correlation between T-cell responses *in vitro* and protection *in vivo,* and the overall data suggest that the arteriviruses probably directly, or indirectly, manipulate CMI (see below).

Immune Evasion

Not much is known about the mechanistic details of immune evasion by the arteriviruses, but it is clear that modulation of the immune response occurs on different levels. An expanding body of data documents the suppression of innate immune responses (reviewed for PRRSV in 240) and several reports suggest that arteriviruses also manipulate CMI. Downregulation of major histocompatibility complex class I and II (MHC-I and MHC-II) molecules on the surface of antigen-presenting cells (APCs) was shown for PRRSV,[43,125] and co-infection with LDV causes a delay of the CD8+ T-cell–mediated immune response to Friend virus in mice, suggesting manipulation of the MHC-I presentation pathway.[162]

With regard to the molecular mechanisms underlying immune suppressive activities, few data are available at present. Several reports previously suggested that PRRSV significantly induces IL-10 production in pigs during the first 2 weeks of infection. This immunosuppressive cytokine interacts with a wide array of immune cells, including the PRRSV target cells from the monocyte/macrophage lineage, to downregulate in particular cell-mediated innate and adaptive immunity. Recent experiments suggest that PRRSV N may be responsible for IL-10 upregulation during infection, and this may be achieved through induction of specific regulatory T-cell populations.[172,192,233,240]

In addition to N, three nonstructural proteins have been implicated in arterivirus immune evasion: nsp1 (nsp1α and nsp1β in PRRSV), nsp2 (PRRSV and EAV), and nsp11 (PRRSV). All three proteins were suggested to suppress innate immune signaling induced by the RLR- or TLR-innate sensors, or TNF-α, which lead to IFN-β and/or nuclear factor kappa B (NF-κB) expression.[16,240] PRRSV nsp1α and nsp1β both inhibit the expression of IFN-β after induction of innate responses by Sendai virus or double-stranded DNA (dsRNA),[16] and nsp1β also inhibits signaling downstream of type 1 IFNs by inhibiting nuclear translocation of STAT1.[31] Furthermore, both nsp1α and nsp1β suppress NF-κB activation.[16,181] Kim et al.[96] showed degradation of cAMP response element-binding (CREB)-binding protein induced by PRRSV nsp1 during infection, causing inhibition of interferon regulatory transcription factor 3 (IRF3) transcription factor activity in the nucleus. Besides localizing to the perinuclear region with other nsps, nsp1 is partially transported to the nucleus,[96,197] which may be connected to at least some of its immune evasive activities.

Arterivirus nsp2 contains a papain-like cysteine protease (PLP2) in its N-terminal domain that cleaves the nsp2/nsp3 junction in the replicase polyproteins. This protease is distantly related to the OTU family of deubiquitinating enzymes (DUB).[123] Upon overexpression, EAV and PRRSV PLP2 showed a general DUB activity toward cellular ubiquitin conjugates, and also cleaved the IFN-induced ubiquitin homolog ISG15, which is thought to have antiviral activity.[76] Indications that these DUB activities could be functional in the suppression of innate immune responses were obtained from experiments in which the EAV PLP2-DUB suppressed TNFα-induced NF-κB signaling in 293T cells. In addition, the PLP2-DUB of PRRSV inhibited the NF-κB signaling pathway, as well as the IRF3-dependent IFN-β pathway induced by Sendai virus infection.[109,187] PRRSV PLP2-DUB appears to remove K48-linked polyubiquitin from IκBα to prevent its proteasomal degradation and thereby downstream signaling toward NF-kB activation. Besides the PLP2 domain of PRRSV nsp2, also the variable regions in the central part of this large protein could influence antiviral responses.[33] Recent data suggest that PLP2 of all arteriviruses suppresses RLR-mediated IFN-β induction by removing K63-linked polyubiquitin from RIG-I, which results in inhibition of downstream signaling.[213]

Probably too few data are available at present to firmly establish the suppression of IFN-β production by arterivirus nsp11.[16] The RNase activity of the NendoU domain in PRRSV nsp11 has been implicated in this activity,[171,240] but it is unclear whether nsp11 confers specific activity targeting certain innate immune responses or might attack the overall mRNA population of the cell on the basis of its RNase activity, thus inducing a translational shut-off.

RELEASE FROM THE HOST AND TRANSMISSION

In nature, EAV and PRRSV are transmitted primarily via the respiratory route.[199,226] Both viruses may persist in the semen of infected male animals, and are shed in milk of infected female animals, making vertical transmission an important secondary route of infection. In addition, LDV is efficiently transmitted from mother to fetus,[250] and also sexual transmission was reported.[23] PRRSV was shown to replicate in testicular germ cells such as spermatids and spermatocytes[188]; infectious EAV is excreted in semen by persistently infected "carrier" stallions and can be transmitted to broodmares.[5,199] Both EAV and PRRSV are furthermore shed in virtually all body secretions, including saliva, respiratory tract secretions, oropharyngeal secretions, urine, and feces (reviewed in 38,88). PRRSV can also be mechanically transmitted in pig herds through aerosols, infected needles, contaminated boots and coveralls, and carrier insects like houseflies.[38,144,151] In contrast to the other arteriviruses, SHFV is not transmitted transplacentally from mother to offspring.[85]

VIRULENCE

Sequence comparisons revealed that the highly pathogenic PRRSV strain causing the "porcine high fever disease" in Asia since 2006 originated from Chinese domestic type II viruses (which are related to the VR-2332 genotype II prototype strain).[236] They all have the same striking deletions of a conserved leucine and a 29-amino acid stretch in nsp2,[107,170,194] but these typical differences were found to be unrelated to the increased virulence.[247]

Infectious full-length cDNA clones were constructed of both cell culture–adapted[208] and virulent[7] EAV isolates, which can be used to study the determinants of virulence. Comparative sequence analysis of EAV strains that differ in virulence identified potentially relevant amino acid substitutions in both structural and nonstructural proteins. Reverse genetics experiments then showed that substitutions in the structural proteins may lead to more severe attenuation than those in the nonstructural proteins.[244] Collectively, interactions of both major (GP5 and M) and minor (GP2, GP3, and GP4) envelope proteins seem to influence tropism, and mutations in these proteins can therefore affect virulence.[80]

PERSISTENCE

Typical for natural EAV infections is the persistence that occurs in about 35% of the infected stallions.[199] The virus persists in the reproductive tract of these "carrier stallions" and is continuously shed into the semen for a long time. In contrast, persistent infection in mares generally does not last longer than one month.[88] The establishment and maintenance of persistent infection is testosterone-dependent in stallions, and high serum titers of neutralizing antibodies are insufficient to clear the virus.[5,199] A study of EAV evolution in persistently infected stallions strongly suggested that neither defective interfering particles nor immune evasion from B-cell responses are involved in persistence.[9]

Persistence of PRRSV has been commonly observed for up to 150 days in pigs, and up to 210 days in congenitally infected piglets.[35] Although the mechanisms underlying the failure to promptly clear PRRSV infection are poorly understood, it appears that a major reason is the inability of pigs to develop effective protective immune responses, which is probably due to the concerted immune evasion strategies exploited by the virus.[117,125]

SHFV appears to be endemic among several species of African monkeys, in which it causes asymptomatic acute or persistent infections depending on the virus strain.[113] LDV is also able to establish a largely asymptomatic persistent infection.[155]

EPIDEMIOLOGY

EAV

Despite its worldwide distribution, EAV has not caused many disease outbreaks. The first recognized and most severe epizootic occurred in 1953 in Bucyrus, Ohio, U.S.A.[62] Milder outbreaks have been reported from elsewhere in the United States, Canada, and a variety of European countries, with recent epizootics occurring in Normandy (France, 2006) and New Mexico (U.S.A., 2007).[88] The apparent discrepancy between the high incidence of the virus and the relatively low number of recorded disease outbreaks is explained by the predominantly subclinical course of infection.

A recent genome-wide association study pin-pointed genetic differences within and among horse populations that are associated with susceptibility of CD3+ T lymphocytes to EAV infection *in vitro*.[78] The genomic region identified encodes proteins (potentially) involved in virus entry, cytoskeletal organization, and antiviral innate responses, and the association of a specific haplotype (ECA11) with susceptibility to EAV infection will allow the development of a targeted molecular test for diagnostic purposes and large-scale studies.

PRRSV

PRRS was first detected in 1987 in the United States,[36] and the first outbreaks in Europe were recognized in Germany in 1990.[225,227] Today, PRRSV infection is ubiquitous in all swine-producing areas of the world, including North and South America, Europe, and Asia. Severe abortion storms had a resurgence in 1996 to 1998 in the United States. Subsequently, the number of acute disease outbreaks decreased until atypical PRRSV variants emerged in China in 2006, causing outbreaks of fatal PRRSV that were unparalleled in severity. The novel variant usually spread through a herd within 3 to 5 days, causing morbidity between 50% and 100%. Mortality rates in the 2006 outbreak were high, with a mean around 20%, and they could be as high as 100% in suckling piglets, 70% in nursery pigs, and 20% in finishing pigs. More than 40% of pregnant sows suffered abortion and 10% of these sows themselves succumbed to the disease.[111,194,246] In the following years, this highly pathogenic PRRSV spread to all Chinese swine-producing areas as well as surrounding Asian countries. About 60% of the Chinese pigs were infected with PRRSV over the 5 years after the virulent virus emerged.[107] To improve infection control, porcine genetic markers associated with PRRSV susceptibility are being sought, which can be used in breeding programs to optimize virus resistance, in balance with other traits of economic importance in pig production such as feeding efficiency, meat production, and leanness (reviewed in 116).

LDV

LDV was first discovered in laboratory mice.[155,161] The virus was also isolated from wild mice in several countries, although the worldwide incidence is not known. Despite a life-long viremia and virus secretion in urine, feces, and saliva, horizontal transmission is inefficient, except in the case of fighting males. In contrast, transmission from mother to offspring is much more efficient, as long as anti-LDV immune responses have not yet been elicited.[155]

SHFV

SHFV appears to be endemic among several species of African monkeys (*Erythrocebus patas, Ceropithecus aethiops, Papio anubus, and Papio cyanocephalus*).[85,103,113] Nevertheless, the virus was first isolated from Asian macaques, during outbreaks of fatal hemorrhagic fever in research centers in the Soviet Union and the United States.[189] These epizootics were probably caused by inadvertent transmission by humans from African monkeys to the macaques. During these outbreaks, SHFV was readily transmitted from the initially infected rhesus monkeys (*Macaca mulatta*) to other macaque species (*Macaca fascicularis* and *Macaca arctoides*), most likely by direct contact and via aerosols, whereas members of other monkey genera did not show clinical symptoms. Subsequently, similar epizootics among macaques occurred in various other primate centers.

CLINICAL FEATURES

EAV

The manifestations of EAV infection after an incubation period of 2 to 14 days range from subclinical to flu-like symptoms in adult animals, abortion in pregnant mares (e-Fig. 29.10A), persistent infection in stallions, and interstitial pneumonia in neonates.[5,62,88] As with most infectious diseases, old, debilitated, or immunosuppressed horses and very young foals are predisposed to more severe disease.[88] Clinical features are characteristic vascular lesions, necrosis of small muscular arteries (from which the name of the family prototype EAV was derived), acute anorexia, and fever, usually accompanied by palpebral edema, conjunctivitis, nasal catarrh, and edema of legs, genitals, and abdomen (62, e-Fig. 29.10). Virulence and clinical signs are strain dependent, but the genetic basis for these differences has not been established.[199]

PRRSV

At 12 to 24 hours after exposure to PRRSV, young pigs, sows, and boars become viremic, a state that can last from 1 to 2 weeks in mature animals to 8 weeks in young pigs. Clinical manifestations of PRRSV include occasional discoloring and blotching of the skin, most often on the ears (which gave PRRS the name "blue ear disease") and vulva, and occasionally on the trunk. Further symptoms are fever, anorexia, breathing difficulties, lymphadenopathy, gross and microscopic lesions in the lung, and reproductive failure characterized by delivery of weak or stillborn piglets (e-Fig. 29.11A), or autolyzed fetuses.[225]

The clinical features of the highly pathogenic PRRSV variants that emerged in China in 2006 are strikingly more severe than those reported for the older isolates (e-Fig. 29.12). The new variant affected pigs of all ages and was characterized by high fever (40 to 42°C), depression, anorexia, lethargy, and rubefaction of the skin and ears. Most diseased pigs showed obvious respiratory distress, such as sneezing, coughing, and asthma, as well as intestinal problems including diarrhea. At autopsy, the severe lesions in skin, lung, gastrointestinal tract, and brain were considered unique for this atypical form of PRRS[194,246] (e-Fig. 29.12F). Mortality rates ranged from 20% to 100%, depending on the age and health of the infected animals.

LDV

Infection of mice with LDV leads to a life-long viremia, but the infection is asymptomatic. It is maintained by continuous rounds of cytocidal virus replication in a renewable subpopulation of macrophages.[142] By 24 h after infection, LDV titers of 10^{10} infectious dose $(ID)_{50}$/ml are present in the plasma, which then decrease to a level of 10^4 to 10^6 ID_{50}/ml. These titers remain present throughout the life of the mouse, together with elevated levels of lactate dehydrogenase and other serum enzymes, which is due to the destruction of the macrophages that play a role in their clearance. LDV can be detected in the spleen, lymph nodes, thymus, and liver of persistently infected mice. Neurovirulent LDV variants can cause a fatal age-dependent poliomyelitis in certain inbred mouse strains that are of the Fv-$1^{n/n}$ genotype and carry N-tropic, ecotropic murine leukemia virus (MuLV)proviruses[37] (e-Fig. 29.13). The replication of these ecotropic MuLVs in the glial cells of the spinal cord was proposed to render the anterior horn neurons susceptible to cytocidal LDV infection. Consequently, the development of age-dependent poliomyelitis may result from a combination of increased expression of ecotropic MuLVs and a decreasing ability to mount a motor neuron-protective anti-LDV response. LDV can also induce severe thrombocytopenia in animals that have been treated with antiplatelet antibodies at a dose that in itself was insufficient to induce clinical disease.[135,136] The mechanism is unknown, but macrophage activation by virus-induced IFN-γ production is likely to play an important role.

SHFV

Depending on the virus strain, SHFV causes asymptomatic acute or persistent infections in several species of African monkeys,[85,113] whereas in captive macaques fatal hemorrhagic fever was reported upon SHFV infection[189] (e-Fig. 29.14). Clinical signs in the latter animals consist of early fever, mild facial erythema, and edema, followed by anorexia, dehydration, and various hemorrhagic manifestations. The macaques usually die within 2 weeks, with mortality rates approaching 100%. Very little is known about SHFV pathogenesis in macaques. Macrophages are the primary target cells for SHFV, and a causal relationship exists between the cytocidal infection of these cells and the clinical symptoms of hemorrhagic fever.[84]

PREVENTION AND CONTROL

Diagnosis

Diagnosis of EAV or PRRSV infections on the basis of clinical signs alone is generally very difficult, and therefore not reliable. This is due to the often subclinical or mild symptoms that resemble the symptoms of other respiratory diseases of horses and swine. Differential diagnosis of EAV- or PRRSV-induced abortions are also not straightforward, although these are generally characterized by (partial) autolysis of the fetuses and a lack of pathognomonic lesions, which is for example different for equine herpesvirus-induced abortions where aborted fetuses are usually fresh.[88]

For laboratory diagnosis of EAV, nasopharyngeal swabs or washings, conjunctival swabs, and blood samples can be used. Several reverse transcriptase polymerase chain reaction (RT-PCR) assays are available for detection of EAV RNA in such clinical samples. In addition, immunohistochemistry using monoclonal antibodies to EAV proteins is a reliable method for EAV diagnosis in tissues. A virus neutralization assay remains the gold standard for detection of serum antibodies against EAV.[88]

PRRSV infection can be diagnosed from pig serum or semen samples from boars, umbilical cords from piglets at birth, or serum samples from weaned sows, using fluorescence microscopy, enzyme-linked immunosorbent assay (ELISA), or an RT-PCR test. Recent studies established that PRRSV detection in oral fluids of boars is an alternative to serum and semen sampling, since it gave very similar results, but with far less invasive sampling procedures. These oral samples were collected from cotton ropes impregnated with apple juice and sugar, which the animals were allowed to chew for approximately 20 minutes. Subsequently, fluids were mechanically extracted from the wet ropes and used to measure the presence of PRRSV RNA[98,102] or PRRSV-specific antibodies.[102a]

Disease Control

Equine viral arteritis is a manageable disease. Effective strategies for prevention and control have been designed, and uniform methods and rules have been published by the U.S. Department of Agriculture–Animal and Plant Health Detection Service (USDA-APHIS). These include directions to prevent spread of the virus in horse breeding populations, which usually suffice to suppress the further spread of infection.

Since 2006, the outbreaks of highly virulent PRRSV variants in Asia have boosted research aimed at the development of efficient control strategies against all variants of this virus, which continues to cause significant economic losses worldwide. Changes in swine management have been proven effective in preventing PRRSV outbreaks and are presently thought to be key to controlling the disease in the less intensive swine industry. The method of herd closure, for example, involves the uniform exposure of a confined herd to PRRSV, followed by a continued isolation of the herd for more than 200 days. This effectively eliminates PRRSV, as long as no new animals, and thereby possibly new PRRSV strains, are introduced from outside. In addition, strict biosecurity protocols, including air filtration, have been shown effective (reviewed in 38,46,133 and references therein). In areas with highly intensive pig farming this type of relatively costly strategies are often difficult to implement, and the need for better PRRSV vaccines than those currently available is high (see below).

Because arteriviruses generally infect production or laboratory animals, low priority has been given to the development of antiviral treatments. Infected animals either die quickly of the disease, or are culled as a way to prevent further spread.

Vaccines

For EAV, several genetically engineered candidate vaccines have been developed and tested in experimental infections. Some promising results were obtained with a vaccine based on Venezuelan equine encephalitis virus replicon particles expressing both EAV GP5 and M. Horses vaccinated with this recombinant vaccine produced neutralizing antibodies, shed little or no virus, and developed only mild symptoms after a challenge with virulent EAV.[4] An EAV candidate live marker vaccine was developed on the basis of the deletion of the immunodominant domain of GP5, for which a peptide-specific ELISA is available.[29] This recombinant virus caused an asymptomatic infection in ponies and induced neutralizing antibodies, albeit only against the recombinant and not against the wild-type virus. The vaccinated animals were fully protected against disease following a challenge with virulent EAV.[29] The ELISA for the deleted immunodominant domain can be used to distinguish between vaccinated and naturally infected animals.

For PRRSV, a variety of live-attenuated and killed vaccines are commercially available. The MLV vaccines induce long-lasting protection, but when derived from a single PRRSV vaccine strain they do not fully protect against heterologous PRRSV infection.[97] Furthermore, MLV vaccines do not completely prevent reinfection with wild-type virus and virus transmission. In some situations, it is impossible to discriminate between vaccinated and naturally infected animals. Either a subunit vaccine or a genetically modified live marker vaccine could overcome this problem, although the use of recombinant viruses in the field continues to be debated between vaccine developers, swine practitioners, and animal health authorities.

Adverse effects of vaccination of Danish pig herds with a modified live PRRS vaccine have been described, which were probably caused by reversion of the vaccine virus to virulence. Acute PRRS-like symptoms, including an increasing number of abortions and stillborn piglets, were experienced in vaccinated herds. Furthermore, vaccine virus was transmitted from vaccinated to nonvaccinated boars in several cases, resulting in viremia and shedding of vaccine virus in the semen.[17,89,120,183] In addition, in Thai swine farms, vaccine-derived viruses were found to spread[2] and homologous recombination with circulating virus was observed in China.[108] In this respect, the killed vaccines are safer but they are less efficacious in the induction of protection.[217,252] In general, it is believed that the strong immunomodulatory capabilities of PRRSV prevent the mounting of an efficient vaccine-induced immune response, and that the limited level of immunity that can be induced is insufficient to protect against challenging viruses.[89,192]

Some promising results were obtained in DNA vaccination experiments with plasmids expressing PRRSV GP5.[10,97,150] Neutralizing antibodies and lymphocyte proliferation were detected in DNA-vaccinated pigs, and the spread and clinical signs of challenge virus were reduced. This DNA immunization protocol was, however, not sufficient to prevent virus persistence and shedding in the respiratory tract. Combination with plasmids encoding M or GP3 in some cases increased the immune efficacy of candidate PRRSV DNA vaccines, as did co-delivery with plasmids encoding IFN-γ and IL-2.[92,93,163,239] These results suggest that PRRSV GP5 may at least be a basis for a DNA-based subunit vaccine. Protection against clinical disease and reduction of pathogenic lesions were also observed with a recombinant pseudorabies virus vaccine expressing PRRSV GP5[159] and a recombinant transmissible gastroenteritis coronavirus expressing GP5 and M.[42] Nevertheless, the genetic instability of heterologous genes inserted in these vaccine vectors remains to be solved. Using reverse genetic systems, chimeric infectious cDNA clones have been engineered aimed at developing attenuated modified live virus (marker) vaccines. Chimeric infectious clones in which sequences from virulent field strains were combined with attenuated vaccine strains gave some promising results.[221] The possibility to engineer marker vaccines was demonstrated by the removal of one or multiple conserved immunodominant B-cell epitopes from PRRSV nsp2, which resulted in viable marker viruses eliciting useful immune responses.[49] These deletions themselves, however, did not attenuate the virus, unless a green fluorescent protein marker gene was inserted at the site of the deletion. In this manner, an attenuated virus with both a negative and a positive marker was engineered, although the foreign insert proved to be genetically instable.[73]

A novel approach to increase the immunogenicity of viral subunits is to facilitate their uptake into dendritic cells

(DCs) by inducing the expression of appropriate surface receptors (reviewed in 89). Proof of principle for this approach was recently obtained for CD169, one of the surface receptors for PRRSV, using anti-CD169 monoclonal antibodies as test ligands, which indeed induced *in vitro* T-cell proliferation at 100-fold lower concentrations than the nontargeting control ligand.[160] When more data will become available about the induction of regulatory T cells by PRRSV, this knowledge could be applied to improve vaccine efficacy as well. Removal of viral activities that suppresses innate immune responses is a strategy that is being developed for other viruses like influenza virus, where the innate immune "evasin" NS1 can be removed to produce a viable, attenuated vaccine virus. However, for arteriviruses, this may be far more difficult, since the viral proteins presently thought to suppress innate immunity are indispensable for virus viability.[89]

PERSPECTIVES

A variety of important issues remain to be addressed in future studies of arteriviruses. Most of the viral proteins have been defined in basic terms only, and understanding the molecular details of their role in the viral life cycle is one of the major challenges for arterivirus research. For example, the characterization of the now eight structural proteins and their functional interactions during particle assembly and disassembly promises to be a highly complex issue, which also links to the many unanswered questions regarding host cell functions relevant for arterivirus attachment and entry.

In recent years, prompted in particular by the enormous PRRSV problems in Asia, determinants of arterivirus pathogenesis and virulence have received a lot of attention. The outline of a highly complex interplay between arterivirus and host is emerging, which will undoubtedly prove to be a critical factor in future vaccine development as well. Reverse genetics will continue to be a crucial tool for both basic and applied research in this area.

Our understanding of arterivirus epidemiology and evolution must be improved to prevent problems like the Asian PRRS outbreak in the future, and this field also connects to the interesting question of the potential for arterivirus cross-species transmission. On a different evolutionary level, that of the order *Nidovirales,* arteriviruses continue to be part of a unique group of positive-strand RNA viruses that is characterized by having the largest and most complicated replication machinery among currently known RNA viruses. In anticipation of systems allowing the complete *in vitro* reconstitution of arterivirus RNA synthesis, progress will continue to depend on successfully combining bioinformatics, biochemistry, and structural and molecular biology. This powerful approach has already provided detailed insights in some of the intricacies of arterivirus RNA synthesis, replication structures, and virus–host interactions, which will also be key to the design of antiviral strategies to combat diseases caused by known or currently unknown arteriviruses. Modern virus hunting techniques are increasingly likely to identify such additional family members in the years to come. This might compensate for the fact that—based on the inapparent and persistent infections frequently caused by currently known arteriviruses—clinical symptoms may not be the most direct indicator for arterivirus infections in other species.

REFERENCES

All cited references are available in the e-book.

1. Ammann CG, Messer RJ, Peterson KE, et al. Lactate dehydrogenase-elevating virus induces systemic lymphocyte activation via TLR7-dependent IFNalpha responses by plasmacytoid dendritic cells. *PLoS One* 2009;4:e6105.
2. Amonsin A, Kedkovid R, Puranaveja S, et al. Comparative analysis of complete nucleotide sequence of porcine reproductive and respiratory syndrome virus (PRRSV) isolates in Thailand (US and EU genotypes). *Virol J* 2009;6:143.
4. Balasuriya UB, Heidner HW, Davis NL, et al. Alphavirus replicon particles expressing the two major envelope proteins of equine arteritis virus induce high level protection against challenge with virulent virus in vaccinated horses. *Vaccine* 2002;20:1609–1617.
5. Balasuriya UB, Maclachlan NJ. The immune response to equine arteritis virus: potential lessons for other arteriviruses. *Vet Immunol Immunopathol* 2004;102:107–129.
6. Balasuriya UB, Patton JF, Rossitto PV, et al. Neutralization determinants of laboratory strains and field isolates of equine arteritis virus: Identification of four neutralization sites in the amino-terminal ectodomain of the GL envelope glycoprotein. *Virology* 1997;232:114–128.
7. Balasuriya UB, Snijder EJ, Heidner HW, et al. Development and characterization of an infectious cDNA clone of the virulent Bucyrus strain of Equine arteritis virus. *J Gen Virol* 2007;88:918–924.
8. Balasuriya UBR, Dobbe JC, Heidner HW, et al. Characterization of the neutralization determinants of equine arteritis virus using recombinant chimeric viruses and site-specific mutagenesis of an infectious cDNA clone. *Virology* 2004;327:318–319.
9. Balasuriya UBR, Hedges JF, Smalley VL, et al. Genetic characterization of equine arteritis virus during persistent infection of stallions. *J Gen Virol* 2004;85:379–390.
11. Barrette-Ng IH, Ng KKS, Mark BL, et al. Structure of arterivirus nsp4 - The smallest chymotrypsin-like proteinase with an alpha/beta C-terminal extension and alternate conformations of the oxyanion hole. *J Biol Chem* 2002;277:39960–39966.
13. Beerens N, Selisko B, Ricagno S, et al. De novo initiation of RNA synthesis by the arterivirus RNA-dependent RNA polymerase. *J Virol* 2007; 81:8384–8395.
15. Beerens N, Snijder EJ. An RNA pseudoknot in the 3′ end of the arterivirus genome has a critical role in regulating viral RNA synthesis. *J Virol* 2007;81:9426–9436.
16. Beura LK, Sarkar SN, Kwon B, et al. Porcine reproductive and respiratory syndrome virus nonstructural protein 1beta modulates host innate immune response by antagonizing IRF3 activation. *J Virol* 2010;84: 1574–1584.
17. Botner A, Strandbygaard B, Sorensen KJ, et al. Appearance of acute PRRS-like symptoms in sow herds after vaccination with a modified live PRRS vaccine. *Vet Rec* 1997;141:497–499.
21. Butler JE, Wertz N, Weber P, et al. Porcine reproductive and respiratory syndrome virus subverts repertoire development by proliferation of germline-encoded B cells of all isotypes bearing hydrophobic heavy chain CDR3. *J Immunol* 2008;180:2347–2356.
23. Cafruny WA, Bradley SE. Trojan horse macrophages: studies with the murine lactate dehydrogenase-elevating virus and implications for sexually transmitted virus infection. *J Gen Virol* 1996;77:3005–3012.
24. Cafruny WA, Chan SP, Harty JT, et al. Antibody response of mice to lactate dehydrogenase-elevating virus during infection and immunization with inactivated virus. *Virus Res* 1986;5:357–375.
25. Cafruny WA, Plagemann PGW. Immune response to lactate dehydrogenase-elevating virus: serologically specific rabbit neutralizing antibody to the virus. *Infect Immun* 1982;37:1007–1012.
26. Calvert JG, Slade DE, Shields SL, et al. CD163 expression confers susceptibility to porcine reproductive and respiratory syndrome viruses. *J Virol* 2007;81:7371–7379.
27. Cancel-Tirado SM, Evans RB, Yoon KJ. Monoclonal antibody analysis of porcine reproductive and respiratory syndrome virus epitopes associated with antibody-dependent enhancement and neutralization of virus infection. *Vet Immunol Immunopathol* 2004;102:249–262.

29. Castillo-Olivares J, Wieringa R, Bakonyi T, et al. Generation of a candidate live marker vaccine for equine arteritis virus by deletion of the major virus neutralization domain. *J Virol* 2003;77:8470–8480.
31. Chen Z, Lawson S, Sun Z, et al. Identification of two auto-cleavage products of nonstructural protein 1 (nsp1) in porcine reproductive and respiratory syndrome virus infected cells: nsp1 function as interferon antagonist. *Virology* 2010;398:87–97.
32. Chen Z, Rowland RRR, Anderson GW, et al. Coexistence in lactate dehydrogenase-elevating virus pools of variants that differ in neuropathogenicity and ability to establish a persistent infection. *J Virol* 1997;71: 2913–2920.
33. Chen Z, Zhou X, Lunney JK, et al. Immunodominant epitopes in nsp2 of porcine reproductive and respiratory syndrome virus are dispensable for replication, but play an important role in modulation of the host immune response. *J Gen Virol* 2010;91:1047–1057.
34. Chirnside ED, Francis PM, de Vries AAF, et al. Development and evaluation of an ELISA using recombinant fusion protein to detect the presence of host antibody to equine arteritis virus. *J Virol Methods* 1995;54:1–13.
35. Cho JG, Dee SA. Porcine reproductive and respiratory syndrome virus. *Theriogenology* 2006;66:655–662.
36. Collins JE, Benfield DA, Christianson WT, et al. Isolation of swine infertility and respiratory syndrome virus (isolate ATCC VR-2332) in North America and experimental reproduction of the disease in gnotobiotic pigs. *J Vet Diagn Invest* 1992;4:117–126.
37. Contag CH, Plagemann PGW. Age-dependent poliomyelitis of mice: expression of endogenous retrovirus correlates with cytocidal replication of lactate dehydrogenase-elevating virus in motor neurons. *J Virol* 1989; 63:4362–4369.
38. Corzo CA, Mondaca E, Wayne S, et al. Control and elimination of porcine reproductive and respiratory syndrome virus. *Virus Res* 2010;154: 185–192.
39. Costers S, Lefebvre DJ, Delputte PL, et al. Porcine reproductive and respiratory syndrome virus modulates apoptosis during replication in alveolar macrophages. *Arch Virol* 2008;153:1453–1465.
41. Costers S, Vanhee M, Van Breedam W, et al. GP4-specific neutralizing antibodies might be a driving force in PRRSV evolution. *Virus Res* 2010; 154:104–113.
42. Cruz JL, Zuniga S, Bécares M, et al. Vectored vaccines to protect against PRRSV. *Virus Res* 2010;154:150–160.
43. Darwich L, Diaz I, Mateu E. Certainties, doubts and hypotheses in porcine reproductive and respiratory syndrome virus immunobiology. *Virus Res* 2010;154:123–132.
44. Das PB, Dinh PX, Ansari IH, et al. The minor envelope glycoproteins GP2a and GP4 of porcine reproductive and respiratory syndrome virus interact with the receptor CD163. *J Virol* 2010;84:1731–1740.
45. Das PB, Vu HL, Dinh PX, et al. Glycosylation of minor envelope glycoproteins of porcine reproductive and respiratory syndrome virus in infectious virus recovery, receptor interaction, and immune response. *Virology* 2011;410:385–394.
46. Dee S, Otake S, Deen J. Use of a production region model to assess the efficacy of various air filtration systems for preventing airborne transmission of porcine reproductive and respiratory syndrome virus and Mycoplasma hyopneumoniae: results from a 2-year study. *Virus Res* 2010; 154:177–184.
48. deLima M, Ansari IH, Das PB, et al. GP3 is a structural component of the PRRSV type II (US) virion. *Virology* 2009;390:31–36.
49. deLima M, Kwon B, Ansari IH, et al. Development of a porcine reproductive and respiratory syndrome virus differentiable (DIVA) strain through deletion of specific immunodominant epitopes. *Vaccine* 2008;26:3594–3600.
50. Delputte PL, Nauwynck HJ. Porcine arterivirus infection of alveolar macrophages is mediated by sialic acid on the virus. *J Virol* 2004;78: 8094–8101.
51. Delputte PL, Vanderheijden N, Nauwynck HJ, et al. Involvement of the matrix protein in attachment of porcine reproductive and respiratory syndrome virus to a heparinlike receptor on porcine alveolar macrophages. *J Virol* 2002;76:4312–4320.
52. den Boon JA, Faaberg KS, Meulenberg JJM, et al. Processing and evolution of the N-terminal region of the arterivirus replicase ORF1a protein: identification of two papainlike cysteine proteases. *J Virol* 1995;69: 4500–4505.
54. den Boon JA, Snijder EJ, Chirnside ED, et al. Equine arteritis virus is not a togavirus but belongs to the coronaviruslike superfamily. *J Virol* 1991; 65:2910–2920.
55. de Vries AAF, Chirnside ED, Bredenbeek PJ, et al. All subgenomic mRNAs of equine arteritis virus contain a common leader sequence. *Nucleic Acids Res* 1990;18:3241–3247.
56. de Vries AAF, Chirnside ED, Horzinek MC, et al. Structural proteins of equine arteritis virus. *J Virol* 1992;66:6294–6303.
57. de Vries AAF, Post SM, Raamsman MJB, et al. The two major envelope proteins of equine arteritis virus associate into disulfide-linked heterodimers. *J Virol* 1995;69:4668–4674.
58. Diaz I, Darwich L, Pappaterra G, et al. Immune responses of pigs after experimental infection with a European strain of Porcine reproductive and respiratory syndrome virus. *J Gen Virol* 2005;86:1943–1951.
59. Doan DNP, Dokland T. Structure of the nucleocapsid protein of porcine reproductive and respiratory syndrome virus. *Structure* 2003;11: 1445–1451.
60. Dobbe JC, van der Meer Y, Spaan WJM, et al. Construction of chimeric arteriviruses reveals that the ectodomain of the major glycoprotein is not the main determinant of equine arteritis virus tropism in cell culture. *Virology* 2001;288:283–294.
61. Dokland T. The structural biology of PRRSV. *Virus Res* 2011;154:86–97.
62. Doll ER, Bryans JT, McCollum WH, et al. Isolation of a filterable agent causing arteritis of horses and abortion by mares. Its differentiation from the equine abortion (influenza) virus. *Cornell Vet* 1957;47:3–41.
64. Duan X, Nauwynck HJ, Favoreel HW, et al. Identification of a putative receptor for porcine reproductive and respiratory syndrome virus on porcine alveolar macrophages. *J Virol* 1998;72:4520–4523.
65. Duan X, Nauwynck HJ, Pensaert MB. Effects of origin and state of differentiation and activation of monocytes/macrophages on their susceptibility to porcine reproductive and respiratory syndrome virus (PRRSV). *Arch Virol* 1997;142:2483–2497.
66a. Dunowska M, Biggs PJ, Zheng T, Perrott MR. Identification of a novel nidovirus associated with a neurological disease of the Australian brushtail possum (Trichosurus vulpecula). *Vet Microbiol* 2012 156:418–424.
67. Even C, Rowland RRR, Plagemann PGW. Cytotoxic T cells are elicited during acute infection of mice with lactate dehydrogenase-elevating virus but disappear during the chronic phase of infection. *J Virol* 1995;69:5666–5676.
68. Faaberg KS, Balasuriya UB, Brinton MA, et al. Familiy Arteriviridae. In: King A, Adams M, Carstens E, Lefkowitz EJ, eds. *Virus Taxonomy, the 9th Report of the International Committee on Taxonomy of Viruses.* London: Academic Press; 2012:796–805.
69. Faaberg KS, Even C, Palmer GA, et al. Disulfide bonds between two envelope proteins of lactate dehydrogenase-elevating virus are essential for viral infectivity. *J Virol* 1995;69:613–617.
70. Faaberg KS, Plagemann PGW. The envelope proteins of lactate dehydrogenase-elevating virus and their membrane topography. *Virology* 1995; 212:512–525.
72. Fang L, Jiang Y, Xiao S, et al. Enhanced immunogenicity of the modified GP5 of porcine reproductive and respiratory syndrome virus. *Virus Genes* 2006;32:5–11.
73. Fang Y, Christopher-Hennings J, Brown E, et al. Development of genetic markers in the non-structural protein 2 region of a US type 1 porcine reproductive and respiratory syndrome virus: implications for future recombinant marker vaccine development. *J Gen Virol* 2008;89:3086–3096.
74. Fang Y, Snijder EJ. The PRRSV replicase: Exploring the multifunctionality of an intriguing set of nonstructural proteins. *Virus Res* 2010;154:61–76.
75. Firth AE, Zevenhoven-Dobbe JC, Wills NM, et al. Discovery of a small arterivirus gene that overlaps the GP5 coding sequence and is important for virus production. *J Gen Virol* 2011;92:1097–1106.
76. Frias-Staheli N, Giannakopoulos NV, Kikkert M, et al. Ovarian tumor domain-containing viral proteases evade ubiquitin- and ISG15-dependent innate immune responses. *Cell Host Microbe* 2007;2:404–416.
77. Fukunaga Y, Imagawa H, Tabuchi E, et al. Clinical and virological findings in experimental equine viral arteritis in horses. *Bull Equine Res Inst* 1981;18:110–118.
78. Go YY, Bailey E, Cook DG, et al. Genome-wide association study among four horse breeds identifies a common haplotype associated with in vitro CD3+ T cell susceptibility/resistance to equine arteritis virus infection. *J Virol* 2011;85:13174–13184.

79. Go YY, Snijder EJ, Timoney PJ, et al. Characterization of equine humoral antibody response to the nonstructural proteins of equine arteritis virus. *Clin Vaccine Immunol* 2011;18:268–279.
80. Go YY, Zhang J, Timoney PJ, et al. Complex interactions between the major and minor envelope proteins of equine arteritis virus determine its tropism for equine CD3+ T lymphocytes and CD14+ monocytes. *J Virol* 2010;84:4898–4911.
81. Godeny EK, de Vries AAF, Wang XC, et al. Identification of the leader-body junctions for the viral subgenomic mRNAs and organization of the simian hemorrhagic fever virus genome: evidence for gene duplication during arterivirus evolution. *J Virol* 1998;72:862–867.
83. Gorbalenya AE, Enjuanes L, Ziebuhr J, et al. Nidovirales: Evolving the largest RNA virus genome. *Virus Res* 2006;117:17–37.
84. Gravell M, London WT, Leon ME, et al. Differences among isolates of simian hemorrhagic fever (SHF) virus. *Proc Soc Exp Biol Med* 1986;181:112–119.
85. Gravell M, London WT, Leon ME, et al. Elimination of persistent simian hemorrhagic fever (SHF) virus infection in patas monkeys. *Proc Soc Exp Biol Med* 1986;181:219–225.
86. Han J, Rutherford MS, Faaberg KS. The porcine reproductive and respiratory syndrome virus nsp2 cysteine protease domain possesses both trans- and cis-cleavage activities. *J Virol* 2009;83:9449–9463.
88. Holyoak GR, Balasuriya UB, Broaddus CC, et al. Equine viral arteritis: current status and prevention. *Theriogenology* 2008;70:403–414.
89. Huang YW, Meng XJ. Novel strategies and approaches to develop the next generation of vaccines against porcine reproductive and respiratory syndrome virus (PRRSV). *Virus Res* 2010;154:141–149.
90. Hwang Y-K, Brinton MA. A 68nt sequence within the 3′ noncoding region (NCR) of simian hemorrhagic fever virus negative-strand RNA binds to four MA104 cell protein. *J Virol* 1998;72:4341–4351.
92. Jiang W, Jiang P, Wang X, et al. Enhanced immune responses of mice inoculated recombinant adenoviruses expressing GP5 by fusion with GP3 and/or GP4 of PRRS virus. *Virus Res* 2008;136:50–57.
93. Jiang Y, Xiao S, Fang L, et al. DNA vaccines co-expressing GP5 and M proteins of porcine reproductive and respiratory syndrome virus (PRRSV) display enhanced immunogenicity. *Vaccine* 2006;24:2869–2879.
94. Johnson CR, Griggs TF, Gnanandarajah J, et al. Novel structural protein in porcine reproductive and respiratory syndrome virus encoded by an alternative ORF5 present in all arteriviruses. *J Gen Virol* 2011;92:1107–1116.
95. Johnson CR, Yu W, Murtaugh MP. Cross-reactive antibody responses to nsp1 and nsp2 of Porcine reproductive and respiratory syndrome virus. *J Gen Virol* 2007;88:1184–1195.
96. Kim O, Sun Y, Lai FW, et al. Modulation of type I interferon induction by porcine reproductive and respiratory syndrome virus and degradation of CREB-binding protein by non-structural protein 1 in MARC-145 and HeLa cells. *Virology* 2010;402:315–326.
97. Kimman TG, Cornelissen LA, Moormann RJM, et al. Challenges for porcine reproductive and respiratory syndrome virus (PRRSV) vaccinology. *Vaccine* 2009:27(28)3704–3718.
98. Kittawornrat A, Prickett J, Chittick W, et al. Porcine reproductive and respiratory syndrome virus (PRRSV) in serum and oral fluid samples from individual boars: will oral fluid replace serum for PRRSV surveillance? *Virus Res* 2010;154:170–176.
99. Knoops K, Bárcena M, Limpens RWAL, et al. Ultrastructural characterization of arterivirus replication structures: Reshaping the endoplasmic reticulum to accommodate viral RNA synthesis. *J Virol* 2012;86:2474–2487.
101. Kreutz LC, Ackermann MR. Porcine reproductive and respiratory syndrome virus enters cells through a low pH dependent endocytic pathway. *Virus Res* 1996;42:137–147.
102. Kroese MV, Zevenhoven-Dobbe JC, Bos-de Ruijter JN, et al. The nsp1alpha and nsp1 papain-like autoproteinases are essential for porcine reproductive and respiratory syndrome virus RNA synthesis. *J Gen Virol* 2008;89:494–499.
102a. Langenhorst RJ, Lawson S, Kittawornrat A, et al. Development of a fluorescent microsphere immunoassay for detection of antibodies against porcine reproductive and respiratory syndrome virus using oral fluid samples as an alternative to serum-based assays. *Clin Vaccine Immunol.* 2012;19:180–189.
103. Lauck M, Hyeroba D, Tumukunde A, et al. Novel, divergent simian hemorrhagic fever viruses in a wild Ugandan red colobus monkey discovered using direct pyrosequencing. *PLoS One* 2011;6:e19056.
105. Lee C, Hodgins D, Calvert JG, et al. Mutations within the nuclear localization signal of the porcine reproductive and respiratory syndrome virus nucleocapsid protein attenuate virus replication. *Virology* 2006;346:238–250.
106. Lee C, Hodgins D, Calvert JG, et al. The small envelope protein of porcine reproductive and respiratory syndrome virus possesses ion channel protein-like properties. *Virology* 2006;355:30–43.
107. Li B, Fang L, Guo X, et al. Epidemiology and evolutionary characteristics of the porcine reproductive and respiratory syndrome virus in China between 2006 and 2010. *J Clin Microbiol* 2011;49:3175–3183.
108. Li B, Fang L, Xu Z, et al. Recombination in vaccine and circulating strains of porcine reproductive and respiratory syndrome viruses. *Emerg Infect Dis* 2009;15:2032–2035.
109. Li H, Zheng Z, Zhou P, et al. The cysteine protease domain of porcine reproductive and respiratory syndrome virus non-structural protein 2 antagonizes interferon regulatory factor 3 activation. *J Gen Virol* 2010;91:2947–2958.
110. Li K, Chen Z, Plagemann PGW. The neutralization epitope of lactate dehydrogenase-elevating virus is located on the short ectodomain of the primary envelope glycoprotein. *Virology* 1998;242:239–245.
111. Li Y, Wang X, Bo K, et al. Emergence of a highly pathogenic porcine reproductive and respiratory syndrome virus in the Mid-Eastern region of China. *Vet J* 2007;174:577–584.
112. Loemba HD, Mounir S, Mardassi H, et al. Kinetics of humoral immune response to the major structural proteins of the porcine reproductive and respiratory syndrome virus. *Arch Virol* 1996;141:751–761.
113. London WT. Epizootiology, transmission, and approach to prevention of fatal simian hemorrhagic fever in rhesus monkeys. *Nature* 1977;268:344–345.
114. Lopez OJ, Osorio FA. Role of neutralizing antibodies in PRRSV protective immunity. *Vet Immunol Immunopathol* 2004;102:155–163.
115. Lu J, Gao F, Wei Z, et al. A 5′-proximal stem-loop structure of 5′ untranslated region of porcine reproductive and respiratory syndrome virus genome is key for virus replication. *Virol J* 2011;8:172.
116. Lunney JK, Chen H. Genetic control of host resistance to porcine reproductive and respiratory syndrome virus (PRRSV) infection. *Virus Res* 2010;154:161–169.
117. Lunney JK, Fritz ER, Reecy JM, et al. Interleukin-8, interleukin-1beta, and interferon-gamma levels are linked to PRRS virus clearance. *Viral Immunol* 2010;23:127–134.
118. Maclachlan NJ, Balasuriya UB, Hedges JF, et al. Serologic response of horses to the structural proteins of equine arteritis virus. *J Vet Diagn Investig* 1998;10:229–236.
122. Maines TR, Young M, Dinh NNN, et al. Two cellular proteins that interact with a stem loop in the simian hemorrhagic fever virus 3′ (+) NCR RNA. *Virus Res* 2005;109:109–124.
124. Markine-Goriaynoff D, Hulhoven X, Cambiaso CL, et al. Natural killer cell activation after infection with lactate dehydrogenase-elevating virus. *J Gen Virol* 2002;83:2709–2716.
125. Mateu E, Diaz I. The challenge of PRRS immunology. *Vet J* 2008;177:345–351.
126. Meier WA, Galeota J, Osorio FA, et al. Gradual development of the interferon-gamma response of swine to porcine reproductive and respiratory syndrome virus infection or vaccination. *Virology* 2003;309:18–31.
129. Meulenberg JJM, van Nieuwstadt AP, van Essen-Zandbergen A, et al. Posttranslational processing and identification of a neutralization domain of the GP4 protein encoded by ORF4 of Lelystad virus. *J Virol* 1997;71:6061–6067.
130. Molenkamp R, Rozier BCD, Greve S, et al. Isolation and characterization of an arterivirus defective interfering RNA genome. *J Virol* 2000;74:3156–3165.
131. Molenkamp R, van Tol H, Rozier BCD, et al. The arterivirus replicase is the only viral protein required for genome replication and subgenomic mRNA transcription. *J Gen Virol* 2000;81:2491–2496.
132. Moore BD, Balasuriya UBR, Watson JL, et al. Virulent and avirulent strains of equine arteritis virus induce different quantities of TNF-alpha and other proinflammatory cytokines in alveolar and blood-derived equine macrophages. *Virology* 2003;314:662–670.
133. Murtaugh MP, Stadejek T, Abrahante E, et al. The ever-expanding diversity of porcine reproductive and respiratory syndrome virus. *Virus Res* 2010;154:18–30.
134. Murtaugh MP, Xiao ZG, Zuckermann F. Immunological responses of swine to porcine reproductive and respiratory syndrome virus infection. *Viral Immunol* 2002;15:533–547.

135. Musaji A, Cormont F, Thirion G, et al. Exacerbation of autoantibody-mediated thrombocytopenic purpura by infection with mouse viruses. *Blood* 2004;104:2102–2106.
137. Nauwynck HJ, Duan X, Favoreel HW, et al. Entry of porcine reproductive and respiratory syndrome virus into porcine alveolar macrophages via receptor-mediated endocytosis. *J Gen Virol* 1999;80:297–305.
138. Nedialkova DD, Gorbalenya AE, Snijder EJ. Arterivirus nsp1 modulates the accumulation of minus-strand templates to control the relative abundance of viral mRNAs. *PLoS Pathog* 2010;6:e1000772.
139. Nedialkova DD, Ulferts R, van den Born E, et al. Biochemical characterization of arterivirus nonstructural protein 11 reveals the nidovirus-wide conservation of a replicative endoribonuclease. *J Virol* 2009;83:5671–5682.
140. Nga PT, del Carmen Parquet M, Lauber C, et al. Discovery of the first insect nidovirus, a missing evolutionary link in the emergence of the largest RNA virus genomes. *PLoS Pathog* 2011;7:e1002215.
141. Nitschke M, Korte T, Tielesch C, et al. Equine arteritis virus is delivered to an acidic compartment of host cells via clathrin-dependent endocytosis. *Virology* 2008;377:248–254.
142. Onyekaba CO, Harty JT, Plagemann PGW. Extensive cytocidal replication of lactate dehydrogenase- elevating virus in cultured peritoneal macrophages from 1–2-week- old mice. *Virus Res* 1989;14:327–338.
143. Ostrowski M, Galeota JA, Jar AM, et al. Identification of neutralizing and nonneutralizing epitopes in the porcine reproductive and respiratory syndrome virus GP5 ectodomain. *J Virol* 2002;76:4241–4250.
146. Pasternak AO, Spaan WJM, Snijder EJ. Nidovirus transcription: how to make sense.? *J Gen Virol* 2006;87:1403–1421.
147. Pasternak AO, van den Born E, Spaan WJM, et al. Sequence requirements for RNA strand transfer during nidovirus discontinuous subgenomic RNA synthesis. *EMBO J* 2001;20:7220–7228.
148. Pasternak AO, van den Born E, Spaan WJM, et al. The stability of the duplex between sense and antisense transcription- regulating sequences is a crucial factor in arterivirus subgenomic mRNA synthesis. *J Virol* 2003;77:1175–1183.
149. Pedersen KW, van der Meer Y, Roos N, et al. Open reading frame 1a-encoded subunits of the arterivirus replicase induce endoplasmic reticulum-derived double-membrane vesicles which carry the viral replication complex. *J Virol* 1999;73:2016–2026.
150. Pirzadeh B, Dea S. Immune response in pigs vaccinated with plasmid DNA encoding ORF5 of porcine reproductive and respiratory syndrome virus. *J Gen Virol* 1998;79:989–999.
152. Plagemann PGW. Porcine reproductive and respiratory syndrome virus: Origin hypothesis. *Emerg Infect Dis* 2003;9:903–908.
154. Plagemann PGW. The primary GP5 neutralization epitope of North American isolates of porcine reproductive and respiratory syndrome virus. *Vet Immunol Immunopathol* 2004;102:263–275.
155. Plagemann PGW, Moennig V. Lactate dehydrogenase-elevating virus, equine arteritis virus, and simian hemorrhagic fever virus: a new group of positive-strand RNA viruses. *Adv Virus Res* 1992;41:99–192.
156. Plagemann PGW, Rowland RRR, Faaberg KS. The primary neutralization epitope of porcine respiratory and reproductive syndrome virus strain VR-2332 is located in the middle of the GP5 ectodomain. *Arch Virol* 2002;147:2327–2347.
157. Posthuma CC, Nedialkova DD, Zevenhoven-Dobbe JC, et al. Site-directed mutagenesis of the nidovirus replicative endoribonuclease NendoU exerts pleiotropic effects on the arterivirus life cycle. *J Virol* 2006; 80:1653–1661.
158. Posthuma CC, Pedersen KW, Lu Z, et al. Formation of the arterivirus replication/transcription complex: a key role for nonstructural protein 3 in the remodeling of intracellular membranes. *J Virol* 2008;82: 4480–4491.
159. Qiu HJ, Tian ZJ, Tong GZ, et al. Protective immunity induced by a recombinant pseudorabies virus expressing the GP5 of porcine reproductive and respiratory syndrome virus in piglets. *Vet Immunol Immunopathol* 2005; 106:309–319.
160. Revilla C, Poderoso T, Martinez P, et al. Targeting to porcine sialoadhesin receptor improves antigen presentation to T cells. *Vet Res* 2009;40:14.
161. Riley V, Lilly F, Huerto E, et al. Transmissible agent associated with 26 types of experimental mouse neoplasms. *Science* 1960;132:545–547.
162. Robertson SJ, Ammann CG, Messer RJ, et al. Suppression of acute anti-friend virus CD8+ T-cell responses by coinfection with lactate dehydrogenase-elevating virus. *J Virol* 2008;82:408–418.
163. Rompato G, Ling E, Chen Z, et al. Positive inductive effect of IL-2 on virus-specific cellular responses elicited by a PRRSV-ORF7 DNA vaccine in swine. *Vet Immunol Immunopathol* 2006;109:151–160.
164. Rowland RRR, Schneider P, Fang Y, et al. Peptide domains involved in the localization of the porcine reproductive and respiratory syndrome virus nucleocapsid protein to the nucleolus. *Virology* 2003;316:135–145.
168. Sawicki SG, Sawicki DL, Siddell SG. A contemporary view of coronavirus transcription. *J Virol* 2007;81:20–29.
169. Seybert A, van Dinten LC, Snijder EJ, et al. Biochemical characterization of the equine arteritis virus helicase suggests a close functional relationship between arterivirus and coronavirus helicases. *J Virol* 2000;74:9586–9593.
170. Shi M, Lam TT, Hon CC, et al. Molecular epidemiology of PRRSV: a phylogenetic perspective. *Virus Res* 2010:154(1-2):7–17.
171. Shi X, Wang L, Li X, et al. Endoribonuclease activities of porcine reproductive and respiratory syndrome virus nsp11 was essential for nsp11 to inhibit IFN-ß induction. *Mol Immunol* 2011;48:1568–1572.
172. Silva-Campa E, Flores-Mendoza L, Reséndiz M, et al. Induction of T helper 3 regulatory cells by dendritic cells infected with porcine reproductive and respiratory syndrome virus. *Virology* 2009;387:373–379.
173. Snijder EJ, Bredenbeek PJ, Dobbe JC, et al. Unique and conserved features of genome and proteome of SARS-coronavirus, an early split-off from the coronavirus group 2 lineage. *J Mol Biol* 2003;331:991–1004.
174. Snijder EJ, Dobbe JC, Spaan WJM. Heterodimerization of the two major envelope proteins is essential for arterivirus infectivity. *J Virol* 2003;77: 97–104.
175. Snijder EJ, Meulenberg JJM. The molecular biology of arteriviruses. *J Gen Virol* 1998;79:961–979.
176. Snijder EJ, van Tol H, Pedersen KW, et al. Identification of a novel structural protein of arteriviruses. *J Virol* 1999;73:6335–6345.
178. Snijder EJ, Wassenaar ALM, Spaan WJM. Proteolytic processing of the replicase ORF1a protein of equine arteritis virus. *J Virol* 1994;68:5755–5764.
179. Snijder EJ, Wassenaar ALM, Spaan WJM, et al. The arterivirus nsp2 protease. An unusual cysteine protease with primary structure similarities to both papain-like and chymotrypsin-like proteases. *J Biol Chem* 1995;270:16671–16676.
180. Snijder EJ, Wassenaar ALM, van Dinten LC, et al. The arterivirus nsp4 protease is the prototype of a novel group of chymotrypsin-like enzymes, the 3C-like serine proteases. *J Biol Chem* 1996;271:4864–4871.
181. Song C, Krell P, Yoo D. Nonstructural protein 1alpha subunit-based inhibition of NF-kappaB activation and suppression of interferon-beta production by porcine reproductive and respiratory syndrome virus. *Virology* 2010;407:268–280.
182. Spilman MS, Welbon C, Nelson E, et al. Cryo-electron tomography of porcine reproductive and respiratory syndrome virus: organization of the nucleocapsid. *J Gen Virol* 2009;90:527–535.
185. Suarez P, Diaz Guerra M, Prieto C, et al. Open reading frame 5 of porcine reproductive and respiratory syndrome virus as a cause of virus-induced apoptosis. *J Virol* 1996;70:2876–2882.
186. Sun Y, Xue F, Guo Y, et al. Crystal structure of porcine reproductive and respiratory syndrome virus leader protease Nsp1alpha. *J Virol* 2009; 83:10931–10940.
188. Sur JH, Doster AR, Christian JS, et al. Porcine reproductive and respiratory syndrome virus replicates in testicular germ cells, alters spermatogenesis, and induces germ cell death by apoptosis. *J Virol* 1997;71:9170–9179.
189. Tauraso NM, Shelokov A, Palmer AE, et al. Simian hemorrhagic fever. III. Isolation and characterization of a viral agent. *Am J Trop Med Hyg* 1968;17: 422–431.
190. Thaa B, Kabatek A, Zevenhoven-Dobbe JC, et al. Myristoylation of the arterivirus E protein: the fatty acid modification is not essential for membrane association but contributes significantly to virus infectivity. *J Gen Virol* 2009;90:2704–2712.
191. Thanawongnuwech R, Halbur PG, Thacker EL. The role of pulmonary intravascular macrophages in porcine reproductive and respiratory syndrome virus infection. *Anim Health Res Rev* 2000;1:95–102.
192. Thanawongnuwech R, Suradhat S. Taming PRRSV: revisiting the control strategies and vaccine design. *Virus Res* 2010;154:133–140.
193. Tian D, Wei Z, Zevenhoven-Dobbe JC, et al. Arterivirus minor envelope proteins are the major determinant of viral tropism in cell culture. *J Virol* 2012;86:3701–3712.
194. Tian K, Yu X, Zhao T, et al. Emergence of fatal PRRSV variants: unparalleled outbreaks of atypical PRRS in China and molecular dissection of the unique hallmark. *PLoS One* 2007;2:e526.

195. Tian X, Lu G, Gao F, et al. Structure and cleavage specificity of the chymotrypsin-like serine protease (3CLSP/nsp4) of Porcine Reproductive and Respiratory Syndrome Virus (PRRSV). *J Mol Biol* 2009;392:977–993.
197. Tijms MA, van der Meer Y, Snijder EJ. Nuclear localization of non-structural protein 1 and nucleocapsid protein of equine arteritis virus. *J Gen Virol* 2002;83:795–800.
200. van Aken D, Benckhuijsen WE, Drijfhout JW, et al. Expression, purification, and in vitro activity of an arterivirus main proteinase. *Virus Res* 2006; 120:97–106.
201. van Aken D, Snijder EJ, Gorbalenya AE. Mutagenesis analysis of the nsp4 main proteinase reveals determinants of arterivirus replicase polyprotein autoprocessing. *J Virol* 2006;80:3428–3437.
202. van Aken D, Zevenhoven-Dobbe JC, Gorbalenya AE, et al. Proteolytic maturation of replicase polyprotein pp1a by the nsp4 main proteinase is essential for equine arteritis virus replication and includes internal cleavage of nsp7. *J Gen Virol* 2006;87:3473–3482.
203. Van Breedam W, Delputte PL, Van GH, et al. Porcine reproductive and respiratory syndrome virus entry into the porcine macrophage. *J Gen Virol* 2010;91:1659–1667.
204. Van Breedam W, Van GH, Zhang JQ, et al. The M/GP5 glycoprotein complex of porcine reproductive and respiratory syndrome virus binds the sialoadhesin receptor in a sialic acid-dependent manner. *PLoS Pathog* 2010;6:e1000730.
205. van den Born E, Gultyaev AP, Snijder EJ. Secondary structure and function of the 5′-proximal region of the equine arteritis virus RNA genome. *RNA* 2004;10:424–437.
207. van der Meer Y, van Tol H, Krijnse Locker J, et al. ORF1a-encoded replicase subunits are involved in the membrane association of the arterivirus replication complex. *J Virol* 1998;72:6689–6698.
208. van Dinten LC, den Boon JA, Wassenaar ALM, et al. An infectious arterivirus cDNA clone: identification of a replicase point mutation which abolishes discontinuous mRNA transcription. *Proc Natl Acad Sci U S A* 1997;94:991–996.
209. van Dinten LC, Rensen S, Spaan WJM, et al. Proteolytic processing of the open reading frame 1b-encoded part of arterivirus replicase is mediated by nsp4 serine protease and is essential for virus replication. *J Virol* 1999;73:2027–2037.
211. Van Gorp H, Van Breedam W, Delputte PL, et al. Sialoadhesin and CD163 join forces during entry of the porcine reproductive and respiratory syndrome virus. *J Gen Virol* 2008;89:2943–2953.
212. van Hemert MJ, de Wilde AH, Gorbalenya AE, et al. The in vitro RNA synthesizing activity of the isolated arterivirus replication/transcription complex is dependent on a host factor. *J Biol Chem* 2008;283:16525–16536.
213. van Kasteren PB, Beugeling C, Ninaber DK, et al. Arterivirus and nairovirus ovarian tumor domain-containing deubiquitinases target activated RIG-I to downregulate innate immunity. *J Virol* 2012;86:773–785.
215. van Nieuwstadt AP, Meulenberg JJM, van Essen-Zandbergen A, et al. Proteins encoded by open reading frames 3 and 4 of the genome of Lelystad virus (Arteriviridae) are structural proteins of the virion. *J Virol* 1996;70:4767–4772.
216. Vanderheijden N, Delputte PL, Favoreel HW, et al. Involvement of sialoadhesin in entry of porcine reproductive and respiratory syndrome virus into porcine alveolar macrophages. *J Virol* 2003;77:8207–8215.
217. Vanhee M, Delputte PL, Delrue I, et al. Development of an experimental inactivated PRRSV vaccine that induces virus-neutralizing antibodies. *Vet Res* 2009;40:63.
218. Verheije MH, Olsthoorn RCL, Kroese MV, et al. Kissing interaction between 3′ noncoding and coding sequences is essential for porcine arterivirus RNA replication. *J Virol* 2002;76:1521–1526.
219. Verheije MH, Welting TJM, Jansen HT, et al. Chimeric arteriviruses generated by swapping of the M protein ectodomain rule out a role of this domain in viral targeting. *Virology* 2002;303:364–373.
220. Vu HL, Kwon B, Yoon KJ, et al. Immune evasion of porcine reproductive and resporatory syndrome virus through glycan shielding involves both glycoprotein 5 as well as glycoprotein 3. *J Virol* 2011;85:5555–5564.
221. Wang Y, Liang Y, Han J, et al. Attenuation of porcine reproductive and respiratory syndrome virus strain MN184 using chimeric construction with vaccine sequence. *Virology* 2008;371:418–429.
222. Wassenaar ALM, Spaan WJM, Gorbalenya AE, et al. Alternative proteolytic processing of the arterivirus replicase ORF1a polyprotein: evidence that NSP2 acts as a cofactor for the NSP4 serine protease. *J Virol* 1997;71:9313–9322.
223. Weiland E, Wieczorek-Krohmer M, Kohl D, et al. Monoclonal antibodies to the GP5 of porcine reproductive and respiratory syndrome virus are more effective in virus neutralization than monoclonal antibodies to the GP4. *Vet Microbiol* 1999;66:171–186.
224. Welch SK, Calvert JG. A brief review of CD163 and its role in PRRSV infection. *Virus Res* 2010;154:98–103.
226. Wensvoort G, de Kluyver EP, Pol JM, et al. Lelystad virus, the cause of porcine epidemic abortion and respiratory syndrome: a review of mystery swine disease research at Lelystad. *Vet Microbiol* 1992;33:185–193.
227. Wensvoort G, Terpstra C, Pol JM, et al. Mystery swine disease in the Netherlands: the isolation of Lelystad virus. *Vet Q* 1991;13:121–130.
228. Wieringa R, de Vries AAF, Post SM, et al. Intra- and intermolecular disulfide bonds of the Gp(2b) glycoprotein of equine arteritis virus: Relevance for virus assembly and infectivity. *J Virol* 2003;77:12996–13004.
230. Wieringa R, de Vries AAF, Rottier PJM. Formation of disulfide-linked complexes between the three minor envelope glycoproteins (GP(2b), GP(3), and GP(4)) of equine arteritis virus. *J Virol* 2003;77:6216–6226.
231. Wieringa R, de Vries AAF, van der Meulen J, et al. Structural protein requirements in equine arteritis virus assembly. *J Virol* 2004;78:13019–13027.
235. Wootton SK, Rowland RRR, Yoo D. Phosphorylation of the porcine reproductive and respiratory syndrome virus nucleocapsid protein. *J Virol* 2002;76:10569–10576.
236. Wu J, Li J, Tian F, et al. Genetic variation and pathogenicity of highly virulent porcine reproductive and respiratory syndrome virus emerging in China. *Arch Virol* 2009;154:1597.
237. Xiao ZG, Batista L, Dee S, et al. The level of virus-specific T-cell and macrophage recruitment in porcine reproductive and respiratory syndrome virus infection in pigs is independent of virus load. *J Virol* 2004; 78:5923–5933.
238. Xue F, Sun Y, Yan L, et al. The crystal structure of porcine reproductive and respiratory syndrome virus nonstructural protein Nsp1beta reveals a novel metal-dependent nuclease. *J Virol* 2010;84:6461–6471.
239. Xue QN, Zhao YG, Zhou YJ, et al. Immune responses of swine following DNA immunization with plasmids encoding porcine reproductive and respiratory syndrome virus ORFs 5 and 7, and porcine IL-2 and IFN gamma. *Vet Immunol Immunopathol* 2004;102:291–298.
240. Yoo D, Song C, Sun Y, et al. Modulation of host cell responses and evasion strategies for porcine reproductive and respiratory syndrome virus. *Virus Res* 2010;154:48–60.
241. Yoon KJ, Wu LL, Zimmerman JJ, et al. Antibody-dependent enhancement (ADE) of porcine reproductive and respiratory syndrome virus (PRRSV) infection in pigs. *Viral Immunol* 1996;9:51–63.
243. Zevenhoven-Dobbe JC, Greve S, van Tol H, et al. Rescue of disabled infectious single-cycle (DISC) Equine arteritis virus by using complementing cell lines that express minor structural glycoproteins. *J Gen Virol* 2004;85:3709–3714.
244. Zhang J, Go YY, Maclachlan NJ, et al. Amino acid substitutions in the structural or nonstructural proteins of a vaccine strain of equine arteritis virus are associated with its attenuation. *Virology* 2008;378:355–362.
245. Zhang J, Timoney PJ, Maclachlan NJ, et al. Persistent equine arteritis virus infection in HeLa cells. *J Virol* 2008;82:8456–8464.
246. Zhou L, Yang H. Porcine reproductive and respiratory syndrome in China. *Virus Res* 2010;154:31–37.
247. Zhou L, Zhang J, Zeng J, et al. The 30-amino-acid deletion in the Nsp2 of highly pathogenic porcine reproductive and respiratory syndrome virus emerging in China is not related to its virulence. *J Virol* 2009;83: 5156–5167.
248. Ziebuhr J, Snijder EJ, Gorbalenya AE. Virus-encoded proteinases and proteolytic processing in the *Nidovirales*. *J Gen Virol* 2000;81:853–879.
249. Zirkel F, Kurth A, Quan PL, et al. An insect nidovirus emerging from a primary tropical rainforest. *MBio* 2011;2:e00077.
250. Zitterkopf NL, Haven TR, Huela M, et al. Transplacental lactate dehydrogenase-elevating virus (LDV) transmission: immune inhibition of umbilical cord infection, and correlation of fetal virus susceptibility with development of F4/80 antigen expression. *Placenta* 2002;23:438–446.
252. Zuckermann FA, Garcia EA, Luque ID, et al. Assessment of the efficacy of commercial porcine reproductive and respiratory syndrome virus (PRRSV) vaccines based on measurement of serologic response, frequency of gamma-IFN-producing cells and virological parameters of protection upon challenge. *Vet Microbiol* 2007;123:69–85.

CHAPTER 30

Robert A. Lamb

Mononegavirales

Host Range
Morphology
Lipids
Proteins
Nucleic Acid, Genome Organization, and Replication

The Eighth Report of the International Committee on the Taxonomy of Viruses (ICTV) (2005)[1] has recognized a hierarchy of viral taxa as follows: (order), family, (subfamily), genus, and species. Only three recognized orders of viruses are listed: *Caudovirales, Nidovirales,* and *Mononegavirales.* To avoid duplication of literature citations with the chapters on *Paramyxoviridae* (Chapter 33), *Rhabdoviridae* (Chapter 31), *Filoviridae* (Chapter 32), and *Bornaviridae* (Chapter 39) only the minimal list of references that are unique to this chapter are cited. For full documentation of facts discussed here, see the specific chapters describing each family of the *Mononegavirales.* Table 30.1 lists nomenclature derivations relevant to this material.

The order *Mononegavirales* is composed of four families that have a phylogenetic relationship. Examples of the members of the *Mononegavirales* are shown in Table 30.2. These enveloped viruses possess linear, nonsegmented, negative-sense, single-stranded RNA (ssRNA) genomes. The four families are *Paramyxoviridae, Rhabdoviridae, Filoviridae,* and *Bornaviridae.* The common features of three families—*Paramyxoviridae, Rhabdoviridae,* and *Filoviridae*—include the negative strandedness of the monopartite RNA genome; a similar gene order (3′-untranslated region [UTR]-core protein genes-envelope protein genes—a large polymerase gene–5′ UTR) (Table 30.3);

TABLE 30.1 Nomenclature Derivations

Borna	From Borna, a town in Saxony, Germany
Cyto	From Greek, *kytos,* "cell"
Ebola	From the river Ebola, Zaire
Ephemero	From Greek, *ephemeros,* "ephemeral"
Filo	From Latin, *filo,* "thread-like"
Lyssa	From Greek, *lyssa,* "rage, fury, canine madness"
Marburg	From the city of Marburg, Germany
Meta	From Greek, *meta,* "after"
Mono	From Greek, *monos,* "single"
Morbilli	From Latin *morbillus,* diminutive of *morbus,* "disease"
Nega	Modern invention from negative-sense RNA
Novi	Modern invention (no- and vi-) to describe a characteristic of the genus
Nucleo	From Latin *nux,* "nut"
Paramyxo	From Greek *para,* "by the side of," and *myxo,* "mucus"
Pneumo	From Greek, *pneuma,* "breathe"
Respiro	From Latin, *respirare,* "to breathe"
Rhabdo	From Latin, *rhabdos,* "rod"
Rubula	From Latin, *rubber,* "red"; *rubula inflans* was the old name for mumps.
Vesiculo	From Latin, *vesicula,* diminutive of *vesica,* "blister"
Virales	From Latin, "viruses"

TABLE 30.2 Taxonomic Structure of the Order *Mononegavirales*

Order	***Mononegavirales***
Family	*Bornaviridae*
Genus	*Bornavirus*
Family	*Rhabdoviridae*
Genus	*Vesiculovirus*
Genus	*Lyssavirus*
Genus	*Ephemerovirus*
Genus	*Novirhabdovirus*
Genus	*Cytorhabdovirus*
Genus	*Nucleorhabdovirus*
Family	*Filoviridae*
Genus	*Marburgvirus*
Genus	*Ebolavirus*
Family	*Paramyxoviridae*
Subfamily	*Paramyxovirinae*
Genus	*Rubulavirus*
Genus	*Avulavirus*
Genus	*Respirovirus*
Genus	Aquaparamyxovirus
Genus	Ferlavirus
Genus	*Henipavirus*
Genus	*Morbillivirus*
Subfamily	*Pneumovirinae*
Genus	*Pneumovirus*
Genus	*Metapneumovirus*

Adapted from Pringle CR. Mononegavirales. In: Fauquet CM, Mayo MA, Maniloff J, et al., eds. *Virus Taxonomy. Eighth Report of the International Committee on the Taxonomy of Viruses.* London: Elsevier/Academic Press; 2005:609–614, with permission.[3]

TABLE 30.3 Representation of the 3′ to 5′ Arrangement of the Transcriptional Units in the Genomes of the *Mononegavirales*

Family Subfamily	Genus	Virus 3′									Gene Order						5′
Bornaviridae	*Bornavirus*	BDV	le			N	(P)		(M)				(G)			L	tr
Rhabdoviridae	*Vesiculovirus*	VSV	le			N	P		M				G			L	tr
	Lyssavirus	RV	le			N	P		M				G	Ps		L	tr
	Cytorhabdovirus	LNYV	le			N	P	4b	M				G			L	tr
	Nucleorhabdovirus	SYNV	le			N	P	Sc4	M				G			L	tr
	Novirhabdovirus	IHNV	le			N	P		M				G	NV		L	tr
	Ephemerovirus	BEFV	le			N	P		M				G	Gus (α1.α2., β.,γ)		L	tr
	Ephemerovirus	ARV	le			N	P		M				G	Gus (α1,α2,β)		L	tr
Filoviridae	*Ebolavirus*	ZEBOV	le			N	P		(M1)				GP/SP	?	(M2)	L	tr
	Marburgvirus	MARV	le			N	P		(M1)				G	?	(M2)		
Paramyxoviridae																	
Parantyxovirinae	*Avulavirus*	NDV	le			N	P/V		M	F			H			L	tr
	Henipavirus	HeV	le			N	P/C/V		M	F			H			L	tr
	Morbillivirus	MeV	le			N	P/C/V		M	F			H			L	tr
	Respirovirus	SeV	le			N	P/C/V		M	F			HN			L	tr
	Rubulavirus	MuV	le			N	P/V		M	F		SH	HN			L	tr
Pneumovirinae	*Metapneumovirus*	TRTV	le			N	P		M1	F	M2	SH	G			L	tr
	Pnetunovirus	HRSV	le	NS1	NS2	N	P		M1	SH	G	F	M2			L	tr

Genes encoding proteins of presumed homologous function are aligned vertically.

Virus abbreviations: ARV, Adelaid River virus; BDV, borna disease virus; BEFV, bovine ephemeral virus; HeV, Hendra virus; HRSV, human respiratory syncytial virus; IHNV, infectious hematopoietic necrosis virus; MARV, Lake Victoria Marburgvirus; MeV, measles virus; MuV, mumps virus; RV, rabies virus; SeV, Sendai virus; SYNV, Sonchus yellow net virus; TRTV, turkey rhinotrachitis virus; VSV, vesicular stomatitis virus; ZEBOV, Zaire ebolavirus.

Gene order abbreviations: Le, noncoding leader region; NS, nonstructural protein gene; N, nucleocapsid protein, P, phosphoprotein/N protein chaperone; V protein, interferon antagonist in most cases; C protein, interferon antagonist and involved in virus assembly; Sc4 and 4b, genes of unknown function, M and M1, matrix protein gene; F, fusion protein gene; SH, small integral membrane protein that may block apoptosis; G (or H or HN), attachment protein (hemagglutinin or hemagglutinin-neuraminidase; SP, secreted version of G; M2 envelope protein gene, Ps, pseudogene; NV, nonvirion protein gene; Gns, presumptive duplicated G sequence; L, large (polymerase) protein; tr, noncoding trailer region.

helical nucleocapsids; initiation of transcription by the virion-associated, RNA-dependent RNA polymerase (RdRp) from a single 3′-promoter; utilization of a stop-start transcription mechanism for each cistron; complementarity of the genome at the immediate 3′ and 5′ ends (to act as polymerase promoters); and 93% to 99% of the genome is protein encoding. The ribonucleoprotein (RNP) cores are infectious, but naked RNA is not infectious because it is not in the form of an RNP with its associated RdRp. Maturation is by budding from a cellular membrane and most members of the *Mononegavirales* bud from the plasma membrane, although rabies virus can bud into intracellular membranes and some plant rhabdoviruses are thought to bud from the inner nuclear membrane.

The family *Bornaviridae* has a unique pattern of messenger RNA (mRNA) processing among the *Mononegavirales* as it utilizes the cellular splicing machinery to process precursor RNA to mRNA. The family *Bornaviridae* is included in the order *Mononegavirales* based on the negative strandedness of the monopartite genome ssRNA, similarity of the order of related genes, complementarity of the immediate 3′ and 5′ ends of the genome, and the relatedness of the transcription start and stop signals. Bornaviruses, however, are different from the other three families because their replication and transcription occurs in the nucleus, whereas replication of the families *Paramyxoviridae*, *Rhabdoviridae*, and *Filoviridae* (with the exception of plant viruses in the genus *Nucleorhabdovirus*) occurs in the cytoplasm. The phylogenetic relationship among the families *Paramyxoviridae*, *Rhabdoviridae*, *Filoviridae*, and *Bornaviridae* are illustrated in Figure 30.1. The phylogenetic relationship among members of the family *Paramyxoviridae* is shown in greater detail in Figure 30.2.

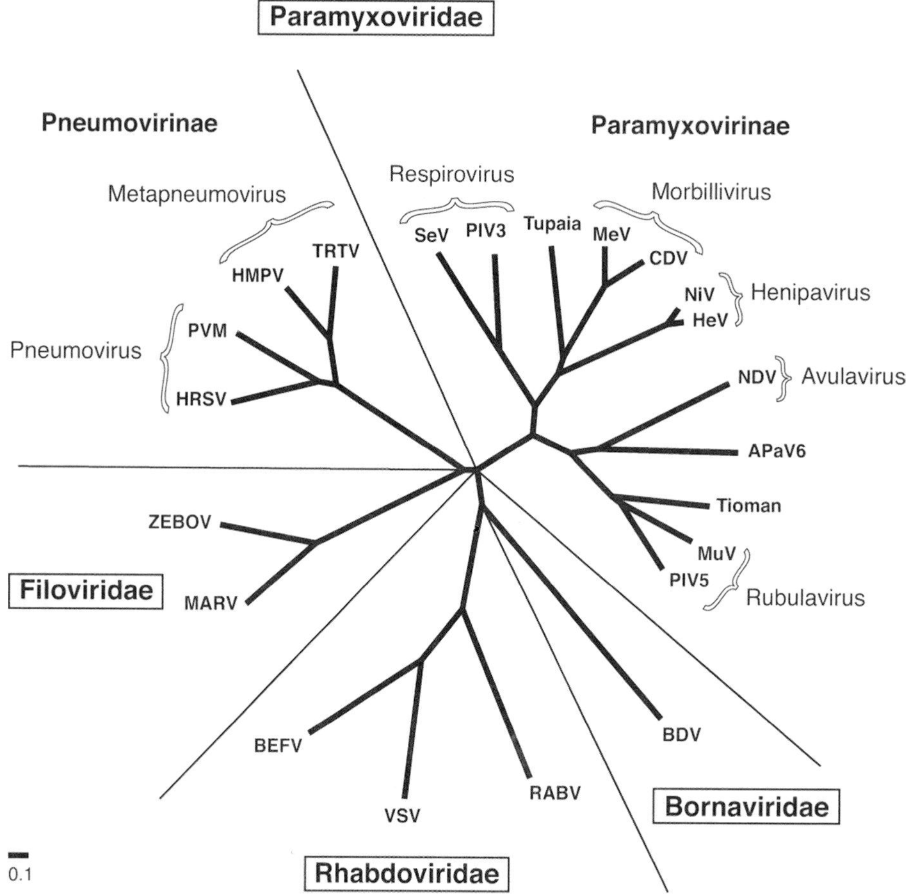

FIGURE 30.1. Unrooted phylogenetic tree of members of the order *Mononegavirales*. The tree was constructed using the CLUSTALX program with the sequences of the conserved domain III of the polymerase proteins. Three paramyxoviruses formerly unclassified by the International Committee on the Classification of Viruses (ICTV) are included: Tupaia paramyxovirus (Tupaia), avian parainfluenza virus type 6 (ApaV6), and Tioman virus (Tioman). BDV–, Borna disease virus; BEFV–, bovine ephemeral fever virus; CDV–, canine distemper virus; HeV–, Hendra virus; HMPV–, human metapneumovirus; HRSV–, human respiratory syncytial virus; MARV–, Marburg virus; MeV–, measles virus; MuV–, mumps virus; NDV–, Newcastle disease virus; NiV–, Nipah virus; PIV3–, parainfluenza virus type 3; PVM–, pneumonia virus of mice; RABV–, rabies virus; SeV–, Sendai virus; PIV5–, parainfluenza virus 5, formerly known as simian virus 5 (SV5); TRTV–, turkey rhinotracheitis virus; VSV–, vesicular stomatitis Indiana virus; ZEBOV–, Zaire Ebola virus. (From Fauquet CM, Mayo MA, Maniloff J, et al., eds. *Virus Taxonomy. Eighth Report of the International Committee on the Taxonomy of Viruses*. London: Elsevier/Academic Press; 2005, with permission.)

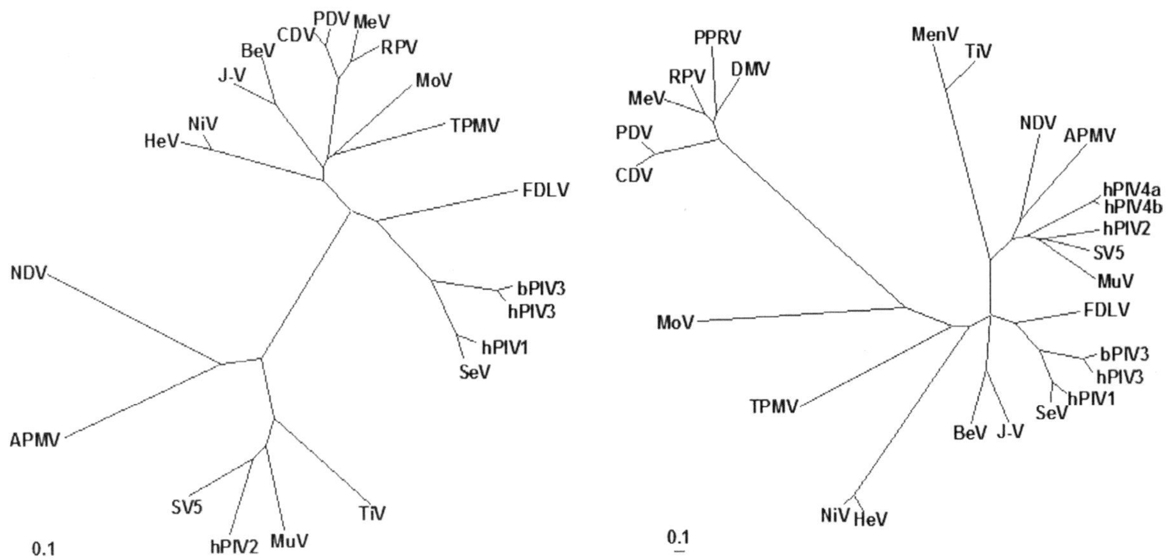

FIGURE 30.2. Unrooted phylogenetic trees based on complete L protein (A) and attachment protein (B) sequences of selected viruses within the subfamily *Paramyxovirinae*. The trees were generated from ClustalW (accurate) protein alignments using distance matrix programs (Protdist and Neighbor) within the PHYLIP software package and drawn in TreeView. Branch lengths represent relative genetic distances. GenBank accession number sequences used to generate the phylogenetic tree are listed below. For viruses in which a full-length genome sequence was not available, individual gene sequences were used and are indicated by the abbreviated gene letter in parentheses followed by the accession number. Avian paramyxovirus type 6 (APMV6) AY029299; BeV DQ100461; bovine parainfluenza virus 3 (bPIV3) AF178654; bovine respiratory syncytial virus (bRSV) AF092942; canine distemper virus (CDV) AF014953; Cetacean morbillivirus (CMV) strain Dolphin morbillivirus (DMV) X75961(N), Z47758(P/V/C), Z30087(M), Z30086(F), Z36978(H); Fer-de-Lance virus (FDLV) AY141760; Hendra virus (HeV) AF017149; human parainfluenza virus 1 (hPIV1) AF457102; human parainfluenza virus 2 (hPIV2) X57559; human parainfluenza virus 3 (hPIV3) AB012132; human parainfluenza virus 4a (hPIV4a) M32982(N), M55975(P/V), D10241(M), D49821(F), M34033(HN); human parainfluenza virus 4b (hPIV4b) M32983(N), M55976 (P/V) D10242(M), D49822(F), AB006958(HN); human respiratory syncytial virus (hRSV) AF013254; J virus (J-V), AY900001; measles virus (MeV) AB016162; Menangle virus (MenV) AF326114 (N,P/V,M,F,HN); Mossman virus (MoV) AY286409; mumps virus (MuV) AB040874; Newcastle disease virus (NDV) strain Beaudette C AF064091(N), X60599(P/V), X04687(M), X04719(F), X04355(HN), X05399(L); Nipah virus (NiV) AF212302; Peste-des-petits-ruminants virus (PPRV) X74443(N), AJ298897(P/V/C), Z47977(M), Z37017(F), Z81358(H); Phocine distemper virus (PDV) X75717(N), D10371(P/V/C, M, F, H), Y09630(L); Rinderpest virus (RPV) Z30697; Salem virus (SalV) AF237881(N,P/V/C); Sendai virus (SeV) AB005795; simian virus 5 (SV5) AF052755; Tioman virus (TiV) AF298895; Tupaia paramyxovirus (TPMV) AF079780. (Adapted from Li Z, Yu M, Zhang H, et al. Beilong virus, a novel paramyxovirus with the largest genome of non-segmented negative-stranded RNA viruses. *Virology* 2006;346:219–228.) PHYLIP software package available from Joseph Felsenstein, Department of Genome Sciences, University of Washington, Seattle, Washington.

HOST RANGE

The host range of *Mononegavirales* varies from restricted to unrestricted. Filoviruses have been isolated from primates only. Paramyxoviruses are found only in vertebrates and there are no known vectors. In contrast, rhabdoviruses infect invertebrates, vertebrates, and plants. Some rhabdoviruses multiply in both invertebrates and vertebrates, some in invertebrates and plants, but no known example exists of a rhabdovirus that replicates in vertebrates and plants. In humans the families *Paramyxoviridae, Rhabdoviridae*, and *Filoviridae* can cause mild to severe morbidity and mortality, for example: hemorrhagic fever (Ebola and Marburg), neurologic disease (rabies virus), respiratory and neurologic disease (paramyxoviruses: measles virus, mumps virus, parainfluenza viruses 1 to 4, Nipah virus and Hendra virus, respiratory syncytial disease virus, and human metapneumovirus). The paramyxoviruses—parainfluenza virus 5, Newcastle disease virus, canine distemper virus, phocine distemper virus, Nipah virus, Hendra virus, pneumonia-like virus of mice, turkey rhinotrachitis virus and the rhabdoviruses, vesicular stomatitis virus, and rabies virus—cause disease in animals. Bornaviruses have been isolated from horses, cattle, sheep, rabbits, rats, cats, and humans. Infection of some model animals is associated with behavioral disturbances to severe nonpurulent encephalomyelitis. There has been great debate concerning whether bornaviruses can cause psychological disease in humans.

MORPHOLOGY

The defining characteristic of all members of *Mononegavirales,* except the family *Bornaviridae,* is that the virions are large, enveloped structures containing a visible fringe of spike glycoproteins. The families exhibit very different shapes, however. Members of the family *Paramyxoviridae* are filamentous or pleomorphic (somewhat) spherical particles (200 to 300 nm in diameter), whereas members of the family *Filoviridae* are bacilliform, forming long threads (800 nm). Viruses within the family *Rhabdoviridae* are regular bullet-shaped particles or bacilliform. The viral nucleocapsid (ribonucleoprotein [RNP]) is often observed in ruptured virion particles on an electron microscopy (EM) grid and the nucleocapsids have a diameter of 13 to 20 nm and characteristic morphologies, depending on the particular virus family.

LIPIDS

The lipid composition of the *Mononegavirales* reflects that of the host cell membrane from where the virions bud. Some of the spike glycoproteins have fatty acid covalently linked to their cytoplasmic tails.

PROTEINS

Members of the *Mononegavirales* contain five to seven structural proteins: the envelope glycoproteins; a matrix protein that underlies the lipid envelope; a major RNA binding protein often called the nucleocapsid protein (N or NP); other nucleocapsid-associated proteins; and a very large protein that has RdRp activity and capping, methylating, and polyadenylate transferase activities. The viruses also encode several nonstructural proteins, several of which are involved in antagonizing the innate immune system. Some viruses have a single glycoprotein that mediates both attachment of the virion to the cellular receptor and fusion of the viral envelope to a cellular membrane for viral entry into the cell. Other viruses have two major spike glycoproteins, one of which has attachment activity and the other of which has membrane fusion activity. When the receptor is sialic acid, the attachment protein usually has a neuraminidase activity that acts as a receptor-destroying activity.

NUCLEIC ACID, GENOME ORGANIZATION, AND REPLICATION

Members of the *Mononegavirales* contain one molecule of negative-sense ssRNA that varies from 8.9 to 19 kilobases (kb). The RNA is not infectious; by definition, a negative-sense RNA has to be copied to a plus-sense RNA to be translated to protein and the naked RNA of the *Mononegavirales* has to be packed into an RNP with its associated RdRp. The 5′ end of the genome RNA is not modified by a cap structure or addition of a covalently linked protein and the 3′ end of the genome RNA is not polyadenylated. The immediate 5′- and 3′-termini exhibit inverse complementarity and are used as promoters by the RdRp for synthesis of both the antigenomic full-length positive RNA strand and the new genome RNA. The genome is composed of a series of genes with limited overlaps in some viruses (e.g., respiratory syncytial virus). The RdRp transcribes the genes in sequential order from the 3′ end of the genome to make a series of mostly monocistronic mRNA. Transcription is polar with step-wise attenuation. Examples of the use of overlapping translational reading frames are found. Mostly, the genes have short 5′ and 3′ UTR (notable exceptions are found for Nipah virus, Hendra virus, J virus, and Beilong virus[2] of the paramyxovirus family). Conserved nucleotide sequence motifs define the transcriptional gene start with addition of a cap structure to the mRNA and conserved nucleotide sequence motifs that define the gene end and cause the addition of poly(A) to the mRNA in all families. A region of genome RNA between the gene-end and gene-start sequences is found, which is called the intercistronic region. This region is not transcribed into mRNA and can range from two nucleotides to hundreds of nucleotides. Members of the subfamily *Paramyxovirinae* undergo an insertion of nontemplated nucleotides at a pseudo-poly(A) addition site within their "*P*" gene to give rise to additional mRNA encoding extra proteins. A related event occurs in the glycoprotein gene of Ebola virus, giving rise to two versions of the glycoprotein. Splicing of mRNA only occurs for bornaviruses. In the subfamily *Paramyxovirinae* of the family *Paramyxoviridae,* the genome length in nucleotides has to be a number divisible by six (the so-called "rule of six"). It is thought that this constraint is because each nucleocapsid protein subunit binds to precisely six nucleotides to form the RNP.

REFERENCES

1. Fauquet CM, Mayo MA, Maniloff J, et al., eds. *Virus Taxonomy. Eighth Report of the International Committee on the Taxonomy of Viruses.* London: Elsevier/Academic Press; 2005.
2. Li Z, Yu M, Zhang H, et al. Beilong virus, a novel paramyxovirus with the largest genome of non-segmented negative-stranded RNA viruses. *Virology* 2006;346:219–228.
3. Pringle CR. Mononegavirales. In: Fauquet CM, Mayo MA, Maniloff J, et al., eds. *Virus Taxonomy. Eighth Report of the International Committee on the Taxonomy of Viruses.* London: Elsevier/Academic Press; 2005:609–614.

CHAPTER 31

Douglas S. Lyles • Ivan V. Kuzmin • Charles E. Rupprecht

Rhabdoviridae

The family *Rhabdoviridae* consists of more than 185 different viruses isolated from both plants and animals. They are enveloped viruses that have helical nucleocapsids containing single-stranded, negative-sense RNA and share a common elongated, rod-like or bullet-like shape. This distinctive morphology separates rhabdoviruses from other taxa in the order *Mononegavirales*, the *Bornaviridae*, the *Filoviridae*, and the *Paramyxoviridae*. Rhabdoviruses can replicate in plants, invertebrates, or vertebrates. The family *Rhabdoviridae* contains many members that are significant medical, veterinary, and agricultural pathogens. Currently, animal rhabdoviruses include four genera: *Lyssavirus*, *Vesiculovirus*, *Ephemerovirus*, and *Novirhabdovirus* (Table 31.1). Many other rhabdoviruses have not received adequate study and are assigned to the family solely on the basis of morphology.

HISTORY

Lyssaviruses

Rabies is an archaic entity, one of the oldest recognized infectious diseases. The continuing biomedical preoccupation with rabies is understandable because of its "alarming manifestations in man and dog alike . . . and its almost inevitable progression to a fatal outcome have ensured unparalleled notoriety".[772] These concerns extend beyond the material to the spiritual plane, as revealed by the following prayer: "San Roque, San Roque, que este perro no me toque!" This supplication for protection to the patron saint against pestilence, taught to children in both the Old and the New World for invocation whenever they encountered a dog on the street, literally translates to "St. Roque, St. Roque, do not allow this dog to touch me!"—classically linking dogs, bites, and resulting misfortune.

Ancient civilizations were familiar with rabies. An early passage mentions the dangers of dog bites, in the pre-Mosaic

TABLE 31.1 Taxonomy of *Rhabdoviridae*

Virus species	Example GenBank accession numbers for genome sequences
Genus *Vesiculovirus*	
Carajas virus	FW339542
Chandipura virus	GU212856
Cocal virus	EU373657
Isfahan virus	AJ810084
Maraba virus	
Piry virus	Z15093, D26175
Spring viremia of carp virus	AJ318079
Vesicular stomatitis Alagoas virus	EU373658
Vesicular stomatitis Indiana virus	AF473864
Vesicular stomatitis New Jersey virus	K02379[a]
Other related viruses that have not been approved as species	
BeAn 157575 virus	
Boteke virus	GU816014[a]
Calchaqui virus	
Eel virus American	
Eel virus European X	FN557213
Grass carp rhabdovirus	
Gray Lodge virus	
Jurona virus	GU816024[a]
Klamath virus	
Kwatta virus	
La Joya virus	
Malpais Spring virus	
Perinet virus	AY854652[a]
Pike fry rhabdovirus	FJ872827
Porton virus	GU816013[a]
Radi virus	
Tench rhabdovirus	
Ulcerative disease rhabdovirus	
Yug Bogdanovac virus	
Genus *Lyssavirus*	
Aravan virus	EF614259
Australian bat lyssavirus	AF418014
Duvenhage virus	EU293119
European bat lyssavirus 1	EU293112
European bat lyssavirus 2	EU293114
Irkut virus	EF614260
Khujand virus	EF614261
Lagos bat virus	EU293108, EU293110, EF547454,[a] GU170202
Mokola virus	Y09762
Rabies virus	M13215, M31046, AY705373, EU293115, EU293111, EU311738
West Caucasian bat virus	EF614258
Other related viruses which have not been approved as species	
Shimoni bat virus	GU170201
Genus *Ephemerovirus*	
Adelaide River virus	L09206,[a] L09208,[a] U05987,[a] U10363[a]
Berrimah virus	
Bovine ephemeral fever virus	AF234533
Other related viruses that have not been approved as species	
Kimberley virus	AY854637[a]
Kotonkan virus	AY854638,[a] DQ457009[a]
Malakal virus	
Obodhiang virus	DQ457098[a]
Puchong virus	
Genus *Novirhabdovirus*	
Hirame rhabdovirus	AF104985
Infectious hematopoietic necrosis virus	L40883
Snakehead virus	AF147498
Viral hemorrhagic septicemia virus	Y18263
Other related viruses that have not been approved as species	
Eel virus B12	
Eel virus C26	
Genus *Cytorhabdovirus*	
Barley yellow striate mosaic virus	FJ665628[a]
Broccoli necrotic yellows virus	
Festuca leaf streak virus	
Lettuce necrotic yellows virus	AJ867584
Lettuce yellow mottle virus	EF687738
Northern cereal mosaic virus	GU985153
Sonchus virus	
Strawberry crinkle virus	AY005146,[a] AY250986[a]
Wheat American striate mosaic virus	
Other related viruses that have not been approved as species	
Wheat rosette stunt virus	AF059602-04,[a] AF059677[a]
Soybean blotchy mosaic virus	EU877231[a]
Ivy vein banding virus	GQ249162,[a] GQ249163[a]
Genus *Nucleorhabdovirus*	
Datura yellow vein virus	
Eggplant mottled dwarf virus	AM922319,[a] AM922322[a]
Maize fine streak virus	AY618417
Maize mosaic virus	AY618418[a]
Potato yellow dwarf virus	GU734660
Rice yellow stunt virus	AB011257
Sonchus yellow net virus	L32603
Sowthistle yellow vein virus	
Taro vein chlorosis virus	AY674964
Other related viruses that have not been approved as species	
Cereal chlorotic mottle virus	
Cynodon rhabdovirus	EU650683[a]
Maize Iranian mosaic virus	DQ186554
Sorghum stunt mosaic virus	

[a]Sequences do not compose the complete genome.

Eshnunna Code of Mesopotamia, circa the 23rd century BC: "If a dog is mad and the authorities have brought the fact to the knowledge of its owner; if he does not keep it in, and it bites a man and causes his death, then the owner shall pay two-thirds of a mina [40 shekels] of silver".[41] In *The Iliad* (700 BC), Hector is compared to a rabid dog. Chinese scholars warned of the dangers of rabid dogs in 500 BC, and Aristotle (4th century BC) correctly associated the disease with animals but erroneously exempted humans from contracting it from a mad dog's bite. In Rome, Cordamus guessed that a poison (i.e., a "virus") was present in saliva. Similarly, in the 1st century AD, another Roman, Celsus, described clinical aspects of human infection: "The patient is tortured at the same time by thirst and by invincible repulsion toward water." For prevention, he recommended immediate excision of the bitten tissue, cauterization of the wound by a hot iron, and dunking the victim into a pool. The Hebrew Talmud, also dating from the 1st century, makes several references to the disease. Throughout the ages, ingestion of a wide variety of substances (e.g., the liver from a mad dog, crayfish eyes, a cock's brain or comb, or the cast slough of snakes pounded in wine with a male crab) and carrying sacred talismans or "madstones" were believed to be cures for rabies.[41]

The transition from the medieval era to the Renaissance period of pragmatism and experimentation resulted in a remarkable treatise in 1546, entitled "The Incurable Wound," by Fracastoro. This Italian physician clearly stated that human beings are susceptible to rabies, and he vividly described a clinical case:

> Its incubation [following a bite by a rabid animal] is so stealthy, slow and gradual that the infection is very rarely manifest before the 20th day, in most cases after the 30th, and in many cases not until four or six months have elapsed. There are cases recorded in which it became manifest a year after the bite. [Once the disease takes hold,] the patient can neither stand nor lie down; like a madman he flings himself hither and thither, tears his flesh with his hands, and feels intolerable thirst. This is the most distressing symptom, for he so shrinks from water and all liquids that he would rather die than drink or be brought near to water; it is then that they bite other persons, foam at the mouth, their eyes look twisted, and finally they are exhausted and painfully breathe their last.[360]

His portrayal of human rabies is accurate in that the incubation periods can extend from months to years after initial exposure,[662] but a biting attack on others by a rabid patient with resultant disease is an uncommon event.[218]

Although rabies is known to have been widespread in the Old World for thousands of years, its occurrence in the New World is less understood because of a dearth of records before European arrival. Rabies in the Americas was reported by the Reverend Marmolejo in Mexico as early as 1709, but some suspect that it was present before Columbus's arrival in the 15th century. For example, not long after the discovery of the Americas, the bishop Petrus Martyr-Anglerius wrote in his *De Rebus Oceanicis et de* Orbi Novi Decades Octo, "In several places bats not much smaller than turtle doves used to fly at them [the Spanish sailors and soldiers] in the early evening with brutal fury and with their venomous bites brought those injured to madness ... [and] bats ... come in from the marshes on the river and attack our men with deadly bite".[388] This may have been one of the first descriptions of rabies transmission by vampire bats.

The bite of a rabid animal was considered a likely source of rabies infection by many, but it was only in 1804 that Zinke used dog saliva for transmission.[386] Later in 1879, Galtier is credited with experimental rabies transmission and serial passage in rabbits.[386] Clinical descriptions formed the basis for diagnosis until the advent of light microscopy. A clear description of viral and neuronal interactions was made by Negri in 1903, with the detection of cytoplasmic inclusions (Negri bodies) in neurons of rabid animals.[393] Although the diagnostic value of Negri bodies was established by 1913, their viral composition had to wait until the later development of electron microscopy.

Pasteur's research on rabies is perhaps the most well-known historical achievement in the field. First, through adaptation of "street" (wild-type) virus to laboratory animals, he was able to change its properties. Today, one could apply the term *attenuated* to his "fixed" virus strains. Second, Pasteur and his team developed concepts and experimental approaches to the first protective vaccination against rabies.[388] Desiccated spinal cords from rabies virus–infected rabbits became the first rabies vaccine, and they were supposedly safe, although now it is known that the fixed viruses from which these vaccines were derived were not apathogenic but could actually cause the disease. July 6, 1885, is a milestone in the history of rabies. On that day, 9-year-old Joseph Meister was bitten at multiple sites by a rabid dog and received the first postexposure prophylaxis with Pasteur's vaccine. Remarkably, Joseph survived.[386] Pasteur's vaccine, with all its modifications, became the accepted rabies prophylactic throughout the world in the early 20th century. Problems remained, however, because improperly inactivated virus caused rabies, and animal brain tissue induced allergic reactions leading to neuroparalytic accidents. Moreover, the vaccine was not very effective in cases of severe bites, such as those inflicted on the face and neck by rabid wolves and dogs.

Postexposure prophylaxis against rabies through simultaneous administration of antirabies serum and vaccine was introduced in 1889 by Babes.[29] This approach found few adherents and languished until about 1940, when interest in the use of serum-containing rabies virus (RABV) antibodies was revived. In a trial organized by the World Health Organization in 1954, the combined use of serum and vaccine was found to be more protective than vaccine alone,[288] an observation later corroborated by Chinese findings.[212] Today, the combination of immune globulin and vaccine is the recommended standard for prophylaxis in human rabies exposure.

In the 1960s, an RABV grown in human diploid cells was used to produce a safe and efficacious inactivated vaccine,[385,386] eliminating many of the problems connected with vaccines produced in brain tissue. This vaccine and others derived from cell culture are used widely throughout the world, although for economic reasons, several developing countries still use nervous tissue vaccines. Other RABV strains are used for vaccine production for human and animal use in addition to the original Pasteur virus (PV) strain. Given the progress in biotechnology, improved versions of rabies vaccines are currently under development.

Vesiculoviruses

Vesicular stomatitis virus (VSV) is the best-studied member of the genus *Vesiculovirus*. The extensive body of knowledge about the replication of VSV reflects its status as a widely studied prototype for the nonsegmented, negative-strand RNA viruses. VSV produces an acute disease in cattle, horses, and pigs characterized by fever and vesicles in the mucosa of the oral cavity and in the skin of the coronary band and teat. Clinically, VS is very similar to foot-and-mouth disease (FMD). VSV can also cause an acute febrile disease in humans. Laboratory-adapted strains, however, are rarely pathogenic for humans.

Although VS was first reported in the United States in 1916 during an epidemic in cattle and horses,[695] a clinically similar disease was previously described in army horses in 1862, during the U.S. Civil War.[484] In 1915, French veterinarians described a disease clinically similar to VS in horses imported to Europe from the United States and Canada during World War I. At that time, the etiology of this disease could not be determined with certainty, but it could be transmitted from horse to horse by rubbing the saliva of a sick animal on the tongue of a healthy one, establishing the infectious nature of the disease.[295] In 1925, cattle transported from Kansas City, Missouri, to Richmond, Indiana, initiated an outbreak of VS in the area. The disease was experimentally transmitted to horses and the infectious agent was maintained by serial passages in animals. This strain became the VS-Indiana virus (VSIV) strain.[149] In 1926, an outbreak of VS in cattle occurred in New Jersey. The causative agent was found to be a filterable agent that could infect cattle, horses, and guinea pigs. This virus, serologically different from the VSIV strain, is currently known as the VS-New Jersey virus (VSNJV) strain.[148,149]

The VSIV and VSNJV viruses represent the two serotypes most commonly isolated in the Americas. Most of the commonly studied laboratory-adapted strains of VSV (e.g., Glasgow, Orsay, San Juan, Mudd-Summers) belong to the VSIV serotype. In the United States, the last reported outbreak of the VSIV serotype occurred in 1965.[751] The VSNJV serotype was responsible for outbreaks in the United States in 1944, 1949, 1957, 1959, 1963, 1982–1983, 1985, and 1995.[87] In 1997, isolated cases were diagnosed in several horses in New Mexico, but this did not initiate an outbreak.[21] Between 1946 and 1954, during an outbreak of FMD in Mexico,[270] the joint Mexico–American commission for the control of FMD developed techniques for the differential diagnosis of FMD and VS based on the isolation of the agent and complement fixation methods.[295] The availability of a more efficient diagnostic methodology demonstrated that VS was prevalent throughout the year in the tropical areas of Mexico.[295]

In South America, the disease was reported in 1939 in La Plata, Argentina.[295] Later, VSV was isolated in Barinas, Venezuela, in 1941, and in Colombia in 1943.[295] Currently, VSV is endemic in many Latin American countries and is responsible for important economic losses in the livestock industry. Disease caused by VSV was reported in 11 countries of Latin America in 1996.[788] Although the presence of VS was previously suggested in Africa in 1884 to 1887 and in Asia in 1944,[295] presently the disease is considered enzootic only in the Americas.[788]

Other vesiculoviruses are endemic in the Americas, Asia, and Africa. Piry virus was isolated from an opossum (*Philander opossum*) in Brazil in 1960[701] and caused a febrile disease in humans.[474] Cocal virus (COCV, or Indiana 2) was isolated from mites of the genus *Gigantolaelaps* from rice rats (*Oryzomys laticeps velutinus*) trapped during 1961, on Bush Bush Island in the Nariva swamp in eastern Trinidad.[354] The VS Alagoas virus (VSAV, or Indiana 3) was isolated from domestic animals in the state of Alagoas, Brazil, during a VS outbreak.[700] Later it also was isolated from sand flies and seropositive (but otherwise healthy) livestock in Colombia.[700] Maraba virus (MARAV) was isolated from sand flies (*Lutzomyia* sp.) collected in the state of Pará, Brazil. Although humans are infrequently infected based on serology, the actual public health significance of MARAV has not been assessed.[709]

Vesiculoviruses endemic in Asia include Chandipura virus (CHPV) and Isfahan virus (ISFV). ISFV was isolated from sand flies (*Phlebotomus papatasi*) collected in Dormian, Isfahan Province, Iran, in 1975.[699] From serologic analyses, the presence of ISFV has been detected in India, Iran, Turkmenistan, and other Asian countries.[474] CHPV was obtained from the sera of two patients with a febrile illness in Nagpur City, Maharashtra State, India, in 1965 during an epidemic of chikungunya and dengue.[66] This virus was also isolated from phlebotomine sand flies in West Africa in 1991.[243] CHPV is now known to be a cause of viral encephalitis in children, following its identification as the cause of two recent outbreaks. One outbreak in 2003 in Andhra Pradesh State, India,[580] included 329 cases (183 fatalities), and another in 2004 in Gujarat State, India,[114] included 26 cases (at least 18 fatalities).

Several vesiculoviruses infect fish, and at least one of these, Spring viremia of carp virus (SVCV), has been recognized as a species of the *Vesiculovirus* genus. Dating back possibly to the Middle Ages, common carp *Cyprinus carpio* in European pond culture have been plagued by a complex of infectious diseases variously known as infectious dropsy, rubella, infectious ascites, hemorrhagic septicemia, and red contagious disease.[59,316,621,706] These diseases proved to be of great economic importance, causing serious losses in carp pond fisheries of the central and eastern parts of Europe.[227,228] The proposed causes (nutrition, environment, parasites, bacteria, viruses) for the acute and chronic forms of the epizootics remained controversial for a long time. However, a viral etiology for the acute form of infectious dropsy became evident when a cytopathic agent was isolated,[706] and River's postulates were fulfilled using virus isolated from affected carp.[229] In order to distinguish the viral disease from other etiologic entities within the infectious dropsy complex, the disease was renamed spring viremia of carp (SVC), and the causative virus was termed SVCV (or, initially, *Rhabdovirus carpio*).[229]

SVCV has been identified in different parts of Europe, Russia, and the Middle East, causing mortality of up to 70% of young carps.[9,58,61,99,229,645,698,706] In 2002, SVCV was first reported in U.S. waters at a North Carolina koi hatchery. Unfortunately, there is evidence that koi had been distributed from this hatchery to most of the 48 contiguous states before being confirmed with SVC. The first common carp die-off of wild fish that tested positive for SVC occurred in 2002 at Cedar Lake, Wisconsin,[183] and the virus has rapidly disseminated to other states.

Ephemeroviruses

The first reference to bovine ephemeral fever (BEF) can be found in the book *The Heart of Africa*.[636] Not until the 20th century was the disease reported among ruminants in much of its natural range throughout the tropical and subtropical regions of Africa, Asia, Australia, and the Middle East.[671] The apparent emergence and re-emergence of BEF over 125 years is likely due to the expansive growth of the cattle industry and improved surveillance.[735] Until 1966, when bovine ephemeral fever virus (BEFV) was grown in mice,[723] research on the agent was restricted largely to transmission studies in cattle.[134] Characterization of ephemeroviruses is an ongoing process. For example, viruses Obodhiang (Sudan, 1963) and Kotonkan (Nigeria, 1967), isolated from mosquitoes, were initially suggested as "rabies related," based on a limited antigenic cross-reactivity with lyssaviruses.[60] However, gene sequencing and phylogenetic reconstructions demonstrated that these viruses belong to ephemeroviruses.[401] Likely, more members of the genus will be recovered among other rhabdoviruses, isolated decades ago and awaiting molecular characterization.

Novirhabdoviruses

Infectious hematopoietic necrosis virus (IHNV) was first discovered in sockeye salmon (*Oncorhynchus nerka*) dying at hatcheries in Washington in 1953.[611] Similar outbreaks among hatchery-reared salmonid fish in California were reported in the following decades.[285,777] It was thought that IHNV was confined to salmonid fish in the Pacific coast of North America.[482] However, the virus spread during the 1970s to the eastern United States, Europe, Japan, Korea, Taiwan, and China by shipment of infected fish and eggs.[85,418,617] Electron microscopy of IHNV particles along with physicochemical and serologic analysis demonstrated that IHNV is a member of the *Rhabdoviridae.*[16,314,483] Gene sequencing demonstrated that IHNV has the five structural genes common to rhabdoviruses, with the addition of a nonstructural, nonvirion (NV) gene between the genes for the G and L proteins.[399] Several more fish rhabdoviruses, which demonstrate similar pathobiology and have similar genome organization, have been described, including Hirame rhabdovirus, snakehead virus, and viral hemorrhagic septicemia virus. These viruses were identified not only in North America but also in eastern and southern Asia, where they appear to be endemic.[363,374] These viruses were first assigned into the genus *Novirhabdovirus,* based on the presence of the NV gene, in the Seventh Report of the International Committee on Taxonomy of Viruses (ICTV).[736]

Sigma Virus

This virus, a natural pathogen of *Drosophila* spp. fruit flies, was described in 1937.[407] Sigma virus appears to be distributed worldwide. This is the only arthropod-specific rhabdovirus described to date, with an unusual mode of transmission: it is only transmitted vertically through both eggs and sperm and does not move horizontally between hosts.[145] Sigma virus was initially placed in the *Rhabdoviridae* based on its bullet-shaped viral particles,[64,696] and this has subsequently been confirmed using sequence data.[71] Initially it was believed that Sigma virus infects only *D. melanogaster.* However, additional surveillance identified recently that related variants of Sigma virus infect *D. affinis* and *D. obscura.*[451]

TAXONOMY

The rhabdoviruses share a variety of gross morphologic and functional attributes with other members of the order *Mononegavirales.* For example, the virions are large structures that mature by budding, with membrane-bound spikes and a helical nucleocapsid. They possess single-stranded, nonsegmented, negative-polarity RNA, with a similar gene arrangement. Within the family, recent analyses support the concept of a unified phylogeny and suggest an evolutionary history influenced by host species and transmission dynamics.[83,404] Currently, the ICTV recognizes four genera of animal rhabdoviruses and two genera of plant rhabdoviruses. Furthermore, several rhabdovirus species have been recognized without inclusion into any of the established genera.[177] Figure 31.1 shows phylogenetic relationships among rhabdoviruses.

Within the genus *Lyssavirus* only one major serogroup had been established, although various serotypes were defined.[613] Placement within the genus was determined by serologic cross-reactivity of viral antigens, primarily based on antigenic sites on the nucleoprotein (the N protein). Historically, placement of a species as a rabies or rabies-related virus was determined by recognition of antigenic sites of the glycoprotein (the G protein) via virus neutralization tests. As nucleotide sequence data became available for a number of other *Lyssavirus* species,[44,84,173,377,400,402,405,663] a trend toward genetic classification was established. Currently ICTV recognizes 11 *Lyssavirus* species, and one more representative (*Shimoni bat virus* [SHIBV]) is included in the genus provisionally without established species status (Table 31.1).

In general, demarcation criteria for *Lyssavirus* species include the following: (1) Genetic distances, with the threshold of 80% to 82% nucleotide identity for the complete N gene or 80% to 81% nucleotide identity for concatenated coding regions of N+P+M+G+L genes. Globally, all isolates belonging to the same species have higher identity values than the threshold, except the viruses currently included into the *Lagos bat virus* (LBV) species. For that reason some authors suggested that LBV be subdivided into several genotypes.[173,473] However, as these LBV representatives are segregated into a monophyletic cluster in the majority of phylogenetic reconstructions, in the absence of other sufficient demarcation characters there is currently no possibility to subdivide LBV into several viral species. (2) Topology and consistency of phylogenetic trees, obtained with various evolutionary models. (3) Antigenic patterns in reactions with antinucleocapsid monoclonal antibodies (preceded by serologic cross-reactivity and definition of *Lyssavirus* serotypes, using polyclonal antisera). (4) Whenever available, additional characteristics, such as ecological properties, host and geographic range, and pathologic features, are considered.[177] Moreover, based on genetic distances and serologic cross-reactivity, the genus has been subdivided into two phylogroups. Phylogroup I includes RABV, *European bat Lyssavirus type 1* (EBLV-1), EBLV-2, *Duvenhage virus* (DUVV), *Australian bat Lyssavirus* (ABLV), *Aravan virus* (ARAV), *Khujand virus* (KHUV), and *Irkut virus* (IRKV). Phylogroup II includes *LBV, Mokola virus* (MOKV), and SHIBV. The remaining species of the genus, *West Caucasian bat virus* (WCBV), cannot be included in either of these phylogroups and is suggested to be considered as a representative of independent phylogroup III.[400,402]

Based on the serologic cross-reactivity patterns and sequence analyses of the members of the genus *Vesiculovirus,* a unique VSV serogroup has been established. This serogroup includes VSIV (currently the type species of the genus), VSNJV, VSAV, *Carajas virus,* CHPV, COCV, ISFV, MARAV, and *Piry virus.*[177] Also recognized as a *Vesiculovirus* species is SVCV. Furthermore, 19 viruses are provisionally included in the genus without established species status (Table 31.1).

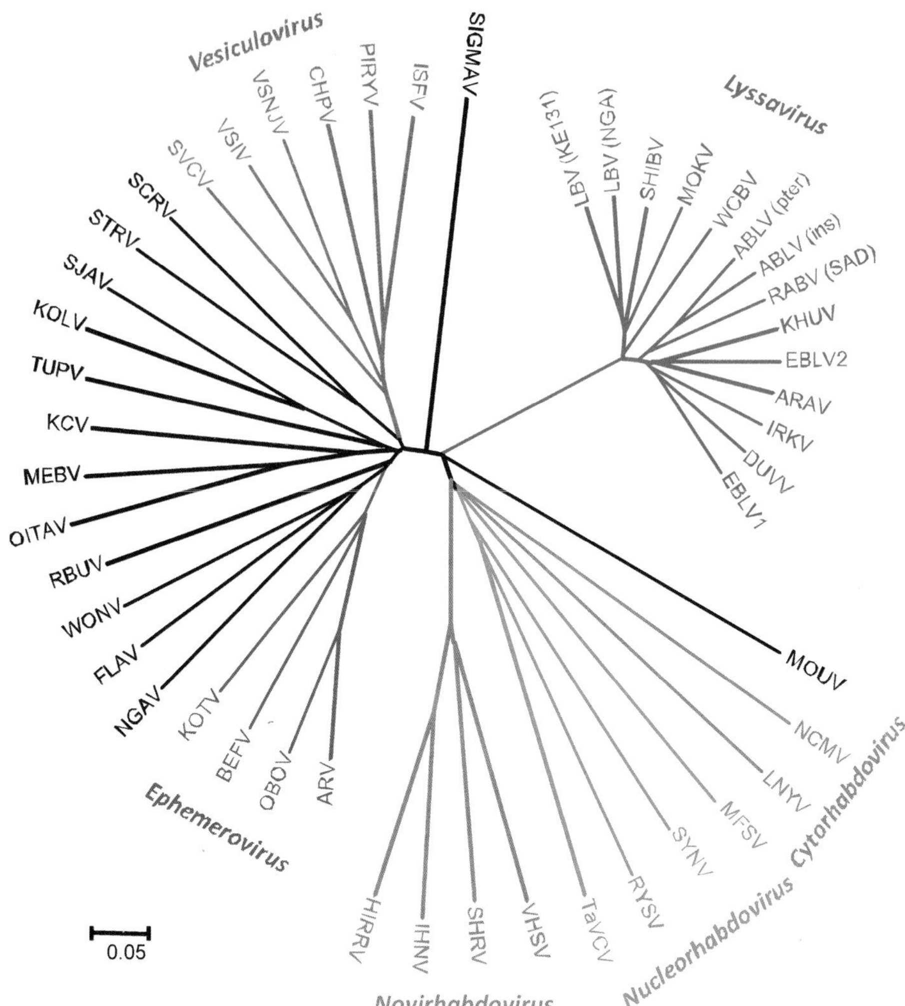

FIGURE 31.1. Phylogenetic relationships among rhabdoviruses.

The members of the genus *Ephemerovirus* show limited cross-neutralization reactivity, but they are highly cross-reactive in complement fixation or indirect immunofluorescence tests. They exhibit similar but distinct genome organization with the common feature of a nonstructural glycoprotein (G_{NS}) gene but variations in the number of accessory protein genes and the location of transcriptional control sequences. Different species may share up to 91% identity in N protein amino acid sequence. Currently the genus includes only three recognized species, but five more viruses are included provisionally[177] (Table 31.1), based on antigenic reactivity and phylogenetic analysis of limited gene fragments.[83,401] Phylogenetic relationships indicate that several intercontinental translocations of ephemeroviruses are likely to have occurred. Adelaide River virus (ARV) (Australia) and Obodhiang virus (OBOV) (Africa) demonstrate more genetic identity to each other than is observed between ARV and BEFV, both circulating in Australia. BEFV also circulates broadly in Africa, the Middle East, and southern areas of Asia, without significant genetic diversity.[401,404,735]

The genus *Novirhabdovirus* was established based on the presence a small NV protein of unknown function. The NV open reading frame (ORF) is located between the G and L genes and is preserved in diverse viruses and strains. The NV protein sequences are significantly less conserved between viruses in different species than sequences of the structural proteins.[317,398] Species within the genus have been distinguished serologically on the basis of cross-neutralization with polyclonal rabbit antisera. Thus, IHNV and hirame rhabdovirus (HIRRV) each constitute single serotypes, and viral hemorrhagic septicemia virus (VHSV) has one major serotype with a small number of associated strains. Viruses from different species do not show cross-neutralization, but in some cases there is a low level of cross-reaction with specific proteins in western blot analyses. Nucleotide sequence data are available for most genes of these viruses and will undoubtedly contribute to the distinction of viral species in the future. For strains within a virus species, the nucleotide sequence divergence ranges up to a maximum of 8% for IHNV G and NV genes and 18% for the G genes of European and North American VHSV. N protein amino acid identity between IHNV and VHSV is approximately 34%.[177]

Members of two genera of the *Rhabdoviridae* infect plants and are transmitted via arthropod vectors, such as leafhoppers, planthoppers, and aphids.[342] The cytorhabdoviruses and nucleorhabdoviruses are primarily distinguished based on their sites of virion maturation, in the cytoplasm and the nucleus, respectively. Genus classification based on sequence diversity has thus far correlated with classification by intracellular virus maturation. The genus *Cytorhabdovirus* currently includes nine recognized species and three provisional members, whereas genus *Nucleorhabdovirus* includes nine and four members, respectively

(Table 31.1). There is no significant sequence similarity (>50%) between analogous genes of the different species analyzed to date. However, nucleotide sequences are available for only a limited number of representatives and at the moment cannot be considered as sufficient to demarcate different species.[177]

Recently, several rhabdoviruses, previously referred to as "unclassified",[707] were recognized by the ICTV as species, without assignment to any particular genus, based on their unique genome structure, phylogenetic and antigenic properties, and sufficient amount of knowledge on their ecology or pathobiology. These include *Flanders, Tupaia, Sigma, Ngaingan,* and *Wongabel* viruses.[177] The recently described *Moussa virus*[575] is another candidate for the establishment of a viral species without inclusion in any recognized genus.

VIRION STRUCTURE

Rhabdoviruses are enveloped, rod- or cone-shaped particles (Fig. 31.2A, B), approximately 100 to 430 nm long and 45 to 100 nm in diameter. Animal rhabdoviruses are usually approximately 180 nm long and 80 nm wide, but those isolated from plants can be longer. The length of the virion is dictated by the length of the RNA genome, so that incorporation of additional genes into the viral genome results in correspondingly longer virions.[629] Typically, mature virions appear either as bullet-shaped particles with one rounded and one flattened end or as bacilliform particles that appear hemispheric at both ends.

The genome RNAs of VSV and RABV, which are 11 to 12 kb, are encapsidated by approximately 1,200 copies of a single major nucleoprotein (N protein), with each molecule of N protein covering nine bases.[277,702] Unlike the paramyxovirus *rule of six*, there is no requirement that the genome size be a multiple of this number. The nucleocapsid also contains 466 copies of the phosphoprotein (P protein, formerly called NS protein)[702] and 50 copies of the large polymerase protein (L protein), which are responsible for the virion-associated RNA polymerase activity. The viral RNA polymerase cannot use naked RNA as a template but instead requires that the virion RNA template be encapsidated by N protein. P protein is responsible for binding L protein to the N protein–RNA template, and L protein is likely responsible for all of the enzymatic activities associated with RNA synthesis.

The structures of N protein–RNA complexes from RABV and VSV have been determined by x-ray crystallography.[11,276] The N protein molecule consists of two lobes, with the RNA inserted between the two lobes (Fig. 31.3). In the nucleocapsid, an amino-terminal extension from each N protein subunit interacts both with the adjacent subunit and with the subunit two positions away (Fig. 31.3, inset). Contacts between the C-terminal lobes also contribute to the stability of the nucleocapsid. N protein forms a stable nucleocapsid-like structure even in the absence of RNA.[278,810] The C-terminal lobes of two N protein molecules in the nucleocapsid form a binding site for the P protein polymerase subunit, which is proposed to bind and dissociate in a processive manner during RNA synthesis.[276]

P protein consists of three domains, an acidic N-terminal domain, a central domain, and a C-terminal domain.[185] P protein forms homo-oligomers, which are necessary for P protein to bind L protein to the nucleocapsid and for subsequent

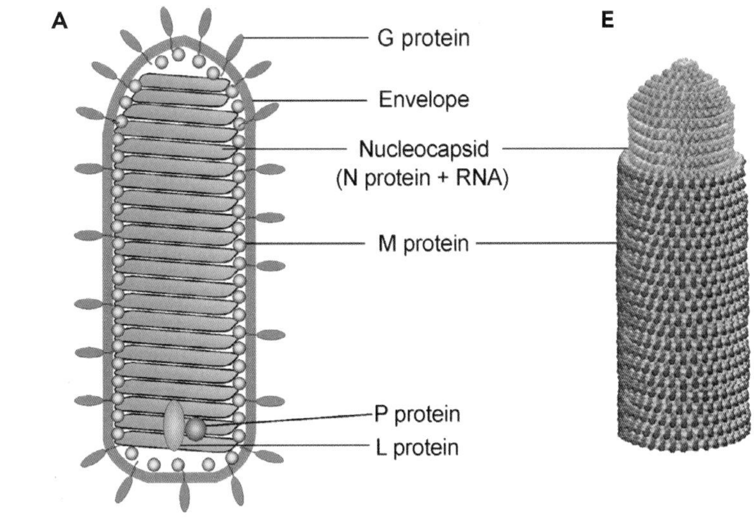

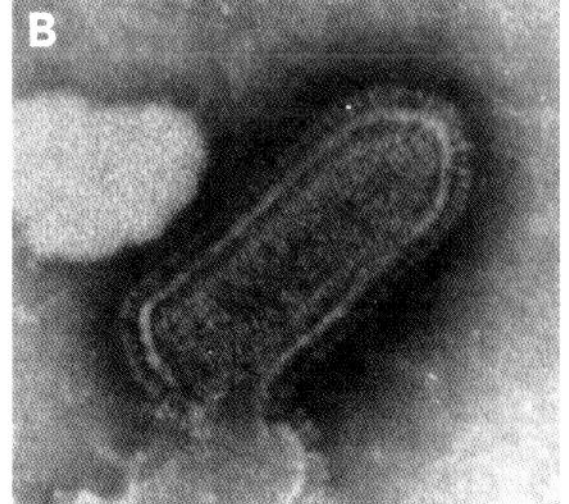

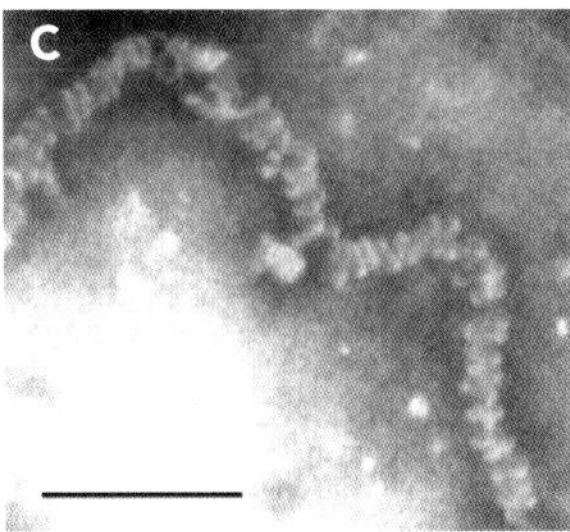

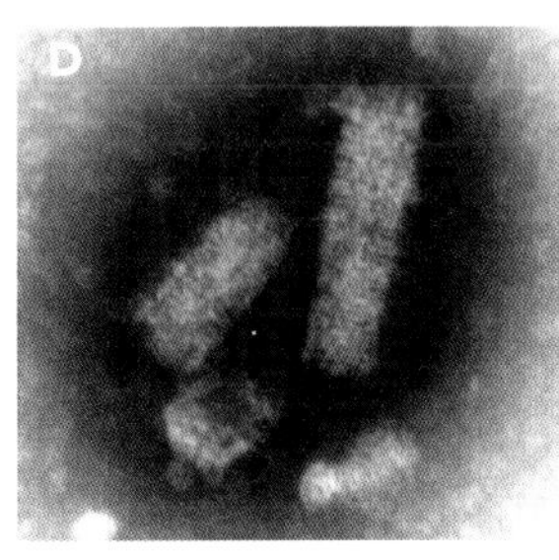

FIGURE 31.2. Structure of rhabdovirus virions. A: Diagram of virion. **B:** Negative stain electron micrograph of vesicular stomatitis virus (VSV) virion. **C:** VSV nucleocapsids prepared by solubilization of virion envelopes with triton X-100 in high-ionic-strength buffer. **D:** VSV nucleocapsid–M protein complexes prepared by solubilization of virion envelopes with triton X-100 in low-ionic-strength buffer. **E:** Model of the VSV nucleocapsid–M protein complex derived from cryoelectron microscopy data of Ge et al.[264] Bar = 100 nm. (Negative stain electron micrographs by E. Alexander Flood, as described in [237].)

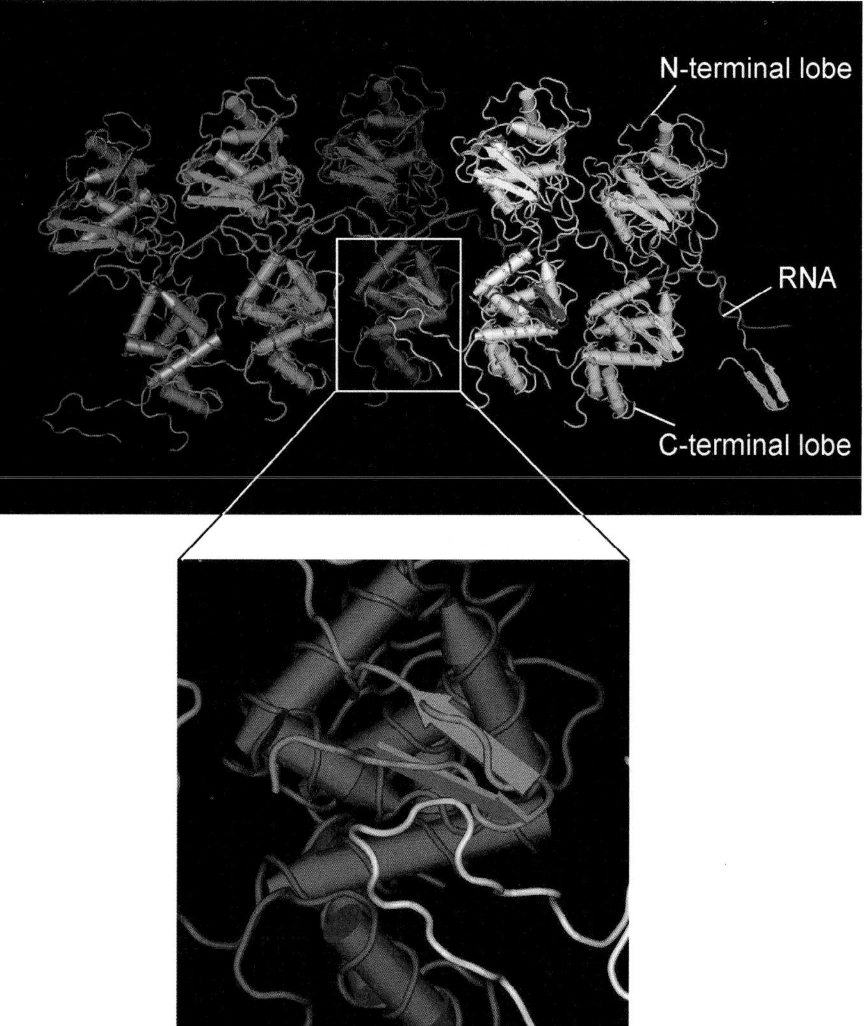

FIGURE 31.3. Structure of the vesicular stomatitis virus (VSV) nucleocapsid. Model of N protein and RNA in the VSV nucleocapsid derived from x-ray crystallography[279] and cryoelectron microscopy.[264] **Inset** shows interaction of the N-terminal extension from the pink N protein subunit with the C-terminal domain of the adjacent subunit (*blue*) as well as the subunit two positions away (*white*). (Assembled from PDB file 2WYY (MMDB ID: 80066) using Cn3D4.2 software.)

transcriptase activity.[256,257] The oligomerization is mediated by the P protein central domain, the structure of which has been determined by x-ray crystallography.[184] Both the isolated central domain and the unphosphorylated full-length P protein form dimers.[184,267] The phosphorylated transcriptionally active form of P protein was originally considered to be a trimer, based on epitope dilution experiments.[256] Reanalysis of those data,[693] however, suggests that P protein forms tetramers, similar to the P proteins of paramyxoviruses. Much of the N-terminal domain of P protein appears to be intrinsically disordered, although it probably adopts a well-defined structure upon binding ligands such as the L protein or soluble N protein (N_0) involved in encapsidation of progeny genomes during genome replication.[268,434] Two sites in the N-terminal domain must be phosphorylated by cellular casein kinase II for P protein to form oligomers and act in transcription.[257,689] The C-terminal domain is responsible for binding the P protein to the nucleocapsid template, as described earlier. A basic region near the C-terminus of P protein is also necessary for interaction with L protein in viral transcription.[164] The structures of the C-terminal domains of RV and VSV P proteins have been determined by x-ray crystallography and NMR spectroscopy.[276,481,588]

The organization of the L protein has been deduced by analysis of sequence homology among members of the order *Mononegavirales,* which identified six conserved regions designated CRI through CRVI. The RNA polymerase activity has been mapped to CRIII.[655] The L protein also has messenger RNA (mRNA) capping and methylation activity, which map to CRV[437] and CRVI,[435] respectively. High-resolution structures of L protein have not been published thus far, but its domain organization has been determined by negative stain electron microscopy combined with proteolytic digestion and deletion mutagenesis.[577] The protein is organized into a ring-like structure that contains the RNA polymerase and an appendage of three globular domains. The capping activity maps to a globular domain attached directly to the ring, and the methylation activity maps to a more distal and flexibly connected domain.

When released from virions by treatment with detergents at high ionic strength, the nucleocapsid is loosely coiled and flexible (Fig. 31.2C), with a total length of 3.6 μm.[702] In virions, however, the nucleocapsid is associated with the matrix (M) protein, which condenses the nucleocapsid into a tightly coiled helical nucleocapsid–M protein complex (Fig. 31.2D), sometimes referred to as the virus *skeleton,*[54,514,515] which gives the virion its bullet-like shape.[54,463,514,515] The structure of the nucleocapsid–M protein complex has been determined to 10.6 Å resolution by analysis of cryoelectron micrographs of VSV virions (Fig. 31.2E).[264] The N and M protein subunits in this structure were identified by fitting the electron density data from electron microscopy to that from x-ray crystallography. The N protein and RNA form an inner helical layer surrounded by an outer helical layer composed of M protein. The orientation of N protein subunits indicated that the 5′ end of the genome RNA is at the tip of the bullet, and the 3′ end is at the base. The conical tip of the bullet is formed by approximately seven successive turns of the N protein helix expanding gradually from 10 subunits per turn to 37.5 subunits per turn, with two turns forming a helical repeat. This pattern continues for approximately 29 turns to form the cylindrical trunk of the bullet. The M protein layer is formed by interaction of each M protein subunit with two successive turns of the N protein helix. The helical structure is held together by the M–N interactions as well as the interaction between M protein subunits in successive turns of the helix.

The amino-terminal 50 to 57 amino acids of M protein appear to be largely disordered in purified M protein.[260,274,362] However, this sequence may form an ordered structure upon binding to the nucleocapsid.[264] The remainder of the M protein sequence forms a compactly folded C-terminal domain, whose structure has been determined by x-ray crystallography.[261,274] Sequences in the amino-terminal region are involved in interaction with N protein in the nucleocapsid–M protein complex, as well as interacting with sequences in the C-terminal domain in M–M interactions in the complex.[144,160,264,274] The C-terminal domain of M protein also appears to interact with the virus envelope, perhaps with the cytoplasmic domain of the envelope glycoprotein.[264]

The structure derived from cryoelectron microscopy accounts for approximately 1,200 of the 1,800 copies of M protein in the virion. The remaining 600 M protein subunits are likely present in a nonhelical arrangement, thus rendering them undetectable in the analysis. One likely location is in association with the envelope lipid bilayer. M protein interacts with the lipid bilayer of the virus envelope, which was shown using lipophilic photoreactive probes.[430,804] The M protein sequences involved in the interaction are present in the N-terminal region, partially overlapping the sequences involved in interaction with the nucleocapsid.[160,430] This supports the idea that there are two populations of M protein in the virion, one involved in the nucleocapsid–M protein complex and the other involved in interaction with the envelope lipid bilayer.

The lipids of the envelope are derived from the host cell membrane during virus assembly by budding. The lipid composition of the envelope generally reflects that of the host membrane from which the virus buds, consisting primarily of phospholipids and cholesterol, although virus envelopes appear to be enriched in cholesterol and sphingomyelin compared with the host membranes from which they were derived.[455] The virus envelope contains approximately 300 to 400 spike-like projections composed of a single species of viral glycoprotein (G protein). The individual spikes are trimers of G protein,[188,262,765] which function in virus attachment and penetration by fusion of the virus envelope with endosome membranes. G protein is anchored in the envelope lipid bilayer by a 20–amino acid hydrophobic transmembrane domain near the C-terminus, which is followed by a 29–amino acid *cytoplasmic domain,* which is inside the virus envelope.[606] The structure of the 446–amino acid external domain (ectodomain) of the VSV G protein has been determined by x-ray crystallography in both the neutral pH ("prefusion") and low pH ("postfusion") conformations (Fig. 31.4).[595,596] Like other viral fusion proteins, the two conformations are dramatically different, indicating that major structural rearrangements must occur during

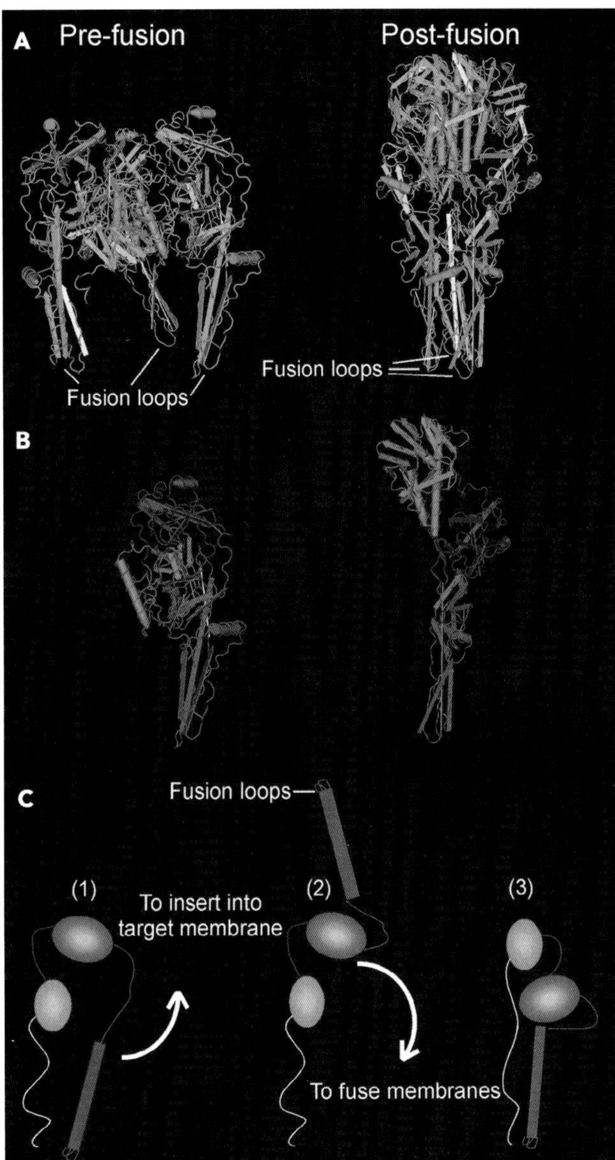

FIGURE 31.4. Structure of the vesicular stomatitis virus (VSV) G protein. A: G protein ectodomain trimers in the prefusion and postfusion state. G protein ectodomain (residues 1 to 422) was generated by limited proteolysis of virions with thermolysin.[595,596] **B:** Comparison of domain organization of a single G protein subunit in the pre- and postfusion states. **C:** Diagram of domain rearrangements in transition from prefusion state **(1)** to proposed intermediate inserted into target membrane **(2)** to postfusion state **(3)**. White line represents G stem leading to membrane anchor sequence that is missing from the crystal structure. (Assembled from PDB files 2CMZ and 2J6J using Cn3D4.2 software.)

the fusion process. The surprising result is that the folding of G protein bears no resemblance to the fusion proteins of other negative-strand or positive-strand RNA viruses that have been determined. Instead, the structure of the VSV G protein is homologous to that of the gB glycoprotein of herpesviruses.[305] This raises interesting questions about the evolutionary origin of these proteins.

GENOME STRUCTURES

Genomes of rhabdoviruses are single-stranded, nonsegmented RNA of negative polarity. They lack 5′ caps and 3′ poly A, consistent with their inability to function as mRNA. Genomes of three genera of *Rhabdoviridae* are shown diagrammatically in Figure 31.5. Genomes of lyssaviruses and vesiculoviruses are similar to each other. The approximately 50 nucleotides at the 3′ and 5′ ends (the leader and trailer sequences, respectively) are partially complementary. They contain important *cis*-acting sequences that serve as promoters for transcription and replication and as signals for encapsidation of genomes and antigenomes during replication, as described later. Although they do not encode proteins, short RNAs of unknown function are generated from these sequences. The five protein-encoding genes are in the order 3′–N–P/C–M–G–L–5′, which is the order of the analogous genes in other nonsegmented, negative-strand RNA viruses, regardless of the number of additional viral genes. Each gene junction contains a conserved sequence specifying the end (E) of the upstream gene, a two-nucleotide intergenic (I) sequence, and the start (S) sequence for the downstream gene. These sequences control the activities of the viral RNA polymerase, which transcribes these genes according to a stop–start mechanism described later. In general, the 5′ and 3′ untranslated regions of the viral mRNA are short (10 to 50 nucleotides) and lack *cis*-acting sequences that control translation or mRNA turnover. The one exception is the P/C gene of vesiculoviruses, which contains alternate start codons. The upstream start codon initiates translation of the P protein, whereas two downstream start codons initiate translation of an alternate reading frame that encodes two small basic proteins, C and C′.[392,667] Analogous proteins encoded by paramyxoviruses often play a role in pathogenesis by altering viral gene expression and suppressing host responses to virus infection. Mutation of the VSV P gene to introduce a stop codon in the C and C′ open reading frame (without altering the sequence of the P protein), however, had no detectable effect on virus replication in cell culture or pathogenesis in mice.[392] This still leaves open the possibility that the C and C′ proteins play a role in replication in other hosts.

The genomes of ephemeroviruses are larger than those of most other rhabdoviruses. The genome of BEFV is 14.8 kb and contains 10 genes (3′–N–P–M–G–G_{NS}–α_1–α_2–β–γ–L-5′) separated by intergenic regions of 26 and 53 nucleotides.[177,735] The genome of the related Adelaide River virus is 14.6 kb in length and contains nine genes (3′–N–P–M–G–G_{NS}–α_1–α_2–β–L–5′) separated by intergenic regions of one to four nucleotides.[742] The G_{NS} gene encodes a glycoprotein, which is synthesized in approximately the same amount as G protein during virus infection,[737] but it is not found in the mature virion. Intracellularly, G_{NS} protein is localized in the endoplasmic reticulum–Golgi complex, and it is associated with amorphous structures in the cell surface but not with viruses in the budding process. It is highly glycosylated, with a molecular weight of 90 kD. G_{NS} protein shares significant amino acid sequence homology with the G protein, but it does not induce *protective* neutralizing antibodies.[312] The function of G_{NS} protein is unknown. It has been proposed that the gene coding for this protein originated by gene duplication by a copy-choice mechanism involving relocation of the polymerase in an upstream position during viral replication.[742]

Genomes of novirhabdoviruses contain an NV gene between the G and L genes. The NV protein (12 to 14 kD) is expressed at variable levels in infected cells but is not detectable in purified virions. The NV protein sequences are significantly less conserved between viruses in different species than sequences of the other structural proteins, such that there is no significant amino acid sequence similarity between the NV proteins of IHNV and VHSV. The specific function of the NV protein is not yet defined, but it is required for efficient virus replication. Results of studies with NV gene deletion mutants generated by reverse genetics are inconsistent in that the NV appears to be required for pathogenicity in IHNV and VHSV but not snakehead virus (SHRV).[317,398]

Rhabdoviruses that have not been assigned to a particular genus have a variety of additional transcription units. For example, the gene order of FLAV is 3′–N–P–pseudogene 1–19K–pseudogene 2–M–G–L–5′. The unique features include the gene encoding a 19-kD protein of unknown function, surrounded by two pseudogenes, about 500 nucleotides each, situated between the P and M genes.[86,177] The gene order of TUPV is 3′–N–P/C–M–SH–G–L–5′. The unique small hydrophobic (SH) transcription unit between M and G genes encodes a protein with two hydrophobic amino acid stretches, including a potential signal sequence at the amino terminus

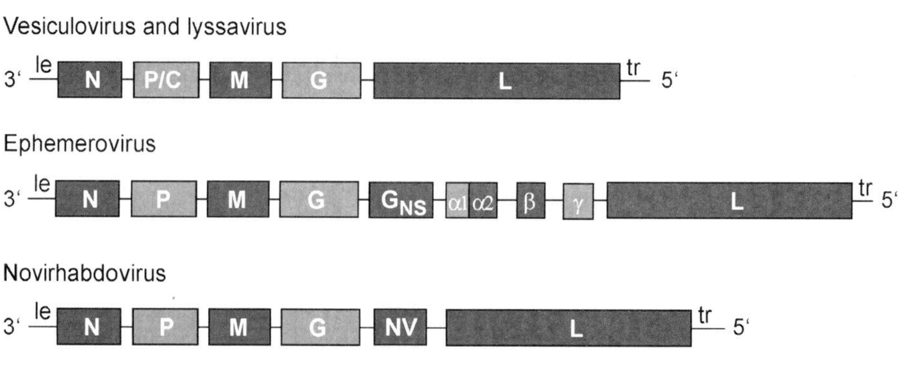

FIGURE 31.5. Diagram of rhabdovirus genomes.

and a potential membrane-spanning sequence near the center. The C protein ORF that overlaps the TUPV P gene has the potential to encode a 221–amino acid basic protein that is more than three times larger than the VSV C protein.[668]

The genome of Ngaingan virus (NGAV) is over 15.7 kb, which is the largest genome yet described for any rhabdovirus, containing 13 ORFs in the order 3′–N–P–U1–U2–U3–M–U4–G–G_{NS}–U5–U6–U7–L–5′. The NGAV P gene contains two alternative ORFs designated P1′ and P2′, analogous to alternative P ORFs referred to as either C or P′ in several other rhabdoviruses. The G_{NS} gene encodes a nonstructural glycoprotein (568 amino acids [aa]) analogous to that of ephemeroviruses. NGAV contains seven additional genes (U1 through U7) with the potential to encode small proteins of unknown function. Although similar in size (81 to 153 aa) to proteins encoded by ORFs located in similar positions in several other rhabdoviruses, they lack significant sequence or structural similarity to any known protein. However, none of the small unique NGAV proteins has yet been detected in infected cells.[283]

The gene order in WONV is 3′–N–U4–P–U1–U2–U3–M–G–U5–L–5′. WONV lacks an alternative ORF in the P gene but contains five additional genes (U1 through U5), each of which encodes a protein that lacks significant amino acid sequence identity with other known proteins. The U1 protein (179 aa) is hydrophilic with numerous potential phosphorylation sites, an N-glycosylation site, an amidation site, and two N-myristoylation sites. The U2 protein (192 aa) contains two predicted N-myristoylation sites and a highly hydrophobic domain of 10 amino acids followed by a mitochondrial energy transfer signature that is characteristic of carrier and transport proteins. The U4 protein (49 aa) contains a single putative N-myristoylation site and shares overall 49% identity with guanosine triphosphate (GTP)-binding proteins of several bacteria. The U5 protein (127 aa) contains a predicted N-terminal extracellular domain, 22-aa transmembrane domain, and highly basic cytoplasmic tail and has overall structural similarity to the α_1 proteins of ephemeroviruses, which have been suggested to be viroporins. Proteins of similar size to the U1, U2, U3, and U5 proteins have been detected in WONV-infected cells by immunoblot analysis using polyclonal mouse ascitic fluid.[284]

The genome of Moussa virus is similar to those of the genera *Lyssavirus* and *Vesiculovirus*. However, the ORFs located in the position of the P (ORF 2) and M (ORF 3) genes in other rhabdoviruses show no nucleotide or amino acid homology to sequences of other rhabdoviruses.[575]

The genomes of Sigma virus and members in the genera *Cytorhabdovirus* and *Nucleorhabdovirus* contain an additional gene between the P and M genes, referred to as "X" or "a." The putative X protein is of unknown function but contains conserved domains found in reverse transcriptases. Another unusual feature is that M and G mRNAs overlap by 33 nucleotides.[106,145]

STAGES OF REPLICATION

The replication cycle of rhabdoviruses is typical of that of most nonsegmented, negative-strand RNA viruses (Fig. 31.6). The initial events of attachment, penetration, and uncoating result in release of the viral nucleocapsid into the cytoplasm of the host cell. The encapsidated parental genome RNA serves as a template for primary transcription by the virion RNA-dependent RNA polymerase, resulting in synthesis of leader (le) RNA and all five viral mRNAs. The accumulation of viral proteins synthesized from primary transcripts leads to replication of the genome, which involves synthesis of full-length positive-strand RNA, or antigenomes. The antigenomes, in turn, serve as templates for synthesis of progeny negative-strand genomes. Encapsidation of genomes and antigenomes occurs concomitantly with their synthesis and, indeed, is a key signal for the RNA polymerase to function as a replicase versus a transcriptase. Progeny nucleocapsids are used for three different purposes: (a) as templates for further rounds of replication; (b) as templates for secondary transcription, which is the major amplification step for viral gene expression; and (c) for assembly into progeny virions, which occurs by budding

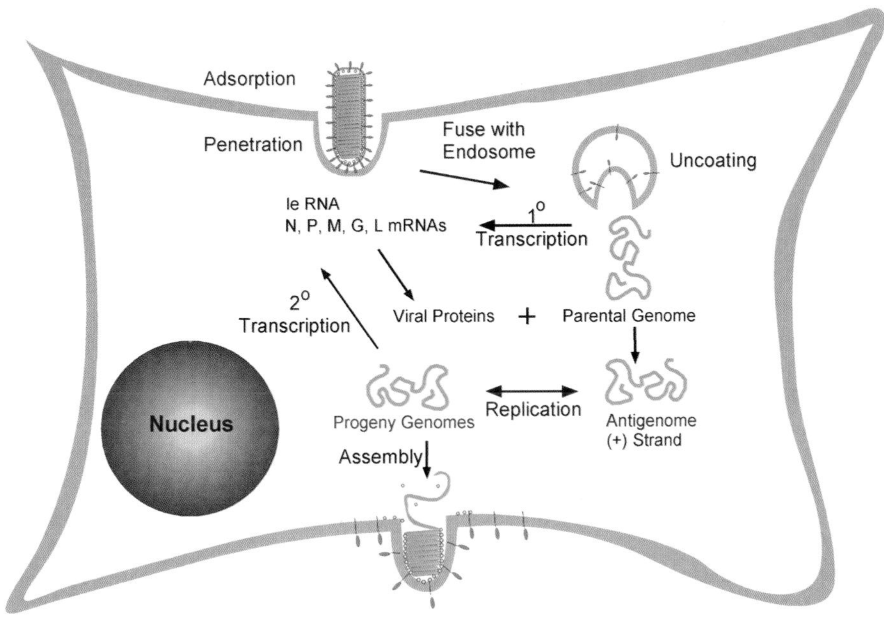

FIGURE 31.6. Diagram of rhabdovirus replication cycle. The steps illustrated are virus adsorption and penetration by endocytosis, envelope fusion with endosome membranes, release of nucleocapsids containing parental genomes into the cytoplasm, primary (1-degree) transcription, genome replication to produce nucleocapsids containing antigenomes and progeny genomes, secondary (2-degree) transcription, and assembly by budding from host plasma membrane. (Drawn by E. Alexander Flood.)

from host membranes. In a single-cycle growth experiment, the early events including attachment, penetration, uncoating, and primary transcription occur within the first few hours postinfection. The processes of genome replication, secondary transcription, and virus assembly occur continuously throughout the remainder of the infectious cycle, which lasts for an additional 12 to 18 hours for VSV or several days for RABV.

Mechanism of Attachment

Rhabdoviruses appear to use a variety of different receptors for attachment to different types of host cells. The RABV G protein binds most effectively to cells of neuronal origin,[713] reflecting the neurotropism of RABV *in vivo.* Several different surface molecules expressed at high levels on neurons have been identified as potential receptors, including the nicotinic acetyl choline receptor,[259,431] the neural cell adhesion molecule (CD56),[704] and the low-affinity nerve-growth factor receptor $p75^{NTR}$.[714,715] Expression of CD56 and $p75^{NTR}$ has been shown to confer susceptibility to RABV on cells that are normally resistant to infection. Transgenic mice that lack CD56 show a delay in RABV spread through the central nervous system (CNS) and in RABV-induced mortality, but the mice still die following virus infection,[704] indicating that other receptors are involved. RABV infection of transgenic mice that lack $p75^{NTR}$ was found to be similar to that of wild-type mice of the same strain,[339] initially indicating that $p75^{NTR}$ was not an important receptor for RABV pathogenesis. However, RABV G protein binds to a region of $p75^{NTR}$ that is present on a splice variant of $p75^{NTR}$ that is still expressed in the transgenic mice.[414] Thus, further experiments are required to fully evaluate the role of $p75^{NTR}$ in RABV pathogenesis.

In addition to the receptors that are enriched on cells of neuronal origin, RABV can also use receptors that are widely distributed among many cell types.[582,685,793] These receptors appear to be of lower affinity than those on neuronal cell surfaces[713] and have been difficult to identify. A similar difficulty exists in identifying receptors for VSV, which also binds to many different cell types in culture by interactions that appear to be of low affinity and often are not easily saturable. For both RABV and VSV, negatively charged lipids have been proposed to be cellular receptors for virus attachment. In the case of RABV, neuraminic acid-containing glycolipids (gangliosides) have been implicated[686] and, in the case of VSV, phosphatidyl serine has been proposed as a cellular receptor,[624] although later experiments have indicated that phosphatidyl serine is not the receptor for VSV.[139] Instead, it seems likely that nonspecific electrostatic and hydrophobic interactions mediate attachment of VSV to cells. Treatment of cells with polycations and polyanions such as diethylaminoethyl-dextran (DEAE-dextran) and dextran sulfate can markedly enhance the efficiency of attachment and infection of cells by both VSV[45] and RABV.[793]

An interesting feature of attachment by both viruses is that binding is markedly enhanced at lower pH in the range from pH 6.5 to 5.6.[248,793] The pH dependence of attachment is similar to that of envelope fusion with cellular membranes (discussed in the next section), although fusion occurs most efficiently at slightly lower pH than does virus attachment. Furthermore, G protein mutations that shift the pH dependence of fusion also shift the pH dependence of attachment.[248] This suggests that attachment to many cell types is mediated by G protein in a conformation that is similar to the fusion-active form of the viral G protein. This idea is supported by experiments with photoactivatable lipid probes, which indicate that the putative *fusion peptide* (described later) is inserted into target membranes under the optimal conditions for both attachment and fusion.[197,542] This would also account for the affinity of the VSV G protein for phosphatidyl serine and other negatively charged phospholipids, because the presence of negatively charged lipids in the target membrane appears to be necessary for virus envelope fusion.[105,199,796]

Mechanism of Penetration

VSV was one of the early examples of a virus shown to penetrate into cells by clathrin-dependent endocytosis.[478] Following attachment to host cell surfaces, virions can either migrate to preformed clathrin-coated pits or nucleate the formation of new coated pits,[157,348] where they undergo endocytosis into coated vesicles (Fig. 31.7). Because VSV virions are longer than the typical diameter of a coated vesicle, the final closure of the endocytic vesicle requires participation of the actin cytoskeleton.[157,158] The endocytic vesicles lose their clathrin coats to become early endosomes. The contents of early endosomes are transported to late endosomes and lysosomes for degradation. During this process, the endosomal vesicles often invaginate to form multiple intraluminal vesicles.[282] Such membranes are referred to as *multivesicular bodies* (MVBs). As virions progress through the endocytic pathway, they are exposed to progressively lower pH. At a pH below 6.5, the G protein mediates fusion of the viral envelope with the endosome membrane. This fusion event releases the internal virion components into the cytoplasm (left side of Fig. 31.7). Most of the available evidence indicates that VSV virions fuse primarily with the membranes of early endosomes.[348,498,648] Other evidence, however, suggests that many fusion events occur within MVBs (right side of Fig. 31.7), releasing the internal virion contents into the cytoplasmic contents trapped within the MVBs and requiring *back-fusion* of internal vesicles with the limiting membrane of the MVBs to release the viral nucleocapsid into the cytoplasm of the cell.[422,460] Viral proteins that fail to be released into the cytoplasm are degraded by proteases and other enzymes in lysosomes.[478]

The mechanism by which rhabdovirus G proteins induce fusion of the virus envelope with cellular membranes shares many features with other viral envelope fusion proteins but is clearly distinct in several respects. The VSV G protein and the structurally similar fusion proteins of herpesviruses and baculoviruses are referred to as class III fusion proteins to distinguish them from class I proteins, which are structurally similar to the influenza virus hemagglutinin, and class II proteins, which include the envelope glycoproteins of the alphaviruses and flaviviruses.[32] As with class I fusion proteins, rhabdovirus G proteins exist as a trimer of subunits held together by noncovalent bonds.[188,262,765] Unlike most viral envelope proteins, however, the subunits of G protein are in a dynamic equilibrium between monomers and trimers because of the rapid dissociation and reassociation of subunits.[464,801,802] As with most low pH-dependent fusion proteins, the effects of low pH are mediated by conformational changes in G protein. Unlike other viral fusion proteins, the conformational changes in G protein are reversible upon returning the pH to neutrality, whereas those of many other viral fusion proteins are not reversible.[188,263,573]

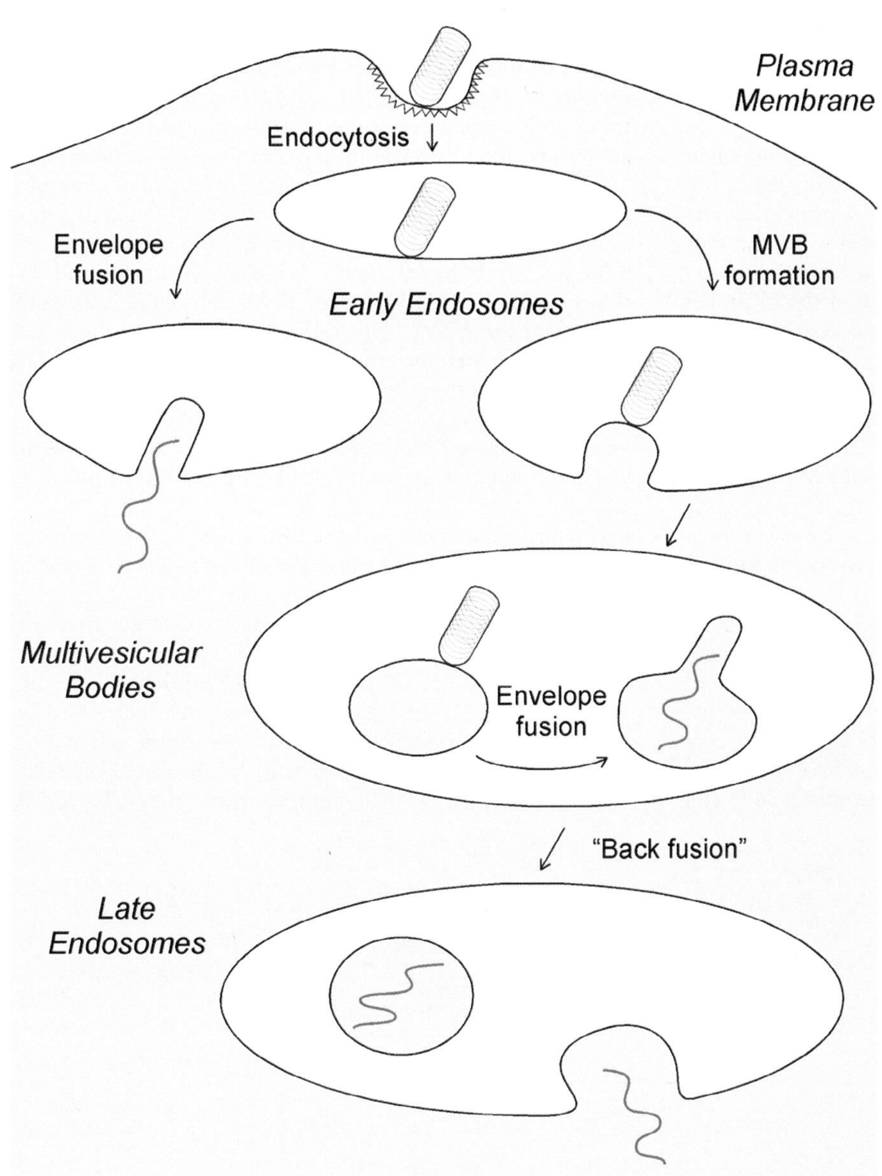

FIGURE 31.7. Diagram of rhabdovirus penetration by endocytosis. Pathway on the **left** shows virus envelope fusion with early endosomes. Pathway on the **right** shows virus envelope fusion with internal vesicles of multivesicular bodies (MVBs) and release of nucleocapsids into the cytoplasm by "back-fusion" with the MVB-limiting membrane.

A general principle by which viral envelope proteins promote fusion is that they must insert into the target membrane through a region of their sequence referred to as the *fusion peptide*. In the class I fusion proteins, such as the influenza virus hemagglutinin (HA) and the paramyxovirus F proteins, the fusion peptide resides at the N-terminus of one of the subunits (HA_2 or F_1, respectively) generated by proteolysis of an inactive precursor. In contrast, proteolysis of rhabdovirus G proteins is not involved in activating fusion. This is similar to the case of the class II fusion proteins, in which the fusion peptide appears to be an internal region of the protein sequence. The regions of G protein that insert into target membranes at low pH have been mapped using photoactivatable lipid probes and mutagenesis studies in both the RABV and VSV G proteins.[197,249,441,684,808] These sequences form two loops containing hydrophobic amino acids that extend from the protein structure ("fusion loops," Fig. 31.4A). In the neutral pH "prefusion" state, the fusion loops are oriented toward the viral membrane (Fig. 31.4A, B). Upon lowering the pH, there is a proposed intermediate, in which the domain containing the fusion loops is reoriented to insert into the target membrane (Fig. 31.4C). Fusion of the viral and target membrane involves another domain rearrangement that brings the two membranes together in the "postfusion" state.

A second region of the G protein sequence functionally involved in fusion is the membrane-proximal ectodomain sequence immediately N-terminal to the membrane anchor sequence. Most of this sequence is not visible in the x-ray structures, because it was cleaved to solubilize the G protein. Mutations in this region dramatically inhibit fusion.[347,647] G protein truncations containing part of this region (amino acids 421 to 461) together with the membrane anchor sequence and the cytoplasmic domain (*G stems*) enhance the fusion activity of other membrane fusion proteins and are able to cause hemifusion (mixing of the outer phospholipid leaflets of the two membranes) in the absence of other fusion proteins.[347] The cooperation of the fusion loops and the membrane-proximal sequence may be analogous to similarly separate sequences in other viral fusion proteins in bringing the viral and host membranes together for fusion.

Uncoating and Primary Transcription

Following fusion of the virus envelope with endosome membranes, which releases the internal virion components into the cytoplasm of the host cell, the viral M protein dissociates from the nucleocapsid.[162,498,590] This step is necessary for viral RNA synthesis to occur, because M protein inhibits viral transcription.[107,136,443,543,775] Binding of most of the M protein to nucleocapsids is readily reversible,[461] and dissociation following envelope fusion is believed to occur spontaneously, although acidification of the virion interior appears to promote M protein dissociation from the nucleocapsid, similar to the M1 protein of influenza virus.[497] Rhabdoviruses do not encode a separate ion channel protein analogous to the M2 protein of influenza viruses. Instead, the G protein is responsible for the permeability of the envelope to protons.[497] Once the M protein has dissociated from the nucleocapsid, no further uncoating is necessary, because the encapsidated RNA is the template for the viral transcriptase complex.

The first biosynthetic step in the viral replicative cycle is primary transcription, mediated by the virion-associated, RNA-dependent RNA polymerase. The mechanism of primary transcription, defined as transcription from parental templates, appears to be identical to that of secondary transcription, or transcription from progeny templates following genome replication. The principal differences are in the much larger quantity of secondary transcripts, because of the larger number of progeny templates, and the brief time of primary transcription, compared with the prolonged period of secondary transcription throughout most of the viral infectious cycle.

The viral RNA polymerase is fully competent to synthesize all of the viral mRNA without new synthesis of viral proteins, as shown by the transcriptase activity of virion cores following solubilization of the envelope.[51,506] Indeed, the first demonstration of a viral RNA-dependent RNA polymerase was made with virions of VSV.[51] This cell-free transcriptase system has been a major tool in determining the mechanisms of viral transcription, establishing the requirement for both the L and P proteins for RNA polymerase activity[203] and the requirement that the template RNA be encapsidated.[70,202] An early insight was that a single entry point exists for the viral RNA polymerase near the 3′ end of the genome, and the viral mRNAs are transcribed sequentially in the order they appear in the genome: N–P–M–G–L. Thus, transcription of each gene depends on prior transcription of all upstream genes.[1,50,201,336,337] This has since been found to be a general property of nonsegmented, negative-strand RNA viruses (see Chapter 30).

The mechanism of sequential transcription is generally considered to be a stop–start mechanism, in which *cis*-acting signals in the template RNA sequence govern the activities of the transcriptase complex at each gene junction (Fig. 31.8). With the exception of the junction between the leader and N

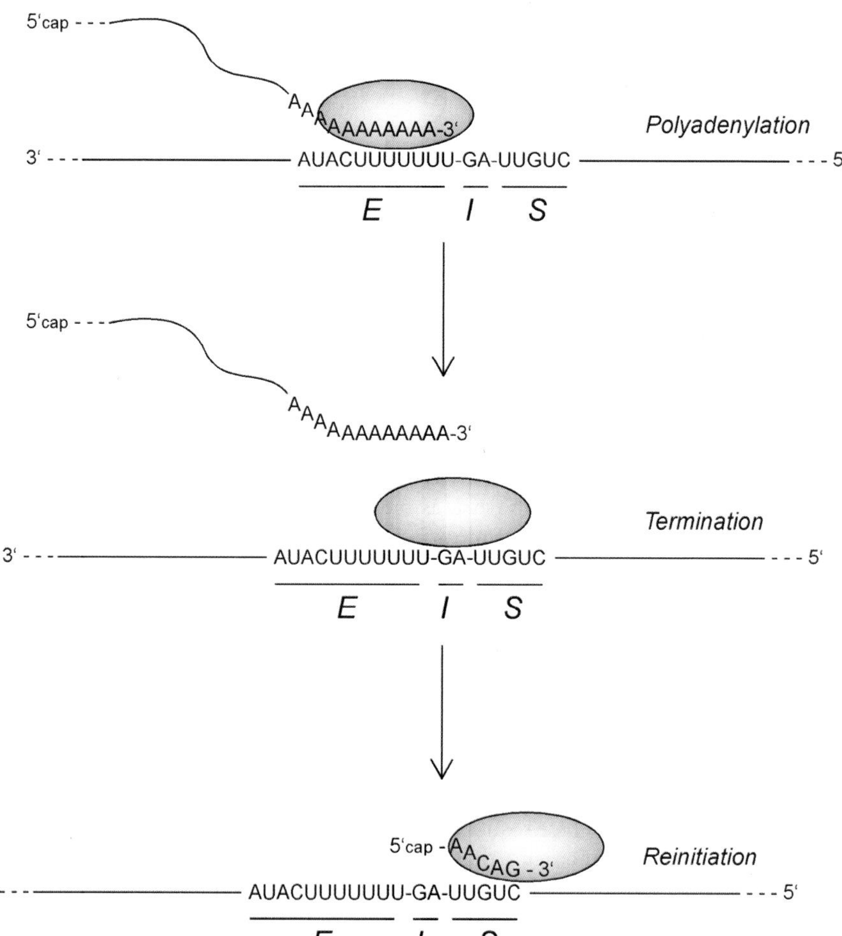

FIGURE 31.8. Diagram of rhabdovirus polymerase activities during transcription in response to gene end (E), intergenic (I), and gene start (S) sequences in the genomic RNA template.

genes (discussed later), each of the VSV gene junctions contains a gene end sequence for the upstream gene (3′AUACUUUUUUU5′); an intergenic dinucleotide (G/CA), which is not transcribed; and a gene start sequence for the downstream gene (3′UUGUC5′).[604] These sequences at each gene junction function as a signal for polyadenylation and termination of the upstream mRNA and also as a signal for the initiation, capping, and methylation of the downstream mRNA.[55–57,315,630,677–679] Whereas the *cis*-acting signals in the template and the resulting modifications to the mRNA have been well defined, the mechanism by which these signals alter the activities of the transcriptase complex to accomplish these different tasks is a major question that remains to be addressed.

Transcript initiation requires both proper termination of the upstream gene and the gene start sequence 3′UUGUC5′.[56,57,315,329,677–679] The requirements of the individual nucleotides in the start sequence for 5′ end modification are more rigorous than the requirements for correct initiation.[679,741] Alterations of the capping and methylation of the transcripts affect the processivity of the polymerase and the extent of polyadenylation of the 3′ end, supporting a model in which the correct initiation and modification of the viral mRNAs play a regulatory role in the subsequent activities of the polymerase.[255,436,741] The mechanism of 5′ end modification of VSV mRNAs and likely those of other negative-strand RNA viruses differs substantially from that of host mRNAs and mRNAs of other virus types. The viral mRNAs are capped by guanosine in a 5′–5′ triphosphate linkage, as are host mRNAs.[2] The capping reaction differs, however, in that both the α- and β-phosphates are derived from the GTP donor, whereas for host capping enzymes, only the α-phosphate is derived from the GTP donor.[2,533] This reaction occurs through an unusual covalent L protein–RNA intermediate.[533] The host translation factor EF-1 is associated with the viral L and P proteins, and it has been proposed that the α-subunit of EF-1 plays a role in the capping reaction through its guanine nucleotide–binding activity.[124,574]

The mechanism of methylation of the viral mRNA cap is also unusual. S-adenosyl methionine is used as a methyl donor,[2] as with host enzymes. However, instead of having separate enzymes that catalyze ribose 2′-O methylation versus guanine-N-7 methylation, both activities appear to reside in a single domain of L.[254,275,435,438] This domain has a single binding site for S-adenosyl methionine and transfers the methyl groups in an unconventional order, in which 2′-O methylation precedes guanine-N-7 methylation.[576]

Following elongation of viral mRNA, the transcriptase complex encounters a termination signal at the end of each gene consisting of the sequence 3′AUACUUUUUUU. This signals the polymerase to "stutter" over the seven Us in the template, resulting in polyadenylation of the viral mRNA.[55,56] Occasionally, the termination signal is ignored, resulting in read-through by the polymerase to give a dicistronic transcript.[56,57,311] Some nonsegmented, negative-strand viruses have gene junctions with a high degree of read-through, which plays a substantial role in regulating the relative levels of the different viral proteins. Because read-through transcripts are rather uncommon for VSV, they are not thought to play a significant role in regulation of viral gene expression.

Following the polyadenylation reaction, which stops after addition of approximately 200 As, two possible fates exist for the transcriptase complex at each gene junction. The most common outcome is that the transcriptase complex traverses the two intergenic nucleotides and resumes transcription at the initiation signal of the downstream gene. Approximately 20% to 30% of transcriptase complexes fail to resume transcription of the downstream gene, however, and presumably dissociate from the template, leading to a 20% to 30% attenuation of expression of the downstream gene at each gene junction.[336,730,757] This transcription attenuation results in a gradient of mRNA and protein expression, such that the abundance of each gene product depends on its distance from the 3′ end of the genome (i.e., N > P > M > G > L). The G–L gene junction is unusual in that the level of attenuation is much higher than that at the other gene junctions,[49] resulting in much lower levels of L protein relative to the other viral proteins. The basis for this difference is not known, because the sequence of the G–L gene junction does not differ from that of the other gene junctions.

Transcription attenuation is a general feature of nonsegmented, negative-strand RNA viruses and is the major mechanism regulating abundance of the individual mRNA. The importance of the gene order in regulating the relative levels of viral proteins was dramatically illustrated by genetic engineering experiments to change the order of the genes of VSV. The resulting changes in relative abundance of the viral proteins resulted in substantial reductions in viral replication and pathogenesis.[49,757] The similarity of the basic mechanisms in virus replication among nonsegmented, negative-strand RNA viruses and their dependence on the relative levels of each viral protein presumably accounts for the conservation of the basic gene order among these viruses.

The initiation and termination of transcription of the leader RNA differs from that of the viral mRNAs. The leader RNA is encoded by the 47 3′-terminal nucleotides of the genome. The leader gene differs from the other genes both in terms of the *cis*-acting signals in the template that initiate transcription[760] and the nature of the product leader RNA, which is phosphorylated at the 5′ end and lacks a cap structure. In addition, the sequence at the leader–N gene junction is distinct from that of the other gene junctions and lacks the U_7 sequence that governs polyadenylation.[760] Correspondingly, leader RNA is not polyadenylated. Another unusual feature of transcriptional regulation at this gene junction is that its behavior is different in the cell-free transcription system versus transcription in infected cells. In the cell-free system, synthesis of leader RNA is required to transcribe the downstream N gene, consistent with the single polymerase entry site and stop–start model.[201,762] In infected cells, however, the viral RNA polymerase can initiate synthesis at the first downstream gene without prior synthesis of leader RNA. This has been shown by inserting a small gene between the leader and N genes and determining the target size for UV inactivation of the inserted gene.[762] This is the only gene junction that shows this behavior, because transcription initiation at all of the other genes requires prior transcription of the upstream gene both in the cell-free assay and in infected cells.

The difference in the site of initiation in infected cells versus that in the cell-free system indicates that host factors can influence the site of initiation. A viral transcriptase complex has been isolated from VSV-infected cells that contains, in addition to P and L proteins, the host proteins EF-1α, heat shock protein 60 (hsp60), and smaller amounts of the host mRNA capping enzyme guanyl transferase.[574] Unlike the virion RNA polymerase, this complex initiates transcription at the N gene and does not transcribe leader RNA.[574] The ability of the polymerase to independently initiate at the first gene downstream of the leader gene appears to account for the phenotype of a VSV mutant (polR1) that synthesizes N mRNA in excess over leader RNA,[128] which would be difficult to achieve if transcription of the N mRNA required prior transcription of the leader RNA. The mutation responsible for the polR phenotype is in the N protein associated with the template,[127] indicating that the nature of the template can influence the site of initiation.

Genome RNA Replication

Requirement for Encapsidation of Newly Synthesized RNA

A fundamental principle in replication of nonsegmented, negative-strand RNA viruses is that the ability of the RNA polymerase to replicate the viral genome depends on new viral protein synthesis to encapsidate the newly synthesized RNA. For example, treating infected cells with inhibitors of protein synthesis (e.g., cycloheximide) allows synthesis of viral mRNA but inhibits replication of genome RNA.[324,756] The critical viral protein required for replication is the N protein, as shown by its ability to support synthesis of genome RNA in the cell-free system.[550] In infected cells, however, a complex of N protein with P protein (often referred to as N_0–P) is likely to be the active complex in promoting genome replication.[555,556] The role of P protein in this complex appears to be to maintain the solubility and proper folding of N protein so that the nascent RNA synthesized by the RNA polymerase can be encapsidated.[167,470,476,477] Analysis of an N_0–P complex expressed in insect cells indicates that the complex contains one N protein and two P proteins.[480]

Encapsidation of nascent RNA appears to constitute a signal for the viral RNA polymerase to ignore the sequences in the genome template at each gene junction that govern the stop–start mechanism for transcription, thereby generating full-length, encapsidated RNA that is complementary to the genome (i.e., antigenomes). Use of antigenomes as templates results in synthesis of progeny genomes. The mechanism of RNA replication appears to be the same regardless of whether genomes or antigenomes are used as templates. In particular, replication of both templates requires that the nascent product RNA be encapsidated to generate full-length products. In addition to serving as a template for progeny genomes, the antigenome can be used as a template to generate a short, noncapped, nonpolyadenylated RNA complementary to the 3′ end of the antigenome that is analogous to the leader RNA. Variously called the *minus strand leader* or *trailer* RNA, this RNA is found in small amounts in infected cells and is the primary product produced in the cell-free system when antigenomes are used as templates in the absence of a source of new viral proteins.[432,755,776]

Cis-Acting Signals and RNA Polymerase Complexes that Govern Replication Versus Transcription

The critical *cis*-acting RNA sequences that govern replication are located at the 3′ ends of the genome and antigenome (Fig. 31.9). These sequences in the templates serve as promoters to initiate RNA synthesis, and their complementary sequences at the 5′ end of the product RNA serve as encapsidation signals, with the resulting encapsidation permitting elongation of the RNA into full-length products. The sequences required for encapsidation have been mapped using synthetic RNA in cell-free encapsidation assays and also in transfected cells using minigenomes (described later).[163,507,548,760] The sequences in the templates that serve as promoters for replication and transcription have been defined by mutagenesis studies using minigenomes.[439,440,548,758,760] The 3′ termini of the genome and antigenome of VSV are identical at 15 of 18 positions. These 18 nucleotides are essential elements of both the genomic and antigenomic promoters. The near identity of the 3′ termini of the genome and antigenome implies that both RNAs display terminal complementarity. This complementarity enhances the activity of these RNA as templates for replication,[758] suggesting that base pairing of the termini is an important element of promoter recognition by the VSV RNA polymerase, similar to promoter recognition by the influenza virus RNA polymerase.

The genomic and antigenomic promoters of VSV differ substantially at positions 19 to 29 and 34 to 46. These

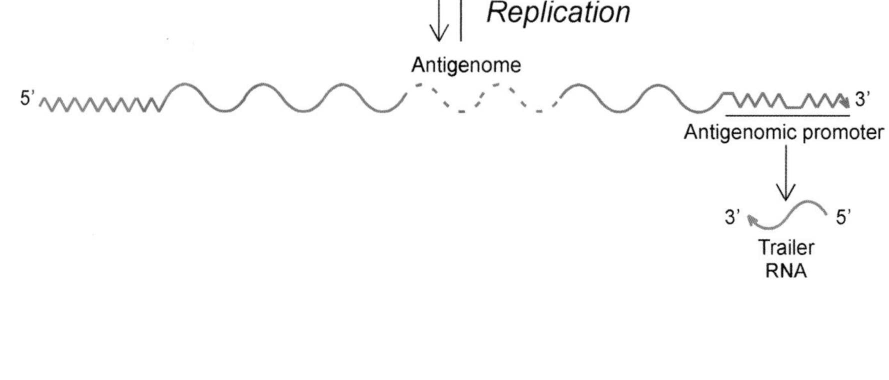

FIGURE 31.9. Diagram of activities of the rhabdovirus genomic and antigenomic promoters in transcription versus replication.

sequences in the genomic promoter are required for mRNA synthesis, but not for replication.[439,760] In contrast, these sequences in the antigenomic promoter serve as an enhancer of replication.[440] As a result of this enhancer activity in the antigenomic promoter, replication of genomes versus antigenomes is asymmetric: many more genomes than antigenomes are synthesized in virus-infected cells.[231,650,666,754] The functional differences between the genomic and antigenomic promoters were dramatically illustrated by engineering an *ambisense* RABV that contained the sequence of the genomic promoter at the 3′ ends of both the genome and antigenome.[231] The promoter in the antigenome of this virus was engineered to drive the transcription of a foreign gene. As a result, both the genome and antigenome of this virus were used as templates for mRNA synthesis—the genome as a template for the five viral mRNAs and the antigenome as a template for the foreign mRNA. Furthermore, the normal asymmetry of replication was abolished, so that genomes and antigenomes were synthesized in approximately equal amounts.

In addition to differences in the *cis*-acting sequences that govern replication versus transcription, differences in the nature of the polymerase complex and the structural requirements of the P protein are also important for replication versus transcription. The C-terminal basic region of P protein that is involved in interaction with L protein is required for transcription, but not replication.[164] Similarly, phosphorylation of serine and threonine residues in the N-terminal domain of P protein by cellular casein kinase II is required for transcription, but not for replication.[550] In contrast, phosphorylation of sites in the C-terminal domain is required for replication, but not transcription.[329] These differences in the structural requirements for P protein are consistent with the idea that the polymerase complex that carries out replication is distinct from that which carries out transcription. In particular, the transcriptase appears to be an L–(P_4) complex, whereas the replicase appears to be an L–N–P_4 complex.[286] Establishing the structural basis for the differences in replication versus transcription, particularly the ability of the two polymerase complexes to respond to *cis*-acting signals in the template and the requirement for encapsidation of the nascent product RNA, is a key issue for understanding RNA synthesis by rhabdoviruses and other nonsegmented, negative-strand viruses.

Secondary Transcription

Once nucleocapsids containing progeny genomes begin to accumulate in infected cells, they are used as templates for secondary transcription, and they are assembled into progeny virions. In the case of VSV, most of the viral nucleocapsids that are made during the infectious cycle remain associated with infected cells and are not released in the form of progeny virions,[379,666] suggesting that use of these nucleocapsids as templates predominates over their use for virion assembly. Although conceptually it is the last step in the virus replication cycle, virus assembly begins at approximately the same time as secondary transcription (for VSV, around 2 to 3 hours postinfection), reaches a maximum rate around 8 to 10 hours postinfection when viral protein synthesis is at its maximum, and declines concomitantly with a decline in viral protein synthesis toward the end of the infectious cycle around 16 to 20 hours postinfection.

Assembly of Progeny Virions

As with most viruses, the individual components of rhabdoviruses are assembled in separate cellular compartments and only come together in the final steps of virus assembly: the nucleocapsid is assembled during the process of RNA replication as described in the previous section, the G protein is assembled in the secretory pathway, and the M protein is synthesized as a soluble protein that then associates with the cytoplasmic surface of the host plasma membrane.

Assembly of G Protein

The assembly of the VSV G protein in the secretory pathway of host cells has been studied for many years by both virologists and cell biologists, not only for its importance for virus assembly, but also as a prototype for the assembly of other host and viral integral membrane proteins. G protein is synthesized by ribosomes bound to the rough endoplasmic reticulum (ER) and is inserted into the ER membrane in the typical *type I* orientation.[605,606] An N-terminal signal sequence of 16 amino acids targets the protein for insertion and is cleaved from the nascent polypeptide.[446] The new N-terminus and most of the protein sequence (446 amino acids) are transferred to the luminal side of the ER membrane to form the protein's ectodomain.[367] A hydrophobic sequence of 20 amino acids near the C-terminus serves as a stop–transfer sequence and becomes the membrane anchor.[606] The 29 C-terminal amino acids remain on the cytoplasmic side of the ER membrane and form the protein's cytoplasmic domain.[367] Two asparagine residues in G protein are glycosylated during translation.[368] The initial oligosaccharides added to G protein are of the high mannose type, which are later modified by enzymes in Golgi membranes to the complex type of oligosaccharides.[581]

Following insertion into the ER, G protein associates with two molecular chaperones, BiP (GRP78) and calnexin,[290,467] which assist in the formation of the proper disulfide bonds and correct folding of the ectodomain. Mutations that prevent correct folding of the ectodomain or that prevent glycosylation, which is required for calnexin binding, result in the formation of aggregates of misfolded G protein together with BiP, which are not transported from the ER.[189,467,468] Therefore, the ability of a mutant protein to be transported from the ER is a minimal criterion by which it can be said to be properly folded. Shortly after release of the properly folded G protein from the chaperones, G protein monomers associate into trimers[189] and are transported to Golgi membranes by membrane vesicles that bud from the ER and subsequently fuse with Golgi membranes.[394,705] G protein is one of the most rapidly transported integral membrane proteins, requiring approximately 15 minutes to be transported from ER to Golgi membranes.[63] This rapid transport is dependent on a six–amino acid sequence in the cytoplasmic domain, which can function to concentrate G protein at the sites of vesicle budding.[520,641]

Once G protein is transported to Golgi membranes, it undergoes further posttranslational modifications, including conversion of its oligosaccharides from the high-mannose type to the complex type, containing additional N-acetyl glucosamine, galactose, and sialic acid.[581] Although these modifications are not required for G protein function, they provide a convenient and widely used marker for transport of G protein through successive Golgi membranes.[635] Another G protein modification that occurs in Golgi membranes is the addition of the fatty acid palmitate to a cysteine residue in the cytoplasmic domain.[606,625] Again, this modification does not appear to be critical, because some strains of VSV lack this modification, and mutation of the target cysteine residue, which abolishes palmitoylation, does not affect G protein function.[766]

Transport of G protein from Golgi membranes to the plasma membrane requires approximately 15 minutes, so that the total time from synthesis in ER to appearance in the plasma membrane is about 30 minutes.[63] In polarized epithelial cells, G protein is selectively transported to the basolateral surface.[82,271,676] The same amino acid sequence in the cytoplasmic domain that promotes the rapid transport of G protein from ER to Golgi membranes is also necessary for the selective transport to the basolateral surface of polarized epithelial cells.[703] Sorting of G protein and other basolaterally targeted proteins from those destined for the apical surface occurs first in Golgi membranes, and from Golgi membranes G protein is transported to the recycling endosome compartment prior to transport to the basolateral plasma membrane.[20,104,155] This intermediate step presumably reflects additional sorting steps by which cells regulate the protein composition of their plasma membranes.

At the plasma membrane of infected cells, G protein is organized into clusters or *microdomains* that are approximately 100 to 150 nm in diameter.[91,92] These G protein–containing microdomains are formed independently of other viral components[92] and appear to be similar to cholesterol- and sphingolipid-rich *lipid rafts* that serve as sites of assembly for other viruses, such as influenza viruses.[455,561] Lipid rafts have been defined in part by their resistance to solubilization with detergents at low temperatures.[90] In contrast to envelope glycoproteins of influenza virus and other viruses that assemble at lipid rafts, G protein in host plasma membranes and in virion envelopes is detergent soluble.[622] Nonetheless, the plasma membrane microdomains (and virus envelopes) that contain G protein resemble lipid rafts in that they are enriched in cholesterol and sphingolipids,[455,561] but these lipids must not be in sufficiently high amounts to confer detergent resistance.[93,622]

The G protein–containing microdomains at the sites of virus budding are somewhat larger (300 to 400 nm) than the microdomains in the plasma membrane outside of virus budding sites (100 to 150 nm), implying that formation of virus budding sites involves clustering of membrane microdomains.[91,93] An interesting feature of the budding process is that envelope glycoproteins from many unrelated viruses, as well as some host integral membrane proteins, can be incorporated into the envelopes of VSV or RABV in a process referred to as *pseudotype formation* or *phenotypic mixing*. Pseudotype formation was originally demonstrated by coinfection of cells with two different viruses.[807] More recently the incorporation of heterologous glycoproteins into the envelopes of VSV and RABV has been demonstrated using recombinant viruses that express the foreign glycoprotein from the viral genome.[101,240,358,391,479,629,690] Incorporation of heterologous glycoproteins into the virus envelope appears to result from clustering of microdomains containing the heterologous glycoprotein together with G protein–containing microdomains at the sites of virus assembly.[93] It is not known what causes microdomains containing G protein or other glycoproteins to cluster at the sites of virus budding, but a model has been proposed in which clustering is driven by formation of the viral nucleocapsid–M protein complex.[93,688]

The efficiency with which heterologous glycoproteins are incorporated into the virus envelope varies over a considerable range, although thus far, none has been found to be incorporated as efficiently as G protein. In the case of RABV, interaction of the G protein cytoplasmic domain with the internal virion components may promote incorporation into the virus budding site, because appending the G protein cytoplasmic domain to foreign glycoproteins enhances their incorporation into RABV virions.[489,490] In the case of VSV, incorporation of glycoproteins into the envelope does not depend on the sequence of the cytoplasmic domain, however, because substituting foreign sequences for the cytoplasmic domain of G protein or deleting the cytoplasmic domain does not alter the efficiency of G protein incorporation,[92,628] and, with one exception (the human immunodeficiency virus [HIV] envelope glycoprotein),[351,539] substituting the G protein cytoplasmic domain into foreign glycoproteins does not promote their incorporation into the virus envelope.[358,594,629] Instead, the ability of a foreign glycoprotein to be incorporated into the VSV envelope may depend on the composition or physical properties of the microdomains containing the foreign glycoprotein. For example, the influenza virus hemagglutinin, which is in detergent-insoluble lipid rafts, is incorporated into the VSV envelope less efficiently than the T-cell antigen CD4, which is present in microdomains that are primarily detergent soluble.[93,391,629]

The presence of G protein in the plasma membrane is not essential for virus budding, as shown by studies with recombinant VSV and RABV in which the G gene has been mutated or deleted.[378,491,594,632,690] In the absence of a complementing source of G protein, these viruses produce noninfectious particles that lack G protein but are otherwise indistinguishable from wild-type viruses. The efficiency of virus budding, however, is reduced by at least an order of magnitude in the absence of G protein, indicating that G protein plays a role in virus assembly to enhance the budding process. Thus, not only is it likely that internal virion components promote incorporation of G protein into the envelope as described earlier, but also it appears that G protein promotes assembly of internal virion components. As with the ability to be incorporated into the envelope, the ability of the VSV G protein to promote assembly is independent of the sequence of the cytoplasmic domain, although a minimal length of eight amino acids in the cytoplasmic domain does appear to be required.[628] Instead of the cytoplasmic domain, the sequences in G protein that are responsible for promoting assembly appear to be in the membrane-proximal amino acids of the ectodomain.[594] This has led to the suggestion that these sequences are responsible for introducing curvature in the membrane that promotes budding.[594] This idea is supported by the observation that G protein expressed in the absence of other viral components is released from cells in membrane vesicles that may form by a process similar to virus budding.[599]

Role of M Protein in Virus Assembly

Unlike G protein, the viral M protein is synthesized as a soluble protein[379,486] and associates with membranes in the manner of peripheral membrane proteins (i.e., through a combination of ionic and hydrophobic interactions and without spanning the membrane lipid bilayer).[430,454,455,532,797,803,804] In virus-infected cells, most of M protein is usually localized in the cytoplasm and is found in the soluble cytosolic fraction in subcellular fractionation experiments, with smaller amounts being membrane associated.[238,379,535,537] This distribution is also observed in transfected cells that express M protein in the absence of other VSV components,[123,124,797] indicating that association of M protein with membranes does not depend on other viral components. In addition, membrane association does not appear to require posttranslational modification, such as phosphorylation or covalent modification with lipids.[361,430] Instead, M protein appears to spontaneously associate with membranes containing negatively charged phospholipids,[454,455,532,797,803] which are enriched on the cytoplasmic surface of host plasma membranes. The N-terminal 20 amino acids of M protein, which are enriched in positively charged residues, appear to be responsible for membrane association, as shown using photoactivatable membrane probes.[430] Mutational analysis has also implicated the N-terminal region of M protein in membrane binding.[123,160,797] The membrane-bound M protein in infected cells is organized into membrane microdomains whose size is similar to G protein microdomains.[688] However, M protein and G protein reside in separate microdomains except at the sites of virus budding.[688]

Both the cytosolic and membrane-bound M protein are recruited into nucleocapsid–M protein complexes at the site of virus budding from host plasma membranes.[237,528] Nucleocapsids clearly get *selected* for assembly with M protein, because most of the intracellular nucleocapsids, which are being used as templates for viral RNA synthesis, are not able to bind M protein.[237,535,537] The only place in infected cells where co-localization of nucleocapsids and M protein is observed is in the nucleocapsid–M protein complexes in the process of budding from the plasma membrane.[485,528,535,537] In the case of VSV, nucleocapsids containing genome RNA are incorporated into virus particles much more efficiently than those containing antigenomes.[610,650,666,756] An RNA sequence near the 5′ end of the genome has been identified that is required for nucleocapsids containing this RNA to be incorporated into virus particles.[761] If such a sequence is present in the RABV genome, it must also be present in the antigenome, because the recombinant ambisense RABV described earlier, which contains the genomic promoter in both the genome and antigenome, incorporates both genome and antigenome RNA into virions with equal efficiency.[231] One of the important questions about virus assembly that needs to be addressed is how this RNA sequence promotes incorporation into virions, because selection of nucleocapsids for virion assembly is a critical step.

Once assembly of nucleocapsid–M protein complexes has begun, the recruitment of M protein into the complex appears to occur spontaneously. This process can be recreated in a cell-free system using purified M protein and virion nucleocapsids that have been stripped of most of their M protein by treatment with high-ionic-strength buffers.[54,461,514,515] Nucleocapsids, from which M protein has been completely removed, however, cannot rebind M protein with the same high affinity observed in virion nucleocapsid–M protein complexes.[237,461] This suggests that addition of the initial one or a few molecules of M protein to nucleocapsids (and, therefore, their removal) is fundamentally different from that of most M protein molecules in the nucleocapsid–M protein complex. Although the basis for this difference has yet to be discovered, it is tempting to think that it may be connected to the process of selection of intracellular nucleocapsids for virus assembly described in the previous paragraph.

Release of Assembled Virions

Following assembly of the nucleocapsid–M protein complex, the final step in virus assembly is release of the budding virion. This process is mediated by interaction of M protein with host proteins involved in MVB formation.[298,299,331,332,345] The MVB machinery is also involved in release of retroviruses and filoviruses mediated by "late budding domains" in their Gag proteins or matrix proteins (VP40), respectively.[564] In the formation of MVBs, vesicles derived from endosome membranes bud into the lumen of the endosome, carrying elements of the cytoplasm as their internal contents (Fig. 31.7). Modification of proteins on the cytoplasmic surface of the endosome membrane by covalent attachment of ubiquitin appears to be an important signal for incorporation of such *cargo* molecules into MVBs. The process of virus budding has the same membrane topology (cytoplasmic contents are internal), except that the process occurs at the plasma membrane rather than at the endosome membrane. A short sequence in M protein (PPPY in VSV, PPEY in RABV) appears to be responsible for redirecting this cellular machinery to the plasma membrane.[298,299,331,332,345,785] No other viral components appear to be required, because expression of M protein in transfected cells in the absence of other viral components results in budding of membrane vesicles containing M protein.[299,357,442] The PPPY sequence interacts with an E3 ubiquitin ligase called *Nedd4*, which is able to ubiquitinate M protein, in a cell-free assay.[298] It has yet to be established whether Nedd4 itself, or one of its numerous family members, ubiquitinate M protein in infected cells, because this is likely to involve only a small proportion of the total M protein. Nonetheless, it is likely that ubiquitination of M protein is critical for release of budding virions, because mutation of the PPPY motif in M protein, or depletion of free ubiquitin in infected cells, dramatically reduces the release of virions and causes the accumulation of budding particles at the plasma membrane because of inhibition of their release.[298,345] One of the questions that needs to be resolved is which cellular factors involved in MVB formation are involved in virus budding? Tsg101, a protein involved in recognizing ubiquitinated cargo proteins, and Vps4a, an adenosine triphosphatase (ATPase) involved in recycling the membrane trafficking machinery, have been implicated in budding of HIV but were reported not to be involved in budding of VSV or RABV.[331,332] However, a more recent report indicated that Vps4a is involved in VSV budding.[694]

MOLECULAR GENETICS OF RHABDOVIRUSES

Rapid Evolution and Existence of Quasispecies

Rhabdoviruses are classic examples of RNA viruses capable of undergoing rapid evolution. This is because of the high error rates of their RNA polymerases and their lack of proofreading activity. As a result, the rate of base substitutions during replication of genome RNA is approximately 1 in 10^4.[190] Because their genomes are only slightly larger than 10^4 bases, this implies that nearly every genome contains at least one base substitution. Thus, even clonal populations of these viruses are actually collections of viruses with closely related sequences (i.e., they are quasispecies). Because of their diversity of genome sequences, these viruses are capable of rapid genetic adaptation when placed under selective pressure of replication under different conditions. These viruses are genetically reasonably stable, however, when replication is maintained under a constant set of conditions.[597] This is because the collection of genome sequences quickly reaches a consensus sequence representing the sequence with the highest level of fitness within a few replication cycles in a new host. This rapid adaptability may be advantageous in nature for viruses that alternate replication among different hosts. For example, VSV replicates both in arthropod hosts, where it establishes persistent infection, and in mammalian hosts, where it causes an acute infection. Transfer from one type of host to the other requires substantial increases in viral fitness to maintain optimal replication in the new host.[806] In principle, this adaptation can occur through random mutation of the consensus sequence from the original host to one with greater fitness in the new host. However, in a virus population undergoing periodic cycling between insect and mammalian hosts, rapid adaptation to the mammalian host likely involves maintenance of a minority population of genomes in the insect host that quickly became dominant during mammalian infection.[524] Replication of RABV is restricted to mammalian hosts, but similar though less drastic adaptation can also occur when RABV is transferred between different hosts.

The high rate of spontaneous mutation makes it feasible to isolate a variety of different types of viral mutants in the laboratory. For example, several large collections of temperature-sensitive mutants of VSV have been isolated, which fall into five or more complementation groups, corresponding to mutants with defects in each of the five viral genes.[234,320,571] Similarly, antigenic variants that escape neutralization with monoclonal antibodies are readily isolated in the laboratory.[410,426,459] Unlike influenza viruses and HIV, however, relatively little *antigenic drift* is found in rhabdoviruses during outbreaks in nature. This may reflect the harmful effects on G protein function of accumulating the multiple mutations necessary to escape neutralization by a polyclonal antibody response in intact animal hosts.[525]

Despite the advantages for rapid adaptation, the high rate of mutation makes these viruses susceptible to the harmful effects of *genetic bottlenecks,* in which only one or a few genomes are selected for further replication. In a process known as *Muller's ratchet,* successive passage under conditions of limited genetic diversity, such as sequential passage by isolation of individual virus plaques, leads to progressive accumulation of base substitutions, most of which decrease virus replication, thus leading to progressively lower viral fitness[192] (see Chapter 11).

Defective Interfering Particles

Besides point mutations generated by nucleotide substitutions during genome replication, the other major mechanism of genetic alteration of rhabdoviruses is the generation of defective interfering (DI) particles. DI particles appear to be generated when the viral RNA polymerase switches from copying one region of the template to copying an alternate template or an alternate region of the same template. Because this inevitably results in generation of defective genomes, DI particles can replicate only in cells co-infected with standard virus to provide a source of viral proteins. If the polymerase switches to copying a distant region of the same template, this generates large deletions of the viral genome, referred to as *internal deletion* DI particles.[140] In other cases, the polymerase will switch to copying the terminal sequences of the nascent product RNA strand, generating RNA products with terminal complementarity, referred to as *panhandle or snap-back* DI particles.[557] Panhandle DI particles derived during synthesis of progeny negative-strand RNA thus have the sequence of the 5′ end of the viral genome, but the 3′ region of terminal complementarity has the sequence of the antigenome, including the antigenomic promoter. Because this is the more powerful of the two viral promoters, such DI genomes have a substantial replicative advantage over standard viral genomes and interfere with the replication of standard virus, resulting in reductions in virus titer.[140] Although they have the same genomic promoter as standard virus, internal deletion DI particles also have a replicative advantage over standard virus, presumably because of their smaller size, and they also interfere with replication of standard virus.

Defective interfering particles are readily generated during virus replication in culture, so that repeated passage at high multiplicity leads to substantial reductions in virus titer because of accumulation of DI particles.[140] Because of the smaller size of their genomes, virions containing DI genomes are shorter than standard virions and can be separated from standard virus by centrifugation in density gradients. This ability to physically separate virions containing DI genomes from those containing standard genomes has proved to be useful in studies of the generation and replication of DI particles. In most experimental situations, however, the presence of DI particles is more of a nuisance, so that virus stocks are usually prepared to minimize the presence of DI particles. This can be accomplished by passaging virus at low multiplicity or by plaque isolation, both of which favor the replication of standard virus over DI particles.

In principle, rhabdoviruses should be able to generate recombinants between genetically distinct viruses in co-infected cells as a result of polymerase *copy choice,* similar to the mechanisms that give rise to DI particles, in which the viral RNA polymerase switches from copying one template to copying another, leading to production of progeny genomes that are recombinants between the two parental genomes. Despite many years of the genetic study of these viruses, no convincing evidence indicates that this type of RNA recombination occurs, although the possibility of rare occurrences in nature has been proposed.[116]

Genetic Engineering of Rhabdoviruses

The methods for genetically engineering viral genomes developed with rhabdoviruses have become the standard methods used for genetic modification of many nonsegmented, negative-strand RNA viruses. A major hurdle is that RNA transcribed from complementary DNA (cDNA) needs to be encapsidated to function as a viral genome. This process, which occurs so efficiently when RNA is replicated by the viral RNA polymerase, occurs inefficiently when RNA is transcribed from cDNA. Shorter RNAs expressed from cDNA appear to be encapsidated more efficiently than longer RNA. Thus, the first viral genomes to be recovered from cDNA were a VSV DI genome[549] and an RABV *minigenome* containing the terminal sequences of the viral genome required for transcription and replication flanking a foreign gene.[146] These genomes were expressed from plasmid cDNA in transfected cells together with plasmids encoding the N, P, and L proteins required for encapsidation and replication. Another hurdle to the recovery of viral genomes from cDNA was the requirement for the 3′ end of the RNA to reflect precisely the sequence of the viral genome (or antigenome) without additional nucleotides, in order to be recognized and replicated by the viral RNA polymerase. This was addressed by incorporating into the cDNA the sequence of the hepatitis delta virus ribozyme engineered to cleave the RNA transcript to generate a precise 3′ end.[549] Apparently, the sequence requirements at the 5′ end of the viral RNA are not as critical, because additional nucleotides derived from cDNA are removed during replication.

The experimental approach used to generate minigenomes from cDNA led to recovery of complete viral genomes from cDNA for RABV[634] and VSV.[421,759] A key insight was that the RNA transcribed from cDNA needed to be the antigenome rather than the genome. Otherwise, the mRNA derived from the helper plasmids encoding N, P, and L proteins would interfere with recovery by hybridization to the genomic RNA transcribed from cDNA. In most recovery experiments, high levels of expression of the antigenome RNA and the mRNA from the helper plasmids have been achieved by infecting cells with a recombinant vaccinia virus encoding T7 RNA polymerase and transfecting them with plasmids driven by T7 promoters.[421,634,759] Because this requires isolation of the recovered virus from contaminating vaccinia virus, methods for isolating recombinant rhabdoviruses without the use of vaccinia virus have been developed.[297,335] Although recovery of infectious recombinant viruses from cDNA has been a major breakthrough, minigenome systems continue to be widely used for studying various aspects of the viral replicative cycle, particularly analysis of mutations that are likely to prevent replication, so that it would be difficult or impossible to isolate viruses containing such mutations.

The ability to engineer specific mutations into viral genomes has become an important tool for studying the mechanistic aspects of virus replication. In addition, it has made possible the use of rhabdoviruses as vectors for expression of foreign genes for potential use as vaccines and therapeutic agents. Several reviews have appeared on the use of rhabdoviruses as potential recombinant vaccines and as cytolytic agents for the treatment of diseases such as cancer.[52,444,488] The basic methodology to express foreign genes is to introduce a new transcription unit containing the gene stop–start signals and the foreign gene between two of the native viral genes, such as between the G and L genes.[492,630] The foreign gene is subject to the same transcriptional attenuation as the other viral genes. Thus, incorporation of a new gene reduces the expression of downstream genes by approximately 20% to 30%. Although this attenuation has the potential to reduce the efficiency of virus replication, incorporation of a single foreign gene usually does not notably reduce virus yields unless the foreign gene product itself has the potential to interfere with virus replication.[629] The processes of genome encapsidation and envelopment are sufficiently flexible that incorporation of new genes into rhabdovirus genomes simply leads to longer nucleocapsids and, therefore, longer virions.[629] In principle, no limit exists for packaging new genetic information, so that multiple foreign genes can be incorporated into genomes of recombinant viruses. Reductions in virus yield owing to multiple new transcription attenuation sites, as well as the difficulty of recovering longer genomes, however, probably places practical limits on the amount of new genetic information that can be incorporated into rhabdovirus genomes.

MOLECULAR AND CELLULAR BASIS OF PATHOGENESIS

Induction and Suppression of Host Antiviral Responses

Two of the major determinants of viral pathogenesis are the nature of the antiviral response mounted by the infected host and the mechanisms used by viruses to suppress or evade this response. In order for cells to mount an antiviral response, viral products have to be recognized by sensors known as pathogen pattern recognition receptors (PRRs). For most cell types, the major PRR that initiates the response to many negative-strand RNA viruses appears to be a cytoplasmic RNA helicase, RIG-I (retinoic acid–inducible gene I).[365,366] The other major PRRs that have been implicated in the host response to these viruses are Toll-like receptors (TLRs). TLRs act either at the plasma membrane or in the endocytic compartment to recognize molecules that may be associated with infection by bacteria, fungi, and protozoa as well as viruses. Activation of RIG-I or TLRs results in formation of signaling complexes through a variety of adapter proteins, which activate protein kinases that turn on the expression of antiviral genes.[512,691] Most of the recent research in this area has focused on the production of type I (α and β) interferons (IFNs) and IFN-stimulated gene products, although other cytokines produced by virus-infected cells also play a major role in innate antiviral responses (Fig. 31.10).

One of the principal ligands for RIG-I is 5′ phosphorylated RNA that is part of a short double-stranded RNA (dsRNA).[322,623] In the normal replication cycle of nonsegmented negative-strand RNA viruses, 5′ phosphorylated RNAs are produced during the process of transcription in the form of leader and trailer RNAs and during genome replication as either genomic or antigenomic RNAs (see earlier). However, the 5′ ends of these RNAs are shielded by the nucleocapsid protein. Thus, removal of the nucleocapsid protein would appear to be necessary to expose free 5′ ends of viral RNA and formation of dsRNA for recognition by RIG-I.[584] Another potential source of such RNAs would be aberrant transcription products that are not capped by the viral polymerase. Thus, the origin of the signals that activate RIG-I is not clear, but to a large extent these signals are coupled to the production of viral RNAs.

Unlike RIG-I–dependent signaling, which is widely distributed among many cell types, the distribution of TLRs and the relative importance of their signaling pathways is often cell type dependent. For example, TLR7 is a major PRR in the response to VSV in plasmacytoid dendritic cells,[458] while TLR13 and perhaps TLR4 are major PRRs in the response to VSV of splenic conventional dendritic cells and macrophages.[266,646] The signal that activates TLR7 appears to be the presence of single-stranded RNA in the endocytic compartment.[176] Such single-stranded RNA can arise during virus penetration by degradation of virions or can be generated from viral RNA in the cytoplasm, which enters the endocytic compartment by autophagy.[425] The signal that activates TLR4 in macrophages appears to be the VSV G protein, which interacts with TLR4 during virus attachment and penetration.[266] The

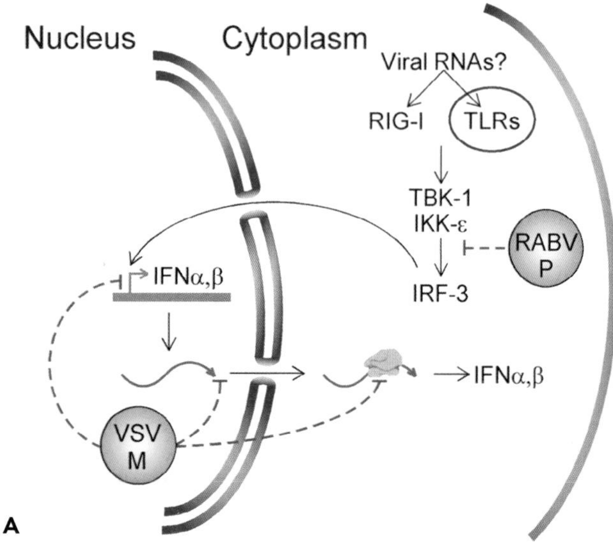

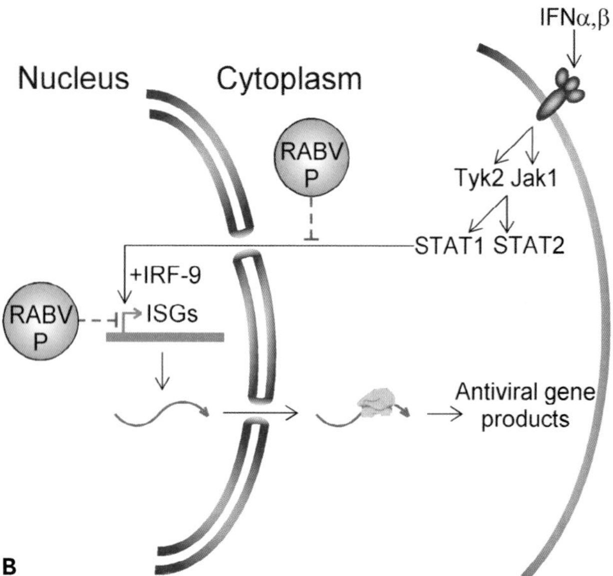

FIGURE 31.10. Induction and suppression of host interferon (IFN) responses by rabies virus (RABV) and vesicular stomatitis virus (VSV). A: Induction of synthesis of type I (α and β) IFN and its suppression by RABV P protein and VSV M protein. **B:** Response to IFN and its suppression by RABV P protein.

signal that activates TLR13 is not known but does not appear to be related to viral RNA.[646]

The only TLR that has been implicated thus far in the innate response to RABV is TLR3.[341,569] TLR3 responds to the presence of dsRNA in the endocytic compartment.[12] As pointed out earlier, dsRNAs are not part of the normal replication cycle but may arise from abnormal replication products. TLR3 may play a role in the antiviral response to RABV, but surprisingly TLR3$^{-/-}$ mice are less susceptible to RABV than their wild-type controls.[493] This appears to be due to a role for TLR3 in the formation of Negri bodies (described later), which are viral inclusions that may play a role in enhancing virus replication.[411,493]

Nearly all viruses have mechanisms to evade or suppress host antiviral responses. This is a critically important aspect of viral pathogenesis. Mutations in viruses that either increase the induction or decrease the suppression of antiviral responses almost inevitably decrease virus replication in susceptible hosts. Vesiculoviruses and lyssaviruses present strikingly different approaches to this aspect of virus replication. If it is possible to generalize, vesiculoviruses usually replicate rapidly and to high levels, generating high levels of potent inducers of host antiviral responses. Correspondingly, they have rapid and potent means of inhibiting these responses, involving the general inhibition of nearly all host gene expression. In contrast, lyssaviruses do not replicate as rapidly and likely are weaker inducers of host responses. As a result, they have more subtle means of inhibiting host responses that do not involve the general inhibition of host gene expression.

Suppression of Interferon Signaling by RABV

The P protein of RABV functions both as a subunit of the viral RNA-dependent RNA polymerase and as a suppressor of IFN production and IFN signaling. P protein inhibits IFN production by preventing the phosphorylation of the transcription factor IRF-3 by two cellular protein kinases, TBK1 and IKK-ε (Fig. 31.10A).[97] Mutations in P protein that inactivate its IFN inhibitory function without affecting its RNA synthesis function have been identified.[589] Recombinant viruses that express either mutant P protein or lower levels of P protein than their wild-type controls[97,230] are less effective in suppressing IFN production. These viruses are able to replicate in cell types that are defective in their IFN responses but are rapidly eliminated from IFN-competent cell types and are less virulent in mice.[97,230,589]

In addition to inhibiting IFN production, RABV P protein inhibits signal transduction in response to IFN (Fig. 31.10B). RABV P is expressed not only as full-length P protein but also as four truncated forms (P2 through P5) that are synthesized from internal start codons.[546] P3, P4, and P5 proteins are found only in the nucleus. The ability of P protein and its truncated derivatives to inhibit IFN signaling is due to their ability to interfere with the transcription factors that activate interferon-stimulated genes (ISGs). Type I IFNs bind to a common receptor that is coupled to two tyrosine kinases, Jak1 and Tyk2.[579] Receptor activation leads to activation of these kinases, which in turn phosphorylate two cytoplasmic proteins, STAT1 and STAT2. Phospho-STAT1 and -STAT2 are transported to the nucleus, where they associate with IRF9 to form the ISGF-3 transcription factor that activates expression of ISGs. RABV P protein does not interfere with STAT phosphorylation. Instead, it binds to phosphorylated STAT1 and STAT2 and inhibits their translocation to the nucleus and binding to target DNAs (Fig. 31.10B).[98,119,504,728,729] This appears to be due to association of the P protein–STAT complex with microtubules in the cytoplasm, which prevents transport to the nucleus.[504] STAT1–STAT2 complexes that do get transported to the nucleus associate with P protein or its truncated derivatives, which interferes with DNA-binding activity.[729]

Inhibition of Host Gene Expression by VSV

VSV inhibits host gene expression at three different levels: (a) transcription of host mRNA, (b) transport of host mRNA from the nucleus to the cytoplasm, and (c) translation of host mRNA into proteins (Fig. 31.10A). The inhibition of all three processes presumably reflects the fact that no single inhibitory mechanism is completely effective in suppressing host antiviral responses. The inhibition of both host transcription and translation generally occurs in parallel and is usually 80% to 90% complete by 4 to 6 hours postinfection.[7,193] Some evidence indicates that the inhibition of nuclear-cytoplasmic RNA transport may occur earlier after infection, although a direct comparison with the inhibition at other levels has not been made.[681,732]

The VSV gene product that is primarily responsible for inhibiting host gene expression is M protein. Expression of VSV M protein in transfected cells in the absence of other viral components inhibits expression of co-transfected genes driven by a wide variety of different promoters.[4,72,225,462,541] This inhibitory activity of M protein is very potent and is evident even when M protein is expressed at 100 to 1,000 times lower levels than those in VSV-infected cells.[462] Viruses containing a variety of M protein mutations are defective in their ability to inhibit host gene expression.[5,7,73,151,175,225,245,346,681] Most of these mutations that render M protein defective in its ability to inhibit host gene expression do not affect its functions in virus assembly. Conversely, M protein mutations such as truncation of the N-terminal sequences that are important for virus assembly do not affect the ability of M protein to inhibit host gene expression.[73,346] Thus, the functions of M protein in the inhibition of host gene expression are genetically separable from its virus assembly functions. Although no separate M protein domains appear to mediate these two classes of functions, the point mutations that affect inhibition of host gene expression do map to one face of the M protein three-dimensional structure. Presumably, this face of M protein is involved in interaction with host components involved in the inhibition.

Because M protein lacks any enzymatic activity, it probably interferes with host gene expression by interacting with cellular proteins to alter their function. Thus far, the only host protein whose binding to M protein is correlated with the inhibition of host gene expression is Rae1.[213] Rae1 was originally implicated in mRNA transport, but more recent experiments suggest its principal function is in mitotic spindle assembly and mitotic checkpoint regulation.[30,79,651,787] M protein and Rae1 form complexes with multiple proteins involved in mRNA transport and other cellular functions, such as Nup98, hnRNP-U, and E1B-AP5.[115,213,732] However, deleting the *Rae1* gene in cultured mouse embryo cells or silencing its expression in *Drosophila* does not lead to mRNA transport inhibition.[30,651] Given the observation that Rae1 is not essential for nuclear-cytoplasmic RNA transport, it is unlikely that the VSV M protein inhibits its host gene expression simply by interfering with Rae1 function. Instead, it is more likely that the complex of M protein and Rae1 interferes with the function of other factors that are essential for host gene expression.

Because Rae1 is distributed throughout the cytoplasm and the nucleus of the cell, M protein–Rae1 complexes may be involved in inhibition of multiple steps in host gene expression. In support of this idea, the inhibition of transcription by host RNA polymerase II involves inactivation of the general transcription factor TFIID,[800] which binds to the TATA box upstream of most RNA polymerase II–dependent promoters and recruits other general transcription factors to these promoters. M protein, however, does not appear to interact directly with TFIID,[799] suggesting that the inactivation is indirect. The mechanisms involved in such an indirect effect have yet to be discovered.

The inhibition of host translation in VSV-infected cells does not result from depletion of cellular mRNA secondary to the inhibition of mRNA transcription and transport. As described earlier, the inhibition of host translation occurs early in the infectious cycle on a time scale too rapid to be caused by turnover of cellular mRNA. Instead, the translation apparatus is reprogrammed such that only new mRNAs are translated.[763] Pre-existing host mRNAs are incorporated into translationally inactive messenger ribonucleoproteins (mRNPs), where they are stably maintained in infected cells.[608,764] Thus, the inhibition of host translation reflects the inhibition of translation of pre-existing mRNAs together with the lack of production of new host mRNAs due to the inhibition of transcription and transport by M protein. The reprogramming of the translation apparatus appears to be due at least in part to alterations in the cap-binding translation factor eIF4F.[142,143,191] How the changes in the eIF4F complex result in the altered translation in VSV-infected cells is a major question that remains to be addressed.

Viral transcription provides a continuous supply of newly synthesized viral mRNAs, which are efficiently translated by the reprogrammed translation apparatus. Translation of viral mRNAs continues until late in the infectious cycle, when translation is inhibited because of phosphorylation of eIF2α by the antiviral kinase PKR, as well as other mechanisms.[142,143,764] Viral mRNAs do not appear to have *cis*-acting sequences that promote their translation analogous to the internal ribosome entry sites in picornavirus mRNAs.[764] Regardless of their sequences, new mRNAs are translated more efficiently in VSV-infected cells than in uninfected cells.[763] This enhancement of translation of new mRNAs appears to involve M protein, because M protein mutant viruses have been identified that inhibit host translation as effectively as their wild-type controls but are defective in promoting translation of viral mRNAs.[144,499]

Induction of Cytopathic Effects

As in the case of suppression of host antiviral responses, lyssaviruses and vesiculoviruses present strikingly different abilities to induce cytopathic effects in infected cells. In the case of most RABV strains, usually few, if any, morphologic changes occur in infected cells that would be interpreted as cytopathic effects until several days after infection. Indeed, some cell types infected with RABV continue to divide and establish persistent infections.[223] In contrast, many strains of VSV are among the most cytocidal of animal viruses, at least in mammalian and avian cells. In many insect cells, however, VSV replication is attenuated and a persistent infection is established with little, if any, cytopathic effect.[794] In most cases, cytopathic effects are a result of host responses to virus infection involving activation of programmed cell death or apoptosis.

Induction of Apoptosis by Vesicular Stomatitis Virus

It is widely appreciated that many viruses induce apoptosis in infected cells, and, in general, apoptosis is a form of antiviral response in which death of the host cell should reduce the number of progeny resulting from the infectious cycle. VSV was one of the early viruses shown to induce apoptosis in infected cells.[389] In fact, most, if not all, of the cytopathic effects of VSV infection are caused by the induction of apoptosis. These effects include nearly all of the morphologic and biochemical changes typical of apoptosis in cell culture.[384,389] One of the earliest effects is cell rounding, followed by membrane blebbing, nuclear condensation and DNA fragmentation, cytoplasmic shrinkage, and cell lysis. Despite the general opinion that apoptosis of infected cells reduces virus yield, little, if any, difference exists in yield of VSV if apoptosis is delayed by overexpression of the antiapoptotic host protein Bcl-2,[383] indicating that the VSV replication cycle is largely complete before the infected cell has a chance to die.

At least two distinct mechanisms exist by which VSV infection can induce apoptosis in infected cells.[109,253,384,553] One appears to be a direct result of the inhibition of host gene expression by M protein, and thus is only activated by viruses with wild-type M protein. The other mechanism appears to be a cellular response to virus replication and is induced by both wild-type and M protein mutant viruses. The relative importance of these two mechanisms varies widely among different cell types, depending on the nature of the proteins that regulate apoptosis pre-existing in the cell before infection and the contribution of newly synthesized proapoptotic protein induced after infection.[109,252,253,383,553,616] Such newly synthesized proapoptotic proteins can contribute to apoptosis induced by M protein mutant viruses but are suppressed by viruses with wild-type M protein.

Wild-type M protein induces apoptosis when expressed in transfected cells in the absence of other viral components.[384] In contrast, mutant M proteins that are defective in their ability to inhibit host gene expression cannot induce apoptosis in the absence of other viral components.[383,384] Induction of apoptosis by M protein appears to be similar to that induced by pharmacologic inhibitors of host gene expression (e.g., actinomycin D). As with most forms of intracellular damage, both M protein and pharmacologic inhibitors of host RNA synthesis activate the *mitochondrial pathway*, involving the release of cytochrome c and other proapoptotic proteins from mitochondria, which activate the upstream caspase, caspase-9.[48,383] As a result, induction of apoptosis by M protein can be inhibited by overexpression of antiapoptotic proteins like Bcl-2 and Bcl-X_L, which prevent release of proapoptotic factors from mitochondria.

Despite the inability of mutant M proteins to induce apoptosis in the absence of other viral components, M protein mutant viruses, which are defective in their ability to inhibit host gene expression, are still very effective inducers of apoptosis in infected cells.[109,252,253,383,384,644] The induction of apoptosis by M protein mutant viruses appears to be part of the antiviral response induced by virus replication. In contrast to apoptosis induced by M protein alone, the death receptor pathway is the major mechanism of cell death, in which caspase-8 is the major upstream caspase, rather than caspase-9.[109,252] The Fas death receptor appears to be the major death receptor involved. In contrast to viruses such as influenza virus, in which Fas signaling is mediated through the adaptor protein FADD,[48] VSV infection appears to activate an alternative adapter protein Daxx, which is involved in the induction of apoptosis.[252] In some cell types, cross-talk between the death receptor and mitochondrial apoptotic pathways is required for efficient induction of cell death. This cross-talk is mediated through caspase-8 cleavage of the pro-apoptotic BH3-only protein Bid. Cleaved Bid (tBid) then promotes destabilization of the mitochondria through activation of pro-apoptotic mitochondrial proteins. Death receptor signaling has been classified as type I or type II depending on whether signaling is independent of the mitochondrial pathway (type I) or depends on amplification by the mitochondrial pathway (type II).[619,620] Cells that respond to death receptor ligands by a type II pathway also respond to VSV infection by a similar pathway.[109]

Induction of Apoptosis by Lyssaviruses

As pointed out earlier, there are cell types in which RABV induces little, if any, cytopathic effect and establishes persistent infections.[223] In other cell types, the infected cells eventually die as a result of induction of apoptosis.[340,718] Furthermore, RABV induces apoptosis in infected neurons *in vivo* during experimentally induced encephalitis in mice.[340] Inhibition of host gene expression does not play a role in the induction of apoptosis by RABV as it does in the case of VSV. Indeed, RABV infection induces the expression of host pro-apoptotic proteins, such as Bax,[718] and in this regard, resembles the induction of apoptosis by M protein mutants of VSV that do not inhibit host gene expression. Also analogous to VSV M protein mutants, the induction of apoptosis depends on activation of the death receptor pathway involving caspase-8, in the case of two other lyssaviruses, MOKV and LBV.[364] In contrast to the activation of the Fas death receptor by VSV M protein mutants, however, MOKV and LBV activate apoptosis through interaction of the death ligand tumor necrosis factor (TNF)-related apoptosis-inducing ligand (TRAIL) with its receptor.[364] Transfection of cells with plasmids encoding lyssavirus M proteins induced apoptosis by the same caspase-8–dependent and TRAIL-dependent mechanism and also through mitochondrial disruption.[269,364] It is unlikely, however, that the lyssavirus M proteins induce apoptosis by a mechanism similar to VSV M protein, because they do not inhibit host gene expression. In addition to M protein, G proteins of some RABV strains also induce apoptosis.[568,570] Thus, it is likely that multiple viral components are involved in the induction of apoptosis in cells infected with lyssaviruses.

MOUSE MODELS OF RHABDOVIRUS INFECTION

Both RABV and VSV are highly neurotropic in mice, and virulence is largely due to virus-induced encephalomyelitis. Laboratory rodents (e.g., mice) have been extensively used for rabies diagnosis, vaccine potency testing, and pathogenic studies, although these taxa are epidemiologically insignificant as lyssavirus vectors or reservoirs,[121,396] compared with the families *Carnivora* and *Chiroptera*. Similarly, rodents are not known to be natural hosts for vesiculoviruses. In fact, the disease induced by VSV in rodents bears little resemblance to the disease in natural hosts, such as horses and cattle (described later). Nonetheless, much of what we know about the mechanisms of pathogenesis and immunity for these viruses is derived from experimental infection of mice.

Entry and Site of Initial Replication

Infection of mice with RABV is usually fatal regardless of the route of inoculation. Intramuscular inoculation is often used as a model for virus transmission by animal bites, and intranasal inoculation is used as a model for the occasional transmission of RABV by inhalation. In contrast to RABV, the ability of VSV to invade the CNS is highly dependent on the age of the mice and route of inoculation,[615] as well as the strain of mice infected.[196,244] In general, adult mice are relatively resistant to VSV inoculated intravenously or intraperitoneally, although systemic virus infection clearly occurs in these mice, as shown by the potent induction of immune responses (described later). In contrast to intravenous or intraperitoneal inoculation, mice are very sensitive to VSV introduced by intranasal or intracerebral inoculation. As an example of strain differences, mice of the 129 strain, which are often used in the generation of transgenic mice, were found to be five orders of magnitude more resistant than strains such as BALB/c, which are often used in studies of immunology and pathogenesis.[196]

Virus entry into the host is accompanied by initial virus replication at the site of entry. In the case of RABV infection of mice, initial replication following intramuscular inoculation can occur in either sensory or motor neurons without apparent replication in muscle,[150,642] although in natural hosts, virus can replicate in muscle tissue before progressing to the peripheral nervous tissue via neuromuscular connections.[117,219,511] In the case of either RABV or VSV infection following intranasal inoculation (Fig. 31.11), the primary site of virus replication is in olfactory receptor neurons and other cells of the olfactory epithelium.[409,563] In addition to olfactory epithelium, VSV can also infect cells of the respiratory epithelium and spread through the respiratory tract to the lungs, although little, if any, pathology is associated with virus replication in the lungs.[244]

Virus Spread and Tissue Tropism

Both RABV and VSV are transmitted to the CNS primarily by neural spread along the tracts served by the initially infected neurons. For example, following intramuscular inoculation, RABV spreads from the initially infected sensory and motor neurons to the spinal cord and sensory ganglia in subsequent rounds of replication.[150] Similarly, following intranasal inoculation (Fig. 31.11), both VSV and RABV quickly spread to the glomerular cells of the olfactory bulb as well as the anterior olfactory nuclei.[327,409] From these sites, the viruses spread to other parts of the CNS that are served by the neurons that innervate the olfactory bulb. These viruses have a clear preference for some classes of neurons over others. For example, RABV can also enter the CNS through neurons of the trigeminal ganglia,[409,642] whereas VSV cannot.[563] Similarly, RABV infects mitral cells of the olfactory bulb and spreads along tracts served by these cells,[409] whereas VSV does not.[327] In addition to neural spread, VSV infects cells lining the ventricular system, where it can be released into the cerebrospinal fluid (CSF) and can spread to other parts of the brain and spinal cord, leading to paralysis.[244,327,563]

The pathology associated with infection of mice by either RABV or VSV is typical of viral encephalomyelitis, involving both death of infected cells and inflammation at the infection sites. The inflammatory changes include activation of resident inflammatory cells (e.g., microglia) and infiltration of inflammatory cells (e.g., monocytes, natural killer [NK] cells, and T cells).[67,126,244,321] The morbidity and mortality associated with virus infection is usually attributed to virus-induced death of infected cells that are critical for the host, rather than to immunopathologic mechanisms, because nearly all experimental manipulations that reduce the immune response to virus infection either enhance mortality by allowing more virus replication or have little effect. For example, virus infection of T-cell–deficient mice results in more extensive spread of virus throughout the brain and higher mortality than in immunocompetent mice.[321,326]

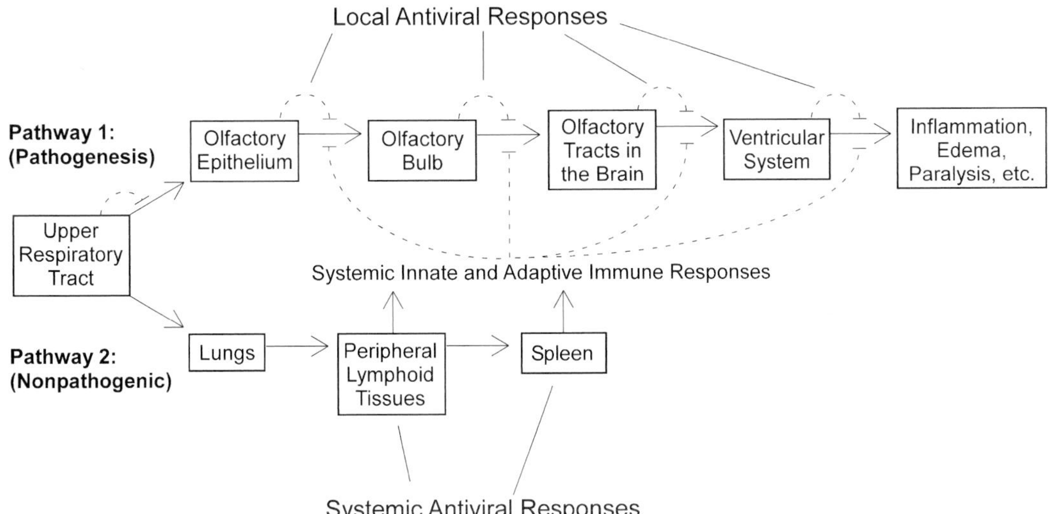

FIGURE 31.11. Diagram of pathogenesis and immune response in mice infected with vesicular stomatitis virus (VSV) by intranasal inoculation. Pathway 1 is the route of virus spread through the central nervous system by neuronal transmission leading to encephalitis.[327] **Pathway 2** is a hypothetical route of spread from the respiratory tract to peripheral and central lymphoid organs. Also shown are sites at which local and systemic antiviral responses exert an inhibitory effect on spread of virus to the next stage. The outcome of infection depends on the relative ability of the virus to replicate and spread versus the ability of the host to inhibit virus replication at each step.

Immune Responses Involved in Recovery from Rhabdovirus Infection

The immune response to VSV infection in mice has been studied for many years by viral immunologists as a prototype immune response to virus infection. In addition, the development of recombinant VSV as a potential vaccine vector[592] has stimulated additional research into the anti-VSV immune response. In most cases, the infection resulting from intraperitoneal or intravenous inoculation has been studied, which often is asymptomatic and results in complete recovery in immunocompetent mice. Less frequently studied is the infection resulting from intranasal inoculation. In this case, nearly all mice develop clinical signs, and only about half of the mice survive. Clearly, differences in the immune responses resulting in resistance or recovery must exist between these two situations. In the case of RABV, there is little incidence of recovery from a productive CNS infection. The immune response to attenuated virus strains is often studied as a model for the immune response to potential live virus vaccine strains.

Immune Response to Vesiculovirus Infection

In the case of VSV infection, elements of both the innate and adaptive immune response are critical for survival (Fig. 31.11). One of the most striking effects on VSV pathogenesis occurs in the absence of a response to type I (α and β) IFN. Mice that lack the type I IFN receptor, or the STAT1 transcription factor that mediates many of the effects of type I IFN, are extremely susceptible to the lethal effects of VSV infection.[195,510] In contrast to immunocompetent mice, in which virus replication occurs primarily in the CNS, in IFN receptor– or STAT1-deficient mice VSV replicates to high titer in all of the tissues tested.[195,510] In fact, the brains of these mice had the lowest titers of any of the organs examined.[510] This result implies that the pronounced neurotropism of VSV in immunocompetent mice is not caused by the inherent ability of different tissues to support virus replication, but rather differences in their ability to produce or respond to type I IFN.

As in the case of most viruses, no single IFN-inducible gene product is responsible for the effect of IFN in protecting nonneural tissues from VSV infection. No deletion of a single IFN-inducible gene has as profound an effect as deficiency of IFN receptor or STAT1. The antiviral protein kinase PKR is notable, however, in that its deletion leads to enhanced virus replication in the lung following intranasal inoculation, leading to enhanced morbidity and mortality caused by respiratory infection.[196]

The major source of type I IFN in mice following systemic inoculation appears to be a subclass of plasmacytoid dendritic cells residing in the marginal zone of the spleen.[53] This would be consistent with the ability of VSV to suppress IFN production by most other cell types, as described in the previous section. Dendritic cells containing TLR7, such as plasmacytoid dendritic cells, appear to be resistant to the inhibition of IFN production following VSV infection.[8,458,734] Other cell types involved in innate immunity also appear to be involved in protecting neural and nonneural tissues from VSV infection. Following systemic inoculation, chemokine-secreting marginal zone macrophages in the spleen are particularly important,[132,529] and following subcutaneous inoculation, subcapsular macrophages in draining lymph nodes are critical for preventing VSV neuroinvasion through peripheral nerves in the lymph nodes.[330]

Whereas the host IFN response and other innate immune mechanisms can protect most nonneural tissues from VSV infection, they do not fully protect the CNS, particularly following intranasal or intracerebral inoculation. This inability to protect the CNS is not because of a failure of neurons to respond to IFN.[710] Instead, the problem appears to reside in the amount of IFN produced in the CNS and the timing of the peripheral IFN response relative to virus invasion.[711] Indeed, treating mice with exogenous IFN can increase their resistance to CNS infection by VSV.[168,281,708] In addition to the IFN response, other innate immune mechanisms affect the susceptibility of the CNS to VSV infection. For example, deficiency in the production of nitric oxide by neuronal nitric oxide synthase-1 (NOS-1) enhances the susceptibility of the CNS to infection.[382] In contrast, deficiency of the inducible NOS (NOS-2) or NOS-3 has little effect on VSV infection of the CNS.

In addition to innate immune responses, adaptive immune responses are critical for recovery from VSV infection. Particularly important is the production of neutralizing antibodies. As with most viruses, the envelope glycoprotein of VSV (G protein) is the viral antigen that elicits neutralizing antibodies.[108,359,427] Induction of antibodies by G protein expressed on the surface of infected cells requires T cells.[31] The high density of G protein in virions is able to induce a T-cell–independent IgM response, however, which is consistent with the induction of T-cell–independent responses by antigens with highly repetitive epitopes.[31] T cells are required for isotype switching to produce immunoglobulin G (IgG) and other isotypes.[428,471] VSV-infected dendritic cells appear to be responsible for transporting the virus to secondary lymphoid organs, such as the spleen (Fig. 31.11), where they present viral antigens to virus-specific T cells and B cells.[131,132,456] The CD4+ T-helper cell (Th) response to VSV infection includes elicitation of both Th1 and Th2 cells. The response is predominantly of the Th1 type, resulting in secretion of IFN-γ and isotype switching in B cells to produce predominantly IgG2a antibodies. Isotype switching to IgG2a is also mediated by IFN-γ–producing γ-Δ T cells.[471] This polarization of the T-cell response presumably reflects secretion of IL-12 by dendritic cells and other antigen-presenting cells. Depletion of phagocytic cells, including marginal zone dendritic cells and macrophages, largely eliminates the Th1 response, although the Th2 response is left largely intact, suggesting that a different class of antigen-presenting cells is responsible for activation of Th2 cells.[132]

VSV infection also effectively elicits CD8+ cytolytic T cells (Tc). In contrast to neutralizing antibodies, which are serotype specific, many of the Tc cells are cross-reactive between Indiana and New Jersey serotypes of VSV.[609] These cells recognize peptides containing conserved sequences derived from G protein or N protein (and perhaps other viral proteins) presented in the context of class I major histocompatibility complex (MHC) molecules on virus-infected cells.[572,722,798] In addition to CD8+ Tc, VSV also elicits CD4+ cytotoxic T cells, which recognize epitopes derived from G protein presented in the context of class II MHC molecules.[94]

The importance of the antibody response in recovery from VSV infection is demonstrated by the observation that mice containing disruptions of the immunoglobulin μ gene are highly susceptible to VSV infection.[95] These mice die from CNS infection, even when infected by intraperitoneal inoculation. In contrast, depletion of either CD4+ or CD8+ T cells has little effect on susceptibility to VSV infection by this route.[428] Depletion of either T-cell subset or both subsets, however, enhances the susceptibility of mice to infection with VSV by intranasal inoculation,[326] indicating that T cells are important for reducing virus replication once infection is established in the CNS.

Immune Response to Lyssavirus Infection

Antibodies induced by vaccination, particularly those with neutralizing activity, play a prominent role in immune defense against RABV infection.[321] On rare occasions, immunity can also be naturally acquired after multiple exposures to virus.[242] The G protein represents the only antigen that induces neutralizing antibodies and is able to confer immunity against a lethal challenge.[153] Antibodies can mediate viral clearance from the CNS without other immune effectors.[180] The presence of other immune mechanisms, including IFN responses, and both CD4+ and CD8+ T cell responses, however, hastens the clearance of virus from the CNS.[321] Although G protein is the only antigen that elicits neutralizing antibodies, the RNP is a major antigenic complex that induces a virus-specific antibody response, and antibodies directed against RNP can contribute to protection against infection.[179,182,448] Animals treated with anti-N sera can be protected against a subsequent challenge with RABV, and anti-N sera can exhibit an antiviral activity *in vitro*.[448] The mechanism by which anti-RNP antibodies inhibit viral replication, however, remains unclear.

Infection with RABV results in the generation of virus-specific CD8+ and CD4+ T cells. The G protein is one of the antigens that induces Tc responses.[465,466] Some mouse strains infected with virus also develop strong Tc responses to the P protein.[417] The role of CD8+ T cells in immune defense is unclear, however. Some investigators report clearance of rabies virus after transfer of RABV-specific T cells and protection against rabies by a Tc clone, whereas other investigators showed that Tc are insufficient to protect against challenge, and *in vivo* depletion of CD8+ T cells had no effect on host resistance to street virus infection.[369,417,558,566] In contrast, Tc may actually be involved in the immunopathology and have been implicated in neuritic paralysis.[683,752] By comparison, the induction of CD4+ T cells is an integral part of the protective immune response against rabies.[178] Elimination of CD4+ cells abrogates the production of IgG neutralizing antibody in response to virus infection.[558] The RNP contains major epitopes that induce CD4+ T-cell responses, and most of these T cells cross-react with other lyssaviruses.[207] The RNP-specific T cells, which can augment the production of neutralizing antibody, are believed to be the major factor that mediates the protective immune response induced by internal viral antigens.[181,251]

Determinants of Viral Virulence

In general, determinants of viral virulence among rhabdoviruses can be classified into those that enhance virus replication and those that enhance the suppression or evasion of host antiviral responses. Mutations in such virulence determinants are of considerable interest, because of their potential to generate live virus vaccines. In the case of RABV, much attention has focused on mutations in G protein that attenuate viral pathogenicity. For example, antigenic variants selected with neutralizing monoclonal antibodies against G protein often display reduced neurovirulence in mice. These variants contain mutations that change R/K333 in G protein to other amino acids. These changes reduce the ability of G protein to attach to neuron-specific receptors,[152,713] although virus replication in nonneuronal cells is not affected. Similarly, mutations in VSV that compromise its ability to replicate often result in attenuated virus strains. For example, truncation of the G protein cytoplasmic domain reduces the efficiency of virus budding, as described earlier. Such mutants are attenuated in their pathogenicity and form the basis for candidate recombinant viral vaccines.[592,607] Likewise, recombinant viruses in which the order of the VSV genes has been altered usually display reduced pathogenicity as a result of reduced virus replication and are candidate recombinant vaccines.[147,236]

An example of the second class of virulence determinants—those that lead to suppression of host antiviral responses—would be the VSV M protein. Mutations in M protein that render it defective in its ability to inhibit host gene expression attenuate viral virulence in mice without compromising the ability of the virus to replicate in cell culture.[3,6,681] In this case, the attenuation is caused by the enhanced innate immune responses elicited in infected cells because of the failure of the virus to suppress host gene expression.[711]

Similar to VSV M protein mutants, RABV P protein mutants have been generated that are defective in their ability to block IRF-3 phosphorylation[589] or STAT1 nuclear translocation.[334] These viruses are also attenuated in their pathogenicity in mice, emphasizing the importance of P protein–mediated suppression of IFN responses as a virulence factor for RABV. However, equally important virulence factors for RABV are viral mechanisms that suppress production of the activators of innate antiviral responses. The difference in pathogenicity of attenuated viruses compared to field strains (i.e., street viruses) is correlated with lower levels of viral gene expression by the more virulent strains.[502,743] This leads to correspondingly lower induction of antiviral responses by the more virulent viruses. Similarly, strain differences in the N protein have been linked to differences in RIG-I signaling and corresponding differences in virulence.[475] Thus, the key to the pathogenicity of RABV is the combination of having a potent suppressive mechanism to inhibit IFN responses in susceptible cells together with a sufficiently low level of viral gene expression to reduce the responses generated in the cells of the innate immune system. In other words, RABV is said to "[use] stealth to reach the brain".[633]

EPIDEMIOLOGY OF RHABDOVIRUS INFECTIONS

Epidemiology of Lyssavirus Infections

Lyssavirus epidemiology is partially influenced by host species distribution, abundance, demographics, behavioral ecology, dispersal, and interactions with humans.[614] Because of its consequences when ignored, rabies is a reportable disease in many countries, although surveillance is inadequate, particularly in sylvatic hosts. Biased epidemiologic information usually derives from clinical reports or the examination of suitable brain material submitted to public health or veterinary diagnostic laboratories only after infectious contact with animals is suspected.

Exposure is generally defined as transdermal contact, typically by a bite, or mucosal contamination with potentially infectious material (e.g., saliva or CNS tissue).[789] The relative risk associated with other scenarios is difficult to define.

The domestic dog is the principal host and major vector of rabies throughout the world,[217,740] currently most prominent in the tropical regions of Asia, Latin America, and Africa. International reporting of both human and animal rabies cases grossly underestimates the magnitude of the problem.[495] Predominant wild reservoirs and maintenance hosts belong to the family *Carnivora*[38,376] and include foxes[74,154] in the Arctic (*Vulpes lagopus*), Canada, central and western Europe, and moderate latitudes of Asia (*V. vulpes, V. corsac*), and scattered foci elsewhere throughout North America (e.g., *Urocyon cinereoargenteus*); the raccoon dog (*Nyctereutes procyonoides*) in eastern Europe, Scandinavia, and portions of Asia[120,395,526]; coyotes, jackals (*Canis* species), and other wild canids in North America, Asia, and Africa[258]; skunks (*Mephitis mephitis, Spilogale putorius*) in North America[118,280]; procyonids, such as the raccoon (*Procyon lotor*), in eastern North America[68,778]; and herpestids (e.g., the yellow mongoose, *Cynictis penicillata;* the small Asian mongoose, *Herpestes javanicus*) and their relatives throughout Africa, Asia, and the Middle East.[725] Additionally, the ferret badger (*Melogale moschata*) was documented as a rabies reservoir in several regions of China.[447,809] Rabies detection in rodents is uniformly rare.[121,396,779]

Bat rabies predominates in the New World, described primarily among insectivorous bats of the United States and Canada (over 40 species) and the three hematophagous vampire species (principally, *Desmodus rotundus*) ranging from northern Mexico to Argentina.[39,122] Many bat species may also be important throughout Latin America.[169,170] Other lyssaviruses are transmitted by bats in Africa, Europe, Asia, and Australia.[17,42,247,400,402,403]

Surveillance efforts in the United States follow changes in indigenous and translocated cases in space and over time. For example, in 2009, 49 states and Puerto Rico reported 6,690 rabid animals and 4 human rabies cases to the Centers for Disease Control and Prevention (CDC). Approximately 92% of reported rabid animals were wildlife. Relative contributions by the major animal groups were 34.8% raccoons, 24.3% bats, 24.0% skunks, 7.5% foxes, 4.5% cats, 1.2% dogs, and 1.1% cattle. Compared with 2008, reported numbers of rabid raccoons and bats decreased, whereas reported numbers of rabid skunks, foxes, cats, cattle, dogs, and horses increased.[75] Historically, Hawaii remained the only rabies-free state, never having reported a case of indigenously acquired rabies.[233,618]

Combined with historical, temporal, and spatial disease surveillance data, antigenic characterization with monoclonal antibodies (MAbs) and nucleotide sequence analysis can assist in the assignment of isolates to different animal reservoirs.[661,663,664] Arctic RABV circulates circumpolarly, although local variability was documented in several areas, such as Alaska and Ontario. Although *V. lagopus* historically has been recognized as the major reservoir of Arctic RABV, *V. vulpes* increasingly participates in circulation of this virus variant due to climate changes. Skunk rabies isolates appear to be distinct variants defining separate outbreaks in the north-central and south-central parts of North America, and California. Additionally, smaller independent foci involve foxes, dogs, and coyotes in Texas, as well as foxes in Arizona and portions of the southwestern United States.[75,135,390,660,661,663]

Analysis of human rabies cases from the United States implicated viruses associated with insectivorous bats as the most frequent source of infection after elimination of canine rabies,[75,390,522] and some bat isolates appear to possess unique pathogenic properties compared with isolates from the family *Carnivora*.[503] During 2003, a first reported occurrence of rabies in a human infected with the raccoon rabies virus variant was documented in Virginia; however, the exposure history was unknown. During 2004, transplantation from an infected donor resulted in four human cases in the United States[669] and three in Germany,[306] demonstrating the devastating consequences when rabies is not suspected.

Host switching from bats to terrestrial mammals during the history of lyssavirus evolution has been inferred from RABV phylogeny.[35] Based on the relatedness of carnivore RABV variants to bat RABV variants, the switch is proposed to have occurred approximately 1,000 to 1,500 years ago. Moreover, relatively frequent spill-over cases and host shifts of bat RABV variants to terrestrial mammals have been documented repeatedly during recent years.[23,433] More controversial is a proposed cross-species shift in lyssaviruses, given that a variety of non-RABV lyssaviruses, but not RABV, have been detected in bats in the Eastern Hemisphere, and only RABV detected in all reservoir hosts, including bats, in the Western Hemisphere.[406]

In western and central Europe, where fox rabies has been largely eliminated via oral vaccination, bat rabies still poses public health concerns. The EBLV-1, first isolated in 1954 in Germany, was later identified across Europe, from Spain to the Ukraine.[17,401] About 95% of EBLV-1 cases have been observed in *E. serotinus* bats.[17,627] However, it has also been reported in numerous other bat species.[627,637,638] Spill-over infections of EBLV-1 were documented in sheep in Denmark,[600] in stone marten in Germany,[509] and in domestic cats in France.[159] In contrast to EBLV-1, distribution of EBLV-2 is limited to northwestern Europe.[406] This virus circulates primarily among bats of the *Myotis* genus. Five human rabies cases of bat origin have been documented in Europe. In one case the virus was identified as EBLV-1, in two others EBLV-2 was identified, and in two cases the virus was not characterized.[406]

Bat lyssavirus surveillance in southeastern Europe and Asia is extremely limited. Nevertheless, such viruses as ARAV and KHUV were isolated from *Myotis* bats in Central Asia,[405] IRKV was isolated from *Murina leucogaster* in Eastern Siberia[81] and later caused a human rabies case in the Far East,[62] and WCBV was isolated in the Caucasus region from *Miniopterus schreibersii*.[400] Historical records indicate isolation of lyssaviruses from bats in India and Thailand,[544,665] and serologic surveys demonstrated the presence of lyssavirus antibodies in bats from the Philippines, Cambodia, Thailand, and Bangladesh.[24,457,587] Presumed human rabies of bat origin was reported from China, although no virological examination was performed.[692] Indeed, significant surveillance efforts are needed in this large part of the world to elucidate ecology and epidemiology of lyssaviruses.

In Africa several divergent lyssavirus species have been documented. Dog rabies is widely distributed and represents the major burden for humans and domestic animals. At least three phylogenetic lineages of dog RABV were described, along with a separate lineage associated with mongooses.[165,473,725] Epizootics in dogs frequently spread to wildlife.[429] Several outbreaks have been described that significantly reduced populations of such endangered species as African wild dog (*Lycaon pictus*)[258,318] and Ethiopian wolf (*Canis simensis*).[353,578] Another African lyssavirus, MOKV, has been sporadically isolated from shrews, domestic cats and dogs, and a rodent in various localities of Sub-Saharan Africa.[370,473,513] MOKV is the only lyssavirus species never documented in bats. However, the principal reservoir host of this virus is still unknown. Two human cases of MOKV infection were documented via active surveillance efforts, both with unknown exposure history.[210,211] In contrast to MOKV, LBV is clearly associated with bats from the *Pteropidae* family, such as *Eidolon helvum, Rousettus aegyptiacus, Micropteropus pussilus, Epomophorus wahlbergi,* and likely others, with only infrequent spill-over infections into terrestrial mammals, such as cats, dogs, and a mongoose.[403,472,473] LBV is broadly distributed in Sub-Saharan Africa and at least once was translocated to France with *R. aegyptiacus* fruit bats, imported from Togo or Egypt.[28] The other two African bat lyssaviruses are less studied. Of the four known isolates of DUVV, three came from humans, who died of rabies after bites of insectivorous bats in South Africa and Kenya, and only one was obtained from a bat, presumably of the *Miniopterus* genus, in Zimbabwe.[375,494,552,724] The last member of the genus, SHIBV, is known by a single isolate, obtained from an insectivorous bat *Hipposideros commersonii* in Kenya.[402] Indeed, more studies are needed to understand ecology and epidemiology of African non-RABV lyssaviruses.

Prior to 1996, Australia had been considered free of rabies and rabies-like viruses. An outbreak of rabies involving several dogs occurred in the island state of Tasmania in 1867 but was quickly eradicated. Since then, only a few imported rabies cases were registered. Following the discovery that flying foxes were a reservoir of Hendra virus, surveillance of these animals was increased, which resulted in the discovery of ABLV in 1996.[247,272] ABLV has been identified in all four flying fox species in continental Australia: *P. alecto, P. poliocephalus, P. scapulatus,* and *P. conspicillatus,* in locations along the eastern coastal territory of the continent, where the surveillance was enhanced.[287] Further, a distinct ABLV variant was identified in insectivorous bats *Saccolaimus albiventris.*[273] Two human cases of ABLV infection have been described to date. The first, documented in 1996, was caused by the insectivorous bat ABLV variant,[14,273] and the other one was caused by the pteropid ABLV variant.[748] Both cases were fatal, and clinical symptoms were compatible with rabies. The distribution range of *P. alecto* bats extends into Papua, New Guinea, and the eastern islands of Indonesia.[247] There is no reason to expect that distribution of ABLV is limited to continental Australia. For example, the presence of antibodies to this virus was demonstrated in 9.5% bat serum samples collected in the Philippines.[24]

Epidemiology of Vesiculovirus Infections

The mechanisms of VSV transmission are not completely understood. Ecologic factors and special conditions regarding the host and the etiologic agent have been implicated in the clinical presentation of the disease.[294–296] Experimental transmission from animal to animal by direct contact has produced irregular results. The virus is unable to penetrate intact skin or mucosa; for a successful transmission, it needs to be introduced beneath the skin and mucous membranes via wounds and abrasions.[295,356] The virus can also be transmitted by the bite of insect vectors such as mosquitoes (*Aedes* spp.),[701,751] sand flies (*Lutzomyia* spp.),[141] blackflies (*Simulium* spp.),[156] and other *Diptera.*[226] Virus isolations from nonbiting insects (e.g., *Musca domestica*) have been reported.[246] Many potential biological vectors of VSV have been suggested, but the phlebotomine sand fly, *Lutzomia shannoni*, is the only one confirmed in the United States.[751]

The disease is present only in the Western Hemisphere, and it is enzootic in southern Mexico, in Central America, in some regions of South America,[750] and on Ossabaw Island, off the coast of Georgia.[673] In temperate zones, VSV outbreaks begin in late summer and end with the arrival of frost.[270] In the United States, the outbreak during 1982–1983 was unusual because it continued throughout the winter months until the following spring.[87] In tropical areas, the disease appears at the end of the rainy season and disappears with the advent of the dry season.[751] Typically, the disease affects only horses, cattle, and swine. During outbreaks, morbidity rates in a herd usually range from 10% to 15%.[750] Cattle generally recover in a few days, but horses and pigs can develop lameness.[295,750] A broad spectrum of wild mammals can also be affected.[750] Factors that influence the disease spread in dairy cattle include coarse roughage, hard pelleted concentrates, poor general and milking hygiene, and insufficient teat sanitation.[294] In the southeastern United States, feral swine had 10% to 100% antibody prevalence from 1979 to 1985[674] and on Ossabaw Island showed 12% and 60% seroconversion between June and September in 1982 and 1983, respectively.[675] In some enzootic areas of Central America, over 80% of the cattle have antibodies against VSV, but only 9% of the animals may present clinical signs in a particular year. In the same regions, wildlife also have a high VSV seroprevalence. In tropical areas where the disease is enzootic, VSV seroprevalence in the human population can be as high as 48%.[352] Serologic studies during outbreaks in Panama demonstrated a seroprevalence of 71% and 34% in personnel working with infected and noninfected cattle, respectively.[89] A similar situation has been observed during VSV outbreaks in Colorado, where personnel (veterinarians, researchers, and regulatory staff) handling sick livestock showed an antibody prevalence of 13%, whereas unexposed humans had a 6% seroprevalence.[586]

The mechanism by which VSV is maintained in enzootic regions is not fully understood. Sand flies may transmit the virus from a reservoir (e.g., plants, wildlife, cattle) to livestock. Alternatively, VSV may be maintained in the sand fly population by transovarial transmission, and the insects infect susceptible animals during feeding.[141] In some enzootic areas, feral swine have been suggested as a potential amplifying host.[673] Molecular epidemiologic studies indicate that enzootic areas may be the origin of the virus responsible for outbreaks in epizootic zones.[517] VSV may be introduced in a particular area by the movement of infected animals, wildlife, or insects, but the actual mechanism is unknown. Viruses circulating in enzootic areas present a high genetic diversity, with several lineages coexisting in the same region.[516] Within enzootic areas, the viruses seem to adapt under selective pressures exerted by ecologic factors. Viruses from different ecologic areas within enzootic regions belong to different genotypes. Viral adaptation to different insect vectors or mammalian reservoirs might be determinant factors for this divergent evolution.[597] Viruses obtained from a particular outbreak are genetically homogeneous.[517]

Epidemiology of Ephemerovirus Infections

Bovine ephemeral fever is distributed throughout Africa, the Middle East, Southeast Asia, and northern Australia.[671] It has never been reported in the Americas. The disease occurs during summer and autumn and disappears with the arrival of the first frosts in subtropical areas. In the tropics, yearly occurrence is associated with the rainy season.[671,735] Although transmission of the virus occurs via insect vectors, the difficulty of isolating the virus from insects hampers the recognition of the vector species involved in its transmission. BEFV was isolated from *Culicoides* spp. and from mosquitoes. In Australia, the geographic range of the disease is greater than that of the *Culicoides* species from which the virus was isolated. Two species of mosquitoes, *Culex annulirostris* and *Anopheles annulipes,* may be implicated in transmission in these areas.[671] In general, morbidity is low, but in some outbreaks, all of the animals in a herd may be affected. In other instances, only 2% or 3% of the animals show clinical signs.[671,735] Natural disease occurs only in cattle and water buffalo. Although seroprevalences of 13% to 38% were reported in cattle in enzootic areas, a higher prevalence of 64% has been observed during outbreaks.[161] The role of wild ruminants in the maintenance of BEFV in nature is not understood. Seroprevalences between 28% and 54% are found in wild ruminants in Kenya, Zimbabwe, and Tanzania.[18,166]

Epidemiology of Novirhabdovirus Infections

Novirhabdoviruses cause severe economic losses to the salmonid farming industries.[317,786] As was described earlier, IHNV is endemic to western North America, and dispersal of the virus outside North America has occurred by inadvertent transport of infected eggs and juvenile fish.[313,373,617] Within North America, dispersal of IHNV is thought to have involved the historical use of unpasteurized salmon viscera in feed for salmon hatcheries, and possibly the historically common practice of salmon transplantations.[102,749,786] Following the introduction to the Eastern Hemisphere, European and Asian IHNV isolates demonstrate relatedness to specific phylogenetic lineages within the endemic area from which they were derived.[372,521,540]

VHSV was first discovered in Western Europe.[786] So far, VHSV has been isolated from over 60 fish species from both marine and freshwater habitats representing North America, Asia, and Europe.[654] VHSV is endemic to numerous marine species in both the Atlantic and Pacific Oceans of the northern hemisphere and could have been introduced into freshwater habitats by marine fish species (e.g., herring, sprat, sand eel) that are used as fresh feed for commercial farming in some countries.[654] The freshwater isolates of VHSV appear to be evolving ~2.5 times faster than the marine isolates.[200] The successful recent viral adaptation in new hosts is one of the possible explanations for such higher evolutionary rates of VHSV in freshwater fish.[505] Alternative explanations for the increased substitution rates in freshwater VHSV are the intensive aquaculture practices and the higher water temperature in culture ponds, which could cause an increase in virus replication rates.[200] A similar pattern has also been observed for IHNV in North America, where the evolutionary rate was found to be three to four times higher in regions with intensive aquaculture, as compared with other regions.[712]

HIRRV was first isolated in Japan from Japanese flounder[374] and subsequently was also reported in Korea.[371,534] It has recently been reported to infect several other fish species endemic to Japan.[374] SHRV was first isolated from snakehead fish in Thailand and has not been reported outside Southeast Asia to date.[363]

CLINICAL FEATURES OF RHABDOVIRUS INFECTIONS

Lyssavirus Infections

Rabies cases are almost always attributable to the bite of a rabid animal. For example, animal bites were the cause of 99.8% of 3,920 human rabies cases examined at various Pasteur Institutes between 1927 and 1946.[487] Nonbite exposures, which rarely cause rabies, include inhalation of aerosols,[325,333,781] licks,[424] transdermal scratches, or other unusual events that lead to contamination of an open wound or mucous membrane,[232] such as tissue or organ transplantation.[344,669] Bat RABV-associated human deaths in the United States may not have a reported exposure source,[112,522] but these cases are most likely caused by bat bites in which either the risk was not appreciated or the bites were not immediately recognized by the patient. Disease development after exposure depends on the location and severity of a bite, the species of animal responsible for the exposure, and the virus variant.[29,40,518,649,726] In the absence of vaccination, the highest mortality tends to occur in persons bitten on the head and face (40% to 80%), with intermediate mortality in those bitten on the hands or arms (15% to 40%), and least in those bitten on the trunk or legs (5% to 10%) or through clothing (less than 5%).[29,637,652,726]

The incubation period (the length of time between exposure to virus and development of clinical signs) is usually 1 to 2 months.[232,744] Because it can vary from less than a week[307,551,560] to several years,[10,33,662,770,774] rabies is one of the most variable infectious diseases. The length of the incubation period may depend on the bite site and relative proximity to the CNS,[10,350,687] severity of the bite, type and quantity of virus introduced, host age, and immune status.[10,19,194,205,301,304,487,519,649]

Development of clinical rabies in humans can be divided into three general phases: a prodromal period, the acute neurologic phase, and coma preceding death.[232,307] During the prodromal period, lasting 2 to 10 days, symptoms are usually mild and almost entirely nonspecific; they include general malaise, chills, fever, headache, photophobia, anorexia, nausea, vomiting, diarrhea, sore throat, cough, and musculoskeletal pain. One specific early symptom is abnormal sensation around the bite site, such as itching, burning, numbness, or paresthesia.[194]

During the acute neurologic phase, patients exhibit signs of nervous system dysfunction such as anxiety, agitation, dysphagia, hypersalivation, paralysis, and episodes of delirium. Occasionally, priapism or increased libido may be observed.[198] Cases in which hyperactivity is predominant are classified as *furious* rabies. When paralysis dominates, it is classified as paralytic or *dumb* rabies.[125,380,727] From 17% to 80% of patients exhibit hydrophobia, a pathognomonic sign of rabies believed to be caused by an exaggerated respiratory tract protective reflex.[10,19,746,774] Hydrophobic episodes, initially triggered by attempts to drink,[307,774] can last from 1 to 5 minutes. In furious rabies, the neurologic period ends after 2 to 7 days with coma or sudden death from respiratory or cardiac arrest.[76]

Paralytic rabies occurs in about 20% of patients and may be more frequent in persons exposed to certain strains, such as vampire bat RABV.[328] In marked contrast to furious rabies, the sensorium is largely spared.[309,328] Patients initially develop paresthesia and weakness, and finally flaccid paralysis, usually in the bitten extremity.[125] Paralysis progresses to paraplegia and quadriplegia. In paralytic rabies, the course is usually less rapidly progressive, with some patients living up to 30 days without intensive care.[453] The final stage of the disease is coma, which lasts 3 to 7 days and results in death.[76] In patients receiving respiratory assistance, survival may be prolonged for weeks,[76,522] with death caused by other complications.[65,204,301]

To date, six cases of human recovery from clinical rabies have been documented. Five had exposure to animal bites,[15,300,565,773] and one occurred after suspected inhalation of rabies virus in the laboratory.[110] Only one of these occurred in a patient who had never been vaccinated,[773] whereas the other five cases were attributed as exposures and vaccination failures. In the nonvaccinated patient, an experimental treatment included induction of ketamine coma in conjunction with antiviral compounds and intensive care.[773] Nevertheless, more than 10 attempts to repeat such experimental treatment (although with deviations and modifications) failed.[338] However, in one vaccination failure case (immunoglobulin was not administered, although all five doses of vaccine were administered on time), the experimental treatment was implemented successfully.[174] In addition, this was the only survival case where the virus variant was identified (vampire bat RABV). In all other survivors neither antigen detection nor virus isolation nor RNA amplification was successful, and rabies diagnosis was based on the history of exposure, compatible incubation period and clinical signs, and serologic tests. Another case of presumptive abortive rabies infection in a human, who never required intensive care, and only once received rabies biologics after establishment of the diagnosis, was reported recently.[113]

Clinical disease in animals is not unlike that of humans, except for the absence of hydrophobia. Signs are variable but can include altered phonation, pica, cranial nerve deficits, altered activity patterns, and loss of fear of humans.[37]

Vesiculovirus Infections

In natural infection, the incubation period of vesiculovirus varies from 2 to 9 days, but usually lesions develop between 2 and 5 days after exposure.[303,356] The lesions of vesiculovirus are indistinguishable from those of FMD. In cattle, the initial lesions are characterized by pink to white papules in the mouth that progress in 1 to 2 days to vesicles. The vesicles can coalesce and rupture, leaving a denuded area that heals in 1 or 2 weeks if no secondary infections occur.[356] These lesions can also occur in the dental pad, lips, gums, muzzle, nose, teats, and feet. In experimental inoculation of horses, vesicles appeared in the mouth 42 hours after inoculation, and 2 days later, part of the dorsal epithelial covering of the tongue sloughed off. Vesicles also appeared on the feet. At necropsy, the spleen was enlarged, but no other lesions were observed in the internal organs.[148] In natural infection of horses, lesions are found in the lips, corners of the mouth, muzzle, nostrils, ears, belly, prepuce, and udder.[303] The lesions in pigs are similar to those described for cattle.[296] Affected animals have increased salivation and a sharp reduction in milk production. Eating is difficult because of the sore mouth, with a consequent decline in physical condition. Lameness develops with foot lesions.

Although development of secondary lesions in places other than the point of inoculation is suggestive of viremia, the virus has not been isolated from blood even at 6 hours after the experimental inoculation of pigs.[133,583,672] The virus is present at its highest titer in the vesicular fluid, which represents a transient but very efficient source of virus for contact transmission. The virus can be isolated from specimens taken from saliva, tonsils, vesicular fluids of feet, and, in some cases, feces.[133,583,672]

Ephemerovirus Infections

After an incubation period of 2 to 4 days, the first clinical sign is fever (40°C to 42°C), accompanied by malaise and a severe drop in milk production. In 12 to 24 hours, fever remits, followed by a second febrile phase. During this second phase, the animals are depressed, are anorexic, and show muscle stiffness and lameness. Ruminal stasis, nasal and ocular discharges, and swelling of one or more joints are present. Subcutaneous emphysema can develop in some animals.[671,735] The clinical signs persist for 1 or 2 days, followed by rapid recovery. Clinical signs are much more severe in adults than in calves. Calves under 6 months of age show no clinical signs.[78]

Novirhabdovirus Infections

Viral hemorrhagic septicemia (VHS) generally occurs at temperatures between 4°C and 14°C. At water temperatures between 15°C and 18°C, the disease generally has a short course with a modest accumulated mortality. VHS rarely occurs at higher temperatures. Low water temperatures (1°C to 5°C) generally result in an extended disease course with low daily mortality but high accumulated mortality. For IHNV, the temperature optimum is slightly greater, 3°C to 18°C. VHS outbreaks occur during all seasons but are most common in spring when water temperatures are rising or fluctuating. For more detailed reviews of the condition see, Smail[656] and Wolf.[786]

VHS progresses in three stages. The acute stage includes a rapid onset of high mortalities (up to 90%, particularly in young fish) often with severe clinical signs such as darkening of body color, exophthalmia (bulging eye), bleeding around eyes and fin bases, pale gills, and petechial (pinpoint) hemorrhaging on the surfaces of the gills and viscera and in the muscle. Virus multiplication in endothelial cells of blood capillaries, hematopoietic tissues, and cells of the kidney underlies the clinical signs. Gross pathology includes generalized petechial hemorrhaging in the skin, muscle tissue (especially in dorsal muscles), and internal organs.[531]

During the second subacute, or chronic, stage, the body continues to darken and exophthalmia may become more pronounced, but hemorrhaging around the eyes and fin bases is often reduced. Fish are severely anemic and paleness is particularly evident in the abdomen. Fish may develop a spiraling swimming motion. The final, nervous stage involves reduced mortality and clinical signs are usually absent, but the corkscrew swimming motion becomes more pronounced. The disease is transmitted horizontally through contact with infected fish or water. Large amounts of virus are shed in the feces, urine, and sexual fluids. There is no vertical transmission of the VHSV. However, vertical transmission has been documented for IHNV.[530] Virus is shed from infected fish via the urine[656] and reproductive fluids and can also be transferred by piscivorous birds as external mechanical vectors.[536,559] Incubation time is dependent on temperature and dose; it is 5 to 12 days at higher temperatures. During and immediately following an outbreak, virus can be isolated readily from kidney, heart, and spleen tissues.

VHSV can also establish a carrier state in freshwater fish species.[206,355] The virological status of such carriers will be dependent on a range of parameters including the length of time following initial exposure and geographical proximity to fish-farm outlets. Based on virus isolation in cell culture, the prevalence of VHSV in marine fish species has been found to be in the range of 0.0% to 16.7%.[654]

DIAGNOSIS OF RHABDOVIRUS INFECTIONS

Lyssavirus Infections

Clinical diagnosis of rabies is not difficult in cases of a documented history of exposure and subsequent compatible clinical signs or symptoms. Because an exposure history may be lacking, rabies should be considered in any acute, unexplained neurologic disease that rapidly progresses to coma and death.[38] Routine diagnosis is established by standard laboratory tests for specific virus isolates, antigens, nucleic acids, or neutralizing antibodies.[293,659,745] Postmortem diagnosis should be performed on CNS specimens, especially the brainstem and cerebellum.[697] The fluorescent antibody test[659] and the avidin-biotin immunohistochemical technique[289] are sensitive and specific methods for detecting virus antigen (Fig. 31.12).

Examination of skin biopsies from the face[96] or hair-covered occipital portions of the neck for virus antigen[77,522] is a rapid method to diagnose human rabies before death. Rabies virus can be isolated from saliva by direct intracerebral inoculation into mice[387] or by infection of neuroblastoma cells.[657] Fluorescent antibody examinations of corneal impressions may occasionally lead to the diagnosis of human rabies.[381] The reverse transcriptase-polymerase chain reaction (RT-PCR) assay has been used to amplify and sequence parts of the lyssavirus genome directly from brain, saliva, and other affected tissues.[138,302,522,659] This allows detection of rabies virus–specific RNA and also permits insights into the identity of the virus variant by genetic sequencing. Detection of specific antibodies in serum[522,662] late in the clinical course can be diagnostic for rabies, if the patient has not been previously vaccinated. Except for certain cases of postvaccinal encephalomyelitis, CSF antibodies are produced only in rabies-infected, not in vaccinated, individuals.[747] Several diagnostic tests have been developed for detection of virus-neutralizing antibodies, such as the rapid fluorescent focus inhibition test (RFFIT) and the fluorescent antibody viral neutralization (FAVN) test, which are recommended by national and international authorities, such as the World Health Organization (WHO), Office International des Epizooties (OIE), and Advisory Commission on Immunization Practices (ACIP).[137,323,658] Recently, lentiviral pseudotypes containing glycoproteins of different lyssaviruses have been developed for replacement of infectious RABV in such virus-neutralizing tests.[791] Several modifications of enzyme-linked immunosorbent assays (ELISAs) have been developed for capture and measure of antiglycoprotein antibodies of RABV.[639,753,810] However, such ELISA-based tests are currently not recommended for the cases where diagnostic accuracy is critical.[501] Other serologic methods have been developed that detect antibodies against other components of RABV, primarily the nucleocapsid, which is most abundant in the infected cells. Of these, the best established is the indirect fluorescent antibody test (IFA). Antibodies detected by IFA appear earlier than virus-neutralizing antibodies and sometimes are the only positive result obtained antemortem.[113,659,662]

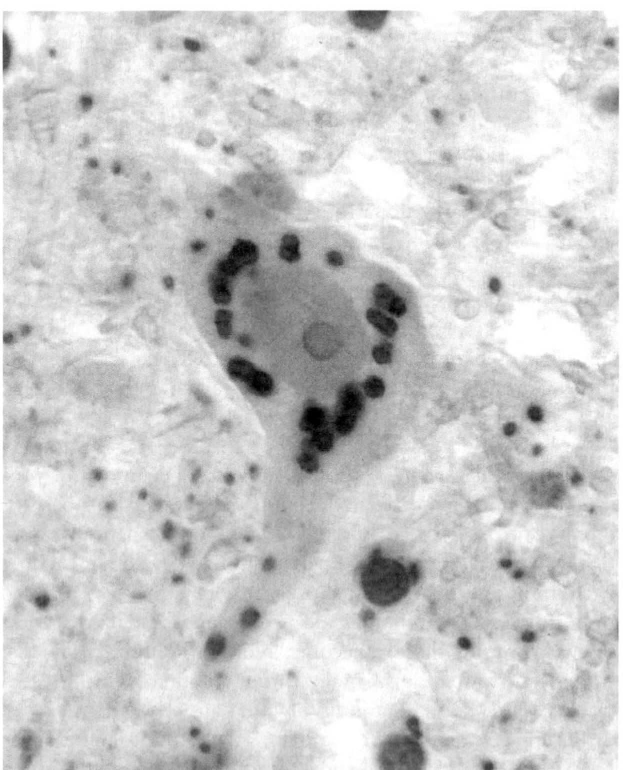

FIGURE 31.12. Immunohistochemical staining of intracytoplasmic viral inclusions in the neuron of a human rabies patient (630×). (Courtesy of M. Niezgoda, CDC/OID/NCEZID/DHPP/PRB.)

Vesiculovirus Infections

Because vesiculovirus is clinically similar to FMD, differential diagnosis between the two diseases is of utmost importance, especially in countries free of the latter disease. VSV can be isolated from vesicular fluid or epithelium of the lesions by inoculation in mice, embryonated eggs, or cell culture.[134] The virus can be identified by virus neutralization, complement fixation, or immunofluorescence.[296] Complement fixation provides a rapid, sensitive, and accurate method for the differentiation of VSV and FMD virus.[295] A rise in virus neutralization or ELISA antibody titer in serum samples taken during the clinical and convalescent phases of the disease is evidence that the infection was caused by VSV.[13] Recently, detection of VSV in clinical samples by RT-PCR has been described. This method is highly sensitive and specific, providing a rapid diagnosis and material for genetic characterization of the virus.[319,598]

Ephemerovirus Infections

Clinical diagnosis of BEF is based on its rapidity of spread and transient nature.[78] For confirmation, virus isolation or the demonstration of an increase in virus neutralization or ELISA antibody in paired serum samples is needed.[187] A blocking ELISA compares favorably with neutralization and does not detect cross-reacting antibodies to Kimberly or Berrimah viruses.[805] Although impractical for routine diagnosis, cattle inoculation with blood from BEFV-affected animals is the most sensitive method for viral isolation. Isolation of BEFV in *Aedes albopictus* cells from the blood of infected animals, followed by direct immunofluorescence to detect the presence of viral antigens, has been used in experimental studies.[720]

Novirhabdovirus Infections

The occurrence of clinical signs of VHS described earlier should suggest the presence of IHNV and VHSV. Gross pathology includes generalized petechial hemorrhaging in the skin, muscle tissue (especially in dorsal muscles), and internal organs. Histopathologic findings reveal degenerative necrosis in the hematopoietic tissues, kidney, spleen, liver, pancreas, and digestive tract. Necrosis of eosinophilic granular cells in the intestinal wall is pathognomic of IHNV infection.[80] The kidney, liver, and spleen show extensive focal necrosis and degeneration—cytoplasmic vacuoles, pyknosis, karyolysis, and lymphocytic invasion. In case of VHSV, diagnosis can involve immunohistochemistry analysis of VHSV-positive endothelial cells in the vascular system.[209] The standard surveillance method to detect carrier fish for IHNV and VHSV is based on direct isolation of the virus in cell culture followed by identification using antibody-based methods (IFA, ELISA) or nucleic acid–based methods (e.g., RT-PCR), followed by gene sequencing. PCR-based detection of viral genomes in fish tissue is still under development. The technique can be used for confirmation of overt infection in fish but has yet to be validated for use in direct surveillance programs.[22,25,172,186,416,784]

PREVENTION AND CONTROL OF RHABDOVIRUS INFECTIONS

Lyssavirus Infections in Humans

Rabies has the highest case-to-fatality ratio of any infectious disease. With rare exceptions, comfort care, sedation, and life support measures may prolong life but do not prevent death. In most situations, use of the term *treatment* is a misnomer and refers to medical aid related to animal bite and disease prevention by postexposure prophylaxis.[767] However, the establishment of a protocol for experimental treatment of clinical rabies[773] has led to more attempts to combat the clinical disease. The majority of these have failed,[338] although at least one positive result, with recovery of the patient, was reported.[174] Indeed, more studies in suitable animal models are needed to investigate different components of the protocol, potential ways of their modifications, and improvements.[338] More than 12 million humans are exposed and may undergo antirabies prophylaxis annually, but in excess of an estimated 50,000 to 100,000 die, primarily from the bite of an infected dog.[495,719] Regional epidemiologic surveillance and knowledge of viral pathogenesis, development of vaccination algorithms, and communication of risk to different occupational groups can significantly reduce human morbidity from inappropriate prophylaxis and rabies mortality.[643,778] Eliminating primary exposure to rabid animals is a fundamental means of rabies prevention. Human rabies deaths are infrequent in regions with controlled canine rabies. Nevertheless, tens of thousands of potential exposure cases are treated annually in Europe and North America because of enzootic wildlife rabies.[293]

Postexposure prophylaxis in humans includes proper wound care and the administration of rabies vaccine and antirabies immune globulin.[111,790] Although the inclusion of antirabies serum or immune globulin in the prophylaxis protocol is not new,[103] it is infrequent. Most cases of human rabies prophylaxis in Africa, Asia, and Latin America are with vaccine only,[496] often a nervous system tissue vaccine.[43,349,415,523,562] Cell culture–based rabies vaccines (e.g., human diploid cell rabies vaccine [HDCV]) are used in much of the developed world and form the standard for historical comparison with the Pasteurian neural vaccines from the 19th century,[731,767] including its later phenolized derivatives (Fermi, Semple, and others). Inactivated cell culture–based vaccines[682] and antirabies immune globulin, which are major improvements over cruder biologicals, decrease the adverse events related to anaphylaxis or serum sickness.[412,769] Other major rabies vaccines are produced in avian embryo fibroblasts (e.g., purified chick embryo cell culture rabies vaccine [PCEC], Rabipur) or in rhesus monkey kidney cells (purified Vero cell rabies vaccine [PVRV], Verorab), with aluminum phosphate as an adjuvant.[790] Production of HDCV is relatively difficult, with limited viral yields, resulting in high production costs. Primary hamster kidney cell vaccines are used in Russia, China, and other parts of Asia.[445] Efficacy trials using reduced doses, different immunization schedules, and alternative routes (e.g., intradermal administration) have been conducted and have demonstrated both high efficacy and safety.[129,130]

At present, no evidence suggests that prophylaxis failure is caused by antigenic variation of RABV.[790] Rather, vaccine failures are usually associated with inadequate wound care, omission of potent serum, failure to infiltrate the wound with immune globulin, delay, or failure to follow recommended procedures.[308,545,585,771] Future tactics for global human rabies prevention will continue to focus on the need for enhanced public health communications; continuing professional education; potent, inexpensive pre- and postexposure vaccines[250,412,413] and new schedules; and viable alternatives to rabies immune globulin (e.g., monoclonal antibodies).[46] Based on the recognition that rabies at its source can be effectively controlled and sometimes eliminated, safer, more effective, and inexpensive veterinary vaccines are a necessity for animal reservoirs, vectors, or victims of the disease.[38,100,220,222,235,780,790]

Although available rabies biologics provide reliable protection against phylogroup I lyssaviruses (RABV, DUVV, EBLV-1, EBLV-2, ABLV, ARAV, KHUV, DUVV), they do not protect against phylogroup II lyssaviruses (LBV, MOKV, SHIBV) or against WCBV, because of the significant antigenic differences.[34,291] Given broad distribution of the latter divergent lyssaviruses in Africa, in southeastern Europe, and perhaps more widely in the world,[81,402,403,473,513] there is a need to develop new biologicals, capable of providing reliable protection against them.

Control of Rabies in Animals

Rabies is not considered a serious candidate for disease eradication at this time because of numerous and diverse wild reservoirs.[112] The correlation between canine rabies and human fatalities, however, has led to the successful application of domestic animal vaccines, particularly in developed countries.[100]

A comprehensive domestic animal program also requires responsible pet ownership. Such a program entails stray animal management; leash law amendments; humane population curtailment (e.g., early spay and neuter programs); animal importation, translocation, and quarantine regulations; schedules for early pre-exposure vaccination of companion animals (in light of potential maternal immune inhibition); and rational postexposure management.[111] Unlike postexposure prophylaxis of humans, euthanasia is usually recommended for the naïve animal exposed to rabies, but this may eventually change with the development of safe and effective biologicals and protocols.

Current veterinary vaccines are more potent than earlier attenuated and inactivated vaccines.[26,567] Because no vaccine is 100% effective, given poor cross-reactivity with some viral species,[291,733] and because correct identification of the properly immunized animal may be confusing, the vaccinated dog or cat is not exempt from confinement and close observation. This strict period of observation of the biting animal applies to dogs, cats, and, in some countries, domestic ferrets.[111] Human prophylaxis may be delayed during this time in areas that are not enzootic for canine rabies.[653] In addition, pet vaccination status does not necessarily alter the need for euthanasia of an offending animal, regardless of vaccine potency or efficacy, if rabies is suspected.

In the case of free-ranging, nondomestic mammals, population reduction of major rabies reservoirs has been practiced for centuries but has not been generally regarded as a humane, long-term, cost-effective, or ecologically sound tool to control widespread lyssavirus infection.[171,293] Anticoagulants, however, have been used successfully to control hematophagous bats in Latin America. Anticoagulants have been applied topically to bite wounds on cattle, followed by systemic treatment of exposed cattle, and finally topical treatment of vampire bats themselves, exploiting their behavior of mutual grooming at the roost.[239] These control efforts can avoid the destruction of beneficial nontarget bat species, perhaps some day to be augmented with novel vaccination strategies.[640]

For more than four decades, efforts have been made to protect free-ranging wildlife against virulent street virus by oral consumption of vaccine contained within bait.[780] Millions of rabies virus vaccine–laden baits have been distributed over rural and urban areas in western Europe, eastern Canada, and the United States for wildlife rabies control.[27,36,235,419,601,602,738] Historically, attenuated rabies virus strains (such as ERA, SAD) were broadly used for oral vaccination of wild carnivores in Western Europe and North America.[626,739] However, sporadically these vaccine strains caused rabies in wildlife.[216,508] A vaccinia–rabies glycoprotein (V-RG) vaccine was the first recombinant rabies vaccine to be constructed, field tested, and considered for regulation in Europe and North America for wildlife rabies control. This vaccine has been extensively reviewed to ensure safety (tested in more than 40 species of mammals and birds) and efficacy (proved against severe rabies challenge in target species). Thermostability of the vaccine has been demonstrated under laboratory and field conditions. Following the success of the V-RG vaccine against fox rabies in Belgium[88] and France, preliminary field trials suggest its potential utility for rabies control in raccoons, foxes, and coyotes in the United States.[215,292,591,603] Other orthopoxviruses have been considered as vectors of lyssavirus antigens, but these have not yet been field tested.[217,450] A number of attenuated and recombinant rabies vaccines have been developed.[36,69,235,408,423,547,612,613,768] Oral vaccines have been successfully developed for red, Arctic, and gray foxes; coyotes; raccoon dogs; raccoons; skunks; and domestic dogs.[88,221,241,526,613] If future recombinant, replication-incompetent, inactivated, or DNA-based vaccines[208,343,420,449,500,538,613,795] prove both efficacious and economical, they may render most previous biosafety concerns obsolete, paving the way for more widespread, free-ranging wildlife and dog rabies control, particularly in developing countries. Another promising approach is combination of rabies vaccination with immunocontraception, which can significantly reduce the population of the disease vectors, particularly stray dogs.[792]

Control of Vesiculovirus Infections

Supportive veterinary care of affected animals helps to prevent complications that can delay recovery from VSV infection. Vaccination against VSV has been practiced to only a limited extent. A modified live vaccine, attenuated in cell culture or chicken embryos, has been used in parts of the United States, Central America, and Peru. This vaccine, administered intramuscularly in cattle, protects from disease for at least 1 year.[296] During the 1985 epizootic in Colorado, an inactivated VSNJV vaccine was used in the field and later tested in an experimental trial. It induced antibodies that lasted for 175 days, but viral challenge was not performed to assess protection.[265] Recently, a recombinant vaccinia virus expressing the VSV-I glycoprotein was developed and used experimentally to immunize cattle. Inoculated animals developed antibodies and resisted intradermal lingual challenge.[469]

Control of Ephemerovirus Infections

Vector control of BEFV is very difficult. International efforts to prevent the introduction of disease and vaccination may be the only practical methods for prevention of BEF.[735] Several attenuated vaccines, produced by serial passage in mouse or cell culture, provided protection against experimental challenge when mixed with adjuvants and given in several doses.[670] Inactivated vaccines were developed in Japan and Australia, but they induced poor and unreliable immunity. Vaccinia virus expressing the G protein elicited neutralizing antibodies in cattle, which were resistant to a subsequent viral challenge.[312] Additionally, an experimental subunit vaccine consisting of purified G protein mixed with Quil adjuvant conferred protection against viral challenge.[721]

Control of Novirhabdovirus Infections

Control methods for IHNV currently rely on avoidance of exposure to the virus through the implementation of strict control policies and sound hygiene practices.[783] The thorough disinfection of fertilized eggs, the use of virus-free water supplies for incubation and rearing, and the operation of facilities under established biosecurity measures are all critical for preventing infectious hematopoietic necrosis at a fish production site.

Vaccination of salmonids against IHNV is at an early stage of development; however, a range of vaccine preparations have shown promise in both laboratory and field trials.[397,782] Both autogenous, killed vaccines and a DNA vaccine have been licensed for commercial use in Atlantic salmon net-pen aquaculture on the West Coast of North America, where such vaccines can be delivered economically by injection. Vaccines against IHNV have not yet been licensed in other countries, where the application of vaccines to millions of small fish will require additional research on novel mass delivery methods. Although research on vaccine development against VHSV has been ongoing for more than three decades, a commercial vaccine is not yet available. DNA-based vaccines have proven to be very promising, inducing good protection from VHS.[452] Several immunostimulants, such as yeast-derived β-glucans, IL-1β–derived peptides, and probiotics, have been assessed for enhancing protection against VHS.[554] Disinfection of eggs is a highly effective method to block egg-associated transmission of novirhabdoviruses in aquaculture settings.[783] The method is widely practiced in areas where the virus is endemic. Other experimental approaches include resistance breeding and restocking with a resistant fish species.[310,783]

PERSPECTIVES

The foreseeable future for rhabdoviruses is for these viruses to occupy essentially the same positions in the science of virology that they have occupied for the past several decades—VSV as a well-studied prototype for the nonsegmented, negative-strand RNA viruses, RABV as a dreaded cause of disease in animals and humans, and the ephemeroviruses and novirhabdoviruses as important animal pathogens. Study of these viruses should continue to provide fundamental insights into the basis for virus–host interactions, neurotropism, and neuropathogenesis. In terms of the basic molecular biology of negative-strand RNA viruses, a number of important questions that have yet to be fully addressed have been pointed out through the course of this chapter. For example, the question of how the large, multifunctional L protein is able to respond to the many different *cis*-acting sequences that regulate its activity and the issue of how different intracellular nucleocapsids are selected for envelopment during the process of virus assembly are fundamental questions. In the area of virus–host interactions, the questions of viral virulence determinants and how rhabdoviruses suppress host responses among the different cell types involved in viral pathogenesis and immunity will be key questions for understanding the basis for viral pathogenesis in intact animals. In terms of the control of rabies, advances will come from the enhanced ability to control the spread of RABV among wild animal populations as well as the development of newer, more effective vaccine strategies.

One of the exciting areas of development with rhabdoviruses is the use of genetically engineered viruses as vaccine vectors or therapeutic agents. The use of recombinant VSV and RABV as vaccine vectors has been mentioned several times throughout the chapter.[147,214,592,593,607,631] In addition, both VSV and RABV have potential use as cytolytic agents for therapeutic purposes. For example, genetically engineered strains of both VSV and RABV for cytolysis of HIV-infected cells have been generated, which lack G protein but express CD4 and chemokine receptors in the virus envelope.[490,632] Another example of use of rhabdoviruses for cytolytic purposes is in the development of oncolytic viruses to treat patients with cancer. These viruses take advantage of the fact that many cancers appear to be defective in their ability to respond to antiviral cytokines, such as IFN.[47,680] Such cancers are susceptible to viruses that induce host antiviral responses (e.g., M protein mutant viruses)[3,681] or viruses that encode antiviral cytokines (e.g., IFN-β, IL-4),[224,527] whereas normal cells are largely resistant. Thus, these genetically engineered viruses have a greater selectivity for replication in cancers compared with normal tissues.

As a result of the efforts in developing recombinant rhabdoviruses as vaccine vectors and as cytolytic agents, it is likely that clinical trials of genetically engineered rhabdoviruses in humans will take place in the near future. For example, at least two genetically engineered VSVs have been considered by the National Institutes of Health Recombinant DNA Advisory Committee for potential oncolytic therapy in humans, a key step toward beginning clinical trials in a variety of cancer types.[716,717] A number of issues need to be considered in the use of such agents, such as their safety for use in humans, as well as the protection of animal populations that may be exposed to such viruses. Nonetheless, the advances in understanding virus replication and pathogenesis should make it feasible to address these issues, so that these viruses that have long been a burden to humanity can instead be a benefit.

REFERENCES

All cited references are available in the e-book.

6. Ahmed M, Marino TR, Puckett S, et al. Immune response in the absence of neurovirulence in mice infected with m protein mutant vesicular stomatitis virus. *J Virol* 2008;82:9273–9277.
8. Ahmed M, Mitchell LM, Puckett S, et al. Vesicular stomatitis virus M protein mutant stimulates maturation of Toll-like receptor 7 (TLR7)-positive dendritic cells through TLR-dependent and -independent mechanisms. *J Virol* 2009;83:2962–2975.
11. Albertini AA, Wernimont AK, Muziol T, et al. Crystal structure of the rabies virus nucleoprotein-RNA complex. *Science* 2006;313:360–363.
23. Arechiga-Ceballos N, Velasco-Villa A, Shi M, et al. New rabies virus variant found during an epizootic in white-nosed coatis from the Yucatan Peninsula. *Epidemiol Infect* 2010;138:1586–1589.
32. Backovic M, Jardetzky TS. Class III viral membrane fusion proteins. *Curr Opin Struct Biol* 2009;19:189–196.
62. Belikov SI, Leonova GN, Kondratov IG, et al. Isolation and genetic characterisation of a new lyssavirus strain in the Primorskiy kray. *East Siberian J Infect Pathol* 2009;16:68–69.
68. Biek R, Henderson JC, Waller LA, et al. A high-resolution genetic signature of demographic and spatial expansion in epizootic rabies virus. *Proc Natl Acad Sci U S A* 2007;104:7993–7998.
75. Blanton JD, Palmer D, Rupprecht CE. Rabies surveillance in the United States during 2009. *J Am Vet Med Assoc* 2010;237:646–657.
98. Brzozka K, Finke S, Conzelmann KK. Inhibition of interferon signaling by rabies virus phosphoprotein P: activation-dependent binding of STAT1 and STAT2. *J Virol* 2006;80:2675–2683.
104. Cancino J, Torrealba C, Soza A, et al. Antibody to AP1B adaptor blocks biosynthetic and recycling routes of basolateral proteins at recycling endosomes. *Mol Biol Cell* 2007;18:4872–4884.
106. Carpenter JA, Obbard DJ, Maside X, et al. The recent spread of a vertically transmitted virus through populations of Drosophila melanogaster. *Mol Ecol* 2007;16:3947–3954.
109. Cary ZD, Willingham MC, Lyles DS. Oncolytic vesicular stomatitis virus induces apoptosis in U87 glioblastoma cells by a type II death receptor mechanism and induces cell death and tumor clearance in vivo. *J Virol* 2011;85:5708–5717.
111. Centers for Disease Control and Prevention. Compendium of Animal Rabies Control, 2008; National Association of State Public Health Veterinarians. *MMWR Morb Mortal Wkly Rep* 2008;57(RR02):1–9.
113. Centers for Disease Control and Prevention. Presumptive abortive human rabies - Texas, 2009. *MMWR Morb Mortal Wkly Rep* 2010;59:185–190.
115. Chakraborty P, Seemann J, Mishra RK, et al. Vesicular stomatitis virus inhibits mitotic progression and triggers cell death. *EMBO Rep* 2009;10:1154–1160.

119. Chelbi-Alix MK, Vidy A, El Bougrini J, et al. Rabies viral mechanisms to escape the IFN system: the viral protein P interferes with IRF-3, Stat1, and PML nuclear bodies. *J Interferon Cytokine Res* 2006;26:271–280.
138. Coertse J, Weyer J, Nel LH, et al. Improved PCR methods for detection of African rabies and rabies-related lyssaviruses. *J Clin Microbiol* 2010;48:3949–3955.
144. Connor JH, McKenzie MO, Lyles DS. Role of residues 121 to 124 of vesicular stomatitis virus matrix protein in virus assembly and virus-host interaction. *J Virol* 2006;80:3701–3711.
145. Contamine D, Gaumer S. Sigma rhabdoviruses. In: Mahy BWJ, van Regenmortel MHV, eds. *Encyclopedia of Virology,* 3rd ed, Vol. 5. London: Elsevier; 2008:576–581.
147. Cooper D, Wright KJ, Calderon PC, et al. Attenuation of recombinant vesicular stomatitis virus-human immunodeficiency virus type 1 vaccine vectors by gene translocations and g gene truncation reduces neurovirulence and enhances immunogenicity in mice. *J Virol* 2008;82:207–219.
155. Cresawn KO, Potter BA, Oztan A, et al. Differential involvement of endocytic compartments in the biosynthetic traffic of apical proteins. *EMBO J* 2007;26:3737–3748.
157. Cureton DK, Massol RH, Saffarian S, et al. Vesicular stomatitis virus enters cells through vesicles incompletely coated with clathrin that depend upon actin for internalization. *PLoS Pathog* 2009;5:e1000394.
158. Cureton DK, Massol RH, Whelan SP, et al. The length of vesicular stomatitis virus particles dictates a need for actin assembly during clathrin-dependent endocytosis. *PLoS Pathog* 2010;6.
159. Dacheux L, Larrous F, Mailles A, et al. European bat Lyssavirus transmission among cats, Europe. *Emerg Infect Dis* 2009;15:280–284.
160. Dancho B, McKenzie MO, Connor JH, et al. Vesicular stomatitis virus matrix protein mutations that affect association with host membranes and viral nucleocapsids. *J Biol Chem* 2009;284:4500–4509.
162. Das SC, Panda D, Nayak D, et al. Biarsenical labeling of vesicular stomatitis virus encoding tetracysteine-tagged m protein allows dynamic imaging of M protein and virus uncoating in infected cells. *J Virol* 2009; 83:2611–2622.
165. David D, Hughes GJ, Yakobson BA, et al. Identification of novel canine rabies virus clades in the Middle East and North Africa. *J Gen Virol* 2007;88:967–980.
173. Delmas O, Holmes EC, Talbi C, et al. Genomic diversity and evolution of the lyssaviruses. *PLoS One* 2008;3:e2057.
174. Departamento de Vigilancia Epidemiologica. Protocolo para Tratamento de Raiva Humana no Brasil. *Epidemiol Serv Saude, Brasilia* 2009;18: 385–394.
177. Dietzgen RG, Calisher CH, Kurath G, et al. Family Rhabdoviridae. In: King AMQ, Adams MJ, Carstens EB, et al., eds. *Virus Taxonomy: Ninth Report of the International Committee on Taxonomy of Viruses.* London: Elsevier; 2011:686.
184. Ding H, Green TJ, Lu S, et al. Crystal structure of the oligomerization domain of the phosphoprotein of vesicular stomatitis virus. *J Virol* 2006;80:2808–2814.
214. Faul EJ, Aye PP, Papaneri AB, et al. Rabies virus-based vaccines elicit neutralizing antibodies, poly-functional CD8+ T cell, and protect rhesus macaques from AIDS-like disease after SIV(mac251) challenge. *Vaccine* 2009;28:299–308.
216. Fehlner-Gardiner C, Nadin-Davis S, Armstrong J, et al. Era vaccine-derived cases of rabies in wildlife and domestic animals in Ontario, Canada, 1989–2004. *J Wildl Dis* 2008;44:71–85.
252. Gaddy DF, Lyles DS. Oncolytic vesicular stomatitis virus induces apoptosis via signaling through PKR, Fas, and Daxx. *J Virol* 2007;81: 2792–2804.
254. Galloway SE, Richardson PE, Wertz GW. Analysis of a structural homology model of the 2′-O-ribose methyltransferase domain within the vesicular stomatitis virus L protein. *Virology* 2008;382:69–82.
255. Galloway SE, Wertz GW. S-adenosyl homocysteine-induced hyperpolyadenylation of vesicular stomatitis virus mRNA requires the methyltransferase activity of L protein. *J Virol* 2008;82:12280–12290.
264. Ge P, Tsao J, Schein S, et al. Cryo-EM model of the bullet-shaped vesicular stomatitis virus. *Science* 2010;327:689–693.
266. Georgel P, Jiang Z, Kunz S, et al. Vesicular stomatitis virus glycoprotein G activates a specific antiviral Toll-like receptor 4-dependent pathway. *Virology* 2007;362:304–313.
267. Gerard FC, Ribeiro Ede A Jr, Albertini AA, et al. Unphosphorylated rhabdoviridae phosphoproteins form elongated dimers in solution. *Biochemistry* 2007;46:10328–10338.
268. Gerard FC, Ribeiro Ede A Jr, Leyrat C, et al. Modular organization of rabies virus phosphoprotein. *J Mol Biol* 2009;388:978–996.
269. Gholami A, Kassis R, Real E, et al. Mitochondrial dysfunction in lyssavirus-induced apoptosis. *J Virol* 2008;82:4774–4784.
274. Graham SC, Assenberg R, Delmas O, et al. Rhabdovirus matrix protein structures reveal a novel mode of self-association. *PLoS Pathog* 2008; 4:e1000251.
276. Green TJ, Luo M. Structure of the vesicular stomatitis virus nucleocapsid in complex with the nucleocapsid-binding domain of the small polymerase cofactor, P. *Proc Natl Acad Sci U S A* 2009;106:11713–11718.
278. Green TJ, Rowse M, Tsao J, et al. Access to RNA encapsidated in the nucleocapsid of vesicular stomatitis virus. *J Virol* 2011;85:2714–2722.
279. Green TJ, Zhang X, Wertz GW, et al. Structure of the vesicular stomatitis virus nucleoprotein-RNA complex. *Science* 2006;313:357–360.
283. Gubala A, Davis S, Weir R, et al. Ngaingan virus, a macropod-associated rhabdovirus, contains a second glycoprotein gene and seven novel open reading frames. *Virology* 2010;399:98–108.
284. Gubala AJ, Proll DF, Barnard RT, et al. Genomic characterisation of Wongabel virus reveals novel genes within the Rhabdoviridae. *Virology* 2008;376:13–23.
305. Heldwein EE, Lou H, Bender FC, et al. Crystal structure of glycoprotein B from herpes simplex virus 1. *Science* 2006;313:217–220.
322. Hornung V, Ellegast J, Kim S, et al. 5′-Triphosphate RNA is the ligand for RIG-I. *Science* 2006;314:994–997.
330. Iannacone M, Moseman EA, Tonti E, et al. Subcapsular sinus macrophages prevent CNS invasion on peripheral infection with a neurotropic virus. *Nature* 2010;465:1079–1083.
334. Ito N, Moseley GW, Blondel D, et al. Role of interferon antagonist activity of rabies virus phosphoprotein in viral pathogenicity. *J Virol* 2010; 84:6699–6710.
338. Jackson AC. Why does the prognosis remain so poor in human rabies? *Expert Rev Anti Infect Ther* 2010;8:623–625.
341. Jackson AC, Rossiter JP, Lafon M. Expression of Toll-like receptor 3 in the human cerebellar cortex in rabies, herpes simplex encephalitis, and other neurological diseases. *J Neurovirol* 2006;12:229–234.
348. Johannsdottir HK, Mancini R, Kartenbeck J, et al. Host cell factors and functions involved in vesicular stomatitis virus entry. *J Virol* 2009; 83:440–453.
353. Johnson N, Mansfield KL, Marston DA, et al. A new outbreak of rabies in rare Ethiopian wolves (Canis simensis). *Arch Virol* 2010;155:1175–1177.
366. Kato H, Takeuchi O, Sato S, et al. Differential roles of MDA5 and RIG-I helicases in the recognition of RNA viruses. *Nature* 2006;441:101–105.
372. Kim WS, Oh MJ, Nishizawa T, et al. Genotyping of Korean isolates of infectious hematopoietic necrosis virus (IHNV) based on the glycoprotein gene. *Arch Virol* 2007;152:2119–2124.
397. Kurath G. Biotechnology and DNA vaccines for aquatic animals. *Rev Sci Tech* 2008;27:175–196.
401. Kuzmin IV, Hughes GJ, Rupprecht CE. Phylogenetic relationships of seven previously unclassified viruses within the family Rhabdoviridae using partial nucleoprotein gene sequences. *J Gen Virol* 2006;87: 2323–2331.
402. Kuzmin IV, Mayer AE, Niezgoda M, et al. Shimoni bat virus, a new representative of the Lyssavirus genus. *Virus Res* 2010;149:197–210.
403. Kuzmin IV, Niezgoda M, Franka R, et al. Lagos bat virus in Kenya. *J Clin Microbiol* 2008;46:1451–1461.
404. Kuzmin IV, Novella IS, Dietzgen RG, et al. The rhabdoviruses: biodiversity, phylogenetics, and evolution. *Infect Genet Evol* 2009;9:541–553.
406. Kuzmin IV, Rupprecht CE. Bat rabies. In: Jackson AC, Wunner WH, eds. *Rabies,* 2nd ed. London: Elsevier; 2007:259–307.
411. Lahaye X, Vidy A, Pomier C, et al. Functional characterization of Negri bodies (NBs) in rabies virus-infected cells: Evidence that NBs are sites of viral transcription and replication. *J Virol* 2009;83:7948–7958.
425. Lee HK, Lund JM, Ramanathan B, et al. Autophagy-dependent viral recognition by plasmacytoid dendritic cells. *Science* 2007;315:1398–1401.
429. Lembo T, Haydon DT, Velasco-Villa A, et al. Molecular epidemiology identifies only a single rabies virus variant circulating in complex carnivore communities of the Serengeti. *Proc Biol Sci* 2007;274:2123–2130.

433. Leslie MJ, Messenger S, Rohde RE, et al. Bat-associated rabies virus in Skunks. *Emerg Infect Dis* 2006;12:1274–1277.
434. Leyrat C, Ringkjobing Jensen M, Ribeiro EA Jr, et al. The N(0)-binding region of the vesicular stomatitis virus phosphoprotein is globally disordered but contains transient alpha-helices. *Protein Sci* 2011;20:452–456.
436. Li J, Rahmeh A, Brusic V, et al. Opposing effects of inhibiting cap addition and cap methylation on polyadenylation during vesicular stomatitis virus mRNA synthesis. *J Virol* 2009;83:1930–1940.
437. Li J, Rahmeh A, Morelli M, et al. A conserved motif in region v of the large polymerase proteins of nonsegmented negative-sense RNA viruses that is essential for mRNA capping. *J Virol* 2008;82:775–784.
438. Li J, Wang JT, Whelan SP. A unique strategy for mRNA cap methylation used by vesicular stomatitis virus. *Proc Natl Acad Sci U S A* 2006;103: 8493–8498.
447. Liu Y, Zhang S, Wu X, et al. Ferret badger rabies origin and its revisited importance as potential source of rabies transmission in Southeast China. *BMC Infect Dis* 2010;10:234.
451. Longdon B, Obbard DJ, Jiggins FM. Sigma viruses from three species of Drosophila form a major new clade in the rhabdovirus phylogeny. *Proc Biol Sci* 2010;277:35–44.
460. Luyet PP, Falguieres T, Pons V, et al. The ESCRT-I subunit TSG101 controls endosome-to-cytosol release of viral RNA. *Traffic* 2008;9: 2279–2290.
472. Markotter W, Kuzmin I, Rupprecht CE, et al. Isolation of Lagos bat virus from water mongoose. *Emerg Infect Dis* 2006;12:1913–1918.
473. Markotter W, Van Eeden C, Kuzmin IV, et al. Epidemiology and pathogenicity of African bat lyssaviruses. *Dev Biol (Basel)* 2008;131: 317–325.
475. Masatani T, Ito N, Shimizu K, et al. Amino acids at positions 273 and 394 in rabies virus nucleoprotein are important for both evasion of host RIG-I-mediated antiviral response and pathogenicity. *Virus Res* 2011;155:168–174.
493. Menager P, Roux P, Megret F, et al. Toll-like receptor 3 (TLR3) plays a major role in the formation of rabies virus Negri Bodies. *PLoS Pathog* 2009;5:e1000315.
497. Mire CE, Dube D, Delos SE, et al. Glycoprotein-dependent acidification of vesicular stomatitis virus enhances release of matrix protein. *J Virol* 2009;83:12139–12150.
498. Mire CE, White JM, Whitt MA. A spatio-temporal analysis of matrix protein and nucleocapsid trafficking during vesicular stomatitis virus uncoating. *PLoS Pathog* 2010;6:e1000994.
499. Mire CE, Whitt MA. The protease-sensitive loop of the vesicular stomatitis virus matrix protein is involved in virus assembly and protein translation. *Virology* 2011;416:16–25.
501. Moore SM, Hanlon CA. Rabies-specific antibodies: measuring surrogates of protection against a fatal disease. *PLoS Negl Trop Dis* 2010;4:e595.
504. Moseley GW, Filmer RP, DeJesus MA, et al. Nucleocytoplasmic distribution of rabies virus P-protein is regulated by phosphorylation adjacent to C-terminal nuclear import and export signals. *Biochemistry* 2007;46: 12053–12061.
508. Muller T, Batza HJ, Beckert A, et al. Analysis of vaccine-virus-associated rabies cases in red foxes (Vulpes vulpes) after oral rabies vaccination campaigns in Germany and Austria. *Arch Virol* 2009;154:1081–1091.
512. Nakhaei P, Genin P, Civas A, et al. RIG-I-like receptors: sensing and responding to RNA virus infection. *Semin Immunol* 2009;21:215–222.
521. Nishizawa T, Kinoshita S, Kim WS, et al. Nucleotide diversity of Japanese isolates of infectious hematopoietic necrosis virus (IHNV) based on the glycoprotein gene. *Dis Aquat Organ* 2006;71:267–272.
524. Novella IS, Ebendick-Corpus BE, Zarate S, et al. Emergence of mammalian cell-adapted vesicular stomatitis virus from persistent infections of insect vector cells. *J Virol* 2007;81:6664–6668.
530. Office International des Epizooties. Infectious haematopoietic necrosis. In: *Manual of Diagnostic Tests for Aquatic Animals 2010* [E-book]. Office International des Epizooties, 2010.
531. Office International des Epizooties. Viral haemorrhagic septicaemia. In: *Manual of Diagnostic Tests for Aquatic Animals 2010* [E-book]. Office International des Epizooties, 2010.
533. Ogino T, Banerjee AK. Unconventional mechanism of mRNA capping by the RNA-dependent RNA polymerase of vesicular stomatitis virus. *Mol Cell* 2007;25:85–97.
540. Padhi A, Verghese B. Detecting molecular adaptation at individual codons in the glycoprotein gene of the geographically diversified infectious hematopoietic necrosis virus, a fish rhabdovirus. *Virus Res* 2008; 132:229–236.
552. Paweska JT, Blumberg LH, Liebenberg C, et al. Fatal human infection with rabies-related Duvenhage virus, South Africa. *Emerg Infect Dis* 2006; 12:1965–1967.
553. Pearce AF, Lyles DS. Vesicular stomatitis virus induces apoptosis primarily through Bak rather than Bax by inactivating Mcl-1 and Bcl-XL. *J Virol* 2009;83:9102–9112.
570. Prehaud C, Wolff N, Terrien E, et al. Attenuation of rabies virulence: takeover by the cytoplasmic domain of its envelope protein. *Sci Signal* 2010;3:ra5.
575. Quan PL, Junglen S, Tashmukhamedova A, et al. Moussa virus: a new member of the Rhabdoviridae family isolated from Culex decens mosquitoes in Cote d'Ivoire. *Virus Res* 2010;147:17–24.
576. Rahmeh AA, Li J, Kranzusch PJ, et al. Ribose 2′-O methylation of the vesicular stomatitis virus mRNA cap precedes and facilitates subsequent guanine-N-7 methylation by the large polymerase protein. *J Virol* 2009;83:11043–11050.
577. Rahmeh AA, Schenk AD, Danek EI, et al. Molecular architecture of the vesicular stomatitis virus RNA polymerase. *Proc Natl Acad Sci U S A* 2010;107:20075–20080.
579. Randall RE, Goodbourn S. Interferons and viruses: an interplay between induction, signalling, antiviral responses and virus countermeasures. *J Gen Virol* 2008;89:1–47.
584. Rehwinkel J, Tan CP, Goubau D, et al. RIG-I detects viral genomic RNA during negative-strand RNA virus infection. *Cell* 2010;140:397–408.
588. Ribeiro EA Jr, Favier A, Gerard FC, et al. Solution structure of the C-terminal nucleoprotein-RNA binding domain of the vesicular stomatitis virus phosphoprotein. *J Mol Biol* 2008;382:525–538.
589. Rieder M, Brzozka K, Pfaller CK, et al. Genetic dissection of interferon-antagonistic functions of rabies virus phosphoprotein: inhibition of interferon regulatory factor 3 activation is important for pathogenicity. *J Virol* 2011;85:842–852.
595. Roche S, Bressanelli S, Rey FA, et al. Crystal structure of the low-pH form of the vesicular stomatitis virus glycoprotein G. *Science* 2006;313: 187–191.
596. Roche S, Rey FA, Gaudin Y, et al. Structure of the prefusion form of the vesicular stomatitis virus glycoprotein G. *Science* 2007;315:843–848.
616. Samuel S, Tumilasci VF, Oliere S, et al. VSV oncolysis in combination with the BCL-2 inhibitor obatoclax overcomes apoptosis resistance in chronic lymphocytic leukemia. *Mol Ther* 2010;18:2094–2103.
623. Schlee M, Roth A, Hornung V, et al. Recognition of 5′ triphosphate by RIG-I helicase requires short blunt double-stranded RNA as contained in panhandle of negative-strand virus. *Immunity* 2009;31:25–34.
633. Schnell MJ, McGettigan JP, Wirblich C, et al. The cell biology of rabies virus: using stealth to reach the brain. *Nat Rev Microbiol* 2010;8:51–61.
639. Servat A, Feyssaguet M, Blanchard I, et al. A quantitative indirect ELISA to monitor the effectiveness of rabies vaccination in domestic and wild carnivores. *J Immunol Methods* 2007;318:1–10.
644. Sharif-Askari E, Nakhaei P, Oliere S, et al. Bax-dependent mitochondrial membrane permeabilization enhances IRF3-mediated innate immune response during VSV infection. *Virology* 2007;365:20–33.
646. Shi Z, Cai Z, Sanchez A, et al. A novel Toll-like receptor that recognizes vesicular stomatitis virus. *J Biol Chem* 2011;286:4517–4524.
684. Sun X, Belouzard S, Whittaker GR. Molecular architecture of the bipartite fusion loops of vesicular stomatitis virus glycoprotein G, a class III viral fusion protein. *J Biol Chem* 2008;283:6418–6427.
688. Swinteck BD, Lyles DS. Plasma membrane microdomains containing vesicular stomatitis virus M protein are separate from microdomains containing G protein and nucleocapsids. *J Virol* 2008;82:5536–5547.
691. Takeuchi O, Akira S. Pattern recognition receptors and inflammation. *Cell* 2010;140:805–820.
694. Taylor GM, Hanson PI, Kielian M. Ubiquitin depletion and dominant-negative VPS4 inhibit rhabdovirus budding without affecting alphavirus budding. *J Virol* 2007;81:13631–13639.
711. Trottier MD, Lyles DS, Reiss CS. Peripheral, but not central nervous system, type I interferon expression in mice in response to intranasal vesicular stomatitis virus infection. *J Neurovirol* 2007;13:433–445.

716. U.S. Department of Health and Human Services. 2008. Minutes of the Recombinant DNA Advisory Committee 9/9–10/08. Recombinant DNA Advisory Committee, U.S. Department of Health and Human Services, Rockville, MD.
717. U.S. Department of Health and Human Services. 2008. Minutes of the Recombinant DNA Advisory Committee 12/3–4/2008. Recombinant DNA Advisory Committee, U.S. Department of Health and Human Services, Rockville, MD.
724. van Thiel PP, van den Hoek JA, Eftimov F, et al. Fatal case of human rabies (Duvenhage virus) from a bat in Kenya: The Netherlands, December 2007. *Euro Surveill* 2008;13:8007.
725. Van Zyl N, Markotter W, Nel LH. Evolutionary history of African mongoose rabies. *Virus Res* 2010;150:93–102.
729. Vidy A, El Bougrini J, Chelbi-Alix MK, et al. The nucleocytoplasmic rabies virus P protein counteracts interferon signaling by inhibiting both nuclear accumulation and DNA binding of STAT1. *J Virol* 2007;81:4255–4263.
734. Waibler Z, Detje CN, Bell JC, et al. Matrix protein mediated shutdown of host cell metabolism limits vesicular stomatitis virus-induced interferon-alpha responses to plasmacytoid dendritic cells. *Immunobiology* 2007;212:887–894.
741. Wang JT, McElvain LE, Whelan SP. Vesicular stomatitis virus mRNA capping machinery requires specific cis-acting signals in the RNA. *J Virol* 2007;81:11499–11506.
753. Welch RJ, Anderson BL, Litwin CM. An evaluation of two commercially available ELISAs and one in-house reference laboratory ELISA for the determination of human anti-rabies virus antibodies. *J Med Microbiol* 2009;58:806–810.
763. Whitlow ZW, Connor JH, Lyles DS. New mRNAs are preferentially translated during vesicular stomatitis virus infection. *J Virol* 2008;82: 2286–2294.
764. Whitlow ZW, Connor JH, Lyles DS. Preferential translation of vesicular stomatitis virus mRNAs is conferred by transcription from the viral genome. *J Virol* 2006;80:11733–11742.
785. Wirblich C, Tan GS, Papaneri A, et al. PPEY motif within the rabies virus (RV) matrix protein is essential for efficient virion release and RV pathogenicity. *J Virol* 2008;82:9730–9738.
787. Wong RW, Blobel G, Coutavas E. Rae1 interaction with NuMA is required for bipolar spindle formation. *Proc Natl Acad Sci U S A* 2006; 103:19783–19787.
791. Wright E, McNabb S, Goddard T, et al. A robust lentiviral pseudotype neutralisation assay for in-field serosurveillance of rabies and lyssaviruses in Africa. *Vaccine* 2009;27:7178–7186.
792. Wu X, Franka R, Svoboda P, et al. Development of combined vaccines for rabies and immunocontraception. *Vaccine* 2009;27:7202–7209.
809. Zhang S, Liu Y, Zhang F, et al. Competitive ELISA using a rabies glycoprotein-transformed cell line to semi-quantify rabies neutralizing-related antibodies in dogs. *Vaccine* 2009;27:2108–2113.
810. Zhang X, Green TJ, Tsao J, et al. Role of intermolecular interactions of vesicular stomatitis virus nucleoprotein in RNA encapsidation. *J Virol* 2008;82:674–682.

CHAPTER 32

Heinz Feldmann • Anthony Sanchez • Thomas W. Geisbert

Filoviridae: Marburg and Ebola Viruses

CLASSIFICATION

Taxonomy

Filoviruses are taxonomically classified within the order *Mononegavirales,* a large group of enveloped viruses whose genomes are composed of a nonsegmented, negative-strand (NNS) RNA molecule.[98] Following their discovery, filoviruses were initially grouped with rhabdoviruses, based primarily on the appearance of virus particles. However, subsequent morphologic, genetic, physiochemical, and virologic studies of Marburg virus (MARV) and Ebola virus (EBOV) isolates revealed unique properties and led to their placement into a separate family, the *Filoviridae.*[224] Further characterization of these agents demonstrated that EBOV and MARV represent divergent lineages of filoviruses; their differences were significant enough to warrant the formation of the genera *Marburgvirus* and *Ebolavirus.* According to the International Committee on Taxonomy of Viruses (ICTV) (http://www.ictvonline.org/virusTaxonomy.asp?version=2009&bhcp=1), the *Marburgvirus* genus contains a single species, *Lake Victoria marburgvirus,* because strains exhibit only limited genetic variation. However, the appearance of distinct MARV lineages may lead to further speciation.[401] There is a greater divergence within the *Ebolavirus* genus, five species having been recognized: *Zaire ebolavirus* (type species; ZEBOV), *Sudan ebolavirus* (SEBOV), *Reston ebolavirus* (REBOV), *Tai Forest ebolavirus* (formerly Ivory Coast or *Cote d'Ivoire ebolavirus,* ICEBOV or CIEBOV), *and Bundibugyo ebolavirus* (BEBOV), of which BEBOV has still to be approved.[403] A distinct filovirus sequence has recently been obtained from bats in Spain, but no virus has yet been isolated. This new "putative virus" (designated Lloviu virus) is proposed to represent the single species *Lloviu cuevavirus* in the new genus *Cuevavirus* of the *Filoviridae* family.[299]

Biosafety and Biosecurity

Because of their high mortality rate, their potential for person-to-person transmission, and a lack of an approved vaccine or antiviral therapy, MARV and EBOV are classified as biosafety level 4 (BSL-4; risk group 4) pathogens, for which maximum containment facilities are required when handling the infectious agent (http://www.cdc.gov/biosafety/publications/bmbl5/BMBL.pdf). Filovirus infectivity is quite stable at room temperature (20°C), but is largely inactivated in 30 minutes at 60°C; MARV is somewhat resistant to desiccation. Infectivity is greatly reduced or destroyed by high doses of ultraviolet light and gamma irradiation, lipid solvents, β-propiolactone, photo-induced alkylating probe 1,5-iodonaphthylazide, guanidinium isothiocyanate, and commercial hypochlorite and phenolic disinfectants.

The threat of bioterrorism in the aftermath of the September 11, 2001 and anthrax attacks against the United States has prompted governments to implement countermeasures. This has led to greater restrictions on the acquisition and use of a variety of agents that pose serious threats to public health. Filoviruses have been classified as Centers for Disease Control and Prevention (CDC) Category A Agents (http://www.bt.cdc.gov/agent/agentlist-category.asp#a), as part of a system for prioritizing initial public health preparedness efforts and grading the potential of agents for large-scale dissemination. Filoviruses are also classified as "select agents" by the CDC Select Agent Program. This program is mandated by federal law to regulate activities involving these agents within the United States and to register laboratories and entities handling one or more select agents (http://www.cdc.gov/od/sap/).

HISTORY

Table 32.1 lists the documented occurrences of MARV and EBOV disease, along with information regarding these outbreaks. Additional details of these episodes are described in the following sections.

TABLE 32.1 Outbreaks of Filovirus Disease

Filovirus (species)	Year	Outbreak location	Place of origin	Human cases (% mortality)
LVMARV	1967	Marburg/Frankfurt, Germany; Belgrade, Serbia	Uganda	32 (23)
	1975	Johannesburg, South Africa	Zimbabwe	3 (33)
	1980	Nzoia and Nairobi, Kenya	Western Kenya	2 (50)
	1987	Kisumu, Kenya	Western Kenya	1 (100)
	1998–2000	Durba/Watsa, DRC	DRC	154 (83)
	2004–2005	Uíge, Angola	Angola	252 (90)
	2007	Uganda (western)	Uganda	4 (25)
	2008	The Netherlands	Uganda	1 (100)
	2008	United States	Uganda	1 (0)
ZEBOV[a]	1976	Yambuku, DRC	DRC	318 (88)
	1977	Tandala, DRC	DRC	1 (100)
	1994	Ogooué-Invindo province, Gabon	Gabon	52 (60)
	1995	Kikwit, DRC	DRC	315 (79)
	1996	Mayibout, Gabon	Gabon	37 (57)
	1996	Booue, Gabon and Johannesburg, South Africa	Gabon	60 (75)[b]
	2001–2002	Ogooué-Invindo province, Gabon; Cuvette region, RC	Gabon?	124 (79)
	2002–2003	Cuvette region, RC; Ogooué-Invindo province, Gabon	RC?	143 (90)
	2003	Mboma and Mbandza, RC	RC	35 (83)
	2005	Etoumbi and Mbomo in Cuvette region, RC	RC	12 (75)
	2007	Kasai Occidental province, DRC	DRC	264 (71)
	2008–2009	Kasai Occidental province, DRC	DRC	32 (47)
SEBOV	1976	Nzara, Maridi, Tembura, Juba, Sudan	Southern Sudan	284 (53)
	1979	Nzara, Yambio, Sudan	Southern Sudan	34 (65)
	2000–2001	Gulu District, Mbarrara, and Masindi, Uganda	Uganda	425 (53)
	2004	Yambio County, Sudan	Southern Sudan	17 (41)
	2011	Uganda (central)	Uganda	1 (100)
BEBOV	2007	Bundibugyo district, Uganda	Uganda	149 (25)[c]
ICEBOV (CIEBOV)	1994	Tai Forest, Ivory Coast, and Basel, Switzerland	Ivory Coast	1 (0)
	1995	Liberia	Liberia?	1 (0)
REBOV	1989	Reston, Virginia (also Pennsylvania and Texas)	Philippines[d]	4 (0)
	1992	Siena, Italy	Philippines	0 (0)
	1996	Alice, Texas	Philippines	0 (0)
	2008	Philippines	Philippines	0 (0)

Note, in 2012, Uganda has reported two EHF and one MHF outbreak; another EHF outbreak was reported from DRC. The EHF outbreaks were caused by SEBOV and BEBOV. The border region between Uganda and DRC seems to be a new "hot spot" for filovirus HF. For more information, please see the CDC and WHO websites.

[a]From approximately 1998 to the present time, there have been partially confirmed reports of transmission of ZEBOV among great apes in Gabon and the Republic of Congo (RC), which has severely impacted gorilla and chimpanzee populations.

[b]Included an imported case in South Africa where an ill Gabonese physician (survivor) infected a nurse who died.

[c]Case fatality rate (CFR) was much higher if one considered only laboratory-confirmed cases.

[d]REBOV has only been traced to a single monkey-breeding facility in the city of Calamba, Philippines, which was depopulated in 1996 and is no longer in operation.

DRC, Democratic Republic of Congo; RC, The Republic of Congo.

Marburg Hemorrhagic Fever (MHF)

The first identified instance of filovirus disease occurred in 1967, when MARV caused severe cases of hemorrhagic fever in Europe.[274,275,276] The epidemic started in mid-August in Marburg, Germany with three laboratory workers who contracted the disease after processing organs from African green monkeys (*Cercopithecus aethiops*) imported from Uganda. Seventeen more patients were hospitalized and two medical personnel contracted the disease while attending to patients. The last patient, who apparently had been infected by her husband during the convalescent period, was admitted in November 1967.[276] Six cases (including two secondary infections) occurred in Frankfurt, Germany concomitant with the Marburg infections.[372] In September, two cases were identified in Belgrade, former Yugoslavia, in which a veterinarian was infected while performing a necropsy on a dead monkey and transmitted the virus to his wife, who nursed him early in his illness.[276] A total of 31 cases (including six secondary infections) were identified, with seven fatalities in primary infections (23%). Subsequent serologic investigations have suggested that there was one additional primary case in Marburg.[370]

MHF remained an obscure medical curiosity until 1975, when three cases were reported in Johannesburg, South Africa.[122] The index case was a white male who just prior to his infection had traveled in Zimbabwe. Seven days after onset, his travel companion also became ill and transmitted the disease to an attending nurse; the index case was the only fatality. An investigation was conducted along the travel route of the index case, but the source of the virus was not determined.[66] Two further episodes of MHF were reported from Kenya in 1980 and 1987. The index case in 1980 became ill in western Kenya and died in Nairobi, where an attending physician was infected but survived the disease.[371] In 1987, a fatal case occurred in the same region of western Kenya.[218] The 1980 and 1987 index cases both traveled to the Mt. Elgon region, which is located close to Lake Victoria and was the source of the monkeys that initiated the original 1967 outbreak (trapped near Lake Kyogo, Uganda).

The first outbreak of MHF in a community setting of central Africa started in October 1998 in Durba/Watsa, located in the northeastern region of the Democratic Republic of Congo (DRC). Its remote location and the hazards of an ongoing armed conflict hampered efforts to study this outbreak, but an investigation was initiated after the death of an attending physician in 1999. Sporadic cases continued and were directly or indirectly linked to activity in the vicinity of an underground gold mine. Primary cases were mainly gold miners who started multiple, usually short chains of human-to-human transmission within their families. Overall, 154 cases were reported with a case fatality rate (CFR) of 83%. Analysis of viral sequences derived from clinical specimens and virus isolates showed nucleotide diversity up to approximately 20%.[22,23,65,400,401] The largest outbreak of MHF (252 cases with 227 deaths; CFR of 90%) took place in northern Angola, Uige province. The first cases date back to October/November 2004, but initial diagnostic tests were negative for filoviruses. The main outbreak started in February/March 2005 and the last confirmed case died in July. Initial infections were linked to a Uige hospital and included a high number of pediatric cases. Sequence analysis of virus isolates suggested a single introduction into the community.[151,211,401] The latest MHF episode dates to 2007, with four documented cases associated with a single mine in western Uganda.[400] In addition, two imported cases were reported from the United States (nonlethal) and the Netherlands (lethal), who independently visited the same cave in Uganda in 2008.[6,396]

Ebola Hemorrhagic Fever (EHF)

EHF was first reported in 1976, when EBOV appeared simultaneously in the DRC (at that time Zaire) and Sudan with 318 (CFR of 88%) and 284 cases (CFR of 53%), respectively. These epidemics were determined to have been caused by two distinct species (ZEBOV and SEBOV), a fact not recognized until years later. Viruses were isolated from patients of both outbreaks and named after a small river in northwestern DRC.[36,449,450]

No index case was clearly identified in the Sudan outbreak in 1976, although initial cases originating in Nzara, Sudan, involved six cotton factory workers and their close relatives. The epidemic was augmented by the spread of cases to neighboring areas (Maridi, Tembura, and Juba). High levels of transmission occurred in the hospital of Maridi (a teaching center for student nurses), primarily through the use of contaminated needles and a lack of barrier nursing practices. At the same time, a larger outbreak in the DRC, centered around a Belgian mission hospital in Yambuku, Equateur Region, was being fueled by similar circumstances. During a 7-week period of the outbreak, the single most significant factor in the spread of infection in the hospital was the reuse of contaminated syringes and needles, although secondary transmission to family members caused 45% of all recorded infections. The outbreak ended with closure of the hospital and quarantining of infected patients.

In 1977, a single fatal ZEBOV case was reported from Tandala, DRC, about 325 km from the original focus of the 1976 Yambuku outbreak.[179] SEBOV reemerged in 1979 in Nzara and Yambio, Sudan. The index case worked in the same textile factory cited as the potential source of infection in the 1976 Sudan outbreak. Hospitalization of the patient led to four nosocomial infections and further transmission to five families (34 cases with 22 fatalities).[451]

No further cases of EHF were reported until 1994, when a novel EBOV (ICEBOV [CIEBOV]) was isolated from an ethnologist who had become ill while working in the Tai Forest reserve of Ivory Coast. The infection was determined to have occurred while performing a necropsy on a dead chimpanzee (whose troop had lost several members to EHF).[114,243] Later, a single seroconversion suggested a second nonfatal human case in nearby Liberia. This episode extended the geographic distribution of known EBOV cases to include most of the African rain forest and was the first case in West Africa.

In 1995, a strain of ZEBOV very similar to the original 1976 virus reemerged in the DRC, causing a large hospital and community outbreak of EHF in and around Kikwit.[223,453] The presumed index case was a charcoal worker, but transmission escalated following two consecutive laparotomies performed on an infected male laboratory worker at Kikwit General Hospital. About three-quarters of the first 70 patients within the subsequent developing epidemic were health care workers. In total, there were 315 cases and 250 deaths (CFR of 81%). Major risk factors for contracting disease were involvement in patient care in hospitals and households and preparations of bodies for burial.

Beginning in 1994, ZEBOV became active in or adjacent to the central African rain forest on both sites of the border between Gabon and the Republic of Congo (RC).[5,148] Almost all outbreaks in this region described in this section were associated with hunting and butchering of wildlife, often great apes. The first epidemic was reported in 1994 from the Ogooué-Ivindo Province in northeast Gabon with a total of 52 cases (CFR of 60%).[147] In 1996, two more outbreaks were reported from the same province.[147] The first epidemic started in early February and included 37 cases (CFR of 57%); the second episode began in July/August and resulted in 60 cases (CFR of 75%). The latter epidemic included an imported case in South Africa where an ill Gabonese physician infected a nurse who died with EHF (2 cases; CFR of 50%). The first reported epidemic that crossed the border into the RC began in late November of 2001 with the index case again reported from Ogooué-Ivindo Province in northeast Gabon. The epidemic spread to Mekambo and Makokou and from there into the RC by ill Gabonese who sought medical care by traditional healers. In total, there were 65 (CFR of 82%) and 59 (75%) cases from Gabon and the RC, respectively.[251] The next occurrence of EHF was a large epidemic reported from the districts of Mbomo and Kelle in Cuvette Ouest Region, RC, in late 2002 to May 2003 with 143 cases (CFR of 90%), followed in late 2003 by a smaller episode in the district of Mbomo with 35 cases (CFR of 83%).[115] A neighboring area (Etoumbi) was affected in 2005 by a small outbreak of EHF with 12 cases (CFR of 75%) (http://www.who.int/csr/don/2005_06_16/en/index.html) (Table 32.1). This has so far been the last reported outbreak in this region.

In 2000 to 2001, the largest known epidemic of filovirus disease occurred in Uganda, with 425 cases and 224 deaths. The causative agent was closely related to SEBOV from the Sudan 1976 and 1979 outbreaks, and marked the first appearance of EBOV in Uganda. The CFR of 53% was in line with the generally lower mortality associated with the SEBOV species.[454] The epidemic was mainly concentrated in the Gulu district, a savannah area located in the north of the country close to the Sudanese border, with person-to-person transmission including nosocomial infections. The index case was never identified. During the epidemic, the virus spread to the neighboring Masindi district and more distantly to the town of Mbarara in southwestern Uganda.[31] During this outbreak a high number of health care workers were infected after barrier nursing procedures were instituted. It was also the first time that laboratory diagnostics were performed in the field to assist in outbreak management.[454] In 2004, southern Sudan was again affected by a small SEBOV outbreak with 17 cases, of which 7 died (CFR of 41%).[455] The index case had butchered a monkey and human-to-human transmission was mainly by contact.

The last reported ZEBOV outbreaks occurred in the Kasai Occidental province of the DRC in 2007 and 2008/09. The first larger outbreak included 264 reported cases with a CFR of 71%[457]; the second smaller outbreak had 32 cases, of which 15 died (CFR of 47%).[458] Both outbreaks affected rural communities in the vicinity of the city of Luebo and are thought to be related to hunting and handling of migratory fruit bats.[248]

A new EBOV species, designated *Bundibugyo ebolavirus* (BEBOV), has been identified as the causative agent for an outbreak that occurred in the Bundibugyo district in western Uganda in 2007.[403,423] In total, there were 149 reported cases, with 37 deaths (CFR of 25%); of these, 56 cases were laboratory confirmed. This single outbreak had the lowest reported CFR among all EBOV that have caused outbreaks in central Africa so far.

Most recently, a single case of SEBOV has been reported from Central Uganda.[7] No further cases have been reported.

EHF in Nonhuman Primates

In November 1989, an EBOV with low or no apparent pathogenicity for humans was recognized in a shipment of cynomolgus monkeys (*Macaca fascicularis*) housed at a quarantine facility in Reston, Virginia. These monkeys were imported from a single supplier in the Philippines, and an unusually high mortality was observed in animals during transportation and quarantine. Simian hemorrhagic fever virus was also circulating in the facility; efforts to culture this virus led to the detection of a new species of EBOV that was named *Reston ebolavirus* (REBOV).[72,203] The actual origin of this novel EBOV was never determined. Resumption of importation of monkeys led to new outbreaks of monkey disease in the United States in 1990 and 1996[336] and in Italy in 1992.[452] Subsequent investigations have traced all shipments except one to a single supplier in the Philippines. The mode of contamination of this exporter's holding compound has never been ascertained, but whether the virus persisted in the facility or was reintroduced from wild-caught animals, the result was a continued movement of infected macaques. A few infected handlers were also identified by serologic methods without reports of severe illness or suspicious deaths among this cohort.[285] Improved shipping, housing, and quarantine regulations regarding importation of monkeys have been implemented to protect the United States from future episodes of EBOV introductions.[74] Recently, REBOV emerged in pigs in the Philippines.[14] The pigs were co-infected with porcine respiratory and reproductive virus (PRRS) and the actual pathogenic potential of REBOV in pigs remains unclear. This discovery certainly raises issues for food production. Six workers from pig farms and slaughterhouses developed antibodies to REBOV, indicating that they became infected but did not develop disease. The potential for REBOV as a human pathogen remains unanswered but should not be totally dismissed. As of yet, REBOV infections/exposures have never resulted in clinical disease in humans.

Note, in 2012, Uganda has reported two EHF and one MHF outbreak; another EHF outbreak was reported from DRC. The EHF outbreaks were caused by SEBOV and BEBOV. The border region between Uganda and DRC seems to be the new "hot spot" for filovirus infections. For more information, please see the CDC and WHO websites.

Laboratory Infections/Exposures

A single laboratory infection of EHF occurred in the United Kingdom in 1976. Treatment with human leukocyte interferon and human convalescent plasma was initiated and the patient survived.[87] In the past two decades there have been at least three laboratory infections with MARV (1 fatal) in Russia.[282] In 2004, accidental ZEBOV exposures via needlesticks while working with animals occurred in the United States and Russia, but only the latter became infected (fatally).[196,233] In 2009, a German researcher had an accidental ZEBOV exposure via needlestick while working with animals. The person was treated with a recombinant vesicular stomatitis virus (VSV)–based vaccine expressing the ZEBOV glycoprotein. It could not be determined if the exposure resulted in infection.[158]

VIRION STRUCTURE

Initial electron microscopic (EM) observations of filoviruses revealed distinctive bacilliform to filamentous virus particles; it was this highly characteristic morphology that inspired their name (Latin filum, *thread*).[294,316] The virions of MARV and EBOV produced in tissue culture are pleomorphic, appearing as either U-shaped, 6-shaped, or circular (torus) configurations, or as elongated filamentous forms of varying length (up to 14,000 nm), all from the same culture fluid (Figs. 32.1A–C). The filamentous forms can also be seen to form branched structures (Fig. 32.1C, *arrow*). The unit length associated with peak infectivity for MARV and EBOV was measured to be 860 and 1,200 nm, respectively.[139] Virions have a uniform diameter of 80 nm, contain a helical ribonucleoprotein complex or nucleocapsid (NC) roughly 50 nm in diameter (Figs. 32.1 and 32.2), and have a central axial space (~20 nm in diameter) running the length of the particle. The NC has a helical periodicity of ~5 nm (Fig. 32.1G), and is surrounded by a matrix protein and a closely apposed outer envelope derived from the host-cell plasma membrane. The virion surface is studded with membrane-anchored peplomers projecting ~10 nm from the surface (Figs. 32.1E and 32.1F). Virions can often appear ragged or "moth-eaten" (Fig. 32.1D) (especially late in the infection). The density of virions has been determined to be 1.14 g/mL by centrifugation in a potassium tartrate gradient.

GENOME STRUCTURE AND ORGANIZATION

The single-stranded, negative-sense RNA molecule that makes up a filovirus genome constitutes ~1% of the virion mass.[330] The genomes of filoviruses are very similar in their organization, which generally conform to those of paramyxoviruses and rhabdoviruses, but their complexity is more akin to those of paramyxoviruses. Filovirus genomes are approximately 19,000 bases in length, making them the largest in the order *Mononegavirales* (Fig. 32.2), and contain seven sequentially arranged genes in the order nucleoprotein (NP)–viron protein (VP) 35–VP40—glycoprotein (GP)–VP30–VP24—polymerase (L). Genes are delineated by conserved transcriptional signals, and begin close to the 3′ end of the genomic sequence with a start site and end with a stop (polyadenylation) site. For rhabdo- and paramyxoviruses, genes are usually separated by short intergenic regions of one or more nucleotides, which are also seen in filovirus genomes. An unusual feature of all filovirus genomes is the presence of gene overlaps, which have been identified in the genomes of some paramyxo- and rhabdoviruses, but do not resemble those of filoviruses. As seen in Figure 32.2, the stop site of an upstream (3′) gene overlaps the start of the downstream gene, and overlapping sequences are limited to the conserved transcriptional signals and are centered on a 3′-UAAUU pentanucleotide sequence common to start and stop sites.[49,98,103,157,192,347] There is one overlap in the MARV genome (VP30–VP24), but the characterized EBOV genomes contain at least two overlaps (VP35–VP40, GP–VP30, and VP24–L; REBOV lacks the GP–VP30 overlap). Intergenic regions of filovirus genomes are generally short, although all genomes have a single lengthy sequence (>120 bases) separating the GP and VP30 genes of MARV and the VP30 and VP24 genes of EBOV. The positioning of the MARV overlap and a long intergenic region (that precedes the VP30 gene) appears to be shifted one gene (in the 3′ direction) with respect to the genome of the EBOV. The significance of this arrangement and how it may have been generated are unknown. The extragenic sequences at the 3′ end of all filovirus genomes (leader) are short, ranging in length from 50 to 70 bases, while the length of the 5′ end (trailer) sequences are variable. The extreme 3′ and 5′ ends of the filovirus genomes are conserved, show a high degree of complementarity, and potentially form stem-loop structures.[67,290,352,414] Filovirus trailer sequences are more variable in length, the longest being that of ZEBOV (677 bases), followed by BEBOV (475 bases), ICEBOV (474 bases), SEBOV (381 bases), MARV (76–95 bases), and REBOV (25 bases).

The evolutionary profile of the family *Filoviridae* (Fig. 32.3) indicates that EBOV and MARV represent distinct filovirus lineages, the five species of EBOV also represent distinct lineages, and there is an extraordinary level of genetic stasis within the lineages of EBOV. Nucleotide and amino acid differences between MARV and EBOV are both approximately 55%, whereas EBOV species show 32% to 41% differences in nucleotide and amino acid sequences.[98,353,400] These same levels of sequence variation are also seen when other genes are compared. Within species of EBOV, however, there is a remarkable degree of genetic stability, indicating that these viruses have most likely reached a high degree of fitness as they have adapted to their respective niches. MARV isolates have not shown the degree of variation seen among EBOV species, but two lineages of MARV have been described that are genetically distinct by more than 20% genetic diversity.[98,354,400]

VIRUS PROTEINS

Filovirus structural proteins can be subdivided into two categories, those that form the NC and those that are associated with the envelope (Fig. 32.2 and Table 32.2). The NC-associated proteins are involved in the transcription and replication of the genome, whereas the envelope-associated proteins have a role in either the assembly of the virion or virus entry. Shown in Figure 32.4 are the characteristic migration patterns of purified filovirus proteins separated by SDS-PAGE.

Nucleoproteins

The NP and VP30 proteins of filoviruses are the major and minor nucleoproteins, respectively, are phosphorylated, and interact strongly with the genomic RNA molecule to form the viral NC (along with VP35 and L).[27,261] Expression of recombinant NP alone in mammalian cells results in the formation of inclusions and nonspecific association with cellular RNA to form helical structures.[306,435] Analysis of NP amino acid sequences has identified a conserved, hydrophobic N-terminal half that contains all the cysteine residues, and a divergent, hydrophilic C-terminal half that contains most of the proline residues and is extremely acidic.[348,349] The N-terminal 450 amino acids of the ZEBOV NP have been linked with self-assembly of NP into tube-like structures that may function as a platform for NC formation.[435] Predicted mass values for NP molecules are approximately 20 kd smaller than estimated sizes derived from SDS-PAGE migration, possibly as a result of reduced binding of SDS molecules to the negatively charged NP. This hypothesis is supported by a study of recombinant

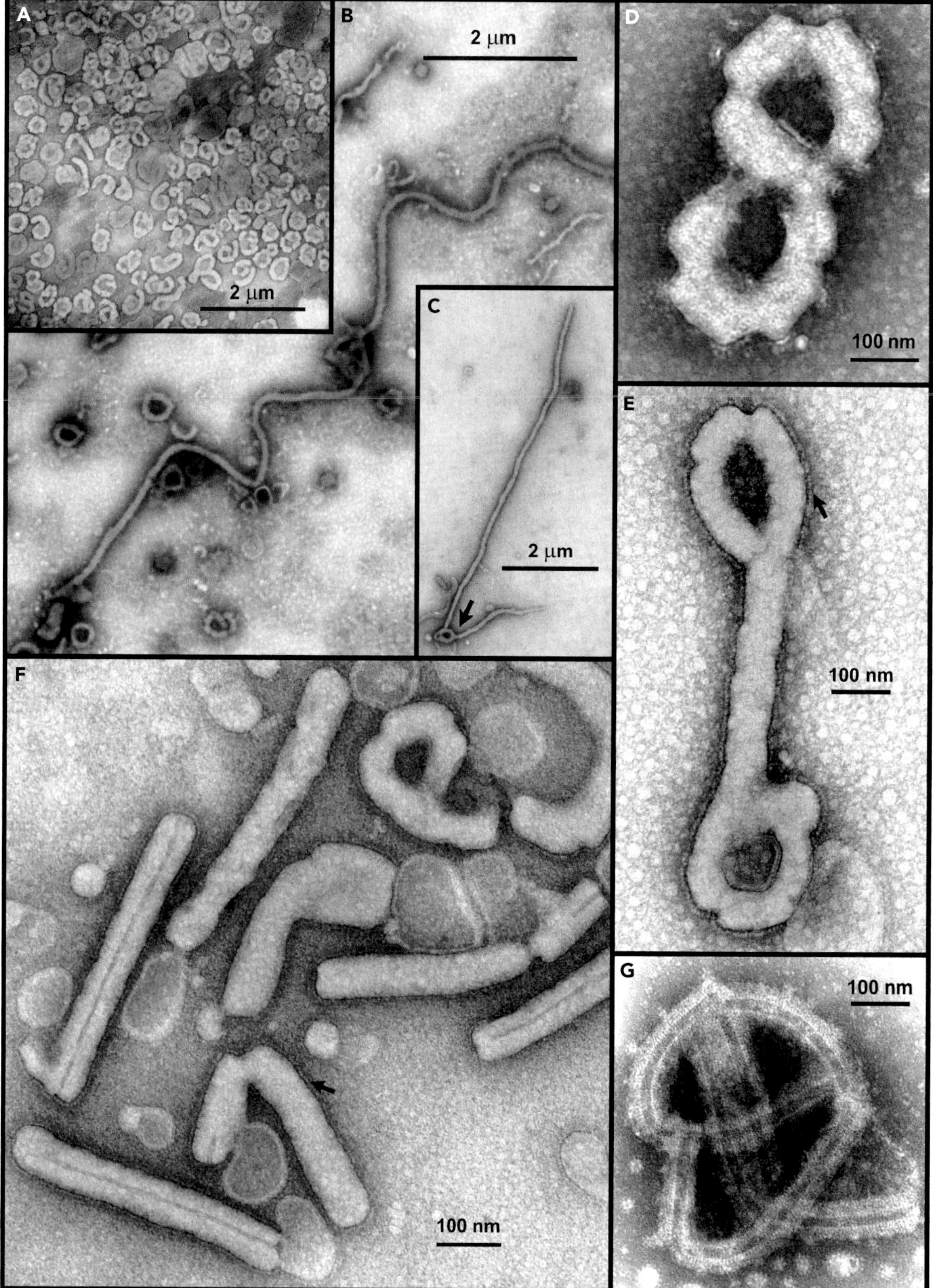

FIGURE 32.1. Transmission electron microscopy (negative stains) of filovirus virions (A–F) and nucleocapsids (G) derived from the culture medium of infected Vero E6 cells. Shown are low magnifications of MARV (strain Angola 2005) **(A)**, SEBOV (strain Yambio 2004) **(B)**, and MARV (strain Yambio 2005) **(C)**, and higher magnification images of ZEBOV (strain Mayinga 1976) **(D, E)**, MARV (strain Ravn 1987) **(F)**, and SEBOV (strain Yambio 2004) **(G)**. *Arrows* indicate a branch point in a filamentous particle (C) and peplomers on the surface of virions **(E, F)**. (Courtesy of A. Sanchez and C. Humphrey, Centers for Disease Control and Prevention, Atlanta, GA.)

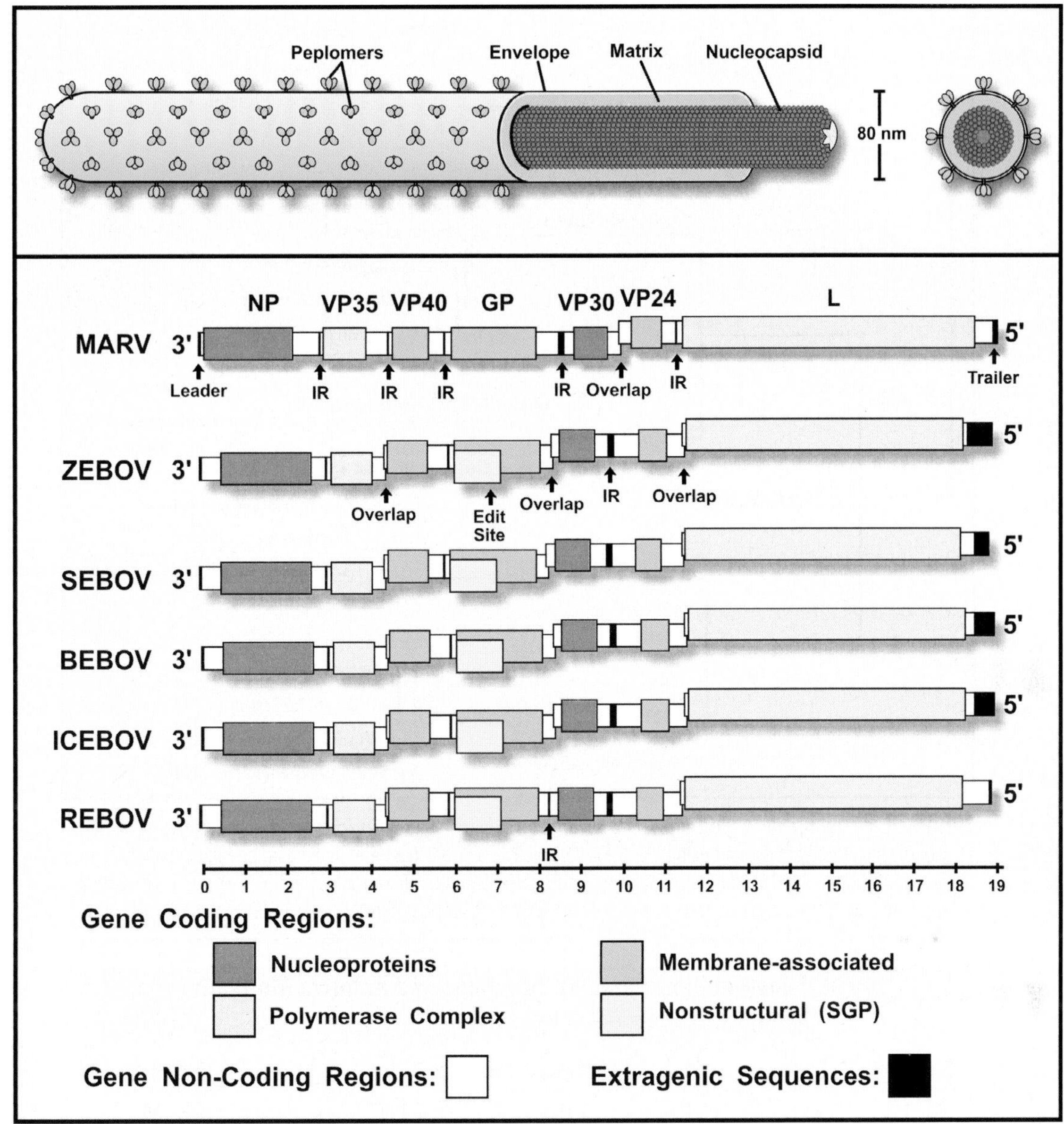

FIGURE 32.2. Schematic representation of a filovirus particle (*top*) and the organization of filovirus genomes (*bottom*).

ZEBOV NP[363] that mapped this property to two C-terminal domains (aa 439–492 and 589–739). In the central region of the NPs of filoviruses is a highly conserved region that shows some homology with nucleoprotein sequences of paramyxoviruses, and to a lesser extent rhabdoviruses, and likely has a similar structure and function.[183,349]

The VP30 protein of ZEBOV is also capable of binding RNA, particularly a stem-loop structure located near the leader sequence; this property mapped to residues 26 to 40 that is arginine rich.[214] This region may have an additional role of binding to the acidic C-terminal half of NP. VP30 contains a zinc-finger motif ~70 to 80 residues from the N-terminus that is highly conserved in filoviruses (consensus = $CX_8CX_4CX_3H X_2D/E$),[286] and RNA binding activity is increased by Zn^{2+}.[214] Immediately C-terminal to this sequence (separated by six residues) is a conserved tetraleucine sequence linked to co-translational homo-oligomerization of VP30.[168] Additional studies have shown that the C-terminal half of VP30 also contains a homo-oligomerization domain and that hexamerization occurs via an N-terminal domain.[169] A functional study of recombinant ZEBOV VP30 has revealed that it behaves as a transcription activator[169,440] regulated by its phosphorylation state,[287] but this property appears to be absent from the VP30 of MARV.[289] The ZEBOV VP30 also interacts with L; a role of bridging NP and L in the NC complex has been postulated.[154] Recently, the ZEBOV VP30 (along with VP35 and VP40) has been implicated in suppressing antiviral immunity through its antagonistic effect on the host cellular RNA interference (RNAi) pathway.[91]

Polymerase Complex Proteins

The L and VP35 proteins form the polymerase complex, which transcribes and replicates the filovirus genome. The

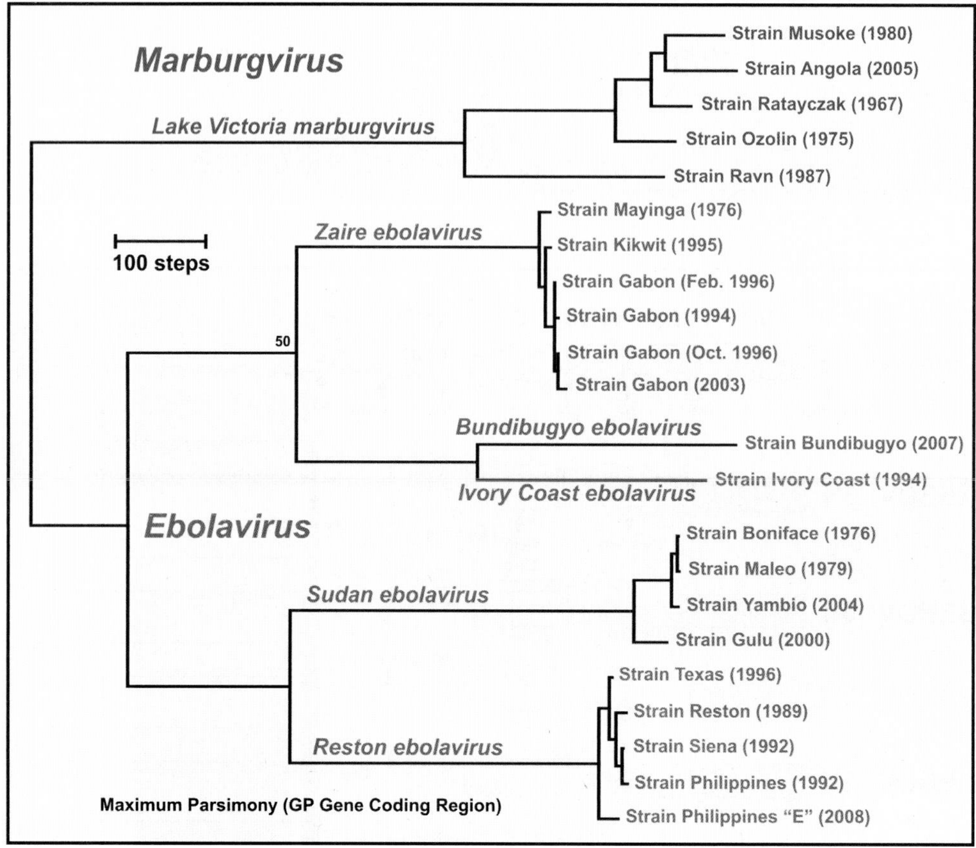

FIGURE 32.3. Phylogeny of the family *Filoviridae.* Nucleotide sequences for the GP gene coding region (ORF) of filovirus isolates were aligned using Clustal X version 2.0, and phylogenetic (maximum parsimony) analysis was performed using the MEGA5 computer program. Sequences were obtained from GenBank. The tree represents the most parsimonious tree, and confidence values at branch points were generated from 1,000 bootstrap replicates.

TABLE 32.2 Filovirus Genes and the Functions and Relative Molecular Weights of Their Gene Products

Gene order	Gene	Protein function	MW (kd)[a]
1	Nucleoprotein (NP)	Major nucleoprotein; RNA encapsidation	90–104
2	Virion protein (VP) 35	Polymerase complex cofactor; interferon antagonist	35
3	VP40	Matrix protein; virion assembly and budding; interferon antagonist[e]	35–40
4	Glycoprotein (GP)	Virus entry (surface peplomer); receptor binding and membrane fusion	150–170[b]
	Soluble glycoprotein (sGP)	unknown	50–55[c]
	Small soluble glycoprotein (ssGP)	unknown	50–55[c]
5	VP30	Minor nucleoprotein; RNA encapsidation and transcription activation	27–30
6	VP24	Minor matrix protein; virion assembly; interferon antagonist[d]	24–25
7	Polymerase (L)	RNA-dependent RNA polymerase; enzymatic component of polymerase complex	~270

[a]Molecular weights (MW) are approximated and based on SDS-PAGE migration.

[b]MW is for the monomeric heterodimer.

[c]Expressed only by EBOV; MW is for the monomeric form.

[d]Only shown for EBOV.

[e]Only shown for MARV.

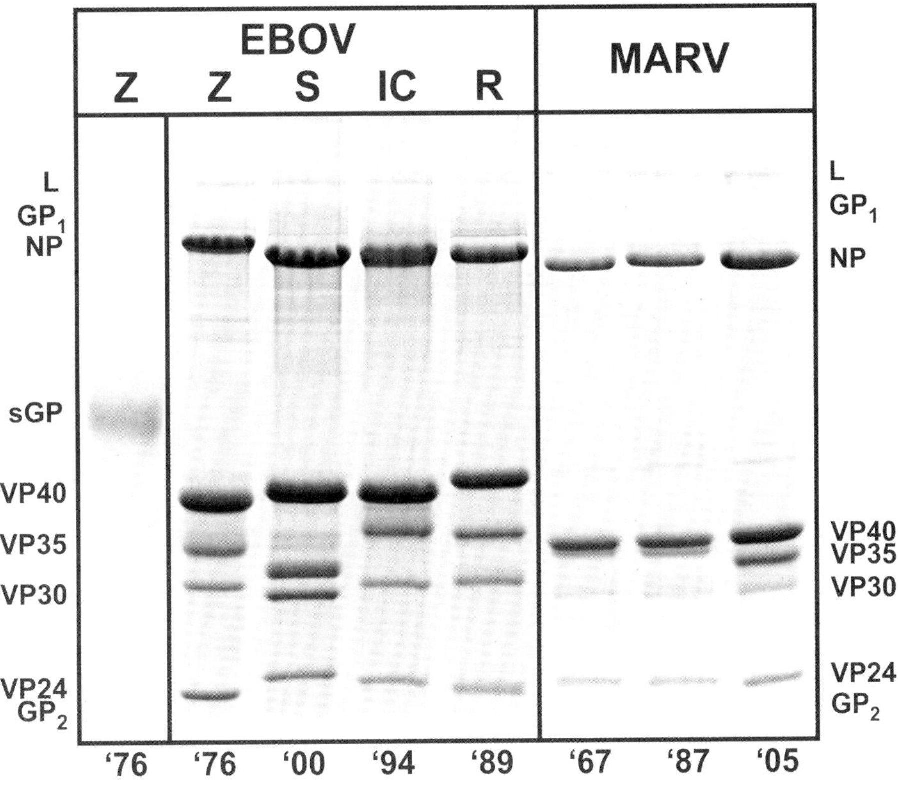

FIGURE 32.4. Migration patterns of filovirus proteins separated by SDS-PAGE on a 10% acrylamide gel (stained with Coomassie blue). The far left lane contains highly purified ZEBOV sGP, while the other lanes contain proteins from purified virion preparations from various filovirus isolates. Approximate migration locations for EBOV and MARV proteins are shown at the left and right margins, respectively, and year of isolate/outbreak is shown along the bottom.

L protein provides the RNA-dependent RNA polymerase activity of the complex; motifs linked to RNA (template) binding, phosphodiester bonding (catalytic site), and a ribonucleotide triphosphate binding have been described.[290,414] Conserved regions or "blocks" of sequences have been identified in filovirus L proteins, but there are also areas of divergence (particularly within the C-terminal quarter of the molecule) and sequences that are unique to the larger MARV L protein.

VP35 has an essential role as a cofactor that affects the mode of RNA synthesis (transcription or replication), similar to that of the P proteins of other NNS viruses[290,292,321,415]; VP35 acts as a link between L and NP.[28] Basic residues in the C-terminal region have been identified as critical to viral RNA synthesis.[321] The ZEBOV VP35 has also been shown to be a virulence factor through its inhibitory effect on the host innate immune system.[255] VP35 has an antagonistic effect on the interferon type I pathway (see Host Immune Response section) by binding virus-generated double-stranded RNA (dsRNA) and by directly interfering with pathway kinases[19,20,21,54,90,170,171,253,322,323]; as noted previously, it also acts as a suppressor of RNA silencing.[91,162] A C-terminal domain in VP35 confers its dsRNA binding property[171] and X-ray crystallography studies of ZEBOV and REBOV VP35 have shown that it forms an asymmetrical dimer, the units of which separately bind and "end-cap" dsRNA[226,253,254,255] (Fig. 32.5). Additionally, the ZEBOV VP35 interacts with the 8kDa dynein light chain, a component of the microtubule transport system,[237] which may have an effect on the virus life cycle.

Structural (Surface) Glycoprotein

As noted earlier, the surface of the filovirus virion is covered with peplomers (spike structures) composed of the structural glycoprotein, GP, and is anchored in the envelope in a type I orientation (Figs. 32.1 and 32.2). GP has been the most studied of the filovirus proteins, due in large part to its role in virus entry, its influence on pathogenesis, its antigenicity, and its attractiveness as an immunogen in vaccine development. The GP of EBOV species is encoded in two reading frames and expressed through transcriptional editing ([353,410]; see Stages of Replication, next section), while the GP of MARV is encoded in a single ORF.[49,103] Despite this difference, the features of their amino acid sequences are very similar. A schematic representation of the EBOV GP is depicted in Figure 32.6 and illustrates the general characteristics of a filovirus GP molecule.

The glycoproteins of filoviruses are translocated into the endoplasmic reticulum (ER) by a signal sequence at the N-terminus of GP_0 (precursor molecule) and are anchored by a membrane-spanning sequence at the C-terminus (Fig. 32.6); the cytoplasmic tail is extremely short (3 residues for EBOV and 7 for MARV). As GP_0 is transported through the ER and Golgi apparatus, it is glycosylated with both N-linked glycans (hybrid and complex) and O-linked glycans.[104,107,149,409] An extremely divergent, mucin-like region (rich in threonine, serine, and proline residues) is located in the middle of GP_0 and is heavily glycosylated; all O-linked glycans are located in this region. Analysis of the carbohydrate composition of GP has shown that MARV isolates lack terminal sialic acid when grown in Vero E6 or MA-104 cells, unlike the GP of EBOV species, which contain abundant α(2–6) and/or α(2–3) linked sialic acids.[104,149] Differences in sialic acid addition may be caused by differences in targeting as they are directed though the *trans*-Golgi apparatus. In addition, no neuraminidase activity has been found with any filovirus. The MARV GP (Musoke strain) is also phosphorylated by Golgi protein

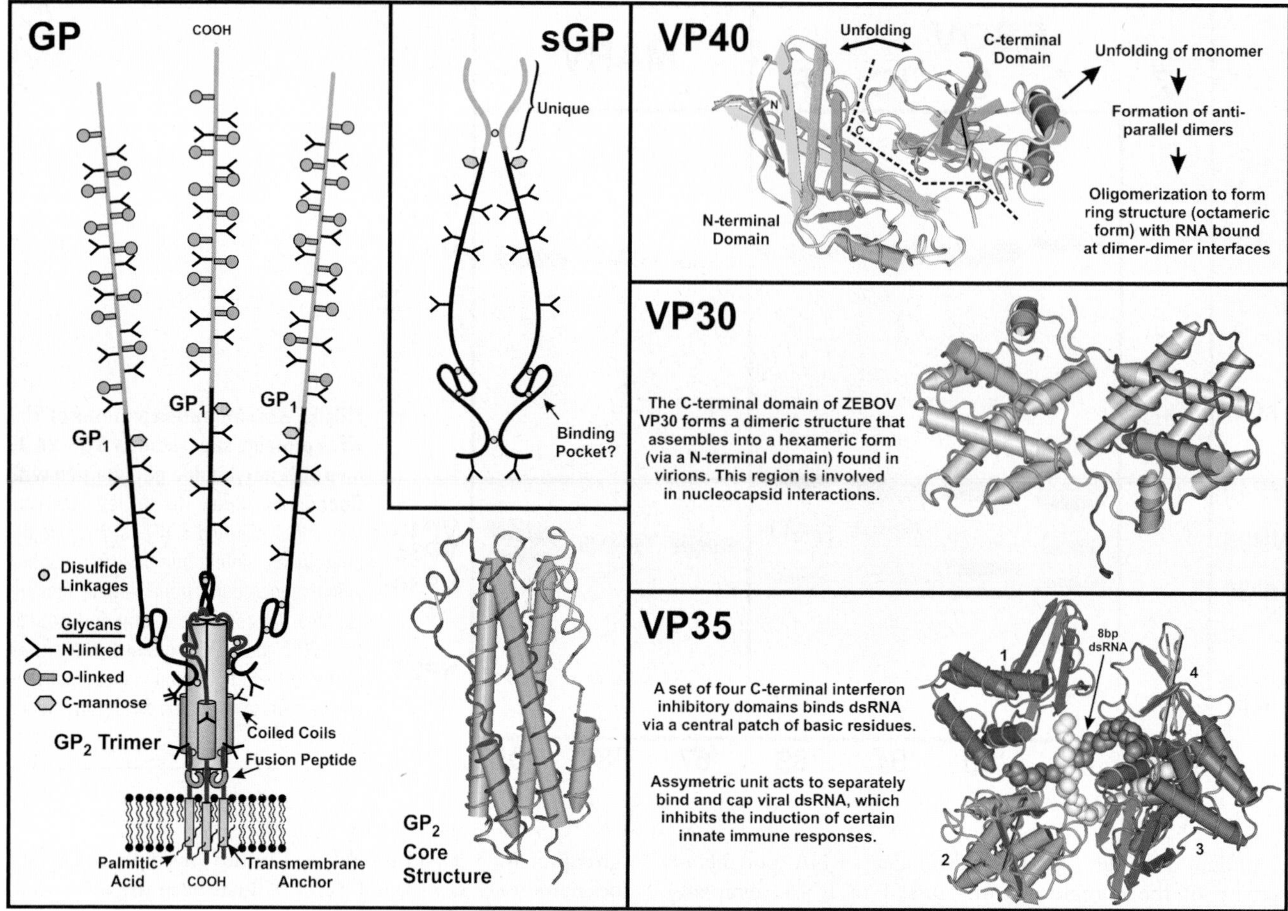

FIGURE 32.5. Structural features of the ZEBOV GP, sGP, VP40, VP30, and VP35 molecules. The left panel shows schematic structures for GP and sGP. The basic features of GP are essentially the same for all filoviruses, as are those of sGP for all EBOV species. Structural depictions of the GP_2 trimer and the C-termini of VP40, VP30 (dimer), and VP35 (four molecules bound to dsRNA) were generated from Research Collaboratory for Structural Bioinformatics (RCSB) Protein Data Bank files (PDB ID = 2EBO, 1ES6, 2I8B, and 3L25, respectively; http://www.rcsb.org/pdb). Structures were rendered using Cn3D 4.1 (http://www.ncib.nlm.nih.gov/Structure/CNeD/cn3d.shtml)

kinases, putatively at serine residues near the center of GP_1 (^{260}**SS**DDEDLAT**S**G**S**G**S**^{273})[357] the C-terminal set of 3 serines is conserved in MARV.[354] The implications of this processing are unknown, but could influence the trafficking of MARV GP.

GP_0 is cleaved by furin, a subtilisin/kexin-like convertase localized in the *trans* Golgi, or a furin-like endoprotease at a site just C-terminal to a long, variable, mucin-like region.[356,413,417] Cleavage leads to the formation of a $GP_{1,2}$ heterodimer that is held together by a single disulfide bond formed between the most N-terminal cysteine of GP_1 (cysteine at position 53 in ZEBOV) and the fifth cysteine from the N-terminus GP_2 (predicted) (Fig. 32.6). The MARV cleavage site is located ~70 residues N-terminal to that of the EBOV site, and a second conserved furin/furin-like cleavage sequence is located immediately after the second cysteine from the N-terminus of GP_2 (just within the first heptad repeat), but there is no evidence that this sequence is cleaved. It should be noted that cleavage of GP_0 to form the $GP_{1,2}$ heterodimer is not required for virus entry in tissue culture, as mutation of the furin cleavage site does not prevent entry by pseudotyped virus,[199,448] nor does it significantly affect infection and subsequent spread by a recombinant ZEBOV or virulence in nonhuman primates.[301,302] Nevertheless, cleavage may be required for efficient maintenance in the natural host.

Peplomers are composed of trimerized $GP_{1,2}$ heterodimers, and X-ray crystallography studies of a recombinant-expressed portion of GP_2 have shown that trimerization occurs when heptad repeat sequences form coiled coils in a rod-shaped structure (Figs. 32.5 and 32.6) similar to those of the HA_2 of influenza, the transmembrane (TM) of retroviruses, and SNAREs.[269,442,443] Two conserved cysteine residues at the C-terminal end of the membrane spanning sequence are palmitoylated,[119,200] which could stabilize the anchorage of the peplomer and may influence virus entry, although GP pseudotyping studies suggests that these cysteines are not essential for infectivity.[200,209] The TM region of GP_2 has been linked to increased permeability of infected cells with the 667ALF669 sequence particularly important.[165] A fusion peptide is internally positioned near the N-terminus of GP_2 and is flanked by two conserved cysteines that are predicted to form a disulfide bond; this arrangement is very similar to the TM of Rous sarcoma virus and avian leukosis virus.[120,209] The fusion peptide of ZEBOV inserts efficiently

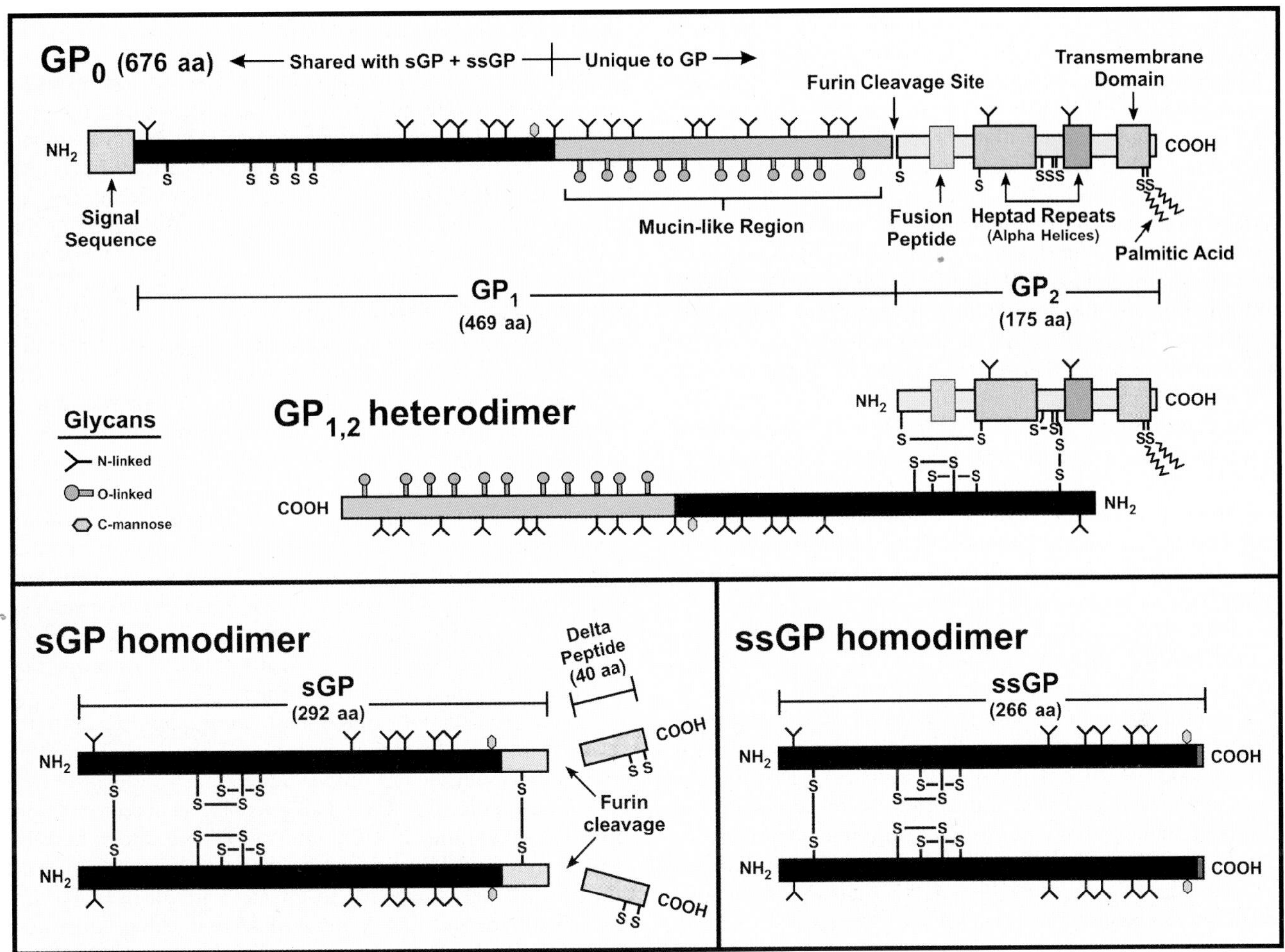

FIGURE 32.6. Features of the GP (*top*), sGP (*bottom left*) and ssGP (*bottom right*) proteins of ZEBOV. N-linked glycosylation sites (Y) and cysteine residues (S) are identified along the sequences. The basic features of GP are essentially the same for all filoviruses, as are those of sGP and ssGP for all EBOV species.

into synthetic membranes containing phosphatidylinositol and promotes fusion of lipid vesicles.[1,200,341,375]

Sequence analysis of the GP gene coding regions indicates that the N-terminal end (~200 residues) of GP_1 and most of GP_2 are conserved and have regions of increased hydrophobicity. The N-terminal region of EBOV GP_1 contains conserved cysteine residues that are closely positioned and form intramolecular disulfide bonds (C108–C135, C121–C147), which are also found in the sGP molecule[15,209,418] and likely form an important structural feature. The MARV GP has conserved cysteines that correspond to the C108–C135 linkage of EBOV, but the other two closely positioned cysteines appear to be shifted towards the center of the molecule (and likely form a disulfide bridge). The abundant O-glycans of the mucin-like region confers an extended structure and its heavy glycosylation makes it very hydrophilic. The mucin-like region is located at the C-terminus of GP_1, and was predicted to project away from the virion membrane (toward the aqueous environment) with the N-terminal end (linked to GP_2) contributing to the stalk structure of the peplomer (Fig. 32.5). X-ray crystallography of GP_1 has verified this prediction.[241] In tissue culture, it has been shown that the ectodomain portion of the ZEBOV peplomer is released from cells (separate from virions) through proteolytic cleavage by tumor necrosis factor α-converting enzyme (TACE; zinc-dependent metalloprotease) near the transmembrane anchor (residue D637 of ZEBOV).[78] GP can also be released into the medium as peplomers anchored in vesicles extruded from the plasma membrane.[416]

Nonstructural Glycoproteins

The expression of a nonstructural soluble glycoprotein (sGP) as the primary product of the GP gene of EBOV is unusual and an important distinction from MARV.[353,410] The N-terminal ~300 amino acids of sGP are identical to those of the structural GP, but the C-terminus is unique in sequence (Fig. 32.6). sGP is produced from a precursor molecule that is also cleaved by furin (or a furin-like endoprotease) near the C-terminus to release a short peptide that seems to contain exclusively O-linked glycans and has been named delta peptide.[409,419] No biologic activity has been attributed to delta peptide. Biochemical and antigenic analyses of the ZEBOV sGP have shown that it is structurally distinct from GP[15,356,418,419] and is secreted from infected cells as a homodimer that is likely formed in the ER. Initial structural studies indicated an antiparallel orientation for sGP molecules in the dimer by disulfide bonding between cysteine residues C53 and C306.[418] However, subsequent MALDI-TOF MS analysis of sGP peptide fragments have unequivocally demonstrated a parallel orientation for the homodimer, which is held together by disulfide bonds between the N-terminal (C53–C53′) and C-terminal (C306–C306′) cysteines that fix the orientation of the molecules.[15,95] The intramolecular disulfide bonds are similar in topology and spacing to the fibronectin type II module (binding site for collagen and gelatin), and may form a binding pocket for an as-of-yet unidentified ligand. Biophysical characterization of ZEBOV sGP has also revealed that the tryptophan residue at position 288 is C-mannosylated,[16,94] an unusual form of glycosylation, at the specific motif W-X-X-W (first W is C-mannosylated) that is in the shared N-terminal region and is conserved in all EBOV species. GP_1 is presumed to have this same type of glycosylation. It is possible that sGP could contribute to disease progression, because large amounts circulate through the blood of acutely infected humans,[350] but there has been no evidence linking sGP to a role in pathogenesis.

Recently, another ZEBOV nonstructural glycoprotein, termed small soluble glycoprotein (ssGP), has been identified and partially characterized,[281] and outwardly appears to be a truncated version of sGP. As with GP, ssGP is expressed through transcriptional editing. This glycoprotein is expressed at a low level (~1/20 that of sGP+GP) and has structural properties similar to that of sGP, in that it has N-linked glycans (no O-linked) and exists as a homodimer (disulfide bond between cysteines at position 53). As with sGP, the function of ssGP has yet to be adequately defined, but ssGP appears to lack an anti-inflammatory property reported for sGP.[281]

Matrix Proteins

The VP40 protein functions as the matrix protein and the VP24 protein may have a secondary/minor matrix protein function.[164] VP40 is the most abundant protein in the virion, while only small amounts of VP24 are incorporated into virus particles (Fig. 32.4). Both proteins have an affinity for membranes and are associated with the virion envelope (no membrane-spanning regions),[208,340,362] and are easily released from virions by nonionic detergents under low-salt conditions.[85,225] VP40 is critical to the budding process, as it initiates and drives the envelopment of the NC by the plasma membrane.[207] In addition, it has been reported that both VP40 and VP24 of EBOV contribute to regulation of genome replication and transcription.[180]

VP24 has a decidedly hydrophobic profile, and a study of a recombinant-expressed form (ZEBOV) indicates that it has an affinity for the plasma membrane and perinuclear region of infected cells.[164] VP24 is capable of forming homotetramers, which is influenced by pH and divalent cation changes. Because disulfide-bonded oligomers of VP24 are not evident in the virion,[352] the formation of multimers is likely due to ionic and/or hydrophobic interactions. The precise role of VP24 in the replication of filoviruses is still unclear and direct interactions with other virus proteins have not been described, but a role in formation of nucleocapsid-like structures has been described.[164] The VP24 of EBOV has also been reported to antagonize the interferon type I signalling pathway, similar to that of VP35 (see Host Immune Response section).[20]

STAGES OF REPLICATION

Recent studies have provided valuable insights into filovirus entry into host cells and the mechanisms leading to the production and release of infectious progeny. Although very much incomplete, the details of this complicated series of molecular events are slowly being revealed. The current understanding of this process is illustrated in Figure 32.7 and described in the following sections.

Mechanism of Attachment

In filovirus infections a variety of host organs and cell types are involved; this broad tropism is related in large part to the binding properties of the peplomers that populate the surface of the virion. Because GP is the only filovirus protein involved in initiating infection, it has been intensely studied for its ability to bind cellular receptors. Much of the work directed at receptor binding (and subsequent entry processes) has utilized recombinant pseudotyping systems, which provide a safer and easier approach to characterizing these properties and eve nts.[56,58,200,390,447,448,467] However, these results need to be verified using infectious filoviruses, as interactions of GP with VP24 and/or VP40 need to be considered along with other properties that may be peculiar to filovirus virions.

Identification of attachment molecules (receptors?) involved in filovirus entry is complicated by the ability of GP trimers to specifically or nonspecifically bind a variety of host-cell surface molecules. The asialoglycoprotein receptor found on hepatocytes binds MARV,[29] yet EBOV also infects hepatocytes despite its GP having sialylated glycans. The $\beta 1$ group of integrins has been suggested to interact with ZEBOV GP on the cell surface and during intracellular trafficking (when co-expressed),[393] although cells that express this molecule (such as Jurkat cells) are not easily infectible. The folate receptor alpha has been implicated as a cofactor in filovirus entry,[56] but virus entry independent of this molecule has been shown to take place.[366,369] C-type lectins (DC-SIGN and DC-SIGNR; bind oligosaccharide ligands)—present on certain forms of dendritic cells, macrophages, and endothelial cells—are also capable of binding filovirus peplomers,[3,12,279,365] especially when N-linked glycans contain high mannose carbohydrates.[213,258] However, there are indications that DC-SIGN may not act as an EBOV receptor, but instead acts to promote attachment and other host factors are involved in entry.[280] One study has shown that macrophages are more susceptible to virus entry by ZEBOV GP-pseudotyped HIV-1 particles than are monocytes, and that HUVEC cultures pretreated with TNF-α showed increased entry over untreated cells.[467] These results imply that changes in cellular gene expression can alter the makeup of surface attachment molecules (and cofactors?). Antibody binding to peplomers might also enhance infectivity through its interaction with the Fc portion of the complement protein C1q bound to the surface of host cells.[391] Very recently, T-cell Ig and mucin domain 1 (TIM-1) has been described as a potential binding protein for EBOV GP and enhances virus entry into cells.[232]

Results of site-directed mutagenesis studies of ZEBOV GP have shown that individual glycosylation sites are not critical to virus entry,[209,270] and deletion of the entire mucin-like region can actually increase virus entry *in vitro*.[209] A role in receptor binding or increased binding has yet to be attributed to the mucin-like region. Further deletion of the GP_1 C-terminal

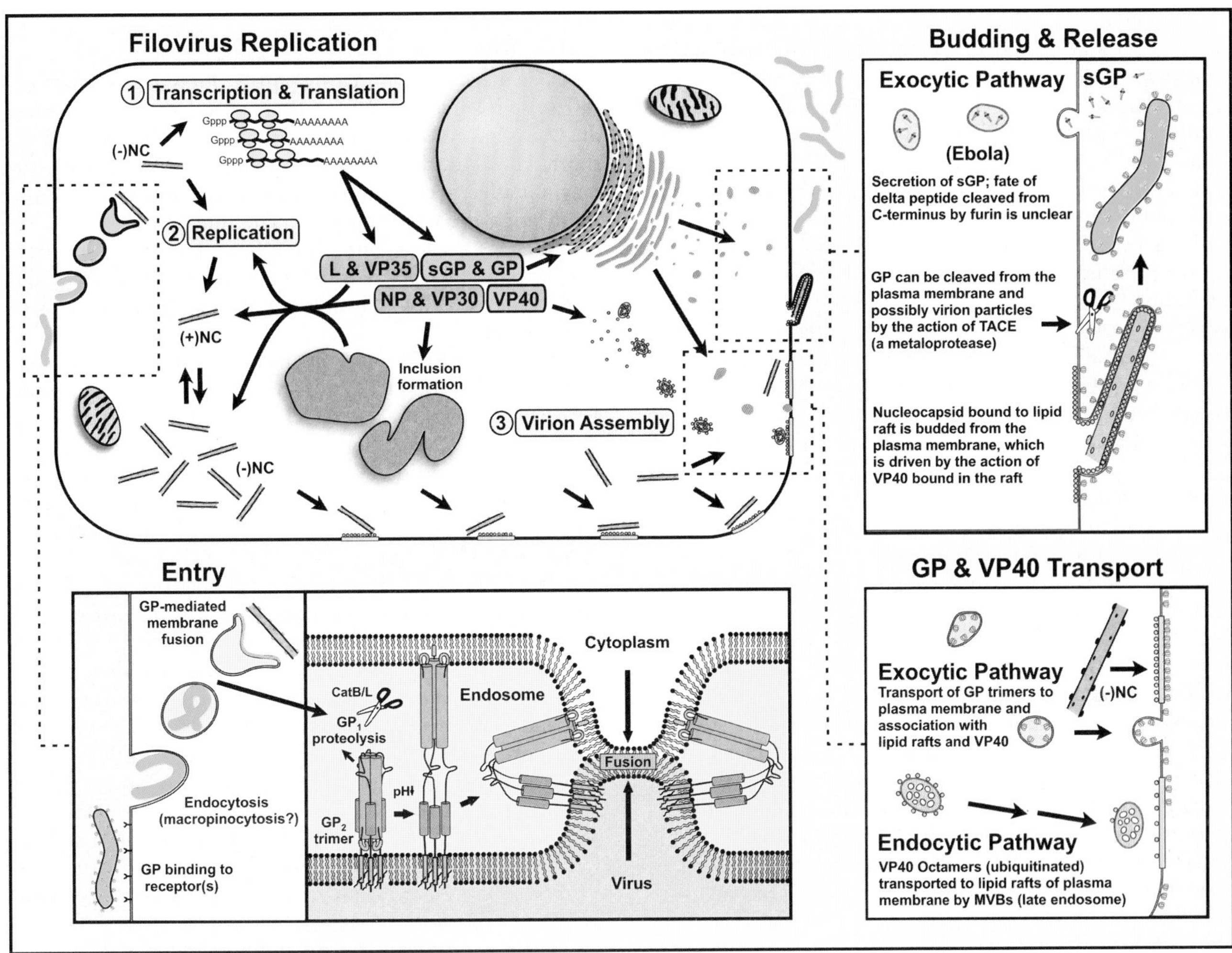

FIGURE 32.7. Schematic view of the processes associated with filovirus entry, synthesis of viral molecules, and the production of infectious virions in a susceptible eukaryotic cell.

sequences (past the mucin-like region), together with mutagenesis of N-terminal residues, has localized the entry function to ~150 residues at the N-terminus (residues 33–185).[270] It should be noted that this region also contains the same intramolecular disulfide bonds as sGP, which potentially forms a binding pocket that is involved in cell attachment and/or receptor binding. If this is the case, then the corresponding region of MARV GP_1 would likely have distinctive binding characteristics due to a differing disulfide bonding pattern. In contrast, another study identified approximately the same region as the potential receptor binding site for both viruses, indicating that EBOV and MARV utilize a common receptor.[239]

Mechanism of Entry and Intracellular Trafficking

Following attachment, virions are presumed to enter the cell by a process of endocytosis, acidification of the endocytic vesicle, and fusion of virus and host membranes resulting in the release of the NC into the cytoplasm. ZEBOV GP-mediated entry and fusion are affected by the treatment of host cells with agents that disrupt microtubules or inhibit the function of microfilaments.[467] These cytoskeletal components are key to clathrin-dependent and caveolae-mediated internalization, and support the theory that filoviruses enter the cell through endocytosis. However, studies examining the type of endocytic pathway utilized by filoviruses are conflicting. One study has demonstrated that disruption of the caveola vesicular system (via cholesterol binding compounds) inhibited ZEBOV and MARV entry and that filovirus GP-pseudotyped virus co-localized with the caveolin-1 (cholesterol binding protein) marker.[88] However, cells lacking caveolae are infectible and co-expression of folate receptor alpha and caveolin-1 in a T-cell line did not increase infectivity.[366] Clathrin-mediated endocytosis and GP-dependent macropinocytosis or a macropinocytosis-like mechanism for EBOV internalization and an involvement of lipid rafts.[2,298,344] It should be noted that inhibitors of macropinocytosis (amiloride) and the lipid raft-caveolae endocytosis pathway did not significantly affect ZEBOV entry.[345] Latest, it was reported that EBOV entry was dependent on Niemann-Pick CI (NPC1), a protein known to function in cholesterol transport.[53] It thus appears that the entry of ZEBOV (and possibly other filoviruses) occurs through multiple routes.

A filovirus virion internalized in a vesicle at the plasma membrane traffics through the endosomal pathway, and at some point in time the NC is released into the cytoplasm by GP_2-mediated fusion of the virus envelope and endosomal membrane. Membrane fusion is dependent on endosomal acidification,[392,447] and endosomal proteolysis of the GP_1 subunit peplomer by the cysteine proteases CatL and CatB (active in acidic pH environments) can enhance ZEBOV entry.[44,59,222,345] CatL removes the glycan cap and mucin-like domain, exposing core residues of a recombinant peplomer and increasing infectivity.[182,222] Removal of GP_1 is believed to set off a conformational change in the GP_2 trimer that triggers the deployment of the fusion machinery, resulting in the insertion of the GP_2 fusion peptides into the endosomal membrane. This event would link and draw viral and host membranes together to induce fusion and the release of the NC into the cytoplasm.[436] The minimum number of peplomers needed to induce fusion has not been determined.

Transcription and Translation

Following filovirus entry, negative-strand RNA genetics dictates that transcription is the first (and obligatory) viral process, similar to paramyxoviruses and rhabdoviruses. Once the nucleocapsid is released into the cytoplasm, polyadenylated monocistronic messenger RNAs (mRNAs) are synthesized from virus genes in a 3′ to 5′ direction (with polar attenuation) from the encapsidated genomic RNA template. Transcription seems to involve a process of starting and stopping as the polymerase complex encounters conserved start (initiation) and stop (termination/polyadenylation) sites along the genome. Synthesis of the "leader" sequence is postulated to occur, but intergenic sequences and the "trailer" sequence seem to be ignored, although this has not been shown experimentally. NP mRNA can be detected as early as 7 hours postinfection, and peaks around 18 hours.[346] It is assumed that transcripts are capped at the 5′ end ($^{7Me}G^{5'}$-ppp$^{5'}$-R) by the L protein, as it contains conserved motifs associated with this enzymatic activity.[108]

Analyses of defective interfering particles of ZEBOV have shown that promoters for initiating RNA synthesis are contained within 156 and 177 nucleotide regions of the genomic and antigenomic RNA 3′ termini, respectively.[52] Subsequent to these studies, it was shown that a bipartite promoter is located within the first 128 nucleotides of the 3′ end of the ZEBOV genome.[441] One element is located at the extreme 3′ end and the other within the nontranslated region of the NP gene. These elements are separated by a nonspecific sequence (nucleotides 56–80) that acts to provide proper spacing and also contains the NP gene transcription start site. This bipartite promoter is similar to that of various paramyxoviruses (i.e., Sendai virus) and obeys the "rule of 6".[441]

Transcriptional start sites are 12 or 14 nucleotides in length and end in the consensus sequence 3′-CUUCUAAUU for EBOV and 3′-CUURUAAUU for MARV, while stop sites are 11 or 12 nucleotides long with the conserved sequence 3′-UAAUUC(U)$_{5/6}$. Polyadenylation is believed to occur by slippage or stuttering of the polymerase at the 5 to 6 uridines ending the stop site. A characteristic that is unique to the transcriptional signals of filoviruses is a common pentanucleotide sequence, 3′-UAAUU, present at the 5′ end of start sites and at the 3′ end of stop sites[103]; the stop sites of ZEBOV and REBOV polymerase genes deviate slightly from this sequence (3′-UAAUA).

The mechanism initiating transcription of a downstream (5′) gene involved in a gene overlap and the consequences of this arrangement are unknown. Because the overlaps are short (18–21 nucleotides), the proximity of the polymerase may not affect recognition of the start site as it finishes polyadenylating the upstream gene. The function of these overlaps remains unclear, but attenuation of transcription does not appear to take place, as the transcription of the VP40 and VP30 genes of ZEBOV is substantial and expression of VP40 is very strong.

Filovirus mRNA molecules have characteristics that make them somewhat unique. They contain long noncoding regions at their 3′ and/or 5′ ends, which contribute to the increased length of the genome and may function in the stability of transcripts. In addition, the 5′ ends of filovirus transcripts have the potential to form stable, stem-loop structures, which might affect their stability and ribosome binding capacity/translation.[291,347,352]

The ZEBOV VP30 has a transcription activation property that is linked to an RNA secondary structure formed at the 5′ end of the NP gene transcript as it is synthesized[168,169,286]; the presence of VP30 is required for transcription of downstream genes. This property is impaired by phosphorylation at six serines and one threonine at the N-terminus, and restored by the action of cellular phosphatases.[286] Because ZEBOV VP30 in the virion is at least partly phosphorylated,[85] the action of phosphatases on the NC may be required before transcription proceeds efficiently. Thus, the phosphorylation state of VP30 may be a critical component in regulating EBOV RNA synthesis; a corresponding mechanism has not been shown for MARV.

The organization and transcription of the GP genes of EBOV are unusual and provide an important distinction between MARV and EBOV. The MARV GP gene encodes a single product, GP, in a conventional open reading frame (ORF), whereas all EBOV species encode their GP in two ORFs (-0 and -1 frames). Expression of the EBOV GP requires a transcriptional editing event[281,353,410] comparable to the editing described for the phosphoprotein gene of certain paramyxoviruses. Translation of the unedited transcript of the EBOV GP gene results in the production of sGP, a smaller, nonstructural, secreted glycoprotein, the primary gene product (Figs. 32.4 and 32.6). The transcriptional editing event that leads to GP expression occurs at a series of seven uridines on the genomic RNA template and results in the insertion of an additional adenosine, which connects the GP open coding frames; approximately 20% to 25% of the transcripts are edited. The mechanism of insertion most likely evolved out of the polymerase's ability to polyadenylate by stuttering on a poly(U) template. However, insertion of a single nucleotide at the editing site appears to occur with a high degree of fidelity, but insertion of two adenosines can occur (in ~5% of GP gene transcripts), which leads to the synthesis of low levels of ssGP.[281] The editing of EBOV GP gene transcripts is the only example of a virus glycoprotein that is expressed through this type of mechanism. Sequence analysis of the GP genes of MARV isolates indicates that a nucleotide sequence that corresponds to the editing region of EBOV GP genes is totally absent.[49,103,356,445] The difference in filovirus GP gene organization provides important evidence pointing to a divergent evolution for EBOV and MARV.

Replication of Genomic Nucleic Acid

In addition to transcription, the promoter at the 3′ end of the genomic RNA also drives the synthesis of full-length complementary/antigenomic RNA from the encapsidated template. As with other NNS RNA viruses, the ends of the genome have a high degree of sequence complementarity,[67,352] and stem-loop structures are predicted to form at the 3′ and 5′ ends of genomic and antigenomic RNAs. These structures are believed to be essential to the replication of filoviruses.[67] The initial expression of virus genes leads to a buildup of viral proteins (especially NP), which is thought to trigger a switch from transcription to replication. This switch results in the synthesis and encapsidation of antigenomic RNA molecules, which in turn serve as templates for genomic RNA that is also rapidly encapsidated. Depletion of capsid proteins is believed to cause a return to transcription, and eventually an equilibrium is established wherein transcription and replication are concurrent processes. As replication progresses in the infected cell, NC particles containing genomic RNA accumulate and are directed to the plasma membrane for virion assembly.

The development of reverse genetics systems based on EBOV and MARV genetics has provided significant advances in understanding filovirus replication[32,89,156,289,292,301,395,415] and has allowed the production/reconstitution of recombinant ZEBOV and MARV (Musoke strain) from plasmid DNA.[89,301,415] For MARV, the NP, VP35, and L proteins are all that is required to transcribe and replicate minigenomes,[298] but systems developed for ZEBOV also required VP30.[301,395,415] When components of minigenome reporter gene systems for REBOV and ZEBOV were switched, it was noted that *cis*-acting signals and nearly all combinations of proteins were exchangeable.[32] Rescue of recombinant ZEBOV using NC-associated proteins from REBOV or MARV has also shown that exchanging of these heterologous proteins can lead to recovery of recombinant virus.[395]

Assembly and Release

When sufficient levels of negative-sense nucleocapsids and envelope-associated proteins are reached, a coalescing of these components occurs at the plasma membrane,[207] or to a lesser extent at membranes forming intracellular vacuoles.[96] Filovirus-infected cells develop prominent inclusion bodies, easily visualized by light, immunofluorescent, and electron microscopy.[183,294] Inclusions are induced by NP, but also contain other proteins that form the NC.[28] Inclusions may be a source of components for forming NCs, which can be seen associated with inclusions (Fig. 32.8A). Recombinant-derived, NC-like structures form in cells expressing NP, which may be facilitated by the expression of VP35 and VP24.[183,305] NC particles are believed to interact with VP40 molecules in the budding process.

Membrane/lipid rafts have been identified as platforms for the assembly of filovirus virions.[24,310] Membrane rafts are rigid microdomains (containing sphingolipids and cholesterol) present in biological membranes and are isolated from the fluid phospholipids surrounding them. GP trimers conveyed to the plasma membrane have an affinity for these lipid rafts, which is associated with palmitoylation of the membrane-spanning anchor sequence.[24]

Structural and functional studies of VP40 have provided important insights into the assembly of filovirus virions.[75,173,198,207,229,230,257,461] Posttranslational processing and intracellular trafficking of VP40 result in the deposition of VP40 at the plasma membrane via the vacuolar protein sorting/endosomal pathway. By itself, ZEBOV VP40 is capable of mediating its own release from mammalian cells to form enveloped virus-like particles (VLPs),[208,256,307,399] which are more efficiently produced when GP and NP are present[256]; VP40 interacts with the C-terminal 50 amino acids of NP.[257] ZEBOV VP40 determines VLP morphology and density,[219] and likely has the same influence on infectious filovirus particles. A structural study of ZEBOV VP40 demonstrated that it associates with lipid bilayers containing a high level of L-α-phosphatidyl-L-serine (abolished by 1 M NaCl).[340] It was also found that this property maps to the C-terminal ~110 residues, which contains basic and hydrophobic regions that could bind membranes.[397] In addition, the N-terminal region is involved in oligomerization, and deletion of the C-terminal region of VP40 allowed it to hexamerize into ring structures. The crystal structure of monomeric ZEBOV VP40 is composed of similar/related β sandwich domains (N-terminal and C-terminal) connected by a hinge region, which unfolds upon interaction with membranes and dimerizes in an antiparallel orientation (Fig. 32.5).[362] These dimers form octomeric rings (~84 Å diameter) with a central pore and RNA binding properties[152] that may be essential for replication.[181] Late (L) domain motifs are positioned near the N-terminus of filovirus VP40 molecules, and are important in posttranslational processing and tracking events that facilitate virus budding.[173,405] The VP40 of EBOV contains overlapping PT/SAP and PPXY motifs (PTAPPE/AY), while MARV contains only the PPXY motif (PPPY). These L domain motifs on the ZEBOV VP40 interact with cellular proteins (with WW domains) associated with the endocytic pathway of mammalian cells[229,230,257,272,398,465]; for ZEBOV the PPXY domain appears to have a greater role in budding efficiencies.[300] Results of *in vitro* studies have suggested that VP40 is bound as an oligomeric form at its PPXY motif by Nedd4 and ubiquitinated, is subsequently targeted to endosomes or multivesicular bodies (MVB) by Tsg101 and VPS-4 (components of the vacuole sorting pathway), and is recruited to membrane rafts through Tsg101 interactions with VP40 and raft proteins (Fig. 32.7). The finding that small interfering RNA (siRNA)-silencing of Rab9, an enzyme important in late endosome transport, inhibits filovirus replication in Vero cells,[60,297] as well as the observation that Rab11 is incorporated into MARV virions,[231] support the involvement of the endosomal sorting machinery in filovirus assembly. However, the details of VP40 transport from the late endosome to the plasma membrane have not been defined. In addition, mutation of L domains from VP40 did not prevent recovery of a recombinant ZEBOV, nor did it significantly reduce virus production in cell culture.[300] This information suggests that VP40 can be transported to the plasma membrane through a process separate from endosomal trafficking. Raft-associated VP40 is believed to associate with NCs, drawing them tightly to the membrane where they are enveloped and extruded from the host cell as infectious virions (Figs. 32.7 and 32.8). Electron tomography studies of MARV budding indicate that the entire length of nucleocapsids associate laterally with the plasma membrane (much like a rising submarine), which is followed by its protrusion and release of

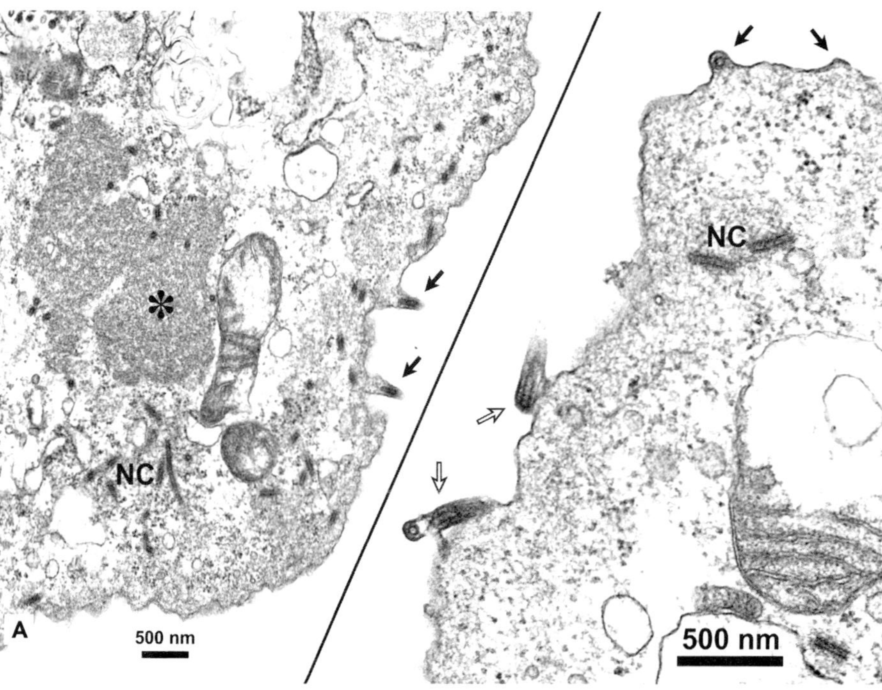

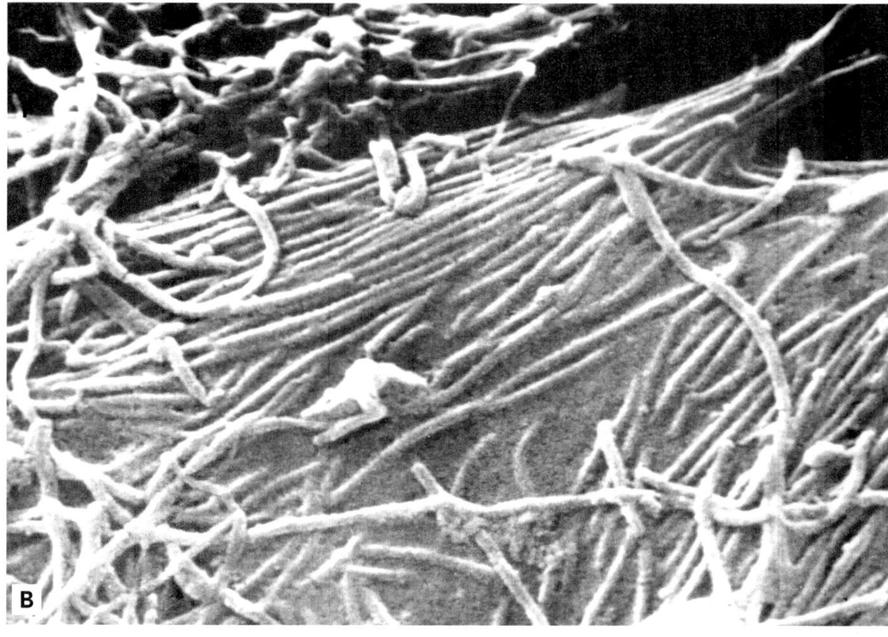

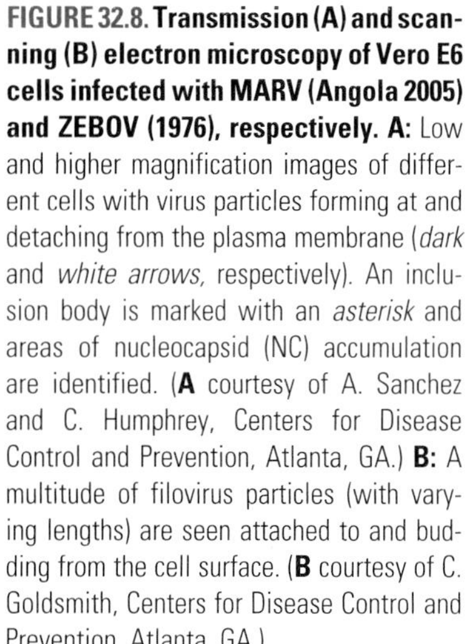
FIGURE 32.8. Transmission (A) and scanning (B) electron microscopy of Vero E6 cells infected with MARV (Angola 2005) and ZEBOV (1976), respectively. A: Low and higher magnification images of different cells with virus particles forming at and detaching from the plasma membrane (*dark* and *white arrows,* respectively). An inclusion body is marked with an *asterisk* and areas of nucleocapsid (NC) accumulation are identified. (**A** courtesy of A. Sanchez and C. Humphrey, Centers for Disease Control and Prevention, Atlanta, GA.) **B:** A multitude of filovirus particles (with varying lengths) are seen attached to and budding from the cell surface. (**B** courtesy of C. Goldsmith, Centers for Disease Control and Prevention, Atlanta, GA.)

the mature virion particle by being pinched off at the trailing end.[405,444]

Effects on Host Cell Cultures

The growth of adapted strains of MARV and EBOV in cultured cells can be striking. Intracytoplasmic vesiculation and mitochondrial swelling are followed by a breakdown of organelles and terminal cytoplasmic rarification or condensation. In African green monkey kidney cell lines infected with filoviruses, cytopathic effects (CPE) are evidenced by a rounding and detachment of cells (without syncytia formation), which can result in a total loss of the monolayer (~5 days). However, replication of REBOV and ICEBOV is slow in tissue culture, and CPE is usually less evident and generally does not develop until after 7 to 9 days incubation. Persistent REBOV infection with continued production of large amounts of virus particles can be established in Vero E6 cells (A. Sanchez, unpublished observations) and ZEBOV can establish persistent infection under partial immunity.[161] Filovirus infection does not lead to the shutdown of host-cell protein synthesis, but expression levels diminish as the infection progresses and virus proteins accumulate. The expression of GP has a cytotoxic effect that is associated with the mucin-like region.[117,415,463] Elevated expression would likely impact the function of host-cell adhesion proteins by downregulating and/or displacing them,[367,380,393] and could also cause cell detachment without cell death through a phosphorylation-dependent signal cascade.[57] Using a reverse genetics system, it was further demonstrated that cytotoxicity depends on the level of GP expression, with overexpression leading to an early detachment and cytotoxicity of infected cells.[415] The effects of filovirus infections on endothelial cells and immunocompetent cells will be discussed in the next section.

PATHOLOGY AND PATHOGENESIS

Clinical investigations from episodes and outbreaks of human EBOV and MARV infections have provided important descriptive information on the pathology and pathogenesis of these agents; however, the available data are sparse, often fragmentary and sometimes paradoxical. Comprehensive studies have been carried out to a much greater extent in laboratory animals. Rodents—including guinea pigs, mice, and hamsters—have been employed to study viral hemorrhagic fever (VHF) caused by filoviruses.[26,38,343,428,472] Because filovirus isolates derived from primates do not typically produce severe disease in rodents upon initial exposure, serial adaptation is required to produce a uniformly lethal infection. Mice and guinea pigs have served well as early screens for evaluating antiviral drugs and candidate vaccines, and genetically engineered mice clearly have utility for dissecting out specific host–pathogen interactions. However, the disease pathogenesis in rodent models is far less faithful in portraying the human condition than disease observed in nonhuman primates.[40,143] As data derived from studies using rodents may not correlate with human disease or may be deficient in identifying certain processes, this section primarily focuses on data obtained from human clinical studies and experimental infections of nonhuman primates (Fig. 32.9).

Entry into Host

Little is known regarding what constitutes a typical dose and route of exposure in human filovirus infections. Viruses enter the host through mucosal surfaces, breaks or abrasions in the skin, or by parenteral introduction. While a recent study has suggested that exposure to fruit bats may have initiated a ZEBOV outbreak in the DRC in 2007,[248] most cases that propagate outbreaks are thought to occur by direct contact with infected patients or cadavers.[79,223,449,450] Infectious filoviruses and/or RNA have been isolated from semen and genital secretions[275,333,338] and detected in skin in human cases[470]; they have also been demonstrated in skin, body fluids, and nasal secretions of nonhuman primates.[137,205,368]

Laboratory exposure through needlestick and filovirus-infected blood has been reported.[87,196] Reuse of contaminated needles played an important role in the 1976 EBOV outbreaks in Sudan and Zaire,[449,450] and the question of whether reuse of contaminated needles contributed to some of the cases in the 2004 to 2005 outbreak of MARV in Angola was raised.[456] A needlestick exposure involving an acute-phase patient would likely entail a dose of 1,000 plaque-forming units (pfu) or more if viremias associated with terminal patients are comparable to viremias in infected nonhuman primates, which often reach levels as high as 10^7 to 10^8 pfu/mL of serum.[83,126,127,137,174,204,220,328] The generation of human viremia data has been notoriously problematic,[235] but levels are thought to exceed 10^6 pfu/mL of serum in outbreaks of SEBOV and ZEBOV.[402,450] The fact that circulating EBOV and MARV particles are readily observed by direct electron microscopic inspection of postmortem fluids and tissues[76,86,138,294,468] supports this view, considering that the lower limit for ultrastructural detection of virus particles is generally on the order of 10^6 pfu/mL of fluid or gram of tissue.

Butchering of a chimpanzee for food was linked to outbreaks of ZEBOV in Gabon[148] with contact exposure the likely route of transmission. While proper cooking of foods should inactivate infectious filoviruses, ingestion of contaminated foods cannot completely be ruled out as a possible route of exposure in natural infections. Organ infectivity titers in filovirus-infected nonhuman primates are frequently in the 10^7 to 10^9 pfu/g range[126,127,137,174,204,220]; thus, it is likely that exposure through the oral route would invariably be associated with very high infectious doses. In fact, ZEBOV is highly lethal when orally administered to rhesus macaques.[201]

The role of aerogenic transmission in outbreaks is unknown, but is thought to be rare.[315] Aerosol transmission in nonhuman primates was inferred in the 1989 to 1990 epizootic of REBOV,[205] although it is thought that aerosols may have been created mechanically by workers cleaning the facility. High concentrations of REBOV in nasal secretions and ultrastructural detection of large numbers of viral particles in alveoli were reported.[205] Filoviruses are reasonably stable in aerosols,[25,61] and reports of intercage transmission of ZEBOV and MARV between monkeys[202,319,368] suggest that virus spread was mediated by small-particle aerosols. Moreover, ZEBOV and SEBOV are highly infectious by aerosol exposure in cynomolgus[126,320,328] and rhesus[217,328] macaques and African green monkeys,[328] as is MARV in cynomolgus and rhesus macaques[4,126,264] and African green monkeys.[25] Rhesus macaques were also lethally infected with ZEBOV by conjunctival exposure.[201]

Host-Cell Pathology

The pathologic changes seen in patients dying with all filovirus infections seem similar, with extensive necrosis in parenchymal cells of many organs, including liver, spleen, kidney, and gonads; little inflammation is seen within infected tissues.[76,294,295,468] The most characteristic histopathologic features are seen in the liver (Fig. 32.10), where hepatocellular necrosis is widespread with intact, hyalinized, ghost-like cells often remaining in place amid large amounts of karyorrhectic debris. Often, extraordinary numbers of virions are present in this debris. Characteristic intracytoplasmic inclusion bodies are present in intact hepatocytes. Light microscopic, electron microscopic, immunohistochemistry (IHC), and *in situ* hybridization studies show concordance between tissue damage, the presence of viral antigens and nucleic acid, and sites of virus replication, suggesting that direct viral damage is one major element in the pathogenesis of the disease (Figs. 32.9 and 32.10).

EBOV and MARV have a broad cell tropism, infecting a wide variety of cell types. IHC and *in situ* hybridization analyses of tissues from fatal human cases or experimentally infected nonhuman primates show that monocytes, macrophages, dendritic cells, endothelial cells, fibroblasts, hepatocytes, adrenal cortical cells, and several types of epithelial cells all support replication of these viruses.[4,18,73,127,137,138,141,146,174,201,296,342,468,470] The sequence of infection, however, has not been fully elucidated. Temporal studies in nonhuman primates experimentally infected with either ZEBOV or MARV suggest that monocytes, macrophages, and dendritic cells are early and preferred replication sites of these viruses.[137,174] These cells appear to play pivotal roles in dissemination of the virus as it spreads

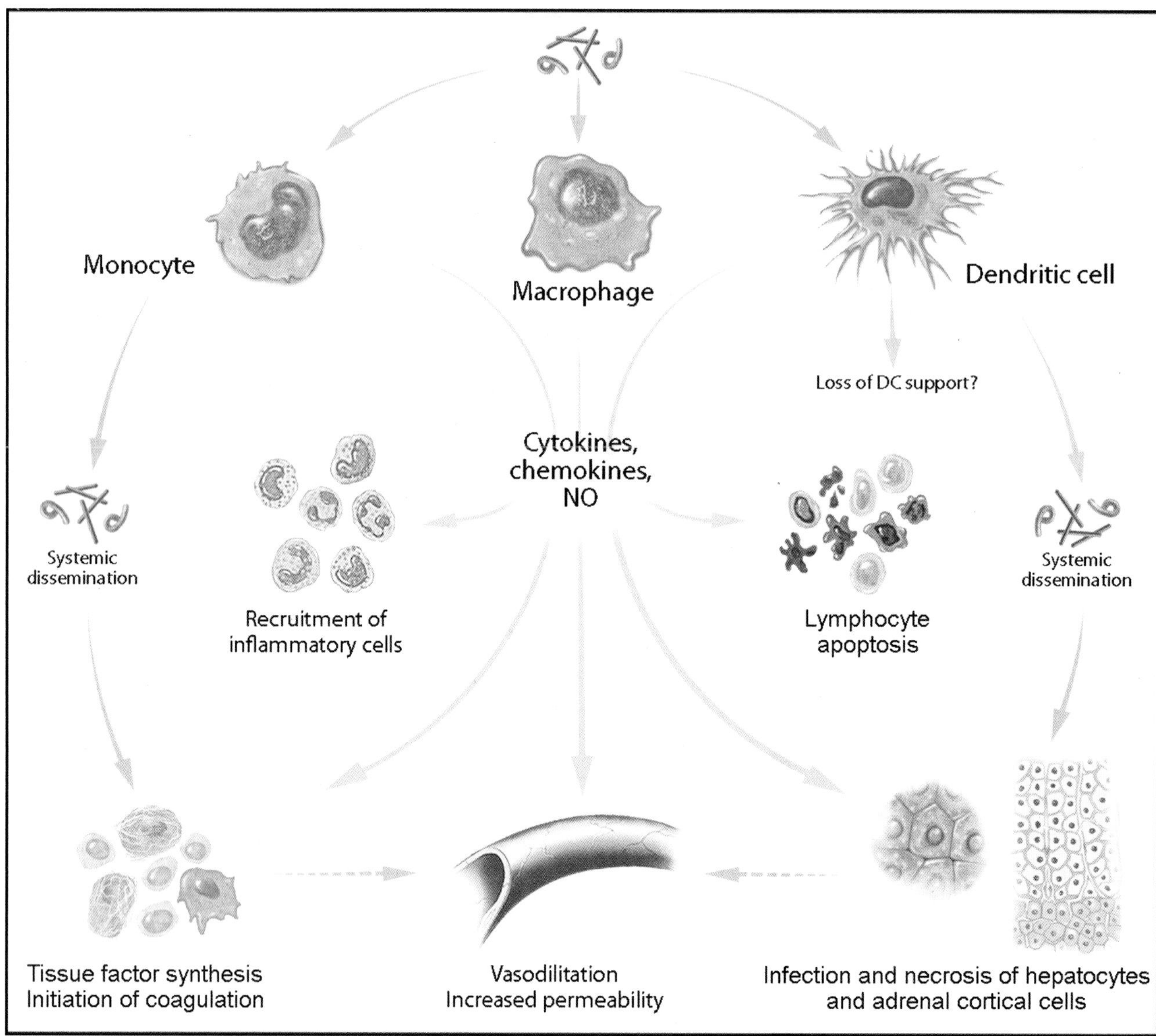

FIGURE 32.9. Model of filovirus pathogenesis in primates. Monocytes, tissue macrophages, and dendritic cells appear to be early and preferred sites of filovirus replication. Soluble factors released from virus-infected mononuclear cells act locally and systemically. Release of chemokines from these virus-infected cells recruits additional monocytes and macrophages to sites of infection, making more target cells available for viral exploitation and further amplifying an already dysregulated host response. In addition, these soluble factors contribute to the impairment of the vascular system. Although filoviruses do not productively infect lymphocytes, the rapid loss of lymphocytes by the process of apoptosis is a noted feature of disease. This lymphocyte loss is probably due to a combination of factors including virus-induced impairment of dendritic cell function, release of proapoptotic soluble factors from virus-infected monocytes and macrophages, and possibly direct interaction between viral antigens and lymphocytes. Coagulation abnormalities are consistent features of filovirus disease and are caused by a number of factors, particularly during the later stages of disease; recent data strongly implicate a role for tissue factor. The hemodynamic and coagulation disorders are exacerbated by infection of hepatocytes and adrenal cortical cells, resulting in impairment in the synthesis of important clotting factors. At the same time, impaired secretion of steroid-synthesizing enzymes by virus-infected adrenal cortical cells leads to hypotension. DC, dendritic cell; NO, nitric oxide. (Adapted from a prior publication by Bray M, Geisbert TW. Ebola virus: the role of macrophages and dendritic cells in the pathogenesis of Ebola hemorrhagic fever. *Int J Biochem Cell Biol* 2005;37:1560–1566.)

from the initial infection site via monocytes/macrophages and dendritic cells to regional lymph nodes, likely by way of lymphatics, and to the liver and spleen through blood. At these locations, filoviruses infect resident macrophages and dendritic cells. Several lines of evidence suggest that filovirus-infected monocytes/macrophages release various soluble factors that then recruit additional monocytes/macrophages to areas of infection; this makes more target cells available for viral exploitation, further amplifying the infection.[39,137,174]

In addition to the macrophage-rich lymphoid tissues such as spleen, the liver and adrenal gland also appear to be important target organs for both EBOV and MARV; this

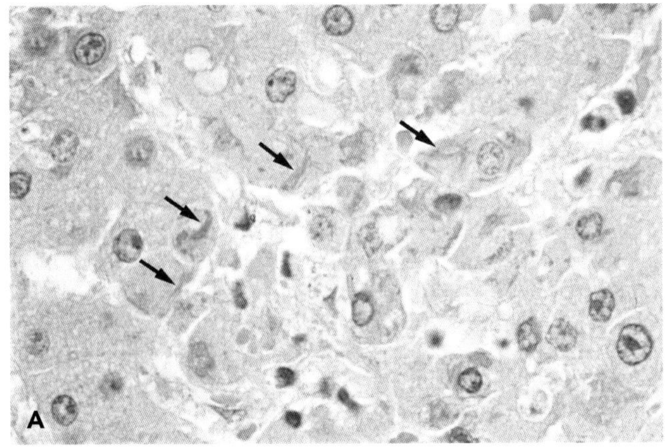
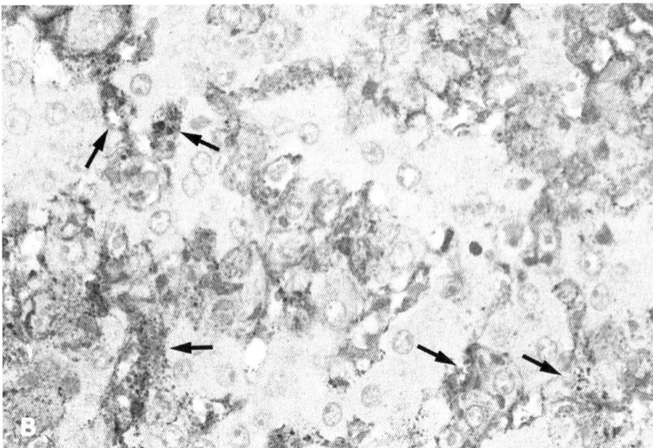
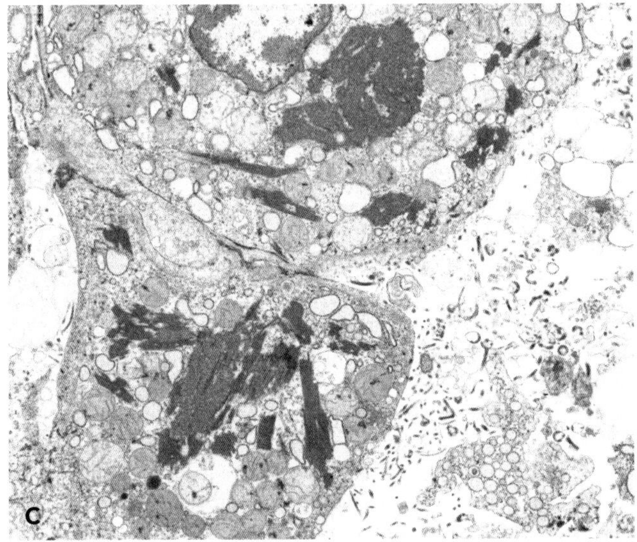

FIGURE 32.10. Pathologic features seen in the liver of an EBOV-infected human. A: Sinusoidal dilation and congestion and hepatocellular necrosis (H&E, 250X). Numerous filamentous intracellular ZEBOV inclusions (arrows) are seen in association with an area of coalescent hepatic necrosis. (B) Heavy immunohistochemical staining of ZEBOV antigens are seen in sinusoids, sinusoidal lining cells, and hepatocytes (arrows) (immunoalkaline phosphatase staining, naphthol fast red substrate with light hematoxylin counterstain, 158×). **C:** Electron micrograph of liver showing several large EBOV inclusions within infected hepatocytes (uranyl acetate and lead citrate stain, 6,600×). Abundant extracellular EBOV particles are also seen in hepatic sinusoids. Note variation in size and shape of viral particles associated with necrotic debris. (Courtesy of S. Zaki, Centers for Disease Control and Prevention, Atlanta, GA.)

tropism likely plays an equally important role in the disease pathogenesis. Elevations in liver enzymes are prominent findings in most filovirus infections.[109,135,137,174,175,201,273,342] Various degrees of hepatocellular degeneration and necrosis have been reported in filovirus infections of humans and nonhuman primates.[4,122,127,137,174,201,294,296,342,468,471] The hepatocellular lesions are generally not significant enough to explain the cause of death. However, impairment of the liver could contribute to the overall pathogenesis as hemorrhagic tendencies in some cases may be related to decreased synthesis of coagulation factors and other plasma proteins as a result of severe hepatocellular necrosis.

Adrenocortical infection and necrosis were also reported in filovirus infections of humans and nonhuman primates.[127,137,138,174,342] The adrenal cortex plays an important role in blood pressure homeostasis. Impaired secretion of steroid-synthesizing enzymes leads to hypotension and sodium loss with hypovolemia, which are important elements that have been noted in nearly all cases of filovirus disease. This suggests that impairment of adrenocortical function by viral infection may contribute to the development of shock that typifies late stages of disease.

Host Immune Response

For both EBOV and MARV, lymphoid depletion and necrosis are commonly seen in spleen, thymus, and lymph nodes of fatal cases and in experimentally infected nonhuman primates.[4,118,122,123,137,138,174,296,342,468,471] Although lymphoid tissues are primary sites of filovirus infection, there is usually little inflammatory cellular response in these tissues or other infected tissues. Lymphopenia is a consistent finding among filovirus infections of humans and nonhuman primates.[83,110,112,127,137,174,201,328,351,368] Despite the massive die off and loss of lymphocytes during filovirus infection, the lymphocytes themselves have not been shown to be infected. For both EBOV and MARV, large numbers of lymphocytes undergo apoptosis in humans and experimentally infected nonhuman primates[4,9,11,134,137,174,327,438] in part, explaining the progressive lymphopenia and lymphoid depletion at death. In the 2000 outbreak of SEBOV in Uganda, numbers of T lymphocytes were lower in fatal cases than in nonfatal cases.[351] In the ZEBOV and MARV macaque models, the lymphocyte loss appears to be greatest among the T-lymphocyte and NK-cell populations.[118,137,327]

The mechanism(s) for the underlying apoptosis and loss of "bystander" lymphocytes during the course of filovirus illness is unknown but is thought to be provoked through several different agonists or pathways. These pathways or processes may include the TNF-related apoptosis-inducing ligand (TRAIL) and Fas death receptor pathways,[137,177,438] impairment of dendritic cell function,[34,35,137,174,177,268] abnormal production of soluble mediators such as nitric oxide (NO) that have pro-apoptotic properties,[10,137,177,351] or possibly by direct interactions between lymphocytes and filovirus proteins. Severe cases of EHF have a prolonged high virus load, and one study of SEBOV-infected humans reported peripheral blood mononuclear cell unresponsiveness during the acute phase of disease.[351] The recognition of an immunosuppressive motif in the C-terminal region of the EBOV and MARV glycoproteins[48,411,460] supports the premise that filovirus particles/proteins may contribute in part to the dysfunction and/or loss of lymphocytes.[63] A recent study has also suggested that the dramatic loss of lymphocytes that occurs during filovirus infection may be a result of the superantigen activity of filoviruses.[247] In this study, human ZEBOV infection was associated with mRNA down-regulation of three T-cell receptor (TCR) Vβ subsets, indicating either anergy or deletion of these T-lymphocyte populations.

Filovirus infection of humans and nonhuman primates triggers the expression of a number of inflammatory mediators including the interferons, interleukin (IL)-6, IL-8, IL-10, IL-12, interferon-inducible protein (IP)-10, monocyte chemoattractant protein-1 (MCP-1), regulated upon activation, normal T-cell expressed and secreted (RANTES), TNF-α, and reactive oxygen and nitrogen species.[9,10,83,135,137,174,177,186,187,351,408,438] Infection of various primary human cells *in vitro* also shows that filovirus infection can trigger the production of many of these same inflammatory mediators.[96,146,159,160,177,374] Overall, it appears that virus-induced expression of these mediators results in an immunologic imbalance that contributes to the progression of disease. However, information regarding the inflammatory response after filovirus infection has not been fully delineated and there are some differences in data among studies. For example, high levels of circulating interferon (IFN)-α were noted in acute-phase sera of patients infected with ZEBOV in one study[408] but not detected in a subsequent similar study.[10] Such differences complicate interpretation of some *in vitro* data as well. The differences in profiles of circulating cytokines and chemokines may be due to factors other than the differences among the filovirus species or strains assessed such as genetic differences among patient populations, and in particular, differences related to the disease phase when the samples were obtained.

For ZEBOV, there has been a report of patients with asymptomatic, nonfatal infections.[244,246] It was proposed that these infections are controlled by an initial increase in cytokines including IL-1β, IL-6, and TNF-α that is followed by a return to baseline levels. Results of this study suggest that protection from development of a fatal infection may depend on an early and robust cytokine response; however, this remains to be proven. On the other hand, disease severity may also be increased by an inappropriate proinflammatory response early in the course of infection; therefore, the balance between protective and detrimental proinflammatory responses remains to be defined.

Inhibition of the type I IFN response appears to be a feature of filovirus pathogenesis, and was initially indicated by studies of ZEBOV-infected endothelial cells.[166,167] Subsequently, the EBOV protein VP35 was shown to function as a type I IFN antagonist[19,20–21] by blocking interferon regulatory factor (IRF-3) activation and possibly preventing transcription of IFN-β.[19] This activity of the ZEBOV VP35 has been linked to a C-terminal motif (^{305}RACQKSLR^{312})[172] that is similar in sequence to the RNA-binding domain of the influenza A NS1 protein (interferon antagonist). In addition to VP35, other studies suggest that EBOV VP24 expression interferes with type I IFN signaling[20,329]; mutations in VP24 have also been linked to adaptation of ZEBOV to produce lethal disease in mice[84] and guinea pigs.[412] Interestingly, MARV utilizes a different mechanism to evade the host IFN response. Recent studies have shown that MARV VP40 blocks the phosphorylation of Janus kinases and their target STAT proteins in response to type I and type II interferon and IL-6.[406] Mutations in VP40 have been linked to adaptation of MARV to produce lethal disease in mice[263] and guinea pigs.[262]

Several studies indicate an important role for reactive oxygen and nitrogen species in filovirus disease pathogenesis. Increased blood levels of NO were reported in nonhuman primates experimentally infected with ZEBOV[137,177] and were also noted in ZEBOV- and SEBOV-infected patients.[10,351] Significantly, increased blood levels of NO in patients was associated with mortality.[351] Abnormal NO production has been associated with a number of pathologic conditions including apoptosis of bystander lymphocytes (as noted previously), tissue damage, and loss of vascular integrity, which may contribute to virus-induced shock. NO is known to have both protective and caustic effects; this autotoxic overproduction may represent the host's endogenous counter-regulatory mechanism of protection against noxious agents, in this case the filoviruses. In general, microbes induce monocytes and macrophages to produce NO in an attempt to control infection. However, in the case of the filoviruses, monocytes and macrophages are preferred host cells for viral replication. Enhanced replication in these cells may in turn exacerbate disease by producing large amounts of NO, resulting in deleterious effects such as suppressive effects on lymphocyte proliferation and damage to other cells. NO is an important mediator of hypotension, a prominent finding in most VHFs including those caused by filoviruses.[140]

Together, the information collected to date suggests that an impaired and ineffective immune response leads to high levels of virus and proinflammatory mediators in the late stages of disease, which are important for the pathogenesis of hemorrhage and shock. Indeed, the prevailing hypothesis at this time is that infection and activation of monocytes/macrophages is fundamental to the development of EHF and MHF, and that it is the release of proinflammatory cytokines, chemokines, and other mediators that causes impairment of the vascular and coagulation systems (discussed in the following section) leading to multiple organ failure and a syndrome that in some ways resembles septic shock.[39,41,135,137,140,145,160,174,177,267,358,359,360,374,420]

Impairment of the Vascular System

The endothelium is thought to play an important role in the pathogenesis of EBOV and MARV, although studies defining the molecular mechanisms of endothelial impairment are incomplete. It was speculated that EBOV GP is the primary determinant of vascular cell injury and that EBOV infection of endothelial cells induces structural damage,[463] which could contribute to hemorrhagic diathesis. Human and nonhuman primate endothelial cells are susceptible to EBOV and MARV infection,[135,166,167,360,361] but while *in vitro* studies have reported some cytopathic effects associated with filovirus replication, in general, filovirus replication in nonhuman primates did not induce overt cytopathology. In fact, in one study using primary human endothelial cells, ZEBOV infection induced an upregulation of protective antiapoptotic genes.[146]

EBOV and MARV infection of endothelial cells *in vivo* has been documented, as noted previously, but human data is sparse. ZEBOV antigens were readily detected in endothelial cells of a variety of tissues during the 1995 Kikwit outbreak.[468] On the other hand, an immunohistochemical survey of a fatal case of MARV infection showed infrequent infection of endothelial cells in the tissues examined.[138] Clearly, disturbance of the blood tissue barrier is an important component of filovirus disease, and direct infection and destruction of endothelial cells cannot completely be dismissed as contributing to the hemorrhagic diathesis. However, histologic observations of autopsy tissues from several of the early filovirus outbreaks failed to identify the presence of vascular lesions[294] and there have been no reports of vascular lesions in any subsequent studies to date. There is also no evidence of significant vascular lesions in filovirus-infected nonhuman primates.[17,18,73,135,174,201,342]

In temporal studies in nonhuman primates, ZEBOV and MARV infection of endothelial cells was infrequent and primarily restricted to the terminal stages of disease.[135,174] In these animals, the endothelium remained relatively intact morphologically, although increased vascular permeability was observed. This is consistent with the imbalance of fluid between the intravascular and extravascular tissue spaces observed in patients. Using *in vitro* systems, increased endothelial permeability was associated temporally with the release of TNF-α from MARV-infected human monocytes/macrophages.[96] Subsequent studies showed that EBOV-induced cytokine release led to activation of the endothelium, as demonstrated by a breakdown of barrier function,[421] providing further evidence that endothelium may be affected indirectly by a mediator-induced inflammatory response of primary target cells more so than by direct filovirus replication-induced cytopathology. It is important to keep in mind, when comparing results among studies, that differences in findings could represent differences between macaque models and human disease possibly through the divergence of endothelial cell receptors such as DC-SIGNR. Nonetheless, and as noted previously, most studies indicate that changes in integrity of the endothelium are influenced primarily by local or systemic increases in levels of cytokines and other host-cell factors triggered by infection.

Impairment of the Coagulation System

Defects in blood coagulation and fibrinolysis during EBOV and MARV infections are manifested as petechiae (Fig. 32.11), ecchymoses, mucosal hemorrhages, congestion, and uncontrolled bleeding at venipuncture sites. However, massive loss of blood is infrequent and, when present, is primarily limited to the gastrointestinal tract. In fact, even in these cases, the amount of blood that is lost is not significant enough to account for death. Thrombocytopenia, consumption of clotting factors, and increased levels of fibrin degradation products are other indicators of the coagulopathy that characterizes EBOV and MARV infections.

Although disseminated intravascular coagulation (DIC) is often viewed as a prominent manifestation of filovirus infection in primates, evidence of DIC in human filovirus infections is sparse primarily due to difficulties encountered in performing studies in inaccessible geographic settings. Clinical laboratory data suggest that DIC is an important feature of human EHF.[197,334,449] D-dimer levels were substantially increased in all patients with SEBOV infections but were four times higher in patients with fatal disease than in patients who survived.[334] The coagulation picture is clearer for nonhuman primates. Numerous studies have shown histologic and biochemical evidence of DIC syndrome during EBOV infection in a variety of nonhuman primate species.[17,40,73,83,109,111,112,141,145,146,176,201,342] For MARV, histologic or biochemical evidence of DIC has been reported in a handful of available cases[122,138] and in a few studies of experimentally infected monkeys.[127,174,471]

Despite any differences between humans and nonhuman primates regarding DIC, impairment of coagulation ostensibly contributes to the disease pathogenesis of EHF and MHF (Figs. 32.9 and 32.11). The mechanism(s) responsible for triggering the coagulation disorders is not completely understood. Several studies suggest that development of coagulation abnormalities might occur much earlier than previously thought. For example, in one study, markedly elevated levels of D-dimers were detected one day after experimental infection of cynomolgus monkeys with ZEBOV, which occurred two days before the detection of viremia in these animals.[145] Although it is likely that the coagulopathy seen during filovirus infections is caused by a number of factors, particularly during the later stages of disease, data strongly implicate tissue factor expression/release from EBOV-infected monocytes/macrophages as a key factor that induces the development of coagulation irregularities.[145] Of course, as noted previously, other factors may also contribute to the coagulopathy associated with filovirus infections. For example, impairment of the fibrinolytic system was documented by rapid declines in plasma levels of protein C during the course of ZEBOV infection of cynomolgus and rhesus monkeys.[83,145,176]

Virulence

The virulence of filoviruses in humans is highly variable depending primarily on the species or strain; a similar variability seems to recapitulate well in nonhuman primates. Among the EBOV species, ZEBOV is the most virulent and REBOV appears to be the least virulent. Infection of nonhuman primates with ZEBOV usually progresses rapidly and is uniformly lethal, with as little as one infectious unit being required to cause disease. The course of disease appears to be influenced by the dose of filovirus used. As an example, cynomolgus macaques exposed by intramuscular injection with a low challenge dose of ZEBOV (10 pfu) succumbed to infection 8 to 12 days after challenge,[377] but when exposed to a high dose (1,000 pfu) died 5 to 8 days after challenge.[137,143] Likewise, a similar protraction of disease course in nonhuman primates concurrent with serial dilution was noted for MARV.[153]

In human cases, route of infection ostensibly affects the disease course and the outcome. The mean incubation period for cases of ZEBOV known to be due to injection was 6.3 days, versus 9.5 days for contact exposures.[43] Moreover, the CFR in this 1976 ZEBOV outbreak was 100% (85 of 85) in cases associated with injection compared with ~80% (119 of 149) in cases of known contact exposure.[43] Although the nonhuman primate models appear to be exquisitely sensitive to the filoviruses compared to humans, particularly for ZEBOV, this observation in part could relate to the fact that most nonhuman primate studies involve intramuscular injection with very high challenge doses.

Fewer studies have evaluated the pathogenesis of SEBOV in nonhuman primates.[86,109] The disease course in experimentally infected rhesus and cynomolgus macaques appears much

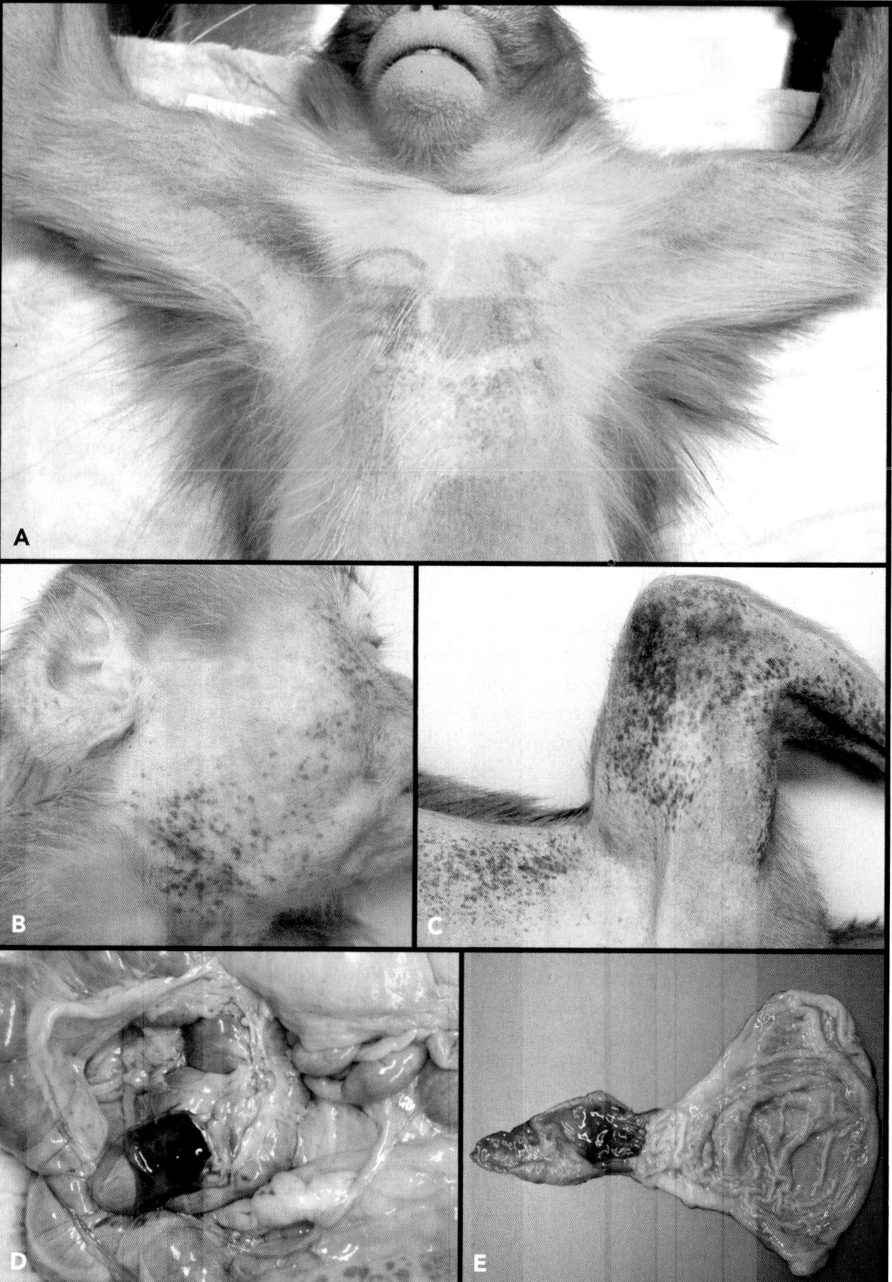

FIGURE 32.11. Hemorrhagic manifestations seen in nonhuman primates acutely infected with filoviruses. Shown are examples of petechiae evident on **(A)** the upper torso and arms of a rhesus macaque infected with ZEBOV (strain Mayinga 1976) **(A)**, the head and neck of a rhesus macaque infected with MARV (strain Angola 2005) **(B)**, and the lower trunk and leg of a cynomolgus macaque infected with SEBOV (strain Gulu 2000) **(C)**. Also shown are a gastroduodenal lesion **(D)** and hemorrhage in the ileum **(E)** of a SEBOV-infected cynomolgus macaque (Courtesy of A. Sanchez and P. Rollin (A), Centers for Disease Control, Atlanta; T.W. Geisbert (B, C) US Army Medical Research Institute for Infectious Diseases (USAMRIID), Frederick; and T. Larsen (D,E), USAMRIID, Frederick).

slower than that seen in ZEBOV infections, and the rates of survival appear consistent with human disease. SEBOV infection was not lethal in a small cohort of African green monkeys nor was REBOV.[109] Similar to SEBOV, the disease course in REBOV-infected cynomolgus monkeys is protracted.[205] Experimental infection of cynomolgus macaques by intramuscular injection with 1,000 pfu of SEBOV results in 50% to 100% mortality, with deaths typically occurring 7 to 12 days after infection. In comparison, experimental infection of cynomolgus macaques with 1,000 pfu of REBOV results in 80% to 100% mortality, with deaths usually occurring 8 to 21 days after infection. Recent studies have shown similar results for CIEBOV and BEBOV. Specifically, experimental infection of cynomolgus macaques with 1,000 pfu of CIEBOV resulted in 60% mortality, with deaths occurring 12 to 14 days after infection[131] while infection with 1,000 pfu of BEBOV resulted in 75% mortality, with deaths occurring 11 to 14 days after infection.[92,175]

There appears to be some difference in virulence among the strains of MARV. Historically, virulence of the MARV strains in humans has been comparable to SEBOV. However, virulence of the recently isolated Angola strain appears to be more consistent with ZEBOV. Most strains of MARV produce near uniformly lethal infections in cynomolgus and rhesus macaques. Among the MARV strains, infections of macaques with the Angola strain appear to progress more rapidly than other strains. For example, challenge of rhesus macaques by intramuscular injection with 1,000 pfu of the Musoke strain produces a uniformly lethal infection, with deaths occurring 10 to 12 days after infection, whereas an identical challenge of rhesus macaques with 1,000 pfu of the Angola strain resulted in deaths occurring 6 to 8 days after challenge.[127]

Currently, the variability in virulence in primates within and between species of filoviruses is unclear, but for EBOV there has been some speculation that the GP has a major influence on virulence.[463] Studies have shown that unlike ZEBOV, expression of the GP from REBOV did not disrupt the vasculature of human blood vessels. It was initially reported that the expression of the EBOV GP caused significant cell death in cultured cells[462,463]; however, subsequent studies showed that most of the detached cells (>90%) were still viable,[57,367] suggesting that GP expression may interfere with cell attachment without triggering cell death. It has been speculated that EBOV may control GP cytotoxicity by regulating its expression through RNA editing,[415] but this mechanism needs to be studied in cells derived from the natural host and reconciled with the importance/role of sGP expression.

EBOV produces five soluble glycoproteins during infection: sGP, Δ-peptide, GP_1, $GP_{1,2\Delta}$, and the newly identified ssGP.[281] MARV produces GP_1 and presumably $GP_{1,2\Delta}$.[105] Upon the discovery of sGP, it was logical to attempt to correlate the higher pathogenicity of EBOV with its expression; however, the EBOV-like virulence and mortality rates associated with the Angola strain of MARV[55] dispel any such associations. Additionally, the lower virulence of REBOV and CIEBOV does not support a role in virulence for sGP.[105] The contribution of the secreted GPs to the disease pathogenesis of EBOV and MARV remains largely unknown, but recent studies have begun to examine the effects of EBOV GPs on the host response to infection. Initial studies suggested that the EBOV sGP interfered with innate immunity by binding to CD16b and inhibiting neutrophil activation.[227,462] However, subsequent studies questioned these findings and in contrast showed that neutrophils do not express a receptor for EBOV sGP.[376] Other studies have evaluated the role of the secreted GPs in activating macrophages and endothelial cells. For example, studies using primary human macrophages and endothelial cells concluded that the presentation of the EBOV $GP_{1,2}$ in a membrane-bound form (on virions or VLPs) is sufficient for activation of these cells.[420,421] However, these studies also showed that none of the four secreted EBOV GPs was capable of activating human macrophages, and neither sGP nor delta peptide were capable of activating endothelial cells. In fact, sGP protected endothelial cell barrier function[420] and could counteract or lessen the cytotoxicity caused by EBOV GP. Furthermore, it has been proposed that soluble glycoproteins circulating in the blood of virus-infected animals may play an important role in pathogenesis by efficiently blocking the activity of virus-neutralizing antibodies.[78,105,200]

Host Genetics

Recent studies have shown that the outcome of filovirus infection could in part be determined by host genetics. Sequence-based HLA-B typing was performed on patients from the 2000 outbreak of SEBOV in Uganda.[355] In this study, statistically significant associations were found between certain sets of alleles and either fatal or nonfatal disease outcomes. Alleles B*67 and B*15 were associated with fatal outcomes, whereas B*07 and B*14 were associated with nonfatal outcomes. In a different study, the association of KIR genotype with disease outcome was determined by comparing genotypes of a Gabonese control population, IgG+ contacts, survivors, and fatalities of ZEBOV infection.[439] In this study, the activating KIR2DS1 and KIR2DS3 genes were associated with fatal outcome.

Persistence

As noted earlier, mortality rates for EBOV and MARV are high and few patients survive infection. In survivors, levels of circulating virus in the blood decline as the patient recovers.[235,351] However, during the recovery phase several lines of evidence suggest that EBOV and MARV may persist in humans in immunologically privileged sites. In one laboratory-acquired infection, EBOV was isolated from semen samples 39 and 61 days after the onset of illness.[87] After the 1995 outbreak of ZEBOV in Kikwit, infectious virus was recovered from seminal fluid of one patient 82 days after disease onset, while viral RNA was detected in semen samples of three additional patients between 63 and 101 days after the onset of illness.[333,338] For MARV, sexual transmission was reported in one case during the original outbreak in Marburg, Germany in 1967, with semen apparently containing infectious virus more than 12 weeks after clinical recovery.[275]

EPIDEMIOLOGY

Because much of the early serosurvey data has been based on the fluorescent antibody test, a subjective and unreliable assay, identification of the geographic range of filoviruses is more accurately determined from filovirus outbreaks. ZEBOV, SEBOV, and CIEBV and BEBOV are found in the African tropical forest or nearby savanna and occasionally emerge often during the rainy season.[155] REBOV has been linked only to a single export nonhuman primate facility in the Philippines and more recently to a few pig farms in the country.[14,285] Based on current data and the new discovery of REBOV on pig farms in the Philippines,[14] REBOV is most likely an Asian filovirus, possibly derived from certain fruit bat species in the forests of the Philippines.[69] Alternatively, the REBOV strains could represent derivates from a single introduction (most likely Africa) through bat migration or importation, and subsequent establishment and circulation in the Philippines. MARV has apparently been contracted in forested and derived areas of Kenya, Uganda, Zimbabwe, the DRC, and recently Angola, but in several cases the epidemiologic information does not provide an adequate description of the environment where infections were suspected to have occurred. The European outbreak from 1967 was initiated through imported infected African green monkeys and could be traced to a source in Uganda. The animals were compounded in Entebbe (central holding station at Lake Victoria) and shipped via London (where they had potential contact with other animals) to Germany and the former Yugoslavia.

The epidemiology of human infections in nature, besides the internationally recognized outbreaks, is unknown. However, the time elapsed between occurrence of the index cases and the recognition of the subsequent large outbreaks suggests that sporadic cases of unrecognized filovirus infections could readily pass unnoticed.[212] The number of such identified clusters in the past decade may represent a combination of unidentified ecologic factors and increasing diagnostic interest. Serologic surveys revealed EBOV antibody prevalence from 10.2% among gold panners in Gabon to 9.3% among rural villagers in the

DRC using enzyme-linked immunoabsorbent assay (ELISA)-based technology. EBOV infection, potentially with nonpathogenic strains/variants or strains/variants of low pathogenicity, may be frequent in select rural African populations.[147,216]

Whatever the source of the initial index case, person-to-person transmission is the means by which human filovirus outbreaks have been propagated. This generally involves intimate contact; secondary attack rates have not exceeded 10% to 15%, indicating that transmission is not efficient. However, this risk increases as a function of contact. For example, during the 1976 SEBOV outbreak 23% of family members sleeping in the same room as the patient were infected, compared to 81% of persons providing active nursing care to a patient.[13] The need for this intimacy is reflected in the relative paucity of infected children, who are less likely to be primary care givers for ill family members.[79] Nosocomial transmission is a special problem and hospitals have often served as a source of disease amplification into the community and to health care workers. A quarter of all cases during the 1995 ZEBOV outbreak were among health care workers. Extreme care should be taken with infected blood, secretions, excretions, tissues, and hospital materials and waste. Well-documented and surreptitious reuse of needles and syringes has also played a role in these outbreaks. No person whose contact was exclusively parenteral during the 1976 ZEBOV outbreak survived. Sexual transmission has been reported with MARV and can also be assumed for EBOV (discussed earlier).

There is a striking difference in the ZEBOV epidemics in Gabon/RC compared to those caused by most other filoviruses including ZEBOV outbreaks at other sites. Most of the epidemics in this area are limited in case numbers and are related to contact with wildlife (chimpanzees, gorillas, and other species). Epidemiologic and genetic investigations showed that outbreaks resulted from the introduction of distinct strains, indicating that multiple ZEBOV strains were co-circulating in this region. All index cases (mainly hunters) were infected by handling dead or wounded animals, and subsequently led to person-to-person transmission within their families. In many instances human infections have been preceded by disease in wildlife, and these infected animals acted as either dead-end hosts or interim/amplification hosts.[106,250] Multiple introductions of MARV lineages were also noticed in the MARV outbreak in Durba/Watsa.[22,23,65,400,401]

Filoviruses are transmissible to nonhuman primates in the laboratory by aerosols,[25,217] and virions have been identified in alveoli of infected monkeys and humans.[141,202,469,470] Furthermore, the outbreak caused by REBOV among quarantined monkeys in 1989/1990 was strongly suggestive of droplet and/or small-particle aerosol transmission. However, these animals were housed in a poorly ventilated building in which aerosols could have been generated by cleaning procedures.[205] Aerosol transmission has not been unequivocally implicated in human outbreaks to date. Interestingly, extremely efficient person-to-person transmission has been attributed to two individuals who may have been the source of infection for over 50 cases in the 1995 ZEBOV outbreak.[223] The mechanism of this heightened transmission was not identified, although contact with the patient and/or cadaver was strongly implicated. Despite little evidence for aerosol transmission in nature, this is the most likely route used for delivery of filoviruses in a deliberate act.

ECOLOGY

The natural reservoir(s) of filoviruses remains elusive despite increased numbers of outbreaks and opportunities to investigate their origins.[106,155,318] As classical zoonotic agents, these viruses likely persist in an animal (or several animals) or arthropods, which transmit the virus directly to humans, great apes, nonhuman primates, or an interim amplifying host.[113,288]

Lack of replication in arthropod cells or inoculated arthropods[404] argues against such an intermediary for filoviruses, and extensive arthropod field surveys have failed to detect the presence of EBOV. It has been suggested that human contact with filovirus-infected bats may have initiated the early SEBOV outbreaks in Sudan,[8] the ZEBOV outbreak in the DRC in 2007[248] and the MARV infections in Kenya.[218,371] In addition, the outbreak of MHF in the northeast region of the DRC had some connection, directly or indirectly, with a bat-infested gold mine.[22] Interestingly, experimental infection of wild African fruit and insectivorous bats has shown that these animals are capable of supporting the replication of EBOV without becoming ill, despite high levels of circulating virus.[383] Recent findings of asymptomatic EBOV and MARV infections in fruit bats are additional evidence that such animals are capable of harboring filoviruses and may serve as reservoir species; in particular Rousettus *aegyptiacus* for MARV.[249,400] Because persistently infected hosts are postulated for zoonotic diseases, chronic infection in bats or other small animal species is likely involved in the ecology of filoviruses.[317,318]

The epizootics caused by REBOV have raised the question as to whether nonhuman primates act as reservoirs for filoviruses.[285] This seems unlikely for the African filoviruses, which are highly pathogenic for nonhuman primates, and this trait is generally incongruous with the concept of a reservoir host. In addition, there has been no evidence for latent virus infection in these animals.[109,113] If monkeys are not the reservoir, they at least act to amplify the virus in the wild, and unexplained disease/mortality in these animals could be an indicator of impending transmission in humans. This is supported by reported deaths in monkey species prior to outbreaks of CIEBOV in the Tai Forest,[243] several of the ZEBOV outbreaks occurring since 1996 in Gabon,[250,252] and a more recent outbreak of ZEBOV in the RC.[115] Investigations into the outbreaks in Gabon/RC confirmed this concept and showed multiple introductions of different ZEBOV strains from an unknown reservoir into wildlife that then served as sources of initial human infections.[250,337] In contrast, filovirus sequences from patients involved in a distinct epidemic chain of human cases were conserved, indicating that these episodes were mainly caused by single-source introductions.[245,250,333] Thus, it appears that distinct filovirus strains have evolved to occupy undefined ecologic niches throughout the forests of Central Africa, and that the potential for human contact with these agents is greatly increased when viruses are circulating in indigenous nonhuman primate populations.

Beginning in 1994, the frequency of filovirus outbreaks in Africa increased and shows no sign of diminishing. Future episodes of EBOV and MARV transmission are unavoidable, which poses a serious risk to human populations, but also threatens to decimate the world's largest populations of gorillas and chimpanzees.[100,250,422] This dangerous situation makes the identification of the natural reservoir an important objective for the scientific community, which needs to improve and formulate new working hypotheses and strategies. Efforts at ecologic niche modeling from data gleaned from outbreaks and sporadic cases have revealed a different Afrotropic distribution for filoviruses, with EBOV more likely to occur in the humid rain forests of Central and Western Africa and MARV in the drier and more open areas of Central and East Africa.[155,317] Future surveillance at existing field sites (e.g., Tai Forest, Ivory Coast; Watsa/Durba, DRC; Gabon, DC; Uíge, Angola) should focus on affected animal populations, such as great apes, and possibly include the use of sentinel animals. Experimental studies of potential reservoir species should be initiated and/or intensified to better understand filovirus persistence and transmission.

CLINICAL FEATURES

Filovirus infections are generally the most severe of the VHFs, but only limited information is derived from close observations of acute human cases. Differences in the clinical syndromes caused by filoviruses may exist, but there have been few opportunities for close observation of the diseases under favorable conditions.[13,51,97,102,114,122,197,210,211,276,282,312] The abrupt onset follows an incubation period of 2 to 21 days, averaging 4 to 10 days, and is characterized by flu-like symptoms (fever, chills, malaise, and myalgia; Fig. 32.12). The subsequent signs and symptoms indicate multisystem involvement and include systemic (prostration), gastrointestinal (anorexia, nausea, vomiting, abdominal pain, diarrhea), respiratory (chest pain, shortness of breath, cough), vascular (conjunctival injection, postural hypotension, edema), and neurologic (headache, confusion, coma) manifestations. Hemorrhagic manifestations develop during the peak of the illness and include petechiae, ecchymoses, uncontrolled oozing from venipuncture sites, mucosal hemorrhages, and postmortem evidence of visceral hemorrhagic effusions. Often a macropapular rash associated with varying degrees of erythema appears by days 5 to 7 of the illness; this is a valuable differential diagnostic feature and is usually followed by desquamation in survivors. Abdominal pain is sometimes associated with hyperamylasemia and true pancreatitis. In later stages, shock, convulsions, severe metabolic disturbances, and, in more than half the cases, diffuse coagulopathy supervenes (Fig. 32.12).

Laboratory parameters are less characteristic but the following findings are associated with the disease. There is an early leukopenia (as low as 1,000/μL) with lymphopenia and subsequent neutrophilia, left shift with atypical lymphocytes, thrombocytopenia (50,000–100,000/μL), markedly elevated serum transaminase levels (AST typically exceeding ALT), hyperproteinemia, and proteinuria. Prothrombin and partial thromboplastin times are prolonged and fibrin split products are detectable. In a later stage, secondary bacterial infection may lead to elevated white blood counts.

Nonfatal cases have fever for about 5 to 9 days and improvement typically occurs around days 7 to 11, about the time the humoral antibody response is noted.[235] Convalescence is prolonged and sometimes associated with myelitis, recurrent hepatitis, psychosis or uveitis.[97,102,276,282,338] There is an increased risk of abortion for pregnant women, and clinical observations indicate a high death rate for children of infected mothers. Fatal cases develop clinical signs early during infection and demise typically occurs between days 6 and 16, due to hemorrhage and hypovolemic shock. The mortality from ZEBOV infections is high (60–90%), SEBOV and BEBOV somewhat lower (50–60% and 25–35%, respectively), and MARV probably around 70% to 85%, with the exception of the outbreak in Europe (only 23%).[97,282] The single observed Ivory Coast infection case survived, as did a second serologically diagnosed case. The few REBOV infections/exposures identified so far in Reston, Virginia and in the Philippines had no symptoms, but one patient (accidentally infected during a necropsy of an infected monkey) yielded a serum virus isolate. Thus, it is generally assumed that REBOV has a reduced pathogenicity or is apathogenic for humans, but this judgement may be premature and needs further investigation.

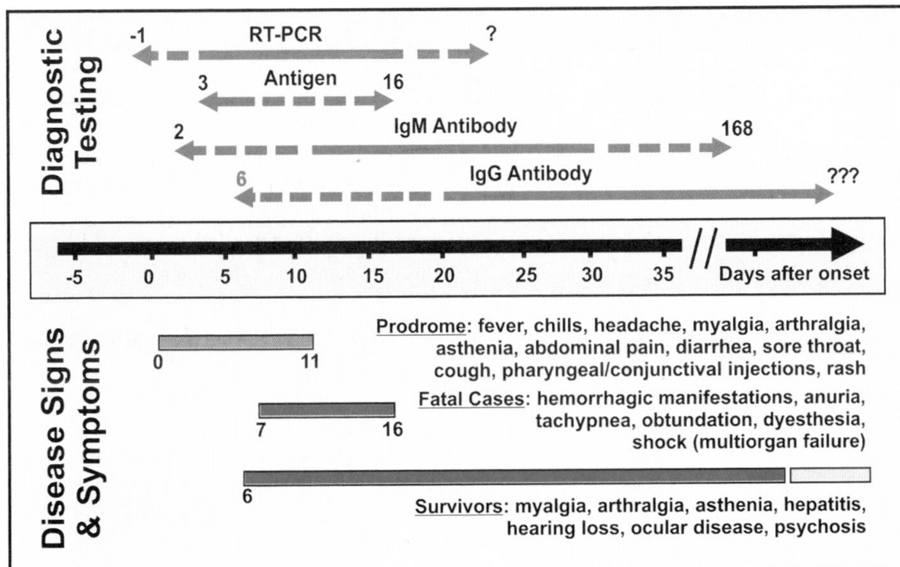

FIGURE 32.12. **Graph showing time frames, relative to the time of disease onset, for the sensitivity of diagnostic assays and the development of signs and symptoms associated with severe filovirus infections.** *Dashed areas on arrows* indicate approximate times where clinical features of disease or assay targets can be negative/absent or difficult to detect.

DIAGNOSIS

Clinical Diagnosis

Filovirus disease can be suspected in acute febrile patients with symptoms, as described earlier, and a history of travel to an endemic area. Identification may be difficult, due to a wide variety of infectious diseases causing similar clinical symptomatology. The most common causes of severe, acute, febrile diseases in filovirus-endemic areas are malaria and typhoid fever. A wide range of infectious diseases must also be considered, such as shigellosis, meningococcal septicemia, plague, leptospirosis, anthrax, relapsing fever, typhus, murine typhus, yellow fever, Chikungunya fever, and fulminant viral hepatitis. Rural travel, jungle or cave exposure, treatment in local hospitals, contact with sick persons or wild and domestic animals, particularly monkeys and apes, are useful historical features, especially in travelers returning from Africa. For patients with filovirus disease, prostration, lethargy, wasting, and diarrhea seem to be more severe than is seen with other VHF infections; the appearance of a characteristic rash is useful in narrowing the differential diagnosis. Diagnosis of single cases is extremely difficult, but the occurrence of clusters of cases with prodromal fever followed by hemorrhagic diatheses and person-to-person transmission are suggestive of VHF and require the implementation of containment procedures.

Laboratory Diagnosis

Despite the capabilities of laboratory diagnostics, it should be kept in mind that initial diagnosis of filovirus infections will be based on clinical assessment. Clinical microbiology and public health laboratories are generally ill equipped to diagnose VHF infections, particularly those caused by filoviruses, so specimens should be sent to national and/or international reference laboratories capable of performing the required testing. In addition, many nations encounter difficulties in sample transport, which can cause substantial delays in laboratory response. Once samples are received by appropriate reference laboratories, response is fairly efficient.

During outbreaks health care workers, who have direct contact with patients, are at high risk for infection; adequate barrier nursing precautions should be implemented in the collection of samples.[314,373] Special care should be taken to avoid needle sticks and to immediately dispose of contaminated material in an appropriate manner. Collection of specimens should be done facilitating sterility and prevention of cross-contamination of specimens. This has become particularly important for ultrasensitive techniques such as reverse transcriptase–polymerase chain reaction (RT-PCR).[373] Filoviruses are relatively stable and infectious particles can survive less than favorable handling and shipping for months. Care should be taken to ensure the physical integrity for biosafety reasons and to maintain an adequate refrigerated or frozen state for biologic integrity of the sample to maximize the reliability of diagnostic results.

Laboratory diagnosis of filovirus infections can be achieved in two ways: measurement of host-specific immune responses to infection and detection of virus particles or particle components (RNA and protein) in infected individuals (Table 32.3). Today, RT-PCR[81,151,350,373,402] and antigen detection ELISA[193,234,235,265,266,304,373] are the primary test systems to diagnose an acute infection. For antibody detection the most commonly used assays are direct IgG and IgM ELISAs and IgM capture ELISA.[195,235,236,373] RT-PCR, antigen detection, and serology can be performed on materials that have been rendered noninfectious by radiation or chemicals. Gamma irradiation is an efficient means of inactivating specimens prior to antigen detection and serology and is achieved by exposure to a cobalt-60 source. Samples for RT-PCR (nucleic acid extraction) can be treated with guanidinium isothiocyanate, a chaotropic agent that denatures proteins and renders the sample noninfectious. These methods of inactivation allow the safe manipulation of material outside of the containment laboratory, where work can be carried out more expediently.

Other serologic tests that have been used in filovirus diagnosis are the western blot assay (can be used as a confirmatory assay) and the indirect immunofluorescence assay (IFA; occasionally used as a screening assay) on gamma-inactivated, fixed

TABLE 32.3 Laboratory Assays Used in the Diagnosis of Filovirus Infections

Test	Target	Source	Remarks
A. Primary Assays			
Polymerase chain reaction (PCR)	Viral nucleic acid	Blood, serum, tissues	Rapid and sensitive; requires special equipment
Antigen enzyme-linked immunosorbent assay (ELISA)	Viral antigen	Blood, serum, tissues	Rapid and sensitive; requires special equipment, but capable of high throughput
ELISA (IgM capture, IgG)	Antiviral antibodies	Serum	Rapid, specific, and sensitive; slower than IFA when testing small numbers of specimens
B. Confirmatory Assays			
Indirect immunofluorescence assay (IFA)	Antiviral antibodies	Serum	Rapid and simple to perform, but prone to nonspecific positives and subjective interpretation
Western blot	Antiviral antibodies	Serum	Protein specific; interpretation sometimes difficult
Immunohistochemistry	Viral antigen	Tissues (e.g., skin, liver)	Slow; material inactivated
Fluorescence assay (FA)	Viral antigen	Tissues (e.g., liver)	Rapid and easy, but interpretation is subjective
Electron microscopy	Viral particle	Blood, tissues	Unique morphology (immunostaining possible); insensitive and requires expensive equipment
Virus isolation	Viral particle	Blood, tissues	Slow; virus isolate available for studies

cells infected with EBOV or MARV or containing expressed recombinant filovirus proteins.[194,215,216,373] Due to relatively high viremia levels in humans, electron microscopy has been helpful in diagnosis of filovirus infections but is not generally used.[139,144,203,294,364] Filovirus particles present in sera and cell culture fluids (primary isolation) can be directly visualized by negative staining, and can be easily detected in thin sections of infected tissues, especially the liver and spleen. IHC on formalin-fixed material and paraffin-embedded tissues can be used for detection of filoviruses[203,470] as well as immunofluorescence (IF) on impression smears of tissues.[335] IHC is a very useful surveillance assay especially when no other specimens are available during an outbreak. Advantages of IHC testing include its simplicity and specificity but also lack of a need for enhanced biocontainment,[260,469,470] as formalin-fixed biopsy specimens are not infectious, are easily generated, and can be transported without special precautions or refrigeration.

Isolation of infectious virus from serum or other clinical material is a relatively simple and sensitive procedure and should always be attempted if BSL-4 containment is available. Filoviruses grow well in a large variety of cell lines, although Vero cells (or the Vero E6 clone) have been most used, but often upon primary isolation the development of CPE may be subtle or lacking. Guinea pigs can be used for primary isolation of those filoviruses that initially do not grow well in tissue culture, but repeated passaging is usually required to produce severe/fatal disease. In addition, broad clinical syndrome–based technologies have been developed on the basis of multiplex PCR and pan-microbial oligonucleotide array technologies.[259,309] These assays, however, have yet to be implemented into common diagnostic settings.

Of the available techniques for diagnosis, antigen-capture ELISA and RT-PCR are today the most useful for making a diagnosis in an acute clinical setting. Viral antigen/nucleic acid can be detected in blood as early as day –1 until past day 16 post-onset of symptoms (Fig. 32.12).[97,282,338] RT-PCR assays seem to be favored by many investigators because BSL-4 biocontainment is not necessary after proper inactivation, as well as the sensitivity/specificity and rapidity of the technique.[151,373] However, the diagnosis of index cases of outbreaks or of single imported cases should not be solely based on RT-PCR. Confirmation by an independent assay such as antigen-capture ELISA should always be attempted. When case confirmatory techniques and biocontainment (virus isolation) are not available, RT-PCR on an independent target gene and/or independent sample should be the minimum confirmation.[151] In such instances it may be useful to seek confirmation through another reference laboratory, which is always preferred.

Serology can be useful for confirmation, but it should be kept in mind that a negative serology is inconclusive because filovirus-infected individuals often die without seroconversion. Based on past investigations, IgM antibodies can appear as early as 2 days post-onset of symptoms and disappear between 30 and 168 days after infection. IgG-specific antibodies develop between days 6 and 18 after onset and persist for many years (Fig. 32.12).[97,282,338] A rising IgM or IgG titer constitutes a strong presumptive diagnosis. However, a single positive result should be confirmed on a follow-up sample, preferably at least a week apart. Decreasing IgM and/or increasing IgG titers (fourfold) in successive paired sera are highly suggestive of a recent infection.

Standardization and evaluation of diagnostic procedures for filoviruses is difficult because of the restricted availability of virologic and clinical material. The European Network for Imported Viral Diseases (ENIVD) provides external quality assurance for filovirus RT-PCR diagnostic procedures.[303] Continued and extended quality assurance studies are required to maximize the robustness of filovirus diagnostic procedures.

Filovirus outbreaks usually occur in remote areas where sophisticated medical support systems are limited and timely diagnostic services are extremely difficult to provide. Provision of a fieldable laboratory offering basic diagnostics for filoviruses and other agents that may be confounding to the diagnosis could aid in the management of patients specifically and the outbreak in general. The development of truly portable real-time thermocyclers and fieldable immunologic assays has made the deployment of a field diagnostic laboratory a reasonable undertaking. In setting up field diagnostics, the initial and most important consideration is to minimize the exposure of workers to infectious materials. This can be accomplished by setting up a portable class III biosafety cabinet, but the use of personal protective equipment, such as powered air-purifying respirators (PAPRs) is perhaps a more convenient and realistic means of protecting workers processing infectious material in the field. Clinical and other specimens can be safely heat inactivated (together with an appropriate ionic or nonionic detergent) for serologic analysis and with guanidinium isothiocyanate buffers for RNA isolation.[151,402]

PREVENTION AND CONTROL

Patient Management

Devising a strategy for the prevention of primary filovirus infections of humans is problematic, as the natural reservoirs and factors that affect filovirus movement in the wild are still largely unknown. Assuming that bats serve as a reservoir, proper education seems the most feasible way of prevention.[248] Except for instances in which infected great apes have been the source of infections, it is difficult to identify a human index case, let alone the type of contact that initiated the infection. However, once it enters a human or nonhuman primate population, it is clear that the virus is spread through close contact with acutely infected members. Isolation of patients and use of strict barrier nursing procedures, including the use of protective clothing and respirators, have been sufficient to rapidly interrupt transmission in the hospital.[65,211] Cadavers from fatal cases represent a residual risk for community members, and unprotected handling of corpses should be avoided.[332] Under specific circumstances, the use of full-face respirators or PAPRs for protection against aerosols may be indicated (79; http://www.cdc.gov/ncidod/dvrd/spb/mnpages/vhfmanual.htm); an N95/N100 mask with face shielding can provide a good level of protection. Methods for implementing barrier nursing, waste disposal, and other key elements (inexpensive and practical in Africa) have been devised, and a field-tested manual is available.[260] One of the important elements is provision of sterile equipment for injections, which are remarkably and tragically lacking in Africa today.

Therapeutic Options

Filovirus infections are currently managed solely with supportive therapy, which is directed towards maintenance of effective blood volume and electrolyte balance. Shock, cerebral edema,

TABLE 32.4 Selected Promising Treatment Options

Treatment option	Success	Issues/concerns
Antibody therapy	Efficacy in rodents and nonhuman primates	Escape mutants; genetic variability; antibody-dependent enhancement (ADE)
Antisense oligonucleotides		
Phosphorodiamidate morpholino oligonucleotides (PMOs)	Efficacy in rodents and nonhuman primates (NHPs) (prophylactic only)	Genetic variation; delivery
Small interfering RNAs (siRNAs)	Efficacy in rodents and NHPs	Genetic variation; delivery
Inflammatory modulators		
Type I interferons	Efficacy in rodents but not in NHPs	Manipulation of immune system
S-adenosylhomocysteine hydrolase (SAH) inhibitors	Efficacy in rodents but not in NHPs	Manipulation of immune system
Coagulation modulators		
Heparin sulfate	Efficacy in humans questionable; not tested in animals	Manipulation of coagulation
Tissue factor pathway inhibitors	Not tested in rodents; partial protection in NHPs	Manipulation of coagulation
Activated protein C	Not tested in rodents; partial protection in NHPs	Manipulation of coagulation
Postexposure vaccination		
Vesicular stomatitis virus (VSV)	Efficacy in rodents and NHPs	Efficacy dependent on species and treatment start

Note: Only approaches that have shown *in vivo* efficacy have been listed.

renal failure, coagulation disorders, and secondary bacterial infection may be life threatening and have to be managed. Antipyretics and pain medication should be provided as needed. At present, there is no proof that any strategy has been successful; however, detailed knowledge of filovirus replication, pathogenesis, and host responses to infections has steadily identified new targets for therapeutic intervention (Table 32.4). Although no single treatment is likely to be sufficiently potent to offset the severe and rapid progression of EHF and MHF, a combination of therapies (with different mechanistic actions) may be a more effective approach to treating infections. Slowing disease progression may provide enough time for the adaptive immune response to develop enough momentum to clear the infection.[42,97,101,282]

Over the years, several experimental therapeutic approaches that target the virus or the host immune response have been evaluated in different animal models.[30,42,97,282] The use of specific antisera as a therapy for filovirus infections (Table 32.4) has been investigated since their discovery,[33,238] but their development has been complicated by lack of efficacy and reports on the potential of antibody-dependent enhancement (ADE) of infection as demonstrated *in vitro*[388,394] but not yet confirmed *in vivo*.[132] Convalescent blood and serum have been administered to human patients,[87,293] but any beneficial results from these treatments are either unsupported or conflicting. Antibody therapy with equine anti-EBOV immunoglobulin has failed to protect nonhuman primates from fatal outcomes.[206,284] However, more recently, the first successful IgG transfer that protected rhesus macaques from lethal MARV and EBOV challenge was reported,[82] which might indicate that antibody therapy could be more beneficial. *In vitro* neutralizing EBOV GP-specific monoclonal antibodies generated from different species, including human, showed distinct protective and therapeutic properties in rodent and nonhuman primate models.[277,308,311,325a,389,446] Although no definite therapeutic conclusion can yet be drawn from the current studies, passively acquired antibodies can to a certain extent reduce the viral burden during infection, which could be useful in combination with other pharmaceutical agents.

Because filoviruses inhibit the expression of type I interferons (discussed earlier), treatment with exogenous IFN would seem to be an obvious therapeutic approach (Table 32.4). However, despite efficacy in the mouse model, IFN-α treatment was less effective in guinea pigs and failed to increase survival rate in nonhuman primates, despite a delay in disease onset, viremia, and death.[204] The beneficial effect of S-adenosylhomocysteine hydrolase (SAH) inhibitors on EBOV infection in mice[185] has been partially associated with a mechanistically unexplained strong increase of IFN-α production. Therefore, improved formulations, selective use of IFN types and IFN-α subtypes, and the combination with other treatment options may be useful.

The viral transcription and replication machinery is an important antiviral target (Table 32.4). Unfortunately, ribavirin (1-β-D-ribofuranosyl-1,2,4-triazole-3carboxamide), a broad-spectrum synthetic guanosine analog with virustatic activity against a number of RNA viruses including arenaviruses and bunyaviruses, has no *in vitro* or *in vivo* effect on filoviruses.[184,190] Recent strategies to interfere with transcription and replication include antisense oligonucleotides, phosphorodiamidate morpholino oligomers (PMOs) and RNA interference (RNAi).[90,116,136,142,387,431,433,434] These approaches are promising, but may be limited by sequence specificity (genetic variation of species), production (high costs) and the administration route (mainly intravenous).

Vaccine vectors based on recombinant vesicular stomatitis virus (VSV) expressing EBOV or MARV GP[121,130] have shown remarkable utility when administered to nonhuman primates 30 minutes and up to 48 hours following lethal EBOV and MARV infection, respectively.[71,99,129,133] This strategy was used in a recent needle stick injury with high-risk exposure to ZEBOV. It is currently unclear whether the treatment prevented infection or the incident did not lead to infection, but there were no adverse effects noted with the administration of the vaccine vector.[158] Postexposure vaccination with VSV-based vectors is species specific due a lack of cross-protection among the various EBOV species.[93,130]

The targeting of host gene products might also prove to be beneficial in treating filovirus disease. The production of TNF-α can develop into a deleterious host response during infection, and the therapeutic use of anti-TNF-α neutralizing antibodies has been partially successful in rodent models,[189,190,191] but has not been evaluated in nonhuman primates. Furthermore, inhibitors of apoptosis of lymphocytes during EBOV infection[134,177] might be a possible intervention strategy. There have been relatively few attempts to modulate the dysregulated cytokine/chemokine response that is a consistent feature of many VHFs. Treating MARV-infected guinea pigs with Desferal, an IL-1 and TNF-α antagonist, partially protected these animals.[190,191] In another study, treating MARV-infected guinea pigs with IL-1 receptor antagonist (IL-1RA) or anti-TNF-α serum decreased the concentration of circulating TNF-α and protected 50% of the animals from lethal infection.[189]

Coagulation abnormalities are a hallmark of filovirus infections and considered a key factor in pathogenesis. The nematode-derived anticoagulation protein (rNAPc2) was used to treat ZEBOV-infected nonhuman primates and resulted in 33% survival in an otherwise uniformly lethal animal model.[135] The same treatment has shown reduced efficacy when administered to animals infected with MARV, Angola strain, but other less virulent strains have not been tested yet[127] (Table 32.4). D-dimer formation has been identified as an early event during EBOV infection in nonhuman primates and could be used as a marker for treatment.[135] As rNAPc2 primarily targets signaling through the extrinsic blood coagulation pathway, additional benefits might be realized by using inhibitors of Factor X, targeting the common pathway, thereby blocking signaling through both the extrinsic and intrinsic blood coagulation pathways. A recent study showed that treatment of ZEBOV-infected nonhuman primates with recombinant human activated protein C resulted in partial protection consistent with survival seen with rNAPc2.[176] Both drugs have been approved for different applications in humans and could be more easily and safely considered under emergency use protocols.

Given the severe and rapid progression of filovirus infections, monotherapy is unlikely to be effective versus combination approaches that interfere with disease progression to allow innate and adaptive immune responses to overcome infection.[42,101] Viremia levels below $1 \times 10^{4.5}$ pfu/mL are strongly associated with survival of patients and experimentally infected nonhuman primates.[97]

Prophylaxis

Protective EBOV and MARV vaccines would be extremely valuable for at-risk medical personnel, first responders, military personnel, researchers, and populations affected during a filovirus outbreak. Attempts to produce vaccines from cell culture–derived filovirus particles (inactivated with formalin, heat, or gamma irradiation) have not been effective in stimulating protective immune responses.[93] More recently, vaccine development has concentrated on the use of subunit vaccines based on a single, or combination of, viral structural proteins to induce protective immunity against an EBOV challenge. Aside from minor efforts to use the viral structural proteins VP24, VP30, VP35, and VP40 as immunogens, GP and to a lesser extent NP are the key viral proteins used for vaccination approaches. The following different delivery/expression systems have been evaluated in established animal models[30]: naked DNA[80,271,283,407,459,464]; virus-like particles (VLPs)[382,385,386,427,429,430,432,437,466]; replication-deficient vectors such as adenovirus[68,125,228,240,313,320,331,339,377,378,381,424,425,426,464]; Venezuelan equine encephalitis virus (VEEV) replicons[178,242,324,325]; and replication-competent live attenuated vectors such as vaccinia virus,[62,150] vesicular stomatitis virus (VSV),[70,126,128,131,220,221] human parainfluenza virus type 3 (HPIV3),[45,46,47,50] and New Castle disease virus (NDV).[77] Recently, a new concept based on replication-deficient ZEBOV (lacking VP35) generated through "reverse genetics" has shown promising protective efficacy in rodent models,[163] but remaining safety issues need to be addressed prior to generating proper vaccine candidates.

Most of the vaccine approaches showed protective efficacy in rodent models, but several failed to protect nonhuman primates.[93,143,130] Currently, at least five different vaccine systems (based on adenovirus serotype 5 [Ad5], VEEV, VSV, HPIV3, and VLPs) have demonstrated complete protection against lethal filovirus infections in nonhuman primates, the gold standard animal model. Of those, the replication-deficient Ad5 system is the furthest developed platform and has already been in phase I clinical trials.[240] This platform has been further developed by others using a multivalent adenovirus technology for the development of a panfilovirus vaccine that provides protection against several filovirus species.[384] In addition, effective mucosal delivery seems possible. The Ad5 platform seems safe and robust but suffers from preexisting immunity in the world population and the recent failure in an AIDS/HIV trial.[37,64] Preexisting immunity might be bypassed through mucosal delivery, which would also be beneficial for mass vaccination and for administration in rural Africa.[68,313] The VLP platform, generated by co-expression of the viral proteins VP40, NP, and GP[429,432] seems to best address safety issues but may require adjuvant and booster immunization for potent efficacy in nonhuman primates, which is less favorable for emergency use. Other issues are associated with the costs and production of the VLP-based vaccine compared to viral vector–based platforms.

Live attenuated recombinant vaccine vectors may be of advantage over nonreplicating vectors because of their ease in production and their more potent stimulation of innate and adaptive (humoral and cellular) immune responses. It would be difficult to ensure the safety of live attenuated EBOV and MARV strains, because of the high level biohazard of filoviruses. However, promising live attenuated filovirus vaccine vectors have recently been developed based on the backgrounds of VSV and HPIV3.[93,124,130] The VSV-based vectors are more advanced and have demonstrated efficacy in nonhuman primate models.[93,124,130] However, the vectors are associated with safety issues despite having a clean record in experimental animal models including immunocompromised animals[93,128,130,221] As with Ad5 and HPIV3 vectors, preexisting immunity is negligible for VSV. Both the HPIV and VSV vaccine platforms may have potential for needleless delivery.[47,326] The VSV-based platform has the potential for a multivalent vaccine protecting against several species of EBOV and MARV[131] and is the only filovirus vaccine platform with postexposure efficacy in the nonhuman primate model.[71,99,129,133]

It should be noted here that vaccine efforts for filoviruses have been largely based on ZEBOV and MARV strain Musoke immunogens. In particular, cross-species protection has only been achieved in a few attempts.[92,93,131,175,278]

Despite largely good to excellent protective efficacy in animal models, correlates and mechanisms of protection have not been well defined for most of the vaccine candidates. Current data on antibody responses, T-cell proliferation, and CTL responses indicate that antibody and T-helper cell memory are essential for protection and that cell-mediated immunity, while possibly important, is not an absolute requirement. Total antibody response is thought to be a correlate for protection for filovirus vaccines.[379]

REFERENCES

All cited references are available in the e-book.

2. Aleksandrowicz P, Marzi A, Biedenkopf N, et al. Ebola virus enters host cells by macropinocytosis and clathrin-mediated endocytosis. *J Infect Dis* 2011;204(Suppl 3):S957–S967.
3. Alvarez CP, Lasala F, Carrillo J, et al. C-type lectins DC-SIGN and L-SIGN mediate cellular entry by Ebola virus in *cis* and in *trans*. *J Virol* 2002;76:6841–6844.
9. Baize S, Leroy EM, Georges-Courbot MC, et al. Defective humoral responses and extensive intravascular apoptosis are associated with fatal outcome in Ebola virus-infected patients. *Nat Med* 1999;5:423–426.
10. Baize S, Leroy EM, Georges AJ, et al. Inflammatory responses in Ebola virus-infected patients. *Clin Exp Immunol* 2002;128:163–168.
11. Baize S, Leroy EM, Mavoungou E, et al. Apoptosis in fatal Ebola infection. Does the virus toll the bell for immune system? *Apoptosis* 2000;5:5–7.
12. Baribaud F, Pöhlmann S, Leslie G, et al. Quantitative expression and virus transmission analysis of DC-SIGN on monocyte-derived dendritic cells. *J Virol* 2002;76:9135–9142.
14. Barrette RW, Metwally SA, Rowland JM, et al. Discovery of swine as a host for the Reston ebolavirus. *Science* 2009;325:204–206.
16. Barrientos LG, Martin AM, Wohlhueter RM, et al. Secreted glycoprotein from Live Zaire ebolavirus-infected cultures: preparation, structural and biophysical characterization, and thermodynamic stability. *J Infect Dis* 2007;196(Suppl 2):S220–S231.
19. Basler CF, Mikulasova A, Martinez-Sobrido L, et al. The Ebola virus VP35 protein inhibits activation of interferon regulatory factor 3. *J Virol* 2003;77:7945–7956.
21. Basler CF, Wang X, Mülberger E, et al. The Ebola virus VP35 protein functions as a type I IFN antagonist. *Proc Natl Acad Sci U S A* 2000;97:12289–12294.
22. Bausch DG, Borchert M, Grein T, et al. Risk factors for Marburg hemorrhagic fever, Democratic Republic of the Congo. *Emerg Infect Dis* 2003;9:1531–1537.
23. Bausch DG, Nichol ST, Muyembe-Tamfum JJ, et al. Marburg hemorrhagic fever associated with multiple genetic lineages of virus. *N Engl J Med* 2006;355:909–919.
28. Becker S, Rinne C, Hofsass U, et al. Interactions of Marburg virus nucleocapsid proteins. *Virology* 1998;249:406–417.
29. Becker S, Spiess M, Klenk HD. The asialoglycoprotein receptor is a potential liver-specific receptor for Marburg virus. *J Gen Virol* 1995;76:393–399.
30. Bente D, Gren J, Strong JE, et al. Disease modeling for Ebola and Marburg viruses. *Dis Model Mech* 2009;2:12–17.
34. Bosio CM, Aman MJ, Grogan C, et al. Ebola and Marburg viruses replicate in monocyte-derived dendritic cells without inducing the production of cytokines and full maturation. *J Infect Dis* 2003;188:1630–1638.
35. Bosio CM, Moore BD, Warfield KL, et al. Ebola and Marburg virus-like particles activate human myeloid dendritic cells. *Virology* 2004;326:280–287.
38. Bray M, Davis K, Geisbert T, et al. A mouse model for evaluation of prophylaxis and therapy of Ebola hemorrhagic fever. *J Infect Dis* 1998;178:651–661.
39. Bray M, Geisbert TW. Ebola virus: the role of macrophages and dendritic cells in the pathogenesis of Ebola hemorrhagic fever. *Int J Biochem Cell Biol* 2005;37:1560–1566.
40. Bray M, Hatfill S, Hensley L, et al. Haematological, biochemical and coagulation changes in mice, guinea-pigs and monkeys infected with a mouse-adapted variant of Ebola Zaire virus. *J Comp Pathol* 2001;125:243–253.
41. Bray M, Mahanty S. Ebola hemorrhagic fever and septic shock. *J Infect Dis* 2003;188:1613–1617.
42. Bray M, Paragas J. Experimental therapy of filovirus infections. *Antiviral Res* 2002;54:1–17.
44. Brindley MA, Hughes L, Ruiz A, et al. Ebola virus glycoprotein 1: identification of residues important for binding and postbinding events. *J Virol* 2007;81:7702–7709.
47. Bukreyev A, Rollin PE, Tate MK, et al. Successful topical respiratory tract immunization of primates against Ebola virus. *J Virol* 2007;81(12):6379–6388.
48. Bukreyev AA, Volchkov VE, Blinov VM, et al. The GP-protein of Marburg virus contains the region similar to the "immunosuppressive domain" of oncogenic retrovirus P15E proteins. *FEBS Lett* 1993;323:183–187.
50. Bukreyev A, Yang L, Zaki SR, et al. A single intranasal inoculation with a paramyxovirus-vectored vaccine protects guinea pigs against a lethal-dose Ebola virus challenge. *J Virol* 2006;80(5):2267–2279.
51. Bwaka MA, Bonnet M, Calain P, et al. Ebola hemorrhagic fever in Kikwit, Democratic Republic of Congo: Clinical observations in 103 patients. *Infect Dis* 1999;179(suppl 1):S1–S7.
53. Carette JE, Raaben M, Wong AC, et al. Ebola virus entry requires the cholesterol transporter Niemann-Pick C1. *Nature* 2011;477:340–343.
54. Cardenas WB, Loo YM, Gale M Jr, et al. Ebola virus VP35 protein binds double-stranded RNA and inhibits alpha/beta interferon production induced by RIG-I signaling. *J Virol* 2006;80:5168–5178.
57. Chan SY, Ma MC, Goldsmith MA. Differential induction of cellular detachment by envelope glycoproteins of Marburg and Ebola (Zaire) viruses. *J Gen Virol* 2000;81:2155–2159.
59. Chandran K, Sullivan NJ, Felbor U, et al. Endosomal proteolysis of the Ebola virus glycoprotein is necessary for infection. *Science* 2005;308:1643–1645.
63. Chepurnov AA, Tuzova MN, Ternovoy VA, et al. Suppressive effect of Ebola virus on T cell proliferation *in vitro* is provided by a 125-kd GP viral protein. *Immunol Lett* 1999;68:257–261.
65. Colebunders R, Tshomba A, Van Kerkhove MD, et al. Marburg hemorrhagic fever in Durba and Watsa, Democratic Republic of the Congo: clinical documentation, features of illness, and treatment. *J Infect Dis* 2007;196(Suppl 2):S148–S153.
68. Croyle MA, Patel A, Tran KN, et al. Nasal delivery of an adenovirus-based vaccine bypasses pre-existing immunity to the vaccine carrier and improves the immune response in mice. *PLoS One* 2008;3(10):e3548.
71. Daddario-DiCaprio KM, Geisbert TW, Ströher U, et al. Postexposure protection against Marburg haemorrhagic fever with recombinant vesicular stomatitis virus vectors in non-human primates: an efficacy assessment. *Lancet* 2006;367:1399–1404.
72. Dalgard DW, Hardy RJ, Pearson SL, et al. Combined simian hemorrhagic fever and Ebola virus infection in cynomolgus monkeys. *Lab Anim Sci* 1992;42:152–157.
75. Dessen A, Volchkov V, Dolnik O, et al. Crystal structure of the matrix protein VP40 from Ebola virus. *EMBO J* 2000;19:4228–4236.
77. DiNapoli JM, Yang L, Samal SK, et al. Respiratory tract immunization of non-human primates with a Newcastle disease virus-vectored vaccine candidate against Ebola virus elicits a neutralizing antibody response. *Vaccine* 2010;29(1):17–25.
78. Dolnik O, Volchkova V, Garten W, et al. Ectodomain shedding of the glycoprotein GP of Ebola virus. *EMBO J* 2004;23:2175–2184.
79. Dowell SF, Mukunu R, Ksiazek TG, et al. Transmission of Ebola hemorrhagic fever: A study of risk factors in family members, Kikwit, Democratic Republic of the Congo, 1995. *J Infect Dis* 1999;179(suppl 1):S87–S91.

84. Ebihara H, Takada A, Kobasa D, et al. Molecular determinants of Ebola virus virulence in mice. *PLoS Pathog* 2006;2:e73.
89. Enterlein S, Volchkov V, Weik M, et al. Rescue of recombinant Marburg virus from cDNA is dependent on nucleocapsid protein VP30. *J Virol* 2006;80:1038–1043.
93. Falzarano D, Geisbert TW, Feldmann H. Progress in filovirus vaccine development: evaluating the potential for clinical use. *Expert Rev Vaccines* 2011;10(1):63–77.
94. Falzarano D, Krokhin O, Van Domselaar G, et al. Ebola sGP-the first viral glycoprotein shown to be C-mannosylated. *Virology* 2007;368:83–90.
96. Feldmann H, Bugany H, Mahner F, et al. Filovirus-induced endothelial leakage triggered by infected monocytes/macrophages. *J Virol* 1996; 70:2208–2214.
97. Feldmann H, Geisbert TW. Ebola haemorrhagic fever. *Lancet* 2011;377: 849–862.
99. Feldmann H, Jones SM, Daddario-DiCaprio KM, et al. Effective postexposure treatment of Ebola infection. *PLoS Pathog* 2007;3(1):e2.
100. Feldmann H, Jones S, Klenk HD, et al. Ebola virus: from discovery to vaccine. *Nat Rev Immunol* 2003;3:677–685.
101. Feldmann H, Jones ST, Schnittler HJ, et al. Therapy and prophylaxis of Ebola virus infections. *Curr Opin Investig Drugs* 2005;6:823–830.
109. Fisher-Hoch SP, Brammer TL, Trappier SG, et al. Pathogenic potential of filoviruses: Role of geographic origin of primate host and virus strain. *J Infect Dis* 1992;166:753–763.
110. Fisher-Hoch SP, Lloyd G, Platt GS, et al. Haematological and biochemical monitoring of Ebola infection in rhesus monkeys: Implications for patient management. *Lancet* 1983;2:1055–1058.
112. Fisher-Hoch SP, Platt GS, Neild GH, et al. Pathophysiology of shock and hemorrhage in a fulminating viral infection (Ebola). *J Infect Dis* 1985;152:887–894.
115. Formenty P, Libama F, Epelboin A, et al. Outbreak of Ebola hemorrhagic fever in the Republic of the Congo, 2003: a new strategy? *Med Trop (Mars)* 2003;63:291–295.
117. Francica JR, Matukonis MK, Bates P. Requirements for cell rounding and surface protein down-regulation by Ebola virus glycoprotein. *Virology* 2009;383(2):237–247.
124. Geisbert TW, Bausch DG, Feldmann H. Prospects for immunisation against Marburg and Ebola viruses. *Rev Med Virol* 2010;20(6):344–357.
126. Geisbert TW, Daddario-Dicaprio KM, Geisbert JB, et al. Vesicular stomatitis virus-based vaccines protect nonhuman primates against aerosol challenge with Ebola and Marburg viruses. *Vaccine* 2008;26:6894–6900.
128. Geisbert TW, Daddario-Dicaprio KM, Lewis MG, et al. Vesicular stomatitis virus-based ebola vaccine is well-tolerated and protects immunocompromised nonhuman primates. *PLoS Pathog* 2008;4:e1000225.
130. Geisbert TW, Feldmann H. Recombinant vesicular stomatitis virus-based vaccines against Ebola and Marburg virus infections. *J Infect Dis* 2011;204(Suppl 3):S1075–S1081.
131. Geisbert TW, Geisbert JB, Leung A, et al. Single-injection vaccine protects nonhuman primates against infection with Marburg virus and three species of Ebola virus. *J Virol* 2009;83:7296–7304.
134. Geisbert TW, Hensley LE, Gibb TR, et al. Apoptosis induced *in vitro* and *in vivo* during infection by Ebola and Marburg viruses. *Lab Invest* 2000;80:171–186.
135. Geisbert TW, Hensley LE, Jahrling PB, et al. Treatment of Ebola virus infection with a recombinant inhibitor of factor VIIa/tissue factor: a study in rhesus monkeys. *Lancet* 2003;362:1953–1958.
137. Geisbert TW, Hensley LE, Larsen T, et al. Pathogenesis of Ebola hemorrhagic fever in cynomolgus macaques: evidence that dendritic cells are early and sustained targets of infection. *Am J Pathol* 2003;163:2347–2370.
142. Geisbert TW, Lee AC, Robbins M, et al. Postexposure protection of non-human primates against a lethal Ebola virus challenge with RNA interference: a proof-of-concept study. *Lancet* 2010;375:1896–1905.
145. Geisbert TW, Young HA, Jahrling PB, et al. Mechanisms underlying coagulation abnormalities in Ebola hemorrhagic fever: overexpression of tissue factor in primate monocytes/macrophages is a key event. *J Infect Dis* 2003;188:1618–1629.
147. Georges A, Leroy EB, Renaut AA, et al. Ebola hemorrhagic fever outbreaks in Gabon, 1994–1997: Epidemiologic and health control issues. *J Infect Dis* 1999;179(suppl 1):S65–S75.
151. Grolla A, Jones SM, Fernando L, et al. The use of a mobile laboratory unit in support of patient management and epidemiological surveillance during the 2005 Marburg outbreak in Angola. *PLoS Neg Trop Dis* 2011;5:e1183.
154. Groseth A, Charton JE, Sauerborn M, et al. The Ebola virus ribonucleoprotein complex: a novel VP30-L interaction identified. *Virus Res* 2009;140:8–14.
155. Groseth A, Feldmann H, Strong JE. The ecology of Ebola virus. *Trends Microbiol* 2007;15:408–416.
160. Gupta M, Mahanty S, Ahmed R, et al. Monocyte-derived human macrophages and peripheral blood mononuclear cells infected with Ebola virus secrete MIP-1alpha and TNF-alpha and inhibit poly-IC-induced IFN-alpha *in vitro*. *Virology* 2001;284:20–25.
163. Halfmann P, Ebihara H, Marzi A, et al. Replication-deficient ebolavirus as a vaccine candidate. *J Virol* 2009;83(8):3810–3815.
164. Han Z, Boshra H, Sunyer JO, et al. Biochemical and functional characterization of the Ebola virus VP24 protein: implications for a role in virus assembly and budding. *J Virol* 2003;77:1793–1800.
166. Harcourt BH, Sanchez A, Offermann MK. Ebola virus inhibits induction of genes by double-stranded RNA in endothelial cells. *Virology* 1998; 252:179–188.
169. Hartlieb B, Muziol T, Weissenhorn W, et al. Crystal structure of the C-terminal domain of Ebola virus VP30 reveals a role in transcription and nucleocapsid association. *Proc Natl Acad Sci U S A* 2007;104:624–629.
170. Hartman AL, Bird BH, Towner JS, et al. Inhibition of IRF-3 activation by VP35 is critical for the high level of virulence of Ebola virus. *J Virol* 2008;82:2699–2704.
173. Harty RN, Brown ME, Wang G, et al. A PPxY motif within the VP40 protein of Ebola virus interacts physically and functionally with a ubiquitin ligase: implications for filovirus budding. *Proc Natl Acad Sci U S A* 2000;97:13871–13876.
175. Hensley LE, Mulangu S, Asiedu C, et al. Demonstration of cross-protective vaccine immunity against an emerging pathogenic Ebolavirus Species. *PLoS Pathog* 2010;6:e1000904.
176. Hensley LE, Stevens EL, Yan SB, et al. Recombinant human activated protein C for the postexposure treatment of Ebola hemorrhagic fever. *J Infect Dis* 2007;196(Suppl 2):S390–S399.
177. Hensley LE, Young HA, Jahrling PB, et al. Proinflammatory response during Ebola virus infection of primate models: possible involvement of the tumor necrosis factor receptor superfamily. *Immunol Lett* 2002;80: 169–179.
181. Hoenen T, Volchkov V, Kolesnikova L, et al. VP40 octamers are essential for Ebola virus replication. *J Virol* 2005;79:1898–1905.
182. Hood CL, Abraham J, Boyington JC, et al. Biochemical and structural characterization of cathepsin L-processed Ebola virus glycoprotein: implications for viral entry and immunogenicity. *J Virol* 2010;84: 2972–2982.
199. Ito H, Watanabe S, Sanchez A, et al. Mutational analysis of the putative fusion domain of Ebola virus glycoprotein. *J Virol* 1999;73:8907–8912.
200. Ito H, Watanabe S, Takada A, et al. Ebola virus glycoprotein: proteolytic processing, acylation, cell tropism, and detection of neutralizing antibodies. *J Virol* 2001;75:1576–1580.
201. Jaax NK, Davis KJ, Geisbert TJ, et al. Lethal experimental infection of rhesus monkeys with Ebola-Zaire (Mayinga) virus by the oral and conjunctival route of exposure. *Arch Pathol Lab Med* 1996;120:140–155.
203. Jahrling PB, Geisbert TW, Dalgard DW, et al. Preliminary report: Isolation of Ebola virus from monkeys imported to USA. *Lancet* 1990; 335:502–505.
204. Jahrling PB, Geisbert TW, Geisbert JB, et al. Evaluation of immune globulin and recombinant interferon alpha-2b for treatment of experimental Ebola virus infections. *J Infect Dis* 1999;179(suppl 1):S224–S234.
207. Jasenosky LD, Kawaoka Y. Filovirus budding. *Virus Res* 2004;106:181–188.
210. Jeffs B. A clinical guide to viral haemorrhagic fevers: Ebola, Marburg and Lassa. *Trop Doct* 2006:36:1–4.
214. John SP, Wang T, Steffen S, et al. Ebola virus VP30 is an RNA binding protein. *J Virol* 2007;81:8967–8976.
220. Jones SM, Feldmann H, Ströher U, et al. Live attenuated recombinant vaccine protects nonhuman primates against Ebola and Marburg viruses. *Nat Med* 2005;11:786–790.

224. Kiley MP, Bowen ETW, Eddy GA, et al. Filoviridae: A taxonomic home for Marburg and Ebola viruses? *Intervirology* 1982;18:24–32.
226. Kimberlin CR, Bornholdt ZA, Li S, et al. Ebolavirus VP35 uses a bimodal strategy to bind dsRNA for innate immune suppression. *Proc Natl Acad Sci U S A* 2010;107:314–319.
228. Kobinger GP, Feldmann H, Zhi Y, et al. Chimpanzee adenovirus vaccine protects against Zaire Ebola virus. *Virology* 2006;346(2):394–401.
230. Kolesnikova L, Berghöfer B, Bamberg S, et al. Multivesicular bodies as a platform for formation of the Marburg virus envelope. *J Virol* 2004; 78:12277–12287.
232. Kondratowicz AS, Lennemann NJ, Sinn PL, et al. T-cell immunoglobulin and mucin domain 1 (TIM-1) is a receptor for Zaire Ebolavirus and Lake Victoria Marburgvirus. *Proc Natl Acad Sci U S A* 2011;108: 8426–8431.
235. Ksiazek TG, Rollin PE, Williams AJ, et al. Clinical virology of Ebola hemorrhagic fever (EHF): Virus, virus antigen, and IgG and IgM antibody findings among EHF patients in Kikwit, Democratic Republic of the Congo, 1995. *J Infect Dis* 1999;179(suppl 1):S177–S187.
239. Kuhn JH, Radoshitzky SR, Guth AC, et al. Conserved receptor-binding domains of Lake Victoria marburgvirus and Zaire ebolavirus bind a common receptor. *J Biol Chem* 2006;281:15951–15958.
240. Ledgerwood JE, Costner P, Desai N, et al. VRC 205 Study Team. A replication defective recombinant Ad5 vaccine expressing Ebola virus GP is safe and immunogenic in healthy adults. *Vaccine* 2010;29(2): 304–313.
241. Lee JE, Saphire EO. Ebolavirus glycoprotein structure and mechanism of entry. *Future Virol* 2009;4:621–635.
243. LeGuenno B, Formenty P, Wyers M, et al. Isolation and partial characterisation of a new strain of Ebola virus. *Lancet* 1995;345:1271–1274.
246. Leroy EM, Baize S, Volchkov VE, et al. Human asymptomatic Ebola infection and strong inflammatory response. *Lancet* 2000;355:2210–2215.
248. Leroy EM, Epelboin A, Mondonge V, et al. Human Ebola outbreak resulting from direct exposure to fruit bats in Luebo, Democratic Republic of Congo, 2007. *Vector Borne Zoonotic Dis* 2009;9:723–728.
249. Leroy EM, Jumulungui B, Pourrut A, et al. Fruit bats as reservoirs of Ebola virus. *Nature* 2005:438:575–576.
250. Leroy EM, Rouquet P, Formenty P, et al. Multiple Ebola virus transmission events and rapid decline of central African wildlife. *Science* 2004; 303:387–390.
251. Leroy EM, Souquiere S, Rouquet P, et al. Re-emergence of Ebola haemorrhagic fever in Gabon. *Lancet* 2002;359:712.
254. Leung DW, Ginder ND, Fulton DB, et al. Structure of the Ebola VP35 interferon inhibitory domain. *Proc Natl Acad Sci U S A* 2009;106:411–416.
257. Licata JM, Simpson-Holley M, Wright NT, et al. Overlapping motifs (PTAP and PPEY) within the Ebola virus VP40 protein function independently as late budding domains: involvement of host proteins TSG101 and VPS-4. *J Virol* 2003;77:1812–1819.
258. Lin G, Simmons G, Pühlmann S, et al. Differential N-linked glycosylation of human immunodeficiency virus and Ebola virus envelope glycoproteins modulates interactions with DC-SIGN and DC-SIGNR. *J Virol* 2003;77:1337–1346.
259. Lipkin WI, Palacios G, Briese T. Diagnostics and discovery in viral hemorrhagic fevers. *Ann N Y Acad Sci* 2009;1171(Suppl 1):E6–E11.
260. Lloyd ES, Zaki SR, Rollin PE, et al. Long-term disease surveillance in Bandundu region, Democratic Republic of the Congo: A model for early detection and prevention of Ebola hemorrhagic fever. *J Infect Dis* 1999; 179(suppl 1):S274–S280.
263. Lofts LL, Wells JB, Bavari S, et al. Key genomic changes necessary for in vivo lethal mouse marburgvirus variant selection process. *J Virol* 2011; 85:3905–3917.
267. Mahanty S, Bray M. Pathogenesis of filoviral haemorrhagic fevers. *Lancet Infect Dis* 2004;4:487–498.
269. Malashkevich VN, Schneider BJ, McNally ML, et al. Core structure of the envelope glycoprotein GP_2 from Ebola virus at 1.9-Å resolution. *Proc Natl Acad Sci U S A* 1999;96:2662–2667.
272. Martin-Serrano J, Zang T, Bieniasz PD. HIV-1 and Ebola virus encode small peptide motifs that recruit Tsg101 to sites of particle assembly to facilitate egress. *Nat Med* 2001;7:1313–1319.
274. Martini GA, Knauff HG, Schmidt HA, et al. Über eine bisher unbekannte, von Affen eingeschleppte Infektionskrankheit: Marburg-Virus-Krankheit. *Dtsch Med Wochenschr* 1968;93:555–571.
276. Martini GA, Siegert R, eds. *Marburg Virus Disease.* Berlin: Springer-Verlag; 1971.
280. Marzi A, Moller P, Hanna SL, et al. Analysis of the interaction of Ebola virus glycoprotein with DC-SIGN (dendritic cell-specific intercellular adhesion molecule 3-grabbing nonintegrin) and its homologue DC-SIGNR. *J Infect Dis* 2007;196(Suppl):S237–S246.
281. Mehedi M, Falzarano D, Seebach J, et al. A new Ebola virus nonstructural glycoprotein expressed through RNA editing. *J Virol* 2011;85:5406–5414.
282. Mehedi M, Groseth A, Feldmann H, et al. Clinical aspects of Marburg hemorrhagic fever. *Future Virol* 2011;6(9):1091–1106.
285. Miranda ME, Ksiazek TG, Retuya TJ, et al. Epidemiology of Ebola (subtype Reston) virus in the Philippines, 1996. *J Infect Dis* 1999;179 (suppl 1):S115–S119.
286. Modrof J, Becker S, Mühlberger E. Ebola virus transcription activator VP30 is a zinc-binding protein. *J Virol* 2003;77:3334–3338.
289. Mühlberger E, Lotfering B, Klenk HD, et al. Three of the four nucleocapsid proteins of Marburg virus, NP, VP35, and L, are sufficient to mediate replication and transcription of Marburg virus-specific monocistronic minigenomes. *J Virol* 1998;72:8756–8764.
292. Mühlberger E, Weik M, Volchkov VE, et al. Comparison of the transcription and replication strategies of Marburg virus and Ebola virus by using artificial replication systems. *J Virol* 1999;73:2333–2342.
296. Murphy FA, Simpson DIH, Whitfield SG, et al. Marburg virus infection in monkeys. *Lab Invest* 1971;24:279–291.
298. Nanbo A, Imai M, Watanabe S, et al. Ebolavirus is internalized into host cells via macropinocytosis in a viral glycoprotein-dependent manner. *PLoS Pathog* 2010;6:e1001121.
299. Negredo A, Palacios G, Vázquez-Morón S, et al. Discovery of an Ebolavirus-like Filovirus in Europe. *PLoS Pathog* 2011;7:e1002304.
300. Neumann G, Ebihara H, Takada A, et al. Ebola virus VP40 late domains are not essential for viral replication in cell culture. *J Virol* 2005;79: 10300–10307.
302. Neumann G, Geisbert TW, Ebihara H, et al. Proteolytic processing of the Ebola virus glycoprotein is not critical for Ebola virus replication in nonhuman primates. *J Virol* 2007;81:2995–2998.
305. Noda T, Aoyama K, Sagara H, et al. Nucleocapsid-like structures of Ebola virus reconstructed using electron tomography. *J Vet Med Sci* 2005;67:325–328.
307. Noda T, Sagara H, Suzuki E, et al. Ebola virus VP40 drives the formation of virus-like filamentous particles along with GP. *J Virol* 2002;76: 4855–4865.
312. Pattyn SR. *Ebola Virus Haemorrhagic Fever.* Amsterdam: Elsevier/North Holland; 1978:1–280.
314. Peters CJ, Jahrling PB, Khan AS. Patients infected with high-hazard viruses: Scientific basis for infection control. *Arch Virol Suppl* 1996;11: 141–168.
317. Peterson AT, Bauer JT, Mills JN. Ecologic and geographic distribution of filovirus disease. *Emerg Infect Dis* 2004;10:40–47.
320. Pratt WD, Wang D, Nichols DK, et al. Protection of nonhuman primates against two species of Ebola virus infection with a single complex adenovirus vector. *Clin Vaccine Immunol* 2010;17(4):572–581.
323. Prins KC, Delpeut S, Leung DW, et al. Mutations abrogating VP35 interaction with double-stranded RNA render Ebola virus avirulent in guinea pigs. *J Virol* 2010;84:3004–3015.
325a. Qiu X, Audet J, Wong G, et al. Successful treatment of ebola virus-infected cynomolgus macaques with monoclonal antibodies. *Sci Transl Med.* 2012;4:138ra81. doi: 10.1126/scitranslmed.3003876. PubMed PMID:22700957.
328. Reed DS, Lackemeyer MG, Garza NL, et al. Aerosol exposure to Zaire ebolavirus in three nonhuman primate species: differences in disease course and clinical pathology. *Microbes Infect* 2011;13:930–936.
329. Reid SP, Leung LW, Hartman AL, et al. Ebola virus VP24 binds karyopherin alpha1 and blocks STAT1 nuclear accumulation. *J Virol* 2006;80: 5156–5167.
334. Rollin PE, Bausch DG, Sanchez A. Blood chemistry measurements and D-Dimer levels associated with fatal and nonfatal outcomes in humans

infected with Sudan Ebola virus. *J Infect Dis* 2007;196(Suppl 2):S364–S371.

338. Rowe AK, Bertolli J, Khan AS, et al. Clinical, virologic, and immunologic follow-up of convalescent Ebola hemorrhagic fever patients and their household contacts, Kikwit, Democratic Republic of the Congo. *J Infect Dis* 1999;179(suppl 1):S28–S35.
340. Ruigrok RW, Schoehn G, Dessen A, et al. Structural characterization and membrane binding properties of the matrix protein VP40 of Ebola virus. *J Mol Biol* 2000;300:103–112.
342. Ryabchikova EI, Kolesnikova LV, Luchko SV. An analysis of features of pathogenesis in two animal models of Ebola virus infection. *J Infect Dis* 1999;179(suppl 1):S199–S202.
344. Saeed MF, Kolokoltsov AA, Albrecht T, et al. Cellular entry of Ebola virus involves uptake by a macropinocytosis-like mechanism and subsequent trafficking through early and late endosomes. *PLoS Pathog* 2010;6: e1001110.
346. Sanchez A, Kiley MP. Identification and analysis of Ebola virus messenger RNA. *Virology* 1987;157:414–420.
351. Sanchez A, Lukwiya M, Bausch D, et al. Analysis of human peripheral blood samples from fatal and nonfatal cases of Ebola (Sudan) hemorrhagic fever: cellular responses, virus load, and nitric oxide levels. *J Virol* 2004;78:10370–10377.
353. Sanchez A, Trappier SG, Mahy BW, et al. The virion glycoproteins of Ebola viruses are encoded in two reading frames and are expressed through transcriptional editing. *Proc Natl Acad Sci U S A* 1996;93:3602–3607.
355. Sanchez A, Wagoner KE, Rollin PE. Sequence-based human leukocyte antigen-B typing of patients infected with Ebola virus in Uganda in 2000: identification of alleles associated with fatal and nonfatal disease outcomes. *J Infect Dis* 2007;196(Suppl 2):S329–S336.
356. Sanchez A, Yang ZY, Xu L, et al. Biochemical analysis of the secreted and virion glycoproteins of Ebola virus. *J Virol* 1998;72:6442–6447.
360. Schnittler HJ, Feldmann H. Viral hemorrhagic fever–a vascular disease? *Thromb Haemost* 2003;89:967–972.
362. Scianimanico S, Schoehn G, Timmins J, et al. Membrane association induces a conformational change in the Ebola virus matrix protein. *EMBO J* 2000;19:6732–6741.
363. Shi W, Huang Y, Sutton-Smith M, et al. A filovirus-unique region of Ebola virus nucleoprotein confers aberrant migration and mediates its incorporation into virions. *J Virol* 2008;82:6190–6199.
367. Simmons G, Wool-Lewis RJ, Baribaud F, et al. Ebola virus glycoproteins induce global surface protein down-modulation and loss of cell adherence. *J Virol* 2002;76:2518–2528.
373. Strong JE, Grolla A, Jahrling PB, et al. Filoviruses and arenaviruses. In: Detrick B, Hamilton RG, Folds JD, eds. In Manual of Molecular and Clinical Laboratory Immunology. 7th ed. Washington, DC: ASM Press; 2006:774–790
374. Ströher U, West E, Bugany H, et al. Infection and activation of monocytes by Marburg and Ebola viruses. *J Virol* 2001;75:11025–11033.
377. Sullivan NJ, Geisbert TW, Geisbert JB, et al. Accelerated vaccination for Ebola virus haemorrhagic fever in non-human primates. *Nature* 2003; 424:681–684.
379. Sullivan NJ, Martin JE, Graham BS, et al. Correlates of protective immunity for Ebola vaccines: implications for regulatory approval by the animal rule. *Nat Rev Microbiol* 2009;7:393–400.
381. Sullivan NJ, Sanchez A, Rollin PE, et al. Development of a preventive vaccine for Ebola virus infection in primates. *Nature* 2000;408: 605–609.
383. Swanepoel R, Leman PA, Burt F, et al. Experimental inoculation of plants and animals with Ebola virus. *Emerg Infect Dis* 1996;2:321–325.
384. Swenson DL, Wang D, Luo M, et al. Vaccine to confer to nonhuman primates complete protection against multistrain Ebola and Marburg virus infections. *Clin Vaccine Immunol* 2008;15(3):460–467.
385. Swenson DL, Warfield KL, Larsen T, et al. Monovalent virus-like particle vaccine protects guinea pigs and nonhuman primates against infection with multiple Marburg viruses. *Expert Rev Vaccines* 2008;7(4):417–429.
388. Takada A, Feldmann H, Ksiazek TG, et al. Antibody-dependent enhancement of Ebola virus infection. *J Virol* 2003;77:753975–753944.
390. Takada A, Fujioka K, Tsuiji M, et al. Human macrophage C-type lectin specific for galactose and N-acetylgalactosamine promotes filovirus entry. *J Virol* 2004;78:2943–2947.
392. Takada A, Robison C, Goto H, et al. A system for functional analysis of Ebola virus glycoprotein. *Proc Natl Acad Sci U S A* 1997;94:14764–14769.
398. Timmins J, Schoehn G, Ricard-Blum S, et al. Ebola virus matrix protein VP40 interaction with human cellular factors Tsg101 and Nedd4. *J Mol Biol* 2003;326:493–502.
400. Towner JS, Amman BR, Sealy TK, et al. Isolation of genetically diverse Marburg viruses from Egyptian fruit bats. *PLoS Pathog* 2009;5:e1000536.
401. Towner JS, Khristova ML, Sealy TK, et al. Marburgvirus genomics and association with a large hemorrhagic fever outbreak in Angola. *J Virol* 2006;80:6497–6516.
403. Towner JS, Sealy TK, Khristova ML, et al. Newly discovered Ebola virus associated with hemorrhagic fever outbreak in Uganda. *PLoS Pathog* 2008;4:e1000212.
405. Urata S, Noda T, Kawaoka Y, et al. Interaction of Tsg101 with Marburg virus VP40 depends on the PPPY motif, but not the PT/SAP motif as in the case of Ebola virus, and Tsg101 plays a critical role in the budding of Marburg virus-like particles induced by VP40, NP, and GP. *J Virol* 2007;81:4895–4899.
406. Valmas C, Grosch MN, Schumann M, et al. Marburg virus evades interferon responses by a mechanism distinct from Ebola virus. *PLoS Pathog* 2010;6(1):e1000721.
408. Villinger F, Rollin PE, Brar SS, et al. Markedly elevated levels of interferon (IFN)-gamma, IFN-alpha, interleukin (IL)-2, IL-10, and tumor necrosis factor-alpha associated with fatal Ebola virus infection. *J Infect Dis* 1999;179(suppl 1):S188–S191.
410. Volchkov VE, Becker S, Volchkova VA, et al. GP mRNA of Ebola virus is edited by the Ebola virus polymerase and by T7 and vaccinia virus polymerases. *Virology* 1995;214:421–430.
411. Volchkov VE, Blinov VM, Netesov SV. The envelope glycoprotein of Ebola virus contains an immunosuppressive-like domain similar to oncogenic retroviruses. *FEBS Lett* 1992;305:181–184.
413. Volchkov VE, Feldmann H, Volchkova VA, et al. Processing of the Ebola virus glycoprotein by the proprotein convertase furin. *Proc Natl Acad Sci U S A* 1998;95:5762–5767.
415. Volchkov VE, Volchkova VA, Mühlberger E, et al. Recovery of infectious Ebola virus from complementary DNA: RNA editing of the GP gene and viral cytotoxicity. *Science* 2001;291:1965–1969.
417. Volchkov VE, Volchkova VA, Stroher U, et al. Proteolytic processing of Marburg virus glycoprotein. *Virology* 2000;268:1–6.
420. Wahl-Jensen VM, Afanasieva TA, Seebach J, et al. Effects of Ebola virus glycoproteins on endothelial cell activation and barrier function. *J Virol* 2005;79:10442–10450.
425. Wang D, Raja NU, Trubey CM, et al. Development of a cAdVax-based bivalent ebola virus vaccine that induces immune responses against both the Sudan and Zaire species of Ebola virus. *J Virol* 2006;80:2738–2746.
427. Warfield KL, Bosio CM, Welcher BC, et al. Ebola virus-like particles protect from lethal Ebola virus infection. *Proc Natl Acad Sci U S A* 2003; 100:15889–15894.
428. Warfield KL, Bradfute SB, Wells J, et al. Development and characterization of a mouse model for Marburg hemorrhagic fever. *J Virol* 2009; 83(13):6404–6415.
432. Warfield KL, Swenson DL, Olinger GG, et al. Ebola virus-like particle-based vaccine protects nonhuman primates against lethal Ebola virus challenge. *J Infect Dis* 2007;196(Suppl 2):S430–S437.
433. Warren TK, Warfield KL, Wells J, et al. Antiviral activity of a small-molecule inhibitor of filovirus infection. *Antimicrob Agents Chemother* 2010:54:2152–2159.
434. Warren TK, Warfield KL, Wells J, et al. Advanced antisense therapies for postexposure protection against lethal filovirus infections. *Nat Med* 2010;16:991–994.
436. Watanabe S, Takada A, Watanabe T, et al. Functional importance of the coiled-coil of the Ebola virus glycoprotein. *J Virol* 2000;74:10194–10201.
437. Watanabe S, Watanabe T, Noda T, et al. Production of novel Ebola virus-like particles from cDNAs: an alternative to Ebola virus generation by reverse genetics. *J Virol* 2004;78:999–1005.
439. Wauquier N, Padilla C, Becquart P, et al. Association of KIR2DS1 and KIR2DS3 with fatal outcome in Ebola virus infection. *Immunogenetics* 2010;62(11-12):767–771.

441. Weik M, Modrof J, Klenk HD, et al. Ebola virus VP30-mediated transcription is regulated by RNA secondary structure formation. *J Virol* 2002;76:8532–8539.
442. Weissenhorn W, Calder LJ, Wharton SA, et al. The central structural feature of the membrane fusion protein subunit from the Ebola virus glycoprotein is a long triple-stranded coiled coil. *Proc Natl Acad Sci U S A* 1998;95:6032–6036.
443. Weissenhorn W, Carfi A, Lee KH, et al. Crystal structure of the Ebola virus membrane fusion subunit, GP_2, from the envelope glycoprotein ectodomain. *Mol Cells* 1998;2:605–616.
446. Wilson JA, Hevey M, Bakken R, et al. Epitopes involved in antibody-mediated protection from Ebola virus. *Science* 2000;287:1664–1666.
447. Wool-Lewis RJ, Bates P. Characterization of Ebola virus entry by using pseudotyped viruses: Identification of receptor-deficient cell lines. *J Virol* 1998;72:3155–3160.
460. Yaddanapudi K, Palacios G, Towner JS, et al. Implication of a retrovirus-like glycoprotein peptide in the immunopathogenesis of Ebola and Marburg viruses. *FASEB J* 2006;20:2519–2530.
462. Yang Z, Delgado R, Xu L, et al. Distinct cellular interactions of secreted and transmembrane Ebola virus glycoproteins. *Science* 1998;279:1034–1037.
463. Yang Z, Duckers HJ, Sullivan NJ, et al. Identification of the Ebola virus glycoprotein as the major determinant of viral toxicity and vascular injury. *Nat Med* 2000;6:886–889.
468. Zaki SR, Goldsmith CD. Pathologic features of filovirus infections in humans. *Curr Top Microbiol Immunol* 1999;235:97–116.
471. Zlotnik I. Marburg agent disease: Pathology. *Trans R Soc Trop Med Hyg* 1969;63:310–323.

CHAPTER 33

Robert A. Lamb • Griffith D. Parks

Paramyxoviridae

The *Paramyxoviridae* include some of the great and ubiquitous disease-causing viruses of humans and animals, including one of the most infectious viruses known (measles virus), some of the most prevalent viruses known (measles virus, parainfluenza viruses [PIVs], mumps virus, respiratory syncytial virus [RSV], and metapneumovirus), a virus that has been targeted by the World Health Organization for eradication (measles virus; however, to date, eradication has failed), a virus that has been eradicated (rinderpest virus), viruses that have a major economic impact on poultry rearing (Newcastle disease virus [NDV]), and many recently identified viruses (pinniped morbilliviruses, Hendra virus, Nipah virus, J virus and Beilong virus), some of which cause deadly diseases (Hendra and Nipah viruses). The *Paramyxoviridae* are enveloped negative-stranded RNA viruses that have special relationships with two other families of negative-strand RNA viruses, namely the *Orthomyxoviridae* (for the biological properties of the envelope glycoproteins) and the *Rhabdoviridae* (for the similarity of organization of the nonsegmented genome and its expression). The *Paramyxoviridae* are defined by having a protein (F) that causes viral–cell membrane fusion, in most cases at neutral pH. The genomic RNA of all negative-strand RNA viruses has to serve two functions: first as a template for synthesis of messenger RNAs (mRNAs) and second as a template for synthesis of the antigenome positive strand. Negative-strand RNA viruses encode and package their own RNA polymerase (RNAP); however, mRNAs are only synthesized once the virus has been uncoated in the infected cell. Viral replication occurs after synthesis of the mRNAs and requires the continuous synthesis of viral proteins. The newly synthesized antigenome positive strand serves as the template for further copies of the negative-strand genomic RNA.

CLASSIFICATION

The family *Paramyxoviridae* is classified into two subfamilies: the *Paramyxovirinae* and the *Pneumovirinae*. The *Paramyxovirinae* contains seven genera: *Respirovirus, Rubulavirus, Morbillivirus, Henipavirus, Aquaparamyxovirus, Avulavirus,* and *Ferlavirus*. The *Pneumovirinae* contains two genera *Pneumovirus* and *Metapneumovirus*. The classification is based on morphologic criteria, the organization of the genome, the biological activities of the proteins, and the sequence relationship of the encoded proteins now that all of the genome sequences have been obtained. The more recently identified tree shrew (*Tupaia*) paramyxovirus, J virus, Beilong virus, Salem virus, Menangle virus, Mossman virus, Fer-de-Lance virus, and Tioman virus have yet to be officially classified within the *Paramyxovirinae* by the International Committee on the Taxonomy of Viruses.

The morphologic distinguishing feature among enveloped viruses for the subfamily *Paramyxovirinae* is the size and shape of the nucleocapsids (diameter 18 nm, 1 μm in length, a pitch of 5.5 nm), which have a left-handed helical symmetry. The biological criteria are (a) antigenic cross-reactivity between members of a genus and (b) the presence (*Respirovirus* and *Rubulavirus*) or absence (*Morbillivirus* and *Henipavirus*) of neuraminidase (NA) activity. In addition, the differing coding potentials of the *P* genes are considered, and there is the presence of an extra gene (*SH*) in some rubulaviruses as well as J virus and Beilong virus. The pneumoviruses can be distinguished from *Paramyxovirinae* morphologically, as they contain narrower nucleocapsids. In addition, the *Pneumovirinae* have major differences in the number of encoded proteins and an attachment protein that is very different from that of *Paramyxovirinae*. Examples of members of various genera are shown in Table 33.1.

TABLE 33.1 Examples of Members of the Family *Paramyxoviridae*

- Family *Paramyxoviridae*
  - Subfamily *Paramyxovirinae*
    - Genus *Rubulavirus*
      - Mumps virus (Mu V)
      - Parainfluenza virus type 5 (previously called simian virus 5 [SV5] (PIV5))
      - Human parainfluenza virus type 2, types 4a and 4b (HPIV2/4a/4b)
      - Mapuera virus
      - Porcine rubulavirus (La-Piedad-Michoacan-Mexico virus)
    - Genus *Avulavirus*
      - Newcastle disease virus (avian paramyxovirus 1) (NDV)
    - Genus *Respirovirus*
      - Sendai virus (mouse parainfluenza virus type 1) (SeV)
      - Human parainfluenza virus type 1 and type 3 (HPIV1/3)
      - Bovine parainfluenza virus type 3 (bPIV3)
    - Genus *Henipaviruses*
      - Hendra virus (HeV)
      - Nipah virus (NiV)
    - Genus *Ferlavirus*
      - Fer-de-Lance virus (FDLV)
    - Genus *Aquaparamyxovirus*
      - Atlantic salmon paramyxovirus
    - Genus *Morbillivirus*
      - Measles virus (MeV)
      - Cetacean morbillivirus
      - Canine distemper virus (CDV)
      - Peste-des-petits-ruminants virus
      - Phocine distemper virus
      - Rinderpest virus
  - Subfamily *Pneumovirinae*
    - Genus *Pneumovirus*
      - Human respiratory syncytial virus A2, B1, S2 (HRSV)
      - Bovine respiratory syncytial virus (BRSV)
      - Pneumonia virus of mice (PVM)
    - Genus *Metapneumovirus*
      - Human metapneumovirus (HMPV)
      - Avian metapneumovirus
  - Unclassified paramyxoviruses
    - *Tupaia* paramyxovirus (TPMV)
    - Menangle virus (MenV)
    - Tioman virus (TiV)
    - Beilong virus
    - J virus
    - Mossman virus (MoV)
    - Salem virus (SaV)
    - Nariva virus

THE STRUCTURE AND REPLICATION STRATEGY OF THE *PARAMYXOVIRIDAE*

Paramyxoviruses contain nonsegmented single-stranded RNA genomes of negative polarity and replicate entirely in the cytoplasm. Their genomes are 15 to 19 kB in length, and the genomes contain 6 to 10 tandemly linked genes. A lipid envelope containing two surface glycoproteins (F and a second glycoprotein variously referred to as HN, or H or G) surrounds the virions. Inside the envelope lies a helical nucleocapsid core containing the RNA genome and the nucleocapsid (N), phospho- (P), and large (L) proteins, which initiate intracellular virus replication. Residing between the envelope and the core lies the viral matrix (M) protein that is important in virion architecture, and which is released from the core during virus entry. In addition to the genes encoding structural proteins, paramyxoviruses contain "accessory" genes that are found mostly as additional transcriptional units interspersed with the tandemly linked invariant genes. For the *Paramyxovirinae,* the accessory genes are found mostly as open reading frames (ORFs) that overlap within the *P* gene transcriptional unit.

Intracellular replication of paramyxoviruses begins with the viral RNA–dependent RNAP (minimally a homo-tetramer of P and a single L protein) transcribing the N-encapsidated genome RNA (N:RNA) into 5′ capped and 3′ polyadenylated mRNAs. The viral RNA-dependent polymerase (vRNAP)begins RNA synthesis at the 3′ end of the genome and transcribes the genes into mRNAs in a sequential (and polar) manner by terminating and reinitiating at each of the gene junctions. The junctions consist of a gene-end (GE) sequence, at which polyadenylation occurs by the reiterative synthesis of adenylates directed by a template of four to seven uridylates (followed by release of the mRNA), a short nontranscribed intergenic (IG) region, and a gene-start (GS) sequence that specifies mRNA initiation as well as capping. The vRNAP occasionally fails to reinitiate the downstream mRNA at each junction, leading to the loss of transcription of further downstream genes; hence, there is a gradient of mRNA synthesis that is inversely proportional to the distance of the gene from the 3′ end of the genome. After primary transcription and translation, when sufficient amounts of unassembled N protein are present, viral RNA synthesis becomes coupled to the concomitant encapsidation of the nascent [+] RNA chain. Under these conditions, vRNAP ignores all of the junctions (and editing sites) to produce an exact complementary antigenome chain in a fully assembled nucleocapsid.

VIRION STRUCTURE

The *Paramyxoviridae* contain a lipid bilayer envelope that is derived from the plasma membrane of the host cell in which the virus is grown.[59] *Paramyxoviridae* are generally spherical, 150 to 350 nm in diameter, but can be pleomorphic in shape, and filamentous forms can be observed. Inserted into the envelope are glycoprotein spikes that extend approximately 8 to 12 nm from the surface of the membrane, and that can be readily visualized by electron microscopy. Inside the viral membrane is the nucleocapsid core (sometimes referred to as the ribonucleoprotein [RNP] core) that contains the 15,000 to 19,000 nucleotide single-stranded RNA genome. Figure 33.1 shows a highly stylized schematic diagram of the virion. F and HN are trimers and tetramers, respectively. No attempt has been made to represent the real abundance of F, HN, SH, or N subunits in the virion. The pleomorphic nature of virus particles is illustrated in the electron micrograph in Figure 33.2, and a comparison of the RNPs of influenza virus, rabies virus, and Sendai virus is shown in Figure 33.3.

The helical nucleocapsid, rather than the free genome RNA, is the template for all RNA synthesis. For Sendai virus,

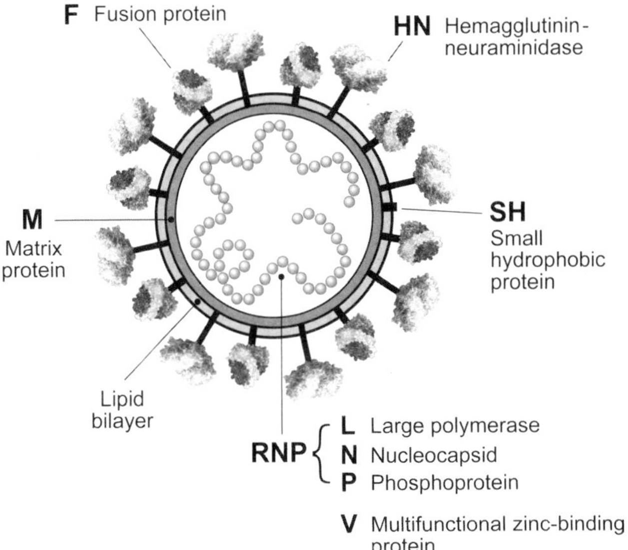

FIGURE 33.1. Schematic diagram of a paramyxovirus (not drawn to scale). The lipid bilayer is shown as the *gray concentric circle*, and underlying the lipid bilayer is the viral matrix protein shown as a dark *gray circle*. Inserted through the viral membrane are the hemagglutinin-neuraminidase (HN) attachment protein and the fusion (F) protein. The relative abundance of HN and F is not illustrated by the diagram. The small hydrophobic protein, SH, is found only in certain rubulaviruses, such as parainfluenza virus type 5 (PIV5). The HN protein is thought to have a stalk region and a globular head, and the F protein consists of two sulfide-linked chains F_1 and F_2. The HN protein is a tetramer, and the F protein a trimer. Inside the virus is the negative-strand virion RNA that is encapsidated with the nucleocapsid protein (N). Associated with the nucleocapsid are the L and P proteins, and together this complex has RNA-dependent RNA transcriptase activity (vRNAP). For the rubulaviruses, the cysteine-rich protein V is found as an internal component of the virion, whereas for other members of the family, the V protein is only found in virus-infected cells. The nature of possible interactions between the cytoplasmic tails of the glycoprotein spikes and the matrix protein, as well as the interactions between the matrix protein and the nucleocapsid, have not been fully elucidated, and no attempt has been made to illustrate them.

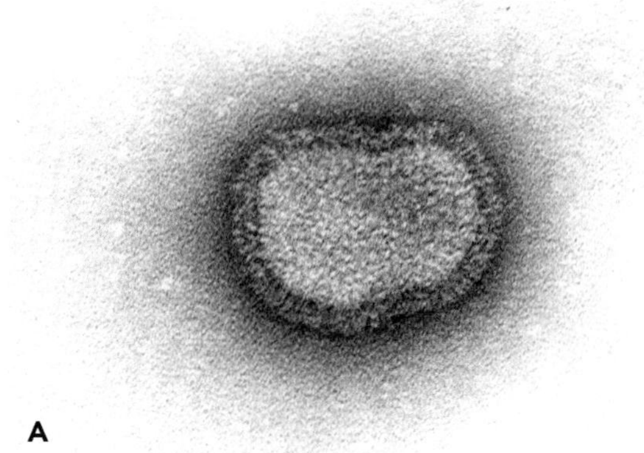

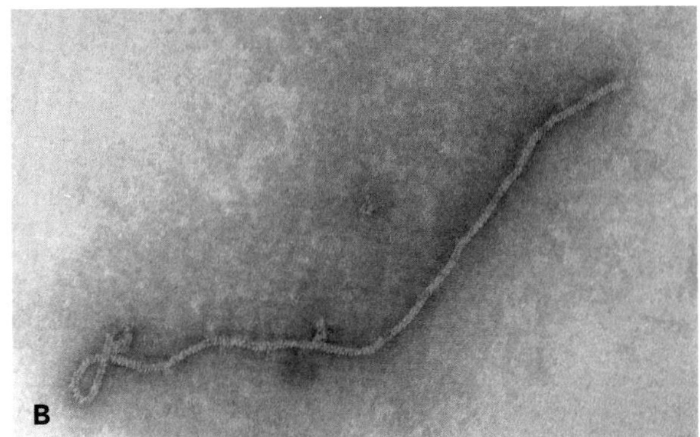

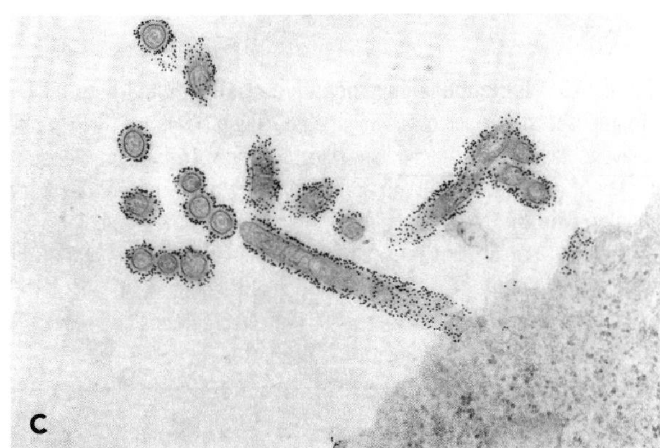

FIGURE 33.2. Ultrastructure of parainfluenza virus type 5 (PIV5; formerly simian virus type 5 [SV5]) virions revealed by negative staining. A: Negatively stained PIV5 particle: The glycoprotein spikes on intact 150- to 300-nm virus particles can be observed (226,280 x). **B:** Negatively stained PIV5 nucleocapsid (74,570 x). **C:** Budding PIV5 virions particles from the surface of CV-1 cells: Colloidal gold staining of hemagglutinin-neuraminidase (HN) is shown (24,700 x). (Micrographs courtesy of George Leser, Northwestern University. Copyright © G. D. Park and R. A. Lamb, 2006.)

each nucleocapsid is composed of approximately 2,600 N, 300 P, and 50 L proteins.[214] The N and genome RNA together form a core structure, to which the P and L proteins are attached. This nucleocapsid core is remarkably stable, as it withstands the high salt and gravity forces of cesium chloride (CsCl) density gradient centrifugation. In the electron micrograph of nucleocapsids, the P and L proteins are not observed and have only been visualized with the aid of antibodies.[327] Holo-nucleocapsids (N:RNA plus P and L) have the capacity to transcribe mRNAs *in vitro*, presumably mimicking primary transcription in infected cells, and they are thought to be the minimum unit of infectivity.

When negatively stained preparations of paramyxovirus nucleocapsids are viewed in the electron microscope, the most tightly coiled forms resemble the *Tobamovirus* tobacco mosaic virus (TMV)—a relatively rigid coiled rod 18 nm in diameter, with a central hollow core of 4 nm and a helical pitch of nearly 5 nm.[68,115] Unlike TMV, however, in which the nucleocapsid must disassemble so its positive RNA genome can function as a template, paramyxovirus nucleocapsids function without disassembling their nucleocapsids.

Sendai virus nucleocapsids exist in several distinct morphologic states at normal salt concentration.[101,156] The most prevalent form in negatively stained preparations is the most tightly coiled one, with a helical pitch of 5.3 nm. Two other forms—one with a slightly larger pitch of 6.8 nm and another with a much larger pitch of 37.5 nm—have also been noted.

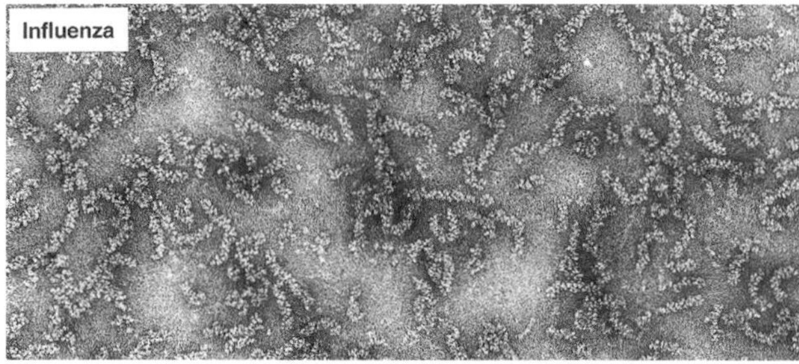

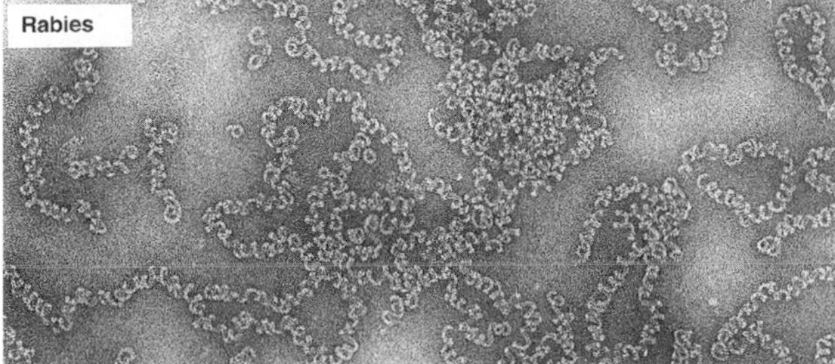

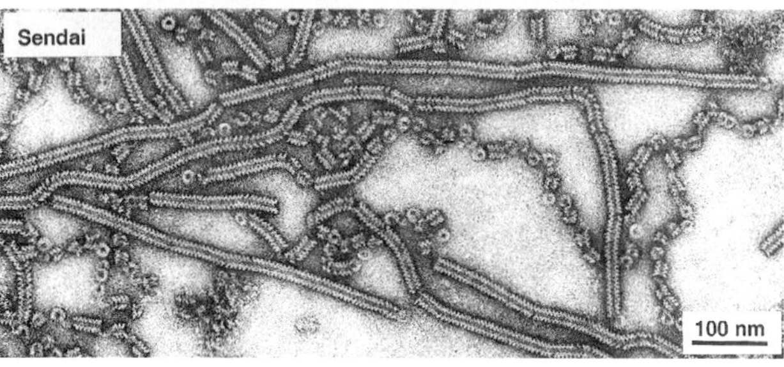

FIGURE 33.3. Nucleocapsids of negative-strand RNA viruses. Electron micrographs of the nucleocapsids of three negative-strand RNA viruses, negatively stained with 1% sodium silicotungstate. **Top:** Ribonucleoprotein particles of influenza virus with a stoichiometry of 24 nucleotides per NP monomer. **Middle:** Nucleocapsids of rabies virus with a stoichiometry of 9 nucleotides per N monomer. **Bottom:** Nucleocapsids of Sendai virus with a stoichiometry of 6 nucleotides per N monomer. All micrographs have the same magnification; bar = 100 nm. (Micrographs courtesy of Rob Ruigrok, EMBL, Grenoble, France.)

The fact that no structures of intermediate pitch have been found indicates that these are distinct states. It is thought that the template is copied without dissociation of N protein from the nucleocapsid and the uncoiling of the nucleocapsid may be necessary for the polymerase to gain access to the RNA bases. It is possible that the vRNAP traverses the nucleocapsid template by uncoiling the helix in front of it and recoiling it once the polymerase has passed a given position, much the same as cellular RNAP generates its template "bubble" in traversing double-stranded DNA (dsDNA).

As expected, the diameter of the nucleocapsid decreases as the pitch increases and the nucleocapsid lengthens; for Sendai virus, the diameter is 3.5 nm less for the 6.8 nm form than for the 5.3 nm pitch form. These latter values are very similar to those of *Pneumovirus* nucleocapsids, which also have a pitch of 7 nm. As discussed earlier, these differences in nucleocapsid morphology are used to distinguish the different *Paramyxoviridae;* however, they probably relate mainly to which form predominates in negatively stained preparations.

THE *PARAMYXOVIRIDAE* GENOMES AND THEIR ENCODED PROTEINS

The complete genome sequence for all known members of the *Paramyxoviridae* has been obtained (available at http://www.ncbi.nlm.nih.gov/). The 15,000 to 19,000 nucleotide genomic RNA contain a 3′ extracistronic region of approximately 50 nucleotides known as the leader and a 5′ extracistronic region of 50 to 161 nucleotides known as the trailer (or [–] leader). These control regions are essential for transcription and replication, and flank the six genes (seven for certain rubulaviruses and eight to ten for pneumoviruses). (Note: By the convention used for paramyxoviruses, the term *gene* refers to the genome sequence encoding a single mRNA, even if that mRNA contains more than one ORF and encodes more than one protein). The coding capacity of the genome of *Paramyxovirinae* is extended by the use of overlapping ORFs in the *P* gene. The gene order of a representative member of each subfamily is shown in Figure 33.4. At the beginning and end of each gene are conserved transcriptional control sequences that are copied into mRNA. Between the gene boundaries are intergenic regions (Fig. 33.5). These are precisely three nucleotides long for the respiroviruses and morbilliviruses but are quite variable in length for the rubulaviruses (1–47 nucleotides) and pneumoviruses (1–56 nucleotides) (see Fig. 33.5).

The Nucleocapsid Protein

The nucleocapsid (N) protein is present as the first transcribed gene in the viral genome for all paramyxoviruses except the pneumoviruses and ranges in size from 489 to 553 amino acids (molecular weight ~53–57 kDa). N is an RNA-binding protein that coats full-length viral negative sense genomic and positive sense antigenomic RNAs to form the helical nucleocapsid template, which is the only biologically active form of these viral RNAs. Electron microscopy and three-dimensional image reconstruction for Sendai virus nucleocapsids reveals that N binds approximately six consecutive nucleotides and 13 N subunits constitute each turn of the nucleocapsid helix.[101] In general, these parameters apply to other paramyxovirus nucleocapsids as well, although there can be slight differences in the number of N subunits per helix turn and in the pitch of the helix.[15] The binding of N to RNA to form a helical structure is thought to serve several functions, including protection from nuclease digestion, minimizing the annealing of mRNA to complementary genomic RNA, alignment of distal RNA segments to create a functional 3′-end promoter, and most likely providing interaction sites for assembly of progeny nucleocapsids into budding virions.

Expression of paramyxovirus N proteins in the absence of other viral components results in the formation of nucleocapsid-like structures, suggesting that N has inherent self-assembly properties and that N–N interactions drive nucleocapsid assembly.[116,277,287] Biochemical and mutational studies have shown that the N protein can be generally divided into two main structural regions: Ncore, an N-terminal domain representing approximately three-fourths of the protein and is conserved in sequence among related viruses, and Ntail, a C-terminal nonconserved acidic domain. Approximately 400 residues of the Sendai virus Ncore are essential for self-assembly, RNA binding, and activity in RNA replication.[76]

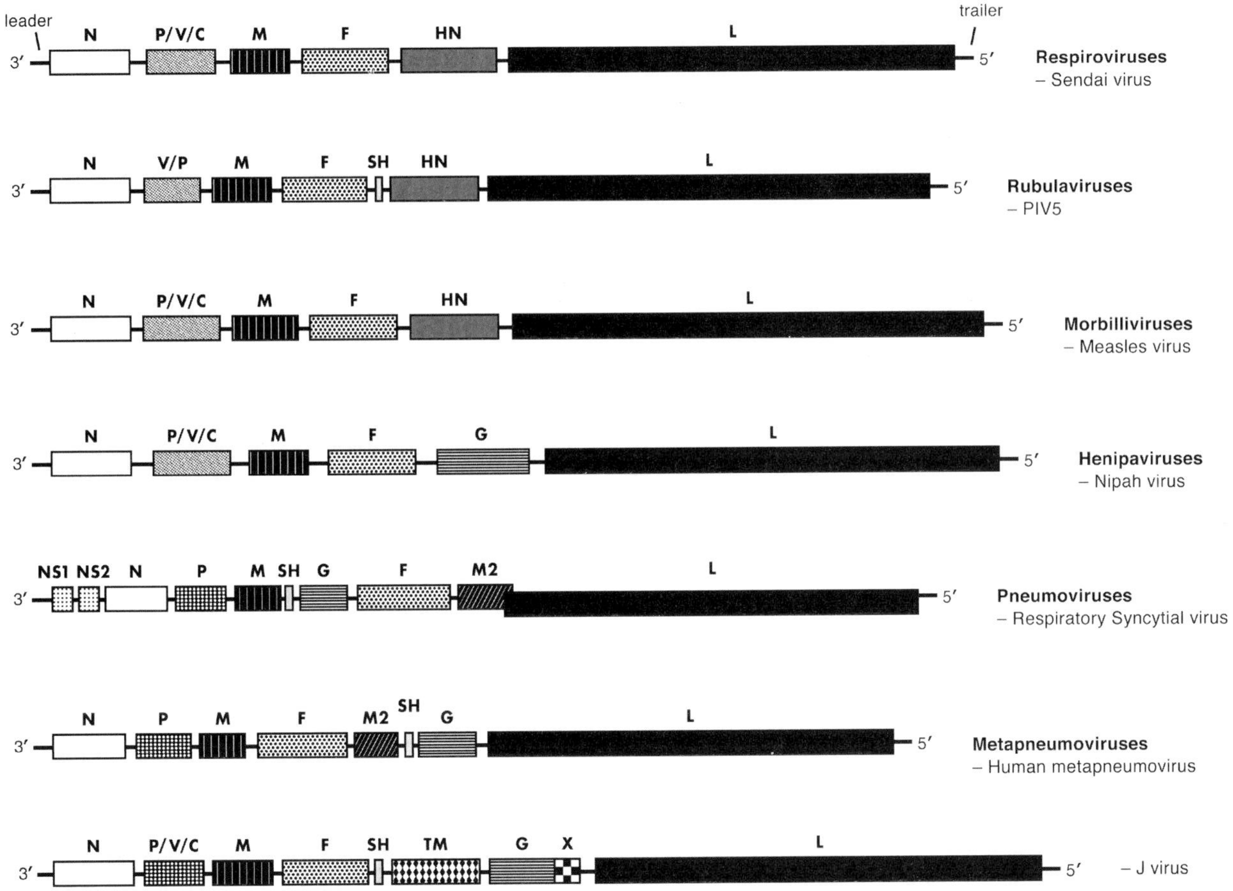

leader
trailer
3′ N P/V/C M F HN L 5′
Respiroviruses
– Sendai virus

3′ N V/P M F SH HN L 5′
Rubulaviruses
– PIV5

3′ N P/V/C M F HN L 5′
Morbilliviruses
– Measles virus

3′ N P/V/C M F G L 5′
Henipaviruses
– Nipah virus

3′ NS1 NS2 N P M SH G F M2 L 5′
Pneumoviruses
– Respiratory Syncytial virus

3′ N P M F M2 SH G L 5′
Metapneumoviruses
– Human metapneumovirus

3′ N P/V/C M F SH TM G X L 5′
– J virus

FIGURE 33.4. Genetic map of a typical member of six genera of the *Paramyxoviridae*. The gene sizes are shown as *boxes* that are drawn to approximate scale, with 3′-leader and 5′-trailer regions indicated for Sendai virus only. Gene boundaries are shown by *thin horizontal lines*. Note that the beginning of the human respiratory syncytial virus *L* gene overlaps the end of the *M2* gene by 68 nucleotides, whereas human metapneumoviruses do not have an *L*-gene overlap. For J virus, *X* denotes an internal open reading frame in the *G* gene of unknown function.

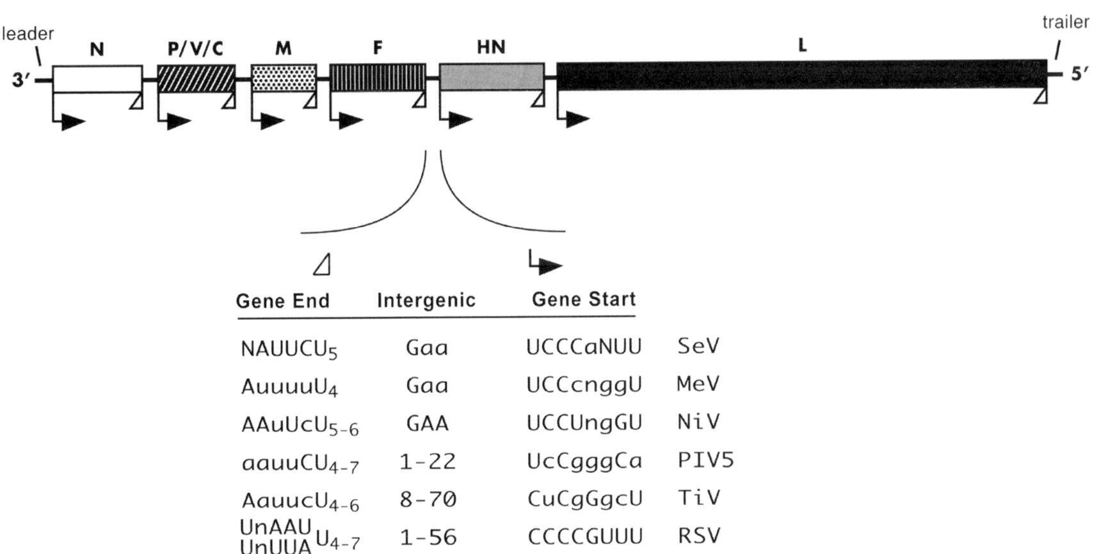

Gene End	Intergenic	Gene Start	
NAUUCU$_{5}$	Gaa	UCCCaNUU	SeV
AuuuuU$_{4}$	Gaa	UCCcnggU	MeV
AAuUcU$_{5-6}$	GAA	UCCUngGU	NiV
aauuCU$_{4-7}$	1-22	UcCgggCa	PIV5
AauucU$_{4-6}$	8-70	CuCgGgcU	TiV
UnAAU / UnUUA U$_{4-7}$	1-56	CCCCGUUU	RSV

FIGURE 33.5. Schematic diagram of a paramyxovirus genome with the transcriptional gene-end, intergenic, and transcription gene-start sequences. The positions of the extragenic 3′-terminal leader, 5′-terminal trailer, and gene junctions are shown as *thin horizontal lines*. The conserved gene-end (*open triangle*) and gene-start (*rightward arrow*) transcription regulatory sequences at the boundaries between genes are indicated. Consensus sequences for the gene-end, intergenic, and gene-start regions of representative viruses are listed as negative sense genomic RNA. Nucleotides that are strictly conserved at each viral junction are shown as *capital letters;* nucleotides that are mostly conserved (3/6 junctions or better) are shown in *lowercase letters*. SeV, Sendai virus; MeV, measles virus; NiV, Nipah virus; PIV5, parainfluenza virus 5; TiV, Tioman virus; RSV, respiratory syncytial virus.

For RSV, the N-terminal 92 residues are sufficient for assembly with RNA.[271] A central region of Ncore that is highly conserved for all members of the *Paramyxovirinae* (residues 258–369 for Sendai virus) contains an F-X4-Y-X3-φ–S-φ-A-M motif (where X is any residue and φ is an aromatic amino acid). This region is essential for self-assembly of N with RNA[276] and may be involved in N–N or N–RNA interactions.

The C-terminal Ntail region is less well conserved among related paramyxoviruses. Treatment of purified nucleocapsids with trypsin removes a portion of the C-terminal Ntail to yield a more rigid structure,[155] suggesting that this domain may confer flexibility in the coiling of the native nucleocapsid. In contrast to the essential role of the N-terminal Ncore in all N functions, the C-terminal Ntail (124 residues for Sendai virus N) is dispensable for binding RNA and for assembly of newly synthesized N-RNA complexes during replication of defective interfering particle RNAs.[76] However, nucleocapsids that are assembled with N that lacks this C-terminal Ntail are not functional as templates for the viral RNAP.[76] Structural studies have shown that the C-terminal Ntail is intrinsically disordered,[26] consistent with a proposed role for this domain in multiple protein–protein interactions. One of these essential interactions with P protein is thought to tether the L-P polymerase complex to the nucleocapsid template.[37] For example, the measles virus C-terminal Ntail has been shown to interact with a C-terminal domain of the P protein, undergoing an induced folding in some parts of this N segment.[26,186] In the case of measles virus, Ntail has also been shown to bind to the cellular chaperone protein Hsp72[455]—an interaction that could influence nucleocapsid morphologies and the synthesis of viral RNAs.[455]

The paramyxovirus nucleocapsid protein is an unusual RNA-binding protein, as it has an overall acidic charge (net charge of –7 to –12, with exception of mumps virus [+2]) and does not contain conventional RNA-binding motifs that are typically found on cellular RNA-binding proteins. The interactions of N with RNA are remarkable stable, and nucleocapsid-associated RNA is protected from nucleases even at very high salt concentrations, or when the hypersensitive C-terminal Ntail is removed by protease digestion.[155] N binding to RNA is thought to be independent of nucleotide sequence and, through interactions with the phosphodiester backbone,[181] a mechanism that would leave the nucleoside bases accessible to the viral RNAP during RNA synthesis. The Sendai virus nucleocapsid-associated RNA shows hyperreactivity to chemical treatment at cytidine residues predicted to be at positions one and six of a hexamer of nucleotides.[181] Together with the finding that the Sendai virus N protein binds six nucleotides,[101] these results have led to the proposal that the accessibility of the viral RNAP to bases within the nucleocapsid-associated genomic RNA may be controlled by their position within a hexamer of N-bound nucleotides.[181,203]

N protein exists in at least two forms in infected cells: one stably associated with RNA in a nucleocapsid structure and a second unassembled soluble form termed N^0. This latter form of N has been found to be associated with P in several viruses, including Sendai virus,[169] PIV5 (formerly known as simian virus 5 [SV5]),[331] measles virus,[379] and RSV.[121] N^0 is thought to be the functional form of N that encapsidates the nascent RNA strand during genome and antigenome replication.[78,169] N-terminal regions of Ncore are important for formation of the N^0-P complex,[166] and these domains are distinct from those involved in binding of P to N in the assembled nucleocapsid.

The *P* Gene and Its Encoded Proteins

The *Paramyxovirinae P* gene is a remarkable example of exploiting the coding capacity within a viral gene. The Sendai virus *P/V/C* gene is the most diverse of the paramyxovirus *P* genes,

TABLE 33.2 Examples of Identified *P* Gene Open Reading Frames

Paramyxovirus		mRNA insertion 0	+1G	+2G	Alternative ORFs
Rubulavirus	PIV5 (SV5); MuV; HPIV2; HPIV4	V	W	P	
Avulavirus	NDV	P	V	I	
Respirovirus	SeV	P	V	W	C′ C Y1 Y2
	BPIV3	P	V	D	C
	HPIV3	P	V	D	C
	HPIV1	P			C′ C
Henipavirus	NiV; HeV	P	V	W	C
Morbillivirus	MeV; CDV	P	V	W	C
Unclassified	J virus; TPMV; MoV	P	V	W	C
	MenV; TiV	V	W	P	
	FDLV	V	W	P	

mRNA, messenger RNA; ORFs, open reading frames; PIV5, paramyxovirus type 5; SV5, simian virus 5; MuV, mumps virus; HPIV2, human parainfluenza virus type 2; HPIV4, human parainfluenza virus type 4; NDV, Newcastle disease virus; SeV, Sendai virus; BPIV3, bovine parainfluenza virus type 3; HPIV3, human parainfluenza virus type 3; HPIV1, human parainfluenza virus type 1; NiV, Nipah virus; HeV, Hendra virus; MeV, measles virus; CDV, canine distemper virus; TPMV, *Tupaia* paramyxovirus; MoV, Mossman virus; MenV; Menangle virus; TiV, Tioman virus; FLDV, Fer-de-Lance virus.

directing the expression of at least seven polypeptides, including the P, V, W, C′, C, Y1, and Y2 proteins. Whereas other paramyxoviruses express fewer proteins from the *P/V/C* gene than Sendai virus, the *P* gene always produces more than one polypeptide species (Table 33.2). Expression of P/V/C proteins can involve two main mechanisms, with members of a paramyxovirus genus having a characteristic combination of these expression strategies. The first expression mechanism, which produces the P, V, and W/I/D proteins, has been termed *RNA editing* or pseudotemplated addition of nucleotides.[307,408,419] This mechanism involves the production of mRNAs whose ORFs are altered by insertion of G residues at a specific position in the mRNA. As described later, the second expression mechanism involves ribosome initiation at alternative translation codons and produces the family of C proteins.

The P and V proteins, as well as virus-specific proteins variously referred to as W, I, and D, are produced as a co–N-terminal nested set of proteins. These polypeptides are translation products from distinct mRNAs that differ only by inserted G nucleotides that shift the translational reading frame at the site of insertion. As shown in Figure 33.6, the *P* gene of the respiro-, morbilli-, and henipaviruses codes for a long N-terminal ORF shared by all three proteins and three shorter ORFs starting at approximately base 400 in the mRNA. During transcription of the nucleocapsid template, the viral RNAP is directed to make an accurate copy of the *P* gene template or to insert one or two G residues at a precise site in the nascent mRNA. The result is that the accurate transcription product encodes the full-length P ORF, whereas the mRNAs with insertions of +1G and +2G have a shift in the translational ORF such that the 5′ end P ORF is fused at the site of insertion in the mRNA coding sequence to a more 3′ ORF encoding V (+1G) or W (+2G). Thus, the P, V, and W/I/D proteins that are produced as a result of RNA editing share a common N-terminal region but differ in their C-terminal regions starting at the site of G insertion.

All viruses of the *Paramyxovirinae* (with the exception of human parainfluenza virus type 1 [HPIV1]) [250] encode a characteristic editing site in the *P* gene, and the number of inserted G residues, as well as the frequency of inserting G nucleotides, is determined by sequences surrounding and within the editing site. For example, Sendai virus encodes the P protein as the translation product from the unedited mRNA (+0 G; see Fig. 33.6). The V

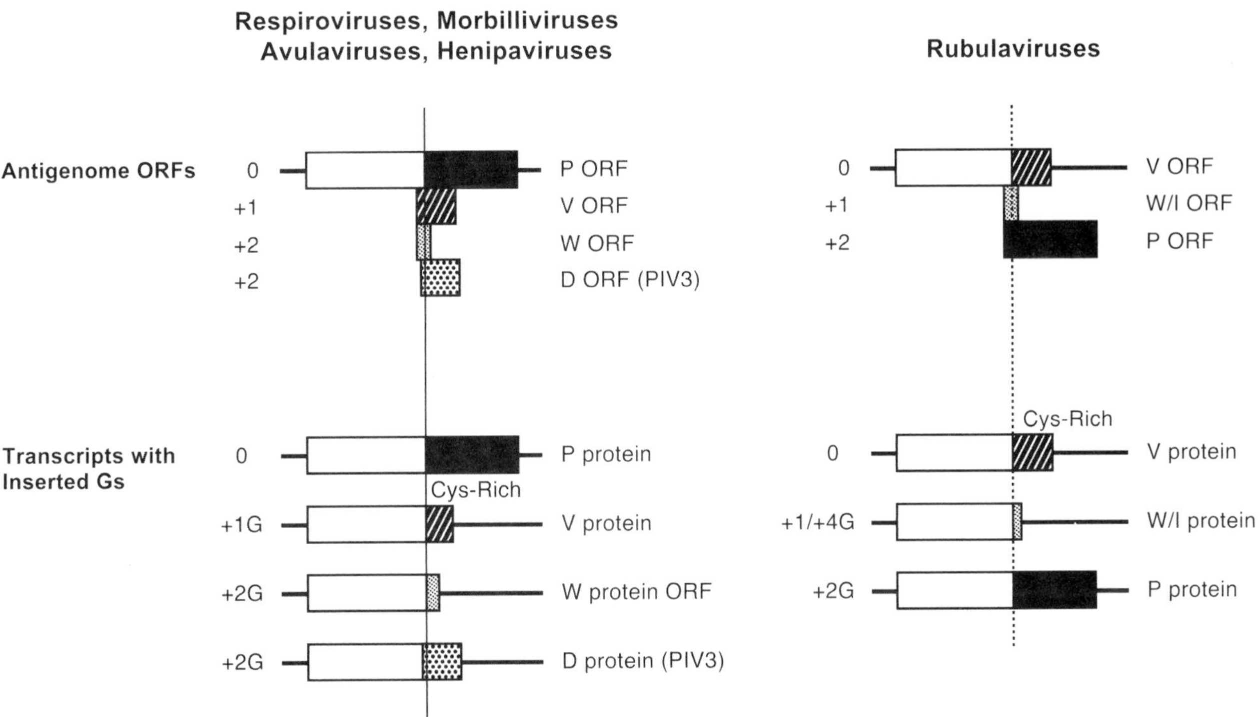

FIGURE 33.6. Schematic diagram of translational open reading frames (ORFs) generated by RNA editing during *P* gene transcription for representative paramyxoviruses. Antigenome ORFs, which span the editing site in the *P* gene, are indicated at the top by *boxes*. The shared N-terminal ORF is shown as a *white box*. The RNA editing site, at which nontemplated nucleotides are added to the messenger RNA (mRNA) is indicated by the *vertical line*. At the bottom, RNA transcripts are shown to contain insertions of zero, one, or two G residues at the editing site, with *shaded boxes* indicating unique C-terminal ORFs fused to the common N-terminal ORF shown in *white*. For the respiro-, morbilli-, avula-, and henipaviruses, the mRNA for the P protein is transcribed faithfully (unedited) from the viral genome and is shown as a *white box* fused to a *black box*. Transcriptional RNA editing with the addition of one G nucleotide at the editing site produces an mRNA that encodes the V protein, in which the common N-terminal domain shown in *white* is fused to a different ORF. Addition of two G nucleotides at the editing site produces an mRNA that encodes the W or D or I proteins (depending on the virus). For rubulaviruses, the unedited mRNA encodes the V protein, the addition of either one or four G nucleotides produces mRNA encoding the W or I protein, and the addition of two G nucleotides produces the mRNA encoding the P protein. The cysteine-rich domain of the V protein is indicated by a *striped box*.

protein is produced from a transcript containing a single G residue at the insertion site (+1 G), which fuses the common N-terminal ORF to the V-specific ORF. The Sendai virus transcript with two inserted G nucleotides codes for the W protein (+2 G). As shown in Figure 33.6, rubulaviruses differ from other paramyxoviruses in that V protein is produced by translation of the unedited mRNA (+0 G), and P is produced by translation of an mRNA containing a two-G insertion (+2 G).

Insertion of G residues into *P* gene mRNA transcripts is a co-transcriptional event catalyzed by the vRNAP[419] and is usually limited to insertions of between 0 and 2 nucleotides, depending on the virus. Human and bovine parainfluenza virus type 3 (HPIV3 and BPIV3) are exceptions to this general rule, and mRNAs with one to six inserted G residues are almost equally abundant.[120]

The Phosphoprotein

The P protein is the only *P/V/C* gene product that is essential for viral RNA synthesis.[78] P is generally 400 to 600 amino acids long and is heavily phosphorylated at serine and threonine residues, predominantly within the N-terminal region. P protein contains regions of high intrinsic disorder,[25] consistent with the requirement for interacting with multiple partners during the viral growth cycle. P is an essential component of both the vRNAP enzyme[141] and the N^0 nascent chain assembly complex that functions to encapsidate RNA during replication.[169] Extensive mutational analyses have identified distinct modular C- and N-terminal domains within the P protein that play essential roles as a polymerase cofactor and in nascent chain assembly, respectively.

The C-terminal polymerase cofactor module is relatively well conserved in predicted secondary structure for all viruses of the *Paramyxovirinae*, and all P proteins carry this essential module as the C-terminal segment of fusion protein with the shared P/V domain; this module is never naturally expressed by itself. The P protein C-terminal region contains domains for P-P multimerization, for interactions with L protein, and for binding to the N:RNA template. P protein functions as a multimer, and structural analysis suggests that the Sendai virus P protein is a tetramer.[402] For Sendai virus, the P-carboxy region is sufficient for catalyzing viral RNA synthesis, as this protein fragment by itself (residues 325–568) can substitute for intact P protein in all aspects of mRNA transcription.[79] Although the L protein is thought to contain all vRNAP catalytic activities, L binds to the nucleocapsid template via the P protein.[169] This P–L interaction requires a domain in P that maps to the C-terminal end of the coiled-coil P-P multimerization region.[32,80] At the end of the C-terminal domain, P also contains a region that binds to the N:RNA template,[32,80] providing the bridge to link L with the N:RNA template. In the case of Sendai virus, structural data indicate that this C-terminal region of P binds through weak hydrophobic interactions to the C-terminal tail of N, inducing folding of the intrinsically disordered Ntail.[232] The ability of P and Ntail to form transient weak interactions between intrinsically disordered domains may be important for the dynamic functions of P during movement of the viral RNAP across the N:RNA template or in the flexibility of the nucleocapsid template.[17,25,200]

In contrast to viral transcription, genome replication requires an N-terminal region of P (defined by deletion of Sendai virus residues 33–41). A short segment of the P protein N-terminal domain is thought to facilitate interactions with unassembled N^0 to prevent N aggregation and to ensure specificity in assembly.[78,169] The rest of the N-terminal domain of P protein is apparently dispensable for genome RNA synthesis and assembly, as a P protein in which residues 78 through 324 have been deleted is still active for minigenome replication in transfected cells.[74]

The V Protein

The V protein is an approximately 25- to 30-kDa polypeptide that shares an N-terminal domain with the P protein but has a distinct C-terminal domain as a result of RNA editing.[48,303,408,419] The C-terminal V-specific domain is highly conserved among related paramyxoviruses (Fig. 33.7), with invariantly

		* * * * * * * *
Respiro-	SeV	316...KG**H**RREHIIYERDGYIVDESW**C**NPV**C**SRIRIIPRREL**C**V**C**KT**C**PKV**C**KL**C**RD...367
	BPIV3	346...RG**H**RREHSIYREGDYIITESW**C**NPI**C**SKIRPVPRQES**C**V**C**GE**C**PKQ**C**GY**C**IE...397
Rubula-	PIV5	169...GF**H**RREYSIGWVGDEVKVTEW**C**NPS**C**SPITAAARRFE**C**T**C**HQ**C**PVT**C**SE**C**ER...220
	HPIV2	172...GN**H**RREWSIAWVGDQVKVFEW**C**NPR**C**APVTASARKFT**C**T**C**GS**C**PSI**C**GE**C**EG...223
	MuV	168...GG**H**RREWSLSWVQGEVRVFEW**C**NPI**C**SPITAAARFHS**C**K**C**GN**C**PAK**C**DQ**C**ER...219
Avula-	NDV	175...PG**H**RREHSISWTMGGVTTISW**C**NPS**C**SPIRAEPRQYS**C**T**C**GS**C**PAT**C**RL**C**AS...226
Morbilli-	MeV	230...KG**H**RREISLIWDGDRVFIDRW**C**NPM**C**SKVTLGTIRAR**C**T**C**GE**C**PRV**C**EQ**C**RT...281
	CDV	230...KG**H**RREVSLTWNGDSCWIDKW**C**NPI**C**TQVNWGIIRAK**C**F**C**GE**C**PPT**C**NE**C**KD...281
	RPV	230...KG**H**RREIDLIWNDGRVFIDRW**C**NPT**C**SKVTVGTVRAK**C**I**C**GE**C**PRV**C**EQ**C**IT...281
Henipa-	HeV	404...KG**H**RREVSICWDGRRAWVEEW**C**NPV**C**SRITPQPRKQE**C**Y**C**GE**C**PTE**C**SQ**C**CH...455
	NiV	404...KG**H**RREISICWDGKRAWVEEW**C**NPA**C**SRITPLPRRQE**C**Q**C**GE**C**PTE**C**FH**C**G....456
Unclassified	SalV	250...SR**H**RREYSIIWDSEGIQIESW**C**NPV**C**SKVRSTPRREK**C**R**C**GK**C**PAR**C**SE**C**GD...301
	TPMV	228...KG**H**RREYSMVWSNDGVFIESW**C**NPM**C**ARIRPLPIREI**C**V**C**GR**C**PLK**C**SK**C**LL...279
	MenV	164...GG**H**RREIAIDWIGGRPRVTEW**C**NPI**C**HPISQSTFRGS**C**R**C**GN**C**PGI**C**SL**C**ER...215
	TiV	162...GG**H**RREIAISWATGTPRVTEW**C**NPI**C**HPISQFTYRGT**C**R**C**GC**C**PDV**C**SL**C**ER...213
	J virus	234...KG**H**RREFCIDNFGGKTYIREW**C**NPQ**C**APITVTPTQSR**C**T**C**GE**C**PKV**C**AR**C**IK...285

FIGURE 33.7. Amino acid sequence alignment of the conserved cysteine-rich C-terminal region of selected paramyxovirus V proteins. Numbers indicate the amino acid position within the respective proteins. Positions of the conserved histidine and seven conserved cysteine residues that are involved in coordinating Zn^{2+} are indicated by *bold lettering.* Additional areas of sequence identity are *shaded.*

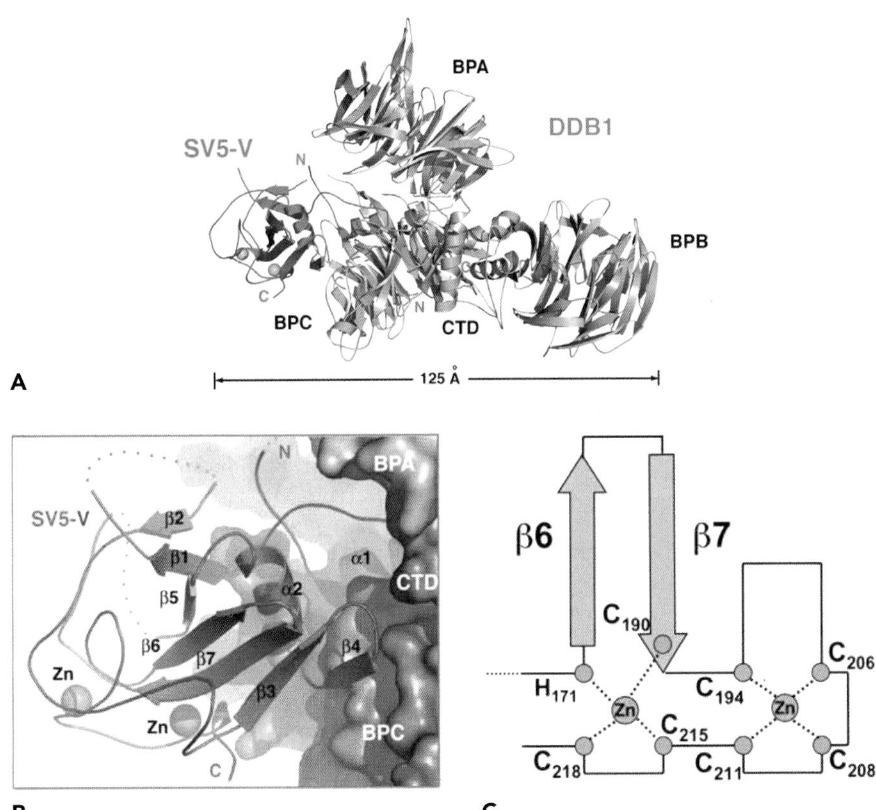

FIGURE 33.8. Atomic structure of the parainflenza virus type 5 (PIV5) V protein in complex with damage-specific DNA-binding protein 1 (DDB1). The PIV5 V protein binds to DDB1, which adopts a four-domain structure consisting of a three-propeller cluster and a helical C-terminal domain. **A:** Overall view of the DDB1-simian virus 5 (SV5)-V complex with DDB1 in *blue* and the PIV5 (SV5) V protein in *red*. The zinc ions in SV5-V are shown as *orange spheres*. The four DDB1 domains are labeled BPA, BPB, BPC, and CTD. The longest dimension of the complex is indicated. **B:** The PIV5 (SV5) V protein adopts a bipartite structure upon interacting with the DDB1 BPC domain. DDB1 and SV5-V are shown in surface and ribbon representation, respectively. The N-terminal part of the V protein, which is also found in the viral P protein, is colored in *red*. The rest of the V protein, including the zinc-binding sequence, is colored in *gray*. **C:** A novel zinc-finger fold found in the SV5-V protein. (Adapted from Li T, Chen X, Garbutt KC, et al. Structure of DDB1 in complex with a paramyxovirus V protein: Viral hijack of a propeller cluster in ubiquitin ligase. *Cell* 2006;124:105–117.)

spaced histidine and cysteine residues forming a novel domain that binds two zinc molecules per V protein.[118,225,231,304] Despite the high level of intracellular synthesis, paramyxovirus particles typically contain little V protein,[304] and the degree of incorporation of V into virions varies among paramyxoviruses.[75,431]

V protein plays several important roles in the virus replication cycle, as evidenced by recombinant viruses that have been engineered to disrupt expression of the V protein Cys-rich domain.[12,153,191,412] In many cases, these mutant viruses display an elevated RNA synthesis phenotype, although they generally grow well in many tissue culture cell lines.[82,192] However, in many cases, these viruses are severely attenuated for growth *in vivo* or are cleared more rapidly than wild-type viruses from lungs of infected animals.[94,192,418] These results suggest that V is an accessory protein that plays a role in viral pathogenesis, perhaps involving a counteracting of host cell antiviral responses that occur early after infection and that can lead to enhanced clearance of virus.

V protein has also been shown to inhibit viral RNA synthesis in transfection experiments involving model RNA genomes.[78,168,229] Recombinant viruses that are engineered with V protein mutations often show increased viral RNA synthesis.[81,191,360,412,430] This has led to the proposal that V protein serves as a negative regulator of viral RNA synthesis. V protein shares the amino-terminal domain of P protein that can interact with N^0 to form the assembly competent P-N^0. Thus, the mechanism of V inhibition may involve interactions with N that result in a form of a V-N^0 complex that is not competent to function during the RNA encapsidation step of replication. This V–N^0 interaction has been detected in the case of PIV5, Sendai virus, and measles virus,[168,331,412] and a model whereby V and P compete for soluble N^0 has been proposed.[78,168] The V protein is also capable of binding RNA,[226] and it has been proposed that this function is involved in inhibiting RNA synthesis for the Sendai virus V protein.[300]

In addition to binding viral components, V protein also has been detected in interactions with cellular proteins. For several paramyxoviruses, V protein interacts in the cytoplasm with the cellular damage-specific DNA-binding protein 1 (DDB1).[4,227] In the case of the PIV5 V protein, interaction with DDB1 is important for the function of blocking signaling through the type I interferon pathway (see later discussion). Interaction of V with DDB1 and the ability of V to inhibit host cell antiviral responses depends on the C-terminal Cys-rich domain but can also be disrupted by alterations to the common N-terminal P/V region.[4,227] The structural analysis of PIV5 V protein complexed with DDB1 shows that V protein has a bi-partite structure,[225] with a core domain built around a central seven-stranded β sheet, which is in turn sandwiched between one alpha helix and two long loops (see Fig. 33.8). The unique C-terminal domain forms the middle two β sheets and part of the central core, and this structure is anchored through the Cys-rich zinc-binding region. Thus, despite sharing a 164 amino acid N-terminal domain, the PIV5 P and V proteins can adopt very different structures owing to the unique properties of the C-terminal Cys-rich region. V protein from several paramyxoviruses has been shown to interact through the Cys-rich domain with the cellular protein MDA-5, an IFN-inducible host cell DExD/H box helicase that is involved in signaling to initiate host cell antiviral responses.

The W/D/I Proteins

The W and D ORFs of respiro-, morbilli- and henipaviruses are expressed from mRNAs with two inserted G residues (see Fig. 33.6). For most of these viruses, the insertion of two G residues into the mRNA is relatively rare, and the ORF is closed by a stop codon shortly after the editing site, resulting in the ORF for the W protein. Thus, the W protein is essentially a truncated P protein, containing the N-terminal N^0 assembly module of the P protein alone. W protein is abundantly expressed in Sendai virus–infected cells[73] and has been found to interact with unassembled N^0, suggesting an inhibitory role in viral RNA synthesis.[168] In the case of BPIV3 and HPIV3, the +2 ORF extends for 131 residues from the editing site, and the protein that links the amino-terminal P domain to this ORF is called *D protein.*[120] The *Rubulavirus* I protein is generated when the upstream N-terminal P region is fused to a downstream ORF by the insertion of either one or four G residues during RNA editing.[303,408] The role that the W/D/I proteins play in the viral growth cycle has not been established.

The C Proteins

In addition to RNA editing, some paramyxoviruses use a second mechanism to express *P* gene polypeptides that involves the use of alternative translation initiation codons to yield the C proteins (Fig. 33.9). The Sendai virus C′, C, Y1, and Y2 proteins comprise a nested set of carboxy–co-terminal polypeptides that range in size from 175 to 215 residues. These proteins are expressed independently from a P/V mRNA through the use of alternative start codons (Fig. 33.9), with the C protein ORF being in the +1 reading frame relative to the P ORF. The C′ and C proteins are translated by a leaky scanning mechanism, being initiated at an unconventional ACG triplet at base 81 and AUG at base 114, respectively.[77] By contrast, translation of the Y1 and Y2 proteins occurs through a scanning-independent ribosome shunting mechanism that is directed by a 5′ noncoding RNA segment, resulting in ribosomes initiating at AUG codon bases 183 and 201, respectively. Translation of each of the C′, C, Y1, and Y2 ORFs is initiated at a different site, although translation is terminated at the same downstream stop codon; thus, these proteins share a common C-terminal region. The C protein is abundantly expressed in infected cells at levels higher than C′, Y1, and Y2; however, virions contain only very low levels of these polypeptides.[217] Morbilliviruses express one C protein,[13] as do the henipaviruses,[427] whereas the respiroviruses such as Sendai virus and HPIV1 express all four C′, C, Y1, and Y2 polypeptides.[128] Rubula- and avulaviruses do not express C proteins (see Table 33.2).

C proteins are small basic polypeptides that play multiple functions in the viral growth cycle, being involved in the control of viral RNA synthesis, counteracting host cell antiviral pathways, and facilitating release of virus from infected cells. Although nonessential for infectivity, Sendai virus mutants engineered to express only a subset of C proteins or lacking expression of all four proteins show defects in virus growth.[209] The C proteins have been shown to inhibit mRNA transcription and suppress RNA replication in a promoter-specific manner.[193,238,399] Consistent with this, viral mutants that are engineered to lack C protein expression show elevated synthesis of viral mRNA and protein.[147] The inhibition of RNA synthesis by C proteins correlates with the ability to bind to the

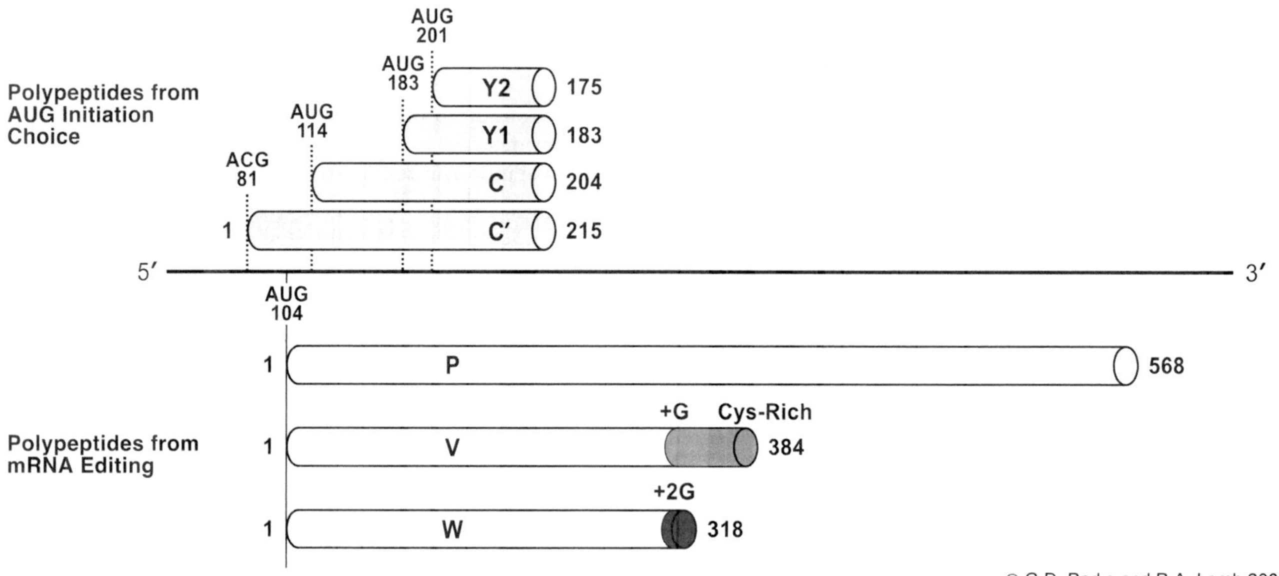

FIGURE 33.9. Representation of the Sendai virus P messenger RNA (mRNA) to illustrate the mechanisms of producing P, V, and C proteins. The position of four unique initiation codons for the C′, C, Y1, and Y2 open reading frames (ORFs) are shown above the *horizontal black line* representing the *P* gene mRNA. The position of the common initiation codon for the P, V, and W ORFs at base 104 is shown below the mRNA. The *gray cylinder* indicates the V protein Cys-rich C-terminal domain, which is fused to the shared P N-terminal domain by addition of a G residue during viral transcription; the *black cylinder* indicates the short W domain, which is accessed by insertion of two G residues. Numbers denote the amino acids contained within each polypeptide chain. Note that the initiation codon for C′ is ACG.

L subunit of the viral polymerase,[170] and in the case of Sendai virus, naturally occurring variant C proteins can have differential effects on inhibition of virus RNA synthesis.[10]

The role of paramyxovirus C proteins in pathogenesis and in counteracting host cell IFN responses is best understood in the cases of Sendai virus and measles virus. For Sendai virus, the C′, C, Y1, and Y2 proteins can antagonize IFN signaling when assayed in stably transfected HeLa cells[193]; however, there may be more subtle differences in the functions of each polypeptide in the context of viral mutants.[124] In the case of measles virus, recombinant viruses defective for C protein expression grow well in certain culture cells but are defective for growth in peripheral blood mononuclear cells[104] and are less virulent *in vivo*.[310] Changes in pathogenesis of C-mutant viruses may be related to the ability of the C proteins to inhibit type I IFN responses.[368] This proposal is further supported by a naturally occurring mutation in the Sendai virus C protein (phenylalanine 170 to serine) that eliminates the ability of C protein to block IFN signaling,[124] and a mutant Sendai virus harboring this altered C protein is attenuated for growth in mice. The mechanism by which C proteins attenuate IFN signaling has not been elicited but may involve binding of C to STAT1[124] or altering STAT1 phosphorylation patterns.[205]

An additional role for C proteins in virus release became evident with the analysis of mutant Sendai virus that cannot express any of the four C proteins.[209] Whereas viral RNA and protein synthesis was high for this mutant virus, production of infectious virions was low, and heterogeneous noninfectious particles were produced.[147] C protein expression enhances release of virus-like particles (VLPs), possibly through interactions with AIP1/Alix—a cellular protein involved in apoptosis and endosomal trafficking.[347]

The Large Protein

The large (L) protein is an essential subunit of the paramyxovirus RNAP. Consistent with a catalytic role in viral RNA synthesis, the L protein is invariably encoded as the most promoter-distal gene in the paramyxovirus genome (see Fig. 33.4). L protein is generally found in only very low amounts in infected cells or associated with nucleocapsids and virions.[214] A paramyxovirus particle typically contains only about 50 copies of L,[214] where it is found on the nucleocapsid in clusters that co-localize with P protein.[327] L is thought to possess all of the enzymatic activities needed for synthesis of functional viral mRNA, including nucleotide polymerization as well as 5′-end capping and methylation and 3′-end polyadenylation of mRNAs.[137,158,289] Polyadenylation of viral mRNAs occurs co-transcriptionally, where L is thought to add poly A tails to nascent viral mRNAs through a mechanism that involves stuttering at a stretch of template U residues at the end of each viral gene (see Fig. 33.5). L protein is also responsible for the replication of viral genomic and antigenomic RNA; however, this form of RNA synthesis differs from mRNA transcription by having a strict requirement for soluble N^0 to allow encapsidation of the nascent genomic RNA.[139,169]

The paramyxovirus L protein is generally approximately 2,200 amino acids in length (~250 kDa). Although the N- and C-terminal regions of the L proteins are diverse, sequence comparisons among L proteins have identified six highly conserved domains (I–VI) near the middle of the polypeptide. It was originally proposed that these domains may be individually responsible for each of the multiple L functions.[319] Domain II is proposed to be an RNA-binding domain owing to the high net positive charge. In domain III, mutational analyses are consistent with the proposal of a conserved GDNQ motif as the active site for nucleotide polymerization.[237] Based on sequence homologies, domain VI of the rhabdovirus L protein has been implicated in playing a major role in 5′ cap formation, perhaps as a methyltransferase domain.[114,319] The precise roles of the remaining domains I, IV, and V in individual steps of RNAP activity are not clear; however, for Sendai virus, mutations in some of these domains result in L proteins that can transcribe viral mRNA but are defective in RNA replication.[56,113] In the case of the L proteins of Sendai virus and rinderpest virus, sequence alignment has identified nonconserved hinge regions that can be modified by insertions of green fluorescent protein (GFP), and remarkably, viable recombinant viruses encoding these L-GFP hybrid proteins have been isolated and used to identify sites of L localization during infection.[35,92]

L protein activity in RNA synthesis highly depends on protein–protein interactions, involving self-assembly as well as binding to other viral and cellular proteins. Biochemical evidence and genetic complementation studies indicate that the Sendai and measles virus L proteins function as homomultimers that interact through an N-terminal self-assembly domain.[54,376] L also binds to the viral P protein—an interaction that is essential for formation of the active enzyme complex and can lead to enhanced stability of L.[141,169] L–P interaction domains generally map to an N-terminal domain of L that is distinct from the L-L assembly domain.[165] Within the L-P complex, P protein serves as the bridge to link the L polymerase to the nucleocapsid template.[80,169] In addition to L–L and L–P interactions, L protein also interacts with host cell proteins.[269,375] In the case of measles virus and Sendai virus, L interactions with tubulin are thought to promote L activity.[269] Other cellular proteins have also been shown to promote viral RNA synthesis (e.g., β-catenin for HPIV3),[22] although the precise role that these proteins play in viral RNA synthesis has not been determined.

Whereas interactions of L with P are generally thought to promote activity, L protein can also interact with other viral components that inhibit the vRNAP. For both rinderpest virus and Sendai virus, L protein has been found to bind the viral C proteins.[170,390] The Sendai virus L–C interactions are through a domain of L that maps to the first 895 residues (domains I–III),[170] and this binding correlates with inhibition of RNA synthesis.[138] Other proteins encoded in the viral *P/V/C* gene (C′, Y1, and Y2) also interact with L and inhibit defective interfering RNA synthesis *in vitro*[138] and *in vivo*.[193]

The Matrix Protein

The paramyxovirus matrix (M) protein is the most abundant protein in the virion. The M proteins contain 341 to 375 residues (M_r ~38,500–41,500), are quite basic proteins (net charge at neutral pH of +14 to +17), and are somewhat hydrophobic, although there are no domains of sufficient length to span a lipid bilayer. In electron micrographs of virions, an electron-dense layer is observed underlying the viral lipid bilayer, and this is thought to represent the location of this protein. Fractionation studies of virions indicate that the M protein is peripherally associated with membranes and is not an intrinsic membrane protein. Reconstitution studies of purified

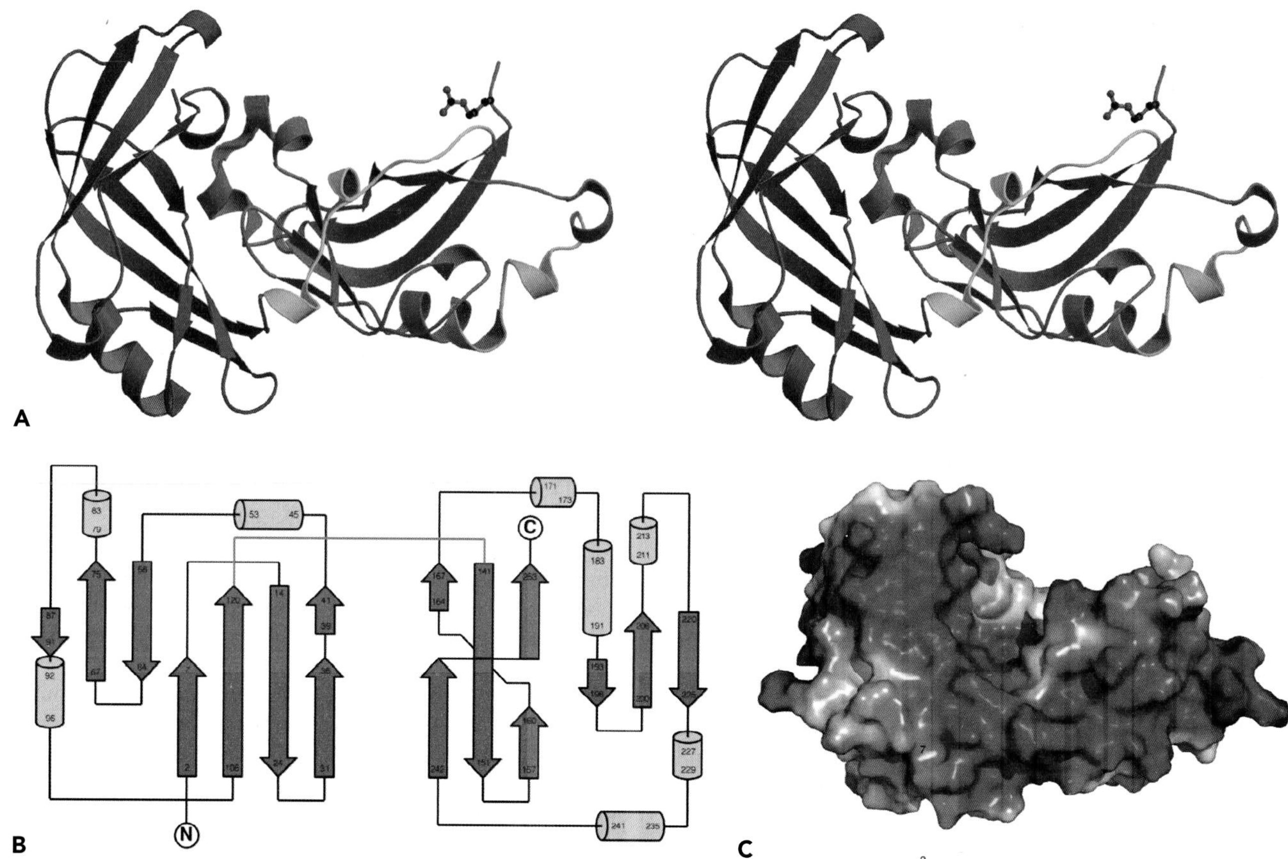

FIGURE 33.10. Three-dimensional structure of the RSV M protein. The crystal structure of M (resolution 1.6 Å) shows two domains composed largely of β-sheets. **A:** Divergent (wall-eyed) stereoview of M colored according to domain with the linker shown in *cyan*, the N-terminal domain in *blue*, and the C-terminal domain in *red*. Residue R254 is shown in ball-and-stick representation. **B:** A topology diagram of the protein. The linker between the N- and C-terminal domains is shown in *magenta*. Residues (numbers refer to Met as +1) in β-sheets are represented by *broad arrows* and helices as *cylinders*. **C:** Electrostatic surface potential (calculated with APBS) for M, presented in a color range from *red* to *blue* (−5 to +5 kT/e); uncharged residues are uncolored. (From Money VA, McPhee HK, Mosely JA, et al. Surface features of a Mononegavirales matrix protein indicate sites of membrane interaction. *Proc Natl Acad Sci U S A* 2009;106:4441–4446.)

M protein and fractionation studies of infected cells indicate that the M protein can associate with membranes.[105,212,280]

As a purified protein, the Sendai virus M protein can self-associate and form two-dimensional paracrystalline assays (sheets and tubes) in low salt conditions.[7,157] There is a paracrystalline array of identical periodicity at the inner surface of the plasma membrane of infected cells when examined by freeze-fracture techniques in the electron microscopy.[7] In addition, the M protein is associated with nucleocapsids.[386] As of January 2011 the only atomic structure of M to be obtained is that of RSV M.[264] It shows that the protein has extensive β-sheets and a continuously charged region covering approximately 600 Å, which probably interacts with a negatively charged surface on the RNP (Fig. 33.10). Genetically engineered recombinant measles virus and PIV5 that lack glycoprotein cytoplasmic tails show a subcellular redistribution of the matrix protein,[46,357] which implies that there is an interaction of the F and HN cytoplasmic tails with the M protein. Thus, the M protein is considered to be the central organizer of viral morphogenesis interacting with the cytoplasmic tails of the integral membrane proteins, the lipid bilayer, and the nucleocapsids. The self-association of M and its contact with the nucleocapsid may be the driving force in forming a budding virus particle.[311] The relative abundance of basic residues in the M protein may reflect their importance in ionic interactions with the acidic N proteins.

For several enveloped viruses, it has been shown that budding occurs by using components of the endosomal sorting complexes required for transport (ESCRTs)—proteins involved in multivesiculate body formation. Protein–protein interaction domains called *late domains* have been identified in the matrix proteins of several viruses; for the paramyxoviruses, a late domain has been identified in PIV5 M protein.[358] This topic is discussed further in the Assembly of the Envelope section.

Consistent with its central role in virus budding, M is often inactivated in persistent paramyxovirus infections where budding fails to occur. For example, in subacute sclerosing panencephalitis (SSPE)—a rare, progressive, and invariably fatal persistent measles virus infection of the brain—the M protein is either absent for various reasons[47] or, when present, is not associated with budding structures *in vivo* and is unable to bind to viral nucleocapsids *in vitro*.[162] Although a genetically engineered recombinant measles virus that lacks a matrix protein has been obtained,[45] it produces approximately 4 logs lower titer of released infectious particles than wild-type virus and remains mostly cell associated. Therefore, it is reasonable to conclude that the M protein does play a very important function in virus assembly. Moreover, in model systems of persistent Sendai virus infection in culture, the normally lytic infection is converted to a persistent one using defective interfering particles. This change correlates mainly with M protein instability and an absence of budding structures.[341]

The M protein of several paramyxoviruses is phosphorylated. For Sendai virus, a large proportion of the M protein is phosphorylated, whereas the M protein found in virions is not phosphorylated.[212] However, a Sendai virus could be rescued from an infectious complementary DNA (cDNA) in which the single phosphorylation site in Sendai virus M protein had been eliminated.[348] This M protein phosphorylation-minus mutant did not show an altered phenotype from wild-type virus in either cultured cells or mice.

Envelope Glycoproteins

All *Paramyxoviridae* possess two integral membrane proteins, and some rubulaviruses and all pneumoviruses encode a third integral membrane protein (Fig. 33.11). One glycoprotein (HN, H, or G) is involved in cell attachment and the other glycoprotein (F) in mediating pH-independent fusion of the viral envelope with the plasma membrane of the host cell. The *Rubulavirus* and *Pneumovirus* third integral membrane protein is referred to as SH; for PIV5, this 44 amino acid integral membrane protein is thought to block virus-induced apoptosis. The assignment of specific biological activities of F and HN was originally made on the basis of purification and reconstitution studies, mainly for the Sendai virus and PIV5 proteins.[353,354] The attachment proteins (HN, H, or G) are all type II integral membrane proteins, and bioinformatics and structural predictions indicate that the proteins will all exhibit a related propeller-like fold despite having different receptors and the presence or absence of NA activity.

For the respiroviruses and rubulaviruses, the attachment glycoprotein binds to cellular sialic acid–containing receptors, and these can be glycoproteins or glycolipids. The binding is probably of fairly low affinity but of sufficiently high avidity that these viruses agglutinate erythrocytes (hemagglutination). The attachment proteins of respiroviruses and rubulaviruses also have NA activity (receptor-destroying activity), and the proteins have been designated hemagglutinin-neuraminidase (HN). However, a possible role of a specific protein–protein involvement in infection of host cells has not been ruled out.

The restricted host range of measles virus for primate cells and the lack of NA or esterase activity make it unlikely that sialic acid is the primary receptor for measles virus. Nonetheless, the *Morbillivirus* attachment protein (H) can cause agglutination of primate erythrocytes, most likely owing to receptor binding: the designation of measles and CDV glycoprotein as H is thus a misnomer. In 1993, human CD46 was identified as a cellular receptor for Edmonston and Halle strains of measles virus.[91,282] Edmonston and Vero cell-isolated strains of measles virus are capable of infecting any $CD46^+$ primate cell. However, viruses isolated from B- and T-cell lines do not grow in $CD46^+$ cells. A second receptor was identified—human CD150 (SLAM), a membrane glycoprotein involved in lymphocyte activation.[404,442] It is now thought that CD150 is the principle receptor for unadapted isolates of lymphotropic measles virus.[291]

Very recently, a third receptor for measles virus has been identified, known as poliovirus receptor-like (PVRL4; Nectin 4) or adherens junction protein nectin 4. It is proposed that this new receptor is the epithelial receptor for measles virus that

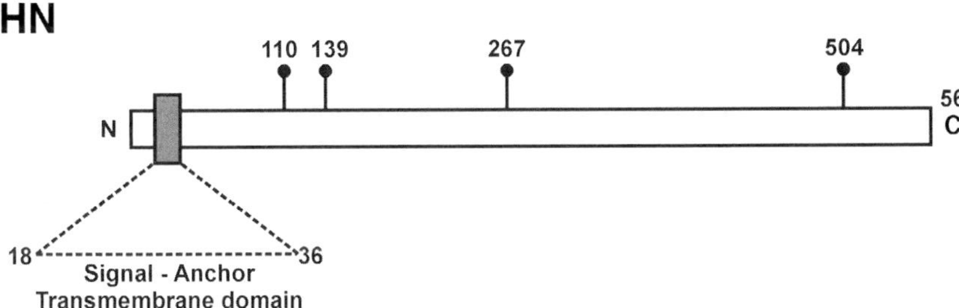

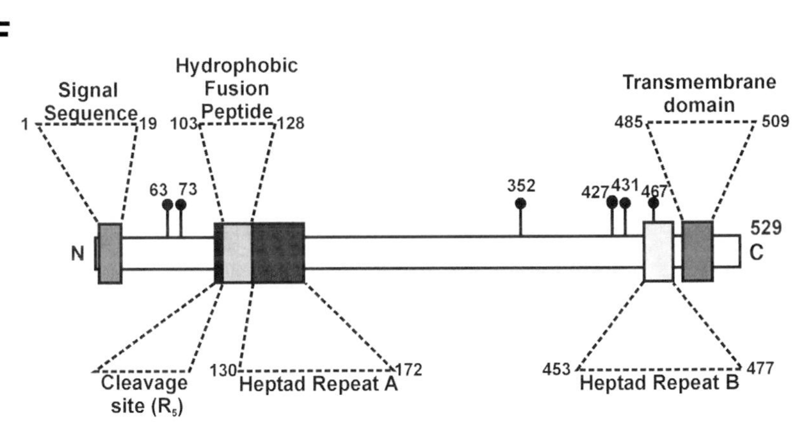

FIGURE 33.11. Schematic diagram showing the orientation and domains of paramyxovirus integral membrane proteins. A: Hemagglutinin-neuraminidase (HN) attachment protein (based on the predicted sequence of the parainfluenza virus type 5 [PIV5] *HN* gene.[159] The signal anchor transmembrane domain and the sites used for addition of N-linked carbohydrate (*lollipops*)[285] are indicated. **B:** Fusion protein (based on the predicted sequence of the PIV5 *F* gene). The position of the signal sequence, the transmembrane domain, the cleavage site, the hydrophobic fusion peptide, and the heptad repeats A and B are indicated. The sites used for addition of N-linked carbohydrate (*lollipops*)[8] are indicated. R_5 indicates the five arginine residues site for cleavage activation.

is used to transfer virus from the basolateral surface of epithelial cells to the lumenal side of the airway.[270,288]

The receptor for Hendra virus and Nipah virus G glycoprotein has been shown to be ephrin-B2 or ephrin-B3. In one approach, direct binding of Nipah G to receptor was obtained and the identity of the receptor determined by protein sequencing and bioinformatics.[284] In another approach, microarray analysis was used to identify mRNAs that were expressed in henipavirus-susceptible cells and not in cells refractory to henipavirus infection.[20] Ephrin-B2 and -B3 are members of a family of cell surface glycoprotein ligands that bind to ephrin (Eph) receptors—a large family of tyrosine kinases. The identification of ephrin-B2/B3 as the cellular receptor for both Hendra virus and Nipah viruses and the widespread occurrence of ephrin-B2/3 in vertebrates, particularly in arterial endothelial cells and in neurons, provides an explanation for the wide host range of henipaviruses and their systemic infection.[98]

The *Pneumovirus* RSV does not cause detectable hemagglutination, and the cellular receptor for RSV is not completely understood but involves interactions with heparan sulfate—a glycosaminoglycan that is part of the extracellular matrix. Interestingly, the G protein of RSV and human metapneumovirus (HMPV) can be deleted from the viral genome,[189] and Sendai virus–like particles devoid of HN can infect cells via the asialoglycoprotein receptor.[224] Both of these cases suggest that some paramyxovirus F proteins may have a binding activity. After attachment of a *Paramyxoviridae* particle to the host cell receptor, the viral envelope fuses with the host cell plasma membrane, and the major viral protein involved in this process is the F glycoprotein.

Paramyxovirus Attachment Protein

The *Respirovirus* and *Rubulavirus* surface glycoprotein HN is a multifunctional protein and the major antigenic determinant of the paramyxoviruses. HN has three activities: (a) receptor binding to sialic acid; (b) cleavage of sialic acid from complex carbohydrate chains (NA activity); and (c) fusion promotion—that is, co-expression of HN and F is required for cell–cell fusion (see later discussion). By analogy to the role of influenza virus NA, it seems likely that the role of this NA activity is to prevent self-aggregation of viral particles during budding at the plasma membrane. These dual activities of HN can be modulated by pH.[258] Whereas the pH of the extracellular environment is optimal for hemagglutination, paramyxovirus NAs have an acidic pH optima (pH 4.8–5.5), suggesting that NA acts in the acidic *trans*-Golgi network to remove sialic acid from the HN carbohydrate chains and from the F protein carbohydrate chains.

The HN polypeptide chain ranges from 565 to 582 residues. For some strains of NDV, HN is synthesized as a biologically inactive precursor (HN_o), and 44 residues from the C-terminus are removed to activate the molecule.[278,279] HN is a type II integral membrane protein that spans the membrane once and contains an N-terminal cytoplasmic tail, a single N-terminal transmembrane (TM) domain, a membrane-proximal stalk domain, and a large C-terminal globular head domain.[159] The globular head domain contains the receptor-binding and enzymatic activity.[301,353,410] HN is glycosylated and contains from four to six potential sites for the addition of N-linked carbohydrate chains. For PIV5 and NDV HN, it is known that four sites are used.[253,285] HN is noncovalently associated to form a dimer of dimers, based on biochemical, cross-linking, electron microscopy, and structural studies that, depending on the paramyxovirus, can be composed of two disulfide-linked dimers.[72,148,218,252,285,286,409,450,451] The covalent linkage occurs through a cysteine residue at the C-terminal end of the stalk domain, just prior to the beginning of the head domain. The stalk domain appears to play an essential role in the formation of the tetramer,[451] and head domains when expressed without the stalk are often monomeric.[72,218,451]

The structure of the enzymatically active head domain of HN is similar to other NAs or sialidases, such as influenza NA,[103] with the globular head composed of identical subunits. Each NA domain exhibits the six-blade propeller fold typical of other NA/sialidase structures from viral, protozoan, or bacterial origin.[41,216,405] Atomic structures of soluble head domains of NDV, HPIV3, PIV5 (liganded and bound to a receptor/substrate sialyllactose), measles virus H (unliganded and bound to its receptor CD150/SLAM), and Hendra and Nipah virus G (unliganded and bound to its receptor ephrin-B2 or ephrin-B3) have been obtained,[30,31,60,72,148,149,218,441,451,453] and it shows the typical sialidase fold consisting of six antiparallel β-strands organized as a super barrel with a centrally located active site (Fig. 33.12). The seven highly conserved active site residues found in NA and sialidases are found in the paramyxovirus HN structures. However, these key active site residues are mutated in the measles H and Nipah/Hendra G proteins, rendering these proteins enzymatically dead. Superimposition of the NDV, HPIV3, and PIV5 HN monomer structures indicates a high degree of conservation on one face of the molecule, with the other face containing more variability and additional protein loops.[451]

It has long been debated whether the hemagglutinin and NA activities of HN involve one or two separate sialic acid binding sites.[72,329,453] The disparate theories of one site with dual function or of two distinct sites that are intimately related are both consistent with the observation that sialic acid–derived NA inhibitors interfere with receptor binding.[177,275,355] A single site can provide both hemagglutinin and NA activities by binding sialic acid tightly and hydrolyzing the molecules slowly.[355] For NDV HN, two sialic acid sites have been observed in the x-ray structures: one is the active site, and a second site is located at the dimer interface.[453] Strong biological evidence supports the notion of a second sialic acid binding site in NDV.[29,323] Mutagenesis of a key residue involved in the dimer interface sialic acid binding site abolishes sialic acid binding to the second site.[29] However, virus containing this key residue mutation is only marginally affected in growth properties.[29] For HPIV3, the second sialic acid binding site is blocked by a carbohydrate chain that prevents its function,[261] although mutagenesis to ablate the carbohydrate chain allows the HPIV3 second site to bind sialic acid. The growth curve of HPIV3 with or without the carbohydrate chain that shields the second sialic acid binding site is very similar, suggesting no major biological importance.

For PIV5 HN, not only was a second sialic acid binding site not observed, the molecule could not form the second sialic acid binding site between two monomers owing to changes in sequence and conformation.[218,451] Thus, the biological importance of the second sialic acid binding sites in NDV HN and the one created in HPIV3 by removal of the carbohydrate addition site are a conundrum.[261,322,325]

From the structural studies of NDV HN, it was also suggested that the NA domain could form two distinct dimeric

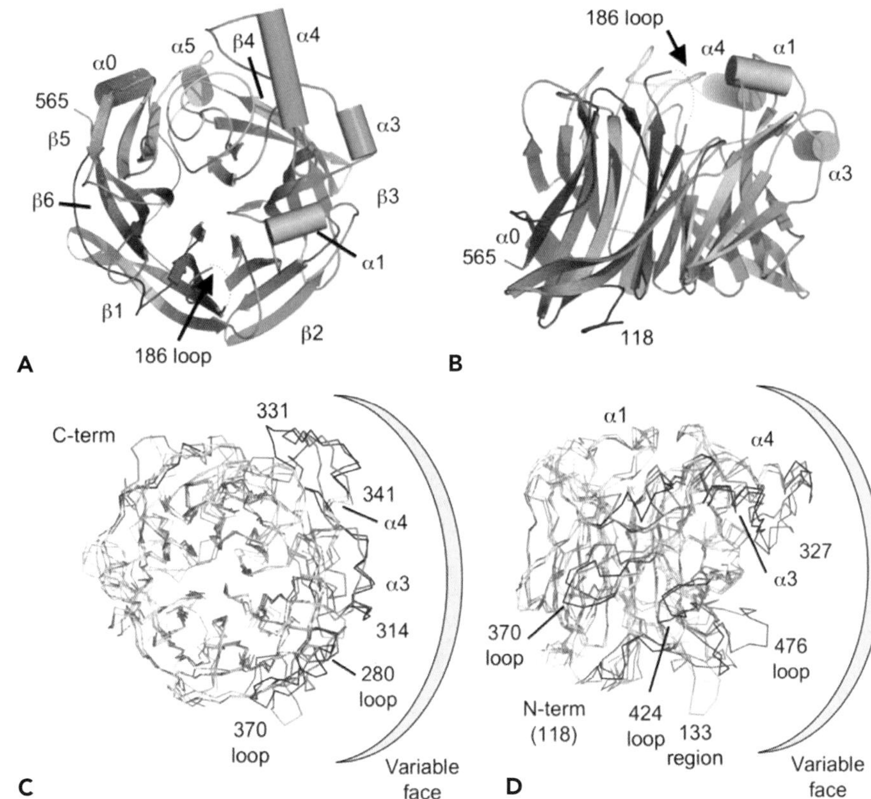

FIGURE 33.12. Parainfluenza virus type 5 (PIV5) hemagglutinin-neuraminidase (HN) monomer structure and comparison with Newcastle disease virus (NDV) HN and human parainfluenza virus type 3 (HPIV3) HN. A, B: Schematic cartoon diagrams showing top and side views of PIV5 HN. Helices are shown in *cylinders,* and β-strands are shown in *arrowed belts.* The N-terminus is shown in *blue,* and the C-terminus is shown in *red.* The missing loop from residues 186 through 190 is indicated as a *dashed blue line.* **C, D:** $C\alpha$ ribbon diagram of the superposition of PIV5 HN with NDV and HPIV3 HN, shown in top and side views. Major differences in the PIV5, NDV, and human parainfluenza virus (HPIV) HN structures are colored *red, blue,* and *green,* respectively. Areas of major structural differences are labeled, and the highly variable face of the HN monomer is highlighted. (Adapted from Yuan P, Thompson T, Wurzburg BA, et al. Structural studies of the parainfluenza virius 5 hemagglutinin-neuraminidase tetramer in complex with its receptor, sialyllactose. *Structure* 2005;13:1–13.)

assemblies that were ligand dependent.[72] One of the dimers, observed after co-crystallization with ligand, formed an extensive buried interface, whereas the second dimer, crystallized in the absence of ligand and at low pH, formed a much smaller interface. Conformational changes were observed in the active site of the HN protein upon ligand binding that were correlated with changes in the dimer interface, suggesting a possible mechanism for coupling ligand recognition to changes in the oligomeric assembly of the HN protein. However, engineered disulfide bonds block dimer dissociation and do not affect fusion, rendering major HN rearrangements unlikely.[234]

Structural studies of HPIV3 and PIV5 HN also do not support the notion that there are ligand-dependent conformational changes within the monomeric protein structure.[218,451] The dimer of HN that is observed in the HPIV3 and PIV5 structures occurs in the absence of ligand binding, and there is no crystallographic evidence that monomeric ligand binding influences the oligomeric structure of these HN proteins.

The HN tetrameric arrangement[451,453] is unusual, because rather than having fourfold rotational symmetry as might be anticipated, it is arranged with two twofold symmetry axes (Fig. 33.13) that are orientated at approximately 90 degrees

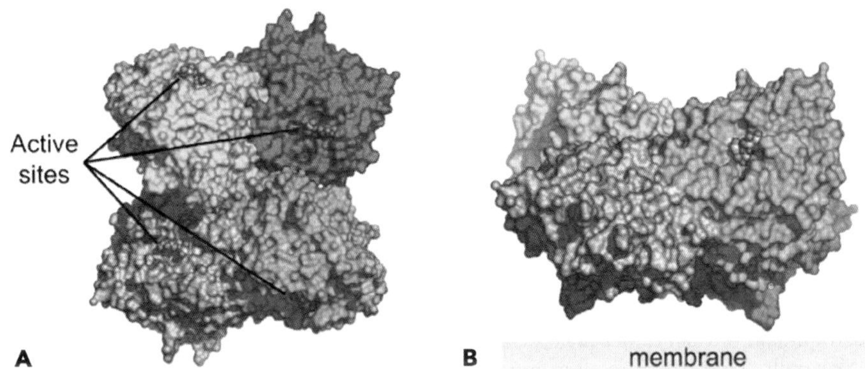

FIGURE 33.13. Parainfluenza virus type 5 (PIV5) hemagglutinin-neuraminidase (HN) tetramers. Active sites are marked by space-filling representations of the ligand sialyllactose. The four subunits are shown in different colors. **A:** Top view of the PIV5 HN tetramer arrangement. **B:** Side view of the PIV5 HN tetramer arrangement, with a 60-degree packing angle between dimers. (Adapted from Yuan P, Thompson T, Wurzburg BA, et al. Structural studies of the parainfluenza virius 5 hemagglutinin-neuraminidase tetramer in complex with its receptor, sialyllactose. *Structure* 2005;13:1–13.)

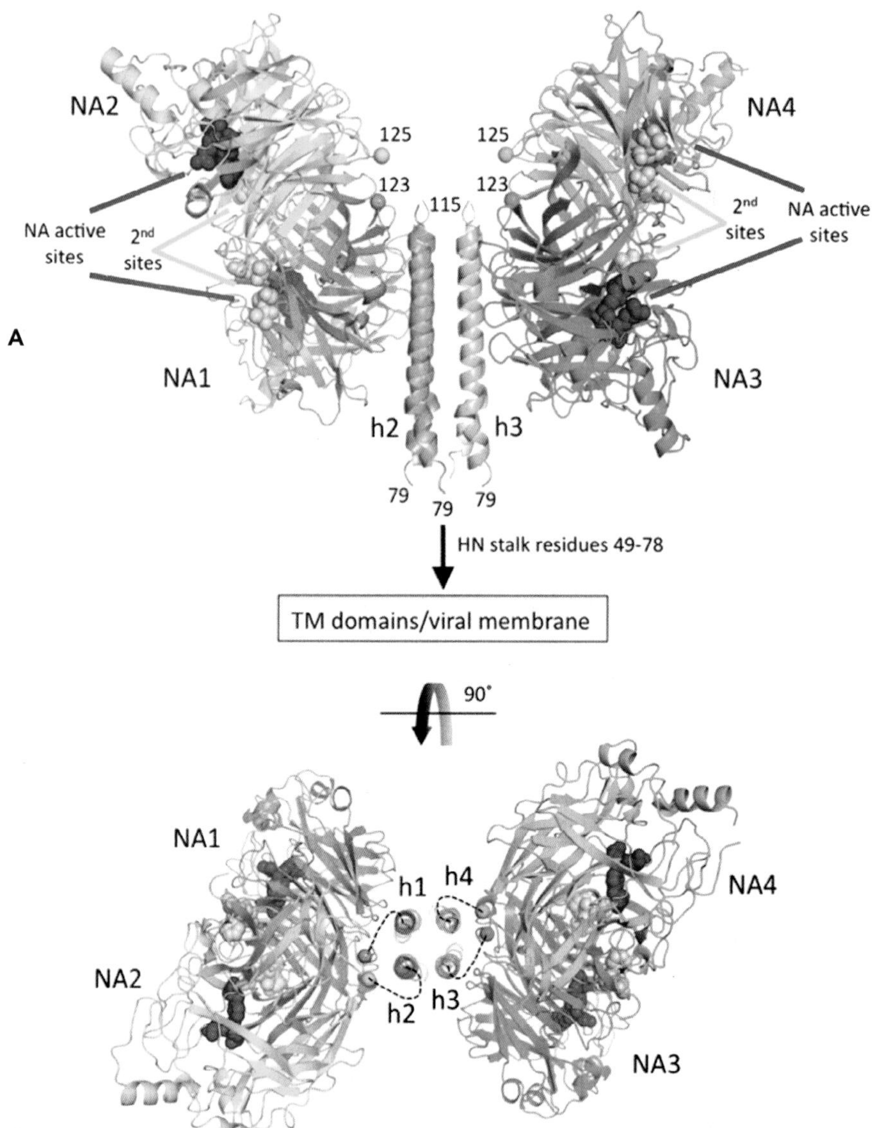

FIGURE 33.14. Structure of the Newcastle disease virus (NDV) hemagglutinin-neuraminidase (HN) (Stain Australian–Victoria) ectodomain. A: Two dimers of the NDV HN neuroaminidase (NA) domains flank the four-helix bundle in the stalk. The four NA domains are labeled NA1 through NA4. The active sites are marked by three residues shown as *blue* CPK spheres (E400, R415, and Y525) and labeled accordingly. The secondary sialic acid binding sites located at the NA domain dimer interfaces are marked by residues shown as *orange* CPK spheres and labeled (second sites). The N-termini of the four NA domains, residues 123 and 125, are labeled and indicated by their α atoms shown in CPK format colored by chain. The connections of the N-terminal region of the stalk to the HN transmembrane domains and viral membrane are indicated. **B:** End-on view of the packing of the HN stalk tetramer between two NA domain dimers rotated through 90 degrees as indicated by the *curved arrow.* Although no electron density was observed to connect the HN stalk helices with the individual NA domains, the *dotted lines* indicate possible linkages between these domains, with NA1/NA2 and NA3/NA4 forming covalently linked dimers through C123. The four-stalk helices are indicated as h1 through h4. (Adapted from Yuan P, Swanson KA, Leser GP, et al. Structure of the Newcastle disease virus hemagglutinin-neuraminidase [HN] ectodomain reveals a four-helix bundle stalk. *Proc Natl Acad Sci U S A* 2011;108:14920–14925.)

to each other and in the crystal lattice, allowing neighboring dimers and tetramers to associate in infinitely long oligomers. The dimer places the two HN active sites at nearly 90 degrees to each other. The calculated buried surface area for each monomer in the PIV5 HN dimer is 1,818 A^2. In contrast to the dimer interaction, the dimer-of-dimers interface is much smaller, involving only 10 residues and burying only 657 A^2. The small surface of interaction suggests that the arrangement is not very strong and that the dimers may dissociate.

Recently, the atomic structure of the NDV head domain with a tetrameric stalk has been obtained[450] (Fig. 33.14). The stalk forms a four-helix bundle, and on either side are dimers of head domains. One head domain of each dimer makes extensive interactions with the stalk. This structure, as compared with the head-only tetramer,[451] suggests plasticity in the stalk/head-connecting region.

The structure of the *Pneumovirus* attachment protein (G) is very different from the attachment protein of the *Paramyxovirinae.* The RSV G protein has neither hemagglutinating nor NA activity. The nucleotide sequence of the RSV *G* gene predicts that the protein is of 289 to 299 amino acids (M_r)[32,587] and is a type II integral membrane protein with a single N-terminal hydrophobic signal/anchor domain.[352,435] The G protein is found in virus-infected cells in both membrane-bound and proteolytically cleaved soluble forms. The distinguishing feature of the RSV G protein is the extent of its carbohydrate modification. On SDS-PAGE, the protein migrates with an apparent M_r of approximately 84,000 to 90,000, and the dramatic increase in molecular weight over that predicted for the polypeptide chain is because 8 to 12 kDa is owing to addition of N-linked carbohydrate (four potential addition sites) and 40 to 50 kDa is owing to the addition of O-linked glycosylation (77 potential acceptor serine or threonine residues; 30% of total residues) (61 and references therein). Quite remarkably, it appears that the RSV G protein is not essential for virus assembly or growth in tissue culture or animals, although it does confer a growth advantage. A virus that had been extensively passaged in cells was found to contain a spontaneous deletion of the *G* and *SH* genes,[189] yet the virus replicated in Vero cells. In addition, the *G* gene has been deleted from recombinant virus recovered from an infectious cDNA clone (see Chapter 38). These findings suggest that RSV has an alternate mechanism for attachment to cells that does not involve G protein, and evidence has been obtained that RSV lacking G protein can bind to heparan sulfate and possibly other molecules.[111,140,406] Similar observations have been made for HMPV.[57]

Paramyxovirus Fusion Protein

The paramyxovirus fusion (F) proteins mediate viral penetration by fusion between the virion envelope and the host cell plasma membrane, and this fusion event occurs at neutral pH for all family members except a few isolates of HMPV, where low pH appears to have some role in fusion activation.[249,362] The consequence of the fusion reaction is that the nucleocapsid is delivered to the cytoplasm. Later in infection, the F proteins expressed at the plasma membrane of infected cells can mediate fusion with neighboring cells to form syncytia (giant cell formation), which is a cytopathic effect that can lead to tissue necrosis *in vivo* and might also be a mechanism of virus spread.

The F proteins are homotrimers[58,346,444,445] that are synthesized as inactive precursors (F0). To be biologically active, they have to be cleaved by a host cell protease at the cleavage activation site. Cleavage releases the new N-terminus of F1, thus forming the biologically active protein consisting of the disulfide-linked chains F1 and F2.[167,354] The paramyxovirus *F* genes encode 540 to 580 residues (see Fig. 33.11). The F proteins are type I integral membrane proteins that span the membrane once and contain at their N-terminus a cleavable signal sequence that targets the nascent polypeptide chain synthesis to the membrane of the endoplasmic reticulum. At their C-termini, a hydrophobic stop-transfer domain (TM domain) anchors the protein in the membrane, leaving a short cytoplasmic tail (~20–40 residues). Sequences adjacent to the fusion peptide and the TM anchor domain typically reveal a 4–3 (heptad) pattern of hydrophobic repeats and are designated HRA and HRB, respectively. Approximately 250 residues separate HRA and HRB (Fig. 33.15A).

Evidence has been presented that there is a second polytopic form of the NDV F protein that is 10% to 50% of the total F protein.[254] The proposed second polytopic form of F has not been found for other paramyxovirus F proteins, and it is unclear why NDV F protein would be different from other F proteins. Because the second form of NDV F is only partially membrane translocated, it would have a very different protein fold from prefusion F (see Fig. 33.15), and it is unclear why NDV would uniquely require this form of F for the viral replication cycle.

The F protein is thought to drive membrane fusion by coupling irreversible protein refolding to membrane juxtaposition, initially folding into a metastable form that subsequently undergoes discrete/stepwise conformational changes to a lower energy state.[183,211] The F protein found on virions is considered to be in a prefusion form; after membrane fusion has occurred, the F protein is considered to be in a postfusion form. Cleavage of F0 primes the protein for membrane fusion. The varying nature of the residues found at the cleavage site, the enzymes involved in cleavage, and the role of cleavage in pathogenesis will be discussed later.

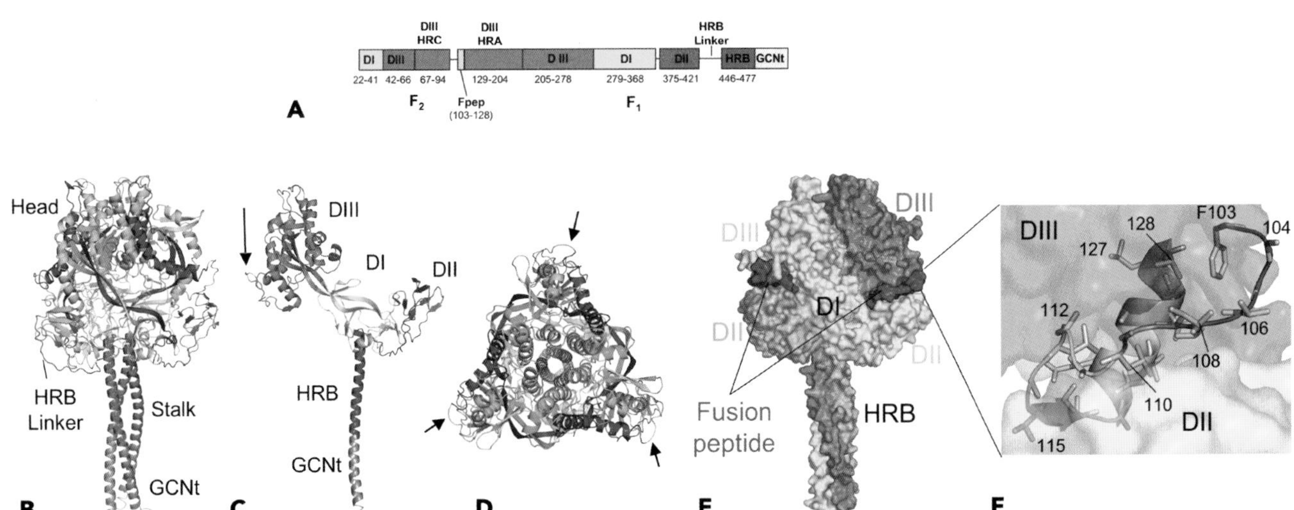

FIGURE 33.15. The fusion (F) protein prefusion structure. A: Schematic diagram of the F-GCNt domains. Important domains are colored and their corresponding residue ranges indicated. **B:** Ribbon diagram of the F trimer, with each chain colored by residue number in a gradient from *blue* (N-terminus) to *red* (C-terminus). The head and stalk regions are indicated. HRB linker residues 429 through 432 could not be modeled in one subunit and had high temperature factors in the other two. **C:** Ribbon diagram of one subunit of the F trimer colored by domain. The domains are labeled, and the colors correspond to those used in **A.** The cleavage/activation site is indicated with an *arrow.* **D:** Top view of the trimer colored as in **A.** Cleavage/activation sites are indicated by *arrows.* **E:** Surface representation of the F trimer colored by subunit. The fusion peptide exposed surface is colored *blue.* **F:** Close-up view of the fusion peptide (residues 103–128). The peptide is folded back on itself with a small hydrophobic core and contains a mixture of extended chain, one β-strand and a C-terminal α-helix. The fusion peptide is sandwiched between two subunits of the trimer, between DII and DIII domains. (Adapted from Yin HS, Wen X, Paterson RG, et al. Structure of the parainfluenza virus 5 F protein in its metastable, prefusion conformation. *Nature* 2006;439:38–44.)

Comparison of the amino acid sequences of paramyxovirus F proteins (reviewed in 267) does not show overall major regions of sequence identity, with the exception of the fusion peptide, which has a conserved sequence (up to 90% identity). However, the overall placement of cysteine, glycine, and proline residues suggests a similar structure for all F proteins. The *Respirovirus* and *Rubulavirus* F2 and F1 subunits are glycosylated, and there are a total of 3 to 6 potential sites for the addition of N-linked carbohydrate. For PIV5 F protein, it is known that all four potential sites for addition of N-linked carbohydrate are used.[8] The measles virus F protein contains three sites in the F2 subunit for N-linked carbohydrate addition, and all three sites are used; there are no sites in F1 for N-linked carbohydrate addition.[1]

Class I Viral Fusion Proteins

The paramyxovirus F proteins belong to the class I viral fusion protein type, of which the longest standing member is the influenza virus hemagglutinin. Class I also includes the fusion proteins from retroviruses including human immunodeficiency virus type 1 (HIV-1; Env/gp160), coronaviruses (S), and Ebola virus (G).[67,96,97,183,213] Models for class I viral fusion protein-mediated membrane merger have been developed, until recently, primarily from the structural studies of hemagglutinin.[373] The general mechanism for class I viral fusion proteins posits the folding of the uncleaved protein to a metastable state, which can be activated to undergo large conformational changes to a more stable fusogenic or postfusion state. The attainment of the prefusion conformation, its regulation, and relative free energy as compared to the postfusion form are all key to the process by which class I viral fusion proteins function.

Class I Viral Fusion Proteins and the Helical Hairpin (Core Trimer)

Biophysical data has indicated that HRA and HRB form a complex, and crystallographic studies have shown that HRA and HRB form a helical hairpin or six-helix bundle (6HB) structure (core trimer) that is related to that observed for the low-pH induced proteolytic fragment of hemagglutinin (TBHA2). For example, the core trimers of PIV5 and human RSV F,[9,187,456] human immunodeficiency virus (HIV) gp41,[42,55,396,432] Moloney murine leukemia virus envelope protein,[107] Ebola GP2,[235,433] and human T-cell leukemia virus type 1 (HTLV-1)[202] fusion proteins all share this similarity in structure (Fig. 33.16A). Although the structural details vary, all reveal a trimeric, coiled-coil beginning near the C-terminal end of the hydrophobic fusion peptide. The C-terminal segment abutting the TM domain is also often helical and packs in an antiparallel direction along the outside of the N-terminal coiled-coil, placing the fusion peptides and TM anchors at the same end of a rod-like structure (for PIV5 6HB, see Fig. 33.16A). These 6HBs typically represent a relatively small fraction of the intact fusion protein, yet their structures are generally highly thermostable, with melting temperatures near 100°C. Intermediates along the pathway of membrane fusion can be trapped by the addition of peptides derived from either the N-terminal (HRA) or C-terminal (HRB) heptad repeat regions for many class I fusion proteins,[97,100,106,344,449] indicating that the intact protein undergoes conformational changes that expose both HR regions prior to refolding to the final 6HB. The intermediates are thought to represent partially refolded forms of the fusion protein, with a hydrophobic fusion peptide anchored in the target cell membrane and the TM domains

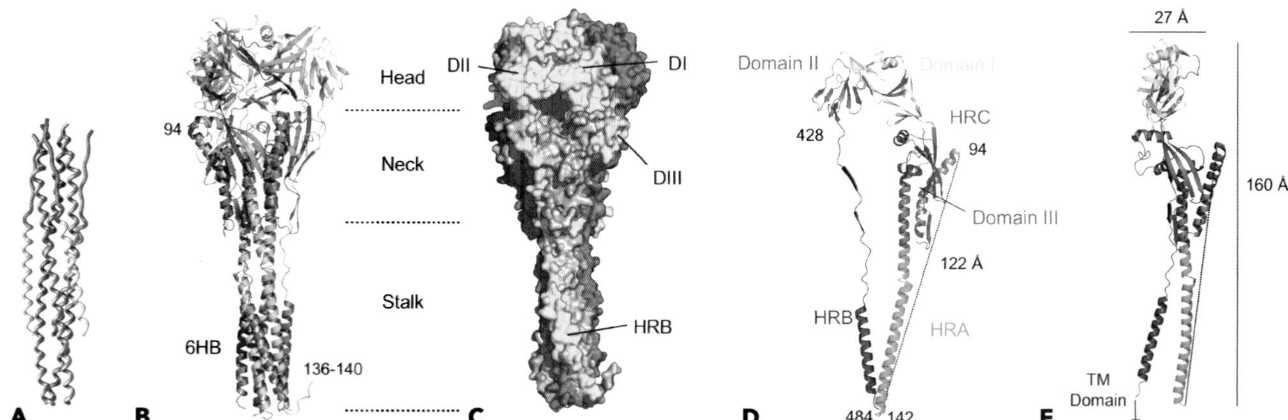

FIGURE 33.16. The F protein postfusion structure. A: The complete parainfluenza virus type 5 (PIV5) F1 core trimer is shown with the N1 helix colored *gray* and the C1 peptide colored *blue* except for the extended-chain N-terminal residues of C1 that are colored *red*. **B:** Ribbon diagram of the HPIV3 solF0 trimer. The three chains are colored similarly from *blue* (N-terminus) to *red* (C-terminus). Residues 95 through 135 are disordered in all chains. Residue 94 is labeled in one chain, and residues 136 through 140 at the base of the stalk are ordered in one chain owing to crystal packing interactions. **C:** Surface representation of the solF0 trimer. Each chain is a different color, and domains I through III and HRB for one chain (*yellow*) are indicated by the DI, DII, DIII, and HRB labels. One radial channel is readily apparent below domain I and II of the yellow chain and above domain III of the red chain. **D:** Ribbon diagram of the solF0 protein monomer colored by domain. The direct distance within one monomer between residue 94 at the end of HRC and residue 142 at the base of the stalk region is 122 Å. **E:** Ribbon diagram of the monomer rotated by 90 degrees, indicating the width and height of the solF0 monomer. An *arrow* at the C-terminus of the HRB segment points toward the likely position of the transmembrane anchor domain that would be present in the full length protein. (Adapted from Yin H-S, Paterson RG, Wen X, et al. Structure of the uncleaved ectodomain of the paramyxovirus [HPIV3] fusion protein. *Proc Natl Acad Sci U S A* 2005;102:9288–9293.)

anchored to the viral membrane. The formation of the 6HB is tightly linked to the merger of lipid bilayers and is thought likely to couple the free energy released on protein refolding to membrane fusion.[257,344]

Atomic Structures of the Paramyxovirus F Protein

Structure of the Prefusion F Protein. The atomic structure of the PIV5 F protein in its uncleaved metastable prefusion form has been determined.[445] To solve the atomic structure, the secreted F protein was stabilized by the addition of a soluble trimeric TM domain (GCNt) that supplants the hydrophobic TM domain. The F trimer has a large globular head attached to a three-helix coiled-coil stalk formed by HRB (see Fig. 33.15B–E) orienting the head away from the viral membrane. The F head contains three domains (DI–DIII) per subunit that extend around the trimer axis, making extensive intersubunit contacts. A large cavity is present at the base of the head, with the bottom and sides formed by DI and DII. DIII (residues 42–278) covers the top of the cavity, HRA, and the fusion peptide (see Fig. 33.15B–D). At the C-terminus of DII, an extended linker to HRB wraps around the outside of the trimer and into the center of the base of the head where the stalk begins. The structure has three lateral vertices projecting from the trimer axis, exposing the cleavage/activation sites adjacent to the fusion peptides (see Fig. 33.15C,D). Helices line the central threefold axis at the top and bottom of the trimer. In DIII, two sets of six helices form rings sealing the top of the head, whereas the HRB three-helix bundle seals the bottom (see Fig. 33.15D).

In the prefusion PIV5 F structure, the hydrophobic fusion peptide (residues 103–128) is wedged between two subunits of the trimer (see Fig. 33.15E). The N-terminal end of the fusion peptide is exposed at the F surface and then proceeds inward, becoming more buried from solvent. The fusion peptide adopts a partly extended, partly β-sheet, and partly α-helical conformation and is sandwiched between DIII of its own subunit and DII of another. Residues 107 through 117 pack against the hydrophobic edge of the neighboring DII domain. The fusion peptide folds back on itself, forming a small hydrophobic core between its N-terminal and C-terminal ends, making less extensive contacts with DIII (see Fig. 33.15E,F). Proteolytic cleavage of F0 might allow the N-terminus of the fusion peptide to make additional contacts with DII and to affect intersubunit interactions.

Structure of the Postfusion Form of the F Protein. The atomic structure of intact F protein in its postfusion form has been determined for HPIV3, NDV, and RSV.[255,388,389,444] The structure of the HPIV3 F protein was solved by molecular replacement, using as a model the structure of a proteolytic fragment of NDV F,[58] now known to be in its postfusion form.

HPIV3 F forms a trimer, with distinct head, neck, and stalk regions (Fig. 33.17A–D). The only part of the structure lacking electron density is the fusion peptide and cleavage site; however, the residues would be draped flexibly on the exterior of the stalk region. Given that the uncleaved F ectodomain was secreted from cells by removal of the TM domain, it was initially unexpected that the structure contained a 6HB (see Fig. 33.17A–D) that represents the postfusion conformation of the protein. It had been widely anticipated that cleavage of F at the cleavage site was a requirement for conversion to the postfusion form. Nonetheless, many lines of evidence suggested that the observed HPIV3 conformation represented the postfusion form, although the polypeptide chains were intact in the crystal and the fusion peptide was not located at the appropriate end of the 6HB.

The observation that the soluble, secreted HPIV3, NDV F, and RSV F proteins were in the postfusion conformation was unexpected, and there are at least two possible explanations for this finding. First, the TM anchor (and potentially the cytoplasmic tail)[428] could be an important determinant of the stability of the prefusion conformation, providing a

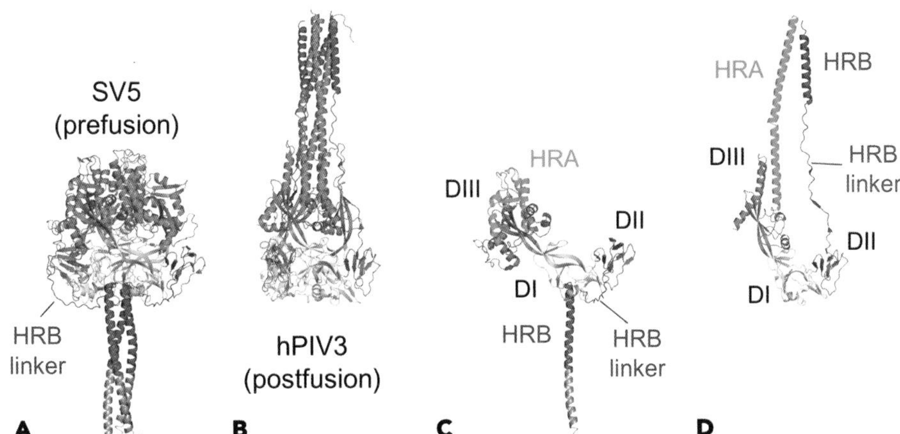

FIGURE 33.17. Structural changes between the pre- and postfusion F protein conformations. **A:** Ribbon diagram of the parainfluenza virus type 5 (PIV5) F-GCNt trimer. DI is colored *yellow*, DII is colored *red*, DIII is colored *magenta*, HRB is colored *blue*, and GCNt is colored *gray*. **B:** Ribbon diagram of the human parainflenza virus type 3 (HPIV3) (postfusion) trimer, colored as in **A**. **C:** Ribbon diagram of a single subunit of the PIV5 F-GCNt trimer, colored as in **A**, except for HRA residues, which are colored *green*. **D:** Ribbon diagram of a single subunit of the HPIV3 F trimer, colored as in **C**. (Adapted from Yin HS, Wen X, Paterson RG, et al. Structure of the parainfluenza virus 5 F protein in its metastable, prefusion conformation. *Nature* 2006;439:38–44.)

significant fraction of the energy barrier that traps the protein in a metastable state. In this case, the secreted protein may fold to the prefusion form transiently but then refold to the postfusion form. A second possible explanation for the structural results is that the TM domain is important for the protein to attain the prefusion metastable state and that in the absence of this region, the soluble F protein folds directly to the final, most stable postfusion conformation. In either case, it appears that the amino acids comprising the intact F protein ectodomain are not sufficient for the protein to fold to and maintain a metastable conformation. Hence, to trap a soluble form of the F protein in its metastable form, the F protein was stabilized by the addition of a soluble trimeric TM domain (GCNt) that supplants the hydrophobic TM domain.

Comparison of the Prefusion and Postfusion F Structures

The PIV5 prefusion F and HPIV3 postfusion F structures are in strikingly different conformations (see Fig. 33.17), consistent with a transition from pre- to postfusion forms. None of the intersubunit contacts are conserved in the pre- and postfusion forms. The two F structures are related by flipping the stalk and TM domains relative to the F head. Substantial compacting of the head is observed in HPIV3 postfusion F compared to PIV5 prefusion F. DI domains pivot slightly inward, shearing intersubunit contacts, and DII domains swing across, contacting neighboring subunits. Individual DI and DII domains in the two structures remain similar. Potentially related forms of the F protein have been observed in electron micrographs of RSV F.[44,130,342,343]

DIII undergoes major refolding between the two structures, projecting a new coiled coil (HRA) upward and away from DI, the prefusion stalk, and the viral membrane. The fusion peptide, located at the top of the HRA coiled coil, moves approximately 115Å from its initial position between subunits in the prefusion conformation, allowing DII domains to reposition. None of the postfusion HRA intersubunit coiled-coil contacts are observed in F-GCNt. Instead, they are replaced by two sets of six-helix rings at the DIII interfaces (see Fig. 33.15D). For the HRA coiled coil to form, DIII must rotate and collapse inward, further compacting the head.

The F protein refolding also requires the opening and translocation of the HRB stalk (see Fig. 33.17). In the prefusion form, HRB is located at the base of the head region. During the conversion to the postfusion conformation, HRB segments must separate and swing around the base of the head to pack against the HRA coiled coil. In the prefusion conformation, HRA is broken up into four helices, two β-strands, and five loop, kink, or turn segments. Thus, the conformational changes in HRA involve the refolding of 11 distinct segments into a single, extended α-helical conformation (Fig. 33.18).

The Mechanism of Paramyxovirus–Mediated Membrane Fusion

The prefusion and postfusion F structures suggest how discrete refolding intermediates are coupled to the activation and progression of F-mediated membrane fusion. Whereas proteolytic cleavage of the paramyxovirus F protein is required for membrane fusion activity, it is not required for the formation of the postfusion conformation. A model for membrane fusion is as follows. In the first step, the HRB helices melt (open-stalk form, Fig. 33.19), breaking interactions at the base of the head but leaving HRA in the prefusion conformation. This intermediate is consistent with effects of mutations of PIV5 residues 443, 447, and 449 as well as peptide inhibition data.[305,344,345] HRA-derived peptides, which likely bind to the endogenous HRB segment, inhibit an early intermediate along the fusion

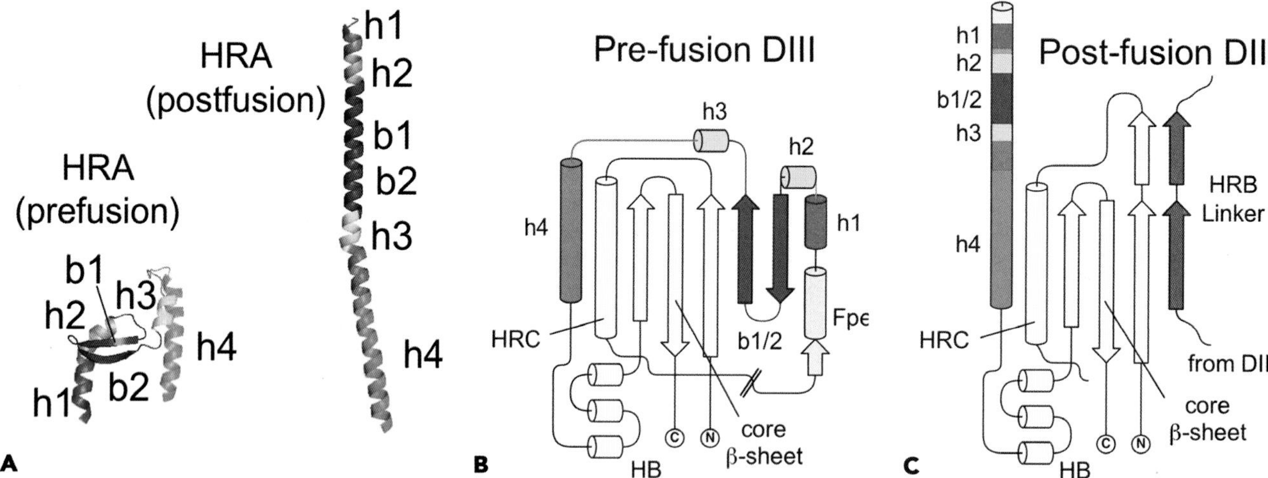

FIGURE 33.18. F protein refolding: the role of DIII in HRA folding and transformation. A: HRA refolds from 11 distinct segments (h1, h2, b1, b2, h3, h4, and the intervening residues) in the prefusion conformation into a single, nearly 120 Å long helix in the postfusion form. **B:** Secondary structure diagram for DIII in the prefusion (parainfluenza virus type 5) conformation. The "DIII core" includes three antiparallel strands, HRC, a helical bundle (HB), and h4 of HRA. HRA segments are colored as in **A,** and the cleavage site (//) and fusion peptide are indicated. The DIII core sheet is extended by the b1 and b2 strands from HRA. **C:** Secondary structure diagram for DIII in the postfusion (human parainfluenza virus type 3) conformation. The DIII core sheet is extended by one strand from HRB linker from a neighboring subunit (*dark violet*). (Adapted from Yin HS, Wen X, Paterson RG, et al. Structure of the parainfluenza virus 5 F protein in its metastable, prefusion conformation. *Nature* 2006;439:38–44.)

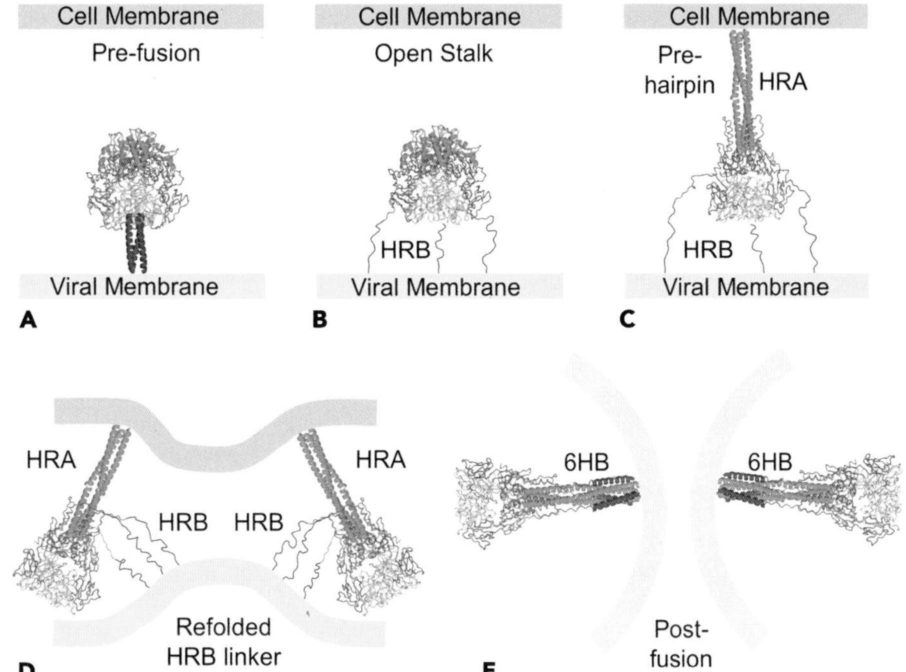

FIGURE 33.19. A model for F-mediated membrane fusion. A: Structure of the prefusion conformation. HRB is colored *blue*, HRA is colored *green*, and domains I, II, and III are colored *yellow*, *red*, and *magenta*, respectively. **B:** An open-stalk conformation, in which the HRB stalk melts and separates from the prefusion head region. HRB is shown as three extended chains because the individual segments are unlikely to be helical. This conformation is consistent with a low-temperature intermediate that is inhibited by HRA peptides but not HRB peptides. Mutations of the switch peptide residues 443, 447, and 449 would influence the formation of this intermediate by affecting stabilizing interactions between the prefusion stalk and head domains. **C:** A pre-hairpin intermediate can form by refolding of DIII, allowing the formation of the HRA coiled coil and insertion of the fusion peptide into the target cell membrane. This intermediate can be inhibited by peptides derived from both HRA and HRB regions. **D:** Prior to forming the final six-helix bundle, the close approach of viral and cellular membranes may be trapped by folding of the HRB linker onto the newly exposed DIII core, with the formation of two β-strands (see Fig. 33.15D,F). **E:** The formation of the postfusion six-helix bundle is tightly linked to membrane fusion and pore formation, juxtaposing the membrane interacting fusion peptide and transmembrane domains. (Adapted from Yin HS, Wen X, Paterson RG, et al. Structure of the parainfluenza virus 5 F protein in its metastable, prefusion conformation. *Nature* 2006;439:38–44.)

pathway, whereas HRB-derived peptides inhibit a later intermediate by binding the endogenous HRA coiled coil. Opening of the HRB stalk could initiate further changes in F by affecting the packing of DII and the fusion peptide (through the HRB linker) and by affecting the stability of the head intersubunit contacts, which shift during the conformational transition. It seems possible that transient dissociation of the F trimer could occur, analogous to the dimer-to-trimer transition characterized in alpha- and flavivirus fusion proteins (Chapter 3). The open-stalk intermediate is then likely followed by refolding of DIII, the assembly of the HRA coiled coil, and the translocation of the fusion peptide toward the target cell membrane (see Fig. 33.19). This pre-hairpin intermediate has been trapped and co-precipitated with HRB peptides[344] and imaged by electron microscopy.[198] Removal of the fusion peptide from the intersubunit interfaces would enable an inward swing of DII and the formation of new contacts with DI of a neighboring subunit, compacting the head. The refolding of DIII HRA would also expose its core β-sheet, and together with the inward movement of DII allow the HRB linker (at the C-terminus of DII) to form parallel β-strands with the DIII core, likely preceding and initiating the final positioning of HRB (see Fig. 33.19). The assembly of the final 6HB completes the conformational change and membrane merger.

HN Activates the F Protein for Membrane Fusion

The triggering mechanism that regulates the F protein conformational changes such that it occurs at the right place and the right time is not fully understood, although as described later for most paramyxoviruses, there is a requirement for the receptor-binding protein (HN, H, or G) in mediating the fusion reaction.[215,268] The precise role of the HN, H, or G protein in stimulating the F conformational change remains to be understood; however, the emerging picture indicates a regulated complex biological machine.[178,222,318]

For all paramyxoviruses, co-expression of F and HN (H or G) is either required for fusion or co-expression of HN (H or G) makes fusion more efficient.[51,99,173,176,266,349,438,443] Furthermore, the homotypic HN (i.e., of the same virus), not a heterotypic HN, has to be co-expressed in the same cell as the F protein to promote fusion.[173,176,365] However, expression of the F of PIV5, measles virus, or RSV alone causes some syncytium formation,[1,173,188,293,302,306] although it is important to note that it is likely that many more cells express the F protein than are found in multinucleated cells.[306] Furthermore, point mutations within NDV F render the protein HN independent for fusion.[367] Thus, it seems likely that there are different activation energies for triggering fusion for the different paramyxovirus F proteins. This is highlighted by the observation that PIV5 F-GCNt soluble protein can be converted to the postfusion form by using heat (55°C) as a surrogate for HN activation.[69]

It was hypothesized that a type-specific interaction would occur between the HN and F protein.[176,211,366] Immunoprecipitation assays show that F and HN co-precipitate, indicating that they can associate[86,256,381,443]; for HPIV3, F and HN undergo antibody-induced co-capping, indicative of a protein complex formation.[443] A great deal of effort has been spent to map the regions of F and HN that interact. One of the difficulties in the work in studying HN is that mutations often affect more than one of the three known biological activities of hemadsorption, NA activity, and fusion promotion. Mutations have been identified in the HN globular domain,[84,260] the HN stalk,[23,86,256,295,324,366,382,397,452] and TM anchor[28,252] that decrease or abolish fusogenic activity with no or little effect on receptor recognition. Analysis of the fusion-promoting activity of chimeric HN molecules derived from different paramyxoviruses largely suggests that the stalk domain and, in some cases, parts of the globular head impart F specificity.[86,397,414] A point mutation was found in the NDV HN globular head that abolishes both its receptor recognition and NA activity, and that also abolishes its ability to interact with F in co-immunoprecipitation assays.[85] Based on the view that HRB in F mediates an interaction with HN, it was found that a peptide mimicking HRB bound to a fragment of HN (residues 124–152) when the HN fragment was expressed as an artificial fusion protein.[136] However, other biological data argues against HN residues 124 through 152 as being part of the F-interactive domain in HN.[256]

No one model for fusion activation has been universally embraced, and data obtained from studying measles virus and Nipah virus fusion suggest different mechanisms of F protein activation.[222,318] There are two major models for F activation, with the constant factor being that the HN stalk is required for activation. The *clamp* model (or dissociation model) posits that F and HN/H/G associate with each other in the endoplasmic reticulum and reach the cell surface as a complex that holds F in its metastable prefusion state. Once the attachment protein binds to its receptor, the attachment protein undergoes a conformational change that causes release of F, enabling F to be fusion active. A corollary of the clamp model is that when F is expressed in cells from cDNA without HN/H/G expression, it should be in its postfusion form. The *provocateur* (or association model) posits that F and HN/H/G are transported to the cell surface independently, and on the HN/H/G-binding receptor, there is a conformational change in the receptor-binding protein that leads to complex formation with F, most likely through the HN/H/G stalk, hence triggering fusion activation.[69,178] Although it is no longer thought that there is a conformational change within an HN/H/G monomer, there is accumulating evidence for more than one form of dimer–dimer interaction[149,283,450,451] and evidence for the association of the NDV HN dimer with its stalk.[450]

Cleavage Activation

As discussed previously, the precursor F0 molecule is biologically inactive and cleavage of F0 to the disulfide-linked chains F1 and F2 activates the protein, rendering the molecule fusion active and permitting viral infectivity. It is important to note that F2 and F1 are not separate domains in the atomic structure of F and thus are not individual parts of the protein. Cleavage of F0 is a candidate to be a key determinant for infectivity and pathogenicity; for certain viruses, this appears to be the case. Proteolytic activation of F0 involves the sequential action of two enzymes: the host protease that cleaves at the carboxyl side of an arginine residue and a host carboxypeptidase that removes the basic residues. The *Paramyxoviridae* can be divided into two groups: those that have F proteins with multibasic residues at the cleavage site and those with F proteins that have a single basic residue at the cleavage site (see Table 33.3). Cleavage of F proteins containing multibasic residues at the cleavage site occurs intracellularly during transport of the protein through the *trans*-Golgi network.

Furin is a cellular protease localized to the *trans*-Golgi network, and its sequence specificity for cleavage is R-X-K/R-R. The available evidence suggests that furin, a subtilisin-like endoprotease, is the (or one of the) protease(s) that cleaves most F proteins intracellularly.[201,294]

Paramyxoviruses that have F proteins with single basic residues in the cleavage site (e.g., Sendai virus) are not usually cleaved when grown in tissue culture, and thus only a single cycle of growth is obtained. However, the F0 precursor that is expressed at the cell surface and incorporated into released virions can be cleavage activated by the addition of exogenous protease,[354] leading to multiple rounds of replication. Purification of a protease from the allantoic fluid of embryonated chicken eggs has indicated that the endoprotease responsible for Sendai virus activation is homologous to the blood clotting factor Xa, which is a member of the prothrombin family.[132,134] A protease with a similar substrate specificity is secreted from Clara cells of the bronchial epithelium in rats and mice, and this enzyme is probably responsible for activating paramyxoviruses in the respiratory tract. For NDV, the nature of the cleavage site correlates with virulence of the virus. Those strains with multibasic residues in the F0 cleavage site are virulent strains and readily disseminate through the host, whereas those strains with F0 molecules having single basic residues are avirulent and tend to be restricted to the respiratory tracts where the necessary secreted protease can be found.[278]

A variation on the cleavage theme is found with Hendra virus, as its F protein does not contain a multibasic cleavage site, and yet Hendra F is cleaved in expressing cells at the sequence HDLVDGVK↓,[71] but the K residue is not essential for cleavage.[262] In the search for the cleavage enzyme, it was found that inhibition of cathepsin L blocks cleavage,[296] suggesting that cleavage occurs in the endocytic pathway.[89,259] Recent evidence suggests that Hendra F protein is expressed at the cell surface in an uncleaved F0 form, internalized, cleaved by cathepsin in the late endosome, and recycled to the cell surface.[321]

Another variation on the cleavage theme is found for RSV F protein. The RSV F protein contains two consensus sequences for furin cleavage. One is located at the F2-F1 junction and the other in F2, 27 residues N-terminal to the F2-F1 junction.[130] Cleavage at both sites is required for fusion activity.[457]

Other Envelope Proteins

The rubulaviruses PIV5 and mumps virus both contain a small gene located between F and HN designated SH.[160,161] The PIV5

TABLE 33.3 Amino Acid Sequences Upstream of the F Protein Cleavage Site of Some Members of the *Paramyxoviridae*

Sendai virus		G-V-P-Q-S-R↓
HPIV1		D-N-P-Q-S-R↓
HPIV3		D-P-**R**-T-**K**-**R**↓
PIV5		T-R-**R**-R-**R**-**R**↓
Mumps		S-R-**R**-H-**K**-**R**↓
NDV (virulent strain)		**R** G-R-**R**-Q—**R**↓ **K**
NDV (avirulent strain)		G K G —G—Q—R↓ E R S
Measles		S-R-**R**-H-**K**-**R**↓
Hendra virus		HDLVDGVK↓
RSV	**R**-A-**R**-**R**↓ 109	ELPRFMNYTLNNTKKTNVTLS**KKRKRR**↓ 136

HPIV1, human parainfluenza virus type 1; HPIV3, human parainfluenza virus type 3; PIV5, parainfluenza virus type 5; NDV, Newcastle disease virus; RSV, respiratory syncytial virus.

Consensus sequence for furin protease cleavage is **R**-X—**R**↓
K

Adapted from Hosaka M, Nagahama M, Kim W-S, et al. Arg-X-Lys/Arg-Arg motif as a signal for precursor cleavage catalyzed by furin within the constitutive secretory pathway. *J Biol Chem* 1991;266:12127–12130.

SH protein is a 44-residue, type II integral membrane protein that is expressed at the plasma membrane and is packaged in virions. The mumps virus SH protein is a 57-residue integral membrane protein orientated in membranes in the opposite direction from the PIV5 SH protein with a C-terminal cytoplasmic domain.[102,393] Owing to the variability in sequence among different strains of mumps virus, the *SH* gene sequence has been used as marker to identify mumps isolates.[394] PIV5 lacking SH (PIV5ΔSH) grows as well as wild-type in tissue culture cells; however, the virus is attenuated *in vivo.*[151] PIV5ΔSH induces apoptosis in L929 and MDCK cells (but not in HeLa cells) through a tumor necrosis factor alpha-mediated extrinsic apoptotic pathway in the PIV5ΔSH-infected cells.[152,228] The *SH* gene has been found in all strains of mumps virus, although expression of the SH protein does not seem to be required for mumps virus replication in tissue culture,[393] because in the Enders strain of mumps virus, a monocistronic mRNA encoding SH is not found. Mumps SH may have a similar role as PIV5 SH, considering replacement of PIV5 *SH* gene with the mumps *SH* gene behaves like wild-type PIV5.[439] It has been proposed that the attenuating phenotype of viruses with deletions in SH (e.g., PIV5-ΔSH) reflects an altered gradient of transcription rather than a loss of critical function.[236]

Members of the *Pneumovirinae* encode a small hydrophobic protein, also designated SH protein. However, this does not necessarily mean that there is a commonality in function with the *Rubulavirus* SH protein. The RSV SH protein contains 64 amino acids and is expressed at the plasma membrane of RSV-infected cells as a type II integral membrane protein and is packaged in virions.[66,292] In RSV-infected cells, four SH-related polypeptide species have been identified: M_r 4,800; M_r 7,500; M_r 13,000 to 15,000; and M_r 21,000 to 30,000. The M_r 4,800 species is thought to result from the initiation of protein synthesis at an internal AUG codon, the M_r 7,500 species is unglycosylated SH, the M_r 13,000 to 15,000 species is SH containing one high-mannose N-linked carbohydrate chain, and the M_r 21,000 to 30,000 species is generated by the addition of polylactosaminoglycan to the N-linked carbohydrate chain.[2,292] The *SH* gene was found to be deleted spontaneously from a virus passaged extensively *in vitro,*[189] and it has been deleted from recombinant RSV[40] with only minor alterations in virus growth properties in tissue culture cells or the respiratory tract of mice or chimpanzees. Thus, the role of the SH protein in the RSV life cycle is not understood.

Pneumovirus M2 Gene

The RSV *M2* gene contains two partially overlapping ORFs, designated M2-1 and M2-2, which give rise to two proteins M2-1 (194 amino acids) and M2-2 (90 amino acids), respectively.[64] The mechanism for translating the M2-2 ORF is not clear but may involve a ribosomal stop-restart mechanism analogous to that used for synthesis of the influenza B virus BM2 protein[174] (see Chapter 40). The M2-1 protein is an essential transcriptional elongation factor,[62,109] and in its absence, the polymerase does not transcribe beyond the *NS1* and *NS2* genes.[109] The *M2-1* gene also increases RNAP processivity across the gene junctions, attenuating transcriptional termination.[109,142,143] The *M2-2* gene is not essential for RSV growth, as it can be deleted from a recombinant RSV.[14,185] However, the ΔM2-2 virus grows slowly in tissue culture, and there is an increase in transcription and decrease in RNA replication,[14,185] suggesting that M2-2 protein is involved in regulating transcription and RNA replication. The *M2* gene products of human metapneumoviruses also play a role in controlling viral RNA synthesis, as recombinant HMPV with deletions in the *M2-2* gene showed elevated levels of viral mRNAs.[38]

Pneumovirus NS1 and NS2 Genes

RSV NS1 (139 amino acids) and NS2 (124 amino acids) are considered to be nonstructural proteins, although the difficulty in purifying virions from contaminating infected cell debris for this poorly growing virus makes this assignment provisional. Neither protein is thought to be essential for virus growth in cultured cells or in chimpanzees, as the genes can be deleted from a recombinant RSV, although growth *in vitro* and *in vivo* is reduced substantially.[39,407,437] In a minireplicon system, when NS1 was expressed, it was inhibitory to both transcription and replication,[6] and expression of NS2 at high levels had a small inhibitory effect on transcription and replication.[407] Thus, the role of these accessory proteins in controlling RNA synthesis remains to be fully understood. In addition, however, the human RSV and bovine RSV *NS1* and *NS2* gene products have been shown to be important viral suppressors of type I IFN induction[24,377] as described later.

STAGES OF REPLICATION

General Aspects

As far as is known, all aspects of the replication of *Paramyxoviridae* take place in the cytoplasm. An overview of the life cycle of the virus is shown schematically in Figure 33.20, and a

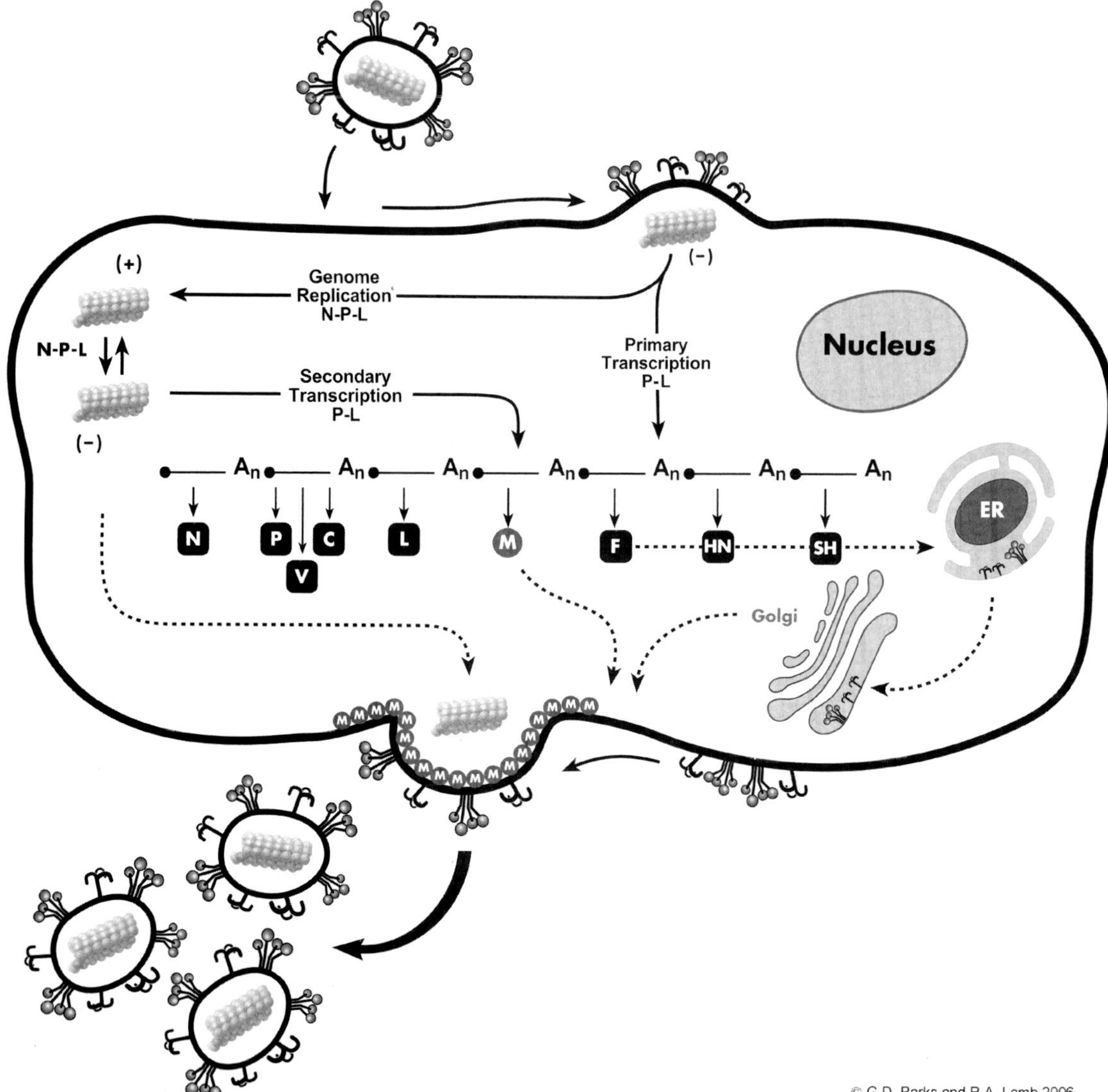

FIGURE 33.20. Schematic representation of the paramyxovirus life cycle. (Refer to the text for details of the viral life cycle.) The top of the figure shows an incoming virion that fuses with the plasma membrane to release the negative sense nucleocapsid in the cytoplasm. Viral messenger RNAs (mRNAs) are indicated by *lines* with the 5′ mRNA cap denoted by a *filled circle* and 3′ poly A tail by A_n. The gradient of decreasing molar abundance of the mRNAs from N to L owing to polar transcription is not illustrated. Also not illustrated is the relative abundance of genomic (negative sense) nucleocapsid versus antigenomic (positive sense) nucleocapsid. *Solid lines* denote primary and secondary transcription carried out by a P-L complex and genome replication carried out by an N-P-L complex. *Dotted lines* denote intracellular transport of nucleocapsid and M protein to the plasma membrane and the viral glycoproteins F, HN, and SH from the endoplasmic reticulum to Golgi to plasma membrane. The *large arrow* denotes release of progeny virions from the plasma membrane by a budding process.

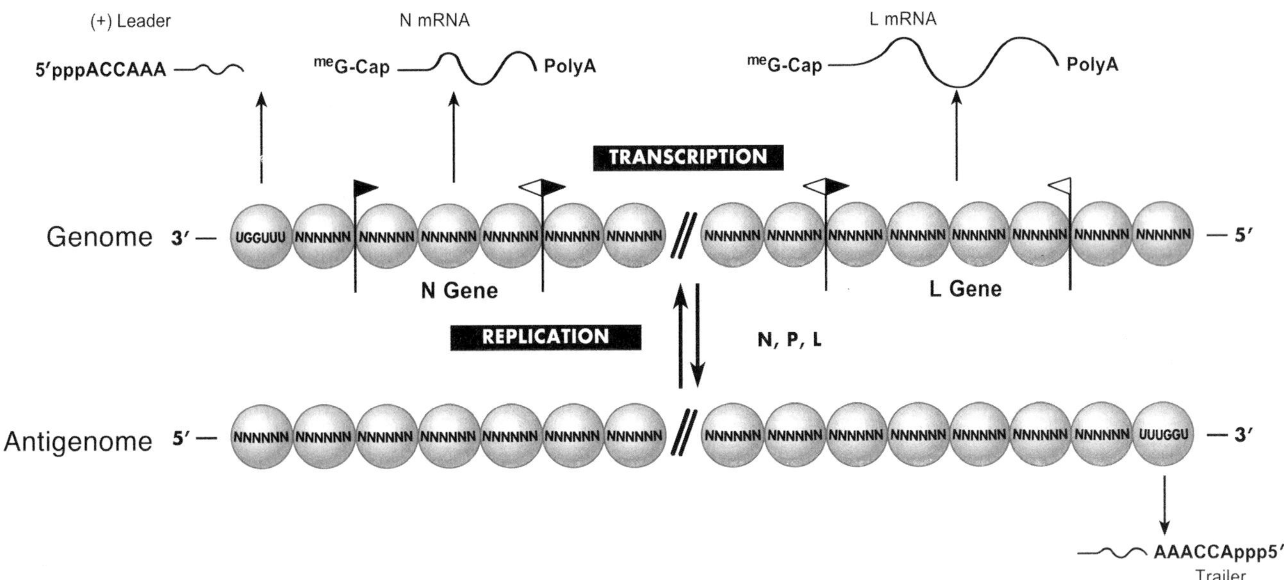

FIGURE 33.21. Paramyxovirus RNA synthesis. Viral nucleocapsids—the templates for RNA synthesis—are shown as a linear array of N subunits (*ovals*), with *arrowheads* indicating the gene junctions. Note that N protein binds six nucleotides, resulting in complete encapsidation of the RNA if it has a chain length that is an even multiple of six. The viral polymerase (P-L) transcribes the genome template, starting at its 3′ end, to generate the positive leader RNA and the successive capped (meG-Cap) and polyadenylated (PolyA) mRNAs, by stopping and restarting at each junction. Once these primary transcripts have generated sufficient viral proteins, unassembled N (as a P-N complex) begins to assemble the nascent leader chain, and the coordinate assembly and synthesis of the RNA causes the polymerase to ignore the junctions, yielding the antigenome nucleocapsid **(bottom)**. The P-L polymerase can also initiate RNA synthesis at the 3′ end of the antigenome in the absence of sufficient P-N; however, only a 5′ trailer RNA is made in this case. Note that positive leader RNA is not capped or polyadenylated and that genomic and antigenomic RNAs never appear as naked RNAs.

diagram indicating the differences between transcription and replication is shown in Figure 33.21. Unlike the situation for influenza viruses, *Paramyxoviridae* mRNA synthesis is insensitive to DNA-intercalating drugs such as actinomycin D,[59] and the *Paramyxoviridae* can replicate in enucleated cells.[316] In cell culture, single-cycle growth curves are generally of 14 to 30 hours duration but can be as short as 10 hours for virulent strains of NDV. The effect of viral replication on host macromolecular synthesis is quite variable, ranging from almost complete shut-off late in infection for NDV to no obvious effect with PIV5.

Virus Adsorption and Entry

For the respiroviruses and rubulaviruses, it has long been accepted that molecules containing sialic acid (sialoglycoconjugates) serve as cell surface receptors. This is based on the fact that sialidase of *Vibrio cholerae* acted as a "receptor destroying enzyme" and protected the host cell from infection.[244] Sialic acid, the acyl derivative of neuraminic acid, is found on both glycoproteins and on lipids (sialoglycolipids or gangliosides). For Sendai virus, gangliosides function as both the attachment factor and the receptor for the virus.[243,245,246] As described earlier, the cellular receptor for the *Morbillivirus* measles virus is the cell surface protein CD150 (SLAM), and the cellular receptor for pneumoviruses, although not proven, seems to involve binding to glycosaminoglycans containing the disaccharide heparan sulfate and chondroitin sulfate B.[112] On adsorption of the virus to the cellular receptor, the viral membrane fuses with the cellular plasma membrane at the neutral pH found at the cell surface, the consequence of which is the release into the cytoplasm of the helical nucleocapsids.

In the virus particle, the M protein shell is thought to make numerous contacts with the nucleocapsid. On fusion of the viral envelope with the cell plasma membrane and release of the nucleocapsid into the cytoplasm, a mechanism needs to exist to disrupt the M-N contacts. With influenza A virus, the factor that alters the equilibrium between self-assembly and disassembly is thought to be the difference in pH between the acidic uncoating compartment (endosomes) and the assembly site (plasma membrane). The driving force for paramyxovirus uncoating is not known.

Viral RNA Synthesis

Paramyxoviruses have evolved mechanisms to control both the level and type of viral RNA that is synthesized during the course of an infection, largely through the use of *cis*-acting RNA sequences. The relationship between RNA sequences and the vRNAP functions that they control is particularly complex, because these *cis*-acting signals are only recognized when they are in the context of the nucleocapsid structure (see Fig. 33.21). Paramyxoviruses also encode *trans*-acting accessory proteins that control activities of the viral RNA. Recently, experimental systems have been developed that reconstitute RNA synthesis from model synthetic minigenomes using cDNA-derived viral components, allowing the functional analysis of *cis*-acting sequences or *trans*-acting proteins.

Viral Transcription (Messenger RNA Synthesis)

Early in virus infection, before the viral translation products have accumulated to high levels (or in the presence of drugs that inhibit protein synthesis at any stage of the infection), vRNAP is restricted to the production of leader RNAs and mRNAs from the incoming virion nucleocapsid in a growth phase called *primary transcription* (see Fig. 33.20). At later times following infection, this input nucleocapsid is used as a template to produce positive sense antigenomes that in turn are used as templates to produce new negative sense genomic RNA. When abundant progeny genomes have been produced, they can serve as additional templates in the growth phase, called *secondary transcription,* to produce much higher levels of viral mRNA transcripts (see Fig. 33.20).

The paramyxovirus RNAP is thought to gain access to the viral genes through a single entry site at or near the 3′ end of the genome. For the *Paramyxovirinae,* the *N* gene is transcribed as the first coding gene, and more than 90% of vRNAP that have initiated the Sendai virus N mRNA complete transcription of the entire N mRNA.[420] This processive vRNAP responds to the *cis*-acting sequences at the end of the *N* gene (open triangles in Fig. 33.21) to produce capped and polyadenylated viral mRNAs. The vRNAP then reinitiates mRNA synthesis at the start site of the next downstream gene (closed triangles in Fig. 33.21), and this sequential "stop-start" mechanism continues across the viral genome in a 3′ to 5′ direction.

The viral gene junctions that modulate transcription can be divided into three segments: a GE region at the 3′ end of the upstream gene, the IG region between the two genes that is normally not transcribed, and a GS region for the downstream 5′ gene (see Fig. 33.5). The GE region contains a signal directing the vRNAP to terminate transcription and a stretch of four to seven uridine residues (U tract) that acts as a template for polyadenylation of the nascent mRNA by a mechanism that involves stuttering by the vRNAP. After termination of transcription, the vRNAP is thought to remain attached to the template as it moves across the IG nucleotides. Reinitiation of transcription is directed by sequences at the downstream GS site, which also directs the addition of a methylated 5′ guanine cap to the nascent mRNA. The frequency of reinitiation is not perfect, and not every vRNAP that terminates at a GE remains on the template to reinitiate transcription at the next GS. This imperfect reinitiation frequency leads to a gradient of mRNA abundance that decreases according to distance from the genome 3′ end, with N mRNAs being found in higher abundance that L mRNA.[50] Initiation at a downstream GS site depends on termination at the upstream GE site,[208] consistent with a single entry site for the vRNAP at the 3′ end of the genome.

In addition to synthesizing monocistronic mRNAs, the vRNAP can also ignore the GE sequences for polyadenylation/termination and synthesize a transcriptional read-through product that consists of a fusion of the upstream and downstream mRNAs. While read-through transcription is generally an infrequent event, for several paramyxoviruses, such as HPIV types 1 through 3, measles virus, and PIV5, read-through transcription is highest at the M-F junction, and approximately 50% to 80% of the F mRNA is locked into an M-F read-through product.[27,49,334,380] An extreme example of this is seen with simian virus 41 (SV41), where the M mRNA is seen exclusively as an M-F read-through product owing to a deletion of the M GE,[413] and F mRNA is found in both mono- and dicistronic forms.[414] The basis for this elevated M-F read-through for some paramyxoviruses is owing to GE insertions[380] or substitutions[334] that alter the efficiency of termination signals. The selective pressure to maintain elevated M-F read-through for some paramyxoviruses is not known but could reflect a need to increase access of a transcribing polymerase to the more 3′ distal genes (e.g., HN or L) or a mechanism to down-regulate F protein expression, as this ORF would be locked into a dicistronic mRNA that would presumably not be translated.[190,334]

Paramyxoviruses can be divided into two groups based on whether the viral GE and IG sequences are highly conserved across the genome or have a high degree of variability. The GE and IG regions of Sendai virus, HPIV1, and HPIV3 have a high degree of genetic conservation.[203] For example, each of the Sendai virus GE sequences consist of a 3′-AUUCU$_5$-5′ motif, and the IG region is 3′-GAA-5′ (except the HN-L junction, which is 3′-GGG-5′). By contrast, the GE and IG regions of RSV, human parainfluenza virus type 2 (HPIV2), mumps virus V, SV41, and PIV5 are highly diverse and provide an additional level of transcriptional control beyond that which results from the distance of a gene from the 3′-end promoter. This diversity is reflected in the combinations of GE and IG sequences that can act together to differentially control vRNAP activities.[144,333] RSV GE sequences are more diverse than their GS sequences and operate at variable efficiency in transcription termination and read-through.[142,207] Moreover, for RSV, the L GS sequence is actually located upstream of the GE sequence of the upstream *M2* gene[65] (see Fig. 33.4). Thus, the RSV polymerase terminates at the M2 GE; however, it is thought to scan backward on the template to reinitiate at the upstream L GS site.[108]

Trans-acting viral proteins can also contribute to the control of stop-start transcription. For example, the RSV M2-1 protein is an essential transcription elongation factor that is necessary for high processivity of the vRNAP.[63] M2-1 can also modulate vRNAP activities at the diverse gene junction sequences,[142] resulting in junction-specific changes in transcriptional read-through versus termination and in the relative abundance of mono- and dicistronic mRNAs.

P Gene Messenger RNA Editing

Pseudo-templated addition of nucleotides, popularly known as RNA editing, is a mechanism for obtaining more coding potential from a gene, and it was first identified for PIV5.[307,408] It is now known that most paramyxovirus *P* genes contain a functional editing site within the coding region of the *P* gene (see Fig. 33.6). In addition to a faithful (unedited) mRNA, transcription across of the *P/V/C* gene yields edited versions that contain variable numbers of inserted G residues. The number of G insertions can differ for each virus group and mirrors their requirements for mRNAs that encode the individual P/V/W/I/D proteins (see Fig. 33.6). For the morbilliviruses, respiroviruses, and NDV, a single G is added to transcripts as the predominant editing event, resulting in an mRNA that shifts from the genome-encoded P ORF to the V ORF (see Fig. 33.6). For the rubulaviruses, which encode the V ORF as the unedited faithful copy of the *P/V* gene, the insertion of 2 Gs constitutes a high proportion of editing events, producing an mRNA that encodes the P protein subunit of the vRNAP. For BPIV3 and HPIV3, where both the V and D ORF overlap the middle of the genome-encoded P ORF, one to six G residues are added at roughly equal frequency so that mRNAs encoding all three overlapping ORFs are transcribed.

As the paramyxoviruses replicate in the cytoplasm, they must provide enzymes for all aspects of their mRNA synthesis. Paramyxovirus vRNAPs polyadenylate their mRNAs by stuttering on a short run of template U residues (four to seven nucleotides long) at the end of each gene. By analogy to the polyadenylation mechanism, it was suggested that the G insertions at the specific site in the *P* gene would occur similarly by pseudo-templated transcription,[408] and there is now strong experimental evidence that the insertions occur by a co-transcriptional stuttering mechanism.[150,419] The efficiency of G insertion by the stuttering polymerase depends on the relative position of an editing site within the N-bound hexamer of nucleotides,[181,203] suggesting that polymerase function is directed by a combination of RNA sequence and N protein structure within the template.

Genome Replication

A schematic diagram of transcription and RNA replication in the paramyxovirus growth cycle is shown in Figure 33.20, and the role of genomes and antigenomes as templates for these phases of RNA synthesis is shown in Figure 33.21. At early times of infection, the genome directs the synthesis of positive leader and viral mRNAs. After translation of the primary transcripts and accumulation of the viral proteins, the negative sense genome is replicated to produce a full-length complementary copy, called the *antigenome,* which is found only in a form that is assembled with N protein. Here, it is thought that the same vRNAP copies the same template that had been used for transcription, although now all of the gene junction signals (and editing sites) are ignored and an exact complementary copy of the template is generated. In infected cells, antigenomes are typically found in lower levels than genomes, and they do not code for any known functional ORFs or mRNAs. The sole function of the antigenome is thought to be as an intermediate in genome replication; however, the short trailer RNAs expressed from the antigenome 3′ end (see Fig. 33.21) may also play a role in preventing the host cell from undergoing programmed cell death.[182]

It has long been known that when infected cells are treated with drugs that inhibit protein synthesis, mRNA synthesis continues normally but genome synthesis is lost very quickly. As genome synthesis and encapsidation appear to occur concomitantly,[139] this requirement for ongoing protein synthesis during RNA replication is thought to reflect the need for a continued supply of unassembled N for genome encapsidation. Similar to the model for vesicular stomatitis virus (VSV), this coupling of genome assembly and synthesis also leads to a self-regulatory system for controlling the relative levels of viral transcription and replication. Because the leader sequences contain the N encapsidation site, the leader must be separated from the body of the first mRNA (by termination and reinitiation at the leader-N junction) to prevent the first mRNA from ending up in an assembled and untranslatable form. Thus, when unassembled N is limiting, such as early times in the growth cycle, vRNAP is preferentially engaged in mRNA synthesis, and this results in an increase in intracellular levels of all the viral proteins, including unassembled N. When unassembled N levels are sufficiently high, some vRNAP would be switched to replication, thereby lowering the levels of unassembled N, as each initiation of encapsidation would commit approximately 2,600 N monomers to finish the assembled genome chain.[420] The level of unassembled N may not be the only mechanism controlling transcription versus RNA replication, because higher levels of N protein have not affected the ratio of replication to transcription for RSV minigenomes.[110]

Paramyxoviruses employ additional mechanisms to control genome and antigenome replication, including the expression of viral accessory proteins that are not essential for virus growth but play a role in control of viral RNA synthesis. For example, the Sendai virus V protein is thought to inhibit RNA replication through binding to N^0, the assembly-competent form of nucleocapsid protein.[168] The RSV M2-2 protein appears to play a role in regulation of transcription versus replication,[14] and the RSV NS1 protein is a potent inhibitor of RNA replication in a minigenome system.[6]

After synthesis, the antigenomic RNA is used as a template to direct synthesis of genomic RNA by a mechanism similar to that for antigenome synthesis, in that the promoter at the 3′ end of the antigenome directs synthesis of the short trailer RNA, also referred to as negative leader (see Fig. 33.21). Under conditions of sufficient intracellular concentrations of unassembled N (and perhaps other viral proteins), encapsidation of the nascent trailer chain would quickly begin and lead to the synthesis of encapsidated minus-strand genomes. As shown in Figure 33.20, these progeny negative sense genomes can serve three subsequent functions: as a template for mRNA synthesis in a phase called *secondary transcription,* as a template to produce additional antigenomes, or for incorporation into progeny virions during the budding process.

Paramyxovirus Replication Promoter

The 3′-end promoter in the antigenome directs the synthesis of progeny genomes and is thought to be a stronger promoter for RNA replication than the genomic 3′-end promoter in the genome that directs the synthesis of both mRNAs and antigenomes (see Fig. 33.21). Thus, the relative strength of genomic and antigenomic promoters in RNA replication can contribute to the relative ratio of these full-length RNAs in infected cells.[221] Extensive mutagenesis studies with model minigenomes have identified three factors that contribute to promoter function: the rule of six chain length requirement, nucleotide sequences within the bipartite promoter, and proper spacing of promoter elements.

It was found that changes in the overall length of a paramyxovirus N-RNA complex can profoundly affect the efficiency of RNA replication.[40] This RNA chain length requirement, called the *rule of six,* dictates that efficient replication of a viral genomic or antigenomic RNA will only occur when the total number of nucleotides in the RNA is an even multiple of six.[43] This surprising requisite is thought to reflect the precise nature with which the genomic RNA must be encapsidated by N to form a nucleocapsid template for the viral polymerase.[43,315] The hexamer requirement emerged from microscopy studies of Sendai virus nucleocapsids, which revealed that each Sendai virus N molecule contacts six bases of RNA.[101] During replication, N-RNA assembly is thought to initiate with the 5′ end of the nascent RNA chain as it emerges from the vRNAP complex, and encapsidation proceeds in a 5′ to 3′ direction.[139,420] As shown schematically in Figure 33.21, a genome whose length is an even multiple of six nucleotides will be precisely encapsidated by N, with no unencapsidated nucleotides protruding from the 3′ end of the nucleocapsid.[315]

There is large variability in the stringency to which various groups of paramyxoviruses adhere to the rule of six requirement. Sendai virus RNA replication highly depends on the rule of six,[43] whereas there is no replicative advantage to RSV genome analogs having genome lengths that are a multiple of any particular integer.[350] RNA replication for PIV5, NDV, and HPIV3 is most efficient for 6N-length genomes, although this is not as stringent a requirement as found for Sendai virus.[95,242,273]

The rule of six was originally proposed to reflect the need to have a functional nucleocapsid template with a precisely encapsidated 3′ end and no "dangling" free bases. However, extensions to the 3′ end of Sendai virus DI RNAs do not result in a decrease in RNA replication, regardless of whether these extensions were multiples of six or not.[425] As shown in Figure 33.22B, an alternative hypothesis emerged by the observation that the phase of a particular base in the promoter can range from position 1 to 6 within a hexamer of N-bound sequences.

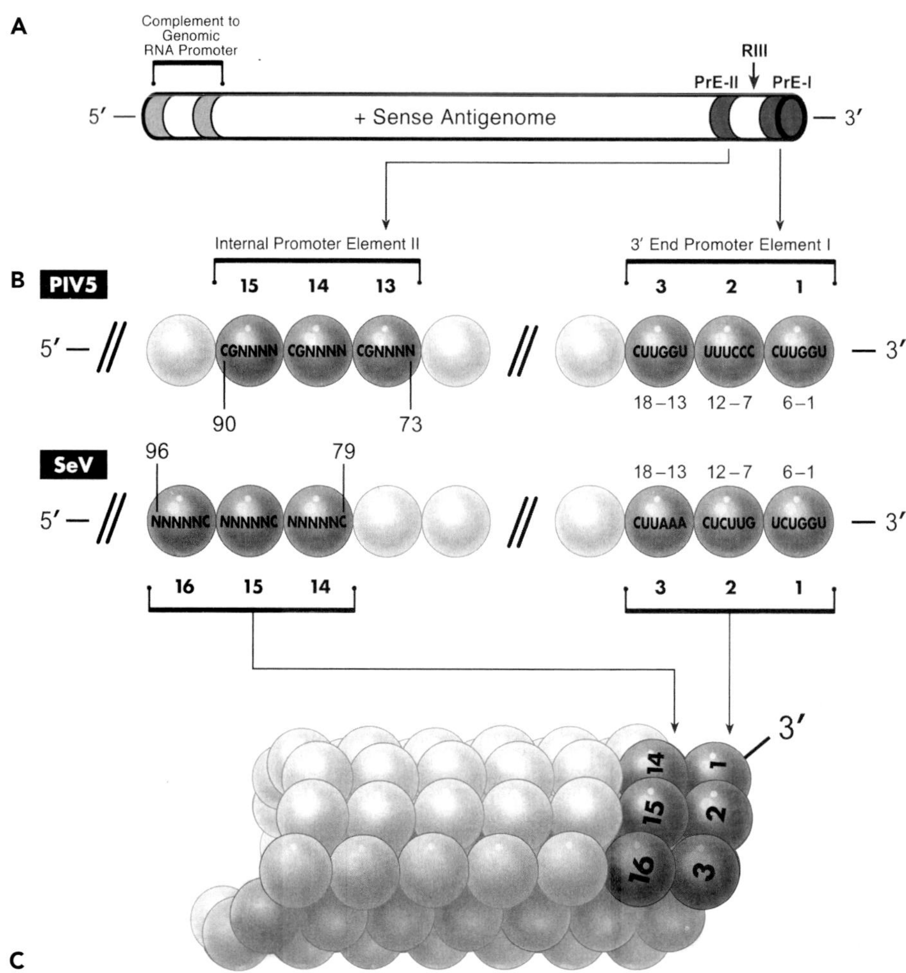

FIGURE 33.22. Nucleocapsid structure, hexamer phasing of nucleotide sequences, and the bipartite replication promoters of the *Paramyxovirinae*. A: Schematic of the paramyxovirus positive sense antigenomic RNA. The location of the 3′-end promoter element I (PrE-I) and internal promoter element II (PrE-II) are indicated by *shaded* areas, with location of the intervening nonessential region III replication element (RIII) shown by an *arrow*. The 5′ end of the antigenome contains sequences that are the complement to the genomic RNA promoter and are partially complementary to the 3′ region of the antigenomic RNA. **B:** Expanded view of a portion of the first 16 N protein subunits (drawn as *ovals*) of the antigenome nucleocapsid. Numbers above the ovals indicate the position of each N monomer, and numbers below the ovals refer to the nucleotide sequence relative to the 3′ end of the RNA. The position of nucleotides within the 3′-end PrE-I and internal PrE-II elements for parainfluenza virus type 5 (PIV5) and Sendai virus are shown relative to the N subunits, with each subunit containing precisely six nucleotides. Note that for the internal PrE-II element, essential C residues are located in the first position of each hexamer for Sendai virus, whereas GC residues are located in the fifth and sixth positions for PIV5. **C:** A model for the Sendai virus and PIV5 nucleocapsid as an assembly of single N protein subunits (*shaded spheres*), in the form of a left-handed helix with N binding six nucleotides and 13 N subunits per turn. Numbers refer to the position of each N subunit from the RNA 3′ end. Note that both PrE-I and PrE-II of the bipartite replication promoter are found on the same face of the helix.

Experimentally altering the predicted phase of nucleotides in the antigenomic promoter reduces RNA replication.[315] This finding is consistent with a model for the rule of six requirement based on critical *cis*-acting promoter sequences that can only be recognized when they are in the correct positions within their encapsidating N monomers.[203] Further support for this hypothesis comes from the finding that the Sendai virus promoter can function when located at an internal position in a viral N-RNA complex, but only when the hexamer phase of promoter elements is correct.[425]

A second primary determinant of replication promoter strength resides in the nucleotide sequence in the leader RNA at the 3′ terminus of the genome and in the trailer complement RNA at the 3′ terminus of the antigenome.[164,242,272,400,401] As shown in Figure 33.22, two discontinuous sequence-specific elements have been identified within the 3′-terminal 90 bases of the antigenomic promoter. In the two original descriptions of this requirement, these elements have been termed conserved region I (CRI) and conserved region II (CRII) for PIV5[272,274] and promoter element I (PrE-I) and promoter element II (PrE-II) for Sendai virus.[400]

PrE-I is located at the 3′ end of viral genomic and antigenomic RNA (see Fig. 33.22), and the specific sequence is highly conserved between members of a paramyxovirus genus. The internal PrE-II sequence is located within the L gene for the antigenomic promoter or within the *N* gene for the genomic promoter.[164,272,400,426] Paramyxoviruses fall into two groups based on the distance of their critical PrE-II bases from the 3′ end of the viral RNA and the sequence and the position of essential bases within an N hexamer. As diagrammed in Figure 33.22B, the internal PrE-II element for PIV5 and related rubulaviruses is located between 72 and 90 bases from the 3′ end of the viral RNA.[272] By contrast, the PrE-II element for Sendai virus and related respiro- and morbilliviruses is located between 79 and 96 bases from the 3′ end.[400,426] The sequence requirements within PrE-II are remarkably simple; however, they differ for PIV5 and Sendai virus RNA replication. For PIV5, extensive mutational analyses[274] indicated that the PrE-II requirements consisted of a CG motif located in the first two positions of three sequential hexamers of nucleotides (5′-CGGGAU CGAUGG CGAGAA-3′, template sense, see Fig. 33.22B). By contrast, the Sendai virus PrE-II requirements consisted of three copies of a 5′-(NNNNNC)-3′ motif (see Fig. 33.22B; shown as template sense). An additional element located between antigenomic PrE-I and the internal PrE-II has been identified for PIV5 (bases 51–66) and HPIV3 (bases 13–55), which is thought to act as a nonessential enhancer of replication.[164,196]

A third factor in RNA replication was identified during mutational analyses of the PIV5 and Sendai virus antigenomic promoters, where it was found that deletions or insertions in the RNA segment located between the 3′-terminal PrE-I and the internal PrE-II resulted in templates that were not competent for RNA replication.[272,400] The template defect was not attributed to disruption of an important *cis*-acting segment or the rule of six. As described in the next section, it is thought that the sensitivity of RNA replication to changes in the length of the region between PrE-I and PrE-II reflects a requirement for these two RNA segments to align to the same face of the nucleocapsid template.[274,400]

Image reconstruction of electron micrographs indicates that Sendai virus N binds six nucleotides and that 13 N monomers constitute a turn of the nucleocapsid helix.[101] Together with extensive mutational analysis of minigenome analogs, these data suggest a model for the paramyxovirus promoters.[220,272,400] As shown in Figure 33.22B,C, nucleotides within the 3′ PrE-I and internal PrE-II elements are separated along the linear RNA sequence by 55 to 60 bases; however, in the N-encapsidated form, these RNA elements are aligned to the same face of the nucleocapsid template by the helical winding. Alignment of PrE-I and PrE-II may form a binding site for the polymerase complex to initiate RNA synthesis at the 3′ end of the template, although formal proof of this hypothesis is not currently available. Taken together, the available evidence indicates that promoter strength is a major factor dictating level of RNA replication, and promoter strength is in turn affected by (a) changes in the phase of nucleotides within the N-induced hexamer phase of PrE-I or PrE-II (rule of six requirement); (b) changes in the RNA sequences themselves; or (c) changes in the spacer region between PrE-I and PrE-II, which alter their alignment on one face of the nucleocapsid template.

Virion Assembly and Release

Paramyxoviruses viruses, like other enveloped viruses, are formed by a budding process. Buds emerge from sites on the plasma membrane where viral components have assembled, then pinch off resulting in the release of particles. Assembly of paramyxoviruses is thought to require coordinated localization of multiple but distinct virus components, including viral glycoproteins, which are transported to the plasma membrane by the exocytic pathway, and soluble viral components, such as the RNP. This coordination appears to be accomplished through a series of protein–protein and protein–lipid interactions, many of which involve the viral matrix protein that could potentially interact with both glycoproteins via their cytoplasmic tails and with the RNPs in the cytoplasm of the infected cell, and also interactions between viral components and the host machinery that allows bud formation and membrane fission. Those *Paramyxovirinae* that have NA activity contain glycoproteins that lack sialic modification of their carbohydrate chains, and it is thought that the HN NA activity serves the same purpose as NA of influenza virus—to prevent self-binding and to prevent reattachment to the infected cell.

Assembly of the Nucleocapsid

Nucleocapsids assemble in the cytoplasm in two steps: first, association of free N subunits with the genome or template RNA to form the helical RNP structure, and second, the association of the P-L protein complex.[199] By analogy to the mechanism of assembly of TMV nucleocapsid, which uses a defined nucleation site for the association of the first coat protein subunit with the RNA, and the observation that the paramyxovirus mRNAs are not encapsidated in contrast to antigenomes, it has been assumed that the positive leader (5′ end of the antigenome) and negative trailer (5′ end of the genome) regions contain specific sequences for initiating encapsidation.[19]

Assembly of the Envelope

The assembly of the second part of the virus—the envelope—is at the cell surface. In polarized epithelial cells, the *Paramyxovirinae* bud only from the apical surface. For a long time, it has been thought that the matrix proteins of negative-strand RNA viruses have important roles in virus assembly and budding.

Matrix proteins are positioned in virions beneath the lipid envelope, so that they have the potential to contact both RNP cores and envelope glycoprotein cytoplasmic tails, and are therefore likely to be the key organizers of virus assembly that induce separate viral components to concentrate together at defined budding sites on the plasma membranes of infected cells. Matrix proteins bind to viral RNPs *in vitro* and are found stably attached to RNPs when purified from virions, they bind to lipid membranes both *in vitro* and in living cells, and they self-assemble into ordered structures as purified proteins *in vitro* and in virus-infected cells. Studies using reverse genetics techniques have aided in understanding the role of the matrix protein in assembly. The M proteins of measles virus and Sendai virus had previously been implicated in budding based on analysis of viruses derived from persistent viral infections. Cells persistently infected with Sendai virus were found to express an unstable M protein, and lack of stable M protein correlated with a reduction in virus particle formation.[341] A role for the measles virus M protein in budding was suggested based on analysis of viruses isolated from patients with SSPE. SSPE viruses are defective for the production of progeny virus particles. Nucleotide sequence analysis has revealed extensive defects in the *M* genes of SSPE measles virus strains.[53,440] Recombinant measles viruses were generated having defective or deleted *M* genes.[45,309] Both of these viruses were shown to be severely defective in budding: Indeed, the infectivity was so low that the particles may represent adventitious vesicles with RNPs.

The Use of Virus-like Particles to Study Assembly

The importance of the matrix protein for virus budding has been investigated using the assembly of VLPs from proteins expressed from cDNAs. For PIV5, although M protein expressed by itself does not induce efficient budding of particles, when M is coexpressed with N protein and a viral glycoprotein (either F or HN), budding of particles becomes very efficient, approaching the budding efficiency observed in virus-infected cells.[359] VLP budding that is normally observed on expression of the Sendai virus M protein alone can be made more efficient by co-expressing the Sendai virus F glycoprotein.[395]

Glycoprotein Cytoplasmic Tails and Assembly

It has long been thought that the glycoprotein cytoplasmic tails would be used in recognizing the M protein. Early studies using a temperature-sensitive mutant of Sendai virus (ts271) demonstrated that the Sendai virus HN protein is dispensable for budding of virus particles.[326,328,387,415] VLP budding was observed on expression of M protein alone and the efficiency of budding was found to be stimulated on co-expression of F protein; however, co-expression of HN protein had no effect on budding efficiency.[395] Recombinant Sendai viruses with altered glycoprotein cytoplasmic tails have been generated, and truncation of the F protein cytoplasmic tail resulted in poor budding. Release of particles on expression of F protein alone was found to depend on the amino acid sequence TYTLE, comprising amino acids 542 to 546 of the F protein cytoplasmic tail.[395] Recombinant PIV5 were recovered harboring HN proteins with truncated cytoplasmic tails, and budding was found to be inefficient on HN protein cytoplasmic tail deletion.[357] The same approach was used to define the role of the PIV5 F protein cytoplasmic tail in virus budding, and it was found that recombinant viruses with deleted F protein cytoplasmic tails replicated in tissue culture and were released from infected cells with similar efficiency to wild-type virus.[429] This result was surprising in light of work with Sendai virus suggesting that F protein is in fact quite important for proper paramyxovirus budding. To investigate further the relative roles of the HN and F glycoproteins for paramyxovirus budding, a VLP system was developed for PIV5.[359] Here, efficient budding of VLPs from transfected cells was observed only on co-expression of multiple PIV5 proteins. Thus, expression of M protein alone did not lead to substantial particle budding, and neither of the PIV5 glycoproteins was found to have an autonomous exocytosis activity. However, co-expression of M protein with N protein and either the HN or F glycoprotein led to budding of VLPs with an efficiency comparable to that found in virus-infected cells. Budding decreased more than 25-fold when neither of the PIV5 glycoproteins were included, and the HN and F proteins were found to be completely interchangeable for VLP budding. This result suggested that the two PIV5 glycoproteins might have redundant functions for budding. Consistent with this idea, recombinant PIV5 lacking both HN and F protein cytoplasmic tails was found to have a greater defect in particle production and release than PIV5 lacking only the HN protein cytoplasmic tail.[429] From VLP experiments, the importance of the glycoprotein cytoplasmic tails for efficient budding was confirmed; VLPs containing wild-type HN or wild-type F as the only glycoprotein bud efficiently, whereas those containing only cytoplasmic tail–deleted HN or cytoplasmic tail–deleted F protein bud poorly.[359] SSPE measles virus strains contain drastic sequence alterations not only in their *M* genes, as discussed previously, but also in their F protein cytoplasmic tail sequences.[52] Truncations or other alterations to the F protein cytoplasmic tail led to more rapid and extensive cell-to-cell fusion of virus-infected cells, consistent with a shift in the mode of virus spread to one that is independent of budding.[46,263] Very recently, for RSV, it was shown that a critical phenylalanine residue in the F protein cytoplasmic tail mediates assembly of internal viral proteins into viral filaments and particles.[369]

Budding and Interactions with the Multivesiculate Body Formation Machinery

For several enveloped viruses, it has been shown that budding occurs in a way that requires the manipulation of host machinery. Protein–protein interaction domains called *late domains* have been defined in retroviral Gag proteins and in the matrix proteins of some negative-strand RNA viruses. These late domains function to recruit host factors to viral assembly sites where they assist in virus release.[117,265] Disruption of viral late domains often leads to phenotypes in which virus particles assemble normally but fail to be released by membrane fission and instead accumulate as tethered particles on cellular membranes.[83,127,135,184]

Several types of late domain have ben identified: P(T/S)AP, PPxY, and YP(x)$_n$L. Each of these late domain sequences likely functions to bind with a different host factor to facilitate virus budding. P(T/S)AP late domains mediate binding to TSG101,[127,248] and the host partner protein for YP(x)$_n$L late domains appears to be AIP1.[247,383,421,424] Both TSG101 and AIP1 are part of the cellular vacuolar protein sorting (VPS) pathway (ESCRT) that allows formation of multivesicular bodies (MVBs), an observation that is significant owing to the fact that virus budding and vesicle budding into MVBs are similar processes, in which cytoplasmic cargo is packed into vesicles that bud outward from the cytoplasm. PPxY-type late domains have been shown to interact with WW domains from a variety of proteins, such as Nedd4-related E3 ubiquitin ligases.[146,197,411] It has been proposed that recruitment of Nedd4 family members may allow indirect recruitment of other host proteins, including those involved in MVB formation.[384]

Budding of PIV5 and PIV5-like particles was reduced by treatment of cells with the proteasome inhibitor MG-132.[358] Proteasome inhibitors also reduce virus budding of retroviruses such as HIV-1[363] and RSV[308]—viruses that use PTAP and PPxY late domains for budding. Inhibition of proteasome function prevents recycling of ubiquitin that is attached to proteins targeted for degradation, thereby depleting free ubiquitin levels in the cell.[423] It has been found that the PIV5 M protein is targeted for monoubiquitination in transfected cells at three lysine residues. Mutation of the lysine residues leads to altered ubiquitination and impaired VLP production. Analysis of these mutations in recombinant viruses suggest that monoubiquitination of PIV5 M protein is needed for virus assembly and budding.[145]

There have been several attempts to discover cell proteins that interact with viral proteins during budding. Production of PIV5 and PIV5-like particles is reduced on expression of a dominant-negative VPS4A adenosine triphosphatase (ATPase).[358] Interestingly, substantial incorporation of the dominant negative VPS4A mutant into VLPs was noted, despite the relatively small amount of VLPs produced under these conditions. VPS4 mutants disrupt the cellular MVB formation pathway, likely because adenosine triphosphate (ATP) hydrolysis is required for release of class E proteins from late endosomal membranes. The PIV5 M protein lacks previously defined late domains (e.g., P[T/S]AP, PPxY, YPDL) to recruit cellular factors. However, a new late domain for budding (core sequence FPIV) that can compensate functionally for lack of a PTAP late domain in budding HIV-1 VLPs was identified.[358] Mutagenesis experiments suggested the more general sequence Ø-P-x-V. The proline residue was found to be critically important for function of this late domain, as substitution of this proline in PIV5 M protein resulted in poor budding of PIV5 VLPs and failure of recombinant PIV5 virus to replicate normally. Adaptation of mutant virus harboring an altered FPIV domain occurred rapidly, resulting in new proline residues elsewhere in the M protein.[358] Yeast two-hybrid screening identified angiomotin-like 1 (AmotL1) as a host factor that interacts with PIV5 M protein. Overexpression of M-binding AmotL1-derived polypeptides potently inhibited production of PIV5 VLP budding and small interfering RNA (siRNA)-mediated depletion of AmotL1 reduced PIV5 budding.[313] Yeast two-hybrid screening also identified a protein designated as 14-3-3 as a binding partner of PIV5 M, and it was found that 14-3-3 negatively affects virus particle formation.[314] However, it is not known if AmotL1 and 14-3-3 are involved in the ESCRT pathway.

For Sendai virus, a sequence YLDL has been found in the M protein that acts as a late domain and is required for budding.[180] Curiously, YLDL of Sendai virus M protein is not replaceable by other late domains, perhaps because of structural constraints. It has been found that the Sendai virus M late domain interacts with the N-terminus of the cellular protein Alix/AIP1, a component of the ESCRT pathway. Mutagenesis of M protein YLDL to ALDA abolished budding and the interaction with Alix/AIP1. A revertant virus was obtained with the sequence ALDV, and budding was restored together with the interaction of the M protein with Alix/AIP1.[179] The Sendai virus C protein also interacts with Alix/AIP1, and C protein expression enhances budding. It is thought that C protein recruits Alix/AIP1 to the plasma membrane and enhances the efficiency of the utilization of the ESCRT machinery for efficient VLP budding.

Budding of Paramyxoviruses from Membrane Rafts

It has recently become clear that lipid molecules within the plasma membrane are not distributed homogenously in each leaflet of the bilayer, but rather participate in lateral associations to form subcompartments within the membrane. One type of lipid microdomain is the membrane raft, which preferentially contains sphingolipids and cholesterol as well as certain integral membrane proteins.[34,372] Membrane rafts can be separated biochemically from other membrane components based on their resistance to solubilization by certain nonionic detergents such as TX-100 at low temperatures. Some viral proteins have been found to be enriched within membrane rafts of infected cells, suggesting that virus assembly can occur on rafts. For example, in influenza A virus–infected cells, the glycoproteins hemagglutinin and NA, as well as the matrix protein, are found associated predominantly with TX-100–insoluble lipids.[223,339,340,374,454] Assembly of viral proteins on raft membranes does not appear to be a universal strategy for negative-strand RNA virus assembly, however, as in the cases of VSV and rabies virus infections, the viral proteins are found excluded from raft membranes in the infected cells. Paramyxovirus proteins in many cases have been found to be associated with raft membranes in infected cells, including the HN and F glycoproteins of Sendai virus,[351] F and HN proteins of NDV,[90,210] the measles virus proteins H, F, M, and N,[239,422] and the RSV glycoproteins F and G.[36]

Polarized Budding from Epithelial Cells

The paramyxoviruses Sendai virus, PIV5, and measles virus have been found to bud preferentially from the apical membranes of polarized cells.[18,338] Polarized budding may have important consequences for viral pathogenesis, as budding from the apical surface could favor restriction of the infection to the epithelial cell layer, whereas budding from the basolateral surface allows viral access to underlying tissue and could favor development of a systemic infection. Consistent with this view, Sendai virus and PIV5 both produce localized infections of the respiratory tract *in vivo,* whereas VSV and Marburg virus both produce systemic infections *in vivo.* Furthermore, a mutant Sendai virus has been characterized in which polarized budding from the apical membrane is lost and virus is instead released in a nonpolar fashion from both the apical and basolateral cell surfaces, and this virus causes a systemic infection and is more virulent than wild-type Sendai virus.[403] The correlation between pathogenicity and virus budding from the basolateral cell surface is not absolute, however, because measles virus is released apically yet produces a systemic infection *in vivo.*

MOLECULARLY ENGINEERED GENETICS (REVERSE GENETICS)

The study of viruses and their interactions with host cells and organisms has benefited greatly from the ability to engineer

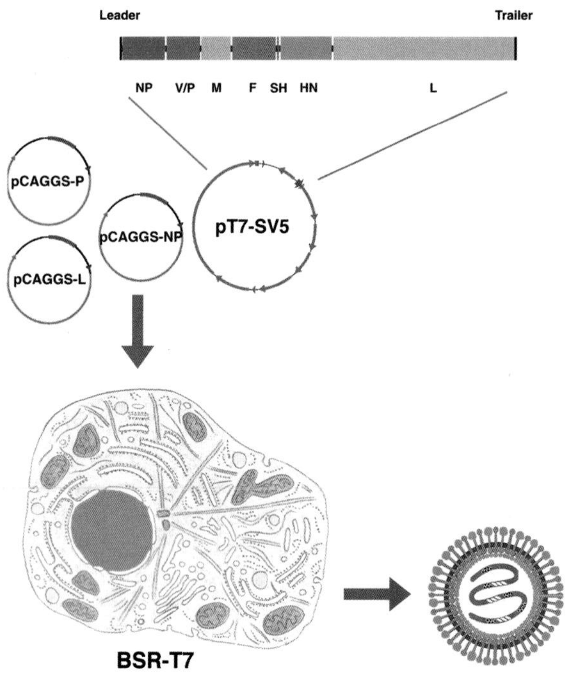

© G.D. Parks and R.A. Lamb 2006

FIGURE 33.23. Rescue of paramyxoviruses from cloned complementary DNA (cDNA). Nonsegmented negative-strand virus rescue involves the transfection of plasmids encoding the viral P, N, and L proteins (and sometimes other viral proteins depending on the virus), as well as the viral antigenome, all under control of the T7 promoter. The bacteriophage T7 RNA polymerase is provided by either infection with a vaccinia virus expressing T7 polymerase (in this case, modified vaccinia virus Ankara, MVA-T7) or by transfecting into cell lines that stably express the protein (e.g., BSR-T7 cells). pT7-SV5 contains a complete copy of the parainfluenza virus type 5 (PIV5) genome (15,246 nucleotides) and is flanked at one end by a bacteriophage T7 RNA polymerase (T7 RNAP) promoter and at the other end by a hepatitis delta virus ribozyme and T7 transcriptional terminator. The plasmids pT7-L, pT7-P, and pT7-N each contain the cDNA for the PIV5 L, P, and N proteins, respectively, under the control of T7 RNAP promoters such that messenger RNA transcripts encoding L, P, and N can be transcribed using T7 RNAP. (Adapted from He B, Paterson RG, Ward CD, et al. Recovery of infectious SV5 from cloned DNA and expression of a foreign gene. *Virology* 1997;237:249–260.)

specific mutations into viral genomes—a technique known as reverse genetics.[434] For RNA viruses, genome manipulation of the positive sense RNA bacteriophage $Q\beta$ was the first to be performed.[398] The negative-stranded RNA viruses, in contrast to positive sense RNA viruses, require that the virion RNA is assembled into an active transcriptase-replicase complex in order for the genome to initiate virus replication. Nonetheless, techniques to manipulate the genomes of nonsegmented negative-strand RNA viruses have now been developed.[335] The development of the system originally proved quite frustrating. Several laboratories studying various rhabdoviruses and paramyxoviruses worked over a period of several years to establish the methods of reconstructing functional nucleocapsids from transfected cells. The concept of replicating minigenomes using support plasmids providing N, P, and L proteins in *trans* was key to the development of the technology. This culminated in the successful recovery of infectious rabies virus in 1994, followed several months later by VSV, and several months later by Sendai, human RSV, and measles virus.

Rabies virus was rescued when plasmids encoding L, P, and N protein, as well as a plasmid containing the viral antigenome, all under control of the bacteriophage T7 RNAP promoter, were transfected into cells infected with a recombinant vaccinia virus expressing the bacteriophage T7 RNAP protein (vac-T7).[361] As an example, the following viruses have been rescued: VSV,[219,436] measles virus,[332] human RSV,[62] Sendai virus,[126,194] rinderpest virus,[11] HPIV3,[93,163] PIV5 (SV5),[154] NDV,[312] and bovine RSV.[39] A schematic diagram showing the general scheme for rescue is illustrated for PIV5 in Figure 33.23. Some refinements to the original technique have been made, such as the use of stably transfected cell lines expressing the bacteriophage T7 RNAP (in lieu of vac-T7 infection), or one or more of the viral proteins required for genome replication.[39,332]

VIRAL ACCESSORY GENES AND THEIR INTERACTIONS WITH THE HOST

Type I IFN is one of the most important antiviral cytokines that can be a major determinant of tropism, pathogenesis, and viral dissemination. As shown in Figure 33.24, the cellular IFN response involves two general phases: the induction of IFN synthesis in a primary transcriptional phase and signaling through the type I IFN signaling pathway to activate a secondary transcriptional phase (see Chapter 8).[16] A large body of work has emerged recently on the role of paramyxovirus accessory proteins in counteracting the host cell IFN pathways at the level of IFN synthesis or IFN signaling.[70,122]

Antagonists of Interferon Synthesis

As shown in Figure 33.24, synthesis of IFN-β can be induced by by-products of virus replication such as viral double-stranded RNA (dsRNA) or 5′-triphosphate RNAs, which are recognized by cellular pattern recognition receptors (PRRs). These PRRs include the dsRNA-activated protein kinase R (PKR), toll-like receptors (TLRs), and two cytoplasmic RNA helicases retinoic acid inducible gene-I (RIG-I), and melanoma differentiation-associated gene 5 (MDA5).[3,446] Many PRRs signal through a mitochondrion-associated protein called *mitochondrial antiviral signaling protein* (MAVS) or IFN-β promoter stimulator 1 (IPS-1)[195] to activate cytoplasmic kinases including TANK-binding kinase 1 (TBK-1)/inhibitor of κB kinase ε (IKKε). Ultimately, this leads to dimerization and phosphorylation of latent transcription factors such as NFκB and members of the family of interferon regulatory factors (IRFs), which can translocate to the nucleus and activate cellular promoters that drive expression of IRF responsive genes such as IFN-β. Results from transfection assays and the study of viruses that have been engineered to encode altered or deleted genes have identified viral antagonists of pathways that lead to IFN-β induction. These antagonists include the respirovirus and morbillivirus V and C proteins, the rubulavirus V protein, and the henipavirus V and W proteins.[24,153,204,320,337,370,377] The pneumovirus NS1 and NS2 proteins also limit induction of IFN-β and are discussed elsewhere in this text.[230,377]

For many paramyxoviruses, PKR is not activated to a large extent during infection except in the case where viral

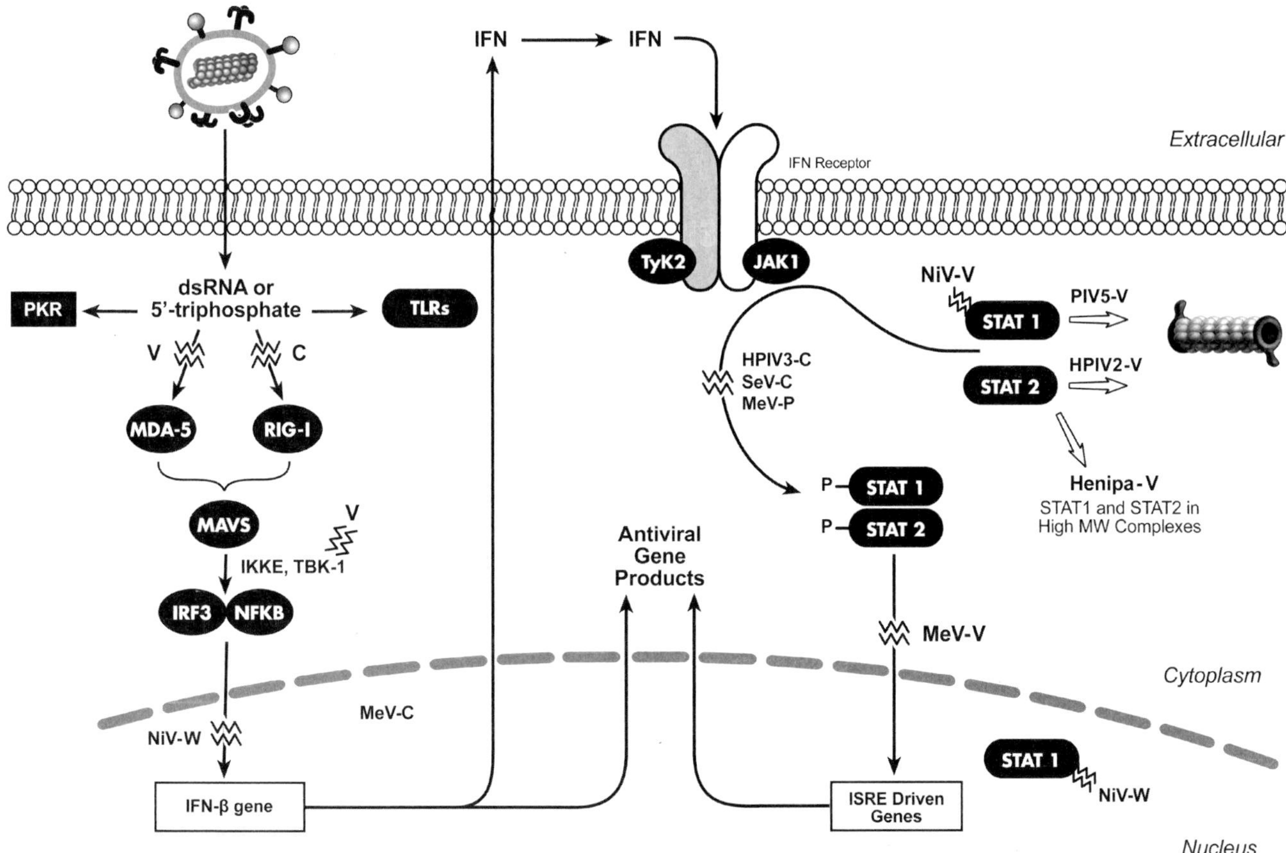

FIGURE 33.24. Interferon (IFN) induction, IFN signaling, and sites of antagonism by paramyxovirus accessory proteins. Schematic diagram of IFN induction **(left)**, binding of IFN to extracellular receptors (**top** and **middle**), and signal tranducers and activators of transcription (STAT)-mediated signaling **(right)** to activate transcription from cellular genes containing an interferon-stimulated response element. Sites of inhibition by a paramyxovirus antagonist are indicated by two *wavy lines* or by an *open arrow.*

antagonist proteins such as V and C proteins are altered.[21,251,391] In the case of these viral mutants, PKR activation results in a global inhibition of both viral and cellular translation, and there is an amplification of IFN-β synthesis.[251] Expression of wild-type viral proteins *in trans* can in some cases suppress activation of the PKR. These results have been interpreted by some as evidence that the V and C proteins directly inhibit PKR activation. A more likely mechanism is that the wild-type proteins act to control viral RNA synthesis, which is deregulated in the case of the mutants, and this indirectly prevents PKR activation.[21,251,391] This is further supported by the finding that PKR activation by a PIV5 P/V mutant is suppressed by expression of the wild-type P protein—a component of the viral RNAP with no known antiviral activity.[119]

The V protein has been shown to be an inhibitor of MDA-5–mediated IFN production for numerous paramyxoviruses.[131] The highly conserved V protein Cys-rich domain is both necessary and sufficient (in transfection experiments) for V protein to limit dsRNA-induced activation of the IFN-β promoter.[204,320] This inhibition is thought to occur through direct interaction of V protein with multiple sites on MDA-5, a competition with dsRNA for MDA-5 binding, and an inhibition of MDA-5 multimerization to the active form.[3] Despite this well-documented inhibition, MDA-5 can still contribute to IFN induction *in vivo.*[129] In the case of Nipah virus, both V and W proteins can block IFN-β promoter activation. This inhibition may result from targeting of different steps in the IFN induction pathway or different cellular sensors, because Nipah virus V and W proteins appear to localize to the cytoplasm and nucleus, respectively,[370] and the W protein completely lacks the Cys-rich C-terminal domain found in the V protein.

In addition to targeting MDA-5, V proteins from a select group of paramyxoviruses have been reported to also act as a decoy substrate for the cellular kinases IKKε/TBK-1 (in the case of rubulaviruses[233]) or IKKα (in the case of measles virus[317]), resulting in a second mechanism for blocking activation of IRF-3 and IRF-7 through a range of PRRs. This would predict that rubulaviruses would have the potential to inhibit many cellular pathways, including TLR3, TLR4, RIG-I, and other activators of IRFs that depend on TBK-1. While intriguing, this would be inconsistent with previous work showing that PIV5 is unable to block signaling through TLR3 and TLR4[5] and that RIG-I function is very likely also not blocked in PIV5-infected cells.[241] An interesting possibility is that these kinases are targeted in a cell-type–specific manner, as evidenced by the finding that V protein acts as a decoy for IKKα kinase to facilitate measles virus inhibition of IRF-7 in plasmacytoid cells.[317] The measles virus V protein is reported to bind to the p65 subunit of NFκB[364]; however, it is unclear how widespread this is among other paramyxoviruses.

The C proteins that are expressed by some but not all paramyxoviruses can play a role in blocking IFN responses through mechanisms distinct from that of V protein.[281] Stable cell lines expressing the Sendai virus C proteins have reduced capacity to activate the IFN-β promoter in response to dsRNA.[204] Sendai virus, measles virus, and HPIV1 mutants that are defective in C (or Y) protein expression are strong inducers of the IFN-β promoter.[21,204,251] Whereas some data support a model whereby the C proteins directly block IFN induction,[33,204,385] other studies indicate that C proteins modulate the viral polymerase to limit production of dsRNA[21,391] and thus indirectly limit IFN induction. This latter model is supported by the finding of high levels of dsRNA in cells infected with C protein mutants compared to infections with wild-type virus.[21,391] Inhibition of IFN-β synthesis by the measles virus C protein appears to depend on the ability of C protein to shuttle between the cytoplasm and nucleus,[378] suggesting an additional mechanism to limit IFN-β transcription.

There is relatively little current available data on the role of RNA-activated TLRs in IFN responses to paramyxovirus infections. The Nipah virus W protein appears to block TLR3 signaling through a mechanism that depends on nuclear localization.[370] Measles virus has been shown to block TLR7- and TLR9-mediated IFN production from human plasmacytoid dendritic cells[356] through V protein targeting the cellular kinase IKKα to inhibit IRF-7 phosphorylation.[317] By contrast to the inhibition seen by measles virus, PIV5 is a potent activator of IFN-α secretion in human plasmacytoid dendritic cells through a mechanism that depends on TLR7 signaling and autophagy pathways.[240]

Antagonists of Interferon Signaling Pathways

As shown in Figure 33.24, IFN signaling is initiated when secreted IFN binds to its receptor on the cell surface, resulting in the phosphorylation of latent transcription factors STAT1 and STAT2 (signal transducers and activators of transcription) by the cellular Janus kinases (JAK) Tyk2 and Jak1. STAT1 and STAT2 heterodimerize and associate with IRF-9 to form the transcription factor ISGF3, which translocates to the nucleus to bind to interferon-stimulated response elements (ISRE) located in the promoter region of IFN-inducible genes.[16,171] Paramyxoviruses employ a remarkably diverse range of mechanisms to circumvent IFN signaling.[172,448]

For some paramyxoviruses, the V protein blocks IFN signaling by targeting one of the STAT proteins for degradation: the PIV5, mumps virus, and SV41 V proteins target STAT1 degradation, whereas the HPIV2 V protein directs STAT2 degradation.[4,88,172,448] V-dependent targeting of STAT to the proteosome involves the assembly of a cytoplasmic ubiquitin ligase complex, which for PIV5 contains V protein, STAT1, STAT2, the ultraviolet (UV)-DNA damage repair binding protein DDB1, and a member of the Cullin family of ubiquitin ligase subunits.[227,330,416,417] The PIV5 V protein specifically targets STAT1 and not STAT2 for degradation, although this STAT1 specificity requires the presence of the nontargeted STAT2 protein.[298] PIV5 V protein degradation of STAT1 occurs in human cells but not mouse cells, and PIV5 growth in mouse cells is restricted.[88] However, efficient STAT1 degradation and higher PIV5 replication levels can be restored in mouse cells engineered to express human STAT2.[298] Similarly, PIV5 replicated to higher levels in lungs of transgenic mice that were engineered to express human STAT2.[206] A single amino acid substitution in the PIV5 V protein N-terminal domain is sufficient to allow targeted degradation of mouse STAT1, leading to a block in IFN signaling.[447] Thus, the ability to assemble specific STAT degradation complexes and disrupt IFN signaling may be a factor in determining the host range of some paramyxoviruses such as PIV5 and NDV,[298,299] which can be restricted for growth in cells from particular species.

IFN signaling is blocked by some paramyxoviruses through mechanisms that do not involve targeted degradation, but rather by binding of V to STAT proteins and preventing phosphorylation or transport to the nucleus. For example, the Hendra virus and Nipah virus V proteins induce the formation in the cytoplasm of high molecular weight complexes consisting of STAT1, STAT2, and IRF-9,[337] and these underphosphorylated complexes are unable to function in signaling. The Nipah virus V and W proteins are both capable of blocking IFN signaling through binding to STAT1 but apparently do so in the cytoplasm and nucleus, respectively.[371] Nipah virus V protein can also bind to STAT2[336]; however, the importance of this binding relative to STAT1 interactions is not entirely clear. By a different mechanism, the measles virus V protein prevents IFN signaling by blocking translocation of both STAT1 and STAT2 into the nucleus,[297] and cytoplasmic aggregates can be detected where STATs co-localize with nucleic acids and viral nucleocapsid protein. Remarkably, the measles virus P protein binds to STAT1 to prevent phosphorylation[87] through interactions involving a specific tyrosine residue that is associated with some attenuated vaccine strains.[290]

The respiro- and morbilliviruses utilize the C proteins to block IFN signaling,[123,133,193,368] and viral C protein mutants can be highly attenuated for growth.[94,124,310] Recent evidence indicates that in different experimental systems, the C proteins can alter STAT phosphorylation patterns,[133] can be detected as an interacting partner with STAT1,[123,392] and can induce ubiquitination and degradation of STAT1 in some types of cells.[125] Thus, the mechanisms by which the C proteins block IFN signaling are not completely understood and may differ depending on a particular cell type and virus.

REFERENCES*

All cited references are available in the e-book.

3. Andrejeva J, Childs KS, Young DF, et al. The V proteins of paramyxoviruses bind the IFN-inducible RNA helicase, mda-5, and inhibit its activation of the IFN-beta promoter. *Proc Natl Acad Sci U S A* 2004;101:17264–17269.
4. Andrejeva J, Poole E, Young DF, et al. The p127 subunit (DDB1) of the UV-DNA damage repair binding protein is essential for the targeted degradation of STAT1 by the V protein of the paramyxovirus SV5. *J Virol* 2002;76:11379–11386.
5. Arimilli S, Johnson JB, Alexander-Miller MA, et al. TLR-4 and -6 agonists reverse apoptosis and promote maturation of simian virus 5-infected human dendritic cells through NFκB-dependent pathways. *Virology* 2007;365:144–156.

*References for the print version were limited by the publisher to 200 references. Thus, referencing could not be all-inclusive, and the authors apologize to colleagues whose work has not been cited. References for the print version were selected on the basis of (a) works published within the past 5 years, (b) journal impact factor, and (c) studies considered by the authors to be (historically) significant.

6. Atreya PL, Peeples ME, Collins PL. The NS1 protein of human respiratory syncytial virus is a potent inhibitor of minigenome transcription and RNA replication. *J Virol* 1998;72:1452–1461.
9. Baker KA, Dutch RE, Lamb RA, et al. Structural basis for paramyxovirus-mediated membrane fusion. *Mol Cell* 1999;3:309–319.
11. Baron MD, Barrett T. Rescue of rinderpest virus from cloned cDNA. *J Virol* 1997;71:1265–1271.
14. Bermingham A, Collins PL. The M2-2 protein of human respiratory syncytial virus is a regulatory factor involved in the balance between RNA replication and transcription. *Proc Natl Acad Sci U S A* 1999;96: 11259–11264.
16. Biron CA, Sen GC. Innate responses to viral infection. In: Knipe DM, Howley PM, eds. *Fields Virology.* 5th ed. Philadelphia: Lippincott Williams & Wilkins; 2005:249–278.
19. Blumberg BM, Leppert M, Kolakofsky D. Interaction of VSV leader RNA and nucleocapsid protein may control VSV genome replication. *Cell* 1981;23:837–845.
20. Bonaparte MI, Dimitrov AS, Bossart KN, et al. Ephrin-B2 ligand is a functional receptor for Hendra virus and Nipah virus. *Proc Natl Acad Sci U S A* 2005;102:10652–10657.
21. Boonyaratanakornkit J, Bartlett E, Schomacker H, et al. The C proteins of human parainfluenza virus type 1 limit double-stranded RNA accumulation that would otherwise trigger activation of MDA5 and protein kinase R. *J Virol* 2011;85:1495–1506.
23. Bose S, Welch BD, Kors CA, et al. Structure and mutagenesis of the parainfluenza virus 5 hemagglutinin-neuraminidase stalk domain reveals a four-helix bundle and the role of the stalk in fusion promotion. *J Virol* 2011;85:12855–12866.
24. Bossert B, Marozin S, Conzelmann KK. Nonstructural proteins NS1 and NS2 of bovine respiratory syncytial virus block activation of interferon regulatory factor 3. *J Virol* 2003;77:8661–8668.
25. Bourhis JM, Canard B, Longhi S. Structural disorder within the replicative complex of measles virus: functional implications. *Virology* 2006; 344:94–110.
27. Bousse T, Matrosovich T, Portner A, et al. The long noncoding region of the human parainfluenza virus type 1 F gene contributes to the read-through transcription at the M-F gene junction. *J Virol* 2002;76:8244–8251.
29. Bousse TL, Taylor G, Krishnamurthy S, et al. Biological significance of the second receptor binding site of Newcastle disease virus hemagglutinin-neuraminidase protein. *J Virol* 2004;78:13351–13355.
30. Bowden TA, Aricescu AR, Gilbert RJ, et al. Structural basis of Nipah and Hendra virus attachment to their cell-surface receptor ephrin-B2. *Nat Struct Mol Biol* 2008;15:567–572.
31. Bowden TA, Crispin M, Harvey DJ, et al. Dimeric architecture of the Hendra virus attachment glycoprotein: evidence for a conserved mode of assembly. *J Virol* 2010;84:6208–6217.
39. Buchholz UJ, Finke S, Conzelmann KK. Generation of bovine respiratory syncytial virus (BRSV) from cDNA: BRSV NS2 is not essential for virus replication in tissue culture, and the human RSV leader region acts as a functional BRSV genome promoter. *J Virol* 1999;73:251–259.
40. Bukreyev A, Whitehead SS, Murphy BR, et al. Recombinant respiratory syncytial virus from which the entire SH gene has been deleted grows efficiently in cell culture and exhibits site-specific attenuation in the respiratory tract of the mouse. *J Virol* 1997;71:8973–8982.
43. Calain P, Roux L. The rule of six, a basic feature for efficient replication of Sendai virus defective interfering RNA. *J Virol* 1993;67:4822–4830.
44. Calder LJ, Gonzalez-Reyes L, Garcia-Barreno B, et al. Electron microscopy of the human respiratory syncytial virus fusion protein and complexes that it forms with monoclonal antibodies. *Virology* 2000;271: 122–131.
45. Cathomen T, Mrkic B, Spehner D, et al. A matrix-less measles virus is infectious and elicits extensive cell fusion: consequences for propagation in the brain. *EMBO J* 1998;17:3899–3908.
47. Cattaneo R, Billeter MA. Mutations and A/I hypermutations in measles virus persistent infections. *Curr Top Microbiol Immunol* 1992;176:63–74.
48. Cattaneo R, Kaelin K, Baezko K, et al. Measles virus editing provides an additional cysteine-rich protein. *Cell* 1989; 56:759–764.
50. Cattaneo R, Rebmann G, Schmid A, et al. Altered transcription of a defective measles virus genome derived from a diseased human brain. *EMBO J* 1987;6:681–688.
53. Cattaneo R, Schmid A, Eschle D, et al. Biased hypermutation and other genetic changes in defective measles virus in human brain infections. *Cell* 1988;55:255–265.
57. Chang A, Masante C, Buchholz UJ, et al. Human metapneumovirus (HMPV) binding and infection are mediated by interactions between the HMPV fusion protein and heparan sulfate. *J Virol* 2012;86:3230–3243.
58. Chen L, Gorman JJ, McKimm-Breschkin J, et al. The structure of the fusion glycoprotein of Newcastle disease virus suggests a novel paradigm for the molecular mechanism of membrane fusion. *Structure* 2001;9: 255–266.
59. Choppin PW, Compans RW. Reproduction of paramyxoviruses. In: Fraenkel-Conrat H, Wagner RR, eds. *Comprehensive Virology.* Vol. 4. New York: Plenum Press; 1975:95–178.
60. Colf LA, Juo ZS, Garcia KC. Structure of the measles virus hemagglutinin. *Nat Struct Mol Biol* 2007;14:1227–1228.
62. Collins PL, Hill MG, Camargo E, et al. Production of infectious human respiratory syncytial virus from cloned cDNA confirms an essential role for the transcription elongation factor from the 5′ proximal open reading frame of the M2 mRNA in gene expression and provides a capability for vaccine development. *Proc Natl Acad Sci U S A* 1995;92:11563–11567.
63. Collins PL, Hill MG, Cristina J, et al. Transcription elongation factor of respiratory syncytial virus, a nonsegmented negative-strand RNA virus. *Proc Natl Acad Sci U S A* 1996;93:81–85.
65. Collins PL, Olmsted RA, Spriggs MK, et al. Gene overlap and site-specific attenuation of transcription of the viral polymerase L gene of human respiratory syncytial virus. *Proc Natl Acad Sci U S A* 1987;84:5134–5138.
66. Collins PL, Wertz GW. The envelope-associated 22K protein of human respiratory syncytial virus: nucleotide sequence of the mRNA and a related polytranscript. *J Virol* 1985;54:65–71.
67. Colman PM, Lawrence MC. The structural biology of type I viral membrane fusion. *Nat Rev Mol Cell Biol* 2003;4:309–319.
69. Connolly SA, Leser GP, Jardetzky TS, et al. Bimolecular complementation of paramyxovirus fusion and hemagglutinin-neuraminidase proteins enhances fusion: implications for the mechanism of fusion triggering. *J Virol* 2009;83:10857–10868.
70. Conzelmann KK. Transcriptional activation of alpha/beta interferon genes: interference by nonsegmented negative-strand RNA viruses. *J Virol* 2005;79:5241–5248.
72. Crennell S, Takimoto T, Portner A, et al. Crystal structure of the multifunctional paramyxovirus hemagglutinin-neuraminidase. *Nat Struct Biol* 2000;7:1068–1074.
73. Curran J, Boeck R, Kolakofsky D. The Sendai virus P gene expresses both an essential protein and an inhibitor of RNA synthesis by shuffling modules via mRNA editing. *EMBO J* 1991;10:3079–3085.
77. Curran J, Kolakofsky D. Ribosomal initiation from an ACG codon in the Sendai virus P/C mRNA. *EMBO J* 1988;7:245–251.
78. Curran J, Marq JB, Kolakofsky D. An N-terminal domain of the Sendai paramyxovirus P protein acts as a chaperone for the NP protein during the nascent chain assembly step of genome replication. *J Virol* 1995;69: 849–855.
85. Deng R, Wang Z, Mahon PJ, et al. Mutations in the Newcastle disease virus hemagglutinin-neuraminidase protein that interfere with its ability to interact with the homologous F protein in the promotion of fusion. *Virology* 1999;253:43–54.
88. Didcock L, Young DF, Goodbourn S, et al. The V protein of simian virus 5 inhibits interferon signalling by targeting STAT1 for proteasome-mediated degradation. *J Virol* 1999;73:9928–9933.
89. Diederich S, Moll M, Klenk HD, et al. The Nipah virus fusion protein is cleaved within the endosomal compartment. *J Biol Chem* 2005;280: 29899–29903.
91. Dorig RE, Marcil A, Chopra A, et al. The human CD46 molecule is a receptor for measles virus (Edmonston strain). *Cell* 1993;75:295–305.
92. Duprex WP, Collins FM, Rima BK. Modulating the function of the measles virus RNA-dependent RNA polymerase by insertion of green fluorescent protein into the open reading frame. *J Virol* 2002;76:7322–7328.
96. Dutch RE, Jardetzky TS, Lamb RA. Virus membrane fusion proteins: biological machines that undergo a metamorphosis. *Biosci Rep* 2000; 20:597–612.

99. Ebata SN, Cote MJ, Kang CY, et al. The fusion and hemagglutinin-neuraminidase glycoproteins of human parainfluenza virus 3 are both required for fusion. *Virology* 1991;183:437–441.
101. Egelman EH, Wu SS, Amrein M, et al. The Sendai virus nucleocapsid exists in at least four different helical states. *J Virol* 1989;63:2233–2243.
108. Fearns R, Collins PL. Model for polymerase access to the overlapped L gene of respiratory syncytial virus. *J Virol* 1999;73:388–397.
109. Fearns R, Collins PL. Role of the M2-1 transcription antitermination protein of respiratory syncytial virus in sequential transcription. *J Virol* 1999;73:5852–5864.
111. Feldman SA, Audet S, Beeler JA. The fusion glycoprotein of human respiratory syncytial virus facilitates virus attachment and infectivity via an interaction with cellular heparan sulfate. *J Virol* 2000;74:6442–6447.
115. Finch JT, Gibbs AJ. Observations on the structure of the nucleocapsids of some paramyxoviruses. *J Gen Virol* 1970;6:141–150.
117. Freed EO. Viral late domains. *J Virol* 2002;76:4679–4687.
119. Gainey MD, Dillon PJ, Clark KM, et al. Paramyxovirus induced shut off of translation: role of P and V proteins in limiting activation of PKR. *J Virol* 2008;83:828–839.
128. Giorgi C, Blumberg BM, Kolakofsky D. Sendai virus contains overlapping genes expressed from a single mRNA. *Cell* 1983;35:829–836.
129. Gitlin L, Benoit L, Song C, et al. Melanoma differentiation-associated gene 5 (MDA5) is involved in the innate immune response to Paramyxoviridae infection in vivo. *PLoS Pathog* 2010;6:e1000734.
130. Gonzalez-Reyes L, Ruiz-Arguello MB, Garcia-Barreno B, et al. Cleavage of the human respiratory syncytial virus fusion protein at two distinct sites is required for activation of membrane fusion. *Proc Natl Acad Sci U S A* 2001;98:9859–9864.
131. Goodbourn S, Randall RE. The regulation of type I interferon production by paramyxoviruses. *J Interferon Cytokine Res* 2009;29:539–547.
132. Gotoh B, Ogasawara T, Toyoda T, et al. An endoprotease homologous to the blood clotting factor X as a determinant of viral tropism in chick embryo. *EMBO J* 1990;9:4189–4195.
136. Gravel KA, Morrison TG. Interacting domains of the HN and F proteins of Newcastle disease virus. *J Virol* 2003;77:11040–11049.
142. Hardy RW, Harmon SB, Wertz GW. Diverse gene junctions of respiratory syncytial virus modulate the efficiency of transcription termination and respond differently to M2-mediated antitermination. *J Virol* 1999; 73:170–176.
145. Harrison MS, Schmitt PT, Pei Z, et al. Role of ubiquitin in PIV5 particle formation. *J Virol* 2012;86:3474–3485.
146. Harty RN, Paragas J, Sudol M, et al. A proline-rich motif within the matrix protein of vesicular stomatitis virus and rabies virus interacts with WW domains of cellular proteins: implications for viral budding. *J Virol* 1999;73:2921–2929.
147. Hasan MK, Kato A, Muranaka M, et al. Versatility of the accessory C proteins of Sendai virus: contribution to virus assembly as an additional role. *J Virol* 2000;74:5619–5628.
148. Hashiguchi T, Kajikawa M, Maita N, et al. Crystal structure of measles virus hemagglutinin provides insight into effective vaccines. *Proc Natl Acad Sci U S A* 2007;104:19535–19540.
149. Hashiguchi T, Ose T, Kubota M, et al. Structure of the measles virus hemagglutinin bound to its cellular receptor SLAM. *Nat Struct Mol Biol* 2011;18:135–141.
150. Hausmann S, Gardin D, Morel A-S, et al. Two nucleotides immediately upstream of the essential A_6G_3 slippery sequence modulate the pattern of G insertions during Sendai virus mRNA editing. *J Virol* 1999;73: 343–351.
151. He B, Leser GP, Paterson RG, et al. The paramyxovirus SV5 small hydrophobic (SH) protein is not essential for virus growth in tissue culture cells. *Virology* 1998;250:30–40.
152. He B, Lin GY, Durbin JE, et al. The SH integral membrane protein of the paramyxovirus simian virus 5 is required to block apoptosis in MDBK cells. *J Virol* 2001;75:4068–4079.
153. He B, Paterson RG, Stock N, et al. Recovery of paramyxovirus simian virus 5 with a V protein lacking the conserved cysteine-rich domain: the multifunctional V protein blocks both interferon-beta induction and interferon signaling. *Virology* 2002;303:15–32.
154. He B, Paterson RG, Ward CD, et al. Recovery of infectious SV5 from cloned DNA and expression of a foreign gene. *Virology* 1997;237:249–260.
155. Heggeness MH, Scheid A, Choppin PW. Conformation of the helical nucleocapsids of paramyxoviruses and vesicular stomatitis virus: reversible coiling and uncoiling induced by changes in salt concentration. *Proc Natl Acad Sci U S A* 1980;77:2631–2635.
157. Heggeness MH, Smith PR, Choppin PW. *In vitro* assembly of the non-glycosylated membrane protein (M) of Sendai virus. *Proc Natl Acad Sci U S A* 1982;79:6232–6236.
158. Hercyk N, Horikami SM, Moyer SA. The vesicular stomatitis virus L protein possesses the mRNA methyltransferase activities. *Virology* 1988;163:222–225.
159. Hiebert SW, Paterson RG, Lamb RA. Hemagglutinin-neuraminidase protein of the paramyxovirus simian virus 5: nucleotide sequence of the mRNA predicts an N-terminal membrane anchor. *J Virol* 1985;54:1–6.
160. Hiebert SW, Paterson RG, Lamb RA. Identification and predicted sequence of a previously unrecognized small hydrophobic protein, SH, of the paramyxovirus simian virus 5. *J Virol* 1985;55:744–751.
163. Hoffman MA, Banerjee AK. An infectious clone of human parainfluenza virus type 3. *J Virol* 1997;71:4272–4277.
167. Homma M, Ohuchi M. Trypsin action on the growth of Sendai virus in tissue culture cells. III. Structural differences of Sendai viruses grown in eggs and tissue culture cells. *J Virol* 1973;12:1457–1465.
168. Horikami S, Smallwood S, Moyer SA. The Sendai virus V protein interacts with the NP protein to regulate viral genome RNA replication. *Virology* 1996;222:383–390.
170. Horikami SM, Hector RC, Smallwood S, et al. The Sendai virus C protein binds the L polymerase protein to inhibit viral RNA synthesis. *Virology* 1997;235:261–270.
171. Horvath CM. STAT proteins and transcriptional responses to extracellular signals. *Trends Biochem Sci* 2000;25:496–502.
173. Horvath CM, Paterson RG, Shaughnessy MA, et al. Biological activity of paramyxovirus fusion proteins: factors influencing formation of syncytia. *J Virol* 1992;66:4564–4569.
174. Horvath CM, Williams MA, Lamb RA. Eukaryotic coupled translation of tandem cistrons: identification of the influenza B virus BM2 polypeptide. *EMBO J* 1990;9:2639–2647.
176. Hu X, Ray R, Compans RW. Functional interactions between the fusion protein and hemagglutinin-neuraminidase of human parainfluenza viruses. *J Virol* 1992;66:1528–1534.
178. Iorio RM, Melanson VR, Mahon PJ. Glycoprotein interactions in paramyxovirus fusion. *Future Virol* 2009;4:335–351.
179. Irie T, Inoue M, Sakaguchi T. Significance of the YLDL motif in the M protein and Alix/AIP1 for Sendai virus budding in the context of virus infection. *Virology* 2010;405:334–341.
180. Irie T, Shimazu Y, Yoshida T, et al. The YLDL sequence within Sendai virus M protein is critical for budding of virus-like particles and interacts with Alix/AIP1 independently of C protein. *J Virol* 2007;81:2263–2273.
182. Iseni F, Garcin D, Nishio M, et al. Sendai virus trailer RNA binds TIAR, a cellular protein involved in virus-induced apoptosis. *EMBO J* 2002;21:5141–5150.
187. Joshi SB, Dutch RE, Lamb RA. A core trimer of the paramyxovirus fusion protein: parallels to influenza virus hemagglutinin and HIV-1 gp41. *Virology* 1998;248:20–34.
189. Karron RA, Buonagurio DA, Georgiu AF, et al. Respiratory syncytial virus (RSV) SH and G proteins are not essential for viral replication in vitro: clinical evaluation and molecular characterization of a cold-passaged, attenuated RSV subgroup B mutant. *Proc Natl Acad Sci U S A* 1997;94:13961–13966.
192. Kato A, Kiyotani K, Sakai Y, et al. The paramyxovirus, Sendai virus, V protein encodes a luxury function required for viral pathogenesis. *EMBO J* 1997;16:578–587.
195. Kawai T, Takahashi K, Sato S, et al. IPS-1, an adaptor triggering RIG-I- and Mda5-mediated type I interferon induction. *Nat Immunol* 2005;6:981–988.
198. Kim YH, Donald JE, Grigoryan G, et al. Capture and imaging of a prehairpin fusion intermediate of the paramyxovirus PIV5. *Proc Natl Acad Sci U S A* 2011;108:20992–20997.
203. Kolakofsky D, Pelet T, Garin D, et al. Paramyxovirus RNA synthesis and the requirement for hexamer genome length: the rule of six revisited. *J Virol* 1998;72:891–899.

209. Kurotani A, Kiyotani K, Kato A, et al. Sendai virus C proteins are categorically nonessential gene products but silencing their expression severely impairs viral replication and pathogenesis. *Genes Cells* 1998;3:111–124.
211. Lamb RA. Paramyxovirus fusion: a hypothesis for changes. *Virology* 1993;197:1–11.
213. Lamb RA, Jardetzky TS. Structural basis of viral invasion: lessons from paramyxovirus F. *Curr Opin Struct Biol* 2007;17:427–436.
214. Lamb RA, Mahy BW, Choppin PW. The synthesis of Sendai virus polypeptides in infected cells. *Virology* 1976;69:116–131.
218. Lawrence MC, Borg NA, Streltsov VA, et al. Structure of the haemagglutinin-neuraminidase from human parainfluenza virus type III. *J Mol Biol* 2004;335:1343–1357.
219. Lawson N, Stillman E, Whitt M, et al. Recombinant vesicular stomatitis viruses from DNA. *Proc Natl Acad Sci U S A* 1995;92:4477–4481.
222. Lee B, Ataman ZA. Modes of paramyxovirus fusion: a Henipavirus perspective. *Trends Microbiol* 2011;19:389–399.
227. Lin GY, Paterson RG, Richardson CD, et al. The V protein of the paramyxovirus SV5 interacts with damage-specific DNA binding protein. *Virology* 1998;249:189–200.
229. Lin Y, Horvath F, Aligo JA, et al. The role of simian virus 5 V protein on viral RNA synthesis. *Virology* 2005;338:270–280.
234. Mahon PJ, Mirza AM, Musich TA, et al. Engineered intermonomeric disulfide bonds in the globular domain of Newcastle disease virus hemagglutinin-neuraminidase protein: implications for the mechanism of fusion promotion. *J Virol* 2008;82:10386–10396.
240. Manuse MJ, Briggs CM, Parks GD. Replication-independent activation of human plasmacytoid dendritic cells by the paramyxovirus SV5 requires TLR7 and autophagy pathways. *Virology* 2010;405:383–389.
241. Manuse MJ, Parks GD. A role for the paramyxovirus genomic promoter in limiting host cell antiviral responses and cell killing. *J Virol* 2009;83: 9057–9067.
243. Markwell MA, Portner A, Schwartz AL. An alternative route of infection for viruses: entry by means of the asialoglycoprotein receptor of a Sendai virus mutant lacking its attachment protein. *Proc Natl Acad Sci U S A* 1985;82:978–982.
250. Matsuoka Y, Curran J, Pelet T, et al. The P gene of human parainfluenza virus type 1 encodes P and C proteins but not a cysteine-rich V protein. *J Virol* 1991;65:3406–3410.
252. McGinnes L, Sergel T, Morrison T. Mutations in the transmembrane domain of the HN protein of Newcastle disease virus affect the structure and activity of the protein. *Virology* 1993;196:101–110.
254. McGinnes LW, Reitter JN, Gravel K, et al. Evidence for mixed membrane topology of the Newcastle disease virus fusion protein. *J Virol* 2003;77:1951–1963.
255. McLellan JS, Yang Y, Graham BS, et al. Structure of respiratory syncytial virus fusion glycoprotein in the postfusion conformation reveals preservation of neutralizing epitopes. *J Virol* 2011;85:7788–7796.
256. Melanson VR, Iorio RM. Addition of N-glycans in the stalk of the Newcastle disease virus HN protein blocks its interaction with the F protein and prevents fusion. *J Virol* 2006;80:623–633.
261. Mishin VP, Watanabe M, Taylor G, et al. N-linked glycan at residue 523 of human parainfluenza virus type 3 hemagglutinin-neuraminidase masks a second receptor-binding site. *J Virol* 2010;84:3094–3100.
264. Money VA, McPhee HK, Mosely JA, et al. Surface features of a Mononegavirales matrix protein indicate sites of membrane interaction. *Proc Natl Acad Sci U S A* 2009;106:4441–4446.
270. Muhlebach MD, Mateo M, Sinn PL, et al. Adherens junction protein nectin-4 is the epithelial receptor for measles virus. *Nature* 2011;480: 530–533.
272. Murphy SK, Ito Y, Parks GD. A functional antigenomic promoter for the paramyxovirus simian virus 5 requires proper spacing between an essential internal segment and the 3′ terminus. *J Virol* 1998;72:10–19.
273. Murphy SK, Parks GD. Genome nucleotide lengths that are divisible by six are not essential but enhance replication of defective interfering RNAs of the paramyxovirus simian virus 5. *Virology* 1997;232:145–157.
274. Murphy SK, Parks GD. RNA replication for the paramyxovirus simian virus 5 requires an internal repeated (CGNNNN) sequence motif. *J Virol* 1999;73:805–809.
278. Nagai Y, Klenk H-D. Activation of precursors to both glycoproteins of Newcastle disease virus by proteolytic cleavage. *Virology* 1977;77:125–134.
279. Nagai Y, Klenk HD, Rott R. Proteolytic cleavage of the viral glycoproteins and its significance for the virulence of Newcastle disease virus. *Virology* 1976;72:494–508.
282. Naniche D, Varior-Krishnan G, Cervoni F, et al. Human membrane cofactor protein (CD46) acts as a cellular receptor for measles virus. *J Virol* 1993;67:6025–6032.
283. Navaratnarajah CK, Oezguen N, Rupp L, et al. The heads of the measles virus attachment protein move to transmit the fusion-triggering signal. *Nat Struct Mol Biol* 2011;18:128–134.
284. Negrete OA, Levroney EL, Aguilar HC, et al. EphrinB2 is the entry receptor for Nipah virus, an emergent deadly paramyxovirus. *Nature* 2005;436:401–405.
286. Ng DT, Randall RE, Lamb RA. Intracellular maturation and transport of the SV5 type II glycoprotein hemagglutinin-neuraminidase: specific and transient association with GRP78-BiP in the endoplasmic reticulum and extensive internalization from the cell surface. *J Cell Biol* 1989;109:3273–3289.
288. Noyce RS, Bondre DG, Ha MN, et al. Tumor cell marker PVRL4 (nectin 4) is an epithelial cell receptor for measles virus. *PLoS Pathog* 2011; 7:e1002240.
293. Olmsted RA, Elango N, Prince GA, et al. Expression of the F glycoprotein of respiratory syncytial virus by a recombinant vaccinia virus: comparison of the individual contributions of the F and G glycoproteins to host immunity. *Proc Natl Acad Sci U S A* 1986;83:7462–7466.
296. Pager CT, Dutch RE. Cathepsin L is involved in proteolytic processing of the Hendra virus fusion protein. *J Virol* 2005;79:12714–12720.
297. Palosaari H, Parisien JP, Rodriguez JJ, et al. STAT protein interference and suppression of cytokine signal transduction by measles virus V protein. *J Virol* 2003;77:7635–7644.
299. Park MS, Garcia-Sastre A, Cros JF, et al. Newcastle disease virus V protein is a determinant of host range restriction. *J Virol* 2003;77:9522–9532.
302. Paterson RG, Hiebert SW, Lamb RA. Expression at the cell surface of biologically active fusion and hemagglutinin-neuraminidase proteins of the paramyxovirus simian virus 5 from cloned cDNA. *Proc Natl Acad Sci U S A* 1985;82:7520–7524.
303. Paterson RG, Lamb RA. RNA editing by G-nucleotide insertion in mumps virus P-gene mRNA transcripts. *J Virol* 1990;64:4137–4145.
304. Paterson RG, Leser GP, Shaughnessy MA, et al. The paramyxovirus SV5 V protein binds two atoms of zinc and is a structural component of virions. *Virology* 1995;208:121–131.
305. Paterson RG, Russell CJ, Lamb RA. Fusion protein of the paramyxovirus SV5: destabilizing and stabilizing mutants of fusion activation. *Virology* 2000;270:17–30.
307. Paterson RG, Thomas SM, Lamb RA. Specific nontemplated nucleotide addition to a simian virus 5 mRNA: prediction of a common mechanism by which unrecognized hybrid P-cysteine-rich proteins are encoded by paramyxovirus "P" genes. In: Kolakofsky D, Mahy BWJ, eds. *Genetics and Pathogenicity of Negative Strand Viruses.* London: Elsevier; 1989:232–245.
313. Pei Z, Bai Y, Schmitt AP. PIV5 M protein interaction with host protein angiomotin-like 1. *Virology* 2010;397:155–166.
314. Pei Z, Harrison MS, Schmitt AP. Parainfluenza virus 5 M protein interaction with host protein 14-3-3 negatively affects virus particle formation. *J Virol* 2011;85:2050–2059.
318. Plemper RK, Brindley MA, Iorio RM. Structural and mechanistic studies of measles virus illuminate paramyxovirus entry. *PLoS Pathog* 2011;7:e1002058.
320. Poole EL, He B, Lamb RA, et al. The V proteins of simian virus 5 and other paramyxoviruses inhibits induction of interferon-beta. *Virology* 2002;303:33–46.
321. Popa A, Carter JR, Smith SE, et al. Residues in the Hendra virus fusion protein transmembrane domain are critical for endocytic recycling. *J Virol* 2012;86:3014–3026.
322. Porotto M, Devito I, Palmer SG, et al. Spring-loaded model revisited: paramyxovirus fusion requires engagement of a receptor binding protein beyond initial triggering of the fusion protein. *J Virol* 2011;85:12867–12880.
323. Porotto M, Fornabaio M, Greengard O, et al. Paramyxovirus receptor-binding molecules: engagement of one site on the hemagglutinin-neuraminidase protein modulates activity at the second site. *J Virol* 2006; 80:1204–1213.

325. Porotto M, Palmer SG, Palermo LM, et al. Mechanism of fusion triggering by human parainfluenza virus type III: communication between viral glycoproteins during entry. *J Biol Chem* 2012;287:778–793.
332. Radecke F, Spielhofer P, Schneider H, et al. Rescue of measles viruses from cloned DNA. *EMBO J* 1995;14:5773–5784.
335. Roberts A, Rose JK. Recovery of negative-strand RNA viruses from plasmid DNAs: a positive approach revitalizes a negative field. *Virology* 1998;247:1–6.
336. Rodriguez JJ, Cruz CD, Horvath CM. Identification of the nuclear export signal and STAT-binding domains of the Nipah virus V protein reveals mechanisms underlying interferon evasion. *J Virol* 2004;78:5358–5367.
338. Rodriguez-Boulan E, Sabatini DD. Asymmetric budding of viruses in epithelial monolayers; a model system for study of epithelial polarity. *Proc Natl Acad Sci U S A* 1978;75:5071–5075.
340. Rossman JS, Jing X, Leser GP, et al. Influenza virus M2 protein mediates ESCRT-independent membrane scission. *Cell* 2010;142:902–913.
342. Ruiz-Arguello MB, Gonzalez-Reyes L, Calder LJ, et al. Effect of proteolytic processing at two distinct sites on shape and aggregation of an anchorless fusion protein of human respiratory syncytial virus and fate of the intervening segment. *Virology* 2002;298:317–326.
344. Russell CJ, Jardetzky TS, Lamb RA. Membrane fusion machines of paramyxoviruses: capture of intermediates of fusion. *EMBO J* 2001;20: 4024–4034.
345. Russell CJ, Kantor KL, Jardetzky TS, et al. A dual-functional paramyxovirus F protein regulatory switch segment: activation and membrane fusion. *J Cell Biol* 2003;163:363–374.
346. Russell R, Paterson RG, Lamb RA. Studies with cross-linking reagents on the oligomeric form of the paramyxovirus fusion protein. *Virology* 1994;199:160–168.
347. Sakaguchi T, Kato A, Sugahara F, et al. AIP1/Alix is a binding partner of Sendai virus C protein and facilitates virus budding. *J Virol* 2005; 79:8933–8941.
348. Sakaguchi T, Kiyotani K, Kato A, et al. Phosphorylation of the Sendai virus M protein is not essential for virus replication either in vitro or in vivo. *Virology* 1997;235:360–366.
350. Samal SK, Collins PL. RNA replication by a respiratory syncytial virus RNA analog does not obey the rule of six and retains a nonviral trinucleotide extension at the leader end. *J Virol* 1996;70:5075–5082.
351. Sanderson CM, Avalos R, Kundu A, et al. Interaction of Sendai viral F, HN, and M proteins with host cytoskeletal and lipid components in Sendai virus-infected BHK cells. *Virology* 1995;209:701–707.
353. Scheid A, Caliguiri LA, Compans RW, et al. Isolation of paramyxovirus glycoproteins. Association of both hemagglutinating and neuraminidase activities with the larger SV5 glycoprotein. *Virology* 1972;50:640–652.
354. Scheid A, Choppin PW. Identification of biological activities of paramyxovirus glycoproteins. Activation of cell fusion, hemolysis, and infectivity of proteolytic cleavage of an inactive precursor protein of Sendai virus. *Virology* 1974;57:475–490.
355. Scheid A, Choppin PW. The hemagglutinating and neuraminidase protein of a paramyxovirus: interaction with neuraminic acid in affinity chromatography. *Virology* 1974;62:125–133.
357. Schmitt AP, He B, Lamb RA. Involvement of the cytoplasmic domain of the hemagglutinin-neuraminidase protein in assembly of the paramyxovirus simian virus 5. *J Virol* 1999;73:8703–8712.
358. Schmitt AP, Leser GP, Morita E, et al. Evidence for a new viral late-domain core sequence, FPIV, necessary for budding of a paramyxovirus. *J Virol* 2005;79:2988–2997.
359. Schmitt AP, Leser GP, Waning DL, et al. Requirements for budding of paramyxovirus simian virus 5 virus-like particles. *J Virol* 2002;76: 3952–3964.
361. Schnell MJ, Mebatsion T, Conzelmann K-K. Infectious rabies viruses from cloned cDNA. *EMBO J* 1994;13:4195–4203.
362. Schowalter RM, Chang A, Robach JG, et al. Low-pH triggering of human metapneumovirus fusion: essential residues and importance in entry. *J Virol* 2009;83:1511–1522.
366. Sergel T, McGinnes LW, Peeples ME, et al. The attachment function of the Newcastle disease virus hemagglutinin-neuraminidase protein can be separated from fusion promotion by mutation. *Virology* 1993;193:717–726.
369. Shaikh FY, Cox RG, Lifland AW, et al. A critical phenylalanine residue in the respiratory syncytial virus fusion protein cytoplasmic tail mediates assembly of internal viral proteins into viral filaments and particles. *MBio* 2012;3:e00270–00211.
370. Shaw ML, Cardenas WB, Zamarin D, et al. Nuclear localization of the Nipah virus W protein allows for inhibition of both virus- and toll-like receptor 3-triggered signaling pathways. *J Virol* 2005;79:6078–6088.
371. Shaw ML, Garcia-Sastre A, Palese P, et al. Nipah virus V and W proteins have a common STAT1-binding domain yet inhibit STAT1 activation from the cytoplasmic and nuclear compartments, respectively. *J Virol* 2004;78:5633–5641.
373. Skehel JJ, Wiley DC. Receptor binding and membrane fusion in virus entry: the influenza hemagglutinin. *Annu Rev Biochem* 2000;69:531–569.
374. Skibbens JE, Roth MG, Matlin KS. Differential extractability of influenza virus hemagglutinin during intracellular transport in polarized epithelial cells and nonpolar fibroblasts. *J Cell Biol* 1989;108:821–832.
381. Stone-Hulslander J, Morrison TG. Detection of an interaction between the HN and F proteins in Newcastle disease virus-infected cells. *J Virol* 1997;71:6287–6295.
388. Swanson K, Wen X, Leser GP, et al. Structure of the Newcastle disease virus F protein in the post-fusion conformation. *Virology* 2010;402: 372–379.
389. Swanson KA, Settembre EC, Shaw CA, et al. Structural basis for immunization with postfusion respiratory syncytial virus fusion F glycoprotein (RSV F) to elicit high neutralizing antibody titers. *Proc Natl Acad Sci U S A* 2011;108:9619–9624.
393. Takeuchi K, Tanabayashi K, Hishiyama M, et al. The mumps virus SH protein is a membrane protein and not essential for virus growth. *Virology* 1996;225:156–162.
395. Takimoto T, Murti KG, Bousse T, et al. Role of matrix and fusion proteins in budding of Sendai virus. *J Virol* 2001;75:11384–11391.
398. Taniguchi T, Palmieri M, Weissmann C. $Q\beta$ DNA-containing hybrid plasmids giving rise to $Q\beta$ phage formation in the bacterial host. *Nature* 1978;274:223–228.
400. Tapparel C, Maurice D, Roux L. The activity of Sendai virus genomic and antigenomic promoters requires a second element past the leader template regions: a motif (GNNNNN)3 is essential for replication. *J Virol* 1998;72:3117–3128.
402. Tarbouriech N, Curran J, Ebel C, et al. On the domain structure and the polymerization state of the Sendai virus P protein. *Virology* 2000; 266:99–109.
404. Tatsuo H, Ono N, Tanaka K, et al. SLAM (CDw150) is a cellular receptor for measles virus. *Nature* 2000;406:893–897.
408. Thomas SM, Lamb RA, Paterson RG. Two mRNAs that differ by two nontemplated nucleotides encode the amino coterminal proteins P and V of the paramyxovirus SV5. *Cell* 1988;54:891–902.
417. Ulane CM, Kentsis A, Cruz CD, et al. Composition and assembly of STAT-targeting ubiquitin ligase complexes: paramyxovirus V protein carboxyl terminus is an oligomerization domain. *J Virol* 2005;79:10180–10189.
419. Vidal S, Curran J, Kolakofsky D. Editing of the Sendai virus P/C mRNA by G insertion occurs during mRNA synthesis via a virus-encoded activity. *J Virol* 1990;64:239–246.
420. Vidal S, Kolakofsky D. Modified model for the switch from Sendai virus transcription to replication. *J Virol* 1989;63:1951–1958.
425. Vulliemoz D, Roux L. "Rule of six": how does the Sendai virus RNA polymerase keep count? *J Virol* 2001;75:4506–4518.
428. Waning DL, Russell CJ, Jardetzky TS, et al. Activation of a paramyxovirus fusion protein is modulated by inside-out signaling from the cytoplasmic tail. *Proc Natl Acad Sci U S A* 2004;101:9217–9222.
429. Waning DL, Schmitt AP, Leser GP, et al. Roles for the cytoplasmic tails of the fusion and hemagglutinin-neuraminidase proteins in budding of the paramyxovirus simian virus 5. *J Virol* 2002;76:9284–9297.
430. Wansley EK, Parks GD. Naturally occurring substitutions in the P/V gene convert the noncytopathic paramyxovirus simian virus 5 into a virus that induces alpha/beta interferon synthesis and cell death. *J Virol* 2002;76:10109–10121.
436. Whelan SP, Ball LA, Barr JN, et al. Efficient recovery of infectious vesicular stomatitis virus entirely from cDNA clones. *Proc Natl Acad Sci U S A* 1995;92:8388–8392.
441. Xu K, Rajashankar KR, Chan YP, et al. Host cell recognition by the Henipaviruses: crystal structures of the Nipah G attachment glycoprotein

and its complex with ephrin-B3. *Proc Natl Acad Sci U S A* 2008;105: 9953–9958.

443. Yao Q, Hu X, Compans RW. Association of the parainfluenza virus fusion and hemagglutinin-neuraminidase glycoproteins on cell surfaces. *J Virol* 1997;71:650–656.
444. Yin H-S, Paterson RG, Wen X, et al. Structure of the uncleaved ectodomain of the paramyxovirus (hPIV3) fusion protein. *Proc Natl Acad Sci U S A* 2005;102:9288–9293.
445. Yin HS, Wen X, Paterson RG, et al. Structure of the parainfluenza virus 5 F protein in its metastable, prefusion conformation. *Nature* 2006; 439:38–44.
447. Young DF, Chatziandreou N, He B, et al. Single amino acid substitution in the V protein of simian virus 5 differentiates its ability to block interferon signaling in human and murine cells. *J Virol* 2001;75:3363–3370.
448. Young DF, Didcock L, Goodbourn S, et al. Paramyxoviridae use distinct virus-specific mechanisms to circumvent the interferon response. *Virology* 2000;269:383–390.
450. Yuan P, Swanson KA, Leser GP, et al. Structure of the Newcastle disease virus hemagglutinin-neuraminidase (HN) ectodomain reveals a four-helix bundle stalk. *Proc Natl Acad Sci U S A* 2011;108:14920–14925.
451. Yuan P, Thompson T, Wurzburg BA, et al. Structural studies of the parainfluenza virius 5 hemagglutinin-neuraminidase tetramer in complex with its receptor, sialyllactose. *Structure* 2005;13:1–13.
453. Zaitsev V, Von Itzsteine M, Groves D, et al. Second sialic acid binding site in Newcastle disease virus hemagglutinin-neuraminidase: implications in fusion. *J Virol* 2004;78:3733–3741.
456. Zhao X, Singh M, Malashkevich VN, et al. Structural characterization of the human respiratory syncytial virus fusion protein core. *Proc Natl Acad Sci U S A* 2000;97:14172–14177.

CHAPTER 34

Ruth A. Karron • Peter L. Collins

Parainfluenza Viruses

HISTORY

The four serotypes of human parainfluenza virus types 1 to 4 (HPIV1 to HPIV4) were first recovered between 1956 and 1960, following the application of cell culture and hemadsorption techniques to the study of pediatric respiratory tract disease.[48,49,175] HPIV1, HPIV2, and HPIV3 were initially isolated from infants and children with lower respiratory tract illness (LRI), and HPIV4 was recovered from children and young adults with mild upper respiratory tract illness (URI). Soon after their discovery, these viruses were shown to be a major cause of croup (HPIV1, 2, and 3) as well as pneumonia and bronchiolitis (HPIV3).[45,115,283] As a group, HPIV1, HPIV2, and HPIV3 are second only to human respiratory syncytial virus (HRSV) as a cause of serious viral respiratory tract disease in infants and children, whereas disease due to HPIV4 is less frequent and less serious.

There also are a number of parainfluenza viruses (PIVs) that infect animals. Indeed, the first PIV to be identified was the avian pathogen Newcastle disease virus (NDV). This virus was isolated following outbreaks in 1926 in Java, Indonesia, and Newcastle-upon-Tyne, England, of a seemingly new poultry disease with high mortality.[91] The origin of this then-emerging pathogen remains obscure. This virus, or a close progenitor, may have been indigenous in wild birds, and its appearance or evolution as a "new" disease entity may have been associated with the increasing scale of poultry farming at that time. Nine distinct serotypes of avian PIVs (now usually called avian paramyxoviruses, or APMVs) are now recognized, of which NDV constitutes serotype 1.[5] Another PIV was recovered in 1952 in Japan from mice inoculated with an autopsy specimen from an infant with respiratory disease.[216,264] The natural history of this virus, Sendai virus (SeV), is not well understood, but it appears to be a murine virus that is closely related to HPIV1 but is not a human pathogen. Its antigenic relatedness to HPIV1 led to some confusion when it was used in serologic studies of patients with acute respiratory disease. Bovine parainfluenza type 3 (BPIV3), a close bovine relative of HPIV3, was isolated in 1959 from cattle with respiratory tract disease called shipping fever.[1,2] PIV5, previously known as simian virus 5 (SV5), was first isolated in 1954 as a common contaminant of primary monkey kidney tissue cultures (hence its name).[163] This was at a time when these cultures were being used to prepare poliovirus vaccine material, and a number of new viruses were recovered and identified from the primary tissue. PIV5 was shown to be related to HPIV2 and was identified as a cause of croup ("kennel cough") in dogs.[21,22,44] Simian virus 41 (SV41) was isolated in 1961, also as a contaminant of primary monkey kidney cell culture.[251] SV41 was found to be even more closely related to HPIV2 than PIV5.[377] Therefore, there are four known human PIVs (HPIV1–4) and 13 known animal PIVs (SeV, BPIV3, PIV5, SV41, NDV/APMV1, and APMV2–9). This number may increase: virus that appears to represent a 10th APMV serotype was recently isolated from penguins from the Falkland Islands.[250]

The name *parainfluenza* originally was coined because some of the disease signs are influenza-like and because, like influenza, the particle is medium-sized, has a lipid envelope, and has hemagglutination and neuraminidase activities. This name was first used in 1959 for the four viruses now known as HPIV1, HPIV2, HPIV3, and SeV.[10] Therefore, the term parainfluenza refers to the four serotypes of HPIV and their close animal relatives, and also includes the APMVs, even though these lack close human relatives. Another common human virus, mumps virus (MuV, Chapter 35), is related to the PIVs (most closely to HPIV2) and shares their physical and morphologic properties, but its hallmarks of parotitis and orchitis render it distinct.

Because they can readily be grown to high titer, the animal PIVs SeV, PIV5, and NDV have been used extensively in studies spanning several decades that have defined many of the basic molecular and biological properties of Family *Paramyxoviridae:* this information is described in detail in Chapter 33. The present chapter focuses on PIV biology and in particular the HPIVs.

INFECTIOUS AGENT

Classification, Relationships, and Diversity

The PIVs are enveloped, cytoplasmic viruses (Fig. 34.1) with single-stranded, nonsegmented, negative-sense RNA genomes of 14.9 to 17.3 kb (Fig. 34.2). They are distributed among three genera (namely *Respirovirus, Rubulavirus,* and *Avulavirus*)

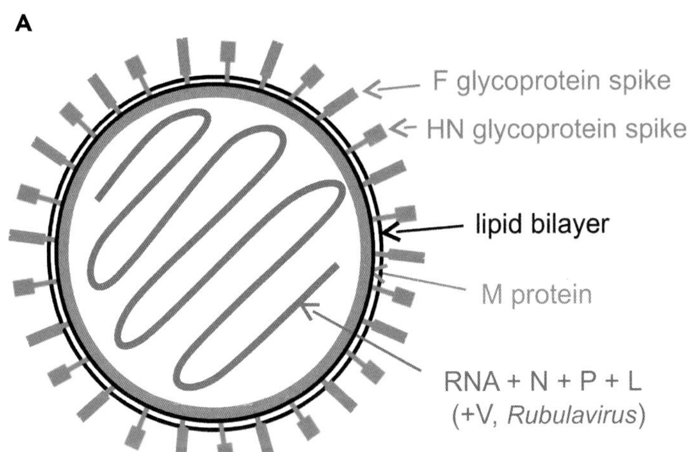

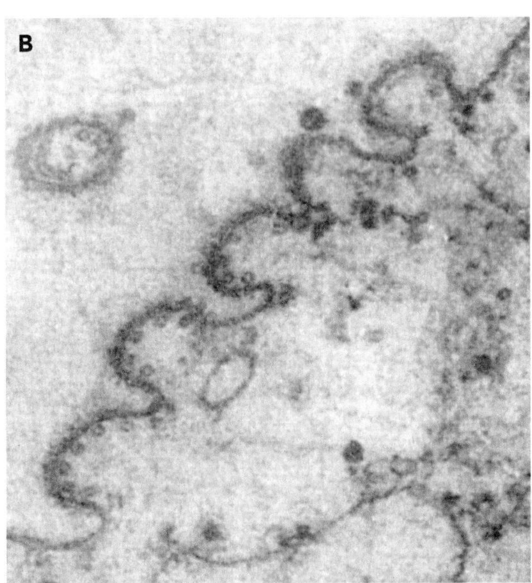

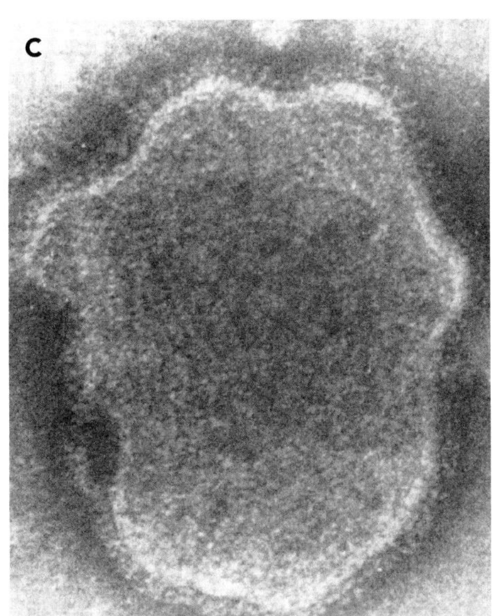

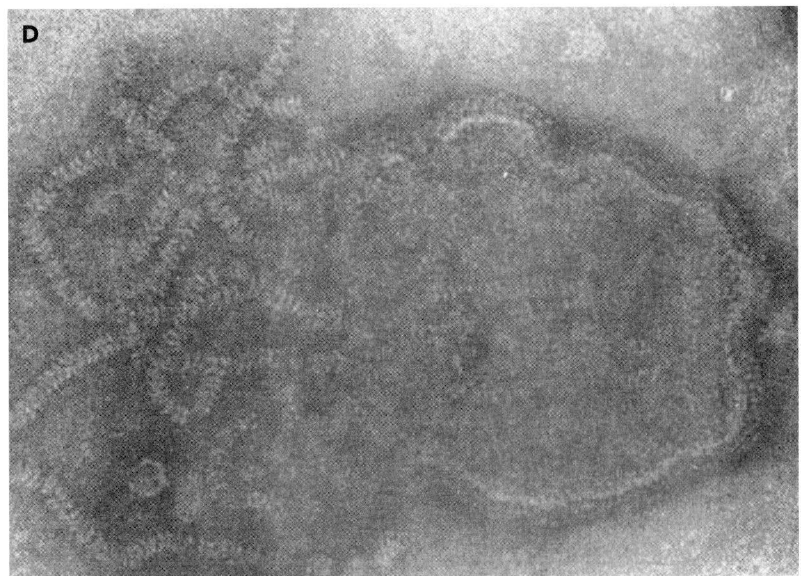

FIGURE 34.1. Schematic diagram (A) and electron photomicrographs (B–G) of parainfluenza virus (PIV) virions. **A:** Idealized diagram of a PIV virion, not to scale and not intended to imply relative molar amounts or exact spatial relationships. The V protein (not shown) is found as a structural protein only in *Rubulavirus.*[284] The C protein (not shown) of the *Respirovirus* Sendai virus (SeV) also has been reported to be present associated with the virion nucleocapsid (not shown).[403] **B:** PIV5 virions budding from the surface of a cultured cell.[58] Intact **(C)** and disrupted **(D)** HPIV2 virions that were fixed and negatively stained; envelope spikes can be seen in both **C** and **D,** and the helical nucleocapsid is evident in **D.**[156] *(continued)*

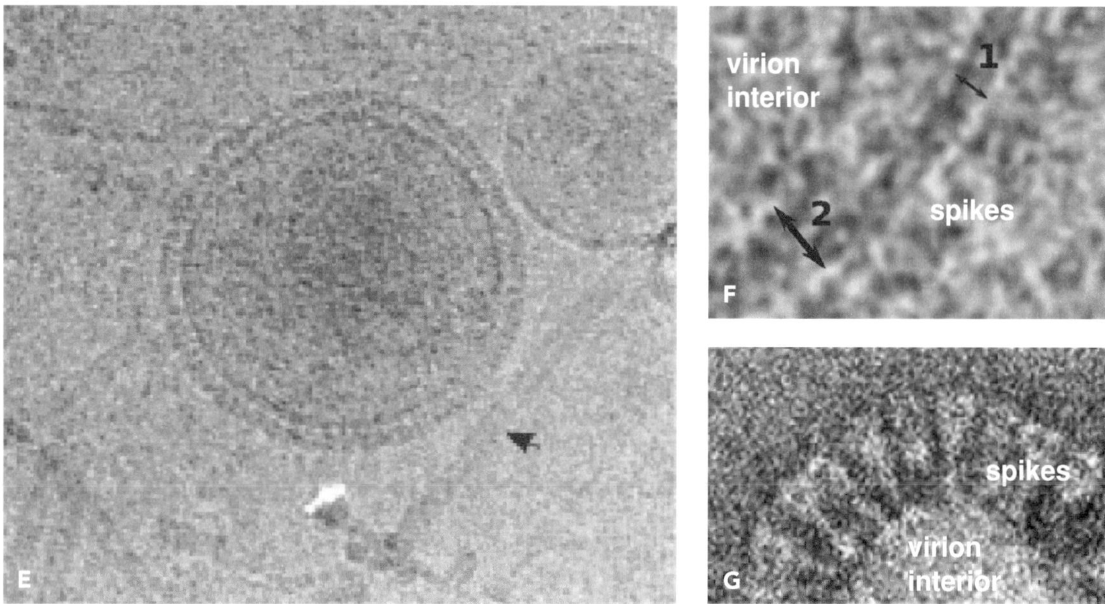

FIGURE 34.1. *(continued)* **E** and **F:** Cryomicrographs of ice-embedded PIV5.[369] **E:** Intact PIV5 virions and free nucleocapsids (*arrow*), and **(F)** higher-magnification images showing the thickness of the lipid bilayer (*double arrow 1*) and areas of the lipid bilayer with underlying matrix M protein (*double arrow 2*).[369] **G:** Negatively stained cryomicrographs of a portion of a PIV5 virion showing distinct envelope spikes.[237]

of subfamily *Paramyxovirinae,* family *Paramyxoviridae,* order *Mononegavirales.*[218] (The other subfamily is *Pneumovirinae,* which contains HRSV, human metapneumovirus [HMPV], and their relatives). HPIV1 and HPIV3, and their respective murine and bovine relatives SeV and BPIV3, constitute the genus *Respirovirus* (Fig. 34.3). HPIV2, its relatives PIV5 and SV41, and HPIV4 are part of the genus *Rubulavirus. Rubulavirus* is a diverse genus that also contains related viruses that are not considered PIVs, such as MuV, Mapuera virus, and porcine rubulavirus. The various APMV serotypes constitute the genus *Avulavirus.*

The relationships between the PIVs are illustrated in Figure 34.3 by alignment of the amino acid sequences of the L proteins. Representative viruses from *Morbillivirus* and *Henipavirus,* two other genera of the subfamily *Paramyxovirinae,* are included for comparison. This shows that the PIVs as a whole are broadly divergent and are not clearly demarcated by sequence relatedness as a group distinct from the non-PIV members of *Paramyxovirinae.* This comparison also shows the close relatedness between some of the human and animal PIVs, such as between HPIV1 and SeV and between HPIV3 and BPIV3. It is likely that these closely related viruses arose from transmission across host species.

The relationships between the PIVs also are illustrated in Tables 34.1 to 34.3 by the percent amino acid sequence identity for the two major surface antigens, namely the fusion F glycoprotein (Table 34.1) and the hemagglutinin-neuraminidase HN glycoprotein (Table 34.2), as well as for the large polymerase L protein (Table 34.3). This illustrates, for example, that the HPIV serotype distinctions are associated with

TABLE 34.1 Percent Amino Acid Sequence Identity Between the F Proteins of the Indicated PIVs[a]

	HPIV1	SeV	HPIV3	BPIV3	HPIV2	SV41	HPIV4A	HPIV4B	NDV
HPIV1		**67**[a]	**43**	**42**	22	23	24	23	23
SeV			**41**	**41**	23	23	24	23	23
HPIV3				**82**	24	23	25	25	23
BPIV3					24	23	24	24	23
HPIV2						***59***	***34***	***35***	29
SV41							***33***	***33***	27
HPIV4A								***95***	33
HPIV4B									33

[a]Comparisons within *Respirovirus* or *Rubulavirus* are in bold or bold italics, respectively.

PIV, parainfluenza virus; HPIV, human parainfluenza virus; SeV, Sendai virus; BPIV, bovine parainfluenza virus; SV41, Simian virus 41; NDV, Newcastle disease virus.

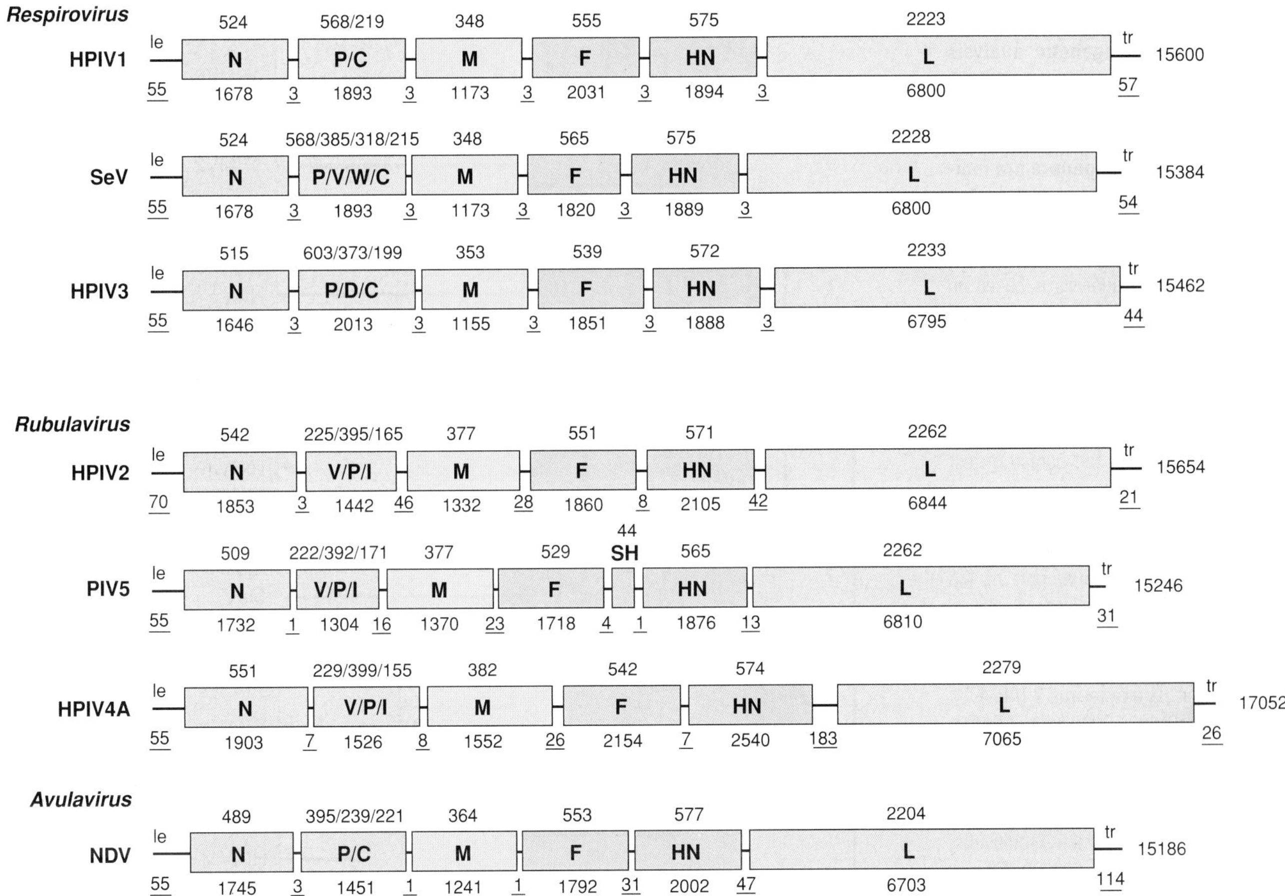

FIGURE 34.2. Gene maps of selected parainfluenza viruses (PIVs), not to exact scale. Each negative-sense genome is drawn 3′ to 5′, which is the direction of transcription. Genes are shown as rectangles: those encoding nucleocapsid-associated and accessory proteins are in blue; those encoding the transmembrane surface glycoproteins are in red; and those encoding the matrix protein of the inner envelope are in brown. The letters within each rectangle identify the encoded protein(s); for P and V, the protein encoded by the unedited messenger RNA (mRNA) is shown first. Nucleotide lengths are shown under each diagram; those representing the extragenic leader (le), trailer (tr), and intergenic regions are underlined. Amino acid sequence lengths are shown above the diagrams. The maps are generally similar, and there is general similarity in genome, gene, and protein lengths, although some differences exist: (a) the P and V proteins are encoded by unedited and edited mRNA, respectively, for *Respirovirus* and *Avulavirus*, whereas for *Rubulavirus* the situation is the converse; (b) there are differences among the PIVs in other proteins encoded by P gene; (c) PIV5 and APMV6 (the latter not shown here) have the additional SH gene; (d) the intergenic regions of *Respirovirus* are conserved trinucleotides, whereas those of the other genera are variable; (e) the P proteins of *Rubulavirus* and *Avulavirus* are shorter compared to those of *Respirovirus;* and (f) human parainfluenza virus 4 (HPIV4) has a substantially longer genome. Maps are based on the Washington/1964 strain of HPIV1 (NC_003461), the Z strain of Sendai virus (SeV) (M30202), the JS strain of HPIV3 (X11575), the V94 strain of HPIV2 (AF533010), PIV5 (NC_006430), the Toshiba/M-25/1966 strain of HPIV4A (AB543336), and the LaSota strain of Newcastle disease virus (NDV) (AF077761).

amino acid sequence identities of less than 50% for F and HN. The APMV serotypes are not shown in these tables, but they also usually (but not always) have less than 50% amino acid sequence identity between F and HN of the different serotypes.[43,172,213,214,265,318,353,401,402] For example, the percent amino acid sequence identity between APMV5 versus serotypes 1, 2, 3, 4, 6, 7, 8, and 9 is, respectively: 41, 47, 31, 33, 55, 37, 46, and 37 for the F protein; and 35, 42, 33, 30, 56, 43, 41, and 31 for the HN protein.[319]

Antigenic reactivity based on binding assays can be detected between PIVs within a genus with polyclonal sera and, less frequently, with monoclonal antibodies (MAbs).[167,203,271] A lower level of reactivity between genera sometimes is detected with polyclonal sera, although there is no group antigen encompassing the three PIV genera.

HPIV4 has been segregated into two variants, A and B, based on antigenic differences detected by hemadsorption-inhibition (HI) and MAb reactivity.[204] Sequence analysis shows that these two subgroups are very closely related: the percent identity between the F, HN, and L proteins is 95, 87, and 97, respectively (Tables 34.1 to 34.3), and they likely would not be distinguishable in neutralization assays with postinfection sera. Variation within the other HPIV serotypes appears to be somewhat less. For HPIV2, the percent amino acid sequence

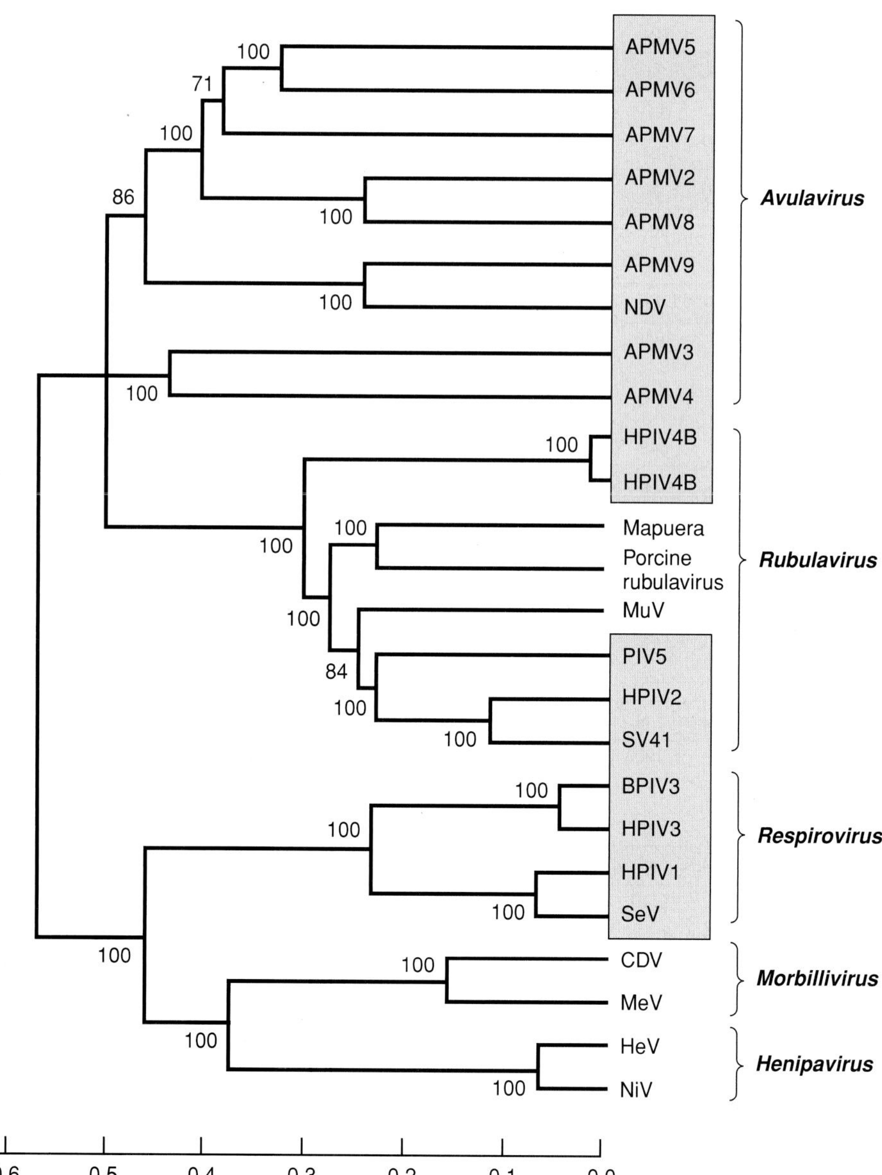

FIGURE 34.3. Phylogenetic analysis of the amino acid sequences of the L proteins of the parainfluenza viruses (PIVs) and other selected members of *Paramyxovirinae* (genera are indicated on the right). PIVs are boxed. The scale at the bottom indicates evolutionary distance as the number of substitutions per site. The analysis is based on the neighbor-joining method[313] and was performed with Molecular Evolutionary Genetics Analysis (MEGA)4.[361] The numbers at branch points indicate the percentage in which the associated taxa clustered together in the bootstrap test (500 replicates). The L protein sequence was chosen for analysis because it is one of the more conserved proteins, accounts for a substantial part of the viral coding sequence, and is similar in size for each virus. The sequences were as in Figure 34.2 or were from the following: avian paramyxovirus 2 (APMV2), EU338413; APMV3, EU403085; APMV4, EU877976; APMV5, GU206351; APMV6, EU622637; APMV7, FJ231524; APMV8, FJ215863; APMV9, EU910942; Mapuera virus, NC_009489; porcine rubulavirus, NC_009640; MuV, NC_002200; Simian virus 41 (SV41), NC_006428; BPIV3, NC_002161; SeV, NC_001552; CDV, canine distemper virus, NC_002728; MeV, measles virus, AF266288; HeV, hendra virus, NC_001906; NiV, Nipah virus, NC_001906. This analysis was kindly provided by Drs. Sachin Kumar and Siba Samal, University of Maryland at College Park.

TABLE 34.2 Percent Amino Acid Sequence Identity Between the HN Proteins of the Indicated PIVs[a]

	HPIV1	SeV	HPIV3	BPIV3	HPIV2	SV41	HPIV4A	HPIV4B	NDV
HPIV1		**73**[a]	**47**	**46**	22	23	24	24	22
SeV			**45**	**46**	22	23	22	22	23
HPIV3				**76**	23	24	22	23	22
BPIV3					22	25	22	22	22
HPIV2						***61***	***38***	***38***	31
SV41							***36***	***36***	33
HPIV4A								***87***	29
HPIV4B									29

[a]Comparisons within *Respirovirus* or *Rubulavirus* are in bold or bold italics, respectively.

PIV, parainfluenza virus; HPIV, human parainfluenza virus; SeV, Sendai virus; BPIV, bovine parainfluenza virus; SV41, Simian virus 41; NDV, Newcastle disease virus.

TABLE 34.3 Percent Amino Acid Sequence Identity Between the L Proteins of the Indicated PIVs[a]

	HPIV1	SeV	HPIV3	BPIV3	HPIV2	SV41	HPIV4A	HPIV4B	NDV
HPIV1		**86**[a]	**60**	**61**	28	29	29	29	26
SeV			**60**	**60**	28	29	28	28	26
HPIV3				**89**	28	28	29	29	25
BPIV3					28	28	29	29	26
HPIV2						***77***	***51***	***50***	35
SV41							***51***	***51***	34
HPIV4A								***97***	35
HPIV4B									35

[a]Comparisons within *Respirovirus* or *Rubulavirus* are in bold or bold italics, respectively.

PIV, parainfluenza virus; HPIV, human parainfluenza virus; SeV, Sendai virus; BPIV, bovine parainfluenza virus; SV41, Simian virus 41; NDV, Newcastle disease virus.

identity between the V94 strain versus the V98 and Greer strains was, respectively, 98 and 99 for F, 95 and 96 for HN, and 99 and nearly 100 for L.[337] For HPIV3, comparison of the F protein sequence of prototype strain Washington/47885/57 with seven clinical strains revealed 98% or more identity,[62] and comparison of HN with six clinical strains revealed 97% or more identity.[385] For HPIV1, comparison of 40 strains showed that the percent amino acid sequence identity for the HN protein was 95% or greater.[146] For NDV, comparison of 50 strains from various times and places of isolation showed that the percent identity between F and HN was 91% and 90% or greater, respectively.[317] Some of the other animal PIVs, such as APMV2,[352] APMV3,[214] APMV6,[402] and BPIV3,[152] have been found to have somewhat greater diversity (i.e., intraserotype amino acid sequence identity for F and HN of 75% to 79% for APMV2, 70% to 73% for APMV3, 81% to 86% for APMV6, and 86% to 89% for BPIV3), resulting in distinct genotypes or subgroups within a serotype. In the case of APMV2, APMV3, and APMV6, this has been shown to be associated with a modest degree of antigenic difference detectable with postinfection sera.

NDV is notable because the many highly related naturally occurring isolates and strains that have been recovered for this single serotype exhibit a broad spectrum of virulence, ranging from nonvirulent or mildly virulent (lentogenic), to moderately virulent (mesogenic), to highly virulent (velogenic). Lentogenic strains are associated with subclinical infection or can cause mild respiratory tract disease, and the more attenuated natural isolates are used as live vaccines. At the other extreme, velogenic strains can be highly virulent and, depending on the strain, can cause hemorrhagic lesions in the intestines (viscerotropic) or neurologic disease (neurotropic).[317] In contrast, there is no evidence of differences in virulence among the various isolates of each of the four serotypes of HPIV, although this has not been studied extensively. Little is known about the possible diversity of disease within the other animal PIVs.

Virion Morphology and Activities

The virions of PIVs are medium-sized particles of 150 to 200 nm. Fixed, negatively stained virions typically appear in electron micrographs as pleomorphic (irregularly shaped) round particles (Fig. 34.1).[58,156,253,324,369] Filamentous virions have been described in some cases, such as for HPIV2.[405] Cryoelectron microscopy of ice-embedded SeV and PIV5 provided images of virions as predominantly perfect spheres of varied diameters.[153,233,369] This suggests that the irregular shapes of particles observed with conventional electron microscopy are artifacts of sample fixation and dehydration, whereas the variations in size were observed using both methods and thus may be authentic. Seventy-one percent of the ice-embedded PIV5 virions consisted of spheres of 129 to 360 nm (average 217 nm), and the remainder were elongated particles of up to 445 nm.[369]

PIVs replicate in the cytoplasm and bud through the plasma membrane (Fig. 34.1B). The virion consists of a nucleocapsid that is packaged in a lipid envelope derived from the host cell plasma membrane during budding (Fig. 34.1). In the nucleocapsid, the viral genome is tightly bound along its entire length with the nucleoprotein N at a ratio of one protein molecule per six nucleotides (2,484 to 2,877 protein molecules, depending on the length of the viral genome). Associated with the nucleocapsid in the virus particle are approximately 300 copies of the phosphoprotein P and approximately 40 copies of the major polymerase protein L, based on studies with SeV.[200,219] *Rubulaviruse* virions contain an additional nucleocapsid-associated protein called V,[284] and the virion of the *Respirovirus* SeV has been reported to contain 40 copies of a small protein called C, also associated with the nucleocapsid.[403] Electron micrographs of nucleocapsids released from PIV virions indicate a length of approximately 1.0 to 1.1 μm.[65,233] The nucleocapsid with its associated proteins has RNA-dependent RNA polymerase activity.[134] Purified virions can be activated for cell-free transcription by disruption of the envelope with detergent and can transcribe the viral genome in its entirety into messenger RNAs (mRNAs).[64]

The envelope bears spike-like surface projections composed of homotrimers and tetramers of the F and HN glycoproteins, respectively. Based on cryoelectron microscopy, PIV5 virions were estimated to contain approximately 2,000 glycoprotein spikes per 200 nm particle, with an average spike length of 14.2 nm.[369] PIV5 and AMPV6 have a third, small transmembrane protein, SH ("small hydrophobic"). The nonglycosylated matrix M protein is associated with the inner surface of the envelope. The hemagglutination activity of the HN protein mediates adsorption of virus to the host cell to initiate infection. The cellular receptor for the PIVs is N-acetylneuraminic acid (sialic acid) in a terminal linkage to cellular glycoproteins and glycolipids.[356,411] In the case of HPIV3, cell surface nucleolin also has been reported to serve as a receptor co-factor.[29] Viral attachment can be measured experimentally by the agglutination of erythrocytes by virus in suspension (hemagglutination) or by the adsorption of erythrocytes to infected cell monolayers expressing HN (hemadsorption) as was used in the original detection of the HPIVs. Late in infection, the neuraminidase activity of HN cleaves sialic acid to facilitate release of progeny virions. Neuraminidase activity can be quantified using sialic acid derivatives as substrates in a colorimetric or fluorometric assay. The F protein mediates fusion between the viral envelope and the host cell plasma membrane, an activity that can be measured *in vitro* by lysis of erythrocytes (hemolysis).

RNA

The PIV genome is a single strand of negative-sense RNA that ranges in length from 14,904 (APMV2) to 17,262 (APMV5) nucleotides (nt). The differences in genome length between the different PIVs are mostly due to differences in the lengths of noncoding sequences rather than substantial differences in the lengths of open reading frames (ORFs). The PIV genome is not capped or polyadenylated. It contains, in 3′ to 5′ order: a short 3′ extragenic leader region of 55 nt (except in the case of HPIV2, for which the leader region is 70 nt), followed by six genes encoding the N, P, M, F, HN, and L proteins, followed by an extragenic trailer region of 21 to 291 nt (Fig. 34.2; note that the longest, 291-nt trailer region is that of APMV-3 and is not shown in this figure). Sequences of the leader regions of selected PIVs are shown in e-Fig. 34.1A. As noted below, the P gene also encodes one or more accessory proteins—namely C, V, W, I, and D—depending on the virus (Fig. 34.2). PIV5 and APMV-6 each contain a seventh small gene that is located between F and HN and encodes the SH protein. In the case of *Respirovirus,* the PIV genes are separated by intergenic (IG) regions that are conserved trinucleotides (usually 3′-GAA in genome-sense); in the case of *Rubulavirus* and *Avulavirus* the IG regions have nonconserved sequences of variable length (0 to 183 nt) (Fig. 34.2; also, see e-Fig. 34.1B for gene junction sequences of selected PIVs).

Transcription and RNA replication occur in the cytoplasm and follow the *Mononegavirales* model. Briefly, the genes are transcribed sequentially in their 3′ to 5′ order to yield separate nonoverlapping mRNAs that are polyadenylated, capped, and methylated. RNA synthesis also yields short nonpolyadenylated and noncapped transcripts of the leader and trailer regions. Transcription is guided by short conserved gene-start (GS) and gene-end (GE) transcription signals that flank each gene (see e-Fig. 34.1B for gene junction sequences of selected PIVs). For RNA replication, the polymerase ignores the GS and GE signals and produces a complete positive-sense copy of the genome that is called the antigenome. Like the genome, the antigenome is not capped or polyadenylated. Both the genome and antigenome are completely bound with N protein.[199] Encapsidation of nascent genomes and antigenomes is thought to drive chain elongation during RNA replication. The tightly encapsidated nature of the nucleocapsid likely shields the uncapped and nonpolyadenylated genome/antigenome from degradation. It also likely shields the genome/antigenome from recognition by the cytoplasmic helicases retinoic acid-inducible gene 1 (RIG-I) and Melanoma Differentiation-Associated protein 5 (MDA5), which detect triphosphorylated RNA and double-stranded RNA (dsRNA) and initiate signaling to activate the cellular transcription factors interferon regulatory factor 3 (IRF3) and nuclear factor kappa B (NF-κB) to induce type I interferon (IFN) and proinflammatory cytokines. This also reduces activation of protein kinase R (PKR), which is triggered through dsRNA to activate NF-κB as well as to phosphorylate eukaryotic translation initiation factor eIF-2a and thereby inhibit translational initiation as part of host defense. As another example of how viral RNA can affect host cell responses, one of the products of SeV RNA replication is a 55-nt aborted RNA representing the 5′ trailer region that contains a U-rich sequence that inhibits apoptosis by binding to the proapoptotic factor T-cell intracellular antigen 1 related (TIAR).[166]

The nucleotide lengths of the genomes and antigenomes of the PIVs (and of all of subfamily *Paramyxovirinae*) are even multiples of six. This property is essential for efficient RNA replication and is called the "rule of six".[199–200,201,337] This is thought to reflect an obligatory nucleocapsid organization in which each N protein monomer associates with exactly six nucleotides. In experiments to recover recombinant HPIV2 and HPIV3 viruses whose nucleotide lengths were designed to not be even multiples of six, the recovered viruses contained genomes that had mutated to conform to the rule.[336,337]

Each PIV gene encodes—via transcribed mRNA—a single major protein, with the exception of the P gene that can encode additional proteins in two ways that are described briefly here and in greater detail for the HPIVs in e-Fig. 34.2. First, all of the PIVs in the genus *Respirovirus* contain a C ORF that initiates near the 5′ end of the P mRNA, closely overlapping the start of the P ORF. Depending on the virus, the C ORF has from one to four different translational start sites that are utilized to give rise to up to four carboxy–co-terminal C proteins. *Rubulavirus* and *Avulavirus* do not have a C ORF. Second, the P genes of most PIVs encode additional proteins by "RNA editing".[199,201,388] This involves the co-transcriptional insertion of 1 or more G residues into the nascent mRNA by polymerase stuttering at an editing motif midway along the P gene. An array of mRNAs is produced: they include the unedited form as well as subpopulations that contain 1, 2, or more G residues inserted at the editing site. The insertion of 1 G residue (or 3+1, and so on) or 2 residues (or 3+2, and so on) creates frameshifts that access ORFs in the two other reading frames. For the PIVs of *Respirovirus* and *Avulavirus,* the unedited mRNA encodes the P protein,[286,348,388] and the addition of a single G by RNA editing fuses the upstream half of the P ORF to an internal ORF encoding a domain with a conserved cysteine-rich domain: the resulting protein is called V. The addition of 2 G residues fuses the upstream half of the P ORF to an ORF in the third reading frame: this downstream ORF encodes only a few added amino acids and results in a protein called W, except in the case of HPIV3 and BPIV3 in which the number of added amino acids is substantially more and the resulting protein is called D (e-Fig. 34.2). HPIV1 is an exception because it does not appear to engage in RNA editing.[245,307] In addition, although HPIV3 does engage in RNA editing, the V ORF is separated from the editing site by two or more (depending on the strain) stop codons in the same reading frame that may preclude expression of V (see e-Fig. 34.2).[108] For the PIVs of *Rubulavirus,* the exact-copy mRNA encodes the V protein, whereas an edited version containing two inserted G residues encodes P.[192,208,276,342,370] An edited version containing one inserted residue encodes the I protein, which is the *Rubulavirus* equivalent of W. [See the ebook for more information on coding assignments and RNA editing.)

Several factors control the relative efficiency of transcription of the various PIV genes. As is typical for *Mononegavirales,* there is a gradient of transcription in which promoter-proximal genes are expressed somewhat more efficiently than promoter-distal genes.[64,138] This is thought to be due to polymerase fall-off at the gene junctions.[168] However, with the exception of L, the gradient of expression is not continuous or steep; in the case of SeV, for example, the P, M, F and HN mRNAs accumulate at 0.30, 1.15, 0.61, and 0.38 times the level of N.[148] Accumulation of the L mRNA is much lower (0.02 that of N). Differences in transcription signals also influence transcription. In PIV5, the efficiency of transcription across the different gene junctions, measured by the relative level of expression of the downstream versus upstream gene, was found to vary over a fourfold range, indicative of regulation at the level of the termination/re-initiation at the gene junctions.[138] However, the HN-L junction was not associated with a particularly high level of fall-off.[138] This suggests that the low level of expression of L relative to the other genes is due to some other factor such as polymerase fall-off during L gene transcription or instability of the L mRNA.

A number of PIVs have evolved mechanisms for downregulating expression of the F gene. The M GE signal of HPIV3 contains an apparent eight-nucleotide insertion that causes increased M-F readthrough (see e-Fig. 34.1B).[344] The M GE signal of PIV5 contains a single nucleotide substitution that has the same effect.[300] In SV41, the M GE signal is lacking altogether and M is expressed solely as an M-F readthrough mRNA.[376] Interestingly, the F gene of SV41 also is expressed as a monocistronic mRNA by initiation at its GS signal, but this occurs at a reduced level because the majority of the polymerase molecules are already engaged in reading across the M-F junction. In HPIV1, the same effect of increased production of M-F mRNA at the expense of monocistronic F mRNA was observed, and studies with recombinant viruses mapped the effect to a combination of features, namely the intergenic sequence, the F GS signal, and the long upstream nontranslated region of the F gene.[31] Therefore, various features in these different viruses result in the synthesis of an M-F readthrough mRNA at the expense of a monocistronic F mRNA. In these M-F readthrough mRNAs, the F ORF would not be efficiently accessed by ribosomes due to its internal position.[211] Finally, SeV downregulates expression of its F gene by yet another mechanism, namely through a suboptimal GS signal.[188] Therefore, each of these strategies results in reduced expression of this fusogenic factor. In the case of SeV, this was shown to reduce the virulence of the virus.[188] It might be that, by reducing morbidity and mortality in the host, the virus increases its opportunities for shedding and spread.

Proteins

All PIVs encode six common proteins: N, P, M, F, HN, and L, all of which are essential for virus replication. All members encode at least one additional protein from the P gene (C, V, D, W, and I, depending on the virus). PIV5 and APMV-6 also encode a small hydrophobic transmembrane SH protein.

HN Glycoprotein

The PIV HN glycoprotein (Fig. 34.4) mediates attachment by binding to host cell sialic acid. This activity is responsible for the ability of the virus to agglutinate erythrocytes. HN also functions late in infection to cleave sialic acid residues on the virus and nearby cell surface proteins to facilitate release of progeny virions. The dual hemagglutinin/neuraminidase functions of HN appear to be modulated by halide ion concentration and pH.[248] Hemagglutination activity appears to be favored by the halide ion concentration and pH of the extracellular environment, consistent with the role of HN in binding to extracellular receptors, whereas neuraminidase activity is optimal at lower pH and halide ion concentration, consistent with the role of HN in stripping sialic acid from newly formed

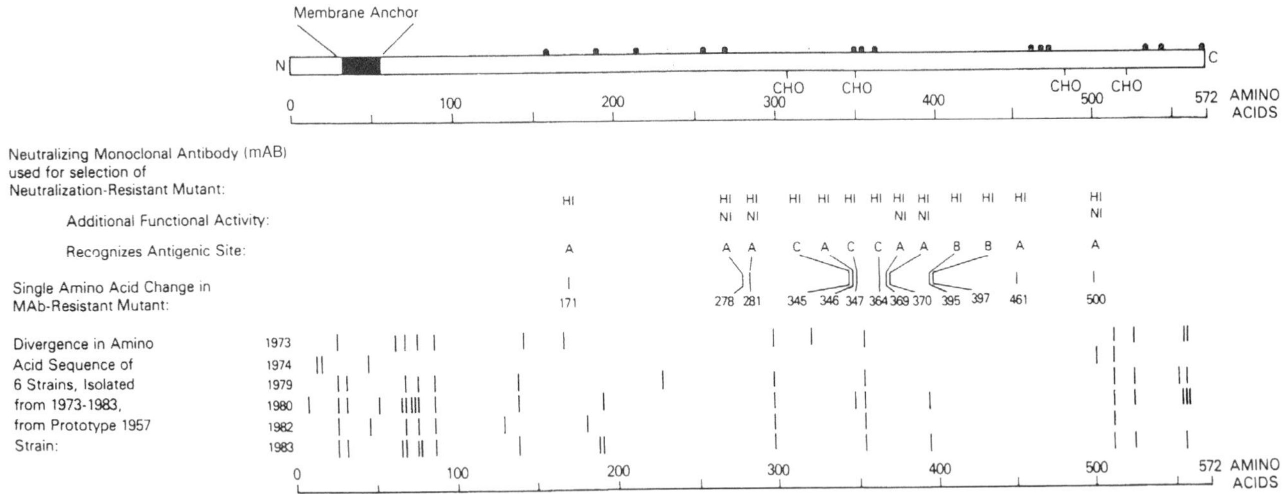

FIGURE 34.4. Linear diagram and antigenic organization of the human parainfluenza virus 3 (HPIV3) HN glycoprotein (strain 47885/57[61]). • Denotes cysteine; CHO denotes a potential site for N-glycan; HI (hemagglutinin-inhibiting) and NI (neuraminidase-inhibiting) denote positions of amino acid substitutions identified in neutralization-resistant mutants selected with HI and NI monoclonal antibodies (MAbs), and the amino acid positions and antigenic sites (A-C) are indicated; bars indicate positions of amino acid variability among natural isolates.

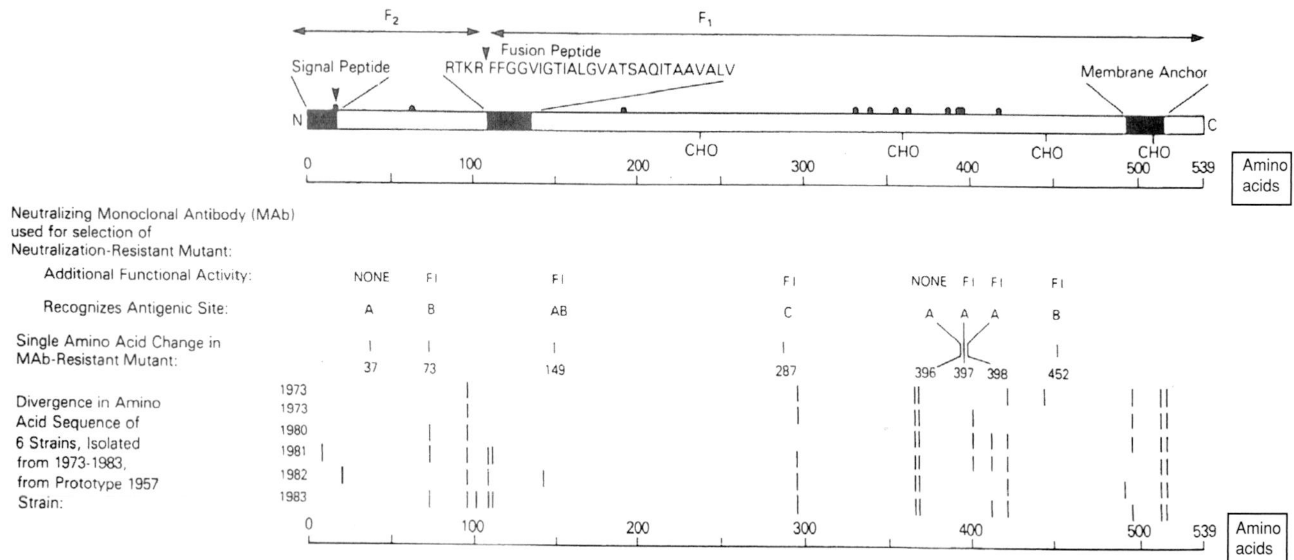

FIGURE 34.5. Linear diagram and antigenic organization of the human parainfluenza virus 3 (HPIV3) F protein (strain 47885/57[61]). • Denotes cysteine; CHO denotes a potential site for N-glycan; FI (fusion-inhibiting) denotes amino acid substitutions identified in neutralization-resistant mutants selected with FI MAbs, and the amino acid positions and antigenic sites are indicated; bars indicate positions of amino acid variability among natural isolates.

viral and host cell glycoproteins in intracellular vesicles during transport to the cell surface. The HN proteins of PIVs and indeed most of *Paramyxovirinae* also play an essential role by interacting with the F protein to promote fusion.[66,256,290,292,311]

HN is a type II glycoprotein that contains an uncleaved signal/anchor sequence located near the N-terminus (Fig. 34.4). HN assembles into homotetramers that contain a stalk that is sensitive to trypsin cleavage and a globular head that represents most of the extracellular domain. The globular head retains the HA and NA biologic activities and the major antigenic sites. On a gross level, the globular head has a box-shaped structure in which the four identical subunits exhibit fourfold symmetry. Crystal structures have been determined for the HN proteins of HPIV3, NDV, and PIV5, both free and complexed with its receptor or inhibitors[32,69,222,312,409]: these are described in Chapter 33.

The HN protein of some avirulent strains of NDV is synthesized as a longer precursor, HN_0, in which the hemagglutinin and neuraminidase are inactive.[263,316] Activation requires an endoproteolytic cleavage that results in the loss of a small, 9-kD glycopeptide from the carboxy terminus and a change in conformation.[198,263] Like the F_0 precursor protein of the avirulent strains (see below), HN_0 is resistant to intracellular cleavage in most cell types and presumably is cleaved by extracellular secretory proteases, but unlike F_0 it does not have a marked trypsin-like specificity and can be activated *in vitro* by a variety of proteases.[263] It might be that the shorter HN proteins of virulent NDV strains that lack this extension and do not require cleavage arose evolutionarily from longer cleaved ancestral ORFs by the introduction of translational stop codons. This is suggested by the finding that the ORFs of certain virulent NDV strains retain the apparent relic of an in-frame C-terminal extension beyond the nonsense codon terminating the current ORF.[249] A counterpart to HN_0 has not been described for any other PIV, although the sequence of the HN gene of HPIV4 has been interpreted as containing a relic of such an extension.[13]

F Glycoprotein

The fusion (F) glycoprotein (Fig. 34.5) mediates penetration of the host cell by fusion of the viral envelope to the plasma membrane. Late in infection, when newly synthesized F glycoprotein has accumulated on the surface of the infected cell, it also can mediate fusion with contiguous uninfected cells. This results in the formation of syncytia, a prominent cytopathic effect in monolayer cultures *in vitro*. At least in the case of SeV, the F protein also can act as an auxiliary attachment protein that binds to cells via the hepatocyte-specific asialoglycoprotein receptor,[24] although the significance of this *in vivo* is not known.

F is a typical type I glycoprotein (Fig. 34.5), with a cleaved N-terminal hydrophobic signal peptide and a C-proximal membrane anchor. The F protein is synthesized as an inactive precursor, F_0, which is converted into the fusogenic form by cleavage by a host endoprotease to yield two subunits: F_2, which contains the N-terminal 20% of the molecule, and F_1, which contains the remainder of the molecule and is anchored in the membrane. F_1 and F_2 remain linked by a disulfide bond.[170,198] The F_1 amino terminus created by cleavage is a hydrophobic region called the fusion peptide that is thought to insert into the target membrane to initiate fusion. Crystal structures have been determined for the F proteins of HPIV3, NDV, and PIV5.[52,357,406,407] The structure and function of F is described in detail in Chapter 33.

Cleavage of F_0 is a prerequisite for PIV infectivity and can be an important determinant of tissue tropism and pathogenesis for NDV and possibly other PIVs (see below and Pathogenesis and Pathology).[262,374] Most velogenic (highly virulent) and mesogenic (moderately virulent) strains of NDV have a cleavage site with the sequence R/K-R-Q-R/K-R↓F (Table 34.4). This multibasic

TABLE 34.4 Cleavage Sites of the F_0 Proteins of Selected PIVs

Virus	Cleavage site sequence[a]							
HPIV1	Asp	Asn	Pro	Gln	Ser	**Arg**	↓	Phe
SeV	Gly	Val	Pro	Gln	Ser	**Arg**	↓	Phe
HPIV3 (prototype and five clinical isolates)[62]	Asp	Pro	**Arg**	Thr	**Arg/Lys**	**Arg**	↓	Phe
HPIV3 (two clinical isolates)[62]	Asp	Pro	**Arg**	Thr	Glu	**Arg**	↓	Ser
HPIV2 (prototype strains)[12]	Thr/**Lys**	Thr	**Arg**	Gln	**Lys**	**Arg**	↓	Phe
HPIV2 (nine clinical isolates)[12]	Thr/Ala	Thr/Pro	**Arg**	Gln	Glu	**Arg**	↓	Phe
HPIV4	Ser	Glu	Ile	Gln	Ser	**Arg**	↓	Phe
NDV (virulent strains, consensus)[249,317,374]	Gly	**Arg/Lys**	**Arg**	Gln	**Arg/Lys**	**Arg**	↓	Phe
NDV (avirulent strains, consensus)[249,317,374]	Gly	Gly/Glu	**Arg/Lys**	Gln	Gly/Glu	**Arg**	↓	Leu

[a]Arg/Lys residues are bold, and Arg/Lys residues consistent with the preferred furin motif (Arg-X-Arg/Lys-Arg↓) are underlined. BPIV3, PIV5, and SV41 are not shown, but all contain the preferred furin motif. For the sources of the sequences, see the legends to Figures 34.2 and 34.3, references,[26,62,158,202,247,346,387] and the other references cited in this table.

PIV, parainfluenza virus; HPIV, human parainfluenza virus; SeV, Sendai virus; BPIV, bovine parainfluenza virus; SV41, Simian virus 41; NDV, Newcastle disease virus.

(basic residues are underlined) cleavage site conforms to the favored cleavage site R-X-R/K-R↓ for the ubiquitous intracellular protease furin,[308] providing for efficient intracellular cleavage. Cleavage by furin or a furin-like protease allows the virus to replicate in cell culture without the need to supply exogenous protease in the culture medium. *In vivo,* it provides the potential for systemic spread and replication in a wide range of tissues, resulting in increased virulence. In comparison, the cleavage site sequence found in most avirulent NDV strains, G/E-K/R-Q-G/E-R↓L, has fewer basic residues and does not conform to the furin cleavage site. These strains are not cleaved by furin and require added protease (typically trypsin or allantoic fluid added to the culture medium) for replication *in vitro,* and are restricted *in vivo* to mucosal tissue of the lungs or intestines where secreted protease capable of cleaving the F_0 precursor is found. Furin reportedly also may cleave at a "minimal" motif R-X-X-R↓,[308] but apparently does not do so for the avirulent NDV strains.

Prototype strains of most of the PIVs have F_0 cleavage sites that contain the furin cleavage motif, including HPIV3, BPIV3, HPIV2, SV41, and PIV5 (examples are shown in Table 34.4), and these viruses do not require added protease for replication *in vitro.* On the other hand, the F_0 proteins of HPIV1, SeV, and HPIV4 lack the furin motif, and these viruses do require added protease *in vitro.* However, for viruses other than NDV, the lack of intracellular cleavage by furin does not necessarily indicate reduced virulence; for example HPIV1 and SeV can be highly virulent *in vivo* despite the lack of furin cleavage. Analysis of clinical isolates of HPIV3 showed that, although five of seven isolates contained the consensus furin motif observed in the prototype strains, two other isolates had the sequence D-P-R-T-E-R↓,[62] which has the same arrangement of basic residues as avirulent NDV strains. However, these strains were fully competent for replication and the production of infectious virus *in vitro* without added protease, and did not exhibit any restriction for replication in the respiratory tract of rhesus monkeys. Similarly, several clinical isolates of HPIV2 were found to have the cleavage site sequence T/A-T/P-R-Q-E-R↓,[12] which does not match the preferred furin motif. In this case, restricted growth by these clinical strains *in vitro* was observed in simian Vero cells but not in primary cultures of primate cells. Therefore, the presence of the preferred furin cleavage motif is not essential for intracellular cleavage or virulence in HPIVs.

Nucleocapsid-Associated N, P, and L Proteins

The N, P, and L proteins, together with the RNA genome, are the viral components that are necessary and sufficient to assemble the nucleocapsid and to direct transcription and RNA replication.[94,134,365]

The N protein is one of the more conserved PIV proteins. It associates with genomic and antigenomic RNAs to form highly stable, RNase-resistant helical nucleocapsids. Monomeric N is maintained in a soluble complex with the P protein prior to assembly into nucleocapsids. The N-terminal 75% of N is the more highly conserved part and is involved in forming the soluble complex with P as well as in subsequently associating with other N monomers and with RNA to form the nucleocapsid. The more variable C-terminal 25% of the molecule is not required to form the nucleocapsid but is essential for it to function as a template.[34,199]

The P protein is not highly conserved within a genus and has little or no significant sequence identity between genera. The P protein consists of N- and C-terminal functional modules separated by a divergent spacer that spans the RNA editing site.[199] P is found as a homotetramer.[366] P is the most heavily phosphorylated viral protein, although the bulk of constitutive phosphorylation can be ablated by mutation in recombinant SeV without effect.[159] The N-terminal module of P is responsible for binding to free N protein and maintaining it as a soluble monomer necessary for nucleocapsid formation during RNA replication.[74,149] The C-terminal module contains the homo-oligomerization domain and the polymerase co-factor domain, and is the only region of P necessary for transcription. This C-terminal module mediates binding of P to the nucleocapsid. It also binds L protein and mediates its association with the nucleocapsid.[149,199]

The L protein is a large multifunctional protein responsible for nucleotide polymerization and mRNA capping and methylation.[275] The N-terminal half of L contains blocks of highly conserved amino acids that are thought to be polymerase domains.[287,288] The L protein forms a complex with the P protein that appears to serve as the RNA polymerase.[149,199]

The matrix M protein is a conserved, nonglycosylated species that is the most abundant virion protein and is located on the inner face of the virion envelope. In the infected cell, M associates with the inner face of the plasma membrane and plays key roles in virion assembly, budding, and release.[326,360] Depending on the virus, expression of M alone (e.g., HPIV1) or together with N and HN or F (e.g., PIV5) triggers the formation and release of virus-like particles.[67,354] The M protein of PIV5 was recently shown to contain a domain that mediates interaction with the host ubiquitin-proteasome pathway during the late stage of budding.[326] M may also play a role in directing the transport of viral components to the plasma membrane.[277,360]

Accessory C, V, D, W, and I Proteins

These are products of the P gene, and the various PIVs differ as to which of these proteins are expressed, with the general pattern being genus specific. These proteins are not essential for virus replication (and thus are termed accessory), although the C and V proteins in particular can substantially increase the efficiency of growth *in vitro* and *in vivo*. As noted, C is encoded by a separate ORF in the P gene of *Respirovirus*, and is not found in *Rubulavirus* or *Avulavirus*. The V, D, W, and I proteins are produced by various PIVs (see Fig. 34.2) by frame shifts introduced by RNA editing (except in the case of *Rubulavirus*, where the V protein is produced from unedited mRNA while P depends on editing). These proteins are summarized below, and additional information on the expression and functions of these proteins in HPIVs is in e-Fig. 34.2. (The complexity of the proteins encoded by the P gene is even greater for SeV, for which the last ~95 codons of the P ORF also are translated independently to yield a small nonstructural protein called X[73,76]; this protein is almost equimolar to P in infected cells, but its function is unknown and it will not be considered further.)

The C protein is an abundant small basic protein whose sequence is not well conserved between viruses. C is expressed into one or more carboxy-co-terminal forms, depending on the virus, by utilization of one or more translational start sites in the ORF: for example, SeV and HPIV1 produce four C proteins (C′, C, Y1, and Y2, in order of decreasing size), whereas HPIV3 produces one C protein (see e-Fig. 34.2). The different forms of the C proteins of SeV have been reported to have functional differences.[75,111,112,220] C has historically been considered to be nonstructural, but the C protein of SeV was reported to co-localize with nucleocapsids in the infected cell and to be tightly associated with the virion-bound nucleocapsid, at 40 molecules per nucleocapsid.[403] The functions of the C proteins have been investigated in detail for SeV. Deletion or mutation of the SeV C proteins results in strong induction of type I IFN and the establishment of an IFN-mediated antiviral state that restricts viral replication in IFN-competent cell culture and *in vivo*.[110,215] The SeV C proteins were reported to inhibit activation of the transcription factors IRF-3 and NF-κB that leads to induction of IFN-β.[206] The C proteins also inhibit signaling from the type I IFN receptor by binding to the signal transducer and activator of transcription protein 1 STAT1 and inhibiting phosphorylation of both STAT1 and STAT2.[112,122,207,359] Another function of the SeV C proteins is to downregulate production of viral RNA at the level of transcription[75] and RNA replication.[37,150,364] By preventing overly robust RNA synthesis, this regulatory activity appears to prevent the formation of dsRNA and unencapsidated triphosphorylated replicative RNAs during SeV infection, thus reducing activation of MDA-5/RIG-I and PKR involved in innate immunity.[358] This regulatory activity also prevents the overproduction of antigenomes, which otherwise can result in the packaging of antigenomes into progeny virions that would be noninfectious.[165] The SeV C proteins inhibit apoptosis[209] and have been reported to play a role in budding.[136,315,354] Expression and functions of the C proteins of the HPIVs are described in e-Figure 34.2.

The V protein consists of the N-terminal half of P fused to a C-terminal V-specific domain that contains a sequence motif that is highly conserved in *Paramyxovirinae* and includes seven invariant cysteine residues (e-Fig. 34.2).[140,272,299,322] The cysteine-rich domain has been shown to coordinate with two zinc atoms per protein molecule.[227,284,347] V is a structural component of the nucleocapsid in the case of *Rubulavirus*, whereas V does not appear to be a structural component in *Respirovirus* virions and may be present in small amounts in *Avulavirus* virions.[72,284,348] The clearest characterization of the functions of the V protein has come from studies with PIV5 and HPIV2, in which the absence of C protein facilitates evaluation. V has been shown to bind to MDA-5 and inhibit induction of IFN-β, whereas it did not appear to inhibit RIG-I.[8,54,289,322] In addition, the V protein inhibits IFN-mediated signaling by mediating degradation of STAT1 or STAT2, depending on the virus and the host cell.[9,161,272,320] PIV5-mediated degradation of STAT1 has been studied in detail and involves the V-protein binding to ubiquitin ligase and hijacking this cellular complex to target STAT1 for ubiquitination and proteosome-dependent degradation.[85,227] The cysteine-rich domain must be present in order for V to inhibit IFN induction and signaling.[140] The V protein also delays apoptosis during viral infection,[355] and downregulates viral transcription and RNA replication.[230] The mechanism for the effect on RNA synthesis was studied with minireplicons of SeV and HPIV2 and was found to be different for the two viruses.[151,270] With SeV, the presence of the N-terminal domain of P allows the V protein to bind to soluble N protein and thus interfere with nucleocapsid assembly,[151] whereas with HPIV2, the inhibitory activity of the V protein was associated with binding to the L protein, and involved the unique C-terminal domain of V.[270] The V protein of PIV5 also has been shown to slow progression of the cell cycle.[228]

Therefore, the PIV C and V proteins have a number of similarities in their general effects, even though they are completely distinct proteins that appear to operate by distinct mechanisms. Two major common functions involve interference with host innate immunity—especially the type I IFN response—and downregulation of viral RNA synthesis. These functions may be related: as noted above for the C protein, reducing viral RNA synthesis can reduce activation of MDA-5/RIG-I, PKR, and other sensors that trigger innate immunity. The V protein is particularly important for members of *Rubulavirus* and *Avulavirus* given their lack of C proteins. For *Respiroviruses*, which encode the potent C proteins, some of the host-antagonist functions of the V protein may be redundant or less robust. For example, although the V protein of SeV has been shown to bind MDA-5 and inhibit induction of IFN-β,[53,54,206,289] the magnitude of this effect may be minor.[123,314,350] Nonetheless, loss of expression of the SeV V protein significantly reduces the efficiency of viral replication *in vivo,* indicating a contribution that is additional to that of the C proteins.[189,190] Exactly what this contribution is remains unclear.[314] For the human *Respiroviruses,* V is more dispensable: as noted, HPIV1 does not encode a V protein due to a lack of RNA editing and the presence of translational stop codons within the V ORF, and HPIV3 likely expresses, at most, only low levels of V due to the presence of stop codons upstream of the V domain (see e-Fig. 34.2 for details on the expression and functions of the V proteins of the human PIVs). The presence of relict V ORFs interrupted by stop codons suggests that predecessors of the present HPIV1 and HPIV3 expressed V proteins, but that this ability became compromised by mutations that introduced these stop codons. Their animal relatives, SeV and BPIV3, respectively, retain the ability to efficiently express V.

The W (present in SeV and *Avulavirus*), I (*Rubulavirus*), and D (HPIV3 and BPIV3) proteins are created when RNA editing fuses the upstream end of the P ORF to a short internal ORF in the remaining reading frame. In the case of W and I, this internal ORF adds only a few amino acids; in the case of the D proteins of HPIV3 and BPIV3 the extension is longer (see e-Fig. 34.2). In general, the functions of the W, I, and D proteins are poorly understood. In the case of SeV, the W protein (like V, as noted above) was reported to downregulate viral genome replication in a reconstituted minireplicon system, an effect that was mediated by its P-related domain.[71,151] The HPIV3 D protein was shown to accumulate in the nucleus of HPIV3-infected cells, but the significance of this is unclear.[398]

SH Protein

Among the PIVs, only PIV5 and AMPV6 encode SH proteins, which are 44 and 142 amino acids in length, respectively. MuV (Chapter 36) and all members of subfamily *Pneumovirinae* (Chapter 38) also encode SH proteins. In each case, SH is a transmembrane virion envelope protein with an externally oriented C-terminus. SH can be deleted without much effect on the magnitude of virus replication *in vitro.* However, deletion of SH from recombinant PIV5 resulted in increased cytopathology in cell culture due to increased apoptosis, although overall replication was not reduced, and the virus was attenuated *in vivo.*[139,229] Further results indicated that infection with the ΔSH virus was associated with increased production of, and signaling by, tumor necrosis factor α, leading to the observed increase in apoptosis.[229]

Antigenic Composition and Determinants

Postinfection sera from animals and humans contain antibodies against most or all of the major PIV proteins. However, the HN and F proteins are the only antigens that have been shown to induce antibodies that neutralize infectivity, and they have been shown to be major independent protective antigens. *In vivo,* the parenteral administration of polyclonal or monoclonal antibodies specific to SeV HN or F mediated resistance to challenge with SeV.[302] Sera obtained from children following HPIV3 infection that contain antibodies specific to the HN and F proteins have been shown to have virus-neutralizing activity.[185] Infection of rodents with vaccinia virus recombinants expressing the HPIV3 HN or F glycoprotein, or immunization with purified HN and F glycoprotein, showed that either protein induced a high level of resistance to HPIV3 challenge, with HN being more protective than F.[7,33,303,345]

The "internal" PIV proteins also induce a protective response. This was demonstrated in experiments in hamsters using a recombinant version of HPIV3 in which the HN and F surface antigen genes were replaced by those of HPIV1. This made it possible to compare the relative contributions of the "internal" proteins and the surface glycoproteins to protection.[363] The HN and F proteins induced a high level of protection (in this case specific to HPIV1) that was long-lived. In contrast, the HPIV3-specific protection attributed to the internal proteins—which presumably was mediated by major histocompatibility class I-restricted, CD8+ cytotoxic T lymphocytes (CTLs)—was weaker and waned over a period of several months.[363] This suggests that cellular immunity can contribute significantly to protection for a short period following infection, but is not effective in providing long-term protection.

Antibodies to HN can be measured by HI and neuraminidase-inhibition (NI) assays, which are based on the ability of the antibodies to block these activities of purified virions *in vitro.* Antibodies specific to the F protein can also be measured by inhibition of syncytium formation (fusion inhibition, FI) in cell culture, as well as by inhibition of hemolysis of erythrocytes by purified virions *in vitro.* However, since F activity also depends upon HN; as already noted, HN-specific antibodies also inhibit these activities.

The antigenic sites in the HN protein of HPIV3 were investigated by competitive-binding assays with pair-wise combinations of MAbs.[384] Six antigenic sites were defined; five of the sites (A, B, D, E, and F) did not overlap, whereas site C overlapped sites A and B. Three of the sites (A, B, and C) reacted with MAbs that neutralize virus and inhibit hemagglutination.[61] Amino acid residues important for the structures of the neutralization epitopes of HPIV3 HN were identified by sequence analysis of neutralization-resistant mutants selected with MAbs to sites A, B, or C (see Fig. 34.4).[60] Each of the mutants sustained a single amino acid substitution that in most cases was located in the C-terminal half of the molecule. Different MAbs directed to the same site selected amino acid sequence substitutions that were widely separated on the HN molecule, suggesting that these sites are formed by juxtaposition of distant regions in the folded structure. Consistent with this interpretation is the observation that boiling and reduction of the HN protein of HPIV3 or NDV markedly reduced reactivity with a panel of MAbs, and that neutralization epitopes could not be mimicked by synthetic peptides.[144] Many of the antigenic sites defined by the murine MAbs for HPIV3 HN (and F) are recognized by antibodies in postinfection human sera.[386]

The antigenic and functional organization of the HPIV3 F protein was elucidated by the same strategy. Competitive binding of a panel of HPIV3 F-specific MAbs identified seven nonoverlapping antigenic sites (A to F) and one site (AB) that bridged sites A and B.[61] Neutralizing MAbs reacted with sites A, B, C, and AB, and at least some of the neutralizing MAbs represented by each site also inhibited fusion. The remaining sites reacted with MAbs that did not neutralize infectivity or inhibit fusion, and site A also reacted with a nonneutralizing MAb. Sequence analysis of neutralization-resistant mutants selected with individual MAbs showed that they contained single amino acid substitutions; those representing sites A or

B contained substitutions located in both the F_1 and F_2 subunits (Fig. 34.5).[61,382] As was the case with the HN protein, this suggests that distant regions of the linear protein are folded into proximity to create antigenic sites. Consistent with this, F-specific MAbs that neutralize infectivity and inhibit fusion usually do not react efficiently with denatured F protein, such as in Western blots.

The primary antibody response to HPIV1, HPIV2, and HPIV3 is relatively specific to the infecting virus, consistent with their status as distinct serotypes.[92] Although HPIV1, HPIV2, and HPIV3 each appear to be monotypic based on reactivity with postinfection sera, antigenic polymorphism within serotypes can be detected with MAbs. For example, analysis of 38 HPIV3 strains recovered over a 26-year interval in widely separated locations (United States and Australia) indicated that 6 of the 11 neutralization epitopes on HN, as well as 3 of 14 such epitopes on F, were completely conserved among all strains.[60,61] The observed variation in HN and F neutralization epitopes did not seem to involve progressive accumulation of changes with time because variation detected in early isolates was not consistently conserved in later strains. Rather, it appears that the heterogeneity that exists results from random mutations that are not subject to strong immunologic selective pressure.[61] Sequence analysis of HPIV1, HPIV2, and NDV has documented the apparent progressive accumulation of sequence differences, resulting in distinct "lineages," but antigenic changes have been noncumulative and nonprogressive, and they do not correlate with the genetic lineages.[147,301,316] Conversely, the detection of subgroups of APMV2, APMV3, and APMV6 that can be distinguished by reactivity with postinfection sera suggests that immune-driven divergent evolution can occur.[214,352,402] The introduction of a vaccine against any of the HPIVs will provide an opportunity to evaluate the capability of circulating virus to accumulate antigenic differences compared to the vaccine strain.

Healthy adult humans tested for memory CD8+ CTL against HPIV1 demonstrated strong responses to HN, P, and N, a weak response to M, and an insignificant response to F in this particular subject group.[78] CTL lines that had been stimulated *in vitro* with HPIV1 showed high reactivity with the closely related SeV, and several cell lines recognized an N peptide that was conserved between HPIV1 and SeV. Remarkably, lower but clearly demonstrable reactivity also was detected against HPIV3 by the HPIV1-stimulated lines. Therefore, the human CTL response is directed against multiple HPIV proteins (as would be expected), and cross-reactivity between serotypes can occur.

Propagation and Assay of HPIVs in Cell Culture

The HPIVs grow well in primary simian or human kidney cell cultures, which allows efficient recovery of these viruses from clinical specimens. They also grow well and can be recovered in a number of established cell lines, including LLC-MK2 rhesus monkey kidney, Vero African green monkey kidney, and NCI-H292 human lung carcinoma cells.[41] Growth of HPIV1 and HPIV4, but not HPIV2 or HPIV3, requires the addition of trypsin (1–5 μg/ml) to the medium for cleavage of the F_0 protein. Virus infection of cultured cells can be monitored by hemadsorption or by immunofluorescence staining. HPIV2 and HPIV3 produce a cytopathic effect that is characterized by syncytia formation, particularly in heteroploid cell lines, whereas that of HPIV1 and HPIV4 is less. HPIV3 can readily be quantitated by plaque assay or by limiting dilution and direct observation of cytopathology, whereas plaque production or growth following limiting dilution by the other HPIVs usually is visualized by hemadsorption or immunostaining. Typical yields in tissue culture for HPIV1, HPIV2, and HPIV3 are 10^7 to 10^8 50% tissue culture infectious dose ($TCID_{50}$) per milliliter of medium, whereas replication of HPIV4 is substantially less efficient.[41]

The ability of a PIV to replicate efficiently in a given cell culture depends in part on whether it can interfere with type I IFN production and signaling in that particular host. For example, SeV efficiently blocks IFN production and signaling in mouse cells and efficiently grows in those cells. In contrast, PIV5 does not efficiently antagonize the IFN system in murine cells, and growth is inefficient; however, efficient growth is achieved if IFN is depleted by adding IFN-specific antibodies to the medium or if the cells are from a genetically manipulated mouse that lacks the type I IFN receptor.[84] Typically, a virus can antagonize the IFN system in its native host but not necessarily in heterologous hosts.

The Nature of Cell Injury

The nature of cell injury *in vivo* is not fully understood and seems to involve different pathways for different PIVs. Some viruses, particularly PIV5, can cause a persistent, productive infection in primary cell culture that does not kill cells or shut off cellular RNA or protein synthesis.[57] In contrast, syncytia formation leading to cell death is a prominent feature of infection of monolayer cell cultures with HPIV2 or HPIV3. As noted, a number of viral products, including the C, V, and SH accessory proteins and the SeV trailer RNA, modulate and reduce cytopathology by inhibiting apoptosis and preventing activation of PKR that otherwise inhibits translation. In some situations, the persistence of PIV5 may also be related to its ability to form cytoplasmic bodies that sequester viral nucleocapsids and may provide for prolonged low-grade infection.[40]

Recently, the characteristics of HPIV infection were studied in a culture system of primary human airway cells that are differentiated into a pseudostratified mucociliary epithelium that closely models the epithelium of the conducting airways (Fig. 34.6).[411] HPIV3 infection was highly specific to ciliated cells on the apical surface of the tissue, and virus release occurred exclusively from the same face. Interestingly, there was no evidence of cell-to-cell fusion or spread to underlying cells, and the tissue remained intact over the 2-week duration of the experiment,[411] in contrast to influenza A virus, which was rapidly cytopathic in this system.[412] Therefore, HPIV3 is not inherently a highly cytotoxic virus. Similar observations have been made with HPIV1 and HPIV2 infections in this *in vitro* model,[15,323] as well as with HRSV (Chapter 38).[412] It may be that much of the cytopathology observed *in vivo* is the result of the host response to infected cells rather than direct viral damage. When the HPIV3-infected cultures were maintained over a course of 2 weeks, most of the infected cells were shed into the medium, possibly by an acceleration of the normal mechanism of cell shedding and replacement. In addition, there was a substantial increase in mucin-containing cells, which is consistent with the increased mucus production observed in infected individuals.

In the *in vitro* model of human airway epithelium, the lack of cell-to-cell fusion appeared to be a consequence of the

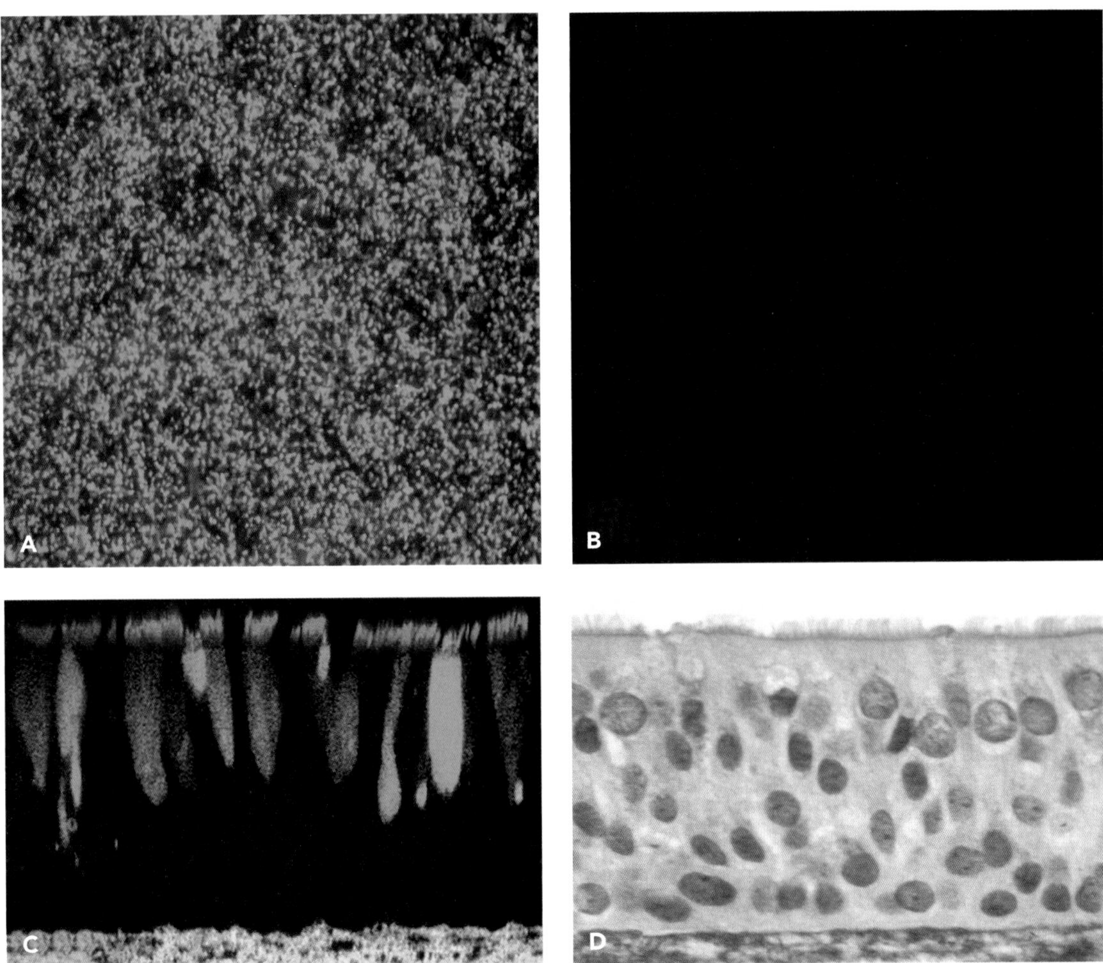

FIGURE 34.6. **Infection of an *in vitro* model of human airway epithelium by HPIV3.** Primary cultures of human airway epithelium, consisting of pseudostratified mucociliary tissue that closely resembles authentic airway epithelium, were infected with approximately 3 plaque-forming units (PFU) per cell of recombinant HPIV3 expressing green fluorescent protein (GFP) from an added gene and were viewed 48 hours postinfection. **A** and **B**: GFP expression in cultures that were infected on the **(A)** apical or **(B)** basolateral surface, viewed *en face* (i.e., from the top) by fluorescence microscopy at low magnification. **C** and **D**: Cross sectional images of infected cultures at higher magnification. **C**: Fluorescence microscopy reveals GFP-expressing parainfluenza virus 3 (PIV3)–infected cells, with counterstaining by antibodies against β-tubulin to identify cilia (*red*). **D**: Infected cells stained with hematoxylin and eosin, illustrating the lack of syncytia and cytopathic effects.[411] Bar, 20 μm.

tightly polarized nature of the apical cells: surface expression of the F glycoprotein was localized to the apical surface and probably was restricted from contact with neighboring cells. Therefore, the syncytium formation that is prominent in nonpolarized monolayer cultures might not be significant in the airway epithelium. Whether it occurs in the alveolar epithelium is unknown. In humans, the pathology of fatal HPIV disease usually does not include giant-cell formation unless the patient has a severe defect in T-lymphocyte function[82,171] or is profoundly immunosuppressed.[395]

Infection of HPIVs in Experimental Animals and Other Laboratory Hosts

Hamsters are readily infected by HPIV1, HPIV2, or HPIV3 and support moderate levels of virus replication. However, infection usually is asymptomatic, and pulmonary pathology is minimal or undetectable. Guinea pigs, cotton rats, and ferrets also undergo a semipermissive silent infection with these viruses, but mice are poorly permissive. Chimpanzees and a variety of monkeys can be infected with HPIV1, HPIV2, and HPIV3, but only HPIV3 has been reported to cause symptomatic illness that sometimes occurs in both chimpanzees and African green monkeys.[59,92] The absence of significant disease in most experimental animals is associated with limited virus replication.

Some strains of HPIV1, HPIV2, or HPIV3 replicate in the embryonated chicken egg, whereas others do not, and eggs are less reliable and sensitive for the isolation of virus from patients than are monkey kidney cells.

Genetics and Reverse Genetics

As is typical for RNA viruses, PIVs have a high rate of nucleotide misincorporation of approximately 10^{-3} to 10^{-4}. This provides the potential for rapid evolution and, indeed, PIVs readily "evolve" under selective pressure *in vitro*.[133] However, these viruses appear to evolve very slowly in nature. For example, the HPIV3 F and HN glycoproteins have undergone little variation (1.5% to 2.4% amino acid sequence differences) since the first strain was recovered from humans.[61] With NDV, sequence analysis of the F and HN genes from strains collected over a 50-year period identified what appeared to be the progressive accumulation of a small number of sequence changes, but these did not correlate with antigenic differences and overall the sequences remained highly conserved.[316,373]

Like other paramyxoviruses, PIVs readily produce defective interfering (DI) particles when virus is passaged *in vitro* at high multiplicities of infection.[304] DI genomes contain large deletions created by polymerase jumping during RNA replication. The polymerase can reinitiate further down the genome to produce an internally deleted molecule containing unaltered 3′ and 5′ ends, or, more commonly, can reinitiate on the nascent strand to produce a copy-back RNA in which the ends are exact complements. In either case, DI genomes lack most or all of the viral genes, are dependent on complementation by standard virus, and interfere with its replication. For this reason, care is taken to avoid high-multiplicity passage of PIVs. DI particles have been proposed to be a mechanism of downregulating standard virus replication based on their effects in cell culture, but the significance of this for infections *in vivo* is unclear. Copy-back DI genomes of SeV have been shown to be highly effective inducers of type I IFN, and the presence of such DI particles in PIV vaccine preparations may increase immunogenicity due to the adjuvant effect of IFN.[16,349] In addition, copy-back DI genomes typically have antigenomic promoters on both the positive and negative strands and are particularly active in expressing the anti-apoptotic trailer-RNA noted above, which may aid virus infection and viral persistence.

It is generally thought that recombination between coinfecting viruses to produce mosaic genomes containing segments from each parent is very rare for *Mononegavirales*.[50,295,316] Early attempts to demonstrate the generation of a mosaic recombinant virus during mixed infections, such as with NDV, were unsuccessful.[77,126,127] A mosaic virus has been produced experimentally only once for *Mononegavirales*, with HRSV.[343] However, there have been reports of viral genomes with sequence discontinuities that may be indicative of RNA recombination.[63] Among the PIVs, this has been noted in particular for NDV, perhaps because the widespread use of live vaccines provides the potential for recombination with endemic wild strains.[56,135,141,298] This evidence remains indirect, and at least some of the cases were found to be PCR artifacts rather than real mosaic genomes.[341] Recombination probably is a rare event that occurs mostly between closely related viruses, and there is no evidence that it is an important force in PIV evolution.[50,63,316]

Complete infectious PIV can be produced entirely from cloned complementary DNA (cDNA) by the reverse genetics strategy that has been developed for *Mononegavirales*.[93,138,267,285,325,337,351] This involves transfecting cells with plasmids that express an RNA copy of the genome or antigenome together with the N, P, and L proteins. These components assemble into a nucleocapsid that launches a productive infection. Reverse genetics provides a method to engineer predetermined changes into infectious virus for use in a variety of studies, including vaccine development.

A second type of reverse genetics system involves minireplicons, which are short cDNA-encoded versions of genomic or antigenomic RNA. In some cases, the minireplicons are modeled after DI genomes; in other cases they resemble genomic RNA in which the viral genes have been replaced by one or more marker genes such as luciferase.[94,365] When complemented by the appropriate mix of viral proteins supplied by co-transfected plasmids, the minireplicon is encapsidated and undergoes efficient RNA replication and transcription and packaging. A minireplicon system has advantages for detailed mutational analysis of *cis*-acting RNA signals or *trans*-acting viral proteins because of its smaller, simpler construction and because mutations that might have drastic effects on infectious virus can be studied in this transient system.

Natural Histories of the Animal PIVs

As noted, SeV was first detected in mice that had been inoculated with material from a fatal case of pediatric pneumonia, but the virus is recognized as a pathogen of rodents rather than humans.[264] SeV replicates and causes disease in the respiratory tract of mice, and also readily infects hamsters, guinea pigs, and rats. SeV has been detected in mouse colonies worldwide, but is infrequently detected in wild mice, which makes its natural history somewhat unclear.[101,281] In addition, SeV has been recovered from pigs experiencing outbreaks of influenza-like disease, but pigs are not thought to be a natural host.[101] In experimental infections, SeV replicated in the respiratory tract of African green monkeys and chimpanzees with an efficiency similar to that of HPIV1, and thus may not have a substantial host range restriction in primates.[335] This raises the possibility that SeV can initiate zoonotic infections in humans, which is one possible explanation for its original isolation from a human autopsy specimen. However, if this indeed ever occurred, it appears to be a rare event. The virus was well tolerated when administered experimentally to healthy adult humans,[339] although it is not clear whether this reflects restriction by host range or by HPIV1-specific immunity present in most adults. SeV presently is being developed as a potential vaccine vector for human use,[164,410] as a vector for gene therapy in the airway,[129] and as an oncolytic agent.[176]

BPIV3 is a common cause of respiratory infections in cattle, and usually is associated with mild disease. However, it can promote secondary bacterial infection resulting in severe respiratory disease (shipping fever). Both inactivated and live attenuated vaccines against BPIV3 are available. BPIV3 is highly restricted in rhesus monkeys[333] and in humans,[128] in which it has been evaluated as a potential live vaccine against HPIV3 (see Prevention and Control). The host range restriction of BPIV3 was investigated using reverse genetics to exchange each gene of HPIV3 with its counterpart from BPIV3. Evaluation of the resulting chimeras in rhesus monkeys showed that all of the BPIV3 genes contribute to the host range restriction, with N and P (the latter including all of the multiple ORFs) making the greatest contribution.[333]

PIV5 is a natural pathogen of dogs[21,22] and causes acute self-limiting tracheobronchitis with the potential to progress to pneumonia, particularly since infection can promote opportunistic bacterial infection. In addition, PIV5 was recovered from a dog with posterior paralysis in 1978, and this isolate was neurotropic and caused acute encephalitis when inoculated intracerebrally in gnotobiotic puppies.[17] Vaccination of puppies against PIV5 is routine. Although PIV5 was first isolated as a contaminant of primary rhesus monkey kidney cells, it does not appear to infect monkeys in the wild.[157] However, captive monkeys readily seroconvert, implying that they are exposed to the virus during captivity, perhaps by human handlers. When inoculated intranasally into nonhuman primates, PIV5 was shed from the upper and lower respiratory tract for a week with mild or no illness. In some animals, the virus was reported to be isolated from the kidneys up to 113 days postinfection, although no viremia was detected.[157] PIV5 also has been isolated from the lungs of a stillborn piglet.[143]

PIV5 has reportedly been isolated from a variety of human tissues, leading some researchers to suggest that the virus naturally infects humans and may establish persistent infections.[51,120,121,157] PIV5 also has reportedly been detected in association with a number of human diseases ranging from the common cold to neurologic diseases (multiple sclerosis, subacute panencephalitis, and Creutzfeldt-Jakob disease). However, infection and possible persistence of PIV5 in humans remain to be clearly demonstrated, and the virus has not been clearly associated with any human disease.[51] Detection of PIV5-specific antibodies in human populations is confounded by its antigenic relatedness to common human pathogens such as HPIV2 and MuV. In addition, the ability of PIV5 to readily contaminate cell cultures raises doubts about reports of its detection and possible association with various diseases. Therefore, the possible status of PIV5 as a common infectious agent in humans—either benign or pathogenic—remains unresolved but is generally considered unlikely. Comparison of partial genome sequences of PIV isolates from human, canine, simian, and porcine sources did not reveal any striking differences, and the isolates did not differ in the species specificity of their IFN antagonists.[51] This suggests that these isolates represent a single viral species rather than a series of host-specific relatives. PIV5 is presently being investigated as a possible vaccine vector for human use,[371] although the unresolved issue of possible long-term infections in humans should be cause for caution.

Evidence of PIV infection in an unexpected host must be viewed critically. As noted, antigenic cross-reactivity between PIVs complicates serologic studies. The high prevalence of circulating PIVs in human and animal populations raises the possibility of contamination of tissue specimens and cell cultures, leading to false "isolations." For example, antigens to HPIV1 and HPIV3—in addition to PIV5—were reported in a large fraction of bone marrow cell specimens,[120] indicating either that all three viruses persistently infect bone marrow cells (which seems unlikely), or that contamination had occurred. In addition, PIVs in general are highly infectious and sometimes can readily infect other species that are not necessarily natural hosts. An APMV2-like virus was isolated from cynomolgus monkeys with respiratory tract disease.[217] An APMV3-like virus was isolated from pigs in Israel.[231] Nonhuman primates are readily infected in captivity with HPIVs from their handlers. A paramyxovirus isolated from a wild Samango monkey was shown by sequence analysis to be HPIV3, and did not exhibit any evidence of divergence compared to a number of human isolates and thus likely was a virus of human rather than simian origin.[212] HPIV3 was isolated from a pig with respiratory tract disease, and serologic studies provided evidence of infection on some farms.[125] More recently, analysis of PIV-like isolates from swine indicated that they were variants of BPIV3 that infected swine but did not become established in that host.[297] Taken together, these incidents suggest that the PIVs, being highly prevalent and infectious viruses, sometimes can infect and cause disease in certain nonnatural hosts without becoming established.

As noted, SV41 is a relative of HPIV2 and PIV5 that was isolated from cynomolgus monkey kidney cell cultures. Its natural history remains unclear. When SV41 was inoculated intracerebrally into suckling mice, adult mice, hamsters, guinea pigs, 2-week-old chicks, and rhesus monkeys, it caused central nervous system disease signs in all of the animals and killed most of them.[251] Approximately 2% of tested human sera had antibodies that reacted with SV41, which was confirmed by immunoprecipitation of the SV41 HN protein by positive sera. This raises the possibility that the virus may sometimes infect humans.[271] The natural host(s) for SV41 remains unknown.

NDV (APMV1) is among the most important pathogens of poultry worldwide.[317] As noted, the many isolates or strains of NDV exhibit a broad spectrum of virulence. Vaccines against NDV are in widespread use, and North America, Australia, and New Zealand are relatively free of the disease.[317] Velogenic and mesogenic strains of NDV are classified by the Centers for Disease Control and Prevention (CDC) and the U.S. Department of Agriculture (USDA) as Select Agents—necessitating strict regulation of the possession and transfer of the virus—due to the potential risk for poultry farming. NDV infects more than 240 species of birds, with disease varying greatly depending on the virus strain and the host species. In addition, NDV can infect humans, particularly poultry farmers or laboratory workers working with the virus, but usually causes only mild conjunctivitis.[39] However, NDV was the apparent etiologic agent of fatal pneumonia in an adult who had been a recipient of a peripheral blood stem-cell transplant and as a consequence had increased susceptibility to infection.[119] There are no reports of human-to-human infection. NDV can replicate in the respiratory tract of nonhuman primates, but is highly restricted.[35,36] Lentogenic and mesogenic strains of NDV are being developed as vaccine vectors to express the protective antigens of other agricultural pathogens[114,160,266,280] and human pathogens.[35,36,86,87] In addition, NDV is being developed as a potential oncolytic agent.[96,97,99,296,389]

Eight other serotypes (serotypes 2–9) of APMV have been identified based on antigenic differences measured by HI and NI assays,[317] and as noted there is new evidence for an additional, 10th serotype.[250] Some serotypes exhibit limited cross-reaction and cross-protection, such as between serotypes 1 and 3. APMV serotypes 2 to 9 have been isolated worldwide from various wild and domesticated birds, although their natural histories are generally unknown. APMV serotypes 2, 3, 6, and 7 have been associated with mild disease in poultry, whereas the others have not been associated with poultry disease. There is serologic evidence in commercial poultry for all of the APMV serotypes except for 5 and 10, although this analysis may be complicated by cross-reactivity and the use of NDV vaccines.[391] As noted, complete genome sequences have been determined for one or more representatives of each APMV serotype.

PATHOGENESIS AND PATHOLOGY

The HPIVs replicate in epithelial cells that line the respiratory tract, causing rhinitis, pharyngitis, laryngitis, tracheobronchitis, bronchiolitis, and pneumonia (Table 34.5). Early during HPIV infection, the mucous membranes of the nose and throat are involved. Obstruction of the paranasal sinuses and eustachian tube may also occur and lead to sinusitis and otitis media. Many

TABLE 34.5 Infections[a] Caused by Parainfluenza, Influenza, or Respiratory Syncytial Virus in Pediatric Inpatients[b]

		Patients with evidence of infection with virus indicated (%)							
Illness	**No. tested**	**HRSV**	**HPIV3**	**HPIV1**	**HPIV2**	**Any HPIV[c]**	**Flu A H2N2[c]**	**Flu A[d] H3N2**	**Flu B**
Pneumonia	1,162–1,742	25.0	11.2	3.5	1.6	14.4	3.5	5.4	1.0
Bronchiolitis	873–1,186	43.1	9.4	2.4	1.1	10.9	0.9	2.5	0.4
Croup	593–776	9.8	18.3	20.3	12.2	41.4	7.7	24.1	1.9
Pharyngitis/bronchitis	895–1,337	10.6	11.0	3.7	2.0	14.7	2.0	4.6	0.9
Total respiratory	3,523–5,104	23.3	11.5	6.0	3.2	17.9	3.2	7.1	1.0
Inpatient control	1,237–2,155	5.4	5.0	1.9	1.2	7.5	0.5	0.9	0.5

[a]Infection documented by virus isolation and/or a complement-fixing antibody response.

[b]Studies performed at Children's Hospital National Medical Center from 1957 to 1976.[194,195,260] Data were summarized by Murphy et al.[260]

[c]Tested from 1957 to 1968.

[d]Tested from 1968 to 1976.

HPIV, human parainfluenza virus; HRSV, human respiratory syncytial virus.

patients with mild disease may have limited involvement of the bronchi as well. In more extensive infections there is a tendency for HPIV1 and HPIV2 to involve the larynx and upper trachea, resulting in the croup syndrome; such infections may extend also to the lower trachea and bronchi, with accumulation of inspissated mucus and resultant atelectasis and pneumonia.[283] When HPIV3 produces severe disease, infection of the small air passages is likely, with the development of bronchopneumonia, bronchiolitis, and/or bronchitis.[283,397]

An intensive longitudinal study of infants and children in a semiclosed nursery indicated that 80% of individuals undergoing primary infection with HPIV3 developed a febrile illness; in one third of the illnesses, there was involvement of the lower respiratory tract, resulting in either pneumonia or bronchiolitis.[46] When infants and children were studied less intensively in a family setting, the estimate for lower respiratory tract involvement during primary HPIV3 infection was 13%.[118] Longitudinal nursery studies also indicated that one half of initial HPIV1 infections and two thirds of initial HPIV2 infections produced a febrile illness.[46] Lower respiratory tract involvement also occurs commonly during primary HPIV1 infection; about 25% of primary infections produced bronchitis or pneumonia.[117] Severe acute laryngotracheobronchitis (croup), which is the most dramatic and serious manifestation of initial HPIV infection, was noted in only 2% to 3% of primary HPIV1 or HPIV2 infections in longitudinal studies of healthy children,[46,116] although HPIV1 and HPIV2 are the major etiologic agents detected among children who develop croup.

The magnitude of viral replication *in vivo* in the natural host appears to be a major factor in pathogenesis. For example, clinical trials of two candidate live-attenuated HPIV3 vaccines indicated that a virus that was highly restricted in replication was well-tolerated in young children, whereas a virus that was less restricted in replication produced fever and LRI in some vaccinees.[19,184] Similar observations have been made with HRSV vaccines.[182]

A possible role of the immune response in pathogenesis was suggested by the observation that infants and children who develop croup associated with HPIV infection produce local, virus-specific immunoglobulin E (IgE) antibodies earlier and in larger amount than patients of comparable age with HPIV URI.[396] In addition, histamine is detected in nasopharyngeal secretions of croup patients more often than in secretions from patients with URI caused by the same virus.[396] Based on these observations, it was proposed that more rapid and increased production of HPIV-specific IgE antibodies mediates histamine release in the trachea and the subglottic region, which in turn produces the symptoms of croup.[396] However, it is not clear whether a more pronounced virus-specific IgE response plays a role in pathogenesis of croup or whether it merely reflects more extensive production of viral antigens and consequent increased antibody response during severe disease. Measurement of proinflammatory cytokines in nasal washes obtained from children with HPIV infections demonstrated increased levels of interleukin 6 (IL-6), CC chemokine ligand (CCL)3, CCL4, CCL5, CXC chemokine ligand (CXCL)8, and CXCL9 compared to nasal washes from control subjects, and increased levels of CXCL8 in children with HPIV LRI compared to those with URI.[95] Cell-mediated immune responses to HPIV antigens, as well as HPIV-specific IgE antibody responses, have also been reported to be greater among infants with HPIV bronchiolitis than among infected infants who developed only URI.[396] These observations have been interpreted as evidence for a role of immunologic factors in HPIV bronchiolitis, but the caveat cited before also applies. Infection of epithelial cells with HPIV2 was reported to increase adhesion of, and concomitant cell damage by, neutrophils, suggesting another potential factor in immune-mediated pathology.[372]

PIVs have been used in a number of animal models to study airway responsiveness to various stimuli following infection. In the guinea pig, which undergoes a brief, self-limited, and asymptomatic bronchiolitis after intratracheal inoculation of BPIV3, hyperresponsiveness to both histamine and a choline receptor agonist, arecoline, was seen from day 4 until day 16 after infection.[103] The effect lasted through the full recovery of the epithelium but was accompanied by airway hypercellularity and depletion of mucosal mast cells. Similar responses to PIV5 have been observed in beagle puppies.[226]

Older children or adolescents who had severe croup as infants or young children may exhibit bronchial hyperactivity following exercise or inhalation of methylcholine.[131,234] It is not known whether heightened airway reactivity is a preexisting condition that contributes to the pathogenesis of croup or whether inflammatory damage during croup produces a prolonged state of increased reactivity. Clearly, an enhanced IgE and histamine response would assume greater importance if preexisting heightened airway reactivity, especially in the trachea and subglottic region, played a role in pathogenesis of croup.

The susceptibility of an individual to severe disease probably is influenced by that individual's genetic background. Studies with HRSV indicate that genetic differences in IL-4, IL-8, and other aspects of host immunity may be associated with a greater frequency of severe disease (see Chapter 38).[252] The same may be true for the HPIVs.

Microscopic pathology is not well defined, as very few fatal cases of HPIV disease have been studied. Syncytium formation was observed in the lungs of two infants with severe immune deficiency who died of HPIV3 pneumonia; however, syncytium formation is not a feature of fatal HPIV disease occurring in immunocompetent individuals.[3,82,90] As with HRSV bronchiolitis, the pathogenesis of HPIV3 bronchiolitis in young infants may involve mechanical events, such as mucus plugging and air trapping in the distal airways, but this has not been clearly defined.

The cleavage-activation of the F_0 precursor can be a major determinant of virulence for NDV, with the presence of a polybasic sequence containing the favored furin cleavage site (R-X-R/K-R↓) being associated with the ability to spread beyond the respiratory and enteric tracts and cause increased disease.[262] For example, natural outbreaks of virulent NDV in Australia in 1998 to 2000 appeared to arise from a low-virulence strain by mutation at the F_0 cleavage site that introduced a furin motif, R-R-Q-G-R↓L to R-R-S/Q-R-R↓F.[124] Serial passage of avirulent NDV strains in chicken eggs and brain resulted in the progressive mutation to a polybasic/furin cleavage site and the acquisition of a highly virulent phenotype.[81,329] Mutation by reverse genetics of the cleavage site in avirulent NDV to be polybasic with a furin motif resulted in a dramatic increase in viral virulence.[279,285,309] However, in this latter case, the engineered strains did not gain the full velogenic phenotype, suggesting that other factors contributed to the difference between the lentogenic and velogenic phenotypes. Other studies have found instances where the cleavage site sequence did not predict the virulence phenotype. For example, highly virulent NDV strains from China have been described with the nonfurin cleavage sequence G-R-Q-G-R↓L.[362] Conversely, some strains from Africa had cleavage sequences containing the furin motif (R-R-Q-K-R↓F) and yet were isolated from healthy chickens,[328] and NDV strains from pigeons with a polybasic/furin cleavage site R-R-K-K-R↓F were avirulent.[88a] Recent studies of the other APMV serotypes have provided additional examples of incongruity between the F_0 protein cleavage site sequence and viral virulence.[317] For example, APMV2 has a nonfurin cleavage sequence (D-K-P-A-S-R↓F) and is avirulent in chickens, and mutation of this site into a variety of polybasic/furin sequences resulted in substantially increased replication *in vitro* but did not increase the virulence of the virus in chickens.[351] Therefore, the presence of a furin motif at the cleavage site can be a major determinant of APMV virulence in some situations but not others. The presence of phenylalanine versus leucine or isoleucine as the first residue of the F1 subunit also has been suggested to be associated with intracellular cleavage[254] and pathogenesis,[191] but there are many exceptions to this association, some of which include examples noted above.

SeV is another PIV that depends on secreted protease for cleavage of its F_0 protein. SeV is considered to be strictly pneumotropic in mice, and the basis for this phenotype was investigated using a mutant, F1-R, which had acquired the ability to cause systemic infection.[277,367,368] Characterization of F1-R and a series of related mutants identified the following three acquired abilities that were necessary in combination for the pantropic phenotype: (a) the ability of F_0 to be cleaved intracellularly, due to mutations near the cleavage site; (b) the ability of the virus to bud from the basolateral surface in addition to the normal apical budding, due to mutations in M; and (c) the ability of the virus to cause depolymerization of microtubules, which also mapped to M.[277,367] The acquisition of intracellular cleavability was sufficient to confer the pantropic phenotype if the virus was administered systemically, confirming the idea that intracellular cleavability confers the ability to replicate widely. The further requirement for basolateral budding provides for delivery of the virus into subepithelial tissues and into the blood, providing for escape from the respiratory tract. It is not yet understood how microtubule depolymerization is related to the pantropic phenotype.

It is not clear how directly one can extrapolate from these observations made with animal PIVs to the HPIVs. For example, it is tempting to speculate that the ability of the F_0 protein of HPIV3 to be cleaved intracellularly, in contrast to HPIV1, might explain the greater predilection of HPIV3 to cause pneumonia. This could be evaluated experimentally by altering F_0 cleavability in recombinant virus. It also is not clear whether other determinants, such as polarity of budding, are significant for the HPIVs. HPIV3 buds exclusively from the apical surface and generally is pneumotropic. However, it readily spreads beyond the respiratory tract under suitable conditions. This was demonstrated experimentally by studies in which immunosuppression of HPIV3-infected cotton rats resulted in dissemination of the virus and productive infection in other organs (G. A. Prince, B. R. Murphy, and R. M. Chanock, unpublished observations). HPIV3 viremia also has been reported during infection of untreated hamsters.[173] Similarly, in children with severe combined immunodeficiency disease, systemic, fatal infection with HPIV3 has occurred, with dissemination to the liver, myocardium, and cerebrospinal fluid.[102,106] The rare isolation of HPIV3 from cerebrospinal fluid associated with aseptic meningitis in infants and children,[68] and a single case report of HPIV3 viremia in humans, also indicates that these viruses can (rarely) disseminate from the respiratory tract in immunocompetent individuals. Therefore, host immunity, rather than viral tropism, seems to be a major factor in restricting HPIV3 to the respiratory tract.

Other factors involved in the differences in virulence among the NDV strains have also been identified. Reciprocal swaps of the HN protein between a virulent and an avirulent strain showed that the HN of the latter was associated with reduced receptor recognition, reduced neuraminidase activity, and reduced virulence, indicating that HN can contribute to tissue tropism and virulence.[162] However, in another study, swaps involving HN from a velogenic strain did not confer increased virulence,[98] suggesting that the contribution of HN depends on the strain. Other studies identified contributions to strain-specific differences in virulence by the NDV N, P, V, L, and, to a lesser extent, M protein.[4,89,310] A limited comparison of virulent and avirulent strains of NDV indicated that reduced virulence was associated with reduced viral RNA synthesis.[238]

IMMUNITY

PIV infections of experimental animals and adults induce potent systemic and local humoral and cellular responses. However, immune responses to HPIV infections in infants and very young children are qualitatively and quantitatively deficient. For example, young infants undergoing primary infection with wild-type HPIV produce local nasal IgA antibodies that neutralize virus infectivity poorly or not at all,[404] and infants infected with live-attenuated HPIV3 vaccines exhibit reduced serum antibody responses to the HN glycoprotein compared to older infants and children.[180] This is likely the result of immunologic immaturity, which is most evident during the first 6 months of life,[70] and suppression of the humoral response to virus infection by maternally derived, virus-specific serum antibodies present in young infants.[70] The production of poorly neutralizing local antibodies and the poor serum antibody response in this young age group may partially explain why symptomatic reinfection (especially with HPIV3) occurs during early childhood.

The ability of serum neutralizing antibodies to confer resistance to pulmonary replication by PIVs has been well documented in experimental animals, where parenteral administration of polyclonal or monoclonal virus-neutralizing antibodies conferred a high level of resistance to virus replication in the lower respiratory tract and a lower level of resistance in the upper respiratory tract.[278,303] Studies of HRSV have demonstrated that significant resistance in the respiratory tract requires high titers of serum antibodies (approximately 1:390 and 1:3,500 for 99% reduction of virus titer in the lungs and nasal turbinates, respectively, of cotton rats),[294,330] and this likely also is the case for HPIVs. High titers of serum antibodies are likely required because there is no specific mechanism for transporting serum IgG to the mucosal surface of the lumen of the respiratory tract.

In a longitudinal study of HPIV3 outbreaks in infants and young children residing in a semiclosed nursery, preexisting serum neutralizing antibodies correlated with resistance to infection and illness.[46] However, resistance associated with serum neutralizing antibodies was only partial. One third of infants and children with a high serum antibody level became infected. Although reinfection occurred, a partial effect of immunity from previous infection was indicated by a shorter period of virus shedding compared to that observed during primary infection. Moderate levels of serum antibody were not associated with complete protection against febrile illness, which occurred approximately 40% as often as during first infection. A somewhat greater reduction of LRI was observed during second infections with HPIV3 in a longitudinal family study.[118]

The protective effect of serum antibodies against the HPIVs is also suggested by the relative sparing of young infants—who possess serum IgG antibodies acquired passively from their mother—from HPIV infection and associated disease. For example, the risk of infection with HPIV3 during the first 4 months of life is inversely related, in the aggregate, to the level of neutralizing antibodies present in cord blood.[118] However, the protective effect of passive immunity to HPIV3 appears to be less than that observed for HPIV1 and HPIV2, as some infants with a moderately high level of maternally derived serum antibodies become infected with HPIV3 and develop illness.[118]

Experimental HPIV1 and HPIV2 infection of adults possessing varying levels of local nasal secretory IgA neutralizing antibodies and relatively high levels of serum neutralizing antibodies indicated that resistance to infection and URI was mainly a function of mucosal antibodies.[340,375] Adults respond to reinfection by developing an increase in local nasal secretory IgA antibodies that neutralize virus infectivity (Fig. 34.7).[340] In

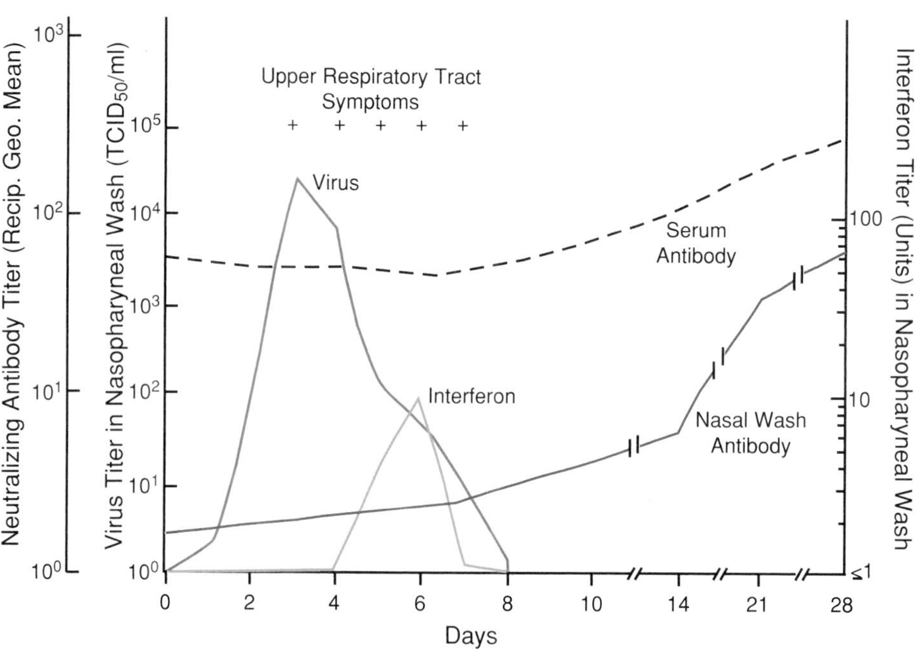

FIGURE 34.7. Experimental infection of adults with wild-type human parainfluenza virus 1 (HPIV1). Adult volunteers, all of whom had evidence of previous natural infection with HPIV1, were administered 10^5 median tissue culture infective doses ($TCID_{50}$) of HPIV1 by the intranasal route, and the indicated parameters were monitored.[261]

addition, the efficacy of IgA in mediating resistance has been demonstrated in studies in experimental animals. IgA and IgG were equally effective in providing resistance to SeV challenge in mice when administered directly into the respiratory tract.[246] However, in the natural situation, IgA has the advantage of being specifically transported through the epithelium to the surface of the lumen as well as being able to neutralize virus within infected epithelial cells.[246]

The role of CD4+ and CD8+ T cells in recovery from pulmonary SeV infection was demonstrated in mice, the putative natural host.[155,186,187] Intranasal infection resulted in a rapid increase in pulmonary CD8+ CTLs, whose appearance coincided with the decrease in titer of pulmonary virus and resolution of infection.[155] However, possible participation of other effectors such as secretory or serum antibodies was not defined. Immunization of mice with a peptide bearing a major epitope for CD8+ CTLs induced a high level of resistance to a short-term virus challenge.[187] Mice that had a mutant nonresponder class I restriction element failed to develop a virus-specific CD8+ CTL response upon infection, whereas serum antibody, delayed-type hypersensitivity, and natural killer (NK) cell responses were unimpaired. These mice cleared infection, but the LD_{50} of SeV in these animals was 10-fold lower than that for wild-type congenic mice. In a situation in which infection was not lethal, removal of CD8+ cells, either through antibody depletion or disruption of the β2-microglobulin gene, resulted in delayed viral clearance and 20% mortality.[155] In comparison, antibody-mediated depletion of CD4+ cells, which inhibited antibody production but did not affect the CD8+ CTL response, delayed viral clearance only marginally with no mortality. Removal of both subsets resulted in a failure to clear the virus and 100% mortality.[155] Pulmonary virus-specific CD8+ cells exhibited efficient cell-killing activity *in vitro,* suggesting that this is a likely effector function *in vivo.* CD4+ cells isolated from normal SeV-infected mice did not have significant *in vitro* cell-killing activity, nor did they seem to have a critical role in promoting the CD8+ response.[155] It seems likely that the major antiviral activity of CD4+ cells was to provide T-cell help for antibody-producing B cells.[155,186]

The importance of virus-specific CD4+ and CD8+ T cells in recovery from HPIV infection has not been formally established. However, as already noted, immunization of hamsters with a recombinant chimeric HPIV3–HPIV1 virus containing the HN and F from HPIV1 and internal protein genes from HPIV3 afforded short-lived protection against HPIV3, presumably involving cell-mediated immunity.[363] The importance of cell-mediated immunity in recovery from HPIV infections is also suggested by the experience of immunodeficient individuals (see Clinical Features).

Evaluation of the role of innate immunity in PIV infections has been limited mostly to identifying the mechanisms by which PIVs interfere with the induction of and signaling by IFN-α/β, as has already been described. As noted, these IFN-antagonist mechanisms are important for efficient infection, and the deletion of the viral proteins involved can be severely attenuating. However, IFN production and action usually are not completely blocked by these viral mechanisms and likely contribute to host defense. A significant proportion (30%) of young patients with HPIV1 infection develop a detectable IFN response (geometric mean titer of 23.5 units) during the acute stage of illness.[132] This frequency is somewhat less than that observed during influenza A virus infection of children (55%) but is decidedly greater than that observed during HRSV infection of infancy and childhood (4%).

In summary, innate immunity, antibodies, and cellular effectors such as CTLs play important independent roles in restricting and clearing an infection. With regard to virus-specific immunologic determinants that confer resistance against re-infection, local IgA plays a key role, but this protective effect can be relatively short-lived, especially following primary infection. Cellular immunity also confers short-lived resistance to reinfection. These short-lived effectors might be important in restricting reinfection during an ongoing epidemic season. Serum antibodies provide long-term protection that is more effective in the lower versus upper respiratory tract. Serum antibodies probably play the major role in resistance to lower respiratory tract infection observed in older children, adolescents and adults. Long-term resistance in the upper respiratory tract is less complete, and reinfection of the upper respiratory tract can occur throughout life. It also should be noted that the immunologic determinants of clearance and protection in the young infant, for whom severe PIV disease is most common, are not well understood.

EPIDEMIOLOGY

Morbidity, Mortality, Age

HPIV1, HPIV2, and HPIV3 have a worldwide distribution and cause acute respiratory illness in individuals of all ages, with the greatest impact in infants and young children. Historically, HPIV4 has been isolated less frequently, likely due in part to the greater difficulty of recovering this serotype in cell culture. However, serologic studies and recent studies using reverse transcription–polymerase chain reaction (RT-PCR) suggest that HPIV4 also is a ubiquitous pathogen that can infect and cause disease in both children and adults.[100,137,306] Each of the four HPIV serotypes has been recovered more often from patients with respiratory diseases than from healthy individuals,[45,46–47,193,282] and each has produced upper respiratory tract infection and illness when administered to adult volunteers.[177,375,378,379]

HPIV infection generally occurs early in life. Serologic surveys indicate that at least 60% of children have been infected with HPIV3 by 2 years of age and that approximately 80% have been infected by 4 years of age.[282,283] A longitudinal study of 121 infants and young children indicated that the incidence of HPIV3 infection was approximately 67 per 100 per year during the first 2 years of life.[118] Infection with HPIV1 or HPIV2 generally occurs somewhat later, but by 5 years of age a majority of children have been infected with HPIV2, and more than 75% have been infected with HPIV1.[282,283] Pneumonia and bronchiolitis associated with HPIV3 infection typically occur during the first 6 months of life, whereas severe illness caused by HPIV1 or 2 is rare in early infancy.[45,46,115] The incidence of croup, which is principally caused by HPIV1 and HPIV2, peaks between 1 and 2 years of age, but croup remains an important cause of LRI in children up to 6 years of age.[145,197]

In infants and young children, disease caused by HPIV1, HPIV2, and HPIV3 can range from mild URI to life-threatening LRI. Table 34.5 shows typical data on the frequency of detection of various respiratory viruses in pediatric inpatients with respiratory tract disease, as well as the association between these viruses and various clinical manifestations, from a prospective study from 1957 to 1976 in Washington DC.[260] In this study, the percentage of pediatric hospitalizations attributable to HPIV1, HPIV2, and HPIV3 was 6.0, 3.2, and 11.5, respectively, compared to 23.3 for HRSV. It should be noted that these data are more than 35 years old, and the now-routine treatment of croup with steroids in outpatient and emergency room settings has markedly reduced hospitalizations for this illness, which is mainly caused by HPIV1 and HPIV2. A more recent study in the United States estimated that HPIV1, HPIV2, and HPIV3 were responsible in aggregate for 6.8% of all hospitalizations for fever and/or acute respiratory illnesses in children younger than 5 years of age, with the different serotypes being responsible for 38%, 12%, and 50% of the HPIV-associated cases, respectively.[393] Therefore, HPIV1, HPIV2, and HPIV3 differ in their contribution to severe respiratory tract disease, with HPIV3 having the greatest impact. One retrospective review of the pediatric medical burden of HPIV3 in the United States estimated that, in children younger than 5 years of age, the virus was responsible yearly for up to 3.24 million cases of medically attended acute respiratory illness (MAARI; rate of 16.9% in that age cohort), 1.08 million cases of LRI (rate of 5.6%), and 29,000 hospitalizations (rate of 0.15%),[223] although a limitation of this study was that rates of outpatient MAARI were extrapolated from rates of LRI. The rate of medically attended HPIV3 disease and LRI was more than threefold greater for those younger than 2 years of age compared to 2 to 5 years of age, and the rate of HPIV3 hospitalization was nearly fivefold greater for those younger than 1 year of age compared to 2 to 5 years of age.

In addition, Table 34.5 illustrates that HPIV1, HPIV2, and HPIV3 each has diversity in its clinical manifestations, with considerable overlap between viruses. However, there are differences in the frequency of association of specific HPIVs with specific illnesses. HPIV1 is the principal cause of croup in children: studies that utilized virus isolation for diagnosis indicate that HPIV1, HPIV2, and HPIV3 are associated with approximately 50% to 75% of cases of croup,[83,197,305] with HPIV1 responsible for 40% to 65% of all cases.[83] In contrast, the principal serious illnesses caused by HPIV3 are pneumonia and bronchiolitis.[45,47,49,83,282] HPIV2 closely resembles HPIV1 in clinical manifestations, but severe illness occurs less frequently.

Pediatric illness associated with HPIV4 is generally thought to be less severe than with the other HPIV serotypes, although the virus has been found in association with a broad spectrum of clinical manifestations including severe LRI.[100,306,338] HPIV4 may account for approximately 10% of pediatric HPIV infections, a prevalence that is less than that of HPIV1 and HPIV3 and may be similar to that of HPIV2.[100,306,338]

The HPIVs commonly reinfect children and adults. However, illness in healthy older children and adults usually is limited to URI; LRI associated with re-infection is rare, although this does occur on occasion and can result in hospitalization.[243] Although the frequency of reinfection is not known, it is probable that most individuals have repeated experience with HPIV1, HPIV2, and HPIV3. In a series of three outbreaks of HPIV3 infection in a semiclosed nursery population, it was observed that 17% of the children infected during one outbreak were reinfected during a subsequent outbreak, although the interval between the first and last outbreaks was only 9 months.[46] Reinfection by HPIV3 of preschool children living at home also occurs with high frequency, and usually is associated with a lower incidence and severity of disease compared to primary infection.[118] HPIV4 also has been detected in adults with medically attended influenza-like illness.[137]

HPIVs are readily spread in the family setting. In a longitudinal study of families with young children, the overall rate of HPIV infection as estimated by serology (HI and complement-fixation assays) was 44.4 infections per 100 person-years.[104] The rate of HPIV infection varied from 59% for children 2 to 5 years of age to 40% for adults. Spread of virus within infected families was extensive, as indicated by serologic studies: following infection of an index case, 64% of family members developed a serum HI antibody response. HPIVs are typically introduced into the family by preschool children.[104]

Nosocomial HPIV infections are particularly problematic in hospitalized children and in immunocompromised patients.[259] Nucleic acid sequence analysis has been used to analyze hospital outbreaks, and it is clear that, although outbreaks caused by a single genotypically uniform strain can occur, much of the problem is due to sporadic spread of multiple strains within the hospital or community.[181] Infection in hospital staff can occur and may be a factor in spread.[331] Transmission may also occur among immunocompromised patients in an outpatient department.[269]

Mortality due to the HPIVs has not been carefully studied but is thought to be uncommon in otherwise healthy individuals (see Clinical Features in this chapter for information on immunodeficient individuals). Although estimates of the fatality rates for the HPIVs are not available, the aggregate rate is thought to be substantially less than for HRSV, another common viral cause of severe pediatric respiratory tract disease (Chapter 38). In one study in Brazil, immunohistochemical analysis of necropsy samples from fatal respiratory infections (200 subjects, aged 1 month to 14 years, median age 7 months) detected HPIV1, HPIV2, and HPIV3; HRSV; and influenza A in 6.5, 8.0, 15.5, 21, and 10.5 percent of cases, with many cases having more than one virus.[88] Another report described a fatal case of HPIV1-confirmed laryngotracheitis, with no evidence of bacterial superinfection, in a 15-month-old toddler.[236] Therefore, infection with the HPIVs can be fatal, although this is uncommon.

The seasonality of HPIV infections has been most clearly defined in temperate climates, principally in the United States. From 1957 to 1961, HPIV1 appeared to be endemic; infection occurred sporadically and without a definite seasonal pattern.[45,46] Beginning in 1962, a different pattern developed, in which sharp outbreaks of HPIV1 occurred every 2 years in the autumn of even-numbered years. In contrast, HPIV2 caused outbreaks in the autumn of odd-numbered years.[46,116] At present, HPIV1 epidemics occur during the fall of odd-numbered years. HPIV2 epidemics occur annually in the fall,[169] but infection with HPIV2 can also occur at other times.[394] For many years, HPIV3 exhibited an endemic pattern, with infection occurring in all seasons of the year. Within the last 15 years, there has been a shift toward yearly epidemics of HPIV3 infection in the spring and summer. In North America, the seasonality of croup primarily mirrors the seasonality of HPIV1, with large peaks occurring in odd-numbered years in the fall[83,244,327] and smaller peaks occurring in the winter, reflecting influenza and HRSV as additional causes of the syndrome.

One of the hallmarks of the HPIVs is that they persist in the population without undergoing significant antigenic change. This persistence is likely the result of reinfection and subclinical infection in older children and adults throughout life. HPIV infections induce potent systemic and local humoral and cellular responses (except in young infants) that are thought to completely resolve the acute infection. Serum antibody responses are durable, but local respiratory tract IgA and cellular responses can be more transient, which may contribute to the ease of reinfection. In addition, reinfection is facilitated by the ability of the HPIVs to block the host IFN response. A number of PIVs readily establish persistent infection in cell culture[57,113,257] raising the possibility that persistent infection might be another mechanism for maintaining virus in the population. However, although prolonged infection by HPIVs can occur in immunocompromised individuals, evidence for persistence of HPIVs in healthy hosts is lacking.

Spread and Infectivity

Transmission of HPIVs is by direct person-to-person contact or by large-droplet spread; however, the viruses do not persist long in the environment. These viruses spread rapidly following introduction into day care, family, and institutional settings. There is evidence from studies in adult volunteers that the infectious dose of HPIV1 is small. For example, in one study, two thirds of adults who possessed a moderately high level of preexisting serum-neutralizing antibodies became infected and developed a "common cold–like" illness following intranasal instillation of 80 $TCID_{50}$ of HPIV1.[340] In addition, reinfected individuals appear to be infectious. HPIV3 appears to be the most efficient of the HPIVs in its ability to spread from person to person. HPIV3 generally infects all susceptible individuals in a semiclosed population (such as a nursery) in a relatively short time.[46] In contrast, HPIV1 and HPIV2 appear to be less effective in this regard, infecting 40% to 69% of susceptible individuals in semiclosed populations.[46] During experimental infection of adult volunteers, the interval between administration of HPIV1, HPIV2, or HPIV3 and onset of upper respiratory tract symptoms ranges from 3 to 6 days (see Fig. 34.7).[177,340,378,379] The incubation period in pediatric infections has not been defined; however, in several institutional outbreaks of HPIV3 infection, the interval between exposure and the onset of virus shedding was 2 to 4 days.[46]

The interval during which an individual infected with an HPIV can infect another person is not known. Longitudinal studies indicate that HPIV3 is usually shed from the oropharynx for 3 to 10 days (median of 8 days) during primary infection, whereas during reinfection the virus is detected during a shorter interval.[46] On occasion, infants and young children may shed HPIV3 during primary infection for as long as 3 to 4 weeks.[105] Prolonged shedding of HPIV3 has also been observed occasionally in adults with underlying chronic lower respiratory tract disease.[130] It is not clear whether chronic damage to the respiratory tract is responsible for this unusual manifestation of adult reinfection.

CLINICAL FEATURES

Most primary infections with the HPIVs result in respiratory illness. In children, the most common type of illness consists of rhinitis, pharyngitis, cough, and hoarseness, usually with fever.[282,283] The cough may be croupy, but respiratory distress is not present. Approximately three fourths of such ill children have a temperature above 100°F; fever usually lasts 2 to 3 days. Coarse breath sounds, rhonchi, erythema of the pharyngeal mucous membranes, and rhinitis are the characteristic physical findings. Cervical adenopathy is uncommon.[283] Otitis media occurs frequently in HPIV infections, and virus can be detected in the middle ear fluids of patients with otitis media.[142]

When acute laryngotracheobronchitis (LTB; croup) develops, the initial symptoms of rhinitis, pharyngitis, fever, and cough progress. After several days, the cough worsens and becomes brassy, "seal-like," or barking, and stridor ensues. The illness typically varies in intensity, with the worst symptoms frequently observed in the evening and at night. Most children recover after 48 to 72 hours. In some children, however, air hunger develops, with cyanosis, sternal and intercostal retractions, and progressive airway obstruction. The anteroposterior (AP) radiograph of the neck (which should be obtained under carefully controlled medical supervision, if at all) shows glottic and subglottic narrowing (the "steeple sign") and differentiates this disease from epiglottitis.

When bronchiolitis or pneumonia develops, fever persists and the cough progresses and becomes somewhat productive. It is accompanied by wheezing, tachypnea, retractions, and, in severe cases, cyanosis. The chest radiograph shows interstitial or perihilar infiltrates and air trapping. In some patients, a combined bronchopneumonia–croup syndrome occurs. There are also case reports of children who have developed severe pulmonary disease resembling the adult respiratory distress syndrome following HPIV infection.[154]

HPIVs may cause prolonged and severe infections in patients with congenital and acquired immunodeficiencies, including those with severe combined immunodeficiency and those who have undergone hematopoietic stem cell transplantation (HSCT) or lung transplantation. In these patients, HPIV3 is the most frequently isolated serotype. In one large study of HSCT recipients, HPIV infection was documented in 7.1% of subjects: all four serotypes were detected, but HPIV3 accounted for 90% of the isolates.[269] Of the HPIV3 cases, 24% developed pneumonia, and 35% of those died within 30 days. Steroid use was a risk factor for development of pneumonia. Co-pathogens were isolated from 53% of those with pneumonia and increased the risk of mortality.[268] HPIV3 also causes LRI in lung transplant recipients and has reported associations with both acute allograft rejection and later development of bronchiolitis obliterans, an often fatal complication.[390] In wealthy countries, prior infection with human immunodeficiency virus (HIV) does not appear to increase the morbidity and mortality associated with HPIV infection in children, although prolonged viral excretion has been reported.[196] In resource-limited countries, HPIVs have been reported to be associated with greater morbidity and mortality in HIV-infected than HIV-noninfected children, although the contribution of other illnesses cannot be excluded.[239]

DIAGNOSIS

Differential

In croup, other viral causes must be considered. Influenza A viruses (particularly H3N2 viruses) cause up to one third of croup cases (Table 34.5), but these are usually confined to epidemic periods. HRSV also occasionally causes croup. In resource-limited settings, measles virus may also produce severe laryngeal inflammation. In regions where *Haemophilus influenzae* type B (HiB) vaccine is not used, epiglottitis becomes the most important differential diagnosis, although this disease is becoming increasingly rare with the global use of HiB vaccines. In contrast to croup, epiglottitis is usually of sudden onset, without a prodrome of rhinitis, hoarseness, or cough, and is accompanied by high fever, leukocytosis, a "toxic" appearance, and drooling. The AP radiograph of the neck is characteristic, as is the cherry-red enlargement of the epiglottis, which should be examined only as part of the intubation procedure or when preparations for nasotracheal intubation have been made. Another bacterial infection that must be differentiated from viral croup is bacterial tracheitis. This disease is usually caused by *Staphylococcus aureus* and may be a complication of viral croup rather than a primary bacterial infection. Intubation for bacterial tracheitis is frequently necessary, as well as antistaphylococcal antibiotic therapy. In bronchiolitis or pneumonia of infancy, other viruses (particularly HRSV and HMPV) and *Chlamydia trachomatis* are the most frequent etiologic agents to be considered.

Laboratory

Definitive diagnosis of HPIV infection requires viral isolation by conventional methods or spin-enhanced culture,[224] identification of viral antigens in respiratory tract secretions by immunofluorescence, or detection of viral RNA in nasal secretions by reverse transcription followed by RT-PCR. For viral culture or immunofluorescence, specimens are best collected by nasal aspirate or nasal wash, but nose and throat swabs appear to be adequate for RT-PCR. To enhance recovery by culture, specimens should be transported to the lab on wet ice or "snap" frozen on dry ice and stored at -80°C. Increasingly, RT-PCR is being used as the diagnostic method of choice in both pediatric and adult populations because the sensitivity of these assays allows detection of even small quantities of virus (adults typically shed less virus than children). RT-PCR can be used in multiplex formats capable of detecting multiple pathogens, and several such assays are currently available. Immunocompromised subjects may shed HPIVs for prolonged periods, which may make it difficult to correlate detection with specific disease states.

PREVENTION AND CONTROL

Treatment

Symptomatic treatment of croup usually includes humidification of air by ultrasonic nebulizer. Nebulized or systemic corticosteroids have been shown to decrease the frequency of intubation and hospitalization in moderate to severe croup.[11,174] A single dose of oral dexamethasone in children with mild croup has been shown to shorten the duration of symptoms, improve patient sleep, and decrease parental stress.[25] Treatment with nebulized epinephrine is usually reserved for patients in severe respiratory distress.[25] Steroids act to reduce inflammation, whereas epinephrine relieves airway constriction through relaxation of smooth muscles.

Specific antiviral treatment is not available. The nucleoside analog ribavirin exhibits *in vitro* activity against the HPIVs, but is not recommended for use in otherwise healthy individuals because its effectiveness is unclear; the same is true for HRSV. Ribavirin does find use in the treatment of HRSV and HPIV infections in HSCT recipients, although its effectiveness in this setting also is unclear.[42,268] A number of potential inhibitors of the HPIVs that target various steps in the replicative cycle are in preclinical development. The neuraminidase inhibitor 4-GU-DANA (zanamivir) that was developed as an antiviral drug for influenza virus inhibits HPIV3 neuraminidase activity. However, it also interferes with HN binding to the cellular receptor and has the undesired effect of promoting HPIV3 release, which makes it unsuitable for therapy of HPIV infections.[255,291] Using the crystal structure of NDV as a guide, neuraminidase inhibitors BCX 2798 and 2855 were developed and shown to be active in inhibiting HPIV1 in cell culture, and were effective in prophylaxis and treatment in mice against a recombinant SeV in which the SeV HN gene had been replaced with that of HPIV1.[6,392] Another strategy has been to use recombinant sialidase to enzymatically remove sialic acid receptor molecules from target cells to block infection by HPIVs and influenza virus: this strategy has been shown to inhibit infection by HPIVs in cell culture and in cotton rats.[258] Structure-based "virtual screening" for compounds predicted to interact with the active sites on the HPIV3 HN protein identified a small molecule that interacts with the HN protein and triggers premature activation of the F protein, with the result that entry is blocked.[258] Fusion is driven by interaction between heptad repeats in the F protein (see Chapter 33), and synthetic peptides derived from these repeats have been shown to block this interaction and inhibit HPIV3 infection *in vitro*.[293] This strategy is based on earlier work with HIV that resulted in the HIV fusion inhibitor enfuvirtide presently in use in anti-HIV therapy. The addition of cholesterol to HIV or HPIV3 peptides targeted them to the membrane and increased their antiviral activity.[293] A novel small molecule LJ001 was recently described that intercalates into viral membrane and irreversibly blocks virus–cell fusion, and is active against a wide array of enveloped viruses including PIVs.[399] Small molecules that inhibit HPIV3 transcription in cell culture have recently been described.[242] In addition, small interfering RNA (siRNA) targeting the HPIV3 N gene was reported to have antiviral activity in cell culture and in mice (with the caveat that HPIV3 replicates poorly in mice)[23]; a similar strategy against HRSV has been shown to reduce virus infection and replication in clinical studies (Chapter 38). Recently, DAS 181, a recombinant sialidase containing the catalytic domain of Actinomyces viscosus, has been shown to have *in vitro* activity against all of the human PIVs[258] and has been associated with viral clearance and clinical improvement when delivered via inhalation to stem cell or lung transplant patients with HPIV3 LRI.[52a,91a,131a] Clinical evaluation of DAS181 is ongoing.

Vaccines

The primary need for HPIV vaccines is in the pediatric population, with the need being greatest for HPIV3 followed by HPIV1 and HPIV2. Given the epidemiology of the viruses, immunization against HPIV3 should begin by the second month of life (ideally given in combination with an HRSV vaccine), whereas immunization against HPIV1 and HPIV2 could begin in late infancy or early childhood. A major obstacle to developing pediatric vaccines is that antibody responses to live respiratory viral vaccines are frequently limited in infants at or below 6 months of age[70,109] (see Immunity, above).

In early work, inactivated vaccines prepared with virus from infected embryonated eggs or primary monkey kidney cell culture were developed for HPIV1, HPIV2, and HPIV3 and shown to be immunogenic in children, as indicated by the development of serum HI and neutralizing antibodies. Unfortunately, parenteral administration of these vaccines failed to induce resistance to HPIV disease.[55,107] Effective immunization against HPIV disease using a killed virus vaccine has not been demonstrated and is not an active area of research.

Subunit vaccines have also been evaluated, namely, preparations of the HPIV3 HN and F glycoproteins isolated from purified HPIV3 or from insect cells infected with recombinant baculoviruses expressing the HN or F protein or a chimeric form of HN and F encoded by an engineered cDNA.[7,225,302,383] Parenteral immunization of cotton rats with these viral glycoproteins induced satisfactory levels of neutralizing, HI, and FI antibodies, and the immunized animals were highly resistant to intranasal challenge with HPIV3. In addition, intranasal administration of the purified glycoproteins was effective in inducing a local IgA response.[303] However, none of these strategies has been validated in nonhuman primates or in clinical trials, which pose a more stringent test of vaccine efficacy, since HPIVs do not replicate efficiently in rodents and thus are readily restricted.

A major focus of current research is the development of live-attenuated intranasal vaccines for HPIV1, HPIV2 and HPIV3, either using attenuated versions of the native human HPIVs, or by using related nonhuman PIVs as vectors to express HPIV HN and F glycoproteins. Information about specific experimental vaccines is detailed below. Importantly, live attenuated respiratory viruses administered intranasally are infectious and moderately immunogenic even in the presence of maternal serum antibodies.[400] Furthermore, these intranasally administered vaccines induce both local and systemic immunity.

HPIV3 Vaccines

Two biologically derived HPIV3 experimental vaccines that have been evaluated in clinical trials have served as prototypes for the development of live-attenuated HPIV3 vaccines. HPIV3 cp45 (cp45) was derived from the JS wild-type strain of HPIV3 by 45 passages in primary African green monkey kidney cells at low temperatures.[18] This cp45 mutant exhibited three interesting properties: (a) cold adaptation (*ca*) (i.e., an ability to replicate efficiently at 20°C, a temperature restrictive for wild-type PIV3); (b) temperature sensitivity (*ts*) (i.e., a decreased ability to produce plaques at the high end of the normal temperature range); and (c) reduction in the level of replication ("attenuation" or *att*) in hamsters, monkeys, and humans.[133] The cp45 virus contains 20 point mutations that differentiate it from the JS wild-type strain, 10 of which are silent, without a change in amino acid sequence. Of the remaining 10 mutations, the ones associated with attenuation involve amino acid substitutions in the C, F, HN, and L proteins, with the L mutations playing the major role.[332,334] The second candidate is BPIV3, which is naturally attenuated in humans, as already noted.[60] BPIV3 and HPIV3 are 25% related antigenically by cross-neutralization assays, which would reduce the effectiveness of BPIV3-specific immunity in restricting HPIV3. Both cp45 and BPIV3 have been evaluated in phase I and phase II trials in adults, HPIV3 seropositive children, HPIV3 seronegative children, and infants as young as 1 month (cp45) or 2 months (BPIV3) of age. Both candidates were over-attenuated in adults and in seropositive children but were highly infectious in seronegative children and infants.[20,59,178,183,184] There were no significant differences in the incidence of respiratory or febrile illnesses among seronegative vaccinees and placebo recipients, suggesting that the vaccines were well tolerated. Otitis media occurred more frequently among seronegative children vaccinated with HPIV3 cp45 in phase I trials than among placebo recipients, but this was not observed in infants vaccinated with HPIV3 cp45, or in phase II trials of HPIV3 cp45 in seronegative children. A recombinant form of the cp45 vaccine, designated rcp45, has been recently developed. rcp45 has the advantage of having a short, well-defined passage history using qualified cells and reagents. rcp45 was recently assessed in phase I and II trials in HPIV3-naïve children to determine the optimal dosage and dosing interval (clinicaltrials.gov NCT01021397, NCT01254175, and NCT01150799), and has been found to be comparable to the biologically derived cp45 vaccine with respect to tolerability, infectivity, and immunogenicity.[179 and unpublished observations]

Although both HPIV3 cp45 and BPIV3 elicited HI antibody responses against HPIV3 in most vaccinated seronegative children, the magnitude of the HPIV3-specific response was lower in children who received BPIV3, consistent with the antigenic differences between BPIV3 and HPIV3.[60] For this reason, recombinant bovine/human PIV3 candidate vaccines containing the HPIV3 HN and F genes and one or more BPIV3 internal genes have been developed by reverse genetics (see below). These viruses were constructed either through replacement of the HN and F genes of BPIV3 with their counterparts from HPIV3[325] or through replacement of individual "internal" protein genes (e.g., N or P genes) of HPIV3 with their counterparts from BPIV3. Two of these vaccines, rHPIV3-N_B (consisting of HPIV3 in which the N gene was replaced with its BPIV3 counterpart) and rB/HPIV3 (consisting of BPIV3 in which the F and HN genes were replaced with their HPIV3 counterparts), have recently been evaluated in phase I clinical trials (clinicaltrials.gov NCT00366782). Each candidate was highly attenuated in adults and seropositive children, but was infectious and immunogenic in seronegative children. An additional candidate, a chimeric vaccine designated MEDI-534, is a version of rB/HPIV3 that also expresses the HRSV F protein from an added gene placed between the N and P genes. This strategy thus provides a bivalent vaccine virus against HPIV3 and HRSV. MEDI-534 has been evaluated in a phase I trial in HRSV and HPIV3 doubly seronegative children ages 6 to 23 months (clinicaltrials.gov NCT00493285). Preliminary data from this trial indicate that all children who received the highest dose of vaccine (10^6 $TCID_{50}$) were infected with vaccine virus, and that seroconversion to HRSV and HPIV3 occurred in 67% and 100%, respectively, of recipients of this vaccine dose.

HPIV1 and HPIV2 Vaccines

SeV, the murine relative of HPIV1, has been evaluated as a HPIV1 vaccine candidate in nonhuman primates and healthy adults. SeV was highly immunogenic and protective against HPIV1 challenge when administered intranasally to African green monkeys, and was well tolerated in adult human recipients and immunogenic in three of nine individuals.[339]

The replication of SeV was not significantly restricted in African green monkeys and chimpanzees compared to

HPIV1,[335] which raises the possibility that it might not be satisfactorily attenuated in infants and children. However, SeV was attenuated in adults and is currently being evaluated as an experimental intranasal vaccine in young children (clinicaltrials.gov NCT00186927).

Live-attenuated candidate vaccines for HPIV1 and HPIV2 have also been developed based on the introduction of known attenuating mutations into cDNA-derived HPIV1 and HPIV2 by reverse genetics. In some cases, mutations were designed to have increased genetic stability, such as by choosing codons that could not revert by a single nucleotide substitution, or by deleting the relevant codon(s). One vaccine candidate, rHPIV1 84/del170/942A, contains mutations in the C, HN, and L proteins. Replication of this virus is highly restricted in adults and HPIV1 seropositive children. Evaluation of this vaccine in HPIV1 seronegative children is in progress (clinicaltrials.gov NCT00641017). Similarly, rHPIV2-15C/948L/Δ1724, an HPIV2 vaccine candidate, contains a mutation in the extragenic leader region of the genome, and an amino acid substitution and a deletion in the L gene. rHPIV2-15C/948L/Δ1724 is highly attenuated in African green monkeys yet protects against challenge with wt HPIV2.[274] Replication of rHPIV2-15C/948L/Δ1724 is highly restricted in adults, and evaluation in HPIV2 seropositive children is in progress (clinicaltrials.gov NCT01139437).

PERSPECTIVE

The HPIVs continue to be an important cause of pediatric respiratory illness. There still are no approved antiviral therapies or vaccines for any of these viruses. The pathogenesis of serious HPIV disease such as croup, bronchiolitis, and pneumonia is still not well understood. Indeed, most of our understanding of HPIV infection, pathogenesis, and the host response is by inference from HRSV. In recent years, we have gained an understanding of the role of HPIV proteins in inhibiting the type I IFN response. Fewer advances have been made in characterizing the adaptive immune response to HPIVs, especially in infants and young children. However, significant progress has been made in the treatment of croup and in the development of HPIV vaccines. The natural histories of most of the animal PIVs remain poorly understood.

ACKNOWLEDGMENTS

R.A.K. was partially funded by NIH NIAID contract HHSN272200900010C. P.L.C. was funded by the Intramural Program of NIAID, NIH.

REFERENCES

All cited references are available in the e-book.

3. Aherne W, Bird T, Court SD, et al. Pathological changes in virus infections of the lower respiratory tract in children. *J Clin Pathol* 1970;23:7–18.
8. Andrejeva J, Childs KS, Young DF, et al. The V proteins of paramyxoviruses bind the IFN-inducible RNA helicase, MDA-5, and inhibit its activation of the IFN-beta promoter. *Proc Natl Acad Sci U S A* 2004; 101:17264–17269.
9. Andrejeva J, Young DF, Goodbourn S, et al. Degradation of STAT1 and STAT2 by the V proteins of simian virus 5 and human parainfluenza virus type 2, respectively: consequences for virus replication in the presence of alpha/beta and gamma interferons. *J Virol* 2002;76:2159–2167.
11. Ausejo M, Saenz A, Pham B, et al. The effectiveness of glucocorticoids in treating croup: meta-analysis. *BMJ* 1999;319:595–600.
15. Bartlett EJ, Hennessey M, Skiadopoulos MH, et al. Role of interferon in the replication of human parainfluenza virus type 1 wild type and mutant viruses in human ciliated airway epithelium. *J Virol* 2008;82:8059–8070.
18. Belshe RB, Hissom FK. Cold adaptation of parainfluenza virus type 3: induction of three phenotypic markers. *J Med Virol* 1982;10:235–242.
20. Belshe RB, Newman FK, Tsai TF, et al. Phase 2 evaluation of parainfluenza type 3 cold passage mutant 45 live attenuated vaccine in healthy children 6–18 months old. *J Infect Dis* 2004;189:462–470.
23. Bitko V, Musiyenko A, Shulyayeva O, et al. Inhibition of respiratory viruses by nasally administered siRNA. *Nat Med* 2005;11:50–55.
25. Bjornson CL, Klassen TP, Williamson J, et al. A randomized trial of a single dose of oral dexamethasone for mild croup. *N Engl J Med* 2004; 351:1306–1313.
27. Boonyaratanakornkit J, Bartlett E, Schomacker H, et al. The C proteins of human parainfluenza virus type 1 limit double-stranded RNA accumulation that would otherwise trigger activation of MDA5 and protein kinase R. *J Virol* 2011;85:1495–1506.
28. Boonyaratanakornkit JB, Bartlett EJ, Amaro-Carambot E, et al. The C proteins of human parainfluenza virus type 1 (HPIV1) control the transcription of a broad array of cellular genes that would otherwise respond to HPIV1 infection. *J Virol* 2009;83:1892–1910.
29. Bose S, Basu M, Banerjee AK. Role of nucleolin in human parainfluenza virus type 3 infection of human lung epithelial cells. *J Virol* 2004; 78:8146–8158.
37. Cadd T, Garcin D, Tapparel C, et al. The Sendai paramyxovirus accessory C proteins inhibit viral genome amplification in a promoter-specific fashion. *J Virol* 1996;70:5067–5074.
38. Caignard G, Komarova AV, Bourai M, et al. Differential regulation of type I interferon and epidermal growth factor pathways by a human Respirovirus virulence factor. *PLoS Pathog* 2009;5:e1000587.
39. Capua I, Alexander DJ. Human health implications of avian influenza viruses and paramyxoviruses. *Eur J Clin Microbiol Infect Dis* 2004;23:1–6.
40. Carlos TS, Young DF, Schneider M, et al. Parainfluenza virus 5 genomes are located in viral cytoplasmic bodies whilst the virus dismantles the interferon-induced antiviral state of cells. *J Gen Virol* 2009;90:2147–2156.
46. Chanock R, Parrott R, Johnson K, et al. Myxoviruses: parainfluenza. *Am Rev Respir Dis* 1963;88:152–166.
47. Chanock R, Vargosko A, Luckey A, et al. Association of hemadsorption viruses with respiratory illness in childhood. *JAMA* 1959;169:548–553.
48. Chanock RM. Association of a new type of cytopathogenic myxovirus with infantile croup. *J Exp Med* 1956;104:555–576.
49. Chanock RM, Parrott RH, Cook K, et al. Newly recognized myxoviruses from children with respiratory disease. *N Engl J Med* 1958;258:207–213.
50. Chare ER, Gould EA, Holmes EC. Phylogenetic analysis reveals a low rate of homologous recombination in negative-sense RNA viruses. *J Gen Virol* 2003;84:2691–2703.
54. Childs KS, Andrejeva J, Randall RE, et al. Mechanism of MDA-5 inhibition by paramyxovirus V proteins. *J Virol* 2009;83:1465–1473.
55. Chin J, Magoffin RL, Shearer LA, et al. Field evaluation of a respiratory syncytial virus vaccine and a trivalent parainfluenza virus vaccine in a pediatric population. *Am J Epidemiol* 1969;89:449–463.
56. Chong YL, Padhi A, Hudson PJ, et al. The effect of vaccination on the evolution and population dynamics of avian paramyxovirus-1. *PLoS Pathog* 2010;6:e1000872.
59. Clements ML, Belshe RB, King J, et al. Evaluation of bovine, cold-adapted human, and wild-type human parainfluenza type 3 viruses in adult volunteers and in chimpanzees. *J Clin Microbiol* 1991;29:1175–1182.
61. Coelingh KL. Antigenic variation among human parainfluenza type 3 viruses: Comparative and epidemiologic aspects. In: Kurstak E, Marusyk R, Murphy V, Van Regenmortel M, eds. *Applied Virology Research: Virus Variation*, vol. 2. New York: Plenum Press; 1989:143–157.
62. Coelingh KV, Winter CC. Naturally occurring human parainfluenza type 3 viruses exhibit divergence in amino acid sequence of their fusion protein neutralization epitopes and cleavage sites. *J Virol* 1990;64:1329–1334.
63. Collins PL, Bukreyev A, Murphy BR. What are the risks - hypothetical and observed - of recombination involving live vaccines and vaccine vectors based on nonsegmented negative-strand RNA viruses? *J Virol* 2008;82:9805–9806.

67. Coronel EC, Murti KG, Takimoto T, et al. Human parainfluenza virus type 1 matrix and nucleoprotein genes transiently expressed in mammalian cells induce the release of virus-like particles containing nucleocapsid-like structures. *J Virol* 1999;73:7035–7038.
69. Crennell S, Takimoto T, Portner A, et al. Crystal structure of the multifunctional paramyxovirus hemagglutinin-neuraminidase. *Nat Struct Biol* 2000;7:1068–1074.
80. de Breyne S, Stalder R, Curran J. Intracellular processing of the Sendai virus C′ protein leads to the generation of a Y protein module: structure-functional implications. *FEBS Lett* 2005;579:5685–5690.
82. Delage G, Brochu P, Pelletier M, et al. Giant-cell pneumonia caused by parainfluenza virus. *J Pediatr* 1979;94:426–429.
83. Denny FW, Murphy TF, Clyde WA Jr, et al. Croup: an 11-year study in a pediatric practice. *Pediatrics* 1983;71:871–846.
85. Didcock L, Young DF, Goodbourn S, et al. The V protein of simian virus 5 inhibits interferon signalling by targeting STAT1 for proteasome-mediated degradation. *J Virol* 1999;73:9928–9933.
86. DiNapoli JM, Nayak B, Yang L, et al. Newcastle disease virus-vectored vaccines expressing the hemagglutinin or neuraminidase protein of H5N1 highly pathogenic avian influenza virus protect against virus challenge in monkeys. *J Virol* 2010;84:1489–1503.
88a. Dortmans JC, Koch G, Rottier PJ, Peeters BP. Virulence of pigeon paramyxovirus type 1 does not always correlate with the cleavability of its fusion protein. *J Gen Virol* 2009;90:2746–2750.
90. Downham MA, Gardner PS, McQuillin J, et al. Role of respiratory viruses in childhood mortality. *Br Med J* 1975;1:235–239.
93. Durbin AP, McAuliffe JM, Collins PL, et al. Mutations in the C, D, and V open reading frames of human parainfluenza virus type 3 attenuate replication in rodents and primates. *Virology* 1999;261:319–330.
95. El Feghaly RE, McGann L, Bonville CA, et al. Local production of inflammatory mediators during childhood parainfluenza virus infection. *Pediatr Infect Dis J* 2010;29:e26–e31.
102. Fishaut M, Tubergen D, McIntosh K. Cellular response to respiratory viruses with particular reference to children with disorders of cell-mediated immunity. *J Pediatr* 1980;96:179–186.
104. Fox J, Hall C. Infections with other respiratory pathogens: influenza, parainfluenza, mumps and respiratory syncytial viruses; mycoplasma pneumoniae. In: Fox J, Hall C, eds. *Viruses in Families*. Littleton, MA: PSG Publishing Company; 1980:335–381.
105. Frank AL, Taber LH, Wells CR, et al. Patterns of shedding of myxoviruses and paramyxoviruses in children. *J Infect Dis* 1981;144:433–441.
106. Frank JA Jr, Warren RW, Tucker JA, et al. Disseminated parainfluenza infection in a child with severe combined immunodeficiency. *Am J Dis Child* 1983;137:1172–1174.
107. Fulginiti VA, Eller JJ, Sieber OF, et al. Respiratory virus immunization. I. A field trial of two inactivated respiratory virus vaccines; an aqueous trivalent parainfluenza virus vaccine and an alum-precipitated respiratory syncytial virus vaccine. *Am J Epidemiol* 1969;89:435–448.
108. Galinski MS, Troy RM, Banerjee AK. RNA editing in the phosphoprotein gene of the human parainfluenza virus type 3. *Virology* 1992;186:543–550.
111. Garcin D, Marq JB, Iseni F, et al. A short peptide at the amino terminus of the Sendai virus C protein acts as an independent element that induces STAT1 instability. *J Virol* 2004;78:8799–8811.
115. Glezen P, Denny FW. Epidemiology of acute lower respiratory disease in children. *N Engl J Med* 1973;288:498–505.
118. Glezen WP, Frank AL, Taber LH, et al. Parainfluenza virus type 3: seasonality and risk of infection and reinfection in young children. *J Infect Dis* 1984;150:851–857.
122. Gotoh B, Takeuchi K, Komatsu T, et al. The STAT2 activation process is a crucial target of Sendai virus C protein for the blockade of alpha interferon signaling. *J Virol* 2003;77:3360–3370.
128. Greenberg DP, Walker RE, Lee MS, et al. A bovine parainfluenza virus type 3 vaccine is safe and immunogenic in early infancy. *J Infect Dis* 2005;191:1116–1122.
132. Hall CB, Douglas RG Jr, Simons RL, et al. Interferon production in children with respiratory syncytial, influenza, and parainfluenza virus infections. *J Pediatr* 1978;93:28–32.
136. Hasan MK, Kato A, Muranaka M, et al. Versatility of the accessory C proteins of Sendai virus: contribution to virus assembly as an additional role. *J Virol* 2000;74:5619–5628.
140. He B, Paterson RG, Stock N, et al. Recovery of paramyxovirus simian virus 5 with a V protein lacking the conserved cysteine-rich domain: the multifunctional V protein blocks both interferon-beta induction and interferon signaling. *Virology* 2002;303:15–32.
142. Heikkinen T, Thint M, Chonmaitree T. Prevalence of various respiratory viruses in the middle ear during acute otitis media. *N Engl J Med* 1999;340:260–264.
144. Henrickson KJ, Kingsbury DW, van Wyke Coelingh KL, et al. Neutralizing epitopes of human parainfluenza virus type 3 are conformational and cannot be imitated by synthetic peptides. *Vaccine* 1991;9:243–249.
146. Henrickson KJ, Savatski LL. Antigenic structure, function, and evolution of the hemagglutinin-neuraminidase protein of human parainfluenza virus type 1. *J Infect Dis* 1997;176:867–875.
150. Horikami SM, Hector RE, Smallwood S, et al. The Sendai virus C protein binds the L polymerase protein to inhibit viral RNA synthesis. *Virology* 1997;235:261–270.
151. Horikami SM, Smallwood S, Moyer SA. The Sendai virus V protein interacts with the NP protein to regulate viral genome RNA replication. *Virology* 1996;222:383–390.
164. Hurwitz JL. Development of recombinant Sendai virus vaccines for prevention of human parainfluenza and respiratory syncytial virus infections. *Pediatr Infect Dis J* 2008;27:S126–S128.
165. Irie T, Nagata N, Yoshida T, et al. Paramyxovirus Sendai virus C proteins are essential for maintenance of negative-sense RNA genome in virus particles. *Virology* 2008;374:495–505.
166. Iseni F, Garcin D, Nishio M, et al. Sendai virus trailer RNA binds TIAR, a cellular protein involved in virus-induced apoptosis. *Embo J* 2002;21:5141–5150.
169. Iwane MK, Edwards KM, Szilagyi PG, et al. Population-based surveillance for hospitalizations associated with respiratory syncytial virus, influenza virus, and parainfluenza viruses among young children. *Pediatrics* 2004;113:1758–1764.
174. Johnson DW, Jacobson S, Edney PC, et al. A comparison of nebulized budesonide, intramuscular dexamethasone, and placebo for moderately severe croup. *N Engl J Med* 1998;339:498–503.
177. Kapikian A, Chanock R, Reichelderfer T, et al. Inoculation of human volunteers with parainfluenza virus type 3. *JAMA* 1961;183:537–541.
178. Karron RA, Belshe RB, Wright PF, et al. A live human parainfluenza type 3 virus vaccine is attenuated and immunogenic in young infants. *Pediatr Infect Dis J* 2003;22:394–405.
181. Karron RA, O'Brien KL, Froehlich JL, et al. Molecular epidemiology of a parainfluenza type 3 virus outbreak on a pediatric ward. *J Infect Dis* 1993;167:1441–1445.
183. Karron RA, Wright PF, Hall SL, et al. A live attenuated bovine parainfluenza virus type 3 vaccine is safe, infectious, immunogenic, and phenotypically stable in infants and children. *J Infect Dis* 1995;171:1107–1114.
184. Karron RA, Wright PF, Newman FK, et al. A live human parainfluenza type 3 virus vaccine is attenuated and immunogenic in healthy infants and children. *J Infect Dis* 1995;172:1445–1450.
185. Kasel JA, Frank AL, Keitel WA, et al. Acquisition of serum antibodies to specific viral glycoproteins of parainfluenza virus 3 in children. *J Virol* 1984;52:828–832.
186. Kast WM, Bronkhorst AM, de Waal LP, et al. Cooperation between cytotoxic and helper T lymphocytes in protection against lethal Sendai virus infection. Protection by T cells is MHC-restricted and MHC-regulated; a model for MHC-disease associations. *J Exp Med* 1986;164:723–738.
201. Kolakofsky D, Roux L, Garcin D, et al. Paramyxovirus mRNA editing, the "rule of six" and error catastrophe: a hypothesis. *J Gen Virol* 2005;86:1869–1877.
206. Komatsu T, Takeuchi K, Yokoo J, et al. C and V proteins of Sendai virus target signaling pathways leading to IRF-3 activation for the negative regulation of interferon-beta production. *Virology* 2004;325:137–148.
221. Latorre P, Kolakofsky D, Curran J. Sendai virus Y proteins are initiated by a ribosomal shunt. *Mol Cell Biol* 1998;18:5021–5031.
222. Lawrence MC, Borg NA, Streltsov VA, et al. Structure of the haemagglutinin-neuraminidase from human parainfluenza virus type III. *J Mol Biol* 2004;335:1343–1357.

223. Lee MS, Walker RE, Mendelman PM. Medical burden of respiratory syncytial virus and parainfluenza virus type 3 infection among US children. Implications for design of vaccine trials. *Hum Vaccin* 2005;1:6–11.
227. Li T, Chen X, Garbutt KC, et al. Structure of DDB1 in complex with a paramyxovirus V protein: viral hijack of a propeller cluster in ubiquitin ligase. *Cell* 2006;124:105–117.
228. Lin GY, Lamb RA. The paramyxovirus simian virus 5 V protein slows progression of the cell cycle. *J Virol* 2000;74:9152–166.
229. Lin Y, Bright AC, Rothermel TA, et al. Induction of apoptosis by paramyxovirus simian virus 5 lacking a small hydrophobic gene. *J Virol* 2003;77:3371–3383.
233. Loney C, Mottet-Osman G, Roux L, et al. 2009. Paramyxovirus ultrastructure and genome packaging: cryo-electron tomography of Sendai virus. *J Virol* 83:8191–8197.
234. Loughlin GM, Taussig LM. Pulmonary function in children with a history of laryngotracheobronchitis. *J Pediatr* 1979;94:365–369.
235. Lu LL, Puri M, Horvath CM, et al. Select paramyxoviral V proteins inhibit IRF3 activation by acting as alternative substrates for inhibitor of kappaB kinase epsilon (IKKe)/TBK1. *J Biol Chem* 2008;283: 14269–14276.
240. Malur AG, Chattopadhyay S, Maitra RK, et al. Inhibition of STAT 1 phosphorylation by human parainfluenza virus type 3 C protein. *J Virol* 2005;79:7877–7882.
243. Marx A, Gary HE Jr, Marston BJ, et al. Parainfluenza virus infection among adults hospitalized for lower respiratory tract infection. *Clin Infect Dis* 1999;29:134–140.
244. Marx A, Torok TJ, Holman RC, et al. Pediatric hospitalizations for croup (laryngotracheobronchitis): biennial increases associated with human parainfluenza virus 1 epidemics. *J Infect Dis* 1997;176:1423–1427.
248. Merz DC, Prehm P, Scheid A, et al. Inhibition of the neuraminidase of paramyxoviruses by halide ions: a possible means of modulating the two activities of the HN protein. *Virology* 1981;112:296–305.
255. Moscona A. Entry of parainfluenza virus into cells as a target for interrupting childhood respiratory disease. *J Clin Invest* 2005;115:1688–1698.
256. Moscona A, Peluso RW. Fusion properties of cells persistently infected with human parainfluenza virus type 3: participation of hemagglutinin-neuraminidase in membrane fusion. *J Virol* 1991;65:2773–2777.
258. Moscona A, Porotto M, Palmer S, et al. A recombinant sialidase fusion protein effectively inhibits human parainfluenza viral infection in vitro and in vivo. *J Infect Dis* 2010;202:234–241.
260. Murphy BR, Prince GA, Collins PL, et al. Current approaches to the development of vaccines effective against parainfluenza and respiratory syncytial viruses. *Virus Res* 1988;11:1–15.
262. Nagai Y. Virus activation by host proteinases. A pivotal role in the spread of infection, tissue tropism and pathogenicity. *Microbiol Immunol* 1995;39:1–9.
263. Nagai Y, Klenk HD. Activation of precursors to both glycoporteins of Newcastle disease virus by proteolytic cleavage. *Virology* 1977;77: 125–134.
268. Nichols WG, Corey L, Gooley T, et al. Parainfluenza virus infections after hematopoietic stem cell transplantation: risk factors, response to antiviral therapy, and effect on transplant outcome. *Blood* 2001;98:573–578.
270. Nishio M, Ohtsuka J, Tsurudome M, et al. Human parainfluenza virus type 2 V protein inhibits genome replication by binding to the L protein: possible role in promoting viral fitness. *J Virol* 2008;82:6130–6138.
273. Nishio M, Tsurudome M, Ito M, et al. Human parainfluenza virus type 4 is incapable of evading the interferon-induced antiviral effect. *J Virol* 2005;79:14756–14768.
280. Park MS, Steel J, Garcia-Sastre A, et al. Engineered viral vaccine constructs with dual specificity: avian influenza and Newcastle disease. *Proc Natl Acad Sci U S A* 2006;103:8203–8208.
283. Parrott RH, Vargosko A, Luckey A, et al. Clinical features of infection with hemadsorption viruses. *N Engl J Med* 1959;260:731–738.
289. Poole E, He B, Lamb RA, et al. The V proteins of simian virus 5 and other paramyxoviruses inhibit induction of interferon-beta. *Virology* 2002; 303:33–46.
290. Porotto M, Fornabaio M, Kellogg GE, et al. A second receptor binding site on human parainfluenza virus type 3 hemagglutinin-neuraminidase contributes to activation of the fusion mechanism. *J Virol* 2007;81: 3216–3228.
293. Porotto M, Yokoyama CC, Palermo LM, et al. Viral entry inhibitors targeted to the membrane site of action. *J Virol* 2010;84:6760–6768.
297. Qiao D, Janke BH, Elankumaran S. Complete genome sequence and pathogenicity of two swine parainfluenzavirus 3 isolates from pigs in the United States. *J Virol* 2010;84:686–694.
299. Ramachandran A, Horvath CM. Dissociation of paramyxovirus interferon evasion activities: universal and virus-specific requirements for conserved V protein amino acids in MDA5 interference. *J Virol* 2010; 84:11152–11163.
302. Ray R, Glaze BJ, Compans RW. Role of individual glycoproteins of human parainfluenza virus type 3 in the induction of a protective immune response. *J Virol* 1988;62:783–787.
305. Reed G, Jewett PH, Thompson J, et al. Epidemiology and clinical impact of parainfluenza virus infections in otherwise healthy infants and young children < 5 years old. *J Infect Dis* 1997;175:807–813.
309. Romer-Oberdorfer A, Werner O, Veits J, et al. Contribution of the length of the HN protein and the sequence of the F protein cleavage site to Newcastle disease virus pathogenicity. *J Gen Virol* 2003;84:3121–3129.
315. Sakaguchi T, Kato A, Sugahara F, et al. AIP1/Alix is a binding partner of Sendai virus C protein and facilitates virus budding. *J Virol* 2005;79: 8933–8941.
317. Samal SK. Newcastle disease and related avian paramyxoviruses. In: Samal SK, ed. *The Biology of Paramyxoviruses.* Norwich, UK: Caister Academic Press; 2011.
319. Samuel AS, Paldurai A, Kumar S, et al. Complete genome sequence of avian paramyxovirus (APMV) serotype 5 completes the analysis of nine APMV serotypes and reveals the longest APMV genome. *PLoS One* 2010;5:e9269.
322. Schaap-Nutt A, Higgins C, Amaro-Carambot E, et al. Identification of human parainfluenza virus type 2 (HPIV-2) V protein amino acid residues that reduce binding of V to MDA5 and attenuate HPIV-2 replication in nonhuman primates. *J Virol* 2011;85:4007–4019.
323. Schaap-Nutt A, Scull MA, Schmidt AC, et al. Growth restriction of an experimental live attenuated human parainfluenza virus type 2 vaccine in human ciliated airway epithelium in vitro parallels attenuation in African green monkeys. *Vaccine* 2010;28:2788–2798.
325. Schmidt AC, McAuliffe JM, Huang A, et al. Bovine parainfluenza virus type 3 (BPIV3) fusion and hemagglutinin- neuraminidase glycoproteins make an important contribution to the restricted replication of BPIV3 in primates. *J Virol* 2000;74:8922–8929.
326. Schmitt AP, Leser GP, Morita E, et al. Evidence for a new viral late-domain core sequence, FPIV, necessary for budding of a paramyxovirus. *J Virol* 2005;79:2988–2997.
327. Segal AO, Crighton EJ, Moineddin R, et al. Croup hospitalizations in Ontario: a 14-year time-series analysis. *Pediatrics* 2005;116:51–55.
329. Shengqing Y, Kishida N, Ito H, et al. Generation of velogenic Newcastle disease viruses from a nonpathogenic waterfowl isolate by passaging in chickens. *Virology* 2002;301:206–211.
331. Singh-Naz N, Willy M, Riggs N. Outbreak of parainfluenza virus type 3 in a neonatal nursery. *Pediatr Infect Dis J* 1990;9:31–33.
332. Skiadopoulos MH, Durbin AP, Tatem JM, et al. Three amino acid substitutions in the L protein of the human parainfluenza virus type 3 cp45 live attenuated vaccine candidate contribute to its temperature-sensitive and attenuation phenotypes. *J Virol* 1998;72:1762–1768.
333. Skiadopoulos MH, Schmidt AC, Riggs JM, et al. Determinants of the host range restriction of replication of bovine parainfluenza virus type 3 in rhesus monkeys are polygenic. *J Virol* 2003;77:1141–1148.
334. Skiadopoulos MH, Surman S, Tatem JM, et al. Identification of mutations contributing to the temperature-sensitive, cold-adapted, and attenuation phenotypes of the live-attenuated cold- passage 45 (cp45) human parainfluenza virus 3 candidate vaccine. *J Virol* 1999;73:1374–1381.
335. Skiadopoulos MH, Surman SR, Riggs JM, et al. Sendai virus, a murine parainfluenza virus type 1, replicates to a level similar to human PIV1 in the upper and lower respiratory tract of African green monkeys and chimpanzees. *Virology* 2002;297:153–160.
337. Skiadopoulos MH, Vogel L, Riggs JM, et al. The genome length of human parainfluenza virus type 2 follows the rule of six, and recombinant viruses recovered from non-polyhexameric-length antigenomic cDNAs contain a biased distribution of correcting mutations. *J Virol* 2003;77: 270–279.

338. Slavin KA, Passaro DJ, Hacker JK, et al. Parainfluenza virus type 4: case report and review of the literature. *Pediatr Infect Dis J* 2000;19:893–896.
339. Slobod KS, Shenep JL, Lujan-Zilbermann J, et al. Safety and immunogenicity of intranasal murine parainfluenza virus type 1 (Sendai virus) in healthy human adults. *Vaccine* 2004;22:3182–3186.
340. Smith CB, Purcell RH, Bellanti JA, et al. Protective effect of antibody to parainfluenza type 1 virus. *N Engl J Med* 1966;275:1145–1152.
341. Song Q, Cao Y, Li Q, et al. Artificial recombination may influence the evolutionary analysis of Newcastle disease virus. *J Virol* 2011;85:10409–10414.
344. Spriggs MK, Collins PL. Human parainfluenza virus type 3: messenger RNAs, polypeptide coding assignments, intergenic sequences, and genetic map. *J Virol* 1986;59:646–654.
345. Spriggs MK, Murphy BR, Prince GA, et al. Expression of the F and HN glycoproteins of human parainfluenza virus type 3 by recombinant vaccinia viruses: contributions of the individual proteins to host immunity. *J Virol* 1987;61:3416–3423.
349. Strahle L, Garcin D, Kolakofsky D. Sendai virus defective-interfering genomes and the activation of interferon-beta. *Virology* 2006;351:101–111.
351. Subbiah M, Khattar SK, Collins PL, et al. Mutations in the fusion protein cleavage site of avian paramyxovirus serotype 2 that increase cleavability and syncytia formation but do not increase viral virulence in chickens. *J Virol* 2011;85:5394–5405.
360. Takimoto T, Portner A. Molecular mechanism of paramyxovirus budding. *Virus Res* 2004;106:133–145.
363. Tao T, Davoodi F, Cho CJ, et al. A live attenuated recombinant chimeric parainfluenza virus (PIV) candidate vaccine containing the hemagglutinin-neuraminidase and fusion glycoproteins of PIV1 and the remaining proteins from PIV3 induces resistance to PIV1 even in animals immune to PIV3. *Vaccine* 2000;18:1359–1366.
365. Tapparel C, Maurice D, Roux L. The activity of Sendai virus genomic and antigenomic promoters requires a second element past the leader template regions: a motif (GNNNNN)3 is essential for replication. *J Virol* 1998;72:3117–3128.
369. Terrier O, Rolland JP, Rosa-Calatrava M, et al. Parainfluenza virus type 5 (PIV-5) morphology revealed by cryo-electron microscopy. *Virus Res* 2009;142:200–203.
372. Tosi MF, Stark JM, Hamedani A, et al. Intercellular adhesion molecule-1 (ICAM-1)-dependent and ICAM-1-independent adhesive interactions between polymorphonuclear leukocytes and human airway epithelial cells infected with parainfluenza virus type 2. *J Immunol* 1992;149:3345–3349.
374. Toyoda T, Sakaguchi T, Imai K, et al. Structural comparison of the cleavage-activation site of the fusion glycoprotein between virulent and avirulent strains of Newcastle disease virus. *Virology* 1987;158:242–247.
375. Tremonti LP, Lin JS, Jackson GG. Neutralizing activity in nasal secretions and serum in resistance of volunteers to parainfluenza virus type 2. *J Immunol* 1968;101:572–577.
376. Tsurudome M, Bando H, Kawano M, et al. Transcripts of simian virus 41 (SV41) matrix gene are exclusively dicistronic with the fusion gene which is also transcribed as a monocistron. *Virology* 1991;184:93–100.
378. Tyrrell D, Bynoe M, Birkum K, et al. Inoculation of human volunteers with parainfluenza viruses 1 and 3 (HA 2 and HA 1). *Br Med J* 1959; 2:909–911.
382. van Wyke Coelingh K, Tierney EL. Antigenic and functional organization of human parainfluenza virus type 3 fusion glycoprotein. *J Virol* 1989;63:375–382.
384. van Wyke Coelingh KL, Winter C, Murphy BR. Antigenic variation in the hemagglutinin-neuraminidase protein of human parainfluenza type 3 virus. *Virology* 1985;143:569–582.
385. van Wyke Coelingh KL, Winter CC, Murphy BR. Nucleotide and deduced amino acid sequence of hemagglutinin-neuraminidase genes of human type 3 parainfluenza viruses isolated from 1957 to 1983. *Virol* 1988;162:137–143.
386. van Wyke Coelingh KL, Winter CC, Tierney EL, et al. Antibody responses of humans and nonhuman primates to individual antigenic sites of the hemagglutinin-neuraminidase and fusion glycoproteins after primary infection or reinfection with parainfluenza type 3 virus. *J Virol* 1990;64:3833–3843.
390. Vilchez RA, Dauber J, Kusne S. Infectious etiology of bronchiolitis obliterans: the respiratory viruses connection - myth or reality? *Am J Transplant* 2003;3:245–249.
393. Weinberg GA, Hall CB, Iwane MK, et al. Parainfluenza virus infection of young children: estimates of the population-based burden of hospitalization. *J Pediatr* 2009;154:694–699.
397. Welliver RC, Wong DT, Sun M, et al. Parainfluenza virus bronchiolitis. Epidemiology and pathogenesis. *Am J Dis Child* 1986;140:34–40.
399. Wolf MC, Freiberg AN, Zhang T, et al. A broad-spectrum antiviral targeting entry of enveloped viruses. *Proc Natl Acad Sci U S A* 2010;107:3157–3162.
406. Yin HS, Paterson RG, Wen X, et al. Structure of the uncleaved ectodomain of the paramyxovirus (hPIV3) fusion protein. *Proc Natl Acad Sci U S A* 2005;102:9288–9293.
407. Yin HS, Wen X, Paterson RG, et al. Structure of the parainfluenza virus 5 F protein in its metastable, prefusion conformation. *Nature* 2006; 439:38–44.
409. Yuan P, Thompson TB, Wurzburg BA, et al. Structural studies of the parainfluenza virus 5 hemagglutinin-neuraminidase tetramer in complex with its receptor, sialyllactose. *Structure* 2005;13:803–815.
410. Zhan X, Slobod KS, Krishnamurthy S, et al. Sendai virus recombinant vaccine expressing hPIV-3 HN or F elicits protective immunity and combines with a second recombinant to prevent hPIV-1, hPIV-3 and RSV infections. *Vaccine* 2008;26:3480–3488.
411. Zhang L, Bukreyev A, Thompson CI, et al. Infection of ciliated cells by human parainfluenza virus type 3 in an in vitro model of human airway epithelium. *J Virol* 2005;79:1113–1124.

CHAPTER 35

Steven A. Rubin • Christian J. Sauder • Kathryn M. Carbone

Mumps Virus

HISTORY

In the 5th century BC, Hippocrates described a mild epidemic illness associated with nonsuppurative swelling near the ears and, variably, with painful swelling of one or both testes. These descriptions of parotitis and orchitis, respectively, are the hallmarks of mumps virus (MuV) infection. The name *mumps* may derive from an old English verb that means to grimace, grin, or mumble. Hamilton, a physician of the late 18th century, is credited as being the first to associate central nervous system (CNS) involvement with mumps in his description of the neuropathology of a fatal case. Later studies would reveal MuV as a highly neurotropic agent and a leading cause of virus-induced aseptic meningitis and encephalitis.[20,42,190]

A number of laboratory investigations suggested that a filterable, transmissible agent was responsible for mumps[141,281,423]; however, a viral etiology was not proven until 1935 when Johnson and Goodpasture, using bacteria-free parotid secretions, successfully transmitted the disease between monkeys and children and then back to naïve monkeys, fulfilling Koch's postulates.[186,187]

The demonstration by Habel[145] and Enders[108] in 1945 that MuV could be isolated and propagated in embryonated eggs enabled the demonstration of the hemagglutinating, hemolytic,[268] and neuraminidase[182] properties of the virus, leading to the development of an inactivated vaccine in 1946[144] and to the first live virus vaccine in 1958.[353] The introduction of tissue culture as a practical alternative for the propagation and study of the virus in 1948[414] was pivotal for advancing studies of the epidemiology and pathogenesis of the disease as well as the molecular biology of the virus, permitting the development of cell-based vaccines.

Although historically a benign disease of childhood, mumps was viewed as a major concern for the military, particularly in times of mobilization. Mumps was a notable issue during the Civil War of the United States,[166] World War I,[138] and during World War II,[253,302] and continues to occur in military settings.[13,218,316] During World War I, mumps was a leading cause of days lost from active duty in the United States Army in France, exceeded only by losses due to influenza and gonorrhea infections.

Use of live, attenuated mumps vaccines have nearly eliminated the disease from countries with high vaccine coverage rates of a two-dose regimen,[126,301] although sporadic and sometimes large mumps outbreaks continue to occur even in highly vaccinated populations.[98]

INFECTIOUS AGENT

Classification

MuV is a nonsegmented, negative-strand RNA virus in the family *Paramyxoviridae,* subfamily *Paramyxovirinae,* genus *Rubulavirus.* See Chapter 33 for a detailed overview of the *Paramyxoviridae.*

Virion Morphology and Structure

Mumps virions are pleomorphic particles ranging from 100 to 600 nm in size, consisting of a helical ribonucleoprotein (RNP) core surrounded by a host cell–derived lipid envelope (Fig. 35.1). The RNP consists of a single-stranded RNA

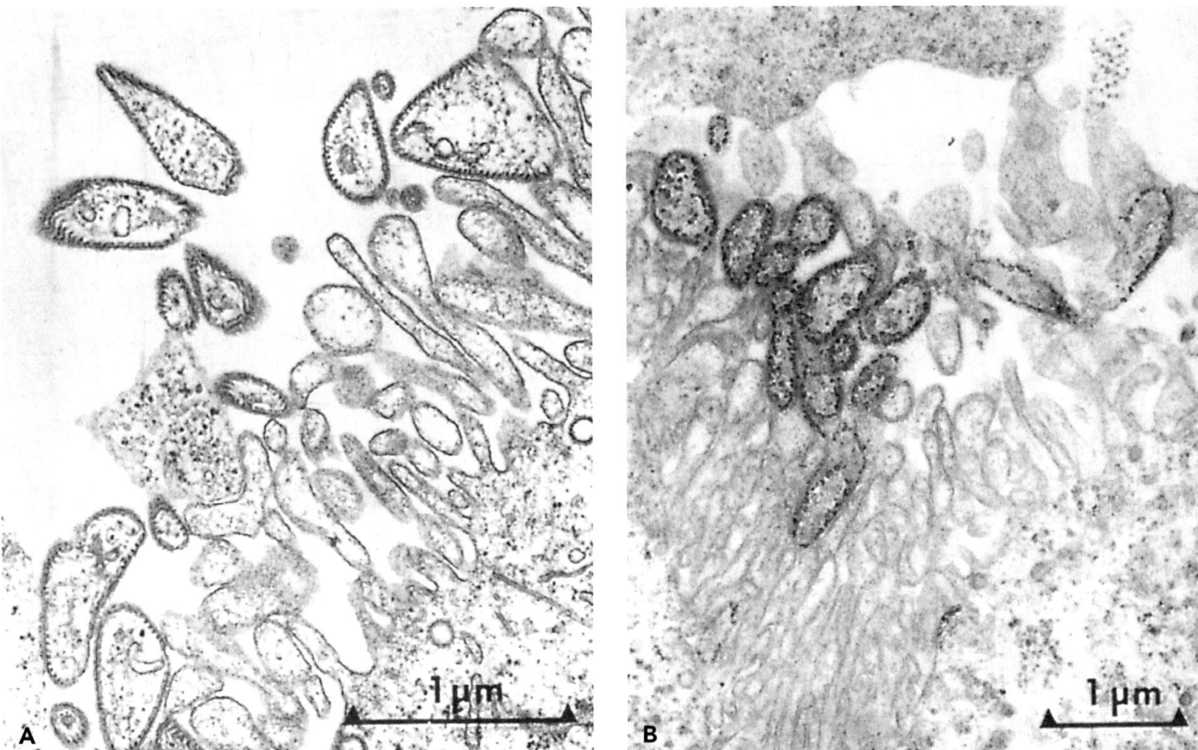

FIGURE 35.1. A: Pleomorphic mumps virions budding from a choroid plexus epithelial cell. **B:** A subjacent section processed for post-embedding localization of the major nucleocapsid-associated protein using monoclonal anti-N antibody. The N is localized by punctate, electron-dense reaction products below the surface membranes of the cell.

(ssRNA) molecule coated by the viral nucleoprotein.[82] The RNP appears to be a hollow tube with a unit length of approximately 1 μm, a diameter of 17 to 20 nm, and a central core of 5 to 6 nm.[168,169,251] The viral host cell–derived envelope contains the viral glycoproteins that project 12 to 15 nm from the virion surface.

Full-length genomic RNA (gRNA) is an unsegmented, single-stranded macromolecule of negative polarity that consists of 15,384 nucleotides. The presence of multiploid virions in MuV preparations has been reported, but only one of the genomes is believed to be biologically active.[250]

Genomic Organization

The MuV genome contains 7 tandemly linked transcription units: the nucleo- (N), V/phospho-/I (V/P/I), matrix (M), fusion (F), small hydrophobic (SH), hemagglutinin-neuraminidase (HN), and large (L) protein genes. The gene order is 3′-N-V/P/I-M-F-SH-HN-L-5′.[105,107] The MuV genome is flanked at the 3′ end by an extracistronic leader sequence of 55 nucleotides[370] and at the 5′ end by a trailer sequence of 24 nucleotides,[288] of which the last 10 share inverse complementarity. These regions are essential for transcription and replication. Unlike most other paramyxoviruses, MuV does not have identical gene-start and gene-end sequences. The consensus gene-start sequence is 3′-U-U/C-C-G/U-G/U-N-C/U-U/C-U and that of the stop sequence is 3′-A-A/U-U/A-U-C/A-U6-7,[105] separated from each other by intergenic sequences of 1 to 7 nucleotides.

Each gene encodes a single protein, with the exception of the V/P/I gene (conventionally referred to as the *P* gene), which gives rise to additional mRNA species as a result of the cotranscriptional insertion of nontemplated G nucleotides between positions 461 to 466.[107,297] Faithful transcription of the gene produces the V protein (formerly referred to as NS1 protein), whereas insertion of two G residues within the editing site produces an mRNA encoding the P protein and insertion of one or four G residues produces an mRNA encoding the I protein (formerly referred to as NS2 protein and analogous to the W protein reported in related paramyxoviruses). Thus, the V, P, and I proteins have the same amino-terminal segment but different C-terminal regions.

Genome transcription occurs by a stop-start mechanism in which the viral polymerase produces a decreasing gradient of monocistronic mRNA for genes located further from the 3′-end promoter (see Chapter 33). Due to the occasional failure of the viral RNA–dependent RNA polymerase (RdRp) to recognize the intragenic stop signals, bi-, tri-, tetra-, penta- and hexacistronic read-through transcripts can be detected in MuV-infected cells, from which only the first cistron is translated.[5,89,106] The size of the monocistronic mRNAs as well as the number of amino acids and molecular weights of the MuV proteins are provided in Table 35.1.

Virus Proteins and Replication

N, P and L Proteins

The first translated transcriptional unit of the virus, the N protein, complexes with the gRNA to form the RNP, the template for RNA synthesis. Only encapsidated RNA, not naked

TABLE 35.1 Mumps Genes and Gene Products

Gene	mRNA[a]	Amino acids	MW in kd Predicted	MW in kd Observed[b]	Biological activity
N	1,845	549	61.4	69–73[c]	• Encapsidates genomic RNA • Protects RNA from nucleases • Confers helical structure of RNP • Binds to RdRp
P	1,314	391	41.6	45–47	• Part of the RdRp • Tethers RdRp to RNP
V	1,312	224	24.2	22–28	• Antagonizes IFN-β induction • Inhibits IFN-α/β and INF-γ signaling
I	1,313/1,315	170–171	18.3	16–19	Unknown
M	1,253	375	41.6	39–42	Virus assembly and budding
F_0	1,721	538	58.8	65–74	Fusion protein precursor
F_1		436	47.4	58–61	Viral attachment and entry
F_2		83[d]	9.4	10–16	Viral attachment and entry
SH	310	57	6.71	6	Anti-apoptotic activity
HN	1,887	582	64	74–80	Viral attachment, entry, and release
L	6,925	2261	256.6	160–200	Part of the RdRp

[a]Without polyA tail.

[b]Approximate molecular weight as observed by gel electrophoresis.

[c]Difference between calculated and observed weight likely due to phosphorylation.

[d]Without the cleaved 10 amino acid signal sequence.

RNA, can be transcribed. RNA synthesis begins with the binding of the RdRp, a complex of the P and L proteins, to the RNP, as inferred from other studies of highly homologous viruses.[140,147]

The MuV N protein is a bipartite molecule consisting of a globular N-terminal assembly domain (amino acids 1 to 398) mediating RNA binding (to form the RNP), and an unstructured hypervariable C-terminal tail believed, based on studies of related viruses, to interact with the MuV M protein during virion assembly.[35,88,342]

The MuV P protein forms homotrimers via a centrally located coiled-coil domain[87] and complexes with the L protein to form the RdRp. The C-terminal 48 amino acids of the P protein is a nucleocapsid-binding domain (NBD), responsible for tethering of the RdRp to the RNP by binding to the assembly domain of the N protein (amino acids 1 to 398).[207] The three-dimensional structure of the NBD has been deciphered using X-ray crystallography and revealed formation of a compact bundle of three α-helices, a feature that appears to be conserved among paramyxovirinae.[208] Unlike the NBD of measles virus and Sendai virus, that of MuV lacks defined tertiary structure and is fundamentally unstable.[207] As indicated by its name, the MuV P protein is heavily phosphorylated,[278] an action believed to regulate polymerase activity, but this has not been clearly demonstrated for MuV.[123,361,362]

Six functional domains have been identified in the MuV L protein based on sequence similarity with L proteins from related viruses.[308,350] These domains have been ascribed all catalytic functions such as execution of transcription and replication, as well as methylation, capping, and polyadenylation of mRNAs (see Chapter 33). A detailed functional and structural analysis of the MuV L protein has not yet been carried out.

Matrix Protein

The MuV M protein orchestrates virus assembly and budding. Only the MuV M protein when expressed alone is sufficient for virus-like particle production, although in the absence of co-expression with other viral proteins, efficiency is low.[234] Evidence indicates that the M protein binds to the cytoplasmic tails of the F and HN glycoproteins assembled at distinct locations on cellular membranes, presumably lipid raft microdomains. There, the M protein functions as an adapter, physically linking the region of host-cell membrane expressing the viral F and HN glycoproteins with the viral RNP via its interaction with the N protein.[152,234] Budding appears to be mediated by an interaction between the MuV M protein and the cellular endosomal sorting complex for transport (ESCRT) machinery.[234] The MuV M protein has also been shown to interact with host proteins angiomotin-like 1 (AmotL1) and 14-3-3.[298,299] Whereas the AmotL1–M protein interaction appears to promote MuV VLP production, based on studies of PIV5, M protein interaction with 14-3-3 decreases the efficiency of virus budding. Interestingly, the MuV M 14-3-3 binding site is adjacent to a sequence motif conserved among rubulaviruses, presumably functioning as a binding site for the host protein caveolin 1 (Cav-1), an essential structural component of caveolae that are considered a subset of lipid rafts. It is therefore likely that MuV budding, like that of PIV5, occurs from caveolae. The close proximity of the 14-3-3 and postulated Cav-1 binding sites raises the possibility that the MuV

M protein switches between either binding to 14-3-3 or Cav-1, thereby regulating the amount of M that can participate in virus budding.[299]

Surface Glycoproteins

The F and HN are transmembrane glycoproteins of types I and II, respectively. The F glycoprotein is synthesized as an inactive precursor, F_0, that is targeted to the rough endoplasmic reticulum via a 19 amino acid signal peptide, which is subsequently cleaved.[408] Following N-glycosylation, the precursor is transported to the trans-Golgi network where it is proteolytically cleaved between amino acids 102 and 103 by the host cell protease furin at the R-R-H-K-R motif to produce two disulfide-linked heterodimers F_1 and F_2.[162,257,278,409] Cleavage of F_0 is essential for virus-to-cell and cell-to-cell membrane fusion and for virus infectivity. The amino terminus of the F_1 subunit possesses the fusion peptide, a conserved hydrophobic domain exposed by the cleavage event (see Chapter 33). Evidence indicates that a second cleavage event occurs during which F_1 is processed into two subunits, F_{1a} and F_{1b}; this event is important in mediating fusion activity.[400]

At least two heptad repeat (HR) domains are found in the F1 ectodomain: HR1 at the amino terminus adjacent to the fusion peptide and HR2 at the carboxyl terminus adjacent to the transmembrane domain.[239] The MuV F protein forms homotrimers and the HR1 and HR2 domains interact to form a stable six-helix bundle structure.[239,249] The HR2 domain is also involved in the binding of F with HN. In related viruses, additional HR domains have been identified, although this has not been confirmed for MuV.[131,270] The specific processes involved in MuV fusion have not been delineated; however, based on similarity with the six-helix bundle structural of the PIV5 F protein, the events that mediate MuV fusion are likely similar to those for PIV5 (see Chapter 34).

In its native state, the HN protein is a disulfide-bonded oligomer assembled as homotetramers. The protein is held in the lipid bilayer by a hydrophobic domain of 19 residues near the amino terminal, a domain that probably also serves as a signal sequence in a manner similar to other paramyxovirus HN proteins. HN monomers display a membrane proximal stalk that supports a globular head, forming a six-blade propeller structure.[84,219] The globular head is responsible for attachment and neuraminidase activity[182,291]; the stalk region, in conjunction with the F protein, mediates virus-to-cell and cell-to-cell fusion.[371,382] Based on inference from related viruses, a single site is believed to mediate both neuraminidase and receptor binding activity using a protein conformational switch mechanism to toggle activity.[77,84,226] There may also be a second sialic acid binding site within the globular head region, theorized to stabilize viral–cellular membrane interactions in addition to the large binding pocket that fluxes between neuraminidase and receptor binding activity.[37,314,437] Two competing models on the HN-assisted mechanism of F protein activation have emerged[78] (see Chapter 34 for details). Briefly, the "clamp model" proposes that the HN protein associates with F intracellularly, stabilizing the prefusion conformation of the protein. Upon binding of HN protein to its receptor, the F protein is released, allowing for the conformational change required for fusion activity. In the "provocateur model," a change in the structure of the HN itself is postulated to promote fusion activity. In this model, the HN protein either is preassociated with the F protein or associates with the protein following receptor binding, at which point the HN protein undergoes a conformational change leading to destabilization of the F protein, which confers fusion activity. Results from recent studies using PIV5 HN and F proteins support the "provocateur model." Whether this model applies to MuV awaits confirmation.

V Protein

The MuV V protein, as reported for other rubulaviruses, is involved in inhibiting IFN production and signaling (see Chapter 33). The 69 aa C-terminal cysteine-rich domain of the MuV V protein appears to be the key player in these activities. This region directly interacts with MDA5 (melanoma differentiation–associated gene 5), a pattern recognition receptor that recognizes cytosolic viral RNA, and with the TBK-1 (TANK-binding kinase 1)/IKKε (inhibitor of kB kinase-ε) kinases responsible for interferon regulatory factor-3 (IRF-3) phosphorylation. MuV V protein interaction with MDA5 inhibits its ability to induce transactivation of the IFN-β promoter,[12,320] and in the case of TBK-1/IKKε, leads to their ubiquitination and subsequent proteasomal degradation,[243] preventing IRF-3 phosphorylation, an event required for transcription of IFN and IFN-stimulated genes. The C-terminus of the MuV V protein also interacts with the cellular signal transducer and activator of transcription (STAT) proteins, STAT-1, STAT-2, and STAT-3.[151,282,434,435] STAT-1 and STAT-2 play a central role in the IFN signal transduction pathway that eventually leads to activation of IFN-induced genes. STAT 3 has also been implicated in cellular antiviral responses.[318,389] Binding of MuV V leads to the ubiquitination and subsequent degradation through the proteasomal pathway of STAT-1 and STAT-3, but not of STAT-2; however, the latter is required for targeting of STAT-1 for degradation.[216,388,389,435] The C-terminus of the MuV V protein is not the only region important in these interactions, as exemplified in a study demonstrating that a single point mutation at amino acid position 95 abrogates the ability of the MuV V protein to degrade STAT3, while retaining the virus's ability to target STAT 1.[318]

The observation that the MuV V protein can oligomerize and form spherical particles suggests that the MuV protein provides a scaffold for coordinating the assembly of the cellular components (e.g., UV-damaged DNA binding protein 1 [DDB1], cullin 4A [Cul4A], and regulator of cullin 1 [Roc1]) involved in ubiquitination, collectively referred to as V-dependent degradation complexes (VDC).[388] For more details on VDC, see Chapter 33.

SH Protein

The SH protein consists of 57 amino acids, 25 of which are highly hydrophobic and clustered at the amino terminus serving as a membrane anchor region with its C-terminus facing the cytoplasm.[104,106,367] The predicted SH mRNA exhibits two AUG start codons, the second of which represents the actual AUG for the SH open reading frame. The first AUG, located at positions 4 to 6, gives rise to a minicistron with a stop codon at nucleotides 19 to 21.[106,367] Due to the immediate proximity of the first cistron to the cap of the mRNA, it is predicted that with a frequency of about 50%, the ribosomes will skip the first AUG and initiate at the second cistron,[212] thus enabling translation of the SH protein, although at reduced efficiency. The biological significance of this minicistron and its proposed role in reducing the amount of SH protein synthesized is unknown.

In certain MuV strains, such as the Enders and Rubini strains, a point mutation exists in the putative F gene polyadenylation signal resulting in an F-SH bicistronic mRNA,[220,367,368] from which only the F protein is made. This demonstrates that the SH protein is not essential for virus replication, which has been confirmed for PIV5.[156]

Studies of PIV5 demonstrated that the SH protein facilitates evasion of the host antiviral response via blocking the TNF-α-mediated apoptosis pathway.[156,157] The MuV SH protein appears to be functionally similar, based on recombinant DNA studies in which PIV5 SH gene was then replaced with that of MuV.[418] Yeast two-hybrid and co-immunoprecipitation studies identified ataxin-1 ubiquitin-like interacting protein (A1Up) as a cellular target of the MuV SH protein. This protein plays a role in proteasomal degradation, but the biological significance of its interaction with the MuV SH protein is not clear.[427]

I Protein

Expression of the I protein in infected cells was confirmed, but its role in the life cycle of the virus is unknown.[297]

Virus Infection of Host Cells

Sialic acid, an acyl derivative of neuraminic acid, is found on cellular glycoproteins and lipids and serves as the receptor for MuV. Following attachment of the virus to its receptor, the viral and cellular membranes fuse, permitting entry of the viral RNP followed by its transcription and replication. These events occur in a manner common to most paramyxoviruses (see Chapter 33 for a detailed description of these and other events such as viral assembly and release).

Because the MuV receptor is ubiquitously expressed on mammalian cells, the virus infects most cell types. The presence of MuV is typically detected in cell cultures by the induction of syncytia, large homogeneous masses of cytoplasm enclosing numerous nuclei (Fig. 35.2), followed by lysis of infected monolayers; however, the cytopathic effects of MuV can vary considerably among isolates and substrates, and in some instances, there is little evident morphologic change.[4,142,250] The type of cytopathic effect produced *in vitro* does not correlate with the *in vivo* behavior of the virus.

PATHOLOGY AND PATHOGENESIS

Infection in Experimental Animals

Humans are the only natural host of MuV, although experimental infection has been induced in laboratory animals, including monkeys,[230,327,334] hamsters,[192,295,419] mice,[205,295] and rats.[315,331] Experimental infection of animals has mostly been used to study the pathogenesis of MuV neurotropism and neurovirulence. Intracerebral inoculation of MuV into the suckling hamster results in a massive inflammatory response, including meningitis, encephalitis, and ventriculitis. Intraperitoneal inoculation of virulent strains into suckling hamsters also leads to CNS infection.[420] Associated neuropathology includes hydrocephalus, Chiari type I cerebellar malformation, and neuronal necrosis.[204,295,366,369,421] Many of these are reported features of CNS infection in humans, suggesting the applicability of the hamster model for studying the pathogenesis of MuV infection in man. Similar findings have also been reported in monkeys.[70,241,326,334,436] Very little, if any, work has been accomplished in mice because MuV infection in this species tends to be abortive, thereby limiting the value of this model system.[155,317,383] Early studies also indicated mumps infection to be abortive in rats, unless adapted by serial passage in brain.[315] Subsequent studies, however, determined that intracerebral inoculation of the virus into newborn rats resulted in inflammation of the ventricular system (choroiditis, ependymitis) and hydrocephalus, but not meningitis or encephalitis.[331] Interestingly, the severity of hydrocephalus in rats was found to correlate well with the virus strain-specific neurovirulence potential for humans, suggesting the relevance of such a model of disease in examining the pathogenesis and molecular basis of MuV neurovirulence.[332] The severity of virus-induced neuropathology in marmosets, but not other monkey species, was also found to correlate with virus neurovirulence potential for humans.[328]

Infection in Humans

Transmissibility after nasal or buccal mucosal inoculation of virus[187] suggests that natural infection is initiated by droplet spread. The incubation period is 16 to 18 days,[167,259] during which the virus multiplies in the upper respiratory mucosa before spreading to draining lymph nodes. Based on studies involving experimental infection of hamsters, virus disseminates via a transient plasma viremia,[420] potentially infecting multiple tissues and

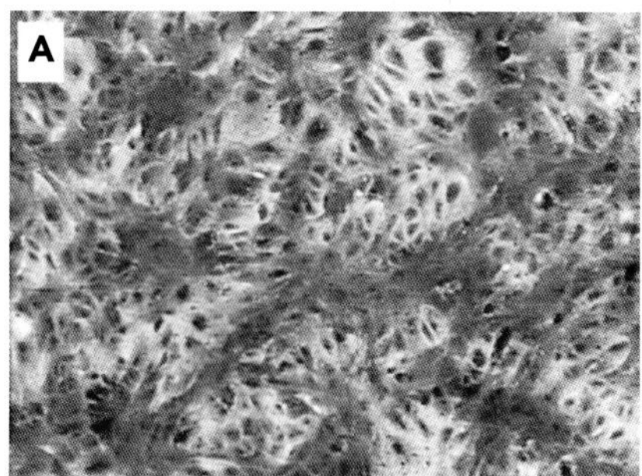

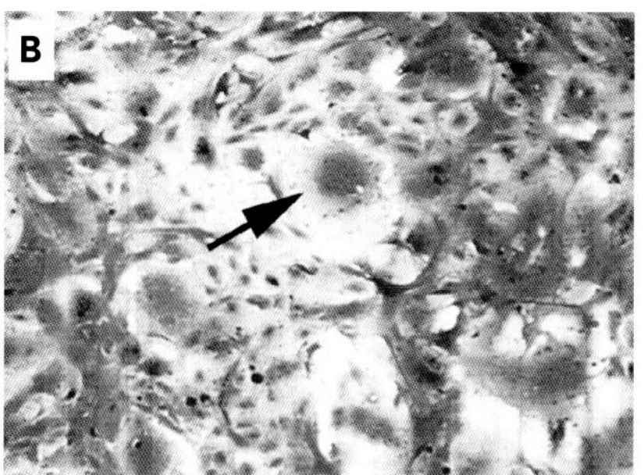

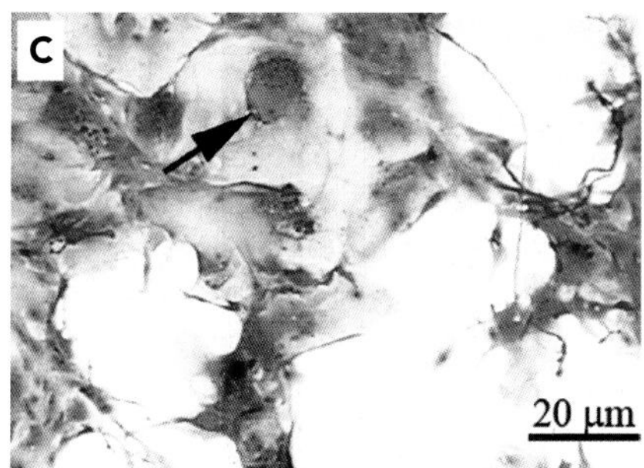

FIGURE 35.2. Phase contrast image showing the progression of typical cytopathic effects of a mumps virus clinical isolate after incubation on Vero cells for 1 (A), 4 (B), and 7 (C) days. The classic cytopathic effect of cell-to-cell fusion and syncytia formation (*arrows*) appear within a few days of culture, followed by cell lysis. By day 7 nearly the entire cell monolayer is consumed by syncytia and lysis. Acetone fixation, cresyl violet stain.

organ systems.[172] The most common sites of virus dissemination are glandular tissues (parotid glands, testes, breasts, and pancreas), and the CNS. If viruria is used as an indication of kidney infection, then kidney involvement is common in mumps, although clinical nephritis is rarely diagnosed.[392,394] In rare cases, MuV can be transmitted transplacentally.

Virus is shed in saliva as early as 6 days before the onset of parotitis.[159] Termination of viral shedding correlates with the local appearance of virus-specific secretory IgA and IgM, as early as a few days after disease onset.[67,304] Fewer than 15% of patients continue to shed virus beyond day 4 of symptom onset.[310] Thus, patients with mumps are capable of spreading virus by the respiratory route over a 10-day interval.

Plasma viremia disappears coincident with the development of MuV–specific antibody, which can be detected in serum as early as 11 days after infection of humans.[159] Animal models suggest that circulating infected lymphocytes provide a means for the spread of virus in the face of mounting humoral immunity.[420] Despite the apparent high frequency of viremia during mumps, MuV has only rarely been detected in blood.[183,201,294]

Parotid Gland

Initial clinical symptoms usually relate to infection of the parotid gland, but viral involvement of this gland is neither a primary nor obligate step in the infection.[202] Virus infects the ductal epithelium, resulting in desquamation of involved cells, periductal interstitial edema, and a local inflammatory reaction primarily involving lymphocytes. Swelling, inflammation, and tissue damage in the parotid gland can produce elevation of serum and urine amylase levels.[346]

Central Nervous System

MuV CNS invasion, as demonstrated by cerebrospinal fluid (CSF) pleocytosis, occurs in greater than one third of patients presenting with clinical mumps.[20,42,46,112] Symptomatic CNS infection (i.e., meningitis) is less common, occurring in approximately 10% of cases.[20,149,198] Encephalitis occurs in less than 0.5% of cases. In the prevaccine era, MuV was a leading cause of viral meningitis and encephalitis in most developed countries and continues to be a leading cause in unvaccinated populations worldwide.[18,125,160,258] Neurologic manifestations appear with a 3:1 or greater male–female ratio[30,210,228] and are generally preceded by parotitis by 4 to 5 days but can occur before or in the total absence of detectable salivary gland swelling.

As inferred from animal studies, viral invasion of the CNS occurs across the choroid plexus.[420] Blood-borne infected mononuclear cells, and possibly cell-free virus, can cross the fenestrated endothelium of the choroid plexus stroma and serve as a source for subsequent infection of the choroidal epithelium. Maturation of virus from the ventricular surfaces of choroidal cells provides progeny virions that are widely distributed through ventricular pathways and the subarachnoid space by CSF (Fig. 35.3). Virus can penetrate brain parenchyma and infect neurons by contiguous spread from infected ependymal cells that line the ventricular cavities of the brain. Once within neurons, virus most likely spreads along neuronal pathways, as reported in nonhuman primates.[230] Although primary encephalitis is typically the response to direct viral invasion of neural cells, cases of postinfectious encephalitis, an autoimmune attack on CNS myelin sheaths, also occurs. Symptoms of primary encephalitis appear before or during the development of parotitis; symptoms of postinfectious encephalitis and associated demyelination appear 1 to 3 weeks after the onset of parotitis.[238,372]

Typical CNS pathology of MuV encephalitis includes edema and congestion throughout the brain with hemorrhage, lymphocytic perivascular infiltration, perivascular gliosis, and demyelination. Findings in the spinal cord include early degenerative changes in the anterior horn cells and perineuronal edema.[102,264,372] When seen, the selective periventricular myelin loss with relative sparing of axons is typical of parainfectious autoimmune encephalitis.

Rarely is CNS infection fatal and most cases resolve without sequelae. In some instances, however, electroencephalographic changes, ataxia, and behavioral disturbances may take months to resolve[173,210] and permanent neurologic damage—such as obstructive hydrocephalus,[286] deafness,[236] and myelitis[284,395]—can occur.

Hydrocephalus can develop days to years after initial MuV infection and can lead to progressively worsening headaches, mental status changes, and gait abnormalities.[71,137,286] The pathogenesis of hydrocephalus is inferred from animal studies that have suggested that desquamation of virus-infected ventricular ependymal cells blocks egress of CSF through the aqueduct of Sylvius. Abnormally restricted flow of CSF to adsorptive sites over the cerebral convexities results in progressive enlargement of the lateral and third ventricles.[191,192] The presence of ependymal cell debris in the CSF of humans presenting with MuV CNS infection suggests a similar mechanism of hydrocephalus induction in humans.[161,286,380] Hydrocephalus, however, has also been observed before, or in the total absence of, aqueductal stenosis.[189,364,365,419] This indicates that stenosis of the aqueduct could be a secondary consequence of external compression by surrounding edematous tissue and not causally related to the pathogenesis of hydrocephalus.

MuV is the most frequent cause of acquired sensorineural hearing loss in children. Transient, high-frequency deafness is the most common form, occurring in approximately 4% of mumps cases.[402] Permanent deafness occurs in less than 1 per 20,000 cases[27,153] and is usually unilateral. Deafness is believed to be the result of direct viral invasion of the cochlea, likely via the perilymph, which freely communicates with the CSF[146,254,352,415]; however, evidence indicates a hematogenous route exists.[265] Pathology includes degeneration of the stria vascularis, tectorial membrane, and organ of Corti and collapse of Reissner's membrane.[111] Hearing loss caused by indirect effects of virus infection (e.g., immune-mediated damage) have also been suggested.[390] Deafness is not disproportionately seen with other complications, suggesting no specific pathogenic link with parotitis, meningitis, or other complications. Deafness has also been observed in otherwise asymptomatic patients.[287,390]

Gonads

Orchitis, usually unilateral, occurs in approximately 20% of postpubertal men who develop mumps.[16,124,224] Orchitis rarely occurs in children, suggesting that certain hormonal factors, such as receptors for luteinizing hormone and follicle-stimulating hormone expressed during adolescence, might promote testicular tropism of the virus.[376] Virus has been isolated from testicular biopsies of the affected gland within the first 4 days of symptoms, and from semen,[29,179] strongly suggesting that symptomatic gonadal involvement reflects local virus replication. The

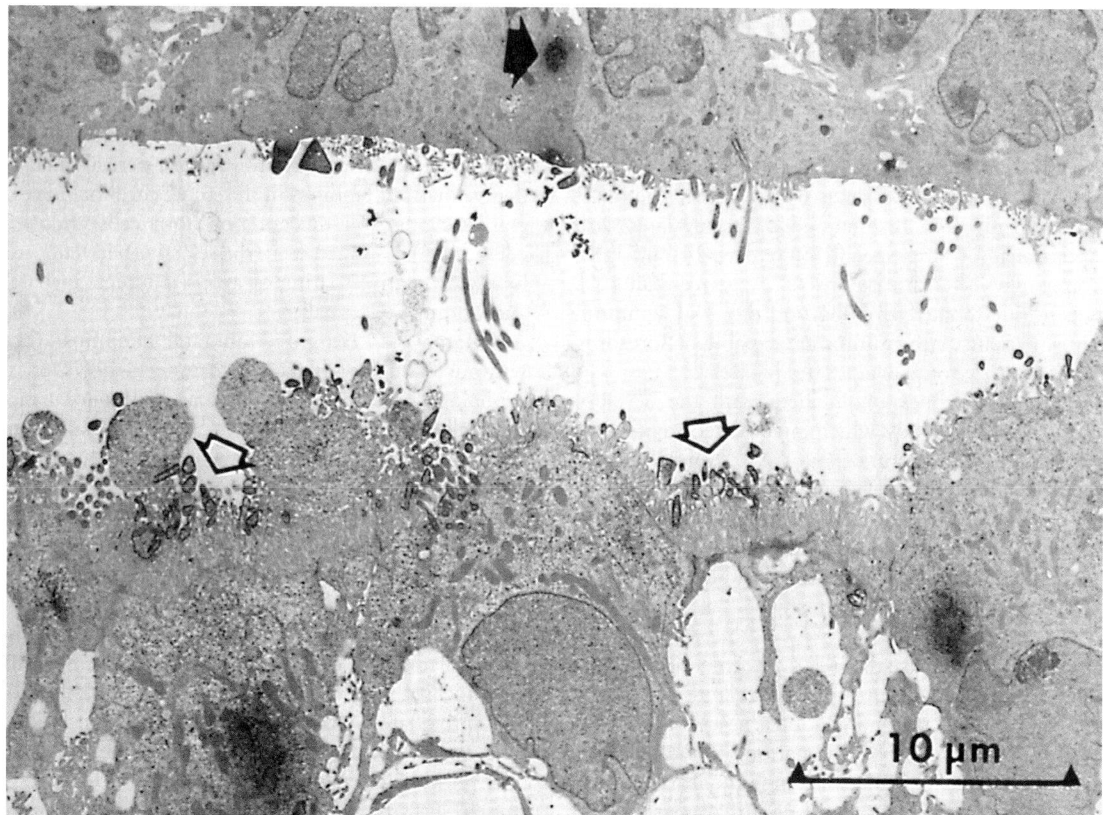

FIGURE 35.3. Post-embedding electron-microscopic immunocytochemical staining of a region of the lateral ventricle of a hamster 5 days after intraperitoneal infection with the Kilham strain of MuV. Anti-N monoclonal antibody was used as the primary reagent. The reaction product defines nucleocapsids located below the cytoplasmic membranes at sites of virion budding along both the ependymal and choroidal (*unfilled arrows*) surfaces. Intracytoplasmic nucleocapsid inclusions are also demarcated by the reaction product in both choroid plexus and individual ependymal (*filled arrow*) cells.

seminiferous tubules may be the primary site of viral replication, with local lymphocytic infiltration and edema of interstitial tissues.

Ovary infection is diagnosed in less than 5% of postpubertal women who develop mumps,[38,64,97,199,248,360] which may be an underestimate because unless a pelvic examination is performed, abdominal or pelvic pain from inflamed ovaries might be attributed to pancreatic infection.

Kidneys

Based on the frequency of viruria, virus frequently disseminates to the kidneys, where epithelial cells of the distal tubules, calyces, and ureters appear to be primary sites of virus replication.[413] Viruria can be detected in most patients, sometimes for as long as 14 days after the onset of clinical symptoms.[392,393] Mild abnormalities of renal function have been described, but they are usually of little clinical importance.[392] Although virus dissemination to, and replication in, the parotid gland and kidney can occur simultaneously, replication in renal tissue is more prolonged and continues well beyond the appearance of neutralizing antibody in serum.

Pancreas

Pancreatic involvement, diagnosed in 1% to 27% of cases,[38,47,64,232,296,345,356,376,416] is usually expressed as mild epigastric pain, but severe hemorrhagic pancreatitis[114] and transient exocrine function abnormalities[92] have been reported. MuV infects human pancreatic beta cells *in vitro,*[403] and virus infection of the pancreas has been demonstrated in hamsters inoculated intraperitoneally.[420] Viral infections have been considered a possible precipitating event leading to the onset of about one third of all cases of juvenile-onset or type I insulin-dependent diabetes mellitus (IDDM); however, whether MuV causes IDDM is unclear.[83,127,136,344] No association has been found between mumps and type II diabetes.[240]

Heart and Joint Tissues

Myocardial invasion occurs frequently in mumps, as indicated by electrocardiographic abnormalities.[14] Although it is seldom symptomatic, interstitial lymphocytic myocarditis and mild pericarditis may occur following mumps replication in cells of the myocardium and pericardium.[43] MuV myocarditis can lead to the rare but serious sequelae of endocardial fibroelastosis.[279]

Mild to moderately severe mono- or polyarticular and, often, migratory arthritis has rarely been associated with mumps.[139] MuV has not been isolated from joint fluids or synovial tissues, and no evidence exists for significant immune complex deposition.

Fetus and Newborn

MuV can be transmitted transplacentally as demonstrated in nonhuman primates[357] and by the isolation of the virus from the human fetus following spontaneous first-trimester abortion during maternal mumps.[221,433] The virus can produce a fetal wastage in humans, with or without subsequent spread of virus to involve fetal tissues directly.[433] MuV has also been isolated from fetal tissues following planned therapeutic abortion of seronegative women 1 week after vaccination with live, attenuated MuV, although it is unclear if the virus detected was vaccine virus, or wild-type virus coincidentally contracted at or shortly before the time of vaccination.[430] A proliferative necrotizing villitis with decidual cells containing intracytoplasmic inclusions has been described in the products of spontaneous and induced abortions.[129] Late-gestation intrauterine infection was reported in an infant born to a mother who developed mumps more than 4 weeks before delivery, diagnosed by reverse transcription polymerase chain reaction (RT-PCR) testing of the infant's cord blood cells.[363] This infant developed severe pulmonary symptoms, including hypertension and hemorrhage.

MuV is excreted in breast milk,[203] but few cases of perinatal mumps have been described[195,222] and it is not clear if breast milk was responsible for these cases. There appears to be a somewhat different mode of pathogenesis of mumps in newborns. In the first year or two of life, infants may have only pulmonary involvement without evidence of parotitis.[195,363] Split immunologic recognition in the infants can follow maternal parotitis, resulting in MuV-specific cell-mediated immune responses without a concomitant antibody response.[1,357,378]

Molecular Basis of Virulence

While comprehensive studies on the molecular basis of MuV virulence have yet to be performed, it is clear that the genetic basis of MuV neurotropism and neurovirulence does not lie within any one gene[7,329,339,348,428] and no simple pattern of genomic mutations capable of discriminating virulent from attenuated MuV strains has been identified.[8,177,339]

CLINICAL FEATURES

The clinical features of mumps reflect the pathogenesis of the infection, as reviewed here. Approximately one third of all MuV infections occur without recognized symptoms.[44,79,112,305,321] Moderate fever is often present at the onset of disease, with defervescence a few days later. The feature most characteristic of mumps is salivary gland swelling, particularly the parotid glands (Fig. 35.4),[305] which constitutes the basis of a clinical diagnosis. Submaxillary gland enlargement and involvement of the sublingual glands also occur. Enlargement of individual glands is painful, usually lasting 2 to 3 days, but may persist 10 days or longer.[158] Virus is present in the saliva for several days before the onset of clinical disease[159] and for up to 5 days later.[67] The virus can be detected in urine for several weeks after the onset of mumps.[393]

Various organs and tissues can be symptomatically involved during mumps, including the testes, CNS, mammary glands, ovary, pancreas, kidneys, and heart.[172] Parotitis usually precedes manifestations of involvement of other sites of virus infection, but the latter can be clinically evident before, during, or even in the absence of parotitis.

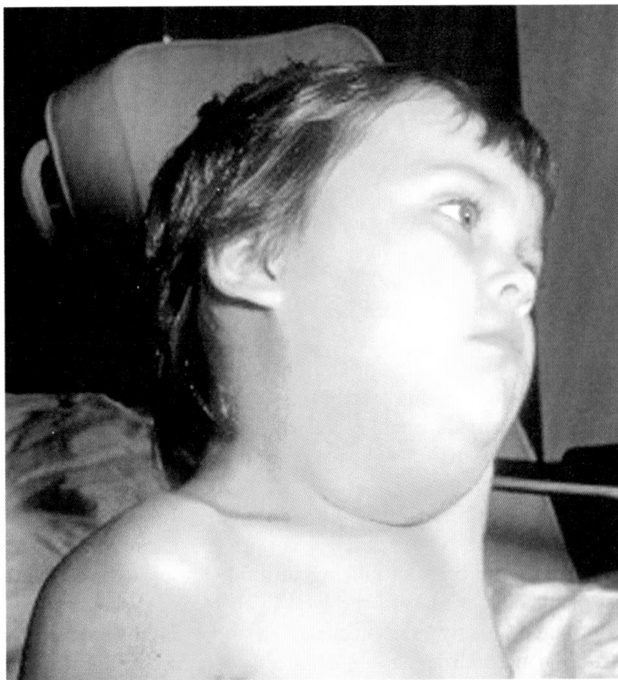

FIGURE 35.4. Child with parotitis. (Courtesy of Centers for Disease Control and Prevention, Atlanta, GA.)

The most common complication of mumps (aside from parotitis) is epididymo-orchitis. Testicular pain and swelling has a time course similar to that of the parotid gland. Mumps orchitis often leads to testicular atrophy of the involved and, occasionally, the clinically uninvolved gland.[25] Atrophy after mumps orchitis is rarely implicated as a cause of male sterility.[349] About 15% of females complain of breast swelling and tenderness. As with orchitis in men, the incidence of mastitis is significantly higher after puberty.[305]

Nausea and vomiting with or without epigastric or left upper-quadrant pain are frequent features of mumps, occurring in approximately half of all cases during the St. Lawrence Island epidemic.[305] It is unclear whether these symptoms reflect involvement of the pancreas or other viscera. Some of these generalized features of the illness may reflect the effects of circulating IFN, which can be found in serum early in the clinical course of mumps.[269,404]

More than one third of mumps cases develop CSF pleocytosis, but symptomatic CNS involvement is far less frequent.[20,42,305] Mumps meningitis may precede parotitis, but it typically develops 5 days following parotitis. However, as many as half of those with mumps meningitis may not have detectable salivary gland enlargement.[193,202]

IMMUNE RESPONSES

Humoral Immunity

Virus-specific salivary IgM and IgA and serum IgA, IgM, IgG, and neutralizing antibody are all detectable at the time of symptom onset. During natural infection, salivary IgM appears to be the first detectable immunoglobulin class, followed by salivary

IgA. The latter is capable of virus neutralization and is detectable for approximately 10 weeks after symptom onset.[68,119,120] Levels of serum IgA and IgM peak approximately 1 to 2 weeks after symptom onset and decline to undetectable levels by week 8 after symptom onset.[41,387] MuV-specific IgG has been detected as early as 4 days before symptom development,[280] peaking 4 to 8 weeks later and detectable for decades.[41,387] In naïve individuals, IgG is of low avidity[277] and IgG3 antibodies predominate early in the course of disease, whereas in later stages isotypes IgG1 and IgG2 predominate. Upon a second exposure to MuV, serum IgM and IgA antibodies are typically absent or are produced at very low levels; the IgG1 subclass, typically of high avidity, predominates.[143]

Virus-neutralizing antibodies, which are a correlate of protection, are detectable as early as day 2 after symptom onset, peaking 4 to 8 weeks later, and are detectable for decades. Studies conducted during the prevaccine era indicate that neutralizing antibody titers in the range of 1:4 to 1:8 confer protection,[23,44,109,260] however, it is not clear if such low levels of vaccine-induced neutralizing antibody are protective. Studies of the effectiveness of the Jeryl Lynn mumps vaccine strain conducted shortly after licensure in the United States indicate that neutralizing antibody titers as low as 1:2 are protective.[410,411] However, in a more recent study conducted among Jeryl Lynn vaccinees involved in a mumps outbreak, many confirmed mumps cases had neutralizing antibody titers in excess of 1:8 in preoutbreak blood samples.[80]

Only antibodies directed against the F and HN protein have been definitively shown to neutralize the virus and protect against infection.[170,235,242,354] Use of polyclonal antisera in virus neutralization assays demonstrates a broad cross-reactivity among different MuV genotypes.[176,291,293,333,431] However, neutralizing antibody titers can differ substantially against different MuV strains, suggesting the existence of virus strain–specific neutralizing epitopes. Despite such demonstrations in the laboratory, MuV appears serologically monotypic in clinical situations as suggested empirically by the dramatic reductions in mumps incidence in countries with high two-dose vaccine coverage.[126,300,351,407]

The role of antibody in arresting the infection cannot be underestimated. Seropositive patients challenged intravenously with up to 10^9 plaque-forming units of MuV showed only transient fever and no symptoms of reinfection developed, although an anamnestic rise in antibody titer was seen 4 to 5 days later.[289] Animals are protected from otherwise lethal viral challenge by neutralizing monoclonal antibody administered several days after primary virus inoculation.[422] The development of hemagglutination-inhibition and virus-neutralizing antibody responses in the hamster model correlates well with the fall in peak virus titers in infected organs. In hamsters, however, viral antigens continue to be expressed, and clinical CNS disease actually occurs, after virus titers have fallen considerably.[420]

Cell-Mediated Immunity

In vitro lymphocyte-proliferative responses to MuV antigens are readily measured in seropositive individuals.[174] CD8+ and γ/δ cytotoxic T lymphocytes have been demonstrated in blood and CSF following infection with wild-type or vaccine MuV strains.[26,69,116,215] Mononuclear cell inflammation in MuV-infected tissues is well developed at the time of onset of clinical disease, suggesting that specific cellular responses develop during the incubation period. The presence of major histocompatibility (MHC) antigen (e.g., MHC Ia)-restricted T lymphocytes and specifically sensitized cells in both the blood and the CSF of some patients with active mumps meningitis support this view.[121] After immunization, peak cell-mediated immune responses are found 2 to 4 weeks later and can last for decades.[69,150,194] Circulating cytotoxic T-cell responses restricted to autologous infected target cells are found within the first few weeks of mumps meningitis.

Although the presence or absence of MuV-specific cell-mediated responses often correlates with the presence or absence of virus-specific antibody, the magnitude of the two types of immune responses do not correlate[66,324]; in some instances, cell-mediated immune responses have been detected in seronegative persons.[150,194] Immunologic studies of related viruses (e.g., measles) indicate the importance of the cellular response in the recovery and long-term protection from disease,[24,128,180,181,303,405] but this has not been established for MuV. For example, levels of interferon-γ induced by MuV infection do not correlate with illness severity[223,404] and patients with severely compromised T-cell responses experience a course of disease that does not differ from that seen in healthy individuals.[99] Similarly, neither severe symptoms of mumps nor a protracted course of illness has been reported in persons with AIDS.

Considering data demonstrating that MuV targets mda-5 and STAT proteins for degradation (discussed earlier), MuV may impede cytotoxic T lymphocyte (CTL) activation, by suppressing IFN production and signaling, which regulate MHC class-I expression.[49]

EPIDEMIOLOGY

Age

Before widespread vaccine use, mumps was most commonly seen in children between 5 and 9 years of age[76]; by 15 years of age, greater than 90% of most populations had serologic evidence of infection with MuV.[52,271] Despite a high seroprevalence in older individuals in the prevaccine era, large outbreaks were common, particularly in high-density, close-contact environments, such as military settings.[138,302]

In the years following mumps vaccine licensure in 1967, a gradual shift was seen in the typical age of infection in the general U.S. population from young children towards those 10 to 19 years of age, likely reflecting protection of younger children by vaccination, while older children and young adults not eligible for vaccination at the time remained susceptible.[54,396] By 1992, the highest age-specific incidence in the United States shifted back to the 5- to 9-year-old age group, where it remained until a large multi-state mumps outbreak occurred in 2006, predominantly on university campuses.[255,256] In the years following the 2006 mumps outbreak, the age-specific incidence returned to the younger age group,[58,59] until the recent mumps outbreaks in New York and New Jersey in 2009–2010, where again most cases occurred in young adults.[64] A similar pattern has been observed in many other countries and the occurrence of mumps predominantly in young adults is now common.

Mumps is rarely seen in children younger than 1 year of age, most likely because of acquisition of immunity by placental transfer of maternal antibody. In premature infants born to seropositive mothers, little maternal antibody can be detected at birth; by 3 months of age, no antibody can be detected in these babies.[133] Thus, premature infants may be particularly susceptible to MuV infection.

Morbidity and Mortality

The major morbidity from mumps results from meningitis, encephalitis, and orchitis. These occur as age- and sex-specific hazards, with peak risk in postpubertal boys.[10] With the case fatality ratio for mumps between 1.6 and 3.8 per 10,000,[51] and with 0.5% to 2.3% of all mumps encephalitis cases being fatal,[266] it is apparent that most fatal mumps cases have CNS infection.

Origin and Spread of Epidemics

Humans are the only natural host for MuV infection; there is no known animal reservoir. MuV, as with measles virus, requires a population of about 200,000 people to sustain its continued transmission. Such population densities were first achieved some four to five millennia ago,[31] so it follows that MuV first evolved about 5,000 years ago. Presently, mumps is a geographically unrestricted disease, except for its absence among a few remote tribes or isolated small-island populations. In modern-day urban populations and in the absence of immunization, mumps is endemic, with peak incidence rates in the winter and spring months.[266] In the prevaccine era, preschool-aged children were an important source of virus introduced into families, given that inapparent infections are common in children of this age.[79,305]

In the present era of high vaccine coverage of children, most cases now occur among young adults, suggesting waning immunity. Indeed, levels of MuV-specific antibody decline significantly with time after vaccination,[36,40,94,96,227,263] and time since last vaccination has been identified as a factor in decreased vaccine effectiveness[75,122,345] and in increased odds of contracting disease.[48,81,397]

Prevalence and Seroepidemiology

Data on the incidence of mumps are complicated by the fact that approximately 30% of all MuV infections are subclinical.[44,79,112,233,246,305,321] Furthermore, only 25% of all cases are seen by a clinician and fewer than 30% are reported to public health agencies.[112,233] Annual incidence rates vary, with an interepidemic period of approximately 3 years.[10,22,283]

The highest incidence of mumps reported in the United States since 1922 was almost 250 per 100,000 population in 1941. In 1968, when mumps vaccine was introduced, the yearly incidence was 76 per 100,000 population, steadily declining to less than 1 case per 100,000 population by 1993 and then to an all-time low of less than 0.1 case per 100,000 population by 2003 (Fig. 35.5).[51,56] Mumps incidence remained low until 2006 when the United States experienced its largest mumps outbreak in 19 years, with 6,584 cases reported, representing a 20-fold increase in disease incidence from the prior year. Mumps incidence rapidly returned to baseline, before another large outbreak occurred in 2009,[63] suggestive of a possible return to the 3-year interepidemic cycle.

In the prevaccine era, or in countries not incorporating mumps vaccine in national immunization programs, most persons become seropositive by adolescence. In the United States, where vaccination is required for school entry, by 1996, approximately 90% of 19- to 35-month-old children had received at least one dose of mumps-containing vaccine[50,57,62] and among adolescents aged 13 to 17 years, by 2006 coverage with two or more doses was 89%.[61] These figures are close to the herd immunity threshold, estimated to be 90% to 92% based on theoretical studies,[11,306] but are lower than the 95% figure based on evidence from the experience in Finland where indigenous mumps has been eliminated.[95]

MuV was the most common cause of viral encephalitis in the United States until 1975, following attainment of high coverage rates of vaccination.[55] In unvaccinated populations,

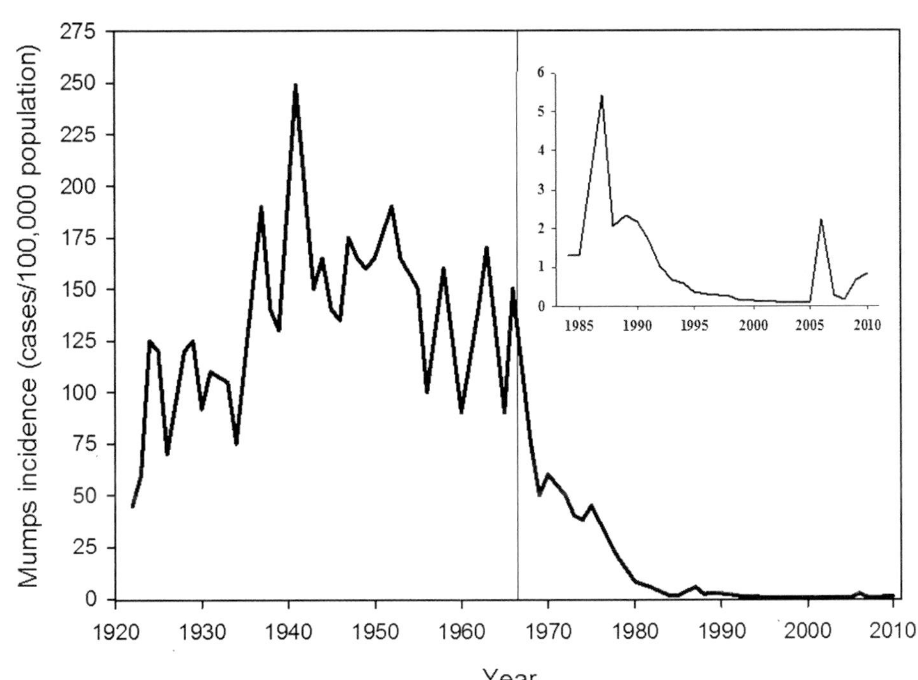

FIGURE 35.5. Mumps cases per 100,000 population in the United States from 1922 to 2010. Vertical line indicates year of vaccine introduction (1967). **Inset:** Larger scale showing disease incidence between 1985 and 2010, with large outbreaks in 1987–1989, 2006, and 2009–2010.

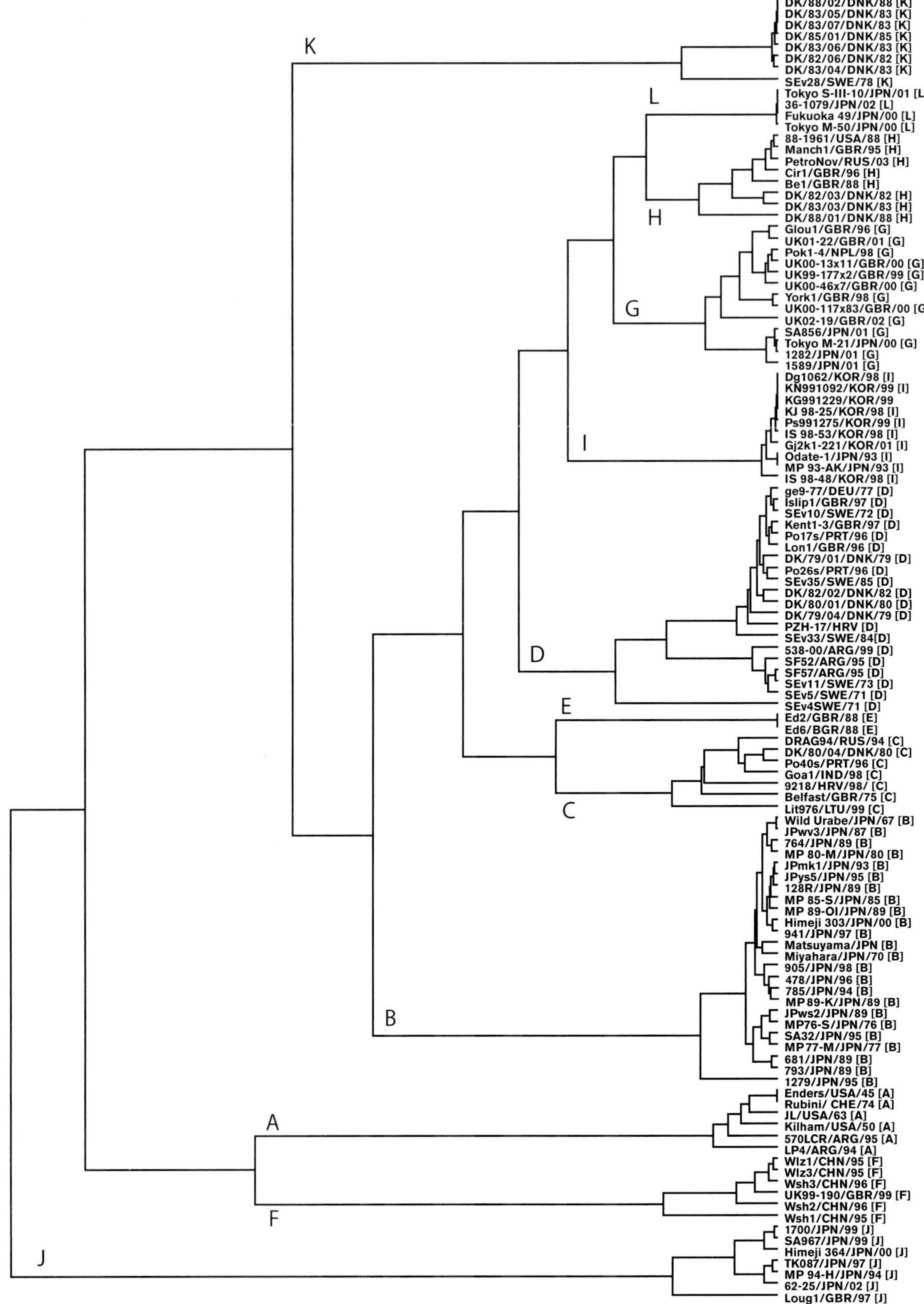

FIGURE 35.6. Phylogenetic tree showing the 12 MuV genotypes, A through L, based on the *SH* gene nucleotide sequence. Strains in bold type have been suggested as international reference strains for the respective genotypes.[184] The tree was constructed based on comparison of coding sequences of *SH* gene using the OligoScan (Micro-Tech, S. Hutchinson, KS) custom computer software package. The algorithm uses nucleotide distance matrix and clustering based on the Pearson correlation coefficient between lines of the matrix. (Tree constructed courtesy of Dr. Konstantin Chumakov, FDA/CBER.)

mumps accounts for up to half of all encephalitis cases.[311] In an epidemic setting, 11% of clinical mumps cases have CNS disease, 90% with meningitis and 10% with encephalitis.[305] Severe mumps meningitis or encephalitis is most common between the ages of 5 and 9 years, with a clear male predominance in all age groups.[30]

New Epidemiologic Approaches

The most significant molecular epidemiology advance has been RT-PCR to identify and group individual virus strains by related genomic sequences. RT-PCR analysis has become a key element in mumps surveillance and is a definitive means of identifying transmission pathways. MuV genotyping is conventionally performed based on the nucleotide sequence of the *SH* gene, the most variable sequence in the genome. Phylogenetic analyses of these sequences place the virus strains into distinct clusters that form the basis for genotype assignment.[432] Virus strains belonging to the same SH genotype vary at the nucleotide level within the SH gene by up to 4%, whereas intergenotype variation is typically on the order of 8% to 19%.[184,185] It has been suggested that establishment of new genotypes be based on variation from existing genotypes by greater than 5% at the nucleotide level, among other criteria.[184,185] Currently, 12 MuV genotypes exist, designated A through L (Fig. 35.6). A provisional genotype M has been proposed.[336] Because of the lack of a central body for assigning genotype designations, some confusion exists to which strains are members of genotype J and which are members of genotype K. Genotypes A, C, D, G, and H are predominantly observed in the Western hemisphere, whereas genotypes B, F, I, J/K, and L are typically found in countries of the Asia-Pacific region.[272] Cocirculation of multiple genotypes within a region, or even within an outbreak, is not uncommon. There is no established association between genotype designation and specific virus characteristics,[8,177,339] although some have suggested that virus genotypes C, D, H, and J are more neurotropic than other genotypes.[319,373,375]

Relationships among MuV strains have also been inferred from nucleotide sequence analyses of the *N*,[178] *P*,[335,429] *F*,[118,374,385] and *HN*[229,330,431] genes. While these genes are more conserved in sequence and, thus, their use in discriminating among virus strains is not as powerful, phylogenetic analyses of these sequences may prove useful. For example, because the HN protein is the major cell surface target of neutralizing antibody,[291,292,347] it stands to reason that HN-based genotyping will provide valuable information on antigenic diversity and protective immunity.[91,211,293] Sequence analysis of this and other genes may also provide valuable information on the evolution of MuV.

RT-PCR and sequencing of viruses has proved particularly useful in investigation of possible vaccine-associated adverse events, such as aseptic meningitis. It was not until the availability of this technology that reports of this complication of vaccination could be confirmed.[17,196,273,275,340,377,401]

DIAGNOSIS

Clinical Diagnosis

A clinical diagnosis of mumps is made on the basis of fever and constitutional symptoms (e.g., parotitis) usually developing within 3 weeks after known exposure. Meningeal symptoms include headache, vomiting, fever, and nuchal rigidity, usually appearing 3 to 5 days after the onset of parotitis with a range of 1 week before to 2 weeks afterward.[20,322] Seizures occur in 20% to 30% of patients with CNS symptoms.[19,132] Meningeal involvement is also suggested by positive Brudzinski's and Kernig's signs and can be differentiated from encephalitis by a normal electroencephalogram (EEG), although the EEG findings can be normal in subjects with encephalitis, even when clinical seizures occur.[132] In many cases, the diagnosis can be confirmed by an elevated CSF-to-serum antibody ratio.[269,387] Mumps meningitis is generally a benign condition with complete recovery in 3 to 4 days. Frank delirium and focal neurologic deficits are uncommon. Patients with mumps meningitis and encephalitis without focal deficits, prolonged or recurrent focal seizures, or papilledema have marked clinical improvement of neurologic function within 2 to 4 days. Even with profound obtundation, patients recover with few sequelae.[19,42,46]

Laboratory confirmation is often required because a number of infectious agents, drugs, and conditions can cause mumps-like symptoms (see Differential Diagnosis below).

Laboratory Diagnosis

Laboratory diagnosis presently rests on infectious virus isolation (typically using Vero cells), detection of viral genome by RT-PCR, and appropriate serologic studies of acute and convalescent sera.

Infectious virus and virus genome can be detected in several clinical fluid specimens, including oral fluid samples (e.g., saliva, throat swabs, and buccal swabs), CSF, and urine. Specimens should be collected as early in the disease as possible (within the first week) with storage at –70°C or below until testing can occur. Success rates are highest with oral fluid samples and lowest with urine and blood samples, despite the apparent high frequency of viruria and viremia.

Studies using oral fluid specimens demonstrate that MuV isolation by cell culture is as sensitive as detection by RT-PCR.[33,213,267,325] For urine, however, success rates are higher for virus isolation as compared to RT-PCR detection, possibly due to the presence of PCR inhibitors in urine,[3,154,213,267,426] and for CSF, for reasons that are not clear, success rates are higher for RT-PCR.[309,384]

The relative success of virus detection also appears to depend on vaccination status. Whereas the success rate of virus detection in cases with a history of 0 or 1 dose of vaccine typically exceeds 70%,[3,90,267] in persons with a history of 2 doses of vaccine, virus could only be detected in approximately 30% of clinically apparent cases.[28,325]

Many of the viruses in the differential diagnosis of mumps cause cellular pathology indistinguishable from that induced by MuV, and not all MuV strains produce cytopathic effects *in vitro*. Therefore, cultures must be tested for the presence of virus antigen by immunocytochemistry on cells inoculated with clinical specimens, or for viral genome by RT-PCR. Direct testing of clinical specimens by RT-PCR without an intervening cell culture step is commonly practiced.

Mumps humoral immune responses are most commonly measured by ELISA or virus neutralization. Other once commonly performed serologic tests, including complement fixation, immunofluorescence assay, hemagglutination-inhibition and hemolysis-in-gel are no longer widely used due to inferior sensitivity and specificity (i.e., cross-reactivity with other paramyxoviruses). Because most people either have a history of vaccination or natural infection, simple detection of MuV antibodies in patient serum is not sufficient for a diagnosis of acute infection or reinfection. Rather, a significant rise in antibody titer relative to that in serum drawn before or at the onset of symptoms (e.g., as neutralizing antibody or ELISA-based IgG) needs to be demonstrated in convalescent serum drawn 2 to 4 weeks after the onset of clinical symptoms. Alternatively, MuV IgM and IgG levels can be compared when only acute-phase serum is available. The MuV-specific IgM response will exceed the IgG response early in the infection before diminishing over the next few weeks to months.[387] In the present era of high vaccine coverage, reliance only on IgM detection is no longer advised, given the difficulty of its detection in anamnestic immune responses.[154,337,338] Thus, in vaccinees, the absence of MuV-specific IgM is not confirmation of the absence of MuV infection. Furthermore, testing of sera too early or too late in the course of disease can also yield false-negative IgM results.[86,214,406]

Because of its ease of use and high throughput, ELISA is more often performed than the labor-intensive virus neutralization assay. However, antibodies without known biological activity (e.g., those directed against the MuV nonstructural proteins) as well as cross-reactive anti-parainfluenza virus antibodies yield a positive result in the MuV ELISA, raising concern with interpretation of ELISA-based results in certain settings.

White blood cell (WBC) and differential counts are usually normal although leukocytosis is common in cases presenting with meningitis, orchitis, or pancreatitis. Serum amylase levels are elevated in cases of parotitis or pancreatitis, the latter being differentiable from parotitis by isoenzyme analysis or serum pancreatic lipase determinations.[238]

In cases of CNS invasion, lymphocytes are the predominant cell type found in the CSF, with WBC counts averaging 250/mm^3.[202,424] Cells counts peak around the third day of neurologic symptoms and then gradually decline over a period of several weeks.[121,417] In some instances, CSF pleocytosis can persist for as long as a year.[398] The CSF is usually under normal pressure[46] and the protein content in the CSF is elevated in 60% to 70% of all cases.[121,202] Protein levels up to 100 mg/dL can be seen; on occasion, they exceed 700 mg/dL. This appears to reflect damage to the blood–brain barrier, as indicated by elevated albumin indices that do not normalize for several weeks to months after the onset of CNS symptoms.[237] The CSF glucose content is modestly depressed to 17% to 41% of the serum value in 6% to 29% of all cases.[101,193,417] About one third of all patients have evidence of intrathecal IgG synthesis and demonstrable oligoclonal immunoglobulins during the first week of CNS symptoms; this oligoclonal antibody can persist for more than 2 years.[121] More than one half show increased IgG indices by the third month following mumps meningitis.[121,237,399] Up to 90% of patients with acute mumps meningitis produce virus-specific IgG within the CNS compartment,[237,387,399] and one half show MuV–specific IgM.[117] Because mumps antibodies are uncommon in the CSF during other CNS infections,[100] in many instances of mumps meningitis, a diagnosis can be confirmed by elevated CSF-to-serum antibody ratios using samples taken during illness.[269,387]

Of all cases of mumps with symptoms sufficiently severe to warrant hospitalization, less than 10% can be expected to show transient electrocardiograph abnormalities consistent with myocardial damage. These usually consist of ST-segment depression, but patients can show evidence of atrioventricular conduction defects, including complete heart block.[14] Seldom is the cardiac involvement acutely symptomatic. MuV myocarditis can be linked, however, to serious long-term sequelae, such as endocardial fibroelastosis.[279]

DIFFERENTIAL DIAGNOSIS

When parotitis is present, the clinical diagnosis of mumps is straightforward, even if the disease is not epidemic. Nonetheless, other causes of parotitis should be considered. These include parainfluenza virus types 1 and 3, influenza A virus, coxsackievirus, lymphocytic choriomeningitis virus, human immunodeficiency virus (HIV), and suppurative infections including *Staphylococcus aureus* and atypical mycobacteria. All can be easily differentiated from MuV by serology or culture. Starch ingestion, drugs (e.g., phenylbutazone, thiouracil, iodides and phenothiazines), metabolic disorders (e.g., diabetes mellitus, cirrhosis, and uremia), and malnutrition can also cause parotitis. Rare conditions such as Mikulicz's, Parinaud's, and Sjogren's syndromes can also be confused with mumps.[238] Other possible causes of parotid swelling include tumors, cysts, and salivary stones. Without parotitis or with inconspicuous salivary gland enlargement, symptoms of other visceral organ or CNS involvement may predominate, thus laboratory confirmation of the diagnosis is required, even during an epidemic.

TREATMENT

Treatment of mumps and its various complications is generally symptomatic. In a controlled study, adult men presenting with parotitis were alternatively given either an intramuscular injection of 20 mL of gammaglobulin prepared from human convalescent serum or simply confined to a hospital for routine, nonspecific symptomatic therapy.[130] Orchitis developed in 4 of 51 antibody-treated and 14 of 51 symptomatically treated patients ($P < 0.01$). No protective effect was seen with gammaglobulin obtained from a normal donor serum pool.[130] This study suggests that immunotherapy with high-titer polyvalent or monoclonal antibody preparations could be useful in selected cases but should be used very early in the course of the illness. Notably, immunoglobulin for the treatment of mumps is no longer available in most countries.

PREVENTION AND CONTROL

The apparent ineffectiveness of passive protection and the near impossibility of preventing virus spread by case isolation (considering that virus is shed before the appearance of clinical symptoms and a significant portion of infected individuals are asymptomatically infected) leaves vaccination as the only practical control measure.

Vaccines and Adverse Events

Two general types of MuV vaccines have been used, formalin-inactivated (killed) vaccines and live, attenuated vaccines. Use of formalin-inactivated MuV vaccines (used in the

TABLE 35.2 Mumps Virus Vaccine Strains in Current Use

Vaccine strain	Genotype	Manufacturer	Vaccine name	Main area of use
Hoshino	B	Kitasato Institute	Hokken, Hoshino	Japan, Korea
NK M-46		Chiba Serum Institute	NK M-46	Japan
Torii		Takeda Pharmaceutical	Torii	Japan
Urabe		Sanofi-Pasteur	Trimovax® (trivalent)	Worldwide
Leningrad-3	Classification pending	Moscow State Facility for Bacterial Preparations	Leningrad-3	Russia
Leningrad-Zagreb	Classification pending	Inst. of Immunol., Zagreb	Leningrad-Zagreb	Croatia, Slovenia
		Serum Institute of India	Tresivac® (trivalent)	Worldwide
Jeryl Lynn	A	Merck/Aventis Pasteur MSD	MMRII® (trivalent)	Worldwide
			MMR-Vaxpro® (trivalent)	Europe
			ProQuad® (quadrivalent)	Worldwide
		GlaxoSmithKline	Priorix® (trivalent)	Worldwide
		(RIT 4385 strain)	PriorixTetra® (quadrivalent)	Europe
		Netherlands Vaccine Inst.	BMR vaccine® (trivalent)	Netherlands
		Sevapharma Inc.	Pavivac®	Czech Republic
			Trivivac® (trivalent)	Slovak Republic
		Dalian Jinjang-Andi Bioproducts	S79	China
S-12	H	Razi State Serum and Vaccine Institute	S-12	Iran
		Crucell Vaccines (formerly Berna Biotek)	BBM-18[a]	Europe

[a]In development

United States from 1950 to 1978) has been discontinued worldwide due to short-lived (<1 year) immunity and relatively poor efficacy.[175,307] All mumps vaccines currently in use are composed of live, attenuated virus (Table 35.2) and have been responsible for the remarkable decline in the incidence of mumps and related sequelae.

Live, attenuated virus mumps vaccines were developed through continuous serial passage of wild-type isolates. At present, no clear distinguishing marker exists for attenuation of MuV strains apart from the failure of a passaged isolate to produce clinical symptoms in vaccinees, although various animal tests of mumps vaccine virulence are under evaluation. In the United States, the only licensed mumps vaccine is the Jeryl Lynn strain and currently is only available in combination with measles and rubella vaccines (MMR) or measles, rubella, and varicella vaccines (ProQuad [Merck, West Point, PA] in the United States). Monovalent Jeryl Lynn vaccine is no longer manufactured.

Because of demonstrated and theoretical considerations about spread of virus to placenta and fetal tissues, administration of vaccines containing live MuV three months before or during pregnancy is not advised.[307]

Prelicensure studies demonstrated that a single dose of the Jeryl Lynn vaccine strain induces protective levels of virus neutralizing antibodies in greater than 95% of recipients.[165,359,412] Similar results have been found for other mumps vaccine strains licensed for use elsewhere.[103,276] Although antibody titers after vaccination develop more slowly and are lower than those following natural infection, protection from natural mumps appears complete,[45,110] and neutralizing antibody persists for decades.[94] However, waning and loss of neutralizing antibody has been reported as early as 4 years postvaccination.[40,93,263]

The Jeryl Lynn vaccine is composed of two distinct but genetically related viruses, designated Jeryl Lynn-5 (JL-5) and Jeryl Lynn-2 (JL-2), existing in an approximate 5:1 ratio.[6] These two viruses differ from each other at 414 nucleotides (3%), leading to 87 amino acid substitutions.[9] Over 500 million doses of the Jeryl Lynn–based MuV vaccines have been distributed worldwide, with few serious adverse effects noted.[164] Most reported complications (e.g., rash, pruritus, and purpura) have been allergic in nature; these complications are both uncommon and usually mild and self-limited.[55] Approaches for the immunization of egg-allergic children have been detailed.[225] A comprehensive survey of the literature by the Vaccine Safety Committee of the Institute of Medicine failed to find adequate information to establish or reject a causal relationship between the administration of Jeryl Lynn MuV–containing vaccines and the development of encephalopathy, encephalitis, residual seizure disorders, optic neuritis, transverse myelitis, Guillain-Barré syndrome, IDDM, or sterility caused by orchitis, all of which have been extensively reviewed elsewhere.[32,358] Parotitis following Jeryl Lynn vaccination occurs in approximately 1% of vaccinees.[115,261,313]

Other widely distributed vaccine strains include the RIT 4385, Urabe AM9, Leningrad-Zagreb, and Rubini (discontinued). The RIT 4385 strain, produced by GlaxoSmithKline (Philadelphia, PA), was derived from the Jeryl Lynn strain by clonally isolating the JL-5 population.[379] The Jeryl Lynn and RIT 4385 strains of vaccine appear to have similar safety and efficacy profiles.[85,262,391]

In contrast to the Jeryl Lynn–based strains, most other strains have been linked to aseptic meningitis,[72,171,200,206,247,274,285,386] occurring 15 to 21 days after vaccination, with a male predominance in those affected. The rate of vaccine-associated aseptic meningitis ranges from more than 1 case per 400 doses to less than 1 case per 100,000 doses, a range influenced by vaccine manufacturer, stringency of adverse event reporting, method of surveillance, study size, clinical definition, and background rates of aseptic meningitis.[34] The course of illness is mild, with no sequelae noted. Other, less frequent adverse events following vaccination include orchitis[2,73,217] and pancreatitis.[113,381] Vaccine-associated sensorineural deafness has been reported but is exceedingly rare.[15] Symptomatic transmission of certain vaccine viruses, including the Leningrad-3, Leningrad-Zagreb, and Urabe strains, has been reported.[17,196,340] Although mumps and its complications are usually mild, most analyses of cost-to-benefit ratios favor an intensive vaccination program for developed nations.[126,199,209,355,438]

The Rubini vaccine strain, which was extensively passaged in embryonated hens' eggs and WI-38 and MRC-5 human diploid cells,[134] was found to offer little protection against mumps.[135,290,312,341] As of 2001, the World Health Organization (WHO) no longer recommended its use for national immunization programs.[425]

Vaccine Use

The Advisory Committee on Immunization Practices (ACIP) recommends administration of the first dose of MMR at 12 to 15 months of age and administration of a second dose at 4 to 6 years of age. The 1-dose schedule was instituted in 1977 and modified to a 2-dose schedule in 1989.[53] ProQuad (quadrivalent measles, mumps, rubella, and varicella vaccine) can be used in place of MMR for the second dose at any age, or for the first dose at 48 months of age or older.[244] Studies suggest that vaccination as early as 9 months of age[197,343] and a second dose at 9 to 13 years of age[55,188,227] may be equally effective.

Vaccination in the face of recent chemotherapy or radiation therapy is unlikely to induce adequate serologic responses and should be delayed for at least 3 months following such treatment.[307] Studies of MuV–containing vaccines in nonimmunocompromised HIV–infected patients, primarily in the form of trivalent mumps, measles, and rubella vaccines, have not documented serious or unusual adverse effects and therefore vaccination is recommended.[60,252]

After many years of steadily declining disease incidence in the United States following the institution of mumps vaccination, a transient reversal in the number of reported cases of mumps occurred between 1986 and 1987 (Fig. 35.5). This appeared to be a reflection of the pool of susceptible children, teenagers, and young adults who were not immunized aggressively for mumps,[39,65,74,163,199,355] especially during the first decade following introduction of the vaccine. Models of the effects of mass vaccination programs suggest that the average age of disease can be anticipated to rise with the level of induced immunity, with the additional paradoxical result of increased relative risk of serious consequences of mumps infection (e.g., orchitis in susceptible postpubertal males).[10]

Following the outbreaks in the late 1980s, the incidence of mumps rapidly returned to preoutbreak levels and then precipitously declined over the next two decades to record low levels before a resurgence in 2006 and then in 2009 (Fig. 35.5). In contrast to the 1986 and 1987 mumps outbreaks, most cases occurring in 2006 and 2009 involved persons with a history of 2 doses of vaccine.[21,38,64,81,93,245,323,325] As discussed earlier, recent outbreaks appear to be facilitated by waning of vaccine-induced immune responses, which may be a consequence of the success of the mumps vaccination program itself in reducing wild-type virus circulation, resulting in reduced opportunities for periodic boosting, which in the past may have served to maintain immunity.[97]

ACKNOWLEDGMENTS

This research was supported in part by the Intramural Research Program of the NIH, NIDCR.

REFERENCES

All cited references are available in the e-book.

5. Afzal MA, Elliott GD, Rima BK, et al. Virus and host cell-dependent variation in transcription of the mumps virus genome. *J Gen Virol* 1990; 71(Pt 3):615–619.
6. Afzal MA, Pickford AR, Forsey T, et al. The Jeryl Lynn vaccine strain of mumps virus is a mixture of two distinct isolates. *J GenVirol* 1993; 74(Pt 5):917–920.
10. Anderson RM, Crombie JA, Grenfell BT. The epidemiology of mumps in the UK: a preliminary study of virus transmission, herd immunity and the potential impact of immunization. *Epidemiol Infect* 1987;99:65–84.
12. Andrejeva J, Childs KS, Young DF, et al. The V proteins of paramyxoviruses bind the IFN-inducible RNA helicase, mda-5, and inhibit its activation of the IFN-beta promoter. *Proc Natl Acad Sci U S A* 2004;101: 17264–17269.
17. Atrasheuskaya AV, Neverov AA, Rubin S, et al. Horizontal transmission of the Leningrad-3 live attenuated mumps vaccine virus. *Vaccine* 2006;24:1530–1536.
20. Bang HO, Bang J. Involvement of the central nervous system in mumps. *Acta Med Scand* 1943;113:487–505.
22. Barskey AE, Glasser JW, LeBaron CW. Mumps resurgences in the United States: A historical perspective on unexpected elements. *Vaccine* 2009;27:6186–6195.
23. Bashe WJ Jr, Gotlieb T, Henle G, et al. Studies on the prevention of mumps. VI. The relationship of neutralizing antibodies to the determination of susceptibility and to the evaluation of immunization procedures. *J Immunol* 1953;71:76–85.
28. Bitsko RH, Cortese MM, Dayan GH, et al. Detection of RNA of mumps virus during an outbreak in a population with a high level of measles, mumps, and rubella vaccine coverage. *J Clin Microbiol* 2008;46:1101–1103.
32. Black S, Shinefield H, Ray P, et al. Risk of hospitalization because of aseptic meningitis after measles-mumps-rubella vaccination in one- to two-year-old children: an analysis of the Vaccine Safety Datalink (VSD) Project. *Pediatr Infect Dis J* 1997;16:500–503.
34. Bonnet MC, Dutta A, Weinberger C, et al. Mumps vaccine virus strains and aseptic meningitis. *Vaccine* 2006;24:7037–7045.
35. Boriskin YS, Booth JC, Yamada A. Sequence variation within the carboxyl terminus of the nucleoprotein gene of mumps virus strains. *Clin Diagn Virol* 1994;2:79–85.
38. Boxall N, Kubinyiova M, Prikazsky V, et al. An increase in the number of mumps cases in the Czech Republic, 2005–2006. *Eurosurveillance* 2008;13.
39. Briss PA, Fehrs LJ, Parker RA, et al. Sustained transmission of mumps in a highly vaccinated population: assessment of primary vaccine failure and waning vaccine-induced immunity. *J Infect Dis* 1994;169:77–82.
40. Broliden K, Abreu ER, Arneborn M, et al. Immunity to mumps before and after MMR vaccination at 12 years of age in the first generation offered the two-dose immunization programme. *Vaccine* 1998;16: 323–327.
42. Brown JW, Kirkland HB, Hein GE. Central nervous system involvement during mumps. *Am J Med Sci* 1948;215:434–441.
46. Bruyn HB, Sexton HM, Brainerd HD. Mumps meningoencephalitis. A clinical review of 119 cases with one death. *Calif Med* 1957;86:153–160.
54. Centers for Disease Control and Prevention. Summary of notifiable diseases, United States, 1996. *MMWR Morb Mortal Wkly Rep* 1996;45: 1–88.
55. Centers for Disease Control and Prevention. Measles, mumps, and rubella—Vaccine use and strategies for the elimination of measles, rubella, and congenital rubella syndrome and control of mumps: Recommendations of the Advisory Committee on Immunization Practices (ACIP). *MMWR Morb Mortal Wkly Rep* 1998;47:1–48.

56. Centers for Disease Control and Prevention. Summary of notifiable diseases, 2003. *MMWR Morb Mortal Wkly Rep* 2005;52:17–72.
60. Centers for Disease Control and Prevention. 2010. Guide to vaccine contraindications and precautions. Available at: http://www.cdc.gov/vaccines/recs/vac-admin/downloads/contraindications-guide-508.pdf.
63. Centers for Disease Control and Prevention. Notifiable diseases and mortality tables. *MMWR Morb Mortal Wkly Rep* 2010;59:1658–1671.
64. Centers for Disease Control and Prevention. Update: mumps outbreak—New York and New Jersey, June 2009–January 2010. *MMWR Morb Mortal Wkly Rep* 2010;59:125–129.
65. Cheek JE, Baron R, Atlas H, et al. Mumps outbreak in a highly vaccinated school population. *Arch Pediatr Adolesc Med* 1995;149:774–778.
66. Chiba Y, Dzierba JL, Morag A, et al. Cell-mediated immune response to mumps virus infection in man. *J Immunol* 1976;116:12–15.
67. Chiba Y, Horino K, Umetsu M, et al. Virus excretion and antibody response in saliva in natural mumps. *Tohoku J Exp Med* 1973;111:229–238.
75. Cohen C, White JM, Savage EJ, et al. Vaccine effectiveness estimates, 2004–2005 mumps outbreak, England. *Emerg Infect Dis* 2007;13:12–17.
81. Cortese MM, Jordan HT, Curns AT, et al. Mumps vaccine performance among university students during a mumps outbreak. *Clin Infect Dis* 2008;46:1172–1180.
89. Curran JA, Quinn JP, Hoey EM, et al. cDNA cloning of the nucleocapsid and nucleocapsid-associated protein genes of mumps virus. *J Gen Virol* 1985;66(Pt 5):977–985.
93. Date AA, Kyaw MH, Rue AM, et al. Long-term persistence of mumps antibody after receipt of 2 measles-mumps-rubella (MMR) vaccinations and antibody response after a third MMR vaccination among a university population. *J Infect Dis* 2008;197:1662–1668.
94. Davidkin I, Jokinen S, Broman M, et al. Persistence of measles, mumps, and rubella antibodies in an MMR-vaccinated cohort: a 20-year follow-up. *J Infect Dis* 2008;197:950–956.
95. Davidkin I, Kontio M, Paunio M, et al. MMR vaccination and disease elimination: the Finnish experience. *Expert Rev Vaccines* 2010;9:1045–1053.
98. Dayan GH, Rubin S. Mumps outbreaks in vaccinated populations: are available mumps vaccines effective enough to prevent outbreaks? *Clin Infect Dis* 2008;47:1458–1467.
104. Elango N, Kovamees J, Varsanyi TM, et al. mRNA sequence and deduced amino acid sequence of the mumps virus small hydrophobic protein gene. *J Virol* 1989;63:1413–1415.
105. Elango N, Varsanyi TM, Kovamees J, et al. Molecular cloning and characterization of six genes, determination of gene order and intergenic sequences and leader sequence of mumps virus. *J Gen Virol* 1988;69(Pt 11):2893–2900.
106. Elliott GD, Afzal MA, Martin SJ, et al. Nucleotide sequence of the matrix, fusion and putative SH protein genes of mumps virus and their deduced amino acid sequences. *Virus Res* 1989;12:61–75.
107. Elliott GD, Yeo RP, Afzal MA, et al. Strain-variable editing during transcription of the P gene of mumps virus may lead to the generation of non-structural proteins NS1 (V) and NS2. *J Gen Virol* 1990;71:1555–1560.
109. Ennis FA. Immunity to mumps in an institutional epidemic. Correlation of insusceptibility to mumps with serum plaque neutralizing and hemagglutination-inhibiting antibodies. *J Infect Dis* 1969;119:654–657.
119. Frankova V, Sixtova E. Specific IgM antibodies in the saliva of mumps patients. *Acta Virol* 1987;31:357–364.
120. Friedman MG. Salivary IgA antibodies to mumps virus during and after mumps. *J Infect Dis* 1981;143:617.
122. Fu C, Liang J, Wang M. Matched case-control study of effectiveness of live, attenuated S79 mumps virus vaccine against clinical mumps. *Clin Vaccine Immunol* 2008;15:1425–1428.
126. Galazka AM, Robertson SE, Kraigher A. Mumps and mumps vaccine: a global review. *Bull World Health Organ* 1999;77:3–14.
138. Gordon JE, Heeren RH. The epidemiology of mumps. *Am J Med Sci* 1940;200:338–359.
143. Gut JP, Lablache C, Behr S, et al. Symptomatic mumps virus reinfections. *J Med Virol* 1995;45:17–23.
152. Harrison MS, Sakaguchi T, Schmitt AP. Paramyxovirus assembly and budding: building particles that transmit infections. *Int J Biochem Cell Biol* 2010;42:1416–1429.
154. Hatchette T, Davidson R, Clay S, et al. Laboratory diagnosis of mumps in a partially immunized population: The Nova Scotia experience. *Can J Infect Dis Med Microbiol* 2009;20:e157–e162.
157. He B, Lin GY, Durbin JE, et al. The SH integral membrane protein of the paramyxovirus simian virus 5 is required to block apoptosis in MDBK cells. *J Virol* 2001;75:4068–4079.
159. Henle G, Henle W, Wendell K, et al. Isolation of mumps virus from human being with induced apparent or inapparent infections. *J Exp Med* 1948;88:223–232.
163. Hersh BS, Fine PE, Kent WK, et al. Mumps outbreak in a highly vaccinated population. *J Pediatr* 1991;119:187–193.
165. Hilleman MR, Weibel RE, Buynak EB, et al. Live attenuated mumps-virus vaccine. IV. Protective efficacy as measured in a field evaluation. *N Engl J Med* 1967;276:252–258.
170. Houard S, Varsanyi TM, Milican F, et al. Protection of hamsters against experimental mumps virus (MuV) infection by antibodies raised against the MuV surface glycoproteins expressed from recombinant vaccinia virus vectors. *J Gen Virol* 1995;76(Pt 2):421–423.
179. Jalal H, Bahadur G, Knowles W, et al. Mumps epididymo-orchitis with prolonged detection of virus in semen and the development of anti-sperm antibodies. *J Med Virol* 2004;73:147–150.
182. Jensik SC, Silver S. Polypeptides of mumps virus. *J Virol* 1976;17:363–373.
184. Jin L, Rima B, Brown D, et al. Proposal for genetic characterisation of wild-type mumps strains: Preliminary standardisation of the nomenclature. *Arch Virol* 2005;150:1903–1909.
186. Johnson CD, Goodpasture EW. An investigation of the etiology of mumps. *J Exp Med* 1934;59:1–19.
187. Johnson CD, Goodpasture EW. The etiology of mumps. *Am J Hyg* 1935;21:46–57.
191. Johnson RT, Johnson KP. Hydrocephalus following viral infection: the pathology of aqueductal stenosis developing after experimental mumps virus infection. *J Neuropathol Exp Neurol* 1968;27:591–606.
194. Jokinen S, Osterlund P, Julkunen I, et al. Cellular immunity to mumps virus in young adults 21 years after measles-mumps-rubella vaccination. *J Infect Dis* 2007;196:861–867.
196. Kaic B, Gjenero-Margan I, Aleraj B, et al. Transmission of the L-Zagreb mumps vaccine virus, Croatia, 2005–2008. *Euro Surveill* 2008;13(16):18843.
201. Kilham L. Isolation of mumps virus from the blood of a patient. *Proc Soc Exp Biol Med* 1948;69:99–100.
202. Kilham L. Mumps meningoencephalitis with and without parotitis. *Am J Dis Child* 1949;78:324–333.
207. Kingston RL, Baase WA, Gay LS. Characterization of nucleocapsid binding by the measles virus and mumps virus phosphoproteins. *J Virol* 2004;78:8630–8640.
208. Kingston RL, Gay LS, Baase WS, et al. Structure of the nucleocapsid-binding domain from the mumps virus polymerase; an example of protein folding induced by crystallization. *J Mol Biol* 2008;379:719–731.
209. Koplan JP, Preblud SR. A benefit-cost analysis of mumps vaccine. *Am J Dis Child* 1982;136:362–364.
213. Krause CH, Eastick K, Ogilvie MM. Real-time PCR for mumps diagnosis on clinical specimens–comparison with results of conventional methods of virus detection and nested PCR. *J Clin Virol* 2006;37:184–189.
214. Krause CH, Molyneaux PJ, Ho-Yen DO, et al. Comparison of mumps-IgM ELISAs in acute infection. *J Clin Virol* 2007;38(2):153–156.
216. Kubota T, Yokosawa N, Yokota S, et al. C terminal CYS-RICH region of mumps virus structural V protein correlates with block of interferon alpha and gamma signal transduction pathway through decrease of STAT 1-alpha. *Biochem Biophys Res Commun* 2001;283:255–259.
221. Kurtz JB, Tomlinson AH, Pearson J. Mumps virus isolated from a fetus. *Br Med J (Clin Res Ed)* 1982;284:471.
227. LeBaron CW, Forghani B, Beck C, et al. Persistence of mumps antibodies after 2 doses of measles-mumps-rubella vaccine. *J Infect Dis* 2009;199:552–560.
231. Levens J, Enders JF. The hemagglutinative properties of amniotic fluid from embryonated eggs infected with mumps virus. *Science* 1945;102:117–120.
234. Li M, Schmitt PT, Li Z, et al. Mumps virus matrix, fusion, and nucleocapsid proteins cooperate for efficient production of virus-like particles. *J Virol* 2009;83:7261–7272.

236. Lindsay JR, Davey PR, Ward PH. Inner ear pathology in deafness due to mumps. *Ann Otol Rhinol Laryngol* 1960;69:918–935.
237. Link H, Laurenzi MA, Fryden A. Viral antibodies in oligoclonal and polyclonal IgG synthesized within the central nervous system over the course of mumps meningitis. *J Neuroimmunol* 1981;1:287–298.
238. Litman N, Baum SG. Mumps Virus. In: Mandell GL, Bennett JE, Donlin R, eds. *Principles and Practice of Infectious Diseases.* 7th ed. Philadelphia: Churchill Livingstone; 2010:2201–2206.
239. Liu Y, Zhu J, Feng MG, et al. Six-helix bundle assembly and analysis of the central core of mumps virus fusion protein. *Arch Biochem Biophys* 2004;421:143–148.
242. Love A, Rydbeck R, Utter G, et al. Monoclonal antibodies against the fusion protein are protective in necrotizing mumps meningoencephalitis. *J Virol* 1986;58:220–222.
243. Lu LL, Puri M, Horvath CM, et al. Select paramyxoviral V proteins inhibit IRF3 activation by acting as alternative substrates for inhibitor of kappaB kinase epsilon (IKKe)/TBK1. *J Biol Chem* 2008;283: 14269–14276.
244. Marin M, Broder KR, Temte JL, et al. Use of combination measles, mumps, rubella, and varicella vaccine: recommendations of the Advisory Committee on Immunization Practices (ACIP). *MMWR Recomm Rep* 2010;59:1–12.
245. Marin M, Quinlisk P, Shimabukuro T, et al. Mumps vaccination coverage and vaccine effectiveness in a large outbreak among college students–Iowa, 2006. *Vaccine* 2008;26:3601–3607.
251. McCarthy M, Lazzarini RA. Intracellular nucleocapsid RNA of mumps virus. *J Gen Virol* 1982;58(Pt 1):205–209.
257. Merz DC, Server AC, Waxham MN, et al. Biosynthesis of mumps virus F glycoprotein: non-fusing strains efficiently cleave the F glycoprotein precursor. *J Gen Virol* 1983;64(Pt 7):1457–1467.
259. Meyer MB. An epidemiologic study of mumps; its spread in schools and families. *Am J Hyg* 1962;75:259–281.
263. Miller E, Hill A, Morgan-Capner P, et al. Antibodies to measles, mumps and rubella in UK children 4 years after vaccination with different MMR vaccines. *Vaccine* 1995;13:799–802.
266. Modlin JF, Orenstein WA, Brandling-Bennett AD. Current status of mumps in the United States. *J Infect Dis* 1975;132:106–109.
272. Muhlemann K. The molecular epidemiology of mumps virus. *Infect Genet Evol* 2004;4:215–219.
277. Narita M, Matsuzono Y, Takekoshi Y, et al. Analysis of mumps vaccine failure by means of avidity testing for mumps virus-specific immunoglobulin G. *Clin Diagn Lab Immunol* 1998;5:799–803.
282. Nishio M, Garcin D, Simonet V, et al. The carboxyl segment of the mumps virus V protein associates with Stat proteins in vitro via a tryptophan-rich motif. *Virology* 2002;300:92–99.
284. Nussinovitch M, Brand N, Frydman M, et al. Transverse myelitis following mumps in children. *Acta Paediatr* 1992;81:183–184.
287. Okamoto M, Shitara T, Nakayama M, et al. Sudden deafness accompanied by asymptomatic mumps. *Acta Otolaryngol Suppl* 1994;514:45–48.
288. Okazaki K, Tanabayashi K, Takeuchi K, et al. Molecular cloning and sequence analysis of the mumps virus gene encoding the L protein and the trailer sequence. *Virology* 1992;188:926–930.
289. Okuno Y, Asada T, Yamanishi K, et al. Studies on the use of mumps virus for treatment of human cancer. *Biken J* 1978;21:37–49.
290. Ong G, Goh KT, Ma S, et al. Comparative efficacy of Rubini, Jeryl-Lynn and Urabe mumps vaccine in an Asian population. *J Infect* 2005;51: 294–298.
291. Orvell C. Immunological properties of purified mumps virus glycoproteins. *J Gen Virol* 1978;41:517–526.
292. Orvell C. The reactions of monoclonal antibodies with structural proteins of mumps virus. *J Immunol* 1984;132:2622–2629.
293. Orvell C, Alsheikhly AR, Kalantari M, et al. Characterization of genotype-specific epitopes of the HN protein of mumps virus. *J Gen Virol* 1997;78(Pt 12):3187–3193.
294. Overman JR. Viremia in human mumps virus infections. *Arch Intern Med* 1958;102:354–356.
297. Paterson RG, Lamb RA. RNA editing by G-nucleotide insertion in mumps virus P-gene mRNA transcripts. *J Virol* 1990;64:4137–4145.
305. Philip RN, Reinhard KP, Lachman DB. Observations on a mumps epidemic in a "virgin" population. *Am J Hyg* 1959;69:91–111.
307. Plotkin SA, Rubin SA. Mumps Vaccine. In: Plotkin SA, Orenstein WA, Offit PA, eds. *Vaccines.* 5th ed. Philadelphia: Saunders Elsevier; 2008:435–465.
310. Polgreen PM, Bohnett LC, Cavanaugh JE, et al. The duration of mumps virus shedding after the onset of symptoms. *Clin Infect Dis* 2008;46:1447–1449.
321. Reed D, Brown G, Merrick R, et al. A mumps epidemic on St. George Island, Alaska. *JAMA* 1967;199:113–117.
325. Rota JS, Turner JC, Yost-Daljev MK, et al. Investigation of a mumps outbreak among university students with two measles-mumps-rubella (MMR) vaccinations, Virginia, September-December 2006. *J Med Virol* 2009;81:1819–1825.
328. Rubin SA, Afzal MA. Neurovirulence safety testing of mumps vaccines-historical perspective and current status. *Vaccine* 2011;29(16)2850–2855.
330. Rubin SA, Mauldin J, Chumakov K, et al. Serological and phylogenetic evidence of monotypic immune responses to different mumps virus strains. *Vaccine* 2005;24:2668.
332. Rubin SA, Pletnikov M, Taffs R, et al. Evaluation of a neonatal rat model for prediction of mumps virus neurovirulence in humans. *J Virol* 2000;74:5382–5384.
333. Rubin SA, Qi L, Audet SA, et al. Antibody induced by immunization with the Jeryl Lynn mumps vaccine strain effectively neutralizes a heterologous wild-type mumps virus associated with a large outbreak. *J Infect Dis* 2008;198:508–515.
337. Sanz JC, Mosquera MM, Echevarria JE, et al. Sensitivity and specificity of immunoglobulin G titer for the diagnosis of mumps virus in infected patients depending on vaccination status. *APMIS* 2006;114:788–794.
339. Sauder CJ, Zhang CX, Link MA, et al. Presence of lysine at aa 335 of the hemagglutinin-neuraminidase protein of mumps virus vaccine strain Urabe AM9 is not a requirement for neurovirulence. *Vaccine* 2009; 27:5822–5829.
340. Sawada H, Yano S, Oka Y, et al. Transmission of Urabe mumps vaccine between siblings. *Lancet* 1993;342:371.
348. Shah D, Vidal S, Link MA, et al. Identification of genetic mutations associated with attenuation and changes in tropism of Urabe mumps virus. *J Med Virol* 2009;81:130–138.
353. Smorodintsev AA, Klyatchko NS. Live anti-mumps vaccine. I. Results of tests of the immunogenic properties of live vaccine when administered intradermally to susceptible children. *Acta Virol* 1958;2:137–144.
367. Takeuchi K, Tanabayashi K, Hishiyama M, et al. The mumps virus SH protein is a membrane protein and not essential for virus growth. *Virology* 1996;225:156–162.
368. Takeuchi K, Tanabayashi K, Hishiyama M, et al. Variations of nucleotide sequences and transcription of the SH gene among mumps virus strains. *Virology* 1991;181:364–366.
371. Tanabayashi K, Takeuchi K, Okazaki K, et al. Expression of mumps virus glycoproteins in mammalian cells from cloned cDNAs: both F and HN proteins are required for cell fusion. *Virology* 1992;187:801–804.
376. Ternavasio-de la Vega HG, Boronat M, Ojeda A, et al. Mumps orchitis in the post-vaccine era (1967–2009): a single-center series of 67 patients and review of clinical outcome and trends. *Medicine (Baltimore)* 2010;89:96–116.
377. Tesovic G, Poljak M, Lunar MM, et al. Horizontal transmission of the Leningrad-Zagreb mumps vaccine strain: a report of three cases. *Vaccine* 2008;26:1922–1925.
380. Timmons GD, Johnson KP. Aqueductal stenosis and hydrocephalus after mumps encephalitis. *N Engl J Med* 1970;283:1505–1507.
387. Ukkonen P, Granstrom ML, Penttinen K. Mumps-specific immunoglobulin M and G antibodies in natural mumps infection as measured by enzyme-linked immunosorbent assay. *J Med Virol* 1981;8:131–142.
388. Ulane CM, Kentsis A, Cruz CD, et al. Composition and assembly of STAT-targeting ubiquitin ligase complexes: paramyxovirus V protein carboxyl terminus is an oligomerization domain. *J Virol* 2005;79: 10180–10189.
392. Utz JP, Houk VN, Alling DW. Clinical and laboratory studies of mumps. IV. Viruria and abnormal renal function. *N Engl J Med* 1964;270: 1283–1286.
395. Vaheri A, Julkunen I, Koskiniemi ML. Chronic encephalomyelitis with specific increase in intrathecal mumps antibodies. *Lancet* 1982;2:685–688.

397. Vandermeulen C, Roelants M, Vermoere M, et al. Outbreak of mumps in a vaccinated child population: a question of vaccine failure? *Vaccine* 2004;22:2713–2716.
408. Waxham MN, Server AC, Goodman HM, et al. Cloning and sequencing of the mumps virus fusion protein gene. *Virology* 1987;159:381–388.
410. Weibel RE, Buynak EB, McLean AA, et al. Long-term follow-up for immunity after monovalent or combined live measles, mumps, and rubella virus vaccines. *Pediatrics* 1975;56:380–387.
412. Weibel RE, Stokes J Jr, Buynak EB, et al. Live attenuated mumps-virus vaccine. 3. Clinical and serologic aspects in a field evaluation. *N Engl J Med* 1967;276:245–251.
416. Wharton M, Cochi SL, Hutcheson RH, et al. A large outbreak of mumps in the postvaccine era. *J Infect Dis* 1988;158:1253–1260.
418. Wilson RL, Fuentes SM, Wang P, et al. Function of small hydrophobic proteins of paramyxovirus. *J Virol* 2006;80:1700–1709.
420. Wolinsky JS, Klassen T, Baringer JR. Persistance of neuroadapted mumps virus in brains of newborn hamsters after intraperitoneal inoculation. *J Infect Dis* 1976;133:260–267.
422. Wolinsky JS, Waxham MN, Server AC. Protective effects of glycoprotein-specific monoclonal antibodies on the course of experimental mumps virus meningoencephalitis. *J Virol* 1985;53:727–734.
425. World Health Organization. Mumps virus vaccines: WHO position paper. *Wkly Epidemiol Rec* 2001;76:346–355.
428. Wright KE, Dimock K, Brown EG. Biological characteristics of genetic variants of Urabe AM9 mumps vaccine virus. *Virus Res* 2000;67:49–57.
431. Yates PJ, Afzal MA, Minor PD. Antigenic and genetic variation of the HN protein of mumps virus strains. *J Gen Virol* 1996;77(Pt 10):2491–2497.
438. Zhou F, Reef S, Massoudi M, et al. An economic analysis of the current universal 2-dose measles-mumps-rubella vaccination program in the United States. *J Infect Dis* 2004;189(Suppl 1):S131–S145.

CHAPTER 36

Diane E. Griffin

Measles Virus

Measles is a highly contagious disease characterized by a prodromal illness of fever, coryza, cough, and conjunctivitis followed by the appearance of a generalized maculopapular rash. Introduction of measles into virgin populations and endemic transmission in populations with inadequate medical care are associated with high mortality. Despite the development of a successful live attenuated vaccine, measles remains a major cause of mortality in children, particularly in developing countries, and a cause of continuing outbreaks in industrialized nations.

HISTORY

Measles is a relatively new disease of humans and probably evolved from an animal morbillivirus. Phylogenetically, measles virus (MeV) is most closely related to rinderpest virus (RPV), a pathogen of cattle (Fig. 36.1), and it is postulated that MeV evolved in an environment where cattle and humans lived in close proximity.[444] Because large numbers of people are required to generate sufficient susceptible individuals to maintain measles in a population, measles may have evolved in the early centers of civilization in the Middle East where populations attained sufficient densities to sustain continued transmission.[444]

Abu Becr, an Arab physician known as Rhazes of Baghdad, is generally credited with distinguishing smallpox from measles in the 9th century. He dated its first description to the 6th century. Rhazes referred to measles as *hasbah* (eruption) and regarded it as a modification of smallpox with the distinction that "anxiety of mind, sick qualms and heaviness of heart oppress more in the measles than in the smallpox".[585] Repeated epidemics of illnesses characterized by a rash are recorded in European and Far Eastern populations between 1 and 1200 AD.[444] It appears that measles spread across the Pyrenees into France with the Saracen invasion of the 8th century.[600] Repeated epidemics identified as measles were recorded in the 11th and 12th centuries, and it is first mentioned as a childhood disease in 1224.[444]

In the European literature the name applied was "morbilli," derived from the Italian "little diseases" to distinguish it from plague, "il morbo," but morbilli included several exanthemata. Sanvages in 1763 defined morbilli as measles but called it rubeola (derived from the Spanish[600]), leading to a common confusion with rubella that persists to the present. Introduction of measles into previously unexposed populations has been associated with high morbidity and mortality.[68,600,655,667] Epidemics of rash illnesses were associated with episodes of depopulation in China, India, and the Mediterranean region. Introduction of measles into the Fiji Islands in 1875 resulted in 26% mortality.[600] Approximately 56 million people died as a result of European exploration of the New World, largely due to the introduction into native Amerindian populations of Old World diseases, notably smallpox and measles. Decreases in population are likely to have facilitated the transfer of Spanish culture to South America.[444]

Many of the basic principles of measles epidemiology were elucidated by Peter Panum, a Danish physician who worked in the Faroe Islands during a large measles epidemic in 1846.[530] Panum deduced the highly contagious nature of the disease, the 14-day incubation period, and the lifelong immunity present in older residents and postulated a respiratory route of transmission.

Complications of measles were first described in the 18th century. In 1790, James Lucas, an English surgeon, described the first case of postmeasles encephalomyelitis in a young woman who developed paraparesis as the rash was fading.[412] Nineteenth-century medical textbooks associated measles with the exacerbation of tuberculosis, and in 1908, while working at a tuberculosis hospital in Vienna, von Pirquet recorded the disappearance of

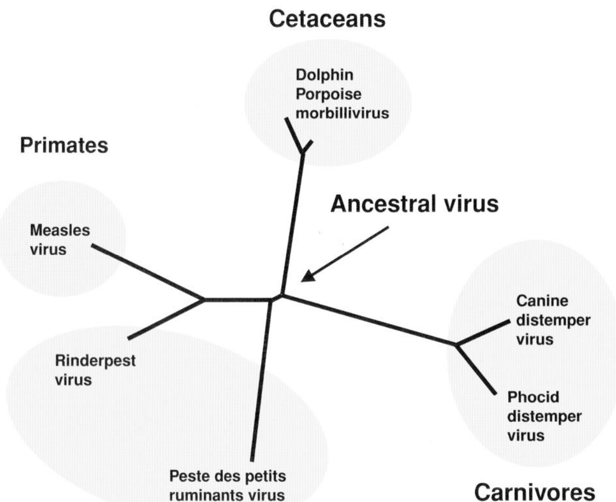

FIGURE 36.1. Genetic relationships between morbilliviruses based on comparison of the nucleotide sequences of the N genes. The tree was derived using PHLIP, DNADIST, and FITCH programs. The branch lengths are proportional to the mutational differences between the viruses and the hypothetical common ancestor that existed at the nodes in the tree. (From Barrett T. Morbillivirus infections, with special emphasis on morbilliviruses of carnivores. *Vet Microbiol* 1999;69:3–13, with permission.)

delayed-type hypersensitivity skin test responses to tuberculin,[750] the first experimental evidence of measles-induced immune suppression.

In 1933, Dawson described subacute sclerosing panencephalitis (SSPE) in a 16-year-old boy with progressive neurologic deterioration. Histologic examination of the brain showed eosinophilic intranuclear and intracytoplasmic inclusions in neurons and glial cells.[142] After reports of paramyxovirus-like particles in the inclusions,[717] observations of elevated levels of MeV antibody in serum and cerebrospinal fluid (CSF) and the reactivity of the inclusions with antibody to MeV identified the paramyxovirus as MeV.[130]

INFECTIOUS AGENT

In 1757, an infectious agent was formally shown to be the cause of measles when the Scottish physician Francis Home, attempting immunization, transmitted the disease to naive individuals using blood taken from measles patients during the early stages of the rash.[297] In 1905, Hektoen transmitted disease to volunteers with blood "free of bacteria" taken from measles cases in the acute stage and observed an incubation period of 13 days.[280] In 1911, Goldberger and Anderson transmitted measles to rhesus macaques with filtered respiratory tract secretions from measles patients and successfully passaged disease from one monkey to another.[238,531]

Propagation and Assay in Cell Culture

Primary Isolation

In 1954, Enders and Peebles first isolated MeV in tissue culture by inoculating primary human kidney cells with the blood of David Edmonston, a child with measles.[184] Isolates were also made using primary monkey kidney cells[184] and later continuous monkey kidney cell lines (e.g., Vero, CV-1).[677] However, isolation of wild-type strains of MeV is most often successful using an Epstein-Barr virus–transformed marmoset B-lymphocyte line, B95-8[365]; a human T-cell line from cord blood, COBL-a[364]; or Vero cells engineered to express the MeV receptor signaling lymphocyte activation molecule (SLAM).[521] Generally, the first observable sign of virus growth is cell–cell fusion and syncytia formation (Fig. 36.2).

Laboratory Propagation and Assay

Growth of MeV led to the development of live-attenuated vaccine strains by adaptation of MeV to growth in cells from foreign hosts, such as the chick embryo and canine and bovine kidney cells.[349] Most experimental work is done with tissue culture–adapted strains so virus stocks are generally grown in Vero cells using a low multiplicity of infection to avoid accumulation of defective interfering (DI) particles. Vero and Vero/SLAM cells are useful for virus titration by plaque formation.[10] The virus replicates slowly and 3 to 5 days of culture are often needed for plaques to become visible. Wild-type strains can also be assayed by syncytia formation in B95-8 or human cord blood mononuclear cells.

Biological Characteristics

The morbilliviruses form two genetically distinct groups of viruses related either to canine distemper virus (CDV) or to RPV (Fig. 36.1)[50] and differ from other paramyxoviruses in formation of intranuclear inclusion bodies. Virions are pleomorphic and range in size from 100 to 300 nm. The envelope carries surface projections that are composed of the viral transmembrane hemagglutinin (H) and fusion (F) glycoproteins (Fig. 36.3). The matrix (M) protein lines the interior of the virion envelope. The helical ribonucleocapsid (total length of 1.2 μm) formed from the 16 kb genomic RNA wrapped with the nucleocapsid (N) protein is packed within the envelope in the form of a symmetrical coil with the phosphoprotein (P) and large polymerase (L) proteins attached.

Proteins

Nucleocapsid Protein

The N protein messenger RNA (mRNA) is the first transcribed from the genome and the N protein (525 amino acids [aa]) is the most abundant of the viral proteins. N appears as a 60-kD band on polyacrylamide gels and can self-assemble but usually surrounds viral genomic or antigenomic RNAs to form helical ribonucleocapsid structures.[100] This conformationally flexible structure[62,643] is the required template for both replication and transcription. Each N monomer binds six nucleotides, and viral genomes must be multiples of six for replication.[367] Monomeric N (N^0) can be transported into the nucleus but is usually retained in the cytoplasm by binding to P.[309,679] Phosphorylation regulates oligomer formation and activation of transcription.[243,267]

N is organized into two functionally distinct regions. The N-terminal portion of the protein (aa 1 to 400, N_{CORE}) is conserved and is required for self-assembly into nucleocapsids and for RNA binding[44,242,342,403,679] (Fig. 36.4). N_{CORE} forms a globular domain located toward the helical axis of the nucleocapsid,[643] includes a nuclear localization signal,[628] and

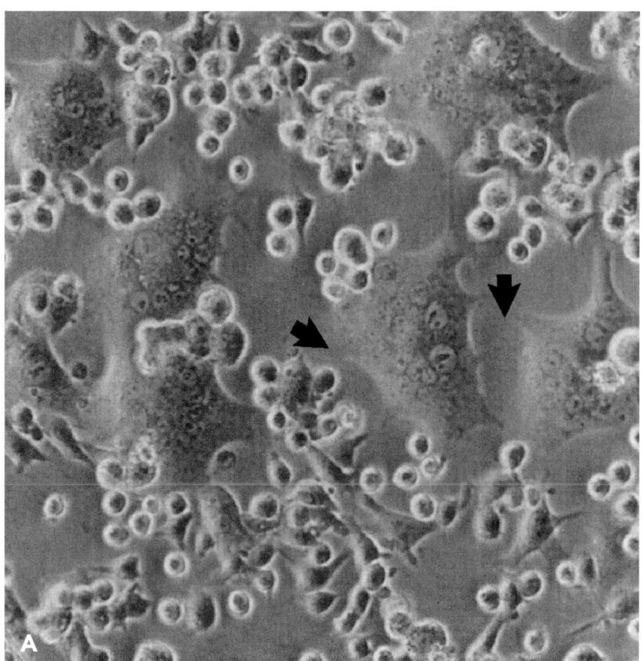

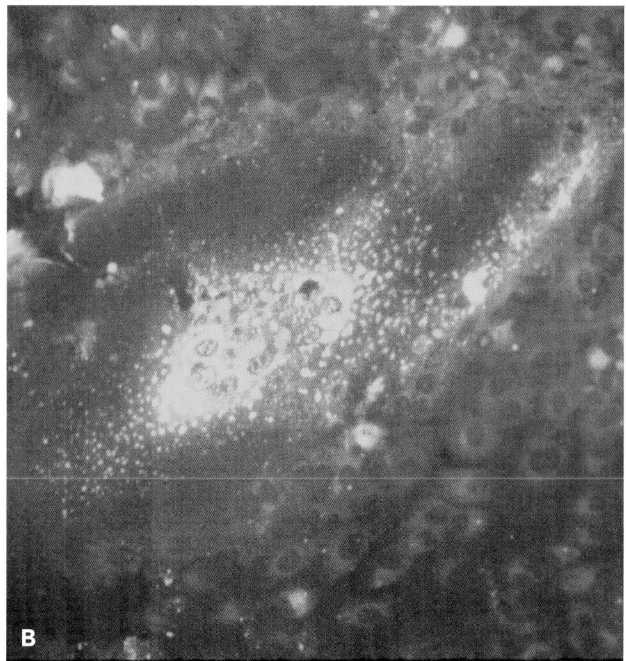

FIGURE 36.2. Typical cytopathic effects of syncytia formation associated with measles virus (MeV) replication in Vero cells. A: Unstained cells in culture. (**A** courtesy of William Bellini, Centers for Disease Control and Prevention, Atlanta, Georgia.) **B:** Cells stained with a fluorescently labeled antibody to MeV.

can also react with the cell surface through FcγRII.[579] The C-terminal portion of the protein (aa 401 to 525, N_{TAIL}) is more variable, intrinsically disordered, acidic, and phosphorylated.[40,110,267,341,408,567] N interacts with P through residues in N_{CORE} and N_{TAIL}.[44,77,356,792] N_{TAIL} is required for nucleocapsid flexibility,[62] but its location in the nucleocapsid structure is not clear.[151] N_{TAIL} contains an α-helical molecular recognition element (α-MoRE, aa 488 to 499) reversibly involved in induced α-helical folding upon interaction with the X domain (XD) in the C-terminus of P (PCT) that likely positions the polymerase

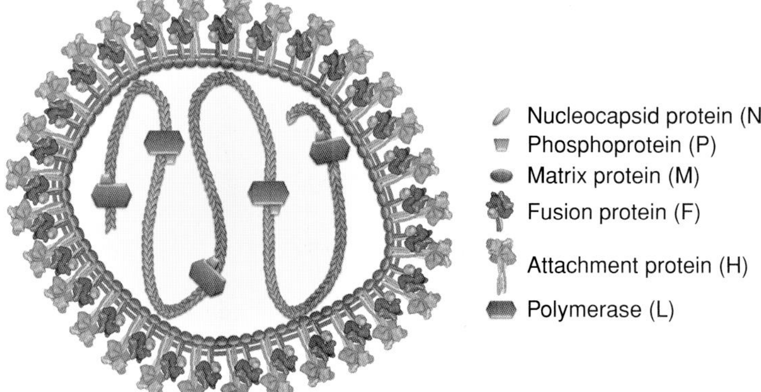

FIGURE 36.3. Schematic diagram of measles virus. The lipid bilayer of the pleomorphic particle is represented by blue lines, under which the matrix protein layer (red) resides. The viral membrane is densely packed with envelope glycoprotein complexes consisting of fusion protein trimers (shades of blue) and attachment protein tetramers (shades of green). The negative-strand RNA genome and the nucleocapsid protein (orange) form the nucleocapsid, which interacts with the phosphoprotein (light blue) and the polymerase (purple). In addition to contacts between the nucleocapsid and matrix proteins,[325] the luminal tails of the glycoproteins are thought to contact the matrix layer. Individual viral components are not drawn to scale. Structural renderings of the glycoprotein complexes are based on original crystal structures (H head domains[277]); homology models of measles virus (MeV) F[386,552] derived from coordinates reported for pre- and postfusion PIV5 and PIV3 F, respectively[794,795]; or hypothetical structural models (F prehairpin intermediate). High-resolution structural models were aligned at the level of the transmembrane domain (viral envelope) as described[527] and then morphed into low-resolution images using the Sculptor (resolution 12, voxel size 3) package.[64] (Adapted from Plemper RK, Brindley MA, Iorio RM. Structural and mechanistic studies of measles virus illuminate paramyxovirus entry. *PLoS Pathog* 2011;7:e1002058; courtesy of M. A. Brindley and R. K. Plemper.)

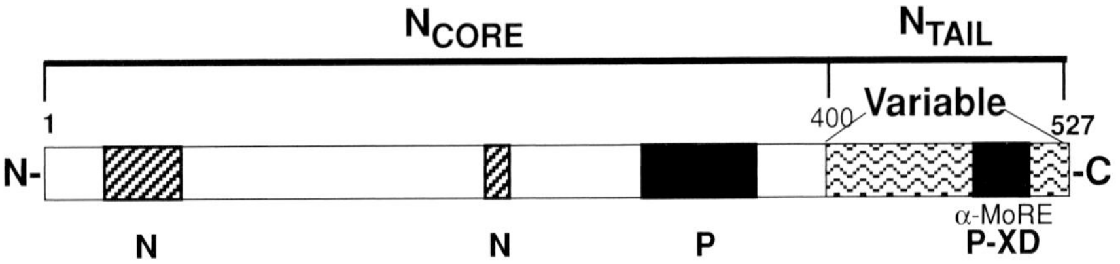

FIGURE 36.4. Schematic diagram of the nucleocapsid (N) protein. The N-terminal region (N_{CORE}) contains the RNA-binding domain and the oligomerization domain and is sufficient for nucleocapsid formation. The C-terminal region (N_{TAIL}) is unstructured and acidic, binds C-terminal domain of P (PCT), and contains the region of sequence variability that is used for identification of measles virus (MeV) clades. Regions of interaction with N and P are indicated.

complex near the RNA in the nucleocapsid.[44,76,77,151,333,408,468] The intrinsic disorder of N_{TAIL} provides a structural plasticity that allows strain- and cell type–specific interactions with several host proteins including heat shock protein (Hsp) 72, interferon regulatory factor (IRF)-3, the cellular protein responsible for nuclear export of N, the p40 subunit of eukaryotic initiation factor 3, cyclophilins A and B, and an unidentified cell surface nucleocapsid receptor.[128,379,627,718,760,803]

P, C and V Proteins

The P (phospho) protein (507 aa) is a polymerase co-factor that is activated by phosphorylation, forms tetramers, and links L to N to form the replicase complex.[135] While the 72-kD P protein is abundant in the infected cell, only small amounts are present in the packaged virus. P is a multifunctional protein with a modular organization (Fig. 36.5). The N-terminus (PNT) is poorly conserved, intrinsically unstructured, acidic, phosphorylated, and required for replication. PNT binds to N_{CORE} and this interaction induces folding of PNT.[343] PNT is a chaperone for N^0 that prevents binding to cellular RNAs, illegitimate N self-assembly, and nuclear translocation. PNT initiates encapsidation of genomic viral RNA by sequence-specific binding of the leader RNA.[135,309] Elongation of the nucleocapsid structure is sequence independent. PNT also interacts with cellular proteins to regulate the response to interferon (IFN) (see discussion of V later).

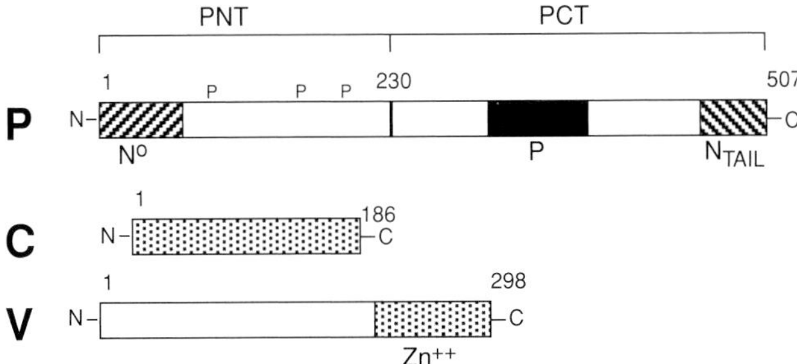

FIGURE 36.5. Schematic diagram of the phospho (P), C, and V proteins. Diagram of the proteins encoded in the P gene. P and C are initiated at AUGs in different reading frames. The N-terminal region of P (PNT) is acidic, unstructured, and phosphorylated on serines and binds N^0. The C-terminal region of P (PCT) has the P oligomerization domain and the X domain that binds and induces folding of N_{TAIL}. V is translated from an edited RNA with a nontemplated G at nucleotide 751 that results in a distinct cysteine-rich zinc-binding C-terminus.

PCT is conserved[45] and contains all domains required for transcription. The region between amino acids 204 and 321 contains the α-helical domain that binds to N_{TAIL} as part of the nucleocapsid structure and is responsible for tethering the polymerase L to its template.[309,356] A coiled-coil domain between aa 344 to 411 is sufficient for P oligomerization.[135] The unique XD portion of PCT (aa 459 to 507) has three α-helices arranged in an antiparallel triple helix bundle that binds the N_{TAIL} α-MoRE with 1:1 stoichiometry and induces its folding.[65,229,336,356,408] Binding affinity is weak, consistent with a model in which XD is responsible for tethering L to the ribonucleocapsid in a way that allows it to progress during RNA synthesis.[356,792] XD also interacts with and stabilizes the ubiquitin ligase p53-induced-RING-H2.[118]

The P gene of MeV, like other members of the *Paramyxoviridae,* encodes proteins in addition to P that, together with P, regulate the innate response to infection (Fig. 36.5). The C protein is a basic protein of 186 amino acids encoded by the same mRNA but translated using an initiator methionine codon 19 nucleotides downstream from that for P and an overlapping reading frame.[60] The V protein shares the initiator methionine and the amino terminal 231 amino acids of the P protein, but RNA editing adds an extra non-template-directed guanosine (G) residue at position 751. This shifts the reading frame and results in a different 68–amino acid cysteine-rich C-terminus with zinc-binding properties.[105,404] Neither C nor V is necessary for MeV replication in Vero cells,[572,636] but both C and V interact with cellular proteins and regulate the response to infection.[155,405,646,722]

C interferes with innate immune responses by inhibition of IFN signaling, modulates viral polymerase activity, and has been implicated in prevention of cell death.[47,584,654,711] Deletion of C decreases MeV replication in monkeys, peripheral blood mononuclear cells (PBMCs), and thymic epithelial cells and decreases neurovirulence for CD46 transgenic mice, suggesting that C has an important *in vivo* role.[155,194,537,711,731] In some cells decreased replication is associated with inhibition of translation and induction of IFN.[491] C suppresses IFN induction by regulating viral RNA synthesis[490] and preventing the activation of the cellular protein kinase PKR.[435,723]

Matrix (M) Protein

The envelope of the virion (Fig. 36.3) consists of the M protein (335 aa) and the two transmembrane glycoproteins F and H. M is a basic protein with several conserved hydrophobic domains.[59] The mRNAs for morbillivirus M proteins contain approximately 400 nucleotides of noncoding sequence at the 3′

end that increases M protein production.[59,705] In infected cells M is associated with nucleocapsids and with detergent-resistant regions of the inner layer of the plasma membrane where it regulates MeV RNA synthesis and assembly.[291,325,556] M also interacts with the intracytoplasmic regions of one or both transmembrane glycoproteins, modulates the targeting and fusogenic capacity of the envelope glycoproteins, and directs release of virus from the apical surface of polarized epithelial cells.[71,487,556,618] Deletion of M increases cell-to-cell fusion and decreases production of infectious virus.[102] These properties are often defective in the mutated M proteins of viruses causing persistent infection.[290,693]

Fusion (F) Protein

F is a highly conserved type I transmembrane glycoprotein synthesized as an inactive precursor (F_0) of about 60 kD. The mRNAs for morbillivirus F_0 proteins contain unusually long (460 to 585 nucleotides) G-C rich 5′ nontranslated regions (NTRs) that are predicted to have extensive secondary structure and are followed by clusters of three to four AUGs.[588] The 5′ NTR influences the choice of AUG and decreases translation of F, virus production, and cytopathogenicity.[101,705] There is a 28-residue signal sequence and after translation, F is glycosylated and trimerized in the endoplasmic reticulum (ER).[550] F_0 is cleaved at a multibasic site (108 to 112: Arg-Arg-His-Lys-Arg) by furin in the trans-Golgi to yield the 41-kD (F_1) and 18-kD (F_2) disulfide-linked fusion-competent mature protein.[73,761] Mutation of Arg 112 results in a reduced rate of F transport to the cell surface, aberrant cleavage, and abolition of the fusogenic activity necessary for infection.[13,761] Restricted processing of F is associated with persistent infection.[447] The 33-residue cytoplasmic tail of F_1 possesses basolateral sorting and endocytosis signals.[461] F_2 has all of the predicted N-linked glycosylation sites (aa 29, 61, and 67). Mutation of any of these asparagines decreases transport to the cell surface and impairs proteolytic cleavage, stability, and the fusion capacity of F, perhaps because F_2 is an integral part of the prefusion F head.[14,746]

F_1 contains a highly conserved stretch of hydrophobic amino acid residues at the new N-terminus (aa 113 to 145) that constitutes the fusion peptide. Oligopeptides that mimic this segment of F_1 inhibit fusion.[587] Mutants resistant to the fusion inhibitory effect of these oligopeptides have amino acid alterations in a cysteine-rich region (aa 337 to 381) of F_1 important for interaction with H[311] (Fig. 36.6). There are two predicted heptad repeat amphipathic α-helices: one adjacent to the fusion peptide and another N-terminal to the transmembrane region. Partial membrane-proximal cleavage between the heptad repeat and the transmembrane region enhances fusion.[748] Synthetic peptides representing the heptad repeat regions inhibit fusion,[381] as does mutagenesis of the leucines in the zipper region.[83] F_2 possesses a third heptad repeat region that modulates fusogenicity through a microdomain around residue 94.[548]

Fusion requires the expression of both H and F, with a predicted interaction of the F head with the H stalk (Fig. 36.6), and binding of H to a cell surface receptor (Fig. 36.7).[385,527,802] Modeling of pre- and postfusion conformations of the F trimer indicates large conformational changes that result in formation of a six-helical bundle.[568] Basolateral expression of H and F is important for syncytia formation and increases cell-to-cell spread *in vitro* and *in vivo.*[461] In polarized epithelial cells transport is directed by interaction of the F luminal tail with M to the apical surface where virus is released.[71,487] F tail mutations in viruses causing persistent infection include premature stop codons, missense mutations, altered reading frames, and

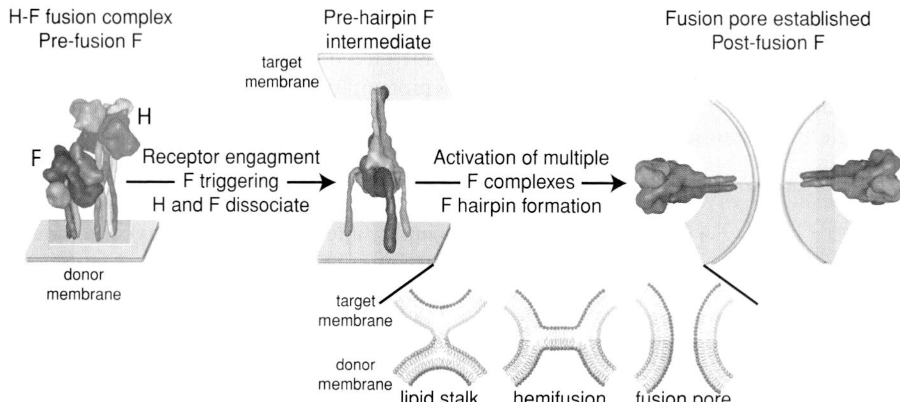

FIGURE 36.6. Schematic of measles virus (MeV) membrane fusion. MeV H and F envelope glycoproteins exist as hetero-oligomeric complexes on the surface of infectious viral particles **(left panel)**. Receptor binding by the H protein triggers major conformational changes in prefusion F, resulting in insertion of the F fusion peptide domain into the target membrane in a hypothetical prehairpin intermediate conformation **(center)**. Most likely, the concerted refolding of several prehairpin F complexes into the thermodynamically stable postfusion conformation is required to open a fusion pore and enable infection **(right panel)**. For clarity, MeV H is represented as a single tetramer and F as a single trimer in the hetero-oligomeric fusion complex. More than one F trimer may interact with each individual H tetramer. The **insert** shows enlarged representations of hypothetical lipid mixing intermediates. Formation of a local fusion nipple is thought to be followed by merger of the outer lipid layers (lipid stalk; hemifusion stage) and ultimately merger of the inner lipid layers and the opening of a fusion pore. F complexes have been eliminated from the lipid mixing representation. Structural renderings were prepared as described in Figure 36.3. (Adapted from Plemper RK, Brindley MA, Iorio RM. Structural and mechanistic studies of measles virus illuminate paramyxovirus entry. *PLoS Pathog* 2011;7:e1002058; courtesy of M. A. Brindley and R. K. Plemper.)

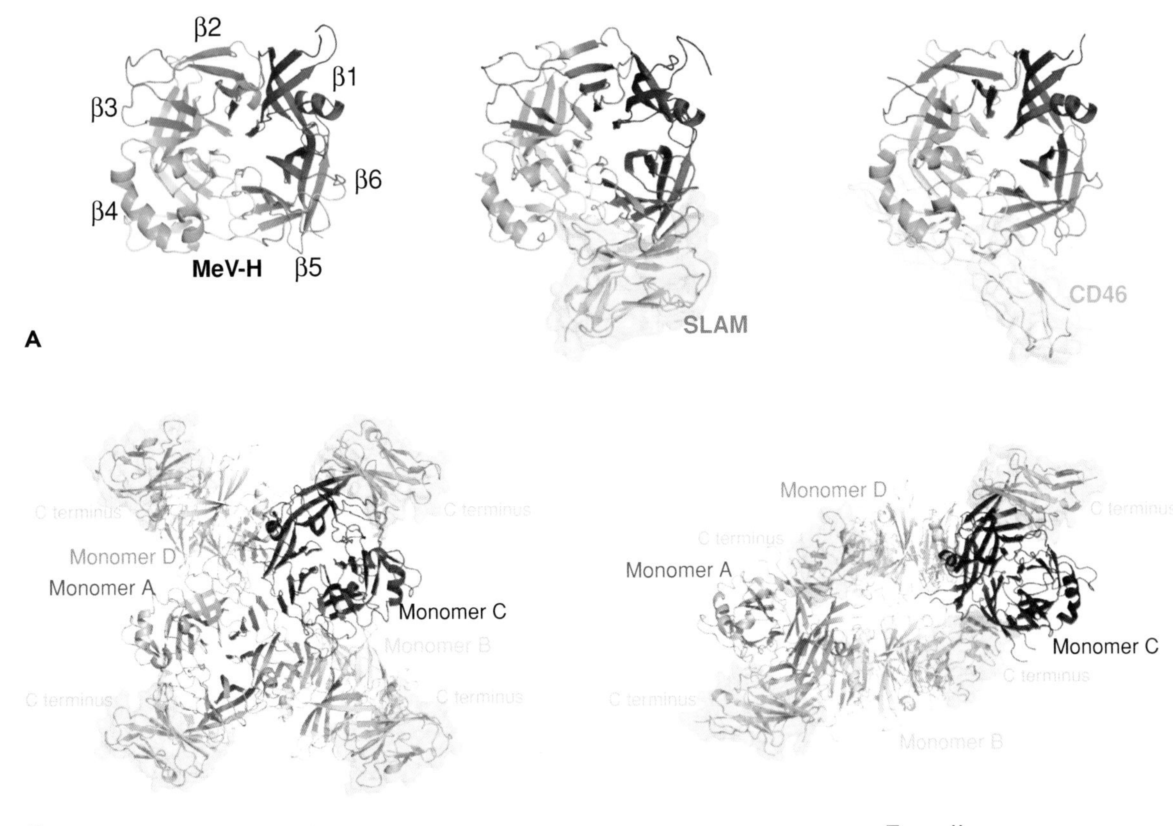

FIGURE 36.7. Crystal structures of the measles virus hemagglutinin (MeV-H) in complex with its receptors. A: The H head domain (monomer) unbound **(left)** and bound to signaling lymphocyte activation molecule (SLAM) **(middle)** or CD46 **(right)**. The H head domain as viewed downward from top is illustrated as a cartoon model. It exhibits the six-bladed β-propeller fold (β1 through β6, rainbow colors). This structure is topologically similar to the hemagglutinin neuraminidase of other paramyxoviruses and the influenza virus neuraminidase. The SLAM V domain (cyan) and CD46 SCR1 and 2 domains (pink) are shown in surface models. **B:** Two forms of H tetramer (dimer of dimers) with each monomer bound to the SLAM V domain as observed in the crystals of the H-SLAM complex. H monomers A (violet) and B (light pink) form one dimer, while monomers C (dark gray) and D (light gray) form another. Each dimer (AB or CD) constituting a tetramer has essentially the same structure within and between the two forms and is likely the basic unit of MeV-H. In Form I **(left)**, monomers A and C largely form the interface of two dimers, whereas in Form II **(right)**, monomers B and D do so. SLAM is shown in cyan. PDB ID: MV-H receptor free form (2ZB6), MV-H-SLAM Form I (3ALZ) and Form II (3ALX), MV-H-CD46 (3INB). (Courtesy of Takao Tashiguchi, Katsumi Maenaka, and Yusuke Yanagi.)

nonconservative amino acid substitutions.[104,635] These changes interfere with virus envelope assembly and budding and increase cell-to-cell fusion and neurovirulence in hamsters.[36,103]

Hemagglutinin (H) Protein

H (617 aa) is the receptor-binding and hemagglutinating (HA) protein and an important determinant of morbillivirus cellular tropism. H is a type II transmembrane glycoprotein that resides on the surfaces of infected cells and virions as disulfide-linked homodimers that associate in the ER to form tetramers (Figs. 36.3 and 36.7).[79,277,550] The mature H protein has a cytoplasmic tail of 34 amino acids preceding a single hydrophobic transmembrane region and a large C-terminal ectodomain with 13 strongly conserved cysteines. The cytoplasmic tail is essential for efficient transport to the cell surface and includes signals for basolateral sorting and endocytosis. However, H can be redirected to the apical surface for efficient particle formation and virus release.[71,462,463]

The H protein of the Edmonston strain of MeV has five predicted N-linked glycosylation sites clustered between positions 168 and 238 (Fig. 36.8). The first four of these sites are used.[305] More recent MeV isolates often have an additional glycosylation site at residue 416, and this correlates with a loss of HA activity.[615] Glycosylation is necessary for proper folding, antigenicity, dimerization, and export of H from the Golgi.[305] H processing and intracellular transport is relatively slow, taking approximately 30 minutes for oligomerization and an hour to reach the medial Golgi.[306] During persistent infections H proteins often accumulate mutations that affect glycosylation, oligomerization, and intracellular transport.[104]

Structural studies of H indicate that the N-terminus forms an α-helical stalk supporting a cubic-shaped six-blade β-propeller head structure (Fig. 36.7).[127,276,385] Each of the blade modules contains four antiparallel β-strands connected sequentially through extended loops. In the dimer, N-linked carbohydrates cover the top pocket of the head domain and

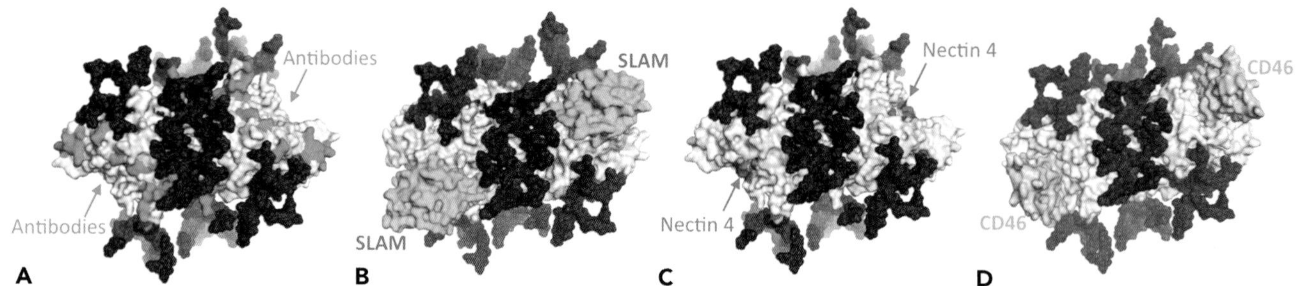

FIGURE 36.8. Structural relationships between glycans, antibody epitopes, and receptor binding sites on the hemagglutinin protein. Measles virus hemagglutinin (MeV-H) dimer (blue white) as viewed downward from top is illustrated as surface presentation with plausible N-linked sugars (black), which cover large surface areas of H. Epitopes for anti-H monoclonal antibodies (magenta) are mapped onto the sugar-uncovered surface of H **(A)**. This area also includes binding sites for signaling lymphocyte activation molecule (SLAM) (cyan, **B**), nectin 4 (red, **C**), and CD46 (pink, **D**). Because the structure of the H-nectin 4 complex has not been determined, the putative binding sites for nectin 4 are indicated, based on mutagenesis analysis. Most neutralizing antibodies bind to sites that overlap or are located very close to the receptor binding sites, which are unlikely to mutate. This may explain why measles virus has never escaped immune responses induced by natural infection or vaccination and why there is only a single serotype. PDB ID: MV-H receptor free form (2ZB6), MV-H-SLAM (3ALX), MV-H-CD46 (3INB). (Courtesy of Takao Tashiguchi, Katsumi Maenaka, and Yusuke Yanagi.)

cause the two molecules to tilt away from each other, optimizing exposure of neutralizing epitopes and the receptor-binding sites away from the dimer interface on the lateral surface (Fig. 36.8)[276,308,749,751] (see section on Cellular Receptors). Cysteine residues at 139 and 154 are responsible for intermolecular disulfide bonding of monomeric H glycoproteins.[549]

H acts in conjunction with F for budding and for cell-to-cell fusion and entry (Fig. 36.6). Fusion occurs through conformational changes in both proteins triggered by the binding of H to a cellular receptor (Fig. 36.7).[277,321,499,500,624] Hetero-oligomerization occurs in the ER.[550] Mutagenesis has identified separate regions in the H stalk required for interacting with F and for triggering F fusion.[385,527,547] MeV fusogenicity correlates inversely with the strength of the interaction between F and H[133,134,189,321,551] (see section on Entry).

L Protein

The L (large) protein (2,183 aa) is a multidomain protein with several highly conserved regions. One contains the Gly-Asp-Asn-Gln motif common to the RNA polymerases of negative-strand viruses.[174,669] L is present in small quantities in the infected cell, interacts with and functions in association with P, and is part of the viral nucleocapsid both in the cell and in the virion. A domain in the N-terminal 408 amino acids binds to a trihelical binding domain in PCT that links it to the nucleocapsid for transcription and replication.[300,357]

Cellular Receptors

MeV can infect several types of cells and uses multiple receptors in a virus strain and cell type–specific manner. Three of these receptors have been identified: membrane co-factor protein or CD46,[168,497] SLAM or CD150,[715] and polio virus receptor–related 4 (PVRL4) or nectin 4.[479,508] The binding sites for these cellular receptors are all found on the lateral surface of the head structure of H[277,622] (Figs. 36.7 and 36.8).

CD46

CD46 is a widely distributed human complement regulatory protein expressed on all nucleated cells and preferentially on the apical surface of polarized epithelial cells.[71,445] It normally acts as a co-factor in the proteolytic inactivation of C3b/C4b by factor I.[591] Monkeys have a CD46 homolog that is expressed on erythrocytes, but such a protein has not been identified in mice. Multiple mRNAs are produced by alternative splicing of CD46 transcripts. All code for proteins that contain an N-terminal signal peptide, four short consensus repeats (SCRs), a transmembrane region, and an anchor. Isoforms differ in the length and composition of an extracellular serine/threonine/proline domain near the transmembrane segment and in having one of two alternative cytoplasmic tails.[591] The cytoplasmic tail of CD46 is associated with intracellular kinases and adaptor proteins, and cross-linking of CD46 can induce autophagy and regulate inflammatory responses.[338,591] The four isoforms common on human cells can all serve as receptors for MeV.[231,423] SCR1 and SCR2 interact with the MeV H protein, while SCRs 2, 3, and 4 bind C3b/C4b.[591] MeV infection of cells or expression of the H protein alone can lead to rapid internalization of CD46 from the cell surface.[373] In persistently infected cells CD46 down-regulation is accomplished through a membrane-proximal Tyr-X-X-Leu motif in the cytoplasmic domain.[791]

The H binding site involves one planar face of SCR1 and SCR2 with an important role for the N-linked carbohydrates on SCR2.[99,304,417] Most vaccine strains use CD46 efficiently, while wild-type strains often do not.[191,790] A tyrosine at position 481 of H and glycine at 546 are key determinants of the affinity of H for CD46,[53,660] but several additional residues are also important.[432,603,637,695] The crystal structure of Edmonston H with SCR1 and SCR2 shows that CD46 binds to the side of the β-propeller through three contact regions on blades 4 and 5 (Figs. 36.7 and 36.8).[622]

SLAM

SLAM/CD150 is a 70-kD glycoprotein expressed on cells of the immune system including immature thymocytes, activated T and B lymphocytes, activated monocytes, and mature dendritic cells.[124] SLAM is a member of a family of immunomodulatory type I transmembrane proteins[93,153] and is the most important receptor for MeV infection of lymphoid tissue.[143]

A recombinant MeV that interacts inefficiently with SLAM is attenuated in macaques.[389] CDV, RPV, and peste des petits ruminants virus also use SLAM as a receptor, suggesting that this is a common feature of morbilliviruses.[5,49,716,749]

SLAM has two highly glycosylated immunoglobulin-like domains (V and C2) and structural features of the CD2 family of membrane proteins.[670,790] The cytoplasmic domain has immunoreceptor tyrosine-based switch motifs that bind small SH2 (src homology 2) domain adaptor proteins, such as SLAM-associated protein (SAP) and Ewing sarcoma–associated transcript-2 (EAT-2), important for cell signaling.[93,153,515,670,790] MeV H binds to the V domain of human, but not mouse, SLAM,[515] and this results in down-regulation of SLAM expression on the surface of infected cells.[767] Mutagenesis studies have identified MeV H residues Ile194, Asp505, Asp507, Asp530, Arg533, Phe552, and Pro554 as important for binding SLAM.[431,500,751] The crystal structure of H with the V domain of SLAM shows that these residues contribute to four components of the binding interface located primarily on the side of H blade 5 contiguous to the binding site for CD46[277] (Fig. 36.7).

Studies of different strains of MeV have shown that both vaccine and wild-type strains can use SLAM as a receptor and that most H proteins can bind both CD46 and SLAM, but receptor affinity and efficiency of entry differ.[191,422,432,521,621,637,751,790] In general, binding to SLAM is of higher affinity than binding to CD46.[432] Viruses with asparagine at H481 use SLAM and enter PBMCs more efficiently than viruses with tyrosine at this position.[191,637] Differences in efficient receptor usage likely involve interactions with MeV proteins in addition to H.[370,710]

Nectin 4

The distributions of SLAM and CD46 in tissues do not account for MeV replication in epithelial cells *in vivo* or *in vitro.*[18,197,278,460,519,661,696,708–710] Recently, poliovirus receptor–like 4/nectin 4, an adherens junction protein of the immunoglobulin superfamily, has been identified as a receptor on epithelial cells.[479,508] This is consistent with previous studies that indicated that an epithelial receptor is expressed on the basolateral surface of polarized cells and involved in formation of tight junctions.[665,674] Nectin 4 is a transmembrane protein with two C2-type immunoglobulin domains and a V domain that interacts with H.[479]

Other Receptors

Several pieces of information suggest that MeV uses additional receptors. The currently known receptors do not account for the ability of MeV to infect endothelial cells in acute infections[197] or cells of the central nervous system in chronic infections.[445,661] Receptors used by attenuated vaccine strains adapted to growth in cells from nonsusceptible hosts (e.g., chickens) probably represent an additional category of MeV receptors that have yet to be identified.[193]

Other cell surface molecules interact with MeV but do not serve as entry receptors. For instance, MeV H can bind Toll-like receptor 2 (TLR2) and induce signaling.[63] Dendritic cell–specific intercellular adhesion molecule 3 (ICAM-3) grabbing nonintegrin (DC-SIGN) is an attachment receptor that enhances infection and modulates function of DCs.[31,147,263] Incorporation of cyclophilin B into MeV virions by binding to N leads to interaction with the cyclophilin ligand CD147/EMMPRIN, a multifunctional transmembrane protein expressed on epithelial and neural cells.[760]

Hemagglutination, Hemadsorption, and Hemolysis

Some strains of MeV bind to and agglutinate the erythrocytes of Old World monkeys, particularly African green, patas, and rhesus macaques. HA occurs optimally at physiologic pH and 37°C. Infected cells can also adsorb monkey erythrocytes (hemadsorption). Both HA and hemadsorption are properties of the H glycoprotein. Many wild-type MeV isolates require high salt or have little HA activity.[594] HA of monkey erythrocytes is indicative of binding to CD46, is improved by adaptation to growth in Vero cells, and is dependent on the C-terminal 18 amino acids of H, amino acids 451 and 481, and absence of glycosylation at 416.[616,630,660] This is consistent with the distribution of the CD46 molecule, which is not present on human red blood cells, and with the molecular characteristics of primate CD46.[303] In baboons, lack of HA is due to an amino acid substitution in SCR2 and in New World monkeys to an absence of SCR1.[303] HA is followed within a few hours by lysis of the agglutinated erythrocytes. Hemolysis is a consequence of fusion and dependent on F, as well as H.[14,108,779]

Entry

H attachment to a cellular receptor is followed by fusion of the virus envelope with the plasma membrane and delivery of the viral ribonucleocapsid into the cytoplasm for initiation of infection (Fig. 36.6). The H dimer of dimers (tetramer) associates with the prefusion F trimer in the secretory system of the host cell and exists as H-F hetero-oligomer on the virion surface (Fig. 36.3). The oligomers cooperate to induce fusion at neutral pH.[516] Fusion requires H and F to be from compatible virus species and prior cleavage of F_0 into F_1 and F_2.[478] The MeV H protein stalk interacts directly with the MeV F protein head, suggesting that the metastable F trimer is shorter than the H tetramer, resulting in a staggered head domain arrangement on the virion surface (Figs. 36.3 and 36.6).[385,527,547] The strength of H and F binding determines fusogenicity. More avid binding decreases fusion, indicating the need for H and F dissociation during the process of entry and productive infection.[189] Separate regions on the H stalk have been identified for F interaction and for F triggering, suggesting that these are discrete functions.[79,547] It is postulated that interaction of H with its receptor on the cell membrane induces a reorganization of the dimer–dimer head domains that transmit receptor binding to the F contact zone in the H stalk to trigger refolding of F and membrane fusion.[277,499,624] This H reorganization may be represented in the crystal structure of H with SLAM that shows two forms of the H dimer with the orientation shifted with respect to each other[277,547] (Fig. 36.7).

Cytopathic Effects

MeV replication in cell culture results in cytopathic changes of three varieties: multinucleated giant cells (syncytia), altered cell shape, and inclusion bodies.[185] Cell-to-cell fusion occurs at neutral pH and syncytia formation occurs *in vitro* (Fig. 36.2) and *in vivo*[184] presumably using fusion mechanisms similar to those for virus entry (Fig. 36.6). Syncytia formation is facilitated by basolateral expression of H and F and the actin filament–plasma membrane cross-linker moesin and is inhibited by cytochalasin B.[167] Fusion of infected cells with uninfected cells may produce syncytia with 50 or more nuclei. Nuclei in the center of the syncytia have marginated chromatin[184] and are often undergoing apoptotic cell death[196] leading to plaque

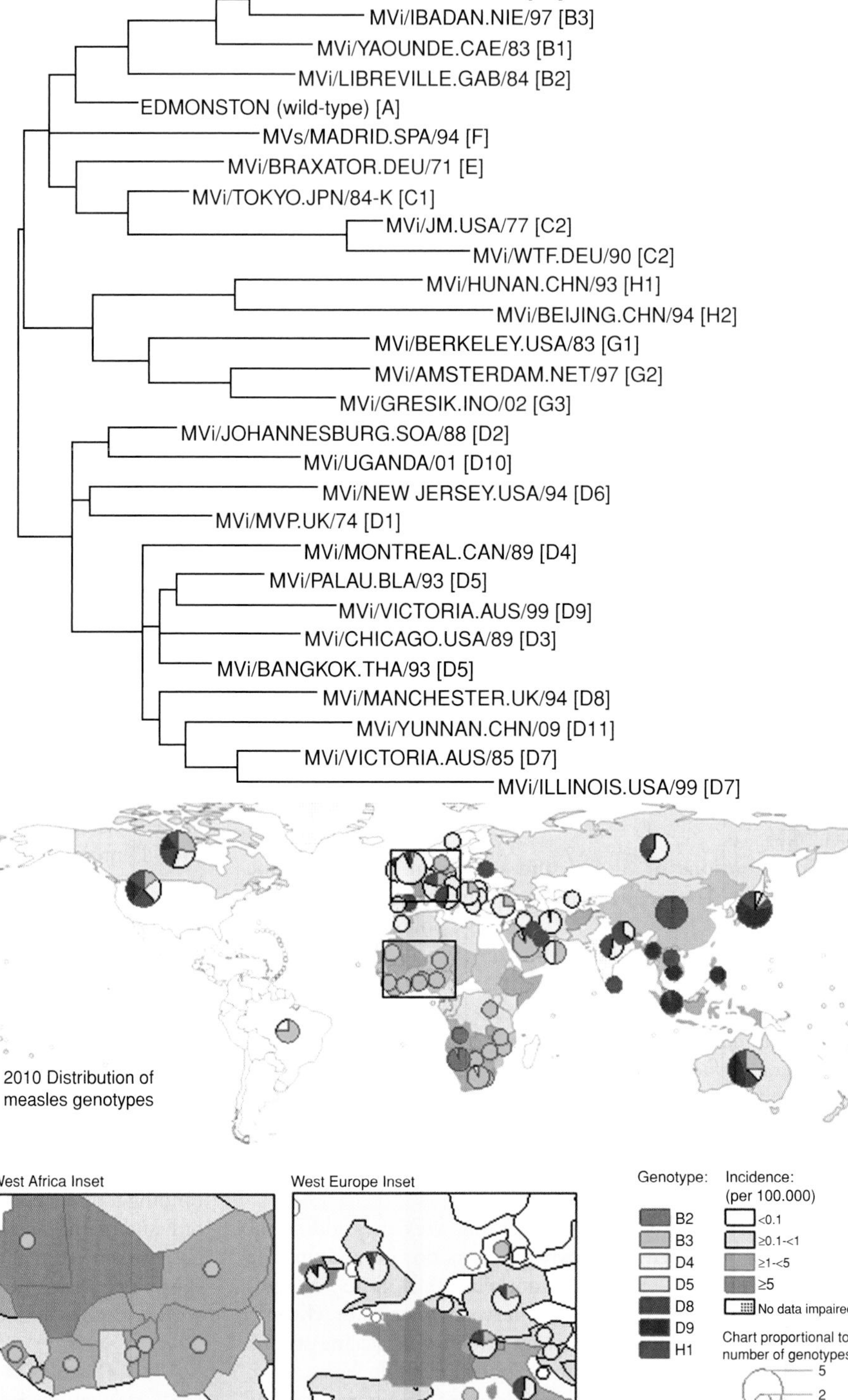

FIGURE 36.9. Genetic variation in wild-type measles viruses (MeV) and geographic distribution of MeV genotypes. The World Health Organization (WHO) currently recognizes 23 genotypes and one provisional genotype of wild-type MeV. The phylogenetic tree **(top)** is based on the sequences of the N genes of the WHO reference strains for each genotype[775] and the provisional genotype.[804] Map **(bottom)** shows the global distribution of MeV genotypes and measles incidence in 2010. Colored circles indicate MeV genotypes reported to the WHO database for the year 2010, and the size of the circles is proportional to the number of genotypes reported for the indicated areas. Two areas, Western Africa and Eastern Europe, are also shown as inserts to provide more resolution. The boundaries and names shown and the designations used on this map do not imply the expression of any opinion whatsoever on the part of the WHO concerning the legal status of any country, territory, city, or area or of its authorities, or concerning the delimitation of its frontiers of boundaries. Dotted lines on maps represent approximate borderlines for which there may not yet be full agreement. (Courtesy of David Featherstone, WHO, and Paul Rota, Centers for Disease Control and Prevention.)

formation *in vitro.* Infected cells may also change from a normal polygonal shape to a stellate, dendritic, or spindle shape with increased refractility to light. This type of "strand-forming" cytopathic effect appears after several passages and may be related to the production of DI particles.[443]

Both spindle-shaped cells and syncytial cells may contain intracytoplasmic and intranuclear inclusion bodies. Cytoplasmic inclusions are generally larger than nuclear inclusions and contain N-encapsidated RNA decorated with P, producing *fuzzy* or *granular* nucleocapsids.[72] Intranuclear Cowdry type A inclusion bodies are characteristic of morbillivirus infections and occur late in infection. CDV intranuclear inclusion bodies are usually complex nuclear bodies derived from nucleoli that contain N and a cellular heat shock protein.[511,513] MeV N, when expressed alone, migrates to the nucleus[309,680] where it can assemble into nucleocapsids that lack P and viral RNA and appear "smooth" by electron microscopy.[140,512] Because binding of P to assembled nucleocapsids leads to cytoplasmic retention,[309] it has been postulated that the amount of P may be limiting late in infection, allowing N to move into the nucleus.[72,309]

Budding

M plays a central role in virus assembly and release. In the absence of M, infectious particles are not released and expression of M alone leads to release of virus-like particles.[102,109,556,611] To initiate virus assembly, M associates with the nucleocapsid, is co-transported to the plasma membrane,[325] and interacts with the cytoplasmic domains of the F/H glycoprotein oligomers to promote virus budding.[461,462,697] Proteins associate with detergent-resistant microdomains[425,556,743] and budding is independent of the cellular endosomal sorting complex required for transport (ESCRT) system.[618] In polarized epithelial cells, budding is directed to the apical surface by the M protein despite the intrinsic glycoprotein targeting to the basolateral surface,[418,487] and loss of apical targeting by M enhances cell–cell fusion at the expense of virus production.[102,103,610]

Evolution, Antigenic Composition, and Strain Variation

Antigenically, MeV is a relatively stable virus. Antisera from individuals infected decades ago retain the ability to neutralize current wild-type strains of MeV and vice versa, although with varying efficiency.[144,361,659] The observed rate of mutation of H in virus circulating in defined geographic locations is low, estimated at 5×10^{-4} per year for a given nucleotide,[594] while the rate of mutation during growth *in vitro* is higher, estimated at 9×10^{-5} per replication for a nucleotide.[644] Although historical accounts date the emergence of measles to approximately the 6th century (see History earlier), phylogenetic analysis of morbillivirus sequences suggests a more recent divergence from a common ancestor with RPV.[222] However, this more recent estimate may reflect the effects on sequence evolution of population bottlenecks after outbreaks and purifying selection to maintain protein function.[222,561,769] The structure of H with carbohydrates masking the top surface and exposed receptor-binding sites on the side (Fig. 36.8) is postulated to constrain acquisition of mutations.[276,608] Evidence of vaccine-induced selective pressure on wild-type strains of MeV has been identified in the noose and receptor-binding regions of H.[209,236,623,658,659,713]

Nucleotide sequence variability, primarily in the N, P, and H genes, has been a useful tool for the MeV genotyping needed for molecular epidemiologic studies of transmission pathways.[353,594,602] N genes differ by up to 7% in the C-terminal N_{TAIL} region, the region most often used for strain identification[82,236] (Fig. 36.4). The P gene is most variable in the shared PV_{NTD},[45] and P gene sequencing has provided increased power to identify transmission routes when the N_{TAIL} sequences are identical.[353] The H gene nucleotide sequence is most variable between residues 167 and 241 where the N-linked glycosylation sites are located, but can become regionally fixed.[353,602]

Strains examined to date separate into eight different clades (A to H) and at least 24 different genotypes based on sequencing of the C-terminal 450 nucleotides of the N gene or the entire coding region of H[590,605,606,775,804] (Fig. 36.9). New genotypes are designated if the nucleotide sequence differs from the closest reference sequence by more than 2.5% in N or 2.0% in H.[776] Some genotypes are found in one geographic region, others are co-circulating, while others are inactive and may be extinct[590] (Fig. 36.9). Live attenuated vaccines were all derived from genotype A wild-type strains and are quite similar.[46]

PATHOGENESIS AND PATHOLOGY

Classic Measles

Measles is typically a childhood infection of humans spread by the respiratory route. Disease is characterized by a latent period of 10 to 14 days and a 2- to 3-day prodrome of fever, coryza, cough, and conjunctivitis followed by the appearance of a characteristic maculopapular rash (Fig. 36.10).[362] The onset of the rash coincides with the appearance of the immune response and initiation of virus clearance (Fig. 36.11). Recovery is accompanied by lifelong immunity to reinfection.[530] Macaques exposed to infected humans or experimentally infected with wild-type strains of MeV develop a similar disease, and much of our more detailed understanding of pathogenesis, immune responses, and sites of virus replication come from studies of nonhuman primates, often facilitated by the use of engineered reporter viruses.[29,143,146,441,735]

Entry and Sites of Primary Replication

MeV is efficiently transmitted over short distances by respiratory droplets and over longer distances by small-particle aerosols.[119,617] High MeV infectivity suggests that the cellular sites of initial virus replication are very susceptible to infection. However, the nature of these cells is unclear because it has been difficult to identify MeV-positive cells in the respiratory tract at early times after infection.[143,388] Although autopsy studies have shown abundant infection of respiratory epithelial cells,[460,617] detailed studies of experimentally infected monkeys early after infection have only identified infected alveolar macrophages and subepithelial DCs.[143,146,388] Because *in vitro* studies suggest that MeV infects epithelial cells from the basolateral

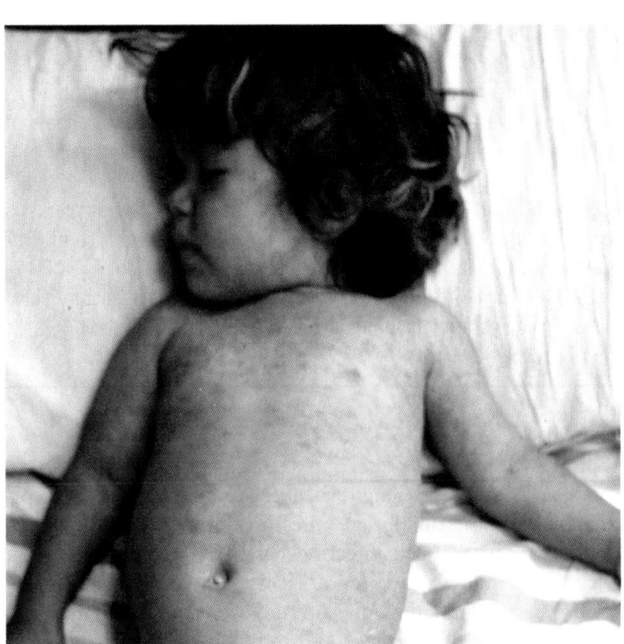

FIGURE 36.10. Measles virus rash.

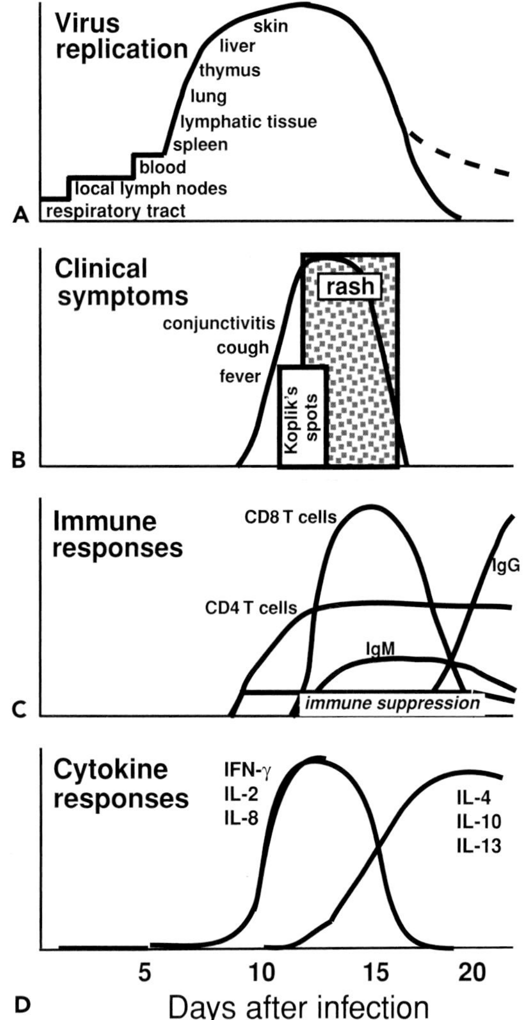

FIGURE 36.11. Pathogenesis of measles. Measles virus (MeV) is spread by the respiratory route and replication begins in the respiratory tract and spreads to lymphocytes, monocyte/macrophages, endothelial cells, and epithelial cells in the blood, thymus, spleen, lymph nodes, liver, skin, and lung and to the conjunctivae and mucosal surfaces of the gastrointestinal, respiratory, and genitourinary tracts. The rash appears at the time of the virus-specific immune response with activation of MeV-specific CD4+ and CD8+ T cells and synthesis of MeV-specific immunoglobulin M (IgM) and IgG antibody. Clearance of infectious virus is approximately coincident with fading of the rash, but clearance of RNA is slower. Cytokines produced are consistent with activation of Th1 CD4+ and CD8+ T cells, followed by Th2 CD4+ T cells and regulatory cells. Immune suppression is initiated during the rash and persists for weeks after its resolution.

surface[414,674] and MeV engineered not to infect respiratory epithelial cells can still initiate infection after intranasal inoculation,[390] epithelial cell infection has been postulated to be a late, rather than an early, event. It is possible that pulmonary macrophages and DCs take up and transport MeV to local lymphoid tissue where virus is amplified, leading to viremia and subsequent systemic spread of infection to many tissues, including the lung.[703]

Spread

MeV interaction with DC-SIGN leads to up-regulation of SLAM on DCs, MeV entry,[31] and likely transport from the respiratory tract to local lymphatic tissues in lung and draining lymph nodes.[339,652,663] *In vitro* and *in vivo* studies suggest that DCs can transfer infection to susceptible T cells.[143,148,663] Replication in lymphatic tissue is efficient, and infected CD150-expressing monocytes, T cells, and B cells are detected in peripheral blood within 4 to 7 days after infection.[29,198,264,439,736] Only rarely has infectious virus been isolated from plasma,[538] but viral RNA can be detected by reverse transcriptase-polymerase chain reaction (RT-PCR). MeV-infected mononuclear cells increase expression of the integrins LFA-1 ($\alpha_L\beta_2$) and VLA-4 ($\alpha_4\beta_1$) and transmigratory cups that promote adherence to endothelial cells and cell-to-cell transmission of infection.[26,166,313,413] These properties likely facilitate virus dissemination. The viremia is accompanied by leukopenia due either to death of infected cells or to changes in leukocyte trafficking.[29,517,613]

Target Cells and Tissues

From the blood, infection is spread to distal lymphoid tissue and to epithelial cells, endothelial cells, and macrophages in multiple organs.[197,460] Transmigration across an endothelial barrier is impaired for MeV-infected lymphocytes,[166] so entry of MeV into tissues may occur primarily from endothelial cells infected by circulating leukocytes or by movement of other types of infected cells, such as monocytes, across blood vessel walls.[413] Once within tissue, spread is cell type and virus strain dependent and occurs by cell–cell fusion or by release of infectious virus. Tyrosine residues in the cytoplasmic tails of F (aa 549) and H (aa 12) are important for basolateral glycoprotein sorting and determine the fusogenic spread of MeV in epithelial cells.[462,463] However, only the H sorting signal determines wild-type MeV release versus cell–cell fusion in lymphocytes.[609,610]

Lymphoid organs and tissues (e.g., thymus, spleen, lymph nodes, appendix, and tonsils) are prominent sites of virus replication[617] where infection results in the appearance of lymphoid or reticuloendothelial giant cells first described by Warthin[759] and Finkeldey.[208] These cells can be 100 μm or more in diameter and contain up to 100 nuclei aggregated near the center. Inclusion bodies are not generally present. Warthin-Finkeldey cells tend to be located in or near germinal centers, in the thymus, and in submucosal lymphoid tissue.[279,509] In the thymus, infection of epithelial cells and thymocyte apoptosis lead to a prolonged decrease in the size of the thymic cortex, while other lymphoid tissues recover promptly.[772]

MeV also spreads to the skin, conjunctivae, kidney, lung, gastrointestinal tract, respiratory mucosa, genital mucosa, and liver (Fig. 36.11). In these nonlymphoid sites the virus replicates primarily in endothelial cells, epithelial cells, and macrophages.[197,198,460,699] Endothelial cell infection may be accompanied by vascular dilatation, increased vascular permeability, mononuclear cell infiltration, and infection of surrounding tissue.[150] The histopathology of the measles rash suggests that the initial event is infection of dermal endothelial cells[355] followed by spread of infection into the overlying epidermis with infection of keratinocytes in the stratum granulosum leading to focal keratosis and edema.[699] Epithelial giant cells form and mononuclear cells accumulate around vessels.[150] Koplik spots found on the oral mucosa are pathologically similar and involve the submucous glands.[150]

On rare occasions there is spread to the nervous system. *In vitro* studies have demonstrated infection of brain microvascular endothelial cells by adherent MeV-infected T lymphocytes,[166] and infection of endothelial cells has been demonstrated in the brains of children dying of measles.[197,358] Polarized endothelial cells can release virus from both the apical and basolateral cell surfaces, allowing access to the brain parenchyma, as well as the blood.[166] If neurons become infected, virus can spread through the central nervous system (CNS) from neuron to neuron without the release of infectious particles.[177] It has been suggested that the F protein interacts at the synapse with the substance P receptor neurokinin-1 to mediate transsynaptic spread.[419]

Immune Responses

The immune responses to MeV are important for clearance of virus and recovery from infection and are directly responsible for several of the clinical manifestations of measles. Although infectious virus cannot be isolated after the rash is cleared, viral RNA can be detected for many weeks, indicating that complete viral clearance is a prolonged process.[529,542,734] The roles of various components of the immune response in recovery from infection have been deduced from *experiments of nature* in which the outcome of MeV infection in patients with deficiencies of immunologic function has been documented and from the studies of monkeys depleted of specific components of the immune system.[244,539,540,542] In general, deficits in antibody production permit recovery, while deficits in cellular immune responses may lead to slowed clearance and progressive disease (see Measles in the Immunocompromised Host later). In immunologically normal individuals, the onset of clinically apparent disease coincides with the appearance of the MeV-specific adaptive immune response. There is also marked activation of the immune system that is coincident with the appearance of immune suppression (Fig. 36.11). Immune suppression and immune activation continue for many weeks after apparent recovery.

Early Innate Responses

Innate responses may contribute to control of virus replication during the incubation period, but determining the role and importance of specific components of the innate response in measles has been complicated. *In vitro* studies have shown that innate responses triggered by interaction of MeV RNA or proteins with pathogen recognition receptors at the cell surface or in the cytoplasm to activate signaling pathways involving transcription factors nuclear factor-κB (NFκB) and IRF-3 differ with the strain of virus, are cell type specific, and are highly regulated by the viral P, C, and V proteins.[63,172,284,345,625,646,718] Epithelial cells show activation of NFκB and activator protein-1 (AP-1)[320] and production of the chemokine CXCL8 (interleukin-8 [IL-8])[629] after MeV infection. However, monocytes respond differently than epithelial cells, and interaction of H with TLR2 at the monocyte cell surface stimulates induction of IL-6 and increases surface expression of CD150,[63] while interaction with CD46 inhibits IL-12 production.[344] The NFκB pathway and tumor necrosis factor-α (TNF-α) production are suppressed in MeV-infected monocytes, potentially as a result of MeV P protein–induced up-regulation of the ubiquitin-modifying enzyme TNFAIP3 (A20), a negative regulator of NFκB.[393,629,756]

Some inflammatory cytokines and chemokines are induced *in vivo* during measles. Levels of IL-1β and IL-8 are increased in plasma of children during measles,[629,807] and infected macaques show increases in IL-6 and IL-8.[626] IL-1β mRNA and protein are increased in MeV-infected monocyte-derived cells and in PBMCs cultured from patients after rash onset.[393,756] Transcriptional analysis of PBMCs from children with measles has shown increases in mRNAs for cytokines IL-1β and TNF-α and chemokines CCL4 (MIP-1β), CXCL2 (MIP-2α), and IL-8.[807] The mRNA for CIAS-1 (NALP3), a component of the inflammasome responsible for processing proIL-1β to its active form, is also increased.[807]

Type I IFN is an important component of the innate response to many virus infections, and MeV replication is sensitive to the inhibitory effects of IFN-α/β.[391,640,714] MeV replication is required for induction of IFN-β transcription in most responsive cells.[288] Two induction mechanisms have been identified. In epithelial cells, MeV leader RNA can interact with and activate RIG-I and, to a lesser extent, MDA5,[318,555] and N can interact with and activate IRF-3 in concert with an unidentified cellular co-factor.[128,718] Induction of IFN by MeV may also occur at the cell surface through interaction of the virus with CD46 or TLR2.[63,345] *In vitro*, MeV infection of epithelial cells and DCs leads to rapid production of IFN-β and many IFN-αs followed by induction of IFN-responsive genes.[463,625,633,714,808] On the other hand, MeV infection of mitogen-stimulated PBMCs does not usually stimulate IFN production.[498] In fact, MeV suppresses type I IFN production and signaling in CD4+ T cells[625] and has a variable effect on plasmacytoid DC IFN production.[169,633]

Many of the reported effects of MeV on immune cell function *in vitro* are secondary to the effects of IFN. For instance, MeV induction of IFN inhibits development of DCs but stimulates maturation of immature DCs and terminal differentiation of cortical thymic epithelial cells.[270,741] IFN also plays a role in suppressing proliferation of T cells in cultures of MeV-infected PBMCs.[619] However, interpretation of investigations related to IFN induction and its role in measles pathogenesis has been confounded by the frequent presence of 5′ copy-back DI RNAs in the stocks of the virus strains studied.[352,662] Vaccine strains are more likely to induce IFN-α/β than wild-type strains,[498] but this may be related to the efficiency with which they generate DI RNAs,[352,662,701] which are potent inducers of IFN through activation of MDA5.[688,800]

It is not clear whether IFN-α/β is induced during MeV infection *in vivo*. Transcriptional analysis of PBMCs during measles shows no evidence of up-regulation of IFN-induced genes.[807] No IFN-α/β has been detected during natural infection in humans or experimental infection of macaques.[259,262,476,664,801] Biologically active IFN has been detected occasionally, but IFN-γ produced by T cells is produced in response to infection, and the protein responsible for IFN activity (type I or II) was not identified.[543,626] A recombinant wild-type MeV that cannot interfere with STAT1 translocation is attenuated in macaques, suggesting some role for this signaling pathway in the response to infection.[156]

Natural killer (NK) cells constitute another potentially important early defense mechanism, but studies of NK activity indicate that NK cell function is actually lower than normal during measles.[262] These studies were performed using samples collected at, or after, the rash, so they do not exclude NK cell activation at earlier stages of infection.

MeV and MeV-infected cells activate the factor B–dependent alternative complement pathway, rendering the cells susceptible to complement-mediated lysis.[675] This is a property of F_1

and results in deposition of C3b on the virion and infected cell surface independent of virus use of the complement regulatory protein CD46 as a receptor.[154] In infected cells, the complement regulators CD46 and CD55 are segregated into separate membrane microdomains from F.[233]

Antibody

Antibodies are first detectable when the rash appears[55,75,249] (Fig. 36.11). The isotype of MeV-specific antibody is initially IgM followed by a switch first to immunoglobulin G2 (IgG2) and IgG3 and then, in the memory phase, to IgG1 and IgG4.[75,322] IgG is initially of low avidity and this improves steadily over several months.[488,726] IgA, IgM, and IgG antibodies to MeV are found in secretions and sampling of saliva has provided a noninvasive method for determining immune status.[81,317]

Antibodies are eventually produced to most viral proteins (Fig. 36.12). The most abundant and most rapidly produced antibody is to N.[249] Because of the abundance of anti-N antibody, absence of this antibody is an indicator of seronegativity. The M protein elicits only small amounts of antibody, except in atypical measles.[249,415] Antibodies to H are the primary antibodies that neutralize virus infectivity.[144,145,237] Neutralization is generally measured by plaque reduction of the Edmonston strain of MeV on CD46-expressing Vero cells,[125] but this assay may not reflect neutralization of the infection of wild-type MeV strains on SLAM-expressing cells.[559] Neutralizing epitopes have been mapped by competitive binding of monoclonal antibodies and by analysis of different strains and escape mutants (Fig. 36.8).[307,312,396,658] Human convalescent sera show reactivity to linear epitopes, as well as to epitopes dependent on conformation and glycosylation.[305,451,482] A highly conserved linear neutralizing epitope is in the H noose (aa 379 to 410).[570] Major conformational epitopes have been localized to regions between amino acids 368 and 396 and in the SLAM-binding region.[192,396] Essentially all of these epitopes are on exposed surfaces on the sides of H (Fig. 36.8).[276,622] Antibodies to F induced by regions encompassing amino acid 73 and amino acids 388 to 402 contribute to virus neutralization, probably by preventing fusion of the virus membrane with the cell membrane at the time of virus entry.[25,144,201,420,420,557] Human sera also recognize linear epitopes in six to seven regions spread over much of the F protein frequently close to T-cell epitopes.[481,778]

Antibody can protect from MeV infection, may contribute to recovery from infection, and may play a role in establishing persistent infection.[9,186,577] Antibody-dependent cellular cytotoxicity correlates temporally with cessation of cell-associated viremia,[212] and failure to mount an adequate antibody response carries a poor prognosis.[770] However, in monkey studies transient depletion of B cells does not affect clearance of infectious virus.[539] Antibody binding to infected cells alters intracellular virus replication and may contribute to control of infection.[218,240,639] The role of antibody in protection from infection is discussed under Vaccination and the role in establishing persistence is discussed under Persistent Infection.

Cellular Immunity

The ability to recover from measles was postulated by Burnet to be an indication of the adequacy of T-lymphocyte–mediated immune responses,[86] and depletion of CD8+ T cells in infected monkeys impairs control of virus replication and slows clearance.[540] MeV-specific, proliferating, and clonally expanded CD8+ T cells are present in blood at the time of the rash and in bronchoalveolar lavage fluid during pneumonitis.[331,464,476,485,732,757] IFN-γ, soluble CD8, and β_2-microglobulin, a component of

Percent Antibody Positive

A Day after rash

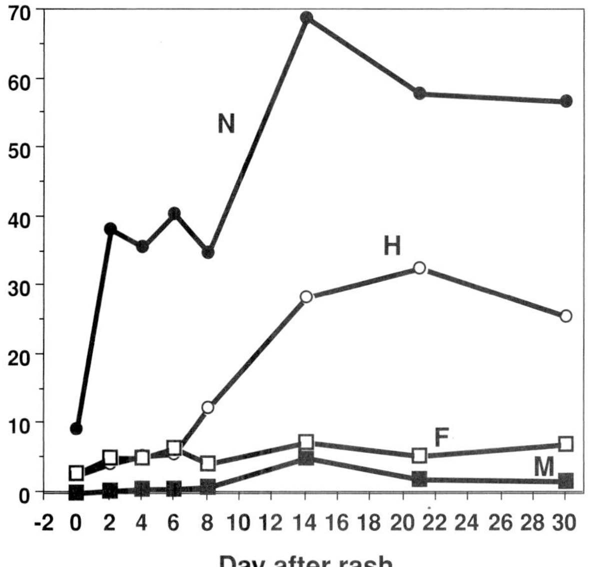

FIGURE 36.12. Production of antibody to measles virus (MeV) proteins during natural infection. A: Percent of individuals positive for antibody to each protein. **B:** Relative amounts of antibody to each protein. Antibody was measured by immunoprecipitation. (Adapted from Graves MC, Griffin DE, Johnson RT, et al. Development of antibody to measles virus polypeptides during complicated and uncomplicated measles virus infections. *J Virol* 1984;49:409–412.)

the major histocompatibility complex (MHC) class I molecule, are increased in plasma.[259,260,261,476] The H and M proteins can be processed and presented to CD8+ T cells in a transporter associated with antigen processing (TAP)-independent fashion.[502] Cultures of PBMCs with autologous MeV-infected or MeV peptide-pulsed cells after recovery show expanded CD8+ T cells that are cytotoxic and produce IFN-γ, demonstrating that effector CD8+ T-cell memory is established by infection.[331,332,492,732] CD8+ T-cell responses in humans show a broad pattern of reactivity with epitopes identified in all viral proteins, except V.[289,330,331,523,737–739]

CD4+ T cells are also activated in response to MeV infection. *In vitro,* binding of H to CD46 targets virion proteins to an endosomal compartment for efficient presentation by MHC class II molecules.[232] CD4+ T cells are proliferating during the rash.[757] Soluble CD4 becomes elevated in plasma and remains so for several weeks after recovery.[258] Classic CD4+ T-cell responses, such as MeV-specific proliferation and production of cytokines, and regulatory T cells are stimulated during measles.[476,732,801] In immune individuals, most MeV proteins can induce lymphocyte proliferation.[430,480,737]

Cytokines produced by CD4+ T cells determine their function. Type 1 CD4+ T (Th1) cells produce IFN-γ that activates macrophages and IL-2 that promotes T-cell proliferation. These are the primary mediators of classical delayed-type hypersensitivity. Type 2 CD4+ T (Th2) cells produce IL-4, IL-5, IL-10, and IL-13 that are important for B-cell growth and differentiation and for macrophage deactivation. Th17 cells are associated with autoimmunity and produce IL-17, while T-regulatory cells produce IL-10 and transforming growth factor-β (TGF-β). In measles, IFN-γ, neopterin (a product of IFN-γ–activated macrophages), and soluble IL-2 receptor rise during the prodrome, prior to the appearance of the rash.[259,261] This is followed by elevation of IL-2, soluble CD4, and soluble CD8 at the time of the rash.[260,261,476] As the rash fades, IL-4, IL-10, and IL-13 increase, and elevation of these cytokines persists in some individuals for weeks[260,476,801] (Fig. 36.11). This pattern of cytokine production suggests early activation of CD8+ (IFN-γ) and type 1 CD4+ (IFN-γ and IL-2) T cells during the rash followed by activation of type 2 CD4+ T cells (IL-4, IL-13) and regulatory T cells (IL-10) during recovery.

IFN-γ may have an important direct antiviral effect. IFN-γ can suppress MeV replication in epithelial and endothelial cells *in vitro* through induction of indoleamine 2,3-dioxygenase[510] and inhibits MeV replication in the brains of infected rodents.[534,764]

Longevity of the Immune Response

Epidemiologic studies have documented that long-term protection from reinfection does not require re-exposure.[530] Immunologic memory includes both continued production of antibody and circulation of MeV-specific memory T cells.[69,302,493,732,784] The role of the slow or potentially incomplete process of MeV clearance from lymphoid tissue in establishing lifelong immunity to reinfection is unknown.[542,589] Extensive replication of MeV in lymphoid tissue may maximize the interaction of viral antigen with antigen-retaining follicular dendritic cells in germinal centers,[441] leading to long-term antibody production.

Immune Suppression

MeV can suppress immune responses *in vivo* during measles, *in vitro* when immune cells are cultured with virus or viral proteins, and in some animal models. It has not yet been possible to synthesize information from these various sources into a coherent understanding of increased susceptibility to other infections, the important clinical correlate of immune suppression.

During Measles. Measles was the first disease recognized to increase susceptibility to other infections, and most measles deaths are caused by other infections.[56] Increased susceptibility continues for weeks after the rash has cleared.[247] Clemens von Pirquet first quantified the immunosuppressive effects of measles in his study of tuberculin delayed-type hypersensitivity skin test responses during a measles outbreak in a tuberculosis sanitarium,[750] and this response is suppressed for weeks after the rash has cleared and recovery appears complete[712] (Fig. 36.13). Reactivation of tuberculosis and remission of immunologically mediated diseases such as nephrotic syndrome, juvenile rheumatoid arthritis, and idiopathic thrombocytopenic purpura have been reported to follow measles[121,401] but not always confirmed.[384] Production of antibody and cellular immune responses to new antigens is impaired.[131] *In vitro,* PBMCs from patients with measles have suppressed lymphoproliferative responses to mitogens and abnormal lymphokine production.[294,756]

Immune suppression is probably a multifactorial process. Evidence of immunosuppression begins during a period of intense immune activation associated with the onset of the

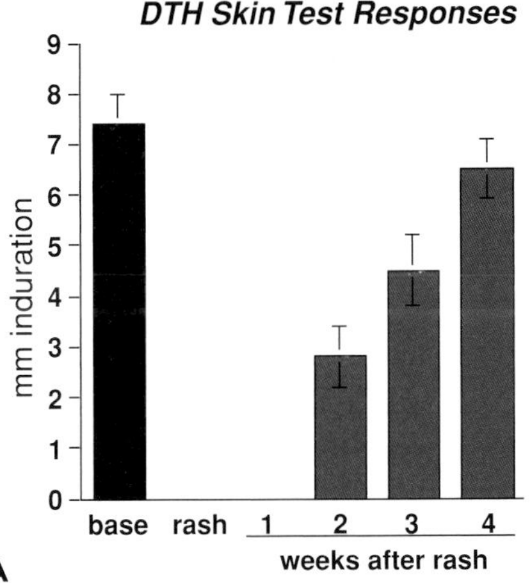

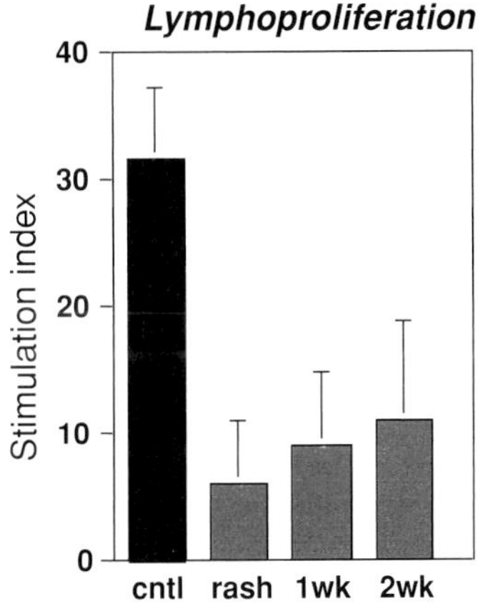

FIGURE 36.13. Immune suppression during measles. A: Changes during measles in tuberculin-induced delayed-type hypersensitivity (DTH) skin test responses in children with measles who had previously received bacille Calmette-Guérin (BCG) immunization against tuberculosis. **B:** Changes in proliferation of peripheral blood mononuclear cells to the mitogen phytohemagglutinin. (Data from Tamashiro VG, Perez HH, Griffin DE. Prospective study of the magnitude and duration of changes in tuberculin reactivity during complicated and uncomplicated measles. *Pediatr Infect Dis J* 1987;6:451–454; and Hirsch RL, Griffin DE, Johnson RT, et al. Cellular immune responses during complicated and uncomplicated measles virus infections of man. *Clin Immunol Immunopathol* 1984;31:1–12.)

measles rash and generation of the immune response to MeV that eventually results in virus clearance and in lifelong immunity to reinfection (Fig. 36.11). *In vitro* studies suggest defects in the responses of both monocytes and lymphocytes. Monocytes and macrophages are infected during measles,[196] and monocyte function is abnormal with low levels of IL-12 and TNF-α production during both acute and convalescent phases of the disease.[24,255,546,560] B cells and T cells, particularly CD4+ memory T cells, are also infected,[143,441] with decreased numbers in circulation and reduced CD4:CD8 ratios during the acute phase of measles.[23,141,256,613,757,773] Lymphocytopenia may be due to death of infected cells or to fever-induced changes in lymphocyte trafficking and is more marked in girls and in malnourished children.[3,196,613] More severe disease has been associated with decreased CD4+ T cells.[354] Induction of bystander lymphocyte apoptosis by MeV-infected cells may contribute to lymphocyte loss.[27,217,379,517,752] Ligation of CD150 also favors CD95-mediated apoptosis.[187,670] However, numbers of T cells in circulation rapidly return to normal during recovery, and output of naive CD4+ and CD8+ T cells from the thymus is sustained,[28,541,729] while other immunologic abnormalities persist.[29,253,613,756]

One of the reasons for low T-cell proliferation to mitogens *in vitro,* especially during convalescence, is inadequate production of IL-2, and supplementation supports spontaneous proliferation and improves mitogen responses of lymphocytes.[256] There is persistent suppression of IL-12 production, lymphocyte expression of CD30, and elevation of IL-4, IL-10, and IL-13 after resolution of the rash (Fig. 36.11).[96,258,546,742] Lack of IL-12 and induction of IL-10 may contribute to the type 2 cytokine responses that develop during recovery.[258,476] *In vitro* production of IFN-γ is low to normal and IL-4 is high compared to controls,[258,756] suggesting that type 2 CD4+ T cells are preferentially activated. The suppressive effects of IL-4 and IL-10 on type 1 CD4+ T cells and macrophages may contribute to suppression of delayed-type hypersensitivity during measles. The role of persistent MeV RNA in these PBMC defects has not yet been evaluated.

Th2 cytokine predominance produces an environment favoring B-cell maturation that facilitates the establishment of humoral memory important for lifelong protection from reinfection while depressing macrophage activation and induction of type 1 responses that may be required for combating new pathogens. Infection of monkeys with an IL-12–producing recombinant MeV increased production of IFN-γ and suppressed production of MeV-specific antibody, but there was no improvement in lymphocyte proliferation.[295] Similarly, infection of cotton rats with an IL-4–producing recombinant MeV did not affect mitogen-induced lymphocyte proliferation.[96] These data suggest that the MeV-induced Th2 cytokine milieu may alter responses to other pathogens and thus contribute to increased susceptibility to infection, but do not explain the characteristic measles-induced defect in lymphoproliferation.

***In vitro* Infection of Immune Cells.** *In vitro* infection of leukocytes and leukocyte cell lines with MeV induces abnormalities of DC, monocyte/macrophage, B-cell, T-cell, and epithelial cell function. T-cell proliferation to mitogens and soluble antigens,[437] cytotoxic function,[98] and B-cell production of immunoglobulin[98,438] are suppressed by *in vitro* infection, and bone marrow stromal cells do not support development of hematopoietic stem cells.[424] In addition, both B and T cells can produce a soluble factor that inhibits proliferation of uninfected cells.[692,755] These abnormalities may be relevant to immune suppression during measles, although some can be attributed to production of type I IFN in the MeV-infected cultures.

Infection of monocytes or macrophage-lineage cells *in vitro* stimulates production of IFN-α/β, inhibits production of TNF-α and IL-12, and may interfere with expression of peptide-loaded MHC class II complexes.[344,393,619,793] Virus production decreases as macrophages mature.[217,283] MeV infection of immature DCs induces maturation,[642,653] but MeV replication impairs CD40L signaling necessary for terminal differentiation.[653] Mannose receptor–mediated endocytosis is not affected.[265]

Monocytes and DCs exposed to MeV or N protein have impaired production of IL-12 but preserved or increased production of the regulatory cytokine IL-10.[217,269,344,427,653] MeV interaction with CD46 increases nitric oxide and decreases IL-12 production,[292,344] and interaction with DC-SIGN during infection of DCs increases IL-10 transcription by inducing acetylation of TLR-activated NFκB subunit p65.[263] Suppression of IL-12 production in response to TLR4 ligation is facilitated by H interaction with SLAM.[269] N_{CORE} interacts with FcγRII on B cells to inhibit antibody production *in vitro* and can trigger apoptosis.[579] N_{TAIL} binds to thymic epithelial cells and activated T cells through an unidentified receptor to induce cell cycle arrest.[579]

Analysis of antigen-presenting function has shown that MeV-infected monocytes can present MeV, but not an unrelated antigen, to T-cell clones.[392] DC antigen-presenting function has been assessed primarily with the mixed leukocyte reaction (MLR) that measures proliferation of heterologous CD4+ T cells.[642,681] The ability to stimulate this allogeneic T-cell response is lost after MeV infection, and the cells become apoptotic when co-cultured with T cells.[217,265] MeV-exposed T cells are recruited into conjugates with DCs *in vitro* but have impaired clustering and maintenance of immune synapse proteins needed for sustained T-cell activation,[666] in part due to sphingomyelinase activation and accumulation of ceramide.[227,483,725]

The importance of the *in vitro* deficiencies identified in DC function is unclear. Microarray analysis of the transcriptional changes in DCs infected with MeV in comparison with other pathogens revealed that many of the changes postulated to be responsible for MeV-induced immune suppression were also induced by pathogens that are not associated with immune suppression[808] and may be associated with IFN production. A vigorous MeV-specific cellular and humoral immune response is mounted to infection. This response results in rapid clearance of infectious virus, gradual clearance of viral RNA, and establishment of lifelong protective immunity.

Lymphocytes infected with MeV *in vitro* can be activated by mitogen but proliferate poorly because entry into S phase and progression through the cell cycle are impaired.[57,225,437,440,496,641,789] Suppression of T-cell proliferation can also be induced without infection through direct inhibitory signaling to T cells by the viral glycoprotein complex of H and F_1–F_2 on virions or infected cells.[170,360,634,642,766] This contact-dependent inhibitory signal prevents S phase entry of T cells for several days with accumulation of cells in the G_0/G_1 phase[503,634,766] and is not dependent on cell death, membrane fusion, production of soluble inhibitors, or T-cell infection.[170,188,505,641,765] Blocking the interaction of H with antibody to SLAM or CD46 does not interfere with suppression of lymphocyte proliferation,[190] but antibody to H or F can reverse the inhibition.[170]

MeV interaction with lipid rafts on the surface of T cells affects association of signaling molecules and their regulators with lipid rafts and interferes with T-cell activation of phosphatidylinositol 3 (PI3) kinase/Akt necessary for cell cycle progression in response to ligation of the T-cell receptor or the IL-2 receptor.[30,33] Binding of the MeV glycoprotein complex to lipid rafts on resting T cells inhibits degradation of the cytoplasmic inhibitory protein Cbl-b and recruitment of Akt kinase and Vav.[33] In addition, induction of SIP110 phosphatase decreases availability of phosphatidylinositol-3,4,5-trisphosphate (PIP3) needed for phospholipid signaling.[32] Determination of the relevance of this process to *in vivo* suppression of lymphoproliferation requires further study, but ongoing interaction of T cells in lymphatic tissue or in circulation with MeV-infected cells could induce this refractory state and result in suppressed proliferation in response to stimulation *ex vivo.*

Animal Models. Small animal models, primarily cotton rats and CD46 and SLAM transgenic mice, have also been used to study immunosuppression *in vivo* after MeV infection. Respiratory infection of cotton rats results in decreased proliferation of cultured T cells.[504] Intravenously or intraperitoneally infected CD46 transgenic mice have impaired T-cell cytotoxicity and antibody production, and this is associated with increased susceptibility to bacterial infection.[520,676] MeV infection of SLAM transgenic mice inhibits differentiation of DCs from bone marrow precursors through STAT1-independent, STAT2-dependent actions of type I IFN.[96,270] N_{CORE} interacts with FcγRII on DCs to inhibit cutaneous hypersensitivity in mice.[579] The relevance of these observations to the immune suppression that occurs during human infection is a matter of continued investigation.

Autoimmunity

An autoimmune demyelinating disease, postinfectious or acute disseminated encephalomyelitis (ADEM), is an important complication of measles[457] (Fig. 36.14) and is associated with an immune response to myelin basic protein[337] similar to that seen in animals with experimental autoimmune encephalomyelitis. The similarity of these diseases and lack of MeV in the brain have led to the current understanding that ADEM is an autoimmune disease[337] induced during measles.

The mechanism of induction of autoimmune disease is not clear. Hypotheses have included altered presentation of myelin antigens due to MeV infection of oligodendrocytes, "molecular mimicry" of myelin antigens by MeV, and dysregulation of immune responses.[294,328] There is little evidence for MeV infection of cells in the nervous system.[230,337,460,460] The possibility of molecular mimicry between myelin basic protein and an MeV protein has been explored. Neither cross-reactive antibodies nor cross-reactive T-cell clones have been identified in humans or rats with demyelinating disease induced in conjunction with MeV infection.[397] Genetic susceptibility to ADEM has been postulated, but the numbers of patients studied have been insufficient to clearly identify a link between MHC antigens or other genetic markers and disease.[383]

Studies of immune regulation have shown that patients with encephalomyelitis differ from patients with uncomplicated disease by having a distinct pattern of immunologic abnormalities. IgE is more persistently elevated and soluble IL-2 receptor is lower.[254,261] The timing of autoimmune disease suggests that immune dysregulation during measles may play a role in allowing activation and expansion of autoreactive lymphocytes.

Release and Transmission

Epidemiologic data suggest that infected individuals become infectious for nonimmune contacts a few days before the onset of the rash.[362] At this time virus can be cultured from the mucous membranes of the nasopharynx, conjunctivae, and mouth,[180] suggesting that the respiratory tract is the site of virus release. Multinucleated epithelial giant cells are readily demonstrated in nasal secretions and the conjunctivae during the prodrome and first days of the rash and are also shed into the urine.[400,632] A recombinant virus that cannot infect epithelial cells is not shed from the respiratory tract of infected macaques, further suggesting that epithelial cells are the source of virus that is transmitted.[390]

Virulence

Strains of MeV can clearly differ in virulence because attenuated vaccine strains cause little disease in humans and wild-type strains cause measles. Sequences of these strains have been compared and several changes that may contribute to attenuation have been identified, but *in vivo* testing of virulence is difficult because of the lack of a good small animal model.[707] Because adaptation of wild-type MeV to growth in Vero cells selects for a virus that no longer causes a rash in monkeys,[43,365] many studies of virulence have focused on the sequence changes required for wild-type viruses to grow in Vero cells. Vaccine strains tend to use the CD46 receptor efficiently, while wild-type strains do not (determined in part by H aa residues at 390, 416, 446, 481, and 492), but this alone does not determine virulence.[695] In addition to changes in H, attenuation and improved growth in Vero cells or chicken embryo fibroblasts are also associated with amino acid changes in the P/C/V, M, F, and L genes.[42,169,346,489,656,697,698,704,706,788]

Virulence has also been assessed by the study of replication of MeV in human tissues explanted into culture or implanted into immunodeficient mice. In thymic implants wild-type

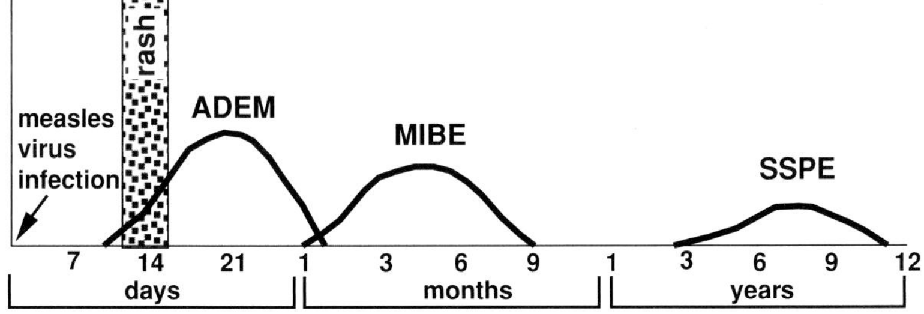

FIGURE 36.14. Time after infection of the occurrence of the three neurologic complications of measles: postinfectious or acute disseminated encephalomyelitis (ADEM), measles inclusion body encephalitis (MIBE), and subacute sclerosing panencephalitis (SSPE).

viruses grow more rapidly, to higher titer, and cause more extensive thymocyte apoptosis than attenuated strains.[28,730] In human mononuclear cell implants and tonsil explants, wild-type strains grow better than vaccine strains.[129,312] Attenuated vaccine strains infect naive T cells (express CD46, but little SLAM) more efficiently than virulent wild-type strains but infect B cells, macrophages, and NK cells less efficiently.[129] Again, the regions of the genome and the specific amino acid substitutions associated with these changes in replication and tissue destruction have not yet been defined.

Persistent Infection

MeV can establish persistent infection of cells *in vitro* and *in vivo*. A number of cell lines persistently infected with MeV have been established. Neurologic disease can be caused by persistent infection of neurons and glial cells.

Persistently Infected Cells in Culture

Replication of MeV usually causes death of cells in culture, but this is not necessarily the case *in vivo*. The elements determining persistent noncytopathic versus lytic infection are not completely understood, but properties of both the infected cell and the infecting virus contribute. Methods used to establish persistently infected cell lines include (a) passage of virus at high multiplicity with generation of DI particles,[592] (b) passage of infected cells in the presence of antibody,[612] (c) cultivation of cells surviving lytic infection,[204,612] and (d) co-cultivation of cells with MeV-infected brain cells from patients with SSPE or animals with persistent infection.[450]

Persistent noncytopathic infection is most easily established in neuronal cells but has also been established in lymphoid, epithelial, and glial cell lines.[456,593] Cellular factors that influence persistence include expression of heat shock proteins, cyclic adenosine monophosphate (cAMP), IFN-inducible proteins, and altered regulation of lipid metabolism.[456,593,597,640,700] Cellular protein synthesis is relatively unaffected by MeV infection, but specific cellular proteins (e.g., cell surface receptors) and functional responses (e.g., signal transduction, expression of transcription factors) may be altered, particularly in neural cells.[54,210]

Strains of MeV and CDV differ in their ability to establish persistent nonlytic infection in the same host cell.[204] Replication of variants likely to cause persistent infection is often temperature sensitive.[574] Persistent infection is usually accompanied by a marked decrease in the amount of infectious virus released and by intranuclear and intracytoplasmic accumulation of nucleocapsids with decreased virus-induced cytopathic effect. Some cell lines produce no infectious virus,[87] and infection is maintained by passage of encapsidated viral RNA to daughter cells during cell division.

Limited expression of viral proteins on the surface of persistently infected cells has led to the suggestion that defects in synthesis of viral envelope proteins or processing of F may be an important component of persistent infection.[450,797] Defects in glycoprotein expression may be due in part to limited mRNA production associated with steep transcriptional gradients and an increase in bicistronic messages.[107] However, mutations in these genes also lead to proteins with altered expression or function. For instance, defects in the M protein facilitate persistence and hinder association of N with the viral glycoproteins.[535]

Subacute Sclerosing Panencephalitis

SSPE is a rare (approximately 1 in 10,000) late complication of measles for which the pathogenesis remains poorly understood.[61,702] The route of virus entry into the CNS is unknown, but infection of cerebral endothelial cells is one possibility.[197,358] SSPE is most likely to occur when MeV infection occurs under the age of 2 years when the immune system is immature and maternal antibody may still be present.[61,152,272,326,455,458]

There is no clustering of cases to suggest that the wild-type virus causing the initial infection is different from the virus causing uncomplicated disease. Extensive sequence analysis of viral RNA from various parts of the brain in SSPE suggests that the virus in the CNS is clonal,[37] implying that virus entered the brain at one time (presumably during the original acute infection), was not cleared, and then gradually spread throughout the nervous system. The typical incubation period is 7 to 10 years[458] (Fig. 36.14). There may also be a genetic predisposition to developing persistent infection.[323,324]

Studies of Brain and Brain-Derived Cell Lines

At the time that neurologic symptoms occur, neurons and glia contain nuclear and cytoplasmic viral inclusion bodies, antibody responses to virus are vigorous and evident both in serum and CSF, and there is an extensive mononuclear inflammatory reaction in the CNS.[80,142,287] Both white matter and gray matter are affected.[142] No virus is seen budding from the surface of infected cells, and nuclear inclusions are filled with "smooth" nucleocapsids.[171,287] The cytoplasm contains "fuzzy" nucleocapsids that extend into neuronal processes, suggesting that virus can spread within the CNS by synaptic transmission of the ribonucleoprotein from cell to cell, a process that has been observed both *in vivo* and *in vitro*.[175,177,382,631] Neurokinin-1, the substance P receptor, may interact with the MeV F protein at the synapse for neuronal transmission.[419] In CDV infection, astrocytes participate in rapid noncytolytic spread from cell to cell to establish persistence.[787]

Alterations in any of the MeV envelope proteins that in some way interfere with assembly and budding of infectious virus can be associated with persistent infection and SSPE.[38,108,110,635] Extensive sequence analysis of viral RNAs from tissue has shown that SSPE viruses are related to wild-type strains circulating at the time of the primary infection but frequently have mutations in the viral genes encoding the M, F, and H proteins.[38,110,335,635]

In general, expression of M, a protein particularly important for assembly of infectious virus, is low.[395] This may be due either to lack of M protein synthesis or instability or mislocalization of the synthesized protein.[334,657,682] A variety of defects have been encountered in the mRNAs encoding M extracted from SSPE brain.[110] Mutations occur throughout the gene, and the frequent U-to-C sequence changes noted in some viruses may suggest mutation of double-stranded RNA in persistently infected cells by adenosine deaminase (biased or A/I hypermutation).[104,783] M transcripts often lack initiator AUGs necessary for expression and, when expressed, the proteins have defects in binding to viral nucleocapsids and in down-regulating transcription.[290,693] H proteins are often defective in intracellular transport and protein–protein interactions important for cell–cell fusion.[108] Truncations, mutations, and deletions in the cytoplasmic domain of F are almost universal and some enhance fusion and thus interfere with virus budding.[35,108,635]

Immune Responses

The possibility that the development of SSPE is due to an immune defect has been investigated. The antibody response to MeV is accentuated with significant production of MeV-specific antibody by plasma cells residing in the CNS and present in CSF.[85,526] Levels of CSF immunoglobulin, much of which is MeV specific, are elevated.[195,724] Antibody produced in the CNS is of restricted heterogeneity, leading to the appearance of oligoclonal immunoglobulin bands on electrophoretic analysis of CSF. Antibodies against the N and P proteins present in the ribonucleoprotein complex are particularly abundant, and antibody against the M protein is particularly deficient.[271]

Antibody to MeV has been postulated to play a role in establishing persistent CNS infection either through alteration of the induction of the primary immune response at the time of infection[577] or through modulation of infection once virus is in the nervous system.[218] Treatment with antibody after intracerebral infection of small mammals with neuroadapted strains of MeV attenuates acute disease but increases the incidence of subacute or chronic encephalitis.[576] Cases of SSPE have been associated with passive transfer of immune globulin, and persistent infection has been induced experimentally by passive transfer of antibody.[577]

Studies of cellular immunity have been less extensive. MeV-specific lymphoproliferation is not impaired, but MeV-specific cytotoxic T-cell activity and production of IFN-γ are decreased compared with healthy seropositive individuals.[158,275] General measures of cellular immunity, such as skin test responses to various recall antigens and proliferative responses to mitogens, are normal. The mononuclear inflammatory response in the brain includes CD4+ and CD8+ T cells, as well as monocytes and Ig-secreting B cells.[20,195] Class I and class II MHC expression is increased in brain, and β_2-microglobulin, soluble IL-2 receptor, and soluble CD8 are increased in CSF.[448] Thus, there is no evidence for a global defect in immune responses, but these immune responses are ineffective in clearing virus from the CNS.

Other Chronic Diseases

In addition to a clear role in SSPE, MeV in combination with genetic factors has also been implicated in the pathogenesis of Paget disease,[216,376,673] otosclerosis,[442,645] chronic active hepatitis,[596] and multiple sclerosis.[15] For most of these diseases an etiologic link to measles is controversial[282,434,453,575,777] and for none has a definitive role for MeV been identified.

Veterinary Correlates

Canine Distemper

Canine distemper was first described by Carre in 1905 as an infectious disease of young dogs associated with gastroenteritis, pneumonitis, conjunctivitis, and encephalomyelitis.[94] The disease has been recognized for centuries and epidemics were recorded in the 17th century.[70] Canine distemper was shown to be of viral etiology in 1926,[378] and the virus was isolated in primary canine kidney cells in 1959.[598] CDV causes disease in both domestic dogs and wild canids.[16,245,465] Through adaptive mutation in the H gene, CDV has acquired a broader host range than many morbilliviruses and can cause disease in monkeys and all families of terrestrial carnivores.[149,436,465,571] Canine distemper has many similarities to measles in humans, but infection of the CNS and neurologic disease are more common with glial cells as a primary target.[740] CDV is spread by aerosol and the disease is characterized by fever, coryza, conjunctivitis, gastroenteritis, and pneumonitis.[173] Using ferrets as a model system, researchers showed that CDV appears first in bronchial lymph nodes followed by a cell-associated viremia and spread to multiple lymphoid organs.[747] Later, infection spreads to epithelial tissues and enters the brain by infecting endothelial cells or through infiltration of infected monocytes.[34] Like measles, canine distemper is associated with profound short- and long-term immune suppression, and much of the mortality is due to secondary infections.

Dogs, ferrets, and lions may develop neurologic complications characterized by gait abnormalities and seizures.[173] Neurologic disease is most common in young animals[372] and can occur either early after infection or 3 to 4 weeks later associated with demyelination.[740] Persistence of virus in neural cells and in epithelial cells of the feet leads to chronic diseases known as old dog encephalitis and hard pad disease.[21,371] Some cases of old dog encephalitis have defective virus, with intranuclear inclusions in the CNS co-existing with high levels of antiviral antibody, features in common with SSPE.

Rinderpest

Rinderpest virus was first recognized as a distinct clinical entity causing severe gastroenteritis in cattle during a 4th-century European epizootic.[553] The causal agent of this disease was reported to be filterable in 1902[4] and was isolated in bovine embryonic kidney cells in 1957.[554] RPV has been an important veterinary pathogen[51] and causes a highly contagious disease of ruminants and swine characterized by inflammation, hemorrhage, necrosis, and erosion of the gastrointestinal tract.[4] RPV replicates in lymphocytes and macrophages, leading to lymphoid necrosis, and in epithelial cells of the gastrointestinal, respiratory, and urinary tracts and endocrine and exocrine glands, but not the brain or spinal cord.[687,780] Vaccination has recently succeeded in eradicating this disease from its last sites in Africa.[301,467]

Peste des Petits Ruminants

Peste des petits ruminants virus (PPRV) causes an economically important disease of sheep, goats, buffalo, and camels in Africa, the Middle East, and Asia.[157,377] The disease was first discovered in West Africa in 1942 and is characterized by fever, erosive stomatitis, pneumonitis, diarrhea, and lymphoid cell depletion.[470] PPRV replicates in epithelial cells, pneumocytes, macrophages, and lymphocytes.[375] PPRV is related to RPV[41] (Fig. 36.1), and four lineages are recognized. Disease in northern and eastern Africa is increasing, perhaps due to the introduction of a more virulent Asian strain into the region.[377]

Morbillivirus Infections of Aquatic Mammals

In 1987, an epizootic of respiratory disease with high mortality due to secondary infections occurred in seals in the Baltic and North Seas.[745] Serology suggested infection with a morbillivirus related to CDV, and the causal agent, phocid distemper virus (PDV), was isolated in 1988 (Fig. 36.1).[351] Infection has since spread to otters in the Pacific Ocean and seals along the East Coast of the United States.[241,545] The disease is characterized by fever, nasal and ocular discharge, and severe respiratory, gastrointestinal, and CNS symptoms. In the CNS there is neuronal infection with inflammation.[683] Disease is complicated by a variety of secondary viral, bacterial, and parasitic infections, suggesting the type of immune suppression seen in measles and canine distemper virus.[522] Similar epizootics of severe respiratory disease were subsequently recognized in porpoises and dolphins, and distinct morbilliviruses (PMV and DMV, now grouped together as cetacean morbillivirus [CeMV]) were isolated from these animals[52] (Fig. 36.1). PDV and CeMV cause giant cell pneumonia, encephalitis, and lymphoid depletion with virus demonstrable in lung, brain, spleen, and bladder.[161]

Experimental Infection in Animals

Nonhuman primates can be infected naturally or experimentally with MeV and provide the only experimental model for the pathogenesis of human disease. Small laboratory mammals generally are not susceptible to wild-type strains of MeV, although replication has been reported in the respiratory tract of cotton rats[785] and in transgenic mice expressing the human MeV receptor CD46[421] and/or SLAM.[663] Several neurotropic strains of MeV have been developed by repeated intracerebral passage in hamsters, mice, and rats. These strains do not produce acute disease similar to that seen in humans, but rather serve as models for neurologic diseases such as SSPE.

Nonhuman Primates

Natural MeV infection occurs only in humans. However, a number of species of monkeys are susceptible to measles and can contract the disease through contact with humans.[583,735] Experimentally, monkeys can be infected by intranasal, intratracheal, or subcutaneous inoculation.[29,735] Disease is generally similar to that seen in humans, and when deaths occur they are often caused by secondary infections.[583] Rhesus and cynomolgus macaques have served as animal models for studies of measles pathogenesis, immune suppression, virus virulence, response to vaccines, and protective immunity.[29,178,182,389,402,439,441,528,735]

Marmosets and tamarins are also susceptible to natural and experimental MeV infection by the respiratory route but develop a fulminant disease with high mortality characterized by interstitial pneumonitis, gastroenterocolitis, and bacteremia.[409] Infection with vaccine strains produces little disease.[409] Intracerebral inoculation with the most virulent strains of MeV produces encephalitis, while attenuated strains do not.[11]

Cotton Rats

The respiratory tract of cotton rats (*Sigmodon hispidus*) can be infected with vaccine and wild-type strains of MeV.[544,785] Virus replicates in the lungs and wild-type strains can spread to mediastinal lymph nodes and induce immunosuppression as measured by decreased proliferation of spleen cells to mitogen stimulation.[544] Cotton rats have been used for studies of pathogenesis, immune suppression, vaccine-induced immune responses, and protection from infection.[96,359,463,544,569,785,786]

Rats

The hamster neurotropic (HNT) strain of MeV can infect laboratory rats after intracerebral inoculation. The CAM strain of MeV was adapted by serial passage to replicate in rat brain and causes fatal encephalitis in newborn rats.[399] The type of disease produced in older rats is determined by the strain of rat. In Brown Norway rats, 10% to 20% develop acute encephalitis and there is no late disease in survivors. In Lewis rats, 80% to 90% develop acute fatal encephalitis and the rest develop subacute disease. Infectious, cell-free virus can be recovered during acute, but not subacute, disease.[399] Unlike mice, transgenic expression of human CD46 does not increase the permissiveness of rats for MeV infection.[506]

Rats have been used to identify determinants of neurovirulence and the role of the immune response in MeV-associated neurologic disease and persistent infection.[416,459,581] Acute encephalitis in newborn rats can be modulated by passive transfer of antibody to the H protein that results in persistent infection and a late onset of disease.[396] Features of subacute disease that are similar to SSPE include an inability to recover virus by routine methods, restricted expression of MeV envelope protein mRNAs in the brain, and intrathecal synthesis of oligoclonal MeV-specific antibody.[399,638] Demyelination is not a feature of subacute encephalitis; however, demyelinating disease can be more easily induced in previously infected animals.[398]

Hamsters

Newborn hamsters are susceptible to CNS infection with wild-type, vaccine, and SSPE strains of MeV; develop hyperirritability leading to death within a few days; and have been used to assess determinants of neurovirulence.[36,329] Brains from these young animals show giant cell encephalitis with intranuclear and intracytoplasmic inclusion bodies and a polymorphonuclear inflammatory response.[753] Older animals develop myoclonus with infection of cortical, thalamic, and hippocampal neurons without giant cell formation.[691,753] Ependymal infection may lead to hydrocephalus.[329] Cell-free virus can be easily recovered from the brains of newborn, but not older, hamsters.[90] Demyelination is uncommon,[753] but some hamsters inoculated as newborns with the LEC SSPE strain develop myelitis weeks later.[95]

Mice

Several strains of MeV have been adapted to grow in the brains of newborn mice and cause fatal disease after intracerebral, but not peripheral, inoculation.[319,501] Histopathology and immunocytochemical staining show neuronal and glial infection and giant cell encephalitis.[257,410,501] Maturation of CNS cells converts the production of MeV from the infectious form in newborn mice to a defective form in weanling mice.[257,286] In weanling mice, MeV antigen–positive neurons have only smooth nucleocapsid structures and no detectable H, F, or M proteins.[286,410] Disease consists of hyperexcitation and seizures associated with production of excitotoxic amino acids and destruction of pyramidal cells in the hippocampus that can be prevented by administration of glutamate receptor antagonists.[257,410] The genetic background of the mouse influences susceptibility,[763] with C3H/He mice most susceptible and SJL mice most resistant.[501] Mice with deficiencies in cellular immunity are more susceptible than immunocompetent mice.[207,727]

A number of investigators have produced mice engineered, either by grafting human cells or by transgenic expression of human genes, to provide better murine systems for studying measles pathogenesis. Mice with severe combined immunodeficiency have been grafted with human PBMCs[315] or implanted with human fetal thymus and liver.[28] In thymic implants MeV shows strain-specific differences in virus growth and thymocyte apoptosis that have been useful for assessing virulence and determinants of replication *in vivo*.[28,730,731] Immunologically normal mice with transplanted human leukocytes develop graft versus host disease and can also be infected with MeV.[315]

Transgenic mice expressing human CD46 or SLAM have been produced using genomic DNA or complementary DNA (cDNA) with promoters designed to provide generalized or cell type–specific expression of the receptor transgene.[270,421,536,663,768] In general, only low levels of infectious virus can be recovered from the mice and this is age dependent, with neonatal mice much more susceptible than older mice.[536] MeV replication in transgenic mice is enhanced by the absence of components of the innate or adaptive immune response,[421,514,663] but blocks to MeV replication in mice are at multiple levels.[744] These mice and cells from these mice have been used for studies of pathogenesis, virulence, immunosuppression, and CNS infection.[205,268,270,366,518,649,650,706]

Ferrets

Intracerebral inoculation of ferrets with cells infected with certain SSPE strains of MeV causes acute encephalitis.[347] Subacute or chronic encephalitis is established if animals are immunized prior to intracerebral injection with infected cells.[720] Pathologic and clinical features in animals with chronic disease resemble SSPE with cerebral inflammation, gliosis and intranuclear inclusion bodies, electroencephalographic changes, bound immunoglobulin in brain, and high titers of antibody to MeV in serum and CSF.[347,720]

EPIDEMIOLOGY

Classic Measles

In the Absence of Vaccination

The study of island populations was important in establishing many of the principles of measles epidemiology. Pioneering observations on the transmissibility, incubation period, and lifelong immunity of measles were made by Panum during the 1846 epidemic in the Faroe Islands.[530] Measles is one of the most infectious of communicable diseases. It is estimated that 76% of household exposures of susceptible persons lead to measles[299] and that the reproductive number (R_o), or average number of secondary cases produced by an infectious individual in a totally susceptible population, is approximately 12 to 18.[466,694] Transmission is most efficient through direct exposure to an infected symptomatic individual, but MeV can survive for hours in respiratory droplets, and direct contact is not required.[119] Individuals are most infectious from 4 to 5 days before through 4 days after the appearance of the rash.[121]

There is no animal reservoir or evidence of latent or epidemiologically significant persistent infection. Therefore, maintenance of MeV in the human population requires a continuous supply of susceptible individuals. Because older members of a community are immune through previous exposure to the virus, endemic measles is primarily a disease of childhood. If the population is too small to establish endemic transmission, the virus cannot be maintained.[66] Mathematical calculations and studies of islands and cities with populations of different sizes have shown a requirement for a population of 250,000 to 500,000 to establish measles as an endemic disease.[67,350] This is approximately the population of the earliest urban civilizations in ancient Sumaria around 3000 BCE where measles is postulated to have emerged.

In large population centers, measles is endemic with occasional epidemics as the numbers of susceptible individuals increase. These epidemics spread in waves from large cities to smaller cities and then to rural areas over time.[252] In temperate climates measles is more frequent in the winter and early spring. The frequency of epidemics is determined by numbers of susceptible individuals, the duration of infectiousness, and patterns of population mixing.[350] The size of the population is also a primary determinant of the age of seroconversion. The average age of infection is earlier in urban than in rural areas in both developed and developing countries.[139] In countries with high birth rates, infection occurs at an early age. Very young infants are protected from measles (and from response to vaccine) by maternal antibody.[9] The duration of protective antibody in the infant is dependent on the level of maternal antibody. The source of maternal immunity (vaccine vs. natural measles), gestational age, and presence of maternal infection (e.g., human immunodeficiency virus [HIV], malaria) are determinants of the amount of antibody passively transferred and, therefore, the length of time required for initial levels of antibody to decay to the point that an infant will become susceptible to measles.[91] In small isolated populations measles epidemics are controlled by extinction and chance reintroduction of the virus that leads to infection at older ages on average.[121,586]

Effect of Vaccination

Immunization alters the epidemiology of measles by reducing the susceptible individuals in the population. In countries with high rates of vaccination, the average age for measles is increased because herd immunity reduces transmission and indirectly protects children from infection. Vaccination also lengthens the interepidemic period.[139] When outbreaks occur in areas of sustained high vaccine coverage, an increasingly large portion of the cases will be in older individuals who are susceptible due to primary or secondary vaccine failure. In contrast to prevaccination populations, outbreaks are increasingly likely to be local and dependent on social networks.[754] Because of the infectiousness of MeV and the high R_0, it is estimated that 95% or more of the population needs to be immune to interrupt endemic transmission.[228] However, even highly immunized populations are vulnerable to localized outbreaks associated with importation from areas where measles remains endemic.[228,607] These risks are increased in communities that include individuals who refuse vaccination for philosophical or religious reasons.[202]

Molecular Epidemiology

Sequence analysis of the variable C-terminus of the N (N_{TAIL}), P, and H genes has been useful for identification of genotypes and analysis of the molecular epidemiology of measles.[605] Several lineages of MeV that have characteristic temporal and geographic distributions have been identified.[595,604] Some are localized to specific regions of the world and some are extinct, but most are widely distributed. Currently 8 distinct clades with 24 genotypes are recognized (see section on antigenic composition and strain variation) (Fig. 36.9). Assembly of this increasingly large database of MeV genotypes has aided in the identification of global measles transmission pathways.[353,606] Identification of the source of the MeV-causing disease in a particular location has become increasingly important as control programs are implemented, and identification of cases as imported or indigenous is necessary.[607]

Subacute Sclerosing Panencephalitis

SSPE occurs preferentially in boys from rural areas with a history of measles at an early age.[272,326,458] In developing countries with high birth rates, measles often occurs in young infants,[247,272,472,475] and these countries have a high burden of SSPE.[426,614,702] This is further exacerbated when there is a high prevalence of HIV infection because children of HIV-infected mothers are more likely to acquire measles at an early age.[179,475] Several studies have identified exposure to birds as a risk factor, but this relationship has not yet been explained.[272] The incidence has decreased dramatically with the introduction of measles vaccination,[61,92] and there is no evidence that the vaccine virus can cause SSPE.[458]

CLINICAL FEATURES

Classic Measles and Its Complications

Measles has an incubation period of 10 to 14 days spanning the time from exposure to the appearance of clinical disease (Fig. 36.11). The first prodromal symptoms of measles are fever, malaise, and anorexia followed by cough, coryza, and conjunctivitis. The prodrome lasts 2 to 3 days, and during this time small bright red spots with a bluish-white speck at the center, Koplik spots, may become visible on the buccal mucosa, providing early diagnostic evidence of measles.[368,721] The prodrome ends as the maculopapular rash appears, first on the face and behind the ears and then on the trunk and extremities (Fig. 36.10). It begins to fade within 3 to 4 days. In malnourished children the rash may desquamate.[469] Generalized involvement of lymphoid tissue may result in lymphadenopathy, mild splenomegaly, and appendicitis. In uncomplicated measles clinical recovery begins soon after appearance of the rash.

Respiratory Disease

The prominent respiratory symptoms are manifestations of diffuse mucosal inflammation in response to widespread infection of epithelial cells. Interstitial pneumonitis due to MeV replication and inflammation in the lower respiratory tract is common in uncomplicated disease but frequently is detectable only by x-ray or by measuring the alveolar–arterial oxygen gradient.[251,285] Pneumonitis is more likely to be clinically severe during pregnancy.[12] Symptomatic giant cell pneumonia is seen primarily in immunocompromised individuals.[183,429] Most of the severe pneumonia that complicates measles and leads to chronic pulmonary disease is caused by secondary bacterial and viral infections.[56,251] Other common respiratory complications caused by secondary infections are otitis media and laryngotracheobronchitis.[56] In addition to increasing susceptibility to new infections, previously latent viral and bacterial infections may be reactivated.[121,690]

Gastrointestinal Disease

MeV replication in the liver, particularly the bile duct epithelium, is common in all ages, but clinically evident hepatitis is most frequent in adults.[235,387] Diarrhea is a common complication of measles, particularly in young patients requiring hospitalization.[250] Many epithelial surfaces are infected with MeV and this may lead directly to gastrointestinal symptoms. However, diarrhea is frequently associated with secondary bacterial and protozoal infections[250] that compound the borderline nutritional status of young children in developing countries.

Myocardial Disease

Electrocardiographic abnormalities, including prolongation of the P-R interval and ST-segment and T-wave changes, can be detected in 20% to 30% of children with uncomplicated measles.[239] However, symptomatic cardiac disease is uncommon and is most often related to transient conduction abnormalities. In autopsy studies, myocardial and pericardial lesions are usually attributable to systemic bacterial infections.

Neurologic Disease

There is little evidence that the brain parenchyma is an important target tissue for MeV replication during acute disease in immunologically normal individuals.[446,460] However, apparently uncomplicated measles is frequently accompanied by a CSF pleocytosis and changes in the electroencephalogram,[234,274] suggesting the possibility of CNS infection. The occasional appearance of slowly progressive neurologic disease (measles inclusion body encephalitis [MIBE]) in immunosuppressed individuals[8,214,484] and the occurrence of late neurologic disease (SSPE) in immunologically normal individuals infected at a young age (Fig. 36.14) attests to the ability of MeV occasionally to enter the brain and replicate in neurons and glial cells.

ADEM complicates 1 in 1,000 cases of measles, with the highest attack rate in children older than the age of 5 years,[457] and usually occurs within 2 weeks after the onset of the rash[406] (Fig. 36.14). The disease is characterized by an abrupt onset of fever and obtundation, accompanied by seizures and multifocal neurologic signs. The majority of survivors have neurologic sequelae.[337,406] Pathologic studies show that this is a perivenular demyelinating disease, not inclusion body encephalitis like MIBE and SSPE.[406] The pattern of perivenular inflammation and demyelination suggests that it is immunologically mediated.[230,799] There is little evidence for virus in the brain as assessed either directly by virus isolation or detection of viral antigen or RNA[230,460] or indirectly by the appearance of MeV-specific antibody in the CSF.[337] There is, however, the induction of an autoimmune response to myelin protein similar to that seen in animals with experimental autoimmune encephalomyelitis and humans with Semple rabies vaccine–induced encephalomyelitis.[78,162,337,380]

Eye Disease

Measles is considered to be an important cause of childhood blindness associated with corneal lesions. In areas of vitamin A deficiency, the two problems are synergistic and corneal ulceration resembling keratomalacia is a frequent complication of measles.[620]

Determinants of Morbidity and Mortality

Measles remains one of the most important causes of child morbidity and mortality worldwide.[473,494,781] Predictors of poor outcome are severe lymphopenia and poor antibody response.[132,770] Mortality is highest at the extremes of age, in girls, in those with low socioeconomic status, and in those without access to medical care.[121,163,226,599] Mortality is also increased in malnourished individuals[48] and secondary cases in a household.[1,369] Malnutrition affects the immune responses to MeV, impairs virus clearance, and may lead to lower rates of diagnosis.[141,564] Vitamin A is a particularly important nutrient influencing outcome.[48] Low serum retinol is common in severe measles due either to prior dietary deficiency or to impaired mobilization from hepatic stores.[48,89] Case-fatality rates range from 0.1% in places with good access to medical care to 6% in developing countries and up to 25% in refugee camps and virgin populations.[139,247,471,494,655,781]

Atypical Measles

A severe form of measles with unusual clinical features was seen in individuals who had previously received an inactivated measles vaccine used in the mid-1960s. Atypical measles differs from typical measles by having higher and more prolonged fever, unusual skin lesions, and severe pneumonitis.[221,486] The rash often is accompanied by evidence of hemorrhage or vesiculation and begins on the extremities and spreads to the trunk. Pneumonitis is associated with distinct nodular parenchymal lesions and hilar adenopathy.[251,798] Abdominal pain, hepatic dysfunction, headache, eosinophilia, pleural effusions, and edema are also described. Cases of atypical measles were reported up to 16 years after administration of the inactivated vaccine. Administration of live virus vaccine after two to three doses of killed vaccine did not eliminate subsequent susceptibility to atypical measles and was often associated with severe local reactions.[88,117,220]

Hypotheses about the pathogenesis of atypical measles included an abnormally intense cellular immune response,[220] an inability of the inactivated vaccine to induce local respiratory tract immunity,[58] and a lack of production of antibody to F, which allowed virus to spread from cell to cell despite the development of antibody to H.[452,507] In rhesus macaques the formalin-inactivated vaccine induces transient neutralizing and fusion-inhibiting antibodies, but there is a poor T-cell response and antibodies induced do not mature. Subsequent infection with MeV induces an anamnestic response of low-avidity antibody that cannot neutralize wild-type virus. This leads to immune complex deposition, vasculitis, and pneumonitis.[559]

Measles in the Immunocompromised Host

Children with hypogammaglobulinemia appear to recover uneventfully from MeV infection, while those with deficiencies in cellular immune responses may not.[244] Virus clearance is delayed,[542] and two types of progressive disease, giant cell pneumonia and MIBE, may complicate infection, often in the absence of the typical rash or other characteristic features of measles.[84,183,429]

Giant cell pneumonia is characterized by increasing respiratory insufficiency beginning 2 to 3 weeks after a history of exposure to measles. Virus can be isolated from lung tissue and bronchial and nasopharyngeal washings.[183] Pathology shows multinucleated epithelial alveolar and bronchiolar giant cells with intranuclear and intracytoplasmic inclusion bodies.[22] There is often evidence of systemic disease with giant cells visualized in multiple organs.[22,183]

MIBE occasionally accompanies giant cell pneumonia[340] but is more often present as an isolated primary manifestation of progressive MeV infection in immunocompromised adults and children.[8,214,310,484,782] Neurologic disease usually becomes evident within 6 to 12 months after exposure to measles (Fig. 36.14). Initial signs and symptoms include altered mental status, focal seizures or epilepsia partialis continua, and occasionally blindness or hearing loss.[6,8,273] The course is typically rapid with progression to coma and death within weeks to months.[484] Pathology shows gliosis with inclusions in glial cells and neurons.[246] Giant cell formation is unusual and little inflammation is present.[6,484] MeV protein and RNA are abundant and detectable by immunocytochemical staining or *in situ* hybridization. MeV can occasionally be recovered from brain, but the virus is usually defective, as it is in SSPE.[6,39,601] Viral nucleocapsids without budding particles are seen intracellularly by electron microscopy.[6,601] The mRNAs for genes encoding the H, M, and F envelope proteins are reduced, and these proteins are often undetectable.[39,106] MIBE may be fundamentally similar to SSPE, but clinical symptoms are manifested earlier after infection and are more rapidly progressive in the absence of an immune response.[601]

Subacute Sclerosing Panencephalitis

SSPE most commonly occurs in individuals younger than the age of 20 who present many years after measles with neurologic disease. The average time to onset of SSPE after measles is 6 to 10 years (Fig. 36.14) but ranges from 1 to 24 years.[92,458] The onset is insidious and the diagnosis is often not suspected early in disease.[298,565] The typical presentation is with mental deterioration and personality changes (stage I). Subsequently, there is myoclonus and often seizures (stage II) followed by progressive neurologic deterioration marked by rigidity (stage III), optic atrophy, akinetic mutism, and coma (stage IV).[327] Death occurs within months to years after onset.[215] Antibody to MeV is elevated in both serum and CSF, and inclusions are present in glial cells and neurons.[287] Perinatal infection can be associated with SSPE that has an accelerated onset and a fulminant course.[92,672]

DIAGNOSIS

The classical clinical features of measles—Koplik spots, fever, erythematous maculopapular rash, coryza, cough, and conjunctivitis—are generally sufficient to make the diagnosis, especially in the setting of a community outbreak, but laboratory confirmation should be obtained. The clinical case definition for measles includes (a) a generalized maculopapular rash of 3 days or more; (b) fever of 38.3°C (101°F); and (c) one of the following: cough, coryza, or conjunctivitis.[111] However, not all of these signs and symptoms may be present in measles and many are shared with other diseases. The differential diagnosis includes all causes of rash and fever including scarlet fever, rubella, alphavirus infection, parvovirus B19, human herpesvirus-6, human herpesvirus-7, meningococcemia, Kawasaki disease, toxic shock syndrome, and dengue.[81,563] Fever and/or rash may be absent during measles in very young infants, immunocompromised patients, malnourished children, and previously immunized individuals.[176,564]

Laboratory diagnostic procedures consist of isolation of virus; direct detection of the virus, viral RNA, or viral antigens in secretions; detection of IgM or low-avidity IgG antibody by enzyme immunoassay (EIA); or documentation of seroconversion using hemagglutination inhibition (HI), complement fixation (CF), virus neutralization, or IgG-specific EIA on serum taken during the acute and convalescent phases of disease. In immune-compromised patients, the diagnosis is difficult, often not suspected, and usually dependent on biopsy to detect MeV in tissue.[8,484,562]

Isolation or Detection of Virus

Virus can be cultured from PBMCs, respiratory secretions, conjunctival swabs, and urine, but culture is rarely used as the means of diagnosing acute disease. Cell lines vary in their susceptibility to infection by wild-type strains, with human cord blood leukocytes, the COBL-a cord blood T-cell line, marmoset B95-8 or B95a cells, and Vero cells expressing SLAM being most sensitive.[211,364,365,521] Epithelial cells from the nasopharynx, buccal mucosa, conjunctivae, or urine can be used for direct cytologic examination for giant cells and inclusions and for antigen detection.[400,677] Generally, the most useful antibody for staining is one directed to N because this protein is most abundant in the infected cell and N antibody reactivity is retained using a wide variety of fixation methods.[677] Direct examination for virus is of particular importance for diagnosis in immunocompromised individuals where antibody responses may not be present. The detection of MeV RNA by RT-PCR using primers targeted to highly conserved regions of the N, M, or F genes has been successfully applied to a variety of clinical samples[7,198,317,542,719] and to most morbilliviruses.[248,394,668]

Detection of Antibody

The clinical diagnosis of measles is most often confirmed by serology. Samples ideally consist of acute and convalescent serum pairs, but detection of MeV-specific IgM in serum or saliva or low-avidity IgG in serum is diagnostic and may require only a single sample.[81,206,317,726] IgM antibody appears at the time of the rash and can be detected by 3 days and for up to 4 weeks after the onset of the rash in most individuals.[281] MeV-specific IgG peaks approximately 2 weeks later and gradually increases in avidity. EIA allows for differential detection of IgM and IgG and is widely used because of its convenience. Plates may be coated with lysates of MeV-infected cells or with recombinant MeV proteins.[74,314]

The HI test detects antibody to HA and correlates well with the neutralization test. The major limitations of the HI test are the requirement for fresh sensitive monkey erythrocytes, the difficulty of producing sufficient antigen for large numbers of tests, and the possible presence of nonspecific HA inhibitors in serum. The CF test has also been used to determine measles immunity, but titers are less stable over time. Neither of these tests is in common use. The virus plaque reduction neutralization assay remains the standard against which other tests are measured. It is more sensitive than HI or EIA tests[10,126] and provides the best correlate for protection from infection[120] and therefore remains the best measure of response to vaccination.[9]

PREVENTION AND CONTROL

Treatment

There is no standard antiviral treatment for measles. Ribavirin inhibits MeV replication *in vitro*; however, immunocompromised patients with pneumonitis have shown no clear evidence of improvement after treatment with aerosolized ribavirin. Newer approaches to therapy that are effective *in vitro* include nonnucleoside polymerase inhibitors[771,796] and fusion inhibitors.[568] Administration of high doses of vitamin A during acute measles decreases morbidity and mortality even in the absence of clinical evidence of vitamin A deficiency by an unknown mechanism.[48,221,316] In areas of vitamin A deficiency and xerophthalmia, supplementation prevents blindness due to measles-induced corneal destruction. The World Health Organization recommends two doses of vitamin A for all children with measles.[774]

Numerous therapeutic agents, including amantadine, IFN, isoprinosine, ribavirin, and transfer factor, have been used for the treatment of SSPE. Evaluation of the efficacy of any of these regimens is difficult because the disease is rare, the course is variable, reports are anecdotal, and the benefits are at best short term.[266]

Vaccination

History

The earliest attempts at vaccination against measles by Home in 1749 were based on the principles of variolation[297] with the reasoning that introduction of disease through the skin would lessen the effects on the lung. "Morbillization" was in general unsuccessful.[280] Subsequent approaches between 1920 and 1940 designed to inactivate or attenuate the virus by culture in chick embryos also met with limited success.[428] The isolation of MeV in tissue culture opened the way for a more concerted approach to vaccine development using the Edmonston strain of virus.[184] Killed virus vaccines were developed using formalin and tween-ether for inactivation.[758] Simultaneously, attenuated vaccines based on adaptation of MeV to growth in chick cells were developed and are now widely used.[349] The attenuated live virus vaccine has dramatically decreased the incidence of measles in all countries in which it has been effectively delivered.

The live attenuated MeV vaccine induces both neutralizing antibody and cellular immune responses that are long-lasting, but the immune responses necessary for protection from infection or disease have not been completely defined. Antibody is sufficient for protection because infants are protected by maternal antibody[9] and passive transfer of immune serum can modify or interfere with measles vaccination and partially protect children from measles after exposure.[582] The role of the cellular immune response in protection has been more difficult to study but is induced more readily than antibody in young infants and in the presence of maternal antibody.[224]

Inactivated Vaccines

The alum-precipitated inactivated vaccine was used in a three-dose regimen.[97,758] Recipients developed moderate levels of neutralizing and HI antibodies and low levels of CF antibody.[97,203,507] Studies in rhesus macaques have shown that the inactivated vaccine induces no CD8+ T-cell response and that the avidity of the MeV antibody induced does not mature.[558,559] The vaccine was protective when exposure to measles occurred soon after immunization.[203,219] However, antibody titers declined rapidly, and recipients again became susceptible to measles[219,578]; when infected, they had a tendency to develop the more severe disease, atypical measles,[486,578] discussed previously, and the vaccine was withdrawn.

Attenuated Live Virus Vaccines

The first attenuated live measles vaccine was developed by adaptation of the Edmonston strain of MeV to chick embryos and subsequently to chick embryo fibroblasts after passage in primary renal and amnion cells to produce the Edmonston B virus.[181] Inoculation of this virus produced no detectable viremia and no spread to the respiratory tract or disease in monkeys, but it did induce antibody and protected from subsequent challenge. This vaccine was efficacious[374] and licensed in 1963 but produced fever and rash in a large proportion of immunized children.[348] Reactions were reduced when MeV antibody was given at the same time as the vaccine. Further passage of the Edmonston B virus in chick embryo fibroblasts produced a more attenuated virus that was licensed in 1965.[647] The Moraten strain used in the United States was licensed in 1968 and is closely related to Schwarz.[603] Other Edmonston-derived vaccine strains (e.g., Zagreb, AIK-C) and attenuated strains developed independently (e.g., CAM, Leningard-16, Shanghai-191) are also successful vaccines. Few differences have been described among MeV vaccine strains (all genotype A) regardless of the geographic origin of the parent virus.[603] The lyophilized vaccine is relatively stable but rapidly loses infectivity at room temperature after reconstitution.[449]

The recommended age of initial vaccination varies from 6 to 15 months. The probability of seroconversion and the levels of antibody induced are determined by the level of persisting MeV-specific maternal antibody and by the age of the infant.[137,223,224,580] The recommended age of immunization is determined by a region-specific balance between the optimum age for seroconversion and probability of acquiring measles before that age.[137] In areas where measles remains prevalent, measles vaccination is routinely performed at 9 months (85% response), whereas in areas with little measles, vaccination is often at 12 to 15 months of age (95% response).[139] The standard route of administration is either subcutaneous or intramuscular, but there is substantial interest in alternative routes that would avoid the need for needles and syringes. Transcutaneous delivery has not yet been successful,[200] and intranasal administration of reconstituted liquid vaccine elicits a local, but not a systemic, immune response.[671] However, respiratory delivery of aerosolized liquid vaccine has shown promise in older children,[136,164,165,293,411] and respiratory delivery of a small-particle dry powder vaccine induces protective immunity in macaques.[402]

Host genetic differences affect the likelihood of seroconversion and level of antibody induced,[164,573] and several specific polymorphisms that affect responses have been identified.[123,159,160,524,525] The effect of common childhood illnesses on seroconversion is unclear,[454] and any potential decrease in seroconversion must be balanced against the loss of the opportunity for vaccination and the consequent risk of the child acquiring measles. Overall, the efficacy of a single dose of measles vaccine in infancy is estimated at 77% to 84% when administered at 9 to 11 months, 92% when administered at 12 months or older, and 94% after two doses.[224,728] Compromises must also be considered with respect to immunizing individuals with HIV infection.[138] Progressive fatal infection has been occasionally associated with measles vaccine in severely immunocompromised children and adults.[19] However, in general, measles vaccine has been well tolerated in HIV-seropositive children,[648] although the seroconversion rate is lower, antibody is of lower avidity, and titers wane more quickly than in HIV-uninfected children.[213,477,488] Because of the potential severity of measles in these individuals, the vaccine is recommended for routine administration to infants without respect to HIV serostatus in most countries, unless the CD4+ T-cell count is known to be low.

The dose of MeV routinely used for immunization is between 10^3 and 10^4 plaque-forming units. Ten- to 100-fold higher doses improved seroconversion in younger infants, but subsequent follow-up of children receiving high-titered vaccines in countries with high childhood mortality showed an increased mortality in girls over the subsequent 2 to 3 years.[296,363] Mortality was not due to measles, but rather to a relative increase in the deaths due to other infections.[2] The pathogenesis of delayed increased mortality after high-titered vaccine is not understood but occurred primarily in those who developed a rash after vaccination and may be related to long-term suppression of immune responses similar to that induced by measles.[651]

The immune response to the live attenuated vaccine is similar to that induced by natural disease. However, the duration of vaccine-induced immunity appears to be more variable. In general, levels of antibody are lower after vaccination than after recovery from natural disease, and MeV-specific antibody and CD4+ T cells decay with time.[122,495] Secondary vaccine failure rates have been estimated at approximately 5% 10 to 15 years after immunization but are probably lower when vaccination is given after 12 months.[17,433] A second dose of vaccine is necessary to immunize persons who did not respond to the first dose.[114,138,228] The second dose can be delivered as a part of a routine vaccination program or in national or regional supplementary immunization campaigns. The two-dose strategy has been credited with elimination of indigenous measles in a number of countries.[138]

Experimental Vaccines

Development of new vaccines has been hampered by an incomplete understanding of protective immunity and of the priming for enhanced disease by the inactivated vaccine. Nevertheless, a number of experimental vaccines have been developed. The primary motivations for development of a new vaccine are to increase thermostability, to provide a vaccine that can be given to young infants, and to avoid the hazards associated with the use of needles and syringes. Vaccination with the H, F, and/or N protein expressed in bacterial, poxvirus, adenovirus, or bacille Calmette-Guérin (BCG) vectors or as DNA, peptides, or proteins can induce cellular and humoral immunity in mice and cotton rats.[116,199,407,532,678,684,762] Monkeys are the most relevant model system, and studies have shown different degrees of protection after vaccination with H, F, and/or N expressed with BCG, alphavirus replicon particles, vaccinia virus, immune-stimulating complexes, and variously formulated DNAs.[529,533,557,566,685,686,733,805,806]

Prospects for Eradication

Theoretically, measles is an ideal virus for eradication through vaccination: there is only one serotype; most cases are clinically identifiable; there is no animal reservoir; and a vaccine is available.[473] However, measles remains a leading cause of vaccine-preventable childhood mortality.[115] In 1979, eradication was identified as a goal for the United States, but it was 20 years before endemic transmission was interrupted.[112] In 2010, the World Health Assembly endorsed 2015 targets of greater than 90% national coverage with one dose of vaccine, reduction of measles incidence to less than 5 cases per million, and mortality reduction of greater than 95% compared to

2000 estimates. The highly communicable nature of the virus requires continued maintenance of high vaccine coverage to prevent outbreaks, with 95% to 98% seropositivity needed for herd immunity. The role of asymptomatic infection of partially immune individuals in maintaining transmission is unclear. Global programs, such as the Expanded Program for Immunization and the Measles Initiative, have increased vaccine coverage worldwide and have resulted in significant decreases in measles and measles mortality.[139,474] However, delivery remains difficult in many areas due to civil strife, the need to maintain a cold chain, decreasing donor support, and religious or philosophical resistance to vaccination.[113,474] Eradication remains a worthy but difficult goal.[689]

REFERENCES

All cited references are available in the e-book.

6. Aicardi J, Goutieres F, Arsenio-Nunes ML, et al. Acute measles encephalitis in children with immunosuppression. *Pediatrics* 1977;59:232–239.
9. Albrecht P, Ennis FA, Saltzman EJ, et al. Persistence of maternal antibody in infants beyond 12 months: mechanism of measles vaccine failure. *J Pediatr* 1977;91:715–718.
17. Anders JF, Jacobson RM, Poland GA, et al. Secondary failure rates of measles vaccines: a metaanalysis of published studies. *Pediatr Infect Dis J* 1996;15:62–66.
19. Angel JB, Walpita P, Lerch RA, et al. Vaccine-associated measles pneumonitis in an adult with AIDS. *Ann Intern Med* 1998;129:104–106.
24. Atabani S, Byrnes A, Jaye A, et al. Natural measles causes prolonged suppression of interleukin-12 production. *J Infect Dis* 2001;184:1–9.
29. Auwaerter PG, Rota PA, Elkins WR, et al. Measles virus infection in rhesus macaques: altered immune responses and comparison of the virulence of six different virus strains. *J Infect Dis* 1999;180:950–958.
30. Avota E, Avots A, Niewiesk S, et al. Disruption of Akt kinase activation is important for immunosuppression induced by measles virus. *Nat Med* 2001;7:725–731.
37. Baczko K, Lampe J, Liebert UG, et al. Clonal expansion of hypermutated measles virus in a SSPE brain. *Virology* 1993;197:188–195.
39. Baczko K, Liebert UG, Cattaneo R, et al. Restriction of measles virus gene expression in measles inclusion body encephalitis. *J Infect Dis* 1988; 158:144–150.
45. Bankamp B, Lopareva EN, Kremer JR, et al. Genetic variability and mRNA editing frequencies of the phosphoprotein genes of wild-type measles viruses. *Virus Res* 2008;135:298–306.
48. Barclay AJG, Foster A, Sommer A. Vitamin A supplements and mortality related to measles: a randomised clinical trial. *Br Med J (Clin Res Ed)* 1987;294:294–296.
51. Barrett T, Rossiter PB. Rinderpest: the disease and its impact on humans and animals. *Adv Virus Res* 1999;53:89–110.
56. Beckford AP, Kaschula ROC, Stephen C. Factors associated with fatal cases of measles: a retrospective autopsy study. *S Afr Med J* 1985;68: 858–863.
60. Bellini WJ, Englund G, Rozenblatt S, et al. Measles virus P gene codes for two proteins. *J Virol* 1985;53:908–919.
61. Bellini WJ, Rota JS, Lowe LE, et al. Subacute sclerosing panencephalitis: more cases of this fatal disease are prevented by measles immunization than was previously recognized. *J Infect Dis* 2005;192:1686–1693.
67. Black FL. Measles endemicity in insular populations: critical community size and its evolutionary implication. *J Theor Biol* 1966;11:207–211.
71. Blau DM, Compans RW. Entry and release of measles virus are polarized in epithelial cells. *Virology* 1995;210:91–99.
76. Bourhis JM, Johansson K, Receveur-Brechot V, et al. The C-terminal domain of measles virus nucleoprotein belongs to the class of intrinsically disordered proteins that fold upon binding to their physiological partner. *Virus Res* 2004;99:157–167.
79. Brindley MA, Plemper RK. Blue native PAGE and biomolecular complementation reveal a tetrameric or higher-order oligomer organization of the physiological measles virus attachment protein H. *J Virol* 2010; 84:12174–12184.
84. Budka H, Urbanits S, Liberski PP, et al. Subacute measles virus encephalitis: a new and fatal opportunistic infection in a patient with AIDS. *Neurology* 1996;46:586–587.
85. Burgoon MP, Keays KM, Owens GP, et al. Laser-capture microdissection of plasma cells from subacute sclerosing panencephalitis brain reveals intrathecal disease-relevant antibodies. *Proc Natl Acad Sci U S A* 2005;102:7245–7250.
86. Burnet FM. Measles as an index of immunological function. *Lancet* 1968;2:610–613.
89. Butler JC, Havens PL, Sowell AL, et al. Measles severity and serum retinol (Vitamin-A) concentration among children in the United States. *Pediatrics* 1993;91:1176–1181.
91. Caceres VM, Strebel PM, Sutter RW. Factors determining prevalence of maternal antibody to measles virus throughout infancy: a review. *Clin Infect Dis* 2000;31:110–119.
92. Campbell H, Andrews N, Brown KE, et al. Review of the effect of measles vaccination on the epidemiology of SSPE. *Int J Epidemiol* 2007; 36:1334–1348.
101. Cathomen T, Buchholz CJ, Spielhofer P, et al. Preferential initiation at the second AUG of the measles virus F mRNA: a role for the long untranslated region. *Virology* 1995;214:628–632.
104. Cattaneo R, Billeter MA. Mutations and A/I hypermutations in measles virus persistent infections. *Curr Top Microbiol Immunol* 1992;176: 63–74.
105. Cattaneo R, Kaelin K, Baczko K, et al. Measles virus editing provides an additional cysteine-rich protein. *Cell* 1989;56:759–764.
113. Centers for Disease Control. Global measles mortality, 2000–2008. *MMWR Morb Mortal Wkly Rep* 2009;58:1321–1326.
119. Chen RT, Goldbaum GM, Wassilak SG, et al. An explosive point-source measles outbreak in a highly vaccinated population. Modes of transmission and risk factors for disease. *Am J Epidemiol* 1989;129:173–182.
120. Chen RT, Markowitz LE, Albrecht P, et al. Measles antibody: reevaluation of protective titers. *J Infect Dis* 1990;162:1036–1042.
125. Cohen BJ, Audet S, Andrews N, et al. Plaque reduction neutralization test for measles antibodies: description of a standardised laboratory method for use in immunogenicity studies of aerosol vaccination. *Vaccine* 2007;26:59–66.
126. Cohen BJ, Dobias D, Andrews N. Comparison of plaque reduction neutralisation test (PRNT) and measles virus-specific IgG ELISA for assessing immunogenicity of measles vaccination. *Vaccine* 2008;26: 6392–6397.
127. Colf LA, Juo ZS, Garcia KC. Structure of the measles virus hemagglutinin. *Nat Struct Mol Biol* 2007;14:1227–1228.
129. Condack C, Grivel JC, Devaux P, et al. Measles virus vaccine attenuation: suboptimal infection of lymphatic tissue and tropism alteration. *J Infect Dis* 2007;196:541–549.
136. Cutts FT, Clements CJ, Bennett JV. Alternative routes of measles immunization: a review. *Biologicals* 1997;25:323–338.
137. Cutts FT, Grabowsky M, Markowitz LE. The effect of dose and strain of live attenuated measles vaccines on serological responses in young infants. *Biologicals* 1995;23:95–106.
144. de Swart RL, Yuksel S, Langerijs CN, et al. Depletion of measles virus glycoprotein-specific antibodies from human sera reveals genotype-specific neutralizing antibodies. *J Gen Virol* 2009;90:2982–2989.
145. de Swart RL, Yuksel S, Osterhaus AD. Relative contributions of measles virus hemagglutinin- and fusion protein-specific serum antibodies to virus neutralization. *J Virol* 2005;79:11547–11551.
146. de Vries RD, Lemon K, Ludlow M, et al. In vivo tropism of attenuated and pathogenic measles virus expressing green fluorescent protein in macaques. *J Virol* 2010;84:4714–4724.
148. de Witte L, de Vries RD, van der Vlist M, et al. DC-SIGN and CD150 have distinct roles in transmission of measles virus from dendritic cells to T-lymphocytes. *PLoS Pathog* 2008;4:e1000049.
149. Deem SL, Spelman LH, Yates RA, et al. Canine distemper in terrestrial carnivores: a review. *J Zoo Wildl Med* 2000;31:441–451.
156. Devaux P, Hudacek AW, Hodge G, et al. A recombinant measles virus unable to antagonize STAT1 function cannot control inflammation and is attenuated in rhesus monkeys. *J Virol* 2011;85:348–356.

164. Dilraj A, Cutts FT, de Castro JF, et al. Response to different measles vaccine strains given by aerosol and subcutaneous routes to schoolchildren: a randomised trial. *Lancet* 2000;355:798–803.
166. Dittmar S, Harms H, Runkler N, et al. Measles virus-induced block of transendothelial migration of T lymphocytes and infection-mediated virus spread across endothelial cell barriers. *J Virol* 2008;82:11273–11282.
168. Dorig RE, Marcil A, Chopra A, et al. The human CD46 molecule is a receptor for measles virus (Edmonston strain). *Cell* 1993;75:295–305.
177. Ehrengruber MU, Ehler E, Billeter M, et al. Measles virus spreads in rat hippocampal neurons by cell-to-cell contact and in a polarized fashion. *J Virol* 2002;76:5720–5728.
178. El Mubarak HS, Yuksel S, van Amerongen G, et al. Infection of cynomolgus macaques (*Macaca fascicularis*) and rhesus macaques (*Macaca mulatta*) with different wild-type measles viruses. *J Gen Virol* 2007;88:2028–2034.
180. Enders JF. Measles virus: historical review, isolation and behavior in various systems. *Am J Dis Child* 1962;103:282–287.
181. Enders JF, Katz SL, Holloway A. Development of attenuated measles-virus vaccines. *Am J Dis Child* 1962;103:335–340.
183. Enders JF, McCarthy K, Mitus A, et al. Isolation of measles virus at autopsy in cases of giant cell pneumonia without rash. *N Engl J Med* 1959; 261:875–881.
184. Enders JF, Peebles TC. Propagation in tissue cultures of cytopathic agents from patients with measles. *Proc Soc Exp Biol Med* 1954;86:277–286.
191. Erlenhofer C, Duprex WP, Rima BK, et al. Analysis of receptor (CD46, CD150) usage by measles virus. *J Gen Virol* 2002;83:1431–1436.
195. Esiri MM, Oppenheimer DR, Brownell B, et al. Distribution of measles antigen and immunoglobulin containing cells in the CNS in subacute sclerosing panencephalitis (SSPE) and atypical measles encephalitis. *J Neurol Sci* 1982;53:29–43.
197. Esolen LM, Takahashi K, Johnson RT, et al. Brain endothelial cell infection in children with acute fatal measles. *J Clin Invest* 1995;96: 2478–2481.
202. Feikin DR, Lezotte DC, Hamman RF, et al. Individual and community risks of measles and pertussis associated with personal exemptions to immunization. *JAMA* 2000;284:3145–3150.
212. Forthal DN, Landucci G, Habis A, et al. Measles virus-specific functional antibody responses and viremia during acute measles infection. *J Infect Dis* 1994;169:1377–1380.
218. Fujinami RS, Oldstone MBA. Antiviral antibody reacting on the plasma membrane alters measles virus expression inside the cell. *Nature* 1979;279:529–530.
221. Fulginiti VA, Eller JJ, Downie AW, et al. Altered reactivity to measles virus: atypical measles in children previously immunized with inactivated measles virus vaccines. *JAMA* 1967;202:1075.
223. Gans HA, Arvin AM, Galinus J, et al. Deficiency of the humoral immune response to measles vaccine in infants immunized at age 6 months. *JAMA* 1998;280:527–532.
226. Garenne M. Sex differences in measles mortality: a world review. *Int J Epidemiol* 1994;23:632–642.
228. Gay NJ. The theory of measles elimination: implications for the design of elimination strategies. *J Infect Dis* 2004;189(Suppl 1):S27–S35.
230. Gendelman HE, Wolinsky JS, Johnson RT, et al. Measles encephalitis: lack of evidence of viral invasion of the central nervous system and quantitative study of the nature of demyelination. *Ann Neurol* 1984;15: 353–360.
234. Gibbs FA, Gibbs EL, Carpenter PR, et al. Electroencephalographic abnormality in uncomplicated childhood diseases. *J Am Med Assoc* 1959; 171:1050–1055.
244. Good RA, Zak SJ. Disturbances in gammaglobulin synthesis as "experiments of nature". *Pediatrics* 1956;18:109–149.
250. Greenberg BL, Sack RB, Salazar-Lindo LE, et al. Measles-associated diarrhea in hospitalized children in Lima, Peru: pathogenic agents and impact on growth. *J Infect Dis* 1991;163:495–502.
252. Grenfell BT, Bjornstad ON, Kappey J. Travelling waves and spatial hierarchies in measles epidemics. *Nature* 2001;414:716–723.
253. Griffin DE. Immunologic abnormalities accompanying acute and chronic viral infections. *Rev Infect Dis* 1991;13:S129–S133.
258. Griffin DE, Ward BJ. Differential CD4 T cell activation in measles. *J Infect Dis* 1993;168:275–281.
265. Grosjean I, Caux C, Bella C, et al. Measles virus infects human dendritic cells and blocks their allostimulatory properties for CD4+ T cells. *J Exp Med* 1997;186:801–812.
266. Gutierrez J, Issacson RS, Koppel BS. Subacute sclerosing panencephalitis: an update. *Dev Med Child Neurol* 2010;52:901–907.
274. Hanninen P, Arstila P, Lang H, et al. Involvement of the central nervous system in acute, uncomplicated measles virus infection. *J Clin Microbiol* 1980;11:610–613.
276. Hashiguchi T, Kajikawa M, Maita N, et al. Crystal structure of measles virus hemagglutinin provides insight into effective vaccines. *Proc Natl Acad Sci U S A* 2007;104:19535–19540.
277. Hashiguchi T, Ose T, Kubota M, et al. Structure of the measles virus hemagglutinin bound to its cellular receptor SLAM. *Nat Struct Mol Biol* 2011;18:135–141.
294. Hirsch RL, Griffin DE, Johnson RT, et al. Cellular immune responses during complicated and uncomplicated measles virus infections of man. *Clin Immunol Immunopathol* 1984;31:1–12.
296. Holt EA, Moulton LH, Siberry GK, et al. Differential mortality by measles vaccine titer and sex. *J Infect Dis* 1993;168:1087–1096.
301. Horzinek MC. Rinderpest: the second viral disease eradicated. *Vet Microbiol* 2011;149:295–297.
309. Huber M, Cattaneo R, Spielhofer P, et al. Measles virus phosphoprotein retains the nucleocapsid protein in the cytoplasm. *Virology* 1991; 185:299–308.
316. Hussey GD, Klein M. Routine high-dose vitamin A therapy for children hospitalized with measles. *J Trop Pediatr* 1993;39:342–345.
318. Ikegame S, Takeda M, Ohno S, et al. Both RIG-I and MDA5 RNA helicases contribute to the induction of alpha/beta interferon in measles virus-infected human cells. *J Virol* 2010;84:372–379.
321. Iorio RM, Mahon PJ. Paramyxoviruses: different receptors - different mechanisms of fusion. *Trends Microbiol* 2008;16:135–137.
326. Jabbour JT, Duenas DA, Sever JL, et al. Epidemiology of subacute sclerosing panencephalitis: a report of the SSPE registry. *JAMA* 1972; 220:959–962.
331. Jaye A, Magnusen AF, Sadiq AD, et al. Ex vivo analysis of cytotoxic T lymphocytes to measles antigens during infection and after vaccination in Gambian children. *J Clin Invest* 1998;102:1969–1977.
333. Jensen MR, Communie G, Ribeiro EA Jr, et al. Intrinsic disorder in measles virus nucleocapsids. *Proc Natl Acad Sci U S A* 2011;108:9839–9844.
336. Johansson K, Bourhis JM, Campanacci V, et al. Crystal structure of the measles virus phosphoprotein domain responsible for the induced folding of the C-terminal domain of the nucleoprotein. *J Biol Chem* 2003;278:44567–44573.
337. Johnson RT, Griffin DE, Hirsch RL, et al. Measles encephalomyelitis - clinical and immunologic studies. *N Engl J Med* 1984;310:137–141.
343. Karlin D, Longhi S, Receveur V, et al. The N-terminal domain of the phosphoprotein of morbilliviruses belongs to the natively unfolded class of proteins. *Virology* 2002;296:251–262.
344. Karp CL, Wysocka M, Wahl LM, et al. Mechanism of suppression of cell-mediated immunity by measles virus. *Science* 1996;273:228–231.
348. Katz SL, Enders JF, Holloway A. Studies on an attenuated measles-virus vaccine. II. Clinical, virologic and immunologic effects of vaccine in institutionalized children. *N Engl J Med* 1960;263:159–160.
365. Kobune F, Sakata H, Sugiura A. Marmoset lymphoblastoid cells as a sensitive host for isolation of measles virus. *J Virol* 1990;64:700–705.
377. Kwiatek O, Ali YH, Saeed IK, et al. Asian lineage of peste des petits ruminants virus, Africa. *Emerg Infect Dis* 2011;17:1223–1231.
381. Lambert DM, Barney S, Lambert AL, et al. Peptides from conserved regions of paramyxovirus fusion (F) proteins are potent inhibitors of viral fusion. *Proc Natl Acad Sci U S A* 1996;93:2186–2191.
388. Lemon K, de Vries RD, Mesman AW, et al. Early target cells of measles virus after aerosol infection of non-human primates. *PLoS Pathog* 2011;7:e1001263.
389. Leonard VH, Hodge G, Reyes-Del VJ, et al. Measles virus selectively blind to signaling lymphocytic activation molecule (SLAM; CD150) is attenuated and induces strong adaptive immune responses in rhesus monkeys. *J Virol* 2010;84:3413–3420.
390. Leonard VHJ, Sinn PL, Hodge G, et al. Measles virus blind to its epithelial cell receptor remains virulent in rhesus monkeys but cannot cross the airway epithelium and is not shed. *J Clin Invest* 2008;118:1–11.

392. Leopardi R, Ilonen J, Mattila L, et al. Effect of measles virus infection on MHC class II expression and antigen presentation in human monocytes. *Cell Immunol* 1993;147:388–396.
402. Lin WH, Griffin DE, Rota PA, et al. Successful respiratory immunization with dry powder live-attenuated measles virus vaccine in rhesus macaques. *Proc Natl Acad Sci U S A* 2011;108:2987–2992.
404. Liston P, Briedis DJ. Measles virus V protein binds zinc. *Virology* 1994; 198:399–404.
408. Longhi S, Receveur-Brechot V, Karlin D, et al. The C-terminal domain of the measles virus nucleoprotein is intrinsically disordered and folds upon binding to the C-terminal moiety of the phosphoprotein. *J Biol Chem* 2003;278:18638–18648.
411. Low N, Kraemer S, Schneider M, et al. Immunogenicity and safety of aerosolized measles vaccine: systematic review and meta-analysis. *Vaccine* 2008;26:383–398.
414. Ludlow M, Rennick LJ, Sarlang S, et al. Wild-type measles virus infection in primary epithelial cells occurs via the basolateral surface without syncytium formation or release of infectious virus. *J Gen Virol* 2009; 91:971–979.
421. Manchester M, Rall G. Model systems: transgenic mouse models for measles pathogenesis. *Trends Microbiol* 2001;9:19–23.
426. Manning L, Laman M, Edoni H, et al. Subacute sclerosing panencephalitis in Papua New Guinean children: the cost of continuing inadequate measles vaccine coverage. *PLoS Negl Trop Dis* 2011;5:e932.
431. Masse N, Ainouze M, Neel B, et al. Measles virus (MV) hemagglutinin: evidence that attachment sites for MV receptors SLAM and CD46 overlap on the globular head. *J Virol* 2004;78:9051–9063.
433. Mathias RG, Meekison WG, Arcand TA. The role of secondary vaccine failures in measles outbreaks. *Am J Public Health* 1989;79: 475–478.
439. McChesney MB, Fujinami RS, Lerche NW, et al. Virus-induced immunosuppression: infection of peripheral blood mononuclear cells and suppression of immunoglobulin synthesis during natural measles virus infection of rhesus monkeys. *J Infect Dis* 1989;159:757–760.
444. McNeill WH. *Plagues and Peoples.* Garden City, NY: Anchor Press/ Doubleday; 1976.
445. McQuaid S, Cosby SL. An immunohistochemical study of the distribution of the measles virus receptors, CD46 and SLAM, in normal human tissues and subacute sclerosing panencephalitis. *Lab Invest* 2002;82: 403–409.
449. Melnick JL. Thermostability of poliovirus and measles vaccines. *Dev Biol Stand* 1996;87:155–160.
457. Miller DL. Frequency of complications of measles, 1963. *Br Med J* 1964;2:75–78.
458. Modlin JF, Jabbour JT, Witte JJ, et al. Epidemiologic studies of measles, measles vaccine, and subacute sclerosing encephalitis. *Pediatrics* 1977;59: 505–512.
460. Moench TR, Griffin DE, Obriecht CR, et al. Acute measles in patients with and without neurological involvement: distribution of measles virus antigen and RNA. *J Infect Dis* 1988;158:433–442.
463. Moll M, Pfeuffer J, Klenk HD, et al. Polarized glycoprotein targeting affects the spread of measles virus in vitro and in vivo. *J Gen Virol* 2004; 85:1019–1027.
469. Morley D. Severe measles in the tropics. *Br Med J* 1969;1:297–300.
471. Moss WJ. Measles still has a devastating impact in unvaccinated populations. *PLoS Med* 2007;4:e24.
473. Moss WJ, Griffin DE. Global measles elimination. *Nat Rev Microbiol* 2006;4:900–908.
474. Moss WJ, Griffin DE. Measles. *Lancet,* in press.
476. Moss WJ, Ryon JJ, Monze M, et al. Differential regulation of interleukin (IL)-4, IL-5, and IL-10 during measles in Zambian children. *J Infect Dis* 2002;186:879–887.
477. Moss WJ, Scott S, Mugala N, et al. Immunogenicity of standard-titer measles vaccine in HIV-1-infected and uninfected Zambian children: an observational study. *J Infect Dis* 2007;196:347–355.
479. Muhlebach MD, Mateo M, Sinn PL, et al. Measles virus targets adherens junction protein nectin-4 to emerge in the airways. *Nature,* in press.
483. Muller N, Avota E, Schneider-Schaulies J, et al. Measles virus contact with T cells impedes cytoskeletal remodeling associated with spreading, polarization, and CD3 clustering. *Traffic* 2006;7:849–858.
487. Naim HY, Ehler E, Billeter MA. Measles virus matrix protein specifies apical virus release and glycoprotein sorting in epithelial cells. *EMBO J* 2000;19:3576–3585.
490. Nakatsu Y, Takeda M, Ohno S, et al. Measles virus circumvents the host interferon response by different actions of the C and V proteins. *J Virol* 2008;82:8296–8306.
496. Naniche D, Reed SI, Oldstone MBA. Cell cycle arrest during measles virus infection: a G_0-like block leads to suppression of retinoblastoma protein expression. *J Virol* 1999;73:1894–1900.
497. Naniche D, Varior-Krishnan G, Cervoni F, et al. Human membrane cofactor protein (CD46) acts as a cellular receptor for measles virus. *J Virol* 1993;67:6025–6032.
498. Naniche D, Yeh A, Eto DS, et al. Evasion of host defenses by measles virus: wild-type measles virus infection interferes with induction of alpha/beta interferon production. *J Virol* 2000;74:7478–7484.
508. Noyce RS, Bondre DG, Lin L-T, et al. Tumor cell marker PVRL4 (Nectin 4) is an epithelial cell receptor for measles virus. *PLoS Pathog* 2011;7:1002240.
514. Ohno S, Ono N, Seki F, et al. Measles virus infection of SLAM (CD150) knockin mice reproduces tropism and immunosuppression in human infection. *J Virol* 2007;81:1650–1659.
517. Okada H, Kobune F, Sato T, et al. Extensive lymphopenia due to apoptosis of uninfected lymphocytes in acute measles patients. *Arch Virol* 2000;145:905–920.
520. Oldstone MB, Lewicki H, Thomas D, et al. Measles virus infection in a transgenic model: virus-induced immunosuppression and central nervous system disease. *Cell* 1999;98:629–640.
525. Ovsyannikova IG, Pankratz VS, Vierkant RA, et al. Human leukocyte antigen haplotypes in the genetic control of immune response to measles-mumps-rubella vaccine. *J Infect Dis* 2006;193:655–663.
530. Panum P. Observations made during the epidemic of measles on the Faroe Islands in the year 1846. *Med Classics* 1938;3:829–886.
540. Permar SR, Klumpp SA, Mansfield KG, et al. Role of CD8(+) lymphocytes in control and clearance of measles virus infection of rhesus monkeys. *J Virol* 2003;77:4396–4400.
542. Permar SR, Moss WJ, Ryon JJ, et al. Prolonged measles virus shedding in human immunodeficiency virus-infected children, detected by reverse transcriptase-polymerase chain reaction. *J Infect Dis* 2001;183:532–538.
547. Plemper RK, Brindley MA, Iorio RM. Structural and mechanistic studies of measles virus illuminate paramyxovirus entry. *PLoS Pathog* 2011;7:e1002058.
551. Plemper RK, Hammond AL, Gerlier D, et al. Strength of envelope protein interaction modulates cytopathicity of measles virus. *J Virol* 2002;76:5051–5061.
555. Plumet S, Herschke F, Bourhis J-M, et al. Cytosolic 5'-triphosphate ended viral leader transcript of measles virus as activator of the RIG I-mediated interferon response. *PLoS One* 2007:2(3):e279.
558. Polack FP, Auwaerter PG, Lee S-H, et al. Production of atypical measles in rhesus macaques: evidence for disease mediated by immune complex formation and eosinophils in the presence of fusion-inhibiting antibody. *Nat Med* 1999;5:629–634.
559. Polack FP, Hoffman SJ, Crujeiras G, et al. A role for nonprotective complement-fixing antibodies with low avidity for measles virus in atypical measles. *Nat Med* 2003;9:1209–1213.
572. Radecke F, Billeter MA. The nonstructural C protein is not essential for multiplication of Edmonston B strain measles virus in cultured cells. *Virology* 1996;217:418–421.
577. Rammohan KW, McFarland HF, McFarlin DE. Subacute sclerosing panencephalitis after passive immunization and natural measles infection: role of antibody in persistence of measles virus. *Neurology* 1982;32: 390–394.
589. Riddell MA, Moss WJ, Hauer D, et al. Slow clearance of measles virus RNA after acute infection. *J Clin Virol* 2007;39:312–317.
593. Rima BK, Duprex WP. Molecular mechanisms of measles virus persistence. *Virus Res* 2005;111:132–147.
599. Rodgers DV, Gindler JS, Atkinson WL, et al. High attack rates and case fatality during a measles outbreak in groups with religious exemption to vaccination. *Pediatr Infect Dis J* 1993;12:288–292.
601. Roos RP, Graves MC, Wollmann RL, et al. Immunologic and virologic studies of measles inclusion body encephalitis in an immunosuppressed

host: the relationship to subacute sclerosing panencephalitis. *Neurology* 1981;31:1263–1270.

603. Rota JS, Wang ZD, Rota PA, et al. Comparison of sequences of the H, F, and N coding genes of measles virus vaccine strains. *Virus Res* 1994; 31:317–330.
605. Rota PA, Brown K, Mankertz A, et al. Global distribution of measles genotypes and measles molecular epidemiology. *J Infect Dis* 2011;204 (Suppl 1):S514–S523.
608. Ruigrok RW, Gerlier D. Structure of the measles virus H glycoprotein sheds light on an efficient vaccine. *Proc Natl Acad Sci U S A* 2007;104: 20639–20640.
609. Runkler N, Dietzel E, Carsillo M, et al. Sorting signals in the measles virus wild-type glycoproteins differently influence virus spread in polarized epithelia and lymphocytes. *J Gen Virol* 2009;90:2474–2482.
620. Sandford-Smith JH, Whittle HC. Corneal ulceration following measles in Nigerian children. *Br J Ophthalmol* 1979;63:720–724.
621. Santiago C, Bjorling E, Stehle T, et al. Distinct kinetics for binding of the CD46 and SLAM receptors to overlapping sites in the measles virus hemagglutinin protein. *J Biol Chem* 2002;277:32294–32301.
622. Santiago C, Celma ML, Stehle T, et al. Structure of the measles virus hemagglutinin bound to the CD46 receptor. *Nat Struct Mol Biol* 2010; 17:124–129.
634. Schlender J, Schnorr J-J, Spielhofer P, et al. Interaction of measles virus glycoproteins with the surface of uninfected peripheral blood lymphocytes induces immunosuppression in vitro. *Proc Natl Acad Sci U S A* 1996;93:13194–13199.
646. Schuhmann KM, Pfaller CK, Conzelmann KK. The measles virus V protein binds to p65 (RelA) to suppress NF-kappaB activity. *J Virol* 2011;85:3162–3171.
647. Schwarz AJF. Preliminary tests of a highly attenuated measles vaccine. *Am J Dis Child* 1962;103:216–219.
648. Scott P, Moss WJ, Gilani Z, et al. Measles vaccination in HIV-infected children: systematic review and meta-analysis of safety and immunogenicity. *J Infect Dis* 2011;204(Suppl 1):S164–S178.
649. Sellin CI, Horvat B. Current animal models: transgenic animal models for the study of measles pathogenesis. *Curr Top Microbiol Immunol* 2009; 330:111–127.
662. Shingai M, Ebihara T, Begum NA, et al. Differential type I IFN-inducing abilities of wild-type versus vaccine strains of measles virus. *J Immunol* 2007;179:6123–6133.
666. Shishkova Y, Harms H, Krohne G, et al. Immune synapses formed with measles virus-infected dendritic cells are unstable and fail to sustain T cell activation. *Cell Microbiol* 2007;9:1974–1986.
677. Smaron MF, Saxon E, Wood L, et al. Diagnosis of measles by fluorescent antibody and culture of nasopharyngeal secretions. *J Virol Methods* 1991;33:223–229.
689. Strebel PM, Cochi SL, Hoekstra E, et al. A world without measles. *J Infect Dis* 2011;204(Suppl 1):S1–S3.
695. Tahara M, Takeda M, Seki F, et al. Multiple amino acid substitutions in hemagglutinin are necessary for wild-type measles virus to acquire the ability to use receptor CD46 efficiently. *J Virol* 2007;81:2564–2572.
696. Tahara M, Takeda M, Shirogane Y, et al. Measles virus infects both polarized epithelial and immune cells by using distinctive receptor-binding sites on its hemagglutinin. *J Virol* 2008;82:4630–4637.
705. Takeda M, Ohno S, Seki F, et al. Long untranslated regions of the measles virus M and F genes control virus replication and cytopathogenicity. *J Virol* 2005;79:14346–14354.
711. Takeuchi K, Takeda M, Miyajima N, et al. Stringent requirement for the C protein of wild-type measles virus for growth both in vitro and in macaques. *J Virol* 2005;79:7838–7844.
712. Tamashiro VG, Perez HH, Griffin DE. Prospective study of the magnitude and duration of changes in tuberculin reactivity during complicated and uncomplicated measles. *Pediatr Infect Dis J* 1987;6:451–454.
715. Tatsuo H, Ono N, Tanaka K, et al. SLAM (CDw150) is a cellular receptor for measles virus. *Nature* 2000;406:893–898.
728. Uzicanin A, Zimmerman L. Field effectiveness of live attenuated measles-containing vaccines: a review of published literature. *J Infect Dis* 2011; 204(Suppl 1):S133–S148.
732. Van Binnendijk RS, Poelen MCM, Kuijpers KC, et al. The predominance of CD8+ T cells after infection with measles virus suggests a role for CD8+ class I MHC-restricted cytotoxic T lymphocytes (CTL) in recovery from measles. *J Immunol* 1990;144:2394–2399.
736. Van Binnendijk RS, van der Heijden RWJ, van Amerongen G, et al. Viral replication and development of specific immunity in macaques after infection with different measles virus strains. *J Infect Dis* 1994;170:443–448.
740. Vandevelde M, Zurbriggen A. Demyelination in canine distemper virus infection: a review. *Acta Neuropathol (Berl)* 2005;109:56–68.
743. Vincent S, Gerlier D, Manie SN. Measles virus assembly within membrane rafts. *J Virol* 2000;74:9911–9915.
747. von Messling V, Milosevic D, Cattaneo R. Tropism illuminated: lymphocyte-based pathways blazed by lethal morbillivirus through the host immune system. *Proc Natl Acad Sci U S A* 2004;101:14216–14221.
750. Von Pirquet C. Verhalten der kutanen tuberkulin-reaktion wahrend der Masern. *Deutsch Med Wochenschr* 1908;34:1297–1300.
756. Ward BJ, Johnson RT, Vaisberg A, et al. Cytokine production in vitro and the lymphoproliferative defect of natural measles virus infection. *Clin Immunol Immunopathol* 1991;61:236–248.
757. Ward BJ, Johnson RT, Vaisberg A, et al. Spontaneous proliferation of peripheral mononuclear cells in natural measles virus infection: identification of dividing cells and correlation with mitogen responsiveness. *Clin Immunol Immunopathol* 1990;55:315–326.
760. Watanabe A, Yoneda M, Ikeda F, et al. CD147/EMMPRIN acts as a functional entry receptor for measles virus on epithelial cells. *J Virol* 2010;84:4183–4193.
766. Weidmann A, Maisner A, Garten W, et al. Proteolytic cleavage of the fusion protein but not membrane fusion is required for measles virus-induced immunosuppression in vitro. *J Virol* 2000;74:1985–1993.
775. WHO. New genotype of measles virus and update on global distribution of measles genotypes. *Wkly Epidemiol Rec* 2005;80:347–351.
779. Wild TF, Malvoisin F, Buckland R. Measles virus: both the haemagglutinin and fusion glycoproteins are required for fusion. *J Gen Virol* 1991;72:439–442.
781. Wolfson LJ, Grais RF, Luquero FJ, et al. Estimates of measles case fatality ratios: a comprehensive review of community-based studies. *Int J Epidemiol* 2009;38:192–205.
788. Xin JY, Ihara T, Komase K, et al. Amino acid substitutions in matrix, fusion and hemagglutinin proteins of wild measles virus for adaptation to vero cells. *Intervirology* 2011;54:217–228.
801. Yu XL, Cheng YM, Shi BS, et al. Measles virus infection in adults induces production of IL-10 and is associated with increased CD4+ CD25+ regulatory T cells. *J Immunol* 2008;181:7356–7366.
807. Zilliox MJ, Moss WJ, Griffin DE. Gene expression changes in peripheral blood mononuclear cells during measles virus infection. *Clin Vaccine Immunol* 2007;14:918–923.

CHAPTER 37

Lin-Fa Wang • John S. Mackenzie • Christopher C. Broder

Henipaviruses

HISTORY

Hendra virus (HeV), the first known member of the genus *Henipavirus* in the family *Paramyxoviridae,* came to light in September 1994 as the causative agent of a sudden outbreak of acute respiratory disease in thoroughbred horses at a stable in Brisbane, Australia. A total of 21 horses and 2 humans (a horse trainer and a stable hand) became infected. The horse trainer and 14 horses died, and 7 horses with mild or subclinical infection were killed.[130] A virus was isolated, called *equine morbillivirus* but later named *Hendra virus* after the Brisbane suburb where the outbreak occurred. A second person died from HeV infection 13 months after the Brisbane outbreak, a farmer from Mackay, nearly 1000 km north of Brisbane. Unlike the first case, however, the man succumbed to encephalitis caused by HeV infection.[107] A forensic investigation found that the farmer had suffered a mild meningitic illness 14 months earlier after assisting at the necropsy of two horses that had died of severe respiratory distress—later found to have been caused by HeV[125]—and that he became infected at that time. After initial serologic evidence suggested that fruit bats (flying foxes) of the genus *Pteropus* in the suborder *Megachiroptera* were the reservoir hosts,[165] HeV was isolated from two species of flying fox.[56] In total, there have been 14 recognized occurrences of HeV in Australia between 1994–2010, with at least one occurrence per year since 2006.[5,10] Every occurrence of HeV has involved horses as the initial infected host, causing lethal respiratory disease and encephalitis, along with a total of seven human cases arising from exposure to infected horses, among which four have been fatal and the most recent in 2009.[6,10,115]

Nipah virus (NiV), the second known member of the genus *Henipavirus,* emerged as the cause of an outbreak of disease in pigs and humans in Peninsular Malaysia in 1998 through 1999. The epidemic started in Perak State as clusters of cases of encephalitis among pig farmers. It was initially believed to be caused by Japanese encephalitis virus; however, various features of the outbreak, including a high proportion of cases in direct contact with pigs and illness and deaths in pigs, differed from those expected with Japanese encephalitis.[30] Indeed, respiratory illness and encephalitis in pigs preceded human cases in the same district.[97] The epidemic spread south to the intensive pig-farming areas of Negeri Sembilan in December 1998 and subsequently peaked between February and April 1999. More than 1 million pigs were destroyed to halt the spread of the epidemic, and by late May, 265 human cases of acute encephalitis with 105 deaths were recorded.[29,30] A cluster of 11 cases with 1 death occurred among abattoir workers in Singapore.[114] In early March 1999, a virus was isolated from the cerebrospinal fluid (CSF) of a patient with encephalitis and identified as the etiologic agent.[29,30] Named *Nipah virus* after the village from which the patient had come, it was shown to be closely related to HeV. NiV was subsequently isolated from the urine of Malaysian flying foxes.[33] The virus re-emerged in Bangladesh in 2001,[68] and outbreaks of NiV-related encephalitis have occurred in people from that country almost every year since, along with two reports of NiV encephalitis in India[23,60] and the most recent occurrence in early 2011 in Bangladesh.[7] The human case fatality rate of these occurrences of NiV has approached 75%.[68,85]

INFECTIOUS AGENT

Classification

When HeV was first isolated in 1994, partial sequencing of the matrix gene (M) revealed that it most closely resembled members of the genus *Morbillivirus* in the subfamily *Paramyxovirinae.*[104] Subsequent characterization of the full-length genome, however, revealed that many of the genetic features of HeV were unique among paramyxoviruses and that the virus did not fit within any of the three genera existing at that time, *Morbillivirus, Respirovirus,* and *Rubulavirus.*[147,148] When NiV was isolated in 1999, it was initially described as Hendra-like on the basis of its strong reactivity with anti-HeV antibodies. Later it was shown that sera raised against HeV were able to neutralize NiV and vice versa, and that both viruses shared a high degree of similarity in genome organization and protein size and sequence.[29,58,59,146] In 2002, the genus *Henipavirus* was created to accommodate these novel paramyxoviruses, and HeV was designated the type species.[75] Currently, the genus *Henipavirus* contains two virus species and several strains isolated from humans, bats, horses, and pigs over a wide geographic area and spanning a period of 15 years (Table 37.1). The susceptibility of humans, the virulence of the viruses, and absence of therapeutics and vaccines led to classification of HeV and NiV as biosafety level 4 (BSL4) pathogens.

Propagation in Cell Culture and Cytopathic Effect

The ultrastructural characteristics of henipavirus-infected cells resemble those found in cells infected by other members of the *Paramyxovirinae.* Shared features include generation of large syncytia and the presence of viral nucleocapsids in cytoplasmic inclusion bodies and underlying electron-dense areas of the plasma membrane.[49,69] In Vero cells, NiV-induced syncytia are significantly larger than those generated by HeV and nuclei and nucleocapsids are frequently located at the cell periphery, compared with HeV-induced syncytia, where they tend to be more centrally located or distributed randomly throughout the cytoplasm (Fig. 37.1). Henipavirus-infected cells also contain structures that are not seen with other paramyxoviruses—specifically a network of membrane-like reticular structures in the cytoplasm and long tubules that appear to be continuous with the plasma membrane in NiV-infected cells. Tubules can also be observed in NiV virions (Fig. 37.2A). *In situ* hybridization suggests that

TABLE 37.1 Summary of Henipaviruses Isolated from Different Species and Geographic Locations

Virus	Isolate name and number	Isolation details			Reference
		Year	Country	Host species/tissue	
Hendra	Horse-1	1994	Australia	Horse/spleen, lung	104
	VR-1	1994	Australia	Human/lung, liver, kidney, spleen	104
	Bat-1-1	1996	Australia	Grey-headed flying fox (*Pteropus poliocephalus*)/uterine fluid	56
	Bat-1-2	1996	Australia	Grey-headed flying fox (*P. poliocephalus*)/fetus	56
	Bat-2	1996	Australia	Black flying fox (*Pteropus alecto*)/fetal lung	56
	Murwillumbah	2006	Australia	Horse/lung	90
	Clifton Beach	2007	Australia	Horse/lung	90
	Peachester	2008	Australia	Horse/blood	90
	Redlands	2008	Australia	Horse/lung	90
	Proserpine	2008	Australia	Horse/lung	90
Nipah	PKL	1999	Malaysia	Human/cerebral spinal fluid	29, 30
	EKK	1999	Malaysia	Human/cerebral spinal fluid	29, 30
	WWS	1999	Malaysia	Human/cerebral spinal fluid	29, 30
	UMMC1	1999	Malaysia	Human/cerebral spinal fluid	24
	UMMC2	1999	Malaysia	Human/throat secretion	24
	UM-0128	1999	Malaysia	Human	2
	VRI-0626	1999	Malaysia	Pig/lung	2
	VRI-1413	1999	Malaysia	Pig/lung	2
	VRI-2794	1999	Malaysia	Pig/lung	2
	B13/6-18	2000	Malaysia	Bat/pooled urine	33
	B13/6-43	2000	Malaysia	Bat/pooled urine	33
	JA13/6-4	2000	Malaysia	Bat/partially eaten jambu air fruit	33
	Rajbari-1	2004	Bangladesh	Human/oropharyngeal	57
	Rajbari-2	2004	Bangladesh	Human/cerebral spinal fluid	57
	Faridpur	2004	Bangladesh	Human/urine	57
	Rajshahi	2004	Bangladesh	Human/urine	57
	CSUR381	2004	Cambodia	Flying fox (*Pteropus lylei*)/urine	120
	CSUR382	2004	Cambodia	Flying fox (*P. lylei*)/urine	120

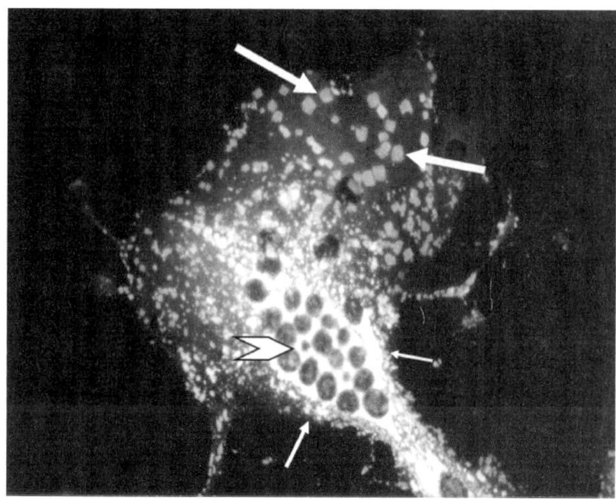
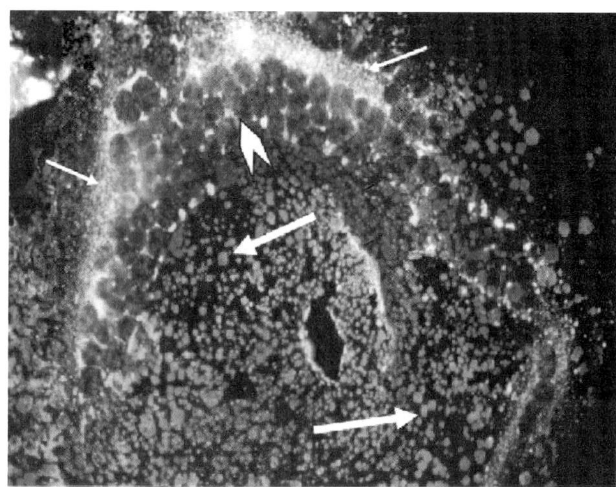

FIGURE 37.1. Syncytia induced in vero cells 24 hours after infection by Hendra virus (HeV) (A) and Nipah virus (NiV) (B). Methanol-fixed infected cells were labeled with rabbit monospecific antiserum to the HeV P protein and fluorescein-conjugated goat antirabbit immunoglobulin G. P protein is detected in extensive perinuclear ribonucleoprotein complexes (*small arrow*) and in discrete regularly shaped arrays (*large arrow*) distributed throughout the cytoplasm and believed to be sites of virus egress from the cell. Nuclei are indicated by *chevrons.*

these reticular structures contain viral RNA and may play a role in viral transcription.[49]

Virus Morphology

Henipavirus particles are pleomorphic, varying from spherical to filamentous and ranging in size from 40 to 1,900 nm.[49,69,104] Nucleocapsids have a diameter of 18 to 19 nm with an average pitch of 5 nm. When examined by electron microscopy (EM), HeV has a unique double-fringed appearance, caused by the presence of surface projections 15 ± 1 nm and 8 ± 1 nm in length (see Fig. 37.2B). Approximately 95% of virions contain the double fringe, and the remaining 5% display a uniform fringe length of 15 ± 1 nm. Unlike HeV, NiV possesses a single layer of surface projections with an average length of 17 ± 1 nm, and NiV particles released into the culture medium are difficult to image because they are routinely penetrated by negative stains. This suggests that the viruses may differ in the physical nature of their envelope.[69]

Genome Length and Organization

In the subfamily *Paramyxovirinae,* the genome length of all characterized viruses is divisible by six, an observation caused by the requirement of each N protein in the viral ribonucleoprotein to bind 6 nucleotide (nt) residues.[76] This is also true

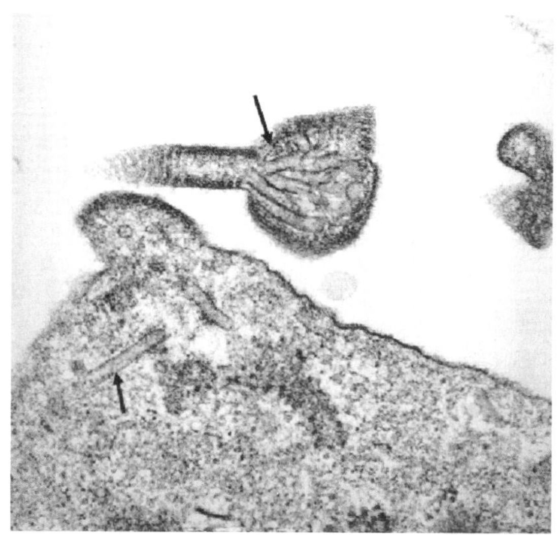
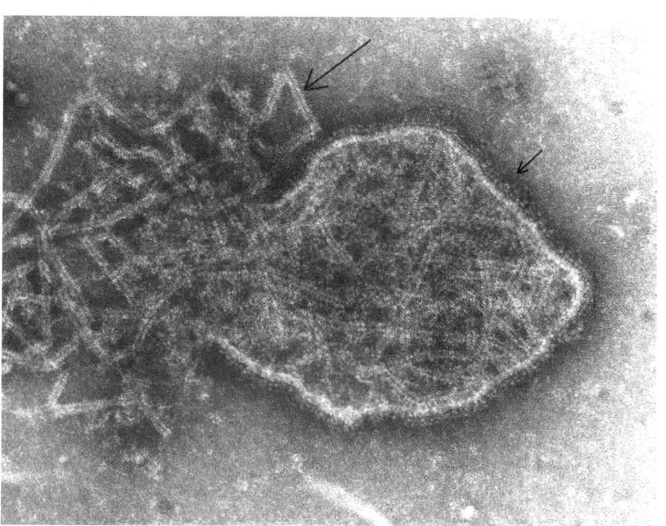

FIGURE 37.2. A: Electron micrograph of Nipah virus (NiV)-infected Vero cells showing tubule-like structures, both in the cytoplasm and in a maturing virus particle (*arrows*). **B:** Electron micrograph of negatively stained Hendra virus (HeV) displaying the double fringe at the virus envelope (*small arrow*) and the herringbone nucleocapsids (*large arrow*). (Courtesy of Dr. Alex Hyatt, CSIRO Australian Animal Health Laboratory.)

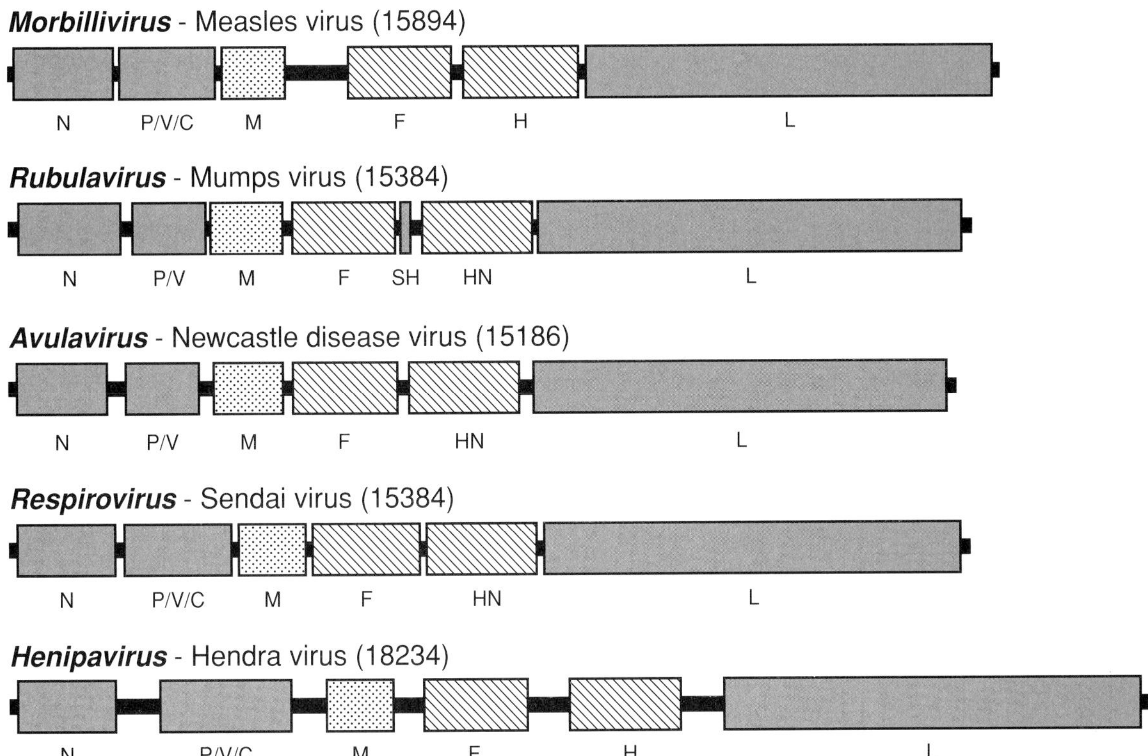

FIGURE 37.3. Genome size and organization of Hendra virus compared with type species of each of the other four classified genera in the subfamily *Paramyxovirinae*. Genome lengths (in nucleotides) are given in brackets after each virus.

for HeV and NiV despite their much larger genome sizes.[146] The genomes of the Malaysian and Bangladesh strains of NiV differ by 6 nt because of a 6-nt increase in the 3′ untranslated region of the *F* gene.[57] A minigenome replicon study confirms that NiV complies with the rule of six.[55] When the complete genome sequence of HeV was determined, its length (18,234 nt) was more than 2,700 nt, or 15% longer than the genomes of all other paramyxoviruses known at that time.[148] The size of the NiV genome at 18,246 nt to 18,252 nt is slightly larger than that of HeV.[57–59] The extra length of the henipavirus genome is in the form of unique, long untranslated sequences at the 3′ end of five of the six genes. A comparison of genome length and untranslated regions of representative members of the *Paramyxovirinae* is shown in Figure 37.3.

The genome organization of henipaviruses resembles that in the genera *Respirovirus* and *Morbillivirus*. The first 12 nt of the 3′ and 5′ genomic terminal sequences of paramyxoviruses are highly conserved and complementary, containing promoter elements for replication and transcription.[76] The first 3 nt of the henipavirus genome termini are 5′-ACC-3′—a sequence that is absolutely conserved in members of the subfamily *Paramyxovirinae* but different from that found in the *Pneumovirinae*.

Genetic Diversity

Partial genome sequencing revealed that HeV isolated from equine and human sources during the outbreak in Brisbane appears identical and differs little from HeV isolated from flying foxes 2 years later.[56,104] Sequencing of five additional horse isolates from five different locations from the 2006 to 2008 HeV occurrences has demonstrated a very high genetic similarity.[90] Similar observations were made in Malaysia, where it was demonstrated that NiV isolated from pigs at the height of the outbreak and at its geographic focus were essentially identical to human isolates made at that time and isolates obtained from flying foxes several years later.[2,24,33,58,59]

In Bangladesh, four human isolates obtained in 2004 demonstrate significant genetic heterogeneity and suggest multiple spillovers of NiV from flying foxes into the human population.[57] The NiV sequence detected from lung tissue of human patients in India was more related to NiV from Bangladesh than NiV from Malaysia.[9,23] On the other hand, NiV isolated from the flying fox *Pteropus lylei* in Cambodia[120] represents an evolutionary lineage that is separated from the Malaysia or Bangladesh/India cluster (Fig. 37.4). Partial *N* gene sequences detected in *Pteropus lylei* in Thailand indicate the circulation of at least two lineages of NiV—one related to the Bangladesh NiV and the other more related to the Malaysian NiV.[144]

The presence of henipavirus-reactive (but not neutralizing) antibodies in bats from other regions of the world (see Epidemiology section) predicts that a much greater genetic diversity of henipaviruses exists in different bat populations. This also suggests the existence of henipaviruses with different transmissibility and pathogenicity in nonbat hosts.

Virus Proteins and Their Properties

Analysis of purified viruses by polyacrylamide gel electrophoresis reveals L, P, G, F_0, N, F_1, and F_2 proteins,[146,147] where F_0 is the uncleaved and F_1 and F_2 the cleaved products of the *F* gene. Interestingly, F_0 is more readily detected in HeV compared with other paramyxoviruses, including NiV.[93,146] Overall, the proteins

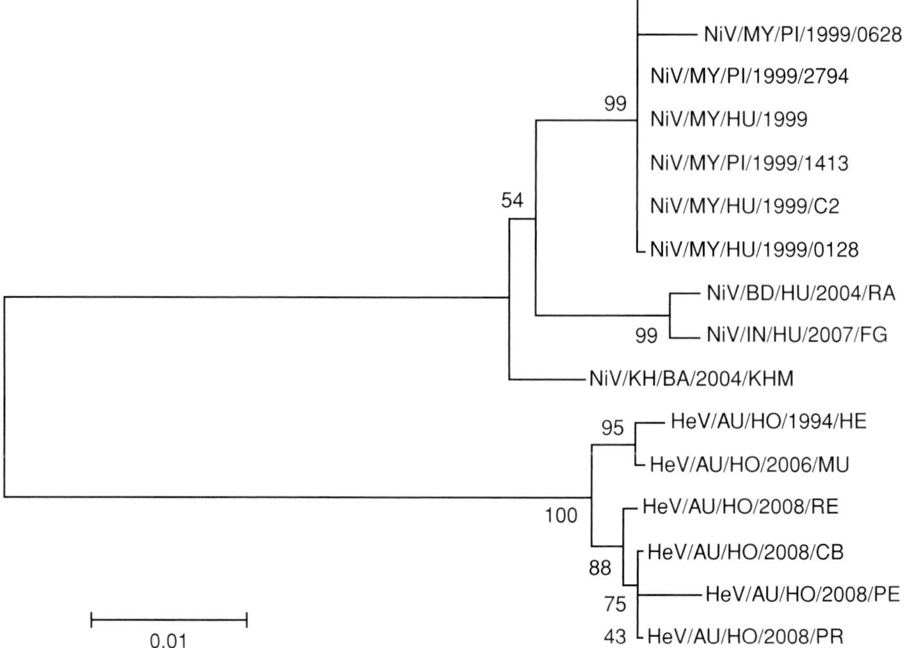

FIGURE 37.4. Phylogenetic relationship between the N protein sequences of henipavirus isolates from different geographic locations. The virus nomenclature abbreviation follows the following format: virus/country origin/host/year/isolate name. For example, NiV/KH/BA/2004/KHM represents a Nipah virus isolated from bats in Cambodia in 2004 with KHM as its isolate name.

of henipaviruses are typical of those of the subfamily *Paramyxovirinae,* with the exception of the P protein, which is significantly larger than cognate proteins in the subfamily.[147] The P protein is translated from messenger RNA (mRNA) that is co-linear with genomic RNA. The *P* gene also encodes V and W proteins, produced from mRNA in which one and two nontemplated G residues, respectively, are inserted at the RNA editing site during transcription. The P, V, and W proteins, therefore, are identical for the first 405 amino acid residues. A C protein is encoded by the 5′ end of the gene in an overlapping reading frame and is produced by an internal translational initiation mechanism, which is common to other members of *Paramyxovirinae,* except for rubulaviruses.[76] The P, V, and the C proteins predicted from the coding regions in the *P* gene are present in HeV-infected cells.[146] The functional expression of W in NiV-infected cells has recently been demonstrated.[84]

Paramyxovirus N, P, and L proteins are necessary and sufficient for replication of viral RNA both *in vitro* and *in vivo,*[76] and this has been confirmed for henipaviruses by reverse genetics. Using a minigenome replicon containing leader and trailer sequences of the NiV genome with its entire coding region replaced with a reporter gene, it was shown that efficient genome replication was achieved only when all three proteins were expressed in the same cell.[55] NiV N, P, and L proteins were also able to rescue a minigenome constructed from the leader and trailer sequences of the HeV genome, further demonstrating the close genetic relationship between the viruses.

The L protein of nonsegmented, negative-stranded RNA (NNR) viruses in the order *Mononegavirales* contains a highly conserved GDNQ motif, believed to be important for polymerase activity.[116] Henipaviruses were the first NNR viruses in which GDNQ was replaced by GDNE. It was speculated that this motif might be unique to paramyxoviruses with relatively large genomes[146,148]; however, the GDNE motif has since been found in the L protein of Mossman virus that has a genome length of 16,650 nt.[96]

The cell attachment proteins of the *Paramyxovirinae* display hemagglutination (H) and neuraminidase (N) activities in a predominantly genus-specific manner. Viruses in the genera *Respirovirus, Avulavirus,* and *Rubulavirus* possess both activities,[76] whereas viruses in the genus *Morbillivirus* do not behave uniformly and only some possess hemagglutination activity.[77] In contrast, henipavirus attachment proteins have neither of these activities[146,166]; rather, they utilize the host cell expressed ephrin-B2 and ephrin-B3 molecules as attachment and entry receptors.[11,13,105,106] Recent solution structures of the henipavirus G glycoprotein alone and in complex with the ephrin-B2 and ephrin-B3 receptors have revealed the details of the virus–host cell binding process, distinguishing it from other paramyxovirus receptor strategies.[20,21,163]

Proteolytic processing of paramyxovirus F proteins is essential for the generation of a fusogenic form of the protein. For most paramyxoviruses that generate systemic infections, cleavage is catalyzed by the cellular protease furin at a multibasic cleavage site.[76] Surprisingly, henipavirus F proteins are cleaved without the involvement of furin and, although cleavage occurs at a single basic residue—lysine for HeV and arginine for NiV[98]—activation of the NiV F protein does not require a basic amino acid at the cleavage site.[93] It has been shown that the lysosomal cysteine protease cathepsin L is responsible for the cleavage of the HeV F protein.[108] The cytoplasmic tails of henipavirus F proteins contain the endocytosis consensus motif YXX ø.[92,143] Endocytosis is required for cleavage activation of the F protein,[35,92] consistent with identification of cathepsin L as the enzyme responsible for cleavage.

Host Range

For most paramyxoviruses, host range is limited and interspecies transmission is rare. In contrast, henipaviruses display a broad species tropism. In addition to at least three flying fox species, two nonpteropid fruit bat species, and an insectivorous species, NiV has naturally infected pigs, humans, dogs, horses, and cats,[29,63,97,120,164] whereas HeV infects four Australian flying fox species and has naturally infected humans and horses.[42,104] Confirmation of the wide host range of henipaviruses and the identical cell tropism of HeV and NiV were obtained early using an *in vitro* cell fusion system that relies on vaccinia virus–mediated cell surface expression of G and F glycoproteins.[17,18,136] Guinea pigs, hamsters, ferrets, squirrel monkeys, and African green monkeys are also susceptible to experimental NiV infection.[19,46,88,94,157] Laboratory studies have added cats, guinea pigs, hamsters, and African green monkeys to the list of HeV-susceptible species,[53,121,151,156] along with ferrets (J. Pallister and L.-F. Wang, unpublished results).

PATHOGENESIS AND PATHOLOGY

Cell and Tissue Tropism

The primary site of NiV replication and the dynamics of virus spread in humans are unknown. However, the distribution and time of appearance of lesions throughout the vasculature and in the brain and lung in NiV encephalitis suggest that secondary infection probably arises via hematogenous spread of the virus, with secondary replication occurring in vascular endothelium.[159] Inflammation of blood vessels occurs in most organs but is particularly prominent in the brain, lung, heart, and kidney.[30,159,160] Vasculitis is limited to small arteries, arterioles, and capillaries where NiV antigen is found in both endothelial cells and the smooth muscle of the tunica media. The pattern and time of appearance of vasculitis and viral antigen distribution are consistent with endothelial cell infection occurring before infection of the smooth muscle. Syncytial endothelial cells are present in blood vessels of various organs and represent a pathognomonic but insensitive feature of henipavirus infections found in only 25% of human NiV infections.[159] Syncytial endothelial cells were also observed in the single human case of encephalitis caused by HeV.[107] NiV antigen is also found in neurons and, less frequently, in bronchiolar and renal epithelial cells. The 5-day interval between maximal vasculitis in the brain and parenchymal infection in acute NiV encephalitis suggests that primary virus replication occurs in endothelial cells, with infection of neurons occurring as a result of vascular damage. The presence of inclusion bodies and viral antigen in neurons suggests that neurologic impairment in encephalitis may be caused by both the effects of ischemia and infarction and viral infection of neurons.[30,114,159] Human HeV encephalitis has been described as widespread cortical, subcortical, and deep white matter involvement in two cases in 2008[115] and similar to those described in a previous HeV encephalitis case[82,107] and NiV encephalitis cases.[82,127]

Although NiV antigen is found less frequently in bronchiolar and renal epithelial cells compared with vascular and neuronal locations, replication in epithelial locations may play a role in virus dissemination, because NiV is found in urine and in tracheal and nasopharyngeal secretions of infected patients in the early phase of their illness.[31,48] Despite this, human-to-human transmission in Malaysia was extremely rare.[100]

The identification of ephrin-B2 and ephrin-B3 as functional receptors for henipaviruses in cultured cells provides an explanation for the observed distribution of viral antigen in arterial endothelial cells, smooth muscle, neurons, and some epithelial cells.[11,13,105,106] Ephrin-B2 is found in arteries, arterioles, capillaries in multiple organs, and tissues including arterial smooth muscle and human bronchiolar epithelial cells[135] but is absent from venous components of the vasculature.[45] Ephrin-B3 is found predominantly in the nervous system as well as the vasculature.[113] The ephrins engage Eph receptors and mediate bidirectional cell–cell signaling events and are modulators of cell remodeling events, especially within the nervous and vascular systems.[113]

Immune Response

In patients with encephalitis, anti-NiV antibodies were observed more frequently in the serum than the CSF. Immunoglobulin M (IgM) antibodies occurred more frequently than immunoglobulin G (IgG) antibodies in both locations.[30,114,159] The appearance of specific IgM antibodies in serum preceded their appearance in the CSF, a sequence consistent with viremia preceding central nervous system (CNS) infection. Anti-NiV antibodies were present in most patients with clinical NiV encephalitis; however, no difference was observed in clinical features, laboratory results, or mortality between seropositive and seronegative patients.[27,48] Seroconversion of IgG against HeV was seen in two human cases of HeV infection, one fatal, in 2008,[115] following an influenza-like illnesses and before progressing to encephalitis.

Inhibition of the Interferon Response

In henipaviruses, as in other paramyxoviruses,[66] anti-interferon (IFN) activities are encoded by the *P* gene and *in vitro* studies indicate that *P* gene products inhibit both IFN induction and signaling.[37] In IFN induction, viral double-stranded RNA (dsRNA) is detected by intracellular RNA helicase enzymes[3,79] and by toll-like receptor 3 (TLR-3).[12] Both of these dsRNA signaling pathways lead to activation of the pre-existing transcription factors interferon regulatory factor 3 (IRF-3) and nuclear factor kappa B (NF-kB),[50] and the synthesis of IFN-α and a subset of IFN-β proteins.[89] HeV inhibits dsRNA signaling by using a strategy adopted by other paramyxoviruses in which the V protein binds to the intracellular RNA helicase sensor and prevents downstream signaling[3] but does not abrogate dsRNA signaling through TLR-3.[132] In an additional strategy unique to henipaviruses, the W protein, by virtue of a nuclear localization signal located in the unique carboxy terminal, inhibits dsRNA signaling in the nucleus by targeting a process that is part of both helicase-dependent and TLR-3–dependent signaling pathways.[132]

In the IFN signaling pathway, IFN binds to cell surface receptors in a paracrine manner and initiates a signaling sequence that leads to activation of members of a family of proteins called *signal transducers and activators of transcription* (STAT).[1,50] Henipaviruses inhibit IFN signaling by sequestering STAT proteins in high molecular weight complexes.[123,124] The anti-IFN signaling activity is a property of the V protein, as has been observed for other paramyxoviruses, but also of the W and P proteins.[123,124,133] The P, V, and W proteins of henipaviruses have an N-terminal extension of 100 to 200 amino acids compared with cognate proteins in the subfamily,[59,147] and the STAT binding domain of NiV V maps to this region.[122] The V and P proteins bind STAT in the cytoplasm, whereas the W protein, with its nuclear localization signal, co-localizes with STAT in the nucleus.[132,133] The W protein is the most and P protein the least efficient IFN antagonist.[112] The NiV

C protein also displays a modest inhibition of IFN signaling, although the mechanism and target are unknown.[112]

It should be noted that most, if not all, studies described previously were carried out *in vitro* using single-gene transfection expression systems. A recent study conducted using live virus infection indicated that IFN signaling remains functional during henipavirus infection of human cell lines, whereas IFN production was inhibited.[142]

Infections of Animals

Only limited data are available on the minimal lethal and infectious doses of henipaviruses. In golden hamsters (*Mesocricetus auratus*), the NiV lethal dose 50% (LD_{50}) following intraperitoneal and intranasal administration was 270 and 47,000 plaque-forming units (pfu), respectively,[157] and was calculated to be 12 pfu for HeV by intraperitoneal injection.[53] The NiV minimal infectious dose in hamsters is 100 pfu if the intraperitoneal route is used and 10^3 pfu if the virus is administered intranasally. Guinea pigs and pigs are also more resistant to infection by HeV and NiV, respectively, when the viruses are administered by the oronasal route compared with the subcutaneous route.[95,154] In contrast, both HeV and NiV appear to be equally infectious for cats following either parenteral (5,000 tissue culture infectious dose 50% [$TCID_{50}$] virus) or oronasal (50,000 $TCID_{50}$ virus) administration.[64,91,95,101,151]

Experimental infection of horses with HeV by parenteral or oronasal routes is almost uniformly fatal, with death or euthanasia usually occurring 5 to 10 days after infection. Several horses in the original outbreak in Hendra survived infection, however, some asymptomatically.[103,104,156] In horses, HeV displays a predominantly respiratory tropism, and infection is characterized by pulmonary edema and congestion.[64,104,156] In field cases, the airways are often filled with a blood-tinged frothy exudate. Neurologic signs do exist, but they have been observed infrequently in terminally ill horses and in horses that recovered from respiratory infection.[125,156] Infection is associated with virus replication and with the appearance of viral antigen in endothelial cells in a wide variety of organs, including lungs, lymph nodes, kidneys, spleen, bladder, and meninges. The subsequent degeneration of small blood vessels is accompanied by the appearance of syncytial endothelial cells.[63] Virus can be recovered from several internal organs, including lung, and from saliva and urine.[64,156]

In contrast, NiV infection of pigs is frequently asymptomatic, particularly following natural infection and after experimental administration of the virus by the ocular and oronasal route.[95,97,150] When symptoms are present, they vary according to the age of the pig, with older animals presenting primarily with a neurologic syndrome, whereas a respiratory syndrome predominates in young animals. The virus manifests respiratory and neurologic tropisms in both asymptomatic and clinical infections.[95,149] Neurologic signs include trembling and neurologic twitches, muscle spasms, and uncoordinated gait.[97] After experimental NiV infection of young pigs by the ocular and oronasal routes, virus replication occurs in the oropharynx and spreads sequentially to the upper respiratory tract and submandibular lymph nodes, the lower respiratory tract, and additional lymphoid tissues.[149] Here, viral antigen is widespread and syncytia are common in clinically affected animals as a result of replication in the endothelial and smooth muscle cells of medium to large veins as well as in the arteries of the central nervous, lymphoid, and respiratory systems.[63,95,149] NiV invades the CNS via the cranial nerves and by crossing the blood–brain barrier.[149] Virus is recovered from a range of tissues, including tonsil, nasal, and throat swabs and lung, but is recovered infrequently from urine.[34,95,149] Experimental HeV infection of pigs (Landrace and Gottingen minipig breeds) via oronasal or nasal inoculations has shown both to be susceptible to infection,[80] with virus detected mainly in tissues from respiratory and lymphoid systems, and could be isolated from nasal, oral, and rectal swabs, indicating the possible routes for virus shedding.

Laboratory Animal Models

In hamsters, the pathologic features following NiV infection resemble those found in humans.[157] Hamsters die 5 to 9 days after intraperitoneal administration of 100 to 10,000 infectious particles and 24 hours after the appearance of tremors and limb paralysis. In contrast, hamsters inoculated intranasally with doses as high as 10^3 to 10^6 infectious particles die between 9 and 15 days later, displaying progressive deterioration with limb paralysis, lethargy, limb twitching, and breathing difficulties. Vascular pathology is observed in a range of organs, including brain, lung, liver, kidney, and heart, and viral antigen and genome are found in endothelial cells. The brain is the most severely affected organ, with the vascular and parenchyma lesions consistent with CNS-mediated clinical signs.[159] HeV infection of hamsters also resembled the pathology seen in acute human cases, including both respiratory and brain pathology.[53] HeV-induced pathology in the hamster was similar to that of NiV[157] and consisted of endothelial infection and vasculitis with thrombosis and microinfarction, with evidence of direct parenchymal cell infection, notably in the CNS.

In cats, the first clinical signs, which are observed on days 4 to 8 after parenteral or oronasal administration of HeV and NiV, include depression, fever, and an increased rate of respiration.[65,101,151,152] Most infected animals die 1 day after the appearance of respiratory distress. The disease caused by HeV and NiV in cats closely resembles that seen in HeV-infected horses, with copious frothy sanguineous fluid in the bronchi and hemorrhage or congestion of the tracheal epithelium.[64] Vaculitis affects both arteries and arterioles, and syncytial cells are observed in endothelia, predominantly in the lungs but also in gastrointestinal, spleen, and lymphoid organs. A major difference between NiV and HeV infection of cats is the extensive degree to which NiV, but not HeV, infects the respiratory epithelium.[95] Henipaviruses are found in the urine and bladder of experimentally infected cats, and NiV can transplacentally infect and replicate in fetal tissues with high levels of recoverable virus from the placenta and uterine fluid.[102]

In guinea pigs, the clinical response to henipavirus infection is frequently mild and often variable, ranging from inapparent to sudden death, with only a proportion of animals displaying signs such as transient weight loss, depression, ataxia, lethargy, and twitching.[154,157] The vascular tropism of HeV in guinea pigs is evident in many organs.[65] Death appears to result from vascular disease in a variety of organs.[65] Only a proportion of infected animals develop encephalitis with virus observed in blood vessels and neurons.[154]

A ferret model of henipavirus infection and pathogenesis has also been developed.[19,110] The ferret exhibits both severe respiratory and neurologic disease as well as generalized vasculitis following an oronasal challenge with NiV with doses as low as 500 $TCID_{50}$ within 6 to 10 days postinfection. Clinical signs in affected ferrets included various combinations of severe depression, cough, serous nasal discharge, dyspnea, subcutaneous edema of the head, cutaneous ecchymoses, and obtundation with tremor and hind limb paresis depending on the challenge dose. Clinical disease in the ferret included vascular fibrinoid necrosis in multiple organs, necrotizing alveolitis, and syncytia of endothelium and alveolar epithelium. Histopathologic lesions included severe focal necrotizing alveolitis, vasculitis, degeneration of glomerular tufts, and focal necrosis in a wide range of other tissues. High levels of viral antigen were noted in blood vessel walls, and syncytial cells were frequently present. Viral antigen was present in neurons, and infectious NiV was isolated from multiple organs including the brain. Overall, NiV-mediated disease observed in the ferret model manifested with all the hallmarks seen among NiV-infected humans, and essentially identical results have been observed with HeV infection of ferrets (J. Pallister and L.-F. Wang, unpublished results).

A nonhuman primate model of henipavirus infection has been developed using the African green monkey,[46,121] which yields a uniformly lethal disease with doses as low as approximately 2×10^4 pfu (NiV) or 4×10^5 $TCID_{50}$ of HeV. Monkeys, following intratracheal inoculation with either NiV or HeV, reveal a rapid spread of the virus (3–4 days postinfection) to numerous organ systems. NiV-infected monkeys developed a severe acute respiratory distress syndrome (ARDS)-like disease, associated with copious amounts of sanguineous fluid and froth. The lungs are enlarged with multifocal areas of congestion and hemorrhage, and immunohistochemical and histopathologic examination revealed significant amounts of polymerized fibrin and NiV antigen.[46] Endothelial syncytial cells were prominent in most of the tissues, and vasculitis was widespread. NiV antigen was present in endothelial and arterial smooth muscle cells in most examined tissues. Respiratory disease development could be seen within 7 days postinfection with either NiV or HeV following intratracheal inoculation by radiologic examination[46,121] progressing to severe congestion and infiltration in the lung fields.

NiV and HeV could be found in virtually every organ system sampled at the time of death in the African green monkey. Immunohistochemical and histopathologic analysis revealed the presence of NiV antigen, predominantly in endothelial cells and smooth muscle cells, along with associated pathology. Most animals showed evidence of henipavirus-induced neurologic disease,[46,121] with severe congestion and evidence of meningeal hemorrhaging and edema. NiV and HeV antigen was detected in endothelial cells in brain, with infection of neurons often widespread in the brain stem.[46,121] NiV infection of squirrel monkeys has also been examined.[88] Although some animals demonstrated limited similarities to NiV pathogenesis in humans, only 50% of challenged animals exhibited any clinical signs, with most remaining well even following intranasal or intravenous delivery of doses as high as 10^7 pfu of NiV.

Unlike the cat, guinea pig, hamster, and squirrel monkey models of NiV or HeV infection, severe respiratory pathology, neurologic disease, and generalized vasculitis all occur in henipavirus-infected African green monkeys, providing an accurate reflection of what is observed in henipavirus-infected humans.

EPIDEMIOLOGY

Age

The age of patients with encephalitis in the Malaysian outbreak ranged from 9 to 76 years, with almost 50% of cases occurring in those 40 to 44 years.[27,28,48,111,159] The male-to-female ratio was approximately 3:1, and more than 80% of the patients were Chinese, with statistics reflecting the increased risk to those working with infected pigs.[48,111] In Bangladesh, the age of patients ranged from 4 to 60 years, and males constituted 47% and 67% of the cases in the 2001 and 2003 outbreaks, respectively.[43,68] The recent outbreak in early 2011 in Bangladesh claimed at least 35 lives, including many children and infants, with ages ranging from 2 to 56 years.[8]

Morbidity and Mortality

In Malaysia, between September 1998 and June 1999, 256 patients who developed acute NiV encephalitis were admitted to Malaysian hospitals and 105 died, a mortality rate of approximately 40%.[30,111] The rate of subclinical infection in households and farms where cases of NiV encephalitis occurred was calculated to be 8% and 11%, respectively.[111,139] In Singapore, where 11 patients were confirmed to have acute NiV encephalitis, a further 2 asymptomatic abattoir workers were serologically positive, representing a rate of subclinical infection of 15%.[25] Subsequently, 89 individuals were identified on the basis of positive serology as having experienced either an asymptomatic or mildly symptomatic NiV infection.[138] This increases the number of people infected with NiV to 345 and decreases the mortality rate to approximately 30%.[160] In Bangladesh, 98 of 135 patients died in eight outbreaks from 2001 to 2008, giving a combined case fatality rate of 73%.[43,62,85] There have only been seven known human cases of HeV infection in Australia in the past 16 years, four of which have been fatal (three acute and one case of relapsed encephalitis).[6,104,107,115]

Origin and Spread of Epidemics

Fruit bats (flying foxes) in the genus *Pteropus,* family *Pteropodidae,* suborder *Megachiroptera* are main reservoir hosts of HeV and NiV.[33,56,164,165] In Australia, HeV has been shown to occur in four flying fox species, with the crude seroprevalence of 47%, indicating an endemic pattern of infection throughout Australia.[42] Serologic tests show that NiV is widely dispersed in pteropid bats in Malaysia, especially the Island flying fox (*Pteropus hypomelanus*) and the Malayan flying fox (*Pteropus vampyrus*).[164] NiV was first isolated from the urine of Island flying foxes and from the saliva on partially eaten fruit[33] and has since been isolated from Lyle's flying foxes (*Pteropus lylei*) in Cambodia.[120] The Indian flying fox (*Pteropus giganteus*) is the only pteropid species throughout Bangladesh and the Indian subcontinent with a high seroprevelence of henipavirus-specific antibody.[39,68,86,87] Additional serologic and limited nucleic acid evidence has suggested that related henipaviruses are circulating in other regions, including Thailand, Indonesia, China, Madigascar, and West Africa.[36,61,70,81,131,145]

Neither HeV nor NiV appear to cause clinical disease in flying foxes infected naturally,[42,43,119,164] and experimental infection with doses of HeV, consistently shown to be lethal in horses, generates only sporadic vasculitis in the lung, spleen, meninges, kidney, and gastrointestinal tract and only in a proportion of infected bats.[156] Viral antigen is detected in the tunica media rather than endothelial cells, a fact that may spare the flying fox from the clinical effects associated with vasculitis.[37] In infected pregnant flying foxes, antigen was observed in similar locations and in the placenta.[155] The mode of transmission between flying foxes is unknown. Transplacental transmission has also been observed experimentally without apparent harm to the fetus.[155] Experimental infection of flying foxes with NiV produced a subclinical infection with a transient presence of virus within selected viscera along with periodic viral excretion in bat urine and seroconversion with neutralizing antibody present.[94]

The spillover and epidemic hosts of HeV and NiV were horses in Australia and pigs in Malaysia. All human infections with HeV in Australia and NiV in Malaysia have only occurred through transmission from these domestic animal hosts.[30,111] No evidence exists of direct transmission from pteropid bats to humans in Australia or Malaysia, despite many opportunities in Australia for transmission to bat carers.[127,129] In contrast, flying foxes apparently play a direct role in the transmission of NiV to humans in the many recent outbreaks of disease in Bangladesh, where epidemiologic evidence in support of a role for pigs was lacking.[43,68] Three pathways of NiV transmission from bats to people have been identified based on epidemiologic investigations in Bangladesh.[85] Consumption of fresh date palm sap appears to be the predominant risk factor, and infrared camera studies have confirmed that *P. giganteus* bats frequently visit date palm sap trees and consume sap during collection.[126] In the 2005 NiV outbreak in Tangail District, Bangladesh, drinking raw date palm sap was the only activity significantly associated with illness (64% among cases vs. 18% among controls).[87] Another route of transmission for NiV from bats to people in Bangladesh could be via domestic animals. Contact with a sick cow in Meherpur, Bangladesh, in 2001 was strongly associated with NiV infection,[68] and contact with pigs and diseased goats have also been implicated in other occurrences of NiV in Bangladesh.[85] Transmission via direct contact with NiV-infected bat secretions also appears possible from evidence in the Goalando outbreak in 2004, where individuals who climbed trees were more likely to develop NiV infection than controls.[99]

The mode of transmission from bats to spillover hosts in Australia and Malaysia remains to be determined. Three principal hypotheses exist. One is that masticated pellets of virus-contaminated, residual fruit pulp spat out by flying foxes are ingested by horses or pigs.[164] The second is that urine from infected animals contaminates pastures or pigsties. The third is that infected fetal tissues or fluids contaminate pastures or sties and are ingested. The latter is based largely on the fact that the HeV outbreaks have occurred during the birthing period of some species of flying fox and is supported by the isolation of virus from a pregnant flying fox and its fetus.[56]

HeV has been transmitted from horse to man on seven occasions from 1994 to 2009, twice during the initial outbreak in Brisbane,[4] twice during necropsy of horses that died in the field,[125,130] twice during either daily nasal cavity lavage and participating in a necropsy,[115] and once from performing an endoscopy on an infected horse.[6] HeV is rarely found in the bronchi or bronchioles of infected horses, which suggests that aerosol transmission to either man or horses is less likely[64] and horse-to-horse transmission of HeV has not been demonstrated.[156] The presence of HeV in equine saliva, however, suggests that close contact with infected horses, such as might occur during manual feeding of the animals, may facilitate horse-to-human transmission.[130] The presence of virus in a wide range of tissues and in the nasal discharge commonly found at the terminal stage of infection offers a range of sources for virus transmission during necropsy.[103,104] As shown in Figure 37.5A, high level of viral antigen can be detected in the nasal cavity of HeV-infected horses.

In the Malaysian NiV outbreak, contact with pigs or fresh pig products was required for transmission of the virus to humans, with greater likelihood of transfer to those in direct contact with sick or dying pigs on farms or in abattoirs.[30,111] The presence of NiV in the respiratory epithelium of naturally and experimentally infected pigs (Fig. 37.5B) indicated that

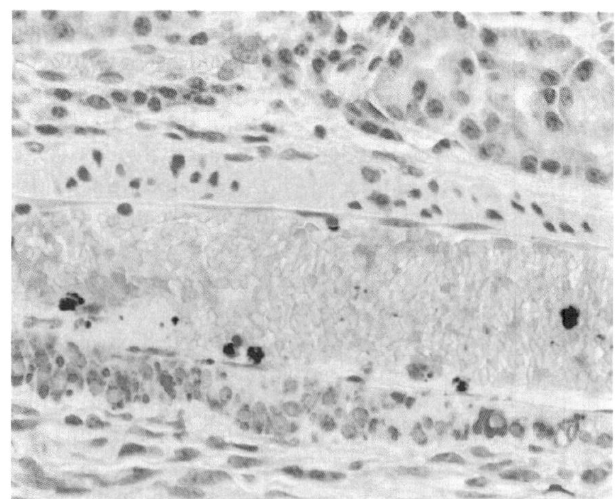

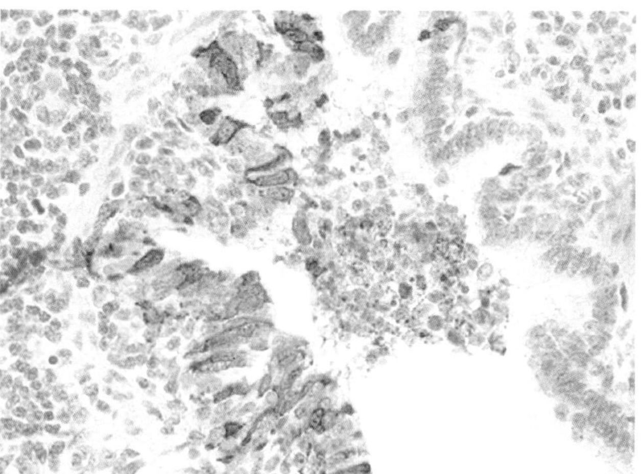

FIGURE 37.5. Immunoperoxidase detection of viral antigen in henipavirus-infected tissues. A: Staining of Hendra virus (HeV) antigen (N protein-specific antibody) within the wall of superficial arteriole in the submucosa of the nasal cavity in a HeV-infected horse. **B:** Immunolabeling (using anti–Nipah virus rabbit serum) within the lung of a pig infected with Nipah virus. Involvement of bronchial epithelium and airway debris is noted. (Courtesy of Dr. Deborah Middleton, CSIRO Australian Animal Health Laboratory.)

virus probably spread to humans and within the pig population by aerosol or by direct contact with oropharyngeal or nasal secretions.[95,97,149] The presence of the virus in a wide range of organs indicates that humans may also have been infected during processes such as slaughtering or farrowing. In Bangladesh, pigs were excluded as potential sources of NiV on epidemiolog grounds, and human-to-human transmission was observed.[54,62] The virus may have been transmitted to human index cases directly through contact with fruit bat secretions in contaminated fruit or date palm sap before circulation in the human population.[33,43,68,85] Nosocomial transmission has been detected in some of the Bangladesh and India outbreaks.[9,23,85]

CLINICAL FEATURES

Incubation Period

Based on the time interval between the last exposure to pigs and onset of disease, the incubation period for NiV ranged from 2 to 45 days; however, for 90% of patients, it was 2 weeks or less.[27,28,48] An estimate of 2 to 3 weeks was made based on the time interval between importation of pigs from NiV-affected areas of Malaysia and development of human disease at a Singaporean abattoir.[25] A mean incubation period of 9.4 days was calculated for four patients who had a fixed period of exposure.[27] In the occurrence of HeV in Australia in 2008, a detailed examination of exposure histories from two infected patients (one fatal) suggested a likely incubation period of 9 to 16 days, with exposure occurring some 3 days before the onset of symptoms of HeV infection in the horse.[115]

Acute Clinical Features

The first two patients infected with HeV presented with myalgia, headaches, lethargy, and vertigo. One patient recovered; however, the other developed pneumonitis, respiratory failure, renal failure, and arterial thrombosis, and died of cardiac arrest 7 days after admission to the hospital. Findings at autopsy were consistent with a viral infection; both lungs were congested, hemorrhagic, and filled with serous fluid, and the histology revealed focal necrotizing alveolitis with many giant cells, some syncytial formation, and viral inclusions.[130] A third case of HeV infection presented first with meningitis and a 12-day history of sore throat, headache, drowsiness, vomiting, and neck stiffness. After an apparent full recovery, this patient developed fatal encephalitis 13 months later and was admitted to the hospital with a generalized tonic-clonic seizure after 2 weeks of irritable mood and low back pain. Recurrent focal motor seizures occurred over the next 7 days, as did secondarily generalized seizures and low-grade fever, followed by dense right hemiplegia, signs of brain stem involvement, and depressed consciousness requiring intubation. The patient remained comatose and died 25 days after admission.[107] Two patients in 2008[115] presented with initial influenza-like illness, although soon after apparent clinical improvement and an absence of fever, encephalitis developed in both. Magnetic resonance imaging (MRI) revealed widespread cortical, subcortical, and deep white matter involvement, similar to the previous late-onset case of HeV encephalitis[107] and to NiV encephalitis cases.[78,127]

With NiV, the mean duration of illness from the onset of symptoms to the nadir was 3 to 31 days, with an average of 6.9 days.[48] Most patients presented with acute encephalitis characterized by fever, headache, drowsiness, dizziness, myalgia, and vomiting, and more than 50% had a reduced level of consciousness.[27,30,48,114] The major clinical signs included drowsiness, areflexia, segmental myoclonus, tachycardia, hypertension, pinpoint pupils, and an abnormal doll's eye reflex. Such clinical features as these suggested involvement of the brain stem and upper cervical spinal cord, and were observed more frequently in patients with a reduced level of consciousness.[48,139] Patients who retained normal levels of consciousness throughout their illness recovered fully; however, only 15% with reduced levels of consciousness survived. Such neurologic manifestations are consistent with vasculitis-induced thrombosis in the brain and the direct infection of neurons.[29,30,114,159] The multiple discrete lesions 1 to 5 mm in diameter in the cerebral white matter detected by MRI may be the site of such microinfarctions and are distinct from lesions caused by other viruses.[30,82,114,127,159] Although the predominant clinical features of NiV encephalitis derive from CNS involvement, a proportion of patients displayed pulmonary involvement, which presented as an atypical pneumonia with fever, cough, and headache.[27,48,114] The clinical presentation of NiV infections in Bangladesh is also predominantly a severe respiratory disease.[67]

Outcome of Infection

Most patients who survived acute NiV encephalitis made a full recovery; however, approximately 20% had residual neurologic deficits.[27,48,83] Neurologic sequelae included cognitive difficulties, tetraparesis, cerebellar signs, nerve palsies, and clinical depression. A few patients remained in a vegetative state. In patients with encephalitis who recovered, most brain lesions revealed by MRI disappeared or became smaller over a period of 12 to 18 months, although some remained unchanged during this period.[83] Approximately 7.5% of patients who recovered from acute encephalitis and 3.4% of those who experienced nonencephalitic or asymptomatic infection developed late neurologic disease.[48,127,138,161] Relapse encephalitis and late-onset encephalitis presented several months to 4 years after the initial infection. Relapsed cases had elevated IgG, but not IgM, and no vasculitis, and unlike the situation in acute encephalitis, virus was not isolated from throat and nasal secretions.[30–32,127,159,161]

The clinical features associated with relapse and late-onset encephalitis resembled those found with acute NiV encephalitis, although decreased incidence was seen of fever, coma, segmental myoclonus, and meningism and an increased occurrence of seizures and focal cortical signs compared with the acute manifestation of the disease.[138] The clinical, radiologic, and pathologic features of relapse NiV encephalitis resembled those of the patient who became infected with HeV, suffered mild, transient aseptic meningitis, and recovered but died of a fatal meningoencephalitis 13 months later.[107,158] Most patients with relapse and late-onset encephalitis had only one neurologic episode, although some patients experienced two episodes separated by a mean of 7.6 months (6 weeks to 1 year).[138] The mortality rate associated with relapse and late-onset encephalitis at 18% was lower than that associated with acute encephalitis, at 30% to 40%. However, 61% of patients with relapse and late onset had further neurologic sequelae compared with 22% after acute encephalitis. Among NiV survivors in Bangladesh, some 30% have moderate to severe persistent neurologic dysfunction for years following acute infection.[128]

The demographics, clinical features, serology, and MRI of patients with relapsed and late-onset encephalitis were similar, suggesting that the two diseases have identical pathogenesis[138] and that the initial infection in late-onset encephalitis patients may not have been sufficiently severe to cause neurologic symptoms. MRI abnormalities similar to those observed in patients with acute encephalitis were also seen in 16% of asymptomatic patients, although the lesions were fewer in number.[139] The involvement of the cortex in relapse and late-onset encephalitis suggests a different pathologic mechanism compared with acute encephalitis. Relapse and late-onset encephalitis are considered to be caused by the recrudescence and rapid replication of virus that had persisted following acute or asymptomatic NiV infection.[138] NiV, however, was not isolated from CSF and brain tissue of patients with relapse and late-onset encephalitis.[138]

DIAGNOSIS

Laboratory Diagnosis

Virus isolation, EM, immuno-EM, immunohistochemistry (IHC), serology, and polymerase chain reaction (PCR) played key roles in the initial discovery of HeV[104] and NiV,[29] and they remain essential elements in a repertoire of procedures for the rapid and specific diagnosis of henipavirus infections in humans and animals.

During investigation of a suspected disease outbreak, attempts to grow henipaviruses may be initiated in a BSL3 laboratory. However, if a cytopathic effect (CPE) is observed and the growth of henipavirus is confirmed by PCR or immune staining, infected cultures should be handled under BSL4 conditions and subsequent work with live virus restricted to BSL4. Both HeV and NiV replicate in various cell lines—a feature that contributed to the efficiency with which they were isolated during the initial disease outbreak investigations.[29,104] Vero cells are commonly used, generating titers of virus as high as 10^8 infectious virions per milliliter.[28,34] In fatal cases, attempts should be made to isolate virus from brain, lung, kidney, and spleen.[34] For tissue specimens containing a high virus load, direct examination by immuno-EM and IHC can be very useful in providing early diagnosis. Various antibody reagents have been developed for this purpose, including polyclonal antisera, monospecific antibodies raised against recombinant antigens,[147] and monoclonal antibodies (mAb) raised against whole virions or vaccinia virus–expressed viral proteins.[71,140,141,153] Using HeV- or NiV-specific mAb, it is possible to differentiate between the two viruses.[141,153] Quantitative real-time PCR (TaqMan assay) has been the method of choice to detect viral materials in infected tissues because of its speed, specificity, and sensitivity. The first-generation henipavirus TaqMan assays are either HeV specific[134] or NiV specific.[52] Recently, several consensus henipavirus real-time PCR assays have been developed that target different conserved regions of the viral genome.[41] It should be cautioned that the current PCR tests may not work with new henipaviruses yet to be discovered, especially those from African bats, owing to expected greater genetic divergence than those detected in Australia and Asia.

For henipaviruses, serologic tests are important both during outbreak investigation and for disease surveillance. The virus neutralization test (VNT) is accepted as the reference standard.[34] Few laboratories, however, can conduct neutralization tests because of the requirement to handle live virus at BSL4. For surveillance and diagnostic purposes, three types of tests that do not require BSL4 containment have been developed:

1. *Enzyme-linked immunosorbent assay (ELISA):* Several ELISA-based tests have been reported for the detection of henipavirus antibodies.[34,40,73] For diagnosis of human infections, two different ELISA tests have been applied: an IgM capture ELISA for early diagnosis of infection and an indirect ELISA for detection of IgG antibodies.[34]
2. *Liquid protein array multiplex test:* A Luminex-based test based on recombinant soluble G proteins of HeV and NiV was developed that is capable of mimicking VNT with great sensitivity and differentiating between antibody responses of HeV versus NiV infection.[15]
3. *Pseudotype virus:* Different pseudotype systems carrying the henipavirus F and G proteins have been developed as a surrogate VNT for detecting henipavirus-specific antibodies.[72,74,137] Incorporation of reporter genes in these systems resulted in greater sensitivity and reproducibility.[72,137]

PREVENTION AND CONTROL

Treatment

Ribavirin, which inhibits replication of HeV *in vitro,*[162] was used during the NiV outbreak in Malaysia in an open-label study in which 140 patients with encephalitis were given the drug, and 54 patients who presented before ribavirin became available or who refused treatment acted as controls.[26] Mortality in the treated group was 32% compared with 54% in the control group, representing a 35% reduction ($P = 0.011$). Duration of ventilation and total hospital stay were both significantly shorter in the ribavirin group ($P = 0.0002$ and <0.0001, respectively). In the absence of other therapies, ribavirin may be an option for treatment of henipavirus infections. However, two HeV-infected patients in 2008[115] were given a high-dose intravenous regimen of ribavirin, although basal concentrations appeared inadequate given the results of *in vitro* susceptibility testing of HeV, and the efficacy of ribavirin as therapy or prophylaxis in people remains at best uncertain. Chloroquine, an antimalarial drug, was first demonstrated to block the critical proteolytic processing needed for HeV F maturation and function.[109] Not surprisingly, the drug was later shown to inhibit NiV and HeV infection in cell culture experiments.[117] Chloroquine was administered along with ribavirin to one HeV-infected individual in 2009[6] with no apparent clinical benefit.

In vivo, ribavirin only delayed but did not prevent deaths caused by NiV and had no effect on HeV infection in a hamster model.[44,47] Ribavirin treatment also only delayed disease onset by 1 to 2 days in African green monkeys challenged with HeV with no significant benefit for disease progression or outcome.[121] Chloroquine administration, either alone or in combination with ribavirin, had no therapeutic benefit in ferrets challenged with NiV or hamsters challenged with either NiV or HeV.[44,110]

Vaccines and Passive Immunotherapy

No henipavirus vaccines are available at this time; however, studies suggest that vaccination may offer several viable anti-henipavirus strategies.[22,38] NiV F and G glycoproteins expressed from vaccinia virus elicit neutralizing antibodies in mice and hamsters,[51,136] with higher antibody titers generated in response to the G glycoprotein compared with the F glycoprotein. Hamsters were protected from lethal challenge with NiV following vaccination with vaccinia virus expressing either NiV F or G glycoprotein.[51] The challenge virus was capable of hyperimmunizing vaccinated animals, indicating that although the virus replicated, the presence of neutralizing antibodies ameliorated replication to an extent that limited infection and prevented clinical disease. Further, the protection afforded hamsters by passive transfer of anti-G and anti-F antibodies before a lethal NiV or HeV challenge confirmed both the importance of a humoral protective immune response to NiV.[51,53]

HeV G glycoprotein has been expressed in a soluble form (sG-HeV) that retains many native characteristics and can elicit a potent cross-reactive neutralizing antibody response in rabbits.[14] Rabbit anti-HeV G antibodies neutralize both HeV and NiV in cell culture, displaying a slightly higher titer against the homologous virus. The nature and location of the neutralizing epitopes on the F glycoprotein have not been reported, although preliminary information is available for the HeV G glycoprotein.[153] Four neutralizing epitopes have been mapped on the globular head of the HeV G protein. Two are located on the base of the head and two on the top, in locations resembling those identified as neutralizing sites in other paramyxoviruses.

Immunization and challenge studies using recombinant sG-HeV in the cat model have demonstrated that the protein can illicit a completely protective immune response against NiV challenge,[101] even at a low-dose formulation with CpG and Alhydrogel and a two-dose protocol followed by oronasal challenge with 50,000 $TCID_{50}$ of NiV.[91] Further sG-HeV immunization studies have been completed in the ferret with a HeV challenge (J. Pallister and L-F. Wang, in submission) and in the African green monkey with a NiV challenge (T. Geisbert and C. Broder, in submission). In both of these investigations, complete protection from henipavirus-induced disease was achieved. The potential application of sG-HeV as an equine vaccine is being evaluated in Australia (D. Middleton, personal communication). These data suggest that a single vaccine (sG-HeV) may be effective against both HeV and NiV. Analysis of the antibody responses in sera from naturally infected or immunized sources has also shown that HeV-infected sources had high levels of NiV G cross-reactive antibodies, whereas NiV-infected individuals had limited cross-reactive antibodies to HeV G. Together, these data suggested that the HeV G stimulates a more cross-reactive immune response.[15]

The sG-HeV glycoprotein was also used to isolate HeV G-specific human mAbs. One human mAb (m102.4) was HeV and NiV cross-reactive and possessed extremely potent virus neutralizing activity.[167,168] *In vivo* studies have demonstrated that m102.4 can protect animals from a lethal challenge with henipavirus as a postexposure application in the ferret model with NiV[19] and in the African green monkey model with HeV (T. Geisbert and C. Broder, in submission). In August 2009, m102.4 was used on a compassionate basis to save the life of an HeV-infected individual while in a coma (G. Playford, personal communication). Unfortunately, delivery and intravenous administration of only 100 mg of available antibody occurred after the onset of encephalitis, and the individual died shortly thereafter. During the 2010 HeV emergence, 11 people had potential exposure and 2 individuals considered at high risk. In this instance, the m102.4 antibody was given to 2 individuals prior to HeV diagnosis or the onset of clinical disease[5] at doses sufficient to achieve a high serum concentration. Both individuals have remained healthy. Altogether, these findings highlight the therapeutic potential of antibody-based passive transfer modalities for treating henipavirus exposure.

Peptide Inhibitors

The first potential henipavirus-specific therapeutic was shown to be a heptad peptide-based fusion inhibitor[17] analogous to the human immunodeficiency virus type 1 (HIV-1)-specific peptide, enfuvirtide (Fuzeon) approved by the Food and Drug Administration (FDA) in March 2003. The henipavirus F_1 glycoprotein resembles other fusion glycoproteins in having α-helical heptad repeat (HR) domains proximal to both the fusion peptide at the amino (N) terminus and the transmembrane domain near the carboxy (C) terminus of the protein. The HR domains are involved in the formation of a trimer-of-hairpins structure during or immediately following the fusion of virus and cell membranes that occurs during infection. Addition of exogenous peptide from either HR domain blocks formation of the trimer-of-hairpins and abrogates membrane fusion and entry of the viral genome into the cell.[16,17,38] These observations were followed up with testing cholesterol tagged HR-derived peptides in the hamster model of NiV infection.[118] The *in vivo* efficacy of peptide fusion inhibitors of henipavirus infection merits further investigation.

PERSPECTIVE AND GEOGRAPHIC CONSIDERATIONS

The high virulence of the henipaviruses and the requirement for BSL4 facilities have hampered investigations into the biology and pathogenesis of these novel paramyxoviruses. Recent investigations into the structure and function of henipavirus proteins expressed from cloned genes have provided insight into the functions of many henipavirus proteins in infected cells. It remains to be determined if all of the functional characteristics of the henipavirus proteins determined *in vitro* accurately reflect the role that they play in the cells of both terrestrial and chiropteran hosts.

Many questions relating to the ecology and biology of henipaviruses remain unanswered. Little doubt exists that *Pteropus* species of fruit bats are the major reservoir host of these viruses. With the wide geographic range of *Pteropus* species as overlapping populations, extending from islands in the South Pacific through Australia, and southern Asia to Pakistan, and with additional species on islands off the eastern coast of Africa, together with the cross-reactive serologic evidence of henipavirus presence,[61,81] it would seem that several other related viruses may remain to be identified.[43,56] The emergence of these and related viruses is probably associated with the destruction of the flying fox native habitats, driving the animals to seek food from orchards and ornamental trees in urban and periurban areas. Thus, with continued deforestation, undoubtedly further outbreaks of HeV, NiV, and novel related members of the genus will occur. The mechanisms by which henipaviruses are transmitted between fruit bats and maintained within their colonies, as well as the pathways leading to the infection of spillover hosts, remain to be elucidated.

REFERENCES

1. Aaronson DS, Horvath CM. A road map for those who don't know JAK-STAT. *Science* 2002;296(5573):1653–1655.
2. AbuBakar S, Chang LY, Ali AR, et al. Isolation and molecular identification of Nipah virus from pigs. *Emerg Infect Dis* 2004;10(12):2228–2230.
3. Andrejeva J, Childs KS, Young DF, et al. The V proteins of paramyxoviruses bind the IFN-inducible RNA helicase, mda-5, and inhibit its activation of the IFN-beta promoter. *Proc Natl Acad Sci U S A* 2004; 101(49):17264–17269.
4. Anonymous. *Hendra virus—Australia (Queensland).* ProMED archive no. 20041214.3307. Brookline, MA: International Society for Infectious Diseases; 2004.
5. Anonymous. *Hendra virus, equine—Australia (05): (QL) human exposure.* ProMED archive no. 20100527.1761. Brookline, MA: International Society for Infectious Diseases; 2010.
6. Anonymous. *Hendra virus, human, equine—Australia (05): Queensland.* ProMED archive no. 20090910.3189. Brookline, MA: International Society for Infectious Diseases; 2009.
7. Anonymous. *Nipah encephalitis, human—Bangladesh (03).* ProMED archive no. 20110218.0539. Brookline, MA: International Society for Infectious Diseases; 2011.
8. Anonymous. *Nipah encephalitis, human—Bangladesh: Rangpur (05).* ProMED archive no. 20110308.0756. Brookline, MA: International Society for Infectious Diseases; 2011.
9. Arankalle VA, Bandyopadhyay BT, Ramdasi AY, et al. Genomic characterization of Nipah virus, West Bengal, India, during an intrafamilial outbreak. *Emerg Infect Dis* 2011;17(5):907–909.
10. Bishop KA, Broder CC. Hendra and Nipah: lethal zoonotic paramyxoviruses. In: Scheld WM, Hammer SM, Hughes JM, eds. *Emerging Infections.* Washington, DC: American Society for Microbiology; 2008: 155–187.
11. Bishop KA, Stantchev TS, Hickey AC, et al. Identification of Hendra virus G glycoprotein residues that are critical for receptor binding. *J Virol* 2007;81(11):5893–5901.
12. Boehme KW, Compton T. Innate sensing of viruses by toll-like receptors. *J Virol* 2004;78(15):7867–7873.
13. Bonaparte MI, Dimitrov AS, Bossart KN, et al. Ephrin-B2 ligand is a functional receptor for Hendra virus and Nipah virus. *Proc Natl Acad Sci U S A* 2005;102(30):10652–10657.
14. Bossart KN, Crameri G, Dimitrov AS, et al. Receptor binding, fusion inhibition and induction of cross-reactive neutralizing antibodies by a soluble G glycoprotein of Hendra virus. *J Virol* 2005;79(11):6690–6702.
15. Bossart KN, McEachern JA, Hickey AC, et al. Neutralization assays for differential henipavirus serology using Bio-Plex protein array systems. *J Virol Methods* 2007;142(1–2):29–40.
16. Bossart KN, Mungall BA, Crameri G, et al. Inhibition of Henipavirus fusion and infection by heptad-derived peptides of the Nipah virus fusion glycoprotein. *Virol J* 2005;2:57.
17. Bossart KN, Wang LF, Eaton BT, et al. Functional expression and membrane fusion tropism of the envelope glycoproteins of Hendra virus. *Virology* 2001;290(1):121–135.
18. Bossart KN, Wang LF, Flora MN, et al. Membrane fusion tropism and heterotypic functional activities of the Nipah virus and Hendra virus envelope glycoproteins. *J Virol* 2002;76(22):11186–11198.
19. Bossart KN, Zhu Z, Middleton D, et al. A neutralizing human monoclonal antibody protects against lethal disease in a new ferret model of acute nipah virus infection. *PLoS Pathog* 2009;5(10):e1000642.
20. Bowden TA, Aricescu AR, Gilbert RJ, et al. Structural basis of Nipah and Hendra virus attachment to their cell-surface receptor ephrin-B2. *Nat Struct Mol Biol* 2008;15(6):567–572.
21. Bowden TA, Crispin M, Harvey DJ, et al. Dimeric architecture of the Hendra virus attachment glycoprotein: evidence for a conserved mode of assembly. *J Virol* 2010;84(12):6208–6217.
22. Broder CC. Therapeutics and vaccines against Hendra and Nipah viruses. In: Levine MM, Dougan G, Good MF, et al, eds. *New Generation Vaccines.* 4th ed. New York: Informa Healthcare USA; 2010:885–894.
23. Chadha MS, Comer JA, Lowe L, et al. Nipah virus-associated encephalitis outbreak, Siliguri, India. *Emerg Infect Dis* 2006;12(2):235–240.
24. Chan YP, Chua KB, Koh CL, et al. Complete nucleotide sequences of Nipah virus isolates from Malaysia. *J Gen Virol* 2001;82(Pt 9):2151–2155.
25. Chew MH, Arguin PM, Shay DK, et al. Risk factors for Nipah virus infection among abattoir workers in Singapore. *J Infect Dis* 2000;181(5): 1760–1763.
26. Chong HT, Kamarulzaman A, Tan CT, et al. Treatment of acute Nipah encephalitis with ribavirin. *Ann Neurol* 2001;49(6):810–813.
27. Chong HT, Kunjapan SR, Thayaparan T, et al. Nipah encephalitis outbreak in Malaysia, clinical features in patients from Seremban. *Can J Neurol Sci* 2002;29(1):83–87.
28. Chua KB. Nipah virus outbreak in Malaysia. *J Clin Virol* 2003;26(3): 265–275.
29. Chua KB, Bellini WJ, Rota PA, et al. Nipah virus: a recently emergent deadly paramyxovirus. *Science* 2000;288(5470):1432–1435.
30. Chua KB, Goh KJ, Wong KT, et al. Fatal encephalitis due to Nipah virus among pig-farmers in Malaysia. *Lancet* 1999;354(9186):1257–1259.
31. Chua KB, Lam SK, Goh KJ, et al. The presence of Nipah virus in respiratory secretions and urine of patients during an outbreak of Nipah virus encephalitis in Malaysia. *J Infect* 2001;42(1):40–43.
32. Chua KB, Lam SK, Tan CT, et al. High mortality in Nipah encephalitis is associated with presence of virus in cerebrospinal fluid. *Ann Neurol* 2000;48(5):802–805.
33. Chua KB, Lek Koh C, Hooi PS, et al. Isolation of Nipah virus from Malaysian Island flying-foxes. *Microbes Infect* 2002;4(2):145–151.
34. Daniels P, Ksiazek T, Eaton BT. Laboratory diagnosis of Nipah and Hendra virus infections. *Microbes Infect* 2001;3(4):289–295.
35. Diederich S, Moll M, Klenk HD, et al. The Nipah virus fusion protein is cleaved within the endosomal compartment. *J Biol Chem* 2005; 280(33):29899–29903.
36. Drexler JF, Corman VM, Gloza-Rausch F, et al. Henipavirus RNA in African bats. *PLoS One.* 2009;4(7):e6367.
37. Eaton BT, Broder CC, Middleton D, et al. Hendra and Nipah viruses: different and dangerous. *Nat Rev Microbiol* 2006;4(1):23–35.
38. Eaton BT, Broder CC, Wang LF. Hendra and Nipah viruses: pathogenesis and therapeutics. *Curr Mol Med* 2005;5(8):805–816.
39. Epstein JH, Prakash V, Smith CS, et al. Henipavirus infection in fruit bats (Pteropus giganteus), India. *Emerg Infect Dis* 2008;14(8):1309–1311.
40. Eshaghi M, Tan WS, Mohidin TB, et al. Nipah virus glycoprotein: production in baculovirus and application in diagnosis. *Virus Res* 2004; 106(1):71–76.
41. Feldman KS, Foord A, Heine HG, et al. Design and evaluation of consensus PCR assays for henipaviruses. *J Virol Methods* 2009;161(1):52–57.
42. Field H, Young P, Yob JM, et al. The natural history of Hendra and Nipah viruses. *Microbes Infect* 2001;3(4):307–314.
43. Field HE, Mackenzie JS, Daszak P. Henipaviruses: emerging paramyxoviruses associated with fruit bats. *Curr Top Microbiol Immunol* 2007; 315:133–159.
44. Freiberg AN, Worthy MN, Lee B, et al. Combined chloroquine and ribavirin treatment does not prevent death in a hamster model of Nipah and Hendra virus infection. *J Gen Virol* 2010;91(Pt 3):765–772.
45. Gale NW, Baluk P, Pan L, et al. Ephrin-B2 selectively marks arterial vessels and neovascularization sites in the adult, with expression in both endothelial and smooth-muscle cells. *Dev Biol* 2001;230(2):151–160.
46. Geisbert TW, Daddario-DiCaprio KM, Hickey AC, et al. Development of an acute and highly pathogenic nonhuman primate model of Nipah virus infection. *PLoS One* 2010;5(5):e10690.
47. Georges-Courbot MC, Contamin H, Faure C, et al. Poly(I)-poly(C12U) but not ribavirin prevents death in a hamster model of Nipah virus infection. *Antimicrob Agents Chemother* 2006;50(5):1768–1772.
48. Goh KJ, Tan CT, Chew NK, et al. Clinical features of Nipah virus encephalitis among pig farmers in Malaysia. *N Engl J Med* 2000;342(17): 1229–1235.
49. Goldsmith CS, Whistler T, Rollin PE, et al. Elucidation of Nipah virus morphogenesis and replication using ultrastructural and molecular approaches. *Virus Res* 2003;92(1):89–98.
50. Goodbourn S, Didcock L, Randall RE. Interferons: cell signalling, immune modulation, antiviral response and virus countermeasures. *J Gen Virol* 2000;81(Pt 10):2341–2364.
51. Guillaume V, Contamin H, Loth P, et al. Nipah virus: vaccination and passive protection studies in a hamster model. *J Virol* 2004;78(2):834–840.

52. Guillaume V, Lefeuvre A, Faure C, et al. Specific detection of Nipah virus using real-time RT-PCR (TaqMan). *J Virol Methods* 2004;120(2): 229–237.
53. Guillaume V, Wong KT, Looi RY, et al. Acute Hendra virus infection: analysis of the pathogenesis and passive antibody protection in the hamster model. *Virology* 2009;387(2):459–465.
54. Gurley ES, Montgomery JM, Hossain MJ, et al. Person-to-person transmission of Nipah virus in a Bangladeshi community. *Emerg Infect Dis* 2007;13(7):1031–1037.
55. Halpin K, Bankamp B, Harcourt BH, et al. Nipah virus conforms to the rule of six in a minigenome replication assay. *J Gen Virol* 2004; 85(Pt 3):701–707.
56. Halpin K, Young PL, Field HE, et al. Isolation of Hendra virus from pteropid bats: a natural reservoir of Hendra virus. *J Gen Virol* 2000; 81(Pt 8):1927–1932.
57. Harcourt BH, Lowe L, Tamin A, et al. Genetic characterization of Nipah virus, Bangladesh, 2004. *Emerg Infect Dis* 2005;11(10):1594–1597.
58. Harcourt BH, Tamin A, Halpin K, et al. Molecular characterization of the polymerase gene and genomic termini of nipah virus. *Virology* 2001; 287(1):192–201.
59. Harcourt BH, Tamin A, Ksiazek TG, et al. Molecular characterization of Nipah virus, a newly emergent paramyxovirus. *Virology* 2000; 271(2):334–349.
60. Harit AK, Ichhpujani RL, Gupta S, et al. Nipah/Hendra virus outbreak in Siliguri, West Bengal, India in 2001. *Indian J Med Res* 2006;123(4): 553–560.
61. Hayman DT, Suu-Ire R, Breed AC, et al. Evidence of henipavirus infection in West African fruit bats. *PLoS One* 2008;3(7):e2739.
62. Homaira N, Rahman M, Hossain MJ, et al. Nipah virus outbreak with person-to-person transmission in a district of Bangladesh, 2007. *Epidemiol Infect* 2010;138(11):1630–1636.
63. Hooper P, Zaki S, Daniels P, et al. Comparative pathology of the diseases caused by Hendra and Nipah viruses. *Microbes Infect* 2001;3(4):315–322.
64. Hooper PT, Ketterer PJ, Hyatt AD, et al. Lesions of experimental equine morbillivirus pneumonia in horses. *Vet Pathol* 1997;34(4):312–322.
65. Hooper PT, Westbury HA, Russell GM. The lesions of experimental equine morbillivirus disease in cats and guinea pigs. *Vet Pathol* 1997; 34(4):323–329.
66. Horvath CM. Silencing STATs: lessons from paramyxovirus interferon evasion. *Cytokine Growth Factor Rev* 2004;15(2–3):117–127.
67. Hossain MJ, Gurley ES, Montgomery JM, et al. Clinical presentation of nipah virus infection in Bangladesh. *Clin Infect Dis* 2008;46(7): 977–984.
68. Hsu VP, Hossain MJ, Parashar UD, et al. Nipah virus encephalitis reemergence, Bangladesh. *Emerg Infect Dis* 2004;10(12):2082–2087.
69. Hyatt AD, Zaki SR, Goldsmith CS, et al. Ultrastructure of Hendra virus and Nipah virus within cultured cells and host animals. *Microbes Infect* 2001;3(4):297–306.
70. Iehle C, Razafitrimo G, Razainirina J, et al. Henipavirus and Tioman virus antibodies in pteropodid bats, Madagascar. *Emerg Infect Dis* 2007; 13(1):159–161.
71. Imada T, Abdul Rahman MA, Kashiwazaki Y, et al. Production and characterization of monoclonal antibodies against formalin-inactivated Nipah virus isolated from the lungs of a pig. *J Vet Med Sci* 2004;66(1):81–83.
72. Kaku Y, Noguchi A, Marsh GA, et al. A neutralization test for specific detection of Nipah virus antibodies using pseudotyped vesicular stomatitis virus expressing green fluorescent protein. *J Virol Methods* 2009; 160(1–2):7–13.
73. Kashiwazaki Y, Na YN, Tanimura N, et al. A solid-phase blocking ELISA for detection of antibodies to Nipah virus. *J Virol Methods* 2004; 121(2):259–261.
74. Khetawat D, Broder CC. A functional henipavirus envelope glycoprotein pseudotyped lentivirus assay system. *Virol J* 2010;7:312.
75. Lamb RA, Collins PL, Kolakofsky D, et al. Family Paramyxoviridae. In: Fauquet CM, Mayo J, Maniloff J, et al, eds. *Virus Taxonomy: 8th Report of the International Committee on Taxonomy of Viruses.* San Diego: Elsevier Academic Press; 2005:655–668.
76. Lamb RA, Parks GD. *Paramyxoviridae:* the viruses and their replication. In: Knipe DM, Griffin DE, Lamb RA, et al, eds. *Fields Virology.* Philadelphia: Lippincott Williams & Wilkins; 2007:1449–1496.
77. Langedijk JP, Daus FJ, van Oirschot JT. Sequence and structure alignment of Paramyxoviridae attachment proteins and discovery of enzymatic activity for a morbillivirus hemagglutinin. *J Virol* 1997;71(8):6155–6167.
78. Lee KE, Umapathi T, Tan CB, et al. The neurological manifestations of Nipah virus encephalitis, a novel paramyxovirus. *Ann Neurol* 1999; 46(3):428–432.
79. Levy DE, Marie IJ. RIGging an antiviral defense—it's in the CARDs. *Nat Immunol* 2004;5(7):699–701.
80. Li M, Embury-Hyatt C, Weingartl HM. Experimental inoculation study indicates swine as a potential host for Hendra virus. *Vet Res* 2010; 41(3):33.
81. Li Y, Wang J, Hickey AC, et al. Antibodies to Nipah or Nipah-like viruses in bats, China. *Emerg Infect Dis* 2008;14(12):1974–1976.
82. Lim CC, Lee KE, Lee WL, et al. Nipah virus encephalitis: serial MR study of an emerging disease. *Radiology* 2002;222(1):219–226.
83. Lim CC, Lee WL, Leo YS, et al. Late clinical and magnetic resonance imaging follow up of Nipah virus infection. *J Neurol Neurosurg Psychiatry* 2003;74(1):131–133.
84. Lo MK, Miller D, Aljofan M, et al. Characterization of the antiviral and inflammatory responses against Nipah virus in endothelial cells and neurons. *Virology* 2010;404(1):78–88.
85. Luby SP, Gurley ES, Hossain MJ. Transmission of human infection with Nipah virus. *Clin Infect Dis* 2009;49(11):1743–1748.
86. Luby SP, Hossain MJ, Gurley ES, et al. Recurrent zoonotic transmission of Nipah virus into humans, Bangladesh, 2001–2007. *Emerg Infect Dis* 2009;15(8):1229–1235.
87. Luby SP, Rahman M, Hossain MJ, et al. Foodborne transmission of Nipah virus, Bangladesh. *Emerg Infect Dis* 2006;12(12):1888–1894.
88. Marianneau P, Guillaume V, Wong T, et al. Experimental infection of squirrel monkeys with nipah virus. *Emerg Infect Dis* 2010;16(3): 507–510.
89. Marie I, Durbin JE, Levy DE. Differential viral induction of distinct interferon-alpha genes by positive feedback through interferon regulatory factor-7. *EMBO J* 1998;17(22):6660–6669.
90. Marsh GA, Todd S, Foord A, et al. Genome sequence conservation of Hendra virus isolates during spillover to horses, Australia. *Emerg Infect Dis* 2010;16(11):1767–1769.
91. McEachern JA, Bingham J, Crameri G, et al. A recombinant subunit vaccine formulation protects against lethal Nipah virus challenge in cats. *Vaccine* 2008;26(31):3842–3852.
92. Meulendyke KA, Wurth MA, McCann RO, et al. Endocytosis plays a critical role in proteolytic processing of the hendra virus fusion protein. *J Virol* 2005;79(20):12643–12649.
93. Michalski WP, Crameri G, Wang L, et al. The cleavage activation and sites of glycosylation in the fusion protein of Hendra virus. *Virus Res* 2000; 69(2):83–93.
94. Middleton DJ, Morrissy CJ, van der Heide BM, et al. Experimental Nipah virus infection in pteropid bats (Pteropus poliocephalus). *J Comp Pathol* 2007;136(4):266–272.
95. Middleton DJ, Westbury HA, Morrissy CJ, et al. Experimental Nipah virus infection in pigs and cats. *J Comp Pathol* 2002;126(2–3):124–136.
96. Miller PJ, Boyle DB, Eaton BT, et al. Full-length genome sequence of Mossman virus, a novel paramyxovirus isolated from rodents in Australia. *Virology* 2003;317(2):330–344.
97. Mohd Nor MN, Gan CH, Ong BL. Nipah virus infection of pigs in peninsular Malaysia. *Rev Sci Tech* 2000;19(1):160–165.
98. Moll M, Diederich S, Klenk HD, et al. Ubiquitous activation of the nipah virus fusion protein does not require a basic amino acid at the cleavage site. *J Virol* 2004;78(18):9705–9712.
99. Montgomery JM, Hossain MJ, Gurley E, et al. Risk factors for Nipah virus encephalitis in Bangladesh. *Emerg Infect Dis* 2008;14(10):1526–1532.
100. Mounts AW, Kaur H, Parashar UD, et al. A cohort study of health care workers to assess nosocomial transmissibility of Nipah virus, Malaysia, 1999. *J Infect Dis* 2001;183(5):810–813.
101. Mungall BA, Middleton D, Crameri G, et al. Feline model of acute Nipah virus infection and protection with a soluble glycoprotein-based subunit vaccine. *J Virol* 2006;80(24):12293–12302.
102. Mungall BA, Middleton D, Crameri G, et al. Vertical transmission and fetal replication of Nipah virus in an experimentally infected cat. *J Infect Dis* 2007;196(6):812–816.

103. Murray K, Rogers R, Selvey L, et al. A novel morbillivirus pneumonia of horses and its transmission to humans. *Emerg Infect Dis* 1995;1(1):31–33.
104. Murray K, Selleck P, Hooper P, et al. A morbillivirus that caused fatal disease in horses and humans. *Science* 1995;268(5207):94–97.
105. Negrete OA, Levroney EL, Aguilar HC, et al. EphrinB2 is the entry receptor for Nipah virus, an emergent deadly paramyxovirus. *Nature* 2005;436(7049):401–405.
106. Negrete OA, Wolf MC, Aguilar HC, et al. Two key residues in EphrinB3 are critical for its use as an alternative receptor for Nipah virus. *PLoS Pathog* 2006;2(2):e7.
107. O'Sullivan JD, Allworth AM, Paterson DL, et al. Fatal encephalitis due to novel paramyxovirus transmitted from horses. *Lancet* 1997;349(9045):93–95.
108. Pager CT, Dutch RE. Cathepsin L is involved in proteolytic processing of the Hendra virus fusion protein. *J Virol* 2005;79(20):12714–12720.
109. Pager CT, Wurth MA, Dutch RE. Subcellular localization and calcium and pH requirements for proteolytic processing of the Hendra virus fusion protein. *J Virol* 2004;78(17):9154–9163.
110. Pallister J, Middleton D, Crameri G, et al. Chloroquine administration does not prevent Nipah virus infection and disease in ferrets. *J Virol* 2009;83(22):11979–11982.
111. Parashar UD, Sunn LM, Ong F, et al. Case-control study of risk factors for human infection with a new zoonotic paramyxovirus, Nipah virus, during a 1998–1999 outbreak of severe encephalitis in Malaysia. *J Infect Dis* 2000;181(5):1755–1759.
112. Park MS, Shaw ML, Munoz-Jordan J, et al. Newcastle disease virus (NDV)-based assay demonstrates interferon-antagonist activity for the NDV V protein and the Nipah virus V, W, and C proteins. *J Virol* 2003;77(2):1501–1511.
113. Pasquale EB. Eph-ephrin bidirectional signaling in physiology and disease. *Cell* 2008;133(1):38–52.
114. Paton NI, Leo YS, Zaki SR, et al. Outbreak of Nipah-virus infection among abattoir workers in Singapore. *Lancet* 1999;354(9186):1253–1256.
115. Playford EG, McCall B, Smith G, et al. Human Hendra virus encephalitis associated with equine outbreak, Australia, 2008. *Emerg Infect Dis* 2010;16(2):219–223.
116. Poch O, Blumberg BM, Bougueleret L, et al. Sequence comparison of five polymerases (L proteins) of unsegmented negative-strand RNA viruses: theoretical assignment of functional domains. *J Gen Virol* 1990;71(Pt 5):1153–1162.
117. Porotto M, Orefice G, Yokoyama CC, et al. Simulating henipavirus multicycle replication in a screening assay leads to identification of a promising candidate for therapy. *J Virol* 2009;83(10):5148–5155.
118. Porotto M, Rockx B, Yokoyama CC, et al. Inhibition of Nipah virus infection in vivo: targeting an early stage of paramyxovirus fusion activation during viral entry. *PLoS Pathog* 2010;6(10):e1001168.
119. Rahman SA, Hassan SS, Olival KJ, et al. Characterization of Nipah virus from naturally infected Pteropus vampyrus bats, Malaysia. *Emerg Infect Dis* 2010;16(12):1990–1993.
120. Reynes JM, Counor D, Ong S, et al. Nipah virus in Lyle's flying foxes, Cambodia. *Emerg Infect Dis* 2005;11(7):1042–1047.
121. Rockx B, Bossart KN, Feldmann F, et al. A novel model of lethal Hendra virus infection in African green monkeys and the effectiveness of ribavirin treatment. *J Virol* 2010;84(19):9831–9839.
122. Rodriguez JJ, Cruz CD, Horvath CM. Identification of the nuclear export signal and STAT-binding domains of the Nipah virus V protein reveals mechanisms underlying interferon evasion. *J Virol* 2004;78(10):5358–5367.
123. Rodriguez JJ, Parisien JP, Horvath CM. Nipah virus V protein evades alpha and gamma interferons by preventing STAT1 and STAT2 activation and nuclear accumulation. *J Virol* 2002;76(22):11476–11483.
124. Rodriguez JJ, Wang LF, Horvath CM. Hendra virus V protein inhibits interferon signaling by preventing STAT1 and STAT2 nuclear accumulation. *J Virol* 2003;77(21):11842–11845.
125. Rogers RJ, Douglas IC, Baldock FC, et al. Investigation of a second focus of equine morbillivirus infection in coastal Queensland. *Aust Vet J* 1996;74(3):243–244.
126. Salah Uddin Khan M, Hossain J, Gurley ES, et al. Use of infrared camera to understand bats' access to date palm sap: implications for preventing Nipah virus transmission. *Ecohealth* 2010;7(4):517–525.
127. Sarji SA, Abdullah BJ, Goh KJ, et al. MR imaging features of Nipah encephalitis. *AJR Am J Roentgenol* 2000;175(2):437–442.
128. Sejvar JJ, Hossain J, Saha SK, et al. Long-term neurological and functional outcome in Nipah virus infection. *Ann Neurol* 2007;62(3):235–242.
129. Selvey L, Taylor R, Arklay A, et al. Screening of bat carers for antibodies to equine morbillivirus. *Commun Dis Intell* 1996;20(22):477–478.
130. Selvey LA, Wells RM, McCormack JG, et al. Infection of humans and horses by a newly described morbillivirus. *Med J Aust* 1995;162(12):642–645.
131. Sendow I, Field HE, Curran J, et al. Henipavirus in Pteropus vampyrus bats, Indonesia. *Emerg Infect Dis* 2006;12(4):711–712.
132. Shaw ML, Cardenas WB, Zamarin D, et al. Nuclear localization of the Nipah virus W protein allows for inhibition of both virus- and toll-like receptor 3-triggered signaling pathways. *J Virol* 2005;79(10):6078–6088.
133. Shaw ML, Garcia-Sastre A, Palese P, et al. Nipah virus V and W proteins have a common STAT1-binding domain yet inhibit STAT1 activation from the cytoplasmic and nuclear compartments, respectively. *J Virol* 2004;78(11):5633–5641.
134. Smith IL, Halpin K, Warrilow D, et al. Development of a fluorogenic RT-PCR assay (TaqMan) for the detection of Hendra virus. *J Virol Methods* 2001;98(1):33–40.
135. Su AI, Wiltshire T, Batalov S, et al. A gene atlas of the mouse and human protein-encoding transcriptomes. *Proc Natl Acad Sci U S A* 2004;101(16):6062–6067.
136. Tamin A, Harcourt BH, Ksiazek TG, et al. Functional properties of the fusion and attachment glycoproteins of Nipah virus. *Virology* 2002;296:190–200.
137. Tamin A, Harcourt BH, Lo MK, et al. Development of a neutralization assay for Nipah virus using pseudotype particles. *J Virol Methods* 2009;160(1–2):1–6.
138. Tan CT, Goh KJ, Wong KT, et al. Relapsed and late-onset Nipah encephalitis. *Ann Neurol* 2002;51(6):703–708.
139. Tan KS, Sarji SA, Tan CT, et al. Patients with asymptomatic Nipah virus infection may have abnormal cerebral MR imaging. *Neurol J Southeast Asia* 2000;5:69–73.
140. Tanimura N, Imada T, Kashiwazaki Y, et al. Monoclonal antibody-based immunohistochemical diagnosis of malaysian Nipah virus infection in pigs. *J Comp Pathol* 2004;131(2–3):199–206.
141. Tanimura N, Imada T, Kashiwazaki Y, et al. Reactivity of anti-Nipah virus monoclonal antibodies to formalin-fixed, paraffin-embedded lung tissues from experimental Nipah and Hendra virus infections. *J Vet Med Sci* 2004;66(10):1263–1266.
142. Virtue ER, Marsh GA, Wang LF. Interferon signaling remains functional during henipavirus infection of human cell lines. *J Virol* 2011;85(8):4031–4034.
143. Vogt C, Eickmann M, Diederich S, et al. Endocytosis of the Nipah virus glycoproteins. *J Virol* 2005;79(6):3865–3872.
144. Wacharapluesadee S, Hemachudha T. Duplex nested RT-PCR for detection of Nipah virus RNA from urine specimens of bats. *J Virol Methods* 2007;141(1):97–101.
145. Wacharapluesadee S, Lumlertdacha B, Boongird K, et al. Bat Nipah virus, Thailand. *Emerg Infect Dis* 2005;11(12):1949–1951.
146. Wang L, Harcourt BH, Yu M, et al. Molecular biology of Hendra and Nipah viruses. *Microbes Infect* 2001;3(4):279–287.
147. Wang LF, Michalski WP, Yu M, et al. A novel P/V/C gene in a new member of the Paramyxoviridae family, which causes lethal infection in humans, horses, and other animals. *J Virol* 1998;72(2):1482–1490.
148. Wang LF, Yu M, Hansson E, et al. The exceptionally large genome of Hendra virus: support for creation of a new genus within the family Paramyxoviridae. *J Virol* 2000;74(21):9972–9979.
149. Weingartl H, Czub S, Copps J, et al. Invasion of the central nervous system in a porcine host by nipah virus. *J Virol* 2005;79(12):7528–7534.
150. Weingartl HM, Berhane Y, Caswell JL, et al. Recombinant nipah virus vaccines protect pigs against challenge. *J Virol* 2006;80(16):7929–7938.
151. Westbury HA, Hooper PT, Brouwer SL, et al. Susceptibility of cats to equine morbillivirus. *Aust Vet J* 1996;74(2):132–134.

152. Westbury HA, Hooper PT, Selleck PW, et al. Equine morbillivirus pneumonia: susceptibility of laboratory animals to the virus. *Aust Vet J* 1995;72(7):278–279.
153. White JR, Boyd V, Crameri GS, et al. Location of, immunogenicity of and relationships between neutralization epitopes on the attachment protein (G) of Hendra virus. *J Gen Virol* 2005;86(Pt 10):2839–2848.
154. Williamson MM, Hooper PT, Selleck PW, et al. A guinea-pig model of Hendra virus encephalitis. *J Comp Pathol* 2001;124(4):273–279.
155. Williamson MM, Hooper PT, Selleck PW, et al. Experimental hendra virus infectionin pregnant guinea-pigs and fruit Bats (Pteropus poliocephalus). *J Comp Pathol* 2000;122(2–3):201–207.
156. Williamson MM, Hooper PT, Selleck PW, et al. Transmission studies of Hendra virus (equine morbillivirus) in fruit bats, horses and cats. *Aust Vet J* 1998;76(12):813–818.
157. Wong KT, Grosjean I, Brisson C, et al. A golden hamster model for human acute Nipah virus infection. *Am J Pathol* 2003;163(5):2127–2137.
158. Wong KT, Robertson T, Ong BB, et al. Human Hendra virus infection causes acute and relapsing encephalitis. *Neuropathol Appl Neurobiol* 2009;35(3):296–305.
159. Wong KT, Shieh WJ, Kumar S, et al. Nipah virus infection: pathology and pathogenesis of an emerging paramyxoviral zoonosis. *Am J Pathol* 2002;161(6):2153–2167.
160. Wong KT, Shieh WJ, Zaki SR, et al. Nipah virus infection, an emerging paramyxoviral zoonosis. *Springer Semin Immunopathol* 2002;24(2): 215–228.
161. Wong SC, Ooi MH, Wong MN, et al. Late presentation of Nipah virus encephalitis and kinetics of the humoral immune response. *J Neurol Neurosurg Psychiatry* 2001;71(4):552–554.
162. Wright PJ, Crameri G, Eaton BT. RNA synthesis during infection by Hendra virus: an examination by quantitative real-time PCR of RNA accumulation, the effect of ribavirin and the attenuation of transcription. *Arch Virol* 2005;150(3):521–532.
163. Xu K, Rajashankar KR, Chan YP, et al. Host cell recognition by the henipaviruses: crystal structures of the Nipah G attachment glycoprotein and its complex with ephrin-B3. *Proc Natl Acad Sci U S A* 2008; 105(29):9953–9958.
164. Yob JM, Field H, Rashdi AM, et al. Nipah virus infection in bats (order Chiroptera) in peninsular Malaysia. *Emerg Infect Dis* 2001;7(3):439–441.
165. Young PL, Halpin K, Selleck PW, et al. Serologic evidence for the presence in Pteropus bats of a paramyxovirus related to equine morbillivirus. *Emerg Infect Dis* 1996;2(3):239–240.
166. Yu M, Hansson E, Langedijk JP, et al. The attachment protein of Hendra virus has high structural similarity but limited primary sequence homology compared with viruses in the genus Paramyxovirus. *Virology* 1998;251(2):227–233.
167. Zhu Z, Bossart KN, Bishop KA, et al. Exceptionally potent cross-reactive neutralization of Nipah and Hendra viruses by a human monoclonal antibody. *J Infect Dis* 2008;197(6):846–853.
168. Zhu Z, Dimitrov AS, Bossart KN, et al. Potent neutralization of Hendra and Nipah viruses by human monoclonal antibodies. *J Virol* 2006;80(2):891–899.

CHAPTER 38

Peter L. Collins • Ruth A. Karron

Respiratory Syncytial Virus and Metapneumovirus

HISTORY

Human respiratory syncytial virus (HRSV) was first isolated in 1955 from a laboratory chimpanzee with illness resembling the common cold.[398] Shortly thereafter, the same virus was recovered from infants with respiratory illness, and serologic studies indicated that infection in infants and children was common.[86,87] HRSV is now recognized as the most important viral agent of pediatric lower respiratory tract illness (LRI) worldwide. In many areas it outranks other microbial pathogens as a cause of pneumonia and bronchiolitis in infants. In addition, HRSV can infect and cause disease in individuals of all ages and severe disease in the elderly and in profoundly immunosuppressed individuals.[146,163,233] Worldwide, acute respiratory infection (ARI) is the leading cause of mortality due to infectious disease, and HRSV remains one of the pathogens deemed most important for vaccine development. HRSV research is hampered by its poor growth *in vitro* and its physical instability. HRSV has a single serotype with two antigenic subgroups A and B.

Human metapneumovirus (HMPV) was first described in 2001 following its isolation from infants and children experiencing HRSV-like disease of unknown etiology.[572] There is serologic evidence of extensive pediatric infection dating back more than 50 years, and thus HMPV is newly discovered rather than newly emerged.[572,608,610] The virus had been overlooked because it grows slowly *in vitro,* has a delayed cytopathic effect, and usually requires added trypsin for activation of the fusion F protein. HMPV is recognized as an important agent of respiratory tract disease worldwide, especially in the pediatric and elderly populations, although its impact is less than that of HRSV.[608] HMPV also has a single serotype with two subgroups A and B.[515]

INFECTIOUS AGENT

Classification

HRSV and HMPV are enveloped, cytoplasmic viruses with single-stranded nonsegmented negative-sense RNA genomes. They are members of the family *Paramyxoviridae* (Chapter 33) of the order *Mononegavirales* (Chapter 30). *Paramyxoviridae* has two subfamilies: *Paramyxovirinae,* which includes the human and animal parainfluenza viruses (PIVs, Chapter 34), mumps virus (Chapter 35), and measles virus (Chapter 36) among others, and *Pneumovirinae,* which consists of HRSV and HMPV and their animal relatives. There are two genera in *Pneumovirinae:* Genus *Pneumovirus* consists of HRSV, bovine RSV (BRSV), and pneumonia virus of mice (PVM), and genus *Metapneumovirus* consists of HMPV and avian metapneumovirus (AMPV, formerly called turkey rhinotracheitis virus [TRTV] or avian pneumovirus [APV]). Comparisons of

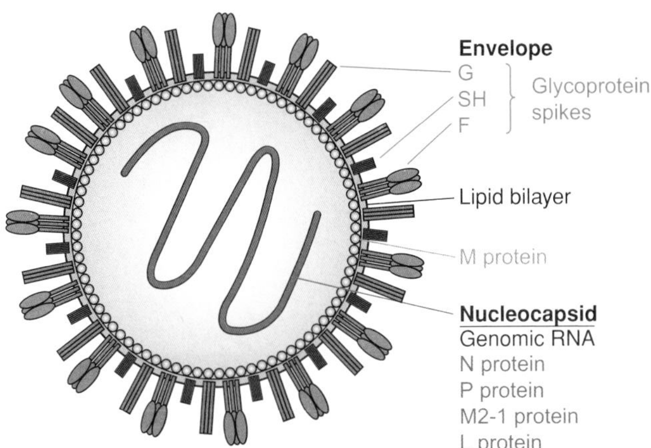

FIGURE 38.1. Idealized diagram of the human respiratory syncytial (HRSV) particle. The G, SH, and F proteins are present in homo-oligomers that constitute the glycoprotein spikes. The M protein underlies the lipid bilayer. The proteins of the nucleocapsid are not depicted individually. The human metapneumovirus (HMPV) particle is similar.

these viruses based on gene maps and nucleotide sequences are shown e-Figures 38.1 and 38.2.

(Note that the descriptions in the following sections usually will begin with HRSV followed by HMPV.)

Virion

The HRSV virion consists of a nucleocapsid that is packaged in a lipid envelope derived from the host cell plasma membrane during budding (Fig. 38.1 and Fig. 38.2C). When visualized by electron microscopy (Fig. 38.2C and E), virions appear as irregular spherical particles of 100 to 350 nm in diameter and long filamentous forms that often predominate and are 60 to 200 nm in diameter and up to 10 μm in length. Despite the variability in size and shape, the ultraviolet (UV) inactivation kinetics of infectivity indicates that most particles contain a single functional genome.[140] Both forms of the virion mostly remain cell associated. The filaments can be visualized as projections from the surface of infected cells by fluorescence photomicroscopy[19,270,423,475] (Fig. 38.2B). The nucleocapsid appears in electron micrographs as a herringbone structure that is characteristic of *Paramyxoviridae*. However, the HRSV nucleocapsid is narrower than those of prototype members of *Paramyxovirinae* (12 to 16 nm compared to 17 to 20 nm) and has a steeper pitch.[19,42,423]

The HRSV envelope contains three virally encoded transmembrane surface glycoproteins: the major attachment protein G, the fusion protein F, and the small hydrophobic (SH) protein (Figs. 38.3A and 38.4). In addition, there is a nonglycosylated matrix M protein that is thought to form a layer on the inner face of the envelope. The viral glycoproteins are present as transmembrane homooligomers that are visualized as short (11 to 20 nm), closely spaced (intervals of 6 to 10 nm) surface projections or "spikes." HRSV lacks a neuraminidase or a hemagglutinin; PVM alone agglutinates murine erythrocytes, via its G protein.[339]

The viral RNA is associated with four nucleocapsid/polymerase proteins: the nucleoprotein N, the phosphoprotein P, the transcription processivity factor M2-1, and the large polymerase subunit L (Fig. 38.3A). However, polymerase activity in purified virions, an activity found in prototypic members of *Mononegavirales,* has not been demonstrated for HRSV preparations.

HRSV virions can readily lose infectivity during handling, presumably reflecting particle instability. This can be partly overcome by agents such as sugars that reduce aggregation and improve thermal stability.[17] When recombinant HRSV was engineered to contain a foreign attachment protein from baculovirus in place of the HRSV glycoproteins, the stability of infectivity was improved,[491] suggesting that the lability of the particle may reside in one or more of the glycoproteins. Other data have implicated the F protein in thermo instability.[469] The long filamentous shape of the particle may also contribute to fragility and loss of infectivity.

HMPV virions were visualized by electron microscopy as pleomorphic spheres and filaments that appear to have general similarity to those of HRSV[443,572] (Fig. 38.2F). The spherical particles had a reported diameter of 150 to 600 nm with envelope spikes of 13 to 17 nm. The nucleocapsid diameter was reported as 17 nm, suggesting a possible difference compared to HRSV.[443] HMPV appears to lack a hemagglutinin[572]; other virion-associated activities have not been reported. HMPV has the same array of structural proteins as HRSV (Fig. 38.3B). The infectivity of HMPV particles is markedly more stable than that of HRSV.[557]

RNA

The HRSV genome (Fig. 38.3C) is a single negative-sense strand of RNA ranging in length from 15,191 to 15,226 nucleotides for six sequenced strains including the subgroup A strains A2 (15,222 nucleotides; GenBank accession number M74568), Long (15,226 nucleotides; AY911262), S2 (15,191 nucleotides; NC_001803), and line 19 (15,191 nucleotides; FJ614813), and the subgroup B strains B1 (15,225 nucleotides; NC_001781) and 9320 (15,225 nucleotides; AY353550). More recently, complete sequences were reported and analyzed for 60 and four additional subgroup A and B strains, respectively.[313a,491a,538a] In addition, extensive sequence information and extensive inter-subgroup comparison is available for subgroup B strain 18537.[274,276,278] The genome is neither capped nor polyadenylated. Both in virions and intracellularly, the genome is tightly and completely bound by N protein to create an RNase-resistant nucleocapsid, as is typical of *Mononegavirales.* This tight encapsidation likely protects the genome, which lacks stabilizing features of capping and polyadenylation, from degradation. It also likely shields the genome from recognition by host cell pattern recognition receptors, especially (a) the cytoplasmic helicases retinoic acid–inducible gene I (RIG-I) and melanoma differentiation–associated protein (MDA-5), which detect triphosphorylated RNA and double-stranded RNA (dsRNA) and activate the cellular transcription factors interferon regulatory factor 3 (IRF3) and nuclear factor kappa B (NF-κB) to induce type I interferon (IFN) and proinflammatory cytokines, and (b) RNA-inducible protein kinase R (PKR), which also activates NF-κB and phosphorylates eukaryotic translation initiation factor 2a (eIF-2a) to inhibit translational initiation as part of antiviral defense.

The HRSV genome contains 10 genes in the order 3′ NS1-NS2-N-P-M-SH-G-F-M2-L (Fig. 38.3C) that are transcribed sequentially into 10 separate messenger RNAs (mRNAs).[95,99,107,140,388] Each gene begins with a highly conserved nine-nucleotide gene-start (GS) transcription signal and ends with a moderately conserved 12- to 13-nucleotide

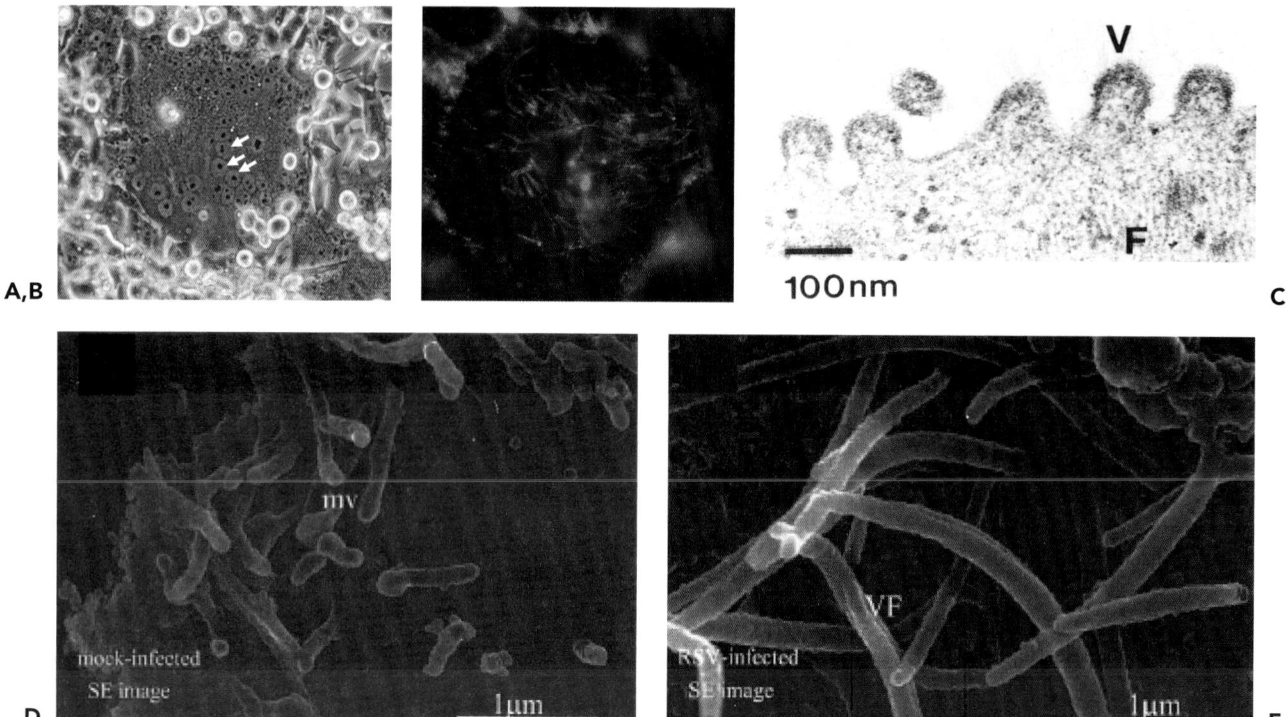

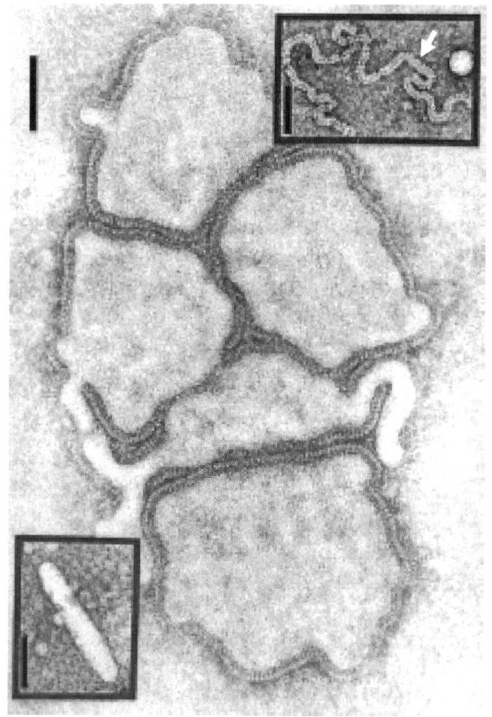

FIGURE 38.2. Photomicrographs (A and B) and electron micrographs (C–F) of human respiratory syncytial virus (HRSV)–infected cells (A–E) and human metapneumovirus (HMPV) virions (F). A: Photomicrograph of an HRSV-infected cell monolayer showing a virus-induced syncytium (several nuclei are indicated with *arrows*). (Courtesy of Dr. Alexander Bukreyev.) **B:** Fluorescence photomicrograph of an HRSV-infected syncytium (not the same one as in **A**) stained with an antibody specific to the F protein, showing filamentous viral projections. (Courtesy of Dr. Ursula J. Buchholz.) **C:** Negatively stained electron micrograph of budding HRSV virions: *V* indicates a budding virion and *F* indicates filamentous cytoplasmic structures that likely are nucleocapsids. (Courtesy of Dr. Robert M. Chanock[284]) **D** and **E:** Field emission scanning electron micrographs of the surface of uninfected **(D)** and HRSV-infected **(E)** cells, illustrating viral filamentous structures (*VF* in **E**) that are thought to form at sites of virus budding and may yield filamentous particles; also shown are microvilli (*mv* in **D**) that are found in uninfected cells. (**D** and **E** reprinted from Jeffree CE, Rixon HW, Brown G, et al. Distribution of the attachment (G) glycoprotein and GM1 within the envelope of mature respiratory syncytial virus filaments revealed using field emission scanning electron microscopy. *Virology* 2003;306:254–267; copyright 2003, with permission from Elsevier.) **F:** Negatively stained electron micrograph of HMPV (bar markers represent 100 nm): the **main panel** shows spherical-type particles, the **upper insert** shows a free nucleocapsid (*arrow*), and the **lower insert** shows a filamentous or rod-like particle. (Reprinted from Peret T C, Boivin G, Li Y, et al. Characterization of human metapneumoviruses isolated from patients in North America. *J Infect Dis* 2002;185:1660–1663, by permission of Oxford University Press.)

gene-end (GE) signal[275,315] (e-Fig. 38.3A). The first nine genes are separated by intergenic regions that vary in length from 1 to 58 nucleotides for the strains sequenced to date.[275] These lack any conserved motifs, are poorly conserved between strains, and appear to be unimportant spacers. The last two HRSV genes, M2 and L, overlap by 68 nucleotides[106] (Fig. 38.3C and e-Fig. 38.3A). Specifically, the GS signal for the L gene is located upstream, rather than downstream, of the M2 GE signal. The same overlap occurs in BRSV; overlapping genes are not found in any other members of *Paramyxoviridae,* but sometimes are found in *Rhabdoviridae* and *Filoviridae*. The 3′ and 5′ ends of the genome consist of short extragenic leader and trailer regions (44 and 155 nucleotides long, respectively, in strain A2).

The HRSV mRNAs contain a methylated 5′ cap structure $m^7G[5']ppp[5']Gp$[24] and are polyadenylated by reiterative copying on a U tract in the GE signal. Each HRSV mRNA encodes a single major protein except for M2, which has separate open reading frames (ORFs) for the M2-1 and M2-2 proteins. The M2-1 ORF is located in the upstream part of the mRNA, whereas the M2-2 ORF is located downstream and

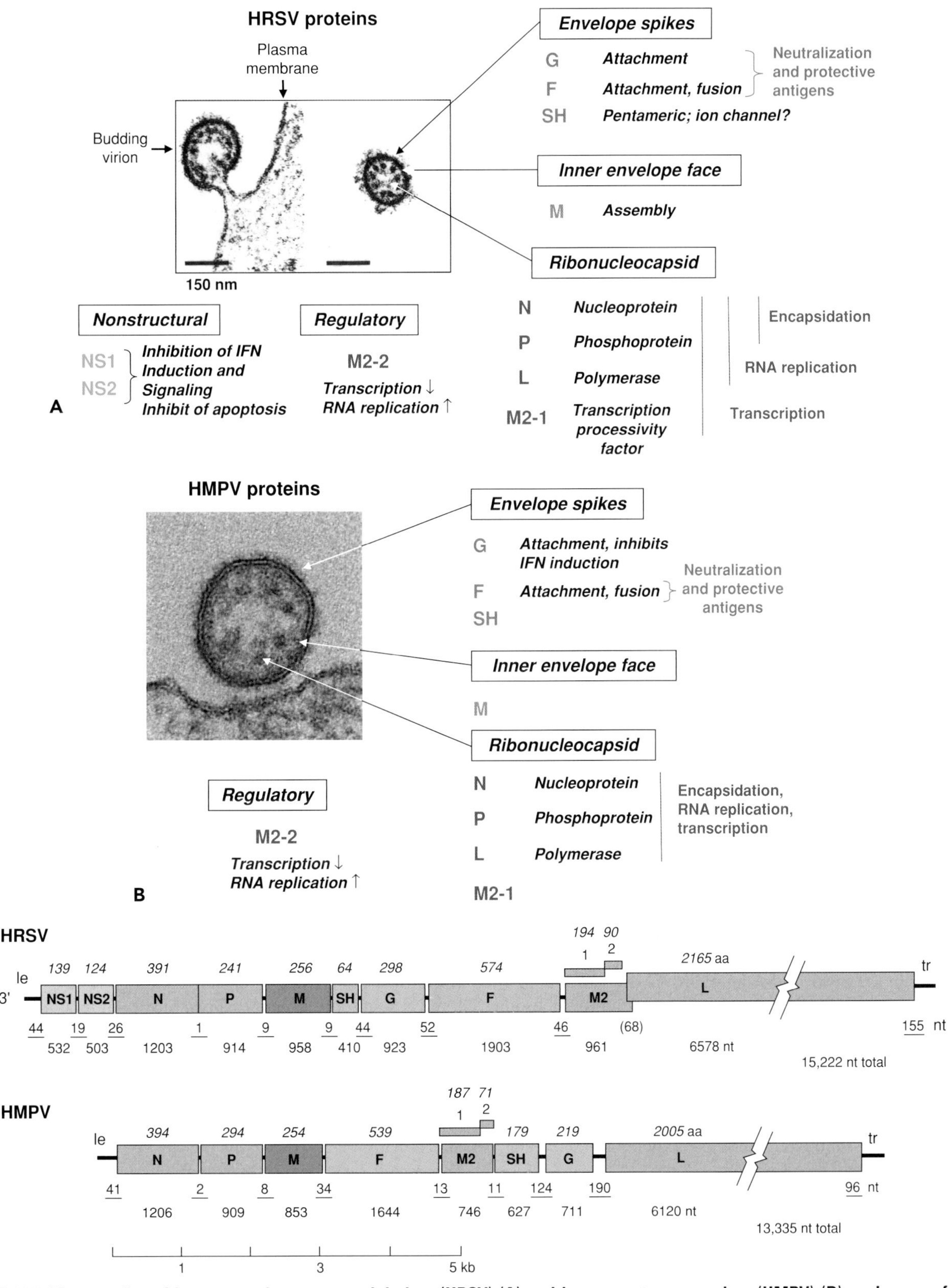

FIGURE 38.3. The proteins of human respiratory syncytial virus (HRSV) (A) and human metapneumovirus (HMPV) (B), and maps of the viral genomic RNAs (C). A and **B:** Locations of the proteins in the virus particle and major functions are indicated when known. **A–C:** Color-coded: proteins/genes of the nucleocapsid and polymerase complex or that are involved in RNA synthesis are in blue, surface glycoproteins in red, matrix protein in magenta, and the two HRSV nonstructural proteins in brown. The maps in **panel C** are approximately to scale and show the 3′ to 5′ negative-sense genomes of HRSV strain A2 and HMPV strain CAN97-83. The overlapping open reading frames (ORFs) of the M2 messenger RNAs (mRNAs) are illustrated over the M2 genes. Numbers beneath each map indicate nucleotide (nt) lengths; those of the extragenic leader (le), trailer (tr), and intergenic regions are *underlined*, and that of the HRSV gene overlap is in *parentheses*. *Italicized numbers* above each map indicate amino acid (aa) lengths.

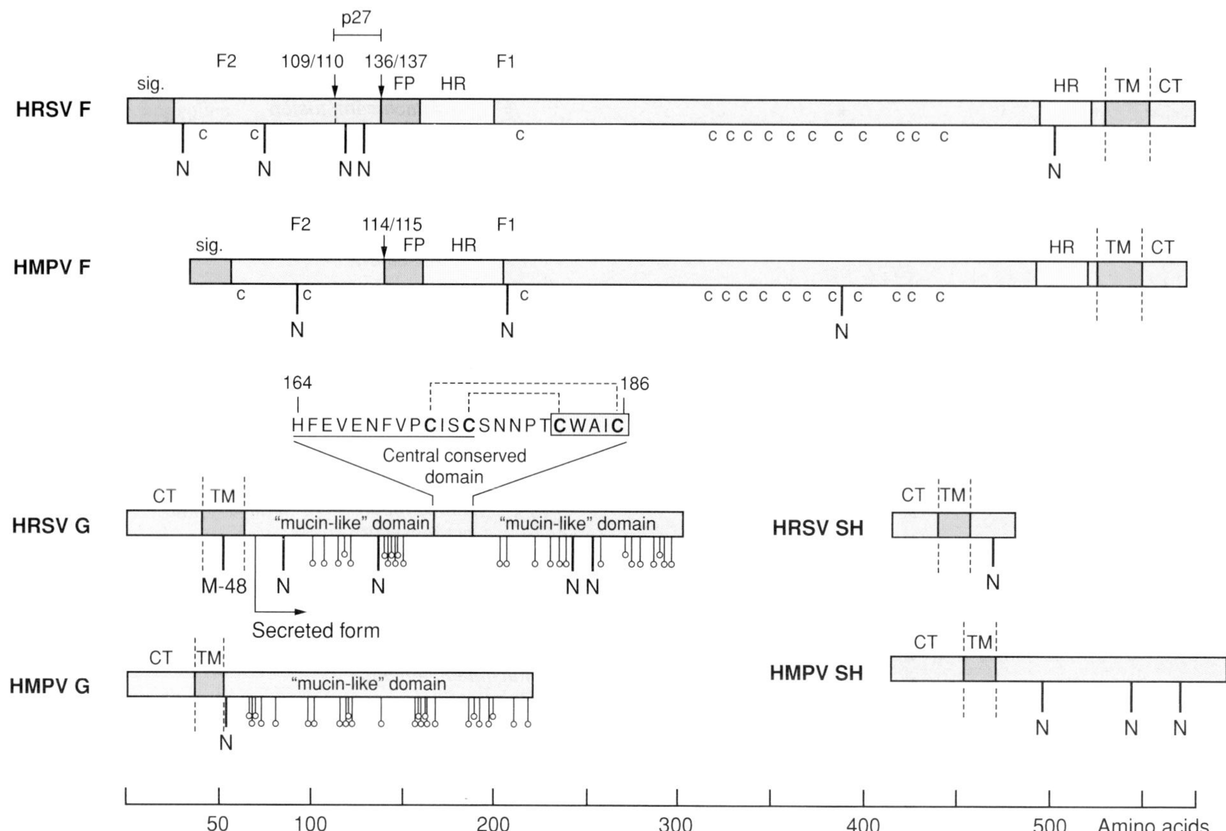

FIGURE 38.4. Primary structures (approximately to scale) of the F, G, and SH surface glycoproteins of human respiratory syncytial virus (HRSV) strain A2 and human metapneumovirus (HMPV) strain CAN97-83. Hydrophobic domains are *brown bars:* Sig., signal peptide; FP, fusion peptide; TM, transmembrane anchor; CT, cytoplasmic tail. Heptad repeats (HR) in the F protein are *green* and cysteine residues conserved between the F proteins of HRSV and HMPV are indicated underneath (indicated as c). *Downward-facing arrows* identify the cleavage-activation site(s) in the F protein. Potential acceptor sites for N-linked carbohydrate are indicated as *downward facing stalks* with N. For each G protein, the 25 potential acceptor sites for O-linked sugars predicted by NetOGlyc 2.0 to be the most likely to be utilized are indicated as *downward facing stalks with small circles.* The sequence excerpt above the HRSV G protein shows the conserved segment (*underlined*) and cystine noose; cysteine residues are *bold;* the disulfide bonding pattern is indicated by *dotted lines*[201]; and the fractalkine CX3C motif is *boxed.* M-48 in the HRSV G protein is the translational start site for the secreted form, and the mature secreted form is indicated.[476]

overlaps by 32 nucleotides in strain A2. Translation of the downstream M2-2 ORF depends on reinitiation by ribosomes exiting the upstream M2-1 ORF, a process that appears to be influenced by the structure of a region of RNA located ~150 nucleotides upstream of the M2-2 translational start site.[202,203] Whereas the P genes of *Paramyxovirinae* encode additional accessory proteins by overlapping ORFs, alternative translational start sites, and RNA editing (Chapter 33), the P gene of HRSV (and HMPV) encodes only P.

HRSV transcription follows the general *Mononegavirales* model[111,140,316] (Chapters 31 and 33), involving initiation at a single 3′ promoter and a start-stop-restart sequential mechanism guided by the GS and GE signals. RNA sequences important in transcriptional initiation are shown in e-Fig. 38.4. Capping seems to be an essential step for efficient mRNA elongation: when capping was blocked using a novel HRSV-specific inhibitor, transcription produced uncapped abortive RNAs of ~45 to 50 nt.[343] Termination at the various GE signals typically is somewhat inefficient, resulting in readthrough transcription that creates mRNAs representing two or more adjacent genes and their intervening intergenic regions.[107] These readthrough mRNAs account for approximately 10% of total mRNA.

The M2/L gene overlap raises two questions for the model of sequential transcription: (a) how do polymerases that exit the M2 gene find the upstream L GS signal (or does polymerase enter independently at that site), and (b) how do polymerases that initiate at the L GS signal avoid premature termination when they cross the M2 GE signal? Studies with a minireplicon system showed that when polymerase completes transcription of the M2 gene, it efficiently gains access to the L gene by retrograde scanning.[170] The polymerase appeared to scan in both directions. This led to the realization that scanning may be a common function of the polymerase, and may occur at each gene junction as well as prior to the initiation of transcription and RNA replication. The M2 GE signal within the L gene indeed causes premature termination for 90% of L gene transcripts, producing a 68-nucleotide polyadenylated RNA that does not appear to encode a protein and is not known to have any further significance.[106] The synthesis of full-length L mRNA depends on polymerase readthrough at the M2 GE signal. Therefore, the "error" of reading through a GE signal is necessary for synthesis of this essential mRNA.[106] Premature termination of 90% of L gene transcripts might be expected to severely downregulate the production of full-length mRNA, but the ability of the polymerase to recycle back to the L GS signal apparently relieves much of this effect, and the amount of L mRNA produced for HRSV relative to the other mRNAs appears to be about the same as for other members of *Paramyxoviridae.* The gene overlap does not seem to be of any particular benefit to the virus, and may be an accidental arrangement that can be tolerated due to the scanning function of the polymerase.

RNA replication by HRSV also follows the general *Mononegavirales* model (Chapters 31 and 33). RNA sequences important in the initiation of RNA replication are shown in e-Fig. 38.4. The replicating polymerase ignores the GS and GE signals and produces a complete positive-sense copy of the viral genome that is called the antigenome and that also is tightly encapsidated. The antigenome serves in turn as the template for producing progeny genomes. Chain elongation of nascent genomes and antigenomes depends on concurrent encapsidation.[373] For viruses in the subfamily *Paramyxovirinae,* the nucleotide length of the genome must be an even multiple of six in order for efficient RNA replication to occur ("rule of six"; Chapter 33), reflecting a requirement for nucleocapsid organization, but there appears to be no comparable requirement for members of *Pneumovirinae.*[303,488]

The HMPV genome is approximately 13.2 kb—nearly 2 kb shorter than that of HRSV—and lacks the NS1 and NS2 genes (Fig. 38.3C). In addition, the order of the SH, G, F, and M2 genes differs between HRSV (SH-G-F-M2) and HMPV (F-M2-SH-G). Correcting for the lack of NS1 and NS2 for HMPV and the difference in gene order, the genomes of HRSV and HMPV share 50% nucleotide sequence identity. Strains for which complete sequences have been reported include the following: CAN97-83 (13,335 nt, GenBank accession AY297749) and NL/00/1 (13,350, AF371337) of subgroup A, and CAN98-75 (13,280, AY297748) and NL/1/99 (13,293, AY525843) of subgroup B.[46,259]

Features of the structure, encapsidation, transcription, and replication of the HMPV genome are generally similar to those described above for HRSV. The cis-acting signals of HMPV have considerable similarity to those of HRSV[46,571] (e-Fig. 38.3B). The HMPV intergenic regions can be longer than those of HRSV, up to 190 nt in the case of CAN97-83 (Fig. 38.3C and e-Fig 38.3B). Unlike HRSV, the HMPV M2-2 protein appears to be translated independently of the upstream M2-1 ORF.[66]

Proteins

HRSV encodes 11 separate proteins (Fig. 38.3A). HMPV encodes nine proteins (Fig. 38.3B) that generally correspond to those of HRSV except for the lack of NS1 and NS2.[46,571] Table 38.1 shows amino acid sequence relatedness between viruses within subfamily *Pneumovirinae.*

Fusion F Glycoprotein

The HRSV F and L proteins are the ones that most closely resemble their counterparts in *Paramyxovirinae.* As is typical for *Paramyxoviridae,* the HRSV F protein directs viral penetration by fusion between the virion envelope and the host cell plasma membrane. Later in infection, F protein expressed on the cell surface can mediate fusion with neighboring cells to form syncytia (Fig. 38.2A). Recent findings suggest that the HRSV F protein also plays a major role in viral attachment involving interaction with the cellular protein nucleolin.[543]

F is a type I transmembrane surface protein that has a cleaved signal peptide at the N-terminus and a membrane anchor near the C-terminus[100] (Fig. 38.4). A predicted three-dimensional structure of the prefusion form of the HRSV F protein has been described based on homology modeling with the crystal structure of the Newcastle disease virus F protein,[517] and crystal structures representing the postfusion form have recently been published.[378,536] The structure of the *Paramyxoviridae* F protein is described in detail in Chapter 33.

As is typical for *Paramyxoviridae,* F is synthesized as an inactive F0 precursor that assembles into a homotrimer.[74] HRSV F is activated by cleavage in the trans-Golgi complex by furin or a furin-like cellular endoprotease to yield two

TABLE 38.1 Percent Amino Acid Sequence Identity between the Proteins of HRSV Subgroup A (HRSV-A) or HMPV Subgroup A (HMPV-A) and the Indicated Viruses[a]

Viruses compared		% Amino acid sequence identity for the indicated protein										
		NS1	NS2	N	P	M	SH	G	F	M2-1	M2-2	L
HRSV-A versus:	HRSV-B	87	92	96	91	91	76	53	89	92	72	93
	BRSV	69	84	93	81	89	38	30	81	80	42	84
	PVM	16	20	60	33	42	23	12	43	43	10	53
	HMPV-A	—[b]	—[b]	42	35	38	23	15	33	36	17	45
	AMPV-A	—[b]	—[b]	41	32	38	19	16	35	37	12	43
HMPV-A versus:	HMPV-B	—[b]	—[b]	96	85	97	59	37	95	96	89	94
	AMPV-C	—[b]	—[b]	88	68	87	24	23	81	83	56	80
	AMPV-A	—[b]	—[b]	70	58	77	20	12	68	73	25	64
	AMPV-B	—[b]	—[b]	69	53	76	20	13	67	71	27	ND[c]

HRSV, human respiratory syncytial virus; BRSV, bovine RSV; PVM, pneumovirus of mice; HMPV, human metapneumovirus; AMPV, avian metapneumovirus.

[a]Viruses are listed in order of decreasing relatedness to HRSV-A or HMPV-A.

[b]Does not encode NS1 or NS2.

[c]ND, not done.

disulfide-linked subunits: NH2-F2–F1-COOH.[103,531] The N-terminus of the F1 subunit that is created by this cleavage contains a hydrophobic domain (the fusion peptide) that inserts directly into the target membrane to initiate fusion. The F1 subunit also contains two areas of heptad repeats that associate during fusion, driving a conformational shift that brings the viral and cellular membranes into proximity[100,633] (Chapter 33). HRSV F protein can direct efficient fusion independent of other viral proteins.[283] This differs from the situation for most members of *Paramyxovirinae,* for which efficient fusion requires interaction with the homologous attachment protein (Chapter 33).

The F proteins of HRSV and BRSV are unique in *Paramyxoviridae* in having two cleavage sites, rather than one cleavage site[200,636] (Fig. 38.4). The site that is immediately upstream of the fusion peptide (with cleavage between residues 136/137 in HRSV strain A2) is the one that corresponds to other *Paramyxoviridae.* This site in HRSV contains six tandem Arg and Lys residues (Lys-Lys-Arg-Lys-Arg-Arg↓). The second, novel site is located 27 amino acids upstream (with cleavage between residues 109/110) and has the sequence Arg-Ala-Arg-Arg↓. Therefore, both sites contain the preferred furin cleavage motif (Arg-X-Arg/Lys-Arg↓). HRSV F appears to be readily cleaved during intracellular processing, although some of the F protein packaged in virions remained uncleaved at site 109/110. There is indirect evidence that the double-cleavage site in the F protein is associated with a hyperfusogenic character that is linked to reduced thermostabilty and the ability to fuse independent of a cognate attachment protein.[469]

Cleavage at the two sites in F0 releases a short peptide of 27 amino acids (p27) that contains two (strain A2) or three (strain Long) potential acceptor sites for N-linked sugars, of which at least two are utilized in strain Long.[636] (Note that the remainder of the F protein has three acceptor sites for N-linked sugars, two in F2 and one in F1, all of which are utilized.[639]) For BRSV, this peptide contains a tachykinin sequence motif and is processed and released from BRSV-infected cells to yield a virokinin that induced smooth muscle contraction *in vitro,* which is a property of tachykinins.[638] Tachykinins also have proinflammatory and immunomodulatory activities. Recombinant BRSV in which most of p27 was deleted, or in which the upstream cleavage site was mutated, replicated as efficiently as the wild-type parent in calves, but induced less pulmonary inflammation and a somewhat lower titer of serum neutralizing antibody.[567,637] Therefore, p27 of BRSV has the potential to augment viral disease by effects on smooth muscle contraction and pulmonary inflammation, and might also stimulate the host immune response. In contrast, the sequence of p27 of HRSV does not resemble a tachykinin, and HRSV p27 did not have tachykinin-like properties *in vitro.*[638]

The HMPV F protein shares a moderate level of amino acid sequence identity with HRSV (33%)[46,571] and is similar in general organization (Fig. 38.4). As with HRSV, HMPV F directs fusion involved in penetration and syncytium formation, and does so efficiently without need of the G and SH proteins.[48] HMPV F also appears to play a role in attachment via interaction with cellular $\alpha v\beta 1$ integrin.[118] This integrin characteristically binds to a specific recognition sequence, Arg-Gly-Asp, and this motif is present in the HMPV F protein and mediates its binding to cells.

The HMPV F0 precursor contains only a single cleavage activation site (Fig. 38.4). The sequence at this site, Arg-Gln-Ser-Arg↓, does not conform to the consensus furin motif and, consistent with this, clinical isolates typically require exogenous trypsin for growth *in vitro. In vivo,* cleavage of the HMPV F protein presumably depends on secreted protease present in the lumen of the respiratory tract. Several observations indicate that this is not a limiting factor in pathogenesis. For example, in some cases, serial passage of HMPV clinical isolates in cell culture resulted in the emergence of mutants that no longer required added trypsin, but these did not exhibit increased replication in hamsters.[492] These mutants contained the substitution of Pro in place of Ser in the –2 position of the cleavage activation site (Arg-Gln-Pro-Arg↓), which conferred intracellular cleavability even though it did not create a furin motif. Similarly, when the F cleavage site of recombinant HMPV was engineered so that it was multibasic and cleaved intracellularly, this did not increase its replication in African green monkeys (AGMs).[45]

Glycoprotein G

The HRSV G protein was originally thought to be the sole viral attachment protein,[334] but it now appears that the F protein also plays a role, as noted. The HRSV G protein has no apparent relatedness by sequence or structure to the attachment HN, H, and G proteins of *Paramyxovirinae* and has only half the amino acid length.[278,597] HRSV G is a type II transmembrane glycoprotein, with a hydrophobic signal/anchor located near the N-terminus (amino acids 38-63 in strain A2) and the C-terminal two thirds of the molecular oriented extracellularly (Fig. 38.4). A secreted version of G is produced by translational initiation at the second ATG in the ORF (codon 48), which lies within the signal/anchor sequence.[255,476] This truncated form is then trimmed by proteolysis, removing the remainder of the signal/anchor and creating a new N-terminus at Asn-66 for the final secreted form. The secreted form constituted approximately 20% of the total G protein expressed in HRSV-infected cells *in vitro,* but because of its rapid secretion it accounted for 80% of the G protein released in cell culture by 24 h post infection, the remainder being virion associated.[255]

The polypeptide backbone of HRSV G has an Mr of approximately 32,000. In the case of strain A2, an estimated four N-linked sugar side chains are added co-translationally, increasing the Mr to 45,000.[102,598] G assembles in the endoplasmic reticulum into oligomers that probably are trimers or tetramers, and O-linked sugars are added subsequently in the trans-Golgi compartment or network.[102,598] Mature G migrates in gel electrophoresis as a broad, seemingly heterogeneous band of Mr 80,000-90,000. Analysis of an F/G fusion protein (created as a potential vaccine) expressed in insect cells by a recombinant baculovirus indicated that G contains approximately 24-25 O-linked side chains.[592] However, when HRSV was grown in an *in vitro* model of human airway epithelium (HAE)—specifically, a differentiated pseudostratified mucociliary tissue that closely resembles the authentic airway epithelium[631]—the Mr observed for the G protein was 180,000.[319] Because these cells would be considered to be a more authentic substrate than typical immortalized monolayer cultures, this suggests that the amount of carbohydrate present on G is substantially greater than previously thought. The presence of a sheath of host-specified sugars might shield the G protein from immune recognition, and might interfere with antigen processing and presentation. The secreted form of G appears to be processed in a similar fashion to the membrane-anchored form except that it is secreted as a monomer, and no antigenic differences were detected when the secreted and membrane-bound forms were analyzed with an extensive panel of monoclonal antibodies (MAbs).[155]

Most of the ectodomain of HRSV G consists of two large domains that are highly divergent between strains and have a "mucin-like" structure. Like mucin, these domains have a high content of serine, threonine, and proline residues; are heavily glycosylated; and are thought to have an extended, nonglobular secondary structure. Because there are more than 75 serine and threonine residues in the mucin-like domains as potential acceptor sites for O-linked sugars, there may be heterogeneity in site usage that could provide additional antigenic heterogeneity. The significance of this mucin-like character remains unknown. One possibility is that it somehow helps the virus penetrate the protective mucous layer overlying the respiratory epithelium.

The two mucin-like domains flank a central conserved domain that includes a 13-residue segment (positions 164–176 in strain A2) that is completely conserved among HRSV strains, as well as an overlapping segment containing four closely spaced invariant cysteine residues (positions 173, 176, 182, and 186)[278] (Fig. 38.4). Disulfide linkages occur between Cys-173 and Cys-186, and between Cys-176 and Cys-182, to create a cystine noose.[201] The cysteine-rich segment contains a Cys-X_3-Cys (CX3C) motif involving Cys-182 and Cys-186 embedded in a region of limited sequence relatedness with the CX3C chemokine called fractalkine.[561] A peptide containing this sequence mimicked the leukocyte chemoattractant activity of fractalkine in an *in vitro* assay.

The HRSV G protein participates in viral attachment *in vitro* by binding to glycosaminoglycans (GAGs), which are long unbranched chains of repeating disaccharide subunits that are part of the glycocalyx present on the outer surface of the cell. The conserved central domain of G seemed like an obvious candidate to be involved in attachment. However, this domain can be deleted from recombinant HRSV with little effect on virus replication in HEp-2 cells or in mice.[548] A study that probed for possible GAG-binding domains by evaluating interaction between peptides spanning the ectodomain of G and the GAG heparin identified a potential binding site shortly downstream from the central conserved domain,[175] but this also could be deleted with little effect on HRSV infection and replication *in vitro* or in mice.[548] More recently, cleavage of the C-terminal domain of G was found to result in virus that bound less efficiently to GAGs and had reduced infectivity in HAE cultures, suggesting that this domain is important for the attachment function of G.[319]

Extensive passage of a subgroup B strain of HRSV in AGM Vero cells—in an attempt to attenuate the virus—resulted in mutants with various spontaneous deletions involving most of the G and SH genes.[288] One such mutant virus that was evaluated as a potential vaccine replicated efficiently in Vero cells but was highly restricted in humans. Recombinant HRSV strain A2 from which the G gene was deleted (ΔG) also replicated efficiently in Vero cells. However, the ΔG virus was restricted in HEp-2 cells, with defects at the levels of virus binding, fusion, and assembly.[544,545,547,550] In addition, the ΔG virus was highly restricted in mice and might not have replicated at all.[550] Therefore, HRSV G is dispensable for replication in Vero cells but it is essential for efficient replication in HEp-2 cells and *in vivo*.

The HMPV G protein (Fig. 38.4) has a number of similarities with HRSV G, although it lacks significant sequence identity[46,571] (Table 38.1). HMPV G has a comparable N-terminal proximal signal/anchor domain and a high content of serine/threonine/proline residues concentrated in the ectodomain.[46,571] In addition it is modified by the addition of N-linked and O-linked sugars to yield a mature form that migrates in gel electrophoresis as a diffuse band of Mr 97,000.[341] Its amino acid sequence also is highly divergent between the HMPV subgroups. However, HMPV G lacks the conserved central domain and cystine noose mentioned above for HRSV and is correspondingly shorter in length. A secreted form of HMPV G has not been described, and the amino acid sequence gives no suggestion that such a species exists. As with HRSV, the HMPV G protein binds to cell surface GAGs, which may reflect its role in attachment.[551] Peptide binding studies suggested that two closely spaced clusters of basic amino acids at positions 149–155 and 159–166 may mediate binding to GAGs.[551]

Deletion of G from recombinant HMPV was less attenuating than for HRSV. Deletion of G had little effect on HMPV replication *in vitro*, and the HMPV ΔG mutant had a low-to-moderate level of replication in hamsters and AGMs.[44,48] Interestingly, infection of epithelial cells *in vitro* with the ΔG mutant resulted in increased activation of the transcription factors IRF3 and NF-κB and increased expression of type I IFN and proinflammatory cytokines compared to wild-type HMPV, implying that the G protein otherwise inhibits these responses.[21] The HMPV G protein was found to bind to the RIG-I cytoplasmic RNA recognition receptor, which explains its inhibitory effect.

Small Hydrophobic SH Protein

The HRSV SH protein (Fig. 38.4) is a short (64 amino acids for strain A2) transmembrane protein that is anchored by a hydrophobic signal-anchor sequence near the N-terminus, with the C-terminus oriented extracellularly.[101,427] Most of the SH protein remains unglycosylated (Mr ~7,500), but there are also forms that contain a single N-linked side chain (resulting in Mr ~13,000 to 15,000), as well as the further addition of polylactosaminoglycan (Mr ~21,000 to 60,000 or more), as well as N-terminally truncated forms that arise from translational initiation at the second methionine codon in the ORF.[9,427] However, the significance of these multiple forms is not known.

Chemical cross-linking studies indicated that the HRSV SH protein associates into pentamers.[101] When SH was expressed in bacteria, it was incorporated into the membrane, resulting in increased membrane permeability.[446] Incorporation of partial or full-length SH into artificial membranes *in vitro* resulted in the formation of pentameric and hexameric pore-like structures and the acquisition of cation-selective channel-like activity.[81,183] Therefore, the SH protein may have properties of a viroporin, which typically are small proteins that modify membrane permeability and can have roles in budding and apoptosis.

Recombinant HRSV from which SH was deleted replicates with wild-type efficiency *in vitro* and appears to be fully fusogenic.[69,544] The SH protein was reported to reduce apoptosis, but the effect was small.[181] SH also appeared to inhibit signaling from tumor necrosis factor (TNF)-α.[181] The ΔSH virus was slightly attenuated in mice and chimpanzees,[69,603] but deletion of the SH gene in an experimental live vaccine strain did not increase its level of attenuation in seronegative children.[290] Therefore, the function(s) and impact of the HRSV SH protein seem unclear.

The SH protein of HMPV is nearly three times longer (177–183 amino acids) than its HRSV counterpart[46,571] (Fig. 38.4). It has the same membrane orientation and a similar array of nonglycosylated and glycosylated forms. Passage of HMPV frequently results in mutations that ablate SH expression,[43] suggesting that the protein may be somewhat toxic in cell culture. Infection of epithelial cells and mice with the ΔSH virus resulted in a modest increase in NF-κB activation and expression of proinflammatory proteins compared to wild-type virus, suggesting that the SH protein downregulates the innate response, but the effect may be small.[20] *In vivo*, deletion of SH had little or no effect on HMPV replication in hamsters or in AGMs.[44,48]

Matrix M Protein

The HRSV M protein is a nonglycosylated internal virion component that is smaller than its *Paramyxovirinae* counterparts (256 amino acids versus 335–375 amino acids), with little apparent amino acid sequence relatedness. HRSV M appears to play two roles typical for *Mononegavirales:* it helps organize virion components at the plasma membrane for budding,[254,547] and it may silence viral RNA synthesis in preparation for packaging into the virus particle.[191] A crystal structure determined for the HRSV M protein revealed a monomer that is organized into compact N-terminal (residues 1 to 126) and C-terminal (residues 140–255) domains joined by a 13-residue linker.[394] The surface of M was found to contain a large positively charged area that extends across the two domains and the linker and may mediate association with the negatively charged membrane as well as with nucleocapsids.[394] The HMPV M protein (254 amino acids) likely is a close functional counterpart.

Nucleocapsid/Polymerase Proteins N, P, L, and M2-1

The N, P, and L proteins of HRSV appear to be close functional analogs of their counterparts in other members of *Paramyxoviridae.* The N protein binds tightly along the entire length of genomic RNA and antigenomic RNA to form separate RNase-resistant nucleocapsids that are templates for RNA synthesis. The P protein is a multifunctional adapter that helps mediate interactions between components of the nucleocapsid/polymerase complex. The L protein contains the polymerase catalytic domains. Studies with HRSV minireplicons showed that N, P, and L are necessary and sufficient to direct RNA replication.[98,215,626] N, P, and L alone also have transcriptase activity, but fully processive transcription requires in addition the M2-1 protein.[98,171]

The 391 amino acid HRSV N protein is shorter than its counterparts in *Paramyxovirinae* (approximately 490–555 amino acids), and sequence relatedness is limited to several conserved segments located towards the C-terminus.[27,542] HRSV N protein produced in bacteria was recovered in decamer rings bound to bacterial RNA, and a crystal structure was obtained[542] that is described in e-Figure 38.5.

The HRSV P protein (241 amino acids) is shorter than its *Paramyxovirinae* counterparts (approximately 390–605 amino acids) and lacks evident sequence relatedness. However, it is thought to have the same general array of functions. Like its counterparts in *Paramyxovirinae,* HRSV P operates as a stable homotetramer formed through a multimerization domain in the middle of the molecule.[15,82,344] The C-terminal region of the P tetramer interacts with N protein in the nucleocapsid by binding to a hydrophobic pocket surrounded by positively charged residues made up from discontinuous segments within amino acids 46-151 of the N protein, a structure distinct from that of other members of *Mononegavirales*[182a] (e-Fig. 38.5). Soluble P also binds to free N protein monomers—probably through the N-terminal domain of P—and delivers N to nascent genomes/antigenomes during RNA replication. P thus prevents N from self-aggregating or binding to nonviral RNA.[82] In addition, P binds to the L[294] and M2-1[12,559] proteins and helps mediate their interactions with the nucleocapsid. P is an essential polymerase co-factor. It may contribute to conformational changes that help the polymerase access the RNA template[82] and appears to be necessary for promoter clearance and chain elongation by the viral polymerase.[147] It also appears to have a role in dissociating the M protein from the nucleocapsid during uncoating to initiate infection.[13]

P is the major phosphorylated HRSV protein and contains phosphate 10 to 12 or more sites, with different sites exhibiting differing rates of turnover: the C-terminal domain contains low-turnover phosphates and accounts for most of the total phosphate, the middle domain contains intermediate-turnover phosphates, and the N-terminal domain contains high-turnover phosphates.[14,418] Many of the activities of P described above appear to be directed by dynamic phosphorylation and dephosphorylation of P at a subset of these sites, usually involving a small percentage of the total phosphate content.[12,13,14–15,580] Most of the constitutive phosphorylation, involving five sites, could be ablated in recombinant HRSV with only modest effects on virus growth.[350]

The 194 amino acid HRSV M2-1 protein is an essential transcription processivity factor; in its absence, the viral polymerase terminates prematurely and nonspecifically within several hundred nucleotides of the 3′ end of the genome, and downstream genes are not significantly transcribed.[94,97,98,171] M2-1 also decreases the efficiency of termination at the GE transcription signals—possibly a reflection of the same processivity activity—resulting in increased production of readthrough mRNAs.[245] HRSV M2-1 accumulates in phosphorylated and nonphosphorylated forms[244] and forms a homotetramer via an oligomerization domain at residues 32 to 63.[559] M2-1 contains a cysteine–histidine zinc finger motif (C-X_7-C-X_5-C-X_3-H) near its N-terminus (residues 7 to 25) that is essential for its activity[244]; this motif is conserved in *Pneumovirinae.*[571] The HRSV M2-1 protein binds RNA, and may be delivered to the RNA template by the P protein.[80,120,559] M2-1 is unique to *Pneumovirinae,* although VP30 of Family *Filoviridae* has some similarities.

The 2,165 amino acid HRSV L protein is similar in length to its *Paramyxovirinae* counterparts and has low but unambiguous sequence relatedness along nearly its entire length.[527] Specific segments of L are conserved within and beyond *Mononegavirales* and appear to include polymerase motifs.[451] A putative nucleotide-binding domain involved in capping mRNA was identified in the central region of the L protein based on sequence analysis of HRSV mutants selected for resistance to novel capping inhibitors, in which resistance was associated with an amino acid substitution at position 1381, 1269, or 1421.[343] In separate work, an amino acid substitution at position 1049 or 1169 in the L protein was associated with reduced efficiency of termination at the GE signals, resulting in increased synthesis of polycistronic mRNAs and reduced growth efficiency.[79,282]

The HMPV N, P, L, and M2-1 proteins are similar in size to their HRSV counterparts and share significant amino acid sequence identity[46,571] (Table 38.1). One notable difference is that, whereas M2-1 appears to be essential for HRSV, recombinant HMPV in which the M2-1 ORF has been silenced is viable and replicates *in vitro* with an efficiency that is only marginally reduced.[66] HMPV lacking M2-1 appeared to execute processive transcription efficiently, although the level of RNA accumulation was somewhat reduced. Therefore, in contrast to HRSV, HMPV M2-1 appears to be a nonessential accessory protein of unknown function.[66] However, in the hamster model, replication of HMPV lacking M2-1 could not be detected, indicating that M2-1 is important for replication *in vivo.*

M2-2 Protein

HRSV M2-2 is a small (90 amino acids for strain A2) protein that is expressed at a low level that may reflect inefficiency of the stop–restart mechanism of translation noted previously.[5] It is not known whether M2-2 is packaged in the virion. Recombinant HRSV in which the M2-2 ORF has been silenced grows more slowly *in vitro* than wild-type HRSV, although it eventually achieves a similar titer.[41,271] In ΔM2-2 virus–infected cells, the accumulation of mRNA was increased, whereas that of the genome and antigenome was decreased compared to wild-type virus. Conversely, when M2-2 was overexpressed during HRSV infection—using a co-transfected plasmid or a recombinant HRSV in which expression of M2-2 was upregulated by engineering it to be a separate gene[89]—HRSV replication was inhibited. Expression of M2-2 also was inhibitory to HRSV RNA synthesis by a minireplicon.[98] These observations indicate that M2-2 plays a role in shifting RNA synthesis from transcription to RNA replication, that M2-2 can be inhibitory to RNA synthesis, and that the inhibitory activity occurs with increased M2-2 expression. The ΔM2-2 virus retained the ability to replicate in mice and chimpanzees, but it was attenuated approximately 500- to 1,000-fold compared to wild-type HRSV.[41,271,549]

HMPV encodes a 71 amino acid M2-2 protein from a comparable internal ORF in its M2 mRNA[46,571] (Fig. 38.3C). The HMPV M2-2 protein co-immunoprecipitated with the L protein and inhibited RNA synthesis by a mini-replicon, an activity that was lost by short deletions at the N- or C-terminus of M2-2.[301] Deletion of HMPV M2-2 from recombinant virus resulted in an attenuated virus in which transcription is increased and RNA replication decreased.[66]

Nonstructural Proteins NS1 and NS2

The NS1 and NS2 proteins (139 and 124 amino acids, respectively) are unique to the genus *Pneumovirus.* NS1 and NS2 can be co-immunoprecipitated[537] and may occur in complexes of various stoichiometries.[156] Monomeric NS2 was unstable with a half-life of 30 minutes.[156]

NS1 and NS2 strongly interfere with the induction and signaling of type I IFN and type III IFN (the latter comprising λ1, λ2, and λ3; also known as IL-29, IL-28A, and IL-28B, respectively) in human epithelial cells, macrophages, and dendritic cells. This suppresses a major component of host innate defense. The steps at which NS1 and NS2 act are summarized in e-Figure 38.6.

Deletion of NS2 from recombinant HRSV decreased its ability to induce activation of transcription factor NF-κB,[524] and small interfering RNA (siRNA)–mediated knockdown of the expression of either NS1 or NS2 in HRSV-infected cells reduced activation of NF-κB and the serine-threonine kinase AKT (also known as protein kinase B), with the effect of speeding the onset of apoptosis.[50] Therefore, the two NS proteins appear to activate prosurvival pathways, thereby prolonging the life of the cell and increasing the viral yield.[50]

In a minireplicon system, coexpression of NS1—and, to a lesser extent, NS2—inhibited transcription and RNA replication, affecting both the genomic and antigenomic promoters.[16] These effects remain to be defined. The V and C accessory proteins of some members of *Paramyxovirinae* also have been shown to downregulate viral RNA synthesis (Chapters 33 and 34). This may be a general viral mechanism to prevent excessive RNA synthesis and avoid the accumulation of naked genomic/antigenomic RNA and the formation of dsRNA, which otherwise would activate the RIG-I/MDA5/PKR pattern recognition molecules.

As might be expected from the results described above, HRSV lacking NS1 and/or NS2 replicates to reduced titer in cultured cells competent for producing type I IFN, as well as in experimental animals, with the level of attenuation increasing in the order ΔNS2<ΔNS1≤ΔNS1+NS2.[272,523,546,549,603]

Replicative Cycle

Efficient infection of cell lines *in vitro* by HRSV involves binding to cellular GAGs, especially heparan sulfate and chondroitin sulfate B.[238] The G and F proteins each appear able to bind to GAGs.[174,175,239,545] A number of additional potential receptor molecules for HRSV have been tentatively identified, including intracellular adhesion molecule (ICAM)-1,[33] RhoA,[438] the CX3CR1 fractalkine receptor,[561] and annexin II.[358] More recently, efficient HRSV infection *in vitro* and in the mouse model was shown to depend on binding to the cellular protein nucleolin,[543] which also has been identified as a co-receptor for human parainfluenza virus 3 (HPIV3).[58] Somewhat unexpectedly, binding to nucleolin is mediated by the F protein rather than by the G protein. This suggests that efficient attachment and infection by HRSV depends on two different binding events mediated by G and F, but the details of this process remain unclear.

HRSV entry occurs by fusion of the viral envelope with the cell plasma membrane[283,526] or with endosomal membranes following clathrin-mediated endocytosis.[304] However, HRSV entry does not require endosomal acidification, suggesting that there is no mechanistic difference between entry at the plasma versus endosomal membrane.[304,526] When infection was monitored by video microscopy, the initiation of fusion by attached virions appeared to be a slow step, but once started the process was rapid.[18] Genome transcription and replication occur in the cytoplasm and the virus can grow in enucleated cells and in the presence of actinomycin D, indicating a lack of essential nuclear involvement.

HRSV mRNAs and proteins can be detected intracellularly at 4 to 6 h after infection and reach a peak accumulation by 15 to 20 hours. The release of progeny virus begins by 10 to 12 h postinfection, reaches a peak after 24 hours, and continues until the cells deteriorate by 30 to 48 hours. Transcription and RNA replication occur concurrently but, as noted, the low-abundance M2-2 protein accumulates during infection and shifts the balance of RNA synthesis from transcription to RNA replication.[41] In minireplicon experiments, increasing the level of accumulation of the N and P proteins did not shift the balance between RNA replication and transcription, indicating that the availability of protein to encapsidate replicative RNA does not control this balance.[172]

Several factors influence the relative levels of expression of the various HRSV genes. Like other *Mononegavirales,* sequential transcription has a polar gradient due to polymerase fall-off, and thus promoter-proximal genes are expressed more efficiently. This gradient of expression is not very steep, with the exception of the L mRNA.[107,307] The greatly reduced accumulation of L mRNA compared to the other mRNAs appears to be due to a posttranscriptional effect rather than polymerase fall-off, with one possibility being mRNA stability.[318] Differences in the termination efficiency of the various GE signals may also have effects on the relative levels of gene expression.[246,399] For example, if a GE signal is particularly inefficient, a greater fraction of the polymerase continues synthesis into the next downstream gene to produce a readthrough transcript, rather than terminating and reinitiating to produce an individual transcript of the next gene. Because ORFs in internal positions in eukaryotic mRNAs generally are not efficiently translated,[306] this would have the effect of downregulating expression of the protein from the downstream gene. HMPV in particular has considerable variation in the efficiency of its GE signals, and in particular this appears to sharply downregulate the production of monocistronic SH mRNA, contributing to the observed low level of expression of SH protein.

HRSV assembly and budding occur at the plasma membrane. In polarized cells, this occurs at the apical surface.[475,631] Video microscopy showed that budding occurs within circumscribed regions on the cell surface and appeared visually to be the reverse of fusion.[18] These regions contain localized virus-modified lipid rafts involving all three viral surface proteins and the M protein.[254,270,371,372,623] The minimum viral protein requirements for the formation of virus-like particles capable of delivering the viral genome to target cells are the F, M, N, and P proteins,[547] and expression of these proteins induced the formation of viral filaments.[564]

As has been observed for other members of *Paramyxoviridae,* HRSV utilizes the host cytoskeleton in its replicative cycle. Viral substructures are associated with polymerized actin throughout the infectious cycle.[269] Actin is packaged in the virion and was required, in combination with profilin (an actin-binding protein involved in restructuring actin polymers), for efficient RNA synthesis by intracellular nucleocapsids in a cell-free reaction.[72] HRSV appears to hijack cellular apical recycling endosomes (ACEs) for budding, a pathway that is distinct from that described for a number of other enveloped RNA viruses.[65,564]

Efficient infection by HMPV *in vitro* depends on binding to cell surface GAGs and $\alpha v\beta 1$ integrin.[118,551] The F proteins of some strains of HMPV depend on acidification for activation, indicating a dependence on endosomal uptake rather than fusion at the plasma membrane: this requirement mapped to the presence of glycine at position 294.[260,496,497] However, this was observed for only 6% of subgroup A strains and not for subgroup B, indicating an unexpected diversity in entry mechanisms. Finally, one notable difference between HRSV and HMPV is that the kinetics of infection of the latter in cell culture are slower, with the peak of intracellular protein expression occurring at 48 to 72 hours postinfection.

Propagation *In Vitro*

HRSV replicates most efficiently *in vitro* in immortalized cell lines derived from human epithelial cells, but can infect and replicate to a significant extent in a wide variety of cell lines representing various tissues from various hosts, including humans, monkeys, bovines, hamsters, and mice. The most commonly used cell line is human HEp-2, now thought to have been contaminated historically with, and outgrown by, the HeLa cell line.[368] Virus is usually quantified by plaque titration; immunostaining is often used to enhance visualization of plaques. Fresh clinical isolates of HRSV may undergo some sort of adaptation to cell culture,[361] but this is poorly understood. However, passaged laboratory strains retain their virulence for chimpanzees and humans.[291,606]

In cell culture, 90% of progeny HRSV virions remain associated with the cells, attached in a manner that suggests a failure to complete the budding process. To make virus stocks, cell-associated virus is dislodged by freeze-thawing, sonication, or vortexing. The yield is low, typically ten plaque-forming units (pfu) per cell. Virion preparations commonly have substantial contamination by cellular debris. A large fraction of released virions appeared to be empty and presumably noninfectious.[19] Less than 5% of the infectivity of a preparation of HRSV passed through a 0.45-mm filter, whereas more than 85% passed through a 3-μm filter, consistent with the infectious particles being filaments[475]; similar findings had been reported for BRSV.[433]

HMPV is more restricted in its *in vitro* host range than HRSV, but is readily propagated in rhesus LLC-MK2 or AGM Vero cells.[134,557] HMPV typically requires added trypsin to support cleavage of the F protein, although some strains mutate during passage to become trypsin independent, as noted.[492] HMPV replicates more slowly than HRSV, its cytopathic effect is less prominent, and the yield of infectious virus is similarly low. Like HRSV, HMPV tends to remain cell-associated but is more stable.

Genetics and Reverse Genetics

HRSV (and presumably HMPV) has a high rate of nucleotide substitution, as is typical for RNA viruses. The rate of nucleotide substitution in RSV was estimated to be 6.47×10^{-4} substitutions/site/year, and the G gene had the elevated rate of $10^{-2.7}$ substitutions/site/year, reflecting relaxed selective constraints, as already noted.[538a,641] HRSV and HMPV, like other *Mononegavirales,* also engage in nonhomologous recombination caused when the polymerase jumps from one template to another during synthesis. This can create defective interfering (DI) genomes,[569] or deletion of parts of genes,[288] or sequence duplications.[560] Foreign sequence also can be acquired, as evidenced by a 1,015-nucleotide insert of unknown origin in the G gene of certain AMPV-C isolates.[38] Recombination between co-infecting viruses appears to be rare, although potential mosaic genomes within a viral species are identified occasionally by sequence analysis.[634] One study detected a single case of recombination between two co-infecting HRSV mutants in cell culture, involving both homologous (i.e., guided by sequence relatedness) and nonhomologous recombination[522]: this is the only such report for *Mononegavirales.* In addition, the difference in the gene orders of HRSV and HMPV may be evidence of past recombination, within one or the other species, resulting in gene rearrangement.

As with other *Mononegavirales,* HRSV and HMPV can be produced entirely from cloned cDNA by reverse genetics, involving co-transfection of plasmids encoding a copy of the genome or antigenome as well as the proteins of the nucleocapsid/polymerase complex. The viral protein requirements for recovering HRSV are N, P, L, and M2-1, but M2-1 is not required for HMPV.[47,66,97,259] A second type of reverse genetics system that has been used extensively for HRSV in particular is based on cDNA-encoded minireplicons in which the viral genes in the genome or antigenome cDNA have been replaced by one or more foreign marker genes, with the system driven by viral proteins supplied from co-transfecting plasmids. Depending on the supplied proteins, this system can recreate genome encapsidation, transcription, RNA replication, and particle morphogenesis.[98,170,373,424,547] This system is ideal for detailed structure-function studies. In addition, mutations that might have drastic or lethal effects on infectious virus can readily be studied in the transient context.

Infection of Experimental Animals

A number of animal species can be infected in the respiratory tract by intranasal administration of HRSV, including cotton rats, mice, ferrets, guinea pigs, hamsters, marmosets, lambs, and various nonhuman primates.[35,73,210,460,521,606] Among experimental animals, only the chimpanzee approaches the human in being highly susceptible to infection by contact, in supporting moderate to high levels of virus replication, and in exhibiting rhinorrhea and cough resembling that of humans. The most widely used experimental animals, cotton rats and mice, support a low to moderate level of virus replication that peaks on day 4 and is cleared quickly. *In situ* hybridization of lung tissue from cotton rats at the peak of virus replication showed that only scattered cells were infected.[413] Inbred strains of mice can vary 100-fold in permissiveness for replication.[460] The BALB/c mouse is one of the more permissive strains, but it is less permissive than cotton rats. Rodents do not exhibit overt HRSV respiratory tract disease, although pulmonary histopathologic changes are evident and disease can be monitored by weight loss and changes in pulmonary function. More recently, newborn lambs have been used as models in detailed studies of neonatal HRSV disease.[521]

Intranasal administration of HMPV has been reported to infect guinea pigs, ferrets, mice, cotton rats, and hamsters, and several species of nonhuman primates.[6,241,353] BALB/c mice and hamsters may be more permissive for HMPV than for HRSV. Among nonhuman primates, cynomolgus macaques and AGMs support moderate levels of virus replication that peak on days 5 to 6 and are mostly resolved by day 10.[311,515] Captive cynomolgus macaques, AGMs, and chimpanzees have a high seroprevalence for HMPV, suggesting that they can be infected readily from their handlers and possibly by animal-to-animal transmission.

Antigenic Subgroups and Diversity

HRSV has a single serotype with two antigenic subgroups, A and B. These exhibit a three- to fourfold reciprocal difference in neutralization by polyclonal convalescent serum.[92] Studies with MAbs have demonstrated extensive antigenic difference in the G protein with substantially less difference in the other viral proteins.[10,400] Analysis of glycoprotein-specific responses in cotton rats or human infants by enzyme-linked immunosorbent assay (ELISA) with purified F and G glycoproteins (the HRSV neutralization antigens) showed that F has 50% antigenic relatedness between subgroups compared to 1% to 7% relatedness for G.[256] Consistent with this, F protein expressed from a recombinant vaccinia virus was equally protective in cotton rats against infection with either subgroup, whereas the G protein was 13-fold less effective against the heterologous subgroup virus.[277] Therefore, the F protein is responsible for most of the observed HRSV cross-subgroup neutralization and protection.

The genomes of the two HRSV subgroups share 81% nucleotide identity. The various proteins vary considerably in their level of subgroup divergence, with M2-2, SH, and G being the most divergent (Table 38.1). The divergence is greatest for the ectodomains of SH and G, which exhibit only 50% and 44% sequence identity between subgroups, respectively.[105,278] The genome-wide nature of the sequence differences indicates that the two subgroups represent two lines of divergent evolution, rather than being variants that differ only at a few major antigenic sites. The divergence of the two HRSV subgroups has been estimated to have occurred approximately 350 years ago.[640] In addition, there is considerable variation within each subgroup: for example, the G glycoprotein can have 20% difference between strains from the same subgroup.

The HRSV F protein is relatively stable antigenically, consistent with its high level of sequence conservation between the two HRSV subgroups. For example, analysis of 18 subgroup A strains and five subgroup B strains recovered from geographically diverse regions over 30 years using F-specific murine MAbs representing 16 separate neutralization epitopes in four antigenic sites showed that seven epitopes were conserved in all but one of the strains.[32] Similarly, a major epitope in the N protein for $CD8^+$ cytotoxic T lymphocytes (CTLs) was highly conserved in field strains.[578]

The G protein appears to be subject to greater change, although this occurs incrementally over a period of years. In one study, analysis of HRSV isolates collected over 47 years suggested that positive selection occurred at 13 codons in the G ectodomain, a number of which involved known epitopes.[641] A second study of isolates collected over 38 years provided evidence of progressive amino acid changes at an average rate of 0.25% per year that were paralleled by changes in reactivity with MAbs.[76] The mucin-like domains in G are unusual in that they are more divergent at the amino acid level than at the nucleotide level,[278] which is the converse of what is observed for most proteins. This suggests that there is a selective pressure for amino acid substitutions, presumably driven by immune pressure. These regions in G may be relatively tolerant of amino acid change because of their proposed extended, nonglobular structure. In contrast, although F would be subjected to the same selective immune pressure, it likely is less tolerant of amino acid substitutions due to constraints from its folded structure and functional requirements. Analysis of BRSV isolates, including those from countries in which vaccination was in wide use, provided evidence of modest progressive changes not only in G, but also in N and F.[568]

HMPV also has a single serotype with two antigenetic subgroups, A and B, which have extensive cross-reactivity and cross-protection.[55,259,442,572,574] The level of genome nucleotide sequence identity (80%) and the relatedness between the various proteins is similar to that described for HRSV (Table 38.1). The HMPV F protein is somewhat more conserved than that of HRSV and plays a major role in the high level of cross-neutralization and protection between the two subgroups.[515] Vaccination against AMPV appears to drive antigenic drift in the field, especially in the G and SH genes, resulting in virus that is sufficiently divergent from the vaccine strain that it is less restricted by vaccination.[84]

Animal Counterparts

The BRSV gene map is very similar to that of HRSV.[67,627] The genome of BRSV strain A51908 (NC_001989 and AF295543) contains 15,140 nucleotides and has 73% nucleotide identity with HRSV. Amino acid sequence identity ranges from 30% (G protein) to 93% (N protein) (Table 38.1), and there is extensive antigenic cross-reactivity. BRSV and HRSV have broadly overlapping host ranges in cell culture; however, *in vivo,* BRSV is highly restricted in nonhuman primates.[68] Ovine and caprine RSV also have been described. Sequence analysis suggests that ovine RSV and BRSV represent two branches of ruminant RSV with a degree of divergence similar to that between the HRSV antigenic subgroups. Caprine RSV appears to be more closely related to BRSV than to ovine RSV.[112]

PVM was first identified during experiments in which clinical material was passaged in mice in an effort to identify new human pathogens, and an apparent mouse virus present in the animals became evident.[264] PVM is a respiratory pathogen that readily infects mice and other rodents and can be highly virulent. However, the natural host of PVM is unclear: the virus occasionally appears in colonies of laboratory mice, but serologic studies usually find little evidence of PVM-specific antibodies in wild rodents under conditions where there is extensive seropositivity for other common rodent viruses.[31,516] Serologic studies suggested that a substantial proportion of the human population has antibodies that react with PVM.[464] However, further analysis suggested that infection of humans by PVM or a closely related virus is unlikely.[64a] A virus that was recently isolated from dogs with acute respiratory disease appears to be a strain of PVM (e.g., the percent amino acid sequence identity between the isolate and PVM strain 15 ranged from a low of 90.2% [SH] to a high of 98.1% [M]).[473,474] Whether PVM commonly infects and causes respiratory tract disease in dogs remains unknown. The PVM gene map[308] is essentially the same as that of HRSV and BRSV except that (a) the M2 and L genes of PVM do not overlap, and (b) the PVM P gene contains a second ORF that encodes a 137-amino acid product that represents a novel, 12th PVM protein.[26] The complete nucleotide sequence of PVM strain 15 (AY729016) is 14,886 nucleotides in length and has 52% identity with that of HRSV.[308] The level of amino acid sequence identity ranges from 10% (M2-2 protein) to 60% (N protein) (Table 38.1).

BRSV and PVM in their respective hosts are used as models for HRSV,[190,285,441,481,614] although a review of these studies is beyond the scope of this chapter. The BRSV model is limited by the inconvenient nature of the large host. PVM differs from HRSV in that lethal infections are typical rather than an infrequent outcome, but it can serve as a model for severe pneumovirus disease and has the advantage of the many available murine immunologic reagents and inbred mouse strains.

AMPV causes respiratory tract disease of economic importance in turkeys and also infects chickens and other birds.[421] Four AMPV antigenic subgroups have been described: subgroups A and B have been found in South Africa, Europe, Israel and Asia; subgroup C in North America; and subgroup D in France.[421] Complete genomic sequences have been determined for strains of subgroup A (AY640317) and subgroup C (AY590688 and AY579780). These range in length from 13,134 to 14,150 nucleotides, have the same general gene map as HMPV, and share 61% to 68% nucleotide sequence identity with HMPV subgroup A. Subgroups A, B, and D are more closely related to each other than to C[205,504] (e-Fig. 38.2B). Surprisingly, AMPV-C is more closely related to HMPV than to the other AMPV subgroups[571,572] (e-Fig. 38.2B). Sequence analysis of isolates collected over a 25-year period suggested that the most recent common ancestor for AMPV-C and HMPV existed approximately 200 years ago, implying a cross-species jump.[127] There is substantial host range restriction between human and avian MPV. AMPV-C (the subgroup most closely related to HMPV) is highly restricted in nonhuman primates.[447] HMPV has been reported to be unable to infect chickens and turkeys,[572] or to transiently infect turkeys.[577]

PATHOGENESIS AND PATHOLOGY

In typical monolayer cultures of immortalized cells, infection with HRSV or HMPV results in long surface filaments that bear viral antigen and probably give rise to filamentous virus particles[489] (Fig. 38.2B and E). The formation of HRSV filaments and filamentous virus depends on activation of RhoA and actin rearrangement: when activation is blocked, the production of infectious virus shifted to the nonfilamentous form.[71,206,371] HRSV-infected cells develop large electron-dense cytoplasmic inclusion bodies of up to several microns in diameter that include the N, P, M2-1, and L proteins and presumably contain active nucleocapsids[78,185]; HMPV forms similar inclusions.[136] Recently, the HRSV inclusion bodies were found to sequester a number of cellular proteins involved in intracellular signaling pathways, with the effect of inhibiting innate immunity and stress responses.[179a] HRSV infection has slight inhibitory effects on cellular DNA and RNA synthesis and little effect on gross protein synthesis.[335] As one factor in the lack of inhibition of protein synthesis, the HRSV N protein binds to PKR and prevents it from phosphorylating eIF-2a and inhibiting protein synthesis.[216] Apoptosis of HRSV-infected cells occurs slowly and is inhibited by the NS1, NS2, and SH proteins, as already noted. HRSV blocks the formation of stress granules, which may otherwise restrict HRSV replication.[179a, 242] The formation of syncytia (Fig. 38.2A) is a major factor in cell death in typical nonpolarized monolayer cell cultures, but usually is not a prominent histopathologic finding *in vivo* (below).

HRSV and HMPV are highly infectious viruses. Humans are their only natural host, although HRSV and HMPV can readily spread to nonhuman primates and are pathogenic in some situations.[305] The major mode of spread by HRSV is by large droplets or through contaminated objects and depends on close contact with infected individuals or contact of contaminated hands to nasal or conjunctival mucosa (self-inoculation). It is generally thought that small-particle aerosols (which can remain airborne for extended periods and also can be inhaled deeply into the respiratory tract) are not an important mode of HRSV transmission,[222,224] although there are contrary data.[338] The incubation period from time of infection to onset of illness for HRSV is about 3 to 5 days[137,286,291] (Fig. 38.5). The incubation period for HMPV is not defined, but is thought to be similar.

HRSV replicates initially in the nasopharynx. Signs of LRI, when it occurs, usually appear 1 to 3 days following the onset of rhinorrhea (Fig. 38.5). Viral spread to the lower respiratory tract likely involves aspiration of secretions. Infants hospitalized

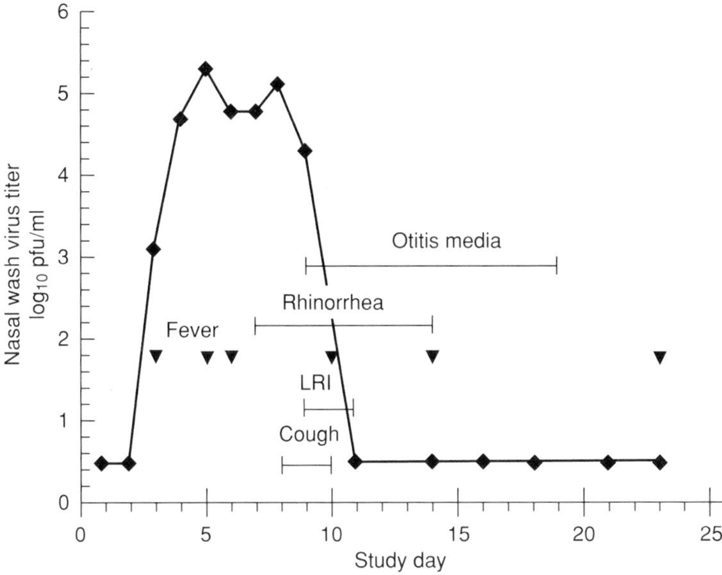

FIGURE 38.5. Time course of viral shedding and disease signs following experimental infection of a young seronegative vaccinee with 10^4 pfu of an investigational live partially attenuated human respiratory syncytial virus (HRSV) vaccine called *cpts*248/955. Fever was intermittent. (Adapted from Karron RA, Wright PF, Crowe JE, Jr, Clements ML, et al. Evaluation of two live, cold-passaged, temperature-sensitive respiratory syncytial virus (RSV) vaccines in chimpanzees, adults, infants and children. *J Infect Dis* 1997;176:1428–1436.)

for HRSV disease shed infectious virus in nasal secretions with peak titers of 10^4 to 10^6 infectious units per ml.[138,139,225,615] Many infants continue to shed virus at hospital discharge and a few can continue to shed virus for weeks following clinical recovery. With the use of quantitative reverse transcription polymerase chain reaction (RT-PCR), the period of detection of HRSV shedding is prolonged, suggesting that virus is present but is neutralized by secretory antibodies made in response to the infection.[137,351] Limited data suggest that the titer of virus in the lower respiratory tract, sampled in bronchoalveolar lavage fluids of ventilated patients, is similar to that in the upper respiratory tract. Infectious virus has been difficult to recover from adults during symptomatic infection despite positive serologic or RT-PCR tests, probably due to the presence of neutralizing antibodies.

HRSV principally exhibits tropism for the airways and lung tissues. Studies in human adenoid or HAE epithelium models *in vitro* showed that HRSV preferentially infected ciliated cells. Infection was limited to the apical surface and did not spread to underlying cells, and virus was released from the apical surface[562,616,631] (Fig. 38.6). In experimental HAE infections lasting several weeks, infected cells were shed and replaced with little visible alteration of the microscopic appearance of the tissue, although ciliary beating usually was impaired.[616,631] Syncytia were not observed, probably because the F glycoprotein was expressed on the apical surface and did not contact adjacent cells. HRSV contrasted sharply with influenza A virus examined in parallel, which was rapidly destructive and quickly spread to underlying cells.[616,631] HRSV infection of epithelial cells induces a rapid inhibition of Na^+ transport, resulting in apical fluid accumulation.[314] This might be a host mechanism to dilute and remove irritants, but also might contribute to excess fluid and virus spread. This effect was not unique to HRSV, and was observed with parainfluenza and influenza viruses as well as with bacterial pathogens.

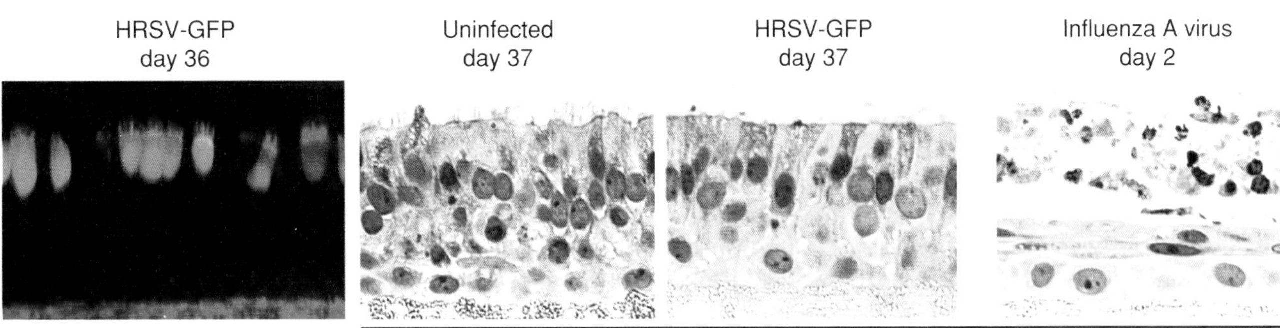

FIGURE 38.6. Infection of an *in vitro* model of human airway epithelium (HAE) with human respiratory syncytial virus (HRSV) and influenza A virus, shown in cross-section. The **left hand panel** is a fluorescence photomicrograph of cells 36 days following infection with HRSV expressing green fluorescent protein (GFP), and also stained with antibody specific to cilia (*red;* note that this antibody also stained the filter support underlying the cells). The three panels to the right show mock-infected, HRSV-infected, and influenza A virus–infected cultures visualized 37 (mock and HRSV) or 2 (influenza) days postinoculation.[631] In the three right-hand panels, the cells were stained with hematoxylin and eosin.

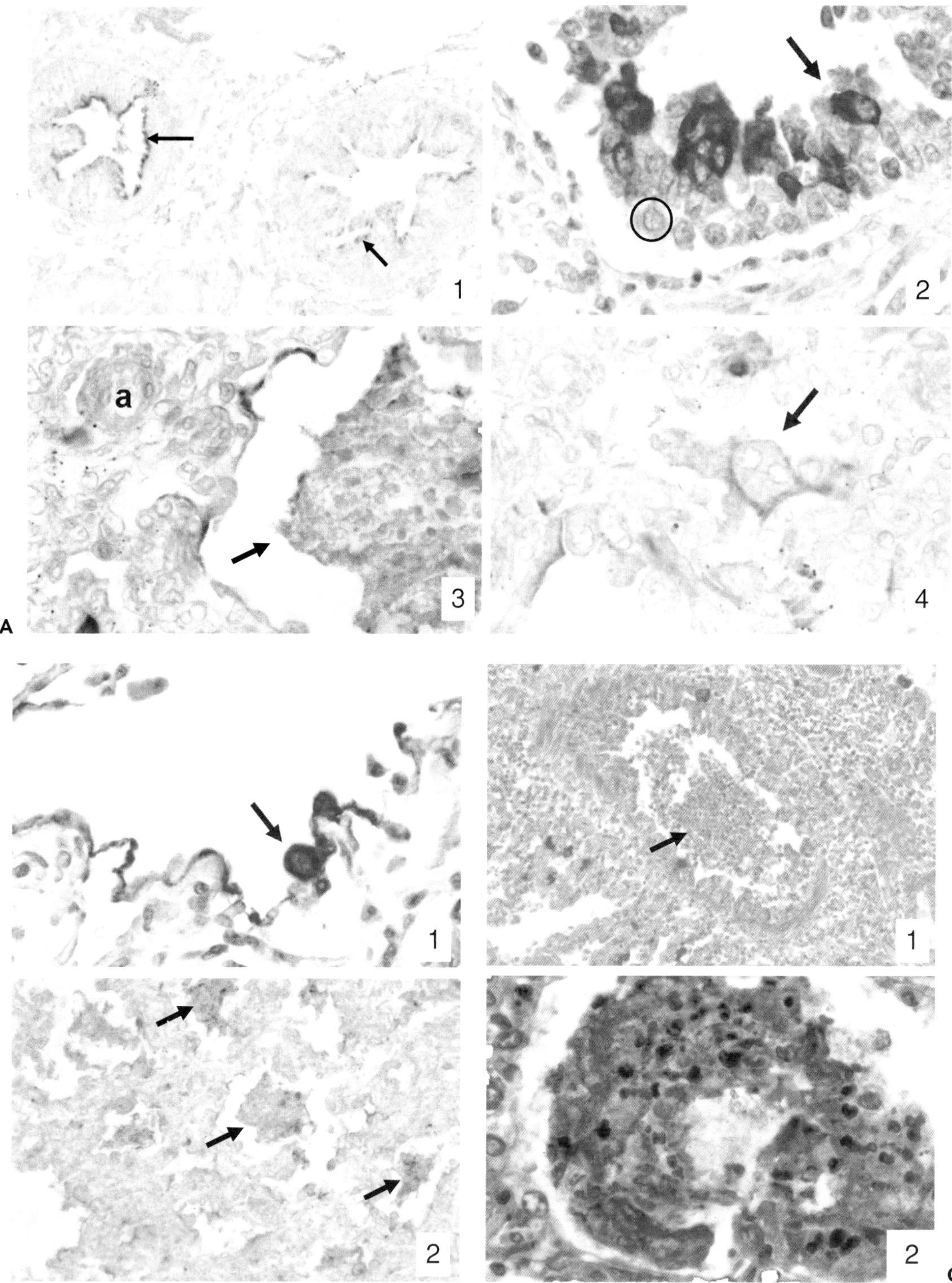

FIGURE 38.7. Histopathology of human respiratory syncytial virus (HRSV) infection in children. A: Bronchiolar localization of HRSV antigen (stained brown) detected by immunohistochemistry. (1) HRSV antigen localized in the luminal epithelium of two bronchioles (*arrows* indicate examples of staining). (2) Higher magnification of infected ciliated cells of the luminal surface of the bronchiole (an example is indicated with the *arrow*), also showing that the basal progenitor cells (an example is *circled*) are not infected. (3) Intraluminal debris (the *arrow* indicates a large debris plug) in a small airway, staining positively for HRSV antigen (an arteriole is marked with "a"). (4) A small syncytium (*arrow*). **B (left):** Alveolar localization of HRSV antigen (brown) detected by immunohistochemistry. (1) HRSV-infected alveolar cells (the *arrow* indicates an infected cell). (2) Alveolar lumens and small airways clogged with debris (examples are indicated with the *arrows*) that stains positively for HRSV antigen. **C (right):** Histopathologic features of bronchiolar inflammation, with periodic acid-Schiff (PAS) staining of carbohydrate macromolecules. (1) Bronchiole occluded with an intraluminal plug of debris and inflammatory cells (*arrow*). (2) Higher magnification image of intraluminal debris. (Reprinted by permission from Macmillan Publishers Ltd. From Johnson JE, Gonzales RA, Olson SJ, et al. The histopathology of fatal untreated human respiratory syncytial virus infection. *Mod Pathol* 2007;20:108–119; copyright 2007.)

Histopathology of fatal HRSV infections indicates that infection is limited to the superficial cells of the respiratory tract, consistent with the findings in HAE cultures, although it is likely that nonciliated cells also are infected[4,187,273,596] (Fig. 38.7). There is necrosis and destruction of ciliated cells and occasional proliferation of the bronchiolar epithelium, but basal cells are spared. Ciliated epithelial cells rarely reappear before 2 weeks postinfection, and complete restoration requires 4 to 8 weeks,[220] similar to the duration of postinfection altered lung function and airway reactivity in adults.[237] There is an early influx of polymorphonuclear cells, and a peribronchiolar infiltrate of lymphocytes, plasma cells, and macrophages develops, with migration of the lymphocytes among the mucosal epithelial cells. Submucosal and adventitial tissues become edematous, and secretion of mucus is excessive, which combines with cell debris and inflammatory cells to obstruct the bronchioles and alveoli, causing either collapse or emphysema of distal portions of the airway. HRSV infects both type I and type II alveolar cells.[273] In those instances in which pneumonia occurs, the interalveolar walls thicken as a result of mononuclear cell infiltration, and the alveolar spaces may fill with fluid. There is usually a patchy appearance of these pathologic changes, even though disease may be widespread. Immunostaining identified virus-infected cells in the bronchial, bronchiolar, and alveolar epithelium.[273,419] Syncytia are sometimes observed, but are not prominent. However, syncytium formation and giant cell pneumonia are hallmarks of infection in individuals with extreme T-cell deficiency. HRSV antigen can be relatively abundant in lower respiratory tract infection, although the staining is usually focal, and in some cases of fatal HRSV bronchiolitis, antigen was present only in small amounts.[187,419] The histopathology of HMPV infection is not well known but has been reported to involve a characteristic enlarged, darkly staining pneumocyte or "smudge cell" that is not seen with other respiratory paramyxoviruses.[532] Studies in nonhuman primates indicate that HMPV has a similar tropism for the superficial cells of the respiratory epithelium.[311]

Infection by HRSV and HMPV is largely limited to the respiratory tract. Infectious virus has not been recovered from the blood of HRSV- or HMPV-infected humans. However, viral nucleic acid can frequently be detected in the blood of HRSV-infected infants,[478] and there are isolated reports of HRSV RNA in cerebrospinal fluid and myocardium.[149] HRSV antigen has been detected in circulating mononuclear leukocytes.[143] HRSV, HMPV, and influenza viral RNA have been detected in sera of immunosuppressed individuals infected with the respective viruses with high viral loads in the respiratory tract.[75] When immunosuppressed cotton rats are infected with HRSV, infectious virus was cultured from the liver and kidneys in a small proportion of animals.[279] HRSV has been cultured from the myocardium of an infected infant with combined immunodeficiency as well as from a liver biopsy from an infected immunocompetent infant.[149,178] This suggests that HRSV (and these other respiratory viruses) has some potential to spread beyond the respiratory tract, but usually is restricted by host immunity. A possible role in extrapulmonary disease manifestations has been suggested.[149]

HRSV is not thought to cause a latent or persistent infection, and the virus is rarely recovered in the absence of respiratory disease. However, some reports suggest the prolonged persistence of virus or viral material. Infectious virus has been recovered from guinea pigs 60 to 100 days postinfection,[124] and was recovered sporadically from mice 100 days postinfection upon T-cell depletion.[499] BRSV RNA and proteins have been detected in bovine pulmonary lymph nodes 71 days following infection, and there was indirect evidence for *in vitro* infectivity from isolated bovine B lymphocytes.[565] There is conflicting evidence as to whether HRSV might persist in some individuals with stable chronic obstructive pulmonary disease.[161,511] HRSV was shed for 199 days, largely without disease, in a child infected with human immunodeficiency virus (HIV),[299] and persistent symptomless shedding of HMPV has been described in a number of hematopoietic stem cell transplant (HSCT) recipients.[133]

The available information suggests that there are not marked differences in replication or virulence among HRSV isolates. Some reports have suggested that subgroup A, or a particular genotype of subgroup A, is associated with increased replication and virulence, but a number of studies have not found such a link.[63,251,363,518] Recently, an HRSV strain called line 19 was shown to induce increased lung IL-13 expression and mucous secretion in BALB/c mice, an effect that mapped to the F gene,[395] raising the possibility that clinically relevant heterogeneity in strain virulence may be uncovered by further investigation. With HMPV, there presently is no indication that specific genotypes are associated with increased disease.[1,60]

Primary HRSV disease is usually symptomatic, but disease manifestations can vary greatly, and may include upper respiratory tract illness (URI), fever, otitis media, LRI ranging from mild disease to bronchiolitis and/or pneumonia with or without subsequent long-term abnormalities in pulmonary function (see *Clinical Features*), and death in rare cases. Infection in immunosuppressed individuals ranges from asymptomatic to highly lethal, probably reflecting the extent of T cell deficiency. In otherwise healthy individuals, a number of factors are thought to contribute to HRSV (and HMPV) pathogenesis and the observed heterogeneity of disease, including direct viral damage, the host immune response, and other host factors including age, immune status, underlying disease, and genetic polymorphisms affecting host defense.[96] These are discussed below and in subsequent sections.

Because HRSV can readily infect and cause disease during the first months of life, young age must be considered as a factor in pathogenesis (e-Fig. 38.7). Maternal antibody and immunologic immaturity result in reduced immune responses during infancy (see Immunity section in this chapter), reducing the ability to control the infection. Immune responses in the neonate and young infant can have a reduced Th1 component, which is protective for the fetus prior to birth but can contribute to a Th2 bias in early infancy,[3,121] and which may contribute to an inflammatory response in the lower airways. The small diameter of bronchioles in infants makes them particularly susceptible to obstruction by edema, secretions, and immune and exfoliated cells.[262] Infancy is a time of considerable lung growth and development.[189] Developing lungs may be more susceptible to disease and to long-term effects on lung function. For example, infants with severe HRSV infection express increased levels of neurotrophic factors and receptors.[558] Studies in a rodent model suggest that this can lead to remodeling of neural networks that innervate the respiratory mucosa, contributing to recurrent airway inflammation and hyperreactivity.[449] Children with a history of HRSV bronchiolitis early in life were found to have higher obstructive sleep

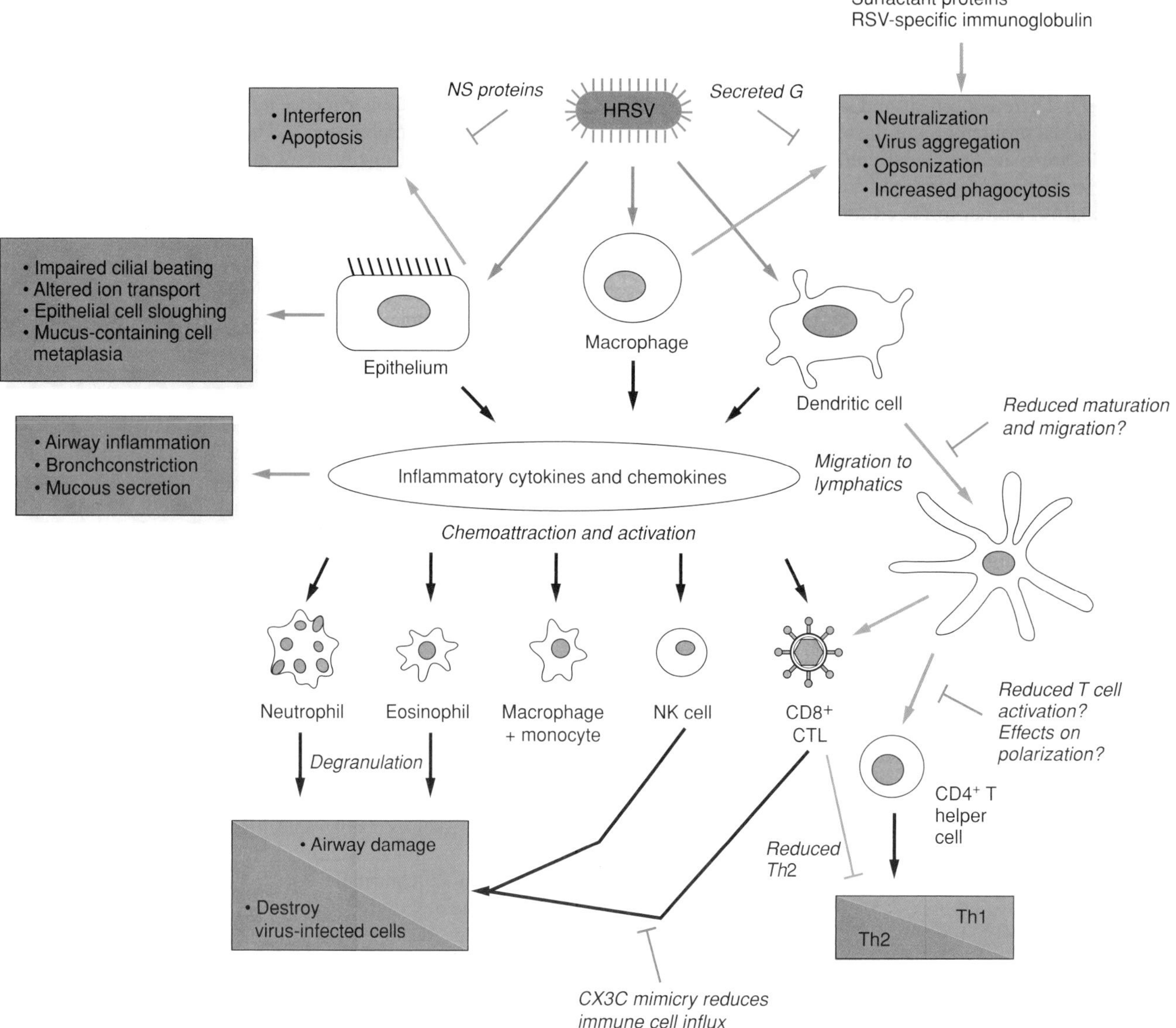

FIGURE 38.8. Factors in human respiratory syncytial virus (HRSV) infection, disease, and immune evasion. In the respiratory tract, the virus **(top)** infects epithelial cells (the major site of virus replication), macrophages, and dendritic cells. Effects that increase virus replication and pathogenesis and/or decrease immune protection are in red; factors favoring protection are in green. **Top right:** surfactant proteins, virus-specific antibodies, and macrophages help restrict infection and spread; antibody-mediated clearance is inhibited by secreted G protein. **Top left:** in infected cells, the viral NS proteins inhibit IFN production and signaling and delay apoptosis. **Center left:** virus infection in epithelial cells impairs their function in maintaining airway fluid level and mucous flow and eventually leads to cell sloughing. **Center:** infected epithelial cells, macrophages, and dendritic cells produce inflammatory cytokines and chemokines that promote airway reactivity and mucous production, attract and activate immune cells, and in some cases may directly induce antiviral effects. **Bottom:** immune cell influx is reduced by viral CX3C fractalkine mimicry. Degranulation by neutrophils (a major inflammatory cell in the airway) and eosinophils, and cell killing by natural killer (NK) cells and $CD8^+$ T cells, help restrict infection but also may contribute to disease. **Right:** antigen encounter by dendritic cells leads to their maturation and migration to secondary lymphatic tissue: infection of dendritic cells by HRSV is inefficient and subsequent maturation and migration may be suboptimal. **Bottom right:** dendritic cells induce $CD4^+$ and $CD8^+$ T-cell activation, polarization, and proliferation: these steps may be reduced due to HRSV exposure. Th2 responses may be suppressed by $CD8^+$ T cells and NK cells. (Adapted from Brearey SP, Symth RL. Pathogenesis of RSV in children, In Cane P, ed. *Respiratory Syncytial Virus*. Elsevier: Amsterdam; 2007;141–162.)

apnea and hypopnea indices than control children, which also is associated with increased expression of neurotrophic factors and receptors.[519] There also is evidence from the mouse model that HRSV infection early in life can result in skewed primary and recall immune responses.[121,541] Other host risk factors are described in the section entitled Epidemiology.

A number of studies, including prospective studies of natural infection, experimental infection of adults with wild-type HRSV, and clinical studies with live HRSV vaccine candidates, have indicated a positive correlation between virus load and disease severity,[137,138,291,362] although there also are contradictory data.[37,225,226,615] High nasopharyngeal viral load also was associated with disease severity for HMPV.[60,362] However, it is not clear whether this correlation reflects pathogenesis due to direct viral damage or a heightened immune response. As noted, studies with *in vitro* human epithelium models indicate that HRSV is not very cytopathic or invasive, compared to influenza virus for example (Fig. 38.6). However, impaired ciliary function and increased cell shedding resulting from HRSV infection would facilitate clogging of bronchioles and alveoli. In experimental infection in adults, the timing of HRSV disease coincided with the timing of viral shedding, suggesting that direct viral damage contributes to disease.[137] The observation that HRSV (and HMPV) can cause severe disease in immunocompromised cotton rats[613] and humans[146,163,233] indicates that severe disease does not depend on an intact adaptive immune system. However, in humans with HRSV LRI, treatment with virus-neutralizing antibodies or the antiviral drug ribavirin that reduced virus replication resulted in limited improvement (see Treatment section), suggesting that factors in addition to direct viral damage are important in pathogenesis, especially by the time that LRI occurs.

It is widely thought that host immunity plays a major role in HRSV (and presumably HMPV) disease. In HRSV-infected cotton rats, treatment with HRSV-neutralizing antibodies rapidly reduced pulmonary titers but had little effect on lung histopathology.[463] In contrast, treatment with antiinflammatory glucocorticoids reduced lung histopathology, even though clearance of the virus was slowed, suggesting that the host immune response played the major role in pathogenesis in this model.[463] However, the situation is less clear in humans, where treatment with corticosteroids does not significantly reduce disease[309,439] (see Treatment section). Immune factors that have been suggested to contribute to HRSV disease include (a) an excessive inflammatory response, (b) an overly robust $CD8^+$ T-cell response, resulting in excessive tissue damage, and (c) a Th2-biased $CD4^+$ T-cell response that is not optimally effective against intracellular pathogens and results in excessive mucous production, airway reactivity, and other effects (see Immune Response). There are supporting and contrary data in each case, as will be shown, and it may be that the contributions of various factors vary in different individuals. Host and viral factors that are suspected to contribute to restriction of HRSV replication and/or to disease pathogenesis, as well as some of the viral mechanisms that subvert or inhibit host immunity, are depicted in Figure 38.8 and discussed throughout this chapter. These general themes likely also apply to HMPV.

IMMUNE RESPONSE

HRSV and HMPV cause acute infections that are restricted and resolved by innate and adaptive immunity. Immune responses to HRSV and HMPV are broadly similar to those against other respiratory viruses such as influenza and the HPIVs. Infection induces mucosal and systemic virus-neutralizing antibody responses as well as cell-mediated responses. Cellular immunity is particularly important in resolving infection. Secretory and serum antibodies play the primary role in protection against reinfection. With the exception of passively acquired HRSV-neutralizing antibodies, correlates of protection in young infants are difficult to measure and are poorly understood.

Antigens

Postinfection sera from experimental animals or humans contain antibodies that recognize a number of HRSV proteins. However, the F and G proteins are the only virus neutralization antigens and are major, independent protective antigens.[108] This was demonstrated in experiments in which cotton rats or mice were immunized with vaccinia virus recombinants expressing individual HRSV proteins and subsequently challenged with HRSV.[108,428] F and G were the only proteins that induced neutralizing antibody responses and conferred long-lasting protection. F was more immunogenic and protective than G[108,428]; the apparent poorer immunogenicity of G may be a consequence of its unusual structure and heavy glycosylation.

A large fraction of MAbs raised against the HRSV F protein neutralize infectivity efficiently, and many inhibit fusion.[32,349] Analysis of viral mutants selected to be resistant to individual MAbs mapped five major antigenic sites that mainly involve the F1 subunit.[113,349] In some cases, mapping has been extended by visualization of antigen–antibody complexes by electron microscopy[74] or by crystallographic analysis,[377] and sites have been mapped on a predicted three-dimensional model of the F protein.[517] Operationally, most of the epitopes of F appear to be conformation dependent, since most monoclonal and polyclonal antibodies raised against native F react poorly with denatured protein, such as in Western blots, and synthetic peptides designed from F are inefficient in inducing neutralizing antibodies or protective immunity.

In contrast, HRSV G has a very different antigenic nature. Most G-specific MAbs bind efficiently to denatured G, such as in Western blots, and many bind efficiently to synthetic peptides, suggesting that reactivity does not depend on a complex folded structure.[186] Most MAbs against the G protein are inefficient in neutralizing RSV infectivity *in vitro* when tested individually, although neutralization can be achieved with mixtures of MAbs.[365,367] Most G-specific MAbs react with some HRSV strains but not others within an antigenic subgroup and thus are "strain-specific": these MAbs often react only with glycosylated G, and their epitopes mostly are in the mucin-like domain in the C-terminal third of the molecule. Other MAbs react broadly within a subgroup, and a small number react with viruses from both subgroups: these MAbs typically do not depend on glycosylation of G for binding, and their epitopes usually are located in the central conserved region of G.[365,384] A synthetic peptide representing this central region was protective in mice and calves,[29] confirming its importance in immunogenicity and antigenicity. Postinfection human serum antibodies to the G protein were found to be enriched for the immunoglobulin G2 (IgG2) subclass, consistent with G being recognized in part as a polysaccharide antigen.[583]

Most of the HRSV proteins stimulated memory $CD8^+$ CTL from seropositive humans.[90] However, in both mice and humans, the G protein is a poor CTL antigen, possibly due to its skewed amino acid content and extensive glycosylation. In the commonly used BALB/c mouse model, the F, N, and M2-1 proteins (of HRSV strain A2) have been shown to induce CD8+ CTL responses: the dominant CTL epitope is contained in amino acids 82 to 90 of the M2-1 protein, accounting for approximately 40% of the primary CTL response.[312] Immunization of mice with vaccinia virus recombinants expressing the N or M2-1 proteins provided protective immunity that was not mediated by neutralizing antibodies and, in the case of M2-1, was confirmed to be mediated by CD8+ CTLs.[108,312] However, protection waned within weeks, suggesting that pulmonary protection by CTLs is short-lived.

For HMPV, the F protein also is a major neutralization and protective antigen, which was shown in studies in which F was expressed by a HPIV1 vector in rodents and nonhuman primates,[515,539] or by an alphavirus replicon evaluated in mice and cotton rats.[392] Surprisingly, vectors that individually expressed the G and SH proteins did not induce detectable neutralizing antibodies or protection in rodents.[392,514] Similarly, purified HMPV G protein administered to cotton rats did not induce neutralizing antibodies or protection.[485] Therefore, HMPV may differ from other members of *Paramyxoviridae* in having only a single surface glycoprotein as a major neutralization and protective antigen.

Innate Immunity and Inflammation

The first line of host defense includes the physical barriers of the glycocalyx of the superficial epithelial cells, the secreted mucous layer, and ciliary sweeping. A number of studies have highlighted the role of pulmonary surfactant proteins (SPs), specifically SP-A, SP-C, and SP-D, in restricting HRSV. SPs are lipoprotein complexes produced by type II alveolar cells. SP-A and SP-D have been shown to bind to HRSV, neutralize infectivity (in the case of SP-A), and promote phagocytosis.[25,192,332] Mice with targeted disruption of SP-A, SP-C, or SP-D exhibited increased pulmonary HRSV titers and disease, which was ameliorated by topical administration of the missing surfactant.[195,332,333] Genetic polymorphisms in SP-A, SP-B, and SP-D have been associated with severe pediatric HRSV disease.[150,389,466] Infants with severe HRSV disease were found to have reduced surfactant concentration and function, although it is not known whether this was a cause or a result of severe disease.[293]

Toll-like receptors (TLRs) present on the plasma membrane and endosomes[302] play a significant role in the host response to HRSV. The HRSV F protein stimulates TLR4 on leukocytes independent of viral replication, leading to activation of the NF-κB pathway to produce cytokines such as IL-6 and IL-8 and activation of IRF3 to induce type I IFN.[317] TLR4-deficient mice are less efficient than normal mice in resolving HRSV infection.[302,317] A number of studies have linked severe pediatric HRSV disease with genetic polymorphisms in TLR4 that reduce its signaling capacity, although other studies did not detect this association.[302] HRSV has also been shown to activate signaling from the TLR2/TLR6 heterodimer complex on the surface of leukocytes, resulting in the expression of proinflammatory cytokines, neutrophil influx, and dendritic cell activation in mice.[407] Mice lacking TLR2 or TLR6 were less able to restrict HRSV challenge compared to normal mice. HRSV also activates TLR3 in epithelial cells, resulting in the production of inflammatory cytokine and chemokines.[483] Studies in TLR3 knockout mice indicated that TLR3 did not make a significant contribution to restricting HRSV replication, but helped prevent IL-13 upregulation and increased mucous production.[484] Excessive stimulation of TLRs can potentially contribute to pathogenesis: viral infection increases the expression of TLR3 and TLR4, promoting sensitivity both to HRSV and to possible co-infecting viruses or bacteria. In addition to TLRs, the cytoplasmic receptor RIG-I plays a major role in innate responses.[348,625] Of course, as noted, HRSV and HMPV have mechanisms that suppress activation of these signaling pathways (e-Fig. 38.6).

Infection of epithelial cells by HRSV (or HMPV) alters the cell transcriptional profile markedly, resulting in changes in expression (mostly upregulation) of 900 genes or more.[22,266,366,632] This was mostly dependent on viral replication. These genes represented multiple biological pathways, showing a broad effect of viral infection. Proteomic profiling of the proteins expressed in A549 epithelial cell cultures following infection with HRSV identified changes in expression for more than 100 cellular proteins, similarly indicating a complex cellular response to infection (the greater number of responding species detected by transcriptional versus proteomic profiling reflects the greater sensitivity of the former method).[81,402] Comparison of the responses in A549 epithelial cells infected with HRSV, HMPV, HPIV3, and measles virus identified a common core response that mainly involved defense against endoplasmic reticulum stress and induction of apoptosis.[576]

Airway epithelial cells and macrophages exposed to HRSV *in vitro* produce a broad array of proinflammatory cytokines, including IL-1, IL-8/CXCL8, RANTES/CCL5, IL-10, MIP-1α/CCL3, MCP-1/CCL2, IP-10/CXCL10, IL-6, TNFα, and type I and type III IFNs.[30,385,386,523] Many of these cytokines have been found in secretions from the upper and lower respiratory tracts of infants with HRSV bronchiolitis.[56,248] One consequence is the recruitment of immune cells to the infected lung (Fig. 38.8). The total number of immune cells recovered in washes from the upper and lower respiratory tracts of infants was several fold higher in cases of severe HRSV disease compared with uninfected controls.[157,249,380] Neutrophils were by far the most abundant immune cells present in the airway, comprising 76% to 93% of recovered cells from the upper and lower respiratory tracts, with lymphocytes and mononuclear cells being present at ≤10% each and eosinophils at <1%.[157,380] Incoming immune cells become activated to express cytokines and other proinflammatory molecules such as cysteinyl leukotrienes that can heighten the inflammatory response.

Inflammation helps control infection but may also contribute to disease (Fig. 38.8), although the picture remains unclear. Studies in mice showed that natural killer (NK) cells are prominent in the early response to infection, are an important source of IFNγ, and have cytotoxic activity against infected cells.[267] Granulocytes release factors, such as neutrophil elastase and eosinophil-associated ribonucleases, which can be antimicrobial but also may damage tissue.[57,480] Increased levels of eosinophil cationic protein and neutrophil elastase have been observed in respiratory washes from infants with severe HRSV disease, indicating the presence and activation of these granulocytes.[2,188] Mice with eosinophilia due to increased IL-5 expression had increased viral clearance, indicating that eosinophils can be protective.[448] The amount of mRNA for IL-8—a cytokine that promotes neutrophil chemotaxis and survival—measured in nasal aspirates of children with bronchiolitis correlated with the severity of disease,[518] and an IL-8 haplotype characterized by increased IL-8 gene transcription was associated with increased susceptibility to HRSV disease.[219] Bronchoalveolar washes from infants with severe HRSV disease had increased levels of mRNA for IL-9, which is secreted by neutrophils and other cells and promotes inflammation and increased mucous production.[379] In infants with severe HRSV disease, the appearance of neutrophil precursors in peripheral blood, preceding their influx into the airways, closely followed the peak of viral load and was coincident with clinical symptoms[351] (e-Fig. 38.8). These findings suggest that neutrophils in particular have the potential to contribute to both viral clearance and disease. Conversely, however, there also is evidence that, although HRSV may indeed induce high levels of inflammatory cytokines in children hospitalized with HRSV disease, this may not be the dominant factor in severe disease and indeed may be protective.[37,503] Furthermore, a prospective study of primary HRSV and HMPV infections in infants showed that, although infants infected with either virus had similar disease signs, the levels of inflammatory cytokines induced by HMPV were significantly lower than with HRSV.[321] Therefore, although these viruses exhibited similar patterns of disease, they do not share a common pattern of overly robust innate immune responses that might be expected if that is the major determinant of disease.

Macrophages are abundant in the respiratory tract and play important roles in restricting virus replication and modulating the host response. Mice that are genetically deficient in macrophage function, or in which macrophages have been depleted, are less able to restrict HRSV infection and exhibit increased lung inflammation.[472] This illustrates a key role for these phagocytic cells in restricting the virus as well as in clearing the lung of debris that can cause further damage and inflammation. Macrophages also play an important role in the early response to HRSV infection by producing an immediate release of proinflammatory cytokines.[457] Studies in mice suggest that macrophages are the primary producers of type I IFN in response to viral respiratory infection in general, with myeloid dendritic cells (DCs) also contributing, whereas pDCs can play a role later in infection if virus replication is not controlled.[313]

Type I IFN has well-known antiviral effects mediated by signaling through its ubiquitous receptor IFNAR. Type I IFN also is considered to stimulate both innate and adaptive immunity, although these effects can be complex.[403] Studies in which bovines were immunized with mutants of BRSV provided evidence of increased humoral and cellular immune responses associated with deletion of NS2, which is the major IFN antagonist of BRSV.[566] Type III IFN is less well characterized but also has antiviral effects. It generally is produced from the same cell types that produce type I IFN. However, its receptor is expressed mainly on the epithelial cells of the respiratory and gastrointestinal tracts, and thus its effects may be largely limited to those sites.[144,396] Studies in mice lacking the receptor for either or both type I and III IFN showed that each is involved in restricting replication of respiratory viruses including HRSV,[396] although a study with PVM suggested that type I IFN has a greater antiviral role.[252]

IFNα/β were detected less frequently and at lower levels in nasal secretions from infants, young children, and adults infected with HRSV, compared to influenza and parainfluenza viruses.[228,229,374] HRSV infection and replication are more resistant to prophylaxis or treatment with IFN-α compared to influenza and parainfluenza viruses.[184,534] Therefore, HRSV may be particularly effective at inhibiting the host IFN response. HMPV induces higher levels of IFN-α/β in mice and is more sensitive to IFN-α than HRSV.[217]

Antibodies

Both serum and secretory antibodies are made in response to HRSV infection. In young infants, the appearance of secretory IgA antibodies usually corresponds with a decrease in HRSV shedding during infection, suggesting a contribution to resolving infection.[376] Secretory IgA antibodies are thought to be particularly efficient in restricting HRSV replication. The secretory antibody response is not long-lasting following primary infection, but as individuals grow older and are reinfected, the response is more sustained.[292] Experimental infections in adults showed that resistance to reinfection correlated with the titer of HRSV-specific secretory or serum antibodies,[235,387] and there are similar findings for natural infection.[585]

Studies of prophylaxis in high-risk infants with either intravenous immunoglobulin containing high titers of HRSV-neutralizing antibodies (RSV-IGIV) or HRSV-neutralizing F MAbs (palivizumab, motavizumab) have demonstrated the protective effect of serum HRSV-neutralizing antibodies against severe HRSV disease[77,214,434] (see Prevention, below). Studies in experimental animals and observations with maternal serum antibodies also illustrate the protective effect of HRSV-neutralizing antibodies (below). The serum antibody response is long-lived (except early in life, as noted below), and peak titers of antibodies detected by ELISA were reached following the second infection in life.[582] However, serum IgG antibodies gain access to the respiratory tract primarily by the relatively inefficient process of passive transudation. As a consequence, high serum antibody titers are necessary to achieve protection in the respiratory tract. For example, in studies of passively transferred antibodies in the cotton rat model, neutralizing serum titers of 1:390 and 1:3,500 were required to achieve a 99% reduction in HRSV replication in the lower and upper respiratory tracts, respectively.[462] As another indication of the concentration gradient between the circulation and the lumen of the respiratory tract, the therapeutic effect of passive antibodies in reducing HRSV replication in cotton rats was 160-fold greater when administered directly to the respiratory tract versus systemically.[459] Studies in humans suggested an antibody concentration gradient of approximately 350:1 between sera and nasal washes.[581] Therefore, protection conferred by serum antibodies obtained by maternal transfer, or prior infection, or passive antibody prophylaxis, depends on a high titer of HRSV-neutralizing antibodies and is less efficient in the upper versus the lower respiratory tract.

Young infants possess maternally derived serum IgG antibodies against HRSV, HMPV, and other common pathogens.[114] Epidemiologic studies indicate that HRSV disease in infants born with higher levels of maternal HRSV-neutralizing antibodies was milder and occurred at an older age than in infants with lower antibody levels, suggesting a protective effect.[196] Maternal antibodies are obtained from the mother during gestation by active transport across the placenta beginning at ~26 weeks of gestation and continuing until birth (Fig. 38.9). Infants who are born prematurely have lower titers, increasing their susceptibility to infection and disease. The IgG1 subclass is preferentially

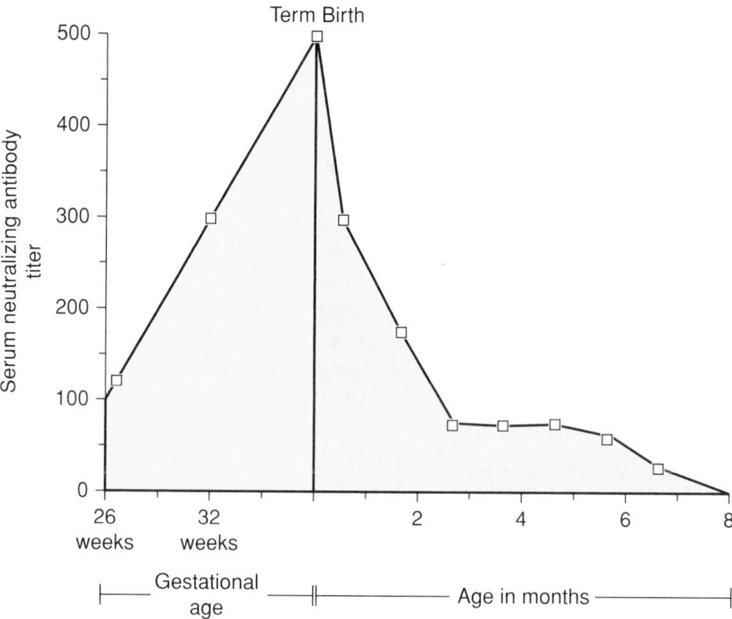

FIGURE 38.9. An idealized diagram based on experimental data illustrating the titer of human respiratory syncytial virus (HRSV)–neutralizing maternal serum antibodies in the fetus[129] and newborn human infant[437] as a function of gestational and postnatal age. This illustration depicts the transplacental transfer of serum antibodies and the subsequent decrease in titer following birth; this diagram shows only the HRSV-neutralizing component of the multivalent maternal antibodies. Courtesy of Dr. James E. Crowe, Jr. Note that absolute neutralizing antibody titers achieved at birth can vary substantially between individual infants depending upon maternal titers.

transferred, but otherwise the titer and specificity of maternally derived IgG antibodies in the full-term neonate are similar to or slightly higher than those of the mother. Thereafter, these antibodies decay with a half-life of approximately 21 to 26 days and protection diminishes. Breast milk may also contribute protective antibodies, although this has not been clearly documented and likely is a minor effect.

In hospitalized infants, HRSV-specific serum IgA and IgG responses were detected 10 days following the onset of illness, and peak titers were achieved at 3 to 4 weeks.[594] The magnitude of serum and secretory antibody responses to HRSV in young infants typically is reduced compared to older individuals. For example, in a study of infants and young children with a primary HRSV infection, the titers of serum antibodies that bound to the F or G glycoprotein or that neutralized HRSV were 8- to 10-fold lower in individuals of 4 to 8 months versus 9 to 21 months of age.[409] The frequency of a detectable secretory IgA response to HRSV in infected infants was directly related to age, and these antibodies often were nonneutralizing *in vitro*.[292,376] The effect of age on the response of serum and nasal wash antibodies to a live attenuated HRSV vaccine is illustrated in e-Figure 38.9. In addition, antibody responses in the young infant are short-lived compared to older individuals: the increases in HRSV-specific IgA and IgG antibodies observed shortly after infection in infants were absent or at very low titer 1 year later.[594] Therefore, secretory and serum antibody responses are reduced in young infants (<~6 months of age) compared to older individuals with respect to magnitude, neutralizing activity, and longevity. This is particularly relevant to HRSV, since HRSV infection is very common in infancy (*Epidemiology*). Responses to HMPV are assumed to be similar.

Reduced immune responses to HRSV (and HMPV) early in life are due to immunologic immaturity[3,336] and the immunosuppressive effects of maternal antibodies.[114,507] Immunologic immaturity has been characterized for a variety of antigens and has been shown to limit innate, antibody, and cellular responses during the first year of life, although these effects are not absolute and adult-like responses can be elicited under some circumstances.[3,336] Examination of the human neonatal B cell response to HRSV revealed a bias in the repertoire of antibody gene expression and a dramatically reduced frequency of somatic mutations compared to individuals older than 3 months, which likely contributes to the poorly neutralizing nature of the response in the young infant.[611] Immunosuppression by HRSV-specific maternal or passive serum antibodies has been documented in natural infection,[408] in experimental animals,[410,411] and in the setting of clinical evaluation of live HRSV vaccines in infants.[617] For example, in the case of live-attenuated vaccines, the titer of maternal antibody had little effect on virus replication in the upper respiratory tract, but suppressed the serum and secretory antibody responses.[617] In mice, passive HRSV-specific serum antibodies suppressed both serum and secretory antibody responses to infection with wild-type HRSV but did not suppress the cell-mediated response and priming for a secondary antibody response.[117] Surprisingly, in a cohort of infants younger than 6 months of age who were identified as having very low titers of HRSV-specific maternal antibodies, natural wild-type HRSV infection induced neutralizing serum antibody titers that were indistinguishable from those of individuals aged 6 to 24 months.[505] This indicates that young infants are capable of mounting a substantial antibody response when maternal antibodies are not present to exert their suppressive role. Therefore, maternal antibodies are beneficial in providing some disease sparing early in life, but also suppress antibody responses.

In adults, natural HRSV infection induced an approximately eightfold rise in serum HRSV-neutralizing antibodies, which declined fourfold during the subsequent year.[165] Titers in uninfected control subjects did not decline during this period, suggesting that there may be a relatively stable set-point, whereas postinfection rises are more short-lived. Interestingly, elderly individuals exhibited a more robust antibody response to infection with HRSV or HMPV compared to younger adults.[162,584] This indicates that the increased susceptibility that comes with aging is not due to a defect in the ability to produce virus-neutralizing antibodies.

It has been suggested that, in some individuals, HRSV infection induces IgE that may contribute to HRSV disease. IgE—whose production is promoted by the Th2 cytokines IL-4 and IL-13—is bound by receptors on mast cells, and contact with antigen induces the release of mediators including histamine and leukotrienes that stimulate inflammation, rhinorrhea, cough, and wheezing. Increased HRSV-specific IgE and histamine were detected in respiratory secretions from HRSV-infected infants with wheezing in concentrations that correlated with the degree of hypoxia.[595] However, other groups have not found convincing evidence of HRSV-specific IgE,[126] and its significance remains uncertain.

T Lymphocytes

Experience with patients with deficiencies in cell-mediated immunity has demonstrated its importance in restricting HRSV and other enveloped respiratory viruses.[178,233,299,600] Immunodeficient children fail to clear HRSV and can shed virus for months rather than the typical interval of 1 to 3 weeks. Severely immunocompromised adults, such as HSCT recipients or individuals with leukemia, are readily infected with HRSV and have a high incidence of serious disease and death. In addition, HMPV can cause severe disease in HSCT recipients,[75] although there also can be prolonged shedding without disease.[133]

In the mouse model for HRSV, depletion of the $CD4^+$ and $CD8^+$ T-lymphocyte subsets individually or together showed that both are important in clearing a primary infection.[209] Both subsets also contributed to disease, with $CD8^+$ cells having the greater effect.[209] In contrast, depletion of B lymphocytes indicated that HRSV-specific antibodies are not required for clearance of a primary infection in mice, although they reduced disease and were important for restricting secondary infection.[207] Although treatment with HRSV-neutralizing antibodies can greatly reduce viral replication in HRSV-infected mice, it was inefficient in eliminating the virus, illustrating the importance of cellular immunity for viral clearance.[431]

In humans, robust $CD8^+$ T-cell responses have been documented in the peripheral blood of infants and children during primary and secondary HRSV infections (e-Fig. 38.8), which precedes the migration of these cells to the respiratory tract.[249,250] Infants with severe HRSV disease have increased numbers of T lymphocytes in the airways, with a greater abundance of the $CD8^+$ versus $CD4^+$ subset, and a greater proportion of airway $CD8^+$ T cells compared with rhinovirus-infected children.[157,250,380] However, although the number of $CD8^+$ T cells was increased by infection, they did not constitute a particularly abundant cell population either in fluid recovered from the airways of infants with severe HRSV disease[157,250,380] or in pulmonary tissue from infants that experienced severe or fatal RSV infection.[273,596] Increased disease was observed in a severely immunocompromised child with a long-term HRSV infection following transfer of donor lymphocytes.[151] However, in infants and children with HRSV LRI, the timing of the $CD8^+$ T-cell response did not correlate with disease: specifically, the appearance of virus-specific $CD8^+$ T cells in peripheral blood peaked during recovery 9 to 15 days following the onset of symptoms[249,351] (e-Fig. 38.8). In addition, the magnitude of the systemic virus-specific $CD8^+$ T-cell response did not correlate with disease severity.[249] Therefore, although studies in mice suggest that $CD8^+$ T cells make an important contribution to HRSV disease, this is less evident from observations in humans.

An increased response of Th2 versus Th1 $CD4^+$ lymphocytes (defined by the signature cytokines IL-4 and IFNγ, respectively) may contribute to pathogenic responses to HRSV infection and reinfection. The clinical picture of severe HRSV disease, including airway plugging, wheezing, and long-lasting effects on lung function, has some similarity with asthma, which involves a Th2 bias. As noted, young infants can have a Th2 bias lingering from the prenatal period. In addition, studies in rodents indicate that a Th2-biased response was involved in the enhanced HRSV disease that was associated with a formalin-inactivated HRSV vaccine evaluated in the 1960s (see *Prevention*). However, analogies to asthma and the formalin-inactivated vaccine are inexact because disease in those examples depends on prior sensitization, whereas HRSV disease during natural infection is most severe during the initial exposure and is less severe with repeat exposures.

The evidence for Th2-biased responses in HRSV disease is mixed. In some studies, peripheral blood mononuclear cells from infants hospitalized with HRSV disease exhibited a Th2-biased HRSV-specific recall response when stimulated *in vitro*.[36,479] However, other studies documented Th1-biased responses[62] or heterogeneity in responses, with some infants having Th1-biased responses and others Th2.[328,390] Th2-biased cytokine responses detected in respiratory washes from infants infected with HRSV were significantly higher than from influenza virus-infected infants.[533] A positive association was found between HRSV disease and a genetic polymorphism in the IL-4 gene that increases gene expression.[389] Other studies detected Th2-biased responses predominantly in individuals with a history of asthma or allergy, suggesting that Th2 involvement is linked to those with this predisposition.[296,330] In another study, Th2-biased responses were observed with influenza and parainfluenza virus in addition to HRSV and were greater in individuals $\leq$3 months of age compared to those >3 months of age, suggesting that this reflects a Th2 bias during the first few months of life but is not specific to HRSV.[310]

Studies in mice suggest that NK cells and HRSV-specific $CD8^+$ CTLs play an important role in enhancing Th1 and limiting Th2 responses to HRSV antigens during infection, an effect mediated by secretion of IFNγ and probably other regulatory molecules.[267,429,525] IFN-α/β also appeared to enhance Th1 and suppress Th2 responses.[148,403] In addition, HRSV-specific $CD8^+$ T cells may reduce virus-induced inflammation through the secretion of IL-10.[529]

Viral Inhibition and Evasion of Host Immunity

HRSV is able to readily reinfect symptomatically throughout life without need for significant antigenic change, and symptomatic reinfection by HMPV also appears to be common (*Epidemiology*). This is in contrast to influenza A virus, for which symptomatic reinfection usually depends on significant antigenic change. This is widely interpreted as evidence that HRSV (and HMPV) inhibits or skews the development of long-term protective immunity. However, the evidence for this is unclear.

HRSV and HMPV indeed have a number of mechanisms that inhibit host innate and adaptive immunity. Some of these have already been noted for HRSV in particular, including very effective (for HRSV) inhibition of type I and type III IFN production and signaling, inhibition of apoptosis, inhibition of TNFα and NF-κB signaling, and inhibition of PKR activation and stress granule formation. HRSV also inhibits signaling from type II IFN (IFNγ) in macrophages.[500]

In addition, studies in the mouse model with HRSV mutants showed that the presence of the fractalkine motif in the G protein has the effect of reducing the pulmonary influx of CX3CR1-bearing leukocytes, including subsets of NK cells and CD4+ and CD8+ T cells, and thus reduces both innate and adaptive responses to infection.[243] In a separate effect, the central conserved domain of G was shown to reduce activation of TLR2, TLR4, and TLR9 in human monocytes, thus suppressing innate immune responses.[453]

As another example, presentation of HRSV and HMPV antigens by myeloid dendritic cells (mDCs) may be inefficient. HRSV and HMPV infect human mDCs inefficiently *in vitro* and induce a low-to-moderate level of mDC maturation.[128,218,325] In the case of HRSV, maturation was partly suppressed by the NS proteins,[404] but reduced maturation also appeared to be due to insufficient stimulation rather than strong inhibition.[325] In addition, expression of NS1 was associated with a shift toward Th2 polarization, reduced Th17 polarization, and reduced activation of CD8+ T cells bearing CD103, a homing integrin that directs CD8+ T cells to mucosal epithelial cells.[403] In mDCs infected with HRSV or HMPV, upregulation of the CCR7 receptor that is necessary for mDC migration to lymphatic tissue was inefficient.[324] Some studies demonstrated reduced activation and altered polarization of CD4+ T lymphocytes *in vitro* in response to HRSV-exposed human mDCs,[128,218,482] although other results suggest that HRSV does not differ significantly from HMPV, HPIV3, and influenza A virus in this regard.[323,325] HRSV also can suppress T-cell proliferative responses *in vitro* by direct contact mediated by the F protein.[494] These observations suggest a variety of mechanisms that might reduce/alter antigen presentation and activation, polarization, and proliferation of CD4+ and CD8+ T cells, but also suggest that some of these effects may not be unique to HRSV.

However, although HRSV has mechanisms that inhibit host immune responses, this likely is true of most viruses, and it is not clear that this is more pronounced with HRSV. It also is not clear that protective responses to HRSV and HMPV are inherently weak or skewed. As noted, the weak and short-lived immune responses observed in young infants are particular to that population rather than to the virus, and brisk serum antibody responses were observed when the suppressive effect of maternal antibodies was minimized.[505] Primary infection of seronegative mice and cotton rats with HRSV induces robust antibody and cellular immune responses and long-lived protective immunity.[208,461] Infection of seronegative chimpanzees with wild-type HRSV or with strongly attenuated live vaccine candidates induced very robust serum antibody titers and protection.[115,549,603,606] With HMPV, infection of mice or cotton rats results in a brisk neutralizing serum antibody response and clearance of the virus, although there was one report of prolonged virus replication for 60 days.[6,241] In another report, infection of cynomolgus macaques with HMPV resulted in neutralizing serum antibody responses that waned substantially over the course of several months, and provided poor protection against a homologous challenge 8 months later.[573] However, in human adults, titers of neutralizing antibodies to HMPV and HRSV are quite high.[162,165] Importantly, reinfection with either virus usually is associated with substantially reduced disease (see *Epidemiology* section), indicating that prior infections induce substantial protection against clinically significant disease. Therefore, the extent to which HRSV and HMPV inhibit or subvert the host protective response remains unclear.

The ability of HRSV and HMPV to reinfect might also reflect evasion of protective immunity. For example, the secreted form of the HRSV G protein was shown to help the virus escape antibody-mediated neutralization, serving as an antigen decoy to spare the virus from neutralizing antibodies, and acting to reduce antibody-mediated clearance by immune cells.[70] Because other common respiratory viruses do not appear to encode secreted forms of a major protective antigen, this may help explain the relative insensitivity of HRSV to restriction by maternal antibodies in HRSV-naïve young infants, and also would facilitate reinfection later in life.

Features of the major viral protective antigens may help evade immunity. As noted, HRSV G is less efficient than F as a neutralization antigen, and HMPV G does not appear to induce neutralizing antibodies or protection. HRSV G also generally appears to be a poor inducer of CD8+ CTLs. Clonal analysis of the human antibody response to HRSV F showed that half of the repertoire was against nonnative protein, suggesting that a substantial proportion of F is produced in an unfolded form that may divert and reduce the immune response to the folded, functional form that is packaged in the virion.[487] Although antigenic differences in HRSV or HMPV are not necessary for reinfection, they do increase its efficiency.[589]

The tropism of HRSV (and HMPV) also may help evade immunity. Restriction of virus replication to the superficial layer of the epithelium, apical budding, and low invasiveness and low cytopathogenicity likely delay and reduce the exposure of viral antigen to the host immune system[631] (Fig. 38.6). Dendritic cells can sample antigen in the respiratory lumen, but poor infectivity and poor induction of CCR7, as noted, would reduce antigen presentation. As noted, serum antibodies are not efficiently transported to the lumen, and local secretory antibodies can be short-lived. In addition, a number of reports have indicated that CD8+ CTLs are functionally downregulated in the lung. This was originally suggested to reflect immune inhibition by HRSV,[85] but further studies showed that this effect does not appear to be specific to HRSV but rather is a property of the tissue.[141,211,570] This probably is a mechanism to reduce lung injury, but would also reduce immune protection. Therefore, evasion of host immune responses likely contributes to infection and reinfection by HRSV and HMPV.

EPIDEMIOLOGY

Infection of Infants and Young Children

HRSV is the most important global cause of severe acute viral LRI in infants and young children. In a benchmark surveillance study from 1957 to 1976 in Washington, DC, HRSV was detected in 23.3% of hospitalizations for respiratory tract disease in infants and young children, compared with 11.5%, 6%, 3.2%, and 5.2% of hospitalizations with HPIV3, HPIV1, HPIV2, and influenza A virus, respectively.[297,412] Similar values for the proportion of ARI hospitalizations attributable to HRSV in infants and young children were obtained in more recent studies.[258,263] HRSV infection was detected in 43% of those hospitalized with a diagnosis of bronchiolitis and in 25% of those with pneumonia, compared to 11% of those hospitalized with bronchitis and 10% of those with croup.[297,412] HRSV infection is more likely to result in pediatric LRI compared to influenza or HPIV1, HPIV2, or HPIV3.[179] Shay et al.[502] estimated that there are 73,400 to 126,306 annual hospitalizations for HRSV pneumonia and bronchiolitis in infants younger than 1 year of age in the United States; more recent estimates by Hall et al.[236] and Lee et al.[329] for annual hospitalizations for HRSV disease in children younger than 5 years of age were 57,527 and 113,000, respectively. The burden of HRSV disease is not confined to hospitalization. In the United States, an estimated 2.1 to 4.2 million children younger than the age of 5 years (representing 10% to 20% of that age group) receive medical care each year for HRSV-related illness.[236,329] Hall et al.[236] estimated that this involves 517,747 (1 of 38) visits to the emergency room and 1,534,064 (1 of 13) primary care office visits, in addition to the hospitalizations already noted.

Although less is known about the burden of HMPV disease, a prospective study of infants hospitalized for ARI or fever without localizing symptoms in Nashville, TN, and Rochester, NY, found that 3.8% of 1,104 such hospitalizations were associated with HMPV.[607] Other retrospective studies at referral hospitals suggested that approximately 5% to 10% of specimens from children hospitalized with ARI or fever were positive for HMPV RNA by RT-PCR. In a cohort of more than 2,000 subjects aged 0 to 5 years followed during a 25-year period at Vanderbilt University Medical Center, approximately 12% of outpatient LRI was associated with HMPV infection, which was second only to HRSV in this population.[608]

Worldwide, HRSV was estimated to cause 33.8 million new cases of LRI in children younger than 5 years of age in 2005, accounting for 22% of all LRI in that age group.[221,417] This resulted in an estimated 3.4 million hospitalizations and 66,000 to 199,000 deaths due to HRSV-associated LRI. These are probably underestimates, since HRSV testing was incomplete and community LRI was undercounted. Although the contribution of HRSV to morbidity and mortality in resource-limited settings is less well understood, a recent study in coastal Kenya showed that HRSV was the predominant virus detected among hospitalized children with severe pneumonia.[39]

HRSV infection is more common in infancy than is infection with other respiratory viruses. Prospective studies have demonstrated that 50% to 69% of infants are infected during the first year of life,[197,253,297] and virtually all are infected by age 2.[197] Primary infection is usually symptomatic, and 25% to 40% of primary infections result in LRI.[197,286] Hospitalization for severe HRSV disease is most frequent between 6 weeks and 6 months of life, with a peak incidence at 1 to 3 months of life (Fig. 38.10). HRSV also causes a substantial disease burden in children beyond the first year of life: of the primary care visits for HRSV disease in infants and children younger than 5 years of age, 61% occurred between the ages of 2 and 5 years.[236] Primary infections with HMPV typically occur slightly later than HRSV, with peak hospitalization occurring at about 6 months of life.[59,401,575] HMPV seropositivity is almost universal by age 5 years.[572]

Reinfection with HRSV is frequent during the first few years of life, more so than with other respiratory viruses. For example, in the prospective study noted above,[197] 47% and 45% of the children during the second and third years of life, respectively, were re-infections. In a day care center study in which 98% of HRSV-naïve infants and young children were infected when exposed to HRSV during an outbreak, the frequency of reinfection during the two subsequent yearly epidemics was 74% and 65%, respectively.[253] Therefore, children often are infected two or more times with HRSV during the first few years of life. Reinfection is usually symptomatic. One study found that LRI could occur during either the first or second infection early in life, whereas for subsequent infections there was a considerable reduction in disease severity reflecting increasing protective immunity.[253] Recurrent infection with HMPV also is thought to be common. In infants, the second HMPV infection can present with upper or lower respiratory tract disease.[610]

Mortality due to HRSV is uncommon in children in developed countries, although mortality is increased substantially in infants with congenital cardiac or pulmonary disease, or immunodeficiency or immunosuppression. There are no

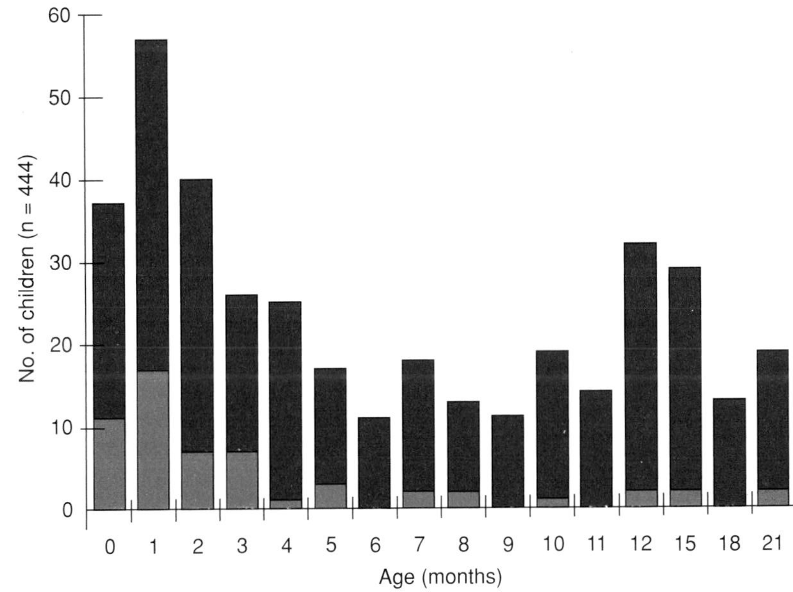

FIGURE 38.10. Age at time of hospitalization for human respiratory syncytial virus (HRSV) disease at the Johns Hopkins Hospital during 1993–1996. The red bars indicate more severe disease. (Adapted from Karron RA, Singleton RJ, et al. Severe respiratory syncytial virus disease in Alaska native children. RSV Alaska Study Group. *J Infect Dis* 1999;180:41–49.)

exact determinations of the overall death rate, but the estimates appear to have dropped over time. A survey from the mid-1970s estimated the fatality rate at 0.5% to 2.5% of hospitalized children with HRSV infection,[91] and in 1985 HRSV was estimated to be responsible for 4,500 pediatric deaths annually in the United States.[381] More recent estimates are as low as 0.3% of hospitalized children. In the United States, the pediatric mortality rate was estimated to be 5.3 and 0.9 per 100,000 per year for individuals younger than 1 year of age and 1 to 4 years of age, respectively, totaling approximately 300 deaths per year.[553] This likely reflects improvement in supportive care.

Major risk factors for pediatric HRSV infection and disease include increased exposure (day care attendance, siblings younger than 5 years of age, and admission to the hospital during HRSV season), low titers of maternal antibodies, lack of previous HRSV infection, premature birth (<36 months gestation, and especially <28 months),[40,122] young age, chronic lung disease,[212] congenital heart disease,[352] neuromuscular diseases, and primary immunodeficiency disorders.[178,375] Other factors include asthma or a family history of asthma, poverty, exposure to tobacco smoke, and male gender. In one study, the estimated number of HRSV hospitalizations per 1,000 during the first year of life was 388 for infants with chronic lung disease, 92 for those with congenital heart disease, 66 for those born at 29 to less than 33 weeks, and 30 for term infants with no underlying disease.[61] Fatality rates for children born prematurely or having underlying pulmonary or cardiac disease were similarly elevated.[593] However, it is important to note that 50% to 70% of HRSV hospitalizations occur in previously healthy full-term infants.[61,455]

Very high rates of hospitalization can occur in certain populations. In American Indian and Alaska Native children, the risk of hospitalization for HRSV is 3 to 5 times greater than that of the general United States pediatric population,[51,289] and high rates of severe HRSV disease have been observed in other aboriginal populations.

Various host genetic factors have been implicated in susceptibility to pediatric HRSV disease. A recent study found an increased concordance of severe pediatric HRSV infection in identical versus fraternal twins.[554] A number of studies have described positive or negative associations of severe pediatric HRSV disease with polymorphisms in a variety of host genes, notably ones involved in innate immunity and the Th2 subclass of $CD4^+$ T lymphocytes. These include genes for surfactant proteins, TLR4, IL-4, IL-8, IL-9, IL-10, IL-13, IL-18, RANTES (CCL5), CX3CR1, vitamin D receptor, nitric oxide synthetase, transcription factor Jun, IFNα5, and other innate immunity genes.[268,346,389,498,508] These gene-association studies remain preliminary and are sometimes contradictory, probably because the study sizes were too small to validate associations, but they suggest that a number of genes contribute to resistance or susceptibility to severe HRSV disease.

Infection of Adults

HRSV reinfects adults at a rate of approximately 5% to 10% per year.[159,163] Reinfection is more frequent in adults with increased exposure to the virus: during a typical HRSV season, 25% to 50% of health care workers are reinfected, and family members of sick children are readily reinfected. It is likely that adults become susceptible to re-infection as titers of secretory and serum HRSV-neutralizing antibodies from previous exposure decline with time.[166,235,387] HRSV is considered to be second to influenza as a cause of medically significant respiratory tract disease in adulthood. For example, in a study in the United Kingdom using RT-PCR to identify pathogens in various age groups with medically attended respiratory disease, in individuals 15 years of age or older, HRSV was identified in 11% to 22% (depending on the year) of cases compared to 16% to 43% with influenza virus.[629] Hospitalization of healthy, nonelderly adults for HRSV disease is rare. However, severe disease and even death due to HRSV can rarely occur in young, previously healthy adults.[501] HMPV reinfection occurs in 1% to 9% of adults each year, with a wide disease spectrum ranging from asymptomatic to severe respiratory disease.[158,586]

HRSV is an important cause of morbidity and mortality in the elderly (>65 years of age). In one study, HRSV infection was associated with 10.6% of hospitalizations in the elderly for pneumonia, 11.4% for chronic obstructive pulmonary disease, 5.4% for congestive heart failure, and 7.2% for asthma.[163] Low serum neutralizing antibody titer was associated with increased risk of hospitalization.[587] HRSV is estimated to cause on average 17,358 deaths annually in the United States, with 78% of these deaths in adults older than age 65.[553] Therefore, in more affluent countries, deaths due to HRSV are much more frequent in the elderly than in the pediatric population, whereas in less affluent countries the pediatric burden is likely to be greater. HMPV also afflicts the elderly. In one study of adult patients hospitalized for cardiopulmonary conditions, 11% had evidence of HMPV infection, and the frail elderly appeared to be at increased risk of severe disease.[160] In another study of elderly adults hospitalized for respiratory tract disease, HMPV was identified in 8% of cases (ranging from 4.4% to 13.2%, depending on the year), compared to 10.5% for influenza A and 9.6% for HRSV.[158] Immune senescence,[440] resulting in a reduced ability to control infection, presumably is an important factor in the increased severity of HRSV and HMPV disease in the elderly.

Other High-Risk Populations

HRSV is important in adults and older children with underlying pulmonary or cardiac disease or who are severely immunocompromised, especially with T-cell deficiencies.[406,600] Patients with congenital immunodeficiencies such as severe combined immunodeficiency diseases are at high risk. The mortality rate associated with severe HRSV disease in adults with profound immunosuppression due to leukemia or HSCT can be as high as 80% to 100%.[600] The severity of disease depends on the type and magnitude of immunosuppression.[247,599] For HSCT recipients, HRSV infection that occurs preengraftment is associated with the highest risk of pneumonia and death, but mortality also is high in those who develop pneumonia postengraftment.[247] HMPV also can cause severe disease in individuals with hematologic malignancies and in HSCT recipients,[609] although mild or asymptomatic infections also can occur. Both HRSV and HMPV can cause severe LRI in lung transplant recipients, and HRSV has also been associated with chronic rejection and the development of bronchiolitis obliterans in these patients.[612] HRSV is the leading viral cause of hospitalization and reduction in pulmonary function for children with cystic fibrosis.[11,220,261] The relationship between HIV infection and HRSV disease appears to vary by setting. In the United States, prior infection with HIV does not appear

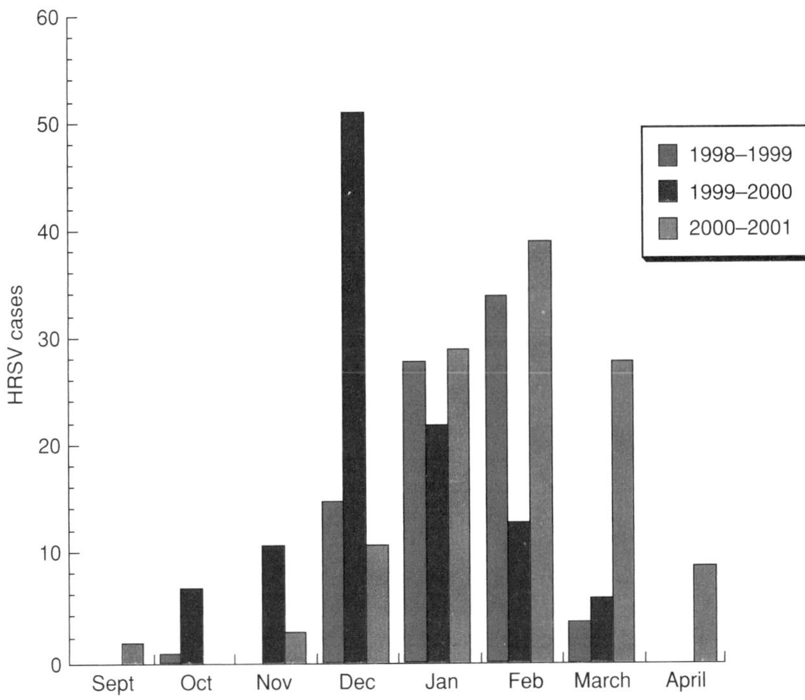

FIGURE 38.11. Variation in human respiratory syncytial virus (HRSV) epidemics during three successive years at the Johns Hopkins Hospital, based on pediatric hospitalizations for HRSV disease.

to increase the morbidity and mortality associated with HRSV infections in children, although prolonged viral shedding has been reported.[299] However, in South Africa, HRSV has been reported to cause greater morbidity and mortality in HIV-infected than HIV-uninfected children, although the contribution of other illnesses cannot be excluded.[357]

Epidemics

In temperate climates, HRSV occurs primarily in yearly epidemics of 4 to 5 months duration in the winter and early spring (Fig. 38.11), although continuous activity also has been reported.[240] Elsewhere in the world, the HRSV season varies from location to location.[628] Globally, HRSV activity is greatest during periods of moderate humidity and either cool (2°C to 6°C) or warm (24°C to 30°C) temperature.[628] HMPV also occurs primarily in annual epidemics during the late winter and early spring in temperate climates, often overlapping in part or in whole with the annual HRSV epidemic.[1,426] However, long-term studies have shown that sporadic HMPV infection occurs year round in temperate areas.[426,608]

HRSV is highly infectious and easily spread by contact, especially in settings of close interaction such as day care facilities, hospitals, and families. HRSV is introduced into families primarily by a young school-aged child, after which infection spreads to siblings and adults with high frequency. In one prospective study, approximately 40% of all family members older than 1 year were infected after the introduction of HRSV.[230] HRSV is a major cause of nosocomial infection. The rate of hospital-acquired infection for infants and children during an HRSV season was reported to range from 26% to 47% in newborn units and from 20% to 40% for older children. Hospital staff members appear to play a major role in nosocomial spread of HRSV infection. The likelihood that an individual infant or child will acquire nosocomial HRSV infection increases with the duration of stay and the number of individuals housed in his or her room.[227] Outbreaks in units caring for immunocompromised patients can be devastating.[370] Outbreaks producing LRI in facilities housing institutionalized adults also have been reported.[177]

An evaluation of the HRSV strains circulating in distinct geographic regions during the same years found that five to seven distinct lineages or genotypes representing both antigenic subgroups circulated during the same season in a given location.[444,445] In a given year, the pattern of genotypes frequently is different in different locations. The pattern of local strains gradually changes in successive years. There typically are one or two dominant local genotypes that are replaced in dominance in successive years. In addition, there can be shifts in the predominance of subgroup A versus B occurring in 1- or 2-year cycles.[589] This presumably reflects an advantage of the heterologous strain in evading previously induced immunity,[602] but reinfection by the same subgroup also frequently occurs. Therefore, HRSV epidemics do not involve spread of a predominant new strain, as is the case with influenza A virus. Rather, epidemics appear to involve local endemic strains as well as new genotypes introduced from other regions. The introduction and spread of new strains were illustrated by the appearance in 1998 of a new subgroup B strain called BA that contains a 60-nucleotide duplication in the G gene, and which subsequently disseminated across five continents and underwent further evolution.[560] The pattern of circulation of HMPV is similar: strains from the two subgroups can co-circulate, and there are several reports of an alternating pattern of dominance by the different subgroups.[1,426]

CLINICAL FEATURES

In the previously healthy term infant who encounters HRSV for the first time at age 6 weeks to 9 months, HRSV infection usually causes URI, sometimes accompanied by fever. In 25% to 40% of such infections, however, the respiratory tract below the larynx also becomes involved.[197] Bronchiolitis and pneumonia are the primary manifestations of HRSV and HMPV LRI, with laryngotracheobronchitis (croup) occurring less frequently. In those infants in whom LRI develops, there is a prodromal phase of rhinorrhea often accompanied by a decrease in appetite. Cough may appear simultaneously, but occurs more often after an interval of 1 to 3 days. At that time, there also may be sneezing and a low-grade fever. Soon after the cough has developed, the child may begin to wheeze; if the disease is mild, the symptoms may not progress beyond this stage. Examination usually shows moderate tachypnea, diffuse inspiratory crackles, and expiratory wheezes. There is profuse rhinorrhea, intermittent fever, and frequently otitis media.[251] In most instances, uneventful recovery occurs after an illness of 7 to 12 days (Fig. 38.5). Among infants and children who require hospitalization with HRSV or HMPV, clinical manifestations range from bronchiolitis or asthma exacerbation to severe pneumonia.[54,401,435] Cough is present in most, fever in 52% to 86%, and wheezing in about half of cases.[608] In more severe cases, the coughing and wheezing progress, and the child becomes dyspneic. Hyperexpansion of the chest is evident, and there may be intercostal and subcostal retractions. Infants often feed poorly, because they are obligate nose breathers and nasal obstruction and tachypnea prevent adequate respiration during feedings. Severe tachypnea is common, even in the absence of visible cyanosis. In advanced disease, the child tires and hypoxia becomes more extreme, and then listlessness and respiratory failure occur.

Bacterial sepsis and lobar pneumonia are unusual complications of HRSV[234] or HMPV infection, although simultaneous bacterial–viral co-infection does occur.[555] Trials of pneumococcal vaccine in infants significantly reduced the incidence of severe HRSV LRI[355] and HMPV LRI,[356] suggesting that there are bacterial–viral interactions that may not be appreciated clinically. In contrast, bacterial otitis media is a common complication of HRSV and HMPV upper respiratory tract infection. HRSV and HMPV are two of the most common precipitating factors associated with otitis media. Most of this disease is due to eustachian tube dysfunction, resulting in bacterial stasis in the middle ear and subsequent otitis media. HRSV and HMPV antigens and nucleic acids have been reported in middle ear fluids.[425,490]

Most infants who require hospitalization for HRSV or HMPV infection are hypoxemic on admission; in fact, a low reading on pulse oximeter is often cited as the criterion for admission. This hypoxemia is probably due to an abnormally low ventilation/perfusion ratio. In those with underlying cardiac or respiratory disease, the progression of symptoms may be rapid, especially in those with cyanotic congenital heart disease or chronic lung disease.[212] In these instances, respiratory failure requiring intubation and ventilation may develop on the second or third day of illness. In children younger than 2 years with cystic fibrosis, the consequence of HRSV infection may be prolonged respiratory morbidity.[261]

In the newborn infant, most HRSV infections produce only URI,[232] probably reflecting the protective effects of maternal HRSV-specific serum antibodies against LRI. Bronchiolitis is rare, and severe infection is more often characterized by lethargy, irritability, and fever or temperature instability than by specific respiratory signs.[232] Symptomatic HMPV infection is rare in newborns. In infants who were born prematurely, and sometimes in normal infants younger than 6 weeks, frequent apneic spells may occur in response to HRSV infection.[556] Apnea often is seen even in the presence of minimal respiratory signs and may be the predominant symptom bringing the infant to medical attention. Such apneic spells, although often recurrent during the acute infection, are usually self-limited and rarely cause neurologic or systemic damage. Exceptions to this occur, however, and such episodes should be an indication for hospitalization and careful medical supervision with respiratory monitoring.

HRSV has been detected in the lungs of a percentage of children dying suddenly and unexpectedly (sudden infant death syndrome [SIDS]). However, there is no statistically significant association between HRSV and SIDS, and the detection of HRSV in some SIDS cases likely reflects its prevalence as well as the historic concurrence of the peak incidence of both HRSV infection and SIDS in winter months.[119] An association between HMPV and SIDS has not been reported.

Abnormalities in pulmonary function are common after HRSV bronchiolitis or pneumonia and may persist for 7 to 10 years or even into adulthood.[231,280,347,422,509,528] Recurrent wheezing may be common after HRSV bronchiolitis or pneumonia and has been reported in 10% to 50% of former patients,[83] but is rarely of great severity. A large case–control study of 200 children hospitalized for bronchiolitis or pneumonia (half of which was due to HRSV) showed that 7 years later there was a significant tendency toward decreased pulmonary function, recurrent cough, wheezing, school absenteeism, asthma, and bronchitis in both of the previously hospitalized groups.[393] Postexercise or pharmacologically induced bronchial lability also is increased, despite an absence of symptoms.[513] The pulmonary function deficit is partially responsive to bronchodilators, indicating a bronchospastic component.[83] Most of these studies did not observe a link between these lingering respiratory abnormalities and allergic sensitization and the development of persistent asthma, but other studies have suggested such a link,[509,510] and this remains an area of controversy. To date, no such epidemiologic links have been reported for HMPV.

It remains unclear whether infection with HRSV (and possibly HMPV) causes subsequent abnormal pulmonary function, or whether the abnormalities observed existed before infection and indeed may have contributed to disease. For example, Martinez et al. measured pulmonary function in infants at birth or shortly thereafter and found a strong correlation between prior reduced function and the development of bronchiolitis with wheezing on HRSV infection.[364] This correlation persisted in children in whom at least one additional lower respiratory infection developed during the first 3 years of life.[364] It is likely that respiratory disease and recurrent abnormalities in children are due to multiple factors. These include prior underlying anatomic or functional abnormality that might predispose to initial and recurrent acute bronchiolitis, a tendency to airway hyperreactivity that might predispose to recurrent wheezing, and infection by HRSV or other airway pathogens. Environmental factors such as family smoking may trigger episodes of lower respiratory dysfunction and aggravate long-term or recurrent airway pathology. There is evidence that preventing severe HRSV infections early in life reduces the incidence of recurrent wheezing, suggesting that HRSV can play a causal role.[512] Most pulmonary abnormalities associated with prior respiratory tract infection resolve by 8 to 12 years of age.

Symptomatic HRSV infections are common in normal adults, particularly in medical personnel or in individuals caring for small children.[227,230] Such episodes are usually characterized by rhinorrhea, pharyngitis, cough, bronchitis, constitutional symptoms of headache and fatigue, and fever. Disease usually lasts about 5 days but may be more prolonged. In contrast, HMPV infection in adults is often asymptomatic, although the spectrum of clinical illness in symptomatic individuals is similar to HRSV, with hoarseness being particularly prominent in young adults.[586] In older persons, particularly those with underlying disease, severe LRI may occur with HRSV or HMPV, requiring hospitalization and intensive care. HRSV infection in severely immunocompromised individuals usually starts with URI for 5 or 6 days, with symptoms similar to those of a normal host, but frequently evolves into LRI.

DIAGNOSIS

Differential Diagnosis

The differential diagnosis of HRSV and HMPV infection in young infants must include all other causes of acute LRI. This includes parainfluenza viruses, particularly HPIV3, adenoviruses, influenza viruses, rhinoviruses, coronaviruses, and enteroviruses. In infants younger than 4 months, *Chlamydia trachomatis* also must be considered, which causes afebrile interstitial pneumonia with cough and, in some cases, wheezing. In HIV-infected children, infection with *Pneumocystis carinii* should be considered. Differentiation from bacterial pneumonia may occasionally be difficult, although wheezing is almost never present during infection with pyogenic bacteria, and infants with bacterial pneumonia typically have lobar pneumonia and may have systemic illness associated with bacteremia. In older infants, infections with HRSV or HMPV must be differentiated from other causes of mild respiratory tract infection as well as causes of acute bronchospastic disease, including environmental allergens and aspiration of a foreign body.

In the elderly, HRSV or HMPV infection should be suspected in any patient (with or without underlying cardiopulmonary disease) who has acute bronchitis, pneumonia, or wheezing accompanied with or without a low-grade fever, particularly when such an event occurs as part of a cluster of cases in the winter season.

Presumptive diagnosis of HRSV infection in infants can often be made on the basis of the clinical syndrome combined with the time of year and other epidemiologic features. It is common to observe that other members of the family have respiratory illness at the time of, or just preceding, an episode of HRSV bronchiolitis or pneumonia in an infant. Usually the infant has far more serious illness than other members of the family.[230]

Radiographic findings for HRSV and HMPV are common but relatively nonspecific. The radiologic findings on chest radiographs of HRSV and HMPV pneumonia are similar to those of bronchiolitis and reactive airways disease and include hyperaeration, diffuse prominent lung markings due to bronchial wall thickening, and focal areas of atelectasis.

Laboratory Diagnosis

Definitive diagnosis of HRSV and HMPV depends on laboratory tests. Rapid detection of HRSV or HMPV is desirable to guide the use of appropriate infection-control measures and to potentially limit unnecessary antibiotic use. In practice, however, while diagnostic testing is typically performed in academic centers, it may be used less frequently in community hospitals even in wealthy countries. Few hospitals in resource-limited settings have the capacity for such testing.

The gold standard is isolation of virus in cell culture from nasal swabs, nasal washes, or nasopharyngeal aspirates; however, the lability of HRSV, the slow growth characteristics of HMPV, the expense of the technique, and the increasing availability of assays that rely on nucleic acid detection have made cell culture an increasingly infrequent choice, even for diagnostic virology laboratories in academic centers.

More rapid diagnosis can be made by the detection of viral antigen in nasal swabs or washes. In the direct immunofluorescence assay (DFA), exfoliated cells and other debris are concentrated from secretions by centrifugation, reacted with virus-specific fluorescence-labeled antibodies, and visualized by microscopy. This has the advantage that a knowledgeable technician can confirm that the signal has the pattern expected for infected cells, but the method is time-consuming and requires expertise and a fluorescence microscope. Alternatively, antigen in secretions can be detected by antigen-capture enzyme-linked immunoassay (EIA), in which the sample is incubated with immobilized virus-specific antibodies to capture viral antigen, which is then detected with a second, enzyme-linked antibody. Both DFA and EIA for HRSV are commercially available (with the former being more sensitive than the latter), and DFA is commercially available for HMPV. Another HRSV rapid antigen test available commercially is based on lateral flow immunochromatography.[194,337] The test sample of secretions is solubilized, mixed with a colored gold-labeled HRSV MAb, and applied to a test membrane on which antibody-antigen complexes migrate laterally and are captured by a line of immobilized HRSV-specific antibody to produce a visible band. The sensitivity of these rapid commercial tests, which produce results in less than 30 minutes, generally is lower than that of DFA, and negative results should be confirmed by DFA. In addition, antigen-based tests in general often have reduced sensitivity in adults due to low levels of viral shedding.[159]

RT-PCR of viral RNA for detection of HRSV or HMPV in nasal swabs, nasopharyngeal aspirates, or nasal washes is a useful method of diagnosis for both pediatric and adult populations, because the sensitivity of these assays allows detection of even small quantities of virus. RT-PCR can be used in multiplex formats capable of detecting multiple pathogens. HRSV and HMPV RT-PCR multiplex assays are commercially available, although the procedure is somewhat time-consuming (3 to 6 hours) and requires technical expertise and specialized equipment.[337,360] RT-PCR is more sensitive than virus culture or antigen assay.[257]

Serologic methods are used infrequently and provide only retrospective information, since antibody rises are detected by analysis of sera collected 2 to 4 weeks postinfection. Typically, serum antibodies are detected by ELISA or microneutralization assay, with fourfold or greater increases considered indicative of infection.

TREATMENT AND PREVENTION

Treatment

Most infants and children with mild HRSV LRI can be managed as outpatients. Treatment of more severe LRI can be guided by measurement of oxygenation, monitoring respiratory rate and the trend in respiratory rate, and evaluation of dehydration. Severe respiratory distress, hypoxia, and dehydration are among the indications for hospitalization.

The American Academy of Pediatrics (AAP) has issued evidence-based recommendations for the diagnosis and management of bronchiolitis,[7] most cases of which can likely be attributed to HRSV or HMPV. Where appropriate, AAP recommendations are cited below.

Symptomatic Interventions and Supportive Care

Inpatient treatment of HRSV infection requires considerable supportive care: mechanical removal of secretions, proper positioning of the infant, administration of humidified oxygen, intravenous fluids, and, in the most severe cases, respiratory assistance with mechanical ventilation. Antibiotic therapy does not improve the outcome in viral pneumonia, does not alter the risk of bacterial complication of viral pneumonia as a superinfection, and should not be used unless there are indications that a bacterial co-infection is present.[7] The youngest infants infected with HRSV may require monitoring for apnea. Improvements in supportive care clearly have had a major impact on mortality from severe HRSV disease, resulting in the current overall low mortality rate in high-resource settings. Current AAP guidelines advocate the use of supplemental oxygen if the oxyhemoglobin saturation (SpO_2) falls below 90%.[7] Of all the potential therapeutic modalities described here for severe HRSV disease, supplemental oxygen may be the most accessible for infants in resource-limited settings.[552]

Corticosteroids have been used in therapy for HRSV bronchiolitis since the 1960s, based in part on their effectiveness in the treatment of acute asthma and on the premise that much of HRSV disease is immune-mediated. However, a meta-analysis of placebo-controlled studies indicated that systemic glucocorticoids on their own provided no improvement in oxygenation, respiratory rate, or length of hospitalization,[439] and a large controlled study indicated that inhaled glucocorticoids provided no improvement in wheezing following HRSV bronchiolitis.[154] Current AAP guidance suggests that corticosteroids should not be routinely used in the management of bronchiolitis.[7]

Other antiinflammatory approaches for the treatment of HRSV have also been considered. Acute HRSV bronchiolitis is associated with elevations of cysteinyl leukotrienes in respiratory secretions[123]; however, the leukotriene receptor antagonist montelukast was not shown to be effective in ameliorating acute bronchiolitis.[8] Assessment of the utility of montelukast for prevention of post-HRSV wheezing episodes has yielded conflicting results[49,295,465] and further studies may be warranted.

Drugs used to treat reversible airway smooth muscle constriction in asthma have also been used to treat HRSV infection. Hospitalized infants in the United States frequently are treated with inhaled bronchodilators, but systematic reviews indicate that they provide only modest short-term improvement.[182,331] This suggests that, in some infants, increased airway resistance is not predominantly due to reversible smooth muscle constriction, but rather is a consequence of obstruction of small airways with mucus, immune cells, and sloughed epithelial cells. Current AAP recommendations are that trial of a bronchodilator may be considered, but that inhaled bronchodilators should be used only if there is a demonstrated objective benefit in an individual child.[7]

Antiviral Interventions

Ribavirin, a nucleoside analog, is a broad spectrum antiviral compound the mode of action of which remains unclear,[506] but which exhibits potent activity against HRSV and HMPV in cell culture and experimental animals.[621] Ribavirin was approved in 1986 in the United States for use in the treatment of HRSV infection.[579] A recent review stated that some improvement in subjectively or objectively measured outcome was observed in 7 of 11 published randomized clinical trials of ribavirin, although the size and quality of the trials were highly variable.[300] In addition, the drug is difficult to administer via aerosol, can cause anemia, and concerns have been raised about health risks for caregivers.[477] Currently, the AAP recommends that ribavirin not be used routinely for the management of bronchiolitis, although it could be considered for use in children at risk with severe disease (e.g., those who are immunocompromised or who have "hemodynamically significant cardiopulmonary disease").[7] Ribavirin has been used empirically for the management of HRSV LRI in HSCT or lung transplant patients,[52] and was administered intravenously to a lung transplant patient with HMPV.[470]

HRSV disease in young infants can be reduced by prophylaxis with HRSV-neutralizing antibodies (see *Prevention*). Therefore, these antibodies also have been evaluated for therapy of established infection. The most recent studies have utilized the HRSV F MAb palivizumab and the more potent motavizumab administered intravenously.[320,359] In these studies, palivizumab and motavizumab reduced viral shedding by 10-fold, but a clear effect on clinical outcome has not been demonstrated.[265] It is possible that these small studies were not sufficiently powered to observe differences in clinical outcome; alternatively, it may be that much of the LRI observed by the time infants reach the hospital (usually several days into their illnesses) is immune mediated and will not be ameliorated by antiviral treatment. However, antibodies sometimes are used empirically for treating severely immunocompromised individuals, in whom infection can be prolonged,[164,322] although definite evidence of efficacy is lacking.

Small molecule antiviral drugs specific for HRSV have been developed that target the F, G, N, or L proteins.[153,343,430,506,530] Four different small molecule inhibitors are undergoing clinical trials for HRSV (www.clinicaltrials.gov, accessed June, 2011). A drug specific to the N protein (AA-60444, previously RSV604)[88] was evaluated in 2006 in a phase 2 clinical trial in HRSV-infected adult HSCT recipients (clinicaltrials.gov NCT00232635), although the results have not been published. An siRNA that targets the N gene (ALN-RSV01) was evaluated in a phase 2 challenge study in 85 healthy adults (clinicaltrials.govNCT00496821).[137] The drug was administered daily by nasal spray for 2 days before and 3 days after HRSV challenge. This resulted in a 38% decrease in the number of individuals infected, and modest but insignificant decreases in viral load in those who were infected.[137] It will be important to evaluate efficacy in a situation where the drug is administered after, rather than beginning before, infection. This drug also was evaluated in a phase 2 trial of 24 lung transplant recipients with HRSV infection, in which three daily doses were associated with reduced symptom scores and significantly reduced incidence of bronchiolitis obliterans syndrome.[630] An orally administered inhibitor specific to the F protein (BTA9881) was recently evaluated for safety and tolerability (clinicaltrials.govNCT00504907). Reports in the lay press indicated that its safety was unsatisfactory and that further preclinical development is planned. A phase 1 study is planned for 2011 to assess safety, tolerability, and pharmacokinetics for another F protein–specific inhibitor (MDT-637, previously VP14637)[145,622] that is delivered by a dry powder inhaler (clinicaltrials.gov NCT01355016). Small molecule inhibitors are under preclinical development for HMPV.

Other antisense strategies also have been explored against HRSV. Conventional antisense oligonucleotides probably have little potential when administered on their own, but they also have been chemically linked to the 2-5A molecule of the host IFN system.[326] This serves to recruit the cellular antiviral nuclease RNase L to cleave the hybridized RNA. A 2-5A-antisense molecule that targets the conserved GS signals in the viral genome reduced nasal HRSV replication up to 10,000-fold in AGMs when the drug was administered intranasally shortly after infection and during the following 5 days,[326] but further development has not been reported.

Combination therapies also are being developed, involving either the combination of two different antiviral drugs to achieve a higher level of inhibition of viral replication, or the combination of one or more antiviral drugs with an antiinflammatory drug to restrict replication and reduce immune-mediated disease. This latter combination strategy effectively resolved viral replication and disease in the cotton rat model.[463] Similarly, early and aggressive combined therapy involving ribavirin, corticosteroids, and antibodies is being explored for severely immunocompromised adults.[342,601] In the more usual setting of acute HRSV infection of otherwise healthy individuals, antiviral therapy of a rapidly progressing infection such as HRSV is challenging because by the time the viral agent is identified, it may be too late to control disease solely by inhibiting virus replication.

Prevention

Infection Control

Infection by HRSV (and HMPV) can be reduced by hand washing, limiting exposure to infected individuals, and avoiding self-inoculation of nasal and conjunctival mucosa. Nosocomial spread of HRSV has been shown to be reduced by the use of gloves and gowns by caregivers, strict observance of hand washing, active surveillance for HRSV infection, limiting visitors during the HRSV season, and cohorting of infected patients and caregivers.[223,327,354,416,520]

Passive Immunoprophylaxis Against HRSV

Based on experimental data in animals[461,462,588] and epidemiologic data in humans[197] indicating that HRSV-neutralizing serum antibodies protected against HRSV LRI, products containing high titers of HRSV-neutralizing antibodies were developed for clinical administration. These products do not necessarily prevent HRSV infection completely, but can proactively restrict replication sufficient to reduce disease. The first product, RSV Immune Globulin Intravenous (RSV-IGIV; RespiGam™, MedImmune), consisted of immunoglobulin purified from human donor sera that had been screened for high HRSV-neutralizing activity. It was licensed in 1996 for use in infants and young children at high risk for severe HRSV disease due to prematurity or underlying disease. Administered in monthly intravenous infusions during the HRSV season, RSV-IGIV reduced the frequency of hospitalization for HRSV disease by 55% or more and reduced days spent in intensive care by 97%.[214,471] However, it had the disadvantages of involving an intravenous infusion, the theoretical risk of adventitious agents, and potential interference with live pediatric vaccines due to the presence of antibodies against common pathogens. RSV-IGIV (RespiGam™) has been superseded by the development of the MAb palivizumab (see below) and has not been commercially available since 2004.

Palizumab (Synagis™; MedImmune) is an HRSV-neutralizing MAb directed against the F glycoprotein that was licensed in 1998. Palivizumab is based on a murine MAb[32] that was "humanized" by recombinantly transferring its complementarity-determining regions (~5% of the molecule) onto a human IgG1 backbone (95% of the molecule). Palivizumab is 50- to 100-fold more effective on a weight basis than RSV-IGIV, and accordingly is administered in a much smaller volume by monthly intramuscular injection. Its clinical efficacy is similar to that of RSV-IGIV.[434] In infants with cyanotic heart disease, RSV-IGIV was associated with an increased incidence of adverse events[214]—likely due to its large volume and high protein content—but a phase III study demonstrated that palivizumab was safe and effective in preventing hospitalizations for HRSV in children with congenital heart disease.[176] Currently the AAP recommends that high-risk infants receive prophylaxis with palivizumab during the HRSV season. Phase 1 trials also showed that palivizumab was well tolerated based on evaluation in a small number of HSCT recipients.[53] There is continued discussion of the cost-effectiveness of palivizumab due to its expense,[456] but antibodies remain the only effective prophylaxis available for HRSV disease other than infection control. The emergence of antibody-resistant mutants in association with the use of palivizumab has not been a significant problem: they are detected in ~5% of treated individuals from whom HRSV was recovered and appear to have a modest reduction in growth fitness *in vitro*.[635]

More recently, palivizumab was modified by *in vitro* affinity maturation to create a more potent derivative called motavizumab (MEDI-524 or Numax, MedImmune). Compared to palivizumab, motavizumab differs at 13 amino acid positions. It exhibits a 70-fold increase in antigen binding and a 20-fold increase in neutralization activity *in vitro*, and is substantially more protective in cotton rats and also protects the upper respiratory tract.[382,620] In a clinical study comparing palivizumab and motavizumab in a group of 6635 preterm infants, infants who received motavizumab had 26% and 55% reductions in HRSV hospitalization and medically attended HRSV LRI (MALRI), respectively, relative to palivizumab.[77,193] Motavizumab also was evaluated in a placebo-controlled trial in healthy Native American populations (clinicaltrials.govNCT00121108). In this study of more than 2,000 infants, motavizumab was found to reduce HRSV hospitalizations by 83% and outpatient MALRIs by 71%. However, this product was associated with a slight increase in the incidence of hypersensitivity reactions and antidrug antibodies in clinical trials, and its further development for HRSV prophylaxis has been suspended as of this writing. Motavizumab also was evaluated for the treatment of infants hospitalized for HRSV disease (clinicaltrials.govNCT00421304). Prior to the problematic clinical data, motavizumab had been engineered to increase its serum half-life by increasing its affinity for a receptor involved in recycling and sparing antibodies that have been taken up intracellularly for degradation.[125] This increased the antibody's serum half-life in cynomolgus monkeys fourfold, but it seems unlikely that this derivative will be developed further. Other approaches have sought to develop fully human HRSV-neutralizing MAbs using recombinatorial phage display libraries,[23,397] or from libraries of transformed B cells.[93] This latter study is noteworthy because it was able to produce G-specific MAbs with high neutralizing activities.

Vaccines

The need for an HRSV vaccine is greatest for infants and the elderly, although a vaccine for toddlers and preschool children might have a substantial impact on emergency room and primary care visits for respiratory illness.[236,329] Immunization with a pediatric HRSV vaccine ideally should be initiated during the first weeks of life. Because the reduced immune responses characteristic of infancy likely will reduce vaccine immunogenicity and efficacy, multiple vaccine doses will likely be required.

Development of a pediatric HRSV vaccine has been complicated by the phenomenon of enhanced disease that occurred in association with a formalin-inactivated HRSV (FI-RSV) vaccine evaluated in infants and children in the 1960s.[287,458] This vaccine consisted of concentrated, formalin-inactivated virus that was mixed with alum adjuvant and administered intramuscularly. Immunization with FI-RSV was well-tolerated but proved to be poorly protective. Unexpectedly, upon subsequent natural infection, vaccinees experienced much greater frequency and severity of HRSV disease: 80% of FI-RSV vaccinees required hospitalization compared to 5% in the control group, and two toddlers (ages 14 and 16 months) died of enhanced RSV disease. Autopsies of the two fatalities provided evidence of HRSV replication and pulmonary inflammation.[458]

Subsequent studies, which had the advantage of improved methods and the development of experimental animals models, showed that the immune response to FI-RSV differed markedly from that to HRSV infection. The serum antibodies induced by FI-RSV in the original vaccinees or in experimental animals bound efficiently to HRSV antigen in ELISA but were inefficient in neutralizing infectivity.[415] Studies in experimental animals showed that FI-RSV did not induce a significant CTL response, reflecting its noninfectious nature. Peripheral blood lymphocytes from the original vaccinees exhibited an exaggerated proliferative response to HRSV antigen *in vitro,* suggestive of a heightened CD4$^+$ T-cell response to FI-RSV compared to natural infection.[298] Consistent with this, subsequent studies in experimental animals showed that FI-RSV induces a disproportionately increased stimulation of the Th2 subset of CD4$^+$ T cells compared with HRSV infection.[109,130,591] These findings indicated that FI-RSV primed for an aberrant, pathologic secondary immune response that occurred upon subsequent infection and viral antigen expression.

The poor neutralizing activity of the serum antibodies induced by FI-RSV likely was a major factor in the lack of protective efficacy, and probably reflects denaturation of neutralization epitopes in the vaccine. It also may reflect deficient antibody affinity maturation due to poor TLR stimulation by the nonreplicating vaccine.[135] The formation of antibody–antigen complexes and complement fixation also appears to have contributed to disease, a consequence of the induction of antibodies that did not restrict infection but bound efficiently to antigen.[383] The Th2-biased response also played a key role, demonstrated by the finding that disease enhancement was not observed when FI-RSV-immunized rodents were treated with antibodies to deplete either CD4$^+$ T cells or selected Th2 cytokines prior to HRSV challenge.[110] The bias toward Th2 appeared to be favored by the lack of stimulation of NK cells and CD8$^+$ CTLs, which otherwise downregulate Th2 responses to HRSV antigens, at least in the mouse model,[267,429] and may also have other immunomodulatory effects.[429,529] The Th2-bias may also have been enhanced by the presence in FI-RSV of carbonyl groups arising from the formalin treatment.[391] Therefore, the major elements of disease enhancement include an inadequate protective response, an altered antibody response, and a heightened Th2 response. Similar phenomena of vaccine-related disease enhancement have been described in the clinical use of formalin-inactivated measles virus vaccine[452] and in experimental animals receiving formalin-inactivated HPIV3[432] and HMPV[131,624] vaccines, and thus does not appear to be specific to HRSV or to *Pneumovirinae.*

Disease enhancement has also been observed in experimental animals that have been immunized with purified HRSV F and G glycoproteins as experimental vaccines.[414] This cautionary finding needs to be strongly considered if nonreplicating HRSV vaccines are developed as potential immunogens for HRSV-naïve infants and children. In contrast, disease enhancement is not observed with natural HRSV infection and reinfection, or in most cases with viral or DNA vectors expressing HRSV antigens. This distinction between killed-virus/subunit HRSV vaccines versus live/vectored HRSV vaccines likely reflects the greater efficiency of the latter in broadly stimulating innate and adaptive immunity, including stimulation of TLRs, NK cells, and CD8$^+$ CTLs important in regulating HRSV-specific immune responses. It also is noteworthy that priming for enhanced disease appears to be limited to HRSV-naïve infants and children and has not been observed when nonlive vaccines are used in HRSV-experienced individuals. This has been demonstrated in experimental animals[590] and in clinical studies described below. Therefore, although a subunit vaccine is contraindicated for RSV-naïve recipients, it could be safely used to boost immunity in older children and adults.

Because of disease enhancement, efforts in recent years to develop an HRSV vaccine for HRSV-naïve infants and young children have focused on live attenuated vaccines. The absence of disease enhancement by live HRSV vaccines has been confirmed in clinical trials in HRSV-naïve infants.[618] Studies in experimental animals including chimpanzees showed that the intranasal route of administration is surprisingly immunogenic and highly protective. It also partially avoids the immunosuppressive effects of serum antibodies.[116] Beginning in the 1960s, a series of live attenuated HRSV strains was developed by classic biological methods, notably multiple passages at increasingly low, suboptimal temperature[180] followed by chemical mutagenesis and selection for temperature-sensitive mutants.[115] None of the viruses produced by these methods had a satisfactory level of attenuation in 1- to 2-month-old HRSV-naïve infants, although one virus (called *cpts*248/404) was well-tolerated and immunogenic in an older age group, namely seronegative infants and children 6 months of age or older.[617] Further efforts to obtain satisfactory derivatives by biological means were unsuccessful, and all subsequent vaccine candidates have been made by reverse genetics.

Reverse genetics provides a number of advantages for developing live vaccines, including the means of identifying attenuating mutations in existing viruses,[104,604] developing new mutations or strategies for attenuation,[28,41,68,420,549,603] producing viruses with short, well-defined passage histories important for safety,[535] increasing genetic stability,[369] introducing mutations in desired combinations to incrementally increase attenuation,[605] and other possibilities such as rearranging the gene order to increase the expression of protective antigens.[307]

Several attenuated HRSV strains produced by reverse genetics have been evaluated in clinical trials.[290,619] The lead candidate, a virus called rA2cp248/404/1030ΔSH (e-Fig. 38.10), was well-tolerated in 1- to 2-month-old infants and was moderately immunogenic and highly protective against a second vaccine dose.[290] This virus contains a series of point mutations and deletion of the SH gene, is strongly temperature sensitive, and does not form plaques at temperatures higher than 35°C. This degree of temperature sensitivity would preferentially restrict replication in the warmer lower respiratory tract. This virus presently is in phase 1/2 clinical trials. Other attenuated HRSV strains also are in development. One example is the ΔM2-2 virus, which lacks most of the coding sequence for the M2-2 protein. This virus exhibits reduced RNA replication and increased gene transcription and antigen production, which may provide for increased immunogenicity.[41]

Another type of live attenuated HRSV vaccine recently evaluated in clinical trials (clinicaltrials.gov NCT00686075, NCT00686075 NCT00493285) uses an attenuated chimera of bovine PIV3, in which the F and HN genes are derived from HPIV3, as a vector to express the HRSV F and/or G proteins from one or two added genes[495,540] (e-Fig. 38.10). This provides a bivalent intranasal vaccine against these two important pediatric pathogens. Importantly, BPIV3 and HPIV3 replicate more efficiently and are more stable physically than HRSV. This might facilitate vaccine manufacture and use. However, recent data indicate that the antibody response to RSV F was inferior to the antibody response to HPIV3,[41a] perhaps resulting from sequence variation in the RSV F transgene (unpublished observations). An analogous approach is being pursued using Sendai virus as vector.[281] Sendai virus is a murine relative of HPIV1 that has sufficient antigenic cross-reactivity that intranasal immunization protects AGMs against HPIV1 challenge. Sendai virus was well-tolerated in adults and has been engineered to express HRSV antigens as a potential bivalent vaccine against HPIV1 and HRSV.[281] Other vectored approaches, such as using replication-defective adenoviruses or alphaviruses, also may have promise for pediatric use.

There also is a need for an HRSV vaccine in older children and the elderly, especially for individuals at increased risk due to underlying disease or old age. Live vaccines appear to be too restricted in replication in HRSV-experienced older individuals due to existing immunity.[199] Vectors might not be suitable for repeated vaccinations due to the development of vector-neutralizing antibodies. However, subunit protein vaccines could be suitable, since they do not prime for enhanced disease in RSV-experienced individuals. In addition, prior immunity can be partially overcome by increased dose.[411] A number of HRSV-subunit vaccines have been evaluated in clinical trials. A series of preparations of purified F protein (PFP) isolated from HRSV-infected cells has been evaluated in healthy adults, in children older than 12 months of age with and without underlying chronic pulmonary disease (chronic lung disease of prematurity or cystic fibrosis), in institutionalized and ambulatory elderly subjects, and in pregnant women (immunization during pregnancy had the goal of increasing the titer of HRSV-neutralizing maternal antibodies in the newborn).[34,167,168,213,405,436,450,563] The PFP vaccines were well tolerated in these populations: acute reactions were minimal, and enhanced disease was not observed. However, HRSV-neutralizing antibody responses were unsatisfactorily low. More recently, a vaccine based on the HRSV F, G, and M proteins purified from HRSV-infected cells was evaluated in an elderly population in conjunction with the inactivated seasonal influenza virus vaccine.[169] This vaccine was moderately immunogenic with or without an alum adjuvant, but is no longer in clinical development.

Another experimental protein-based vaccine, called BBG2Na, consists of a bacterially expressed fragment containing the central conserved domain of the HRSV G protein fused to the albumin-binding domain of the streptococcal G protein. However, in HRSV-naïve infant macaques it was associated with a low level of pulmonary eosinophilia in some animals upon challenge,[132] and in clinical trials in adults it induced low levels of HRSV-neutralizing antibodies,[454] with hypersensitivity observed in some vaccine recipients.

Increasing knowledge of the structure and antigenic properties of the HRSV F protein and improved methods of expression and purification may allow for the production of more stable and more immunogenic HRSV F vaccine preparations. As of this writing, the only HRSV subunit vaccine currently being evaluated in clinical trials is an F protein particle vaccine developed by Novavax (clinicaltrials.gov NCT01290419), which is currently undergoing phase 1 evaluation in healthy adults. In other recent work, the HRSV F protein was engineered to remove the fusion peptide, transmembrane region, and cytoplasmic tail, yielding an expressed protein that formed a postfusion trimeric structure that was homogeneous, stable, and highly immunogenic.[378,536]

Numerous additional approaches to an HRSV vaccine continue to be evaluated in preclinical studies, including synthetic peptides, engineered multiepitope vaccines, antigen expressed by recombinant baculoviruses or produced in plants, antigen fused to carrier proteins such as cholera toxin B subunit, immune-stimulating complexes containing HRSV antigens, liposome-encapsidated HRSV antigen, the use of adjuvants such as CpG oligonucleotides or biopolymer nanoparticles, and vectors including vesicular stomatitis virus, vaccinia virus (Modified Vaccinia Ankara), rhinovirus, Newcastle disease virus, *Mycobacterium bovis* BCG (Bacillus Calmette-Guerin), and *Salmonella typhimurium.* Whether any of these offer advantages remains to be seen. Realistic evaluation of candidate vaccines for HRSV (and HMPV) is complicated by the semipermissive nature of infection of convenient experimental rodent models, which thus gives overly optimistic appraisals of efficacy.

Recombinant HMPVs that lack the M2-2 ORF or G gene have been developed by reverse genetics. These viruses were highly attenuated in rodents and AGMs while retaining a satisfactory level of immunogenicity.[44,48,66] The ΔM2-2 and

ΔG viruses have levels of attenuation and immunogenicity suitable to be evaluated clinically as candidate live intranasal vaccines. Another approach has been to replace individual genes of HMPV with their AMPV counterparts to create chimeric viruses that are attenuated in primates due to host incompatibility effects of the AMPV gene. A chimera in which the HMPV P gene was replaced by its AMPV counterpart replicated efficiently *in vitro* and appeared to have a satisfactory level of attenuation in AGMs,[447] and presently is being evaluated in phase 1 clinical trials for safety and immunogenicity (clinicaltrials.govNCT01255410). An attenuated HPIV3 vaccine virus also has been used as a vector to express the F protein of HMPV as a bivalent HPIV3-HMPV vaccine in preclinical studies.[515,539]

PERSPECTIVE

HRSV is one of the more complex members of *Mononegavirales.* We have general information on many of the roles of the viral proteins and RNAs in the viral replicative cycle, and have some information on how they affect the host cell and host immune system. Continued research is needed to identify and elucidate these mechanisms and their significance to viral biology and the host response.

HRSV is one of the most common and widespread human viruses. HRSV is notable for a historic and tragic vaccine failure, namely the formalin-inactivated vaccine. It also is notable for the development of the successful strategy of antibody immunoprophylaxis against HRSV, which contributed to widespread interest in the development of products based on MAbs. Although the importance of HRSV has been known for more than 50 years, we lack effective vaccines or antiviral therapeutic drugs. There is a need for both, but developing these products for young infants is challenging. A substantial reduction in serious HRSV disease would be a major advance for human health. Vaccines may be improved by new adjuvants, and antiviral drugs may be improved by combination with antiinflammatory therapy.

HRSV is unusual in its ability to efficiently infect and cause disease in early infancy even in the presence of maternal antibodies. The consequences of severe HRSV infection in the context of the immature lung and immature immune system are poorly understood. Severe HRSV disease early in life frequently is associated with lingering abnormalities in pulmonary function, although the causal relationship is uncertain. It also has been speculated that early infection in life can result in long-term deficiencies in the immune response to this virus in some individuals. Further studies of infants who receive passive or (when available) active immunoprophylaxis against HRSV may help to resolve these issues. The relative contributions of direct viral damage and immune factors to HRSV disease remain unclear and likely will vary among individuals, due in part to genetic differences that are being identified. HRSV can reinfect symptomatically throughout life in the absence of significant antigenic change. The extent to which this reflects virus-mediated inhibition or subversion of protective responses remains controversial.

HMPV is a close relative to HRSV that infects somewhat less early in life and causes severe disease less frequently. Many of the questions regarding disease mechanisms, immune response, and long-term consequences of HRSV infection early in life also apply to HMPV. Research into these important causes of severe LRI in infants and the elderly should yield new insights into pathogenesis and host responses at both extremes of age.

ACKNOWLEDGMENTS

P.L.C. was funded by the NIAID Intramural Program. R.A.K. was partially funded by NIH NIAID contract HHSN272200900010C.

REFERENCES

All cited references are available in the e-book.

2. Abu-Harb M, Bell F, Finn A, et al. IL-8 and neutrophil elastase levels in the respiratory tract of infants with RSV bronchiolitis. *Eur Respir J* 1999;14:139–143.
10. Anderson LJ, Hierholzer JC, Tsou C, et al. Antigenic characterization of respiratory syncytial virus strains with monoclonal antibodies. *J Infect Dis* 1985;151:626–633.
13. Asenjo A, Gonzalez-Armas JC, Villanueva N. Phosphorylation of human respiratory syncytial virus P protein at serine 54 regulates viral uncoating. *Virology* 2008;380:26–33.
18. Bachi T. Direct observation of the budding and fusion of an enveloped virus by video microscopy of viable cells. *J Cell Biol* 1988;107:1689–1695.
21. Bao X, Liu T, Shan Y, et al. Human metapneumovirus glycoprotein G inhibits innate immune responses. *PLoS Pathog* 2008;4:e1000077.
37. Bennett BL, Garofalo RP, Cron SG, et al. Immunopathogenesis of respiratory syncytial virus bronchiolitis. *J Infect Dis* 2007;195:1532–1540.
39. Berkley JA, Munywoki P, Ngama M, et al. Viral etiology of severe pneumonia among Kenyan infants and children. *JAMA* 2010;303: 2051–2057.
41. Bermingham A, Collins PL. The M2-2 protein of human respiratory syncytial virus is a regulatory factor involved in the balance between RNA replication and transcription. *Proc Natl Acad Sci U S A* 1999;96: 11259–11264.
50. Bitko V, Shulyayeva O, Mazumder B, et al. Nonstructural proteins of respiratory syncytial virus suppress premature apoptosis by an NF-kappaB-dependent, interferon-independent mechanism and facilitate virus growth. *J Virol* 2007;81:1786–1795.
55. Boivin G, Mackay I, Sloots TP, et al. Global genetic diversity of human metapneumovirus fusion gene. *Emerg Infect Dis* 2004;10:1154–1157.
56. Bonville CA, Rosenberg HF, Domachowske JB. Macrophage inflammatory protein-1alpha and RANTES are present in nasal secretions during ongoing upper respiratory tract infection. *Pediatr Allergy Immunol* 1999; 10:39–44.
60. Bosis S, Esposito S, Osterhaus AD, et al. Association between high nasopharyngeal viral load and disease severity in children with human metapneumovirus infection. *J Clin Virol* 2008;42:286–290.
61. Boyce TG, Mellen BG, Mitchel EF Jr, et al. Rates of hospitalization for respiratory syncytial virus infection among children in medicaid. *J Pediatr* 2000;137:865–870.
64. Brearey SP, Symth RL. Pathogenesis of RSV in children. In: Cane P, ed. *Respiratory Syncytial Virus.* Amsterdam: Elsevier; 2007:141–162.
66. Buchholz UJ, Biacchesi S, Pham QN, et al. Deletion of M2 gene open reading frames 1 and 2 of human metapneumovirus: effects on RNA synthesis, attenuation, and immunogenicity. *J Virol* 2005;79:6588–6597.
68. Buchholz UJ, Granzow H, Schuldt K, et al. Chimeric bovine respiratory syncytial virus with glycoprotein gene substitutions from human respiratory syncytial virus (HRSV): Effects on host range and evaluation as a live-attenuated HRSV vaccine. *J Virol* 2000;74:1187–1199.
70. Bukreyev A, Yang L, Fricke J, et al. The secreted form of respiratory syncytial virus G glycoprotein helps the virus evade antibody-mediated restriction of replication by acting as an antigen decoy and through effects on Fc receptor-bearing leukocytes. *J Virol* 2008;82:12191–12204.

73. Byrd LG, Prince GA. Animal models of respiratory syncytial virus infection. *Clin Infect Dis* 1997;25:1363–1368.
75. Campbell AP, Chien JW, Kuypers J, et al. Respiratory virus pneumonia after hematopoietic cell transplantation (HCT): associations between viral load in bronchoalveolar lavage samples, viral RNA detection in serum samples, and clinical outcomes of HCT. *J Infect Dis* 2010;201: 1404–1413.
81. Carter SD, Dent KC, Atkins E, et al. Direct visualization of the small hydrophobic protein of human respiratory syncytial virus reveals the structural basis for membrane permeability. *FEBS Lett* 2010;584:2786–2790.
84. Catelli E, Lupini C, Cecchinato M, et al. Field avian metapneumovirus evolution avoiding vaccine induced immunity. *Vaccine* 2010;28: 916–921.
87. Chanock RM, Roizman B, Myers R. Recovery from infants with respiratory illness of a virus related to chimpanzee coryza agent. I. Isolation, properties and characterization. *Am J Hyg* 1957;66:281–290.
89. Cheng X, Park H, Zhou H, et al. Overexpression of the M2-2 protein of respiratory syncytial virus inhibits viral replication. *J Virol* 2005;79: 13943–13952.
93. Collarini EJ, Lee FE, Foord O, et al. Potent high-affinity antibodies for treatment and prophylaxis of respiratory syncytial virus derived from B cells of infected patients. *J Immunol* 2009;183:6338–6345.
96. Collins PL, Graham BS. Viral and host factors in human respiratory syncytial virus pathogenesis. *J Virol* 2008;82:2040–2055.
98. Collins PL, Hill MG, Cristina J, et al. Transcription elongation factor of respiratory syncytial virus, a nonsegmented negative-strand RNA virus. *Proc Natl Acad Sci U S A* 1996;93:81–85.
106. Collins PL, Olmsted RA, Spriggs MK, et al. Gene overlap and site-specific attenuation of transcription of the viral polymerase L gene of human respiratory syncytial virus. *Proc Natl Acad Sci U S A* 1987;84: 5134–5138.
107. Collins PL, Wertz GW. cDNA cloning and transcriptional mapping of nine polyadenylylated RNAs encoded by the genome of human respiratory syncytial virus. *Proc Natl Acad Sci U S A* 1983;80:3208–3212.
108. Connors M, Collins PL, Firestone CY, et al. Respiratory syncytial virus (RSV) F, G, M2 (22K), and N proteins each induce resistance to RSV challenge, but resistance induced by M2 and N proteins is relatively short-lived. *J Virol* 1991;65:1634–1637.
109. Connors M, Giese NA, Kulkarni AB, et al. Enhanced pulmonary histopathology induced by respiratory syncytial virus (RSV) challenge of formalin-inactivated RSV-immunized BALB/c mice is abrogated by depletion of interleukin-4 (IL-4) and IL-10. *J Virol* 1994;68:5321–5325.
111. Cowton VM, McGivern DR, Fearns R. Unravelling the complexities of respiratory syncytial virus RNA synthesis. *J Gen Virol* 2006;87: 1805–1821.
114. Crowe JE Jr. Influence of maternal antibodies on neonatal immunization against respiratory viruses. *Clin Infect Dis* 2001;33:1720–1727.
117. Crowe JE Jr, Firestone CY, Murphy BR. Passively acquired antibodies suppress humoral but not cell-mediated immunity in mice immunized with live attenuated respiratory syncytial virus vaccines. *J Immunol* 2001; 167:3910–3918.
118. Cseke G, Maginnis MS, Cox RG, et al. Integrin alphavbeta1 promotes infection by human metapneumovirus. *Proc Natl Acad Sci U S A* 2009; 106:1566–1571.
128. de Graaff PM, de Jong EC, van Capel TM, et al. Respiratory syncytial virus infection of monocyte-derived dendritic cells decreases their capacity to activate CD4 T cells. *J Immunol* 2005;175:5904–5911.
131. de Swart RL, van den Hoogen BG, Kuiken T, et al. Immunization of macaques with formalin-inactivated human metapneumovirus induces hypersensitivity to hMPV infection. *Vaccine* 2007;25:8518–8528.
133. Debiaggi M, Canducci F, Terulla C, et al. Long-term study on symptomless human metapneumovirus infection in hematopoietic stem cell transplant recipients. *New Microbiol* 2007;30:255–258.
135. Delgado MF, Coviello S, Monsalvo AC, et al. Lack of antibody affinity maturation due to poor Toll-like receptor stimulation leads to enhanced respiratory syncytial virus disease. *Nat Med* 2009;15:34–41.
137. DeVincenzo J, Lambkin-Williams R, Wilkinson T, et al. A randomized, double-blind, placebo-controlled study of an RNAi-based therapy directed against respiratory syncytial virus. *Proc Natl Acad Sci U S A* 2010; 107:8800–8805.
149. Eisenhut M. Extrapulmonary manifestations of severe respiratory syncytial virus infection–a systematic review. *Crit Care* 2006;10:R107.
157. Everard ML, Swarbrick A, Wrightham M, et al. Analysis of cells obtained by bronchial lavage of infants with respiratory syncytial virus infection. *Arch Dis Child* 1994;71:428–432.
159. Falsey AR. Respiratory syncytial virus infection in adults. *Semin Respir Crit Care Med* 2007;28:171–181.
162. Falsey AR, Hennessey PA, Formica MA, et al. Humoral immunity to human metapneumovirus infection in adults. *Vaccine* 2010;28: 1477–1480.
163. Falsey AR, Hennessey PA, Formica MA, et al. Respiratory syncytial virus infection in elderly and high-risk adults. *N Engl J Med* 2005;352: 1749–1759.
165. Falsey AR, Singh HK, Walsh EE. Serum antibody decay in adults following natural respiratory syncytial virus infection. *J Med Virol* 2006;78: 1493–1497.
169. Falsey AR, Walsh EE, Capellan J, et al. Comparison of the safety and immunogenicity of 2 respiratory syncytial virus (rsv) vaccines–nonadjuvanted vaccine or vaccine adjuvanted with alum–given concomitantly with influenza vaccine to high-risk elderly individuals. *J Infect Dis* 2008;198:1317–1326.
170. Fearns R, Collins PL. Model for polymerase access to the overlapped L gene of respiratory syncytial virus. *J Virol* 1999;73:388–397.
171. Fearns R, Collins PL. Role of the M2-1 transcription antitermination protein of respiratory syncytial virus in sequential transcription. *J Virol* 1999;73:5852–5864.
179. Fisher RG, Gruber WC, Edwards KM, et al. Twenty years of outpatient respiratory syncytial virus infection: a framework for vaccine efficacy trials. *Pediatrics* 1997;99:E7.
189. Gern JE, Rosenthal LA, Sorkness RL, et al. Effects of viral respiratory infections on lung development and childhood asthma. *J Allergy Clin Immunol* 2005;115:668–674; quiz 675.
190. Gershwin LJ. Bovine respiratory syncytial virus infection: immunopathogenic mechanisms. *Anim Health Res Rev* 2007;8:207–213.
197. Glezen WP, Taber LH, Frank AL, et al. Risk of primary infection and reinfection with respiratory syncytial virus. *Am J Dis Child* 1986;140: 543–546.
198. Gomez M, Mufson MA, Dubovsky F, et al. Phase-I study MEDI-534, of a live, attenuated intranasal vaccine against respiratory syncytial virus and parainfluenza-3 virus in seropositive children. *Pediatr Infect Dis J* 2009;28:655–658.
200. Gonzalez-Reyes L, Ruiz-Arguello MB, Garcia-Barreno B, et al. Cleavage of the human respiratory syncytial virus fusion protein at two distinct sites is required for activation of membrane fusion. *Proc Natl Acad Sci U S A* 2001;98:9859–9864.
203. Gould PS, Easton AJ. Coupled translation of the second open reading frame of M2 mRNA is sequence dependent and differs significantly within the subfamily Pneumovirinae. *J Virol* 2007;81:8488–8496.
206. Gower TL, Pastey MK, Peeples ME, et al. RhoA signaling is required for respiratory syncytial virus-induced syncytium formation and filamentous virion morphology. *J Virol* 2005;79:5326–5336.
209. Graham BS, Bunton LA, Wright PF, et al. Role of T lymphocyte subsets in the pathogenesis of primary infection and rechallenge with respiratory syncytial virus in mice. *J Clin Invest* 1991;88:1026–1033.
214. Groothuis JR, Simoes EA, Levin MJ, et al. Prophylactic administration of respiratory syncytial virus immune globulin to high-risk infants and young children. The Respiratory Syncytial Virus Immune Globulin Study Group. *N Engl J Med* 1993;329:1524–1530.
220. Hall CB. Respiratory syncytial virus and parainfluenza virus. *N Engl J Med* 2001;344:1917–1928.
222. Hall CB. The spread of influenza and other respiratory viruses: complexities and conjectures. *Clin Infect Dis* 2007;45:353–359.
226. Hall CB, Douglas RG Jr, Geiman JM. Respiratory syncytial virus infections in infants: quantitation and duration of shedding. *J Pediatr* 1976; 89:11–15.
231. Hall CB, Hall WJ, Gala CL, et al. Long-term prospective study in children after respiratory syncytial virus infection. *J Pediatr* 1984;105: 358–364.
232. Hall CB, Kopelman AE, Douglas RG Jr, et al. Neonatal respiratory syncytial virus infection. *N Engl J Med* 1979;300:393–396.

233. Hall CB, Powell KR, MacDonald NE, et al. Respiratory syncytial viral infection in children with compromised immune function. *N Engl J Med* 1986;315:77–81.
236. Hall CB, Weinberg GA, Iwane MK, et al. The burden of respiratory syncytial virus infection in young children. *N Engl J Med* 2009;360: 588–598.
238. Hallak LK, Collins PL, Knudson W, et al. Iduronic acid-containing glycosaminoglycans on target cells are required for efficient respiratory syncytial virus infection. *Virology* 2000;271:264–275.
241. Hamelin ME, Yim K, Kuhn KH, et al. Pathogenesis of human metapneumovirus lung infection in BALB/c mice and cotton rats. *J Virol* 2005;79:8894–8903.
242. Hanley LL, McGivern DR, Teng MN, et al. Roles of the respiratory syncytial virus trailer region: Effects of mutations on genome production and stress granule formation. *Virology* 2010;406:241–252.
243. Harcourt J, Alvarez R, Jones LP, et al. Respiratory syncytial virus G protein and G protein CX3C motif adversely affect CX3CR1+ T cell responses. *J Immunol* 2006;176:1600–1608.
245. Hardy RW, Wertz GW. The product of the respiratory syncytial virus M2 gene ORF1 enhances readthrough of intergenic junctions during viral transcription. *J Virol* 1998;72:520–526.
249. Heidema J, Lukens MV, van Maren WW, et al. CD8+ T cell responses in bronchoalveolar lavage fluid and peripheral blood mononuclear cells of infants with severe primary respiratory syncytial virus infections. *J Immunol* 2007;179:8410–8417.
250. Heidema J, Rossen JW, Lukens MV, et al. Dynamics of human respiratory virus-specific CD8+ T cell responses in blood and airways during episodes of common cold. *J Immunol* 2008;181:5551–5559.
252. Heinze B, Frey S, Mordstein M, et al. Both nonstructural proteins 1 and 2 of pneumonia virus of mice are inhibitors of the interferon type I and III response in vivo. *J Virol* 2011;85:4071–4084.
253. Henderson FW, Collier AM, Clyde WA Jr, et al. Respiratory-syncytial-virus infections, reinfections and immunity. A prospective, longitudinal study in young children. *N Engl J Med* 1979;300:530–534.
256. Hendry RM, Burns JC, Walsh EE, et al. Strain-specific serum antibody responses in infants undergoing primary infection with respiratory syncytial virus. *J Infect Dis* 1988;157:640–647.
263. Holberg CJ, Wright AL, Martinez FD, et al. Risk factors for respiratory syncytial virus-associated lower respiratory illnesses in the first year of life. *Am J Epidemiol* 1991;133:1135–1151.
268. Janssen R, Bont L, Siezen CL, et al. Genetic susceptibility to respiratory syncytial virus bronchiolitis is predominantly associated with innate immune genes. *J Infect Dis* 2007;196:826–834.
269. Jeffree CE, Brown G, Aitken J, et al. Ultrastructural analysis of the interaction between F-actin and respiratory syncytial virus during virus assembly. *Virology* 2007;369:309–323.
273. Johnson JE, Gonzales RA, Olson SJ, et al. The histopathology of fatal untreated human respiratory syncytial virus infection. *Mod Pathol* 2007; 20:108–119.
277. Johnson PR Jr, Olmsted RA, Prince GA, et al. Antigenic relatedness between glycoproteins of human respiratory syncytial virus subgroups A and B: evaluation of the contributions of F and G glycoproteins to immunity. *J Virol* 1987;61:3163–3166.
278. Johnson PR, Spriggs MK, Olmsted RA, et al. The G glycoprotein of human respiratory syncytial viruses of subgroups A and B: extensive sequence divergence between antigenically related proteins. *Proc Natl Acad Sci U S A* 1987;84:5625–5629.
281. Jones B, Zhan X, Mishin V, et al. Human PIV-2 recombinant Sendai virus (rSeV) elicits durable immunity and combines with two additional rSeVs to protect against hPIV-1, hPIV-2, hPIV-3, and RSV. *Vaccine* 2009;27:1848–1857.
287. Kapikian AZ, Mitchell RH, Chanock RM, et al. An epidemiologic study of altered clinical reactivity to respiratory syncytial (RS) virus infection in children previously vaccinated with an inactivated RS virus vaccine. *Am J Epidemiol* 1969;89:405–421.
288. Karron RA, Buonagurio DA, Georgiu AF, et al. Respiratory syncytial virus (RSV) SH and G proteins are not essential for viral replication in vitro: clinical evaluation and molecular characterization of a cold-passaged, attenuated RSV subgroup B mutant. *Proc Natl Acad Sci U S A* 1997;94:13961–13966.
290. Karron RA, Wright PF, Belshe RB, et al. Identification of a recombinant live attenuated respiratory syncytial virus vaccine candidate that is highly attenuated in infants. *J Infect Dis* 2005;191:1093–1104.
292. Kaul TN, Welliver RC, Wong DT, et al. Secretory antibody response to respiratory syncytial virus infection. *Am J Dis Child* 1981;135: 1013–1016.
304. Kolokoltsov AA, Deniger D, Fleming EH, et al. Small interfering RNA profiling reveals key role of clathrin-mediated endocytosis and early endosome formation for infection by respiratory syncytial virus. *J Virol* 2007;81:7786–7800.
308. Krempl CD, Lamirande EW, Collins PL. Complete sequence of the RNA genome of pneumonia virus of mice (PVM). *Virus Genes* 2005;30: 237–249.
310. Kristjansson S, Bjarnarson SP, Wennergren G, et al. Respiratory syncytial virus and other respiratory viruses during the first 3 months of life promote a local TH2-like response. *J Allergy Clin Immunol* 2005;116:805–811.
311. Kuiken T, van den Hoogen BG, van Riel DA, et al. Experimental human metapneumovirus infection of cynomolgus macaques (Macaca fascicularis) results in virus replication in ciliated epithelial cells and pneumocytes with associated lesions throughout the respiratory tract. *Am J Pathol* 2004;164:1893–1900.
317. Kurt-Jones EA, Popova L, Kwinn L, et al. Pattern recognition receptors TLR4 and CD14 mediate response to respiratory syncytial virus. *Nat Immunol* 2000;1:398–401.
319. Kwilas S, Liesman RM, Zhang L, et al. Respiratory syncytial virus grown in Vero cells contains a truncated attachment protein that alters its infectivity and dependence on glycosaminoglycans. *J Virol* 2009;83:10710–10718.
323. Le Nouen C, Hillyer P, Munir S, et al. Effects of human respiratory syncytial virus, metapneumovirus, parainfluenza virus 3 and influenza virus on CD4+ T cell activation by dendritic cells. *PLoS One* 2010;5:e15017.
324. Le Nouen C, Hillyer P, Winter CC, et al. Low CCR7-mediated migration of human monocyte derived dendritic cells in response to human respiratory syncytial virus (HRSV) and metapneumovirus (HMPV). *PLoS Pathog* 2011;17:e1002105.
329. Lee MS, Walker RE, Mendelman PM. Medical burden of respiratory syncytial virus and parainfluenza virus type 3 infection among US children. Implications for design of vaccine trials. *Hum Vaccin* 2005;1:6–11.
332. LeVine AM, Elliott J, Whitsett JA, et al. Surfactant protein-d enhances phagocytosis and pulmonary clearance of respiratory syncytial virus. *Am J Respir Cell Mol Biol* 2004;31:193–199.
336. Levy O. Innate immunity of the newborn: basic mechanisms and clinical correlates. *Nat Rev Immunol* 2007;7:379–390.
340. Ling Z, Tran KC, Teng MN. Human respiratory syncytial virus nonstructural protein NS2 antagonizes the activation of beta interferon transcription by interacting with RIG-I. *J Virol* 2009;83:3734–3742.
342. Liu V, Dhillon GS, Weill D. A multi-drug regimen for respiratory syncytial virus and parainfluenza virus infections in adult lung and heart-lung transplant recipients. *Transpl Infect Dis* 2010;12:38–44.
343. Liuzzi M, Mason SW, Cartier M, et al. Inhibitors of respiratory syncytial virus replication target cotranscriptional mRNA guanylylation by viral RNA-dependent RNA polymerase. *J Virol* 2005;79:13105–13115.
345. Lo MS, Brazas RM, Holtzman MJ. Respiratory syncytial virus nonstructural proteins NS1 and NS2 mediate inhibition of Stat2 expression and alpha/beta interferon responsiveness. *J Virol* 2005;79:9315–9319.
349. Lopez JA, Bustos R, Orvell C, et al. Antigenic structure of human respiratory syncytial virus fusion glycoprotein. *J Virol* 1998;72:6922–6928.
351. Lukens MV, van de Pol AC, Coenjaerts FE, et al. A systemic neutrophil response precedes robust CD8(+) T-cell activation during natural respiratory syncytial virus infection in infants. *J Virol* 2010;84:2374–2383.
357. Madhi SA, Venter M, Madhi A, et al. Differing manifestations of respiratory syncytial virus-associated severe lower respiratory tract infections in human immunodeficiency virus type 1-infected and uninfected children. *Pediatr Infect Dis J* 2001;20:164–170.
364. Martinez FD, Morgan WJ, Wright AL, et al. Initial airway function is a risk factor for recurrent wheezing respiratory illnesses during the first three years of life. Group Health Medical Associates. *Am Rev Respir Dis* 1991;143:312–316.
373. McGivern DR, Collins PL, Fearns R. Identification of internal sequences in the 3′ leader region of human respiratory syncytial virus that enhance transcription and confer replication processivity. *J Virol* 2005;79:2449–2460.

377. McLellan JS, Chen M, Kim A, et al. Structural basis of respiratory syncytial virus neutralization by motavizumab. *Nat Struct Mol Biol* 2010; 17:248–250.
378. McLellan JS, Yang Y, Graham BS, et al. Structure of the respiratory syncytial virus fusion glycoprotein in the post-fusion conformation reveals preservation of neutralizing epitopes. *J Virol* 2011;85:7788–7796.
379. McNamara PS, Flanagan BF, Baldwin LM, et al. Interleukin 9 production in the lungs of infants with severe respiratory syncytial virus bronchiolitis. *Lancet* 2004;363:1031–1037.
382. Mejias A, Ramilo O. Review of palivizumab in the prophylaxis of respiratory syncytial virus (RSV) in high-risk infants. *Biologics* 2008;2: 433–439.
384. Melero JA, Garcia-Barreno B, Martinez I, et al. Antigenic structure, evolution and immunobiology of human respiratory syncytial virus attachment (G) protein. *J Gen Virol* 1997;78:2411–2418.
389. Miyairi I, DeVincenzo JP. Human genetic factors and respiratory syncytial virus disease severity. *Clin Microbiol Rev* 2008;21:686–703.
391. Moghaddam A, Olszewska W, Wang B, et al. A potential molecular mechanism for hypersensitivity caused by formalin-inactivated vaccines. *Nat Med* 2006;12:905–907.
392. Mok H, Tollefson SJ, Podsiad AB, et al. An alphavirus replicon-based human metapneumovirus vaccine is immunogenic and protective in mice and cotton rats. *J Virol* 2008;82:11410–11418.
394. Money VA, McPhee HK, Mosely JA, et al. Surface features of a Mononegavirales matrix protein indicate sites of membrane interaction. *Proc Natl Acad Sci U S A* 2009;106:4441–4446.
395. Moore ML, Chi MH, Luongo C, et al. A chimeric A2 strain of respiratory syncytial virus (RSV) with the fusion protein of RSV strain line 19 exhibits enhanced viral load, mucus, and airway dysfunction. *J Virol* 2009;83:4185–4194.
398. Morris JA, Blount RE, Savage RE. Recovery of cytopathic agent from chimpanzees with coryza. *Proc Soc Exp Biol Med* 1956;92:544–550.
400. Mufson MA, Orvell C, Rafnar B, et al. Two distinct subtypes of human respiratory syncytial virus. *J Gen Virol* 1985;66:2111–2124.
403. Munir S, Hillyer P, Le Nouen C, et al. Respiratory syncytial virus interferon antagonist NS1 protein suppresses and skews the human T lymphocyte response. *PLoS Pathog* 2011;7:e1001336.
409. Murphy BR, Graham BS, Prince GA, et al. Serum and nasal-wash immunoglobulin G and A antibody response of infants and children to respiratory syncytial virus F and G glycoproteins following primary infection. *J Clin Microbiol* 1986;23:1009–1014.
410. Murphy BR, Olmsted RA, Collins PL, et al. Passive transfer of respiratory syncytial virus (RSV) antiserum suppresses the immune response to the RSV fusion (F) and large (G) glycoproteins expressed by recombinant vaccinia viruses. *J Virol* 1988;62:3907–3910.
414. Murphy BR, Sotnikov AV, Lawrence LA, et al. Enhanced pulmonary histopathology is observed in cotton rats immunized with formalin-inactivated respiratory syncytial virus (RSV) or purified F glycoprotein and challenged with RSV 3–6 months after immunization. *Vaccine* 1990; 8:497–502.
415. Murphy BR, Walsh EE. Formalin-inactivated respiratory syncytial virus vaccine induces antibodies to the fusion glycoprotein that are deficient in fusion-inhibiting activity. *J Clin Microbiol* 1988;26:1595–1597.
417. Nair H, Nokes DJ, Gessner BD, et al. Global burden of acute lower respiratory infections due to respiratory syncytial virus in young children: a systematic review and meta-analysis. *Lancet* 2010;375:1545–1555.
422. Noble V, Murray M, Webb MS, et al. Respiratory status and allergy nine to 10 years after acute bronchiolitis. *Arch Dis Child* 1997;76:315–319.
425. Okamoto Y, Kudo K, Ishikawa K, et al. Presence of respiratory syncytial virus genomic sequences in middle ear fluid and its relationship to expression of cytokines and cell adhesion molecules. *J Infect Dis* 1993; 168:1277–1281.
429. Olson MR, Varga SM. CD8 T cells inhibit respiratory syncytial virus (RSV) vaccine-enhanced disease. *J Immunol* 2007;179:5415–5424.
434. Palivizumab, a humanized respiratory syncytial virus monoclonal antibody, reduces hospitalization from respiratory syncytial virus infection in high-risk infants. The IMpact-RSV study group. *Pediatrics* 1998;102:531–537.
442. Peret TC, Abed Y, Anderson LJ, et al. Sequence polymorphism of the predicted human metapneumovirus G glycoprotein. *J Gen Virol* 2004; 85:679–686.
444. Peret TC, Hall CB, Hammond GW, et al. Circulation patterns of group A and B human respiratory syncytial virus genotypes in 5 communities in North America. *J Infect Dis* 2000;181:1891–1896.
449. Piedimonte G, Hegele RG, Auais A. Persistent airway inflammation after resolution of respiratory syncytial virus infection in rats. *Pediatr Res* 2004;55:657–665.
453. Polack FP, Irusta PM, Hoffman SJ, et al. The cysteine-rich region of respiratory syncytial virus attachment protein inhibits innate immunity elicited by the virus and endotoxin. *Proc Natl Acad Sci U S A* 2005; 102:8996–9001.
457. Pribul PK, Harker J, Wang B, et al. Alveolar macrophages are a major determinant of early responses to viral lung infection but do not influence subsequent disease development. *J Virol* 2008;82:4441–4448.
458. Prince GA, Curtis SJ, Yim KC, et al. Vaccine-enhanced respiratory syncytial virus disease in cotton rats following immunization with Lot 100 or a newly prepared reference vaccine. *J Gen Virol* 2001;82:2881–2888.
459. Prince GA, Hemming VG, Horswood RL, et al. Effectiveness of topically administered neutralizing antibodies in experimental immunotherapy of respiratory syncytial virus infection in cotton rats. *J Virol* 1987;61: 1851–1854.
462. Prince GA, Horswood RL, Chanock RM. Quantitative aspects of passive immunity to respiratory syncytial virus infection in infant cotton rats. *J Virol* 1985;55:517–520.
463. Prince GA, Mathews A, Curtis SJ, et al. Treatment of respiratory syncytial virus bronchiolitis and pneumonia in a cotton rat model with systemically administered monoclonal antibody (palivizumab) and glucocorticosteroid. *J Infect Dis* 2000;182:1326–1330.
472. Reed JL, Brewah YA, Delaney T, et al. Macrophage impairment underlies airway occlusion in primary respiratory syncytial virus bronchiolitis. *J Infect Dis* 2008;198:1783–1793.
476. Roberts SR, Lichtenstein D, Ball LA, et al. The membrane-associated and secreted forms of the respiratory syncytial virus attachment glycoprotein G are synthesized from alternative initiation codons. *J Virol* 1994; 68:4538–4546.
484. Rudd BD, Smit JJ, Flavell RA, et al. Deletion of TLR3 alters the pulmonary immune environment and mucus production during respiratory syncytial virus infection. *J Immunol* 2006;176:1937–1942.
485. Ryder AB, Tollefson SJ, Podsiad AB, et al. Soluble recombinant human metapneumovirus G protein is immunogenic but not protective. *Vaccine* 2010;28:4145–4152.
494. Schlender J, Walliser G, Fricke J, et al. Respiratory syncytial virus fusion protein mediates inhibition of mitogen-induced T-cell proliferation by contact. *J Virol* 2002;76:1163–1170.
495. Schmidt AC, Wenzke DR, McAuliffe JM, et al. Mucosal immunization of rhesus monkeys against respiratory syncytial virus subgroups A and B and human parainfluenza virus type 3 using a live cDNA-derived vaccine based on a host range-attenuated bovine parainfluenza virus type 3 vector backbone. *J Virol* 2002;76:1089–1099.
499. Schwarze J, O'Donnell DR, Rohwedder A, et al. Latency and persistence of respiratory syncytial virus despite T cell immunity. *Am J Respir Crit Care Med* 2004;169:801–805.
502. Shay DK, Holman RC, Newman RD, et al. Bronchiolitis-associated hospitalizations among US children, 1980–1996. *JAMA* 1999;282: 1440–1446.
503. Sheeran P, Jafri H, Carubelli C, et al. Elevated cytokine concentrations in the nasopharyngeal and tracheal secretions of children with respiratory syncytial virus disease. *Pediatr Infect Dis J* 1999;18:115–122.
505. Shinoff JJ, O'Brien KL, Thumar B, et al. Young infants can develop protective levels of neutralizing antibody after infection with respiratory syncytial virus. *J Infect Dis* 2008;198:1007–1015.
507. Siegrist CA. Mechanisms by which maternal antibodies influence infant vaccine responses: review of hypotheses and definition of main determinants. *Vaccine* 2003;21:3406–3412.
508. Siezen CL, Bont L, Hodemaekers HM, et al. Genetic susceptibility to respiratory syncytial virus bronchiolitis in preterm children is associated with airway remodeling genes and innate immune genes. *Pediatr Infect Dis J* 2009;28:333–335.
509. Sigurs N, Aljassim F, Kjellman B, et al. Asthma and allergy patterns over 18 years after severe RSV bronchiolitis in the first year of life. *Thorax* 2010;65:1045–1052.

512. Simoes EA, Carbonell-Estrany X, Rieger CH, et al. The effect of respiratory syncytial virus on subsequent recurrent wheezing in atopic and nonatopic children. *J Allergy Clin Immunol* 2010;126:256–262.
515. Skiadopoulos MH, Biacchesi S, Buchholz UJ, et al. The two major human metapneumovirus genetic lineages are highly related antigenically, and the fusion (F) protein is a major contributor to this antigenic relatedness. *J Virol* 2004;78:6927–6937.
517. Smith BJ, Lawrence MC, Colman PM. Modelling the structure of the fusion protein from human respiratory syncytial virus. *Protein Eng* 2002; 15:365–371.
518. Smyth RL, Mobbs KJ, O'Hea U, et al. Respiratory syncytial virus bronchiolitis: disease severity, interleukin-8, and virus genotype. *Pediatr Pulmonol* 2002;33:339–346.
521. Sow FB, Gallup JM, Olivier A, et al. Respiratory syncytial virus is associated with an inflammatory response in lungs and architectural remodeling of lung-draining lymph nodes of newborn lambs. *Am J Physiol Lung Cell Mol Physiol* 2011;300:L12–L24.
522. Spann KM, Collins PL, Teng MN. Genetic recombination during coinfection of two mutants of human respiratory syncytial virus. *J Virol* 2003; 77:11201–11211.
524. Spann KM, Tran KC, Collins PL. Effects of nonstructural proteins NS1 and NS2 of human respiratory syncytial virus on interferon regulatory factor 3, NF-kappaB, and proinflammatory cytokines. *J Virol* 2005;79: 5353–5362.
525. Srikiatkhachorn A, Braciale TJ. Virus-specific $CD8^+$ T lymphocytes downregulate T helper cell type 2 cytokine secretion and pulmonary eosinophilia during experimental murine respiratory syncytial virus infection. *J Exp Med* 1997;186:421–432.
528. Stein RT, Sherrill D, Morgan WJ, et al. Respiratory syncytial virus in early life and risk of wheeze and allergy by age 13 years. *Lancet* 1999;354: 541–545.
529. Stevens WW, Sun J, Castillo JP, et al. Pulmonary eosinophilia is attenuated by early responding CD8(+) memory T cells in a murine model of RSV vaccine-enhanced disease. *Viral Immunol* 2009;22:243–251.
536. Swanson KA, Settembre EC, Shaw CA, et al. Structural basis for immunization with post-fusion RSV F to elicit high neutralizing antibody titers. *Proc Natl Acad Sci U S A* 2011;108:9619–9624.
537. Swedan S, Musiyenko A, Barik S. Respiratory syncytial virus nonstructural proteins decrease levels of multiple members of the cellular interferon pathways. *J Virol* 2009;83:9682–9693.
541. Tasker L, Lindsay RW, Clarke BT, et al. Infection of mice with respiratory syncytial virus during neonatal life primes for enhanced antibody and T cell responses on secondary challenge. *Clin Exp Immunol* 2008; 153:277–288.
542. Tawar RG, Duquerroy S, Vonrhein C, et al. Crystal structure of a nucleocapsid-like nucleoprotein-RNA complex of respiratory syncytial virus. *Science* 2009;326:1279–1283.
543. Tayyari F, Marchant D, Moraes TJ, et al. Identification of nucleolin as a cellular receptor for human respiratory syncytial virus. *Nat Med* 2011; 17:1132–1135.
548. Teng MN, Collins PL. The central conserved cystine noose of the attachment G protein of human respiratory syncytial virus is not required for efficient viral infection in vitro or in vivo. *J Virol* 2002;76: 6164–6171.
550. Teng MN, Whitehead SS, Collins PL. Contribution of the respiratory syncytial virus G glycoprotein and its secreted and membrane-bound forms to virus replication in vitro and in vivo. *Virology* 2001;289: 283–296.
551. Thammawat S, Sadlon TA, Hallsworth PG, et al. Role of cellular glycosaminoglycans and charged regions of viral G protein in human metapneumovirus infection. *J Virol* 2008;82:11767–11774.
553. Thompson WW, Shay DK, Weintraub E, et al. Mortality associated with influenza and respiratory syncytial virus in the United States. *JAMA* 2003;289:179–186.
558. Tortorolo L, Langer A, Polidori G, et al. Neurotrophin overexpression in lower airways of infants with respiratory syncytial virus infection. *Am J Respir Crit Care Med* 2005;172:233–237.
560. Trento A, Casas I, Calderon A, et al. Ten years of global evolution of the human respiratory syncytial virus BA genotype with a 60-nucleotide duplication in the G protein gene. *J Virol* 2010;84:7500–7512.
561. Tripp RA, Jones LP, Haynes LM, et al. CX3C chemokine mimicry by respiratory syncytial virus G glycoprotein. *Nat Immunol* 2001;2:732–738.
564. Utley TJ, Ducharme NA, Varthakavi V, et al. Respiratory syncytial virus uses a Vps4-independent budding mechanism controlled by Rab11-FIP2. *Proc Natl Acad Sci U S A* 2008;105:10209–10214.
566. Valarcher JF, Furze J, Wyld S, et al. Role of alpha/beta interferons in the attenuation and immunogenicity of recombinant bovine respiratory syncytial viruses lacking NS proteins. *J Virol* 2003;77:8426–8439.
567. Valarcher JF, Furze J, Wyld SG, et al. Bovine respiratory syncytial virus lacking the virokinin or with a mutation in furin cleavage site RA(R/K) R109 induces less pulmonary inflammation without impeding the induction of protective immunity in calves. *J Gen Virol* 2006;87:1659–1667.
570. Vallbracht S, Unsold H, Ehl S. Functional impairment of cytotoxic T cells in the lung airways following respiratory virus infections. *Eur J Immunol* 2006;36:1434–1442.
571. van den Hoogen BG, Bestebroer TM, Osterhaus AD, et al. Analysis of the genomic sequence of a human metapneumovirus. *Virology* 2002;295:119–132.
572. van den Hoogen BG, de Jong JC, Groen J, et al. A newly discovered human pneumovirus isolated from young children with respiratory tract disease. *Nat Med* 2001;7:719–724.
576. van Diepen A, Brand HK, Sama I, et al. Quantitative proteome profiling of respiratory virus-infected lung epithelial cells. *J Proteomics* 2010; 73:1680–1693.
579. Ventre K, Randolph A. Ribavirin for respiratory syncytial virus infection of the lower respiratory tract in infants and young children. *Cochrane Database Syst Rev* 2004:CD000181.
582. Wagner DK, Muelenaer P, Henderson FW, et al. Serum immunoglobulin G antibody subclass response to respiratory syncytial virus F and G glycoproteins after first, second, and third infections. *J Clin Microbiol* 1989;27:589–592.
586. Walsh EE, Peterson DR, Falsey AR. Human metapneumovirus infections in adults: another piece of the puzzle. *Arch Intern Med* 2008;168: 2489–2496.
589. Waris M. Pattern of respiratory syncytial virus epidemics in Finland: two-year cycles with alternating prevalence of groups A and B. *J Infect Dis* 1991;163:464–469.
590. Waris ME, Tsou C, Erdman DD, et al. Priming with live respiratory syncytial virus (RSV) prevents the enhanced pulmonary inflammatory response seen after RSV challenge in BALB/c mice immunized with formalin-inactivated RSV. *J Virol* 1997;71:6935–6939.
593. Welliver RC, Checchia PA, Bauman JH, et al. Fatality rates in published reports of RSV hospitalizations among high-risk and otherwise healthy children. *Curr Med Res Opin* 2010;26:2175–2181.
594. Welliver RC, Kaul TN, Putnam TI, et al. The antibody response to primary and secondary infection with respiratory syncytial virus: kinetics of class-specific responses. *J Pediatr* 1980;96:808–813.
596. Welliver TP, Garofalo RP, Hosakote Y, et al. Severe human lower respiratory tract illness caused by respiratory syncytial virus and influenza virus is characterized by the absence of pulmonary cytotoxic lymphocyte responses. *J Infect Dis* 2007;195:1126–1136.
598. Wertz GW, Krieger M, Ball LA. Structure and cell surface maturation of the attachment glycoprotein of human respiratory syncytial virus in a cell line deficient in O glycosylation. *J Virol* 1989;63:4767–4776.
605. Whitehead SS, Firestone CY, Karron RA, et al. Addition of a missense mutation present in the L gene of respiratory syncytial virus (RSV) cpts530/1030 to RSV vaccine candidate cpts248/404 increases its attenuation and temperature sensitivity. *J Virol* 1999;73:871–877.
607. Williams JV, Edwards KM, Weinberg GA, et al. Population-based incidence of human metapneumovirus infection among hospitalized children. *J Infect Dis* 2010;201:1890–1898.
608. Williams JV, Harris PA, Tollefson SJ, et al. Human metapneumovirus and lower respiratory tract disease in otherwise healthy infants and children. *N Engl J Med* 2004;350:443–450.
611. Williams JV, Weitkamp JH, Blum DL, et al. The human neonatal B cell response to respiratory syncytial virus uses a biased antibody variable gene repertoire that lacks somatic mutations. *Mol Immunol* 2009;47:407–414.
612. Wolf DG, Greenberg D, Kalkstein D, et al. Comparison of human metapneumovirus, respiratory syncytial virus and influenza A virus lower respiratory tract infections in hospitalized young children. *Pediatr Infect Dis J* 2006;25:320–324.

615. Wright PF, Gruber WC, Peters M, et al. Illness severity, viral shedding, and antibody responses in infants hospitalized with bronchiolitis caused by respiratory syncytial virus. *J Infect Dis* 2002;185:1011–1018.

617. Wright PF, Karron RA, Belshe RB, et al. Evaluation of a live, cold-passaged, temperature-sensitive, respiratory syncytial virus vaccine candidate in infancy. *J Infect Dis* 2000;182:1331–1342.

619. Wright PF, Karron RA, Madhi SA, et al. The interferon antagonist NS2 protein of respiratory syncytial virus is an important virulence determinant for humans. *J Infect Dis* 2006;193:573–581.

620. Wu H, Pfarr DS, Johnson S, et al. Development of motavizumab, an ultra-potent antibody for the prevention of respiratory syncytial virus infection in the upper and lower respiratory tract. *J Mol Biol* 2007;368: 652–665.

630. Zamora MR, Budev M, Rolfe M, et al. RNA interference therapy in lung transplant patients infected with respiratory syncytial virus. *Am J Respir Crit Care Med* 2011;183:531–538.

631. Zhang L, Peeples ME, Boucher RC, et al. Respiratory syncytial virus infection of human airway epithelial cells is polarized, specific to ciliated cells, and without obvious cytopathology. *J Virol* 2002;76:5654–5666.

637. Zimmer G, Conzelmann KK, Herrler G. Cleavage at the furin consensus sequence RAR/KR(109) and presence of the intervening peptide of the respiratory syncytial virus fusion protein are dispensable for virus replication in cell culture. *J Virol* 2002;76:9218–9224.

638. Zimmer G, Rohn M, McGregor GP, et al. Virokinin, a bioactive peptide of the tachykinin family, is released from the fusion protein of bovine respiratory syncytial virus. *J Biol Chem* 2003;278:46854–46861.

CHAPTER 39

Christiane Herden • Thomas Briese • W. Ian Lipkin • Jürgen A. Richt

Bornaviridae

HISTORY

The syndrome we know as Borna disease (BD) was first described in European veterinary textbooks in the 1700s[331,358] as a disease of farm horses using various names like Hitzige Kopfkrankheit (German; "hot-headed disease") or Seuchenhafte Gehirn-Rückenmarksentzündung (German; "epidemic encephalomyelitis"). The contemporary name Borna disease was coined after the occurrence of major outbreaks in the years 1894–1896 in the district around the town of Borna in Saxony, Germany.[358] The name contains the "classifying" letters "RNA," a classification that was only justified at the end of the 20th century, when the etiologic agent Borna disease virus (BDV) was identified as an RNA virus. BD predominantly affects horses and sheep but other Equidae, certain farm and zoo animals, or companion animals are occasionally also diagnosed with natural BD (reviewed in[67,113,253,262,310]).

During the first decades of the 20th century, studies of BD focused primarily on defining the etiology, pathology, and pathophysiology of the disease. Initial evidence for a viral etiology was presented by Zwick[358] by reproducing the disease with bacteria-free filtrates of brain homogenates from affected horses. Histopathologic studies demonstrated a nonpurulent encephalomyelitis characterized by massive lymphohistocytic infiltrates affecting the gray, and to a lesser extent, the white matter of the central nervous system (CNS), reactive astrogliosis, and intranuclear eosinophilic, so-called "Joest-Degen," inclusion bodies (described in detail in[88,141,142,294]). Pathologic changes were preferentially localized in the limbic system, most likely resulting in the observed behavioral disturbances.[135,262] Detailed studies have been performed on the spectrum of susceptible host species and on the manifestations of the infection. Transmission experiments between naturally infected horses and sheep as well as other host species—including rabbits, guinea pigs, rats, chickens, and monkeys—established the infectious nature of the BD agent and confirmed that the same agent afflicted horses and sheep.[113,181,205,223,262,358,359]

Interest in BD and its causative virus lapsed until the late 1970s/early 1980s, when the optimization of tissue and cell-culture techniques for propagating the agent paved the way for work on the identification of the agent and on mechanisms of its pathogenesis in rabbit, rat, and tree shrew models.[177,191,203,308] Milestones in pathogenesis included the adaptation to Lewis and Wistar rats, the demonstration of an age-dependent outcome in experimentally infected rats,[128,203,206] and the recognition of T-cell–dependent immunopathology.[128,203,204,257,258,313,318] Narayan's observations of a biphasic disease in adult-infected rats characterized by initial hyperactivity and followed by hypoactivity prompted efforts to determine whether humans were infected with a related agent. Serologic findings suggestive of a potential role for BDV in affective disorders[263] intrigued many investigators (including the authors of this chapter), resulting in new efforts to identify the causative agent and explore the pathobiology and epidemiology/epizootiology of BDV infection.

However, the causative agent remained elusive until the late 1990s, when BDV was isolated and classified as a negative, single-stranded, nonsegmented RNA virus, the first member of the new family *Bornaviridae* in the order *Mononegavirales*.[27,44,51,176,258,277,281,326] With the advent of reverse genetics systems to produce infectious cDNA clones, detailed molecular analyses of the BDV genome and its gene products, regulation of their expression, and detailed pathogenicity studies using constructs stably expressing fluorescent proteins became possible.[1,52,220,282,286,353]

In the first decade of the 21st century, a novel BDV, now designated avian bornavirus (ABV), was identified in parrots with proventricular dilatation disease (PDD).[131,152] PDD is a progressive, variably contagious and often fatal disease of domesticated and wild psittacine birds worldwide. Typical clinical signs such as gastrointestinal (GI) dysfunction and associated wasting with or without neurologic symptoms are caused by nonpurulent inflammation of the enteric, autonomic, and central nervous system (CNS). A viral etiology for PDD has been assumed for over 40 years; recent work provides evidence for the etiologic role of ABV in the development of clinically manifest PDD. ABV has been detected worldwide in many captive parrots but also in other nonpsittacine species.[55,112,132,217,343]

Until recently, it has been believed that no endogenous nonretroviral viruses exist in animal genomes. Surprisingly, endogenous elements homologous to BDV genes were detected in the genomes of bats, elephants, fish, lemurs, rodents, squirrels, primates, and humans.[11,133] Although phylogenetic analyses indicate that bornaviruses infected primates at least 40 million years ago, there is only controversial data to support current infection of humans. Indeed, a recently published multicenter study used a wide range of molecular and serologic methods to analyze well characterized samples from subjects with schizophrenia and affective disorders, finding no evidence for human infection with a virus similar to either of the two currently known bornaviruses, BDV and ABV.[134]

THE VIRUS

Taxonomy

Although the syndrome known as BD has been described since the 1700s, its causative agent, BDV, eluded characterization until the late 1980s, when the application of a novel technique, subtractive cDNA cloning, yielded the first cDNA clones of the agent.[176,326] Thereafter, analysis of concentrated, partially purified virus preparations[24,251] led to the identification of BDV as a nonsegmented, negative-strand RNA virus, distantly related to rhabdo-, paramyxo-, and filoviruses.[27,44] Identification of distinctive features including nuclear replication and transcription,[24,42,258] differential use of transcription initiation and termination signals,[27,276] and the use of alternative mRNA splicing[27,45,281] resulted in the creation of a new family *Bornaviridae* within the order *Mononegavirales* in 1996.[243] BDV is the prototype of the family and was its sole member until a new species, ABV, was discovered in 2008.[131,152]

Morphology and Physical Characteristics

Spherical, enveloped particles of 80 to 100 nm with an electron dense core have been visualized by electron microscopy (EM) in extracts of BDV-infected cultured cells.[159,356] ABV viral particles of 83 to 104 nm in diameter have been detected in the brain, eye, or small intestine of ABV-infected birds and detection of comparable particles 25 years ago led to the conclusion that PDD is due to a virus infection.[132,185,352] Smaller structures also identified in these extracts presumably represent defective particles. No similar structures have been reported in tissues or fluids from infected mammals.[3,40,270] The virion M_r and the S_{20},ω are not known; partially purified virus has a buoyant density of 1.15 to 1.22 g/cm^3 in CsCl, 1.18 to 1.22 g/cm^3 in sucrose, and 1.13 g/cm^3 in renografin.[47,84,216,251,356] Virus infectivity is only marginally affected after 24 hours in serum or by incubation at 37°C. In tissues and cell-free virus preparations the virus can be more stable than in culture extracts, and depending on the mode of desiccation, dried preparations can remain infectious for months (tissue at ambient temperature) to years (brain suspension under vacuum).[47,177,179,205,358,360] At 4°C BDV infectivity is stable for more than 3 months. BDV can withstand both alkaline and acidic environments, but is most stable at neutral pH.[47,70,114] Heating to 56°C for more than 3 hours inactivates the virus and common disinfection methods are appropriate as BDV is sensitive to organic solvents, detergents, pH below 4, and to UV light.[47,63,113,114,203,205,216,358]

Genome

The bornaviral genome is a negative sense, single-stranded, nonsegmented RNA comprising approximately 8,900 nucleotides (nt) that includes six major open reading frames (ORF) with structural proteins in a 3′ and the viral polymerase in a 5′ position.[27,131,152,208,230] Short noncoding complementary sequences are found at the termini. Unlike other nonsegmented negative-strand (NNS) RNA viruses, bornaviruses lack specific intergenic regions and instead have mostly overlapping ORFs (Fig. 39.1). The first transcription unit encodes the nucleocapsid protein (N). N exists in two isoforms, p40 (40 kDa) and p38 (38 kDa), that differ in the presence or absence of an amino terminal basic sequence that mediates nuclear localization.[156,245] Although nucleocytoplasmic shuttling can be deduced from immunohistochemical and *in situ* hybridization results for ABV,[340,341] there is no proof for the existence of N isoforms in ABV.[92,327,328] The viral phosphoprotein (P, p23) and the regulatory X protein (X, p10) are encoded by the second transcription unit.[339] The 5′ end of the P ORF overlaps with the 3′ portion of the X ORF in the +1 reading frame, an organization that resembles the P/C/C′ organization of the second gene of vesiculoviruses.[167,307] However, BDV X is the first ORF in the RNA transcript and there is no evidence of co-transcriptional mRNA editing, a mechanism used by some paramyxoviruses to regulate expression of multiple reading frames from their second transcription unit.[160,321] The first and second transcription units of bornaviruses overlap, because the transcription start S2 is located upstream of the termination/polyadenylation signal T1 (Fig. 39.1).[276] The start S3 of the third transcription unit is located 2 nt downstream of T2 and generates multiple transcripts for the matrix protein (M, p16), the type I surface glycoprotein (G, p57), and the L-polymerase (L, p190). The G ORF overlaps the M ORF in the +1 reading frame. The L gene initiates with a short ORF of 6 amino acids (aa) that is spliced to the large 5′ ORF (Fig. 39.1).[281,334]

Bornaviruses are phylogenetically distinct from other taxa. Sequence divergence between strains of BDV and ABV is less than 20%, while divergence between BDV and ABV is greater than 30%; thus, they are classified as different species.[131,152] The only region where bornaviruses have significant sequence

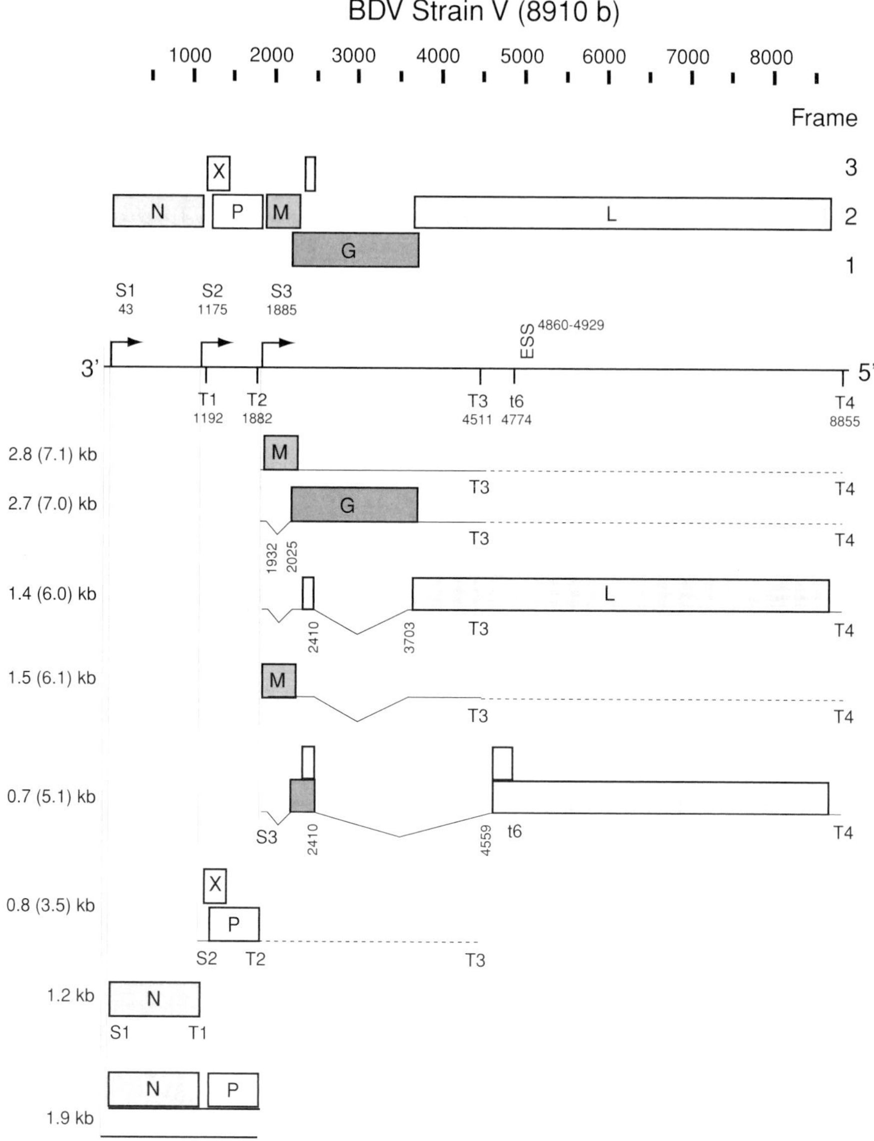

FIGURE 39.1. Genome and subgenomic transcript map of BDV. S1 through S3, transcriptional initiation sites; T1 through T4, and t6, transcriptional termination sites; ESS, exon-splicing suppressor. Dashed lines indicate readthrough at termination sites T2 and T3. See text for details.

similarity to other known viruses is in the conserved signature motifs of RNA-dependent RNA polymerases (RdRp).[234,235] The closest phylogenetic relations exist to rhabdo- and paramyxoviruses,[27,44] with the N-terminal half of the L sequence being closer to rhabdoviruses, whereas the C-terminal half is more closely related to paramyxoviruses.

Sequences distantly related to BDV L, M, and N sequences were recently identified in the genomes of several animal species, including bats, elephants, fish, lemurs, rodents, squirrels, primates, and man.[11,133] Detailed phylogenetic analyses suggest multiple ancient independent integration events. An intriguing example is a BDV N-related sequence that likely integrated before the separation of marmosets and macaques 40 million years ago.[11,133] In some instances, the endogenous Borna-like (EBL) element comprises a complete ORF that includes BDV-like transcription initiation and termination signals. The finding of mRNA transcripts of such EBL elements suggests potential functional roles that may include protection from BDV infection.[11,81]

Genetic Diversity

BDV isolates reveal a remarkably high degree of genetic stability and homology. Among wild-type and experimentally host-adapted viruses, sequence identity is about 95% at the nucleotide level, and 1.5% to 3% at the predicted amino acid level.[18,27,44,123,161,208,230,278,310] Phylogenetic analysis of wild-type and laboratory strains of BDV indicates distinct clusters, which correspond to the different endemic areas in Central Europe.[161] Geographical virus clusters exhibited a higher degree of identity to each other than to BDV isolates from distant regions, independent of host species or year of isolation. There is only one highly divergent BDV strain, No/98, which originated from Styria in Austria where Borna disease is not endemic.[208]

ABV displays remarkable genetic variability in contrast to the high genome conservation of BDV. At present, 7 different genotypes (ABV1, ABV2, ABV3, ABV4, ABV5, ABV6, ABV of canaries) have been identified that share less than 70% sequence identity to any of the described BDV isolates.[131,152,217,340,343] The ABV genotypes vary considerably in their gene sequences with a homology range of 50% to 90% without clustering according to country of origin or avian species.[131,132,152,153,259,309,340,343] ABV4 appears to be the most abundant genotype in natural PDD cases but also in healthy carriers. Recently, a distinct ABV genotype has been detected in wild geese and trumpeter swans.[55,217]

Proteins

Nucleocapsid Protein (N)

In BDV, N exists as a 40-kDa and 38-kDa isoform;[26,156,245] N isoforms have not yet been observed in ABV.[92,327,328] The 40-kDa variant (p40) is derived from the full length ORF, while the 38-kDa variant (p38) initiates at a second in-frame AUG, resulting in the lack of 13 aa at the amino terminus (Fig. 39.2). Although an RNA with coding information for p38 has been found that starts downstream of S1,[245] it is unknown whether p40 and p38 can both be translated from mRNA transcripts starting at the S1 transcriptional initiation site. The 13 aa amino terminal sequence present in p40 contains a nuclear localization signal (NLS; P_3KRRLVDDA$_{11}$) compatible with the differential cellular distribution of the two isoforms seen in cells transfected with constructs expressing only one of the isoforms; while p40 is primarily nuclear, p38 is primarily cytoplasmic.[156,245] However, both, p38 and p40 bind to P. As P contains potent NLS (Fig. 39.2), the *in vivo* significance of the two N isoforms is unknown; p38 may enter the nucleus through interaction with P. Experimental evidence with expression constructs indicates that p38 can accumulate in the nucleus to levels similar to those of p40; however, p38 alone cannot support transcription/replication of BDV (mini-)genomes.[220] Thus, the amino terminal sequence of p40 may have functions in addition to N protein translocation. Both p40 and p38 bind to P through two motifs (K_{51}–Y_{100}, and L_{131}–I_{158}; Fig. 39.2).[13,155] p38 appears to regulate cellular levels of free p40 by blocking the respective binding site on P, thus modulating cellular ratios of free p40 to P.[284] In addition, p38 and p40 contain a nuclear export signal (NES; L_{128}TELEISSIFSHCC$_{141}$)[155] that overlaps the binding motif for P (Fig. 39.2). It is therefore hypothesized that p38, which lacks the NLS motif, may redistribute to the cytosol after dissociation from bound P, possibly once assembled in ribonucleoprotein (RNP) complexes.[155] As indicated by purification experiments and co-localization studies, both p38 and p40, as well as P and M, are included with genomic RNA in the RNP.[35,189] Association of genomic RNA with N relies on basic amino acid residues located in a cleft formed between the amino- and carboxy-terminal helical domains of N.[129,267] However, binding to N in the multimeric RNP appears not to shield the genomic RNA from enzymatic attack.

Together with P, N constitutes the BDV s-antigen, a complex found in the noninfectious supernatant fluid obtained after high-speed centrifugation of sonicated infected brain tissue or cultured cells. Characterization of the s-antigen provided the

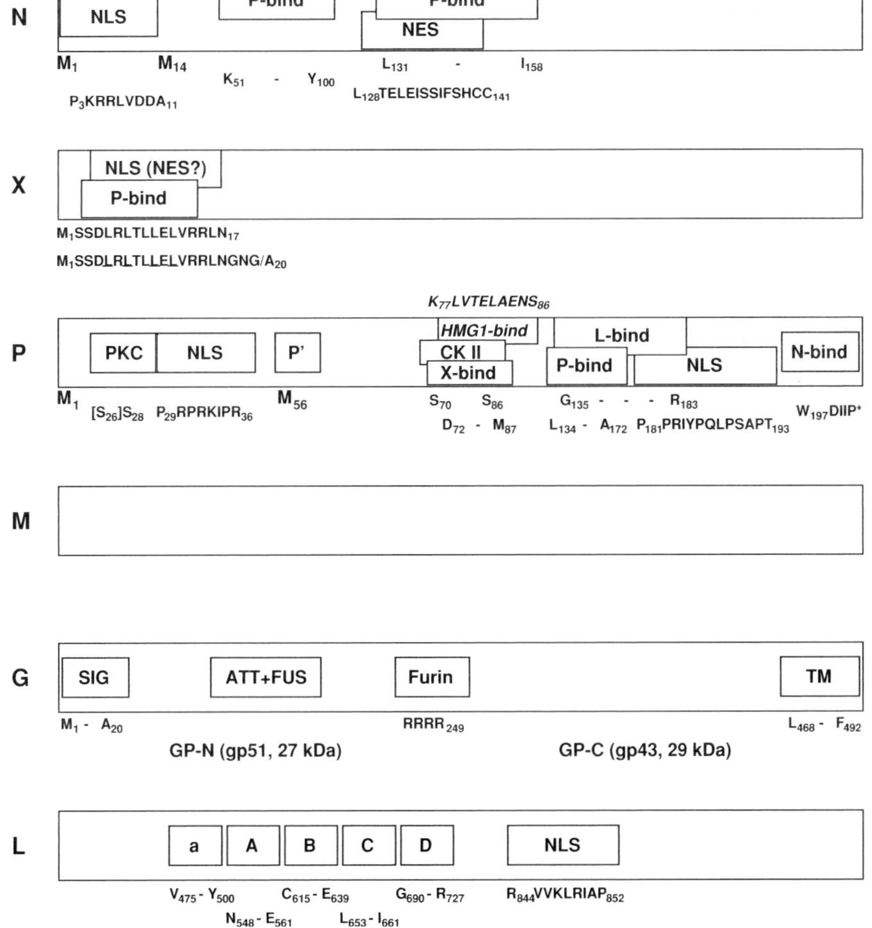

FIGURE 39.2. Map of motifs identified in BDV proteins. M1 and M14 in N, and M1 and M56 in P indicate start sites of p40 and p38, or P and P′, respectively; NLS, nuclear localization signal; NES, nuclear export signal; P-bind, site of interaction with P; X-bind, site of interaction with X; L-bind, site of interaction with L; N-bind, site of interaction with N; HMG1-bind, site of interaction with host-cell protein amphoterin; PKC, protein kinase Cε phosphorylation; CK II, casein kinase II phosphorylation; SIG, signal peptide; TM, transmembrane domain; ATT+FUS, attachment and fusion domain; Furin, Furin cleavage site; "*", stop codon a, A, B, C, D, conserved L-polymerase motifs. See text for further details.

first evidence of protein-protein interactions,[8,96,177] and until the development of molecular assays, served as the critical diagnostic marker for infection.[211,332,333]

X Protein (X)

BDV X or p10[339] is a nonstructural protein[189,288] that, together with P, modulates BDV polymerase activity as a function of the relative abundance of the two proteins.[237,288] X effects appear to be differently pronounced in different cell types.[353] Although X is not essential for the formation of infectious particles,[219] it does perform crucial functions during the BDV life cycle because recombinant BDV constructs carrying a nonfunctional X ORF are not viable.[239] Mammalian two-hybrid and co-immunoprecipitation experiments indicate an interaction between X and P,[293] and recombinant BDV systems showed that X inhibited BDV RNA replication and transcription through binding to P[220,238,285] in the absence of viral M and G.[219] The site of X interaction with P has been mapped to the N-terminal motif S_3DLRLTLLELVRRL$_{16}$, with aa 7 through 15 being probably most essential.[184,350] X is small (10 kDa) and can be found in the nucleus and cytoplasm. A leucine-rich amino-terminal motif with primary sequence similarity to the NES of cellular and viral export proteins like HIV-1 Rev or PKI (Fig. 39.2, underlined leucines) led to the speculation that X may mediate nucleocytoplasmic shuttling through its interaction with the viral RNP via P. However, X has not been shown to be part of the RNP,[35,189,219] and other data suggest that this motif functions as an NLS rather than an NES (R_6LTLLELVRRNGN$_{19}$).[351] These experiments also showed that transport of X through the nuclear pore complex is mediated by direct binding to importin-alpha.

Phosphoprotein (P)

P, a cofactor of the L viral polymerase, is phosphorylated at multiple serine residues by two different cellular kinases.[289,320] P is phosphorylated predominantly by protein kinase Cε (PKCε) at Ser28 (and Ser26, which is not present in all BDV strains), and to a lesser extent by casein kinase II (CK II) at Ser 70 and Ser 86 (Fig. 39.2). As in other NNS virus phosphoproteins, phosphorylation status may regulate P's ability to form homomultimers, bind to other viral proteins, and serve as a transcriptional activator. P interacts with itself, X, N, M, and L as shown by mammalian two-hybrid and co-immunoprecipitation analyses. Regions of interaction of P with P (aa 135–172), with N (aa 197–201),[293] with M (aa 1–11),[35] and with X (aa 72–87)[158] were mapped through analysis of truncation mutants of P. A region of interaction with L (aa 135–183) overlaps that identified for homo-oligomerization; however, the sites are functionally separated as shown by analyses of P mutants that bound to L but had lost the ability to oligomerize.[283] These analyses also demonstrated that P-oligomerization is essential for polymerase activity. Overlap also exists between the CK II phosphorylation sites and the region of interaction with X, as well as between the PKCε phosphorylation site(s) and the amino-terminal NLS of P; two NLS have been mapped at the amino- and carboxyl-terminus of P (Fig. 39.2).[292,295] Thus, it is conceivable that P phosphorylation may influence nuclear trafficking of P (and possibly of X through its interaction with P). In this context it is intriguing that PKCε is highly concentrated in limbic circuitry,[268] as it suggests that PKCε phosphorylation may be important to the limbic distribution of BDV. BDV infection of neurons interferes with synaptic vesicle recycling through blockade of PKC-phosphorylation of myristoylated alanine-rich C kinase substrate (MARCKS) and mammalian uncoordinated-18 (Munc-18). There is speculation that P may contribute to BDV pathogenesis by competing with neuronal substrates for phosphorylation by PKC.[241,330]

Matrix Protein (M)

Like the BDV s-antigen, a 14.5-kDa protein purified from infected brain homogenate had been linked to the unidentified BD agent prior to molecular characterization of BDV.[274] Once genome sequence data became available, microsequencing indicated that this protein is the product of the 16-kDa ORF of BDV (p16).[154] Subsequent analyses showed that p16 forms noncovalently linked tetramers and constitutes a nonglycosylated viral matrix protein.[165,166] M is a component of the viral RNP and can bind to P. However, in contrast to other NNS RNA virus M proteins, BDV M appears to have no inhibitory effect on polymerase activity.[35,189]

Glycoprotein (G)

The BDV glycoprotein is a classical type I membrane protein that is generated from the 57-kDa ORF and posttranslationally modified by N-glycosylation to yield a 94-kDa primary product (gp94).[252,279] The primary product is processed by cellular furin protease into an amino-terminal GP-N (27 kDa, gp51) and a carboxy-terminal GP-C (29 kDa, gp43) through cleavage after arginine$_{249}$[151,252] (Fig. 39.2). Whereas the gp94 precursor contains only high-mannose glycans, analysis of the cleaved fragments indicated glycan maturation by showing mixtures of high-mannose and complex-type glycans on both GP-N and GP-C.[151] Anchored by its transmembrane domain, GP-C is transferred to the cell membrane, while the gp94 precursor predominantly accumulates in the endoplasmic reticulum. The final composition of mature virions is not clear; gp94 as well as GP-C and GP-N have been found in infectious particles,[38,68,84] but GP-N and GP-C were also demonstrated in infectious particles that lacked the gp94 precursor after virus purification.[151] Computational analyses indicate an arrangement of structural features of BDV G that is co-linear to rhabdoviral G, suggesting that BDV G also belongs to the class III viral fusion proteins.[80]

RNA-Dependent RNA Polymerase (L)

The large polymerase protein (L) of BDV is the product of alternative splicing, a mechanism unique among NNS RNA viruses.[27,281] The generated continuous ORF translates a 190-kDa protein[334] that displays motifs characteristic of RNA-dependent RNA polymerases (RdRp). L interacts with P and, analogous to other NNS L-polymerases, it is phosphorylated by cellular kinases (Fig. 39.2).[334] Plasmid constructs directing expression of the continuous 190-kDa protein that supported replication of recombinant BDV genomes confirmed the polymerase activity of the protein.[187,220,285,286,353] Translocation of L to the nucleus of the infected cell appears to be promoted by an NLS motif (R_{844}VVKLRIAP$_{852}$; Fig. 39.2) located toward the center of L,[335] or in association with BDV P.[285]

Cycle of Infection

Attachment and Entry

BDV attachment and entry appear to be analogous to the pH-dependent entry via intracellular vesicles described for rhabdo- and filoviruses, as opposed to the pH-independent surface fusion mechanism used by paramyxoviruses.[229,260,269] BDV G binds to one or more still unidentified cellular surface receptor(s).[84,279] Receptor interaction of G triggers BDV internalization through energy-dependent, clathrin-mediated endocytosis and subsequent pH-dependent membrane fusion leads to release of the RNP from intracellular vesicles into the cytosol.[37,83] Protease inhibitor studies indicate that cleavage of the precursor gp94 is essential for infectivity.[252] Whereas the amino-terminal 244 aa of gp94 and/or GP-N are involved in receptor binding, the hydrophobic amino-terminus of GP-C is hypothesized to initiate membrane fusion upon a conformational change induced by acidification in the early to intermediate endosome.[37,68,83,221,279] No data are available regarding trafficking of the released nucleocapsid after membrane fusion.

Despite its predilection for neuronal cell types *in vivo*, BDV has the capacity to infect a wide variety of cultured neuronal as well as nonneuronal cell types from many species. Only hematopoietic cells[264] and mouse cell lines[74] have been reported as resistant to infection *in vitro*. This may indicate potential exploitation of secondary receptors, and has also led to hypotheses about a nonreceptor–mediated cell-to-cell spread of BDV that is supported by *in vitro* as well as *in vivo* observations.[86,180] More recent studies with a CHO cell line that apparently was resistant to infection by BDV virions, and with furin protease-deficient CHO cells, indicated that BDV can disseminate by G-receptor–independent pathways.[38] However, correct G maturation enhanced the proposed receptor independent cell-to-cell spread, and is mandatory for the formation of infectious progeny virions.

Transcription, Replication and Gene Expression

Recombinant virus systems confirm that BDV N, P, and L are essential and sufficient for transcription and replication of the viral genome.[187,219,220,285,286,353] As with other negative-strand RNA viruses, genomic RNA packaged by N constitutes the RNP that serves as a template for the associated polymerase complex components L and P.[129,189] The BDV X protein, although not part of the incoming RNP complex,[189,288] appears to modulate the formation and activity of functional polymerase complexes later in infection by buffering the crucial N-to-P ratio and likely attenuating the enzymatic activity of the polymerase.[219,237,337] Furthermore, BDV is unique among known animal NNS RNA viruses in its nuclear location for transcription and replication.[24,42] To generate its proteins, BDV uses predominantly polycistronic mRNAs that are transcribed from three transcriptional initiation sites characterized by a CUU consensus sequence and terminate at four AU_6 termination/polyadenylation sites (Fig. 39.1).[27,276]

The first and second transcription units overlap such that the initiation signal S2 lies upstream of the termination signal T1.[27,44,240,276] A similar organization was postulated to serve as an attenuation signal for the control of polymerase expression in respiratory syncytial virus.[39] However, attenuation appears not to take place in BDV as the two transcription units are found at similar levels,[27] in contrast to the usual transcriptional gradient observed in the other viruses of the order. Other factors may modify mRNA levels beyond effects attributable to the typical 3′-to-5′ transcriptional gradient, including the incorporation of regulatory sequences in spliced introns.[296]

Read-through at termination/polyadenylation signals is a vital feature of BDV transcription, leading to primary, subgenomic RNA transcripts of 0.8, 1.2, 1.9, 2.8, 3.5, and 7.1 kb. The 1.2-kb transcript is the only monocistronic product. It is co-linear with the p40 ORF and directs translation of the p40 and p38 isoforms of BDV N from alternative in-frame AUG codons.[156,245] The second transcription unit generates the 0.8-kb transcript that codes for the X and the P protein in overlapping ORFs. There is no evidence of splicing to eliminate the AUG initiating translation of X.[27,276,339] Thus, it is likely that P is expressed through a leaky scanning mechanism, possibly analogous to the termination-mediated reinitiation of X translation from the small upstream ORF included in the 0.8-kb transcript. The expression of X may be further modulated by cellular protein interactions with the long 5′-untranslated region (UTR) of this BDV transcript.[338] The long 5′-UTR region also includes poorly defined regulatory elements controlling polymerase read-through at the T1 signal.[237,240] Interestingly, the region containing the AUG of the upstream small ORF has been found deleted in sequenced psittacine ABV genomes but not in sequences derived from geese.[217,259] In BDV, a truncated 16-kDa P′ product of undefined function may result from initiation at a downstream in-frame AUG.[157]

Read-through at T2 produces an elongated 0.8-kb derivative of 3.5 kb. Two primary transcripts of 2.8 and 7.1 kb are generated from the third transcription unit through differential read-through at T3. The 2.8- and 7.1-kb transcripts include the p16 and p57, or the p16, p57, and pol ORF, respectively; in addition, several secondary transcripts are derived from these RNAs through alternative splicing (Fig. 39.1).

Transcripts of the third transcription unit include two intron sequences, intron-1 and intron-2, that are subject to alternative splicing.[281] Whereas the 2.8- and 7.1-kb transcripts direct translation of M, the expression of G likely requires removal of intron-1. Although G may also be expressed *in vitro* from unspliced transcripts by leaky ribosomal scanning, splicing of intron-1 creates a stop-codon after the 13th aa of the p16 ORF that facilitates translational initiation at the AUG of G.[280] Splicing of intron-2 removes almost the complete p57 ORF and fuses a small 17 nt ORF located upstream of the splice donor site to the large downstream ORF that, in the case of the 2.8-kb RNA, terminates at T3, generating a truncated L protein of unknown function (Fig. 39.1). Expression of L is, analogous to G, likely facilitated by splicing of intron-1. In addition, an alternative splice acceptor site, controlled by a downstream exon-splicing suppressor, has been identified at nt 4559.[322] Splicing of this potential intron-3 (nt 2410–4559), and transcriptional read-through at t6,[27] may result in expression of two additional BDV-specified proteins.[43,322] However, the splice acceptor side at nt 4559 is not strictly conserved throughout sequenced BDV isolates. The lack of conservation in BDV No/98[230] as well as in ABV isolates indicates that the potential gene products are unlikely to fulfill essential functions in the bornavirus life cycle.

There have been reports of multiple types of BDV 1.9-kb RNA transcripts with unspecified function. Analyses based on RNA circularization and sequencing over the junction indicated the presence of a noncapped RNA complementary to position 1 to 1882 of the BDV genome that interacted with oligo(dT)-beads, but was not fully polyadenylated.[276] Such transcripts may represent abortive replication intermediates or subgenomic

RNAs analogous to leader RNAs found in other mononegaviruses. On the other hand, studies employing precipitation with a cap-specific antibody characterized a capped 1.9-kb mRNA with a long poly(A)-tail, extending from S1 to T2[240] (Fig. 39.1).

Initiation of transcription and replication in negative-strand RNA viruses is commonly mediated by sequences located in the UTR. A single transcriptional promoter located in the 3′-UTR of the genome generates the usual transcriptional gradient, and promoter sequences driving genome replication are located in both the complementary 3′- and 5′-genomic termini. However, BDV analyses indicated remarkable terminal heterogeneity.[230] Kinetic analyses comparing the genomic termini in acute and persistent BDV infection showed an accumulation of terminal truncations in the course of infection, which in several cases resulted in strongly attenuated replicational and transcriptional promoter activity, possibly contributing to BDV's persistent lifestyle.[261] In addition, rescue of infectious recombinant BDV constructs demonstrated trimmed 5′ genomic termini generated from originally perfectly complementary constructs.[286] In this system, when recessed 5′ ends aligned to the 3′ terminus were generated, there was strong attenuation of replication while transcriptional activity appeared to be unaffected. This finding is compatible with the high antigen levels in conjunction with low levels of infectious virus that are observed during persistent BDV infection. The four 5′ terminal bases of genome and antigenome appear to be copied from internal template motifs through backfolding of the termini followed by specific elongation and termination on the template motifs.[186] This allows later cleavage of these terminal bases to generate monophosphorylated 5′ termini of progeny strands without the loss of genetic information. Trimming of the termini in BDV may support its persistent infection by escape from innate immune responses through RIG-I–mediated recognition of triphosphorylated genomic termini.[97] It is not known whether viral and/or host functions are responsible for the terminal trimming. Further characterization of these unique BDV transcriptional and replicational promoter sequences may help to resolve results obtained in various recombinant test systems.

Assembly and Release

As with other negative-strand RNA viruses, a first step in the production of BDV progeny is packaging of the replicated nascent genomic RNA by N. The 5′-trailer RNA specifically promotes its association with N via basic residues in the cleft between the amino- and carboxy-terminal domains of the protein.[129,267] Formation of the RNP complex includes association of P via its carboxy-terminal aa residues, and the inclusion of L is hypothesized to occur via its characterized protein–protein interaction sites (Fig. 39.2). Based on NLS located in N, P, L, and X, and NES in the two N isotypes and possibly X, various hypotheses concerning nucleocytoplasmic shuttling of BDV RNP have been proposed, but experimental confirmation is lacking. Co-localization studies suggest that M is also an integral part of the BDV RNP.[35] M, but not X, has been demonstrated in purified RNP,[189] a finding consistent with the observation that in recombinant BDV mini-genome systems the expression of M and G, but not X, is required for the formation of infectious BDV-like particles.[219] The processing of BDV G by protease digestion appears to be crucial to the assembly of infectious virions.[5,38] Distinct packaging signals are not defined.

EPIDEMIOLOGY OF BDV INFECTION

Host Range

BD is reported most commonly in horses and sheep; but disease has also been reported in other *Equidae,* farm animals (cattle and goats), rabbits, lynx, zoo animals (alpacas, sloths, various monkeys, hippopotamuses), and rarely in companion animals (dogs and cats).[21,31,46,54,67,113,138,140,182,192,262,310,344,358] Experimental infections have been achieved in various animal species ranging from chickens to nonhuman primates.[4,46,87,113,148,188,201,212,255,262,266,308,314] Infection in horses leads to death 1 to 4 weeks after onset of signs in 80% to 90% of animals.[67,89,91,253] In 72% of stables with equine BD cases, only individual animals develop clinically manifested BD. In cattle and sheep, death was noted after 1 to 6 weeks or 1 to 3 weeks in more than 50% of animals, respectively.[21,255]

Geographic Distribution and Potential Reservoir

Natural BD is endemic in areas of central Europe such as southern and eastern Germany, Switzerland, Liechtenstein, and Austria.[30,46,66,113,120,193,344,358] Reports of natural BD outside these endemic areas suggest a wider distribution of the disease.[78,98,99,144,147,354] Virus-specific serum antibodies and/or nucleic acids in absence of disease or in association with unusual clinical signs have been reported in animals from different geographic areas, including European countries, such as France, Sweden, Finland, and Italy, as well as Turkey, Israel, Japan, Iran, China, Australia, and the United States.[66,78,98,99,144,147,178,253,262,354] However, as some of these data are debated and require more confirmation, further epidemiologic studies are warranted.

A seasonal accumulation of BD cases in April, May, and June—with a significant decrease in late fall and winter—is quite characteristic and argues, in combination with the geographically limited occurrence, for a natural reservoir.[66,67,89,113,181,325] Recently, BDV infection has been detected in bicolored shrews (*Crocidura leucodon*) in endemic areas in Switzerland. These animals had a disseminated virus distribution in the absence of overt disease and represent a potential reservoir for BDV.[127,244] Whether other species can serve as reservoir species is currently unknown.

Prevalence and Seroepidemiology

In contrast to the epidemic course of BD at the end of the 19th century, the incidence of BD decreased significantly during recent decades; usually less than 100 horses or sheep are diagnosed with BD per year.[66,120,199] However, BDV infections in horses and sheep can be inapparent as indicated by seroepidemiologic surveys in Germany. The average seroprevalence of BDV-specific antibodies in clinically healthy horses in Germany is approximately 11.5%[120] and increases in endemic areas up to 22.5%, reaching 50% in stables with a history of clinical BD.[91] There is a higher frequency of BD on farms with mixed stock of horse, sheep, and cattle, operating under lower hygiene standards.[66] Repeated outbreaks of BD within the same premises have been noted but usually spaced several months or years apart.[91,253] The reason for the discrepancy between the high BDV seroprevalence and the low BD incidence remains unknown but may relate to age, immune status, genetic background, virus strain, and/or dose of infection.

Route of Infection and Transmission

There is evidence that nerve endings in the nasal and pharyngeal mucosa represent the most likely natural route of entry.[142,188,197] Experimental BDV infection of neonatal rats results in virus persistence and disseminated virus distribution with presence of viral gene products and infectious virus in saliva, urine, and feces.[188,197] Such secreta or excreta are important in transmission of other pathogenic viruses (e.g., lymphocytic choriomeningitis virus and hantaviruses). This finding further supports the concept of a natural reservoir of BDV, which is substantiated by stable geographic virus clusters,[18,161,325] despite substantial horse movement and trade. This was recently confirmed by a case of natural BD in Great Britain that was traced back to a likely origin of infection in Germany.[242] It seems that widespread horse-to-horse or sheep-to-sheep transmissions do not occur.[16,66,254,310] The infectious dose for natural infections is unknown.

EPIDEMIOLOGY OF ABV INFECTION

The epidemiology of ABV infections is less well understood. Since its first description in the United States and Israel in 2008, ABV infections have been reported from various European countries, for example, Germany, Austria, Switzerland, Hungary, Spain, Italy, United Kingdom, and Denmark, but also from Canada, Australia, and Japan,[112,131,152,172,209,246,259,340] indicating a worldwide distribution of ABV.

Within the order *Psittaciformes,* ABV infections have been reported in captive psittacines of 34 different genera as well as in a canary (*Serinus canaria*), and recently in a toco tucan (*Ramphastos toco*) and wild waterfowl (Canada geese, [*Branta canadensis*], and trumpeter swans, [*Cygnus buccinator*]) in Canada and the United States.[55,112,132,218,343] Whether wild birds might serve as a natural reservoir for ABV remains to be further investigated. The transmissibility of ABV in natural infections has also been confirmed.[111,153] The natural route of ABV infection is unclear but detection of ABV RNA in feces, cloacal and crop swabs argues for oronasal entry and bird-to-bird transmission. The possibility of vertical transmission has to be further investigated.[173]

HUMAN INFECTION

Much of the impetus for characterization of BDV came from concerns that it infected humans and might be implicated in psychiatric syndromes, including major depressive disorder, bipolar disorder, schizophrenia, and autism, as well as chronic fatigue syndrome, AIDS encephalopathy, multiple sclerosis, motor neuron disease, and brain tumors (glioblastoma multiforme) (Tables 39.1 and 39.2). Over a period of three decades investigators reported evidence for human infection using primarily PCR and serologic assays, including the detection of circulating immune complexes.[23] However, there were also reports of infectious virus isolated from humans or BDV gene products detected in human brain by *in situ* hybridization and immunohistochemistry.[53,202] Failure to independently replicate positive results in the majority of laboratories undermined confidence in the association of BDV with human disease.[175,349] Another concern was the possibility of cross-contamination suggested by sequence similarity of putative human BDV sequences with those of the laboratory strains and field isolates handled in the laboratories reporting the human sequences.[65,134,250,291,310,349] A recent blinded multicenter analysis failed to find either molecular or serologic evidence for human BDV infection using methods established by investigators reporting links between BDV and human neuropsychiatric disease.[134] Thus, although the potential for human infection has not been excluded it is exceedingly unlikely that a bornavirus similar to those identified to date is responsible for a significant burden of human disease.

BDV NEUROPATHOGENESIS

Experimental Infection of Animals with BDV

Early virus detection and isolation experiments by Zwick and colleagues were performed in rabbits,[358] which has served since then as the most sensitive small-animal model for BDV infection. Rabbits are highly susceptible and after early weight loss develop neurologic disease about 3 weeks after infection with BDV-infected brain homogenates. Symptoms include slow movement, depression, and somnolence followed by flaccid back musculature, paresis starting from the hind limbs, and trismus.[179] Comparable to BD in ungulates, infection of rabbits is not characterized by excessive hyperactivity, as seen in infected rats. Nevertheless, most insights into pathogenesis have been obtained after adaptation of BDV to the rat.[128,203,204,206] Susceptibility to disease in rats is genetically determined. Wistar rats and black-hooded rats show less severe disease than Lewis rats, a strain with deficiencies in the hypothalamic–pituitary-adrenal axis associated with enhanced susceptibility to immune-mediated disorders.[36,128,312] Resistance to BD is inherited as a dominant trait independent of MHC genes in black-hooded and Lewis hybrids.[121,128] Serial passage in rat brain may enhance the virulence of BDV strains for rats.[206] BDV infection of susceptible adult rats results in a biphasic disorder that manifests approximately 10 to 20 days after intracerebral infection as an acute immunopathologic disease, presenting clinically as hyperactivity and exaggerated startle responses.[203,204] The onset of acute disease coincides with infiltration of mononuclear cells into the brain, particularly in areas of high viral burden such as the hippocampus, amygdala, and other limbic structures.[32] After the initial acute phase, the animals enter a chronic disease phase characterized by somnolence, apathy, paralysis, dystonias, dyskinesias, stereotyped and self-mutilation behaviors, and blindness.[203,204,299,301] Chronic disease is paralleled by widespread distribution of virus in the limbic system and prefrontal cortex, and 5% to 10% of animals become obese, developing up to 3 times the weight of normal rats.[179] BDV variant strains have been described that cause primarily an obesity syndrome without obvious neurologic disease. The obese phenotype is correlated with inflammation and viral antigen expression in the septum, hippocampus, amygdala, and ventromedian tuberal hypothalamus.[116]

Initially, the unique neuropathogenesis of BDV was mostly studied in the adult rat model, in which infection is associated with behavioral changes and disturbances in monoamine neurotransmitter systems and limbic circuitry. However, disease in immunocompetent adults is characterized by marked CNS inflammation, loss of brain mass, and gliosis. In contrast, neonatally infected rats present with hippocampal and cerebellar

TABLE 39.1 Serum Immunoreactivity to Borna Disease Virus in Subjects with Various Diseases

Disease	Prevalence		Assay	Reference
	Disease (%)	Control (%)		
Psychiatric (various)	0.6 (4/694)	0 (0/200)	IFA	Rott et al. (1985) *Science* 228:755
	2 (13/642)	2 (11/540)	IFA	Bode et al. (1988) *Lancet* 2:689
	4–7 (200–350/5000)	1 (10/1000)	WB/IFA	Rott et al. (1991) *Arch Virol* 118:143
	12 (6/49)		IFA	Bode et al. (1993) *Arch Virol* S7:159
	30 (18/60)		WB	Kishi et al. (1995) *FEBS Lett* 364:293
	14 (18/132)	1.5 (3/203)	WB	Sauder et al. (1996) *J Virol* 70:7713
	24 (13/55)	11 (4/36)	IFA	Igata-Yi et al. (1996) *Nat Med* 2:948
	0 (0/44)	0 (0/70)	IFA/WB	Kubo et al. (1997) *Clin Diagn Lab Immunol* 4:189
	2.8 (35/1260)	1.1 (10/917)	ECLIA	Yamaguchi et al. (1999) *Clin Diagn Lab Immunol* 6:696
	9.8 (4/41)		IFA	Bachmann et al. (1999) *J Neurovirol* 5:190
	15 (4/27)	0 (0/13)	IFA	Vahlenkamp et al. (2000) *Vet Microbiol* 76:229
	0 (0/89)	0 (0/210)	IFA/WB	Tsuji et al. (2000) *J Med Virol* 61:336
	5.5 (5/90)	0 (0/45)	WB (N[a])	Fukuda et al. (2001) *J Clin Microbiol* 39:419
	2.1 (17/816)		ECLIA	Rybakowski et al. (2001) *Eur Psychiatry* 16:191
	2.4 (23/946)	1.0 (4/412)	ECLIA	Rybakowski et al. (2002) *Med Sci Monit* 8:CR642 Rybakowski et al. (2001) *Psychiatr Pol* 35: 819
	13 (11/87)	16 (45/290)	IFA	Lebain et al. (2002) *Schizophr Res* 57:303
	15 (26/171)	2 (1/50)	RLA	Matsunaga et al. (2005) *Clin Diagn Lab Immunol* 12:671
	23 (39/171)	0 (0/9)	WB	Matsunaga et al. (2005) *Clin Diagn Lab Immunol* 12:671
	29 (24/84)	20 (77/378)	RLA	Matsunaga et al. (2008) *J Clin Virol* 43:317
	67 (26/39)	22 (28/126)	CIC	Rackova et al. (2009) *Neuro Endocrinol Lett* 30:414
	4.5 (12/265)	0 (0/105)	IFA	Amsterdam et al. (1985) *Arch Gen Psych* 42:1093
Affective disorders	4.2 (12/285)	0 (0/200)	IFA	Rott et al. (1985) *Science* 228:755
	38 (53/138)	16 (19/117)	WB (P[a])	Fu et al. (1993) *J Affect Disord* 27:61
	37 (10/27)		IFA	Bode et al. (1993) *Arch Virol* S7:159
	12 (6/52)	1.5 (3/203)	WB	Sauder et al. (1996) *J Virol* 70:7713
	0–0.8 (0–1/122)	0 (0/70)	IFA/WB	Kubo et al. (1997) *Clin Diagn Lab Immunol* 4:189
	2.2 (1/45)	0 (0/45)	WB	Fukuda et al. (2001) *J Clin Microbiol* 39:419
	93 (26/28)	32 (21/65)	CIC	Bode et al. (2001) *Mol Psychiatry* 6:481
	27 (9/33)	4 (1/25)	WB	Terayama et al. (2003) *Psychiatry Res* 120:201
	19 (25/129)	20 (77/378)	RLA	Matsunaga et al. (2008) *J Clin Virol* 43:317
	4.8 (5/104)	0 (0/42)	ELISA	Flower et al. (2008) *APMIS Suppl* (124):89
	0 (0/138)	0 (0/60)	IFA	Na et al. (2009) *Psychiatry Investig* 6:306
Schizophrenia	25 (1/4)		IFA	Bode et al. (1993) *Arch Virol* S7:159
	32 (29/90)	20 (4/20)	WB	Waltrip et al. (1995) *Psychiat Res* 56:33
	17 (15/90)	15 (3/20)	IFA	Waltrip et al. (1995) *Psychiat Res* 56:33
	14 (16/114)	1.5 (3/203)	WB	Sauder et al. (1996) *J Virol* 70:7713
	20 (2/10)		WB	Richt et al. (1997) *J Neurovirol* 3:174
	0–1 (0–2/167)	0 (0/70)	IFA/WB	Kubo et al. (1997) *Clin Diagn Lab Immunol* 4:189
	14 (9/64)	0 (0/20)	WB	Waltrip et al. (1997) *Schizoph Res* 23:253
	36 (24/67)	0 (0/26)	WB (P[a])	Iwahashi et al. (1997) *Acta Psych Scand* 96:412
	12 (38/276)		WB	Chen et al. (1999) *Mol Psychiatry* 4:33
	10 (3/29)	23 (6/26)	IFA	Selten et al. (2000) *Med Microbiol Immunol* 189:55
	8.9 (4/45)	0 (0/45)	WB	Fukuda et al. (2001) *J Clin Microbiol* 39:419
	13 (11/87)	16 (45/290)	IFA	Lebain et al. (2002) *Schizoph Res* 57:303
	8.6 (10/116)	0 (0/54)	WB	Yang et al. (2003) *Zhonghua Shi Yan He Lin Chuang Bing Du Xue Za Zhi* 1:85
	22 (7/32)	4 (1/25)	WB	Terayama et al. (2003) *Psychiatry Res* 120:201
	23 (21/91)	20 (77/378)	RLA	Matsunaga et al. (2008) *J Clin Virol* 43:317
	0 (0/60)	0 (0/60)	IFA	Na et al. (2009) *Psychiatry Investig* 6:306
Childhood neuro-psychiatric disorder	56 (93/166)	51 (50/98)	CIC	Donfrancesco et al. (2008) *APMIS Suppl* (124):80

TABLE 39.1 Serum Immunoreactivity to Borna Disease Virus in Subjects with Various Diseases (*continued*)

Disease	Prevalence: Disease (%)	Prevalence: Control (%)	Assay	Reference
CFS	24 (6/25)		WB	Nakaya et al. (1996) *FEBS Lett* 378:145
	34 (30/89)		WB	Kitani et al. (1996) *Microbiol Immunol* 40: 459 Nakaya et al. (1997) *Nippon Rinsho* 55: 3064
	0 (0/69)	0 (0/62)	WB	Evengard et al. (1999) *J Neurovirol* 5:495
	100 (7/7)	33 (1/3)	WB	Nakaya et al. (1999) *Microbiol Immunol* 43:679
	11 (7/61)	0 (0/73)	WB	Li et al. (2003) *Zhonghua Shi Yan He Lin Chuang Bing Du Xue Za Zhi* 17:330
	21 (17/82)	0 (0/73)	WB	Li et al. (2005) *Zhonghua Yi Xue Za Zhi* 85:701
MS	13 (15/114)	2.3 (11/483)	IP/IFA	Bode et al. (1992) *J Med Virol* 36:309
	0 (0/50)		IFA	Kitze et al. (1996) *J Neurol* 243:660
HIV-positive	7.8 (36/460)	2.0 (11/540)	IFA	Bode et al. (1988) *Lancet* ii:689
HIV-early	8.1 (61/751)	2.3 (11/483)	IP/IFA	Bode et al. (1992) *J Med Virol* 36:309
HIV-LAP	14 (34/244)	2.3 (11/483)	IP/IFA	Bode et al. (1992) *J Me. Virol* 36:309
Schisto/malaria	9.8 (19/193)	2.3 (11/483)	IP/IFA	Bode et al. (1992) *J Med Virol* 36:309
SSPE associated BDV antibody	22 (39/174)	23 (39/173[b])	ELISA	Güngör et al. (2005) *Pediatr Infect Dis J* 24: 833
Mental healthcare workers	9.8 (8/82)	2.9 (8/277)	WB	Chen et al. (1999) *Mol Psychiatry* 4:33
Family of schizophrenic patients	12 (16/132)	2.9 (8/277)	WB	Chen et al. (1999) *Mol Psychiatry* 4:33
Living near horse farms	15 (16/108)	1 (1/100)	ELISA	Takahashi et al. (1997) *J Med Virol* 52:330
Ostrich exposure	46 (19/41)	10 (4/41)	ELISA	Weisman et al. (1994) *Lancet* 344:1232
Veterinarians	0.7 (1/138)		IFA	Kinnunen et al. (2007) *J Clin Virol* 38: 64
Suspected hanta virus infection	0.2 (1/361)		IFA	Kinnunen et al. (2007) *J Clin Virol* 38:64
Alcohol and drug addiction	37 (15/41)	37 (47/126)	CIC	Rackova et al. (2010) *BMC Psychiatry* 10: 70
Multi-transfused	8.3 (14/168)	0 (0/42)	ELISA	Flower et al. (2008) *APMIS Suppl.* (124):89
Pregnant women	0.9 (2/214)		ELISA	Flower et al. (2008) *APMIS Suppl.* (124):89
Blood donors	2.3 (5/219)		ELISA	Flower et al. (2008) *APMIS Suppl.* (124):89
Normal population	59 (1204/2101)		TELISA	Patti et al. (2008) *APMIS Suppl* (124):70
	37 (591/1588)		TELISA	Patti et al. (2008) *APMIS Suppl* (124):74
	50 (130/258)		TELISA	Patti et al. (2008) *APMIS Suppl* (124):77

CFS, chronic fatigue syndrome; CIC, circulating immune complexes; ECLIA, enhanced chemiluminescence immunoassay; ELISA, enzyme-linked immunosorbent assay; HIV, human immunodeficiency virus; IFA, immunofluorescence assay; IP, immunoprecipitation; LAP, lymphadenopathy; MS, multiple sclerosis; RLA, radioligand assay; Schisto/malaria, schistosomiasis and malaria; SSPE, subacute sclerosing panencephalitis; TELISA, triple ELISA–CIC, Ab, Ag; WB, western immunoblot.

[a]Immunoreactivity to BDV N and P was measured and the higher prevalence is given.

[b]Epilepsy, headache, and cerebral palsy.

dysgenesis and display behavioral changes in the absence of appreciable inflammation, which offers an alternative, potentially more relevant model to study consequences of viral infection of the CNS. Rats inoculated as neonates with low passage virus during the first day of life become persistently infected, are smaller than uninfected littermates, and display only mild behavioral disturbances manifest as cognitive, emotional or social deficits.[10,33,61,135,169,231,232,265]

In addition to rats, BDV has been experimentally transmitted to a variety of other animal species. Susceptibility to infection varies according to species and virus strain. Compared to the highly susceptible rabbits, guinea pigs, gerbils, and rats, other species, such as mice, cattle, chickens, monkeys, and tree shrews, appear to be less susceptible to disease.[4,46,87,148,179,188,201,255,262,266,308,314] Ferrets, pigeons, dogs, and hamsters develop no disease symptoms although they usually become persistently infected.[46,262]

BDV Infection of the Adult Rat

Intracranial, intraocular, or intranasal inoculation routes have been used to infect adult rats. However, all routes that give the virus access to nerve terminals appear successful and produce infection of the CNS and symptomatic disease after varying incubation periods. Onset of disease correlates with distance from the inoculation site to the CNS,[32] indicating that BDV spreads primarily through neural networks. This is supported by the finding that sciatic nerve transection after footpad infection prevents CNS infection.[32] Further, after olfactory, ophthalmic, or intraperitoneal inoculation, viral proteins or nucleic

TABLE 39.2 Borna Disease Virus Nucleic Acid in Subjects with Various Diseases

Disease	Tissue	Prevalence: Disease (%)	Prevalence: Control (%)	Divergence[a]	Reference
Psychiatric (various)	PBMC	67 (4/6)	0 (0/10)	0–3.6	Bode et al. (1995) *Nat Med* 1:232
	PBMC	37 (22/60)	6.5 (5/77)	4.2–9.3	Kishi et al. (1995) *FEBS Lett* 364:293 Kishi et al. (1996) *J Virol* 70:635
	PBMC-coculture	9.1 (3/33)	0 (0/5)	0.07–0.83	Bode et al. (1996) *Mol Psych* 1:200 de la Torre et al. (1996) *Virus Res* 44:33
	PBMC	1.9 (2/106)	0 (0/12)		Kubo et al. (1997) *Clin Diagn Lab Immunol* 4:189
	PBMC	0 (0/24)	0 (0/4)		Richt et al. (1997 *J Neurovirol* 3:174
	PB	0 (0/159)			Lieb et al. (1997) *Lancet* 350:1002
	Blood	(1/1)			Planz et al. (1998) *Lancet* 352:623
	PBMC	4 (5/126)	2.4 (2/84)		Iwata et al. (1998) *J Virol* 72:10044
	PBMC	20 (3/15)	0 (0/3)		Planz et al. (1999) *J Virol* 73:6251
	PBMC	0 (0/81)			Kim et al. (1999) *J Neurovirol* 5:196
	PBMC	0 (0/27)			Bachmann et al. (1999) *J Neurovirol* 5:190
	CSF	0 (0/27)			Bachmann et al. (1999) *J Neurovirol* 5:190
	PBMC	1.8 (1/56)	0.6 (1/173)		Tsuji et al. (2000) *J Med Virol* 61:336
	PBMC	37 (10/27)	15 (2/13)		Vahlenkamp et al. (2000) *Vet Microbiol* 76:229
	PBMC	1.1 (1/90)	0 (0/45)		Fukuda et al. (2001) *J Clin Microbiol* 39:419
	PBMC	33 (10/30)	13 (4/30)		Miranda et al. (2006) *J Affect Disord* 90:43
Affective disorders	PBMC	33 (1/3)	0 (0/23)		Sauder et al. (1996) *J Virol* 70:7713
	PBMC	17 (1/6)	0 (0/36)		Igata-Yi et al. (1996) *Nat Med* 2:948
	PBMC	0 (0/9)			Richt et al. (1997) *J Neurovirol.* 3:174
	Brain	40 (2/5)	0 (0/10)		Salvatore et al. (1997) *Lancet* 349:1813
	PBMC	4.1 (2/49)	2.4 (2/84)	0–5.1	Iwata et al. (1998) *J Virol* 72:10044
	CSF	4.6 (3/65)	0 (0/69)	[Protein]	Deuschle et al. (1998) *Lancet* 352:1828
	PBMC	2.2 (1/45)	0 (0/45)		Fukuda et al. (2001) *J Clin Microbiol* 39:419
	PBMC	11 (6/53)	0 (0/32)		Wang et al. (2006) *Zhonghua Liu Xing Bing Xue Za Zhi* 27(6):479
	PBMC	0 (0/138)	0 (0/60)		Na et al. (2009) *Psychiatry Investig* 6:306
Schizophrenia	Brain	0 (0/3)	0 (0/3)		Sierra-Honigman et al. (1995) *Br J Psych* 166:55
	CSF	0 (0/48)	0 (0/9)		Sierra-Honigman et al. (1995) *Br J Psych* 166:55
	PBMC	0 (0/9)	0 (0/9)		Sierra-Honigman et al. (1995) *Br J Psych* 166:55
	PBMC	64 (7/11)	0 (0/23)		Sauder et al. (1996) *J Virol* 70:7713
	PBMC	10 (5/49)	0 (0/36)		Igata-Yi et al. (1996) *Nat Med* 2:948
	PBMC	0 (0/26)	0 (0/14)		Richt et al. (1997) *J Neurovirol* 3:174
	Brain	53 (9/17)	0 (0/10)		Salvatore et al. (1997) *Lancet* 349:1813
	PBMC	9.8 (6/61)	0 (0/26)		Iwahashi et al. (1997) *Acta Psych Scand* 96:412
	PBMC	3.9 (3/77)	2.4 (2/84)	0–5.1	Iwata et al. (1998) *J Virol* 72:10044
	PBMC	14 (10/74)	1.4 (1/69)		Chen et al. (1999) *Mol Psychiatry* 4:566
	Brain	25 (1/4)		[RNA, virus, and protein]	Nakamura et al. (2000) *J Virol* 74:4601
	PBMC	14 (4/29)	35 (9/26)		Selten et al. (2000) *Med Microbiol Immunol* 189:55
	PBMC	0 (0/45)	0 (0/45)		Fukuda et al. (2001) *J Clin Microbiol* 39:419
	PBMC	12 (3/25)		6.0–14	Nakaya et al. (1996) *FEBS Lett* 378:145 Kitani et al. (1996) *Microbiol Immunol* 40:459
	PBMC	12 (7/57)	4.9 (8/172)		Nakaya et al. (1997) *Nippon Rinsho* 55:3064
	PBMC	0 (0/18)			Evengard et al. (1999) *J Neurovirol* 5:495
	PBMC	0 (0/60)	0 (0/60)		Na et al. (2009) *Psychiatry Investig* 6:306

TABLE 39.2 Borna Disease Virus Nucleic Acid in Subjects with Various Diseases (*continued*)

Disease	Tissue	Prevalence		Divergence[a]	Reference
		Disease (%)	Control (%)		
Schizoaffective	PBMC	44 (12/27)	15 (4/27)		Nunes et al. (2008) *J Clin Lab Analysis* 22: 314
Viral encephalitis	CSFMC	12 (6/52)	0 (0/32)		Wang et al. (2006) *Zhonghua Liu Xing Bing Xue Za Zhi* 27(6): 479
	PBMC	14 (6/43)	0 (0/98)	2.3–4.5	Wang et al. (2008) *Zhonghua Liu Xing Bing Xue Za Zhi* 29:1213
	PBMC	15 (6/40)	0 (0/46)		Li et al. (2009) *Eur J Neurol* 16:399
	PBMC	10 (6/59)	0 (0/60)	4.7	Ma et al. (2009) *Zhonghua Liu Xing Bing Xue Za Zhi* 30:1284
FMS	CSF	0 (0/18)	0 (0/6)		Wittrup et al. (2000) *Scand J Rheumatol* 29:387
CFS	PBMC	12 (3/25)		6.0–14	Nakaya et al. (1996) *FEBS Lett* 378:145
	Brain	80 (4/5)			de la Torre et al. (1996) *Virus Res* 44:33
Hippocampal sclerosis	Brain	15 (3/20)	0 (0/85)		Czygan et al. (1999) *J Infect Dis* 180:1695
Epilepsy	Brain	0 (0/106)			Hofer et al. (2006) *J Clin Virol* 36:84
MS	CSF	11 (2/19)	0 (0/69)	[Protein]	Deuschle et al. (1998) *Lancet* 352:1828
	PBMC	0 (0/34)	0 (0/40)		Haase et al. (2001) *Ann Neurol* 50:423
	PBMC	22 (2/9)	0 (0/98)	2.3–4.5	Wang et al. (2008) *Zhonghua Liu Xing Bing Xue Za Zhi* 29:1213
	PBMC	0 (0/9)	0 (0/46)		Li et al. (2009) *Eur J Neurol* 16:399
Peripheral neuropathy	PBMC	0 (0/7)	0 (0/98)		Wang et al. (2008) *Zhonghua Liu Xing Bing Xue Za Zhi* 29:1213
	PBMC	0 (0/16)	0 (0/46)		Li et al. (2009) *Eur J Neurol* 16:399
Parkinson's disease	PBMC	0 (0/5)	0 (0/98)		Wang et al. (2008) *Zhonghua Liu Xing Bing Xue Za Zhi* 29:1213
HIV infection	PBMC	13 (11/82)			Cotto et al. (2003) *J Clin Microbiol* 41:5577
Immunosuppressive treatment	PBMC	1.3 (1/80)			Cotto et al. (2003) *J Clin Microbiol* 41:5577
Multiple transfusions	PBMC	0.8 (1/127)	2 (2/200)		Lefrere et al. (2004) *Transfusion* 44:1396
Mental health-care workers	PBMC	15 (7/45)	1.4 (1/69)		Chen et al. (1999) *Mol Psychiatry* 4:566
Normal controls	PBMC		4.7 (8/172)		Kishi et al. (1995) *Med Microbiol Immunol* 184:135
	Brain		6.7 (2/30)		Haga et al. (1997) *Brain Res* 770:307
	PBMC		0 (0/100)		Davidson et al. (2004) *Vox Sang* 86:148
	Plasma		0 (0/275[b])		Davidson et al. (2004) *Vox Sang* 86:148

CFS, Chronic fatigue syndrome; CSF, cerebrospinal fluid; PBMC, peripheral blood mononuclear cells; PB, peripheral blood; FMS, fibromyalgia syndrome; MS, multiple sclerosis.

[a]Divergence of P gene nucleotide sequence from Borna disease virus strain V and He/80.

[b]Plasma minipools of 91 individual samples.

acids move centripetally via synaptic connections.[32] Analogous to rabies virus, spread of viral RNPs instead of mature virus within neural networks has been hypothesized for BDV[86]; and the possibility of G-receptor–independent dissemination of BDV has been described *in vitro*.[38,180] Although viral RNA can be found in peripheral blood mononuclear cells (PBMC) of infected animals, viremia is currently not considered to play a significant role in the pathogenesis and dissemination of BDV.

BDV infection of adult Lewis rats results in severe CNS immunopathology and pronounced behavioral disturbances.[203,204,257,313] Monocyte infiltration, glial activation and Th_1-type cytokines in limbic structures coincide with the onset of hyperactivity and exaggerated startle responses 2–3 weeks after infection and persist until the animals enter the chronic phase approximately 12 weeks later. This is associated with a switch of the Th1 to a Th2 response.[104] Microglial activation precedes astroglial reaction but seems to depend on persistent infection of neurons and activation of astrocytes.[118,214] In many other viral CNS infections, the presence of an intact immune response results in viral clearance or death of the host. However, in BDV infection the virus persists at high titer in the presence of a robust cellular immune response during the acute phase, and also during the chronic phase when Th_2-type cytokines increase while immune cell infiltrates decline in the presence of almost unchanged viral load in the CNS and continued glial activation.[104] While lymphocytes isolated from the brains of acutely infected rats had potent cytolytic activity *in vitro* and can recreate BD-specific pathology after adoptive transfer into healthy, immunosuppressed BDV-infected rats, the lymphocytes isolated from brains of chronically infected rats failed to lyse BDV-infected target cells *in vitro* or to induce pathology after adoptive transfer.[297] Furthermore, levels of IgG antibodies produced intrathecally increase during the chronic disease phase, accompanied by high titer neutralizing antibodies in peripheral blood,[105,106] in addition to the nonneutralizing anti-N and anti-P serum antibodies generated during the acute phase.[25,77] Although the increasing titer of neutralizing antibodies does not result in viral clearance, it is likely restricting the virus to the nervous system. Passive immunization of immunoincompetent rats restricts viral replication to cells of the central, peripheral, and autonomic nervous system, whereas rats not passively immunized showed viral replication outside of the nervous system.[315]

Infection of immunoincompetent, immunosuppressed, or athymic animals does not result in overt disease, and combined with the fact that BDV does not show cytopathic effects in cultured cells suggested a primarily immune-mediated pathology in immunocompetent adult rats.[125,203,204,318] This was further supported by the finding that adoptive transfer of spleen cells from diseased rats, or of BDV-specific CD4$^+$ T-cell lines, triggered classical disease in such animals.[203,226,249,256,257,297] Infiltrating cells in infected animals include CD4$^+$ and CD8$^+$ T cells, macrophages and B cells, with CD4$^+$ cells accumulating primarily in perivascular cuffs and CD8$^+$ cells distributing in the parenchyma.[17,57,225] A crucial role for CD8$^+$ cells has been deduced from the effects of antibody treatment against CD4$^+$ and CD8$^+$ cells, which led in both cases to neuroprotection and abrogation of severe immunopathology.[17,226,317] However, the ultimate mechanisms of immune-mediated pathologic cell death remain undefined. Both CD4$^+$cell lines possessing or lacking cytotoxic capacity have been established, and although current evidence is compatible with an involvement of classical cytotoxic T-cell action,[207] a role of indirect mechanisms elaborated through proinflammatory cytokines and their potentially cytotoxic effects, particularly in neuronal cell death, is also possible.[215] The immunopathology in adult infected rats represents a delayed-type hypersensitivity response with contribution of both CD8$^+$ and CD4$^+$ T cells in the immunopathologic events.

Behavioral and movement disturbances in adult infected rats have been linked to dysfunction of the dopamine (DA) neurotransmitter system.[299,300,301–302,303] Both pre- and postsynaptic sites appear to be damaged. DA reuptake sites are reduced in the caudate-putamen and nucleus accumbens.[302,303] DA receptor losses vary by receptor subtype and brain region. D2-receptor binding is markedly reduced in the caudate-putamen. Both D2 and D3 receptor binding are reduced in nucleus accumbens.[300,301–302] In contrast, postsynaptic DA receptors (D1, D2, D3) are intact in the prefrontal cortex.[300] Selective losses of D2 receptors and resultant D1 receptor hypersensitivity may be implicated in behavioral disturbances. Whereas treatment with D1 receptor antagonists such as SCH23390, or clozapine—an atypical antipsychotic with mixed D1, D2, D3 and D4 antagonist activity—reduces repetitive and self-injurious behaviors, D2-selective antagonists such as raclopride do not.[301] Neurochemical studies indicate a lesion in DA transmission consistent with partial DA deafferentation and compensatory metabolic hyperactivity in nigrostriatal and mesolimbic DA systems.

In addition to disturbances in the DA system, decreased mRNA levels for somatostatin, cholecystokinin, and glutamic acid decarboxylase have been recorded in adult infected rats during the acute phase of disease, while recovery to normal levels was observed during the chronic phase.[174] Decreases are also evident in choline acetyltransferase-positive fibers of the cholinergic system involved in learning and memory. Losses in cholinergic fibers become evident by 6 days postinfection (dpi), and almost complete absence of choline acetyltransferase-positive fibers is reported in the hippocampus and neocortex by 15 dpi.[82] Infected animals also respond abnormally to the opiate antagonist naloxone with hyperkinesis and seizures.[305] Normal rats show increased levels of the endogenous cannabinoid anandamide in hippocampus and amygdala after naloxone treatment, and develop no seizures. In virus-infected rats seizures develop after naloxone treatment, while anandamide levels remain comparable to baseline levels recorded in the same structures of mock-treated BDV-infected or normal rats.[298] Blockade of anandamide transport in infected rats prevented naloxone-induced seizures. Furthermore, levels of mRNA encoding the opioid precursor preproenkephalin were elevated in striatum of infected rats 14, 21, and 45 dpi, and virus and met-enkephalin co-localized in a high percentage of cells.[75,304] Induction of enkephalin expression in infected cells may relate to increased levels of phosphorylated cyclic AMP response element binding (phosphoCREB) protein due to activation of the mitogen-activated protein kinase (MAPK) pathway.[162] Indeed, interaction of BDV with MAPK signaling has been demonstrated in cell culture systems.[103,227] The marked CNS inflammation in adult infected rats makes it difficult to determine to what extent monoamine, cholinergic, and opiatergic dysfunction results from direct effects of the virus, indirect effects on resident cells of the CNS, or cellular immune responses to viral gene products.

BDV Infection of the Neonatal Rat

The neonatal rat model is not characterized by overt immunopathology as described for the adult rat; instead, lifelong persistence of high virus load in the brain correlates with only mild behavioral disturbances that are compatible with the observed cerebellar and hippocampal dysgenesis.[33,136,204] Infected animals exhibit learning deficits, increased motor activity, decreased anxiety responses, stereotypic behaviors, reduced initiation of and response to play interactions, and a preference for salt solutions.[10,61,136,233,265] Compared to normal littermates, rats neonatally infected with BDV show an altered circadian rhythm, and have a smaller size, although food ingestion and levels of glucose, growth hormone, and insulin-like growth factor 1 appear to remain at normal levels.[9,10,33] Neuropathologic, physiologic, and neurobehavioral features of the neonatal BDV infection are therefore suitable for exploring the mechanisms by which viral and immune factors may damage developing neurocircuitry.

Despite significant astrocytosis and microgliosis, the overall CNS architecture of neonatally infected rats appears maintained, although losses in distinct structures such as the granule cells of the dentate gyrus after formation of mossy fibers, Purkinje cell subsets of the cerebellum in a temporal pattern, and pyramidal neurons of the cortex, are recorded.[69,136,265,290,342,346,347] Consistent with Purkinje cell loss in the cerebellum, testing of cerebellar function demonstrated deficits in motor coordination and postural stability.[136] Neuronal loss in the dentate gyrus correlates with the severity of the spatial learning and memory deficiencies observed.[231,265]

BDV infection in neonates does not cause immunopathology, but transient and modest immune responses are observed. Serum antibody titers measured in an immunofluorescence assay are low in comparison to adult infected rats, but persist for more than 10 months.[33] In the CNS a brief surge of T-cell infiltration is observed starting at 4 weeks and resolving by 6 weeks postinfection, paralleled by elevated expression of proinflammatory cytokine, chemokine, and chemokine receptor transcripts,[136,248,271,272,357] whereas the observed neuropathology parallels regions and time course of microglial proliferation and expression of MHC class I and class II, ICAM, CD4 and CD8 molecules.[342]

Abnormal regulation of apoptosis also contributes to the disturbance of CNS architecture in neonatal BDV infection. Excitotoxic stimulation, including activation of glutamatergic circuitry, is one factor that might trigger neuronal apoptosis. There are complex alterations in mRNAs for apoptosis mediators in the hippocampus, amygdala, prefrontal cortex, nucleus accumbens, and cerebellum consistent with prolonged promotion of apoptosis throughout the brains of rats neonatally infected with BDV.[136] Levels of mRNAs for FAS and ICE (caspase-1), two promotors of apoptosis, were increased. Levels of mRNA for bcl-x, a factor that inhibits apoptosis, were decreased. Maximal shifts were observed at 4 and 6 weeks postinfection, closely paralleling the increases in proinflammatory cytokines noted earlier. Terminal deoxynucleotidyl transferase dUTP-biotin nick end labeling (TUNEL) was shown in cerebral cortex and dentate gyrus, and in the granule cell layer of the cerebellum.[136,342] Degeneration of cells in the hippocampal formation is related to activation of caspase 3, PARP-1, and deregulation of zinc homeostasis.[346] Although apoptosis is described in the normally developing rat hippocampus as late as days 7 to 10 of postnatal life, it is normally not found at later time points.[323] The anatomic location of apoptotic cells and the absence of inflammatory cells in the hippocampus and cerebellum suggest that apoptotic processes may play a more important role than cell-mediated immunity to BDV in neonatal BDV infections.

CNS dysfunction in neonatally infected animals may be linked to direct viral effects on morphogenesis of the hippocampus and cerebellum, two structures that continue to mature postnatally in rodents. BDV-induced down-regulation of the neuronal gap junction protein connexin 36 occurs first throughout the hippocampal formation and at 8 weeks postinfection also in the cerebellum; this indicates reduced electrical coupling and impaired neuronal functioning in these structures.[163] Further studies are needed to evaluate the mechanisms by which early postnatal exposure to BDV induces apoptotic losses and morphogenic damage in cerebellar and limbic circuitry.

BDV Infection of Tree Shrews

Nonacute infection in a phylogenetically higher species has been reported in the prosimian tree shrew (*Tupaia glis*). In this model, intracerebral inoculation establishes a persistent infection and transient mild encephalitis, resulting in a disorder characterized primarily by hyperactivity and alterations in sociosexual behavior rather than motor dysfunction.[308] Housing of animals as mating pairs revealed pronounced disturbances in social and breeding behavior.[308] Females, not males, initiated mating and despite increased sexual activity the infected animals failed to reproduce. The behavioral changes were attributed to dysfunction of the limbic system, although neuroanatomic analyses were not performed.

BDV Infection of Nonhuman Primates

The only reported studies of experimentally infected primates employed adult immunocompetent rhesus macaques (*Macaca mulatta*). Following intracerebral infection, an acute neurologic syndrome ensued, during which animals were initially hyperactive and subsequently became apathetic and hypokinetic, similar to BDV-infected adult rats. Pathologic changes were remarkable and severe meningoencephalitis and retinopathy were observed.[34,205,223,314,358]

BDV Infection of Mice

Adult mice develop high virus titers in the CNS after BDV inoculation, but most strains do not develop encephalitis.[148] However, disease may be induced by infection of certain mouse strains during the neonatal period[100] or by adaptation of virus through multiple passages in mice.[266] Serial passage results in adaptive mutations in the viral polymerase that may contribute to pathogenicity.[2] The reason for the different course of experimental BDV infection in adult vs. newborn mice, and in rats, remains unclear, but might be associated with the time point of antigen presentation in the periphery.[107]

The incidence and severity of BDV-induced clinical manifestations varies considerably between different mouse strains. Similar to the adult rat model, occurrence of clinical signs is associated with immune cell infiltration in the brain and glial activation, mainly in the cerebral cortex and hippocampus. An immunopathologic syndrome mediated by MHC class I–restricted $CD8^+$ T cells in a $CD4^+$ T-cell–dependent manner is most pronounced in mouse strains such as MRL with the MHC H-2k allele.[100,108] This MHC I–haplotype is associated with severity of clinical disease, but the incidence of disease is most likely associated with other, to date unknown, genetic factors.[100] The BDV N peptide T_{129}ELEISSI was the dominant epitope shown to sensitize cytotoxic T cells.[275] Transgenic expression of BDV-N in neurons or astrocytes in B10.BR mice did not result in clinical disease and prevented induction of BDV-N specific $CD8^+$ T-cells.[247] Moreover, downregulation of the functional avidity of virus-specific $CD8^+$ T cells in experimentally infected mice seemed to be involved in controlling the inflammatory reaction and facilitating viral persistence.[71] Overexpression of cytokines such as IL-12 or TNF in mice less susceptible to BDV-induced disease sensitize the mice to develop an immune-mediated disorder and clinical disease, for example, epileptic seizures in the case of TNF overexpression.[73,100,130,164] The IL-12 effect seems to be mediated via IFN-γ, which also exerts neuroprotective effects in the mouse model.[109,130]

A behavioral syndrome similar to that of neonatally infected rats has been described after expression of an individual BDV gene product in transgenic mice. High glial expression of BDV-P decreases synaptic density, serotonin receptors, and levels of brain-derived neurotropic factor (BDNF), resulting in behavioral disturbances.[145] Thus, at least one viral product interferes with neural function (see below), but in natural disease, replication of the virus itself and other viral components are also likely to contribute.[236]

Tissue Culture Models

Studies in cell culture systems are beginning to provide further insights into the mechanisms by which BDV interferes with cellular functions and induces neuropathology. Interference with basic cellular signalling pathways and modulation of cellular protein functions through direct binding by, or indirect interaction with, individual viral proteins has been recognized. The N-terminal portion (aa 13-171) of BDV N binds to the Cdc2-cyclin B1 complex and delays cell cycle progression in primary rat and mouse fibroblasts.[228] Direct protein-protein interaction was also shown between BDV P and the neurite outgrowth factor amphoterin (also designated HMG1).[146] Complex formation between amphoterin's A-box and BDV P (aa 77-86) leads to competitive inhibition of p53 binding to amphoterin, resulting in downregulation of cyclin G promoter activity.[355] Through interference with the transcriptional activity of p53, BDV may affect cell-cycle regulation as well as apoptosis. BDV P interaction with amphoterin also causes altered intracellular distribution of amphoterin in infected cells, leading to an inhibition of neurite outgrowth and migration that has been ascribed to interference with the normal interaction between amphoterin and its receptor RAGE (Receptor for Advanced Glycation End-products).[146] Studies of neuronal differentiation of PC12 cells indicate an interaction of BDV with cellular MAPK signaling pathways.[103] Persistently infected PC12 cells demonstrate constitutive phosphorylation of MAPK/ERK kinase (MEK), extracellular signal-regulated kinase (ERK), and the E 26 (ETS)–like transcription factor 1 (Elk-1); however, nuclear translocation of ERK is impaired, contributing to the failure of the cells to differentiate with nerve growth factor (NGF) treatment. Activation of MAPK signaling is evident within 1 hour after acute infection, suggesting that gene expression is not required for BDV's activation of the MAPK cascade, whereas sustained MAPK activation appears essential to virus transmission. Chemical blockade of MEK inhibited virus spread to neighboring cells.[227] BDV impairment of ERK-mediated neurotrophin signaling also modulates synaptic functioning by interfering with synaptogenesis and synaptic protein synthesis.[102] Analogous to findings in the neonatal rat,[85] BDV infection of neuronal cells specifically downregulates the expression of proteins related to synaptic plasticity, such as synaptophysin and growth-associated protein 43 (GAP-43).[103] In addition, infection interfered with synaptic activity by inhibiting synaptic vesicle recycling in response to stimulus-induced potentiation in hippocampal neuronal cultures.[330] Several cellular kinases participate in the phosphorylation events involved in synaptic vesicle recycling, including protein kinase C (PKC), the epsilon isoform of which phosphorylates BDV P.[289] Thus, it is conceivable that the high levels of BDV P that are expressed in the cytoplasm as well as in the nucleus of BDV-infected cells may act as a decoy substrate for PKC, analogous to the BDV P phosphorylation by Traf family member-associated NF-κB (TANK)–binding kinase 1 (TBK-1) that results in the suppression of TBK-1–dependent interferon (IFN) expression in non-neuronal cells.[324] However, species-specific differences appear to exist in the susceptibility of BDV to the antiviral action of IFNγ. Human IFNγ efficiently prevented BDV infection of human and monkey cell lines, whereas rat IFN interfered only ineffectively with the infection of rat cell lines or rat hippocampal slice cultures.[273] Moreover, experiments in mouse brain slice cultures indicated a tissue-specific action of IFNγ, with a more pronounced effect of IFNγ on BDV proliferation in cerebellar than in hippocampal cultures.[74]

NATURAL INFECTION WITH BDV

Clinical Signs

In the main natural hosts, horse and sheep, infection with BDV typically causes a severe neurologic disorder.[29,30,67,89,91,113,139,179,181,193,253,262] Death within 1 to 4 weeks after onset of clinical signs is common. However, inapparent infections occur more frequently in both horses and sheep.[120,199,253] Clinical recovery or recurrence of acute disease is observed only rarely.[46,67,89,91,113,149,190,193,223,253] A few animals may also develop a chronic disease course with low-level viral persistence. The incubation period for natural BD has been estimated to range from 2 weeks to several months.[181,262] This is substantiated by recent cases of natural BD in a horse in the United Kingdom and an alpaca in Germany that had likely been infected in their endemic home areas before transport to the new housing areas outside endemic regions, where clinical signs were noted approximately 3 to 4 months later.[140,242] In experimental studies, the incubation period for 3 ponies after intracerebral inoculation was 15 to 26 days.[149]

Neurologic signs of BD in horses may vary between individual animals depending on the brain area affected by inflammatory lesions and on the course of the disease (Fig. 39.3).[67,89,91,181,253,358] Clinical hallmarks are simultaneous or consecutive changes in psyche, sensorium, sensibility, motility, and in the autonomous nervous system.[67,89,91,113,181,253,262,358,361] Recurrent therapy-resistant fever, lethargy, somnolence and stupor, hyperexcitability, fearfulness, and aggressiveness accompanied by repetitive motor activities, slow-motion eating, and "Pfeifenrauchen" (pipe smoking, eating arrest with chewing movements, Fig. 39.3A) are typically recorded. Disturbances of mental status could be attributed to impairment of the limbic system, mainly the hippocampus, which usually shows the most pronounced inflammatory lesions.[15,89,91,117,253] With disease progression, postural instability, unawareness, hyporeflexia, hypokinesia, head tilt, hypoesthesia with disturbances in proprioceptive sensory functions, and ataxia can appear (Fig. 39.3B). Finally, food intake ceases; torticollis, compulsive circular walking, head tremor with subsequent convulsions and head pressing, coma, and possibly blindness are characteristic (Fig. 39.3C).[15,91,126] Depending on brain inflammation localization, cranial nerve disturbances might lead to dysphagia, salivation, trismus, and facial nerve paresis, as well as nystagmus, strabismus, or miosis.[91,253] Besides neurologic signs, a variety of atypical symptoms have been reported, for example, mental, behavioral or gait disturbances, recurrent colic, emaciation, and chronic lameness.[12,22,58,66,178]

Sheep can develop similar clinical signs as horses, with disturbances in behavior and movement.[30] The few cases of natural BD in cattle exhibited a classical neurologic disorder analogous to horses.[21,31] Rabbits, analogous to experimental

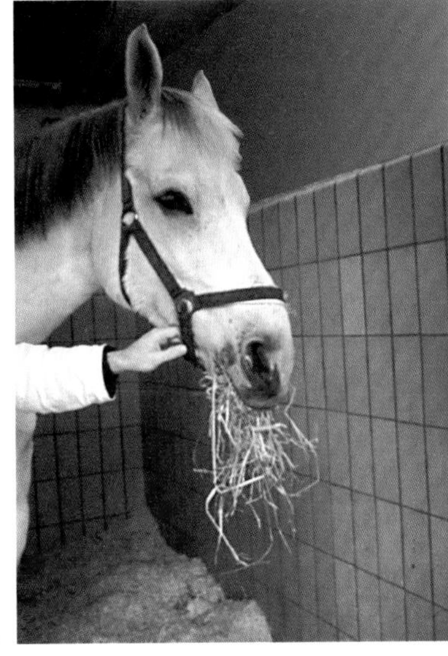

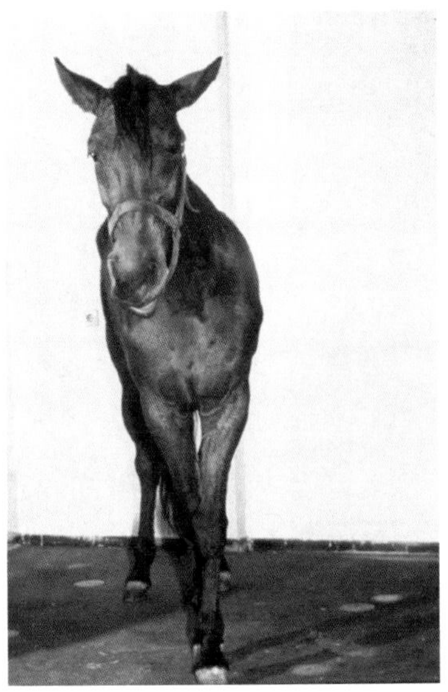

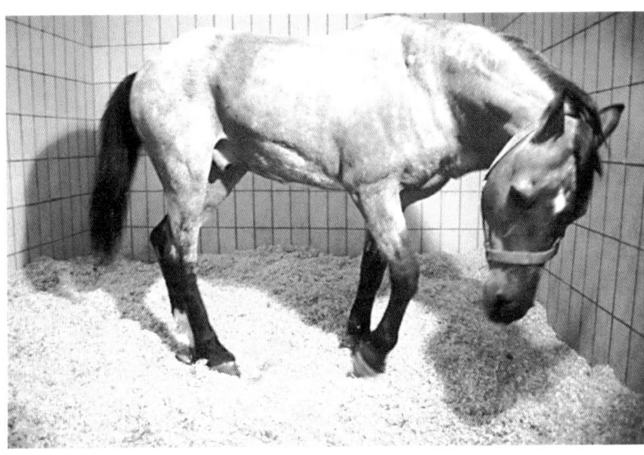

FIGURE 39.3. Clinical signs of Borna disease in horses in different stages of disease. A: Early stage of BD. The BDV-infected horse exhibits somnolence and eating arrest with chewing movements (so-called "Pfeifenrauchen" or "pipe smoking"). **B:** More advanced stage of BD. The BDV-infected horse displays abnormal posture as sign of disturbed proprioception and facial nerve paralysis. **C:** Final stage of BD. The BDV-infected horse presents neurogenic torticollis and compulsive circular walking. (From Richt JA, Grabner A, Herzog S, et al. Borna disease in horses. *Vet Clin North Am Equine Pract* 2000;16:579–595, with permission.)

infection, develop an acute and fatal paralytic disease accompanied by blindness.[181,192,212,262]

Pathogenesis

In horses, gross findings are mostly sparse and consist of leptomeningeal hyperemia, brain edema, or hydrocephalus internus in later disease stages.[113,149,358,361] Viral antigen and RNA are present in neurons, astrocytes, and occasionally in ependymal cells and oligodendrocytes as described for experimental infections of rodents (Fig. 39.4). In contrast to the variability of lesion severity and affected organs in ABV infections (see below), histopathologic changes after BDV infection are similar in all mammalian species and mainly restricted to gray matter areas of the CNS, spinal cord, and retina. A severe nonpurulent poliomeningoencephalomyelitis with perivascular and parenchymal immune cell infiltrates accompanied by activation of astrocytes and microglia is characteristic. Diagnosis can be completed if pathognomonic intranuclear "Joest-Degen" inclusion bodies are present in neurons (Fig. 39.5). A loss of pyramidal cells of the hippocampus is noted occasionally but neuronal necrosis and neuronophagia are not regular features. The main affected brain areas are the olfactory bulb, basal cortex, caudate nucleus, thalamus, hippocampus, and periventricular areas of the medulla oblongata.

Despite the detection of viral antigen and infectious BDV in the retina in most affected horses, the retina is microscopically mostly unaffected, indicating central blindness.[15,117] However, degeneration of retinal neurons resulting in blindness has been reported.[60] In contrast, BDV-infected rats and rabbits typically develop blindness caused by a nonpurulent chorioretinitis with degeneration of rods and cones.[168,203,204]

Naturally infected horses display a similar composition of infiltrating immune cells (macrophages, $CD4^+$ and $CD8^+$ T cells, and plasma cells in chronic stages) and increased expression of MHC class I– and class II–antigens as described for experimentally infected rats.[16,29,57,117] Thus, it can be assumed that the underlying neuropathogenesis is also immunopathologic in naturally infected hosts.

NATURAL INFECTION WITH ABV

Clinical Signs

Reports of natural cases and experimental studies provide evidence that ABV infections are the cause of PDD; ABV has been detected in 60% to 100% of PDD-affected birds investigated.[79,92,112,131,132,152,213,218,246,259,309,340] Interestingly, ABV infections, as shown either by detection of viral RNA and/or

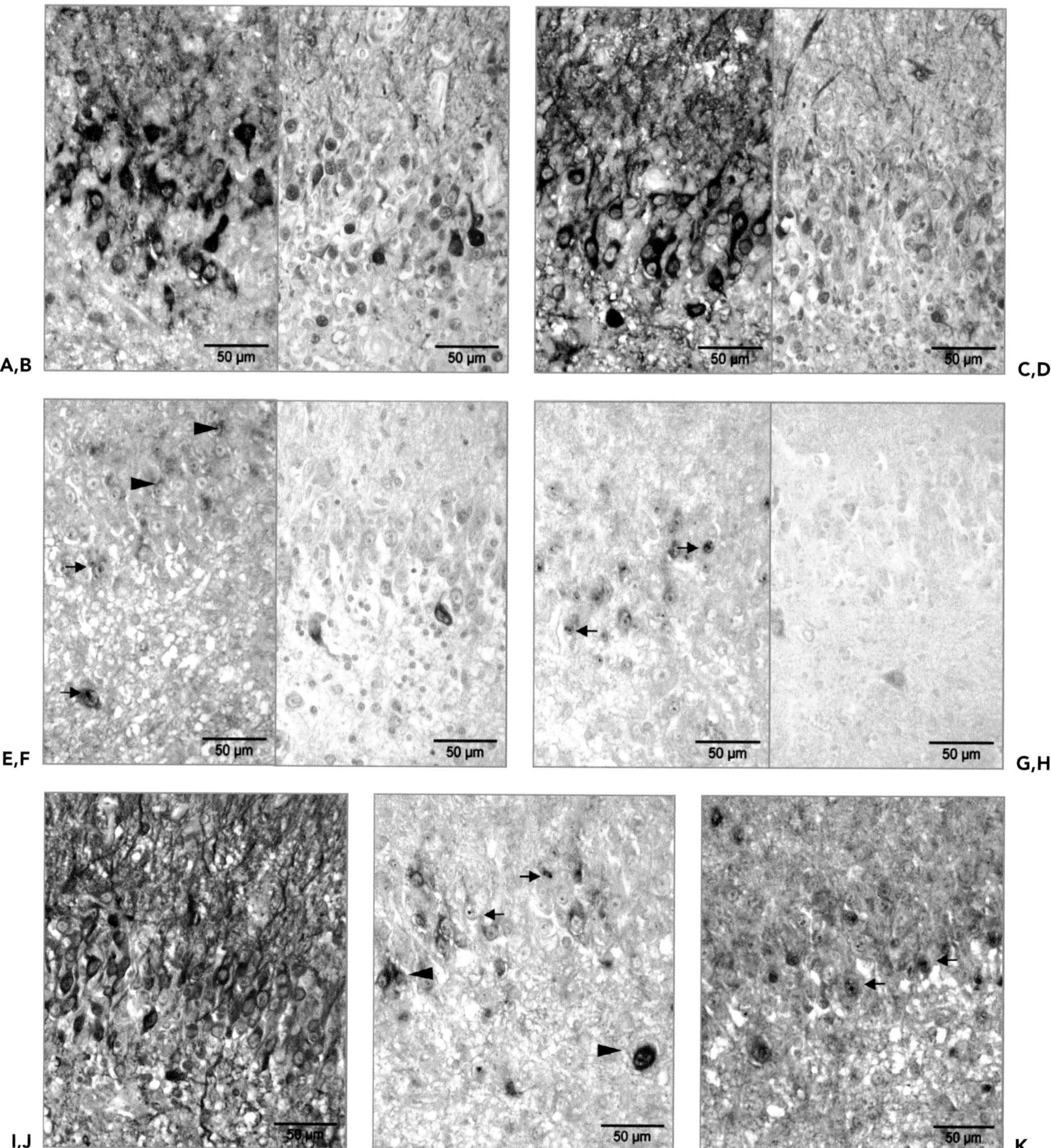

FIGURE 39.4. Demonstration of BDV RNAs and proteins in a horse with typical BD by *in situ* hybridization and immunohistochemistry. A, C, E, G, J, K: Demonstration of BDV-specific RNAs by *in-situ* hybridization (ISH). **B, D, F, H, I:** Demonstration of BDV-specific proteins by immunohistochemistry (IHC). **A:** Widespread BDV N mRNA mainly in the cytoplasm and processes of neurons. **B:** Widespread BDV N (monoclonal antibody Bo 18) in the cytoplasm and nuclei of infected neurons and in the neuropil. **C:** Widespread BDV P mRNA mainly in the cytoplasm and processes of neurons. **D:** Widespread BDV-P (polyclonal monospecific anti-BDV P antibody) in the cytoplasm and a few nuclei of neurons and in the neuropil. **E:** Demonstration of BDV M mRNA in the cytoplasm (*arrowhead*) and few nuclei as dot-like signal (*arrow*) in some neurons. **F:** Detection of the BDV M (polyclonal anti-BDV M antibody) mainly in the cytoplasm of some neurons. **G:** Demonstration of BDV G mRNA mainly in the nuclei as dot-like signal (*arrow*) in some neurons. **H:** Detection of the BDV G (monospecific polyclonal anti-BDV G antibody) only in the cytoplasm of a few neurons. **I:** Detection of BDV X (polyclonal anti-BDV X antibody) mainly in the cytoplasm of neurons and the neuropil. **J:** Demonstration of BDV L mRNA in the cytoplasm (*arrowhead*) and nuclei as dot-like signal (*arrow*) in some neurons. **K:** Demonstration of genomic BDV RNA mainly in the nuclei as dot-like signal (*arrow*) in some neurons. N, nucleoprotein; P, phosphoprotein; X, X protein; M, matrix protein; G, glycoprotein; L, polymerase; Bar, 50 μm. (From Herden C, Richt JA. Equine Borna disease. *Equine Vet Educ Manual* 2009;8:113–127, with permission.)

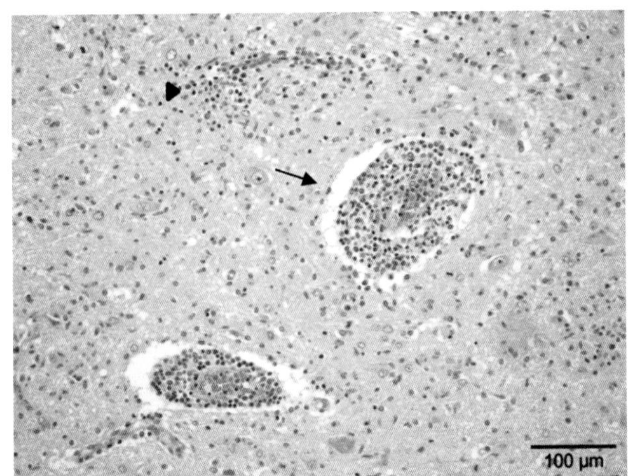

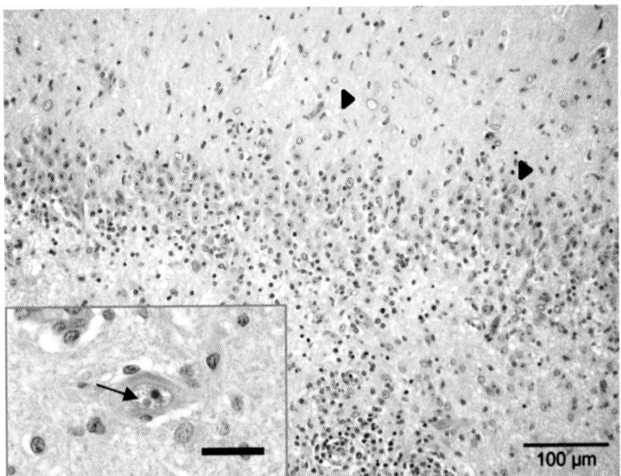

FIGURE 39.5. Characteristic histopathologic lesions in a horse suffering from BD. A: Severe perivascular (*arrow*) and moderate parenchymal (*arrowhead*) mononuclear immune cell infiltrates in the CNS. **B:** Moderate to severe parenchymal immune cell infiltrates with astroglial and microglial activation (*arrowhead*) in a more advanced stage of BD. **Insert:** Intranuclear Joest-Degen inclusion body (*arrow*). **Bar:** a, b: 100 μm, **Insert:** 25 μm. (From Herden C, Richt JA. Equine Borna disease. *Equine Vet Educ Manual* 2009;8:113–127, with permission.)

viral antigen, were also found in psittacines without clinical signs of PDD.[50,111,119,132,172,218,327,352] Clinically healthy animals that only show ABV-specific antibodies are also described.

PDD was initially reported in macaws in the late 1970s and several synonyms—for example, macaw wasting disease, neuropathic gastric dilatation of psittacines, and myenteric ganglioneuritis—have been used.[14,62,95,185] Up to now, PDD has been found in approximately 60 psittacine species that belong to 20 different genera, but also in some nonpsittacine species.[48,55,95,132,222,343] Large parrots, including endangered species, seem to be affected most frequently and severely. Typical clinical signs of PPD are GI dysfunction and associated wasting with or without neurologic signs.[14,95,132,185,309] Affected animals develop decreasing GI motility until stasis resulting in anorexia, lethargy, undigested seeds in the feces, regurgitation, diarrhea, weight loss leading to cachexia, and vomiting. Finally, affected birds die. Interestingly, there are also cases displaying only neurologic signs such as depression, ataxia, tremor, seizures, and motor or proprioceptive deficits. Blindness has been described in a few cases,[311] and the mortality rate approaches 100%.[95]

Pathogenesis

The incubation period of natural ABV infection is unknown and varied in experimental infections from approximately 20 to 60 days, up to 200 days.[79,92,218,224] In these experiments, ABV-specific serum antibodies were detected between 7 and approximately 60 DPI and ABV RNA was detected in swabs between 20 and 72 DPI, depending on the route of inoculation (intracerebral, intramuscular, intravenous) and the bird species used, with the earliest detection of virus after intracerebral infection in cockatiels.[79,92,218,224] Surveillance studies in aviaries with PDD cases revealed that birds displaying high viral RNA loads and high ABV-specific antibody titers are more likely to develop clinical PDD.[111] It should be noted that, similar to BDV infection, ABV-specific antibodies do not have any protective effect.[111,218,224] A wide variation in the clinical status of infected animals has been noted, including healthy animals that show typical histologic lesions at necropsy, clinically inconspicuous birds with widespread ABV distribution or restriction of viral RNA to the nervous tissue and any variation thereof.[50,172,224,246,327,352] Asymptomatic carriers may contribute to virus dissemination. However, animals that did not become infected despite close contact to ABV-infected birds also exist.[111,246]

Typical gross findings consist of emaciation with atrophy of pectoral muscles, dilatation or rupture of the proventriculus, and atrophy of the proventricular muscle (Fig. 39.6).[95,185] Clinically manifest PDD is associated with characteristic mononuclear (lymphocytes, macrophages, plasma cells) infiltrates in ganglia and nerves of the enteric autonomous nervous system of crop, proventriculus, gizzard, and duodenum and, in most cases, nonpurulent encephalitis, myelitis and/or ganglioradiculoneuritis of spinal nerves (Fig. 39.7).[14,95,132,150,153,213,224,246,352] Gliosis and inflammation in peripheral nerves, myocardium, cardiac conductive tissue, and adrenal glands or eyes may also occur.

ABV shows a strong affinity for nervous tissue comparable to BDV, but broad peripheral tissue distribution is also seen. ABV RNA or antigen is most frequently found in the brain, spinal cord, and GI tract (crop, proventriculus, gizzard, small intestine) but often also in many other organs, for example, adrenal gland, eye, heart, liver, kidney, spleen, pancreas, lungs, gonads, thyroid, and skin (Fig. 39.8).[119,153,218,224,246,259,340,341,352]

Many factors may contribute to the variability of the clinical picture and *in vivo* dissemination of ABV. Viral properties and host-specific features such as species, genetic background, age, immune competence, and the extent of contact with ABV-infected animals may influence the outcome of infection. It is unknown whether clinically apparent disease is due to similar immunopathologic processes as those in BD. Although similar inflammatory infiltrates and possibly virus persistence occurs, striking differences between ABV and BDV infection exist regarding the variability of clinical outcome, tissue tropism, and virus distribution.

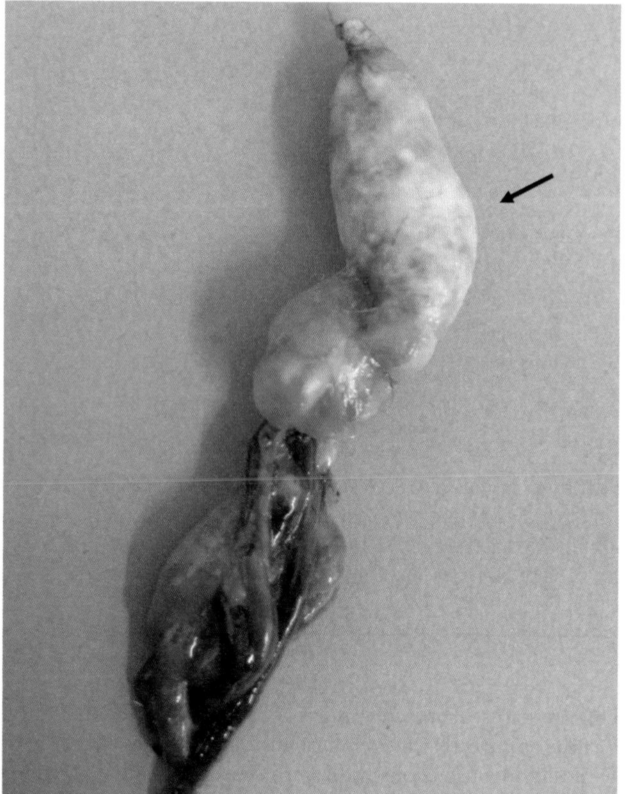

FIGURE 39.6. Gross findings in an African grey parrot suffering from proventricular dilation disease (PDD). Note the thin-walled, filled and dilated proventriculus (*arrow*). (Courtesy of A. Piepenbring and M. Lierz, Clinic for Birds, Reptiles, Amphibians and Fish, Faculty of Veterinary Medicine, Justus Liebig University Gießen, Germany.)

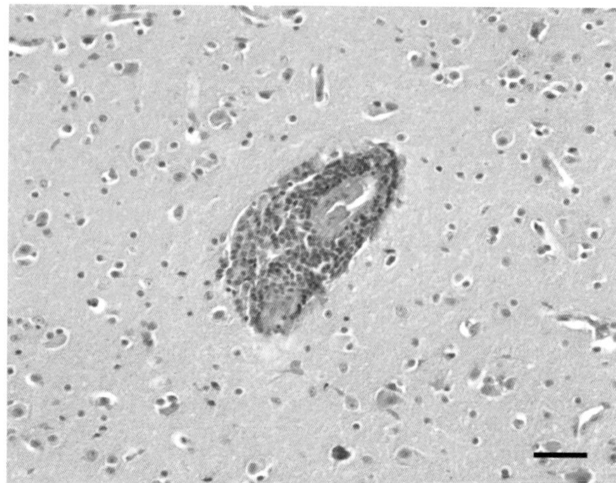

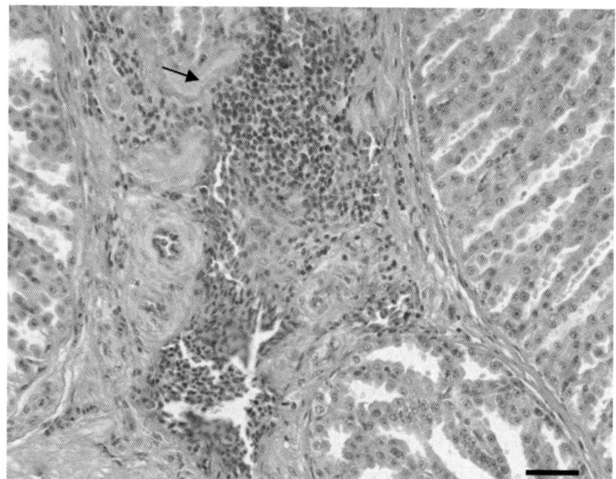

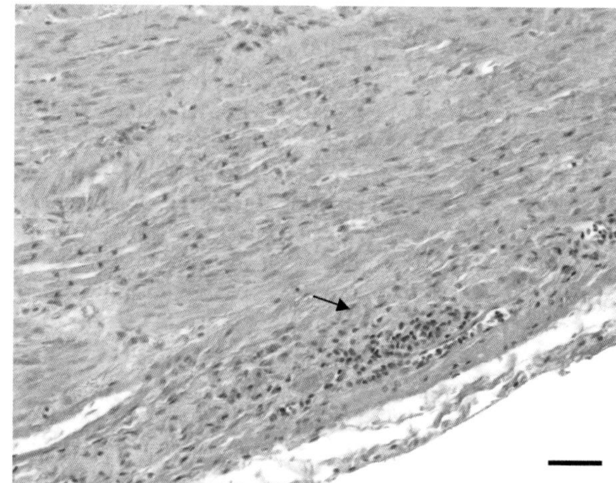

FIGURE 39.7. Typical histopathologic lesions in PDD. A: Perivascular lymphohistiocytic infiltrate in the brain. **B:** Severe lymphohistiocytic infiltrate in the proventriculus (*arrow*). **C:** Lymphohistiocytic infiltrate in and around ganglia of the gizzard (*arrow*). **Bar:** 50 μm.

DIAGNOSIS

Differential Diagnoses

Neurologic signs of BD of mammals can be complex and variable so that a variety of CNS infections can result in a comparable clinical picture. Due to this lack of specificity, further laboratory tests are needed for a confirmed diagnosis. The differential diagnosis includes other neurotropic virus infections such as equine herpesviruses,[348] rabies,[93] tick-borne encephalitis,[198] as well as bacterial diseases such as botulism[345] and bacterial meningitis,[72] and parasitic infections such as verminous myeloencephalitis[64] and equine protozoal myeloencephalitis (EPM).[183] In certain geographic regions, arthropod-borne flaviviruses (e.g., West Nile virus) and alphaviruses (e.g. western, eastern, Venezuelan equine encephalitis viruses) must also be considered.

Reliable *ante mortem* diagnosis of PDD and ABV infection has been problematic since clinical signs resembling PDD can also occur in other diseases such as bacterial, parasitic, or mycotic infection of the GI tract, ingestion of foreign bodies, intoxications or neoplasia, and the detection of ABV might be only intermittently possible.[95,112,132,218] Thus, ABV infection and a diagnosis of PDD have to be confirmed by laboratory investigation.

Intra Vitam Diagnosis

BD can be confirmed by the demonstration of BDV-specific antibodies in the serum and CSF,[89,91] or BDV-specific antigens, RNA, or virus in blood or CSF specimens. As serologic test

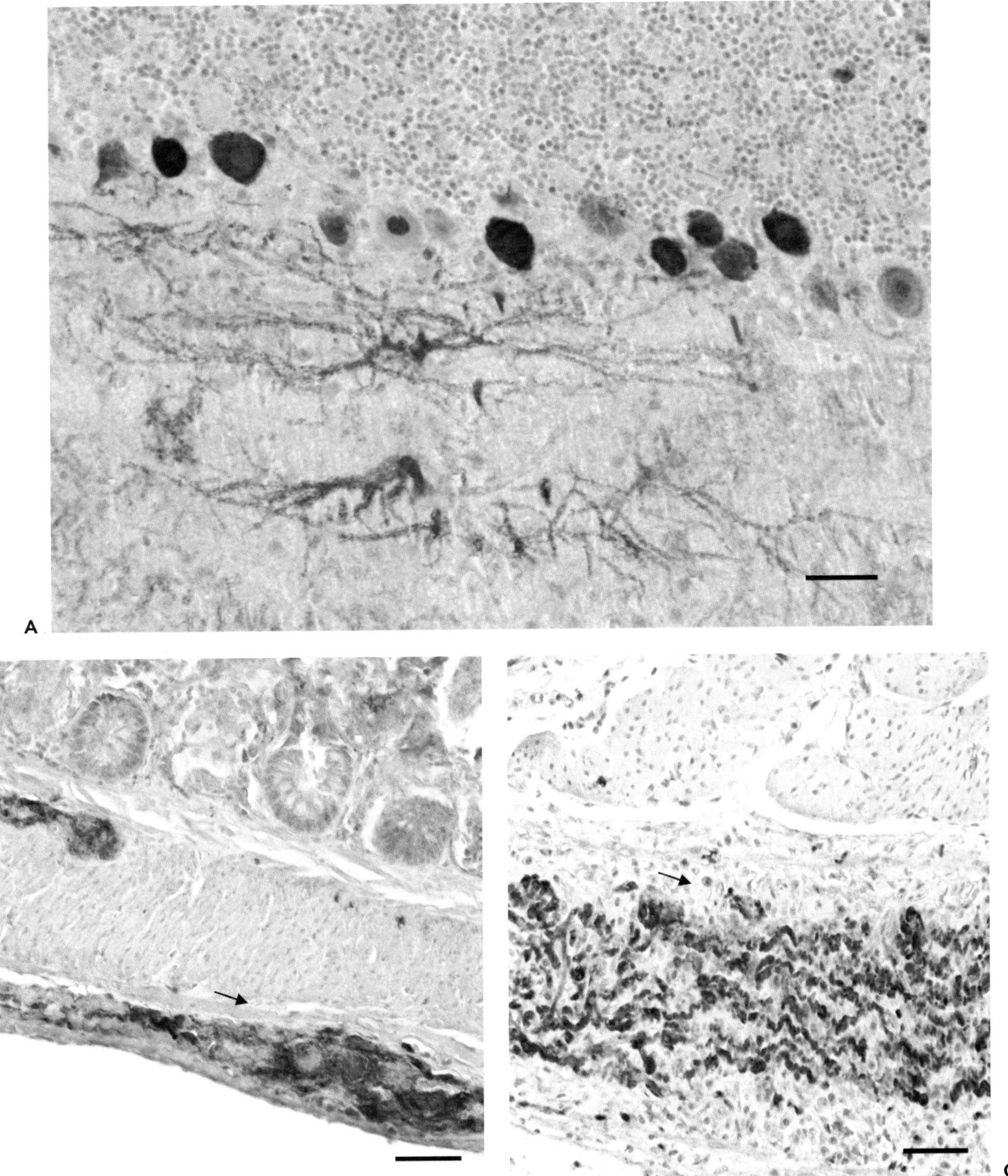

FIGURE 39.8. Demonstration of ABV phosphoprotein (P) by immunohistochemistry (IHC) in psittacines. A: Expression in the nucleus, cytoplasm, and processes of numerous Purkinje cells and a few granule cells in the cerebellum. **B:** Expression in ganglia (*arrow*) of the small intestine. **C:** Expression in nerve fibers (*arrow*) of the gizzard. **Bar:** 50 μm.

systems, Western blot (WB) analysis, enzyme-linked immunosorbent assay (ELISA) and an indirect immunofluorescence assay (IFA) have been established (Fig. 39.9).[23,91,120,122,124] IFA with BDV-infected and control cells is considered to be the most reliable method for the detection of BDV-specific antibodies with high sensitivity and specificity.[122] Titers of BDV-specific antibodies vary widely from 1:2 to 1:1280 in serum and CSF, and do not correlate with the clinical course of the infection.[91,120] In very early stages of acute BD, or after treatment with corticosteroids, BDV-specific antibodies may

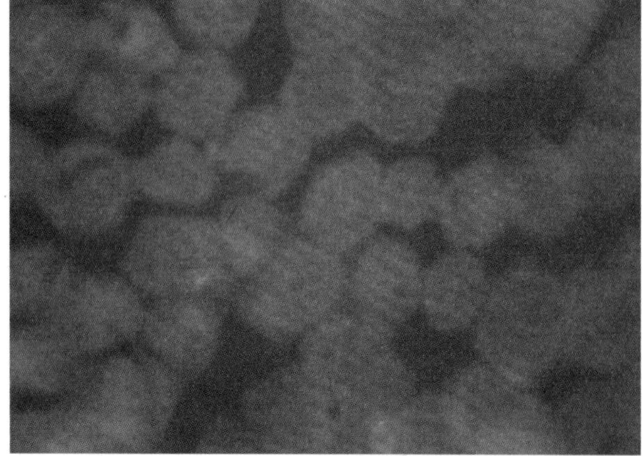
A

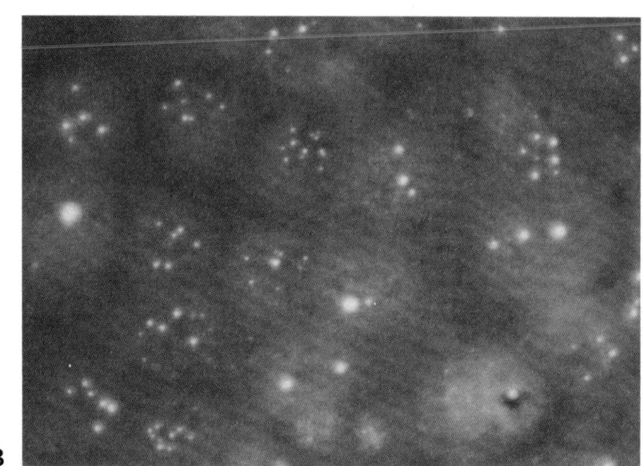
B

FIGURE 39.9. Indirect immunofluorescence assay (IFA) for the demonstration of BDV-specific antibodies in horse sera employing Madin-Darby canine kidney (MDCK) cells. A: BDV-positive serum incubated with uninfected MDCK cells. **B:** BDV-positive serum incubated with BDV-infected MDCK cells. (From Richt JA, Grabner A, Herzog S, et al. Borna disease in Equines. In: Sellon DC, Long M, eds. Equine Infectious Diseases, St Louis: Saunders Elsevier, 2007:201–216, with permission.)

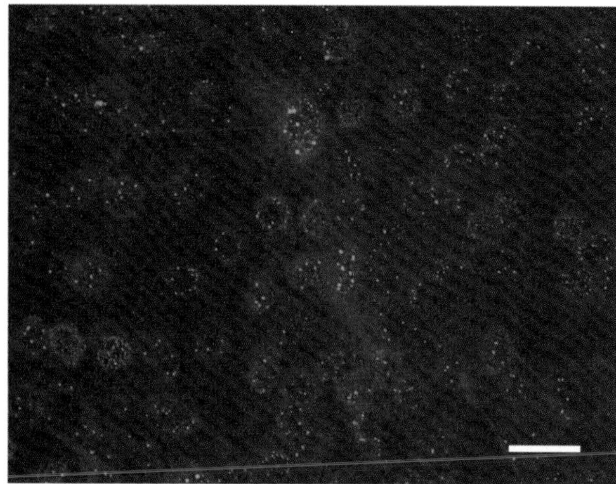
A

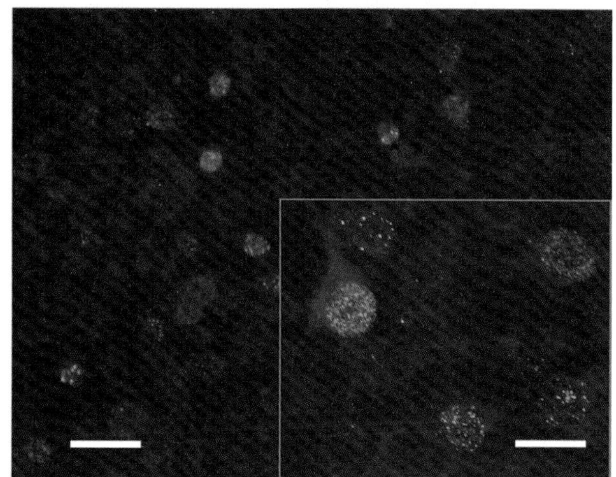
B

FIGURE 39.10. Indirect immunofluorescence assay for the demonstration of ABV-specific antibodies. A: IFA for demonstration of ABV-specific antibodies employing BDV-infected MDCK cells. Note the brilliant granular fluorescence in the nucleus. **Bar:** 50 μm. **B:** IFA for demonstration of ABV-specific antibodies employing ABV-infected CEC cells. Note the brilliant granular fluorescence in the nucleus. **Bar:** 100 μm; **Insert:** 50 μm. (From Herzog S, Enderlein D, Heffels-Redmann U, et al. Indirect immunofluorescence assay for intra vitam diagnosis of avian bornavirus infection in psittacine birds. *J Clin Microbiol* 2010;48:2282–2284, with permission.)

not be detectable. Clinically healthy horses can have BDV-specific antibodies in the serum but not in the CSF.[91,120] In acute BD, the quantity of CSF protein content can be elevated and a mononuclear pleocytosis is regularly present.[91] Evidence of infection including BDV RNA or BDV antigen in PBMC, or circulating immune complexes, has been presented by some investigators,[23,58,200] but has been questioned by others.[91,122] BD is reliably diagnosed *ante mortem* by neurologic signs combined with CSF pleocytosis and BDV-specific antibodies in serum and/or CSF.

As with BD in horses and sheep, signs and symptoms of PDD are not pathognomonic of ABV infection. Dilatation of the proventriculus and possibly other parts of the upper GI tract can be visualized by radiography/imaging techniques.[56] A definite diagnosis of PDD has to be substantiated by histopathologic examination of upper GI tract biopsies, which is hampered by the inconsistent distribution of lesions. Only the presence of mononuclear infiltrates of ganglia are confirmatory. In one study, crop biopsies revealed false negative results in approximately 24% of cases.[94] ABV-specific serum antibodies can be demonstrated by WB assay,[50,172,327] ELISA,[50] and IFA (Fig. 39.10).[92,119] ABV infection has also been diagnosed by detection of ABV RNA in feces, swabs of crop and cloaca, blood, and feather calami using RT-PCR.[49,92,153,172,259] The diversity of different ABV genotypes may require several RT-PCR assays. ABV genotypes 4 and 2 have been detected most frequently.[79,92,153,194,224] Due to the possible intermittent presence of RNA in swabs and presence of ABV RNA and/or ABV-specific antibodies in clinically healthy virus carriers, repeated testing and the combined demonstration of ABV-specific serum antibodies and ABV RNA in crop and cloacal swabs currently represent the most reliable diagnostic approach.[50,111,119,153,172,327]

Postmortem Diagnosis

For the postmortem diagnosis of natural BD, typical histopathologic lesions (Fig. 39.5), infectious virus and/or viral proteins and RNA in the CNS are usually demonstrated. Viral proteins are demonstrated by monoclonal or polyclonal antibodies recognizing the BDV N, P, M, X, or G proteins in immunohistochemical (IHC) approaches (Fig. 39.4) or WB analysis.[15,91] Histopathology, IHC, WB, and nested RT-PCR gave identical diagnostic results in a comparative study of over 150 horses with or without BD.[117] Furthermore, isolation of infectious BDV and demonstration of BDV RNA by *in situ* hybridization (ISH) (Fig. 39.4) can be used with adequately preserved tissue specimens.

Postmortem investigations in PDD show typical histopathologic lesions predominantly in the GI tract and CNS (Fig. 39.7). ABV RNA can be demonstrated not only in the nervous system and GI tract, but often in many other tissues.[92,112,131,152,153,172,246,259,327,352] ABV RNA may be visualized by ISH[341] and ABV protein by IHC, applying either cross-reactive anti-BDV antibodies against the N, P, or X-protein, or ABV-specific antibodies against the N protein (Fig. 39.8).[119,213,224,246,259,340,352] However, the monoclonal anti-BDV N antibody Bo18 that is widely used for diagnosis of mammalian BDV infections consistently gives negative results with ABV. Virus isolation has been successful in the quail cell lines CEC-32 and QM7[119,259] or duck embryo fibroblasts.[92]

THERAPY AND CONTROL

Vaccination

Although there is only limited experience with vaccines in BD, better success has been reported with live attenuated than with killed virus vaccines.[46,210] A lapinized live vaccine[362] was used for many years in the eastern federal states of Germany. Because efficacy was questionable, and there were concerns regarding the possible post-vaccination shedding of infectious virus as well as potential establishment of a persistent virus reservoir, the vaccine was abandoned in 1992.[196,287] High virus titer may be important for the successful implementation of live vaccines.[196,287] Cell-culture attenuated BDV protected rats against intracerebral challenge with a virulent inoculum only when administered at high titer (10^5–10^6 vs. 10^2–10^4).[210] Similarly, a high dose of another extensively passaged virus resulted in strong humoral and cellular immunity. A lower dose inoculum did not provide this protection.[76] Neither of these studies investigated virus shedding by the vaccinated animals or the biology of progeny virus.

There have been several efforts to develop recombinant BDV vaccines. A vaccinia virus recombinant expressing BDV N primed rats for enhanced viral clearance after challenge, but also for aggravated disease due to increased immunopathology.[171] More recently, expression of BDV N by a parapoxvirus vector system was reported to protect rats from challenge.[115] No data are available on vaccines based on BDV G; however, the observation that a monoclonal anti-G antibody was protective in rats suggests that such an approach could be successful.[77]

Therapeutics

Amantadine sulfate (AS), a drug with antiviral activity against influenza A,[110] inhibits replication of certain human and horse BDV isolates in cell culture and improves the clinical course in some subjects with affective disorders.[19,20,59] However, the efficacy of AS for treatment of persistently BDV-infected cell cultures and animals is controversial.[41,101,316] In a small clinical study of horses with acute BD, AS (2 mg/kg orally) had no effect in 8 out of 9 animals.[90]

Ribavirin inhibits transcription and replication of both He/80 and strain V BDV in a variety of cell lines.[143,195] In addition to its antiviral effects through depletion of cellular GTP pools, interference with mRNA capping, and direct interaction with viral polymerases, ribavirin can promote a Th_1-type immune response.[137,319] This led to concerns that enhancement of cellular immunity might aggravate immunopathology of BD.[104,171,297] In one study, the efficacy of ribavirin administered directly to the brain by intraventricular injection was assessed in the rat model. Although ribavirin had no effect on viral load, treated animals had less inflammation and milder disease presumably due to antimitotic effects on microglia.[306] In another animal model, the Mongolian gerbil, in which BDV can cause direct neuronal damage independent of immunopathology,[336] ribavirin at a higher dosage than tolerated in the rat model reduced virus load in the brain.[170]

1-β-D-arabinofuranosylcytosine (Ara-C) inhibits BDV replication in cultured cells and inhibits viral replication, improving clinical outcome in infected rats.[6,47] Ara-C is a DNA polymerase inhibitor and has no effect on polymerases of influenza or measles viruses, but has antiviral activity against rabies virus.[28] In BDV, Ara-C appears to act as a competitive inhibitor of cytidine.[329] A related cytosine nucleoside, 2′-fluoro-2′-deoxycytidine, shows similar antiviral activity *in vitro* and may be preferable due to its reduced cytotoxicity.[7]

At present, there is no curative therapy for PDD or ABV infection; symptomatic treatment is the only option. Methods for ABV infection control and prevention include appropriate management practices in aviaries such as isolation of ABV-infected birds, sanitation, and disinfection.[132] Control of traffic and trading may help to impede spread in the pet bird population.

PERSPECTIVES AND PUBLIC HEALTH CONSIDERATIONS

In the last 20 years, substantial progress in BD research has been achieved regarding the molecular characterization of the causative agent, underlying immunopathogenesis, mechanism of viral persistence, and natural distribution of BD. However, we still know little about its ecology and epidemiology, especially the identity of reservoirs and mechanisms for natural transmission. Also, a novel bornavirus, ABV, was discovered in a variety of avian species. The worldwide epidemiology of BD in various warm-blooded animals remains controversial. Virulence of the virus and genetic predisposition of the host or other exogenous and endogenous factors might play a role in the outcome of infection. Although the genomic fossil record indicates infection of primates, including human ancestors up to 40 million years ago, there is no convincing evidence of human infection. The intriguing properties of BDV are providing insights into cellular trafficking, neural circuitry, neural development, and immunopathology of CNS infections. Further investigations will improve our understanding of the complexity of the disease mechanisms, BDV-associated disorders, and the epidemiology of BD.

REFERENCES

All cited references are available in the e-book.

1. Ackermann A, Guelzow T, Staeheli P, et al. Visualizing viral dissemination in the mouse nervous system, using a green fluorescent protein-expressing Borna disease virus vector. *J Virol* 2010;84:5438–5442.
2. Ackermann A, Staeheli P, Schneider U. Adaptation of Borna disease virus to new host species attributed to altered regulation of viral polymerase activity. *J Virol* 2007;81:7933–7940.
5. Bajramovic JJ, Munter S, Syan S, et al. Borna disease virus glycoprotein is required for viral dissemination in neurons. *J Virol* 2003;77:12222–12231.
7. Bajramovic JJ, Volmer R, Syan S, et al. 2′-fluoro-2′-deoxycytidine inhibits Borna disease virus replication and spread. *Antimicrob Agents Chemother* 2004;48:1422–1425.
10. Bautista JR, Schwartz GJ, De La Torre JC, et al. Early and persistent abnormalities in rats with neonatally acquired Borna disease virus infection. *Brain Res Bull* 1994;34:31–40.
11. Belyi VA, Levine AJ, Skalka AM. Unexpected inheritance: multiple integrations of ancient bornavirus and ebolavirus/marburgvirus sequences in vertebrate genomes. *PLoS Pathog* 2010;6(7):e1001030.
16. Bilzer T, Planz O, Lipkin WI, et al. Presence of CD4+ and CD8+ T cells and expression of MHC class I and MHC class II antigen in horses with Borna disease virus-induced encephalitis. *Brain Pathol* 1995;5:223–230.
20. Bode L, Dietrich DE, Stoyloff R, et al. Amantadine and human Borna disease virus in vitro and in vivo in an infected patient with bipolar depression. *Lancet* 1997;349:178–179.
21. Bode L, Durrwald R, Ludwig H. Borna virus infections in cattle associated with fatal neurological disease. *Vet Rec* 1994;135:283–284.
24. Briese T, de la Torre JC, Lewis A, et al. Borna disease virus, a negative-strand RNA virus, transcribes in the nucleus of infected cells. *Proc Natl Acad Sci U S A* 1992;89:11486–11489.
26. Briese T, Lipkin WI, de la Torre JC. Molecular biology of Borna disease virus. *Curr Top Microbiol Immunol* 1995;190:1–16.
27. Briese T, Schneemann A, Lewis AJ, et al. Genomic organization of Borna disease virus. *Proc Natl Acad Sci U S A* 1994;91:4362–4366.
29. Caplazi P, Ehrensperger F. Spontaneous Borna disease in sheep and horses: immunophenotyping of inflammatory cells and detection of MHC-I and MHC-II antigen expression in Borna encephalitis lesions. *Vet Immunol Immunopathol* 1998;61:203–220.
31. Caplazi P, Waldvogel A, Stitz L, et al. Borna disease in naturally infected cattle. *J Comp Pathol* 1994;111:65–72.
32. Carbone KM, Duchala CS, Griffin JW, et al. Pathogenesis of Borna disease in rats: evidence that intra-axonal spread is the major route for virus dissemination and the determinant for disease incubation. *J Virol* 1987;61:3431–3440.
33. Carbone KM, Park SW, Rubin SA, et al. Borna disease: association with a maturation defect in the cellular immune response. *J Virol* 1991; 65:6154–6164.
35. Chase G, Mayer D, Hildebrand A, et al. Borna disease virus matrix protein is an integral component of the viral ribonucleoprotein complex that does not interfere with polymerase activity. *J Virol* 2007;81:743–749.
37. Clemente R, de la Torre JC. Cell entry of Borna disease virus follows a clathrin-mediated endocytosis pathway that requires Rab5 and microtubules. *J Virol* 2009;83:10406–10416.
38. Clemente R, de la Torre JC. Cell-to-cell spread of Borna disease virus proceeds in the absence of the virus primary receptor and furin-mediated processing of the virus surface glycoprotein. *J Virol* 2007;81:5968–5977.
44. Cubitt B, Oldstone C, de la Torre JC. Sequence and genome organization of Borna disease virus. *J Virol* 1994;68:1382–1396.
45. Cubitt B, Oldstone C, Valcarcel J, et al. RNA splicing contributes to the generation of mature mRNAs of Borna disease virus, a non-segmented negative strand RNA virus. *Virus Res* 1994;34:69–79.
46. Danner K. *Borna-Virus und Borna-Infektionen.* Enke Copythek, Stuttgart; 1982.
49. De Kloet AH, Kerski A, de Kloet SR. Diagnosis of Avian bornavirus infection in psittaciformes by serum antibody detection and reverse transcription polymerase chain reaction assay using feather calami. *J Vet Diagn Invest* 2011;23:421–429.
50. De Kloet SR, Dorrestein GM. Presence of avian bornavirus RNA and anti-avian bornavirus antibodies in apparently healthy macaws. *Avian Dis* 2009;53:568–573.
51. De la Torre JC. Molecular biology of borna disease virus: prototype of a new group of animal viruses. *J Virol* 1994;68:7669–7675.
52. De la Torre JC. Reverse-genetic approaches to the study of Borna disease virus. *Nat Rev Microbiol* 2006;4:777–783.
53. De La Torre JC, Gonzalez-Dunia D, Cubitt B, et al. Detection of borna disease virus antigen and RNA in human autopsy brain samples from neuropsychiatric patients. *Virology* 1996;223:272–282.
55. Delnatte P, Berkvens C, Kummrow M, et al. New genotype of avian bornavirus in wild geese and trumpeter swans in Canada. *Vet Rec* 2011; 169:108.
57. Deschl U, Stitz L, Herzog S, et al. Determination of immune cells and expression of major histocompatibility complex class II antigen in encephalitic lesions of experimental Borna disease. *Acta Neuropathol* 1990;81:41–50.
58. Dieckhöfer R. Infections in horses: Diagnosis and therapy. *APMIS Suppl* 2008;124:40–43.
61. Dittrich W, Bode L, Ludwig H, et al. Learning deficiencies in Borna disease virus-infected but clinically healthy rats. *Biol Psychiatry* 1989;26: 818–828.
63. Duchala CS, Carbone KM, Narayan O. Preliminary studies on the biology of Borna disease virus. *J Gen Virol* 1989;70(Pt 12):3507–3511.
65. Durrwald R, Kolodziejek J, Herzog S, et al. Meta-analysis of putative human bornavirus sequences fails to provide evidence implicating Borna disease virus in mental illness. *Rev Med Virol* 2007;17:181–203.
66. Durrwald R, Kolodziejek J, Muluneh A, et al. Epidemiological pattern of classical Borna disease and regional genetic clustering of Borna disease viruses point towards the existence of to-date unknown endemic reservoir host populations. *Microbes Infect* 2006;8:917–929.
67. Durrwald R, Ludwig H. Borna disease virus (BDV), a (zoonotic?) worldwide pathogen. A review of the history of the disease and the virus infection with comprehensive bibliography. *Zentralbl Veterinarmed B* 1997;44:147–184.
68. Eickmann M, Kiermayer S, Kraus I, et al. Maturation of Borna disease virus glycoprotein. *FEBS Lett* 2005;579:4751–4756.
71. Engelhardt KR, Richter K, Baur K, et al. The functional avidity of virus-specific CD8+ T cells is down-modulated in Borna disease virus-induced immunopathology of the central nervous system. *Eur J Immunol* 2005;35:487–497.
74. Friedl G, Hofer M, Auber B, et al. Borna disease virus multiplication in mouse organotypic slice cultures is site-specifically inhibited by gamma interferon but not by interleukin-12. *J Virol* 2004;78:1212–1218.
76. Furrer E, Bilzer T, Stitz L, et al. High-dose Borna disease virus infection induces a nucleoprotein-specific cytotoxic T-lymphocyte response and prevention of immunopathology. *J Virol* 2001;75:11700–11708.
79. Gancz AY, Kistler AL, Greninger AL, et al. Experimental induction of proventricular dilatation disease in cockatiels (Nymphicus hollandicus) inoculated with brain homogenates containing avian bornavirus 4. *Virol J* 2009;6:100.
81. Geib T, Sauder C, Venturelli S, et al. Selective virus resistance conferred by expression of Borna disease virus nucleocapsid components. *J Virol* 2003;77:4283–4290.
83. Gonzalez-Dunia D, Cubitt B, de la Torre JC. Mechanism of Borna disease virus entry into cells. *J Virol* 1998;72:783–788.
84. Gonzalez-Dunia D, Cubitt B, Grasser FA, et al. Characterization of Borna disease virus p56 protein, a surface glycoprotein involved in virus entry. *J Virol* 1997;71:3208–3218.
85. Gonzalez-Dunia D, Watanabe M, Syan S, et al. Synaptic pathology in Borna disease virus persistent infection. *J Virol* 2000;74:3441–3448.
91. Grabner A, Herzog S, Lange-Herbst H, et al. Die intra-vitam-Diagnose der Bornaschen Krankheit (BD) bei Equiden. *Pferdeheilkunde* 2002;18.

92. Gray P, Hoppes S, Suchodolski P, et al. Use of avian bornavirus isolates to induce proventricular dilatation disease in conures. *Emerg Infect Dis* 2010;16:473–479.
94. Gregory CR, Latimer K, Campagnoli R, et al. Histologic evaluation of the crop for diagnosis of proventricular dilatation syndrome in psittacine birds. *J Vet Diagn Invest* 1996;8:76–80.
95. Gregory CR, Latimer KS, Niagro FD, et al. Review of proventricular dilatation syndrome. *J Assoc Avian Vet* 1994;8:68–75.
96. Haas B, Becht H, Rott R. Purification and properties of an intranuclear virus-specific antigen from tissue infected with Borna disease virus. *J Gen Virol* 1986;67(Pt 2):235–241.
97. Habjan M, Andersson I, Klingstrom J, et al. Processing of genome 5′ termini as a strategy of negative-strand RNA viruses to avoid RIG-I-dependent interferon induction. *PLoS One* 2008;3:e2032.
100. Hallensleben W, Schwemmle M, Hausmann J, et al. Borna disease virus-induced neurological disorder in mice: infection of neonates results in immunopathology. *J Virol* 1998;72:4379–4386.
101. Hallensleben W, Zocher M, Staeheli P. Borna disease virus is not sensitive to amantadine. *Arch Virol* 1997;142:2043–2048.
102. Hans A, Bajramovic JJ, Syan S, et al. Persistent, noncytolytic infection of neurons by Borna disease virus interferes with ERK 1/2 signaling and abrogates BDNF-induced synaptogenesis. *FASEB J* 2004;18:863–865.
103. Hans A, Syan S, Crosio C, et al. Borna disease virus persistent infection activates mitogen-activated protein kinase and blocks neuronal differentiation of PC12 cells. *J Biol Chem* 2001;276:7258–7265.
104. Hatalski CG, Hickey WF, Lipkin WI. Evolution of the immune response in the central nervous system following infection with Borna disease virus. *J Neuroimmunol* 1998;90:137–142.
106. Hatalski CG, Kliche S, Stitz L, et al. Neutralizing antibodies in Borna disease virus-infected rats. *J Virol* 1995;69:741–747.
107. Hausmann J, Baur K, Engelhardt KR, et al. Vaccine-induced protection against Borna disease in wild-type and perforin-deficient mice. *J Gen Virol* 2005;86:399–403.
108. Hausmann J, Hallensleben W, de la Torre JC, et al. T cell ignorance in mice to Borna disease virus can be overcome by peripheral expression of the viral nucleoprotein. *Proc Natl Acad Sci U S A* 1999;96:9769–9774.
109. Hausmann J, Pagenstecher A, Baur K, et al. CD8 T cells require gamma interferon to clear borna disease virus from the brain and prevent immune system-mediated neuronal damage. *J Virol* 2005;79:13509–13518.
111. Heffels-Redmann U, Enderlein D, Herzog S, et al. Follow-up investigations on different courses of natural avian bornavirus infections in psittacines. *Avian Dis* 2012;56:153–159.
112. Heffels-Redmann U, Enderlein D, Herzog S, et al. Occurrence of avian bornavirus infection in captive psittacines in various European countries and its association with proventricular dilatation disease. *Avian Pathol* 2011;40:419–426.
113. Heinig A. Die Bornasche Krankheit der Pferde und Schafe. In: Röhrer H, ed. Handbuch der Virusinfektionen bei Tieren, vol. Band 4. VEB G. Fischer, Jena; 1969:83–148.
116. Herden C, Herzog S, Richt JA, et al. Distribution of Borna disease virus in the brain of rats infected with an obesity-inducing virus strain. *Brain Pathol* 2000;10:39–48.
117. Herden C, Herzog S, Wehner T, et al. Comparison of different methods of diagnosing Borna disease in horses post mortem. In: Equine Infectious Diseases VIII. Wernery U, Wade J, Mumford JA, Kaaden OR (Hrsg.), R&W Publications, Newmarket; 1999:286–290.
119. Herzog S, Enderlein D, Heffels-Redmann U, et al. Indirect immunofluorescence assay for intra vitam diagnosis of avian bornavirus infection in psittacine birds. *J Clin Microbiol* 2010;48:2282–2284.
120. Herzog S, Frese K, Richt JA, et al. Ein Beitrag zur Epizootiologie der Bornaschen Krankheit der Pferde. *Wien Tierärztl Mschr* 1994;81:374–379.
122. Herzog S, Herden C, Frese K, et al. Borna disease of horses: contradictory results between antemortem and postmortem investigations. *Pferdeheilkunde* 2008;24:766–774.
127. Hilbe M, Herrsche R, Kolodziejek J, et al. Shrews as reservoir hosts of borna disease virus. *Emerg Infect Dis* 2006;12:675–677.
130. Hofer M, Hausmann J, Staeheli P, et al. Cerebral expression of interleukin-12 induces neurological disease via differential pathways and recruits antigen-specific T cells in virus-infected mice. *Am J Pathol* 2004;165:949–958.
131. Honkavuori KS, Shivaprasad HL, Williams BL, et al. Novel borna virus in psittacine birds with proventricular dilatation disease. *Emerg Infect Dis* 2008;14:1883–1886.
132. Hoppes S, Gray PL, Payne S, et al. The isolation, pathogenesis, diagnosis, transmission, and control of avian bornavirus and proventricular dilatation disease. *Vet Clin North Am Exot Anim Pract* 2010;13:495–508.
133. Horie M, Honda T, Suzuki Y, et al. Endogenous non-retroviral RNA virus elements in mammalian genomes. *Nature* 2010;463:84–87.
134. Hornig M, Briese T, Licinio J, et al. Absence of evidence for bornavirus infection in schizophrenia, bipolar disorder and major depressive disorder. *Mol Psychiatry* 2012;17(5):486–493.
135. Hornig M, Briese T, Lipkin WI. Bornavirus tropism and targeted pathogenesis: virus-host interactions in a neurodevelopmental model. *Adv Virus Res* 2001;56:557–582.
136. Hornig M, Weissenböck H, Horscroft N, et al. An infection-based model of neurodevelopmental damage. *Proc Natl Acad Sci U S A* 1999;96:12102–12107.
140. Jacobsen B, Algermissen D, Schaudien D, et al. Borna disease in an adult alpaca stallion (Lama pacos). *J Comp Pathol* 2010;143:203–208.
142. Joest E, Degen K. Untersuchungen über die pathologische Histologie, Pathogenese und postmortale Diagnose der seuchenhaften Gehirn-Rückenmarksentzündung (Bornasche Krankheit) des Pferdes. *Z Infkrankh Haustiere* 1911;9:1–98.
143. Jordan I, Briese T, Averett DR, et al. Inhibition of Borna disease virus replication by ribavirin. *J Virol* 1999;73:7903–7906.
145. Kamitani W, Ono E, Yoshino S, et al. Glial expression of Borna disease virus phosphoprotein induces behavioral and neurological abnormalities in transgenic mice. *Proc Natl Acad Sci U S A* 2003;100:8969–8974.
146. Kamitani W, Shoya Y, Kobayashi T, et al. Borna disease virus phosphoprotein binds a neurite outgrowth factor, amphoterin/HMG-1. *J Virol* 2001;75:8742–8751.
147. Kao M, Hamir AN, Rupprecht CE, et al. Detection of antibodies against Borna disease virus in sera and cerebrospinal fluid of horses in the USA. *Vet Rec* 1993;132:241–244.
148. Kao M, Ludwig H, Gosztonyi G. Adaptation of Borna disease virus to the mouse. *J Gen Virol* 1984;65(Pt 10):1845–1849.
149. Katz JB, Alstad D, Jenny AL, et al. Clinical, serologic, and histopathologic characterization of experimental Borna disease in ponies. *J Vet Diagn Invest* 1998;10:338–343.
150. Keller DL, Honkavuori KS, Briese T, et al. Proventricular dilatation disease associated with Avian bornavirus in a scarlet macaw (Ara macao). *J Vet Diagn Invest* 2010;22:961–965.
152. Kistler AL, Gancz A, Clubb S, et al. Recovery of divergent avian bornaviruses from cases of proventricular dilatation disease: identification of a candidate etiologic agent. *Virol J* 2008;5:88.
153. Kistler AL, Smith JM, Greninger AL, et al. Analysis of naturally occurring avian bornavirus infection and transmission during an outbreak of proventricular dilatation disease among captive psittacine birds. *J Virol* 2010;84:2176–2179.
155. Kobayashi T, Kamitani W, Zhang G, et al. Borna disease virus nucleoprotein requires both nuclear localization and export activities for viral nucleocytoplasmic shuttling. *J Virol* 2001;75:3404–3412.
156. Kobayashi T, Shoya Y, Koda T, et al. Nuclear targeting activity associated with the amino terminal region of the Borna disease virus nucleoprotein. *Virology* 1998;243:188–197.
159. Kohno T, Goto T, Takasaki T, et al. Fine structure and morphogenesis of Borna disease virus. *J Virol* 1999;73:760–766.
161. Kolodziejek J, Durrwald R, Herzog S, et al. Genetic clustering of Borna disease virus natural animal isolates, laboratory and vaccine strains strongly reflects their regional geographical origin. *J Gen Virol* 2005;86:385–398.
163. Koster-Patzlaff C, Hosseini SM, Reuss B. Loss of connexin36 in rat hippocampus and cerebellar cortex in persistent Borna disease virus infection. *J Chem Neuroanat* 2009;37:118–127.
165. Kraus I, Bogner E, Lilie H, et al. Oligomerization and assembly of the matrix protein of Borna disease virus. *FEBS Lett* 2005;579:2686–2692.
166. Kraus I, Eickmann M, Kiermayer S, et al. Open reading frame III of borna disease virus encodes a nonglycosylated matrix protein. *J Virol* 2001;75:12098–12104.

168. Krey HF, Ludwig H, Boschek CB. Multifocal retinopathy in Borna disease virus infected rabbits. *Am J Ophthalmol* 1979;87:157–164.
169. Lancaster K, Dietz DM, Moran TH, et al. Abnormal social behaviors in young and adult rats neonatally infected with Borna disease virus. *Behav Brain Res* 2007;176:141–148.
171. Lewis AJ, Whitton JL, Hatalski CG, et al. Effect of immune priming on Borna disease. *J Virol* 1999;73:2541–2546.
172. Lierz M, Hafez HM, Honkavuori KS, et al. Anatomical distribution of avian bornavirus in parrots, its occurrence in clinically healthy birds and ABV-antibody detection. *Avian Pathol* 2009;38:491–496.
173. Lierz M, Piepenbring A, Herden C, et al. Vertical transmission of avian bornavirus in psittacines. *Emerg Infect Dis* 2011;17:2390–2391.
174. Lipkin WI, Carbone KM, Wilson MC, et al. Neurotransmitter abnormalities in Borna disease. *Brain Res* 1988;475:366–370.
175. Lipkin WI, Hornig M, Briese T. Borna disease virus and neuropsychiatric disease–a reappraisal. *Trends Microbiol* 2001;9:295–298.
176. Lipkin WI, Travis GH, Carbone KM, et al. Isolation and characterization of Borna disease agent cDNA clones. *Proc Natl Acad Sci U S A* 1990; 87:4184–4188.
178. Ludwig H, Bode L. Borna disease virus: new aspects on infection, disease, diagnosis and epidemiology. *Rev Sci Tech* 2000;19:259–288.
179. Ludwig H, Bode L, Gosztonyi G. Borna disease: a persistent virus infection of the central nervous system. *Prog Med Virol* 1988;35:107–151.
181. Ludwig H, Kraft W, Kao M, et al. [Borna virus infection (Borna disease) in naturally and experimentally infected animals: its significance for research and practice]. *Tierarztl Prax* 1985;13:421–453.
182. Lundgren AL, Lindberg R, Ludwig H, et al. Immunoreactivity of the central nervous system in cats with a Borna disease-like meningoencephalomyelitis (staggering disease). *Acta Neuropathol* 1995;90: 184–193.
183. MacKay RJ. Equine protozoal myeloencephalitis. *Vet Clin North Am Equine Pract* 1997;13:79–96.
184. Malik TH, Kishi M, Lai PK. Characterization of the P protein-binding domain on the 10-kilodalton protein of Borna disease virus. *J Virol* 2000;74:3413–3417.
185. Mannl A, Gerlach H, Leipold R. Neuropathic gastric dilatation in psittaciformes. *Avian Dis* 1987;31:214–221.
186. Martin A, Hoefs N, Tadewaldt J, et al. Genomic RNAs of Borna disease virus are elongated on internal template motifs after realignment of the 3′ termini. *Proc Natl Acad Sci U S A* 2011;108:7206–7211.
187. Martin A, Staeheli P, Schneider U. RNA polymerase II-controlled expression of antigenomic RNA enhances the rescue efficacies of two different members of the Mononegavirales independently of the site of viral genome replication. *J Virol* 2006;80:5708–5715.
190. Mayr A, Danner K. Persistent infections caused by Borna virus. *Infection* 1974;2:64–69.
194. Mirhosseini N, Gray PL, Hoppes S, et al. Proventricular dilatation disease in cockatiels (Nymphicus hollandicus) after infection with a genotype 2 avian bornavirus. *J Avian Med Surg* 2011;25:199–204.
196. Möhlmann H. 10 Jahre Forschungsinstitut für Impfstoffe Dessau. *Arch Exp Veterinarmed* 1965;19:253–260.
197. Morales JA, Herzog S, Kompter C, et al. Axonal transport of Borna disease virus along olfactory pathways in spontaneously and experimentally infected rats. *Med Microbiol Immunol* 1988;177:51–68.
199. Muller-Doblies D, Baumann S, Grob P, et al. The humoral and cellular immune response of sheep against Borna disease virus in endemic and non-endemic areas. *Schweiz Arch Tierheilkd* 2004;146:159–172.
202. Nakamura Y, Takahashi H, Shoya Y, et al. Isolation of Borna disease virus from human brain tissue. *J Virol* 2000;74:4601–4611.
203. Narayan O, Herzog S, Frese K, et al. Behavioral disease in rats caused by immunopathological responses to persistent borna virus in the brain. *Science* 1983;220:1401–1403.
204. Narayan O, Herzog S, Frese K, et al. Pathogenesis of Borna disease in rats: immune-mediated viral ophthalmoencephalopathy causing blindness and behavioral abnormalities. *J Infect Dis* 1983;148:305–315.
207. Noske K, Bilzer T, Planz O, et al. Virus-specific CD4+ T cells eliminate borna disease virus from the brain via induction of cytotoxic CD8+ T cells. *J Virol* 1998;72:4387–4395.
208. Nowotny N, Kolodziejek J, Jehle CO, et al. Isolation and characterization of a new subtype of Borna disease virus. *J Virol* 2000;74:5655–5658.
209. Ogawa H, Sanada Y, Sanada N, et al. Proventricular dilatation disease associated with avian bornavirus infection in a Citron-crested Cockatoo that was born and hand-reared in Japan. *J Vet Med Sci* 2011;73:837–840.
210. Oldach D, Zink MC, Pyper JM, et al. Induction of protection against Borna disease by inoculation with high-dose-attenuated Borna disease virus. *Virology* 1995;206:426–434.
213. Ouyang N, Storts R, Tian Y, et al. Histopathology and the detection of avian bornavirus in the nervous system of birds diagnosed with proventricular dilatation disease. *Avian Pathol* 2009;38:393–401.
215. Ovanesov MV, Sauder C, Rubin SA, et al. Activation of microglia by borna disease virus infection: in vitro study. *J Virol* 2006;80:12141–12148.
217. Payne S, Covaleda L, Jianhua G, et al. Detection and characterization of a distinct bornavirus lineage from healthy Canada geese (Branta canadensis). *J Virol* 2011;85:12053–12056.
218. Payne S, Shivaprasad HL, Mirhosseini N, et al. Unusual and severe lesions of proventricular dilatation disease in cockatiels (Nymphicus hollandicus) acting as healthy carriers of avian bornavirus (ABV) and subsequently infected with a virulent strain of ABV. *Avian Pathol* 2011; 40:15–22.
220. Perez M, Sanchez A, Cubitt B, et al. A reverse genetics system for Borna disease virus. *J Gen Virol* 2003;84:3099–3104.
221. Perez M, Watanabe M, Whitt MA, et al. N-terminal domain of Borna disease virus G (p56) protein is sufficient for virus receptor recognition and cell entry. *J Virol* 2001;75:7078–7085.
222. Perpiñán D, Fernández-Bellon H, López C, et al. Lymphoplasmacytic myenteric, subepicardial, and pulmonary ganglioneuritis in four nonpsittacine birds. *J Avian Med Surg* 2007;21:210–214.
224. Piepenbring AK, Enderlein D, Herzog S, et al. Pathogenesis of avian bornavirus in experimentally infected cockatiels. *Emerg Infect Dis* 2012; 18:234–241.
225. Planz O, Bilzer T, Sobbe M, et al. Lysis of major histocompatibility complex class I-bearing cells in Borna disease virus-induced degenerative encephalopathy. *J Exp Med* 1993;178:163–174.
227. Planz O, Pleschka S, Ludwig S. MEK-specific inhibitor U0126 blocks spread of Borna disease virus in cultured cells. *J Virol* 2001;75:4871–4877.
230. Pleschka S, Staeheli P, Kolodziejek J, et al. Conservation of coding potential and terminal sequences in four different isolates of Borna disease virus. *J Gen Virol* 2001;82:2681–2690.
231. Pletnikov MV, Rubin SA, Carbone KM, et al. Neonatal Borna disease virus infection (BDV)-induced damage to the cerebellum is associated with sensorimotor deficits in developing Lewis rats. *Brain Res Dev Brain Res* 2001;126:1–12.
236. Poenisch M, Burger N, Staeheli P, et al. Protein X of Borna disease virus inhibits apoptosis and promotes viral persistence in the central nervous systems of newborn-infected rats. *J Virol* 2009;83:4297–4307.
238. Poenisch M, Unterstab G, Wolff T, et al. The X protein of Borna disease virus regulates viral polymerase activity through interaction with the P protein. *J Gen Virol* 2004;85:1895–1898.
241. Prat CM, Schmid S, Farrugia F, et al. Mutation of the protein kinase C site in borna disease virus phosphoprotein abrogates viral interference with neuronal signaling and restores normal synaptic activity. *PLoS Pathog* 2009;5:e1000425.
242. Priestnall SL, Schoniger S, Ivens PA, et al. Borna disease virus infection of a horse in Great Britain. *Vet Rec* 2011;168:380b.
244. Puorger ME, Hilbe M, Muller JP, et al. Distribution of Borna disease virus antigen and RNA in tissues of naturally infected bicolored white-toothed shrews, Crocidura leucodon, supporting their role as reservoir host species. *Vet Pathol* 2010;47:236–244.
246. Raghav R, Taylor M, Delay J, et al. Avian bornavirus is present in many tissues of psittacine birds with histopathologic evidence of proventricular dilatation disease. *J Vet Diagn Invest* 2010;22:495–508.
247. Rauer M, Gotz J, Schuppli D, et al. Transgenic mice expressing the nucleoprotein of Borna disease virus in either neurons or astrocytes: decreased susceptibility to homotypic infection and disease. *J Virol* 2004; 78:3621–3632.
249. Richt J, Stitz L, Deschl U, et al. Borna disease virus-induced meningoencephalomyelitis caused by a virus-specific CD4+ T cell-mediated immune reaction. *J Gen Virol* 1990;71(Pt 11):2565–2573.

250. Richt JA, Alexander RC, Herzog S, et al. Failure to detect Borna disease virus infection in peripheral blood leukocytes from humans with psychiatric disorders. *J Neurovirol* 1997;3:174–178.
252. Richt JA, Furbringer T, Koch A, et al. Processing of the Borna disease virus glycoprotein gp94 by the subtilisin-like endoprotease furin. *J Virol* 1998;72:4528–4533.
253. Richt JA, Grabner A, Herzog S, et al. *Borna Disease.* St. Louis: Saunders Elsevier; 2007.
256. Richt JA, Schmeel A, Frese K, et al. Borna disease virus-specific T cells protect against or cause immunopathological Borna disease. *J Exp Med* 1994;179:1467–1473.
257. Richt JA, Stitz L, Wekerle H, et al. Borna disease, a progressive meningoencephalomyelitis as a model for CD4+ T cell-mediated immunopathology in the brain. *J Exp Med* 1989;170:1045–1050.
259. Rinder M, Ackermann A, Kempf H, et al. Broad tissue and cell tropism of avian bornavirus in parrots with proventricular dilatation disease. *J Virol* 2009;83:5401–5407.
261. Rosario D, Perez M, de la Torre JC. Functional characterization of the genomic promoter of borna disease virus (BDV): implications of 3′-terminal sequence heterogeneity for BDV persistence. *J Virol* 2005; 79:6544–6550.
262. Rott R, Becht H. Natural and experimental Borna disease in animals. *Curr Top Microbiol Immunol* 1995;190:17–30.
263. Rott R, Herzog S, Fleischer B, et al. Detection of serum antibodies to Borna disease virus in patients with psychiatric disorders. *Science* 1985; 228:755–756.
265. Rubin SA, Sylves P, Vogel M, et al. Borna disease virus-induced hippocampal dentate gyrus damage is associated with spatial learning and memory deficits. *Brain Res Bull* 1999;48:23–30.
266. Rubin SA, Waltrip RW 2nd, Bautista JR, et al. Borna disease virus in mice: host-specific differences in disease expression. *J Virol* 1993;67:548–552.
270. Sasaki S, Ludwig H. In borna disease virus infected rabbit neurons 100 nm particle structures accumulate at areas of Joest-Degen inclusion bodies. *Zentralbl Veterinarmed B* 1993;40:291–297.
271. Sauder C, de la Torre JC. Cytokine expression in the rat central nervous system following perinatal Borna disease virus infection. *J Neuroimmunol* 1999;96:29–45.
273. Sauder C, Herpfer I, Hassler C, et al. Susceptibility of Borna disease virus to the antiviral action of gamma-interferon: evidence for species-specific differences. *Arch Virol* 2004;149:2171–2186.
274. Schadler R, Diringer H, Ludwig H. Isolation and characterization of a 14500 molecular weight protein from brains and tissue cultures persistently infected with borna disease virus. *J Gen Virol* 1985;66(Pt 11): 2479–2484.
275. Schamel K, Staeheli P, Hausmann J. Identification of the immunodominant H-2K(k)-restricted cytotoxic T-cell epitope in the Borna disease virus nucleoprotein. *J Virol* 2001;75:8579–8588.
276. Schneemann A, Schneider PA, Kim S, et al. Identification of signal sequences that control transcription of borna disease virus, a nonsegmented, negative-strand RNA virus. *J Virol* 1994;68:6514–6522.
277. Schneemann A, Schneider PA, Lamb RA, et al. The remarkable coding strategy of borna disease virus: a new member of the nonsegmented negative strand RNA viruses. *Virology* 1995;210:1–8.
278. Schneider PA, Briese T, Zimmermann W, et al. Sequence conservation in field and experimental isolates of Borna disease virus. *J Virol* 1994; 68:63–68.
279. Schneider PA, Hatalski CG, Lewis AJ, et al. Biochemical and functional analysis of the Borna disease virus G protein. *J Virol* 1997;71:331–336.
281. Schneider PA, Schneemann A, Lipkin WI. RNA splicing in Borna disease virus, a nonsegmented, negative-strand RNA virus. *J Virol* 1994; 68:5007–5012.
285. Schneider U, Naegele M, Staeheli P, et al. Active borna disease virus polymerase complex requires a distinct nucleoprotein-to-phosphoprotein ratio but no viral X protein. *J Virol* 2003;77:11781–11789.
286. Schneider U, Schwemmle M, Staeheli P. Genome trimming: a unique strategy for replication control employed by Borna disease virus. *Proc Natl Acad Sci U S A* 2005;102:3441–3446.
289. Schwemmle M, De B, Shi L, et al. Borna disease virus P-protein is phosphorylated by protein kinase Cepsilon and casein kinase II. *J Biol Chem* 1997;272:21818–21823.
291. Schwemmle M, Jehle C, Formella S, et al. Sequence similarities between human bornavirus isolates and laboratory strains question human origin. *Lancet* 1999;354:1973–1974.
292. Schwemmle M, Jehle C, Shoemaker T, et al. Characterization of the major nuclear localization signal of the Borna disease virus phosphoprotein. *J Gen Virol* 1999;80(Pt 1):97–100.
293. Schwemmle M, Salvatore M, Shi L, et al. Interactions of the borna disease virus P, N, and X proteins and their functional implications. *J Biol Chem* 1998;273:9007–9012.
296. Siemetzki U, Ashok MS, Briese T, et al. Identification of RNA instability elements in Borna disease virus. *Virus Res* 2009;144:27–34.
299. Solbrig MV, Fallon JH, Lipkin WI. Behavioral disturbances and pharmacology of Borna disease. *Curr Top Microbiol Immunol* 1995;190: 93–101.
301. Solbrig MV, Koob GF, Fallon JH, et al. Tardive dyskinetic syndrome in rats infected with Borna disease virus. *Neurobiol Dis* 1994;1:111–119.
302. Solbrig MV, Koob GF, Joyce JN, et al. A neural substrate of hyperactivity in borna disease: changes in brain dopamine receptors. *Virology* 1996;222:332–338.
308. Sprankel H, Richarz K, Ludwig H, et al. Behavior alterations in tree shrews (Tupaia glis, Diard 1820) induced by Borna disease virus. *Med Microbiol Immunol* 1978;165:1–18.
309. Staeheli P, Rinder M, Kaspers B. Avian bornavirus associated with fatal disease in psittacine birds. *J Virol* 2010;84:6269–6275.
310. Staeheli P, Sauder C, Hausmann J, et al. Epidemiology of Borna disease virus. *J Gen Virol* 2000;81:2123–2135.
313. Stitz L, Bilzer T, Planz O. The immunopathogenesis of Borna disease virus infection. *Front Biosci* 2002;7:d541–555.
315. Stitz L, Noske K, Planz O, et al. A functional role for neutralizing antibodies in Borna disease: influence on virus tropism outside the central nervous system. *J Virol* 1998;72:8884–8892.
317. Stitz L, Sobbe M, Bilzer T. Preventive effects of early anti-CD4 or anti-CD8 treatment on Borna disease in rats. *J Virol* 1992;66:3316–3323.
320. Thiedemann N, Presek P, Rott R, et al. Antigenic relationship and further characterization of two major Borna disease virus-specific proteins. *J Gen Virol* 1992;73(Pt 5):1057–1064.
324. Unterstab G, Ludwig S, Anton A, et al. Viral targeting of the interferon-{beta}-inducing Traf family member-associated NF-{kappa}B activator (TANK)-binding kinase-1. *Proc Natl Acad Sci U S A* 2005;102:13640–13645.
325. Vahlenkamp TW, Konrath A, Weber M, et al. Persistence of Borna disease virus in naturally infected sheep. *J Virol* 2002;76:9735–9743.
326. VandeWoude S, Richt JA, Zink MC, et al. A borna virus cDNA encoding a protein recognized by antibodies in humans with behavioral diseases. *Science* 1990;250:1278–1281.
327. Villanueva I, Gray P, Mirhosseini N, et al. The diagnosis of proventricular dilatation disease: use of a Western blot assay to detect antibodies against avian Borna virus. *Vet Microbiol* 2010;143:196–201.
334. Walker MP, Jordan I, Briese T, et al. Expression and characterization of the Borna disease virus polymerase. *J Virol* 2000;74:4425–4428.
335. Walker MP, Lipkin WI. Characterization of the nuclear localization signal of the borna disease virus polymerase. *J Virol* 2002;76:8460–8467.
336. Watanabe M, Lee BJ, Yamashita M, et al. Borna disease virus induces acute fatal neurological disorders in neonatal gerbils without virus- and immune-mediated cell destructions. *Virology* 2003;310:245–253.
339. Wehner T, Ruppert A, Herden C, et al. Detection of a novel Borna disease virus-encoded 10 kDa protein in infected cells and tissues. *J Gen Virol* 1997;78(Pt 10):2459–2466.
340. Weissenbock H, Bakonyi T, Sekulin K, et al. Avian bornaviruses in psittacine birds from Europe and Australia with proventricular dilatation disease. *Emerg Infect Dis* 2009;15:1453–1459.
341. Weissenbock H, Fragner K, Nedorost N, et al. Localization of avian bornavirus RNA by in situ hybridization in tissues of psittacine birds with proventricular dilatation disease. *Vet Microbiol* 2010;145:9–16.
342. Weissenböck H, Hornig M, Hickey WF, et al. Microglial activation and neuronal apoptosis in Bornavirus infected neonatal Lewis rats. *Brain Pathol* 2000;10:260–272.
343. Weissenbock H, Sekulin K, Bakonyi T, et al. Novel avian bornavirus in a nonpsittacine species (Canary; Serinus canaria) with enteric ganglioneuritis and encephalitis. *J Virol* 2009;83:11367–11371.

346. Williams BL, Hornig M, Yaddanapudi K, et al. Hippocampal poly(ADP-Ribose) polymerase 1 and caspase 3 activation in neonatal bornavirus infection. *J Virol* 2008;82:1748–1758.
349. Wolff T, Heins G, Pauli G, et al. Failure to detect Borna disease virus antigen and RNA in human blood. *J Clin Virol* 2006;36:309–311.
351. Wolff T, Unterstab G, Heins G, et al. Characterization of an unusual importin alpha binding motif in the borna disease virus p10 protein that directs nuclear import. *J Biol Chem* 2002;277:12151–12157.
352. Wunschmann A, Honkavuori K, Briese T, et al. Antigen tissue distribution of Avian bornavirus (ABV) in psittacine birds with natural spontaneous proventricular dilatation disease and ABV genotype 1 infection. *J Vet Diagn Invest* 2011;23:716–726.
353. Yanai H, Hayashi Y, Watanabe Y, et al. Development of a novel Borna disease virus reverse genetics system using RNA polymerase II promoter and SV40 nuclear import signal. *Microbes Infect* 2006;8:1522–1529.
355. Zhang G, Kobayashi T, Kamitani W, et al. Borna disease virus phosphoprotein represses p53-mediated transcriptional activity by interference with HMGB1. *J Virol* 2003;77:12243–12251.
358. Zwick W. Bornasche Krankheit und Enzephalomyelitis der Tiere. In: Gildemeister E, Haagen E, Waldmann O, eds. Handbuch der Viruskrankheiten, 2. Band. G. Fischer, Jena; 1939:254–354.
361. Zwick W, Seifried O, Witte J. Weitere Untersuchungen über die seuchenhafte Gehirn- und Rückenmarksentzündung der Pferde (Bornasche Krankheit). *Z Infkrankh Haustiere* 1927;32:150–179.

CHAPTER 40

Megan L. Shaw • Peter Palese

Orthomyxoviridae

Influenza viruses were probably responsible for the disease described by Hippocrates in 412 BC,[275] and thus they have been with us for a long, long time. Influenza remains a major cause of morbidity and mortality worldwide, and large segments of the human population are affected every year. In addition, many animal species can be infected by influenza viruses, and some of these viruses may give rise to pandemic strains in humans, as in the case of the 2009 H1N1 pandemic. Most threatening is the possibility of another pandemic similar to that experienced in 1918, which is estimated to have caused on the order of 50 million deaths worldwide.[319]

CLASSIFICATION

The family of *Orthomyxoviridae* is defined by viruses that have a negative-sense, single-stranded, and segmented RNA genome. The definition of negative-sense RNA viruses came from work by David Baltimore, who showed that the packaged genome of this class of viruses is complementary to the messenger RNA (mRNA), which is defined as positive.[21] There are six different genera in the family of *Orthomyxoviridae:* the *Influenzaviruses A, B,* and *C; Thogotovirus; Isavirus;* and a new genus, *Quaranfilvirus*[526] (Fig. 40.1). Members belonging to any of the three different genera of influenza viruses can undergo genetic reassortment (see below), and thus readily exchange genetic information. However, reassortment between members of different genera (types) has never been reported. This absence of genetic exchange between viruses of different genera (types) is one manifestation of speciation as a result of evolutionary divergence.

Different influenza virus strains are named according to their genus (type), the species from which the virus was isolated (omitted if human), location of the isolate, the number of the isolate, the year of isolation, and, in the case of the influenza A viruses, the hemagglutinin (H) and neuraminidase (N) subtypes. For example, the 220th isolate of an H5N1 subtype virus isolated from chickens in Hong Kong in 1997 is designated influenza A/chicken/Hong Kong/220/97(H5N1) virus. There are now 17 different hemagglutinin (H1 to H17) subtypes and 9 different neuraminidase (N1 to N9) subtypes for influenza A viruses as well as a new N10 neuraminidase,[186,668,721] while the influenza B virus hemagglutinins and neuraminidases are each classified into two lineages (Fig. 40.2).

VIRION STRUCTURE

Influenza A viruses have a complex structure and possess a lipid membrane derived from the host cell (Fig. 40.3A). This envelope harbors the hemagglutinin (HA), the neuraminidase (NA), and the M2 proteins that project from the surface of the virus. The matrix protein (M1) lies just beneath the envelope, and the core of the virus particle is made up of the RNP (**r**ibo**n**ucleo**p**rotein) complex, consisting of the viral RNA segments, the polymerase proteins (PB1 [**p**olymerase **b**asic 1], PB2 [**p**olymerase **b**asic 2], and PA [**p**olymerase **a**cid]), and the nucleoprotein (NP).[601] The NEP/NS2 (**n**uclear **e**xport **p**rotein/**n**on**s**tructural protein **2**) protein is also present in purified viral preparations.[556] The overall composition of virus particles is about 1% RNA, 5% to 8% carbohydrate, 20% lipid, and approximately 70% protein.[2,116,188] However, these results will have to be revisited using more quantitative approaches. Specifically, it will be important to get more quantitative data on the presence of individual viral components as well as cellular components that are packaged into the virus.[602] Excellent analyses have already been performed using electron

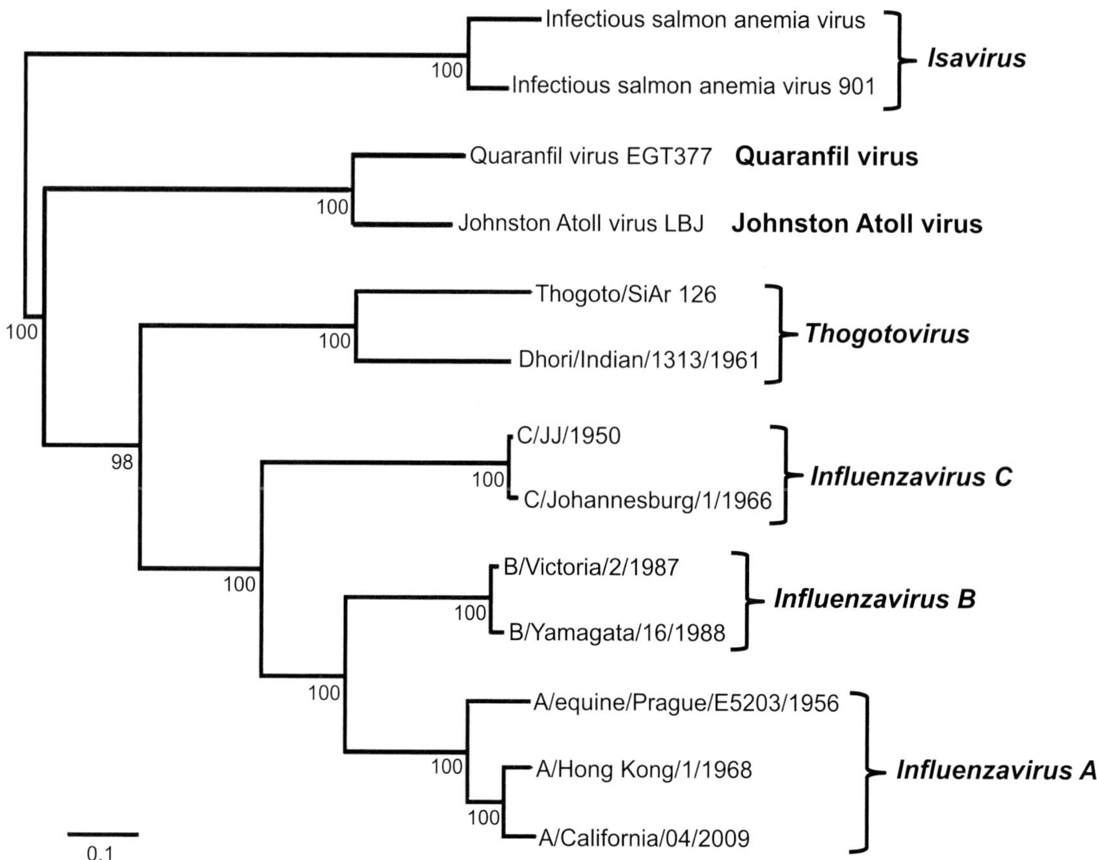

FIGURE 40.1. Phylogenetic relationships within the family *Orthomyxoviridae*. Nucleotide sequences of the polymerase basic 1 proteins (PB1) were aligned using transAlign and CLUSTAL W, and their phylogenetic relationships were determined by the neighbor-joining method (HKY model) using PAUP* (version 4.0b). The tree was midpoint rooted and bootstrap values (1,000 replicates) are indicated on the branches. The GenBank accession numbers for the sequences used for comparison were (top to bottom) AF404346, GU830904, FJ861695, FJ861697, AF004985, M65866, M28060, AF170575, CY018763, CY018771, GU053121, CY044267, and FJ966080. (Adapted from Perez D, Rimstad E, Smith G, et al. Orthomyxoviridae. In: King AMQ, Adams MJ, Carstens EB, et al, eds. *Virus Taxonomy*. Oxford, UK: Elsevier, 2011:749–762.)

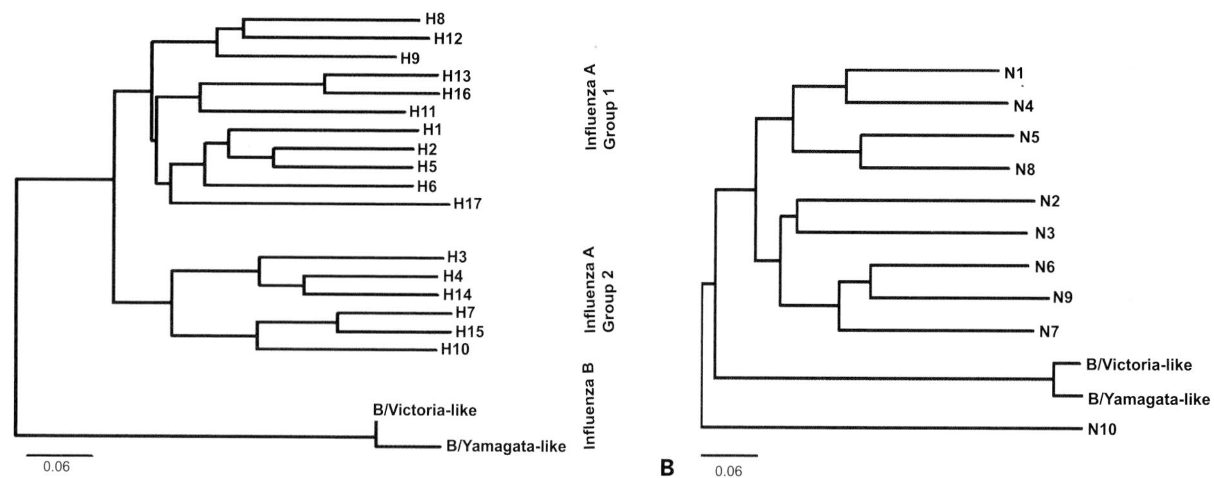

FIGURE 40.2. Phylogeny of influenza A and B virus hemagglutinins (HAs) and neuraminidases (NAs). Rooted phylogenetic trees are based on amino acid sequences of HA **(A)** and NA **(B)** segments from influenza A and B viruses. Representative viruses were selected from GenBank and then aligned using ClustalW. Phylogenetic trees were constructed using FigTree software. The scale bars represent approximately 6% amino acid changes between close relatives. (Courtesy of Natalie Pica.)

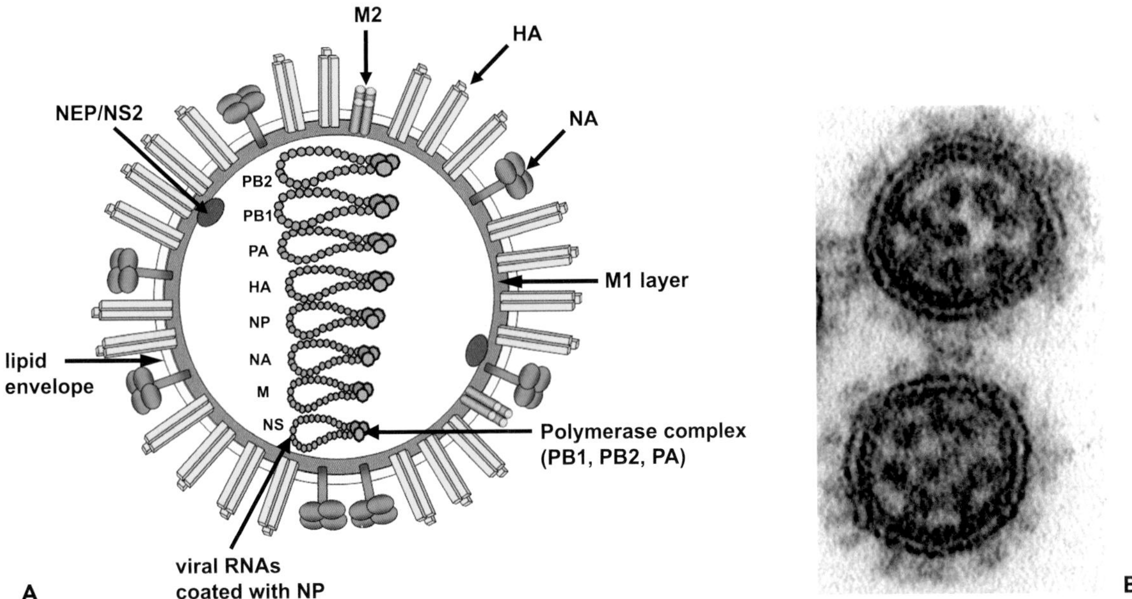

FIGURE 40.3. Schematic diagram and electron micrograph of influenza virus particles. A: The hemagglutinin (HA), neuraminidase (NA), and M2 proteins are inserted into the host-derived lipid envelope. HA is found as a trimer and NA and M2 both as tetramers. The matrix (M1) protein underlies the lipid envelope. A nuclear export protein (NEP/NS2) is also associated with the virus. The viral RNA segments are coated with nucleoprotein and are bound by the polymerase complex. **B:** Electron micrograph thin section image of influenza virus particles (diameter ~100 nm) with the HA and NA spikes visible on the surface and the eight ribonucleoprotein (RNP) segments visible in the interior of each particle. (Courtesy of Yi-ying Chou.)

microscopy (EM) of negatively stained or frozen-hydrated (cryoelectron microscopy) particles and tomographic reconstructions.[80,192,256,464,489] The morphology of influenza A virus particles is characterized by distinctive spikes that are readily observable in electron micrographs of negatively stained virus particles (Fig. 40.3B). These spikes, made up of HA and NA, have lengths of ~10 to 14 nm, with an approximate ratio of four HA to one NA. Influenza viruses are pleomorphic. The spherical particles have a diameter of about 100 nm, but filamentous particles with elongated viral structures (more than 300 nm) have frequently been observed, particularly in fresh clinical isolates[102] and in preparations of viruses with specific M1 or M2 proteins (e-Fig. 40.1).[55,77,159,571]

Less is known about the internal structures of influenza viruses. However, the underlying M1 layer can be visualized and reveals a helical superstructure.[80,575,577] The RNP complexes were first separated by Duesberg[147] on sucrose gradients and were visualized by electron microscopy using positive staining with uranyl acetate.[115] These RNP structures appear to consist of a strand that is folded back on itself to form a double-helical arrangement.[115] Most recently, attempts have been made to visualize RNPs or individual RNA segments by electron microscopy of thin sectioned virus particles[489] (for review see (488)).

Influenza B viruses are mostly indistinguishable from the A viruses by electron microscopy. They have four proteins inserted in their lipid envelopes: the HA, NA, NB, and BM2.[38,62,491,757] The M1 and the RNP complexes make up the interior of the particle. It has also been shown that the influenza B virus NEP/NS2 is associated with purified virus preparations.[304]

Influenza C viruses have been found to possess hexagonal reticular (net-like) structures on the surface[10] and to form unusually long (500 μm) cord-like structures on the surface of infected cells.[461,484] Influenza C viruses also contain a core of three polymerase proteins and the NP, which are associated with seven RNA segments. The influenza C virus M1 appears to have a similar role to those of influenza A and B viruses. The major glycoprotein, HEF (**h**emagglutinin-**e**sterase-**f**usion), combines the functions of the HA and NA (and thus influenza C viruses contain one less RNA segment than do the A and B viruses). The HEF is inserted into the lipid membrane, as is the glycosylated CM2, which is structurally analogous to the M2 of influenza A viruses and the NB of influenza B viruses.[466,467,524]

GENOME STRUCTURE AND ORGANIZATION

Influenza Viruses

All A- and B-type influenza viruses possess eight RNA segments, whereas influenza C viruses only have seven RNAs (Fig. 40.4 and e-Figs. 40.2 to 40.4). This was first shown by using polyacrylamide gel electrophoresis of isolated RNAs from two parent influenza A virus strains and their reassortants. Identifying the derivation of an RNA segment (by gel electrophoresis) in a reassortant and simultaneous protein analysis (by serologic or gel analysis) allowed the assignment of individual RNAs to specific viral proteins[508,513,514] (for review, see (509)) (Fig. 40.5 and e-Fig. 40.4). Interestingly, influenza A viruses increase the coding capacity of their genomes via both splicing and use of alternative open reading frames. The M and NS genes each give rise to a spliced mRNA encoding the M2 and the NEP/NS2 proteins, respectively.[354,355] The PB1-F2 and PB1 N40 proteins are expressed from alternative open reading frames

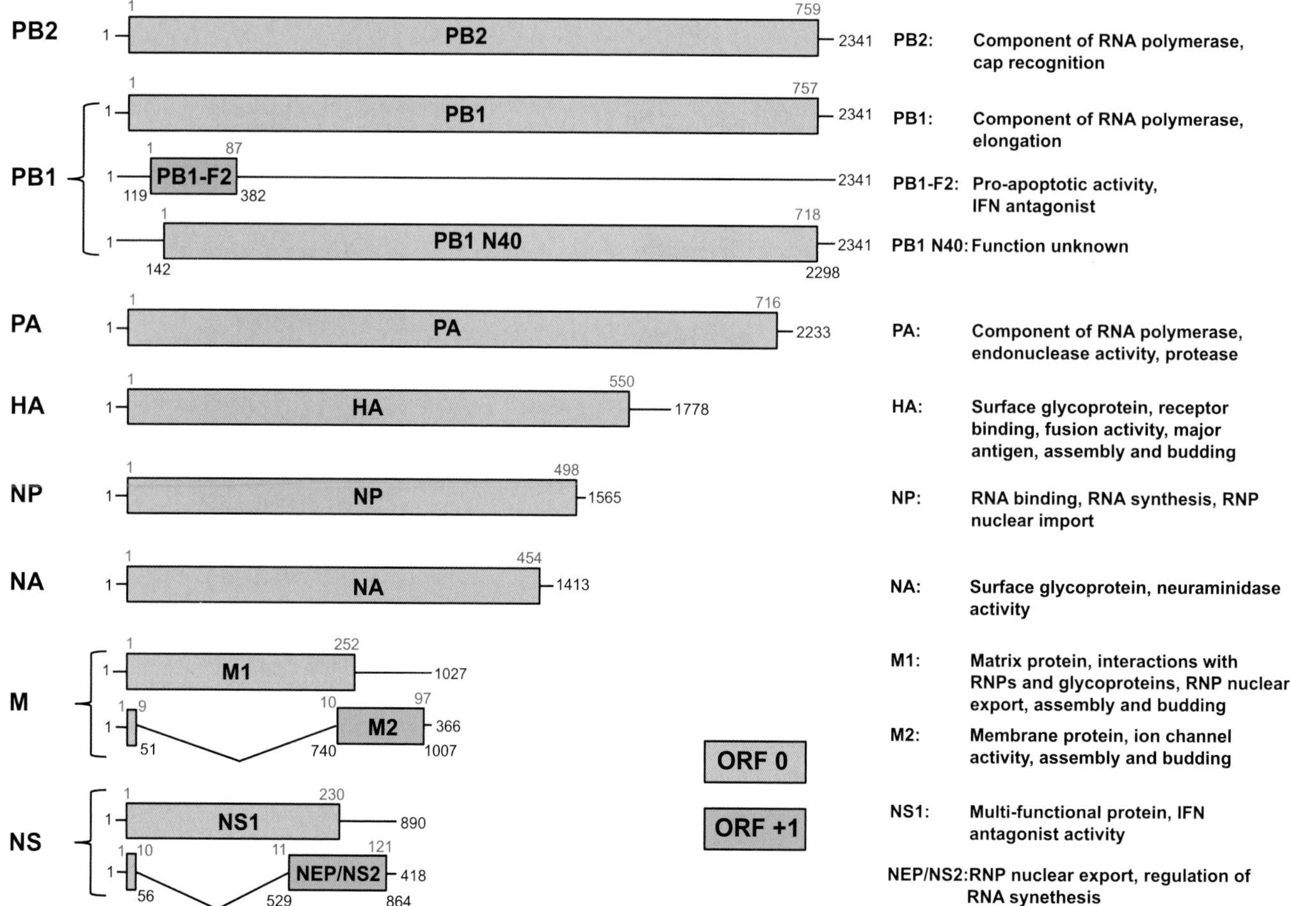

FIGURE 40.4. Genome structure of influenza A/Puerto Rico/8/34 virus. RNA segments (nucleotides in black) shown in positive sense and their encoded proteins (amino acids in red). The lines at the 5′ and 3′ termini represent the noncoding regions. The polymerase basic 1 protein (PB1) segment contains a second open reading frame (ORF) in the +1 frame resulting in the PB1-F2 protein and a third ORF in the 0 frame resulting in the PB1 N40 protein. The M2 and nuclear export protein (NEP/NS2) proteins are encoded by spliced messenger RNAs (mRNAs) (the introns are indicated by the V-shaped lines). (Courtesy of Heinrich Hoffmann.)

within the *PB1* gene[93,726] (Fig. 40.4), although not all influenza A virus strains encode these proteins, making them true accessory proteins. Each viral segment contains noncoding regions at both the 5′ and 3′ ends. The extreme ends are conserved among all segments of influenza A viruses and this is followed by a segment-specific noncoding region.

The influenza B virus genome is similar to that of influenza A virus. Again, eight RNA segments code for one or more viral proteins (e-Figs. 40.2 and 40.4) with the three largest RNAs coding for the polymerase proteins, the fourth RNA for the HA, and the fifth and sixth RNAs for the NP and NA, respectively.[550] The NA gene codes for the NB protein as well as for the NA. The NB protein is encoded by a −1 open reading frame seven nucleotides upstream (…AUGAACAAUG…) of the NA coding frame.[603] The seventh RNA codes for the M1 protein (248 amino acids in length). Its termination codon (…UAAUG) overlaps with the initiation codon (UAAUG…) for the BM2 (109 amino acids in length), which allows for a "stop–start" translation mechanism.[288] The eighth RNA codes for the NS1 as well as for the NEP/NS2 protein, the latter via a spliced mRNA. Cognate PB1-F2 and PB1 N40 proteins have not yet been identified in influenza B viruses. The noncoding regions of the influenza B virus genome are longer than those in influenza A virus.

The genome of influenza C viruses has only seven RNA segments, with the three largest RNAs each coding for one of the polymerase proteins (e-Figs. 40.3 and 40.4). The PB1 and PB2 proteins are homologous to the corresponding influenza A and B virus proteins. The third influenza C virus polymerase protein is named P3 because it does not display acid charge features at neutral pH, as do the corresponding PA proteins of influenza A and B viruses.[740] The fourth RNA codes for the HEF protein,[271] combining the hemagglutinin, receptor-destroying, and fusion activities. The NP is encoded by the fifth RNA. The sixth RNA codes for the M protein, which is expressed from a spliced mRNA, and from the unspliced mRNA a long precursor is translated (p42), which is then processed by signal peptide cleavage into CM2. This 115-amino acid (aa)-long protein consists of an amino-terminal extracellular domain (with a carbohydrate chain), a hydrophobic transmembrane domain, and an

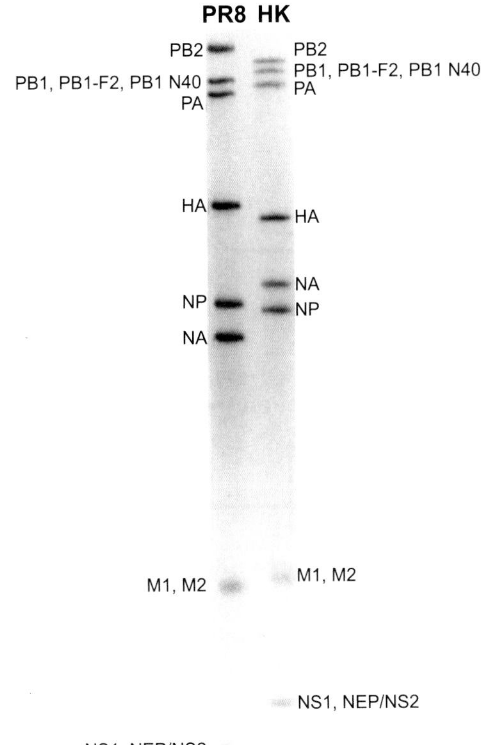

FIGURE 40.5. RNA segments of influenza A/Puerto Rico/8/34 (H1N1) and A/Hong Kong/8/68 (H3N2) viruses. The viral RNAs are separated on a polyacrylamide gel and the proteins encoded by the RNAs are indicated. (Adapted from Palese P. The genes of influenza virus. *Cell* 1977;10[1]:1–10.)

intracellular cytoplasmic tail.[523,524,741] Finally, RNA 7 codes for the NS1 protein (246 amino acids),[467] and via a spliced mRNA, for the NEP/NS2 protein (182 amino acids).[5,284]

Evolutionarily, influenza A, B, and C viruses have a common precursor, and it is also likely that influenza A and B viruses diverged from each other more recently than influenza C viruses. Based on comparative sequencing studies using the hemagglutinin molecules, it has been postulated that the influenza A viruses diverged about 2,000 years ago, and the influenza B and C viruses about 4,000 and 8,000 years ago, respectively.[653] Clearly, these numbers are based on a series of unproveable assumptions, including a steady rate of evolution over time, and therefore must be taken *cum grano salis.*

Thogoto Virus

The genomes of Thogoto viruses possess only six single-stranded RNA segments of negative polarity, with a total coding capacity for seven proteins. As with the influenza viruses, three proteins make up the RNA-dependent RNA polymerase complex. The NP, the glycoprotein (G), the matrix protein (M), and one non-essential accessory protein (ML) are coded for by the remaining three RNAs. The M and ML proteins are both encoded by the shortest RNA, with the M protein being derived from a spliced mRNA.[242,339] The 304-aa-long ML protein has been shown to possess interferon antagonist activity[69,242,316] and is virion associated.[241] It appears that Thogoto viruses do not possess a nonstructural protein.

Infectious Salmon Anemia Virus

The genome of infectious salmon anemia virus consists of eight negative-sense, single- stranded RNA segments.[122,447] Segment 1 most likely encodes a protein analog of the influenza virus PB2.[626] The second segment appears to code for a PB1 analog because it carries the PB1-specific polymerase motifs.[626] Segments 3 and 4 code for the NP and PA proteins, respectively.[15,169] Segment 5 encodes the 50-kD F (fusion) protein, and segment 6 encodes the HA (**h**emagglutinin-**a**cetylesterase) protein.[16,169,526] The 42-kD HA has been demonstrated to bind to 4-O-acetylated sialic acid (i.e., to use it as a receptor) and also to hydrolyze the acetyl group.[267] This activity is similar to the binding and receptor-destroying enzyme (RDE) activities previously observed for the HEF protein of influenza C viruses and the HE glycoprotein of coronaviruses.[267,271,685–687] Segment 7 encodes two proteins via an alternative splicing mechanism.[40] The larger protein is expressed from the unspliced transcript and has interferon antagonist activity.[211,430] Segment 8 encodes two proteins of 27.6 kD and 22 kD, the larger of which has interferon antagonist activity.[122,211] The smaller protein is a structural protein, presumed to be the equivalent of the influenza virus matrix protein.[169]

Quaranfil Virus

The genome of *Quaranfil virus,* which is the type species of the new *Quaranfilvirus* genus, consists of six negative-sense, single-stranded RNA segments.[526] The ends of each segment are conserved and partially complementary. Segments 1, 2, and 3 encode the PB2, PA, and PB1 polymerase subunits, respectively, while segment 5 codes for a protein that is distantly related to the Thogoto virus glycoprotein, and thus is likely the attachment protein.[544] The predicted protein products of segments 4 and 6 do not show any homology with known proteins.

STAGES OF VIRAL REPLICATION

An overview of the influenza virus life cycle is illustrated in Figure 40.6 and in the following pages we will discuss each stage of this life cycle in order.

Mechanism of Attachment

Influenza viruses bind to neuraminic acids (sialic acids) on the surface of cells to initiate infection and replication. The interaction of influenza viruses with a ubiquitous molecule such as sialic acid is constrained by the fact that the HAs of viruses that replicate in different species show specificity toward sialic acids with different linkages. Human viruses preferentially bind to N-acetylneuraminic acid attached to the penultimate galactose sugar by an α2,6 linkage (SAα2,6Gal), whereas avian viruses mostly bind to sialic acid with an α2,3 linkage[120] (e-Fig. 40.5). In agreement with this finding is the fact that human tracheal epithelial cells contain mostly SAα2,6Gal, while the gut epithelium from ducks possesses mostly SAα2,3Gal sugar moieties.[123,307] It should be noted, however, that this viral specificity is not absolute and that avian and human cells can contain both neuraminic acid linkages (2,3 as well as 2,6). Studies on ciliated cells in the human airway epithelium have shown that sialylated proteins with α2,3 linkages are present and that these cells can be infected with avian influenza viruses.[425] Furthermore, glycan structure is far more complex than just the terminal sialic acid

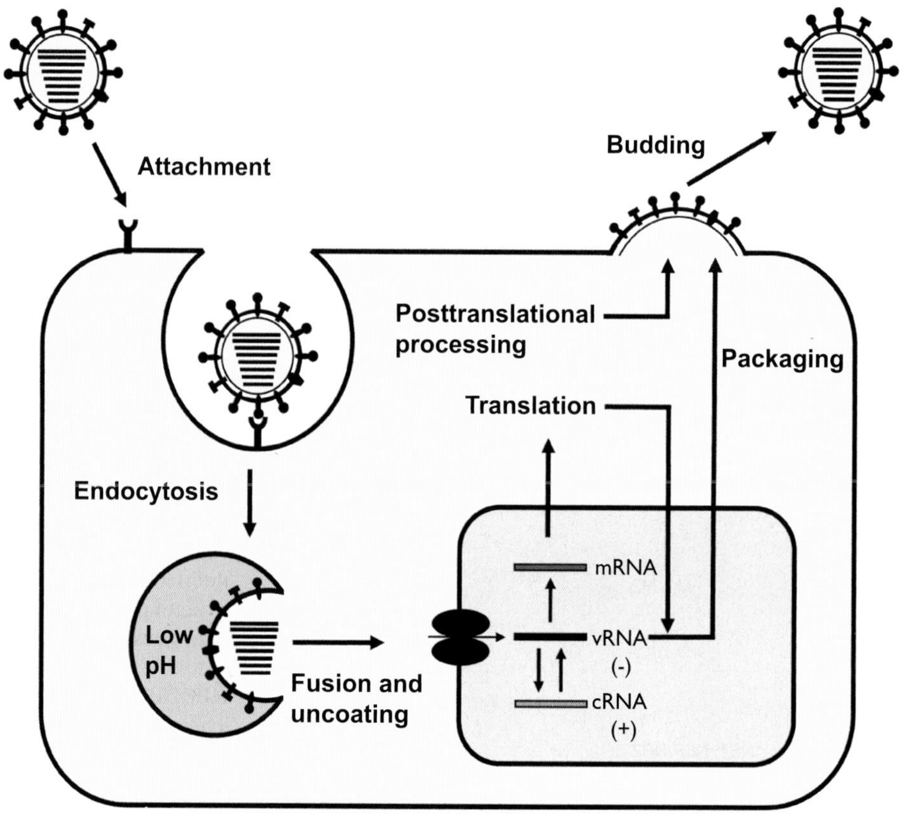

FIGURE 40.6. Illustration of the influenza virus replication cycle. Upon binding at the cell surface, the virus is internalized by receptor-mediated endocytosis. The low pH in the endosome triggers fusion of the viral and endosomal membranes, releasing the viral ribonucleoproteins (vRNPs) into the cytoplasm. vRNPs are imported into the nucleus where they serve as the template for transcription. New proteins are synthesized from viral mRNA. The viral genome (vRNA) is replicated through a positive-sense intermediate (complementary RNA [cRNA]). Newly synthesized viral RNPs are exported from the nucleus to the assembly site at the apical plasma membrane, where virus particles bud and are released.

linkage, and evidence suggests that factors such as the type of backbone, chain length, and branching pattern as well as sulfation and fucosylation may also influence the interactions with HA.[99,639] Glycan microarrays that contain a wide spectrum of glycan structures are now being used as tools to better understand the specificity of receptor binding.[638] Also, when viruses are passaged in a particular host, they can adapt to that host by mutating the receptor-binding site in the viral HA.[202,448] In a study of the A/New York/1/1918 virus HA, it was shown that the binding specificity can be changed by a single amino acid mutation (D190E) to a preference for α2,3-linked sialic acids. It is thus hypothesized that the HA gene of the 1918 influenza virus has its origin in avian species and that a single amino acid change (E190D) allowed the hemagglutinin to recognize the α2,6-linked sialic acids prevalent in human cells.[222,637]

Mechanism of Entry

While some viruses (e.g., paramyxoviruses and herpes viruses) can enter cells directly through the plasma membrane by a pH-independent fusion process, influenza viruses require a low pH to initiate fusion and are therefore internalized by endocytic compartments. There are four internalization mechanisms: (a) via clathrin-coated pits; (b) via caveolae; (c) through nonclathrin, noncaveolae pathways; and (d) through macropinocytosis (for review, see (119,353,443,613)). Clathrin-mediated endocytosis has traditionally been the model for influenza virus entry.[424] However, a non-clathrin, non-caveolae-mediated internalization mechanism has also been described for influenza viruses.[612] The latter pathway is dependent on low pH and trafficking to late endosomes, as it requires protein kinase C, Rab5, and Rab7 functions.[611] More recently, through the use of specific inhibitors and RNA interference (RNAi), it has been shown that in addition to entering via a dynamin-dependent, clathrin-driven pathway, influenza viruses can also enter via a dynamin-independent pathway that is characteristic of macropinocytosis.[133] Potential differences in the entry pathways defined in polarized versus nonpolarized cells should also be appreciated, as, for example, the actin cytoskeleton appears to be critical for uptake of influenza viruses into polarized cells but not nonpolarized cells.[651] The requirement of specific host proteins during influenza virus entry will help to further define the cellular pathways utilized by the virus. Genome-wide RNAi screens have identified multiple factors that are required for efficient entry mediated by the influenza virus glycoproteins[341]; however, the ability of the virus to enter via different routes means that this approach is unlikely to capture factors that are specific to one endocytic route. A more focused approach, such as that which shows the requirement of epsin 1 for clathrin-mediated uptake of influenza virus, is needed.[90] The epidermal growth factor receptor (EGFR) has also been demonstrated to play a role during influenza virus entry,[154] and it is thought that virus attachment to the cell stimulates EGFR, which leads to activation of signaling cascades such as phosphatidylinositol 3 kinase (PI3K) signaling, which is known to promote influenza virus entry.[152] There are also questions over whether sialic acid is the only attachment molecule. Lec-1 cells, which are deficient in N-linked glycosylation (but still contain sialylated proteins), are unable to internalize influenza viruses.[103] Similarly, cells deficient in sialic acid can be made to support influenza virus entry if they express one of the C-type lectins, DC-SIGN or L-SIGN.[398]

Mechanism of Fusion and Uncoating

Influenza viruses and other enveloped viruses (including rhabdo-, flavi-, bunya-, and filoviruses) require low pH to fuse with endosomal membranes. After binding to the target cell surface and endocytosis, the low pH of the endosome activates fusion of the viral membrane with that of the endosome. This fusion activity is induced by a structural change in the HA of influenza viruses, but in order for this to occur, the HA0 precursor must first be cleaved into two subunits, HA1 and HA2. Once in the acid environment of the endosome, the cleaved HA molecule undergoes a conformational change and this exposes the fusion peptide at the N-terminus of the HA2 subunit, enabling it to interact with the membrane of the endosome (for review, see (128,258,632) and for details see the following section on Hemagglutinin). The transmembrane domain of the HA2 (inserted into the viral membrane) and the fusion peptide (inserted into the endosomal membrane) are in juxtaposition in the low pH–induced HA structure. The concerted structural change of several hemagglutinin molecules then opens up a pore, which releases the contents of the virion (i.e., viral RNPs) into the cytoplasm of the cell. The precise timing and the location of uncoating (maturity of the endosome) depends on the pH-mediated transition of the specific HA molecule involved.

The uncoating of influenza viruses in endosomes is blocked by changes in pH caused by weak bases (e.g., ammonium chloride or chloroquine) or ionophores (e.g., monensin) (for review, see (418)). Effective uncoating is also dependent on the presence of the M2 protein, which has ion channel activity.[532,534] Early on it was recognized that amantadine and rimantadine inhibit replication immediately following virus infection.[617] Later it was found that the virus-associated M2 protein allows the influx of H^+ ions from the endosome into the virus particle, which disrupts protein–protein interactions and results in the release of RNP free of the M1 protein[424,767] (for review, see (534)). Amantadine and rimantadine have been shown to block the ion channel activity of the M2 protein and thus uncoating.[100,281,532,648,699] The HA-mediated fusion of the viral membrane with the endosomal membrane and the M2-mediated release of the RNP result in the appearance of free RNP complexes in the cytoplasm. This completes the uncoating process.[421] The time frame for the uncoating process was examined by inhibiting virus penetration with ammonium chloride. The majority of virus particles showed a half time for penetration of about 25 minutes (after adsorption). Barely 10 minutes later (half time of 34 minutes after adsorption) RNP complexes are found in the nucleus.[421] The process for uptake of RNP molecules through nuclear pores is an active one, involving the nucleocytoplasmic trafficking machinery of the host cell (for details, see Nuclear Import of RNPs).

Much less is known about the uptake and uncoating of influenza B and C viruses. Influenza B viruses are more like influenza A viruses as both recognize N-acetylneuraminic acid as receptors, while influenza C viruses bind to 9-O-acetylated neuraminic acid derivatives.[272] Like influenza A viruses, the B- and C-type viruses go through an endosome-mediated uncoating process, which requires proteolytic activation (cleavage) of the HA or HEF proteins and subsequent fusion of the viral and endosomal membranes. Although the viral glycoproteins of both viruses are dependent on a low pH–triggered fusion process, the influenza C virus HEF-mediated fusion/uncoating may occur at a higher pH in early endosomes.[184,767] At this point, the role of CM2 in uncoating of influenza C viruses is less well established than that of the BM2 protein of influenza B viruses, which is the homolog of the influenza A virus M2 protein.[193,253,262,283,455,701]

The Hemagglutinin

STRUCTURAL FEATURES

Much is known about the HA molecule and excellent reviews are available.[150,204,258,613,618,633,658] In fact, the influenza virus HA has become a model for studies of protein folding and trafficking, protein quality control, membrane fusion, protein–receptor interactions, and antigen–antibody complexes and, last but not least, for investigating how the immune system reacts to a foreign protein. The major functions of the HA are the receptor-binding and fusion activities, but there may also be a structural role for the HA in budding and particle formation. The HA is a trimeric rod-shaped molecule with the carboxy terminus inserted into the viral membrane and the hydrophilic end projecting as a spike away from the viral surface (i.e., a type I integral membrane protein). Early on it was shown that (a) posttranslational modifications of the precursor molecule (i.e., glycosylation and palmitoylation), (b) cleavage of the signal peptide in the endoplasmic reticulum (ER), and (c) cleavage of the HA0 precursor into HA1 and HA2 subunits are required for the full activity of the molecule.[335,363,542]

The first x-ray crystallographic structure of an HA (the ectodomain released from the virus by bromelain treatment) was resolved in 1981 by Wilson et al.[725] At that time the HA (from A/Aichi/68 [H3N2] virus) was the largest biological molecule for which a structure had been resolved, and it started an unprecedented drive to study the structure/function relationships of biologically important molecules, which continues unabated to this day. The structures of numerous HAs have now been resolved, including the subtype 1 HA molecules of the 1918 and 2009 pandemic influenza viruses[203,640,735] and that of an H2 subtype HA[736] (Fig. 40.7). Remarkably, even though the overall amino acid sequence identity can be less than 50%, the structure and functions of these HAs are highly conserved (e-Fig. 40.6). This represents a case of evolution and sequence variation proceeding to an extreme level while structure and function have remained conserved. Even more surprising is that the structure of the influenza B virus HA is similar to that of influenza A virus HA despite sharing only 25% sequence identity.[703,704]

The crystallographic structure of the uncleaved influenza A virus HA is superimposable onto that of the cleaved HA1 and HA2, with the exception of the amino acids adjacent to the cleavage site. The major features of the structure are (a) a long fibrous stem, which is made up of a triple-stranded coiled coil of α-helices derived from the three HA2 parts of the molecule (helix A and helix B; Fig. 40.7 and e-Fig. 40.6), and (b) the globular head, which is also made up of three identical domains whose sequences are derived from the HA1 portions of the three monomers. The *first major function* of HA is binding to receptors and the receptor-binding site lies within the globular head of the molecule. This site has been defined through crystallization and structure analysis of HA–receptor complexes, as well as by mutational analysis. In the H3-subtype viruses, it appears that within the receptor-binding pocket of an avian HA, a glutamine in position 226 preferentially accommodates the 2,3-linked sialic acid, whereas a leucine in that position in human H3 HAs preferentially accommodates the 2,6-linked sialic acid[239] (e-Fig. 40.7). (See the previous section on Attachment for more details).

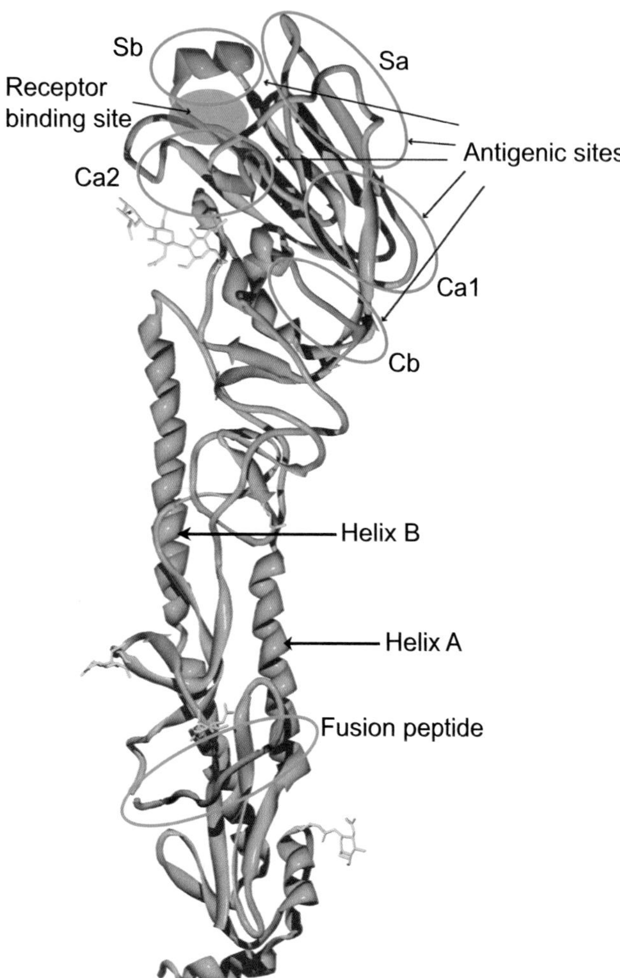

FIGURE 40.7. Ribbon representation of the uncleaved hemagglutinin monomer from the 1918 influenza virus based on x-ray diffraction analysis. The five predicted antigenic sites (Ca2, Sb, Sa, Ca1, and Cb) surround the sialic acid receptor–binding site. Toward the membrane proximal end **(bottom)** is the fusion peptide and helices A and B are indicated. For details see (640). (Courtesy of James Stevens and Ian Wilson.)

The *second major function* of the HA is acid pH–triggered fusion, which is required for the uncoating process. Low pH treatment changes the structure of the HA dramatically. The molecule becomes susceptible to protease digestion, and the disulfide bond linking the HA1 and HA2 subunits becomes susceptible to mercaptoethanol.[232,615] However, the important feature of the acid pH–mediated change is that the fusion peptide becomes aligned antiparallel to the membrane anchor of the HA2 (Fig. 40.8). The end result is that the fusion peptide brings the endosomal membrane into juxtaposition with the viral membrane, leading to fusion. The presence of more than one hemagglutinin then leads to the formation of a fusion pore through which the RNP can enter the cytoplasm (Fig. 40.9). Structures of the postfusion HA as well as an early fusion intermediate have helped to reveal the molecular details of the changes that occur during the transition from pre- to postfusion state.[75,737] Structures of the fusion peptide in lipid environments have been resolved by nuclear magnetic resonance (NMR) and show that the peptide forms a tight helical hairpin structure that angles back on itself[252,351,399] (e-Fig. 40.8). This hook structure may help to pull the endosomal membrane close to the viral membrane, resulting in the initiation of the actual fusion process. These studies represent the first foray into the characterization of the transmembrane region, which so far has proved difficult to analyze.

The third major structural element of the HA, the cytoplasmic tail, is highly conserved among all subtypes. There are three cysteines that are palmitoylated (with one of them located in the transmembrane domain). The role of this cytoplasmic tail (and the palmitates attached to the cysteines) is not entirely clear due to subtype- and cell/host-specific differences.[89,318,439,696,774]

Antigenic Determinants

In addition to having an important role in receptor binding, fusion, and assembly, the influenza virus HA is also the *major determinant* recognized by the adaptive immune system of the host. Following infection and replication, a vigorous immune response is induced, which usually results in the formation of neutralizing antibodies. These antibodies then lead to the selection of "antibody escape" variants. The amino acids undergoing change are almost exclusively on the HA1 (and on the outside of the molecule). Many of these changes get fixed (accumulate over time), defining the antigenic drift of influenza viruses (e-Fig. 40.9). Fab antibody fragments have been shown to bind to different regions of the HA1 (e-Fig. 40.10) and, interestingly, not in all cases do three Fabs bind to one trimeric spike (3:1 ratio). Examples have been found where only one Fab molecule binds to one HA spike (1:1 ratio) or where just two Fab molecules bind to a trimeric spike (2:1 ratio) (e-Fig. 40.10).[336] In the latter case, the two Fab fragments cross-link the two monomers so that the HA molecule cannot undergo an acid pH–induced conformational change.[336] Attempts have also been made to measure antigenic evolution of influenza virus strains by pairwise comparison of hemagglutination inhibition assays.[187,622]

Unexpectedly, broadly cross-reactive monoclonal antibodies have been identified, which do not bind to the tip of the HA molecules but also have neutralizing activity.[121,157,327,495,650,663,730] These antibodies are directed against the conserved stem region of the HA spike and recognize the membrane-proximal part of HA1 in combination with HA2 or the HA2 alone (Fig. 40.10).[707] In general, these antibodies recognize the HAs within either group 1 (for review see (706)) or group 2,[158,707] but recently a human monoclonal antibody was described that binds to the stem of both group 1 and group 2 HAs.[121] The most likely mechanism by which these cross-reactive antistem antibodies neutralize influenza viruses is by blocking conformational rearrangements associated with membrane fusion (antifusion vs. hemagglutination inhibition activity). A broadly neutralizing human monoclonal antibody that recognizes the highly conserved sialic acid–binding site of H1 HAs has also been described.[343] It is hoped that the conserved epitopes identified by these cross-protective antibodies could be utilized as immunogens with the possibility of developing novel vaccine constructs that will result in effective and safe universal influenza virus vaccines.[47,631,708]

The HEF of Influenza C Viruses

In contrast to the HA of influenza A and B viruses, the major glycoprotein of the C viruses has a receptor-destroying activity.

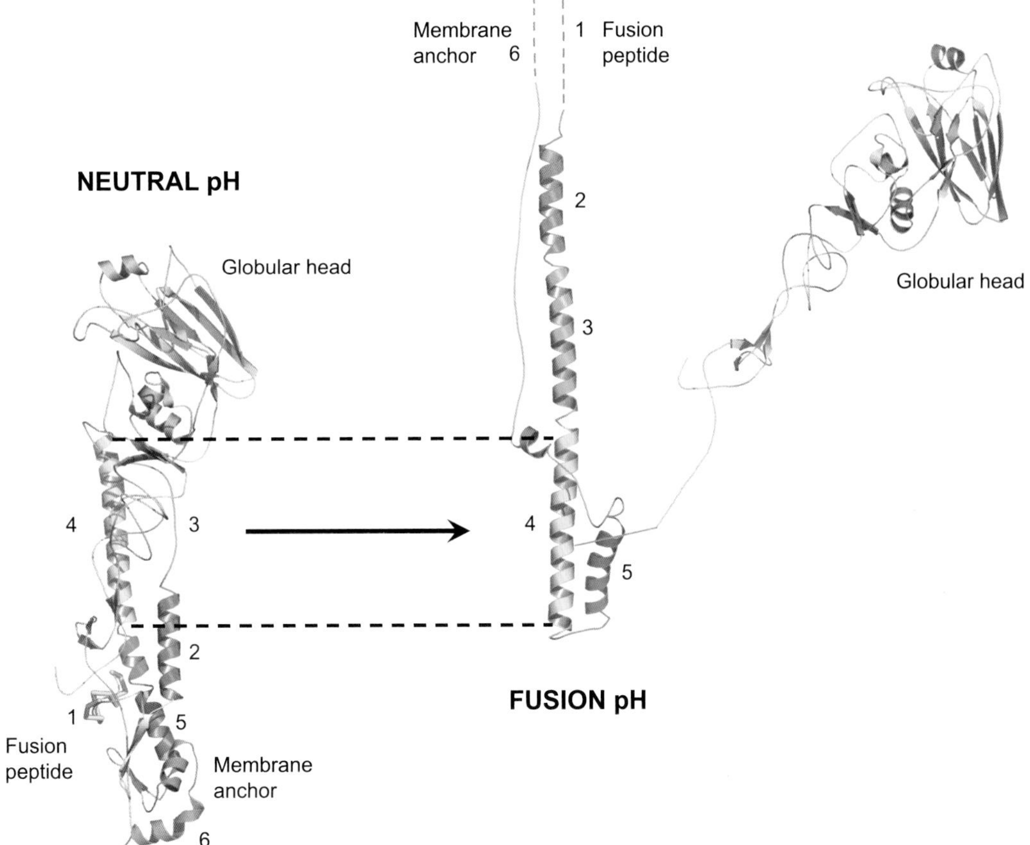

FIGURE 40.8. Ribbon representation of the structural changes that occur in hemagglutinin (HA) at low pH. Bromelain-treated HA monomer with regions of HA2 undergoing conformational changes at low pH as indicated by numbered domains **(left)**. The domains, starting at the fusion peptide (domain 1), are numbered sequentially until the membrane anchor is reached (domain 6). The structure and the position of the region comprising residues 75 to 106 (domain 4) are the same before and after the conformational change (denoted by the dotted lines). The globular head domains retain their structures but detrimerize (falling to the right, away from the HA2 portion). For details see (92) and (616). (Courtesy of John Skehel and Rupert Russell.)

In contrast to the neuraminidase activity of the NA proteins of influenza A and B viruses (see Neuraminidase section), HEF has esterase activity, which cleaves off an acetyl group at position 9 of the neuraminic (sialic) acid receptor, eliminating the ligand (for review, see (644)). This activity is important for entry of the virus, implying a role in releasing the incoming virus from the receptor so that the uncoating process can begin.[688] Thus, in addition to receptor-binding (**h**emagglutination) and **f**usion activities, the molecule also has **e**sterase activity, hence the name HEF. Although there is only about a 12% sequence identity between HAs and HEF, the overall structure of the molecule is similar, as was shown by x-ray crystallographic analysis.[569] Even more surprising are structural and sequence similarities between the esterases of influenza C viruses and some coronaviruses.[758]

The M2 Protein

The M2 protein of influenza A viruses is a tetrameric type III (lacking a signal peptide sequence) integral membrane protein. It has a short ecto-domain, a transmembrane domain, and a cytoplasmic domain with palmitate and phosphate modifications (for review, see (531,534)). M2 has been shown to possess ion channel activity, and its major role is thought to be that of conducting protons from the acidified endosomes into the interior of the virus to dissociate the RNP complex from the rest of the viral components, thus facilitating the uncoating process (see earlier section on Fusion and Uncoating). The structural and genetic analysis of the M2 protein has revealed that the ion channel is acid gated (but not voltage gated) and highly selective for H^+ ions.[86,100,453,454,485] The structures of the transmembrane regions of M2 and of those that include the cytoplasmic sequences reveal a good understanding of the mechanism of proton conductance, which is controlled by the histidine-37 and tryptophan-41 cluster.[1,79,291,482,589,599,643] The transmembrane region, when viewed from the top, shows four helices that sit at an angle in the lipid bilayer, forming a pore (Fig. 40.11). Structural studies on M2 in complex with adamantine drugs indicate two potential sites of interaction. In the x-ray structure, a single drug molecule binds to the core of the pore.[643] In contrast, the NMR structure shows four drug molecules binding to the lipid-exposed surface of the channel close to the cytoplasmic ends of the helices.[589] More recent data confirm the existence of these two interaction sites and propose that both drug-binding mechanisms may have physiologic

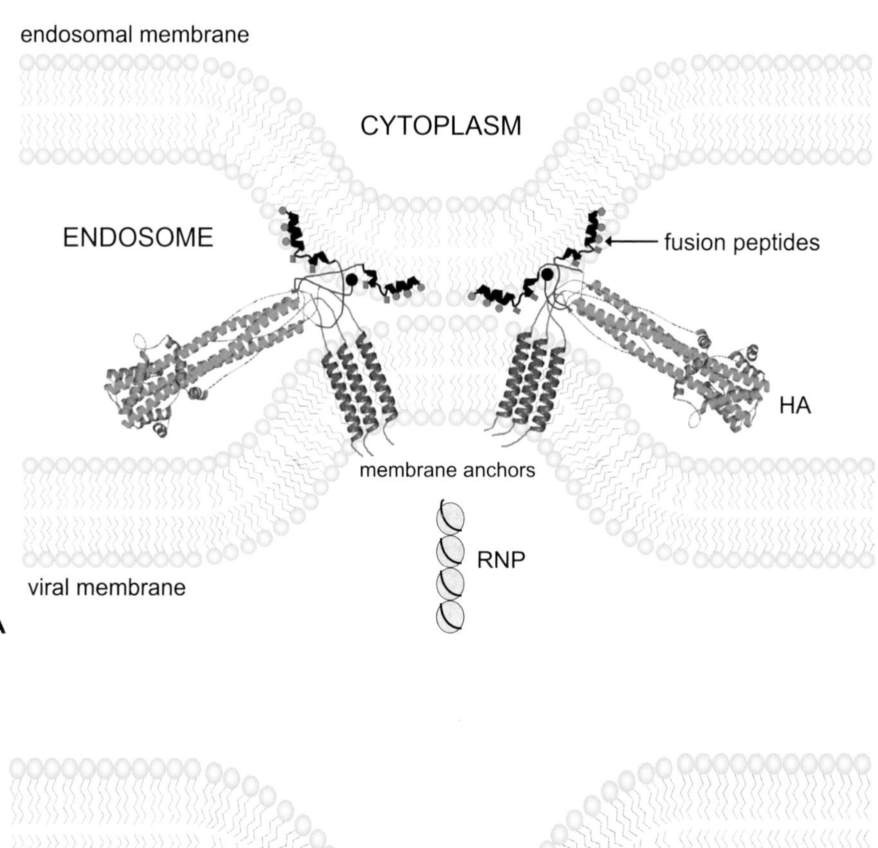

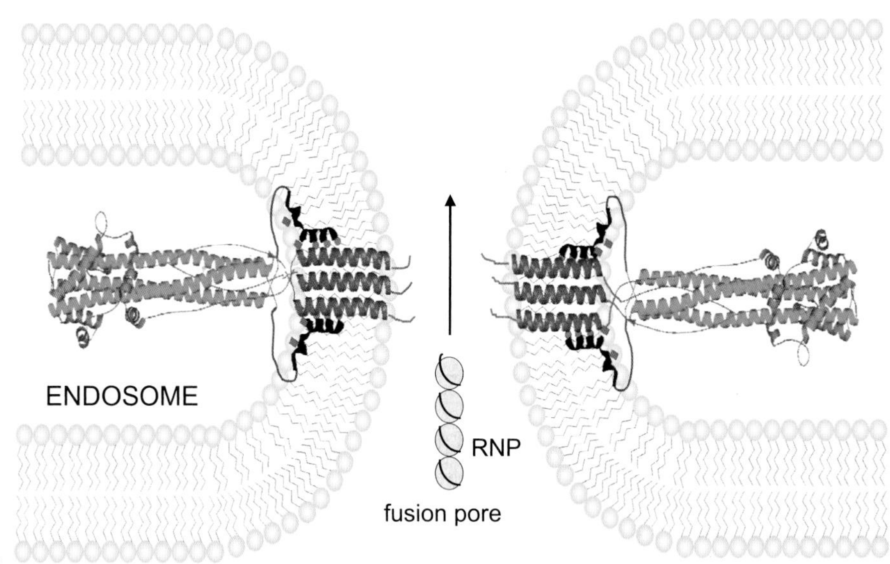

FIGURE 40.9. Model for juxtaposition of viral and endosomal membranes resulting in formation of a fusion pore and release of ribonucleoproteins (RNPs). Structures of influenza virus hemagglutinins in their postfusion state modeled into a possible fusion intermediate **(A)** and into a fusion pore **(B)**. The fusion peptides are shown inserted into the endosomal membrane, while the transmembrane domains remain anchored in the viral membrane. Note the large conformational changes of the ecto- and fusion domains when compared to their prefusion structures (see Figs. 40.7 and 40.8). The small spheres (pink) on the fusion peptide denote glycines that may mediate helix interactions and the small squares (blue) denote glutamates that may be responsible for the pH dependence of the fusion peptide penetration into lipid bilayers. Following the formation of a pore, the RNPs are released from the interior of the virus particle into the cytoplasm, completing the uncoating process. (Courtesy of Lukas Tamm.)

significance.[79,342] The structure and the precise function of the extracellular portion of the M2 protein remain to be resolved. This external portion of M2 has been considered as the basis of a universal influenza virus vaccine approach because the M2 protein maintains a highly conserved sequence over long periods of time.[590]

The ion channel activity of M2 has also been implicated in stabilizing HAs from premature low pH transitions in the trans-Golgi network, but this second function may only come into play for viruses carrying highly acid-sensitive HAs.[104] This is the case for H5 and H7 HAs, which have a multibasic cleavage site that can be cleaved by ubiquitous proteases and are therefore more susceptible to a premature low pH–induced conformational change. Further functions attributed to the M2 protein include roles in particle morphology,[231,310,564,571] genome packaging,[231,310,432] membrane scission[572] (see Assembly and Release), and inhibition of autophagy.[205]

Influenza Virus Transcription and Replication

Overview

After uncoating, the viral ribonucleoproteins (vRNPs) are transported into the nucleus and the incoming negative-sense viral RNAs (vRNAs) are transcribed into mRNA by a primer-dependent mechanism. These mRNA products are incomplete copies of the vRNA templates and are capped and polyadenylated, unlike vRNA. Replication occurs via a two-step process. A full-length, positive-sense copy of the vRNA is first made, which is referred to as complementary RNA (cRNA), and is in turn used as a template to produce more vRNA (Fig. 40.12).

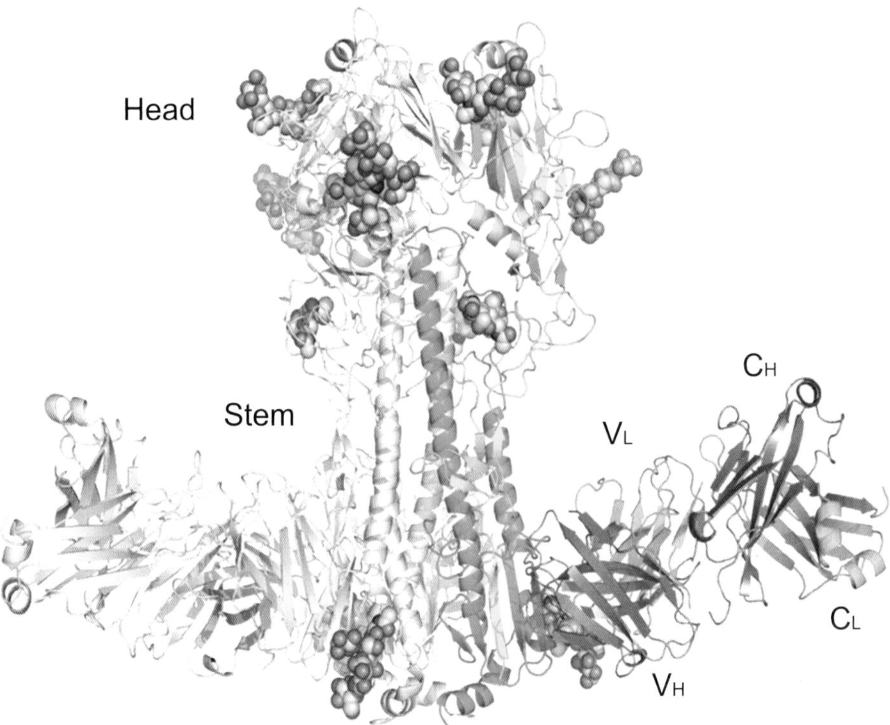

FIGURE 40.10. Crystal structure of antibody CR8020 bound to the H3 hemagglutinin. CR8020 binds an epitope on the hemagglutinin (HA) stem and has broad neutralizing activity against multiple group 2 influenza A viruses, including H3, H7, and H10. One monomer from the HA trimer is depicted in yellow and green (HA1 and HA2 subunits, respectively) and CR8020 is colored blue and cyan (heavy chain and light chain, respectively). N-linked carbohydrates are represented as pink van der Waals spheres. See (158) for details. (Courtesy of Damian Ekiert and Ian Wilson.)

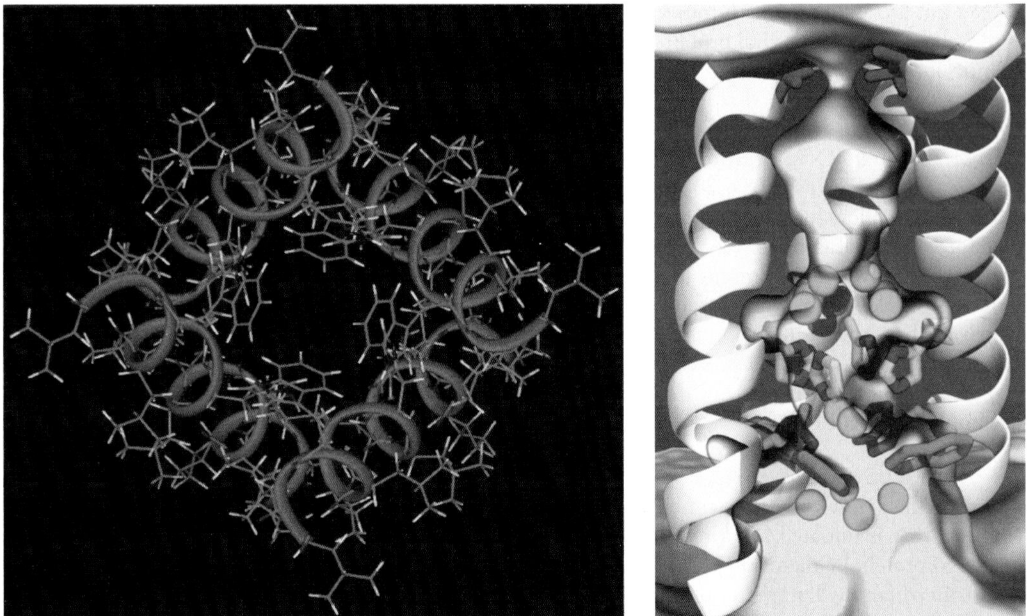

FIGURE 40.11. Structure of the tetrameric M2 ion channel. A: As seen from the top, four helices sit at an angle in the lipid membrane forming a pore. The backbone structure was determined by solid-state nuclear magnetic resonance (NMR) spectroscopy of the aligned bilayers. The histidine 37 and the tryptophan 41 side chains form the bottom of the pore in the closed state at neutral pH. For details see (485). (Courtesy of Tim Cross.) **B:** X-ray structure of the transmembrane section of the M2 proton channel. The protein backbone is shown as a cartoon, viewed from across the viral membrane (lipid molecules and one of the monomers are hidden). Cyan spheres represent crystallographically resolved water molecules, which are stepping stones in possible proton conduction pathways. The three most important groups of side chains (the Val27-valve [blue], the His37-box [orange], and the Trp41-basket [magenta]) are shown in sticks. The three-dimensional density of water at 37°C, calculated from molecular dynamics simulations, is drawn as a white contour. See (1) for details. (Courtesy of Giacomo Fiorin.)

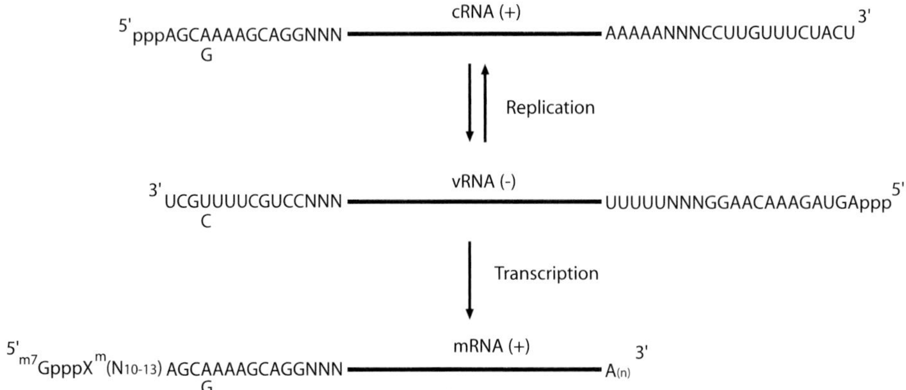

FIGURE 40.12. Influenza virus RNA synthesis. The incoming negative-sense RNA is shown in the middle with the conserved noncoding sequences at either end, adjacent to the segment-specific nucleotides (NNN). The polyadenylation signal consisting of a poly-uridine stretch is at the 5′ end of the viral RNA (vRNA). The messenger RNA (mRNA) derives its cap and 10 to 13 5′ nucleotides from host mRNAs and has a 3′ poly(A) tail. The complementary RNA (cRNA) is an exact positive-sense copy of the incoming virion vRNA. The variation at position 4 in the 3′ vRNA noncoding region is indicated.

Nuclear Import of Ribonucleoproteins

One of the characteristics of the influenza virus life cycle, and one that is unusual for an RNA virus, is its dependence on nuclear functions. All viral RNA synthesis occurs in the nucleus, and the trafficking of the viral genome into and out of the nucleus is a tightly regulated process (reviewed in (54,127)). The eight influenza virus genome segments never exist as naked RNA but are associated with four viral proteins to form vRNP complexes. The major viral protein in the RNP complex is the nucleocapsid protein (NP), which coats the RNA. The remaining proteins are the three polymerase proteins (PB1, PB2, and PA), which bind to the partially complementary ends of the viral RNA, creating the distinctive panhandle structure.[290] These RNPs (10 to 20 nm wide)[115,419] are considered too large to allow for passive diffusion into the nucleus and therefore, once released from an incoming particle, they must rely on an active nuclear import mechanism. All proteins in the RNP complex possess nuclear localization signals (NLSs), which mediate their interaction with the nuclear import machinery.[320,456,470,483,625,702,720] However, it is the signals on NP that have been shown to be both sufficient and necessary for the import of viral RNA[73,126,496,503] (e-Fig. 40.11).

NP Interactions with Karyopherin α

The transport of proteins across the nuclear membrane is an energy-driven process that is initiated upon recognition of an NLS-containing cargo protein by members of the karyopherin α (also called importin α) family. Karyopherin α binds directly to the NLS and then recruits karyopherin β into a trimeric complex, which docks at the nuclear pore (e-Fig. 40.12). Prior to the identification of a definitive NLS within NP, the human homolog of yeast SRP-1 was identified as an NP-interacting partner.[497] This uncharacterized protein was subsequently identified as karyopherin $\alpha 1$ and NP was also shown to interact with another family member, karyopherin $\alpha 2$.[496] The minimal karyopherin α–binding site was used to identify the unconventional NLS in NP, so named because it does not contain a cluster of basic residues.[702] As described earlier,[126] this NLS has been shown to be essential for RNP import, and this implicates karyopherin α as a critical component of RNP nuclear import. Interestingly, the NP NLS-binding site on karyopherin α is distinct from that of classical NLS-containing proteins.[126,437] One could postulate that this serves to avoid competition for karyopherin α binding with host proteins and may explain the use of an unconventional NLS. There is also evidence that differential interactions with human versus avian karyopherin α proteins may determine species specificity of influenza viruses.[197,198]

The Viral Ribonucleoprotein Template

Each viral RNA segment exists as an RNP complex in which the RNA is coated with NP and forms a helical hairpin that is bound on one end by the heterotrimeric polymerase complex (reviewed in (554)). NP is an arginine-rich protein and has a net positive charge (at pH 6.5), which reflects its RNA-binding activity and its primary role in encapsidation (reviewed in (541)). The RNA/NP interaction is thought to be mediated by the positively charged residues on NP and the negatively charged phosphate backbone of the RNA, and thus there is no apparent sequence specificity to the interaction.[30,161] The RNA within the influenza virus RNP also remains sensitive to digestion with RNase,[147] supporting the model that the RNA is wrapped around the outside of the NP with its bases exposed so that they can be accessed by the polymerase without disrupting the RNP structure.[30] Approximately 24 nucleotides of RNA are bound by each NP monomer,[502] and NP also has homo-oligomerization properties,[547] which adds a higher-order structure to the RNP complex. This is maintained even in the absence of RNA[147,576] and has been shown to be crucial for maintaining the RNP in a transcriptionally active form.[83,160] Crystal structures of NP show that it is composed of a head domain and body domain and that a flexible tail loop mediates oligomerization.[481,745] A potential RNA-binding groove, which is highly positively charged, has been identified between the head and body domains.[745] Structural data based on electron microscopy also provide evidence that NP makes direct contact with the bound polymerase complex on the RNP[13,113,419] (e-Fig. 40.13A), which may reflect the previously reported interaction of free NP with both PB1 and PB2.[41] Detailed mutagenesis of conserved residues in NP indicates regions that are involved in genome replication/transcription and also genome packaging.[388]

The RNA Polymerase Complex

The influenza virus RNA-dependent RNA polymerase is a 250-kD complex of three proteins: PB1, PB2 and PA.[59] A three-dimensional image of the complex obtained by electron microscopy indicates that the three subunits are tightly associated to form a compact structure[13,669] (e-Fig. 40.13B). Protein interaction studies have shown that PB1 binds to both PA and PB2, through its N- and C-terminal domains, respectively,[228,492] and that the N-terminus of PA interacts with PB2.[268] The details of how the newly synthesized polymerase is assembled are still under debate. One model proposes that PB1 and PA enter the nucleus as a dimer through interactions with RanBP5 and then bind to PB2, which is imported independently via a karyopherin α interaction.[135,183,300,555,661] This is supported by fluorescent spectroscopy data in live cells.[295] However, another model suggests that PB1-PB2 dimer is transported into the nucleus (via the chaperone Hsp90) and that PA traffics separately.[465] It has also been shown that vRNA can bind to the PB1-PA dimer *in vitro* prior to PB2 binding as well as to the preformed trimeric complex.[136]

The PB1 Protein

The PB1 protein catalyzes the sequential addition of nucleotides during RNA chain elongation[59] and contains the conserved motifs characteristic of RNA-dependent RNA polymerases.[42] The active site for the polymerization activity is an S-D-D motif at positions 444 to 446,[42] but we currently lack structural information for this region. In fact, only small regions encompassing the extreme N- and C-termini of PB1 have been crystallized in complex with portions of PA and PB2, respectively. Two studies have provided x-ray structures of either residues 1 to 81 or 1 to 25 of PB1 in complex with the C-terminal portion of PA,[265,490] and it has been shown that synthetic peptides corresponding to this region of PB1 can compete with full-length PB1 for PA binding and inhibit virus replication.[219] The PB1 C-terminus (residues 678 to 757) has been shown to mediate an interaction with residues 1 through 37 of PB2, and structural analysis of this complex indicates that both peptides form three helices whose folding is dependent on the presence of each partner.[646] PB1 is also responsible for binding to the terminal ends of both vRNA[226,377] and cRNA[227] for initiation of transcription and replication.

The PB2 Protein

The PB2 protein plays a critical role in the initiation of transcription as it is responsible for binding the cap on host pre-mRNA molecules.[43,674] Despite earlier discrepancy in the position of the binding site, it has now been shown that a domain encompassing PB2 residues 318 to 483 is sufficient for cap binding[236] and confirms the findings of a mutagenesis study that identified two aromatic residues (F363 and F404) as being important for the interaction.[171] An x-ray structure of this minimal domain bound to cap analog m^7GTP reveals that the cap is sandwiched between phenylalanine 404 and histidine 357 in a mode similar to that described for other cap-binding proteins, although the involvement of a histidine is unique.[236] In fact, in influenza B and C virus PB2 proteins, the histidine is replaced with a more traditional tryptophan. Both NMR and x-ray structures of the C-terminal domain (aa 678 to 759) of PB2 have been obtained, the latter in complex with karyopherin α1.[661] Within this domain the authors report the presence of a bipartite nuclear localization signal, and in the co-crystal it is shown how this region unfolds to allow for interaction with karyopherin α1. PB2 has also been shown to localize to the mitochondria, and this is determined by an N-terminal mitochondrial-targeting signal.[81] However, avian influenza viruses have a polymorphism in this signal, so it appears that mitochondrial localization of PB2 is unique to human influenza viruses.[229] Finally, as well as interacting with PB1 via its N-terminus (see PB1 section earlier), PB2 is also reported to interact with PA; however, the region of PB2 involved has not yet been defined.[268] PB2 also participates in genome replication as mutations affecting this activity but not transcription have been reported.[215]

The PA Protein

Until recently, the specific function of PA was unknown, but crystal structures of the N-terminal domain revealed that the endonuclease activity of the polymerase, which is required to generate the capped primer, resides in the PA protein.[139,752] Previous work had mistakenly attributed this function to the PB1 protein. In the structure, the fold and position of the active site identifies the PA endonuclease as a member of the PD-(D/E)XK family of nucleases. The catalytic site involves residues His 41, Glu 80, Asp 108, Glu 119, and Lys 134 and harbors two $Mn^{(2+)}$ ions.[124,139] Mutation of these residues abolishes the transcriptional activity of the trimeric polymerase but replication activity is unaffected, confirming the specific role of the endonuclease in viral transcription.[124,752] PA does, however, participate in genome replication as mutations affecting this process have been described.[179,294] In addition to encoding nuclease function, the N-terminus of PA (aa 1 to 100) is also reported to be involved in an interaction with PB2,[268] while the C-terminus makes contact with PB1. Structures of PA residues 257 to 716 show this region forming a "dragon-like head" with the N-terminal peptide of PB1 inserted into the mouth.[265,490] Another function ascribed to PA is that it possesses proteolytic activity.[582] Two residues, S624[255] and T157,[525] have been reported to be involved in the proteolytic function, although viruses containing mutations at position 157 appear to be more severely affected than those mutated at position 624.[294,670] PA has also been shown to be a target for casein kinase II and to be phosphorylated at serine and threonine residues.[583]

The vRNA Promoter

All influenza virus RNA segments contain noncoding sequences at their 5′ and 3′ ends, which flank the coding region. Some of this sequence is segment specific,[766] but the terminal ends are conserved between all segments in all influenza viruses. These conserved 13 nucleotides at the 5′ end and 12 nucleotides at the 3′ end display partial and inverted complementarity, which led to the proposal of a panhandle structure created by base-pairing of the 5′ and 3′ ends.[138,565] This is supported by cross-linking experiments that demonstrated a circular configuration for virion RNAs[290] as well as by more recent structural analysis.[19,419] Studies using *in vitro* transcription of model RNA templates or reporter gene expression *in vivo* have shown that both 5′ and 3′ terminal ends are necessary for promoter activity and that base-pairing is required (reviewed in (177,475)). Furthermore, it has been demonstrated that the polymerase can interact with both 5′ and 3′ ends and that the binding affinity decreases when the duplex is disrupted.[182,226,240,373,664] These data define the vRNA promoter as a double-stranded element formed by the conserved 5′ and 3′ terminal ends of the vRNA molecule.[487] While the need for base-pairing is clear, several models for the secondary structure of the promoter have been proposed based on mutational analyses (e-Fig. 40.14). The original panhandle model predicts extensive Watson-Crick base-pairing, whereas the RNA-fork model proposes that the extreme termini remain single stranded.[181,182,332] The corkscrew model suggests that these single-stranded regions in fact base-pair within themselves to form 5′ and 3′ hairpin loops.[176] The presence of both 5′ and 3′ stem-loops has been shown to be critical for endonuclease activity, and the 5′ stem-loop is also required for polyadenylation.[364,365,545] This favors a model where the stem-loop structures are involved in binding and stabilizing the polymerase complex.[64]

Initiation of Messenger RNA Synthesis

Influenza virus mRNA synthesis is dependent on cellular RNA polymerase II activity. This is because it requires a 5′-capped primer, which it steals from host pre-mRNA transcripts, to initiate its own mRNA synthesis. This process is known as cap snatching and involves the cap-binding function of the PB2 protein and endonuclease function of the PA protein. The initiation of transcription commences with binding of the 5′ end of the vRNA to the PB1 subunit (Fig. 40.13). This induces an allosteric change in the polymerase, which allows the PB2 protein to recognize and bind the cap structure on host pre-mRNAs[106,377] (reviewed in (170)). The change in the polymerase also increases its affinity for the 3′ vRNA end, which is bound by PB1. Binding of the 3′ terminus stabilizes the polymerase complex[64] and also serves to activate the endonuclease function.[106,240,364,377] However, in contrast to this model, one report states that endonuclease activation only requires a bound 5′ end,[551] the difference being that this study used capped RNA fragments with "CA" 3′ termini as primers. Primers with this specific end have previously been shown to be used preferentially for transcription initiation in infected cells.[32,604] Another study indicates that both primer-binding and endonuclease activities are greatly enhanced when the polymerase binds simultaneously to the 5′ and 3′ ends (i.e., in a preformed duplex).[373] Endonuclease activation leads to cleavage of the bound pre-mRNAs. This occurs approximately 10 to 13 nucleotides from their 5′ caps, usually after a purine residue.[32,537] Transcription is then initiated by the addition of a "G" residue to the primer, directed by the penultimate "C" nucleotide at the 3′ end of the vRNA template,[32] although in some instances the incorporation of a "C" that is directed by the "G" at position 3 in the vRNA has also been observed.[181] Unlike influenza viruses, Thogoto viruses lack host-derived sequences at the 5′ end of their capped mRNAs.[719] RNA chain elongation is

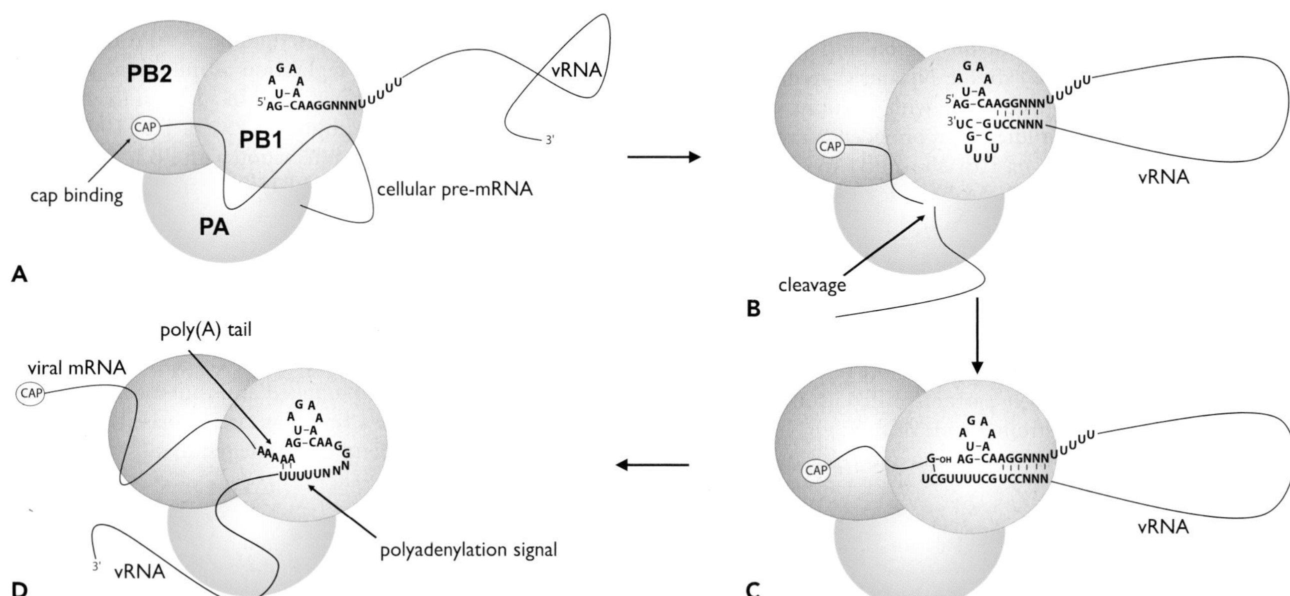

FIGURE 40.13. Proposed model for transcription initiation, elongation, and polyadenylation of influenza virus messenger RNA (mRNA). A: The 5′ end of the viral RNA (vRNA) is shown in the corkscrew configuration bound to the polymerase basic 1 (PB1) subunit of the polymerase complex. This activates the cap-binding activity of the PB2 subunit. **B:** The 3′ end of the vRNA binds to PB1 and forms a duplex with the 5′ end. The endonuclease activity of the polymerase acid (PA) then cleaves the pre-mRNA 10 to 13 nucleotides downstream of the cap structure. **C:** A guanosine residue is added to the 3′ end of the capped primer and base-pairs with the penultimate C residue at the 3′ end of the vRNA. This initiates transcription and chain elongation is catalyzed by the polymerase function of the PB1 subunit. **D:** During elongation the cap detaches from the polymerase. However, the 5′ end of the vRNA remains bound while the template vRNA is read in a 3′ to 5′ direction and consequently the polymerase is unable to read beyond the poly-uridine stretch due to steric hindrance. This causes it to stutter and a poly(A) tail is added to the 3′ end of the nascent mRNA. (Adapted from Fodor E, Brownlee GG. Influenza virus replication. In: Potter CW, ed. *Influenza.* Amsterdam, The Netherlands: Elsevier, 2002:1–29.)

catalyzed by the polymerase function of PB1 and continues until a stretch of uridine residues is encountered approximately 16 nucleotides before the 5′ end of the vRNA.[383,407,566] This is the signal for polyadenylation (Fig. 40.13).

Polyadenylation

Unlike host cells, which use a specific poly(A) polymerase for generating the poly(A) tail on mRNA transcripts, polyadenylation of influenza virus mRNAs is catalyzed by the same polymerase that is used for transcription. This activity is dependent on an uninterrupted stretch of five to seven "U" residues and the adjacent double-stranded region of the vRNA promoter.[383,407,566] The current model proposes that the 5′ end of the vRNA remains bound to the polymerase during elongation while the template is threaded through in a 3′ to 5′ direction (Fig. 40.13). When the polymerase nears the 5′ end to which it is bound, it is blocked by steric hindrance and consequently it stutters on the preceding stretch of uridines, which it repeatedly copies to produce a poly(A) tail.[182,240,539,765] In support of this model, mutations introduced into the 5′ end of the vRNA that prevent or weaken polymerase binding have been shown to also inhibit polyadenylation.[180,540,545,546] The polyadenylation signal is vital for gene expression as replacement of the uridines with adenosines has been shown to result in transcripts with poly(U) tails, which fail to be properly exported from the nucleus.[538]

Splicing

Members of the *Orthomyxovirus* family can extend the coding capacity of their genomes by producing two proteins from one gene via an alternative splicing mechanism. Genome segments that encode proteins from both spliced and unspliced mRNA transcripts are segments 7 and 8 of influenza A virus,[358,360] segment 8 of influenza B virus,[63] segments 6 and 7 of influenza C virus,[468,741] segment 6 of Thogoto virus,[339] and segment 7 of isavirus[40] (see Genome Structure and Organization section). The primary transcripts from these segments have 5′ and 3′ splice sites, which (more or less) fit the consensus sequence for the exon/intron boundaries of cellular transcripts. This, combined with the fact that splicing can be demonstrated in the absence of any viral proteins,[357,359] indicates that the virus is using the cellular splicing machinery. However, unlike cellular splicing, which is extremely efficient, splicing of viral mRNA has to be relatively inefficient because proteins must be expressed from both spliced and unspliced mRNAs. In influenza virus–infected cells, splicing is tightly regulated such that the steady-state level of spliced viral transcripts is only 10% that of the unspliced viral transcripts.[356,360] These control mechanisms may act on several different levels. The rate of nuclear export of the unspliced transcript is certainly crucial as this determines its availability for splicing. It has been proposed that the NS1 protein inhibits both the splicing and nuclear export of NS1 transcripts via negative feedback,[8,209] but contradictory reports[559] suggest that alternative mechanisms may exist for regulating splicing of viral transcripts. Potentially these may involve *cis*-acting sequences in the NS1 transcript that negatively control the rate of splicing.[7,474] Strangely, the influenza C virus NS1 protein has been reported to up-regulate viral mRNA splicing.[458] Splicing of the influenza A virus M1 transcript is controlled by the aforementioned rate of nuclear export[675] as well as by the viral polymerase and a cellular splicing factor, SF2/ASF. The polymerase determines the time at which splicing (and hence production of M2) occurs, and SF2/ASF is required to activate splicing.[605,606]

Replication Products: cRNA and vRNA

Full-length copies of the incoming vRNA have to be made, and these positive-sense cRNAs serve as templates for the synthesis of new negative-sense genomic vRNA. *In vitro* evidence suggests that the *de novo* initiation mode for vRNA synthesis may occur via terminal initiation and elongation, whereas for cRNA synthesis it involves internal initiation and realignment.[137] This is a primer-independent model; however, a primer-dependent mode of vRNA initiation has also been proposed.[528] The cRNA promoter is complementary to the vRNA promoter and has also been reported to assume a corkscrew configuration, albeit with subtle differences.[18,129,519,766] This variation has been implicated in determining whether or not the endonuclease function of the polymerase is activated and therefore may play an important regulatory role.[366]

The Switch from Transcription to Replication

The vRNA serves as a template for both mRNA and cRNA synthesis, and yet the means of initiation and termination for the generation of these two molecules are quite different. In contrast to the primer-dependent mechanism of initiation of mRNA synthesis, initiation of cRNA synthesis occurs without a capped primer and cRNA molecules are full-length copies of the vRNA and thus are not prematurely terminated and polyadenylated as are mRNAs. The different initiation and termination reactions therefore have to be coordinated, but exactly how the polymerase switches between these two modes is not well understood. It has been proposed that the transcription-competent polymerase is structurally different from the replication-competent polymerase, and support for this theory comes from evidence that different domains of PB1 are involved in binding vRNA versus cRNA and that PA is more critical for binding the cRNA than the vRNA promoter.[227,412] One obvious difference is that the cap-binding and endonuclease functions of PB2 and PA are not required when the polymerase is in replication mode.

In contrast to mRNAs, newly synthesized cRNAs and vRNAs are encapsidated, and it has been proposed that the availability of soluble NP (i.e., not associated with RNPs) controls the switch between mRNA and cRNA synthesis. This hypothesis arose from the observation that replication is dependent on *de novo* protein synthesis, which means that the incoming RNPs are only capable of transcription.[263] Indeed, free NP has been shown to be required for production of full-length cRNA (antitermination),[33] and this is consistent with data from temperature-sensitive (ts) NP mutants,[345,435,598] which show that cRNA but not mRNA synthesis is affected at the nonpermissive temperature. However, this model has been challenged by a report demonstrating that overexpressed NP does not promote replication.[457] Another study disputes the existence of a switch, rather suggesting a stabilization role for NP and the polymerase.[694] It claims that the incoming polymerase is able to synthesize both mRNA and cRNA,[690] but until there is a sufficient pool of polymerase and NP to encapsidate the cRNA, it is degraded and therefore at early times postinfection there is a bias toward mRNA accumulation. Also, requirements for higher nucleotide concentrations to initiate cRNA synthesis may determine the timing of transcription versus replication.[693] Furthermore, the accumulation of NEP/NS2 is associated with a decrease in transcription and an increase in replication, suggesting a regulatory role.[74,560] Interestingly, NEP/NS2 is also required for the generation of small viral RNAs (svRNAs), which have been implicated in the initiation of vRNA synthesis.[528] The svRNAs are 22 to 27 nt in length and correspond to the 5′ end of each viral RNA segment. These segment-specific svRNAs are needed for vRNA but not cRNA synthesis, so according to this model the polymerase is in replication mode when these svRNAs are present. It has also been proposed that the switch from transcription to replication is the result of accumulation of a newly synthesized free polymerase complex, which enhances cRNA to vRNA synthesis (and vice versa) over mRNA synthesis.[322] The role of host factors in regulating influenza virus replication, including posttranslational modification of viral proteins, should also not be excluded.[51,323,392,427,449,450]

Regulation of Viral Gene Expression

Early studies have provided evidence for temporal regulation of viral gene expression,[263,624] but the mechanism(s) is still unresolved. Disproportionate accumulation of mRNAs from the eight segments has been observed, but whether this represents specific up-regulation of transcription for these segments[164,260] or reflects different rates of vRNA synthesis[597,624] or RNA stability is unclear. Suffice to say that the synthesis of NP and NS1 mRNAs and protein is favored at early stages, whereas the synthesis of HA, NA, and particularly M1 mRNAs and proteins is delayed.[260,263,597,624] This differential expression is mirrored by the roles these proteins play at different points in the virus life cycle. As discussed earlier, NP is required for replication, and NS1 plays a crucial role in combating the host immune response; thus, both these proteins are needed early in the virus life cycle. M1 has been found to inhibit viral transcription,[527,713] which demands its delayed expression, and at later stages M1 accumulation probably dictates the arrest of viral mRNA synthesis. M1 is also involved in the export of RNPs from the nucleus,[420] which must only occur once replication is complete.

Another control mechanism for differential gene expression resides in the vRNA promoter. A natural variation is found at position 4 from the 3′ vRNA end in an otherwise totally conserved region. The PB1, PB2, and PA RNA segments have a "C" at this position, while the remaining segments usually have a "U." The C4-containing promoter is associated with a down-regulation in transcription and an up-regulation in replication compared to the U4 promoter,[370] which correlates with the lower amounts of polymerase mRNAs and proteins found in infected cells.[263,624] A structural analysis of the C4 and U4 promoters has revealed differences that may alter their interaction with the polymerase and thereby regulate gene expression.[372]

As observed with many other viruses, influenza virus gene expression is also controlled at the level of translation. This is achieved via numerous mechanisms and results in the selective translation of viral genes and suppression of host protein synthesis (reviewed in (200,692,743)). These mechanisms include (a) degradation of host pre-mRNAs following cleavage (due to cap-snatching), (b) inhibition of host mRNA processing, (c) degradation of cellular RNA polymerase II, and (d) preferential translation of viral mRNA transcripts. Several of these processes involve the influenza virus NS1 protein. The NS1-mediated effect on mRNA processing is discussed in a later section (see The Actions of Influenza Virus Nonstructural Proteins on the Host Cell). NS1 is also involved in the specific translational enhancement of viral mRNAs through its association with the 5′ noncoding region of viral mRNA transcripts and with cellular proteins involved in translation initiation.[11,76,520] These include the translation initiation factor eIF4GI and poly(A)-binding protein 1, and it has been proposed that this protein complex acts to specifically recruit ribosomes to the 5′ end of viral mRNA transcript. Another cellular protein that may play a role is GRSF-1, an RNA-binding protein that has been reported to interact with the 5′ end of the NP transcript and to stimulate the specific translation of a template driven by the NP 5′ noncoding region in a cell-free translation system.[326,521] Whether this interaction is relevant *in vivo* remains to be determined.

An interesting model explaining the selective translation of viral mRNAs has been proposed suggesting that the viral polymerase complex remains associated with the viral mRNA transcript in the cytoplasm. It is thought that this interaction eliminates the need for complex formation with eIF4E. As eIF4E is inactivated in influenza virus–infected cells,[172] this would explain the selective translation of viral transcripts over cellular transcripts. Other components of the translation machinery, such as eIF4A and eIF4G, are required for influenza viral protein translation.[742] Although this model is compelling in its simplicity, this mechanism is questioned by the finding that viral mRNAs in the cytoplasm are devoid of viral polymerase but are associated with cellular cap-binding proteins, including eIF4E.[39] Clearly, further investigation is required to explain the selective translation of viral transcripts in infected cells.

An additional host shut-off mechanism is controlled by the viral polymerase at the level of host transcription. It has been shown that the influenza virus polymerase interacts with the C-terminal domain of the large subunit of cellular RNA polymerase II[167] and that this interaction mediates the degradation of RNA polymerase II at late times postinfection.[568,691] This may play a role in viral pathogenicity because attenuated influenza viruses have been shown not to induce RNA polymerase II degradation.[567]

Virus Assembly and Release

Nuclear Export of Ribonucleoproteins

Association of RNP with M1

Following virus replication, newly formed RNP complexes are assembled in the nucleus from where they are exported into the cytoplasm. Two viral proteins, the matrix protein (M1) and the nuclear export protein (NEP/NS2), are involved in directing the nuclear export of RNPs (reviewed in (54,127)). Our present understanding of this process indicates that M1 associates with RNPs in the nucleus and may actually promote the formation of RNP complexes.[293] M1 makes contact with both the vRNA and NP[31,746] (reviewed in (127,472)), and evidence that M1 also binds to nucleosomes[210,769] has led to the hypothesis that M1 interactions cause the dissociation of RNP from the nuclear matrix. This agrees with the significant finding that nuclear import of M1 is required for subsequent export of RNP complexes.[72,420] Furthermore, at high temperatures, heat shock protein 70 is found bound to RNP, which prevents association with M1 and results in a block in RNP export.[273,580] Recently it has been reported that sumoylation of M1 is essential for its nuclear export function.[732]

NEP/NS2 Interacts with the Cellular Export Machinery

Initially these data suggested that M1 alone could control RNP export, but as is the case for import, nuclear export of large molecules involves direct interactions with the cellular export machinery and as yet no such interactions with M1 have been demonstrated. However, NEP/NS2 has been found to interact with the export receptor Crm1[477] and several nucleoporins.[91,498] NEP/NS2 also associates with M1,[4,608,744] so the current model is that an RNP–M1–NEP/NS2 complex is formed in the nucleus and that NEP/NS2 is responsible for recruiting the export machinery and directing export of the complex (e-Fig. 40.15). In support of this role, it has been shown that injection of anti-NEP/NS2 antibodies into the nucleus of infected cells inhibits RNP export,[498] which is also seen in a system using recombinant virus-like particles lacking NEP/NS2.[477] A methionine/leucine-rich nuclear export signal (NES) has been identified in the N-terminus of NEP/NS2[498] and shown to be critical for RNP export and virus growth[309,477]; however, this NES does not appear to mediate the interaction of NEP/NS2 with Crm1.[477] Yet treatment with leptomycin B, a Crm1 inhibitor, completely inhibits RNP export in infected cells, which indicates that export does occur in a Crm1-dependent manner.[162,309,714]

Another viral protein, NP, has also been shown to bind to Crm1[162] and therefore is proposed to play a role in export as well as import. Both this study and another also revealed that RNPs are localized to the periphery of the nucleus after leptomycin B treatment but that M1 and NEP/NS2 retain diffuse nuclear staining.[162,410] The RNPs were shown to co-localize with nuclear lamins just beneath the nuclear pore complex, which may represent an intermediate step prior to export through the pore.[410] The roles of M1 and NEP/NS2 are obviously called into question by their differing staining pattern compared to RNP,[162,410] but this could be explained if only a fraction of the total M1 and NEP/NS2 pool was used for export. Nevertheless, it raises the possibility that redundant export mechanisms may exist.

Regulation of RNP Export

As discussed earlier, the late expression of M1 determines that export takes place only after a full round of replication has occurred, therefore preventing premature exit of RNPs from the nucleus. Similarly, control mechanisms must also exist to stop the re-entry of RNPs into the nucleus following export. Studies with a temperature-sensitive virus (ts51) showed that when grown at the nonpermissive temperature, this virus is unable to retain its RNPs in the cytoplasm following export.[723] This defect mapped to M1,[724] once again demonstrating the vital role of this protein in regulating the nucleocytoplasmic transport of RNPs. It is interesting to note that the NEP/NS2-binding site on M1 maps to the M1 NLS,[4] which suggests that NEP/NS2 may act to mask the NLS on M1 and therefore prevent the complex from re-entering the nucleus. NP is also proposed to cause the cytoplasmic retention of RNPs by binding to filamentous actin and thereby anchoring the RNPs in the cytoplasm.[140] All these processes are likely to be regulated at some level, and protein modification by phosphorylation is probably involved as several studies have reported alterations in M1, NEP/NS2, and NP trafficking in the presence of kinase inhibitors.[70–72,536,553,724]

RNP Export in Influenza B and C Viruses

Few studies concerning export in influenza B and C viruses have been performed, but it has been shown that as with influenza A viruses, the NEP/NS2 proteins possess nuclear export activities.[518] They have both been shown to interact with Crm1 (and a subset of nucleoporins), and NES motifs have been defined in each protein. Interestingly, the influenza C virus NES is composed of two separate leucine-rich domains, both of which are required for full activity.[518] In contrast to influenza A virus where M1 acts as a bridge between NEP/NS2 and the RNP complex, the influenza B NEP/NS2 has been proposed to bind directly to RNP as well as to M1,[304] which suggests that the model for export of influenza B virus RNPs may be slightly different.

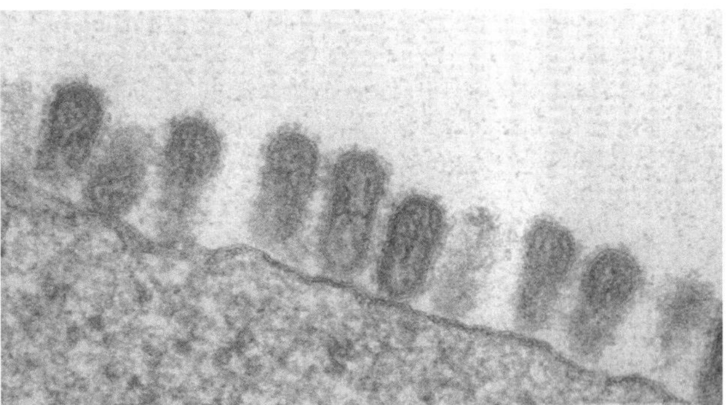

FIGURE 40.14. Budding influenza virus particles. Electron micrograph thin section image of influenza virus particles budding from the apical surface of an infected cell. (Courtesy of Yi-ying Chou.)

The Site of Virus Assembly and Budding

Influenza viruses assemble and bud from the apical plasma membrane of polarized cells (e.g., lung epithelial cells of the infected host)[53] (reviewed in (573,587)) (Fig. 40.14). This asymmetrical process (i.e., apical vs. basolateral) is thought to have an important role in viral pathogenesis and tissue tropism in that viruses that bud from the internal cell surface (e.g., Marburg virus) tend to cause systemic disease, whereas viruses such as influenza virus that bud from the external cell surface generally have a more restricted tissue tropism.[173] The influenza virus HA, NA, and M2 have all been shown to localize to the apical surface of polarized cells when expressed alone,[296,321,574] and apical sorting signals have been identified within the transmembrane domains of HA and NA.

The M1 Protein

M1 is the most abundant virion protein and lies just beneath the lipid envelope where it is believed to make contact with the cytoplasmic tails of the glycoproteins and with the RNPs, thereby forming a bridge between the inner core components and the membrane proteins (reviewed in (471,587)). Structural analyses indicate that the M1 protein consists of two globular helical domains that are linked by a protease-sensitive region.[14,257,595] Rods (6 nm in length) corresponding to M1 monomers have been observed by negative stain electron microscopy of virions with one end in contact with the membrane and the other end pointing toward the interior of the particle.[575] These rods form an ordered structure consistent with the homo-oligomerization properties of M1[80,764] and are arranged such that the positive and negatively charged residues are on opposite sides of the oligomer.[14,257] Several reports have documented the ability of M1 to associate with lipid membranes[163,575,759] (reviewed in (471,587)), and as mentioned previously (see section on Nuclear Export of Ribonucleoproteins), M1 interacts with both RNP and NEP/NS2. M1 also interacts with the cytoplasmic tail of M2.[87] Therefore, it is proposed that M1 plays a vital role in assembly by recruiting the viral components to the site of assembly at the plasma membrane.

Assembly of Viral Components

Following synthesis on membrane-bound ribosomes, the three integral membrane proteins, HA, NA, and M2, enter the ER where they are folded and glycosylated (except for M2) and where HA is assembled into a trimer and NA and M2 into tetramers (reviewed in (141)). They are subsequently transported to the Golgi apparatus where cysteine residues on HA and M2 are palmitoylated in the *cis*-Golgi network.[635,647,681–683] For those HAs that have a multibasic cleavage site (i.e., some H5 and H7 subtypes), furin cleavage of HA into HA1 and HA2 subunits may occur in the *trans*-Golgi network.[642] From here HA, NA, and M2 are all directed to the virus assembly site on the apical plasma membrane via their apical sorting signals. The signals for HA and NA have been described to reside in their transmembrane domains (TMDs).[26,350,393] The TMDs of HA and NA also contain the determinants for association with lipid rafts[26,393] (reviewed in (25)). Lipid rafts are nonionic detergent-resistant lipid microdomains within the plasma membrane that are rich in sphingolipids and cholesterol (reviewed in (499)), and examination of the lipid content of purified virus particles indicates that influenza virus buds preferentially from these domains.[585,760] HA and NA individually also selectively accumulate at and are incorporated into rafts.[350,586] Although the signals for apical sorting and raft association both lie within the TMD, they are not mutually exclusive (reviewed in (25,472)). Raft association of HA has been shown to be essential for efficient virus replication.[655] This is thought to be because of a requirement for concentrated "patches" of HA at the plasma membrane, which governs the level of HA incorporation into budding particles and hence affects fusion. A similar explanation holds for raft association of NA, as an optimal amount of NA must be incorporated to allow for efficient virus release.[24] In contrast to HA and NA, the majority of M2 protein is excluded from lipid rafts,[760] which may reflect its low abundance in virus particles. M2 has been shown to bind cholesterol and this property is suggested to target M2 to the raft periphery where it may act to bridge several raft domains.[591] Mutation of the cholesterol recognition/interaction amino acid consensus (CRAC) motif in M2 is reported to affect membrane targeting but not raft association,[662] and in the context of a recombinant virus it is shown to attenuate the virus *in vivo* but not in tissue culture.[641] There is also evidence that M2 is involved in capturing the RNPs at the assembly site. Experimental evidence for this mechanism was first demonstrated with an influenza B virus that lacked BM2 expression and produced particles devoid of RNPs.[303] Subsequently, mutation or truncation of the influenza A virus M2 cytoplasmic tail has been shown to correspond with decreased incorporation of genome segments into virions.[231,310,431,432]

In comparison to the integral membrane proteins, relatively little is known about how the remaining viral components reach the assembly site. A long-standing hypothesis is that M1 acts as the master recruiter as dictated by its position between the viral envelope and the RNP core. This is supported by evidence that the availability of M1 affects the timing of assembly and maturation, as seen with a virus engineered to express reduced levels of protein from the M segment.[56] This virus showed no defects in virion protein composition but displayed delayed growth kinetics, suggesting that a minimum amount of M1 protein must accumulate before assembly can begin. The association of M1 with the RNP–NEP/NS2 complex is well described (see section on Nuclear Export of Ribonucleoproteins), but the specific interaction of M1 with the membrane-bound glycoproteins has been difficult to prove because of its intrinsic membrane-binding properties and initially resulted in some conflicting reports.[163,344,759] However, it was noted that in influenza virus–infected cells M1 becomes resistant to extraction with Triton X-100 (a marker for lipid raft association), whereas M1 expressed alone remains soluble.[6,759] This suggested a role for other viral proteins, and indeed, coexpression of HA and NA together with M1 has been shown to promote raft association of M1.[6] This requires the TMDs and cytoplasmic tails of HA and NA,[6,760] and in the absence of the cytoplasmic tails of these two proteins, virus particles have been found to be grossly distorted, which perhaps indicates reduced M1 association.[317] The hypothetical model therefore proposes that M1 becomes associated with the glycoproteins during their passage through the exocytic pathway and "hitches a ride" to raft domains in the apical membrane, taking the RNP–NEP/NS2 complex with it. However, alternative models have been suggested, and these include the possibility that the M1/RNP complex may use the cytoskeleton to reach the virus assembly site. This is fueled by the finding that both NP and M1 interact with cytoskeletal components.[17] The M1 interaction is dependent on the presence of RNP and is most likely mediated by direct binding of F-actin by NP.[17,140] However, an intact cytoskeleton has only been found to be necessary for the production of filamentous virus particles,[563,614] so a specific role in assembly *per se* is debatable, although actin does appear to be involved in the organization of lipid rafts.[614] Finally, there is evidence that NP alone is intrinsically targeted to the apical plasma membrane and associates with lipid rafts in a cholesterol-dependent manner, which suggests that RNPs could reach the assembly site independently of the other viral components.[82] Recent studies have shown that the Rab11-dependent recycling endosome is critical for the delivery of RNPs to the plasma membrane.[9,155,451] as is another endosomal protein, human immunodeficiency virus rev-binding protein (HRB), which interacts with NEP.[156]

Packaging of Eight RNA Segments

Correct assembly and packaging of a full complement of RNA genome segments is a requirement for a fully infectious virion. The precise mechanism of packaging of the eight viral RNA segments is not well understood, although two different models have been proposed. The first model, *the random incorporation model,* assumes that a common structural feature is present on all vRNAs (vRNPs), which enables them to be randomly incorporated into budding virions. This model is supported by evidence that virions may possess more than eight vRNPs, ensuring the presence of a full complement of eight vRNPs in a significant percentage of virus particles.[22,166,207] Mathematical analysis of packaging suggests that if eight RNA segments were randomly packaged into budding virions, only 0.24% of released virus particles would be infectious.[166] However, if a greater number of RNA segments were randomly packaged, then the percentage of infectious particles increases (reviewed in (114)). If 12 RNA molecules are packaged per virion, then approximately 10% of the virus particles would be infectious,[166] a number that is compatible with experimental data ((142) and reviewed in (114)).

The second model, *the selective incorporation model,* suggests that each vRNA segment acts independently, allowing each segment to be packaged selectively. A similar model has been reported for the packaging of the 3 double-stranded RNA (dsRNA) segments of bacteriophage $\varphi6$ (reviewed in (446)) and for the packaging of the 11 dsRNA segments of rotavirus (RV) (reviewed in (433)). This model suggests that each vRNA segment contains a unique "packaging signal" and predicts that every virion possesses a full complement of the eight vRNP segments. There is increasing evidence to support this model. First, the precise number of RNAs packaged in a single virion has been determined by imaging of serially sectioned budding virions using electron microscopy.[489] Each virion appears to contain exactly eight vRNPs organized in a distinct pattern: one in the center and seven in the surrounding positions. The eight vRNPs are oriented perpendicular to the budding tip. Second, the existence of packaging signals within the noncoding and coding regions at both the 5′ and 3′ ends of the genomic RNAs has been confirmed (e-Fig. 40.16). Coding regions of the NA[191]; HA[718]; NS[189]; PB2, PB1, and PA[390,462]; NP[503]; and M[505] segments have all been demonstrated to increase the ability of a reporter sequence to be incorporated within assembling virions. Both the coding and noncoding regions of the packaging signals are relatively conserved compared to other parts of the sequences.[194,224] Mutations introduced into the packaging signal region of one segment can result in a decrease in packaging efficiency of the segment itself and other segments,[299,302,391,416,417] suggesting the existence of specific interactions among genomic segments. Interestingly, data also show that efficient packaging of the NS segment does not absolutely require the original sequences of the packaging signal.[190] Segment-specific packaging is hypothesized to occur via specific RNA–RNA or protein–RNA interactions, but exactly how the packaging signals participate during the genome packaging process is yet to be determined. Another piece of evidence supporting the specific packaging model is the generation of a rewired influenza virus carrying the HA packaging signal on the NS segment and the NS packaging signal on the HA segment.[208] The modified virus grew well; however, it lost its ability to independently reassort its rewired HA or NS segment with a wild-type virus, indicating that only viruses containing a full complement of all eight packaging signals will grow to high yields. This model is also supported by data showing specific interference of deleted RNA segments with packaging of the corresponding wild-type RNA segment but not with any other genome segment.[148,149] It will be interesting to define the precise sequences or structures that determine the specific packaging of each segment. Such conserved features must also be compatible with the divergent sequences observed among influenza viruses. For further details about the influenza genome packaging process, please see the reviews by Noda et al[488] and Hutchinson et al.[301]

The Budding Process

Initiation of bud formation requires outward curvature of the plasma membrane. The virus bud is then extruded until the inner core is enveloped. The budding process is completed when the membranes fuse at the base of the bud and the enveloped virus particle is released following fission from the cell membrane (reviewed in (573,587)). It is likely that several of the influenza virus structural proteins contribute to the budding process. HA, NA, and M2, when expressed alone in transfected cells, are all competent to form virus-like particles (VLPs).[88,352,750] Although M1 obviously participates in the formation of virus particles from infected cells, unlike other viral matrix proteins, it does not appear to possess a late domain sequence that mediates interaction with the cellular ESCRT pathway.[66,572,715] It has also been demonstrated that in the absence of other viral proteins, M1 does not associate with membranes.[700] Thus, it appears that there are redundant mechanisms for the initiation of bud formation, and in the context of an infected cell it is presently unclear which of these are dominant. The extent to which the membrane is extruded before pinching off occurs affects the size and shape of the virus particle. Generally, influenza virus particles are either spherical or filamentous, and this characteristic morphology is genetically linked to the M segment[55,159,564,621] (e-Fig. 40.1). It has been further shown that the determinants for a particular filamentous isolate (A/Udorn/72[H3N2]) map to two residues (R95 and E204) in the M1 protein,[55] although other residues in M1 as well as in the cytoplasmic tail of M2 are also involved in regulating morphology.[231,310,564,571] Host factors such as polarization and an intact actin cytoskeleton also play a critical role in determining the morphology of virus particles.[563,614] The final step of the budding process is membrane scission, which may be facilitated by both viral and cellular factors. The amphipathic helix in the cytoplasmic tail of M2 has been demonstrated to mediate membrane curvature and scission.[572] Also, the small guanosine triphosphate (GTP)-binding protein, Rab11, has been implicated in this process.[65]

Release

Influenza virus particles have to be actively released after the viral envelope has separated from the cell membrane during the completion of budding. This is because the HA anchors the virus to the cell by binding to sialic acid–containing receptors on the cell surface. The enzymatic activity of the NA protein is required to remove the sialic acid and thereby releases the virus from its host cell. NA activity is also required to remove sialic acid from the carbohydrates present on the viral glycoproteins themselves so that the individual virus particles do not aggregate. The essential function of NA in particle release has been demonstrated through the use of NA inhibitors,[404,510] ts NA mutant viruses,[516] and NA-deficient viruses.[395] In all cases, the absence of NA enzymatic activity was seen to cause viral particles to amass in clumps at the cell surface (Fig. 40.15), resulting in a loss in infectivity that could be restored by addition of exogenous sialidase.

Due to the fact that both HA and NA recognize the same molecule (sialic acid) but have opposing effects (receptor binding vs. receptor destroying), a delicate balance exists between the HA and NA functions.[697] This is optimized for individual viruses but if disturbed can result in attenuation.[748]

The Neuraminidase

The NA is the second major glycoprotein of influenza A and B viruses and is a type II integral membrane protein with its

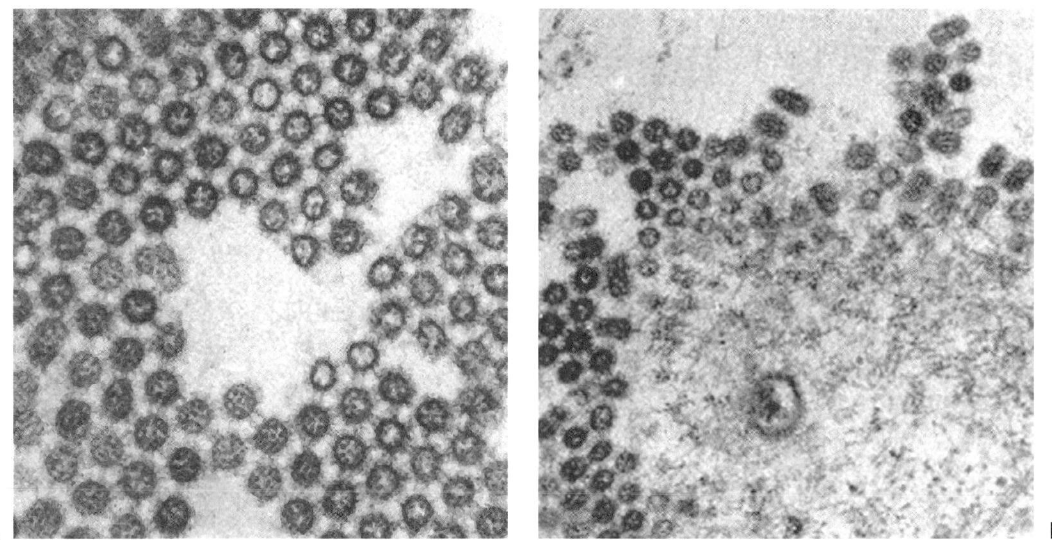

FIGURE 40.15. Aggregate formation of influenza virus particles in the absence of neuraminidase activity. Electron micrograph thin section images showing aggregates of temperature-sensitive neuraminidase (NA) mutant influenza virus grown at nonpermissive temperature **(A)** or grown in the presence of the neuraminidase inhibitor FANA **(B)**. For details see (516) and (510).

N-terminus oriented toward the interior of the virus[109] (for review see (204) and for an interesting personal account see (362)). The nine subtypes of the A virus NA fall into two major groups (N1, N4, N5, N8 and N2, N3, N6, N7, N9) based on sequence comparisons[186] (Fig. 40.2). No subtypes have been found for the NAs of B viruses, possibly because these viruses do not have an animal reservoir. The influenza A virus NAs have a highly conserved short cytoplasmic tail and a hydrophobic transmembrane region, which provides the anchor for the stalk and the head domains. The purified head domain of an N2 NA (obtained by pronase treatment of whole virus) was first crystallized by Graeme Laver and its x-ray crystallographic structure was solved by Peter Colman.[112] The structure of the N1 NA from the 1918 pandemic virus has also been determined.[738] The head of the NA is a homotetramer, each monomer of which is composed of six topologically identical β sheets arranged in a propeller formation. Sugar residues are attached to four of the five potential glycosylation sites in the head (e-Fig. 40.17). The structure of the influenza B virus neuraminidase, similar to that of the A virus, is characterized by the interaction of the sialic acid ligand with nine conserved active site residues.[78] The enzymatic activity of NA was first recognized by George Hirst, who found that red blood cells treated with virus were refractory to reagglutination by another virus preparation.[274] The enzyme was also found to cleave (at position 2 of neuraminic acid) ketosidically bound sugars of alcohols (for review, see (68)), and neuraminidases from different subtypes are described to have different substrate specificities.[385,543] Transition state inhibitors such as 2-deoxy-2,3-dehydro-N-trifluoroacetylneuraminic acid, which mimic the enzymatic substrate, were shown early on to inhibit influenza virus replication,[515] and compounds with the same mechanism of action were later developed for use as highly effective antivirals in humans (for review, see (214,315,434)). Early work had also elucidated the function of the NA in virus replication. Cells infected by temperature-sensitive mutants with defects in the NA were shown by electron microscopy to have large aggregates of intact virus particles accumulating near the cell surface (Fig. 40.15). This finding was interpreted to mean that the viral NA must remove the sialic/neuraminic acid receptor from the surface of the cell as well as from the virus particles to prevent recognition by the HA of the virus. The NA thus has a role in releasing the virus from the infected cell and in cleansing the environment (e.g., mucus and cell surfaces in the respiratory tract) of sialic acid receptors to allow for virus spread.[510,516] In addition, it has been shown that the viral NA may also play a role early in infection, possibly facilitating entry of the virus[426,493] and/or enhancing late endosome/lysosome trafficking.[652] As described earlier (see Budding Process), the NA can also mediate virus budding[352,750] and the cellular restriction factor, tetherin, can influence this step.[716,750] Another function for at least one subtype NA has also been reported. In the case of an N9 NA, a hemadsorption activity was found to be associated with the purified molecule, and x-ray structure analysis revealed a second independent binding site for sialic acid.[678] This activity is only associated with avian neuraminidases and appears to be lost upon adaption to humans.[673]

It is assumed that the function of the influenza B virus NA is similar, if not identical, to that of the A virus NA,[220,405] and the active sites of influenza A and B virus NAs are conserved, which allows for broad-spectrum activity of NA inhibitors. In influenza C viruses, the receptor-destroying role of the NA is played by the esterase activity of the viral HEF. By removing the acetyl group from 9-O-acetylneuraminic acid, the HEF facilitates the release and spread of virus from infected cells. In addition, it appears that the enzyme is needed for virus entry, suggesting that there is a need for the HEF to be released from cell receptors during the endosomal uptake and fusion/uncoating process.[688]

Like the HA, NA molecules are antigenic and variants are selected in nature. Antibodies directed against the NA are usually not neutralizing, but immunization with NA preparations has been proposed as an infection-permissive, disease-suppressive vaccine approach against influenza.[330,654]

Interactions of Influenza Virus with the Host Cell

Cellular Functions Required for Influenza Virus Replication

A virus with a small coding capacity, such as influenza virus, relies on numerous host cell functions in order to complete its replication cycle. In comparison to our understanding of the role of each viral protein in the influenza virus life cycle, we know relatively little about the contribution of host cell proteins. Some well-characterized interactions between viral and host proteins are noted in the sections covering specific viral proteins (e.g., NP and karyopherin α, NEP/NS2 and Crm1, NS1 and CPSF30), but these probably represent only a small fraction of the molecular interactions that occur between influenza virus and its host cell during the viral life cycle. More recent efforts to expand our knowledge of these cellular binding partners have involved a comprehensive yeast two-hybrid analysis of 10 influenza virus proteins (all except PB1-F2), which identified interactions with 87 human proteins.[596] These interactions exist in a tightly connected network, as 24 of the human proteins interact with two or more viral proteins and there are 51 known interactions occurring between the 87 human proteins. Other studies have examined interacting partners of viral protein complexes rather than individual proteins, and particularly those that retain functionality such as the RNP or trimeric polymerase complexes. Forty-one human proteins were reported to interact with the viral RNP complex of influenza A/WSN/33 (H1N1) virus,[427] and 13 interacting proteins were identified in two studies on the WSN polymerase complex.[323,427] A recent large-scale proteomic analysis of an H5N1 influenza virus polymerase complex has revealed an astonishing 859 human proteins that are associated with either the full polymerase complex or PA-containing subcomponents thereof.[60] In their analyses, the authors also distinguished between those interactions that are dependent on RNA and those that are not. In summary, 166 PA interacting proteins, 23 that bind to the PB1-PA dimer and 10 that associate with the full polymerase, were identified irrespective of the presence of RNA. Notably, a number of the PA-interacting host proteins are localized to the mitochondria and may be linked to apoptosis. Functional studies are now required to determine if these interacting proteins are required for efficient replication of influenza virus or whether they perhaps play an antiviral role. Using RNAi, 31 proteins known for interacting with the vRNP or polymerase complex were assessed for their role in polymerase activity.[51] Eighteen were shown to facilitate the activities of both H1N1 and H5N1 polymerases, while two antagonized both polymerases, supporting the idea that interacting proteins are likely to play functional roles. Moreover, Bortz et al[51] showed that an interaction with human DDX17 is specifically associated with promoting activity of the mammalian adapted H5N1 polymerase (PB2 627K), while the chicken homolog is required by the avian H5N1 polymerase (PB2 627E). Thus, knowledge of these interactions provides a molecular basis for host adaptation and contributes to our understanding of differing pathogenicity phenotypes.

Completion of the human genome and the discovery of RNAi have made it possible to query the participation of each human gene product in functional assays using genome-wide small interfering (siRNA) libraries. Using this powerful tool, genome-wide RNAi screens have been performed on influenza virus–infected cells to identify those genes that are required for efficient virus growth (reviewed in (636,717)). These five studies[61,254,325,341,596] identified a total of 1,077 unique genes that when targeted by siRNAs lead to decreased influenza virus replication. Each study employed different assay conditions and this likely contributes to the finding that only 85 genes were common to two or more of the screens (34 of these were validated with at least two different siRNAs and with wild-type influenza virus [Fig. 40.16]). However, a greater degree of concordance is seen when one analyzes the results at the level of cellular function rather than gene name.[600,636,717] Host factors involved in kinase-mediated signaling, pre-mRNA processing, nucleocytoplasmic transport, the COPI complex, and the vacuolar-type H+ ATPase (vATPase) complex are all significantly enriched (Fig. 40.16), indicating that these processes are critical for influenza virus replication. Depending on the design of the assay used for the RNAi screen, it is also possible to detect factors that have antiviral activity and thus enhance virus replication when they are depleted. The interferon-inducible transmembrane (IFITM) proteins were identified in this manner and are thought to inhibit entry of influenza virus as well as several other viruses.[61,292]

Future progress in this area will depend on integrating the data obtained from these global approaches (e.g., proteomics, RNAi, microarray) to build a clearer picture of the cellular networks that govern efficient influenza virus growth. Such information may address questions concerning species specificity and also provide new avenues to explore for drug discovery (see section on Inhibition of Cellular Factors).

The Actions of the NS1 Protein

When a virus infects a cell, it has to contend with the rapid onset of the host innate immune response, whose mission it is to establish an antiviral state within the cell and prevent virus replication. A critical component of this response is type I interferon (IFN-α/β), which is secreted from virus-infected cells. A characteristic feature of all orthomyxoviruses is their sensitivity to the inhibitory effect of IFN-inducible Mx GTPases.[251] In fact, IFN was first described as a factor induced by heat-inactivated influenza virus,[305] although interestingly, live influenza virus was found to inhibit the induction of IFN by inactivated virus.[394] The reason for this observation did not become clear until almost 40 years later when, with the benefit of reverse genetics technology, it was possible to engineer an influenza A virus that lacked the *NS1* gene (delNS1).[213] This virus displayed unusual growth properties as it was severely attenuated in IFN-competent systems but grew well in IFN-deficient systems such as Vero cells and 6-day-old embryonated eggs and was lethal in STAT1$^{-/-}$ mice[213,657] (e-Fig. 40.18). Thus, in the absence of an IFN response, NS1 appears to be dispensable, whereas in the context of an immune-competent host, it is essential. Microarray analysis has demonstrated that infection with delNS1 virus leads to enhanced expression of IFN and IFN-regulated genes compared to wild-type influenza virus infection,[218] and NS1 is therefore termed an *IFN antagonist* because it acts to suppress the virus-induced host IFN response (reviewed in (245,727)). These findings have given rise to a new concept for the design of live-attenuated vaccines based on mutations in the NS1 gene[657] (reviewed in

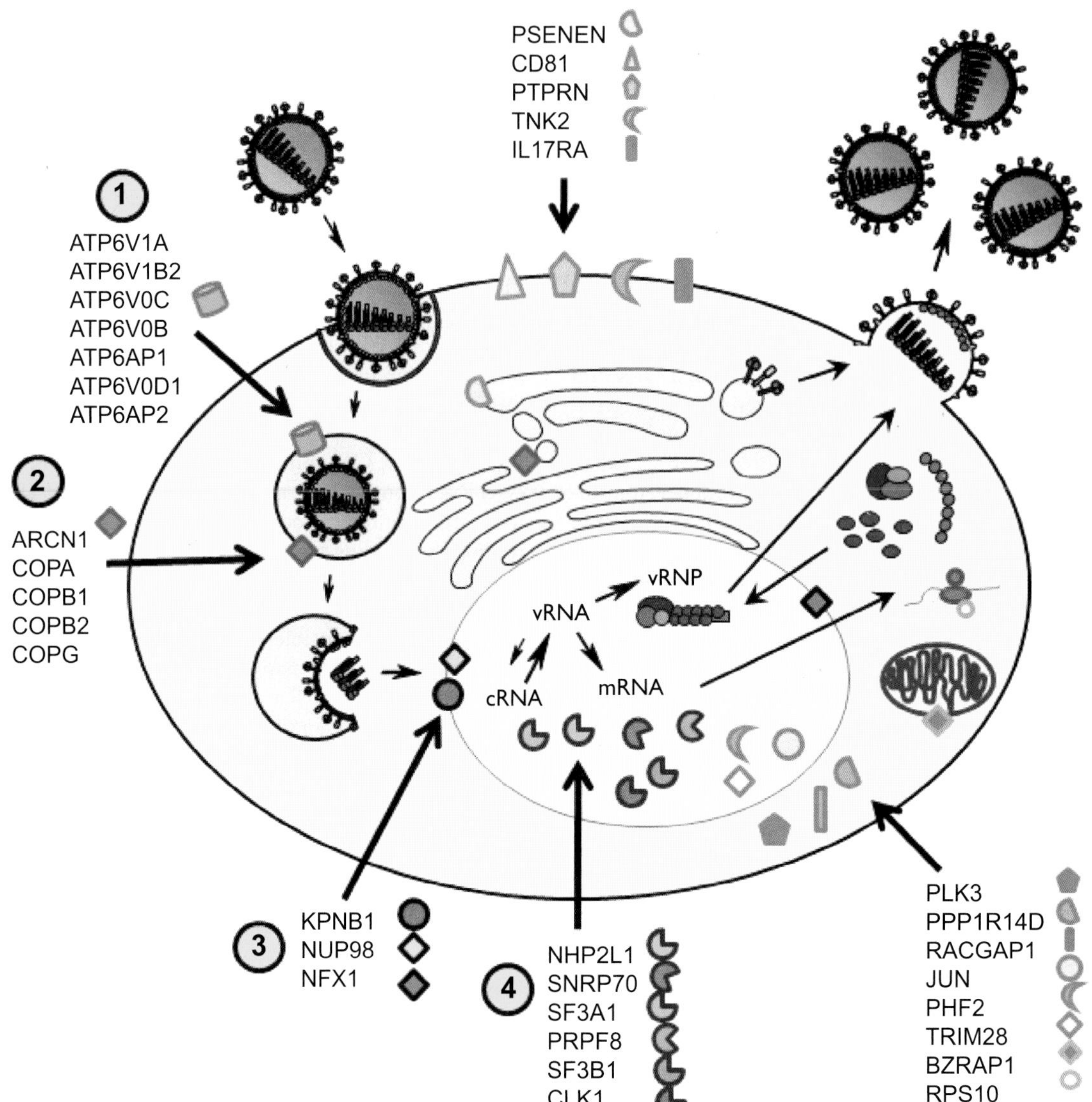

FIGURE 40.16. Graphical representation of the 34 best validated host factors identified in the influenza virus RNA interference (RNAi) screens. Analysis of the validated hits from the RNAi screens by Brass et al,[61] Karlas et al,[325] and König et al[341] resulted in a list of 34 genes that were identified in at least two screens. These 34 host cell factors are shown with regards to their localization within the cell and in context of the viral replication cycle. The four different groups of host proteins with known function in the viral life cycle are depicted in colored symbols: (1) components of the viral adenosine triphosphatase (vATPase) complex, (2) COPI proteins, (3) nucleocytoplasmic transport factors, and (4) members of the splicing machinery. The host factors with as yet unknown function are illustrated with gray symbols. See (636) for details. (Reprinted from Stertz S, Shaw ML. Uncovering the global host cell requirements for influenza virus replication via RNAi screening. *Microbes Infect* 2011;13[5]:516–525; with permission from Elsevier.)

(511,512,557)). Studies on viruses expressing truncated forms of NS1 have shown that the level of attenuation is determined by the amount of IFN induced by the virus (i.e., highly attenuated viruses induce larger quantities of IFN),[27,174,549,627,657] and immunization with these mutant viruses produced protective immunity in mice, chickens, swine, horses, and macaques (reviewed in (557)).

Structural Features of the NS1 Protein

NS1 is a nuclear, dimeric protein that is highly expressed in infected cells and has a dsRNA-binding domain, an effector domain, and a disordered tail (reviewed in (250)). The RNA-binding domain lies within the N-terminal 73 amino acids (548), for which both NMR and crystal structures have been obtained.[96,97,397,749] These data indicate that the NS1 RNA-binding domain forms a symmetric homodimer with a six-helical fold and that conserved tracks consisting of basic and hydrophilic residues on each monomer mediate interactions with dsRNA. Mutational analysis has further demonstrated that dimer formation is crucial for RNA binding as are residues R38, R35, and R46.[96,710] Residue K41 strongly enhances the binding affinity[710] and residues S42 and T49 also participate in dsRNA binding.[96] It is suggested that the basic residues make contact with the phosphate backbone of the RNA via electrostatic interactions,[98,710,749] which is consistent with the observed lack of sequence specificity.[259,548] Structural data indicate that the NS1 dimer spans the major groove of canonical A-form dsRNA in a length-independent mode.[96] Structures of the influenza B virus NS1 RNA-binding domain indicate a similar binding mode.[749]

The remaining portion of NS1 has been termed the effector domain and includes binding sites for several host factors (as reviewed in (250)) (e-Fig. 40.19). Crystallographic structures of the NS1 effector domain have been determined for several influenza A virus strains. While the monomer conformation is very similar, different dimer interfaces have been determined, specifically, one that is mediated by a helix–helix interaction[12,246,328,733] and another mediated by a strand–strand interaction.[49,329] The helix–helix interaction is dependent on residue W187 in each monomer,[246,734] and it has been proposed that the monomer interface can twist and therefore the dimer can exist in both open and closed conformations.[328] Finally, one structure of a full-length NS1 protein has been reported.[50] Strikingly, instead of individual dimers, NS1 is shown to form a chain with alternating interactions occurring via the dsRNA-binding and effector domains. Moreover, three of these chains are shown to interact with one another to form a tubular structure that can accommodate dsRNA in its center. This chain-like structure opens up questions regarding how interactions between NS1 and its cellular partners can be accommodated, but models for how this may occur in the context of an individual NS1 dimer have been proposed.[328]

Inhibition of Interferon Synthesis

Wild-type (WT) influenza virus infection induces far less IFN than does delNS1 virus, and this difference lies at the level of mRNA molecules.[218,656,712] This implies that NS1 either acts to prevent the synthesis of IFN mRNA or destabilizes IFN mRNA. The transcriptional activation of IFN-β in response to virus infection is regulated by transcription factors including interferon regulatory factor-3 (IRF-3), nuclear factor-κB (NF-κB), and activator protein-1 (AP-1). Each one of these transcription factors has been shown to be activated in delNS1 virus–infected cells but not in WT virus–infected cells,[403,656,712] which corresponds with the differential induction of IFN-β by these viruses. Moreover, expression of NS1 alone inhibits the activation of the IFN-β promoter in response to infection with a heterologous virus or even delNS1 virus.[403,712] Substantial progress has been made to understand the precise mechanism by which NS1 suppresses IFN synthesis (reviewed in (245,250)) (Fig. 40.17). First, dsRNA binding is important as

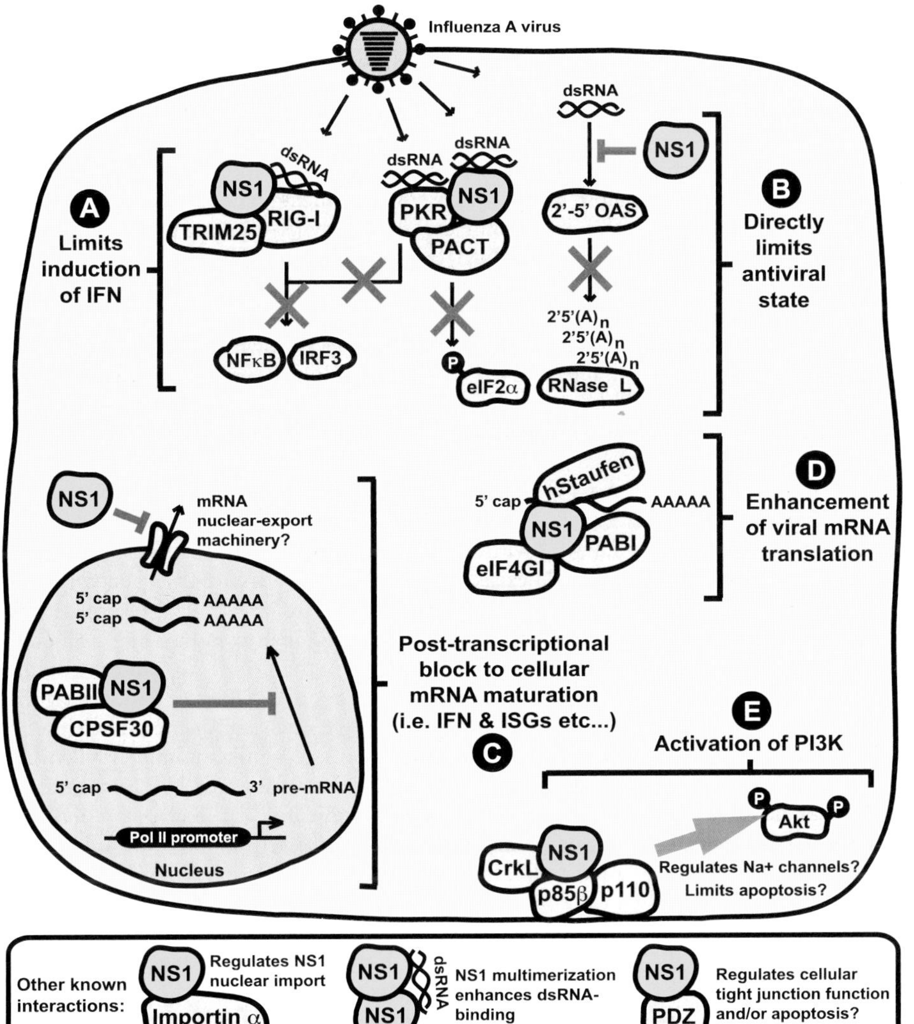

FIGURE 40.17. Schematic diagram of the multiple functions of NS1 within infected cells. A: Pretranscriptional limitation of interferon-β (IFN-β) induction. **B:** Inhibition of the antiviral properties of protein kinase R (PKR) and 2′-5′-oligoadenylate synthetase (OAS)/RNase L. **C:** Posttranscriptional block to processing and nuclear export of all cellular messenger RNAs (mRNAs). **D:** Enhancement of viral mRNA translation. **E:** Activation of phosphatidylinositol 3 kinase (PI3K). Some other interactions that have been characterized are detailed in the **lower box**. See (250) for details. (Adapted from Hale BG, Randall RE, Ortin J, et al. The multifunctional NS1 protein of influenza A viruses. *J Gen Virol* 2008;89[Pt 10]:2359–2376; courtesy of Ben Hale.)

expression of the RNA-binding domain alone is sufficient to block virus induction of IFN.[712] However, a virus expressing only the first 73 residues is still attenuated in mice (with a phenotype intermediate to that of delNS1 and WT virus), pointing to a role for the effector domain *in vivo*.[174,657,711] Alanine substitution of the residues involved in RNA binding (R38 and K41) was found to significantly reduce the ability of NS1 to inhibit IRF-3 and NF-κB activation[656,712] and, hence, IFN-β synthesis.[143] In the context of a virus, these mutations resulted in increased IFN-β production and, therefore, an attenuated phenotype in mice.[143] Second, NS1 is found in complex with the cytoplasmic sensor RIG-I and acts to prevent RIG-I signaling and IFN-β production.[238,444,501,530] This interaction appears to depend on the same residues implicated in dsRNA binding, indicating that it is potentially mediated by RNA.[530] Third, NS1 interacts with TRIM25 via residues E96 and E97.[199] TRIM25 is responsible for ubiquitinating and activating RIG-I and the presence of NS1 blocks this activity.

Inhibition of Protein Kinase R and the RNase L Pathway

Protein kinase R (PKR) is activated in the presence of dsRNA (i.e., during virus infection) and is responsible for the phosphorylation of the eIF2α subunit, which causes protein translation to cease and thus prevents further viral replication. Not surprisingly, many viruses have devised ways of blocking the activation of PKR, and influenza virus does so via two different mechanisms. PKR expression is induced by IFN and therefore the NS1-induced block in IFN synthesis will reduce the levels of PKR in infected cells. In addition, NS1 has been shown to inhibit PKR activation by sequestering its activator, dsRNA,[261,401] and NS1 has also been observed to form a complex with PKR,[659] which inhibits its activation in response to both dsRNA and the cellular PACT protein.[378] The role of NS1 in PKR inhibition has been demonstrated *in vivo*, as seen by restoration of delNS1 virus replication in $PKR^{-/-}$ mice with an accompanying increase in pathogenicity.[37] Via a similar mechanism (i.e., sequestration of dsRNA), NS1 can prevent activation of the 2′-5′-oligoadenylate synthetase (OAS)/RNase L pathway.[445]

Inhibition of Host mRNA Processing

Influenza virus–infected cells harbor pre-mRNAs in their nuclei that do not undergo efficient 3′-end processing and therefore cannot be exported.[94,607] This is thought to be an NS1-mediated effect that occurs via interaction of the NS1 effector domain with two components of the 3′-end processing machinery: the 30-kD subunit of the cleavage and polyadenylation specificity factor (CPSF)[131,338,473] and the poly(A)-binding protein II (PABII)[94] (reviewed in (245,250,346)). The NS1 interaction effectively inhibits these processing factors and results in pre-mRNAs that either remain uncleaved[473,607] or only acquire short poly(A) tails.[94] NS1 also inhibits splicing of pre-mRNAs, which also results in their retention in the nucleus,[185,400] and evidence for the requirement of CPSF in splicing suggests that both of these mRNA-processing defects in influenza virus–infected cells may be related to the inhibition of CPSF.[386] NS1 also interferes with mRNA export via complex formation with several components of the nuclear export machinery.[584] As the induction of the host antiviral response relies so heavily on transcriptional up-regulation of genes, this global posttranscriptional inhibition may aid in aborting or at least delaying the onset of this response. This is reflected in data from a CPSF-binding mutant virus, which is attenuated in tissue culture and which causes an earlier induction of antiviral gene products compared to WT virus.[486] It should be noted, however, that the delNS1 virus shows shutoff of host protein synthesis at levels similar to that of wild-type virus.[581] This suggests that other (or additional) factors may be responsible for inhibition of general gene expression.

Additional NS1 Interactions with Host Cell Factors

The influenza A virus NS1 protein binds directly to the p85β regulatory subunit of PI3K via its C-terminal effector domain, and NS1 expression is sufficient to activate PI3K signaling.[153,248,610] Specifically, residues Y89, M93, P164, P167, L141, and E142 in the NS1 protein, which are located in predicted src homology 2 (SH2)- and SH3-binding motifs, have been implicated in the interaction with p85β.[248,384,609,610] The NS1-binding site on p85β is located in an inter-SH2 domain,[247] and a co-crystal of the NS1 effector domain in complex with this region of p85β shows that residues Y89 and P167 of NS1 are at the binding interface.[249] Furthermore, a model of a heterotrimeric complex consisting of NS1–p85β–p110 predicts that the presence of NS1 would disrupt the inhibitory contact between p85β and p110.[249] This explains the PI3K-activating properties of NS1, which theoretically serve to delay apoptosis at late stages of infection.[151] However, recombinant viruses expressing NS1 proteins that fail to activate PI3K were not seen to induce any more apoptosis than wild-type virus, so the biological significance of NS1-mediated PI3K activation remains unclear.[314] It also should be noted that a pro-apoptotic activity of NS1 has been reported.[592]

NS1 has also been reported to interact with several other host factors (e-Fig. 40.19), including the eukaryotic translation initiation factor 4GI, poly (A)-binding protein I, staufen, NS1-I and NS1-BP, nucleolin, hnRNP-F, E1B-AP5, Herc5, PAB-II, importin α, CrkL, scribble, Dlg1, PDLim2, p15, NXF1, Rae1, PACT, and Ubc9.[11,76,94,168,225,266,289,368,396,438,463,584,588,660,728,729,751,763] It has been shown that disruption of the staufen-1/NS1 interaction inhibits influenza virus replication, indicating that this virus–host interaction is required for optimal virus growth.[369]

Anti-interferon Proteins of Influenza B and C Viruses, Thogoto Virus, and Isavirus

Like its A virus counterpart, the NS1 protein of influenza B virus (B/NS1) exists as a dimer and has RNA-binding activity in its N-terminal domain (residues 1 to 93).[144,709,753] A virus lacking B/NS1 has also been demonstrated to induce larger amounts of IFN than WT virus,[132] and the B/NS1 protein can complement the growth of influenza A delNS1 virus,[144] indicating that A/NS1 and B/NS1 are functional equivalents. Therefore, as described for influenza A virus, recombinant influenza B viruses either lacking NS1 or expressing truncated NS1 proteins have been proposed as vaccine candidates.[244,731] Expression of B/NS1 has been shown to inhibit virus activation of the IFN-β promoter,[132,144] but interestingly, both N- and C-terminal domains of the protein encode this inhibitory activity and hence RNA binding was found not to be essential for inhibition of IFN-β synthesis.[144] However, in the context of the N-terminal domain alone, RNA binding was required. Similarly, both portions of B/NS1 were shown to independently inhibit virus activation of the transcription factor, IRF-3.[144] B/NS1 is also an inhibitor of PKR, but unlike A/NS1 it does not interfere with mRNA processing.[709] B/NS1 does possess the unique ability to bind to *ISG15* (an IFN-inducible gene) and prevent its conjugation to target proteins,[754] which it does through its N-terminal domain independently of RNA binding.[753] Structural analysis shows that a dimer of the B/NS1 N-terminal domain interacts with two ISG15 molecules, with each ISG15 binding distinct regions of each NS1 monomer.[233] ISG15 conjugation or ISGylation has been shown to regulate the IFN signaling pathway and to be critical for host antiviral defense.[413,558,762] Interestingly, B/NS1 inhibits ISGylation in a species-specific manner, binding only to human and nonhuman primate ISG15.[628,684] This likely contributes to the fact that influenza B infections are restricted to humans. The influenza B virus NS1 protein may also have a role in virus replication as the virus lacking B/NS1 grows to lower titers, even in IFN-deficient cells.[132] It has also been shown that B/NS1 associates with nuclear speckles and that this is linked to residues in its N-terminal region.[588]

The influenza C virus NS1 protein (C/NS1) has been shown to inhibit RIG-I–mediated activation of the IFN-β promoter through a region located in its C-terminus.[507] C/NS1 has also been shown to up-regulate splicing of viral mRNAs.[458]

Unlike the influenza viruses, Thogoto virus does not have an NS segment and instead its anti-IFN activity is encoded by the M segment.[242] The M segment produces the M protein from a spliced transcript and the ML protein from an unspliced transcript, of which the latter has been shown to be an IFN antagonist protein.[242,339] As seen with the delNS1 influenza virus, a recombinant Thogoto virus lacking the ML protein was shown to induce far greater levels of IFN in infected cells than WT virus[242] and was remarkably attenuated in mice expressing functional Mx1 (an IFN-inducible protein that protects against orthomyxovirus infection).[529] ML has also been demonstrated to inhibit virus-induced activation of IRF-3 but in a manner distinct from that of NS1.[316] Another striking difference between ML and NS1 is that ML is a structural protein.[241] Because expression of ML is controlled by the same promoter as that of the M protein (which is expressed late in infection), this strategy ensures that ML is present at the initial stages of virus infection when it can most effectively exert its effect on the host immune response.

The isavirus IFN antagonist proteins are expressed from the unspliced transcript of RNA segment 7 and the larger open reading frame (ORF) of RNA segment 8.[122,211]

The Actions of the PB1-F2 Protein

Influenza A viruses can express an 11th protein, PB1-F2, which is encoded by the +1 alternate ORF in the *PB1* gene.[93] PB1-F2 is 87 to 90 aa long, depending on the virus strain, and is expressed by most human H3N2 viruses, while a large number of human H1N1 isolates have a premature stop codon in the PB1-F2 ORF. Of note, the pandemics that occurred in 1918, 1957, and 1968 were all caused by influenza viruses that express full-length PB1-F2. The protein has been shown to contribute to influenza virus pathogenicity through several mechanisms. Initially, a pro-apoptotic function was described for PB1-F2. It was found to localize to mitochondria and disturb the mitochondrial membrane potential, leading to the efflux of cytochrome c into the cytoplasm.[93,221] The induction of apoptosis by PB1-F2 is thought to occur specifically in immune cells in a strain-dependent manner and thus contribute to immune evasion by influenza viruses.[93,428,756] It was demonstrated that PB1-F2 triggers an apoptotic response by interacting with the mitochondrial adenine nucleotide translocase 3 (ANT3) and voltage-dependent anion channel 1 (VDAC1) proteins[755] and/or form pores via self-oligomerization[67,84,269] (Fig. 40.18).

In addition to its pro-apoptotic activity, PB1-F2 was reported to have pro-inflammatory properties. Specifically, it was observed that PB1-F2–expressing viruses increase the levels of several cytokines and chemokines, enhance cell infiltration, and exacerbate lung injury in infected mice.[117,118,428,429] Notably, it was found that a serine (S) at position 66 in the PB1-F2 protein dramatically increases immunopathology and mortality caused by the 1918 pandemic strain and by highly pathogenic H5N1 viruses.[118] Transcriptional profiling of mice infected with a PB1-F2 N66S-expressing virus revealed an early suppression of interferon-stimulated genes (ISGs)[117] and *in vitro* studies demonstrated an anti-interferon activity of PB1-F2 at the level of the MAVS adaptor protein[677] (Fig. 40.18). Interestingly, PB1-F2 N66S, which is associated with increased pathogenicity, inhibited the induction of IFN more efficiently than a wild-type PB1-F2 protein.[677] It is hypothesized that there may be a possible link between the pro-apoptotic and anti-interferon functions of PB1-F2 through the MAVS protein.[676]

REVERSE GENETICS

Because the *Orthomyxoviridae* are negative-strand RNA viruses, introduction of the genomic RNAs into cells does not result in the formation of infectious virus (as it does in the case of positive-strand RNA viruses). Initial experiments eventually leading to the genetic engineering of influenza viruses involved the reconstitution of functional RNP complexes *in vitro*[282,522] and transfection of functional RNPs into cells. In these experiments, cDNA-derived RNA for a specific segment was mixed with purified virion NP and polymerase proteins and transfected into cells before or after infection with a helper influenza virus in order to provide the remaining vRNP segments.[409] Rescue of infectious virus containing the cDNA-derived RNA required selection of the novel virus against the helper virus.[165] Alternatively, cells were transfected with a plasmid construct containing the gene of interest flanked by an RNA polymerase I promoter and terminator sequences. Cellular RNA polymerase I normally transcribes rRNA (which lacks a 5′ cap and 3′ poly[A] tail), and therefore the RNA synthesized from the plasmid construct is an exact replica of the vRNA. The viral polymerase proteins were supplied by transfection with polymerase II–driven expression plasmids, and the remaining genomic segments were provided by infection with a helper influenza virus.[480,535] A disadvantage of these early systems was the need for helper virus, which must be selected against in order to isolate the rescued virus.

In 1999, a decade after the initial influenza reverse genetics system had been described, Fodor et al[178] and Neumann et al[479] reported the generation of influenza viruses entirely from cloned cDNAs. In the system reported by Fodor et al, cDNA from each of the eight genome segments was cloned in negative orientation between a truncated human RNA polymerase I promoter and the hepatitis delta virus ribozyme.[178] Transfection of the eight vRNA-encoding plasmids into Vero cells along with four polymerase II–driven plasmids expressing NP and the polymerase complex (PB1, PB2, PA) resulted in

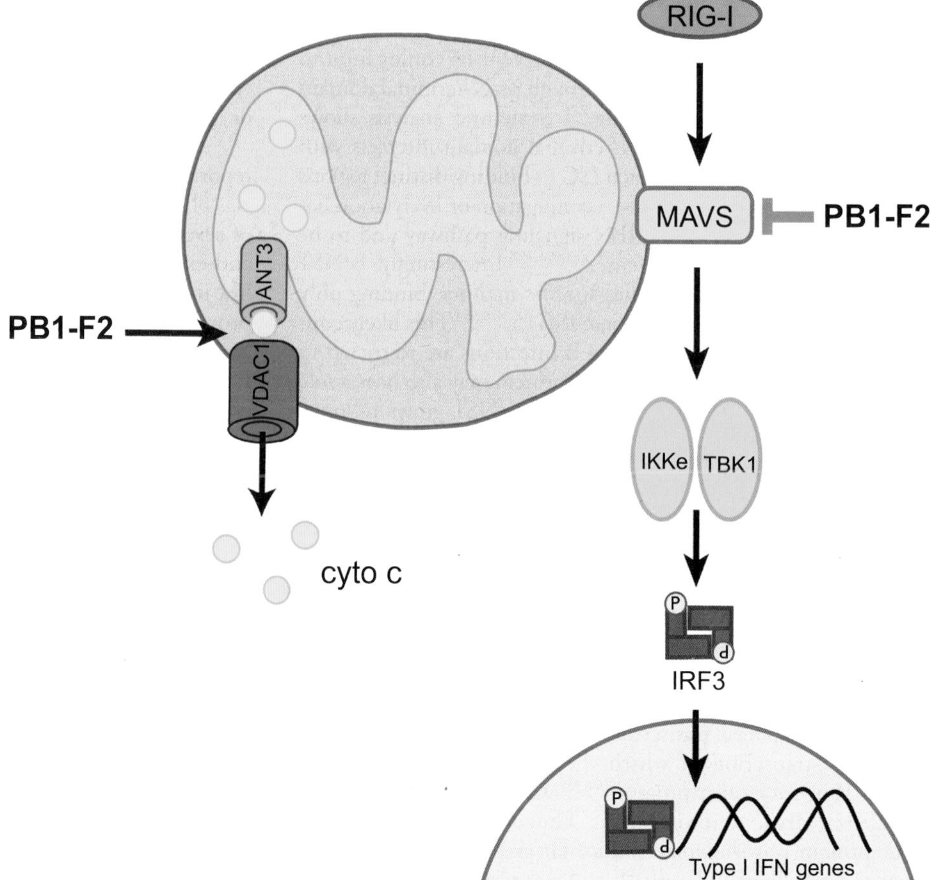

FIGURE 40.18. The pro-apoptotic and anti-interferon activities of the influenza A virus protein PB1-F2. The protein promotes apoptosis by interacting with the mitochondrial VDAC1 and ANT3 proteins and interferes with the induction of interferon at the level of the MAVS adaptor protein. Cyto c: cytochrome c. (Courtesy of Zsuzsanna T. Varga.)

recovery of infectious virus (Fig. 40.19). As helper virus is not required for the generation of recombinant virus, the cumbersome selection process was unnecessary. Improvements to this system now include the transfection of co-cultured 293T cells (necessary due to the human RNA polymerase I promoter) and Madin Darby Canine Kidney (MDCK) cells, which support high levels of virus replication (for review, see (478)).

Further improvements to these systems were reported in which only eight plasmids were required.[278,279] The plasmids contained cDNAs of genomic segments cloned in negative

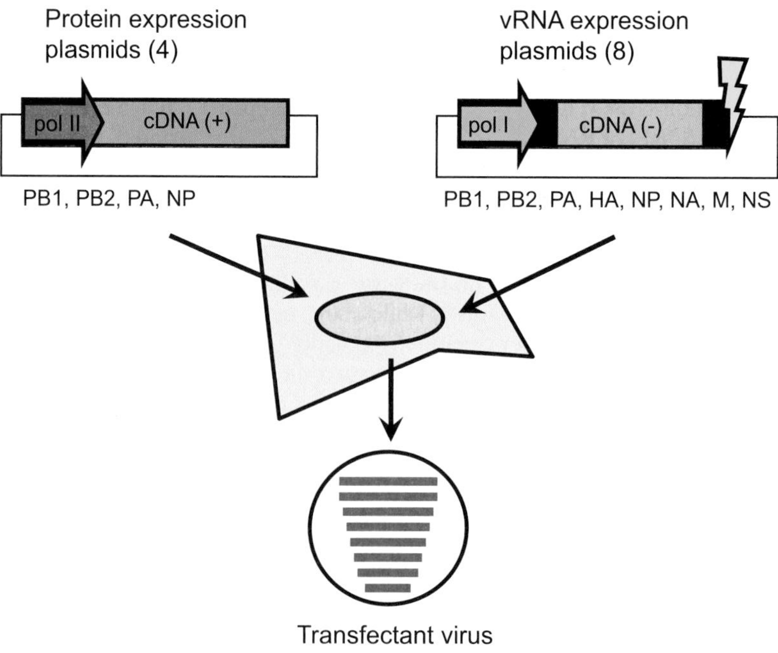

FIGURE 40.19. Schematic representation of the plasmid-based rescue system for influenza A virus. The negative-sense complementary DNA (cDNA) for each viral segment is cloned between a polymerase I promoter and the hepatitis delta virus ribozyme or polymerase I terminator. These eight plasmids are transfected into mammalian cells along with four expression plasmids for the polymerase proteins and nucleoprotein (NP). The resulting transfectant virus is then passaged on fresh cells. For details see (178). (Courtesy of Adolfo García-Sastre.)

orientation with a human RNA polymerase I promoter at the 5′ end and the mouse RNA polymerase I terminator at the 3′ end. The cellular RNA polymerase I was responsible for the copying of the cDNA into vRNA. Downstream of the RNA polymerase I terminator was a CMV immediate-early promoter. A polyadenylation sequence was inserted at the other end, giving rise to a polymerase II–driven mRNA transcript from the opposite DNA strand. Expressed viral proteins and vRNAs then assembled in the transfected cells and resulted in the formation of infectious virus derived entirely from only eight plasmids. A single plasmid containing the cDNAs of all eight RNAs resulted in the generation of infectious virus when transfected into human cells.[476] Most likely, transcription of mRNA-like molecules occurred from this plasmid, which then gave rise to the formation of the complementing viral polymerase proteins. These proteins, together with the full-length vRNA segments (also transcribed from the plasmid), allowed rescue of fully infectious virus. Another one-plasmid system was developed for the rescue of influenza A viruses in chicken cells.[761] Other modifications of the rescue system involve the use of uncloned PCR-amplified products, which obviates possible problems in cloning toxic sequences,[772,773] and the use of adenovirus as a vector to deliver the required plasmid constructs.[504] Finally, de Wit et al[134] designed a rescue system built on transcription by the T7 polymerase, which allows the rescue of influenza viruses in practically all cells independent of the species origin.

Influenza viruses expressing foreign genes have also been generated, demonstrating the use of influenza virus as a vector to deliver foreign antigens to the immune system. Numerous approaches have been successful for the expression of foreign antigens by influenza viruses. These include (a) replacement of the antigenic domains of either the influenza HA or NA glycoproteins with epitopes from foreign proteins.[379,380] (b) Modification of existing viral genomic segments to express influenza viral proteins fused to foreign proteins. These polyproteins can subsequently be cleaved into two proteins. Also reported was the rescue of an influenza virus that expresses an uncleaved chimeric HA with a 140–amino acid insertion of the receptor-binding domain of the *Bacillus anthracis* protective antigen (PA).[389] (c) Replacement of ectodomains of surface glycoproteins with those of foreign glycoproteins.[175] (d) Preparation of viruses with foreign antigens encoded by a ninth RNA segment (for review, see (212,478)).

Advantages of influenza viruses over other viruses for the expression of foreign proteins include the fact that influenza virus is extremely safe as a nonintegrating, nononcogenic virus. Infection with influenza viruses also elicits a strong and long-lasting immune response, and thus recombinant influenza viruses may be useful vaccine vectors in the future. The limitations related to the use of influenza viruses for expression of foreign antigens include the limited (but not yet well-defined) capacity of influenza viruses to express foreign sequences and the requirement of packaging signals on both the 5′ and 3′ ends of the vRNA, which may interfere with the expression of foreign genes.

The advances of reverse genetics techniques have been of great benefit to the study of structure/function of different influenza virus genes and their proteins. In many cases, the definitive role of a gene or of a domain (or even of a single amino acid) can only be explored by introducing appropriate mutations into the genome of the virus and then analyzing the phenotype of the rescued virus. As discussed, rescue systems have been described for influenza A viruses (for review see (212,367,422)) and B viruses[277,312] (for review see (313)). Also, rescue systems have now been developed for influenza C viruses[125,460,506] (for review see (459)). Influenza viruses have been generated that express chimeric (type A/B) HAs and NAs. For example, such viruses may express, in a type A genetic background, the extracellular portion (ectodomain) of an influenza B HA and/or NA.[175,285,287] These findings show that the HA and NA of an influenza A virus can be functionally replaced with the corresponding protein from an influenza B virus. In turn, viruses have been made in the influenza B virus background expressing proteins derived from influenza A viruses.[243] By taking advantage of the knowledge about packaging sequences, influenza A viruses have been made to contain nine segments expressing an H1 and an H3 HA[207] or only seven segments.[206] In the latter virus the HA and the NA have been replaced by the HEF protein of an influenza C virus. Whole organ imaging and analysis of infected cells is now facilitated by chimeric influenza viruses that express a green fluorescent protein (GFP) molecule for visualization of influenza virus–infected cells.[414] Reverse genetics has also been successfully used to rescue an influenza virus expressing all eight genes of the "extinct" 1918 pandemic virus, which has allowed its extraordinary virulence to be studied.[517,671]

Reverse genetics has also helped in designing improved influenza virus vaccines. The live attenuated pH1N1 2009 vaccine was made from a plasmid-generated strain, into which HA gene mutations were introduced to give high yields without changing the antigenicity of the strain.[95] Also, killed and live pandemic H5N1 virus vaccines were prepared using reverse genetics, allowing the removal of the basic peptide from the HA cleavage site, in order to make the strains used for manufacturing less virulent (for review (286)).

Thogoto virus, which has six negative-strand RNA segments, has also been rescued by a reverse genetics system.[337,695] The viral RNAs were transcribed from the plasmids under the control of a polymerase I promoter and the structural proteins were expressed from six plasmids driven by a T7 polymerase promoter in the presence of a T7 vaccinia recombinant.

INHIBITORS OF INFLUENZA VIRUSES

Because influenza viruses remain a constant health threat, major efforts have been directed at discovering effective antivirals over the past several decades. Presently there are four Food and Drug Administration (FDA)-approved drugs available for use in humans: amantadine, rimantadine, oseltamivir, and zanamivir (Fig. 40.20). Past and current approaches to antiviral therapy are briefly discussed here (according to the step in virus replication targeted by each drug). Extensive reviews cover the vast literature on this subject.[28,36,46,110,216,264,315,406,408,562]

Inhibition of Attachment and Uncoating

While vaccination, in essence, targets the HA so that specific antibodies are generated that block attachment of the virus to the receptor, drugs that interfere with the HA–sialic acid interaction have not been successfully developed. This is perhaps surprising because the x-ray crystallographic structures of the HA and of HA–ligand complexes have now been known for more than two decades. In principle, such an approach could work,[101,223] but this strategy, using sialic acid analogs (or polymers bearing sialic acids), has not led to an FDA-approved

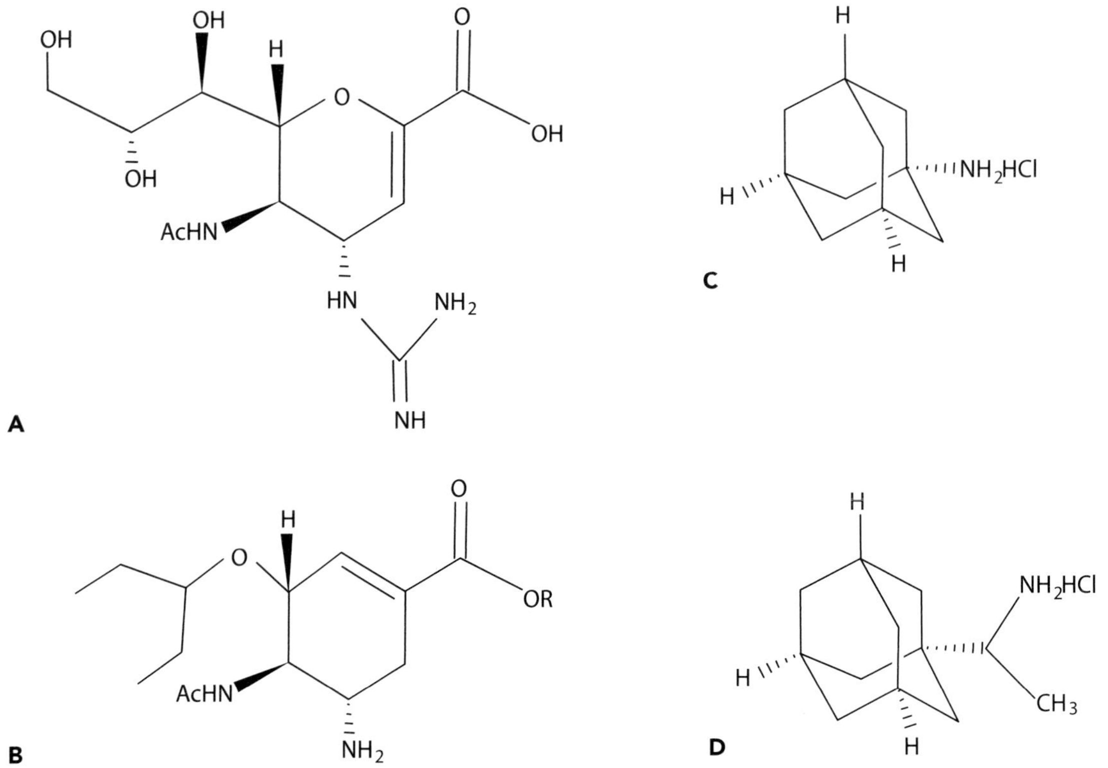

FIGURE 40.20. Anti-influenza virus compounds. The chemical structures of **(A)** zanamivir (Relenza), **(B)** oseltamivir (Tamiflu), **(C)** amantadine (Symmetrel), and **(D)** rimantadine (Flumadine) are shown.

drug. Whether removal of receptor molecules from the respiratory tract by administration of exogenous sialidase/neuraminidase is a viable antiviral approach remains to be seen. A sialidase fusion protein, DAS181, has been shown to be an effective antiviral strategy in tissue culture and animal models.[35,361] However, it seems doubtful that receptors could be (safely) denuded for extended periods of time in order to prevent infection by influenza viruses.

Quinone derivatives that prevent the first stage of the conformational change of the HA and thus inhibit infection were discovered in 1993,[45] and other compounds with a similar mechanism showed inhibition for some strains but not for others.[106,630] Compounds have also been identified that appear to push the HA into an inactive state[276] or that associate with the N-terminal heptad-repeat trimer, thus interfering with the *trimer of hairpins* (helix bundle) formation.[105] This latter approach would be similar to that successfully applied for human immunodeficiency virus (HIV) using the fusion inhibitor T-20.[331] In addition, several other approaches aimed at preventing virus attachment have been reported.[201,237,374,579,620,629] Nitazoxanide (a thiazolide) is reported to prevent terminal glycosylation of HA and thereby impair HA maturation and trafficking to the cell surface.[570] So far, none of the influenza virus HA inhibitors has advanced beyond the experimental stage.

Another approach concerns the inhibition of the posttranslational cleavage of the HA, which results in a molecule unable to undergo the conformational change required for fusion/uncoating. Several exogenous protease inhibitors have been investigated,[34,52,371,770,771] of which aprotinin has been found to be effective in humans.[768] Drugs belonging to this general class have been successful against HIV but have not been further developed for widespread therapeutic or prophylactic use against influenza in humans.

Amantadine, which has been known for many decades to inhibit most influenza A viruses, has been found to target the M2 ion channel (for details see M2 Protein). During uptake, virus enters endosomes where the acid pH activates the ion channel, resulting in the transport of protons into the viral interior. This process, which is required for the dissociation of the RNP complex from the M1 protein and subsequent release of the RNP into the cytoplasm, is blocked by amantadine and its derivatives (including rimantadine),[722] (for review see (533)). In addition, amantadine can affect the pH regulation of vesicles involved in the transport of viral glycoproteins to the cell surface during assembly.[634] Thus, there are two possible steps at which amantadine can exert an antiviral effect: uncoating and HA stability (in some strains) during transport in vesicles. Unfortunately, resistance to amantadine and to its 10-fold more active derivative, rimantadine, develops with increased use in humans and animals (for review see 452). In fact, according to Centers for Disease Control and Prevention (CDC) guidelines, adamantanes are not recommended for clinical use as of 2010/2011.

Inhibitors of the Viral Replication Complex

The viral RNA-dependent RNA polymerase is a good antiviral target as it possesses unique features not found in the cell. Tomassini et al[665,666] reported that 2,4-dioxobutanoic acid and

2,6-diketopiperazine derivatives selectively inhibit the endonuclease activity (PA) of the influenza virus polymerase. Recent knowledge of the PA structure will encourage investigation of endonuclease inhibitors.[130]

Ribavirin (which is approved for treatment of hepatitis C) and several other nucleotide analogs are known to inhibit influenza in humans, but toxicity remains a problem (for review see (376,406)). For RNA viruses, most of the antiviral effects of ribavirin are likely due to incorporation as a purine analog, resulting in lethal mutations. Similarly, T-705 (favipiravir) inhibits influenza virus RNA polymerase activity by acting as a purine analog and has been shown to be effective against several RNA viruses.[195,196,334] Also, capped and uncapped RNA fragments interfering with cap binding, capped-RNA primed transcription, or panhandle formation have been reported (for review see (406)), but these compounds would have pharmacologic limitations because of difficulties in getting charged molecules into cells. Recent high-throughput screens of small molecules have uncovered novel inhibitors of influenza virus replication that target the NP and PB1 proteins.[324,645]

Antisense Oligonucleotides and siRNAs

Synthetic oligodeoxynucleotides in the phosphorothioate series corresponding to sequences in the *PB1* gene of influenza A and C viruses were found to inhibit virus replication,[375] possibly mediated through an antisense RNA mechanism (for review see (408)). More recently, siRNA inhibition has become a promising route to interfere with influenza virus replication in tissue culture and in animals (for review see (23,36,216,594)). RNAi is a process by which small molecules of double-stranded RNA direct the sequence-specific degradation of mRNA molecules. Theoretically, viral mRNA as well as cRNA and vRNA could be targets for an siRNA approach, and several siRNA molecules directed against specific influenza virus genes have been shown to successfully inhibit influenza virus replication in tissue culture and mice.[217,297,382,649,667] Challenges of this approach remain: First, the effective delivery of these molecules defies standard approaches. Second, contradictory results have been reported regarding the induction of interferons and cytokines by siRNAs, which may represent an obstacle to their use as specific and nontoxic inhibitors.[411,561,619]

NS1 Inhibitors

The NS1 protein is being considered as a possible antiviral target due to its role as a pathogenicity factor. Loss of NS1 activity should restore normal immune function to influenza virus–infected cells and promote viral clearance. For this reason small-molecule inhibitors that are able to reverse NS1-mediated inhibition of the innate immune response are being sought. One such molecule has been described that is dependent on an intact IFN response and, specifically, RNAse L.[29,698] Some screens have focused specifically on compounds that may act by disrupting the interaction of NS1 with RNA,[3,415] while others have examined NS1-mediated inhibition of host gene expression.[423]

Neuraminidase Inhibitors

The study of temperature-sensitive mutants with defects in the NA of influenza viruses has shown that the function of this enzyme is to release the newly formed virus from the cell surface.[516] Also, it was shown that neuraminic acid analogs inhibit influenza virus replication in tissue culture and that aggregates of virus are formed at the cell surface in the presence of these drugs[510,515] (Fig. 40.15). By relying on the three-dimensional x-ray structure, von Itzstein et al[689] designed a derivative of neuraminic acid that had a guanidino group at C atom 4 instead of the OH group of the previously studied neuraminidase inhibitor, DANA (e-Fig. 40.20).[436] This compound, zanamivir (Fig. 40.20), is not orally bioavailable and is FDA approved for administration by inhalation or by nasal spray. Most recently intravenous administration has been investigated.[552] In numerous studies, this compound has been shown to be a potent anti-influenza drug, both prophylactically and therapeutically (for review, see (108,214,315,434)). Peramivir is another neuraminidase inhibitor that can be administered intravenously.[340] It received emergency approval in the United States during the 2009 H1N1 pandemic and is already approved in several Asian countries. A long-acting neuraminidase inhibitor (laninamivir), which requires a single administration for the entire course of treatment, was recently developed.[739] A search for compounds that are orally active led to oseltamivir.[381] Its prodrug is an ethyl ester of a compound that has the three OH groups of C atoms 7, 8, and 9 of sialic acid replaced by a hydrophobic side chain, thus making the drug pass through the gut into the bloodstream (Fig. 40.20). This systemically active compound has been shown to be highly effective against both influenza A and B viruses, including strains containing the NA gene of the 1918 pandemic virus,[672] (for review see (306,315,434)). Although oseltamivir-resistant variants had been described with escape mutations in the HA as well as the NA,[20,111,234,311,333] it was still unexpected that such widespread resistance would be seen among the seasonal H1N1 viruses by the 2009 season.[298,500] Prior to 2007, the presence of the NA H274Y mutation was associated with a cost to viral fitness.[270,308] By 2008/2009, this mutation had a fitness advantage even in the absence of oseltamivir and these resistant viruses were shown to be highly transmissible in a guinea pig model.[58] It has been proposed that compensating mutations in the NA resulted in a more stable molecule with enhanced expression at the cell surface than was observed for a mutant with only the H274Y mutation.[44] Interestingly, for the H3N2 viruses, oseltamivir resistance is associated with a loss of fitness and is detrimental to transmissibility of these viruses.[57,747] However, resistant H3N2 viruses have been isolated particularly from immunocompromised patients undergoing therapy.[442,494] Similarly, oseltamivir-resistant isolates of the 2009 pandemic virus have been observed in these patients but not in the community.[230,441] Based on experiments in animal models, it is predicted that an H275Y change in the NA of the 2009 pandemic virus would not be associated with any substantial loss in fitness or transmissibility.[146,440,593] With this virus already being resistant to the adamantanes, acquisition of oseltamivir resistance would make it a multidrug-resistant virus and a significant threat. Fortunately, mutations associated with oseltamivir resistance do not generally confer zanamivir resistance, and there are rare reports of zanamivir resistance in patients.[235] Structures of oseltamivir-resistant NAs that remain sensitive to zanamivir show that this is due to an altered hydrophobic pocket in the active site that affects oseltamivir but not zanamivir binding.[107]

Inhibition of Cellular Factors

The identification of host factors that are required for optimal influenza virus replication (see section Cellular Functions Required for Influenza Virus Replication) provides additional targets that can be explored for potential antiviral development (reviewed in (402,600)). There are distinct advantages and disadvantages to this approach. First, the obvious disadvantage is that inhibition of a cellular activity that is essential for cell survival or growth may be detrimental to the host, so such proteins may not be suitable as antiviral targets. However, particularly with acute infections such as influenza, the short duration of therapy may allow for temporary loss of a cellular function without harming the host. The major advantage of targeting a host factor over a viral factor is that resistance is much less likely to develop. Also, there is greater opportunity for host-directed compounds to have broad-spectrum activity as many viruses may rely on the same host function. For example, HSP90 inhibitors have been shown to inhibit influenza virus[85] and other viruses including hepatitis C virus and Ebola virus.[469,623] Several inhibitors of enzymes in the *de novo* pyrimidine synthesis pathway have been shown to inhibit the replication of a wide range of viruses, including influenza virus,[48,280,705] presumably because virus replication is particularly dependent on large pyrimidine pools. Inhibitors of receptor tyrosine kinases have also been shown to inhibit influenza virus replication as well as other viruses.[348,349] The identification of the target of a novel compound is not always easy, but a cellar target is strongly suggested if the compound can inhibit viruses belonging to different families and/or shows species-specific activity. This is the case with a compound shown to block replication of both influenza viruses and several paramyxoviruses,[347] and future identification of the target may reveal an important virus–host interaction. Likewise, known inhibitors of host factors or signaling pathways identified as critical for influenza virus replication could be repurposed as antivirals or at least chemical probes for investigating the function of the virus–host interaction. Inhibitors of the following cellular factors have all been shown to inhibit influenza virus growth: MEK, CAMK2B, vATPase, and CLK1.[145,325,341,536] Rather than inhibiting the activity of a required host protein, it is also feasible for an antiviral compound to act by activating a cellular factor with antiviral activity, as shown by chemical activation of REDD1 expression, which decreases growth of both influenza and vesicular stomatitis viruses.[423]

PERSPECTIVES

Human influenza viruses were first isolated in 1933, and since that time they have been studied extensively. Extraordinary progress has been made in elucidating the components of the virus and in understanding the medical consequences of an influenza virus infection. Many of these discoveries have had implications far beyond the influenza virus field and have sparked new developments in disciplines such as immunology and protein structure as well as furthering our basic understanding of viruses in general. For example, the ability of virus to agglutinate red blood cells (hemagglutination) was first recognized as a property associated with influenza virus, hence the name of its major surface glycoprotein. With the discovery that this phenomenon extends to other viruses (e.g., measles virus, rubella virus), it became the basis for viral diagnostic tests, allowing for easy detection of virus or of protective antibody (hemagglutination inhibition) in patient sera. The influenza virus neuraminidase was also the first enzyme found to be associated with any animal virus, even before it was recognized that viruses encode their own polymerases, including those with reverse transcriptase activity. The discovery of interferon by Isaacs and Lindenmann in 1957 was as a result of studying infection with heat-inactivated influenza virus, and structural analyses of the HA and NA proteins helped to lay the foundation for the exploration of structure/function relationships of large, biologically active proteins. Today, the intensity of studying influenza and influenza viruses has not diminished and a PubMed search yields approximately 65,000 entries (at the time this chapter was written).

Many approaches that served us well in the past have now been superseded by newer techniques, but their contribution to our current knowledge should not be overlooked. The superb collections of temperature-sensitive mutants obtained and characterized by Akira Sugiura in Japan and by Christoph Scholtissek and Rudolf Rott in Germany made it possible to study the genetics of the virus on a gene-by-gene level, and thus allowed the field to take a giant step forward. The sequencing of these influenza virus proteins and RNAs was an effort of months, if not years. Now this can be done in a matter of hours, and since the last edition of this book, there has been a 20-fold increase in the number of influenza virus sequences submitted to GenBank, which now number almost 200,000. We also have exciting new molecular technologies (including reverse genetics) that have allowed us to obtain an excellent understanding of the virus on a molecular level and to learn how it has changed over the years. Using this technology, we have even been able to resurrect the 1918 pandemic influenza virus from sequenced RNA fragments and to study its pathogenicity in an animal model.

What are the challenges for the future? With the threat of yet another pandemic influenza virus emerging, a detailed molecular understanding of virus–host interactions is needed in order to know how best to disable the virus. Perhaps one of the most pressing questions is, what makes an influenza virus transmissible from human to human and from animal to animal? This aspect has been notoriously difficult to study and will require the use of complex animal models. On a molecular level it will be important to learn more about the cell's signaling pathways and how they are modulated during influenza virus replication. What makes the virus a pathogen in one species and not in another? How does the virus affect the host immune response, and is it in turn affected in any way? What role does the age of a person (child, adult, elderly) and conditions/diseases (pregnancy, obesity, diabetes) play in influenza virus replication? What are the complicating factors (coinfection with other viral/bacterial agents, environmental changes) in an influenza virus infection? And last but not least, we need to address the question of host genetics in influenza virus infection and in virus infections in general. Which genetic makeup (polymorphisms and gene expression profiles) determines susceptibility to (and recovery from) influenza virus infection in humans and animals?

These efforts will need to be accompanied by the development of reliable and rapid diagnostic tests and safe and broadly effective antivirals. As we begin to obtain a better understanding of the host factors involved in influenza virus replication, it presents the opportunity to use these host factors as new antiviral drug targets. Potentially, this approach can lead to the development of broad-spectrum antivirals that can be used to treat not only influenza but also other viral diseases. Since the isolation and characterization of broadly protective monoclonal antibodies directed against conserved portions of the HA, it is now possible to design new immunogens that may serve as vaccine constructs. Such universal influenza vaccines may avoid annual revaccinations against influenza and provide protection against intrasubtype variants and possibly even against strains belonging to different subtypes. In a new pandemic outbreak the availability of such tools will be imperative. It is likely that answers to these challenges will come from a vigorous basic science enterprise, which has brought us a long way in the past several decades of influenza virus research.

REFERENCES

All cited references are available in the e-book.

1. Acharya R, Carnevale V, Fiorin G, et al. Structure and mechanism of proton transport through the transmembrane tetrameric M2 protein bundle of the influenza A virus. *Proc Natl Acad Sci U S A* 2010;107(34):15075–15080.
9. Amorim MJ, Bruce EA, Read EK, et al. A Rab11- and microtubule-dependent mechanism for cytoplasmic transport of influenza A virus viral RNA. *J Virol* 2011;85(9):4143–4156.
12. Aramini JM, Ma LC, Zhou L, et al. Dimer interface of the effector domain of non-structural protein 1 from influenza A virus: an interface with multiple functions. *J Biol Chem* 2011;286(29):26050–26060.
13. Area E, Martin-Benito J, Gastaminza P, et al. 3D structure of the influenza virus polymerase complex: localization of subunit domains. *Proc Natl Acad Sci U S A* 2004;101(1):308–313.
21. Baltimore D. Expression of animal virus genomes. *Bacteriol Rev* 1971; 35(3):235–241.
23. Barik S. Intranasal delivery of antiviral siRNA. *Methods Mol Biol* 2011; 721:333–338.
39. Bier K, York A, Fodor E. Cellular cap-binding proteins associate with influenza virus mRNAs. *J Gen Virol* 2011;92(Pt 7):1627–1634.
44. Bloom JD, Gong LI, Baltimore D. Permissive secondary mutations enable the evolution of influenza oseltamivir resistance. *Science* 2010; 328(5983):1272–1275.
46. Boltz DA, Aldridge JR Jr, Webster RG, et al. Drugs in development for influenza. *Drugs* 2010;70(11):1349–1362.
47. Bommakanti G, Citron MP, Hepler RW, et al. Design of an HA2-based Escherichia coli expressed influenza immunogen that protects mice from pathogenic challenge. *Proc Natl Acad Sci U S A* 2010;107(31):13701–13706.
48. Bonavia A, Franti M, Pusateri Keaney E, et al. Identification of broad-spectrum antiviral compounds and assessment of the druggability of their target for efficacy against respiratory syncytial virus (RSV). *Proc Natl Acad Sci U S A* 2011;108(17):6739–6744.
49. Bornholdt ZA, Prasad BV. X-ray structure of influenza virus NS1 effector domain. *Nat Struct Mol Biol* 2006;13(6):559–560.
50. Bornholdt ZA, Prasad BV. X-ray structure of NS1 from a highly pathogenic H5N1 influenza virus. *Nature* 2008;456(7224):985–988.
51. Bortz E, Westera L, Maamary J, et al. Host- and strain-specific regulation of influenza virus polymerase activity by interacting cellular proteins. *MBio* 2011;2(4):e00151-11.
54. Boulo S, Akarsu H, Ruigrok RW, et al. Nuclear traffic of influenza virus proteins and ribonucleoprotein complexes. *Virus Res* 2007;124(1–2):12–21.
55. Bourmakina SV, Garcia-Sastre A. Reverse genetics studies on the filamentous morphology of influenza A virus. *J Gen Virol* 2003;84:517–527.
58. Bouvier NM, Rahmat S, Pica N. Enhanced mammalian transmissibility of seasonal influenza A/H1N1 viruses encoding an oseltamivir-resistant neuraminidase. *J Virol* 2012;86(13):7268–7279.
60. Bradel-Tretheway BG, Mattiacio JL, Krasnoselsky A, et al. Comprehensive proteomic analysis of influenza virus polymerase complex reveals a novel association with mitochondrial proteins and RNA polymerase accessory factors. *J Virol* 2011;85(17):8569–8581.
61. Brass AL, Huang IC, Benita Y, et al. The IFITM proteins mediate cellular resistance to influenza A H1N1 virus, West Nile virus, and dengue virus. *Cell* 2009;139(7):1243–1254.
65. Bruce EA, Digard P, Stuart AD. The Rab11 pathway is required for influenza A virus budding and filament formation. *J Virol* 2010;84(12):5848–5859.
79. Cady SD, Schmidt-Rohr K, Wang J, et al. Structure of the amantadine binding site of influenza M2 proton channels in lipid bilayers. *Nature* 2010;463(7281):689–692.
80. Calder LJ, Wasilewski S, Berriman JA, et al. Structural organization of a filamentous influenza A virus. *Proc Natl Acad Sci U S A* 2010;107(23):10685–10690.
83. Chan WH, Ng AK, Robb NC, et al. Functional analysis of the influenza virus H5N1 nucleoprotein tail loop reveals amino acids that are crucial for oligomerization and ribonucleoprotein activities. *J Virol* 2010; 84(14):7337–7345.
87. Chen BJ, Leser GP, Jackson D, et al. The influenza virus M2 protein cytoplasmic tail interacts with the M1 protein and influences virus assembly at the site of virus budding. *J Virol* 2008;82(20):10059–10070.
88. Chen BJ, Leser GP, Morita E, et al. Influenza virus hemagglutinin and neuraminidase, but not the matrix protein, are required for assembly and budding of plasmid-derived virus-like particles. *J Virol* 2007; 81(13):7111–7123.
90. Chen C, Zhuang X. Epsin 1 is a cargo-specific adaptor for the clathrin-mediated endocytosis of the influenza virus. *Proc Natl Acad Sci U S A* 2008;105(33):11790–11795.
93. Chen W, Calvo PA, Malide D, et al. A novel influenza A virus mitochondrial protein that induces cell death. *Nat Med* 2001;7(12):1306–1312.
95. Chen Z, Wang W, Zhou H, et al. Generation of live attenuated novel influenza virus A/California/7/09 (H1N1) vaccines with high yield in embryonated chicken eggs. *J Virol* 2010;84(1):44–51.
96. Cheng A, Wong SM, Yuan YA. Structural basis for dsRNA recognition by NS1 protein of influenza A virus. *Cell Res* 2009;19(2):187–195.
99. Childs RA, Palma AS, Wharton S, et al. Receptor-binding specificity of pandemic influenza A (H1N1) 2009 virus determined by carbohydrate microarray. *Nat Biotechnol* 2009;27(9):797–799.
107. Collins PJ, Haire LF, Lin YP, et al. Crystal structures of oseltamivir-resistant influenza virus neuraminidase mutants. *Nature* 2008;453(7199):1258–1261.
110. Colman PM. New antivirals and drug resistance. *Annu Rev Biochem* 2009;78:95–118.
113. Coloma R, Valpuesta JM, Arranz R, et al. The structure of a biologically active influenza virus ribonucleoprotein complex. *PLoS Pathog* 2009; 5(6):e1000491.
117. Conenello GM, Tisoncik JR, Rosenzweig E, et al. A single N66S mutation in the PB1-F2 protein of influenza A virus increases virulence by inhibiting the early interferon response in vivo. *J Virol* 2011;85(2):652–662.
118. Conenello GM, Zamarin D, Perrone LA, et al. A single mutation in the PB1-F2 of H5N1 (HK/97) and 1918 influenza A viruses contributes to increased virulence. *PLoS Pathog* 2007;3(10):1414–1421.
121. Corti D, Voss J, Gamblin SJ, et al. A neutralizing antibody selected from plasma cells that binds to group 1 and group 2 influenza A hemagglutinins. *Science* 2011;333(6044):850–856.
127. Cros JF, Palese P. Trafficking of viral genomic RNA into and out of the nucleus: influenza, Thogoto and Borna disease viruses. *Virus Res* 2003; 95(1–2):3–12.
130. Das K, Aramini JM, Ma LC, et al. Structures of influenza A proteins and insights into antiviral drug targets. *Nat Struct Mol Biol* 2010;17(5):530–538.
131. Das K, Ma LC, Xiao R, et al. Structural basis for suppression of a host antiviral response by influenza A virus. *Proc Natl Acad Sci U S A* 2008; 105(35):13093–13098.
133. de Vries E, Tscherne DM, Wienholts MJ, et al. Dissection of the influenza A virus endocytic routes reveals macropinocytosis as an alternative entry pathway. *PLoS Pathog* 2011;7(3):e1001329.
134. de Wit E, Spronken MI, Vervaet G, et al. A reverse-genetics system for Influenza A virus using T7 RNA polymerase. *J Gen Virol* 2007;88(Pt 4):1281–1287.

135. Deng T, Engelhardt OG, Thomas B, et al. Role of ran binding protein 5 in nuclear import and assembly of the influenza virus RNA polymerase complex. *J Virol* 2006;80(24):11911–11919.
139. Dias A, Bouvier D, Crepin T, et al. The cap-snatching endonuclease of influenza virus polymerase resides in the PA subunit. *Nature* 2009; 458(7240):914–918.
145. Droebner K, Pleschka S, Ludwig S, et al. Antiviral activity of the MEK-inhibitor U0126 against pandemic H1N1v and highly pathogenic avian influenza virus in vitro and in vivo. *Antiviral Res* 2011;92(2):195–203.
146. Duan S, Boltz DA, Seiler P, et al. Oseltamivir-resistant pandemic H1N1/2009 influenza virus possesses lower transmissibility and fitness in ferrets. *PLoS Pathog* 2010;6(7):e1001022.
151. Ehrhardt C, Ludwig S. A new player in a deadly game: influenza viruses and the PI3K/Akt signalling pathway. *Cell Microbiol* 2009;11(6):863–871.
154. Eierhoff T, Hrincius ER, Rescher U, et al. The epidermal growth factor receptor (EGFR) promotes uptake of influenza A viruses (IAV) into host cells. *PLoS Pathog* 2010;6(9):e1001099.
155. Eisfeld AJ, Kawakami E, Watanabe T, et al. RAB11A is essential for transport of the influenza virus genome to the plasma membrane. *J Virol* 2011;85(13):6117–6126.
156. Eisfeld AJ, Neumann G, Kawaoka Y. Human immunodeficiency virus rev-binding protein is essential for influenza a virus replication and promotes genome trafficking in late-stage infection. *J Virol* 2011;85(18): 9588–9598.
157. Ekiert DC, Bhabha G, Elsliger MA, et al. Antibody recognition of a highly conserved influenza virus epitope. *Science* 2009;324(5924): 246–251.
158. Ekiert DC, Friesen RH, Bhabha G, et al. A highly conserved neutralizing epitope on group 2 influenza A viruses. *Science* 2011;333(6044): 843–850.
170. Fechter P, Brownlee GG. Recognition of mRNA cap structures by viral and cellular proteins. *J Gen Virol* 2005;86:1239–1249.
178. Fodor E, Devenish L, Engelhardt OG, et al. Rescue of influenza A virus from recombinant DNA. *J Virol* 1999;73(11):9679–9682.
186. Fouchier RA, Munster V, Wallensten A, et al. Characterization of a novel influenza A virus hemagglutinin subtype (H16) obtained from black-headed gulls. *J Virol* 2005;79(5):2814–2822.
190. Fujii K, Ozawa M, Iwatsuki-Horimoto K, et al. Incorporation of influenza A virus genome segments does not absolutely require wild-type sequences. *J Gen Virol* 2009;90(Pt 7):1734–1740.
194. Furuse Y, Oshitani H. Evolution of the influenza A virus untranslated regions. *Infect Genet Evol* 2011;11(5):1150–1154.
197. Gabriel G, Herwig A, Klenk HD. Interaction of polymerase subunit PB2 and NP with importin alpha1 is a determinant of host range of influenza A virus. *PLoS Pathog* 2008;4(2):e11.
198. Gabriel G, Klingel K, Otte A, et al. Differential use of importin-alpha isoforms governs cell tropism and host adaptation of influenza virus. *Nat Commun* 2011;2:156.
199. Gack MU, Albrecht RA, Urano T, et al. Influenza A virus NS1 targets the ubiquitin ligase TRIM25 to evade recognition by the host viral RNA sensor RIG-I. *Cell Host Microbe* 2009;5(5):439–449.
204. Gamblin SJ, Skehel JJ. Influenza hemagglutinin and neuraminidase membrane glycoproteins. *J Biol Chem* 2010;285(37):28403–28409.
205. Gannage M, Dormann D, Albrecht R, et al. Matrix protein 2 of influenza A virus blocks autophagosome fusion with lysosomes. *Cell Host Microbe* 2009;6(4):367–380.
207. Gao Q, Lowen AC, Wang TT, et al. A nine-segment influenza a virus carrying subtype H1 and H3 hemagglutinins. *J Virol* 2010;84(16): 8062–8071.
208. Gao Q, Palese P. Rewiring the RNAs of influenza virus to prevent reassortment. *Proc Natl Acad Sci U S A* 2009;106(37):15891–15896.
213. Garcia-Sastre A, Egorov A, Matassov D, et al. Influenza A virus lacking the NS1 gene replicates in interferon-deficient systems. *Virology* 1998; 252(2):324–330.
224. Gog JR, Afonso Edos S, Dalton RM, et al. Codon conservation in the influenza A virus genome defines RNA packaging signals. *Nucleic Acids Res* 2007;35(6):1897–1907.
225. Golebiewski L, Liu H, Javier RT, et al. The avian influenza virus NS1 ESEV PDZ binding motif associates with Dlg1 and Scribble to disrupt cellular tight junctions. *J Virol* 2011;85(20):10639–10648.
231. Grantham ML, Stewart SM, Lalime EN, et al. Tyrosines in the influenza A virus M2 protein cytoplasmic tail are critical for production of infectious virus particles. *J Virol* 2010;84(17):8765–8776.
233. Guan R, Ma LC, Leonard PG, et al. Structural basis for the sequence-specific recognition of human ISG15 by the NS1 protein of influenza B virus. *Proc Natl Acad Sci U S A* 2011;108(33):13468–13473.
236. Guilligay D, Tarendeau F, Resa-Infante P, et al. The structural basis for cap binding by influenza virus polymerase subunit PB2. *Nat Struct Mol Biol* 2008;15(5):500–506.
239. Ha Y, Stevens DJ, Skehel JJ, et al. X-ray structure of the hemagglutinin of a potential H3 avian progenitor of the 1968 Hong Kong pandemic influenza virus. *Virology* 2003;309(2):209–218.
243. Hai R, Garcia-Sastre A, Swayne DE, et al. A reassortment-incompetent live attenuated influenza virus vaccine for protection against pandemic virus strains. *J Virol* 2011;85(14):6832–6843.
244. Hai R, Martinez-Sobrido L, Fraser KA, et al. Influenza B virus NS1-truncated mutants: live-attenuated vaccine approach. *J Virol* 2008;82(21): 10580–10590.
245. Hale BG, Albrecht RA, Garcia-Sastre A. Innate immune evasion strategies of influenza viruses. *Future Microbiol* 2010;5(1):23–41.
246. Hale BG, Barclay WS, Randall RE, et al. Structure of an avian influenza A virus NS1 protein effector domain. *Virology* 2008;378(1):1–5.
247. Hale BG, Batty IH, Downes CP, et al. Binding of influenza A virus NS1 protein to the inter-SH2 domain of p85 suggests a novel mechanism for phosphoinositide 3-kinase activation. *J Biol Chem* 2008;283(3): 1372–1380.
248. Hale BG, Jackson D, Chen YH, et al. Influenza A virus NS1 protein binds p85beta and activates phosphatidylinositol-3-kinase signaling. *Proc Natl Acad Sci U S A* 2006;103(38):14194–14199.
249. Hale BG, Kerry PS, Jackson D, et al. Structural insights into phosphoinositide 3-kinase activation by the influenza A virus NS1 protein. *Proc Natl Acad Sci U S A* 2010;107(5):1954–1959.
250. Hale BG, Randall RE, Ortin J, et al. The multifunctional NS1 protein of influenza A viruses. *J Gen Virol* 2008;89(Pt 10):2359–2376.
251. Haller O, Staeheli P, Kochs G. Protective role of interferon-induced Mx GTPases against influenza viruses. *Rev Sci Tech* 2009;28(1):219–231.
254. Hao L, Sakurai A, Watanabe T, et al. Drosophila RNAi screen identifies host genes important for influenza virus replication. *Nature* 2008; 454(7206):890–893.
256. Harris A, Cardone G, Winkler DC, et al. Influenza virus pleiomorphy characterized by cryoelectron tomography. *Proc Natl Acad Sci U S A* 2006; 103(50):19123–19127.
258. Harrison SC. Viral membrane fusion. *Nat Struct Mol Biol* 2008;15(7): 690–698.
264. Hayden F. Developing new antiviral agents for influenza treatment: what does the future hold? *Clin Infect Dis* 2009;48(Suppl 1):S3–S13.
265. He X, Zhou J, Bartlam M, et al. Crystal structure of the polymerase PA(C)-PB1(N) complex from an avian influenza H5N1 virus. *Nature* 2008;454(7208):1123–1126.
266. Heikkinen LS, Kazlauskas A, Melen K, et al. Avian and 1918 Spanish influenza a virus NS1 proteins bind to Crk/CrkL Src homology 3 domains to activate host cell signaling. *J Biol Chem* 2008;283(9): 5719–5727.
268. Hemerka JN, Wang D, Weng Y, et al. Detection and characterization of influenza A virus PA-PB2 interaction through a bimolecular fluorescence complementation assay. *J Virol* 2009;83(8):3944–3955.
269. Henkel M, Mitzner D, Henklein P, et al. The proapoptotic influenza A virus protein PB1-F2 forms a nonselective ion channel. *PLoS One* 2010;5(6):e11112.
280. Hoffmann HH, Kunz A, Simon VA, et al. Broad-spectrum antiviral that interferes with de novo pyrimidine biosynthesis. *Proc Natl Acad Sci U S A* 2011;108(14):5777–5782.
286. Horimoto T, Kawaoka Y. Designing vaccines for pandemic influenza. *Curr Top Microbiol Immunol* 2009;333:165–176.
289. Hrincius ER, Wixler V, Wolff T, et al. CRK adaptor protein expression is required for efficient replication of avian influenza A viruses and controls JNK-mediated apoptotic responses. *Cell Microbiol* 2010;12(6): 831–843.
290. Hsu MT, Parvin JD, Gupta S, et al. Genomic RNAs of influenza viruses are held in a circular conformation in virions and in infected

cells by a terminal panhandle. *Proc Natl Acad Sci U S A* 1987;84(22):8140–8144.

291. Hu F, Luo W, Hong M. Mechanisms of proton conduction and gating in influenza M2 proton channels from solid-state NMR. *Science* 2010;330(6003):505–508.
292. Huang IC, Bailey CC, Weyer JL, et al. Distinct patterns of IFITM-mediated restriction of filoviruses, SARS coronavirus, and influenza A virus. *PLoS Pathog* 2011;7(1):e1001258.
298. Hurt AC, Holien JK, Parker MW, et al. Oseltamivir resistance and the H274Y neuraminidase mutation in seasonal, pandemic and highly pathogenic influenza viruses. *Drugs* 2009;69(18):2523–2531.
301. Hutchinson EC, von Kirchbach JC, Gog JR, et al. Genome packaging in influenza A virus. *J Gen Virol* 2010;91(Pt 2):313–328.
302. Hutchinson EC, Wise HM, Kudryavtseva K, et al. Characterisation of influenza A viruses with mutations in segment 5 packaging signals. *Vaccine* 2009;27(45):6270–6275.
305. Isaacs A, Lindenmann J. Virus interference. I. The interferon. *Proc R Soc Lond B Biol Sci* 1957;147(927):258–267.
313. Jackson D, Elderfield RA, Barclay WS. Molecular studies of influenza B virus in the reverse genetics era. *J Gen Virol* 2011;92(Pt 1):1–17.
315. Jackson RJ, Cooper KL, Tappenden P, et al. Oseltamivir, zanamivir and amantadine in the prevention of influenza: a systematic review. *J Infect* 2011;62(1):14–25.
322. Jorba N, Coloma R, Ortin J. Genetic trans-complementation establishes a new model for influenza virus RNA transcription and replication. *PLoS Pathog* 2009;5(5):e1000462.
323. Jorba N, Juarez S, Torreira E, et al. Analysis of the interaction of influenza virus polymerase complex with human cell factors. *Proteomics* 2008;8(10):2077–2088.
324. Kao RY, Yang D, Lau LS, et al. Identification of influenza A nucleoprotein as an antiviral target. *Nat Biotechnol* 2010;28(6):600–605.
325. Karlas A, Machuy N, Shin Y, et al. Genome-wide RNAi screen identifies human host factors crucial for influenza virus replication. *Nature* 2010;463(7282):818–822.
327. Kashyap AK, Steel J, Rubrum A, et al. Protection from the 2009 H1N1 pandemic influenza by an antibody from combinatorial survivor-based libraries. *PLoS Pathog* 2010;6(7):e1000990.
328. Kerry PS, Ayllon J, Taylor MA, et al. A transient homotypic interaction model for the influenza A virus NS1 protein effector domain. *PLoS One* 2011;6(3):e17946.
334. Kiso M, Takahashi K, Sakai-Tagawa Y, et al. T-705 (favipiravir) activity against lethal H5N1 influenza A viruses. *Proc Natl Acad Sci U S A* 2010;107(2):882–887.
338. Kochs G, Garcia-Sastre A, Martinez-Sobrido L. Multiple anti-interferon actions of the influenza A virus NS1 protein. *J Virol* 2007;81(13):7011–7021.
341. Konig R, Stertz S, Zhou Y, et al. Human host factors required for influenza virus replication. *Nature* 2010;463(7282):813–817.
342. Kozakov D, Chuang GY, Beglov D, et al. Where does amantadine bind to the influenza virus M2 proton channel? *Trends Biochem Sci* 2010;35(9):471–475.
343. Krause JC, Tsibane T, Tumpey TM, et al. A broadly neutralizing human monoclonal antibody that recognizes a conserved, novel epitope on the globular head of influenza H1N1 virus hemagglutinin. *J Virol* 2011;85(20):10905–10908.
348. Kumar N, Liang Y, Parslow TG. Receptor tyrosine kinase inhibitors block multiple steps of influenza a virus replication. *J Virol* 2011;85(6):2818–2827.
352. Lai JC, Chan WW, Kien F, et al. Formation of virus-like particles from human cell lines exclusively expressing influenza neuraminidase. *J Gen Virol* 2010;91(Pt 9):2322–2330.
362. Laver WG. Influenza virus surface glycoproteins, haemagglutinin and neuraminidase: a personal account. In: Potter CW, ed. *Influenza.* Vol 7. Amsterdam: Elsevier Science B.V.; 2002:31–48.
367. Lee CW, Suarez DL. Reverse genetics of the avian influenza virus. *Methods Mol Biol* 2008;436:99–111.
368. Lee JH, Kim SH, Pascua PN, et al. Direct interaction of cellular hnRNP-F and NS1 of influenza A virus accelerates viral replication by modulation of viral transcriptional activity and host gene expression. *Virology* 2010;397(1):89–99.
391. Liang Y, Huang T, Ly H, et al. Mutational analyses of packaging signals in influenza virus PA, PB1, and PB2 genomic RNA segments. *J Virol* 2008;82(1):229–236.
392. Liao TL, Wu CY, Su WC, et al. Ubiquitination and deubiquitination of NP protein regulates influenza A virus RNA replication. *EMBO J* 2010;29(22):3879–3890.
396. Liu H, Golebiewski L, Dow EC, et al. The ESEV PDZ-binding motif of the avian influenza A virus NS1 protein protects infected cells from apoptosis by directly targeting Scribble. *J Virol* 2010;84(21):11164–11174.
398. Londrigan SL, Turville SG, Tate MD, et al. N-linked glycosylation facilitates sialic acid-independent attachment and entry of influenza A viruses into cells expressing DC-SIGN or L-SIGN. *J Virol* 2011;85(6):2990–3000.
399. Lorieau JL, Louis JM, Bax A. The complete influenza hemagglutinin fusion domain adopts a tight helical hairpin arrangement at the lipid:water interface. *Proc Natl Acad Sci U S A* 2010;107(25):11341–11346.
409. Luytjes W, Krystal M, Enami M, et al. Amplification, expression, and packaging of foreign gene by influenza virus. *Cell* 1989;59(6):1107–1113.
414. Manicassamy B, Manicassamy S, Belicha-Villanueva A, et al. Analysis of in vivo dynamics of influenza virus infection in mice using a GFP reporter virus. *Proc Natl Acad Sci U S A* 2010;107(25):11531–11536.
416. Marsh GA, Hatami R, Palese P. Specific residues of the influenza A virus hemagglutinin viral RNA are important for efficient packaging into budding virions. *J Virol* 2007;81(18):9727–9736.
417. Marsh GA, Rabadan R, Levine AJ, et al. Highly conserved regions of influenza a virus polymerase gene segments are critical for efficient viral RNA packaging. *J Virol* 2008;82(5):2295–2304.
419. Martin-Benito J, Area E, Ortega J, et al. Three-dimensional reconstruction of a recombinant influenza virus ribonucleoprotein particle. *EMBO Rep* 2001;2(4):313–317.
422. Martinez-Sobrido L, Garcia-Sastre A. Generation of recombinant influenza virus from plasmid DNA. *J Vis Exp* 2010;42:2057.
423. Mata MA, Satterly N, Versteeg GA, et al. Chemical inhibition of RNA viruses reveals REDD1 as a host defense factor. *Nat Chem Biol* 2011;7(10):712–719.
427. Mayer D, Molawi K, Martinez-Sobrido L, et al. Identification of cellular interaction partners of the influenza virus ribonucleoprotein complex and polymerase complex using proteomic-based approaches. *J Proteome Res* 2007;6(2):672–682.
428. McAuley JL, Chipuk JE, Boyd KL, et al. PB1-F2 proteins from H5N1 and 20 century pandemic influenza viruses cause immunopathology. *PLoS Pathog* 2010;6(7):e1001014.
429. McAuley JL, Hornung F, Boyd KL, et al. Expression of the 1918 influenza A virus PB1-F2 enhances the pathogenesis of viral and secondary bacterial pneumonia. *Cell Host Microbe* 2007;2(4):240–249.
440. Memoli MJ, Davis AS, Proudfoot K, et al. Multidrug-resistant 2009 pandemic influenza A(H1N1) viruses maintain fitness and transmissibility in ferrets. *J Infect Dis* 2011;203(3):348–357.
443. Mercer J, Schelhaas M, Helenius A. Virus entry by endocytosis. *Annu Rev Biochem* 2010;79:803–833.
445. Min JY, Krug RM. The primary function of RNA binding by the influenza A virus NS1 protein in infected cells: inhibiting the 2′-5′ oligo (A) synthetase/RNase L pathway. *Proc Natl Acad Sci U S A* 2006;103(18):7100–7105.
451. Momose F, Sekimoto T, Ohkura T, et al. Apical transport of influenza A virus ribonucleoprotein requires Rab11-positive recycling endosome. *PLoS One* 2011;6(6):e21123.
459. Muraki Y, Hongo S. The molecular virology and reverse genetics of influenza C virus. *Jpn J Infect Dis* 2010;63(3):157–165.
471. Nayak DP, Balogun RA, Yamada H, et al. Influenza virus morphogenesis and budding. *Virus Res* 2009;143(2):147–161.
476. Neumann G, Fujii K, Kino Y, et al. An improved reverse genetics system for influenza A virus generation and its implications for vaccine production. *Proc Natl Acad Sci U S A* 2005;102(46):16825–16829.
487. Noble E, Mathews DH, Chen JL, et al. Biophysical analysis of influenza A virus RNA promoter at physiological temperatures. *J Biol Chem* 2011;286(26):22965–22970.
488. Noda T, Kawaoka Y. Structure of influenza virus ribonucleoprotein complexes and their packaging into virions. *Rev Med Virol* 2010;20(6):380–391.

489. Noda T, Sagara H, Yen A, et al. Architecture of ribonucleoprotein complexes in influenza A virus particles. *Nature* 2006;439(7075): 490–492.
490. Obayashi E, Yoshida H, Kawai F, et al. The structural basis for an essential subunit interaction in influenza virus RNA polymerase. *Nature* 2008;454(7208):1127–1131.
499. Ono A, Freed EO. Role of lipid rafts in virus replication. *Adv Virus Res* 2005;64:311–358.
500. Operario DJ, Moser MJ, St George K. Highly sensitive and quantitative detection of the H274Y oseltamivir resistance mutation in seasonal A/H1N1 influenza virus. *J Clin Microbiol* 2010;48(10):3517–3524.
505. Ozawa M, Maeda J, Iwatsuki-Horimoto K, et al. Nucleotide sequence requirements at the 5′ end of the influenza A virus M RNA segment for efficient virus replication. *J Virol* 2009;83(7):3384–3388.
506. Pachler K, Mayr J, Vlasak R. A seven plasmid-based system for the rescue of influenza C virus. *J Mol Genet Med* 2010;4:239–246.
509. Palese P. The genes of influenza virus. *Cell* 1977;10(1):1–10.
510. Palese P, Compans RW. Inhibition of influenza virus replication in tissue culture by 2-deoxy-2,3-dehydro-N-trifluoroacetylneuraminic acid (FANA): mechanism of action. *J Gen Virol* 1976;33(1):159–163.
516. Palese P, Tobita K, Ueda M, et al. Characterization of temperature sensitive influenza virus mutants defective in neuraminidase. *Virology* 1974;61(2):397–410.
517. Pappas C, Aguilar PV, Basler CF, et al. Single gene reassortants identify a critical role for PB1, HA, and NA in the high virulence of the 1918 pandemic influenza virus. *Proc Natl Acad Sci U S A* 2008;105(8): 3064–3069.
526. Perez D, Rimstad E, Smith G, et al. Orthomyxoviridae. In: King AMQ, Adams MJ, Carstens EB, et al, eds. *Virus Taxonomy.* Oxford: Elsevier; 2011:749–762.
528. Perez JT, Varble A, Sachidanandam R, et al. Influenza A virus-generated small RNAs regulate the switch from transcription to replication. *Proc Natl Acad Sci U S A* 2010;107(25):11525–11530.
530. Pichlmair A, Schulz O, Tan CP, et al. RIG-I-mediated antiviral responses to single-stranded RNA bearing 5′-phosphates. *Science* 2006;314(5801): 997–1001.
533. Pinto LH, Lamb RA. Controlling influenza virus replication by inhibiting its proton channel. *Mol Biosyst* 2007;3(1):18–23.
534. Pinto LH, Lamb RA. The M2 proton channels of influenza A and B viruses. *J Biol Chem* 2006;281(14):8997–9000.
554. Resa-Infante P, Jorba N, Coloma R, et al. The influenza virus RNA synthesis machine: advances in its structure and function. *RNA Biol* 2011;8(2):207–215.
557. Richt JA, Garcia-Sastre A. Attenuated influenza virus vaccines with modified NS1 proteins. *Curr Top Microbiol Immunol* 2009;333:177–195.
559. Robb NC, Jackson D, Vreede FT, et al. Splicing of influenza A virus NS1 mRNA is independent of the viral NS1 protein. *J Gen Virol* 2010;91 (Pt 9):2331–2340.
560. Robb NC, Smith M, Vreede FT, et al. NS2/NEP protein regulates transcription and replication of the influenza virus RNA genome. *J Gen Virol* 2009;90(Pt 6):1398–1407.
567. Rodriguez A, Perez-Gonzalez A, Hossain MJ, et al. Attenuated strains of influenza A viruses do not induce degradation of RNA polymerase II. *J Virol* 2009;83(21):11166–11174.
571. Rossman JS, Jing X, Leser GP, et al. Influenza virus m2 ion channel protein is necessary for filamentous virion formation. *J Virol* 2010;84(10): 5078–5088.
572. Rossman JS, Jing X, Leser GP, et al. Influenza virus M2 protein mediates ESCRT-independent membrane scission. *Cell* 2010;142(6):902–913.
573. Rossman JS, Lamb RA. Influenza virus assembly and budding. *Virology* 2011;411(2):229–236.
584. Satterly N, Tsai PL, van Deursen J, et al. Influenza virus targets the mRNA export machinery and the nuclear pore complex. *Proc Natl Acad Sci U S A* 2007;104(6):1853–1858.
589. Schnell JR, Chou JJ. Structure and mechanism of the M2 proton channel of influenza A virus. *Nature* 2008;451(7178):591–595.
593. Seibert CW, Kaminski M, Philipp J, et al. Oseltamivir-resistant variants of the 2009 pandemic H1N1 influenza A virus are not attenuated in the guinea pig and ferret transmission models. *J Virol* 2010;84(21): 11219–11226.
594. Seth S, Templin MV, Severson G, et al. A potential therapeutic for pandemic influenza using RNA interference. *Methods Mol Biol* 2010;623: 397–422.
596. Shapira SD, Gat-Viks I, Shum BO, et al. A physical and regulatory map of host-influenza interactions reveals pathways in H1N1 infection. *Cell* 2009;139(7):1255–1267.
599. Sharma M, Yi M, Dong H, et al. Insight into the mechanism of the influenza A proton channel from a structure in a lipid bilayer. *Science* 2010;330(6003):509–512.
600. Shaw ML. The host interactome of influenza virus presents new potential targets for antiviral drugs. *Rev Med Virol* 2011;21(6):358–369.
601. Shaw ML, Palese P. Orthomyxoviruses: molecular biology. In: Mahy B, van Regenmortel M, eds. *Encyclopedia of Virology.* Vol 3. 3rd ed. Oxford, UK: Elsevier; 2008:483–489.
602. Shaw ML, Stone KL, Colangelo CM, et al. Cellular proteins in influenza virus particles. *PLoS Pathog* 2008;4(6):e1000085.
608. Shimizu T, Takizawa N, Watanabe K, et al. Crucial role of the influenza virus NS2 (NEP) C-terminal domain in M1 binding and nuclear export of vRNP. *FEBS Lett* 2011;585(1):41–46.
622. Smith DJ, Lapedes AS, de Jong JC, et al. Mapping the antigenic and genetic evolution of influenza virus. *Science* 2004;305(5682):371–376.
628. Sridharan H, Zhao C, Krug RM. Species specificity of the NS1 protein of influenza B virus: NS1 binds only human and non-human primate ubiquitin-like ISG15 proteins. *J Biol Chem* 2010;285(11):7852–7856.
631. Steel J, Lowen AC, Wang TT, et al. Influenza virus vaccine based on the conserved hemagglutinin stalk domain. *MBio* 2010;1(1):e00018–00010.
636. Stertz S, Shaw ML. Uncovering the global host cell requirements for influenza virus replication via RNAi screening. *Microbes Infect* 2011; 13(5):516–525.
637. Stevens J, Blixt O, Glaser L, et al. Glycan microarray analysis of the hemagglutinins from modern and pandemic influenza viruses reveals different receptor specificities. *J Mol Biol* 2006;355(5):1143–1155.
638. Stevens J, Blixt O, Paulson JC, et al. Glycan microarray technologies: tools to survey host specificity of influenza viruses. *Nat Rev Microbiol* 2006;4(11):857–864.
640. Stevens J, Corper AL, Basler CF, et al. Structure of the uncleaved human H1 hemagglutinin from the extinct 1918 influenza virus. *Science* 2004;303(5665):1866–1870.
641. Stewart SM, Wu WH, Lalime EN, et al. The cholesterol recognition/interaction amino acid consensus motif of the influenza A virus M2 protein is not required for virus replication but contributes to virulence. *Virology* 2010;405(2):530–538.
643. Stouffer AL, Acharya R, Salom D, et al. Structural basis for the function and inhibition of an influenza virus proton channel. *Nature* 2008; 451(7178):596–599.
645. Su CY, Cheng TJ, Lin MI, et al. High-throughput identification of compounds targeting influenza RNA-dependent RNA polymerase activity. *Proc Natl Acad Sci U S A* 2010;107(45):19151–19156.
646. Sugiyama K, Obayashi E, Kawaguchi A, et al. Structural insight into the essential PB1-PB2 subunit contact of the influenza virus RNA polymerase. *EMBO J* 2009;28(12):1803–1811.
650. Sui J, Hwang WC, Perez S, et al. Structural and functional bases for broad-spectrum neutralization of avian and human influenza A viruses. *Nat Struct Mol Biol* 2009;16(3):265–273.
653. Suzuki Y, Nei M. Origin and evolution of influenza virus hemagglutinin genes. *Mol Biol Evol* 2002;19(4):501–509.
657. Talon J, Salvatore M, O'Neill RE, et al. Influenza A and B viruses expressing altered NS1 proteins: a vaccine approach. *Proc Natl Acad Sci U S A* 2000;97(8):4309–4314.
660. Tang Y, Zhong G, Zhu L, et al. Herc5 attenuates influenza A virus by catalyzing ISGylation of viral NS1 protein. *J Immunol* 2010;184(10): 5777–5790.
661. Tarendeau F, Boudet J, Guilligay D, et al. Structure and nuclear import function of the C-terminal domain of influenza virus polymerase PB2 subunit. *Nat Struct Mol Biol* 2007;14(3):229–233.
662. Thaa B, Levental I, Herrmann A, et al. Intrinsic membrane association of the cytoplasmic tail of influenza virus M2 protein and lateral membrane sorting regulated by cholesterol binding and palmitoylation. *Biochem J* 2011;437(3):389–397.

671. Tumpey TM, Basler CF, Aguilar PV, et al. Characterization of the reconstructed 1918 Spanish influenza pandemic virus. *Science* 2005;310(5745):77–80.
677. Varga ZT, Ramos I, Hai R, et al. The influenza virus protein PB1-F2 inhibits the induction of type I interferon at the level of the MAVS adaptor protein. *PLoS Pathog* 2011;7(6):e1002067.
684. Versteeg GA, Hale BG, van Boheemen S, et al. Species-specific antagonism of host ISGylation by the influenza B virus NS1 protein. *J Virol* 2010;84(10):5423–5430.
691. Vreede FT, Chan AY, Sharps J, et al. Mechanisms and functional implications of the degradation of host RNA polymerase II in influenza virus infected cells. *Virology* 2010;396(1):125–134.
692. Vreede FT, Fodor E. The role of the influenza virus RNA polymerase in host shut-off. *Virulence* 2010;1(5):436–439.
693. Vreede FT, Gifford H, Brownlee GG. Role of initiating nucleoside triphosphate concentrations in the regulation of influenza virus replication and transcription. *J Virol* 2008;82(14):6902–6910.
698. Walkiewicz MP, Basu D, Jablonski JJ, et al. Novel inhibitor of influenza non-structural protein 1 blocks multi-cycle replication in an RNase L-dependent manner. *J Gen Virol* 2011;92(Pt 1):60–70.
700. Wang D, Harmon A, Jin J, et al. The lack of an inherent membrane targeting signal is responsible for the failure of the matrix (M1) protein of influenza A virus to bud into virus-like particles. *J Virol* 2010;84(9):4673–4681.
701. Wang J, Pielak RM, McClintock MA, et al. Solution structure and functional analysis of the influenza B proton channel. *Nat Struct Mol Biol* 2009;16(12):1267–1271.
704. Wang Q, Tian X, Chen X, et al. Structural basis for receptor specificity of influenza B virus hemagglutinin. *Proc Natl Acad Sci U S A* 2007;104(43):16874–16879.
706. Wang TT, Palese P. Biochemistry. Catching a moving target. *Science* 2011;333(6044):834–835.
707. Wang TT, Tan GS, Hai R, et al. Broadly protective monoclonal antibodies against H3 influenza viruses following sequential immunization with different hemagglutinins. *PLoS Pathog* 2010;6(2):e1000796.
708. Wang TT, Tan GS, Hai R, et al. Vaccination with a synthetic peptide from the influenza virus hemagglutinin provides protection against distinct viral subtypes. *Proc Natl Acad Sci U S A* 2010;107(44):18979–18984.
716. Watanabe R, Leser GP, Lamb RA. Influenza virus is not restricted by tetherin whereas influenza VLP production is restricted by tetherin. *Virology* 2011;417(1):50–56.
717. Watanabe T, Watanabe S, Kawaoka Y. Cellular networks involved in the influenza virus life cycle. *Cell Host Microbe* 2010;7(6):427–439.
725. Wilson IA, Skehel JJ, Wiley DC. Structure of the haemagglutinin membrane glycoprotein of influenza virus at 3 A resolution. *Nature* 1981;289(5796):366–373.
727. Wolff T, Ludwig S. Influenza viruses control the vertebrate type I interferon system: factors, mechanisms, and consequences. *J Interferon Cytokine Res* 2009;29(9):549–557.
730. Wrammert J, Koutsonanos D, Li GM, et al. Broadly cross-reactive antibodies dominate the human B cell response against 2009 pandemic H1N1 influenza virus infection. *J Exp Med* 2011;208(1):181–193.
731. Wressnigg N, Voss D, Wolff T, et al. Development of a live-attenuated influenza B DeltaNS1 intranasal vaccine candidate. *Vaccine* 2009;27(21):2851–2857.
732. Wu CY, Jeng KS, Lai MM. The SUMOylation of matrix protein M1 modulates the assembly and morphogenesis of influenza A virus. *J Virol* 2011;85(13):6618–6628.
733. Xia S, Monzingo AF, Robertus JD. Structure of NS1A effector domain from the influenza A/Udorn/72 virus. *Acta Crystallogr D Biol Crystallogr* 2009;65(Pt 1):11–17.
735. Xu R, Ekiert DC, Krause JC, et al. Structural basis of preexisting immunity to the 2009 H1N1 pandemic influenza virus. *Science* 2010;328(5976):357–360.
739. Yamashita M. Laninamivir and its prodrug, CS-8958: long-acting neuraminidase inhibitors for the treatment of influenza. *Antivir Chem Chemother* 2010;21(2):71–84.
743. Yanguez E, Nieto A. So similar, yet so different: selective translation of capped and polyadenylated viral mRNAs in the influenza virus infected cell. *Virus Res* 2011;156(1–2):1–12.
745. Ye Q, Krug RM, Tao YJ. The mechanism by which influenza A virus nucleoprotein forms oligomers and binds RNA. *Nature* 2006;444(7122):1078–1082.
748. Yen HL, Liang CH, Wu CY, et al. Hemagglutinin-neuraminidase balance confers respiratory-droplet transmissibility of the pandemic H1N1 influenza virus in ferrets. *Proc Natl Acad Sci U S A* 2011;108(34):14264–14269.
750. Yondola MA, Fernandes F, Belicha-Villanueva A, et al. Budding capability of the influenza virus neuraminidase can be modulated by tetherin. *J Virol* 2011;85(6):2480–2491.
751. Yu J, Li X, Wang Y, et al. PDlim2 selectively interacts with the PDZ binding motif of highly pathogenic avian H5N1 influenza A virus NS1. *PLoS One* 2011;6(5):e19511.
752. Yuan P, Bartlam M, Lou Z, et al. Crystal structure of an avian influenza polymerase PA(N) reveals an endonuclease active site. *Nature* 2009;458(7240):909–913.
755. Zamarin D, Garcia-Sastre A, Xiao X, et al. Influenza virus PB1-F2 protein induces cell death through mitochondrial ANT3 and VDAC1. *PLoS Pathog* 2005;1(1):e4.
758. Zeng Q, Langereis MA, van Vliet AL, et al. Structure of coronavirus hemagglutinin-esterase offers insight into corona and influenza virus evolution. *Proc Natl Acad Sci U S A* 2008;105(26):9065–9069.
761. Zhang X, Kong W, Ashraf S, et al. A one-plasmid system to generate influenza virus in cultured chicken cells for potential use in influenza vaccine. *J Virol* 2009;83(18):9296–9303.
762. Zhao C, Denison C, Huibregtse JM, et al. Human ISG15 conjugation targets both IFN-induced and constitutively expressed proteins functioning in diverse cellular pathways. *Proc Natl Acad Sci U S A* 2005;102(29):10200–10205.
763. Zhao C, Hsiang TY, Kuo RL, et al. ISG15 conjugation system targets the viral NS1 protein in influenza A virus-infected cells. *Proc Natl Acad Sci U S A* 2010;107(5):2253–2258.
773. Zhou B, Jerzak G, Scholes DT, et al. Reverse genetics plasmid for cloning unstable influenza A virus gene segments. *J Virol Methods* 2011;173(2):378–383.

CHAPTER 41

Peter F. Wright • Gabriele Neumann • Yoshihiro Kawaoka

Orthomyxoviruses

INTRODUCTION

Influenza viruses (family *Orthomyxoviridae*) cause highly contagious respiratory disease with potentially fatal outcomes. Symptoms include fever, headache, cough, sore throat, nasal congestion, sneezing, and body aches. Influenza viruses also cause local epidemics or pandemics (worldwide outbreaks) with significant infection rates. Although the economic burden of influenza is most prominent during pandemics, the combined annual costs of seasonal epidemics due to sick days, emergency department visits, and medications are significant. With the realization that avian influenza viruses can be directly transmitted to humans, influenza viruses are now considered a major, global health threat.

Technologies such as reverse genetics[1496] have allowed the routine manipulation of influenza viral genomes. In addition, large-scale sequencing of viral genomes in combination with improved tools for sequence analysis, and other technologies—including yeast two-hybrid screens, small interfering RNA (siRNA)–mediated screens, and transcriptomics, proteomics, metabolomics, and lipidomics studies—are being used to discover the viral and cellular factors that control influenza virus replication, interspecies transmission, and pathogenesis. Despite recent advances, much still needs to be learned about the molecular determinants of these events.

NOMENCLATURE

Influenza viruses belong to the *Orthomyxoviridae* family. This family comprises five genera: *Influenzavirus A; Influenzavirus B; Influenzavirus C; Thogotovirus,* which includes *Thogoto virus* and *Dhori virus;* and *Isavirus,* which includes infectious salmon anemia virus (ISAV; see the International Committee on Taxonomy of Viruses website: http://www.ictvonline.org).[520,1358] Influenza A viruses are further classified into subtypes based on the antigenicity of their HA and NA molecules; currently, 17 HA subtypes (H1–H17) and 9 NA subtypes (N1–N9) are known. The present nomenclature system[1] includes type of virus, host of origin (except for humans), geographic site of isolation, strain number, and year of isolation, followed by the antigenic description of the HA and NA subtypes in parenthesis; for viruses isolated before 2000, the year should be given as two digits; for viruses isolated in 2000 or later, the year should be given as four digits. For example, A/swine/Iowa/15/30 (H1N1) describes an influenza A virus isolated from a pig in Iowa in 1930 with a strain number of 15 and an H1N1 subtype. Antigenic subtypes have not been identified for influenza B and C viruses. Thogoto virus, Dhori virus, and ISAV do not cross-react antigenically.

Seroarcheology

Retrospective seroepidemiologic analysis, or seroarcheology, has provided information about influenza virus outbreaks that preceded the virologic techniques currently used to unequivocally identify infectious agents. Early studies suggested that the pandemic of 1889 to 1891 was caused by a virus of the H2N2 subtype, whereas that of 1900 had been attributed to an H3N8 strain.[1326,1327,1435,1531,1719] More recent re-evaluation of the data indicates that the 1889 to 1891 pandemic was caused by an H3-like virus, and there is no compelling evidence that links the H2 subtype to a pandemic other than that of 1957.[442] The latter conclusion is substantiated by the lack of protection among those who were at least 80 years old during the 1957 H2 pandemic. Seroarcheology has also linked the 1918/1919 pandemic to an H1 virus, a finding that has been confirmed by sequence determination of influenza virus RNA from the lung tissues of victims.[1712] Studies using antibodies to the NA protein suggest that in the late 1800s, viruses of the N8 subtype were circulating and later replaced by N1 and N2 subtype viruses. Thus, during the 1900s, only a limited number of virus subtypes (H1N1, H2N2, H3N2, H3N8) was established in humans. Reassortant H1N2 viruses emerged in humans in 2001 and circulated in 2002 and 2003, but have not been isolated from humans since early 2004.

Virus Isolation

In 1930, the first swine influenza virus, A/swine/Iowa/30, was isolated,[1863] but it was not until 1933 that the first human virus was isolated by Wilson Smith, Sir Christopher Andrewes, and Sir Patrick Laidlaw of the National Institute for Medical Research in London, England. These investigators inoculated ferrets intranasally with human nasopharyngeal washes from an influenza patient. The animals exhibited an influenza-like disease, and the virus was transmitted to cage mates. One of their junior colleagues (later Sir Charles Stuart-Harris) became infected by these experimentally infected animals; the virus was subsequently isolated from him.[1907] Because it was the first human influenza virus, it was named influenza A virus. In 1940, an antigenically distinct virus was isolated and named type B virus (B/Lee/40).[551] The first influenza C virus was isolated in 1947.[2054] "Fowl plague" was first described in 1878 as a disease that affected chickens in Italy. The causative agent was isolated in 1902 (A/chicken/Brescia/1902 [H7N7]); however, it was not until 1955 that Schafer recognized fowl plague virus as an influenza virus.[1792]

Virus Propagation

Influenza viruses were first propagated in embryonated hens' eggs,[202] which continue to be the most widely used system for vaccine production, although cell-culture systems are now also in use (see later discussion). Avian and equine strains of influenza A viruses can be isolated from the allantoic cavity of 10- to 11-day-old embryonated eggs after 2 to 3 days of incubation at 33°C to 37°C. Human influenza viruses have also been isolated from clinical samples inoculated into the allantoic or amniotic cavity of eggs and incubation at 33°C to 34°C. However, recent human viruses are difficult to isolate from embryonated eggs. Influenza virus growth in embryonated eggs leads to the selection of antigenic variants that are characterized by mutations in the HA protein[202,992,1738,1739,1800] (see also Host Cell-Mediated Selection of Antigenic Variants section). Influenza C viruses amplify in the amniotic, but not allantoic, cavity of eggs and are usually grown for 5 days in 7- to 8-day-old embryonated eggs.

Influenza viruses can also be propagated in cell culture. Madin-Darby canine kidney (MDCK) cells support the efficient replication of many influenza A and B viruses and are used to isolate viruses from humans.[2071,2072] Although many influenza viruses can grow in African green monkey kidney (Vero) cells,[660] they do so less efficiently than in MDCK cells. Cell culture systems based on MDCK,[730] Vero,[1055] and PER.C6 (human primary embryonic retinoblast)[1197,1620] cells have been developed for influenza virus vaccine production, and MDCK and Vero cell–based vaccines are approved in Europe for use in humans; MDCK cell-based vaccines are now also approved in the U.S. Influenza viruses also replicate in a number of primary cell cultures, including monkey, calf, hamster, and chicken kidney cells, as well as in chicken embryo fibroblasts and primary human epithelial cells. With the exception of primary human airway epithelium and kidney cells, most cell culture systems require the addition of trypsin to cleave the HA protein of human viruses (except highly pathogenic H5N1 viruses), a prerequisite for efficient replication.

Replication of influenza viruses in eggs or cell culture is measured by testing the ability of the viruses to agglutinate erythrocytes[814] or by use of molecular biology techniques, such as reverse transcriptase (RT)-polymerase chain reaction (PCR).

EVOLUTION OF INFLUENZA VIRUSES

Influenza viruses evolve via a complex process that involves the accumulation of mutations over time and the rearrangement of viral RNA segments in cells infected with two (or more) different viruses (known as "reassortment"). In wild aquatic birds, avian influenza viruses evolve slowly; while mutations occur, most are not sustained in viral populations since they do not provide an evolutionary advantage. The exceptions are avian viruses in terrestrial poultry, including highly pathogenic H5N1 viruses, which evolve rapidly [see Outbreaks of Highly Pathogenic Avian Influenza (HPAI) Virus section]. In contrast to most avian influenza viruses, human influenza viruses show detectable net evolution over time.

Evolutionary Rates of Influenza A Viruses

Phylogenetic analyses, together with the finding that viruses of all known HA and NA subtypes are maintained in wild aquatic birds, led to the hypothesis that all mammalian influenza A viruses are derived from one avian influenza virus pool[647,648–649,881,1864,2214,2221] (Fig. 41.1). At the nucleotide level, the reported mutation rates range from $\sim 5 \times 10^{-4}$ to $\sim 8 \times 10^{-3}$ nucleotide substitutions per site per year.[198,288,397,538,548,562,648,1233,1870,1985,2214,2221,2289,2359]

At the amino acid level, viruses from wild aquatic birds evolve slower than those from terrestrial poultry, swine, or humans.[562,647,648–649,1870,1995,2214,2246] The fact that in wild aquatic birds most avian influenza A viruses seem to evolve slowly suggests that they are well adapted to their hosts.[91,2214] Thus, although mutations may occur with similar frequency compared to other hosts, they do not result in many amino acid changes.[647] Among avian influenza A viruses, the evolutionary rates are highest for the HA, NA, and NS1 proteins,[288,1110] possibly reflecting their immunogenic or immunomodulatory functions.

Proteins of mammalian and terrestrial poultry viruses continuously accumulate amino acid substitutions. For human influenza A viruses, the evolutionary rates differ among the proteins, likely reflecting differences in the selective pressure of the host.[527,1870,2214] For example, the HA protein evolves faster than the PB2, PB1, PA, NP, and M1 proteins, because HA variants may confer a selective advantage by allowing the virus to evade the host immune response. The human M1 and M2 proteins, encoded by overlapping reading frames, are under different selective pressures: For the M1 protein, a higher percentage of changes is silent than for the M2 protein.[562,881,2214] The M1 protein thus appears to be well adapted to its mammalian

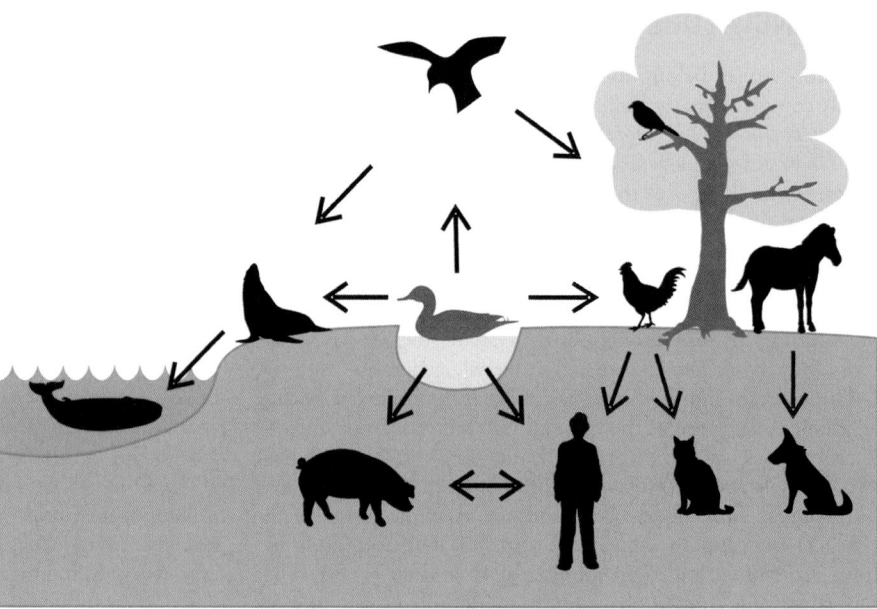

FIGURE 41.1. Influenza A virus reservoir. Wild aquatic birds are the main reservoir of influenza A viruses. Virus transmission has been reported from wild waterfowl to poultry, sea mammals, pigs, horses, and humans. Viruses are also transmitted between pigs and humans, and from poultry to humans. Equine influenza viruses have been transmitted to dogs.

hosts, whereas the M2 protein is under stronger selective pressure. The biologic reason for the selective pressure on the M2 protein is unknown. The two proteins encoded by the NS gene also differ in their evolutionary rates, with NS1 showing more variation between alleles than NS2.[1000,1987] High evolutionary rates have been reported during the establishment of new virus lineages, for example, the introduction of avian H1N1 influenza viruses into European pigs in 1977,[1274] the emergence of highly pathogenic avian H5N2 influenza viruses in poultry in Mexico in 1993/1994,[603] and the emergence of highly pathogenic avian H5N1 influenza viruses in Hong Kong in 1997,[2375] which may reflect preferential selection of mutants that provide an advantage in a new host. This process may be facilitated by so-called mutator mutants that lead to increased error rates in the viral replication complex.[1274,1812,1984,1990]

Host-Specific Lineages, and Geographic Segregation of Influenza A Viruses

Extensive phylogenetic analyses have revealed host-specific virus lineages for several viral genes (e-Fig. 41.1). The phylogenetic trees of the PB2, PA, NP, M, and NS genes are similar in that they can be divided into two major branches consisting of avian and avian-like swine, or classic swine and human influenza viruses, respectively.[90,562,592,647,648,682,881,1559,1901,2214]

The phylogenetic tree of the PB1 gene differs from those of other influenza virus genes. The PB1 genes of human H1N1 viruses cluster with classic swine viruses, whereas the PB1 genes of human H2N2 and H3N2 viruses form a different sublineage that reflects the introduction in 1957 and 1968 of avian virus PB1 genes into human influenza viruses.[682,1001,1813,1901,2214] The genes other than the HA and NA of equine H7N7 viruses do not cluster with avian, human, or swine influenza viruses,[1901] suggesting their early separation into a separate lineage.

The phylogenetic tree of the NS gene is divided into two alleles: A and B.[1000,1987] All mammalian virus NS genes belong to allele A, whereas avian influenza virus NS genes can belong to allele A or B.[1000,2091]

The H1 HA genes can be separated into a branch consisting of avian and avian-like swine influenza viruses versus a branch consisting of human and classic swine viruses.[961,1901] The phylogenetic tree of the H3 HA gene consists of two major branches[1901]: one branch splits into two major subbranches that represent equine/canine and North American avian virus isolates. The second branch can be separated into Eurasian avian viruses, and human and swine H3 HAs that separated from the avian viruses in the 1960s. The human H3 gene has evolved in a single lineage since its introduction into the human population in 1968.[527,682,2214]

The phylogenetic tree of N1 NA genes shows two major branches that separate into human and classic swine, or Eurasian swine and avian N1 NA genes, respectively.[516,548,1901] The phylogenetic tree of the N2 NA gene can be divided into a North American avian clade, and a second clade that evolved into Eurasian avian and human virus genes at the beginning of the last century.[1901]

These analyses also reveal that influenza virus genes can be separated by their geographic origin, with a North American and a Eurasian gene pool.[438,456,1446,1545,1569,2246] These gene pools appear to evolve largely independently, although reassortment between North American and Eurasian viruses has been reported.[456,1050,1094,1248,1305,2181,2210,2246,2263]

Host-Specific Amino Acids

Recent large-scale sequencing efforts have generated thousands of full-genome influenza viral sequences[1545] (www.ncbi.nlm.nih.gov/genomes/FLU/FLU.html; www.fludb.org; www.gisaid.org). The comparison of viral proteins derived from different host species has revealed signature amino acids at specific positions that distinguish human, avian, and swine virus isolates.[10,19,276,516,533,562,603,648,881,1037,1205,1233,1399,1400,1559,1603,1686,1812,1840,1986,2214] In particular, comparative studies have identified a number of human-like signature amino acids in highly pathogenic avian H5N1 influenza viruses,[19,276,533,1037,1205,1400,1686,1840] the pandemic 1918 virus[276,533,1399,1603,1713,2049] and 2009 pandemic H1N1 viruses,[1603] which may play a role in adaptation to humans. For some of these signature amino acids, a role in pathogenicity has been demonstrated (see Molecular Determinants of Host Range Restriction and Pathogenesis section).

Computational analyses of viral sequences have also identified differences in mutation patterns and codon usage between human and avian influenza viruses.[460,663,927,1698,2258] Such approaches may improve our understanding of influenza virus evolution.

Quasispecies

The high error rate of the replication complex of RNA viruses results in the generation and co-circulation of different genetic variants within a host organism.[433] If the biologic fitness of a quasispecies is comparable to that of the predominant variant, the minor variant may be maintained in virus populations at low frequencies.[1149] In the event of host or environmental pressure (including innate and adaptive immune responses, and selective pressure resulting from a host change or antiviral pressure), greater genetic diversity may increase the probability for variants that are better adapted to the changed environment. In such a scenario, quasispecies may be selected and become the dominant virus population. In the past, the detection of quasispecies was cumbersome due to the detection limits of conventional sequencing techniques. With advances in deep sequencing and mass spectrometry analyses, minor sequence variants can be detected more easily. These techniques are now used to assess the levels of quasispecies and mixed infections,[620,1118,1786,2318] which may provide critical information on the emergence of novel variants. For example, deep sequencing revealed that variants of the 2009 pandemic H1N1 virus possessed mutations in the antigenic site[1118]; it will be interesting to assess whether these variants become dominant in the future.

Evolution in Influenza B and C Viruses

Significant differences in evolutionary rates exist for influenza A, B, and C viruses.[289,527,812,1000,1100,1236,1534] Type B viruses, and especially type C viruses, evolve more slowly than influenza A viruses. Type B and C viruses seem to be near or at an evolutionary equilibrium in humans; in contrast, the genes of type A human viruses were introduced from birds[2214] and have not reached an equilibrium in humans. Influenza A viruses in humans evolve along single lineages, which suggests evolution by clonal selection[196] and limited co-circulation of sublineages. Co-circulation of sublineages has been shown over only limited periods.[372,527] In contrast, the evolution of influenza B and C viruses is characterized by the co-circulation of antigenically and genetically distinct lineages over extended periods of time.[197,2305] For influenza B viruses, two lineages—B/Victoria (represented by B/Victoria/2/87) and B/Yamagata (represented by B/Yamagata/16/88)—have been co-circulating for about 25 years with changing patterns of prevalence and geographic distribution.[812,960,1236,1360,1488,1623,1757,1759]

INFLUENZA VIRUS GENETICS

Reassortment

Reassortment is the rearrangement of viral gene segments in cells infected with two (or more) different influenza viruses (Fig. 41.2). Reassortment between two viruses can theoretically result in 256 2^8 different gene variations (i.e., the two parental genotypes and 254 new gene combinations). Reassortment occurs for influenza A, B, and C viruses, but has not been observed among the different types of influenza viruses.

The importance of reassortment to the generation of new influenza virus strains is highlighted by the last three pandemics: reassortant viruses that contained HA, PB1, and NA, or HA and PB1 segments of avian virus origin in a human genetic background, caused the so-called Asian Influenza in 1957 and Hong Kong Influenza in 1968.[1001,1155,1813] The H1N1 pandemic in 2009 was caused by a reassortant virus that possessed North American avian-like PB2 and PA segments, Eurasian avian-like swine NA and M segments, a human H3N2-like PB1 segment, and classic swine H1N1-like HA, NP, and NS segments.[388,604,1903,2094] Six of these segments (all but the NA and M segments) were derived from triple human/avian/swine reassortant viruses that emerged in 1997/1998 and have spread throughout the North American pig populations[972,1570,2209,2373] (see Influenza in Swine section). These viruses caused a few cases of self-sustained human infections without further spread.[78,2055,2163] Hence, at least two sequential reassortment events were critical in the emergence of the new pandemic strain: first, the generation of a triple reassortment swine virus; and second, the introduction into this virus of Eurasian avian-like NA and M segments. In addition, the highly pathogenic H5N1 viruses currently circulating in Southeast Asia arose from multiple reassortment events among avian influenza viruses, and continue to reassort[278,279,281,449,677,678,681,826,1089,1205,1247,1296,1491,1902,2157,2290] [see Outbreaks of Highly Pathogenic Avian Influenza (HPAI) Viruses section].

In addition to reassortment events that create new lineages or pandemics, reassortment can create novel viruses that circulate for a limited time period.[752,846,873,1034,1174,1182,2005,2187,2277,2285,2358] For human influenza viruses, intrasubtypic reassortment may be more important than previously thought,[829,1235,1479,1481,1482,1700] and may have led to the epidemics observed with reassorted H1N1 viruses in 1947 and 1951,[1030,1482] reassorted H2N2 viruses in 1967,[1235] and reassorted H3N2 viruses in 1997 and 2003.[829,1700]

In experimental settings, multiple reassortants can be generated between highly pathogenic avian H5N1 and human H3N2[284,905,1198,1301] or 2009 pandemic H1N1 viruses[1548]; between 2009 pandemic H1N1 and seasonal H1N1[1547] or avian H9N2 viruses[2006]; or between human H3N2 and genetically distant equine H7N7 viruses.[1199] However, not all gene combinations can be generated experimentally, and others may not be compatible in nature. Nonetheless, these studies demonstrate the propensity of influenza viruses for reassortment.

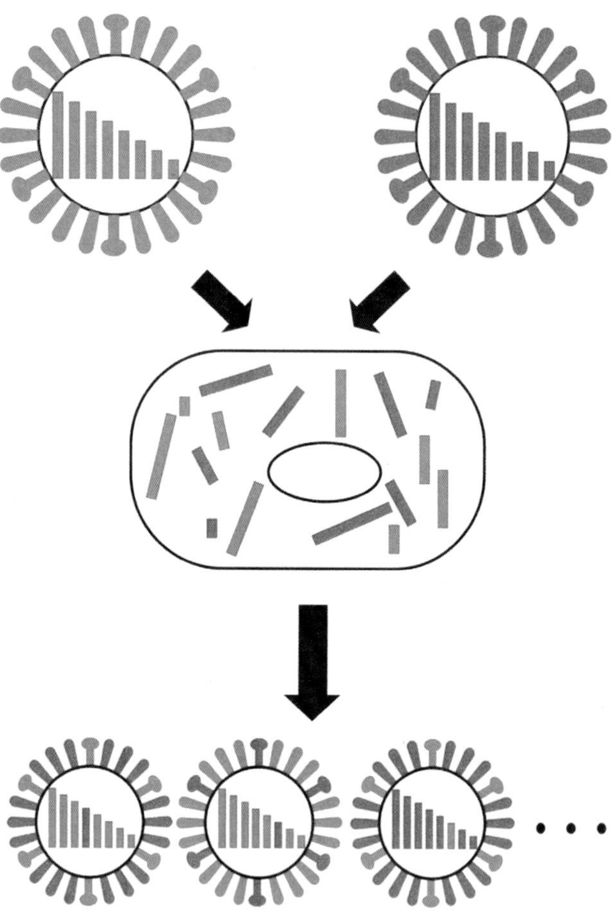

FIGURE 41.2. Reassortment. Co-infection of cells with two different influenza A viruses can theoretically result in 256 different genotypes (2^8, i.e., the two parental genotypes and 254 new genotypes). Reassortment is a major mechanism for the generation of pandemic influenza viruses, as demonstrated in 1957 (Asian influenza), 1968 (Hong Kong influenza), and 2009 [A(H1N1)pdm09].

Recombination

Recombination has been detected in influenza virus segments that contain genetic material from more than one origin. For negative-sense RNA viruses, homologous recombination is uncommon; however, recombination by "template switching" can occur and lead to increased biologic fitness of the virus. For example, the insertion of 54 nucleotides of 28S ribosomal RNA into the A/turkey/Oregon/71 HA gene increased HA cleavability.[1020] Similarly, an A/seal/Massachusetts/1/80 variant contained a 60-nucleotide insertion (likely derived from the NP gene) in the HA gene, which also enhanced HA cleavability.[1576] Avian influenza viruses of low pathogenicity have converted to high pathogenicity following the insertion of 21 nucleotides of the M segment[161,815,1614] or 30 nucleotides of the NP segment[1989] into the HA segment. Serial egg passages of an A/WSN/33 virus containing a 24-amino-acid deletion in the NA stalk led to variants that replicated efficiently in eggs.[1401] The NA stalk of these variants contained sequences that originated from the PB1, PB2, and NP genes. In another example, a virus contained an NP gene that likely resulted from intracistronic recombination between two NP segments.[1747] In this case, it is unclear whether the recombination event provided a selective advantage to the virus. Moreover, attempts to generate influenza virus by providing an *in vitro* synthesized RNA encoding a viral segment yielded several recombinant viruses.[121] Recently, computational analyses of influenza viral sequences identified several potential recombination events among influenza viral genes[152,770,771]; however, some of these may in fact represent laboratory-generated artifacts.

Reverse Genetics

Highly efficient systems are now in place for the artificial generation of influenza A,[542,1496] B,[824,897] and C[362,1448] viruses, and of Thogotovirus.[2173] These systems rely on the intracellular synthesis of influenza viral RNAs by a cellular enzyme, RNA polymerase I, that transcribes ribosomal RNA in the nucleus of eukaryotic cells. The influenza viral segments are encoded by cDNAs flanked by the RNA polymerase I promoter and the RNA polymerase I terminator or a ribozyme sequence. RNA polymerase I transcription in transfected cells results in the efficient synthesis of RNA transcripts with defined 5′ ends, whereas the integrity of the 3′ ends is achieved by using the nucleotide-specific RNA polymerase I terminator[1496] or a self-cleaving ribozyme.[542] To generate influenza viruses, cells are transfected with eight plasmids to provide all eight viral RNAs, as well as with four plasmids for the expression of the polymerase and NP proteins that are required to initiate viral replication. Although this approach requires the co-transfection of cells with 12 plasmids, it is highly efficient, routinely yielding 10^8 plaque-forming units of influenza A virus per mL of cell culture supernatant. In one modification, both the RNA polymerase I transcripts (for viral RNA synthesis) and the RNA polymerase II transcripts (for mRNA synthesis) are derived from the same template,[825] which reduces the number of plasmids required for virus generation to eight. In another modification, the eight RNA polymerase I transcription units for the eight viral RNAs are combined,[1490] allowing the generation of the entire viral genome from a single plasmid. In addition, a reverse genetics system based on T7 RNA polymerase has been established.[407] These systems have revolutionized influenza virus research [reviewed in[1492–1494,1497]] in that they allow researchers to study the functions of viral proteins in the viral life cycle, as well as their roles in pathogenesis and host range restriction. Moreover, these systems are now invaluable tools for the generation of influenza virus vaccines and vaccine vectors. In fact, reverse genetics has permitted the generation of inactivated and live vaccine strains for H5N1 viruses that could not have been produced by conventional approaches.

INFLUENZA IN HUMANS—PAST PANDEMICS AND THE H5N1 EPIDEMIC

Pandemics are outbreaks that impact large geographic areas and large portions of the population in a short period of time. Pandemics are the most dramatic manifestation of influenza, attacking 20% to 40% of the world population and causing significant mortality. Influenza pandemics have occurred in 10- to 40-year intervals, although reliable records only date back to the 1918/1919 pandemic (Fig. 41.3). The cumulative death toll of epidemics in interpandemic periods, although less dramatic, parallel those of pandemics.

The Pandemic of 1918/1919—Spanish Influenza (H1N1)

The pandemic of 1918/1919 remains unprecedented in its severity. It killed more people than World War I and reduced life expectancy in the United States by 10 years. AIDS has killed 25 million people in its first 25 years—the Spanish influenza killed an equal number in 25 weeks (from September 1918 to March 1919). This pandemic occurred in three waves. In the spring of 1918, a mild respiratory disease started at Fort Funston, Kansas (now Fort Riley), attributed to a soldier that had been cleaning pig pens.[366] There is no mention of the presence of poultry in the camp at that time. The disease spread among soldiers from Fort Funston along the rail lines to other military bases and cities in the United States and on troopships to Europe.[1619] This first wave was highly contagious but caused few deaths and received limited attention in most parts of the world. In Spain, a neutral country without news censorship, the outbreak was covered extensively by news media and was soon referred to as the "Spanish influenza." In late August, a second wave with a higher mortality rate started, probably in western France, from where it spread around the world; this wave peaked between September and November. During that time, death tolls reached more than 10,000 people per week in some US cities. About one-third of the US population became sick,[557] and the mortality rate was estimated to be over 2.5%, compared to less than 0.1% in typical influenza outbreaks. These figures reflect the impact of the pandemic on the developed world; death rates are believed to have been significantly higher in African and Asian countries. In some isolated populations, the mortality rate reached 70%, likely because of the lack of previous exposure to influenza virus. A third wave of similar impact to that of the second wave struck in late 1918/early 1919.

Typically, the onset of symptoms was sudden, with high fever, severe headache and myalgia, cough, pharyngitis, and coryza. Pathologic findings were mostly restricted to the respiratory tract; death was due to pneumonia and respiratory failure.[2255] There was no evidence of systemic viral infection.[2255] Most patients died of secondary bacterial pneumonia,[190,302,1272,1420] but some showed massive acute pulmonary hemorrhage or pulmonary edema,[2255] indicating the extreme virulence of the virus. The high rate of bacterial complications may be attributed to the lack of antibiotics in 1918 and 1919.

Age-specific morbidity was similar to that of other pandemics, with children younger than 15 years experiencing the highest infection rates.[940] The mortality pattern, however, differed significantly from that of other influenza virus outbreaks. In typical influenza outbreaks, the highest death rates are observed in very young children and in the elderly. In 1918 and 1919, many deaths occurred among young adults. The death rate for the 15- to 35-year-old age group was 20 times higher in 1918 than in previous years[1229,1880] and persons younger than 65 years accounted for more than 99% of excess deaths.[1880]

The origin of the 1918/1919 virus remains an enigma. In 1927, E. Jordan[940] published a comprehensive review of the origin of the pandemic. He found no evidence that the disease had originated in China. He also evaluated two reports that described local outbreaks of respiratory infections associated with high mortality and heliotrope cyanosis, which was

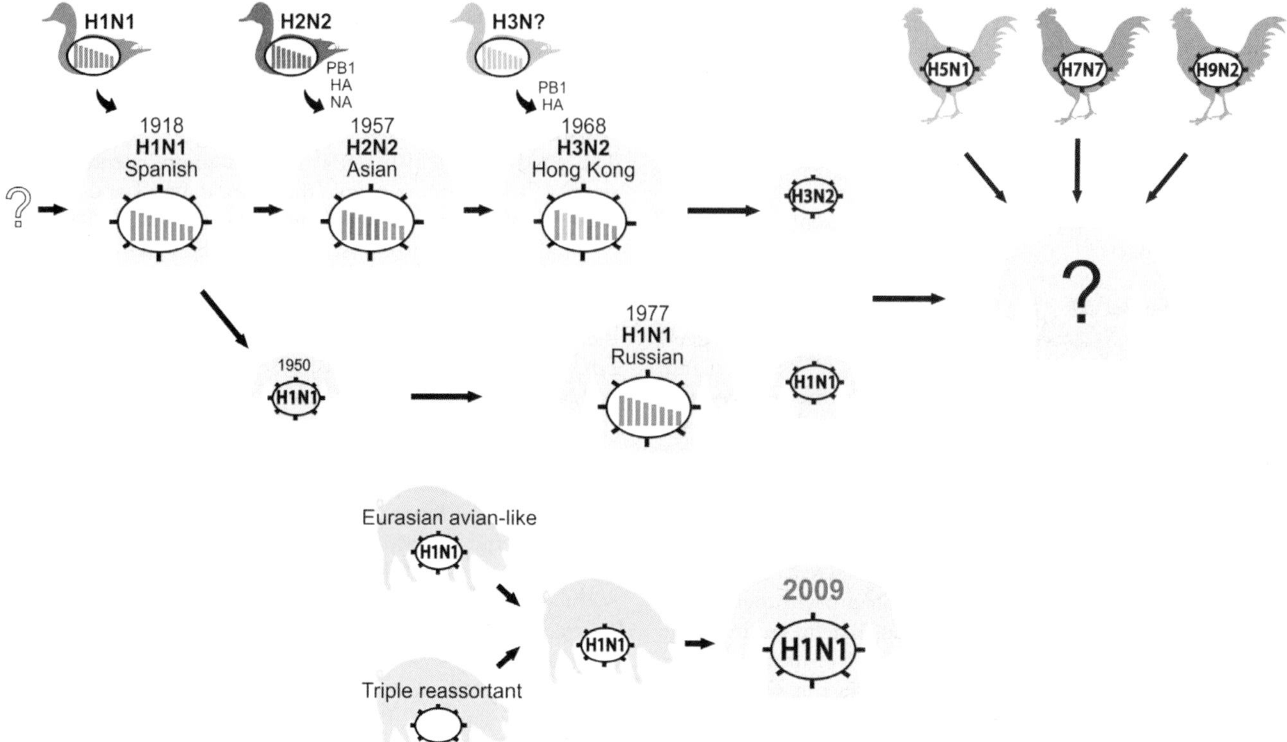

FIGURE 41.3. Evolution of influenza A viruses circulating in humans. An avian H1N1 virus caused the Spanish influenza in 1918. Its descendants circulated until the mid-1950s and reemerged in 1977, causing the Russian influenza. Viruses of this lineage continued to circulate in human populations until 2009. The Asian influenza in 1957 was caused by an H2N2 virus that acquired its HA, NA, and PB1 genes from an avian H2N2 virus. A similar reassortment event in 1968 resulted in the introduction of avian virus HA and PB1 genes into the human population, causing the Hong Kong influenza. H3N2 viruses circulate in humans to this day. In 2009, reassortment of triple-reassortant swine viruses and Eurasian avian-like swine viruses (which donated the NA and M segments) resulted in the A(H1N1)pdm09 virus (see Fig. 41.5 for more details), which replaced the then-circulating H1N1 viruses.

observed during the 1918/1919 outbreak, in army camps in Étaples in Northern France in the winter of 1916 and in Aldershot barracks in March 1917. He dismissed both reports because the disease did not spread but disappeared after short episodes. The most likely origin of the pandemic was Haskell County, Kansas, where Dr. L. Miner noticed an outbreak of influenza in early February 1918 that differed from other influenza outbreaks in that it attacked young, healthy adults, who developed pneumonia that often led to sudden death.[75] Dr. Miner's observations were published in *Public Health Reports* (now *Morbidity and Mortality Weekly Reports*) and appear to be the first reference to the 1918/1919 pandemic. Men from Haskell County reported to Fort Funston for military training, where they arrived between February 26 and March 2, 1918. On March 4, the first soldier at the camp was reported ill; within a 3-week period, more than 1,100 soldiers at the camp required hospitalization.

Seroarcheology suggests that the causative agent was an H1N1 virus. This was confirmed by Taubenberger et al., who recovered viral RNA from formalin-fixed, paraffin-embedded tissues from two soldiers who died in 1918,[1712,2048] and from an Inuit female of unknown age whose body was exhumed from a mass grave in the permafrost of Alaska.[1712] RT-PCR amplification of the viral RNAs provided viral gene sequences.[2048] Phylogenetic analyses revealed that 1918 Spanish influenza virus proteins contain both "avian-like" and "human-like" signature amino acids (see Host-Specific Amino Acids section).[2049] Further analysis suggested that the 1918 virus genes were not directly transmitted from an avian species, but likely circulated in a mammalian host for several years before causing the pandemic outbreak in 1918.[33,1901,2258]

Reconstitution of the 1918 Spanish influenza virus by use of reverse genetics demonstrated its high pathogenicity in mice, ferrets, and nonhuman primates.[1068,2102,2107,2206] In nonhuman primates, the virus caused severe respiratory disease with extensive edema and hemorrhagic exudates,[1068] similar to reports of human infections. Rapid recruitment of macrophages and neutrophils was observed in the lungs of infected mice,[1068,1639,2105] in line with findings of altered immune responses in infected mice[983] and nonhuman primates.[1068] Further studies indicated a role in virulence for several viral proteins (see later discussion and Molecular Determinants of Host Range Restriction and Pathogenesis section): HA,[981,1070,1607,2103,2104–2105] the polymerase proteins, particularly PB1,[1607,2102,2131,2206] NS1,[132,612] and PB1-F2.[1356] Two viral proteins, HA and PB2, are critical for the transmissibility of this virus in ferrets.[2131] In contrast to its high virulence in humans, mice, ferrets, and nonhuman primates, the 1918 virus is of low pathogenicity in pigs,[2231] chickens, and mallard ducks.[53]

Unlike contemporary human viruses, reassortants possessing the 1918 HA, or HA and NA, genes are highly pathogenic in mice.[981,1070,1607,2103,2104–2105] Reassortant viruses containing the 1918 HA gene induce high levels of macrophage-derived cytokines and chemokines, which stimulate inflammatory cell infiltration and hemorrhage[981,1070,2105]—hallmarks of Spanish influenza infection. The underlying mechanism is unknown. Structural analysis of the HA protein revealed that although most of the amino acids of the receptor-binding pocket are avian-like, the amino acid at position 190 (an aspartic acid as found in human viruses) is responsible for HA binding to human respiratory cell-surface receptors,[590,1972] as previously predicted.[1330] Consistent with this structural finding, the 1918 HA protein preferentially recognizes human-type receptors in receptor-binding assays.[628] The replacement of two amino acids in the 1918 HA (D190E and D225G) abolished respiratory droplet transmission in ferrets, although the mutant virus maintained its lethal phenotype in infected animals.[2107]

The NS1 protein is an interferon antagonist and, as such, is considered a determinant of pathogenicity. A recombinant virus containing the 1918 virus NS gene in the background of A/WSN/33 (H1N1) virus[77] is attenuated in mice; however, microarray studies of samples obtained from mice infected with this virus indicate that the 1918 virus NS gene blocks the expression of interferon (IFN)-regulated genes more efficiently than does the parental A/WSN/33,[132,612] suggesting a role for NS1 in viral pathogenicity. This is further supported by the finding that the PDZ ligand domain motif of the 1918 NS1 protein (formed by the four C-terminal amino acids of this protein; see Molecular Determinants of Host Range Restriction and Pathogenesis section) increased the virulence in the background of A/WSN/33 virus.[898] In addition, the PB1-F2 protein (see Molecular Determinants of Host Range Restriction and Pathogenesis section for more information) of the 1918 virus contributes to virulence.[340,1356] Further studies using recombinant viruses found no significant contributions of the 1918 M and NP genes to viral pathogenicity.[2103,2104]

The Pandemic of 1957—Asian Influenza (H2N2)

This pandemic originated in the Southern Chinese province of Guizhou in February 1957 and spread to Hunan Province and to Singapore and Hong Kong in March and April, respectively.[1980] In May 1957, the causative agent of the outbreak, an influenza A virus of the H2N2 subtype, was isolated in Japan. A first wave struck the United States and United Kingdom in October 1957, and was followed by a second wave in January 1958. The infection rate was highest in 5- to 19-year-olds,[630] where it exceeded 50%. Both waves were characterized by heightened mortality, with about 70,000 deaths in the United States[1531,1880] and more than 1 million deaths worldwide.

Genetic and biochemical analyses indicated that the 1957 pandemic virus originated from reassortment between human and avian viruses (Fig. 41.3). It contained H2 HA and N2 NA genes of avian virus origin.[1791,1813] Because the pandemic virus did not appear to be extraordinarily pathogenic, the increased mortality is attributed to the lack of preexisting immunity among humans to the new surface glycoproteins of this virus. In addition to avian virus HA and NA genes, the 1957 pandemic virus also possessed a PB1 gene of avian virus origin.[1001] The contribution of this gene segment to the pathogenicity of the pandemic 1957 virus is unknown.

Influenza viruses of the H2 subtype continue to be isolated from avian species, and were isolated from pigs in 2006.[1292] Since vaccination against H2N2 viruses was discontinued in the late 1960s, only individuals 40 years of age or older have protective antibodies against this subtype,[1461] suggesting that a new pandemic by an H2 virus would cause appreciable excess morbidity and mortality in a large section of the population. However, avian H2N2 viruses have evolved slowly, so that the pandemic H2N2 vaccine from 1957 still protects mice against recently circulating avian or swine H2 strains[274,997]; this vaccine may thus provide a first line of defense in the event of an H2N2 pandemic.

The Pandemic of 1968—Hong Kong Influenza (H3N2)

Eleven years after their emergence, viruses of the H2N2 subtype were completely replaced by those of the H3N2 subtype (Fig. 41.3). The first signs of a new pandemic emerged in southern Asia in the summer of 1968.[330] A virus of the H3N2 subtype was isolated in Hong Kong in July 1968, which soon spread around the world. The attack rates reached 40% and were highest in 10- to 14-year-olds. The excess mortality was estimated to be 33,800 in the United States.[1531]

The 1968 pandemic virus contained an avian virus HA protein of the H3 subtype that shared less than 30% sequence homology with its predecessor. However, preexisting antibodies to the N2 protein in human populations likely accounted for the moderate severity of the outbreak. In addition to an avian H3 gene,[1813] the 1968 pandemic strain also acquired an avian virus PB1 gene,[1001] as did the 1957 pandemic strain. It is unknown whether the introduction of an avian virus PB1 gene into the human population contributed to the pathogenicity of the 1968 pandemic virus. The HA and PB1 genes originated from viruses of the Eurasian avian lineage, consistent with epidemiologic findings that southern China was the likely origin of the pandemic.

The Reemergence of H1N1 Viruses in 1977—Russian Influenza

The first signs of a new influenza virus outbreak were noted in Tianjin, China, in May 1977. From November 1977 through the end of 1978, young adults around the world suffered from an influenza virus outbreak in the Union of Soviet Socialist Republics and in China.[1114,2361] The United States experienced a similar outbreak in mid-January 1978, and outbreaks in other countries occurred during the following winter. Among school-age children, the attack rates were more than 50%. Morbidity was almost exclusively limited to persons younger than 25 years, suggesting that older individuals were protected by preexisting immunity. This assumption was proven when the causative agent was identified as an influenza H1N1 virus (A/USSR/77) closely related to strains that had circulated in the early 1950s[1016,1091,1469,1814] (Fig. 41.3). This close relationship and the lack of mutations that are typically acquired during replication argue against maintenance of the virus in a nonhuman species. It is now believed that accidental release of this virus started the pandemic. In contrast to 1968, when the newly emerging H3N2 viruses replaced the circulating H2N2 viruses, replacement of H3N2 viruses did not occur in 1977 with the reemergence of H1N1 viruses. Instead, both H1N1 and H3N2 viruses continue to circulate to this day.

The H5N1 Outbreak

Although not yet a pandemic, the outbreak of H5N1 viruses across Asia and the Middle East deserves discussion here because of its socioeconomic implications and clinical threat. The virus first emerged on geese farms in 1996 in Guangdong Province, China.[1883,2290] In May 1997 in Hong Kong, a 3-year-old boy was infected and succumbed to the infection.[320,322,1993] The causative agent was an H5N1 virus of entirely avian origin. This incident marked the first reported transmission of a wholly avian influenza virus to a human with fatal outcome.[320,322] In November and December 1997, 17 additional cases were reported, 5 of which had fatal outcomes. No conclusive evidence of human-to-human transmission exists. These human cases accompanied an outbreak of influenza in live bird markets in Hong Kong. Because most infected individuals had contact with poultry prior to their illness, officials ordered the culling of all poultry in Hong Kong's live bird markets, resulting in appreciable economic losses. This intervention proved successful, and no further cases were reported until 2003. Further human infections were probably prevented when poultry stocks were depopulated again in May 2001 and February and April 2002, after highly pathogenic H5N1 viruses reemerged in live bird markets. However, in February 2003, two Hong Kong residents were infected with H5N1 virus.[1625] A 9-year-old boy became sick when his family traveled to Fujian Province in mainland China and was hospitalized in Hong Kong. He recovered from an H5N1 virus infection, but his 33-year-old father succumbed to the disease. The 7-year-old daughter died in a hospital in China during the family's travels; the cause of her death was not determined.

A new outbreak of H5N1 virus started in July 2003 in poultry in Vietnam, Indonesia, and Thailand, although it lacked official recognition at the time. It has since spread to more than 60 Asian, European, Middle Eastern, and African countries, and has led to the depopulation or death of more than 100 million poultry. H5N1 viruses are now enzootic in poultry populations in China, Indonesia, Vietnam, Egypt, India, and Bangladesh[432] (http://www.fao.org/news/story/en/item/66118/icode/), and continue to cause outbreaks in the Middle East and sporadic infections in Europe. In addition to far-reaching economic consequences, direct avian-to-human transmission of highly pathogenic avian viruses has caused widespread public apprehension. As of February 1, 2013, 615 cases with 364 fatalities had been reported, resulting in a mortality rate of ~60% (http://www.who.int/influenza/human_animal_interface/EN_GIP_20130201CumulativeNumberH5N1cases.pdf). Most human infections have occurred in Indonesia, Egypt, and Vietnam. The number of reported human infections was highest in 2006 (115 infections that resulted in 79 fatalities), and has declined to 48 cases (with 24 fatalities) in 2010. It is not known if this decline can be attributed to changes in human behavior and/or viral properties, or represents a random fluctuation.

Although H5N1 viruses have not yet acquired the ability to spread efficiently among humans, isolated cases of human-to-human transmission may have occurred.[626,958,959,1573,1574,1829,2084,2116,2118,2191,2245] However, most of these clusters involved family members living in the same household, and infection may have occurred through exposure to a common source (such as sick or dead poultry), rather than human-to-human transmission. Overall, transmission of H5N1 viruses to humans appears to be rare and primarily associated with contact with sick or dead poultry,[32,38,283,426,519,957,1429,2084,2133,2371] although other modes of infection (for example, through virus-contaminated feces or water) have been considered as well.[398,958,1829,2169,2170,2244]

During the 1997 and 2003 H5N1 outbreaks in Hong Kong, there was no evidence of systemic viral infection in infected individuals.[1625,2069] More recent H5N1 viruses, however, appear to cause systemic infection in humans[398,399,676,2112,2113]: virus has been recovered from not only respiratory organs, but also stool and cerebrospinal fluid (CSF), while viral sequences and/or antigens have been detected in brain neurons; in epithelial cells of the intestinal tract; in heart, spleen, kidney, and liver; and in the placenta and fetus of a pregnant women infected with an H5N1 virus. The detection of viral sequences and antigen in the intestinal tract is consistent with the expression of avian-like virus receptors in the human gut,[1873] the *ex vivo* infection of gut tissue with an H5N1 virus,[1873] and reports of gastrointestinal symptoms.[37,797,2084,2345] In H5N1 virus-infected patients, acute respiratory distress syndrome (ARDS) with diffuse alveolar damage is common.[38,95,310,591,676,1087,1509,1650,1662,2069,2084,2112,2331,2357] Virus and/or antigen binding has been detected to nonciliated epithelial cells in the bronchioles, and type II pneumocytes and macrophages in the alveoli.[413,676,1219,1521,1662,2113,2139] Type II pneumocytes differentiate to type I pneumocytes, which are critical for gas exchange in the alveoli; the infection of type II pneumocytes may thus result in more severe lung damage. The observed pattern of virus binding is also in accordance with the detection of avian-type receptors on some bronchiolar and alveolar cells.[1521,1662,1854,2139] However, H5N1 viruses also replicate in *ex vivo* organ cultures of the upper respiratory tract.[1521] The levels of proinflammatory cytokines are higher in individuals infected with H5N1 viruses than in those infected with seasonal influenza virus, and higher in fatal than in nonfatal cases of H5N1 infection.[399,1625] The pathology in humans is in line with cell-culture studies that demonstrate increased levels of proinflammatory cytokines upon H5N1 infection,[266,298,300,611,848,1131,1180,2190,2368] animal infection studies that show increased pathology, viral targeting of type II pneumocytes,[1064,1733,2139] and stronger innate immune responses upon H5N1 virus infection compared to infection with control viruses [see Outbreaks of Highly Pathogenic Avian Influenza (HPAI) Virus section]. Collectively, the available data suggest that the high mortality in humans results from a combination of high virus loads and the induction of high levels of proinflammatory pathways, which may culminate in extensive alveolar damage.

Some of the currently circulating H5N1 viruses are resistant to the antiviral drugs amantadine and rimantadine.[299,1686] Most H5N1 viruses are sensitive to the NA inhibitors oseltamivir and zanamivir[1186]; however, oseltamivir-resistant viruses have been isolated from H5N1 virus–infected patients treated with this drug[400,1164] (http://www.emro.who.int/csr/media/pdf/ai_press_22_01_07.pdf). These viruses contain an amino acid substitution at position 274 or 294 of the NA protein. It is of major concern that two patients treated with oseltamivir subsequently shed drug-resistant viruses and eventually died.[400]

The H1N1 Pandemic in 2009

The first reports of an influenza-like outbreak in a small Mexican town can be dated to mid-February 2009 (http://www.guardian.co.uk/world/2009/apr/27/swine-flu-search-outbreak-source).

In early April, Mexican public health authorities began investigating and informed international agencies of a possible outbreak. In mid-April, genetically similar swine-origin H1N1 influenza A viruses were detected in several specimens collected in southern California[253,388] and Mexico.[249,258,331,332] The novel virus spread rapidly among humans across different continents, prompting the World Health Organization (WHO) to declare Phase 6 (pandemic phase, which is characterized by community-level outbreaks with human-to-human spread in at least two countries in more than one WHO region) on June 12, 2009.[333,2351] The WHO soon adopted the name "pandemic (H1N1) 2009" for the novel virus (http://www.who.int/csr/disease/swineflu/en/index.html) but now suggests A(H1N1) pdm09 (http://afludiary.blogspot.com/2011/10/who-call-it-ah1n1pdm09.html). This outbreak marked the first pandemic in more than 4 decades. Viruses of the H1N1 subtype have circulated in humans since 1977; hence, pandemics are not limited to viruses with novel HA subtypes (i.e., those not recently circulating in humans), but can be caused by viruses possessing HA subtypes that are circulating in human populations, as long as the novel HA is antigenically distantly enough from its predecessor to escape human immune responses.

The pandemic virus spread rapidly.[189] The southern hemisphere (where the influenza season lasts from May to September) experienced significant pandemic influenza activity from May to mid-July of 2009; the United States experienced a first wave in May and June, and a second wave that started in late August and peaked during the second week of October. The novel virus soon dominated the previously circulating seasonal H1N1 viruses; in fact, more than 99% of influenza A viruses subtyped during the winter of 2009/2010 were novel A(H1N1)pdm09 viruses.[256] For the United States, the Centers for Disease Control and Prevention (CDC) estimated a total of 61 million infections with 274,000 hospitalizations and 12,470 deaths between April 2009 and April 2010 (http://www.cdc.gov/h1n1flu/estimates_2009_h1n1.htm). However, about 30,000 influenza-related deaths occur in the United States during each interpandemic season, indicating a low case-fatality rate for infections with the A(H1N1)pdm09 virus. Morbidity and mortality rates differed significantly between age groups[311,469,556,705,1676,1677,1770,2310]: children experienced a low case-fatality rate. Nonetheless, an appreciable number of small children died from infection with the A(H1N1)pdm09 virus. In contrast to seasonal influenza epidemics, the elderly experienced a low infection, but high case-fatality rate. The low infection rate among the elderly can be explained by serum cross-reactivity between A(H1N1) pdm09 viruses and close descendants of the pandemic 1918 virus,[252,311,705,734,864,890] which is a consequence of shared antigenic epitopes between the HA proteins of these two viruses.[604,664,860,890,1093,1309,1903,2229,2287,2307] Those aged 5–59 years accounted for the highest absolute numbers of deaths and cases of pneumonia, in contrast to seasonal outbreaks.[311,469] Epidemiologic data identified several factors associated with an increased risk of severe disease, including pregnancy (particularly in the last trimester), underlying chronic conditions, and obesity.[57,244,246,259,388,469,705,706,909,910,1254,1261,2351]

Human infections with A(H1N1)pdm09 viruses typically caused mild upper respiratory tract illnesses with fever, cough, sore throat, shortness of breath, headache, and rhinorrhea.[223,244,259,388,469,705,706,1635] In addition, gastrointestinal symptoms (which are unusual with seasonal influenza infections) were reported in some cases. In some patients, respiratory and multiorgan failure occurred, leading to death. These severe infections caused diffuse alveolar damage, hemorrhagic interstitial pneumonitis, and peribronchiolar and perivascular lymphocytic infiltrates[86,625,684,705,706,1635,1847,1927] (Fig. 41.4), similar to human infections with avian H5N1 viruses (see The H5N1 Outbreak section). These findings are in line with animal infection studies that demonstrated more severe lung lesions and higher lung virus titers in mice, ferrets, and nonhuman primates infected with A(H1N1) pdm09 virus compared with seasonal influenza virus infections.[101,890,1302,1442,1637,1772,2126] In nonhuman primates, viral antigen was detected in type I and II pneumocytes,[890] as has been reported for some human cases of A(H1N1)pdm09 infection,[684] and for nonhuman primates infected with avian H5N1 influenza virus.[76] Efficient replication in the lungs with infection of type I and II pneumocytes (which likely contributes to the observed alveolar damage) may thus be a hallmark of severe influenza virus infections. In many human A(H1N1)pdm09 cases, bacterial co-infections were detected[243,625,705,706,914,1254,1345,1599,1635] (Fig. 41.4), a finding that has rekindled interest in the contribution of bacterial infections to influenza-related morbidity and mortality.

Sequence and phylogenetic analyses revealed that the A(H1N1)pdm09 virus possesses PB2 and PA genes of North American avian virus origin; a PB1 gene of human H3N2 virus origin; HA (H1), NP, and NS genes of classic swine virus origin; and NA (N1) and M genes of Eurasian avian virus origin[388,604,1903,2094] (Figs. 41.3 and 41.5). A(H1N1)pdm09 viruses do not possess amino acids associated with high virulence in mammals.[388,556,604,1495,1903,1931] In line with its presumed porcine origin, the virus replicates efficiently, but without symptoms, in experimentally infected miniature pigs[890] and transmits efficiently among pigs.[178] Other studies have demonstrated efficient transmission of A(H1N1)pdm09 viruses in ferrets.[890,1302,1442,1637] In nature, A(H1N1)pdm09 viruses have also infected turkeys,[123] cats,[1256,1362,1935] dogs,[459] and ferrets.[2015] The widespread circulation of A(H1N1)pdm09 viruses may lead to reassortment with other human, swine, or avian influenza viruses. In fact, the pandemic virus has infected pigs[511,827,1417] and reassortment with swine influenza viruses has been repo rted.[1418,1949,2158] Experimental studies demonstrated ready reassortment of A(H1N1)pdm09 viruses with avian H5N1,[1548,1921] avian H9N2,[2006] or contemporary human influenza viru ses[1547,1819,1921]; some of these reassortants showed increased replicative ability than the A(H1N1)pdm09 parental viruses.[1547,1819,1921]

Concerns over a potentially severe pandemic spurred the development of vaccines for the new pandemic virus. In the United States and Europe, the first vaccines were approved in September 2009.[251,254,933] These vaccines proved to be safe and efficacious. Protective antibody titers were obtained with a single dose of vaccine, despite earlier concerns that two doses may be required; however, two doses were recommended for children younger than 10 years of age, due to lack of preexisting immunity.[1215,1664,2376] A(H1N1)pdm09 viruses have now replaced seasonal H1N1 virus as part of annual, trivalent influenza vaccines (see also Vaccines section). On August 10, 2011, the WHO declared an end to the pandemic (http://www.who.int/mediacentre/news/statements/2010/h1n1_vpc_20100810/en/index.html). The A(H1N1)pdm09

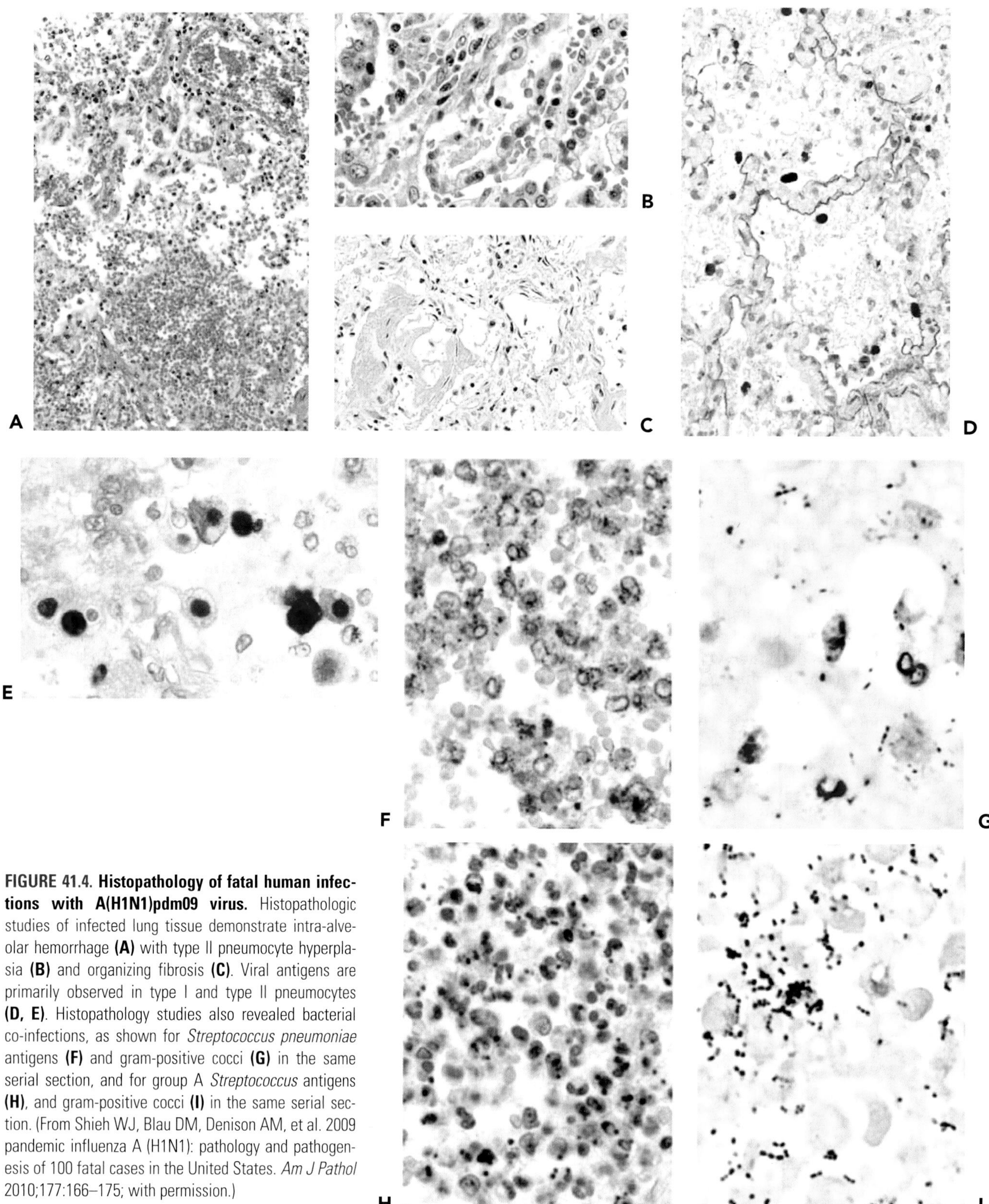

FIGURE 41.4. Histopathology of fatal human infections with A(H1N1)pdm09 virus. Histopathologic studies of infected lung tissue demonstrate intra-alveolar hemorrhage **(A)** with type II pneumocyte hyperplasia **(B)** and organizing fibrosis **(C)**. Viral antigens are primarily observed in type I and type II pneumocytes **(D, E)**. Histopathology studies also revealed bacterial co-infections, as shown for *Streptococcus pneumoniae* antigens **(F)** and gram-positive cocci **(G)** in the same serial section, and for group A *Streptococcus* antigens **(H)**, and gram-positive cocci **(I)** in the same serial section. (From Shieh WJ, Blau DM, Denison AM, et al. 2009 pandemic influenza A (H1N1): pathology and pathogenesis of 100 fatal cases in the United States. *Am J Pathol* 2010;177:166–175; with permission.)

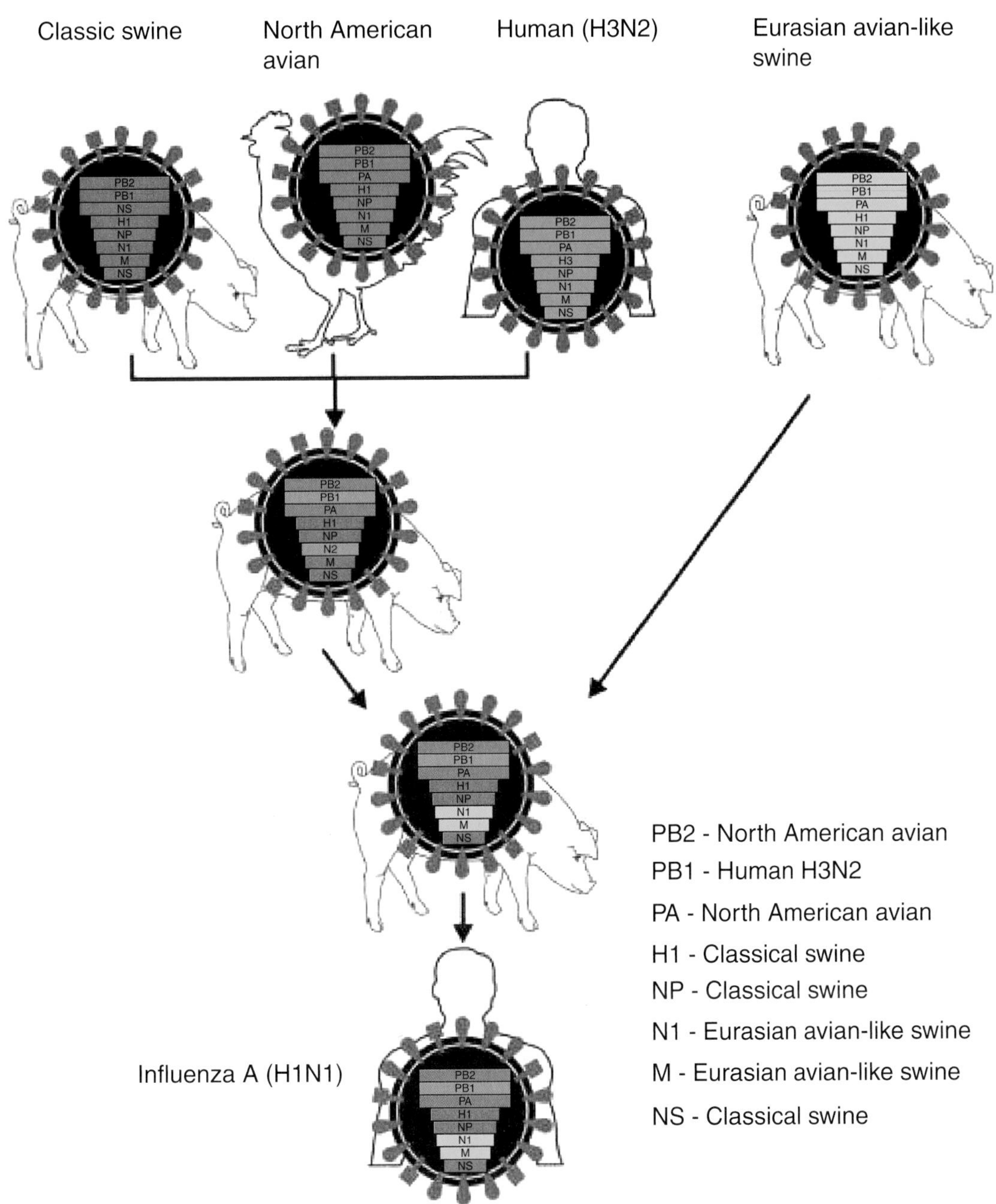

FIGURE 41.5. Genesis of A(H1N1)pdm09 virus. In the late 1990s, reassortment between classical swine, North American avian, and human H3N2 viruses resulted in triple-reassortant H3N2 and H1N2 swine viruses that became established in North American pig populations (see Influenza in Swine—North America section). Reassortment of these viruses with a Eurasian avian-like swine virus led to the emergence of the A(H1N1)pdm09 virus. (From Neumann G, Noda T, Kawaoka Y. Emergence and pandemic potential of swine-origin H1N1 influenza virus. *Nature* 2009;459:931–939, with permission.)

virus will likely continue to circulate as a seasonal influenza virus.

INFLUENZA IN HUMANS—EPIDEMIOLOGY

Since 1977, seasonal H1N1 and H3N2 viruses have been circulating together with influenza B viruses; in 2009, the seasonal H1N1 viruses were largely replaced by A(H1N1)pdm09 viruses. The prevalence of these groups of viruses varies geographically and temporally, making influenza virus epidemiology complex.

Several studies have assessed the global circulation patterns of influenza viruses[532,1480,1700]; some analyses indicate that human H3N2 and H1N1 epidemic strains originate from Southeast Asia, from where they are seeded into temperate regions.[94,263,1766] Temporally overlapping epidemics in Southeast Asia result in continuous virus circulation.[1766] Even though influenza viruses circulate in tropical regions throughout the year,[1766,2155,2257] seasonality has been observed in these areas, although it is less pronounced than in temperate climates.[1430,1610,1766] In the temperate regions of North America and Europe, multiple variants may circulate during the early epidemic period, which are replaced by a dominant variant at the peak of an epidemic.[361]

The epidemiology of human influenza viruses is defined by their constant antigenic variation to escape the host immune response. In contrast to most other respiratory viruses, influenza viruses possess two different mechanisms that allow them to reinfect humans and cause disease—antigenic drift and antigenic shift.

Antigenic Drift

Antigenic drift occurs as a result of point mutations in influenza A and B viruses and refers to minor, gradual, antigenic changes in the HA or NA proteins. Influenza A virus drift variants result from the positive selection of spontaneous mutants by neutralizing antibodies.[204,1666] These variants can then no longer be neutralized by antibodies to the "parental" strains. Antigenic drift has also been observed among influenza viruses in terrestrial poultry, although to a lesser extent than in humans.[1170]

Mutations in the human virus HA or NA amino acid sequence occur at a frequency of less than 1% per year. Nevertheless, antigenic drift variants can cause epidemics and typically prevail for 1 to 5 years before being replaced by a different variant.

Antigenic Drift of the HA Protein

The HA protein is the major antigenic component of the virus. Its function and structure are described in more detail in Chapter 40. X-ray crystallography, comparative sequence analysis, and the characterization of escape mutants have identified five antigenic domains (A–E) for H3 HAs[619,1066,2223,2247,2248] (Fig. 41.6A): Site A is formed by a protruding loop (amino acids 140–146); site B is formed by another loop (amino acids 155–160) and an α-helix (amino acids 188–198) and is situated at the membrane distal end of HA; site C is located at the base of the globular domain in the antiparallel sheet of HA1; site D is situated near the trimeric interface of the globular head domains; and site E lies near the bottom of the globular distal domain between sites C and A. For H1 viruses, the antigenic sites are designated Ca1, Ca2, Cb, Sa, and Sb[239] (Fig. 41.6B). Some overlap exists among antigenic sites.[239,374] For H5 HAs, X-ray crystallographic structures have been resolved for the HA proteins of an H5N1[1970] and an H5N3[707] virus, which allowed the mapping of antigenic escape variants obtained with H5N2,[995,996] H5N9,[1649] and H5N1[995,1204,1762] viruses. Depending on the virus and antibodies used for the analysis, three to five antigenic sites that confer neutralization were identified, some of which overlap with antigenic sites in H3 or H1 HA proteins.

Numerous studies have analyzed antigenic drift in nature.[156,157,395,1100,1150,1387,1472,1634,1799,1801,1892,2293,2294] Minor antigenic heterogeneity among the viruses is detectable at any time,[64,395,1586,1888,1967] whereas larger differences, detectable in hemagglutination-inhibition tests, usually require the accumulation of mutations over a 1- to 5-year period.[930,1363,2150] However, single point mutations in one HA antigenic site can be sufficient for antigenic variation.[2247,2248,2252] The H3 HA has drifted more rapidly than the H1 and H2 HAs,[527] resulting in the frequent replacement of antigenic variants. Although human H1 and H3 HAs evolve in single lineages,[204,2085] H1 antigenic drift variants co-circulate, yielding a phylogenetic tree with more side branches.[527,2085] The faster evolution of H3 HAs has necessitated the update of the H3 vaccine component 23 times since 1972, whereas the H1 component has been replaced only eight times[236,756] (http://www.who.int/csr/disease/influenza/vaccinerecommendations1/en/index.html). The HA of A(H1N1)pdm09 viruses has not yet drifted significantly,[563] presumably due to the lack of selective pressure in a predominantly naïve population.

In the laboratory, antigenic drift can be mimicked by virus propagation in the presence of monoclonal antibodies to a single site, with a frequency of variant selection of 1 in 10^5.[328,618,1137,1151–1153,1470,1471,2144,2215,2222,2223,2224] The selection of variants in the presence of antibodies to several antigenic sites is likely a rare event. Accordingly, the selection of drift variants in humans who have polyclonal responses is difficult to imagine. Postinfection human sera have a limited antibody repertoire,[2193] and some animal sera are essentially monoclonal.[1136] Therefore, the selection of antigenic drift variants may be a sequential event with the stepwise accumulation of mutations through different individuals.

Recently, a new hypothesis has been proposed for antigenic drift.[784] Escape variants selected with neutralizing antibodies showed increased affinity to cellular receptors; passage of such variants in naïve mice resulted in the loss of high-affinity receptor binding, while this property was maintained in immune mice. These findings suggest interplay between selection by antibody and receptor recognition, at least in the mouse model.

Over the past decade, computational bioinformatics approaches have become an invaluable tool for studying and predicting antigenic drift. Most notably, antigenic cartography now provides an interpretation of antigenic clusters and their relationships, as well as the extent and directionality of antigenic drift[547,1900] (Fig. 41.7). Antigenic cartography suggests that antigenic drift of human H3N2 viruses occurs in clusters: while nucleotide changes continue to occur, clusters of antigenically similar variants exist for several years until they are replaced by a new cluster, founded by an antigenic variant that necessitates an update of the vaccine strain.[58,1077,1078,1766,1900] Hence, the genetic evolution of H3 HA genes is continuing, while its antigenic evolution is punctuated. The same pattern of antigenic jumps likely also exists for human H1 viruses. Antigenic cartography as developed by Smith et al. is now routinely used by the WHO for the selection of vaccine strains.[499] Other groups have developed similar approaches.[212,843,2279]

Antigenic drift has also led to the diversification of recent H5 HA proteins into several antigenically and genetically distinguishable clades and subclades; these are described in the Outbreaks of Highly Pathogenic Avian Influenza (HPAI) Virus section.

Antigenic cartography and computational modeling have provided new insight into antigenic drift of human influenza viruses. Computational approaches have also been used to analyze mutation patterns in HA, and have demonstrated that most positively selected amino acid changes map to the antigenic sites.[41,140,204,638,844,1842,1843,1848]

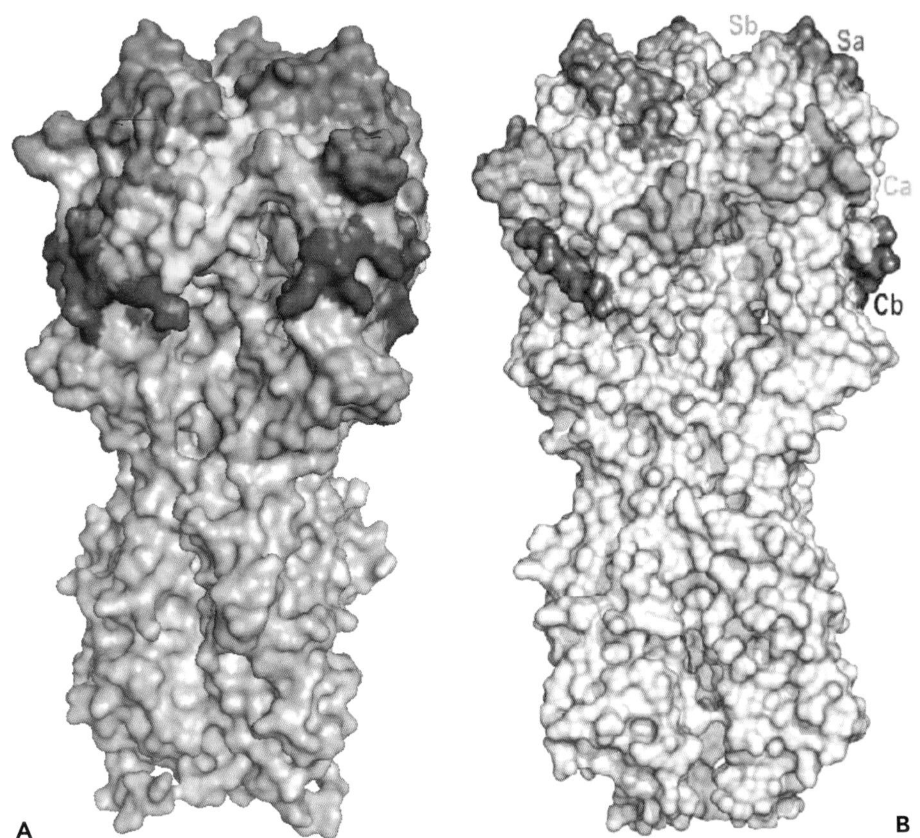

FIGURE 41.6. Crystallographic structures of influenza A virus H3 and H1 HA proteins. A: Crystallographic structure of the trimer complex of influenza A virus H3 HA protein (Protein Data Bank #1HGD) showing the locations of the five antigenic epitopes: antigenic site A (amino acids 122, 124, 126, 130–133, 135, 137, 138, 140, 142–146, 150, 152, 168), *red;* antigenic site B (amino acids 128, 129, 155–160, 163–165, 186–190, 196–198), *green;* antigenic site C (amino acids 44–48, 50, 51, 53, 54, 273, 275, 276, 278–280, 294, 297, 299, 300, 304, 305, 307–312), *blue;* antigenic site D (amino acids 96, 102, 103, 117, 121, 167, 170–177, 179, 182, 201, 203, 207–209, 212–219, 226–230, 238, 240, 242, 244, 246–248, *yellow;* antigenic site E (amino acids 57, 59, 62, 63, 67, 75, 78, 80–83, 91, 92, 94, 109, 260–262, 265), *purple.* **B:** Crystallographic structure of the HA protein of A(H1N1)pdm09 virus. Shown is the trimer complex with the antigenic sites Ca (amino acids 140–145, 169–173, 206–208, 224, 225, 238–240), *orange;* Cb (amino acids 79–84), *dark blue;* Sa (amino acids 128, 129, 156–160, 162–167), *red;* Sb (amino acids 187–198), *light blue.* (**B** reproduced from Xu R, Ekiert DC, Krause JC, et al. Structural basis of preexisting immunity to the 2009 H1N1 pandemic influenza virus. *Science* 2010;328:357–360, with permission.)

Antigenic Drift of the NA Protein

The function and structure of this protein are discussed in detail in Chapter 40. In addition to HA, antigenic drift has also been reported for NA[367,1286,1350,1605,1802] and correlated with amino acid differences in the molecule.[338] Studies with monoclonal antibodies and amino acid sequence analyses have revealed two to three antigenic sites.[11] The NA of most influenza A virus subtypes and of influenza B viruses has been crystallized.[12,1226,2050,2291] The structure contains two major antigenic sites located on the upper surface of the molecule, where they flank the sialic acid-binding site. A possible third antigenic site resides on the bottom of the head; however, it is difficult to imagine how antibodies binding to this site would result in the selection of escape mutants. A more detailed structural analysis of the Fab fragment of a monoclonal antibody (NC41) to N9 NA showed that five peptide loops, located at the rim of the enzyme active site, constitute the epitope.[2100] The second epitope, characterized with monoclonal antibodies to N8 NA, is located at the interface of two adjacent monomers in the tetrameric NA and involves peptide loops on both monomers.[1779] Antibodies with this epitope bind only to NA tetramers.

Antigenic Shift

Antigenic shift involves major antigenic changes in which an HA or NA that is antigenically distinct from the circulating variant is introduced into the human population. Typically, antigenic shift is caused by an HA or NA of a new subtype, that is, one that did not circulate in humans prior to the pandemic. The H1N1 pandemic in 2009 was a notable exception since it was caused by a virus of the H1N1 subtype, even though viruses of this subtype had been circulating in humans since 1977. These newly introduced proteins are immunologically distinct from the previously circulating strains and result in

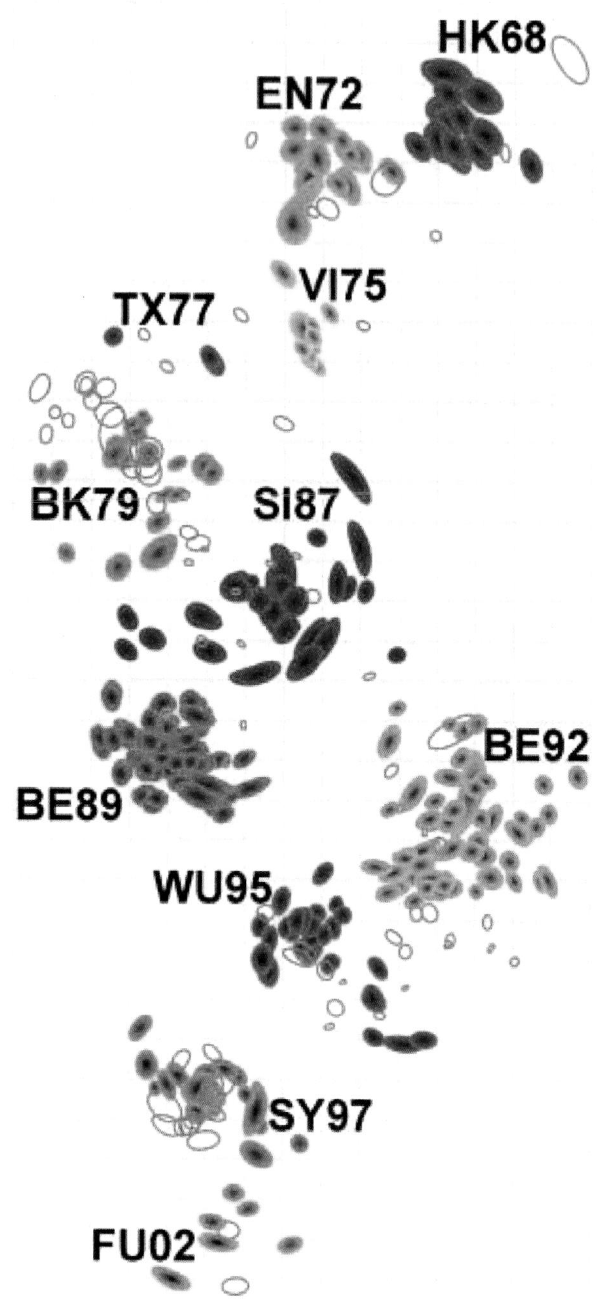

FIGURE 41.7. Antigenic cartography. The map shows seasonal H3N2 viruses from 1968 to 2003. Each *open circle* represents an antiserum used for analysis. Each *colored circle* represents an H3N2 strain tested by using the hemagglutination inhibition assay against the selected antisera. The distances between strains and/or antisera are relative to their antigenic distances (in HI units). The spacing between the grid lines is equivalent to a twofold dilution of antiserum in the HI assay. Typically, fourfold changes in HI titers (i.e., two gridlines in the map) require an update of the vaccine. The different colors represent the antigenic clusters to which the strains belong (HK68, Hong Kong 1968; EN72, England 1972; VI75, Victoria 1975; TX77, Texas 1977; BK79, Bangkok 1979; SI87, Sichuan 1987; BE89, Beijing 1989; BE92, Beijing 1992; WU95, Wuhan 1995; SY97, Sydney 1997; FU02, Fujian 2002). (From Smith DJ, Lapedes AS, de Jong JC, et al. Mapping the antigenic and genetic evolution of influenza virus. *Science* 2004;305:371–376, with permission.)

high infection rates of the novel virus in the immunologically naïve population, leading to pandemics.

Since the beginning of the last century, five antigenic shifts have occurred: in 1918, with the appearance of H1N1 viruses that caused the Spanish influenza; in 1957, when the H1N1 subtype was replaced with H2N2 viruses, causing the Asian influenza; in 1968, when H3N2 viruses replaced the H2N2 subtype, leading to the Hong Kong influenza; in 1977, when the H1N1 subtype reappeared (Russian influenza); and in 2009, when a novel, antigenically distinct H1N1 virus caused a pandemic that largely replaced seasonal H1N1 viruses (see The H1N1 Pandemic in 2009 section). These new subtypes occurred suddenly and at irregular and unpredictable intervals.

The antigenic shift that caused the pandemics in 1957 and 1968 resulted from reassortment between human and avian viruses. By contrast, the A(H1N1)pdm09 virus resulted from reassortment events among swine, avian, and human influenza viruses (see The H1N1 Pandemic in 2009 section). Although not conclusive, phylogenetic evidence suggests that the Spanish influenza was caused by the introduction of an avian-origin virus into the human population.[77,1712,1713–1715,2048,2049]

Transmission of Avian Influenza Viruses to Humans

Prior to 1997, the direct transmission of avian influenza viruses to humans was not considered a serious human health threat. This assumption was based on findings that avian viruses do not replicate efficiently in experimentally infected humans[92] and that no severe cases of human infections had been reported during any outbreaks of highly pathogenic avian influenza (HPAI). The differences in receptor-binding specificities between human and avian viruses (for details, see Molecular Determinants of Host Range Restriction and Pathogenesis section) were believed to provide a host range barrier that limited the transmission of avian viruses to humans. Until 1997, only three cases of direct avian-to-human transmission of influenza viruses had been described: (1) an HPAI virus of the H7N5 subtype isolated from a patient with hepatitis in 1959,[219,409] (2) an H7N7 HPAI virus isolated from a laboratory worker who developed conjunctivitis,[2053] and (3) an H7N7 virus of low pathogenicity isolated from a woman who developed conjunctivitis and was likely infected from ducks she kept.[60,1119] These cases, together with serologic studies,[1864,1872,2345,2372] demonstrated the potential for avian influenza viruses to be transmitted to humans; however, the true threat of avian-to-human virus transmission was not fully realized until 1997, when avian H5N1 viruses were transmitted to humans in Hong Kong and killed 6 of 18 patients.[320,322,394,1993,2345]

In 1998 and 1999, H9N2 viruses transmitted from birds to pigs and humans. Five human infections were reported in southern China[698] and, in March 1999, two children were infected in Hong Kong.[1227,1626] Both presented with symptoms of typical influenza and recovered. The isolates were genetically similar to those from quail (A/quail/Hong Kong/G1/97 [H9N2]). There was, however, no evidence of human-to-human transmission.[2119] During an outbreak of HPAI H7N7 viruses in poultry in the Netherlands in February/March 2003, 89 people were infected, 83 of whom developed conjunctivitis.[546,1085] Most cases were mild and self-limiting, although a veterinarian developed acute respiratory distress and an ultimately fatal pneumonia.[2135] In three cases, human-to-human transmission was documented and antibodies were detected in 59% of those who had contact with infected poultry workers. Also in 2003, a young child in Hong Kong was infected with an H9N2 virus but recovered uneventfully.[207,297] In November 2003, an H7N2 virus was isolated from an adult in New York who was hospitalized for upper and lower respiratory tract illness, but eventually recovered.[255,463] In 2004, two people developed conjunctivitis and mild respiratory symptoms after an outbreak of an HPAI H7N3 virus in poultry in Canada.[815,2111] Additional cases of human infection with avian influenza viruses were detected in the United Kingdom in 2006 and 2007, when H7N3 and H7N2 viruses caused conjunctivitis in one[1510] and four individuals,[463] and in Hong Kong in 2008 and 2009, when genetically different H9N2 viruses were isolated from two immunocompromised patients.[297] These findings underscore the potential of H7 and H9 viruses to infect humans, although human-to-human transmission has thus far been limited. In 2004, two cases of human infection with H10N7 virus were reported in Egypt (http://www.paho.org/english/ad/dpc/cd/eid-eer-07-may-2004.htm); this subtype has not been isolated in humans before or since.

Highly pathogenic H5N1 viruses have thus far claimed 364 lives in several countries (for more details see The H5N1 Outbreak section). The recent increase in the number of human infections with avian influenza viruses may be a consequence of better surveillance and reporting infrastructure, and/or increased human contacts with poultry and other bird populations.

Vaccines for use in humans for H5 (see Vaccines section), H7,[275,357,405,906,944,1608] and H9[275,977] viruses are currently in development. In the United States, the first H5N1 vaccine for human use was approved in April 2007 (http://www.fda.gov/BiologicsBloodVaccines/Vaccines/ApprovedProducts/ucm112838.htm). However, due to the antigenic drift of the H5 HA, the cross-protection among the antigenic clades is not optimal without an adjuvant. Likewise, human infections with H7 viruses have been caused by antigenically distinct viruses of the North American and Eurasian lineages, which may necessitate the development of several vaccines based on antigenically different viruses.

Transmission Among Humans

Influenza viruses do not cause persistent or latent infections in immunocompetent individuals; they are maintained in human populations by direct person-to-person spread during acute infections. Seasonal disease patterns have been reported for temperate climate regions[444,1242,1255]: In the northern hemisphere, epidemics generally peak between January and April, but may flare up as early as December or as late as May.[532,830,1531] In the southern hemisphere, outbreaks occur between May and September. The low relative indoor humidity during the winter months may prolong the survival of influenza in aerosols[735,780,781,1263,1793] and contribute the seasonal pattern in the northern hemisphere. However, seasonality is also observed in tropical and subtropical climates[23,376,402,1181,1431,1766,2155,2308] where increased influenza activity appears to coincide with the onset of the rainy season.[301,402,440,1431,1703,1704] On a global scale, influenza virus activity is detectable throughout the year,[1531,1766] and viruses can be isolated in large cities year-round.

The incubation period is 1 to 3 days for influenza A viruses and 1 to 4 days for influenza B viruses.[550,1191] The most effective means of spread among humans are aerosols.[1428,2056] Most aerosol droplets formed during sneezing or coughing are less than 2 μm in diameter and are preferentially deposited in the lower airways of the lung[46,290,1231,1232,1513,2309]; however, normal breathing also produces aerosols.[471,512,529] Volunteers are readily infected by aerosol transmission[17]; the human infectious dose of influenza A virus infection is 0.6 to 3 $TCID_{50}$ (dose required to infect 50% of tissue culture) when delivered by aerosol,[17] but 127 to 320 $TCID_{50}$ when delivered intranasally.[347] Ferrets are an established animal model for influenza virus transmission studies (reviewed in[1341,1542]). Recently, guinea pigs have been established as a model for aerosol transmission,[1265,1434] and have been used to assess the importance of temperature and humidity for influenza virus transmission.[1264,1266]

Influenza-Related Morbidity and Mortality

The collective burden of interpandemics can be substantial and depends on a variety of factors, as indicated in this section. The average annual death toll during interpandemic seasons is about 20,000 in the United States.

Morbidity

Influenza virus is estimated to cause about 50 million illnesses annually in the United States. Excess hospitalizations of between 50,000 and 200,000 Americans per season have been reported.[670,1436,1879,1882,2063] The H1N1 pandemic in 2009 is estimated to have caused 274,000 hospitalizations in the United States alone. Direct costs include hospitalizations, medical fees, drugs, and testing, and were estimated in 1986 to be about $1 billion annually, while indirect costs such as loss of productivity reached $2 to $4 billion annually.[1806] The temporal curves of individual pandemics are similar in that virus introduction into a community is followed by a relatively sharp, single peak that represents school and workplace absenteeism, which is followed by excess mortality slightly later.[1531] Notable exceptions are the pandemics in 1918 and 1957, both of which were characterized by a second, more severe wave.[941,2047,2185]

A number of studies have documented how influenza virus epidemics reduce school attendance and work productivity, increase doctor's visits and hospitalizations, and can cause increased mortality, particularly among high-risk groups.[1504,1505,1506] Children younger than two years of age and the elderly have the highest hospitalization rates,[631,895,1506,1641] reaching 1 per 270 for those older than 65 years, compared to 1 per 2,900 for the 1- to 44-year-old age group.[68,69] The impact of influenza on the elderly extends beyond influenza and pneumonia to all respiratory conditions as well as to congestive heart failure.[1516] It is an important cause of respiratory infections in nursing homes.[69] Among children, 14% to 16% of those seeking medical care for acute respiratory illness or fever are infected with influenza virus.[635,1668,2272]

During interpandemic seasons, the overall infection rates range from 10% to 20% but can reach 50% in selected age groups or populations. The rate and severity of infection depend on the level of preexisting immunity, age of an individual, and virulence of the virus, all of which vary greatly among outbreaks.[304,549,629,942,1724] Age-specific attack rates are highest in school-age children, and symptoms in this age group are usually more severe than in young adults.[549,629,632,1411,2018] Often, increases in school absenteeism mark the beginning of a new epidemic,[631] suggesting that school-age children play a critical role in disseminating influenza viruses. Increases in school absenteeism are typically followed by increases in workplace absenteeism. Influenza A viruses of the H1N1 and H3N2 subtypes, as well as influenza B viruses, all cause similar symptoms[555,1522,1934]; however, the frequency of severe infections is higher with H3N2 viruses.[2063] Reinfection with a closely related variant can occur,[384,385,549,553,554,1924] although the symptoms are usually less severe than those that follow the initial encounter with a particular virus strain.[384,385,629,1924]

The H1N1 pandemic in 2009 showed a similar pattern to previous pandemics since elderly people (who typically suffer high attack rates) were infected in relatively small numbers; their exposure to the descendants of the 1918 pandemic virus which circulated until 1957 may have provided partial protection against the A(H1N1)pdm09 virus[252,311,705,734,864,890] (see The H1N1 Pandemic in 2009 section).

Mortality

The increase in mortality during pandemics and epidemics is a hallmark of influenza virus infection. The term "excess mortality" was introduced by William Farr and describes the number of deaths observed during an outbreak in excess of the number of expected mortalities. The number of influenza virus–related deaths, however, is difficult to determine because the death certificate may not indicate influenza as a primary cause of death or because a laboratory diagnosis may not have been performed.

Excess mortality was estimated to be between 20 and 50 million deaths for Spanish influenza worldwide,[1619] and 70,000, 33,800, and 12,470 deaths in the United States for the Asian influenza, Hong Kong influenza, and H1N1 pandemic in 2009, respectively. Although excess mortality is highest during a pandemic, the cumulative deaths of interpandemic seasons usually exceed those of pandemic years[1531,1881] (Fig. 41.8). During epidemics, excess mortality is estimated to be more than 20,000 in the United States alone but can exceed 40,000 deaths. In the United States, the annual excess mortality appears to have increased over the last decades, perhaps because of an increasing number of elderly and/or immunocompromised individuals.[2063] Excess mortality is typically highest with H3N2 virus infections, whereas H1N1 and type B viruses contribute to smaller extents.[168,667,1881,2063]

Excess mortality affects all age groups but is highest in those older than 65 years, who account for approximately 90% of excess mortalities during interpandemic seasons.[69,71,483,1936] This age group has a 100-fold higher mortality rate than those younger than age 65.[1879] During the 1968 pandemic, however, people younger than 65 accounted for 50% of influenza virus-related deaths,[354] and during the 1918 pandemic, excess mortality rates were extremely high not only in the elderly, but also in young adults.[1531] The reasons for these unusual patterns are unknown. The highest risk for pneumonia is seen in the elderly who have cardiovascular and pulmonary conditions[71]; other risk factors include metabolic or neoplastic diseases and pregnancy.[69,70,665,1505] Several other factors associated with increased risk of severe disease have been identified for infections with A(H1N1)pdm09 viruses (see The H1N1 Pandemic in 2009 section).

EPIZOOLOGY AND PATHOGENESIS IN ANIMALS

Influenza A viruses infect a variety of animals, including humans, birds, swine, horses, and dogs. Occasionally, influenza viruses have been isolated from cats, tigers and leopards, stone martens and Owston civets, whales, seals, mink, and camels. Serologic evidence also suggests exposure of several ruminant, reptile, and amphibian species to immunogens related to influenza viruses (reviewed in[1723]).

Viruses of all known HA and NA subtypes are maintained in aquatic birds, generally without causing disease; therefore, aquatic birds are considered the natural reservoir of influenza A viruses.[465,807,809,1749,1755,1864,1894,2214,2221] Nonpathogenic viruses of the H5 and H7 subtypes can evolve into highly pathogenic avian strains that cause significant losses to the poultry industry.[62,225,834,836,1002,1748] Viruses of the H5, H6, and H9 subtypes have established or may be establishing lineages in chickens.[432,1182,2220] Although human pandemics have been associated with viruses of the H1 to H3 subtypes, the ability of avian viruses of the H5, H7, and H9 subtypes to infect humans has flagged viruses of these subtypes as potential candidates for future influenza pandemics. Influenza B viruses typically replicate in humans but have been isolated from seals.[1550,1582] Influenza C virus infects humans, swine,[701,1558,2303,2344] and dogs.[1310,1558]

Influenza in Birds

The natural reservoir of influenza A viruses are the orders *Anseriformes* (ducks, geese, swans) and *Charadriiformes* (gulls, terns, shorebirds),[445,1894,2214] although influenza A viruses have been isolated from at least 105 different avian species from 26 different families.[466,1340,1489,1569,1943,1945] Almost all HA and NA subtypes have been detected in dabbling ducks (*Anas* spp.),[999,1095,1147,1560,1569,1837,1838,1947,2182,2225] suggesting that these species are the major reservoir of influenza A viruses. In mallard ducks (*Anas platyrhynchos*), viruses of the H3, H4, and H6 subtypes are isolated most frequently; the most prevalent subtypes are H4N6 and H6N2.[737,1095,1441,1838,2182] In addition, several HA subtypes (including H1, H2, H5, H7, and H9–H12), in combination with several NA subtypes, have been detected in waders of the *Charadriidae* family, suggesting a role for these species in the perpetuation of influenza A viruses. Viruses of the H13 and H16 subtypes appear to circulate only in *Laridae* (gull and tern) species.[262,999,1094,1441,1569,1633,2142] This observation is consistent with the finding that a gull influenza virus did not replicate efficiently in ducks,[802] perhaps due to differences in receptor-binding preferences between viruses derived from ducks or *Laridae* species.[2306] For the NA gene, N2, N6, and N8 subtypes predominate in ducks, whereas N6 and N9 are prevalent in shorebirds and gulls. Poultry play a critical role in the perpetuation of influenza A viruses; thus, most HA and NA subtypes can be isolated from poultry in live-bird markets.[195,308,1249,1511,1932,1986,2214,2319]

Surveillance studies have demonstrated seasonal patterns in prevalence; the infection rate of mallard ducks reaches 60%

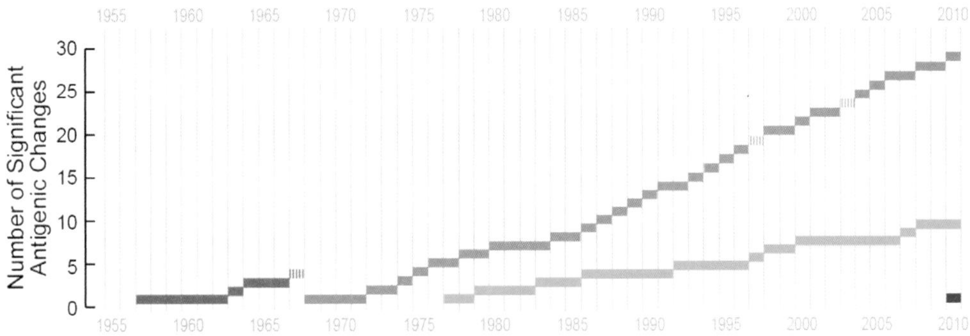

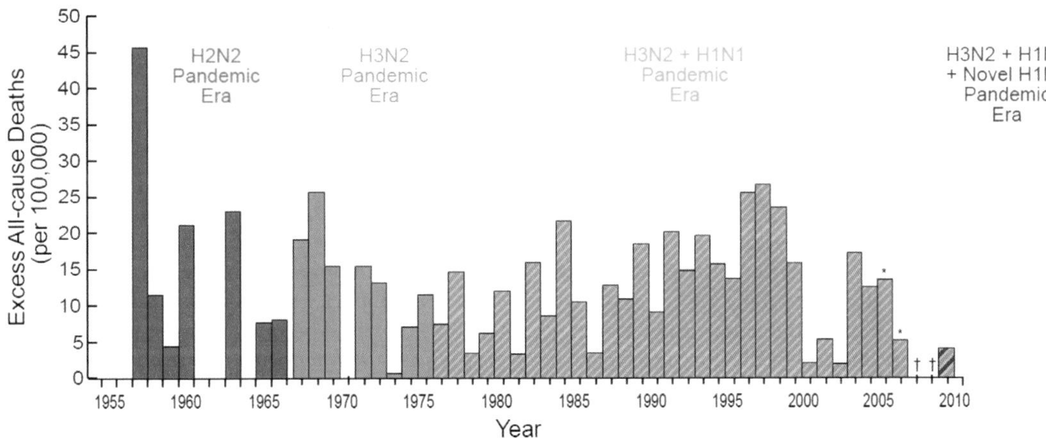

FIGURE 41.8. Influenza virus mortality rates in the United States from 1957 to 2010. Shown are the excess mortality rates per 100,000 persons. *Estimates are given since data are unavailable; †, data unavailable. (Modified from Morens, DM, Taubenberger JK, Fauci AS. 2010. The 2009 H1N1 Pandemic Influenza Virus: What Next? *MBio* 1(4):e00211–10; with permission.)

before the autumn migration, and declines to less than 10% in spring and summer.[809,811,1095,1441,1560,1569,1945,2182,2214] This pattern may represent the influx of immunologically naïve juveniles every summer, and/or the high population density in marshalling areas before the migration. By contrast, in North American shorebirds, the infection rate is highest in late spring and early summer.[1095] Since the prevalence of infection declines along the migration route and is relatively low at the wintering grounds of mallard ducks, geographic patterns in prevalence can be observed (i.e., infection rates are higher at the marshalling areas in the North than at the wintering grounds in the South). Moreover, the prevalence of virus subtypes in the same species changes from year to year.[811,1095,1838,1945] In particular, cyclic patterns exist in which high rates of prevalence for one subtype in a certain population may be followed by low detection rates in this population in subsequent seasons,[1095,1838] perhaps due to herd immunity to viruses of the respective subtype.

Reassortment may play a critical role in the evolution of avian influenza viruses with significant contributions of both intrasubtypic reassortment (i.e., reassortment between viruses of the same subtype) and intersubtypic reassortment (i.e., reassortment between viruses of different subtypes),[278,449,677,678,752,805,1089,1205,1296,1491,2157,2187] and of reassortment between the North American and Eurasian gene pools, which evolve largely independently, as described earlier.[388,456,752,1050,1094,1248,1305,2181,2210,2246,2263]

Avian Influenza Viruses of High or Low Pathogenicity

Based on their pathogenicity in chickens, avian influenza viruses are classified as highly pathogenic avian influenza (HPAI) or low pathogenicity avian influenza (LPAI) viruses. LPAI viruses cause mild respiratory disease, depression, and/or a decrease in egg production. For outbreak control purposes, the Office International des Epizooties (OIE) classifies an avian influenza virus as HPAI if it is "lethal for six, seven, or eight of eight 4- to 8-week-old susceptible chickens within 10 days following intravenous inoculation with 0.2 ml of a 1/10 dilution of a bacteria-free, infective allantoic fluid" (OIE Manual of Diagnostic Tests and Vaccines for Terrestrial Animals 2010; accessible at: http://www.oie.int/en/international-standard-setting/terrestrial-manual/access-online/), or if it has an intravenous pathogenicity index (IVPI) greater than 1.2 (the IVPI is the mean clinical score of ten 6-week-old chickens intravenously infected). All H5 and H7 viruses of low pathogenicity in chickens with a multibasic sequence at the HA cleavage site are considered highly pathogenic.

Most HPAI viruses have a series of basic amino acids at the HA cleavage site; however, exceptions exist in which viruses with multiple basic amino acids at this site are not highly pathogenic in chickens,[1002,1171,1257,2012] or highly pathogenic viruses do not possess a conventional HA cleavage site.[1614,1989] All HPAI viruses known to date belong to the H5 or H7 subtype; however, only a small proportion of all H5 and H7 viruses are highly pathogenic. Historically, disease caused by HPAI viruses was called "Fowl plague." Viruses that are highly pathogenic for chickens often cause high mortality in turkeys and Japanese quail, but are usually nonpathogenic for ducks and geese, with the exception of some of the recently circulating HPAI H5N1 viruses.

The infection of aquatic birds with LPAI is typically asymptomatic, although even LPAI viruses can cause mild disease in mallards[945,1147] and swans.[2128] In ducks, avian viruses replicate in the epithelial cells in the intestinal tract and, to a substantially lesser extent, in cells of the respiratory tract.[489,2218,2228] These viruses are resistant to the low pH environment they encounter during their passage through the digestive tract. Avian species shed influenza viruses in high concentrations in feces.[1023,1893,2225,2228] The viruses are relatively stable in water[1944,1946] and have been isolated from water samples of lakes where wild birds have nested or congregated before migration.[731,809,810,886] Contaminated water and feces may, therefore, serve as major routes of transmission of LPAI among feral birds.[810,1885] By contrast, highly pathogenic H5N1 viruses replicate efficiently in the upper respiratory tract of infected birds.[1006,1982] Human influenza viruses also replicate in the upper respiratory, but not in the intestinal, tract of ducks,[2218] because they do not recognize efficiently the receptors in duck intestine [sialic acid (Sia) linked to galactose by α2,3 linkages (Siaα2,3Gal)].[1744]

Infection of ducks with some highly pathogenic H5N1 influenza viruses results in systemic infections with high virus titers in the respiratory organs; neurologic symptoms may also be observed.[488,1049,1982,2148] However, infected birds may die without clinical symptoms.[488] In experimental infections of several bird species, HPAI H5N1 were not uniformly lethal, and infected animals shed appreciable amounts of viruses, which could facilitate virus spread.[185,279,1006,1147,1983] A characteristic feature of HPAI H5N1 infection in ducks is that virus titers in oropharyngeal swabs are higher than those in cloacal swabs.[1006,1983] In chickens, influenza virus infections can result in mortality rates of up to 100%.

Occasionally, avian influenza viruses infect mammalian species. Most of these infections are self-limiting and stable lineages have emerged rarely, such as in pigs in 1979 with the introduction of an avian H1N1 virus.[1630] In mammals, LPAI viruses cause bronchitis, bronchiolitis, and/or pneumonia. Infection with HPAI results in severe, systemic infection (see following discussion and The H5N1 Outbreak section).

Outbreaks of Highly Pathogenic Avian Influenza (HPAI) Viruses

With only three exceptions [A/tern/South Africa/61(H5N3),[93] a highly pathogenic H7N1 virus that caused an outbreak in a backyard flock of geese and Muscovy ducks in Italy in 1999/2000,[228] and the so-called Qinghai Lake HPAI H5N1 viruses,[279,281,1247]], all HPAI outbreaks have occurred in poultry (Table 41.1). However, H5N2 viruses isolated from an apparently healthy duck and goose possessed an HA cleavage sequence characteristic of HPAI viruses,[573] demonstrating that HPAI viruses may emerge in aquatic birds without apparent signs of infection. HPAI is controlled by depopulation and vaccination. Although LPAI viruses had long been considered of negligible risk, it is now clear that HPAI arise from LPAI by mutations.[62,225,834,836,1002,1748] The major recent outbreaks of HPAI are discussed in the sections that follow (Table 41.1).

H5N1

HPAI H5N1 viruses were first isolated from sick domestic geese in 1996 in Guangdong province.[1883,2290] Outbreaks of H5N1 HPAI occurred in poultry in Hong Kong from March to May 1997 and again in November 1997.[1865,1869] These viruses caused high mortality rates (70–100%) in experimentally infected chickens.[1988,1993] The causative agent was identified as an H5N1 reassortant virus that had acquired its HA gene from an A/goose/Guangdong/1/96 (H5N1,Gs/Gd)-like virus,[2290] its NA gene from another avian N1 virus, and its remaining six genes (i.e., PB2, PB1, PA, NP, M, and NS) from other avian viruses.[681,826] H5N1 HPAI viruses have in common an HA protein with a multibasic sequence at the cleavage site (a characteristic of highly pathogenic viruses).[1869] By the same token, many H5N1 isolates possess a shortened NA stalk,[2367] a characteristic of viruses adapted in terrestrial poultry.[116,1331,1869,1988] The H5N1 viruses isolated from Hong Kong patients in 1997 fell into two groups of either high or low pathogenicity in mice.[593,990,1269,1869] The outbreaks in poultry were accompanied by the first transmissions of wholly avian influenza viruses to humans with fatal outcomes.[320,322,394,1993] These events, together with the finding that H5N1 infections were widespread in poultry markets in Hong Kong (close to 20% in chickens)[1865] prompted the slaughter of all poultry in Hong Kong in late December 1997/early January 1998. The mass slaughter of poultry eliminated HPAI H5N1 viruses from the Hong Kong poultry markets, and no further cases of human infections were reported. However, HPAI H5N1 viruses with an HA gene belonging to the Gs/Gd lineage continued to circulate in avian species in mainland China.[1205] They reappeared in poultry in Hong Kong in 2001 and 2002, and have been isolated from both aquatic and terrestrial poultry since 2001.[677,1205] The outbreaks in poultry in Hong Kong in 2001 and 2002 were controlled by depopulation, and by vaccination with an H5N2 strain in April 2002. These strict surveillance and vaccination measures have reduced the number of outbreaks of HPAI H5N1 viruses in Hong Kong.

Waterfowl are usually resistant to HPAI viruses; however, in late 2002, waterfowl in Kowloon and Penfold Park, Hong Kong, showed signs of neurologic disease as they succumbed to H5N1 influenza virus infection.[488,1982] With the exception of A/tern/South Africa/61(H5N3)[93] and a highly pathogenic H7N1 virus that caused an outbreak in Muscovy ducks in Italy in 1999/2000,[228] influenza viruses were not known to cause disease in aquatic birds. At the same time as the Kowloon Park outbreak, H5N1 viruses were isolated from dead chickens in retail poultry markets and a local chicken farm.

In April/May 2005, more than 6,000 birds—mostly bar-headed geese, but also brown- and black-headed gulls, ruddy

TABLE 41.1 Outbreaks of Highly Pathogenic Avian Influenza Viruses Since 1955

Virus[a]	Subtype	Comments
A/chicken/Scotland/59	H5N1	Two chicken flocks
A/tern/South Africa/61	H5N3	1,300 common terns
A/turkey/England/63	H7N3	29,000 breeder turkeys
A/turkey/Ontario/7732/66	H5N9	8,100 breeder turkeys
A/chicken/Victoria/76	H7N7	25,000 laying chickens, 17,000 broilers, and 16,000 ducks
A/chicken/Germany/79	H7N7	Outbreaks in former East Germany; numbers unknown
A/turkey/England/199/79	H7N7	3 commercial turkey farms
A/chicken/Pennsylvania/1370/83	H5N2	17 million birds, mostly chickens or turkeys
A/turkey/Ireland/1378/83	H5N8	800 infected turkeys died; 8,640 turkeys, 28,020 chickens and 270,000 ducks were culled
A/chicken/Victoria/85	H7N7	24,000 broiler breeders, 27,000 laying chickens, 69,000 broilers, and 118,518 unspecified chickens
A/turkey/England/50-92/91	H5N1	8,000 turkeys
A/chicken/Victoria/92	H7N3	12,700 broiler breeders and 5,700 ducks
A/chicken/Queensland/95	H7N3	22,000 laying chickens
A/chicken/Puebla/8623-607/94 A/chicken/Queretaro/14588-19/95	H5N2	Millions of birds died or were culled; exact numbers are not available
A/chicken/Pakistan/447/95 A/chicken/Pakistan/1369-CR2/95	H7N3	3.2 million broilers and broiler breeder chickens
A/chicken/Hong Kong/220/97	H5N1	1.5 million chickens and other domestic birds; 6 human fatalities (among 18 infected individuals)
A/chicken/New South Wales/1651/97	H7N4	128,000 broiler breeders, 33,000 broilers, and 261 emus
A/chicken/Italy/330/97	H5N2	Chickens, turkeys, guinea fowl, ducks, quail, pigeons, geese, pheasant (all in small numbers)
A/turkey/Italy/4580/99	H7N1	8.1 million laying chickens, 2.7 million meat and breeder turkeys, 2.4 million broiler breeders and broilers, 247,000 guinea fowl, 260,000 quail, ducks, and pheasants; also backyard poultry and ostriches
A/chicken/Chile/4957/2002	H7N2	2 million birds died or were culled
A/grey heron/Hong Kong/861.1/2002	H5N1	Outbreak in wild birds in Hong Kong; over 800,000 domestic birds were culled
A/chicken/Netherlands/1/2003	H7N7	Virus was isolated from 241 poultry farms in The Netherlands, two farms in Belgium, and one farm in Germany; outbreak was controlled by killing more than 30 million birds; one human fatality
A/chicken/Canada/AVFV1/2004 A/chicken/Canada/AVFV2/2004	H7N3	Spread to more than 40 commercial poultry farms; outbreak was controlled by culling all 19 million domestic birds in Fraser Valley, British Columbia
A/ostrich/South Africa/2004	H5N2	Outbreak in ostriches; 26,000 ostriches were culled to control virus spread
Various H5N1 viruses (since 2003)	H5N1	Outbreak started in July 2003 in poultry in Vietnam, Indonesia, and Thailand and has since spread to a number of Southeast Asian, European, Middle Eastern, and African countries; more than 100 million domestic birds have died or have been culled; mortality has also been observed among wild birds; as of February 1, 2013, 364 human fatalities had been reported (among 615 infected individuals)
A/chicken/North Korea/2005	H7N7	Approximate number of birds affected: 219,000
A/chicken/Saskatchewan/HR-00011/2007	H7N3	Outbreak on a broiler breeding farm in Saskatchewan, Canada; depopulation of all animals on the premise (53,000)
A/chicken/England/1158-11406/2008	H7N7	Outbreak in a laying flock of chickens; death or depopulation of 25,000 animals
A/chicken/Spain/6279-2/2009	H7N7	Outbreak in a layer hen farm; outbreak was stopped through death (~30,000) and depopulation (~278,000) of all animals on the farm

[a]Outbreaks that caused significant economic losses (defined as outbreaks that killed or resulted in the slaughter of more than 1 million birds) are shown in bold.

(Modified from Swayne DE, Halvorson DA. Influenza. In: Saif YM, Barnes HJ, Fadly AM, et al., eds. *Diseases of Poultry.* 11th ed. Ames: Iowa State University Press; 2003:135–160.)

shelducks, and great cormorants—died from HPAI H5N1 virus infection at the Qinghai Lake Nature Reserve in Gangcha County, Qinghai Province, China.[279,281,1247] Although viruses of several genotypes were detected during the outbreak, one genotype was dominant.[279,281,1247,2370] HPAI H5N1 viruses closely related to the Qinghai Lake isolates have spread through Russia, into Europe, the Middle East, and several African countries. Two factors likely contributed to the dissemination of these viruses: movement of infected poultry and virus spread through migratory birds.[280,522,1031,1444,1645,1680,1722,1876,2125,2212,2253]

Recent HPAI H5N1 viruses have expanded their geographic range, become enzootic in poultry populations in different parts of the world, more pathogenic in ducks than isolates from 1997,[1606,1647,1982] and have a broad host range. While HPAI infections are typically limited to terrestrial poultry, the currently circulating H5N1 viruses have been isolated from a number of different wild birds including water birds (order *Anseriformes*) such as ducks, geese, and swans; shore birds (order *Charadriiformes*) such as gulls and waders; small songbirds (order *Passeriformes*) such as sparrows and crows; large wading birds (order *Ciconiiformes*) such as herons, storks, and egrets; several *Ratites* species including ostriches,[390] emu, and rhea; and species of several other birds orders.[279,281,454,488,1082,1221,1247,1287,1839,1982] In addition, HPAI H5N1 viruses have been isolated from carnivores including dogs,[29,206,325,624,1923] cats,[29,1064,1104,1105,1733,1922,2120] tigers,[28,2058] leopards,[1005] a stone marten,[1065,1735] Owston civets[1735] (www.promedmail.org, Archive no. 20080312.0991), and raccoon dogs.[1688] Moreover, HPAI H5N1 viruses have been isolated from pigs on several occasions[1202,1526,1846,2378]; these animals can also be infected experimentally with HPAI H5N1 viruses.[306,1241,1869] However, pigs do not show symptoms upon infection with HPAI H5N1 viruses.[1241] The experimental infection of calves was limited to subclinical seroconversion,[955] and no HPAI H5N1 infections have been reported in horses to this point.

Past outbreaks of HPAI originated from one virus strain. However, antigenic drift and reassortment have resulted in a diversification of HPAI H5N1 viruses, both genetically and antigenically. Based on the HA sequence, ten clades (clade 0–9) are currently recognized, some of which are divided into second- and third-order clades.[547,674,675] Recently, only viruses of clades 1, 2, and 7 have been isolated (http://www.who.int/influenza/gisrs_laboratory/201101_h5n1evoconceptualdiagram.pdf): clade 2.1 represents Indonesian H5N1 viruses, whereas Qinghai Lake H5N1 viruses[279,281,1247] and their European, Middle Eastern, and African descendants form clade 2.2. Clade 2.3 viruses have become dominant in southern China, but have also been isolated in Hong Kong, Vietnam, Thailand, Laos, Malaysia, and Japan. Other Japanese H5N1 viruses belong to clade 2.5, which also includes viruses from Korea and China. Clade 2.4 is formed predominantly by chicken viruses from southern China (Yunnan and Guangxi Provinces). Human infections have been caused by viruses of clades 0, 1, 2.1, 2.2, 2.3, and 7. Viruses of clade 2.2 have spread to three continents and continue to infect humans. The evolution of these viruses has been studied intensively.[281,451–454,1054,1409,1785,1948] The NA genes of HPAI H5N1 viruses can be divided into two lineages: one possesses a 19-amino-acid deletion in the stalk region (amino acids 54–72); the second comprises viruses with a full-length NA stalk or with a 20-amino-acid deletion spanning amino acids 49–68.

Since their first appearance, multiple genotypes have been isolated that are indicative of frequent reassortment with viruses of other genotypes or subtypes.[278,449,677,678,1089,1205,1296,1491,2157] One genotype became dominant in 2002[280,1129,1205]; its descendants continue to circulate in Indonesia and have spread westward into the Middle East. In southern China and other parts of Southeast Asia, however, this genotype was replaced by viruses of another genotype (the Fujian-like viruses).[1902]

Reassortment between HPAI H5N1 and circulating human influenza viruses could create highly pathogenic viruses that transmit among humans. While such an event (which would likely result in a devastating pandemic) has not occurred yet, experimental studies have demonstrated a high propensity of HPAI H5N1 viruses for reassortment with A(H1N1) pdm09[1548] or with seasonal H3N2 viruses.[284,905,1198,1301] While viruses possessing the HPAI HA and NA genes in combination with human H3N2 internal genes failed to transmit among ferrets,[1301] other reassortants were more pathogenic than either parent virus.[1198]

HPAI H5N1 viruses have been extensively studied in primary human cells[264,265–266,300,369,611,848,1180,1405,1410,1639,1780,2354,2368,2369] and in several animal models including mice, ferrets, guinea pigs, and nonhuman primates.[76,186,279,292,319,515,1097,1106,1731,1825,2075] In alveolar epithelial cells[264,266,2354] and macrophages,[300,611,848,1180,1410,1639,1780,2368,2369] HPAI H5N1 viruses typically—but not always—elicit higher levels of proinflammatory cytokines than are observed upon infection with contemporary human viruses. Upregulated factors include IFN-β, IP-10, RANTES, and IL-6 in alveolar epithelial cells, and TNF-α, IFN-α and -β, IP-10, RANTES, MIP-1, and MCP-1 in macrophages. Many of these factors are also upregulated in the lungs of infected mice,[232,318,339,1148,1239,1640,1784,2017,2106] ferrets,[216] and nonhuman primates.[76,186,319] In these animal models, HPAI are highly pathogenic and cause diffuse alveolar damage with massive infiltration of immune cells and infection of pneumocytes. In nonhuman primates, HPAI H5N1 viruses are more pathogenic than the 1918 virus, or reassortants possessing 1918 virus genes (HA and NA, or HA, NA, and NS) in the background of a contemporary human virus.[76,186,2075]

H5N2

Pennsylvania Outbreak. In April 1983, a low virulent H5N2 virus (A/chicken/Pennsylvania/1/83) emerged in chickens in Pennsylvania. By October, this virus had mutated into a highly pathogenic variant (A/chicken/Pennsylvania/1370/83) with a mortality rate of more than 80% in chickens. The virus was eventually eradicated by the slaughter of more than 17 million birds. The avirulent predecessor was unusual in that it had multiple basic amino acids at the HA cleavage site. The virulent strain differed from its predecessor by only a few nucleotides[1002] including one that caused the loss of the HA glycosylation site,[415,1002] thereby exposing the multibasic HA cleavage site to ubiquitous cellular proteases, furin, and PC6.[1002]

Mexican Outbreak. In May 1994, a mildly pathogenic H5N2 virus was isolated from Mexican chickens (A/chicken/Mexico/26654-1374/94). This virus was not eradicated by mass slaughter because it had already spread widely. Stepwise accumulation of mutations over several months yielded moderately (A/chicken/Puebla/8624-602/94) and highly (A/chicken/Queretaro/14588-19/95) pathogenic strains with a series of basic residues at the HA cleavage site.[602,836,2011,2013] Vaccination was implemented in 1995 and by 2001, more than 1 billion doses of inactivated vaccine had been used. Between 1998 and 2001, 459 million doses of recombinant fowl poxvector vaccine were also administered. Cases of HPAI have not occurred since 1996; however, low pathogenic H5N2 strains continue to circulate, as do genetically related viruses in the neighboring countries of Guatemala and El Salvador. In 2005, an H5N2 virus with low pathogenicity emerged in chickens in Japan. This virus is a descendant of the virus responsible for the Mexican outbreak and is closely related to a virus isolated from Guatemala. The origin of the Japanese strain remains unknown.

H7N1

In March 1999, an LPAI virus of the H7N1 subtype was isolated from a poultry farm in Italy.[226,227,229] The virus was not eradicated and the infection spread, resulting, in December, in the emergence of a highly pathogenic isolate. More than 13 million birds were destroyed to control the outbreak. The reappearance of this LPAI in August 2000 was controlled by additional depopulation followed by a vaccination campaign from November 2000 to May 2002. The vaccine was based on inactivated H7N3 virus to allow *d*ifferentiation of *i*nfected and *v*accinated *a*nimals (DIVA).[231] Vaccination in combination with intensive monitoring led to the eradication of this H7N1 virus.

H7N3

An outbreak of HPAI H7N3 viruses occurred in poultry farms in Pakistan in 1995. This outbreak killed 3.2 million birds and was brought under control by vaccination.[1462] In 2001, H7N3 viruses of both high and low pathogenicity were again identified, and despite further vaccination, HPAI H7N3 viruses reappeared in 2003 and 2004, causing the death of an estimated 10 million birds. Outbreaks of LPAI and HPAI H7N3 viruses also occurred in Chile in 2002[1750] and Canada in 2004,[122,161,815,1613] leading to the slaughter of 2 million and 19 million birds, respectively. In Canada, two workers involved in the depopulation developed symptoms of influenza virus infection, including conjunctivitis, headache, and coryza.[815,2111] H7N3 viruses isolated from these individuals had increased binding affinity for human-type receptors (as did other recent North American H7 viruses tested in this study).[99] Both the Chilean and 2004 Canadian isolates arose from LPAI viruses by recombination events that inserted 10 amino acids from the NP protein[1989] (Chilean virus) or 7 amino acids from the M1 protein[161,815,1614] (Canadian virus) into the HA cleavage site.

Again in Canada, an HPAI H7N3 virus caused another outbreak in 2007 among roosters in a broiler hatching egg farm. After hundreds of roosters in one of the barns died, all animals on the premise (53,000) were culled.[122,1613] The source of the outbreaks is not known, although serologic data indicate that a low pathogenic H7N3 had circulated in some birds on the premise prior to the outbreak. Phylogenetic analysis indicates that the HPAI H7N3 virus was similar to North American H7 viruses isolated from waterfowl.

H7N7

In 2003, an HPAI of the H7N7 subtype caused outbreaks in layer farms in The Netherlands, resulting in the death or culling of more than 30 million birds.[1955] Experimental infection of chickens confirmed the highly pathogenic phenotype of the virus.[486,487,2141] The outbreak spread to Belgium and Germany but was brought under control by mass slaughtering. In The Netherlands, the outbreak was associated with one fatal human case, a veterinarian who contracted the disease, and with conjunctivitis in 78 individuals who either directly handled affected poultry or had family members who did.[546,1085] These data suggest human-to-human transmission, and experimental infection of cats demonstrated that the virus isolated from the fatal case caused alveolar damage with infection of type II pneumocytes and nonciliated bronchial cells, comparable to infection with an HPAI H5N1 virus.[2140] The virus isolated from the fatal case differed by 14 amino acids from a virus isolated from an individual with conjunctivitis; the acquisition of PB2-627K (a known determinant of pathogenicity in mammals; see Molecular Determinants of Host Range Restriction and Pathogenesis section) was critical for increased pathogenicity and tissue tropism.[1443] Depopulation of infected poultry and the treatment of at-risk individuals with NA inhibitors likely prevented further spread to or among humans.

Further outbreaks of H7N7 HPAI occurred in the United Kingdom in 2008 and in Spain in 2009. In the United Kingdom in 2008, mild disease was first noted in a laying flock of chickens, followed by the death of approximately 10,000 birds (http://www.oie.int/wahid-prod/public.php?page=weekly_report_index&admin=0). The remaining 15,000 chickens in the flock were culled. In Spain in 2009, an outbreak of H7N7 HPAI in a layer hen farm resulted in the death of approximately 30,000 birds, while the remaining 278,640 birds on the farm were culled (http://www.oie.int/wahis/public.php?page=single_report&pop=1&reportid=8521).[861]

Despite the typically mild symptoms of human infection with H7 viruses, these viruses cause systemic infections in experimentally infected mice and ferrets without prior adaptation.[100,405]

Low Pathogenic H9N2 Avian Influenza Viruses

LPAI viruses of the H9N2 subtype became panzootic in the mid-1980s among chickens, ducks, turkeys, pheasants, quail, and ostriches in Europe, Africa, North America, Asia, and the Middle East.[14,15,61,224,1200,1636,1864] Since the mid-1990s, several sublineages have become established in Asia, represented by the prototype viruses A/chicken/Beijing/1/94, A/duck/Hong Kong/Y280/97, and A/quail/Hong Kong/G1/97.[307,679,1206] These viruses appear to evolve rapidly through reassortment and antigenic drift.[846,873,1034,1174,1182,2005,2277,2285,2358] A recent computational analysis of available H9N2 sequences revealed multiple different genotypes that likely originated from frequent reassortment with viruses of various subtypes.[437]

H9N2 viruses were detected in approximately 5% of birds in live poultry markets in Hong Kong in 1997. These viruses were not highly pathogenic but caused respiratory symptoms and decreased egg production. Between 2001 and 2003, H9N2 viruses were the most prevalent subtype in live poultry markets in Hong Kong, presenting in various different genotypes.[307] Viruses of the A/quail/Hong Kong/G1/97 lineage share six internal genes with the H5N1 viruses isolated from humans in Hong Kong in 1997, and reassortants between H9N2 and H5N1 viruses have been described.[771,873,2285,2358] On several occasions, H9N2 viruses of the A/duck/Hong Kong/Y280/97 lineage have been isolated from pigs in China,[342,1624,2332] and seem to reassort frequently in these animals.[2337] In an experimental study, multiple reassortants were generated between avian H9N2 and A(H1N1)pdm09 viruses, some of which were more pathogenic in mice than the parental viruses,[2006] as has been observed for reassortants between HPAI H5N1 and seasonal H3N2 viruses.[1198]

In animal experiments, H9N2 viruses replicate in chickens and mice without adaptation[307,2277]; subsets of these viruses cause acute respiratory distress syndrome with high lethality in mice.[307,412]

Some H9N2 viruses bind to Siaα2,3Gal (preferentially recognized by most avian viruses) and also to Siaα2,6Gal (preferentially recognized by human viruses).[1335,2332] This is consistent with the finding that a virus possessing avian H9N2-derived HA and NA genes in the genetic background of a human H3N2 virus requires little adaptation for transmission among ferrets.[1926]

Continued circulation of H9N2 viruses in poultry populations, combined with frequent reassortment, occasional transmission to pigs, and recognition of human-type receptors, emphasize the pandemic potential of the currently circulating H9N2 viruses.

Vaccines for Avian Influenza Viruses

The increasing number of outbreaks caused by HPAI H5 and H7 viruses, the fact that H5 and H9 viruses are now enzootic in poultry populations in parts of the world, and the increasing number of human infections with H5, H7, and H9 viruses have spurred the development of avian vaccines for these viruses, and the vaccination of poultry flocks. Most approved vaccines for H5, H7, and H9 viruses are based on inactivated whole-virus preparations, although some live recombinant vaccines based on Newcastle disease and fowl pox virus are in use (reviewed in[230,277,432,559,1072,1763]; for an overview of currently available avian influenza vaccines, see ftp://ftp.fao.org/docrep/fao/011/ai326e/ai326e00.pdf).

Official vaccination programs against H5N1 viruses have been carried out in Hong Kong, Indonesia, China, Vietnam, Russia, India, Pakistan, Egypt, and Côte d'Ivoire, but failed to eradicate H5N1 viruses in some of these countries. Possible reasons include limited coverage of vaccination campaigns, failure to induce sterilizing immunity that may result in undetected virus spread and evolution, and limited cross-reactivity with viruses of different clades.

Influenza in Swine

Since the isolation of the first influenza virus from pigs in 1930 (A/swine/Iowa/15/30 [H1N1]),[1863] swine influenza has become enzootic and is a prevalent respiratory disease in these animals. Avian and human viruses of several subtypes (or reassortants thereof) have caused local outbreaks or become enzootic in pigs (Table 41.2). Until 2009, human influenza viruses contributed to the establishment of several new lineages in pigs (Table 41.2), whereas swine influenza viruses only infected humans occasionally, and without sustained human-to-human transmission (reviewed in[1459]; see also[78,1081,2055,2163]). This situation changed dramatically with the H1N1 pandemic in 2009, which originated from pigs.[388,604,1903]

Collectively, the prominent role for pigs in the emergence of pandemic influenza viruses is supported by several findings: (1) pigs can be naturally (Table 41.2) or experimentally[306,876,1021,1869,2180] infected with avian or human viruses; (2) swine influenza viruses can play a critical role in the emergence of new pandemic viruses,[388,556,604,1903] although most (reassortant) swine viruses cause self-limiting infections in humans (see previous discussion), which, however, can be fatal[315,607,1042,1618,1758,1906,2235,2236]; (3) epithelial cells in pig trachea contain both human- and avian-type receptors (i.e., Siaα2,6Gal- and Siaα2,3Gal, respectively)[880]; (4) frequent reassortment (both intra- and intersubtypic) has been described for viruses isolated from pigs, suggesting repeated mixed infections of swine, avian, and/or human viruses; and (5) in nature, continued replication of an avian virus in pigs leads to variants that preferentially recognize human-type receptors.[880] These observations support the "mixing vessel" hypothesis that pigs are simultaneously infected with avian and human influenza viruses, which allow for the generation of reassortants capable of causing pandemics.[1810]

In pigs, influenza virus infections cause high morbidity, but typically low mortality. Signs of infection include inactivity, nasal discharge, coughing, fever, labored breathing, weight loss, and conjunctivitis. Infections are limited to the respiratory tract with tracheobronchial lesions. During the Spanish influenza of 1918/1919,[1079] pigs presented with symptoms similar to those observed in humans.[1863] Phylogenetic analyses indicate that the 1918/1919 human and swine viruses were genetically similar and likely originated from a common ancestor.[647,1717]

Influenza in Swine—North America

The descendants of the H1N1 1918/1919 isolates, now referred to as "classic swine viruses," circulated in pig populations for more than 6 decades.[181,1285,1532,1572,1841,2161] However, serologic studies in 1988 and 1989 also indicated a low prevalence of H3N2 viruses.[260] In North America, this changed in 1997 and 1998, when H3N2 double human/swine reassortant and triple human/avian/swine reassortant viruses emerged[2373] (Fig. 41.9). The double reassortant virus possessed human-like HA, NA, and PB1 genes, while the remaining genes were of classic swine virus origin. This virus did not establish a stable lineage but was soon replaced by human/avian/swine triple reassortant viruses that contain HA, NA, and PB1 polymerase genes of human virus origin; PB2 and PA polymerase genes of avian virus origin; and NP, matrix (M), and nonstructural (NS) genes of classic H1N1 swine virus origin.[972,1570,2209,2373] These triple reassortants have spread widely throughout the swine population,[972,1570,2209,2373] and have been linked to respiratory disease in pigs and abortion in pregnant sows. The major difference between the double and triple reassortant viruses was the presence of avian-origin PB2 and PA genes, suggesting that these genes may have contributed to the genetic stability of the novel reassortant virus; however, no mechanistic explanation is currently available. Although the biologic significance remains unknown, it is interesting that the HA and PB1 polymerase genes share the same origin, because this occurred with the 1957 and 1968 human pandemic viruses.[1001] The triple reassortant H3N2 viruses evolved into four HA clades and continue to circulate in North American pig populations along with several reassortants that carry the same internal genes (PB2, PB1, PA, NP, M, NS), but different HA and NA genes (Table 41.2). These reassortants include several different H3N2 viruses possessing human-like HA genes[1729,2208,2209]; an H1N1 virus possessing classic swine HA and NA genes[2208] (cH1N1); an H1N2 virus possessing a classic swine HA gene (cH1N2)[305,970,971]; an H1N2 virus possessing a human-like HA gene[969] (huH1N2); and an H1N1 virus possessing human-like

TABLE 41.2 Overview of Major Swine Virus Lineages

Geographic distribution	Subtype	Designation	Date	Currently circulating	Origin of HA	Origin of NA	Origin of internal genes	Comments
North America	H1N1	Classic swine	1918	Yes	Classic swine	Classic swine	Classic swine	Descendants of 1918 pandemic virus
	H3N2	Triple reassortant H3N2	1997/1998	Yes	Human H3	Human N2	Avian, human, swine (TRIG)	PB1: human; PB2, PA: avian; NP, M, NS: classic swine (triple reassortant internal genes = TRIG)
	H1N1	cH1N1	1999	Yes	Classic swine	Classic swine	TRIG	Reassortants of classic swine H1N1 × triple reassortant H3N2 viruses
	H1N2	cH1N2	1999	Yes	Classic swine	Human N2	TRIG	Reassortants of classic swine H1N1 × triple reassortant H3N2 viruses
	H1N2	huH1N2	2003–2005	Yes	Human H1	Human N2	TRIG	Reassortants of human H1N1 × TRIG virus
	H1N1	huH1N1	2003–2005	Yes	Human H1	Human N1	TRIG	Reassortants of human H1N1 × TRIG virus
Europe	H1N1	Classic swine	1976	No	Classic swine	Classic swine	Classic swine	Descendants of 1918 pandemic virus
	H1N1	Eurasian avian-like swine H1N1	1979	Yes	Avian	Avian	Avian	Wholly avian virus
	H1N1	Reassortant swine H1N1	2001, 2006	Unknown	Human	Avian	Avian	Reassortants of Eurasian avian-like swine H1N1 × human-like swine H3N2
	H3N2	Human-like swine H3N2	1970s	No	Human	Human	Human	Wholly human viruses
	H3N2	Eurasian reassortant human-like swine H3N2	1984	Yes	Human	Human	Avian	Reassortants of human-like swine H3N2 × Eurasian avian-like swine H1N1
	H1N2	Reassortant human-like swine H1N2	1994	Yes	Human	Human	Avian	Reassortants of Eurasian reassortant human-like swine H3N2 × human-like swine H1N1
	H1N2	Reassortant human-like swine H1N2	2000	Yes	Human	Human	Avian	Reassortants of reassortant human-like swine H1N1 × Eurasian avian-like swine H1N1
Asia	H3N2	Human-like swine H3N2	Early 1970s	Yes	Human	Human	Human	Wholly human viruses
	H1N1	Classic swine	Late 1970s	Yes	Classic swine	Classic swine	Classic swine	Descendants of 1918 pandemic virus
	H1N2	cH1N2	1978	Yes	Classic swine	Human N2	Classic swine	Reassortants of classic swine H1N1 × human H3N2
	H1N1	Eurasian avian-like swine H1N1	1993	Yes	Avian	Avian	Avian	Wholly avian virus
	H3N2	Double reassortant H3N2	1999	Unknown	Human	Human	Avian	
	H3N2	Triple reassortant H3N2	2001	Unknown	Human	Human	Avian, swine	PB2, PB1, PA, M, NS: avian; NP: swine
	H9N2		2002	Yes	Avian	Avian	Avian	Wholly avian virus

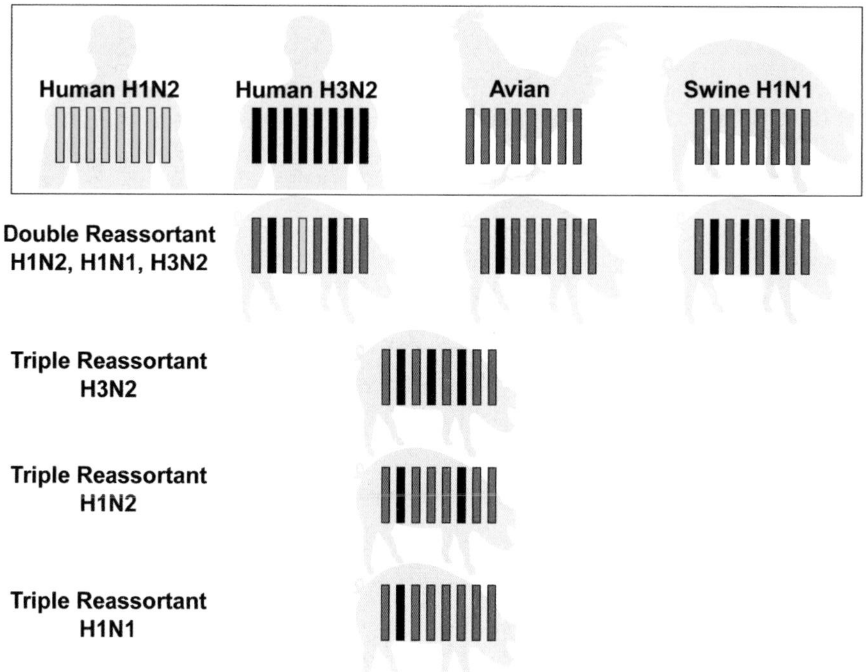

FIGURE 41.9. Recent reassortment events among North American swine viruses. In 1998, triple reassortant viruses emerged in North American pig populations that contained PB2 and PA genes of avian origin; PB1, HA, and NA genes of human origin; and NP, M, and NS genes that originated from classical H1N1 swine viruses. Subsequent reassortment events resulted in triple reassortant H1N2 and H1N1 viruses. In addition, human/swine reassortants of different genotypes have been isolated from North American pigs since 1998. The eight viral RNA segments are arranged from left to right according to their lengths, starting with the longest segment (i.e., PB2, PB1, PA, HA, NP, NA, M, and NS).

HA and NA genes[2162] (huH1N1). Hence, while the HA and NA genes have been replaced frequently with genes of human or swine origin (further supporting the role of pigs as "mixing vessels"), the constellation of the internal genes (now referred to as TRIG—triple reassortant internal genes) has been stable. Moreover, experimental co-infection of pigs with classic H1N1 and triple reassortant H3N2 viruses resulted in the selection of the TRIG cassette in most viruses characterized.[1291] The reason for the biologic fitness of the TRIG cassette in pigs is not known. In 2009, the introduction of NA and M genes of Eurasian avian-like swine virus origin into a triple reassortant swine virus created the A(H1N1)pdm09 virus. In addition, a reassortant between triple reassortant and seasonal H1N1 viruses infected three individuals in Canada in 2009, but did not spread further.[78]

Several other wholly avian or reassortant viruses have been isolated from pigs in North America, but did not establish new lineages; these include avian viruses of the H1N1,[973] H3N3,[973] and H4N6[968] subtypes, and reassortant viruses of the H1N1 and H1N2,[969] H3N2,[2374] H2N3,[1292] and H3N1[1185,1290] subtypes. The H4N6 virus isolated from pigs in Canada possessed two amino acid changes,[968] one of which confers binding to Siaα2,6Gal.[79] The H2N3 virus isolated from pigs in the United States was transmitted among experimentally infected pigs and ferrets, and its HA amino acid sequence suggests the ability to recognize mammalian-type receptors.[1292]

Influenza in Swine—Europe

In Europe, three virus subtypes—H1N1, H3N2, and H1N2—are currently circulating in pig populations.[1121,2137] Influenza viruses were first isolated from European pigs in 1938 and 1940.[141,1139] Classic swine H1N1 viruses were detected in pigs in Czechoslovakia in 1950.[435] These viruses were reintroduced in 1976 into pigs in Italy (Table 41.2), probably by pigs imported from the United States.[1476] In 1979, a wholly avian H1N1 virus, closely related to a duck virus, was introduced into European pigs[1630] and replaced the classic H1N1 viruses in the 1990s.[237,1274,1809,1824] These so-called Eurasian avian-like swine H1N1 viruses still circulate in European pig populations. New antigenic variants of this lineage have caused multiple outbreaks throughout European pig populations.[183,396,1319] In 2001 and 2006, reassortant swine H1N1 viruses were isolated in France that arose from the reassortment of Eurasian avian-like swine H1N1 viruses with reassortant human-like swine H1N2 viruses (see later discussion[1116]).

Human H3N2 viruses were introduced into pig populations in the early 1970s, where they established a new lineage.[741,1670,1787] Multiple introductions of human H3N2 viruses into pigs occurred,[51,237,1319,1388,1583,2067] and these so-called human-like swine H3N2 viruses circulated over the next decade. In 1984, severe disease among Italian and French pigs was traced to a novel reassortant H3N2 strain that possessed human-like HA and NA genes, while the internal genes were derived from Eurasian avian-like H1N1 swine viruses.[220,238,1736,2101] The novel virus (referred to as Eurasian reassortant human-like swine H3N2 virus, Table 41.2) soon became enzootic and replaced the human-like swine H3N2 viruses. Viruses of this lineage continue to circulate to this day. Also, Eurasian reassortant human-like H3N2 swine viruses were transmitted to two children in The Netherlands,[321] and to a child in Hong Kong.[668]

Since the mid-1990s, H1N2 viruses have been isolated frequently that contain an HA gene similar to a human H1N1 virus introduced into pigs in 1977 (human-like swine H1N1, Table 41.2), and the remaining genes from Eurasian reassortant human-like swine H3N2 viruses.[184] These so-called reassortant human-like swine H1N2 viruses spread throughout European pig populations and established a new lineage.[182,184,656,1306,1319,1817,2138] Since their emergence, the reassortant human-like swine H1N2 viruses have reassorted with avian-like swine H1N1 viruses or reassortant human-like swine H3N2 viruses.[1319,2353]

Influenza in Swine—Asia

Some of the viruses detected in European and North American pig populations have also been isolated from swine in Asia. In the early 1970s, human H3N2 viruses were isolated from pig populations in Asia[1113,1868] (Table 41.2), where they continue to circulate.[1624,2332,2333] From the late 1970s onwards, human H3N2 viruses have co-circulated with classic swine H1N1 viruses in pig populations in several Southeast Asian countries.[40,948,1867,1871,2301] During this time, multiple introductions of human H3N2 virus into Asian pig populations must have occurred, since the human H3N2 viruses detected in pigs typically resembled human epidemic viruses circulating at the time.[652,956,989,1403,1485,1705,1866,1871,1872] Influenza H1N2 viruses (cH1N2) that resulted from reassortment of classic H1N1 swine viruses and human H3N2 viruses were first isolated in Japan in 1978[1487,1994] and have since spread in the Japanese swine population.[39,885,1484,1486,1584,1778,2316] H1N2 viruses of the same and different genotypes also circulate in other parts of Asia, including Taiwan, China, and Korea.[932,946,948,1689,2096] Eurasian avian-like H1N1 viruses were first detected in Asian pigs in 1993[680] and may be enzootic in pig populations in parts of Asia.[1245,2027] A recent study also demonstrated the circulation of double and triple reassortant H3N2 viruses in pigs in China.[2333] These viruses possess human-like HA and NA genes in combination with avian-like internal genes (double reassortants), while the NP gene of the triple reassortant viruses is of swine virus origin,[2333] The gene constellation of these viruses is thus different from that of the North American double and triple reassortant swine viruses.

In 1998, avian H9N2 viruses were first detected in swine in Hong Kong but did not establish a stable lineage.[1624] However, different H9N2 viruses may now be circulating in pigs in Asia[342,2282,2332,2337] (Table 41.2). Based on their HA sequences, some of the swine H9N2 viruses may bind to human-type receptors.[2332]

HPAI H5N1 viruses have been isolated from pigs in Asia on several occasions,[306,1526,1846,2026] although the prevalence of HPAI H5N1 viruses in pigs appears to be low.[306] Moreover, H9N2 viruses have been isolated from pigs that possess HPAI H5N1-like sequences, suggesting reassortment between H5N1 and H9N2 viruses.[341]

In addition to the established lineages, human H1N1 viruses have been isolated occasionally from pigs in Japan[988] and China.[2335,2338] In Korea in 2006, a novel H3N1 virus was isolated from pigs[1850] that possessed an HA gene from a human-like H3N2 virus, an NA gene from a swine H1N1 virus, and internal genes from swine H1N2 viruses. The H3N1 virus likely circulated for some time, since it donated the PB2, PA, NP, and M segments to an H5N2 virus isolated from pigs in 2008.[1176] Another H5N2 virus isolated in the same study was a wholly avian virus. In addition, numerous reassortant viruses have been isolated from pigs in Asia,[2002,2027,2158,2283,2336] suggesting frequent reassortment between swine, avian, and human influenza viruses.

Interspecies Transmission

The first report of interspecies transmission involving pigs dates back to 1938, when Shope presented serologic evidence for the transmission of a human virus to pigs.[1862] Further evidence for virus transmission between these two species came in 1976, when an H1N1 swine virus was isolated from a soldier who had died of influenza at Fort Dix, New Jersey.[607,642,819,1013] This virus was subsequently isolated from five other soldiers; serologic studies suggest that more than 500 personnel were infected.[443,607,819] As stated earlier, more than 50 cases of human infection with swine influenza virus had occurred until 2009 (reviewed in[78,1081,1459,2055,2163]), some of which resulted in fatal outcomes.[315,607,1042,1618,1758,1906,2235,2236] Although the A(H1N1)pdm09 virus was not isolated from pigs prior to the 2009 pandemic, sequence and phylogenetic analyses strongly suggest that this virus originated from pigs.[388,604,1903] Recently, A(H1N1)pdm09 viruses have been reintroduced into pigs in several countries (http://www.oie.int/wahis/public.php?page=weekly_report_index&admin=0),[1615,1919,2158,2232] and have reassorted with swine viruses.[1304,1949,2158] It remains to be seen if these viruses will establish novel virus lineages in pigs.

Several other reports indicate the sporadic transmission of swine viruses to avian species, or *vice versa:* classic swine H1N1[1404,2259] or triple reassortant H3N2 viruses have been isolated from turkeys[2314]; surveillance studies suggest infection of ducks with swine H1N1[208] or H1N2 viruses[1571]; avian H3N2 viruses likely transmitted to pigs[1022,2315]; and serologic evidence also suggests the infection of Chinese pigs with H4, H5, and H9 influenza viruses.[1529] Moreover, two equine H3N8 viruses were isolated from pigs in China.[2098]

Influenza in Horses

Two different subtypes of influenza A viruses are recognized in horses: H7N7, historically referred to as equine 1, and H3N8,[2172] referred to as equine 2. Equine influenza is typically associated with fever, nasal discharge, dry hacking cough, loss of appetite, muscular soreness, and tracheobronchitis. The disease is usually more severe with equine 2 (i.e., H3N8) viruses and can include inflammation of the heart muscle. Secondary bacterial infections can be fatal.

The first equine influenza virus (A/equine/Prague/56 [H7N7]) was isolated in 1956 during a widespread pandemic of respiratory disease among horses in Eastern Europe. The last confirmed outbreak of this subtype occurred in 1979.[2213] Anecdotal reports of equine H7N7 outbreaks in Egypt[875] and India,[1884] and the sporadic detection of H7-specific antibodies in reportedly unvaccinated horses, suggest that the viruses may have still circulated in small geographic pockets and/or in a subclinical form since their last isolation. In 1963, an equine influenza virus of the H3N8 subtype (A/equine/Miami/63 [H3N8]) was isolated in the United States[2172] and caused a major epidemic. It was later found to have been introduced into North American horses via the importation of horses from Argentina. Another enzootic with an H3N8 virus occurred in China in 1989. This virus caused morbidity rates of up to 80% and mortality rates of up to 20%.[702] Based on sequence analysis, the virus was of avian origin and unrelated to the H3N8 virus already established in horse populations.[699,2217] It remained confined to the Chinese horse population and was not isolated after the mid-1990s.[700] Several studies suggested reassortment between H7N7 and H3N8 horse viruses while they were co-circulating,[8,90,884,1450] and intrasubtypic reassortment among H3N8 horse viruses.[1450] Moreover, phylogenetic separation of the Eurasian and American lineages has been observed in the equine H3 HA proteins since 1987; within the American lineage, three clades (original strains, Florida clade 1, Florida clade 2) are currently recognized (reviewed in[371]).

An H3N8 virus isolated from a horse did not replicate in ducks but caused disease in experimentally infected mice and ferrets.[699] More importantly, an equine H3N8 horse virus transmitted to dogs in North America in 2004,[359] and has been circulating in domestic dogs since then. Inactivated vaccines against the H7N7 and H3N8 subtypes are widely used; however, with H7N7 viruses seemingly extinct in horses, the H7N7 vaccine component is no longer critical. Studies suggested that immunity conferred by inactivated vaccines is short lived.[1437] Therefore, between 1978 and 1981, and again in 1989, widespread epidemics of H3N8 viruses occurred in Europe and North America, affecting both unvaccinated and vaccinated horses. Outbreaks of equine H3N8 continue to occur throughout the world, probably supported by the international transportation of vaccinated horses, in which virus replicates in a subclinical form. For example, international transportation of vaccinated horses likely led to the introduction of equine influenza into Australia in 2007.[215] A cold-adapted, temperature-sensitive, modified live equine influenza virus vaccine has been licensed for use in the United States. Although this vaccine is safe and efficacious, it does not provide sterilizing immunity.[261,1284,2082,2328] In addition, a recombinant canarypox virus vaccine expressing H3 HA is now licensed in several countries.[470]

Influenza in Dogs and Cats

Two reports demonstrated the natural infection of dogs with human influenza viruses.[269,1753] However, these viruses did not establish stable lineages in dogs, in line with surveillance studies that show low levels of seropositivity to influenza viruses in dogs.[459,1195,1651]

In 2004, outbreaks of respiratory disease occurred in racing greyhounds in Florida.[359] The causative agent was an influenza A virus (A/canine/Florida/43/04 [H3N8]) closely related to contemporary H3N8 equine viruses, suggesting interspecies transmission. The virus spread among greyhound populations, indicating that the equine influenza viruses replicated in and transmitted among greyhounds. Serologic studies indicate that the virus has spread to other breeds, although it has not spread widely within the general dog population. The canine H3N8 influenza virus appears to be largely confined to animal shelters in some large cities in the United States where the turnover of dogs and introduction of new susceptibles has allowed this apparently inefficiently spread virus to be maintained for the past 11 years.[359] The H3N8 viruses circulating in horses and dogs in North America have become genetically distinguishable and no interspecies transmission from horses to dogs or back to horses has been reported.[1734,2300] Infection of dogs with an equine H3N8 virus was also reported in Australia in 2007.[1046] A retrospective study suggested that an outbreak of respiratory disease in English foxhounds in the United Kingdom in 2002 was also caused by an equine H3N8 virus.[370] In experimental studies, horses infected with the canine virus seroconverted but showed little signs of disease.[2299,2300] The infection of dogs with equine influenza viruses may be facilitated by the presence on canine respiratory epithelium cells of Siaα2,3Gal receptors, which are preferentially bound by equine influenza viruses.[370,1449] Experimental infection of chickens, turkeys, and ducks with the canine virus did not cause infection.[1369]

In 2007, three genetically similar avian H3N2 influenza viruses were isolated in Korea from domestic dogs with severe respiratory symptoms.[1915] Experimental testing showed that these viruses cause tracheobronchitis and bronchiolitis in dogs,[947,1916] and are transmitted to contact animals.[1916] Surveillance studies demonstrated that avian H3N2 viruses circulate at low but detectable levels in dog populations in Korea[31,1169] and China.[1209]

Recently, domestic cats and zoo tigers died after eating poultry infected with HPAI H5N1 viruses,[28,500,1005] and probable virus transmission was reported among tigers.[2058] Several other reports now also indicate the infection of dogs[206,325,624,1923] and cats[1064,1104,1105,1733,1922,2120] with HPAI H5N1 viruses. Cats and dogs can also be infected with HPAI H5N1 viruses in experimental settings.[624,1105,1733]

Influenza in Seals and Whales

The most significant epizootic in seals occurred in 1979 and 1980, when approximately 20% of the harbor seal (*Phoca vitulina*) population of the northeast coast of the United States died of a severe respiratory infection with consolidation of the lungs typical of primary viral pneumonia.[613] Antigenic and genetic analyses[1143,2219] revealed that the influenza virus isolated from the lungs and brains of dead animals (A/seal/Massachusetts/1/80 [H7N7]) was of avian origin. This virus replicated to high titers in ferrets, cats, and pigs,[2219] and caused conjunctivitis in humans.[2216,2219] The death of an experimentally infected squirrel monkey[1454] and recovery of the virus from several of its organs demonstrated systemic spread of this virus. From June 1982 to March 1983, harbor seals along the New England coastline again died of viral pneumonia,[804] which was caused by an avian H4N5 virus that was antigenically and genetically related to avian viruses and replicated in the intestinal tracts of ducks, a characteristic of avian influenza viruses. Serology and direct virus isolation revealed infection of seals with influenza A viruses of the H3N3[214] and H4N6 subtypes,[214] as well as influenza B virus.[1550,1582] Further surveillance studies identified antibodies to influenza A[375,391,1527,1549,1550,1981] and B viruses in several seal species.[1550]

Influenza viruses of the H13N2 and H13N9 subtypes were isolated from the lungs and hilar nodes of a stranded pilot whale.[803] It is not known whether the influenza virus infection caused or contributed to the stranding of this whale. In addition, H1N3 viruses have been isolated from lung and liver samples of whales from the South Pacific.[1288]

Influenza in Mink

Mink are naturally susceptible to infection with human and avian influenza viruses.[1063,1562] Avian influenza viruses of the H10N4 subtype killed mink in Sweden and spread to contact animals.[118,494,1063] In 2006, respiratory problems were noticed among mink in mink ranches in Canada; subsequently, an influenza A virus was isolated from one animal with clinical signs. Further analysis identified the virus as a swine triple reassortant H3N2 virus.[572] Influenza viruses of human, swine, avian, and equine origin replicate in experimentally infected mink,[118,494,495,1343] and transmission to cage mates has been observed for human and avian viruses,[118,1343,1561,2292] as well as for equine and swine viruses.[2292]

Experimental Infections

Mice

Although mice are not naturally infected, they can be experimentally infected with influenza A or B viruses. Most human influenza viruses cause indiscernible infection of the upper and lower respiratory tract and do not cause lethal disease without adaptation, although A(H1N1)pdm09 viruses are more pathogenic than other human viruses.[101,890,1302] By contrast, most avian influenza viruses will replicate in respiratory organs (but not cause lethal infections) without prior adaptation (reviewed in[1542]), most likely because of the presence of Siaα2,3Gal receptors in murine respiratory tissues.[856,1528] Notable exceptions include the recently isolated H5N1 viruses, which can cause lethal infections without prior adaptation.[593,1269,2106] Most laboratory strains are susceptible to infection with influenza A viruses and have been used widely to study the pathogenesis of and the immune response to influenza viruses. Knock-out mice are useful tools for deciphering the molecular basis of virus–host interactions. However, most laboratory strains lack the Mx gene, which plays a role in the innate host defense,[838,1941] and data obtained from laboratory strains may not therefore be strictly comparable to natural virus infections. Recent studies have identified appreciable differences in susceptibility between mouse strains.[153,1938] The comparison of influenza virulence and pathogenicity in different mouse strains may lead to a better understanding of the contribution of host genetics to infections with influenza viruses.

Guinea Pigs

Influenza virus propagation in guinea pigs was first reported in 1938,[2264] then in the 1970s.[1648,2014] Recently, guinea pigs have been established as a transmission model for influenza viruses.[1264–1266,1434,1830,2004] Human, swine, and avian influenza viruses can be isolated from the lungs and nasal turbinates of infected animals, suggesting efficient virus replication; however, signs of disease such as weight loss and increased temperature are largely missing,[1265] and no mortality was observed upon infection with HPAI H5N1 or pandemic 1918 virus.[2130] The nasal tract and trachea of guinea pigs possess both avian-type (Siaα2,3Gal) and human-type (Siaα2,6Gal) receptors, whereas the lungs contain predominately avian-type receptors.[2004]

Ferrets

Ferrets infected with influenza A or B viruses develop a febrile rhinitis. Upon infection with human influenza viruses, the lesions are usually confined to the nasal mucosa, but infection of the lower respiratory tract has been demonstrated. The pathologic changes of bronchitis and pneumonia resemble those seen in humans,[1904] which makes ferrets a valuable animal model to study various aspects of influenza virus infection. Unlike mice, ferrets can also be used to study the transmissibility of influenza viruses. The high susceptibility of ferrets to human influenza viruses may be due to the predominance of Siaα2,6Gal receptors in their upper respiratory tract.[1184]

Nonhuman Primates

Influenza viruses infect various Old and New World primates, such as chimpanzees, gibbons, and baboons, as well as rhesus, squirrel, African green, and cynomolgus monkeys.[1458] Several species (e.g., gibbons, baboons) can be infected and develop illness.[934] Illness has also been observed in other species (e.g., cynomolgus, rhesus) experimentally infected with influenza virus.[671] Several human viruses known to be virulent in humans also produce illness in squirrel monkeys,[1455,1458] indicating that nonhuman primates may be a useful animal model for the study of influenza virus infections. Nonhuman primates have been used to test the pathogenicity of (reassortant) 1918 viruses,[76,186,319,1068] HPAI H5N1 viruses,[76,186,279,292,319,1106,1731,2075] and A(H1N1)pdm09 virus.[890,1772]

MOLECULAR DETERMINANTS OF HOST RANGE RESTRICTION AND PATHOGENESIS

Four influenza virus proteins—HA, PB2, NS1, and PB1-F2—are known determinants of host-range restriction and pathogenicity. Other viral proteins also participate in these events.

The HA Protein

The HA protein is responsible for virus attachment and the subsequent fusion of viral and cellular membranes. It is synthesized as a single polypeptide chain (HA0) that undergoes posttranslational cleavage by cellular proteases. This cleavage is essential for infectivity because it exposes the hydrophobic N-terminus of HA2, which mediates fusion between the viral envelope and the endosomal membrane.[1060,1159,2241]

HA Cleavage

HA is a critical determinant of the pathogenicity of avian influenza viruses, with a clear link between HA cleavability and virulence.[833,1059,1959,2227] The HA proteins of highly pathogenic H5 and H7 viruses contain multiple basic amino acids at the cleavage site (Table 41.3), which are recognized by ubiquitous proteases such as furin,[1973] PC6,[835] mosaic serine protease large (MSPL)[1025,1564] and transmembrane protease 13 (TMPRSS13).[1025,1564] For this reason, these viruses can cause systemic infections in poultry. In cell culture, the HAs of these viruses do not need exogenous proteases to form plaques. In contrast, the HA proteins of avirulent avian and nonavian influenza A viruses, with the exception of H7N7 equine influenza viruses,[998] contain a single arginine residue at the HA cleavage site[154,155] and are cleaved in only a few organs. These viruses, therefore, produce localized infection of the respiratory and/or intestinal tract that is usually asymptomatic or mild. The tissue tropism of viruses is thus partly determined by the availability of host proteases to recognize and cleave the two types of amino acid sequences found at the HA cleavage site. The significance of HA cleavability for pathogenicity of avian influenza viruses is underscored by the finding that the acquisition of a highly cleavable HA can convert avirulent strains to virulent ones, as occurred in Pennsylvania in 1983 (H5N2),[1002] in Mexico in 1994 (H5N2),[602] in Italy in 1999 (H7N1),[62] in Chile in 2002 (H7N3),[1989] and in Canada in 2004 (H7N3)[1614] (Table 41.3).

Two groups of proteases are responsible for HA cleavage. The first group recognizes a single arginine and cleaves all HAs. Members of this group include plasmin,[1160] blood-clotting factor X-like proteases,[654] tryptase Clara,[1026] mast-cell tryptase,[293] ectopic anionic trypsin I,[2081] tryptase TC30,[1789] miniplasmin,[1024] HAT (human airway trypsin-like protease),[159] TMPRSS2 (transmembrane protease serine S1 member 2),[159] and bacterial proteases.[1577,2043] *In ovo,* a protease similar to the blood-clotting factor Xa that is present in allantoic fluid cleaves HA, which explains why influenza viruses grow efficiently in eggs.[654] Tryptase Clara is secreted from specialized respiratory

TABLE 41.3 Sequence at HA Cleavage Site Determines Pathogenicity

Virus isolate	Pathogenicity	Sequence at HA cleavage site	Reference
A/chicken/Pennsylvania/1/83 (H5N2)	Avirulent	PQ-----------KKKR/G	(1002)
A/chicken/Pennsylvania/1370/83 (H5N2)	Virulent	PQ-----------KKKR/G[a]	(1002)
A/chicken/Mexico/31381–7/94 (H5N2)	Avirulent	PQ-----------RETR/G	(602,836)
A/chicken/Queretaro/14588–19/95 (H5N2)	Virulent	PQ---------RKRKTR/G	(602,836)
A/turkey/Italy/99 (H7N1) consensus	Avirulent	PEIPKG----------R/G	(62)
A/turkey/Italy/99 (H7N1) consensus	Virulent	PEIPKG------SRVRR/G	(62)
A/chicken/Chile/176822/02 (H7N3)	Avirulent	PEKPK----------TR/G	(1989)
A/chicken/Chile/4957/02 (H7N3)	Virulent	PEKPKTCSPLSRCRKTR/G	(1989)
A/chicken/Chile/4322/02 (H7N3)	Virulent	PEKPKTCSPLSRCRETR/G	(1989)
Isolate CN6/04	Avirulent	PENPK----------TR/G	(1614)
A/chicken/BC/CN12/04 (H7N3)	Virulent	PENPK---QAYQKRMTR/G	(1614)
A/chicken/BC/NS1337–1/04 (H7N3)	Virulent	PENPK---QAYKKRMTR/G	(1614)
A/chicken/BC/NS–1319–2/04 (H7N3)	Virulent	PENPK---QAYHKRMTR/G	(1614)
A/chicken/BC/CN7–3/04 (H7N3)	Virulent	PENPK---QAYRKRMTR/G	(1614)
A/chicken/BC/NS–1390–2/04 (H7N3)	Virulent	PENPK---QAHQKRMTR/G	(1614)
A/chicken/BC/NS–2035–12/04 (H7N3)	Virulent	PENPK---QACQKRMTR/G	(1614)
A/goose/Guangdong/1/96 (H5N1)	Virulent	PQRE-------RRRKKR/G	(2290)
A/Hong Kong/156/97 (H5N1)	Virulent	PQRE-------TRRKKR/G	(322,1993)
A/Hong Kong/486/97 (H5N1)	Virulent	PQRE-------RRRKKR/G	(322,1993)
H5N1 HPAI[b]	Virulent	PQRE-------RRRKKR/G	Influenza Sequence Databases
H5N1 HPAI	Virulent	PQGE-------RRRKKR/G	Influenza Sequence Databases
H5N1 HPAI	Virulent	PQRE-------RRRRKR/G	Influenza Sequence Databases
H5N1 HPAI	Virulent	PLRE-------RRRKKR/G	Influenza Sequence Databases
H5N1 HPAI	Virulent	PQRE-------GRRKKR/G	Influenza Sequence Databases
H5N1 HPAI	Virulent	PQRE-------SRRKKR/G	Influenza Sequence Databases
H5N1 HPAI	Virulent	PQGE-------RRRRKR/G	Influenza Sequence Databases
H5N1 HPAI	Virulent	PLRE-------RRRRKR/G	Influenza Sequence Databases
H5N1 HPAI	Virulent	PQREREGG----RRRKR/G	Influenza Sequence Databases

/, HA cleavage site.

[a]HA cleavability is enhanced by a single amino acid substitution that abrogates glycosylation near the HA cleavage site.

[b]For H5N1 HPAI viruses, there are numerous cleavage site motifs; several examples are listed here.

epithelial cells in rats and mice[1026]; mast-cell tryptase is found in mast cells,[293] whereas ectopic anionic trypsin I is present is stromal cells in the peribronchiolar region.[2081] The tissue tropism of tryptase TC30 is currently unknown. The type II transmembrane serine proteases HAT and TMPRSS2 localize to human airways and support influenza virus replication in cell culture.[125,158,159] Miniplasmin is a trypsin-type serine protease in the epithelial cells of the bronchia that cleaves HA downstream of the consensus motif Gln(Glu)-X-Arg.[1024,1447] Cleavage of HA by plasmin can be augmented by the ability of the A/WSN/33 (H1N1) NA protein to sequester its protease precursor, plasminogen.[651] Bacterial proteases can also activate HA, either directly or indirectly by activating plasminogen, a property that may explain the development of pneumonia after mixed infections with viruses and bacteria.[2043]

The second group of proteases that cleaves HA proteins[834,1973] comprises the ubiquitous intracellular subtilisin-related endoproteases furin and PC6.[835,1973,2178] These enzymes are calcium dependent, have an acidic pH optimum, and are located in the Golgi and/or *trans*-Golgi network.[1058,1061,2179] Recently, two other ubiquitous type II membrane serine proteases (mosaic serine protease large form, MSPL, and transmembrane protease 13, TMPRSS13) were identified that do not require calcium for enzymatic activity,[1025] and support the replication of an HPAI H5N1 virus in cell culture.[1564] The cleavage efficiency of these ubiquitous proteases is determined by the sequence at the cleavage site and absence or presence of a nearby carbohydrate chain on the HA molecule.[415,640,831,832,834,1002,1003,1025,1426,1556,1577,2003,2154,2177] The proposed sequence required for HA cleavage is Q-R/K-X-R/K-R (X, nonbasic amino acid) in the absence of a nearby carbohydrate chain. The presence of a nearby carbohydrate chain requires insertion of two additional residues, Q-X-X-R-X-R/K-R, or alteration of the conserved glutamine at position –5 or the proline at position –6, B(X)-X(B)-R/K-X-R/K-R (B, basic residue). The presence of direct repeats of basic amino acid insertions of various lengths in the HA proteins of several H5 and H7 viruses suggests that these sequences arose from polymerase stuttering,[1631] likely caused by secondary structure in the template RNA. HA cleavage efficiency can also be affected by the nature of the amino acid immediately downstream of the cleavage site, that is, the N-terminal amino acid of HA2.[832]

Introduction of multibasic HA cleavage sites into low-pathogenic avian H6N1[1445] or H9N2[639] viruses created highly pathogenic variants. However, this finding is not universally applicable, as the introduction of multibasic HA cleavage sites into low-pathogenic H5N1[149] or H3N8 viruses,[1951] or into a human H3N2[1818] virus did not create highly pathogenic viruses. Thus, a multibasic HA cleavage site seems to be necessary, but not always sufficient for high pathogenicity.

Sialic Acid Receptors

Influenza viruses bind to sialic acids, that is, negatively charged 9-carbon sugars that typically occupy the terminal positions of glycoproteins or glycolipids. The term sialic acid is now usually used for the most common member of the group, *N*-acetylneuraminic acid (NeuAc). Another sialic acid species that is not synthesized in humans, *N*-glycolylneuraminic acid (NeuGc), is also recognized by some influenza viruses; in fact, influenza viruses differ in their recognition of these two sialic acid species.[798] Most sialic acids are linked to galactose (Gal) or *N*-acetylgalactosamine (GalNAc) by α2,3- or α2,6-linkages (Siaα2,3/6Gal, Siaα2,3/6GalNAc), or to *N*-acetylglucosamine (GlcNAc) by α2,6-linkages (Siaα2,6GlcNAc).[1795,2147]

Sialic Acid Receptors in Humans

Early studies demonstrated that epithelial cells in human trachea contain Siaα2,6Gal sialyloligosaccharides on their cell surface but lack those with α2,3-linkage.[345] Consequently, viruses with Siaα2,6Gal specificity (i.e., human virus isolates, which preferentially bind to Siaα2,6Gal), but not those with Siaα2,3Gal specificity (i.e., avian virus isolates, which preferentially bind to Siaα2,3Gal), bind to the epithelial cells lining the human trachea.[345] Recent data obtained with *in vitro* differentiated human epithelial cells from tracheal/bronchial tissues suggest a more complex situation: Nonciliated epithelial cells express Siaα2,6Gal oligosaccharides and are predominantly infected by human virus isolates, whereas ciliated cells contain Siaα2,3Gal oligosaccharides and are preferentially infected by avian virus isolates.[1336] Additional studies of human respiratory tissue have shown that while Siaα2,6Gal oligosaccharides are dominant on epithelial cells in nasal mucosa, paranasal sinuses, pharynx, trachea, and bronchi, Siaα2,3Gal oligosaccharides are found on nonciliated cuboidal bronchiolar cells at the junction between the respiratory bronchiole and alveolus, and on type II cells lining the alveolar wall[85,1521,1854,2311] (Fig. 41.10). Attachment and infection data for viruses of known receptor specificity are consistent with this distribution of Siaα2,3Gal and Siaα2,6Gal oligosaccharides.[1854,2139] These findings offer an explanation for the severe pneumonia observed after infection of humans with some avian influenza viruses[320,322,546,1993] and suggest that the limited human-to-human transmission of highly pathogenic avian H5N1 viruses likely reflects the restrictive replicative efficiency of these viruses in the upper portion of the respiratory tract, where transmission could occur via droplets generated by coughing and sneezing (Fig. 41.11). Conversion to preferential recognition of the human-type receptor thus is required for efficient human-to-human transmission, an assumption supported by the finding that the earliest isolates in the 1918, 1957, and 1968 pandemics preferentially recognized Siaα2,6Gal, rather than Siaα2,3Gal, sialyloligosaccharides.[1330] One study found higher amounts of Siaα2,3Gal in the respiratory tract of children compared to adults,[1520] a finding that may suggest higher susceptibility of children to infection with avian influenza viruses. Another study reported predominant expression of Siaα2,3Gal in epithelial cells of the human eye,[1567] which may explain the conjunctivitis associated with H7 influenza virus infections.

Sialic Acid Receptors in Other Mammals

Epithelial cells in pig trachea contain both Siaα2,3Gal and Siaα2,6Gal,[80,880,1478,1939,2136] which may explain why this species can be infected by both avian and human influenza viruses.[1021] For mice, one study reported the expression of both types of receptors in the trachea, lung, and other organs,[1528] while another study did not detect human-type receptors in these animals.[856] Ferrets express predominantly Siaα2,6Gal on cells of the upper respiratory tract.[85,1184] Equine viruses prefer Siaα2,3Gal sialyloligosaccharides, which predominate in horse trachea.[887,1449,2010] These studies also demonstrated that epithelial cells in horse trachea express NeuGc in addition to NeuAc, and that influenza viruses isolated from horses bind to oligosaccharides possessing NeuGc. Siaα2,3Gal is also found on epithelial cells in the respiratory tract of dogs,[370,1293,1449] and in the lungs of seals and whales.[883] The nasal tract and trachea of guinea pigs possess avian-type (Siaα2,3Gal) and human-type (Siaα2,6Gal)

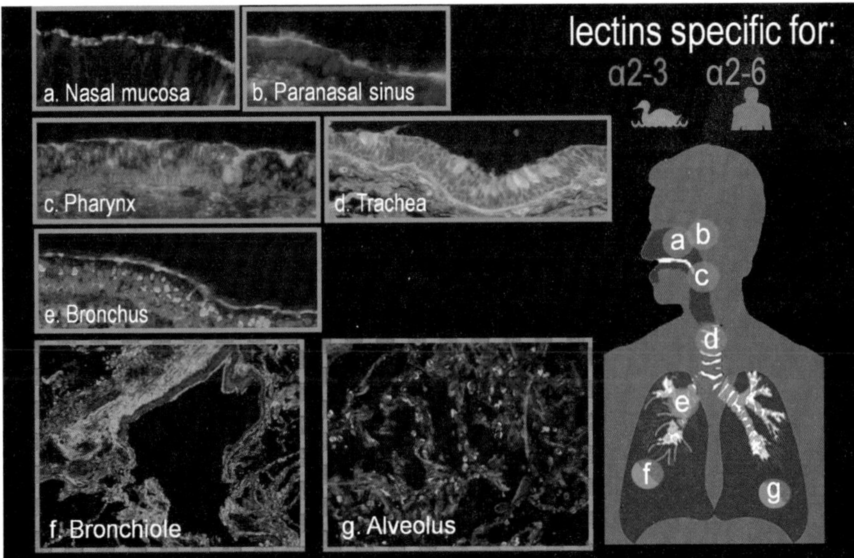

FIGURE 41.10. Expression of human virus (Siaα2,6Gal) and avian virus (Siaα2,3Gal) receptors in human respiratory tissue. The indicated tissues were tested with *Sambucus nigra* lectin (*green*), indicating the presence of sialic acid linked to galactose by an α2,6-linkage (Siaα2,6Gal), or with *Maackia amurensis* lectin (*red*), indicating the presence of Siaα2,3Gal. Cells were counterstained with DAPI (4,6-diamidino-2-phenylindole; *blue*). In the nasal mucosa, paranasal sinuses, pharynx, trachea, and bronchus, Siaα2,6Gal dominated. In the bronchiole and alveolus, both Siaα2,6Gal and Siaα2,3Gal were detected. (From Shinya K, Ebina M, Yamada S, et al. Avian flu: influenza virus receptors in the human airway. *Nature* 2006;440:435–436, with permission.)

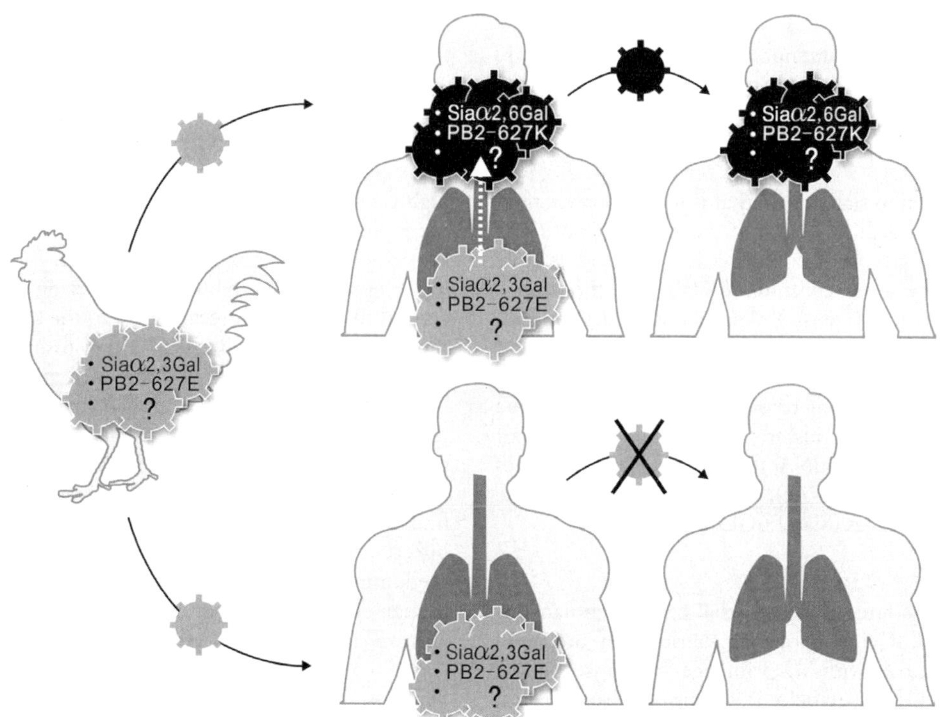

FIGURE 41.11. Model for the emergence of avian-derived influenza A viruses capable of being transmitted efficiently among humans. Avian influenza viruses preferentially bind to Siaα2,3Gal oligosaccharides and contain Glu at position 627 of their PB2 protein (see The Replication Complex section). After transmission to humans, these viruses can infect epithelial cells in the lower respiratory tract that contain Siaα2,3Gal oligosaccharides on their surface. However, due to their limited replication in mammalian cells (determined by PB2-627E) and their restriction to the lower respiratory tract, viruses do not efficiently spread among humans. The current working model predicts at least two changes for the generation of avian-derived viruses that are efficiently transmitted among humans: **(A)** mutations (e.g., PB2-627E to PB2-627K) that increase the viruses' replicative ability in mammalian cells and also provide a growth advantage at the lower temperature in the upper respiratory tract, and **(B)** changes in HA that allow the virus to bind to Siaα2,6Gal oligosaccharides that are prevalent on epithelial cells of the upper respiratory tract. These two changes are likely required but not sufficient for the generation of a pandemic H5N1 virus. Additional, yet unknown, mutations may be required for efficient transmission among humans.

receptors, whereas the lungs contain predominately avian-type receptors.[2004]

Sialic Acid Receptors in Avian Species

The epithelial cells of duck intestine (where avian influenza viruses replicate) express predominantly Siaα2,3Gal,[882] although small amounts of Siaα2,6Gal have been detected in the intestinal and respiratory tract.[578,580,586,1041,1103,1654,2339] The duck intestinal tract also possesses NeuGc, which appears to be absent in chickens.[888] In the respiratory and intestinal tract of chickens, Siaα2,6Gal and Siaα2,3Gal are expressed.[578,580,586,695,1036,1103,1654,2339] Similarly, both Siaα2,3Gal and Siaα2,6Gal are expressed on tracheal and intestinal cells of quail, turkey, pheasant, and guinea fowl,[580,695,1041,1654,2186,2339] that is, species that may play a role in the adaptation of avian influenza viruses to mammalian species (see Role of Terrestrial Poultry in the Emergence of New Influenza Viruses section). However, differences exist among poultry species in the relative abundances of influenza virus receptors in the different organs and cell types tested.[578,586,695,1036,1041,1103,1654,2339] Substantial amounts of Siaα2,6Gal were detected in the respiratory tract of pigeons,[1250] which are not known to play a significant role in influenza virus ecology.

Receptor Specificity of Influenza Viruses

The specificity of HA for the different sialyloligosaccharides is responsible for the host-range restriction of influenza virus. Human and classical H1N1 swine influenza viruses bind preferentially to Siaα2,6Gal, whereas most avian and equine viruses have higher binding affinity for Siaα2,3 Gal.[343,589,882,1330,1333,1533,1743,1744,1746,1889,1969]

Receptor specificity is determined by the amino acids that form the receptor-binding pocket. For H2 and H3 HAs, glutamine at position 226 and glycine at position 228 (found in avian viruses) determine the specificity for Siaα2,3Gal oligosaccharides, whereas leucine and serine at these positions (found in human viruses) confer Siaα2,6Gal specificity in H2 and H3 viruses[343,1330,1463,1745,2034,2164] (Fig. 41.12). For H1 viruses, aspartate at positions 190 and 225 (found in human viruses) confers binding to α2,6, while aspartate and glycine at these positions (found in swine viruses) allow binding to both α2,6 and α2,3 linkages; glutamate and glycine at positions 190 and 225 (found in avian viruses) are responsible for the interaction with α2,3-linked sialic acids.[590,1070,1330,1333,1716,1937,1969,1972,2034,2107] In addition to these key residues, the amino acids at several other positions also affect receptor-binding

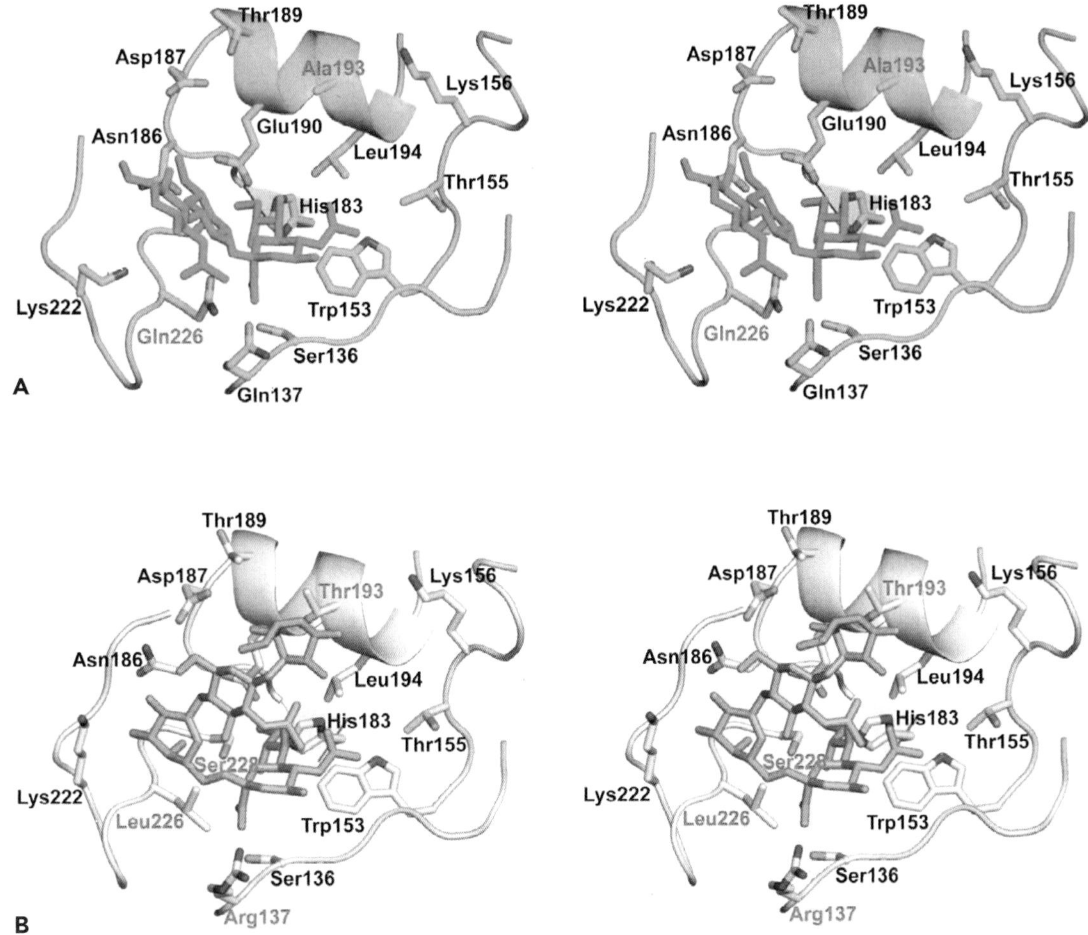

FIGURE 41.12. Structural models of HA–glycan receptor complexes. A: Interaction of avian H2 HA receptor-binding site (*magenta*) with avian-type receptor (*green*). **B:** Interaction of human H2 HA receptor-binding site (*gray*) with human-type receptor (*orange*). (From Viswanathan K, Koh X, Chandrasekaran A, et al. Determinants of glycan receptor specificity of H2N2 influenza A virus hemagglutinin. *PLoS One* 5:e13768, with permission.)

properties.[1330,1333,1372,1380,1627,1743] X-ray crystallographic structures of HA proteins in complex with receptor analogs are available for human H1–H3 HAs,[484,590,1246] avian H1–H3 and H5 HAs,[590,708,709,1246] and swine H1 and H9 HAs,[590,709] and provide detailed insights into the role of individual HA amino acids in receptor binding.

With the use of synthetic sialylglycopolymers,[584] glycan arrays that allow the simultaneous testing of hundreds of carbohydrates and glycoproteins,[1969] and surface plasmon resonance assays,[2029] a more complex picture of influenza viral receptor specificities has emerged. Binding of influenza viruses to their receptor is not only determined by the linkage between the sialic acid and the penultimate sugar residue (α2,3 vs. α2,6) but also by the nature of the penultimate sugar (Gal, GalNAc, or GlcNAc), the length of the carbohydrate chain, and the inner core of the carbohydrate (such as the linkage between the second and third sugar residue, modifications such as sulfation, or other sugar residues such as fucose).[268,579–581,586–588,795,1112,1216,1332–1334,1768,1937,1969,1971,2306] Noteworthy differences exist between human and avian influenza viruses, and among avian viruses. For example, viruses isolated from ducks, chickens, and gulls differ in their preference for the inner core structure of the receptor.[581] Avian influenza viruses favor NeuAcα2,3 attached to shorter carbohydrate chains over the same sialic acid attached to a long chain; by contrast, seasonal human H1 and H3 influenza viruses bind to α2,6 linkages preferentially in the context of long oligosaccharides[795,1112,1969]; thus, avian virus HAs bind to their receptors in a narrow cone-like topology, whereas human virus HAs bind in a more flexible umbrella-like topology.[268,1937] These differences in receptor-binding specificities can be correlated with specific differences in the HA sequence and/or structure.[343,373,583,585,740,1330,1333,1533,1745,1968–1969,1970,2288]

Receptor Specificity of Avian Influenza Viruses

HPAI H5N1 viruses bind efficiently to Siaα2,3Gal.[579,1331] Mutations at position 190 or 225 that change the receptor-binding specificity of H1 HAs do not confer H5N1 virus binding to Siaα2,6Gal; however, the introduction of human-type amino acids at positions 226 and 228 increases binding to Siaα2,6Gal, while retaining substantial binding to Siaα2,3Gal.[746,1970]

HPAI H5N1 viruses isolated from infected individuals typically retain specificity for Siaα2,3Gal.[579,1331,1969,2297] However, several HPAI H5N1 viruses have been isolated that recognize Siaα2,6Gal and Siaα2,3Gal.[48,579,1856,1968,2196,2297,2320] This change in binding properties can be linked to several specific amino acid changes in HA, most notably a serine-to-asparagine mutation at position 227, with or without a mutation at position 158 that results in the loss of a glycosylation site. Passage in ducks of a virus possessing asparagine at position 227 resulted in reversion to serine and reduced human-type receptor-binding specificity,[1857] suggesting that the human-adapting mutation is not stably maintained in ducks. One study tested all naturally or experimentally identified mutations that alter H5 receptor-binding specificity in the same genetic background and noted differences in their effect on binding to Siaα2,6Gal.[314]

Poultry H9N2 viruses isolated in China in 1999 possessed mutations at positions 190 and 226[1227] that conferred binding to Siaα2,6Gal.[1335,1776] These viruses, which also infected humans,[1227,1626] demonstrated that variants with human-type receptor-binding properties can emerge in avian species. Similarly, several low pathogenic H7 viruses isolated from avian species and humans in the United States in 2002 to 2003 and in Canada in 2004 showed increased binding to Siaα2,6Gal, although they retained their ability to bind to avian-type receptors.[99]

Receptor Specificity of Human Influenza Viruses

The HA proteins of the pandemic 1918, 1957, and 1968 viruses originated from avian influenza viruses; nonetheless, the earliest available human isolates of these pandemic viruses already possessed Siaα2,6Gal receptor-binding specificity,[343,628,1330,1969] indicative of strong selective pressure. However, early pandemic H3N2 viruses differ from more recent isolates in their amino acid sequence and their binding affinity to nonciliated cells.[1234,1329,1333,2061]

For the pandemic 1918 virus, two variants have been identified that differ at amino acids 190 and 225: A/South Carolina/1/18 (possessing aspartate at positions 190 and 225 as typically found in human influenza viruses) binds to Siaα2,6Gal and transmits efficiently among ferrets, whereas A/New York/1/18 (possessing aspartate at position 190 but glycine at position 225) binds to both Siaα2,6Gal and Siaα2,3Gal and transmits with reduced efficiency compared to A/South Carolina/1/18.[628,1937,1969,2107] Replacement of aspartate at positions 190 and 225 with the avian-like amino acids at these position—that is, glutamate and glycine—abolishes binding to Siaα2,6Gal and transmission in ferrets.[2107] The X-ray crystallographic structure of a 1918 HA protein in complex with receptor analogs demonstrates how this overall avian-like protein interacts with human-type receptors.[590]

The A(H1N1)pdm09 viruses possess aspartate at positions 190 and 225 and bind efficiently to Siaα2,6Gal,[285,1302,2307] although one study reported dual recognition of both Siaα2,6Gal and Siaα2,3Gal.[303] Molecular dynamics simulation of H1 proteins of the 1918 pandemic, a swine virus from 1930, a seasonal human H1N1 virus from 2005, and the A(H1N1)pdm09 virus showed that lysine at position 145 and glutamate at position 227 [found in the A(H1N1)pdm09 virus] increased the binding affinity to a human-type receptor, and that aspartate 225 increased the number of hydrogen-bonding interactions compared to glycine at this position.[1540] An aspartate-to-glycine change at position 225 (H3 numbering; position 222 in H1 numbering) has been found in some A(H1N1)pdm09 viruses and appears to correlate with more severe disease outcomes in humans.[34,282,448,637,863,1027,1168,1303,1389,1593,1671] Few transmission events have been reported for this variant,[1687] suggesting that it does not transmit efficiently among humans. The aspartate-to-glycine change at position 225 arises during passage in eggs or adaptation to mice and increases virulence *in vitro* and *in vivo.*[868,1781,2286,2362] Experimental infection of pigs with a mixed population of viruses encoding glycine or glutamate at position 225 resulted in the selection of glutamate in viruses isolated from nasal secretions, but glycine in viruses isolated from the lower respiratory tract.[178]

Glycan arrays in combination with X-ray crystallographic structures of pandemic 1957 H2 HAs highlight the significance of position 226 for H2 HA receptor-binding specificity.[2288] This is further supported by the finding that A/El Salvador/2/57, possessing glutamine and glycine at positions 226 and 228, preferentially binds avian-type receptors and transmits poorly among ferrets, while A/Albany/6/58, possessing leucine and serine at position 226 and 228, recognizes human- and avian-type receptors and transmits efficiently in ferrets.[1609] Moreover, a mutational study demonstrated a critical role for the amino acids at positions 226 and 228 in converting an avian H2N2 virus into one that binds human-type receptors.[2166] The amino acids at position 137 and 193 also contributed to receptor-binding specificity.[2166]

Glycosylation

Influenza virulence and host range are also affected by the number and location of oligosaccharide side chains, which are not conserved among strains or subtypes.[859,1533] HAs typically contain 5 to 11 glycosylation sites that affect receptor-binding affinity and/or specificity,[404,583,694,1216,1331,1555,2097,2189] antigenicity,[3,52,379,1656,1777,2196,2200] innate immune responses,[298,1709,2045] replication,[59,2174] fusion activity,[1557] virulence,[744,1342,1463,1632,1708,2156] and host range.[1752] For efficient virus replication, a functional balance between HA and NA is critical.[55,2175] Growth restrictions due to the lack of HA glycosylation site(s) can be partially overcome by amino acid substitutions in NA.[55,2175]

Role of Terrestrial Poultry in the Emergence of New Influenza Viruses

Terrestrial poultry, such as chickens and quail, are susceptible to infection with influenza viruses. Most influenza viruses circulating in wild birds are typically asymptomatic in poultry, but their continued circulation among terrestrial poultry could lead to viruses with increased virulence in these birds.

Adaptation of waterfowl viruses in terrestrial poultry may lead to the emergence of viruses that are better able to replicate in humans or pigs than their original counterparts[580,695,1041,1654,2186,2339] due to altered receptor specificity.[841,1331,1335,1925] Support for this hypothesis comes from the finding that viruses isolated from terrestrial poultry resemble human viruses in their low affinity for Siaα2,3Gal compared to viruses isolated from wild birds[1331] and that the receptor specificity of H9N2 viruses isolated from terrestrial poultry, but not that of viruses isolated from aquatic birds, is similar to the receptor specificity of human isolates.[1335,1776] The H5N1 viruses isolated from terrestrial poultry are characterized by an additional glycosylation site in HA that reduces the affinity for the receptor and, in some instances, by a deletion in the NA stalk that reduces NA functionality and balances the functions of these two proteins. The presence of additional glycosylation sites and a deletion in the NA stalk are typical for human viruses[1331] and have also been found in different virus subtypes isolated from terrestrial poultry.[55,62,116,145,146,221,622,1331,1335,1401,1776,1932] Collectively, these data suggest that waterfowl viruses acquire certain mutations in terrestrial poultry, such as NA stalk deletions and additional HA glycosylation sites that may facilitate their transmission to humans or other mammals such as pigs.

Host Cell-Mediated Selection of Antigenic Variants

In 1942, Burnet and Clarke[203] first described "O" (original) and "D" (derived) variants that differed in their ability to agglutinate human or guinea pig erythrocytes after passage in eggs. Subsequent studies established that the antigenicity of influenza A and B viruses grown in embryonated chicken eggs differs from that of viruses propagated in cell culture, including chicken embryo fibroblasts.[583,991,993,1335,1738,1800] For minor populations of egg isolates, however, the antigenic properties remained identical to those of cell culture isolates.[1589] The HA sequences of cell culture–grown but not egg-grown viruses are identical to those of the original isolates, demonstrating that HA variants arise during virus replication in eggs.[202,296,582,583,585,589,605,992,1277,1278,1699,1739,1800,1971,2028] Moreover, human isolates tend to grow better in cell culture than in eggs,[458,1415] further suggesting that human viruses undergo selection in eggs. Historically, human viruses were isolated by inoculation of samples into the amniotic cavity of embryonated eggs, followed by virus amplification in the allantoic cavity. Some recent human viruses do not grow in eggs when inoculated into the allantoic cavity. Mutations in the HA of egg-grown viruses cluster around the receptor-binding pocket, likely reflecting an adaptation to selective pressure in eggs. This selective pressure can be attributed to the fact that in addition to Siaα2,3 sialyloligosaccharides, Siaα2,6 sialyloligosaccharides exist on amniotic cells, whereas only Siaα2,3 sialyloligosaccharides are found on allantoic cells.[889]

Currently, influenza vaccine viruses are propagated in embryonated chicken eggs. In animal models, however, vaccines prepared from cell culture–grown viruses induce better protective immunity than those grown in eggs,[26,993,994,1394,1508,2261] a finding that was substantiated when these vaccines were tested in humans.[27,1508] Influenza vaccine production in cell culture rather than eggs thus may be preferable.

The NS1 Protein

The NS1 protein functions as an IFN antagonist that allows efficient virus replication in IFN-competent hosts,[599–600,601,1406,1978] in addition to roles in the splicing and nuclear export of viral mRNAs[22,513,596] and the enhancement of viral mRNA translation.[401,490] NS1 targets the production of type I IFN (IFN-α, IFN-β), and interferes with IFN-induced antiviral factors. These functions are described in the Innate Immune Responses section.

The Replication Complex

The influenza viral replication complex comprises the three polymerase proteins—PB2, PB1, and PA—and the nucleoprotein NP. The PB2 protein recognizes and binds to type I cap structures of cellular mRNAs. It has emerged as an important determinant of virulence and host-range restriction. Early studies suggested that the PB2 segment,[21,327,1991] in particular the amino acid at position 627,[1991] was involved in host-range restriction.[21,327,1991] The significance of this finding in the context of interspecies transmission was not recognized, however, until 2001, when a substitution at position 627 of PB2 from glutamic acid (found in most avian isolates) to lysine (found in all contemporary human isolates) was shown to enhance the pathogenicity of an HPAI H5N1 virus in mice.[753]

Multiple lines of evidence now suggest that PB2-627K is a major determinant of pathogenicity in mammals: (1) PB2-627K leads to increased virulence of HPAI H5N1 viruses[593,753,1037,1783,1855]; (2) PB2-627K is selected during virus replication in humans[1165]; (3) PB2-627K was critical for the pathogenicity of an H7N7 virus isolated from a fatal infection in The Netherlands in 2003[406,546,1443]; by contrast, viruses isolated from nonfatal cases and chickens contained glutamic acid; (4) HPAI H5N1 viruses with PB2-627K have been isolated from tigers (A/tiger/Suphanburi/Thailand/Ti-1/04 [H5N1])[28] and a cat in Thailand in 2004 (A/cat/Thailand/KU-02/04 [H5N1]); (5) viruses possessing PB2-627K were isolated after adaptation of H5N1, H7N7, and H9N2 viruses to mice,[841,1203,1322,1860,2278] and after virus replication in pigs[1312]; (6) PB2-627K increases virus transmission in the guinea pig model[1952]; (7) PB2-627K is selected during HPAI H5N1 virus replication in ostrich cells and ostriches[1858] and has been found in viruses isolated from turkeys, ostriches, emu, rhea, and quail, suggesting that PB2-627K selection can occur in some avian species, which may facilitate the adaptation of avian influenza viruses to mammals (see Role of Terrestrial Poultry in the Emergence of New Influenza Viruses section); and (8) PB2-627K increases replicative ability in mammalian cells,[363,1324,1464,1855] particularly at the lower temperatures of the upper respiratory tract[754] (Fig. 41.11). Collectively, these findings suggest that PB2-627K provides a replicative advantage in mammals and is hence selected in these species. However, PB2-627K also emerged in HPAI H5N1 viruses isolated from wild waterfowl at Qinghai Lake in 2005 (see The H5N1 Outbreak section)[279,281,1247] and is maintained in descendants of the Qinghai Lake viruses to this day.

Considering the significance of PB2-627K for influenza virus replication in humans, the finding of PB2-627E (i.e., the avian-type amino acid) in A(H1N1)pdm09 viruses was unexpected. Two studies demonstrated that the lack of PB2-627K is compensated for by a basic amino acid at position 591.[1373,2296] In fact, PB2-627K does not provide a replicative advantage in the background of A(H1N1)pdm09 viruses.[785,907,2296,2377] Structural analyses demonstrated that positions 591 and 627 are in close proximity,[1120,2041] and that a basic amino acid at position 591 alters both the shape and charges on the surface of the protein,[2296] which may affect the interaction of PB2 with other host and/or viral factors.[543,1374,1407] For example, one study suggested that the amino acid at PB2-627 affects the association of the polymerase complex with NP.[1125,1701]

A second amino acid in PB2—at position 701—was first identified as a virulence factor of HPAI H5N1 viruses in mice,[1212] and is now known to facilitate viral adaptation to mammalian species. Replacement of aspartic acid (found in most avian influenza viruses) with asparagine at residue 701 enhances binding of PB2 to the cellular nuclear import factor importin α and facilitates PB2 nuclear import and replicative ability in mammalian cells.[566,568,569] This amino acid change was found upon adaptation of an avian H7N7 virus to mice[567]; it also proved to be critical for virus transmission in guinea pigs.[595,1952] In addition, mouse-adapted human H3N2 viruses possessed the PB2-D701N mutation.[1655] Like PB2-627K, PB2-701N is selected during HPAI H5N1 virus replication in humans[1165] and ostriches,[1858] but does not provide a replicative advantage to A(H1N1)pdm09 viruses.[785,2296]

Replacement of the avian-type threonine residue at position 271 of PB2 with alanine (i.e., the residue typically found in human influenza viruses) increases virus replication in mammalian cells and mice.[205] The PB2 protein of the A(H1N1) pdm09 virus (which is of avian-virus origin) encodes alanine at position 271, suggestive of human adaptation.

The PB1 protein possesses conserved motifs found in all RNA-dependent RNA polymerases[137] and is considered critical for the polymerase enzymatic function. In a minireplicon system, reporter gene expression was more efficient with avian than with human virus PB1 protein.[1464] Avian virus PB1 protein may hence provide a replicative advantage over its human counterpart, an attractive hypothesis since both the 1957 and 1968 pandemic strains contained avian PB1 genes (in combination with avian HA, or HA and NA genes[1001,1813]). Moreover, in reassortment studies between HPAI H5N1 and human H3N2 viruses, one of the most pathogenic reassortants possessed the avian PB1 gene.[284] Reassortment studies also demonstrated a critical role for the pandemic 1918 PB1 gene in virulence in animal models.[1607,2206]

The PA protein is an integral part of the influenza viral replication complex with a role in the cap-snatching process.[418] Recent studies now also suggest a role for PA in the virulence of the A(H1N1)pdm09 virus[1781,1921,2006] and in the adaptation of an avian H5N2 virus to mice.[1920]

In addition to the polymerase genes, the NP gene may play a role in host range restriction.[592,1810,1811,2066]

A large body of information demonstrates that the composition of the replication complex affects viral pathogenicity.[284,905,1192,1198,1199,1300,1464,1548,1607,1819,2006,2019,2203,2206] As a general trend, more efficient replication in minireplicon assays translates into increased pathogenicity in animal models.

The PB1-F2 Protein

PB1-F2 is a short protein of 87 to 90 amino acids that was discovered in 2001.[291] It is expressed from the +1 reading frame of the PB1 gene of most avian and human influenza viruses; however, human H1N1 viruses isolated after 1950 encode a truncated version of 57 amino acids.[291,2352] Most swine virus isolates (particularly classical H1N1 swine influenza viruses) do not encode a functional PB1-F2 peptide, due to several in-frame stop codons. These stop codons are also found in the reading frames of A(H1N1)pdm09 virus PB1-F2s, which likely originated from pigs; therefore, human pandemic viruses do not encode a functional PB1-F2 protein. Reconstitution of full-length PB1-F2 expression in the background of A(H1N1)pdm09 viruses had only minor effects on replicative ability and virulence in mice and ferrets,[273,711,1592] suggesting that PB1-F2 is not critical for the pathogenicity of A(H1N1) pdm09 viruses. Phosphorylation of PB1-F2 may be critical for its function.[1402] The role of PB1-F2 in viral pathogenicity is discussed in more detail in the Innate Immune Responses section.

The NA Protein

The sialidase activity of the NA protein removes sialic acid from sialyloligosaccharides, thereby serving two functions: (1) the removal of sialic acid from HA, NA, and the cell surface, facilitating virus release; and (2) the removal of sialic acid from the mucin layer, which likely allows the virus to reach the surface of the epithelial cells.[1331,1602] The NA protein may also have a role in host-range restriction[808] and pathogenicity.[651,1607,1819] Notably, the NA activity of some avian viruses is more resistant to the low pH of the upper digestive tract than that of human- or swine-derived NA,[2009,2025] a feature that may contribute to host-range restriction. Interestingly, low-pH stability has also been reported for the NA protein of the pandemic 1918 virus.[2024] The NA protein of A/WSN/33 (H1N1) virus is critical for plaque formation in Madin-Darby bovine kidney cells and for neurovirulence[1473,1821,1996]; these two phenotypes are linked to the loss of a carbohydrate chain on NA and the presence of a C-terminal lysine residue.[1208] The lack of the carbohydrate chain at position 146 of NA (N2 numbering) allows the NA protein to bind to and sequester plasminogen, a plasmin precursor. This function facilitates HA cleavage and, thereby, virus pathogenicity in mice.[651,653,1208]

Multiple studies now indicate that the length of the NA stalk affects virulence and pathogenicity[55,62,116,145,146,221,622,1331,1335,1342,1401,1439,1776,1869,1932,1988,2367]; deletions in the NA stalk have been observed after virus replication in eggs and in poultry, and among recent HPAI H5N1 viruses.

Like HA, the NA protein shows preference for certain types of sialyloligosaccharides according to the host species. Avian virus NAs cleave α2,3-linked, but not α2,6-linked, sialic acids. After their introduction into the human population, N2 NAs acquired the ability to cleave α2,6-linked sialic acids in addition to α2,3-linked sialic acids[84]; however, the enzymatic activity for α2,6-linked sialic acids is significantly lower than that for α2,3-linked sialic acids. This acquired ability likely represents adaptation to the respective recognition pattern of the HA protein. NA substrate specificity is determined by the amino acid at position 275.[1069]

CLINICAL FEATURES AND PATHOGENESIS IN HUMANS

Pattern of Virus Shedding

Human influenza viruses replicate almost exclusively in superficial cells of the respiratory tract. Influenza virus is released from the apical surface of the cell, which may limit more systemic spread but facilitate accumulation of virus in the lumen of the respiratory tract for transmission to the next susceptible host. Alveolar macrophages and dendritic cells can also be infected. Their role is in initiating the innate and cognate immune response to influenza virus by processing antigens and presenting them for recognition (see Innate Immune Cells and Cellular Immunity sections). Influenza virus replicates throughout the respiratory tract, with virus being recoverable from the upper and lower tracts of people naturally or experimentally infected with virus. The site of optimal growth in the respiratory tract for influenza viruses is, in part, determined by the prevalence of the Siaα-2,3Gal or Siaα-2,6Gal receptors (see the HA Protein section).

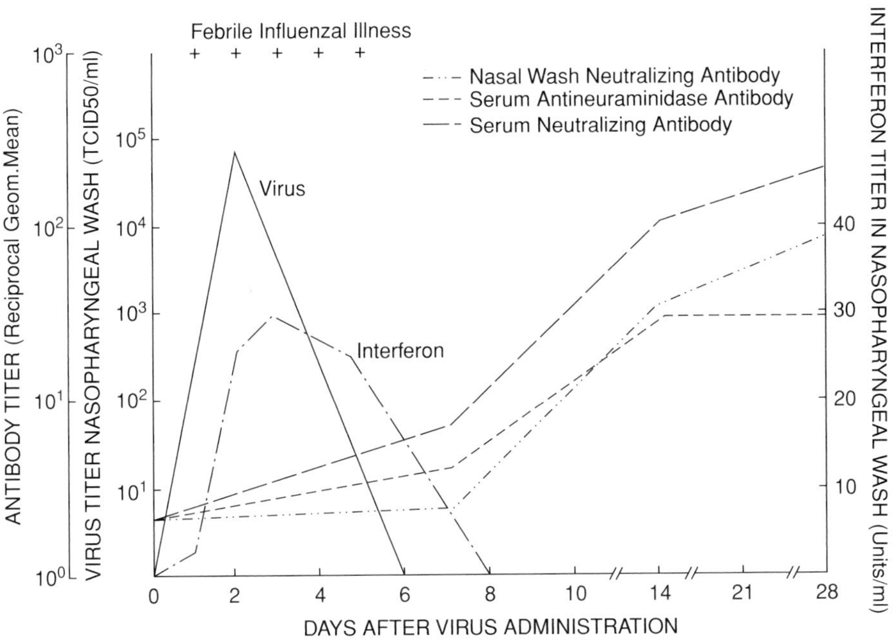

FIGURE 41.13. Six seronegative volunteers received $10^{4.0}$ $TCID_{50}$ of wild-type A/Bethesda/1015/68 virus intranasally on day 0.

The pattern of virus replication in six adult volunteers administered an influenza A/Hong Kong/68-like H3N2 virus, in relation to the onset of clinical symptoms, IFN response, and serum and nasal wash antibody responses, is presented in Figure 41.13.[1728] More recent work has defined the patterns of local and systemic chemokine and cytokine responses seen with experimental influenza infection.[764]

Virus replication peaks about 48 hours after inoculation and declines slowly thereafter, with little shedding after days 6 to 8. Peak virus titers in symptomatic adult volunteers range from $10^{3.0}$ to $10^{7.0}$ $TCID_{50}$/mL of nasopharyngeal wash. There was a positive correlation between the amount of virus shed and the severity of the clinical illness. Individuals who shed less than $10^{3.0}$ $TCID_{50}$/mL were either asymptomatic or had only minor upper respiratory tract symptoms. Even after infectious virus can no longer be recovered, viral antigen can be detected for several days in cells and secretions of infected individuals.[119,467,2046] Viral antigen is detectable in conjunctival cells and secretions.[2046] In children, virus can be found for up to 13 days after the onset of symptoms.[555] The higher titers and more prolonged shedding in children contribute to the important role of this population in the spread of influenza.

The duration of shedding of A(H1N1)pdm09 virus is similar to that of seasonal influenza viruses. In immunocompetent patients, the A(H1N1)pdm09 virus is typically shed from the day prior to the onset of symptoms to 5 to 7 days after the onset of illness.[131,2070,2334] The highest amounts of virus are shed within the first two days of illness. In a study of elementary school children (median age, 8 years), A(H1N1)pdm09 virus was isolated for a median 2 days after fever resolution.[131] Early oseltamivir treatment within 48 hours of symptom onset significantly reduced the duration of shedding.[1237,2334] More prolonged shedding of A(H1N1)pdm09 virus can occur in young children,[1201] immunocompromised individuals,[1145] and in patients with severe disease such as acute respiratory distress syndrome or fatal infection.[2070]

Pathology

Influenza A virus induces changes throughout the respiratory tract, but the most clinically important pathology develops in the lower respiratory tract.[688,791–792,793,2183] During bronchoscopy in uncomplicated influenza infections, acute diffuse inflammation of the larynx, trachea, and bronchi are observed with mucosal inflammation and edema. Light microscopic studies of infected cells show that columnar ciliated cells become vacuolated, edematous, and lose cilia before desquamating down to a one-cell-thick basal layer. Submucosal edema and hyperemia occur with the infiltration of neutrophils and mononuclear cells.[1320] In more severe primary viral pneumonia, there is an interstitial pneumonitis with marked hyperemia and broadening of the alveolar walls, with a predominantly mononuclear leukocyte infiltration and capillary dilation and thrombosis. Influenza virus–specific antigen is present in types 1 and 2 alveolar epithelial cells, as well as in intra-alveolar macrophages[685,1847] (Fig. 41.4). The pathologic changes associated with HPAI H5N1 viruses include a hemophagocytic syndrome, renal tubular necrosis, lymphoid depletion, and diffuse alveolar damage with interstitial fibrosis.[267,310,1087,1101,1625,1993,2069,2116] Similarly, infection with A(H1N1)pdm09 virus leads to diffuse alveolar damage, hemorrhagic interstitial pneumonitis, and peribronchiolar and perivascular lymphocytic infiltrates[86,625,684,705,706,1635,1927] (see The H5N1 Outbreak section).

Necrotizing changes may occur with rupture of alveoli and bronchiole walls. Influenza virus has been obtained from lungs at autopsy in titers of $10^{2.0}$ to $10^{5.7}$ 50% egg infectious doses per gram of tissue.[1262]

At the cellular level, influenza virus shuts off cell protein synthesis and induces apoptosis as an additional mechanism of cell destruction.[806,1130,1267,1424,1822,2355,2356] From the third to fifth day after onset of illness, mitoses appear in the basal cell layer, and regeneration of the epithelium begins. During this time, reparative and destructive processes may be present simultaneously. Complete healing of the epithelial damage takes up to 1 month.

Clinical Features

Adults

Infection with influenza A viruses results in clinical responses ranging from asymptomatic infection to primary viral pneumonia that rapidly progresses to a fatal outcome. The typical uncomplicated influenza syndrome is a tracheobronchitis with some involvement of small airways.[200,441] The incubation period ranges from 1 to 5 days (reviewed in[468]). The onset of illness is usually abrupt, with headache, chills, and dry cough, which are rapidly followed by high fever, myalgias, malaise, and anorexia. Substernal tightness and soreness can accompany the cough. The most prominent sign of infection is fever that often peaks within 24 hours at 38°C to 40°C. The fever begins to decline on the second or third day of illness and has usually abated by the sixth day.[441] The elderly can have high fever, lassitude, and confusion without respiratory signs.

Physical findings in influenza are confined to the respiratory tract. Nasal obstruction, rhinorrhea, sneezing, and pharyngeal inflammation without exudate are common. Conjunctival inflammation and excessive tearing may occur. Conjunctivitis was the hallmark of an H7N7 outbreak in poultry workers in the Netherlands.[546] Small cervical nodes can be felt in a minority of cases. Chest radiograph and auscultatory findings are usually normal, although occasionally patchy rales and rhonchi are heard.

As the fever declines, the respiratory signs and symptoms may become more prominent. The cough frequently changes from dry and hacking to one that produces small amounts of mucoid or purulent sputum. After the fever and upper respiratory tract symptoms resolve, cough and weakness can persist for 1 to 2 additional weeks. Illness is more frequent and more severe in cigarette smokers.[974] The loss of the mucociliary blanket is a factor in a predisposition to secondary sinusitis and bacterial pneumonia. Although airflow in large airways is usually unaltered in uncomplicated influenza, there is an increase in bronchial reactivity to chemical and particulate stimuli during infection.[2117] Small peripheral airways are often affected even in otherwise uncomplicated influenza A virus infections.[721] This small airway abnormality can persist after symptomatic illness has subsided. Alterations in pulmonary gas exchange are seen, with a depression of the diffusing capacity of carbon dioxide and an increase in the alveolar-arterial oxygen tension gradient.[839] Tracheobronchial clearance of radiolabeled particles is depressed during acute influenza virus infections but returns to normal levels about 1 month later.[217] Although significant abnormalities in large and small airways can be demonstrated during acute infection and early convalescence, uncomplicated influenza appears to cause little permanent damage in the lung, even in patients with chronic obstructive lung disease.[336,1167]

Clinical symptoms of A(H1N1)pdm09 virus infections in adults were similar to those of seasonal influenza, although gastrointestinal manifestations—including vomiting and diarrhea—occurred at higher rates (approximately 20–30%)[86,1261] (see The H1N1 Pandemic in 2009 section). In addition, adults with A(H1N1)pdm09 infection were more likely to have radiographically confirmed pneumonia (4.0%) compared with those with seasonal H1N1 (2.3%) or H3N2 (1.1%) infection.[97]

Children

The clinical manifestations of influenza in children are similar to those in adults, but there are some distinct differences. There is a proportionally greater burden of illness in children than in adults.[1668] Children have higher fevers that may be accompanied by febrile convulsions.[1678] At least 14% of fevers with respiratory tract symptoms that result in a pediatrician visit are caused by influenza viruses.[629,633,635,2268,2271]

Otitis media, croup, pneumonia, and myositis are more frequent in children than in adults.[782,1035] Otitis media develops in approximately 12% of influenza-infected seronegative children.[2272] Between 24% and 33% of children hospitalized with influenza A virus infection have otitis media.[1595] Although less well documented in children than in adults, bacterial sinusitis may follow acute influenza.

Studies in children have shown that some influenza A viruses are important causes of laryngotracheobronchitis (croup).[1035] Croup occurs predominantly in children younger than 1 year. Influenza-associated croup can be especially severe and occasionally requires intubation of the patient.[193] In a prospective study of 121 susceptible (seronegative) young children seen during an H3N2 virus outbreak, 5 of 60 infected infants had clinical and radiographic evidence of pneumonia.[2270] Influenza A virus infection has been shown to exacerbate asthma.[1083,1395] Children (especially those younger than 3 years) have a higher incidence of gastrointestinal manifestations such as vomiting and abdominal pain. Infection of neonates can present as unexplained fever[1375] and can be life threatening.[81,1375] With HPAI H5N1 infections, acute respiratory distress syndrome is observed frequently (see The H5N1 Outbreak section).[95] Influenza A and B viruses are significant causes of serious lower respiratory tract disease that often lead to hospitalization of children[398,634,1238,1503,1581,2062] and rarely to death.[130,353]

Lower Respiratory Tract Complications

Three distinct syndromes of severe pneumonia can follow influenza infection in children or adults. Complications are most common in the elderly.[1279]

Primary Viral Pneumonia

Primary influenza virus pneumonia was first described in fatal cases caused by the 1957 Asian influenza A virus (H2N2),[1297,1320] although retrospectively, it occurred during previous influenza A epidemics.[645] Primary viral pneumonia occurs predominantly in individuals at high risk for the complications of influenza virus infection (i.e., the elderly or patients with cardiopulmonary disease), but 25% of cases are in individuals without risk factors and an additional 13% are in pregnant women. The typical case of primary viral pneumonia develops abruptly after the onset of influenza illness. It progresses within 6 to 24 hours to a severe pneumonia with rapid respiration rate (30 to 60 respirations per minute), tachycardia (greater than 120 beats/min), cyanosis (in 80% of patients), high fever (average of 39°C), and hypotension. The illness may progress rapidly to hypoxemia and death in 1 to 4 days; the presence of frothy hemoptysis, tachypnea, and cyanosis portends a fatal outcome. Auscultatory findings include bilateral crepitant inspiratory rales. Examination by radiograph reveals mottled densities in two or more lobes. Diffuse symmetric interstitial infiltrates or areas of consolidation, cavitation, or pleural effusion suggest bacterial superinfection. Pathologic findings in the trachea and bronchi are similar to those previously seen during acute uncomplicated disease, but bronchiolitis and alveolitis are also present.[1320] The laboratory findings in primary viral pneumonia are not specific. The erythrocyte sedimentation rate and the complete blood count are usually within normal ranges.

In nonfatal cases, initial improvement occurs from 5 to 16 days after onset of pneumonia. Resolution of radiographic changes can take up to 4 months.[2254] Survivors can develop diffuse interstitial fibrosis with decreases in diffusion capacity of carbon dioxide and in arterial oxygen tension.[1146,1657,2254] Influenza B virus can cause severe disease but does not seem to be associated with fatal primary viral pneumonia in normal individuals.[534,2095]

Avian H5N1 influenza appears to follow a clinical pathway of primary viral pneumonia, although with a striking mortality of ~60% (updated regularly at http://www.who.int/csr/disease/avian_influenza/en/). As of February 1, 2013, 615 cases with 364 fatalities had been reported, resulting in a mortality rate of ~60%.[95]

During the H1N1 pandemic in 2009, a small number of patients developed rapidly progressive primary viral pneumonia that led to acute respiratory distress syndrome and multiple organ failure, which was associated with high mortality[86,625,684,705,706,1635,1927] (see The H1N1 Pandemic in 2009 section). Histopathologic findings included diffuse alveolar damage (DAD) with hyaline membranes and septal edema, DAD with intense alveolar hemorrhage, and necrotizing bronchiolitis.[625,1345,1847]

Combined Viral–Bacterial Pneumonia

Combined viral–bacterial pneumonia is quite common. The bacteria most often involved are *Streptococcus pneumoniae*, *Staphylococcus aureus*, and *Haemophilus influenzae*, although other micro-organisms can play a role[614,1320,1644,1827] (Fig. 41.4). Clinically, this syndrome may be indistinguishable from primary viral pneumonia, except that the symptoms of pneumonia appear somewhat after the influenza symptoms and chest radiographs are more likely to show pleural effusions. Virus has been recovered from the lungs and pleural fluid.[1320,1347] The erythrocyte sedimentation rate is more frequently elevated than in primary viral pneumonia. Because there is no effective distinction between the two syndromes, the diagnosis depends solely on the demonstration of bacteria in the sputum, in fluid obtained at bronchoscopy, or in the pleural fluid. The case fatality rate for combined viral–bacterial pneumonia is 10% to 12%.[136,510,1262,1644] Co-infection with influenza and *S. aureus* can have a fatality rate of up to 42%.[1741]

The available data suggest that bacterial pneumonia contributed significantly to the high mortality rate associated with the 1918 pandemic[190,302,1272,1420] (see The Pandemic of 1918/1919—Spanish Influenza (H1N1) section). Bacterial superinfections were frequently observed with A(H1N1)pdm09 infections, in particular with fatal cases[243,625,705,706,914,1254,1345,1599,1635,1847] (Fig. 41.4). The most common bacterial pathogens were *S. pneumoniae, S. aureus, H. influenzae*, and group A *Streptococcus,* similar to those found with seasonal influenza.

Influenza virus–infected mice experience a higher mortality rate upon *S. aureus* infection compared to mice not infected with influenza viruses.[891] In ferrets, influenza virus infections increase the susceptibility to *S. pneumoniae* infection.[1359] The magnitude of this effect may vary among the influenza (sub)types: 9 out of 10 ferrets infected with an H3N2 virus and subsequently infected with pneumococcus developed sinusitis or otitis media, in contrast to only 1 of 11 ferrets infected with an influenza A H1N1 or influenza B virus.[1628]

There are strains of *S. aureus* that secrete proteases capable of activating the infectivity of influenza virus by proteolytic cleavage of the HA. These strains play a synergistic role in experimental pneumonia in mice.[2043,2044] Such protease-secreting bacterial strains could be an added pathogenic factor in combined viral–staphylococcal pneumonias in humans. An apparent increase in combined viral–bacterial pneumonias was being noted with the 2003–2004 influenza A H3N2 epidemic, perhaps coincident with the rapidly increasing impact of staphylococcal disease and emergence of methicillin-resistant *S. aureus.*[1667]

Secondary Bacterial Pneumonia

In this syndrome, an individual recovering from a typical influenza illness develops shaking chills, pleuritic chest pain, and an increase in cough productive of bloody or purulent sputum.[1262] Cyanosis and a marked increase in respiratory rate are less common than with primary viral pneumonia. Radiographic examination reveals local areas of lung consolidation but not diffuse pneumonia. Often, influenza virus is no longer recoverable, leukocytosis is common, and the erythrocyte sedimentation rate is elevated. This condition is generally amenable to antibiotic therapy, although a case fatality rate of about 7% has been described.[1262]

Extrapulmonary Manifestations

Viremia

Viremia is highly unusual in influenza virus infections.[1028,1397] Virus was isolated from the blood at low levels (present only in undiluted blood specimens) from a patient on the fourth day of influenza illness.[1465] Virus was present in barely detectable amounts in the blood of two patients with fatal primary viral pneumonia on the sixth day after the onset of illness and was recovered at necropsy from the liver and spleen of one patient.[1183] In addition, the presence of viremia has been inferred because virus was present in low titer in extrapulmonary tissues such as heart, liver, spleen, kidney, adrenal glands, and meninges of patients dying of pneumonia.[954,1737]

During the H1N1 pandemic in 2009, viremia (detected by RT-PCR) occurred rarely and was only observed in severe and fatal cases.[1585,2070] Viremia and systemic spread is more common with avian H5N1 influenza, with PCR detection of virus from the blood in each of six patients tested.[95]

Myositis

In adults, a diffuse myositis can occur with generalized pain, tenderness, and weakness of muscles, increased serum levels of muscle enzymes, myoglobinemia, and myoglobinuria.[1396] Acute renal failure sometimes follows. The pathogenesis of myositis remains uncertain.[1018,1396] Although influenza virus has been recovered from muscle, the relation between the virus and myositis remains unclear. In children, myositis is usually localized to the gastrocnemius and soleus muscles and is characterized by pain on walking. Onset of myositis occurs as respiratory illness wanes—the muscles are tender and swollen, serum levels of muscle enzymes are elevated, the course is usually benign and reversible, and light microscopic changes of muscle necrosis and inflammatory cell infiltrates are seen.[421]

Cardiac Involvement

Influenza recovery from the heart of patients with myocarditis associated with fatal pulmonary infection is rare.[1320,1581] Clinical findings and cardiac function studies in patients with severe pulmonary infection suggest that myocardial dysfunction is not a direct result of influenza A virus infection.[200,1262,2070]

Reye Syndrome

Reye syndrome is a rapidly progressive noninflammatory encephalopathy and fatty infiltration of the viscera, especially the liver, which results in severe hepatic dysfunction with elevated serum transaminase and ammonia levels. This syndrome is seen following respiratory, varicella, and gastrointestinal viral infections. The onset of the central nervous system (CNS) and hepatic symptoms usually begins as respiratory tract symptoms wane. The case fatality rate varied between 22% and 42%.[855] The etiology and pathogenesis of this syndrome are unknown. There is electron microscopic evidence of mitochondrial swelling.[1612] Influenza B virus infection is the most common antecedent infection. The disease associated with influenza B virus infection occurs in children ages 0 to 18 years (median age, 11 years) and is more frequently seen in rural than in urban areas.[855] Salicylate administration is a critical cofactor in the development of Reye syndrome. The incidence of Reye syndrome after influenza virus infection in the salicylate era was estimated to be between 0.37 and 0.88 cases per 100,000 children younger than 18 years. This may have been underestimated because milder forms of Reye syndrome have been described.[1218] There has been a dramatic decrease in Reye syndrome cases in the United States associated with reduced use of salicylates, which are now widely recognized to be contraindicated in influenza virus infection.

Central Nervous System Involvement

A wide spectrum of CNS disease has been observed during influenza A and B virus infections in humans,[635,759] ranging from irritability, drowsiness, boisterousness, and confusion to serious manifestations such as psychosis, delirium, and coma. Febrile convulsions leading to hospitalization occur in children with and without underlying CNS abnormalities. The pathogenesis of these CNS symptoms is unclear. Nonspecific metabolic effects such as hypoxia resulting from severe pulmonary infection may contribute to the CNS signs and symptoms.

Two specific CNS syndromes accompany influenza infection: influenzal encephalopathy and postinfluenzal encephalitis.[541] Encephalopathy occurs at the height of influenza illness and may be fatal.[410] The cerebrospinal fluid (CSF) is usually normal, the brain at autopsy shows severe congestion, and histologic changes are minimal. Lungs of such patients show changes typical of influenza and yield virus in high titer. A subset of influenza encephalopathy has been described extensively in Japan and seen in other countries as an acute necrotizing encephalopathy with bilateral thalamic and cerebellar involvement.[2234]

The postinfluenzal encephalitic syndrome is extremely rare, occurring from 2 to 3 weeks after recovery from influenza. Recovery is achieved in most cases. The association of postencephalitic syndrome with influenza virus infection is less certain because virus is no longer recoverable and initial serum specimens may already reflect a rising antibody titer.[541] Influenza A virus has only rarely been recovered from the brain or cerebrospinal fluid, and attempts to isolate it from the CNS of individuals dying of primary viral pneumonia have been unsuccessful.[1320]

The syndrome of encephalitis lethargica followed by postinfluenzal encephalitic Parkinson disease was associated with the influenza epidemics of 1918 and the epidemics that followed.[1707] The epidemics of encephalitis lethargica followed the epidemics of influenza, which were followed, in turn, by postencephalitic Parkinson disease about 1 decade later.[1707] Experiments in animals suggest that avian H5N1 viruses can cause pathology similar to Parkinson disease.[911]

An increase in the incidence of Guillain-Barré syndrome (GBS), an acute neurologic disorder that causes muscle weakness and partial paralysis, has not been seen after influenza A or B virus epidemics (see the Reactogenicity of Seasonal Influenza Vaccines and Vaccines to A(H1N1)pdm09 Virus sections).

Infection During Pregnancy

Pregnant women in the second or third trimester have an increased risk of developing fatal influenza disease.[1505] The increased mortality is generally seen during the years after introduction of a new pandemic strain, as in 1918, 1957, and 2009,[665,1807,2134,2265] although using a large data set, the impact can be appreciated in the interpandemic period.[1505] During the H1N1 pandemic in 2009, an increased risk of complication, hospitalization, and death was observed among pregnant and postpartum women, when compared to the general population.[1261,1427,1887] Based on a systematic review, pregnant women infected with A(H1N1)pdm09 virus accounted for 6.3%, 5.9%, and 5.7% of hospitalizations, intensive care unit admissions, and deaths, respectively, although only approximately 1% of the population is pregnant at any given time.[1427] The risk for complications is greater during the later stages in pregnancy; among 56 pregnant women who died from A(H1N1)pdm09 virus infection in the United States from April through December 2009, four (7.1%) were in the first trimester of pregnancy, 15 (26.8%) in the second, and 36 (64.3%) in the third.[1887] Increased risks of adverse neonatal outcomes including preterm delivery and low birth weight were observed, particularly with severe maternal illness due to A(H1N1)pdm09 influenza.[360,1887]

Virus is typically not recovered from the fetus, although in one case viral RNA was detected in the fetus of a woman who succumbed to infection with HPAI H5N1.[676] Influenza virus itself has not been implicated as a cause of congenital defects.[975,1297,1408] Although an increase in congenital anomalies and hematologic malignancies has been reported after influenza virus infection in pregnancy, no consistent association between specific defects or malignancies and influenza epidemics has emerged.[49,669,712,1702]

Infection in Immunosuppressed Patients

Influenza viruses can cause severe disease in immunocompromised individuals,[348,1251,1742,2240] but more often the illness resembles that seen in immunocompetent persons.[1393] Somewhat prolonged shedding of virus occurs in immunosuppressed persons.[877,878,1742,2240]

In adults infected with human immunodeficiency virus (HIV)—most of whom were on antiretroviral therapy and had well controlled-HIV infections—the clinical outcomes of infection with A(H1N1)pdm09 virus (including the frequency of severe illness and death) were similar between HIV-infected and noninfected patients.[1643,1730] In the United States, however, the hospitalization rate among patients co-infected with HIV and A(H1N1)pdm09 virus (3.4%) was higher compared to the HIV prevalence rate in the US adult population (0.45%).[1643] Among recipients of hematopoietic stem cell transplants or solid organ transplants, A(H1N1)pdm09 influenza caused an increased risk of severe illness with a high incidence of lower respiratory tract complications, and an increased risk of mortality.[508,1109,1911]

Influenza B and C Virus Infections

Influenza B virus causes the same spectrum of disease as influenza A but there are less frequent epidemics so that its total impact in a pediatric population is roughly one-third that of influenza.[986] Severe illness can occur[56,1035,2268]; however, the frequency of serious influenza B virus infections requiring hospitalization is about fourfold less than that of influenza A virus. Influenza B virus illness predominantly involves adolescents and school-age children, but adults and the elderly can also be affected.[56,323,629,633,635,722,1536] Myositis, Reye syndrome, and gastrointestinal symptoms appear to occur more commonly with influenza B than A virus infection.[323,518,1017,1140]

Influenza C virus causes sporadic upper respiratory tract illness and is rarely associated with severe lower respiratory tract disease.[1422] By early adulthood, most individuals (96%) have antibody to influenza C virus.[1541] Administration of influenza C virus to volunteers induced mild coryza with some systemic symptoms.[938] Of 170 children infected with influenza C virus, most (92%) were younger than 6 years of age.[1344] In infants and young children (particularly <2 years of age), complications of bronchitis, bronchiolitis, and bronchopneumonia that may require hospitalization have been reported[655,1344]; nevertheless, influenza C virus is not a major cause of lower respiratory tract infection in children.

IMMUNOLOGY

The respiratory tract has multiple nonspecific protective mechanisms against influenza virus infection—including the mucin layer, ciliary action, and protease inhibitors—that may prevent effective cell entry and virus uncoating. The extremely short incubation period between infection and clinical illness implies that innate immunity or preformed cognate recognition components are important. Much of what we know about the protective components of immunity and events that terminate primary influenza infection is from murine models. To better understand immune responses to influenza infection and vaccination, systems biology approaches are now employed.[169,192,738,939,976,1084,1348,1467,1468,1474,1836,1998,2205]

INNATE IMMUNE RESPONSES

In vertebrates, innate immune responses are a critical first line of defense against microbes. Innate immune responses can broadly be divided into three steps: (1) microbe recognition by a pathogen recognition receptor (PRR), resulting in the production of type I IFN, chemokines, and cytokines; (2) activation of IFN-signaling pathways leading to the upregulation of IFN-stimulated genes, many of which have antimicrobial functions; and (3) the actions of cellular proteins with antimicrobial functions. Recent data also demonstrate high induction of IFN-λ upon influenza virus infection,[924] suggesting a role for type III IFN in innate immune responses to influenza virus infections.

Pathogen Recognition Receptors (PRRs)

Microbes are recognized by PRRs, including Toll-like receptors (TLRs), RIG-I-like receptors, and NOD-like receptors (NLRs). Recognition of pathogen-associated molecular patterns by PRRs results in the activation of signaling pathways that ultimately converge on the expression of antimicrobial genes. Influenza virus infection is sensed by TLR3 in airway epithelium[693,1161,1386,2281] and TLR7 in plasmacytoid dendritic cells,[419,610,1214,1283,1386,2281] upregulating their expression. For example, high levels of TLR3 were found in the lungs of individuals who died after infection with A(H1N1)pdm09 virus.[1345]

TLR3 (gene name: *TLR3*) senses double-stranded RNA (dsRNA) and acts through the adaptor molecule TRIF, thereby leading to the activation of IRF3, NFκB, and the activator protein 1 (AP1) transcription factors. These three factors are critical in stimulating the expression of type I IFN and of pro-inflammatory cytokines. TLR7 (gene name: *TLR7*) recognizes single-stranded RNA (ssRNA), and relies on the adaptor protein MyD88 to induce NFκB and IRF7, which subsequently induce the expression of type I IFN and pro-inflammatory cytokines. TLR7 is expressed in high amounts in plasmacytoid dendritic cells, and hence, may be critical for abundant IFN-α secretion, which is observed in response to influenza virus infection.[419,951,1338,1339] By contrast, TLR3 may play a more significant role in the induction of NFκB-dependent proinflammatory cytokines.[1162] Compared to wild-type mice, TLR3$^{-/-}$ mice infected with influenza virus showed reduced levels of proinflammatory cytokines and increased virus titers in the lungs, but reduced mortality.[1161] This suggests that TLR3-dependent gene expression, potentiated in airway epithelium, may contribute to immunopathology associated with influenza virus infections.

Stimulation with TLR2 and TLR4 prior to influenza virus infection increases resistance to virus infection,[1859] and TLR4 signaling has been implicated in influenza viral pathogenicity.[329,870] Immunization of mice with nanoparticles containing influenza HA protein in combination with ligands that signal through TLR4 and TLR7 induced higher levels of neutralizing antibodies and better protection against viral challenge than treatment with antigen and one ligand only[985]; hence, the interplay of B-cell responses and TLR4/7 signaling seemed to confer robust protection from influenza virus infection. TLR7 has also been shown to play a critical role in Th1-mediated immunogenicity triggered by inactivated whole influenza virus vaccine.[610] Despite these findings, the exact roles of TLRs in the induction of B- and T-cell responses to influenza virus infection remain somewhat controversial.[774,1090,1260,1833]

RIG-I (gene name: *DDX58*) is activated by 5′-triphosphate groups on influenza viral RNAs.[82,83,1652,1711] Once activated,

RIG-I interacts with the interferon β promoter stimulator-1 (IPS-1) protein at the mitochondrial membrane,[1551] which leads to the stimulation of IRF3, IRF7, and NF-κB activity. RIG-I expression increases in response to influenza virus infection; the expression of both RIG-I and IPS-1 is essential for the induction of type I IFN and upregulation of IFN-stimulated antiviral genes in mouse embryo fibroblasts.[1259] RIG-I is critical for virus recognition and type I IFN production in fibroblasts, conventional dendritic cells, and epithelial cells.[987,1575]

The inflammasome, a complex of a NOD-like receptor and the ASC adaptor protein, is also activated by influenza virus infection, in a mechanism that may involve M2 ion channel activity.[18,857,858,2059] Inflammasome activation leads to the cleavage and activation of procaspase-1, which in turn cleaves and activates certain cytokines, particularly IL-18 and IL-1β. In human macrophages infected with influenza virus, IL-18 and IL-1β release occurs in a caspase-1–dependent manner, consistent with inflammasome activation in response to infection.[1661] In addition, these two cytokines are upregulated in bronchoalveolar lavage fluids of mice infected with influenza virus, an effect that was not observed in mice deficient in NLRP3 (the prototype NLR), ASC, or caspase-1.[18,857,2059] Mice lacking different components of the inflammasome show increased mortality and delayed viral clearance after influenza virus infection.[18,857,858,2059]

NS1 Interferes with the Activation of PRRs

The activation of PRRs stimulates the synthesis of type I IFN, chemokines, and cytokines. Influenza viruses, primarily through their NS1 protein, have evolved mechanisms to counteract the induction of antiviral responses. Viruses with truncated, deleted, or mutated NS1 proteins induce higher levels of IFN than their wild-type counterparts.[241,380,381,474,703,767,1074,1075,1385,1507,1575,1652,1914,2032] Early studies suggested that NS1 may accomplish this function by sequestering dsRNA, which activates transcription factors such as ATF-2/c-Jun, NFκB, and IFN regulatory factors (IRFs) that stimulate IFN-β production.[1271,1275,2032,2198] However, little dsRNA seems to be produced in influenza virus infected cells,[1652,2211] and mutation of the NS1 amino acids that are critical for dsRNA binding have only limited effects on IFN levels.[381] Rather, NS1 seems to regulate IFN production through two other mechanisms: interference with RIG-I activation and signaling, and interference with the processing of cellular pre-mRNAs.

The NS1 protein interferes with RIG-I activation,[703,1385,1575,1652] most likely by interacting with RIG-I directly,[1385,1652] and/or by interacting with TRIM25,[570] a factor that is required for RIG-I ubiquitination and activation. Moreover, influenza virus infection prevents the activation of IRF-3[436,1073,1575,2032] and blocks IPS-1 (a function that is carried out by the viral polymerase complex[894]). Interestingly, chickens seem to lack RIG-I,[65] which may, at least in part, explain their high susceptibility to influenza virus infections.

NS1 also controls IFN levels by blocking splicing,[545,1270,1694] polyadenylation, and nuclear export of cellular pre-mRNAs (including IFN-β mRNA).[545,1530,1690,1693] This function requires the interaction of NS1 with the 30-kDa subunit of the cleavage and polyadenylation specificity factor (CPSF; gene name: *CPSF4*).[295,378,1073,1483,1530] Two amino acids in NS1 at positions 103 and 106 are critical for CPSF binding and affect virulence.[378,952,1073] Strain-specific differences in the ability to interfere with the maturation of pre-mRNA[952,1073] may contribute to viral pathogenicity. For example, the NS1 of the A(H1N1)pdm09 virus does not efficiently block host gene expression,[719,952] a function that was restored upon the introduction of three human virus-like amino acids at positions 108, 125, and 189, which also increased binding to CPSF.[719] Interestingly, however, these mutations attenuated the virus in mice.[719]

IFN Signaling

Type I IFN acts in an autocrine and paracrine manner through the ubiquitously expressed IFN-α/β receptor (IFNAR). IFNAR loss results in high susceptibility to influenza virus infection[600,1080] but, interestingly, increases survival of mice to secondary bacterial infections.[1835] Activation of IFNAR by type I IFN stimulates the Janus kinase (JAK)/signal transducers and activators of transcription (STAT) pathway. JAK/STAT signaling induces the formation of a transcription factor complex that upregulates the expression of IFN-stimulated genes. The suppressor of cytokines signaling (SOCS) proteins 1 and 3 are upregulated upon influenza virus infection[1621,1672] and counteract type I IFN signaling, likely by interfering with the JAK/STAT pathway. As a consequence, reduced levels of SOCS-3 or lack of this protein reduce influenza virus titers in cell culture.[1621]

Proteins with Antiviral Activity

IFN-induced stimulation of the JAK-STAT pathway results in the induction of IFN-stimulated genes, including those encoding TLRs (suggesting positive feedback loops), PKR, OAS, RNaseL, ISG15, Mx proteins, Viperin, and IFITM.

PKR

Activation of dsRNA-activated protein kinase R (PKR; gene name: *EIF2AK2*) leads to the phosphorylation of the translation initiation factor eIF2α and the subsequent shutdown of protein synthesis. Influenza viruses inhibit PKR activation,[120,749,1271,1280] and a mutant virus lacking NS1 was virulent in PKR$^{-/-}$ mice, but not in wild-type mice.[120] NS1 may block PKR activation through direct binding[1207,1391,2037] and/or sequestration of dsRNA.[749,1271] However, as stated earlier, little dsRNA has been detected in influenza virus–infected cells; in addition, PKR is now also known to be activated by ssRNA with 5′-triphosphate groups,[1475] suggesting that influenza viral RNAs may activate both RIG-I and PKR. PKR activity may also be affected by the influenza virus M2 protein, which binds to the cellular PKR inhibitor p58(IPK), resulting in increased PKR phosphorylation.[683] The role of p58(IPK) in the regulation of PRK activity and influenza pathogenesis is underscored by the finding of increased lung pathology and mortality in influenza virus–infected p58(IPK)$^{-/-}$ mice, compared to wild-type mice.[644]

OAS and RNase L

Two members of the 2′-5′-oligoadenylate synthetase (OAS) family, the OAS1 (gene name: *OAS1*) and OAS-like (gene name: *OASL*) genes are induced upon influenza virus infection.[1381,1390] Activated OAS stimulates RNase L (gene name: *RNASEL*), a single-strand–specific nuclease that degrades cellular and viral RNA, resulting in antiviral activity. Pretreatment of cells with IFN-β had no significant effect on a wild-type virus, but restricted a virus with a mutation in the RNA-binding domain of NS1.[1390] This restriction was relieved in RNase L$^{-/-}$ mouse cells or in cells treated with siRNA to RNase L.[1390] These findings demonstrate that the RNA-binding domain in NS1 controls the antiviral functions of OAS/RNase L.

ISG15

Interferon-stimulated gene 15 (ISG15; gene name: *ISG15*) is conjugated (ISGylated) to its target proteins; this alteration may interfere with the normal (enzymatic) function of the target protein. For example, ISG conjugation promotes IRF3 activation by preventing ubiquitination and subsequent degradation of the transcription factor.[1845] ISG15$^{-/-}$ mice are more susceptible to infection with influenza A and B viruses than are control mice,[1127,1187] and treatment of cells with siRNAs to ISG15 partially impairs IFN-induced antiviral activity.[842] Mechanistically, conjugation of ISG15 to NS1 appears to interfere with NS1 function in several ways: it impairs dimerization of the NS1 RNA-binding domain; disrupts NS1 binding to dsRNA, U6 snRNA, and PKR; interferes with NS1-mediated disruption of antiviral gene expression; and inhibits NS1 association with importin α.[2038,2360] In contrast to the influenza A virus NS1 protein, the influenza B virus NS1 protein blocks the antiviral activity of ISG15 by interfering with E1 ligase for ISG15 modification activity.[2342,2343]

Mx Proteins

Mx proteins are IFN-induced GTPases of the dynamin superfamily. They confer resistance to influenza virus infection[598,723,1228,1942] by interfering with viral replication.[725,727,2383] In particular, they interfere with the replicative activity of the viral ribonucleoprotein complex,[427,2110] perhaps by interacting with and wrapping around the nucleoprotein.[724,2110] Mx proteins have been identified in several mammalian and avian species; most, but not all, inhibit influenza viruses (reviewed in[726]).

Of note, influenza viruses differ in their sensitivity to Mx proteins: in general, avian influenza viruses are more sensitive to inhibition by Mx proteins than human influenza viruses.[427] The replication complex of an HPAI H5N1 virus was significantly affected by human MxA protein,[427] and mice expressing murine Mx1 protein were protected against infection with HPAI H5N1.[2108]

Most conventional laboratory mice, including most commercially available knock-out mice, lack a functional Mx gene.[1940] This fact should be taken into account when interpreting data obtained with such mice.

IFITM

The interferon-induced transmembrane (IFITM) proteins 2 and 3 (gene names: *IFITM2* and *IFITM3*) are ubiquitously expressed cellular proteins with roles in immune cell signaling, oncogenesis, and cell adhesion. Overexpression of IFITM2 and 3 inhibits influenza virus, most likely during cell entry.[169] IFITM3 is modified by palmitoylation; deletion of its palmitoylation site abrogates its antiviral activity against influenza virus.[2329] The underlying mechanism is currently not known.

Viperin

Viperin (gene name: *RSAD2*) is an IFN-stimulated, ER-associated protein expressed in many species from fish to mammals. It inhibits several viruses, including influenza virus, most likely by disrupting lipid rafts, the sites of influenza virus budding.[2197]

Other Strategies to Counteract Innate Immune Responses

The PDZ Domain of the NS1 Protein

A large-scale sequencing project of avian influenza viruses identified a PDZ ligand domain motif at the carboxy-terminal four amino acids of NS1.[1545] This motif is recognized by PDZ domain proteins, a large family of proteins that play multiple roles in cellular processes. Most human influenza viruses possess an RSKV motif, in contrast to the ESEV motif found in most avian influenza viruses. When tested in the background of a laboratory-adapted human H1N1 virus (A/WSN/33), the PDZ ligand domain motifs of pandemic 1918 and HPAI H5N1 viruses conferred increased virulence to viruses in mice,[898] demonstrating the significance of this sequence for influenza viral pathogenicity. Interestingly, the observed differences in virulence did not correlate with IFN expression levels,[898] suggesting that the PDZ ligand domain motif in NS1 affects pathogenicity through a currently unknown mechanism. By contrast, the PDZ ligand domain motif had little effect on the virulence of an HPAI H5N1 in mice and chickens.[2380] Replacement of the avian virus ESEV motif with the human virus RSKV motif in a low pathogenic avian H7N1 virus attenuated the virus in mice.[1930] The ESEV motif binds to the PDZ domain proteins Scribble, Dlg1, and MAGI-1, -2, and -3.[1244] Scribble possesses proapoptotic function and interaction of NS1 with Scribble reduces apoptosis,[1244] suggesting that the PDZ ligand domain motif may regulate the induction of apoptosis in virus-infected cells. Moreover, the PDZ ligand domain motif affects Mx levels,[1930] suggesting a role in the regulation of innate immune responses.

The A(H1N1)pdm09 viruses encode a truncated NS1 protein that lacks the 11 C-terminal amino acids. Reconstitution of this region and thus the PDZ domain does not significantly affect replication, pathogenicity, or transmission in animal models.[718,1592]

NS1 Activates the PI3K/Akt Pathway

PI3K (phosphoinositide-3-kinase) and its most prominent substrate, the serine/threonine protein kinase Akt, regulate many different cellular events including apoptosis, cell metabolism, and proliferation. In addition, PI3K plays a role in the transcriptional regulation of IFN-stimulated genes, and in the regulation of TLR-mediated cytokine production.

The NS1 proteins of influenza A,[475–477,713,714,717,1211,1852,1853] but not influenza B viruses,[476] activate the PI3K/Akt pathway. Although this pathway was believed to have antiviral function, its activation is also required for efficient influenza virus replication.[475,1852] NS1 binds to p85β, a regulatory subunit of PI3K; several residues in NS1 have been identified that are critical for this interaction.[713–715,1211,1851,1853] One study demonstrated that NS1 interacts with phosphorylated Akt, resulting in increased Akt activity.[1337] Activation of the PI3K/Akt pathway may delay the induction of apoptosis,[476,1268,1851,2363,2365] although another study suggested that this process is not regulated through the PI3K pathway.[899] Two recent studies also suggest roles for PI3K in clathrin-independent endocytosis[560] and endosomal acidification,[1316] suggesting that PI3K activation may facilitate virus infection through these processes.

Additional Roles of NS1 in Pathogenicity

In addition to the described functions and key amino acids, several studies have identified amino acids in NS1 that contribute to virulence and possibly also innate immune responses through currently unknown mechanisms.[869,926,1213,1681,1788,1831,1832,1956] For example, the differences in pathogenicity in pigs between NS genes derived from HPAI H5N1 or a non-H5N1 virus were traced to a single amino acid at position 92 of NS1, with glutamic acid at this position conferring higher pathogenicity than aspartic acid.[1831,1832]

Two internal deletions in NS1 affect pathogenicity. Since 2000, most HPAI H5N1 viruses possess a deletion of amino acids 80 to 84 in their NS1 proteins, which enhances virulence.[1258] Of note, during the generation of viruses possessing this deletion, the D92E mutation was co-selected,[1258] suggesting a functional relationship between these two potential virulence determinants. In addition, HPAI H5N1 viruses isolated in 2004 to 2005 in Thailand possessed both the 5-amino-acid deletion at positions 80 to 84 and the D92E mutation.[2007] In virus-infected cells, the 5-amino-acid deletion and the D92E mutation affected responses to TNF-α, or the induction of IFN, respectively.[1210] The other deletion in NS at nucleotides 612 to 626 (resulting in amino acid deletions in both the NS1 and NS2 proteins) also affects IFN induction and virulence.[2378]

Differences Between NS1 Proteins in Their Ability to Affect Innate Immune Responses

NS proteins differ in their ability to counteract cellular IFN responses. Compared to the NS1 proteins of human viruses, the NS1 proteins of HPAI H5N1 viruses induce higher levels of proinflammatory cytokines, such as TNF-α and IFN-β,[300] and confer higher pathogenicity in pigs.[1831] These findings suggest that the NS1 protein of highly pathogenic viruses may cause the cytokine imbalance that was observed in victims of H5N1 infection in Hong Kong in 1997.[95,399,2069,2345] The NS gene of the 1918 pandemic virus interfered with the transcription of IFN-regulated genes more efficiently than did a control virus possessing an NS gene derived from a human virus.[132,612]

Role of Mitogen-Activated Protein Kinase (MAPK) Signaling Pathways in Influenza Virus Infection

Currently, four MAPK signaling pathways are recognized including the extracellular signal regulated kinases 1/2 (ERK1/2), the c-jun-N-terminal kinase (JNK), p38, and ERK5. Activation by external stimuli leads to the phosphorylation of kinases in the signaling cascades, and the phosphorylation of transcription factors such as c-Jun or ATF-2, which are critical for the upregulation of IFN-β, RANTES, and other factors with functions in innate immune responses and apoptosis.

All four MAPK pathways are activated upon influenza virus infection.[611,794,1107,1223,1273,1321,1421,1665,2280] The p38 and ERK1/2 MAPK pathways are strongly activated by HPAI H5N1 viruses, in contrast to H1N1 viruses.[1172] ERK1/2 is important for efficient viral replication[1276,1316,1568,1665,2280] since the influenza HA protein-mediated activation of ERK1/2[1315,1317] appears to be critical for efficient nuclear export of viral ribonucleoprotein complexes.[1665] In addition, ERK1/2 may phosphorylate NS1, which might be critical for efficient virus replication.[716] By contrast, JNK, p38, and ERK5 have antiviral activity through their roles in the regulation of apoptosis and the expression of cytokines and chemokines; p38 may also play a role in influenza virus internalization.[1314]

The PB1-F2 Protein

For some influenza viruses, PB1-F2 increases viral pathogenicity, inflammation, and the frequency and severity of bacterial co-infections in mice.[340,891,1356,1899,2349] These phenotypic differences likely result from the currently known functions of PB1-F2 in the induction of apoptosis and replicative ability.

PB1-F2 localizes to mitochondria,[291,623,2295] where it interacts with the ANT3 (adenine nucleotide translocator 3) and VDAC1 (voltage-dependent anion channel 1) proteins,[2348] and induces the formation of membrane pores with subsequent changes in mitochondrial permeability.[271,783] The resulting induction of apoptosis, which is primarily observed in immune cells,[291,623,2348] may contribute to the increased virulence upon PB1-F2 expression. However, one study suggests that this induction of apoptosis is strain specific and may not be the major function of PB1-F2.[1355]

PB1-F2 enhances inflammatory responses, as demonstrated by an increased influx of inflammatory cells in lungs of mice infected with an influenza virus expressing the PB1-F2 protein from the 1918 pandemic influenza virus.[1356] Enhanced inflammatory responses were observed with PB1-F2 peptides (encompassing the 27 C-terminal amino acids) of an HPAI H5N1 virus and the pandemic 1918, 1957, and 1968 viruses, but not for that of a recent human H3N2 virus.[1355] The PB1-F2 protein of the 1918 pandemic virus encodes serine at position 66, instead of the asparagine commonly found among human influenza viruses at this position. Serine at position 66 of PB1-F2 increased virus titers and pathogenicity, immunopathology, cytokine levels, and the severity of secondary bacterial pneumonia in mice, resulting in higher mortality.[339,340] The increased pathogenicity of the serine variant likely resulted from delayed immune responses, as assessed by transcriptional profiling studies.[339]

PB1-F2 co-localizes and interacts with the polymerase PB1 protein. Lack of PB1-F2 expression results in altered intracellular localization of PB1 and decreased viral polymerase activity,[1352] which may affect virulence. These effects are strain specific and cell type specific.[1357]

Innate Immune Cells

Innate immune cells—including macrophages, neutrophils, dendritic cells, and natural killer (NK) cells—play an important role in the control of influenza virus infections. These cells contribute to virus clearance through phagocytosis or lysis of infected cells, the production of cytokines and chemokines, and/or the stimulation of adaptive immune response. Macrophages and neutrophils phagocytose infected cells and produce chemokines and cytokines. Macrophages also act as professional antigen-presenting cells.[561,748,1033] Infection with highly pathogenic influenza viruses leads to pronounced infiltration of macrophages and neutrophils into the lungs of infected individuals[95,2345] or animals.[76,1068,1639,2105] Inhibition of macrophage and neutrophil phagocytosis,[748] or depletion of alveolar macrophages,[2105] increases virus titers and mortality in mice. By contrast, mice lacking CXCR2 (a receptor on neutrophils) can clear influenza viruses, although they fail to recruit neutrophils to the lung.[2202] Macrophages may also contribute to excessive inflammation and immunopathology since they produce high levels of cytokines/chemokines upon infection with highly pathogenic influenza viruses.[300,848,1180,1405,2340,2368] In addition, macrophages produce nitric oxide synthetase 2 (NOS2), which exacerbates influenza virus infections.[913,1912]

Dendritic cells (DC) present antigens to other immune cells, acting as messengers between the innate and adaptive arms of the immune system. Upon influenza virus infection, they are the major professional antigen-presenting cell and, hence, CD4 and CD8 T cell–stimulating cell population.[128,129,1538] DCs can acquire antigen through direct infection by influenza viruses[114,128,733,1538] or through the phagocytosis of infected epithelial cells.[13,128,739,1790] DCs also produce type I IFN and various cytokines and chemokines.[739] In particular, large amounts of type I IFNs are produced by plasmacytoid dendritic cells, a subset of DCs that is rapidly recruited into the lungs of mice infected with influenza viruses.[2256] The maturation and type I IFN production of respiratory dendritic cells are affected by the NS1 protein.[420,528,767]

NK cells release perforin and granzymes that lead to the lysis of infected cells; in addition, they produce chemokines and cytokines. A large body of data indicates a role for NK cells in innate immunity to influenza virus infections,[7,43,446,608,697,817,1088,1243,1308,1384,1886,1957,1958] and NK cell depletion renders mice and hamsters more susceptible to influenza infections.[1958] NK cells detect influenza viruses through interaction of the NK receptor NKp46 with HA,[7,43,1308,1384] and mice lacking NKp46 show increased morbidity and mortality upon influenza virus infection.[608] The HA proteins of different subtypes may trigger different activation programs in NKs: while an H1 HA triggered NK cell–mediated lysis, additional activation signals for killing were required with an H5 HA.[7] Influenza viruses appear to interfere with NK functions by infecting them[696,1313]: infected NK cells have reduced killing capacity, produce lower amounts of chemokines and cytokines, and eventually die. In several cases of influenza virus infection, low levels of peripheral NK cells were detected[414,779]; however, it is not clear if these cells were killed by influenza viruses or migrated to respiratory organs.

In summary, several immune cell populations have functions that may in parallel dampen and aggravate influenza virus infection. Most likely, a fine balance between temporal, spatial, and quantitative regulation of these cell populations and regulatory factors will contribute to infection outcome.

ADAPTIVE IMMUNE RESPONSES

Mice that lack both B and T cells succumb to influenza virus infection,[428,2060,2230] whereas those lacking either immune cell type can control, although not necessarily clear, influenza virus infections.[115,480,481,1222,1726] These findings demonstrate that adaptive antibody- and T cell–mediated immune responses are important to clear influenza virus infections.

Strain-specific immunity to influenza can be of long duration as reflected in the age-specific attack rates of pandemics with reemergence of a strain, as in the A/USSR H1N1 pandemic in 1977, recall cellular immunity to distant infection,[1158] and neutralizing antibodies to the pandemic 1918 virus or its descendants that were detectable 90 years later.[734,890,1070,1309,1890,2341]

Although murine models clearly demonstrate immune responses that are cross-reactive among influenza strains of the same subtype, the classic teaching in humans based on experiencing recurrent influenza infections is that adaptive immunity is quite strain specific. The rapid drift of B-cell epitopes in influenza viruses due to immune selection suggests that there is strong evolutionary pressure exerted by the collective population immunity. Similar pressure on T-cell epitopes has been suggested, but there appears to be less variability in these sites.[2167]

However, two recent observations suggest immunity that is cross-reactive among influenza viruses of different subtypes in humans. The first is the demonstration of common neutralizing epitopes in the stem of the hemagglutinin.[485,1565,1897,1999,2230] The second is a strong resistance to infection of adults with live, attenuated vaccines with the HA and NA of potentially pandemic strains—for example, H5N1, H7N7, H9N2—that vaccinees have never been infected with.[978]

Humoral Immunity

Serum antibodies play an important role in resistance to and recovery from influenza illness in humans, or at the very least are a strong correlate of immunity.[346,349,616,617,1282,1452] Indicative of the importance of antibody is that immunization of mothers during pregnancy provides protection in infancy through placental transfer of antibody.[2347] Upon infection with influenza viruses, antibodies to the HA, NA, NP, and M proteins are produced, of which antibodies to HA are the most important for virus neutralization.[364,615,616,1674] HA and NA are the primary protective antigens, and antibodies against these glycoproteins are the main mediators of resistance to virus challenge.[346,349,503,1452]

The level of serum antibody to HA and NA correlates with resistance to illness and with restriction of influenza virus replication in the respiratory tract of humans.[326,351,923,980,1456] In addition to the levels of serum antibodies, their avidity is likely important for optimal protection.[187,525,900,1067,1808]

HA antibodies can prevent infection by neutralizing the infectivity of the virus, typically by interfering with HA-mediated receptor binding or fusion.[66,485,1067,1999,2035,2051,2052,2165,2326] Most neutralizing antibodies are believed to bind conformational epitopes. The X-ray crystallographic structures of several HA/antibody complexes have been resolved now[138,485,540,1999] and allow the structural interpretation of antibody binding to HA (for more information on the HA antigenic sites, refer to the Antigenic Drift of the HA Protein section). Although antibodies to HA play the primary role in protection against influenza virus infections, NA antibodies mediate an antiviral effect by limiting virus release and hence restricting virus spread.[350,1029,1456,1675,2226] NA-specific antibodies may have thus ameliorated the severity of the Hong Kong influenza in 1968,[1414] when an H3N2 influenza virus emerged following a reassortment event with a previously circulating H2N2 virus.

Passively transferred monoclonal antibodies to M2 are protective in mice[1433,2077] and M2 antibodies develop in naturally infected humans,[139,526,2092] although the titers are typically low. M2 is highly conserved among influenza A viruses, suggesting its potential as a universal influenza vaccine (see later discussion and Vaccines section). Antibodies to NP have been detected in individuals,[498,685,2000,2302] and vaccination with NP leads to faster virus clearance and reduced mortality in mice.[67,491,502,504,558,1138,1252,1796,2036,2068,2114,2115,2266,2366] Information on the three-dimensional structure of NP[2317] allowed the mapping of several monoclonal antibodies onto NP.[2146] Infection with influenza viruses also elicits antibodies to M1.[364,1019]

A protective effect of transplacentally acquired antibody has been inferred from the correlation between age at the time of symptomatic influenza A virus infection in infants and level of maternally transmitted antibody measured in cord serum.[1682] In addition, vaccination of pregnant women against A(H1N1) pdm09 virus increased the percentage of newborns with protective immunity to influenza virus compared to babies born to unvaccinated mothers,[1683,2382] further suggesting vertically acquired passive immunity.

A vaccine that elicits heterosubtypic immunity against influenza A viruses of different subtypes would no longer require frequent changes in the composition of influenza vaccines. Heterosubtypic immunity was first demonstrated in the 1960s when infection with an influenza virus was shown to reduce virus titers and pathology of a challenge virus belonging to a different subtype in mice.[1820] In contrast, sequential heterotypic infections have been demonstrated in children in a single season[2271]; the prior receipt of a heterotypic cold-adapted vaccine did not alter the pattern of virus shedding with subsequent vaccination while the second dose of the same strain shows no evidence of reinfection. Broadly neutralizing antibodies to HA have been described[344,485,984,1565,1566,1898,1999,2065,2195,2230] that bind to a highly conserved region in the stem region of HA2, and block the low pH–induced conformational changes that mediate membrane fusion. Their broad neutralizing activities and the apparently low rate of escape mutants[344,1999,2195] make HA2 an interesting target for a universal vaccine (see Vaccines section). Cross-protective antibodies against the ectodomain of M2 have also been described.[393,506,514,530,849,1432,1477,2077] Although M2 is immunogenic and antibodies to it are protective in mice,[393,506,514,849,1432,1477,2077] the potential of M2 vaccines in other animal models[514,1706] and humans[1816] is less well established.

A potent antibody-dependent cellular cytotoxicity (ADCC) response has been demonstrated following influenza infection,[747] but it has not been integrated into our conceptualization of the protective immune response to influenza.

Cellular Immunity

The role of cellular immunity in clearance of influenza virus has been well defined in the murine model but is less well understood in humans.[979,1370]

There are two major subsets of effector lymphocytes in humans. The first subset mediates cytotoxicity that is restricted by class I histocompatibility antigens and has the CD8$^+$ phenotype. CD8$^+$ T cells (cytotoxic lymphocyctes, CTLs) eliminate virus through two mechanisms: direct killing of virus-infected cells, and the production of proinflammatory cytokines.[1124] CTLs appear in the blood of infected individuals or those vaccinated with a live virus on days 6 to 14 and largely disappear by day 21.[497] Most studies have examined memory CTLs, which are detected *in vitro* by stimulation of peripheral blood lymphocytes with antigen. These CTLs can exhibit a cross-reactive pattern of virus specificity (i.e., they lyse target cells infected with influenza A viruses belonging to any subtype, but not target cells infected with influenza B virus).[165,473,501,1096,1370,2313,2325,2385] The cross-reactivity of CTL responses likely contributed to the lower infection rate of the elderly with A(H1N1)pdm09 virus, as 50% of influenza-derived T cell epitopes are similar between the pandemic 1918 and 2009 viruses.[662,664] Indeed, both CD8$^+$[2099] and CD4$^+$[609] cells reactive with A(H1N1) pdm09 virus were present prior to infection with this virus. However, a more specific subpopulation of CTLs lyses only cells infected with homologous virus. Depending on human leukocyte antigen (HLA) haplotype, individuals differ considerably in the peptides that their CTLs can recognize.[1371] Memory CTLs characterized after infection or vaccination of humans have the cross-reactive pattern of cytotoxicity. The pre-challenge level of memory CTLs did not correlate with susceptibility to infection or illness after experimental administration of wild-type virus, but did correlate with accelerated clearance of virus from the respiratory tract of humans.[1370]

The other class of T cells is restricted by histocompatibility class II antigens and has the CD4$^+$ phenotype[965,1966]; thus, it belongs to the T-helper class of T cells. CD4$^+$ T cells are helper T cells, providing help to B cells for antibody production and to class I–restricted CTLs for their proliferation.[1132–1134,2325] Helper T cells specific for M or NP antigen can provide help to B cells secreting HA antibody[1132–1134,1798] and, in this manner, can augment the antibody response to protective antigens. CD4$^+$ T cells also have cytolytic activity[661,1979] that is most likely mediated through perforin, rather than Fas:FasL.[179,180]

The important role of CD4$^+$ T cells in immunity to influenza virus infection has been defined by studies in CD8$^+$ T cell–deficient animals, which can clear influenza A virus by a CD4$^+$ T cell–dependent mechanism.[115,480,481,1222] Passively transferred influenza virus–specific CD4$^+$ T-cell clones require functional B cells to clear an ongoing influenza virus infection. Thus, the primary antiviral activity of the CD4$^+$ T cell is probably to help B cells produce antiviral antibodies. Because CD4$^+$ T cells recognize many epitopes on influenza viral proteins, a large number of T cells are available to provide such help.[240]

CD8$^+$ T cells can mediate clearance of influenza A virus infection in CD4$^+$ T cell–deficient animals.[481,1726] In mice lacking CD4$^+$ T cells, primary CD8$^+$ T cell responses are not significantly affected,[1726] in contrast to CD8$^+$ T cell memory formation and recall.[112] Animals deficient in both CD4$^+$ and CD8$^+$ T cells succumb to infection,[428,2060] indicating that nonspecific mediators of immunity are not sufficient in the absence of T cells to contain and clear influenza A virus infection. The number of CD8$^+$ T cell epitopes on viral proteins is much more restricted than the number of B-cell or CD4$^+$ T cell epitopes. Cytolysis of influenza virus–infected cells can also be mediated by antibody plus complement and antibody-armed lymphocytes.[747,1697,1760] While CD8$^+$ T cells play a critical role in virus elimination, they may induce significant immunopathology.[429,1123]

Lymphoproliferation is another measure of the cellular response to influenza. Lymphocytes responsive to influenza virus antigens have been isolated from the blood and lower respiratory tract secretions of influenza virus–infected humans, but only the former have been studied extensively.[949,2325] Lymphocyte blastogenic responses to influenza antigens in humans increase after influenza A virus infection, beginning between the third and sixth day after infection,[430] and return to baseline levels by day 28.

Invariant NKT (iNKT) cells (also referred to as type I NKT cells) are the most prevalent NKT cells in mice. Their name reflects the invariant T cell receptor α chain expressed by these cells. Activated iNKT cells appear to play roles in both cell- and antibody-mediated immunity,[1108] and produce large amounts of interferons and cytokines such as IFN-γ and

IL-4.[2109] Stimulation of iNKT in mice reduced virus titers compared to control mice,[818] and mice lacking iNKT cells show a higher mortality rate than wild-type mice.[403] Moreover, use of an iNKT activator as an adjuvant for influenza vaccination results in increased immunogenicity and protection.[1086] These findings suggest a contribution of iNKT cells to immunity against influenza viruses.

Influenza A virus infection can depress skin test reactivity to common antigens used to assess cutaneous delayed hypersensitivity.[1710] In addition, depression of the peripheral blood lymphocyte blastogenic responses to mitogenic and antigenic stimulation[430,1196] is seen during the acute stage of infection and early convalescence. Despite this transient depression of delayed hypersensitivity and blastogenic responses to noninfluenza antigens or mitogens, influenza virus–specific cellular responses develop. The mechanisms underlying the depression in the function of lymphocytes in influenza virus infection indicated earlier have not been defined, but influenza A virus infection can abortively infect human lymphocytes *in vitro*[188] and possibly *in vivo*.[2251]

Mucosal Antibody Response

Francis[552] was the first to detect neutralizing activity to influenza in nasal secretions. He subsequently showed that resistance to experimental influenza A virus infection in mice was mediated by an antibody in bronchial secretions. The neutralizing antibody in the nasal secretions of humans is primarily locally produced IgA.[44,1756] Antibody to both HA and NA can be detected in local secretions, but the former is easier to detect.[349] It has been proposed that IgA antibodies can act intracellularly during transcytosis to the apical surface to inhibit virus replication and thus participate in clearance of infectious virus from the epithelial cells and lumen of the respiratory tract.[1351,1720] IgA and IgG may switch in relative importance between the upper and lower respiratory tract as shown in a murine model of the protective role of passive neutralizing antibody.[1721]

During primary viral infection, IgA, IgG, and IgM hemagglutinin-specific antibodies can be detected in nasal washes by use of an enzyme-linked immunosorbent assay (ELISA). IgA and IgM antibodies are detected more frequently than IgG antibody.[1457] Most of the HA-specific IgA and IgM antibodies are actively secreted locally, whereas local secretion has been demonstrated only infrequently for IgG antibody, although a receptor for IgG transport is present on bronchial epithelial cells.[2327] Individuals with a local IgA response also have a serum IgA response. Local IgA antibody stimulated by natural infection is detectable for 3 to 5 months after infection, and there is local IgA memory for influenza antigen.[1452] After secondary infection, local antibody is also primarily of the IgA isotype, those with a local IgA response also have a serum IgA response, and the magnitude of the serum IgA HA antibody response correlates with that of the local response.

The presence of local IgA antibody induced by infection with an attenuated virus correlates with resistance of volunteers to infection and illness after challenge with a virulent wild-type virus.[935] Challenge of children with an attenuated live vaccine shows similar findings.[162,163] Resistance to experimental wild-type infection also correlates with the level of local HA antibody present at the time of virus administration, with IgG and IgA each contributing to resistance.[326]

SURVEILLANCE

Surveillance efforts in humans have increased considerably in recent years. These efforts are coordinated by the WHO through the Global Influenza Surveillance and Response System (GISRS; formerly the Global Influenza Surveillance Network, GISN) that was founded in 1952 and currently includes five Collaborating Centres (in Atlanta, Beijing, London, Melbourne, and Tokyo), 136 National Influenza Centres in 106 countries, 11 H5 Reference Laboratories, and four Essential Regulatory Laboratories (http://influenzacentre.org/centre_GISN.htm). The National Influenza Centres collect more than 175,000 samples each year from patients with influenza-like illness and submit approximately 2,000 representative samples per year to the Collaborating Centres for antigenic and genetic characterization. These data are used to monitor antigenic drift and resistance to antiviral compounds. Based on surveillance, antigenic, and genetic data, vaccine viruses are recommended by the WHO each February and September for the Northern and Southern Hemispheres, respectively.

Summaries of influenza activity are published in the *Morbidity and Mortality Weekly Report* from the Centers for Disease Control and Prevention (CDC) during the influenza season and in the *Weekly Epidemiologic Record* published by the WHO. An even more current report of influenza epidemiology is available at the CDC FluView website (www.cdc.gov/flu/weekly). These reports are linked with reports of pneumonia and influenza deaths in 121 US cities to monitor the emergence of an influenza epidemic. Surveillance in the face of highly pathogenic H5N1 viruses has focused not only on human illness, but also on causes of mortality in domestic and wild birds. There continues to be a strengthening of routine surveillance particularly in China and Southeast Asia to identify the emerging strains that inform the choice of vaccine components for the coming influenza season. The threat has propelled countries around the world to prepare for an influenza pandemic. The US plan can be found at www.hhs.gov/nvpo/pandemicplan; since its release in 2005, the plan has been updated to reflect the guidelines established during the H1N1 pandemic in 2009.

DIAGNOSIS

Several diagnostic tests are available to detect influenza A and B viruses, including viral culture, reverse transcriptase-polymerase chain reaction (RT-PCR), immunofluorescence assays, and rapid antigen testing. Growth of samples in eukaryotic cells is still considered the gold standard but requires 3 to 10 days (pertinent cell lines are described in the Virus Propagation section). This time can be reduced to 1 to 3 days. Influenza virus in culture can be detected by using immunoassays or RT-PCR. PCR-based diagnosis is significantly more sensitive than culture. RT-PCR is now the method of choice in many diagnostic labs since it combines several attractive features: it is highly sensitive (which, on the other hand, requires good laboratory practices and stringent controls to avoid or monitor for cross-contamination); it has reasonable test times since data can be obtained within 1 day; and it can be designed to distinguish between different types and subtypes, depending on the sets of oligonucleotides used. In addition, multiplexing is possible to test multiple samples at once, or to test for more than one viral RNA segment in one reaction.

In recent years, multiple rapid influenza diagnostic tests have been developed and approved for the analysis of human samples. Most of these are immunoassays that detect the NP antigen. Some of these can distinguish between influenza A and B viruses. Currently available rapid influenza diagnostic tests provide results within 5 to 30 minutes, but have a low sensitivity rate of about 40% to 70%. Indirect immunofluorescence assays are not widely used for routine diagnostics since they are not conducive to high-throughput testing or multiplexing. Overviews of currently recommended diagnostic tests and rapid tests can be found at http://www.cdc.gov/flu/professionals/diagnosis/, http://www.cdc.gov/flu/professionals/diagnosis/rapidlab.htm, and http://www.who.int/csr/disease/avian_influenza/guidelines/RapidTestInfluenza_web.pdf. The standard protocols for the diagnosis of influenza viruses from avian species (some of which are also used for the diagnosis of human samples) can be found in the OIE Manual of Diagnostic Tests and Vaccines for Terrestrial Animals 2010 (http://www.oie.int/international-standard-setting/terrestrial-manual/access-online/).

The available tests can be carried out with nasopharyngeal or throat swabs, bronchial washes, nasal or endotracheal aspirate, or sputum. The tests can differ in their sensitivity and specificity for different types of specimens. In general, nasopharyngeal specimens collected with a swab are more sensitive than throat swab samples. Samples should be collected as soon as possible after the onset of symptoms. In adults, virus shedding typically declines on days 4 to 5 after the onset of symptoms, making virus detection difficult. Children typically shed virus for longer periods of time.

Serologic testing to assess influenza A virus subtypes and HA antigenic drift variants is typically carried out by using hemagglutination inhibition (HI) or microneutralization assays. These assays are used by the WHO because of their reliability, but are not recommended for standard diagnostic testing because of their complexity.

ANTIVIRALS

Four antiviral compounds—the M2 ion channel inhibitors amantadine and rimantadine, and the neuraminidase inhibitors oseltamivir and zanamivir—are currently approved in many countries for use in humans. Additional neuraminidase inhibitors such as peramivir and laninamivir received temporary emergency approval during the H1N1 pandemic in 2009, and/or are licensed in Japan and Korea. Most H1N1 and H3N2 viruses currently circulating in humans are sensitive to neuraminidase inhibitors; in contrast, more than 90% of currently circulating H1N1 and H3N2 viruses are resistant to the ion channel inhibitors. Accordingly, this latter class of compounds is no longer recommended for use in humans.[535]

Amantadine and Rimantadine

Amantadine hydrochloride and rimantadine, an analog of amantadine, were licensed for prophylactic and therapeutic use against influenza A virus in humans in the United States in the 1960s. These compounds are active against all subtypes of influenza A virus, but not against influenza B or C viruses.[209]

Amantadine and rimantadine are adamantane derivatives. Both compounds have a tricyclic structure with an amine side group. They inhibit virus replication by blocking the acid-activated ion channel formed by the virion-associated M2 protein.[110,757,758,872,1659,1660,1997,2192,2239] The primary antiviral action of these compounds results from blocking the flow of H^+ ions from the acidified endosome into the interior of the virion, a process necessary for release of ribonucleoprotein complexes into the cytosol for transport to the nucleus. These compounds also inhibit the replication of viruses that have multiple basic amino acids at their HA cleavage site by inhibiting M2 ion channel activity in the *trans*-Golgi network, which prevents the premature low pH-induced conformational change of HAs cleaved by furin.[316,1764,1782]

Until 2004, amantadine and rimantadine were used to treat infections caused by seasonal influenza A viruses.[25,575,720,1056,1057] Symptomatic improvement, including accelerated clearance of local symptoms and fever, occurs about 1 day earlier in treated than in untreated patients, and peripheral airway dysfunction also resolves more quickly. Accelerated clearance of symptoms was seen in children infected with an H3N2 virus treated with rimantadine compared with control children who received an antipyretic.[720]

Amantadine and rimantadine have also been used for prophylaxis against seasonal influenza A virus infections.[25,36,387,431,915,1141,1412,1622,1646,1725,1828,1908–1910,2073,2074,2381] During an epidemic involving both influenza A H1N1 and H3N2 viruses, amantadine and rimantadine protected against influenza-like illness (78% and 65%, respectively), documented influenza illness (91% and 85%, respectively), and influenza A virus infection (74% and 66%, respectively).[431] Lower efficacy rates against documented illness (70%) and infection (39%) were observed for amantadine prophylaxis during an H1N1 virus epidemic in 1977.[1412]

At the recommended adult dose of amantadine or rimantadine (i.e., 100 mg twice daily orally), significant adverse effects have not been reported (reviewed in[904]).

Resistance to adamantanes is conferred by mutations at position 26, 27, 30, 31, 34, or 38 of M2, with mutations at position 27, 30, or 31 found most frequently.[110,757,758,1658,2008] Structural studies of the M2 ion channel in the absence and presence of amantadine[210,1805,1976] show that the channel is relatively narrow at position Val27, but opens into a wider cavity that is lined by Ala30 and Ser31 (among other amino acids), providing structural information on the effect of mutations at these critical positions.

In experimental settings, resistant variants emerge rapidly and frequently.[788,1587,1588,1590,2176] Until 2004, the rates of resistance among seasonal influenza viruses remained low,[102,389,2379] although adamantane-resistant variants had been isolated from infected individuals.[408,493,765,776,893,1325,1587,1629,1774,1775,1803,1861] During the 2003 to 2004 season, the rate of adamantane-resistant seasonal H3N2 viruses increased to 12.3%.[175] One year later, more than 90% of seasonal H3N2 viruses had acquired adamantine resistance,[176,416,761,799,1175,1383,1773] typically conferred by a Ser-to-Asn mutation at position 31 of M2. At that time, many seasonal H1N1 viruses remained sensitive to ion channel inhibitors.[73,416,799] In 2009, the seasonal H1N1 viruses were largely replaced by the novel A(H1N1)pdm09 viruses, which are resistant to adamantanes.[253] Hence, the H1N1 and H3N2 viruses circulating in humans since 2009 are resistant to adamantanes, thus use of these compounds is no longer recommended.[535,537]

Several avian H5 viruses isolated before the emergence of the currently circulating HPAI H5N1 viruses were found to be resistant to amantadine.[2176] For HPAI H5N1 viruses, the rate of adamantine resistance varies greatly depending on their geographic origin.[199,299,772,801,853,866,1163,1686] Based on sequence analysis, avian H6 viruses should be sensitive to amantadine[866]; among H7 and H9 viruses, some were identified with mutations known to confer resistance to adamantanes.[866] Many European swine viruses of several lineages are resistant to adamantanes,[1099,1804] likely because their M genes belong to the same phylogenetic lineage.[1099] The pandemic 1918 virus is sensitive to ion channel inhibitors.[1714,2103]

Neuraminidase Inhibitors

The neuraminidase inhibitors oseltamivir and zanamivir were approved in the United States in 1999.[1460] They are effective against influenza A and B viruses and are currently recommended for "all persons with suspected or confirmed influenza requiring hospitalization or who have progressive, severe or complicated illness regardless of previous health or vaccination status".[535]

The recommended treatment differs by age group (summarized in[535]). Five-day courses are recommended for therapeutic treatment, while longer courses may be used for prophylactic treatment. Oseltamivir is administered orally as a granulated powder in capsules. The standard dose for adults is 75 mg, twice daily. Oseltamivir is currently approved for persons aged 1 year and older. During the H1N1 pandemic in 2009, emergency approval was granted in the United States (http://www.cdc.gov/h1n1flu/recommendations.htm), Europe (http://www.ema.europa.eu/docs/en_GB/document_library/EPAR_-_Product_Information/human/000402/WC500033106.pdf), and several other countries for the use of oseltamivir in infants younger than 1 year of age. Zanamivir is provided as a powder and administered by inhalation. For adults, two daily inhalations (5 mg each) are recommended for the treatment of infections, whereas one daily inhalation of 10 mg is recommended for prophylactic purposes. Zanamivir is approved for persons aged 7 years or older. Adverse effects to neuraminidase inhibitors include vomiting, abdominal pain, and nausea, but are generally mild[762,763,1642,2171] (reviewed in[462]).

The first NA inhibitors included DANA (2-deoxy-2,3-dihydro-*N*-acetylneuraminic acid; Neu5Ac2en) and its *N*-trifluoroacetyl analog FANA, which were effective *in vitro*[1379,1600] but did not inhibit replication of influenza viruses in animals.[1601] After resolution of the NA structure,[338,2145] DANA served as the lead compound in the rational design of drugs targeting the NA protein. Replacement of the 4-hydroxyl group on DANA with a guanidino group filled the unoccupied pocket in the NA active site with an inhibition constant (K_i) of 2×10^{-10} mol/L,[2168,2262] resulting in zanamivir (5-(acetylamino)-4-[(aminoiminomethyl)-amino]-2,6-anhydro-3,4,5-trideoxy-D-glycero-D-galacto-non-2-enonic acid, also called 4-guanidino-Neu5Ac2en).

An additional NA inhibitor, oseltamivir, was developed during the following years. This was achieved through the discovery and use of a hydrophobic pocket in the enzyme-active center that could accommodate lipophilic groups necessary to improve the inhibitor's oral bioavailability.[1032,1834] The resulting compound, oseltamivir, is administered in the form of a prodrug, oseltamivir phosphate; in the liver, oseltamivir phosphate is converted into the active form, oseltamivir carboxylate (reviewed in[383]). Finally, an intravenously administered NA inhibitor, peramivir, was approved for emergency use in hospitalized patients during the H1N1 pandemic in 2009 but is not presently considered an option (except for Japan and Korea).[908]

The efficacy of oseltamivir and zanamivir in the treatment and prevention of influenza A and B virus infections have been assessed in a number of studies.[25,201,461,535,904,916–918,1328,1875,2040] Both compounds are also effective against A(H1N1)pdm09 viruses.[704,909,1887] In general, the initiation of treatment within 48 hours of the onset of symptoms is critical[360,434,517,1177,1179,1261,1887,2334]; however, treatment later in infection may still provide some benefit.[1173,1177–1179,1365,1887]

For uncomplicated infections with seasonal influenza viruses, both drugs reduce the duration of illness by about 1 day (if treatment is started early). In addition, the amount of virus shed appears to be reduced. Several studies suggest that neuraminidase inhibitors also reduce the risk of severe complications.[272,736,778,936,953,1177–1179,2243]

Oseltamivir is effective against HPAI H5N1 viruses. It improves the outcome of mice[659,1186,2324] and ferrets[151,658] infected with highly pathogenic viruses. Data from infected individuals suggest that treatment with NA inhibitors improves survival rates; early treatment was again noted as a critical factor.[2,796,957,959,1220,1829] Based on these findings, NA inhibitors are recommended by the WHO as the primary treatment for human HPAI H5N1 virus infections (http://www.who.int/csr/disease/avian_influenza/guidelines/pharmamanagement/en/index.html). Although treatment with NA inhibitors improves the outcome of HPAI H5N1 infections in humans, a significant percentage of individuals still succumb to the infection; in one example, even early treatment of infected individuals resulted in the emergence of resistant variants (see later discussion) and death of the treated patients.[400] Higher doses and prolonged treatment with neuraminidase inhibitors have shown additional benefits in animal studies[151,2324] and also in infected individuals.[2]

Oseltamivir may also be efficacious in the prophylaxis or treatment of human infections with avian viruses of the H7 subtype. During the H7N7 virus outbreak in The Netherlands in 2003 (see Transmission of Avian Influenza Viruses to Humans section), health care workers and their close contacts were prophylactically treated with oseltamivir, which likely prevented severe infections[1376]; the reported cases of conjunctivitis[546,1085] and death[2135] were limited to individuals who did not take oseltamivir.

Treatment with neuraminidase inhibitors does not appear to prevent the development of humoral antibodies, which is critical to protect against reinfection with antigenically similar viruses. Ferret studies have demonstrated protection against reinfection,[151,658] and seroconversion has also been noted in individuals.[171,257]

Resistance to Neuraminidase Inhibitors

Variants with reduced sensitivity to oseltamivir or zanamivir can be selected experimentally,[72,143,334,687,691,1368,1383,1950,2021] and have been isolated from patients treated with neuraminidase inhibitors (see later discussion). Mutations that confer resistance to neuraminidase inhibitors are summarized in e-Table 41.1; most of these mutations map to catalytic sites in NA (R118, D151, R152, R224, E276, R292, R371, and Y406;

N2 numbering),[2145] or framework sites (E119, R156, W178, S179, D/N198, I222, E227, H274, E277, N294, and E425; N2 numbering)[2145] that stabilize the active site. The most frequently identified mutations are R292K or E119V for H3N2 viruses,[35,686,1367,2064] and H274Y for H1N1 viruses.[35,686,1367,2064] Most oseltamivir-resistant viruses remain sensitive to zanamivir.

Resistance to zanamivir is extremely rare in treated patients,[690] likely because of the structural differences between zanamivir and oseltamivir.[337,1767] However, several viruses have been isolated that are resistant to both zanamivir and oseltamivir (e-Table 41.1), including these following 5 viruses. (1) An A(H1N1)pdm09 virus isolated from an immunocompromised child possessing H274Y and I222R mutations that were acquired during treatment with oseltamivir, and subsequent treatment with zanamivir, respectively; the I222R mutation rendered the virus less susceptible to zanamivir, oseltamivir, and peramivir (see Other Antivirals Against Influenza section).[2127] (2) Another A(H1N1)pdm09 virus with H274Y and I222R mutations was isolated from an immunocompromised child sequentially treated with oseltamivir and zanamivir; retrospective analysis revealed that both mutations had emerged before the initiation of zanamivir treatment.[1512] (3) H274Y/I222V mutations were reported for oseltamivir-resistant viruses isolated from two individuals who developed A(H1N1)pdm09 virus infection after prophylactic treatment with oseltamivir.[247] (4) In an infant with no history of neuraminidase inhibitor treatment, an influenza B variant possessing a D197E (D198E in N2 numbering) mutation in NA was detected, in addition to wild-type virus.[1544] While viruses with a D197N mutation are known to confer resistance to oseltamivir,[686,751,879] the D197E mutation had not been described. Of note, the D197E mutation conferred resistance to oseltamivir, zanamivir, and peramivir (see Other Antivirals Against Influenza section).[1544] The crystal structures of the D197 (wild-type) and D197E (resistant) variants have been resolved with and without inhibitor,[1544] and revealed that the D197E mutation affects the interaction with the *N*-acetyl group of sialic acid and NA inhibitors. (5) Zanamivir treatment of a ferret experimentally infected with an HPAI H5N1 virus yielded a zanamivir-resistant variant possessing a Q136L mutation in NA.[852] This mutation also conferred reduced sensitivity to oseltamivir.[852]

Overall, the rate of resistance to oseltamivir remained relatively low until 2007 to 2008, and resistance was observed more often with H1N1 viruses[689,1961,2233] than with H3N2[88,377,879,1051,1563,1961] or influenza B viruses.[879] Only 8 of 2287 influenza A and B isolated from humans during routine surveillance between 1999 and 2002 showed reduced susceptibility to oseltamivir.[1416] Another analysis of 1050 viruses isolated during surveillance in 2000 to 2002 found no mutations at positions known to confer resistance to neuraminidase inhibitors.[1438] A Japanese study reported resistance rates of 0.3% to 2.2% for viruses isolated in 2003 to 2007,[1289] whereas a global surveillance study of viruses isolated in 2004 to 2007 reported a resistance rate of 0.4% (12/3261).[1844] Another study of almost 2,000 patients treated with oseltamivir found resistance rates of 0.33% and 4.0% for viruses isolated from adults or children, respectively.[35] Resistance emerges frequently after prolonged treatment of immunocompromised patients, in whom the viruses replicate for extended periods of time.[88,248,352,457,690,800,879,1382,1543,1563,2233]

During the 2007 to 2008 season, an increase in the number of oseltamivir-resistant H1N1 viruses was noted: in the United States, 6.4% of isolates were resistant,[1844] while this number was even higher in Europe (with a resistance rate of ~20%) (http://ecdc.europa.eu/en/activities/surveillance/EISN/Newsletter/SUN_EISN_INFL_Bulletin_2008week16.pdf). In Europe, large differences were reported from country to country, with resistance rates between 1% in Italy and 68% in Norway.[1092,1377] In 2008, 64% of seasonal H1N1 viruses tested in the Southern Hemisphere were resistant to oseltamivir,[851] and by March 2009, 1291 of 1362 seasonal H1N1 viruses analyzed had acquired resistance (http://www.who.int/csr/disease/influenza/H1N1webupdate20090318%20ed_ns.pdf). Clinical data indicate that oseltamivir-resistant H1N1 viruses are comparable in their severity to oseltamivir-sensitive viruses,[194,317,417,755,1377] a finding that is consistent with studies in ferrets.[732]

In 2009, the oseltamivir-resistant H1N1 viruses were largely replaced by A(H1N1)pdm09 viruses. Most A(H1N1)pdm09 viruses are sensitive to neuraminidase inhibitors; however, up to 1% of viruses are oseltamivir resistant.[89,218,222,247,248,352,457,745,871,1166,1382,1512,1933,2057,2064,2083,2127,2188]

Currently, most HPAI H5N1 viruses are sensitive to neuraminidase inhibitors, although several resistant variants have been isolated.[400,464,606,636,800,801,853,1164] Of particular concern, avian surveillance studies have identified a number of HPAI H5N1 viruses with NA mutations that are known to confer resistance to neuraminidase inhibitors.[1578]

Early studies indicated that viruses resistant to oseltamivir are attenuated in animal models, as demonstrated for lab-adapted H1N1 viruses,[5,142] seasonal H1N1[787,892] and H3N2 viruses,[160,234,786,2021] an avian H4N2 virus,[691] and artificially generated viruses.[2321] Based on these findings, viruses resistant to neuraminidase inhibitors were not expected to out-compete the viruses circulating at the time. This assumption was consistent with the finding that oseltamivir-resistant viruses isolated from treated individuals did not transmit efficiently among humans (exceptions include an oseltamivir-resistant influenza B virus that may have arisen spontaneously or was transmitted from a treated patient,[751] and a community cluster of oseltamivir-resistant A(H1N1)pdm09 viruses.[1166] Therefore, the rapid spread of oseltamivir-resistant seasonal H1N1 viruses in 2007 to 2008 was unexpected. However, these viruses possess additional mutations in NA (V234M and R222Q) that compensate for the loss of viral fitness due to the H274Y mutation.[147]

In animal models, some oseltamivir-resistant A(H1N1)pdm09 viruses appear attenuated,[450] while others are comparable in their pathogenicity and transmissibility to oseltamivir-sensitive A(H1N1)pdm09 viruses[732,1052,1830]; the latter finding raises concerns that the resistant variants may supersede sensitive viruses, as was observed in 2007 to 2008 with seasonal H1N1 viruses. This concern is potentiated by increasing numbers of A(H1N1)pdm09 viruses possessing an S247N mutation that confers reduced sensitivity to oseltamivir and zanamivir.[850] In an oseltamivir-treated patient, this mutation was found in combination with the H274Y mutation, resulting in extremely high resistance to oseltamivir.[850]

Combination Therapy

Although a number of influenza viruses have acquired resistance to adamantane or neuraminidase inhibitors, HPAI H5N1 viruses remain largely sensitive to both classes of compounds. Therefore, the combined use of adamantanes and neuraminidase inhibitors has been assessed in several *in vitro* and *in vivo* studies.[574,657,865,867,1323,1425] The combination of amantadine and oseltamivir was well tolerated in volunteers,[1425] and superior to monotherapy in terms of efficacy in mice.[867,1323] Similarly, the combination of rimantadine with oseltamivir, zanamivir, or peramivir provided additive effects in cell culture[657] and mice.[574] Combination therapy could reduce the rate of emergence of resistant variants, as demonstrated in one study in cell culture.[865]

Other Antivirals Against Influenza

Peramivir, a neuraminidase inhibitor that is administered intravenously, received market authorization in Japan and Korea in 2010. In several other countries, including the United States, peramivir is currently in clinical trials[54] (http://www.clinicaltrials.gov/ct2/show/NCT00958776?term=biocryst%2C+peramivir&rank=1; accessed 06/05/2011). During the H1N1 pandemic in 2009, peramivir was available in the United States by Emergency Use Authorization (which expired in June 2010).[135,789] Its efficacy has been assessed in mice and ferrets,[1878,2346] and limited data on peramivir use in humans suggest a reduction in the duration of symptoms.[74,213,789] Several mutations that confer resistance to oseltamivir also render those viruses resistant to peramivir (e-Table 41.1).

Laninamivir, a long-lasting inhaled NA inhibitor, is effective against oseltamivir-resistant influenza viruses.[2204,2304] It is licensed in Japan[1102,2304] and is in clinical trials in other countries.[2204,2304]

T-705 (favipiravir) is an antiviral compound currently in phase II clinical trials in the United States (http://www.fujifilmholdings.com/en/pdf/investors/library/ff_announcement_20100215_001.pdf); in Japan, a phase III clinical trial has been completed (http://www.clinicaltrials.jp/user/showCteDetailE.jsp?japicId=JapicCTI-090934). It has favorable pharmacokinetics in cell culture[1895] and is effective against influenza A, B, and C viruses,[564,1877,2023] including HPAI H5N1 viruses sensitive or resistant to oseltamivir.[1053,1891,1896] T-705 inhibits the viral polymerase[565] but, unlike ribavirin, does not affect cellular DNA or RNA polymerases.[565] T-705 may be attractive for combination therapy with a neuraminidase inhibitor.[1896] Other targets include both viral and host pathways involved in influenza replication.[760] An example would be the host-encoded proteases that cleave the influenza HA[2364] (see HA cleavage section).

VACCINES

Vaccination is one of the most effective methods for preventing influenza virus infections and complications.[355] Both inactivated and live attenuated vaccines are available against seasonal influenza viruses. These vaccines are currently trivalent, that is, they contain influenza A virus components of the H1N1 and H3N2 subtypes, and an influenza B virus component. Trivalent inactivated vaccines can be used for persons older than 6 months of age, while live attenuated vaccine is currently approved in the United States for healthy, nonpregnant individuals 2 to 49 years of age. In 2009, monovalent vaccines to A(H1N1)pdm09 virus were used widely. In the 2010 to 2011 season, A(H1N1)pdm09 virus became part of the trivalent vaccine and replaced the former seasonal H1N1 component. In addition, several vaccines to HPAI H5N1 viruses have been approved. Other vaccines to H5, H7, and H9 viruses are in development.

Seasonal Inactivated Vaccines

Based on the immune status of the populations, and on antigenic and genetic information about circulating viruses (obtained through surveillance studies), the vaccine strains are recommended each year by the WHO (see Surveillance section). Since this decision has to be made more than 6 months prior to the influenza season, the selected vaccine strains occasionally differ antigenically from the viruses circulating during the subsequent influenza season. Limited antigenic match between the selected vaccine strains and the actually circulating strains may result in low efficacy (see Efficacy of Seasonal Influenza Vaccines section). After vaccine virus selection, so-called seed strains are generated that possess at least the HA and NA genes of the selected vaccine strains, and the remaining genes from the A/Puerto Rico/8/34 (A/PR/8/34; H1N1) virus, which confers a high level of growth in eggs.[1740] Traditionally, these seed viruses were generated by co-infecting cells with A/PR/8/34 virus and the donor virus of the HA and NA genes, and subsequent selection with antibodies to select viruses with the desired gene constellation. Although not yet used widely, reverse genetics methods (see Reverse Genetics section) can be used to accomplish this task faster and in a more controlled manner. As an alternative to these reassortant vaccine viruses, some countries use the WHO-recommended wild-type viruses for vaccination.

Most vaccine viruses are grown in the allantoic cavity of embryonated chicken eggs; in this system, however, they may acquire mutations in HA that can change the antigenic properties of the virus (see Virus Propagation and Host Cell–Mediated Selection of Antigenic Variants sections). In Europe and in the U.S., vaccines produced in MDCK cells are now also marketed. Several theoretical advantages exist for preparation of vaccine in mammalian cells including maintaining the mammalian HA phenotype and relative easiness of capacity expansion compared to egg-based vaccine production.[2267]

For vaccine virus production in embryonated chicken eggs, virus present in the allantoic fluid is purified and concentrated by zonal centrifugation or column chromatography and inactivated with formalin or beta-propiolactone. The resulting preparations are referred to as whole virus vaccine; due to their reactogenicity, whole virus vaccines are no longer used widely. Vaccine virus preparations may be further disrupted by treatment with chemicals (split vaccine) and partially purified to remove viral ribonucleoprotein complexes (subunit vaccine). Split and subunit vaccines are often collectively referred to as subvirion vaccines. In addition, so-called virosomal subunit vaccines can be generated by treating viruses with detergent, followed by ultracentrifugation to remove viral ribonucleoprotein complexes. After the extraction of detergent, membrane vesicles form that contain the HA and NA proteins.[2250] Collectively, these purification procedures have greatly reduced the incidence of local and systemic reactions.

The quantity of immunoreactive HA in each dose is standardized to contain the amount recommended by the Advisory Committee on Immunization Practices, which is usually 15 μg per component for adults and older children or 7.5 μg for children younger than 3 years. The quantity of NA is not standardized because this glycoprotein is highly labile during purification and storage.[1012,1015] Each 0.5-mL dose of vaccine contains approximately 10 billion virus particles, and one egg yields one to three doses of vaccine. Vaccine also contains variable but small quantities of endotoxin, egg-derived protein, free formaldehyde, and most have thiomersal preservative, all of which do not appear to contribute to the reactogenicity or toxicity of the vaccines for humans. Inactivated vaccines are administered intramuscularly or, less often, subcutaneously or intradermally.

Seasonal Live Attenuated Vaccines

A live attenuated vaccine based on the A/Ann Arbor/6/60 (A/AA/6/60; H2N2) and B/Ann Arbor/1/66 (B/AA/1/66)[108,472,1294,1451] viruses was developed in the United States and approved in 2003.[108,1517,2080] A different live attenuated vaccine based on the A/Leningrad/134/17/57 and B/USSR/60/69 viruses has been used in the Russian Federation since the 1960s.[16,1011,1014]

The A/AA/6/60 master donor virus was developed by passage of the wild-type virus at progressively lower temperatures in primary chicken kidney cell cultures until a mutant was identified that replicated efficiently at 25°C, a temperature restrictive for the replication of wild-type virus.[1294,1295] The donor virus is temperature sensitive (*ts;* i.e., restricted in its replication at 38°C to 39°C, temperatures permissive for the replication of wild-type virus); cold adapted (*ca;* i.e., replicates efficiently at 25°C); and attenuated (*att;* i.e., restricted in its replication in the upper and lower respiratory tract of ferrets). The attenuated B/AA/1/66 master donor virus was developed by using a similar approach.

For the A/AA/6/60 master donor virus, the *ts* and *att* phenotypes are each defined by mutations in the PB2, PB1, and NP proteins,[929,931] while the mutations that define the *ca* phenotype have not been identified. For the B/AA/1/66 master donor virus, the *att, ts,* and *ca* phenotypes are defined by mutations in the PA, NP, and M1 proteins[823]; the PA and NP[823] proteins; or the PB2, PA, and NP proteins,[294] respectively. The type A and type B master donor viruses differ by only seven or eight amino acids from the respective wild-type viruses; however, each of the characterized phenotypes is conferred by at least two mutations in different proteins, and reversion to wild type has not been observed.[1010,1453,2152]

The attenuated A/Leningrad/134/17/57 virus was developed through 17 sequential passages in embryonated chicken eggs at 25°C. It differs by eight amino acids from the parental virus, which map to the PB2, M1, M2, and NS2 proteins (one amino acid change each), and the PB1 and PA proteins (two amino acid changes each).[1062] The *ts* phenotype is conferred by mutations in the polymerase proteins.[874,1047] The *ts* phenotype of the attenuated B/USSR/60/69 virus is defined by mutations in the PB2 and PA genes.[1048]

Originally, seed viruses for vaccine production were generated by co-infecting, for example, the A/AA/6/60 master donor virus with the recommended vaccine viruses, followed by selection of reassortant progeny viruses at 25°C (restrictive for replication of wild-type virus) in the presence of an H2N2 antiserum, which inhibits replication of viruses bearing the surface antigens of the attenuated A/AA/6/60 master donor virus. In the United States, live attenuated vaccine viruses are now generated by using reverse genetics methods. Vaccine viruses are then grown in embryonated eggs, filtered, and concentrated. The vaccine is administered intranasally by spray.

Shedding of live attenuated viruses on days 1 to 2 postvaccination is frequent in young children, but decreases with age.[111,144,1043,1045,1194,1307,2031,2152] So far, only one case of virus transmission has been reported.[2152]

Reactogenicity of Seasonal Influenza Vaccines

For inactivated vaccines, local or systemic allergic reactions to vaccine components are rare,[126,1460,1594] and are primarily due to residual egg protein.[1460,1594] Reactions generally occur within the first 24 hours and last for 1 to 2 days; they include systemic manifestations such as fever, malaise, myalgia, and headache, as well as local manifestations such as pain, erythema, induration, and tenderness at the inoculation site. The reactogenicity of influenza B virus vaccine is similar to that of influenza A virus.[20,643,1156,1546] In children, whole virus vaccines cause more systemic reactions than subvirion vaccines[127,166,382,1154,2273]; for children younger than 12 years of age, subvirion vaccines are therefore recommended. Cell culture–grown vaccines are comparable in their reactogenicity to egg-grown vaccines.[27,673,1597,1598,1718] More recently developed adjuvants, MF59 and AS03, have increased local reactogenicity. For live attenuated vaccines, mild symptoms including stuffy or runny nose, sore throat, and/or mild fever have been reported.[103,108,536,902,1517,1553,1554,2080]

An increase in reported cases of GBS (see Central Nervous System Involvement section) occurred in the United States in 1976 to 1977 during vaccination to the swine H1N1 virus that infected recruits in New Jersey[1318,1754,1771,1815,2260] (see Interspecies Transmission section). About 1 in 100,000 individuals who received the vaccine against the 1976 swine H1N1 influenza virus developed GBS, with a relative risk in vaccine recipients about four- to eightfold greater than that in unvaccinated subjects[1318,1771,1815]; these findings led to the cessation of the vaccination program. Typically, the risk of GBS after influenza virus vaccination is very small.[710,950,966,1928,1929] Preliminary data from the A(H1N1)pdm09 vaccination program in 2009 suggests a definable but minimal risk of GBS.[250]

In vaccinated individuals, exacerbated illness (as observed after measles or respiratory syncytial virus vaccination) does not occur. There has been a single instance in which vaccinated school-aged children had more influenza-related lower respiratory tract illness than their unvaccinated counterparts.[912] Inactivated influenza virus vaccines otherwise have a consistent record of efficacy and safety.

Immunogenicity of Seasonal Influenza Vaccines

The immunogenicity of a vaccine is significantly affected by prior exposure to the antigen. In unprimed individuals (such as children or persons with no or limited previous exposure to the respective antigen), higher amounts of antigen are required to elicit satisfactory levels of antibody. Thus, two doses of inactivated vaccine are recommended for children in their first year of vaccination.[537,1500,1502,2184] In the elderly, serum antibody responses are typically lower than in younger subjects,[646,1364,1596] which spurred the development of a high-dose vaccine (containing 60 μg of HA per component) that is now available for adults 65 years of age and older.[245,537,2001]

Whole virion vaccines are more immunogenic and cross-protective than subvirion vaccines,[127,170,496,610,1224,1579,1673,1964,2269,2273] likely because the RNA content of whole virus preparations stimulates TLR7[610] (see Pathogen Recognition

Receptors section); however, due to their higher reactogenicity, they are not used widely.

Live attenuated vaccine viruses replicate primarily in epithelial cells of the nasopharyngeal mucosa where they induce mucosal IgA antibodies, serum IgG antibodies, and cellular immunity, overall stimulating better cross-protection than inactivated viruses[30,106,107,356,544,773,2076,2129] (reviewed in[2080]). Compared to inactivated vaccines, vaccination with live attenuated vaccine more closely resembles a natural infection, stimulating both arms of the immune system and providing better heterosubtypic immunity.[356,1519,1962]

The addition of adjuvants to seasonal vaccines [and to avian virus vaccines and A(H1N1)pdm09 vaccines] increases their immunogenicity, particularly in immunologically naïve individuals[126,577,1524] [see also Vaccines to Avian Influenza Viruses and Vaccines to A(H1N1)pdm09 Virus sections].

Controlled studies comparing the antibody response after intradermal and parenteral administration of vaccine containing comparable amounts of HA antigen indicated that intradermal administration offers a dose-sparing advantage over parenteral administration.[1117,1695,1696,2143] Such approaches may be particularly important in the face of a pandemic when estimates indicate that vaccine supply will be a rate-limiting step.

The duration of immunity after inactivated influenza vaccination has not been evaluated systematically, but a relatively rapid decline in antibody levels suggests that protective immunity is of short duration. At any rate, antigenic changes in the influenza virus predicate annual immunization with current vaccines.

Efficacy of Seasonal Influenza Vaccines

Vaccination with influenza A and B viruses reduces infection and influenza-related illness.[50,472,523,921,1378,1422,1423] The timing of vaccination is important since protective levels of antibodies are usually not reached until 2 weeks after vaccination.[177,1157]

For inactivated vaccines, the levels of neutralizing antibodies against the infecting strain correlate well with the level of protection.[326,813,1499,1591,1674] For live attenuated vaccines, the hemagglutination inhibition antibody test is not an optimal correlate, as seroconversion rates often remain low,[109,544,978,2086] and protection has been observed in the absence of significant levels of antibody responses.[472,2089]

Vaccine efficacy, defined as the reduction of cell culture–confirmed influenza illness, ranges from 70% to 90% in years in which the vaccine strains closely match the circulating viruses, and 50% to 80% in years when the vaccine is not well matched.[98,172,411,536,790,919,1515,1517,1553,1874,1977,2160] Several meta-analyses have clearly established the benefits of vaccination.[790,920,1515,2160] In healthy adults, inactivated and live attenuated vaccines provide similar levels of protection.[172,411,472,482,1514,1515,1553,1554,1977,2080,2089,2199]

In the elderly, vaccine efficacy is significantly lower than that in young adults,[69,70,672,1769] ranging from 20% to 40% in years of good antigenic match, and little protection in years of poor antigenic match.[335,903,1217,1413,1518,1552] Limited data suggest that live attenuated and inactivated vaccines are of similar efficacy in the elderly.[650,2042]

In children, influenza vaccines are efficacious.[105,108,164] In this age group, live attenuated vaccine is more efficacious than inactivated vaccine,[45,103,539,919,1514,2080,2151] and also provides better protection against antigenically mismatched strains.[106,571,728,729] Compliance with the currently recommended two doses of vaccine for children may be low; however, several studies demonstrated that even a single dose of live attenuated vaccine elicits protective immune responses in more than half of the children tested.[108,164,2033]

Vaccination protects the vaccine recipient, but unvaccinated individuals can also benefit if the extent of vaccination is sufficient to dampen the epidemic spread of virus in the community (herd effect).[386,509,621,854,1039,1044,1411,1501,1653,2201,2238]

Vaccination of high-risk groups, including pregnant women,[742,895,1230,1440,1505,2347] patients with impaired immunity due to cancer,[191,348,524,1115,1253,1353,1580,1797,1849,1974,2330] organ transplants,[9,133,134,148,173,242,455,492,597,769,1004,1040,1111,1115,1346,1354,1794,1913,2159] HIV infections,[1043,1045,1115,1194,1225,1398,1498,2298] or patients with chronic heart disease[392,1298] is efficacious, although the antibody responses may be lower than those in healthy individuals.

Recommendations for Seasonal Influenza Vaccines

Recommendations for vaccination in the United States have continued to expand. Currently, annual vaccination is recommended for all over 6 months of age.[537] Protection of persons at higher risk for influenza-related complications should continue to be a focus of vaccination efforts as providers and programs transition to routine vaccination of all persons aged 6 months or older. A summary of current influenza vaccination recommendations follows (modified after[537]):

When vaccine supply is limited, vaccination efforts should focus on delivering vaccination to person who:

- Are aged 6 months to 4 years (59 months)
- Are aged ≥50 years
- Have chronic pulmonary (including asthma), cardiovascular (except hypertension), renal, hepatic, neurologic, hematologic, or metabolic disorder (including diabetes mellitus)
- Are immunosuppressed (including immunosuppression caused by medications or by human immunodeficiency virus
- Are or will be pregnant during the influenza season
- Are aged 6 months to 18 years and receiving long-term aspirin therapy and who therefore might be at risk for experiencing Reye syndrome after influenza virus infection
- Are residents of nursing homes and other chronic-care facilities
- Are American Indians/Alaska Natives
- Are morbidly obese (body mass index ≥ 40)
- Are health-care personnel
- Are household contacts and caregivers of children aged less than 5 years and adults aged 50 years or older, with particular emphasis on vaccinating contacts of children aged <6 months
- Are household contacts and caregivers of persons with medical conditions that put them at higher risk for severe complications from influenza

Vaccines to A(H1N1)pdm09 Virus

Based on the initial characterization of A(H1N1)pdm2009 viruses, the WHO recommended a vaccine strain (A/California/07/2009) on May 26, 2009 (http://www.who.int/csr/resources/publications/swineflu/H1N1Vaccinevirus recommendation26May2009.pdf). Early studies indicated that the candidate vaccines grew poorly in eggs (http://www.thelancet.com/H1N1-flu/egmn/0c03c805), and that two doses of vaccine might be needed to elicit protection against the novel virus.[439,1071] However, several egg- and cell culture–grown, inactivated and live attenuated vaccines became available that grew to reasonable titers and, more importantly, triggered robust immune responses after one vaccination[254,324,666,1215,1535,1664,1751,2122,2124,2249,2376] (for an overview of clinical trials, see[627]). Overall, seroconversion rates were lower in children,[1215,1664,2376] although one dose of vaccine induced protective immune responses in some children.[1535] The robust immune responses in adults likely resulted from partial immunity due to prior infection with an antigenically similar strain (see The H1N1 Pandemic in 2009 section); in the United States, vaccination with the 1976 swine H1N1 virus also contributed to partial immunity to the A(H1N1)pdm09 virus.[982,1361]

Vaccines against A(H1N1)pdm09 virus became available in China, Europe, Australia, and the United States in the fall of 2009[251,254,933,1975] (http://www.ema.europa.eu/influenza/vaccines/home.htm; http://www.tga.gov.au/alerts/medicines/h1n1vaccine.htm). By February 2010, about 30 A(H1N1)pdm09 vaccines had been approved.[627] In the United States, nonadjuvanted subvirion vaccines and a live attenuated vaccine were available; one dose was recommended for adults, and two doses for children between the age of 6 months and 9 years. In Europe, only inactivated (whole virus and subvirion) vaccines have been approved, and two doses are recommended for all age groups; both nonadjuvanted vaccines and preparations adjuvanted with MF-59 or ASO3 received market authorization. MF-59 greatly enhanced the responses to A(H1N1)pdm09[324] and HPAI H5N1[1960] vaccines. A similar dose-sparing and enhanced response to novel antigens has been seen with AS03 in adults[2] and children.[233]

The safety of the A(H1N1)pdm09 vaccines has been monitored closely, particularly for cases of GBS (see Reactogenicity of Seasonal Influenza Vaccines section). While a few cases of GBS have been reported after vaccination with A(H1N1)pdm09 vaccines,[845] the frequency of reported GBS cases does not exceed the baseline number of cases reported annually (http://vaers.hhs.gov/resources/2010H1N1Summary_June03.pdf).

Vaccines to Avian Influenza Viruses

For most vaccines to highly pathogenic avian influenza viruses, the multibasic cleavage site in the HA protein is replaced with a low-pathogenic motif[834,837,1525,1992,2207] (see HA Cleavage section) to generate attenuated vaccine viruses. This step is critical to increase the biosafety of vaccine production, and to avoid low vaccine virus yields in eggs resulting from the killing of the chicken embryo by the highly pathogenic avian viruses.

The first clinical trials of vaccines to HPAI H5N1 viruses indicated that very high amounts of antigen[2087] and/or two doses of antigen, possibly in combination with adjuvant,[170] may be required to elicit protective immune responses. Since then, a number of candidate vaccines have been tested in clinical trials, including inactivated whole virus vaccines,[478,479,521,862,1224,2020,2121,2123,2275,2276] inactivated subvirion vaccines,[63,96,104,117,124,167,309,312,313,422,777,840,1007,1008,1144,1188–1190,1193,1466,1537,1617,1761,1765,1826,1905,2153,2275,2276,2350] and live attenuated viruses.[978,1761] Most of these candidate vaccines were grown in eggs; however, several were propagated in Vero,[479] MDCK,[1007] or primary monkey kidney cells.[766] In addition, a DNA vaccine,[1905] virus-like particle vaccine (http://www.medicalnewstoday.com/articles/139352.php), and vaccines composed of recombinant M2 protein expressed in *Escherichia coli* (http://www.who.int/vaccine_research/immunogenicity/immunogenicity_table.xls2009), or recombinant HA protein expressed in insect cells,[766,2093] have been tested in clinical trials. For an overview of clinical trials, see http://www.who.int/vaccine_research/diseases/influenza/flu_trials_tables/en/ (last modified: 06/08/2010; accessed 05/30/2011).

These studies tested various virus strains, vaccine preparations, and vaccination regimens, including different amounts of antigen administered in one to three doses at different intervals, with or without adjuvants. Generally, nonadjuvanted vaccines are of low antigenicity in humans[124,167,170,309,1008,1189,1193,1311,2087]; the addition of aluminum salts as adjuvants (currently the only adjuvant approved in the United States for use in influenza vaccines) provided little or no increase in immunogenicity,[124,170,1009,1189,1190,1311] whereas oil-in-water emulsions such as MF-59 (approved in Europe for use with inactivated vaccines) and ASO3 [approved in Europe for use with A(H1N1)pdm09 vaccine] increased the immunogenicity of experimental H5N1 vaccines more noticeably.[63,124,1189,1193,1311,1765] By 2010, several egg-derived, inactivated H5N1 influenza vaccines had been approved in different countries, including four whole virus vaccines adjuvanted with aluminum and one split virus vaccine adjuvanted with ASO3 (reviewed in[1679]).

Other vaccine approaches are in different stages of development. These include inactivated low-pathogenic surrogate H5N3[576,1269,1524,1960,1963] or H5N4[1240,2022] virus; H5 HA or NP protein expressed by baculovirus,[641,2090,2093] adenovirus,[594,820–822,828,1616,1706,2132,2149] alphavirus,[847,1823] poxviruses,[24,967,1097,1098,1122,1349,1669,1691,1692,1732,1954] or Newcastle disease virus.[423,424] Virus-like particles generated by expressing the influenza virus HA, NA, M1, and/or M2 proteins have been tested,[42,174,365,368,425,766,768,962–964,1142,1299,1638,1917,2016,2039,2274] and a VLP vaccine is now in clinical trials (http://www.medicalnewstoday.com/articles/139352.php). DNA vaccines to H5 HA, NP, NA, and/or M2[270,286,287,425,502,505,743,1038,1076,1126,1128,1281,1604,1706,2079,2284,2312] have been tested, but often suffered from suboptimal immune responses; however, several DNA vaccines are now in clinical trials.[447,928,937,1905] Delivery of a DNA construct by small-particle aerosol has proven highly immunogenic in nonhuman primates.[1918]

The rapid evolution of HPAI H5N1 viruses might result in suboptimal cross-protection against viruses from different clades, and several H5N1 vaccines may have to be prepared to cover the currently circulating clades (for an overview of recently circulating clades and their antigenic properties, and an overview of current candidate vaccines, see http://www.who.int/csr/disease/avian_influenza/guidelines/2011_02_h5_h9_vaccinevirusupdate.pdf). However, recent data indicate that vaccination with an antigenically distinct H5N1 vaccine has a priming effect that leads to a faster and stronger response upon revaccination.[576,1965] Hence, prepandemic priming,[922] potentially limited to high-risk groups, may be considered to prepare for a possible H5N1 pandemic.

Similar vaccine strategies are being applied to viruses of the H7[358,405,906,925,943,944,1392,1608,1611,2016,2078,2242] and H9 subtypes.[47,211,775,977,1684,1685,1964] Clinical trials have been conducted for live attenuated H7N3[2030] and H9N2[977] viruses. A cell culture–grown H7N1 split virus vaccine,[357] and H9N2 whole virus and subunit vaccines[1964] have also been evaluated.

Universal Vaccines and Other Approaches to Influenza Vaccination

Universal influenza A vaccines that protect against viruses of all subtypes are highly desirable. Antibodies against the highly conserved ectodomain of the M2 ion channel protein are broadly cross-reactive (see Humoral Immunity section), but a DNA/adenovirus vaccine expressing M2 is suboptimal in ferrets.[1706] A vaccine in which the M2 ectodomain is expressed as a fusion peptide of the hepatitis B virus core protein is now in clinical trials.[531,1816] Broadly neutralizing antibodies to a conserved region in HA2 (see Humoral Immunity section) are attractive as broad-acting therapeutics, while the HA2 stalk region may be an attractive vaccine candidate because of its broad protective efficacy.[1953,2194] These approaches have not been tested yet in clinical trials. In another approach, a universal vaccine composed of a synthetic protein encoding conserved linear epitopes from the HA, NP, and M1 proteins is undergoing trials in humans.[113] Other approaches to improving our current influenza vaccines include changes in the substrate for vaccine preparation, vector-based vaccines, DNA vaccines, recombinant proteins, virus-like particles (VLPs) and newer adjuvants (see review in[1135]).

PERSPECTIVES

Over the last decade, we have witnessed several important developments in influenza virology. Highly pathogenic avian influenza viruses, which in the past caused transient, local outbreaks, have now become enzootic in parts of Asia in the form of H5N1 viruses. It is unlikely that these viruses will be eradicated in the near future. More likely, they will continue to circulate in—and transmit between—wild bird and domestic poultry populations, with ample opportunity for reassortment with other avian influenza viruses. In 2007 to 2008, oseltamivir-resistant H1N1 viruses became dominant around the world. This event reminds us that novel antiviral compounds, ideally targeted at different viral proteins and/or steps in the viral life cycle, are urgently needed. Finally, the H1N1 pandemic in 2009 caught most researchers by surprise, since the next pandemic was believed to be caused by a virus of an HA subtype that is not circulating in humans. Hence, while the next pandemic was thought to be caused by a virus of the H5, H7, or H9 subtype (scenarios that should not be dismissed), the H1N1 pandemic in 2009 has renewed the awareness for the pandemic potential of H1, H2, and H3 viruses. In particular, H2 viruses, which have not circulated in humans since 1968, are now receiving more attention.

Techniques are in place to rapidly sequence, analyze, generate, and test novel influenza virus strains and potential vaccine candidates. The development of additional adjuvants and the transition to cell culture systems for vaccine production will provide more flexibility for scale-up in case of a pandemic. However, significant administrative and regulatory challenges in the development of novel vaccines and antivirals remain.

In summary, the most important lesson may be that influenza pandemics do occur, will continue to occur, and will continue to challenge our ability to respond.

REFERENCES

All cited references are available in the e-book.

17. Alford RH, Kasel JA, Gerone PJ, et al. Human influenza resulting from aerosol inhalation. *Proc Soc Exp Biol Med* 1966;122:800–804.
62. Banks J, Speidel ES, Moore E, et al. Changes in the haemagglutinin and the neuraminidase genes prior to the emergence of highly pathogenic H7N1 avian influenza viruses in Italy. *Arch Virol* 2001;146:963–973.
95. Beigel JH, Farrar J, Han AM, et al. Avian influenza A (H5N1) infection in humans. *N Engl J Med* 2005;353:1374–1385.
108. Belshe RB, Mendelman PM, Treanor J, et al. The efficacy of live attenuated, cold-adapted, trivalent, intranasal influenzavirus vaccine in children. *N Engl J Med* 1998;338:1405–1412.
170. Bresson JL, Perronne C, Launay O, et al. Safety and immunogenicity of an inactivated split-virion influenza A/Vietnam/1194/2004 (H5N1) vaccine: phase I randomised trial. *Lancet* 2006;367:1657–1664.
202. Burnet FM. Influenza virus on the developing egg. I. Changes associated with the development of an egg-passage strain of virus. *Br J Exp Pathol* 1936;17:282–293.
209. Current status of amantadine and rimantadine as anti-influenza-A agents: memorandum from a WHO meeting. *Bull World Health Organ* 1985;63:51–56.
239. Caton AJ, Brownlee GG, Yewdell JW, et al. The antigenic structure of the influenza virus A/PR/8/34 hemagglutinin (H1 subtype). *Cell* 1982;31:417–427.
243. Centers for Disease Control and Prevention. Bacterial coinfections in lung tissue specimens from fatal cases of 2009 pandemic influenza A (H1N1)—United States, May-August 2009. *MMWR Morb Mortal Wkly Rep* 2009;58:1071–1074.
244. Centers for Disease Control and Prevention. Hospitalized patients with novel influenza A (H1N1) virus infection—California, April-May, 2009. *MMWR Morb Mortal Wkly Rep* 2009;58:536–41.
249. Centers for Disease Control and Prevention. Outbreak of swine-origin influenza A (H1N1) virus infection—Mexico, March-April 2009. *MMWR Morb Mortal Wkly Rep* 2009;58:467–470.
250. Centers for Disease Control and Prevention. Preliminary results: surveillance for Guillain-Barre syndrome after receipt of influenza A (H1N1) 2009 monovalent vaccine—United States, 2009–2010. *MMWR Morb Mortal Wkly Rep* 2010;59:657–661.
252. Centers for Disease Control and Prevention. Serum cross-reactive antibody response to a novel influenza A (H1N1) virus after vaccination with seasonal influenza vaccine. *MMWR Morb Mortal Wkly Rep* 2009;58:521–524.
253. Centers for Disease Control and Prevention. Swine influenza A (H1N1) infection in two children–Southern California, March-April 2009. *MMWR Morb Mortal Wkly Rep* 2009;58:400–402.
254. Centers for Disease Control and Prevention. Update on influenza A (H1N1) 2009 monovalent vaccines. *MMWR Morb Mortal Wkly Rep* 2009;58:1100–1101.
258. Centers for Disease Control and Prevention. Update: novel influenza A (H1N1) virus infection—Mexico, March-May, 2009. *MMWR Morb Mortal Wkly Rep* 2009;58:585–589.
265. Chan MC, Chan RW, Yu WC, et al. Tropism and innate host responses of the 2009 pandemic H1N1 influenza virus in ex vivo and in vitro cultures of human conjunctiva and respiratory tract. *Am J Pathol* 2010; 176:1828–1840.
266. Chan MC, Cheung CY, Chui WH, et al. Proinflammatory cytokine responses induced by influenza A (H5N1) viruses in primary human alveolar and bronchial epithelial cells. *Respir Res* 2005;6:135.
275. Chen GL, Subbarao K. Live attenuated vaccines for pandemic influenza. *Curr Top Microbiol Immunol* 2009;333:109–132.
279. Chen H, Li Y, Li Z, et al. Properties and dissemination of H5N1 viruses isolated during an influenza outbreak in migratory waterfowl in western China. *J Virol* 2006;80:5976–5983.

280. Chen H, Smith GJ, Li KS, et al. Establishment of multiple sublineages of H5N1 influenza virus in Asia: implications for pandemic control. *Proc Natl Acad Sci U S A* 2006;103:2845–2850.
281. Chen H, Smith GJ, Zhang SY, et al. Avian flu: H5N1 virus outbreak in migratory waterfowl. *Nature* 2005;436:191–192.
291. Chen W, Calvo PA, Malide D, et al. A novel influenza A virus mitochondrial protein that induces cell death. *Nat Med* 2001;7:1306–1312.
311. Chowell G, Bertozzi SM, Colchero MA, et al. Severe respiratory disease concurrent with the circulation of H1N1 influenza. *N Engl J Med* 2009;361:674–679.
320. Claas EC, de Jong JC, van Beek R, et al. Human influenza virus A/HongKong/156/97 (H5N1) infection. *Vaccine* 1998;16:977–978.
322. Claas EC, Osterhaus AD, van Beek R, et al. Human influenza A H5N1 virus related to a highly pathogenic avian influenza virus. *Lancet* 1998;351:472–477.
337. Collins PJ, Haire LF, Lin YP, et al. Structural basis for oseltamivir resistance of influenza viruses. *Vaccine* 2009;27:6317–6323.
338. Colman PM, Ward CW. Structure and diversity of influenza virus neuraminidase. *Curr Top Microbiol Immunol* 1985;114:177–255.
339. Conenello GM, Tisoncik JR, Rosenzweig E, et al. A single N66S mutation in the PB1-F2 protein of influenza A virus increases virulence by inhibiting the early interferon response in vivo. *J Virol* 2011;85: 652–662.
343. Connor RJ, Kawaoka Y, Webster RG, et al. Receptor specificity in human, avian, and equine H2 and H3 influenza virus isolates. *Virology* 1994;205:17–23.
345. Couceiro JN, Paulson JC, Baum LG. Influenza virus strains selectively recognize sialyloligosaccharides on human respiratory epithelium; the role of the host cell in selection of hemagglutinin receptor specificity. *Virus Res* 1993;29:155–165.
349. Couch RB, Kasel JA. Immunity to influenza in man. *Annu Rev Microbiol* 1983;37:529–549.
354. Cox NJ, Subbarao K. Global epidemiology of influenza: past and present. *Annu Rev Med* 2000;51:407–421.
388. Dawood FS, Jain S, Finelli L, et al. Emergence of a novel swine-origin influenza A (H1N1) virus in humans. *N Engl J Med* 2009;360:2605–2615.
394. de Jong JC, Claas EC, Osterhaus AD, et al. A pandemic warning? *Nature* 1997;389:554.
398. de Jong MD, Bach VC, Phan TQ, et al. Fatal avian influenza A (H5N1) in a child presenting with diarrhea followed by coma. *N Engl J Med* 2005; 352:686–691.
399. de Jong MD, Simmons CP, Thanh TT, et al. Fatal outcome of human influenza A (H5N1) is associated with high viral load and hypercytokinemia. *Nat Med* 2006;12:1203–1207.
400. de Jong MD, Tran TT, Truong HK, et al. Oseltamivir resistance during treatment of influenza A (H5N1) infection. *N Engl J Med* 2005;353:2667–2672.
419. Diebold SS, Kaisho T, Hemmi H, et al. Innate antiviral responses by means of TLR7-mediated recognition of single-stranded RNA. *Science* 2004;303:1529–1531.
429. Doherty PC, Turner SJ, Webby RG, et al. Influenza and the challenge for immunology. *Nat Immunol* 2006;7:449–455.
438. Donis RO, Bean WJ, Kawaoka Y, et al. Distinct lineages of influenza virus H4 hemagglutinin genes in different regions of the world. *Virology* 1989;169:408–417.
442. Dowdle WR. Influenza A virus recycling revisited. *Bull World Health Organ* 1999;77:820–828.
443. Dowdle WR, Millar JD. Swine influenza: lessons learned. *Med Clin North Am* 1978;62:1047–1057.
456. Dugan VG, Chen R, Spiro DJ, et al. The evolutionary genetics and emergence of avian influenza viruses in wild birds. *PLoS Pathog* 2008; 4:e1000076.
468. Eccles R. Understanding the symptoms of the common cold and influenza. *Lancet Infect Dis* 2005;5:718–725.
469. Echevarria-Zuno S, Mejia-Arangure JM, Mar-Obeso AJ, et al. Infection and death from influenza A H1N1 virus in Mexico: a retrospective analysis. *Lancet* 2009;374:2072–2079.
535. Fiore AE, Fry A, Shay D, et al. Antiviral agents for the treatment and chemoprophylaxis of influenza—recommendations of the Advisory Committee on Immunization Practices (ACIP). *MMWR Recomm Rep* 2011;60:1–24.
537. Fiore AE, Uyeki TM, Broder K, et al. Prevention and control of influenza with vaccines: recommendations of the Advisory Committee on Immunization Practices (ACIP), 2010. *MMWR Recomm Rep* 2010;59:1–62.
538. Fitch WM, Bush RM, Bender CA, et al. Long term trends in the evolution of H(3) HA1 human influenza type A. *Proc Natl Acad Sci U S A* 1997;94:7712–7718.
542. Fodor E, Devenish L, Engelhardt OG, et al. Rescue of influenza A virus from recombinant DNA. *J Virol* 1999;73:9679–9682.
546. Fouchier RA, Schneeberger PM, Rozendaal FW, et al. Avian influenza A virus (H7N7) associated with human conjunctivitis and a fatal case of acute respiratory distress syndrome. *Proc Natl Acad Sci U S A* 2004;101:1356–1361.
552. Francis T Jr, Quilligan JJ Jr, Minuse E. Identification of another epidemic respiratory disease. *Science* 1950;112:495–497.
556. Fraser C, Donnelly CA, Cauchemez S, et al. Pandemic potential of a strain of influenza A (H1N1): early findings. *Science* 2009;324:1557–1561.
589. Gambaryan AS, Tuzikov AB, Piskarev VE, et al. Specification of receptor-binding phenotypes of influenza virus isolates from different hosts using synthetic sialylglycopolymers: non-egg-adapted human H1 and H3 influenza A and influenza B viruses share a common high binding affinity for 6′-sialyl(N-acetyllactosamine). *Virology* 1997;232:345–350.
590. Gamblin SJ, Haire LF, Russell RJ, et al. The structure and receptor binding properties of the 1918 influenza hemagglutinin. *Science* 2004; 303:1838–1842.
601. Garcia-Sastre A, Egorov A, Matassov D, et al. Influenza A virus lacking the NS1 gene replicates in interferon-deficient systems. *Virology* 1998; 252:324–330.
604. Garten RJ, Davis CT, Russell CA, et al. Antigenic and genetic characteristics of swine-origin 2009 A(H1N1) influenza viruses circulating in humans. *Science* 2009;325:197–201.
619. Gerhard W, Yewdell J, Frankel ME, et al. Antigenic structure of influenza virus haemagglutinin defined by hybridoma antibodies. *Nature* 1981;290:713–717.
627. Girard MP, Katz J, Pervikov Y, et al. Report of the 6th meeting on the evaluation of pandemic influenza vaccines in clinical trials World Health Organization, Geneva, Switzerland, 17–18 February 2010. *Vaccine* 2010;28:6811–6820.
628. Glaser L, Stevens J, Zamarin D, et al. A single amino acid substitution in 1918 influenza virus hemagglutinin changes receptor binding specificity. *J Virol* 2005;79:11533–11536.
631. Glezen WP. Serious morbidity and mortality associated with influenza epidemics. *Epidemiol Rev* 1982;4:25–44.
648. Gorman OT, Bean WJ, Kawaoka Y, et al. Evolution of the nucleoprotein gene of influenza A virus. *J Virol* 1990;64:1487–1497.
649. Gorman OT, Donis RO, Kawaoka Y, et al. Evolution of influenza A virus PB2 genes: implications for evolution of the ribonucleoprotein complex and origin of human influenza A virus. *J Virol* 1990;64:4893–4902.
666. Greenberg ME, Lai MH, Hartel GF, et al. Response to a monovalent 2009 influenza A (H1N1) vaccine. *N Engl J Med* 2009;361:2405–2413.
676. Gu J, Xie Z, Gao Z, et al. H5N1 infection of the respiratory tract and beyond. *Lancet* 2007;370:1137–1145.
677. Guan Y, Peiris JS, Lipatov AS, et al. Emergence of multiple genotypes of H5N1 avian influenza viruses in Hong Kong SAR. *Proc Natl Acad Sci U S A* 2002;99:8950–8955.
705. Human infection with new influenza A (H1N1) virus: clinical observations from Mexico and other affected countries, May 2009. *Wkly Epidemiol Rec* 2009;84:185–189.
706. Human infection with pandemic A (H1N1) 2009 influenza virus: clinical observations in hospitalized patients, Americas, July 2009—update. *Wkly Epidemiol Rec* 2009;84:305–308.
726. Haller O, Staeheli P, Kochs G. Protective role of interferon-induced Mx GTPases against influenza viruses. *Rev Sci Tech* 2009;28:219–231.
734. Hancock K, Veguilla V, Lu X, et al. Cross-reactive antibody responses to the 2009 pandemic H1N1 influenza virus. *N Engl J Med* 2009;361: 1945–1952.

751. Hatakeyama S, Sugaya N, Ito M, et al. Emergence of influenza B viruses with reduced sensitivity to neuraminidase inhibitors. *JAMA* 2007;297:1435–1442.
753. Hatta M, Gao P, Halfmann P, et al. Molecular basis for high virulence of Hong Kong H5N1 influenza A viruses. *Science* 2001;293:1840–1842.
757. Hay AJ, Wolstenholme AJ, Skehel JJ, et al. The molecular basis of the specific anti-influenza action of amantadine. *EMBO J* 1985;4:3021–3024.
760. Hayden F. Developing new antiviral agents for influenza treatment: what does the future hold? *Clin Infect Dis* 2009;48(Suppl 1):S3–S13.
784. Hensley SE, Das SR, Bailey AL, et al. Hemagglutinin receptor binding avidity drives influenza A virus antigenic drift. *Science* 2009;326:734–736.
793. Hers JF, Mulder J. Broad aspects of the pathology and pathogenesis of human influenza. *Am Rev Respir Dis* 1961;83(2)Pt 2:84–97.
798. Higa HH, Rogers GN, Paulson JC. Influenza virus hemagglutinins differentiate between receptor determinants bearing N-acetyl-, N-glycollyl-, and N,O-diacetylneuraminic acids. *Virology* 1985;144:279–282.
833. Horimoto T, Kawaoka Y. Pandemic threat posed by avian influenza A viruses. *Clin Microbiol Rev* 2001;14:129–149.
834. Horimoto T, Kawaoka Y. Reverse genetics provides direct evidence for a correlation of hemagglutinin cleavability and virulence of an avian influenza A virus. *J Virol* 1994;68:3120–3128.
836. Horimoto T, Rivera E, Pearson J, et al. Origin and molecular changes associated with emergence of a highly pathogenic H5N2 influenza virus in Mexico. *Virology* 1995;213:223–230.
858. Ichinohe T, Pang IK, Iwasaki A. Influenza virus activates inflammasomes via its intracellular M2 ion channel. *Nat Immunol* 2010;11:404–410.
880. Ito T, Couceiro JN, Kelm S, et al. Molecular basis for the generation in pigs of influenza A viruses with pandemic potential. *J Virol* 1998;72:7367–7373.
888. Ito T, Suzuki Y, Suzuki T, et al. Recognition of N-glycolylneuraminic acid linked to galactose by the alpha2,3 linkage is associated with intestinal replication of influenza A virus in ducks. *J Virol* 2000;74:9300–9305.
890. Itoh Y, Shinya K, Kiso M, et al. In vitro and in vivo characterization of new swine-origin H1N1 influenza viruses. *Nature* 2009;460:1021–1025.
958. Kandun IN, Wibisono H, Sedyaningsih ER, et al. Three Indonesian clusters of H5N1 virus infection in 2005. *N Engl J Med* 2006;355:2186–2194.
981. Kash JC, Basler CF, Garcia-Sastre A, et al. Global host immune response: pathogenesis and transcriptional profiling of type A influenza viruses expressing the hemagglutinin and neuraminidase genes from the 1918 pandemic virus. *J Virol* 2004;78:9499–9511.
1001. Kawaoka Y, Krauss S, Webster RG. Avian-to-human transmission of the PB1 gene of influenza A viruses in the 1957 and 1968 pandemics. *J Virol* 1989;63:4603–4608.
1002. Kawaoka Y, Naeve CW, Webster RG. Is virulence of H5N2 influenza viruses in chickens associated with loss of carbohydrate from the hemagglutinin? *Virology* 1984;139:303–316.
1003. Kawaoka Y, Webster RG. Sequence requirements for cleavage activation of influenza virus hemagglutinin expressed in mammalian cells. *Proc Natl Acad Sci U S A* 1988;85:324–328.
1013. Kendal AP, Goldfield M, Noble GR, et al. Identification and preliminary antigenic analysis of swine influenza-like viruses isolated during an influenza outbreak at Fort Dix, New Jersey. *J Infect Dis* 1977;136(Suppl):S381–S385.
1027. Kilander A, Rykkvin R, Dudman SG, et al. Observed association between the HA1 mutation D222G in the 2009 pandemic influenza A(H1N1) virus and severe clinical outcome, Norway 2009–2010. *Euro Surveill* 2010;15(9):pii=19498.
1028. Kilbourne ED. Studies on influenza in the pandemic of 1957–1958. III. Isolation of influenza A (Asian strain) viruses from influenza patients with pulmonary complications; details of virus isolation and characterization of isolates, with quantitative comparison of isolation methods. *J Clin Invest* 1959;38:266–274.
1051. Kiso M, Mitamura K, Sakai-Tagawa Y, et al. Resistant influenza A viruses in children treated with oseltamivir: descriptive study. *Lancet* 2004;364:759–765.
1060. Klenk HD, Rott R, Orlich M, et al. Activation of influenza A viruses by trypsin treatment. *Virology* 1975;68:426–439.
1066. Knossow M, Daniels RS, Douglas AR, et al. Three-dimensional structure of an antigenic mutant of the influenza virus haemagglutinin. *Nature* 1984;311:678–680.
1068. Kobasa D, Jones SM, Shinya K, et al. Aberrant innate immune response in lethal infection of macaques with the 1918 influenza virus. *Nature* 2007;445:319–323.
1070. Kobasa D, Takada A, Shinya K, et al. Enhanced virulence of influenza A viruses with the haemagglutinin of the 1918 pandemic virus. *Nature* 2004;431:703–707.
1085. Koopmans M, Wilbrink B, Conyn M, et al. Transmission of H7N7 avian influenza A virus to human beings during a large outbreak in commercial poultry farms in the Netherlands. *Lancet* 2004;363:587–593.
1135. Lambert LC, Fauci AS. Influenza vaccines for the future. *N Engl J Med* 2010;363:2036–2044.
1155. Laver WG, Webster RG. Studies on the origin of pandemic influenza. 3. Evidence implicating duck and equine influenza viruses as possible progenitors of the Hong Kong strain of human influenza. *Virology* 1973;51:383–391.
1164. Le QM, Kiso M, Someya K, et al. Avian flu: isolation of drug-resistant H5N1 virus. *Nature* 2005;437:1108.
1165. Le QM, Sakai-Tagawa Y, Ozawa M, et al. Selection of H5N1 influenza virus PB2 during replication in humans. *J Virol* 2009;83:5278–5281.
1166. Le QM, Wertheim HF, Tran ND, et al. A community cluster of oseltamivir-resistant cases of 2009 H1N1 influenza. *N Engl J Med* 2010;362:86–87.
1198. Li C, Hatta M, Nidom CA, et al. Reassortment between avian H5N1 and human H3N2 influenza viruses creates hybrid viruses with substantial virulence. *Proc Natl Acad Sci U S A* 2010;107:4687–4692.
1205. Li KS, Guan Y, Wang J, et al. Genesis of a highly pathogenic and potentially pandemic H5N1 influenza virus in eastern Asia. *Nature* 2004;430:209–213.
1247. Liu J, Xiao H, Lei F, et al. Highly pathogenic H5N1 influenza virus infection in migratory birds. *Science* 2005;309:1206.
1261. Louie JK, Acosta M, Jamieson DJ, et al. Severe 2009 H1N1 influenza in pregnant and postpartum women in California. *N Engl J Med* 2010;362:27–35.
1294. Maassab HF. Biologic and immunologic characteristics of cold-adapted influenza virus. *J Immunol* 1969;102:728–732.
1301. Maines TR, Chen LM, Matsuoka Y, et al. Lack of transmission of H5N1 avian-human reassortant influenza viruses in a ferret model. *Proc Natl Acad Sci U S A* 2006;103:12121–12126.
1302. Maines TR, Jayaraman A, Belser JA, et al. Transmission and pathogenesis of swine-origin 2009 A(H1N1) influenza viruses in ferrets and mice. *Science* 2009;325:484–487.
1330. Matrosovich M, Tuzikov A, Bovin N, et al. Early alterations of the receptor-binding properties of H1, H2, and H3 avian influenza virus hemagglutinins after their introduction into mammals. *J Virol* 2000;74:8502–8512.
1336. Matrosovich MN, Matrosovich TY, Gray T, et al. Human and avian influenza viruses target different cell types in cultures of human airway epithelium. *Proc Natl Acad Sci U S A* 2004;101:4620–4624.
1356. McAuley JL, Hornung F, Boyd KL, et al. Expression of the 1918 influenza A virus PB1-F2 enhances the pathogenesis of viral and secondary bacterial pneumonia. *Cell Host Microbe* 2007;2:240–249.
1373. Mehle A, Doudna JA. Adaptive strategies of the influenza virus polymerase for replication in humans. *Proc Natl Acad Sci U S A* 2009;106:21312–21316.
1390. Min JY, Krug RM. The primary function of RNA binding by the influenza A virus NS1 protein in infected cells: Inhibiting the 2′-5′ oligo (A) synthetase/RNase L pathway. *Proc Natl Acad Sci U S A* 2006;103:7100–7105.
1419. Morens DM, Taubenberger JK, Fauci AS. The 2009 H1N1 Pandemic Influenza Virus: What Next? *MBio* 2010;1.
1420. Morens DM, Taubenberger JK, Fauci AS. Predominant role of bacterial pneumonia as a cause of death in pandemic influenza: implications for pandemic influenza preparedness. *J Infect Dis* 2008;198:962–970.

1435. Mulder J, Masurel N. Pre-epidemic antibody against 1957 strain of Asiatic influenza in serum of older people living in the Netherlands. *Lancet* 1958;1:810–814.
1442. Munster VJ, de Wit E, van den Brand JM, et al. Pathogenesis and transmission of swine-origin 2009 A(H1N1) influenza virus in ferrets. *Science* 2009;325:481–483.
1457. Murphy BR, Nelson DL, Wright PF, et al. Secretory and systemic immunological response in children infected with live attenuated influenza A virus vaccines. *Infect Immun* 1982;36:1102–1108.
1459. Myers KP, Olsen CW, Gray GC. Cases of swine influenza in humans: a review of the literature. *Clin Infect Dis* 2007;44:1084–1088.
1460. Neuraminidase inhibitors for treatment of influenza A and B infections. *MMWR Recomm Rep* 1999;48:1–9.
1469. Nakajima K, Desselberger U, Palese P. Recent human influenza A (H1N1) viruses are closely related genetically to strains isolated in 1950. *Nature* 1978;274:334–339.
1483. Nemeroff ME, Barabino SM, Li Y, et al. Influenza virus NS1 protein interacts with the cellular 30 kDa subunit of CPSF and inhibits 3′ end formation of cellular pre-mRNAs. *Mol Cell* 1998;1:991–1000.
1495. Neumann G, Noda T, Kawaoka Y. Emergence and pandemic potential of swine-origin H1N1 influenza virus. *Nature* 2009;459:931–939.
1496. Neumann G, Watanabe T, Ito H, et al. Generation of influenza A viruses entirely from cloned cDNAs. *Proc Natl Acad Sci U S A* 1999;96: 9345–9350.
1505. Neuzil KM, Reed GW, Mitchel EF, et al. Impact of influenza on acute cardiopulmonary hospitalizations in pregnant women. *Am J Epidemiol* 1998;148:1094–1102.
1512. Nguyen HT, Fry AM, Loveless PA, et al. Recovery of a multidrug-resistant strain of pandemic influenza A 2009 (H1N1) virus carrying a dual H275Y/I223R mutation from a child after prolonged treatment with oseltamivir. *Clin Infect Dis* 2010;51:983–984.
1520. Nicholls JM, Bourne AJ, Chen H, et al. Sialic acid receptor detection in the human respiratory tract: evidence for widespread distribution of potential binding sites for human and avian influenza viruses. *Respir Res* 2007;8:73.
1521. Nicholls JM, Chan MC, Chan WY, et al. Tropism of avian influenza A (H5N1) in the upper and lower respiratory tract. *Nat Med* 2007;13: 147–149.
1531. Noble GR. Epidemiological and clinical aspects of influenza. In: Beare AS, ed. *Basic and Applied Influenza Research.* Boca Raton: CRC Press; 1982:11–50.
1535. Nolan T, McVernon J, Skeljo M, et al. Immunogenicity of a monovalent 2009 influenza A(H1N1) vaccine in infants and children: a randomized trial. *JAMA* 2010;303:37–46.
1545. Obenauer JC, Denson J, Mehta PK, et al. Large-scale sequence analysis of avian influenza isolates. *Science* 2006;311:1576–1580.
1575. Opitz B, Rejaibi A, Dauber B, et al. IFNbeta induction by influenza A virus is mediated by RIG-I which is regulated by the viral NS1 protein. *Cell Microbiol* 2007;9:930–938.
1593. Preliminary review of D222G amino acid substitution in the haemagglutinin of pandemic influenza A (H1N1) 2009 viruses. *Wkly Epidemiol Rec* 2010;85:21–22.
1607. Pappas C, Aguilar PV, Basler CF, et al. Single gene reassortants identify a critical role for PB1, HA, and NA in the high virulence of the 1918 pandemic influenza virus. *Proc Natl Acad Sci U S A* 2008;105:3064–3069.
1625. Peiris JS, Yu WC, Leung CW, et al. Re-emergence of fatal human influenza A subtype H5N1 disease. *Lancet* 2004;363:617–619.
1635. Perez-Padilla R, de la Rosa-Zamboni D, Ponce de Leon S, et al. Pneumonia and respiratory failure from swine-origin influenza A (H1N1) in Mexico. *N Engl J Med* 2009;361:680–689.
1638. Perrone LA, Ahmad A, Veguilla V, et al. Intranasal vaccination with 1918 influenza virus-like particles protects mice and ferrets from lethal 1918 and H5N1 influenza virus challenge. *J Virol* 2009;83:5726–5734.
1652. Pichlmair A, Schulz O, Tan CP, et al. RIG-I-mediated antiviral responses to single-stranded RNA bearing 5′-phosphates. *Science* 2006; 314:997–1001.
1658. Pinto LH, Holsinger LJ, Lamb RA. Influenza virus M2 protein has ion channel activity. *Cell* 1992;69:517–528.
1664. Plennevaux E, Sheldon E, Blatter M, et al. Immune response after a single vaccination against 2009 influenza A H1N1 in USA: a preliminary report of two randomised controlled phase 2 trials. *Lancet* 2010;375:41–48.
1711. Rehwinkel J, Tan CP, Goubau D, et al. RIG-I detects viral genomic RNA during negative-strand RNA virus infection. *Cell* 2010;140:397–408.
1712. Reid AH, Fanning TG, Hultin JV, et al. Origin and evolution of the 1918 "Spanish" influenza virus hemagglutinin gene. *Proc Natl Acad Sci U S A* 1999;96:1651–1656.
1728. Richman DD, Murphy BR, Baron S, et al. Three strains of influenza A virus (H3N2): interferon sensitivity in vitro and interferon production in volunteers. *J Clin Microbiol* 1976;3:223–226.
1731. Rimmelzwaan GF, Kuiken T, van Amerongen G, et al. A primate model to study the pathogenesis of influenza A (H5N1) virus infection. *Avian Dis* 2003;47:931–933.
1744. Rogers GN, Paulson JC. Receptor determinants of human and animal influenza virus isolates: differences in receptor specificity of the H3 hemagglutinin based on species of origin. *Virology* 1983;127:361–373.
1745. Rogers GN, Paulson JC, Daniels RS, et al. Single amino acid substitutions in influenza haemagglutinin change receptor binding specificity. *Nature* 1983;304:76–78.
1766. Russell CA, Jones TC, Barr IG, et al. The global circulation of seasonal influenza A (H3N2) viruses. *Science* 2008;320:340–346.
1767. Russell RJ, Haire LF, Stevens DJ, et al. The structure of H5N1 avian influenza neuraminidase suggests new opportunities for drug design. *Nature* 2006;443:45–49.
1799. Schild GC, Henry-Aymard M, Pereira MS, et al. Antigenic variation in current human type A influenza viruses: antigenic characteristics of the variants and their geographic distribution. *Bull World Health Organ* 1973;48:269–278.
1800. Schild GC, Oxford JS, de Jong JC, et al. Evidence for host-cell selection of influenza virus antigenic variants. *Nature* 1983;303:706–709.
1801. Schild GC, Oxford JS, Dowdle WR, et al. Antigenic variation in current influenza A viruses: evidence for a high frequency of antigenic 'drift' for the Hong Kong virus. *Bull World Health Organ* 1974;51:1–11.
1813. Scholtissek C, Rohde W, Von Hoyningen V, et al. On the origin of the human influenza virus subtypes H2N2 and H3N2. *Virology* 1978; 87:13–20.
1831. Seo SH, Hoffmann E, Webster RG. Lethal H5N1 influenza viruses escape host anti-viral cytokine responses. *Nat Med* 2002;8:950–954.
1847. Shieh WJ, Blau DM, Denison AM, et al. 2009 pandemic influenza A (H1N1): pathology and pathogenesis of 100 fatal cases in the United States. *Am J Pathol* 2010;177:166–175.
1854. Shinya K, Ebina M, Yamada S, et al. Avian flu: influenza virus receptors in the human airway. *Nature* 2006;440:435–436.
1862. Shope RE. Serological Evidence For The Occurrence of Infection With Human Influenza Virus In Swine. *J Exp Med* 1938;67:739.
1863. Shope RE. Swine Influenza : I. Experimental Transmission and Pathology. *J Exp Med* 1931;54:349–359.
1864. Shortridge KF. Pandemic influenza: a zoonosis? *Semin Respir Infect* 1992;7:11–25.
1893. Slemons RD, Easterday BC. Type-A influenza viruses in the feces of migratory waterfowl. *J Am Vet Med Assoc* 1977;171:947–948.
1900. Smith DJ, Lapedes AS, de Jong JC, et al. Mapping the antigenic and genetic evolution of influenza virus. *Science* 2004;305:371–376.
1901. Smith GJ, Bahl J, Vijaykrishna D, et al. Dating the emergence of pandemic influenza viruses. *Proc Natl Acad Sci U S A* 2009;106:11709–11712.
1902. Smith GJ, Fan XH, Wang J, et al. Emergence and predominance of an H5N1 influenza variant in China. *Proc Natl Acad Sci U S A* 2006; 103:16936–16941.
1903. Smith GJ, Vijaykrishna D, Bahl J, et al. Origins and evolutionary genomics of the 2009 swine-origin H1N1 influenza A epidemic. *Nature* 2009;459:1122–1125.
1915. Song D, Kang B, Lee C, et al. Transmission of avian influenza virus (H3N2) to dogs. *Emerg Infect Dis* 2008;14:741–746.
1970. Stevens J, Blixt O, Tumpey TM, et al. Structure and receptor specificity of the hemagglutinin from an H5N1 influenza virus. *Science* 2006;312:404–410.
1972. Stevens J, Corper AL, Basler CF, et al. Structure of the uncleaved human H1 hemagglutinin from the extinct 1918 influenza virus. *Science* 2004;303:1866–1870.

1982. Sturm-Ramirez KM, Ellis T, Bousfield B, et al. Reemerging H5N1 influenza viruses in Hong Kong in 2002 are highly pathogenic to ducks. *J Virol* 2004;78:4892–4901.
1991. Subbarao EK, London W, Murphy BR. A single amino acid in the PB2 gene of influenza A virus is a determinant of host range. *J Virol* 1993; 67:1761–1764.
1993. Subbarao K, Klimov A, Katz J, et al. Characterization of an avian influenza A (H5N1) virus isolated from a child with a fatal respiratory illness. *Science* 1998;279:393–396.
2040. Tappenden P, Jackson R, Cooper K, et al. Amantadine, oseltamivir and zanamivir for the prophylaxis of influenza (including a review of existing guidance no. 67): a systematic review and economic evaluation. *Health Technol Assess* 2009;13:iii, ix–xii, 1–246.
2048. Taubenberger JK, Reid AH, Krafft AE, et al. Initial genetic characterization of the 1918 "Spanish" influenza virus. *Science* 1997;275:1793–1796.
2049. Taubenberger JK, Reid AH, Lourens RM, et al. Characterization of the 1918 influenza virus polymerase genes. *Nature* 2005;437:889–893.
2069. To KF, Chan PK, Chan KF, et al. Pathology of fatal human infection associated with avian influenza A H5N1 virus. *J Med Virol* 2001; 63:242–246.
2070. To KK, Hung IF, Li IW, et al. Delayed clearance of viral load and marked cytokine activation in severe cases of pandemic H1N1 2009 influenza virus infection. *Clin Infect Dis* 2010;50:850–859.
2084. Tran TH, Nguyen TL, Nguyen TD, et al. Avian influenza A (H5N1) in 10 patients in Vietnam. *N Engl J Med* 2004;350:1179–1188.
2099. Tu W, Mao H, Zheng J, et al. Cytotoxic T lymphocytes established by seasonal human influenza cross-react against 2009 pandemic H1N1 influenza virus. *J Virol* 2010;84:6527–6535.
2102. Tumpey TM, Basler CF, Aguilar PV, et al. Characterization of the reconstructed 1918 Spanish influenza pandemic virus. *Science* 2005;310: 77–80.
2104. Tumpey TM, Garcia-Sastre A, Taubenberger JK, et al. Pathogenicity and immunogenicity of influenza viruses with genes from the 1918 pandemic virus. *Proc Natl Acad Sci U S A* 2004;101:3166–3171.
2105. Tumpey TM, Garcia-Sastre A, Taubenberger JK, et al. Pathogenicity of influenza viruses with genes from the 1918 pandemic virus: functional roles of alveolar macrophages and neutrophils in limiting virus replication and mortality in mice. *J Virol* 2005;79:14933–14944.
2107. Tumpey TM, Maines TR, Van Hoeven N, et al. A two-amino acid change in the hemagglutinin of the 1918 influenza virus abolishes transmission. *Science* 2007;315:655–659.
2113. Uiprasertkul MP, Puthavathana K, Sangsiriwut P, et al. Influenza A H5N1 replication sites in humans. *Emerg Infect Dis* 2005;11:1036–1041.
2116. Ungchusak K, Auewarakul P, Dowell SF, et al. Probable person-to-person transmission of avian influenza A (H5N1). *N Engl J Med* 2005;352:333–340.
2131. Van Hoeven N, Pappas C, Belser JA, et al. Human HA and polymerase subunit PB2 proteins confer transmission of an avian influenza virus through the air. *Proc Natl Acad Sci U S A* 2009;106:3366–3371.
2139. van Riel D, Munster VJ, de Wit E, et al. H5N1 Virus attachment to lower respiratory tract. *Science* 2006;312:399.
2145. Varghese JN, Laver WG, Colman PM. Structure of the influenza virus glycoprotein antigen neuraminidase at 2.9 A resolution. *Nature* 1983;303:35–40.
2150. Verhoeyen M, Fang R, Jou WM, et al. Antigenic drift between the haemagglutinin of the Hong Kong influenza strains A/Aichi/2/68 and A/Victoria/3/75. *Nature* 1980;286:771–776.
2158. Vijaykrishna D, Poon LL, Zhu HC, et al. Reassortment of pandemic H1N1/2009 influenza A virus in swine. *Science* 2010;328:1529.
2166. Viswanathan K, Koh X, Chandrasekaran A, et al. Determinants of glycan receptor specificity of H2N2 influenza A virus hemagglutinin. *PLoS One* 2010;5:e13768.
2168. von Itzstein M, Wu WY, Kok GB, et al. Rational design of potent sialidase-based inhibitors of influenza virus replication. *Nature* 1993; 363:418–423.
2206. Watanabe T, Watanabe S, Shinya K, et al. Viral RNA polymerase complex promotes optimal growth of 1918 virus in the lower respiratory tract of ferrets. *Proc Natl Acad Sci U S A* 2009;106:588–592.
2214. Webster RG, Bean WJ, Gorman OT, et al. Evolution and ecology of influenza A viruses. *Microbiol Rev* 1992;56:152–179.
2218. Webster RG, Hinshaw VS, Bean WJ Jr, et al. Influenza viruses from avian and porcine sources and their possible role in the origin of human pandemic strains. *Dev Biol Stand* 1977;39:461–468.
2223. Webster RG, Laver WG. Determination of the number of nonoverlapping antigenic areas on Hong Kong (H3N2) influenza virus hemagglutinin with monoclonal antibodies and the selection of variants with potential epidemiological significance. *Virology* 1980;104:139–148.
2230. Wei CJ, Boyington JC, McTamney PM, et al. Induction of broadly neutralizing H1N1 influenza antibodies by vaccination. *Science* 2010; 329:1060–1064.
2247. Wiley DC, Skehel JJ. The structure and function of the hemagglutinin membrane glycoprotein of influenza virus. *Annu Rev Biochem* 1987; 56:365–394.
2248. Wiley DC, Wilson IA, Skehel JJ. Structural identification of the antibody-binding sites of Hong Kong influenza haemagglutinin and their involvement in antigenic variation. *Nature* 1981;289:373–378.
2252. Wilson IA, Skehel JJ, Wiley DC. Structure of the haemagglutinin membrane glycoprotein of influenza virus at 3 A resolution. *Nature* 1981; 289:366–373.
2267. Wright PF. Vaccine preparedness–are we ready for the next influenza pandemic? *N Engl J Med* 2008;358:2540–2543.
2271. Wright PF, Thompson J, Karzon DT. Differing virulence of H1N1 and H3N2 influenza strains. *Am J Epidemiol* 1980;112:814–819.
2287. Xu R, Ekiert DC, Krause JC, et al. Structural basis of preexisting immunity to the 2009 H1N1 pandemic influenza virus. *Science* 2010; 328:357–360.
2296. Yamada S, Hatta M, Staker BL, et al. Biological and structural characterization of a host-adapting amino acid in influenza virus. *PLoS Pathog* 2010;6(8):e1001034.
2297. Yamada S, Suzuki Y, Suzuki T, et al. Haemagglutinin mutations responsible for the binding of H5N1 influenza A viruses to human-type receptors. *Nature* 2006;444:378–382.
2345. Yuen KY, Chan PK, Peiris M, et al. Clinical features and rapid viral diagnosis of human disease associated with avian influenza A H5N1 virus. *Lancet* 1998;351:467–471.
2373. Zhou NN, Senne DA, Landgraf JS, et al. Genetic reassortment of avian, swine, and human influenza A viruses in American pigs. *J Virol* 1999; 73:8851–8856.

CHAPTER 42

Richard M. Elliott • Connie S. Schmaljohn

Bunyaviridae

HISTORY

The family *Bunyaviridae* takes its name from Bunyamwera virus (BUNV), which was isolated originally from *Aedes* mosquitoes in the Semliki Forest, Uganda, during a yellow fever study in 1943.[499] Following the isolation of BUNV, several additional arboviruses were discovered that clearly did not fit into the classic arbovirus group A and B antigenic groups (which now are included in the *Flaviviridae* family or the *Alphavirus* genus of the *Togaviridae* family) and were assigned to what became known as group C arboviruses.[83] During the next decade, further virus discovery and detailed serologic studies, together with biochemical and morphologic analyses,[363] led to the concept of a Bunyamwera supergroup consisting of groups of viruses that could be linked by repeatable serologic cross-reactions. Serogroups (viruses related by their reactivity in any serologic test) and complexes (closely related members of a serogroup) were further defined for these viruses.[73]

The family *Bunyaviridae* was formally established in 1975.[423] The International Committee on Taxonomy of Viruses (ICTV) approved the creation of the *Bunyavirus* genus in 1980, along with viruses morphologically and biochemically similar but antigenically distinct, that formed the *Uukuvirus, Phlebovirus*, and *Nairovirus* genera.[46] The discovery of a novel group of rodent-borne viruses and another group of plant infecting viruses with conforming molecular properties respectively led to the additions of the *Hantavirus* genus in 1985, and the *Tospovirus* genus in 1991. Further studies demonstrated a close biochemical similarity between uukuviruses and phleboviruses, resulting in their combination into the *Phlebovirus* genus in 1991.[71] To prevent confusion when discussing viruses in the *Bunyavirus* genus as opposed to the family as a whole, the former was renamed *Orthobunyavirus* in 1995.[142] Viruses within each genus are thus referred to as hantaviruses, nairoviruses, orthobunyaviruses, and so on, whereas the term "bunyavirus" is used to refer to any member of the family. Currently more than 350 named viruses are included in the family, making it one of the largest families of RNA viruses.

Except for the hantaviruses, which are transmitted in aerosolized rodent excreta, bunyaviruses are carried and

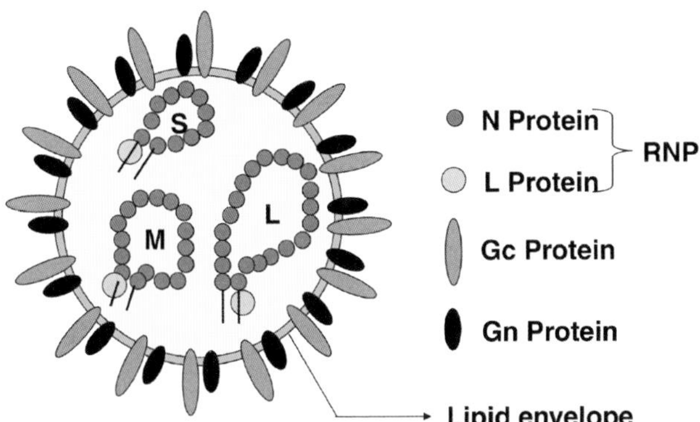

FIGURE 42.1. Schematic of a bunyavirus virion. The three genome segments (L, M, and S) are encapsidated by nucleocapsid protein to form ribonucleoprotein complexes (RNPs), and together with the viral L protein (RNA dependent RNA polymerase, RdRp) are packaged within a host cell–derived lipid envelope modified by insertion of the viral glycoproteins Gn and Gc. Note that there is no matrix protein.

transmitted by arthropods, primarily mosquitoes, ticks, sand flies, or thrips.

BUNV is the prototype of the family, and remains an important research model. It was the first bunyavirus whose genome was completely sequenced,[141,306] and significantly was the first segmented genome negative-sense RNA virus that was recovered (rescued) entirely from cloned complementary DNA (cDNA).[62,450]

CLASSIFICATION

The essential criteria for inclusion in the family are enveloped virions of 80 to 120 nm diameter (Fig. 42.1), containing a tripartite, single-stranded RNA genome of negative- or ambi-sense polarity, which replicate in the cytoplasm, and usually assemble at the Golgi complex. Assignment to one of the five genera is based on lack of serologic cross-reactivity with members of other genera, the patterns of sizes of virion proteins (Table 42.2) and genome segments (Table 42.1), gene expression strategy (Fig. 42.2), and conserved terminal nucleotide sequences of the genomic RNAs (Table 42.3). The ICTV, through the *Bunyaviridae* Study Group, describes criteria for the designation of individual species within each genus.[372] These designations, which are based on rather limited molecular data, should be treated with caution and as being fluid. The field requires large-scale, organized sequencing projects to more accurately understand the relationships between these viruses, and in particular to investigate the extent of genome segment reassortment among isolated viruses.[65,378,390,391] A potential prototype of a sixth genus, Gouleako virus, has recently been described.[329] This virus is most similar to phleboviruses but appears restricted to mosquitoes and could not infect vertebrate cells in culture. Table 42.4 lists the most notable members in the currently defined genera, and a brief introduction to each genus follows.

Orthobunyavirus Genus

The largest genus of bunyaviruses is the *Orthobunyavirus* genus, which contains more than 170 named viruses that are found throughout the world. Almost all of these viruses are transmitted by mosquitoes and have amplification cycles in a variety of vertebrate hosts.[73,372] Among important orthobunyavirus pathogens in humans are La Crosse virus (LACV) that causes pediatric encephalitis, Oropouche virus (OROV) that causes a debilitating febrile illness, and Ngari virus that causes hemorrhagic fever, whereas Aino, Akabane, and Cache Valley viruses are examples of viruses causing disease in domestic animals (Table 42.4).

Classification of orthobunyaviruses has proven to be a complex issue. The majority of viruses have been placed in one of 18 serogroups based on serologic relatedness of complement fixing antibodies (mediated by the N protein) and hemagglutinating and neutralizing antibodies (mediated by the glycoproteins), although a number of viruses classified into the *Orthobunyavirus* genus are currently not assigned to any of these serogroups.[73,372] The 18 serogroups are Anopheles A, Anopheles B, Bakau, Bunyamwera, Bwamba, Group C, Capim, California, Gamboa, Guama, Koongol, Minatitlan, Nyando, Olifanstlei, Patois, Simbu, Tete, and Turlock. Serologic relatedness varies within a serogroup and is further complicated by the occurrence of natural reassortant viruses (e-Fig. 42.1), such that viruses may be more related to members of one group or another depending on the assay used.[72]

The latest report of the ICTV delineates the orthobunyaviruses into 44 species,[372] although as described above such classification should be regarded as fluid because of the paucity of molecular data. Comprehensive molecular genetic studies have involved viruses in only 4 serogroups, namely Bunyamwera, Group C, California, and Simbu,[57,126,378,457] but S segment nucleotide sequences have been obtained for one or two representatives of the Anopheles A, Anopheles B, Bakau, Bwamba, Nyando, Tete, and Turlock serogroups.[292,351,588] In most cases the S genome segment encodes two proteins, N and, in an overlapping reading frame, a small nonstructural protein termed NSs. N and NSs proteins are translated from the same

TABLE 42.1 Pattern of Sizes of Viral RNA Segments in *Bunyaviridae* Genera

Genus RNA segment	*Orthobunyavirus*	*Hantavirus*	*Nairovirus*	*Phlebovirus*	*Tospovirus*
L	6.9	6.5	12.2	6.4	8.9
M	4.5	3.6	4.9	3.5	4.8
S	1.0	1.7	1.7	1.7	2.9
Total	12.4	11.8	18.8	11.6	16.6

Sizes given in kb.

TABLE 42.2 Pattern of Sizes of Viral Structural Proteins in *Bunyaviridae* Genera

Genus protein	*Orthobunyavirus*	*Hantavirus*	*Nairovirus*	*Phlebovirus*	*Tospovirus*
L	260	250	460	250	330
Gc	110	55	75	65	75
Gn	35	70	35	55–70	50
N	25	50	50	30	30

Sizes given in kD.

viral messenger RNA (mRNA) species as the result of alternate AUG-initiation codon selection.[48,144] However, viruses in the Anopheles A, Anopheles B, and Tete serogroups do not show evidence of having an NSs ORF. In addition, these viruses have rather longer N proteins than those in the other serogroups.[351]

Phlebovirus Genus

The *Phlebovirus* genus contains more than 80 viruses, with about half classified into nine antigenic complexes that are regarded as species, whereas 33 are considered as tentative species in the genus. The viruses of the genus *Phlebovirus* are present throughout the world, with the exception of Australia, and are more diverse in terms of arthropod vector than those of the other arthropod-borne genera. Most virus members are associated with phlebotomine sandflies, hence the genus name *Phlebovirus* (see Table 42.4). However, there are prominent exceptions, such as Rift Valley fever virus (RVFV), a medically and agriculturally important virus in Africa, which is primarily associated with *Aedes* species mosquitoes. In addition, Uukuniemi virus (UUKV), which has been used in a number of laboratory studies, is associated with the tick *Ixodes ricinus*. Recently a newly emerged phlebovirus was described in China (Huaiyangshan virus or severe fever with thrombocytopenia syndrome virus) that is associated with significant human mortality, and is transmitted by *Haemaphysalis* ticks.[595]

RVFV was first isolated in 1930 by Daubney et al. from an infected newborn lamb as part of an investigation of a large epizootic of disease causing abortion and high mortality in sheep.[113] Large RVFV epizootics in various areas of sub-Saharan Africa have been noted since that time, and clinically compatible outbreaks have been retrospectively identified as far back as 1912.[133] Several decades passed before serologic and molecular similarities to phlebotomine fever viruses were noted. Sandfly fever Sicilian and Naples viruses (SFSV, SFNV) were first isolated from American troops with febrile illness in the Palermo region of Sicily, Italy in 1943 and Naples, Italy in 1944, respectively, by inoculation of acute-phase sera into human volunteers and passage in newborn mice.[456] Outbreaks of compatible human illness in the Mediterranean region date back to the time of the Napoleonic Wars, and association of the disease with sandflies was suggested as early as 1905.[203]

TABLE 42.3 Consensus 3′ and 5′ Terminal Nucleotide Sequences of Genome RNAs

Orthobunyavirus	3′ UCAUCACAUGA......UCGUGUGAUGA 5′
Hantavirus	3′ AUCAUCAUCUG...........AUGAUGAU 5′
Nairovirus	3′ AGAGUUUCU............AGAAACUCU 5′
Phlebovirus	3′ UGUGUUUC................GAAACACA 5′
Tospovirus	3′ UCUCGUUAG...........CUAACGAGA 5′

Nairovirus Genus

The nairoviruses are almost exclusively tick-borne viruses, although a few isolations have been made from *Culicoides* flies and mosquitoes (Table 42.4). Several serogroups exist, but the most important ones are the Crimean-Congo hemorrhagic fever (CCHF) group, which includes CCHF virus (CCHFV) and Hazara virus, and the Nairobi sheep disease (NSD) group, which includes NSD virus (NSDV) and Dugbe virus (DUGV).

The *Nairovirus* genus was named after NSDV, which was originally isolated in Nairobi, Kenya in 1910 by inoculation of sheep with the blood of sheep with acute gastroenteritis.[354] The virus is now known to be present throughout various parts of Africa, and possibly India. CCHF was first recognized in the Crimean peninsula in the mid-1940s, when a large outbreak of severe hemorrhagic fever among agricultural workers was identified. The outbreak included more than 200 cases and a case fatality of about 10%.[99] Similar disease cases were later reported throughout the European and central Asian republics of the former Soviet Union, Romania, and Bulgaria. However, the virus was first isolated from a patient with a one-day fever in Kisangani, Democratic Republic of Congo, in 1956.[494] It was some years before the connection was established, but subsequent serologic studies and virus isolations from Asia and Europe revealed that the viruses from the different outbreaks and geographic regions were essentially the same virus, which then became named CCHFV.[82,100]

Hantavirus Genus

The discovery of hantaviruses traces back to 1951 to 1953, when United Nations troops were deployed during the border conflict between North and South Korea. More than 3,000 cases of an acute febrile illness were seen among the troops, about one third of which exhibited hemorrhagic manifestations, and an overall mortality of 5% to 10% was seen.[129,305] The disease was initially termed Korean hemorrhagic fever but is now referred to as hemorrhagic fever with renal syndrome (HFRS). Despite considerable efforts, it took about 25 years until the field mouse, *Apodemus agrarius*, was identified as the rodent reservoir, and the virus was eventually isolated. At that

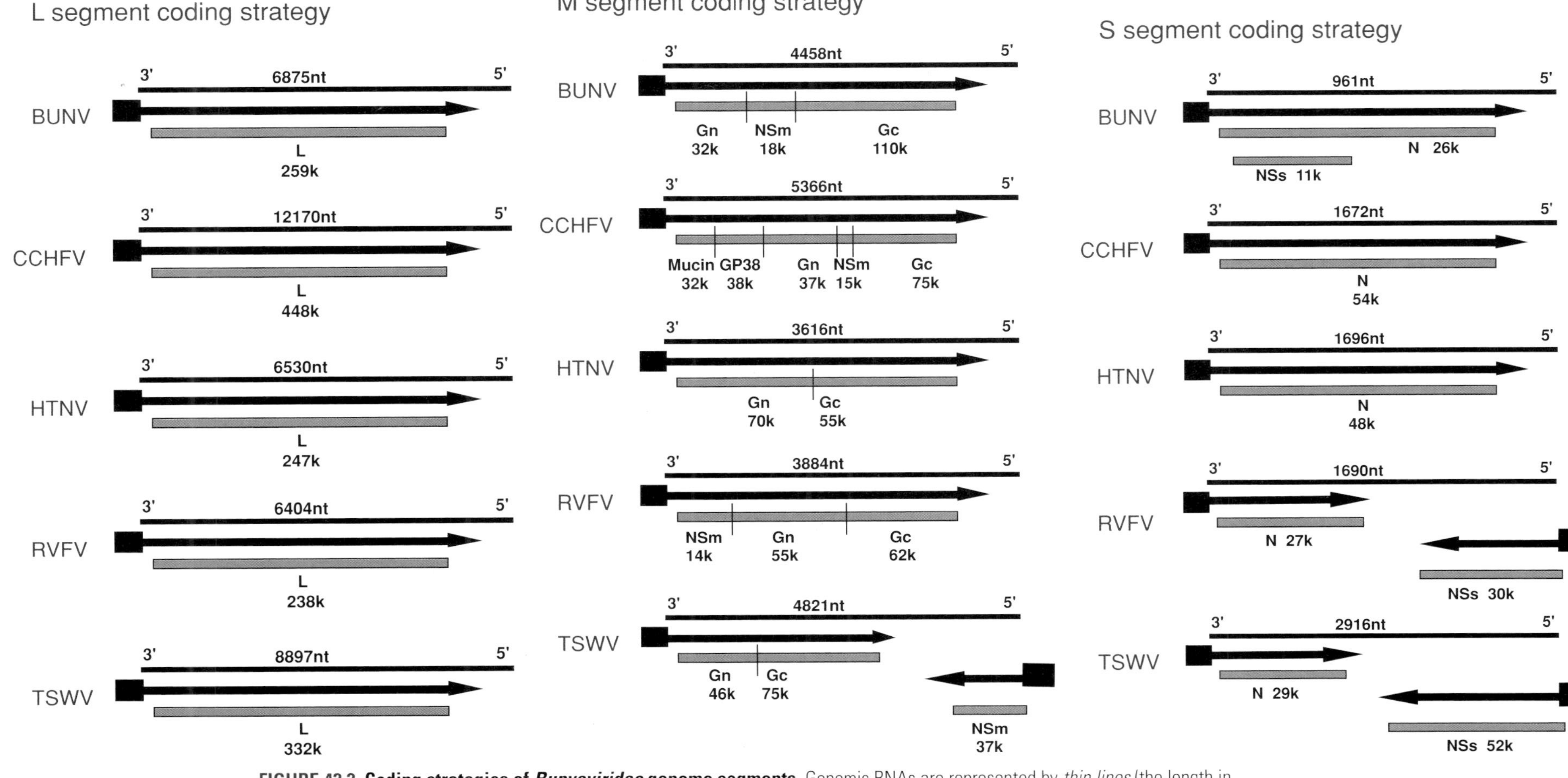

FIGURE 42.2. Coding strategies of *Bunyaviridae* genome segments. Genomic RNAs are represented by *thin lines* (the length in nucleotides is given above each segment) and the mRNAs are shown as *arrows* (■ indicates host-derived sequences at 5′ end). Gene products, with their apparent M_r, are represented by colored boxes. BUNV, Bunyamwera orthobunyavirus; CCHFV, Crimean-Congo hemorrhagic fever nairovirus; HTNV, Hantaan hantavirus; RVFV, Rift Valley fever phlebovirus; TSWV, tomato spotted wilt tospovirus. In the CCHFV M segment, mucin represents mucin-like region.

TABLE 42.4 Species in the Family *Bunyaviridae*

Genus	Species	Notable virus	Geographic distribution	Principal vector	Disease
Orthobunyavirus	*Acara virus*	Acara virus	SA/ NA	Mosquitoes	
	Akabane virus	Akabane virus	Africa, Asia, Australia	Mosquitoes, culicoid flies	Cattle
	Alajuela virus	Alajuela virus	NA	Mosquitoes	
	Anopheles A virus	Anopheles A virus	SA	Mosquitoes	
	Anopheles B virus	Anopheles B virus	SA	Mosquitoes	
	Bakau virus	Bakau virus	Asia	Mosquitoes	
	Batama virus	Batama virus	Africa	N.D.	
	Benevides virus	Benevides virus	SA	Mosquitoes	
	Bertioga virus	Bertioga virus	SA	N.D.	
	Bimiti virus	Bimiti virus	SA	Mosquitoes	
	Botambi virus	Botambi virus	Africa	Mosquitoes	
	Bunyamwera virus	Bunyamwera virus	Africa	Mosquitoes	Human
		Batai virus	Asia, Europe	Mosquitoes	Human
		Cache Valley virus	NA	Mosquitoes	Sheep, Cattle, Human
		Fort Sherman virus	SA	Mosquitoes	Human
		Germiston virus	Africa	Mosquitoes	Human
		Ilesha virus	Africa	Mosquitoes	Human
		Ngari virus	Africa	Mosquitoes	Human
		Shokwe virus	Africa	Mosquitoes	Human
		Xingu virus	SA	Mosquitoes	Human
	Bushbush virus	Bushbush virus	SA	Mosquitoes	
	Bwamba virus	Bwamba virus	Africa	Mosquitoes	Human
		Pongola virus	Africa	Mosquitoes	Human
	California encephalitis virus	California encephalitis virus	NA	Mosquitoes	Human
		Inkoo virus	Europe	Mosquitoes	Human
		Jamestown Canyon virus	NA	Mosquitoes	Human
		La Crosse virus	NA	Mosquitoes	Human
		Lumbo virus	Africa	Mosquitoes	Human
		Snowshoe hare virus	NA	Mosquitoes	Human
		Tahyna virus	Europe	Mosquitoes	Human
	Capim virus	Capim virus	SA	Mosquitoes	
	Caraparu virus	Caraparu virus	SA, NA	Mosquitoes	Human
		Apeu virus	SA	Mosquitoes	Human
		Ossa virus	NA	Mosquitoes	Human
	Catu virus	Catu virus	SA	Mosquitoes	Human
	Estero Real virus	Estero Real virus	NA	Ticks	
	Gamboa virus	Gamboa virus	NA	Mosquitoes	
	Guajara virus	Guajara virus	SA, NA	Mosquitoes	
	Guama virus	Guama virus	SA, NA	Mosquitoes	Human
	Guaroa virus	Guaroa virus	SA, NA	Mosquitoes	Human
	Kairi virus	Kairi virus	SA	Mosquitoes	Horse
	Kaeng Khoi virus	Kaeng Khoi virus	Asia	Nest bugs	
	Koongol virus	Koongol virus	Australia	Mosquitoes	
	Madrid virus	Madrid virus	NA	Mosquitoes	Human
	Main Drain virus	Main Drain virus	NA	Mosquitoes, culicoid flies	Horse
	Manzanilla virus	Ingwavuma virus	Africa, Asia	Mosquitoes	Pig
	Marituba virus	Marituba virus	SA	Mosquitoes	Human
		Murutucu virus	SA	Mosquitoes	Human
		Nepuyo virus	SA, NA	Mosquitoes	Human
		Restan virus	SA	Mosquitoes	Human

TABLE 42.4 Species in the Family *Bunyaviridae* (*continued*)

Genus	Species	Notable virus	Geographic distribution	Principal vector	Disease
	Minatitlan virus	Minatitlan virus	NA	Mosquitoes	
	M'Poko virus	M'Poko virus	Africa	Mosquitoes	
	Nyando virus	Nyando virus	Africa	Mosquitoes	Human
	Olifantsvlei virus	Olifantsvlei virus	Africa	Mosquitoes	
	Oriboca virus	Oriboca virus	SA	Mosquitoes	Human
		Itaqui virus	SA	Mosquitoes	Human
	Oropouche virus	Oropouche virus	SA	Mosquitoes, culicoid flies	Human
	Patois virus	Patois virus	NA	Mosquitoes	
	Sathuperi virus	Sathuperi virus	Africa, Asia	Mosquitoes, culicoid flies	
	Simbu virus	Simbu virus	Africa	Mosquitoes, culicoid flies	
	Shamonda virus	Shamonda virus	Africa	Culicoid flies	
	Shuni virus	Shuni virus	Africa	Mosquitoes, culicoid flies	
	Tacaiuma virus	Tacaiuma virus	SA	Mosquitoes	Human
	Tete virus	Tete virus	Africa	N.D.	
		Weldona virus	NA	culicoid flies	
	Thimiri virus	Thimiri virus	Africa, Asia	N.D.	
	Timboteua virus	Timboteua virus	SA	Mosquitoes	
	Turlock virus	Turlock virus	NA, SA	Mosquitoes	
	Wyeomyia virus	Wyeomyia virus	SA	Mosquitoes	Human
	Zegla virus	Zegla virus	NA	N.D.	
Hantavirus	*Andes virus*	Andes virus	SA	*Oligoryzomys longicaudatus*	Human
		Bermejo virus	SA	*Oligoryzomys chacoensis*	Human
		Lechiguanas virus	SA	*Oligoryzomys flavescens*	Human
		Maciel virus	SA	*Bolomys obscurus*	
		Oran virus	SA	*Oligoryzomys longicaudatus*	Human
		Pergamino virus	SA	*Akadon azarae*	
	Bayou virus	Bayou virus	NA	*Oryzomys palustris*	Human
	Black Creek Canal virus	Black Creek Canal virus	NA	*Sigmodon hispidus*	Human
	Cano Delgadito virus	Cano Delgadito virus	SA	*Sigmodon alstoni*	
	Dobrava-Belgrade virus	Dobrava virus	Europe	*Apodemus flavicollis*	Human
	El Moro Canyon virus	El Moro Canyon virus	NA	*Reithrodontomys megalotis*	
	Hantaan virus	Hantaan virus	Asia	*Apodemus agrarius coreae*	Human
	Isla Vista virus	Isla Vista virus	NA	*Microtus californicus*	
	Khabarovsk virus	Khabarovsk virus	Asia	*Microtus maximowiczii, Microtus fortis*	
	Laguna Negra virus	Laguna Negra virus	SA	*Calomys laucha*	Human
	Muleshoe virus	Muleshoe virus	NA	*Sigmodon hispidus*	
	New York virus	New York virus	NA	*Peromyscus leucopus*	Human
	Prospect Hill virus	Bloodland Lake virus	NA	*Microtus ochrogaster*	
		Prospect Hill virus	NA	*Microtus pennsylvanicus*	
	Puumala virus	Puumala virus	Europe, Asia	*Myodes glareolus*	Human
	Rio Mamore virus	Rio Mamore virus	SA	*Oligoryzomys microtis*	
	Rio Segundo virus	Rio Segundo virus	NA, SA	*Reithrodontomys mexicanus*	
	Saaremaa virus	Saaremaa virus	Europe	*Apodemus agrarius agrarius*	Human
	Seoul virus	Seoul virus	Worldwide	*Rattus norvegicus*	Human
	Sin Nombre virus	Blue River virus	NA	*Peromyscus leucopus*	
		Monongahela virus	NA	*Peromyscus maniculatus*	Human
		Sin Nombre virus	NA	*Peromyscus maniculatus*	Human
	Thailand virus	Thailand virus	Asia	*Bandicota indica*	
	Thottapalayam virus	Thottapalayam virus	India	*Suncus murinus*	
	Topografov virus	Topografov virus	Asia, Europe	*Lemmus sibiricus*	
	Tula virus	Tula virus	Europe	*Microtus arvalis, M. rossiaemeridionalis*	

(*continued*)

TABLE 42.4 Species in the Family *Bunyaviridae* (*continued*)

Genus	Species	Notable virus	Geographic distribution	Principal vector	Disease
Nairovirus	*Crimean-Congo hemorrhagic fever virus*	Crimean-Congo hemorrhagic fever virus	Africa, Asia, Europe	Culicoid flies, ticks	Human
		Hazara virus	Asia	Ticks	
	Dera Ghazi Khan virus	Dera Ghazi Khan virus	Asia	Ticks	
	Dugbe virus	Dugbe virus	Africa	Ticks	Human, cattle
		Nairobi sheep disease virus (Ganjam virus)	Africa, Asia	Ticks, culicoid flies, mosquitoes	Human, cattle
	Hughes virus	Hughes virus	NA, SA	Ticks	Seabirds
	Qalyub virus	Qalyub virus		Ticks	
	Sakhalin virus	Sakhalin virus	Asia	Ticks	
	Thiafora virus	Erve virus	Europe	N.D.	Human
Phlebovirus	*Bujaru virus*	Bujaru virus	SA	N.D.	
	Candiru virus	Alenquer virus	SA	N.D.	Human
		Candiru virus	SA	N.D.	Human
	Chilibre virus	Chilibre virus		Phlebotomines	
	Frijoles virus	Frijoles virus		Phlebotomines	
	Punta Toro virus	Punta Toro virus	NA, SA	Phlebotomines	Human
	Rift Valley fever virus	Rift Valley fever virus	Africa	Mosquitoes	Human, cattle
	Salehabad virus	Salehabad virus	Asia	Phlebotomines	
	Sandfly fever Naples virus	Sandfly fever Naples virus	Europe, Africa, Asia	Phlebotomines	Human
		Sandfly fever Sicilian virus	Europe	Phlebotomines	Human
		Toscana virus	Europe	Phlebotomines	Human
	Uukuniemi virus	Uukuniemi virus	Europe	Ticks	Seabirds
Tospovirus	*Groundnut bud necrosis virus*	Groundnut bud necrosis virus (Peanut bud necrosis virus)	Asia	*Frankliniella schultzei, Thrips palmi*	Plant
	Groundnut ringspot virus	Groundnut ringspot virus	SA, Africa	*F. occidentalis, F. schultzei, F. gemina*	Plant
	Groundnut yellow spot virus	Groundnut yellow spot virus (Peanut yellow spot virus)	Asia	N.D.	
	Impatiens necrotic spot virus	Impatiens necrotic spot virus	NA, Europe	*F. occidentalis*	Plant
	Tomato spotted wilt virus	Tomato spotted wilt virus	Worldwide	*F. bispinosa, F. cephalica F. gemina, F. fusca, F. intonsa, F. occidentalis, F. schultzei, F. setosus, T. tabaci*	Plant
	Watermelon silver mottle virus	Watermelon silver mottle virus	Asia	*T. palmi*	Plant
	Zucchini lethal chlorosis virus	Zucchini lethal chlorosis virus	SA	*F. zucchini*	Plant

NA, North America; SA, South America; N.D., not determined.

time, all identified viruses of the family *Bunyaviridae* were known to be arthropod-borne viruses. Therefore, it was a big surprise when this rodent-borne virus was shown to share characteristics of viruses of the family *Bunyaviridae.* The virus was named Hantaan virus (HTNV), after the Hantaan river close to the location of some of the initial Korean cases, and became the prototype of the *Hantavirus* genus.[305]

During the course of the early studies in Korea, it became clear that HFRS cases were also occurring in urban areas. Years of investigation finally demonstrated that the urban cases in Korea, China, and Japan were associated with infection with Seoul virus, which is hosted by the rats *Rattus norvegicus* and *R. rattus.*[300,305,514] For more than 50 years, a similar, but generally milder, disease termed nephropathia epidemica (NE) was described in various parts of Scandinavia.[375] Following the isolation of HTNV, the virus was shown to react with sera from patients with convalescent phase NE.[375] This led to the discovery of Puumala virus (PUUV) as the cause of this form of HFRS and the bank vole, *Clethrionomys glareolus,* as the virus host.

The most recent major event in the history of hantaviruses was the discovery of hantavirus pulmonary syndrome (HPS) in the southwestern United States in 1993.[373] A cluster of cases was identified in the Four Corners region, which presented with a flu-like illness (i.e., fever, headache, muscle aches, chills, and so on), but rapidly progressed to a more severe respiratory disease with bilateral pulmonary infiltrates, respiratory failure, shock, and death, occurring approximately 2 to 10 days after onset of illness in almost 50% of the cases.[257] Within a couple of weeks of the initial outbreak, a newly identified virus, Sin Nombre virus (SNV), was shown to be the cause of HPS, and the rodent reservoir was shown to be the common deer mouse, *Peromyscus maniculatus.*[96,373] Within the next several years, HPS was shown to occur throughout the Americas from Canada to Patagonia, and was found to be caused by least 10 hantaviruses, each associated with a different rodent species. During the study of the hantaviruses associated with HPS and HFRS, many additional hantaviruses not known to be associated with human illness were discovered in a wide variety of rodent hosts (Table 42.4).

In addition to rodents, a number of hantaviruses have been isolated from insectivores. In fact the first hantavirus isolated was Thottapalayam virus, from the Asian house shrew, in Southern India,[79] although it was not recognized as a hantavirus until several years later.[594] Very recently a number of other insectivore-associated hantaviruses have been identified; interestingly, prevalence in these animals is much higher than in rodents. The insectivore-borne viruses are widely distributed across the globe and display greater genetic diversity than the rodent-borne hantaviruses.[434]

Tospovirus Genus

The tospoviruses are plant viruses that are transmitted propagatively by thrips.[579] At least 13 species of thrips, in the *Frankliniella* and *Thrips* genera, are reported to transmit these viruses.[384,575] Several of these viruses are now recognized as being of significant agricultural importance.[427]

The history of the tospoviruses goes back to 1915, with the recognition of spotted wilt of tomatoes in Australia,[66] and then the subsequent isolation in 1930 of tomato spotted wilt virus (TSWV),[460] from which the genus gained its name.[275] By the late 1940s, TSWV infections were greatly reduced in the United States and Western Europe due to pesticide use controlling the onion thrips, *Thrips tabaci,* which was likely the primary vector at that time. The geographic spread during the 1960s and 1970s of the Western flower thrips, *Frankliniella occidentalis,* another efficient vector of TSWV, led to a rapid expansion of TSWV.[543,575] The virus is now known to be global in distribution, and it is found throughout agricultural areas in warmer climate zones and prevalent in greenhouse cultivations in more temperate areas. In contrast to the other genus members, TSWV has an unusually wide host range, with more than 925 plant species, including 82 botanical families, reported to be susceptible to infection. These include several important crops such as peanuts, peppers, tobacco, potatoes, peas, tomatoes, celery, lettuce, and ornamental flowers, with crop losses amounting to more than a billion dollars.[393] There are 21 viruses assigned to the *Tospovirus* genus, with currently eight recognized species.[200,372]

VIRION STRUCTURE

Morphology

Under the electron microscope, negatively stained bunyaviruses appear spherical or pleomorphic, 80 to 120 nm in diameter, and display surface glycoprotein (GP) projections of 5 to 10 nm, which are embedded in a lipid bilayered envelope approximately 5 to 7 nm thick. (Fig. 42.3). With use of cryoelectron microscopic techniques, which more accurately preserve particle integrity, LACV particles were reported to be 75 to 115 nm in diameter,[522] whereas particles of RVFV and Uukuniemi

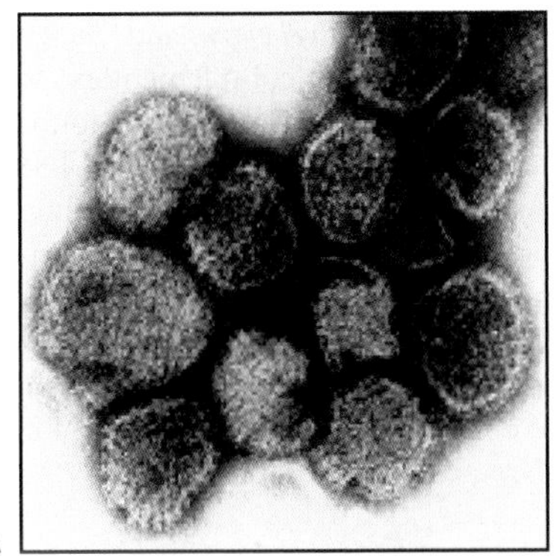

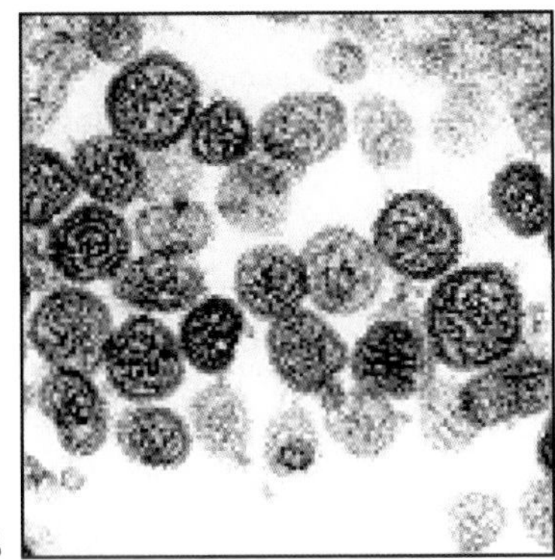

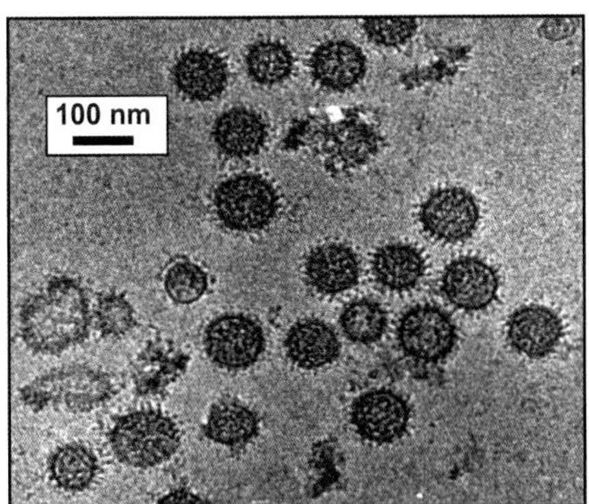

FIGURE 42.3. Morphology of bunyaviruses. A: Electron micrograph of glutaraldehyde fixed negatively stained Hantaan virions (*Hantavirus* genus). The morphologic units on the surface form a grid-like pattern. As described in the text, viruses in other genera show different surface characteristics. **B:** Thin-section electron micrograph of Puumala virus (*Hantavirus* genus). The interior of the virion has a filamentous or coiled bead appearance, presumably due to the presence of the ribonucleoprotein complexes (RNPs). **C:** Cryoelectron micrographs of purified vitrified-hydrated La Crosse virions (*Orthobunyavirus* genus). The glycoproteins spikes are clearly visible. (**A** and **B,** courtesy of Geisbert T, Kuhl K,White JS, U.S. Army Medical Research Institute of Infectious Diseases, Frederick, MD; **C,** courtesy of Prasad BVV, Baylor College of Medicine, Houston, TX.)

(UUKV) phleboviruses had mean diameters of 100 nm and 125 nm, respectively,[162,386] and Tula and Hantaan hantaviruses had mean diameters of 130 to 135 nm.[35,216] The spikes are thought to mostly consist of heterodimers of the two viral GPs, and biochemical analysis of purified LACV particles indicated that the two GP species were equimolar and present at about 650 copies per virion. The GPs interact to form surface morphologic units that vary among viruses in different genera.[333] Virions in the *Orthobunyavirus* genus have surfaces covered with closely packed, knoblike morphologic units with no detectable order. Similarly, no obvious order was found for the small surface structures with central cavities observed on viruses in the *Nairovirus* genus.[333] The appearances of viruses in the *Tospovirus* genus have been likened to that of the nairoviruses.[344] Other than the presence of GP projections, which are observed as a fringe on negatively stained virions, distinctive surface structure has not been noted for these viruses.

Viruses in the *Phlebovirus* genus have round, closely packed morphologic units, approximately 10 to 11 nm in diameter, with central cavities approximately 5 nm in diameter.[333] Negative staining of glutaraldehyde-fixed particles, freeze-etching techniques, and/or cryoelectron tomography demonstrated that the glycoprotein spikes of UUKV and RVFV are organized on a T-12 icosahedral lattice, an arrangement so far unique to phleboviruses.[162,386,557] For UUKV, two pH-dependent conformations of the glycoproteins were observed: tall spikes at pH7 and flat spikes at pH6. It is suggested that at low pH the conformational change exposes hydrophobic regions on the GP, possibly on Gc, that facilitate fusion between the viral and endosomal membrane during viral entry,[386] a mechanism observed for other enveloped viruses that enter cells via the endocytic pathway.

The surface structure of viruses in the *Hantavirus* genus also are distinctly ordered but have a square grid-like appearance (Fig. 42.3).[571] Electron cryotomography[35,216] confirms that the Gn-Gc spike complex has fourfold symmetry. Each spike is likely composed of four Gn-Gc heterodimers that form lattices on the virion surface. Specific lateral interactions between spike complexes are thought to induce membrane curvature during the budding process.

The interior of virions, as observed by thin-section electron microscopy, has a filamentous or coiled bead appearance, presumably due to the presence of the ribonucleocapsids (Fig. 42.3).[122] From single particle reconstructions of tomograms, internally virions contained parallel thread or rod-like structures assumed to be ribonucleoprotein complex (RNP); some were located very close to the membrane suggesting interaction with the cytoplasmic tails of one or both of the glycoproteins.[35,216,386,440]

Biochemical and Biophysical Properties

The composition and structure of virions has been inferred from biochemical and morphologic studies. An overall chemical content of 2% RNA, 58% protein, 33% lipid, and 7% carbohydrate was estimated for UUKV.[380] Sedimentation coefficients of virions range from 400 to 500 S, and their buoyant densities in sucrose are 1.16 to 1.18 g/cm^3, and in CsCl, 1.20 to 1.21 g/cm^3. Treatment with lipid solvents or nonionic detergents removes the viral envelope and results in loss of infectivity for arthropods and mammals.[380] For plants, the envelope is not required for infectivity, as demonstrated in studies with TSWV, for which repeated mechanical passage among plants resulted in a defective virus that was unable to produce enveloped particles but was able to replicate in plant cells.[116]

GENOME STRUCTURE AND ORGANIZATION

Viral Genome

Virions contain three single-stranded RNA genome segments designated as large (L), medium (M), and small (S). All three RNA segments of a virus have the same complementary nucleotides at their 3′ and 5′ termini. The terminal nucleotide sequences are highly conserved among viruses within a genus, but differ from those of viruses in other genera (Table 42.3). Base-pairing of the terminal nucleotides is predicted to form stable panhandle structures and noncovalently closed circular RNAs. Direct support for base-pairing comes from electron microscopy of RNA extracted from virions, in which three sizes of circular RNAs were evident.[204]

The RNA segments are complexed with N to form individual L, M, and S nucleocapsids, which were generally assumed to have helical symmetry,[379] but analysis of isolated RVFV nucleocapsids did not show this pattern but rather a string-like appearance.[440] Nucleocapsids released by nonionic detergent treatment of virions often also appear as circular structures in electron micrographs,[411] suggesting that the complementary RNAs can base-pair even when complexed with protein in an estimated ratio of 4% RNA to 96% protein.[431] This hypothesis is supported by data showing cross-linking of the ends of nucleocapsid-enclosed RNAs by treatment with psoralens, which are photoreactive, nucleic acid, cross-linking agents.[431]

At least one each of the L, M, and S ribonucleocapsids must be contained in a virion for infectivity; however, equal numbers of nucleocapsids may not always be packaged in mature virions, as suggested by various reports of equimolar or nonequimolar ratios of L, M, and S RNAs.[49,218] Unequal complements of the ribonucleocapsids may contribute to the size differences of virions observed by electron microscopy.[35,522]

In addition to ribonucleocapsids containing virion-sense RNA (vRNA), certain viruses in the *Phlebovirus* and *Tospovirus* genera encapsidate small amounts of complementary sense (cRNA or antigenome). The phlebovirus UUKV was found to have S but not M segment cRNA, and the tospovirus TSWV had both M and S cRNAs in virions.[274,491] For the orthobunyavirus, LACV, S segment cRNA was detected in virions synthesized in insect cells, but not in mammalian cells.[431] Interestingly, the phlebovirus RVFV encapsidated all three cRNA gene segments, and, as will be described later (see "S segment products"), at least one of the cRNA genes may have a role in early replication processes.[225]

Coding Strategies of Viral Genes

Both similarities and noteworthy differences in the coding strategies of viruses in the family *Bunyaviridae* are known. Viruses in each genus encode all structural proteins in their cRNA. Certain viruses also encode nonstructural proteins in their cRNA or in their vRNA. Therefore, some viruses in the family *Bunyaviridae* use only a negative-sense coding strategy and others use a combination of negative-sense and ambisense coding strategies (Fig. 42.2).

S Segment Strategies

Viruses in the *Orthobunyavirus* genus have smaller S segments than those of viruses in other genera (Table 42.1). Some orthobunyaviruses encode two polypeptides, the nucleocapsid protein (N) and a nonstructural protein (NSs), in ORFs in cRNA[48] (Fig. 42.2), whereas others only encode N protein.[351] The presence of NSs in virus-infected cells was demonstrated for several members of the genus.[140] Only one S segment mRNA species can be found in orthobunyavirus-infected cells[84]; therefore, N and NSs are generated by alternative start codon recognition by ribosomes.[126,144]

Hantaviruses and nairoviruses encode larger N proteins than viruses in other genera, (Table 42.2, Fig. 42.2).[332,470] Some hantaviruses (e.g., SNV, PUUV, Tula [TULV] and Prospect Hill [PHV] viruses), have ORFs within the N ORF, and an NSs protein has been detected in PUUV- and TULV-infected cells.[227] No NSs protein has been detected in nairovirus infected cells. Only one S-segment mRNA, similar in size to the coding region for N, was identified in hantavirus- or nairovirus-infected cells, indicating that transcription termination occurs shortly after the translation stop codon.[469,563] Certain hantaviruses (e.g., SNV) have long 3′ noncoding regions (of greater than 700 nucleotides) containing numerous repeated sequences. These repeats may result from polymerase slippage on the vRNA template.[505]

The ambisense coding strategy of the S segments of phleboviruses and tospoviruses produces N from a subgenomic mRNA that is complementary to vRNA, and NSs from a subgenomic mRNA of the same polarity as vRNA (Fig. 42.2).[118,220] Evidence that the mRNA for NSs is copied from cRNA (after genome replication) comes from time-course studies. For the phlebovirus UUKV, N was detected at 4 to 6 hours after infection, whereas NSs did not appear until 8 hours after infection.[492,542] Likewise, the mRNA for NSs of the tospovirus TSWV was detected in infected plant cells 15 hours later than for N.[507] In addition, studies with the phlebovirus Punta Toro virus (PTV) demonstrated that protein synthesis inhibitors arrest production of NSs mRNA, but not N mRNA.[222] These results suggest that protein synthesis must occur before the NSs mRNA can be made. In contrast, studies with the phlebovirus RVFV demonstrated the presence of cRNAs to all three RNA segments in purified virions. Moreover, mRNA for the NSs protein was detected as early as 20 minutes after infection, concomitant with the appearance of mRNA for N, suggesting that the ambisense-encoded NSs mRNA are transcribed from the incoming antiviral sense RNA.[225]

M Segment Strategies

Sizes of M segments range from ~3,600 nucleotides to ~4,900 nucleotides (Table 42.1). All bunyavirus M segments encode the two envelope GPs in a single ORF of cRNA (Fig. 42.2). Previous designations of G1 and G2, which were based on relative migration of the proteins in polyacrylamide gels, have been replaced by designations of Gn and Gc, referring to the amino-terminal or carboxy-terminal coding of the proteins.[294] As described below, it is becoming increasingly clearer that the functions of the Gn and Gc proteins are conserved among the five genera.

Some viruses encode NSm proteins, and others do not. Except for the tospoviruses, which use an ambisense strategy to generate NSm from a subgenomic mRNA, a single mRNA, nearly equivalent in size to the cRNA ORF has been detected in virus-infected cells. For tospoviruses, separate, subgenomic messages for the Gn-Gc precursor and for NSm were identified.[273,295] NSm is readily detected in infected plants and is the only M segment nonstructural protein in the *Bunyaviridae* family to have a clearly defined role (i.e., it is a movement protein [see "M Segment Products," below]). Another possible role for NSm for some viruses may be as a virulence factor. For example, a genetically engineered RVFV lacking NSm induced more extensive apoptosis than did one with NSm and the expression of NSm significantly inhibited the cleavage of caspase 8 and 9 induced by staurosporine, indicating that the NSm protein suppresses apoptosis.[582]

L Segment Strategies

The L segments of hantaviruses, orthobunyaviruses, and phleboviruses are of similar size, (~6,500 nucleotides), whereas those of tospoviruses and nairoviruses are considerably larger (~9,000 and 12,000 nucleotides, respectively; Table 42.1). All L segments of viruses in the family use conventional negative-sense coding strategies (Fig. 42.2). For each L segment described thus far, there are fewer than 200 nucleotides of total noncoding information, and there is no evidence for additional coding regions in either the cRNA or vRNA.[117,141,143,209,360,465]

STAGES OF REPLICATION

The principal stages of the replication process for viruses in the *Bunyaviridae* are illustrated in Figure 42.4 and are summarized in the following:

1. Attachment, mediated by an interaction of viral proteins and host receptors
2. Entry, by receptor-mediated endocytosis
3. Uncoating, by acidification of endocytic vesicles, and fusion of viral membranes with endosomal membranes
4. Primary transcription of viral-complementary mRNA species from genome templates using host-cell–derived primers and the virion-associated polymerase
5. Translation of L, M, and S mRNAs
   - co-translational cleavage of M-segment polyprotein and postranslational cleavage of precursors for some viruses
   - dimerization of Gn and Gc in the endoplasmic reticulum (ER)
6. Membrane-associated RNA replication
   - synthesis and encapsidation of cRNA to serve as templates for vRNA or, for ambisense genes, templates for subgenomic mRNA
   - genome replication
7. Morphogenesis
   - localization of N in budding compartments
   - transport of dimerized Gn and Gc to the Golgi
   - glycosylation
   - acquisition of modified host membranes, generally by budding into the Golgi cisternae
8. Fusion of cytoplasmic vesicles containing viruses with the plasma membrane and release of mature virions
   - more rarely, some viruses in some cell types have been observed to bud directly from the host cell's plasma membrane

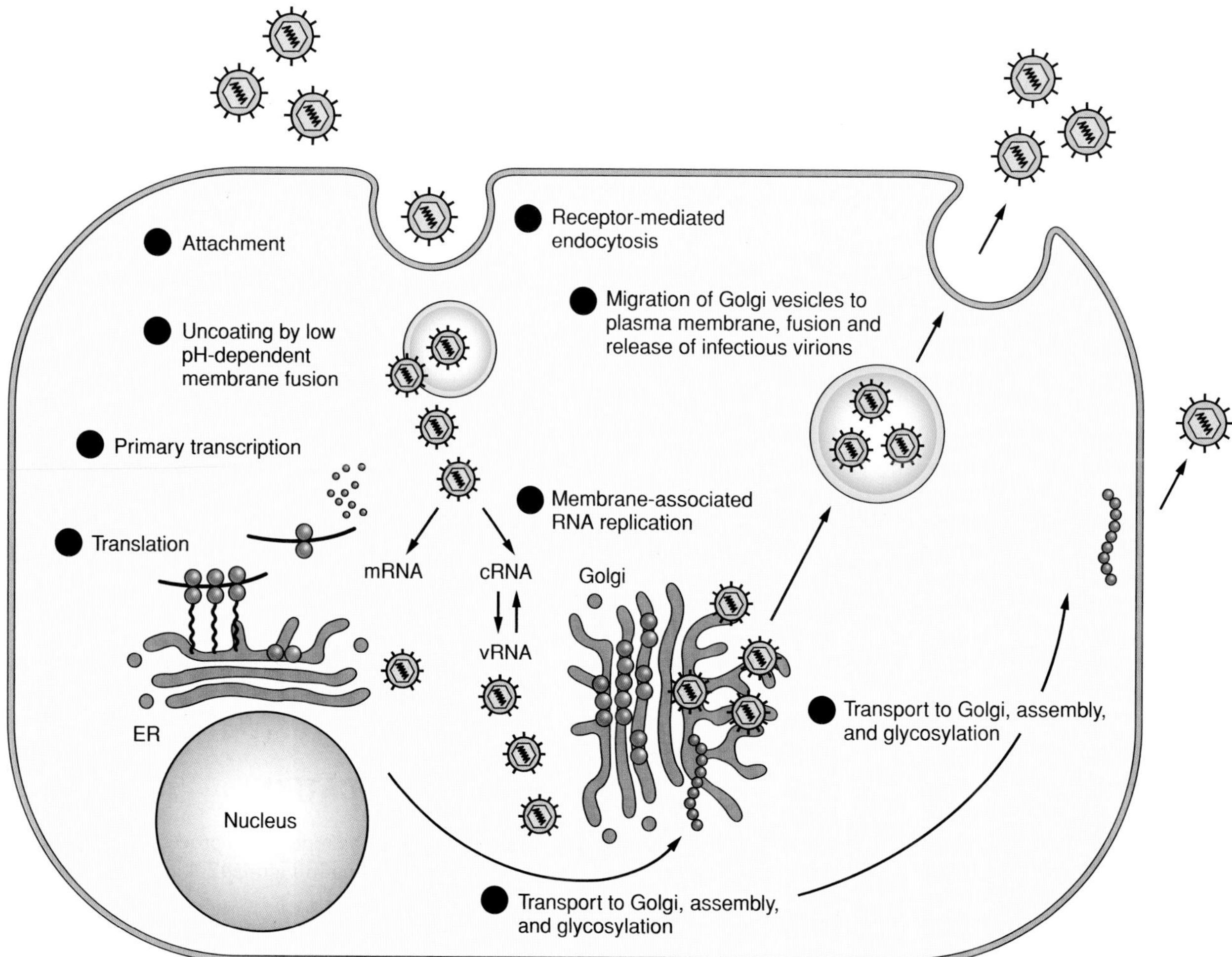

FIGURE 42.4. Replication cycle of viruses in the family *Bunyaviridae*. Steps in the replication cycle are the following: 1. Attachment, mediated by an interaction of viral proteins and host receptors; 2. Receptor-mediated endocytosis; 3. Uncoating, by acidification of endocytic vesicles, and fusion of viral membranes with endosomal membranes; 4. Primary transcription of viral-complementary messenger RNA (mRNA) species from genome templates using host-cell–derived primers and the virion-associated polymerase; 5. Translation of L, M, and S mRNAs, co-translational cleavage of the M-segment polyprotein, dimerization of Gn and Gc in the endoplasmic reticulum (ER); 6. Membrane-associated RNA replication, synthesis, and encapsidation of cRNA to serve as templates for vRNA or, for ambisense genes, templates for subgenomic mRNA, genome replication; 7. Morphogenesis including transport of the structural proteins to the Golgi, glycosylation of Gn and Gc, budding into the Golgi cisternae; 8. Migration of Golgi vesicles containing viruses to the cell surface, fusion of vesicular membranes with the plasma membrane, and release of infectious virions. Some viruses in some cell types can bud both into intracellular vesicles and also from the plasma membrane.

Attachment and Entry

Viral Attachment Proteins and Cellular Receptors

The mechanisms by which members of the family *Bunyaviridae* gain access to the host cell's cytoplasm appear similar to those reported for many other enveloped viruses. The first step involves an interaction between cell surface receptors and viral attachment proteins, Gn and/or Gc. The presence of neutralizing and hemagglutination-inhibiting sites on both the Gn and Gc proteins of phleboviruses and hantaviruses[27,252] suggests that both proteins may be involved in attachment. Although it is possible that both are directly involved, it is more likely that both are required due to conformational requirements that depend on dimerization of Gn and Gc.

In general, Gc appears to be the primary attachment protein for orthobunyaviruses in mammalian cells, mosquito cells, and mosquitoes.[193,261,515] Consistent with this view, expression of M-segment products of three orthobunyaviruses demonstrated that Gc, but not Gn, could effect attachment and entry when tested in a cell-to-cell fusion assay and a pseudotype transduction assay.[419] However, the amino terminal half of BUNV Gc ectodomain is not required for infection of cultured mammalian cells,[483] and this region can be replaced by green fluorescent protein (GFP) allowing the creation of viable viruses expressing chimeric Gc-GFP in their virions.[486]

For tospoviruses, the envelope GPs are required only for infection of their arthropod vectors, as evidenced by the ability of envelope-deficient mutants to replicate in plants after mechanical transmission, but their inability to infect thrips.[445] In addition, analysis of reassortant viruses demonstrated that mutations that disrupted the Gn-Gc ORF of TSWV ablated transmissibility by thrips.[495] These studies provide indirect evidence that the L-polymerase protein remains associated with ribonucleocapsids and is active despite the absence of intact virions.

Although there are no specific reports of Gc being the attachment protein of tospoviruses, functional homology to the Gc proteins of other bunyaviruses was proposed based on amino acid sequence homologies detected for iris yellow spot virus.[106] In contrast, however, a study with a soluble, truncated form of TSWV Gn expressed in baculoviruses showed binding of this protein to epithelial cells in the midguts of thrips, suggesting that Gn could mediate attachment in thrips.[573] Similar results were reported earlier with the orthobunyavirus LACV, in that virions treated with a protease that cleaved Gc but not Gn exhibited increased binding to the insect vector midgut, but reduced binding to cultured mammalian or mosquito cells.[324] Given that both of these systems use a Gn protein in the absence of Gc, it remains to be determined whether Gn functions for attachment when in its native conformation on virions.

Host cell receptors have not been identified for most viruses in the family; however, pathogenic and nonpathogenic hantaviruses were shown to use $\beta 3$ and $\beta 1$ integrins, respectively, to enter endothelial cells.[170] This finding was suggested to relate to pathogenesis, in that binding of hantaviruses to integrins might disrupt their ability to regulate cell-to-cell adhesion and result in the vascular permeability characteristic of hantaviral diseases.[171] In addition, decay accelerating factor (DAF)/CD55 a glycosylphosphatidylinositol (GPI)-anchored protein, has been shown to mediate HTNV and PUUV entry across the apical membrane of polarized epithelial cells,[277] and gC1qR/p32, a 32-kD glycoprotein that interacts with complement protein C1q, binds HTNV and mediates infection of cultured A549 lung cells.[98]

Entry of the Viral Genome into the Host Cytoplasm

Shortly after attachment, viruses in the *Phlebovirus* and *Nairovirus* genera were observed in phagocytic vacuoles.[145,455] This suggested a mode of viral entry similar to that first described for alphaviruses in which the virus is endocytosed in coated vesicles, and inhibitor studies have confirmed this to be so for the animal-infecting bunyaviruses. Orthobunyaviruses, hantaviruses, and nairoviruses enter by endocytosis into clathrin-coated pits,[239,463,490] and HTNV proteins were shown to colocalize with clathrin in confocal immunofluorescence studies.[239] In addition, CCHFV requires functional microtubules for infection.[489] By contrast, entry of UUKV phlebovirus is predominately in a clathrin-independent manner, and viruses enter Rab5a+ early endosomes and subsequently Rab7+ and LAMP-1+ late endosomes.[323] After endocytosis, acidification of the endocytic vesicles is thought to promote a conformational change in Gn and/or Gc that facilitates fusion of the viral and cellular membranes, thereby allowing the viral genome and polymerase access to the cytoplasm. Infection is blocked if cells were treated with ammonium chloride, which prevents acidification.[229,419,463,484] Additional indirect support for membrane fusion as a mode of entry came from experiments demonstrating the ability of viruses in the family to mediate syncytia formation at low pH.[153,183,229,383,419,484,574]

Computational studies revealed that the Gc proteins have characteristics similar to those of class II fusion proteins identified for viruses in the *Flaviviridae* and *Togaviridae* families.[169] Such proteins have internal fusion domains, as opposed to terminal domains found for the class I fusion proteins. Experimental support for this finding was obtained by demonstrating interaction of the fusion peptide postulated for the Gc protein of the hantavirus, Andes virus (ANDV), with artificial membranes.[537] In addition, several lines of evidence indicate that the Gc of orthobunyaviruses is involved in membrane fusion. Protease sensitivity assays, detergent partitioning experiments, and antibody-binding studies suggest that Gc undergoes a conformational change at pH conditions where fusion is observed.[182] Mutational analyses of a hydrophobic region (residues 1,066–1,087) of LACV Gc that is well conserved among different orthobunyaviruses[106] supported this notion,[229,420] and the residues flanking the predicted fusion peptide in BUNV Gc (residues 1,058–1,079) were shown to be structurally critical for the conformational change in Gc that occurs during the fusion process.[483] LACV Gc alone, however, when expressed from recombinant vaccinia viruses, could not cause cell fusion, suggesting that an association of the two GPs may be needed for membrane fusion,[229] and mutations in the cytoplasmic tail of BUNV Gn severely affected membrane fusion indicating that Gn must also play an important role in the fusion process.[484] Likewise for HTNV, both Gn and Gc were required to achieve surface expression and cell-to-cell fusion activity.[383] Recombinant LACV carrying mutations in the Gc fusion peptide was impaired for growth in both mammalian and insect cells but were still neurotoxic to neuronal cells, implying that the fusion peptide is a determinate of neuroinvasiveness but not necessarily neurovirulence.[501]

Transcription and Replication

After uncoating of viral genomes, primary transcription of negative-sense vRNA to mRNA is initiated by interaction of the virion-associated L protein, which is an RNA-dependent RNA polymerase (RdRp), and the three viral ribonucleocapsids.[55] Studies with hantavirus N protein suggest that N participates in transcription initiation by facilitating dissociation of the RNA panhandle and by subsequently remaining attached to the 5′ terminus of the RNA, thereby freeing the 3′ terminus for RdRp interactions. Furthermore, N was suggested to be important for replication by acting as an RNA chaperone and transiently and continuously unfolding the RNA to allow it to form more stable structures.[347] A role for N in both transcription and replication is also evident by analysis of the behavior BUNV N proteins carrying specific mutations, either in a minigenome assay or in the context of virus infection.[135,560] Four BUNV temperature sensitive mutants, carrying single amino acid substitutions in N, could be divided into two groups, those that were defective in antigenome synthesis but not mRNA transcription, and those that were replication defective but transcription competent, suggesting that different domains within N are associated with different RNA synthesis activities.[135] The mechanism by which residues in N modulate template activity requires elucidation; one possibility is that transcription and replication require different cellular cofactors that bind to distinct regions on the N protein.

Because only L and N are needed for RNA synthesis,[127] the location of these proteins must correlate with the site of RNA synthesis. For nairoviruses and hantaviruses, N (or L and N) proteins were found to localize to the perinuclear region and to have a peripheral association with perinuclear membranes.[283] In cells infected with a recombinant BUNV expressing an epitope-tagged L protein immunofluorescence microscopy showed L to have a punctate to reticular staining pattern, with concentration of staining in the perinuclear region, whereas cell fractionation studies showed L to be distributed in both cytosolic and microsomal fractions.[481] Together, these data suggest that bunyavirus RNA replication is membrane-associated, similar to that described for flaviviruses.

The L Protein

To mediate replication, the RdRp must affect numerous enzymatic functions. For primed synthesis of mRNA from genomic templates and nonprimed synthesis of vRNA from cRNA templates (as will be described), the RdRp performs endonuclease, transcriptase, replicase, and probably RNA helicase activities. Motifs common to polymerases in general are conserved in the bunyaviral RdRps, most notably a catalytic core motif.[26,237,282,360] The N-terminal domain of orthobunyavirus L proteins contains a conserved PD-(D/E)xK amino acid nuclease motif and the isolated domain of LACV L exhibited nuclease activity *in vitro;* furthermore, bioinformatic analyses indicated that viruses in all the other *Bunyaviridae* genera contain a similar domain.[442] The nuclease domain of LACV bears structural similarities to that of the PA subunit of the influenza A virus polymerase, suggesting a common origin of the cap-snatching process of segmented negative sense viruses. None of the other functions has been definitively localized to a region of the RdRp gene or gene product; however, comparison of two nairovirus L proteins with functionally defined regions of other polymerases revealed potential helicase, topoisomerase, and gyrase coding regions as well as an N-terminal cysteine-protease motif typical of the ovarian tumor (OTU) protein superfamily and protease.[262] Biochemical and structural analyses demonstrate that in addition to the deubiquitinase activity as shown by cellular OTU proteases, the nairovirus OTU also targets ISG15 modification and thus enhances its role in overcoming host innate immune defenses.[5,77,165,230] The OTU domain is not required for the RNA polymerase activity by CCHFV in a minigenome system.[43]

Genome Promoters

The template for bunyavirus transcription and replication is not naked RNA but RNA in the form of ribonucleocapsid.[127,319] The 3′ and 5′ nontranslated complementary nucleotides contain signals for both mRNA synthesis and antigenome synthesis, and thus are the genome promoters. For the phleboviruses RVFV and UUKV, the first 13 or the first 10 nucleotides, respectively, of the 3′ end of the genome are sufficient for RNA synthesis activity.[156,424]

For the orthobunyavirus BUNV, a minigenome reporter system was used to demonstrate that optimal transcription required exact complementarity at the 3′ and 5′ termini; however, one to three nucleotide deletions could be tolerated at the 3′ terminus, but not the 5′ terminus.[268] Although sequence changes at several positions could be tolerated as long as complementarity was maintained, some changes did reduce transcription. Interestingly, mutagenesis experiments indicated that the single exception to complementarity (a U residue at 3′ position 9) was critical for transcription from the genomic promoter, whereas the corresponding 5′ position 9 could be changed without influencing transcription.[33] Therefore, the mismatch itself is not important, but the nucleotide is. This nucleotide, however, does not have to be maintained for transcription activity of the antigenomic promoter.[33] Together, these data suggest that the structure of the panhandles is more important than the sequence, but that the sequence also plays a role in promoter strength and activity.

To further investigate promoter regions in an authentic replication system, S segments with shortened complementary termini were introduced into a BUNV reverse genetics system, and rescued viruses were screened to determine the minimal terminal complementary region needed for virus production.[322] The minimal 3′ and 5′ deletion mutant viable in this system maintained 29 of the 85 untranslated nucleotides on the 3′ end and 112 of the 174 untranslated nucleotides on the 5′ end, whereas those with shorter untranslated regions were not viable. Therefore, although only the complementary regions are needed for promoter activity *in vitro,* actual virus production also requires some of the unique sequences in the untranslated regions at the 3′ and 5′ termini of BUNV.[322]

The *in vivo* importance of intact termini was also suggested by a study in which terminally deleted RNAs were shown to accumulate during the establishment of persistent infections with the hantavirus, Seoul virus (SEOV). It was hypothesized that as deletions accrued, fewer replication-competent genomes were present, leading to a downregulation of the replication processes, and possibly to persistence.[342] Similar deletions were found on the termini of ANDV M and L, but not S genes, leading to a speculation that differences observed in the relative abundance of Gn and Gc compared to N could reflect down regulation of M-segment expression from genes without intact termini.[389]

Primed mRNA Synthesis (Cap Snatching)

Like influenza viruses, viruses in the family *Bunyaviridae* prime mRNA synthesis with capped oligonucleotides that are scavenged from host mRNAs (Fig. 42.5). Cleavage of the capped primers is accomplished by endonuclease activity found in virions and associated with the L protein.[398,442] Unlike influenza viruses, which take primers from newly synthesized mRNAs in the host cell's nucleus, members of the *Bunyaviridae* family use primers cleaved from cytoplasmic host cell mRNAs. Evidence has been presented that the hantavirus N protein binds to the 5′ cap of cellular mRNAs to protect them from cell-mediated degradation, and that N accumulates in cytoplasmic processing bodies (P bodies) where protected 5′ caps are sequestered, and hence can serve as a pool of primers to initiate mRNA synthesis.[346] A result of this mode of mRNA transcription is the presence of 5′ terminal extensions of approximately 10 to 20 heterogeneous nucleotides that are not found in vRNA.[47] Studies using anticap antibodies to immunoselect mRNAs[192] have provided direct proof for the presence of caps on the scavenged primers. Further evidence for capped extensions of mRNAs was provided by a study of tospoviruses, in which plants were co-infected with TSWV and with a positive-strand RNA virus (alfalfa mosaic virus). The tospovirus acquired 5′ mRNA extensions with nucleotide sequences that matched those of the other virus with a preference for cleaving at an A residue.[125] It was suggested that this

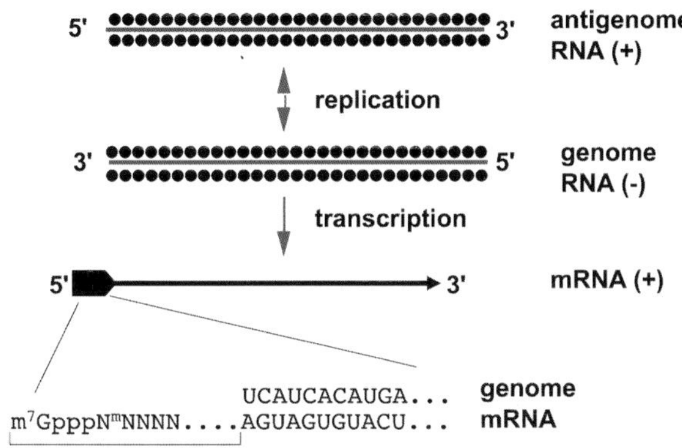

FIGURE 42.5. Transcription and replication scheme of negative-sense bunyavirus genome segments. The genome RNA and the positive-sense complementary RNA known as the antigenome RNA are found only as ribonucleoprotein complexes and are encapsidated by N protein (●). The messenger RNA (mRNA) species contain host-derived primer sequences at their 5′ ends (■) and are truncated at the 3′ end relative to the virion RNA (vRNA) template; the mRNAs are neither polyadenylated nor encapsidated by N protein. The sequence at the 5′ end of an orthobunyavirus mRNA is shown.

preference is due to a need for base-pairing at the ultimate U residue of the gene segments. Consistent with this, later studies indicated that double and triple base complementarity to nucleotides at the ends of the tospovirus gene segments were preferred, even more than the single complementary residue.[545] Interestingly, it was also found that newly synthesized mRNAs can serve as cap donors *in vitro* for tospoviruses, suggesting a "resnatching" mechanism.[544]

Other viruses in the family also have nucleotide or nucleotide motif preferences for endonuclease cleavage of capped primers. These preferences vary among the genera, and sometimes among viruses within a genus. A preferred primer sequence, or a favored nucleotide at the site of cleavage due to a need for limited base pairing with the viral genome, appears to be a common feature of primed transcription for bunyaviruses. In one study, the 3′-terminal nucleotides of the scavenged host primers often were similar to the 5′-terminal viral nucleotides.[238] It was proposed that after transcription of two or three nucleotides of the nascent mRNA, the viral polymerase might slip backward on the template before further elongation, resulting in a partial reiteration of the 5′-terminal sequence. An extension of this concept, termed "prime and realign," was proposed for mRNA transcription of hantaviruses.[168] According to this model (e-Fig. 42.2), priming by host oligonucleotides with a terminal G residue would initiate transcription by aligning at the third nucleotide of the viral RNA template (C residue). After synthesis of a few oligonucleotides, the nascent RNA could realign by slipping backward two nucleotides on the repeated terminal sequences (AUCAUCAUC) (Table 42.3), such that the G becomes the first nucleotide of the nontemplated 5′ extensions (e-Fig. 42.2). The frequent deletion of one or two of the triplet repeats in hantaviral mRNA supports this sort of slippage mechanism and suggests that sometimes the initial priming might start at the C residue of the third triplet in the conserved sequence rather than at the C of the second triplet.[168]

Bunyavirus transcription is unique among negative-sense RNA viruses in that functional viral mRNA synthesis requires ongoing protein synthesis,[31,400,430,432,433,553] a finding that at face value appears incompatible with the presence of a virion transcriptase. In the absence of protein synthesis, only short transcripts are produced *in vivo* and *in vitro*. If the *in vitro* reaction is supplemented with rabbit reticulocyte lysate, however, full-length RNAs are synthesized. The translational requirement is not at the level of mRNA initiation, but rather during elongation or, more precisely, to prevent the transcriptase from terminating prematurely. A model to account for these observations proposed that in the absence of ribosome binding and protein translation, the nascent mRNA chain and its template can base-pair, thereby preventing progression of the transcriptase enzyme.[37] Recently this model (e-Fig. 42.3) has been tested using BUNV model templates containing translational stop codons,[31] and the results showed that translation of nascent mRNAs prevented transcription termination. Thus orthobunyaviruses couple transcription and translation, a feature commonly found in prokaryotes, but rare in eukaryotic cells.

Transcription Termination

For gene segments with simple negative-sense coding, synthesis of M- and S-segment mRNAs terminates about 40 to 100 nucleotides before the end of the genome RNA template.[109,148,235,399] Although most other negative-strand RNA viruses use a stretch of nucleotides rich in U residues to signal transcription termination and polyadenylation, no such tract has been consistently identified for members of the family *Bunyaviridae*. This is supported by experimental evidence showing that bunyavirus mRNAs are not 3′ polyadenylated,[1,400,542] but many have the potential to form stem-loop structures that are probably involved in enhancing translation of viral mRNAs.[53,551]

By using a reporter system that involved mutated S segments, the transcription termination signal for the orthobunyavirus BUNV was mapped to a 33-nucleotide region within the 5′ nontranslated region of the S segment.[32] Within this region, a 6-nucleotide motif, 3′-GUCGAC-5′ was critical to transcription termination. In addition, changing the nucleotides in this transcription termination signal revealed a second downstream transcription termination signal, which had a 5-nucleotide motif, 3′-UGUCG′-5′, that was also found within the 33-nucleotide region of the upstream site, and that partially overlapped the critical 6-nucleotide motif. The finding that there are no U-rich regions in the transcription termination signal of BUNV is consistent with the absence of poly-A tails on the mRNAs.

Comparison of these S-segment sequences with those of other orthobunyaviruses revealed a high degree of conservation, suggesting that similar motifs also function for transcription termination throughout the genus, at least for S segments. A motif similar to that on the BUNV S segment was observed within the BUNV L, but not the M segment.[32] Experimental mapping of BUNV L and M mRNA termination sites has not been reported.

Analysis of the L mRNAs of SNV hantavirus[218] and RVFV and Toscana (TOSV) phleboviruses[7] showed they were co-terminal with the L vRNA template, suggesting L mRNA synthesis terminates by run-off of the RNA template.

A U-rich motif was proposed as the site of termination for the M mRNA and a C-rich motif (CCCACCC) as termination site for the S mRNA of SNV hantavirus.[218] Fine mapping of M-segment mRNA termination sites for three phleboviruses (RVFV, TOSV, and SFSV) showed that termination occurred immediately following a C-rich domain in the template at a conserved motif 3′-C_{1-3} GUCG/A-5′.[7] Although previously it was thought the C-rich region itself was involved in transcript termination[178] deletion of this region in template RNA did not affect specific termination at the identified motif.[7]

The mechanism of transcription termination of the ambisense genes of phleboviruses and tospoviruses was initially thought to involve RNA secondary structure in the intergenic region.[103,118,146,187,188,493] However, reanalysis of computer predictions of hairpin formation in these intergenic regions suggest that they are unlikely to form because of their complexity or low energy.[7] Detailed mapping of mRNA termination sites for the N and NSs mRNA of RVFV, TOSV, and SFSV phleboviruses showed that the 3′ ends of the mRNAs contained most of the intergenic sequence and indeed overlapped each other.[7] Furthermore, termination occurred for both messages at the same motif, 3′-C_{1-3}GUCG/A-5′, as in the M segment. Two copies of this motif are thus present, one in vRNA (genome) and one in the cRNA (antigenome). The conservation of this motif in viral genomes that display considerable sequence diversity suggests a similar mechanism for transcription–termination in the M and S segments. Deletion of either copy of the motif in RVFV S segment did not prevent correct termination of unaffected N or NSs mRNA, but the mutant viruses were attenuated in growth compared to wild-type.[7]

Genome Replication

The change from primary transcription to replication requires that the RdRp, either acting alone or in concert with undefined viral or cellular factors, must at some point, switch from primed mRNA synthesis to independently initiating transcription at the precise 3′ end of the template to produce a full-length transcript. The processes involved in making that switch from primary transcription to genome replication have not been defined completely for any member of the family. Presumably, some viral or host factor is required to signal a suppression of the transcription termination signal responsible for generation of truncated mRNA and also to prevent the addition of the capped and methylated structures to the 5′ termini of the cRNAs. There is no question that genome replication and subsequent secondary transcription are prevented by translational inhibitors such as cycloheximide. These results indicate that continuous protein synthesis is required for replication of the genome. Although not proven, it is likely that synthesis of N is required for genome replication, as described for other negative-strand RNA viruses such as the rhabdovirus, vesicular stomatitis virus, and the paramyxovirus Sendai virus. For these viruses, encapsidation by N seems to serve as an antitermination signal, thus allowing full-length genome synthesis.

A prime-and-realign model was also postulated for the nonprimed transcription of hantaviral vRNA and cRNA, except that transcription would initiate with pppG alignment at the third nucleotide (C residue) of the template RNA. After synthesis of several nucleotides, polymerase slipping would realign the nascent RNA such that the initial priming G residue would overhang the template. It was further theorized that nucleolytic activity of the L protein might remove the overhanging G, leaving a monophosphorylated U residue at the nascent 5′ end. The presence of the monophosphorylated U on HTNV RNA was experimentally demonstrated[168] (e-Fig. 42.2).

Indirect evidence suggesting that a prime-and-realign method of initiation is used by phleboviruses was obtained by using a reconstituted transcription system to study the polymerase recognition sequence at the 3′ termini of the ambisense S segment RNA of RVFV. In those studies, mutational analysis of the terminal nucleotides revealed that the first 13 nucleotides are required for polymerase recognition, but that one of the two terminal dinucleotides (UGUG) could be removed without deleterious effects on transcription.[424] These data also suggested that realignment is not a prerequisite for transcription initiation. In contrast, a recent study using the BUNV minigenome system showed that the viral polymerase was able to repair both insertions and deletions in model template RNAs, although this did not appear to involve the prime-and-realign mechanism.[559]

Schematics of transcription and replication based on information above are presented in Figures 42.5 and 42.6.

Encapsidation Signals

Signals for the encapsidation of the vRNAs and cRNAs of orthobunyaviruses, phleboviruses, nairoviruses, and hantaviruses were found entirely within the noncoding 3′ and 5′ regions of minireplicon reporters.[52,154,155,157,321,345,348,382] Mutational

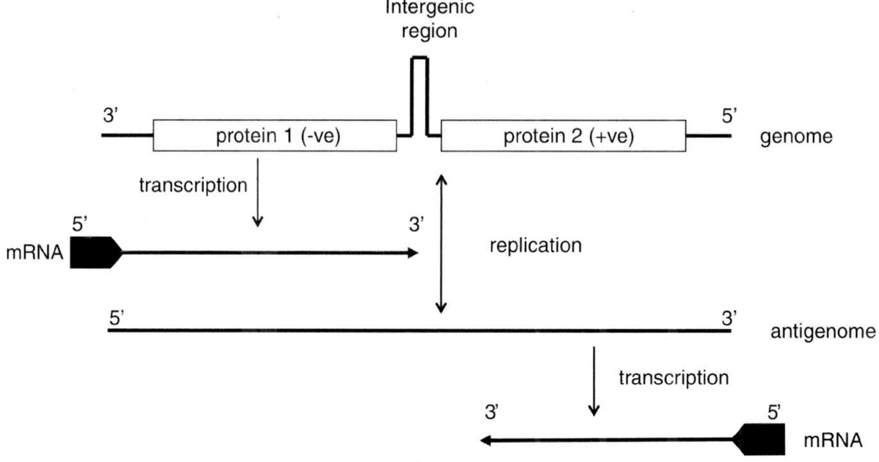

FIGURE 42.6. Transcription and replication scheme of ambisense-sense bunyavirus genome segments. The genome RNA encodes proteins in both negative- and positive-sense orientations, separated by an intergenic region that for some viruses has the potential to form a hairpin structure. The proteins are translated from specific subgenomic messenger RNAs (mRNAs), with the mRNA encoding protein 2 transcribed from the antigenome RNA after the onset of genome replication.

analysis of these terminal regions for BUNV revealed a conserved sequence within nucleotides 20–33 of the 5′ end of vRNA that was critical for packaging.[270] Variable packaging efficiencies were noted for the L, M, and S segment–derived minireplicons, and packaging appeared to be independent for each.

Host Factors

Beyond the need for host-derived primers for initiating mRNA synthesis, little is known about the role that host factors might play in viral replication. One putative host transcription factor is an ~40-kD protein isolated from the main insect vector of TSWV, and it was shown to bind to the viral RdRp at its C-terminus and to the viral RNA at its N-terminus.[119] Both this protein and reticulocyte lysates were needed for RNA synthesis *in vitro,* indicating that other cellular factors are also required. Expression of this protein in mammalian cells rendered them permissive to TSWV replication.[119] As is the case for a number of other negative-strand RNA viruses, heat-shock protein 90 (Hsp90) appeared essential for La Crosse virus replication in that virus yields were diminished in cells treated with Hsp90 inhibitors like geldanamycin due to destabilization of the viral L protein.[105]

Translation and Processing of Viral Proteins

Viral polypeptides are synthesized shortly after infection, with S and L mRNAs translated on free ribosomes and M mRNAs translated on membrane-bound ribosomes. Expression products vary among the genera, and even within a genus.

S Segment Products: N and NSs

The N protein is the most abundant viral product in virions and infected cells. N plays several important roles in viral replication. In addition to protecting the RNA from degradation, N also interacts with L and Gn and Gc, although the exact interactions have not been defined. A critical step in N interaction with RNA appears to be the ability of the proteins to oligomerize. Oligomerization characteristics of the N proteins are likely different among the genera, which is probably not surprising, given the size differences of the N proteins, which range from approximately 19kD for orthobunyaviruses to 54kD for hantaviruses and nairoviruses (Table 42.2).

Chemical cross-linking studies indicated that the ribonucleocapsids of the phlebovirus RVFV, either from authentic virions or reconstituted from bacterially expressed protein, contain dimers of N as the basic oligomer.[297,440] The crystal structure of RVFV N has been determined to 1.93Å resolution, which revealed that it has a novel all-helical fold without a positively charged surface RNA binding cleft as seen for other negative-sense RNA virus nucleocapsid proteins.[440] Extensive ribonuclease digestion of authentic or reconstituted RNAs released heterogenous N-RNA multimers, consistent with the lack of observed helical symmetry. In contrast, hantaviral N proteins form stable trimers, which are postulated to assemble on the viral RNA, followed by further protein–protein interactions that encapsidate the entire RNA.[249] The N–N interactions are likely to be electrostatic, with both amino- and carboxy-terminal residues participating.[250] The N-terminal residues of hantaviral N proteins are predicted to form a coiled coil domain, providing a trigger for trimerization, and containing charged residues important for intermolecular interactions.[9,10,13,562] For TULV, carboxy-terminal amino acids 393 to 398 were shown to be crucial for trimerization, and amino acids 1 to 43 provided a secondary interaction region.[249] These data are in agreement with those obtained with other hantaviruses (e.g., SNV and HTNV, for which carboxy-terminal and amino-terminal regions were shown to be involved in the homotypic interactions of N).[9,589]

Orthobunyaviruses and tospoviruses, in contrast to hantaviruses, do not appear to assemble preformed trimers, but instead multimerize by adding one N protein at a time. This hypothesis comes from chemical cross-linking experiments, which showed that the N protein of the orthobunyavirus BUNV was able to form a range of multimers from dimers to high–molecular-weight structures, with a preponderance of tetramers.[308] Deletion of N- or C-terminal portions of N prevented multimerization and also resulted in loss of functionality in a minireplicon system. The data were interpreted to indicate a head-to-head and tail-to-tail multimerization model of individual N proteins. Likewise, for the tospovirus TSWV, analysis of deletion mutants identified binding regions both at the amino- and carboxy-termini of N, and although the type of multimers formed was not examined closely, it appears to be a continuous addition process, like that proposed for the orthobunyaviruses.[242,540]

In addition to protein–protein interaction, the amino- and carboxy-terminal regions of the tospovirus N were also implicated in RNA binding.[447] In contrast, the RNA-binding site of hantaviral N was localized to a central, conserved region of the protein.[474] For hantaviruses and bunyaviruses, RNA-binding studies with bacterially expressed, hexahistidine-tagged N proteins indicated that N preferentially interacts with the 5′ end of the vRNA.[385,475] In another study, high-affinity binding of hantaviral N to panhandle RNA was demonstrated, and it was suggested that such binding is related specifically to the trimers, which were able to discriminate viral from nonviral RNA, whereas monomer or dimer subunits bound nonspecifically to RNA.[348] These data suggest a requirement for multimerization of N for effective RNA binding and encapsidation, and implicate the panhandle structure as the trigger for encapsidation. Hantavirus N is also able to bind 5′ capped mRNAs (to generate a source of primers for transcription initiation; see above), and the cap and vRNA binding sites have been mapped to separate domains within the protein.[349] Furthermore, binding to the mRNA cap induces a conformational change in N, and the structurally altered N loaded with the capped primer binds specifically to the conserved 3′ terminus of vRNA.

The S segments of viruses in the *Phlebovirus* and *Tospovirus* genera and some viruses in *Orthobunyavirus* and *Hantavirus* genera produce NSs proteins as well as N proteins. Sizes of NSs range from 10 kD for orthobunyaviruses and hantaviruses to more than 50 kD for tospoviruses (Fig. 42.2). The NSs protein of the phlebovirus RVFV is phosphorylated and accumulates in the nuclei of infected cells, where it forms fibrillar structures (e-Fig. 42.4).[513] The major phosphorylation sites of the RVFV NSs were mapped to serine residues located near the carboxy-terminus of the protein.[267] Expression studies revealed that fibrils could form in the absence of other viral proteins; however, if the carboxy-terminal region of NSs was removed, NSs were still transported to the nuclei, but did not coalesce into fibrils.[584] Similar fibrillar structures of NSs were observed for some strains of TSWV, but the structures appeared only in the cytoplasm.

Comparing the deduced amino acid sequences of NSs for five different phleboviruses revealed homologies of only 17% to 30%.[178] However, comparison of the NSs gene sequences for a number of strains of a single phlebovirus RVFV showed that certain areas were highly conserved.[459] These data suggest that there may be a strong evolutionary pressure to maintain distinct portions of the NSs for individual viruses, but that the remainder of the protein can diverge without affecting the function of NSs.

Earlier work suggested that the NSs of phleboviruses and tospoviruses were only synthesized after viral replication; that is, after the ambisense vRNA has been copied to cRNA and mRNA was transcribed from cRNA. Recent work with RVFV, however, indicates that at least for this phlebovirus, virions can encapsidate cRNA and that the incoming cRNA ribonucleocapsids can serve as templates for NSs mRNA.[225] The outcome of this is that NSs are present early in infection and might have a role in early replication. The NSs of three orthobunyaviruses all inhibited BUNV RNA synthesis in a dose-dependent manner in a minireplicon system.[567] The results were suggested to indicate a function for NSs in regulating the activity of the RdRp. In addition to a possible role for NSs in early replication processes, NSs proteins have other important roles in viral infection, such as interferon antagonism, host-range determination, and gene silencing. These effects will be described in the context of effects on host cells.

M Segment Products: Gn, Gc, and NSm

The viral envelope GPs Gn and Gc are translated from a single mRNA complementary to vRNA. The polyprotein precursor of Gn and Gc is not seen in infected cells, and has been observed only by *in vitro* translation of RNA transcripts in the absence of microsomal membranes.[542] For most viruses, both Gn and Gc are preceded by signal sequences; therefore, cleavage of the polyprotein precursor is likely mediated by host signalase.[150] A pentapeptide motif, WAASA, which is highly conserved among hantaviruses, was shown to be the polyprotein cleavage site for HTNV, by mutational analysis of the signal sequence preceding Gc.[318]

M-segment gene products have a cysteine content of approximately 4% to 7%. Positions of these residues are highly conserved in the M-segment products of related viruses, suggesting that extensive disulfide-bridge formation may occur and that the positions may be crucial for determining correct polypeptide folding. The secondary structure of the proteins is also involved in immunogenicity, as indicated by the finding that neutralizing or protective epitopes are often nonlinear.

All M-segment polyproteins display variable numbers of predicted transmembrane regions, and a hydrophobic sequence at the carboxy-terminus, indicative of a membrane anchor region. Therefore, the M-segment translation products of viruses in the family *Bunyaviridae* are typical class 1 membrane proteins, with the amino terminus exposed on the surface of the virion and the carboxy-terminus anchored in the membrane.

The Gn and Gc proteins of all viruses in the family possess asparagine-linked oligosaccharides. Examination of the oligosaccharides attached to the Gn and Gc proteins of orthobunyaviruses revealed that Gc has mostly high-mannose glycans, whereas Gn contains both complex and a novel intermediate-type oligosaccharide.[326,377,479] In contrast, the GPs of hantaviruses were found to be mostly of the high-mannose type.[467] These findings indicate that the proteins are incompletely processed through the Golgi. This is likely related to retention of Gn and Gc in the Golgi, where assembly occurs, and which will be discussed more fully.

Nairoviruses appear unique among viruses in the family in that they have both N-linked and a region of heavily O-linked carbohydrates (a mucin-like domain, as will be described).[461]

The M-segment gene-product processing events differ among the genera. Hantaviruses produce only Gn and Gc,[471] whereas some viruses in the *Phlebovirus* and *Orthobunyavirus* genera produce NSm from the same M-segment mRNA as Gn and Gc. The NSm protein of orthobunyaviruses is encoded between the Gn and Gc proteins.[149] Its hydropathy profile suggests that it is a membrane-bound protein, and expression studies demonstrated that it localizes to the Golgi along with Gn and Gc.[301] Although a function for this protein has not been identified, it was suggested that it might be involved in facilitating virion assembly in the Golgi.[301]

For the phlebovirus RVFV, a NSm of approximately 14 kD is cleaved from the amino-terminus of the polyprotein translation product (e-Fig. 42.5). Sequence studies revealed five in-frame translation initiation codons (AUG) upstream of the amino-terminus of Gn. Mutational analysis of those codons indicated the fourth and the fifth AUGs to translate Gn and Gc. Whilst NSm was found to originate from the second AUG and a 78-kD polypeptide, representing uncleaved NSm and Gn, was translated from the first AUG.[198] Pulse-chase experiments revealed no precursor–product relationship between the 78- and 14-kD proteins; therefore, it appears that use of the first and second AUGs, respectively, is what dictates generation of these proteins.[77] Both the 14-kD NSm and the 78-kD polypeptide are found in abundance in RVFV-infected cells,[78] suggesting that they might play a role in replication or morphogenesis.

An even larger NSm (~30 kD) is cleaved from the amino terminus of the M-segment polyprotein of the phlebovirus, PTV (e-Fig. 42.5). *In vitro* expression studies indicated that both envelope GPs could be produced in the absence of the NSm coding region,[335] but other studies to evaluate the use of the 13 potential translation initiation codons present in the NSm coding information have not been reported. No homology between the NSm proteins of PTV and RVFV was apparent.[221]

In contrast to the mosquito-borne phleboviruses PTV and RVFV, the tick-borne phlebovirus UUKV does not produce an NSm (e-Fig. 42.5). The first (and only) initiation codon preceding sequences of the envelope GPs is located 17 amino acids upstream of the amino terminus of Gn[449]; hence, the Gn protein of UUKV appears to be analogous to the 78-kD NSm–Gn fusion product produced by RVFV (although there is no obvious sequence homology of these predicted products). Until a function can be assigned to NSm, it is impossible to determine whether UUKV replicates in the absence of such a function or accomplishes whatever function is required without removal of a portion of the amino terminus of Gn.

M-segment polyprotein processing events for nairoviruses are more complicated and appear to differ from those of other viruses in the family (e-Fig. 42.6). Nucleotide sequences of DUGV, CCHFV, and NSDV revealed a coding strategy similar to other viruses in the family, that is, a single ORF.[331] Studies on CCHFV demonstrated the polyprotein is co-translationally cleaved into 140-kD PreGn and 85-kD PreGc precursors and a 15-kD NSm protein.[14,44,461,462,555] PreGn is processed to the mature 37-kD Gn by cleavage with a cellular secretory pathway protease, SKI-1, following a consensus motif, RRLL, early in the secretory pathway.[461] SKI-1 cleavage generates a subprecursor of the other two polypeptides that is cleaved by a furin-like protease late in the secretory pathway.[461] This cleavage site is completely conserved among several CCHFV strains, suggesting that it has importance for viral replication or pathogenicity.[461] The amino-terminal portion of this subprecursor is a highly variable (among CCHFV strains) polypeptide with mucin-like characteristics, including numerous serines, threonines, and prolines and predicted extensive O-linked glycosylation. The carboxy-terminal portion of the subprecursor is a 38-kD nonstructural polypeptide. After furin cleavage, secreted proteins GP38, GP85, GP160, and the mucin-like protein are produced; presumably these products reflect extensive O-linked glycosylation differences. Although the PreGc precursor also possesses a SKI-1–like cleavage motif, SKI-1 cleavage could not be demonstrated for this protein, so it is likely that a related enzyme is responsible for the processing to yield mature Gc.[461]

Unlike all other viruses in the family, the NSm protein of tospoviruses is translated from an ambisense mRNA.[274] It is also the only NSm protein in the family to have a definitively assigned function. By subcellular fractionation of infected plants, or in thin-section immunoelectron microscopy studies, the NSm of TSWV was found to be present in cell wall–containing fractions or associated with aggregates of nucleocapsids and with the plasmodesmata.[275] Expression of the NSm protein in plant cells or insect cells revealed that the protein first appeared near the cell surface and later as tubular structures protruding from the cell surface. In infected leaf tissues, the tubules were observed only in the plasmodesmata.[510] These data are characteristic of proteins able to aggregate into plasmodesmata-penetrating tubules that allow cell-to-cell movement of the virus across the cell walls in infected plants. In several other studies, the TSWV NSm protein was shown to have additional characteristics of plant movement proteins, including sequence similarity, expression during the early stages of infection, and RNA-binding activity. Formal proof of this function was obtained from experiments in which NSm of TSWV was able to complement cell-to-cell movement of a movement-defective tobacco mosaic virus vector.[311] This expression system was also used to show that NSm alone induced tubule formation in protoplasts and induced TSWV-like symptoms in *Nicotiana benthamiana*. Separate domains within NSm have been mapped for each of these functions.[312] NSm was found to be expressed in its natural thrip insect vector, but did not aggregate into tubules, leading to the suggestion that NSm might only have a role in the plant portion of the tospovirus replication cycle.[511]

L Segment Product: L Polymerase Protein

The L proteins of bunyaviruses range in size from about 237 kD for phleboviruses, to 459 kD for nairoviruses (Fig. 42.2). There are no known processing or posttranslational modifications to the L proteins.[546] Although structural analysis of an L protein from the family *Bunyaviridae* is not yet available, several features common to other polymerase proteins have been observed.[282]

The overall shape of the polymerase is compared to that of a right hand, with fingers, palm, and thumb domains. Four major conserved motifs in the palm region, designated as A–D are shared by many viral polymerases. Motifs A and C are involved in divalent cation use, whereas motifs A and B may be involved in sugar and nucleoside triphosphate selection. Motif C contains the catalytic core of the protein. For BUNV, site-directed mutagenesis demonstrated the importance of amino acids in motif C for polymerase activity.[237] Alignment of the amino acid sequences of L proteins of several viruses in the family *Bunyaviridae* demonstrate the presence of A–D motifs in these proteins. In addition, two novel regions, found at the amino-terminus of the L protein of the phlebovirus RVFV, were shown to be conserved only in the polymerases of viruses in the *Bunyaviridae* and *Arenaviridae* families.[361]

The function of the L protein as an RNA-dependent RNA polymerase was first confirmed by using L protein expressed from vaccinia virus recombinants to transcribe authentic orthobunyavirus ribonucleocapsid templates.[236] Endonuclease activity was demonstrated *in vitro* with expressed BUNV L protein, providing evidence that the L protein is also responsible for generating the capped primers needed for transcription,[236] and this was confirmed by expression of an N-terminal fragment of LACV L protein.[442]

Morphogenesis

Transport of Viral Proteins

In contrast to other negative-strand RNA viruses, bunyaviruses usually mature within cells by budding at smooth membranes of the Golgi (e-Fig. 42.7). The plant-infecting members of the family, the tospoviruses, also appear to assemble in the Golgi; however, it was suggested that instead of budding, there is a coalescence of Golgi membranes around the ribonucleocapsids.[258] Budding at membranes other than those associated with the Golgi have been reported for some viruses; for example, the hantaviruses, SNV, and Black Creek Canal virus (BCCV), and the phlebovirus RVFV were found to bud from the plasma membrane as well as in the Golgi in some cells.[17,437] The reason(s) for maturation of viruses in the family *Bunyaviridae* in the Golgi complex as opposed to the more usual mode of viral morphogenesis (budding at the plasma membrane) are not understood completely; however, important clues have been obtained by studying the viral proteins, transport to and retention in the Golgi.

Golgi Targeting and Retention

Expression of M gene segments of representative bunyaviruses demonstrated that Gn and Gc are targeted to the Golgi in the absence of other viral components. When expressed individually, Gn is able to exit the ER, but Gc remains in the ER for the orthobunyaviruses, phleboviruses, nairoviruses, and tospoviruses.[45,262,294,334] For hantaviruses, neither protein exits the ER when expressed separately.[454,482] For all studies to date, the signal for Golgi transport has been localized to Gn and complexing of Gn and Gc in the ER is necessary for efficient transport of Gc to the Golgi.

Although ER retention signals have not been identified on Gc for most viruses, the phleboviruses have a characteristic carboxy-terminal ER retention motif (KKXX, where K = lysine and X = any amino acid).[176] Evidently, this signal can be overcome when Gn and Gc oligomerize.

To map the Golgi targeting and retention signal(s) on Gn of orthobunyaviruses or phleboviruses, a series of deleted and/or chimeric genes were constructed and their expression products were examined for Golgi targeting and retention. For BUNV, the Golgi localization and retention signal was mapped to the transmembrane domain of Gn.[485] The Golgi localization signal for the phleboviruses PTV and RVFV were identified within the transmembrane domain plus 10 (PTV) or 28 (RVFV) amino acids of the cytoplasmic tail.[176,334] The Golgi localization signal of another phlebovirus, UUKV, was found to be within a 30 amino acid peptide of the cytoplasmic tail.[18]

Similar expression studies with M-segment constructs of HTNV indicated that the ability of Gn to transport Gc to the Golgi requires the presence of the complete signal sequence of Gc. This suggests that the Gc signal peptide remains attached to the Gn cytoplasmic tail. This signal alone, however, is apparently not sufficient for Golgi targeting because M segment constructs that maintained the Gc signal peptide but had other internal deletions in Gn or Gc failed to reach the Golgi. These results were interpreted to indicate that the correct conformation of the oligomerized Gn and Gc is also important for Golgi targeting.[471] Consistent with this is the observation that overexpression of SNV Gn resulted in the apparent accumulation of misfolded proteins in aggresomes.[504] In addition, the cytoplasmic tail of Gn was found to be polyubiquitinated when expressed alone, suggesting that it would undergo proteasomal degradation if not complexed with Gc.[172]

For the nairovirus, CCHFV, removal of the transmembrane domain and cytoplasmic tail of Gn did not prevent Golgi targeting, and this soluble truncated Gn was still able to dimerize with Gc and transport both proteins to the Golgi.[45] In another study, Golgi targeting was dependent both on a signal found in the hydrophobic region of the cytoplasmic tail, as well as in the ectodomain[196]; therefore, unlike other bunyaviruses, nairoviruses appear to have at least part of their Golgi-targeting signal in the ectodomain, rather than only in the transmembrane or cytoplasmic tail regions of Gn.

Clearly, although there are definite signals targeting the viral glycoproteins to the Golgi, there is no consensus motif or even region of Gn conserved among viruses in the family.

Trafficking Through the Golgi

The Golgi complex consists of several subcompartments, including the cis-, medial-, and trans-Golgi.[264] By using the fungal antibacterial reagent Brefeldin A, which inhibits transport of proteins out of the ER and causes a redistribution of the Golgi component to the ER, the GPs of the phlebovirus PTV were found to be localized in the cis and medial Golgi membranes.[93] Similar redistribution of Gn and Gc from the Golgi to the ER were observed following Brefeldin A treatment of cells infected with vaccinia virus recombinants expressing the M segment of BUNV.[366] Immunohistochemical and electron microscopy studies of the phlebovirus UUKV demonstrated that budding may begin as early as the pre-Golgi intermediate compartment and that virus budding continues in the Golgi stack.[232,458]

Examination of the type and amount of oligosaccharides attached to viral proteins influences trafficking and provides clues regarding the transit of the proteins through the Golgi compartments. For example, shortly after primary glycosylation of nascent proteins at the ER, oligosaccharides are susceptible to cleavage by endoglycosidase H (endo-H), an enzyme that cleaves only high-mannose residues. Later, after removal of glucose residues at the rough ER, migration of the GPs to the smooth ER and Golgi, trimming of residues, and attachment of peripheral sugars, the oligosaccharides are no longer susceptible to endo-H cleavage. Therefore, acquired resistance to endo-H generally indicates that the proteins have been processed through specific Golgi compartments as described earlier (see "M segment products"). For the nairovirus CCHFV and the hantavirus HTNV the GPs remain endo-H sensitive, suggesting that they have not been processed through the medial Golgi.[45,480] In contrast, the GPs of the orthobunyavirus, BUNV become endo-H–resistant, so they can be assumed to have moved through the trans-Golgi.[377]

To identify the roles of specific glycosylation sites on trafficking of HTNV GPs, a series of expression constructs were created in which each of the four glycosylation sites that are used on Gn and the single site used on Gc were mutated. Removal of the glycosylation site closest to the amino-terminus of Gn resulted in its inability to exit the ER and for a loss of reactivity with monoclonal antibodies to native Gn.[480] Mutating the third glycosylation site in Gn was also poorly tolerated, and resulted in inefficient Golgi targeting and loss of monoclonal antibody reactivity. In contrast, mutating the single site on Gc or two of the other three sites of Gn were well tolerated. A similar study with BUNV indicated that the single Gn glycosylation site is absolutely required for correct protein folding, trafficking, and infectivity.[479] These data are consistent with results from another study, which will be described below, indicating that the processing of sugars plays a key role in maturation of BUNV.[377]

The time required to convert between endo-H susceptibility and resistance correlates with the time needed for protein transport from the ER to the Golgi. For the phlebovirus PTV, heterodimerization occurred between newly synthesized Gn and Gc within 3 minutes after protein synthesis, and the dimers were found to be linked by disulfide bonds. The dimeric Gn–Gc proteins were observed both during transport and after accumulation in the Golgi complex.[93] For another phlebovirus, UUKV, it was found that the transport of Gn and Gc from their site of synthesis on the rough ER through the Golgi occurred at an estimated two to three times slower rate than that of most viral membrane GPs destined to be transported to the plasma membrane.[166] That is, endo-H resistance was achieved at 45 and 90 to 150 minutes for Gn and Gc of UUKV,[281] compared to 15 to 20 minutes for the hemagglutinin protein of influenza virus or the G protein of vesicular stomatitis virus. The finding that UUKV Gn and Gc have different transport kinetics (i.e., Gn is incorporated into virions 20 minutes faster than Gc) suggests that the dimers may arise from different precursor proteins, possibly because faster-folding Gn cannot dimerize with slower-folding Gc until Gc has reached its correct conformation.[580] In this same study, the Gn and Gc proteins of UUKV were found to exit the ER quickly, but did not enter the Golgi for 15 to 20 minutes. These findings suggest that the Gn and Gc proteins may dimerize in an intermediate compartment between the ER and Golgi.[580]

The NSm proteins are not known to play a role in transport or Golgi retention. For representative phleboviruses and orthobunyaviruses, expression of Gn and Gc in the absence of NSm had no effect on their transport to the Golgi; however, when the entire M segments were expressed, NSm co-localized to the Golgi with Gn and Gc, suggesting an interaction of these proteins before their exit from the ER.

Assembly

For assembly to occur, N as well as Gn and Gc must move to the same intracellular location. For the hantavirus, SEOV, N could first be observed approximately 2 hours after infection and accumulated as scattered granules in the cytoplasm. Although N was not observed in the Golgi, it could be observed to surround the Golgi by 24 hours after infection.[247] The N proteins of the nairovirus CCHFV and the hantavirus BCCV were both observed in the perinuclear region of infected cells, and both were found to bind to actin.[21,436] Disrupting the cellular actin network by treatment with cytochalasin D, reduced the assembly of infectious CCHFV, suggesting a role for actin in transporting N to the site of virion assembly. For BCCV, the N protein was found to be peripherally associated with Golgi membranes, suggesting that the ribonucleocapsids are recruited to the Golgi for assembly.[504] In contrast, the CCHFV N protein was not found in association with Golgi membranes; therefore, it is unclear where the actual assembly site is for nairoviruses, and it was suggested that some sort of novel structure close to the nucleus might be involved in bunyavirus assembly.[21]

This was confirmed by detailed electron microscopic analysis of BUNV-infected cells, which identified viral replication occurring in a "viral factory" that is built around the Golgi complex (Fig. 42.7) and comprises repetitive units of Golgi stacks, mitochondria, components of the rough ER, and virus-derived tubular structures with a globular head.[458] The viral polymerase and N protein were found mainly in the globular head, and viral RNPs were released from disrupted, purified tubes.[159] Viral tubes contain cellular proteins such as actin and myosin I, and both tube assembly and viral morphogenesis were sensitive to drugs that affect actin. Advanced imaging and three-dimensional (3D) reconstruction of infected cells showed that the tubes link cellular organelles, for example, mitochondria, to the Golgi and interact with intracellular viral forms, thereby providing a route for cellular factors required for genome replication. Based on these observations a model has been proposed (e-Fig.42.8) whereby viral RNPs are transported from sites of replication in the globular domain to the cytoplasm where they condense on Golgi membranes modified by the insertion of Gn and Gc, and promote budding of immature particles into Golgi-derived vesicles.

Unlike most other negative-strand RNA viruses, members of the *Bunyaviridae* do not have an M protein to link the integral viral envelope proteins and their nucleocapsids and to act as the nucleating step for assembly. The absence of M protein suggests a direct interaction between the ribonucleocapsids, which accumulate on the cytoplasmic side of vesicular membranes, and viral envelope proteins, which are displayed on the

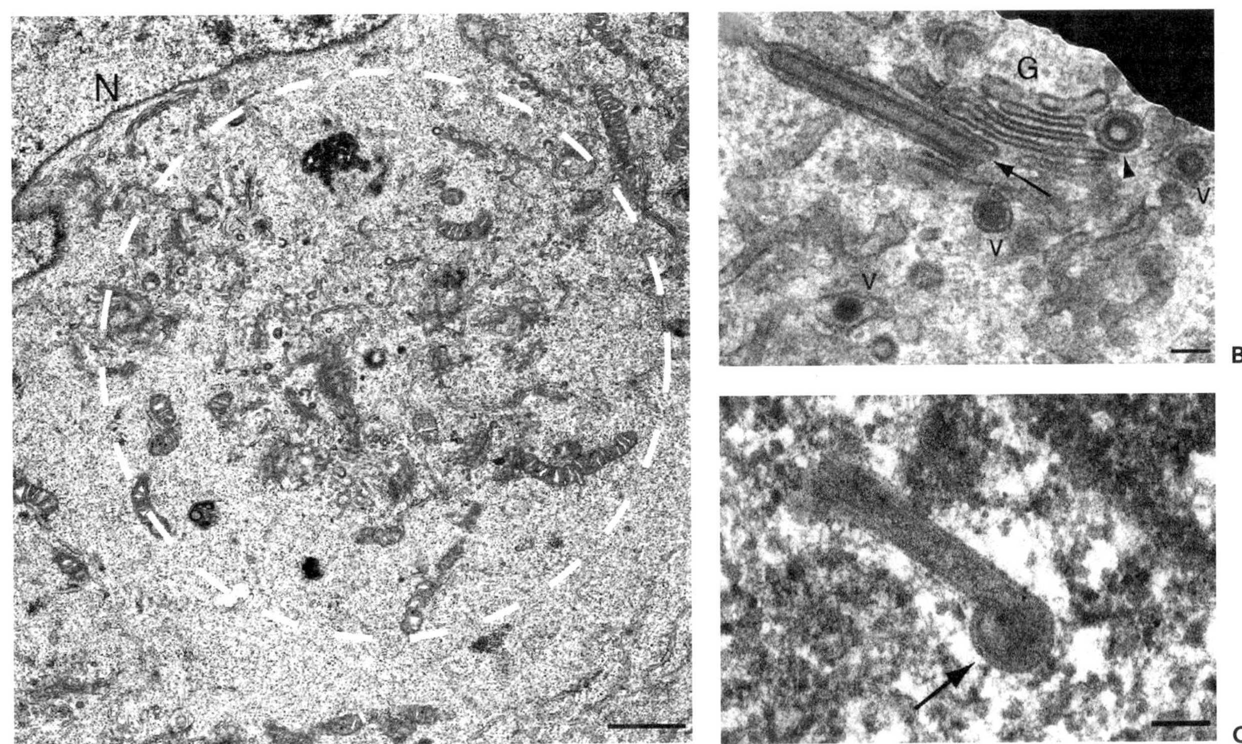

FIGURE 42.7. Visualization of viral factory in Bunyamwera virus (BUNV)–infected BHK cells by electron microscopy. **A:** Viral factory (*dashed white circle*) shows groups of organelles near the nucleus (N). **B:** Higher magnification shows longitudinal (*arrow*) and transverse (*arrowhead*) sections of tubular structures in Golgi stacks (G). Virus particles (V) are also seen. **C:** Tubular assembly with a bigger globular domain (*arrow*). N, nucleus; G, Golgi stack; V, virus particle; scale bar represents 1 μm in **(A)**. (Modified from Fontana J, Lopez-Montero N, Elliott RM, et al. The unique architecture of Bunyamwera virus factories around the Golgi complex. *Cell Microbiol* 2008;10:2012–2028.)

luminal side. Electron microscopy of cells infected with the phleboviruses PTV or Karimabad virus, revealed that ribonucleocapsids and spike structures (i.e., viral envelope GPs) were present only in regions of Golgi membranes where budding appeared to be occurring, and not on adjacent areas of the same membrane, suggesting a transmembranal interaction of N with Gn or Gc.[497] Direct evidence for the requirement of the cytoplasmic tails of both glycoproteins has been obtained using virus-like particle production assays.[484]

The signal directing the ribonucleocapsids to the budding compartment has not been identified for most viruses in the family. For hantaviruses, however, N was shown to interact with the cellular proteins, SUMO-1 (small ubiquitin-like modifier-1) and Ubc9 (SUMO-1 conjugating enzyme 9) in yeast two-hybrid systems.[251,301,327] For HTNV, the interaction occurred at a four amino acid motif, MAKE, located at amino acid positions 188 and 189 of N, and mutation of this motif prevented transport of N to the perinuclear region, suggesting a role for this interaction in directing N to the site of assembly.

Excess ribonucleocapsids of hantaviruses, tospoviruses, and nairoviruses were found to accumulate in large cytoplasmic inclusions, suggesting that only ribonucleocapsids that interact with the envelope proteins are transported to the Golgi. Although not yet defined, it is likely that the transmembrane domains of Gn or Gc that are exposed on the cytoplasmic face of the membrane are involved in this interaction. Candidate transmembrane regions have been predicted from hydropathic characteristics of derived amino acid sequences representing the envelope proteins of all bunyaviruses examined to date. Direct examination of a phlebovirus by enzymatic digestion of exposed proteins embedded in intracellular membranes, demonstrated that approximately 12% of Gn or Gc was exposed on the cytoplasmic face of membranes in infected cells and was accessible to digestion. A large protease-resistant fragment was identified, which was presumably sequestered in the membrane in a manner that rendered it safe from enzymatic digestion.[497] These enzyme-resistant fragments may therefore represent transmembrane regions of proteins, which could provide the interaction between ribonucleocapsids and the cellular membranes required for envelopment. The predicted cytoplasmic tails on Gn have also been suggested to be logical candidates for interacting with the ribonucleocapsids.[444]

Tospovirus assembly and release in plants may differ from those processes of other viruses in the family. A model was proposed in which Golgi membranes with integral viral envelope proteins wrap around ribonucleocapsids. These particles may then fuse with each other or with ER membranes to release single enveloped particles into the cisternae.[258] Mature virions accumulated within the ER cisternae likely remain there until ingested by thrips.

For BUNV, the complete suite of L, M, and S packaging signals was not required for generation of infectious virus as a virus lacking the L segment UTRs (the L ORF was flanked by the complete UTRs from the M segment) was created by reverse genetics.[321] In contrast, a recent study on RVFV packaging suggested M-segment UTRs, particularly a region in the 5′UTR, was critical for co-packaging of the L and S segments.[526]

Transport and Release

After budding into the Golgi cisternae, virions apparently are transported to the cell surface within vesicles analogous to those in the secretory pathway. The release of virus from infected cells presumably occurs when the virus-containing vesicles fuse with the cellular plasma membrane (i.e., by normal exocytosis). Numerous viruses in the family have been observed late in infection within vesicles or in the process of exocytosis by electron microscopy, and more recently by light microscopy of BUNV expressing a Gc-GFP fusion protein (Fig. 42.8). In polarized cells, the phleboviruses PTV and RVFV show differing release characteristics, in that no marked polarized release could be detected for RVFV, whereas PTV was released primarily from the basolateral surfaces.[94,177] In contrast to these phleboviruses, the hantavirus BCCV was released from the apical surface.[437] Such polarized release of viruses might be important for disseminating virus during natural infection to produce a systemic disease. Release of tospoviruses from insect cells probably occurs via secretory exocytosis similar to that of animal-infecting members of the family.[579]

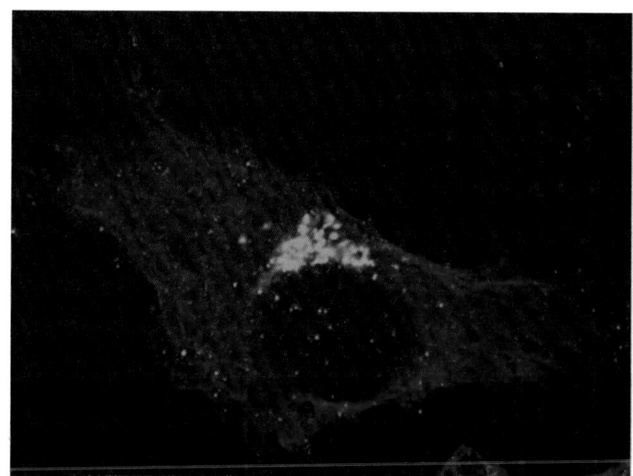

FIGURE 42.8. Bunyavirus transport by exocytosis. BSR-T7/5 cells were infected for 8 h with a recombinant Bunyamwera virus (BUNV) expressing a Gc-GFP (green fluorescent protein) fusion protein and co-stained with an anti-tubulin antibody (*in red*). Progeny virions in vesicles en route to the plasma membrane are visible as *green dots*. (From Shi X, van Mierlo JT, French A, et al. Visualizing the replication cycle of Bunyamwera orthobunyavirus expressing fluorescent protein-tagged Gc glycoprotein. *J Virol* 2010;84:8460–8469.)

EFFECTS OF VIRAL REPLICATION ON HOST CELLS

Cytopathic Effects

The cytopathic effects observed in cultured cells infected with members of the family *Bunyaviridae* vary widely, depending both on the virus and the type of host cell studied. Viruses in all genera except for the *Hantavirus* genus are capable of alternately replicating in vertebrates (or plants for tospoviruses) and arthropods, and generally they are cytolytic for their vertebrate/plant hosts but cause little or no cytopathogenicity in their invertebrate hosts. Some viruses display a narrow host range, especially for arthropod vectors. Although the reason for this has not been defined completely, studies on variant and revertant LACV orthobunyaviruses have suggested that the specificity was related to Gc, probably at the level of viral attachment to susceptible cells.[515] In natural infections of mammals, viruses are often targeted to a particular organ or cell type. For example, orthobunyaviruses such as LACV appear to be neurotropic[396]; the phlebovirus RVFV is primarily hepatotropic[407]; and the hantavirus HTNV persists in rodent lungs.[304] It will be interesting to determine whether this targeting is due solely to host-cell receptors or to other factors such as differences in effects on host-cell metabolism in targeted cell types versus the unnatural situation in cultured vertebrate cell lines.

Host-Cell Metabolism

In vertebrate cells, orthobunyaviruses and some phleboviruses were found to cause a reduction in host-cell protein synthesis, which became more prominent as the infection progressed. For example, by 5 hours after infection, cells infected with BUNV at high multiplicity showed reduced levels of host protein synthesis, and by 7 hours there was almost no synthesis.[402] RVFV-infected cells displayed reduced host protein synthesis, which gradually became more pronounced from 4 to 20 hours after infection.[394] In contrast, a reduction in host protein synthesis did not occur, even late in infection, with another phlebovirus, UUKV, or with the nairovirus DUGV,[410,542] both of which are transmitted by ticks rather than mosquitoes. Hantaviruses not only cause no detectable reduction in host macromolecular synthesis,[466] but routinely establish persistent, noncytolytic infections in susceptible mammalian host cells, a finding consistent with their nonpathogenic persistence in their natural rodent hosts.[304]

The arthropod-borne members of the family, like most other arboviruses, cause little detectable cytopathology in mosquito cell cultures, and viral persistence is readily established. Unlike cultured vertebrate cells, mosquito cells infected with the orthobunyavirus, Marituba virus, displayed no reduction in host macromolecular synthesis; therefore, viral infection apparently does not drastically interfere with normal cellular processes.[81] One suggested reason for this is that, in arthropod cells, excess viral proteins do not accumulate in the cells but rather are more efficiently processed into mature virions.[369] Another possibility is that viral transcriptase may be less active in arthropod cells than in mammalian cells and that the endonuclease activity of the polymerase (which is used to acquire transcriptional primers) is detrimental to host-cell messages. A reduced level of activity of the viral transcriptase would, therefore, produce less damage to host-cell messages and consequently to protein synthesis.[451]

Persistence, both in insect and mammalian cells, can be mediated by defective interfering (DI) viruses. Conventional DI particles, which displayed deletions only in L, were described for orthobunyaviruses and tospoviruses. The L deletions identified both in the TSWV and BUNV DI particles were in-frame, thus allowing translation of truncated L polypeptides.[116,397] Persistent infections of viruses in the family have also been described that do not involve typical DI particles, but instead are caused by infection with temperature-sensitive and plaque morphology mutants.

Host-Cell Responses and Viral Suppression

Interferon-Stimulated Genes and Gene Products

A first line of host defense against viruses is the innate immunity mechanism mediated by the type I interferon (IFN) pathway. Type I IFN (also called IFNα/β) is produced in, and secreted from, infected cells, and in neighboring cells activates the expression of hundreds of IFN-stimulated genes (ISGs) whose gene products directly or indirectly inhibit virus replication. IFN induction is mediated by the recognition of pathogen-associated molecular patterns (PAMPs) by cellular receptors.[412] Two RNA helicases, RIG-I and MDA5, are intracellular receptors that are activated by RNA, though the double-stranded RNA (dsRNA)–binding protein kinase PKR may also assist.[413,435,443,473] RIG-I binds short dsRNAs and also the 5′ triphosphate groups on uncapped viral single-stranded RNA (ssRNA), whereas MDA5 recognizes long dsRNA. Negative-sense RNA viruses do not produce much dsRNA,[568] although they are strong activators of RIG-I, probably because of the 5′ triphosphate groups on their genomes. Activation of RIG-I by binding of RNA initiates a signaling cascade that leads to phosphorylation of the transcription factor IFN regulator factor 3 (IRF-3)[205]; phosphorylated IRF-3 dimerizes, enters the nucleus, and initiates IFN-β mRNA synthesis. Virus replication also activates other transcription factors such as IRF-7, NF-kB, and AP-1, which enhance IFN gene expression. IFN-induced proteins have a myriad of functions, some of which have been characterized with respect to their specific antiviral activity. The three major antiviral defence mechanisms are the Mx protein, PKR, and the 2′-5′ oligoadenylate synthase (2′-5′-OAS)/RNaseL system.

The Mx proteins are interferon-induced cytoplasmic proteins, which belong to a family of large GTPases that function in intracellular trafficking. After viral infection, Mx proteins are rapidly induced and accumulate in the cytoplasm. Human MxA has been shown to inhibit the replication of representative members of the *Orthobunyavirus, Hantavirus, Nairovirus,* and *Phlebovirus* genera.[61,163,245,254] Both inhibition of primary transcription and genome replication have been observed.[163,190,444] The MxA protein was shown to bind to the N proteins of LACV, BUNV, RVFV, ANDV, and CCHFV[19,254,265,444] and in LACV infected cells to redistribute it into membrane-associated perinuclear cytoplasmic complexes, thus removing the protein from use in viral replication[265,444]). For the orthobunyavirus LACV, MxA inhibits replication in mammalian cell cultures, in mosquito cells expressing the human MxA gene, and in MxA-transgenic mice that lack a functional IFN system.[163,202,350]

Inhibition of the replication of several hantaviruses by MxA protein has been described. ANDV infection of human vein endothelial cells (HUVECs) was found to upregulate transcription of MxA RNA and expression of MxA protein. Virus replication was required for the induction of MxA, and the virus was found to replicate best in cells with low or no expressed MxA. Comparison of induction of MxA protein for pathogenic and nonpathogenic hantaviruses in HUVECs demonstrated that the nonpathogenic hantaviruses (PHV or TULV) induced an early and vigorous onset of MxA expression, whereas the pathogenic hantaviruses (ANDV or HTNV) induced MxA relatively late (48 hours) after infection.[174,276] In contrast, Vero E6 cells, which lack IFN genes, supported the growth of both viruses. These results suggest that pathogenic, but not nonpathogenic hantaviruses, can delay the IFN-β induced antiviral MxA response and allow efficient viral replication early in infection.[276]

To determine whether MxA would be active against tospoviruses in plants, transgenic tobacco plants expressing MxA were created and then challenged with TSWV. No increased resistance to viral replication was observed in the transgenic plants, indicating that expression of human MxA alone is not sufficient to impart virus resistance to plants.[164]

In MxA-deficient systems bunyavirus replication can still be impaired, implying that other ISGs have anti-bunyaviral activity.[20,56,191,381] PKR was shown to contribute to host resistance to BUNV, whereas 2′-5′ OAS and RNaseL had no effect,[512] and RVFV lacking its NSs protein is sensitive to PKR *in vitro* and *in vivo*.[191,224] Other IFN-stimulated genes have been identified in hantavirus-infected cells. These studies were conducted mostly with the idea of understanding pathogenic mechanisms involved in disease and are discussed in more detail later. In one study, gene microarray analysis and reverse transcription-PCR revealed that a variety of ISGs, but not IFN genes, were turned on in response to infection or to treatment with ultraviolet-inactivated SNV.[426] Because there was no IFN gene upregulation, it was suggested that IFN-independent pathways mediated the induction of the ISG, perhaps by binding of the viral particles to the $\beta 3$ integrin receptor that has been shown to be used by SNV and other pathogenic hantaviruses for entry via receptor-mediated endocytosis. Consistent with this, and with the aforementioned MxA study, differences in ISGs were observed at early times after infection of human endothelial cells with pathogenic or nonpathogenic hantaviruses, with the nonpathogenic hantavirus inducing much higher levels of ISGs as compared to pathogenic hantaviruses.[174]

Interferon Antagonism

Because the IFN response induces an antiviral state in cells, most or all viruses encode one or more IFN antagonistic proteins, which allows them to overcome the effects of IFN early in infection. Evasion of the IFN response by viruses can occur by preventing IFN release or by inhibiting IFN-signaling and/or the activity of ISGs.

IFN antagonism has been demonstrated for the NSs proteins of the phlebovirus RVFV, the orthobunyaviruses BUNV and LACV, and the hantaviruses PUUV and TULV.[227] For the phleboviruses and orthobunyaviruses, NSs were identified as IFN antagonists by comparing wild-type and mutant viruses that do not express NSs. A RVFV mutant, called Clone 13, was naturally occurring, whereas the BUNV and LACV mutants were created by reverse genetics.[51,63,362] The wild-type viruses induced little IFN and were virulent in mice, whereas the NSs-defective viruses were potent inducers of IFN and attenuated in mice. In genetically altered mice that are nonresponsive to type 1 IFN, the mutant viruses were just as virulent as the wild-type parents, indicating that type 1 IFN is the target of NSs.[53,63,265,566]

Although the orthobunyavirus and phlebovirus NSs have no sequence similarity and are expressed by different coding strategies, they both appear to antagonize host IFN at the level of cellular transcription. For BUNV and LACV, NSs was shown to inhibit phosphorylation of the C-terminal domain of the RNA polymerase II complex, leading to a downregulation of host mRNA synthesis.[266,533,552] This effect was seen only in mammalian cells, not in insect cells, suggesting that IFN antagonism by NSs might be involved in the lytic infections observed in mammalian cells as opposed to viral persistence in insects.[269] BUNV NSs was shown to interact with the protein MED8, a component of the Mediator complex that is essential for mRNA synthesis.[307] LACV NSs selectively targets the RPB1 subunit of the elongating form of RNA polymerase II for proteasome-mediated degradation, an event similar to that seen during the cellular DNA damage response.[552] RVFV NSs inhibits transcription of IFN mRNA in two ways, firstly by interacting with, and degrading, the p44 subunit of the TFIIH transcription factor,[296] and secondly by recruiting the SAP30 repressor factor to the IFN-β promoter.[298] The NSs proteins of the phleboviruses PTV and SFSV also block IFN induction[191,404] whereas that of TOSV only blocked induction when expressed in a heterologous context.[184] In addition to interfering with the IFN response, BUNV NSs was also reported to delay apoptosis, probably by inhibiting some downstream effect of IRF-3 activation. This effect, however, was independent of the IFN response, in that the NSs-deleted BUNV also induced rapid apoptosis in a cell line that was not responsive to IFN. In a cell line that produces low levels of IRF-3, induction of apoptotic cell death by the wild-type and NSs deletion mutant was similar, suggesting that IRF-3 is involved in the BUNV-induced apoptotic pathways and that NSs somehow counteracts this effect.[266] Orthobunyaviruses in the Anopheles A, Anopheles B, and Tete serogroups do not encode an NSs protein, and most behaved like a recombinant BUNV with the NSs gene deleted in failing to prevent induction of IFN-β mRNA.[351] However, Tacaiuma virus in the Anopheles A serogroup inhibited IFN induction similar to wild-type BUNV, suggesting that TCMV has evolved an alternative mechanism, not involving a typical NSs protein, to antagonize the host innate immune response.

Some hantaviruses have an additional ORF in the S segment,[421] and evidence for the expression of an NSs protein has been obtained for PUUV and TULV.[227] The NSs protein was shown to be weakly antagonistic to IFN when overexpressed in cell culture, and the presence of a full-length NSs gave a growth advantage to TULV strains in IFN-competent cells.[228] Both hantaviruses and nairoviruses have 5′monophosphorylated nucleotides on their genomes, thereby avoiding recognition by RIG-I and hence inducing IFN,[189] although the viruses also encode other countermeasures to innate immunity. The OTU domain in the nairovirus L protein deconjugates ubiquitin and ISG15 from cellular targets, thus antagonizing the antiviral effects of ISG15 and inhibiting NF-κB dependent signaling.[77,165,230] Certain hantaviruses have also been shown to interfere with TNF-α induced activation of NF-κB signaling through an interaction between the viral N protein and karyopherin molecules that normally transport the NF-κB subunits from the cytoplasm to the nucleus, thus preventing their use to activate ISG.[523]

As described above, it has been reported that pathogenic hantaviruses do not efficiently activate the IFN response as compared to nonpathogenic hantaviruses, suggesting the presence of an IFN antagonistic gene in pathogenic hantaviruses.[174] The cytoplasmic tail of the Gn glycoprotein (Gn-T) from pathogenic hantaviruses has been shown to downregulate IFN induction by interacting with TNF receptor-associated factor 3 (TRAF3), an adaptor protein for IRF-3 and NF-kB signaling, whereas Gn-T from PHV fail to inhibit IFN induction.[11,12] However, a recent paper demonstrates that the Gn-T of nonpathogenic TULV can also downregulate IFN induction, but does so in a manner not involving interaction with TRAF3.[336] These data suggest that the pathogenic potential of hantaviruses does not depend on their ability to downregulate IFN alone. The situation is further complicated by the demonstration that for ANDV, IFN induction is inhibited by co-expression of the glycoprotein precursor (GPC) and N protein, whereas downstream IFN signaling may be inhibited by either protein.[309] In addition, hantavirus infection of VeroE6 cells was reported to result in induction and secretion of type III IFN (IFN-γ).[425,509] Furthermore, the induction of ISGs in epithelial cell lines (e.g., A549 cells) infected with Vero cell grown virus was found to be due to the presence of IFN-γ rather than to virus infection.[425]

Cytokines/Chemokines/ITAMs

The host cells' responses to hantaviral infection have been studied in an attempt to understand the mechanism of disease. Hantaviruses cause two serious human disease syndromes: HFRS and HPS. Both HFRS and HPS are believed to result from host immune responses to viral infection, rather than damage caused by the viruses themselves.[255] In both syndromes, vascular endothelial cells show increased permeability, which is believed to contribute greatly to the diseases. Several studies have measured the types of cytokines and chemokines released in response to disease, and these are discussed in the context of viral pathogenesis below. Of note is the presence of immunoreceptor tyrosine-based activation motifs (ITAMs) within the cytoplasmic tails of the Gn protein of hantaviruses. ITAMS are cell-signaling elements involved in regulating endothelial cell function. The presence of these elements in hantaviruses has also been suggested to relate to the dysregulation of endothelial cells during hantaviral infection.[172,173]

Apoptosis

Apoptosis, or programmed cell death has been described for hantaviruses, orthobunyaviruses, and phleboviruses. Apoptosis usually results from activation of a proteolytic system involving caspases, a group of cysteine proteases that cleave cellular substrate proteins.

Apoptosis caused by a virus in the family *Bunyaviridae* was first noted in cultured cells and brains of newborn mice infected with the orthobunyavirus LACV.[401] The NSs proteins of LACV were found to have an amino acid sequence similar to that of a *Drosophila* protein, Reaper, which is involved in regulating caspase activity and can induce apoptosis.[104] Reaper is one of several proteins that are able to bind to a group of proteins, known as inhibitors of apoptosis, which function to control caspase activity.[487] Like Reaper, BUNV NSs proteins were shown to both inhibit cellular protein translation and activate caspase in cell-free extracts. To demonstrate *in vivo* apoptosis, a Sindbis replicon expressing NSs was injected into the brains of young mice. The mice developed neuronal apoptosis and died 6 days after infection. A similar mechanism of action for inducing apoptosis by Reaper and orthobunyavirus NSs was proposed because both were shown to bind to and counteract the effects of a protein known as Scythe, which is an apoptosis regulator.[104] Mosquito cells persistently infected by LACV do not undergo apoptosis.[51] Oropouche orthobunyavirus (OROV) induces apoptosis in HeLa cells that is dependent on virus uncoating and replication, and treatment of cells with a pan-caspase inhibitor did not affect virus production although apoptosis was prevented.[3] The results indicated that the intrinsic apoptosis pathway was triggered by virus replication but apoptosis was not necessary for efficient virus production.

Apoptosis was also observed in the brains of adult Balb/c mice infected with a neurotropic strain of the phlebovirus TOSV, but the mechanism of apoptotic triggering was not investigated.[110]

For several hantaviruses, apoptosis was observed in infected cultured monkey kidney (Vero E6) cells,[246,313] in cultured human embryonic kidney cells (HEK-293),[330] and in lymphocytes of HFRS patients.[4] Unlike most infections with hantaviruses, which are generally noncytolytic and persistent, cytopathic effects were observed in the HEK-293 cells infected with hantaviruses, and apoptosis was observed almost entirely in cells adjacent to those actively infected with the hantavirus.[330] In another report, apoptosis was not seen in confluent Vero E6 cells infected with various hantaviruses, and only a few apoptotic cells could be seen when subconfluent cells were infected.[198] Likewise, infection of primary immature dendritic cells or HUVECs with HTNV did not induce cell lysis or apoptosis.[429] These differing results remain to be resolved, but it is likely that they can be attributed to differences in the cells or the condition and passage histories of the cells.

The factors triggering apoptosis for hantaviruses are not generally known. In TULV-infected Vero E6 cells, caspase 8 activation was observed and apoptosis could be inhibited with a caspase inhibitor.[313] Caspase 8 is one of several caspases that can be induced by the binding of a specific ligand to "death receptors," such as tumor necrosis factor 1 (TNF1) and Fas (also called CD95), which are found on certain cells.[29] Consistent with this, TNF1 was upregulated at times when apoptosis was apparent in the TULV-infected cells and a Fas-mediated apoptosis enhancer, Daxx, was found to bind to PUUV N proteins.[315] However, in another study, no significant increase in the mRNAs of the TNF superfamily was observed in hantavirus-infected HEK-293 cells.[330]

Stress on the host cell ER is another cellular condition that can trigger apoptosis. TULV infection of Vero E6 cells was noted to activate markers of ER stress, including induction of the chaperone protein, Grp78/bip, which was suggested to be induced by the accumulation of misfolded proteins in the ER.[314] Another cellular stress-response protein, heat shock protein 70, was found to be abundant in postmortem tissues of hantavirus-infected patients and to be upregulated in VeroE6 cells infected with HTNV.[589] In this study, it was not clear what role the stress protein played in host-cell response to infection. Additional work is needed to identify the many possible factors that can contribute to cellular stress and apoptosis in bunyavirus-infected cells.

RNA Silencing

RNA silencing, or RNA interference (RNAi) was first described for plants as a mechanism to defend against viral infection, but is now known to occur in most eukaryotes. The gene silencing is mediated by short interfering RNAs (siRNAs), which arise from cleavage of dsRNAs, including the replication intermediates of RNA viruses by a host enzyme known as Dicer. The 21 to 25 nucleotide siRNAs become part of a protein complex known as the RNA-induced silencing complex, which recognizes and degrades sequence-specific mRNAs. Some viruses have been shown to produce suppressors to counteract the gene silencing mechanism. In the family *Bunyaviridae*, the NSs protein of the tospovirus TSWV was found to act as a suppressor of gene silencing.[68,521] In addition to the plant-infecting bunyaviruses, siRNA suppression has been observed with the orthobunyavirus LACV, both in mammalian and insect cells, and with the nairovirus Hazara virus (HAZV) in tick cells. As for the tospoviruses, the LACV-suppressing activity was localized to NSs, despite the completely different coding strategy used for this protein (i.e., ambisense vs. ORFs).[502] For HAZV, which does not produce an NSs protein, the activity was observed with the S-segment gene in either the sense or antisense orientation.[167]

Although not yet demonstrated, it was suggested that the similarities of the ambisense-encoded NSs proteins of tospoviruses and phleboviruses would suggest similar functions in viral replication. It will be interesting to see whether the NSs of phleboviruses will have both interferon antagonistic activity (as described earlier) as well as RNAi activity. Such dual-pathogenic activity is known to occur for other viral proteins, for example, the NS1 protein of influenza virus.[197]

PATHOGENESIS AND PATHOLOGY

Orthobunyavirus Genus

Human infections with California encephalitis, LACV, or Jamestown Canyon (JCV) viruses are initiated by the bite of a virus-infected mosquito. The course of the infection has been extensively modeled in mice.[396] Similar to the human infection, the outcome of the infection in mice is dependent on the age of the animal and strain of virus used, with subcutaneous challenge of newborn mice most closely mimicking the natural human infection. The virus initially spreads from the site of inoculation into striated muscle, which is the major site of replication. It spreads to the plasma, presumably through the lymphatic channels, and the resulting high viremia allows the virus to cross the blood–brain barrier.[231] Mice inoculated intraperitoneally with LACV showed high levels of replication in nasal turbinates, suggesting the virus could enter the central nervous system (CNS) by olfactory neurons.[38] Once in the CNS, the virus replicates in neurons and glial cells, causing considerable neuronal necrosis. Death occurs 3 or 4 days postinfection. In contrast, although rhesus monkeys were highly susceptible to LACV infection, the animals remained asymptomatic and developed neutralizing antibodies.[38] High viremia is essential for neuroinvasion. A monoclonal antibody escape mutant of LACV (V22) showed decreased replication in striated muscle, and hence did not generate sufficient viremia to permit neuroinvasion, but V22 was as neurovirulent as wild-type LACV when inoculated intracranially.[182] A similar distinction between neurovirulence and neuroinvasiveness is implied from observations on recombinant LACV with mutations in the fusion peptide domain of Gc, which showed reduced replication in muscle cells but retained the ability to cause neuronal loss in culture.[501] The lesions observed in the brains of fatal La Crosse encephalitis cases differ from those in infected suckling mice. In humans, and to a large extent in adult mice infected intracerebrally, cerebral edema, perivascular cuffing, glial nodules, mild leptomeningitis, and occasional areas of focal necrosis that are typical of acute severe viral encephalitis are observed. Lesions are mostly in the cerebral cortex, with some in the brainstem.[243] Studies with Tahyna virus and JCV showed strain differences in neuroinvasiveness and neurovirulence in a Swiss Webster mouse model, whereas in rhesus monkeys no clinical disease was observed but the animals mounted strong neutralizing antibody responses.[39,40]

Infection of natural vertebrate amplifying hosts of these viruses, such as adult chipmunks (LACV) or snowshoe hares (snowshoe hare virus), results in inapparent infection and viremia sufficient to infect mosquitoes.[477] *Aedes triseriatus* mosquitoes are the principal vector of LACV, and their experimental infection with California encephalitis serogroup viruses has been studied in detail.[36,529,535,564] Viruses ingested via a viremic bloodmeal infect the epithelial layer surrounding the mosquito midgut. Replication of the virus results in release of the virus across the basal lamina into the hemocele, allowing transport of the virus to tissues throughout the body. Virus infection of mosquitoes other than the principal vector species usually results in poor penetration of the virus across this midgut barrier. Experimental infections using reassortant viruses have shown that virus M genomic segment (encoding the glycoproteins and NSm protein) is an important component in the correct match between virus and host mosquito, which allows efficient transit across the midgut barrier.[36] Once across the barrier, virus replication occurs in a wide variety of tissues, including the ovaries and salivary glands.[529] Release of virus from the salivary glands allows virus transmission from the female mosquito to the vertebrate host during feeding. Mosquitoes begin to be infectious approximately 1 or 2 weeks after ingestion of virus, an interval referred to as the extrinsic incubation period.

The infection of the ovaries is thought to be crucial for virus maintenance in mosquito populations, in that it results in transovarial transmission of the virus from the female to the offspring and allows the virus to overwinter in infected eggs.[461] In addition, LACV-infected females appear to mate more efficiently than uninfected mosquitoes.[441] Male mosquitoes play no role in the vertical transovarial transmission of the virus, or in the horizontal transmission via amplifying vertebrate hosts, as they do not take a bloodmeal. However, the virus is detected in the gonads of transovarially infected males and can result in venereal transmission of the virus horizontally within the mosquito population.[535] This combination of transmission mechanisms allows efficient maintenance of the LACV in *A. triseriatus* populations. Similar processes are thought to function in host mosquito infections with other California serogroup viruses,[539] and results from studies with these viruses and their arthropod hosts serve as a model for understanding virus maintenance and transmission mechanisms for other family *Bunyaviridae* viruses.

Aino and Akabane virus (AKAV) are important causes of disease in livestock, causing epizootics of abortions and congenital defects in cattle, sheep, and goats.[201,259,538] Experimental infections of pregnant cattle or ewes with either virus have been shown to produce viremia, followed by virus replication in the placenta and fetal tissues, and resulting in congenital defects such as microencephaly, and hydrocephalus.[201,286,395,538] Similarly, experimental infection of pregnant hamsters with AKAV results in death of the fetus.[16]

Phlebovirus Genus

RVFV pathogenesis and disease has been reviewed in-depth recently.[54,226,403] RVFV infections of livestock are often recognized by the onset of "abortion storms," which sweep through livestock-producing areas, with simultaneous acute febrile disease in humans. Most human infections with RVFV result in a mild febrile illness. The incubation period is approximately 2 to 6 days, and is followed by an abrupt onset of fever, chills, and general malaise. Susceptibility of livestock to RVFV infection varies considerably, depending on a variety of factors, including livestock species and age and the strain of the virus. Based on data from experimental infections and analogy with other arbovirus infections, the general pattern of infection likely follows the same course as that following inoculation of the virus by mosquito bite: the virus is transported by lymphatic drainage to the regional lymph node where local replication takes place. The virus spills over into the circulation, causing the primary viremia and spread of the virus to the major organs. Replication in the lymph nodes, spleen, liver, adrenals, lungs, and kidney tissues results in high viremia, and, in severe cases, hepatic necrosis is prominent and necrotic foci can be observed in the brains of cases exhibiting the less frequent encephalitic form of the disease.[355] RVFV replication in cells is highly cytotoxic, suggesting that most cellular destruction in acute illness is likely due to direct virus killing of host cells.

Pathologic features of the disease in livestock vary considerably. Leukopenia is frequently seen during the first 3 or 4 days of infection, when fever and viremia are usually at their highest. Altered serum enzyme levels (e.g., aspartate aminotransferase and sorbitol dehydrogenases) indicative of hepatocyte destruction are often seen during the acute phase. Leukocytosis often occurs in the early phase of recovery. Thrombocytopenia and fibrin thrombi in several organs suggest that disseminated intravascular coagulopathy (DIC) may be a feature of severe disease in livestock, as is seen in hemorrhagic infections in humans.[107,520]

Infection of pregnant animals frequently results in abortion of the fetus. Abortions early in the course of infection are probably the result of the high fever associated with the acute phase of illness; later abortions are more commonly the result of direct infection of the fetus with resulting hepatic necrosis. No clear correlation between RVFV infection and abortion has been seen in human infections.[340]

Nairovirus Genus

Vertebrate Hosts

CCHF and NSD viruses are maintained in nature predominantly in their respective tick hosts. Although the viruses can persist in the ticks through the various life stages (transstadial transmission) and can be passed to the offspring (transovarial transmission), vertebrates are needed to provide blood meals for the ticks, and they can become infected and develop viremia capable of supporting virus transmission to uninfected ticks.[115] In this manner, vertebrates may play an important amplifying role in the virus natural cycle. In the case of CCHFV, a variety of livestock (e.g., sheep, goats, cattle, ostriches), large wild herbivores, hares, and hedgehogs may become infected, resulting in an inapparent or subclinical disease.[210,519] Sheep and goats are implicated as being important vertebrate hosts of NSD virus, and infection often results in severe disease.[115] These animals are presumably subcutaneously infected when bitten by infected ticks. Studies of CCHFV pathogenesis have been hampered by lack of a suitable animal model, and most nonhuman primates do show evidence of disease. Recently, two mouse models have been described, one using type I IFN-receptor knockout mice,[42] the other using Signal Transducer and Activator of Transcription (STAT1) knockout mice[41]; the animals are highly susceptible to infection, and the STAT1 knockout mice display many features of human disease including fever, leukopenia, thrombocytopenia, and highly elevated liver enzymes.

In experimental NSD virus infections of sheep, goats, and suckling mice, the virus replicates to high titers in the lung, liver, spleen, and other organs of the reticuloendothelial system.[527] Vascular endothelium appears to be the primary cell target. Virus replication in the endothelial cells results in edema and necrosis of the capillary walls of the mucosal surfaces of the intestine, gall bladder, and female genital tract, leading to congestion, hemorrhage, and catarrhal inflammation.

Human Infections

In contrast to the inapparent infection characteristic of CCHFV infection of other vertebrate hosts, human infections often result in severe hemorrhagic fevers. On introduction of the virus, there is likely local replication followed by blood- and lymph-borne spread of the virus to the major organs, including the liver, where high levels of replication take place.[518] Congestion, edema, and focal hemorrhage and necrosis are seen in most organs. DIC is evident early, with thrombocytopenia, elevated prothrombin time ratio and activated partial thromboplastin time (APTT) present during the first few days of illness, and likely plays a central role in disease progression. Little is known regarding host-cell receptor use or factors influencing virus virulence. Both IgM and IgG antibodies are usually detectable approximately 7 days after the onset of illness and are detectable in all survivors by day 9.[87,158] Antibody responses are rarely detectable in fatal cases.

NSD virus has been isolated from sick patients in Uganda, as has the identical or closely related Ganjam virus from febrile patients in India, but their importance in terms of human disease is currently unclear.

Hantavirus Genus

Reservoirs

Hantaviruses have been detected in numerous rodents and insectivores (reviewed in 241). To date, all known pathogenic viruses are harbored by rodents, but additional study of the disease potential of the many hantaviruses carried by sorcid and talpid insectivores is needed. Hantaviruses are horizontally transmitted among rodents primarily through exposure to excreta and saliva. Infection of natural reservoirs results in an acute phase with high viremia followed by prolonged or persistent infection with variable durations of virus shedding in the urine feces and/or saliva from days to months or even for the life of the rodent. Hantavirus persistence in rodents was found to relate to increased regulatory T cells that modulate the immune response and prevent clearance of infected cells.[130,131,472] Experimental infection of host rodents indicates that viremia peaks approximately 2 weeks postinfection, and results in dissemination of the virus throughout the animal (e-Fig. 42.9).[371] The cessation of viremia correlates with the induction of hantavirus-specific antibodies, which first become detectable around 14 days postinfection, peak at approximately 50 days postinfection, and remain detectable for the life of the rodent.[304] Although naturally infected rodent reservoirs do not display apparent disease symptoms, reduced winter survival and reduced body weights of infected rodents have been reported.[95,123,244] Aggressive behavior has been correlated with increased infection among rodents in that the highest seropositive rates are seen in older males and animals with more scars.[179] Hantaviruses appear to target primarily endothelial cells of rodents, with the highest concentrations of virus antigen being observed in the lungs and kidneys.[368]

Human Infections

In stark contrast to the asymptomatic hantavirus infection of primary rodent reservoir species, human infections frequently result in HFRS or HPS. Humans are infected by inhalation of aerosols produced from the infected rodent excreta. Virus RNA is usually detectable in patient blood during the early stages of disease. At the time of death, virus antigens are detectable in endothelial cell layers throughout the body, but predominantly in lung endothelial cells in the case of HPS, or kidney endothelial cells in the case of HFRS.[217,591] Pathologic findings in HFRS patient kidney biopsies include mild to moderate interstitial infiltration of lymphocytes, plasma cells, monocytes/macrophages, and polymorphonuclear leukocytes (mainly eosinophilic granulocytes and neutrophils), although the exact mechanism of kidney failure in HFRS patients is unclear.[525] The lung is the primary target organ of HPS. Patients usually develop pulmonary edema, plural effusions, and interstitial mononuclear cell infiltrate, edema, and focal hyaline membranes. Viral antigen is plentiful in lung endothelial cell.[409,591]

In general, both HFRS and HPS result from capillary leakage and fluid loss. A number of studies have implicated immune-modulated processes rather than virus-induced cell death as the primary cause of disease. Hantavirus-specific antibodies and Tcells are detectable at the time of onset of disease symptoms, consistent with immune-pathogenesis (reviewed in 241). For example, in HFRS, the expression of the cytokines tumor necrosis factor α (TNF-α), TGF-β, and platelet-derived growth factor has been observed at the peritubular area of the distal nephron. Similarly, high numbers of cytokine-producing cells can be seen in the lungs (but not the kidneys and livers) of fatal HPS cases, suggesting that local cytokine production may play an important role in pulmonary edema and the high case-fatality rate. Severity of illness in humans has been correlated with specific human lymphocyte antigen (HLA) haplotypes, both HFRS and HPS.[328,365,548,561]

EPIDEMIOLOGY AND ECOLOGY

Orthobunyavirus Genus

Most orthobunyaviruses are transmitted by mosquitoes, although a few have been isolated from tabanids, phlebotomines, tick, and bedbugs, and have been found in every continent except Antarctica.[50]

California Serogroup Viruses

LACV is the most significant of the California encephalitis serogroup viruses in terms of causing human disease in the United States, with an average of 79 cases per year, predominantly in children younger than 15 years of age. There is, however, severe underreporting.[195,240] The primary vector is the forest-dwelling, tree-hole–breeding mosquito, *Aedes triseriatus,* although more recently, and concerning, the virus has also been isolated from the aggressive day-feeing Asian tiger-mosquito, *A. albopictus.*[290] *A. triseriatus* is found throughout the northern Midwestern and Northeastern United States, and LACV is maintained in these mosquitoes by transovarial transmission, which allows overwintering of the virus in mosquito eggs.[565] During the summer months, squirrels, chipmunks, foxes, and woodchucks become viremic following LACV infection, and are important amplifying hosts.[534,590] The majority of La Crosse encephalitis cases occur in the summer and early fall months when risk of bite from infected female mosquitoes is highest. Historically LACV infections mostly occurred in the Mississippi and Ohio river basins, with more than 90% of cases coming from Wisconsin, Minnesota, Iowa, Indiana, Ohio, and Illinois,[50] but since the 1980s, more cases have been reported from Appalachia and eastern Tennessee, and between 1987 to 2009 more than 30% of total cases in the United States were from West Virginia.[194]

Jamestown Canyon virus (including the closely related Jerry Slough variety) is also associated with arboviral encephalitis in the United States. The virus is vectored by *Culex inornata* mosquitoes, and several species of *Aedes* mosquitoes, and is broadly distributed across much of North America. Vertical transmission of the virus has been demonstrated in several *Aedes* species mosquitoes.[199] White-tailed deer are the most likely vertebrate amplifying host. Unlike LACV, which mainly causes encephalitis in children, Jamestown Canyon virus appears to predominantly cause disease in adults, although only 15 human cases have been reported since 2004.[23]

Bunyamwera Serogroup Viruses

Bunyamwera virus is present throughout much of sub-Saharan Africa, and appears to be an important cause of acute febrile illness in humans. The virus has been isolated from humans in Uganda, Nigeria, and South Africa.[181,271,532] More recently, Ngari virus has been identified as a reassortant BUNV, with its M segment derived from the Batai virus (i.e., S_{BUN} M_{BAT} L_{BUN}). This reassortant virus has been associated with hemorrhagic fever cases in Somalia and Kenya and a large outbreak of acute febrile illness in Sudan.[58,64,175,587] In addition, human antibodies reactive with BUNV have been detected in most of sub-Saharan Africa, with high prevalence (up to 82%) being recorded in some locations.[499] Isolation of the virus from several *Aedes* species mosquitoes has implicated them as the primary vector.[271,499] Antibodies reactive with BUNV have been detected in domestic animals, nonhuman primates, rodents, and birds, and viremias capable of supporting mosquito transmission have been recorded in experimentally infected rodents, bats, and primates.[499,576] However, the role of a potential vertebrate amplifying host is currently unclear.

Several additional Bunyamwera serogroup viruses are present in the Americas[370] and are infrequently reported to cause acute febrile illness in humans. Cache Valley virus is found throughout the United States, Canada, and Mexico, and often infects sheep and possibly all ruminants; infections have been associated with embryonic and fetal death, stillbirths, and multiple congenital malformations in sheep.[134,337] The virus has caused a fatal encephalitis in a human.[476] It remains unclear whether Cache Valley and serologically closely related viruses may play a role in syndromes of congenital malformations and embryonic losses in humans in North America.[75]

Simbu Serogroup Viruses

Simbu serogroup viruses are global in distribution, and are principally vectored by biting midges of the genus *Culicoides.* Since the original isolation of OROV from a febrile patient in

Trinidad in the 1950s, the medical importance of the virus, particularly in the Amazon basin regions of northern Brazil and Peru, has become increasingly evident.[418] Between 1960 and 2009, at least 500,000 people are thought to have been infected in more than 30 outbreaks.[550] Most of these outbreaks were in relatively urban areas, leading to the suggestion that there are likely separate urban and sylvatic cycles.[121,448]

The principal urban vector in Brazil appears to be the tiny biting midge, *Culicoides paraensis*.[415,448] which breeds in rotting vegetative matter, and seasonal populations can become high in agricultural areas, where build-up of debris such as banana tree stalks or cacao husks may occur.[417] These midges feed predominantly in the early evening hours and are quite anthropophilic. Infected humans develop viremia sufficiently high to transmit the virus to uninfected midges, and appear capable of serving as the vertebrate amplifying host during urban epidemics.[417] Serologic data also suggest that primates or sloths, or even birds, may be potential hosts in the sylvatic cycle. Recent phylogenetic studies indicate that four distinct OROV lineages are present in different geographic areas, and that OROV emerged in Brazil in around 1790.[550]

AKAV is widely distributed throughout Australasia (Australia, Japan, Korea, Taiwan), the Middle East (occasionally extending as far north as Turkey), and sub-Saharan Africa.[8,15,111,352,524] The virus is an important cause of disease in livestock, with periodic outbreaks of abortions, stillbirths, and congenital malformations recorded in cattle, sheep, and goats in Australia, Japan, Korea, Taiwan, Israel, and Turkey, although intriguingly no disease outbreaks have been observed in Africa, despite the widespread presence of the virus.[8] The virus is vectored by midges of the genus *Culicoides,* and although *C. brevitarsis* is the primary vector in Australia,[364] different species are important in Asia and the Middle East.[6,234,285]

Phlebovirus Genus

The geographic distribution of SFSV and SFNV Naples viruses closely follows that of their sandfly host, *Phlebotomus papataci.*[528] This distribution extends from the Mediterranean basin throughout the Middle East and Arabian peninsula, north up into areas around the Caucus mountains, and as far east as Pakistan and India. Sandflies are most numerous in the warmer months, are found at ground level, and feed in the early evenings. Unfortunately, their small size allows them to pass through untreated mosquito netting.

A related phlebovirus, TOSV, is hosted by *P. perniciocus* and is found in central Italy, Cyprus, Portugal, and Spain. Relatively high (20% to 25%) antibody prevalence rates suggest that human infections with TOSV are widespread and frequent in endemic areas.[60,136] In addition, many acute lymphocytic meningitis and meningoencephalitis cases, particularly those in children, occurring in the summer months are attributable to TOSV infection.[59,136,341,374] These viruses replicate in their sandfly hosts, and virus transstadial and transovarial transmission have been demonstrated.[531] Sexual transmission of TOSV among sandflies has also been shown.[530] The relatively low efficiency of transovarial transmission demonstrated in experimental infections suggests that vertebrate amplifying hosts are required to maintain these viruses in endemic areas. However, although antibodies to TOSV are present in many domestic animals, virus isolation has been unsuccessful, suggesting that these animals do act as reservoirs,[367] and the identity of amplifying hosts remains uncertain. Data showing that viremic humans can infect *P. papatasi,* together with attack rates as high as 75% and records of urban outbreaks of sandfly fever, suggest that humans can on occasion serve as the amplifying vertebrate host.[456]

The ecology and epidemiology of RVFV is complex and poorly understood. The geographic distribution of RVFV covers much of Africa, from Senegal to Madagascar and from Egypt to South Africa, with most reported epizootics in livestock being reported in East and Southern Africa.[288,403] Mosquitoes have long been known to play an important role in RVFV epizootics, with epizootics frequently occurring at times of unusually high precipitation.[316] More recent data indicate that floodwater *Aedes* mosquitoes of the subgenera *Aedimorphus* and *Neomelaniconion* are likely the principal vectors. The ecology of RVFV has been best studied in Kenya, Zimbabwe, and South Africa. In these regions, damboes or vleis, which are shallow depressions up to several hundred meters across near streams and fed by ground water, are thought to play a central role.[516] These damboes flood at times of unusually heavy rainfall, which triggers a population explosion in floodwater *Aedes* mosquitoes.

Isolation of RVFV from unfed male and female *A. mcintoshi* mosquitoes hatched at a dambo in the endemic area of Kenya during an interepidemic period demonstrated the maintenance of the virus between epidemics and the transovarial transmission of the virus in such mosquitoes.[317] *A. mcintoshi* is thought to be the principal maintenance vector in Kenya and Zimbabwe.[517] The biology of these mosquitoes is such that they are among the earliest mosquitoes to hatch from eggs following flooding. If the eggs contain virus (via transovarial transmission), infected mosquitoes hatch and feed on nearby livestock, potentially initiating a local epizootic. Viremic livestock act as amplifying hosts that transmit the virus to other floodwater *Aedes,* and also other species of mosquitoes including culicines and anophelines, promoting further amplification and spread of the virus. When such a cycle gets initiated at damboes throughout a livestock producing area, it could give rise to a regional, relatively synchronous eruption of RVFV activity with an associated abortion storm, such as those observed in livestock at various intervals in East and Southern Africa.[403] Although such a scenario is an attractive explanation of the dynamics of RVFV epizootics, more data are necessary to confirm this is the case.

Hemorrhagic fever cases in humans are usually seen 1 or 2 weeks after the appearance of abortions and disease in livestock. Cases are usually among farmers and others living in proximity to livestock. Humans likely acquire infection through a bite from an infected mosquito when vector densities are high. However, contact transmission seems to be most important with RVFV. People involved in the birth or abortions of livestock, butchering of animals, abattoir workers, and so on, are at high risk of infection during epizootics.[2,88] RVFV is also highly infectious by aerosol, having resulted in many infections of laboratory personnel working with the virus.[161,500] The relative contribution of infectious aerosols or fomites to transmission is unclear. Although less than 1% of human infections result in severe disease (hemorrhagic fever, encephalitis, retinitis), this can add up to a substantial number of cases given the large scale of some epizootics. For instance, an estimated 27,500 RVFV infections occurred during the 1997/1998 outbreak in the Garissa district of Kenya,[583] and approximately 200,000 human cases with 600 deaths were estimated to have occurred during the outbreak in Egypt in 1977 and 1978.[339] The 2008 outbreak of RVFV in Sudan resulted in 698 human cases with 222 deaths, a case fatality rate of 31.8%.[577] The economic effects of RVFV epidemics are huge, with the 2006/2007 outbreak in Kenya resulting in losses from livestock deaths valued at more than 7.6 million US dollars.[446]

In contrast to the long history of periodic RVFV epizootics in East and Southern Africa, the recent large RVFV outbreaks in Egypt in 1977 and 1978 and in West Africa in Mauritania/Senegal in 1987 were different situations.[593] In Egypt, retrospective studies showed that RVFV had not been enzootic prior to 1977.[340] Virus activity disappeared after 1981, only to be reintroduced in 1993.[28] These data suggest that although mosquitoes capable of acting as epizootic vectors (e.g., *Culex* sp.) exist in Egypt, mosquitoes capable of RVFV transovarial transmission are probably lacking. It is thought that RVFV was most likely introduced into Egypt from enzootic areas in Sudan.[339]

The first confirmed RVFV outbreak outside Africa was reported September 2000, in the western coastal plains of Saudi Arabia and Yemen.[488] Unusually heavy rains and flooding of the foothills of the Asir mountains appeared responsible for increased mosquito populations and the explosive outbreak in naïve livestock. Eight hundred eighty-four hospitalized patients were identified in Saudi Arabia, with 124 deaths. In Yemen, 1,087 cases were estimated to have occurred, with 121 deaths. The virus associated with this outbreak was almost identical to those associated with earlier RVFV epidemics in East Africa, consistent with the recent introduction of RVFV into the Arabian Peninsula from East Africa.[488] More recent outbreaks in Madagascar have been linked to importations of infected animals from on-going epidemics in East Africa.[80]

Nairovirus Genus

The epidemiology of CCHFV reflects the complex ecology and geographic distribution of the *ixodid* tick hosts of the virus, particularly those of genus *Hyalomma*.[147,210] Although CCHFV has been isolated from approximately 30 different tick species, evidence is lacking as to whether they truly represent vectors, or merely reflect the isolation of virus from engorged ticks that have fed on a viremic vertebrate host. Only some ticks of three genera, *Hyalomma*, *Dermacentor*, and *Rhipicephalus*, have actually been shown to be capable of transstadial transmission of CCHFV (i.e., passing the virus through the various stages of the life cycle, from larva to nymph to adult) following feeding on a viremic host. Transovarial transmission of CCHFV has also been shown to occur with some of the tick species in these genera. Moreover, the overall global pattern of geographic distribution of CCHFV cases corresponds most closely with the distribution of *Hyalomma* ticks, suggesting their principal role as vector.

There is evidence that CCHFV is present throughout much of sub-Saharan Africa (from Egypt to South Africa, and from Senegal to Madagascar), eastern Europe, the Middle East, and parts of Asia, particularly the former Central Asian republics, and Xinjiang province of NW China.[147] Of note is the emergence of CCHFV in Turkey since 2002,[387] which may be related to climate change influencing tick distribution.[139,558]

Most human infections are acquired by bite from infected ticks, contact with infected ticks during their removal from animals or human body, or contact with blood or tissues of infected livestock. As one would expect, most cases are among individuals (e.g., shepherds, ranchers, and abattoir workers) living or working in close contact with livestock (e.g., sheep, goats, cattle, or ostriches) in endemic areas. Nosocomial outbreaks have also been reported in several regions, with infection of medical personnel following treatment or surgery on an unsuspected CCHFV case.[147]

The distribution of NSD virus mirrors the distribution of the principal tick host, *Rhipicephalus appendiculatus*. The virus is present throughout much of Africa, from as far north as Ethiopia and Somalia, extending through much of East and Central Africa, and as far south as the Mozambique coastal plain.[114,585] The distribution likely extends through parts of the Middle East and into India, based on the detection of the closely related NSD virus Ganjam variant from *Haemaphysalis intermedia* ticks.[112]

Hantavirus Genus

The geographic distribution of hantaviruses and epidemiologic patterns observed for HFRS and HPS reflect the distribution and natural history features of the hantavirus-infected rodent hosts of these viruses. This is because hantavirus infection of the rodent primary reservoir species produces a persistent infection with prolonged shedding of the virus, whereas infection of humans results in an acute infection with quick clearance of virus and recovery in survivors. Epidemiologic data accumulated since the 1950s for a variety of hantaviruses, including HPS-associated hantaviruses, suggest that human-to-human virus transmission does not occur, and that virtually all human infections are acquired by exposure to infected rodent excreta, with the one exception of an ANDV-associated HPS outbreak in Patagonia, Argentina, which clearly demonstrated human-to-human transmission between a patient and her physician, and circumstantial evidence suggested several additional human-to-human virus transmissions during this particular outbreak.[388,570] This does not appear to be a common property of ANDV, as no health care workers became infected in the course of handling ANDV-associated HPS cases in a subsequent large HPS outbreak in Chile.[89]

HTNV is found in various parts of eastern China and Korea and Far Eastern Russia, and is present in *Apodemus agrarius mantchuricus*, a mouse that is common in agricultural fields. Adults in rural areas (e.g., farmers, forest workers, or troops stationed in the field) are the most at risk of infection, and HFRS cases are seen to peak in the fall. This likely reflects a mixture of factors including the increased abundance of virus-infected mice in the fall coinciding with increased human activity in the fields associated with harvest of crops, and movement of rodents into the houses as winter approaches.[299] Most cases are 20 to 50 years in age, and cases in children younger than age 10 are uncommon.[91,303] A greater number of male than female cases is seen, consistent with predominant exposure being in the fields rather than in the homes. HTNV-related HFRS is probably most important in China, where approximately 100,000 cases are reported each year. A range of 300 to 900 HFRS cases are estimated to occur in Korea each year, and approximately the same number of cases are thought to occur in Far Eastern Russia annually.

SEOV is associated with the domestic rats, *R. norvegicus* and *R. rattus*,[305,514] and is worldwide in distribution due to the recent global spread of rats to port cities and beyond through international shipping.[300] Seoul is the only hantavirus known to cause disease in urban areas, as the other hantaviruses are associated with rodents that are predominantly rural in their distribution. SEOV-related HFRS cases appear to be rare outside of China and Korea and institutions housing laboratory rat colonies, the exact reason for which is unclear. SEOV-related HFRS cases in general tend to be more moderate than those associated with HTNV, although mortality rates still range up to approximately 1% to 5%. Although most cases are in cities, SEOV-related HFRS cases are also seen in some rural areas in China. The seasonality of SEOV-related outbreaks are different from HTNV-related HFRS, with most cases occurring in spring and early summer as opposed to fall and early winter.[92] The annual number of cases is unknown, as figures for SEOV- and HTNV-related HFRS are often not separated. However, Chinese reports suggest that SEOV-related HFRS in urban areas of several provinces has been on the increase since its discovery in 1981.[90] A genetically related virus, Thailand virus, is found in *Bandicota indica* rodents in Thailand, but is not known to cause human disease.

In Europe and Scandinavia most cases of HFRS are caused by infection with PUUV. Particularly in Scandinavia, disease is referred to as Nephropathia epidemica (NE). NE is usually milder than HTNV-associated HFRS. The virus is hosted by the bank vole, *Myodes glareolus*. In Sweden and Finland, the number of cases in rural residents usually peaks in November and January, although cases in urban residents appear to peak in August, which likely correlates with vacationing in summer cabins in rural areas. A male-to-female case ratio of approximately 2:1 is seen, and the disease is rare in children.[67] Local epidemics usually reflect increased local bank vole densities, which tend to cycle with a 3- to 4-year periodicity. Approximately 30% of PUUV infections result in reported disease, based on data from areas of Finland with high surveillance for disease.[67] In addition, antibody prevalence rates of up to 20% can be seen in known endemic areas in northern Sweden.[212] Hantaviral disease in Belgium, northeastern France, and Germany occurs mainly in autumn and spring, and the extent of activity reflects the alterations in the size and structure of bank vole communities.[414] Large PUUV-associated HFRS outbreaks are periodically recorded in several areas of European Russia, particularly Udmurtia and Bashkortostan. A genetically distinct PUUV-like virus has also been identified in *C. rufocanus* voles in Far Eastern Russia and on Hokkaido Island, Japan, but is not known to be associated with human disease.[248] Several additional hantaviruses are known to be associated with other subfamily *Arvicolinae* rodents but are not known to cause human disease. Topografov virus is present in lemmings in Arctic regions of Russia, and at least five hantaviruses are associated with various Old and New World rodents of the *Microtus* genus.

Dobrava virus (DOBV) also causes a considerable number of severe HFRS cases in Europe, particularly in the Balkan countries.[30,392] The primary rodent reservoir is *A. flavicollis,* which is widely abundant in this region. However, a variant of DOBV, Saaremaa virus, can be found in *Apodemus agrarius* (a subspecies distinct from that which carries HTNV in Asia), which is of greater abundance in more northern areas.[496] Although *A. flavicollis* does not frequent houses and other manmade structures, it will often enter campsites or places where food may be present. Unlike HTNV-associated HFRS, most DOBV-associated HFRS cases occur in the late spring and summer months when activity in the rural areas is greatest. Epidemics of disease are seen at times when rodent populations are high, and have also been noted to increase in years when military conflicts are ongoing.[325] Seroprevalence rates can be high in rural areas; for instance, antibody positivity rates of up to 14% were seen in mountainous areas of northern and western Greece.[24]

Since the discovery of SNV and HPS in 1993, numerous other hantaviruses have been detected in New World subfamily Sigmodontinae rodents. In North America, SNV is by far the most important cause of HPS.[353] SNV is present in deer mice (*P. maniculatus,* grasslands form) throughout Western and Central United States and Canada.[353] The initial 1993 cluster of HPS cases occurred in the Four Corners region (meeting point of New Mexico, Arizona, Colorado, and Utah), and the majority of subsequent cases have been identified in the southwestern United States. However, HPS cases have now been identified in 32 states in the United States and four provinces of Canada, and SNV-infected deer mice have been detected throughout most of its range, which stretches from the Yukon to Mexico and from California to the Appalachian mountains in the eastern United States and Canada.[343,353] Through December 2010, a total of 560 cases of hantavirus pulmonary syndrome have been reported in the United States with a case fatality rate of 36%. A survey of 2,500 individuals in risk groups, such as those with occupations that would bring them in close contact with rural rodents, found hantavirus-specific antibodies in only approximately 0.5% of those sampled,[556,592] suggesting infection of humans with SNV is rare. It appears that clusters of cases are generally associated with local increases in infected deer mice populations. The peak of HPS cases occurs late spring–early summer, and as of December 2009, in the United States, 63% of cases have been male and 37% female and the mean age of patients is 37 years (range 6 to 83 years). Retrospective studies suggest the disease had gone unrecognized since at least 1959.[160] Several other hantaviruses are capable of causing HPS in the United States. The forest form of deer mice (*P. maniculatus nubiterrae*), which are found predominantly throughout the Appalachian mountain range extending from Georgia to eastern Canada, harbor a genetically distinct SNV-like virus referred to as Monongahela virus.[353,503] This virus has been associated with several HPS cases in the Eastern United States. The white-footed mouse, *P. leucopus* (eastern haplotype) hosts another SNV-like virus, named New York virus. This virus has been responsible for some HPS cases in the Northeastern United States.[208,213] A different hantavirus, Blue River virus, is present in *P. leucopus* (western haplotypes), in the Central and Western United States, but this virus is not known to be associated with human disease.[358] Mitochondrial DNA analysis of the different rodent hosts shows that each of these rodent hosts is genetically distinct.[358] This is in keeping with the general pattern for hantaviruses, whereby each specific hantavirus is hosted by a single different species or subspecies of rodent, and each specific rodent species or subspecies serves as the primary reservoir for only a single specific hantavirus.[371,422]

Other sigmodontine genera harbor HPS-associated hantaviruses in the United States, such as BCCV, which was associated with a single HPS case in southern Florida and is hosted by the cotton rat, *Sigmodon hispidus* (eastern form).[438] The genetically distinct western form of *S. hispidus* hosts a genetically distinct hantavirus, Muleshoe virus.[439] Bayou virus was discovered in 1994, associated with a fatal HPS case in Louisiana.[357] Subsequently the virus was shown to be hosted by the rice rat *Oligoryzomys palustris,* to be present throughout the range of the rodent,[279] and associated with a nonfatal HPS case in Texas.[206] Although the HPS associated with BCCV and Bayou virus is still predominantly a pulmonary disease, there does appear to be more renal involvement than seen in classic SNV-associated HPS.[206,256]

The confirmation of an HPS case in Brazil in late 1993 marked the beginning of a wave of discovery of HPS cases and associated hantaviruses throughout South and Central America. In addition to Brazil, Argentina, Bolivia, Brazil, Chile, Ecuador, Paraguay, Panama, Uruguay and Venezuela have also reported HPS. Rodents carrying viruses similar SNV have been found in Colombia, Costa Rica, and Mexico, but have not been associated with disease in humans.

The finding of high prevalence of hantavirus-specific antibodies in the general population in some areas of South and Central America differs considerably from the epidemiologic picture seen in North America, where seropositivity rates of 0.2% or less are seen. For instance, high rates of hantavirus-specific antibodies have been seen on surveillance of general populations in regions of Paraguay (40%), Salta province in Argentina (17%), and Los Santos province in Panama (13%).[152,581] These data suggest more frequent exposure of people to hantaviruses in these areas and more inapparent or subclinical infections than seen with North American hantavirus infections.

Phylogenetic analysis of hantaviruses and their rodent reservoirs have indicated that their evolutionary trees overlap with only a few exceptions, suggesting that these viruses have co-evolved with their rodent hosts over 20 to 30 million years.[371,373,422] These data show that although HPS and many hantaviruses were only recently discovered, they are actually quite ancient.

CLINICAL FEATURES

Orthobunyavirus Genus

The California serogroup viruses, LACV, Jamestown Canyon, and the prototype California encephalitis virus, all cause a similar encephalitic disease in humans.[453] Indeed, due to serologic cross reactivity, many of the early disease descriptions of California encephalitis cases were likely due to Jamestown Canyon virus or LACV rather than California encephalitis virus, which is now known to be less common.[76,120] The major difference between the viruses is in age-dependence of the spectrum of clinical disease observed, in that LACV infections tend to be more severe in children, whereas Jamestown Canyon virus infection is more severe in adults. The spectrum of disease ranges from inapparent or mild febrile disease through to fatal encephalitis.[101,338,536]

The incubation period is approximately 3 to 7 days. Most cases report sudden onset of fever, followed by stiff neck, lethargy, headache, and nausea and vomiting, and symptoms usually end within 7 days. Approximately half the cases exhibit seizures, and up to 30% develop coma and exhibit a longer disease course. About 65% of patients have meningitis on presentation, with both mononuclear and polymorphonuclear cells present in cerebrospinal fluid. Despite mild neurological symptoms often present at the time of patient discharge, surprisingly little residua is found. The most important sequela is epilepsy, which is observed in approximately 10% to 15% of children, and these are almost always patients who had seizures during acute phase of illness. In addition, about 2% of patients have persistent paresis.[101,194,338]

Several thousand cases of acute febrile illness can occur during Oropouche virus epidemics observed throughout the Amazon basin regions of Brazil and Peru. Humans acquire the infection by bite from infected midges. The incubation period is approximately 4 to 8 days, followed by sudden onset of fever, with arthralgia, myalgia, severe headache, chills, photophobia, and prostration. Occasionally, rash, meningitis, or meningismus are seen.[359,416] Most of the symptoms resolve within 3 to 5 days, although the myalgia may last 1 or 2 weeks. Viremia is detectable in the majority of patients 2 to 3 days after onset of illness. Approximately half of the patients can exhibit recurrence of some disease symptoms 1 to 10 days after initial recovery.[549] Oropouche virus is also suspected to be infectious by aerosol, based on reported laboratory infections.[418]

Phlebovirus Genus

Human infections with sandfly fever viruses results in an acute febrile illness with rapid onset. The incubation period last 2 to 6 days, followed by fever and general malaise, often accompanied by headache, photophobia, and back and joint pain.[34,456] The disease is self-limiting, lasting 2 to 4 days before rapid and complete recovery.

Experimental RVFV infection of newborn lambs and kids suggests that the incubation period is usually 24 to 36 hours, but can be as short as 12 hours.[132] Fever, which is often biphasic, is accompanied by listlessness, lack of appetite, abdominal pain, increased respiration rate, and lack of movement. Mortality rates of greater than 90% can be seen in animals younger than 1 or 2 weeks of age, with animals rarely surviving beyond 24 to 36 hours after onset of illness. Older lambs and kids, and adult sheep and goats are often less susceptible to RVFV infection, ranging from peracute to inapparent infection. Most older animals develop a febrile acute illness similar to the disease seen in 1- to 2-week-old animals, but with morality ranging from 5% to 60%, and a longer incubation period of 1 to 6 days. High and prolonged viremias, widespread tissue damage, vasculitis, and hepatic necrosis are seen in the more severe cases. Abortions in pregnant animals are frequently observed, with rates varying from 40% to 100%.

Human infections rarely lead to severe illness, with most infections resulting in a self-limiting influenza-like illness. However, approximately 0.5% of infections lead to severe hemorrhagic fever. In such cases, it is likely that the reduction of the antithrombotic function of the endothelial cells initiates intravascular coagulation and extensive necrosis of hepatocytes and other infected cells. The release of procoagulants into the circulation, together with the extensive liver damage, which severely impairs synthesis of coagulation factors and removal of circulating activated coagulation factors, are likely important factors resulting in DIC in the hemorrhagic fever cases.[406,407]

In less than 0.5% of human RVFV infections, retinal vasculitis or encephalitis can be observed 1 to 4 weeks after recovery from the acute illness. Encephalitis begins with headache, meningismus, and confusion. Often fever reappears, and symptoms of severe cases include hallucinations, stupor, coma, and death. Focal necrosis, which most likely involves direct cell destruction by the virus, is seen in the brain. In addition, that the onset of encephalitis after viremia has ceased and RVFV-specific antibodies are readily detectable suggests that there may be an immunopathologic component to these late complications.[405] Indeed, polymorphonuclear and mononuclear cell infiltration associated with necrotic lesions implicates delayed hypersensitivity or cytotoxic T cells.[405]

Nairovirus Genus

The incubation period for CCHFV infections is commonly 3 to 7 days, but it varies depending on type of the exposure. Symptoms usually appear abruptly, and can include severe headache, dizziness, nausea, fever, neck and abdominal pain, and chills. Overall myalgia and malaise occur, and hepatomegaly may be seen. Hemorrhage frequently appears by 3 to 6 days postonset of illness, with a petechial rash observable on the trunk and limbs. Patients are often apathetic or obtunded by this stage, with delirium or coma occurring in the more severe cases. Blood may be seen in the urine, and bleeding from the nose, gums, vagina, and other mucosal surfaces or needle puncture sites may occur approximately 5 days after onset. The case fatality rate is approximately 30%, with most deaths occurring 5 to 14 days after onset of illness.[147,518,572]

Hantavirus Genus

Severe HFRS begins with a phase lasting for 3 to 5 days typified by high fever, headache, malaise, chills, and prostration. Flushing of the face and neck, and conjunctival and pharyngeal injection (indicating capillary dilation) are frequently observed. Increased capillary permeability is likely responsible for the retroperitoneal edema and lower back pain often described. This febrile phase is followed by a hypotensive phase lasting several hours to days, characterized by marked thrombocytopenia, and often by petechial hemorrhage. Many patients exhibit low-grade DIC, and approximately 10% to 15% of patients show some degree of shock around this time. Usually shock improves within 12 to 48 hours and blood pressure returns to normal, or the patient becomes hypertensive. Oliguria may occur, and, historically, renal failure contributes to about half of the deaths.[129] Recovering patients will then go through a phase of diuresis that may last several months. Obviously, not all patients go through all the stages described, with some of the more severe cases rapidly progressing through to death in a few days, whereas other cases will skip some phases of the disease or exhibit very mild symptoms and not be recognizable as HFRS. However this tends to be the most severe form of HFRS, with a 5% to 15% case fatality. SEOV-associated HFRS tends to be milder, with a mortality rate of 1% or 2%. In general, the disease course resembles that observed with milder HTNV- and DOVB-associated cases, although more prominent liver involvement often occurs.[260] PUUV-associated HFRS (often referred to as NE), is the mildest form of the disease, with a mortality rate of less than 1%. The phases of the illness are generally less pronounced, and symptoms are milder, with hypotension rather than shock, petechiae instead of more frank hemorrhage, and relatively mild renal involvement.

Similar to HFRS, in HPS there is also a 2- to 3-week incubation period followed by rapid onset of acute disease. The first 4 days often include fever, myalgia, malaise, headache, and gastrointestinal symptoms. Patients frequently present for medical attention with the onset of pulmonary edema, dyspnea, and hypoxemia. These features, together with the hemoconcentration that is frequently observed, are presumably linked to the hantavirus infection of the microvascular endothelial cells surrounding the lungs, which leads to increased permeability and fluid leakage into the lungs. Bilateral pulmonary infiltrates are often visible on chest x-rays. Deterioration of patient condition is often rapid, with death occurring in almost 50% of the cases within 1 to 3 days of hospital admission. Clinical laboratory tests frequently reveal thrombocytopenia and prolonged PTT. Hypotension and shock can be prominent at this stage. Recovery of surviving patients is often remarkably quick, with rapid resolution of the lung lesion and shock within 3 to 6 days. Very similar clinical pictures are seen with HPS cases associated with other viruses found in rodents of the subfamily *Sigmodontinae.* HPS cases have also been associated with SNV-related Monongahela, and New York viruses, Bayou virus, BCCV, ANDV, and related viruses Oran, Lechiguanas and Hu39694, Laguna Negra, Juquitiba, Araraquara, and Castelo dos Sonhos. The clinical picture seen in HPS cases associated with the BCCV and Bayou viruses differs slightly, in that more renal involvement and elevated serum creatine phosphokinase observed. Renal failure also appeared to be common with Oran virus–associated HPS in northern Argentina.[310] Flushing and petechiae and frank hemorrhage were seen in some HPS patients infected with ANDV in Argentina and Chile, respectively.[22]

DIAGNOSIS

Orthobunyavirus Genus

A wide variety of assays have been used in the diagnosis of infections with viruses of the genus *Orthobunyavirus,* including complement fixation (CF), hemagglutination inhibition (HI), neutralization (NT), immunofluorescence assay, IgM capture enzyme-linked immunosorbent assay (ELISA), and reverse transcriptase-polymerase chain reaction (RT-PCR).[74,128,186,284,293,428] Diagnosis of California serogroup virus infections relies on serologic methods, as the virus is generally absent from blood or secretions during the phase of CNS disease. The HI test is considerably more sensitive for these viruses than CF, but NT assay or RT-PCR coupled with multiplex nucleotide sequencing[291] is need for confirmation and subtype identification. The IgM capture ELISA works well for diagnosis of most infections by viruses of the genus *Orthobunyavirus,* but has not been widely applied to date.[128,219,476] Virus isolation attempts complement serologic and genetic assays, and is best achieved by intracerebral (i.c.) inoculation of suckling mice or infection of susceptible cells such as Vero cells.

Phlebovirus Genus

Sandfly fever should be suspected when patients present with a classic "3 day fever" in areas where phlebotomine sandflies are numerous.[136,456] Similarly, TOSV infection should be suspected in patients with acute CNS disease during the summer months in rural or semirural areas where phlebotomine sandflies are present.[60,374] Diagnostic confirmation using acute or early convalescent phase samples is readily achieved by virus isolation by i.c. inoculation of suckling mouse or susceptible tissue culture cells, or IgM capture ELISA.

Differential clinical diagnosis of RVFV varies depending on the region in question. The disease should be suspected in

RVFV-endemic regions following abnormally high precipitation, increased rates of abortion in livestock, and appearance of acute influenza-like illness in persons in close contact with potentially infected livestock (e.g., farmers, veterinarians, and abattoir workers). Virologic diagnosis is usually simple given the high viremias present throughout the acute phase of illness and the ease of growth of the virus when inoculated i.c. into suckling mice, or in a wide variety of susceptible tissue culture cells.[518] Serologic testing is also straightforward, particularly if paired sera (one taken acute and the other 1 or 2 weeks later) are available. IgM and IgG ELISA tests using inactivated RVFV-infected cell lysates or slurries have proven particularly useful in outbreak investigations.[278,356,547,583] RT-PCR protocols have also been developed, although their utility in clinical settings requires further investigation.[569]

Nairovirus Genus

Clinical differential diagnosis of CCHFV varies in the different regions where the disease is known to occur and can be difficult in early stages. In general, the disease can be suspected for patients presenting with a rapid onset of severe influenza-like symptoms, and known exposure to tick bite or contact with blood or tissues of potentially infected livestock or humans. The early stages can be confused with sandfly fevers in regions where the diseases overlap, and leptospirosis, Omsk hemorrhagic fever, other viral hemorrhagic fevers (yellow fever, HFRS, Ebola), tick typhus, and mycotoxicoses can appear similar in the more advanced hemorrhagic phase of the illness. Clinical values can be helpful in diagnosis, with leukopenia and thrombocytopenia both frequently being present early in the disease.[147,518]

Rapid laboratory diagnosis of CCHFV can be achieved by RT-PCR,[70,124] but virus isolation or antigen detection ELISA from patient acute phase sera[69,147] are also performed. The virus and antigen are usually detectable up to 1 to 2 weeks after onset of illness. For CCHFV isolation, i.c. or intraperitoneal inoculation of patient acute phase blood samples into newborn mice is probably most sensitive, although quicker results can be obtained by inoculation into susceptible tissue culture cells, such as LLC-MK2, Vero, and baby hamster kidney (BHK)-21 cells, followed by fluorescent antibody staining.[478] Fatal cases rarely show significant antibody responses. However, in those destined to survive, IgM and IgG antibodies are frequently detectable after about a week of illness.

Hantavirus Genus

Clinical differential diagnosis of HFRS and HPS cases can be difficult due to the nonspecific early symptoms in both types of cases. In areas of China, Korea, Far Eastern Russia, Europe, and Scandinavia where HFRS is known to occur, a febrile patient presenting with thrombocytopenia and renal symptoms should be questioned about potential rodent exposure and tested for evidence of hantavirus infection. The early signs of severe HFRS can be easily confused with those of leptospirosis, typhus, pyelonephritis, poststreptococcal glomerulonephritis, an acute abdominal emergency, or other hemorrhagic fevers. Mild HFRS can be confused with hepatitis A, mild leptospirosis, streptococcal pharyngitis, influenza, or nonsteroidal anti-inflammatory toxicity.

In the Americas, the early stages of HPS are extremely difficult to recognize, being easily confused with influenza. However, fever and myalgia and a history of potential rural rodent exposure, together with the appearance of shortness of breath, and findings of thrombocytopenia, leukocytosis with left shift (higher ratio of immature-to-mature neutrophils), and atypical lymphocytes would be strongly suggestive of HPS.[376]

Antibodies are invariably seen in patient sera around the time of onset of illness. Laboratory analysis of the presence of virus-specific antibodies has historically included indirect fluorescent antibody (IFA) testing. This has good sensitivity, and hantavirus cross-reactivity and use of a representative virus from each of the main rodent subfamilies harboring hantaviruses (i.e., *Murinae, Arvicolinae,* and *Sigmodontinae*) will identify infections caused by virtually all hantaviruses. However, false positives are not uncommon, due to rheumatoid factor problems and overall nonspecific "stickiness" of some patient sera. Some of these difficulties can be controlled for by the inclusion of appropriate negative antigens to detect and remove the effects of problem sera. Although of some utility for acute diagnosis, the inherent nonspecific background and subjectivity problems make the IFA test unsuitable for serologic survey studies. Acute diagnosis is best achieved by IgM capture ELISA using hantavirus-infected cell slurry as antigen and incorporating an uninfected cell slurry control.[280] The use of recombinant nucleocapsid proteins with appropriate negative control protein fractions have also proved useful as antigens in this assay format.[137,151,185] Such assays have been shown to be highly sensitivity, rapid, and inexpensive. Considerable cross-reactivity among related hantaviruses is seen, such that inclusion of a limited number of representative virus antigens (e.g., SNV, PUUV, and HTNV) allow detection of virtually all acute hantavirus infections. The disadvantage of the cross-reactivity of the assay is the inability to precisely identify the virus based on a positive result. Western blot assays utilizing recombinant nucleocapsid proteins or GPs have also been effectively used for acute diagnosis, particularly with New World hantaviruses, and can provide additional insights into virus identity.[207,233]

Virus isolation attempts from acute clinical specimens are almost always negative. The exact reason for difficulty of isolation of hantaviruses is unknown, but it is likely related to the presence of a strong immune response at the time of onset of illness, including serum-neutralizing antibodies. Demonstration of the lack of amino acid substitutions during the isolation of Sin Nombre virus from infected lung material would suggest that virus adaptation to growth in tissue culture is not a major element in the difficulty of isolation of these viruses.[97] Given the frequent difficulty in obtaining infectious virus, RT-PCR assay has been used effectively to complement immunodiagnostic assays and allow detailed genetic comparison of the hantaviruses.[320,373,392,468] Given the potential for false positives due to cross-contamination, RT-PCR is not recommended as the sole means of hantavirus diagnosis.

PREVENTION AND CONTROL

Orthobunyavirus Genus

Prevention and control is difficult for the mosquito-borne California and Bunyamwera serogroup viruses due to the widespread presence of the mosquito vector hosts and relatively sporadic nature of the associated human or livestock diseases. No vaccines are available for human-infecting orthobunyaviruses.

Broad application of insecticides, as carried out in earlier decades, is no longer ecologically acceptable. Relative to human disease, use of fine mesh netting and personal protectants containing N,N-diethyl-meta-toluamide (DEET) are highly recommended in areas with high risk of people being bitten by virus-infected mosquitoes.

Similar vector control challenges exist for the Simbu serogroup viruses vectored by *Culicoides* midges. With the Oropouche virus disease in Brazil and Peru, avoiding the build-up of rotting organic debris such as banana tree stalks or cacao husks in agricultural areas may help curtail population levels of *C. paraensis* and reduce the risk of seasonal epidemics.[417] Avoiding exposure (treated netting, DEET repellents) to these midges during their early evening feeding hours is also recommended. Similar protective measures are recommended for AKAV. In addition, a successful formalin-inactivated AKAV vaccine has been developed in Japan using virus-infected hamster lung cell cultures,[287] and a trivalent-inactivated vaccine protective against AKAV, Aino virus (AINOV), and Chuzan orbivirus has been successfully trialed in Korea.[259] With knowledge of the distribution and seasonality of AKAV disease outbreaks, vaccination of at risk animals prior to pregnancy is feasible.

Phlebovirus Genus

The sandfly hosts of SFSV, SFNV, and TOSV have short flight range, and locomotion is often by hopping, making localized use of insecticide sprays particularly effective around residences. In addition, the use of repellants and treated bed nets and screens is recommended in such areas.

Immunization of livestock remains the most effective way to prevent RVFV epizootics and human cases. Several vaccines exist. Live attenuated viruses based on the mouse neuroadapted Smithburn RVFV strain are used in Kenya and South Africa.[78,498] Formalin-inactivated wild-type viruses have also been used in Egypt and South Africa.[138] The modified live Smithburn vaccine has good efficacy in sheep (but not cattle), with a single dose inducing lasting immunity in sheep 6 to 7 days after vaccination.[102] However, it appears to be only partially attenuated, causing abortions or teratology in some pregnant animals.[223,289] The formalin-inactivated vaccines are safer, but are expensive and induce only short-lived immunity in sheep and cattle. Other candidate live-attenuated vaccines such the mutagen-derived MP12 strain, the naturally occurring clone 13 (which has a large deletion in NSs), and genetically engineered recombinant viruses lacking NSs protein, and perhaps also NSm, are in various stages of evaluation.[54,223,289,403] Other approaches include DNA vaccines, nonreplicating virus-like particles and subunit vaccines. The main livestock vaccination problem is the long periods between epizootics and their irregular appearance, which makes it difficult to convince livestock owners to vaccinate regularly. Recent advances in the use of satellite imagery and surface ocean temperatures to predict regions at higher than usual risk of RVFV activity, may allow the timely vaccination of animals prior to potential epizootics.[25,316,554]

In an African setting, humans are probably best protected by vaccination of livestock to prevent amplification of virus, thus limiting human exposure and epizootic potential. Formalin-inactivated RVFV vaccines have been developed for immunization of laboratory and field workers at risk of exposure[223,288] but are unlikely to be used on a larger scale, given their limited commercial potential. RVFV is highly infectious by aerosol, as shown by numerous infections of laboratory personnel. Workers at risk of exposure wear protective clothing to avoid contact with potentially infectious materials and aerosols. The antiviral drug ribavirin may be of some benefit in the treatment of sandfly fevers and RVFV, although human efficacy data are still lacking.[108,408]

Nairovirus Genus

The best means of prevention is to minimize exposure to the virus. Treatment of clothing with pyrethroid preparations, which repels and even kills ticks, is highly recommended for those persons likely to come into contact with CCHFV-infected ticks (e.g., slaughterhouse workers, sheep shearers, veterinarians, and others involved with livestock). In addition, habits that avoid virus-contaminated blood or tissues contacting the skin should be practiced (e.g., wearing of gloves and avoiding crushing ticks with fingers). Medical personnel should practice standard barrier-nursing techniques during care of suspected CCHFV patients. Formalin-inactivated vaccines have been prepared from virus-infected suckling mouse brains and used in Bulgaria and other parts of Eastern Europe and the former Soviet Union, but their efficacy is currently unclear.[253]

Treatment of patients is by means of supportive and replacement therapy with blood products. Administration of immune plasma has been tried on numerous occasions, but its usefulness remains unclear. Based on the susceptibility of the virus in experimental tissue culture and mouse infections to the antiviral drug ribavirin, several CCHFV cases have been treated with ribavirin and shown encouraging results.[147,253]

Hantavirus Genus

The primary means of prevention is the reduction of rodent exposure. Effective measures include rodent-proofing of homes, correct storage of food, airing of seasonally closed cabins, and disinfection and removal of trapped rodents and rodent droppings.[85,86,180] The lack of nosocomial transmission or person-to-person transmission reported for virtually all hantavirus outbreaks suggests that spread to medical personnel or contacts is usually not a concern. The one exception is the limited person-to-person spread that can occur during ANDV-associated HPS outbreaks.[388,570]

Several different inactivated virus vaccines for HTNV and SEOV have been developed in Asia.[211] These include virus-infected rodent brain–derived antigens inactivated with formalin or beta-propiolactone.[302,586] Although such products would not be suitable for use outside the region, good efficacy has been reported.[211] Several monovalent and bivalent HTNV- and SEOV-tissue culture–derived inactivated vaccines have also been produced in China,[211] some of which may have high efficacy. In addition, a number of recombinant DNA approaches to vaccine development have been investigated, some of which show promise in experimental systems (reviewed in 464). Of these, the only study in humans to date was with DNA vaccines for HTNV and PUUV delivered by gene gun, which showed both vaccines to be immunogenic when delivered alone or in combination (C. S. Schmaljohn, unpublished). The sensitivity of HTNV to the inhibitory effects of the antiviral drug ribavirin on virus replication in tissue culture or in animal models[215] has promoted clinical trials both with HFRS patients and HPS patients, with positive results reported in the case of HFRS.[214,452]

TOSPOVIRUS GENERAL FEATURES

In infected plant cells, several types of aggregates of virus proteins are observed, and mature virus particles accumulate in the endoplasmic reticulum.[263] Although the spread of virus from plant to plant is by ingestion of the cell contents by thrips, acquisition of a virus envelope membrane containing the virus GPs is still thought to be important for virus transmission by thrips. However, once inside the plant, complete virus maturation may be less critical as movement from cell to cell likely involves virus nucleocapsid movement through plasmodesmata cytoplasmic channels.[275,510] In addition to the structural proteins, nucleocapsid (N), glycoproteins (Gn and Gc), and RNA polymerase (L), the tripartite genome of these viruses encode two nonstructural proteins, one from the S genome segment, NSs, and one from the M segment, NSm.[273] The NSs protein accumulates in the salivary gland of infected thrips, suggesting a role in virus transmission.[579] The NSm associates with virus nucleocapsids and localizes to plasmodesmata, where it forms tubular structures thought to be involved in virus cell-to-cell movement.[275,510]

In contrast to the other arthropod-borne members of the family *Bunyaviridae,* adults of the vector thrips do not acquire the virus, only larvae becoming infected when feeding on virus-infected plants.[541,575] Infected male *F. occidentalis* thrips were shown to feed more actively than uninfected thrips, thus increasing the opportunities for virus transmission.[506] TSWV has been shown to be trans-stadially transmitted through molting, pupation, and emergence to the adult stage, and both larvae and adults can transmit the virus to plants.[578] Unlike many of the other arthropod-borne bunyaviruses, there is no evidence of transovarial transmission for any of the tospoviruses. This presumably reflects the widespread and year-round replication of thrips in most climates and the enormous number of susceptible plants, making vertical transmission of the virus in the vector thrips of lesser importance.

Control of tospovirus infections in a field setting is difficult due to problems in eliminating thrips and the fact that many weed species surrounding cultivated fields will serve as a virus reservoirs. Several breeding programs have attempted to increase natural host resistance of plants to tospovirus infection, but with little success to date.[508] Attempts to create genetically engineered host-plant resistance are showing promising results and have been reviewed in detail recently.[272]

PERSPECTIVES

Although unified by shared characteristics such as tripartite ssRNA genome, virion composed of four structural polypeptides, and cytoplasmic site of replication, the bunyaviruses exhibit considerable diversity in RNA and encoded protein sequences, their genome expression strategies, and biological properties. The degree of understanding of different bunyaviruses varies greatly, dependent on their clinical, veterinary, or agricultural importance, or ease of handling. The family affords considerable research opportunities for the future, three of which are considered of immediate importance highlighted in the following. (a) Large scale sequence analyses of bunyavirus genomes to begin to understand their relationships and evolution, with practical implications for robust classification and improved diagnostics. (b) The development of reverse genetic systems that allow rescue of infectious hanta-, nairo-, and tospoviruses, which will enhance the pace of research on these viruses (as evidenced from progress with orthobunya- and phleboviruses for which the technology is well-established) and should provide new opportunities in the generation of vaccine and antivirals. (c) An understanding of how bunyaviruses persist in either their arthropod or rodent hosts. What are the cellular interactions that occur that permit efficient viral replication without damage to the host or clearance from it?

REFERENCES

All cited references are available in the e-book.

7. Albarino CG, Bird BH, Nichol ST. A shared transcription termination signal on negative and ambisense RNA genome segments of Rift Valley fever, sandfly fever Sicilian, and Toscana viruses. *J Virol* 2007;81:5246–5256.
11. Alff PJ, Gavrilovskaya IN, Gorbunova E, et al. The pathogenic NY-1 hantavirus G1 cytoplasmic tail inhibits RIG-I- and TBK-1-directed interferon responses. *J Virol* 2006;80:9676–9686.
12. Alff PJ, Sen N, Gorbunova E, et al. The NY-1 hantavirus Gn cytoplasmic tail coprecipitates TRAF3 and inhibits cellular interferon responses by disrupting TBK1-TRAF3 complex formation. *J Virol* 2008;82:9115–9122.
14. Altamura LA, Bertolotti-Ciarlet A, Teigler J, et al. Identification of a novel C-terminal cleavage of Crimean-Congo hemorrhagic fever virus PreGN that leads to generation of an NSM protein. *J Virol* 2007;81:6632–6642.
17. Anderson G, Smith J. Immunoelectron microscopy of Rift Valley morphogenesis in primary rat hepatocytes. *Virology* 1987;161:91–100.
25. Anyamba A, Chretien JP, Small J, et al. Prediction of a Rift Valley fever outbreak. *Proc Natl Acad Sci U S A* 2009;106:955–959.
26. Aquino VH, Moreli ML, Moraes Figueiredo LT. Analysis of Oropouche virus L protein amino acid sequence showed the presence of an additional conserved region that could harbour an important role for the polymerase activity. *Arch Virol* 2003;148:19–28.
30. Avsic-Zupanc T, Toney A, Anderson K, et al. Genetic and antigenic properties of Dobrava virus: a unique member of the *Hantavirus* genus, family *Bunyaviridae*. *J Gen Virol* 1995;76:2801–2808.
31. Barr JN. Bunyavirus mRNA synthesis is coupled to translation to prevent premature transcription termination. *RNA* 2007;13:731–736.
35. Battisti AJ, Chu YK, Chipman PR, et al. Structural studies of Hantaan virus. *J Virol* 2011;85:835–841.
36. Beaty BJ, Miller BR, Shope RE, et al. Molecular basis of bunyavirus per os infection of mosquitoes: role of the middle-sized RNA segment. *Proc Natl Acad Sci U S A* 1982;79:1295–1297.
37. Bellocq C, Raju R, Patterson J, et al. Translational requirement of La Crosse virus S-mRNA synthesis: in vitro studies. *J Virol* 1987;61:87–95.
38. Bennett RS, Cress CM, Ward JM, et al. La Crosse virus infectivity, pathogenesis, and immunogenicity in mice and monkeys. *Virol J* 2008;5:25.
47. Bishop D, Gay M, Matsuoko Y. Nonviral heterogeneous sequences are present at the 5′ ends of one species of snowshoe hare bunyavirus S complementary RNA. *Nucl Acid Res* 1983;11:6409–6419.
49. Bishop D, Shope R. Bunyaviridae. In: Fraenkel-Conrat H, Wagner RR, eds. *Comprehensive Virology* 1979;14:1–156.
53. Blakqori G, van Knippenberg I, Elliott RM. Bunyamwera orthobunyavirus S-segment untranslated regions mediate poly(A) tail-independent translation. *J Virol* 2009;83:3637–3646.
54. Boshra H, Lorenzo G, Busquets N, et al. Rift Valley Fever-Recent insights into pathogenesis and prevention. *J Virol* 2011;85:6098–6105.
56. Bouloy M, Janzen C, Vialat P, et al. Genetic evidence for an interferon-antagonistic function of rift valley fever virus nonstructural protein NSs. *J Virol* 2001;75:1371–1377.
58. Bowen MD, Trappier SG, Sanchez AJ, et al. A reassortant bunyavirus isolated from acute hemorrhagic fever cases in Kenya and Somalia. *Virology* 2001;291:185–190.
62. Bridgen A, Elliott RM. Rescue of a segmented negative-strand RNA virus entirely from cloned complementary DNAs. *Proc Natl Acad Sci U S A* 1996;93:15400–15404.
63. Bridgen A, Weber F, Fazakerley JK, et al. Bunyamwera bunyavirus nonstructural protein NSs is a nonessential gene product that contributes to viral pathogenesis. *Proc Natl Acad Sci U S A* 2001;98:664–669.

64. Briese T, Bird B, Kapoor V, et al. Batai and Ngari viruses: M segment reassortment and association with severe febrile disease outbreaks in East Africa. *J Virol* 2006;80:5627–5630.
68. Bucher E, Sijen T, De Haan P, et al. Negative-strand tospoviruses and tenuiviruses carry a gene for a suppressor of gene silencing at analogous genomic positions. *J Virol* 2003;77:1329–1336.
73. Calisher CH. History, classification and taxonomy of viruses in the Family Bunyaviridae. In: Elliott RM, ed. *The Bunyaviridae.* New York: Plenum Press; 1996:1–17.
77. Capodagli GC, McKercher MA, Baker EA, et al. Structural analysis of a viral ovarian tumor domain protease from the Crimean-Congo hemorrhagic fever virus in complex with covalently bonded ubiquitin. *J Virol* 2011; 85:3621–3630.
80. Carroll SA, Reynes JM, Khristova ML, et al. Genetic evidence for Rift Valley fever outbreaks in Madagascar resulting from virus introductions from the East African mainland rather than enzootic maintenance. *J Virol* 2011;85(13):6162–6167.
87. Cevik MA, Erbay A, Bodur H, et al. Clinical and laboratory features of Crimean-Congo hemorrhagic fever: predictors of fatality. *Int J Infect Dis* 2008;12:374–379.
93. Chen S, Compans R. Oligomerization, transport, and Golgi retention of Punta Toro virus glycoproteins. *J Virol* 1991;65:5902–5909.
94. Chen S, Matsuoka Y, Compans R. Assembly and polarized release of Punta Toro virus and effects of Brefeldin A. *J Virol* 1991;65:1427–1439.
97. Chizhikov VE, Spiropoulou CF, Morzunov SP, et al. Complete genetic characterization and analysis of isolation of Sin Nombre virus. *J Virol* 1995;69:8132–8136.
113. Daubney R, Hudson JR, Garnham PC. Enzootic hepatitis or Rift Valley fever. An undescribed virus disease of sheep cattle and man from East Africa. *J Path Bact* 1931;34:545–579.
118. de Haan P, Wagemakers L, Peters D, et al. The S RNA segment of tomato spotted wilt virus has an ambisense character. *J Gen Virol* 1990;71:1001–1007.
125. Duijsings D, Kormelink R, Goldbach R. In vivo analysis of the TSWV cap-snatching mechanism: single base complementarity and primer length requirements. *EMBO J* 2001;20:2545–2552.
127. Dunn EF, Pritlove DC, Jin H, et al. Transcription of a recombinant bunyavirus RNA template by transiently expressed bunyavirus proteins. *Virology* 1995;211:133–143.
142. Elliott RM, Bouloy M, Calisher CH, et al. Family Bunyaviridae. In: van Regenmortel MHV, Fauquest CM, Bishop DHL, et al., eds. *Virus Taxonomy: Classification and Nomenclature of Viruses. Seventh report of the International Committee on Taxonomy of Viruses.* San Diego, CA: Academic Press; 2000.
146. Emery VC. Characterization of Punta Toro S mRNA species and identification of an inverted complementary sequence in the intergenic region of Punta Toro phlebovirus ambisense S RNA that is involved in mRNA transcription termination. *Virology* 1987;156:1–11.
147. Ergonul O. Crimean-Congo haemorrhagic fever. *Lancet Infect Dis* 2006; 6:203–214.
149. Fazakerley JK, Gonzalez-Scarano F, Strickler J, et al. Organization of the middle RNA segment of snowshoe hare Bunyavirus. *Virology* 1988; 167:422–432.
158. Flick R, Whitehouse CA. Crimean-Congo hemorrhagic fever virus. *Curr Mol Med* 2005;5:753–760.
159. Fontana J, Lopez-Montero N, Elliott RM, et al. The unique architecture of Bunyamwera virus factories around the Golgi complex. *Cell Microbiol* 2008;10:2012–2028.
162. Freiberg AN, Sherman MB, Morais MC, et al. Three-dimensional organization of Rift Valley fever virus revealed by cryoelectron tomography. *J Virol* 2008;82:10341–10348.
163. Frese M, Kochs G, Feldmann H, et al. Inhibition of bunyaviruses, phleboviruses, and hantaviruses by human MxA protein. *J Virol* 1996; 70:915–923.
164. Frese M, Prins M, Ponten A, et al. Constitutive expression of interferon-induced human MxA protein in transgenic tobacco plants does not confer resistance to a variety of RNA viruses. *Transgenic Res* 2000;9:429–438.
168. Garcin D, Lezzi M, Dobbs M, et al. The 5′ ends of Hantaan virus (Bunyaviridae) RNAs suggest a prime-and-realign mechanism for the initiation of RNA synthesis. *J Virol* 1995;69:5754–5762.
169. Garry CE, Garry RF. Proteomics computational analyses suggest that the carboxyl terminal glycoproteins of Bunyaviruses are class II viral fusion protein (beta-penetrenes). *Theor Biol Med Model* 2004;1:10.
170. Gavrilovskaya IN, Brown EJ, Ginsberg MH, et al. Cellular entry of hantaviruses which cause hemorrhagic fever with renal syndrome is mediated by beta3 integrins. *J Virol* 1999;73:3951–3959.
171. Gavrilovskaya IN, Peresleni T, Geimonen E, et al. Pathogenic hantaviruses selectively inhibit beta3 integrin directed endothelial cell migration. *Arch Virol* 2002;147:1913–1931.
172. Geimonen E, Fernandez I, Gavrilovskaya IN, et al. Tyrosine residues direct the ubiquitination and degradation of the NY-1 hantavirus G1 cytoplasmic tail. *J Virol* 2003;77:10760–10868.
174. Geimonen E, Neff S, Raymond T, et al. Pathogenic and nonpathogenic hantaviruses differentially regulate endothelial cell responses. *Proc Natl Acad Sci U S A* 2002;99:13837–13842.
175. Gerrard SR, Li L, Barrett AD, et al. Ngari virus is a Bunyamwera virus reassortant that can be associated with large outbreaks of hemorrhagic fever in Africa. *J Virol* 2004;78:8922–8926.
177. Gerrard SR, Rollin PE, Nichol ST. Bidirectional infection and release of Rift Valley fever virus in polarized epithelial cells. *Virology* 2002;301: 226–235.
182. Gonzalez-Scarano F, Janssen RS, Najjar JA, et al. An avirulent G1 glycoprotein variant of La Crosse bunyavirus with defective fusion function. *J Virol* 1985;54:757–763.
183. Gonzalez-Scarano F, Pobjecky N, Nathanson N. LaCrosse bunyavirus can mediate pH-dependent fusion from without. *Virology* 1984;132: 222–225.
189. Habjan M, Andersson I, Klingstrom J, et al. Processing of genome 5′ termini as a strategy of negative-strand RNA viruses to avoid RIG-I-dependent interferon induction. *PLoS One* 2008;3:e2032.
191. Habjan M, Pichlmair A, Elliott RM, et al. NSs protein of rift valley fever virus induces the specific degradation of the double-stranded RNA-dependent protein kinase. *J Virol* 2009;83:4365–4375.
193. Hacker JK, Volkman LE, Hardy JL. Requirement for the G1 protein of California encephalitis virus in infection in vitro and in vivo. *Virology* 1995;206:945–953.
204. Hewlett MJ, Pettersson RF, Baltimore D. Circular forms of Uukuniemi virion RNA: an electron microscopic study. *J Virol* 1977;21:1085–1093.
214. Huggins JW, Hsiang CM, Cosgriff TM, et al. Prospective, double-blind, concurrent, placebo-controlled clinical trial of intravenous Ribavirin therapy of hemorrhagic fever with renal syndrome. *J Infect Dis* 1991;164: 1119–1127.
216. Huiskonen JT, Hepojoki J, Laurinmaki P, et al. Electron cryotomography of Tula hantavirus suggests a unique assembly paradigm for enveloped viruses. *J Virol* 2010;84:4889–4897.
218. Hutchinson KL, Peters CJ, Nichol ST. Sin Nombre virus mRNA synthesis. *Virology* 1996;224:139–149.
220. Ihara T, Akashi H, Bishop DH. Novel coding strategy (ambisense genomic RNA) revealed by sequence analyses of Punta Toro Phlebovirus S RNA. *Virology* 1984;136:293–306.
223. Ikegami T, Makino S. Rift Valley fever vaccines. *Vaccine* 2009;27:D69–D72.
224. Ikegami T, Narayanan K, Won S, et al. Rift Valley fever virus NSs protein promotes post-transcriptional downregulation of protein kinase PKR and inhibits eIF2alpha phosphorylation. *PLoS Pathog* 2009;5:e1000287.
225. Ikegami T, Won S, Peters CJ, et al. Rift Valley fever virus NSs mRNA is transcribed from an incoming anti-viral-sense S RNA segment. *J Virol* 2005;79:12106–12111.
226. Ikegani T, Makino S. The pathogenesis of Rift Valley fever. *Viruses* 2011;3:493–519.
236. Jin H, Elliott RM. Expression of functional Bunyamwera virus L protein by recombinant vaccinia viruses. *J Virol* 1991;65:4182–4189.
239. Jin M, Park J, Lee S, et al. Hantaan virus enters cells by clathrin-dependent receptor-mediated endocytosis. *Virology* 2002;294:60–69.
241. Jonsson CB, Figueiredo LT, Vapalahti O. A global perspective on hantavirus ecology, epidemiology, and disease. *Clin Microbiol Rev* 2010;23: 412–441.
253. Keshtkar-Jahromi M, Kuhn JH, Christova I, et al. Crimean-Congo hemorrhagic fever: Current and future prospects of vaccines and therapies. *Antiviral Res* 2011;90:85–92.

254. Khaiboullina SF, Rizvanov AA, Deyde VM, et al. Andes virus stimulates interferon-inducible MxA protein expression in endothelial cells. *J Med Virol* 2005;75:267–275.
258. Kikkert M, Van Lent J, Storms M, et al. Tomato spotted wilt virus particle morphogenesis in plant cells. *J Virol* 1999;73:2288–2297.
265. Kochs G, Janzen C, Hohenberg H, et al. Antivirally active MxA protein sequesters La Crosse virus nucleocapsid protein into perinuclear complexes. *Proc Natl Acad Sci U S A* 2002;99:3153–3158.
276. Kraus AA, Raftery MJ, Giese T, et al. Differential antiviral response of endothelial cells after infection with pathogenic and nonpathogenic hantaviruses. *J Virol* 2004;78:6143–6150.
277. Krautkramer E, Zeier M. Hantavirus causing hemorrhagic fever with renal syndrome enters from the apical surface and requires decay-accelerating factor (DAF/CD55). *J Virol* 2008;82:4257–4264.
284. Kuno G, Mitchell CJ, Chang GJ, et al. Detecting bunyaviruses of the Bunyamwera and California serogroups by a PCR technique. *J Clin Microbiol* 1996;34:1184–1188.
288. LaBeaud AD, Kazura JW, King CH. Advances in Rift Valley fever research: insights for disease prevention. *Curr Opin Infect Dis* 2010;23: 403–408.
289. Labeaud D. Towards a safe, effective vaccine for Rift Valley fever virus. *Future Virol* 2010;5:675–678.
292. Lambert AJ, Lanciotti RS. Molecular characterization of medically important viruses of the genus Orthobunyavirus. *J Gen Virol* 2008;89: 2580–2585.
296. Le May N, Dubaele S, Proietti De Santis L, et al. TFIIH transcription factor, a target for the Rift Valley hemorrhagic fever virus. *Cell* 2004; 116:541–550.
298. Le May N, Mansuroglu Z, Leger P, et al. A SAP30 complex inhibits IFN-beta expression in Rift Valley fever virus infected cells. *PLoS Pathog* 2008;4:e13.
302. Lee H, Ahn C, Song J, et al. Field trial of an inactivated vaccine against hemorrhagic fever with renal syndrome in humans. *Arch Virol* 1990;(Suppl 1):35–47.
306. Lees JF, Pringle CR, Elliot RM. Nucleotide sequence of the Bunyamwera virus M RNA segment: conservation of structural features in the Bunyavirus glycoprotein gene product. *Virology* 1986;148:1–14.
307. Leonard VH, Kohl A, Hart TJ, et al. Interaction of Bunyamwera Orthobunyavirus NSs protein with mediator protein MED8: a mechanism for inhibiting the interferon response. *J Virol* 2006;80:9667–9675.
309. Levine JR, Prescott J, Brown KS, et al. Antagonism of type I interferon responses by new world hantaviruses. *J Virol* 2010;84:11790–11801.
310. Levis S, Morzunov SP, Rowe JE, et al. Genetic diversity and epidemiology of hantaviruses in Argentina. *J Infect Dis* 1998;177:529–538.
311. Lewandowski DJ, Adkins S. The tubule-forming NSm protein from Tomato spotted wilt virus complements cell-to-cell and long-distance movement of Tobacco mosaic virus hybrids. *Virology* 2005;342: 26–37.
318. Lober C, Anheier B, Lindow S, et al. The Hantaan virus glycoprotein precursor is cleaved at the conserved pentapeptide WAASA. *Virology* 2001;289:224–229.
320. Lopez N, Padula P, Rossi C, et al. Genetic identification of a new hantavirus causing severe pulmonary syndrome in Argentina. *Virology* 1996;220:223–226.
321. Lowen AC, Boyd A, Fazakerley JK, et al. Attenuation of bunyavirus replication by rearrangement of viral coding and noncoding sequences. *J Virol* 2005;79:6940–6946.
323. Lozach PY, Mancini R, Bitto D, et al. Entry of bunyaviruses into mammalian cells. *Cell Host Microbe* 2010;7:488–499.
324. Ludwig GV, Christensen BM, Yuill TM, et al. Enzyme processing of La Crosse virus glycoprotein G1: a bunyavirus-vector infection model. *Virology* 1989;171:108–113.
325. Lundkvist A, Hukic M, Horling J, et al. Puumala and Dobrava viruses cause hemorrhagic fever with renal. *J Med Virol* 1997;53:51–59.
326. Madoff DH, Lenard J. A membrane glycoprotein that accumulates intracellularly: cellular processing of the large glycoprotein of LaCrosse virus. *Cell* 1982;28:821–829.
328. Makela S, Mustonen J, Ala-Houhala I, et al. Human leukocyte antigen-B8-DR3 is a more important risk factor for severe Puumala hantavirus infection than the tumor necrosis factor-alpha(-308) G/A polymorphism. *J Infect Dis* 2002;186:843–846.
329. Marklewitz M, Handrick S, Grasse W, et al. Gouleako virus isolated from West African mosquitoes constitutes a proposed novel genus in the family Bunyaviridae. *J Virol* 2011;85(17):9227–9234.
333. Martin ML, Regnery HL, Sasso DR, et al. Distinction between Bunyaviridae genera by surface structure and comparison with Hantaan virus using negative stain electron microscopy. *Arch Virol* 1985;86: 17–28.
334. Matsuoka Y, Chen SY, Compans RW. A signal for Golgi retention in the bunyavirus G1 glycoprotein. *J Biol Chem* 1994;269:22565–22573.
336. Matthys V, Gorbunova EE, Gavrilovskaya IN, et al. The C-Terminal 42 residues of the TULV Gn protein regulate interferon induction. *J Virol* 2011;85(10):4752–4760.
341. Mendoza-Montero J, Gamez-Rueda MI, Navarro-Mari JM, et al. Infections due to sandfly fever virus serotype Toscana in Spain. *Clin Infect Dis* 1998;27:434–436.
342. Meyer BJ, Schmaljohn C. Accumulation of terminally deleted RNAs may play a role in Seoul virus persistence. *J Virol* 2000;74:1321–1331.
343. Mills JN, Johnson JM, Ksiazek TG, et al. A survey of hantavirus antibody in small-mammal populations in selected United States National Parks. *Am J Trop Med Hyg* 1998;58:525–532.
346. Mir MA, Duran WA, Hjelle BL, et al. Storage of cellular 5′ mRNA caps in P bodies for viral cap-snatching. *Proc Natl Acad Sci U S A* 2008; 105:19294–19299.
349. Mir MA, Sheema S, Haseeb A, et al. Hantavirus nucleocapsid protein has distinct m7G cap- and RNA-binding sites. *J Biol Chem* 2010;285: 11357–11368.
350. Miura TA, Carlson JO, Beaty BJ, et al. Expression of human MxA protein in mosquito cells interferes with LaCrosse virus replication. *J Virol* 2001;75:3001–3003.
351. Mohamed M, McLees A, Elliott RM. Viruses in the Anopheles A, Anopheles B, and Tete serogroups in the Orthobunyavirus genus (family Bunyaviridae) do not encode an NSs protein. *J Virol* 2009;83: 7612–7618.
357. Morzunov SP, Feldmann H, Spiropoulou CF, et al. A newly recognized virus associated with a fatal case of hantavirus pulmonary syndrome in Louisiana. *J Virol* 1995;69:1980–1983.
362. Muller R, Saluzzo JF, Lopez N, et al. Characterization of clone 13, a naturally attenuated avirulent isolate of Rift Valley fever virus, which is altered in the small segment. *Am J Trop Med Hyg* 1995;53:405–411.
363. Murphy FA, Harrison AK, Whitfield SG. Morphologic and morphogenetic similarities of Bunyamwera serological supergroup viruses and several other arthropod-borne viruses. *Intervirology* 1973;1: 297–316.
368. Netski D, Thran BH, St Jeor SC. Sin Nombre virus pathogenesis in Peromyscus maniculatus. *J Virol* 1999;73:585–591.
369. Newton SE, Short NJ, Dalgarno L. Bunyamwera virus replication in cultured Aedes albopictus (mosquito) cells: establishment of a persistent viral infection. *J Virol* 1981;38:1015–1024.
371. Nichol ST. Genetic analysis of hantaviruses and their host relationships. In: Saluzzo J, Dodert B, eds. *Factors in the emergence and control of rodent-borne viral disease.* Paris: Elsevier; 1999:99–109.
372. Nichol ST, Beaty BJ, Elliott RM, et al. Bunyaviridae. In: Fauquet CM, Mayo MA, Maniloff J, et al., eds. *Virus taxonomy. Eighth report of the International Committee on Taxonomy of Viruses.* Amsterdam: Academic Press; 2005: 695–716.
373. Nichol ST, Spiropoulou CF, Morzunov S, et al. Genetic identification of a novel hantavirus associated with an outbreak of acute respiratory illness in the southwestern United States. *Science* 1993;262:914–917.
377. Novoa RR, Calderita G, Cabezas P, et al. Key Golgi factors for structural and functional maturation of bunyamwera virus. *J Virol* 2005;79:10852–10863.
379. Obijeski JF, Bishop DH, Palmer EL, et al. Segmented genome and nucleocapsid of La Crosse virus. *J Virol* 1976;20:664–675.
383. Ogino M, Yoshimatsu K, Ebihara H, et al. Cell fusion activities of Hantaan virus envelope glycoproteins. *J Virol* 2004;78:10776–10782.
385. Osborne JC, Elliott RM. RNA binding properties of bunyamwera virus nucleocapsid protein and selective binding to an element in the 5′ terminus of the negative-sense S segment. *J Virol* 2000;74:9946–9952.

386. Overby AK, Pettersson RF, Grunewald K, et al. Insights into bunyavirus architecture from electron cryotomography of Uukuniemi virus. *Proc Natl Acad Sci U S A* 2008;105:2375–2379.
388. Padula PJ, Edelstein A, Miguel SD, et al. Hantavirus pulmonary syndrome outbreak in Argentina: molecular evidence for person-to-person transmission of Andes virus. *Virology* 1998;241:323–330.
390. Palacios G, Tesh R, Travassos da Rosa A, et al. Characterization of the candiru antigenic complex (bunyaviridae: phlebovirus), a highly diverse and reassorting group of viruses affecting humans in tropical America. *J Virol* 2011;85:3811–3820.
393. Pappu HR, Jones RA, Jain RK. Global status of tospovirus epidemics in diverse cropping systems: successes achieved and challenges ahead. *Virus Res* 2009;141:219–236.
395. Parsonson IM, Della-Porta AJ, Snowdon WA. Congenital abnormalities in newborn lambs after infection of pregnant sheep with Akabane virus. *Infect Immun* 1977;15:254–262.
396. Parsonson IM, McPhee DA. Bunyavirus pathogenesis. *Adv Virus Res* 1985;30:279–316.
398. Patterson JL, Holloway B, Kolakofsky D. La Crosse virions contain a primer-stimulated RNA polymerase and a methylated cap-dependent endonuclease. *J Virol* 1984;52:215–222.
401. Pekosz A, Phillips J, Pleasure D, et al. Induction of apoptosis by La Crosse virus infection and role of neuronal differentiation and human bcl-2 expression in its prevention. *J Virol* 1996;70:5329–5335.
403. Pepin M, Bouloy M, Bird BH, et al. Rift Valley fever virus (Bunyaviridae: Phlebovirus): an update on pathogenesis, molecular epidemiology, vectors, diagnostics and prevention. *Vet Res* 2010;41:61.
408. Peters CJ, Reynolds JA, Slone TW, et al. Prophylaxis of Rift Valley fever with antiviral drugs, immune serum, an interferon inducer, and a macrophage activator. *Antiviral Res* 1986;6:285–297.
417. Pinheiro FP, Travassos da Rosa AP, Gomes ML, et al. Transmission of Oropouche virus from man to hamster by the midge Culicoides paraensis. *Science* 1982;215:1251–1253.
418. Pinheiro FP, Travassos da Rosa AP, Travassos da Rosa JF, et al. Oropouche virus. I. A review of clinical, epidemiological, and ecological findings. *Am J Trop Med Hyg* 1981;30:149–160.
419. Plassmeyer ML, Soldan SS, Stachelek KM, et al. California serogroup Gc (G1) glycoprotein is the principal determinant of pH-dependent cell fusion and entry. *Virology* 2005;338:121–132.
420. Plassmeyer ML, Soldan SS, Stachelek KM, et al. Mutagenesis of the La Crosse Virus glycoprotein supports a role for Gc (1066–1087) as the fusion peptide. *Virology* 2007;358:273–282.
421. Plyusnin A. Genetics of hantaviruses: implications to taxonomy. *Arch Virol* 2002;147:665–682.
422. Plyusnin A, Morzunov SP. Virus evolution and genetic diversity of hantaviruses and their rodent hosts. *Curr Top Microbiol Immunol* 2001; 256:47–75.
425. Prescott J, Hall P, Acuna-Retamar M, et al. New World hantaviruses activate IFNlambda production in type I IFN-deficient vero E6 cells. *PLoS One* 2010;5:e11159.
426. Prescott J, Ye C, Sen G, et al. Induction of innate immune response genes by Sin Nombre hantavirus does not require viral replication. *J Virol* 2005;79:15007–15015.
430. Raju R, Kolakofsky D. Inhibitors of protein synthesis inhibit both LaCrosse virus S-mRNA and S genome syntheses in vivo. *Virus Res* 1986;5:1–9.
431. Raju R, Kolakofsky D. The ends of La Crosse virus genome and antigenome RNAs within nucleocapsids are base paired. *J Virol* 1989;63:122–128.
434. Ramsden C, Holmes EC, Charleston MA. Hantavirus evolution in relation to its rodent and insectivore hosts: no evidence for codivergence. *Mol Biol Evol* 2009;26:143–153.
436. Ravkov EV, Compans RW. Hantavirus nucleocapsid protein is expressed as a membrane-associated protein in the perinuclear region. *J Virol* 2001;75:1808–1815.
437. Ravkov EV, Nichol ST, Compans RW. Polarized entry and release in epithelial cells of Black Creek Canal virus, a New World hantavirus. *J Virol* 1997;71:1147–1154.
440. Raymond DD, Piper ME, Gerrard SR, et al. Structure of the Rift Valley fever virus nucleocapsid protein reveals another architecture for RNA encapsidation. *Proc Natl Acad Sci U S A* 2010;107:11769–11774.
442. Reguera J, Weber F, Cusack S. Bunyaviridae RNA polymerases (L-protein) have an N-terminal, influenza-like endonuclease domain, essential for viral cap-dependent transcription. *PLoS Pathog* 2010;6(9):e1001101.
444. Reichelt M, Stertz S, Krijnse-Locker J, et al. Missorting of LaCrosse virus nucleocapsid protein by the interferon-induced MxA GTPase involves smooth ER membranes. *Traffic* 2004;5:772–784.
451. Rossier C, Raju R, Kolakofsky D. LaCrosse virus gene expression in mammalian and mosquito cells. *Virology* 1988;165:539–548.
454. Ruusala A, Persson R, Schmaljohn CS, et al. Coexpression of the membrane glycoproteins G1 and G2 of Hantaan virus is required for targeting to the Golgi complex. *Virology* 1992;186:53–64.
456. Sabin AB. Experimental studies on Phlebotomus (Pappataci, Sandfly) fever during World War II. *Arch Virol* 1951;4:367–410.
458. Salanueva IJ, Novoa RR, Cabezas P, et al. Polymorphism and structural maturation of bunyamwera virus in Golgi and post-Golgi compartments. *J Virol* 2003;77:1368–1381.
461. Sanchez AJ, Vincent MJ, Erickson BR, et al. Crimean-congo hemorrhagic fever virus glycoprotein precursor is cleaved by Furin-like and SKI-1 proteases to generate a novel 38-kilodalton glycoprotein. *J Virol* 2006;80:514–525.
463. Santos RI, Rodrigues AH, Silva ML, et al. Oropouche virus entry into HeLa cells involves clathrin and requires endosomal acidification. *Virus Res* 2008;138:139–143.
464. Schmaljohn C. Vaccines for hantaviruses. *Vaccine* 2009;27(Suppl 4): D61–D64.
468. Schmaljohn CS, Hjelle B. Hantaviruses: a global disease problem. *Emerg Infect Dis* 1997;3:95–104.
472. Schountz T, Prescott J, Cogswell A, et al. Regulatory T cell-like responses in deer mice persistently infected with Sin Nombre virus. *Proc Natl Acad Sci U S A* 2007;104:15496–15501.
479. Shi X, Brauburger K, Elliott RM. Role of N-linked glycans on bunyamwera virus glycoproteins in intracellular trafficking, protein folding, and virus infectivity. *J Virol* 2005;79:13725–13734.
485. Shi X, Lappin DF, Elliott RM. Mapping the Golgi targeting and retention signal of Bunyamwera virus glycoproteins. *J Virol* 2004;78:10793–10802.
486. Shi X, van Mierlo JT, French A, et al. Visualizing the replication cycle of bunyamwera orthobunyavirus expressing fluorescent protein-tagged Gc glycoprotein. *J Virol* 2010;84:8460–8469.
488. Shoemaker T, Boulianne C, Vincent MJ, et al. Genetic analysis of viruses associated with emergence of Rift Valley fever in Saudi Arabia and Yemen, 2000–01. *Emerg Infect Dis* 2002;8:1415–1420.
489. Simon M, Johansson C, Lundkvist A, et al. Microtubule-dependent and microtubule-independent steps in Crimean-Congo hemorrhagic fever virus replication cycle. *Virology* 2009;385:313–322.
490. Simon M, Johansson C, Mirazimi A. Crimean-Congo hemorrhagic fever virus entry and replication is clathrin-, pH- and cholesterol-dependent. *J Gen Virol* 2009;90:210–215.
491. Simons JF, Hellman U, Pettersson RF. Uukuniemi virus S RNA segment: ambisense coding strategy, packaging of complementary strands into virions, and homology to members of the genus Phlebovirus. *J Virol* 1990;64:247–255.
494. Simpson DI, Knight EM, Courtois G, et al. Congo virus: a hitherto undescribed virus occurring in Africa. I. Human isolations–clinical notes. *East Afr Med J* 1967;44:86–92.
497. Smith JF, Pifat DY. Morphogenesis of sandfly viruses (Bunyaviridae family). *Virology* 1982;121:61–81.
498. Smithburn K. Rift Valley fever: the neurotropic adaptation of the virus and the experimental use of this modified virus as a vaccine. *Br J Exp Pathol* 1949:1–16.
499. Smithburn KC, Haddow AJ, Mahaffy AF. A neurotropic virus isolated from Aedes mosquitos caught in the Semliki forest. *Am J Trop Med Hyg* 1946;26:189–208.
501. Soldan SS, Hollidge BS, Wagner V, et al. La Crosse virus (LACV) Gc fusion peptide mutants have impaired growth and fusion phenotypes, but remain neurotoxic. *Virology* 2010;404:139–147.
504. Spiropoulou CF, Goldsmith CS, Shoemaker TR, et al. Sin Nombre virus glycoprotein trafficking. *Virology* 2003;308:48–63.
509. Stoltz M, Klingstrom J. Alpha/beta interferon (IFN-alpha/beta)-independent induction of IFN-lambda1 (interleukin-29) in response to Hantaan virus infection. *J Virol* 2010;84:9140–9148.

510. Storms MM, Kormelink R, Peters D, et al. The nonstructural NSm protein of tomato spotted wilt virus induces tubular structures in plant and insect cells. *Virology* 1995;214:485–493.
512. Streitenfeld H, Boyd A, Fazakerley JK, et al. Activation of PKR by Bunyamwera virus is independent of the viral interferon antagonist NSs. *J Virol* 2003;77:5507–5511.
513. Struthers JK, Swanepoel R. Identification of a major non-structural protein in the nuclei of Rift Valley fever virus-infected cells. *J Gen Virol* 1982;60:381–384.
515. Sundin DR, Beaty BJ, Nathanson N, et al. A G1 glycoprotein epitope of La Crosse virus: a determinant of infection of Aedes triseriatus. *Science* 1987;235:591–593.
522. Talmon Y, Prasad BV, Clerx JP, et al. Electron microscopy of vitrified-hydrated La Crosse virus. *J Virol* 1987;61:2319–2321.
523. Taylor SL, Frias-Staheli N, Garcia-Sastre A, et al. Hantaan virus nucleocapsid protein binds to importin alpha proteins and inhibits tumor necrosis factor alpha-induced activation of nuclear factor kappa B. *J Virol* 2009;83:1271–1279.
533. Thomas D, Blakqori G, Wagner V, et al. Inhibition of RNA polymerase II phosphorylation by a viral interferon antagonist. *J Biol Chem* 2004;279:31471–31477.
535. Thompson WH, Beaty BJ. Venereal transmission of La Crosse virus from male to female Aedes triseriatus. *Am J Trop Med Hyg* 1978;27:187–196.
540. Uhrig JF, Soellick TR, Minke CJ, et al. Homotypic interaction and multimerization of nucleocapsid protein of tomato spotted wilt tospovirus: identification and characterization of two interacting domains. *Proc Natl Acad Sci U S A* 1999;96:55–60.
545. van Knippenberg I, Lamine M, Goldbach R, et al. Tomato spotted wilt virus transcriptase in vitro displays a preference for cap donors with multiple base complementarity to the viral template. *Virology* 2005;335: 122–130.
549. Vasconcelos HB, Azevedo RS, Casseb SM, et al. Oropouche fever epidemic in Northern Brazil: epidemiology and molecular characterization of isolates. *J Clin Virol* 2009;44:129–133.
552. Verbruggen P, Ruf M, Blakqori G, et al. Interferon antagonist NSs of La Crosse virus triggers a DNA damage response-like degradation of transcribing RNA polymerase II. *J Biol Chem* 2011;286:3681–3692.
554. Vignolles C, Tourre YM, Mora O, et al. TerraSAR-X high-resolution radar remote sensing: an operational warning system for Rift Valley fever risk. *Geospat Health* 2010;5:23–31.
555. Vincent MJ, Sanchez AJ, Erickson BR, et al. Crimean-Congo hemorrhagic fever virus glycoprotein proteolytic processing by subtilase SKI-1. *J Virol* 2003;77:8640–8649.
564. Watts D, Pantuwatana S, DeFoliart G, et al. Transovarial transmission of La Crosse virus (California encephalitis group) in the mosquito, *Aedes triseriatus*. *Science* 1973:123–130.
566. Weber F, Bridgen A, Fazakerley JK, et al. Bunyamwera bunyavirus nonstructural protein NSs counteracts the induction of alpha/beta interferon. *J Virol* 2002;76:7949–7955.
569. Weidmann M, Sanchez-Seco MP, Sall AA, et al. Rapid detection of important human pathogenic Phleboviruses. *J Clin Virol* 2008;41: 138–142.
570. Wells RM, Sosa Estani S, Yadon ZE, et al. An unusual hantavirus outbreak in southern Argentina: person-to-person transmission? Hantavirus pulmonary syndrome study group for patagonia. *Emerg Infect Dis* 1997; 3:171–174.
572. Whitehouse CA. Crimean-Congo hemorrhagic fever. *Antiviral Res* 2004; 64:145–160.
575. Whitfield AE, Ullman DE, German TL. Tospovirus-thrips interactions. *Annu Rev Phytopathol* 2005;43:459–489.
582. Won S, Ikegami T, Peters CJ, et al. NSm protein of Rift Valley fever virus suppresses virus-induced apoptosis. *J Virol* 2007;81:13335–13345.

INDEX

Note: Page number followed by "f" and "t" indicates figure and table respectively.

A

B

D

G

J

N

O

P

S

U

W

X

Y

Z